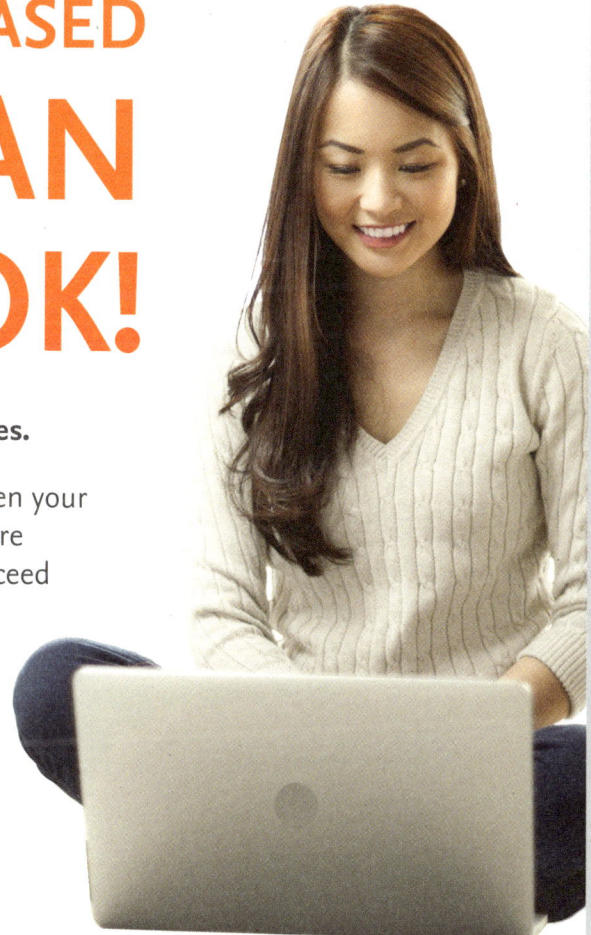
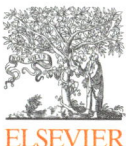

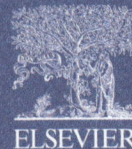

SEVENTH EDITION

POTTER AND PERRY'S
Canadian Fundamentals of Nursing

EDITORS

Barbara J. Astle, RN, PhD, FCAN
Professor & Director of the MSN Program
Director, Centre for Equity & Global
 Engagement (CEGE)
School of Nursing
Trinity Western University
Langley, British Columbia

Wendy Duggleby, RN, PhD
Professor Emerita
Faculty of Nursing
University of Alberta
Edmonton, Alberta

US TENTH EDITION EDITORS

Patricia A. Potter, RN, MSN, PhD, FAAN
Formerly, Director of Research
Patient Care Services
Barnes-Jewish Hospital
St. Louis, Missouri

Patricia A. Stockert, RN, BSN, MS, PhD
Formerly, President, College of Nursing
Saint Francis Medical Center College of Nursing
Peoria, Illinois

Anne Griffin Perry, RN, MSN, EdD, FAAN
Professor Emerita
School of Nursing
Southern Illinois University Edwardsville
Edwardsville, Illinois

Amy M. Hall, RN, BSN, MS, PhD, CNE
Professor and Dean
School of Nursing
Franciscan Missionaries of Our Lady University
Baton Rouge, Louisiana

ELSEVIER

Notice

Practitioners and researchers must always rely on their own experience and knowledge in evaluating
and using any information, methods, compounds, or experiments described herein. Because of rapid
advances in the medical sciences, in particular, independent verification of diagnoses and drug dosages
should be made. To the fullest extent of the law, no responsibility is assumed by Elsevier, authors, editors,
or contributors for any injury and/or damage to persons or property as a matter of products liability,
negligence or otherwise, or from any use or operation of any methods, products, instructions, or ideas
contained in the material herein.

Managing Director, Global ERC: Kevonne Holloway
Director, Content Development: Laurie Gower
Senior Content Strategist (Acquisitions, Canada): Roberta A. Spinosa-Millman
Content Development Specialist: Martina van de Velde
Publishing Services Manager: Catherine Jackson
Specialist: Kristine Feeherty
Cover Design and Design Direction: Brian Salisbury
Cover Image: Elymas/Shutterstock

Printed in Canada

Last digit is the print number: 9 8 7 6 5 4 3 2 1

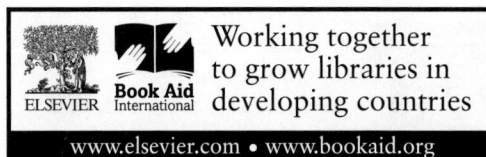

ELSEVIER | Book Aid International | Working together
to grow libraries in
developing countries

www.elsevier.com • www.bookaid.org

CONTENTS

PREFACE TO THE STUDENT

Potter and Perry's Canadian Fundamentals of Nursing provides you with all of the fundamental nursing concepts and skills you will need in a visually appealing, easy-to-use format. As you begin your nursing education, it is very important that you have a resource that includes all of the information required to prepare you for lectures, classroom activities, clinical assignments, and examinations. We've designed this text to meet all of those needs.

Check out the following special learning aids featured in *Potter and Perry's Canadian Fundamentals of Nursing,* Seventh Edition.

Learning Objectives begin each chapter to help you focus on the key information that follows.

Key Terms are listed at the beginning of each chapter and are boldfaced and defined in the text. Page numbers help you quickly find where each term is defined.

Case Study beginning each chapter relates to the chapter topic, and end-of-chapter clinical-judgement review questions refer to this case study.

1

Health and Wellness

Written by Deborah Gibson, RN, MSN

OBJECTIVES

Mastery of content in this chapter will enable you to:
- Define the key terms listed.
- Describe ways that definitions of health have been conceptualized.
- Describe key characteristics of medical, behavioural, and socioenvironmental approaches to health.
- Identify factors that have led to each approach to health.
- Describe contributions of the following Canadian publications to conceptualizations of health and health determinants: *Lalonde Report, Ottawa Charter, Epp Report, Strategies for Population Health, Jakarta Declaration, Bangkok Charter,* and *Toronto Charter.*
- Identify key health determinants and their interrelationships and how they influence health.
- Contrast distinguishing features of health promotion and disease prevention.
- Describe the three levels of disease prevention.
- Identify and give examples of the five health promotion strategies discussed in the *Ottawa Charter.*
- Analyze how the nature and scope of nursing practice are influenced by different conceptualizations of health and health determinants.

KEY TERMS

At-risk population	Health as unity	Prerequisites for health
Behavioural approach	Health disparities	Psychosocial risk factors
Behavioural risk factors	Health equity	Racialization
Determinants of health	Health field concept	Racism
Disease	Health inequalities	Risk factor
Disease prevention	Health inequities	Social determinants of health
Downstream thinking	Health literacy	Socioenvironmental approach
Evidence-informed decision making	Health promotion	Socioenvironmental risk conditions
Food insecurity	Health promotion strategies	Structural vulnerability
Health	Identity politics	Systemic racism
Health as actualization	Illness	Upstream thinking
Health as actualization and stability	Medical approach	Wellness
Health as resource	Physiological risk factors	
Health as stability	Population health approach	

WEBSITE

http://evolve.elsevier.com/Canada/Potter/fundamentals/

CASE STUDY

You are a nurse who is working in a small rural community with a population of 1 200 people, limited resources, and high rates of unemployment. Most of the community consists of families living in small homes. Meet the Lazzer family. There are nine members living in a small two-bedroom house that is a 15-minute drive from town. Joey Lazzer (preferred pronouns: he/him), who is 70 years of age, has been unable to work because of lung problems (chronic obstructive pulmonary disease; COPD) he developed from working in the local mine. Joey indicates that he is happy to have his family around, despite the crowded living circumstances. You notice that the house feels cold and a bit drafty when you enter. Joey informs you that he and his family are often cold, but he does not have the money to buy a new furnace or fix the broken living room window. He tells you that they put a tarp over the window in winter, but it still gets as cold as –20°C. Joey states that he finds it very difficult to breathe in the cold air during winter. His partner, Elsie (preferred pronouns: she/her), who is 68 years

Continued

1

> concept **map**

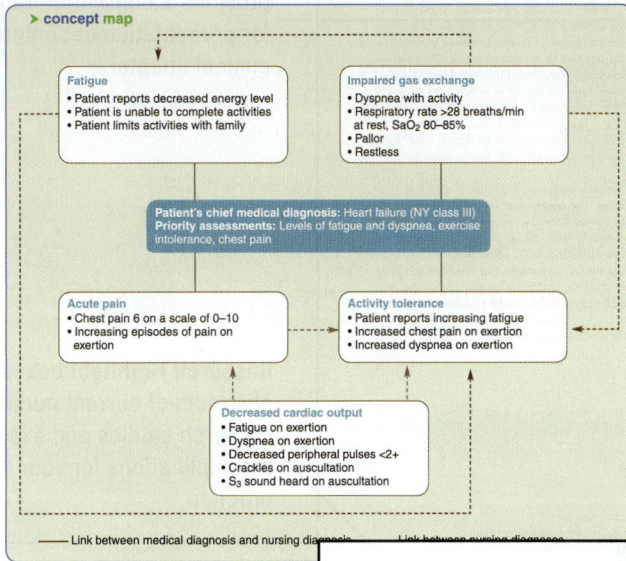

Fatigue
- Patient reports decreased energy level
- Patient is unable to complete activities
- Patient limits activities with family

Impaired gas exchange
- Dyspnea with activity
- Respiratory rate >28 breaths/min at rest, SaO$_2$ 80–85%
- Pallor
- Restless

Patient's chief medical diagnosis: Heart failure (NY class III)
Priority assessments: Levels of fatigue and dyspnea, exercise intolerance, chest pain

Acute pain
- Chest pain 6 on a scale of 0–10
- Increasing episodes of pain on exertion

Activity tolerance
- Patient reports increasing fatigue
- Increased chest pain on exertion
- Increased dyspnea on exertion

Decreased cardiac output
- Fatigue on exertion
- Dyspnea on exertion
- Decreased peripheral pulses <2+
- Crackles on auscultation
- S$_3$ sound heard on auscultation

—— Link between medical diagnosis and nursing diagnosis   ---- Link between nursing diagnoses

FIGURE 37.10 Concept map for a patient

Concept Maps show you the association among multiple nursing diagnoses and their relationship to medical diagnoses.

experienced angina, immediate investigation and treatment of the angina is the priority.

Teamwork and Collaboration

Planning involves understanding a patient's need to maintain function and independence. To ensure comprehensive patient-centred care, nurses need to collaborate with the multidisciplinary team. Contributions from the primary health care provider, physiotherapists, kinesiologists, and occupational therapists are essential in planning care. The nurse must always individualize a care plan to meet the actual and potential needs of the patient (Box 37.9).

Implementation

Health Promotion. A sedentary lifestyle contributes to the development of health-related challenges. As a nurse, you can promote health by encouraging patients to engage in a regular exercise program in any setting (Box 37.10). Discuss the recommendations for physical activity and fitness with the patient (Box 37.11). Design a program of physical activity in collaboration with the patient, taking into account age and developmental (see Box 37.11) and cultural factors. Collaborate with the patient's health care provider, physiotherapist, occupational therapist, and other members of the health care team to ensure patient-centred care.

Before starting an exercise program, teach patients to calculate their maximum heart rate by subtracting their current age in years from 220

The unique **Critical Thinking Model** shows clearly how the nursing process and critical thinking come together to help you provide the best care for your patients.

patient's level of knowledge regarding home safety so that deficiencies can be corrected with an individualized nursing care plan.

CRITICAL THINKING

Successful critical thinking requires a synthesis of a nurse's knowledge and experience, as well as of information gathered from patients, combined with professional standards. Clinical judgements require nurses to anticipate necessary information, analyze the data, and make decisions regarding patient care. Critical thinking is an ongoing process. During an assessment (Figure 38.3), the nurse should consider all critical thinking elements and information about the specific patient to make appropriate nursing diagnoses.

In the case of safety, a nurse integrates knowledge from nursing and other scientific disciplines with previous experiences in caring for patients who were at risk for or had an injury. This is combined with critical thinking attitudes such as responsibility and discipline, and any standards of practice that are applicable. Agency guidelines and professional nursing associations provide standards for nursing activities such as medication administration, fall-prevention steps, and infection control to guide nurses in the provision of safe care. One such set of standards is the Registered Nurses' Association of Ontario (RNAO) (2017) *Preventing Falls and Reducing Injury from Falls.* For example, while assessing a patient's home environment, the nurse needs to

consider typical locations within the home where dangers commonly exist. For a patient who has a visual impairment, the nurse applies previous experience in caring for patients with visual changes to anticipate how to thoroughly assess the patient's needs. Critical thinking directs the nurse to anticipate what needs to be assessed and how to make conclusions about available data.

◆ **SAFETY AND THE NURSING PROCESS**

Nurses are responsible for incorporating critical thinking skills when using the nursing process, assessing each patient and their environment for hazards that threaten safety, and planning and intervening appropriately to maintain a safe environment. The nursing process provides a clinical decision-making approach to develop and implement an individualized plan of safe patient care.

◆ **Assessment**

To conduct a thorough patient assessment, nurses must consider possible threats to a patient's safety, including the patient's immediate environment, as well as any individual risk factors.

Health History. By conducting a health history, the nurse gathers data about the patient's level of wellness to determine if any underlying conditions exist that pose threats to safety. For example, nurses should give special attention to assessing the patient's gait, muscle strength and coordination, balance, and vision. A review of the patient's developmental status must be considered as assessment information is analyzed. A nurse must also review whether the patient has been exposed to any environmental hazards or is taking medications or undergoing procedures that pose risks. For example, the use of diuretics increases the frequency of voiding and may result in the patient having to use toilet facilities more often. This may then increase the likelihood of a fall, as these often occur when patients get out of bed quickly because of urinary urgency.

Patient's Home Environment. When caring for a patient in the home, a home hazard assessment is necessary. The nurse should walk through the home with the patient and discuss how the patient normally conducts daily activities. Key areas to inspect are the bathroom, kitchen, and areas with stairs. For example, when assessing the adequacy of the lighting, the nurse should inspect areas where the patient moves and works, such as outside walkways, steps, interior halls, and doorways. Getting a sense of the patient's routine helps the nurse recognize less obvious hazards.

Health Care Environment. When a patient is being cared for within a health care facility, a nurse must determine if any hazards exist in the immediate care environment. Does the placement of equipment or furniture pose barriers to ambulation? Does the positioning of the patient's bed allow the patient to reach items on a bedside table? Does the patient need assistance with ambulation? Is the patient aware of activity restrictions? Has the patient been taught to use the call bell, and is it within reach? Collaboration with clinical engineering staff is essential to make sure that equipment has been assessed and is in proper functioning condition.

Risk for Falls. Assessment of the patient's fall risk factors is essential in determining specific needs and targeting interventions to prevent falls. A fall assessment tool (Table 38.1) can help determine potential risks before accidents and injuries result. The tool shown in Table 38.1 is the Hendrich II Fall Risk Model. This tool is intended for use in acute care settings and takes into account the patient's ability to move independently

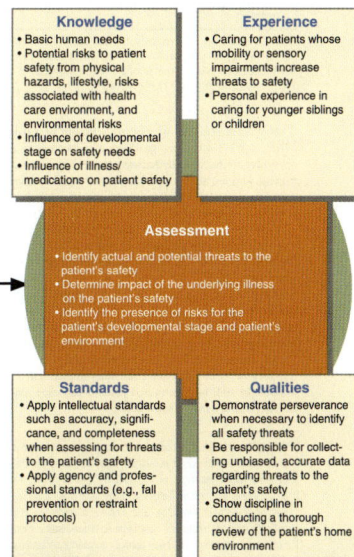

Knowledge
- Basic human needs
- Potential risks to patient safety from physical hazards, lifestyle, risks associated with health care environment, and environmental risks
- Influence of developmental stage on safety needs
- Influence of illness/medications on patient safety

Experience
- Caring for patients whose mobility or sensory impairments increase threats to safety
- Personal experience in caring for younger siblings or children

Assessment
- Identify actual and potential threats to the patient's safety
- Determine impact of the underlying illness on the patient's safety
- Identify the presence of risks for the patient's developmental stage and patient's environment

Standards
- Apply intellectual standards such as accuracy, significance, and completeness when assessing for threats to the patient's safety
- Apply agency and professional standards (e.g., fall prevention or restraint protocols)

Qualities
- Demonstrate perseverance when necessary to identify all safety threats
- Be responsible for collecting unbiased, accurate data regarding threats to the patient's safety
- Show discipline in conducting a thorough review of the patient's home environment

FIGURE 38.3 Critical thinking model for safety assessment.

❖ NURSING PROCESS AND THERMOREGULATION

Knowledge of the physiology of body temperature regulation is essential for assessing and evaluating the patient's response to temperature alterations and for intervening safely. Independent measures can be implemented to increase or minimize heat loss, promote heat conservation, and increase comfort. These measures complement the effects of medically ordered therapies. Many measures can be taught to caregivers and parents of children.

❖ Assessment

Sites. Core and surface body temperature may be measured at several sites. The core temperatures of the pulmonary artery, esophagus, nasopharynx, and urinary bladder are measured in critical care settings. These measurements require the use of invasive devices placed in body cavities or organs that continuously display readings on an electronic monitor.

Intermittent temperature measurements are obtained invasively from the sites of the mouth, rectum, and tympanic membrane or non-invasively from the axilla and temporal artery sites. Chemically prepared thermometer patches can also be applied to the skin. In order to measure oral, rectal, axillary, and skin temperature, blood circulation at the measurement site must be effective so that the heat of the blood is conducted to the thermometer probe. Tympanic temperature relies on the radiation of body heat to an infrared sensor. The temporal artery blood supply is believed to come from the external carotid artery, directly from the heart and centre of the body, which has a relatively high and stable blood flow, indicating the body's central temperature (Mahmoudi et al., 2020, p. 148). Because they share the same arterial blood supply as the hypothalamus, tympanic and temporal artery temperature measurements can be considered core temperatures (Purssell et al., 2009).

Correct measuring technique must be used at each site (Skill 31.1) to ensure accurate readings. The temperature obtained varies according to the site used but should remain between 36.0°C and 38.0°C. Rectal temperatures are usually 0.5°C higher than oral temperatures, and axillary temperatures are usually 0.5°C lower than oral temperatures. Each measurement site has advantages and disadvantages (Box 31.4). The rectal site was traditionally chosen because of the close replication of core body temperature but is now less routinely measured given the availability of less invasive and accurate alternative measurement devices such as the temporal thermometer. The safest and most

---

The five-step Nursing Process provides a consistent framework for presentation of content in clinical chapters.

SKILL 31.1	MEASURING BODY TEMPERATURE

Delegation Considerations

The task of measuring temperature can be delegated to unregulated care providers (UCPs). The nurse is responsible for assessing the impact of changes in body temperature; therefore, when the task of measuring temperature is delegated, it is important to *inform the UCP* about the following:

- The appropriate route and device to measure temperature
- Patient-specific factors that can falsely raise or lower temperature
- Appropriate precautions when positioning the patient
- Frequency of temperature measurement for the patient
- Usual values for patient
- Abnormalities that should be reported to the health care provider

Equipment

- Appropriate thermometer
- Soft tissue or wipe
- Alcohol swabs
- Lubricant (for rectal measurements only)
- Pen and either vital sign flow sheet or documentation form

PROCEDURE

STEPS

1. Identify patient using at least two person specifics (e.g., name and date of birth or name and medical record number) according to employer policy.
2. Assess for signs and symptoms of temperature alterations and for factors that influence body temperature.
3. Determine previous activity that would interfere with accuracy of temperature measurement. Wait before measuring oral temperature in the following situations: 2 minutes after patient has smoked, 5 minutes after patient has chewed gum, and 20 minutes after patient has ingested hot or cold liquids or foods.
4. Determine appropriate temperature site and device for patient.
5. Explain to patient the route by which temperature will be measured and the importance of maintaining the proper position until the reading is complete.
6. Perform hand hygiene.
7. Obtain temperature reading.

Research Highlight boxes provide abstracts of current nursing research studies and explain the implications for your daily practice.

BOX 38.10	RESEARCH HIGHLIGHT

Effects of Nursing Rounds

Research Focus

Hospitalized patients often require assistance with basic activities of daily living such as eating, toileting, and ambulating. Patients usually communicate their needs by use of a call light. Not meeting a patient's needs in a timely fashion decreases patient satisfaction and places them at greater risk for injury. The nurse plays a key role in the prevention of falls and injuries related to falls.

Research Abstract

Christiansen and colleagues (2018) wanted to know the impact of intentional rounding on patient and nursing outcomes and aimed to identify the barriers and facilitators surrounding implementation.

Methods

In their systematic literature review, they found 21 articles that met their inclusion criteria. Six studies reported a reduction in the number of falls, and another five studies reported a reduction in call bell use following the introduction of intentional rounding. Although results were positive, the overall quality of the studies was weak.

Implications for Practice

- Intentional rounding has demonstrated mixed results.
- A robust evaluation plan is needed to measure the impact of intentional rounding.

From Christiansen, A., Coventry, L., Graham, R., et al. (2018). Intentional rounding in acute adult healthcare settings: A systematic mixed-method review. *Journal of Clinical Nursing, 27*(9–10), 1759–1792. https://doi.org/10.1111/jocn.14370

BOX 38.11	Alternatives to Restraints

- Orient patients and families with the care environment; explain all procedures and treatments.
- Provide companionship and supervision; use trained sitters or adjust staffing.
- Offer diversionary activities, such as listening to music or having something to hold; enlist support and input from the family.
- Assign confused or disoriented patients to rooms near the nurses' station; observe these patients frequently.
- Use calm, simple statements and physical cues as needed.
- Use de-escalation, time-outs, and other verbal intervention techniques when managing aggressive behaviours.
- Provide appropriate visual and auditory stimuli (e.g., family pictures, a clock, or a radio).
- Remove cues that promote leaving (e.g., sight of elevators, stairs, or street clothes).
- Promote relaxation techniques and normal sleep patterns.
- Institute exercise and ambulation schedules as allowed by patients' conditions; consult a physiotherapist for mobility and exercise programs.
- Attend to the patient's toileting, food, and fluid needs.
- Camouflage intravenous lines with clothing, a stockinette, or a Kling dressing.
- Evaluate all medications the patients are receiving and ensure effective pain management.
- Reassess the physical status of patients, and review laboratory findings connected with their health.

Adapted from The Joint Commission (TJC). (2020). *Comprehensive accreditation manual for hospitals. Restraint and seclusion—enclosure beds, side rails and mitts.* https://www.jointcommission.org/standards/standard-faqs/hospital-and-hospital-clinics/provision-of-care-treatment-and-services-pc/000001668; American Nurses Association. (2021). Geriatric nursing resources for care of older adults. *Physical restraints.* https://hign.org/consultgeri/resources/protocols/physical-restraints

A physical restraint immobilizes a patient or a patient's extremity (CNO, 2009). The optimal goal with all patients is to avoid the use of physical restraints, and alternatives must always be considered. However, patients who are at risk for injury to self or others may need physical restraints temporarily. Physical restraints do not prevent falls and may actually increase the severity of an injury from a fall (RNAO, 2017).

Whenever patients are physically restrained, there is a natural tendency for them to try to remove the restraint, and this can lead to injury. Restrained patients can easily become entangled in a restraint device when attempting to get out of it. In some cases, death has resulted from strangulation or asphyxiation. As a result, long-term care facilities and many health care facilities have banned the use of the jacket (vest) restraint. The use of any physical restraint is also associated with serious complications, including pressure injuries, constipation, pneumonia, urinary and fecal incontinence, and urinary retention. Contractures, nerve damage, and circulatory impairment are also potential hazards. In addition, restrained patients can experience humiliation, fear, anger, and a loss of self-esteem.

> **SAFETY ALERT** Routine assessment of a patient in a physical restraint is critical to prevent injury. The restraint must be moved and the patient repositioned at regular intervals, according to the agency's policy. Restraints should be used only after other alternatives have been tried, and the least restrictive method of restraint should be used. The use of restraints must be part of the patient's medical treatment. Restraints are considered a short-term intervention, and once they have been applied, regular assessments are needed to determine whether they should be continued. All assessments and interventions must be clearly documented according to the agency's policy.

For legal purposes, nurses must know the agency's policy and procedures for the appropriate use and monitoring of physical restraints. The use of a restraint must be clinically justified and be a part of the patient's prescribed medical treatment and care plan. A physician's order may be required, depending on provincial or territorial legislation and agency policy—in some settings, nurses may order restraints. Requirements for ordering restraints may vary depending on the circumstances of a patient's situation and the type of restraint needed; nurses must comply with the agency's policies. Assessment of patients who are restrained must be ongoing. Proper documentation, including the behaviours that necessitated the application of restraints, the procedure used in restraining, the condition of the body part restrained (e.g., circulation to the patient's hand), and the evaluation of the patient response, is essential. Restraints should be removed periodically and the patient should be assessed to determine if the restraints continue to be needed.

Skill 38.1 includes guidelines for the proper use and application of restraints. Use of restraints must meet the following objectives:

- Reduce the risk of patient injury
- Prevent the interruption of therapy, such as traction, IV infusion, nasogastric tube feeding, or Foley catheterization
- Prevent the confused or combative patient from removing life-support equipment
- Reduce the risk of injury to others by the patient

⊚ BOX 38.6   NURSING CARE PLAN
Risk for Injury

ASSESSMENT

The following is a scenario for developing a nursing care plan to mitigate against the risk of patient injuries. A visiting nurse is seeing Ms. Cohen, an 85-year-old woman, at her home. The patient has been recovering from a mild stroke affecting her left side. Ms. Cohen lives alone but receives regular assistance from her daughter and son, who both live within 16 km. The nurse's assessment includes a discussion of Ms. Cohen's health problem and how the stroke has affected her, as well as a pertinent physical examination.

Assessment Activities	Findings and Defining Characteristics
Ask Ms. Cohen how the stroke has affected her mobility.	She responds, "I bump into things, and I'm afraid I'm going to fall."
Conduct a home hazard assessment.	Cabinets in the kitchen are in disarray and full of breakable items that could fall out. Throw rugs are on floors; bathroom lighting is poor (40-watt bulb); bathtub lacks safety strips and grab bars; and home is cluttered with furniture and small objects.
Observe Ms. Cohen's gait and posture.	Ms. Cohen has kyphosis and has a hesitant, uncoordinated gait. She frequently holds walls for support.
Assess Ms. Cohen's muscle strength.	The left arm and leg are weaker than the right.
Assess visual acuity with corrective lenses.	Ms. Cohen has trouble reading and seeing familiar objects at a distance while wearing current glasses.

NURSING DIAGNOSIS: Risk for injury related to impaired mobility, decreased visual acuity, and physical environmental hazards

PLANNING

Goals (Nursing Outcomes Classification)*	Expected Outcomes
	Risk Control
Home will be free of hazards within 1 month.	Modifiable hazards in kitchen and hallway will be reduced in the home within 1 week. Revisions to bathroom will be completed in 1 month.
	Knowledge: Personal Safety
Patient and family will be knowledgeable of potential hazards for patient's age group within 1 week.	Patient and her daughter or son will identify risks and the steps to avoid them in the home at the conclusion of a teaching session next week.
	Fall Prevention Behaviour
Patient will express greater sense of feeling safe from falls in 1 month.	Patient will report improved vision with the aid of new eyeglasses within 1 week.
Patient will be free of injury within 2 weeks.	Patient will be able to safely ambulate throughout the home and perform personal care activities within 2 weeks.

*Outcome classification labels from Moorhead, S., Swanson, E., Johnson, M., & Maas, M. L (Eds.). (2018). *Nursing outcomes classification (NIC)* (6th ed.). Elsevier

INTERVENTIONS

Interventions (Nursing Interventions Classification)†	Rationale
Fall Prevention	
Review findings from home hazard assessment with patient and her daughter and son.	Fall risks for homebound older persons include visual disturbances, unsteady gait, and postural changes (Meiner & Yeager, 2018). Evaluation of home hazards will highlight extrinsic factors that may lead to falls.
Establish a list of priorities to modify. Have patient's son or daughter assist in installing bathroom safety devices.	Modification of environment reduces fall risk (McCullagh, 2006).
Install lighting (75-W bulbs, nonglare) throughout the home. Have patient's son or daughter install blinds over kitchen windows.	With aging, the pupil loses the ability to adjust to light, causing sensitivity to glare. Glare can make it difficult to clearly see a walking path (Meiner & Yeager, 2018).
Discuss with patient and daughter and son the normal changes of aging, effects of recent stroke, associated risks for injury, and how to reduce risks.	Education regarding management of hazards can reduce fear of falling (Touhy & Jett, 2020).
Encourage daughter or son to schedule patient's vision testing for new prescription within 2–4 weeks.	Improved visual acuity reduces incidence of falls (Dames et al., 2021).
Refer patient to a physiotherapist to assess need for assistive devices for kyphosis, left-sided weakness, and gait.	Exercise often improves gait, balance, and flexibility. Modifying gait problems by increasing lower extremity strength reduces fall risk.

†Intervention classification labels from Bulechek, G. M., Butcher, H. K., McCloskey Dochterman, J. M., et al. (Eds.). (2019). *Nursing interventions classification (NIC)* (7th ed.). Mosby.

EVALUATION

Nursing Actions	Patient Response and Finding	Achievement of Outcome
Ask patient and family to identify risks.	Ms. Cohen and her daughter and son are able to identify risks during a walk through the home and expressed a greater sense of safety as a result of changes made.	Ms. Cohen and her children are more knowledgeable of potential hazards.
Observe environment for elimination of hazards.	Throw rugs have been removed. Lighting has been increased to 75 watts, except in the bathroom and bedroom.	Environmental hazards have been partially reduced.
Reassess Ms. Cohen's visual acuity.	Ms. Cohen has new glasses and says she can read better and see distant objects more clearly.	Ms. Cohen's vision has improved, enabling her to ambulate more safely.
Observe Ms. Cohen's gait and posture.	Ms. Cohen's gait remains hesitant and uncoordinated; she reports that her daughter or son has not had time to take her to the physiotherapist.	The outcome of safe ambulation has not been totally achieved; continue to encourage Ms. Cohen and daughter or son to go to physiotherapy appointment.

Nursing Care Plans feature a format that helps you understand the process of assessment, the relationship between assessment findings and nursing diagnoses, the identification of goals and outcomes, the selection of interventions, and the process for evaluating care.

Rationales for each of the interventions in the care plans help you to understand why a specific step or set of steps is performed.

Evaluation sections explain how to evaluate and determine whether the outcomes have been achieved.

Patient Teaching boxes highlight what and how to teach patients and how to evaluate learning.

---

considered contaminated if touched by any object that is not sterile. When nurses are working with a sterile field or with sterile equipment, they must understand that the slightest break in technique results in contamination. Surgical asepsis should be used in the following situations:

- During procedures that require the intentional perforation of the patient's skin (e.g., the insertion of intravenous catheters or administration of injections)
- When the skin's integrity is broken as a result of trauma, surgical incision, or burns
- During procedures that involve the insertion of catheters or surgical instruments into sterile body cavities

Although surgical asepsis is commonly practised in the operating room, labour and delivery area, and major diagnostic areas, nurses may also use surgical aseptic techniques at the patient's bedside—for example, when inserting intravenous or urinary catheters, suctioning the tracheobronchial airway, or reapplying sterile dressings. In an operating room, nurses must follow a series of steps to maintain sterile technique, including applying a mask, protective eyewear, and a cap; performing a surgical hand scrub; and applying a sterile gown and gloves. In contrast, when performing a dressing change at a patient's bedside, nurses may only perform hand hygiene and apply sterile gloves (see "Principles of Surgical Asepsis" section). When using the principles of surgical asepsis, nurses need to remember that they are trying to prevent infections. For more information on infection control, see Box 34.19.

Patient Preparation. Because surgical asepsis necessitates exact techniques, the nurse must have the patient's cooperation. Therefore, the nurse must prepare the patient before any procedure. Some patients may fear moving or touching objects during a sterile procedure, but others may try to assist. Nurses need to explain how a procedure is to be performed and what the patient can do to avoid contaminating sterile items, including the following:

- Avoid sudden movements of body parts covered by sterile drapes.
- Refrain from touching sterile supplies, drapes, or the nurse's gloves and gown.
- Avoid coughing, sneezing, or talking over a sterile area.

to prevent its transmission. The home environment does not always lend itself to infection prevention—often you must help patients adapt according to the resources available to maintain hygienic techniques. However, patients in a home care setting generally have a lower risk of infection than do patients in a hospital because they have less exposure to resistant organisms and undergo fewer invasive procedures.

Surgical Asepsis. Surgical asepsis, or sterile technique, requires precautions different from those of medical asepsis. Surgical asepsis includes procedures used to eliminate all microorganisms, including spores, from an object or area. In surgical asepsis, an area or object is

---

BOX 34.18   PATIENT TEACHING
Infection Control

Objective
- Patient will perform self-care using proper infection-control techniques.

Teaching Strategies
- Instruct patient to clean equipment using soap and water and to disinfect it with an appropriate disinfectant.
- Demonstrate proper hand hygiene, explaining that it should be done before and after all treatments and when infected body fluids are contacted.
- Inform patient of the signs and symptoms of wound infection.
- For patients who receive tube feedings, explain the importance of following instructions regarding how long formula can be prepared ahead of time and left unrefrigerated. Tell patient that contaminated enteral feedings can cause infections. Teach patient to care for the feeding bag and tubing as per the organization's protocol.
- Instruct patient to place contaminated dressings and other disposable items containing infectious body fluids in impervious plastic bags and to place needles in a puncture-proof and leak-proof container, such as an empty bleach bottle with the opening taped shut or a coffee can with the lid taped closed. Glass containers should not be used. Ensure that the patient knows to contact the local municipality or public health department before disposing of contaminated items (Provincial Infection Control Network of British Columbia [PICNet], 2014).

- Instruct patient (or family) to separate noticeably soiled linen from other laundry, wash it in water that is as hot as the fabric will tolerate, add 250 mL of bleach to detergent, and set the dryer temperature as high as the fabric will allow.

Evaluation
- Ask patient or family member to describe techniques used to reduce the transmission of infection.
- Ask patient to demonstrate select techniques.
- Ask patient to explain the risks for infection, based on the condition.

After patients are at home, nurses need to educate them about infection and techniques to prevent or control its spread, and nurses need to determine patients' adherence to infection-control practices. Family members caring for patients must be involved in the teaching plan: Patients and family members should be taught a common-sense approach to controlling and preventing infection. Topics to address in a teaching session include the following:
- The patient's susceptibility to infection
- The chain of infection, with specific reference to the means of transmission
- Hygienic practices that minimize organism growth and spread; emphasize hand hygiene
- Preventive health care (e.g., proper diet, immunizations, and exercise)
- The proper methods for handling and storage of food
- An awareness of family members who are at risk for acquiring infection

Evidence-Informed Practice boxes provide examples of recent state-of-the-science guidelines for nursing practice.

BOX 41.3 EVIDENCE-INFORMED PRACTICE

Preventing and Responding to Dehydration* in Older Persons

Evidence Summary

- Dehydration is the most common fluid and electrolyte challenge in older persons and has a very high mortality rate (Minooee, 2021).
- Older persons are at increased risk of illness and death from dehydration, overhydration, and salt overload.
- Reduced thirst sensation and diminished appetite contribute to dehydration in older persons. Older people also have diminished capacity to correct volume losses.
- Chronic dehydration contributes to constipation in older persons.
- Adequate hydration in older persons is recommended for the prevention of falls, possibly related to hypotension or postural hypotension.
- Dehydration is a risk factor for delirium. The risk for delirium can be reduced as much as 33% with each additional glass of water consumed (El-Sharkawy et al., 2015a).
- Signs and symptoms of dehydration can be easily confused with normal aging processes; therefore, assessment requires knowledge, skill, and commitment to acting on signs and symptoms.

Nursing Practice Guidelines

- Calculating fluid requirements should take into consideration individual characteristics, including weight, gender, environmental factors, physical activity, and comorbidities, such as renal and cardiac disease.
- Because older persons are more susceptible to dehydration and have a higher rate of mortality from dehydration, early detection of infection and disorders in fluid balance is very important (Shepherd, 2013).
- Identify risk factors for each older person from the following: age over 70 years, female, high or low body mass index, recent hospitalization, new admission to long-term care, situations causing increased insensible loss (pyrexia), decreased access or ability to request fluids, and situations causing decreased intake, such as swallowing disorder (dysphagia), physical frailty, and decreased sentience. Previous malnutrition, dehydration, polypharmacy, and having more than three medical conditions are significant risk factors.
- Establish an assessment, monitoring, and evaluation tool for identifying risk factors for older persons when initiating a caregiving relationship (e.g., on admission to long-term care; with home assessment of older persons; routine health care visits).
- Assessment of hydration status should include physiological measures (urine colour, blood pressure, pulse, and respiration) as well as observed intake patterns and treatments. Recommend blood testing to determine the cause and severity in suspected dehydration.
- Maintain fluid intake through documented planning using the nursing process in home, long-term care, and hospital settings, offering fluids every 1.5 hours (Minooee, 2021) to meet a daily fluid intake goal. Caffeinated beverages can be offered, in addition to water.
- Educate older persons and their family and friends on the importance of hydration.
- Diarrhea and vomiting are key causes of dehydration in older persons. Evaluate acute losses such as diarrhea and vomiting.
- Attend more diligently to fluid balance in the context of medical issues such as diabetes, with the use of diuretics, with decreased cognitive level or functional status, and with reduced level of consciousness.
- Minimize fasting for diagnostics and procedures (Minooee, 2021).
- Ensure availability of adequate fluids, including water, tea, coffee, milk, and other beverages, throughout the day and assist persons who are unable to access their own fluids. Replenish and refresh fluids through the day.
- Advocate for adequate staffing levels in long-term care and acute care facilities, as inadequate staffing is closely linked to increased mortality (Shepherd, 2013).
- Promote audits of hydration practices and barriers or obstacles in health care settings and identify benchmarks for improved practice.
- Ongoing management consists of daily fluid goals, comparing current intake with physiological needs, and monitoring actual consumption of fluids and fluid-rich foods.
- Incorporate the offer of fluids, hot or cold, into regular rounds, socializing, and aspects of care using the "little and often" approach. Offer assistive devices

*Dehydration is defined variably. Shepherd (2013) defines dehydration as
text and Tables 41.3 and 41.4 for exploration of dehydration and tonicity.

that place patients at high risk for fluid, electrolyte, and acid–base alterations. When obtaining a medical history, it is important to review any allergies. Treatment for fluid, electrolyte, and acid–base imbalances may involve exposure to latex in equipment and supplies. With newborns and infants, the nurse needs to assess the mother for known latex allergy to prevent inadvertent exposure to latex sensitization.

Burns. The burned patient can lose body fluids by many routes. The greater the body surface burned, the greater the fluid loss. Burns can result in a plasma-to-interstitial fluid shift. Plasma and interstitial fluids are also lost as burn exudate. Water vapour and heat are lost in proportion to the amount of skin that is burned away, increasing insensible losses. Blood leaks from damaged capillaries, adding to the loss of intravascular fluid volume. Sodium and water shift into the cells, further compromising ECF volume (Lewis et al., 2023). Cell damage is accompanied by a loss of serum proteins, and a release of potassium into the intravascular fluid.

Respiratory disorders. Many alterations in respiratory function predispose the patient to respiratory acidosis. For example, pneumonia or sedative overdose interferes with the elimination of carbon dioxide due to hypoventilation. As the carbon dioxide continues to build up in

branes caused by the presence of desaturated hemoglobin in capillaries, is a late sign of hypoxia. The presence or absence of cyanosis is not a reliable measure of oxygenation status. Central cyanosis, observed in the tongue, soft palate, and conjunctiva of the eye, where blood flow is high, indicates hypoxemia. Peripheral cyanosis, seen in the extremities, nail beds, and earlobes, is often a result of vasoconstriction and stagnant blood flow. Cyanosis may be best observed in racialized persons by assessing mucous membranes and nailbeds (Medline Plus, 2021). Hypoxia is a life-threatening condition. Untreated, it can produce cardiac dysrhythmias that result in death. Hypoxia is managed by administration of oxygen and treatment of the underlying cause, such as airway obstruction.

NURSING KNOWLEDGE BASE

Developmental Factors

According to the Canadian Association of Schools of Nursing (CASN, 2022), foundational knowledge of human development expanding over the lifespan is an essential domain to consider when developing a plan of care. The developmental stage of the patient and the normal aging process can affect tissue oxygenation.

Infants and Toddlers. Infants and toddlers are at risk for upper respiratory tract infections as a result of frequent exposure to other children and exposure to second-hand smoke. In addition, during the teething process, some infants develop nasal congestion, which encourages bacterial growth and increases the potential for respiratory tract infection. Upper respiratory tract infections are usually not dangerous, and infants or toddlers recover with little difficulty.

School-Aged Children and Adolescents. School-aged children and adolescents are exposed to respiratory infections and respiratory

Older Persons. The cardiac and respiratory systems undergo changes throughout the aging process (Box 40.4). These changes are associated with calcification of the heart valves, SA node, and costal cartilages. The arterial system develops atherosclerotic plaques. Osteoporosis leads to changes in the size and shape of the thorax.

The trachea and large bronchi become enlarged from calcification of the airways. The alveoli enlarge, decreasing the surface area available for gas exchange. The number of functional cilia is reduced, causing a decrease in the effectiveness of the cough mechanism, putting the older person at increased risk for respiratory infections (Touhy et al., 2019). Ventilation and transfer of respiratory gases decline with age because the lungs are unable to expand fully, leading to lower oxygenation levels.

Lifestyle Risk Factors

Lifestyle modifications that influence cardiopulmonary functioning are frequently difficult because a patient is being asked to change a habit or behaviour that may be enjoyed, such as cigarette smoking or eating certain foods; however, these changes can be achieved with encouragement, support, and time (Box 40.5). Risk factor modification is important and includes smoking cessation, weight reduction, a low-cholesterol and low-sodium diet, management of hypertension, and moderate exercise. Although it may be difficult to change long-term behaviour, assisting patients with healthy behaviours can slow or halt the progression of cardiopulmonary diseases.

Poor Nutrition. Nutrition affects cardiopulmonary function in several ways. Severe obesity decreases lung expansion, and the increased body weight increases oxygen demands to meet metabolic needs. The malnourished patient may experience respiratory muscle wasting, resulting in decreased muscle strength and respiratory excursion. Cough

Focus on Older Persons boxes prepare you to address the special needs of older persons.

BOX 40.4 FOCUS ON OLDER PERSONS

Changes to Cardiac and Respiratory Systems

- Cardiac problems differ from other chronic conditions in that, when they become acute, symptoms worsen rapidly and necessitate hospitalization, whereas other chronic conditions can be managed in the home (Touhy et al., 2019).
- In existing or developing atherosclerosis or hypertension, there may be increased consequences for older persons (Touhy et al., 2019).
- Mental status changes are often the first signs of respiratory problems and may include forgetfulness and irritability.
- Older persons may not complain of dyspnea until it affects the activities of daily living that are important to them.
- Changes in the older person's cough mechanism may lead to retention of pulmonary secretions, airway plugging, and atelectasis, if cough suppressants are not used with caution.
- Age-related changes in the structure of the chest and muscle strength can affect the older person's ability to cough, thus putting them at increased risk for respiratory infections (Touhy et al., 2019).
- For older persons who are sedentary, a compromised immune system may lead to respiratory complications. It is encouraged that older persons receive an annual influenza immunization and a single pneumococcal vaccine (Touhy et al., 2019).

Focus on Primary Health Care boxes draw attention to principles of primary health care and their application.

BOX 40.5 FOCUS ON PRIMARY HEALTH CARE

Positive Lifestyle Practices for Cardiopulmonary Health Promotion

As part of a primary health care focus, it is important to educate young to older persons about the following lifestyle practices that promote cardiopulmonary health:

- Maintain ideal body weight.
- Eat a low-fat, low-salt, low-sugar, calorie-appropriate diet.
- Engage in regular aerobic exercise 30 to 60 minutes daily.
- Use stress-reduction techniques.
- Reduce exposure to secondary infections.
- Do not smoke.
- Avoid exposure to second-hand smoke and other pollutants.
- Using recreational drugs (e.g., cannabis, cocaine, opioids) can increase the risk of stroke and of developing heart disease.
- Limit the use of alcohol.
- Have annual visits with a health care provider.
- Monitor blood pressure.
- Monitor cholesterol and triglyceride levels.
- Request an annual influenza vaccine, especially if at risk for development of influenza.
- Request a pneumococcal vaccine, if appropriate.

Adapted from Heart and Stroke Foundation of Canada. (2022). *Lifestyle risk factors.* https://www.heartandstroke.ca/stroke/risk-and-prevention/lifestyle-risk-factors

Nursing Skills are presented in a clear, two-column format that includes Steps and Rationales to help you learn how and why a skill is performed.

Delegation Considerations guide you in delegating tasks to assistive personnel.

Critical Decision Points alert you to critical steps within a skill to ensure safe and effective patient care.

CHAPTER 39 Hygiene   927

SKILL 39.2   PERFORMING NAIL AND FOOT CARE

Delegation Considerations

The skill of nail and foot care for the nondiabetic patient can be delegated to a regulated or an unregulated care provider; however, this skill should not be delegated if the patient is diabetic. It is important to discuss the following:

- That nail clipping must be performed by the nurse
- Any special considerations for patient positioning

Equipment

- Wash basin
- Emesis basin
- Washcloth and bath towel
- Nail clippers (the patient's)
- Emery board or nail file
- Unscented lotion
- Disposable bath mat
- Paper towels
- Disposable gloves

PROCEDURE

STEPS	RATIONALE
1. Identify patients at risk for foot or nail conditions:	• Certain conditions increase the likelihood of foot or nail problems.
A. Older person	• Poor vision, lack of coordination, or inability to bend over contributes to difficulty in performing foot and nail care. Normal physiological changes of aging also result in nail and foot conditions (Muchna et al., 2018).
B. Diabetes mellitus	• Vascular changes associated with diabetes mellitus reduce blood flow to peripheral tissues. Breaks in skin integrity place a diabetic patient at high risk for a skin infection. Meticulous foot assessment and care reduce the diabetic patient's risk of debilitating foot conditions (Behroozian & Beckman, 2020).
C. Heart failure or renal disease	• Both conditions can increase tissue edema, particularly in dependent areas (e.g., feet). Edema reduces blood flow to neighbouring tissues.
D. Cerebrovascular accident (stroke)	• The presence of residual foot or leg weakness or paralysis results in altered walking patterns. An altered gait pattern increases friction and pressure on feet.
2. Assess patient's knowledge of foot and nail care practices.	• Det
3. Ask patients about whether they use nail polish and polish remover frequently.	• Che
4. Assess patient's ability to care for nails or feet; consider visual alterations, fatigue, and musculoskeletal weakness.	• Der of a
5. Assess types of home remedies (e.g., aloe vera, herbal preparations) that the patient uses.	• Son exp
A. Over-the-counter chemical preparations to remove corns or calluses	• Che
B. Cutting or shaving of corns or calluses with razor blade or scissors	• Cut incr
C. Use of oval corn pads	• Oval rou
D. Application of adhesive tape	• The tape
6. Assess type of footwear worn by patients: Are socks worn? Are shoes tight or ill fitting? Are garters or knee-high nylons worn? Is footwear clean?	• Son pro me mai
7. Observe patient's walking gait. Have the patient walk down a hall or in a straight line (if able).	• Stru ura
8. Assist an ambulatory patient to sit in a bedside chair. Help a bed-bound patient to a supine position with head of the bed elevated. Place a disposable bath mat on the floor under the patient's feet or place a towel on the mattress.	• Sitti feet

---

928   UNIT VIII Basic Physiological Needs

SKILL 39.2   PERFORMING NAIL AND FOOT CARE—cont'd

STEPS	RATIONALE
9. Obtain a health care provider's order for cutting nails if agency policy requires it.	• The patient's skin may be accidentally cut. Certain patients are more at risk for infection, depending on their medical condition.
10. Explain the procedure to the patient, including the fact that proper soaking requires several minutes.	• The patient must be willing to place their fingers and feet in the basin for 10–20 minutes. Patient may become anxious or fatigued.

CRITICAL DECISION POINT: *Patients with diabetes do not soak hands and feet. Soaking increases their risk of infection due to maceration of the skin.*

STEPS	RATIONALE
11. Perform hand hygiene. Arrange equipment on an overbed table.	• Reduces transmission of microorganisms. Easy access to equipment prevents delays.
12. Fill wash basin with warm water. Test water temperature.	• Warm water softens nails and thickened epidermal cells, reduces inflammation of the skin, and promotes local circulation. Proper water temperature prevents burns.
13. Place basin on bath mat or towel.	• Avoids spills; this maintains safety of the care provider and the patient.
14. Fill emesis basin with warm water, and place basin on paper towels on overbed table.	• Warm water softens nails and thickened epidermal cells.
15. Pull curtain around the bed or close the room door (if desired).	• Maintaining the patient's privacy reduces anxiety.
16. Inspect all surfaces of the fingers, toes, feet, and nails. Pay particular attention to areas of dryness, inflammation, or cracking. Also inspect the areas between toes, heels, and soles of feet.	• The integrity of feet and nails determines the frequency and level of hygiene required. Heels, soles, and sides of the feet are prone to irritation from ill-fitting shoes.

CRITICAL DECISION POINT: *Patients with peripheral vascular diseases or diabetes mellitus, older persons, and patients whose immune system is suppressed may require nail care from a specialist to reduce the risk of infection.*

STEPS	RATIONALE
17. Assess colour and temperature of toes, feet, and fingers. Assess capillary refill. Palpate radial and ulnar pulses of each hand and dorsalis pedis pulses of feet (see Chapter 33).	• Assesses the adequacy of blood flow to extremities. Peripheral vascular disease can contribute to poor wound healing. Patients who are immunocompromised or who have neuropathy or peripheral vascular disease are at increased risk of foot infections (Diabetes Canada, 2020).
18. Instruct patient to place their fingers in the emesis basin and place arms in a comfortable position. Assist patient in placing their feet in the basin.	• Prolonged positioning can cause discomfort unless normal anatomical alignment is maintained. • Patients with muscular weakness may have difficulty positioning their feet.
19. Allow patient's feet and fingernails to soak for 10–20 minutes (unless the patient has diabetes). Rewarm water after 10 minutes.	• Softening of corns, calluses, and cuticles ensures easy removal of dead cells and easy manipulation of cuticles.
20. Clean gently under the fingernails with an orange stick or the wooden end of a cotton-tipped swab while fingers are immersed (see Step 20 illustration). Remove fingers from the emesis basin, and dry thoroughly.	• The orange stick removes debris under nails that harbours microorganisms. Thorough drying impedes fungal growth and prevents maceration of the tissues.
21. Using nail clippers, clip fingernails straight across and even with the tops of fingers (see Step 21 illustration). Using a file, shape the nails straight across. If patient has circulatory problems, do not cut the nail; only file the nail.	• For infection-control purposes, use the patient's own nail clippers. Cutting straight across prevents splitting of the nail margins and the formation of sharp nail spikes that can irritate lateral nail margins. Filing prevents cutting the nail too close to the nail bed.
22. Push cuticle back gently with a wet facecloth. Thoroughly dry the hands.	• Reduces incidence of inflamed cuticles. Thorough drying impedes fungal growth and prevents maceration of the tissues.

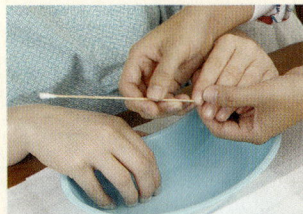

STEP 20 Clean fingernails with the end of a cotton-tipped swab or an orange stick.

STEP 21 Using nail clippers, trim nails straight across.

SKILL 35.2   ADMINISTERING OPHTHALMIC MEDICATIONS—cont'd

STEPS	RATIONALE
16. With the tissue or cotton resting below the lower lid, gently press downward with your thumb or forefinger against the bony orbit.	• Exposes the lower conjunctival sac. Retraction against the bony orbit prevents pressure and trauma to the eyeball and prevents your fingers from touching the eye.
17. Ask the patient to look at the ceiling and explain the steps to the patient.	• Retracts the sensitive cornea up and away from the conjunctival sac and reduces stimulation of the blink reflex.
A. Instill the eye drops: (1) With your dominant hand resting on the patient's forehead, hold the filled medication eyedropper or the ophthalmic solution approximately 1–2 cm above the conjunctival sac (see Step 17A[1] illustration).	• Prevents accidental contact of the eyedropper with eye structures, reducing risk of injury to the eye and transfer of infection to dropper. Ophthalmic medications are sterile.

STEP 17A(1) Hold the eyedropper above the conjunctival sac.

(2) Instill the prescribed number of medication drops into the conjunctival sac.	• The conjunctival sac normally holds one or two drops, which provides even distribution of medication across the eye.
(3) If the patient blinks or closes their eye, or if the drops land on the outer lid margins, repeat the procedure.	• Medication must enter the conjunctival sac to be effective.
(4) After instilling the drops, ask the patient to close the eye gently.	•
(5) When administering medications that cause systemic effects, apply gentle pressure with your finger and a clean tissue on the patient's nasolacrimal duct for 30–60 seconds.	•
B. Instill eye ointment: (1) Ask the patient to look at the ceiling.	•
(2) Holding the ointment applicator above the lower lid margin, apply a thin stream of ointment evenly along the inner edge of the lower eyelid on the conjunctiva (see Step 17B[2] illustration) from the inner canthus to outer canthus.	•

STEP 17B(2) Apply ointment along the lower eyelid.

Clear, close-up **photos** and **illustrations** show you how to perform important nursing techniques.

SKILL 39.2   PERFORMING NAIL AND FOOT CARE—cont'd

STEPS	RATIONALE
23. Move the overbed table away from the patient.	• Provides easier access to the feet.
24. Put on disposable gloves, and scrub callused areas of the feet with a washcloth.	• Gloves help prevent transmission of fungal infection. Friction removes dead skin layers.
25. Clean gently under nails with an orange stick. Remove feet from basin, and dry them thoroughly.	• Removal of debris and excess moisture reduces chances of infection.
26. Clean and trim toenails using the procedures in Steps 21 and 22. Do not file the corners of toenails.	• For infection-control purposes, use the patient's own nail clippers. Shaping corners of toenails may damage tissues.
27. Apply lotion to feet and hands, and assist patient back to bed and into a comfortable position.	• Lotion lubricates dry skin by helping to retain moisture.
28. Remove disposable gloves and place in a receptacle. Clean and return the equipment and supplies to the proper place. Dispose of soiled linen in a hamper. Perform hand hygiene.	• Reduces the transmission of infection.
29. Inspect the nails and surrounding skin surfaces after soaking and nail trimming.	• Determines the condition of skin and nails. Allows caregiver to note any remaining rough nail edges.
30. Ask patient to explain or demonstrate nail care.	• Evaluates patient's level of learning techniques.
31. Observe patient's walk after toenail care.	• Evaluates the level of comfort and mobility achieved.

UNEXPECTED OUTCOMES	RELATED INTERVENTIONS
Inflammation and tenderness of cuticles and surrounding tissues	• Repeated soakings may be needed to relieve inflammation and loosen layers of cells from calluses or corns. • Patients with diabetes or peripheral vascular disease may require referral to a podiatrist. • Antifungal cream may be needed.
Localized areas of tenderness on feet, with calluses or corns at points of friction	• Change in footwear may be needed. • Refer to a podiatrist.
Appearance of ulcer between toes or other pressure areas on foot	• Notify health care provider. • Refer to a podiatrist. • Increase frequency of foot assessment and hygiene.

RECORDING AND REPORTING
• Document the procedure and any observations (e.g., breaks in the skin, inflammation, ulcerations) on the patient's record sheets using the forms provided by your agency or facility.
• Report any breaks in the skin or ulcerations to the person in charge or to the health care provider. These breaks are serious in patients with diabetes, peripheral vascular disease, and illnesses that impair circulation. Special foot care treatments may be needed.

CARE IN THE COMMUNITY CONSIDERATIONS
• If the patient has diabetes or decreased peripheral circulation, alternative therapies or foot soaking should be carried out only after consulting with a health care provider.
• An alternative therapy would be moleskin applied to areas of the feet that are experiencing friction—this is less likely to cause pressure than corn pads. Spot adhesive bandages can guard against friction, but they do not have padding to protect against pressure.
• If the patient is ambulatory, instruct them to soak their feet in a bathtub.
• If the patient's mobility is limited, a large basin or pan can be used for soaking.

affects the health and integrity of tissues of the feet and should be advised to use the following guidelines in a routine foot and nail care program:

Inspect the feet daily, including the tops and soles of the feet, the heels, and the areas between the toes. Use a mirror to help inspect the feet thoroughly or ask a family member to check daily.

Patients with diabetes mellitus should receive a thorough foot examination at least once a year. Patients with one or more high-risk foot conditions should be evaluated more frequently and referred to a specialist as necessary.

Wash the feet daily using lukewarm water; *do not soak the feet.* If there is reduced sensation, a bath thermometer can be used at home to test the water temperature. Thoroughly dry the feet and in between toes.

Do not cut corns or calluses or use commercial removers. Consult a physician, podiatrist, or certified foot nurse.

If the feet perspire excessively, apply a nonallergenic foot powder. If dryness is noted along the sides of the feet, rub a nonallergenic lotion gently into the skin, wiping off any excess. *Do not apply lotion between the toes, as excessive moisture can result in infection.*

Trim the toenails straight across and square; do not use scissors. Consult a podiatrist as needed.

Do not use over the counter preparations or home remedies. Consult a physician, podiatrist, or certified foot nurse.

Recording and Reporting sections provide guidelines for what to chart and report with each skill.

Home Care Considerations explain how to adapt skills for the home setting.

---

744   UNIT VII   Scientific Basis for Nursing Practice

medication calculation or conversion, ensure that another nurse verifies the calculated dose.

After confirming the calculated dose, prepare the medication by using standard measurement devices. Use graduated cups, syringes, and scaled droppers to measure medications accurately. At home, patients should use measuring spoons and cups, not household spoons and cups, which vary in volume.

Only tablets that are scored by the manufacturer should be broken. When a scored tablet needs to be broken, ensure the break is even. A tablet can be cut in half by using a knife or a pill-cutting device. Discard tablets that do not break evenly. Some agencies allow nurses to save the unadministered portion of the scored medication tablet for subsequent doses if the remaining tablet is repackaged and labelled. Nurse should verify with the employer policy before administering a tablet that has been opened, cut, and repackaged. In the community care setting, pill splitting is particularly risky. It is important to determine whether the patient has both the motor dexterity and visual acuity needed to split tablets (Baig et al., 2016). If possible, prescribers need to avoid prescribing medications that require splitting.

Often a nurse prepares a tablet by crushing it so that it can be mixed in food. The crushing device should always be cleaned completely before the tablet is crushed. Remnants of previously crushed medications may increase a medication's concentration or result in the patient receiving a portion of an unprescribed medication. Crushed medications should be mixed with very small amounts of food or liquid but should not be mixed with the patient's favourite foods or liquids because a medication may alter the taste of the food or liquid and thereby decrease the patient's desire for them. This is particularly important when administering crushed medications to pediatric patients.

> **SAFETY ALERT** Not all medications can be crushed. Some medications, such as timed-release or extended-release capsules, are coated with special material to prevent the medication from being absorbed too quickly. Before crushing a medication, refer to a medication manual or another medication reference to ensure that the medication can be safely crushed.

Right Patient. Medication incidents often occur because one patient receives a medication intended for another patient. An important step in administering medications safely is to ensure medications are given to the right patient. Remembering every patient's name and face is difficult. To identify a patient correctly, ask the patient to state their name. Compare the patient's name and another identifier (e.g., hospital identification number) on the MAR against the information on the patient's identification bracelet. Scan the patient's barcode on their identification bracelet, if applicable (see Figure 35.12).

If an identification bracelet is missing or the text is smudged or illegible, acquire a new bracelet for the patient. When asking the patient's name, you should not merely speak the name and assume that the patient's response indicates that they are the right person. Instead, ask the patient to state their full name. To avoid making the patient feel uneasy, simply explain that the question is routine for giving medications.

Right Route. If a prescription does not designate a route of administration, or if the specified route is not the recommended route, always consult with the prescriber.

When administering injections, take precautions to ensure that the medications are given correctly. Prepare injections only from preparations designed for parenteral use. The injection of a liquid designed for oral use can produce local complications, such as a sterile abscess, or

fatal systemic effects. Medication companies label parenteral medications "for injectable use only."

Right Time and Frequency. Nurses must know why a medication is prescribed for certain times of the day and whether the time schedule can be altered. For example, two medications are prescribed: one q8h (every 8 hours) and the other three times a day. Both medications are scheduled three times within a 24-hour period. The prescriber intends the q8h medication to be given around the clock to maintain therapeutic blood levels of the medication. In contrast, the nurse needs to give the three-times-a-day medication during the waking hours. Each institution has a recommended or standard time schedule to guide the administration of medications prescribed for various intervals. Nurses may alter recommended times if necessary or appropriate.

The prescriber often gives specific instructions for the timing of administration of a medication. Medications prescribed to follow an ongoing, consistent, standard dosing schedule are referred to as ROUTINE. As mentioned, when a preoperative medication is to be given ON CALL the nurse needs to administer the medication when notified that the patient can be transferred for surgery by health care providers in the operating room. A medication prescribed pc (after meals) is to be given within half an hour after a meal, when the patient has a full stomach. A STAT medication is to be given immediately. Priority is given to medications that must act at certain times. For example, insulin should be administered at a precise interval before a meal. Antibiotics should be administered on time around the clock to maintain therapeutic blood levels. Medications should be given within 60 minutes of the times for which they are prescribed (i.e., 30 minutes before or after the prescribed time).

Some medications require nurses to use their clinical judgement to determine the proper time for administration. A prn sleeping medication should be administered when the patient is prepared for bed or at another time appropriate for maximum benefit. When administering prn analgesics, nurses need to use their judgement. For example, the nurse may need to obtain a STAT prescription if the patient requires a

Safety Alerts indicate techniques you can use to ensure patient and nurse safety.

CHAPTER 38   Quality and Patient Safety   883

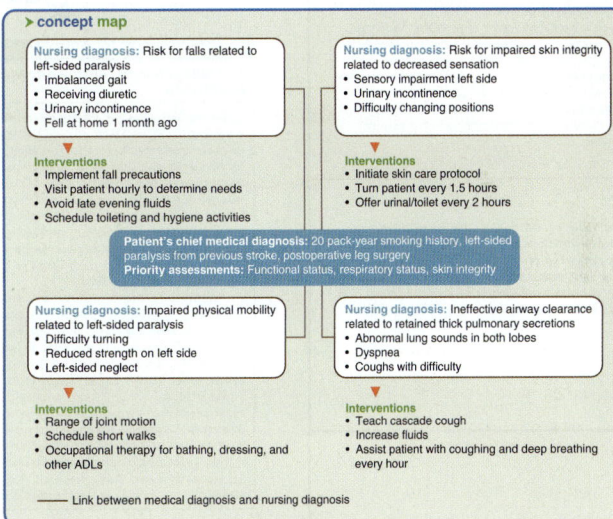

> concept map

FIGURE 38.5 Concept map for a patient with a cerebrovascular accident 3 months previously with left-sided paralysis, 2 days after right femoral–popliteal bypass. *ADLs,* Activities of daily living.

BOX 38.7   CULTURAL ASPECTS OF CARE

Cultural phenomena affecting health and safety include attitudes toward personal space, social organizations, communication, and environmental control. While conducting a home assessment for risks to safety, nurses must remember that they have entered the patient's territory and that the patient's attitude toward their residence and belongings must be appreciated. For example, some patients may be considered aloof and distant when it comes to personal space. It may be very difficult for them to have an outsider in their home who suggests changes regarding their personal belongings to reduce physical hazards. It is particularly difficult to determine a patient's attitude toward their home environment when the patient's primary language and that of the health care provider differ.

Another culturally sensitive issue involves the patient's sense of environmental control. Nurses must be aware of health beliefs and practices that will affect the outcome of interventions. For example, a reliance on family and religious organizations, as opposed to community resources, may affect the patient's adherence to nursing interventions and referrals.

Nurses must learn to ask questions sensitively and to show respect for different cultural beliefs. Adapting to different cultural beliefs and practices requires flexibility. Respect for the belief systems of others and the effects of those beliefs on the patient's well-being are critically important to competent health care. The nurse must have the ability and knowledge to communicate about and to understand health behaviours influenced by culture.

Implications for Practice

- Resistance to change long-standing habits can interfere with a cultural group's acceptance of injury-prevention practices. Nurses should include family members who have a strong influence, such as a dominant man or older woman, when providing safety education.
- Nurses should evaluate the use of traditional ethnic remedies or foods that contain lead, as these can increase a patient's risk for lead poisoning.
- Nurses should remember that living in rural areas and in manufactured housing places the patient at greater risk for fire-related injuries and death.
- Nurses should stress the importance of having fully functioning smoke detectors and a multipurpose fire extinguisher.
- Nurses should assess the patient's smoking and drinking habits. Residential fire deaths are often attributed to the use of cigarettes and alcohol.
- Patients who live in poverty and have low educational levels are at greater risk for injury and disease. Nurses should assist the patient and family in identifying community resources, such as the local health office or clinic.
- Nurses also need to be aware of family patterns and how the patient and family interact with each other. Family disruption and weak intergenerational ties can increase a patient's risk for injury from violent behaviour.

Adapted from Giger, J. N., & Davidhizar, R. (2002). The Giger and Davidhizar transcultural assessment model. *Journal of Transcultural Nursing, 13,* 185.

Cultural Aspects of Care boxes prepare you to care for patients of diverse populations and suggest actions needed to meet different cultural needs and preferences.

Procedural Guideline boxes provide streamlined, step-by-step instructions for performing basic skills.

Case Study boxes tell a real-life story concerning one or more topics in the chapter.

BOX 41.12 PROCEDURAL GUIDELINE
Removing a Short-Peripheral Intravenous Catheter (PIVC)

Delegation Considerations
The skill of removing a PIVC may be delegated to other health care providers if they have had appropriate education, it is within their governing body scope of practice, and it is approved by employer policy. The skill of removing a PIVC cannot be carried out by an unregulated care provider (UCP). The nurse instructs the UCP to report the following immediately:

• Report to the nurse any bleeding at the site after catheter has been removed.
• Report any complaints of pain by the patient or observation of redness at the site.

Equipment
• Clean gloves
• Sterile 5 × 5–cm (2 × 2–inch) or 10 × 10–cm (4 × 4–inch) gauze sponge or small adhesive dressing
• Tape

Procedure
1. Key assessments prior to removal of PIVC include identifying if the patient is on any anticoagulant or antiplatelet therapy or has a disorder that causes slow clotting.
2. Review accuracy and completeness of health care provider's prescription for discontinuation of PIVC, if required.
3. Perform hand hygiene and collect equipment.
4. Identify patient using at least two identifiers (e.g., name and birthday or name and medical record number) according to employer policy. Compare identifiers with information on patient's medication administration record (MAR) or medical record.
5. Perform hand hygiene and apply clean gloves. Palpate catheter site through intact dressing.
6. Assess patient's understanding of the reason for PVAD removal.
7. Explain procedure to patient before you remove the catheter.
8. If PIVC is connected to an administration set, turn administration set roller clamp to "off" position or turn electronic infusion device (EID) off and roller clamp to "off" position.
9. Carefully remove PIVC dressing as per Skill 41.4.
   Critical Decision Point: Never use scissors to remove the tape or dressing because you may accidentally cut the catheter.
10. Place clean, sterile gauze above insertion site and, using your dominant hand, withdraw catheter using a slow, steady motion and keeping the hub parallel to skin (see Step 10 illustration).
    Critical Decision Point: Do not raise or lift catheter before it is completely out of the vein, to avoid trauma or hematoma formation.
11. Apply pressure to site for a minimum of 30 seconds until bleeding has stopped. If patient has increased clotting, maintain pressure until hemostasis occurs.

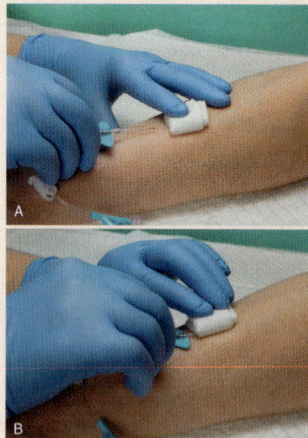

STEP 10 PIVC removal: **A,** Apply pressure and cover site. **B,** Remove catheter. From Cobbett, S. L., Perry, A.G., Potter, P. A., et al. [Eds.]. [2020]. *Canadian clinical nursing skills & techniques.* Elsevier. Photos courtesy Patrick Coble.)

Blood administration tubing with a 70- to 260-micron filter is used, and the nurse needs to determine if the tubing is appropriate for the EID when using one. When priming blood administration tubing, 0.9% normal saline must be used to prevent hemolysis, or breakdown of RBCs. Timing of blood transfusion is extremely important. The infusion is begun within 30 minutes of accessing the blood component

BOX 13.1 CASE STUDY
The Application of Nursing Knowledge to Policy Leadership: Addressing Indigenous-Specific Racism in Health Care

On June 19, 2020, allegations of Indigenous-specific racism in health care in British Columbia (BC) went public when the Minister of Health announced the launch of an independent investigation (Government of British Columbia, 2020). The investigation initially focused on reports of a racist game being played in emergency departments. It was then expanded to broadly encompass reports and experiences of racism in health care from both Indigenous peoples and non-Indigenous people. Led by Mary Ellen Turpel-Lafond, the investigation resulted in the publication of the *In Plain Sight* report (Turpel-Lafond, 2020). In it, Turpel-Lafond documents the stories of Indigenous peoples who have faced racism and discrimination in the health care system and makes recommendations for action to address Indigenous-specific racism.

In Plain Sight is the most recent of many such reports on Indigenous-specific racism and the resilience of Indigenous peoples experiencing genocide, discrimination, and the ongoing impacts of colonialism. Reports by the Truth and Reconciliation Commission of Canada (2015), the National Inquiry Into Missing and Murdered Indigenous Women and Girls (Buller, 2019), and the Public Inquiry Commission on Relations Between Indigenous Peoples and Certain Public Services in Québec (Viens, 2019) are all examples of the intersecting testimonies and recommendations now guiding anti-racism work in health care. As BC health organizations attempted to respond to the recommendations in the *In Plain Sight* report, the need for a systematic analysis of the diverse recommendations emerged to guide decision makers in effectively enacting anti-racism work.

In response to this need, two nurse leaders in a regional health authority were commissioned to undertake a systematic analysis of recommendations from six

intersecting reports, using the *In Plain Sight* report as the reference point. Initial analysis identified for decision makers the ways in which recommendations aligned and diverged between reports. In charting the full landscape for potential policy action, this analysis enabled decision makers, including Indigenous nurse executives, to make meaning out of the recommendations within each report and to make decisions on key areas for immediate action. Secondary analysis, including the development of a logic model, matched recommendations to governance layers, drawing clear lines of accountability and responsibility among interlocking parts of the health system. For example, recommendations that had legislative requirements were aligned to the provincial government's task force rather than to a health authority. This has prevented duplication of effort and supported decision makers in communicating clearly to staff and communities what expectations and responsibilities are within their areas of authority.

As a further measure of its success, the analysis supported the rapid development of an anti-racism strategy for the provincial health authorities and was escalated to the Ministry of Health as a knowledge resource. Critically, the work of these two nurse leaders enabled a major change in the BC health system: instead of asking Indigenous peoples what colonial health systems should do to provide better patient care, health system leaders began to align with and respond to what Indigenous peoples had named for decades. This work has not only supported project coordination, but also cultivated a sense of possibility and strengthened relationships that are the foundation for truth and reconciliation.

BOX 13.2 Entry-Level Registered Nurse Competencies Related to Nursing Leadership Roles

Recently developed national **entry-level competencies** for registered nurses in Canada relate specifically to the roles of collaborator, coordinator, and leader (British Columbia College of Nurses and Midwives [BCCNM], 2020). The role of coordinator of care is becoming increasingly complex as nurses provide leadership at the point of care, ensuring that people receive the right care or service from the provider. Nurses in coordinator roles navigate people's experiences of health and illness transitions across institutional and community-based sectors of care, a role that involves complex consultations and information exchanges (BCCNM, 2020). This role also requires the enactment of competencies related to collaboration, as it involves leading and supporting teams (MacKinnon et al., 2018). Other roles for which nursing students must develop competencies include the role of collaborator and advocate, whereby nurses work with others to advocate and support health equity for all and human rights (BCCNM, 2020). Specific competencies associated with the role of leader appear below.

Leader
Registered nurses are leaders who influence and inspire others to achieve optimal health outcomes for all.

Competencies:
6.1 Acquires knowledge of the Calls to Action of the Truth and Reconciliation Commission of Canada.
6.2 Integrates continuous quality improvement principles and activities into nursing practice.
6.3 Participates in innovative client-centred care models.
6.4 Recognizes the impact of organizational culture and acts to enhance the quality of a professional and safe practice environment.
6.5 Participates in creating and maintaining a healthy, respectful, and psychologically safe workplace.
6.6 Demonstrates self-awareness through reflective practice and solicitation of feedback.
6.7 Takes action to support culturally safe practice environments.
6.8 Uses and allocates resources wisely.
6.9 Provides constructive feedback to promote professional growth of other members of the health care team.
6.10 Demonstrates knowledge of the health care system and its impact on client care and professional practice.
6.11 Adapts practice to meet client care needs within a continually changing health care system.

Adapted from British Columbia College of Nurses and Midwives (BCCNM). (2020). *Entry-level competencies for registered nurses* (pp. 10–11). https://www.bccnm.ca/Documents/competencies_requisite_skills/RN_entry_level_competencies_375.pdf

Historically, nursing leadership often meant clinical operational *management*, where nurses held responsibility for the day-to-day delivery of patient care, upholding standards of professional practice, and stewarding health care resources through financial management (Hibberd et al., 2006). Today, **nursing leadership** also refers to management in clinical operations, but it extends much further to include leadership in knowledge creation through research, policy advocacy and development in governance contexts, executive leadership in executive teams and boards of directors, health care quality leadership in quality improvement and assurance, education as nurse educators and professors, and so much more (Marcellus et al., 2018). To meet the needs of communities and populations, nurse leaders in every domain

SUMMARY

The Canadian health care system will require significant restructuring to meet the complex needs of a diverse population and in response to local and global challenges. In this context, nursing's contributions to health and health care in Canada range from providing direct care to actively participating in the reformation processes, as well as maintaining a continuous presence in the pursuit of equitable access for all patient groups. Nursing has been instrumental in the advancement of nursing practice, interdisciplinary practices, and collaborative efforts for the betterment of society (Turale & Kunaviktikal, 2019). In the future, we must assert our roles as critical stakeholders, partners, and providers within the emerging health care system.

KEY CONCEPTS

- Medicare is a key component of Canada's social safety net.
- All levels of government play a major role in co-funding national health insurance and setting health care policy in accordance with the *Canada Health Act*.
- The *Canada Health Act* articulates the five principles of our national health insurance system—public administration, comprehensiveness, universality, portability, and accessibility—and forbids extra billing and user fees.
- Health care services are provided in institutional, community, and home settings; across all age groups; and for individual, family, group, and community populations.
- The five levels of health care are promotive, preventive, curative, rehabilitative, and supportive.
- Escalating costs, technological innovations, and consumer expectations challenge the health care system in efforts to deliver innovative, efficient, and quality care.
- Equality, equity, access, interdisciplinary approaches, communication, and continuity of care challenge the health care system.
- The primacy of PHC and home care align with the reforming health care environment and cost effectiveness.
- Successful health promotion and disease prevention programs help patients acquire healthier lifestyles and achieve optimal quality of life.
- Sufficient, diverse, and qualified human health resources are essential for a culturally competent workforce attending to a culturally safe Canadian health care system.
- Enhancing the health of the Indigenous population in Canada is a significant challenge to society and to the health care system.
- Nurses must continually seek out information and evidence to remain responsive to providing quality, culturally competent, and safe care.

CRITICAL THINKING EXERCISES

1. Debate the following challenges facing the Canadian health care system: escalating costs, privatization, continuity of care, regionalization/centralization, and digital health.
2. Consider and describe how the economy and technology have changed the Canadian health care system. What are the implications for nursing? For patients and families?
3. Referring to the case study at the beginning of the chapter, describe the types of health care services, safety issues, interprofessional competencies, and technological supports that might play a part in W.W's postsurgical care.

🌐 *Answers to Critical Thinking Exercises appear on the Evolve website.*

REVIEW QUESTIONS

Review Questions 1 to 10 relate to the case study at the beginning of the chapter.

1. During a community health placement, a nursing student interacts with W.W., who tells the student about his upcoming hip replacement surgery. W.W. explains that he went to the preassessment clinic and that they connected him with community services such as Meals on Wheels, home care, and an outpatient physiotherapist. The nursing student understands that these services are important aspects of:
   a. Acute care
   b. Primary health care
   c. Primary care
   d. Ambulatory care
2. During W.W.'s preoperative assessment, the nurse explains the various roles of the interprofessional team members who will be involved in his care after his hip replacement. Which of the following team members would the nurse most likely indicate will be a part of the interprofessional team? *(Select all that apply.)*
   a. Occupational therapist
   b. Physiotherapist
   c. Pharmacist
   d. Translator
   e. Medical-surgical nurse
3. W.W's hip replacement surgery is considered medically necessary in order for W.W. to maintain a good quality of life. The _____ currently ensures that Canadians do not have to pay out of pocket for medically necessary procedures.
   a. Canada Health Act

6. Connecting W.W. with appropriate community-based health services is important because: *(Select all that apply.)*
   a. Community-based services can help to prevent unnecessary and costly hospitalizations.
   b. Community-based services ensure that W.W. can recover at home.
   c. Community-based services can be used instead of hospitalization.
   d. Community-based services are an important element of primary health care.
   e. Community-based services enable W.W. to age in place.
7. W.W. tells the nursing student that he has waited for a long time for this surgery and does not feel that the long wait time was acceptable. W.W. asks the nursing student if anything is being done to address surgical wait times. The nursing student tells W.W. that the following agencies have made efforts to reduce wait times, reduce duplication of tests, and support coordination of care: *(Select all that apply.)*
   a. Canada eHealth
   b. Canadian Institute for Health Information
   c. Canada Health Infoway
   d. Canadian Institutes for Health Research
   e. Consumers' Association of Canada
8. W.W. asks his nurse practitioner why his hip replacement surgery was covered, but his prescription glasses are not. The nurse practitioner explains that there are some health services that are generally not covered under the publicly funded health care system. Some of these noninsured services include: *(Select all that apply.)*
   a. Dental services
   b. Home care
   c. Medical transportation
   d. Medical equipment and appliances (i.e., wheelchairs, prostheses)
   e. Prescription drugs (outside of hospitals)

9. During his hospital stay, W.W. notices that the postoperative surgical unit is often short-staffed. W.W. expresses his concerns about this to the unit manager. This has been one of several similar complaints over the past 6 months, prompting management to request a brief report from the nurse manager on a human resources plan for the next 5 years. Which of the following statements best represents the factors that should be mentioned?
   a. We should be working with our aging nurses to transition them out of full-time work, allowing younger nurses to be mentored into their vacated positions and increasing the number of nurses we are educating.
   b. With all the workplace injuries, we should be hiring an occupational therapist or there will soon be no nurses working.
   c. We will soon be able to replace nurses with robots and technology, so that is where we should be investing.
   d. We are not educating enough nurses, so we may have to recruit from international pools to fill positions.
   e. There are too many variables to be able to predict what will be needed in 5 years, so the best we can do is try to keep the nurses we have.
10. Two months after his hip replacement surgery, W.W. has a minor fall. W.W. is not injured after this incident, but he realizes that he needs to further improve his mobility to return to his previous level of function. W.W. expresses his concern to his nurse practitioner, who refers him to a physiotherapist. This is an example of which level of care?
    a. Level 1: Health Promotion
    b. Level 2: Disease and Injury Prevention
    c. Level 3: Diagnosis and Treatment
    d. Level 4: Rehabilitation
    e. Level 4: Supportive Care

Answers: 1. a; 2. a, b, c; 3. a; 4. e; 5. d; 6. a, b, d; 7. b, c; 8. a, b, c, d, e; 9. a; 10. d.

🌐 *Rationales for the Review Questions appear on the Evolve website.*

RECOMMENDED WEBSITES

Canada Health Infoway: https://www.infoway-inforoute.ca
A not-for-profit corporation created by Canada's first ministers to foster and accelerate development and adoption of digital health innovations across all groups.
Canadian Foundation for Healthcare Improvement: https://www.cfhi-fcass.ca/Home.aspx
This site addresses initiatives of the foundation to advance promising innovations across health care organizations to improve patient care, health outcomes, and efficiencies.
Canadian Institute of Health Information: https://www.cihi.ca
A not-for-profit organization seeking to improve the health care system and the health of Canadians by providing timely and essential health information.

Canadian Patient Safety Institute: https://www.patientsafetyinstitute.ca
This institute was established to build and advance a safer health care system for Canadians. It reports on activities in leadership across health sectors and health care systems, highlights promising practices, and raises awareness with stakeholders and the public about patient safety.
Canadian Public Health Association: https://www.cpha.ca
A national not-for-profit association seeking excellence in public health nationally and internationally and seeking universal and equitable access to basic health-sustaining conditions.
Health Canada: https://www.hc-sc.gc.ca
This website provides links to information about the Canadian health care system, such as the *Canada Health Act* legislation, the federal budget, and federal reports.

🌐 REFERENCES

A full reference list is available on the website for this book at https://evolve.elsevier.com/Canada/Potter/fundamentals/

Review Questions at the end of each chapter help you review and evaluate what you have learned. Answers and rationales are provided at the back of the book.

Key Concepts appear at the end of each chapter to help you review important content.

Recommended Websites provide up-to-date online resources and are annotated to give you some information about each website.

Critical Thinking Exercises encourage you to think creatively and effectively to apply essential content.

PREFACE TO THE INSTRUCTOR

The future of nursing in Canada in a globalized world is dynamic, interconnected, and ever-changing. Our planet's natural systems are changing, which will require all of us to act on the global challenges they present to safeguard the health of our most vulnerable people and of future generations. It is imperative that our student nurses are prepared to have the necessary foundational knowledge of our planet as it relates to their professional nursing practice. The nurses of tomorrow will continue to need to provide evidence-informed nursing practice in order to address the myriad of global and planetary health challenges while maintaining and improving the health of Canadians. Professional nursing practice requires (a) critical thinking and critical reasoning, (b) the ability to collaborate and communicate with diverse clients/patients and the interprofessional team, (c) patient/client advocacy, (d) excellence in clinical decision making, and (e) client/patient and community teaching within a broad spectrum of health services. Moreover, nursing practice will involve engaging in the translation and mobilization of knowledge as well as in leadership development and advocating for health policy change at the local, national, and global levels. *Potter and Perry's Canadian Fundamentals of Nursing* is specifically designed for students at all levels of undergraduate nursing programs. The text provides comprehensive coverage of fundamental nursing concepts, knowledge, research, and skills that are essential to informing nursing practice.

The seventh edition of *Potter and Perry's Canadian Fundamentals of Nursing* has been extensively revised, updated, and thoroughly edited to feature inclusive language that reflects Canada's diverse and multicultural populations, the most current evidence and issues, and future directions for nursing in Canada. All chapters have been written or revised so that they reflect Canadian standards, traditions, research, and practice.

The authors and contributors of the text recognize and acknowledge the diverse histories of the first peoples of the lands now referred to as Canada. It is recognized that individual communities identify themselves in various ways; within this text, the term *Indigenous* is used to refer to all First Nations, Aboriginal, Inuit, Métis, and non-status people within Canada. We also recognize that knowledge and language concerning sex, gender, and identity are fluid and continually evolving. The language and terminology presented in this text endeavour to be inclusive of all people and reflect what is, to the best of our knowledge, current at the time of publication.

Potter and Perry's Canadian Fundamentals of Nursing includes content covering the entire scope of primary, secondary, tertiary, rehabilitative, and end-of-life care. The focus is on the central role of primary health care in all areas of nursing practice. Emphasis is also placed on evidence-informed practice in skills and care plans to foster understanding of how research findings should guide clinical decision making. First-person accounts, in the form of case studies, of issues that have arisen in nursing practice are designed to engage the nursing student's attention and encourage more detailed reading and understanding.

This textbook is the result of the combined efforts of many expert nursing scholars who are committed to excellence. As in our previous editions, we have continued to use expert contributors from across Canada to provide a national perspective. All contributors approached the revisions with enthusiasm and worked hard to ensure that the content is current and reflects the Canadian health care system, Canadian health and social organizations, and uniquely Canadian health care issues in a globalized world. Reviewers scrutinized the chapters and made many helpful suggestions. We appreciate the conscientiousness and commitment of all these dedicated scholars.

CLASSIC FEATURES

- **Comprehensive** coverage and readability of all fundamental nursing content are provided.
- **Full-colour** text is used to enhance visual appeal and instructional value, with many of the images updated.
- **Case Study** boxes present first-person accounts of issues in relation to chapter content.
- **Primary health care and health promotion** issues are discussed throughout the text.
- **Chronic Illness** boxes pertain uniquely to the Canadian health care system.
- **Research Highlight** boxes are integrated throughout the text to provide current and applicable nursing research studies and explain the implications for daily nursing practice.
- **Patient Teaching** boxes highlight patient/client education, listing teaching objectives, strategies, and evaluation for clinical topics throughout the text.
- **Evidence-informed practice** is discussed throughout the text.
- **Evidence-Informed Practice** boxes provide examples of recent state-of-the-science guidelines for nursing practice.
- **Nursing principles** specific to older persons are addressed throughout the text.
- **Nursing Care Plans** guide students in how to conduct an assessment and analyze the defining characteristics that indicate nursing diagnoses. The plans include Nursing Interventions Classification (NIC) and Nursing Outcomes Classification (NOC) labels to familiarize students with this important nomenclature. The evaluation sections of the plans show students how to determine the expected outcomes and evaluate the results of care.
- **Concept Maps** demonstrate the relationships among nursing assessment, diagnosis, planning, intervention, and evaluation.
- **Procedural Guideline** boxes provide step-by-step instructions and photos on how to perform basic skills.
- **End-of-chapter Review Questions** assist students in critically reviewing what they have learned and are based on the case study presented at the beginning of each chapter. Answers and rationales are provided on the Evolve website.
- The annotated **Recommended Websites** section at the end of each chapter directs the student to current resources.
- The **Laboratory Values** appendix (Appendix A) is a concise, up-to-date source of current laboratory values for use in clinical practice.
- Expert contributors and reviewers from across Canada have provided a national perspective.

UPDATED FEATURES

- Each chapter begins with a case study relating to the chapter topic, and end-of-chapter clinical-judgement review questions refer to this case study.
- Language has been updated in all chapters to address cultural and gender diversity and inclusivity.
- **Health and Wellness (Chapter 1)** has been updated to include concepts of health-in-all policies, identity politics, and systemic racism.

- **The Development of Nursing in Canada (Chapter 3)** has been updated to include discussion about decolonizing health care and racism in nursing education and practice.
- A **NEW** chapter, **Practical Nursing in Canada (Chapter 5)**, has been added to provide important information on this nursing role in Canada.
- A revised and updated **Critical Thinking in Nursing Practice (Chapter 7)** was moved into the Foundations Unit of the book to reflect the importance of critical thinking as a foundational skill in nursing practice.
- **Evidence-Informed Practice (Chapter 8)** was updated to include the evidence from systematic reviews as it applies to evidence-informed practice.
- **Global and Planetary Health (Chapter 11)** has been fully updated and expanded, with emphasis on the interconnectedness of the health of humans, other species, and the physical environment related to planetary health; the global COVID-19 pandemic; sustainable development goals (SDGs); environmental sustainability; climate change; climate justice; environmental racism; critical perspectives (health equity, intersectionality, political economy, transnationalism, and relational theory and ethics); immigration; transnationalism; interdisciplinary collaboration; and competencies in global and planetary health.
- **Nursing Leadership and Collaborative Practice (Chapter 13)** has been updated to include a focus on health equity, shared governance, and wellness for nurses.
- **Nursing Informatics and Canadian Nursing Practice (Chapter 17)** has been updated and expanded to discuss "digital health," the use of digital technologies to improve health, as well as consumer health informatics.
- **Family Nursing (Chapter 20)** and **Young to Middle Adulthood (Chapter 24)** have been updated and expanded to fully discuss issues relating to gender identity and gender diversity.
- **Sex, Gender, and Sexuality (Chapter 28)** has been fully updated and expanded, using language from the Canadian LGBTQ2 Secretariat, with added discussion about barriers to access to care and experiences of discrimination among gender minority groups. The chapter also includes information about education and skill-training programs to help student nurses become more aware of potential implicit biases toward LGBTQ2 patients.
- **Spirituality in Health and Health Care (Chapter 29)** has been fully updated and expanded to address diversity and expectations that nurses need to be conversant with and responsive to within a range of spiritual and religions identities. The links between religion or spirituality and positive health outcomes, as well as spiritualty for different age groups in the life journey, are addressed, along with developing and maintaining spirituality as a nurse.
- **Pain Assessment and Management (Chapter 32)** has been updated to focus on pain assessment and management as a multidimensional process. It includes new discussion about the opioid epidemic and stewardship, as well as use of cannabinoids for pain management.
- **Health Assessment and Physical Examination (Chapter 33)** has been expanded to include a new section on telehealth and virtual patient care.
- **Medication Administration and Management (Chapter 35)** has been significantly updated with new Canadian guidelines, revised discussion about scope of practice, medication dose responses, role of authorized prescribers, and medication safety, with revised skills and many new photographs.
- **Cardiopulmonary Functioning and Oxygenation (Chapter 40)** has been updated to include the new terminology for acute coronary syndrome and revised skills.

- **Fluid, Electrolyte, and Acid–Base Balances (Chapter 41)** has been updated to include more discussion about physiological processes, updated emphasis on teamwork and collaboration, more information about safety, and more specific discussion about types of vascular access devices, including updating of related skills.
- **Nutrition (Chapter 43)** includes information from the new *Canada's Food Guide,* and new discussion about diet culture, the Canadian Obesity Guidelines, health promotion and disease prevention, as well as additional case studies and skills.
- **References** have been thoroughly updated throughout the text to include the latest Canadian research and practice standards, such as the best nursing practice guidelines of Health Canada, Public Health Agency of Canada, Statistics Canada, the Canadian Nurses Association (CNA), and the Canadian Association of Schools of Nursing (CASN). References have been organized by chapter and are available on the Evolve website.

LEARNING SUPPLEMENTS FOR STUDENTS

- The **Evolve Student Resources** are available online at http://evolve.elsevier.com/Canada/Potter/fundamentals/ and include the following valuable learning aids, organized by asset:
  - Case Studies
  - Concept Map Creator
  - Content Updates
  - Examination Review Questions
  - Glossary
  - Key Points
  - Skills Performance Checklists
  - Tutorial – Calculations
  - Tutorial – Fluids and Electrolytes
  - Video Clips
- *Sherpath:* Sherpath Book-Organized collections offer digital lessons, mapped chapter-by-chapter to the textbook, so the reader can conveniently find applicable digital assignment content. Sherpath features convenient teaching materials that are aligned with the textbook, and the lessons are organized by chapter for quick and easy access to invaluable class activities and resources.

TEACHING SUPPLEMENTS FOR INSTRUCTORS

- The **Evolve Instructor Resources** (available online at http://evolve.elsevier.com/Canada/Potter/fundamentals/) are a comprehensive collection of the most important tools instructors need, including the following:
  - **TEACH for Nurses Lesson Plans** focus on the most important content from each chapter and provide innovative strategies for student engagement and learning. These new lesson plans provide teaching strategies that integrate textbook content with activities for pre-class, in-class, online, group, clinical judgement, and interprofessional collaboration, all correlated with RN-NGN Clinical Judgement Model and PN Clinical Judgement Skills competencies.
  - The revised **Test Banks** (one for RN-level and one for PN-level students) contain more than 1 300 multiple-choice questions with text page references and answers coded for NCLEX competencies and cognitive level for RN students, and CPRNE and REx-PN competencies and cognitive level for PN students. The ExamView software allows instructors to create new tests; edit, add, and delete test questions; sort questions by category,

cognitive level, and question type; and administer and grade online tests.

- Revised **PowerPoint Presentations** include over 1 500 slides for use in lectures.
- The **Image Collection** contains more than 1 100 illustrations from the text for use in lectures.
- **Simulation Learning System** is an online toolkit that helps instructors and facilitators effectively incorporate medium- to high-fidelity simulation into their nursing curriculum. Detailed patient scenarios promote and enhance the clinical decision-making skills of students at all levels. The system provides detailed instructions for preparation and implementation of the simulation experience, debriefing questions that encourage critical thinking, and learning resources to reinforce student comprehension. Each scenario in the Simulation Learning System complements the textbook content and helps bridge the gap between lectures and clinicals. This system provides the perfect environment for students to practise what they are learning in the text for a true-to-life, hands-on learning experience.

NEXT GENERATION NCLEX

The National Council for the State Boards of Nursing (NCSBN) is a not-for-profit organization whose members include nursing regulatory bodies. In empowering and supporting nursing regulators in their mandate to protect the public, the NCSBN is involved in the development of nursing licensure examinations, such as the NCLEX-RN®. In Canada, the NCLEX-RN® was introduced in 2015 and is, as of the writing of this text, the recognized licensure exam required for practising RNs in Canada.

The NCLEX-RN® will, as of 2023, be changing in order to ensure that its item types adequately measure clinical judgement, critical thinking, and problem-solving skills on a consistent basis. The NCSBN will also be incorporating into the examination what they call the Clinical Judgement Measurement Model (CJMM), which is a framework that the NCSBN has created to measure a novice nurse's ability to apply clinical judgement in practice. These changes to the examination come as a result of research findings indicating that novice nurses have a much higher than desirable error rate with patients (i.e., errors that cause patient harm) and, upon NCSBN's investigation, that the overwhelming majority of these errors were caused by failures of clinical judgement.

Clinical judgement has been a foundation of nursing education for decades, based on the work of a number of nursing theorists. The theory of clinical judgement that most closely aligns with what NCSBN is basing their CJMM is the work by Christine A. Tanner. The new version of the NCLEX-RN® is loosely being identified as the "Next-Generation NCLEX" or "NGN," and will feature the following:

- Six key skills in the CJMM: recognizing cues, analyzing cues, prioritizing hypotheses, generating solutions, taking actions, and evaluating outcomes.

- Approved item types as of March 2021: multiple response, extended drag and drop, cloze (drop-down), enhanced hot-spot (highlighting), matrix/grid bow tie, and trend. More question types may be added.
- All new item types are accompanied by mini–case studies with comprehensive patient information—some of it relevant to the question, and some of it not.
- Case information may present a single, unchanging moment in time (a "single-episode" case study) or multiple moments in time as a patient's condition changes (an "unfolding" case study).
- Single-episode case studies may be accompanied by one to six questions; unfolding case studies are accompanied by six questions.

For more information (and detail) regarding the NCLEX-RN® and changes coming to the exam, visit the NCSBNs website: https://www.ncsbn.org/11447.htm and https://ncsbn.org/Building_a_Method_for_Writing_Clinical_Judgment_It.pdf.

For further NCLEX-RN® examination preparation resources, see *Elsevier's Canadian Comprehensive Review for the NCLEX-RN Examination*, Third Edition, ISBN 9780323810333.

Prior to preparing for any nursing licensure examination, nursing students should refer to their provincial or territorial nursing regulatory body to determine which licensure examination is required in order for them to practise in their chosen jurisdiction.

MULTIMEDIA SUPPLEMENTS FOR INSTRUCTORS AND STUDENTS

- **Nursing Skills Online 5.0** contains 19 modules rich with animations, videos, interactive activities, and exercises to help students prepare for their clinical lab experience. The instructionally designed lessons focus on topics that are difficult to master and pose a high risk to the patient if done incorrectly. Lesson quizzes allow students to check their learning curve and review as needed, and the module exams feed out to an instructor grade book. Modules include Airway Management, Blood Therapy, Bowel Elimination/Ostomy Care, Chest Tubes, Enteral Nutrition, Infection Control, Injections, IV Fluid Administration, IV Fluid Therapy Management, IV Medication Administration, Nonparenteral Medication Administration, Safe Medication Administration, Safety, Specimen Collection, Urinary Catheterization, Vascular Access, Vital Signs, and Wound Care. Nursing Skills Online 5.0 is available alone or packaged with the text.
- **NEW Canadian Clinical Skills: Essentials Collection** covers 161 of the most important nursing skills within fundamentals and health assessment. Each skill in this collection features a consistent seven-part framework to guide students through all aspects of the skill. From high-definition videos that demonstrate each step of the skill to an interactive supply list that visually familiarizes students with related equipment, your students will gain a firm understanding of how to properly perform each skill before they ever step foot in the clinical environment. Best of all, this remarkable training product includes competency checklists and interactive quizzes for each skill to help you easily keep tabs on your students' progress.

ACKNOWLEDGEMENTS

In this seventh edition of *Potter and Perry's Canadian Fundamentals of Nursing*, we would like to acknowledge the expertise of our nursing scholars from across Canada, who ensured that the most up-to-date information was included so that our student nurses will have a fundamental textbook to meet their learning needs throughout their undergraduate nursing program. In addition, it was very important for us that the information provided prepares the student nurse to care for clients in local, national, and global contexts.

The task of updating a textbook of this magnitude is certainly an enormous undertaking that could only be accomplished through the collaborative efforts and commitment of the contributors, educator reviewers, editorial and production professionals, and our professional colleagues. We are so grateful for having the opportunity to collaborate with so many dedicated and committed individuals. We would like to acknowledge the following professionals from Elsevier:

- Martina van de Velde, Freelance Content Development Specialist, who provided outstanding leadership and capable organization of all parts of the developmental process and has been extremely supportive of all the contributors and editors. We were so grateful that we could continue to work with Martina, as this familiarity with each other fostered a sense of respect, collegiality, and warmth that created a high-quality textbook.
- Kristine Feeherty, Specialist, for her dedication to the production of this edition.
- Jerri Hurlbutt and Micheila Storr, Copyeditors, for their tireless dedication to the production of this edition. We are grateful to have worked with both Micheila and Jerri for this 7th edition.
- Roberta A. Spinosa-Millman, Content Strategist (Acquisitions) for Elsevier Canada, who oversaw the entire publication of this edition. We are grateful to have felt so supported, over several years of working with Roberta.
- Daniela Freitas, Editorial Operations Manager for Elsevier's Canadian operations, who ensured that the contracts and queries related to these matters were always attended to.

We are very excited about this seventh edition of *Potter and Perry's Canadian Fundamentals of Nursing*, as it addresses many of the trends and emerging issues for an ever-changing planet that are so important for equipping our next generation of student nurses to provide exemplary professional nursing practice in Canada and to the well-being of the global community.

Barbara J. Astle
Wendy Duggleby

CONTRIBUTORS

CANADIAN EDITORS

Barbara J. Astle, RN, PhD, FCAN
Professor & Director of the MSN
    Program
Director, Centre for Equity & Global
    Engagement (CEGE)
School of Nursing
Trinity Western University
Langley, British Columbia

Wendy Duggleby, RN, PhD
Professor Emerita
Faculty of Nursing
University of Alberta
Edmonton, Alberta

CANADIAN CONTRIBUTORS

Barbara G. Anderson, RN, MN
Assistant Clinical Professor
School of Nursing
McMaster University
Hamilton, Ontario

**Colleen M. Astle, RN, BScN, MN,
CNeph(C), NP**
Nurse Practitioner
University of Alberta Hospital
Edmonton, Alberta

Chantal Backman, RN, MHA, PhD
Assistant Professor
School of Nursing
University of Ottawa
Ottawa, Ontario

**Robin Coatsworth-Puspoky, RN,
PhD**
Professor of Nursing
Lambton College
Sarnia, Ontario

Sherry Dahlke, RN, PhD, GCN(c)
Associate Professor
Faculty of Nursing
University of Alberta
Edmonton, Alberta

**Susan M. Duncan, RN, BScN, PhD,
FCAN**
Professor
School of Nursing
University of Victoria
Victoria, British Columbia

Jennifer Dunsford, RN, MN, MPA
Instructor II
College of Nursing
University of Manitoba
Winnipeg, Manitoba

Pamela Durepos, RN, PhD
Assistant Professor
Faculty of Nursing
University of New Brunswick
Fredericton, New Brunswick

**Nancy A. Edgecombe, RN-NP, BN, MN,
PhD**
Assistant Professor (Retired)
School of Nursing
Dalhousie University
Halifax, Nova Scotia

Joyce Engel, RN, PhD
Adjunct Professor
School of Nursing
Brock University
St. Catharines, Ontario

Jaimee Feldstein, RN, MSN, PhD
Program Head
Bachelor of Science in Nursing Program
BCIT School of Health Sciences
Burnaby, British Columbia

**Laurence Fernandez, RN, MN,
NP(Cand.)**
Renal Vascular Access Nurse
Alberta Kidney Care—North
Edmonton, Alberta

**Caroline Foster-Boucher, RN,
BScN, MN**
Assistant Professor
Faculty of Nursing
MacEwan University
Edmonton, Alberta

Deborah Gibson, RN, MSN
Assistant Professor
School of Nursing
Trinity Western University
Langley, British Columbia

Jennifer Girvin, RN, MN
Nursing Faculty
Bachelor of Science in Nursing Program
College of the Rockies
Cranbrook, British Columbia

Sonya Grypma, RN, PhD
Adjunct Professor
School of Nursing
University of British Columbia
Vancouver, British Columbia

**Kathryn J. Hannah, CM, MScN, PhD,
DSc(HC)**
Professor (ADJ)
School of Nursing
University of Victoria
Victoria, British Columbia

Giuliana Harvey, RN, PhD
Associate Professor
School of Nursing and Midwifery
Mount Royal University
Calgary, Alberta

Selena Hebig, BScN, RN, BSKin
Nursing Faculty
Camosun College
Victoria, British Columbia

Carla T. Hilario, RN, PhD
Assistant Professor
Faculty of Nursing
University of Alberta
Edmonton, Alberta

**Sandra P. Hirst, RN, PhD,
GNC(c)**
Associate Professor Emerita
University of Calgary
Calgary, Alberta

Deborah Hobbs, BScN, RN, CIC
Infection Control Professional
University of Alberta Hospitals
Edmonton, Alberta

**Lorraine Holtslander, RN, MN, PhD,
CHPCN(c)**
Professor
College of Nursing
University of Saskatchewan
Saskatoon, Saskatchewan

**Sonya L. Jakubec, RN, BHScN,
MN, PhD**
Professor
School of Nursing and Midwifery
Mount Royal University
Calgary, Alberta

Darlaine Jantzen, RN, MA, PhD
Associate Professor
School of Nursing
Trinity Western University
Langley, British Columbia

Nicholas Joachimides, RN, BScN, IIWCC, NSWOC, MClSc, MSc, CHE, CpedN(c)
Academic Advisor
Continence Program
Wound, Ostomy, Continence Institute
Ottawa, Ontario;
Manager, Brain Injury Rehabilitation
Hollard Bloorview Kids Rehabilitation
    Hospital
Toronto, Ontario

Sarah L. Johnston, RN, MN
Assistant Professor, Teaching Stream
Lawrence S. Bloomberg Faculty
    of Nursing
University of Toronto
Toronto, Ontario

Harjit Kaur, RCC, PhD
Clinical Supervisor/Clinical Counsellor
Cushna Wellness Centre
Vancouver, British Columbia

Margaret Ann Kennedy, RN, PhD, CPHIMS-CA, FCAN
President
Kennedy Health Informatics Inc.
Halifax, Nova Scotia;
Senior Principal, Strategy & Consulting
Accenture
Halifax, Nova Scotia

Mi-Yeon Kim, RN, PhD
Assistant Professor
School of Nursing
Trinity Western University
Langley, British Columbia

Rosemary Kohr, RN, BA, BScN, MScN, PhD, Tertiary Care Nurse Practitioner Certificate
Program Director
Health Leadership & Learning Network
Faculty of Health
York University
Toronto, Ontario;
Adjunct Associate Professor
Faculty of Health Sciences
University of Western Ontario
London, Ontario

Marnie L. Kramer, RN, MEd, PhD
Assistant Professor
College of Nursing
University of Manitoba
Winnipeg, Manitoba

Mary Ellen Labrecque, NP, PhD
Director of Nurse Practitioner Programs
Assistant Professor
College of Nursing
University of Saskatchewan
Saskatoon, Saskatchewan

Annette M. Lane, MN, PhD
Professor
Faculty of Health Disciplines
Centre for Nursing and Health Studies
Athabasca University
Athabasca, Alberta

Nicole Letourneau, RN, PhD, FCAHS, FCAN, FAAN
Professor & Chair in Parent and Child
    Mental Health
Faculty of Nursing and Cumming School of
    Medicine
Departments of Pediatrics, Psychiatry, and
    Community Health Sciences
University of Calgary
Calgary, Alberta

Carly Lindsay, RN, BNSc, MClSc-WH, NSWOC, WOCC(C)
Academic Advisor – Continence
Nurses Specialized in Wound, Ostomy and
    Continence Canada (NSWOCC)
Ottawa, Ontario;
Clinical Instructor
School of Nursing
Queen's University
Kingston, Ontario;
Nurse Specialized in Wound, Ostomy and
    Continence
Kingston Health Sciences Centre
Kingston, Ontario

Sarah Liva, RN, PhD
Assistant Professor
School of Nursing
Trinity Western University
Langley, British Columbia

Janet Luimes, NP, MScN
Assistant Professor, Academic Programming
College of Nursing
University of Saskatchewan
Saskatoon, Saskatchewan

Heather MacLean, RN, MN, CHSE, CCNE, CCSNE
Associate Professor
School of Nursing & Midwifery
Mount Royal University
Calgary, Alberta

Brenda L. Martelli, RN(EC), BScN, BEd, MEd
Pediatric Nurse Practitioner
Acute Pain Services and Follow-up Clinic
Department of Anesthesiology and Pain Medicine
Ontario Certified Teacher (OCT)
Children's Hospital of Eastern Ontario (CHEO)
Ottawa, Ontario

Salima Meherali, RN, MN, PhD
Assistant Professor
Faculty of Nursing
University of Alberta
Edmonton, Alberta

Megan Meszaros, RN, PhD(c)
College of Nursing
University of Saskatchewan
Saskatoon, Saskatchewan

Heather Meyerhoff, MSN, RN
Associate Professor
School of Nursing
Trinity Western University
Langley, British Columbia

Judee E. Onyskiw, RN, MN, PhD
Associate Professor
Faculty of Nursing
MacEwan University
Edmonton, Alberta

Carole Orchard, BSN, MEd, EdD
Professor Emerita
Adjunct Research Professor
Arthur Labatt Family School of Nursing
Western University
London, Ontario

Tanya Park, RN, PhD
Associate Professor
Faculty of Nursing
University of Alberta
Edmonton, Alberta

Pammla Petrucka, RN, PhD
Professor
College of Nursing
University of Saskatchewan
Saskatoon, Saskatchewan

J. Craig Phillips, RN, PhD, LLM, ACRN, FAAN, FCAN
Professor
School of Nursing
University of Ottawa
Ottawa, Ontario

Katrina Plamondon, RN, MSc, PhD
Assistant Professor
School of Nursing
Faculty of Health & Social Development
University of British Columbia
Kelowna, British Columbia

Shelley Raffin Bouchal, RN, PhD
Associate Professor
Faculty of Nursing
University of Calgary
Calgary, Alberta

Sheryl Reimer-Kirkham, RN, PhD, FCAN
Dean and Professor
School of Nursing
Trinity Western University
Langley, British Columbia

Laura Robbs, RN, MN, NSWOC, WOCC(C), NCA
Lead Academic Advisor
Continence Program
Wound, Ostomy, Continence Institute
Nurses Specialized in Wound, Ostomy and Continence Canada
Toronto, Ontario

Shawna M. Ryan, RN, BN, OHN, MN
BSN Program Coordinator/BSN Faculty
Health and Human Service Programs
College of the Rockies
Cranbrook, British Columbia

Elizabeth M. Saewyc, RN, PhD, FSAHM, FCAHS, FAAN, FCAN
Professor and Director
School of Nursing
University of British Columbia
Vancouver, British Columbia

Bukola (Oladunni) Salami, RN, MN, PhD, FCAN
Professor
Faculty of Nursing
University of Alberta
Edmonton, Alberta

Monakshi Sawhney, NP (Adult), BScN, MN, PhD
Associate Professor
School of Nursing & Department of Anesthesiology and Perioperative Medicine
Queen's University
Kingston, Ontario

Kara Schick-Makaroff, RN, PhD
Associate Professor
Faculty of Nursing
University of Alberta
Edmonton, Alberta

Carla Shapiro, RN, MN
Senior Instructor (Retired)
College of Nursing
University of Manitoba
Winnipeg, Manitoba

Najwa Shbat, RN, BScN, NSWOC, NCA
Skin, Wound and Ostomy Care
Nurse Clinician
Hamilton Health Sciences
Hamilton, Ontario

Savitri Singh-Carlson, RN, PhD, FAAN
Professor of Nursing
San Diego State University
San Diego, California

Candis Spiers, RN, MN
Nursing Faculty
College of the Rockies
Cranbrook, British Columbia

Tracy Stephen, RN, MN
Prince Albert Home Care
Saskatchewan Health Authority
Prince Alberta, Saskatchewan

Holly Symonds-Brown, RN, PhD
Assistant Professor
Faculty of Nursing
University of Alberta
Edmonton, Alberta

Claudette Taylor, RN, PhD, NP (Adult)
School of Nursing
Cape Breton University
Sydney, Nova Scotia

Sally Thorne, RN, PhD, FCAHS, FAAN, FCAN
Professor, School of Nursing
Associate Dean, Faculty of Applied Science
University of British Columbia
Vancouver, British Columbia

Jill Vihos, RN, MN, PhD
Assistant Professor
Faculty of Nursing
MacEwan University
Edmonton, Alberta

Kathryn Weaver, RN, MN, PhD
Honorary Research Professor
Faculty of Nursing
University of New Brunswick
Fredericton, New Brunswick;
Mental Health Professional
Eating Disorder Care & Services
Fredericton, New Brunswick;
Adjunct Professor
Faculty of Nursing
Brandon University
Brandon, Manitoba

Christina H. West, RN, PhD
Associate Professor
College of Nursing
University of Manitoba
Winnipeg, Manitoba

Angela Wignall, RN, BSN, BA, MA, PhD(c)
Director, Professional Practice & Health Policy Implementation
Nurses and Nurse Practitioners of British Columbia (NNPBC)
Burnaby, British Columbia

Lydia Wytenbroek, RN, PhD
Assistant Professor
Co-Director, Consortium for Nursing History Inquiry
School of Nursing
University of British Columbia
Vancouver, British Columbia

US CONTRIBUTORS

Kimberly Diane Baxter, DNP, APRN, FNP-BC
Associate Dean of Undergraduate Programs
Orvis School of Nursing
University of Nevada, Reno
Reno, Nevada

Sharon Ferguson Beasley, PhD, MSN, RN, CNE
Director, Executive
Accreditation Commission for Education in Nursing (ACEN)
Atlanta, Georgia

Carolyn J. Wright Boon, MSN, BSN
Assistant Professor
Nursing
Saint Francis Medical Center College of
    Nursing
Peoria, Illinois

Jessica L. Bower, DNP, MSN, RN
Simulation Lab Coordinator
Nursing Department
Pennsylvania College of Technology
Williamsport, Pennsylvania

Janice C. Colwell, RN, MS, CWOCN, FAAN
Advanced Practice Nurse
Surgery
University of Chicago Medicine
Chicago, Illinois

Bronwyn Doyle, RN, PhD, CNE
Associate Dean of Undergraduate Nursing
School of Nursing
Franciscan Missionaries of Our Lady
    University
Baton Rouge, Louisiana

Jane Fellows, MSN, CWOCN-AP
Wound/Ostomy CNS
Advanced Clinical Practice
Duke University Health System
Durham, North Carolina

Victoria N. Folse, PhD, APRN, PMHCNS-BC, LCPC
Director and Professor; Caroline F. Rupert
    Endowed Chair of Nursing
School of Nursing
Illinois Wesleyan University
Bloomington, Illinois

Lorri A. Graham, DNP-L, RN
Visiting Professor
Nursing
Chamberlain University
Downers Grove, Illinois

Carla Armstead Harmon, PhD (Curriculum & Instruction), MSN, BSN
Associate Professor
School of Nursing
Franciscan Missionaries of Our Lady University
Baton Rouge, Louisiana

Tara Hulsey, BSN, MSN, PhD
Vice-President and Dean
Nursing
West Virginia University
Morgantown, West Virginia

Lenetra Jefferson, PhD, MSN, BSN, LMT
Nurse Educator
JeffCare
Jefferson Parish Human Services
    Authority
Metairie, Louisiana;
Contributing Faculty
School of Nursing
Walden University
Minneapolis, Minnesota;
Adjunct Faculty
School of Nursing
Troy University
Troy, Alabama

Nöel Marie Kerr, PhD
Associate Professor
School of Nursing
Illinois Wesleyan University
Bloomington, Illinois

Shari Kist, RN, PhD, CNE
Project Supervisor
Missouri Quality Initiate for Nursing
    Homes
Sinclair School of Nursing
University of Missouri–Columbia
Columbia, Missouri

Emily McClung, MSN, RN, PhD
Nursing Instructor
Hiram College
Hiram, Ohio

Angela McConachie, FNP, DNP
Associate Professor
Faculty
Goldfarb School of Nursing at Barnes Jewish
    College
St. Louis, Missouri

Emily McKenna, APN, CNS
Illinois Neurological Institute
INI Neurology
OSF St. Francis Medical Center
Peoria, Illinois

Jill Parsons, RN, PhD
Associate Professor
Nursing
MacMurray College
Jacksonville, Illinois

Anne Griffin Perry, RN, MSN, EdD, FAAN
Professor Emerita
School of Nursing
Southern Illinois University
    Edwardsville
Edwardsville, Illinois

Patricia A. Potter, RN, MSN, PhD, FAAN
Formerly, Director of Research
Patient Care Services
Barnes-Jewish Hospital
St. Louis, Missouri

Lynette Savage, BS, BSN, MS, PhD
Associate Professor, Joint
    Appointment
School of Health Professions
University of Providence
Great Falls, Montana

Angela Renee Starkweather, PhD, ACNP-BC, FAAN
Professor and Associate Dean for Academic
    Affairs
School of Nursing
University of Connecticut
Storrs, Connecticut

Patricia A. Stockert, RN, BSN, MS, PhD
Formerly, President, College of
    Nursing
Saint Francis Medical Center College of
    Nursing
Peoria, Illinois

REVIEWERS

Nora Ahmad, RN, BN, DMedSci
Associate Professor
Department of Nursing
Brandon University
Brandon, Manitoba

Liette Brown, LPN
LPN Instructor
Faculty of Nursing
Oulton College
Fredericton, New Brunswick

Joanne Crawford, RN, PhD, CON(C)
Associate Professor
Department of Nursing
Brock University
St. Catharines, Ontario

Trudy F. Gilbert, RN
Practical Nurse Instructor
Northern Lakes College
Grande Prairie, Alberta

Dr. Tracy Hoot, RN, BScN, MSN, DHEd
Associate Dean
School of Nursing
Thompson Rivers University
Kamloops, British Columbia

Amy Jackson, RN, BN, MN, CCCI, CCNE
Manager, Clinical Education Resources & Professor
Faculty of Health Sciences and Wellness
Humber Institute of Technology and Advanced Learning
Toronto, Ontario

Christine Kucava, RN, BScN, MN
Nursing Faculty
McMaster University
Hamilton, Ontario

Alia Lagace, RN
Instructor I
College of Nursing
University of Manitoba
Winnipeg, Manitoba

Asal Makhmour, RN, BSN, PIDP
Nursing Faculty
School of Health Sciences
Vancouver Community College
Vancouver, British Columbia

Cyndee McPhee, RN, MN
Associate Professor
School of Nursing
Cape Breton University
Sydney, Nova Scotia

Laura Pellicciotta, RN, MEd(c)
Nursing Instructor
Department of Nursing
Champlain College
Saint-Lambert, Quebec

Trina Propp, RN, BScN
Nursing Instructor, Practical Nursing Program
School of Health Sciences
Vancouver Community College
Vancouver, British Columbia

Suzee Rocque, RN, BScN, MScN/Ed, CRFN, CPMHN(c)
Professor
Coordinator BScN Collaborative Program
Faculty of Nursing
St. Lawrence College/Laurentian University
Cornwall, Ontario

Sarah Tekatch, RN, MN
Instructor III
Faculty of Nursing
University of Regina
Saskatoon, Saskatchewan

Jody Vaughan, RN, BScN, MEd
Nursing Instructor, Northern Collaborative
Baccalaureate Nursing Program
College of New Caledonia
Prince George, British Columbia

Jess White, RN, BN, ENC(c)
Faculty
School of Nursing
Assiniboine Community College
Winnipeg, Manitoba

Health and Wellness

Written by Deborah Gibson, RN, MSN

OBJECTIVES

Mastery of content in this chapter will enable you to:

- Define the key terms listed.
- Describe ways that definitions of health have been conceptualized.
- Describe key characteristics of medical, behavioural, and socioenvironmental approaches to health.
- Identify factors that have led to each approach to health.
- Describe contributions of the following Canadian publications to conceptualizations of health and health determinants: *Lalonde Report, Ottawa Charter, Epp Report, Strategies for Population Health, Jakarta Declaration, Bangkok Charter,* and *Toronto Charter.*

- Identify key health determinants and their interrelationships and how they influence health.
- Contrast distinguishing features of health promotion and disease prevention.
- Describe the three levels of disease prevention.
- Identify and give examples of the five health promotion strategies discussed in the *Ottawa Charter.*
- Analyze how the nature and scope of nursing practice are influenced by different conceptualizations of health and health determinants.

KEY TERMS

At-risk population
Behavioural approach
Behavioural risk factors
Determinants of health
Disease
Disease prevention
Downstream thinking
Evidence-informed decision making
Food insecurity
Health
Health as actualization
Health as actualization and stability
Health as resource
Health as stability

Health as unity
Health disparities
Health equity
Health field concept
Health inequalities
Health inequities
Health literacy
Health promotion
Health promotion strategies
Identity politics
Illness
Medical approach
Physiological risk factors
Population health approach

Prerequisites for health
Psychosocial risk factors
Racialization
Racism
Risk factor
Social determinants of health
Socioenvironmental approach
Socioenvironmental risk conditions
Structural vulnerability
Systemic racism
Upstream thinking
Wellness

WEBSITE

http://evolve.elsevier.com/Canada/Potter/fundamentals/

CASE STUDY

You are a nurse who is working in a small rural community with a population of 1 200 people, limited resources, and high rates of unemployment. Most of the community consists of families living in small homes. Meet the Lazzer family. There are nine members living in a small two-bedroom house that is a 15-minute drive from town. Joey Lazzer (preferred pronouns: he/him), who is 70 years of age, has been unable to work because of lung problems (chronic obstructive pulmonary disease; COPD) he developed from working in the local mine. Joey

indicates that he is happy to have his family around, despite the crowded living circumstances. You notice that the house feels cold and a bit drafty when you enter. Joey informs you that he and his family are often cold, but he does not have the money to buy a new furnace or fix the broken living room window. He tells you that they put a tarp over the window in winter, but it still gets as cold as −20°C. Joey states that he finds it very difficult to breathe in the cold air during winter. His partner, Elsie (preferred pronouns: she/her), who is 68 years

Continued

CASE STUDY—CONT'D

old, and their three children also live in the house. The eldest child, Sue (she/ her), is currently separated from her partner and has 16-year-old twins named Sam (he/him) and Joe (he/him) living with her. The next child, Tracy (she/her), is a single parent with 13-year-old twins Brian (he/him) and Ethan (he/him). The Lazzers own an older car that is not dependable in the winter. Sue and Tracy were working at the local restaurant but are now unable to work because of COVID-19 and the current public health restrictions, which included the closure of the restaurant. Sam and Joe stopped attending school and started working in the mine (like their grandfather, Joey) to earn money to help support the family. The nearest grocery store and medical facility are 15 minutes away. Joey needs

regular check-ups for his COPD. While there is public transit available, it runs only twice a day (once in the morning and once in the afternoon). There is a community centre and a high school a 20-minute walk from their house. Joey and Elsie try to visit friends at the community centre, but are unable to walk there in the winter. They indicate that they are feeling isolated from friends with the COVID-19 restrictions.

Case Study Reflection: Consider some of the health issues and disparities that rural populations may experience.

Think about this case study as you read this chapter. There are review questions at the end of the chapter about this case study.

Concepts of health and the factors that determine health have changed significantly since the 1970s. These issues have been magnified by the COVID-19 pandemic, the health status of Indigenous peoples, the Black Lives Matter movement, and the health of the lesbian, gay, bisexual, transgender, queer, and Two-Spirit (LGBTQ2) communities. While the COVID-19 pandemic has affected all Canadians, Indigenous peoples, the LGBTQ2 communities, and older persons have been disproportionately impacted (Health Canada, 2021; United Nations, 2020; Villeneuve & Betker, 2020). This conceptual change has major implications for Canadian nursing in the twenty-first century because how a nurse perceives health—and what determines it—influences the nature and scope of nursing practice. The importance of health to nursing is reflected in nursing models and frameworks, in which health is one of the "metaparadigm" concepts along with *person, environment, nursing,* and, more recently, *social justice* (see Chapter 4 for definitions of these concepts). In each framework, health concepts are congruent with the assumptions and focus of the model. Moreover, knowledge of health and health determinants is identified as an essential component of nursing education in Canada (Canadian Association of Schools of Nursing [CASN], 2022).

CONCEPTUALIZATIONS OF HEALTH

Discussions about the nature of health revolve around the relationship of health to *disease, illness,* and *wellness*. Debates often focus on whether health is defined in negative or positive terms. When health is negatively defined as the absence of disease, health and illness are represented on a continuum, with maximum health at one end and death at the other. When health is positively defined, however, health and illness are viewed as distinct but interrelated concepts. Therefore, a person can have disease, such as a chronic pathological condition, yet possess healthy characteristics as well.

Many people use the words *illness* and *disease* interchangeably. Others suggest that **disease** is an objective state of ill health, the pathological process of which can be detected by medical science, whereas **illness** is a subjective experience of loss of health (Jensen & Allen, 1993; Labonte, 1993). Figure 1.1 shows the relationships among health, illness, and disease.

Definitions of health that go beyond the absence of disease usually have multidimensional components, including physical, mental, social, and spiritual health. Some scholars have considered this broad definition of health to be synonymous with wellness (Labonte, 1993; Murdaugh et al., 2019). Others have argued that **health** is an objective process characterized by functional stability, balance, and integrity, whereas **wellness** is a subjective experience (see discussion in Mackey, 2009). The word *health* is derived from the Old English word *hoelth*,

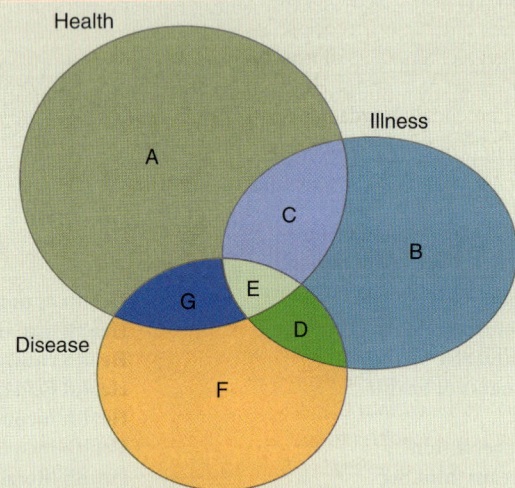

Legend

Circle A represents health or wellness, the clear area being experiences such as feeling vital, enjoying good social relationships, having a sense of purpose in life, and experiencing a connectedness to "community."

Circle B represents experiences of illness, the clear area representing illness that cannot be explained by conventional biomedical concepts and research.

Shaded area C is feeling "so-so," where little is required to tip one into wellness or illness.

Shaded area D is where a diagnosed pathology objectively validates and explains the subjective experience of illness.

Shaded area E represents feeling "so-so," being diagnosed with a pathology, and becoming sick.

Circle F represents diagnosed pathology, the clear area being undiagnosed or silent pathology, such as hypertension, CVD, congenital diseases, or cancers.

Shaded area G represents being diagnosed with a pathology, but still reporting oneself as feeling well or healthy.

FIGURE 1.1 Health, illness, and disease. CVD, cardiovascular disease. (From Labonte, R. [1993]. *Issues in health promotion series. 3. Health promotion and empowerment: Practice frameworks* [p. 18]. Centre for Health Promotion (University of Toronto) and ParticipACTION.)

meaning whole of body. Historically, physical wholeness was important for social acceptance, and people with contagious or disfiguring diseases were often ostracized. Good health was considered natural, whereas disease was considered unnatural. As science progressed, disease was regarded less negatively because it could be countered by scientific medicine. After World War II, the World Health Organization (WHO, n.d.), in its constitution, defined health as "a state of complete physical, mental and social well-being, and not merely the absence of disease or infirmity." This is still the most commonly cited definition of health.

Classifications of Health Conceptualizations

Conceptualizations of individual health have been classified in a variety of ways. One way to organize conceptualizations is by describing the dimensions that make up the whole of a person's life or, alternatively, by treating the whole as a unitary life (i.e., not separable into dimensions):

- **Health as stability.** Health is defined as the maintenance of physiological, functional, and social norms, and encompasses views of health as a state, as a process, as adaptation, and as homeostasis (Murdaugh et al., 2019; Thorne et al., 1998).
- **Health as actualization.** Health is defined as the actualization of human potential (Murdaugh et al., 2019). Scholars and researchers who adhere to this definition often use the terms *health* and *wellness* interchangeably.
- **Health as actualization and stability.** Both actualization and stability concepts are incorporated in the definition of health as "the realization of human potential through goal-directed behaviour, competent self-care, and satisfying relationships with others, while adapting to meet the demands of everyday life and maintain harmony with the social and physical environments" (Murdaugh et al., 2019, p. 13).
- **Health as resource.** The definition of health as a resource or asset emerged in the *Ottawa Charter for Health Promotion* (WHO, 1986) and includes capacities to fulfill roles, meet demands, and engage in the activities of everyday living (Mikkonen & Raphael, 2010; Murdaugh et al., 2019; Williamson & Carr, 2009).
- **Health as unity.** Health is defined as "reflecting the whole person as process and is synonymous with self-transcendence" (Thorne et al., 1998, p. 1261) or actualization.

Most contemporary nursing theorists have conceptualized health as stability or actualization, although some have advanced the conceptualization of health as unity. Interestingly, Nightingale's definition of health reflects both the stability and actualization dimensions (Thorne et al., 1998).

In 1984, the WHO updated its conceptualization of health as follows:

The extent to which an individual or group is able, on the one hand, to realize aspirations and satisfy needs; and, on the other hand, to change or cope with the environment. Health is, therefore, seen as a resource for everyday life, not the objective of living; it is a positive concept emphasizing social and personal resources, as well as physical capacities. (p. 3)

Rather than viewing health as an ideal state of well-being (as in the WHO's 1946 definition of health; WHO, n.d.), this definition, which incorporates both the actualization and stability dimensions, suggests that people in a variety of situations—even those with physical disease or nearing death—could be considered healthy.

Labonte (1993) developed a multidimensional conceptualization of health that reflects both the actualization and stability perspectives. Aspects include the following qualities:

- Feeling vitalized and full of energy
- Having satisfying social relationships

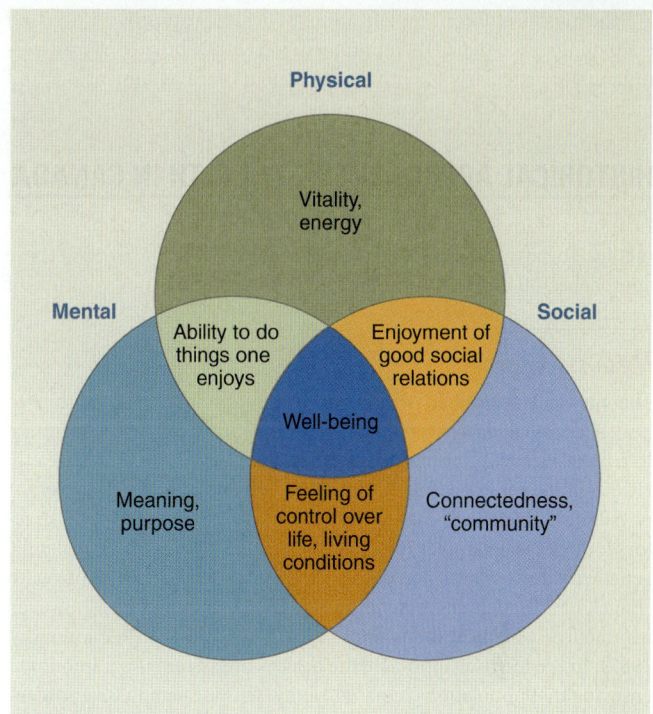

FIGURE 1.2 Dimensions of health and well-being. (From Labonte, R. [1993]. *Issues in health promotion series. 3. Health promotion and empowerment: Practice frameworks* [p. 20]. Centre for Health Promotion [University of Toronto] and ParticipACTION.)

- Having a feeling of control over one's life and living conditions
- Being able to do things that one enjoys
- Having a sense of purpose
- Feeling connected to community.

Using the WHO dimensions of physical, mental, and social well-being, Labonte (1993) categorized these characteristics using a Venn diagram (Figure 1.2). The diagram clearly depicts the concept of holism, whereby health is more than the sum of the component parts in that the interrelationships between and among different components result in different aspects of health.

Scholars conceptualize health in different ways (see Chapter 6 for further information on health). Rootman and Raeburn (1994) view health as a quality enhanced by a sensible lifestyle and equitable access to resources that promote the individual and collective initiative to maintain or improve well-being. Jones and Meleis (1993) articulated health as empowerment:

Health is being empowered to define, seek, and find conditions, resources, and processes to be an effective agent in meeting the significant needs perceived by individuals. (p. 12)

These conceptualizations are congruent with Labonte's (1993) focus and reflect the essence of health promotion discussed later in this chapter. In an attempt to describe health, Card (2017) emphasizes the importance of subjectivity and person-centred assessment by defining health as the experience of physical and psychological well-being. Good health and poor health do not exist as a dichotomy, but as a continuum. The absence of disease or disability is neither sufficient nor necessary to produce a state of good health. This definition of health denotes that health is not a dichotomous variable, that health status is experiential, and that while it is shaped by social influences, an individual's experience of health itself is psychological and physical in nature (p. 131).

The most useful conceptualizations of health are positive (not based on pathology or deficit), comprehensive (with a broad set of determinants), particularly attentive to the mental health dimension, and inclusive of quality of life and spirituality.

HISTORICAL APPROACHES TO HEALTH IN CANADA

In modern times, the three major approaches to health have been medical, behavioural, and socioenvironmental (Labonte, 1993). These approaches offer a useful framework for examining the evolution of health orientations in Canada.

Medical Approach

The **medical approach**, which represents a stability orientation to health, dominated Western thinking for most of the twentieth century. It emphasizes the notion that medical intervention restores health. Health problems are defined primarily as **physiological risk factors**—physiologically defined characteristics that are precursors to or risk factors for disease. Examples include hypertension, hypercholesterolemia, genetic predispositions, and obesity. The biopsychosocial view of health (Engel, 1977) includes psychological and social elements; however, in practice, a medical focus on pathology was retained (Antonovsky, 1987). In the medical approach, the health care system is paramount to ensuring that populations remain healthy. This idea emphasizes **downstream thinking**, an approach to health care intervention that focuses on individual health concerns, treatment, and cure.

Focusing on treatment of disease was strongly supported after World War II, when new technological and scientific medical advances facilitated the medical approach. In Canada, postwar economic growth increased funding to build new hospitals. National health insurance was created to remove financial barriers to care. Many people believed that scientific medicine could solve most health problems and that accessible and quality health care (or, more correctly, illness care) would improve the health of Canadians. This approach placed less emphasis on health promotion and disease prevention.

Behavioural Approach

By the early 1970s, increasingly large amounts of money were spent on health care, but the health status of the population did not improve proportionately. To better understand what contributed to illness and death, the Minister of Health and Welfare, Marc Lalonde, commissioned a study that resulted in the 1974 report *A New Perspective on the Health of Canadians* (Lalonde, 1974). The *Lalonde Report* shifted the emphasis of health care from a medical to a **behavioural approach** to health. The report concluded that the traditional medical approach to health care was inadequate and that "further improvements in the environment, reductions in self-imposed risks, and a greater knowledge of human biology" were necessary to improve the health status of Canadians (Lalonde, 1974, p. 6). The *Lalonde Report* was the first modern government document in the Western world to acknowledge the inadequacy of a strictly biomedical health care system.

The *Lalonde Report* broadly defined health determinants as lifestyle, environment, human biology, and the organization of health care. This **health field concept** was widely used, modified, and expanded by other countries, and its release was a turning point in broadening Canadians' attitudes about factors that contribute to health and acknowledging the role of government in promoting health (Health Canada, 1998). Of the four determinants, lifestyle received the most attention, perhaps because lifestyle behaviours contribute to chronic diseases (such as cancer and heart disease) and to injuries—both of which are the leading causes of morbidity and mortality in Canada (Labonte, 1993). In addition, greater understanding of behavioural social psychology shed

light on the factors that motivated individuals to engage in healthy or unhealthy behaviours. In 1978, the Canadian government established the Health Promotion Directorate in the Department of National Health and Welfare—the first official health promotion undertaking of its kind. Its aim was to decrease **behavioural risk factors** such as smoking, substance use, lack of exercise, and an unhealthy diet. Public health programs such as Operation Lifestyle and ParticipACTION were developed through this department.

The behavioural approach places responsibility for health on the individual, thereby favouring health promotion strategies such as education and social marketing. Strategies are often based on the assumption that if people know the risk factors for disease, then they will engage in healthy behaviours. Indeed, health-enhancing practices among Canadians increased during this time. With the ParticipACTION initiative, for instance, many people increased their physical activity. Antismoking campaigns led to a substantial decrease in tobacco use.

Socioenvironmental Approach

By the mid-1980s, however, the behavioural approach to health and illness prevention was challenged. Studies showed that lifestyle improvements were made primarily by well-educated, well-employed, and higher-income Canadians. The *Lalonde Report* was criticized for deflecting attention from the environment and for how it defined environment and lifestyle. Lifestyle was viewed as being within an individual's control, with health risks considered "self-imposed" behaviours. This supported "victim blaming" and the view that health is largely an individual responsibility. Critics suggested that health-related behaviours could not be separated from the social contexts (environments) in which they occurred. For example, living and working conditions were perceived as barriers to engaging in healthy behaviours (Labonte, 1993).

In the **socioenvironmental approach**, health is closely tied to social structures. For example, poverty and unhealthy physical and social environments, such as air pollution, poor water quality, and workplace hazards, are recognized as direct influences on health. Thus, Canadian public health providers expanded Lalonde's (1974) health field concept to emphasize the social context of health and the relationship between personal health behaviours and social and physical environments (Hancock & Perkins, 1985). This concept is aligned with an **upstream thinking** approach, in which health promotion and prevention strategies are focused on policy interventions that benefit the whole population. An upstream approach may also include primary health care interventions that focus on people's well-being by addressing, and taking action on, the root causes of preventable diseases and injuries (Lind & Baptiste, 2020).

Internationally, more attention was also given to the social context of health. The WHO regional conference in Europe produced a discussion paper identifying the social conditions that influence health (WHO, 1984). Just as Canada led the behavioural approach to health with the *Lalonde Report*, it was now instrumental in focusing on social and environmental conditions. In 1986, the First International Conference on Health Promotion was held in Ottawa, sponsored by the WHO, the Canadian Public Health Association (CPHA), and Health and Welfare Canada. It produced a watershed document—the *Ottawa Charter for Health Promotion*—that supported a socioenvironmental approach. This document has since been translated into more than 40 languages.

Ottawa Charter. The *Ottawa Charter for Health Promotion* (WHO, 1986) identified the **prerequisites for health** as peace, shelter, education, food, income, a stable ecosystem, sustainable resources, social justice, and equity. These prerequisites go well beyond lifestyle factors or

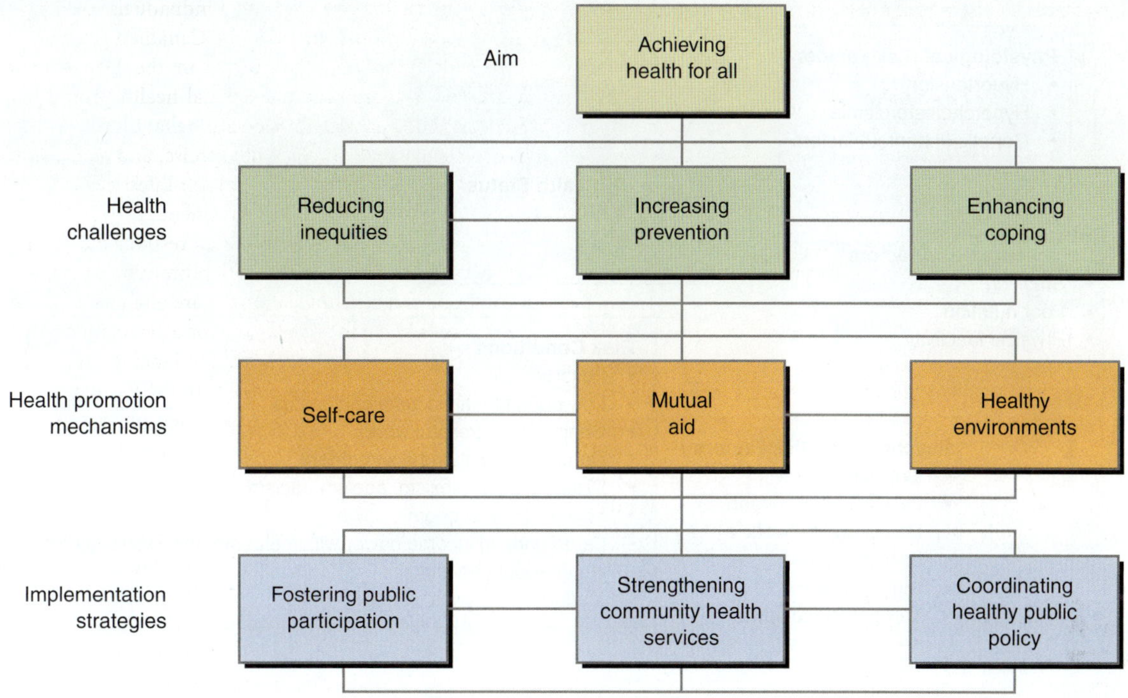

FIGURE 1.3 Achieving Health for All: A Framework for Health Promotion. (© All rights reserved. From Epp, J. [1986]. *Achieving health for all: A framework for health promotion* [p. 8]. Health and Welfare Canada. Adapted and reproduced with permission from the Minister of Health, 2022.)

personal health practices to include social, environmental, and political contexts. This framework placed responsibility for health on society rather than on individuals alone. The *Ottawa Charter's* focus on social justice and equity also incorporated the concept of *empowerment*—a person's ability to define, analyze, and solve problems—as an important goal for health care providers (Registered Nurses' Association of British Columbia, 1994). Indeed, Wallerstein (1992) contended that powerlessness could be the underlying health determinant influencing other risk factors. Subsequently, the health promotion literature began to emphasize the concept of empowerment. The *Ottawa Charter* incorporated the then-new 1984 WHO definition of health (discussed previously), which identified the social and individual dimensions of health, emphasized its dynamic and positive nature, and viewed it as a fundamental human right (Naidoo & Wills, 1994). The *Ottawa Charter* outlined five major strategies to promote health: building healthy public policy, creating supportive environments, strengthening community action, developing personal skills, and reorienting health services (discussed later in this chapter).

Achieving Health for All. Concepts from the *Ottawa Charter* were incorporated into another important Canadian document, *Achieving Health for All: A Framework for Health Promotion* (Epp, 1986). This report, developed under the leadership of Jake Epp, Minister of National Health and Welfare from 1984 to 1989, became Canada's blueprint for achieving the WHO goal of "Health for All 2000" (Figure 1.3).

Epp's (1986) report identified three major health challenges: reducing inequities, increasing prevention, and enhancing coping mechanisms. The report acknowledged disparities in health, particularly between low- and high-income people, and that living and working conditions were critical **determinants of health** (factors that influence the risk for or distribution of health outcomes). The need for effective ways to prevent injuries, illnesses, chronic conditions, and disabilities was emphasized. The health challenge of enhancing people's ability to cope reflected an acknowledgement that the dominant diseases in

Canada were chronic conditions that could not be cured. Thus, people needed to be assisted in managing and coping with chronic conditions to be able to live meaningful and productive lives. The *Epp Report* emphasized society's responsibility for providing supports to people experiencing chronic medical conditions, stress, mental illness, and challenges associated with aging, as well as the need for supports for caregivers. The report identified self-care, mutual aid, and promotion of healthy environments as ways to address the three major health challenges, reflecting both personal and social responsibility. Specific strategies included fostering public participation, strengthening community health services, and coordinating healthy public policy.

The *Ottawa Charter* and the *Epp Report* both reflect a socioenvironmental approach in which health is seen as more than the absence of disease and engaging in healthy behaviours; rather, this approach emphasizes connectedness as well as self-efficacy and the capacity to engage in meaningful activities (see Figure 1.2).

Risk Factors and Risk Conditions. Labonte (1993) categorized the major determinants of health in a socioenvironmental approach as psychosocial risk factors and socioenvironmental risk conditions. A **risk factor** is a condition that increases a person's susceptibility to develop a disease.

- **Psychosocial risk factors** are complex psychological experiences that result from social circumstances such as isolation, lack of social support, limited social networks, low self-esteem, self-blame, and low perceived power.
- **Socioenvironmental risk conditions** are social and environmental living conditions that include poverty, low educational or occupational status, dangerous or stressful work, dangerous physical environments, pollution, discrimination, relative political or economic powerlessness, and inequalities of income or power.

According to a socioenvironmental approach to health, political, social, and cultural forces affect health and well-being both directly and indirectly through their influence on personal health behaviours.

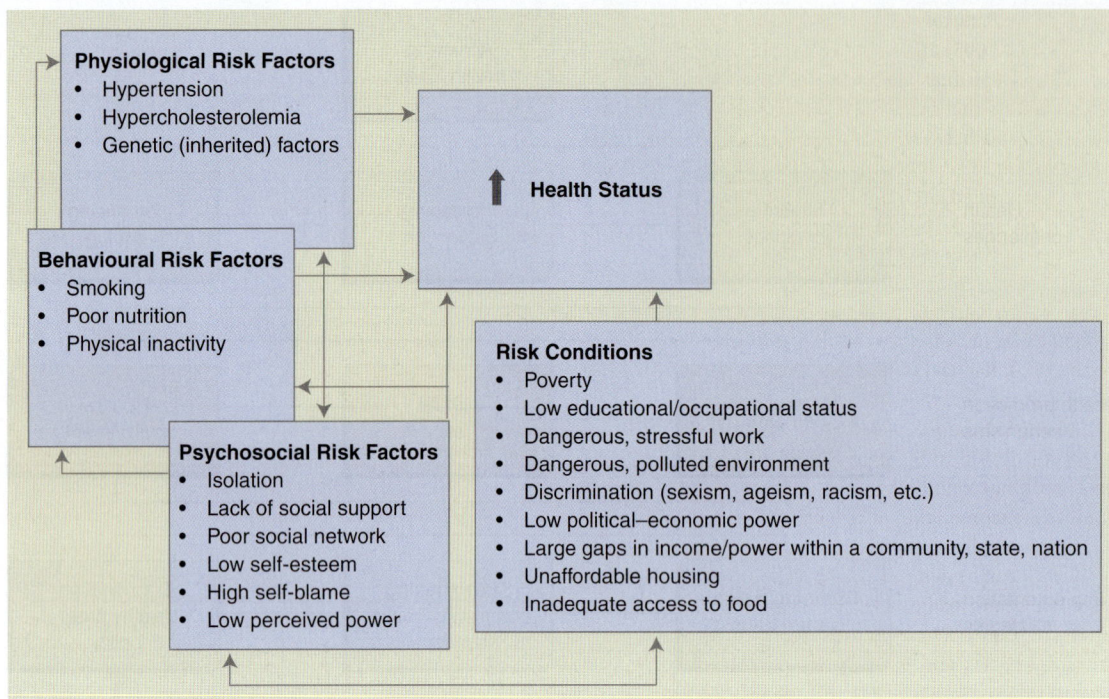

FIGURE 1.4 Socioenvironmental approach to health. (From Labonte, R. [1993]. *Issues in health promotion series. 3. Health promotion and empowerment: Practice frameworks* [p. 11]. Centre for Health Promotion [University of Toronto] and ParticipACTION.)

Socioenvironmental risk conditions can contribute to psychosocial risk factors, which can then lead to unhealthy behaviours (Figure 1.4). This means that health care providers should recognize the influence of environment on personal behaviours, and that "health-inhibiting" behaviours could be coping strategies for managing the stress created by living and working conditions that decrease access to resources. In other words, "to change behaviour it may be necessary to change more than behaviour" (Wilkinson, 1996, p. 64). For example, in addition to working "downstream" to assist people who are experiencing the negative health effects of socioenvironmental conditions, nurses need to work "upstream" by advocating for policies that ensure affordable housing, financial support to patients with low incomes, and safe, fulfilling work environments. This places individuals or populations "at risk for negative health outcomes through their interface with socioeconomic, political and cultural/normative hierarchies" (Bourgois et al., 2017, p. 17). Individuals experience **structural vulnerability** when their location in society powers hierarchies, and policy-level and institutional statuses constrain their ability to access health care in the pursuit of a healthy lifestyle (Bourgois et al., 2017).

Strategies for Population Health. In Canada, the determinants of health have been further emphasized through the **population health approach** (Public Health Agency of Canada [PHAC], 2013a). This approach, initiated by the Canadian Institute for Advanced Research (CIFAR), was officially endorsed by the federal, provincial, and territorial ministers of health in the report titled *Strategies for Population Health: Investing in the Health of Canadians* (Federal, Provincial, and Territorial Advisory Committee on Population Health [ACPH], 1994; PHAC, 2020). In a population health approach, "the entire range of known individual and collective factors and conditions that determine population health status, and the interactions among them, are taken into account in planning action to improve health"

(Health Canada, 1998). The population health approach emphasizes the use of epidemiological data to determine the etiology of health and disease. The following is a list of 14 social determinants of health (CPHA, 2021a):

- Income and income distribution
- Education
- Unemployment and job security
- Employment and working conditions
- Early childhood development
- Food insecurity
- Housing
- Social exclusion
- Social safety network
- Health services
- Indigenous status
- Gender
- Race
- Disability

Jakarta Declaration. The *Jakarta Declaration on Leading Health Promotion Into the 21st Century* (WHO, 1997) emerged from the 4th International Conference on Health Promotion, the first to be held in a developing country and to involve the private sector. The *Jakarta Declaration* affirmed the *Ottawa Charter* prerequisites for health; added four other prerequisites (*empowerment of women, social security, respect for human rights*, and *social relations*); and declared poverty to be the greatest threat to health. The *Jakarta Declaration* identified the following priorities for action: promoting social responsibility for health in the public and private sectors; increasing investments for health in all sectors; consolidating and expanding partnerships for health to all levels of government and the private sector; increasing community capacity and empowering the individual; and securing adequate infrastructure for health promotion.

Bangkok Charter. The *Bangkok Charter for Health Promotion in a Globalized World* (WHO, 2005) affirmed health as a human right and emphasized mental and spiritual well-being as important elements. It identified critical factors that influence health, such as the increasing inequalities within and between countries, global environmental change, and urbanization. The *Bangkok Charter* emphasized strong political action and sustained advocacy, empowering communities with adequate resources, and corporate sector commitment to healthy workplaces and ethical business practices.

Toronto Charter. In the early to mid-1990s, Canadian social and health policies resulted in increased social and economic inequalities (Bryant & Raphael, 2020; Raphael, 2016) and health disparities. These concerns culminated in the *Toronto Charter on the Social Determinants of Health*, which identified the following social determinants as particularly important for health: Indigenous status, early life, education, employment and working conditions, food security, gender, health care services, housing, income and its distribution, social safety net, social exclusion, and unemployment and employment security. **Social determinants of health** can be defined as "the *economic and social conditions* that shape the health of individuals, communities, and jurisdictions as a whole . . . [and] determine the extent to which a person possesses the physical, social, and personal resources to identify and achieve personal aspirations, satisfy needs, and cope with the environment" (Raphael, 2016, p. 3; italics added).

This conceptualization of health determinants emphasizes *societal* responsibility for reducing health disparities because it focuses on how a society distributes economic and social resources through its economic and social policies. A social determinants of health perspective calls attention to the political, economic, and social forces that shape policy decisions, thereby reflecting a critical/structural approach to health (Bryant & Raphael, 2020). The social determinants of health identified in the *Toronto Charter* were chosen because they (a) are important to the health of Canadians, (b) are understandable to Canadians, (c) have clear policy relevance to decision makers and citizens, and (d) are especially timely and relevant (Bryant & Raphael, 2020).

Concern about **health disparities** (i.e., differences in health status among different population groups) has been raised worldwide. The WHO Commission on Social Determinants of Health (WHO, 2008) was charged with developing strategies to narrow health disparities through action on the social determinants of health. In Canada, a report commissioned by PHAC identified socioeconomic status, Indigenous identity, gender, and geographic location as the most important factors contributing to health disparities (Health Disparities Task Group of the Federal/Provincial/Territorial Advisory Committee on Population Health and Health Security, 2005). In 2007, the Senate Subcommittee on Population Health was established to examine the impact of social determinants of health on disparities and inequities in health (Senate Subcommittee on Population Health, 2009). *The Chief Public Health Officer's Report on the State of Public* Health in Canada 2008 (PHAC, 2008) also underscored health inequalities.

Despite Canada's status as one of the healthiest countries in the world, some Canadians are healthier and have more opportunities for a heathier life than others (Health Canada, 2020). These differences in the health status of individuals and groups, referred to as **health inequalities**, are attributed to genes and to people's personal choices. Social determinants of health also influence and contribute to overall health. As such, clear definitions of health equity and health disparities are imperative to ensure that resources are properly allocated to populations in need from a human rights perspective (Phillips & Moss, 2021). **Health equity** is the absence of unfair systems and

policies that cause health inequalities. Health equity seeks to increase access to opportunities and conditions that are conducive to health for all (Health Canada, 2020) (see Chapter 11 for further information on health equity and health inequities).

Health disparities are defined as health differences closely linked to social, economic, and/or environmental disadvantages that adversely affect groups that have systematically experienced greater obstacles to health (Office of Disease Prevention and Health Promotion, n.d., para. 6). Since inequitable access (lack of or unequal access) to health determinants results from economic and social policies, the term **health inequities**, rather than *health inequalities* or *disparities*, more accurately reflects the source and nature of health differences among people (Figure 1.5).

SOCIAL DETERMINANTS OF HEALTH

The following section introduces the social determinants of health (the conditions of our lives that influence our health) that affect Canadians. Figure 1.6 depicts the core determinants of health.

Experiences of racism, discrimination, and historical trauma are significant social determinants of health for specific groups in Canada, namely Indigenous peoples, LGBTQ2 Canadians, and Black Canadians (Bryant & Raphael, 2020; Health Canada, 2021; Hernandez-Cancio & Thompson, 2021; Raphael, 2016; Villeneuve & Betker, 2020). Furthermore, the emergence of SARS-CoV-2, the coronavirus that causes COVID-19, has identified that social inequalities in health profoundly and disproportionately impact morbidity and mortality. For example, several social determinants of health, including poverty, physical environment (smoke exposure, homelessness), and race and ethnicity, have had a considerable effect on COVID-19 outcomes. Homeless families are at higher risk of transmitting and contracting the virus because they live in crowded spaces and have limited access to screening and testing sites. The pandemic has revealed that "the ability to physically distance is a privilege that is not accessible is all communities" (Abrams & Szefler, 2020, p. 1). Although each determinant on its own contributes to health, the determinants are also interrelated and influence each other.

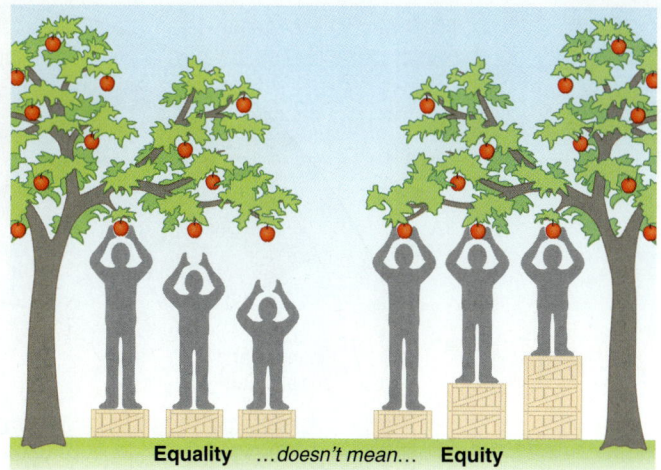

FIGURE 1.5 Equality versus equity. (From Aalhus, M., Oke, B., & Fumerton, R. [2018]. *The social determinants of health impacts of resource extraction and development in rural and northern communities: A summary of impacts and promising practices for assessment and monitoring.* https://www.northernhealth.ca/sites/northern_health/files/services/office-health-resource-development/documents/impacts-promising-practices-assessment-monitoring.pdf)

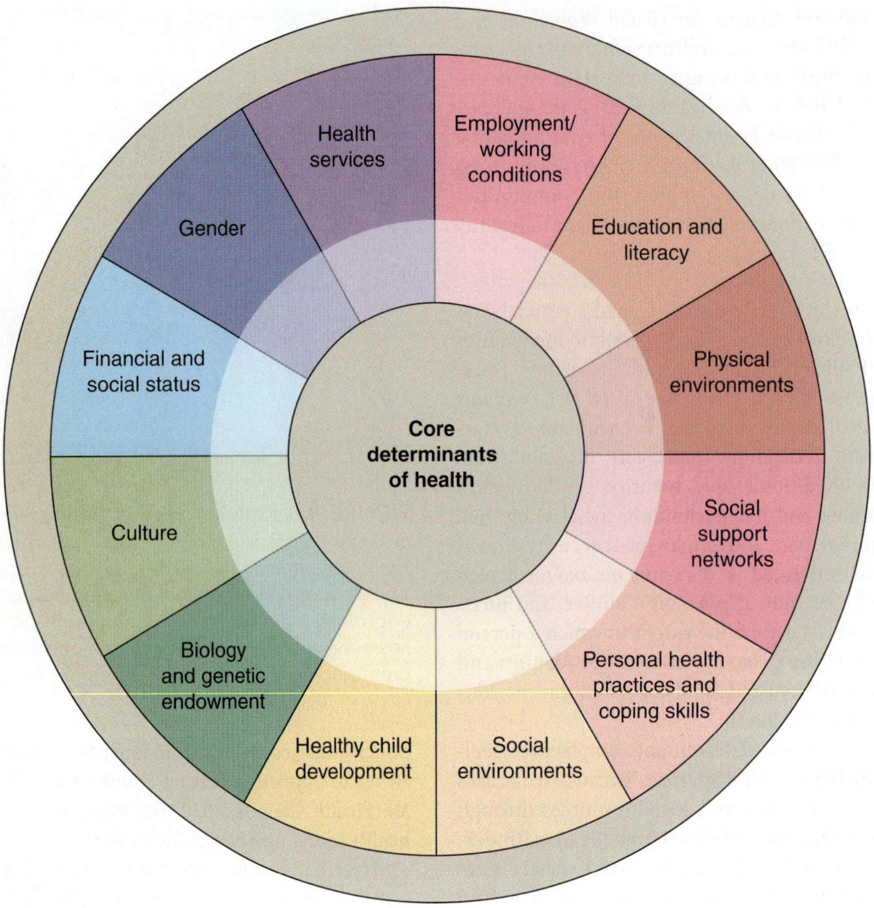

FIGURE 1.6 Core determinants of health. (From Colleaga. [2021]. *What are the determinants of health?* https://www.colleaga.org/article/what-are-determinants-health)

Income and Income Distribution

Income, income distribution, and social status influence most other social determinants of health (Blumenthal & Rothwell, 2018; Bryant & Raphael, 2020). According to Statistics Canada, after-tax low-income cut-offs in 2018 indicate that 12.3% of Canadians were living in poverty, with much higher rates among single mothers and unattached nonelderly women and men (Bryant & Raphael, 2020; Zhang, 2021). Indigenous peoples, racialized people, persons with disabilities, and recent immigrants in urban areas also have much higher rates of poverty compared to the Canadian average (Bryant & Raphael, 2020). Although more persistent in the 2000s than the 1990s, low household income has become less persistent since mid-2010. Zhang (2021) suggests that this decline in poverty and low income before the pandemic resulted from people's moving out of poverty and low income faster than before. Of concern, however, is that the economic impact from the COVID-19 pandemic has not yet been fully realized.

Poverty exerts its effects on health through lack of material resources that support health, through higher levels of psychosocial stress, and through the adoption of health-threatening behaviours to cope with limited resources and stress (Bryant & Raphael, 2020; Raphael, 2016). Low-income and impoverished Canadians, particularly immigrants, racialized people, women, and Indigenous peoples, are more likely to suffer from **food insecurity** (a state of being without reliable access to a sufficient quantity of affordable and nutritious food) and hunger, lack of affordable housing and homelessness, growing inequality, interpersonal violence, substance use, chronic and communicable diseases,

and ill health (Bryant & Raphael, 2020; Raphael, 2016). About 20% of Canadians' premature loss of life can be accounted for by income differences resulting from chronic health problems such as cardiovascular disease, type 2 diabetes, mental health challenges, and substance use (Raphael, 2016). With each step up the economic ladder, Canadians' health status improves, suggesting that this "social gradient" of health is related to more than absolute material deprivation (Raphael, 2016).

Adverse birth outcomes, such as preterm birth, low birth weight, and infant mortality, disproportionately affect families living in low-income neighbourhoods, despite overall improvements in health care quality and access. Jairam et al. (2019) conducted a population-based study examining singleton live births in Ontario, Canada, from 2002 to 2011. They found that women residing in low-income areas were at high risk of having a preterm birth or a severely small-for-gestational-age birth weight.

Income inequality (i.e., the increasing gap between the rich and the poor; Curry-Stevens, 2016) also influences population health, highlighting that people living in countries with greater economic inequality have lower overall health and life expectancies. Although the mechanisms responsible for this association are complex and still being explored, Bryant and Raphael (2020) suggest that income inequality may result in less public investment in sectors that affect health, such as education, health services, transportation, and housing.

Education

Health status improves with education and literacy. The intersectionality between the various determinants of health can impact different population groups' health in various ways. For example, education is closely linked with socioeconomic status. Effective education for children and lifelong learning for adults are key to good health for individuals and the country as a whole because they equip people with the knowledge and skills for employment, income security, job satisfaction, problem-solving skills, and a sense of control and mastery over life circumstances.

Health literacy "describes the skills that enable individuals to obtain, understand, and use information to make decisions, and take actions that will have an impact on health status" (Nutbeam & Muscat, 2020, p. 116). Education and literacy influence health both directly (e.g., access to health services and health information, reading medication prescriptions, or knowing where to go when they have questions about their health) and indirectly (e.g., use of services, personal health practices, income, work environments, and stress levels) (CPHA, 2021a). For example, people with low literacy skills are more likely to be unemployed, receive income support, earn minimum wages in unskilled jobs, and have higher stress levels and less likely to make use of preventive services (Ronson McNicol & Rootman, 2016). By comparison, people with higher education levels tend to smoke less, be more physically active, and have access to healthier foods and physical environments (CPHA, 2021a; Health Canada, 2013).

Through a scoping review (using an Indigenous determinants of health framework and worldview conceptualization of wellness, resilience, well-being, and balance within the concept of aging), Webkamigad and colleagues (2020) examined the health and social care needs and priorities of older Indigenous persons with chronic conditions. The key determinants of health influencing older Indigenous persons' needs are education, literacy, social support, and health promotion and health care. The authors' findings also highlight the importance of using Indigenous knowledge and perspectives to improve accessibility of culturally relevant health and social services (Webkamigad et al., 2020).

As a progression from functional literacy, *interactive literacy* reflects advanced ability to apply new information to changing circumstances. *Critical literacy* reflects further advanced ability to "critically analyze information, and to apply this information to exert greater control over life events and situations that impact health" (Nutbeam & Muscat, 2020, p. 117).

Unemployment and Job Security

Unemployment and job/employment security significantly affect physical, mental, and social health. Paid work provides financial resources, a sense of identity and purpose, social contacts, and opportunities for personal growth (Smith & Polanyi, 2016). Unemployment is linked to material and social deprivation, adoption of health-threatening coping behaviours, psychological stress, and physical and mental health challenges (Bryant & Raphael, 2020).

Employment and Working Conditions

Working conditions can either support health or pose health hazards. Smith and Polanyi (2016) identified the qualities of available, adequate, appropriate, and appreciative work as pillars of workplace health. Healthy workplaces include job and employment security, safe physical conditions, reasonable work pace, low stress, opportunities for self-expression and individual development, participation, and work–life balance (Jackson & Rao, 2016). Risk factors for poor workplace psychological health may include, but are not limited to, high demand and low control, high effort and low reward, unfair treatment, excessive workload, unfulfilling work, low employee engagement, poor physical work environment, limited professional development opportunities, physical violence at work, abuse of authority, discrimination, harassment, and lack of work flexibility (Health Canada, 2016). Additional factors include temporary employees, part-time workers, and people working in low-wage jobs, all of whom have high levels of job insecurity and frequent periods of unemployment without benefits or pensions.

One in five Canadians experience a psychological health concern or illness in any given year, costing the Canadian economy approximately $51 billion per year, $20 billion of which results from work-related causes. Importantly, 47% of Canadian workers find their work to be the most stressful part of daily life, with only 23% of workers reporting that they feel comfortable talking to their employer about a psychological health issue (Health Canada, 2016).

Indeed, the concern regarding negative workplace conditions in the health sector is considerable; nurses have had the highest or second-highest rates of absenteeism of all workers in Canada, particularly in response to the psychological impact of the COVID-19 pandemic and staffing issues, access to appropriate supply of PPE, rapid virus spread and testing, extensive training, and required self-isolation (Stelnicki et al., 2020). Workplace stress is linked to an increased risk for physical injuries, high blood pressure, cardiovascular disease, and depression and increases in tobacco and alcohol use (Jackson & Rao, 2016).

Early Childhood Development

While all health determinants influence child development, early child development is a separate determinant because of its importance to healthy lifelong outcomes. Children who experience disadvantaged conditions are more vulnerable in all areas of early development (PHAC, 2018a). When coupled with a health equity approach to inform decision making at the policy, program, and system levels, the outcomes of early development for at-risk children and families are profoundly improved (De Voe et al., 2019). Experiences from conception to age 6 are the most influential in connecting the brain's neurons (Devoe et al., 2019; Icer, 2020). During development, the brain is highly responsive to environmental cues and undergoes dramatic changes. By the time children reach school age, they have acquired significant cognitive functions, including attention, past experiences, coding, and recall (Icer, 2020).

Healthy child development can be disrupted by excessive or prolonged activation of stress response systems in the body and brain, often referred to as *toxic stress*. Toxic stress has the potential to negatively affect the architecture of the developing brain (Center for the Developing Child, 2021) and can be linked to the determinants of health. Maternal and childhood exposure to environmental stressors such as poverty, violence, conflict, neglect, and food insecurity have been associated with many lifelong health concerns, including cognitive deficits, mental health and behavioural disorders, substance use, hypertension, type 2 diabetes, and coronary heart disease (De Voe et al., 2019; Icer, 2020; PHAC, 2018a). Schools play a role in healthy child development because they can provide an environment in which students feel secure, respected, challenged, and cared for, helping to ensure that children succeed socially and academically.

Conditions that support early childhood development include household income above the poverty line, living in safe housing and communities, ability to afford nutritious foods, supportive parenting, and higher parental education. Quality early childhood education and care are particularly important in early child development, so much so that they have been singled out by some researchers as a combined social determinant of health (Friendly, 2016). These programs promote cognitive development and social competence and support parents in education and employment. Despite the Canadian government's acknowledgement of the importance of early childhood development programs and intervention through its Early Childhood Development Initiative (Health Canada, 2020), Canada does not have a national child care program.

Sixty-two countries, including municipalities throughout Canada, have adopted comprehensive and protective smoke-free policies to improve children's health. Smoking is prohibited in outdoor spaces, such as school grounds, playgrounds, outdoor dining spaces, parks, beaches, indoor common spaces, as well as in cars when children are present. Tobacco use and secondhand tobacco smoke exposure during pregnancy and throughout childhood cause devastating harm, including increasing children's risk for sudden unexpected infant death (SUID), acute respiratory infections, ear problems, and reduced lung development and adults' risk for coronary heart disease and lung cancer (WHO, 2021).

The biological and organic makeup of the human body significantly influences one's overall health. Genetic endowment provides an inherited predisposition to a wide range of individual responses and appears to predispose some individuals to particular diseases or health concerns, ultimately affecting health status (Health Canada, 2013). The social environment has a profound impact upon the function of one's genes, providing the context and stimulus for the variable expression of an inherited code. For example, a child's brain develops optimally under optimal socioenvironmental and political conditions.

Childhood obesity is a major public health issue in Canada. The prevalence of overweight or obesity among 0- to 5-year-olds is 6%. Of concern is that the rate increases to 31% among 6- to 17-year-olds. Poor nutrition, particularly overconsumption of fats, sugars, and salt, is linked to diseases such as certain cancers, cardiovascular diseases, type 2 diabetes, hypertension, osteoarthritis, and gallbladder disease and to functional limitations and disabilities (Tjepkema, 2006). The prevalence of obesity, which is associated with a higher risk of mortality, disability, and reduced quality of life, has risen considerably, creating a significant burden on the Canadian health care system. Obesity is considered a major public health threat, with the 2020 Canadian Community Health Survey (CCHS) revealing that 24.3% of adult Canadians were obese (body mass index [BMI] of 30 or more) and 35.5% were overweight (Statistics Canada, 2020). As BMI increased, so did the likelihood of high blood pressure, diabetes, and heart disease. About 17.4% of children (aged 5–17 years) were considered overweight or obese. Furthermore, 70% of children aged 4–8 years ate fewer than the minimum five recommended daily servings of vegetables and fruits. Moreover, 25% of Canadians overall (and one-third of teenagers aged 14–18) had eaten at fast-food outlets (where they serve foods high in fat and salt) the previous day. Several factors influence food consumption patterns, including household income, food advertising, and availability of nutritious choices.

Food Insecurity

The limited or uncertain availability of nutritious foods (i.e., food insecurity) is a growing public health concern in Canada because it is connected to the health and well-being of children and families (Kozkowski & Wayman, 2021). In 2020–2021, there was a significant spike in food insecurity resulting from the shutdown of businesses and schools due to the COVID-19 pandemic. One in eight households, including 1.15 million children in Canada, were at risk of hunger and food insecurity, with isolated and low-income families, older persons, and individuals with chronic health or compromised immune systems being at particular risk (Canada Helps, 2020). Of note is that food insecurity is 50% greater in off-reserve Indigenous households than in the general population of Canada (Batal et al., 2021; Tarasuk et al., 2019). Food insecurity is significantly associated with poor overall health, quality of life, multiple chronic conditions, distress, anxiety, and depression (Kozkowski & Wayman, 2021).

Environment

Physical environment includes environmental quality. Contaminants in the air, water, food, and soil can cause adverse health effects, including cancer, respiratory and gastrointestinal illness, and birth defects. Furthermore, geographic conditions may contribute to isolation and limit access to health care (McGibbon, 2016). Factors related to housing, indoor air quality, urban development, lighting, and transportation systems can significantly influence physical and psychological well-being. Increases in urbanization (two in three people are predicted to be living in urban areas by 2050) negatively impact social and health inequities including physical and mental health, well-being, and social cohesion (Hunter et al., 2019, p. 1). Children from low-income families, who often live in neighbourhoods located near highways or industrial areas, are particularly likely to be exposed to these contaminants. Benefits to overall health and well-being are achievable by enhancing the provision of parks and urban green space (WHO, 2016, 2017a, 2017b).

Additionally, the effects of climate change on the health of populations and the planet itself have increased in magnitude. The Canadian Nurses Association (CNA) has produced several documents related to nursing's role in addressing climate change (Canadian Nurses Association [Canadian Nurses Association [CNA], 2017) (see Chapter 11 for more information about climate change). The need for sustainable ecosystems, a prerequisite for health first identified in the *Ottawa Charter*, is becoming all the more critical. Nurses are well positioned to evaluate the vulnerabilities within population groups and to support policies that reduce emissions and improve the health and well-being of Canadians (CNA, 2017).

Housing

Housing, an important social determinant of health, includes factors in the built environment, such as safe and affordable housing and community planning with green spaces, as well as factors in the natural environment, such as geography, environmental quality, and climate change.

Lack of affordable, suitable, and adequate housing is a concern, as inadequate and insecure housing can affect health *directly* (e.g., presence of lead, asbestos, poor heating systems, overcrowding, dampness) and *indirectly* through its influence on other determinants (Bryant & Raphael, 2020). Spending a disproportionate amount of income on rent, for example, reduces the amount of money that families can spend on food, clothing, recreation, and health care. Homelessness in Canada is increasing, in part because of reduced government funding of social housing and a lack of affordable rental accommodations (Bryant & Raphael, 2020). Whereas historically homelessness in Canada was experienced primarily by older single men, the current homelessness crisis affects substantial numbers of women, youth, families, veterans, and Indigenous peoples (Health Canada, 2018a, 2018b). Homeless populations are at greater risk for a variety of health problems, including mental illness, substance use, suicide, tuberculosis, injuries and assaults, chronic medical conditions (e.g., respiratory, musculoskeletal), poor oral and dental health, and a shorter lifespan.

Social Exclusion

Experiences of social exclusion such as being isolated, excluded from a group, or disliked by others threaten the basic human need or desire to form strong and stable interpersonal relationships with others (de Gennaro et al., 2020). Social isolation, social exclusion, and lack of supportive relationships directly increase stress and vulnerability to disease, and indirectly increase risk behaviours such as smoking, substance use, and overeating (Xiong et al., 2020).

Social Safety Network

Social safety networks and inclusion are associated with healthy aging through practical, emotional, informational, and affirmational support. The caring, respect, and sense of well-being experienced in social relationships can act as a buffer against health problems. For example, 5.9 million people in Canada were over the age of 65 in 2021, with 12 million older persons projected by 2051. As such, active living, social support, and supportive environments, along with the provision of opportunities for lifelong learning, will be important for maintaining the health and cognitive capacity of older persons (Health Canada, 2013; Statistics Canada, 2022).

The inability to address the influences of social support among other health determinants can lead to chronic conditions that affect health, health behaviours, and health care utilization (Bryant & Raphael, 2020; Reimer-Kirkham et al., 2020). Social support has been linked to positive health outcomes (Bryant & Raphael, 2020). For instance, experiences of social isolation during the COVID-19 pandemic, which resulted from the implementation of necessary physical distancing measures, highlighted that those relationships are essential for good mental health (Xiong, 2020) and are as important to overall health as established risk factors such as obesity, smoking, and high blood pressure (Federal, Provincial, and Territorial ACPH, 1999; Health Canada, 2013).

In general, Canadians have reported high levels of social support (Health Canada, 2013). Four in five Canadians reported that they had someone to confide in whom they could count on in a crisis or for advice, and who made them feel loved and cared for. Nevertheless, men, lone-parent families, and lower-income Canadians generally reported less support than did their respective counterparts. Support from families and friends and from informal and formal groups can provide practical aid during times of crisis and emotional support in times of distress and change. Social support assists in coping and making behavioural changes and can help individuals solve problems and maintain a sense of mastery and control over their lives. A study conducted in Western Canada found that social conditions such as low income, low education, lack of social support, language barriers, and living in rural settings all aggravate symptom burdens that may increase the complexity of symptoms in populations with cancer. Of note is that certain population groups, including homeless individuals, Indigenous peoples, and individuals with a history of mental health concerns or addictions, were more susceptible to complex symptom burden (Santos Salas et al., 2019). It is important to address social support in relation to not only individual behaviours but also the broader social, political, and economic context that shapes community norms, values, and behaviours (Bryant & Raphael, 2020).

Health Services

Health care services account for only 25% of a population's health status; other contributing factors include child benefits, housing, gender equality, equity, reconciliation, and climate change (Health Canada, 2018e). Quality and accessible primary care, hospital care, long-term care, home care, and public health services are therefore important to health. Prenatal care, well-child and immunization clinics, education services about health practices, and services that maintain older persons' health and independence, as well as the COVID-19 vaccine initiative across Canada, are good examples of preventive and primary health care services (discussed further in Chapters 2 and 4). Principles of the *Canada Health Act*—universality, portability, accessibility, comprehensiveness, and public administration—apply to hospital and physician services, which cover only 70% of total health care costs. Medicare does not cover drug costs or dental care, and home care coverage varies across provinces (Bryant & Raphael, 2020), contributing to inequitable

access. Increasingly, the trends in health care services are toward the provision of community-based care rather than institutionalized care, decision making that is based on the best available evidence, and more regional administration. The government has invested considerably in initiatives that incorporate principles of primary health care; however, progress has been relatively slow (Health Canada, 2018e).

Indigenous Status

Indigenous peoples in Canada are more likely to experience health inequities and the burden of disease because of racism and the historical and contemporary discrimination they have experienced as a result of colonization (see Chapter 12) (Batal et al., 2021; The Lancet, 2020; Phillips-Beck, 2020). Over 150 000 Indigenous children were forced into government-funded residential schools from the 1870s until the late 1990s (Box 1.1) to eliminate parental involvement in their intellectual, cultural, and spiritual development (Truth and Reconciliation Commission of Canada [TRC], 2015a; Parks Canada, 2020). The impact of these injustices has been felt for generations and continues to affect the overall health and well-being of Indigenous populations in Canada.

Indigenous peoples are much more likely to suffer acute and chronic diseases and to experience higher infant mortality and shorter life expectancy than the general Canadian population (Batal et al., 2021; The Lancet, 2020; Parks Canada, 2020). For example, Indigenous youth living on reserve who are between the ages of 10 and 29 years are five to

---

BOX 1.1 CASE STUDY

The Truth and Reconciliation Commission of Canada (TRC)

During the 1870s, the Canadian government began to separate Indigenous children from their families and communities and place them in residential schools far from home. This action was implemented as part of the greater colonization effort occurring in Canada. The objective of residential schools was to assimilate Indigenous children into the dominant culture by removing and isolating them from their home, family, and heritage. Children were taken from their homes primarily against their will and the will of their family. It was often stated that the residential schools were established to "kill the Indian" in the child (Truth and Reconciliation Commission of Canada [TRC], 2015a, p. 137).

Residential schools operated in Canada for over 150 years. More than 150 000 Indigenous children attended these schools. Many never returned. Often underfunded and overcrowded, these schools were used as a tool of assimilation by the Canadian state and churches. Thousands of students suffered physical and sexual abuse. All students suffered from loneliness and a longing to be home with their families. The trauma inflicted by these schools continues to be felt to this day (TRC, 2015b).

On June 11, 2008, Prime Minister Stephen Harper issued a statement of apology to all former students of residential schools on behalf of the Government of Canada. In this statement, Harper apologized for the legacy and impact of the residential schools on generations of Indigenous peoples in Canada and supported the establishment of the Indian Residential Schools Settlement Agreement, which began in September 2007. A foundational piece of this agreement was the Truth and Reconciliation Commission of Canada. In 2009, the TRC began a multiyear process to listen to survivors, communities, and others affected by the residential school system. As a result of the TRC's findings, and to facilitate reconciliation efforts to make amends for the legacy of residential schools, the TRC identified 94 Calls to Action to change governmental policies and programs in the areas of child welfare, education, language and culture, health, and justice (TRC, 2015c).

six times more likely to die by suicide than are non-Indigenous youth; 40% of deaths among Inuit youth are the result of suicide, compared to 8% in the rest of the population (TRC, 2015b).

The link between social determinants of health (i.e., culture, social support, employment, income, and early childhood development) and the experiences of many Indigenous peoples highlights the importance of culture in health outcomes, as well as the detrimental effects of racism and racialization on health. The Truth and Reconciliation Commission of Canada's Call to Action 79 called on the federal government to commemorate the history and legacy of residential schools as a defining event in Canadian history that continues to have significant impact today (Parks Canada, 2020). September 30, 2021, marked the first time that Indigenous peoples and Canadians observed the National Day for Truth and Reconciliation (Canadian Heritage, 2021), which is a response to the TRC's Call to Action 80 and coincides with Orange Shirt Day (see Chapter 12 for further information on Indigenous health).

Gender

Gender is "the array of society-determined roles, personality traits, attitudes, behaviours, values, relative power, and influence that society ascribes to the two sexes on a differential basis" (PHAC, 2013b). Many health issues are a function of gender-based social roles, and gender can influence health status, behaviours, and care (Armstrong, 2016). Gender also intersects with and influences all other health determinants, such as income, culture, education, employment, and access to health services (Armstrong, 2016). Adverse social circumstances, including lack of education, poverty, and hazardous working conditions raise morbidity and mortality (Heymann et al., 2019). While all genders face inequities that negatively affect health, women disadvantaged by lower wages, fewer social protections, and less individual agency have fewer household resources and poorer health (Heymann et al., 2019). In Canada, men are more likely than women to experience extreme forms of social exclusion and to die prematurely, largely as a result of heart disease, unintentional fatal injuries, cancer, and suicide. By comparison, women are more likely to experience depression, stress (often resulting from efforts to manage both paid and family work), chronic conditions such as arthritis and allergies, and injuries and death from family violence (Bryant & Raphael, 2020).

The WHO emphasized the need to address gender inequalities through an equity and human rights lens to maintain the "leave no one behind" pledge of the Sustainable Development Goals (WHO, 2019, p. 1678). The WHO notes the importance of gender mainstreaming but emphasizes that gender should be regarded as a relational concept that "includes everyone and intersects with other drivers of inequalities such as poverty, age, sexuality, ethnicity and disability resulting in differential behaviours, exposures to risk factors, vulnerabilities, and health outcomes" (WHO, 2019, p. 1678). An example is the WHO's policy on ethnicity and health (Pan American Health Organization [PAHO] & WHO, 2017), which was developed to address health inequities among Indigenous women such as maternal mortality rates (partly due to stigma and discrimination) and lack of culturally appropriate health services.

Culture, Race, and Racism

Cultural and ethnic factors influence people's interactions with the health care system, their participation in prevention and health promotion programs, their access to health information, their health-related lifestyle choices, and their understanding of health and illness (Health Canada, 2013). Among immigrants and refugees, health is negatively affected by unmet expectations; challenges to successful social integration; and difficulties arising from underemployment or unemployment, low income, and food and housing insecurity (Bryant & Raphael, 2020; Mikkonen & Raphael, 2010; Oppedal et al., 2020; Villeneuve & Betker, 2020). The health of immigrants and refugees is also affected by their experiences in their country of origin, such as exposure to violence, armed conflict, economic challenges, and patterns of migration (Oppedal et al., 2020). Oppedal et al. (2020) have noted that the level of cultural competence of immigrant population groups is affected by length of stay, attitudes toward maintaining the heritage culture, role models, and frequency of interaction and supportive quality of social networks of either culture. These examples represent the complex political influences on the determinants of health that contribute to health inequity as introduced by the Oslo Commission on Global Governance for Health in 2014.

In Canada, racial disparities in health are often attributed to bias, discrimination, and stereotyping in health care delivery (Community Health Nurses of Canada, 2020; Nestel, 2012; PHAC, 2018b; Phillips-Beck et al. 2020). DiAngelo (2018) classifies identity politics as "barriers [that] specific groups face in their struggle for equality" (p. xiii). The most basic cause of racialized health inequities is racism (Allan & Smylie, 2015; Barber, 2020; Curtice & Choo, 2020; DasGupta et al., 2020; Phillips-Beck et al., 2020). Racism, though often subtle, is "an ideology that either directly or indirectly asserts that one group is inherently superior to others" (Ontario Human Rights Commission, n.d.). This ideology is used to represent, interpret, understand, and make sense of social existence. Examples include individualism, superiority, and capitalism, in which—either directly or indirectly—one group believes it is superior to others, and this belief is reinforced throughout society (DiAngelo, 2018).

Systemic racism—racism that is embedded in the laws, regulations, policies, and practices of a society or an organization—can be traced back to colonization and the narrative of cultural hierarchy and white supremacy that still persists and that continues to perpetuate health disparities for Indigenous peoples across Canada (Phillips-Beck et al., p. 3). It manifests as discrimination in areas such as criminal justice, employment, housing, health care, education, and political representation.

Racialization occurs when the dominant group or groups in society construct races as being real, different, and unequal in ways that matter to economic, political, and social life, thus forcing people to seek explanations for racial disparities in health. Racialized individuals in Canada (i.e., visible minorities) are more likely to be unemployed, employed in hazardous work environments, have limited social benefits, and experience job insecurity than are non-racialized Canadians (Nestel, 2012; Phillips-Beck, 2020). Racialization and racism adversely affect health by limiting access to health resources, creating fewer socioeconomic opportunities, and fostering unhealthy coping behaviours. Experiencing racism can cause significant distress, triggering negative psychological states such as anxiety and depression, which in turn initiate harmful physiological and biological processes in the cardiovascular, immune, and endocrine systems (The Lancet, 2020; Phillips-Beck, 2020).

Disability

Disabilities take many forms and are associated with both acute and chronic conditions and situations. Persons with disabilities are more likely to experience social isolation due to accessibility issues (Fergusen & Risling, 2020, p. 294). The use of information and communication technologies such as eHealth and telehealth may help to reduce social isolation by providing people with opportunities to connect with those who have had similar experiences, become better informed, communicate more frequently, and access health information more easily (Fergusen & Risling, 2020).

An individual's health practices and coping skills—the actions by which an individual can prevent diseases and promote self-care, cope with challenges, develop self-reliance, and make choices that enhance health—are directly associated with the social determinants of health. Individuals who have effective coping skills can better face challenges without needing to resort to risk behaviours such as substance use. Some risk behaviours may, in fact, be coping strategies to manage the stress and strain caused by living circumstances. For example, Gori et al. (2020) explored the impact of the COVID-19 pandemic on mental health and found that the relationship between life satisfaction and perceived stress was partially mediated by coping skills, a positive attitude, and defences. This work suggests that positive coping strategies help to provide a protective pathway for mental health outcomes.

There is evidence that rural, low-income women who face multiple barriers smoke as a means of coping with the stress related to feeling isolated, having limited access to social and economic resources, and experiencing poverty and unemployment. A study by Mitchell and colleagues (2021) identified an interconnection between social isolation, stigmatization, and smoking. Participants perceived a sense of rejection from community members and limited social support because of their smoking behaviour, which potentiated further isolation for this population. To mitigate this isolation, the authors emphasized that smoking cessation interventions must be offered in safe environments, thereby enhancing safety, empowerment, and social support.

Three risk behaviours that lead to major detrimental health consequences are physical inactivity, poor nutrition, and tobacco use. Physical inactivity is a major risk factor for some types of cancer, diabetes, cardiovascular disease, osteoporosis, obesity, hypertension, depression, stress, and anxiety. Only 35% of children and youth aged 5 to 17 years meet the physical activity recommendation of at least 60 minutes of moderate to vigorous physical activity per day; 77% participate in organized physical activity; and 21% use inactive modes of transportation (e.g., car, bus) to travel to and from school. Furthermore, children aged 9 to 12 are in the 28th percentile for cardiorespiratory fitness (Barnes et al., 2018).

Tobacco use remains the leading preventable cause of death and disease in Canada and worldwide, with a mortality rate five times higher than that due to traffic injuries, alcohol abuse, murder, and suicide combined (Health Canada, 2018c; Poirier et al., 2019). There are 4.6 million Canadians (15%) who use tobacco; of those, 3.9 million are cigarette smokers (Health Canada, 2018c). Approximately 1 in 10 Canadians smoke cigarettes on a regular basis, and those aged 25 and older are 3.5 times more likely to be current smokers (11%) (Statistics Canada, 2021). Young adult males have the highest prevalence of cigarette smoking (22%), along with 24 to 45% of LGBTQ2 persons. (Health Canada, 2018c). Tobacco is the only legal consumer product that can harm everyone who is exposed to it. For example, tobacco kills more than 8 million people each year—7 million from direct tobacco use, and 1.2 million non-smokers who are exposed to second-hand smoke. Of note is that 80% of the 1.3 billion tobacco users live in low- and middle-income countries (WHO, 2021), with the prevalence among Indigenous peoples being two to five times higher than among the non-Indigenous population in Canada (Health Canada, 2018d).

Vaping—the act of inhaling and exhaling vapours produced by a device such as an e-cigarette, vaporizer, or vape pen—is common among younger Canadians. In 2020, 35% of youth aged 15 to 19 reported having tried vaping at some point in their lives. Vaping products contain nicotine and may lead to addiction as well as increasing the risk of exposure to other harmful chemicals. Reported reasons for vaping included enjoyment, stress reduction, smoking reduction or cessation, and a desire to try it (CPHA, 2021c).

At the end of 2020, 6.2 million or 20% of Canadians aged 15 years and older reported having used cannabis in the past 3 months. Usage, primarily through smoking, has increased since the *Cannabis Act* was enacted by the federal government. Rates of consumption were comparable by gender in 2020. In the first year of legalization, few products that included dried cannabis or cannabis oil were available under the Access to Cannabis for Medical Purposes regulations; however, individuals could make their own products with some conditions. One year after legalization, more women consumed edibles in 2020 than in 2019 (42.5% versus 28.0%), and consumption of edibles was also more prevalent among males aged 25 to 44 than it was in the previous 2 years (Rotermann, 2021; Statistics Canada, 2021).

By now, it should be clear that many factors influence individual health behaviours (e.g., income, education, culture, and social support). Developing and maintaining health-enhancing behaviours requires not only health education but also social policies related to income security, product marketing, and supportive environments that make healthy choices the "easy" choices.

Social Environments (Social Safety Net, Social Exclusion, and Disability)

Social environments are defined as "the array of values and norms of a society [that] influence in varying ways the health and well-being of populations. In addition, social stability, recognition of diversity, safety, good working relationships, and cohesive communities provide a supportive society that shares resources, builds attachments with others, and reduces or avoids many potential risks to good health" (PHAC, 2013b). The social environment is clearly related to other factors and expands on the social support determinant by incorporating broader community characteristics, norms, and values. Healthy social environments include freedom from discrimination and prejudice. The determinant of social environment is also evident in the prerequisites of human rights, social security, and social relations identified in the *Jakarta Declaration* (WHO, 1997). These prerequisites relate to social exclusion—the process by which people have limited opportunities to participate in many aspects of cultural, economic, social, and political life (Galabuzi, 2016; Salma & Salami, 2019).

The people most likely to be excluded are Indigenous peoples, those who are homeless, LGBTQ2 individuals, people living in poverty, single mothers, new Canadians, and members of racialized groups; however, people also experience marginalization on the basis of income, age, gender, activity or ability limitation, ethnicity, and sexual orientation.

Social exclusion limits people's access to the resources that support their health and participation in community life (Herrick & Duncan, 2018; Mitchell et al., 2021; Salma & Salami, 2019). Additionally, a sense of community belonging has been linked to better self-rated general health and mental health. For example, Canadian youth who identify as LGBTQ2 experience worse health and social outcomes than their heterosexual peers. Health and social issues faced by LGBTQ2 individuals may include depression, anxiety, suicidal ideation and attempts at suicide, homelessness, fear of family rejection, fear of violence, eating disorders, and physical abuse (Herrick & Duncan, 2018). A strong public health drive to address the inequities in health and social outcomes experienced by LGBTQ2 youth has led some school boards in Canada to help students create gay–straight alliances in schools as a way to provide community and peer support to LGBTQ2 youth (Day et al., 2020).

Another important aspect of the social environment is the absence of violence, both in the home (child abuse, intimate partner violence, older person abuse) and in the community (youth violence, victimization, bullying, assault by strangers, violence due to property crimes, violence in the workplace) (McIver et al., 2018). In 2018, 60 651 Canadian children and youth were the victims of sexual or physical assault, with 6 out of 10 assaults being perpetrated by a family member. More recently, police in Canada reported that 12 000 (33%) older persons over the age of 65 were victims of a violent crime committed by a family member (Statistics Canada, 2019). In light of the COVID-19 pandemic and the restrictions that were put in place to slow the spread of the virus, many family violence victims were "trapped" in their homes with their perpetrators. Such restrictions can result in further control and isolation. The health effects of family violence are devastating—both for those experiencing or exposed to violence and for the perpetrators—and include negative psychological, physical, behavioural, academic, sexual, interpersonal, self-perceptual, and spiritual consequences, which may appear immediately or over time (Campbell, 2020).

STRATEGIES TO INFLUENCE HEALTH DETERMINANTS

Health Promotion and Disease Prevention

The understanding that health is qualitatively different from disease has led to a differentiation of the concepts of health promotion and disease prevention, although they are interrelated. Pender and colleagues (2015) differentiated between health promotion and disease prevention as follows: **health promotion** is "directed toward increasing the level of well-being and self-actualization" (p. 27), while **disease prevention** (specifically primary prevention) is "action to avoid or forestall illness/disease" (p. 26). On the other hand, Leavell and Clark's (1965) initial conceptualization of levels of prevention considered health promotion one aspect of primary prevention and not necessarily disease specific. In contrast, the *Ottawa Charter*, put forth health promotion as the overarching concept, defining it as "the process of enabling people to increase control over, and improve, their health" (WHO, 1986). The following more comprehensive definition was offered by Nutbeam (1998):

> Health promotion represents a comprehensive social and political process; it not only embraces actions directed at strengthening the skills and capabilities of individuals, but also action directed towards changing social, environmental and economic conditions so as to alleviate their impact on public and individual health. Health promotion is the process of enabling people to increase control over the determinants of health and thereby improve their health. Participation is essential to sustain health promotion action. (p. 351)

Three levels of disease prevention correspond to the natural history of disease:

- *Primary prevention* activities protect against a disease before signs and symptoms occur (prepathogenesis stage of disease). Examples include immunization (to prevent infectious diseases) and reduction of risk factors (such as inactivity, smoking, and exposure to air pollution).
- *Secondary prevention* activities promote early detection of disease once pathogenesis has occurred so that prompt treatment can be initiated to halt disease and limit disability. Examples include preventive screening for cancer (e.g., Pap test, testicular self-examination), blood pressure screening to detect hypertension, and blood glucose screening to detect diabetes.
- *Tertiary prevention* activities are initiated in the convalescence stage of disease and are directed toward minimizing residual disability and helping people to live productively with limitations. An example is a cardiac rehabilitation program after a myocardial infarction.

Nursing strategies guided by a prevention framework focus on assessment and alleviation of risk factors for disease. Health promotion, by contrast, may be viewed more broadly than disease prevention

as it emphasizes participation, empowerment, and equity and goes beyond individual health education to a broader ecological approach that incorporates community development and policy advocacy. Health promotion strategies are therefore often political because they emphasize addressing structural and systemic inequities and have a strong philosophy of social justice. Health promotion is guided by the following principles (CPHA, 1996):

- Health promotion addresses health issues in context.
- Health promotion supports a holistic approach.
- Health promotion requires a long-term perspective.
- Health promotion is multisectoral.
- Health promotion draws on knowledge from social, economic, political, environmental, medical, and nursing sciences, as well as from first-hand experiences.

HEALTH PROMOTION STRATEGIES

The *Ottawa Charter* identified five broad strategies to enhance health. The following is a brief introduction to each of these **health promotion strategies**. For further examples of each of these strategies, see Reutter and Kushner (2010).

1. **Build Healthy Public Policy.** Advocating for healthy public policies is a priority strategy for health promotion in Canada. Indeed, some academics have suggested that this strategy is the foundation of all others because policies shape how money, power, and material resources are distributed to society (CPHA, 1996). Advocating for healthy public policy means focusing on policies that create healthy living conditions. Because the determinants of health are broad, healthy public policy necessarily extends beyond traditional health agencies and government health departments to other sectors such as agriculture, education, transportation, labour, social services, energy, and housing. Therefore, policymakers in all government sectors and organizations should ensure that their policies have positive health consequences. This emphasis is reflected in national documents such as advocacy position statements (CPHA, 2021b) and international documents, including the International Council of Nurses (ICN), whose advocacy places nursing and health policy at the centre of what they do (International Council of Nurses [ICN], 2021).

Advocating for healthy public policy is best achieved through intersectoral collaboration. A nurse might work with others to develop policy options, encourage public dialogue, persuade decision makers to adopt the healthiest option, and follow up to make sure the policy is implemented (ICN, 2021). Cathy Crowe, a Toronto "street nurse," is an excellent example of a nurse who advocates for healthy public policy to reduce homelessness (Box 1.2).

Increasingly, policy advocacy is incorporated into nursing role statements (CNA, 2021; Nurses and Nurse Practitioners of British Columbia [NNPBC], 2021) and nursing education curricula (Turale & Kunaviktikul, 2019). In providing nursing care, the nurse needs to think about what policies have contributed to the health situations of their patients, what policies would help alleviate health problems, and how they can champion public policies. For example, how do current welfare incomes, which are lower than "poverty lines" (low-income cut-offs), influence recipients' abilities to obtain adequate food and shelter and participate meaningfully in Canadian society? An informative resource on policy implications arising from social determinants of health is *Social Determinants of Health: The Canadian Facts* (see the website at the end of the chapter). Turale and Kunaviktikul (2019) provide suggestions for the role of nursing in policy advocacy and outline ways that nurses can engage in policy advocacy.

Cathy Crowe: Advocating for Healthy Public Policy

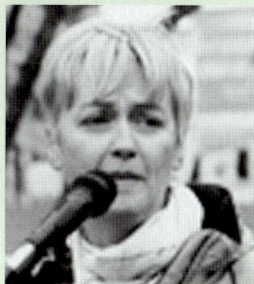

(Photo courtesy https://cathycrowe.ca/.)

Cathy Crowe is a Toronto-based street nurse who has advocated for policies related to a variety of social determinants. Her work as an outreach street nurse in Toronto since the 1980s exemplifies nursing's role in not only attending to the immediate health needs of people who are homeless but also advocating for policies that will provide more adequate and affordable housing to alleviate the root causes of these health problems. Crowe co-founded the Toronto Disaster Relief Committee (TDRC) in 1998, which declared homelessness a national disaster in Canada. The committee advocated a "1% solution," calling on the federal, provincial, and territorial governments to allocate an additional 1% of their budget to fully fund a national affordable housing program. The efforts of the TDRC increased awareness, both in large cities in Canada and at the United Nations, about Canada's housing problem. This awareness led to the appointment of a federal minister responsible for homelessness and federal emergency relief monies (e.g., for shelter beds, food banks, programs for homeless youth). Although monies were also made available to provide housing, the goal of a fully funded national housing strategy has not yet been realized, and homelessness continues to increase across Canada.

Crowe has founded numerous coalitions and advocacy initiatives, working with homeless people and other organizations. The TDRC was involved in fighting the evictions of Toronto's Tent City in 2002 and succeeded in eventually securing housing for many residents. Crowe is currently on the board of directors of a nonprofit organization that is building affordable housing in Toronto. To raise awareness about children who are homeless, she co-produced the film *Home Safe*, which is set in several Canadian cities. As part of this initiative, a children's forum on homelessness was organized to give children the opportunity to voice their concerns to the United Nations Special Rapporteur on Adequate Housing when he visited Canada. Crowe has also written a book, *Dying for a Home*, co-authored with activists who are homeless themselves.

Crowe has received numerous awards for her advocacy work. She sees advocacy as a critical nursing role and responsibility. You are encouraged to view her many speeches and activities on her website, at https://cathycrowe.ca.

2. Create Supportive Environments. The *Ottawa Charter* (WHO, 1986) states that "the overall guiding principle . . . is the need to encourage reciprocal maintenance, to take care of each other, our communities and our natural environment" (p. 2). This strategy helps ensure that physical environments are healthy and safe and that living and working conditions are stimulating and satisfying. Creating supportive environments also means protecting the natural environment and conserving natural resources (WHO, 1986).

An excellent example of an initiative that helps create supportive environments is the Comprehensive School Health Initiative, which focuses on improving school environments by providing health instruction, social support, support services, and positive physical environments (Pan-Canadian Joint Consortium for School Health,

2015). Other examples of supportive environments include flexible workplace policies, quality child care programs that support early child development and parental employment, and baby- and age-friendly community initiatives.

3. Strengthen Community Action. Strengthening communities is a requisite for successful health promotion and community health nursing practices in Canada (CPHA, 2010). In this strategy, often referred to as *community development*, "health promotion works through concrete and effective community action in setting priorities, making decisions, and planning and implementing strategies" (WHO, 1986), often partnering with other community organizations to achieve better health, empowerment of communities, and community ownership and control of development and change (see Chapter 4). Public participation in all phases of community programming is key to community development. Examples of community development projects are community gardens and collective kitchens targeted at enhancing food security.

4. Develop Personal Skills. This strategy, which is probably the most familiar to nurses, helps clients develop personal skills, enhance coping strategies, and gain control over their health and environments so that they can make healthy lifestyle choices. Personal skills development includes health education, but it also emphasizes adequate support and resources. Some examples of interventions to enhance personal skills include early intervention programs for children, home visiting by public health nurses, parenting classes, and fall prevention programs for older persons. On a broader level, examples include province-wide health communication initiatives aimed at improving nutrition and physical activity (e.g., Healthy Food Checker, Alberta Health Services; B.C. First Nations Act Now Toolkit, First Nations Health Council).

5. Reorient Health Services. Health system reform has two objectives: to shift the emphasis from treating disease to improving health, and to make the health care system more efficient and effective (CPHA, 1996). A proactive approach to health requires improved access to primary health care services, increased community development, improved community-based care services, increased family-based care, and public participation. In Canada, there is considerable emphasis on developing the primary health care model, a whole-society approach to health that seeks to help people attain the highest possible level of health and well-being through an accessible and wide range of services.

A recent example is COVID-19 vaccine delivery within various communities to ensure access for all Canadians. Other examples include health promotion, disease prevention, treatment, rehabilitation, and palliative care. Successful implementation of this strategy requires that primary health care delivery be accompanied by empowerment of the population (Chotchoungchatchai et al., 2020; see also Chapters 2 and 4).

POPULATION HEALTH PROMOTION MODEL: PUTTING IT ALL TOGETHER

This chapter has presented two major approaches to health: health promotion and population health. Hamilton and Bhatti (1996) integrated these two concepts into one model that shows their relationship to each other (Figure 1.7). Aimed at developing actions to improve health, the model explores four major questions: "On *what* can we take action?"; "*How* can we take action?"; "With *whom* can we act?"; and "*Why* take action?"

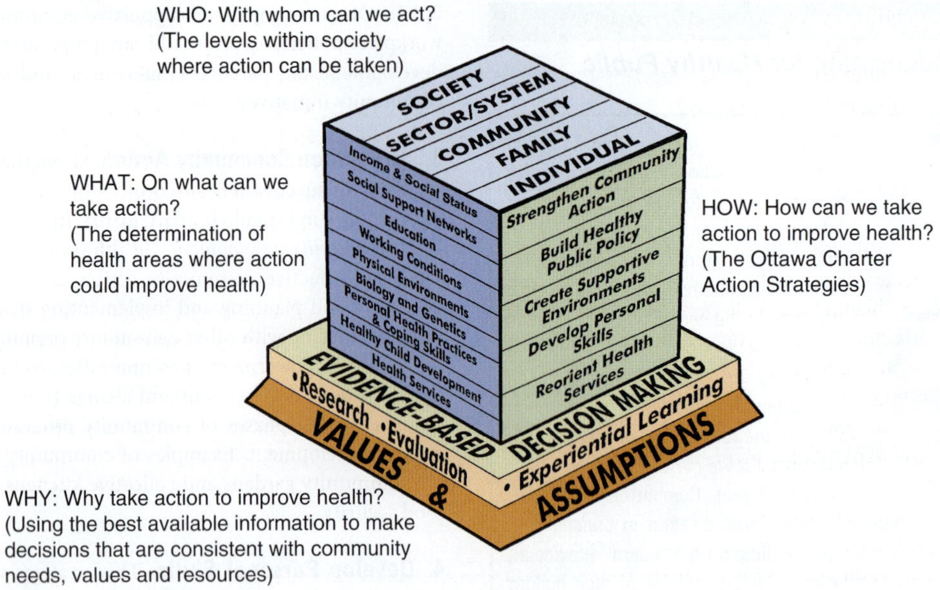

WHO: With whom can we act?
(The levels within society
where action can be taken)

WHAT: On what can we
take action?
(The determination of
health areas where action
could improve health)

HOW: How can we take
action to improve health?
(The Ottawa Charter
Action Strategies)

WHY: Why take action to improve health?
(Using the best available information to make
decisions that are consistent with community
needs, values and resources)

FIGURE 1.7 **Population health promotion model.** (From Hamilton, N., & Bhatti, T. [1996]. *Population health promotion: An integrated model of population health and health promotion.* Health Promotion Development Division, Health Canada. Copyright 1996 by Minister of Public Works and Government Services Canada.)

The document *Strategies for Population Health* (Federal, Provincial, and Territorial Advisory Committee on Population Health, 1994) identifies health determinant actions that could be taken (the "what"). The *Ottawa Charter* provides a comprehensive set of five strategies to enhance health (the "how"). Together, these documents suggest that to enhance population health, action must be taken on a variety of levels (the "who"). Clearly, nurses must direct these strategies toward individuals and families, communities, individual sectors of society (such as health or environmental sectors), and society.

For example, nurses wishing to promote the health of lower-income patients can help them access resources and supports that will enhance their personal skills. Community programs such as school lunch programs, recreational activities, collective kitchens, and support groups can be provided. Nurses can lobby the government sectors responsible for housing and employment to implement healthy public policies pertaining to affordable housing, job creation, child care, income security, and financially accessible health services. On a societal level, nurses can raise awareness about the negative effects of poverty on health and well-being and can advocate for policies that will decrease poverty. The population health promotion model illustrates how **evidence-informed decision making** serves as a foundation to ensure that policy and program leaders focus on the right issues, take effective action, and produce successful results (Hamilton & Bhatti, 1996)—the "why" of action. Evidence is informed by research, experiential learning, and evaluation of programs, policies, and projects. Values and assumptions that are the foundation of the model include the following:

- Stakeholders representing the various determinants must collaborate to address health determinants.
- Society is responsible for its members' health status.
- Health status is a result of people's health practices and their social and physical environments.
- Opportunities for healthy living are based on social justice, equity, and relationships of mutual trust and caring rather than power and status.
- Health care, health protection, and disease prevention complement health promotion.
- Active participation in policies and programs is essential.

SUMMARY

This chapter has provided an introduction to different ways of viewing health, wellness, and health determinants, and briefly discussed the historical development of these concepts within the Canadian context. The content of the chapter challenges you to approach health situations broadly by identifying the myriad determinants that influence health. An increased understanding of health determinants should enable you to provide more sensitive care at the individual level and to consider strategies at the community and policy levels that will address the root causes of health situations.

KEY CONCEPTS

- Health conceptualizations and determinants influence the nature and scope of professional practice.
- Definitions of health can be classified in several ways; recent definitions reflect a multidimensional perspective and a positive orientation.
- Three recent approaches to health are medical, behavioural, and socioenvironmental.
- Behavioural approaches focus primarily on health practices.
- Socioenvironmental approaches emphasize psychosocial factors and socioenvironmental conditions.
- Health determinants are intersectoral and interrelated.
- Health literacy involves functional, interactive, and critical abilities needed to exert control over life events and circumstances that influence health experience and health status.
- Canada is a leader in ever-changing views of health and health determinants.
- Health promotion differs from disease prevention.
- Three levels of disease prevention are primary (protection against disease), secondary (activities that promote early detection), and tertiary (activities directed toward minimizing disability from disease and helping clients learn to live productively with their limitations).

- The *Ottawa Charter* identifies five major categories of health promotion strategies: building healthy public policies; creating supportive environments; strengthening community action; developing personal skills; and reorienting health care services.

CRITICAL THINKING EXERCISES

1. Describe your current level of health. What criteria did you use? Which definition of health discussed in this chapter best matches your understanding of health? Consider another definition of health discussed in this chapter. Does your current level of health change on the basis of this definition? How might your nursing practice differ depending on which conceptualization of health you choose to guide your practice? How might your definition of health change as you experience different life transitions (e.g., aging, parenthood)?
2. What do you consider to be the three most important health problems facing Canadians today? What are the major determinants of these problems? Which health promotion strategies would you consider the most appropriate to address them?
3. Imagine you are a community health nurse working in an area where many low-income individuals smoke. Using a socioenvironmental approach to health, what questions would you need to address to decrease smoking behaviour in your area? How would your approach differ if you were using a behavioural approach to health?

Answers to Critical Thinking Exercises appear on the Evolve website.

REVIEW QUESTIONS

Review Questions 1 to 10 relate to the case study at the beginning of the chapter.

1. As a nurse working in a rural practice, what do you believe are some of the health issues that rural populations may experience? *(Select all that apply.)*
   a. Higher mortality rates
   b. Increased risk for injuries
   c. Decreased cardiovascular disease
   d. Longer lifespans
   e. Lower mortality rates
2. As you work with structurally vulnerable persons or populations who are living in poverty, what factors related to health disparities would you expect to encounter with this population group?
   a. A higher education status
   b. Increased access to health services
   c. Fewer chronic diseases
   d. Lack of food security
3. The majority of the Lazzer family is unable to work because of COVID-19 restrictions or chronic illnesses. What is the immediate primary health care concern for the Lazzer family?
   a. Access to adequate health care
   b. Skin cancer from the sun
   c. Chronic neck pain
   d. Eye problems related to dust

4. Which approach to health should you, as the nurse, focus on when caring for this family?
   a. The behavioural approach to health
   b. A medical approach to health
   c. A socioenvironmental approach to health
   d. Physiological risk factors
5. From a socioenvironmental perspective, what are the most concerning determinants of health for the Lazzer family? *(Select all that apply.)*
   a. Income and social status
   b. Biological and genetic endowment
   c. Healthy child development
   d. Gender
   e. Visibility
6. Which disease prevention level should you focus on to assess Joey Lazzer's COPD?
   a. Primary prevention
   b. Secondary prevention
   c. Tertiary prevention
   d. Risk assessment
7. You inform the Lazzer family that there will be a COVID-19 vaccination clinic in the community next week. What level of prevention is being offered with this clinic?
   a. Primary prevention
   b. Secondary prevention
   c. Tertiary prevention
   d. None of the above. Vaccinations are not considered a level of prevention.
8. Which statement does NOT accurately describe the population health promotion model?
   a. The model suggests that action can address the full range of health determinants.
   b. The model incorporates the health promotion strategies of the *Ottawa Charter*.
   c. The model focuses primarily on interventions at the societal level.
   d. The model attempts to integrate population health and health promotion concepts.
9. The Lazzer family lives 15 minutes away from town and is unable to access fresh produce. Considering their circumstances, which strategy would best improve the health of family members?
   a. Strengthen community action.
   b. Build healthy public policy.
   c. Develop personal skills.
   d. Reorient health services.
10. As a nurse who is a settler, you are aware that you are providing care to Indigenous members of this community who have experienced residential school trauma. Care that is absent of unfair systems and policies that cause health inequalities is referred to as which of the following:
    a. Health disparity
    b. Health equity
    c. Equality
    d. Racism

Answers: 1. b; **2.** d; **3.** a; **4.** c; **5.** a; **6.** c; **7.** a; **8.** c; **9.** b; **10.** b.

Rationales for the Review Questions appear on the Evolve website.

RECOMMENDED WEBSITES

Canadian Institute for Health Information (CIHI): https://www.cihi.ca/en
The CIHI is a not-for-profit Canadian organization working to improve the health of Canadians and the health care system. One of its goals is to generate public awareness about the factors affecting health. This website offers current information and numerous links to government health reports.

Public Health Agency of Canada (PHAC): https://www.phac-aspc.gc.ca
The PHAC website provides excellent information on many aspects of public health, including the population health approach and the determinants of health.

Social Determinants of Health-—The Canadian Facts: https://www.thecanadianfacts.org/The_Canadian_Facts.pdf
This document summarizes the social determinants of health in the Canadian context and includes policy implications, references, and resources.

Social Determinants of Health e-Learning Course: https://nccdh.ca/resources/entry/social-determinants-of-health-online-course
This website from the National Collaborating Centre for Determinants of Health provides an interactive eLearning module about how social and economic conditions influence the health of individuals, communities, and nations.

WHO Commission on Social Determinants of Health: https://www.who.int/teams/social-determinants-of-health
This WHO web page provides a global perspective and many excellent papers pertaining to various determinants of health.

World Health Organization (WHO): https://www.who.int/publications
This website provides links to the publications of the WHO, including the *World Health Report*.

REFERENCES

A full reference list is available on the website for this book at http://evolve.elsevier.com/Canada/Potter/fundamentals/

2

The Canadian Health Care Delivery System

Written by Pammla Petrucka, RN, PhD, and Megan Meszaros, RN, PhD(c)

OBJECTIVES

Mastery of content in this chapter will enable you to:

- Define the key terms listed.
- Describe the evolution of Canada's social safety net and Medicare.
- Identify and define the principles of the *Canada Health Act* and significant legislation related to the Canadian health care system.
- Explain the principal factors influencing ongoing health care reform and the current health care delivery system.
- Describe patients' rights to health care.

- Explain specific issues and opportunities within the health care delivery system related to Indigenous peoples' health.
- Describe the multiple roles and challenges for all categories of regulated nurses in different health care settings.
- Describe the five levels of health care and the associated types of services.
- Identify the various settings and models of care delivery in the Canadian health care system.
- Identify the challenges and initiatives related to enhancing the quality of the Canadian health care delivery system.

KEY TERMS

Accessibility
Acute care
Adult day support programs
Assisted-living facilities
Comprehensiveness
Continuity of care
eHealth
Electronic health record (EHR)
Evidence-informed practice
Health promotion
Home care
Hospice
Inpatient
Insured residents

Levels of health care
Medicare
mHealth
Outpatients
Palliative care
Parish nursing
Portability
Primary care (PC)
Primary health care (PHC)
Public administration
Quality of care
Recentralization
Regional health authorities
Rehabilitation

Remote monitoring
Respite care
Secondary care
Self-care
Social safety net
Supportive care
Sustainability
Tertiary care
Truth and Reconciliation Commission of Canada (TRC)
Universal health care (UHC)
Universality
Voluntary agencies

WEBSITE

https://evolve.elsevier.com/Canada/Potter/fundamentals/

CASE STUDY

W.W., a 68-year-old widower (preferred pronouns: he/him) with no immediate family support, is scheduled to have major hip replacement surgery. W.W. is generally in good health and lives in a seniors-only apartment complex in a rural town. W.W. is concerned about the upcoming surgery and his ability to cope and convalesce at home in the postsurgery recovery phase. Although W.W. has neighbours in the apartment complex, he lives alone and is hesitant to call on them if he needs anything.

Think about this case study as you read this chapter. There are review questions at the end of the chapter about this case study.

Nurses are an essential part of the Canadian health care delivery system. They constitute the largest group of human health resources and are recognized as being invaluable to the health of Canadians. Nursing services are necessary for virtually every patient seeking care. Between 2006 and 2019, the number of regulated nurses (employed and unemployed) in Canada grew by 20.2% (351 048 to 439 975) (Canadian Institute for Health Information [CIHI], 2019a). In 2019, there were 300 669 registered nurses (RNs), 6 159 nurse practitioners (NPs), 127 097 licensed practical nurses (LPNs), and 6 050 registered psychiatric nurses (RPNs), reflecting 68.3%, 1.4%, 25.9%, and 1.4% of Canada's regulated nursing workforce, respectively (CIHI, 2019a) (Box 2.1).

BOX 2.1 **Facts About Nursing in Canada, 2019**

Care Setting
- Registered nurses (RNs): 65% practised in the hospital sector; 15% in community health; 9% in nursing homes/long-term care; and 11% in other settings.
- Licensed practical nurses (LPNs): 45% practised in hospitals; 15% in community health; 32% in nursing homes/long-term care; and 8% in other settings.
- Registered psychiatric nurses (RPNs): 47% practised in hospitals; 27% in community health; 13% in nursing homes/long-term care; and 13% in other settings.
- Nurse practitioners (NPs): 36% practised in hospitals; 36% in community health; 4% in nursing homes/long-term care; and 24% in other settings.

Education
- In 2019, 55% of RNs were degree prepared.
- 9 out of 10 Canadian graduates either remained in or returned to the jurisdiction of graduation to practise, a continuous pattern since 2006.
- Internationally educated nurses in the regulated nursing workforce: 9.4% of RNs, 4.5% of NPs, 7.6% of LPNs, and 7.8% of RPNs.
- 13 833 RNs obtained CNA certification in 1 of 22 specialty areas.
- Between 2019 and 2020, 295 LPNs (or registered practical nurses in some Canadian jurisdictions) obtained CNA certification in gerontological (285) or medical-surgical nursing (10).
- In 2020, CNA certification in gerontological or psychiatric and mental health was made available to RPNs.

Nurses Employed Per Capita
- In 2019, the rate of regulated nurses employed per 100 000 Canadians was 833 for RNs, 17 for NPs, 343 for LPNs, and 51 for RPNs.

Demographics
- By gender: RNs: 91% female, 9% male; NPs: 92% female, 8% male; LPNs: 91% female, 9% male; RPNs: 81% female, 19% male.
- Average age: RNs, 44 years; LPNs, 40.7 years; RPNs, 44.4 years.
- For RNs, 25.5% were aged 55 years or older, 13.5% were aged 60 years or older, and 1.2% were aged 65 years or older. For LPNs, 17.1% were aged 55 or older, and 7.9% were aged 60 or older.

Adapted from Canadian Institute for Health Information. (2019). *Nursing in Canada, 2019: A lens on supply and workforce.* https://www.cihi.ca/sites/default/files/rot/nursing-report-2019-en-web.pdf

Since the late 1990s, the size of the Canadian nursing workforce has remained relatively stable. Building the Future (Kephart et al., 2004) was the first national study to outline a long-term strategy to ensure adequate Canadian nursing human resources. The National Expert Commission of the Canadian Nurses Association sought input on the future of nursing to achieve "better health, better care, better value for all Canadians," producing two reports (Browne et al., 2012; Muntaner et al., 2012) that consider strategies and policies to enable effective use of existing health care providers (HCPs) throughout the health system. The nursing profession is currently facing the challenges of an aging workforce, high retirement rates, ethical international recruitment, and lack of full-time positions.

Nursing is integral to the health care delivery system. Practising nurses ought to appreciate the complexities of a health care delivery system replete with human and fiscal resource challenges and imperatives for quality services. Financial pressures have challenged health care institutions to shift priorities and to contain costs by changing the workforce, often through the use of alternative staff and support

services mixes. Nurses must participate in restructuring delivery systems, toward the uptake of universal health care, and achieving excellence in health care through leadership, advocacy, and reinforcement of the values of safe, quality, ethical, patient- and family-centred, and evidence-informed patient care.

EVOLUTION OF THE CANADIAN HEALTH CARE SYSTEM

Despite significant changes since the 1960s, a network of national, provincial, and territorial social programs, referred to as the **social safety net**, exists to protect the most vulnerable members of Canadian society. Most programs target specific populations (e.g., older persons, children), while a few are universally accessible. Provincial social assistance programs provide income support to those who experience prolonged unemployment or are underemployed; the federal employment insurance program provides income support for short-term employment interruption. Key to Canada's social safety net is the provision of hospital and medical insurance, known as **Medicare**, which is funded by general taxation. Although it is called a "national" program, Medicare is, in fact, an interlocking set of 10 provincial and 3 territorial insurance schemes providing a core palette of medically essential hospital and physician services to individuals registered in their respective province or territory (Marchildon et al., 2020). Medicare is a source of national pride and solidarity as a commitment to the well-being of Canadians. It is also a source of national debate regarding costs, effectiveness, and sustainability.

Early Health Care in Canada

Europeans arriving in Canada in the fifteenth century brought infectious diseases that flourished under conditions of poor sanitation. Settlements enacted public health laws to control the spread of diseases. For years, government care was limited to essential services (e.g., care of "insane" persons, epidemics). Permanent boards of health did not exist; hence, families, churches, and local communities managed medical and social problems.

Canada became a self-governing colony with the passage of the *British North America Act* (also known as the *Constitution Act*) in 1867, which united three colonies into the original four provinces of Ontario, Quebec, Nova Scotia, and New Brunswick. This act accorded powers to the national (federal) and provincial governments. Responsibility for public health (including regulation of hospitals, education, and social services) fell to the provinces, whereas the federal government retained jurisdiction over public policy components such as health care for Indigenous peoples and pharmaceutical safety (Storch, 2006).

As Canada's population grew, urbanized, and industrialized, substandard living conditions and sanitation accelerated. Provinces enacted public health acts to establish local boards of health to hire medical health officers and sanitation inspectors, while nurses (ultimately the first public health nurses) continued working with the community and the poor.

By 1920, health and social programs had expanded, and voluntary agencies formed; the latter included the Children's Aid Society (in 1891), the Red Cross (in 1896), the Victorian Order of Nurses (in 1897), and the Canadian Mental Health Association (in 1918). Municipalities organized services for the poor and established hospitals. Patients who could not pay depended on charity. Fraternal societies (e.g., Knights of Columbus) and unions created trusts that members could access when ill, injured at work, or unemployed, becoming the precursors of modern employment insurance.

As urbanization continued, rural communities experienced difficulty attracting and paying physicians. The federal *Municipality Act,*

1916 allowed communities to levy taxes to pay for physicians. But with the onset of the Great Depression, many people could no longer pay their medical bills and hospital stays caused financial ruin. With increasing needs, many provinces did not have the tax base to fund and ensure parallel services across the country.

These hardships inspired the provincial governments to create a prepaid medical and hospitalization insurance plan. In 1947, Premier Tommy Douglas of Saskatchewan introduced a public, universal hospital insurance plan, the basis of the first major federal initiative for national hospital insurance that led to the *Hospital Insurance and Diagnostic Services Act, 1957* (HIDSA). For provinces establishing universal hospital insurance, HIDSA provided federal funds covering approximately half of service costs. By 1961, all provinces and territories were providing coverage for inpatient hospital care.

To ensure the availability of medical services outside of hospitals, Saskatchewan again took the lead. With the federal government funding half of the hospital insurance, Saskatchewan could afford to provide medical insurance and, in 1962, passed the *Medical Care Insurance Act*. The legislation was opposed by the province's physicians, who went on a 23-day strike. Later, the province and its physicians reached a compromise: the physicians' autonomy to practise was preserved in exchange for their agreeing to a single-payer insurance system to fund their services.

In 1964, the Royal Commission on Health Services studied provision of hospital and medical care to all Canadians and recommended that "strong federal government leadership and financial support for medical care" was needed (Wilson, 1995). The *Hall Commission Report* called for national expansion of the Saskatchewan model on a cost-shared basis, similar to that used by HIDSA (Royal Commission on Health Services, 1965).

These recommendations led to the federal *Medical Care Act, 1966*. Federal grants were awarded on a cost-sharing basis to the provinces for programs meeting the coverage criteria for hospital and physician services. Federal, provincial, and territorial governments agreed to share health care expenses equally. By 1972, all provincial and territorial insurance plans extended coverage to include medical services provided outside of hospitals. Thus began modern Medicare, with all Canadians enjoying free access to hospital and medical care, regardless of ability to pay. During the 1970s, the "social determinants of health" approach emerged, emphasizing the need for the upstream "wellness" initiatives put forth in the 1974 Lalonde Report (Marchildon et al., 2020).

Although the programs prospered, cost sharing did not last. In 1977, the federal government enacted the *Federal–Provincial Fiscal Arrangements and Established Programs Financing Act* to replace cost sharing with block transfers of funds and a complicated formula of transferring tax points. These block transfers decreased federal contributions, which led some provinces to allow extra billing of patients by hospitals and providers above Medicare coverage.

The federal government's response was to enact the *Canada Health Act* in 1984, which amalgamated the HIDSA and *Medical Care Act*, effectively banning extra billing and user fees. The *Canada Health Act* added the principle of accessibility to the principles of public administration, comprehensiveness, universality, and portability (Table 2.1). Recently, a sixth principle—sustainability—has been debated. For a province or territory to fully benefit under the *Canada Health Act*, they cannot participate in extra billing or user charges, must ascribe to the five (or six) principles listed, and must fulfill the two conditions of recognition and information (Health Canada, 2020). Information refers to reporting requirements from the provinces and territories to the federal government, whereas recognition is the public recognition of the federal government's financial contributions to health service (Government of Canada [GOC], 2020). These principles apply to all insured residents (i.e., eligible residents), but exclude members of the

TABLE 2.1	Principles of the *Canada Health Act, 1984*	
Principle	**Mandate**	**Actions/Exceptions**
Public administration	Provincial and territorial plans operate on a nonprofit basis through a public authority	Regional authorities and some agencies (i.e., cancer agencies) are entrusted with delivery of programs and services.
Comprehensiveness	Provincial and territorial plans must cover all insured health care services (i.e., medically necessary services; includes hospital and physician services) Determine medically necessary services (not defined in the Act), so may differ by province or territory	Access to surgical or medical hospital-based care with no out-of-pocket charges is ensured. Charges exist for extraordinary supplies or nonessential care elements (e.g., private duty nursing). Seeing a physician is without direct cost, but certain in-office procedures (e.g., wart removal, completion of medical forms) may involve patient direct payment. Coverage for programs such as long-term care and home care is not included.
Universality	Includes all registered residents and ensures access free of discrimination based on race, gender, income, ethnicity, or religion	Canadians are entitled to receive care that is respectful and embraces diversity. Challenges in achieving equity and equality under Medicare remain.
Portability	Enables insured residents' access to health care services in another province or territory without cost or penalty. Provide continuous coverage for 3 months upon relocation within Canada to secure registration and coverage. Personal coverage required when moving or travelling outside of Canada.	Mobility across the country for purposes of travel, work, relocation and so on is covered, but seeking care in another province or territory is through prior approval from the jurisdiction where the individual holds a health card.
Accessibility	Provide insured residents reasonable access to health care facilities and providers, based on medical need regardless of ability to pay	Reasonable access is difficult to assess and measure. Varying levels of access to services exist for rural or remote people and urban people, often related to distance, health human resource availability, and facility capacities. Some individuals experience significant costs related to transportation (personal or ambulance), arguably a deterrent to access.

Adapted from Health Canada. (2020). *Canada Health Act, Annual report 2019–2020.* https://www.canada.ca/content/dam/hc-sc/documents/services/publications/health-system-services/canada-health-act-annual-report-2019-2020/canada-health-act-annual-report-2019-2020-eng.pdf

TABLE 2.2 Relevant Health-Related Legislation*	
Legislation and Date Passed	**Purpose**
Canadian Environmental Protection Act, 1999 https://laws-lois.justice.gc.ca/eng/acts/c-15.31/	Regulates pollution prevention; promotes environmental protection, contributes to climate control matters, and enhances human health for sustainable development
Canadian Institutes of Health Research Act, 2000 https://www.cihr-irsc.gc.ca/e/9466.html	Strategizes and funds health-related research through 13 virtual institutes and creates networks on topics and challenges that face Canadians and the Canadian health care system, as well as global health and system issues
Cannabis Act, 2018 https://laws-lois.justice.gc.ca/eng/acts/C-24.5/	Protects young persons from access to and advances public awareness of risks associated with cannabis. Shifts personal cannabis use from the criminal justice system and regulates production.
Controlled Drugs and Substances Act, 1996 https://laws-lois.justice.gc.ca/eng/acts/C-38.8/	Controls certain drugs, precursors, and related substances
Bill C-7, *an Act to amend the Criminal Code (medical assistance in dying)* https://www.justice.gc.ca/eng/csj-sjc/pl/charter-charte/c7.html	Expands the 2016 law respecting eligibility criteria for medical assistance in dying (MAiD) to include mature minors, advance requests, and mental health disorder requests
Emergency Management Act, 2007 https://laws-lois.justice.gc.ca/eng/acts/E-4.56	Develops and implements civil emergency plans; facilitates and coordinates across government levels and institutions, foreign governments, and international organizations
Food and Drugs Act, 1985 https://laws-lois.justice.gc.ca/eng/acts/F-27/	Regulates food, drugs, cosmetics, and therapeutic devices
Quarantine Act, 2005 https://laws.justice.gc.ca/eng/acts/Q-1.1/	Controls the introduction and spread of infectious or contagious diseases
Tobacco and Vaping Products Act, 1997 https://laws.justice.gc.ca/eng/acts/T-11.5/	Regulates the manufacture, sale, labelling, and promotion of tobacco and vaping products, especially those targeting young people

*Section contributor: T. McIntosh, PhD.

Canadian Forces, eligible veterans, inmates of federal penitentiaries, and some refugee claimants (Health Canada, 2016a). First Nations and Inuit health services receive special considerations, discussed later in this chapter.

Under previous health acts, access to services took place through physician gatekeepers, but the *Canada Health Act* allowed multiple points of access and insurance through additional HCPs. Despite some opposition, by 1987 all provinces and territories were following the *Canada Health Act* principles "to protect, promote and restore the physical and mental well-being of residents of Canada and to facilitate reasonable access to health services without financial or other barriers" (Health Canada, 2011).

Along with the *Canada Health Act*, other federal legislation (Table 2.2) has influenced the health of Canadians and health services in areas such as tobacco use, environmental health, and health research.

Indigenous Health Care

The *Indian Act, 1985* (see https://laws-lois.justice.gc.ca/eng/acts/i-5/) identified the federal government's role in providing health care services to First Nations and Inuit. Prior to November 2017, the federal government's First Nations and Inuit Health Branch shared responsibility with communities, other federal government departments, and provincial/territorial partners in supporting optimal health outcomes for Indigenous peoples in Canada (Health Canada, 2016b). At that time, two new departments were created—Indigenous Services Canada (ISC) and Crown–Indigenous Relations and Northern Affairs Canada (CIRNAC)—with the former assuming the responsibility for the First Nations and Inuit Health branch, and the latter focusing on renewal of relationships and building structures for self-determination and capacity building (GOC, 2019).

The treaty-making process between First Nations communities and European colonists began in 1701—these agreements were made with the British before Confederation and the Government of Canada after Confederation; modern treaties, known as comprehensive land claim agreements (e.g., the James Bay Claim), consist of an agreement between a First Nations community, the federal government,

and the relevant province or territory (Crown–Indigenous Relations and Northern Affairs Canada, 2015). These treaties outline agreements regarding land, services, and relationships; some (i.e., Treaty 6) included a health care services provision, often referred to as the "medicine chest" clause (Littlechild, 2018). Treaties enable direct delivery of services to Indigenous peoples, regardless of where they live in Canada, including **primary health care** (PHC) and emergency services on remote and isolated reserves where provincial or territorial services are not readily available; community-based health programs both on reserve and in Inuit communities; and noninsured health benefits programs (e.g., pharmaceuticals, dental, and medical transportation).

Between 2008 and 2015, the **Truth and Reconciliation Commission of Canada** (TRC) created a historical record of the residential school system and brought attention to its legacy. Throughout its 5-year mandate, the TRC merged both truth (through over 6 500 stories, testimonials, document reviews, and other information seeking) and reconciliation as a way to rebuild and renew relationships between Indigenous peoples and non-Indigenous people in Canada. The TRC (2015) released a six-volume final report containing 94 Calls to Action, seven of which are directed at health, including the following: provide sustainable funding for healing; embed Indigenous cultural healing practices; deliver cultural competency and safety training for all HCPs; and increase the number of Indigenous professionals in health care (see Chapter 12 for further information regarding Indigenous health).

Indigenous self-governance is enabled through the "inherent right of self-government" under Section 35 of the *Canadian Constitution Act, 1982*. As self-governance models emerge, there will be challenges to HCPs to be "responsive to [Indigenous] political, economic, legal, historical, cultural and social circumstances" (Indian and Northern Affairs Canada, 2015).

ORGANIZATION AND GOVERNANCE OF HEALTH CARE

Under the *Canadian Constitution Act*, the administration and delivery of health care services are primarily provincial and territorial responsibilities. The federal government plays a role in health care financing, enforcing the *Canada Health Act*, delivering services to the previously described targeted groups, and setting national agendas related to public health and safety, pharmaceuticals, and biomedical/health services research.

Federal Jurisdiction

The federal government is charged to do the following:

- Set and administer the principles of the *Canada Health Act.*
- Assist in financing provincial and territorial health care services through transfer payments in alignment with the principles of the *Canada Health Act.*
- Deliver or co-deliver health services for targeted groups.
- Provide national policy and programming to promote health and prevent disease, such as healthy environment, consumer safety, health product regulation, and public health programs.

Provincial and Territorial Jurisdiction

Each provincial and territorial government is charged to do the following:

- Develop and administer its own health care insurance plan.
- Manage, finance, and plan insurable health care services and delivery, in compliance with the principles of the *Canada Health Act* (see Table 2.1).
- Determine the organization and location of health care facilities, mix of the HCP workforce, and fiscal allocations for health care services.
- Reimburse physician and hospital expenses and provide co-payment with users for select rehabilitation and long-term care services.

Each provincial and territorial plan is unique in the coverage it provides, such as for medication taken outside of hospitals, ambulance services, and home care. Health Canada provides general information on the eligibility and availability of programs and services on its website, plus links to all provincial and territorial ministries of health (Health Canada, 2019a). To offset the cost of services not covered by provincial or territorial insurance, Canadians can buy private health insurance or participate in employer-offered plans.

Professional Jurisdiction

Most health professions (i.e., medicine, nursing, pharmacology) in Canada are self-regulated, which allows them to determine, monitor, and manage standards, competencies, codes of ethics, and disciplinary actions for their respective members. Some professions are regulated through governments (e.g., emergency medical technicians in Ontario) or other regulatory mechanisms (e.g., osteopathic physicians in British Columbia). In some cases, omnibus legislation regulates several professions simultaneously (e.g., Alberta's *Health Disciplines Act* of 2000).

HEALTH CARE SPENDING

"Canadians pay, directly or indirectly, for every aspect of our health care system through a combination of taxes, payments to government, private insurance premiums, and direct out-of-pocket fees of varying types and amounts" (Romanow, 2002, p. 24). In 2019, total health care spending reached approximately $265.5 billion (69% public spending; 15.46% out of pocket; 12.4% private insurance; 3.2% other), representing a 4.2% increase from 2018 while maintaining a relatively stable public–private 70–30 split (CIHI, 2019b; Marchildon et al., 2020). Experts have projected an increased shift toward the use of private insurance from the out-of-pocket pool (Marchildon et al., 2020). According to the CIHI (2019b), hospital and health care institutions (28.3%),

medication sales (15.7%), and physician services (15.1%) account for approximately 60% of health care spending. In 2019, $7 064 per person was spent on health care, in comparison to $6 299 in 2016, $5 614 in 2010, and $4 548 in 2006 (CIHI, 2019b). In 2018, trends showed higher per capita spending for infants (at $12 655) and older persons (ranging from $6 807 [age 65–69] to $28 627 [over age 90]) than for younger adults (CIHI, 2020). Although older persons constitute less than 16% of the population, they account for 45.7% of government health care spending (CIHI, 2019b). Projections state that by 2040, older persons will consume 71.4% of total health care expenditures (Globerman, 2021).

Canada has been ranked eleventh in the world for health care spending ($5 418 US per person), which is lower than the first-ranking United States ($11 072 US per person), but greater than the average spent by Organisation of Economic Co-operation and Development (OECD) member countries ($4 224 US per person) (Organisation of Economic Co-operation and Development [OECD], 2019). Canada is seventh among OECD countries with respect to proportion of the gross domestic product spent on health care, and ranks in the mid-range with respect to quality indicators such as life expectancy, self-reported health status, and disease-specific mortality rates (OECD, 2019).

TRENDS AND REFORMS IN CANADA'S HEALTH CARE SYSTEM

Since the 1980s, rapid changes in health care delivery, technologies, and public expectations have challenged all levels of government to reconstruct a health care system that balances current and future political, legal, economic, and social realities. Two influential national reports on Canada's health care system reforms are the *Kirby Report* (Kirby, 2002) and the *Romanow Report* (Romanow, 2002).

In most provinces, restructuring and health reform became entrusted to regional health authorities led by appointed or elected community representatives whose mandates, roles, and responsibilities are provincially legislated (Lewis & Kouri, 2004). Regionalization was intended to streamline health services, reduce fragmentation, respond to local needs, improve public participation, and address the continuum of health care services (McIntosh et al., 2010). Although these principles were initially promising, the process has not lived up to its potential, becoming primarily a fiscal exercise rather than a philosophical or health-motivated reform (McIntosh et al., 2010).

Framed within the determinants of health approach, reforms were intended to deliver better-quality and more appropriate care at a lower cost through the adoption of sound business and managerial strategies. Currently, there is a trend toward recentralization (or consolidation) of health authorities and a gradual shift toward Indigenous self-governance of health care, as discussed earlier in this chapter. In 2005, Prince Edward Island dissolved its longstanding health boards and transferred the responsibility to the Department of Health, which has since morphed into Health PEI (an arm's-length Crown corporation) (Institute of Public Administration in Canada [IPAC], 2013). In 2008, Alberta went from nine regional health authorities to one province-wide health authority known as Alberta Health Services, with the goal of improving governance/accountability, management, health care levels, and standardized services for all Albertans (Healthy Debate, 2013). Other provinces followed suit, with British Columbia reducing its 20 regional boards to 5 regional authorities and 1 provincial authority (IPAC, 2013), Manitoba restructuring from 11 to 5 regional authorities, and Saskatchewan reducing from an initial 32 provincial health boards and 1 authority to a single health authority in 2016 (Abrametz et al., 2016; Marchildon et al., 2020).

Policy reform (such as regionalization) is only one means to change health care delivery. Other catalysts include emerging medical technology, such as new diagnostic approaches (i.e., point-of-care testing in lieu of laboratory drawn tests) or robotics (i.e., remote presence nursing), and information and communication technologies (i.e., wireless devices; eHealth is the secure and cost-effective use of communications and information technologies in support of health and health-related fields (Canada Health Infoway [CHI], 2018; Lazar et al., 2013; WHO, 2022a).

In 2004, the federal government initiated a transfer scheme (i.e., *10-Year Plan to Strengthen Health Care*) to increase the efficiency and sustainability of the Canadian health care system (Health Canada, 2006). This plan furthered the dialogue on shared values such as person-centred, accountable, efficient, and equitable health care, but remained silent on shared and sustainable solutions (Brasset-Latulippe et al., 2011).

For 2017–2018, a new federal funding model was introduced that included Canada Health Transfer (CHT) payments aligned with mandatory requirements per the *Canada Health Act* (GOC, 2017). In the past, CHT was adjusted to address tax bases in each province/territory, but the new model made payments on a per capita basis. Beginning in 2004, the CHT grew by 6% per year; however, in 2017, this amount fell to 3.5% (Council of Canadians, 2016). The 2017 federal budget committed $6 billion over 10 years for home care (including support for home, community, and palliative services as well as informal caregivers) and $5 billion for mental health initiatives (GOC, 2017). Additionally, at that time, 5-year targeted federal funding was announced respecting investments in efforts to access affordable and appropriate medications ($140.3 million); technologically mediated health initiatives ($300 million), such as e-prescribing, virtual care, and eHealth records; and evidence-informed decision making and improved data uptake for health system enhancements ($53 million) (GOC, 2017). An additional $17 million per year for 3 years was to be directed to health care innovations and improvements (GOC, 2017). In 2021–2022, the federal transfer amounts were $83.9 billion, an increase of $2.2 billion from the previous fiscal year (GOC, 2020). In addition, the COVID-19 pandemic period resulted in significant health and infrastructure transfers of nearly $325 billion, with a top-up of $24 billion committed for 2021–2022 (GOC, 2020).

Role of Nurses in Health Care Policy

Individually and collectively, nurses are integral to health care policy advocacy, development, and implementation (Falk-Raphael & Betker, 2012). Nurses need to take a coordinated, integrated approach if they are to inform policy decisions and help shape the country's health care systems (Villeneuve, 2017). Almost continually since the late 1950s, the federal government position of a senior or chief nurse has existed (i.e., Office of Nursing Policy), and many provincial governments have hosted similar positions. In recent years, especially in light of the COVID-19 pandemic, there has been a renewed call for the creation of a Chief Nursing Officer to guide the next generation of nursing practice, research, and policy for Canadians. Representatives from the Registered Nurses' Association of Ontario (RNAO) recently stated that "Canada would be a healthier country if nurses and nursing had a voice in our federal government" (D'Sa, 2020).

RIGHT TO HEALTH CARE

The consensus in Canada is that everyone has a right to health care; however, neither the *Canadian Charter of Rights and Freedoms, 1982* nor the *Canada Health Act* explicitly include health care as a right. Therefore, federal and provincial/territorial legislation must embed legal entitlement. (Only Quebec has legislated health care rights.)

Rights Within the Health Care System

Various sectors have called for a health guarantee (Kirby, 2002) or a patient-centred charter (Collier, 2010) to specify the rights, obligations, and expectations of governments, citizens, and HCPs. A key recommendation of Saskatchewan's independent *Patient First Review* was to "make patient- and family-centred care the foundation and principal aim of the Saskatchewan health system . . . as an overarching guide for health care organizations, professional groups and others to make the Patient First philosophy a reality in all work places" (Dagnone, 2009).

Although, in practice, no statutory requirement exists in Canada to include patient advocacy groups in policy processes, numerous national groups and disease-specific patient groups (e.g., Canadian Cancer Society) are involved. These groups invariably share information, endorse, report on, advocate for, or critique health care policy decisions from the consumer's perspective (Consumers' Association of Canada, 2017).

As for Canadian health care worker rights, expectations include the right to reasonable working conditions, including the right to refuse unsafe work; the right to be informed about actual or potential workplace hazards; the right to freedom from discrimination, abuse, and harassment; and the right to have access to proactive measures (such as personal protective equipment) (Canadian Labour Congress, 2021). Professional associations and unions work to establish and protect the rights of HCPs.

PRIMARY HEALTH CARE

PHC is the foundation of Canada's health care system, serving as the first point of contact in the system for nonurgent/emergent care as well as the vehicle for continuity of care (Health Council of Canada [HCC], 2008; Marchildon et al., 2020). (See Chapter 18 for more on continuity of care.)

Initially, PHC was envisioned as a system addressing nonmedical determinants of health to improve health (HCC, 2008) by connecting health status and social determinants of health (i.e., employment, poverty, lifestyle, environment, and genetic endowment). Other documents, such as the *Alma-Ata Declaration* (World Health Organization [WHO], 1978) and the *Ottawa Charter for Health Promotion* (*Ottawa Charter*) (WHO, 1986), informed population health and health promotion approaches globally. The Canadian federal, provincial, and territorial health departments have all established units that focus on, promote, and fund PHC-based programs and services.

PHC is a philosophy and model for improving health that supports essential health care services. It puts a strong emphasis on the principles of health promotion and disease prevention and has roots in social justice and equity. PHC is a whole-of-society approach to health that aims to optimize health and well-being and their equitable distribution by focusing on people's needs as early as possible along the continuum—from health promotion and disease prevention to treatment, rehabilitation, and palliative care—and as close as feasible to people's everyday environment (WHO & UNICEF, 2021). According to the WHO (2017), the goal of PHC is to achieve better health for all by doing the following:

- Addressing equity issues for health
- Providing patient- and community-relevant and accessible health services and programs
- Situating health intersectorally
- Building collaborative models for program and policy dialogues
- Embedding patient, stakeholder, and partner participation

As an integrated approach, PHC involves building a related spectrum of programs and services (i.e., housing, education) beyond the traditional health care system. The PHC model (Figure 2.1) focuses on

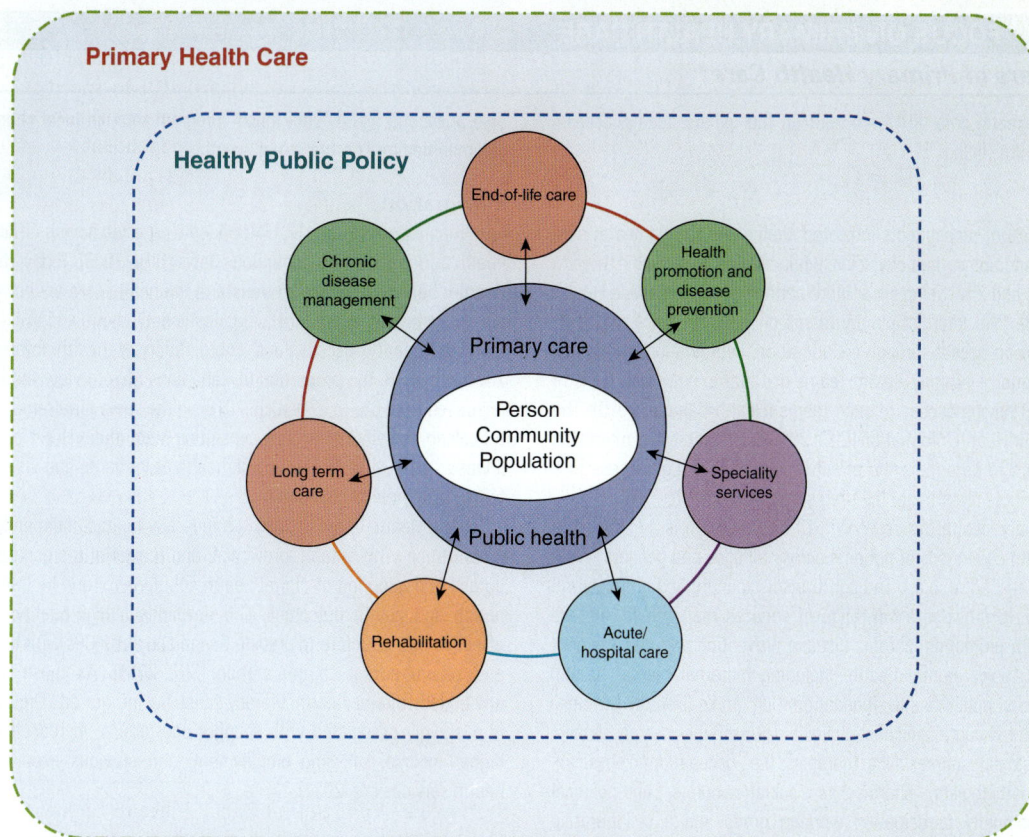

FIGURE 2.1 Hub and spoke model for primary health care. (From Lankshear, S. [2012]. *Primary health care summary report* [p. 15, Figure 2]. Canadian Nurses Association and Canadian Medical Association. From a URL formerly available at https://www.cna-aiic.ca/-/media/cna/page-content/pdf-en/primary_health_care_report_e.pdf. © Canadian Nurses Association. Reprinted with permission. Further reproduction prohibited.)

intersectoral collaboration among HCPs, community members, and others, emphasizing health promotion, development of health policies, and prevention of disease for all. PHC may, and often does, look different in each community, as it is derived from the needs of consumers and patients, access to HCPs, the assets of specific communities (i.e., water supply, school, air quality), and proximity or transport to health care services.

According to the CIHI (2019c), PHC services may include the following:
- Health promotion and disease prevention
- Urgent care for minor or common health problems
- Care across the spectrum, including mental health, maternal–child health, rehabilitation, and end-of-life (EOL) care
- Inter-agency and inter-program referrals and coordination

From 2000 to 2006, the federal Primary Health Care Transition Fund provided opportunities to advance PHC, which was viewed as an integral component of health care renewal. Support was provided for pan-Canadian, provincial/territorial, and multijurisdictional efforts and for Indigenous and minority language projects (Health Canada, 2007) to increase access and coordination of PHC programs, services, and multidisciplinary teams to 24 hours a day, 7 days a week.

An example of PHC programming is currently underway in the Northwest Territories, where six projects are being developed in response to community needs, including same-day access, integrated care teams, and chronic disease management. The projects are client-, family-, and community-centred and adopt a vision of a culturally safe health and social system (Northwest Territories Health and Social Services Authority, 2019). The learning from these programs will impact how communities are informed and engaged in their health, how professionals are educated and function in the field, and how change is implemented through multi-level, multi-sectoral efforts.

Throughout this book, "Focus on Primary Health Care" boxes highlight the vital role that nurses play in providing PHC. Box 2.2 links health care situations to PHC principles. Knowledge of PHC care is identified as an essential component of nursing education in Canada (Canadian Association of Schools of Nursing, 2022).

Barriers to Primary Health Care

The meaning of PHC has caused confusion among health care consumers and even HCPs. The distinction between PHC and **primary care(PC)** is often misunderstood. PC focuses on personal health services, whereas PHC extends beyond PC to include health education, nutrition, maternal and child health care, family planning, immunizations, and control of locally endemic diseases. PHC is a whole-of-society approach that leaves no one behind and engages people and communities in identifying needs, opportunities, and barriers to achieving health (WHO & UNICEF, 2018).

According to Zephyrin et al. (2020), three key barriers in PHC are utilization, delivery, and leadership. Barriers to PHC utilization may include a lack of access or inconsistent PHC, increased uptake of alternatives (such as urgent care or walk-in clinics), shortage of PHC providers, cultural safety, communication barriers (Schwei et al., 2017), and gender issues (e.g., women often defer self-care because of personal obligations) (Kaiser Family Foundation, 2018). Barriers to PHC delivery include time and resource constraints, sex- and gender-based biases, inequity/equity issues (such as income), lack of integrated care

♥ BOX 2.2   FOCUS ON PRIMARY HEALTH CARE

The Four Pillars of Primary Health Care*

Models of primary health care (PHC) are built on four pillars: teams, access, information, and healthy living.

Teams

In a 2018 report, 45% of respondents indicated seeing one to two health care providers (HCPs) in addition to their physician, while another 11% seeing three to five additional HCPs and 2% seeing six or more additional HCPs (Canada Health Infoway [CHI], 2018). PHC interdisciplinary teams or networks deliver patient-centred care, improving access through collaboration, coordination, continuity, and quality (Association of Family Health Teams of Ontario, n.d.). Only 39% of Canadians indicated having access to such teams (Health Canada, 2015). The Canadian Institute for Health Information (CIHI, 2016) has created and measured a series of indicators to determine the effectiveness of PHC (i.e., access to a family physician or nurse practitioner [NP]/registered nurse [RN]).

West Winds Primary Health Centre (WWPHC) in Saskatoon is a PHC centre addressing the health care needs of patients across all ages and genders (West Winds Primary Health Centre, n.d.). Through transdisciplinary and intersectoral collaboration, WWPHC provides a full range of services that include, but are not limited to, health promotion, chronic disease prevention and management (i.e., diabetes education), mental health (including maternal mental health) and addiction services, public health, foundational programs (Healthy Mother–Healthy Baby, Food for Thought), and dental clinics. The staff includes physicians, nutritionists, psychologists, nurses, NPs, therapists (i.e., occupational, physical), speech-language pathologists, pharmacists, social workers, and clinical researchers. A community participation working group and a collaborative practice resource group provide direction and support development of evidence-informed programs.

Access

Although 85% of Canadians reported having access to a regular family physician (Statistics Canada, 2020), slightly more than half report having difficulties accessing after-hours PHC services (Allin et al., 2020).

In urban settings, interprofessional teams often work to bring PHC to the streets. They work with vulnerable groups—individuals in poor health or those who are homeless, malnourished, or lacking support—to assess and monitor health status and provide care "in place." Nurses on "PHC street teams" care for individuals and communities in need. For example, one nurse runs a community program called Having Healthy Babies for young, vulnerable women, co-located at a centre near the train tracks, thereby increasing accessibility; the nurse also advocates for a "chili lunch" program through local church and business communities for "on-the-street" youth.

Information

Less than a decade ago, 17.1% of people reported having difficulty in accessing health information on a continuous basis (CIHI, 2009). Today, the ubiquity of the Internet has the potential to transform the health care environment. Tools (e.g., electronic health record [EHR], diagnostic equipment) and skills (e.g., telehealth) facilitate quality, access, and coordination of health information. Between 2014 and 2018, the proportion of Canadians able to view their medical records increased from 6% to 22% (CHI, 2018). In the same timeframe, only 8% reported e-booking appointments and consulting with their HCPs online (CHI, 2018). (Please visit https://www.fraserhealth.ca/patients-and-visitors/virtual-health for a virtual health example).

Canada Health Infoway (CHI) is a federally funded, independent, not-for-profit organization with federal, provincial, and territorial representation. CHI fosters uptake and adoption of digital health solutions for and by Canadians to impact health and health outcomes. CHI envisions a high-quality, sustainable, and effective info-structure to provide Canadians and HCPs with timely, appropriate, and secure access to information (CHI, 2011). As these solutions become embedded, digital health literacy must be integrated. Digital health literacy is positively associated with younger age groups, increased education levels, higher income, full-time employment, and previous experience with digital health services (Yu, 2021).

Healthy Living

Practitioners within PHC embrace strategies for prevention, chronic illness management, and **self-care** while recognizing that factors outside the health care system (e.g., social, economic, environmental) influence individual and community health. The World Health Organization (WHO, 2022c) defines self-care as "the ability of individuals, families and communities to promote health, prevent disease, maintain health, and to cope with illness and disability with or without the support of a healthcare provider" (para. 1). An example is a public health nurse in southern Ontario running a program that educates low-income mothers about nutrition, child development, and community action. The women shared strategies to meet their families' nutritional requirements on tight budgets. Upon learning that a national bakery was closing its local day-old-bread outlet, the nurse coached the women to call a local newspaper reporter, who in turn contacted the bakery's president. The women persuaded the owner to keep the outlet open, thereby benefitting the entire community.

*Section contributor: V. R. Ramsden, RN, PhD.

---

teams (Canadian Alliance for Sustainable Health Care, 2012), lack of sufficient comprehensive PHC, and digital innovations.

The Canadian Interprofessional Health Collaborative (2010) advocates for and promotes six core competencies (i.e., interprofessional communication; patient-, client-, family-, and community-centred care; role clarification; team functioning; collaborative leadership; and interprofessional conflict resolution) as future areas of training and development (see Chapter 19 for further information about interprofessional collaboration). In terms of PHC leadership, the main issues to address include the shift to PHC-oriented health systems and transformative and community-engaged leadership models (WHO & UNICEF 2018).

FUTURE OF PRIMARY HEALTH CARE

According to the CNA, PHC creates "the conditions that improve the health of all Canadians and [puts] the people who receive health services at the centre of care" (Canadian Nurses Association [CNA], 2015, 2021a). For example, trauma programs will include health promotion activities (road safety education), preventive programming (helmet legislation), secondary care and tertiary care (emergency transportation), and rehabilitation (head injury–related recovery programs). Programs will cover multiple sites, may be defined by a particular disease or population group (e.g., children), and will comprise multiple disciplines and sectors of society (e.g., health care, education, and justice systems).

PHC is a recurring global priority because it is agile and adaptive in our increasingly complex and interrelated world. With the emerging emphasis on universal health care (UHC) (see Table 2.1) and the Sustainable Development Goals, PHC is seen as being an imperative component (WHO & UNICEF, 2018).

Because of its integrated approach and patient-centredness, PHC may hold the key to Canada's looming health care crisis. Embedding

BOX 2.3   CASE STUDY

Primary Health Care

During a community meeting in the core area of a small city, parents, educators, health care providers, and volunteers agree to pilot an integrated program to reduce obesity in children. Social services staff and volunteers run a breakfast program. Fruits and vegetables for twice-daily snacks are donated by a local grocery store. Dietitians and kinesiologists educate teachers how to integrate nutrition and physical fitness into the curriculum. Schools commit to having students and teachers participate in activities for at least 30 minutes every day and establish rules for school lunches (e.g., no soft drinks). Nurse practitioners arrange visits with the parents of children identified as being overweight or at risk. If only 10% of the children in the program develop a healthier lifestyle, future savings to the health care system will pay for program costs.

PHC through evidence-informed policies and programs will contribute from a life course (individual) to a whole-system (societal) approach. By integrating and investing in the health care, education, social services, and voluntary sectors, competition for government monies may decline and each sector will articulate beyond its own boundaries (Box 2.3).

SETTINGS FOR HEALTH CARE DELIVERY

Although health care delivery varies across Canada, three types of delivery agencies are prevalent: institutional, community and voluntary, and private sector.

Institutional Sector

Institutional agencies, including hospitals, long-term care (LTC) facilities, psychiatric facilities, and rehabilitation centres, offer health care services to **inpatients** (a patient who stays at an institution for diagnosis, treatment, or rehabilitation). Most also offer services to **outpatients** (a patient who visits an institution for select services).

Hospitals. Hospitals have traditionally been considered major health care agencies, with most specializing in acute care services. **Acute care** is health care delivered for a short time (usually days to weeks, typically less than 3 months) whereby an immediate health problem is diagnosed, treated, or both. Hospital services may include emergency and diagnostic, inpatient, surgical intervention, intensive care, outpatient, and rehabilitation services.

The numbers of hospitals, hospital beds, and admissions in Canada have decreased significantly since the 1990s, creating increased pressure to deal with patients whose needs are more acute and specialized. In 2019, Canada had 2.52 acute beds per 1 000 people (down from 2.68 beds in 2013), mirroring the situation in the United States (2.46 and 2.93, respectively), but significantly lower than that in Australia (3.84 beds, an increase from 3.75 in 2013) and Japan (12.98 beds, a reduction from 13.32 in 2013) (OECD, 2016, 2021).

Hospitals strive to provide quality care with the newest treatments and technologies and to facilitate appropriate, safe, and timely patient discharge to the appropriate environment in which to manage residual needs. **Quality of care** is the "degree to which health services for individuals and populations increase the likelihood of desired health outcomes" (WHO, 2022b, para. 1). They are distinguished by their size (e.g., community hospitals), service provision (e.g., cancer care hospitals, children's hospitals), and connection to academic institutions (e.g., university health science centres), as well as by their public versus private status. Public hospitals are financed and operated by a local, provincial, or national government entity, whereas private hospitals are owned and operated by groups such as churches, corporations, and charitable organizations. Military hospitals, although limited in Canada, provide medical services to members of the military and their families. Veterans' hospitals provide residential care, extended care, and rehabilitation to aging, injured, and disabled military veterans.

The roles and functions of hospitals and hospital-based nurses have evolved in this era of health care reform. Hospital nurses use critical thinking and clinical judgement skills (see Chapter 7 for further information about critical thinking and critical reasoning); apply the nursing process to coordinate and delegate care (see Chapter 13 for further information about collaborative practice); invoke **evidence-informed practice** (see Chapter 8); and stress patient teaching and post-discharge self-care (see Chapter 21 for further information about patient education). Nurses participate in clinical care rounds and discharge planning as a critical interdisciplinary strategy for continuity of care, facilitating safe transitions of patients between levels of care and the community. Clinical nurse specialists care for patients with specific needs (e.g., palliative) or specific diseases (e.g., cardiovascular). Other hospital roles include nurse manager, infection control coordinator, clinical educator, and clinical nurse researcher.

Long-Term Care Facilities. LTC (extended care) facilities provide accommodations and 24-hour intermediate and custodial care (e.g., nursing, rehabilitation, dietary, recreational, social, and spiritual services) for residents of any age with chronic or debilitating illnesses or disabilities. Most residents are frail, older persons who have multiple health issues (see Chapter 25 for further information about caring for older persons). Some are younger adults with severe, chronic health conditions (see Chapter 24 for further information about chronic conditions in younger adults). LTC facilities function as the resident's temporary or permanent home; therefore, the surroundings are as homelike as possible. The philosophy of care is to provide a planned, systematic, and interdisciplinary approach that helps residents reach and maintain their highest level of function, with all LTC facilities using a needs-based approach to determine eligibility (Allin et al., 2020).

Currently, there are 2 076 LTC homes in Canada that house approximately 5% of Canada's population of older persons (CIHI, 2021b). There is a fairly equal distribution of private for-profit, private not-for-profit, and public LTC facilities in Canada (Tikkanen et al., 2020). LTC facilities are not part of the insured services bundle within the *Canada Health Act*, although many provincial and territorial plans do provide some coverage. According to Health Canada (2019b), nonhospital institutions consume approximately 11% of health expenditures, of which nearly three-quarters comes from public funds. Most jurisdictions require some form of co-payment (Allin et al., 2020). In these settings, nurses plan and coordinate resident care, manage chronic illnesses, conduct rehabilitation programs, and assume roles in education (see Chapter 21 for further information about patient education), communication (see Chapter 18 for further information about relational communication), administration, and family-related interventions (see Chapter 20 for further information about family assessments).

Psychiatric Facilities. Located in hospitals, independent outpatient clinics, or mental health clinics, psychiatric facilities offer inpatient and outpatient services. In a survey of Canadians, 85% indicated that mental health is the most underfunded service in the health care system (Canadian Mental Health Association, 2018), with over 1.6 million Canadians reporting unmet mental health needs. Nurses in these facilities collaborate with doctors, psychologists, social workers, and therapists in co-planning with the patient, their family, and caregivers to enable the patient's return to the community. At discharge from inpatient facilities, patients are usually referred for follow-up services with community-based agencies (see list of resources at Government of British Columbia, n.d.). Nurses working in these settings are especially adept in communication skills, case management, and patient safety (see Chapter 38).

Rehabilitation Centres. A *rehabilitation centre* is a residential institution providing therapy and restorative training to decrease patients' dependence on care. Many centres offer programs to teach the patient, the patient's family, or both to achieve optimal function after an impairment (i.e., stroke, head, or spinal cord injury). Substance rehabilitation centres help patients withdraw from alcohol and drug dependence and return to the community. Nurses in rehabilitation centres collaborate closely with physical and occupational therapists, psychologists, and social workers, working with patients experiencing stress and adapting to challenges to mobility and safety.

Community Sector

Community services are directed at primary and secondary care, described later in this chapter, and should be accessible to patients in locations where they live, work, play, and engage. These agencies focus on empowerment and community development opportunities that effect change at the broadest social level, reducing inequities in access to health services by identifying and removing barriers (Bryant et al., 2019; Raphael et al., 2020). Community health nurses oversee and participate in outreach programs that provide services and locate patients who might not seek care through traditional routes, and "support the health and well-being of individuals, families, groups, communities, populations, and systems" (Community Health Nurses of Canada, 2019). Community health nurses work in diverse rural and urban settings, such as public health units, family practices, schools, and community-based settings. Nurses practising in the community sector are involved in delivering community-based nursing (see Chapter 4) and care throughout the lifespan (see Unit V).

Public Health. Public health is committed to ensuring the conditions and circumstances that foster health through appropriate screening, assessment, development, monitoring, and support (i.e., public policy). Public health differs from many clinical practice settings in its focus on entire populations or subsets of populations rather than on individuals.

Activities related to pandemic planning, planetary health (i.e., the indivisible link of human health and the health of our planet, including issues of climate change) (Canadian Institute for Climate Choices, 2021; Myers & Frumkin, 2020; United Nations, 2021), and global surveillance have put public health at the forefront (Kahn, 2017) of protection and promotion efforts (see Chapter 11). Public health nurses work closely with a range of HCPs, including medical health officers, therapists, psychologists, dietitians, and environmental and public health inspectors. Nurses are the primary professionals in public health clinics offering well-baby clinics, school health programs, sexually transmitted infections surveillance, and screening programs, as well as health promotion (e.g., tobacco reduction) and disease prevention programs.

Physicians' Offices. Most Canadian physicians function as private contractors within the publicly funded health care system, working on a fee-for-service basis. Physicians' offices offer PC focusing on diagnosis and treatment of specific illnesses rather than health promotion. In this setting, nurses record assessments, prepare patients for examination, and collaborate with physicians to conduct physical examinations, document histories, offer health education, and recommend therapies. RNs partnering in PC integrated teams participate in "assessment, screening, healthy lifestyle support, education, and chronic disease management with a goal of improving health outcomes and facilitating access to services" (Canadian Family Practice Nurses Association, 2020). NPs work in a range of settings, such as community care, LTC, hospitals, and autonomous NP-led clinics, providing wellness care; handling minor emergencies; conducting screening; ordering and interpreting diagnostic tests; and prescribing medications (CNA, 2021b).

Community Health Centres and Clinics. Community health centre (CHC) teams plan, manage, and deliver comprehensive services to designated geographic areas or specific at-risk populations. According to the Canadian Association of Community Health Centres (2017), CHCs are the first point of contact for a variety of primary health, social, rehabilitation, and noninstitutional services, delivering integrated, locally relevant patient-centred services and programs.

Increasingly, NPs and nurses are managing CHCs, focusing on enabling patients to assume more responsibility for their health. NPs are integral CHC team members focused on delivering preventive and supportive services rather than traditional practitioner–driven curative and rehabilitative care.

Assisted Living. Assisted-living facilities are community-based residential facilities where adults live and receive a range of support services, including personalized assistance in achieving optimal independence. These facilities usually combine professional and nonprofessional staff on an around-the-clock basis. Personal assistance services promote maximum dignity and independence through meal preparation, personal hygiene practice, mobility, and socialization.

Home Care. Canadian health care is shifting from institution-based care to a system embedding the critical role of community-based care (see Chapter 4). Home care is the provision of health care services (i.e., short-term postoperative recovery, EOL care) and equipment to patients and families in their homes, residential settings, hospitals, and ambulatory clinics (CIHI, 2017a). Home care is an uninsured extended health service (Marchildon et al., 2020). All provinces and territories fund assessment and case management, nursing care, and support services for eligible patients, while patients may pay for extra professional or support services through insurance or pay-for-service arrangements. The federal government delivers home care services to some Indigenous populations (First Nations people living on reserve, Inuit living in designated communities), members of the armed forces, federal inmates, some refugee claimants, and eligible veterans (Allin et al., 2020).

Home care primarily involves nursing care plus adjunct professional and nonprofessional services (i.e., physiotherapy, social work, speech therapy). Support services are nonmedical services and include personal care, assistance with activities of daily living, and assistance with home management. There has been a shift in recent years toward private home care services, which range from basic services (e.g., meals, bathing) to complex nursing care (Marchildon et al., 2020).

Nurses working in home care experience all levels of care within the home setting (see "Levels of Care") as well as complex caseloads. The Canadian Home Care Association (CHCA, 2012) states that home care is a cost-effective alternative to acute care because it maintains patients at optimal levels of functioning, delays institutionalization, and provides a viable substitution for health services (e.g., wound care makes up 50% of home care services). The CHCA's (2014) *Vision 2020* describes an integrated system providing appropriate and accessible services that support individuals and families in their own homes while preserving independence, dignity, safety, and quality of life.

Adult Day Support Programs. As an alternative to hospitalization, **adult day support programs** (ADSPs) may be associated with a hospital or LTC facility or exist independently and provide continuous health care services for specific patients (e.g., those with dementia, those needing physical rehabilitation). In one survey, nearly 45% of Canadians reported that they had provided care to a family member or friend with a long-term health condition, disability, or age-related need (Vanier Institute of the Family, 2016). ADSPs play a critical role in enabling a caregiver's participation in care while they continue working. Nurses in ADSPs provide continuity between the care delivered at home and ADSPs by administering treatments and encouraging patients to adhere to prescribed medication regimens (see Chapter 35), linking patients with community resources (see Chapter 4), and providing counselling services (see Chapter 20).

Community and Voluntary Agencies. National, provincial, and regional voluntary agencies (e.g., Cystic Fibrosis Canada, Diabetes Canada, John Howard Society, United Way) meet needs for target populations, circumstances (i.e., homebound individuals, incarcerated individuals), or conditions (i.e., disease specific). Most **voluntary agencies** offer programs to educate about, prevent, and detect specific conditions rather than treat them. Voluntary agencies depend on the help of professional volunteers (e.g., VON [Victorian Order of Nurses]) and lay volunteers (e.g., Meals on Wheels). Many offer financial support or scholarships for training HCPs and students through fundraising and donations.

Occupational Health. The Canadian Association for Occupational Health Nurses (n.d.) seeks to advance integrated occupational health and safety services to individual and communities of workers. RNs certified in occupational health through the CNA (2021c) have met specific eligibility requirements, passed a written examination, and achieved a national standard of competency.

Hospice and Palliative Care. **Palliative care** is an interdisciplinary EOL approach to care that manages life-threatening or serious illnesses, regardless of a person's age or condition, with the intent of improving quality of life, addressing physical and psychological symptoms, and facilitating a dignified death. It includes caregiver support during and beyond the palliative care involvement. Palliative care—in recognition of diverse needs, capacities, and cultural practices—is available in hospitals, homes, shelters, LTC facilities, and hospices.

Hospice is a family-centred care system that enables a person with a terminal illness to live in comfort and with independence and dignity. Hospice care is palliative, not curative (see Chapter 26). It is an interprofessional approach involving physicians, nurses, social workers, pharmacists, and pastoral care staff. Hospice nurses work in hospitals, free-standing hospices, or homes, caring for the patient and family during the terminal phase of illness, at the time of death, and through the bereavement phase, including by providing counselling and assistance in finding a support network (see Canadian Virtual Hospice at https://www.virtualhospice.ca).

Given Canada's aging population and chronicity trends, there is an imperative for a well-constructed and responsive integrated EOL care system. In 2015, Canada ranked eleventh out of 80 countries on the international Quality of Death index, which considers hospice and palliative care environments as well as other EOL care factors (Economist Intelligence Unit, 2015).

Palliative and hospice care are inconsistently offered across Canada, reflecting the lack of policies, training, and funding related to EOL care as well as variances in delivery based on location and program criteria.

Program offerings, such as palliative medication coverage, nursing/personal care services, and hospice care, are nonstandardized nationally, leading families and charitable entities to frequently bear the significant costs of these services.

EOL care is complex and replete with contradictions. Although most Canadians express a desire to die on their own terms in the presence of loved ones, many Canadians receive a significant proportion of EOL care in hospital (CIHI, 2018).

This disconnect has created the context for greater engagement of all parties (patients, families, HCPs, and politicians) in advance care planning and Medical Assistance in Dying (MAiD) for Canadians. In 2016, the *Criminal Code* was amended to allow for MAiD by physicians or nurse practitioners. Between December 2015 and October 2019, over 10 000 Canadians undertook MAiD (Health Canada, 2019c).

Respite care provides short-term relief or time off for family caregivers by health care providers or trained volunteers in either institutional or home settings.

Parish Nursing. **Parish nursing** (or faith community nursing) is becoming more popular as faith-based communities promote and maintain members' health. According to the Canadian Association for Parish Nursing Ministry (2021), a parish nurse is an RN with specialized knowledge who is called to the ministry and affirmed by a faith-based community to promote health, healing, and wholeness through advocacy, counselling, education, and intersectoral referrals.

LEVELS OF CARE

Five **levels of health care** exist: promotive, preventive, curative (diagnosis and treatment), rehabilitative, and supportive (including home care, LTC, and palliative care) (WHO & UNICEF, 2021).

Level 1: Health Promotion

The first level of health care, **health promotion**, "enables people to have more control over their own health through better health literacy and improved ability to provide self-care and care for others" (WHO & UNICEF, 2021). Although rooted in health education (Fong et al., 2020), health promotion takes an interdisciplinary approach to the provision of wellness services, such as antismoking education, promotion of self-esteem in children and adolescents, and advocacy for healthy public policy.

The *Ottawa Charter* (WHO, 1986) lists five action strategies for health promotion: building healthy public policy, creating supportive environments, strengthening community action, developing personal skills, and reorienting health care services. Furthermore, the foundation of health promotion consists of "the fundamental conditions and resources for health, [which] are peace, shelter, education, food, income, a stable ecosystem, sustainable resources, social justice, and equity" (WHO, 1986) (see Chapter 1). The *Ottawa Charter* details how HCPs enable patients to make decisions that affect their health.

Level 2: Disease and Injury Prevention

The second level includes illness prevention services delivered at both individual and population levels to reduce risk factors for disease and injury (WHO & UNICEF, 2021) (see Chapter 4). Prevention strategies include clinical actions (immunizing), behavioural aspects (support groups), and environmental actions (climate control activism).

Level 3: Diagnosis and Treatment

Diagnosis and treatment focus on recognizing and managing individual patients' existing health problems at three sublevels: primary, secondary, and tertiary.

- *Primary care* (PC) is the first point of contact of a patient with the health care system that leads to a decision regarding a course of action to resolve any actual or potential health problem. PC providers include physicians and NPs in practice settings such as physicians' offices, nurse-managed clinics, community health centres, and schools. The focus is on early detection, routine care, and education to prevent recurrences. (Recall and note the differences between PC and PHC.)
- *Secondary care* usually occurs in hospital or home settings and involves specialized medical services provided by a physician specialist or a hospital on referral from a PC practitioner. Secondary care considers definitive or extended diagnosis.
- *Tertiary care* is specialized technical care involving the diagnosis and treatment of complicated health problems. Tertiary care occurs in regional, teaching, university, or specialized hospitals that house sophisticated diagnostic equipment.

Level 4: Rehabilitation

The aim of rehabilitation nursing is to improve the health and quality of life of individuals who are facing life-altering conditions, regardless of age or circumstances, by promoting and advancing professional rehabilitation nursing practice through education, advocacy, collaboration, and research. Rehabilitation occurs after a physical or mental health illness, injury, or chemical addiction or in response to chronic illness, disability, frailty, and aging. Ideally, rehabilitation begins the moment a patient enters a health care setting as part of an interdisciplinary effort (i.e., therapists [physical, occupational, respiratory], nurses). As a health condition stabilizes, rehabilitation assists patients with returning to their previous level of function or reaching an optimal level of function, establishing quality of life while promoting independence and self-care. For example, some patients undergo physiotherapy before major joint repair to enhance their recovery (see Chapter 37). Nurses have a key role in the continuity-of-care aspects of rehabilitation across agencies and settings. RNs in Canada can gain certification as rehabilitation nurses through the CNA (see list of specialties at CNA, 2021c).

Level 5: Supportive Care

People of all ages who have chronic (i.e., long term) or progressive (i.e., worsen over time) illnesses or disabilities may require supportive care. Supportive care consists of health, personal, and social services provided over a prolonged period to people who are disabled, do not function independently, or have a terminal disease. The demand for supportive care will continue to grow in response to increasing lifespans, escalating chronic conditions, and the expanding diversity of care settings (i.e., institutional, community, and home). Two examples of supportive care include palliative care and respite care (please refer to descriptions in the earlier Hospice and Palliative Care section).

CHALLENGES TO THE HEALTH CARE SYSTEM

While Canada's health care system is often heralded as a prime example of UHC, it is not without its challenges. UHC coverage is an aspiration, rather than a destination, and hence requires a continuous commitment to ensure adequate "depth and scope of coverage that is politically achievable and fiscally feasible" (Martin et al., 2018, p. 1731). A successful health care system must continue to evolve and realign resources to meet changing population needs, foster evidence-informed care, ensure equitable access to care, and contain costs.

Next, we discuss the current major challenges to our health care system that necessitate health system reform and nursing engagement.

Sustainability

Political Economy of Health. While most Canadians assert that health care is a fundamental human right, rising costs and increasing wait times have fueled an ideological debate about how the health care system should be funded and delivered (Valle, 2016). Right-wing political groups assert that health care costs are rising at unsustainable rates and call for privatization, whereas left-wing political groups argue for system restructuring and increased breadth of coverage. Both ideologies have been instrumental in shaping our current system, but the rise of neo-liberalism, especially during the 1990s, has resulted in increased health inequalities and weakened social provisions (Valle, 2016).

The ideological premises of the political group in power dramatically influence health and public policy. Thus, the future of the Canadian health care system is subject to the views and priorities of those in positions of power. Nurses have a professional obligation to be civically engaged and to advocate for equitable and accessible health care services that will meet the current and future needs of Canadians.

Climate Change. Over the coming decades, climate change will pose the biggest threat to human health and well-being worldwide (Canadian Institute for Climate Choices, 2021; Martin & Vold, 2019). Canadians will be faced with increasing extreme cold and heat events, weather-related natural disasters, poor air quality, waterborne and foodborne contamination, exposure to ultraviolet light, and changing patterns of vectorborne and zoonotic diseases (Bush & Lemmen, 2019; Health Canada, 2019d; Warren & Lulham, 2021). The extent of the impacts on human health will depend on how fast our climate changes and how well our health care system can adapt to cope with the associated challenges and health risks (Health Canada, 2019d). Nursing engagement, advocacy, and leadership are urgently needed to mitigate the deleterious health effects of climate change by addressing the vulnerabilities of the health care system and fostering resiliency (see Chapter 11).

Primary Health Care Versus Primary Care Spending. In the 1960s, the major health care needs of Canadians revolved around the treatment of acute injuries and disease. To meet these needs, Canada built a reactive health care system where treatment services dominated and care was primarily delivered in hospitals. The hospital–doctor model worked well for that reality, but Canada's population has changed and so have its health care needs (Simpson et al., 2017). Hospital spending consistently accounts for the largest portion of overall health care costs, with hospital services representing 26.4% of total health expenditures in 2019 (CIHI, 2021a). The bulk of health care spending has been focused on acute care settings rather than PHC. However, unlike in the 1960s, Canadians' health care needs are primarily and increasingly centered on chronic disease management and care. As an increasing number of Canadians are living with chronic diseases, they also require increased community supports to prevent exacerbations and to enable them to appropriately manage their conditions at home. In the absence of these services, many Canadians with chronic conditions require hospitalization, which is not only costly but also further strains our health care system. Nurses must advocate for and lead the establishment of a strong health care system focused on upstream approaches and PHC.

Responsive Health Care Planning and Delivery

Human Health Care Resources. In 2019, more than 1.4 million people in Canada worked directly in health-related occupations compared to 1.7 million people in 2012 (CIHI, 2015, 2020). Despite a growing Canadian population, the number of people employed in the health care sector has decreased, leaving many job vacancies, particularly in rural or remote locations and in specialty areas, which has compromised many Canadians' accessibility to health care services. In 2019, 30% of these vacant positions were nursing positions (Hou & Schimmele, 2020). The shortage of HCPs has been made even more evident during the COVID-19 pandemic. Health human resource planning is a critical component of a successful health care system. Effective planning requires consideration of the broader health care system and its challenges (i.e., wait times, patient safety, bed closures) as well as population demographics and trends (i.e., aging population, urbanization) (Health Canada, 2016c).

Aging Canadian Population. Over the next 20 years, as the baby-boom generation enters its senior years, Canada's population of older persons is expected to grow by 68% (CIHI, 2017b). While the majority of Canadian older persons living in the community report having good physical and mental health and being happy and satisfied with their lives, the aging process can often be characterized by chronic diseases and conditions that prompt older persons to access additional health care services (Public Health Agency of Canada, 2020). To ensure that Canadian older persons can "age in place," or remain at home for as long as possible, we need to guarantee the availability and accessibility of appropriate home-based and community-based services (i.e., home care, independent living support).

Currently, our health care system is primarily designed to deliver acute and emergent services, with a limited number of LTC facilities. While necessary, these services will soon fail to meet the needs of our growing population of older persons. These facilities are therefore at risk of being overwhelmed in the absence of appropriate home and community health care venues. To meet these needs, nurses, in collaboration with other HCPs, will need to advocate for, fulfill, and develop more health care services that meet the needs of older persons wherever they live. This will prevent unnecessary and costly hospital admissions while also empowering older persons to optimize their quality of life while remaining in their own homes (see Chapter 25).

Truth and Reconciliation Calls to Action. By listening to and documenting the stories of residential school survivors, the TRC compelled Canadians to confront our dark history of violence toward Indigenous peoples. As one aspect of the legacy of colonization, Indigenous peoples in Canada disproportionately experience worse access to care, poorer health outcomes, and a higher burden of disease and disparities than their non-Indigenous counterparts (Villeneuve & Betker, 2020). Based on the TRC Calls to Action, engaging in reconciliation to address Indigenous health inequities requires that we promote policy and system changes, engage Indigenous communities, recruit and retain Indigenous HCPs, engage in cultural safety training and anti-racism efforts, and improve Indigenous patient care, access, and outcomes (HealthCareCAN, 2018). Promoting reconciliation within health care remains an ongoing challenge to our health care system, and nurses must commit to addressing these Calls to Action (see Chapter 12).

Geographical Distribution of Services. Approximately 18% of Canadians live in rural or remote communities, and this population is served by only 11.8% of regulated nurses and 8% of physicians (MacLeod et al., 2017; Wilson et al., 2020). The distribution of HCPs and health services does not mirror need, and thus rural and remote Canadians face a greater challenge in accessing health care and experience poorer health outcomes than the general Canadian population (Wilson et al., 2020). Canadians living in remote and rural areas must travel long distances to access services beyond the most basic health care (i.e., labour and delivery, specialty services) (Martin et al., 2018).

In rural and remote locations where health care services do exist, nurses provide the bulk of care and maintain continuity of services. Nurses should leverage technology and establish mobile clinics to ensure that rural and remote Canadians have equitable access to care.

NURSING'S FUTURE IN THE EMERGING HEALTH CARE SYSTEM

As the Canadian health care system evolves to meet the health needs of Canadians, nursing roles must also continue to evolve and diversify. Nursing's presence and critical role in nearly every facet of the health care system provides us with a unique understanding of the current and future needs of those we serve. To date, nursing practice has primarily involved direct care, with a conspicuous absence at the executive and decision-making levels of health care agencies. Now, more than ever, nurses are needed to serve in leadership positions to catalyze health system change by leveraging our unique understanding of Canadians' health care needs. Nurses will be key in developing innovative solutions to the health care challenges identified here, and it is our professional responsibility to expand and forge new nursing roles to meet these needs.

Health care operates within frameworks of health policies that directly affect delivery and availability of health care, health outcomes, health disparities, working conditions of health care workers, and even nursing practice (Turale & Kunaviktikal, 2019). While many nurse leaders are involved in developing and shaping health policy, more often nurses are the recipients and implementers of health policies. Thus, the policy impact of the nursing voice is minimal, often leading to frustration when policies do not align with the needs of our patients, the contexts in which we work, or our scope of practice. By engaging in health policy development and reformation, nurses hold considerable potential to address the pressing health challenges that Canadians face. Nursing voices in decision making are needed at each level of the health care system (Rafferty, 2018). We cannot wait to be asked to take our seat at the table. Nursing has a professional obligation to contribute to health care policy, and we are well positioned to lead and catalyze health system changes that contribute to a better future for all (Rafferty, 2018) (Box 2.4).

BOX 2.4 A Guide for Nurses and Nursing Students to Begin Advocating for Policy Change

Established in 2018, the Nursing Now campaign is a global campaign to improve health by raising the status and profile of nursing. Nursing Now outlined the following essential steps for nurses to begin advocating for policy change:

1. Define your problem and build your case for change.
   - What is the challenge or issue you want to address and what needs to change?
2. Choose the target.
   - Identify the individuals, structures, or organizations that control the problem area and who you need to target to achieve that change
3. Find your allies.
   - Consider other stakeholders who can influence your target decision maker
4. Call for change.
   - Request a meeting, send emails and letters, develop a media campaign, engage champions, and propose policy changes

Adapted from Nursing Now. (2018). *Nurses together.* https://nursingnow.pageflow.io/nurses-together#278163

SUMMARY

The Canadian health care system will require significant restructuring to meet the complex needs of a diverse population and in response to local and global challenges. In this context, nursing's contributions to health and health care in Canada range from providing direct care to actively participating in the reformation processes, as well as maintaining a continuous presence in the pursuit of equitable access for all patient groups. Nursing has been instrumental in the advancement of nursing practice, interdisciplinary practices, and collaborative efforts for the betterment of society (Turale & Kunaviktikal, 2019). In the future, we must assert our roles as critical stakeholders, partners, and providers within the emerging health care system.

KEY CONCEPTS

- Medicare is a key component of Canada's social safety net.
- All levels of government play a major role in co-funding national health insurance and setting health care policy in accordance with the *Canada Health Act.*
- The *Canada Health Act* articulates the five principles of our national health insurance system—public administration, comprehensiveness, universality, portability, and accessibility—and forbids extra billing and user fees.
- Health care services are provided in institutional, community, and home settings; across all age groups; and for individual, family, group, and community populations.
- The five levels of health care are promotive, preventive, curative, rehabilitative, and supportive.
- Escalating costs, technological innovations, and consumer expectations challenge the health care system in efforts to deliver innovative, efficient, and quality care.
- Equality, equity, access, interdisciplinary approaches, communication, and continuity of care challenge the health care system.
- The primacy of PHC and home care align with the reforming health care environment and cost effectiveness.
- Successful health promotion and disease prevention programs help patients acquire healthier lifestyles and achieve optimal quality of life.
- Sufficient, diverse, and qualified human health resources are essential for a culturally competent workforce attending to a culturally safe Canadian health care system.
- Enhancing the health of the Indigenous population in Canada is a significant challenge to society and to the health care system.
- Nurses must continually seek out information and evidence to remain responsive to providing quality, culturally competent, and safe care.

CRITICAL THINKING EXERCISES

1. Debate the following challenges facing the Canadian health care system: escalating costs, privatization, continuity of care, regionalization/centralization, and digital health.
2. Consider and describe how the economy and technology have changed the Canadian health care system. What are the implications for nursing? For patients and families?
3. Referring to the case study at the beginning of the chapter, describe the types of health care services, safety issues, interprofessional competencies, and technological supports that might play a part in W.W.'s postsurgical care.

🌐 *Answers to Critical Thinking Exercises appear on the Evolve website.*

REVIEW QUESTIONS

Review Questions 1 to 10 relate to the case study at the beginning of the chapter.

1. During a community health placement, a nursing student interacts with W.W., who tells the student about his upcoming hip replacement surgery. W.W. explains that he went to the preassessment clinic and that they connected him with community services such as Meals on Wheels, home care, and an outpatient physiotherapist. The nursing student understands that these services are important aspects of:
   a. Acute care
   b. Primary health care
   c. Primary care
   d. Ambulatory care
2. During W.W.'s preoperative assessment, the nurse explains the various roles of the interprofessional team members who will be involved in his care after his hip replacement. Which of the following team members would the nurse most likely indicate will be a part of the interprofessional team? *(Select all that apply.)*
   a. Occupational therapist
   b. Physiotherapist
   c. Pharmacist
   d. Translator
   e. Medical-surgical nurse
3. W.W.'s hip replacement surgery is considered medically necessary in order for W.W. to maintain a good quality of life. The _____ currently ensures that Canadians do not have to pay out of pocket for medically necessary procedures.
   a. Canada Health Act
   b. Emergency Management Act
   c. Canadian Medicare Act
   d. Medical Care Act
   d. Hospital Insurance and Diagnostic Act
4. With his sister's help, W.W. has recently had to start caring for his 89-year-old mother, who is requiring increased assistance with her activities of daily living. At the clinic, W.W. expresses to the nurse that despite taking turns caring for their mother, both he and his sister are nearing exhaustion caring for her. As the nurse opens the dialogue on potential placements for his mother, it is obvious that there is a lack of understanding about the existence of community agencies such as _____, which might provide an alternative for this family.
   a. Home care
   b. Palliative care
   c. Hospital care
   d. Ambulatory care
   e. Adult day support
5. After W.W.'s surgery, he develops a postoperative infection that requires daily dressing changes. W.W. explains to the student nurse that he cannot manage the dressing changes on his own. Which community service should the student nurse communicate with to ensure that W.W. will have assistance with his daily dressing changes?
   a. Adult day services
   b. Ambulatory care
   c. Palliative care
   d. Home care
   e. Hospice care

6. Connecting W.W. with appropriate community-based health services is important because: *(Select all that apply.)*
   a. Community-based services can help to prevent unnecessary and costly hospitalizations.
   b. Community-based services ensure that W.W. can recover at home.
   c. Community-based services can be used instead of hospitalization.
   e. Community-based services are an important element of primary health care.
   e. Community-based services enable W.W. to age in place.
7. W.W. tells the nursing student that he has waited for a long time for this surgery and does not feel that the long wait time was acceptable. W.W. asks the nursing student if anything is being done to address surgical wait times. The nursing student tells W.W. that the following agencies have made efforts to reduce wait times, reduce duplication of tests, and support coordination of care: *(Select all that apply.)*
   a. Canada eHealth
   b. Canadian Institute for Health Information
   c. Canada Health Infoway
   d. Canadian Institutes for Health Research
   e. Consumers' Association of Canada
8. W.W. asks his nurse practitioner why his hip replacement surgery was covered, but his prescription glasses are not. The nurse practitioner explains that there are some health services that are generally not covered under the publicly funded health care system. Some of these noninsured services include: *(Select all that apply.)*
   a. Dental services
   b. Home care
   c. Medical transportation
   d. Medical equipment and appliances (i.e., wheelchairs, prostheses)
   e. Prescription drugs (outside of hospitals)
9. During his hospital stay, W.W. notices that the postoperative surgical unit is often short-staffed. W.W. expresses his concerns about this to the unit manager. This has been one of several similar complaints over the past 6 months, prompting management to request a brief report from the nurse manager on a human resources plan for the next 5 years. Which of the following statements best represents the factors that should be mentioned?
   a. We should be working with our aging nurses to transition them out of full-time work, allowing younger nurses to be mentored into their vacated positions and increasing the number of nurses we are educating.
   b. With all the workplace injuries, we should be hiring an occupational therapist or there will soon be no nurses working.
   c. We will soon be able to replace nurses with robots and technology, so that is where we should be investing.
   d. We are not educating enough nurses, so we may have to recruit from international pools to fill positions.
   e. There are too many variables to be able to predict what will be needed in 5 years, so the best we can do is try to keep the nurses we have.
10. Two months after his hip replacement surgery, W.W. has a minor fall. W.W. is not injured after this incident, but he realizes that he needs to further improve his mobility to return to his previous level of function. W.W. expresses his concern to his nurse practitioner, who refers him to a physiotherapist. This is an example of which level of care?
   a. Level 1: Health Promotion
   b. Level 2: Disease and Injury Prevention
   c. Level 3: Diagnosis and Treatment
   d. Level 4: Rehabilitation
   e. Level 4: Supportive Care

Answers: 1. a; 2. a, b, c, e; 3. a; 4. e; 5. d; 6. a, b, d, e; 7. b, c, d; 8. a, b, c, d, e; 9. a; 10. d.

Rationales for the Review Questions appear on the Evolve website.

RECOMMENDED WEBSITES

Canada Health Infoway: https://www.infoway-inforoute.ca
A not-for-profit corporation created by Canada's first ministers to foster and accelerate development and adoption of digital health innovations across all groups.

Canadian Foundation for Healthcare Improvement: https://www.cfhi-fcass.ca/Home.aspx
This site addresses initiatives of the foundation to advance promising innovations across health care organizations to improve patient care, health outcomes, and efficiencies.

Canadian Institute of Health Information: https://www.cihi.ca
A not-for-profit organization seeking to improve the health care system and the health of Canadians by providing timely and essential health information.

Canadian Patient Safety Institute: https://www.patientsafetyinstitute.ca
This institute was established to build and advance a safer health care system for Canadians. It reports on activities in leadership across health sectors and health care systems, highlights promising practices, and raises awareness with stakeholders and the public about patient safety.

Canadian Public Health Association: https://www.cpha.ca
A national not-for-profit association seeking excellence in public health nationally and internationally and seeking universal and equitable access to basic health-sustaining conditions.

Health Canada: https://www.hc-sc.gc.ca
This website provides links to information about the Canadian health care system, such as the *Canada Health Act* legislation, the federal budget, and federal reports.

REFERENCES

A full reference list is available on the website for this book at https://evolve.elsevier.com/Canada/Potter/fundamentals/

3

The Development of Nursing in Canada

Written by Lydia Wytenbroek, RN, PhD, and Sonya Grypma, RN, PhD

OBJECTIVES

Mastery of content in this chapter will enable you to:
- Define the key terms listed.
- Describe the historical development of professional nursing.
- Describe the historical development of nursing education in Canada.
- Describe the historical development of nursing practice in Canada.

KEY TERMS

Canadian Association of Schools of Nursing (CASN)

Canadian Indigenous Nurses Association (CINA)

Canadian Nurses Association (CNA)

Code of ethics

Education reform

Entry-to-practice requirement

International Council of Nurses (ICN)

World Health Organization (WHO)

🌐 WEBSITE

http://evolve.elsevier.com/Canada/Potter/fundamentals/

CASE STUDY

History is a tool that nurses can use to understand how power and context may operate in health care. In a recent report, In Plain Sight, *which documents the Indigenous-specific racism that exists within British Columbia's health care system, First Nations woman (preferred pronouns: she/her) describes her family's experience in the ICU before her father's death as follows:*

> *"The overall tone of what I can only describe as 'disdain' that was shown to my family day in and day out for taking up space in the hospital. The glances, the glares, the apathy was heavily noted by many of us, as it seemed they would prefer that we not be there . . . Throughout watching the head of our family die, we maintained our dignity, decorum and ensured that we were respectful of all rules and policies, and with all of this 'on our side' we were still met with indifference, intolerance and discrimination."—Turpel-Lafond, 2020, p. 50*

Case Study Reflection: What should have been the outcome of this situation? Why do you think it went the way it did? What could be done to prevent this situation? How do we show culturally competent care? How can history help nurses understand the importance of providing culturally safe care?

Think about this case study as you read this chapter. There are review questions at the end of the chapter about this case study.

Turpel-Lafond, M. E. (2020). *In plain sight: Addressing Indigenous-specific racism and discrimination in BC health care—Full report.* https://engage.gov.bc.ca/app/uploads/sites/613/2020/11/In-Plain-Sight-Full-Report-2020.pdf

A historical lens calls us to think about how the events of the past impact the present. This chapter discusses the history of nursing and health care in Canada, and asks you to consider how current experiences of health inequities and racism might be rooted in historical health approaches, systems, and priorities in Canada. For example, understanding nurses' participation in colonial health care in Canada can help you better understand why health care has not always been a safe and equitable space for all people. Nurses have been part of health care systems and structures that have not always provided equitable and just care. Understanding this history will help you to recognize current structural inequities and stigmatizing assumptions—including your own—that may impact people's health and health care experiences.

Anticipating what nursing practice will look like when current students graduate is an important and challenging aspect of nursing education. One way to anticipate the future of nursing is to track changing social and political trends and related health care policies—something that provincial and national nursing associations do well (see Chapter 2 for further information about health care policies). Another is to stay abreast of cutting-edge research—something that nursing and health care researchers do well (see Chapter 8 for further information about research). A third way is to study nursing's past. By identifying key persons, issues, and events in nursing and how these have changed over time, this chapter intends to help readers envision nursing's future and their role in shaping it.

WHY NURSING HISTORY MATTERS

Early nurse leaders made nursing history a core component of nurses' education (Toman & Thifault, 2012). During the first wave of nursing history (1870–1970), comprehensive works like Nutting and Dock's (1907–1912) four-volume *History of Nursing* was required reading in nursing programs worldwide. By the 1970s, nursing history was set aside to make way for the emerging field of nursing theory. The field sat dormant until the 1990s, when women's historians "discovered" nursing and began to reintroduce nurses to themselves. If the first wave focused on nursing leaders who established associations (Bates et al., 2005), the second wave of nursing history (1990 to the present) includes the lives and experiences of ordinary nurses and the events and social structures that have helped shape nursing into what it is today. Despite the increase in superb historical studies, nursing history had all but disappeared from the curriculum by the end of the twentieth century (Toman & Thifault, 2012). In Canada and elsewhere, small groups of historians are working actively to reintroduce history into nursing curricula (Toman & Thifault, 2012).

History offers the opportunity to engage in historically informed discussions about present-day problems. According to Nelson (2009), historical amnesia is dangerous. As this chapter will demonstrate, nursing history provides context, explains the present, and provides a way to look forward (Grypma, 2017). History provides the basis for developing an informed and critical understanding of our society. It serves as an overarching conceptual framework that allows us to better understand the various meanings of nursing and the different experiences of nurses (D'Antonio, 2003). History explains the present by recognizing that what happens today is not an accident; it has roots in the past (Lynaugh, in D'Antonio & Fairman, 2010).

In 2008, the Canadian Nurses Association (CNA) developed a position statement on promoting nursing history, noting that learning from the lessons of history is "critical to advancing the profession in the interests of the Canadian public" (CNA, 2007). The Canadian Association of Schools of Nursing (CASN) also considers nursing history an essential component of nursing education, emphasizing in the *National Nursing Education Framework* (CASN, 2022) that nursing programs must prepare students to demonstrate "foundational knowledge of nursing including nursing history, nursing theories, and other theories relevant to nursing practice" (p. 10). This chapter introduces readers to historical events and persons in Canadian nursing history, with an emphasis on the twentieth century.

INDIGENOUS CAREGIVERS: RECONSIDERING NURSING NARRATIVES

Nursing in Canada has a much longer history than is typically acknowledged, one that precedes Florence Nightingale and her health care reforms (Wytenbroek & Vandenberg, 2017). Indigenous healers and midwives are often excluded from nursing histories because they fall outside of the boundaries of the concept of the professionally educated nurse. Long before European settlers colonized the land that we now call Canada, Indigenous peoples in North America had extensive healing traditions and health practices, which included knowledge about how to harvest, prepare, and administer medicinal plants to relieve symptoms and treat ailments (Benoit & Carroll, 2005) (see Chapter 12, Indigenous Health)

Indigenous women played essential roles within their own communities and for White settler communities as midwives, nurses, and caregivers (Burnett, 2010). For example, a White settler in Saskatchewan wrote in 1833 that an Indigenous woman had cured his sister-in-law

of dysentery by giving her a tea made from white prairie flowers, after a local physician had been unable to assist her (Burnett, 2010). In this way, Indigenous peoples and settler groups had formalized social structures for caring for ill, injured, birthing, and dying persons long before hospitals were built and "modern" (i.e., hospital-based) nursing was established.

CARE OF STRANGERS: THE CATHOLIC NURSING TRADITION

The history of hospitals in Canada is intimately linked to the history of female religious orders. Catholic nursing sisters built a vast network of nurse-run hospitals, beginning with the establishment of the Hôtel-Dieu de Québec in 1639 in Quebec City. It was Canada's first hospital and the only hospital in North America at that time, other than one located in the Dominican Republic. By 1947, nursing sisters operated at least 146 hospitals across Canada (Paul, 2005). They were guided by a distinct ethos of service and assumed roles of significant influence as hospital administrators and leaders in health care (Wytenbroek & Vandenberg, 2017).

The First Nurses and Hospitals in New France

From the outset, it was nurses rather than physicians who both provided and administered health care in the settlement known as New France. In 1608, Samuel de Champlain selected what is now Quebec (in "New France") as the site for a colony of settlers to support the growing fur trade. The first laywoman to provide nursing care in New France was Marie Rollet Hébert. She and her husband emigrated in 1617 at the request of Champlain. Although she was a layperson, Mme Hébert extended care to Indigenous peoples and settlers who were ill. Indigenous peoples' knowledge of herbs and remedies also benefited European settlers.

The first nurses to tend to the sick in a type of health care centre were male attendants at a "sick bay" established in 1629 at the French garrison in Port-Royal in Acadia (Gibbon & Mathewson, 1947). The Jesuit priests, who were missionaries to New France, also served as nurses. They used the care of the sick to aid their mission of converting Indigenous peoples to Christianity.

The Expansion of Catholic Hospitals Across Canada

Female religious orders had a prominent role in building an impressive hospital system in what is now known as the province of Quebec. Catholic hospitals were founded as charitable institutions that were devoted to the care of the ill. Nursing sisters viewed their work as a spiritual ministry and "were out to win souls through hospital care" (Violette, 2005, p. 60). Catholic hospitals were characterized by a hierarchy in which nuns were assigned to different caregiving roles. The most senior nun was the superintendent of the hospital and was responsible for the administration of the institution. The apothecary was responsible for preparing treatments and remedies, changing dressings, and taking vital signs. Sister Saint Martin, an apothecary at Hôtel-Dieu de Québec in the early 1800s, excelled at surgery. On one occasion, she successfully performed an amputation after a physician failed at the first attempt (Violette, 2005).

The Catholic hospital network expanded across Canada. Nursing sisters' religious identities enabled them to emerge as leaders at a time when women had few other employment options. For example, Mother Joseph, who was born in Quebec in 1823, designed and built more than two dozen hospitals across the Pacific Northwest. She had learned carpentry skills from her father and joined a Catholic order so that she could put these skills to use. She oversaw every facet of hospital construction, even living in a makeshift shelter on construction sites so that she could oversee and give direction to the workmen (Wytenbroek & Vandenberg, 2017).

Florence Nightingale and Nursing Reform

Florence Nightingale has been long hailed as the founder of modern nursing and invoked by nursing leaders as a powerful symbol of the profession. Nightingale spearheaded a movement to improve standards of nursing care in the mid-nineteenth century, initiating a system of nurse training that prevailed globally for over 100 years. Her work has attracted both praise and critique over the years. Today, as nurses work to increase awareness of racism and inequality, it is helpful to also consider Nightingale's legacy in the larger historical context of colonialism and privilege (Smith, 2020), and to ensure that lesser-known nurses also receive the historical recognition they deserve.

Nightingale was born in 1820 to a wealthy, well-connected, upper-class family. She railed against the customs of her time, which did not allow middle- and upper-class women to work outside the home: "Why have women passion, intellect, moral activity—these three—and a place in society where no one of the three can be exercised?" (Nightingale, 1979/2010, p. 25). She was well educated and, against the wishes of her family, travelled to Kaiserswerth, Germany, where she studied to become a nurse at the Institute of Protestant Deaconesses. She returned to London in 1853 and accepted the post of superintendent at the Establishment for Gentlewomen During Temporary Illness.

In 1854, Sidney Herbert, British Secretary of State for War and a personal friend of Nightingale's, asked her to organize a group of nurses to go to Turkey during the Crimean War (1853–1856). Nightingale secured medical supplies, implemented sanitary reforms, improved the hygiene of the army hospital, and visited patients at night. New telegraph technology was key to her rise to fame, as reports about her outstanding efforts to care for British troops were broadcast throughout Britain and the English-speaking world (McPherson, 2005).

By the time Nightingale returned to England, in 1856, she was a national heroine. To honour Nightingale, the English government established a Nightingale Fund, which Nightingale used to establish nurse education programs in several British hospitals. The first Nightingale School of Nursing was established at St. Thomas's Hospital in London in 1860. Nightingale did not work at the school herself, but it followed an administrative model that she created. Nightingale was not the only, or even the first, person to promote education for nurses, but the Nightingale model became the standard model of nursing education around the world, including in Canada, for the next century. This model involved a hospital-based school that was overseen by a trained superintendent, trained staff members who also acted as instructors, and a cadre of nursing students who provided the bulk of the patient care.

Nursing in the Nightingale tradition also carried with it class, imperial, gender, and racial biases (McCallum, 2014). Prior to the introduction of nursing schools, hospital care was carried out by a range of available ward attendants—male and female, religious and lay, paid and unpaid, skilled and unskilled (McPherson, 2005, p. 74). Nightingale raised the status of nursing through her model of apprenticeship training by recasting nursing as a "respectable" profession for women and distinguishing it from untrained caregiving work. Her vision of a good nurse was a woman who was well trained and had "the highest class of character" (Nightingale, 1888, p. 1048). According to Nightingale, nurses had to possess the virtues of purity, honesty, truthfulness, trustworthiness, cheerfulness, and quietness. Nurses were also expected to be "submissive" to physicians (all of whom were male at that time) and obey their directions. While working-class women were paid to attend nursing school, "lady pupils" from the middle and upper classes could pay to attend the school; these "ladies" were prepared to undertake supervisory roles (McPherson, 2005).

Nightingale expressed her opinions and beliefs through voluminous writings and lobbied members of parliament to act on her views. In 1860, she published *Notes on Nursing*. Focused more on health than illness care, her book was designed for use in the home by laywomen and nurses. In it, Nightingale stressed the need for good environmental conditions, like clean air and water, that would allow nature to cure naturally. The nurse's role was to put the patients in the best position for nature to act upon them. She drew her conclusions from health data that she had collected and analyzed, for which she is also celebrated as the first female statistician. The 16-volume *Collected Works of Florence Nightingale* (2001–2012) by Lynn McDonald (2001) makes available the full range of Nightingale's written work.

Mary Seacole and the Crimean War

While Nightingale is a well-known character in nursing history, Mary Seacole (Figure 3.1)—a biracial woman whose reputation after the Crimean War rivalled Nightingale's—is not. Seacole was born in Kingston, Jamaica, in 1805 and raised there. Seacole learned traditional herbal remedies from her mother, a doctress. When the Crimean War broke out, Seacole travelled to London and attempted to join a contingent of nurses that was heading to Crimea to work with Nightingale. However, she was turned away, including by one of Nightingale's companions. Seacole was devastated by this rejection, writing, "Did these ladies shrink from accepting my aid because my blood flowed beneath a somewhat duskier skin than theirs?" (Seacole, 1857). Undeterred, Seacole paid her own way to Turkey and set up the British Hotel to care for convalescing officers.

Seacole was lauded in the press, with newspaper correspondents writing about her skill at treating wounds and broken bones. When the war ended, Seacole was financially bankrupt. However, Queen Victoria, the future King Edward VII, and his brother the Duke of Edinburgh set up a "Seacole Fund" in honour of her service. In 1857, Seacole published her autobiography, *Wonderful Adventures of Mrs. Seacole in Many Lands*, one of the first travel memoirs written by a Black woman. It included a description of her nursing work in Crimea. Her book was popular and quickly went into a second printing. Even so, Seacole's contributions were not recognized in history in the same way as Nightingale's—a dismissive response that was undoubtedly related to her race and class (Pitts, 2018). In 2016, a statue of Seacole was erected outside St. Thomas's Hospital in London.

COLONIAL HEALTH CARE IN CANADA

Colonial Health Care: "Indian Hospitals"

The history of "Indian hospitals" reveals the fact that health care services in Canada were unequal (Meijer-Drees, 2013). Christian orders had been delivering health care in parts of Canada for many centuries, but in the 1800s they became involved in Indigenous health services when the Grey Nuns left Quebec for the West Coast, providing health care in small settler and Indigenous communities along the way. Between the 1890s and 1945, the federal Department of Indian Affairs controlled initiatives related to health and health care for Indigenous peoples (Meijer-Drees, 2013). The expansion of formal, Western-style medical services to Indigenous peoples came in response to public pressure over the widely held opinion that diseases such as tuberculosis spread from Indigenous to non-Indigenous communities.

During that period (1890s to 1945), Indian Affairs patched together Church-run and state-run medical services. For example, when the Grey Nuns built a hospital on the Kainai (Blood) reserve in Alberta in 1893, the federal Department of Indian Affairs paid the salaries of the nursing sisters and provided funds for other operating costs (Meijer-Drees, 1996). Indigenous populations in the southern parts of Canada

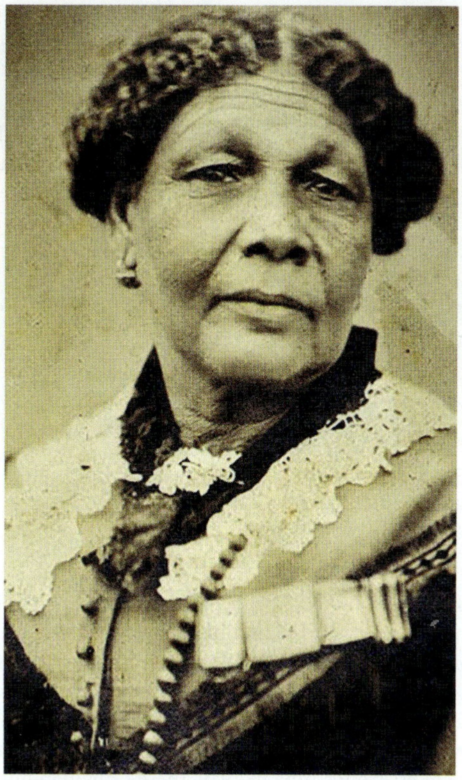

FIGURE 3.1 Mary Seacole. (From https://www.starkefrauen.online/home/wollen-ist-knnen-atybc-5eewc)

were served by federally funded Indian hospitals. Northern locations were served entirely by mission hospitals, which were partially but inconsistently funded through Indian Affairs (Meijer-Drees, 2013).

During this period, the federal government offered Indigenous peoples a health care service that was *separate* from the one available to the non-Indigenous population (Lux, 2016). Indian hospitals were chronically underfunded, overcrowded, and understaffed. Many of the hospitals were housed in redundant residential school buildings or military barracks, and lacked basic facilities such as adequate laundries or kitchens (Lux, 2016). Health conditions were poor: Indigenous peoples had some of the highest mortality and morbidity rates in the country, with tuberculosis at crisis levels. Christian church-run facilities were viewed as an "obstacle to the implementation of a progressive health care system" because health care initiatives were too generalized and were hampered by inter-church competition and proselytizing goals (Meijer-Drees, 2013, p. 14). A campaign was mounted to create a secular system of health care facilities to replace Church-run ones. Through these efforts, the federal government directly controlled and operated 22 Indian hospitals by the 1960s.

One of the most consequential decisions at the time was the Indian Health Services' insistence that northern tuberculosis patients receive treatments in the south. This meant moving Indigenous patients away from their local communities and enhancing the services of southern hospitals instead of investing in the North. Many of those who travelled to the distant south to receive months of tuberculosis treatment had never travelled outside of their local community, and many never returned. This loss had a devastating and lasting impact on Indigenous communities.

The Indian Health Services department had four strategic goals: (1) it sought to provide complete health service for Indigenous peoples to raise the standard of health; (2) it sought to assimilate Indigenous

peoples into mainstream, non-Indigenous societies; (3) it aimed to "correct" the traditional medical and health practices of Indigenous peoples; and (4) its primary interest was public health—particularly reducing the threat of tuberculosis, the rate of which was 10-fold higher in Indigenous communities. In fact, in 1951–1952, tuberculosis patients occupied 75% of the beds in hospitals run by Indian Health Services (Meijer-Drees, 2013).

Like residential schools, Indian hospitals were designed to assimilate Indigenous peoples into Euro-Canadian society by replacing traditional healing practices with biomedicine. Nurses who worked within the Indian hospital system played a role in perpetuating harm against Indigenous patients. Many Indian hospital survivors recall loneliness, vulnerability, fear, and abuse in situations where medical staff did not understand their culture and languages (Truth and Reconciliation Commission of Canada, 2015).

In 2013, historian Ian Mosby published a seminal article revealing that prominent nutrition scientists in Canada had performed highly unethical research on children in residential schools between 1942 and 1952 (Mosby, 2013). Many of these children were already malnourished because of government policies and the terrible conditions in residential schools. In some experiments, leading physicians and nutritional experts withheld essential vitamins and minerals to children in control groups and prevented dental care, arguing that this would impact their study results. While nurses were complicit in colonial health structures, their role in residential schools, Indian hospitals, and the nutritional experiments documented by Mosby remains largely unexplored.

By the 1970s, with the introduction of federally funded medical insurance in Canada, the Canadian government dramatically curbed its commitment to Indian hospitals. Only nursing stations remained as the foundation of health services to serve Indigenous communities directly; these continued to be concentrated in more remote and northern areas (Meijer-Drees, 2013).

The history of Indian hospitals reveals the extent to which racial segregation and colonial practices negatively influenced Indigenous individuals, families, and communities. Their legacy is ongoing. In 2018, health care providers in Quebec launched the #aHand2Hold campaign, which confronted the Quebec government's practice of separating children from their families during medical evacuation airlifts, which disproportionately impacted Cree and Inuit children from remote and northern Indigenous communities (Shaheen-Hussain, 2020). Being aware of the history of colonialism in Canada and its negative impact on Indigenous health and health care experiences can enable nurses to anticipate and develop trauma-informed, culturally safe, and anti-racist approaches to health inequities.

Decolonizing Health Care: The Canadian Indigenous Nurses Association

Indigenous nurses have a long history of working for better health care for Indigenous peoples in Canada. By the late 1950s, Indian Health Services employed 604 graduate nurses—very few of whom were Indigenous—to work at nursing stations, health centres, and Indian hospitals. Indigenous nurses were aware of the failures of the colonial health system and came together in the 1970s to form the Registered Nurses of Canadian Indian Ancestry (RNCIA), now called the Canadian Indigenous Nurses Association (CINA). The RNCIA was the first group of Indigenous professionals to organize as an association. Its founding members—Jean Goodwill (Box 3.1), Jocelyn Bruyere, and Ann Callahan—advocated for Indigenous control over Indigenous health services. The primary aim of the organization was to improve the health of Indigenous communities and expand the participation of Indigenous nurses in the provision of Indigenous health services

Jean Cuthand Goodwill, 1928–1997

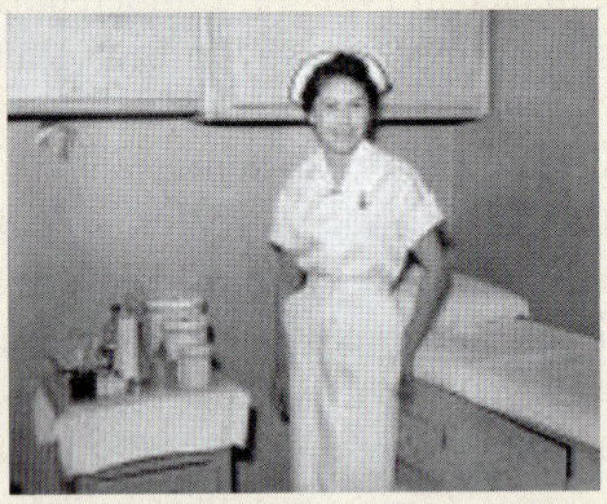

Jean Cuthand Goodwill, head nurse at the nursing station in La Ronge, Saskatchewan. Photo taken in 1958. (Provincial Archives of Saskatchewan/R-B6085.)

Jean Cuthand Goodwill grew up on Little Pine First Nation in Saskatchewan. She was raised by her mother's sister, a midwife and medicine woman. Goodwill developed an interest in nursing that grew after she spent time in a tuberculosis sanatorium as a teenager. She graduated as a registered nurse from the Holy Family Hospital in Prince Albert, and was one of the first Indigenous nurses to break through the colour bar in nursing to attend a mainstream nursing school in the 1950s (McCallum, 2014). After graduation, Goodwill worked for Indian Health Services. This experience informed her view that systemic issues influencing Indigenous health could only be changed through political action and activism, so she pursued leadership positions in government. She worked as a nursing consultant for the medical services division of Health and Welfare Canada in 1978, was appointed special advisor to the Minister of National Health and Welfare in 1981, was president of the Registered Nurses of Canadian Indian Ancestry (RNCIA) from 1982 to 1989, and helped establish an access program for Indigenous students to enter nursing at the University of Saskatchewan. Goodwill exemplified the RNCIA's commitment to improving Indigenous health by fostering Indigenous access to education and Indigenous nurse representation.

From McCallum, M. J. (2014). *Indigenous women, work, and history, 1940–1980*. University of Manitoba Press.

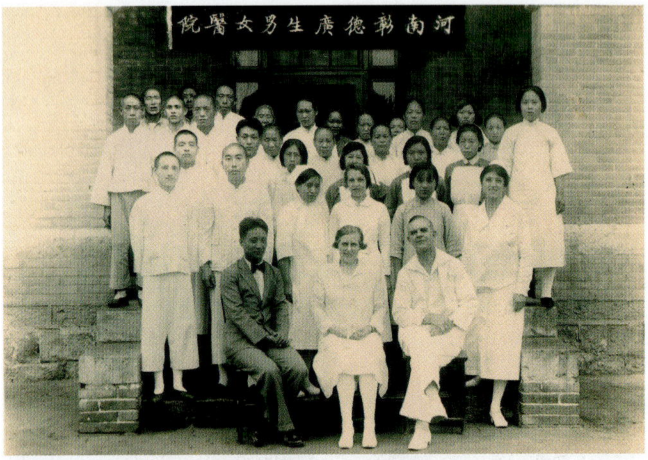

FIGURE 3.2 Canadian missionary nurses in Huaiqing, China, during the 1930s. (United Church of Canada Archives, Toronto. Access #1999.001P-1657.)

(McCallum, 2014). As historian Mary Jane Logan McCallum notes, these goals were revolutionary because the RNCIA sought to "transform the very nature of the relationships between Indigenous people and governments, and to reject the colonization of Indigenous health" (McCallum, 2017). Indigenous nurses remain underrepresented in the nursing workforce, and CINA continues to work to address inequities in nursing and health care.

GLOBALIZATION AND THE EMERGENCE OF MODERN NURSING

The history of modern nursing, at its heart, is a story of globalization (see Chapter 11). Throughout the history of the profession, nurses have travelled across geographic and national boundaries to bring nursing services and training to communities in need (Grypma & Wu, 2012).

Missionary Nursing

While Christian missions played a central role in Canadian nursing for three centuries, their importance peaked during the missionary movement that began in China in the late 1880s and spread across the globe. In the late 1880s, China's defeat in the Opium Wars, the women's suffrage movement, the establishment of professional nursing education, advances in transportation, and the evangelistic student missionary movement converged to provide an unprecedented opportunity for unmarried, ambitious, and intelligent women looking

for a way to express their religion in practical terms—as missionary nurses (Grypma & Wu, 2012). When the Presbyterian Church in Canada commissioned its first missionary nurse, Harriet Sutherland, to China in 1888, it initiated a wave of an estimated 100 Canadian missionary nurses to China (Figure 3.2). Before Mao Zedong's expulsion of foreigners from China in 1949, these Canadian nurses helped to establish hospitals and training schools in at least five provinces in China. They were among the cadre of Western missionaries credited with the birth and growth of modern nursing in China (Grypma, 2008). Although Canadian missionary nursing would continue in other regions, after the closure of the China field in 1949, missionary nursing moved from the centre to the margins of Canadian nursing practice (Grypma, 2007), largely ending the missionary era of nursing.

Canadian nurses' interest in international work continued past the missionary era with the movement of Canadian nurses into postwar organizations such as the **World Health Organization** (WHO), which was established in 1948. The WHO's prime objective, as defined in Article 1 of its original constitution, was "the attainment by all peoples of the highest possible level of health." Nursing was a central component of the WHO from the start, largely due to the lobbying efforts of the International Council of Nurses, an organization that sought to promote nursing and influence health policy worldwide. The WHO formed a nursing section in 1951, and by 1957 there were 155 WHO nurses working in 44 countries (Wytenbroek, 2015). Canadian nurse Lyle Creelman became the chief nursing officer (CNO) of the WHO from 1954 to 1968 (Armstrong-Reid, 2014). A number of other Canadian nurses also worked for the WHO, including Margaret Jackson, who worked as a WHO nurse in Iran from 1954 to 1956 (Wytenbroek, 2015). In 2017, following a 7-year absence of a CNO at the organization, WHO Director-General Dr. Tedros Adhanom Ghebreyesus appointed Elizabeth Iro from the Cook Islands as the new CNO. With this announcement, Dr. Tedros fulfilled a commitment he had made to appoint a nurse to his senior leadership team (World Health Organization [WHO], 2017).

Nursing in Remote Regions

Remote nursing is a distinguishing feature of Canadian nursing. Since the early twentieth century, people living in regions considered too small or too remote for hospitals or physician care have depended on

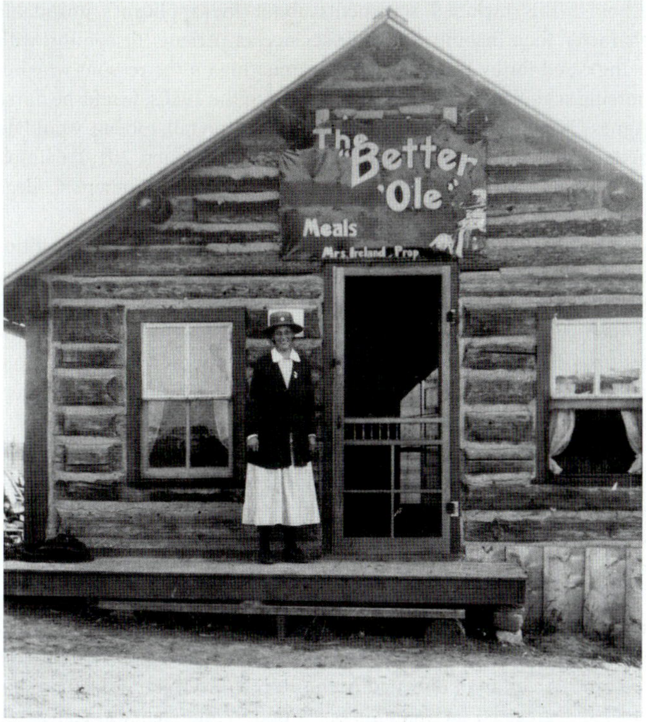

FIGURE 3.3 Red Cross nurse stopping for lunch, Pouce Coupe, British Columbia, circa 1920s. (Glenbow Archives, NA-2903-67.)

nurses for their health care needs. Nursing work in remote regions was crucial and all-encompassing. In the absence of physicians, nurses in outpost and outport nursing stations have provided public health, diagnostic, and emergency medical services.

The Grenfell Mission relied heavily on nurses in its efforts to provide health care for people living along hundreds of kilometres of coastline in Newfoundland and Labrador between 1894 and 1981. In addition to standard nursing duties, the station nurse's responsibilities included operating the dispensary, midwifery, public health, first aid, and dentistry (Coombs-Thorne, 2010). Similarly, nurses working at Red Cross outpost stations in Ontario between 1922 and 1984 acquired diverse skills considered more in the purview of physicians, including suturing wounds, administering anaesthesia, taking X-rays, and diagnosing illnesses (Elliott, 2010) (Figure 3.3).

NURSING EDUCATION IN CANADA

The Nightingale model shaped the development of nursing education in Canada. In the late nineteenth century, hospitals were transformed into sites of modern medicine that required trained nurses. Hospitals began to establish their own nursing schools based on the principles of Nightingale's apprenticeship model. Unlike Nightingale schools in England, which had independent funding, nursing schools established in Canada had no financing and required students to provide nursing service to the hospital in return for their education and living expenses. This enabled hospitals to provide nursing services at minimal cost. The lack of independent funding limited nursing's control over nursing education. Up until 1940, most patient care in hospitals was provided by student nurses. Graduate nurses typically went into private-duty or public health nursing. Historian of nursing Kathryn McPherson argues that the strongest evidence of Nightingale's influence in Canada is "not in the direct application of the

Nightingale blueprint, but in the ideological power of Nightingale's publicly articulated vision for nursing education and in her ability to champion nursing as a respectable occupation for women" (McPherson, 2005, p. 78).

The First Canadian Nursing Schools

In 1874, Theophilus Mack, MD, established a nursing school at St. Catharines General and Marine Hospital in Ontario. He hoped to improve the sanitation and postsurgical mortality rates at the hospital by replacing untrained nurses with trained nurses. He hired two nurses who had trained in the Nightingale system in London to set up the nurse training program. This was the first nursing school in Canada to operate under the Nightingale system, and its bylaws were influenced by Nightingale's ideas. Mack wrote that student nurses were to be "kind and respectful on all occasions," attend to the needs of their patients with the "gentleness and exactitude taught by their superiors," "faithfully carry out the physician's directions," and "never to interfere with or criticize the treatment" (Gibbon & Mathewson, 1947, p. 145). Students were taught to observe patients for changes in temperature, skin condition, pulse, and respirations (Healey, 1990). The Nightingale influence is best captured in the school's motto: "I see and I am silent" (Kirkwood, 2005, p. 184).

The movement to establish hospital schools of nursing swept the country. The School for Nurses at the Toronto General Hospital was established in 1881; Mary Agnes Snively was appointed superintendent in 1884 (Box 3.2). Although working and living conditions were poor, Snively worked hard to improve the program. In 1896, she introduced a 3-year course with 84 hours of practical nursing and 119 hours of instruction by the medical staff (Gibbon & Mathewson, 1947). In 1887, the Winnipeg General Hospital initiated the first Training School for Nurses in Western Canada. During the First World War, 134 of its graduates served as nurses (Gibbon & Mathewson, 1947). By 1890, hospitals in Montreal, Fredericton, Saint John, Halifax, and Charlottetown had opened schools. Vancouver General Hospital began a school in 1891, and in Alberta, a school was opened in Medicine Hat in 1894. By 1930, there were 212 training schools in the 886 hospitals across Canada (Kirkwood, 2005).

Racism in Nursing Education and Practice

Racism has deep historical roots in nursing and health care. Nursing leaders and school administrators used educational, linguistic, and race-related barriers, along with marital status and age, to define nursing as a "respectable" profession for young, unmarried, middle-class, White women (McPherson, 2005). This was part of a wider campaign to elevate the status of nursing and differentiate nursing from untrained domestic service and caregiving work. As a result, men and racialized women were barred from nursing schools. In 1931, 99.8% of Canadian graduate nurses identified as having British, French, or European ancestry (McPherson, 1996, p. 118). Indigenous and Black students were largely excluded from nursing schools until after the Second World War. Small numbers of Chinese Canadian and Japanese Canadian women were admitted to Vancouver General Hospital in the 1930s, but it was on the assumption that they would work in "their own" communities (McPherson, 1996, p. 118). In the 1930s, Vancouver General Hospital had a "foreign ward" for Chinese, South Asian, Mexican, and Japanese patients (Grypma, 2008). Before 1920, the Chinese and Japanese communities organized and financed private hospitals to serve their local communities for both humanitarian and political ends (Vandenberg, 2017).

Some racialized nurses, unable to gain access to nursing schools in Canada, pursued nursing education in the United States. Charlotte

BOX 3.2 | Milestones in Canadian Nursing History

Mary Agnes Snively, 1847–1933

Mary Agnes Snively was a teacher before she was a nurse. Upon graduation from the school of nursing at Bellevue Hospital, New York, in 1894, she was appointed Lady Superintendent of Nurses at Toronto General Hospital and director of the school of nursing. Snively found that there was no organized plan for the students' classes or clinical experience, nor was there a residence (students were housed in various locations in the hospital). Written records of nursing care, medical orders, and client histories were also lacking.

Snively rectified all these deficiencies. A residence was soon built; she developed a curriculum plan, including nursing theory and practice; and she lengthened the education period to 3 years. By the end of her tenure in 1910, the Toronto General Hospital school was thriving as the largest school of nursing in Canada, with hundreds of graduates, a full complement of students, and many more seeking admission.

Snively achieved acclaim for her organizational work. She attended the historic 1899 founding meeting of the International Council of Nurses (ICN) in England, and was elected first honorary treasurer of the ICN, even though Canada did not have the necessary national nursing association to become an ICN member at the time. In 1907, Snively established the Canadian Society of Superintendents of Training Schools for Nurses. Recognizing that a national organization would be needed for Canada to become a member of the ICN, she was the driving force behind the 1908 founding of the Provisional Society of the Canadian National Association of Trained Nurses (CNATN, later the CNA), becoming its first president. She shepherded the entry of the fledgling Canadian organization to membership in the ICN and later served as ICN vice president.

From Gibbon, J. M., & Mathewson, M. S. (1947). *Three centuries of Canadian nursing.* Macmillan; Riegler, N. (1997). *Jean I. Gunn: Nursing leader.* Associated Medical Services with Fitzhenry & Whiteside.

Edith Anderson Monture, from the Six Nations of the Grand River in Ontario, broke many barriers to become the first Indigenous registered nurse in Canada, in 1914. Although Anderson applied to nursing school in Ontario, she was denied admission. The federal *Indian Act* posed an additional barrier, as it restricted "Status Indians" from pursuing higher education. Undeterred, Anderson attended New Rochelle Hospital School of Nursing in New York, graduating first in her class in 1914, and then working as a public health nurse in New York City. She volunteered as a Nursing Sister with the American Expeditionary Force's Army Medical Corps and served overseas at a US Army base hospital in France before returning to the Six Nations reserve in 1919 (Eggertson, 2020). Married with children, she worked as a midwife and nurse at Lady Willingdon Hospital on the reserve until her retirement in 1955. Under the *Military Voters Act, 1917,* Anderson became the first Indigenous women to gain the right to vote in a federal election (Conn, 2017). Throughout her life, she advocated for better health care and the extension of voting rights to Indigenous peoples in Canada.

In the first half of the twentieth century, nursing administrators used unwritten rules to prevent Black students from entering nursing schools. This included statements about the applicant's unsuitable character, their inability to handle science, or patients' discomfort with being cared for by Black nurses. Commenting on the reasons why her nursing school applications were rejected in the 1940s, would-be nurse Agnes Clinton commented, "They said I was too tall, too big, would do better somewhere else, or some other excuse" (Daubs, 2019). Clinton later became the first Black nurse to graduate from Women's College Hospital School of Nursing in Toronto, in 1951.

Similarly, Donna Smith, who became the first Black nurse practitioner (NP) in Nova Scotia, applied to a nursing school in Saint John, New Brunswick, and was accepted. After the school received her picture (which students were often required to submit as part of their application), she was told that she would not be able to attend the school because she had not taken trigonometry (Mount Saint Vincent University Archives, 2005).

In yet another example, a Black woman wrote to Toronto General Hospital in 1940. She indicated that she was Black and requested an application, but was informed that there were no vacancies. She subsequently wrote to the hospital again, this time using a variation of her name in Spanish and omitting her race. She was invited to the hospital for an interview (Flynn, 2009).

Black Canadian nurses who entered nursing in the 1950s had grown up with an awareness of racial discrimination and learned skills to cope. As children, they had been subjected to legal ordinances that created segregated facilities for Black and White Canadians and had watched family members work toward racial justice (Flynn, 2009). Once they were admitted to nursing schools, Black students were separated from White students, placed in segregated residences, and faced racism from patients. Yet, they formed strong bonds with each other and were aware that they were forging a path for future generations of Black nurses, which gave them the strength to endure the racism they experienced.

Historian Karen Flynn notes that Black nurses could never be "just nurses" (Flynn, 2021). Marginalization in nursing, combined with the socioeconomic conditions in Black communities, led them to activism. Lillie Johnson, born in Jamaica in 1922, studied nursing in Scotland in the early 1950s and trained as a midwife in England in 1955. She practised as a nurse in Jamaica and in the United States before working in Canada as a public health nurse, administrator, and volunteer. During this time, she advocated for the improvement of living conditions for Caribbean farm workers in Ontario. From 1974 until 1981, Johnson worked as a nursing consultant for the Ontario Ministry of Health. She founded the Sickle Cell Association of Ontario in 1981, and influenced the Ontario Ministry of Health and Long-Term Care's decision in 2005 to include sickle-cell disease as one of the genetic diseases included in universal newborn screening (Flynn & Armstrong, 2020).

Gloria Clarke Baylis, a British-trained Caribbean migrant nurse, won Canada's first case of discrimination in employment. In 1964, she inquired about a part-time nursing position at the Queen Elizabeth Hotel in Montreal. At her interview, she was told that the position had been filled. The next day, she phoned the hotel and was told that the position was still open and that the hotel was accepting applications. Baylis filed a complaint under Quebec's new *Act Respecting Discrimination in Employment.* A judge ruled that the hotel had violated the act and ordered the hotel to pay a fine. Baylis' activism had much broader implications for Black Canadians, who were empowered to bring attention to discriminatory practices in the workplace (Flynn, 2018).

Nursing is beginning to acknowledge its racist and colonial past and its impact on the present. For example, in 2020, the CASN, in partnership with the CINA, published a framework for responding to the Truth and Reconciliation Commission of Canada's Calls to Action. The document included the recognition that "nursing students need to develop an understanding of the social determinants of health including systemic and interpersonal racism, learn to implement anti-racism interventions, and to provide culturally safe care" (CASN, 2020, p. 10).

The Impact of Nursing Organizations on Nursing Education

The Victorian Order of Nurses. As hospital training schools for nurses were being established, nurses began to advocate for improved educational standards and passage of legislation for their profession. Women's associations were instrumental in the public health care crusade in Canada and in the rise of nursing organizations. The National Council of Women, under the presidency of Lady Ishbel Aberdeen, wife of the governor general of Canada, approved the formation of the Victorian Order of Nurses (VON) in 1898. Lady Aberdeen had conceived the idea of establishing the VON after she discovered the plight of women in Western Canada who had to give birth in remote locations with no assistance. The formation of the VON signified the setting of a professional standard of education for Canadian nurses that recognized the need not only for altruism and compassion but also for nursing knowledge (Figure 3.4).

The International Council of Nurses. The International Council of Nurses (ICN) started out as a small organization in the broader context of the women's movement (Boschma, 2014). The organization was founded in 1899 as the initiative of British nurse and suffragist Ethel Gordon Manson (later Mrs. Bedford Fenwick), who also founded the British Nurses' Association with her husband a decade earlier. The founders of the ICN sought to address the professional welfare of nurses, the interests of women, and the improvement of people's health. The founding members were part of a growing number of women who were active in social and health care reform and who simultaneously sought to improve women's social position, including by seeking the right to vote (Boschma, 2014, p. 115).

When Bedford Fenwick founded the ICN in 1899, the first member organizations to join were Britain, Germany, and the United States—countries without national nursing organizations could not become members. Although Canada did not yet have a national nursing organization, Mary Agnes Snively was elected as the first treasurer of the ICN and held the position until 1904. The formation of the ICN was a catalyst in organizing Canadian nurses. The *Canadian Nurse* journal was established in 1905. While others focused on establishing a national journal, Snively focused on organizing the superintendents of nursing schools. In 1907, she was named the first president of the Canadian Society of Superintendents of Training Schools for Nurses. In 1908, the new Canadian National Association of Trained Nurses (CNATN, later the CNA) was established, with Snively as its first president. In 1909, the CNATN was officially welcomed into the ICN. For almost a century, the ICN has sustained its place as the key organization for uniting nurses around the globe (Boschma, 2014, p. 115). In May 2021, Michelle Acorn, former provincial CNO at the Ontario Ministry of Health and Long-Term Care, was appointed as chief nurse of the ICN (CNA, 2021).

The Origins of the Canadian Nurses Association and Provincial Nursing Associations

After becoming a full-fledged member of the ICN in 1909, the CNATN streamlined its organization when the registration of nurses was established through legislation in each province. The CNATN changed its name to the Canadian Nurses Association (CNA) in 1924, and it

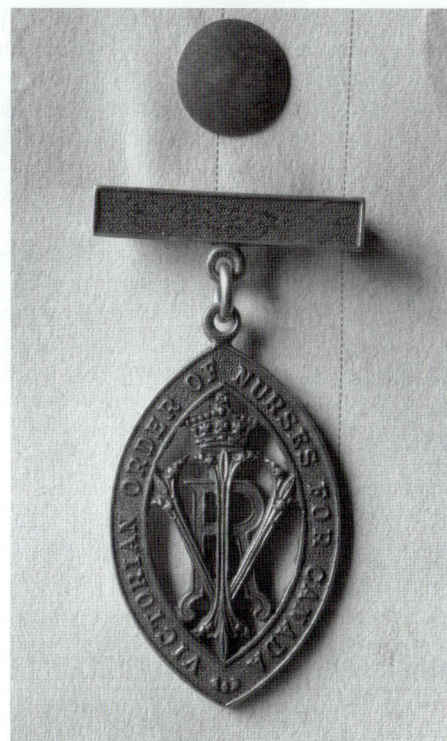

FIGURE 3.4 Victorian Order of Nurses badge, Edmonton, Alberta, 1927. (Glenbow Archives, NC-6-12085.)

became a federation of provincial nursing associations in 1930 (CNA, 1968).

The struggle for women's rights helped nurses to secure laws to regulate their profession. Nurses formed provincial nurses' associations and sought legislation that would set educational standards and improve nursing care. The first province to gain such legislation was Nova Scotia, where a voluntary registration act was passed in 1910. It also allowed nongraduate nurses to register. Initial acts passed in other provinces contained more restrictive standards. Admission criteria and curricula were set for nursing schools, as were rules governing the registration and discipline of practising nurses.

Provincial or territorial legislation and regulations are used to grant qualified nurses the legal authority to use the title "registered nurse" or "RN" (CNA, 2015). The distinguishing feature of *mandatory legislation* is that the statute defines the scope of nursing practice and protects the use of the title "registered nurse," whereas *permissive legislation* only protects the use of the title "registered nurse" (Baker, 2020). Licensure laws are designed to protect the public against unqualified and incompetent practitioners.

In 1979, Sister Simone Roach was appointed by the CNA to develop a new code of ethics for Canadian nurses (Meyers, 2013). Roach identified two underlying values: (1) caring as a unique focus of nursing and (2) respect for persons, and its related principle, the sanctity of human life (Meyers, 2013, p. 238). Approved by the CNA Board of Directors in 1980, the code was intended to provide meaningful guidelines for nurses experiencing ethical conflicts in daily practice. Through its various iterations since then, the *CNA Code of Ethics for Registered Nurses* (CNA, 2017) has remained a value-based, rather than a rule-based, code for Canadian nurses (Storch, in Meyers, 2013).

The First University Programs

The devastating consequences of the First World War and the influenza pandemic of 1918 led to support for public health programs and new patterns of health care delivery. Community health care was promoted, and nurses were seen as central participants who needed university-level education. To this end, the Canadian Red Cross Society awarded grants to several Canadian universities to develop postgraduate courses in public health nursing: the University of Toronto, McGill University, The University of British Columbia, the University of Alberta, Dalhousie University, and the University of Western Ontario (Canadian Red Cross Society, 1962).

The first Canadian undergraduate nursing degree program was established at The University of British Columbia in 1919, with Ethel Johns as director. The operating costs of the new department were to be borne by the hospital, an incentive for the university to support the program. The program was nonintegrated—that is, "the university assumed no responsibility for the two or three years of nursing preparation in a hospital school of nursing" (Bonin, 1976, p. 7). In the 1920s and 1930s, several new 5-year nonintegrated degree programs began at the following Canadian universities: the University of Western Ontario, the University of Alberta, l'Institut Marguerite d'Youville, the University of Ottawa, and St. Francis Xavier University. In 1942, the University of Toronto became the first institution in Canada to approve a degree in nursing.

HEALTH CARE AND EDUCATIONAL REFORM

The *Weir Report*

Between 1874, when the first Canadian nursing school was opened, and the 1930s, when Canada boasted 330 hospital training schools (Paul, 2020), nursing education remained virtually unchanged—hospitals used apprenticeship-style training (Pijl-Zieber et al., 2014). Nursing students were the primary means of staffing hospitals. Hospitals provided a low-cost education, and students provided a low-cost service. Growing concern about the quality of nursing education and exploitation of nursing students led to a nationwide study on nursing education that was jointly funded by the CNA and the Canadian Medical Association(CMA). The resultant *Survey of Nursing Education in Canada* (Weir, 1932), known as the *Weir Report*, confirmed widespread insufficient classroom instruction and lack of variety in clinical experience. The report recommended that nurse preparation be transferred from hospitals to the general education system, and that nurses receive adequate liberal arts as well as technical education at the degree level. Despite these recommendations, by the 1960s, 95% of Canadian nurses were still being trained in hospitals (Pijl-Zieber et al., 2014).

Education Reform

Preparing a sufficient number of graduate nurses became the rallying cry of the 1940s, both during the war and throughout the late 1940s and 1950s. In the expansionist years of the 1960s, nursing leaders called for nursing education reform: better-prepared faculty in schools, and high quality and standards as priorities in nursing education programs. Sparked by an interest in accreditation, the CNA sponsored a second nationwide survey of nursing education, conducted by Helen Mussallem. The resultant 1960 report, *Spotlight on Nursing Education*, found that only 16% of schools met the criteria for accreditation (Pijl-Zieber et al., 2014). Mussallem's recommendation that the CNA focus on upgrading nursing education led to another report in 1964, *A Path to Quality*, intended to serve as a plan to revise nursing education. The 1965 Royal Commission on Health Services, led by Justice Emmett Hall, called for the separation of nursing education from hospital services (Baker, 2014). Both reports recommended a two-tiered education system with baccalaureate-prepared leaders and diploma-prepared bedside nurses (Baker, 2014; Pijl-Zieber et al., 2014). The *Hall Commission Report* successfully initiated the demise of the hospital training schools and launched 10 additional baccalaureate nursing programs.

Baccalaureate as an Entry-to-Practice Requirement

By the 1960s, a movement to separate nursing education programs from the authority of hospitals began in earnest. Two-year programs in nursing began to appear, and Ontario, Quebec, and Saskatchewan developed a system of diploma-granting programs based entirely in community colleges. This transfer of diploma programs to the general education system was in full swing when, in 1975, the Alberta Task Force on Nursing Education recommended that all new graduates be prepared at the baccalaureate level before entering professional practice. The position was endorsed by the Alberta Association of Registered Nurses in 1976. The provincial governments' reluctance for two decades to endorse the baccalaureate as the standard for entry to the practice of nursing reflected the fact that equality in education for women in nursing did not come easily.

In 1982, the CNA passed a resolution that nurses would need to earn a baccalaureate degree as an entry-to-practice requirement. The entry-to-practice position stipulated that by the year 2000, all new graduates in nursing must be qualified at the baccalaureate level when they entered professional practice. Although it was a government committee in Alberta that originally proposed this position in 1975, it took less than a decade for the idea to spread across the country and become a highly valued goal of the nursing profession. When nursing organizations released their own statements in support of this position, they hoped that it would become a reality by the target date. At the same time, they recognized from the outset that achieving the position would be unlikely by the year 2000; it was simply a target date to help them move toward the goal. Contrary to what many believed, the position never had any kind of legal or political mandate.

By 1988, when the New Brunswick Association of Registered Nurses endorsed the position, all provincial associations had declared their support (CNA, 1991). The announcement by the premier of New Brunswick in 1992 that the baccalaureate degree should be a prerequisite to the practice of nursing was the first such endorsement by a first minister of a Canadian province (Nurses Association of New Brunswick, 1992). Implementation of the baccalaureate standard occurred first in Prince Edward Island in 1992, but that would not have been the case without the strong support of its provincial government. Slowly but surely, other provincial governments endorsed the position and made adjustments in the capacity of their provincial degree-granting nursing education programs in order to accommodate all students studying nursing at the undergraduate level. Between 2000 and 2010, baccalaureate education as an entry-to-practice requirement was realized in every province and territory in Canada, except for Quebec (Baker, 2020).

INFLUENCE OF PERIODS OF SOCIAL UPHEAVAL ON NURSING

Public Health, War, and the Emergence of University Nursing Education

Canadian nurses who served in the military during World War I (1914–1918) left an extraordinary legacy (Toman, 2016). During that time, a small cadre of 2 845 women cared for over 750 000 patients in 135 medical units for the duration of the war. Serving mostly in France, England, and the Mediterranean, these nurses worked close to the front lines or along evacuation routes to military hospitals, adapting their nursing to extreme wartime conditions. Although recognized through public memorials, such as the Nurses' Memorial in the Centre Block of

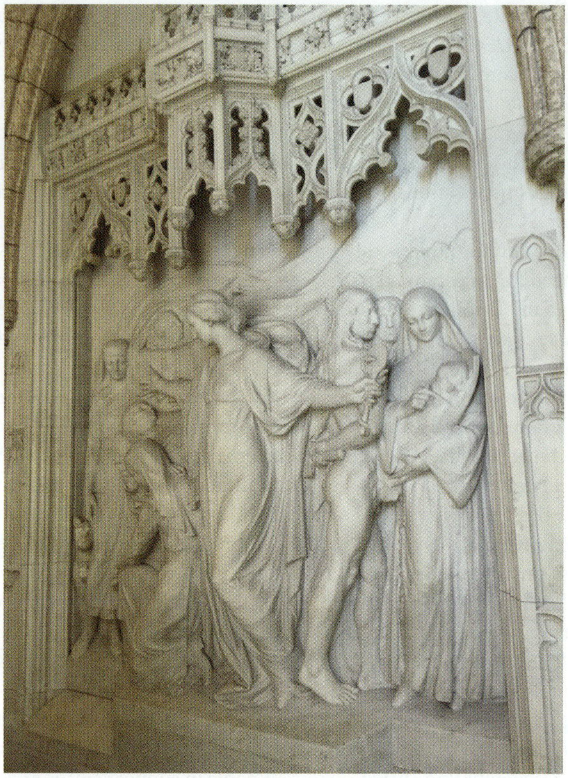

FIGURE 3.5 Nurses' Memorial on Parliament Hill in Ottawa, Canada. The Nurses' Memorial was funded entirely through donations made by nurses from across the country and their provincial associations. (Courtesy Sonya Grypma, RN, PhD.)

the Parliament of Canada, it is only recently that these nurses' work has been a subject of serious study (Toman, 2016) (Figure 3.5).

The devastating consequences of the war were compounded by the worldwide influenza epidemic of 1918 and 1919. The pandemic led to support for public health programs and new patterns of health care delivery to prevent disease and improve the health and well-being of Canadians. The impetus for the introduction of nursing programs to the university, then, was the perceived need for additional and highly capable nursing staff for public health work. In the aftermath of World War I, the impact of casualties and disability led to new value being placed on promoting and maintaining health. The health of mothers and children was seen as particularly critical to the nation because nurturing the health of the young was believed to raise the likelihood that the adult population of the future would be healthier than that of the past. In the new movement to promote health in the community, nurses were seen as central players who needed further university-level preparation for their work.

Because of these issues, the Canadian Red Cross Society became a partner in establishing the League of Red Cross Societies and in planning an international program for peacetime activity in public health. This organization served as a catalyst for the development of university programs in nursing. A national committee was formed with representatives from the CNATN, the Canadian Red Cross Society, and the St. John Ambulance Association, and they endorsed resolutions on September 10, 1919, to approach the universities with a view to supporting the establishment of nursing departments (Canadian Red Cross Society, 1962). The Canadian Red Cross Society then gave 3-year grants to six Canadian universities for the development of postgraduate courses in public health nursing. Funds for the provision of facilities for postgraduate instruction in public health nursing subsidized

special courses for 3 years at the University of Toronto, McGill University, The University of British Columbia, the University of Alberta, and Dalhousie University (Gibbon & Mathewson, 1947, p. 342).

When the first course in public health nursing was offered at the University of Alberta in 1918, shortly after the establishment of the Public Health Nursing Service, it became the first nursing program to be offered by a university in Canada (Department of Public Health Nursing, 1918). This 2-month course began on April 1, 1918 (Stewart, 1979). A second course ran in 1919, and a third in 1921. The *Public Health Nurses' Act*, passed in 1919, formalized the program and designated the University of Alberta as the institution offering the course. The act specified that the program would lead to a certificate or diploma and authorized the graduate to "affix after her name the letters 'PH.'"

From the Great Depression to the Post–World War II Years

The Great Depression "brought unemployment and hardship to nurses" (Allemang, 1974, p. 172). Patients could no longer afford to employ private-duty nurses, the area of employment that had been the most promising for graduate nurses (Gunn, 1933). During the Great Depression, Canadian universities faced reduced revenues, staff layoffs, and difficult working conditions. This period was especially hard on McGill University, which depended on funds from private sources. Raising private funds became next to impossible. Leaders of McGill's nursing school had fought unsuccessfully for years for a degree program. Once the university's finances began to deteriorate, the Board of Governors threatened to close the school altogether. The school's director gave up her salary, the faculty bought books for the library, and nursing alumnae groups all over the country raised funds to ensure the survival of McGill's nursing school (Tunis, 1966).

During World War II, health education again became a priority as doctors and nurses were needed to care for military personnel as well as civilians. Nurses who held critical positions as administrators, supervisors, teachers, and public health nurses were recruited for military service and left their positions. A shortage of nurses soon developed. During and after the war, a new interest in nursing education led to increased external university funding, more scholarships and bursaries from private foundations, the growth of existing schools, and the founding of new programs between 1941 and 1949 (at Queen's, McMaster, Manitoba, Mount Saint Vincent, and Dalhousie).

The new interest in nursing education led to exciting innovations. In 1942, the University of Toronto introduced an integrated basic degree program. Under the leadership of Edith Kathleen Russell (see Chapter 4), courses in the arts and sciences were taught concurrently with nursing courses to enhance student development. Also, university instructors supervised student clinical practice at health care agencies. At McGill, new funds flowed in, and in 1944, supporters of the school were rewarded with a 5-year nonintegrated degree program. In 1946, 4 years after the introduction of the University of Toronto basic degree program, a second basic degree program was developed at McMaster University under Gladys Sharpe's direction.

Emerging From Economic and Military Crises

In the 1960s, existing nursing degree programs expanded, and new programs emerged at other universities. The first master's degree program in nursing was established at the University of Western Ontario in 1959, followed in the 1960s and 1970s by similar programs at universities across the country. In 1962, the Canadian Nurses Foundation was established as an entity separate from the CNA to provide scholarships, bursaries, and fellowships for graduate studies in nursing.

Nursing leaders called for better faculty preparation, more integrated programs, and more university-based opportunities for students, such as student placements and increased enrollments. The movement to separate nursing education programs from the authority of hospitals began in earnest, particularly after the studies on nursing education conducted in the early 1960s identified persistent problems.

Universities resisted introducing basic integrated degree programs because of the costs associated with the low student–teacher ratios required for clinical nursing. It was cheaper for them to let hospitals finance clinical education, but this meant that universities granted degrees for work over which they had no control. In 1964, the Royal Commission on Health Services castigated universities for this practice. By the late 1960s, the basic integrated degree program, modelled on the program at the University of Toronto, finally became the prototype for the establishment of integrated programs in nursing in universities across Canada.

In 1967, Dalhousie University offered the first education program for NPs working at remote nursing stations (Worster et al., 2005). In 1973, the CNA and CMA released a joint statement expressing their agreement on the need for an expanded role for nurses (CNA and CMA, 1973). That same year, a group of NP graduates from two newly established NP education programs at the University of Toronto and McMaster University established the Nurse Practitioners' Association of Ontario. However, these programs were closed in 1983 owing to lack of both funding for positions and legislative support for the role. Despite this outcome, approximately 250 NPs worked in Ontario through the 1980s and early 1990s, primarily at community health centres and northern nursing stations (Worster et al., 2005). In 1995, NP university programs were re-established. In 1997, Ontario passed the *Expanded Nursing Services for Patients Act*, which allowed RNs who hold an extended certificate to provide primary health care services (Bill 127, *Expanded Nursing Services for Patients Act*, 1997).

Throughout the 1970s and 1980s, university faculties and schools of nursing developed research resources so that they could offer graduate programs first at the master's level and then at the doctoral level. The first doctoral nursing program was established at the University of Alberta's Faculty of Nursing on January 1, 1991, and others quickly followed.

Nursing Education Today

With continuing expansion of health care knowledge and technology, beginning practitioners require a broad educational foundation. New curricula and collaborative baccalaureate programs across the country attest to the profession's commitment to maintaining high standards of health care and responding to society's changing health care needs. In collaborative programs, students may take part or all of their degree at a partner institution to the university that is granting the degree, such as a college in another region. The Internet, digital technology, computerized learning and testing programs, and online courses provide practising nurses with many options to complete their degrees. The CNA's website features a database with professional development resources, available to nurses across the country. Some universities have innovative programs at the baccalaureate level, including accelerated programs offered to candidates who already hold a baccalaureate degree in another field. Baccalaureate, master's, and doctoral programs are offered online, in full or in part.

Standards for nursing education are monitored by provincial regulators and associations and by the CASN to ensure that educational programs are of appropriate quality and that they respond to changes in health care. Anyone applying to practise as an RN in Canada must pass the National Council Licensure Examination (NCLEX). This is one of several requirements for entry to practice. On a national level, the CASN has developed the *National Nursing Education Framework*, a national consensus-based framework describing expectations for

baccalaureate, master's, and doctoral programs in nursing education (CASN, 2022). As health professionals, nurses must acquire, maintain, and continuously enhance the knowledge, skills, attitudes, and judgement necessary to meet patient needs in an evolving health care system. The responsibility for educational support for competent nursing practice is shared among individual nurses, professional nursing organizations, educational institutions, and governments (Baker, 2020).

The need for nurses with graduate degrees is rising in tandem with the need for research. A master's degree in nursing (typically a Master of Nursing [MN] or Master of Science in Nursing [MSN]) is required for nurses seeking positions as clinical nurse specialists, nurse administrators, or nurse educators. Most master's programs in Canada now offer streams in nursing leadership, education, and advanced practice. This graduate-level training provides advanced preparation in nursing science, theory, and practice, with emphasis on evidence-informed clinical practice and knowledge translation.

In most provinces, RNs who would like to become NPs will need to complete further education at the graduate level, but this varies across provinces (CASN, 2011a). In British Columbia, NPs were first legislated in 2005 (MacDonald, 2006). NPs in British Columbia work in many practice settings and across three "streams," or populations: family, adult, and pediatrics. NPs are not substitutes for physicians, but their roles complement one another's to improve patient access. NPs bring the nursing focus of teaching, counselling, and support to the diagnostics and treatment they provide (College of Registered Nurses of British Columbia, 2017).

In comparison, Ontario has had primary health care NPs since the 1970s, although the role was first regulated in 1998 through the introduction of the Extended Class designation. Adult and pediatric NPs (formerly known as acute care NPs) have worked in Ontario hospitals since the late 1980s. There are now four NP specialty certificates in the Extended Class: NP-Primary Health Care, NP-Pediatrics, NP-Adult, and NP-Anesthesia (Nurse Practitioners' Association of Ontario, 2020). The Ontario Primary Health Care Nurse Practitioner Program (OPHCNPP) offers a common curriculum across nine university sites, some as part of a master's degree (MN-PHCN) and others as a PHCN certificate (OPHCNPP, n.d.). In Ontario, NPs work in community health, long-term care, palliative care, Indigenous health centres, community-based facilities, and ambulatory care centres as well as on family health teams (OPHCNPP, n.d.).

Doctoral nursing education in Canada consists solely of PhD programs in nursing; there are no profession- or practice-based doctoral programs (CASN, 2011b). Nurses with doctorates can undertake research that advances knowledge and evidence-informed practice (see Chapter 8 for further information about research). This research enhances the quality of nursing care and improves health outcomes for Canadians.

SUMMARY

Organized nursing has been a part of the social fabric of Canada for nearly four centuries. The development of Canadian health care institutions is complex, marked by altruism and racism, inequality and advocacy for equitable care. A fundamental guiding principle of the French-Canadian hospitals that survived largely intact into the twentieth century was that care was available to all people regardless of their background, status in life, or ability to pay. This continues to be a principle for which nurses, through their professional organizations, have argued in national debates on the nature and continuing direction of Canada's national health care insurance program. In the presence of pressure to reshape Medicare, nurses have continued to strongly resist calls for privatization of more aspects of the health system. They have also repeatedly called for all health care providers to be remunerated on a salary or contract basis (Paul, 2005, 2020).

The transformation of both nursing and the nursing education programs that have supported the profession since the nineteenth century has been truly remarkable. Nurses have demonstrated the value of their service, the integrity of their goals, the quality of their education programs, and the strength of their commitment. It is certain that the nursing profession will continue to evolve in the interest of providing high-quality nursing care.

KEY CONCEPTS

- Nursing has responded to the health care needs of society, which have been influenced over time by economic, social, and cultural factors.
- Nurses were involved in the delivery of unequal health care to Indigenous peoples in Canada through colonial medicine, including through the Indian hospital system.
- The Nightingale model of nursing shaped the establishment of the first nursing schools in Canada in the late 1800s.
- The development of a system of nursing education in Canada emerged from the early nursing sisterhoods and from schools of nursing associated with hospitals.
- Baccalaureate as an entry-to-practice requirement for nursing has been fully implemented in English-speaking Canada.
- Basic nursing education is acquired in college, collaborative college–university, or university programs.

CRITICAL THINKING EXERCISES

1. Explain the influence of Florence Nightingale's ideas on the development of nursing education in Canada.
2. Identify some of the ways that racism has shaped the history of nursing and health care in Canada.
3. Describe the Indian hospital system, and discuss its ongoing impact on health care today.
4. Observe various levels of nursing practice, such as a staff nurse, nurse practitioner, and nurse educator. Identify similarities and differences in their roles and educational preparation.
5. Outline some career objectives for yourself after you have completed your nursing program. Think about what you want to do as a practising nurse, and then outline strategies for achieving these goals.

🌐 *Answers to Critical Thinking Exercises appear on the Evolve website.*

REVIEW QUESTIONS

Review Questions 1 to 4 relate to the case study at the beginning of the chapter.

1. The case study described an incident of Indigenous-specific racism in health care. How can knowledge about colonial medicine in Canada assist the nurse with reflecting on experiences like the one described in this case study?
   a. History can assist the nurse to learn important dates about colonial medicine in Canada.
   b. History can provide the nurse with the context needed to understand present-day issues in health care.
   c. History can help to foster new avenues of inquiry in nursing.
   d. History can teach nurses that health care in the past was problematic.
2. Intergenerational trauma is a reality for many Indigenous peoples in Canada because of colonial policies, residential schools, and unequal health care. Which of the following statements best describes your understanding of the Indian hospital system?
   a. Indian hospitals were separate, underfunded, and inadequate facilities for Indigenous patients.
   b. Indian hospitals provided advanced medical care.
   c. Both Indigenous and non-Indigenous patients accessed and used Indian hospitals.
   d. Indian hospitals were adequately funded by the Canadian government.
3. The establishment of the Indian hospital system was motivated by which of the following factors?
   a. Preventing the spread of epidemic disease from Indigenous to settler communities
   b. Providing Indigenous peoples with excellent care
   c. Enabling Indigenous control over Indigenous health care
   d. Creating nursing jobs for newly trained graduate nurses
4. The case study reveals the needs for ongoing efforts to decolonize health care in Canada. Which of the following is a primary goal of the Canadian Indigenous Nurses Association, originally founded in the 1970s?
   a. To achieve better working conditions for all nurses
   b. To create new nursing schools
   c. To create social connections
   d. To improve health care for Indigenous peoples

Answers: 1. b; 2. a; 3. a; 4. d.

🌐 *Rationales for the Review Questions appear on the Evolve website.*

RECOMMENDED WEBSITES

Canadian Association for the History of Nursing (CAHN): https://cahn-achn.ca
An affiliate group of the CNA, the CAHN offers information about Canadian nursing history and promotes historical research.
Canadian Association of Schools of Nursing (CASN): https://www.casn.ca
CASN is the national voice for nursing education, research, and scholarship and represents baccalaureate and graduate nursing programs in Canada.
Canadian Indigenous Nursing Association (CINA): https://indigenousnurses.ca
The mission of the CINA is to improve the health of Indigenous peoples by supporting Indigenous nurses and promoting the development and practice of Indigenous Health Nursing.
Canadian Nurses Association (CNA): https://www.cna-aiic.ca/en

The CNA is the national professional voice of registered nurses in Canada, representing nearly 139 000 members.
Canadian Nursing Students' Association (CNSA): https://cnsa.ca
The CNSA is the national voice of Canadian nursing students.
Canadian Society for the History of Medicine (CSHM): https://cshm-schm.ca
This website provides information about the history of medicine and health care in Canada and promotes historical research.
Coalition of African, Caribbean and Black Nurses in British Columbia (CACBN): https://www.cacbn.ca
The CACBN is a coalition of Black nurses working to address racism and discrimination in nursing and health care.

Consortium for Nursing History Inquiry: https://blogs.ubc.ca/nursinghistory

The Consortium at The University of British Columbia serves as a resource for critical perspectives on nursing and health care history. It includes links to recorded symposia and talks on nursing history.

Nursing History Digitization Project: http://forms.msvu.ca/library/tutorial/nhdp/index.htm

This site explores the history of nursing in Nova Scotia from 1890 until the late twentieth century. Of note is the section on "racial exclusion," which includes interviews with Black women who discuss their experiences of entering the nursing profession.

Nursing History Research Unit (URHN): https://urhn-nhru.com

The URHN at the University of Ottawa is a bilingual, interprofessional research unit focused on academic research on the history of health and nursing.

REFERENCES

A full reference list is available on the website for this book at http://evolve.elsevier.com/Canada/Potter/fundamentals/

4

Community Health Nursing Practice

Canadian content written by Holly Symonds-Brown, RN, PhD, with original chapter contributions by Kaysi Kushner, RN, PhD

OBJECTIVES

Mastery of content in this chapter will enable you to:

- Define the key terms listed.
- Explain the relationship between community health nursing and primary health care.
- Describe the roles and functions of the community health nurse.
- Differentiate between public health nursing, home health nursing, and primary care nursing.
- Explain how structural inequities can lead to marginalization within particular populations.
- Describe the standards, competencies, roles, and activities important for success in community health nursing practice.
- Describe elements of a community assessment.

KEY TERMS

Community
Community-based nursing
Community health nursing
Community health nursing practice
Empowerment
Harm reduction
High-priority populations
Home health nursing
Marginalized populations
Population
Population health
Primary care/Family practice nursing
Primary health care
Public health
Public health nursing
Public health principles
Social justice
Trauma-informed care

WEBSITE

http://evolve.elsevier.com/Canada/Potter/fundamentals/

CASE STUDY

Kira (preferred pronouns: she/her) is a 20-year-old woman who lives in the inner city. Kira has a history of depression, brain injury, hepatitis C, and polysubstance use. She has been living in a temporary shelter for the past 3 months since leaving an abusive relationship. Kira is referred to the outreach nurse from the local harm-reduction program by the shelter staff for help with a sore, reddened area that has developed on her forearm.

Kira is nervous about going to the program space because she has had negative experiences in the past with health care providers judging her for her substance use. Jan (preferred pronouns: she/her), one of the outreach nurses, agrees to meet Kira at the shelter. Jan meets Kira and explains that the harm-reduction service provides lots of different kinds of help and then asks Kira what she would like help with. Kira shows Jan her arm and says that it really hurts but she doesn't want to go to the hospital. Jan takes a look at the arm and asks Kira about any previous history of abscesses or other health problems. Jan asks the questions in a nonjudgemental way that makes Kira feel like an expert about her own body and drug use, making Kira more comfortable with answering the questions. Jan tells Kira that she could help her take care of the sore arm, and, if Kira is interested, she might have some ideas for how to prevent it from happening again. After Kira agrees, Jan reviews safe-injection techniques with Kira and they discuss what might work best for Kira. Jan leaves Kira with enough clean needles, sterile water, and a tourniquet for the week and instructions about using warm compresses. Jan

tells Kira that she will be back at the shelter next week, but if the arm gets redder, Kira can always come by the program and Jan will get the nurse practitioner to give her an antibiotic.

Kira stops by the program 2 days later and sees Jan in the lobby. Jan offers Kira a cup of coffee and introduces her to the other people at the program that day. Kira tells Jan her arm is doing better but she is worried about other things to do with her health. Jan tells her that the program offers health checkups, a safe injection site, needle exchange, STI testing, naloxone kits, a specialized program for pregnant women, and lots of resource referrals. Jan ensures that Kira knows that while the program has lots of options for her, it is Kira who decides for herself what kind of help she wants. Kira asks for help with getting hepatitis medications that she can't afford and also asks about options for more stable housing. At this point, Jan and Kira begin working together toward protecting Kira's health despite her injection drug use and toward decreasing some of the barriers that get in the way of Kira receiving help for other parts of her life.

Later in the year, Jan and the other staff at the program discuss the barriers to health literacy that occur for many of their clients with cognitive impairment or literacy issues. Jan and the other staff work with a small group of clients, including Kira, to design easy-to-read health promotion materials that they then distribute throughout the city.

Think about this case study as you read this chapter. There are review questions at the end of the chapter that relate to the case study.

Today's health care climate is rapidly changing in response to economic pressures, technological and medical advances, and client participation in health care. As a result, many clients are receiving care in the community rather than in hospital. There is a growing need to deliver health care where people live, work, and learn (Community Health Nurses of Canada [CHNC], 2019). Community health nursing care focuses on health promotion and protection, disease and injury prevention, and restorative and palliative care. The goals of community health nursing are to keep individuals healthy, encourage client participation and choice in care, promote health-enhancing social and physical environments, and provide in-home care for ill or disabled patients.

Promoting individual and community health has always been key to the holistic practice of nursing. In the 1730s, the Grey Nuns were established as Canada's first community nursing order. More than a century later, in England, Florence Nightingale articulated a nursing philosophy grounded in knowledge of environmental conditions. By the end of the century, the Victorian Order of Nurses was providing in-home nursing, often in outpost and remote regions of Canada. In the early twentieth century, the civic departments of health employed nurses to establish health education and prevention programs for infant mortality, healthy development of school-aged children, and tuberculosis control (Vukic & Dilworth, 2020).

Canadians such as Kate Brighty Colley and Edith Kathleen Russell pioneered community and public health nursing in Canada. Today, nursing is leading the way in assessing, implementing, and evaluating public and community-based health services needed by patients. Community health nursing is essential for improving the health of the general public.

PROMOTING THE HEALTH OF POPULATIONS AND COMMUNITY GROUPS

Nurses practising in the community face many challenges in promoting the health of populations and community groups. A **population** is a collection of individuals who have in common one or more personal or environmental characteristics (Maurer & Smith, 2005). Examples of populations are Canadians inclusively and, more specifically, older persons or Indigenous peoples. A healthy population is composed of healthy individuals, and the health status of individuals is considered an overall aggregate that reflects an average or general health status. To determine a population's health status, individual characteristics (such as occurrence of illness, disability, and death; lifespan; education; and living conditions) are considered. A **community** is a group of people who share a geographical (locational) dimension and a social (relational) dimension (Diem & Moyer, 2015; Laverack, 2004). The social dimension—which comprises individual relationships, interactions among groups, and shared characteristics among members—distinguishes a community from a population. Examples of communities are geographical groupings (e.g., neighbourhoods) and shared-interest groups (e.g., women's health networks). A healthy community consists of healthy individuals engaged in collective relationships that create a supportive living environment. Both individual and community characteristics are used to determine community health status. Key characteristics of a healthy community include a collective capacity to solve problems; adequate living conditions; a safe environment; and sustainable resources such as employment, health care, and educational facilities.

COMMUNITY HEALTH NURSING PRACTICE

The scope of **community health nursing practice** includes population health promotion, protection, maintenance, and restoration; community, family, and individual health promotion; and individual rehabilitation or palliative care. Community health nurses "promote, protect, and preserve the health of individuals, families, groups, communities, and populations" (CHNC, 2019, p. 8). Practice involves coordinating care and planning services, programs, and policies by collaborating with individuals, caregivers, families, other disciplines, communities, and governments. Practice combines knowledge of nursing theory, including the metaparadigm concepts of person, health, nursing, environment, and social justice as a theoretical foundation, social sciences, and public health science (CHNC, 2019). Figure 4.1 depicts the multiple components of community health nursing practice. **Social justice** is rooted in notions of societal (social) responsibility and fairness (justice). "Social justice is the equitable, or fair, distribution of society's benefits, responsibilities and their consequences. It focuses on the relative position of social advantage of one individual or social group in relation to others in society as well as on the root causes of inequities and what can be done to eliminate them" (Canadian Nurses Association [CNA], 2010, p. 13). Social justice encompasses equity, human rights, democracy and civil rights, capacity building, just institutions, enabling environments, poverty reduction, ethical practice, advocacy, and partnerships (CNA, 2010).

Community health nursing includes the specialties of public health nursing, family practice and primary care nursing, and home health nursing. Within these specialties are a variety of roles, such as community mental health nursing, outpost nursing (Box 4.1), street or outreach nursing, and parish nursing (CHNC, 2019; see also Stamler et al., 2020, for in-depth descriptions of community health nursing roles in Canada). Occupational health nursing has emerged as a distinctive specialized practice, although it is arguably within the inclusive focus of community health nursing.

The community health nursing focus is broad, emphasizing both the community's health and direct care to subpopulations within that community. By focusing on subpopulations, the community health nurse cares for the whole community and considers the individual to be one member of a group. The practice focus of different specialties within community health nursing varies: for example, home health nurses focus on individual clients, then broaden their view to consider family and community, whereas public health nurses more often shift from a broad view of populations to narrow their focus to specific vulnerable groups or families (CHNC, 2019). Regardless of the specific role, function, or setting, community health nursing practice is guided by values of social justice and caring (CHNC, 2019).

Primary health care is defined by the World Health Organization (WHO) and United Nations Children's Fund (UNICEF) as "a whole-of-society approach to health that aims at ensuring the highest possible level of health and well-being and their equitable distribution by focusing on people's needs and as early as possible along the continuum from health promotion and disease prevention to treatment, rehabilitation and palliative care, and as close as feasible to people's everyday environment" (WHO & UNICEF, 2018, p. 2) (see Chapter 2). Primary health care involves the principles of accessibility, public participation, health promotion and appropriate technology, and intersectoral cooperation. These principles guide community health nurses to use empowerment-based models of community practice (CHNC, 2019). **Empowerment** may be most simply described as a psychological, cultural, social, or political process by which people, individually and collectively in organizations and communities, exercise their ability to effect change to enhance control over events in their daily lives (Canadian Public Health Association [CPHA], 2010; Laverack, 2019). Empowerment is both an outcome and a process by which that outcome is achieved. Empowerment exists in dynamic power relations among people, which from a health promotion perspective are expressed as "power with" rather than "power over" relations (Labonte, 1993).

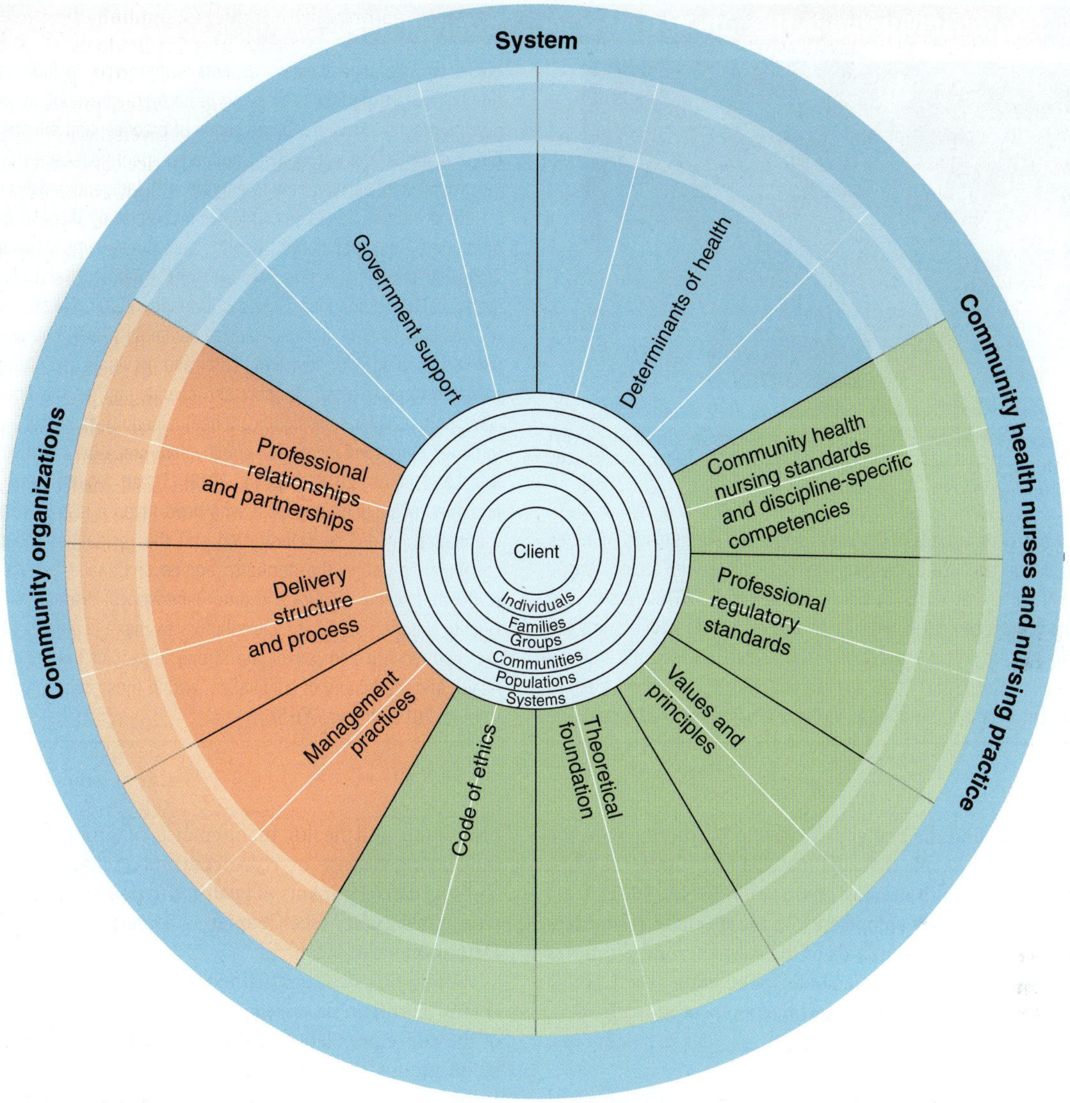

FIGURE 4.1 Canadian community health nursing professional practice model. (From Community Health Nurses of Canada. [2019]. *Canadian community health nursing professional practice model & standards of practice.* [p. 11]. https://www.chnc.ca/en/membership/documents/loadDocument?id=1697&download=1# upload/membership/document/2018-06/canadiancommunityhealthnursingprofessionalpracticecompomentse.pdf. © Community Health Nurses of Canada. Reprinted with permission. Further reproduction prohibited.)

Community empowerment is commonly conceptualized as an interactive process between individuals, family, and the community, through which people organize and take action together toward their goals for social and political change (Laverack, 2019). Criticisms that empowerment is often misinterpreted as increasing individual responsibility but overlooking power and control (Tanekenov et al., 2018) highlight the importance of action to ensure that adequate resources are available for individuals and for groups and communities collectively. Such action needs to be grounded in ethical commitment to inclusion, diversity, participation, social justice, advocacy, and interdependence as a complementary foundation to the Canadian Nurses Association (CNA, 2017) *Code of Ethics* intended to guide all nursing practice.

Empowerment-based skills of patient advocacy and communication and the design of new systems in cooperation with existing systems help make community health nursing practice effective. The Canadian Community Health Nursing Practice Model (CHNC, 2019) articulates how community health nursing care encompasses actions aimed at illness care; illness, disease, or injury prevention; and health promotion. Nursing actions are guided by approaches oriented toward capacity building, participation, collaboration, inclusiveness, equity, social justice, and advocacy. These actions complement one another, even as their underlying aims, approaches to care, and perceptions of clients may differ.

Community health nursing practice requires a distinct set of skills and knowledge. The National Nursing Education Framework (Canadian Association of Schools of Nursing [CASN], 2022) has identified five domains important to undergraduate nursing education that include essential components relevant to preparation for community health nursing practice. These include the foundational skills in communication and collaboration, assessment, planning, and provision of care with diverse patients, along with foundational knowledge of population health, social justice, primary health care, health equity, cultural safety and humility, Indigenous healing practices, and determinants of health (CASN, 2022). Competent community health nurses understand the needs of a population or community through experiences with individuals, families, and groups. They think critically in applying a wide

---

BOX 4.1   **Outpost Nursing in Remote and Northern Communities**

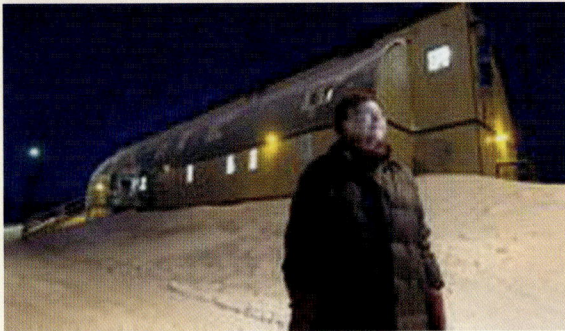

Nurse Cathy Rose stands outside the Resolute Bay Health Centre in Resolute, Nunavut, on November 21, 2013. Ms. Rose, originally from Kitchener, Ontario, had been working in the north for 28 years. (Photo Credit: Peter Power/*The Globe and Mail*.)

Providing health care services to Canada's remote and northern communities has been a challenge because of geographical location as well as Indigenous and northern cultural and linguistic barriers (MacLeod et al., 2018). Health care in these regions is most commonly provided by outpost nurses who assume the role of both primary care provider and primary health care provider. In a study by MacLeod and colleagues (2017), rural and remote outpost nurses were asked to describe what it meant to be a nurse in Canada's Northern territories. The nurses wrote of many positive aspects of their work, including the deep connection between experiences of living in northern communities and those of their nursing practice, having a broad scope of practice, and the ability to use a wide range of skills and autonomy. Challenges identified were related to isolation, geography, and learning how to engage with Indigenous ways of knowing.

Outpost nurses are responsible for incorporating disease prevention, health promotion, and population health and community development practices alongside providing illness management, treatment, and clinical assessment (Berry, 2018; Indigenous Services Canada, 2022). Nurses working in these regions also take on multiple roles of community health nursing by visiting new parents, helping with new baby care, and providing immunization. Provision of these services is often complex and challenging, as the populations in these communities experience significant health inequities related to decreased access to health care, food insecurity, employment precarity, and historical colonialism (MacLeod et al., 2018; Norbye, 2018). These regions tend to be populated primarily by Indigenous people who have faced a loss of cultural identity and traumatization due to colonization and the residential school system. Some communities within the northern regions of Canada experience higher rates of death, suicide, alcohol and drug dependence, disease, and trauma (Health Quality Ontario, 2018). The contributors to these health challenges and issues are multifaceted and reflect the strong impact of the social determinants of health and the history of colonialism within these communities (Health Quality Ontario, 2018; Norbye, 2018).

---

range of knowledge to find the best approaches for partnering with the communities, groups, or people that are their clients. In 2006, the CNA introduced community health nursing certification (CNA, 2021). Certification confirms practitioner competence in the specialty, recognizes nurses who meet the national standards of the specialty, and promotes excellence in nursing care for the Canadian population (see CHNC, 2019 and CNA, 2021 for standards and certification procedures).

Public Health Nursing

Public health nursing merges knowledge from public health science, social and environmental sciences, and primary health care with professional nursing theories to safeguard and improve the health of populations in the community (CHNC, 2019; CPHA, 2010). The goal of public health is to achieve a healthy environment for everyone. To understand public health nursing, it is necessary to know how public health works. The emphasis in **public health** is on the health of the entire population. Historically, government-funded agencies have supported public health programs that improve food and water safety and provide adequate sewage disposal. Public health policy has largely been responsible for the dramatic gain in life expectancy for North Americans during the past century (Fournier & Karachiwalla, 2021; McKay, 2016). **Public health principles** of disease prevention, health promotion and protection, and healthy public policy (CPHA, 2017) can be applied to individuals, families, groups, or communities. Public health practice calls for competencies (i.e., knowledge, skills, attitudes) that cross the boundaries of specific disciplines and are independent of programs and roles (CASN, 2014; Public Health Agency of Canada [PHAC], 2008). These competencies include "public health sciences in nursing practice; population and community health assessment and analysis; population health planning, implementation, and evaluation; partnerships, collaboration and advocacy; and communication in public health nursing" (CASN, 2014, p. 3; see also CHNC, 2019; PHAC, 2008).

A public health focus requires understanding of the needs of a population. Focus may be narrowed to specific target populations with potential risks (e.g., low-income families, recent immigrants). Public health professionals must understand factors influencing the health promotion and health maintenance of groups, trends and patterns influencing disease or risk occurrence within populations, physical and social determinants of health, and political processes used to influence public policy (see Chapter 1, "Determinants of Health and Social Determinants of Health").

Population health is defined by the Public Health Agency of Canada (PHAC, 2013) as "an approach to health that aims to improve the health of the entire population and to reduce health inequities among population groups." The concept was introduced in 1989 by the Canadian Institute for Advanced Research, grounded in the recognition that determinants of health interact in complex ways to influence health. The population health promotion approach (Hamilton & Bhatti, 1996) provides a framework for thinking about health and taking action to improve the health of populations. Action is directed primarily at community levels. Strategies address the determinants of health in order to improve population health and reduce risks (see Chapter 1). Most health determinants involve other sectors of society, such as education, agriculture, business, and government. Multisectoral collaboration between the health sector and other sectors is essential, broadening the scope of nursing practice in the community. Population-based public health programs focus on disease prevention, health protection, and health promotion, which provide a foundation for health care services at all levels (see Chapter 2).

Using public health principles helps public health nurses to understand the environments in which clients live, the factors that influence client health, and the types of interventions supportive of client health. Interventions by public health nurses often include work that is collaborative with the community and often bring a focus on the "bigger picture" of community development, program planning, or policy development and advocacy (CPHA, 2017). Figure 4.2 illustrates a framework for public health programs that provides a means of organizing public health program development in public health practice (Edwards & Moyer, 2000).

Successful public health nursing practice involves capacity-building approaches. This involves using an asset-based approach that focuses on strengths, coalition building, community engagement, and partnerships (CHNC, 2019). The public health nurse is responsive by being

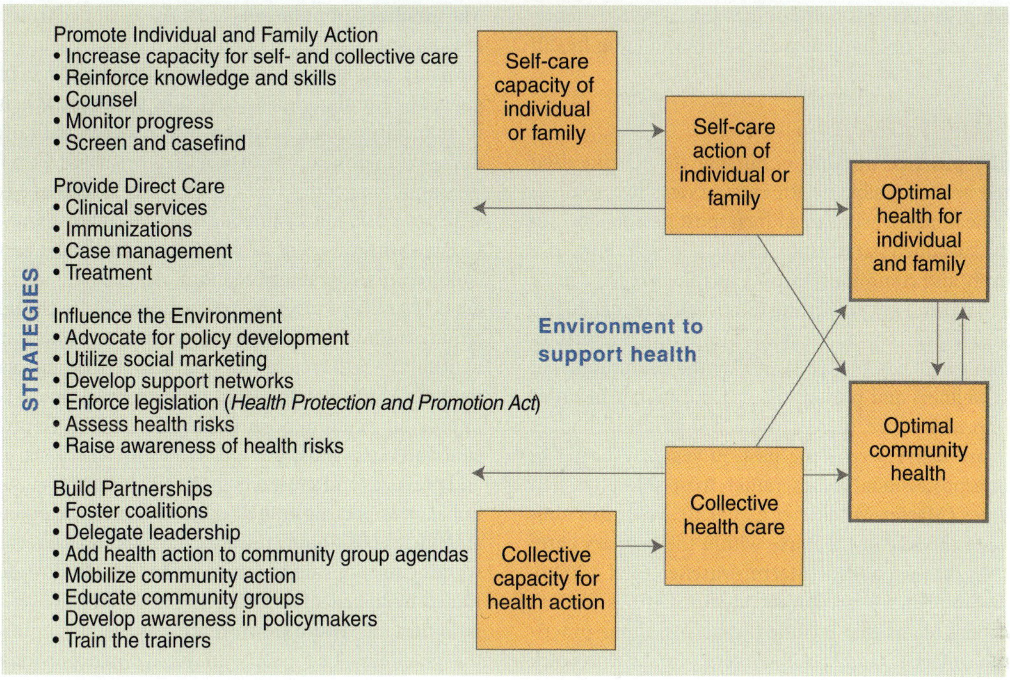

FIGURE 4.2 Framework for public health programs. (From N. Edwards et al. [1995]. *Building and sustaining collective health action: A framework for community health practitioners*. Community Health Research Unit, Pub. No. DP95-1, as cited by Edwards, N. C., & Moyer, A. [2000]. Community needs and capacity assessment: Critical component of program planning. In M. J. Stewart [Ed.], *Community nursing: Promoting Canadians' health* [2nd ed., p. 433]. W. B. Saunders.)

active in the community; knowing its members, needs, and resources; working collaboratively to establish health promotion and disease prevention programs; and advocating for programs and public policies that promote health and build capacity to identify and address health issues among individuals, families, communities, and service providers. This means developing and maintaining relationships with other professional systems and individuals and encouraging them to respond to a population's needs. For example, during the COVID-19 pandemic, Canadian community health nurses worked closely within their communities to advocate for evidence-informed public health approaches; engaged with community partners to ensure equitable access to protective equipment, testing, and vaccines; worked on social messaging campaigns to educate the public; and designed innovative ways to do health promotion and screening under the new circumstances of social distancing (Schofield et al., 2020).

Home Health Nursing

Home health nursing, also known as **community-based nursing**, involves activities related to prevention, health restoration, maintenance, and palliation. The focus of nursing care is on the individual, their designated caregivers, and families, to enhance their day-to-day functioning, capacity for self-care, and promote autonomy in decision making (CHNC, 2019). Nursing takes place in community settings such as the home, assisted living centre, school, or clinic. The nurse's competence is based on critical thinking and decision making in relation to assessing health status, selecting nursing interventions, and evaluating care outcomes. Because they provide care where clients live, work, and play, home health nurses need to be individual- and family-oriented and also need to appreciate the community context (CHNC, 2010).

Components of home health nursing practice include teaching and supports for client and family self-management, preventive care, care within the community context, continuity of care between home and health system services, and collaborative client care among health practitioners (CHNC, 2019). Nurses use their clinical expertise to provide direct care (e.g., a case manager monitors clients recovering from stroke and provides rehabilitation services). Nursing supports and improves clients' quality of life. Illness is seen as one aspect of clients' everyday lives. Nursing tends to be problem focused while also addressing client needs for primary, secondary, and tertiary prevention (CHNC, 2010).

A strong theoretical foundation for home health nursing, and community health nursing broadly, is provided by the ecological model, which conceptualizes human systems as open and interactive with the environment (Bronfenbrenner, 1974; McLeroy et al., 1988). In an ecological model, the individual is viewed within the larger systems of family, social network, community, and society, which are commonly depicted as concentric circles: an innermost circle of the client and the immediate family, a second circle of people and settings that have frequent contact with the client and family, a third circle of the local community and its values and policies, and an outermost circle of larger social systems such as business and government. People's health experiences are shaped by their individual circumstances, social interaction, and organizational processes, all situated in policy and values of the community and society (Keefe et al., 2020) A home health nurse must understand the interaction of all systems while caring for clients and families in the home environment. Nurses typically become involved in the domain of the first three circles. For example, as a home health nurse, you would work closely with a client recently diagnosed with diabetes and with the family to establish a care plan. You would use observations of the client's lifestyle, personal relationships and responsibilities, food security, and access to recreational areas of the neighbourhood when considering an exercise schedule and meal routines. Knowing community resources (e.g., shops with glucose-monitoring supplies, food banks, insulin subsidy programs, or local diabetes support groups) would enable you to provide comprehensive support.

Home health nursing is family-centred care (CHNC, 2010; Hunt, 2013). This care requires knowledge of family theory (see Chapter 20), global health (see Chapter 11), communication (see Chapter 18), and group dynamics. Empowerment-based strategies guide the nurse to work in partnership with clients and families (Sharkey & Lefebre, 2017) in planning, deciding on, implementing, and evaluating health care approaches.

Primary Care or Family Practice Nursing

Primary care/Family practice nursing is nursing that is practised within the integrated and accessible health care services by provided physicians and their health care teams to address most personal health care needs, develop a sustained partnership with patients, and practise in the context of family and community. Most Canadians receive most of their health care in a primary care setting (Statistics Canada, 2019). Accessible and inclusive primary care services are part of the principles of primary health care (see Chapter 2) and are the conditions that improve health and wellness and prevent disease and injury. In order to increase access to primary care, there have been significant changes in organization of care delivery over the past 30 years, resulting in increased use of interprofessional teams rather than sole-physician or provider-run clinics (Martin-Misener et al., 2020). With this shift in health care delivery, the role of the nurse within the primary care/ family practice setting has expanded (Martin-Misener et al., 2020). Often nurses working in primary care/family practice settings work as part of interprofessional teams that include physicians, nurse practitioners, dietitians, pharmacists, and social workers. Nurses who work in primary care/family practice focus on prevention (e.g., fall risk assessment, immunization), health education, assessment, chronic disease management, treatments (e.g., wound care, mental health counselling, insulin management), case management, and medication review (CHCN, 2019). Primary care/family practice nurses use a client-centred approach to work with individuals and families across the lifespan (CHNC, 2019). Case management and system navigation are often part of the role and require strong interprofessional collaboration skills, advocacy, and knowledge of community-level supports.

HIGH-PRIORITY POPULATIONS FOR COMMUNITY HEALTH NURSING

Health promotion can be provided in universal programs where interventions are designed to reach most of the general population (e.g., immunization clinics) or they can target specific populations. Community health nursing, with its roots in social justice and mandate to address health inequity, is frequently focused on delivering specialized programs to reach populations that are deemed to be a high priority due to the lack of protective factors or their increased exposure to risks.

High-Priority Populations: People Most Affected by Health Inequities

High-priority populations are those populations exposed to the most risk through structural barriers of social exclusion, poor access, or dependency on others and who are therefore more likely to develop health problems. Their risks for poor health can be understood in relation to the determinants of health, particularly social determinants that compromise socioeconomic status, literacy, and social inclusion (see Chapter 1). People who live in poverty, people who are homeless, people who live in precarious circumstances (such as women in abusive interpersonal relationships), people with chronic conditions and disabilities, people who engage in stigmatizing risk behaviours (including substance misuse and unsafe sexual practices), as well as Indigenous people, new immigrants and refugees, and people who are LGBTQ2 are all examples of high-priority populations (Beiser & Stewart, 2005). Individuals and their families often belong to more than one of these groups and may live in communities that can be characterized as marginalized by mainstream health and social service practices.

Marginalized populations are those excluded from mainstream social, economic, educational, or cultural life (e.g., groups excluded because of ethnicity, gender identity, sexual orientation, age, physical ability, language, or immigration status). Responding to their distinctive needs in culturally safe and relevant ways is essential for community health nurses in their health care practice.

To provide competent care to people who live in circumstances of structural risk, nurses in community health care practice must be comfortable with diversity as valuable to individual and social well-being. Culture, ethnicity, ability, economic status, gender, and sexual orientation are all aspects of diversity in Canadian society. Comfort with diversity requires more than tolerance of difference, which implies that the dominant culture is the reference point. Chapter 11 addresses factors influencing individual differences within a cultural context and the nurse's role in providing culturally sensitive and safe care. To provide culturally safe care, the nurse must be sensitive to the client's cultural beliefs, values, and practices and must recognize any history of injustice and any power imbalances present in their current context that could affect the client's and nurse's positioning toward each other (Curtis et al., 2019). Whether a working relationship or intervention is culturally safe can only be determined by the client experiencing it, so frequent check-in or evaluation is important. Trauma-informed care is an approach that recognizes the possibility that people may have had previous traumatic experiences in their lives and that processes of care systems can sometimes re-traumatize people by taking away their control and exerting power over them. While not designed specifically as trauma-informed care, practitioners are encouraged to use a strengths-based orientation, have an awareness of effects of trauma, and work *with* clients to determine their needs and the interventions most likely to improve their health (Chang et al., 2021). The nurse should not judge or evaluate a client's beliefs and values about health in terms of the nurse's own culture, beliefs, and values (see Chapter 18 for a more in-depth discussion of communication and relational practice). Communication and caring practices are crucial for understanding clients' perceptions and for planning effective, culturally sensitive, and safe health care. Thus, nurses need to be aware that beliefs about health and medicine are often shaped by one's culture and context. Dominant cultural practices and policies in health care often create barriers for a minority or marginalized population's utilization of services (Browne et al., 2016).

People who live in circumstances of inequity typically experience poorer health outcomes than people with ready access to resources and health care services (Raphael, 2016). Members of marginalized groups frequently experience cumulative risk factors or intersecting risk conditions that can increase the adverse effects of individual risk factors (Raphael, 2016). Community health nurses assessing clients who are marginalized must consider multiple risk factors and the clients' strengths and must work to create services that people find welcoming and supportive. Box 4.2 gives an example of how public health nurses might develop positive spaces for LGBTQ2 individuals, which is one example of a high-priority population that is often marginalized in health care settings.

People Who Live in Poverty or Are Homeless. In Canada, women, children, female lone parents, people with disabilities, older persons without a partner or other family, racialized groups, and recent immigrants are more likely to experience poverty (Raphael, 2016; Statistics Canada, 2021). People who live in poverty are more likely to live in hazardous environments, work at high-risk jobs, have less access to nutritious foods, and experience multiple stressors. They often face practical problems such as limited access to transportation, limited quality child care to support employment, and limited medication or dental coverage from supplementary health benefits. People who are homeless

Adapted from Allwright, K., Goldie, C., Almost, J., et al. (2019). Fostering positive spaces in public health using a cultural humility approach. *Public Health Nursing, 36,* 551–556. https://doi-org.login. ezproxy.library.ualberta.ca/10.1111/phn.12613; Fahlberg, B., Foronda, C., & Baptiste, D. (2016). Cultural humility. *Nursing, 46*(9), 14–16. https://doi.org/10.1097/01.nurse.0000490221.61685.e1

BOX 4.2 Creating Positive Spaces in Public Health

Positive spaces are safe health care environments that are open, accessible, and welcoming to sexually and/or gender-diverse persons (Allwright et al., 2019). This practice should include providing a positive space for both clients and workers that helps to overcome the hetero- and cis-normativity that is often typical in health care environments. Rather than trying to be an expert, public health nurses can use an approach of cultural humility and cultural safety (see Chapter 11) to foster the creation of such places in order to increase accessibility and positive working conditions of people who identify as LGBTQ2. *Cultural humility* is the ongoing process of being curious, self-aware, and reflective of one's interactions with individuals different from oneself (Fahlberg et al., 2016). A public health nurse using cultural humility to create positive spaces would consider ways to do the following:

- Partner with people as experts in their own lives.
- Be curious, listening, and open to learning from clients.
- Practice self-reflection and have an awareness of power imbalances and the limits of previous knowledge and training.
- Evaluate each interaction and consider: What went well? Where were there tensions? What could I have done better?
- Embrace lifelong learning: Ask clients when you don't know; show your willingness to understand and learn from them.
- Recognize the LGBTQ2 population's right to self-determination and involve them in program planning and evaluation.

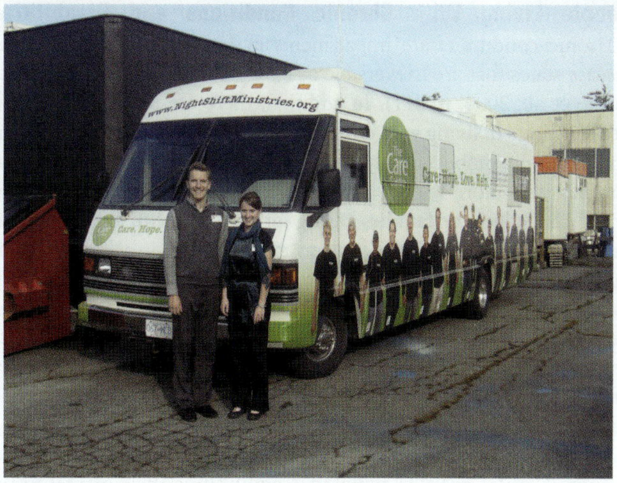

FIGURE 4.3 Nursing students working in a care bus to provide basic health care to the homeless population. (Courtesy Barbara J. Astle, RN, PhD.)

have even fewer resources than do people living on low incomes. Their vulnerability lies in their social condition, lifestyle, and environment, all of which diminish their ability to maintain or improve their health or access to health care. People who are homeless may live on the streets, in temporary accommodation such as shelters and boarding houses, or serially stay with friends (couch surf). They may distrust health and social services as bureaucratic and judgemental, using them only when their health has deteriorated (Omerov et al., 2020). Chronic health problems can worsen because of barriers to supportive self-care and medical care. People who are homeless have a high incidence of mental illness and substance misuse. Nurses can help people identify their capacities and resources, their eligibility for assistance, and interventions to help improve their health (Figure 4.3). For example, Cathy Crowe's work as a street nurse in Toronto includes direct care such as "dressing a wound under a highway overpass" and "treating frostbite" as well as advocacy such as "constantly seeking donations like Gatorade to counter dehydration" and "documenting police-inflicted injuries" (Crowe, 2007, p. 6) (see Box 1.2 in Chapter 1).

People in Precarious Circumstances. Women are at greater risk for problems related to low income, violence, and the stressors associated with unpaid caregiving. Such risks are further complicated for some women who are new immigrants and for those living in geographically isolated settings (Leipert et al., 2015; O'Mahoney & Clark, 2018). Community health nurses' work is guided by their recognition of the need to listen to, respect, and communicate with women in their communities (Leipert et al., 2015).

Physical, emotional, and sexual abuse and neglect are major public health problems, particularly affecting older persons, women, and children (Conroy, 2021; CPHA, 2010). Abuse occurs in many settings, including the home, workplace, school, health care facility, and public areas, and is most often committed by an acquaintance of the victim (CPHA, 2010). When working with clients at risk for or who may have suffered abuse, nurses must seek to provide protection for them. Interviews with clients should occur in private, away from the individual suspected of being the perpetrator. Clients who have been abused often fear retribution if they discuss their problems with a health care provider. Most regions have reporting agencies or hotlines for notification when an individual has been identified as being at risk, and nurses can work with clients to reflect on concerns, identify acceptable alternatives, and make decisions about their situation.

Unintentional injuries, unemployment, depression, and suicide are a concern among youth, particularly young men and those in Indigenous communities. As Gillis noted in 2000, "Community health nurses who are concerned with adolescent health promotion must consider the broad range of factors that affect adolescent health decisions and behaviours. Individual, family and environmental factors must be considered, together with many structural and societal factors" (p. 257). These considerations remain relevant for nurses working with youth today (Russell et al., 2015).

A focus on how the physical environment influences health has re-emerged as a priority for community health nurses, reflecting increasing public concerns about potential exposure to hazardous physical environments. These environments include natural and built environments. The quality of the built environment of daily life—dwellings, schools, workplaces, and community spaces—has an impact on individual and community health. Environmental racism, documented in racialized communities who experienced disproportionate exposure to hazardous waste facilities, landfills, and incinerators (Dodd-Butera et al., 2019), is a form of environmental injustice, encompassing racial and class-based discrimination that underpins such exposures in marginalized communities. An environmental justice perspective can support action to address policies that lead to inequitable distribution of health-promoting amenities, such as walkable neighbourhoods and park space, and of hazardous exposures, such as unsafe housing, toxic industrial sites, and polluted ground waters. Related to environmental justice is the broader field of planetary health, which recognizes the interdependence of human health with earth's ecosystems, and focuses on strategies to mitigate the effects of climate change and protect and build resilient ecosystems for health (Behera et al., 2020; Kalogirou et al., 2020).

People Living With Chronic Conditions and Disabilities. "Chronic conditions are impairments in function, development, or disease states that are irreversible or have a cumulative effect" (Ogden Burke et al., 2000, p. 211). In addition, there are physical and emotional aspects of living with chronic conditions. Societal trends toward greater family mobility, higher rates of maternal employment, smaller families, and more female-headed, lone-parent, low-income families create challenges for families caring for children with chronic conditions (PHAC, 2020). Older persons experience more chronic conditions as they age (PHAC, 2020). The shift in health care service delivery from institutional to community-based care places demands on families, particularly women, to provide caregiving in the community. Nurses need to work with individuals, families, and communities to promote adequate support for family caregivers and access to resources and services.

For a client with a severe mental illness, multiple health and socioeconomic issues must be explored. Complicating their mental health status are a higher risk of poverty, which can result in inadequate housing and food insecurity, as well as increased rates of physical disease comorbidities that lead to decreased functioning and lower employment (Aucoin et al., 2020; Dai et al., 2020). People with severe mental illness often require medication therapy, counselling, housing, and vocational assistance. No longer hospitalized in long-term psychiatric institutions, clients with mental illness are offered resources within their community. However, many communities face continuing difficulties establishing comprehensive, coordinated, and accessible service networks (Loranger & Fleury, 2020). Many clients who lack functional skills are left with fewer, more fragmented services.

Collaboration among community resources is key to helping people with mental illness obtain health care. For example, the "Cool Aid Society" in Victoria, B.C. offers a comprehensive program of services for people who are homeless and living with severe mental illness. Such programs include emergency shelter, permanent housing supports, vocational supports, a food bank, recreational activities, and primary health and dental care (CoolAid Society, 2022).

With the increasing population of older persons, there is a corresponding increase in the number of patients with chronic disease and a greater demand for health care (PHAC, 2020). Healthy aging is achieved through individual, family, community, and societal-level supports that ensure health equity over the life course (WHO, 2020). In providing health care to this population, nurses need to view health promotion from a broad perspective, by understanding what health means to older persons, the ways they can maintain their own health, and the community resources they might need in order to do so. Individuals who feel empowered to control their own health may experience an enhanced engagement with health promotion efforts and a sense of health as a resource for everyday living (McWilliam et al., 2014). Ageism is powerful determinant of health for older persons. Public health nurses and community health nurses can advocate against organizational policies that might be ageist and for increased inclusion of older persons in community activities (WHO, 2020). Through empowering patients to maintain their health and ensuring age-friendly access to community resources, nurses can help improve the quality of life for older persons.

People Who Engage in Stigmatizing Risk Behaviours. Potentially stigmatizing risk behaviours include use of certain substances and certain sexual practices, such as those that do not involve protection or that occur with multiple partners. The social determinants of health provide a holistic perspective to address social and structural conditions that influence behaviour and to challenge the "unprecedented reliance on interventions that focus on addressing what is wrong with the individual" (Shoveller & Johnson, 2006, p. 56). Substance use can range from being helpful to being problematic (CPHA, 2014). *Problematic substance use* occurs when the use of substances has negative effects on the individual, their relationships, or their community (examples include impaired driving, binge drinking, or sharing needles for intravenous administration of drugs). *Dependence* is when people continue to use a substance despite experiencing negative social and health effects (CPHA, 2014). People with problematic use or dependence often have associated health and socioeconomic problems. Socioeconomic problems often result from financial strain, employment loss, and family breakdown. People who use injection drugs have a higher risk of contracting hepatitis C and human immunodeficiency virus (HIV) through sharing injection equipment (Tarasuk et al., 2020). People within this population are also more likely to die from opiate overdose related to a contaminated drug supply (Belzak & Halverson, 2018). Over the past 5 years, deaths and injuries from opiate overdose in Canada has reached epidemic proportions and it is now considered a public health crisis. This situation became further complicated by the conditions of the COVID-19 pandemic, where more people used substances alone, increased their frequency of substance use, and had less access to safe consumption sites (PHAC, 2021).

Poverty, exposure to violence, and disrupted family situations are linked to increased adolescent risk-taking behaviour (Thompson et al., 2018), the consequences of which can be long-lasting for a person's physical and mental health (Phillips et al., 2019). While alcohol and nicotine use has decreased among adolescents in the past decades, problematic polysubstance use and new forms of risk (energy drink overuse, sedentary lifestyles) are increasing among Canadian adolescents (Thompson et al., 2018). In addition, Canadian adolescents are considered to be the most frequent users of cannabis in the world (Thompson et al., 2018).

Community health nurses can partner with clients to assess the circumstances that contribute to substance use, sexual practices that decrease protection, and other risk behaviours and identify strategies to address the often multiple and interrelated concerns. For example, Smith and colleagues (2016) identified strategies such as small-group education, counselling, behavioural training, and self-advocacy skill development within an empowering health promotion framework to prevent sexually transmitted infections (STIs) among gay and bisexual men. Harm reduction is an important approach to health promotion that is based on user input and demand, compassionate pragmatism, and commitment to offering alternatives to reduce risk behaviour consequences, to accept alternatives to abstinence, and to reduce barriers to treatment by providing user-friendly access (Immarino & Pauly, 2021; Pauly et al., 2007). Harm-reduction practices can be used in any setting. Box 4.3 highlights research on the role of nurses in a specific type of harm-reduction intervention for people who use drugs, that of supervised substance-consumption sites.

Standards, Competencies, Roles, and Activities in Community Health Nursing

Nurses in community health practice must have a broad base of knowledge and skills in order to work with clients to meet their health care needs and develop community relationships. Primary health care and health promotion approaches help nurses recognize the interplay between individual experience and social conditions, the value of diversity, and the importance of building capacity to promote health-enhancing change. The CHNC (2019) has identified eight standards of practice for community health nurses: health promotion; prevention and health protection; health maintenance, restoration, and palliation; professional relationships; capacity building; health equity; evidence-informed practice; and professional responsibility and accountability.

BOX 4.3 RESEARCH HIGHLIGHT

Role of Nurses in Supervised Substance-Consumption Sites

Research Focus

There are currently more than 150 supervised consumption sites (SCS) worldwide. These sites offer a much-needed point of contact between the health care system and people who use drugs and, as such, have been proven to effectively reduce harm and improve health. SCS are typically staffed by mental health and harm-reduction workers, social workers, workers with living or lived experience, and nurses. It has been established that the care provided by nurses within SCS falls within their legislated scope of practice, but the actual role of nurses in SCS remains poorly defined and understood. To address this significant practice, policy, and research gap, a consensus statement was developed on the basis of information generated by 17 content experts from 10 countries: Canada, Spain, Australia, France, Denmark, Norway, Ireland, Switzerland, Germany, and Scotland.

Findings

- *Philosophy of Care*: Nurses working in SCS require a broad philosophy of care located between harm reduction, cultural safety, health equity, relational care, social justice, and anti-oppressive practices.

- *Framework*: Nurses working in SCS work in a team-based environment that requires collaboration and relationship building.

- *Nursing Role*: Nurses working in SCS should be prepared to work with complex, dynamic situations and clients. They require strong physical and mental health assessment skills and the ability to perform a variety of interventions, from airway management and health education to community resource referrals. They require autonomy, critical thinking, flexibility, creativity, and leadership.

Websites

Canadian Nurses Association—Harm-Reduction Links. (https://www.canadian-nurse.com/topic/f-m/harm-reduction)
StreetWorks. (http://www.streetworks.ca/pro/index.html)

Harm-reduction nursing practice at Vancouver's Insite, showing an injection kit that contains sterile drug injection supplies (**A**) and the interior of the facility (**B**). http://www.vch.ca/public-health/harm-reduction/supervised-consumption-sites.

Adapted from Gagnon, M., Gauthier, T., Adán, E., et al. (2019). International consensus statement on the role of nurses in supervised consumption sites. *Journal of Mental Health and Addiction Nursing, 3*(1), e22–e31. https://doi.org/10.22374/jmhan.v3i1.35

These standards "define the scope and depth of community nursing practice; establish criteria and expectations for acceptable nursing practice and safe, ethical care; and inspire excellence in and commitment to community nursing practice" in nursing care, education, administration, and research (CHNC, 2019, p. 8). Nurses in community health nursing practice are responsible for meeting these professional nursing standards (CHNC, 2019). In addition, nurses in the specialty practice areas of public health, primary care/family practice, or home health are responsible for meeting relevant competencies (i.e., having required knowledge, skills, and attitudes; see CHNC, 2019).

Community health nurses have multiple important roles in health promotion, disease and injury prevention, health protection, health surveillance, population health assessment, and emergency preparedness and response (CPHA, 2010). A summary of key activities that nurses engage in to meet the responsibilities for these multiple roles was articulated in 1990 and updated in 2010 by the CPHA and is presented in the following sections.

Communication. *Communication* skills support all other activities in community health nursing practice. Skill as an effective communicator is closely related to the leadership and advocacy skills of the facilitator. Nurses may use negotiation and mediation to foster collaboration.

Facilitation. To *facilitate* is to promote. Community health nurses work within a participatory process to identify issues, develop goals for change, and implement strategies for action and evaluation of results. Leadership and advocacy skills are key to these activities.

Leadership. *Leadership* focuses on supporting processes that build capacity among participants, rather than on directing or controlling decision making. To develop proactive approaches to health and environmental issues, nurses need to apply knowledge of professional, community, and political issues and processes.

Advocacy. *Advocacy,* underpinned by commitment to equity and social justice, fosters attention and action to address social determinants of health and accessibility of care, especially among high-priority populations. Community health nurses may help clients become aware of issues that influence their health, build capacity to speak for themselves, and access resources to address issues.

Consultation. Community health nurses *consult* with clients as well as with community members, health care providers, professionals from other disciplines, members of other sectors, policymakers, and government officials. Nurses respond to inquiries about and make referrals to community resources. By developing collaborative relationships, nurses support client access to these resources.

Team Building and Collaboration. *Team building and collaboration* is a way of working together, characterized by recognition of interdependence, collective responsibility, and negotiated equity in relationships (Gray, 1989; Labonte, 1993). Nurses may participate in a team or collective process as a collaborator with clients, community members, agencies, and sectors. This process is supported by developing honest relationships and mutual respect, recognizing many forms of expertise, valuing diversity, and being organized and committed.

Building Capacity. *Building individual and collective capacity* is a means to address health issues and overcome barriers to achieve enhanced quality-of-life outcomes (Labonte et al., 2002). Community health nurses may help community members understand their strengths and abilities, develop leadership, extend social networks, and work together. Group process skills are integral to supporting capacity-building activities.

Building Coalitions and Networks. Community health nurses also use capacity-building skills in situations where there is need for *building coalitions and networks* to support collective action on health issues. Nurses may work with community members to identify the type of coalition or network that best fits their intended purpose, to clarify leadership roles, to create links between the coalition or network and the community at large, and to provide requested support to the coalition or network.

Outreach. *Outreach* supports a holistic approach to community nursing practice and is particularly critical when working with vulnerable populations. Outreach often involves locating services in places that are considered safe or comfortable for potential users, using acceptable approaches to care, and working with clients "where they are at," including using harm-reduction strategies.

Resource Management, Planning, Coordination. *Coordination,* often also involving resource management and planning, has long been associated with nursing practice. Nurses work with clients and diverse agencies to plan and coordinate activities, resources, access, and care to promote client health. These activities complement activities focused on education, care/counselling, and community development.

Case Management. *Case management* skills are closely linked with resource management, planning, and coordination skills and activities. Community health nurses' work will commonly involve case finding, including identification of potential clients who live in circumstances of structural risk, in addition to assessment as a basis for planning, implementing, and evaluating actions to address identified issues. Development of trusting relationships with clients, capacity building, and collaboration are central to effective case management.

Care/Counselling. Community health nurses provide *care/counselling* as they work with clients to promote and protect health and to prevent injury and illness. In many communities, home visiting remains integral to practice, as do services such as health assessment and immunization clinics. Nurses treat illness, monitor risk conditions, educate or guide informed decision making, and support client self-care.

Referral and Follow-Up. Community health nurses work with individuals and families to make decisions about appropriate *referral and follow-up* care, services, or resources. Nurses will need to develop links with other providers, agencies, and networks to support effective and appropriate referral and follow-up.

Screening. *Screening* is used to identify emerging, typically presymptomatic health problems for early treatment and improved health outcomes. Screening contributes to timely case finding. Nurses work to ensure that clients understand and consent to screening activities, that acceptable approaches are used to support culturally safe and competent care, and that appropriate referral and follow-up are completed.

Surveillance. *Surveillance* information is used to enhance understanding of health threats or problems, their natural course, and intervention effectiveness. Nurses may be involved in informal surveillance as well as formal or legally mandated protocols that contribute to documenting, interpreting, and sharing relevant surveillance information.

Health Threat Response. Community health nurses may be involved in *health threat response* procedures, such as when a pandemic or natural disaster occurs in a community. Nurses must understand and follow established procedures that may include case investigation, provision of preventive care, and referral and follow-up for those persons needing treatment.

Health Education. Skillful and effective client education with individuals and groups requires a broad knowledge base, as well as communication and learning process skills. Nurses provide information to support community, family, and individual decision making. Nurses may participate in formal education sessions, such as prenatal classes, or in informal sessions, such as discussions with families during home visits.

Community Development. Community health nurses apply knowledge of *community assessment and development* to support community participation. Participation encourages open identification of issues, shared decision making, egalitarian relationships, and collective ownership of action (Labonte, 1993). Participation and empowerment are closely linked.

Policy Development and Implementation. Activities related to *policy development and implementation* include identifying the need for policy and program development; participating in program development, implementation, and evaluation; helping to establish policies to support practice; and using political processes to promote health. Nurses need to support the collective voice of professional associations (e.g., CNA, CHNC) to advocate for health-enhancing public policy. Falk-Rafael (2005) contends that "nurses, who practice at the intersection of public policy and personal lives, are, therefore, ideally situated and morally obligated to include political advocacy and efforts to influence health public policy in their practice" (p. 212).

Research and Evaluation. *Research and evaluation* are used to generate information, identify issues, determine directions for action, consider strategies to promote change, and assess results. Nurses need to review research and apply knowledge to practice. Nurses may also engage in research and evaluation projects as a participant or investigator to support evidence-informed decisions about practice.

COMMUNITY ASSESSMENT

As a community health nurse, you will need to assess the community, the environment in which people live and work. Without an understanding of that environment, any effort to promote health and to support change is unlikely to succeed, whether you work with an individual, a family, a group, or a community as client.

The community can be seen as having three components: the locale or structure, the social systems, and the people. A complete assessment involves studying each component to understand the health status of the people and the health determinants that influence their health as a basis on which to identify needs for health policy, health program development, and service provision. (For detailed descriptions of community assessment strategies, see community health nursing textbooks such as those by Diem & Moyer, 2015; MacDonald & Jakubec, 2022; Stamler et al., 2020; and Vollman et al., 2017.) To assess the locale or structure, you might travel around the community and observe the physical environment, the location of services, and the places where residents congregate (completing what is referred to as a "windshield" or walking survey). Information about social systems, such as schools, health care facilities, recreation, transportation, and government, may be acquired by visiting various sites and learning about their services (observing activities, interviewing key informants). Community statistics from a local library or health department can help with assessing a population's demographics and health status (reviewing population data). Discussion with community members, including a social and environmental health history (interviewing key informants, holding focus groups), is also helpful to identify priority issues within the community. It is essential to identify community resources and capacities, as well as issues and problems (Stamler et al., 2020).

Recall the determinants of health as you consider the following scenario. As a community health nurse, you wish to familiarize yourself with the local area to help you begin to identify potential health concerns and available resources that will guide your work with the community. Your windshield and walking surveys reveal an older, high-density neighbourhood where pawn shops and bars outnumber grocery stores, schools, and community recreation facilities. You observe a culturally diverse population, including young families and older people who interact with each other at community events sponsored by faith-based groups and social agencies. Your observations are reinforced in discussions as you develop relationships with community leaders and health and social agency staff, whose perspectives are supported by census tract data and regional health statistics. You are alerted to tensions related to high unemployment and language barriers to services. Once you have a good understanding of the community, you may then perform individual or family client assessment against that background. For example, consider assessment of families in a low-income housing complex. Is lighting along walkways and entryways operational? Do they feel comfortable calling on their neighbours for assistance if necessary? Are health and social services easy to reach when needed? Do they feel a sense of belonging in the neighbourhood? No individual or family assessment should occur in isolation from the environment and conditions of the community setting. A collaborative approach to community assessment grounded in an empowerment process helps in establishing working relationships, identifying shared concerns, recognizing collective capacities, and developing effective strategies to enhance health.

PROMOTING CLIENTS' HEALTH

The challenge for nurses in community health practice is how to promote and protect the health of clients, whether within the context of their community or with the community as the focus. Community health nurses may bring together the resources necessary to improve the continuity of client care. In collaboration with clients, health care and social service providers, and other community members, nurses coordinate health care services, locate appropriate social services, and develop innovative approaches to address clients' health issues.

Perhaps the key to being an effective community health nurse is the ability to understand clients' everyday lives. The foundation for this understanding is the establishment of strong, caring relationships with clients (see Chapters 18 and 19) that support empowerment as an active process rooted in cultural, religious, and personal belief systems and awareness of links between personal lives, community experiences, and social political contexts (Falk-Rafael, 2001, 2005). The quasi-insider status of nurses in a community often enables them to identify local patterns and needs that can be addressed through programs, policies, and advocacy (Baisch, 2009; Stamler et al., 2020) that are responsive, supportive, and effective. The day-to-day activities of family and community life and the cultural, economic, and political environment influence how they adapt nursing interventions. Once a nurse acquires an understanding of an individual's or family's life, interventions designed to promote health and prevent disease can be introduced. Similarly, understanding the relationships, activities, and concerns of groups and communities is central to health promotion practice. A continuing challenge for community health nurses is to take up their practice in ways that establish meaningful, respectful engagement with people in their communities and that promote individual, family, and collective empowerment, to enhance health in everyday life.

KEY CONCEPTS

- A successful community health nursing practice involves building relationships with the community members and being responsive to changes within the community.
- The principles of public health nursing practice support assisting individuals in acquiring a healthy environment in which to live.
- The public health nurse cares for the community as a whole and considers the individual or family to be one member of a population or potential group at risk.
- The home health nurse's competence is based on decision making at the level of the individual client and their family.
- Within an ecological model of home health nursing, the individual is viewed within the larger systems of family, social network, community, and society.
- The primary care or family practice nurse collaborates in an interprofessional team, using a client-centred model to promote clients' health and management of illness and their navigation of community resources.
- Marginalized individuals and their families are often made vulnerable by multiple forms of inequity.
- While high-priority populations can be vulnerable to health inequities, they also have capacities that can be protective for them and that should be recognized in any health promotion efforts.
- Exacerbations of chronic health problems are common among homeless people because they have access to fewer protective resources.
- An important principle in working with clients at risk for or who may have suffered abuse is protection of the client.
- Clients who engage in risky behaviours such as substance use may respond to a harm-reduction approach.
- In community health practice, it is important to understand what health means to clients and what clients do to maintain their own health.

- A community health nurse must be competent in fulfilling a multidimensional role, including engaging in communication, facilitation, leadership, advocacy, consultation, team building, and collaboration; building capacity; building coalitions and networks; outreach; resource management, planning, and coordination; case management; care/counselling; referral and follow-up; screening; surveillance; responding to health threats; health education; community development; policy development and implementation; and research and evaluation activities.
- Assessment of a community includes assessing population health status and relevant determinants of health in relation to three elements: locale or structure, the social systems, and the people.
- An important consideration in becoming an effective community health nurse is to strive to understand clients' lives.

CRITICAL THINKING EXERCISES

1. Referring to the case study at the beginning of the chapter, what are some of the strategies Jan uses to engage with Kira? How might this experience be different from Kira's other health care experiences?
2. What community health nursing standards and activities does Jan take on in her work with Kira?
3. Based on the high-priority populations they serve, what other population health-promotion efforts might Jan and her colleagues design?

🌐 *Answers to Critical Thinking Exercises appear on the Evolve website.*

REVIEW QUESTIONS

Review Questions 1 to 10 relate to the case study at the beginning of the chapter.

1. Which of the following examples from the case study demonstrates that the nurse is using a population health approach when working with Kira?
   a. Jan takes a look at the arm and asks Kira about any previous history of abscesses or other health problems.
   b. Jan asks the questions in a nonjudgemental way, which makes Kira feel like an expert about her own body and drug use.
   c. Jan tells Kira that she could help her take care of the sore arm and, if Kira is interested, she can offer some suggestions for how to prevent it from happening again.
   d. Jan and the other staff work with a small group of clients, including Kira, to design easy-to-read health promotion materials that they then distribute throughout the city.
2. What would be important for the nurse to recognize about Kira's health as a marginalized person? *(Select all that apply.)*
   a. Kira is less likely to have health problems because she is young.
   b. Kira is likely to have poorer health outcomes because of poor access to care.
   c. Kira's risk factors may intersect and have cumulative effects on her health.
   d. Kira requires the same health interventions as the general public.
3. Which of the following actions by the nurse demonstrate use of trauma-informed care? *(Select all that apply.)*
   a. Jan ensures that Kira knows that while the program has lots of options for her, it is Kira who decides for herself what kind of help she wants.
   b. Jan leaves Kira with enough clean needles, sterile water, and a tourniquet for the week as well as instructions about using warm compresses.

   c. Jan asks the questions in a nonjudgemental way, which makes Kira feel like an expert about her own body and drug use, making Kira more comfortable with answering the questions.
   d. Jan refers Kira to nurse practitioner for antibiotics.
4. Which of the following actions by the nurse demonstrates that she is implementing the principles of primary health care in her nursing practice? *(Select all that apply.)*
   a. She collaborates with a vocational training agency and the shelter.
   b. She cleans Kira's wound.
   c. She takes a swab culture of Kira's wound.
   d. She meets Kira at the shelter rather than at the health clinic.
5. What actions does the nurse take within her community that demonstrate effective community health nursing practice?
   a. Jan takes a passive role to allow the community to initiate change.
   b. Jan takes time to build relationships with and respond to trends in the community.
   c. Jan spends all of her time doing wound care on individuals who need her help.
   d. Jan insists on standardized approaches to care for everyone seen by the outreach team.
6. The nurse working with the team and the small group of clients to create health promotion materials is an example of a nurse engaging in which community nursing activity?
   a. Screening
   b. Health education
   c. Consultation
   d. Building coalitions and networks
7. Which community nursing activity is the nurse doing when she tells Kira about the vocational program that can help Kira prepare for getting a job?
   a. Outreach
   b. Collaboration
   c. Coordination
   d. Building coalitions and networks
8. If the nurse was doing a community assessment of Kira's community, which of the following would be included?
   a. Locale or structure, social systems, and people
   b. People, neighbourhoods, and social systems
   c. Health care systems, geographical boundaries, and people
   d. Environment, families, and social systems
9. The nurse's provision of syringes, sterile water, and a tourniquet to Kira is an example of which community health nursing intervention?
   a. Maintenance
   b. Treatment
   c. Screening
   d. Prevention
10. Which of the following actions reflects that the nurse is using cultural humility in her work with Kira?
    a. Jan treats Kira and all of her other clients exactly the same.
    b. Jan is curious and open-minded about understanding Kira's substance use patterns and techniques.
    c. Jan is an expert at safe injection and knows lots of tips to help Kira inject safely.
    d. Jan takes extra courses at university about substance use disorder.

Answers: 1. d; **2.** b; **3.** a, c; **4.** a, d; **5.** b; **6.** d; **7.** c; **8.** a; **9.** d; **10.** b.

🌐 *Rationales for the Review Questions appear on the Evolve website.*

RECOMMENDED WEBSITES

Canadian Public Health Association: http://www.cpha.ca
The Canadian Public Health Association (CPHA) is a national, independent, not-for-profit, voluntary association representing public health care in Canada.
Community Health Nurses of Canada: http://www.chnc.ca
Community Health Nurses Canada (CHNC) is a national organization. It provides standards and information on community health nursing.
Fact Sheet: The Primary Health Care Approach: https://hl-prod-ca-oc-download.s3-ca-central-1.amazonaws.com/CNA/2f975e7e-4a40-45ca-863c-5ebf0a138d5e/UploadedImages/documents/FS02_Primary_Health_Care_Approach_June_2000_e.pdf

This Canadian Nurses Association publication defines and describes primary health care in Canada.
Public Health Agency of Canada: Health Promotion: http://www.phac-aspc.gc.ca/hp-ps/index-eng.php
This federal website provides links to many useful health promotion resources and guides that will aid health professionals and community leaders.
Victorian Order of Nurses: http://www.von.ca
The Victorian Order of Nurses (VON) is Canada's leading charitable organization addressing community health and social needs.

REFERENCES

A full reference list is available on the website for this book at http://evolve.elsevier.com/Canada/Potter/fundamentals/

5

Practical Nursing in Canada

Written by Joyce Engel, RN, PhD

OBJECTIVES

Mastery of content in this chapter will enable you to:
- Define the key terms listed.
- Explain how practical nursing has evolved as a regulated nursing category in Canada.
- Discuss the current issues and trends that affect practical nurses in Canada.
- Differentiate the scope of practice of the practical nurse from that of the registered nurse and unregulated care provider.
- Explain how legislation, regulatory bodies, and professional associations govern the practice of practical nurses.
- Predict the future role of practical nurses within the Canadian health care system.

KEY TERMS

Acuity

Authorized act

Canadian Practical Nurse Registration Exam (CPNRE)

Competence

Controlled act (restricted or reserved act)

Credentialling

Delegation

Educational laddering

Entry-level competencies

Epidemiology

Internationally educated nurses (IENs)

Jurisprudence

Licensed practical nurse (LPN)

Practical nursing

Proactive

Protected title

Registered nurse (RN)

Registered practical nurse (RPN)

Registration

Regulatory Exam-Practical Nurse™ (REx-PN™)

Standards of practice

Supervision

Unregulated care provider (UCP)

🌐 WEBSITE

http://evolve.elsevier.com/Canada/Potter/fundamentals/

CASE STUDY

Taylor (preferred pronouns: she/her) has been practising for 11 months since initial licensure as an LPN. She is new to the surgical unit and is caring for a patient who is 2 days postoperative. The team leader, Michelle (preferred pronouns: she/her), is an experienced RN and a helpful colleague. Michelle tells Taylor that the surgeon of her assigned patient reviewed the patient's lab results and prescribed a unit of blood. Taylor indicates that she checked the order, assessed the intravenous site, assembled everything for starting the transfusion, and explained the procedure to the patient, but she has not yet started the infusion. Michelle congratulates Taylor on her timely efficiency and thoroughness of preparation but is hesitant about starting the transfusion. Although Michelle has heard that starting a blood transfusion is within an LPN's scope of practice, she is uncertain that administration of blood by LPNs has been fully approved and about Taylor's experience and educational background.

Think about this case study as you read this chapter. There are review questions at the end of the chapter that relate to the case study.

HISTORY OF PRACTICAL NURSING IN CANADA

Licensed or registered practical nurses use the title of **registered practical nurse (RPN)** in Ontario and **licensed practical nurse (LPN)** in the territories and other provinces in Canada. Of the four categories (**registered nurses [RNs]**, registered psychiatric nurses, L/RPNs, nurse practitioners) of regulated nurses in Canada, LPNs and RPNs form the second largest category in the Canadian nursing workforce (Canadian Institute for Health Information [CIHI], 2020a).

Practical nurses, first called either *nursing aides* (if female) or *orderlies* (if male), numbered 4 700 in Canada in 1931. By 1947, this number had increased to 7 900, largely because of the increased hospital services needed after the Second World War. In 2020, there were 130 710 LPNs in Canada (CIHI, 2020a), which attests to their value and their contributions to health and health care.

Practical nursing became a profession in the late 1930s but was not recognized as a distinct profession that required formal education until the 1970s. Up until the mid-1970s, minimal high school preparation was necessary for admission to a practical nursing program, and the program was likely a short apprenticeship in a hospital setting. No licensure examination was required, and no official **registration**, **protected title**, or professional body existed (Almost, 2021).

The Evolution of Practical Nursing

Practical nursing has evolved in a similar way in most provinces and has followed a pattern of other occupations when they became established as professions, such as initiating self-regulation and increasing formal education to acquire its specialized and complex knowledge (Flexner, 2001). The evolution of practical nursing has also been marked by societal need and overlap between the roles of regulated nurses, including between LPNs and RNs (Almost, 2021).

Canada. The first formal education program specifically for practical nurses began in Manitoba in 1943 (Almost, 2021). Like the earlier changes in education for RNs, practical-nurse programs have become more holistically focused and complex and longer and have moved out of the hospital into colleges.

The first legislative acts regarding practical nursing were introduced in the 1940s and controlled the education, testing, licensing, regulation, and practice of practical nursing. By the 1980s, most provinces had developed regulations to govern practical nursing and required graduates to write a national licensing examination provided by the Canadian Nurses Association Testing Service (CNATS) (see Table 5.1 for historical highlights in selected provinces).

Nationally, the Canadian Council for Practical Nurse Regulators (CCPNR), which was formed in 2004, is a federation of provincial and territorial regulators. It provides leadership in ensuring excellence in regulation of practical nurses and has established national entry-level competencies for LPNs (CCPNR, 2019). Through an overwhelming vote in 2018, LPNs are now also included in the Canadian Nurses Association (CNA), which is the national professional and advocacy organization for nurses. The CNA provides accreditation for RN programs and is currently considering accreditation processes for LPN programs as well (Almost, 2021).

The Demand for Practical Nursing

In the late 1940s and early 1950s, demand for practical nurses increased significantly in most jurisdictions. Several factors were responsible for this increased demand, which included political and economic pressures and changes within the nursing profession.

Political and Economic Pressures. As roles for women expanded after World War II and more opportunities were available in a range of occupations and professions, the number of nurses decreased. This shortage of RNs came at a time when patients' **acuity** (i.e., level of sickness) was increasing in institutions. In addition, the increasing age of the population required more supportive care in communities and long-term care facilities, and private enterprise began exerting a greater economic influence on health care.

Because this public demand for safe and competent practice increased at the same time as economic and personnel challenges, practical nursing became more important within the health care system. Practical nursing offered an economical but highly competent workforce to meet the needs of patients in hospitals and of those requiring long-term care.

Changes Within Nursing
Nursing Education. Nursing shortages brought about by the world wars in the twentieth century led to the development of formalized training and education for practical nurses. In 1941, Ontario began a demonstration program for practical nurses, and in 1943, Manitoba

introduced the St. Boniface School for Practical Nurses (Almost, 2021). The ensuing early programs were run largely by provincial governments and hospitals, and students became a source of free staffing in hospitals and other health care agencies.

When nursing education moved from a hospital base to a postsecondary base (beginning in the early 1970s), the number of staff who were available on hospital units decreased suddenly. Institutions responded by employing greater numbers of less trained health care assistants and aides to provide basic care. This reliance on a less prepared workforce was a concern for the public and also for employers of assistants and aides, whose education was largely determined by their training sites and therefore resulted in inconsistencies in skills and practice. Leaders in practical nursing recognized the need for consistent and upgraded education if practical nurses were to remain employable and to move forward professionally with appropriate acknowledgement of their contribution to health care (College of Licensed Practical Nurses of Alberta [CLPNA], 2016).

Registration Laws. In the early twentieth century, beginning legislation was secured by RNs that outlined aspects of practice and preparation for practice, such as nursing curricula and admission criteria. Permissive registration protected the title of *registered nurse* but not who could use it, and if health care providers did not claim to be registered, they could practise many nursing activities and claim to be a nurse.

After World War II, the public began demanding more qualified practitioners. As a result, mandatory registration was established, which laid out scopes of practice and protected not only titles but also who could use the title of *registered nurse, licensed practical nurse (LPN)* (*registered practical nurse, or RPN,* in Ontario), *nurse practitioner,* and, in the four Western provinces and the Yukon, *registered psychiatric nurse* (Almost, 2021).

Development of Categories Within the Nursing Profession. The evolution of three categories of Canadian nurses (and in Western provinces, four categories with the addition of registered psychiatric nurses) distinguishes nursing from some other professions. The medical profession, for example, essentially has one level of practitioner (a medical doctor), although there are many subspecialties (e.g., pediatrics, ophthalmology, orthopedics). Despite many subspecialities, the function of medical doctors is clear to the public: they diagnose and treat disorders. Nursing, however, has developed a much less definitive practice, and divisions between the knowledge base and functions of the categories of nurses are somewhat unclear to employers, the public, and even to nurses. Basic theory and practice are common to both categories of nurses and are divided only by depth of knowledge and complexity of care required, which leads sometimes to confusion and tensions (Villeneuve, 2021).

PRACTICAL NURSING TODAY: ISSUES AND TRENDS

Educational Preparation and Entry-Level Competencies

Patients' needs are more complex than ever. Practical nurses must respond to increased acuity, multiple comorbidities among patients experiencing chronic disorders, wide cultural and social variations among patients, and a continuing trend toward home and community care. In response, the Canadian Council for Practical Nurse Regulators recognized the need to articulate what competencies might be expected of LPNs upon graduation from a recognized program and initial registration. The compilation of entry-to-practice competencies, initially published in 2013, was reviewed with key stakeholder groups and revised in the *2019 Entry-Level Competencies for LPNs* (CCPNR, 2019) to reflect the changing needs of the health care environment.

TABLE 5.1		History of Practical Nursing in Selected Provinces
Province	**Year**	**Significant Developments and Comments**
Alberta	1945	School for Nursing Aides established in Calgary, sponsored by the Department of Veteran Affairs and Canadian Vocational Training
	1947	*Provincial Nursing Aides Act* is passed, which allowed licensing of the Certified Nursing Aide
	1961	Alberta Certified Nursing Aide Association incorporated
	1972	Alberta Certified Nursing Aide Association, along with eight other practical nursing associations, becomes a founding member of the Canadian Association of Practical Nurses and Nursing Assistants
	1978	*Nursing Assistant Registration Act* combines aides and orderlies in one category of RNA (registered nursing assistant)
	1987	Professional Council of RNAs becomes first health care discipline under the *Health Disciplines Act*. Registered nurse assistants become self-regulatory with a distinct scope of practice. Nursing assistant graduates are required to write the national Canadian Practical Nurse Registration Examination for licensing.
	1990	RNAs change title to Licensed Practical Nurses (LPNs)
		Provincial Council of RNAs becomes Professional Council of LPNs (PCLPN)
	1995	Mandatory educational upgrading instituted as a result of LPN devaluation and membership decline
	1998	*Health Disciplines Act* becomes *Health Professions Act*, which eventually includes all regulated health care professions under their separate provincial colleges
	2003	College of Licensed Practical Nurses of Alberta formally proclaimed
	2004	LPNs in specialized practice are recognized by *Health Professions Act*
	2006	Diploma approved as the entry-to-practice requirement
	2020	Amendments to *Licensed Practical Nurse Profession Regulation* provide authorization and clarity around broader range of nursing tasks
British Columbia	1951	*Practical Nurse Act* passed
	1965	*Practical Nurses Act* legally approved
		Council of LPNs established as the licensing body
	1991	Council of LPNs becomes an independent regulatory body of the Ministry of Health
	1996	Council of LPNs in BC becomes College of LPNs of British Columbia under the *Health Professions Act*
	2018	College of LPNs of British Columbia amalgamates with College of Registered Nurses of British Columbia and College of Registered Psychiatric Nurses to become British Columbia College of Nursing Professionals (BCCNP)
	2020	British Columbia College of Nursing Professionals amalgamates with the College of Midwives of British Columbia to become the British Columbia College of Professional Nurses and Midwives (BCCNM)
Manitoba	1943	First official practical nurse education program in Canada
Ontario	1938	Centres begin offering 6-month courses for nursing assistants
	1941–1945	With approval of Ontario Department of Health, Registered Nurses' Association of Ontario sponsors eight 6-month training programs for nursing assistants
	1947	*Nurses Act* is amended to allow title of certified nursing assistant (CNA)
	1963	CNA title changed to registered nursing assistant (RNA)
	1990	RNA training programs moved to community colleges
	1993	RNA title changed to registered practical nurse (RPN)
	2001	College of Nurses of Ontario (CNO) passes regulation to require all RPNs to obtain their basic diploma through enhanced 2-year programs in provincial colleges as an entry-to-practice requirement beginning January 2005
	2002	All practical nursing programs offered in colleges
New Brunswick	1977	Legislature established act of incorporation, giving the Association of New Brunswick Registered Nursing Assistants the responsibilities of education, registration, and discipline of registered practical nurses
	1987 and 2000	Unsuccessful attempts to change the RNA title to licensed practical nurse through the New Brunswick Legislature
	2002	*Licensed Practical Nurses Act* recognizes the new LPN title
		Association of New Brunswick Licensed Practical Nurses becomes the name of the provincial association
Nunavut	2011	Last jurisdiction in Canada to pass regulations governing LPN practice
Nova Scotia	2016	College of LPNs of Nova Scotia and Council of Registered Nurses of Nova Scotia vote to form a single nursing regulator, the Nova Scotia College of Nursing
	2019	*Nursing Act* proclaimed, which gives regulatory authority to Nova Scotia College of Nursing

Data from Almost, J. (2021). *Regulated nursing in Canada: The landscape*. https://www.cna-aiic.ca/en/nursing/regulated-nursing-in-canada; Association of New Brunswick Licensed Practical Nurses. (2021). *About ANBLPN*. https://www.anblpn.ca/about-anblpn; College of Licensed Practical Nurses of Alberta. (2016). *History of Alberta's licensed practical nurses*. https://www.clpna.com/about-clpna/history-alberta-lpns/; College of Licensed Practical Nurses of Alberta. (2019). *Regulation change for licensed practical nurses enhance continuity of care for Albertans*. https://www.clpna.com/2019/10/regulation-change-for-licensed-practical-nurses-enhances-continuity-of-care-for-albertans; Government of British Columbia. (n.d.). *Nursing professions*. https://www2.gov.bc.ca/gov/content/health/practitioner-professional-resources/professional-regulation/nursing; Nova Scotia College of Nursing. (2021). *Journey to NSCN*. https://www.nscn.ca; Registered Practical Nurses Association of Ontario. (2013). *History of practical nursing and RPNAO*. http://174.142.213.171/about/history; Vancouver Island University. (n.d.). *Twenty-one days: History of nursing and practical nursing*. http://twentyonedays.ca/vancouver-island-university-practical-nursing-program-guide/professional-issues-practical-nursing-study-guide/history-of-nursing-practical-nursing/

These national 76 **entry-level competencies (ELCs)** are applicable in regulatory jurisdictions where they have been approved and enacted. The ELCs reflect minimum standards of knowledge, skills, attitudes, and judgement expected of beginning practical nurses along five categories (CCPNR, 2019):

- Professional practice
- Legal practice
- Ethical practice
- Foundations of practice
- Collaborative practice

The competencies serve to outline what the public can expect of practical nurses and guide educational preparation of practical nurses. They are also used by regulators to approve programs, assess practice competency and applications for registration, and develop practice standards. The competencies also incorporate important assumptions of Canadian practical nursing practice, such as the grounding of LPN practice in primary health care and the capacity of LPNs to work in any health care setting or in situations that involve delivery of health care (CCPNR, 2019).

Entry to a Practical Nurse Program. Early programs required elementary school completion for entry to a practical nurse program (Almost, 2021). Review of admission requirements for Canadian practical nursing programs indicates that applicants need a secondary diploma, with specific courses such as language and one or two sciences. Mature students may be admitted if applicants can demonstrate equivalent learning or can successfully complete pre-entrance student testing. Successful applicants must also submit proof of immunization (which may include COVID vaccination), a criminal record check, cardiopulmonary resuscitation (CPR) certification, and complete mask fit testing.

Location and Length of Program. In most Canadian jurisdictions, practical nursing programs are 16- to 24-month diploma programs and are offered in postsecondary institutions and private colleges. To facilitate student access to nursing education, some educational institutions offer practical nursing programs through nontraditional delivery methods such as distance education and online learning. The trend toward longer and more complex education for practical nurses is driven by the increased complexity of the patient base, legislative changes, new developments in technology, increased public expectations, changing skill mixes, and expanded opportunities for practice (Almost, 2021).

Increased educational requirements for entry to practice have both positive and negative aspects for the individual professional, the profession, the workplace, the government, and society in general. Positive effects include wider employment opportunities, national and international mobility, and enhanced service to the public. Negative effects may include increased educational costs for students and society, delayed entry into the job market, problems in workplace collective agreements, exacerbation of job shortages, and higher expectations of compensation, which creates economic burdens for employers.

Instructors in Practical Nursing Programs. Canadian nursing instructors are usually required to have clinical experience and have current registration as a nurse, as well as educational preparation and experience relevant to what they are teaching (College of Nurses of Ontario [CNO], 2022a). Today, RNs and LPNs who teach in practical nursing programs, particularly in full-time positions, may have a variety of degree preparations, including baccalaureate degrees, master's degrees, or doctorates in nursing, education, or other related areas, and

may be required to take part in teaching workshops or certification programs as an employment condition. Program approval guidelines may set additional conditions for faculty qualifications or program faculty, such as requiring that 15% of faculty are LPNs (CLPNA, 2019). Importantly, practising LPNs serve as role models and support students educationally during preceptorship experiences.

Student Clinical Practice. To prepare students for practice as nurses, it is important to secure clinical settings that provide opportunity for solid practice of knowledge and skills gained in the classroom and laboratory settings. Securing appropriate clinical placements for students can be a challenge for two main reasons:

- Lack of clarity around student scope of practice and contributions of students to care leads to restrictions in placement (Ontario Nurses Association, 2018). This is further compounded in some settings (e.g., acute care areas such as pediatrics or mental health or community) that may not use LPNs in their staffing mix or restrict what LPNs are able to do because of unit or institutional mandates or lack of familiarity with LPN scope of practice.
- Rapid growth in nursing enrollments, short staffing, and funding issues, as well as requests for placements for students in other health disciplines, mean that clinical areas are frequently inundated and sometimes overwhelmed by requests for clinical placements. The impacts of crises such as the COVID-19 pandemic compound these issues as clinical areas struggle to keep up with patient care and programs weigh the risks of clinical learning against the benefits (Dewart et al., 2020). Consequently, practical nursing programs incorporate approaches to clinical learning and placements such as simulation, and extend clinical learning to weekends, across all work shifts, and into the summer months in order to increase availability of clinical settings.

Requirements for Practice as a Licensed Practical Nurse

In order to practise, practical nurses must become registered in the provincial or territorial jurisdiction in which they intend to practise. The regulatory colleges in the provinces and territories are mandated to set requirements for registration or licensing.

Educational Preparation. Applicants for registration must demonstrate successful and recent completion of a nursing education program that prepares them to safely and capably perform the entry-level competencies expected in the jurisdiction to which they are applying. Students who are applying for registration in the jurisdiction where they have taken an approved educational program will satisfy this requirement when their program provides documentation that the students have successfully completed their program. If an applicant is applying from outside the jurisdiction, then the regulatory college evaluates documentation from the applicant to determine if the educational background of the applicant is equivalent to that received by applicants from that jurisdiction. Recent graduates of programs may be able to practise with a provisional or temporary license or graduate practical nurse registration until they write and pass the national licensing exams (British Columbia College of Nurses and Midwives [BCCNM], 2021a).

Evidence of Practice. Applicants for registration must also present evidence of recent practice as a practical nurse. For most applicants, this requirement is met through the recent completion of an approved educational program. Applicants who have already been in practice must provide evidence of recent employment as an LPN, including number of hours worked (BCCNM, 2021a).

Registration Examinations. When the regulatory college is satisfied that recent graduates of programs (or internationally prepared nurses) have met educational, experience, and other requirements, the final step in registration is applying to write the licensing or registration examination, after submitting the application and administration fees. The Canadian Practical Nurse Registration Examination (CPNRE) is currently used in all regulatory jurisdictions in Canada (with the exception of Quebec, which has its own licensing examination) (CNA, 2022a; CNO, 2022b). This examination, which was made available in an online format in 2017, is based on national ELCs and is provided by Yardstick Assessment Inc. It includes approximately 170 multiple-choice questions and is available four times a year in both English and French. In 2022, the exam moved to a computer adaptive format (Almost, 2021; Yardstick Assessment Inc, 2022). Official results of the CPRNE are emailed within approximately 3 to 6 weeks of writing the examination. Unsuccessful examination writers will not be able to register as a practical nurse until they pass the examination. The number of times that the examination may be repeated is directed by the regulatory body of the province or territory in which registration is sought.

The regulatory jurisdictions of Ontario and British Columbia are jointly developing a new entry-to-practice examination, in partnership with the National Council of State Boards of Nursing (NCBSN). This new examination, the Regulatory Exam-Practical Nurse™ (REx-PN™) examination, was offered for the first time in January 2022, thus phasing out the CPNRE in the regulatory jurisdictions of Ontario and British Columbia. The REx-PN™ will give writers the opportunity to write the examination at any time, with no limit on the number of attempts (CNO, 2022b), and will be administered by the NCBSN.

Presently, applicants for registration in Alberta, British Columbia, Manitoba, New Brunswick, and Nova Scotia also need to pass jurisprudence examinations or complete a module. These examinations test knowledge and comprehension of laws and regulations, by-laws, and standards that apply to practice in the province to which application is made, as well as knowledge of relevant federal laws (Almost, 2021; CNO, 2020a).

Usually, the school receives a summary of the passing and failing marks on the registration examination for a class cohort and information about the school's success in relation to other programs in its jurisdiction and in Canada.

Other Requirements. Because professionals have a position of power, concerns inevitably arise that they could take advantage of vulnerable persons, especially young children and older persons. Thus, applicants are required to provide evidence of good character and fitness to practise (BCCNM, 2021a), which includes completion of a criminal record check and disclosure of mental or physical health problems that would have an impact on the ability to practise safely, competently, and ethically. Safe care involves the ability to communicate clearly and accurately; therefore, applicants must also provide information as to fluency in the use of the English language and, possibly, in the French language (depending on the province or territory).

Continuing Education Issues

Laddering. Should health care aides be given the opportunity to become practical nurses? Should practical nurses be given the opportunity to become degree nurses? The concept of educational laddering, or *bridging*, recognizes prior learning and acknowledges that knowledge and expertise are acquired in various ways. It provides a means by which individuals can progress in their careers with reasonable access to other levels or categories of education and nursing. Institutions across Canada offer academic pathways that bridge health care aide (or personal support worker) and practical nursing programs, as well as practical nursing and registered nursing programs.

Postgraduate Certification. Practical nurses can further their education and their contribution to the profession by specializing in specific fields. Practical nurses have plentiful opportunities to obtain certification or complete additional training and education in specialty or advanced practice areas after graduation from a basic program. These certificates may be offered to LPNs or to both registered and practical nurses. Examples of specialty areas are certification in perioperative nursing, foot care, gerontology and geriatric nursing, dialysis, women's health, specialized mental health, and occupational nursing.

The Role of the Practical Nurse

Most jurisdictions recognize that practical nursing is a separate category within the wider field of professional nursing. There is also recognition that LPNs and RNs study from the same body of nursing knowledge. RNs study this content in greater detail and breadth and over a longer period of time, which allows for a deeper base in clinical practice, as well as in decision making, leadership, and research utilization. Practical nurses study for a shorter period, which results in a more focused knowledge and skills base (Almost, 2021).

National data indicate that the LPN proportion of the nursing workforce in long-term care settings has dramatically increased (Table 5.2). The trend toward increasing proportions of LPNs in the nursing workforces of long-term care and geriatrics began in 2007 (CIHI, 2017), which is indicative of the value that employers in these settings place on LPNs. This same data suggest that the number of LPNs working in medical-surgical areas in hospitals is declining. This is perhaps related to the continued rise in acuity and complexity in medical-surgical settings, although LPNs are working in other acute care areas that would not have been previously available to them, such as operating rooms, emergency departments, maternal child nursing, addiction and mental health services, where they work independently or collaboratively with RNs.

While the proportion of LPNs working in medical-surgical settings has decreased, the proportion of LPNs in nursing staffing mixes in community settings has increased. The diversity of responsibilities of LPNs in community settings has also increased as LPNs continue to become integrated into intraprofessional and interprofessional teams. The shift in employment of LPNs into community and long-term care settings parallels major shifts in health care: there is higher demand for community and home-based services and for long-term care (CIHI, 2019) related to an aging population and an increased emphasis on home-based recovery. Addictions and mental health are also growing areas of practice for LPNs, with the number of LPNs in these areas growing faster since 2014 than the number of RNs (CIHI, 2019). Other areas

TABLE 5.2	Licensed Practical Nurses by Percentage of Nursing Staffing Mix in Selected Settings and Years		
	2015	**2016**	**2019**
Hospitals	47.2	21.2	21.6
Long-term care settings	40.2	56.3	58.2
Community settings	12.8	24.1	27.5

From Canadian Institute for Health Information (CIHI). (2016). *Regulated nurses, 2015.* https://www.cihi.ca/sites/default/files/document/pt_highlights_final_en.pdf; CIHI. (2017). *Regulated nurses, 2016.* https://www.cihi.ca/sites/default/files/document/regulated-nurses-2016-report-en-web.pdf; CIHI. (2020). *Nursing in Canada, 2019.* https://www.cihi.ca/sites/default/files/rot/nursing-report-2019-en-web.pdf

of employment for LPNs include health provider offices, education, government offices, occupational health, and industrial settings. LPNs may also be self-employed. Consequently, practical nurse programs are providing instruction in skills and knowledge needed to care for stable patients in acute care settings (e.g., intravenous therapy, oxygen therapy) and long-term care settings, as well as in community and mental health.

Workplace Trends

Supply refers to the number of regulated nurses registered and available to the health care workforce. Predicting and understanding nursing supply and workforce data is important for ensuring that there is adequate access to care and that quality is maintained, as well as for ensuring that policies and practices reflect current health care needs. Supply is influenced by factors such as the number of students enrolled in and graduating from programs, volume of new graduates and **internationally educated nurses (IENs)** entering the workforce, and attrition related to nurses leaving the workforce because of retirement or other reasons. The distribution of supply across provinces and the territories is also influenced by mobility of nurses across jurisdictions. A sufficient and well-prepared nursing workforce is of interest in overcoming the challenges of those who may be inadequately serviced, are underserviced, or have unique vulnerabilities, such as older persons, and will vary with jurisdiction.

Between 2015 and 2019, the supply (nurses registered and available to work) of regulated nurses grew at an annual average of 1.6%, which outpaced the annual 1.2% growth of the Canadian population. During that same period, LPNs had the second largest annual growth rate in supply (CIHI, 2020a), with provinces such Ontario and Alberta showing the greatest growth in the number of L/RPNs and the territories seeing the largest percentage growth in LPNs from 2015 to 2019 (CIHI, 2016, 2017, 2020a). Clearly, the numbers of LPNs have increased in each of the jurisdictions in Canada, suggesting that there may be more hiring in diverse health care settings and even wider acceptance of the roles that LPNs can play in contemporary health care in Canada.

LPNs in Canada are also becoming a younger workforce. Of the four regulated nursing groups in Canada, LPNs have the highest proportion (35.9%) under 35 years of age and the smallest proportion 55 years and older (CIHI, 2020a).

Workforce Issues

While supply growth is positive, a critical indicator of the adequacy of the nursing workforce is the percentage of supply already in the workforce; at 90% of available nurses in the workforce (CIHI, 2020a), limited reserves may be available when crises such as pandemics occur. This limited reserve prompts concern about the retention of nurses. Additionally, the adequacy of nursing workforce numbers in areas such as long-term care, highlighted during the COVID-19 pandemic, and in rural and remote areas, is a concern. Canada currently has fewer health care providers per 100 long-term care residents than other Organisation for Economic Co-operation and Development (OECD) countries and has a more vulnerable population living in this setting (CIHI, 2020b). The number of LPNs, who comprise the majority of nursing staff in long-term care, needs to be given careful consideration to ensure that the needs and safety of this population are appropriately addressed. In rural and remote areas, 14% of Canada's regulated nurses care for 17% of Canada's population (MacLeod et al., 2019), and the increase in nursing supply has not kept pace with growth in these areas, which impacts access to health care. Inconsistent use and acknowledgement of the full scope of LPN practice (Box 5.1) can influence retention of LPNs in rural areas, stability of staffing, and level of team functioning within small rural work groups, which affects access and quality of care.

▲ BOX 5.1 RESEARCH HIGHLIGHT

Rural and Remote Licensed Practical Nurses' Perceptions of Working Below Their Legislated Scope of Practice

Research Focus
A 26-page, cross-sectional survey questionnaire, in English and French, was mailed to a stratified random sample of regulated nurses working in rural and remote areas in all provinces and territories in Canada.

Research Abstract
Over the past two decades, there has been a simultaneous increase in the educational preparation and scope of practice (SOP) of licensed practical nurses (LPNs) and in the number of LPNs employed in rural and remote communities. The aim of this study was to examine factors that predicted the perceptions of LPNs working in rural and remote areas as to whether they were working below their legislated SOP and their reflections on working below their SOP.

Methods
Of 9 622 eligible participants, 3 822 completed the survey, of which 1 370 were LPNs. Bivariate analyses, using a chi-square test for categorical data and t-tests or ANOVA for continuous data, were conducted on a subsample of LPNs whose reported primary position was staff nurse ($n = 1 206$), manager ($n = 32$), or clinical nurse specialist ($n = 98$). The subsample of LPNs ($n = 65$) whose reported SOP was beyond the legislated SOP was excluded from analysis because of low sample size and the priorities of the study.

Logistic regression analysis included 11 independent variables (individual = gender, age, career stage, perceived stress; practice = perceived work confidence and competence; workplace = supervision, recognition and feedback, staffing and time, autonomy and control; job demands = isolation and comfort with working conditions).

Results
Results showed that 17.6% of the LPNs perceived their practice to be below their legislated SOP. LPNs who were under 30 years of age were twice as likely to identify working below SOP than those age 55 years and over, and those who were at early or mid-career were twice as likely to identify working below SOP than LPNs in late career.

Implications for Practice
New understanding of legislated SOPs in terms of knowledge and responsibilities rather than tasks is required to avoid unnecessary gaps and overlaps in care, missed opportunities for appropriate registered nurse (RN) delegation, and intraprofessional collaboration, especially within the context of small rural and remote health care teams and expected shortages of LPNs and RNs.

From MacLeod, M. L. P., Stewart, N. J., Kosteniuk, J. G., et al. (2019). Rural and remote licensed practical nurses' perceptions of working below their legislated scope of practice. *Nursing Leadership, 32*(1), 8–19. https://doi.org/10.12927/cjnl.2019.25852

Indigenous people, many of whom live in rural and remote areas, also experience barriers in access to health care. The Truth and Reconciliation Commission of Canada has called for cultural competence of all health care providers and for increased numbers of Indigenous health professionals to combat racism, facilitate bridging between Western and traditional medicine, and facilitate access and positive health outcomes (CNA, 2014). Indigenous practical nursing programs, such as the one offered by Saskatchewan Independent Institute of Technologies that is designed from a First Nations perspective, offer a way forward to addressing the gaps identified in health care and its access for Indigenous people (Lindquist, 2021).

Despite growth in the numbers of LPNs practising in Canada, the outflow of nurses from the profession, particularly in the first 2 years after graduation, continues to be a concern. Of the four nursing groups, LPNs experienced the largest number of nurses leaving nursing in 2019 (CIHI, 2020a). Nowrouzi and colleagues (2016) reviewed the literature on workplace issues and workplace satisfaction among both RNs and LPNs. These authors suggested several factors that may contribute to nurses' stress, burnout, and, potentially, absenteeism, poor-quality care or productivity, or decision to leave the profession and health care:

- Overtime and long hours
- Long hours, especially 12-hour shifts
- Short staffing
- Situations of ethical distress
- Working for several employers
- Violence in the workplace
- Conflicted or noncollaborative relationships with other nurses or with physicians
- Lack of institutional support or commitment for nursing activities
- Feelings of powerlessness
- Amount of compensation

STANDARDS AND SCOPE OF PRACTICE

Standards of Practice

As a regulated profession, practical nursing is responsible for establishing its own **standards of practice**. While the CCPNR has established a national framework for standards of practice, the regulatory authority for LPNs in each jurisdiction has the legislative responsibility to set, monitor, and enforce the standards. The national framework facilitates interjurisdictional mobility and includes four broad standards that are applicable in any setting (CCPNR, 2021, p. 4):

- Professional accountability and responsibility
- Evidence-informed practice
- Public protection through self-regulation
- Professional and ethical practice

Standards of practice are written statements that outline the expectations and minimum level of performance for which LPNs in a particular jurisdiction are accountable. The practice of any LPN can be continually measured against these standards. They also demonstrate to the public that the profession of practical nursing is dedicated to protecting public safety and providing high-quality care (CCPNR, 2021).

Ethics in Nursing

Ethics refers choices about what is right or wrong; in nursing, these choices are guided by values and ethical standards and codes that guide nurses in their choices. Ethics influences behaviour and relationships with other people, including colleagues. Providing ethical nursing care means that the LPN forms a respectful, caring, helping relationship with the patient in order to help the patient achieve and maintain optimal health (CCPNR, 2013a).

The CCPNR has identified five principles in the Code of Ethics for Practical Nurses in Canada that include responsibility to the public, patients, the profession, colleagues, and oneself (CCPNR, 2013a, p. 3). Regulatory bodies for practical nursing are responsible for establishing and promoting codes of ethics or statements of values that are agreed upon by members of a profession and guide ethical decision making in their own jurisdictions.

Scope of Practice

Nurses practise autonomously within their scopes of practice. *Scope of practice* refers to the legal limits of a professional role as established by statutes or acts and in associated regulations. Scopes of practice generally outline the roles, functions, and accountabilities of professionals (Nova Scotia College of Nursing [NSCN], 2020). Each category of regulated nurse in Canada has its own scope of practice that reflects the education, performance requirements, and legal authority for that category (Table 5.3). Scopes of practice within a category may vary among jurisdictions because they are determined by individual provinces and territories.

TABLE 5.3	Educational Preparation and Decision Making Related to Care Provision for Practical and Registered Nurses	
	Practical Nurse	**Registered Nurse**
Entry-level education	Completion of a recognized practical nursing education program and successful completion of the Canadian Practical Nurse Registration Examination (CPRNE) or Registration Exam-Practical Nurse™ (REx-PN™)	Completion of a recognized baccalaureate program and successful completion of the NCLEX-RN
Patient	Educated to work collaboratively with patients (individuals, families, groups, and communities) and health care providers across the continuum of health	Educated to work collaboratively with patients (individuals, families, groups, populations, and communities) and with members of the health care team across the continuum of health
Context of practice	Focus is primarily on direct care in all settings and provides leadership (e.g., directs unregulated care providers [UCPs], mentors students, represents nursing and nursing care issues).	Works independently or as team member in diverse clinical, administrative, education, and research roles. Provides leadership (e.g., leads interprofessional teams, directs UCPs, makes decisions about resource allocation) in all care settings
Implementation	Coordinates care for patients who are stable, with more predicable outcomes. Provides elements of care for highly complex patients in close consultation with the RN. Initiates certain restricted or controlled activities, providing the LPN has the knowledge and **competence** (or ability) to do so, without an order from an authorized health care provider	Coordinates care of patients regardless of acuity, complexity, variability, or predictability. Directs plans of care for highly complex patients. Researches and uses evidence-informed practice. Initiates restricted or controlled activities that are common to and different from those authorized to the practical nurse, providing the RN has the knowledge and competence to do so, without an order from an authorized health professional. Assists in medical assistance in dying.

From College of Nurses of Ontario (CNO). (2018). *RN and RPN practice: The client, the nurse, and the environment.* https://www.cno.org/globalassets/docs/prac/41062.pdf; Nova Scotia College of Nursing (NSCN). (2020). *Nursing scope of practice: Practice guideline.* https://cdn1.nscn.ca/sites/default/files/documents/resources/Scope_of_Practice2020.pdf

The capacity to optimize legislated scopes of practice in specific working environments is determined by employment scopes of practice, which are outlined in job descriptions and policies and will vary from site to site. Nurses are responsible for knowing their employment as well as their legislated scope of practice and for advocating for changes as patient needs and environmental shifts occur. They must also consider whether it is possible to attain and maintain competence in specific areas of practice when the scope of practice is optimized. Employers must consider whether the expansion of the scope of practice in a specific work setting will benefit patients and minimize possible risks, as well as whether there are clear policies, procedures, and supervision to support optimization of the scope of practice. In addition, it is important to consider the impact on other members of the health care team and stakeholders and whether they have been adequately consulted and informed. Employer convenience is not considered an adequate reason to optimize scopes of practice (NSCN, 2020).

While regulatory bodies and employers place parameters on what LPNs are able to do, it is also important for LPNs to recognize the responsibility that they assume for their individual practice through licensure. What this means is that LPNs are obligated to ensure that they have the necessary knowledge, skills, and judgement to perform safe care, as well as to determine when safe care of a patient is beyond their scope of practice and level of competence and requires consultation with other health care providers or RNs (Almost, 2021).

While specific scopes of practice may differ among jurisdictions, it is common to find that as the complexity and unpredictability of the patient's condition and risk of negative outcomes increase, practical nurses will need more collaboration and support from RNs. This support may involve consultation with the RN, sharing the patient assignment with the RN, or the RN taking complete responsibility for the patient (CNO, 2018; NSCN, 2020) It is essential that LPNs and RNs are aware of each other's scopes of practice because this awareness enhances their ability to work collaboratively to determine and deliver the most appropriate plan of care.

Challenges to Working to Full Scope of Practice. Although graduates of practical nursing programs are prepared with entry-level competencies that are consistent with their scope of practice, there are many factors that can influence their level of practice. For example, practical nurses can and do acquire skills, knowledge, and judgement consistent with the scope of practice for practical nurses beyond what is needed for entry-level practice, such as operating room techniques, special foot care, orthopedic care, dialysis care, and specialized gerontological care.

Whether LPNs can fully apply their expanded skills and knowledge or even skills expected for entry-level competencies is dependent on several enablers and barriers. In reference to RPNs in Ontario, a report by the Registered Practical Nurses Association of Ontario (2014) identified that RPNs were much more likely to understand the role of the RN than RNs were to understand the role of RPNs, which is a concern when many RNs are in positions of leadership and administration within organizations. Optimization of the full scope of practice of LPNs is more likely when there is strong team acceptance of the LPN role, organizational support and policies, and procedures and job descriptions that align with the current regulatory, legislative, and practice guidelines in relation to LPN practice. Barriers to full optimization include confusion and ambiguity about the differences and similarities in the roles of LPNs and RNs. This confusion is further fueled by discussions centred around nursing tasks, where there is considerable overlap between those commonly performed by LPNs and those performed by RNs. These discussions can serve to devalue the depth and breadth of nursing knowledge and to generate further role conflict and ambiguity. Instead, a focus on competencies leads to greater understanding and appropriate utilization of the complex skills, knowledge, and judgement inherent in the practice of all nurses.

Underutilization, overutilization, or inappropriate utilization of the skills and knowledge of LPNs can lead to frustration for both LPNs and RNs, LPN attrition (MacLeod et al., 2019), as well as missed opportunities to build strong, collaborative teams. Outdated conceptions of RN and LPN roles, such as the requirement for RNs to supervise LPNs, mean that the skills and knowledge of both categories of nurses are unable to be optimized, which is a detriment in health care systems that continue to be challenged by fiscal issues and staffing shortages.

Understanding the roles of RNs and LPNs in various care delivery models requires ongoing efforts for dialogue, shared learning, and research among leaders, practitioners, educators, and researchers. Organizational practices such as clear policies and job descriptions and strong leadership that instills and exemplifies respect for the care capacities of nurses is important in reducing ambiguity and conflict in nursing teams. Curriculum in pre-entry programs that provide opportunities for intraprofessional students to learn together and to learn about the roles and competencies of RNs and LPNs can also assist in building collaborative teams.

Interprofessional and Intraprofessional Collaborative Practice

The LPN is a team member and thus should always work in a collaborative manner with other health care personnel. Interprofessional collaboration includes communicating with the patient, the family, and other health care workers to define, implement, and evaluate the plan of care. Good working relationships and intraprofessional collaboration between LPNs and RNs in the team are essential in the delivery of quality patient care. The LPN also makes suggestions and referrals to individual members of the health care team and in team meetings in which patient care and concerns are discussed. Full understanding of all roles and clear and appropriate communication are integral to effective collaboration within a team.

Leadership: Supervising and Delegating

LPNs receive supervision and accept delegation and can themselves supervise and delegate. Commonly, delegation by LPNs involves that of **unregulated care providers (UCPs)**, who can be paid (such as home support workers, resident care attendants, or personal support workers) or family members and who are an increasingly important part of health care delivery. UCPs have no legally defined scope of practice, mandated educational requirements, or practice standards, and their role and position are defined by employers (BCCNM, 2021b).

To supervise and delegate, the LPN must have knowledge and skill in what is being supervised or delegated. Supervision and delegation, although different skills, serve to ensure that a task is performed safely and competently.

Supervision. Supervision is usually required by individuals who are new to a skill or role, such as practical nurse students, new members of a profession, and UCPs, and does not require transfer of authority (CNO, 2020b). The person who is supervising may or may not be a member of the same profession or occupational group.

Supervision is an intervention and usually part of an ongoing and developing relationship. The purposes of **supervision** are to enhance competent functioning of an inexperienced person and to protect the public and the professional practice. Supervision requires indirect or direct observation, monitoring, and evaluation until the task can be safely performed alone (CNO, 2020b). The supervisor provides evaluative information about the task performed as soon as is feasible.

Delegation. In delegation, the authority to perform a task is transferred to another person or group and refers only to transfer of authority for controlled acts or legally restricted procedures. The nurse must make this decision carefully. Before delegating a task to another person, the nurse must ensure that the nurse has the regulated authority to perform the task and whether it can be legally delegated. The nurse must also have the required knowledge, skill, and judgement to perform the task. Other factors that need to be considered when delegating include the following (CNO, 2020b):

- The associated risks and benefits for the patient
- The need for another person to perform the task
- Whether the necessary support (including supervision) and resources are available for the delegatee to safely perform the task
- Whether institutional policies and procedures allow the delegatee to accept delegation

Responsibility does not stop once a task is delegated to another person. The delegating nurse retains ultimate responsibility for the correct completion of the task and for documentation.

Continuing Education and Expanded Competencies

The LPN is expected to continue professional growth and acquire a range of knowledge, skills, and judgement beyond that of the minimal entry-to-practice standards, particularly in changing health care and regulatory environments (CLPNA, 2020). Many educational opportunities are available to the LPN from postsecondary institutions, the CNA, other professional organizations, employers (e.g., in-house to optimize scope), and charitable agencies (e.g., Diabetes Canada).

LEGISLATION, REGULATORY BODIES, AND PROFESSIONAL ASSOCIATIONS

Legislation, regulatory bodies, and professional associations govern the practice of nursing. These have been created to protect public safety and promote ethical practice.

Legislation

In most provinces and territories, nursing practice has similar legal regulatory requirements (education, registration, and complaints and disciplinary processes) and professional standards. Legislation that enables regulation of health professions, including LPNs, serves to protect the best interests of the public (CCPNR, 2021).

Acts That Govern Health Care Professions. In most provinces and territories, health professions have their own governing legislation, called an *act*. These acts, as well as regulations and provisions specific to each health profession (e.g., physicians, nurses, physiotherapists), mandate how professional colleges are to be established and governed and the protection of professional titles. The acts also lay out the rules and processes for initial registration and continuing competence for members of the colleges, handling of grievances and complaints, and what controlled acts individual professions may perform (Government of Manitoba, n.d.). Regulation of LPNs is managed through a combination of legislation and provincial colleges or associations, except in Nunavut, the Northwest Territories, and Yukon, where they are managed through territorial legislation (Almost, 2021).

Some provinces have removed separate acts for individual health care professions and are replacing them with a single, generic umbrella act that applies to all health care professions (e.g., *Regulated Health Professions Act* in Ontario) (Almost, 2021; CNO 2020b, 2020c). Others are replacing acts that govern individual categories of nurses with a single act that encompasses all categories of nurses, such as Nova Scotia's *Nursing Act* (NSCN, 2021). Umbrella acts enable consistency in rules and processes across all aspects of regulation and enable the public to better understand these processes. Umbrella legislation also makes it easier to address issues that may affect all the regulated professions. The nonexclusivity of controlled or reserved acts allows greater practice flexibility and interprofessional care because scopes of practice are no longer exclusive to single professions (CNO 2020b, 2020c; Government of Manitoba, n.d.).

Controlled Acts. Controlled or authorized acts (e.g., in Ontario), restricted acts (e.g., in British Columbia), or reserved acts (e.g., Manitoba) are acts that are harmful unless performed by qualified persons. The *Ontario Nursing Act 1991* defines which of the 13 authorized acts specified in the *Regulated Health Professions Act* nurses are allowed to perform (CNO, 2020b):

- Performing a procedure below the dermis or mucous membrane
- Placing an instrument, hand, or finger into a body opening
- Administering a substance by injection or inhalation
- Dispensing a medication

The complexity of patient care, health care priorities, and advancement of technology have prompted changes in controlled acts that LPNs are able to perform. In Alberta, for example, changes and revisions to the LPN Regulation allow LPNs to administer blood and blood products, providing they have the necessary skills and knowledge to do so, which may depend on year of graduation from a basic practical nurse program or on-the-job training. Revisions to the Alberta LPN Regulation also clarify which restricted activities are considered advanced practice (or specialized practice in other jurisdictions), such as removal of corns and calluses in foot care, and require special authorization from the College (CLPNA, 2020).

Regulatory Bodies

According to the professional and health care acts, each profession must have a regulatory body that governs it. As the health care environment changes, regulatory bodies adapt by modifying practice standards and guidelines accordingly. Depending on the province or territory, regulatory bodies for nurses may be a college, an association, or the government (Nunavut, Northwest Territories, and Yukon) (Almost, 2021).

Functions of the Regulatory Body. The primary mandate of nursing regulatory bodies is protection of the public, which is accomplished through self-regulation. Self-regulation is a legislative privilege and acknowledges that nurses have the knowledge and expertise to regulate themselves as individual practitioners by maintaining competence and fitness to practise. Self-regulation for the profession as a whole involves several processes (Office of the Superintendent of Professional Governance, n.d.), including:

- Establishing entry-to-practice requirements and requirements for registration
- Establishing, promoting, and enforcing practice standards
- Enforcing standards of conduct and investigating complaints and grievances
- Ensuring the continuing competence of its members
- Approving education programs

Protecting or Reserving Titles. Regulatory bodies are usually responsible for ensuring that the professional title (e.g., LPN) of registered members is protected or reserved. This also means that only registered members are authorized to call themselves by the professional title. Protection is usually also extended to other, synonymous terms for the title (Office of the Superintendent of Professional Governance, n.d.). For example, in Ontario, all the following related terms and abbreviations are protected: *nurse, registered practical nurse, LPN,* and their variants.

The Registration Process for the Practical Nurse (Credentialling). The regulatory body (also called a *registering body*) in each province and territory determines whether applicants have sufficient educational background and competency for registration as a practical nurse. To be registered as practical nurses, applicants must prove that their education meets requirements for theoretical and clinical hours in specified topics and clinical areas and pass the licensing examination required by the jurisdiction. The requirement for evidence of successful, current practice is satisfied if an applicant is a recent graduate of a program in the province where registration is sought. Applicants from outside the province, territory, or country or those who are returning to work must provide evidence of recent competent work (usually within the past 3 to 5 years) in the practical nursing field, as well as successful completion of Canadian licensing examinations or their equivalent. If the certification examination, educational preparation, or evidence of competent practice are not accepted by the regulatory body, then applicants may need to write the licensing examination or take theoretical or clinical courses to meet current Canadian standards. As already noted, in many jurisdictions, applicants must also pass a criminal record check before registering to practise (CCPNR, 2013b).

Professional Associations

Professional associations provide a voice for practical nurses to government and other organizations, as well as informed advocacy in issues affecting patient and health care, opportunities for networking, and enhancement of professional knowledge. For example, WeRPN, the former Registered Practical Nurses Association of Ontario and a stand-alone association for practical nurses, has been an active advocate for adequate physical and staffing resourcing, testing, and vaccination during the COVID-19 pandemic and for retention of nurses in remote and rural areas (WeRPN, 2020).

In British Columbia and Manitoba, practical nurses can join associations that are inclusive of other nursing groups, and in New Brunswick, there is a dual regulatory/professional association. LPNs in jurisdictions without associations can access the Canadian Practical Nurses Association, the Canadian Nurses Association, or the Canadian Association of Practical Nurse Educators (Almost, 2021). Unlike membership in the regulatory body, membership in the professional association is usually voluntary.

THE FUTURE OF PRACTICAL NURSING IN CANADA

The health care system in Canada is continually changing, and these changes affect practical nursing. To cope effectively, nurses must be **proactive** and view change as a challenge and an opportunity rather than a threat. By doing so, nursing will maintain and advance its niche position in health care.

General Health Care Trends

Current and projected changes have the potential to affect practical nursing. Reports and data from sources such as the Canadian Institute for Health Information (CIHI, 2020b, 2022), Canadian Medical Association (2019) and Public Health Agency of Canada (PHAC, 2018, 2020a, 2020b) suggest factors, issues, and discussions that affect health care now and in the future:

- Personalized technology that enables continuous monitoring and surveillance outside of clinic and health facilities
- Access to data of individuals and across systems and providers, with ensuing questions about privacy and security of data
- Ongoing public demand for transparency and voice in health decisions

- Significantly rising costs of health care
- Growing population of older persons
- Increasing wait times for some procedures
- Emergence of new infectious diseases (e.g., COVID-19)
- Adequacy of public health care
- Ongoing inequities in access to and quality of health care among rural and remote populations, Indigenous people, persons with lower socioeconomic conditions, and older persons in long-term care
- Increased prevalence of chronic disorders and multiple comorbidities

These trends within the Canadian health care system and in the health of Canadians drive discussions around appropriate staffing mixes and alternative care delivery and funding models. For example, there is increasing interest in how to manage transitions from hospital to home or to long-term care to prevent readmission to hospitals. With the increasing prevalence of chronic disorders, there is also increasing interest in different management strategies and health promotion and education to manage and prevent chronic disorders. Prevention efforts among older persons include measures to reduce the frequency of falls at home as well as the negative health and social effects for caregivers of older persons. Increased awareness about the mental health of caregivers, older persons, children, and others as well as concerns about violence in homes and in the workplace continue to raise concerns about the safety of patients, caregivers, the public, and health care providers. The COVID-19 pandemic highlighted gaps and inequities in care for the most vulnerable persons in the population, especially those who are in long-term care, as well as the need for adequate public health services. Ongoing concerns remain about access to care in communities in remote and rural areas of Canada and for Indigenous people (CNA, 2022b; WeRPN, 2020).

Complex patient needs, evolving technology, and evolving care strategies require that professionals work collaboratively together and with patients, which is acknowledged directly in nursing legislation (Almost, 2021). While interprofessional collaboration is still an emphasis, there is increased interest in intraprofessional teams. Nurses from all categories indicate that intraprofessional collaboration and patient care models that optimize professional competencies are key to safe, quality patient care and healthy work environments (Villeneuve, 2021).

Implications for Practical Nursing

Continuous rapid change and the emergence of new research, innovations, technology, and pandemics requires professionals to respond appropriately in order to cope effectively. Practical nurses need to be lifelong learners and develop increasingly broad-based competencies to adapt to changing occupational demands. This is not the time to focus solely on one narrow skill set or to cling stubbornly only to the knowledge base acquired in pre-entry programs.

Practical nurses have the competencies to contribute significantly within primary care and on interprofessional and intraprofessional teams. The complexity of care and rapid evolution of knowledge will require practical nurses to be increasingly aware of current scopes of practice among other health care providers and to be an advocate for the optimization of these scopes of practice, including their own.

Practical nurses of the future will likely need to have increased knowledge of **epidemiology**, given the demands of the COVID-19 pandemic as well as of their work among vulnerable populations such as older persons in long-term care and in the community. They will assume a greater role in illness prevention, health promotion, and health teaching for patients throughout the lifespan, which will involve teaching about healthy lifestyles, collaboration with the patient and others, and empowerment of patients to make their own health care decisions. In addition, practical nurses will likely become increasingly involved in teaching other health care workers about infection prevention practices, as well as modelling excellence in this area of practice, and thus will be instrumental in the prevention of devastating infections among vulnerable populations.

Technology use has become the norm rather than the exception in most health care institutions and with patient self-management. Practical nurses will need continued competency in technology to appropriately use various tools and applications in direct patient care and to pursue their education.

Nurses work with an increasingly diverse and multicultural population base and will themselves become more diverse. There will be continued emphasis on the preparation of nurses who are Indigenous, who understand both Indigenous and Western approaches to health and wellness. Practical nurses of the future will need more knowledge and skill in applying concepts from the humanities and social sciences, such as psychology, sociology, and anthropology, and will have opportunities to take programs that are designed with Indigenous people and practitioners as a primary focus.

Possible Evolution of the Practical Nurse Role

Changes in Educational Standards for Entry to Practice. In view of the likely expanding roles for the practical nurse, a high school diploma will continue to be the minimum requirement for entry into a practical nursing program. Some knowledge of or fluency in a second language would be useful in our increasingly multicultural society.

Practical nurse education programs need to be at least two academic years in length and must occur in a postsecondary institution that meets general program standards for preparing professionals to meet entry-level requirements. These programs must be academically sound and include components of pure science, social science, and humanities, as well as interprofessional and intraprofessional learning opportunities. Beyond the basic program, there will need to be more opportunities for LPNs to gain partial or full transfer credit into baccalaureate nursing programs. Should a university degree in practical nursing be available? It could assist in increasing access in rural and remote areas and lead to positive outcomes among older persons, such as those in long-term care, although it could also serve only to further blur roles between LPNs and RNs.

Scope of Practice and New Competencies. The practical nursing profession faces an exciting future. The practical nursing scope of practice will continue to evolve in response to changes in the Canadian health care system. Despite changes in roles, collaborative practice between RNs and practical nurses is viewed as important in health care delivery (Villeneuve, 2021).

Practical nurses of the future will continue to acquire separate postgraduate competencies in specific areas such as wound care, orthopedics, leadership, palliative care, and chronic disease management through credentialling, certifications, and other post–basic education and training. This will make them well positioned to work with persons with diverse needs, illness, and cultural experiences, as well as make them increasingly important in the care of underserviced and vulnerable persons such as those who are older or experiencing chronic illness. This will mean ongoing dialogue with RNs, as well as research related to patient care models and intraprofessional relationships, to plan for future roles and scopes of practice that serve all stakeholders in the Canadian health care system.

What Is the Final Answer?

What will happen to practical nursing in the future? No one knows for certain, but the history of practical nurses indicates that it has been able to adapt and change to meet socioeconomic and health demands.

Practical nurses and registered nurses may always maintain separate scopes of practice that together mean that patients with diverse needs and levels of acuity and complexity will experience care that addresses various aspects of their health and illness. Practical nursing will position its significance for health care of the future by developing more diverse and specialized competencies in our changing society. As it has done in the past, it must continue to address the needs of society and change to meet health care demands in this environment of continued rapid change.

KEY CONCEPTS

- Nursing is the largest single group of health care providers in Canada, and licensed practical nurses are the second largest nursing group.
- Practical nursing was recognized in the 1970s as a distinct profession that necessitates formal education.
- Education programs for practical nurses have become longer and more complex and are now diploma programs that are offered in postsecondary institutions.
- Registered nurses and practical nurses differ in the depth and breadth of their knowledge base.
- Licensed practical nurses have a strong foundation in clinical practice, decision making, and critical thinking.
- Competencies, rather than tasks, are useful in differentiating registered nursing and practical nursing practice and in optimizing practice.
- Although primarily involved in direct care, practical nurses work in a range of roles and in increasingly diverse settings.
- Through legislation, licensed practical nurses have autonomous practice and are accountable for their own practice.
- The practice of practical nurses is guided not only by the scope of practice but also by their knowledge and skills, organizational policies and job descriptions, and practice standards.
- Ongoing dialogue with organizations is necessary to create understanding about the current scopes of practice of licensed practical nurses, to optimize care, prevent frustration among practical nurses, and prevent their early departure from the profession.
- Self-regulation is a privilege that is entrusted to the regulatory bodies for the protection of the public interest, which includes ensuring that requirements for licensure and continuing competence are met.
- Practical nurses are expected to continue professional growth and acquire a range of knowledge, skill, and judgement beyond that of minimal entry-level standards.
- Practice includes both interprofessional and intraprofessional considerations.
- Ongoing change in the health care system and crises such as pandemics require the practical nursing profession to continue to adapt entry-level practice competencies and scope of practice.

CRITICAL THINKING EXERCISES

1. The delivery of health care will be different in the future. If RNs begin to play a larger role in primary health care, how will that affect the future roles of L/RPNs and UCPs? How would you design the human resources structure of the Canadian health care system of the future?

2. The manager of a surgical unit is reviewing the staffing complement for the unit. The responsibilities of the practical nurses have not changed on the unit for the last 5 years. Based on what you know about the scope of practice for L/RPNs and delegation, what could be done to optimize the L/RPN scope of practice and patient care? What resources would you suggest the manager access?

3. A newly graduated practical nurse is caring for a patient after a total knee replacement. Eight hours after the patient's return to the unit, he begins to complain of shortness of breath and chest pain on inhalation. The nurse identifies that oxygen saturation levels are falling and air entry is decreased to the patient's left lower lobe. The nurse has never encountered this type of situation before. Describe how the practical nurse and RN can partake in consultation and collaboration in this situation.

🌐 *Answers to Critical Thinking Exercises appear on the Evolve website.*

REVIEW QUESTIONS

Review Questions 1 to 10 relate to the case study at the beginning of the chapter.

1. According to various studies, it is important for Michelle and others in the health care team to understand the full scope of Taylor's practice for which of the following reasons? *(Select all that apply.)*
   a. Lack of understanding can create gaps in the appropriate utilization of LPN knowledge and skills in patient care.
   b. Where there is a difference, professional scopes of practice override the authority of employment scopes of practice and must be followed.
   c. RNs are required to assume accountability when an LPN is unable to practise to the standards set out for LPNs.
   d. Lack of understanding of the scope of practice of LPNs can lead to underutilization, job dissatisfaction, and early departure from nursing.

2. Which of the following BEST explains Michelle's doubt about whether Taylor should start the blood transfusion? *(Select all that apply.)*
   a. Michelle and Taylor may have an interpersonal conflict.
   b. Taylor can no longer continue with the patient assignment because of the patient's complex needs.
   c. Michelle is not fully aware of the current scope of practice for LPNs.
   d. Michelle may be unaware of Taylor's skills and knowledge in this area.

3. Which of the following would be MOST helpful for Taylor to say at this point?
   a. "I am not sure why you are hesitant about me starting the blood transfusion with this patient. The patient is stable, and LPNs started blood at my previous workplace."
   b. "I feel that you are hesitant about whether I should start the blood transfusion with my patient. Could you share your reasons with me?"
   c. "I am not sure why you are hesitating. You indicated that I efficiently prepared for the blood transfusion and, as an LPN, I am an autonomous professional who is knowledgeable and responsible for her own practice."
   d. "Michelle, I see you have doubts about me starting the blood transfusion. You likely don't know, but LPNs who graduate from 2-year programs can now start blood transfusions."

4. Which factors contributed to the inclusion of this and other restricted procedures in the basic preparation of LPNs? *(Select all that apply.)*
   a. The need of the health care systems for better preparation of LPNs
   b. Changes to the scope of practice for RNs
   c. Revisions to entry-level competencies for LPNs
   d. Ceding of restricted activities to LPNs by physicians and RNs

5. Taylor is eager to show Michelle the current legislated scope of practice for LPNs. Together, they search regulatory documents, which clearly outline the expansion of scope of practice for LPNs and accountability of LPNs for their own practice. Which of the following is important to consider about Taylor's individual practice that is relevant in the current situation? *(Select all that apply.)*
   a. How Taylor has maintained skills, knowledge, and judgement in administration of blood products
   b. Whether the curriculum for Taylor's basic practical nursing program was approved by its provincial or territorial regulatory body
   c. Whether the LPN's prior regulatory body had specific requirements for evidence of continuing competence in nursing practice
   d. The level of supervision and mentorship provided to Taylor in prior nursing assignments

6. Taylor indicates to Michelle that she has received further training in blood administration and that Taylor successfully started blood transfusions in her recent past employment. Assuming that the patient is stable at this point, what is the next step?
   a. The RN will administer the blood until the manager is contacted and provides confirmation that LPNs can administer blood.
   b. The RN and the LPN will review organizational policies related to administration of blood.
   c. The RN will ask other staff members on the unit if LPNs can administer blood or blood products.
   d. The LPN will proceed to administer the blood to the patient.

7. To enable LPNs to optimize their scope of practice, which of the following steps does the employer of Taylor and Michelle need to take? *(Select all that apply.)*
   a. Consult with other health care providers and stakeholders regarding impacts of optimization.
   b. Provide information and education to staff regarding current scopes of practice.
   c. Consider the benefits to patients of LPNs administering blood products.
   d. Determine what models of nursing care will support optimization.
   e. Ensure cost savings by replacing RNs with LPNs.

8. Taylor returns to her assigned patient to update the patient about the blood transfusion. Taylor finds the patient nearly unresponsive and quickly assesses the patient, including vital signs (BP 85/40 and falling; P 130 and weak; R 32) and the operative site, which is dry and intact. What follow-up does Taylor need to initiate? *(Select all that apply.)*
   a. Administer an analgesic.
   b. Return in 15 minutes to reassess the patient.
   c. Initiate the blood transfusion.
   d. Call the RN immediately.

9. Taylor eventually decides to focus on the advanced practice area of perioperative nursing. Which of the following would Taylor pursue with this goal in mind?
   a. Completion of a baccalaureate program in nursing
   b. A challenge of the NCLEX-RN examination
   c. A review of procedure and policy manuals
   d. Completion of a certificate course in perioperative nursing

10. A friend of Taylor's and graduate from an international nursing program excitedly proclaims that it is now possible to use the title of LPN. The friend indicates that the only things required for registration were transcripts from the program completed and assessment of work experience, and the provincial regulatory body granted registration. Taylor expresses concern that the friend may not have accurately understood the process of registration. What would be the reason(s) for Taylor's concern? *(Select all that apply.)*

a. Internationally prepared nurses are rarely allowed to register as LPNs in Canada because there are too many LPNs in the workforce.
b. Internationally prepared nurses do not have educational preparation and the job experiences required for registration.
c. After satisfying educational, practice, and other requirements, all applicants for registration must write the registration examination.
d. It is too difficult for regulatory bodies to determine if international applicants from different countries have met the requirements for registration.

Answers to Review Questions: 1. a, d; **2.** c, d; **3.** b; **4.** a, b; **5.** a; **6.** b; **7.** a, b, c, d; **8.** d; **9.** d; **10.** c.

Rationales for the Review Questions appear on the Evolve website.

RECOMMENDED WEBSITES

Association of New Brunswick Registered Practical Nurses: https://www.anblpn.ca.
British Columbia College of Nurses and Midwives: https://www.bccnm.ca.
Canadian Council for Practical Nurse Regulators: https://www.ccpnr.ca. This is a federation of provincial and territorial members responsible for regulation of L/RPNs.
Canadian Nurses Association: https://www.cna-aiic.ca/en. This is the voice of RNs and L/RPNs across Canada, including advocacy and influence regarding public policies and initiatives affecting nursing practice, patient care, and the health care system.
College of Licensed Practical Nurses of Alberta: https://www.clpna.com.
College of Licensed Practical Nurses of Manitoba: https://www.clpnm.ca.
College of Licensed Practical Nurses of Prince Edward Island: https://clpnpei.ca.
College of LPNs of Newfoundland & Labrador: http://www.clpnnl.ca.
College of Nurses of Ontario: https://www.cno.org.

Government of Northwest Territories, Office of the Registrar of Professional Licensing, Health and Social Services: https://www.hss.gov.nt.ca/en/services/professional-licensing.
Government of Yukon, Professional Licensing: https://yukon.ca/en/professional-licensing.
Nova Scotia College of Nurses: https://www.nscn.ca.
Ordre des infirmières et infirmiers auxiliaires du Québec: https://www.oiiq.org.
Saskatchewan Association of Licensed Practical Nurses: https://salpn.com.
WeRPN: Registered Practical Nurses Association of Ontario: https://www.werpn.com.
A professional association for RPNs that engages in advancing the role and expertise of RPNs and patient care, influencing policy and initiatives related to the nursing profession and patient care.

*These are the websites of colleges and associations that regulate practical nurses. They provide information and support related to legislation and regulation related to L/RPNs, education and registration requirements, and practice standards.

REFERENCES

A full reference list is available on the website for this book at http://evolve.elsevier.com/Canada/Potter/fundamentals/

6

Theoretical Foundations of Nursing Practice

Written by Sally Thorne, RN, PhD, FCAHS, FAAN, FCAN

OBJECTIVES

Mastery of content in this chapter will enable you to:

- Define the key terms listed.
- Describe selected theories of nursing practice and differentiate between them.
- Describe the challenges inherent in theorizing about nursing practice.
- Recognize selected conceptual frameworks associated with nursing practice.
- Appreciate the historical development of thought related to nursing practice.
- Interpret current debates surrounding various theories of nursing practice.
- Describe the relationships between theorizing and other forms of nursing knowledge.
- Appreciate the role of "theorizing" about the essence of nursing.

KEY TERMS

Assumption

Concept

Conceptual framework

Conceptualization

Descriptive theory

Grand theory

Metaparadigm concepts

Middle-range theory

Model for nursing

Nursing diagnosis

Nursing process

Nursing science

Nursing theory

Paradigms

Philosophy of science

Praxis

Prescriptive theory

Proposition

Theoretical model

Theory

Ways of knowing

🌐 WEBSITE

http://evolve.elsevier.com/Canada/Potter/fundamentals/

CASE STUDY

Undergraduate students Nassim (preferred pronouns: them/they) and Geertje (preferred pronouns: them/they) have heard about a "nursing theory–practice gap" and want to better understand why that matters. Nassim asks, "Professor Xiao, why is it important to know about nursing theory? What possible role could it play in our nursing practice?" Professor Xiao replies, "You have raised an excellent question, and I hope that throughout your career you will continue to be intrigued by 'why does this matter' questions—and continue to be curious about the answers." As the conversation continues, Professor Xiao explains that nursing theory represents our discipline's best efforts to articulate the complexity of nursing excellence. Nurses may learn tasks and skills in the classroom, but they enact them in the practice world in the context of human lives, complete with their histories and wider social contexts, and under difficult circumstances across the spectrum of health and illness. In fact, nursing done well is so complex that it defies clear definition, but we know it exists, so we theorize various ways of explaining that. By studying the nursing theorists, we uncover layers of understanding about this marvelous profession of ours.

Think about this case study as you read this chapter. There are review questions at the end of the chapter about the case study.

Although many nursing tasks can be mastered by anyone trained to perform them, the hallmark of nursing practice is a unique body of knowledge combined with a set of principles that guide the systematic application of that knowledge in an infinite array of contexts. The aim of **nursing theory** is to organize knowledge about nursing to enable nurses to use it in a professional and accountable manner (Beckstrand, 1978).

A **theory** is a purposeful set of **assumptions** or **propositions** that identify the relationships between **concepts**. Theories are useful because they provide a systematic way of explaining, predicting, and prescribing phenomena. Although nursing theories are not generally propositional, they reflect a **conceptualization** of nursing for the purpose of describing, explaining, predicting, or prescribing care (Meleis, 2018). Theories constitute one aspect of disciplinary knowledge and create vital linkages to how inquiry is approached (Fawcett et al., 2001). Nursing theories provide nurses with a perspective from which to view patient situations, a way to organize data, and a method of analyzing and interpreting information to bring about coherent and informed nursing practice.

EARLY NURSING PRACTICE AND THE EMERGENCE OF THEORY

Although nursing practices have been documented throughout history (Yura & Walsh, 1973), the advent of modern nursing practice, in which the knowledge and practice of nursing are formalized into a professional context, is often attributed to the work of Florence Nightingale, a visionary leader in Victorian England who created systems for nursing education and practice (see Chapter 3). Contemporary scholars now consider Nightingale's work an early theoretical and conceptual **model for nursing**. Her descriptive theory provided nurses with a way to think about nursing practice in a frame of reference that focuses on patients and the environment.

Since Nightingale's era, the status of nursing practice has paralleled that of the authority of women in society. After World War II, major developments in science and technology had a powerful influence on health care, including nursing practice. **Nursing science** came into its own. No longer simply thinking of themselves as applying the knowledge of other disciplines, nurses began to acquire a distinctive body of knowledge about the practice of nursing.

Since the 1960s, scientific knowledge has proliferated across all disciplines. In particular, nursing knowledge has drawn from and contributed to developments in health sciences, basic physical sciences, social and biobehavioural sciences, social theory, ethical theory, and the **philosophy of science** (discussed later in this chapter in the section "Philosophy of Nursing Science"). Each of these sources of knowledge is relevant to the interpretation of nursing care and the synthesis of relevant facts and theories for application to practice.

Several major developments in nursing theory occurred in the late 1960s (Meleis, 2018). The health care system was expanding and changing, influenced by scientific discoveries and technological applications. Disease interventions became more sophisticated and scientifically driven. The focus of society shifted from simply attending to sick and injured people toward the larger problem of curing and eradicating disease, which expanded the influence of physicians over the structure of health care delivery. For the first time, nurses realized the urgency of articulating exactly how their role differed from those of other health care providers (Chinn et al., 2022; Engebretson, 1997; Fawcett, 2013; Newman, 1972).

Early theorizing about the practice of nursing was driven by nurse educators, who noted that the traditional ways of preparing professional nurses were rapidly becoming outdated. Until the 1960s, a nursing apprenticeship model, augmented by lectures offered by physicians,

had seemed sufficient. Around that time, nursing educational leaders became inspired to theorize about nursing in order to structure and define what a curriculum oriented to nursing knowledge might contain (Dean, 1995; Orem & Parker, 1964; Torres, 1974). This meant grappling with large theoretical and philosophical questions, such as the following:

- What are the focus and scope of nursing?
- How is nursing unique and different from other health care professions?
- What should be the appropriate disciplinary knowledge for professional nursing practice?

To answer these questions, early theorists developed **conceptual frameworks** in which they organized core nursing concepts and proposed relationships among these concepts. These conceptual frameworks were "mental maps" whose purpose was to make sense of the information and decisional processes that nurses needed in order to apply knowledge to nursing practice (Ellis, 1968; Johnson, 1974; McKay, 1969; Wald & Leonard, 1964). Expressing knowledge about nursing in scientific language created a context in which nursing science gained stature and began to flourish (Cull-Wilby & Peppin, 1987; Jones, 1997). However, these nursing theories were not the kind of propositional scientific theories that could be confirmed or disproved with empirical evidence (Levine, 1995); rather, they represented ideas about how nurses might organize knowledge, as well as the processes by which they would apply that knowledge to unique practice situations. Table 6.1 defines some of the basic terms that are used in theorizing about scientific issues.

❖ NURSING PROCESS

Early nursing theorists sought to organize the knowledge about the practice of nursing that nurses draw upon to direct their approach to clinical encounters. However, theorists generally lacked ways of systematically explaining how nurses work with knowledge in new situations (Field, 1987). An important early step in the application of knowledge to nursing practice was the development of a problem-solving approach by Orlando (1961) that came to be known as the **nursing process** (Yura & Walsh, 1973). This process originally involved four steps (assessment, planning, intervention, and evaluation), with each step representing a distinct way in which general nursing knowledge could be applied to unique and individual nurse–patient situations (Carnevali & Thomas, 1993; Henderson, 1966; Meleis, 2018; Torres, 1986):

- Assessment phase: Nurses would gather information, including biological, sociocultural, environmental, spiritual, and psychological data, to create an understanding of the patient's unique health or illness experience. Organizing the data would enable the nurses to interpret major issues and concerns (Barnum, 1998) and produce a **nursing diagnosis**—the nurse's perspective on the appropriate focus for the patient (Durand & Prince, 1966).
- Planning phase: Nurses would prioritize the issues raised during assessment in relation to the nursing diagnoses, identify which issues could be supported or assisted by nursing intervention, and create a plan of care.
- Intervention phase: The plan of care would be carried out.
- Evaluation phase: The plan's success or failure would be judged both against the plan itself and against the patient's overall health status; that is, it would be determined whether the intended outcomes had been achieved or whether the nursing intervention strategies required revision. The nursing process was intended as a sequence within which thoughtful interpretation always preceded action, and the effects of action were always evaluated in relation to the original situation.

TABLE 6.1	The Terminology of Scientific Theorizing	
Term	**Description**	**Example**
Concept	A mental formulation of objects or events representing the basic way in which ideas are organized and communicated	Anxiety
Conceptualization	The process of formulating concepts	Framing behavioural patterns as anxiety related
Operational definition	A description of concepts, articulated in such a way that they can be applied to decision making in practice. It links concepts with other concepts and with theories, and it often includes the essential properties and distinguishing features of a concept.	Differentiation and measurement of state and trait anxiety
Theory	A purposeful set of assumptions or propositions about concepts; shows relationships between concepts and thereby provides a systematic view of phenomena so that they may be explained, predicted, or prescribed	Social determinants of illness
Assumption	A description of concepts or connection of two concepts that are accepted as factual or true; includes "taken for granted" ideas about the nature and purpose of concepts, as well as the structure of theory	"Nursing exists to serve a social mandate."
Proposition	A declarative assertion	"Patients who receive appropriate nursing care have better health outcomes."
Phenomenon	An aspect of reality that can be consciously sensed or experienced (Meleis, 2018); nursing concepts and theories represent a theoretical approach to making sense of aspects of reality of concern to nursing	Pain
Theoretical model	Mental representation of how things work. For example, an architect's plan for a house is not the house itself but rather the set of information necessary to understand how all the building elements will be brought together to create that particular house.	Biopsychosocial model of health
Conceptual framework	The theoretical structure that links concepts together for a specific purpose. When its purpose is to show how something works, it can also be described as a theoretical model. Nursing conceptual frameworks link major nursing concepts and phenomena to direct nursing decisions (e.g., what to assess, how to make sense of data, what to plan, how to enact a plan, and how to evaluate whether the plan has had the intended outcome). Conceptual frameworks are also often referred to as nursing models or nursing theories (Meleis, 2018).	Orem's (1971) self-care model for nursing

From Meleis, A. I. (1987). ReVisions in knowledge development: A passion for substance. *Scholarly Inquiry for Nursing Practice, 1*(1), 5–19; Orem, D. E. (1971). *Nursing: Concepts of practice.* McGraw Hill.

The nursing process was widely accepted by nurses because it was a logical way to describe basic problem-solving processes whereby knowledge was effectively used to guide nursing decisions (Henderson, 1982). Nurses quickly adopted the nursing process because it represented a continuous, rapid cycling of information through each of the phases. However, although the nursing process was useful for organizing and applying knowledge to clinical practice (Meleis, 2018), some later theorists began to challenge it as being too linear and rigid for nursing's purposes (Varcoe, 1996).

In current practice, terms such as *clinical judgement* are used to refer to reasoning processes that rely on *critical thinking* and multiple ways of knowing; clinical judgement implies the systematic use of the nursing process to invoke the complex intuitive and conscious thinking strategies that are part of all clinical decision making in nursing (Alfaro-LeFevre, 2019; Benner & Tanner, 1987; Tanner, 1993).

CONCEPTUAL FRAMEWORKS

The conceptual framework builders of the late 1960s and thereafter are usually referred to as the *nursing theorists.* All were fascinated by how nurses systematically organized general knowledge about nursing in order to understand an individual patient's situation and determine which of many available strategies would work best to restore health and ameliorate or prevent disease (Orem & Parker, 1964). This reasoning process differed from linear cause-and-effect reasoning, and it was what the nursing theorists understood to be the hallmark of excellence in nursing practice (Barnum, 1998; Meleis, 2018). Indeed, when

effective nurses made intelligent clinical decisions, it was often difficult to determine the precise dynamics that explained how those nurses applied that knowledge (Benner et al., 2009).

The building of nursing models was an attempt to theorize how all nurses might be taught to organize and synthesize knowledge about nursing so that they would develop these kinds of advanced clinical reasoning skills (Raudonis & Acton, 1997). Theorists who developed frameworks and models sought to depict theoretical structures that would enable a nurse to grasp all aspects of a clinical situation within the larger context of available options for nursing care. Table 6.2 describes four types of theory: **grand theory**, **middle-range theory**, **descriptive theory**, and **prescriptive theory**.

METAPARADIGM CONCEPTS

Each conceptual framework attempted to define nursing by creating a theoretical definition for the substance and structure of the key bodies of knowledge needed to understand clinical situations (Figure 6.1). This collective body of knowledge was called the **metaparadigm concepts** and included the concepts of person, environment, health care, and nursing care (Fawcett, 1992).

Patient, Client, and Person

By the 1960s, professional leaders recognized that nurses did much more than simply care for hospitalized patients. Consequently, many nursing theorists started using the term *client* rather than *patient* to refer to the person at the centre of any nursing process. The term *client*

TABLE 6.2	Types of Theory
Type of Theory	Description
Grand theory	Global conceptual framework that provides insight into abstract phenomena, such as human behaviour or nursing science. Grand theories are broad in scope and therefore require further application through research before the ideas they contain can be fully tested (Chinn et al., 2022). They are intended not to provide guidance for specific nursing interventions but rather to provide the structural framework for broad, abstract ideas about nursing. They are sometimes called paradigms because they represent distinct world views about those phenomena and provide the structural framework within which narrower-range theories can be developed and tested.
Middle-range theory	Encompasses a more limited scope and is less abstract. Middle-range theories address specific phenomena or concepts and reflect practice (administration, clinical, or teaching). The phenomena or concepts tend to cross different nursing fields and reflect a variety of nursing care situations.
Descriptive theory	Describes phenomena (e.g., responding to illness through patterns of coping), speculates on why phenomena occur, and describes the consequences of phenomena. Descriptive theories are able to explain, relate, and, in some situations, predict phenomena of concern to nursing (Meleis, 2018). Descriptive nursing theories are designed not to direct specific nursing activities but rather to help explain patient assessments and possibly guide future nursing research.
Prescriptive theory	Addresses nursing interventions and helps predict the consequences of a specific intervention. A prescriptive nursing theory should designate the prescription (i.e., nursing interventions), the conditions under which the prescription should occur, and the consequences (Meleis, 2018). Prescriptive theories are action oriented, which tests the validity and predictability of a nursing intervention. These theories guide nursing research to develop and test specific nursing interventions (Fawcett, 2013).

From Chinn, P. L., Kramer, M. K., & Sitzman, K. (2022). *Integrated knowledge development in nursing* (11th ed.). Elsevier; Meleis, A. I. (1987). ReVisions in knowledge development: A passion for substance. *Scholarly Inquiry for Nursing Practice, 1*(1), 5–19; Fawcett, J. (1992). Contemporary conceptualizations of nursing: Philosophy or science. In J. F. Kikuchi & H. Simmons (Eds.), *Philosophic inquiry in nursing* (pp. 55–63). Sage.

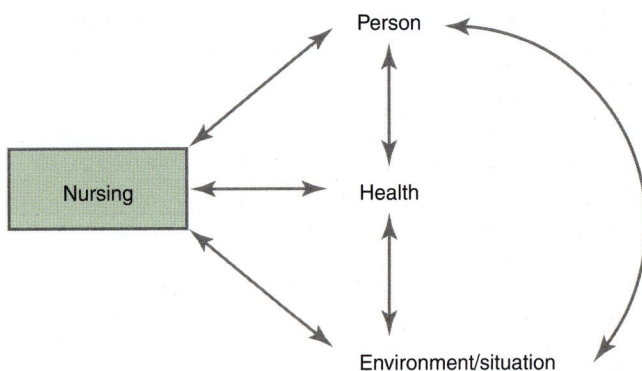

FIGURE 6.1 Nursing's metaparadigm concepts.

signified a range of health states, including both illness and wellness, and an explicitly interactive relationship between the nurse and the persons to whom care was directed. At the same time, nurses were becoming aware of their potential to deliver care beyond the individual—that is, to families, groups, and communities. Although theories to articulate the role of nursing care in families and communities also began to arise around that time, most early conceptual models focused on the individual.

To help nurses systematically organize and make sense of the vast amount of information that might be relevant to the care of a patient or client, most early models were oriented around a clearly defined concept of a person. These theorists variously understood a person as a system of interacting parts, a system of competing human needs, or an entity with biological, psychological, social, and spiritual dimensions. Each framework drew attention to multiple aspects of human experience so that the nurse could understand each instance of wellness and illness for its uniqueness within the context of that individual's body, feelings, and situation. Each model depicted a way of thinking about the whole individual with the aim of helping nurses understand how the implications of any action or intervention could be systematically individualized toward the benefit of all facets of that individual.

Environment

Each conceptual framework reflected an understanding that the person is part of and interacts with a complex environmental system. This environment may involve the person's family and social ties, the community, the health care system, as well as the geopolitical issues that affect health. The early conceptual frameworks helped shape nurses' increasing appreciation of how to work within the larger context of every experience of wellness and illness. In so doing, these frameworks set the stage for a time when nurses would begin spearheading advances in social and health care policy, health promotion, and community development.

Health

Because nursing exists within a social mandate to improve the health of both the individual and society, the early theorists struggled to articulate the overarching goal that drives nursing practice. They defined health as much more than simply the absence of disease or injury but rather as an ideal state of optimal health or total well-being toward which all individuals could strive (see Chapter 1). This definition reflected a vision of nursing care that was relevant to both the individual and society, and that applied to all persons, sick or well. It recognized that persons with chronic disease could strive for better health and that overall health could be compromised by psychosocial or spiritual challenges, even among the most physically fit individuals. Although perfect health was not necessarily achievable, this broad conceptualization guided nurses to help all patients or clients reach outcomes that were productive and satisfying.

Nursing

Each early conceptual framework also included a unique definition of nursing that linked a view of the patient or client with an understanding of the person's environment, life, and health goals. Built on a distinct subset of knowledge, each conceptual framework presented a coherent and complete belief system about nursing practice, albeit using different terms and a different alignment of ideas. Because most nursing scholars of the era assumed that one model would eventually become dominant (Meleis, 2018), competition among the frameworks became somewhat heated. Over time, as enthusiasm for the idea of implementing theory-based nursing practice grew, the application of the frameworks in practice became rigid and codified. Although the original focus had been on guiding nurses to think systematically, the implementation process caused the emphasis to shift toward such aspects as using language in particular ways and filling out assessment forms correctly. Many experienced nurses began to conclude that these frameworks actually inhibited their systematic thinking, and much debate ensued about the utility of the models.

PHILOSOPHY OF NURSING SCIENCE

When nursing theorists began developing their frameworks and models, nurses understood the process of building a knowledge base as a matter of science and discovery. In that context, theories were considered logical propositions that could be rigorously tested for their capacity to answer (or not answer) the hypothetical questions posed by a discipline. However, while creating frameworks for the complex reasoning involved in nursing practice, these early theorists were applying traditional scientific ways of understanding how knowledge works without fully appreciating the limitations of science, especially in relation to complex problems. As thinkers in all disciplines began to move beyond their traditional boundaries, other possibilities related to the development of knowledge about nursing practice began to emerge.

Scientific Revolutions

Thomas S. Kuhn, a philosopher of science, created a way of thinking about science and knowledge that expanded thought in many disciplines. First published in 1962, his book *The Structure of Scientific Revolutions* (Kuhn, 1962) was popularized in the 1970s and 1980s as scholars began to realize the potential of his ideas to support new thinking about how knowledge is built. Kuhn challenged the traditional notion of science as a logical progression of discoveries, arguing that major scientific developments occurred only when scientists thought about problems in radically new ways. These ways of thinking departed from the traditional to such an extent that an entirely different world view, or "paradigm shift," developed.

According to Kuhn, scientific advances happen when people think creatively and look beyond established norms. Such creative thinking could stimulate new understandings of problems that were once considered irresolvable (e.g., quantum physics introduced the idea that the behaviour of very small particles could explain atomic behaviour in ways that defied explanation through conventional Newtonian physics). This new way of thinking about the philosophy of science led nurses to consider their theoretical frameworks as not only theoretical propositions about logical relationships among concepts but also as actual world views, or **paradigms**, that might help them grasp the complexities of nursing (Fry, 1995).

Complexity Science

A second major shift in scientific thinking occurred with the introduction of chaos theory (Gleick, 1987). Originating from observations in physics that predictable patterns existed among factors that could not be predicted scientifically, this theory created a new way of approaching complex situations. In rejecting the simple cause-and-effect relationships used in traditional science, chaos theory led to what has been termed *complexity science*. In this kind of science, dynamic and interactive phenomena are reduced to the smallest properties that can be observed within their natural context so that their interactions can be interpreted with as little interference as possible

from prior assumptions. For example, chaos theory explains how, in sensitive weather systems, minor variations in initial conditions (e.g., barometric pressure) might explain large-scale physical patterns over time (e.g., hurricanes). These ideas created a new language to apply to scientific thinking. Because experiences of health and illness are exceedingly difficult to understand out of their individual context, chaos theory offered a new way to approach nursing science (Coppa, 1993; Ray, 1998).

WAYS OF KNOWING IN NURSING PRACTICE

As ideas shifted, nursing theorists also realized that science was just one of several forms of knowledge necessary for their practice discipline. In 1978, professor of nursing Barbara A. Carper published an influential paper in which she used the expression **ways of knowing** to refer to patterns of knowledge application in nursing practice (Carper, 1978). Carper articulated a critical role in nursing practice not only for empirical science but also for ethical, personal, and aesthetic knowledge; this idea has become foundational to our understanding of the multiple lenses nursing uses to interpret complex phenomena (see Chapter 8 for further information about evidence-informed practice). Later theorists added sociopolitical knowledge (White, 1995), emancipatory knowing (Chinn & Kramer, 2011), and critical thinking (see Chapter 7) to the list of central ways of knowing that are essential to the highest quality of clinical nursing. These ideas contributed to the emergence of discussions in other social and life sciences around *how* nurses know what they know (Chinn et al., 2022).

PARADIGM DEBATES WITHIN NURSING

With the new philosophical approach to scientific knowledge, nurses struggled with how to define their work as both an art and a science and as both applied and practical (Donaldson, 1995; Johnson, 1991; Rodgers, 1991; Sarter, 1990). Ideas about the theoretical foundations of nursing practice shifted. Some scholars began to question conceptual models as a valid form of theorizing (Holden, 1990). The frustration resulting from overly formal and rigid approaches to applying many of these models led to a period of what has been called *model bashing* (Engebretson, 1997). However, the question that had confronted the early theorists remained: How does a nurse organize and make sense of all available knowledge and apply it intelligently to the challenges that arise in an individual clinical case?

In this context, many nurse scholars began to recognize that the original theories were better understood as philosophical statements than as scientific prescriptions. However, one group of theorists, who considered some of the original theories to be overly simplistic and insufficiently holistic, began to categorize various nursing models as reflective of two entirely different paradigms of thinking (Parse, 1987). This group of theorists considered most nursing models and frameworks old fashioned and outdated, coining the term *totality paradigm frameworks* to describe them. They contended that this kind of model reduced an understanding of the human person to fragmented parts out of context. They further proposed the term *simultaneity paradigm frameworks* to depict a set of conceptual frameworks that they considered to be radically different and hence preferable by virtue of being both holistic and philosophically sophisticated (Parse, 1987). Some advocates of simultaneity theories continued to depict the diverse universe of theorizing about nursing as reflecting these two mutually exclusive groupings, positioning one set of conceptual frameworks as philosophically and morally superior to what they understood the other to represent (Cody, 1995; Nagle & Mitchell, 1991; Newman, 1992).

❖ NURSING DIAGNOSIS

Another discussion about nursing theory centred on nursing diagnosis. The scholars who devised conceptual frameworks focused on models to assess and interpret data about individual patient situations. However, the conceptual frameworks were less explicit about how to plan, implement, and evaluate nursing care. To fill this gap, nursing diagnosis emerged as an additional phase in that process. In making explicit the idea that nurses arrived at a clinical judgement about actual or potential health processes, sometimes now referred to as "nursing issues" or "priority problems," it became a discrete focus of theorizing about nursing care.

In the 1970s, some scholars became convinced of the need for precise language to categorize and document nursing diagnoses into a taxonomy (Warren & Hoskins, 1990). This resulted in the formation of the North American Nursing Diagnosis Association (NANDA) (see Chapter 14 for further information about NANDA), which held a series of consensus conferences to establish a list of the common patient problems addressed by practising nurses. The nursing diagnosis movement led to considerable general debate on the merits of using NANDA's fixed list of nursing diagnoses as compared to the theoretically infinite options for nursing care that had been intended by the conceptual models (Fitzpatrick, 1990; Roy, 1982). Although it was recognized as practical rather than theoretical (Fitzpatrick, 1990), NANDA's list became a popular device for organizing nursing care in part because it enabled efficient categorization into electronic databases and the subsequent standardization of nursing care plans (Warren & Hoskins, 1990). However, despite its popularity with health care administrators, NANDA's list is recognized by many nurses as a system that relies entirely upon an agreement about what constitutes average wellness and illness experiences. It can therefore create worrisome barriers to the individualized care of patients (Lee et al., 2006).

REFLECTIONS ON CONCEPTUALIZATIONS OF NURSING

The scientific and philosophical aspects of today's nursing practice are built on the foundation of early theorizing about nursing. The history of "nursing theory" is the story of an enlightened attempt to articulate excellent clinical reasoning in nursing care. How effective nurses actually use knowledge within the complexity of their clinical reasoning is, however, still difficult to determine with any precision. In this context, theorizing about nursing is perhaps best understood as an extended philosophical struggle to make sense of how highly skilled nurses think. Instead of arguing the advantages of one nursing theory over another, nursing scholars of today appreciate the creativity of their predecessors within the constrained conceptual contexts in which they were expected to operate.

MAJOR THEORETICAL MODELS

A chronology of the development of various theoretical models is illustrated in Box 6.1. In Box 6.2, you will find examples of the key ideas upon which some of the early model builders based their thinking. They are categorized here as a way of highlighting some of the differences between them and so you can get a feel for the diverse range of ideas at play. Note, however, that because many nursing theorists based their models on complex combinations of ideas from other disciplines, the categorization used here is somewhat simplistic. Alternatively, these models could have been grouped by way of the larger theories upon which they have been built, such as adaptation theory, systems theory, or human needs theory. Your aim in this context is not

BOX 6.1	Milestones in the Development of Nursing Theory
1859	Florence Nightingale's *Notes on Nursing: What It Is and What It Is Not* was published (updated version published 1946).
1952	*Nursing Research* (the first peer-reviewed scientific journal about nursing care) was established.
1952	Hildegard Peplau's text *Interpersonal Relations in Nursing* was published.
1955	Virginia Henderson's definition of nursing was first published in the 5th edition of Harmer and Henderson's (1955) basic nursing text.
1961	Ida Orlando introduced the nursing process.
1970	Martha Rogers's model was first published.
1970	Callista Roy's model was first published.
1971	Dorothea Orem's model was first published.
1976	The North American Nursing Diagnosis Association (NANDA) list of nursing diagnoses was first published.
1976	The University of British Columbia model of nursing practice was first published (Campbell et al., 1976).
1978	Barbara Carper's paper on fundamental patterns of knowing in nursing practice was published.
1979	Evelyn Adam's model was first published (English version published 1980).
1981	Rosemarie Parse's model was first published.
1987	The McGill model of nursing was first published (Gottlieb & Rowat, 1987).
2000	The Prince Edward Island conceptual model for primary care nursing was published (Munro et al., 2000).
2013	*Strengths-Based Nursing*, building on the McGill model, was published (Gottlieb, 2013).
2014	Canadian Nurses Association articulates integration of Indigenous Ways of Knowing as a policy direction for Canada.

to achieve a full understanding of each theory but rather to appreciate the wide diversity of intellectual tradition that enriched the thinking of these theory-building nursing scholars.

Practice-Based Theories

All conceptual models of nursing are designed to guide and shape practice. Although their theoretical inspiration is derived directly from the practice setting, many conceptual models do not capture all of what might be influencing that practice, such as societal and demographic changes, current health care belief models, therapeutic strategies, and the political struggles inherent in health care delivery. The early practice theories therefore reflect the issues that were shaping the role and context of nursing during those specific time frames.

Florence Nightingale. Whereas most later theorists drew on social and psychological theories, Nightingale was directly inspired by nursing practice. In *Notes on Nursing*, she described the conditions necessary to promote health and healing (Nightingale, 1859/1946). The observations she made during the Crimean War, which led to the first set of principles for nursing practice, acknowledged the particular importance of the environment—namely clean living spaces, fresh air, and the presence of light. The role of nursing care included ensuring that wounded soldiers were warm, comfortable, and adequately fed. Torres (1986) noted that Nightingale demonstrated how to think about patients and their environment. By shifting the focus from treating

BOX 6.2	Examples of Key Ideas Embedded in Various Nursing Theories	
Type of Theory	**Theorist**	**Key Ideas**
Practice-based theories	Nightingale	Practice observations; epidemiology; creating an environment conducive to healing
	McGill	Practice observations; focus on health rather than illness; family as context
Needs theories	Henderson	Basic human needs; assisting the individual, sick or well, to perform those activities that they would perform unaided given the strength, will, or knowledge
	Orem	Philosophy of human capability; maintaining capacity for self-care
	Adam	Basic human needs with biological, physiological, and psychosociocultural dimensions; nursing as a helping process of restoring independence to satisfy basic human needs
Interactionist theories	Peplau	Harry Stack Sullivan's theory of interpersonal relations; nursing as an interpersonal process; understanding the behaviour of others
	Travelbee	Existential philosophy; preventing, coping with, and making meaning of illness and suffering
Systems theories	Johnson	Chinn's theory of behavioural systems; maintaining stability and balance through adjustments and adaptation to the forces that impinge on them
	UBC	von Bertalanffy's general systems theory and Lewin's field theory; nurturing the person as a behavioural system during critical periods of the life cycle
	Neuman	Open system affected by intrapersonal, interpersonal, and extrapersonal stressors; addressing variables affecting the client's response to stressors
	Roy	Helson's adaptation theory; facilitating the individual as an adaptive system
Simultaneity theories	Rogers	Wasserman's energy fields; focus on unitary or irreducible human being and environment as pan-dimensional energy fields
	Parse	Dilthey's human science philosophy; indivisible human beings and environment co-create health, structured around abiding themes of meaning, rhythmicity, and transcendence
	Watson	Phenomenal field/unitary consciousness; nursing as caring; clinical Caritas Processes

BOX 6.3	Milestones in Canadian Nursing History

Moyra Allen, 1921–1996

A creative and independent thinker, Moyra Allen was one of the first Canadian nurses to earn a doctoral degree. She lobbied for collective bargaining rights for nurses and was the founding president of the United Nurses of Montreal. She was also the founder of *Nursing Papers*, later renamed the *Canadian Journal of Nursing Research.*

Allen was a founding member of the World Health Organization committee that developed the criteria for accreditation of nursing schools. She designed an evaluation model for nursing schools and evaluated schools in South America, India, and Ghana.

She joined the faculty of the School of Nursing at McGill in 1954 and became professor emeritus in 1985 upon her retirement.

In demonstrating her model of nursing, now known as the McGill model, Dr. Allen established a community health facility, The Health Workshop, in 1977. There, she put into practice a developmental concept of health and nursing as a prototype of primary health care. The workshop, viewed as complementary to existing services, was staffed with nurses, a community development officer, and a health librarian. The workshop's purpose was to demonstrate the validity of a local health resource managed by nurses that focused on long-term family health. It proved to be an innovative means of improving the health status of families coping with illness and other problems.

Allen received numerous awards, including the Jeanne Mance Award, which recognizes major contributions to the health of Canadians. In 1986, she was named an Officer of the Order of Canada for her outstanding contributions to Canadian nursing.

disease processes to creating an environment conducive to healing, Nightingale's conceptualization clearly differentiated the role of nursing from that of medicine.

The McGill Model. Dr. Moyra Allen (Box 6.3) conceived the McGill model and developed it further with her colleagues (Gottlieb & Rowat, 1987). Systematically studying actual nursing situations, Allen and her colleagues created a way of thinking about nursing that focused on promoting health. They recognized that many patients' health concerns were best approached through changes in lifestyle. The McGill scholars focused on the individual in the context of the family and, like Nightingale, viewed nursing as complementary to medicine. The main features of the McGill model were "a focus on health rather than illness

and treatment, on all family members rather than the patient alone, on family goals rather than on the nurse's, and on family strengths rather than their deficits" (Gottlieb & Feeley, 1999, p. 194). Over time, the model has been further developed to demonstrate its application to a variety of clinical contexts and settings (e.g., Feeley & Gerez-Lirette, 1992; Feeley & Gottlieb, 1998; Gottlieb, 2013).

Needs Theories

Many early theorists organized their thinking by conceptualizing the patient as representing a collection of needs. This reflected a common orientation to studying the nature of people, popularized in the 1960s, in which needs, drives, and competencies were thought to hold potential for explaining human behaviour. Of these theories, Maslow's

(1954) hierarchy of needs was one of the best known and most influential. The idea that complex human behaviour can be best explained as a response to the competing demands of various basic needs is featured prominently in many nursing models.

Virginia Henderson. Henderson (Harmer & Henderson, 1955) conceptualized the patient as a compilation of 14 basic human needs: to breathe, eat and drink, eliminate waste products, move and maintain posture, rest and sleep, dress and undress, maintain body temperature, be clean, avoid danger, communicate, worship, work, play, and learn. Viewing the patient in this way clearly defined the nurse's role. Accordingly, Henderson defined nursing practice as assisting the individual, sick or well, in the performance of activities that contribute to health, recovery, or a peaceful death. Henderson's model has remained popular in practice because its language is familiar and easily comprehensible and because it explains how a person's biological, psychological, social, and spiritual components combine to influence the way illness is experienced and health can be regained.

Dorothea Orem. Orem's (1971) self-care theory, the origins of which lay in Henderson's work, was used widely in both nursing practice and research. Orem's theory addressed the ways in which people are responsible for meeting the following universal self-care requisites:

- Maintaining sufficient intake of air, water, and food
- Maintaining a balance between activity and rest and between solitude and interaction
- Providing for elimination processes
- Preventing hazards to life, functioning, and well-being, and
- Promoting functioning and growth in social groups in accordance with human potential.

Drawing on both human need and developmental theory, Orem's theory focused on the individual's role in maintaining health. This theory emerged at a time when the passive role of the patient was being questioned and the health care system was beginning to shift away from full responsibility for people's health. With increased understanding of illness patterns, Orem acknowledged the effects of multiple lifestyle factors such as smoking, diet, and exercise, reminding nurses that patients can look after their own health and that they must learn to care for themselves within their families and communities. Thus, the role of the nurse, according to Orem, was to act temporarily for the patient until the patient could resume a more independent role in self-care.

Interactionist Theories

Interactionist theories focused on the relationships between nurses and their patients. These theories defined more clearly the specific human communicative and behavioural patterns by which practitioners met their patients' needs. As the theorists reframed definitions of the nursing profession, they drew from the work of psychologists and psychoanalysts such as Harry Stack Sullivan, Abraham Maslow, and Sigmund Freud.

Hildegard Peplau. Peplau, a psychiatric specialist, defined the core of nursing care as the interpersonal relationship between the nurse and the patient. Building upon the ideas of psychoanalyst Harry Stack Sullivan, Peplau depicted the practice of nursing as an interactive therapeutic relationship. Peplau felt that such relationships allowed nurses to challenge the practice of long-term stays in large inpatient psychiatric hospitals and to envision supporting patients to achieve independent living. "The kind of person each nurse becomes makes a substantial difference in what each patient will learn as he is nursed through his experience with illness" (Peplau, 1952, p. vii). Peplau described the nurse as follows:

an investigator, prober, interpreter, and reporter, using the rich data she extracts from the patient concerning his life. She develops insights, his and hers, into the meaning of a patient's behaviour and helps the patient recognize and change patterns that obstruct achievement of his goals.

(Barnum, 1994, p. 217)

An early advocate of an orderly and systematic approach to care, Peplau created a way of thinking about nursing care that directed nurses toward preventing illness and maintaining health.

Joyce Travelbee. Writing in the late 1960s and early 1970s, Travelbee also viewed nursing care as an interpersonal process. In contrast to Peplau's more psychoanalytic orientation, Travelbee drew on a school of thought known as *existential philosophy* to guide her theorizing. Travelbee (1971) viewed the "client" as including not only the individual but also the individual's family and community, and she articulated the role of the nurse as assisting clients to "prevent or cope with the experience of illness and suffering and, if necessary, to find meaning in these experiences" (p. 7). Travelbee emphasized that nurses must recognize the humanity of their clients, suggesting that even the term *patient* should be regarded as a stereotypical categorization. Recognizing the reciprocity of human interaction, Travelbee focused attention on the communication that occurs between nurses and their clients as an important vehicle for finding meaning in illness.

Evelyn Adam. Influenced by Dorothy Johnson, as well as by earlier interactionist theorists (George, 1995), Canadian theorist Evelyn Adam (1979, 1980) articulated the essence of nursing as a helping process. From her perspective, the nurse played a complementary–supplementary role in supporting the patient's strength, knowledge, and will. Adam's model drew on Henderson's framework of basic human needs and extended it into a model that would explain not only how nurses conceptualized the patient but also how they applied that knowledge in the context of a helping relationship characterized by empathy, caring, and mutual respect.

Systems Theories

In the 1970s and 1980s, as conceptual models of nursing became more sophisticated and structured, several theorists drew on general systems theory (von Bertalanffy, 1968) for guidance in conceptualizing the complexity of human health. The main appeal of systems theory was that it accounted for the whole of an entity (the system) and its component parts (subsystems), as well as the complex interactions between the parts and the whole. In this way, systems theory allowed theorists to expand the conceptualization of nursing practice through both structure and process, whereby the individual was viewed as an open system in constant interaction with their environment. Being outside the system, the nurse became one of the many forces to affect that system. Using this perspective, nurses were encouraged to appreciate the interactions of a system with its component parts and with its environment. Systems approaches helped nurses recognize that intervention in any one part of a system would produce consequent reactions in other parts, as well as in the system as a whole. Regardless of how each theorist depicted the nature of the system, these general principles—common to all living systems—were featured in each of the nursing systems models.

Dorothy Johnson. Johnson's theoretical work was popularized in the early 1960s through the distribution of her class notes and speeches, but it remained unpublished until much later (Grubbs, 1980; Johnson, 1980). In her nursing model, Johnson identified the individual as a behavioural system with seven subsystems, each of which has a goal, a set of behaviours, and a choice. The notion of subsystem goals was based on drives that are considered universal and applicable to all patients. However, the meanings attributed to each goal and the set of behaviours for achieving goals were seen as highly individual and unique to each patient. Together with the choices made by the patient in relation to meeting their behavioural system goals, each subsystem also had a function that could be considered analogous to the physiological function of a biological system (Meleis, 2018).

The University of British Columbia Model. The behavioural systems model developed at The University of British Columbia (UBC) School of Nursing was inspired by Johnson's model and developed by a committee led by Margaret Campbell that included several of Johnson's former students. Broadening the view of human experience on the basis of behavioural drives, the UBC model for nursing depicted the behavioural system as being composed of nine basic human needs, each of which is shaped by the psychological and sociocultural environment within which it is expressed (Campbell et al., 1976). Whereas needs were considered universal and therefore fundamental to human experience, the specific goals toward which needs-related human behaviour were directed and the strategies for achieving those goals were recognized as unique to individuals and their particular physiological, psychological, or social circumstances (Thorne et al., 1993). Thus, the UBC model provided a structure by which general knowledge about human health and illness could be combined with specific knowledge about each individual patient. In accordance with the tenets of general systems theory, the goal of nursing practice was to achieve balance of the behavioural system. The nurse's role was to foster, protect, sustain, and teach (Campbell, 1987) and thereby bring about not only system balance but also stability and optimal health.

Betty Neuman. Neuman's approach to theorizing about nursing differed from that of other systems theorists in that it did not rely on concepts concerning needs and drives, nor did it break the system into any component parts. Neuman understood the person to be a physiological, psychological, sociocultural, developmental, and spiritual being (Meleis, 2018) and oriented the attention of the nurse to the "client system" in a health care–oriented and holistic manner (Neuman, 1982). Neuman considered the client system to have innate factors consistent with being human, as well as unique factors that characterized each individual person. According to Neuman, each client had a unique set of response patterns determined and regulated by a core structure. Neuman believed that because the person was vulnerable to environmental stressors, the role of the nurse ought to focus on actual and potential stressors. In this way, Neuman's model focused on prevention.

Sister Callista Roy. In contrast to most other systems theorists, Roy considered the client not as a behavioural system but rather as an adaptive one. She viewed the person as a biopsychosocial being in constant interaction with a changing environment (Roy, 1984). Her model depicted four modes of adaptation: physiological needs, self-concept, role function, and interdependence (Roy, 1974). She conceptualized the person as an adaptive system with two major internal processes by which to adapt: the cognator subsystem and the regulator subsystem (Roy & Andrews, 1999). Roy used these mechanisms to describe and explain the interconnectedness of all aspects of human adaptation and to conceptualize the role of the nurse in managing the stimuli that influence that adaptation (Meleis, 2018).

Simultaneity Theories

The theorists who identified their work as belonging to the simultaneity paradigm considered their theories to be fundamentally distinct from the practice, needs, interactionist, and systems theories. Although simultaneity theories were first articulated long before the paradigm debate arose and before the terms *simultaneity* and *totality* were used to categorize the theories, the language of simultaneity has become prominent in distinguishing this group of nursing theories from others. A characteristic feature of these theories is what Rogers (1970) called the *unitary human being*. Previous theorists had sought to identify aspects of the individual that not only represented an abstract conceptualization of the whole but also provided a comprehensive understanding of the person in terms of their parts (such as problems, needs, or goals). In contrast, the simultaneity theorists viewed the individual as an entirely irreducible whole, inherently and "holographically" connected with the universal environment (Parse, 2004). These theories therefore represented a distinctive approach to articulating an understanding of the client of nursing as well as nursing's role in relation to that client.

Martha Rogers. Martha Rogers's (1970) model was revolutionary in presenting the client not simply as a person but as an energy field in constant interaction with the environment, which in itself was also an irreducible energy field, coextensive with the universe (Meleis, 2018). According to Rogers, who based her theory on her interpretations of evolving ideas in physics, the role of nursing was to focus on the life process of a human being along a time–space continuum (Rogers, 1970). An early proponent of pattern recognition, Rogers believed that pattern gave the energy field its identity and its distinguishing characteristics (Meleis, 2018). The objective of nursing practice became one of helping clients reach their maximum health potential in the context of constant change and developing what Rogers referred to as "homeodynamic unity within diversity."

Rosemarie Parse. Parse's (1981) theory of "man-living-health," later termed *human becoming* theory (Parse, 1997) and over time evolving into the *human becoming* school of thought (Parse, 2007), was another view of the individual as a unitary being who is "indivisible, unpredictable, and everchanging" and "a freely choosing being who can be recognized through paradoxical patterns co-created all-at-once in mutual process with the universe" (Parse, 2004, p. 293). According to Parse's perspective, the caring presence of nurses and their particular patterns of relating support individuals in the human "becoming" process. Within Parse's nursing theory, the goal of nursing is articulated not in traditional definitions of health but rather as the notion of people in a continuous process of making choices and changing health priorities. According to Parse's theory, nurses engage with people in their process of "becoming" through the application of three core processes referred to as explicating, dwelling with, and moving beyond (Parse, 1999).

Jean Watson. Watson (1979) considered the individual to be a totality who can be viewed as a transpersonal self. According to Watson, in contrast to depictions of the individual as a body and an ego, it is more useful to understand the individual as "an embodied spirit; a transpersonal transcendent evolving consciousness; unity of mind body spirit; person-nature-universe as oneness, connected" (Watson, 1999, p. 129). Watson therefore believed that nurses must do far more than deal with physical illness: they must attend to their primary function, which is caring. From Watson's perspective, caring infuses all aspects of a nurse's role and draws attention to nursing acts as embodying an aesthetic that facilitates both healing and growth.

Each of the models just described attracts continual analysis and implementation. In some instances, nurses draw on them holistically as a coherent approach to guide all their practices. More often, nurses today consider themselves informed by the intellectual structure that any good framework provides, but typically expand their thinking beyond the limitations of a single model as their practice develops and progresses.

THEORIZING INTO THE FUTURE

Theoretical knowledge leads us to reflect on "the basic values, guiding principles, elements, and phases of a conception of nursing" (Meleis, 2018). The goals of theoretical knowledge are to stimulate thinking and create a broad understanding of the science and practice of the nursing discipline (King & Fawcett, 1997). Although nurses today can appreciate the inherent complexity of these objectives, the creativity and vision modelled by these early theorists continue to inspire theorizing about the core essence of nursing.

Nursing is solidly established as a distinct health care discipline with its own unique scientific basis. In addition, current theorists draw heavily from philosophy to resolve some of nursing's most complex theoretical challenges. However, as Kikuchi (1999) pointed out two decades ago, much of the theorizing about the purpose of nursing has confused rather than clarified thinking. As nursing scholarship evolves to include stronger philosophical and scientific inquiry, nursing practice must also be conceptualized with increasing clarity (Silva et al., 1995). Nurse philosophers, as well as scientists, are continuing to use new ways of tackling nursing's most complex theoretical feature, which is applying expanding, dynamic, and multiple sources of knowledge to a diverse range of patient situations (Bender, 2018). This problem of understanding the general and applying it to the specific features in the work of many contemporary nursing scholars.

Meleis (1987), a scholar of nursing theory, challenged nurses to direct their theorizing away from the processes by which nurses use knowledge and toward the equally challenging issues associated with the substance of that knowledge. In accepting this challenge, many nursing scholars have shifted their theorizing about nursing to include both theoretical and substantive knowledge. Liaschenko (1997; Liaschenko & Fisher, 1999) oriented this theorizing into three levels of abstraction: knowing the case, knowing the patient, and knowing the person. Engebretson (1997) positioned nursing theory in relation not only to biomedicine but also to Eastern and holistic understandings of health and illness. Canadian theorists Starzomski and Rodney (1997) worked toward articulating the link between definitions of health and more philosophical notions of the greater social good. Campbell and Bunting (1991) explored the possibilities of using critical social and feminist theories for emancipatory theorizing in nursing. Watson (1990; see also Brenwick & Webster, 2000) developed the idea of embedding "caring" as a moral component into nursing theory. Yeo (1989) considered the implications of ethical reasoning for nursing theory.

In Canada, nurses at the Prince Edward Island School of Nursing developed a conceptual framework for nursing grounded in the social determinants of health (Munro et al., 2000). Gottlieb (2013, 2014) developed the McGill model into strengths-based nursing, a comprehensive philosophy of care that "reaffirms nursing's goals of promoting health, facilitating healing, and alleviating suffering by creating environments that work with and bolster patients' capacities for health and innate mechanisms of healing" (Gottlieb 2014, p. 24).

We can expect ongoing refinements to our thinking about nursing as we move into the future. A prime example will be the challenge of integrating Indigenous Ways of Knowing into current practice models and education, first formally proposed by the Canadian Nurses Association in 2014 (Canadian Nurses Association, 2014) and increasingly being taken up by thought leaders across the country.

The capacity to provide a rationale for nursing actions and decisions based on theoretical knowledge is a recognized core competency for nursing practice in Canada (Canadian Association of Schools of Nursing, 2022). However, as this review of the history of theorizing in nursing illustrates, linking theory with practice requires a dynamic and evolving skill set. The inherent complexities underlying the interrelationships between theory and practice are therefore of continuing interest to nursing scholars (Mudd et al., 2020).

A lively dialogue representing the dynamic interaction between theorizing and clinical practice (often termed **praxis**) has also emerged (Clarke et al., 1996; Mitchell, 1995; Newman, 2002; Reed, 1995; Reed & Ground, 1997; Thorne, 1997). This form of theorizing does not seek static truths about nursing practice because it considers apparent truths to be potentially illusory as our understanding evolves. Rather, it seeks to create a coherent foundation upon which nurses can build, challenge, and integrate an infinite range of new ideas, new forms of knowledge, and new paths toward action. For some theorists, this notion of praxis represents a blend of what has been described as the art and science of person-centred care (Taylor et al., 2018). For others, it reflects a call to engaging with knowledge in a reflexive manner that invokes emancipation and fuels social action toward the betterment of health for all (Kagan et al., 2010).

As Levine once wrote, "Theory is the poetry of science" (Levine, 1995, p. 14). In this manner, theorizing in nursing becomes the engine by which ideas about the discipline are advanced over time. It brings the old and familiar concepts of nursing together and shapes them into bold and exciting new configurations, rendering previously disconnected aspects of the human experience part of a greater whole. In so doing, it makes the intellectual excitement of the discipline come alive.

KEY CONCEPTS

- The hallmark of nursing practice is its unique body of knowledge and the way nurses use it.
- Nursing science has evolved within a historical and social context.
- Nursing theory represents attempts by nursing scholars to articulate the ways in which knowledge from multiple sources can be systematically applied in a wide variety of ways to guide professional, accountable, and defensible nursing practice.
- Much of the early theorizing about nursing practice was specifically designed to guide nursing curriculum development so that nursing education would be focused on the knowledge unique to nursing care.
- The nursing process is the fundamental problem-solving process by which new situations are assessed, plans are developed, and interventions are performed and evaluated.
- Nursing care requires the application of general knowledge to an infinite range of unique situations. Nursing process and nursing theory represent strategies to guide the application process.
- The major components of nursing theory, sometimes called the *metaparadigm concepts*, are person, environment, health, and nursing.
- Nurses' understanding of the role of science has changed as more complex forms of science have been articulated by philosophers of science; science is no longer limited to simple relationships such as cause and effect but instead provides strategies for understanding increasingly complex relationships and phenomena.
- Nursing knowledge derives from various sources in addition to science, including aesthetics, personal knowing, sociocultural understanding, and ethics.
- Nursing theorists based their conceptual frameworks on various ways of thinking about human behaviour and experience. Some framed their ideas within theories of human behaviour, such as needs, interaction, or systems, and others drew their primary inspiration from what they observed in excellent nursing practice.

- Conceptual frameworks of nursing include those for understanding both the person as the nurse's patient and the nurse's role in relation to that patient.
- Although each framework may have attempted to organize nursing knowledge and systematic reasoning processes in a different way, each was aiming for a very similar ideal of excellent decision making in nursing practice.
- Although nursing theoretical frameworks are no longer considered useful as prescriptive models for practice, they provide a way of conceptualizing nursing's interests and identifying researchable nursing problems.
- As the practice of theorizing about nursing care evolves, the role of philosophy in helping nurses understand their relationship to knowledge has become increasingly relevant.

CRITICAL THINKING EXERCISES

1. How do you think different ways of conceptualizing the patient might influence the kinds of decisions that nurses might make in their practice? Consider how understanding the person in terms of needs, system theory, or interaction might lead you to notice certain things and not others.
2. What sorts of gaps in information or misunderstandings might occur if nurses failed to use a systematic way of thinking about each person in their care?
3. How do you think conceptual frameworks and nursing theories might be used to generate research questions for developing knowledge for evidence-informed practice?
4. Why is it useful for nurses to question how they know what they think they know?

🌐 *Answers to Critical Thinking Exercises appear on the Evolve website.*

REVIEW QUESTIONS

Review Questions 1 to 11 relate to the case study queries from Nassim and Geertje at the beginning of the chapter.

1. A theory is best understood as a set of assumptions or propositions that becomes useful when it does which of the following?
   a. Helps people meet their self-care needs
   b. Isolates concepts
   c. Helps the nurse implement care
   d. Provides a systematic view of explaining, predicting, and prescribing phenomena
2. The enterprise of early theorizing about nursing practice was primarily driven by:
   a. Physicians
   b. Political leaders
   c. Nursing educators
   d. Policymakers
3. The nursing process in its original form involved which four basic steps?
   a. Assessment, planning, intervention, evaluation
   b. Assessment, nursing diagnosis, planning, intervention
   c. Nursing diagnosis, planning, intervention, evaluation
   d. Planning, assessment, intervention, evaluation
4. The metaparadigm concepts that formed the structure of concepts that nursing theories were concerned about included which of the following:
   a. Person, environment, health, and nursing
   b. Caring, health promotion, and supportive care

   c. Chaos theory and systems theory
   d. Existentialism, phenomenology, and metaphysics
5. The main question on which the early nursing theorists focused their attention was to work out which of the following?
   a. How to differentiate between nursing theories and medical theories
   b. How to reconcile the generalizations of the North American Nursing Diagnosis Association with the unique situations of each patient
   c. How to organize and make sense of general nursing knowledge and apply this knowledge to an individual clinical case
   d. Whether to use theories from other disciplines such as philosophy and apply them to nursing
6. According to Kuhn, scientific advances are most likely to happen when creative individuals do which of the following?
   a. Approach a problem in a new way
   b. Use the cause-and-effect model to solve problems
   c. Use the work of other scientists to solve problems
   d. Use empirical evidence to solve problems
7. The central idea characterizing the McGill model for nursing is that it:
   a. Focuses on health rather than on illness or treatment
   b. Accounts for holistic aspects of the individual rather than component parts
   c. Views the person as an energy field in constant interaction with the environment
   d. Considers the human experience to be based on behavioural drives
8. Building upon a psychoanalytic perspective, theorist Hildegard Peplau considered which of the following as fundamental aspects of nursing practice?
   a. Interacting in a therapeutic manner
   b. Developing the relationship between the nurse and the patient
   c. Investigating the meaning of patient behaviour
   d. All of the above
9. The distinctive contribution that Canadian theorist Evelyn Adam made to nursing's thinking at the time was a conceptualization of the essence of nursing as:
   a. A collaboration with health care providers
   b. A helping process
   c. The management of patients and health care systems
   d. All of the above
10. The idea that nursing theorists drew specifically from systems theories was to consider the human being as:
    a. An irreducible whole
    b. A whole and component parts in intricate interaction with one another
    c. An embodiment of mind, body, and spirit
    d. All of the above
11. The most distinctive feature of Rosemarie Parse's theory is that it considers the individual as a unitary being who is engaged in which of the following?
    a. Seeking health
    b. Engaging in a continuing process of making choices
    c. Striving for homeostasis
    d. All of the above

Answers: 1. d; **2.** c; **3.** a; **4.** a; **5.** c; **6.** a; **7.** a; **8.** d; **9.** b; **10.** b; **11.** b.

🌐 *Rationales for the Review Questions appear on the Evolve website.*

RECOMMENDED WEBSITES

McGill Model of Nursing: https://www.mcgill.ca/nursing/events/model
The McGill model of nursing was developed and refined under the guidance of Dr. Moyra Allen, who envisioned nursing as taking a unique, active, and complementary role in providing health care.

Nursing Theories and Models: https://airtable.com/shrNEpT7s2qsPgT7c/tblb CTW4IIcC8TqB8
This website presents a gallery of nursing theorists and links to their work.

Nursing Theory: https://nursing-theory.org
This website provides a list of major nursing theorists who have contributed to the development of professional nursing practice into what it is today.

Nursing Theory and Research: https://www.sandiego.edu/nursing/research/nursing-theory-research.php
The Nursing Theory page is a collaborative effort by an international group interested in developing a collection of resources about nursing theories throughout the world. This site provides links to pages built and maintained by others who have knowledge about a theory.

Strengths-Based Nursing and Health Care (SBNH):
https://www.mcgill.ca/strengths-based-nursing-healthcare/about/strengths-based-nursing-and-healthcare
SBNH is both a philosophy and a value-driven approach to guide clinicians, leaders, and educators. This website provides a detailed description of the approach, which aims to transform the health care system by humanizing health care through knowledgeable and compassionate care.

The University of British Columbia (UBC) Model for Nursing:
https://nursing.ubc.ca/ubc-model-nursing
The UBC model for nursing is a conceptual framework that guides nursing practice decision making. It was developed by a team of faculty members under the leadership of Dr. Margaret Campbell in the early 1970s. This website provides further information about the model, as well as a link to an interpretive version of the model.

🌐 REFERENCES

A full reference list is available on the website for this book at
http://evolve.elsevier.com/Canada/Potter/fundamentals/

7

Critical Thinking in Nursing Practice

*Canadian content written by Salima Meherali, RN, MN, PhD,
with original chapter contributions by Patricia A. Potter, RN, MSN, PhD, FAAN*

OBJECTIVES

Mastery of content in this chapter will enable you to:

- Define the key terms listed.
- Describe characteristics of a critical thinker.
- Examine the relationship between critical thinking and patient-centred care.
- Describe the components of a critical thinking model for clinical decision making.
- Explain the relationship between clinical experience and critical thinking.
- Describe critical thinking competencies used in nursing practice.
- Describe the nurse's responsibility in making clinical decisions.
- Explain the relationship of the nursing process to critical thinking.
- Describe the critical thinking attitudes used in clinical decision making.
- Explain how professional standards influence a nurse's clinical decisions.
- Describe how case-based learning fosters how to critically think.
- Identify how reflective writing promotes critical thinking.
- Explain how concept maps can improve a nurse's ability to think critically.

KEY TERMS

Case-based learning
Clinical decision-making process
Clinical inference
Clinical reasoning
Concept map
Critical thinking

Decision making
Diagnostic reasoning
Evidence-informed knowledge
Information literacy skills
Nursing process
Patient-centred care

Problem solving
Reflection
Reflective writing
Scientific method

WEBSITE

http://evolve.elsevier.com/Canada/Potter/fundamentals/

CASE STUDY

Joan Walker (preferred pronouns: she/her) is an 84-year-old patient, widowed 6 months ago after 64 years of marriage, who resides in assisted living. The patient has had a productive cough of green phlegm that started 4 days ago and persists. She has a history of chronic obstructive pulmonary disease (COPD). Three days ago the patient started on prednisone 40 mg PO (by mouth) daily and azithromycin 250 mg PO ×5 days prescribed by the clinic physician. The patient has had intermittent chills, a temperature of 38.9°C, and more difficulty breathing during the night so has been using her albuterol inhaler every 1–2 hours, with no improvement. As a result, the patient called 9-1-1 and was brought to the emergency department (ED), where you are the nurse who will be responsible for her care. Your patient's current vital signs are T 39.6°C; P 110/min (regular); R 30/min (laboured); BP 178/96; O₂ sat 86%; and chest pain 5/10. You ask Mrs. Walker about the frequency and type of pain, and she responds, "Intermittent—lasting a few seconds, influenced by deep breaths or relieved with shallow breathing."

Think about this case study as you read this chapter. There are review questions at the end of the chapter that relate to the case study.

Nurses face many complex situations involving patients, family members, and other health care workers. To deal with these experiences effectively, nurses need to develop sound critical thinking skills so that they can approach each new problem with open-mindedness, creativity, confidence, and wisdom. When a patient develops a new set of symptoms, asks the nurse to provide comfort measures, or requires a procedure, it is important to think critically and make prudent clinical judgements so that the patient receives the best nursing care possible. Failure to employ critical thinking results in wasted time and energy, poor-quality patient outcomes, frustration, and anxiety (Paul & Elder, 2020). Critical thinking is not a simple, step-by-step linear process that one can learn overnight. Nurses' ability to think critically will increase as they gain experience and progress from novice to expert nurse (Benner, 1984; Benner et al., 2010). Critical thinking is central to professional nursing practice because it enables the nurse to test and refine nursing approaches, learn from successes and failures, apply nursing research findings, and ensure holistic patient-centred care.

CRITICAL THINKING DEFINED

Critical thinking is a complex phenomenon that can be defined as a process and as a set of skills. Definitions of critical thinking emphasize the use of knowledge and reasoning to make accurate clinical judgements and decisions. Nurses need complex thinking skills to effectively manage the fast-paced and constantly changing health care environments in which they work. Accordingly, nurses recognize that an issue (e.g., patient challenge or health-related concern) exists, analyze information about the issue (e.g., clinical data about the patient), evaluate information (e.g., review assumptions and evidence), and draw conclusions (e.g., decide how to proceed). In consultation with patients, nurses consider what is important in a situation, explore alternative solutions, consider ethical principles, and then make informed decisions about how to proceed. Consider the case study at the beginning of the chapter.

Critical thinking requires purposeful and reflective reasoning to examine ideas, assumptions and beliefs, principles, conclusions, and actions within the context of the situation. In the case study of Mrs. Walker, when you begin planning care for this patient, you would start to think critically by asking questions such as "What do I know about the patient's situation? How do I know it?" "What is the patient's situation now? How might it change?" "What is the patient's perspective on the situation?" "What else do I need to know to understand this situation better or improve it? How can I obtain that information?" "In what way will a specific therapy affect the patient?" "Are other options available?" "What health outcomes are important to the patient?" "How can I work with the patient to attain those outcomes?" By answering these questions, you are able to identify alternative solutions to address the patient's health-related concerns and to involve the patient in making decisions about the care provided. (Box 7.1 illustrates how strategies designed to foster critical thinking can promote patient-centred care.)

As you gain experience in nursing, avoid letting your thinking become routine or standardized. Instead, learn to look beyond the obvious in any clinical situation, explore the patient's unique responses to actual or potential health alterations, and recognize what actions are needed to benefit the patient. Over time, your experience with many patients will help you recognize patterns of behaviour, see commonalities in signs and symptoms, and anticipate reactions to nursing interventions. Reflecting on your experiences will help you determine how the knowledge you gained working with one patient may be applicable to another patient's situation.

In Mrs. Walker's case, based on your experience with patients with the same etiology, you recognize that the patient is likely to have pleuritic chest pain because the characteristics of the patient's pain do not fit a cardiac etiology. Your review of patient observations and the patient's report of pain confirm that this is not a myocardial infarction or angina pain. Based on your clinical decision making, your plan of care will focus on Mrs. Walker's impaired gas exchange due to infection and ineffective airway clearance. Once Mrs. Walker's respiration gets settled, you might also ask Mrs. Walker whether she would like to try some deep-breathing exercises and incentive spirometry, which will promote alveolar expansion and improves gas exchange.

You can begin to learn to think critically early in your practice and use relevant information, knowledge, and communication technologies to support evidence-informed nursing practice (Canadian Association of Schools of Nursing (CASN), 2022). For example, as you learn about administering bed baths and other hygiene measures to your patients, take time to read the nursing literature about the concept of comfort. What are the criteria for comfort? How do patients from other cultures perceive comfort? What are the many factors that promote comfort? The use of **evidence-informed knowledge**—knowledge based on

BOX 7.1   RESEARCH HIGHLIGHT
Promoting Critical Thinking Through an Evidence-Informed Skills Fair Intervention

Research Focus
The lack of critical thinking in new graduates has been a concern to the nursing profession for a number of years. Adopting teaching practice to promote critical thinking is a crucial component of nursing education. The purpose of this research study, undertaken by Gonzalez and colleagues in 2020, was to investigate the effects of an innovative, evidence-informed skills fair intervention on nursing students' achievements and perceptions of critical thinking skills development.

Research Abstract
A skills fair intervention (a 1-day event) was implemented to assist baccalaureate students who had taken the summer off from their studies in nursing, and all faculty participated in operating the stations. This study incorporated evidence-informed practice rationale with critical thinking prompts using Socratic questioning, evidence-informed practice videos, psychomotor skills rubrics, group work, guided discussions, expert demonstration followed by guided practice, and blended learning in an attempt to promote and develop critical thinking in these students.

Implications for Practice
The skills fair intervention enhanced the development of self-confidence and critical thinking by allowing participants to practise previously learned skills in a controlled, safe environment. This information is useful for nurse educators who plan their own teaching practice to promote critical thinking and improve patient outcomes. The findings also provide schools and educators with information that helps review their current approach in educating nursing students. As evidenced in the findings, the importance of developing critical thinking skills is crucial for becoming a safe, professional nurse.

From Gonzalez, H. C., Hsiao, E.-L., Dees, D. C., et al. (2020). Promoting critical thinking through an evidence-based skills fair intervention. *Journal of Research in Innovative Teaching & Learning,* 2397–7604. https://doi.org/10.1108/JRIT-08-2020-0041

research or clinical expertise—makes you an informed critical thinker and improves patient outcomes.

Critical thinking requires not only cognitive skills, such as interpretation, analysis, inference, evaluation, explanation, and self-regulation, but also a nurse's habit (disposition) to ask questions, to be well informed, to be honest in facing personal biases, and to always be willing to reconsider and think differently about issues. Without these dispositions, sound critical thinking is unlikely to occur (Meherali et al., 2015; Noone & Seery, 2018; Paul & Elder, 2020). When applied to nursing, these core critical thinking skills and critical thinking dispositions reveal the complex nature of the **clinical decision-making process** (Table 7.1). Learning to apply these skills and establish critical thinking habits takes time and practice. Being open-minded, inquisitive, and systematic in thinking about practice situations will help you incorporate research findings in your clinical decision making.

Nurses who apply critical thinking in their work consider all aspects of a situation, reflect on knowledge derived from other interdisciplinary subject areas such as the biophysical and behavioural sciences and the humanities, and make well-reasoned judgements about a variety of possible alternative actions in order to provide holistic nursing care (Gonzalez et al., 2020; Noone & Seery, 2018). For example, nurses who work in crisis situations such as child abuse and suicide prevention programs act quickly when patient challenges develop. These nurses must, however, exercise discipline in decision making to avoid premature and

TABLE 7.1	Critical Thinking Skills and Dispositions	
Elements of Decision-Making Process	**Critical Thinking Behaviour**	
Cognitive Skills*		
Interpretation	Be orderly in data collection. Look for patterns to categorize data (e.g., formulate nursing diagnoses [see Chapter 14]). Clarify any data about which you are uncertain.	
Analysis	Be open-minded as you look at information about a patient. Avoid making careless assumptions. Ask whether the data reveal what you believe is true or whether other scenarios are possible.	
Inference	Examine meanings and relationships in the data. Form reasonable hypotheses and conclusions on the basis of the patterns observed.	
Evaluation	Assess all situations objectively. Use criteria (e.g., expected outcomes) to determine the effectiveness of nursing actions. Identify required changes. Reflect on your own behaviour.	
Explanation	Support your findings and conclusions. Use knowledge and experience to select the strategies you use in the care of patients.	
Self-regulation	Reflect on your experiences. Adhere to standards of practice. Apply ethical principles in your nursing practice. Identify in what way you can improve your own performance.	
Dispositions or Habits†		
Truth-seeking	Learn what is actually happening in a situation. Consider scientific principles and evidence, even if they do not support your preconceptions or personal beliefs.	
Open-mindedness	Be receptive to new ideas and tolerant of other points of view. Respect the right of other people to hold different opinions. Be aware of your own prejudices.	
Analyticity	Determine the significance of a situation. Interpret meaning. Anticipate possible results or consequences. Use evidence-informed knowledge in your nursing practice.	
Systematicity	Be organized and focused in data collection. Use an organized approach to problem solving and decision making.	
Self-confidence	Trust your own reasoning processes. Seek confirmation from experts when uncertain.	
Inquisitiveness	Be curious and eager to acquire new knowledge and learn reasoning and explanations.	
Maturity	Accept that multiple solutions are possible. Reflect on your own judgements; be willing to consider other explanations. Use prudence in making, suspending, or revising judgements.	

*Facione, P. (2020). *Critical thinking: What it is and why it counts.* https://www.insightassessment.com/wp-content/uploads/ia/pdf/whatwhy.pdf
†Alfaro-LeFevre, R. (2019). *Critical thinking, clinical reasoning, and clinical judgment: A practical approach* (7th ed., p. 13). Elsevier.

inappropriate decisions. Learning to think critically helps the nurse to care for patients as their advocate and to make better informed choices about their care. Critical thinking is more than just problem solving; it is an attempt to continually improve how one critically analyzes and applies knowledge when faced with problems in patient care.

Cognitive skills are used to (1) interpret problems accurately by using both objective and subjective data from common information sources; (2) analyze ideas and arguments about the problem; (3) infer or assess arguments and draw conclusions; (4) explain the decision; (5) evaluate the information to ascertain its trustworthiness; and (6) self-regulate, or constantly monitor one's own thinking for clarity, precision, accuracy, consistency, logic, and significance (Alfaro-LeFevre, 2019). Hence, in thinking critically, one not only tries to determine thoughtfully what to do or what to believe but also applies the core critical thinking skills to one another. In other words, one analyzes one's own inferences, explains one's own interpretation, or evaluates one's own analysis (Alfaro-LeFevre, 2019).

A CRITICAL THINKING MODEL FOR CLINICAL DECISION MAKING

Thinking critically is a benchmark or standard for professional nursing competence. Kataoka-Yahiro and Saylor (1994) developed a model of critical thinking for nursing judgement based in part on previous work by Paul (1993), Glaser (1941), Perry (1979), and Miller and Malcolm (1990) (Figure 7.1). The model helps explain what is involved as the nurse makes clinical decisions and judgements about their patients. It also defines the outcome of critical thinking: nursing judgement that is relevant to nursing situations in a variety of settings.

Throughout this text, this model is used for applying critical thinking during the **nursing process** (see Chapter 5). Each clinical chapter of the text (Chapters 31 to 49) is organized by the steps of the nursing process and includes both scientific and nursing knowledge. It is your knowledge base (the first critical thinking component) that prepares you to make clinical judgements as a nurse. Figure 7.1 demonstrates how to apply elements of critical thinking in assessing patients, in planning the interventions you provide, and in evaluating the outcomes.

LEVELS OF CRITICAL THINKING IN NURSING

The nurse's ability to think critically grows as they gain new knowledge and experience in nursing practice. Three levels of critical thinking in nursing—basic, complex, and commitment—are incorporated in the critical thinking model developed by Kataoka-Yahiro and Saylor (1994). As a beginning nursing student, you will apply the critical thinking model at the basic level. As you advance in practice, you will adopt complex critical thinking and commitment.

Basic Critical Thinking

At the basic level of critical thinking, thinking is concrete and based on a set of rules or principles. For example, as a student nurse, you use a hospital's procedure manual to confirm how to insert a Foley catheter. In completing this procedure for the first time, you will probably follow the procedure step by step without adjusting the procedure to meet a patient's unique needs (e.g., positioning to minimize the patient's pain or mobility restrictions) because you do not have enough experience to know how to individualize the procedure. At this level, answers to complex problems are seen to be either right or wrong (e.g., the Foley

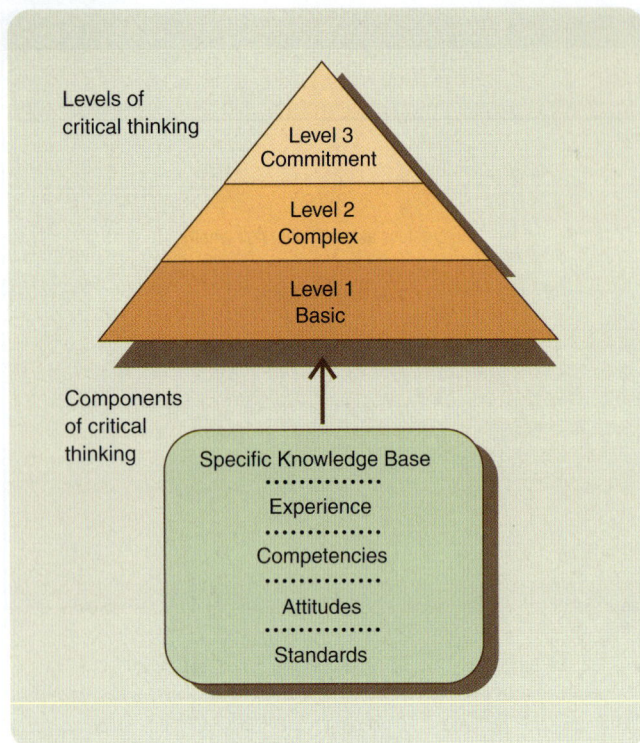

FIGURE 7.1 Critical thinking model for nursing judgement. (Redrawn from Kataoka-Yahiro, M., & Saylor, C. [1994]. A critical thinking model for nursing judgment. *Journal of Nursing Education, 33*[8], 351. Adapted from Glaser, E. [1941]. An experiment in the development of critical thinking. Bureau of Publications, Teachers College, Columbia University; Miller, M., & Malcolm, N. [1990]. Critical thinking in the nursing curriculum. *Nursing & Health Care, 11*, 67; Paul, R. W. [1993]. The art of redesigning instruction. In J. Willsen & A. J. A. Blinker [Eds.], *Critical thinking: How to prepare students for a rapidly changing world*. Foundation for Critical Thinking; and Perry, W. [1979]. *Forms of intellectual and ethical development in the college years: A scheme.* Holt, Rinehart, & Winston.)

catheter balloon contains too much or not enough sterile water), and you may believe that one right answer exists for each problem. As you gain more experience in nursing, you will begin to explore the diverse opinions of expert others (e.g., instructors and staff nurse role models) and engage in more complex critical thinking.

Complex Critical Thinking

When you engage in complex critical thinking, you begin to separate your thinking processes from those of expert others and to analyze and examine choices more independently. Your thinking abilities and initiative to look beyond expert opinion begin to change as you realize that alternative, and perhaps conflicting, solutions to a problem or issue exist.

Consider the following case example:

Mrs. Olsen, 70 years old, and Ms. Christine, 30 years old, both have rheumatoid arthritis. Their disease processes are much the same, and both patients experience persistent pain. Mrs. Olsen views her condition as part of the aging process and is responding with acceptance. Ms. Christine, however, is more concerned about her pain and is refusing to take prescribed steroids and analgesics because of the medication's adverse effects. While discussing the management of persistent pain with Ms. Christine, the nurse, Edwina, learns that Ms. Christine practices mindfulness techniques (such as guided meditation and yoga) at home using a mindfulness mobile app on her phone. In complex critical

thinking, Edwina recognizes that for relief of persistent pain, the patient has options other than pharmacological measures. Edwina decides to also discuss other nonpharmacological interventions with Ms. Christine. Edwina also based this decision on research evidence showing that mindfulness is an evidence-informed approach for dealing with persistent pain that has been tested and proven to be effective.

In complex critical thinking, you are willing to consider other options, including patient preferences regarding care, in addition to routine procedures, when complex situations develop. As a nurse, you learn to weigh the benefits and risks of each potential solution before making a final decision. Thinking becomes more creative, innovative, and patient centred as you explore a broad range of perspectives and alternative solutions.

Commitment

The third level of critical thinking is commitment. The nurse anticipates the need to make choices without assistance from other professionals and then assumes responsibility and accountability for those choices. As a nurse, you do more than just consider the complex alternative solutions that a problem poses. At the commitment level, you choose an action or belief on the basis of the viability of the alternative solutions available, and you stand by your choice. Sometimes an action is to not take action, or you may choose to delay taking action as a result of your experience and knowledge. Because you take responsibility for the decision, you evaluate the results of the decision and determine whether it was appropriate or if a different approach is required.

COMPONENTS OF CRITICAL THINKING IN NURSING

Critical thinking consists of five components: knowledge base, experience, competencies, attitudes, and standards. These elements explain how nurses make clinical judgements that are necessary for safe, competent, and ethical nursing care. (Box 7.2 highlights the components of critical thinking in nursing.)

Specific Knowledge Base

Nurses must possess a sound knowledge base to think critically, formulate accurate clinical judgements and decisions, and improve clinical practice. The nurse's knowledge base includes information and theory from the basic sciences, humanities, behavioural sciences, and nursing. The *Framework for the Practice of Registered Nurses in Canada* describes how nurses use their knowledge base in a way that is different from that of other health care providers and how nurses think holistically about patient situations and health-related matters (Canadian Nurses Association [CNA], 2015). For example, a nurse's broad knowledge base offers a physical, psychological, social, moral, ethical, legal, and cultural view of patients and their health concerns. The breadth and depth of the nurse's knowledge influences their ability to integrate and apply different kinds of knowledge and to think critically about nursing problems in a range of practice settings. Consider this scenario:

Robert Perez (preferred pronouns: he/him) previously earned a bachelor's degree in education and taught high school for 1 year. He has successfully completed the required human and biological science courses in his nursing program as well as those related to health ethics, fundamental nursing concepts, and communication principles. His first clinical course focuses on health promotion, with a clinical assignment in an outpatient primary care clinic. Although he is still new to nursing, his experience as a teacher and his preparation and knowledge base in nursing will help him know how to begin to make clinical decisions about patients' self-care and health promotion practices.

<table>
<tr><td colspan="2">

BOX 7.2 | **Components of Critical Thinking in Nursing**

I. Specific knowledge base
II. Experience in nursing
III. Critical thinking competencies
   A. General critical thinking competencies (scientific method, problem solving, and decision making)
   B. Specific critical thinking competencies in clinical situations (diagnostic reasoning, clinical inference, and clinical decision making)
   C. Specific critical thinking competency in nursing (use of nursing process)
IV. Attitudes for critical thinking
   A. Independence (own thinking, objectivity, and honesty)
   B. Fair-mindedness (neutral judgements without bias)
   C. Aware of self-limits (knowing limits of intellect and experiences)
   D. Integrity (challenging own ideas and methods of providing nursing care)
   E. Perseverance (motivated)
   F. Confidence (trusting the skills and intellect abilities)
V. Standards for critical thinking
   A. Intellectual standards
   B. Professional standards
      1. Ethical criteria for nursing judgement
      2. Criteria for evaluation
      3. Professional responsibility

</td></tr>
</table>

Adapted from Paul, R., & Elder, L. (2020). *The miniature guide to critical thinking concepts and tools* (8th ed.). Thinker's Guide Library; Sullivan, E. A. (2012). Critical thinking in clinical nurse education: Application of Paul's model of critical thinking. *Nurse Education in Practice, 12*(6), 322–327; Falcó-Pegueroles, A., Rodríguez-Martín, D., Ramos-Pozón, S., et al. (2020). Critical thinking in nursing clinical practice, education and research: From attitudes to virtue. *Nursing Philosophy, 22*(1), e12332. https://doi.org/10.1111/nup.12332

The proliferation of digital technologies influences how knowledge is documented, acquired, utilized, and shared in clinical practice. Building a sound knowledge base demands that nurses develop strong **information literacy skills**, which includes proficiency in knowing when information is needed and how to effectively find, retrieve, evaluate, and apply research findings (Melnyk & Fineout-Overholt, 2019). Critical thinking dispositions, such as truth-seeking, being systematic, analytical, open-minded, and inquisitive, enables nurses to become informed consumers of information found in print, through social media, and on the Internet.

Experience

Nursing is a practice discipline, and clinical nursing experiences are necessary for nurses to acquire clinical decision-making skills. In clinical situations, nurses learn from observing, sensing, talking with patients and families, and reflecting actively on their experiences. Clinical experience is the laboratory for evaluating nursing knowledge. As a nurse, you learn that "textbook" approaches form the basis for nursing practice, but you make safe adaptations or revisions in approaches to accommodate the setting, unique characteristics and desires of the patient, and the experience you gained from caring for previous patients. With experience, you begin to understand clinical situations, recognize cues of patients' health patterns, and interpret cues as relevant or irrelevant (Tanner, 2006). As a result, your critical thinking skills advance beyond the basic level. You also learn to seek new knowledge as needed, act quickly when events change, and make quality

decisions that promote the patient's health and well-being. Critical thinkers admit what they do not know and try to acquire the knowledge needed to make correct decisions. A patient's safety and welfare are at risk if you do not admit your inability to deal with a practice problem.

Returning to Robert Perez, during the previous summer he worked as a nurse assistant in a long-term care facility. This experience provided him with valuable experience in interacting with older persons and in giving basic nursing care. He has been able to develop good interviewing skills and understand the importance of the family in an individual's health. He has also learned that older persons often require more time to perform activities of daily living such as eating, bathing, and grooming, and so he has adapted skill techniques to accommodate this requirement. His time spent in the physical assessment laboratory and working in the long-term care facility helped him to become a careful observer. As he reflects on his experiences, Robert also knows that much of what he learned can be applied in promoting health, wellness, and independence among the older patients who attend the outpatient primary care clinic for routine follow-up visits.

Becoming familiar with practice standards developed by clinical experts and professional nursing regulatory bodies assists nurses in enhancing their knowledge base. For example, the Best Practice Guidelines developed by the Registered Nurses' Association of Ontario (RNAO) include standards for patient-centred care and for clinical conditions such as asthma, diabetes, and pain. Others focus on nursing practice issues such as cultural competence, end-of-life care, and intimate partner violence. The aim of the Best Practice Guidelines is to incorporate research into practice, increase consistency of care, eliminate interventions that are of questionable value, and improve health outcomes. Visit the RNAO's website (http://www.rnao.org/bestpractices/) and those of other Canadian professional nursing associations to learn more about the range of practice guidelines that are available to help you develop a sound knowledge base for your nursing practice.

CRITICAL THINKING COMPETENCIES

Kataoka-Yahiro and Saylor (1994) described critical thinking competencies as the cognitive processes that a nurse uses to make judgements about the clinical care of patients. They include general critical thinking, specific critical thinking in clinical situations, and specific critical thinking in nursing.

General Critical Thinking Competencies

General critical thinking competencies are not unique to nursing. They include the scientific method, problem solving, and decision making.

Scientific Method. The **scientific method** is a systematic, ordered approach to gathering data and solving problems that is used in nursing, medicine, and various other disciplines. Research incorporating the scientific method contributes to evidence-informed nursing practice and the development of Best Practice Guidelines. Evidence-informed nursing practice and the research process are described in more detail in Chapter 8.

Problem Solving. Everyone faces problems every day. When a problem arises, people obtain information and then use the information, in addition to what they already know, to find a solution. Patients routinely present problems in nursing practice. For example, a home care nurse visits a patient and learns that the patient cannot describe what medications she has taken for the past 3 days. The nurse must solve the problem of why the patient is not adhering to her medication schedule. The nurse knows the patient was recently discharged from the hospital and five medications were prescribed. When the nurse asks the patient to show the medications that she takes in the morning, the nurse notices that the patient is anxious and has difficulty reading the medication labels. The patient is able to tell the nurse the names of the medications she is to take but is uncertain about the times of administration. The nurse recommends having the patient's pharmacy relabel the medications in larger lettering. In addition, the nurse shows the patient examples of pill organizers that will help her sort her medications by time of day for a period of 7 days.

Effective problem solving also involves evaluating the solution over time to be sure that it is still effective. It becomes necessary to try different options if a problem recurs. As a continuation of the example just described, the nurse finds during a follow-up visit that the patient has organized her medications correctly and is able to read the labels without difficulty. The patient confirms that she is now more confident about her ability to follow her medication regimen. The nurse obtained information that correctly clarified the cause of the patient's problem, and the nurse tested a solution that proved successful. Having solved a problem in one situation adds to the nurse's experience in practice and enables the nurse to apply that knowledge in future situations with patients.

Decision Making. When a person faces a problem or situation and needs to choose a course of action from several options, they are making a decision. Decision making is a product of critical thinking that focuses on problem resolution. Following a set of criteria helps one make a well-reasoned decision. For example, decision making occurs when a new parent chooses an infant car seat. To make a decision, the parent needs to recognize and define the situation (need to protect the infant) and assess all options (consider available models). The parent has to weigh each option against a set of criteria (e.g., safety rating; cost; ease of installation and use), test possible options (e.g., search the Health Canada website for recall notices; seek advice from other parents), consider the consequences of the decision (safety of infant; risk of injury), and then make a final decision. Although the criteria follow a sequence of steps, decision making involves moving back and forth between steps when all criteria are considered. Decision making leads to informed conclusions that are supported by evidence and reason. Other examples of decision making include deciding on the specific dressing to be used for a patient with a surgical wound or selecting the best approach for teaching a family how to assist a patient who is returning home after a stroke. The nurse learns to make sound decisions by approaching each clinical situation thoughtfully and by applying each component of the decision-making process described previously.

Specific Critical Thinking Competencies in Clinical Situations

Specific critical thinking competencies in clinical situations include diagnostic reasoning, clinical inference, and clinical decision making.

Diagnostic Reasoning and Clinical Inference. As soon as the nurse receives information about a patient in a clinical situation, the nurse begins diagnostic reasoning, a process of determining a patient's health status after making physical and behavioural observations and after assigning meaning to the behaviours, physical signs, and symptoms exhibited by the patient. The information that the nurse collects and analyzes leads to a diagnosis of the patient's condition. An expert nurse sees the context of a patient situation (e.g., recognizes that a patient who is feeling lightheaded, has blurred vision, and has a history of diabetes is experiencing a problem with blood glucose levels), observes patterns and themes (e.g., symptoms including weakness, headache, hunger, and visual disturbances that suggest hypoglycemia),

and chooses an appropriate intervention quickly (e.g., offers a food source containing glucose). Considering the context of the situation enhances the nurse's analytical skills (Falcó-Pegueroles et al., 2020) and results in a more accurate diagnosis.

Part of diagnostic reasoning is clinical inference—the process of drawing conclusions from related pieces of evidence. An inference involves forming patterns of information from data before making a diagnosis. Seeing that a patient has lost their appetite and experienced a loss of weight over the past month, the nurse infers that the patient has a nutritional problem. An example of diagnostic reasoning is forming a nursing diagnosis such as imbalanced nutrition, less than body requirements (see Chapter 43).

Often the nurse cannot make a precise nursing diagnosis during their first meeting with a patient. The nurse will sometimes sense that a problem or health concern exists but not have sufficient data to make a specific diagnosis. Some patients' physical conditions limit their ability to tell the nurse about their symptoms. Other patients may choose not to share sensitive and important information during the nurse's initial assessment. For example, patients who live with mental illness or human immunodeficiency virus (HIV) may fear discrimination if they reveal their diagnosis. Other patients' behaviours and physical responses, such as those related to post-traumatic stress disorder (PTSD), may become observable only under certain conditions not present during the initial assessment. When the nurse is uncertain of a diagnosis, they need to continue data collection until they are able to determine the patient's unique situation.

In diagnostic reasoning, the nurse will use patient data that are gathered to logically explain a clinical judgement. For example, after turning a patient over in bed, you see an area of redness and a small blister on their right hip. You palpate the area and note that it is warm to the touch, and the patient complains of tenderness there. You push on the area with your finger, and, after you release pressure, the area does not blanch or turn white. You think about what you know about normal skin integrity and the effects of pressure. You form the conclusion the patient has a stage I pressure injury. As a new student, confirm your judgement with experienced nurses. At times, your clinical judgement may be incorrect (e.g., a blistered area is indicative of a stage II pressure injury [Registered Nurses' Association of Ontario (RNAO), 2016a]); however, nurse experts will give you feedback to build on in future clinical situations.

Nurses do not make medical diagnoses, but they do assess and monitor patients closely and compare the patient's signs and symptoms with those that are common to a medical diagnosis. This type of diagnostic reasoning helps nurses and other health care providers pinpoint the nature of a health problem more quickly and select proper interventions. Similarities and differences between medical and nursing diagnoses are described in more detail in Chapter 14.

Clinical reasoning is a term that is also used to describe the cognitive process of thinking about patient issues, making inferences, and deciding on the actions to be implemented in a particular situation. Engaging in clinical reasoning involves collecting cues, processing information, coming to understand the patient problem or situation, planning and implementing interventions, evaluating outcomes, and reflecting on and learning from the process. As you gain experience in nursing, your ability to identify the salient aspects of patient situations and to differentiate between clinical conditions that require immediate attention (difficulty breathing due to an adverse medication reaction) and those that are less acute (shortness of breath related to chronic pulmonary disease) will increase. As a result, you will be able to accurately identify patients who are at greatest risk of complications, make sound clinical judgements about how to intervene, and manage complex clinical situations effectively (Harding & Snyder, 2018).

Strategies such as "thinking-out-loud" (verbalizing your thinking) as you work through a simulated patient care scenario can be useful in honing your clinical reasoning skills (Downs & Halls, 2020; Falcó-Pegueroles et al., 2020). Using clinical reasoning, nursing knowledge, and other evidence to inform decision making in diverse practice situations enables the nurse to provide safe, competent, compassionate, ethical, and culturally safe care to patients and families (CASN, 2022). Clinical reasoning incorporates critical thinking and is essential to sound clinical decision making.

Clinical Decision Making. Clinical decision making focuses on defining patient problems or situations and selecting appropriate interventions. When the nurse approaches a clinical problem, such as a patient who is experiencing difficulty walking, the nurse makes a decision that identifies the problem (e.g., right-sided weakness) and chooses nursing interventions (e.g., teach the use of appropriate assistive devices) for that patient. Use of clinical decision making distinguishes professional nurses from technical personnel. It is the professional nurse, for example, who takes immediate action when a patient's clinical condition deteriorates, decides whether a patient is experiencing complications that call for notification of a physician, or decides whether a teaching plan for a patient is ineffective and needs revision. Benner (1984) described clinical decision making as judgement that includes critical and reflective thinking and action and the application of scientific and practical knowledge.

Clinical judgement requires that you recognize the salient aspects of a clinical situation, interpret their meanings, and respond appropriately. It includes four components: noticing or grasping the situation; interpreting or developing a sufficient understanding of the situation to respond; responding or deciding on a course of action; and reflecting on or reviewing the actions taken and their outcomes. In making a clinical judgement, you consider the context of the situation and rely on analytical processes, intuition, and narrative thinking (i.e., thinking that occurs as a result of telling and interpreting stories). As you reflect on actions taken, you acquire clinical learning, which contributes to future clinical judgements.

Nurses regularly encounter practice situations in which little is straightforward. Each patient's situation and challenges are unique and products of many factors, including the patient's physical health, lifestyle, culture, relationship with family and friends, living environment, and experiences. Clinical decision making requires careful reasoning so that the nurse chooses the options for the best patient outcomes on the basis of the patient's condition, the priority of the problem, or health concern.

Nurses improve their clinical decision making by knowing their patients. For example, an expert nurse who has worked on a general surgery unit for many years is more likely to detect signs of internal hemorrhage (e.g., fall in blood pressure, rapid pulse, change in consciousness) than is a new nurse. Over time, a combination of knowledge, experience, time spent in a specific clinical area, and the quality of relationships formed with patients allow expert nurses to know clinical situations and quickly anticipate and select the right course of action. As a nurse, spending more time during initial patient assessments to both observe patient behaviour and measure physical findings is a way to better know your patients. Accounts of patients' health challenges can help you learn about their experiences through their eyes and foster empathy. Consistently monitoring patients as problems occur helps you see how clinical changes develop over time. The selection of nursing actions is built on both clinical knowledge and patient data, including the following:

- The identified status and situation of the patient
- Knowledge about the clinical variables (e.g., patient's age, seriousness of the health problem, pathological process of the problem,

patient's pre-existing disease conditions) involved in the situation and how the variables are related
- Knowledge about the usual patterns of any diagnosed health problem or prognosis and a judgement about the likely course of events and outcomes of the diagnosed condition, in view of any coexisting health risks the patient also possesses
- Additional relevant information about the patient's daily living situation, functional capacity, and social resources
- Knowledge about the nursing interventions available and the way in which specific actions will predictably affect the patient's situation
- Knowledge about the patient's desired health outcomes

After determining a patient's nursing care priorities, the nurse selects actions most likely to relieve each health problem or to promote health, wellness, and quality of life. A wide range of choices is often available, from nurse-administered to patient self-care strategies. The nurse collaborates with the patient and then selects, tests, and evaluates the chosen approaches. Making an accurate clinical decision enables the nurse to set priorities for nursing action. Because each situation involves different patients and different variables, a certain activity is sometimes more of a priority in one situation and less of a priority in another. For example, if a home care patient is physically dependent, unable to eat, and incontinent of urine, skin integrity is of higher priority than if the patient were immobile but continent of urine and able to eat a normal diet. Do not assume that certain health situations produce automatic priorities. For example, an adolescent who has embarked on a smoking cessation program is expected to experience some withdrawal symptoms, which often become a priority of care. However, if the patient is experiencing anxiety about potential weight gain that decreases their ability to participate fully in the program, it becomes necessary for the nurse to focus on ways to relieve the anxiety before the smoking cessation measures will be effective.

Nurses make decisions about individual patients and about groups of patients. The nurse needs to use criteria such as the clinical condition of patients, their specific needs, risks involved in treatment delays, and patients' expectations of care to determine which patients have the most urgent priorities for care. For example, a patient in a community care centre who is experiencing a sudden drop in blood pressure along with a change in consciousness requires the nurse's attention immediately, in contrast to a small child who requires a routine immunization or a group of expectant parents attending a prenatal class. In order for nurses to manage the wide variety of health problems and situations associated with groups of patients, skillful, prioritized decision making is crucial. Learning to set priorities effectively takes time and experience. Consulting with more experienced nurses and being aware that priorities may change rapidly can help you identify and deal with unexpected events (Box 7.3).

Nursing Process as a Critical Thinking Competency

Nurses apply the nursing process as a critical thinking competency when delivering patient care. The nursing process is a five-step clinical decision-making approach that consists of assessment, diagnosis, planning, implementation, and evaluation (see Chapters 14 and 15). The purpose of the nursing process is to assist nurses in identifying and treating patients' health-related concerns and help patients attain agreed-upon health outcomes (Figure 7.2). The nursing process incorporates general (e.g., scientific method, problem solving, and decision making) and specific critical thinking competencies (e.g., diagnostic reasoning, inference, and clinical decision making), described earlier in this chapter, in a manner that focuses on a particular patient's unique needs. The format of the nursing process is unique to the discipline of nursing and provides a common language and process for nurses to "think through" patients' clinical issues (Kataoka-Yahiro & Saylor, 1994). Chapter 14 describes the nursing process in more detail.

BOX 7.3   Clinical Decision Making for Groups of Patients

- Identify the nursing diagnosis and collaborative issues of each patient.
- Analyze patients' diagnoses or health problems and decide which are most urgent in light of the patient's basic needs, changing or unstable status, and problem complexity.
- Consider the resources available for managing each health problem, including unregulated care providers assigned to work with you and the patients' family members.
- Consider how to involve patients as decision makers and participants in care.
- Decide how to combine activities to resolve more than one patient situation at a time.
- Decide what, if any, nursing care procedures to delegate to unregulated care providers so that you are able to spend your time on activities requiring professional nursing knowledge.

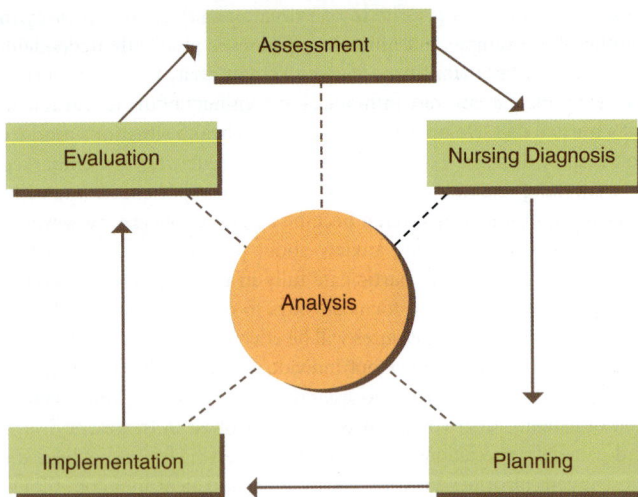

FIGURE 7.2 Five-step nursing process model.

The nursing process is often called a blueprint or plan for care. When you use the nursing process, you identify a patient's health-related concerns, clearly define a nursing diagnosis or collaborative problem, determine priorities of care, and set goals and expected outcomes of care. Then you develop and communicate a plan of care, perform nursing interventions, and evaluate the effects of your care. Involving your patient in each step of the nursing process helps ensure that care is patient centred. As you become more competent in using the nursing process, you will be able to focus on multiple health problems or diagnoses and move back and forth between steps when considering all the information available to you about a patient's concerns.

Several clinical judgement models can be used to learn the nursing process. The United States National Council of State Boards of Nursing (NCSBN) (NCBSN, 2019) Clinical Judgment Measurement Model (CJM) presents the complexities associated with decision making in a simplified manner to enable better assessment of clinical judgement, which is an important component of the nursing process. Detailed information about this model is provided in Chapter 14.

Attitudes for Critical Thinking

The fourth component of the critical thinking model incorporates the attitudes needed to think critically. An important part of critical thinking is interpreting, evaluating, and making judgements about the adequacy of various arguments and available data. Attitudes determine how a successful critical thinker approaches a problem or a situation that necessitates decision making. For example, when a patient complains of anxiety before undergoing a diagnostic procedure, the curious nurse explores possible reasons for the patient's concerns. The nurse also exhibits discipline and perseverance in taking responsibility to complete a thorough assessment to find the sources of the patient's anxiety. Knowing when you need more information, knowing when information is misleading, and recognizing your own knowledge limits and personal biases are examples of how critical thinking attitudes play a key role in decision making.

Standards for Critical Thinking

The fifth component of the critical thinking model includes intellectual and professional standards (Kataoka-Yahiro & Saylor, 1994).

Intellectual Standards. An *intellectual standard* is a guideline or principle for rational thought. Nurses apply such standards when they conduct the nursing process. When the nurse considers a patient's health problem, the nurse applies intellectual standards such as thoroughness, precision, accuracy, and consistency to make sure that all clinical decisions are sound. Efficacious use of the intellectual standards in clinical practice ensures that nurses do not perform critical thinking haphazardly.

Professional Standards. *Professional standards* for critical thinking refer to ethical criteria for nursing judgements, evidence-informed criteria for evaluation, and criteria for professional responsibility. Professional standards promote the highest level of quality nursing care for individuals and groups in institutional and community-based settings.

Ethical Criteria for Nursing Judgement. Effective nursing practice reflects sound ethical principles. Being able to focus on a patient's values and beliefs helps the nurse make clinical decisions that are just, faithful to the patient's choices, and beneficial to the patient's health and well-being. The *Code of Ethics for Registered Nurses* (CNA, 2017) is based on core values that serve as a guide to ethical decision making in nursing practice. Among these values and ethical responsibilities are providing safe, compassionate, competent, and ethical care; promoting health and well-being; promoting and respecting informed decision making; preserving dignity; maintaining privacy and confidentiality; promoting justice; and being accountable. Critical thinkers maintain a sense of self-awareness through conscious awareness of their own values, beliefs, and feelings and of the multiple perspectives of patients, family members, staff, and peers in clinical situations. Chapter 9 summarizes ethical standards to use when you as a nurse are faced with ethical dilemmas or problems, as in the following example.

A patient in a community health clinic is a young man who has signs and symptoms of chlamydia, a sexually transmitted infection. The patient has had the symptoms for more than 3 weeks and voices concern about what it will mean to have the infection. Richard (pronouns: he/him), a nurse, examines the young man and finds that the patient has redness and itching on his penis, with a yellowish discharge. Richard checks further and asks whether the patient has pain on urination. He also assesses the patient for fever. Richard has limited knowledge about chlamydia, and so he consults with the clinic nurse practitioner, who explains the nature of the infection, the risks it poses to the patient, the usual course of treatment, and some of the legal and ethical guidelines that govern nurses' actions when working with patients with sexually transmitted infections. Richard returns to the patient and speaks confidently with him about chlamydia, the reason for his symptoms, the need to tell sex partners about the infection, and the importance of wearing a condom.

Criteria for Evaluation. Nurses routinely use evidence-informed criteria to assess patients' conditions, determine a course of action, and evaluate the efficacy of nursing interventions. For example, accurate assessment of symptoms such as pain or shortness of breath requires use of assessment criteria such as the duration, severity, location, aggravating or relieving factors, and effects on daily lifestyle (see Chapter 32). Assessment criteria enable you to accurately determine the nature of a patient's symptoms, select appropriate interventions, and later evaluate whether the interventions are effective. Another example is the use of the criteria incorporated in Best Practice Guidelines to differentiate between delirium, dementia, and depression in older persons in order to make prudent decisions about the care and services needed by patients and their caregivers to optimize clinical outcomes and reduce caregiver burden (RNAO, 2016b).

Professional Responsibility. The standards of professional responsibility that a nurse strives to achieve are the standards cited in institutional practice guidelines, professional organizations' standards of practice, and legislation governing nursing practice. The nursing practice standards that govern nurses' actions in Canada are found on the websites of provincial and territorial professional nursing organizations. These standards outline the responsibilities and accountabilities that a nurse assumes in providing high-quality health care to the public.

DEVELOPING CRITICAL THINKING SKILLS

To develop critical thinking skills, it is important to learn how to connect knowledge and theory in practice. Making sense of what you learn in the classroom, from reading, or from dialogue with patients, other students, and health providers and then applying it during patient care is challenging. Using strategies such as case-based learning, reflective writing, and concept mapping will help you develop and refine your critical thinking skills.

Case-Based Learning

Case-based learning is a strategy that can help you explore complex problems and engage in decision making without the risk of harming a patient. It includes approaches such as case studies, problem-based learning, simulation, and virtual reality. Simulation and virtual reality can be used to practise psychomotor skills to enhance your knowledge base, respond to unanticipated events in a controlled environment, and receive immediate feedback on your performance. Using these technologies you can identify knowledge gaps, learn from your mistakes in a safe environment, and enhance your ability to solve problems and make clinical judgements in increasingly complex scenarios. Case-based strategies prepare you to apply diagnostic reasoning, inference, and clinical decision making in real-life situations and are a valuable complement to your clinical practice experiences (CASN, 2015).

Reflective Writing

Reflective writing is a tool for developing critical thought that uses the process of reflection to purposefully recall a situation in order to discover its purpose or meaning. Reflective writing gives you the opportunity to describe a clinical experience in your own words, explore your perceptions and understanding of the experience, and become more aware of how you use clinical decision-making skills. It invites to you to consider questions such as "What have I learned from this experience?" and "What could I have done differently?" Reflection promotes knowledge transfer by enabling you to identify how previously acquired knowledge can be applied in another situation. Reflecting on your experiences is also an important component of monitoring your competence in nursing practice.

Reflective writing can also help you learn to know your patients better, even though you may not have had similar experiences. Instead of becoming a source of fear, diversity and difference can become an opportunity for you to come to understand their experience. Reflection allows you to examine your assumptions about what it means to be of a different age, race, or sexual orientation or to live with a mental illness. Similarly, reflecting on visual images, narratives, poetry, music, or drama can offer you opportunities to examine multiple perspectives, challenge your assumptions, and develop self-awareness and empathy (Bjerkvik & Hilli, 2019; Falcó-Pegueroles et al., 2020). Box 7.4 reports on a research study in which reflective writing was used as a tool in getting to know patients and their experiences.

Concept Mapping

As a nurse, you will care for patients with multiple nursing diagnoses. A concept map is a visual representation of patient health problems and interventions that depicts their relationships to one another. Drawing a concept map can help you synthesize relevant data about a patient, including assessment data, health needs, nursing diagnoses, nursing interventions, and evaluation measures. It also helps you move beyond memorizing, recalling facts, and focusing on tasks that need to be done to organizing or linking information in a unique way so that the diverse information you have about a patient begins to connect to

---

BOX 7.4 RESEARCH HIGHLIGHT

Reflective Writing in Undergraduate Clinical Nursing Education: A Literature Review

Research Focus

Reflective writing is one of many tools used to promote critical thinking, analysis, metacognition, and synthesis. It is a way to bridge the gap between thought and action and provides an opportunity to describe internal processes, evaluate challenges, and recognize triumphs in ways that otherwise would remain unarticulated (Allan & Discroll, 2014).

Research Abstract

The aim of this literature review was to explore the evidence of learning from reflective writing in undergraduate clinical nursing education. A combination of 17 quantitative and qualitative studies were included, and three main categories emerged: 1) development of clinical reasoning skills, 2) professional self-development, and 3) facilitators and barriers for learning.

The results revealed that reflective writing enhanced the students' reasoning skills and awareness in clinical situations. However, most students reflected primarily at a descriptive level, showing only limited and varied development of reflective skills. They focused on self-assessment and on their own emotional reactions and ability to cope in clinical situations but had difficulties with reflecting on the process of thinking and learning. Learning was promoted through instructive guidelines, scaffolding, and detailed feedback from a trusted, available, and qualified faculty teacher. Factors that facilitated learning included student maturity, individual cognitive skills, student collaboration, and mixed tools for learning.

Implications for Practice

On the basis of this literature review, the authors concluded that reflective writing is a useful tool for students' professional learning but, above all, for the students' personal development on the pathway to becoming a professional nurse.

From Bjerkvik, L. K., & Hilli, Y. (2019). Reflective writing in undergraduate clinical nursing education: A literature review. *Nurse Education in Practice, 35*, 32–41. https://doi.org/10.1016/j.nepr.2018.11.013

form meaningful patterns and concepts. When you see the relationship between the various patient diagnoses and the assessment data that support them, you gain a holistic understanding of a patient's clinical situation.

Concept maps take many visual forms (see Chapters 40 and 42 for examples). Select a format (e.g., hierarchical, flow chart, spider, system map, etc.) that allows the concept map to become a "living" document that can change as you develop and document your plan of care for the patient over time. The final map gives you a broader and more complex understanding of your patient's health care needs and demonstrates your integration of theory into practice. Save the concept maps you create and use them as a reference as you care for other patients with similar health concerns.

Several apps that can be used on a tablet are available for creating and sharing concept maps. Some apps that now support concept mapping include the following: MindMeister, Popplet, MindGenius, SimpleMind, iMindQ, Ideament, MindNode, bubbl.us, and Notability.

Concept Mapping Example. *Tara Chambler (preferred pronouns: she/her) is a 65-year-old homeless woman who was brought to the emergency department for frostbite on her extremities. She had her fourth and fifth fingers amputated from frostbite in her left hand during this month and a wound debridement of tissue from frostbite on her right lower leg. She has a history of asthma and smokes cigarettes and cannabis; she is malnourished and was hospitalized 6 years ago for a previous infection of a wound on her leg and 2 years ago for pneumonia. She reports 5 out of 10 pain in her hand and you note wheezes in her chest. She reports some difficulty breathing but tells you that it usually passes.*

Current vital signs: B/P 158/90, T 37.9°C, P 94, R 24, O₂ sat 93% on room air.

Figure 7.3 depicts the interrelatedness of the concepts from this case scenario and its attributes in the form of a Spider map.

CRITICAL THINKING SYNTHESIS

Critical thinking is a reasoning process by which nurses use knowledge, reflect on previous experience, and integrate professional practice standards to provide competent and ethical nursing care to patients (Figure 7.4). Thinking critically requires dedication and a desire to grow intellectually. For novice nurses, it is important to learn the steps of the nursing process and to incorporate the elements of the critical thinking model in their practice. The two processes are intertwined in making quality decisions about patient care. The key components of critical thinking are integrated into other chapters in this text to help you better understand its relationship to the nursing process and make quality judgements and decisions about patient care.

KEY CONCEPTS

- Critical thinking is a process acquired through learning and experience.
- Nurses who apply critical thinking in their work focus on options for solving problems and making decisions, rather than rapidly and carelessly adopting solutions.
- Following a procedure step by step without adjusting to a patient's unique needs is an example of basic critical thinking.
- In complex critical thinking, a nurse learns that alternative and perhaps conflicting solutions to problems exist.
- The critical thinking model combines a nurse's knowledge base, experience, competence in nursing process, attitudes, and standards to explain how nurses make clinical judgements that are necessary for safe, effective nursing care.
- In diagnostic reasoning, the nurse collects patient data and then logically develops a clinical judgement, such as a nursing diagnosis.
- When the nurse faces a clinical problem or situation and chooses a course of action from several options, they are making a clinical decision.
- Clinical learning experiences are necessary for you as a beginning nurse to acquire clinical decision-making skills.
- Nurses improve their clinical decision making by knowing their patients and including them in the decision-making process.
- Clinical decision making involves judgement that includes critical and reflective thinking and action and the application of scientific and practical knowledge.
- The nursing process is a blueprint for patient care that involves both general and specific critical thinking competencies in a way that focuses on the patient's unique needs and desired health outcomes.
- Critical thinking attitudes help a nurse to know when more information is needed, to know when information is misleading, and to recognize personal knowledge limits.

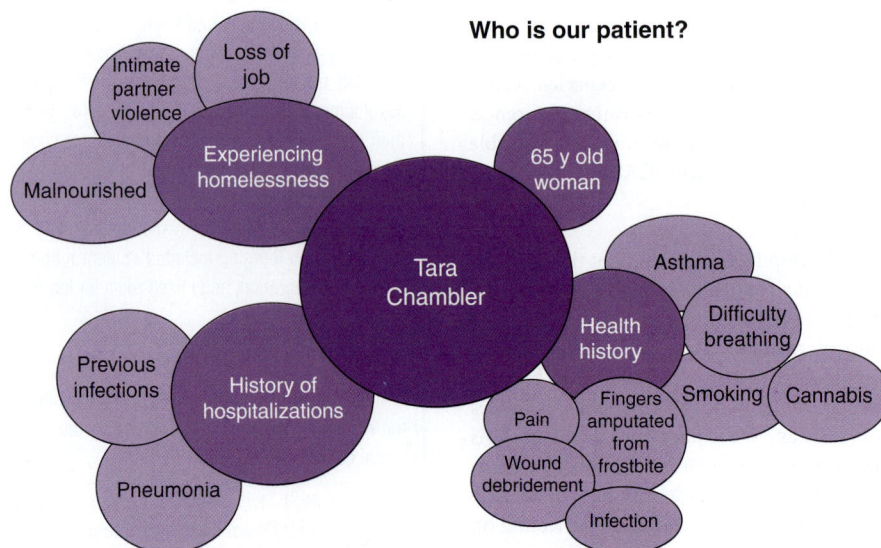

FIGURE 7.3 Spider map for Tara Chambler.

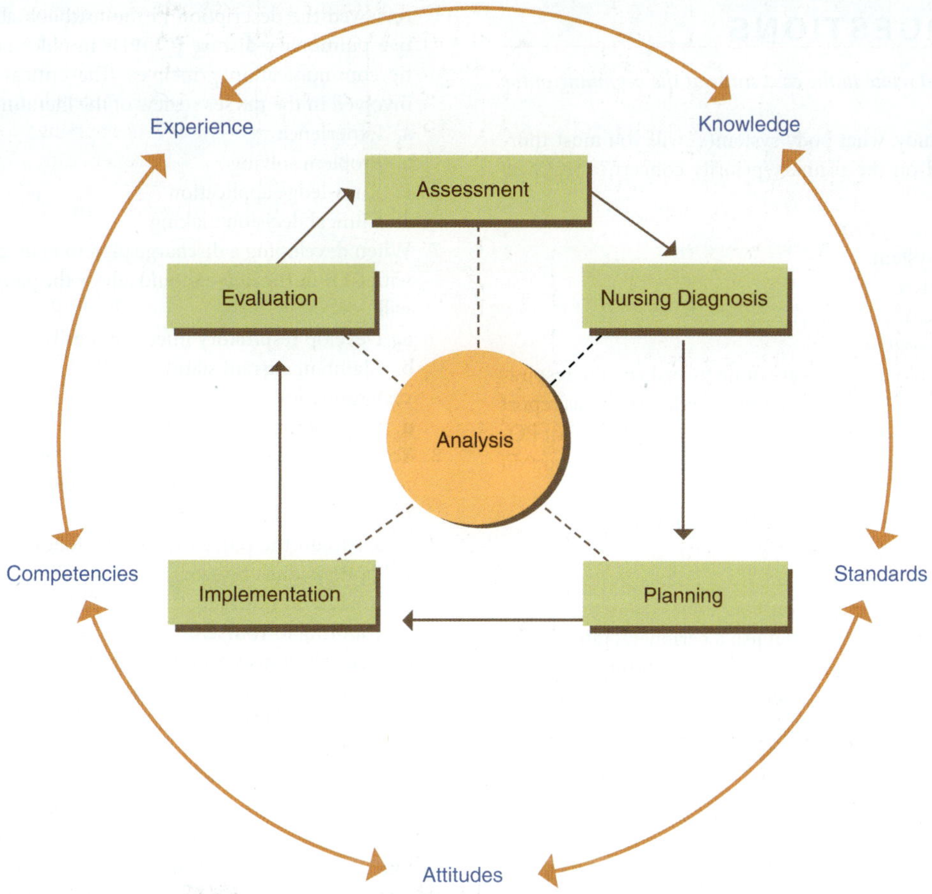

FIGURE 7.4 Synthesis of critical thinking with the nursing process in developing nursing competency.

- Sound information literacy skills help nurses locate, retrieve, evaluate, and apply research findings and are essential to thinking critically.
- The use of intellectual standards during assessment ensures a complete database of information.
- Professional standards for critical thinking refer to ethical criteria for nursing judgements, scientific and practice criteria to be used for evaluation, and criteria for professional responsibility.
- Case-based learning complements, but cannot replace, clinical experience in learning to think critically.
- Reflective writing gives one the opportunity to define and express clinical experiences in one's own words.
- Drawing a concept map enables the nurse to gain a broader and more complex understanding of their patient's complex health care needs.

▌ CRITICAL THINKING EXERCISES

1. You are meeting with a patient with obesity for the first time. She states that she has been successful in losing weight but is frustrated by her inability to maintain her weight loss. She reports having tried "virtually every fad diet" and "multiple exercise programs." She admits that as her weight increases, she tends to be become less active. She has become increasingly reluctant to leave her home because of the negative reactions of other people. In listening to her story, you attempt to imagine what it would be like to be in her situation and begin to examine your biases and assumptions about people with obesity. Your goal is to begin to discuss potential options with her for dealing with her situation. Describe the level of critical thinking that is necessary in this scenario and how it will assist you in helping this patient develop an effective plan of action.

2. Mr. Yousif is a terminally ill patient receiving home care. His wife and son are asking you about his pain control. Mrs. Yousif is requesting that her husband's medication be increased, even if it means he will be less responsive. She does not want her husband to suffer. The son is vehemently opposed to too much narcotic and feels that his father is still able to make decisions for himself. Mr. Yousif remains alert much of the time and is able to talk with you about his pain, his feelings regarding death, and his desire to die at home. How might you use critical thinking to help the family resolve this complex problem?

3. Reflect on a situation in which you needed to provide care to someone from a distinctly different culture. Construct a concept map that illustrates your approach to this situation. What were the key health challenges of concern to the patient? How were they related to each other? How did you approach knowing the patient? How did your beliefs and assumptions about the patient's culture change over time? What factors contributed to this change? Try to incorporate these factors into your concept map.

🌐 *Answers to Critical Thinking Exercises appear on the Evolve website.*

REVIEW QUESTIONS

Review Questions 1 to 10 relate to the case study at the beginning of the chapter.

1. Based on the case study, what body system(s) will you most thoroughly assess, based on the primary/priority concern? *(Select all that apply.)*
   a. Peripheral vascular system
   b. Cardiovascular system
   c. Neurological system
   d. Respiratory system
   e. Gastrointestinal system

2. The patient's arterial blood gases were done to evaluate the respiratory status. As her nurse, you reviewed the arterial blood gas report and found the following results: pH 7.35; PCO_2 62 (8.25 kPa); PO_2 70 (9.31 kPa); HCO_3 34 mmol/L (34 mEq/L). What should you do first?
   a. Apply a 100% nonrebreather mask to the patient.
   b. Assess the patient's vital signs.
   c. Reposition the patient.
   d. Prepare the patient for intubation.

3. The physician orders the nurse to establish a peripheral intravenous (IV) line for IV antibiotics. The nurse uses an institution's procedure manual to confirm how to insert an IV line. Which level of critical thinking is the nurse using?
   a. Commitment
   b. Scientific method
   c. Basic critical thinking
   d. Complex critical thinking

4. As the nurse enters a patient's room, she observes that the IV line is not infusing at the ordered rate. The nurse checks the flow regulator on the tubing, looks to see whether the patient is lying on the tubing, checks the connection between the tubing and the IV catheter, and then checks the condition of the site where the IV catheter enters the patient's skin. She readjusts the flow rate and the infusion begins at the correct rate. This is an example of:
   a. Inference
   b. Reflection
   c. Problem solving
   d. Evidence-informed decision making

5. Match the questions on the right with the appropriate step in the nursing process on the left for the patient.

Stage of Nursing Process	Question
1. Assessment	a. What actions will help the patient achieve their desired outcomes?
2. Nursing diagnosis	b. How will I know if the patient has achieved their desired outcomes?
3. Planning	c. How can I help the patient achieve their desired outcomes?
4. Implementation	d. What is the patient's health-related concern?
5. Evaluation	e. What are the patient's desired health outcomes?

6. The next day of the patient's hospital admission, the nurse asks the patient how she feels now. Before the discussion, the nurse reviewed the description in the textbook about chronic obstructive pulmonary disease (COPD) in older patients and therapeutic communication principles. The critical thinking component involved in the nurse's review of the literature is:
   a. Experience
   b. Problem solving
   c. Knowledge application
   d. Clinical decision making

7. When developing a discharge plan to manage the care of a patient with COPD, the nurse should advise the patient to expect that they will:
   a. Develop respiratory infections easily
   b. Maintain current status
   c. Require less supplemental oxygen
   d. Show permanent improvement

8. To control shortness of breath and provide a quick and easy way to slow the pace of breathing, the nurse has instructed the patient to do pursed-lip breathing. In which order, from first step to last step, should the nurse explain the following steps to the patient? All options must be used:
   a. Breathe in normally through your nose for two counts (while counting to yourself, 1, 2).
   b. Relax your neck and shoulder muscles.
   c. Pucker your lips as if you were going to whistle.
   d. Breathe out through pursed lips for four counts (while counting to yourself, 1, 2, 3, 4).

9. The nurse sits down to speak with the patient, whose husband died 6 months ago. The patient reports that she is unable to sleep, feels very fatigued during the day, and is having trouble concentrating. The nurse asks her to clarify the type of trouble she is having, and the patient explains that she cannot concentrate or even solve simple problems. The nurse records the results of her assessment, describing the patient's condition as *ineffective coping*. This conclusion reflects the nurse's use of:
   a. Inference
   b. Nursing process
   c. Evaluation criteria
   d. General critical thinking competencies

10. Match the clinical thinking skills and dispositions (habits) on the left with the corresponding critical thinking behaviour on the right.

Critical Thinking Skills and Dispositions	Critical Thinking Behaviour
1. Inference	a. Observe patterns and formulate conclusions
2. Evaluation	b. Ask how you can improve your clinical performance
3. Explanation	c. Consider opposing points of view
4. Self-regulation	d. Select criteria to assess the effectiveness of nursing interventions
5. Open-mindedness	e. Defend your conclusions

Answers: 1. b, d; **2.** b; **3.** c; **4.** c; **5.** 1(e), 2(d), 3(a), 4(c), 5(b); **6.** c; **7.** a; **8.** b, a, c, d; **9.** a; **10.** 1(a), 2(d), 3(e), 4(b), 5(c).

🌐 *Rationales for the Review Questions appear on the Evolve website.*

RECOMMENDED WEBSITES

Canadian Nurses Association: https://www.cna-aiic.ca/en
A wide range of valuable resources, including the *Code of Ethics for Registered Nurses* (CNA, 2017), can be found on this website, as well as links to those of each of the provincial and territorial professional nursing associations in Canada. The position papers and other documents found on these websites demonstrate how Canadian nurse leaders have used critical thinking to explore important issues in nursing and nursing practice.
Concept Mapping Tools: https://uwaterloo.ca/centre-for-teaching-excellence/teaching-resources/teaching-tips/teaching-tips-educational--technologies/all/concept-mapping-tools

This site, created by the Centre for Teaching Excellence at the University of Waterloo, provides an overview of the strengths and limitations of several concept mapping tools. Other tools, including examples of nursing-related concept maps, can be accessed via the Internet.
Critical Thinking Community: http://www.criticalthinking.org
The section of this website titled "Begin Here" includes links to a number of short articles specifically related to critical thinking in nursing and in health care. Explore the remainder of the website to locate yet other resources that may be of value to you in developing your critical thinking skills.

REFERENCES

A full reference list is available on the website for this book at http://evolve.elsevier.com/Canada/Potter/fundamentals/

8

Evidence-Informed Practice

Written by Wendy Duggleby, RN, PhD, Barbara J. Astle, RN, PhD, FCAN, and Kara Schick-Makaroff, RN, PhD

OBJECTIVES

Mastery of content in this chapter will enable you to:

- Define the key terms listed.
- Explain the need for evidence to inform nurses' decision making.
- Identify the steps of evidence-informed decision making.
- Discuss methods for developing new nursing knowledge.
- Describe types of literature reviews.
- Explain how nursing research improves nursing practice.
- Discuss the steps of the research process.

KEY TERMS

Evidence-informed decision making
Evidence-informed practice
Informed consent
Nursing research

Qualitative nursing research
Quantitative nursing research
Research
Research literacy

Research process
Research synthesis

🌐 WEBSITE

http://evolve.elsevier.com/Canada/Potter/fundamentals/

CASE STUDY

Natalie (preferred pronouns: she/her) has been a nurse on an acute care medical-surgical unit for more than 5 years. During that time, the nurses have continued to notice that patients often fall, despite a falls-prevention program that has been implemented on the unit. Natalie has noticed for some time that the falls-prevention program is not always used and that new nurses on the unit are often unaware of this program. Natalie raises some questions with the other nurses in the department: "What can we do to prevent our patients from falling?" "What are the best ways to prevent falls?" "What is the best way to implement a fall-prevention guideline so that it is sustainable?"

Natalie then began to look for evidence in the scientific literature to inform her practice and to change policy on the unit. In reading the literature, she was able to find a recent review that described and evaluated an individualized fall-prevention program in an acute care setting (Spano-Szekley et al., 2020). Natalie also found a research study that reported a mentored approach to implementing a fall-prevention program in an acute care setting, which resulted in sustainability of the program (Ploeg et al., 2018). Findings suggested the following recommendations: senior leadership must 1) actively make falls prevention a priority, 2) engage staff as champions who mentor other staff, and 3) engage patients and their families in the program.

Most nurses like Natalie practise nursing according to what they learned in their nursing education, their experiences in practice, and the policies and procedures of their health care agency. In Natalie's case, the evidence from the scientific literature provided a basis for her and her colleagues to make evidence-informed decisions to provide the highest quality of care to their patients and families.

Think about this case study as you read this chapter. There are review questions at the end of the chapter that relate to the case study.

WHY EVIDENCE?

The Canadian Nurses Association's (CNA) 2018 position statement *Evidence-Informed Decision-Making and Nursing Practice* notes that all nurses must use evidence-informed decision making. This means that critically appraised scientific evidence is integrated into the decision making of every nurse. When that happens, quality of care, as well as the health care system as a whole, is improved.

Multiple terms are used to describe the utilization of research by nurses in their practice, such as *research-based nursing practice*, *evidence-based practice*, *evidenced-based decision making*, evidence-informed practice, and *evidence-informed decision making*. Evidence-based practice refers to the use of evidence in a nurse's practice, whereas evidence-informed decision making involves use of evidence as part of the decision-making process, along with other factors beyond evidence, such as resources or cultural values and beliefs (CNA, 2018). Evidence-informed decision making is defined by the CNA as "an ongoing process that incorporates evidence from research findings, clinical expertise, client preferences and other available resources to inform decisions that nurses make about clients" (CNA, 2018, p. 1). As a result, evidence-informed decision making enables nurses to make accurate, timely, and appropriate clinical decisions. In this chapter, we will use the term *evidence-informed decision making*.

Relationship Between Evidence-Informed Decision Making, Research, and Quality Improvement

Nurses conduct research in a variety of settings and with a variety of methods. Student nurses and practitioners participate in investigations of patient outcomes and nursing care specific to their place of practice, commonly called *quality assurance* or *improvement studies*. In these types of studies, data are collected to determine the influence of nurses on achievement of patient care objectives in a particular clinical setting. Because the results usually apply only to one facility, quality improvement (QI) studies are not considered research. However, such studies are important to the facility involved because they can demonstrate the contributions made by nurses to patient care and help the facility to improve processes, if necessary.

Evidence-informed decision making, research, and QI are closely interrelated. All three processes require nurses to use the best evidence to provide the highest quality of patient care. As a nurse, you should know the differences between these terms and know which process to select when you face clinical problems or when you wish to improve patient care. Although you will use all of these in nursing practice, it is important to know the similarities and differences among them (Table 8.1). When implementing evidence-informed decision making, it is important to first review evidence from appropriate research and QI data. This information can help you better understand the extent of a problem in practice and within your organization. QI data inform you about how processes work in an organization and thus offer information about how to make changes.

DEVELOPMENT OF NURSING KNOWLEDGE

Nursing knowledge must be expanded continuously to keep approaches to nursing care relevant and current; it is the foundation of the profession of nursing. Without new knowledge, nursing cannot improve therapies such as infant care, pain management, grief counselling, or patient education. The major source of new knowledge is research, which can provide a solid foundation for nursing practice. It is important to translate the best evidence into best practices at a patient's bedside. Nurses need a sound knowledge base to support practice, and research is essential for building that knowledge.

Professional nurses must stay informed about current evidence. This is not easy to do. Students may diligently read the assigned materials from texts and articles and assume they have the latest information. A good textbook incorporates evidence into the practice guidelines it describes. However, it takes about 2 years for a book to be written, published, and in print; therefore, the scientific literature used in the book can be outdated by the time the book is published. Articles, particularly scientific ones, are more likely to be current, but the findings may not be easily applied. They may be inconclusive, or the particular practice that would incorporate the research may not have been studied yet. Moreover, these articles are not readily available to staff nurses at the bedside. It is a distinct challenge to obtain the best, most current evidence when nurses need it for patient care.

The sources of information about evidence are well-designed, systematically conducted research studies, found in scientific journals, systematic reviews of research studies, and summaries of valid and clinically useful published studies in peer-reviewed journals (CNA, 2018). Nurses need to have the ability to locate, understand, and critically evaluate evidence for application to practice. When no evidence is available, tradition prevails.

Non-research evidence is another source of information to support practice. This includes quality improvement and risk management data; international, national, and local standards; infection control data; chart reviews; and clinical expertise. These sources can be valuable, but their value never approaches that of research evidence.

A third source of evidence that must be incorporated into good clinical decisions consists of individual patients and families, and their values, beliefs, and experience. No efficacious clinical decision can be made without consideration of the uniqueness of the patient. Figure 8.1 illustrates the process for evidence-informed decision making.

Steps to foster success in evidence-informed decision making are summarized in Box 8.1.

TABLE 8.1	Similarities and Differences Among Evidence-Informed Decision Making, Research, and Quality Improvement		
	Evidence-Informed Decision Making	**Research**	**Quality Improvement**
Purpose	Use of information from research, professional experts, personal experience, and patient preferences to determine safe and effective nursing care with the goal of improving patient care and outcomes	Systematic inquiry answers questions, solves problems, and contributes to the generalizable knowledge base of nursing; it may or may not improve patient care.	Improves local work processes to improve patient outcomes and efficiency of health systems; results usually not generalizable
Focus	Implementation of evidence already known into practice	Evidence is generated to find answers for questions that are not known about nursing practice.	Measures effects of practice and/or practice change on specific patient population
Data sources	Multiple research studies, expert opinion, personal experience, patients	Participants have predefined characteristics that include or exclude them from the study; the researcher collects and analyzes data from participants.	Data from patient records or patients who are in a specific area, such as on a patient care unit or admitted to a particular hospital
Who conducts the activity?	Practising nurses and possibly other members of the health care team	Researchers who may or may not be employed by the health care agency and usually are not a part of the clinical health care team conduct it.	Employees of a health care agency, such as nurses, physicians, pharmacists
Is activity part of regular clinical practice?	Yes	No	Yes
Is approval needed from an institutional research review ethics (REB) board?	Sometimes	Yes	Sometimes
Funding sources	Internal, from health care agency	Funding is usually external, such as a grant	Internal, from health care agency

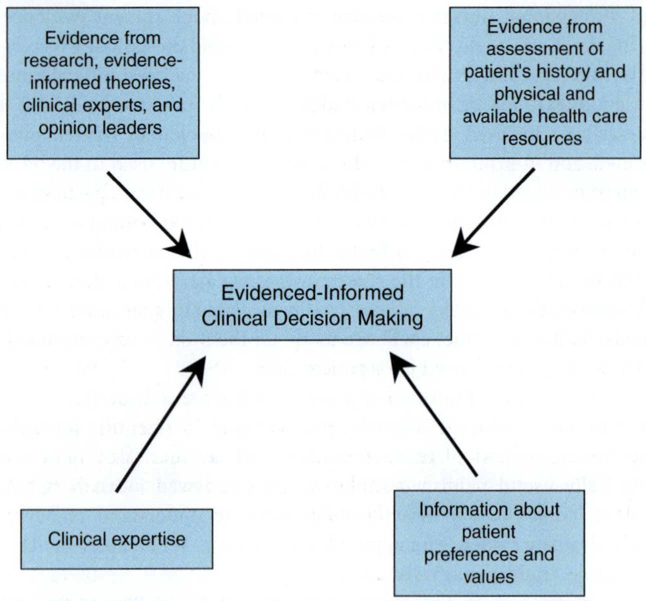

FIGURE 8.1 Processes involved in evidence-informed decision making.

RESEARCHING THE EVIDENCE

Ask the Clinical Question

Clinical questions arise out of your nursing practice and represent problems that you wonder about or things that do not make sense to you. For example, while caring for an unconscious patient, you might wonder, "What is the best cleaner to use when I provide mouth care to this patient?" Or you might notice, like Natalie did, that there has been an increase in patient falls on your unit, leading you to ask, "How can I reduce falls on my unit?"

Clinical questions that arise from your nursing practice should first be addressed by looking to see if the answer is readily available. Important sources of this type of information can be found in practice guidelines available from professional associations. All professions have focused on ensuring that service professionals understand practice guidelines. "Best practices" are guiding principles leading to the most appropriate courses of action in certain standard practice situations. They are based on the accumulated research findings, as well as on evidence from practice. An example is the Best Practice Guidelines developed by the Registered Nurses' Association of Ontario (RNAO). The RNAO has 50 published guidelines, as well as a toolkit and educator's resource to implement these guidelines into practice.

The questions you ask will eventually lead you to the evidence required for an answer. When you consult the empirical literature for an answer, you will want to read the most informative four to six articles that address your practice question specifically, not be mired in hundreds of articles that might have some relationship to your question. This means that your question must be well stated and focused on just the relevant components of the issue. Unfocused questions ("What is the best way to reduce wandering?" "What is the best way to measure blood pressure?") are too vague and will lead to many irrelevant sources of information. The Canadian Institutes of Health Research, in their learning module on evidence-informed decision making (Ciliska, 2020), have suggested using a PICO format to state your question. A PICO question has four components:

BOX 8.1 Steps for Successful Evidence-Informed Practice

1. Ask a question that clearly presents the clinical problem.
2. Search for and collect the most relevant best evidence.
3. Critically appraise the evidence.
4. Integrate all evidence with clinical expertise, patients' preferences, and patients' values to make a practice decision or change.
5. Evaluate the outcome of the practice decision or change and modify it if necessary.
6. Disseminate the outcomes of the decision or change.

Adapted from Melnyk, B. M., & Fineout-Overholt, E. (2019). Making the case for evidence-based practice and cultivating a spirit of inquiry. In B. M. Melnyk & E. Fineout-Overholt (Eds.), *Evidence-based practice in nursing and health care. A guide to best practice* (4th ed., p. 17). Wolters Kluwer.

P = Patient population of interest: What are the age, gender, ethnicity, and disease or health problem of the patients?
I = Intervention of interest: What is the best intervention or health services strategies you are considering?
C = Comparison of interest: What is the usual standard of care or current intervention used now in practice?
O = Outcome: What result (e.g., change in patient behaviour, physical finding) do you want to achieve as a result of the intervention?

For example, a fall-prevention team used PICO to guide their search for evidence-informed fall-prevention programs. The PICO question was "In adult hospitalized medical-surgical patients, does an evidence-based fall prevention program that includes comprehensive assessment and individualized interventions based on patient-specific risks decrease the fall rate?" (Spano-Szekely et al., 2020, p. 128). In this example P = adult hospitalized medical-surgical patients; I = evidence-based fall-prevention program that includes comprehensive assessment and individualized interventions based on patient-specific risks; C = usual care; and O = decrease in rate of falls.

When looking at context or experiences, these questions are best answered by qualitative research, so the PS question frame is used (Ciliska, 2020):

P = Population: Who are the people involved—individuals, families, or populations? Age? Specific problem or prevention issue?
S = Situation: What circumstances or experiences do you want to know about?

Do not be satisfied with clinical routines if they do not improve the patient's quality of life. Always ask questions and use critical thinking to consider better ways to provide patient care. The questions you raise by using a PICO or PS format help you identify knowledge gaps within a clinical situation and assist you in making sound clinical decisions for change.

Collect the Best Evidence

Once you have a clear and concise PICO or PS question, you are ready to search for evidence. You can find the evidence you need in a variety of sources: agency policy and procedure manuals, quality improvement data, existing clinical practice guidelines, or bibliographical databases. Always ask for help to find appropriate evidence. Nursing faculty are always a key resource, as are advanced practice nurses, staff educators, infection control nurses, and librarians.

When you go to the literature for evidence, a librarian can help you locate the appropriate databases. The databases contain published empirical studies, including peer-reviewed research. An article that has undergone peer review has been reviewed by a panel of experts before publication. The search process requires you to come up with keywords or phrases from your question that most accurately describe what you want from the search. The librarian can help you find the language that yields the most informative results. You usually need to adjust the wording of your search criteria until you get the results you want.

The best-known databases for nursing literature are MEDLINE and CINAHL. These are comprehensive databases containing articles from most nursing and health journals. These are usually available at no cost to students through the university or college library. As a guide to help you find the best available research evidence quickly and efficiently, the 6S search pyramid tool was developed (DiCenso et al., 2009). Table 8.2 is based on the 6S search pyramid and explains each of the categories outlined in the pyramid.

Research Literacy—Critique the Evidence

The most difficult step in the evidence-informed practice process is critiquing (appraising) or evaluating the available evidence (Jakubec & Astle, 2022). **Research literacy** is an essential competency for evidence-informed practice; it is the ability to locate, understand, and critically evaluate empirical literature for application in practice (Hines, 2016; Jakubec & Astle, 2022).

The critiquing of evidence involves determining its value, feasibility, and utility for changing practice. When you critique evidence, first evaluate the scientific merit and clinical applicability of each study's findings. Then, with a group of studies and expert opinion, determine what findings have a strong enough basis for use in practice. After critiquing the evidence, you will be able to answer the questions: Do the articles together offer evidence to explain or answer your question? Do the articles show that the evidence is true and reliable? Can you use the evidence in practice? Because you are a student and new to nursing, it will take time to acquire the skills to critique evidence like an expert. When you read an article from the literature, do not let the statistics or technical wording cause you to stop reading the article. Know the elements of an article and use a careful approach when you review each one. Evidence-informed articles include the following elements:

- *Abstract:* An abstract is a brief summary of the article that quickly tells you whether the article is research or clinically based. An abstract summarizes the purpose of the study or clinical query, the major themes or findings, and the implications for nursing practice.
- *Introduction:* The introduction contains information about the purpose of the article and the importance of the topic for the audience who reads the article. Brief supporting evidence is usually presented as to why the topic is important from the author's point of view. Together, the abstract and introduction tell you whether you want to read the entire article. You will know if the topic of the article is similar to your question or related closely enough to provide you with useful information. If it is, continue to read the next elements of the article.

- *Literature review or background:* A useful article has a detailed background of the existing level of science or clinical information about the topic of the article. Therefore, it offers an argument about what led the author to conduct a study or report on a clinical topic. This section of an article is valuable. Perhaps the article itself does not address your question in the way you desire, but it may lead you to other articles that are more useful. A literature review of a research article indicates how past research led to the researcher's question. For example, an article about a study designed to test an educational intervention for older-person family caregivers includes a review of the literature describing characteristics of caregivers, the type of factors influencing caregivers' ability to cope with stressors of caregiving, and any previous educational interventions used with families.
- *Article narrative:* Narratives of articles differ according to the type of evidence-informed article they are describing. For example, a clinical article describes a clinical topic and often includes a description of a patient population, the nature of a certain disease or health alteration, how patients are affected, and the appropriate nursing therapies. Some clinical articles explain how to use a therapy or new technology. A research article will contain several subsections within the narrative, including the following:
  - *Purpose statement:* A purpose statement explains the focus or intent of a study. It identifies what concepts were researched. This includes research questions or hypotheses—predictions made about the relationship or difference between study variables (concepts, characteristics, or traits that vary within or among participants). An example of a research question is as follows: "What characteristics are common among older persons who have annual breast screening?"
  - *Methods or design:* The methods or design section explains how a research study is organized and conducted in order to answer the research question or to test the hypothesis. This explanation includes the type of study to be conducted (e.g., randomized control trial, case–control study, or qualitative study) and how many participants or persons are in a study. In health care studies, "participants" may include patients, family members, or health care staff. The language in the methods section is sometimes confusing because it contains details about how the researcher designs the study to minimize bias and thereby obtain the most accurate results possible. Consult with your instructor or other researchers as a resource to help interpret this section.
  - *Results or conclusions:* Clinical and research articles have a summary section. A clinical article explains the clinical implications for the topic presented, whereas a research article details the results of the study and explains whether a hypothesis is supported or how a research question is answered. For a qualitative study, the article presents a thorough summary of the descriptive themes and ideas that arise from the researcher's analysis of data. A quantitative study will present data using statistical analysis. Read carefully and ask whether the researcher describes the results and whether the results were significant. Have a faculty member assist you in interpreting statistical results. A helpful results section also discusses any limitations to a study. This information on limitations is valuable in helping you decide whether you want to use the evidence with your patients.
- *Clinical implications:* A research article includes a section that explains whether the findings from the study have clinical implications. This section also explains how to apply findings in a practice setting for the type of participants studied.

TABLE 8.2	Sources of Research Evidence
Systems	Sophisticated electronic systems that link to patient records and prompt practitioners about guidelines for care
Summaries	Summaries of synthesized sources of research evidence for a given health issue
Synopses of syntheses	Summaries of the findings from systematic reviews
Syntheses	Synthesis of primary studies by using systematic review methods to answer a focused research question
Synopsis of single studies	A summary of the results and implications of single studies
Studies	Single research studies related to a particular focused question

Adapted from DiCenso, A., Bayley, L., & Haynes, R. B. (2009). Accessing pre-appraised evidence: Fine-tuning the 5S model into a 6S model. *Evidence-Based Nursing, 12*(4), 99–101.

After you have critiqued each article for your question, synthesize or combine the findings from all of the articles to determine the state of the evidence. Use critical thinking to consider the scientific rigour of the evidence and how well it answers your area of interest. Consider the evidence in view of your patients' concerns and preferences. Your review of articles offers a snapshot conclusion that is based on combined evidence about one focused topical area. As a clinician, judge whether to use the evidence for a particular patient or group of patients, who usually have complex medical histories and patterns of responses (Melnyk & Fineout-Overholt, 2019). It is ethically important to consider evidence that benefits patients and does no harm. Decide whether the evidence is relevant, is easily applicable in your setting of practice, and has the potential for improving patient outcomes.

INTEGRATE THE EVIDENCE

Once you decide that the evidence is strong and applicable to your patients and clinical situation, incorporate the recommended evidence into practice. Your first step is to simply apply the research in your plan of care for a patient. Use the evidence you find as a rationale for an intervention you plan to try. For instance, you learned about an approach for preventing falls and you decide to use this information during your next clinical assignment. You use the approach with your own assigned patients, or you work with a group of other students or nurses in revising a policy and procedure or in developing a new clinical protocol.

Evidence is useful in a variety of ways in formulating teaching tools, clinical practice guidelines, policies and procedures, and new assessment or documentation tools. Depending on the amount of change needed to apply evidence in practice, it becomes necessary to involve a number of staff from a given nursing unit. It is important to consider the setting in which you want to apply the evidence: Do all staff members support the change? Does the practice change fit with the scope of practice in the clinical setting? Are resources (time, administrative support, and staff) available to make a change? When evidence is not strong enough to apply in practice, your next option is to conduct a pilot study to investigate your question. A *pilot study* is a small-scale research study or a study that includes a quality or performance improvement project. As a nursing student, along with a nurse leader or nurse researcher, your study begins with searching for and applying the most useful evidence to improve the care you provide directly to your patients. The evidence available within nursing literature gives you almost unlimited access to innovative and effective nursing interventions. Using an evidence-informed practice approach helps you improve your skills and knowledge as a nurse and improve outcomes for your patients.

EVALUATE THE PRACTICE DESIGN OR CHANGE

After applying evidence in your practice, your next step is to evaluate its effect. How does the intervention work? How effective was the clinical decision for your patient or practice setting? Sometimes your evaluation is as simple as determining whether the expected outcomes you set for an intervention are met. For example, when you implement a falls-prevention program, do the number of falls decrease?

When an evidence-informed practice change occurs on a larger scale, an evaluation is more formal. For example, evidence of factors that contribute to pressure injuries might lead a nursing unit to adopt a new skin care protocol. To evaluate the protocol, the nurses track the incidence of pressure injuries over a course of time (e.g., 6 months to a year). In addition, the nurses collect data to describe both the patients who develop pressure injuries and those who do not. This comparative information is valuable for determining the effects of the protocol and whether modifications are necessary.

SUPPORT FOR EVIDENCE-INFORMED DECISION MAKING

Nursing practice is based on theory, professional values, and evidence. Nurses base decisions on these factors, as well on other influences such as individual values, ethics, legislation, patient choice, and practice environments. The CNA position statement on evidence-informed decision making specifies its importance in providing quality nursing care and in effecting change across the health care system. The evidence to be used in practice is derived through research and the scientific evaluation of practice. The CNA believes that individual nurses must read and critique evidence-informed literature in order to provide high-quality care to clients (CNA, 2018).

THE DEVELOPMENT OF RESEARCH IN NURSING

Research is the primary means by which new knowledge is discovered and brought into practice to improve the care that nurses provide to their patients. It is a systematic process in which questions that generate knowledge are asked and answered. This knowledge becomes part of the scientific basis for practice and may be used to validate interventions.

Nursing research is a systematic examination of phenomena important to the nursing discipline, as well as to nurses, their patients, and families. Its purpose is to expand the knowledge base for practice by answering nurses' questions. Nursing research addresses a range of issues related to actual and potential patient populations and to individual and family responses to health problems. Some research tests nursing theories; other research generates theory from findings. This "back-and-forth" relationship between theory and research is the way knowledge develops in any discipline (Polit & Beck, 2021). In the current health care environment, nursing research is frequently undertaken in interprofessional teams, in which nurses examine factors relevant to nursing in the context of the larger health care picture. The scientific knowledge needed for nursing practice is discovered, tested, and enhanced through nursing research. The interprofessional nature of nursing challenges nurses not only to keep up with nursing research but also to know the status of research in other health disciplines, as well as in the behavioural, social, and physical sciences.

Nursing research improves nursing practice, raising the profession's standards. Involvement in research takes many forms, including designing studies, being on a research team, collecting data, and using research findings to change clinical practice, improve patient outcomes, and contain health care costs. Promoting research and using it in practice increases the scientific knowledge base for nursing practice. Patients benefit from these improvements to practice, as is evident in the case study at the beginning of this chapter.

THE HISTORY OF NURSING RESEARCH IN CANADA

During the Crimean War, Florence Nightingale's detailed and systematic observation of nursing actions and outcomes resulted in major changes in nursing practice. Her work demonstrated the importance of systematic observational research to nursing practice.

In Canada, the establishment of university nursing courses starting in 1918, followed by master's degree programs in the 1950s and 1970s and by doctoral programs in the 1990s and 2000s, was crucial to the development of nursing research (see Chapter 3). The first master's degree program, established at the University of Western Ontario

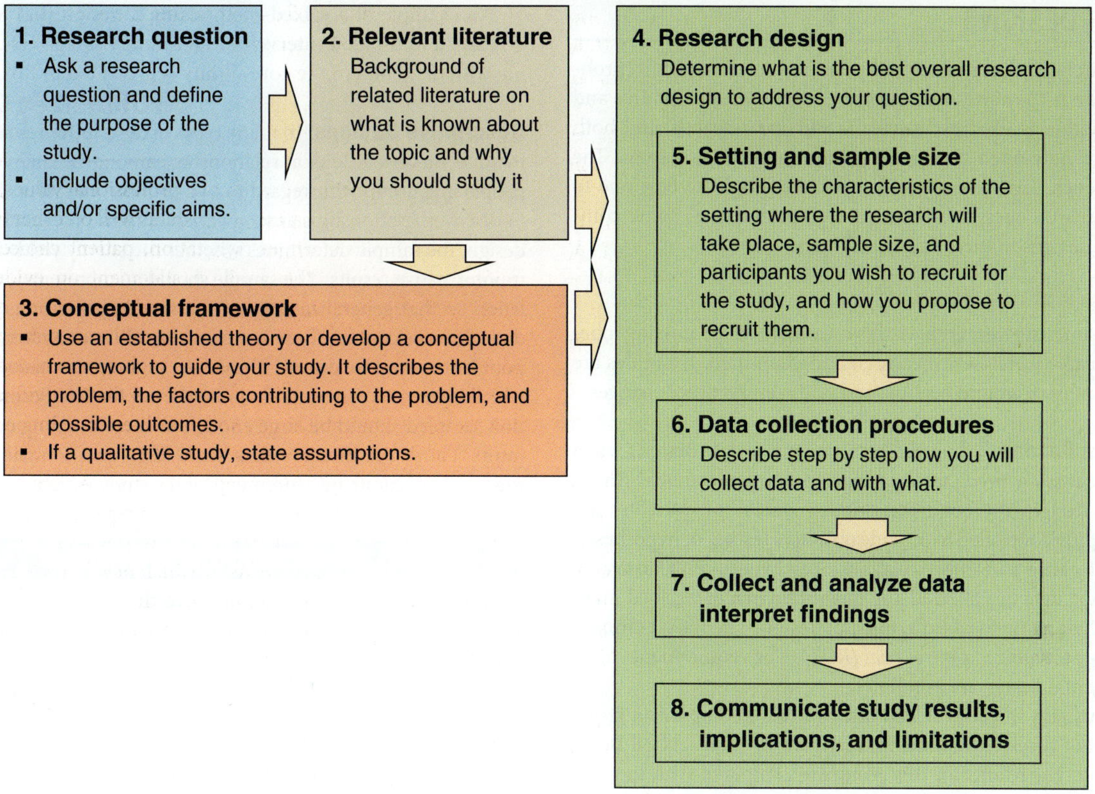

FIGURE 8.2 A visual representation of the research process.

(now Western University) in 1959, highlighted the need for Canadian research capacity in nursing.

The first nursing research journal, *Nursing Research,* was launched in the United States in 1952. The first nursing research journal published in Canada, *Nursing Papers* (later the *Canadian Journal of Nursing Research*), was established at McGill University in 1969. Other journals were later established, and today, nurses publish their research, both within nursing and in interprofessional fields, in hundreds of journals.

Since the 1970s and 1980s, the two major factors in the development of nursing research have been the establishment of research training through doctoral programs and the establishment of funding to support nursing research. Throughout the 1970s and 1980s, university faculties and schools of nursing built their research resources so that they could establish doctoral programs. The first provincially approved doctoral nursing program was established at the University of Alberta Faculty of Nursing in 1991. Another was established at the University of British Columbia School of Nursing later that year, and programs at McGill University and the University of Toronto followed in 1993. Currently there are many doctoral nursing programs in universities across Canada.

Growing awareness of the importance of nursing research gradually led to the availability of research funds. The year 1964 marked the first time that a federal granting agency funded nursing research in Canada (Good, 1969). In 1999, 14 years after the US government had established funding for nursing research under the National Institutes of Health, the Canadian government established the Nursing Research Fund, budgeting $25 million for nursing research ($2.5 million over each of the following 10 years). The research areas targeted for support included nursing policies, management, human resources, and nursing care. Although this funding is no longer available, nurse researchers have been successful at obtaining Tri-Council funding nationally and international funding to support their programs of research.

Tri-Council is a term referring to three federal research agencies: Canadian Institutes of Health Research, National Science and Engineering Research Council of Canada, and the Social Sciences and Humanities Research Council.

NURSING RESEARCH

There are several types of research that can inform nursing evidence-informed decision making. The type of research that is conducted depends on the research question or purpose. The process of nursing research involves seven to eight steps, starting with the research question. This **research process** is outlined in Figure 8.2.

If properly stated, the research question guides the rest of the process; thus, asking the question is a crucial step. Once an initial question has been formulated, the literature is searched to discover what is already known about the topic and to determine whether the question must be revised, in light of prior knowledge.

The research design provides the ground rules for data collection and analysis, ensuring that the research question will have a valid answer. The design steps are systematic and precise in order to control unwanted influences that might affect the answer. For example, in a study of the relationship between diet and heart disease, influences such as stress or smoking must be controlled because they are known to influence heart disease. The design also specifies the type of sample and sample selection techniques that will provide the most useful data for the study.

Data are gathered from the sample through measurement techniques that quantify the variables in the research question. Techniques include interviews, tests of knowledge, and physiological measures such as heart rate and blood pressure. When the evidence is analyzed, the result answers the original question and becomes the basis for discovering new knowledge.

RESEARCH DESIGNS

Nursing research approaches vary, depending on the specific problem to be studied. They are sometimes categorized as quantitative and qualitative. Neither is used exclusively in nursing research, and both approaches are now often combined (mixed-methods research). The research approach used is the one that is considered the best one to answer the research question. The next section describes some common research designs in these three categories.

Quantitative Nursing Research

Quantitative nursing research is the investigation of nursing phenomena that can be precisely measured and quantified. Examples are pain severity, rates of wound healing, and body temperature changes.

Experimental Research.
Experiments are appropriate designs when one variable causes a predictable change in another variable. In an experimental design, the conditions under which the variables are studied are tightly controlled to provide objective testing of hypotheses, which predict cause-and-effect relationships. Experimental research requires that the data be collected and quantified in a prescribed manner. There are many types of experimental design. The most common one is called a *randomized control trial (RCT)*. The requirements of an RCT experimental design are as follows:

- The study usually includes at least one control or comparison group that does not receive the nursing treatment or intervention being investigated. The results for this group are compared with those of the experimental group, which is the group that receives the treatment or intervention. The participants—people selected for the comparison and experimental groups—are randomly assigned to these groups, so that the groups are as similar as possible to each other before the intervention. Random assignment of participants ensures that all participants have the same chance to be in the control or experimental (treatment) group and that variables that could affect the outcome of the study are randomly distributed between the groups and therefore are no more likely to affect experimental participants than to affect control participants.
- An experimental variable must be manipulated by the researcher. For example, in a study of the effect of preoperative teaching on postoperative anxiety, the researcher manipulates preoperative teaching by providing it for the experimental group but not for the control group. The expectation is that the differences in postoperative anxiety measures between the two groups can be attributed to the effect of preoperative teaching because all other factors are under control. However, the researcher cannot control participants' prior experiences, such as hearing other patients' stories about surgery. Psychological factors, which cannot be controlled, may influence a participant's level of anxiety. If participants are randomly assigned to the two groups, however, those with negative prior experiences should be distributed equally between the two groups, and these experiences would affect both groups equally. Thus, differences between the groups in postoperative anxiety can still be attributed to the preoperative teaching intervention.
- The researcher proposes theory-based and statistically tested hypotheses about the action of the variables to answer the research question. For example, in a study of preoperative teaching, the hypothesis might be as follows: "Patients who receive interactive preoperative teaching will have significantly lower postoperative anxiety levels than will patients who receive other teaching methods." The researcher must explain why a lower anxiety level is expected, in a discussion of the theory behind the study.

An example of a mixed-methods RCT design that was utilized to evaluate a web-based intervention for family caregivers of persons living with dementia in the community is presented in Box 8.2.

Descriptive Designs.
In many types of descriptive research, investigators use surveys to look at relationships among variables or to compare people in a group with regard to two or more variables. The purpose is to discover relationships among variables in the population. In a survey design, the sample determines whether the survey yields informative or uninformative results. The sample should be representative of the population so that generalizations can be made on the basis of the sample data. Surveys contain three key elements. First, a random sample of the population must be drawn, if possible, or a representative sample, from which inferences can be made about the population. Second, the population sampled should be large enough to keep sampling error to a minimum. Third, the measurement tools (e.g., questionnaires, interviews) must yield accurate measurements of the study variables.

BOX 8.2   RESEARCH HIGHLIGHT
Evaluation of My Tools 4 Care

Research Focus
Duggleby et al. (2018) used a mixed-methods experimental design to evaluate My Tools 4 Care (MT4C) by collecting quantitative and qualitative data. MT4C is a web-based intervention intended to support carers of community-living persons with Alzheimer's disease and related dementia (ADRD) and multiple chronic conditions (MCC).

Research Abstract
Carers of persons living with ADRD have been found to have poor mental and physical health. The objective of the study was to evaluate the effectiveness of MT4C with respect to increasing hope, self-efficacy, and health-related quality of life (HRQOL) in carers of community-living older persons with ADRD and MCC.

Methods
A total of 199 participants were randomized into either treatment (MT4C) or educational control groups. Those in the treatment group were able to use MT4C for 3 months. At baseline and 1, 3, and 6 months, data were collected on hope (Herth Hope Index [HHI]), self-efficacy (General Self-Efficacy Scale), and HRQOL (Short Form–12 item [version 2] health survey; SF-12v2). Generalized estimating equations were used to identify group differences over time. Qualitative data were analyzed using a descriptive thematic approach and informed the quantitative results.

Results
The carers using MT4C had significantly higher hope scores (HHI-factor 2 [P = .01]) than in the control group. Although there were no significant changes in quality of life, as the participants' hope increased, so did their quality of life. These results were supported by the qualitative data.

Implications for Practice
MT4C increases hope, and as such has a positive influence on the lives of carers. Nurses can share the link for MT4C with family carers as a way to support them. Because hope is an important factor in improving the quality of care for carers, it is important that nurses assess hope and utilize strategies to engender hope.

From Duggleby, W., Ploeg, J., McAiney, C., et al. (2018). Web-based intervention for family carers of persons with dementia and multiple chronic conditions (My Tools 4 Care): Pragmatic randomized control trial. *Journal of Medical Internet Research, 20*(6), e10484. https://doi.org/10.2196/10484

Exploratory Descriptive Designs. Exploratory descriptive designs provide in-depth descriptions of populations or variables not previously studied. Typically, these questions begin with "what"; for example, "What are the health-promoting behaviours of older persons living in subsidized housing?" The results provide a detailed description of the variable or population. No relationships among variables are posited at this stage, although the results might indicate that relationships should be examined in subsequent research.

Data Analysis. All quantitative studies entail the use of statistical analysis. The type of analysis should address the research question. For example, if the research question is asking whether there is a difference between an intervention or control group, then the analysis should be chosen to determine that. The choice of which analysis to use is also based on the type of data that is collected. For example, some statistical tests require that data be normally distributed.

Qualitative Nursing Research

Qualitative nursing research poses questions about nursing phenomena that cannot be quantified and measured. To answer questions about these phenomena, researchers must understand the perspective of the person in the situation. Researchers using qualitative methods can choose one of many design strategies. The research question is the basis for the choice of design. Examples of qualitative designs that may be used in nursing research include ethnography, phenomenology, grounded theory, participatory action research, interpretive descriptive research, and narrative inquiry. In addition, each of the various qualitative methods has its own unique underlying philosophy as well as data collection and analysis approaches. For example, Box 8.3 provides an example of a nursing study using an Indigenous qualitative approach.

Transferability is an important concept to understand when using qualitative research findings in practice. It refers to the extent to which the findings of a qualitative study are thought to be meaningful and applicable to similar cases or other situations (Meadows-Oliver, 2019, p. 210). You can assess transferability by asking the following questions:
1. Do the findings make sense with your own observations?
2. Were the study participants similar to those you care for?

Do the findings provide insights or make you think differently regarding your own experience? Although there is not a hierarchy of evidence for qualitative research, there are systematic reviews and metasyntheses (combining of findings from several qualitative studies) that would help you determine if you wish to use the knowledge from qualitative studies in practice.

Conducting Nursing Research

Clinical nursing research should be undertaken by nurses educated to conduct scientific investigations. An experienced researcher is usually more qualified than a beginner to undertake a complex, long-term project. Nurses new to research may, however, assist with data collection, conduct replication studies (studies previously performed elsewhere), or conduct less complex studies. They may also be involved in knowledge synthesis of published research.

RESEARCH SYNTHESIS

There are some research questions that are best answered by combining and synthesizing the results from multiple research studies that have already been conducted. This is often referred to as research synthesis or *knowledge synthesis*. Because it includes systematic strategies to review, appraise, and synthesize findings from the literature on a specific topic, the approaches are called *systematic reviews*. This is a

BOX 8.3 RESEARCH HIGHLIGHT

Living Stories Through a Sweetgrass Porcupine Quill Box Methodology: An Innovation in Chronic Kidney Disease

Research Focus

Smith et al. (2019) used a qualitative design and an Indigenous approach to study the stories of chronic kidney disease as told by Indigenous people living in a remote Canadian community.

Research Abstract

The purpose of this research was 1) to engage with a distinctive Indigenous methodology and 2) to gather the living stories regarding community health experiences pertaining to chronic kidney disease.

Methods

The Indigenous methodology was artistically inspired by the community, expressed through the art and crafting of a sweetgrass and porcupine quill box. (A sweetgrass and porcupine birch box is a circular container; the walls and bottoms of this container are made of birch bark, bound together through a weaving of sweetgrass that holds the walls to the bottom. The lid is made of different colours of porcupine quills surrounded by intertwined sweetgrass.) The methods respected traditional community protocols and included three sharing circles involving elders and storytelling with 10 people who had chronic kidney disease, knew someone in the community who was receiving dialysis, or had a relative on dialysis. Contextually, they lived in a remote community where access to hemodialysis necessitated lengthy travel to satellite clinics located within hospital environments outside the community.

Results

The living stories illuminated relationality and cultural Indigenous knowledge as a strength amid fears and feelings of mistrust. Additionally, inequitable access and racialized health care emerged as root factors leading to decreased participation in health care. The participants' shared dreams revealed wisdom and interpretations that created living stories where dreams are enmeshed in all daily moments to guide and direct life.

Implications for Practice

Indigenous qualitative methodologies have great potential to improve and identify ways to strengthen health care and education. For people living in remote communities who lack access to necessary health care services to sustain life, such as dialysis, supporting relational ways of knowing and being are a foundational support to well-being.

From Smith, M., McDonald, C., Bruce, A., et al. (2019). Living stories through a sweet grass porcupine quill box methodology: An innovation in chronic kidney disease. *International Journal of Indigenous Health*, *14*(2), 276–292. https://doi.org/10.32799/ijih.v14i2.31059

form of research in its own right; it could also be considered "research of research." All approaches to research synthesis include asking a research question or forming an objective, systematically searching for literature, screening the literature, reading the literature, appraising the literature for quality, analyzing (looking closely at the certain components), and synthesizing (combining components) the results. The literature can include peer-reviewed published texts, or "grey-literature" texts such as reports, websites, policy documents, newsletters, and so on. Because it incorporates multiple studies to answer a research question, it may be used to inform nursing policy, decision making, evidence-informed practice, or knowledge translation (Cooper et al., 2019; Schick-Makaroff et al., 2016).

When systematically synthesizing the literature, a number of approaches are available. A few examples are outlined in Table 8.3.

TABLE 8.3	Examples of Research Syntheses	
Type of Research Synthesis	**Purpose**	**Data Included**
Integrative review	To review, critique, and synthesize literature of a topic to show its depth and breadth (Dhollande et al., 2021)	Diverse data are included, such as experimental and nonexperimental research, qualitative research, or theoretical literature.
Scoping review	To "map" the literature in order to investigate the extent, range, and nature of the research on a topic (Munn et al., 2018)	All types of data may be included, such as qualitative, quantitative, theoretical literature, conceptual literature, or grey literature.
Concept analysis	To clarify, refine, or define the meaning of a concept (Delves-Yates et al., 2018)	All types of data may be included, such as qualitative, quantitative, or theoretical literature.
Qualitative meta-synthesis	Systematic review and synthesis of qualitative research findings using qualitative approaches to develop new knowledge (Finfgeld-Connett, 2018)	Qualitative research findings
Meta-analysis	To integrate the results from primary studies in order to increase the power to detect the effect of interventions (Deeks et al., 2021)	Quantitative research studies and findings, primarily randomized control trials
Mixed-method synthesis	To review and synthesize knowledge from empirical qualitative, quantitative, and mixed-methods studies that address the same areas of research (Howell Smith & Bazis, 2020)	Data from quantitative, qualitative, and mixed-method studies

Choosing which approach to use may be based on your research question or objective, or what type of literature is already available. Systematic reviews are reported in a consistent manner (for examples, see Equator Network, 2021). Research syntheses are often conducted with a team of people and may include researchers, clinicians, a librarian, students, or patient partners. The overarching goal is to generate new knowledge through the process of synthesizing findings across diverse research studies on a similar topic. An example of research synthesis follows.

A nurse had been reading about the importance of using patient- and family-reported outcomes and experience measures when an older person was experiencing transitions from home to hospital. The nurse wondered if these measures had been used and what motivated other nurses to use them. In a search of the literature, the nurse found a narrative synthesis of the empirical literature on this topic (Schick-Makaroff et al., 2020). This synthesis reported that patient- and family-reported outcomes and experience measures were rarely used to inform continuity across transitions of care, but they were used when health care providers wanted to restore the older person's independence and to evaluate health care provided.

ETHICAL ISSUES IN RESEARCH

Research must meet ethical standards in ways that respect the dignity and preserve the well-being of human research participants. In Canada, every health care facility and university receiving public funds for research must meet federal standards for protecting human research participants. The most recent standard is the *Tri-Council Policy Statement* (Canadian Institutes of Health Research et al., 2018), which requires that the institution have in place a research ethics board (REB) to review all research proposals to determine whether ethical principles are being upheld (Box 8.4). The REB focuses on **informed consent** and weighs benefits versus harms from the research. No research may be performed in a university or health care facility without the approval of the REB. All proposals are subject to review. However, if data collection processes (such as quality assurance studies) are a normal part of institutional business, performance reviews, or testing within normal educational requirements and are not for research purposes, they are exempt from REB review.

To refine existing knowledge and develop new knowledge, investigators in clinical research sometimes use new procedures whose

BOX 8.4	Guiding Ethical Principles for Research in Canada

1. *Respect for persons*: All research must be conducted in a manner that values and respects human beings. This includes the obligation to respect autonomy of human research participants and at the same time to protect those with developing, impaired, or diminished autonomy.
2. *Concern for welfare*: Researchers and ethics review boards should aim to protect the welfare of participants and, when possible, promote their welfare. The welfare of a person is the quality of a person's experience in all aspects of their life.
3. *Justice*: This principle reflects the importance of treating people fairly and equitably. This treatment includes ensuring that research participants are not unduly burdened by research or denied access to the benefits of research.

Adapted from Canadian Institutes of Health Research, the Natural Sciences and Engineering Research Council of Canada, & the Social Sciences and Humanities Research Council of Canada. (2018). *Tri-Council policy statement: Ethical conduct for research involving humans (TCPS 2)*. https://ethics.gc.ca/eng/policy-politique_tcps2-eptc2_2018.html

outcome is doubtful or unknown. This research may seem to conflict with the purpose of nursing practice, which is to meet specific patients' needs. In such cases, the investigator must structure the research to avoid or minimize harm to the participants. Although not all undesirable effects can be anticipated, investigators are obligated to inform everyone involved about the known potential risks. Other basic human rights must also be observed. These principles are set forth by the CNA (2017). Procedures for obtaining informed consent must be outlined in the study protocol. The consent form must describe in lay language the purpose of the study, the role of the participants, types of data that are to be obtained, how the data are obtained, the duration of the study, participant selection, procedures, risks to the participant (including financial risks), potential benefits (including the possibility of no benefit), alternatives to participation, and contact information concerning the principal investigator and local REB. The consent process gives participants complete information regarding the study's risks, benefits, and costs so that they can make an informed decision.

The REB also determines whether the investigator has the necessary knowledge and skills to undertake the research, including familiarity with the clinical area in which the data will be collected and sufficient research training and experience. For example, a nurse planning a study of psychiatric patients should be familiar with psychiatric nursing principles and theory, as well as research procedures for data collection and analysis.

Rights of Other Research Participants

Student nurses and practising nurses may be asked to participate in research as data collectors or may be involved in the care of patients participating in a study. All participants, including health care providers, have the right to be fully informed about the study, its procedures (including the consent process and risk factors), and physical or emotional injuries that patients could experience as a result of participation. Often, the physical risks are more obvious than the emotional risks. For example, patients may be asked to give highly personal, intrusive information; some may find this experience stressful. The researcher should prepare all participants, including nurses delivering care, for this possibility and assist them in coping with the effects. Participants also have the right to see review forms from the REB that certify approval of the study. Participants can refuse to perform research procedures if they are concerned about ethical aspects.

APPLYING RESEARCH FINDINGS IN NURSING PRACTICE

Research evidence as a basis for scholarly, professional decision making in clinical practice is essential for providing competent, efficient, and state-of-the art nursing care (Rodgers et al., 2019). As a nurse, you can make links between research findings and nursing care by identifying appropriate clinical problems, reading peer-reviewed literature from numerous sources, and incorporating evidence-informed practice activities into the nursing practice of your nursing unit or agency.

In a policy statement, the CNA (2018) stated that evidence-informed decision making by registered nurses is key to quality nursing practice. Nurses need not only skills to access and appraise existing research but also scientific knowledge and skills to change practice settings and to promote evidence-informed decisions about patient care.

Evidence-informed nursing practice de-emphasizes ritual, isolated, and unsystematic clinical experiences; ungrounded opinion; and tradition as bases for nursing practice. It stresses the use of research findings and, as appropriate, quality improvement data, other evaluation data, and the consensus of recognized experts and affirmed experience to support a specific practice (Melnyk & Fineout-Overholt, 2019, p. 17). Many aspects of health care are not justly served by the research in only one discipline. The expertise of several disciplines must be brought to bear on complex health issues. Just as nurses play a vital role on the health care team, so, too, are they crucial to interprofessional health research. Policymakers in the broader arena of health care must account for nursing practice, which is so essential to patient care. Nurses need a sound knowledge base to support practice, and research is essential for building that knowledge.

KEY CONCEPTS

- Evidence-informed decision making includes knowledge from research, clinical expertise and patient preferences, and values.
- Development of nursing knowledge is essential to the profession of nursing.
- Research literacy is an essential competency for evidence-informed practice.

- Conducting research studies is critical to the development of evidence.
- How a study is conducted (study design) is dependent on the research question being asked.
- When human participants participate in research, the researcher must obtain informed consent of study participants, must maintain the confidentiality of participants, and must protect participants from undue risk or injury.
- When summarizing data reported in a research study, the nurse should note when, how, where, and by whom the investigation was conducted and who and what were studied.
- A researchable clinical nursing problem is one that is not satisfactorily resolved by current nursing interventions, occurs frequently in a particular group, can be measured or observed, and has a possible solution within the realm of nursing practice.
- To determine whether research findings can be used in nursing practice, the nurse considers the scientific worth of the study by substantiating evidence from other studies, the similarity of the research setting to the nurse's own clinical practice setting, the status of current nursing theory, and factors affecting the feasibility of application.

CRITICAL THINKING EXERCISES

1. A nurse is concerned about learning how to properly insert an intravenous catheter. What are the benefits to the patient if the nurse learns how to do this by drawing from information in the research literature rather than from current practice?
2. The research literature reflects many different methods for inserting intravenous catheters. If you wished to determine the best method for doing this, use PICO to clarify the search questions. What would be your PICO question for this clinical issue?
3. If you wanted to design a study to answer a specific research question about the best way to insert intravenous catheters, how would you do this? What steps would you take?

Answers to Critical Thinking Exercises appear on the Evolve website.

REVIEW QUESTIONS

Review Questions 1 to 8 relate to the case study at the beginning of the chapter.

1. Why was Natalie using evidence-informed decision making to improve her practice and the practice of others in preventing falls? Because it:
   a. Is based on current nursing practice
   b. Has been found to improve patient care
   c. Includes information from the Internet
   d. Includes information only from randomized control trials
2. Because Natalie was looking for interventions to prevent falls, she would frame her literature search question using:
   a. PS
   b. MRTT
   c. PICO
   d. RCT
3. It is important that Natalie critically appraise or evaluate any of the literature she finds for quality. This ability is referred to as:
   a. Research literacy
   b. Research design
   c. Research exploration
   d. Research synthesis

4. If Natalie was unable to find the answer to her practice question in the literature, she should consider:
   a. Implementing a quality improvement project on her unit
   b. Working with a researcher to conduct research to answer her practice question
   c. Not addressing the issue of falls prevention
   d. Use literature from falls-prevention programs in long-term care

5. Natalie wanted to learn about the lived experiences and perspectives of older persons who have experienced multiple falls. What type of research would she conduct?
   a. Experimental research
   b. Descriptive design
   c. Qualitative research
   d. Research synthesis

6. Why is evidence-informed decision making important to Natalie?
   a. It enables the transfer of clinical practice techniques into policy.
   b. It requires that evidence be always research based.
   c. It is synonymous with research-based practice.
   d. It entails the use of knowledge based on research studies and takes into account a nurse's clinical experience and patient preferences.

7. Since Natalie was looking for fall-prevention programs that have been evaluated, she could consider a knowledge synthesis project, with the assistance of a nurse researcher. Which type of knowledge synthesis project may be most applicable in addressing her PICO question regarding the effectiveness of falls-preventions programs in acute care?
   a. Scoping review
   b. Meta-synthesis
   c. Meta-analysis
   d. Integrative review

8. Natalie has found a qualitative article that has recommendations for how to implement a falls-preventions program. She would like to determine whether she can use these findings in her own practice. Which question will help her determine this?
   a. What is the generalizability of the study findings?
   b. What is the transferability of the findings?
   c. How much bias has been introduced into the study?
   d. What is the validity of the study findings?

Answers: 1. b; **2.** c; **3.** a; **4.** b; **5.** c; **6.** d; **7.** c; **8.** b.

Rationales for the Review Questions appear on the Evolve website.

RECOMMENDED WEBSITESRECOMMENDED WEBSITES

Canadian Institutes of Health Research (CHIR): https://www.cihr-irsc.gc.ca/e/193.html
This website contains information on evidence-informed decision making, evidence-informed practice, and using research in practice (knowledge translation). It also contains pages for all 13 CIHR institutes.

Canadian Nurses Association: https://www.cna-aiic.ca
This website contains information about policies and position statements for nursing research in Canada, as well as information about research funding.

Canadian Nurses Foundation: https://www.cnf-fiic.ca
This website provides information about available research funding and about scholarships for students.

National Collaborating Center for Methods & Tools: https://www.nccmt.ca
This Canadian website provides information on evidence-informed decision making as well as methods and tools.

REFERENCES

A full reference list is available on the website for this book at http://evolve.elsevier.com/Canada/Potter/fundamentals/

9

Nursing Values and Ethics

Written by Shelley Raffin Bouchal, RN, PhD, and Barbara J. Astle, RN, PhD, FCAN

OBJECTIVES

Mastery of content in this chapter will enable you to:

- Define the key terms listed.
- Explain the role of values in the study of ethics.
- Examine and clarify personal values.
- Describe how values influence patient care.
- Explain the relationship between ethics and professional nursing practice.
- Describe some basic ethical philosophies relevant to health care.
- Apply a method of ethical analysis to a clinical situation.
- Identify contemporary ethical issues in nursing practice.

KEY TERMS

Accountability

Advance care planning

Advocacy

Answerability

Applied ethics

Autonomy

Beneficence

Bioethics

Biomedical ethics

Code of ethics

Consequentialism

Constrained moral agency

Cultural values

Deontology

Descriptive moral theory

Embodiment

Engagement

Environment

Ethical dilemma

Ethics

Futile care

Informed consent

Justice

Medical assistance in dying

Metaethics

Moral distress

Moral integrity

Moral residue

Mutuality

Nonmaleficence

Normative ethics

Relational ethics

Responsibility

Social justice

Teleology

Utilitarianism

Value

Values clarification

WEBSITE

http://evolve.elsevier.com/Canada/Potter/fundamentals/

CASE STUDY

On your unit, a 35-year-old person has been hospitalized in the final stages of brain cancer. Meghan (preferred pronouns: she/her) is a single parent of two young children. Although Meghan has been treated using both conventional and experimental treatments, the tumour has continued to grow, and the medical team has agreed that further treatment would be futile. You have cared for this patient during past hospital admissions, and during an especially open discussion, Meghan had expressed her wish to explore "do not resuscitate" (DNR) orders. During the current admission, Meghan's primary physician is out of town. The attending physician does not know the patient personally, but they have spent time with Meghan. They have reviewed the clinical data and agree that the patient is entering the terminal stage of the disease. In the physician's opinion, however, the patient is not ready to discuss end-of-life issues. The physician states that the patient has declined to discuss DNR orders. You ask the physician to convene a family conference about the issues. The physician refuses, stating that they believe the patient is not ready to participate.

Think about this case study as you read this chapter. There are review questions at the end of the chapter about this case study.

Values and ethics are inherent in all nursing acts. A value is a strong personal belief and an ideal that a person or group (such as nurses) believes to have merit. Ethics is the study of the philosophical ideals of right and wrong behaviour based on what one thinks one ought (or ought not) to do. The term also commonly refers to the values and standards that individuals and professions strive to uphold (e.g., health care ethics, nursing ethics). In other words, ethics reflects what matters most to people or professions. Nurses and other health care providers agree to national codes of ethics that offer guidelines for responding to difficult situations that occur in practice and that give the public an overview of professional practice standards. For example, the Canadian Nurses Association (Canadian Nurses Association [CNA], 2017a) publishes a code of ethics that outlines nurses' professional values and ethical commitments to their patients and the communities they serve. Revisions to the code of ethics normally occur every 5 to 7 years.

Because of their prominent and intimate role in the provision of health care, nurses continually make decisions about the correct course of action in different circumstances. In many situations, no answer or course of action is best. To manage such difficult situations, nurses need a keen awareness of their values and those of their patients, a good understanding of ethics, and a sound approach to ethical decision making. They also must be guided by a broader understanding of ethics through the application of philosophies, theories, and sets of principles. In addition, students should refer to the *National Nursing Education Framework* nursing ethics competencies—cited in the nursing practice (3.1) and professionalism (5.1) domains—to create and maintain a growth and development competency portfolio (Canadian Association of Schools of Nursing, 2022).

VALUES

Values are at the heart of ethics. Values influence behaviour through one's conviction that a certain action is correct in a certain situation. An individual's values reflect cultural and social influences, relationships, and personal needs. Values vary among people, and they develop and change over time. Nurses who seek to understand and respect the important values of others strengthen their role as moral agents and enrich their relationships with others.

In nursing, value statements express broad ideals of nursing care and establish reasonable directions for practice. The CNA (2017a, pp. 8–17) *Code of Ethics for Registered Nurses* is organized around seven values that are central to ethical nursing practice. These values include providing safe, compassionate, competent, and ethical care; promoting health and well-being; promoting and respecting informed decision making; preserving dignity; maintaining privacy and confidentiality; promoting justice; and being accountable. Each provincial nursing association also has shared values, such as those held in position statements and practice standards. These standards reflect the values of the profession and clarify what is expected of you as a practising nurse.

Because of the intimacy of the nurse–patient relationship, you must be aware of your personal values, as well as the values of patients, physicians, employers, or other groups. To understand the values of others, it is important to understand your own values—what they are, where they came from, and how they relate to others' values.

Values Formation

People acquire values in many ways through their upbringing and acculturation. Throughout childhood and adolescence, people learn to distinguish right from wrong and to form values on which to base their actions. This is known as *moral development* (see Chapter 23). Family experiences strongly influence value formation.

Values are also learned outside the family. A person's culture, ethnic background, and religious community strongly influence that person's values, as do schools, peer groups, social media, and work environments. Cultural values are those adopted through immersion in a certain social setting. A basic task of the young adult is to identify personal values within the context of the community. Over time, the person acquires values by choosing some values that are strongly upheld in the community and by discarding or transforming others. A person's experience as well as lack of experience also influences their values.

Values Clarification

Within the context of nursing, several layers of values inform the ethical questions and actions that you as a nurse will consider in your practice. Clarifying your values helps you articulate what matters most and what priorities are guiding your life and decision making. Values influence how you interpret confusing or conflicting information. Values change as you mature and experience new situations. As you become more aware and reflective about who you are, you may consider embracing or modifying your value set. As a result, you may modify your attitudes and behaviour. The willingness to change reflects a healthy attitude and an ability to adapt to new experiences.

To adopt new values, you must be aware of your existing values and how they affect behaviour. Values clarification is the process of appraising personal values (Box 9.1). It is not a set of rules, nor does it suggest that certain values should be accepted by all people; rather, it is a process of personal reflection. When you clarify your values, you make conscious decisions about which values are most important in your practice, and this in turn shapes your professional identity in accordance with the related ethical values of the profession.

By understanding your personal values, you will become more sensitive to the values of others. A *values conflict* occurs when personal values are not congruent with those of a patient, a colleague, or an institution. Values clarification plays a major role in recognizing and identifying ethical issues when they arise. In addition, you can better advocate for a patient when you are able to identify your personal values and the values of the patient.

Relational communication can encourage the patient to examine their personal thoughts and actions. When you make a clarifying response, it should be brief and nonjudgemental. For example, when talking with a patient who exercises only rarely, you might ask, "What is your understanding of the purpose of exercise?" A supportive clarifying response encourages the patient to think about personal values after the exchange is over and does not impose your own values onto the patient. In this way, you respect the patient's values and avoid inappropriately introducing personal values into the conversation.

ETHICS

Ethics is the study of good conduct, character, and motives. It is concerned with determining what is good or valuable for all people. Often the terms *morals* (or *morality*) and *ethics* are used interchangeably (Yeo et al., 2020). Morality is concerned with norms, principles, or what "ought to be," while ethics is focused on reflective analysis about those norms or principles and putting them into action (Yeo et al., 2020). Ethics requires one to be critically reflective, to explore one's moral norms and ideals as they relate to practice decisions (Yeo et al., 2020). In this chapter, the terms *ethics* and *morals* are used interchangeably.

BOX 9.1 | Values Clarification Questions

Describe a situation in your personal or professional experience in which you felt uncomfortable, in which you believed that your beliefs and values were being challenged, or in which you believed your values were different from others'.

- As you record the situation, mention how you felt physically and emotionally at the time you experienced the situation.
- Write down your feelings as you remember the situation. Are your current reactions any different from those when you were actually in the situation?
- What personal values do you identify in the situation? Whose values?
- Who are the significant people involved? How do they interpret the issue?
- What values do you think were being expressed by others involved? Are they similar to or different from your own values?
- What are the main arguments on the different sides of the issue?
- What are the relationships of power involved and the roles they play?
- Are people free to express their views, and do they feel free?
- How do you feel about your response to the situation? If you could repeat the scenario, would you change something about it? Rewrite the scenario with the same changes. What might be the consequences of these same changes?

Adapted from Yeo, M., Moorehouse, A., Khan, P., & Rodney, P. (2020). *Concepts and cases in nursing ethics* (4th ed.). Broadview Press.

Nursing and Ethics

Codes of Ethics. The CNA *Code of Ethics* is a statement of the ethical values of nurses and of nurses' commitments to persons with health care needs and persons receiving care (CNA, 2017a, p. 2). It is intended to guide nurses in all contexts and domains of nursing practice (clinical practice, education, administration, research, and policy; CNA, 2015) and at all levels of decision making (CNA, 2017a, p. 2). In Canada, nursing is a self-regulating profession. As part of being self-regulatory, nurses are bound to a code of ethics to serve and protect the public. The code developed by nurses for nurses serves the profession with practical orientation supported by theoretical diversity (CNA, 2017a).

As stated in the *Code of Ethics*, "the code provides guidance for ethical relationships, responsibilities, behaviours and decision-making and it is to be used in conjunction with professional standards, best practice, research, laws, and regulations that guide practice" (CNA, 2017a, p. 2). The code offers nurses guidance when they are working through ethical challenges that emerge from practice as they care for persons and work with interprofessional colleagues in health care.

The CNA (2017a) and the International Council of Nurses (2021) have established widely accepted codes for nurses that reflect the principles of responsibility, accountability, and advocacy (Boxes 9.2 and 9.3).

Responsibility. **Responsibility** refers to the characteristics of reliability and dependability. It implies an ability to distinguish between right and wrong. In professional nursing, responsibility includes a duty to perform actions adequately and thoughtfully. When administering

---

BOX 9.2 Canadian Nurses Association Code of Ethics (2017)

Part I: Nursing Values and Ethical Responsibilities

There are seven primary values and responsibility statements related to each value:

A. Providing safe, compassionate, competent, and ethical care
B. Promoting health and well-being
C. Promoting and respecting informed decision making
D. Honouring dignity
E. Maintaining privacy and confidentiality
F. Promoting justice
G. Being accountable

Part II: Ethical Endeavours Related to Broad Societal Issues

Part two of the code describes activities that nurses enact to address social inequities. Ethical nursing practice involves striving towards addressing broader elements of social justice that relate to health and well-being.

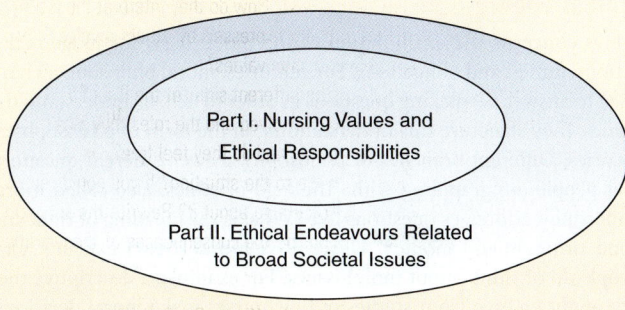

Part I. Nursing Values and Ethical Responsibilities

Part II. Ethical Endeavours Related to Broad Societal Issues

© Canadian Nurses Association. Reprinted with permission. Further reproduction prohibited.

---

a medication, for example, a nurse is responsible for assessing the patient's need for the drug, for administering it safely and correctly, and for evaluating the patient's response to it. By agreeing to act responsibly, the nurse gains trust from patients, colleagues, and society.

Nurses in all domains of practice uphold responsibilities related to all the values in the code of ethics. Nurses are responsible in their interactions with individual patients, families, groups, populations, communities, and society, as well as with students, nursing colleagues, and other health care colleagues. These responsibilities serve as the foundation for articulating nursing values to employers, other health care providers, and the public (CNA, 2017a).

Accountability. Accountability is grounded in the moral principles of fidelity (faithfulness) and respect for the dignity, worth, and self-determination of patients and others with whom nurses work. Fidelity is a guiding principle of relationships based on loyalty, promise-keeping, and truth-telling (veracity). As accountable professionals, "nurses are honest and practise with integrity in all of their professional interactions" (CNA, 2017a, p. 16). **Accountability** means being able to accept responsibility or account for one's actions—to be answerable to someone for something one has done. **Answerability** means being able to offer reasons and explanations to other people for aspects of nursing practice. When explanations are not readily available to patients, the nurse might seek the advice of other health care providers or search for evidence that would support best practice. Nurses need to balance accountability to the patient, the profession, the employer, and society. For example, you may know that a patient who will be discharged soon is confused about how to self-administer insulin. The action that you take in response to this situation is guided by your sense of accountability. The patient, the institution, and society rely on your judgement and trust you to take action in response to this situation. Being ethically accountable does not mean that you will make the "right" decision based on what others believe; rather, it justifies whatever decision you do make (Yeo et al., 2020).

According to the CNA (2017a), nurses who are enacting professional accountability are (1) keeping up with professional standards, laws, and regulations; (2) ensuring that they have the competence to provide these practices; (3) maintaining their fitness to practise, ensuring that they have the necessary physical, mental, and emotional capacity to practise safely and competently; (4) sharing their knowledge with other nurses, nursing students, and other health care providers through mentorship and giving feedback; and (5) advocating for comprehensive and equitable mental health care services.

Professional accountability is also the mandate of professional associations. Professional associations both check unethical practice in a profession and support conscientious professionals who may be under pressure to act unethically or to overlook unethical activity by colleagues. Professional nursing associations have the authority to register and discipline nurses. They also set and maintain professional standards of practice and communicate them to the public. These standards, developed by nursing clinical experts, provide a basic structure against which nursing care is objectively measured.

Advocacy. The ethical responsibility of **advocacy** means acting on behalf of another person, speaking for persons who cannot speak for themselves, or intervening to ensure that views are heard. Advocacy recognizes the need for improvement of systems and societal structures to create equity and better health for all (CNA, 2017a). Individually and collectively, nurses advocate for eliminating social inequities. This includes protecting the patient's right to choice by providing information, obtaining informed consent for all nursing care, and respecting patients' decisions. Nurses should protect patients' right to dignity by

BOX 9.3   International Council of Nurses: The Code of Ethics for Nurses

Nurses have consistently recognized four fundamental nursing responsibilities: to promote health, to prevent illness, to restore health, and to alleviate suffering. The need for nursing is universal. Inherent in nursing care is respect for human rights, including cultural rights, the right to life and choice, the right to dignity, and the right to be treated with respect. Nursing care is respectful of and unrestricted by considerations of age, creed, culture, disability or illness, gender, sexual orientation, nationality, politics, race, religious or spiritual beliefs, and legal, economic, or social status. Nurses render health services to the individual, the family, community, and populations and related groups.

Nurses and Patients or People Requiring Care

The nurse's primary professional responsibility is to people requiring nursing care. In providing care, the nurse promotes an environment in which the human rights, values, customs, and religious and spiritual beliefs of the individual, family, and community are respected and promoted by everyone. The nurse ensures that the individual receives sufficient and timely information in a culturally appropriate manner on which to base consent for care and related treatment. The nurse holds in confidence personal information and respects the privacy, confidentiality, and interests of patients in the lawful collection, use, access, transmission, storage, and disclosure of this information. The nurse shares with society the responsibility for initiating and supporting action to meet the health needs of all people. The nurse advocates for equity and social justice in resource allocation, access to health care, and other social and economic services. The nurse demonstrates professional values such as respect, justice, responsiveness, compassion, empathy, trustworthiness, and integrity.

Nurses and Practice

The nurse carries personal responsibility and accountability for nursing practice and maintaining competence by continual learning. The nurse engages in continuous professional development and lifelong learning. The nurse maintains fitness to not compromise the ability to provide care. The nurse practises within the limits of their individual competence and uses judgement when accepting and delegating responsibility. The nurse at all times maintains standards of personal conduct that reflect well on the profession and enhance its image and public confidence. In their professional role, nurses recognize and maintain personal relationship boundaries. The nurse fosters and maintains a practice culture that promotes ethical behaviour and open dialogue. Nurses may conscientiously object to participating in a particular medical procedure or research study; however, they must still ensure that people receive care. Nurses maintain a person's right to give and withdraw informed consent to access their genetic and genomic-based research. They protect the use, privacy, and confidentiality of genetic information and human genome materials. Nurses are active participants in the promotion of patient safety. They promote ethical conduct when errors or near misses occur, speak up when patient safety is threatened, and work with others to reduce the potential for errors.

Nurses and the Profession

The nurse assumes the major role in determining and implementing acceptable standards of clinical nursing practice, management, research, and education. The nurse is active in developing a core of research-based updated professional knowledge that supports evidence-informed practice. The nurse is active in developing and sustaining a core of professional values. The nurse, through professional organizations, participates in creating a positive practice environment that supports individual practice, ensures safe quality care, and maintains safe, equitable social and economic conditions for nurses. The nurse contributes to positive and ethical organizational environments and challenges unethical practice settings. Nurses engage in the creation, dissemination, and use of research. The nurse prepares for and responds to emergencies, disasters, conflicts, epidemics, and conditions of scarce resources.

Nurses and Global Health

The nurse values access to health care as a human right, affirming the need for universal health coverage. The nurse upholds the dignity, freedom, and worth of all human beings and opposes all forms of exploitation, such as human trafficking and child labour. The nurse leads or contributes to health policy development. The nurse supports and works toward the achievement of the United Nations Sustainable Development Goals. The nurse recognizes the significance of the social determinants of health. Nurses contribute to, and advocate for, policies and programs that address them. The nurse collaborates and practises to preserve, sustain, and protect the natural environment and is aware of its consequences on health. Nurses advocate for initiatives that reduce environmentally harmful practices in order to promote health and well-being. The nurse collaborates with other health professionals and the public to uphold principles of justice by promoting responsibility in human rights, equity and fairness, the public good, and a healthy planet.

Adapted from International Council of Nurses. (2021). *ICN code of ethics for nurses*. https://www.icn.ch/sites/default/files/inline-files/2012_ICN_Co deofethicsfornurses_%20eng.pdf. Reprinted by permission of International Council of Nurses.

advocating for appropriate use of interventions in order to minimize suffering, intervening if other people fail to respect the dignity of the patient, and working to promote health and social conditions that allow patients to live and die with dignity. For example, obtaining **informed consent** means that nurses advocate on behalf of patients to make sure that the patient understands the treatment and has the capacity to give their consent for the treatment. Nurses should protect a patient's right to privacy and confidentiality by helping the patient access their health records (subject to legal requirements), intervening if other members of the health care team fail to respect the patient's privacy, and following policies that protect the patient's privacy. According to the *Code of Ethics*, nurses should also advocate for the discussion of ethical issues among health care team members, patients, and families, and nurses should advocate for health policies that enable fair and inclusive allocation of resources.

Advocacy requires that nurses have a strong awareness of the context in which situations arise, as well as an understanding of the influence of power and politics on how they make decisions. If you, as a nurse, experience **constrained moral agency**—that is, if you feel powerless to act for what you think is right, or if you believe your actions will not effect change—then you will have difficulty being an effective advocate.

Ethical Theory

Ethics concerns the examination of the moral basis for judgements, actions, duties, and obligations. For centuries, moral philosophers have tried to answer perplexing questions in order to help us understand the world. They structure this understanding in the form of philosophical theories. Different branches of philosophy answer different questions that people are grappling with. The field of ethics, also called moral philosophy, addresses questions like "What is the meaning of right and good, or ought and should?" **Descriptive moral theory** explains what people do or think about moral issues. For example, a descriptive theory might emerge from studies of how nurses make moral decisions. Such theory describes the rules, principles, and values that people apply when making moral decisions or judgements in different situations.

Taking this one step further, philosophers ask, "Do we believe this is the right way to make moral decisions, just because many people do it this way?" Metaethics is the field of ethics that analyzes the meanings of key terms such as *right*, *obligation*, *good*, and *virtue*, attempting to distinguish what is moral and what is not. A person studying metaethics might ask if "good" is socially related, an expression of emotion, or the will of a higher power such as God. Is "good" out there to be discovered or is it socially constructed? Is there a true "right," and on what moral basis can moral judgements be assessed as being true or false?

Another branch of moral philosophy is normative ethics. A normative ethical theory is prescriptive in that it tells us how we ought to think about moral questions. Normative ethical theory presents us with moral principles or virtues that allow us to judge the quality and the way we make and evaluate decisions based on our obligations to others. Normative theories question or reveal our obligations as nurses. These are clearly stated in the CNA *Code of Ethics for Registered Nurses*.

In applied ethics (or practical ethics), we look at how decisions should be made in particular situations and ask questions about what moral beliefs and values should apply in specific contexts. Theories that address issues of "right" or "ought" in applied ethics transcend disciplines. Applied ethics in nursing helps us to examine our practice and how our behaviours are shaped by our practice as nurses. A nurse might reflect on how medical technology changes the way they communicate with family members regarding nutrition at the end of life. The following section introduces a variety of contemporary ethical theories. It is neither exclusive nor comprehensive.

Deontology. A traditional ethical theory, deontology is the system of ethics that is perhaps most familiar to practitioners in health care. Its foundations are often associated with the work of the eighteenth-century philosopher Immanuel Kant (1724–1804). In deontology, actions are defined as right or wrong according to moral duties, principles, rules, or imperatives. The role of the moral agent (nurse) is to discern what their duties are and to act consistently with, and in the spirit of, those duties (Yeo et al., 2020). Deontologists specifically do not look to the consequences of actions to determine rightness or wrongness. Instead, they critically examine a situation for the existence of essential rightness or wrongness. Ethical principles such as justice, allowing free choice (autonomy), and doing the greatest good (beneficence) serve to define right or wrong. If an act is just, respects autonomy, and provides good, then the act is ethical. The process depends on a mutual understanding and acceptance of these principles.

Difficulties arise when one must choose among conflicting principles, which is often the case with ethical dilemmas in health care. For example, applying the principle of respect for autonomy can be confusing when dealing with health care for children. The health care team may recommend a treatment, but a parent may disagree with or refuse the recommendation. In discussing the dilemma with your nursing colleagues, you might refer to a guiding principle such as respect for autonomy. However, questions remain: Whose autonomy should receive the respect? That of the parents? Who should advocate for the child's best interest? Society often struggles to understand who should be ultimately responsible for the well-being of children. A commitment to respecting autonomy does not guarantee that controversy can be avoided.

Utilitarianism. According to a utilitarian system of ethics, the value of something is determined by its usefulness. This philosophy, utilitarianism, may also be known as consequentialism because its main emphasis is on the outcome or consequences of an action. A third term associated with this philosophy is teleology (from the Greek word *telos*, meaning "end"), which is the study of ends or final causes. Its philosophical foundations were first proposed by John Stuart Mill

(1806–1873), a British philosopher and social commentator. The greatest good for the greatest number of people is the guiding principle for determining the correct action in this system. The difference between utilitarianism and deontology lies in the focus of the former on consequences and outcomes: utilitarianism concerns the effect that an act will have (outcome), while deontology concerns the presence of principle, regardless of outcome.

Individuals or groups may have conflicting definitions of "greatest good." For example, research suggests that education regarding safer sex practices may reduce the spread of the human immunodeficiency virus (HIV). Some scholars, however, argue that education about sex should be provided by the family and that sex education in public schools diminishes the role and value of family. For them, the greater good is the preservation of family values and the protection of individual choices regarding the sex education of children. Other scholars define the "greater good" as educating the greatest number of people in the most effective way possible. The concepts of utilitarianism provide guidance, but they do not invariably provide for universal agreement.

Bioethics. In the 1970s, a group of ethics scholars concluded that then-current ethical theories were not sufficient for the health care field because they did not provide specific guidance for important moral questions that arose in the context of medicine. Biomedical ethics came to denote ethical reasoning for physicians, whereas bioethics became the general term for principled reasoning across health care professions. Bioethical theory is based on obligation, outcome, and reason (Oberle & Raffin Bouchal, 2009). The central idea of bioethics—also known as *health care ethics*—is that moral decision making in health care should be guided by four principles: autonomy, beneficence, nonmaleficence, and justice. According to this theory, health care providers should examine each situation, determine which of the principles has priority, and use that principle to guide their actions.

Autonomy. Autonomy refers to one's freedom or self-determination. Respect for another person's autonomy is prominent among the foundational principles or values in health care practice. Health care providers express respect for autonomy by assisting patients with deciding on and achieving their own health goals and by ensuring that care plans are consistent with patients' wishes (Yeo et al., 2020). The agreement to respect autonomy requires the recognition that patients are free to make choices and have the capacity to do so. Autonomy assumes the person is competent; has the ability to decide rationally rather than impulsively; and has the ability to act upon those decisions and choices. For example, the purpose of the preoperative consent that patients must read and sign before surgery is to ensure in writing that the health care team respects the patient's choice by obtaining permission to proceed. The consent process implies that a patient may refuse treatment, and in most cases, the health care team must agree to follow the patient's wishes. Health care providers agree to abide by a standard of respect for the patient's autonomy, which comes directly from Kant's ethics and his idea of respect for persons.

Beneficence. Beneficence means promoting someone else's good or well-being. It speaks directly to duty or obligation, as in deontological theories. Commitment to beneficence helps guide difficult decisions concerning whether the benefits of a treatment may be challenged by risks to the patient's well-being or dignity. For example, vaccination may cause temporary discomfort, but the benefits of protection from disease, both for the patient and for society, outweigh the patient's discomfort. The agreement to act with beneficence also requires that the best interests of the patient remain more important than self-interest. For example, as the nurse, you do not simply follow medical orders; you act thoughtfully to understand patient needs and then actively work to meet those needs.

Nonmaleficence. *Maleficence* refers to harm or hurt; thus, **nonmaleficence** is the avoidance of harm or hurt. The health care provider tries to balance the risks and benefits of a plan of care while striving to cause the least harm possible. This principle is often helpful in guiding discussions about new or controversial technologies. For example, a new bone marrow transplantation procedure may provide a chance for a cure. However, the procedure may entail long periods of pain and suffering. These discomforts should be considered in view of the suffering that the disease itself might cause and in view of the suffering that other treatments might cause. The commitment to exercising due care and caution in working to produce benefit illustrates the term *nonmaleficence.* The standard of nonmaleficence promotes a continuing effort to consider the potential for harm even when the action being considered may be necessary to promote health.

Justice. **Justice** refers to fairness and equity (Braveman, 2014; Braveman et al., 2011) (see Chapter 11). Theories of justice focus on how we treat individuals and groups within society, how we distribute benefits and burdens in an equitable way, and how we compensate those who have been unfairly burdened or harmed. In decisions related to the COVID-19 vaccine rollout to the populations that were most in need (e.g., older persons, Indigenous persons, frontline health care workers), it was understood that the vaccine doses would be allocated as fairly as possible (Ismail et al., 2020). Understandings of fairness depend on community and societal values. Choices must often be made between competing resource needs and claims. Of course, the definition of need can be debated, and when two people have equal need, nothing in the theory helps health care providers decide between them. These are ethical questions that require further exploration of values, principles, and priorities to guide decisions in resource allocation.

The literature also mentions other important forms of justice that nurses need to understand, such as **social justice.** Social justice often concerns the equitable distribution of benefits and burdens in society—especially among marginalized individuals and populations—and promotes the view that broad social change is necessary to address the determinants of health and to reduce inequities in health (Commission on Social Determinants of Health, 2008) (see Chapters 1 and 4 for further information about social justice).

In terms of the social justice issues raised by the COVID-19 vaccine rollout, we should be concerned about a reliable supply of needed resources being distributed to the most vulnerable individuals and groups. These discussions are led by experts and publicly available (Yeo et al., 2020).

Other scholars of bioethics, including Canadians Michael Yeo, Anne Moorhouse, Pamela Kahn, and Patricia Rodney (Yeo et al., 2020), who have written about nursing ethics, have incorporated the principles of fidelity (faithfulness), veracity (truth-telling), and confidentiality.

Feminist Ethics. Much of the early work in feminist ethics focused on matters traditionally defined as "women's issues," such as reproduction and gender differences. However, as feminist ethics has developed, the variety of issues that it covers has also expanded. Its scope today recognizes that cultural and institutional dynamics similar to sexism are at work alongside other prejudices and dynamics, such as discrimination on the basis of sexual orientation, race, ethnicity, class, and disability. Feminist analyses of gender prejudices and unjustifiable differential consideration and treatment can be applied to any marginalized group (Yeo et al., 2020).

Relational Ethics. Relationships are the basis of ethics in nursing. According to **relational ethics** theory, ethical understandings are formed in, and emerge from, a person's relationships with others, including patients, families, communities, and colleagues (Bergum & Dossetor, 2020; Doane & Varcoe, 2021. According to Bergum & Dossetor (2020), relational ethics is a way of "being" displayed in everyday interactions rather than a mode of decision making. It influences how a nurse inserts a needle, engages in conversation, shows respect, and behaves with other people. Relational ethics is most helpful in guiding the day-to-day ethical moments that occur between people.

Relational ethics focuses on the role of relational context or the experience of relationships in shaping moral choices. In their research on relational ethics, Bergum and Dossetor (2020) identified four themes: environment, embodiment, mutual respect, and engagement. **Environment** concerns critical elements or characteristics of the health care system within which a nurse works and how the nature of the nurse's relationships is affected by this system. Bergum encourages nurses to consider the entire health care arena as a network or matrix in which each part is connected, either directly or indirectly, to the other. An awareness of this connectedness encourages the nurse to look beyond the immediate situation in order to envision a broader context. It also makes nurses conscious of how power and politics affect the entire system of care (Oberle & Raffin Bouchal, 2009).

Embodiment, in relational ethics, refers to knowledge generated from the mind, body, and spirit; it recognizes that the notion of a mind–body split is an artificial construct, and that healing for both patient and family cannot occur unless scientific knowledge and human compassion are given equal weight. Emotions are respected, and embodied knowledge provides space for these emotions to be explored (Deschenes & Kunyk, 2020). Such recognition requires nurses to become attuned to what other people may be experiencing. Nurses must make this awareness a part of their own experience. The nurse–patient relationship requires that patients are valued and treated with respect. Within the nurse–patient relationship, nursing knowledge is used to enhance the patient's health and well-being. The nurse always considers the patient as an individual with unique needs. Mutual respect is created, with attention to both the nurse's and the patient's needs, wishes, expertise, and experience (Bergum & Dossetor, 2020).

Mutuality, loosely defined as a relationship that benefits both the nurse and the patient (and harms neither), requires the nurse's and the patient's willingness to participate in a relationship that embraces, rather than judges, one another's values and ideas as a means of developing new understandings.

Engagement means connecting with another person in an open, trusting, and responsive manner. Bergum and Dossetor (2020) suggested that it is through this connection that the nurse develops a meaningful understanding of another person's experience. Engagement takes skill and practice as much as it requires a commitment to keeping the relationship caring and respectful. Bergum and Dossetor (2020) have asserted that engagement requires the nurse to come to the relationship with a commitment to exploring what is needed in that specific situation and for the patient to come to the relationship with a desire to share. Engagement requires that the nurse connects with the patient, but at the same time sets appropriate boundaries such that the relationship remains professional. Knowing how much to engage with another person is one of the greatest challenges in nursing.

ETHICAL ANALYSIS AND NURSING

An **ethical dilemma** is a conflict between two sets of human values, both of which are judged to be "good," but neither of which can be fully served. Ethical dilemmas can cause distress and confusion for patients and caregivers. As a nurse, you may well be faced with ethical questions that have not been examined previously and for which no practical wisdom exists. You must be able to examine issues and apply experience and wisdom in each situation. The CNA (2017a) *Code of Ethics*

BOX 9.4	How to Analyze an Ethical Dilemma

Step 1: Determine whether the issue is an ethical dilemma.
Step 2: Gather all the information relevant to the case.
Step 3: Examine and determine your own values on the issues.
Step 4: Verbalize the problem.
Step 5: Consider possible courses of action.
Step 6: Reflect on the outcome.
Step 7: Evaluate the action and the outcome.

identifies the responsibility of nurses to maintain their "fitness to prac-tise" as having the "necessary physical, mental or emotional capacity to practise safely and competently" (p. 17). Such fitness requires nurses to be knowledgeable and skillful as they engage in problem solving. Ethi-cal issues must be analyzed carefully and deliberately. Ethical analysis involves descriptive, conceptual, and normative processes. Analysis of situations begins with acquiring knowledge to gain a sense of what is going on (descriptive analysis), as well as finding out about relevant policies, laws, relationships, and stakeholders. Conceptual analysis is clarifying the meaning of the situation, values, and assumptions of all individuals involved. Normative analysis focuses on what ought to be done, based on the people involved and their respective values (Yeo et al., 2020).

Resolving an ethical dilemma requires deliberate, critical, and sys-tematic thinking (Box 9.4). It also requires the negotiation of differ-ences (between beliefs, values, opinions, and so forth), incorporation of conflicting ideas, and an effort to respect differences of opinion. The process of negotiating ethical dilemmas may in part be the pro-cess of understanding ambiguities. Nurses need to be knowledgeable about and adept at making logical, fair, and consistent decisions. Ethi-cal decision-making models offer a variety of methods for reaching informed conclusions (Figure 9.1).

Documentation of the ethical process can take a variety of forms. Whenever the process involves a family conference or results in a change in the plan of care, the process should be documented in the medical record. At some institutions, the ethics committee may use a formal consultation format whenever a request for discussion arises. If the ethical dilemma does not directly affect patient care, however, the discussion may be documented by minutes from a meeting or in a memorandum to the affected parties. For example, in the case study at the beginning of this chapter, the nursing concerns and the family conferences would be recorded in the medical record and in nursing flow sheets.

Review the case study, then work through the following steps:

Step 1: Is this an ethical dilemma? What may at first appear to be a question of ethics may be resolved by clarifying your knowledge about clinical facts. A review of policy and procedure, or of standards of care, may reveal legal obligations that will determine a course of action, regardless of personal opinion. If the question remains perplexing, and the answer will be profoundly relevant to several areas of human con-cern, then an ethical dilemma may exist.

The single parent's situation meets the criteria for an ethical dilemma. Further review of scientific data will probably not contrib-ute to a resolution of the dilemma, but it is important to review the data carefully to make this determination. The disagreement does not revolve around whether the patient is in a terminally ill state, so fur-ther clinical information will not change the basic question: Should the patient have an opportunity to discuss do-not-resuscitate (DNR) orders at this time? The question is perplexing. Two professional team members disagree on an assessment of a patient's readiness to confront

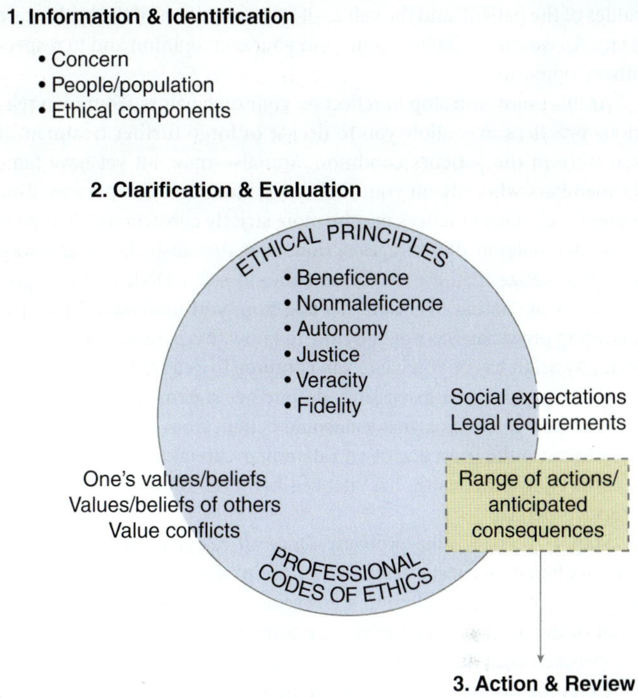

1. Information & Identification

- Concern
- People/population
- Ethical components

2. Clarification & Evaluation

FIGURE 9.1 Ethical Decision-Making Framework. (From Storch, J. L. [2013]. Model for ethical decision making for policy and practice. In J. Storch, P. Rodney, & R. Starzomski [Eds.], *Toward a moral horizon: Nursing ethics for leadership and practice* [p. 538]. Pearson Education.)

the difficult issues related to dying. The answer to the question "Is this patient ready to discuss end of life?" has important implications. If she is not ready, then raising the issue may cause anguish and fear in the patient and her family. If she is ready and the team avoids discussion, she may suffer unnecessarily in silence. If she is very close to death, then in the absence of a DNR order, cardiopulmonary resuscitation (CPR) will be performed in a futile situation. You know that CPR can cause pain. If applied in a situation in which the patient's life is unlikely to be extended or improved, CPR could prolong her suffering and reduce her dignity.

Step 2: Gather as much information as possible that is relevant to the case. Because resolution to ethical dilemmas may arise from unlikely sources, it is important to incorporate as much knowledge as possi-ble at every step of the process. At this point, the information could include laboratory and test results, the clinical state of the patient, and current literature about the diagnosis or condition of the patient. It may include investigation of the psychosocial concerns of the patient as well as those of her significant others. The patient's religious, cultural, and family orientations are part of the nurse's assessment.

You obtain all the clinical information that is pertinent to the ques-tion. It may be helpful to determine whether the patient retains most cognitive functions, even though her tumour is aggressive. You review the chart and discuss this aspect with the physician, and you agree that the patient is fully competent but afraid and overwhelmed by the prog-nosis. Because two professionals disagree on a patient's state of mind, it may be helpful to reassess the patient or request that an independent person assess the patient's readiness to discuss end-of-life issues. Some-times family members or significant others hold important clues to a patient's state of mind.

Step 3: Examine and determine your own values on the issues. This step is important for all participants in the discussion. At this stage, as the patient's nurse, you and the other participants practise values clarification: this involves differentiating between your own values, the values of the patient, and the values of other members of the health care team. An essential aim here is to form your own opinion and to respect others' opinions.

At this point, you stop to reflect on your own values. Your own religious practices may allow you to decide to forgo further treatment if you were in the patient's condition. You also may not yet have family members who rely on you, such as children or older parents. This patient's religious practices may be more strictly constructed than your own. Her religion discourages actions that diminish life in any way, and you realize that she may have come to see a DNR order as giving up or as "acting like God." In addition, you understand that the attending physician has not had time to know this patient as well as her own physician has or you have. You continue to believe that the patient would be capable of a discussion, despite her statements to the physician. In fact, you believe that she would benefit from a discussion, perhaps because the presence of an unfamiliar caretaker, combined with declining physical health, has silenced her, even though her fears and concerns persist.

Step 4: Verbalize the problem. Once all relevant information has been gathered, accurate definition of the problem may proceed. It is helpful to state the problem in a few sentences. By agreeing to a statement of the problem, the health care team, the patient, and the family can proceed with discussion in a focused way.

Here, the problem seems to be whether this patient should discuss DNR at this time. Determine the benefits and risks of a DNR order at this time. Other important questions relate to the patient's current state of mind: Is she afraid to speak? Is she feeling cut off from her normal network (a primary physician)? Are these feelings contributing to confusion about DNR decisions?

Step 5: Consider possible courses of action. What options are available within the context of the situation and the patient's values?

Once you have asked the basic question, other questions and possible courses of action arise. Should you initiate a discussion with the patient independently of the physician? Would you be outside your professional role if you facilitated a DNR order? What if your assessment were incorrect? Would you contribute not to the dignity but to the distress of the patient? The answers to these questions may be elusive because they depend on an understanding of the patient's feelings and values, which are not necessarily obvious. Even if the nurse cannot legally write a DNR order, the nurse can influence a physician's or patient's decision regarding DNR; therefore, troubling questions remain.

Step 6: Reflect on the outcome. This is the most important and delicate step of the process. These negotiations may happen informally at the patient's bedside or in the charting room, or a formal ethics meeting may be necessary. Your point of view represents a unique contribution to the discussion.

In an ethics committee meeting, the discussion is usually interprofessional. A facilitator or chairperson ensures that all points of view are examined and that all pertinent issues are identified. A decision or recommendation is the usual outcome of discussion and the result of a successful discussion. In the best of circumstances, participants discover a course of action that meets criteria for acceptance by all. On occasion, however, participants may leave the discussion disappointed or even opposed to the decision.

The discussion focuses on the disagreement between your assessment and the physician's regarding the patient's readiness to discuss end-of-life issues. The principles mentioned during the discussion include beneficence and nonmaleficence: Which plan would provide this patient with the most good—a DNR order or no order? A separate question addresses the patient's point of view: Would a discussion with the patient promote well-being or induce anguish? Furthermore,

according to the principle of autonomy, a troublesome question remains: Does the patient want something different from the desire she is expressing?

With several members of the health care team present, the discussion proceeds. You present your point of view. You continue to sense that the patient is ready to discuss DNR orders but that she may be reluctant to trust the circumstances of this admission. You respect the attending physician and his analysis and continue to be concerned that the patient may have experienced a change of mind between the last admission and this one. In the end, the team proposes a formal meeting with the patient, in which you, the attending physician, and a supportive family member are present. You support this proposal because you sense that it will maximize the support of the patient's existing network. In addition, you recognize that in a trusting environment, the patient is more likely to express fears, insecurities, and wishes. Team members agree to keep the discussion open ended and exploratory. You suggest that rather than asking whether the patient wants a DNR order, the team could wait for her to bring up the issue. In this way, the team could be assured of her consent and willingness to participate in the discussion.

Step 7: Evaluate the action and the outcome.

At the meeting, the patient does in fact open up. She expresses relief at the chance to explore her options and feelings. Pain management issues are clarified. She wants to discuss a DNR order but requests a visit from her priest before making a final decision.

ETHICAL ISSUES IN NURSING PRACTICE

With increased professional responsibility and accountability, and with changes in the workplace and health care system, nurses are increasingly facing a myriad of ethical issues. Ethical issues arise daily while nurses are caring for patients and families, relating to other health care providers and institutions, and dealing with global societal issues. The following section explores current issues that raise ethical challenges. As a nurse, you have a unique understanding of ethical situations based on the context in which you practise. For example, a home care nurse may recognize the moral dimensions of practice that are particular to that setting and have a way of thinking about ethical challenges that will help the patient and family know how best to act in a situation. In other words, answers to moral problems must be negotiated in the context in which they arise; no two settings are alike.

Patient Care Issues

Futile Care. Futility in health care has been a prevalent topic in the literature since the early 1980s. Current issues such as rising health care costs, an aging population, enhanced life-sustaining technologies, and limited resources have led to academic discussions, debates, and practice policies on health care futility. There are many definitions of **futile care**, but most focus on life-sustaining or life-prolonging technologies in circumstances where care will not return the patient to a productive life, the patient will remain in a persistent vegetative state, or there is no foreseeable benefit to the proposed care. Patients often worry, in the event of their becoming incapacitated and unable to express their wishes, that they will be "hooked up to machines" and receive treatment that they do not desire. At issue is whether clinicians are sufficiently objective to establish that a given intervention is futile, as determinations of futility are often laden with biases.

Although health care providers are best equipped to determine the physical benefits of treatment, only the patient or people who know the patient best can determine whether treatment is advancing the patient's overall well-being. Taylor and Lightbody (2018) identified this issue as "qualitative" futility or determination. In other words, it is not just medical facts but also what the patient (or the patient's surrogate) values as their goals for undergoing treatment that leads decision makers to conclude that a treatment has no benefit according to those values.

Achieving holistic outcomes of care must be based on an interplay of physical facts and subjective values. Hsu et al. (2018) suggested that medical futility involves the following criteria: (1) the chance of success is extremely unlikely; (2) a desirable goal (physiological signs) cannot be achieved; (3) the patient's quality of life is unacceptable to the patient and their significant others; and (4) the extent of resource consumption exceeds the expected benefits. It is evident that these classifications have objective and subjective dimensions, as well as quantitative and qualitative dimensions, and that they constitute a more complete way of viewing the complex notion of futility.

The issue of who has priority in health care decision making remains complex and often troublesome. The potential for futility conflicts is high in situations of critically and chronically ill patients. What, then, is the nurse's role? Nurses play a leading role in working toward pursuing negotiated compromise between health care providers and patients equally, for the best possible outcome for the patient. Nurses can work toward this by communicating with other members of the health care team about patients, families, and health care teams at risk of experiencing conflict about futile care, and then initiating dialogue that may prevent or resolve conflict. Rather than subscribing to categories of levels of futility to drive decision making, many health care agencies have now developed end-of-life guidelines that are tailored to patients' needs. These guidelines include a determination of levels of intervention or goals of care that range from fully acute to palliative/comfort care (Rocker & Dunbar, 2000). Levels of intervention are based on the premise that specific interventions may either be withheld or administered according to individual patient needs and that supportive/palliative care ought to be integrated with all levels. Advance care planning is one way to address this problem.

Advance care planning (ACP) is a multidimensional process through which people share with health care providers their values, goals, and preferences regarding future medical treatments, with the purpose of aligning care received with patient wishes (Shaw et al., 2021). ACP requires open and ongoing conversations between patients, their families, and health care providers. During the ACP process, patients can also identify surrogate decision makers should they become unable to make their own health care decisions (Lum & Sudore, 2016; Lund et al., 2015). ACP, when utilized and implemented effectively, has the potential to improve patient and family experiences during end of life. The number of unwanted medical interventions is reduced, and health care providers are better able to deliver quality care that aligns with patients' wishes following ACP conversations (Lum & Sudore, 2016). Yet, despite its benefits, considerable variability exists in ACP processes between and within clinical settings and health care providers, which is driven by different perceptions of the content and when ACP discussions should occur (Shaw et al., 2021).

Ideally, ACP should be facilitated by multiple health care providers (physicians, nurses, social workers, chaplains, and others). Nurses serve as facilitators, educators, and advocates to help start ACP conversations and ease transitions between care settings, based on thorough discussions. Nurses encourage all individuals in their care (patients and families) "to reflect on, communicate and document their values (i.e., personal, cultural, religious and those that constitute a legacy for enduring and sustaining life), in addition to health and personal care wishes that include end-of-life care" (CNA et al., 2015, p. 5). Nurses are involved in advocating for patients' rights, and nursing research has found that their presence is an important factor in helping patients

to develop advance directives (living wills and identifying a surrogate decision maker; CNA, 2015).

Medical Assistance in Dying. Canada's approach to freedom of choice regarding end-of-life care and decision making has undergone unprecedented change in recent years. One of the most significant changes occurred on January 15, 2016, when the Supreme Court of Canada suspended the operation of its declaration in *Carter v. Canada*, permitting physician-assisted death (CNA, 2017b). This landmark court ruling was followed by a federal statute, Bill C-14, which instituted medical assistance in dying (MAiD) and the legal framework that this procedure could be carried out in Canada in certain circumstances. This legislation revises the Canadian *Criminal Code* to include exemptions (legal protection in accordance with the law) for health care providers, such as registered nurses, who may help to provide MAiD under the direction of a physician or nurse practitioner, and establishes safeguards for individuals. Canada became the first country where nurse practitioners may legally facilitate MAiD in the same capacity as a physician (CNA, 2017b).

MAiD is defined in the Act as (a) the administering by a medical practitioner or nurse practitioner of a substance to a person, at their request, that causes their death, or (b) the prescribing or providing by a medical practitioner or nurse practitioner of a substance to a person, at their request, so that they may self-administer the substance and in doing so cause their own death (Special Joint Committee on Physician-Assisted Death, 2016).

On March 17, 2021, revisions to Canada's MAiD legislation came into effect. These changes to the Canadian *Criminal Code* now allow eligible persons to pursue a medically assisted death whether or not their natural death is foreseeable. However, those individuals solely suffering from mental illness, as well as mature minors, are not currently eligible for MAiD (Department of Justice Canada, 2021).

Each province, based on their shared responsibility for health care, may choose to develop additional legislation and policies to clarify the rules governing the everyday practice of MAiD (CNA, 2017b). Health care providers who choose to participate in MAiD must comply with those additions since, according to the MAiD legislation, "medical assistance in dying must be provided with reasonable knowledge, care and skill and in accordance with any applicable provincial laws, rules or standards" (*Criminal Code*, 1985, c. 3, s. 241.2 [1][7]). Nurses who have a conscientious objection may elect not to participate in MAiD, and what counts as participation may differ as well (CNA, 2017b). Provisions for conscientious objection vary from one jurisdiction to another, and from agency to agency as well (CNA, 2017b).

Nursing regulatory bodies across the country have the legal mandate to protect the public by ensuring that nurses who practise are qualified and provide safe, competent, ethical care. Regulators are responsible for setting standards and guidelines that apply to the scopes of practice (nurse practitioner, registered nurse, registered psychiatric nurse) established for nurses under provincial or territorial legislation (CNA, 2017b). Provincial and territorial governments and health professional regulatory bodies undertook a process of developing policies and procedures to guide MAiD-related practice specific to their jurisdiction. However, even with these developed guidelines, nursing colleagues find MAiD-related scope of practice to be challenging and ever-changing. Restrictions exist within the MAiD process related to the role of the registered nurse, which differs between provinces (Pesut et al., 2019).

One example of these differences is between Alberta and Nova Scotia regarding the way in which registered nurses are to respond to a patients' request for information about MAiD. Nurses in the College of Registered Nurses of Alberta (2021) are required to make a referral to someone who can provide accurate, objective information to the patient if the nurse cannot provide it themselves. In contrast, the Nova Scotia College of Nursing (2021) allows for a distinct choice by registered nurses regarding the way they respond to such a request from a patient, and the registered nurses are not required to make a referral. The resulting differences can result in professional and moral challenges. However, the CNA (2017b) reminds nurses to be aware of responsibilities in their jurisdictions as they exist. A comprehensive review of the regulatory commonalities and differences among nursing associations in Canada related to MAiD is outlined by Pesut et al. (2019).

Nurses are intimately involved in end-of-life care processes, and registered nurses perform key roles in ensuring that patients receiving MAiD receive high-quality care (Pesut et al., 2019). A recent Canadian study showed that MAiD is impactful for nurses, and that for some, it entails intensive and ongoing moral sense-making (Pesut et al., 2020). The CNA (2017b) document *National Nursing Framework on Medical Assistance in Dying in Canada* and the CNA (2017a) *Code of Ethics for Registered Nurses* remain valuable resources that support all nurses and students to gain a greater understanding of MAiD as it unfolds in the Canadian context. In essence, nurses have a unique perspective and bring an important contribution to providing end-of-life care that includes medical assistance in dying (CNA, 2017b).

Issues of Safety and Ethics Related to the Work Environment

Social Networking and Safety. The online presence of social networks presents ethical challenges for nurses. On the one hand, social networks can be a supportive source of information about patient care or professional nursing activities. Nurses can seek and receive emotional support through social media when encountering hardships at work with colleagues or patients. On the other hand, the risk to patient privacy is high. Even if a nurse posts an image of a patient without any obvious identifiers, the nature of shared media reposting can result in the image's surfacing in a place where the mere context of the image provides clues to friends or family to identify the patient.

Slobogian et al. (2017) identified three key themes in their paper on the impact of personal social media use and nursing practice challenges as follows: the onus of boundary maintenance is on health care providers; the most common boundary violations are related to breaches of confidentiality; and there is an obvious gap in organizational policy to assist providers in navigating these issues (p. 394). In a review of policy documents on social media and nurses, Slobogian et al. (2017) identified only one document that provided direct guidance, such as a clear list of "dos and don'ts" (p. 35). The now-dated CNA's (2012) *Ethics in Practice* paper on the challenges and opportunities of social media identifies the central concern as being patient confidentiality and privacy. This important document offers useful social media etiquette for nurses to maintain professional standards while using these technologies (CNA, 2012). The CNA cautions that the "use of social media is not considered in any way 'private' but is firmly within the public domain, with a potential audience of many thousands if not millions" (CNA, 2012, p. 2). Given the nonprivate nature of media platforms such as Facebook, the posting of information with well-intended goals, such as professional consulting purposes, could potentially lead to harm to both the nurse and the patient. A breach in private information can lead to serious legal and disciplinary actions.

Social media, when used sensibly, can also afford potential benefits to nurses. Networking with other nurses who have similar interests can lead to professional growth, learning opportunities, and knowledge transfer of key information to support continuing education. Social media can also be a way of sharing nursing knowledge as a way of offering the public a glimpse of the significance of the nursing role.

Working With a Health Care Team to Promote Safe Care. Nurses are responsible for providing safe, compassionate, competent, and ethical care (CNA, 2017a). In ensuring safety, care must be delivered in such a way that harm is minimized. Lack of control over important aspects of the environment can lead to ethically ambiguous situations. Nurses are at risk from workplace harm related to a complicated work environment and the complex nature of the ethical situations they face in practice. The outcomes of moral distress in these situations may become evident in the form of psychological and physical symptoms, reduced job satisfaction, and even inadequate or inappropriate nursing care. Moral distress occurs within the context of the environment, and the relationships within that environment matter (Deschenes & Kunyk, 2020). Complex life-and-death events, multiple role responsibilities, loyalties and expectations, reduced numbers of skilled health care providers, minimal clinical nursing leadership, interdisciplinary team conflict, and autocratic organizational decision making may all contribute to the creation of personal moral conflict for nurses (Austin, 2016).

Causing harm to patients in the form of pain and suffering from continuing treatment is a source of **moral distress** for nurses that they often believe could be avoided. "Moral distress arises when nurses are unable to act according to their moral judgement" (Rodney, 2017, s-7). Sometimes nurses find it hard to care for a patient when other health care providers, usually physicians, make choices that nurses think are causing more harm than good. For example, the situation of a patient in intensive care who is comatose but seems to experience great pain when turned over can be very upsetting for nurses. The nurse may experience moral distress if they feel that they are, in effect, torturing the patient each time they turn them over. Keeping patients safe from harm can be difficult, and sometimes it requires great ethical sensitivity to be aware of harms that are being caused. In these situations, nurses may lose their sense of **moral integrity** or "wholeness" when they are committed to certain values and beliefs that are not upheld because of situational constraints. If these situations continue and integrity is compromised, nurses may experience **moral residue**—a situation in which they seriously compromise themselves or allow themselves to be compromised (CNA, 2017a, p. 7). In such situations, relational ethics can help you know what the patient considers to be harm, and it is crucial to engage in discussions with your patients and colleagues.

In an interprofessional environment, all health care providers must take responsibility and work with colleagues at all levels of the system for the care provided (Box 9.5). Moral distress can be a very lonely experience, but meeting with co-workers to discuss the conflict, assess others' reactions to the situation, obtain additional information, or seek assistance can be helpful strategies to address the issue causing moral distress. A prime example of this scenario has occurred during the COVID-19 pandemic. Nurses have experienced moral distress when decisions are being made at the system level—a level at which nurses feel they have little input. Moral distress has also been realized for nurses and other clinicians because of their inability to save all who need their care and because of the real worries they have for their colleagues' (and their own families') health.

There is also real concern about the likelihood that nurses may experience post-traumatic stress due to the experiences they encounter (Thorne et al., 2020). As discussed by Rodney (2017), nurses need their practice environments to function as moral communities where ethical values drive practice at all levels. When they know these supports exist, they are better equipped to manage the aftermath of their encounters with difficult ethical situations.

BOX 9.5   **RESEARCH HIGHLIGHT**
Ethics in Nursing Practice

Research Focus
Pesut et al. (2020) explored how nurses construct good nursing practice in the context of medical assistance in dying (MAiD).

Background and Research Design
Nurses play a central role in MAiD; however, we know little about their experiences with this new end-of-life-option. This Canadian study used interpretive description methodology to interview 59 nurses in semi-structured telephone interviews. Data were analyzed inductively using a constant comparative analysis method to determine codes agreed to by all researchers. From these codes, a thematic account of the data was constructed.

Evidence-Informed Practice
Data synthesis and comparison of similarities and differences revealed the following themes:
- Registered nurses and nurse practitioners described creating a person-centered MAiD process that included establishing relationship, planning meticulously, orchestrating the MAiD death, and supporting the family.
- A nursing gaze focused on relationships crosses the moral divides that characterize MAiD. What united participants was a desire to nurse well and compassionately in this new practice context.
- Confidence and competence required structured education, mentored experiences, and supportive briefing.

The authors concluded that the findings illustrated the ways in which nurses constructed artful practice to humanize what was otherwise a medicalized event. Not only is MAiD an extreme change in nursing practice, but it is also morally contentious and has the potential to be divisive for nurses. Some nurses view the act as morally wrong, while others see it as a peaceful end to suffering. These divisive views offer the opportunity to explore nursing's unique perspective with the possibility of asking the question of whether there is some common nursing gaze even across these moral differences. Respecting moral differences is a way to come together in this experience. These findings provide an in-depth look at what constitutes good nursing practice in MAiD that can support the development of best practice in all aspects of MAiD that nurses encounter.

From Pesut, B., Thorne, S., Schillar, C., et al. (2020). Constructing good nursing practice for medical assistance in dying in Canada: An interpretive descriptive study. *Global Qualitative Nursing Research, 7,* 1–11. https://doi.org/10.1177%2F2333393620938686

KEY CONCEPTS

- Values clarification helps nurses explore personal values and feelings and decide how to act on personal beliefs. It also facilitates nurse–patient communication.
- Ethics is the study of philosophical ideals of what is beneficial or valuable for all.
- A code of ethics provides a foundation for professional nursing. Such a code promotes accountability, responsibility, and advocacy.
- Theories of bioethics refer to ethical issues specific to the delivery of health care. They are based on the principles of autonomy, beneficence, nonmaleficence, and justice.
- Relational ethics theory encompasses more than bioethics; it addresses the role of relationships in the ethical delivery of health care. It maintains that the nurse–patient relationship is the foundation of nursing ethics.
- Ethical problems arise from differences in values, from technological advances, from end-of-life experiences, and from changes in work environments.

- A standard process for thinking through ethical dilemmas, including critical thinking skills, helps health care providers resolve conflict or uncertainty about correct actions.

CRITICAL THINKING EXERCISES

1. Complete the values clarification exercise (see Box 9.1) with your classmates or others. Compare the answers and discuss the differences.
2. Yvonne (preferred pronouns: she/her) is an educator in a long-term care facility where Ginnie (preferred pronouns: she/her) works as a nurse. Yvonne is involved in pandemic education, and Ginnie is attending one of the mandatory sessions about personal protective equipment (PPE). During the session, Ginnie is with a group of nurses who voice their mistrust in the supply and proper use of PPE in the facility. They share the belief that the resources will not be sufficient and that the practices of the equipment will not be safe. They also share that if the stress becomes too great to them as nurses, and if they cannot protect themselves or the residents, they will not hesitate to take sick leave without notice. Ginnie feels their concern and is torn about what her next steps should be. Consider the following questions (adapted from the CNA *Code of Ethics*) in working through Ginnie's decisions:
   a. What would be an "unreasonable burden" in relation to providing care and withdrawing or refusing to provide care?
   b. What should the nurse do to prevent further harm?
   c. What information would the nurse need to make a decision to fulfill her duty to provide care?
   d. What duty or courses of action would Yvonne need to uphold to ensure that the risk would be minimal to the nurses?

🌐 *Answers to Critical Thinking Exercises appear on the Evolve website.*

REVIEW QUESTIONS

Review Questions 1 to 10 relate to the case study at the beginning of the chapter.

1. The nurse understands that personal values about death and dying may impact how decision making occurs at the end-of-life (EOL). How might values clarification help in EOL decision making with Meghan?
   a. It will create a set of rules for conduct.
   b. It will identify values that should be accepted by all.
   c. It will resolve issues of "value conflict."
   d. It will help in developing a code of ethics.
2. Nurses often participate in helping patients like Meghan to engage in advance care planning. Which of the following would NOT be considered in the process of completing an advance care plan with Meghan?
   a. The nurse would check with Meghan upon admission whether she has completed an advance care plan.
   b. Nurses would only consider an advance care plan if Megan is at the EOL.
   c. Advance care planning may have opened the EOL discussion and uncovered Meghan's values and beliefs about her EOL care.
   d. Meghan's advance care plan may include her wishes regarding treatment decisions and about who may be her agent in helping to make these decisions.

3. Health care providers, including nurses, agree to "do no harm" to their patients. In Meghan's case, the nurse and physician may be causing harm to Meghan when communication is not open. Which ethical principle espouses "doing no harm"?
   a. Beneficence
   b. Accountability
   c. Nonmaleficence
   d. Respect for autonomy

4. Meghan may be hesitant to discuss her care with a new physician. The nurse carefully assesses her situation and determines that she is fearful. The nurse establishes interventions designed to reduce these fears. How can the nurse be an advocate for Meghan?
   a. By seeking out the nurse supervisor to speak with the patient
   b. By documenting patient fears in the medical record in a timely manner
   c. By working to change the hospital environment
   d. By assessing the patient's point of view and preparing to articulate it

5. Meghan's nurse assesses her pain and then offers a plan to manage the pain. The ethical principle that encourages the nurse to monitor Meghan's perspective about the plan is:
   a. Beneficence
   b. Justice
   c. Nonmaleficence
   d. Respect for autonomy

6. Including Meghan in decision making regarding care and respecting her choices of treatment demonstrate which of the following principles?
   a. Beneficence
   b. Autonomy
   c. Justice
   d. Veracity

7. Nurses agree to be advocates for their patients. In advocating for patients, which nursing action has the highest priority?
   a. Seeking out a nursing supervisor in situations involving conflict
   b. Working to understand the law as it applies to the patient's clinical condition
   c. Assessing the patient's point of view and preparing to articulate this point of view

   d. Documenting all clinical changes in the medical record in a timely manner

8. Which action is *NOT* part of the nurse's role as patient advocate?
   a. Intervening if other people fail to respect the patient's dignity
   b. Protecting the patient's right to confidentiality and privacy
   c. Making nursing care decisions for the patient
   d. Advocating for appropriate use of interventions to minimize suffering

9. Meghan's wait in emergency was lengthy. Her family members, who were extremely anxious about this, approached the triage desk. Which of the following nursing actions best reflects a relational ethics approach?
   a. When approached, the triage nurse comments that the clinic policy is to see people in order of medical priority, not waiting time.
   b. The triage nurse assures the family member that everything will be just fine.
   c. As the family member shares the narrative of needing to be seen, the nurse interrupts to assure them that the best effort will be made to have Meghan seen in a timely manner.
   d. The nurse respectfully listens to the family and explains that, although they cannot predict the time, they will do their best to keep the family member informed.

10. Meghan's nurse has determined that she may have a difference of opinion from the physician about how to proceed with discussing EOL care with Meghan. The priority action to be taken first to negotiate this difference of opinion would be:
    a. Consulting a professional ethicist to ensure that the steps of the process occur in full
    b. Gathering all relevant information regarding the dilemma
    c. Listing the ethical principles that inform the dilemma so that negotiations use a common language during the discussion
    d. Ensuring that the attending physician has written an order for an ethics consultation to support the ethics process

Answers: 1. c; **2.** b; **3.** c; **4.** d; **5.** d; **6.** b; **7.** c; **8.** c; **9.** d; **10.** b.

🌐 *Rationales for the Review Questions appear on the Evolve website.*

RECOMMENDED WEBSITES

Canadian Bioethics Society: https://www.bioethics.ca
Founded in 1988 through the amalgamation of the Canadian Society of Bioethics and the Canadian Society for Medical Bioethics. Members include health care administrators, lawyers, nurses, philosophers, physicians, theologians, and other professionals concerned with the ethical and humane dimensions of health care. The website offers information about the organization's annual conference, national and international ethics organization links, and relevant ethics journals from a variety of disciplines.

John Dossetor Health Ethics Centre at the University of Alberta:
https://www.ualberta.ca/john-dossetor-health-ethics-centre

The John Dossetor Health Ethics Centre is the only interdisciplinary academic health ethics centre in Alberta and one of the first in Canada. The Centre is involved in health ethics education, research, and community engagement at the University of Alberta.

W. Maurice Young Centre for Applied Ethics: https://www.ethics.ubc.ca
Established by The University of British Columbia in 1993, the Centre is primarily an interdisciplinary research centre where researchers study a variety of ethics topics. The website has links to other ethics organizations and ethics resources. The Centre's newsletter is also available on the website.

🌐 REFERENCES

A full reference list is available on the website for this book at
http://evolve.elsevier.com/Canada/Potter/fundamentals/

10

Legal Implications in Nursing Practice

Written by Carla Shapiro, RN, MN, and Jennifer Dunsford, RN, MN, MPA

OBJECTIVES

Mastery of content in this chapter will enable you to:

- Define the key terms listed.
- Differentiate between the governance roles of the four "pillars" of the nursing profession.
- Demonstrate the application of legal concepts in nursing.
- Identify the legal responsibilities and obligations of nurses.
- List sources for standards of care for nurses.
- Define the legal aspects of nurse–patient, nurse–physician, nurse–nurse, and nurse–employer relationships.
- List the elements needed to prove negligence.

KEY TERMS

Advance directive
Adverse occurrence report
Assault
Battery
Civil law
Common law

Euthanasia
Incident report
Informed consent
Intentional torts
Living will
Medical assistance in dying (MAiD)

Negligence
Nursing practice acts
Risk management
Standards of care
Statute law
Tort

WEBSITE

http://evolve.elsevier.com/Canada/Potter/fundamentals/

CASE STUDY

DJ is a student nurse completing a rotation at a long-term care facility. The unit is busy because of a recent influenza outbreak, with numerous residents on isolation precautions, and the resulting increase in assessments for all residents. DJ's assignment includes an elderly resident (preferred pronouns: she/her) with a history of dementia, myocardial infarction, type 2 diabetes, and peripheral vascular disease. During morning rounds, DJ finds the resident appearing well, and notes that her vital signs are as follows: pulse 72, temperature 37° C, respiratory rate 12, and blood pressure 98/67. DJ prepares the resident's medications, which include metoprolol and metformin. Unable to find a preceptor to double check, DJ notes that all medications have been provided daily without interruption and makes the decision to go ahead with medication administration. Checking on the resident an hour later, DJ finds her on the floor of her room, complaining of dizziness and right leg pain. A focused assessment reveals swelling and deformity of the right hip, and blood pressure of 78/56. It is suspected that the resident has a fractured hip from to a fall due to hypotensive syncope. An ambulance is called.

Think about this case study as you read this chapter. There are review questions at the end of the chapter about this case study.

Safe nursing practice requires knowledge of the legal boundaries within which nurses must function. Nurses must understand the law to protect themselves from liability and to protect their patients' rights. Nurses need not fear the law; rather, they should view it as representing what society expects from them. Laws are continually changing to meet the needs of the people they are intended to protect. As technology has expanded the role of the nurse, the ethical dilemmas associated with patient care have increased and often become legal issues as well. As health care evolves, so do the legal implications for health care. Although federal laws apply to all provinces and territories, nurses must be aware that laws do vary across the country. Nurses are responsible for knowing the laws in their province or territory that affect their practice. Being familiar with the law enhances nurses' ability to be patient advocates.

THE PROFESSION OF NURSING

Nursing is a collaborative profession. There are over 400,000 regulated nurses in Canada working in a multitude of settings (Almost, 2021). The profession comprises four designations: registered nurse, licensed or registered practical nurse, registered psychiatric nurse, and nurse practitioner. Each province or territory has legislation that governs the profession of nursing and specifies the regulation of the profession. Licensure or registration as a nurse comes with obligations and privileges. All nurses are required to complete an approved educational program and demonstrate that they meet the entry-level competencies set by their provincial or territorial regulatory body before they can write an entry-to-practice exam and register to practise. Demonstration of a commitment to life-long learning, possession of professional liability protection, and maintenance of good character are conditions

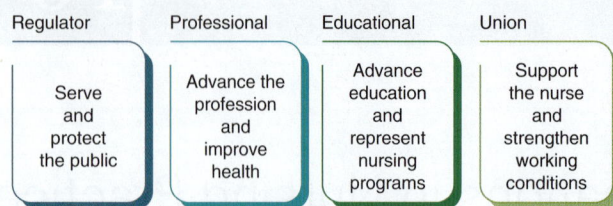

FIGURE 10.1 The four "pillars" of nursing. (From Almost, J. [2021]. *Regulated nursing in Canada: The landscape in 2021* [p. 26, Figure 2]. Canadian Nurses Association. https://www.cna-aiic.ca/en/nursing/regulated-nursing-in-canada. © Canadian Nurses Association. Reprinted with permission. Further reproduction prohibited.)

of licensure. Nurses have a duty to adhere to their code of ethics, to maintain their fitness to practise, and to engage in conduct that is consistent with the values of the profession. The use of the title "nurse" is reserved for those who have met all requirements. The practice of nursing is varied, with employment opportunities being open only to members of the profession.

In addition to nursing regulators, whose focus is the governance of the profession and protection of the public, there are also three other "pillars" of nursing (see Figure 10.1). Many nurses are represented by unions that advocate for suitable compensation and working conditions. Professional associations work to advance the profession at the provincial/territorial, national, and international levels. If current laws, rules and regulations, or policies under which nurses must practise do not reflect reality, nurses must engaged as advocates to see that the scope of nursing practice is accurately defined. Finally, educational institutions work to advance nursing education to ensure all graduates of approved programs can demonstrate the entry-level requirements set by their regulatory bodies. Taken together, the four pillars of regulator, union, professional association, and education provide oversight, governance, and advancement for the profession and contribute to the high level of public trust that nurses and nursing enjoy (Almost, 2021).

LEGAL LIMITS OF NURSING

Nurses have a *fiduciary relationship* with their patients. A fiduciary relationship is one in which a professional (the nurse) provides services that, by their nature, cause the recipient (the patient) to trust in the specialized knowledge and integrity of the professional. In a fiduciary relationship, nurses are obligated to provide knowledgeable, competent, and safe care and to act in the best interests of their patients. Nursing students are subject to the same obligations.

Although legal actions against nurses were once rare, the situation has been changing. The public is better informed now than in the past about their rights to health care and are more likely to seek damages for professional negligence. The courts have upheld the concept that nurses must provide a reasonable standard of care. Thus, it is essential that nurses understand the legal limits influencing their daily practice.

Sources of Law

The Constitution of Canada is the primary source of Canadian law (*Constitution Act*, 1867 to 1982). It divides areas of responsibility between the federal government and the provinces. The federal government has authority over such matters as unemployment insurance, the postal service, and criminal law. The federal law applies across the country. The Constitution gives the provinces authority over matters such as the management of hospitals, the solemnization of marriage, and civil rights. In the constitutional context, civil rights have a broad meaning and refer to private relationships between people, including contract rights, ownership of property, and negligence disputes. In

Canada, there are two systems that deal with private law issues: civil law (based on Roman law) in Quebec and common law (based on British common law) in the rest of the country. The three territories exercise many of the same powers as the provinces by virtue of the authority delegated to them by the federal government.

When either a civil or a criminal case goes to court, rulings are made based on statute law and previous case rulings. How courts rule on the circumstances and facts surrounding the case is called a *precedent*. If legal rulings are made in a case, the court is bound to follow that decision in subsequent similar cases. Not every jurisdiction has case law on a given issue. For example, cases regarding a patient's right to refuse treatment are not found in every province. However, the cases from another province or territory are often consulted. In general, breaches of private law result in the payment of money to compensate the aggrieved party for damages incurred. Violations of some public law statutes such as the *Criminal Code* may result in a range of remedies, including fines or imprisonment.

Statute law is created by elected legislative bodies such as the Parliament of Canada and provincial or territorial legislatures. Federal statutes apply throughout the country, and provincial and territorial statutes apply only in the province or territory in which they were created. Examples of provincial statutes are the *Regulated Health Professions Act* (1991) in Ontario and nursing practice acts throughout the country, which describe and define nursing practice within each province or territory. Examples of federal statutes are the *Criminal Code* (1985), the *Assisted Human Reproduction Act* (2004), the *Controlled Drugs and Substances Act* (1996), and the *Food and Drugs Act* (1985).

Professional Regulation

Like all self-governing professions in Canada, nursing is regulated at the provincial or territorial level. Each province and territory has legislation that grants authority to a nursing regulatory body to operationalize and enforce the laws and regulations that define the profession and its practice. These regulatory bodies are accountable to the public for ensuring safe, competent, and ethical nursing care. Regulatory bodies are responsible for granting certificates of registration, offering practice support, ensuring continuing competence of their members, investigating complaints against members' conduct, and disciplining members when necessary. Regulatory bodies are also responsible for developing codes of ethics, setting standards of practice, and approving nursing education programs that meet the expectations of the Canadian Association of Schools of Nursing (CASN) framework for nursing education (Canadian Association of Schools of Nursing, 2022; McDonald & McIntyre, 2019).

Separate regulatory bodies exist for registered nurses and practical nurses. Some provinces also have regulatory bodies for registered psychiatric nurses. These regulatory bodies are called either the *provincial association* or the *college of nursing* (e.g., the College and Association of Registered Nurses of Alberta, the College of Nurses of Ontario). Most provinces now follow the college model, with a stronger focus on regulation of practice and accountability to the public (Almost, 2021).

Nurses must be registered with the nursing regulator of the province or territory in which they practise. The requirements for registration (or licensure, as applicable) vary across the country, but most provinces and territories require that nurses meet minimum education requirements and pass an examination. Registration (or licensure) enables nurses to practise nursing and use the applicable protected nursing title and initials: registered nurse (RN) or registered practical nurse (RPN). All nurses' credentials must be verified either by the listing of their names on a register or by their holding of a valid licence to practise.

Registration can be suspended or revoked by the regulatory body if a nurse's conduct violates provisions in the registration statute. For example, nurses who perform illegal acts jeopardize their registration status.

Due process must be followed before registration can be suspended or revoked. *Due process* means that nurses must be notified of the charges brought against them and have an opportunity to defend themselves against the charges in a hearing. Such hearings do not occur in courts but are usually conducted by the regulatory body. If the case involves civil or criminal wrongs, then further legal consequences may follow.

Regulation of Nurse Practitioners

Over the years, the roles and responsibilities of nurse practitioners have evolved. The utilization and regulation of nurse practitioners varies from jurisdiction to jurisdiction across Canada. For instance, in Newfoundland and Labrador, the Northwest Territories, and Nunavut, the title "nurse practitioner" is protected, while in Manitoba, the terms used for these nurses are RN(EP) (extended practice) and RN(NP) (nurse practitioner). It is important that nurses communicate their regulated title to their patients, families, and other members of the health care team. The differences in regulatory approaches among jurisdictions can be confusing to consumers and can affect the mobility of nurses across the country as a result (McDonald & McIntyre, 2019).

Standards of Care

Standards of care are legal guidelines for nursing practice. Standards establish the expectation that nurses will provide safe and appropriate patient care. If nurses do not perform their duties within accepted standards of care, they may place themselves at risk of legal action and, more importantly, put their patients at risk for harm and injury. Nursing standards of care arise from a variety of sources, including statutes, case law, and the detailed regulations, practice standards, and codes of ethics that are generated by nursing regulators. Nursing standards are also outlined in the written policies and procedures of employing institutions.

All provincial and territorial legislatures have passed health professions acts or **nursing practice acts** that define the scope of nursing practice. These acts set educational requirements for nurses, distinguish between nursing and medical practice, and generally define nursing practice. The rules and regulations enacted by a provincial or territorial regulatory body define the practice of nursing more specifically. For example, a nursing regulator may develop a rule regarding intravenous therapy. All nurses are responsible for knowing the provisions of the nursing practice or regulated health professions act for the province or territory in which they work, as well as the rules and regulations enacted by the regulatory bodies of their province or territory.

Professional organizations are another source for defining standards of care. The Canadian Nurses Association (CNA, 2015) has developed standards for nursing practice, policy statements, and similar resolutions. The standards delineate the scope, function, and role of the nurse in practice. Nursing specialty organizations also have standards of practice defined for the certification of nurses who work in specific specialty areas, such as the operating room or the critical care unit. The same standards also serve as practice guidelines for defining safe and appropriate nursing care in specialty areas.

Accreditation Canada requires that accredited health care institutions have nursing policies and procedures in writing that detail how nurses are to perform their duties. These internal standards of care are usually quite specific and are found in procedural manuals on most nursing units. For example, a procedure or policy that outlines the steps that should be taken when a dressing is changed or when medication is administered will provide specific information about how nurses are to perform these tasks. Nurses must know the policies and procedures of their employing institution because all institutional policies and procedures must conform to laws and cannot conflict with legal guidelines that define acceptable standards of care.

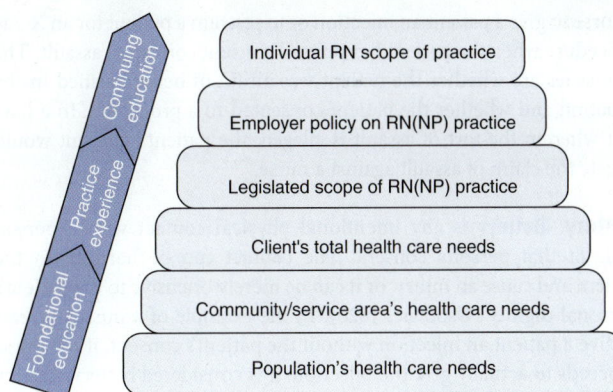

FIGURE 10.2 Individual nurse's scope of practice. (From College of Registered Nurses of Manitoba. [2019]. *Scope of practice for RNs* [p. 4]. https://www.crnm.mb.ca/uploads/document/document_file_254 .pdf?t=1580488652)

In a negligence lawsuit, these standards of care are used to determine whether the nurse has acted as any reasonably prudent nurse in a similar setting with the same credentials would act. A nursing expert is called to testify about the standards of nursing care as applied to the facts of the case. It is recognized and understood that nursing practice differs according to the rural or urban nature of the institutional setting. In addition, home health care, occupational health nursing, and other community-based clinical settings require that the expert be familiar with the standards of care in these settings as opposed to the traditional hospital or institutional setting. The expert must have the appropriate credentials, the appropriate experience, and an understanding of what the standard of care should have been in the specific case. The expert witness is distinguished from the fact witness. Staff nurses may testify in a court proceeding as fact witnesses if they have first-hand personal experience with the facts of the case. The expert witness evaluates the defendant's professional judgements and behaviour under the circumstances being reviewed.

General duty nurses are legally responsible for meeting the same standards as other general duty nurses in similar settings. However, specialized nurses, such as nurses in a critical care unit or nurses who perform dialysis, are held to standards of care and skill that apply to all professionals in the same specialty. Figure 10.2 shows the building blocks that establish an individual nurse's scope of practice. Nursing practice is based on foundational nursing education; it progresses with professional experience and continuing education (College of Registered Nurses of Manitoba, 2019). All nurses must know the standards of care that they are expected to meet within their specific specialty and work setting. Ignorance of the law or of standards of care is not a defence against negligence.

LEGAL LIABILITY ISSUES IN NURSING PRACTICE

Torts

A **tort** is a civil wrong committed against a person or property. Torts may be classified as intentional or unintentional. **Intentional torts** are willful acts that violate another person's rights (Keatings & Adams, 2020). Examples are assault, battery, invasion of privacy, and false imprisonment. Negligence is an example of an unintentional tort.

Intentional Torts

Assault. **Assault** is conduct (such as a physical or verbal threat) that creates in another person apprehension or fear of imminent harmful or offensive contact. No actual contact is necessary for damages for assault to be awarded (Botterell et al., 2020; Osborne, 2020). Threats by a nurse to give a patient an injection or to restrain a patient for an X-ray procedure when the patient has refused consent constitute assault. The key issues are whether the patient was afraid of being harmed in the situation and whether the patient consented to a procedure. In a lawsuit wherein the tort of assault is alleged, the patient's consent would negate the claim of assault against a nurse.

Battery. **Battery** is any intentional physical contact with a person without that person's consent. The contact can be harmful to the patient and cause an injury, or it can be merely offensive to the patient's personal dignity (Osborne, 2020). In the example of a nurse's threats to give a patient an injection without the patient's consent, if the nurse proceeds to actually give the injection, it is considered battery. Battery could even be a life-saving measure, as in the Ontario case of *Malette v. Shulman et al.* (1990). In that case, the plaintiff was unconscious and bleeding profusely. The physician determined that she needed a life-saving blood transfusion. Before the transfusion, a nurse found a signed card in the plaintiff's purse that identified the patient as a Jehovah's Witness and stated that under no circumstances was she to receive blood. Despite knowing this information, the physician chose to administer the blood to preserve the patient's life. The plaintiff survived, recovered from her injuries, and successfully sued the physician for battery (Irvine et al., 2013).

In some situations, consent is implied. For example, if a patient gets into a wheelchair or transfers to a stretcher of their own volition after being advised that it is time to be taken for an X-ray procedure, the patient has given implied consent to the procedure. A patient has the right to revoke or withdraw consent at any time.

Invasion of Privacy. The tort of invasion of privacy protects the patient's right to be free from unwanted intrusion into their private affairs. Patients are entitled to confidential health care. Nursing standards for what constitutes confidential information are based on professional ethics, the common law, and privacy statutes. The ideals of privacy and sensitivity to the needs and rights of patients who may not choose to have nurses intrude on their lives but who depend on nurses for their care guide the nurse's judgement. The nurse's fiduciary duty requires that confidential information not be shared with anyone else except on a need-to-know basis.

One form of invasion of privacy is the release of a patient's medical information to an unauthorized person, such as a member of the press or the patient's employer, or through social media. The information contained in a patient's medical record is a confidential communication. It should only be shared with health care providers for the purpose of medical treatment. The nurse should not disclose the patient's confidential medical information without the patient's consent. For example, a nurse should respect the patient's wish not to inform the patient's family of a terminal illness. Similarly, a nurse should not assume that a patient's spouse or family members know the patient's entire medical history, especially potentially sensitive issues such as mental illness, pregnancy, medical assistance in dying, or sexually transmitted infections.

Confidentiality is not an absolute value, however, and in certain circumstances breaching confidentiality is justifiable. At times, a nurse may be required by law (statutory duty) to breach confidentiality and disclose information to a third party. For example, each province or territory has laws that require health care providers to report suspected child abuse to a local child protection agency. In some jurisdictions, statutes require the notification of the police when a patient has sustained a gunshot or a stab wound (*Gunshot and Stab Wounds Mandatory Reporting Act*, 2008). Nurses may also be required to release information about a patient when they receive a subpoena (a legal order) to testify in court.

Nurses are under no legal obligation to release confidential information to the police except in rare cases in which the life, safety, or health of the patient or an innocent third party is in jeopardy (such as when a patient tells a nurse that they intend to hurt or kill someone). Such a statement should first be reported to the employer's administration or legal counsel before being released to the police (Canadian Nurses Protective Society [CNPS], 2014). Other admissions made by a patient may not have to be disclosed.

The conflict between confidentiality and risk of public harm is not always clear. When a nurse has serious concerns about the welfare of others (e.g., if a patient is infected with human immunodeficiency virus [HIV] and admits to having unsafe sex or donating blood), the nurse should first strongly encourage the patient to disclose this information. If the patient refuses, the nurse should seek consultation with professional colleagues and supervisors. The need for privacy and confidentiality of privileged communication and the need for public safety should be weighed carefully.

Computers and Confidentiality. Most health care facilities use electronic patient records. This system improves accountability and the timeliness of communication, but also introduces legal concerns related to the risk of unauthorized access. Access to confidential patient information is generally controlled by a variety of technological safeguards, including magnetized cards and passwords. These security devices should not be shared with other people, and access cards should be used for file retrieval only when warranted. The improper use of a magnetized card and password to obtain confidential information could lead to legal repercussions or disciplinary action. Care must be taken to protect portable devices, such as laptop computers and flash drives containing health information, as there have been cases where such devices were stolen from offices and cars (Office of the Information and Privacy Commissioner of Alberta, 2020).

Nurses must also be extremely cautious about what information or images they post online, as any information can be easily distributed and make its way into the public domain. There is the mistaken belief that privacy controls are totally secure and that anonymous postings provide protection. Breaches of privacy legislation can lead to disciplinary action by the professional regulatory body or to civil lawsuits (Keatings & Adams, 2020). The best way to avoid the inadvertent disclosure of confidential or private information about patients is by maintaining professional boundaries, following employer policies, not posting or sharing any patient-related information online, and not making disparaging comments about employers or colleagues, as these may be viewed as defamatory (CNPS, 2020a).

False Imprisonment. The tort of false imprisonment serves to protect a person's individual liberty and basic rights. Preventing a patient from leaving a health care facility voluntarily may constitute the tort of false imprisonment. The inappropriate or unjustified use of restraints (e.g., by confining a person to an area, or by using physical or chemical restraints) may also be viewed as false imprisonment. Nurses must be aware of their facility's policies and specific legislation in their jurisdiction (e.g., under the *Mental Health and Consequential Amendments Act*, 1998) relating to when and how restraints can be used (CNPS, 2021a).

Unintentional Torts
Negligence. When nurses are sued, most often the proceedings against them are for the tort of negligence, also referred to as *malpractice* (Irvine et al., 2013). **Negligence** in nursing is conduct that does not meet a standard of care established by law. No intent is needed for negligence to occur. It is characterized chiefly by inadvertence, thoughtlessness, or inattention. Negligence may involve carelessness, such as not checking an identification bracelet, which results in administration

Adapted from Frank, L., & Danks, J. (2019). Perianesthesia nursing malpractice: Reducing the risk of litigation. *Journal of PeriAnesthesia Nursing, 34*(3), 463–468; Keatings, M., & Adams, P. (2020). *Ethical and legal issues in Canadian nursing* (4th ed.). Elsevier Canada.

of the wrong medication. However, carelessness is not always the cause of misconduct. If nurses perform a procedure for which they have not been educated and do so carefully, but still harm the patient, a claim of negligence can be made. In general, courts define *nursing negligence* as the failure to use the degree of skill or learning ordinarily used under the same or similar circumstances by members of the nursing profession (Box 10.1).

Nurses can be found liable for negligence if the following criteria are established: (1) the nurse (defendant) owed a duty of care to the patient (plaintiff); (2) the nurse did not carry out that duty; (3) the patient was injured; and (4) the nurse's failure to carry out the duty caused the injury (Keatings & Adams, 2020).

The ability to predict harm (i.e., the foreseeability of risk) is evaluated in negligence cases. The circumstances surrounding the injury are evaluated to determine whether it was likely that the injury or harm to the patient could have been expected from the care that was or was not provided. In other words, had it not been for what the nurse did or did not do, could an injury have been prevented?

The case of *Downey v. Rothwell* (1974) is an example of nursing negligence. This case involved a plaintiff (preferred pronouns: she/her) who suffered a severe injury while under the care of a nurse. The patient, who had a history of epilepsy, informed the nurse that she was about to have a seizure. The nurse left the patient unattended on an examining table while she left the room for a few moments. During this time, the patient had a seizure, fell onto the floor, and broke her arm. The nurse should have anticipated that the patient could fall during a seizure and ensured her safety either by moving her to the floor or by putting up guardrails on the examining table. This case involved an undertaking by the nurse to provide care, a reliance by the patient on this nurse, and a foreseeable risk. The nurse was found negligent in this case, and the employers were held vicariously liable. Vicarious liability is a legal doctrine that applies in situations where the law holds the employer legally responsible for the acts of its employees that occur within the scope and course of their employment (Botterell et al., 2020).

In the case of *Granger v. Ottawa General Hospital* (1996), two nurses (a staff nurse and the team leader) were found negligent in the care they provided to a labouring patient. During labour, the plaintiff's fetal heart monitor strip showed deep, persistent, variable decelerations. The staff nurse did not appreciate that these were a sign of fetal distress and did not immediately report these findings to other members of the obstetrical team. The ensuing delay in care resulted in severe and permanent brain injury in the baby. In this case, the nurses breached their duty to exercise appropriate skill in making an assessment and to communicate the information to the physicians.

Preventing Negligence. The best way for nurses to avoid being negligent is to follow standards of care; give competent health care; insist on appropriate orientation, continuing education, and adequate staffing; communicate with other health care providers; develop a caring rapport with the patient; and document assessments, interventions, and evaluations fully.

The health care record, or "chart," is a permanent record of the nursing process. The courts consult the patient's chart for a chronological record of all aspects of care provided from admission to discharge. As a legal document, it is the most comprehensive record of the care provided. Careful, complete, and thorough documentation is one of the best defences against allegations of negligence or violations of nursing standards (see Chapter 16). The record can show that even in the event of an adverse patient outcome, the nursing care that was provided met the expected standards. An institution has a legal duty to maintain nursing records. Nursing notes contain substantial evidence needed to understand the care received by a patient. If records are lost or incomplete, the care is presumed to have been negligent and therefore the cause of the patient's injuries. In addition, incomplete or illegible records undermine the credibility of the health care provider.

In the classic case of *Kolesar Estate v. Joseph Brant Hospital* (1977), the Supreme Court of Canada addressed the issue of poor record keeping. A patient underwent major spinal surgery and was transferred to a surgical unit, where the patient was nursed on a Stryker frame. The patient was found dead the following morning. No nursing notes were recorded from 2200 hours the previous evening until 0500 hours the next morning, when the patient was found dead. Although at trial several nurses and nursing assistants testified that they had tended to the patient multiple times throughout the night, the court inferred that "nothing was charted because nothing was done." One of the nurses was held negligent in this patient's death.

Timely documentation is crucial. Any significant changes in the patient's condition must be reported to the physician and documented in the chart (see Chapter 16). Recording nursing care notes on a worksheet and then transferring them to the chart at the end of the shift can be a dangerous practice. If this practice is followed, other health care providers may administer medications or provide care to the patient without up-to-date information. Harm may come to a patient whose record is not accurate and current. Nurses must always follow the style of charting adopted by their employer (CNPS, 2021b).

Truthful documentation is also essential. If an error is made in the documentation, nurses must follow the policies and procedures of the institution to correct it. Errors that are obliterated or erased may give the impression that misconduct is being concealed and lead to charges of fraud. The credibility of a nurse who goes to court is negatively affected if it appears that the nurse's initial charting was changed after an injury occurred to a patient.

This scenario is exemplified in the case of *Meyer v. Gordon* (1981). Nurses did not adequately monitor a labouring patient, and their notes were sloppy and vague. The fetus experienced severe distress, required resuscitation on delivery, and was transferred to another hospital. When a nurse realized that the documentation was deficient, they altered it. However, the original chart had already been photocopied and sent to the second hospital. At trial, it was obvious that the original document had been tampered with. The court held that the nursing staff had been negligent in several ways, and the judge severely condemned the nurse's tampering with the evidence as follows:

> My criticism of the defendant hospital is not confined to the lack of care of its nursing staff. The hospital chart contains alterations and additions which compel me to view with suspicion the accuracy of many of the observations which are recorded.
>
> *Meyer v. Gordon, 1981*

Nurses should also be familiar with the current nursing literature in their areas of practice. They should know and follow the policies and procedures of the institution in which they work. Nurses should be sensitive to common sources of injury to patients, such as falls and medication errors. Nurses must communicate with the patient, explain the tests and treatment to be performed, document that specific explanations were provided to the patient, and listen to the patient's concerns about the treatment.

Nurse–patient relationships are critical not only in ensuring quality care but also in minimizing legal risks. Trust needs to develop between a nurse and patient. Sincere caring for patients is an essential role of the nurse and an effective risk management tool. However, caring does not protect nurses completely if negligent practice occurs. When a patient is injured, the investigation into the incident may implicate the nurses even if the patient feels kindly toward them.

Criminal Liability

Although most nursing liability issues involve negligence claims, criminal law is also relevant. The *Criminal Code* has many offences that could be committed by nurses. For example, Canadian nurses have been charged with criminal offences such as assault, administering a noxious substance, criminal negligence that causes death (a category of manslaughter), and first-degree murder (Gillese, 2019). Many of the acts that can give rise to a tort claim for damages may also give rise to a criminal charge. A nurse who assaults a patient could face a civil suit for damages brought by the patient and a criminal charge of assault laid by the police. Sometimes the difference between the tort and the criminal charge is one of degree. The tort of negligence involves the breach of duty of care expected of a reasonably competent practitioner, whereas the offence of criminal negligence involves actions that reach the level of "wanton or reckless disregard for the lives or safety of other persons" (*Criminal Code*, 1985, s. 219 [1]).

Consent

A signed consent form is required for all routine treatment, procedures such as surgery, some treatment programs such as chemotherapy, and research involving patients. A patient signs general consent forms when admitted to the hospital or other health care facility. The patient or the patient's representative must sign a special consent or treatment form before each specialized procedure or treatment. According to the CNA *Code of Ethics*, "if a person receiving care is clearly incapable of consent, the nurse respects the law on capacity assessment and substitute decision making in the nurse's jurisdiction" (CNA, 2017a, p. 12; see also CNPS, 2018a). Provincial and territorial laws describe what constitutes the legal ability to give consent to medical treatment. Nurses should know the law in their own jurisdiction and be familiar with the policies and procedures of their employing institution regarding consent.

In general, the following factors must be verified for consent to be legally valid:

- The patient must have the legal and mental capacity to make a treatment decision.
- The consent must be given voluntarily and without coercion.
- The patient must understand the risks and benefits of the procedure or treatment, the risks of not undergoing the procedure or treatment, and any available alternatives to the procedure or treatment.

If a patient is Deaf or does not communicate in the language of the health care providers, an official interpreter must be used to explain the terms of consent. A caregiver or acquaintance who can speak a patient's language should not be used to interpret health information except as a last resort. A patient experiencing the effects of a sedative is unable to clearly understand the implications of an invasive procedure. Every effort should be made to assist the patient in making an informed choice.

Nurses must be sensitive to the cultural issues of consent. The nurse must understand the way in which patients and their families communicate and make important decisions. It is essential for nurses to understand the various cultures with which they interact. The cultural beliefs and values of the patient may be very different from those of the nurse. It is important for nurses not to impose their own cultural values on the patient.

Informed Consent

Nurses ensure that nursing care is provided with the person's informed consent. Nurses recognize and support a capable person's right to refuse or withdraw consent for care or treatment at any time.

British Columbia College of Nurses and Midwives, 2020a, p. 1; CNA, 2017a, p. 11

Informed consent is a person's agreement to allow a medical action to happen, such as surgery or an invasive procedure, based on full disclosure of the likely risks and benefits of the action, alternatives to the action, and the consequences of refusal (Garner & Black, 2019; Osborne, 2020). Informed consent creates a legal duty for the physician or other health care provider to disclose material facts in terms that the patient can reasonably understand in order to make an informed choice. The explanation should also describe treatment alternatives, as well as the risks involved in all treatment options. Failure to obtain consent in situations other than emergencies may result in a claim of battery. In the absence of informed consent, a patient may bring a lawsuit against the health care provider for negligence, even if the procedure was performed competently. Informed consent requires the provision of adequate information for the patient to form a decision and the documentation of that decision.

The following elements are required for informed consent to be valid (Health Care Consent Act, 1996; Keatings & Adams, 2020):

- Capacity to consent: The person must be capable of making an informed decision about the specific intervention proposed.
- Information: The person must be provided with enough information to make the decision.
- Voluntariness: The decision must be voluntary and not the result of coercion or undue influence.

A legally capable person's consent is considered informed if they have received adequate information about the nature and purpose of the proposed treatment, its expected benefits, and its material risks—including the risks of possible harm, permanent damage, or death, as well as the risks of not proceeding. An explanation of alternatives to the proposed procedure or treatment is also required. Patients must also be informed of their right to refuse the procedure or treatment without discontinuing other supportive care, and of their right to withdraw their consent even after the procedure has begun.

Informed consent is part of the relationship between health care providers and patients. Because nurses do not perform surgery or direct medical procedures, obtaining patients' informed consent is not *usually* one of nurses' duties unless they are providing the intervention, as a nurse practitioner might. While a nurse may act as witness to the patient's signature on the consent form, *the nurse is not legally responsible for obtaining informed consent for a medical procedure*. The nurse's signature witnessing the consent does not mean that the nurse has provided information about the risks of and alternatives to a particular procedure, only that the patient voluntarily gave consent, that the patient's signature is authentic, and that the patient appears to be competent to give consent (Irvine et al., 2013).

When nurses provide consent forms for patients to sign, the patients should be asked whether they understand the procedures to which they are consenting. If they deny understanding or if the nurse suspects that they do not understand, the nurse must notify the physician or nursing supervisor. Some consent forms also have a line for the physician to sign after explaining the risks and alternatives to a patient. Such a form is helpful in a court case when a patient alleges that consent was not informed. If a patient refuses treatment, this should also be written, signed, and witnessed.

If a patient participates in an experimental treatment program or submits to use of experimental medications or treatments, the informed consent form must be even more detailed and stringently regulated. An organization's institutional review board should review the information in the consent form for research involving human subjects. The patient may withdraw from the experiment at any time (see Chapter 9).

Many of the procedures that nurses perform (e.g., insertion of intravenous or nasogastric tubes) do not require formal written consent; nonetheless, a patient's right to consent to or refuse treatment must be protected. Implied consent to treatment is often involved in nursing procedures. For example, when the nurse approaches the patient with a syringe in hand and the patient exposes the injection site, consent is implied. If the patient resists the injection either verbally or through actions, the nurse must not proceed with the injection. Forcing or otherwise treating a patient without consent could result in criminal or civil charges of assault and battery. Many advanced practice nurses are now autonomously treating patients. It is therefore likely that formal written consent for nursing procedures will also be expected for the treatment patients receive from advanced practice nurse specialists.

Parents are usually the legal guardians of pediatric patients and are therefore responsible for signing the consent forms for treatment. If the parents are divorced, the forms must be signed by the parent who has legal custody. On occasion, a parent or guardian will refuse treatment for a child. In those cases, the court may intervene on the child's behalf. The practice of making the child a ward of the court and administering necessary treatment is relatively common in such cases.

The case of 13-year-old Tyrell Dueck (preferred pronouns: he/him) from Saskatchewan illustrates such a scenario. The teenager received a diagnosis of cancer in 1998. He had completed part of his chemotherapy treatment when he decided that he did not want more treatment or the recommended amputation of his leg, believing that he had been "cured by God" and that further treatment was unnecessary. His statements were consistent with his family's Christian value system. Following his parents' advice, the boy wished to undergo alternative therapy at a clinic in Mexico. The treating physicians maintained that without further conventional treatment, Tyrell would die within a year. A judge concluded that Tyrell had been given inaccurate information by his father about the benefits and risks of the proposed alternative therapy and that Tyrell was therefore unable to give informed consent or refusal. The family's wishes to forgo conventional treatment were legally overruled, and the patient's grandparents were instead assigned responsibility to take him for treatments. Before the enforced treatment could be started, however, tests revealed that the cancer had already spread and the treatment would no longer be helpful. The teenager was returned to the care of his parents, and he died a short time later.

In some instances, obtaining informed consent is difficult or simply not possible. If, for example, the patient is unconscious, consent must be obtained from a person legally authorized to give consent on the patient's behalf. Other surrogate decision makers may have legally been delegated this authority through proxy directives or court guardianship procedures. In emergency situations, if it is impossible to obtain consent from the patient or an authorized person, the procedure required to benefit the patient or save the patient's life may be undertaken without liability for failure to obtain consent. In such cases, the law assumes that the patient would wish to be treated. This is referred to as the emergency doctrine.

Patients with mental health issues and frail older persons must also be given the opportunity to give consent. They retain the right to refuse treatment unless a court has legally determined that they are incompetent to decide for themselves.

Nursing Students and Legal Liability

Nursing students must know their own capabilities and competencies and must not perform nursing actions unless competent to do so. However, if a student nurse performs a nursing action (e.g., medication administration by injection), the student will be held to the same standards as a reasonable, competent professional nurse and may be subject to the same legal consequences for actions that fail to meet those standards (Patton & Lewallen, 2015). In a few reported cases in Canada, nursing students have been sued for negligence in their care of patients. A nursing student in Nova Scotia who caused permanent injury to a patient through an improperly administered intramuscular injection was found negligent, and the hospital was found vicariously liable for the student's actions (*Roberts v. Cape Breton Regional Hospital*, 1997). Thus, nursing students are liable if their actions cause harm to patients. However, if a patient is harmed as a direct result of a nursing student's actions or lack of action, the liability is generally shared by the student, the instructor, the hospital or health care facility, and the university or educational institution.

Nursing students should never be assigned to perform tasks for which they are unprepared, and they should be carefully supervised by instructors as they learn new skills. Although nursing students are not considered employees of the hospital, the institution has a responsibility to monitor their acts. Nursing students are expected to ensure that their student status is known to patients and to perform as professional nurses would in providing safe patient care. Faculty members are usually responsible for instructing and observing students, but in some situations, staff nurses serving as preceptors may share these responsibilities. Every nursing school should provide clear definitions of student responsibility, preceptor responsibility, and faculty responsibility (CNPS, 2012).

When students are employed as aides or unregulated care providers (UCPs) when not attending classes, they should not perform tasks that do not appear in a job description for a UCP. For example, even if a student has learned to administer intramuscular medications in class, this task may not be performed by a nurse aide. If a staff nurse overseeing the UCP knowingly assigns work without regard for the person's ability to safely conduct the task as defined in the job description, that staff nurse is also liable. If students employed as UCPs are requested to perform tasks that they are not prepared to complete safely, this information should be brought to the nursing supervisor's attention so that the needed help can be obtained.

The website of the Canadian Nurses Protective Society (CNPS) (http://www.cnps.ca/, members-only section) is an excellent resource available to nursing students, providing information about the legal risks that nurses face in practice. However, nursing students are not entitled to receive legal consultation services or financial assistance from the CNPS; these services are provided only for the benefit of eligible registered nurses.

Professional Liability Protection

Most nurses in Canada are employed by publicly funded health care facilities that carry malpractice insurance. These facilities are considered employers and thus are vicariously liable for negligent acts of their employees, provided the employees were working within the normal scope and course of practice (Keatings & Adams, 2020).

Because of this legal principle, an employer will generally be liable to those who may have suffered damages because of an employee's negligence. Consequently, a patient who feels they have been injured by the actions of an employee will often look to the employer for compensation (Keatings & Adams, 2020). This legal principle does not apply when the employee is working outside the normal scope of their employment. Accordingly, a nurse who is self-employed or engages in activities that are not related to their employment (even if they are undertaken on the employer's premises) is solely liable for their own negligence. All nurses should be aware of their employment status as well as the availability and extent of their professional liability coverage.

A nurse who is providing emergency assistance at an accident scene may not be covered by an employer's insurance policy because the care given would not fall within the scope of employment. However, some provinces have adopted "Good Samaritan" laws (e.g., Alberta's *Emergency Medical Aid Act*, 2000) that prevent voluntary rescuers from being liable for negligent care provided during a rescue, unless it can be proved that they displayed gross negligence. Nurses must be familiar with these laws in their own province or territory.

As a condition of licensing and registration, nurses are required to obtain professional liability protection through the organization set by their regulator, such as the CNPS. This liability protection is like an insurance policy and provides the nurse with access to resources on legal issues, confidential legal advice, and coverage of financial penalties awarded by the courts in certain legal proceedings.

Abandonment, Assignment, and Contract Issues

Short Staffing. During nursing shortages or periods of staff downsizing, the issue of inadequate staffing may arise. Legal problems may result if the number of nurses is insufficient or if an appropriate mix of staff to provide competent care is lacking. If assigned to care for more patients than is reasonable, nurses and students should bring this information to the attention of the nursing supervisor. In addition, a written protest such as a workload or staffing report form should be completed to document the nurse's concerns about patient safety. Most provinces and territories have some reporting mechanism in place to document heavy workload or staffing situations. Although such a protest may not relieve nurses of responsibility if a patient suffers injury because of inattention, documenting the nurse's concern would show that they were attempting to act reasonably. Whenever a written protest is made, nurses should keep a copy of this document in their personal files. Most administrators recognize that knowledge of a potential problem shifts some of the responsibility to the institution.

Nurses should not walk out when staffing is inadequate because charges of abandonment could be made. A nurse who refuses to accept an assignment may be considered insubordinate, and patients would not benefit from having even fewer staff available. Delegation of appropriate tasks to other health care providers may be necessary in some circumstances. The nurse is responsible for ensuring the competence of the care provider and for providing ongoing supervision (CNPS, 2021c). Nurses should be aware of the institution's policies and procedures and the nursing union's collective agreement on how to handle such circumstances before they arise.

Floating. Nurses are sometimes required to "float" from the area in which they normally practise to other nursing units. Nurses must practise within their level of competence. Nurses should not be floated to areas where they have not been adequately cross-trained. Nurses who float should inform the nursing supervisor of any lack of experience in caring for the type of patients on the nursing unit. They should also request and be given orientation to the unit. A nursing supervisor can be held liable if a staff nurse is given an assignment they cannot safely

perform. In one case (*Dessauer v. Memorial General Hospital*, 1981), an obstetrics nurse was assigned to an emergency room. A patient entered the emergency room, complaining of chest pain. The obstetrical nurse gave the patient too high a dosage of lidocaine, and the patient died after suffering irreversible brain damage and cardiac arrest. The nurse lost the negligence lawsuit.

Prescribers' Orders. The physician is responsible for directing medical treatment. Nurses are obligated to follow physicians' orders unless they believe the orders are in error, violate hospital policy, or would harm patients. Therefore, all orders must be assessed; if an order is found to be erroneous or harmful, further clarification from the prescriber is necessary. If the physician confirms the order and the nurse still believes it to be inappropriate, the supervising nurse should be informed. A nurse should not proceed to perform a prescriber's order if harm to the patient is foreseeable. The nursing supervisor should be informed of and given a written memorandum detailing the events in chronological order; the nurse's reasons for refusing to carry out the order should also be documented to protect the nurse from disciplinary action. The supervising nurse should help resolve the questionable order. A medical or pharmacy consultant may be called in to help clarify the appropriateness or inappropriateness of the order. A nurse carrying out an inaccurate or inappropriate order may be legally responsible for any harm done to the patient.

In a negligence lawsuit against a health care provider and a hospital, one of the most frequently litigated issues is whether the nurse kept the provider informed of the patient's condition. To inform a provider properly, nurses must perform a competent nursing assessment of the patient to determine the signs and symptoms that are significant in relation to the attending provider's tasks of diagnosis and treatment. Nurses must document that the provider was notified as well as the provider's response, the nurse's follow-up, and the patient's response.

For example, nurses noticed that a patient with a cast on his leg was experiencing poor circulation in his foot. The nurses recorded these changes, but did not notify the physician. Gangrene subsequently developed in the patient, and an amputation was required. The hospital, physician, and nursing staff were all charged with negligence (Irvine et al., 2013).

The physician should write all medical orders, including "do not resuscitate" or "allow natural death" orders. The nurse must make sure that orders are transcribed correctly. Verbal orders are not recommended because they increase the possibilities for error. If a verbal order is necessary (e.g., during an emergency), it should be written and signed by the prescriber as soon as possible, usually within 24 hours. The nurse should be familiar with the institution's policy and procedures regarding verbal orders.

Dispensing Advice Remotely. Providing advice over the telephone or by video conferencing is a high-risk activity because it is difficult to assess a patient remotely. The nurse is legally accountable for advice given. The most common allegations of negligence in this area are provision of inadequate advice, improper referrals, and failure to refer (CNPS, 2020b). It is essential that nurses precisely follow institutional guidelines and policies and thoroughly document each interaction to avoid serious repercussions for all parties.

LEGAL ISSUES IN NURSING PRACTICE

Abortion

In the 1988 case of *R. v. Morgentaler*, the Supreme Court of Canada ruled that the *Criminal Code* (1985) regulations on legal access to abortion were unconstitutional. At that time, the *Criminal Code* required that a woman seeking an abortion first needed to secure the approval of a hospital-based committee before the procedure could be performed. By rejecting these *Criminal Code* provisions, the Supreme Court in effect referred the abortion issue to Parliament, but Parliament had not (and has not) rewritten a criminal law policy on abortion. Abortion is thus unregulated by law, which is tantamount to its legalization. However, the legal entitlement to abortion does not mean abortion services are readily available. Because health care facilities are not obliged to offer abortions, many do not do so. Thus, abortion access remains an ongoing issue in Canada.

Prescription Medications and Controlled Substances

Canadian law closely regulates the administration of medications. Two federal acts control the manufacture, distribution, and sale of food, medications, cosmetics, and therapeutic devices in Canada: the *Food and Drugs Act* (1985) and the *Controlled Drugs and Substances Act* (1996). The *Food and Drugs Act* lists the medications that can be sold only by prescription (e.g., antibiotics) and medications that are subject to stringent controls (e.g., barbiturates, amphetamines). The distribution of these medications requires specific handling and record keeping. The *Controlled Drugs and Substances Act* controls the manufacture, distribution, and sale of narcotics (e.g., morphine, codeine). However, it also regulates other medications that are controlled in the same manner as narcotics, such as cocaine. Most institutions have policies about medication administration and record keeping, especially for controlled medications and narcotics. Nurses must be aware of their employer's policies.

Nurses are not legally entitled to prescribe medications except in provinces where the designation of authorized nurse prescriber is available. In that instance, nurses must have completed the necessary education and registration requirements to be granted prescriptive authority for specified medications and devices (Almost, 2021). In several jurisdictions, NPs have the authority to prescribe certain medications specific to their area of practice. Which controlled substances nurse practitioners are authorized to prescribe, and what additional education is required for practising nurse practitioners to prescribe them, differs by province and territory (Almost, 2021).

The administration of medications in accordance with a prescription is a basic nursing responsibility. A competent nurse is expected to know the purpose and effect of any medication administered, as well as potential side effects and contraindications. It is also a nurse's responsibility to question any provider's order that may be incorrect or unsafe. A nurse who follows a prescriber's order that is unclear or incorrect may be found negligent, be disciplined, be dismissed by the employer, or be investigated by the professional regulatory body (CNPS, 2007).

Cannabis. Since 2018, the use of cannabis for medical and recreational purposes has been governed by the *Cannabis Act* (2018) and the associated *Cannabis Regulations* (2018). As use of cannabis grows, it is essential that nurses educate themselves on the federal, provincial, and territorial legislation governing its use and consult the latest evidence about the potential health benefits and risks of cannabinoids (CNPS, 2018b).

Communicable Diseases

The COVID-19 pandemic and outbreaks of other communicable diseases, such as HIV infection, hepatitis, and pandemic influenza, have raised legal implications for nurses (Finch, 2020). Health care providers are at risk for exposure to communicable diseases because of the nature of their work, and employers have an obligation to provide their employees with the necessary protective gear. Despite nurses' best efforts to protect themselves against communicable diseases through

the proper and consistent use of personal protective equipment such as masks and gloves, accidental injuries or life-threatening illnesses can occur. Nurses have an ethical and legal obligation to provide care to all assigned patients, and to mitigate their risks of contracting a work-related illness such as COVID-19 by diligently adhering to guidelines around the proper use of personal protective equipment.

There may be "some circumstances in which it is acceptable for a nurse to withdraw from care provision or to refuse to provide care" (British Columbia College of Nurses and Midwives, 2020b, p. 1). *Unreasonable burden* is a concept raised in relation to duty to provide care and withdrawing from providing or refusing to provide care: "An unreasonable burden exists when a nurse's ability to provide safe care and meet the standards of practice is compromised by unreasonable expectations, lack of resources, or ongoing threats to personal and family well-being" (CNA, 2017a, p. 38). For example, a nurse may be justified in refusing to provide care when there is insufficient protective equipment or staff to provide care safely. However, serious consideration must be given and all options must be exhausted before leaving patients without care, especially when it may mean that the patient will experience severe harm or death.

The courts have upheld an employer's right to fire a nurse who refuses to care for a patient with acquired immunodeficiency syndrome (AIDS). Nurses who flatly refuse to care for a patient with an infectious disease could be reprimanded or fired for insubordination. According to the CNA's (2017a) *Code of Ethics for Registered Nurses*, nurses must not discriminate on the basis of any attribute (p. 15). One limitation outlined in the *Code of Ethics* regarding a nurse's right to refuse care to a patient is that nurses are not obligated to comply with a patient's wishes when those wishes are contrary to the law. If the care requested is contrary to the nurse's personal values, such as assisting with an abortion or medical assistance in dying (MAiD), the nurse must provide appropriate care until alternative care arrangements can be made.

Nurses must be concerned with balancing the right to protect themselves with protection of the patient's rights. Both are afforded protection against discrimination and protection of privacy by human rights legislation. Most current legal cases involving nurses and communicable diseases are related to the protection needed for nurses as employees. Strict adherence with routine practices and the use of transmission-based precautions (e.g., against airborne or droplet transmission) for patients known or suspected of having other serious illnesses is the nurse's wisest strategy (see Chapter 34).

End-of-Life Issues

Many legal issues surround the end of life, one of which is the lack of a basic definition of death. There is no federal legislation in Canada that defines death. Most provinces have legislatively defined death as "the irreversible cessation of brain function" (Keatings & Adams, 2020). This "brain death" definition has become standard medical practice across Canada. Until the 1960s, death was defined as the irreversible cessation of cardiopulmonary function. However, two developments at that time necessitated a shift to consideration of the brain: (1) the emergence of artificial life-support devices that could maintain cardiopulmonary functioning in a brain-dead person, and (2) the emergence of organ transplantation. Death had to be redefined so that organs could be donated.

Homicide or Natural Death? The law draws a distinction between "killing" (an act of homicide) and "letting die." Withholding or withdrawing life-prolonging treatment is considered "letting die." The disease process causes the patient to die a natural death. A mentally competent patient has the legal right to refuse life-prolonging treatment. If, for example, such a patient requests that a ventilator be withdrawn, understanding that they will die as a result, their wishes must be honoured in accordance with the principle of "no treatment without consent."

In the case of *Nancy B. v. Hôtel-Dieu de Québec* (1992), a young, mentally competent patient (preferred pronouns: her/she) who was totally and permanently paralyzed by a neurological disease had twice asked that her ventilator be disconnected. After the second refusal, she sought a court order to enforce her will. The order was granted by the Quebec Superior Court, which ruled that as a mentally competent patient, she could not be treated without consent. Physicians may also terminate life-prolonging treatment when it no longer offers any reasonable hope of benefit to the person—even if the patient has not asked for the termination of life-prolonging treatment, either directly or by way of an advance directive—but must still consult family members before doing so (*Cuthbertson v. Rasouli*, 2013). When a patient rejects life-prolonging treatment, the nurse focuses on the goal of caring versus curing.

Ethical and legal questions are raised by the related issues of euthanasia and assisted suicide. Euthanasia is an act undertaken by one person with the motive of relieving another person's suffering and the knowledge that the act will end that person's life. This term is no longer common in Canada owing to the Supreme Court decision that led to the legalization of euthanasia under specific circumstances, called medical assistance in dying (MAiD). The case that led to MAiD legislation, known as *Carter v. Canada (AG)*, was brought forward by the B.C. Civil Liberties Association and a group of individuals, including Gloria Taylor, who was living with amyotrophic lateral sclerosis (*Carter v. Canada [AG]*, 2011).

In February 2015, the Supreme Court of Canada unanimously ruled in *Carter v. Canada* that some sections of the *Criminal Code* violated the right to life, liberty, and security of the person—a right protected by section 7 of the *Canadian Charter of Rights and Freedoms*—because those sections prohibited mentally competent adults from obtaining medical assistance to end their lives. This led to the tabling of Bill C-14, an Act to amend the *Criminal Code*, which would allow eligible individuals to request MAiD. The amended legislation came into effect on June 17, 2016, making it legally permissible for mentally competent adults who are suffering from a "grievous and irremediable medical illness, disease, or disability" in an advanced state causing intolerable suffering, to request MAiD. Following a court challenge (*Truchon v. Canada*, 2019) in Quebec in 2019, the Act was amended to clarify eligibility criteria (Box 10.2).

Only physicians or nurse practitioners can provide a person with MAiD, either by administering a substance that causes death (euthanasia or clinician-assisted death) or by prescribing a substance (self-administered assisted death). Nurses, however, can assist by participating in discussions with individuals and family members, advocating for aggressive symptom management, and continuing to provide routine care. Nurses are not required to participate in the provision of MAiD should they be morally opposed; however, the right to conscientious objection must be communicated to their supervisor as soon as the nurse anticipates such a conflict arising, and routine care of a patient planning an assisted death must not be abandoned.

It is essential that all health care providers have a thorough understanding of the law and of any related institutional processes and responsibilities (CNA, 2017b; CNPS, 2021d).

Advance Directives and Health Care Proxies

The advance directive is a mechanism that enables a mentally competent person to plan for a time when they may lack the mental capacity to make medical treatment decisions. It takes effect only when the

---

BOX 10.2   Eligibility Criteria for Medical Assistance in Dying (MAiD)

In order to be eligible for medical assistance in dying (MAiD), a person must meet *ALL* of the following criteria:
- The person is eligible for publicly funded health services in Canada.
- The person is at least 18 years of age and capable of making health care decisions.
- The person has a GRIEVOUS and IRREMEDIABLE MEDICAL condition.
- The patient makes a voluntary request (no coercion) in writing (or by proxy, if the patient is unable to write), signed and dated in the presence of two independent witnesses.
- The patient must provide informed consent after being informed of all therapeutic options to relieve their suffering.

The definition of a GRIEVOUS and IRREMEDIABLE MEDICAL condition must meet *ALL* of the following criteria:
- The person must have a serious illness, disease, or disability.
- The person must be in an advanced state of decline that ***cannot*** be reversed.
- The person must experience unbearable physical or mental suffering from the illness, disease, or disability, or a state of decline that ***cannot*** be relieved under conditions that the person considers acceptable.

The following procedural safeguards are required:
- A written request must be made and signed by an independent witness.
- Two independent doctors or nurse practitioners must provide an assessment and confirm that all of the eligibility requirements are met.
- The person must be informed that they can withdraw their request at any time, in any manner.
- The person must be given an opportunity to withdraw consent and must expressly confirm their consent immediately before receiving MAiD.

Furthermore, if the patient's health condition is such that their natural death is not reasonably foreseeable, the patient must also—over a period of at least 90 days—consult with practitioners who have expertise in their health condition to ensure they are aware of all options to relieve their suffering.

From *An Act to amend the Criminal Code and to make related amendments to other Acts (medical assistance in dying)*, SC 2016, c. 3. http://laws-lois.justice.gc.ca/eng/AnnualStatutes/2016_3/FullText.html; *An Act to amend the Criminal Code (medical assistance in dying)*, SC 2021, c. 2. https://laws.justice.gc.ca/eng/AnnualStatutes/2021_2/FullText.html

---

person becomes incapable of speaking for themselves. Advance directives often outline treatment preferences and authorize a particular person to act as a proxy, or substitute decision maker, to make health care decisions on behalf of a patient who is unable to communicate their wishes. The advance directive is a more sophisticated concept than that of the living will, although the two terms are often confused. A living will is a document in which the person makes an anticipatory refusal of life-prolonging measures during a future state of mental incompetence. An advance directive, in contrast, is not restricted to the rejection of life-support measures; its focus is on values and preferences and may include both requests for and refusals of treatment.

If nurses know about the existence of a health care directive, they are required to follow it. Nurses are also required to follow the wishes of a validly appointed proxy (assuming these instructions are legal). A proxy has the right to receive all medical information concerning the patient's condition and proposed plan of care. Failure to comply with a proxy's directions could result in charges of battery.

If another provider ignores the advance directive, the nurse must bring the directive to their attention and document that they did so, along with their response to this information. The nurse should also notify the nursing supervisor, who can then give direction regarding institutional policies and guidelines for such circumstances.

The *psychiatric advance directive* is a new type of advance directive. An individual with mental health issues completes this type of directive during periods of mental stability and competence. The directive outlines how the patient wishes to be treated in the future if the underlying mental illness causes them to lose decision-making capacity. For example, it may specify preferences for and against certain interventions (e.g., electroconvulsive therapy) or medications. The psychiatric advance directive can also designate a surrogate decision maker to act on the person's behalf in the event of an incapacitating mental health crisis.

Organ Donation

Legally competent people are free to donate their bodies or organs for medical use. Every province or territory has legislation that provides for donation of tissues and organs by deceased and living donors. For example, a mentally competent adult can donate a kidney, a lobe of the liver, or bone marrow. If a deceased person has left no direction for postmortem donation, consent is obtained from their family. Nova Scotia is the first province to enact "opt-out" consent for organ donation. The *Human Organ and Tissue Donation Act* (2019), which took effect in 2021, deems consent to donate as granted unless a person has recorded their refusal on a registry. The intent of this deemed or presumed consent is to increase the availability of donor organs. In some provinces, like Manitoba, the statutes contain "required request" provisions that take effect when a deceased person did not consent to organ removal but is considered a good donor candidate (*Human Tissue Gift Act,* 1987). In such an event, the physician is legally obliged to approach the family to consider donation. In many hospitals, a nurse transplantation coordinator performs this function. Since organs cannot be procured for transplant until death has been pronounced, and because of the critical shortage of organs available for transplant, national guidelines for pronouncing cardiac death for organ donation have been developed. Given variation across the country, it is essential that nurses be familiar with relevant provincial or territorial laws as well as institutional regulations (Norris, 2020).

Mental Health Issues

Treating patients with mental health challenges raises legal and ethical issues. Provincial mental health legislation such as the *Mental Health and Consequential Amendments Act* (1998) provides direction for health care providers, protects patient autonomy, and recognizes that some individuals with severe mental health issues may lack the ability to appreciate the consequences of their health condition.

A patient can be admitted to a psychiatric unit involuntarily or voluntarily. Patients admitted voluntarily have the right to refuse treatment and the right to discharge themselves from the hospital. However, provincial or territorial mental health legislation provides that if the patient may cause harm to self or others, police (or other authorized parties) may bring the patient to a health care facility for examination and treatment without the patient's consent (Carver, 2013).

Potentially suicidal patients may be admitted to psychiatric units. If the patient's history and medical records indicate suicidal tendencies, the patient may be kept under supervision. A lawsuit may result if a patient attempts suicide within the hospital. The allegations in the lawsuits would be that the institution failed to provide adequate supervision or safeguard the facilities. Documentation of precautions against suicide is essential.

Public Health Issues

Nurses must understand public health laws, especially if they are employed in community health settings. Public health acts, which have been enacted in all provinces and territories, are directed toward the prevention, treatment, and suppression of communicable disease (Schulz, 2013). They include orders such as those for mandatory quarantine, restriction of public gatherings, and mask-wearing—the same orders that were imposed throughout the COVID-19 pandemic. Community health nurses have the legal responsibility to follow the laws enacted to protect public health. These laws may include reporting suspected abuse and neglect, such as child abuse, elder abuse, or intimate partner violence; reporting communicable diseases; and reporting other health-related issues to protect the public's health.

Some provinces (e.g., Ontario and New Brunswick) have legislation that requires proof of immunization for school entry. However, exceptions in these provinces are permitted on medical or religious grounds and for reasons of conscience (Wilson et al., 2019). Although a signed consent form is not required for immunization, nurses are advised to obtain some documentation (evidence) that they discussed the risks and benefits. Nurses should be aware of their employer guidelines for documentation.

Every province and territory has child abuse legislation that requires the reporting of witnessed or suspected child abuse or neglect directly to child protection agencies. To encourage reports of suspected cases, the laws offer legal immunity for the reporter if the report is made in good faith. Nurses who do not report suspected child abuse or neglect may be held liable for civil or criminal action. Several provinces and territories also have laws that require health care providers to report witnessed or suspected abuse of patients within facilities (e.g., Manitoba *Protection of Persons in Care Act*, 2000). Even if not required by law, nurses should report all suspicions of patient abuse to their nursing supervisors. It is essential for nurses to know their provincial or territorial laws and employer policies regarding the reporting of abuse.

RISK MANAGEMENT

In the health care context, **risk management** is a system that ensures the appropriate delivery of nursing care by identifying potential hazards in order to prevent harm to patients (Keatings & Adams, 2020). The steps involved in risk management include identifying possible risks, analyzing them, acting to reduce them, and evaluating the steps taken.

One tool used in risk management is the **incident report**, or **adverse occurrence report**. When a patient is harmed or endangered by incorrect care, such as a medication error, a nurse completes an incident report (see Chapter 16). Such reports are analyzed to determine how future problems can be avoided. For example, if incident reports show that medication errors commonly involve a new intravenous pump, the risk manager must ensure that staff members have been properly trained in its use. In-service education may be all that is necessary to prevent future errors; however, quality care is the responsibility of both the employer and the individual provider.

Risk management requires sufficient documentation. The nurse's documentation can be the evidence of what was done for a patient and can serve as proof that the nurse acted reasonably and safely. Documentation should be thorough, accurate, and performed in a timely manner. When a lawsuit is being evaluated, the nurse's notes are very often the first record to be reviewed by the plaintiff's counsel. If the nurse's credibility is questioned because of these documents, the nurse faces the risk of greater liability. The nurse's notes act as risk management and quality assurance tools for the employer and the individual nurse.

KEY CONCEPTS

- With increased emphasis on patient rights, nurses in practice today must understand their legal obligations and responsibilities to patients.

- The civil law system is concerned with the protection of a person's private rights, while the criminal law system deals with the rights of individuals and society.
- A nurse can be found liable for negligence if the following criteria are established: the nurse (defendant) owed a duty of care to the patient (plaintiff), the nurse did not carry out that duty, the patient was injured, and the nurse's failure to carry out the duty caused the patient's injury.
- Patients are entitled to confidential health care and freedom from unauthorized release of information.
- Under the law, practising nurses must follow standards of care. These standards originate in nursing practice acts and regulations, the guidelines of professional organizations, and the written policies and procedures of employing institutions.
- Nurses are responsible for confirming that a patient has given informed consent to any surgery or other medical procedure before the procedure is performed.
- Nurses are responsible for performing all procedures correctly and exercising professional judgement as they carry out a prescriber's orders.
- Nurses are obligated to follow a prescriber's orders unless they believe the orders are in error or could be detrimental to patients.
- Staffing standards determine the ratio of nurses to patients. If the nurse is required to care for more patients than is reasonable, a formal protest should be made to the nursing administration.
- Mentally competent adults suffering from a "grievous and irremediable medical illness, disease or disability" in an advanced state may request medical assistance in dying.
- A competent adult can legally give consent to donate specific organs, and nurses may serve as witnesses to this decision.
- All nurses should know the laws that apply to their area of practice.
- Depending on provincial/territorial statutes, nurses are required to report suspected child abuse and certain communicable diseases.
- Nurses are patient advocates and ensure quality of care through risk management and lobbying for safe nursing practice standards.
- Nurses must file incident or adverse occurrence reports in all situations when someone could or did get hurt.

CRITICAL THINKING EXERCISES

1. Nurse Rossi and Nurse Kao are getting on an elevator to go down to the cafeteria. Several visitors are present in the elevator, as are hospital personnel. Nurse Rossi and Nurse Kao are talking about a patient in the critical care unit who has just tested positive for HIV infection. They identify the patient as "the patient in Room 14B." Several visitors in the elevator overhear this information; one of them is the fiancée of the patient in Room 14B.
   a. Have Nurse Rossi and Nurse Kao breached a patient's right to confidential health care?
   b. Would the patient in Room 14B have any legal cause of action against the nurses?
   c. Even though the patient's fiancée may have a right to know the HIV status of their future spouse, do the nurses have any duty to disclose confidential information to the fiancée?
2. Nurse Reyes is caring for a patient with end-stage heart failure. One day, the patient asks Nurse Reyes for information on medical assistance in dying (MAiD). Although she knows it is legal, Nurse Reyes feels that MAiD is unethical. What are her obligations in response to the patient's request?

Answers to Critical Thinking Exercises appear on the Evolve website.

REVIEW QUESTIONS

Review Questions 1 to 8 relate to the case study at the beginning of the chapter.

1. What should the nurse have done when a preceptor or supervisor was unavailable?
   a. Documented their thought process before administering the medication.
   b. Looked for further orders on the resident's medical record.
   c. Waited for a nurse to be available to confirm that the medication should be given.
   d. Provide the medication, but wait with the resident to ensure that she does not have a reaction.
2. If the nurse is found to have made a medication error that results in injury or death, it would be an example of which type of liability?
   a. False imprisonment
   b. Assault
   c. Battery
   d. Negligence
3. After this error, the resident's family names the nurse in a lawsuit. Which of the following statements is correct? *(Select all that apply.)*
   a. The nurse does not need any representation.
   b. The resident must prove that harm or injury occurred.
   c. The resident must show that the nurse provided substandard care.
   d. The resident must show that the nurse's actions or inaction caused the injury.
   e. The burden of proof is always the responsibility of the nurse.
4. If DJ's error resulted in harm and DJ were named in a lawsuit, then who would generally hold liability?
   a. Student
   b. Student's instructor or preceptor
   c. Hospital or health care facility
   d. All of the above
5. The duty of care conferred on DJ by virtue of their being assigned to care for the resident meant that DJ was obligated to administer the resident's medication, unless:
   a. The order was a verbal order issued outside of an emergency situation.
   b. The prescriber's order is illegible.
   c. The nurse has questions or concerns about the order.
   d. The order is in error, violates hospital policy, or would be detrimental to the patient.
   e. All of the above.
6. What should DJ have done when the availability of nursing staff was insufficient to meet the standards of care, such as double-checking a medication prior to its administration? *(Select all that apply.)*
   a. Notify their supervisor and complete a workload or staffing report form.
   b. Take care of the sickest patients and delegate tasks to unregulated health care providers.
   c. Refuse to provide care until safe staffing levels can be restored.
   d. Post their concerns on social media.
7. The resident's family makes a complaint against DJ to the province's nursing regulator. What type of discipline might DJ face?
   a. None. DJ is a student, so the regulator has no jurisdiction.
   b. DJ could be fined or suspended from practising nursing.
   c. DJ's license could be revoked.
   d. DJ could be held liable by the regulator for negligence.

8. What mitigating factors might a court find that reduce DJ's liability for negligence in this case?
   a. Prompt and accurate charting of the administration of the resident's medications.
   b. The resident's history of stable blood pressure that is consistent with DJ's assessment findings.
   c. Completion of the "10 rights" of medication administration.
   d. Testimony that DJ acted with kindness and concern for the resident's well-being.

Answers: 1. c; 2. d; 3. b; c; 4. d; 5. e; 6. a; b; 7. a; 8. b.

🌐 *Rationales for the Review Questions appear on the Evolve website.*

RECOMMENDED WEBSITES

Canadian Council of Registered Nurse Regulators: http://www.ccrnr.ca/members.html
This website provides links to all provincial and territorial nursing colleges and associations.
Canadian Nurses Protective Society (CNPS): http://www.cnps.ca
The CNPS helps nurses manage their professional legal risks by offering legal support and liability protection. The members-only section of the website provides information on a variety of legal topics relevant to nursing practice in Canada.

Department of Justice Canada: https://www.justice.gc.ca
This website provides links to consolidated statutes, including the *Criminal Code, 1985*.
Health Law Institute—End-of-Life Law and Policy in Canada: http://eol.law.dal.ca/?page_id=221
The Health Law Institute at Dalhousie University provides information about Canadian legislation pertaining to various aspects of end-of-life care, including advance directives and the withholding of life-sustaining treatment.

🌐 REFERENCES

A full reference list is available on the website for this book at http://evolve.elsevier.com/Canada/Potter/fundamentals/

11

Global and Planetary Health

Written by Barbara J. Astle, RN, PhD, FCAN, Katrina Plamondon, RN, MSc, PhD, and Bukola (Oladunni) Salami, RN, MN, PhD, FCAN

OBJECTIVES

Mastery of content in this chapter will enable you to:

- Differentiate between global health and planetary health.
- Describe critical perspectives for understanding global and planetary health.
- Describe the interconnectedness between planetary health and the health of humans, other species, and the physical environment.
- Describe the current impact of global and planetary health issues (climate change) on the health care system.
- Recognize and understand epidemiological trends and patterns in the global burden of disease and their relationship to population health.

- Describe the history of the shift from the United Nations Millennium Development Goals to the United Nations Sustainable Development Goals.
- Describe the impact of immigration and migration trends on population health in Canada.
- Describe the concepts of global citizenship and the professional roles of nursing in a global world.
- Describe the role of nurses in responding to global and planetary health challenges.

KEY TERMS

Anthropocene

Asylum seekers

Climate change

Climate justice

Communicable diseases

Coronavirus disease (COVID-19)

Determinants of planetary health from an Indigenous perspective

Displaced persons

Ebola

Environmental justice

Environmental racism

Environmental sustainability

Gender equality

Global burden of disease (GBD)

Global citizen

Global citizenship

Global health

Global health competencies

Global warming

Globalization

Governance

H1N1 virus

Health disparities

Health equity

Health inequities

Intersectionality

Millennium Development Goals (MDGs)

Multiculturalism

Noncommunicable diseases (NCDs)

One Health

Pandemic

Paris Agreement

Planetary citizenship

Planetary health

Planetary Health Education Framework

Political economy

Refugees

Severe acute respiratory syndrome (SARS)

Social and structural determinants of health

Sustainable Development Goals (SDGs)

Transnationalism

Variants

🌐 WEBSITE

http://evolve.elsevier.com/Canada/Potter/fundamentals/

CASE STUDY

Migrant Agricultural Workers' Access to Health Care

Elijah (preferred pronouns: he/him) is a triage nurse working in an emergency room in southern Ontario. Early in the summer, a person (he/him) approaches the triage station wincing in pain and cradling his arm, which appears to be broken. A second person accompanies him. Elijah greets both of them and asks what brings them to the emergency room. The two individuals look at one other, and then the person accompanying the injured man responds by saying, "This is Pablo. He doesn't speak much English. He hurt his arm at home today

and I'll be staying with him to make sure he understands what's going on." Elijah turns to Pablo, acknowledges the injury, and asks him what language he speaks. Pablo responds that he speaks a little English, but mostly Spanish. Elijah invites Pablo to proceed to the waiting area until he can be assessed. Knowing that thousands of seasonal agricultural workers are currently working in the area, and recalling a recent article highlighting what nurses can do to support them, Elijah searches for that article online. He recognizes that there

Continued

Migrant Agricultural Workers' Access to Health Care

are many issues of equity at play in the context of temporary foreign workers who live seasonally in Canada. Finding two relevant articles, he discovers that an important first step is to ask Pablo whether he works in agriculture and how long he will be staying in Canada. Next, to ensure that Pablo receives the care and supports needed, Elijah contacts the hospital's translation team and a local Spanish-speaking outreach worker from an organization that supports migrant workers. Elijah recognizes that Pablo faces many social determinants of health that require specific attention so that he can access care, safely disclose details about his injury, connect with benefits such as worker's compensation, and receive follow-up care.

Think about this case study as you read this chapter. There are Review Questions at the end of the chapter about this case study.

GLOBAL HEALTH—DEFINITIONS AND EXPLANATIONS

As the twenty-first century unfolds, nurses will play a key role in examining global and planetary health issues, developing solutions, and implementing change both locally and internationally. Perhaps more than ever before, the multiple planetary crises facing humanity—the COVID-19 pandemic, climate change, and biodiversity loss—have starkly revealed the ways in which global processes, policies, and issues intimately affect the health of people and the planet (Astle et al., 2020; Intergovernmental Panel on Climate Change [IPCC], 2021; Plamondon, 2021; Potter, 2019; Potter et al., 2021; Salvage & White, 2020). Nurses must be well versed in the key concepts related to a myriad of global health issues (Canadian Association of Schools of Nursing [CASN], 2022) and the emerging field of planetary health (CASN, 2022; Astle, 2021a; Kurth, 2017; Myers & Frumkin, 2020).

Inherently global health issues—including, for example, macroeconomic policy, pandemics, the climate crisis, and migration—transcend national borders and jurisdictions, such that their scope extends beyond the reach of any one country (Labonté et al., 2003). It is imperative that our collective responses to these pressing health and social challenges be informed by an understanding of health equity and social justice in order to develop solutions that meet the needs of diverse populations worldwide (CASN, 2022; International Council of Nurses [ICN], 2021). As António Guterres, the United Nations Secretary-General reminds us, "Making peace with nature is the defining task of the twenty-first century" (United Nations, 2020, p. 3), and "[t]he fallout of the assault on our planet is impeding our efforts to eliminate poverty and imperiling food security" (p. 2). As one of the world's most trusted professions, comprising the majority of the global health care workforce, nurses have an important role to play in responding to inherently global health issues. Nursing's responsibility for global and planetary health is consistent with our history in advocating for social justice, and it is critical that we play a leadership role in minimizing or eliminating health inequities (Astle, 2021a).

Global health refers to "the optimal well-being of all humans from the individual and collective perspective and is considered a fundamental human right, which should be accessible to all" (Canadian Nurses Association [CNA], 2009, p. 1). According to Koplan and colleagues (2009), global health encompasses prevention, treatment, and care while focusing on the improvement of health for all. These authors argue that in addition to transnational health issues, global health is concerned with domestic health disparities. Rather than being tied to geography, "the *global* in global health refers to the scope of problems, not their location" (Koplan et al., 2009, p. 1994). Global health also requires an attentiveness to forces and processes that unfold at an inherently global level and manifest in local experiences. For example, poverty in inner-city neighbourhoods, limited access to health care in rural communities, and high rates of malaria among sub-Saharan African children are all examples of global health issues for which local experiences are connected to processes and policies far beyond the boundaries of a neighbourhood or community. Interprofessional collaboration and authentic partnerships between high-income and low-or middle-income countries are required in order to develop effective solutions to these complex health issues and thus achieve global health (Koplan et al., 2009).

Koplan and colleagues (2009) also suggest that global health overlaps with concepts derived from the disciplines of public health and international health. Though both *international health* and *global health* are terms that remain in use today, the latter began to replace *international health* in the mid-2000s. *International health* becomes global health when the focus of understanding the causes or consequences of a health issue transcend national borders (Lee et al., 2002) and when broad global political, historical, and social contexts and issues are considered (Brown et al., 2006). Each of these domains shares several common characteristics: a population-based and preventative focus, work with marginalized populations, a focus on interprofessional approaches, acknowledgement that health is a public good, an emphasis on systems and structures, and participation with key stakeholders. Most importantly, these terms overlap and more than one term might be relevant in a given context—they are not mutually exclusive.

Global Health Governance and Global Institutions

Governance occurs at local, national, and international levels and involves "efforts societies make to organize and exercise political power in response to challenges and opportunities they face" (Fidler, 2007, p. 2). Global health governance brings together actors from across different sectors to develop mechanisms to respond to complex global issues (Dodgson et al., 2002; Kickbusch & Szabo, 2014). Several international institutions play central roles in global health governance. International financial institutions, such as the World Bank and the World Trade Organization, emerged from the post–World War II Bretton Woods System to govern macroeconomic policy and directly impact social determinants of health worldwide (Kay & Owain, 2009). Also established following WWII, the World Health Organization (WHO) and the United Nations (UN) play important roles in global health governance.

In the twenty-first century, the global health governance landscape has grown increasingly complex. Private-sector actors hold significant power and resources, affording large corporations such as pharmaceutical and tobacco companies a strong voice in trade-related policies that affect health (Lee et al., 2009). Multilateral organizations such as the Global Fund to Fight Aids, Tuberculosis, and Malaria (The Global Fund, 2022) and philanthropic organizations such as the Bill and Melinda Gates Foundation (2022) are now among the influential bodies shaping global health governance. Critical to understanding and working toward improving collective global health, for all people, is recognition that this landscape is being shaped by an uneven and inequitable distribution of power that privileges and amplifies the interests of high-income countries at the expense of low- and middle-income countries, and, arguably, of the planet (Smith et al., 2017; Sparke et al., 2022). Indeed, a complex and interdependent relationship exists between global health and governance.

Millennium Development Goals and Sustainable Development Goals

In 2000, the UN General Assembly established eight Millennium Development Goals (MDGs) to address key health and development issues affecting the global community (United Nations, 2015). A target date of 2015 was established to meet these goals. The MDGs were instrumental in creating a global partnership between all countries of the world and development institutions (United Nations, 2015). While many achievements were made to meet the MDG targets, including a reduction in poverty, educational improvements, a reduction in child and maternal mortality, and improvements in lowering the incidence of human immunodeficiency virus (HIV), tuberculosis, and malaria, gaps between and within countries remain, with vulnerable populations the most at risk.

In September 2015, in an effort to build on the MDGs, the UN General Assembly adopted the Sustainable Development Goals (SDGs) (WHO, 2022a) which focus largely on the social determinants of health, and wellbeing, poverty and sustainability. The SDGs include 17 universal goals (Box 11.1) and 169 targets planned for the next 15 years

| BOX 11.1 | The 17 Sustainable Development Goals Adopted by the UN General Assembly |

1. End poverty in all its forms, everywhere.
2. End hunger, achieve food security and improved nutrition, and promote sustainable agriculture.
3. Ensure healthy lives and promote well-being for all at all ages.
4. Ensure inclusive and equitable quality education and promote lifelong learning opportunities for all.
5. Achieve gender equality and empower all women and girls.
6. Ensure availability and sustainable management of water and sanitation for all.
7. Ensure access to affordable, reliable, sustainable, and modern energy for all.
8. Promote sustained, inclusive, and sustainable economic growth, full and productive employment, and decent work for all.
9. Build resilient infrastructure, promote inclusive and sustainable industrialization, and foster innovation.
10. Reduce inequality within and among countries.
11. Make cities and human settlements inclusive, safe, resilient, and sustainable.
12. Ensure sustainable consumption and production patterns.
13. Take urgent action to combat climate change and its impacts.
14. Conserve and sustainably use the oceans, seas, and marine resources for sustainable development.
15. Protect, restore, and promote sustainable use of terrestrial ecosystems, sustainably manage forests, combat desertification, and halt and reverse land degradation and halt biodiversity loss.
16. Promote peaceful and inclusive societies for sustainable development, provide access to justice for all, and build effective, accountable, and inclusive institutions at all levels.
17. Strengthen the means of implementation and revitalize the global partnership for sustainable development.

From United Nations. (2017). *Sustainable development goals.* https://sdgs.un.org/goals

that address the health and well-being of persons of all ages, including newborns, children, adolescents, and middle-aged and older persons (United Nations, 2017a). What makes the SDGs unique is that they call on all countries to promote prosperity while protecting the planet. Although the SDGs are not legally binding, there is an expectation that governments worldwide will assume ownership and establish national frameworks to achieve the 17 goals (United Nations, 2017b). SDG 3 targets health directly, while five other goals focus on environmental concerns. This approach aligns with a planetary perspective on health. The goals are primarily focused on ending poverty, protecting the planet, and ensuring prosperity (WHO, 2022a). The UN General Assembly has been closely monitoring the progress of member states and will continue doing so until 2030 (WHO, 2022a).

Nurses have an important role in attaining the SDGs, as these goals directly relate to the social determinants of health; the International Council of Nurses has stated that "nurses, as the primary providers of health care to all communities in all settings, are key to the achievement of the SDGs" (ICN, 2021, p. 3).

Global Health Indicators

In order for nurses to address and understand some of the key issues in global health, they must have access to reliable global health indicators. Nurses also need to acknowledge that the indicators used for comparative purposes are not perfect, and that some are more equity-centred than others. Therefore, it is essential to have the most comprehensive sources and updated statistics (Organisation for Economic Co-operation and Development, 2021).

The Global Burden of Disease (GBD) study, led by the Institute for Health Metrics and Evaluation, is an example of using metrics to quantify the health of populations at the regional, country, and other subnational levels (Skolnik, 2021). The GBD study has provided the most comprehensive global observational epidemiological data to date. This information helps track progress between and within countries, informing clinicians, researchers, and policymakers in their efforts to promote accountability and improve lives (The Lancet, 2022). Specific GBD data include estimates of morbidity and mortality by cause, sex, age, and country from 1990 to the present. In global health work, the composite indicator of health status that is most commonly used is called the disability-adjusted life year, or DALY. This indicator is consistently used in GBD studies. The DALY is the sum of years lost due to premature death (YLLs) and years lived with disability (YLDs). For example, for a man in Denmark who dies at age 50 with hypertension, he would have 25 years lost (YLLs), assuming that the highest life expectancy for males in Denmark is 75 years. If this same Danish man lived with this disease for 10 years, and hypertension was assigned a burden of 0.5, then he would have lived with this disability for $10 \times 0.5 = 5$ YLDs. The DALY for this individual would be $25 + 5 = 30$ years.

THEORETICAL PERSPECTIVES ON GLOBAL HEALTH

Health Equity and Health Inequities

Health equity is an aspirational concept that reflects values of social justice (Braveman, 2014; Braveman et al., 2011; Reutter & Kushner, 2010) and is fundamental to understanding and achieving global health (see Chapter 4 for further information social justice and population health). Achieving health equity means that all people (individuals, groups, and communities) are able to reach their full health potential without being disadvantaged by social, economic, or environmental conditions (National Collaborating Centre for Determinants of Health, 2015). Braveman and colleagues (2011) caution that health inequity includes a moral judgement about the causality of differences, and suggest that measurement of health inequities relies on quantifying health disparities. Advancing health equity is recognized as one of the single most important investments in health (Canadian Institutes of Health Research, 2021) and is a critical and necessary element to upholding human rights and achieving health for all.

Researchers have found that the greater the gap between a population's richest and poorest people, the greater the differences in health between them (Marmot & Bell, 2012; Ottersen et al., 2014; Schrecker & Labonté, 2021). **Health disparities** are defined as

> a particular type of health difference that is linked with social, economic, and/or environmental disadvantage. Health disparities adversely affect groups of people who have systematically experienced greater obstacles to health based on their racial or ethnic group; religion; socioeconomic status; gender; age; mental health; cognitive, sensory, or physical disability; sexual orientation or gender identity; geographic location; or other characteristics historically linked to discrimination or exclusion.
>
> ***Healthy People, 2014, para. 5***

By contrast, **health inequities** refer to those inequalities in health that are deemed to be unfair or that stem from some form of injustice. Unequal and unfair systems of power between and within nation-states perpetuate health inequities by disproportionately protecting some lives at the cost of others (Came & Griffith, 2018; Pan American Health Organization [PAHO], 2019). Differences in life trajectories and health outcomes across intersecting social positionalities (such as class, race, ability, gender, etc.) are unjust because they reflect an unfair distribution of the underlying **social and structural determinants of health** (for example, access to educational opportunities, safe jobs, health care, and social self-respect)" (Raphael, 2016). (See Chapter 1 for further information on the social determinants of health.)

Indeed, the influence of the social and structural determinants of health on health outcomes repeatedly reveals the same pattern, regardless of what scale or issue is examined. Whether looking at data about the prevalence of infectious diseases such as HIV/AIDS, noncommunicable diseases (e.g., diabetes, cardiovascular disease), life expectancy, maternal and child health outcomes, or the distribution of hunger and poverty, health inequities consistently reflect patterns of an unfair distribution of power, resources, and wealth. Health inequities place disadvantaged groups at further unearned disadvantage. Importantly, unearned disadvantage can only exist in the presence of unearned advantage, where access to resources is unfairly privileging particular people and excluding others (Nixon, 2019). The inability of all persons living with HIV in sub-Saharan Africa to access care and treatment is an example of a health equity issue.

Reutter and Kushner (2010) argue that nursing has a strong and clear mandate to reduce health inequities among individuals, families, and communities, as well as a mandate to address the social conditions that contribute to health inequities. These authors suggest that nurses must provide sensitive, empowering care to individuals experiencing health inequities and, at the same time, participate in policy analysis and advocacy to promote equity and reduce inequities.

Intersectionality

Intersectionality is a theoretical perspective regarding the influence of different social characteristics—race, ethnicity, gender, class, and socioeconomic status—on a particular phenomenon, such as the experience of health and its outcomes. Intersectionality was first introduced by Kimberlé Crenshaw (1989) as a theory to challenge the idea that race and gender are mutually exclusive categories. Crenshaw (1989) argues that the inclusion of a single-issue framework for addressing discrimination marginalizes Black women and girls. For example, Black women and girls are often excluded from feminist discourse and

anti-racist policy because both are based on distinct sets of experiences that do not consider the interaction of gender and race. Much of anti-racist discourse focuses on what happens to middle-class Black men, and much of feminist discourse focus on what happens to middle-class White women. Intersectionality moves beyond first- and second-wave feminist perspectives that essentialize the experiences of women. It examines the question of sameness and difference and its relation to power (Cho et al., 2013). It conceives of diverse social locations (including gender, race, class, etc.) as being fluid and independent. Diverse social categories are always permeated by other categories and are always changing and in the process of being created and creating dynamics of power.

Crenshaw (1991) subsequently proposed three types of intersectionality: structural intersectionality, political intersectionality, and representational intersectionality. *Structural intersectionality* asserts that intersectionality-based interventions must consider multiple social locations, including gender, race, income, immigration status, and so on, and how these intersect. In Canada, structural barriers experienced by racialized women can include income status, housing, immigration status, and linguistic ability. These can intersect with gender and race to affect the experiences of immigrant women, including in cases of domestic violence. Interventions and strategies based solely on the experiences of women will not be effective for racialized women because these interventions do not consider the structural issues affecting their lives, including poor housing, income, and racism. *Political intersectionality* highlights the fact that women and girls are situated within at least two subordinated social locations (e.g., Black and girl) and these groups often pursue conflicting political agendas. *Representational intersectionality* is concerned with the production of images of Black people across gender lines in a way that ignores the intersectionality interests of Black people.

Intersectionality has been used by Canadian nursing and health researchers to examine global health issues (Clark & Vissandjée, 2019; Hankivsky & Mussell, 2018; Kapilashrami & Hankivsky, 2018; Lane, 2020). Hankivsky and Christoffersen (2008) argue that intersectionality can contribute to our understanding of social determinants of health in Canada. Social determinants of health cannot be reduced to one single determinant or marker of difference; rather, diverse social determinants of health interact to contribute to population health in Canada. Intersectionality can help illuminate how diverse social inequities interact to manifest health inequities. For instance, by examining the interconnections between social relationships, dominance, and oppression, deeper insights may be revealed about a person's mental health status (Hankivsky et al., 2010). Intersectionality helps us to extend the analytical boundaries of what we think we know about the health context of the human condition, to recognize that "these [multiple dimensions of social identity] come together in distinct ways and lead to distinct health outcomes for individuals [and] groups, providing context to health experiences and drawing attention to the dynamic interplay between different system levels" (Van Herk et al., 2011, p. 30).

An understanding of intersectionality is useful to nursing and offers a way to think about and make sense of the complexities of human experience. Intersectionality is useful for building nursing knowledge. Nursing as a discipline pays attention to the needs of underserved or disadvantaged people across the lifespan. Intersectionality offers a way to challenge the status quo and to generate knowledge and action that focuses on improving the welfare of marginalized and at-risk groups. A deeper understanding of poverty, marginalization, subordination, social exclusion, and social injustice will help direct attention toward reducing and eventually eliminating these conditions. Critical reflection related to the health of women, children, and families, as well as solutions to challenges arising from the complexities of gender and its interactions, are needed (Hankivsky, 2012; Hankivsky & Cormier, 2009).

Nurses are well positioned to influence multi-level root causes of health disparities that deny people access to health services. Iyer and colleagues (2008) conducted a literature review of class and gender and argued that a deeper understanding of the intersection of these two concepts was required. The review revealed that the interactions of class and gender played a significant role in the health of women and their access to health services in high- and low-income countries (Iyer et al., 2008). Thus, intersectionality helped the researchers to consider multiple factors to explain health outcomes and understand the interrelationships between these factors.

Postcolonialism

Colonial and neocolonial (i.e., new and present forms of colonial relations) policies continue to shape health outcomes across the globe, including for Indigenous peoples in Canada. For example, Canada's history of slavery of Indigenous peoples and Black people as well as residential schools continue to contribute to health and social disparities in Canada. Cultural genocide of Indigenous peoples in Canada continues to perpetuate health and social inequities for Indigenous populations. Nurse researchers in Canada have used a postcolonial theoretical lens to shed light on health disparities (Anderson, 2002; Browne et al., 2005; Kirkham & Anderson, 2002; Racine, 2003). Postcolonial theory offers insight into how colonial relations, and the unequal relations of power embedded in them, continue to perpetuate inequities across the globe. Furthermore, a postcolonial feminist framework understands the impact of colonialism, imperialism, and gender inequities on health outcomes. A nurse using a postcolonial lens may consider how historical colonial relations with the population they are providing care to may influence the distribution of resources, access to care, and health outcomes for populations. A nurse using this orientation may also critique perspectives related to knowledge and knowledge production. Colonial orientation often views Western knowledge as the most superior knowledge or Western-educated professionals as the most knowledgeable. A postcolonial (or anticolonial) lens challenges this perspective by embracing other forms of knowledge, including Indigenous knowledge systems. A postcolonial theoretical lens also encourages nurses to be antiracist and to continue to reflect on how their own social location may affect the health care that they deliver in a global context.

Political Economy

Global health governance bodies play a role in shaping a political economy of health. **Political economy** involves the intersecting mechanisms, political ideologies, and systems of power that structure public policy to distribute resources (including health resources), wealth, and power and shape health care delivery (Bryant et al., 2019). Global health governance and political economy go hand in hand, with political economy offering a framework for understanding what and how institutions and social structures work to shape the distribution of social, political, and economic resources that affect health inequities and disparities among people. The Commission of the Pan-American Health Organization on Equity and Inequalities in the Americas framework (PAHO, 2019) directly connects structural drivers of health (e.g., histories of colonialism; racism; climate change; political, social, cultural, and economic structures) to conditions of daily life (e.g., early life and education; working life; income; environment; housing; health systems), framing these as instrumental forces that make health equity and dignified lives possible.

Globalization, Transnationalism, and Health

Among the inherently global health issues that nurses need to understand are the processes of globalization and transnationalism, both of which pose important questions for nursing practice, research, and ethics. **Globalization** is a "constellation of processes by which nations, businesses and people are becoming more connected and interdependent via increased economic integration and communication exchange, cultural diffusion (especially of Western culture) and travel" (Labonté & Torgerson, 2005, p. 158). Although the movement of people and ideas around the globe is not new, the speed and depth of economic globalization accelerated beginning in the 1980s and continuing into the twenty-first century in ways that have shaped the social and structural determinants of health.

Neoliberal capitalism has characterized globalization during this time. Some have argued that neoliberalism extends beyond economic policy or governance models to be an "order of reason" (Brown, 2015, p. 20). As the dominant political discourse, neoliberalism directly shapes the policy environments in which people live. Essential elements of neoliberalism include minimization of state involvement in service provision (e.g., privatization of health care, education, and social benefits), unregulated "free" markets and reduced trade barriers, emphasis on so-called "efficiency" and, more recently, the introduction of austerity policy (Brown, 2015; Labonté & Stuckler, 2016; Labonté & Torgerson, 2005). The spread of neoliberal capitalism through globalization has amplified poverty and contributed to environmental degradation and the erosion of health and social infrastructure in lower- to middle-income countries (Falk-Rafael, 2006). Nurses' engagement in advocacy for policy environments that promote and protect health, locally and globally, requires an awareness of the relationship between neoliberal economic globalization as an inherently global issue that shapes individual and population health around the world (see Chapter 1).

For example, in a globalized and deeply interconnected world, **transnationalism** plays a role in shaping social connections, mobility, and exchange across borders. It is defined as the sustained and continuous interaction between networks, groups, organizations, and communities across national borders, extending from individuals, families, communities, and groups to include institutions that hold authority to restrict or enable this interaction (Rosemberg et al., 2016). The concept of transnationalism suggests a weakening of the control a nation-state has over its borders, inhabitants, and territory. Contextualized within a broader political economy and analysis of the influences of globalization, transnationalism is also useful for examining issues related to brain drain and the flow of trained health care providers—including nurses—from lower-income countries to higher-income countries (Harper, 2019; Runnels et al., 2011). The social interactions and contexts arising from highly mobile global populations are situated in an overall net flow of resources from lower-income to higher-income settings, reflecting structural drivers of health that continue to concentrate resources, wealth, and power among already well-resourced countries (Brisbois et al., 2019), thereby contributing to the entrenchment of global health inequities.

Relational Theory and Ethics

Central to understanding the connections between local and global health, between globalization and health, or between social and structural determinants of health and health outcomes is an understanding of relational theory and ethics. Relational theory and ethics support nurses' considerations of the concepts of health equity and inequities, their situatedness in the political economy, and their influence on the social and structural determinants of health. Relational ethics, with its focus on why nurses (and others) should care about global health, provides a moral justification for understanding and responding to health inequities and their causes, both within and between countries. Responding to the structural conditions (political economy of health) that inhibit health equity evokes ethically and morally urgent obligations to act, both as health professionals (CNA, 2009) and as countries (Benatar et al., 2021). For decades, evidence about the impact of social and structural determinants of health (PAHO, 2019; WHO, 1978, 2008, 2011) has underpinned calls to address the complex governance challenges related to advancing more equitable futures worldwide.

Relational theories (Doane, 2014; Doane & Varcoe, 2021) have inspired nurses to embrace the stance of assuming that the connections between people, ideas, organizations, bodies of knowledge, and contexts all include something relational (Plamondon & Caxaj, 2018). Relational ways of thinking are foundational to understanding the complex interactions between global and local health across different scales of the political economy (e.g., local, regional, national, and international). Research on promising practices for advancing health equity shows that working relationally is important. In global health, practices for working relationally to achieve equity include fostering inclusion and connectedness and mitigating power imbalances (Plamondon et al., 2019). Embracing relational theory in our practice as nurses, then, requires being attentive to who and how people are involved in identifying, understanding, and responding to health issues—and working actively to listen for and amplify voices that are often excluded by virtue of the social and structural determinants of health that contribute to inequities in representation.

THE HISTORY OF PLANETARY HEALTH AND CLIMATE CHANGE—DEFINITIONS AND EXPLANATIONS

Environmental Sustainability and One Health

Significant disruptions to the Earth's climate, biodiversity, and ecosystems are impacting the health of our population and that of our planet (Horton & Lo, 2015). The Anthropocene, the unofficial name for the current geological age—a period during which human activity has been the dominant influence on climate and the environment—was first described in 2002 by Paul J. Crutzen, a Dutch atmospheric chemist who proposed this term to describe the dramatic changes detectable in fossils, rock, or both (Crutzen, 2002). Global environmental sustainability is defined as "the responsibility to conserve natural resources and protect global ecosystems to support health and well-being, now and in the future" (Sphera, 2022, para. 3). Environmental risk factors, such as climate change, ultraviolet radiation; air, water, and soil pollution; and chemical exposure, contribute to more than 100 diseases and injuries. As a result, nurses have a role "to promote and support actions to optimize the health of the environment because of the link to human health" (CNA, 2017a, para. 1).

The focus on environmental sustainability has also led to increased attention on the interdependence of humans, plants, and animals. This relationship has been referred to as One Health, an initiative that "recognizes that the health of people is connected to the health of animals and the environment" (Centers for Disease Control and Prevention [CDC], 2022, para. 1). The primary goal of the One Health initiative is to foster collaboration between many disciplines working locally, nationally, and globally to achieve the best health for all people (CDC, 2022; International Development Research Centre, 2021).

Planetary Health

In response to global environmental changes, an emerging movement has arisen that focuses on planetary health. Planetary health is an emerging holistic health field that seeks to foster interdisciplinary collaborations, integrate Indigenous knowledge, facilitate education, and drive public and policy engagement (Faerron Guzman & Potter, 2021;

Faerron Guzman et al., 2021). In 2014, the Rockefeller Foundation–*Lancet* Commission on Planetary Health met in Bellagio, Italy, and defined planetary health as follows:

> *The achievement of the highest attainable standard of health, wellbeing, and equity worldwide through judicious attention to the human systems—political, economic, and social—that shape the future of humanity and the Earth's natural systems that define the safe environmental limits within which humanity can flourish. Put simply, planetary health is the health of human civilization and the state of the natural systems on which it depends . . . The concept of planetary health is based on the "understanding that human health and human civilization depend on flourishing natural systems and the wise stewardship of those natural systems"*
>
> **Whitmee et al., 2015, p. 1974**

For example, deforestation leads to greater human–wildlife contact, which can promote the transmission of various zoonotic diseases. In 2016, Prüss-Ustün and colleagues completed a comprehensive assessment of the burden of disease and reported that premature deaths and disease could be prevented through healthier environments. As a result, knowledge of the influences that environmental hazards and risks have on planetary health is important for nurses to critique and understand if they are to assist in the promotion of healthier environments (Potter, 2019). Myers and Frumkin (2020) state that "perhaps the single largest driver of human sickness and death over the next century will be our own transformation and degradation of Earth's natural life-support systems (p. 329).

With the increasing interest in planetary health as both a social movement and a transdisciplinary field, planetary health leaders have begun focusing their attention on how to restore planetary health (Myers & Frumkin, 2020). The Planetary Health Alliance (PHA) is a consortium of over 300 universities, research institutes, nongovernmental organizations, and government entities globally committed to understanding and addressing global environmental change and its health impacts. The PHA has developed a set of 12 cross-cutting principles as a curriculum development guide for educators (Stone et al., 2018) (Box 11.2).

These principles for planetary health education are important to include alongside an understanding of how Indigenous peoples have also been protecting the Earth for the well-being of the community

---

BOX 11.2   Cross-Cutting Principles for Planetary Health Education

1. A planetary health lens
2. Urgency and scale
3. Policy
4. Organizing and movement building
5. Communication
6. Systems thinking and transdisciplinary collaborations
7. Inequality and inequity
8. Bias
9. Governance
10. Unintended consequences
11. Global citizenship and cultural identity
12. Historical and current global values

From Stone, S. B., Myers, S. S., Golden, C. D., & Planetary Health Education Brainstorm Group. (2018). Cross-cutting principles for planetary health education. *The Lancet: Planetary Health, 2*(5), 192–193. https://doi.org/10.1016/S2542-5196(18)30022-6

through Indigenous sovereignty (Manuel & Derrickson, 2017; Redvers et al., 2022). Redvers and colleagues (2022) have defined **determinants of planetary health from an Indigenous perspective** using an Indigenous process of consensus (Box 11.3). They have proposed 10 main determinants of planetary health under three main interconnected levels: (1) Mother Earth–level determinants, (2) interconnecting-level determinants, and (3) Indigenous peoples–level determinants, illuminating the interconnectedness of these determinants. They argue that addressing planetary health issues calls for the inclusion of solutions with an Earth-centred world view. As a result, it is important that nurse educators employ planetary health concepts alongside Indigenous sovereignty principles in global health curricula, nursing practice, research, and leadership.

Climate Change

The terms *global warming* and *climate change* are often used interchangeably; however, they mean two different things. **Global warming** refers to "the rise in global temperatures due mainly to the increasing concentrations of greenhouse gases in the atmosphere" (US Geological Survey, n.d., para 1). By comparison, **climate change** refers to "long-term shifts in temperatures and weather patterns" (United Nations, n.d.-a, para. 1). The Earth has gone through many such natural cycles throughout its history. However, "since the 1800s, human activities have been the main driver of climate change, primarily due to burning fossil fuels like coal, oil and gas (United Nations, n.d.-a, para. 1).

Today, climate change is considered a major public health threat (Watts et al., 2017). Greenhouse gases that occur naturally in the atmosphere warm the Earth and thus make it livable; however, the generation of greenhouse gas emissions by human beings beginning during the Industrial Revolution has upset this natural balance and led to increased warming of the planet. As a result, greenhouse gases in the atmosphere that are unable to escape from the Earth's system warm the Earth's surface and lower atmosphere. *Canada's Changing Climate Report*, the first report to assess "how Canada's climate has changed, why, and what changes are projected for the future," found that Canada's annual average temperature has warmed by 1.7°C since 1948 (Bush & Lemmen, 2019, p. 428).

BOX 11.3   Determinants of Planetary Health—An Indigenous Consensus Perspective

I. Mother Earth-Level Determinants
- Respect of the feminine
- Ancestral legal personhood designation

II. Interconnecting-Level Determinants
- Human interconnectedness within Nature
- Self and community relationships
- The modern scientific paradigm
- Governance and law

III. Indigenous Peoples'-Level Determinants
- Indigenous land tenure rights
- Indigenous languages
- Indigenous peoples' health
- Indigenous Elders and children

From Redvers, N., Celidwen, Y., Schultz, C., et al. (2022). The determinants of planetary health: An Indigenous consensus perspective. *The Lancet: Planetary Health, 6*(2), E156–E162. https://doi.org/10.1016/s2542-5196(21)00354-5

Therefore, what we are now witnessing in Canada and globally is human-induced climate change, which includes an increase in the Earth's temperature due to greenhouse gas emissions. Globally, the primary sources of these emissions are electricity and heat production, agriculture, transportation, forestry, land use change, and manufacturing; it is estimated that the health care sector in Canada, including hospitals, contributes about 5% of those emissions (Health Care Without Harm & Arup, 2019, p. 10). Along with temperature fluctuations, there have been more unpredictable and extreme weather events; for example, wildfires have resulted in a poorer Air Quality Health Index (AQHI), droughts, increases in precipitation that then cause flooding, heat waves, and melting snow and ice that leads to rising sea levels. These adverse changes in the environment directly impact the health and well-being of the population and the planet (Figure 11.1). For instance, more wildfires can result in worse AQHI values; poor air quality can, in turn, pose a major health risk to individuals with underlying respiratory conditions. The AQHI is based on a scale of 1 to 10+; the higher the number, the greater the health risk (Government of Canada, 2021).

The Paris Agreement. In response to the critical impacts of climate change, on December 12, 2015, the **Paris Agreement**, a "legally binding international treaty on climate change" (United Nations Climate Change, 2022, para. 1), was adopted by 195 participating member states and the European Union at the UN Framework Convention on Climate Change to address the adaptation, mitigation, and finance of greenhouse gas emissions. The Paris Agreement's long-term temperature goal is to keep the global average temperature to well below 2°C above preindustrial levels, and to limit the temperature increase even further to 1.5°C, with the intention of reducing the effects and risks of climate change. In 2021, the United Kingdom hosted the 26th UN Climate Change Conference of the Parties (COP26) to accelerate action toward the goals of the Paris Agreement and the UN Framework Convention on Climate Change. This event resulted in the participants, along with the Secretary-General, outlining a plan for the next 5 years for moving towards implementation of their plan (United Nations Climate Change Conference of the Parties, 2021).

In Canada, the Canadian Association of Nurses for the Environment (2022) and the Canadian Nurses Association (CNA) have emphasized the key role of nurses "to promote climate change adaptation (that is, responding to the effects of climate change) and mitigation (taking action to reduce it)" (CNA, 2017b, para. 3). Taking on an advocacy role in an organization is another way nurses can become involved in collective actions to mitigate the threats to health and well-being posed by climate change (Butterfield et al., 2021; Mitchell, 2021).

Canada's pledge to reduce greenhouse gas emissions is merely one example of our many international commitments to achieve environmental sustainability and improve health for all (IPCC, 2021). Nurses can be instrumental in promoting personal behavioural changes that will reduce greenhouse gas emissions. For example, nurses can educate themselves and make choices that will decrease their carbon footprint, including using electric or hybrid vehicles and other more sustainable forms of transportation such as cycling, walking, and taking public transportation; instead of flying to attend conferences in another province or country, nurses can choose to attend virtual conferences (CNA, 2017b).

As Thomas (2017) explains, a solid understanding of climate change and its connection to natural disasters is a prerequisite for transforming economies and policies that will lead us to a sustainable future. Natural disasters are a rising threat in response to global warming—there is a greater incidence of storms, floods, fires, and droughts across the globe. Achieving our vision of a sustainable world requires a key

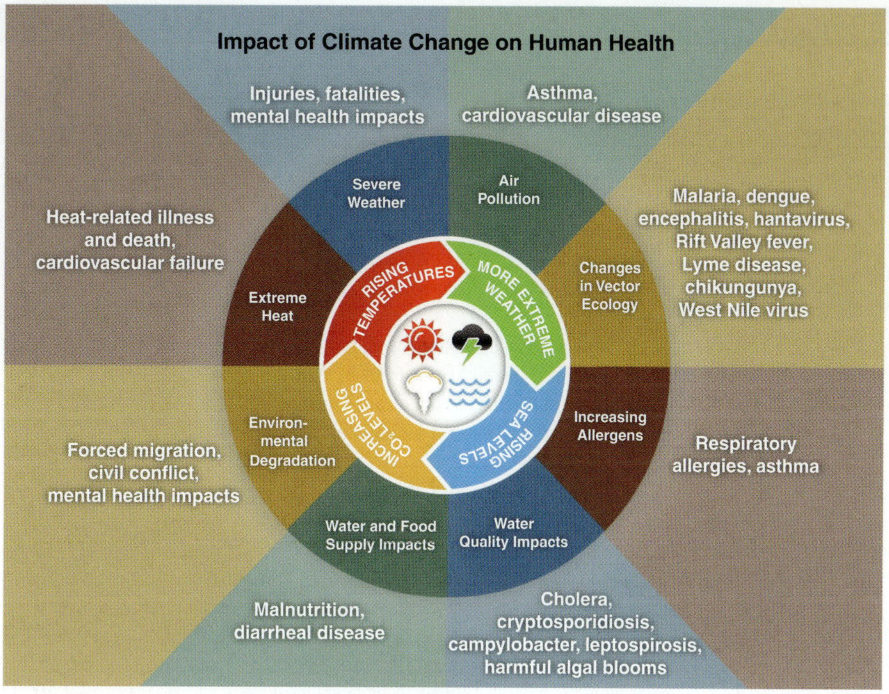

FIGURE 11.1 The impact of climate change on human health. (From Centers for Disease Control for Prevention. [2022]. *Climate effects on health.* https://www.cdc.gov/climateandhealth/effects/default.htm.)

understanding: the material desires of the present must no longer cause environmental destruction in the future.

ISSUES IN GLOBAL HEALTH

Communicable Diseases

Communicable diseases are infectious diseases (such as cholera, hepatitis, influenza, malaria, measles, or tuberculosis) that are "transmissible by contact with infected individuals or their bodily discharges or fluids (such as respiratory droplets, blood, or semen), by contact with contaminated surfaces or objects, by ingestion of contaminated food or water, or by direct or indirect contact with disease vectors (such as mosquitoes, fleas, or mice)" (Merriam-Webster, n.d.).

Pandemics. The significant global health impacts of recent pandemics have illuminated the importance of being better prepared, both at home and globally, to address them. A **pandemic** is defined as the worldwide spread of a new disease (World Health Organization [WHO], 2009). The WHO has a developed a framework that describes the phases of a pandemic along with actions to be taken during each phase (Table 11.1).

The major pandemics of the past couple of decades have been **severe acute respiratory syndrome (SARS)** in 2003, H1N1 virus, Ebola, and COVID-19. SARS is caused by a type of virus known as a coronavirus. This virus is included in the family of viruses that cause mild to moderate upper respiratory illnesses such as the common cold (WHO, 2022d). In 2009–2010, the WHO announced a global pandemic of the influenza A **H1N1 virus**, which originated from animal influenza viruses (WHO, 2022b). Today, the H1N1 virus is included in the vaccines against seasonal influenza because it continues to circulate in the population. In 2014 and 2016, West Africa faced the largest Ebola outbreak since the virus was discovered in 1976 (WHO, 2021a, para. 3). **Ebola** virus disease (EVD), formerly known as Ebola haemorrhagic

fever, is caused by the Ebola filovirus and is a highly infectious and rapidly fatal disease with a high mortality rate (WHO, 2021a). The virus is transmitted to people from wild animals and then spreads through human-to-human transmission.

COVID-19 Pandemic. On March 11, 2020, the director-general of the WHO declared COVID-19 a pandemic (WHO, 2020a). **Coronavirus disease (COVID-19)** is an infectious disease caused by the SARS-CoV-2 virus (WHO, n.d., para. 1), a severe acute respiratory syndrome. The virus can spread from an infected person's nose or mouth in the form of small liquid particles when the person sneezes, speaks, coughs, sings, or breathes. These particles range in size from tiny aerosols to large respiratory droplets.

The virus that causes COVID-19 was first identified in December 2019 in Wuhan, China. The first presumptive case of what would be later called COVID-19 in Canada was reported on January 25, 2020, and the first death in Canada occurred on March 9, 2020 (Government of Canada, 2022). With the COVID-19 virus, it quickly became apparent how such an outbreak can rapidly overwhelm the world. During the course of the global pandemic, it has also become apparent that certain people are at higher risk for more severe forms of COVID-19 and worse outcomes than others. In addition, the risk of getting COVID-19 varies within and between communities in Canada and worldwide. Residents of long-term care in Canada have been disproportionately affected by COVID-19, resulting in increased deaths among older persons (Canadian Institute for Health Information, 2021; Johnson et al. 2020). In addition, there has been gross inequity in the global distribution of approved vaccines (Labonté et al., 2021). For example, in April 2021, the WHO estimated that 87% of approved available vaccines went to high-income and upper middle-income countries, while just 0.2% went to low- and middle-income countries (WHO, 2021b).

Like all viruses, SARS-CoV-2 naturally mutates. These mutations change the genetic material inside the virus and produce what are called **variants**. A concern about some variants of COVID-19

TABLE 11.1	The World Health Organization (WHO) Pandemic Phases			
	Estimated Probability of Pandemic	Description	Main Actions in Affected Countries	Main Actions in Not-Yet-Affected Countries
Phase 1	Uncertain	No animal influenza virus circulating among animals has been reported to cause infection in humans.	Producing, implementing, exercising, and harmonizing national pandemic influenza preparedness and response plans with national emergency preparedness and response plans.	
Phase 2		An animal influenza virus circulating in domesticated or wild animals is known to have caused infection in humans and is therefore considered a specific potential pandemic threat.		
Phase 3		An animal or human–animal influenza reassortment virus* has caused sporadic cases or small clusters of disease in people, but has not resulted in human-to-human transmission sufficient to sustain community-level outbreaks.		
Phase 4	Medium to high	Human-to-human transmission of an animal or human–animal influenza reassortment virus able to sustain community-level outbreaks has been verified.	Rapid containment	Readiness for pandemic response
Phase 5	High to certain	The same identified virus has caused sustained community-level outbreaks in at least two countries in one WHO region.	Pandemic response: each country to implement actions as called for in their national plans	Readiness for imminent response
Phase 6	Pandemic in progress	In addition to the criteria defined in Phase 5, the same virus has caused sustained community-level outbreaks in at least one other country in another WHO region.		
Post-Peak Period		Levels of pandemic influenza in most countries with adequate surveillance have dropped below peak levels.	Evaluation of response; recovery; preparation for possible second wave	
Possible New Wave		Level of pandemic influenza activity in most countries with adequate surveillance is rising again.	Response	
Post-Pandemic Period		Levels of influenza have returned to the levels seen for seasonal influenza in most countries with adequate surveillance.	Evaluation of response; revision of plans; recovery	

*Reassortant is the process by which influenza viruses swap gene segments to form novel genome combinations. Reassortment can occur when two different influenza viruses infect a host at the same time.
Adapted from World Health Organization. (2009). The WHO pandemic phases. In *Pandemic influenza preparedness and response: A WHO guidance document* (p. 11). https://apps.who.int/iris/bitstream/handle/10665/44123/9789241547680_eng.pdf

is that they continue to mutate, resulting in a virus that is not only more infectious, allowing it to spread more easily, but also capable of causing more severe illness. A number of variants have emerged in Canada, including Alpha (B.1.1.7), Beta (B.1.351), Gamma (P.1), Delta (B.1.617.2), and Omicron (B.1.1.529) (Government of Canada, 2022). In Canada, as of August 2022, the total number of COVID-19 cases was 4 179 337.

Noncommunicable Diseases

Noncommunicable diseases (NCDs), also known as *chronic diseases*, are not contagious, meaning that they are not passed from person to person. NCDs such as heart disease, stroke, diabetes, cancer, and chronic lung disease are collectively responsible for almost 70% of all deaths worldwide (WHO, 2022c). The WHO's mission is to continue to provide ongoing evidence and leadership for international action on surveillance, prevention, and control of NCDs. The four major risk factors driving the increase in NCDs are physical inactivity, tobacco use, unhealthy diets, and harmful use of alcohol. As a result, the epidemic of NCDs can result in significant health consequences for a population along with corresponding socioeconomic expenditures. This makes control and prevention of NCDs a necessity for the twenty-first

century. In Canada, NCDs are the leading causes of death (Government of Canada, 2019).

Gender Equality

Gender equality is the view that all people should be given equal treatment and not be discriminated against on the basis of their gender. The Universal Declaration of Human Rights includes gender equality as one of its objectives, such that people are treated equally in social situations, law, democratic activities, politics, the workplace, or any policy-designated realm (United Nations, n.d.-b). Gender inequality is viewed as a major obstacle to human development. Although progress in this area has been made since 1990—for example, in 2021, 25% of all national parliamentarians were female compared with only 11.3% in 1995—continued discrimination against women and girls in education, health, political participation, employment, and the labour market results in negative developmental outcomes, reduced life opportunities, and compromised freedom of choice; globally, on average, women still earn 20% less than men (United Nations, n.d.-b). The UN, along with other global agencies, has accepted several conventions focused on the promotion of gender inequality (United Nations Development Programme, 2020). In addition, SDG 5 is the only one of the goals that recognizes the importance of achieving gender equality and empowering women and girls. With women and girls representing half of the world's population, it is essential that they achieve their full human potential.

IMMIGRATION AND MIGRATION TRENDS—INDIGENOUS PEOPLES AND ETHNOCULTURAL DIVERSITY

In 1971, Canada became the first country in the world to officially adopt multiculturalism as an official policy, "to preserve the cultural freedom of all individuals and provide recognition of the cultural contributions of diverse ethnic groups to Canadian society" (Gagnon et al., n.d., para. 1). Since then, various laws have been passed to protect and promote the rights of minorities in Canada (Box 11.4).

The demographic portrait of Canada is continually evolving (Statistics Canada, 2022). More than 250 ethnocultural backgrounds were reported in the 2016 census of Population (Statistics Canada, 2017a). The most frequently reported non-Canadian origins in 2016, either alone or with other ethnicities, were English, French, Scottish, Irish, German, Italian, Chinese, Indigenous (see Chapter 12 for further information on Indigenous peoples), Ukrainian, Indian, Filipino, Dutch, and Polish.

Indigenous peoples are the fastest growing population in Canada as well as the youngest. According to the 2021 census (Statistics Canada, 2022), the Indigenous population grew by 9.4% between 2016 and 2021. Indigenous peoples were also 8.2 years younger, on average, than the non-Indigenous population (Statistics Canada, 2022). As of 2021, more than 1 million people (1 048 405) in Canada identified as Indigenous—that is, First Nations, Inuit, or Métis (Statistics Canada, 2022). (See Chapter 12 for further discussion of Indigenous health.)

Racialized people (Statistics Canada uses the term *visible minorities*) accounted for 30% of Canada's total population on the 2016 census; of this group, 30% were born in Canada and 65.1% were born outside of the country (Statistics Canada, 2017a). The 2016 census found that 3 of the 20 most commonly reported ethnocultural origins are Asian: Filipino, Indian, and Chinese. In 2016, South Asian Canadians represented 25.1% of all racialized people and 4.8% of the total population, Chinese Canadians accounted for about 20.5% of the racialized population and 4% of the total population, and Black Canadians accounted for 15.6% of the racialized population and represented 3.5% of the population (Statistics Canada, 2017b).

Ethnocultural Diversity

Canada's valuing of multiculturalism is reflected within the ethnocultural diversity of its population: approximately 20% of the total population are immigrants. According to the 2016 census, approximately one in five people in Canada were born outside of the country (Statistics Canada, 2017c). Canada ranks second only to Australia as the country with the highest proportion of foreign-born citizens. The largest groups of immigrants to Canada are from Asian and Middle Eastern countries; this fact has remained virtually unchanged since the 2001 census.

Canada is also home to many refugees, having welcomed more than 1 million since 1980. Refugees are individuals who have been forced to flee their home country in order to escape war, persecution, or natural disaster. In 2020 , the top 10 origin countries of persons claiming refugee status in Canada were India, Mexico, Iran, Colombia, Haiti, Pakistan, China, Nigeria, Turkey, and Sri Lanka (Statista, 2021). Asylum seekers are individuals who have fled their home country and sought international protection (United Nations High Commissioner of Refugees [UNHCR], 2022). Internally displaced persons are individuals who are forced to leave their homes because of conflict, human rights violations, or natural disasters, yet remain in their home country (UNHCR, 2022). Refugees may be relocated without having chosen their destination, while immigrants are able to choose where they wish to live. Refugees tend to experience greater dislocation and deprivation than do immigrants, who have the option of returning to their homelands. Newcomers and refugees both frequently experience language barriers, social isolation, separation from family, loss and grief, and a lack of information and access to available health care resources (Box 11.5).

GLOBAL/PLANETARY HEALTH NURSING—CALLS TO ACTION

Nurses understand the importance of global health, the emerging field of planetary health, and their application to nursing education, practice, research, and advocacy (Astle, 2021a; CASN, 2022; Kalogirou et al., 2020; LeClair & Potter, 2022; Potter et al., 2021). There is also recognition within the profession that global is local and local is global, such that nurses are cognizant of how various urgent global health challenges need to be addressed wherever they may work (Astle, 2021b; Bragadóttir & Potter, 2019).

Planetary health focuses on the linkages between human-caused disruptions of the Earth's natural systems and the health of people. Humans depend on planetary health for safe and healthy food and clean air, land, and water. Nurses have a key role to play as individuals and as a group in taking the lead to mitigate the effects of human-induced climate change and environmental racism in order to advance health equity toward climate justice. Environmental racism is a form of systemic racism related to racial discrimination in policymaking. It includes the enforcement of laws and regulations and actions such as the deliberate siting of toxic waste facilities in predominantly racialized communities, the official sanctioning of the life-threatening presence of poisons and pollutants in certain communities, and the historical exclusion of racialized people from positions of leadership in the environmental movement (MacDonald, 2020).

BOX 11.4 Legislation Recognizing the Diversity of Canadian Society

Official Languages Act (1969; Updated 1988)
This Act recognizes English and French equally as Canada's official languages. The 1988 amendment to this Act outlines the obligations of Canadian federal institutions to commit to promoting full recognition and use of both English and French in Canadian society, as well as supporting the development of anglophone and francophone communities across the country.

Constitution Act (1982)
This Act replaced the *British North America Act* as Canada's Constitution, outlining how Canada governs and structures its society. It also recognizes the "aboriginal peoples" in Canada as "the Indian (Status and Non-Status), Inuit and Métis peoples" (note that this Act has not replaced its outdated terminology with more contemporary terminology: "Indigenous peoples" is preferred over "aboriginal peoples, and "First Nations" over "Indian").

Canadian Charter of Rights and Freedoms (1982)
Written into the *Canadian Constitution* in 1982, this charter is a statement of the basic human rights and freedoms of all Canadians.

Canadian Multiculturalism Act (1985)
In recognition of Canada's cultural diversity, this Act enshrines the enhancement and preservation of multiculturalism in Canada.

BOX 11.5 RESEARCH HIGHLIGHT

Access to Health Care for Immigrant Children in Canada

Research Focus

The aim of the study by Salami et al. (2020) was to understand the factors that contribute to access to health care for immigrants in Canada.

Abstract

Immigrants in Canada experience poorer health outcomes than nonimmigrants for several reasons. A central contributing factor to poor health outcomes for immigrants is access to health care. Previous research on access to health care for immigrants has largely focused on the experience of immigrant adults. The purpose of this study was to investigate how immigrants access health services for their children in Alberta, Canada.

Methods

The study used a descriptive qualitative design. Upon receiving ethics approval from the University of Alberta Research Ethics Board, the authors invited immigrant parents to participate in this study. They interviewed 50 immigrant parents, including 17 fathers and 33 mothers. Interviews were audio recorded, transcribed, and analyzed according to the themes that emerged.

Results

The findings revealed that systemic barriers contributed to challenges in accessing health care for immigrant children. Participants identified several of these barriers—namely system barriers, language and cultural barriers, relationship with health care providers, and financial barriers. These barriers can be addressed by policymakers and service providers by strengthening the diversity of the workforce, addressing income as a social determinant of health, and improving access to language interpretation services.

Implications for Practice

- Nurses must recognize the vital importance of the social determinants of health, especially income, on the health of immigrants in Canada.
- Nurses can bridge language barriers by providing interpretation services. Nurses must also be cognizant of the context and culture of participants when providing interpretation services.
- Showing respect and dedicating time to address the complex health and settlement challenges that immigrants face will improve access to health care.

From Salami, B., Mason, A., Salma, J., et al. (2020). Access to healthcare for immigrant children in Canada. *International Journal of Environmental Research and Public Health, 17*(9), 3320. https://doi.org/10.3390/ijerph17093320

Environmental justice refers to the fair treatment and meaningful participation of all people regardless of national origin, colour, race, or income with respect to the development, implementation, and enforcement of environmental laws, regulations, and policies (US Environmental Protection Agency, 2022). Climate justice was created as a submovement of the environmental justice movement to look at the climate crisis through a human rights lens and environmental justice perspective. The climate justice movement insists on shifting away from the discourse about greenhouse gases and melting ice caps to a focus on the people and communities that are most vulnerable to the impacts of climate change. Climate justice is based on the belief that working together will allow us to create a better future for present and future generations (United Nations, 2019, para. 3), and that with a strong focus on climate action we can ensure a healthy future for the planet (Astle, 2021b; LeClair & Potter, 2022; Mitchell, 2021).

This global/planetary approach underscores the importance of international collaboration between nurses and other health professionals across disciplines in order to address health inequities. The International Council of Nurses (ICN) and the WHO strongly advocate that every nurse can have a direct impact on health and that nurses are key to achieving the SDGs (Catton, 2020; WHO, 2018). By working in partnership with other professionals who possess the skills and expertise to address these health inequities, our health systems can be strengthened (Astle, 2021a).

Global and Planetary Citizenship

A variety of disciplines have advocated for policies that centre **global citizenship**, including education, law, community health, epidemiology (Landorf & Feldman, 2015) and nursing (Burgess et al., 2014; Chavez et al., 2008; Mill et al., 2010; Simpson et al., 2015). Mill and colleagues (2010) have argued that nurses must examine their roles and responsibilities in relation to global citizenship. As a framework, global citizenship is necessary to shift the perspectives of nursing students toward a more critical inquiry of global issues (Burgess et al., 2014). A **global citizen** incorporates not only an *inward* personal awareness and commitment to global issues, but also *outward* actions on local or global issues (Hanson, 2010). Byers (2005) suggests that "global citizenship empowers individuals to participate in the decisions concerning their lives, including the political, economic, social, cultural and environmental conditions in which they live" (p. 37). The common thread in global citizenship is our *interconnectedness* and the acknowledgement that the local and global are intertwined, with one perspective not privileged over the other (Mill et al., 2010). According to Oxfam (2015), the characteristics of a global citizen include (but are not limited to) awareness of the wider world, respecting and valuing diversity, contributing to the community at both local and global levels, striving toward sustainability in the world, taking responsibility for our own actions, and acting on social injustice.

The roots of social responsibility in nursing can be traced back to pioneers such as Florence Nightingale, Margaret Sanger, Lavinia Dock, and Lillian Wald (Kelley et al., 2008). More recently, Rosa (2020) has stated that **planetary citizenship** "is a more inclusive notion than global citizenship" because it "incorporates the idea that human health and well-being are integrally tied to [the health and well-being] of other animal species and the environment at large" (p. 11). While both global and planetary citizenship espouse the importance of interconnectedness, planetary citizenship emphasizes the importance of interconnection for humans living on a vibrant and rich planet. Therefore, keeping global and planetary citizenship front of mind is essential as nurses continue to advocate for social justice, the health of the population, and the health of the planet.

Investing in the Global Nursing Workforce

Our future health care providers will shoulder increasing responsibility for providing health services for some very complex health issues (Frenk et al., 2010). Many health care systems in the world are struggling to oversee unmet health needs, a situation that has reached a crisis point during the global COVID-19 pandemic. The nursing profession is being confronted with a global nursing shortage, the mass traumatization of nurses, an aging nursing workforce, the lack of protection, and increasing workloads and lower salaries, all of which have led to a global call for investing in the nursing workforce to meet current and future health care needs (Buchan et al., 2022).

In 2020, the WHO published the first *State of the World's Nursing* (SOWN) report, which critically examined the nursing workforce, identified important gaps in the nursing workforce, and highlighted priority areas for investing in nursing jobs, education, and leadership in order to strengthen nursing globally and improve the health of our populations (WHO, 2020b). Building on the SOWN report, the WHO developed another report, *Global Strategic Directions for Nursing and Midwifery*. This report provided evidence-informed practices and interrelated policy priorities to help countries ensure that nurses and midwives have strategic directions that contribute to achieving universal health coverage and other health goals (WHO, 2021d). These two global reports by the WHO, alongside reports published by the ICN (Buchan et al., 2022; Stewart et al., 2022), have become the foundation for implementing the suggested directions, priorities, and recommendations. In Canada, there has also been a call to action for investing in Canada's nursing workforce in response to, and to recover from, the COVID-19 pandemic to ensure safe and high-quality patient care (Tomblin Murphy & Sampalli, 2022).

Global and Planetary Health Education

Global Health Competencies and Planetary Health Education Framework. Acknowledgment of the importance of addressing global/planetary health issues has resulted in the rapid growth of undergraduate and graduate programs in global health education (Jogerst et al., 2015), and more recently in planetary health education (Faerron Guzman & Potter, 2021; Faerron Guzmán et al., 2021; Potter, 2019). To address this increased interest, many Canadian nursing programs have integrated global health concepts and developed curricula with courses focusing on global health. Schools of nursing are also increasingly integrating planetary health and climate change content into their nursing curricula. The CASN (2022), as part of its educational framework at the undergraduate level, has emphasized that nurses must demonstrate knowledge of social justice, population health, environmental, and global health issues; the updated CASN National Education Framework includes planetary health as one of the essential components (CASN, 2022).

Curriculum development has accompanied this growth in global health education programs. Initiatives have been undertaken to identify interprofessional global health competencies (Consortium of Universities for Global Health Competency Subcommittee, 2018; Jogerst et al., 2015) and understand host perspectives (Cherniak et al., 2017a, 2017b). Global health competencies refer to the knowledge and skills that a nurse should possess when working in the area of global health. Research continues, however, in nursing and other disciplines that are working collaboratively toward implementation and evaluation of global health competencies in order to critically examine the decolonialization of global health education and to challenge current power asymmetries (Sayegh et al., 2022).

From 2019 to 2021, a group of 24 thought leaders convened to develop a Planetary Health Education Framework (PHEF) to provide a blueprint for all professions and disciplines to integrate this content into their curricula (Faerron Guzman & Potter, 2021; Faerron Guzmán et al., 2021b; Haines & Frumkin, 2021). This framework consists of five core interconnected domains:

1. Interconnection with Nature
2. The Anthropocene and Health
3. Equity and Social Justice
4. Systems Thinking and Complexity, and
5. Movement Building and Systems Change.

The framework gives nurses the background and shared language to collaborate and partner with other disciplines in order to promote planetary health (Potter et al., 2021). It also incorporates the Planetary Health Alliance's 12 cross-cutting principles of planetary health education (Stone et al., 2018). Other areas that require further exploration and integration into nursing education are the concepts of climate justice, environmental racism, and postcolonial critical theories; learning these concepts will allow nurses to better understand and appreciate the injustices experienced by various populations (LeClair & Potter, 2022).

National and International Organizations for Global/Planetary Health. There are a number of local, national, and international organizations that promote interprofessional and transdisciplinary collaborations within nursing to advance global and planetary health. These organizations are listed in Box 11.6.

Implications for Nursing

The nursing profession has acknowledged the important role that nursing practice, education, and research must play in addressing critical global/planetary health issues. Nurses who possess a foundational understanding of a myriad of global/planetary health concepts will be better prepared to care for patients at the local, national, and international levels. Issues that require ongoing critical examination and a call to action by nurses include focusing on leading and promoting change in global/planetary health in practice, education, research, and advocacy; social justice initiatives; human rights; and health equity. To achieve health equity, social justice, and human rights for all, and to build inclusive and sustainable communities, nurses must acquire the necessary knowledge to provide competent and culturally safe care (discussed in Chapter 12), and work in collaboration with community leaders and policymakers in leading the way to ensure the health of the planet.

BOX 11.6 | **National and International Organizations for Global and Planetary Health**

Alliance of Nurses for Healthy Environments: https://envirn.org
Canadian Association for Global Health: https://cagh-acsm.org/en
Canadian Nurses Association: https://www.cna-aiic.ca/en
Canadian Association of Nurses for the Environment: https://cane-aiie.ca
Canadian Red Cross: https://www.redcross.ca
Center for Climate Change, Climate Justice, and Health: https://www.mgihp.edu/climate
Consortium of Universities for Global Health: https://www.cugh.org/
Global Advisory Panel on the Future of Nursing and Midwifery: https://www.sigmanursing.org/connect-engage/our-global-impact/gapfon
Global Alliance of Nurses for Healthy Environments: https://envirn.org
Global Consortium on Climate and Health Education: https://www.publichealth.columbia.edu/research/global-consortium-climate-and-health-education
Global Nursing Caucus: https://www.globalnursingcaucus.org
Immigration, Refugees, and Citizenship Canada: https://www.canada.ca/en/immigration-refugees-citizenship.html
International Council of Nurses: https://www.icn.ch
InVIVO Planetary Health: https://www.invivoplanet.com
The Lancet: Planetary Health: https://www.thelancet.com/journals/lanplh/home
Médecins Sans Frontières (Doctors Without Borders Canada): https://www.doctorswithoutborders.ca
Nurses Climate Challenge: https://nursesclimatechallenge.org
Nurses Drawdown: https://www.nursesdrawdown.org
Planetary Health Alliance: https://www.planetaryhealthalliance.org
United Nations: https://www.un.org/en
United Nations Sustainable Development Goals—Climate justice: https://www.un.org/sustainabledevelopment/blog/2019/05/climate-justice
World Health Organization (WHO)—Nursing: https://www.who.int/health-topics/nursing#tab=tab_1

KEY CONCEPTS

- Global health is concerned with the health needs of people worldwide.
- Health equity is an aspirational concept that reflects values of social justice.
- Intersectionality is a theoretical perspective regarding the influence of different social characteristics—race, ethnicity, gender, class, and socioeconomic status, to name a few—on a particular phenomenon, such as the experience of health and its outcomes.
- Sustainable Development Goals (SDGs) address the well-being of people worldwide, an approach that aligns with a global/planetary perspective of health.
- Planetary health focuses on understanding and addressing human disruption of the Earth's natural systems through a transdisciplinary and inclusive approach.
- Nurses have a key role to play in promoting climate change adaptation, responding to its effects, and taking actions to mitigate its impact.
- Global environmental sustainability relies on intact and healthy ecosystems.
- Global citizenship is the active engagement of nurses in global health issues. As global citizens, nurses identify and act on health inequities in the populations they work with at the local, national, and international levels.
- Planetary citizenship emphasizes the importance of interconnection to humans living on a vibrant and rich planet.
- Nurses require education in global and planetary health in order to provide competent and culturally safe care that promotes human health and the health of the planet.

CRITICAL THINKING EXERCISES

1. Amy (she/her) is a nurse working in the emergency department. She is caring for Munish (he/him), a patient experiencing wheezing and shortness of breath. Munish states that he is having trouble sleeping at night. He explains that he has asthma and that it has gotten increasingly worse during the forest fires that have been burning near his home. You have just been in discussions with other nurses about how the Air Quality Health Index (AQHI) has become worse with the ever-increasing number of wildfires in the area, resulting in more patients coming into the emergency room in respiratory distress. Consider the following questions that you might ask yourself when caring for Munish:
   a. What are the environmental health risks of being chronically exposed to forest fires?
   b. What are the health risks associated with climate change?
   c. What are your nursing priorities when caring for Munish?

🌐 *Answers to Critical Thinking Exercises appear on the Evolve website.*

REVIEW QUESTIONS

Review Questions 1 to 6 relate to the case study at the beginning of the chapter.

1. Which structural determinants of health contribute to the inequities experienced by temporary foreign workers while they are living in Canada?
   a. Poor health hygiene and knowledge about self-care
   b. Inadequate access to water, sanitation, and housing

   c. Low levels of education and therefore low health literacy
   d. Social isolation, stigma, and discrimination
2. In addition to routine triage assessment, what special consideration needs to be included among Elijah's triage assessment priorities?
   a. Pablo's previous experiences with accessing health care in Canada
   b. The companion's account of how Pablo's arm was injured
   c. The relationship between Pablo and the person who brought him to the emergency room
   d. Pablo's vaccination history
3. The translator is not immediately available, and Elijah must complete his triage assessment. In addition to routine triage assessment documentation, what does Elijah need to document about Pablo's presentation to the emergency room?
   a. Observations of relational interaction between Pablo and his companion
   b. Steps taken to find an English–Spanish translator for Pablo
   c. The quality and cleanliness of the clothing Pablo was wearing
   d. Words Pablo said in English about his arm
4. What can Elijah do to mitigate the possibility of an inequitable power balance between Pablo and the person who brought him to the emergency room?
   a. Reassure Pablo that there will be an opportunity to speak through a translator soon, and hand him written Spanish-language patient teaching materials about fractures.
   b. Invite the companion to translate while they wait for formal translation supports, and ask assessment questions through the companion.
   c. With both people present, ask the companion whether Pablo feels comfortable having the companion stay for his assessment.
   d. Briefly invite Pablo into a private space, then use an online translation tool to ask Pablo directly about his relationship to the person who accompanied him to the emergency room.
5. Pablo's ulnar fracture requires surgery. To prepare for transfer, and in addition to physical assessment, what other information needs to be provided in Elijah's handover report from emergency to orthopedic surgery?
   a. The contact information for the person who brought Pablo to the emergency room, and when they will return.
   b. The potential for the injury to be work related and the language barrier.
   c. The risk for infection due to dusty clothing and crowded housing.
   d. The time and date of the next meeting for a Spanish language course.
6. In addition to routine documentation, what additional documentation must Elijah initiate in the patient record in order to protect Pablo's entitlements to care?
   a. Pablo's country of origin and length of stay in Canada.
   b. The country of origin and place of employment of the person who accompanied Pablo.
   c. Pablo's provincial health care and supplementary insurance numbers.
   d. The possibility that the injury occurred in the workplace, and the need for translation supports.

Answers: 1. d; 2. c; 3. a; 4. d; 5. b; 6. d.

🌐 *Rationales for the Review Questions appear on the Evolve website.*

RECOMMENDED WEBSITES

International Council of Nurses (ICN): https://www.icn.ch
The ICN is a federation of more than 130 national nursing associations, representing the more than 27 million nurses worldwide. Founded in 1899, the ICN is the world's first and widest reaching international organization for health professionals. Its mission is to represent nursing worldwide, advance the nursing profession, promote the well-being of nurses, and advocate for health in all policies.

Public Health Agency of Canada: https://www.canada.ca/en/public-health.html
This website provides information on the prevention of diseases and injuries, the promotion of good physical and mental health, and information to support informed decision making.

United Nations (UN): https://www.un.org/en
This website provides updates on maintaining international peace and security, the promotion and protection of human rights globally, as well as publications related to the Sustainable Development Goals (SDGs).

World Health Organization (WHO): https://www.who.int/en
This website provides links to information and publications on a variety of topics related to population health.

WHO Commission on Social Determinants of Health: https://www.who.int/health-topics/social-determinants-of-health#tab=tab_1
This website provides links to publications related to the social determinants of health.

REFERENCES

A full reference list is available on the website for this book at http://evolve.elsevier.com/Canada/Potter/fundamentals/

12

Indigenous Health

Written by Caroline Foster-Boucher, RN, BScN, MN

OBJECTIVES

Mastery of content in this chapter will enable you to:

- Describe the diversity of Indigenous peoples in Canada.
- Examine the Canadian history of colonization, including pre-European and post-European contact.
- Describe the historical timeline of key Indigenous events and legislative changes in Canada.
- Analyze components of colonialism to understand the complexities of the relationship that evolved between Indigenous peoples and Europeans.
- Examine the impact of the residential school system on Indigenous communities across Canada.
- Describe the concepts of structural racism, child welfare, poverty, and the justice system in relation to nursing practice.
- Differentiate between respect, trust, and spirituality in the context of caring for Indigenous peoples.
- Describe components of Indigenous cultural orientations in relation to nursing practice.
- Describe the historical development of the concept of culture, cultural competence, cultural safety, and cultural humility in relation to nursing practice.
- Analyze components of cultural assessment critical to understanding the values, beliefs, and practices of people experiencing cultural transitions.
- Apply research findings to the provision of culturally competent care that incorporates cultural safety and relational practice.
- Apply research findings to the provision of nursing care to Indigenous peoples in Canada, with consideration of assessment and intervention underpinned by cultural safety, health equity, and social justice.
- Examine selected chronic illness experiences relevant to Indigenous peoples in Canada.
- Differentiate between Indigenous health from a global perspective and Indigenous health from a Canadian perspective.

KEY TERMS

Colonialism
Colonization
Cultural awareness
Cultural genocide
Cultural humility
Cultural safety
Cultural sensitivity
Culturally competent care
Culturally congruent care
Distal determinants of health
Historical trauma

Holistic view
Indian Act
Indigenous health
Indigenous peoples
Indigenous world views
Intergenerational trauma
Intermediate determinants of health
Medicine Wheel
Post-European contact
Pre-European contact
Proximal determinants of health

Residential schools
Sixties Scoop
Smudging
Social determinants of health
Structural racism
Theories of Indigenous health
Transcultural assessment model
Transcultural nursing
Truth and Reconciliation Commission of Canada (TRC)
Two-Spirit

🌐 WEBSITE

http://evolve.elsevier.com/Canada/Potter/fundamentals/

CASE STUDY

An older Indigenous person, Helen (preferred pronouns: she/her), is admitted to the medical unit for congestive heart failure and a frequent cough. In her chart, it states that she has congestive heart failure, diabetes, and a history of tuberculosis. She is 70 years old and apparently was brought in from a remote fly-in Cree reserve. She has her daughter with her, who stays as long as she is allowed to that day, and then goes to stay overnight at a local hotel.

Over the next few days, there is a steady stream of visitors to see Helen, including her seven adult children, many grandchildren and great grandchildren, as well as numerous relatives and friends. The nurses have to limit the number of visitors because Helen is in a two-bed hospital room.

Finally, Helen is diagnosed with severe chronic obstructive pulmonary disease. She is discharged because there is nothing more that can be done for her at the hospital, and she is scheduled to fly home the next day.

Think about this case study as you read this chapter. There are Review Questions at the end of the chapter about this case study.

INDIGENOUS DIVERSITY—THE CANADIAN PERSPECTIVE

In order to appreciate the contemporary health issues facing Indigenous peoples in Canada, it is essential to first recognize and respect their diversity of cultural and social histories and current day realities, and ways of knowing (Canadian Nurses Association [CNA], 2018; Canadian Association of Schools of Nursing, 2022). Indigenous peoples are a unique and fast-growing population. In 2021, the number of people who identified as Indigenous (First Nations, Inuit, or Métis) numbered 1.8 million (Statistics Canada, 2022). Since the mid-1990s, the Indigenous population has increased significantly. Between 2006 and 2021, it grew by 56.8%, more than four times faster than the non-Indigenous population (Statistics Canada, 2022). In 2021, Indigenous peoples accounted for 5% of the total population of Canada (Statistics Canada, 2022). Of the three Indigenous groups, the First Nations population increased the most between 2016 and 2021, by 9.7% (Statistics Canada, 2022). The Inuit population increased by 8.5%, and the Métis population increased by 6.3% between 2016 and 2021 (Statistics Canada, 2022).

Indigenous peoples in Canada increasingly live in urban centres. In 2021, 801 045 Indigenous people lived in urban areas (including large cities, or census metropolitan areas, and smaller urban centres); this proportion increased by 12.5% between 2016 and 2021 (Statistics Canada, 2022). Furthermore, the Indigenous population is, on average, 8.2 years younger than the non-Indigenous population. The average age of the Indigenous population was 33.6 years, while the average age of the non-Indigenous population was 41.8 years (Statistics Canada, 2022).

The three Indigenous groups—First Nations, Inuit, and Métis—have their own unique languages, heritages, cultural practices, and spiritual beliefs (Government of Canada, 2022). These groups contain many subgroups, each with their own unique culture. The Government of Canada uses the legal term *Indian* to describe all Indigenous peoples in Canada who are not Inuit. This includes First Nations people, the groups of people who were the original inhabitants of Canada before European explorers began to arrive in the 1600s (pre-European contact), and the Métis, a distinct cultural group formed after Indigenous peoples made contact with Europeans (post-European contact) but before colonization. The legal definitions used to describe Indigenous peoples in Canada include Status Indians, non-Status Indians, and Treaty Indians. *Status* Indians are individuals registered under the Indian Act (AANDC, 2013b), the legislation that regulates the management of reserves and sets out certain federal obligations. A *Treaty* Indian is a Status Indian who belongs to a First Nation that signed a treaty with the Crown (AANDC, 2013b).

Until recently, non-Status Indians and Métis were not included as Indians under section 91(24) of the *Constitution Act*. However, in 1999, four claimants brought action against the federal government seeking a declaration that Métis and non-Status Indians fall within federal jurisdiction. In addition, their actions declared that Métis and non-Status Indians have the right to be consulted by, and to negotiate with, the federal government over needs, rights, and interests as Indigenous peoples. In what is now known as the "Daniels Decision," in 2016 the Supreme Court of Canada ruled in favour of non-Status Indians and Métis as being considered "Indian" under section 91(24) of the *Constitution Act* (Indigenous Services Canada, 2022a; *Daniels v. Canada [Indian Affairs and Northern Development]*, 2016). This ruling resulted in the signing of a political accord by the federal government and the Congress of Aboriginal Peoples. The *Canada and the Congress of Aboriginal Peoples Political Accord* describes objectives, policy priorities, and an implementation process for funding that has been jointly agreed upon, with the goal of decreasing socioeconomic inequity between Indigenous and non-Indigenous peoples in Canada

(Congress of Aboriginal Peoples, n.d.-a.; Crown–Indigenous Relations and Northern Affairs Canada, 2018).

More than 70 Indigenous languages were reported in the 2022 Census of Population, with Cree languages being the most commonly spoken (Statistics Canada, 2022). Many Indigenous languages have identifiable dialects; however, some of these languages are in decline owing to the Canadian government's history of assimilation policies; for example, Indigenous children who were forced to attend residential schools were forbidden from speaking their own language. In 2022, the number of Indigenous people learning an Indigenous language increased by 7% from 2016 to 2021. As well, the federal government signed the *Indigenous Languages Act* into law in 2019, providing the legal mandate for funding for initiatives to "reclaim, revitalize, maintain and strengthen Indigenous languages" (Assembly of First Nations, n.d.-a; Statistics Canada, 2022).

Interpreters who translate for Indigenous patients not only understand and translate the language but also make concepts relevant within the cultural realm, interpreting the Indigenous patient's culture for the health care provider. Health care information translated in an accurate and culturally appropriate way can lead to patient empowerment and better health choices (Eggertson, 2014).

Indigenous peoples in Canada are exceptionally diverse—culturally, linguistically, socially, economically, and historically. The distinct cultural differences between Indigenous groups stem from historical and geographical influences on their day-to-day life. The diversity of Indigenous peoples exists within First Nations communities (or Indian bands, the governing units of First Nations) across Canada (Assembly of First Nations, n.d.-b); within at least two distinct cultures of the Métis; and where differences emanate from particular historical experiences and geographical locations of the Inuit. Connecting diversity to Indigenous health, Waldram et al. (2006, p. 23) have stated the following:

The recognition and acceptance of such diversity is essential to an appreciation of developments in the healthcare field and to an appreciation of the myriad processes that have affected the health status of Indigenous people in both the pre-contact and post-contact periods.

INDIGENOUS HISTORY IN CANADA

Indigenous history is inseparable from the history of European colonization, which includes pre-European and post-European contact (see Table 12.1 for a historical timeline of key Indigenous events and legislation in Canada). Pre-European contact refers to the history of Indigenous peoples before the exploration and settlement of the Americas by Europeans. During that period, Indigenous peoples were composed of distinct cultures from the Arctic, Western Subarctic, Eastern Subarctic, Northeastern Woodlands, Plains, Plateau, and Northwest Coast.

The Inuit have inhabited northern Canada for over 5 000 years. According to the 2021 Census of Population, there were 70 545 Inuit, who make up 3.9% of the Indigenous population (Statistics Canada, 2022). More than two-thirds of Inuit live in the northern part of Canada, in four territories (Inuit Nunangat) that were negotiated in Comprehensive Land Claim Agreements with the federal government (Penny et al., 2012; Statistics Canada, 2022). The four areas of Inuit Nunangat (the Inuit homeland) include Nunatsiavut (Northern Labrador), Nunavik (Northern Quebec), Nunavut, and the Inuvialuit Settlement Region (Northwest Territories) (Crown–Indigenous Relations and Northern Affairs Canada, 2020). Each of the four regions has its own flag and history, as well as distinct geography and regional experiences of its people (Inuit Tapiriit Kanatami, n.d.).

TABLE 12.1	Indigenous Timeline: Key Events and Legislation
1500s and 1600s	**Early contact** made between Indigenous peoples and Europeans. Relationship consists of trading, mutual curiosity, and intermarriage. French settlement develops in Acadia.
1613	**Two-Row Wampum Treaty** established between the Haudenosaunee and the Dutch in Upstate New York—belts said to be created in order to record the agreement, with two rows of purple shells symbolizing two boats (one Indigenous, one European) travelling side by side on the River of Life (Parmenter, 2013).
1664	**Two-Row Wampum Treaty** established between the Haudenosaunee and the British Crown in Albany, New York (Mohawks of the Bay of Quinte, n.d.; Parmenter, 2013).
1670	**Hudson's Bay Company** incorporated by the English Royal Charter. Headquarters at York Factory on Hudson's Bay, controlled fur trade in North America for two centuries (Hudson's Bay Company History Foundation, 2016a, 2016b).
1754–1763	**French and Indian War, Seven Years' War**—French and British colonies and their Indigenous allies are pitted against each other; results in Treaty of Paris; Britain gains control of French Canada and Acadia (Dickason & Newbigging, 2015).
1763	**Royal Proclamation of 1763** issued by King George III to protect the land rights of Indigenous peoples by prohibiting purchase of or settling on Indigenous lands.
1834	**Mohawk Indian Residential School opens in Brantford Ontario** (TRC, 2015b).
1857	*British North America Act* creates Dominion of Canada, giving Canada jurisdiction over "Indians" and lands reserved for "Indians" (Dickason & Newbigging, 2015).
1867	*Gradual Civilization Act* introduces the idea of enfranchisement for Indigenous peoples. Eligible males are aged 21 and up, literate in English or French, with minimal education and "good moral character and free from debt." Accepted males would receive 20 hectares of land but would voluntarily relinquish their treaty rights. Government sees it as an honour that would be sought after; however, it is rejected by Indigenous peoples, with only a single candidate enfranchised by 1867 (Robinson, 2016).
1871–1921	Canadian government enters into 11 numbered **treaties** with Indigenous peoples (Dickason & Newbigging, 2015).
1876	*Indian Act* passed—introduced in 1876 as a consolidation of previous legislation that focused on assimilation of Indigenous peoples into Canadian society. Gives the Government of Canada vast powers over First Nations people with regard to identity, political structures, cultural practices, governance, and education. Amended several times, most notably in 1951 and 1985 (Henderson & Parrott, 2016). (See Box 12.1 for amendments to *Indian Act* up to 1950.) The *Indian Act* is still in use today.
1880	**Department of Indian Affairs** created by the Government of Canada—numerous organizational and name changes since its creation. In 2017, Trudeau government divides it into two departments: Crown–Indigenous Relations and Northern Affairs Canada, and Indigenous Services Canada (Government of Canada, 2020).
1883	**Formal Indian residential school system** established by the Canadian government in partnership with the Roman Catholic and Anglican churches (TRC, 2015a). Three industrial schools opened in Western Canada.
1884	**Attendance at Indian residential schools compulsory** for Indigenous children between 7 and 16 years of age (TRC, 2015b).
1885	**Northwest Rebellion**—Uprising by Métis led by Louis Riel (in what is now Manitoba) against the Government of Canada, with the grievance that Canada has failed to protect the rights, land, and survival of Métis as a distinct people. Riel and the Métis surrender; Riel is found guilty of treason and hanged (Beal et al., 2021).
1948	**Compulsory attendance ends** at Indian residential schools (Canadian Baptists of Western Canada Justice and Mercy Network, 2013).
1951	**Changes to *Indian Act*** lift the ban on traditional practices and ceremonies; women included in band democracy (Dickason & Newbigging, 2015).
1960	**Indigenous peoples given right to vote** (Leslie, 2016).
1969	**White paper** issued by the federal government proposing repeal of the *Indian Act*, abolishment of Department of Indian Affairs, and transfer of responsibility for Indigenous affairs to the provinces in order to assimilate Indigenous peoples into mainstream Canada. Indigenous peoples strongly resist, putting forth their own document, "Citizens Plus" (Red Paper), in which they insist that treaty and inherent rights be respected. The government retracts the white paper (Dickason & Newbigging, 2015).
1973	**Calder case** ruling by the Supreme Court of Canada—legal assertion of Indigenous land rights, which leads to the Comprehensive Land Claims Policy to address Indigenous title claims (Cruickshank, 2020).
	Indian Control of Indian Education paper issued by the National Indian Brotherhood—policy adopted by the federal government (Assembly of First Nations, 2010).
1975	**James Bay Agreement** established between Quebec, Cree, and Inuit communities (Dickason & Newbigging, 2015).
1982	*Constitution Act* **recognizes** Indigenous and treaty rights, and "Aboriginal peoples" defined as Indian, Métis, and Inuit (Dickason & Newbigging, 2015).
1984	*Western Arctic (Inuvialuit) Claims Settlement Act* passed (Dickason & Newbigging, 2015).
1985	*Indian Act* **changes**—Métis and non-Status defined as Indian; **Bill C-31** allows women who have lost their Indian status (because of marriage, widowing, or abandonment) to regain it (Dickason & Newbigging, 2015).
1990	**Oka crisis**—ignited by the town of Oka's plans for a golf course to be built on Mohawk burial grounds in Quebec; crisis lasts for 6 months (Dickason & Newbigging, 2015).
	Meech Lake Accord defeated in part by Elijah Harper in Manitoba legislature (Dickason & Newbigging, 2015).
1991–1996	**Royal Commission on Aboriginal Peoples**—report released in 1996, most in-depth study of Indigenous issues to date (TRC, 2015d)
1992	Parliament passes motion citing **Louis Riel as the founder of Manitoba** (J. Clark, 1992).
1996	**Last federally run Indian residential school in Canada closes** (Gordon Indian Residential School in Punnichy, Saskatchewan).
1997	*Delgamuukw v. British Columbia*—Supreme Court decision regarding principles of Indigenous title, including property rights entitling the holders to exclusive possession and use of land and its resources (Dickason & Newbigging, 2015).
1999	**Nunavut created** (Dickason & Newbigging, 2015).

TABLE 12.1	Indigenous Timeline: Key Events and Legislation—cont'd
2000	**Nisga'a Treaty approved** (Dickason & Newbigging, 2015).
2008	**Formal apology by Prime Minister Stephen Harper, on behalf of Government of Canada, to Indigenous peoples** for Canada's role in residential school system (TRC, 2015b).
	Truth and Reconciliation Commission of Canada officially launched (TRC, 2015d).
2012	**Idle No More movement** forms in response to alleged legislative abuses of Indigenous treaty rights by the federal government, specifically Bill C-45, an omnibus bill that produces sweeping legislative changes, including removal of protections for forests and waterways (T. Marshall, 2015).
2016	Canada removes objector status and officially adopts **United Nations Declaration on the Rights of Indigenous Peoples** (Fontaine, 2016).
	Daniels Decision handed down, in which Supreme Court of Canada rules that the federal government "has constitutional responsibility for Métis, and non-Status Indians" (Congress of Aboriginal Peoples, n.d.-b).
	Truth and Reconciliation Commission of Canada releases their final report with 94 Calls to Action (TRC, 2015d).
	Government of Canada launches official national inquiry into **missing and murdered Indigenous women and girls** (Crown–Indigenous Relations and Northern Affairs Canada, 2022; Kirkup, 2016).
2018	The **Canada–Congress of Aboriginal Peoples Political Accord** signed by the Canadian government and the Congress of Aboriginal Peoples as a result of the Daniels Decision, thereby demonstrating recognition of federal government's jurisdiction and fiduciary responsibility to Métis and non-Status Indians as per Daniels Decision (Congress of Aboriginal Peoples, n.d.-a).
2019	Release of ***Reclaiming Power and Place: Final Report of the National Inquiry into Missing and Murdered Indigenous Women and Girls*** (Volumes 1a and 1b), a 1200-page report that includes 231 recommendations for sweeping changes to colonial policies and structures across the country (Tasker, 2019).
2020	***An Act Respecting First Nations, Métis and Inuit children, youth and families*** came into force on January 1, 2020. This act was co-developed with Indigenous peoples and the provinces/territories to reduce the number of Indigenous children in care by affirming the rights of First Nations, Métis, and Inuit communities to exercise jurisdiction over child and family services.
2020	**Joyce Echaquan** dies in a Quebec hospital; a recording of racist taunts from health care providers, including nurses, is found on her cell phone. The Coroner's inquiry report, released in 2021, states that Echaquan died from pulmonary edema; however, racism and prejudice were factors in her death, which could have been prevented had she been treated differently (Nerestant, 2021).
2020	Review of racism in health care in British Columbia (BC), ***In Plain Sight: Systemic Racism in BC Health Care***, published. Findings include widespread systemic racism across BC health care system. Apology given by leaders of health care provider regulatory colleges. BC government responds with a 5-year plan in 2022, which includes specific actions to address systemic racism (Schmunk, 2021; Skrypnek, 2022).
2021	Using ground-penetrating radar, an anthropologist makes preliminary findings of possible 215 unmarked graves of children—this number is later changed to 200. Across Canada, other First Nations begin searches around Indian residential school sites, with more possible gravesites found.
2021	Government of Canada pledges $320 million to help First Nations search for burial sites around Indian residential school sites and to support residential school survivors, families, and communities.
2021	Senate releases report ***Forced and Coerced Sterilization of Persons in Canada***, which confirms that Indigenous women, among other groups, have been subjected to forced and coerced sterilization in Canada. Senate Committee urges Government of Canada to engage in a larger study in order to identify solutions (Senate of Canada, 2021).
2022	Government of Canada settles class action lawsuit with $40 billion child welfare settlement agreement for children harmed by discriminatory child welfare practices from 1991 to 2017 (Major, 2022; Stefanovich, 2022).
2022	The ***Anishinabek Nation Governance Agreement Act***—the first agreement of its kind in Ontario—receives royal assent, granting five First Nations the power to make their own decisions regarding leadership selection, citizenship, language and culture, and operations and management of government (CBC News, 2022; Migneault, 2022).

The Métis are a distinct Indigenous group borne from the union of Indigenous women and European men during the fur trade era, post-European contact but precolonization. Métis communities became established and remained distinct from other Indigenous communities, with their own culture and way of life, including unique language (Michif), music (fiddling), dance (jigging), transportation (the Red River cart), and clothing (woven Métis sashes) (Métis National Council, n.d.). Ancestral Métis traditional homelands stretch from the Great Lakes to the Mackenzie Delta across the Prairies, as well as reaching into Ontario, British Columbia, and the Northwest Territories (Rupertsland Institute, n.d.).

There are 624 220 Métis living in Canada, with 224 655 people reporting membership in a Métis organization or settlement, and 79.8% reporting being a member of one of the five signatories to the Canada–Métis Nation Accord (Statistics Canada, 2022). In 2017, the Canada–Métis Nation Accord was signed between the Government of Canada and the Métis National Council (MNC) and their five governing members: the Métis Nation of Ontario, the Métis Nation Saskatchewan, the Métis Nation British Columbia, the Manitoba Métis Federation, and the Métis Nation of Alberta. This accord encompassed an agreement to work government to government on issues such as education, health, and employment (Lilley, 2021). Historically, the Métis have suffered great inequity and social exclusion from Canadian society. Currently, there is a lack of sufficiently accurate health statistics about the Métis owing to issues related to identity, interpretation of statistics, and other political pressures that influence the definition of who is Métis and how data are gathered and interpreted (Andersen, 2016). The Métis suffer from disparities in the social determinants of health, poor health outcomes, and health service gaps. The Métis may also be excluded from health care services intended for other Indigenous groups (Monchalin & Monchalin, 2018).

The term *First Nations* is derived from *Indian*, a legal term used in the *Indian Act* to refer to a Status Indian. The *Indian Act* was passed in 1876 and has been amended frequently since then (Box 12.1 lists specific amendments). Its main purpose was to assimilate First Nations people into Canadian society. It delineates federal obligations toward

BOX 12.1   Amendments to the *Indian Act*, 1876–1950

Between 1876 and 1950, a series of amendments were made to the *Indian Act*. Their purpose was to strengthen the philosophy of civilization and assimilation underlying the initial act. Moreover, many of the changes to the act granted the government greater powers to move Indigenous peoples and expropriate their lands for non-Indigenous use.

Key amendments to the *Indian Act* during this period include the following:

- 1885: Prohibition of several traditional Indigenous ceremonies, such as potlatches.
- 1894: Removal of band control over non-Indigenous peoples living on reserve. This power is transferred to the Superintendent General of Indian Affairs.
- 1905: Power to remove Indigenous peoples from reserves near towns with more than 8 000 people.
- 1911: Power to expropriate portions of reserves for roads, railways, and other public works, as well as to move an entire reserve away from a municipality if deemed expedient.
- 1914: Requirement that western Indigenous peoples seek official permission before appearing in Indigenous "costume" in any public dance, show, exhibition, stampede, or pageant.
- 1918: Power to lease out uncultivated reserve lands to non-Indigenous peoples if the new leaseholder will use it for farming or pasture.
- 1927: Prohibition of anyone (Indigenous or otherwise) from soliciting funds for Indigenous legal claims without special license from the Superintendent General. This amendment grants government control over the ability of Indigenous peoples to pursue land claims.
- 1930: Prohibition of pool hall owners from allowing entrance of an Indigenous person who "by inordinate frequenting of a pool room either on or off an Indian reserve misspends or wastes his time or means to the detriment of himself, his family or household."

Adapted from Makarenko, J. (2008). *The Indian Act: Historical overview*. https://repolitics.com/features/the-indian-act-historical-overview

"Indians" and regulates the management of reserves, money, and other resources for "Indians." The term *Indian* is generally not preferred by Indigenous peoples; *First Nation*, by comparison, is a term in widespread use that can refer to either a person or a group of people; legally, a group of First Nations people is known as an *Indian band* (AANDC, 2013b). There are currently 634 First Nations, or Indian bands, in Canada.

A *reserve* is a piece of land that has been set aside by the federal government for the exclusive use of an Indian band or First Nation. Each First Nation may have one or more reserves based on treaty agreement and population. First Nations have a Chief and Council governance structure that was imposed on them through the *Indian Act*. Traditionally, this was not the way Indigenous peoples self-governed (St. Germain & Dyck, 2010), as many Indigenous groups are traditionally matriarchal (Allan & Smylie, 2015).

Historical knowledge of Indigenous peoples in Canada is foundational to understanding how Indigenous people currently view health. This vantage point includes an appreciation of health from a traditional Indigenous view, a Western biomedical view, and a combination view. Historically, Indigenous communities experienced healing and well-being through a holistic view of health that considered the physical, emotional, mental, and spiritual dimensions of illness and treatment. Traditional shamans, herbalists, and specialized healers worked within a holistic framework to heal afflicted persons (Earle, 2011; Waldram et al., 2006). Research demonstrates that Indigenous peoples were generally healthy and well-nourished before contact, with death resulting from injury, accidents, or war. Diseases were minimal, and there is no evidence to date of widespread diffusion of disease pre-European contact (Douglas, 2013).

Colonialism

Colonialism is the ongoing policy of domination that begin with the age of European imperialism in the fifteenth century, during which the monarchs of Europe strove to expand their empires and wealth (Kohn & Reddy, 2017; Truth and Reconciliation Commission of Canada [TRC], 2015a). This expansion was accomplished through exploration of other lands and the resettlement of Europeans globally on lands in use by the original inhabitants. Colonization is the purposeful practice of settling invaders onto foreign lands, plundering the land's resources, and exploiting and marginalizing the inhabitants. Other aspects of colonialism include the development of institutions and policies by European imperial and Euro-American settler governments toward Indigenous peoples (TRC, 2015b, pp. 43–50). In Canada, this history of colonization and ongoing colonial policies and structures have led to a complex and troubled relationship between Indigenous peoples and Canadian society. Nelson (2012) has noted the importance of knowing this history and current-day reality in order to work toward healing the relationship between settlers and Indigenous peoples. Colonialism resulted in overwhelming historical trauma (the nature of trauma as experienced over many years) for Indigenous peoples. Responding to the health challenges that Indigenous peoples experience requires an understanding of the historical, social, and economic contexts in which Indigenous families and communities are situated.

Europeans first encountered Indigenous peoples in 1000 BC, when the Norse made contact with the Inuit. From the 1500s onward, other Europeans began arriving in what is now known as Canada. French explorers and fur traders introduced diseases such as smallpox, tuberculosis (TB), and measles, which killed thousands of Indigenous people. Scarce resources diminished Indigenous livelihoods, and malnutrition, starvation, and alcohol consumption made circumstances worse (Dickason & Newbigging, 2015; Waldram et al., 2006).

During post-European contact, Europeans established relationships with Indigenous peoples, and colonization damaged Indigenous systems of government, trade, and health care. The Canadian government displaced Indigenous peoples from their traditional lands, and government policies both isolated and assimilated Indigenous peoples into Canadian society, resulting in the destruction of Indigenous cultures. These oppressive and suppressive policies and acts had extensive negative effects on Indigenous cultural identities and governance structures (TRC, 2015c, pp. 3–4). The Indian residential school system, for example, which no longer exists in Canada (the last federally run school closed in 1996 [TRC, 2015d]), left a legacy that has persisted over generations; the physical and psychological abuse of Indigenous children at these schools "is reflected in the significant educational, income, health and social disparities between Aboriginal people and other Canadians" (TRC, 2015b, p. 135).

Indian Residential Schools and Indian Day Schools

Residential schools and associated policies were a central element in colonial practices in Canada. Indigenous children as young as 4 years old were separated, often forcibly, from their parents and sent to residential schools to board year-round in order to sever the link between their Indigenous identity and culture. This system was part of the government's policy to eliminate Indigenous peoples as a distinct group and to assimilate them into mainstream Canadian society. The federal government's ulterior motive was to avoid fulfilling its legal and financial obligations to Indigenous peoples as well as to gain control over their lands and resources, thereby eliminating treaties, reserves, and Indigenous rights (TRC, 2015b, p. 3; Union of Ontario Indians, 2013). Indian Day Schools were also operated in a similar manner and for the same reasons; however, students were allowed to go home for the night (McGill Indigenous Initiatives, n.d.). Indian Day Schools were cheaper to run and operated in a greater number and for a longer time period than Indian residential schools. Part of the mandate of Indian Day Schools was to assimilate the community as well as the student (Whitebean, 2019).

The Government of Canada funded the Roman Catholic, Anglican, United, Methodist, and Presbyterian churches to operate at least 139 residential schools beginning in the 1880s, the last of which closed in 1996 (TRC, 2015b, p. 3). At least 150 000 Indigenous children attended these schools over a period of approximately 130 years. The buildings were poorly built and maintained and had limited numbers of inadequately trained staff. Regulations were minimal and weakly enforced. The children were harshly disciplined and forbidden to speak their own language or to practise any part of their own culture, including their spirituality. They received a rudimentary education and were often forced to engage in chores to maintain the schools' operations. Physical and sexual abuse were rampant throughout the schools (TRC, 2015b, pp. 105–110), and if reported, which was rare, little was done other than moving the perpetrator to another school or having the person resign. Few police investigations occurred, and prosecutions were rare.

At least 3 200 children are estimated to have died from malnourishment, diseases such as TB, and abuse; this number includes those who ran away and those who froze to death. The total number of children that died could be 5 to 10 times higher; however, given the schools' poor record keeping, the actual number of deaths may never be known (Mas, 2015; TRC, 2015a, 2015e). In many cases, the schools did not record the names or genders of the children who died. Nor did the schools send children's bodies back to their home communities for burial, a fact that is becoming more apparent with the discovery of potential unmarked graves on the sites of former residential schools (TRC, 2015a, p. 118; TRC, 2015b, p. 100).

Ground-penetrating radar and other noninvasive archeological tools have so far located 1728 unmarked children's graves on the grounds of former residential schools (Deer, 2021b; "One quarter of Canada's Indian Residential Schools," 2022). The discovery of 200 unmarked graves in 2021 at the former Kamloops Indian Residential School attracted international attention (Sterritt & Dickson, 2021) and came as a shock to many Canadians. The search for more graves is planned or ongoing at dozens of former residential school sites (Hopper, 2021; "One quarter of Canada's Indian Residential Schools," 2022).

The legacy of residential schools continues to this day, with devastating consequences for Indigenous communities across Canada. Students at residential schools received no parenting and became institutionalized. As a result of this upbringing, they did not learn how to be parents themselves. Descendants of residential school survivors recall being harshly disciplined by their parents in abusive homes, with minimal affection—experiences similar to those of residential school survivors (Elias et al., 2012; TRC, 2015c, pp. 11–12, 32–33). This legacy is now understood as **intergenerational trauma**, which is defined as shared collective experiences of sustained and numerous attacks on a group that may accumulate over generations (Barker et al., 2017, 2019; Centre for Suicide Prevention, n.d.).

Research is needed to study why suicide rates are so much higher among the children and grandchildren of survivors than among survivors themselves. Some survivors have used alcohol and other substances to cope with post-traumatic stress disorder; the effects of addiction have had a stronghold on some families and communities for decades. Diets have been poor owing to a lack of knowledge about nutrition and because of food pattern issues derived from residential schools. Sexual abuse is rampant in some communities, as evidenced by recent reports (Elias et al., 2012; Kirkup & Ubelacker, 2016; TRC, 2015c, p. 70).

The Government of Canada has failed in its assimilation goal—Indigenous peoples have survived the atrocities of residential schools and maintained their identity and communities. However, the legacy of residential schools is still reflected in the significant health, educational, and income disparities between the Indigenous and non-Indigenous population in Canada. Furthermore, intergenerational trauma is rampant within Indigenous communities, with some children who were abused becoming abusers, developing addictions as a way of coping, and being unable to parent their own children because of lack of experience of being parented (Allen, 2020; TRC, 2015c).

Truth and Reconciliation

Beginning in the 1960s, the assertion of Indigenous rights globally and the United States' civil rights movement led churches to begin examining their relationship with Indigenous peoples in Canada (TRC, 2015d). Some churches apologized in the 1970s, 1980s, and 1990s for their treatment of, and the impact of their work on, Indigenous peoples in Canada (TRC, 2015d). Most recently, Pope Francis travelled to Canada to deliver an apology to Residential school survivors and their descendants for the Catholic Church members' roles in abusing children and attempted erasure of Indigenous cultures. Responses from the Indigenous communities were mixed with some stating that his apology lacked specificity and clarity regarding the role of the Catholic Church in Indian Residential School activities and mandate (Maqbool, 2022; Thompson Reuters, 2022).

During this time, residential school survivors wrote accounts of their experiences, and the Royal Commission on Aboriginal Peoples (RCAP) was established to study the relationship between Indigenous peoples, the Government of Canada, and Canadian society. The final report, released in 1996, contained a chapter dedicated to elucidating the residential school experience. In response to RCAP, the federal government issued an action plan that included an apology and a healing fund—the Aboriginal Healing Foundation (AHF) (TRC, 2015d, pp. 521–579).

Residential school survivors subsequently organized into associations, and by 2005, over 18 000 residential school survivors had filed lawsuits against the involved organizations, churches, the federal government, and individuals who had committed the abuses. The response from the government was insufficient to stem the tide of litigation, and in the early 2000s, over 20 class action lawsuits were filed against the federal government. Eventually, Indigenous organizations, church organizations, and the federal government began talks that would lead to the Indian Residential Schools Settlement Agreement (IRSSA), which came into effect in 2007 (TRC, 2015d).

The five components of the IRSSA include the **Truth and Reconciliation Commission of Canada (TRC)**, which provided opportunities for individuals, families, and communities to share their experiences of residential schools and also created a comprehensive historical record. The other components include the Common Experience Payment (CEP), in which every former student who had resided at a residential school would be eligible for a $10 000 compensation for the first year, plus an additional $3 000 for each year or partial year they attended (TRC, 2015d); the Independent Assessment Process (IAP), which was an out-of-court process for resolving claims of abuse or neglect; $20 million allocated for commemorative projects acknowledging the impact of residential schools; and $125 million set aside for the AHF to address the healing needs of Indigenous peoples affected by residential schools. The Anglican, Presbyterian, United, and Catholic churches were parties to the agreement, and all contributed some funds (TRC, 2015d).

However, the IRSSA covered only those Indigenous peoples who fell within the prior series of lawsuits, and it limited compensation to those who attended schools with a residential component. It failed to address the claims of Métis students and did not compensate those who attended other institutions such as day schools (TRC, 2015d). The matter of compensation is still being dealt with to this day, with a class action lawsuit being filed for First Nations people who attended residential schools as day students but went home at night (CBC News, 2016; Munson, 2016) and another lawsuit for those who were in hospital but attended school during the day.

In 2008, then-Prime Minister Stephen Harper issued a national apology in Parliament to Indigenous peoples in Canada, followed by apologies from leaders of the opposition parties and responses to the apologies from Indigenous leaders, including National Chief Phil Fontaine; Mary Simon, President of the Inuit Tapiriit Kanatami; and others (TRC, 2015d).

The final report of the TRC, released in 2015, comprises 10 volumes that cover the country's history, from early European imperialism to the year 2000; the report also includes survivors' stories and documentation of Inuit and Métis experiences, missing children and unmarked graves, and the legacy of residential schools. The TRC determined that many of the 150 000 children who had attended the residential schools were abused sexually, physically, emotionally, and spiritually, and that Canada was guilty of cultural genocide with respect to Indigenous peoples in Canada. **Cultural genocide** is defined as the "destruction of those structures and practices that allow the group to continue as a group" (TRC, 2015a, p. 3). Instances of destruction of practices and structures included occupying and seizing land; forcing relocation of Indigenous peoples; confining them to reserves; disempowering people through replacement of existing forms of Indigenous government; and denying their basic rights, such as the right to practice their faith, the right to assemble, and the right to legal counsel.

The TRC also released 94 Calls to Action to address the ongoing legacy of residential schools (TRC, 2015b). The Calls to Action target policy and institutional and governmental structures within Canada, including the child welfare, justice, education, and health care systems; language rights; and government funding of Indigenous programs. The TRC further encouraged Canadian citizens to become *settler allies*—teachers and learners who question how non-Indigenous people can change and support Indigenous peoples in their quest for equity and self-governance (Gillmore, 2016; Monkman, 2018) (Box 12.2). In addition, the Calls to Action were directed at the government to take steps to improve its policies and funding practices. This included the commencement and completion of the inquiry into missing and murdered Indigenous women and girls in Canada and adoption of the United Nations Declaration on the Rights of Indigenous Peoples (TRC, 2015c).

Of the Calls to Action addressing Indigenous health, Call to Action 24 specifically addresses medical and nursing schools:

We call upon medical and nursing schools in Canada to require all students to take a course dealing with Aboriginal health issues, including the history and legacy of residential schools, the United Nations Declaration on the Rights of Indigenous Peoples, Treaties and Aboriginal rights, and Indigenous teachings and practices. This will require skills-based training in intercultural competency, conflict resolution, human rights, and anti-racism.

TRC, 2015c, p. 181

As of October 2022, 13 Calls to Action had been completed, 19 had not been started, and 60 were either being proposed or had projects underway (Barrera, 2022; Manitoba Indigenous and Northern Relations, 2020).

Structural Racism

Structural racism is the legitimized and normalized spectrum of attitudes, practices, and policies that consistently result in chronic and continuous substandard outcomes for a group of people—in this case, Indigenous peoples. An example would be the delays in health service provision for on-reserve Status First Nations children due to complexities in funding and delivery of health care services as well as jurisdictional issues. Non-Indigenous children's health care is funded provincially or territorially. Health care services for on-reserve First Nations children, by contrast, are funded through the federal government but regulated through provincial/territorial systems and policies. This complex process often results in denied, delayed, or disrupted services, which can lead to severe health consequences—as it did in the case of 5-year-old Jordan River Anderson, of Norway House First Nation, who died in hospital, having never lived in a family home (despite medical approval to go home 2 years earlier) because of jurisdictional funding disputes between provincial and federal government agencies (Jordan's Principle Working Group, 2015). Jordan's Principle, which was established following his death, states that the government agency that has first contact with the Indigenous child and family must pay for services without delay and resolve financial agreements with other agencies after the child has received services. This action was included in the TRC's 94 Calls to Action (Jordan's Principle Working Group, 2015).

Missing and Murdered Indigenous Women and Girls. Violence toward Indigenous women is another consequence of structural racism. In recent decades, up to and including the present day, a disproportionate number of Indigenous women and girls in Canada have disappeared or been murdered. The Royal Canadian Mounted Police (RCMP) has determined that 16% of all female homicide victims in Canada are Indigenous, even though they represent only 4.3% of the total population. In addition, between 2001 and 2014, the average rate of homicide of Indigenous women and girls was four times higher than that of other female victims in Canada (Royal Canadian Mounted Police, 2015). To identify the root causes of this violence and to develop solutions to resolve the crisis, the Canadian government launched the National Inquiry into Missing and Murdered Indigenous Women and Girls (NI-MMIWG) in 2015 (Crown–Indigenous Relations and Northern Affairs Canada, 2022). The National Inquiry released their two-volume report in 2019. In it, they present information and analysis gleaned from 15 community hearings and statements from 2 380 people, including the family and friends of the missing or murdered Indigenous women and girls, expert witnesses, Elders, and Knowledge Keepers. The National Inquiry concluded that the Canadian government is complicit in the "race-based genocide of Indigenous peoples . . . which especially targets women, girls, and [LGBTQ2 people]" (NI-MMIWG, 2019, p. 50):

This genocide has been empowered by colonial structures evidenced notably by the Indian Act, the Sixties Scoop, residential schools and breaches of human and Indigenous rights, leading directly to the current increased rates of violence, death, and suicide in Indigenous populations.

The National Inquiry determined that it was impossible to estimate the number of MMIWG owing to lack of or improper investigations and the lack of a database until 2010. As well, they found that RCMP reports were inaccurate and there were serious issues in police

BOX 12.2 A Set of Questions for Personal Reflection—Steps to Becoming a Settler Ally

What Is a Settler Ally?

A *settler ally* is someone who collectively considers what steps they can take to advance the Truth and Reconciliation process (94 Calls to Action). All Canadians have been invited by the Truth and Reconciliation Commission of Canada to become settler allies—teachers and learners who want to be informed of Indigenous–non-Indigenous historical relations; of Indigenous world views related to treaties, economic development, environment, community, and negotiations; and of instructional holistic approaches that are inclusive and safe, such as smudging, talking circles, and Indigenous teachings.

Why Do Non-Indigenous Canadians Need to Share the Burden of the Residential School System?

If you have come to help me, you are wasting your time; but if you are here because your liberation is bound up with mine, then let us work together.
—Lilla Watson, Aboriginal Elder, activist, educator (Australia)

Steps to Becoming a Settler Ally

1. Self-awareness
   - Note the circumstances throughout your life that have placed you where you are now—education, social support, family financial situation, and environment. Examine them for aspects that have matched dominant societal expectations—ethnicity, financial situation, dwelling, ability to go to school, clothing, transportation, social support.
   - Consider the history of your family in Canada. Are you settlers from generations back or more recent settlers? What part did your family play in society during key times in the last 150 years in Canada? Were they settlers buying land, building a farm, or building a business? Or were they newcomers that arrived in the last 20 years? Learn about your ancestry and the cultural history of your family.
   - What are your assumptions about what a good life is and how to attain it? What are your assumptions about right and wrong, about what causes the ills in society? Examine your assumptions and how they were formed.

Did you gain them through discussion with family and friends? Through the media? Through school? What alternative viewpoints might there be?

2. Self-education
   - Access resources to learn about the history of Indigenous peoples in Canada.
   - Read about residential schools, treaties, and racism.
   - Watch videos, look at blogs, attend lectures and film screenings.
   - Discuss with Indigenous community members.
   - Discuss with settlers.
3. Create an open and supportive environment
   - Acknowledge and appreciate the similarities and differences among individuals and within groups.
   - Encourage an atmosphere of respect and trust.
   - Be open to feedback regarding yourself, your organization, your workplace, and your community. Create safe spaces and opportunities to receive feedback.
   - Listen carefully and reflect on feedback.
   - Take action to move forward using feedback as a guide.
   - Make mistakes and learn. Be gentle with yourself.
   - Speak for yourself, not for others. Do things for others only if asked to.
4. Action
   - Recognize that your identity as an ally comes from the community, not from yourself.
   - Share knowledge with those around you; help others understand privilege and oppression, colonization and decolonization.
   - Build partnerships with others and develop plans to promote structural change.
   - Stand up against and challenge oppression, racism, and colonization.
   - Stand with Indigenous peoples. Do not lead them. Do not speak for them. Follow rather than lead. Be supportive and offer assistance in whatever way is needed. Recognize that there may be politics and processes that you may not be aware of in the Indigenous arena.

From Gehl, L. (2014). *A colonized ally meets a decolonized ally: This is what they learn.* https://www.lynngehl.com/gehl-blogging/a-colonized-ally-meets-a-decolonized-ally-this-is-what-they-learn; Pinch, S. (2014). *Revolution 101: How to be a settler ally.* https://rabble.ca/indigenous/revolution-101-how-to-be-settler-ally; Theatre Communications Group. (n.d.). *Leadership development in interethnic relations: 4 steps to becoming an ally.* https://www.tcg.org/pdfs/events/fallforum/4_Steps_to_Becoming_an_Ally.pdf; *Unsettling America: Decolonization in theory and practice.* (n.d.). https://unsettlingamerica.wordpress.com

investigations of MMIWG, including lack of communication with families, under-resourcing, under-prioritization of Indigenous communities, as well as institutional and interpersonal racism that impacted how police procedures were carried out.

Child Welfare. The **Sixties Scoop** refers to the apprehension of thousands of Indigenous children from their families and reserves "on the slightest pretext" from the 1960s to the 1990s (Johnston, 1983, p. 23), supposedly to "save them from the effects of crushing poverty, unsanitary health conditions, poor housing and malnutrition" (Johnston, 1983, p. 23). These children were often placed in non-Indigenous homes; however, the devastating effects of removing children from their families and culture were not considered. Some First Nations lost nearly an entire generation of children in this way (Johnston, 1983).

Current discourse has placed the blame for the Sixties Scoop not on the compassion of social workers but instead on the continuation of the assimilation process and devaluation of the cultures of a colonized people. While residential schools were being phased out as the institutional agent of colonization, the child welfare system was still able to remove Indigenous children from families "in the best interest of the child" (Johnston, 1983, p. 24).

Research has found that many of the children who were removed and placed with non-Indigenous families experienced abuse and neglect, and many eventually left their adopted families. Children also experienced the loss of culture and identity, racialized power dynamics, and struggles with identity and low self-esteem, resulting in self-harm and suicide in some cases (Affleck et al., 2020; Carriere, 2005; N. MacDonald & J. MacDonald, 2007; McKenzie et al., 2016; Petrow, 2016; Sinclair, 2007). Johnston (1983) states:

In retrospect, the wholesale apprehension of Native children during the Sixties Scoop appears to have been a terrible mistake. While some individual children may have benefited, many did not, nor did their families. And Native culture suffered one of many severe blows. (p. 62)

Sixties Scoop survivors entered into a class action lawsuit against the federal government, settling for $875 million in 2018. However, the settlement covers only First Nations and Inuit survivors; it does not compensate Métis survivors or non-Status First Nations survivors (Deer, 2021a; Hyslop, 2021).

While the child welfare system in Canada offers services aimed at protecting children and encouraging family stability (Canadian Child

Welfare Research Portal, n.d.), Indigenous children are overrepresented in the system. Indigenous children make up 52.2% of children in foster care from birth to 4 years of age, despite representing only 7.7% of this age group in the population as a whole (Statistics Canada, 2019). Prior to colonization, Indigenous families cared for their children according to their own belief systems and community values, laws, and traditions.

In the 1980s, in response to the concerns of First Nations communities about children in care, First Nations child and family service agencies emerged, numbering 125 agencies across Canada by 2008. However, despite the use of culturally appropriate community-based programming and preventative strategies, the proportion of Indigenous children in out-of-home care remains high. In 2020, the Government of Canada passed Bill C-92, *An Act Respecting First Nations, Inuit and Métis Children, Youth and Families*, in order to reduce the number of youth in care and allow Indigenous communities to formulate their own child welfare systems to help keep children within the community (Indigenous Services Canada, 2022b; Stefanovich & Tasker, 2020).

Poverty. The Indigenous child poverty rate across Canada is about 18%, placing Canada 27th out of 34 countries in the Organisation for Economic Cooperation and Development (Campaign 2000, 2020; D. Macdonald & Wilson, 2016). Indigenous children have much higher rates of child poverty than their non-Indigenous counterparts. In 2016, 53% of Status First Nations children on reserve and 41% of Status First Nations children off reserve lived in poverty, as did 25% of Inuit children and 22% of Métis children (Beedie et al., 2019). In contrast, 12% of nonracialized, non-Indigenous children in Canada live in poverty (Beedie et al., 2019). Manitoba and Saskatchewan have the highest rates of on-reserve Status First Nations child poverty (65% for both provinces; Beedie et al., 2019). These numbers measure income. They do not elucidate other barriers that Indigenous children face, such as poor on-reserve housing, an underfunded education system, and other systemic and structural issues that exacerbate the impact of low income. Currently, there are high levels of violence in some Indigenous communities, severe addiction issues, alarming health statistics, and potable water issues on many reserves (TRC, 2015c).

The Justice System. Incarceration has a negative impact on health. The Canadian justice system has incarcerated a disproportionate number of Indigenous peoples, with an inadequate response to the criminal victimization of Indigenous peoples (TRC, 2015c, p. 186). Despite representing only 4% of the Canadian population, Indigenous peoples accounted for 29% of admissions to federal custody and 31% of admissions to provincial/territorial custody (Statistics Canada, 2020). As well, 40% of all women incarcerated in Canada are Indigenous (S. Clark, 2019).

Given their historical experiences of inequity in justice, Indigenous peoples have viewed the justice system–including the police, the courts, and the prison system—with fear and mistrust (TRC, 2015c). Historically, the police were instrumental in enforcing attendance at residential schools. Furthermore, Indigenous peoples in Canada have been denied access to legal counsel and hence a lack of equitable justice has prevailed, as is seen, for instance, in the inadequate investigations into residential school abuse and the deaths of children.

Incarceration is impacted by health and impacts health: 79% of men and 72% of women who are in prison suffer from mental health issues. Given that Indigenous peoples constitute 30 to 42% of inmates, Indigenous peoples' mental health needs are similar to those of other prisoners (Mental Health Commission of Canada, 2020). Fetal alcohol spectrum disorder (FASD) is a serious condition that plays a role in the increasing incarceration rates of Indigenous peoples. It is estimated that 10 to 25% of all Canadians who are incarcerated suffer from FASD.

For Indigenous peoples, there is often a connection between residential school experiences, addiction, and FASD (TRC, 2015c, p. 222).

Health impacts experienced by Indigenous peoples who have been incarcerated include a high risk of death from drug overdose or suicide within 2 weeks of release, major depression, infections both acute and chronic, and heart disease (Chartrand, 2019). Furthermore, those who are incarcerated lose 2 years of life expectancy for every year spent behind bars (Singh et al., 2019). The families of Indigenous peoples who are incarcerated also are affected, especially their children, who are effectively severed from the incarcerated parent; this traumatic experience echoes the cycle of historical separation of children from their families (McGuire & Murdoch, 2021).

Recommendations have been made to decrease the impact of incarceration and structural racism in the justice system on Indigenous peoples. These include having Indigenous peoples organize their own culturally appropriate justice systems and supporting Indigenous peoples to practise restorative justice, which focuses on the rehabilitation of offenders and reconciliation with the community at large (TRC, 2015c, p. 273).

CULTURAL ORIENTATIONS

Globally, **Indigenous world views** tend to include a strong connection to the land; millennia-old knowledge of the land and its uses; collective cultures focused on the good of the group, not the individual; and an elastic sense of time focused on seasons rather than hours (McCabe, 2008). In Canada, while there is a wide diversity of values, lifestyles, and perspectives within Indigenous communities, such commonalities also exist (Kirmayer et al., 2008). Traditionally, Indigenous peoples have viewed everything as being connected physically and spiritually, including knowledge, which is seen as holistic—there is trust for inherited wisdom and respect for all living things. Knowledge is passed down orally, and spirituality is interwoven into daily life (Barnhardt & Kawagley, 2005).

Many Indigenous cultures are matriarchal (Goettner-Habendroth, 2012). They view humans as being related to the world around them, but not as the most important part of the world. Reality is defined in a relational manner to ancestors, spirits, animals, plants, and rocks (Roy, 2014). By contrast, in Western traditions, human development and other theories often have linear trajectories, moving from lower to higher levels. This is not the case in the Indigenous world view, where health and other aspects of life are based on a circular perspective in which the past, present, and future generations are connected.

In Canada, there are several ways of viewing health and healing. The Medicine Wheel Teachings (Figure 12.1) and the Seven Grandfather Teachings (or Seven Sacred Values)—**theories of Indigenous health**—can be used as a framework when contemplating health and healing strategies (Kotalik & Martin, 2016; Wenger-Nabigon, 2010). These frameworks do not fully integrate Eurocentric concepts. However, they can be used alongside Eurocentric approaches in order to deepen our understanding of parallel ways of seeing health and healing.

The circle is an important symbol in Indigenous healing that represents the interconnectedness of all beings. The **Medicine Wheel**, otherwise known as the Wheel of Life, the Circle of Life, the Hoop, or the Pimatisiwin Circle (McCabe, 2008; Moodley & West, 2005; Wenger-Nabigon, 2010), is a symbolic circular representation of the interconnectedness of life that denotes a philosophical foundation of an Indigenous world view. It is used and presented in a range of ways, depending on who is using and presenting it. Often divided into four realms, the Medicine Wheel can be used to demonstrate the importance of balance or harmony among the four areas (discussed next) in order to achieve wellness. It surrounds the core, which is viewed as

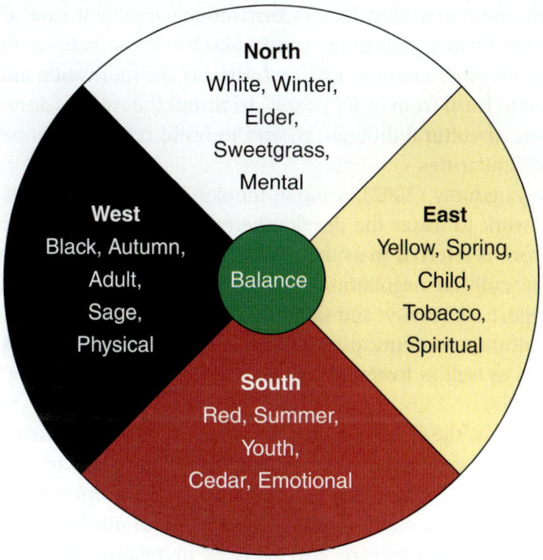

FIGURE 12.1 Ojibwe Medicine Wheel.

the person who requires healing. The Medicine Wheel can be used for teaching and for demonstrating the continuation and phases of the life cycle, as well as the four directions. It has been used in areas such as natural childbirth, mental illness, diabetes, cancer, and other illnesses (Wenger-Nabigon, 2010).

Central to the use of Medicine Wheel Teachings is the core belief of sacredness, which is a fundamental principle of Indigenous theories of healing and wellness. In different Indigenous cultures, colours are ascribed to specific parts of the circle. The four directions are paired with aspects of the person as well as parts of nature, the seasons, and other elements. Indigenous health is traditionally understood to be a balance among the emotional, physical, spiritual, and mental aspects of a person. Poor health results from disharmony or imbalance among the four components (M. Marshall et al., 2015), and the prescribed treatment attends to the imbalance (Nabigon & Wenger-Nabigon, 2012). Traditional Indigenous health systems encompass a variety of modes of treatment, including ceremonial, herbal and medicinal, and storytelling.

The person who prescribes may be a traditional healer, a medicine person, or an Elder who specializes in that area. Elders are not necessarily older persons—they are people upon whom the title has been bestowed by the community because they have become known for their extensive knowledge in an area of specialty, be it medicines, a knowledge of history, or other wisdoms. Elders are highly respected by the community.

Values are passed down through ceremony, teachings, and role modelling by Elders and other community members. Depending on the Indigenous community, these values may include kindness, sharing, noncompetitiveness, noninterference, and accepting responsibility for one's actions.

Indigenous identity has also been attacked through systemic devaluing and essentialism within public institutions and government structures. Popular media continues to frame Indigenous peoples and issues in a paternalistic manner, perpetuating harmful stereotypes (e.g., the stereotype that Indigenous peoples cannot manage their own affairs; Moeke-Pickering et al., 2018). In recent years, however, there has been a push toward reclaiming Indigenous identity through learning about cultures, traditions, traditional knowledge, languages, and medicine ways.

Identity is closely connected to health (Murdoch-Flowers et al., 2019). Research has shown a direct correlation between a decrease in

Indigenous suicide rates and an increase in identity-preserving practices in Indigenous communities (Chandler & Lalonde, 2008; O'Rourke et al., 2019). However, notions of identity involve intersections between historical, cultural, linguistic, geographical, and political dimensions, and not just traditional ways. Indigenous identity is also linked to phenotypes (braids, brown skin) and behavioural attributes; these are shaped by cultural scripts. Indigenous identity is a social construction that can unite or marginalize (Forte, 2013; Kirmayer et al., 2008).

The Sixties Scoop (Hanson, 2009) yielded generations of Indigenous peoples who struggle with identity. Many Sixties Scoop survivors were raised in middle-class White families. Their first point of contact with the Indigenous world was through street services and addiction agencies, where they learned that they were a part of the most marginalized and oppressed group in Canada (Sinclair, 2007). As a result, Indigenous youth who were adopted have shown extremely poor self-esteem and high rates of suicidal ideation as they struggle with reconfiguring their identity.

Many Indigenous peoples have found it therapeutic to be reconnected to cultural teachings and ways of healing. Indigenous healing addresses the spiritual, mental, physical, and emotional dimensions and thus is well suited to helping Indigenous peoples and communities work toward wellness. It is important that health care providers recognize this Indigenous world view and work with Indigenous peoples in using traditional ways to heal.

Place is also an important concept in health for Indigenous peoples, specifically the land. For the Inuit, place is described in terms of flora and fauna, snowdrift patterns, and animal trails. Relationships are built with the land and with all aspects of the land (Tagalik, 2015). When this holistic perspective is lost, the Inuit relate that they become disoriented and disconnected, with a lesser sense of belonging and wellness (Tagalik, 2015).

Environmental dispossession has added to a lack of wellness among Indigenous peoples in Canada. Traditionally, Indigenous peoples' teachings include having strong moral responsibility as protectors of the land. Struggles with the mining of resources and pollution of land and water have caused disruption to the health of Indigenous peoples (Fernandez-Llamazares et al., 2019). Well-being comes from the spiritual relations one has with the land, water, and food, and medicines from the land, as well as the social relationships one has with family and community (Richmond, 2015). Other key aspects in Indigenous conceptions of healing include Indigenous philosophies, cosmologies, ceremonies, identity, knowledge, lands and medicines, and environmental health (Steinhauer & Lamouche, 2015).

HISTORICAL DEVELOPMENT OF THE CONCEPT OF CULTURE

It is important for nurses to understand the historical development of the concept of culture and the shifts in thinking around the provision of culturally competent care. Framed primarily within the Canadian context, this history is also best discussed in terms of culturally appropriate nursing practice and education. The importance of being culturally sensitive and aware of a diverse society has been acknowledged by nurses and continues to evolve. Through a critical cultural analysis of the significance of power relations and structural constraints on health and health care, nurses are conceptualizing new ways to provide culturally competent and culturally safe care (Anderson et al., 2003; Baker, 2007; Browne et al., 2009; Gustafson, 2007; Hartrick Doane & Varcoe, 2015; Racine, 2009; Ramsden, 2002; Smith et al., 2006).

A critical historical view of transcultural nursing, cultural competence, and cultural safety is important for understanding the strengths and limitations of these approaches in nursing practice and education

(Gustafson, 2005; Hartrick Doane & Varcoe, 2015). Nurse scholars are increasingly questioning whether the health needs of ethnocultural groups are being equitably met (Hartrick Doane & Varcoe, 2015). Health equity may be considered one of the prerequisites and conditions for health. Ogilvie and colleagues (2005) explained that "nurses can play a pivotal role by becoming informed advocates, challenging their organizations to incorporate a global health mandate and exercising their rights as citizens to influence policy" (p. 25).

The discipline of anthropology and the seminal work by Leininger (2002a) relative to culture have provided the theoretical foundation for transcultural nursing (Glittenberg, 2004). Leininger (2002a) defined transcultural nursing as a comparative study of cultures, an understanding of similarities (culture universal) and differences (culture specific) across human groups in order to provide meaningful and beneficial delivery of health care. According to Leininger, the goals of transcultural nursing are to provide *culturally congruent* and *culturally competent care.*

Culturally congruent care is "the use of sensitive, creative, and meaningful care practices to fit with the general values, beliefs, and lifeways of clients" (Leininger & McFarland, 2002, p. 12). In other words, nurses must provide care that does not conflict with patients' valued life patterns and sets of meanings, which may be distinct from their own (Leininger, 2002b).

Leininger and McFarland (2002) define culturally competent care as "the explicit use of culturally based care and health knowledge in sensitive, creative, and meaningful ways to fit the general lifeways and needs of individuals or groups for beneficial and meaningful health and well-being or to help them face illness, disabilities, or death" (p. 84). To provide culturally competent care, nurses must bridge cultural gaps in care, work with cultural differences, and enable patients and families to receive meaningful care. Nurses need to exhibit specific ability, knowledge, sensitivity, openness, and flexibility toward the appreciation of cultural difference. They are then able to develop effective and meaningful interventions that promote optimal health for patients, families, and communities.

Leininger's Sunrise Model (Leininger, 2002a) has been a model used in nursing to promote culturally competent care with people from diverse cultures. It has been used as a guide in nursing curricula and practice policies in North America for several decades. In addition, other scholars have developed models of cultural competency in which they have expanded Leininger's work. Davidhizar and Giger (1998) and Giger (2013) developed a transcultural assessment model with a focus on cultural competency that is also used in nursing practice. The underlying premise of their model is that each person is culturally unique and should be assessed according to six cultural phenomena: communication, space, social organization, time, environmental control, and biological variations. This model suggests that these phenomena are apparent in all cultural groups, but their application to practice settings varies. Giger and Davidhizar's (2002) transcultural assessment model offers a means for nurses to assess patients' unique health care needs, including their specific cultural health practices.

Campinha-Bacote (2002) defined *cultural competence* as an ongoing process whereby nurses continuously strive to work within the patient's cultural context. As a result, nurses continually develop cultural competence rather than possess it. This ongoing process involves integrating cultural awareness, knowledge, skills, encounters, and desire. *Cultural awareness* involves an in-depth self-examination to recognize one's biases, prejudices, and assumptions about other people in order to develop insight into one's own background. *Cultural knowledge* refers to knowing about the patient's culture. It involves learning about the values, health beliefs, care practices, and world views of diverse groups. The development of *cultural skills* involves the assessment of social,

cultural, and biophysical factors that influence patient care. *Cultural encounters* involve engaging in cross-cultural interactions that can teach about other cultures. *Cultural desire* is the motivation and commitment to learn from other people, to accept the role of learner, to be accepting of cultural differences, and to build relationships based on cultural similarities.

Narayanasamy (2002), a nurse scholar in Britain, also developed a framework to foster the development of cultural competence. This framework is referred to as the ACCESS model (assessment; communication; cultural negotiation and compromise; establishing respect and rapport; sensitivity; and safety). This model focuses on developing cross-cultural communication, cultural negotiations, diversity, and celebrations as well as fostering cultural safety (Narayanasamy & White, 2005).

In Canada, the CNA (2018) advocates in its position statement that culturally competent care can and should be practised in all clinical settings. Cultural competence is viewed as a key concept in the application of knowledge, skills, attitudes, and personal attributes by nurses providing appropriate care and services in relation to the cultural characteristics of patients. A nurse practising in this way, for instance, values diversity, is interested in and seeks out knowledge about cultural mores and traditions from diverse patients, and is sensitive to these traditions while caring for culturally diverse persons. Although nurses are responsible for providing culturally competent care, nursing regulatory bodies, professional associations, educational institutions, governments, health service agencies, and accreditation organizations share responsibility in supporting culturally competent care. Nurses are in a position to build partnerships with other health care providers, patients, and funding agencies to establish culturally diverse practices that optimize patients' health outcomes.

Cultural Safety and Humility

The provision of culturally competent care has been promoted since the 1960s. Since 2000, however, Canadian nurse scholars have begun to question the limitations of such an approach (Anderson et al., 2003; Kirkham, 2003) and explore the concept of cultural safety as another approach to providing care to diverse groups. This approach is in contrast to the notion of transcultural nursing (Ramsden, 2002). The British Columbia College of Nurses and Midwives' (2021) profile of newly graduated registered nurse practice focuses on the therapeutic caring and culturally safe relationships between patients and health care team members. The cultural safety literature is positioned within a critical social theory and postcolonial framework. The concept of cultural safety evolved over a number of years in New Zealand as nurses tried to identify a way for health care providers to more effectively address the inequity in the health status of the Māori. This was combined with an analysis of the historical, political, social, and economic situations influencing the health of the Māori (Ramsden, 2002). Cultural safety involves considering the redistribution of power and resources in a relationship:

Cultural safety is based on the premise that the term 'culture' is used in its broadest sense to apply to any person or group of people who may differ from the nurse/midwife because of socio-economic status, age, gender, sexual orientation, ethnic origin, migrant/refugee status, religious belief or disability.

Ramsden, 2002, p. 114

In contrast to transcultural nursing, the term *culture* refers to ethnicity. As a result, the philosophy of cultural care has shifted from the notion of cultural sensitivity underpinning the provisions of care irrespective of culture to one of cultural safety with the recognition

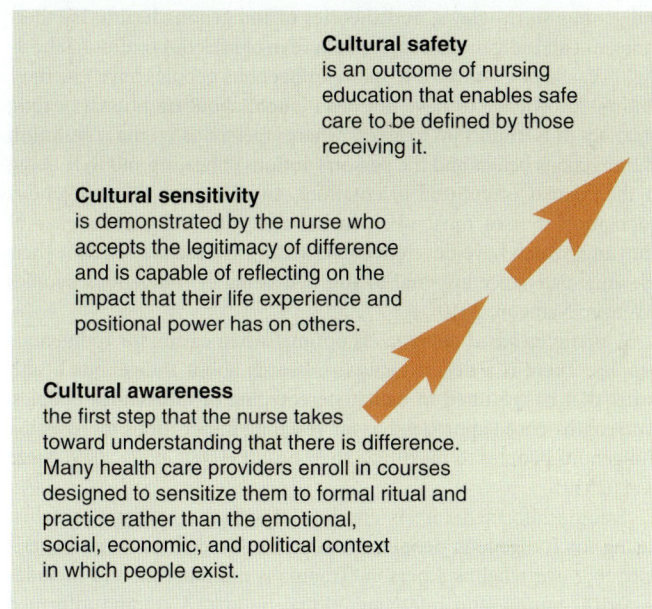

Cultural safety
is an outcome of nursing education that enables safe care to be defined by those receiving it.

Cultural sensitivity
is demonstrated by the nurse who accepts the legitimacy of difference and is capable of reflecting on the impact that their life experience and positional power has on others.

Cultural awareness
the first step that the nurse takes toward understanding that there is difference. Many health care providers enroll in courses designed to sensitize them to formal ritual and practice rather than the emotional, social, economic, and political context in which people exist.

FIGURE 12.2 Steps toward achieving cultural safety in nursing practice. (*Adapted from Ramsden, I. M. [2002]. Cultural safety and nursing education in Aotearoa and TeWaipounamu [Unpublished doctoral dissertation]. Victoria University of Wellington. https://www.croakey.org/wp-content/uploads/2017/08/RAMSDEN-I-Cultural-Safety_Full.pdf)*

BOX 12.3	Using the Ideas of Cultural Safety

1. Start with the organization to inquire at the level of context.
   - How are organizational practices supporting the health of nondominant groups?
   - What policies or organizational practices diminish, demean, or disempower the cultural identity and well-being of any individual or group? How do such policies or practices support discrimination?
   - What policies or organizational practices would recognize, respect, and nurture the unique cultural identities of people and families and safely meet their needs, expectations, and rights?
2. Examine nursing practices to inquire interpersonally.
   - What is the unique identity of this person or family? What are this person's or family's needs and expectations?
   - How can I practise to recognize, respect, and nurture that identity and meet those needs and expectations?
3. Use reflexivity to inquire intrapersonally.
   - How do my own personal and cultural history, values, and beliefs influence my practice?
   - How do my own economic, political, and historical locations shape my practice?

From Hartrick Doane, G., & Varcoe, C. (2015). *How to nurse: Relational inquiry with individuals and families in changing health and health care contexts* (p. 180). Lippincott Williams & Wilkins.

of power imbalances, an understanding of the nature of interpersonal relationships, and an awareness of institutional discrimination (Browne et al., 2009; Canadian Indigenous Nurses Association [CINA] et al., 2009; CNA, 2010; Racine, 2009). Thus, understanding and providing culturally competent and safe care has the potential to make a difference to the health of all culturally diverse groups.

Ramsden (2002) articulated that *cultural awareness* and *cultural sensitivity* are separate concepts and that those terms are not interchangeable with *cultural safety*. Achieving cultural safety is a stepwise progression from cultural awareness through cultural sensitivity to cultural safety (Figure 12.2). The outcome of cultural safety is that safe care, defined as such by patients who receive the care, is provided. According to Ramsden (2002), **cultural sensitivity** "alerts students to the legitimacy of difference and begins a process of self-exploration as the powerful bearers of their own life experience and realities which can have an impact on others" (Ramsden, 2002, p. 117). **Cultural awareness** "is a beginning step toward understanding that there is difference. Many people undergo courses designed to sensitize them to formal ritual and practice rather than the emotional, social, economic and political context in which people exist" (Ramsden, 2002, p. 117). A strategy for achieving cultural awareness is to conduct a self-assessment in order to reflect on one's biases and feelings.

With regard to achieving cultural safety in nursing practice, Ramsden has stated the following:

. . . the skill for nurses does not lie in knowing the customs or even the health-related beliefs of ethno-specific groups. The step before that lies in the professional acquisition of trust. Rather than the nurse determining what is culturally safe, it is consumers or patients who decide whether they feel safe with the care that has been given, that trust has been established, and that difference between the patient, the nurse and the institutions that underpin them can then be identified and negotiated.

Ramsden, 2002, p. 118

As well, Hartrick Doane and Varcoe (2015) have stated that the "ideas of cultural safety are harmonious with a relational approach" (p. 179); the authors emphasize an "understanding of context and culture as inseparable, developing a relational consciousness, and inquiring at all levels" (p. 179). For nurses to integrate cultural safety in their practice, the authors suggest that there are certain questions that are helpful to ask (Box 12.3).

In nursing, and in a wide variety of other disciplines, cultural humility is now viewed as essential (Foronda et al., 2016). Cultural humility includes a variety of core features and consolidating definitions. Worthington et al. (2017) describe **cultural humility** as a lifelong learning experience, value, or virtue that shapes character traits across the lifespan. In addition, cultural humility refers to actions that demonstrate interpersonal respect and interpersonal reflection on one's cultural assumptions and biases. The focus of cultural humility offers something new as we continue to think about and apply cultural competence and safety frameworks. It is especially important to nursing as a profession that involves cross-cultural engagement, with applications across a wide variety of nursing domains (Worthington et al., 2017).

NURSING CONSIDERATIONS AND INDIGENOUS HEALTH

Recently, nursing in Canada has come under scrutiny because of situations in which nurses have engaged in racist behaviour toward Indigenous peoples. An inquiry was ordered after the death of Joyce Echaquan, an Atikamekw woman, in a Quebec hospital. She used her cell phone to record nurses taunting her as she lay dying (Gee, 2021; Page, 2021; Shingler, 2021; Turner, 2021; Zingler, 2019). According to expert testimony during the inquiry held in spring 2021, Echaquan died of pulmonary edema and could have been saved had she been monitored more closely (CBC News, 2021). The nursing profession as a whole has begun to recognize that transformative changes must be made in nursing to ensure that nursing lives up to its ethics and values of social justice and equity. Nurses need to engage in antiracist and anticolonial practice at all times.

Respect is a fundamental aspect of nursing practice and is seen as a human value that addresses dignity and justice. Respect in nursing means acknowledging and appreciating the intrinsic value of others in an active and authentic way (Gallagher, 2007). In a study exploring the meaning of respect to First Nations people, the authors found that respect was seen as a reciprocal process: one respects others by seeing and treating others as being inherently worthy and equal in principle. The First Nations participants felt that respect was demonstrated by a willingness to be accepting and to listen actively, to communicate clearly, sincerely, and kindly, as well as genuinely trying to understand the situations that patients found themselves in. Lack of respect was shown through not ensuring privacy for patients, negative nonverbal behaviours, and discriminatory behaviours (Browne, 1995).

Trust is an essential element of all nurse–patient relationships (Dinc & Gastmans, 2012). Trust requires vulnerability, dependency, and risk taking by the person exhibiting the trusting behaviour. It requires that nurses understand the unequal power relationship between themselves and their patient, as well as the vulnerability and dependency of the patient (Dinc & Gastmans, 2012). Trust is vital in the relationship between an Indigenous patient, family, or community and the health care provider. Nurses can build trust by listening to their patients, accepting them for who they are, understanding their needs, and being willing to adapt to the patient's, family's, or community's ways of being (Zeidler, 2011). Learning about the history of Indigenous peoples and understanding its impact on the behaviours and attitudes of Indigenous patients or families will help shape this relationship.

Although efficiency is paramount in conventional health care settings, within Indigenous communities, relationships come before business. Tending to the relationship first will help to build sufficient trust for the clinical aspects of caring for the patient and family. It is also important to recognize how Indigenous patients are connected to their family, community, and way of life in a holistic paradigm (Zeidler, 2011). Also important is ensuring that the family understands what is happening and that there is space provided for community members who visit. Other important relational aspects include keeping one's word, maintaining confidentiality, and being reliable, kind, and nonjudgemental (Zeidler, 2011).

Spirituality is important to many Indigenous peoples. Traditional Indigenous spirituality is believed to have healing aspects. In the holistic view of health for Indigenous peoples, spirituality is one of the four aspects within a person that must be in balance in order for the person to be healthy. Therefore, it is important that Indigenous patients and families are able to practise their spirituality in a health care setting. Nurses should inquire about where Indigenous peoples can hold ceremonies or practise **smudging**, which involves the use of smoke released from the burning of sweetgrass or other traditional medicines for spiritual cleansing. This may mean locating the Indigenous helper or Elder in the health care setting who can assist the family or patient with tending to their spiritual needs. Items placed in the bed or on the wall or pinned to the patient's gown must not be moved without permission, as these items may hold spiritual and healing significance for the patient and family. Not all Indigenous peoples practise traditional Indigenous spirituality. Other religions followed by Indigenous peoples across Canada include Roman Catholicism, Protestantism, Pentecostalism, and other faiths. The nurse needs to find out what the patient's spiritual needs are and to act accordingly (North American Indigenous Ministries, 2017; Public Safety and Emergency Preparedness Canada, 2006; Todd, 2016; Vancouver Native Pentecostal Church, n.d.).

It is important to recognize that different Indigenous groups have their own interpretations and emphasis on various aspects of belief,

Indigenous world views, and theories of Indigenous health. Furthermore, not all Indigenous peoples believe in or seek out traditional healing. Because of colonization, many Indigenous peoples have lost their cultural knowledge or have not been taught about traditional healing practices. It is important to assess where a person is on the continuum of Indigenous beliefs and the person's notions of healing and well-being in the context of cultural orientations. In caring for the Indigenous population, nurses must work in balance with Indigenous ways of knowing, which have developed over tens of thousands of years; their use and sustenance are vital to the well-being of Indigenous peoples (Wenger-Nabigon, 2010).

A *strengths-based approach* is optimal when caring for Indigenous peoples. There is a deficit focus in research about Indigenous health issues that has resulted in deficit stereotyping of Indigenous peoples. A strengths-based approach has far-reaching implications for assisting Indigenous peoples to maximize their health (Hyett et al., 2019; Njeze et al., 2020)

Trauma-informed care is another important consideration when caring for Indigenous peoples. Trauma can be defined as an experience that overwhelms a person. Trauma is multifaceted and includes historical trauma and intergenerational trauma. A trauma-informed approach to health care recognizes the patient's need for safety, choice, and control (British Columbia Ministry of Children and Family Development, 2017).

ILLNESS EXPERIENCES—CHRONIC DISEASES

Nursing and interdisciplinary scholars continue to research the health challenges faced by Indigenous peoples (see Box 12.4) and to emphasize the importance of culture safety in nursing practice.

Implications for Nursing

The importance of cultural competency, safety, and humility for health care administrators, practitioners, and educators has been recognized by the Canadian Indigenous Nurses Association (CINA; formerly Aboriginal Nurses Association of Canada) in their 2009 document *Cultural Competence and Cultural Safety in Nursing Education*, which describes the impact of cultural competency and safety; a theoretical and methodological approach to cultural safety, an approach that originated with Indigenous peoples; and the importance of its application to health care (CINA et al., 2009).

With regard to the success of an interaction between nurse and patient, Harrowing et al. (2010) emphasize that such an outcome begins with the nurse's reflection on their "personal and cultural history, values, and beliefs and continues with the situating of those understandings within a framework of power imbalances, institutional discrimination, and colonizer–colonized relationships" (p. 246). In situating the professional discipline of nursing in the broader context of colonizing relations, McGibbon et al. (2013) emphasize that nursing must also look toward decolonizing itself, which includes understanding the colonial history of nursing and strategies for increasing the counternarrative.

Indigenous peoples in Canada experience major health disparities, which are caused in part by impaired access to appropriate and adequate housing, income, education, and health care. Health inequities are largely due to historical colonialism and current-day postcolonial institutional racism, demonstrated in the policies and procedures of governmental institutions that negatively impact Indigenous peoples.

It is imperative that nurses understand the social determinants of health through an Indigenous lens, which helps to explain the underlying economic and social conditions that shape health. **Social determinants of health** are the living and working conditions that impact

BOX 12.4	Indigenous Nursing Leader—Madeleine Kétéskwew Dion Stout

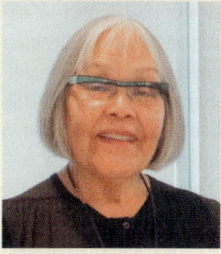

Madeleine Kétéskwew Dion Stout is a Cree speaker who was born and raised on the Kehewin First Nation in Alberta. After graduating from the Edmonton General Hospital nursing program, she earned a bachelor's degree in nursing, with distinction, from the University of Lethbridge and a master's degree in international affairs from Carleton University. She has served on many boards and committees, including the National Collaborating Centre for Indigenous Health and the First Nations Health Authority Board in British Columbia, and was also appointed to the Mental Health Commission of Canada as an inaugural vice-chair of the board of directors. She is past president of the Canadian Indigenous Nurses Association and an appointee to the National Forum on Health. She was a professor in Canadian Studies and founding director of the Centre for Aboriginal Education, Research, and Culture at Carleton University in Ottawa. Now self-employed as the president of Dion Stout Reflections Inc., she adopts a Cree lens in her research, writing, and lectures on First Nations health. Her active involvement in research projects has her shaping the way social, health, and health care equity is best encouraged, cultivated, and disciplined for Indigenous peoples. She is the recipient of many awards, including from the Canadian Indigenous Nurses Association, the University of Lethbridge, The University of British Columbia (honorary Doctor of Laws), the University of Ottawa, and Carleton University, as well as a 2008 Centennial Award from the Canadian Nurses Association. She received a National Aboriginal Achievement Award (now known as the Indspire Awards) in the health category in 2010 and the Order of Canada in 2015.

(Courtesy CARNE. Photograph by vsaranphoto.com.)

From personal communication with Caroline Foster-Boucher, March 29, 2017; Delta Optimist. (2015). *Local nurse Madeleine Dion Stout appointed to the Order of Canada.* https://www.delta-optimist.com/local-news/local-nurse-madeleine-dion-stout-appointed-to-the-order-of-canada-3014647; Thunderbird Partnership Foundation. (n.d.). *Madeleine Dion Stout.* https://thunderbirdpf.org/events/madeleine-dion-stout-2

health (Lucyk, 2020; Raphael et al., 2020). In the Indigenous context, however, social determinants of health need to be viewed through a different lens because the context that Indigenous peoples are situated in has significant differences from that of other Canadians. Indeed, colonialism itself, which is historical, continued, and current, has been identified by Indigenous peoples globally as their most fundamental determinant of health (De Leeuw et al., 2018).

Reading (2018) visualized a tree as a way to understand Indigenous peoples' determinants of health. The **proximal determinants of health**, the leaves and the branches of the tree, include factors such as early childhood development, income and income status, education and literacy, social support networks, employment and working conditions, culture, and gender.

The tree trunk represents the **intermediate determinants of health**, including health promotion and health care, education, justice, social supports, the labour market, and government and private enterprise. These connect the proximal determinants to the distal determinants.

The **distal determinants of health**, as the roots of the tree, are hidden, yet critical. These consist of historical, political, ideological, economical, and social foundations, which feed and strongly influence all the other determinants (Reading, 2018, p. 5). These distal determinants are critical to consider when thinking about Indigenous peoples and determinants of health, because they impact how all other determinants connect, intersect, and thus impact Indigenous peoples.

An example of how these factors determine health can be seen when considering diabetes. Proximal determinants may include weight, income, and health literacy. Intermediate determinants for Indigenous peoples may include access to culturally safe primary care, education level, and sufficient social supports. When we expand our thinking to include the distal determinants, however, we must consider the impact of residential schools and the *Indian Act* and the ongoing impacts of colonization by asking ourselves questions such as the following:

- How have this person's experiences in residential school impacted their ability to earn a living?
- How have this person's ideas around food been shaped when considering the impact of an extremely poor diet and periods of severe hunger throughout a childhood spent in residential school?
- How does racism (social foundations) impact this person's ability to have health literacy, social support or, in fact, even shop for foods?

Structural racism, which has devastating impacts on all other determinants, can also be included in the root system of the "tree" of social determinants of health because it impacts all of the other determinants of health. By looking at the distal aspects for Indigenous peoples, we can see how all the other determinants of health are impacted, and are different from, the determinants of health for other Canadians.

This framework for understanding what influences Indigenous peoples' health is not accurately reflected in other determinants of health frameworks. This framework also allows for incorporation of Indigenous ways of knowing, language, storytelling, and the connection between the past, present, and future that are encompassed by children, the power of place, and the land.

The implications of these social determinants of health for nursing among Indigenous peoples can be summed up by Reutter and Kushner's (2010) statement that "nursing has a clear mandate to ensure access to health and health-care by providing sensitive empowering care to those experiencing inequities and working to change underlying social conditions that result in and perpetuate health inequities" (p. 269). A relational approach to nursing shapes the places of inquiry and practice that determine how to find one's way through relationships, culture, safety, ethics, diversity, power, economics, communication, and history. A deep consideration of relational practice and nursing obligations offers an understanding of experience by which to imagine how one might incorporate reflexivity, intentionality, and openness into practice, education, and research. (Refer to Chapter 18 for information on implementing relational practice, and Chapter 19 for more information on patient-centred care.)

In critically analyzing nursing practice—as clinicians, educators, researchers, and administrators—it is essential that nurses, individually and collectively, enact and refine the role of the nurse in the provision of care to Indigenous peoples. Nurses must also commit to enacting change in nursing practice through antiracist and anticolonial actions and values.

The nursing profession must continue to adapt nursing practice to an Indigenous context, preserve the perspective of Indigenous peoples, sustain the holistic nature of responding to social and health challenges, uphold a strengths-based perspective, and value new ways of forming partnerships in respectful ways.

Diabetes Mellitus

Diabetes mellitus (type 2 diabetes) was a condition unknown before the 1940s, but it has been viewed as an epidemic in progress since the 1970s among Indigenous peoples in Canada (Howard, 2014). Diabetes

BOX 12.5 RESEARCH HIGHLIGHT

Health Care Experiences of Indigenous Peoples Living With Type 2 Diabetes in Canada

A recent study explored Indigenous perspectives on diabetes care. Findings indicated that study participants' experience of diabetes improved when they were able to engage in equitable and positive interactions with care providers and organizations. Participants also cited negative experiences, such as being dismissed and lecturing by physicians. They indicated that negative caregiver actions and attitudes triggered their residential school memories. These issues and lack of access to care were viewed as affecting how often Indigenous patients sought care and how willing they were to share all their symptoms, regardless of their willingness to accept the suggested treatments (Jacklin et al., 2017). Recommendations for improved health care encounters include cultivating a positive relationship with Indigenous patients by tending to power differentials, incorporating a holistic view of health and treatment, and recognizing how important a trustful therapeutic relationship is between patient and health care provider in mitigating historical trauma and colonial history.

From Jacklin, K. M., Henderson, R. I., Green, M. E., et al. (2017). Health care experiences of Indigenous people living with type 2 diabetes in Canada. *Canadian Medical Association Journal, 189*(3), 106–112. https://doi.org/10.1503/cmaj.161098

has a prevalence (dependent on location) that is three to five times higher in the Indigenous population than in the non-Indigenous population (Public Health Agency of Canada [PHAC], 2011). Research has found that the lifetime risk of diabetes at 20 years old is 75.6% for First Nations men and 87.3% for First Nations women, compared with 55.6% and 46.5 % for non-Indigenous men and women, respectively (Turin et al., 2016). First Nations men and women face a greater risk of diabetes at a much younger age than non–First Nations people, and the rates of diabetes are higher among First Nations people living in rural areas versus those in urban settings (Turin et al., 2016).

Researchers think that these high rates of diabetes are linked to a combination of genetic susceptibility, changes associated with transitioning from a physically active lifestyle to a sedentary lifestyle, and the intake of a diet high in sugar, fat, and salt. Other factors that contribute to the prevalence of diabetes include inequities in the social, political, and economic determinants of health, stress, insufficient access to nutritious food, and barriers to appropriate health care, such as lack of comprehensive primary care and lack of specialized care within a reasonable distance (Benedict et al., 2020; Marushka et al., 2018; Rice et al., 2016; Turin et al., 2016) (Box 12.5).

Type 2 diabetes is diagnosed with increasing frequency in Indigenous children and youth (Carino et al., 2021; Dyck et al., 2014; PHAC, 2011). Earlier onset of the disease leads to an earlier onset of complications, as well as excessive mortality rates among young and middle-aged adults. In Inuit communities, the rate of type 2 diabetes is still relatively low, but concerns have been raised that this situation may change if the Inuit alter their traditional eating patterns and lifestyle (Little et al., 2020).

Indigenous Perspective. In considering diabetes in the Indigenous population, it is necessary to view this epidemic through a lens highlighting the impact of colonization and intergenerational trauma on the social determinants of health, such as personal coping habits and patterns of food use (Boxes 12.6 and 12.7). Howard (2014) has noted the impact of the residential school experience on the eating habits of residential school survivors, who associate eating with abuse, trauma, and powerlessness. Wild animal meat and other Indigenous foods were

BOX 12.6 The National Indigenous Diabetes Association

The National Aboriginal Diabetes Association (now the National Indigenous Diabetes Association; NIDA) was formed in 1995 in response to the alarming increase in the rates of diabetes in Indigenous communities (NIDA, 2019). NIDA provides diabetes resources and information for Indigenous peoples in Canada and hosts national conferences to raise awareness and share successes. Its vision is diabetes-free healthy communities. The organization also partners with other groups to support projects focused on reducing the complications of diabetes (NIDA, 2020). NIDA currently receives funding through an annual contribution agreement with Indigenous Services Canada instead of through multiyear funding agreements, which tend to increase the stability of programming for not-for-profit organizations. Despite this challenge in funding and increasing costs, NIDA has focused their strategic plan on a 5-year cycle, from 2016 to 2021, with hopes of achieving increased funding, multiyear funding agreements, and increased partnerships that will help to strengthen its programs.

BOX 12.7 The Aboriginal Diabetes Initiative

In 1999, the First Nations and Inuit Health Branch (now part of Indigenous Services Canada) launched the Aboriginal Diabetes Initiative (ADI) in order to fund health promotion, disease prevention, and screening and treatment services in more than 600 Indigenous communities in Canada (Health Canada, 2011; Indigenous Services Canada, 2021). ADI receives annual funding from Indigenous Services Canada (Casey, 2019) and focuses on the following areas:

- Initiatives for children, youth, parents, and families
- Diabetes in childbearing women and pregnant women
- Community-led food security planning to improve access to healthy foods, including traditional and market foods, and
- Enhanced training for health providers on clinical practice guidelines and chronic disease management strategies.

Using local knowledge, First Nations and Inuit communities are encouraged to develop innovative, culturally relevant approaches aimed at increasing community wellness and ultimately reducing the burden of type 2 diabetes. Community approaches and activities include walking clubs, weight loss groups, diabetes workshops, fitness classes, community kitchens, community gardens, and healthy school food policies. ADI also supports traditional activities, such as traditional food harvesting and preparation, canoeing, drumming, dancing, and traditional games (Indigenous Services Canada, 2021).

denigrated and were replaced with food that was less nutritious (Howard, 2014).

HIV and AIDS

Human immunodeficiency virus (HIV) infections and cases of acquired immune deficiency syndrome (AIDS) among Indigenous peoples in Canada have increased steadily since the 1990s, whereas the annual number of AIDS cases has levelled off in the rest of the population. Indigenous peoples are overrepresented among HIV and AIDS cases in Canada; although Indigenous peoples make up about 4.9% of the Canadian population, it is estimated that they represent about 11.3% of all those living with HIV and AIDS (PHAC, 2018). In addition, the HIV infection rate is about two times higher among Indigenous peoples than among non-Indigenous peoples (PHAC, 2018). Compared with their non-Indigenous counterparts, Indigenous peoples diagnosed with HIV are more likely to be younger (31.6% vs. 22.2%

BOX 12.8 Policy Highlight: Implications for Indigenous Health—HIV/AIDS

Globally, the Joint United Nations Program on HIV and AIDS (UNAIDS) is the main advocate for comprehensive and coordinated global action on the HIV/AIDS epidemic (UNAIDS, 2006, 2021). In 2021, UNAIDS released its latest 5-year plan, which focuses on decreasing inequities in order to reach the goal of ending AIDS as a public health threat by 2030 (UNAIDS, 2021). In Canada, the government has supported the UNAIDS 90-90-90 treatment targets, which focus on ensuring that by 2020, 90% of HIV-positive people will know their status, 90% of people who know their status will be treated, and 90% of those treated will have their viral loads suppressed (Canadian AIDS Society, 2016). There is also a focus on HIV/AIDS research that is community based, specifically in Indigenous communities. However, there have been recent government funding cutbacks to HIV/AIDS organizations across Canada as a result of the government's increased focus on prevention and education rather than on treatment of people who already have HIV/AIDS (Britneff, 2018). The decreased funding is especially relevant for Indigenous peoples, for whom this may have far-reaching consequences (Easton, 2016).

BOX 12.9 CASE STUDY

An Indigenous Man With HIV

James is a 50-year-old Two-Spirit person (preferred pronouns: he/him) from the Muskoday First Nation in northern Saskatchewan. He recently went to see his family doctor in Prince Albert for an HIV test. When he returned to the doctor for his results, he was shocked to learn that his test came back positive. James had lived with his partner, Sam, for more than 10 years; however, they separated 7 months ago, and James is unsure of Sam's HIV status.

James has been referred to the sexually transmitted infections clinic for an assessment with a nurse. During his first visit, James is very quiet and withdrawn, and it is difficult for the nurse to engage him in a conversation. James would like to return to his home community to live, but he is hesitant to do so because he is afraid he will not be accepted. He receives his medical care on the basis of his First Nations status; however, he is worried that his HIV care will not be covered.

1. What does the nurse need to demonstrate in order to provide this patient with compassionate, culturally safe, and relationship-centred care?
2. How could the nurse demonstrate effective and culturally safe communication with this patient?

between 15 and 29 years old), female (47.3% vs. 20.1%), and infected through intravenous drug use (58.1% vs. 13.7%) (PHAC, 2014).

Factors contributing to these high rates of infection and disease include intergenerational and historical trauma, societal and institutional racism, stigma, community violence, and the intersection of health issues (Jongbloed et al., 2019) (see Box 12.8).

Indigenous Perspective. Indigenous peoples diagnosed with HIV/AIDS state that they have been devastated by the diagnosis, a reaction that is similar to that among other HIV-positive groups of people (Cain et al., 2013). The difference for HIV-positive Indigenous peoples, however, is that the diagnosis is often being added to existing layers of trauma, including intergenerational trauma, a history of familial violence, lack of being parented or lack of affection from parents, and loneliness. For many individuals, the diagnosis either triggers or increases depression, along with an increased incidence of self-abusive behaviours. For some Indigenous clients, the diagnosis triggers an evaluation of life, a search for and renewal of culture, and healing from trauma (Cain et al., 2013).

Indigenous women connect their understandings of HIV and wellness within the constructs of gendered violence and negative intimate partner relationships. They also regard the wider family connections and community norms as being important to the discussion of self-care and community education. Barriers to effective HIV prevention and care include denial, stigma, and shame within Indigenous communities (O'Brien et al., 2020).

While research shows that intravenous drug use is a more common method of transmission of HIV for Indigenous peoples, there are currently no data or statistics on the effect of HIV/AIDS on Two-Spirit people (a term used by Indigenous peoples to encompass a range of roles and identities, including cultural, spiritual, gender, and sexual identity). Historically, Indigenous peoples had a fluid view of gender and sexuality, which was deeply affected by colonization, including by residential schools (Hunt, 2016). However, HIV/AIDS has caused Indigenous communities to organize and become active, resulting in the introduction of culturally safe programming and education initiatives that resonate for Indigenous youth, including Two-Spirit youth (Hunt, 2016) (Box 12.9). Factors that promote engagement in HIV/AIDS care include culture, identity, and ceremony as well as social support systems and the personal attributes of strength, resilience, and determination (Jongbloed et al., 2019).

Cancer

Cancer was relatively unknown among Indigenous peoples in Canada a few generations ago. However, studies have found dramatic increases in cancer rates among Indigenous peoples in recent years, and it is now becoming one of the top three causes of death for First Nations people (Beben & Muirhead, 2016). Using statistics from 1991 to 2009, Withrow et al. (2017) found that First Nations people had poorer survival for 14 out of 15 common types of cancers than non-Indigenous people in Canada. This difference could not be explained away by income or location.

For the Métis, bronchus/lung cancer is the leading cause of death, with much higher rates among Métis men than among non-Métis men (Sanchez-Ramirez et al., 2016). Rates of incidence for other types of cancer were not particularly different between the Métis and other population groups in Canada (Sanchez-Ramirez et al., 2016). The circumpolar Inuit population has the highest rate of lung cancer in the world, and the overall rate of cancer has increased especially for lung, colorectal, and female breast cancers. The Inuit are also at extremely high risk for the rare nasopharyngeal cancer (Kue Young et al., 2016). The Inuit have a high prevalence of smoking; almost 63% of Inuit in Canada are daily smokers (Kue Young et al., 2016). The effects of colonization, residential schools, dietary changes, and changes in lifestyle have all been cited as factors increasing the incidence of cancers among Indigenous peoples in Canada (Wakewich et al., 2016).

Indigenous Perspective. There is limited research on cancer from the perspective of Indigenous peoples in Canada. However, researchers have found that, in general, Indigenous peoples from Australia, New Zealand, and Canada are fearful of receiving a cancer diagnosis. In studies focusing on cervical cancer screening, Indigenous women in Canada shared that despite feeling fearful of being screened, owing to the colonial history of health care in Canada, they felt great responsibility to take care of their health given their role as family caretakers. Other women spoke about a lack of time for screening owing to caretaking activities and employment. Barriers to screening included a lack of female physicians, lack of transportation, employment factors, lack of health literacy, and a general mistrust of the health care system (Maar et al., 2013). Spirituality was described as a cultural resource in cancer survivorship (Gifford et al., 2019). Gifford and colleagues

(2020) collaborated with Indigenous groups in five Canadian communities to develop culturally safe cancer survivorship interventions that included focusing on navigating health care, spirituality and ceremony, land and traditional healing, and finding strength together.

Tuberculosis

Although the overall incidence of TB has dropped steadily since the 1960s, in 2016, the incidence rate of active TB disease reported for the First Nations population was 41 times higher than for the Canadian-born non-Indigenous population (Vachon et al., 2018). The rate for the Inuit population was 170.1 cases per 100 000 people, which is 296 times greater than the rate for the Canadian-born non-Indigenous population; for the Métis, the rate was more than three times higher (Vachon et al., 2018). Factors contributing to such a high rate include the historical context of colonialism, insufficient housing leading to overcrowded and often poorly ventilated living conditions, and environmental conditions. Challenges related to the health care system include barriers to access to diagnosis and treatment in remote communities (Alvares et al., 2014; PHAC, 2013).

Indigenous Perspective. Even though historically TB has devastated Indigenous communities, many current patients have little knowledge of the history of TB in their families (M.E. Macdonald et al., 2010). Research participants stated that details were not shared when parents and other family members went away to sanatoriums. Participants with TB also had some knowledge of TB as a lung disease that was serious, contagious, and potentially fatal. They tended to acquire information about TB from health care providers, television, and pamphlets. The TB treatment regimen was seen as a heavy burden that was exacerbated by language difficulties, lack of social support, racism, and mistrust of the health care system. There was also fear of getting a positive result when being screened for TB (M.E. Macdonald et al., 2010). Participants in another study described using many other treatments to manage symptoms, and they attributed symptoms such as coughing and fatigue to other causes. They also indicated that they avoided seeking health care until they had to because of overwhelming symptoms (Abonyi et al., 2017).

Chronic Obstructive Pulmonary Disease and Asthma

Statistics for rates of chronic obstructive pulmonary disease (COPD) among Indigenous peoples in Canada are higher than those for non-Indigenous Canadians; however, exact numbers remain unknown (Turner et al., 2020). Inuit and First Nations people have higher rates of COPD than do Métis. Indigenous peoples, on average, smoke twice as much as the non-Indigenous population. Other factors influencing the incidence of COPD include exposure to environmental contaminants, housing conditions such as mould and poor ventilation, and lower levels of education. Poor nutrition, poverty, remote locations, and childhood exposure to cigarette smoke are additional contributing factors (Gershon et al., 2014; Ospina et al., 2015; Pahwa et al., 2015). Turner and colleagues (2020) led a community-based research project to estimate COPD statistics and burden in rural and remote First Nations communities in Canada because there has been insufficient research in this area, resulting in insufficient health service delivery planning and prevention efforts in communities. There are not enough data at this time to provide an Indigenous perspective.

Asthma is a significant respiratory disease among Indigenous children and youth, affecting 10 to 15.6% and possibly more (Castleden et al., 2016; Rennie et al., 2020; Senthilselvan et al., 2015). Even though the rates are similar to or higher than those for non-Indigenous children in Canada, it is thought that Indigenous children receive fewer health care services related to treatment for asthma because of decreased

access to health care services overall. Factors linked to the incidence and severity of asthma in Indigenous communities include overcrowded or poorly ventilated housing, mould, the presence of tobacco and ceremonial smoke indoors, use of wood-burning stoves, lack of financial resources, and stressful home environments (Castleden et al., 2016; Rennie et al., 2020; Senthilselvan et al., 2015). Asthma among Indigenous children is also associated with having frequent inner-ear infections, low birth weight, and allergies (Senthilselvan et al., 2015). For youth, risk factors for lifetime risk of developing asthma included urban residence, a low socioeconomic status, less educated parents, and having a history of bronchitis (Karunanayake et al., 2019).

In many Indigenous communities, asthma is often underdiagnosed and undertreated because of under-reporting by families, a lack of knowledge about asthma within Indigenous communities (including among health care providers), lack of funding for health promotion related to asthma, and lack of culturally safe and specialized care for families and patients with asthma (Castleden et al., 2016; Filler et al., 2018). Studies demonstrate that breastfeeding is protective for asthma in Indigenous children and should be promoted (Ming et al., 2012).

Indigenous Perspective. In a study completed in five Mi'kmaq communities in Nova Scotia, few Indigenous children self-identified in school as having a diagnosis of asthma owing to fear of stigma, exclusion, and isolation (Castleden et al., 2016). Children noted that they received support from their families as well as from their peers. Families also said that they needed better asthma care in the on-reserve health care centres and were reluctant to seek out medical intervention off reserve because of racism in the health care system, the complexity of the funding for Indigenous health, and the lack of consistency in information from health care providers (Castleden et al., 2016).

Cardiovascular Disease

Indigenous peoples in Canada have more than 10 times the rate of cardiovascular disease relative to the non-Indigenous population. This includes myocardial infarctions, strokes, coronary artery disease, and angina (Foulds et al., 2016). The high rate is attributed to a higher prevalence of diabetes, hypertension, smoking, dyslipidemia, and dysglycemia (Tobe et al., 2015). Also, while First Nations people with out-of-hospital cardiac arrests had similar outcomes to non-Indigenous people, they were on average 19 years younger, which is a significant public health concern (Scheirer et al., 2020). Indigenous communities with better socioeconomic conditions, increased trust among community members, higher levels of education, and social support had a lower burden of cardiovascular risk than other communities. Communities with decreased access to primary health care had a higher burden of cardiovascular risk (Anand et al., 2019).

Indigenous Perspective. In a study examining contextual factors and health behaviours on the Six Nations reserve in Ontario, participants found that the walkability score of the reserve was low owing to lack of street connectivity, aesthetics, and safety (Joseph et al., 2012). Participants also identified high levels of cigarette smoking as an on-reserve problem. Food was bought off reserve because of greater availability and better affordability of produce (Joseph et al., 2012).

Indigenous women have been identified as having the highest levels of cardiovascular disease in the Indigenous population. Indigenous women identified the common themes of disability and loss of life associated with family heart disease, a willingness to use Western medicine for treatment, and a lack of awareness of their own risk factors for heart disease owing to their role as family caregiver—a role often carried out in chaotic circumstances and with insufficient support from the men in the family and community (Medved et al., 2013). Education initiatives that incorporated cultural traditions, relationships among participants, a focus on holistic self-care, and positive messaging have been shown to be effective for cardiac health promotion for Indigenous women (Ziabakhsh et al., 2016).

Otitis Media

It is thought that Indigenous peoples began to experience otitis media (OM) only after colonization and the introduction of new pathogens (Bhutta, 2015). OM has been reported to be more prevalent among Indigenous children, especially Inuit, than among the non-Indigenous population (Bowd, 2005). One study, however, found that a cohort of First Nations children had a lower incidence than non-Indigenous children (Karunanayake et al., 2016).

There is limited information about OM rates among the Indigenous population owing to inconsistent definitions of OM and the inclusion of children of varying ages. Contributing factors to OM rates include lack of access to health care, inconsistency in obtaining a diagnosis, and the remote locations of First Nations communities. Other factors include gender (more common among males), lower socioeconomic status, cigarette smoke exposure, inadequate housing conditions, low birth weight, and day care attendance.

Consequences of OM include hearing loss, which has been reported at rates as high as 44% for adult Inuit and 39% for adult First Nations people. Inuit appear to be more at risk, with contributing factors including exposure to wind, diet, activity in the winter, and increased rates of smoking (Bowd, 2005). Another factor contributing to the greater impact of OM is decreased access to appropriate medical care for children in remote communities. Recommendations for decreasing the incidence of OM include encouraging breastfeeding, having culturally safe, community-driven health promotion programs about OM, appropriate antibiotic use, immunization programs, and decreased infant exposure to cigarette smoke (Bowd, 2005). Insufficient data were found to provide an Indigenous perspective on OM.

Rheumatic Disease

Rheumatic disease rates in Canada are higher in the Indigenous population than in the non-Indigenous population. This includes lupus, rheumatoid arthritis, osteoarthritis, and other connective tissue disorders such as spondyloarthropathies (Barnabe et al., 2017; Hitchon et al., 2019; Levy et al., 2013; McDougall et al., 2017). Osteoarthritis rates for Indigenous peoples range from 6 to 16% compared with 3.4 to 7.4% for the non-Indigenous population (McDougall et al., 2017). Lupus rates in Canada are twice as high in the Indigenous population as in the non-Indigenous population (McDougall et al., 2017). Arthritis is the most common chronic disease among Indigenous peoples in Canada, with estimates indicating that rates among Indigenous peoples are 1.3 to 1.6 times that for non-Indigenous people; high rates of disability have also been noted (Thurston et al., 2014). Smoking and indoor air pollution are associated with an increased risk of rheumatic diseases among the Indigenous population in Canada (McDougall et al., 2017).

Indigenous Perspective. Indigenous people with arthritis have described feelings of anger, frustration, and depression as a result of their experiences with arthritis. However, the use of health care services by the Indigenous population with arthritis is less than that among the non-Indigenous population with arthritis; this difference is related to the normalization of arthritis in the Indigenous population, as well as experiences of racism and other barriers in the health care system (Thurston et al., 2014). Indigenous women have suggested that shared decision making and culturally appropriate care models, such as traditional healing methods, would be beneficial, as well as having

increased accessibility to decision aids and decision coaches related to care for rheumatoid arthritis (Umaefulam et al., 2021).

Mental Health

Mental health issues plague many Indigenous communities in Canada. Indigenous peoples on the whole experience higher rates of substance use disorders, chronic depression, mental illness, and suicide than non-Indigenous people (Graham et al., 2021). These are overwhelming issues within Indigenous communities, mainly owing to historical and intergenerational trauma resulting from colonialism past and present in Canada. Mental wellness is the goal for Indigenous communities; it is a broad concept that is defined by a general state of well-being "in which the individual realizes [their] own potential, can cope with the normal stresses of life, and is able to make a contribution to [their] own community" (Indigenous Services Canada, 2015). Mental health for Indigenous peoples in Canada has been described in statistics and negative terms for many years. However, with a mental wellness focus, a more positive approach is coming into view. While Western treatment can be beneficial for treating mental illness in Indigenous peoples, research shows that "culture as treatment'" is the most effective path toward mental wellness for Indigenous peoples in Canada (Auger, 2019, 2021; Graham et al., 2021; Waddell et al., 2017). This includes culturally grounded activities (e.g., retreat camps, ceremonies, Indigenous language study), Elder and peer mentorship, participation in activities with Elders and peers (e.g., noncompetitive games, sharing a meal, discussion circles), and strengthening connection with family and community (Graham et al., 2021; Waddell et al., 2017).

A mental wellness continuum framework has been developed by First Nations in partnership with Indigenous Services Canada (2015) (Figure 12.3). This framework provides guidance to Indigenous communities for culturally safe mental wellness program development while adapting, optimizing, and realigning services to provide a continuum of quality programs and services. Based on the Medicine Wheel, the framework consists of concentric rings delineating outcomes, community, population, specific population needs, continuum of essential services, supporting elements, partners, Indigenous social determinants of health, themes of mental wellness, and culture as foundation. Mental wellness programs in Indigenous communities may include addiction programs, domestic violence prevention programs, and talking circles to assist with depression and other issues. Residential school survivors and their families have access to counselling through the Residential Schools Resolution Health Support Program (Government of Canada, 2021). Addressing mental health using an Indigenous determinants of health lens and a traditional Indigenous health view lens (hybrid traditional Indigenous–Western health view) requires an understanding of a holistic perspective (emotional, mental, spiritual, and physical dimensions) that is situated within place, family, and community.

Indigenous Peoples in Canada and the COVID-19 Pandemic

Research shows that Indigenous communities have been greatly impacted by the COVID-19 pandemic. Inequities in social determinants of health, such as adequate housing, potable water, and health care access have left communities unprepared to cope with the pandemic. For instance, handwashing becomes difficult when potable water is not accessible. Lack of access to health care and insufficient community buildings for isolation can result in increased morbidity and mortality from the virus. Indigenous peoples are vocal in their request for Indigenous engagement in decision making, support for seniors and Elders, and concern for youth experiencing a lack of employment and interrupted schooling. Food security has been a concern and mental

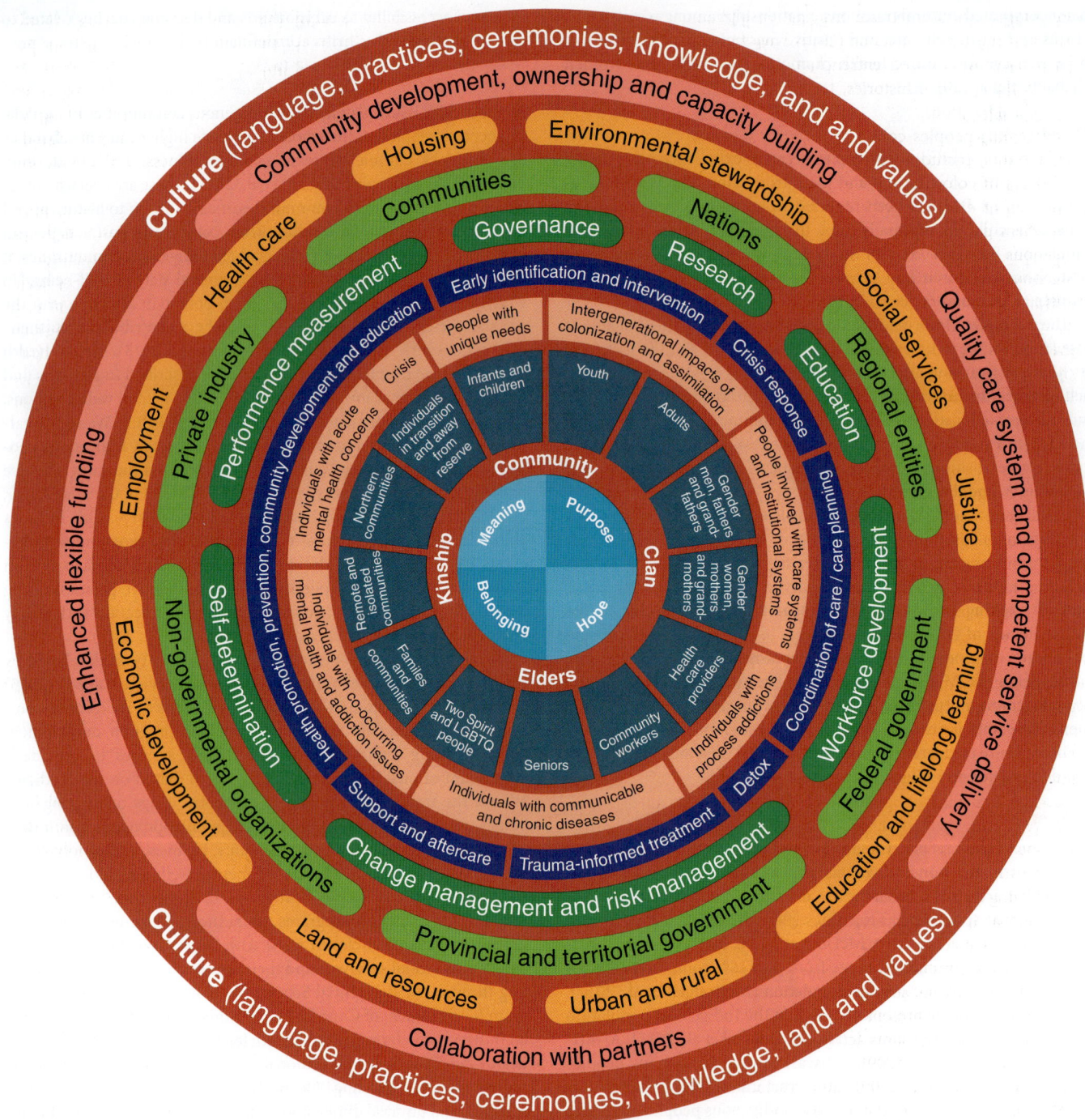

FIGURE 12.3 Visual representation of the First Nations Mental Wellness Continuum. (From Wise Practices. [2019]. *Project summary.* https://wisepractices.ca/project-summary)

wellness has suffered owing to inability to practise traditional aspects of the culture, such as ceremonies and other group activities, and the closing of physical activity programs or facilities for youth. Indigenous communities have responded by supplying traditional foods in communities, involving youth in solution-oriented discussions, and ensuring the safety and care of their Elders. Suggestions for the way forward include government commitment to authentic community engagement with Indigenous communities, providing sufficient pandemic funding and resources, and consideration of the differences among Indigenous communities in terms of their infrastructure and needs (Mashford-Pringle et al., 2021).

INDIGENOUS HEALTH—THE GLOBAL PERSPECTIVE

An Indigenous health global perspective considers an estimated 370 to 500 million Indigenous people who reside in countries on every continent around the world (United Nations, 2018; United Nations Educational, Scientific and Cultural Organization, 2019). Present trends indicate that Indigenous peoples represent approximately 15% of the poorest people globally yet make up only about 5% of the population worldwide (The World Bank, 2021). Poverty within Indigenous groups needs to be eradicated, as it contributes to poor health from malnutrition, prevalent infections, environmental contamination, overcrowding, and inadequate hygiene. In addition, as King et al. (2009) and the United Nations (2018) have highlighted, Indigenous peoples have experienced entrenched discrimination and isolation owing to their unique histories, traditions, cultures, languages, and geographical locations.

Indigenous peoples continue to suffer abuse and the denial of human rights, including their right to health and right to land. The effects of colonization, the barriers of structural racism, and the burden of disease have resulted in long-standing societal and government denial of the complex and serious problems faced by Indigenous peoples. Recognizing the burden of disease among Indigenous groups—thought to be the result of the transition from traditional to modern lifestyles—requires an understanding of the impact of colonialism and how it has resulted in obesity; type 2 diabetes; cardiovascular disease; and mental, social, and physical ailments linked to alcohol and substance misuse (Gracey & King, 2009). Postcolonial theoretical perspectives, social theory, and the work of Indigenous scholars may guide thinking that can result in appreciating the detail and intricacies within Indigenous ways of viewing the world and thus a better understanding of their world. Topics of Indigenous health involve ethical issues related to cultural pluralism and the development of culturally competent and culturally safe knowledge.

Indigenous peoples around the world experience a multitude of common health disparities and inequities. For example, the infant mortality rate among Indigenous peoples in Latin America is 60% higher than it is for the non-Indigenous population (United Nations Interagency Support Group, 2014). In Australia, Indigenous children have a shorter life expectancy and higher burden of poor health compared with non-Indigenous children (United Nations, 2009). Connections between determinants of health and illness patterns and major health concerns such as obesity, type 2 diabetes, and TB as well as substance misuse are more impactful among Indigenous groups than among non-Indigenous populations (United Nations, 2009). The major health problems facing Indigenous peoples are thought to be better understood as illness experiences that vary according to local culture and linguistic membership, geographical placement, and the extent of isolated living circumstances.

The global Indigenous health crisis can be characterized by life expectancies that are lower than those for the general populations living in the same country. Nutritional deficiencies, diseases associated with cigarette smoking, accidents, poisonings, interpersonal violence, homicide, and suicide present similarities in health and illness experiences and their determinants across the great diversity of Indigenous peoples (Gracey & King, 2009).

The United Nations (2009) indicates that the life expectancy of Indigenous peoples in Nepal is approximately 20 years lower than that of the non-Indigenous population; for the Māori in New Zealand, life expectancy is nearly 10 years lower than it is for non-Māori. These findings indicate that when considering Indigenous health worldwide, it is complex, and the variation in high disease burden and poor life outcomes among different Indigenous populations require more attention and research. Advocacy related to the provision of health and social services that benefit Indigenous peoples is even more urgently required. Finally, empirical evidence is still replete with examples of the limited effectiveness of specific Indigenous health approaches that have been adapted to meet the needs of diverse Indigenous peoples globally.

Although global achievements directed at improving population health have been reached, the overall health of Indigenous populations lags far behind that of other populations (United Nations, 2018). In recent years, the health of some Indigenous populations has been considered improved, but access to holistic and culturally appropriate health services remains challenging, as does a deepening response to health problems related to the health of mothers and children, infectious diseases, and diseases related to urbanization and lifestyle (Gracey & King, 2009; United Nations, 2018).

To make progress toward improving Indigenous health, nurses will need to play key roles in examining Indigenous health challenges, developing appropriate responses, and implementing knowledge and action through understanding. In responding to Indigenous health, nurses have participated in huge numbers and will continue to do so, continuing a history of advocacy related to health inequities and social injustices (see Chapter 3). However, as Gracey and King (2009) emphasize, from a politics, policy, and future-directions perspective, assisting Indigenous peoples to build capacity in order to orchestrate effective services and programs and work closely with systems of health care will be part of the next wave of radical reorientation that is urgently needed.

KEY CONCEPTS

- Between 350 and 500 million Indigenous people reside in countries on every continent around the world. As of 2021, the Indigenous population in Canada was 1.8 million people.
- The three Indigenous groups in Canada—First Nations, Métis, and Inuit—have their own unique languages, heritages, cultural practices, and spiritual beliefs.
- Colonialism is the process and practise of European domination across the globe, including in Canada, that began in the fifteenth century. Colonial processes and structures continue to operate in Canada today, as does a fractured and complex relationship between Indigenous peoples and European settlers and their descendants owing to colonial policies, structures, and discrimination.
- The experiences of colonialism have resulted in historical and intergenerational trauma for Indigenous peoples.
- Structural racism is the legitimized and normalized spectrum of attitudes, practices, and policies that consistently result in chronic and continuous substandard outcomes for Indigenous peoples.
- All Canadians have been invited by the Truth and Reconciliation Commission of Canada to become settler allies—teachers and learners that question how non-Indigenous people can change, as opposed to just Indigenous people changing.
- Cultural orientations include theories of Indigenous health, the symbol of the circle, the Medicine Wheel, traditional healers, ceremony, teachings, and role modelling of Elders.
- Nurses need to develop the ability to adapt nursing practice for use in an Indigenous context in order to preserve the perspectives of Indigenous peoples, sustain the holistic nature of responding to social and health challenges, value new ways of forming partnerships in respectful ways, and focus on strengths-based practice. Addressing chronic disease requires appropriate knowledge and skills to create culturally safe chronic disease management programs in collaboration with Indigenous communities.
- Nurses' advocacy can decrease the inequities in determinants of health for Indigenous peoples and help to treat and reduce chronic disease in the Indigenous population in Canada.

CRITICAL THINKING EXERCISES

1. A nurse is caring for a patient with influenza. How would the nurse use Reading's concept of a tree, which represents the Indigenous determinants of health, to ascertain what inequities might have increased the susceptibility of the patient to acquiring illness?

2. A 65-year-old First Nations person (preferred pronouns: he/him) who lives on reserve is scheduled to go for an invasive procedure to treat his liver cancer. He meets with the nurse, who assesses him and gives him all the relevant information. On the day of the procedure, the patient fails to attend and cannot be reached by phone. Two weeks later, the patient contacts the nurse coordinator. The patient relates that he was too scared to go for the procedure.
   a. What could be done to help this patient?
   b. How might colonization have impacted this patient's life in such a way that the patient's fear was triggered?

3. After further discussion and encouragement, the patient goes for the procedure. The patient's niece (preferred pronouns: she/her) calls a week later. She states that her uncle is a spiritual leader in the community and that this was not taken into account when the assessment and patient education was done with him. She offers to come in to further discuss this matter so that future Indigenous patients will not have to go for treatment without their culture and spirituality being taken into account.
   a. Thinking about hospital policies and procedures, staff knowledge, and community connections that the hospital may need to have to improve their care for Indigenous patients, what ideas do you have that could be helpful in tackling any or all of these areas?
   b. Where might you gather more information?
   c. Find an article or two from the nursing literature that might help you make suggestions to the liver transplant unit and the clinical nurse educators in the hospital. Could this information improve policies, procedures, and knowledge of hospital staff related to the care of Indigenous patients?

4. A community health nurse (preferred pronouns: he/him) at the community health centre is waiting for his next client—a single parent with five children. The family is late. The policy is to reschedule patients who are more than 15 minutes late for their appointment. Twenty-five minutes after the family's appointment time, the parent (preferred pronouns: she/her) comes in with her five children. The children, aged 6 months to 10 years, are all behind on their immunizations. The parent tells the nurse that the children were immunized the summer before on reserve and that she has given staff this information. The parent also says she had trouble getting a ride to the clinic and the bus was late. The parent looks exhausted, and the baby has a cough. The desk staff person insists on rescheduling the parent, but the nurse disagrees with this decision.
   a. What could the nurse do about the parent's late appointment?
   b. How have determinants of health impacted this patient and her family?
   c. How can this family best be helped?

🌐 *Answers to Critical Thinking Exercises appear on the Evolve website.*

REVIEW QUESTIONS

Review Questions 1 to 11 relate to the case study at the beginning of the chapter.

1. When Helen, the 70-year-old Cree person, is first admitted, the nurse thinks that Helen must be confused when Helen tells her that she was in hospital for 3 years as a child for TB. Which of the following should the nurse know in order to better understand what Helen is talking about?
   a. That older Indigenous persons get dementia and Helen should be assessed for dementia.
   b. That Helen probably meant 3 months, but maybe her English is poor and she needs a translator.
   c. That Helen likely stayed in an "Indian hospital" in the city for 3 years as a child because she had TB.
   d. That it must have felt like 3 years to Helen because she was only a child, but it was probably only 3 months at most.

2. The nurse is teaching Helen about her diet and making suggestions for meals. Initially, Helen is engaged and tells the nurse about what she eats at home. The nurse suggests a number of alternatives and Helen seems reluctant to agree. What should the nurse know about food in Indigenous communities?
   a. Indigenous peoples prefer the food they had at residential school and are reluctant to change their diets.
   b. Indigenous peoples on reserve may not know how to cook certain foods and so they will not eat them.
   c. Prices for food in northern fly-in communities are very high and can be inaccessible for many people who live there.
   d. Indigenous peoples prefer traditional Indigenous foods and will not eat fruit and vegetables that are not grown on reserve.

3. The nurse who is taking Helen's history writes down "Indigenous" on the sheet under spirituality. She asks Helen whether she would like to see the Indigenous Elder to pray with her. What would have been a better approach for assessing Helen's spirituality?
   a. Ask Helen whether there is a specific Indigenous Elder she would like to see.
   b. Ask Helen whether she would like a sweetgrass ceremony.
   c. Ask Helen whether she practises a specific religion.
   d. Avoid the spirituality question because residential school survivors have been traumatized by priests and nuns.

4. Helen tells the nurse on the current shift that the nurse on the previous shift was racist toward her. She gives some examples of statements made by the previous nurse that sound inappropriate. What should the nurse do about what Helen has told her?
   a. Explain that the previous nurse may have said some inappropriate things, but that she likely meant well.
   b. Reassure Helen that no one on the unit is racist.
   c. Spend some time sitting with Helen and listening to her discuss the situation.
   d. Listen to Helen, take notes, and then discuss the situation with the nursing supervisor.

5. The nurse sees Helen drinking some liquid from a brown bottle. When she asks Helen what the liquid was, Helen becomes evasive and does not provide a response to the nurse. What should the nurse take into consideration when questioning Helen?
   a. That Helen considers it to be a private matter.
   b. That Helen may have some mistrust of the health care system owing to previous experiences with interpersonal and systemic racism.
   c. That Helen is likely drinking something she is not supposed to, because she may not know what interacts with her current medications.
   d. That Helen does not like the nurse and therefore is refusing to answer.

6. The nurse finds out that Helen was drinking a special tea made for her by a healer on her reserve and brought to her by her family. What is the best way to respond to this information?
   a. Gently ask Helen to hand over the tea because other medicines are not allowed.
   b. Ask Helen to get a family member to take the tea away because other medicines are not allowed.
   c. Allow Helen to drink the tea because it is necessary to be open to other healing paradigms.
   d. Have a discussion with Helen about the tea in terms of its possible interaction with other medications.

7. The family is upset that Helen still has serious health issues, and that she may not get better. They request that staff attend a prayer ceremony with them. What would be the most culturally safe action to take?
   a. Let the family know that staff unfortunately cannot attend because they have to maintain a focus on caring for patients, but that there is no problem with the family having a prayer service.
   b. Let the family know that it is unethical for staff to attend because they are not of the same faith, but that it is fine if the family has the prayer service.
   c. Ask the hospital's Indigenous Elder to attend the prayer service on behalf of the unit.
   d. Designate specific willing staff members to attend the prayer service with the family on behalf of the unit.

8. The nurse starts discharge planning for Helen. What should she focus on in her planning? *(Select all that apply.)*
   a. Educating the family about Helen's medications and treatments
   b. Calling the home community's nursing station to arrange continuity of care for Helen
   c. Discussing Helen's strict diabetic diet in terms of what she is allowed to eat
   d. Asking the family how funerals are conducted up north and if they have planned for this outcome
   e. Providing emotional support to the family by listening to their concerns, empathizing, and asking clarifying questions

9. The day before Helen is to be discharged, a large crowd of people wanting to visit Helen forms outside her room. What would be the best way to handle this scenario and why?

   a. Ask the group to designate one or two people to visit with Helen so they can update the rest of the group about Helen's condition.
   b. Tell the group that only immediate family is allowed to visit because of hospital policy.
   c. Find an empty room nearby for the visitors because in Indigenous cultures it is normal for family and community members to visit their loved ones in hospital.
   d. Tell them it is not necessary to visit Helen because she is going home soon and they have all visited her before.

10. Later that same day, Helen confides to one of the nurses that her daughter was murdered 15 years ago by a man who picked her up while she was hitchhiking. What would be the nurse's best response to this information?
    a. "I'm so sorry to hear that. The grief must be so difficult to bear. Can you tell me more about your daughter?"
    b. "I'm sorry to hear that. Were alcohol or drugs involved? I've heard that can be a factor in these cases."
    c. "I'm sorry to hear that. Hitchhiking is so dangerous. Why was she hitchhiking?"
    d. "I'm so sorry to hear that. Let's talk about your discharge plans now. There's no point in dwelling on the past."

11. On her last night in hospital, Helen asks the nurse whether one of her guests can stay in her room with her because she has nowhere else to go. What does the nurse need to know in order to manage this situation in a culturally safe way? *(Select all that apply.)*
    a. Indigenous people who are not patients may need a referral to the social worker.
    b. Indigenous peoples have high poverty rates.
    c. Indigenous peoples do not usually live in the city.
    d. Hospitals need to ensure they have sufficient resources for Indigenous patients and their families in order to provide family-centred and culturally safe care.
    e. In many Indigenous cultures, kindness is an important value that is practised.

Answers: 1. c; **2.** c; **3.** c; **4.** d; **5.** b; **6.** d; **7.** d; **8.** a, b, c, e; **9.** c; **10.** a; **11.** a, b, d, e.

🌐 *Rationales for the Review Questions appear on the Evolve website.*

RECOMMENDED WEBSITES

Alberta Health Services—Trauma Training Initiative: https://www.albertahealthservices.ca/info/page15526.aspx
The Trauma Training Initiative offers professional development to health care providers who support people who have had any traumatic experience. The training focuses on enhancing knowledge of trauma-informed care and developing trauma-focused skills for practice.

Canadian Indigenous Nurses Association (CINA): https://www.indigenousnurses.ca
The CINA works to improve the health of Indigenous peoples by supporting Indigenous nurses and promoting the development and practice of Indigenous nursing. Key objectives include working with communities, health care providers, and government institutions to address elements of the Canadian health care system that affect the health and well-being of Indigenous communities; engaging and conducting research on Indigenous health nursing; and promoting awareness nationally and internationally of the health needs of Indigenous peoples in Canada.

First Nations Child and Family Caring Society of Canada: https://fncaringsociety.com/who-we-are

The First Nations Child and Family Caring Society of Canada is a nonprofit organization that provides reconciliation-based public education, research, and support to promote the safety and well-being of First Nations children, young people, families, and Nations. The organization also works with national and international partners to promote the rights of Indigenous children, youth, and families.

Healthcare Excellence Canada: Canadian Northern and Remote Healthcare Network: https://www.healthcareexcellence.ca/en/what-we-do/all-programs/canadian-northern-and-remote-health-network
This network aims to improve the health status of people living in northern and remote regions of Canada by providing opportunities for practitioners, leaders, and policymakers to network, build leadership, and improve capacity.

In Plain Sight: Addressing Indigenous-Specific Racism and Discrimination in BC Health Care: https://engage.gov.bc.ca/app/uploads/sites/613/2020/11/In-Plain-Sight-Full-Report-2020.pdf
This report contains an in-depth review of Indigenous-specific racism and discrimination in the provincial health care system and makes recommendations to address the issues.

Indigenous Canada Massive Open Online Course:https://www.ualberta.ca/admissions-programs/online-courses/indigenous-canada/index.html

Developed at the University of Alberta from an Indigenous perspective, this free 12-lesson online course provides education on key issues facing Indigenous peoples from a historical and critical lens and explores Indigenous–settler relations.

Institute of Indigenous Peoples' Health (IIPH): https://cihr-irsc.gc.ca/e/8668.html

Part of the Canadian Institutes of Health Research (CIHR), IIPH was developed to help fill in the gaps in our knowledge about the health disparities experienced by Indigenous peoples. The institute leads a national advanced research agenda in the area of Indigenous health and promotes innovative research to improve the health of Indigenous peoples in Canada.

National Collaborating Centre for Indigenous Health: https://www.nccih.ca/en

The National Collaborating Centre for Indigenous Health supports First Nations, Inuit, and Métis health equity and renewal through knowledge translation and exchange. It was established by the government of Canada in 2005, is funded through the Public Health Agency of Canada, and is hosted by The University of Northern British Columbia.

Native Women's Association of Canada: https://www.nwac.ca

The Native Women's Association of Canada is an aggregate of Indigenous women's organizations whose goal is to enhance, promote, and foster the social, economic, cultural and political well-being of Indigenous women, girls, and gender-diverse people in their respective communities and Canadian societies while recognizing, respecting, promoting, defending, and enhancing Indigenous ancestral laws, spiritual belief, language, and Traditions provided by the Creator.

San'yas Anti-Racism Indigenous Cultural Safety Training Program: https://sanyas.ca

Originating in British Columbia, this organization provides a cultural safety training program that based on anti-racist, decolonizing, transformative, and adult education theories. The program can be accessed online or in person and is designed for all sectors, including health care providers.

Walking in Her Moccasins: https://unveilingtruths.ca/walking-in-her-moccasins

An experiential violence prevention resource for Indigenous men and boys that was officially launched across Canada in December 2017. This project is rooted in the rights of Indigenous women and girls to live free from all forms of violence, and it encourages Indigenous men and boys to play positive and culturally relevant roles to promote gender equality.

🌐 REFERENCES

A full reference list is available on the website for this book at http://evolve.elsevier.com/Canada/Potter/fundamentals/

13

Nursing Leadership and Collaborative Practice

Written by Susan M. Duncan, RN, BScN, PhD, FCAN, and Angela Wignall, RN, BSN, BA, MA, PhD(c)

OBJECTIVES

Mastery of content in this chapter will enable you to:

- Define the key terms listed.
- Describe entry-level professional nurse competencies related to leadership and collaborative practice.
- Identify strategies for developing entry-level competencies for nursing leadership and collaborative practice.
- Consider the implications of the *State of World's Nursing* reports and other contextual influences on the nursing profession, including COVID-19.
- Describe the ways in which nursing leadership shapes and contributes to healthy practice environments, patient safety, quality patient care outcomes, and health care system excellence.
- Describe evolving theories of leadership, nursing leadership roles, and the skills nurses use to lead in health systems.
- Understand perspectives on global leadership and leadership within nursing organizations.
- Describe how nurses lead collaborative practice and evidence-informed best practice implementation.
- Describe the ways in which nursing knowledge is applied in team-based care and in leadership.
- Explain principles for delegation and supporting top of scope practice in team-based care.
- Identify nursing leadership accountability and initiatives related to Indigenous-specific and other forms of racism in health care.

KEY TERMS

Accountability
Anti-racism
Authority
Autonomy
Best Practice Guidelines
Career development
Case management
Clinical governance
Collaborative practice
Competencies for safe practice

Continuity of care
Delegation
Entry-level competencies
Health equity
Healthy practice environment
Interprofessional teams
Intraprofessional teams
Mentoring
Models of care
Nurse-sensitive outcome

Nursing leadership
Patient safety
Responsibility
Team-based care
Team nursing
Theoretical perspectives on leadership
Transformational leadership
Trauma-informed leadership

🌐 WEBSITE

http://evolve.elsevier.com/Canada/Potter/fundamentals/

CASE STUDY

K.H. (preferred pronouns: she/her) is a recently graduated registered nurse working at a residential care facility. A.B. (preferred pronouns: she/her), the nurse manager of the facility, is aware of K.H.'s interest in leadership for best practices in the care of older persons.

As a fourth-year student, K.H. had completed a special project on falls prevention in the facility using local statistics on falls and evidence-informed practice guidelines. A.B. recognizes that there is an increased rate of falls among residents in the facility. As such, she wishes to implement a falls prevention program that is based on evidence-informed best practices and that includes the participation of residents, families, and the team of professionals and providers who provide care. Current Canadian statistics indicate that falls are the leading cause of overall injury costs in Canada and that falls continue increasing among older persons in residential care settings, despite a growing

body of evidence about how to prevent them (Public Health Agency of Canada, 2014; Williams-Roberts et al., 2021). *A.B. sees this as an excellent opportunity for K.H. to be involved so that she can continue to develop her leadership skills in the areas of collaborative practice, team nursing, and best practices implementation.*

At A.B.'s invitation, K.H. seeks out resources to guide her work, including the Registered Nurses' Association of Ontario Best Practice Guidelines for falls prevention (RNAO, 2017). *K.H. begins her work by thinking about how she can bring health care team members and other professionals into the project team in order to achieve a broad perspective on the changes required to prevent falls, to create buy-in, and to successfully lead a practice change. She forms a working group that represents the diversity of the care team and facilitates collaborative brainstorming sessions to get every good idea on the table.*

Continued

CASE STUDY—CONT'D

K.H. also knows that the evidence for falls prevention and for quality improvement in patient care suggests that involving patients and families is a critical part of designing patient-centred solutions. She remembers the phrase "nothing about us without us," and wants to make sure the changes she champions are reflective of the needs of the residents she cares for. She decides to create a learning community to engage residents and their families in the initiative. The learning community brings the working group, residents, and family members together to improve patient safety and prevent falls.

As a member of the team, K.H. contributes to leading a collaborative, evidence-informed process that results in high-quality tools for identifying residents at risk for falls. The inclusive process she has facilitated ensures that all care team members as well as residents and families are able to contribute their experiences and ideas to the process of managing risk and improving the quality of care. The result is a change in practice that

team members are excited to implement, and that residents and families understand and support.

An evaluation of the working group and learning community demonstrates a high level of satisfaction and buy-in among participants. Most importantly, the incidence of falls in the facility decreases and the quality of care increases.

K.H. is inspired by this experience and is motivated to further develop her leadership competencies in the areas of inspiring a vision, leading change, facilitating collaborative practice, and developing respectful and supportive relationships in a care community. She begins work with the nurse researcher at the local university to develop a plan for studying the impact of the changes on the incidence of falls over time. A.B.'s mentorship as a leader and K.H.'s willingness to embrace the opportunity sets K.H. up for the next opportunity where her leadership skills can make a difference.

Think about this case study as you read this chapter. There are Review Questions at the end of the chapter about this case study.

In this chapter, you will explore what it means to be a nurse leader in Canada and around the world today. From bedside to boardroom, nurses provide leadership for health systems, organizations and institutions, and patient care environments. Nurses in leadership roles enable quality nursing care and promote health in many roles and settings—from the point of care to organizational leadership, including in government. Nurses also enact leadership by advancing the health of communities and populations through their involvement in nursing organizations, including regulatory bodies, unions, and professional associations. Nurses also perform a critical function in the promotion of health equity, which is the ability to attain one's full health potential and not face any barriers to achieving this potential because of social position or other socially determined circumstances (World Health Organization [WHO], 2020). (See Chapter 11 in the context of rapid social change.)

Within the Canadian context, nursing leadership is shaped by a wide range of influences, including global, national, provincial, and local directives and priorities. In 2020, the WHO released the *State of the World's Nursing 2020*, the first global report on the state of nursing as a workforce and as a profession (WHO, 2020). This report calls for investments in nursing education and leadership as a key strategy for enabling health equity around the world. Strengthening nursing leadership was identified as one of three key areas of advancement required to meet global health needs and achieve the ambitious social policy objectives set out by the United Nation's Sustainable Development Goals (United Nations, 2015) and adopted by Canada as a United Nations member state. The WHO report noted that countries with formal nursing leadership roles (such as Chief Nursing Officers) and programs for nursing leadership development also showed beneficial increases in nursing regulation, including improved working conditions and stronger nursing education (WHO, 2020). The report also identified that investment in nursing leadership is an important policy option for addressing nursing retention, gender-based discrimination in nursing, and the production of healthy public policy (WHO, 2020).

Since the publication of this far-reaching report, the COVID-19 global pandemic has exposed longstanding inequities in health and heath care, and demonstrated in real time the urgent need for an expansive view of nursing leadership. Inequities on a global scale include global vaccine inequity, whereby some countries are immunizing entire populations while those countries hardest hit by the virus have low to no access to vaccines; social injustice, including Indigenous-specific racism in health care; social justice movements such as Black

Lives Matter; growing calls for reform of care for older persons in long-term care settings; and the disadvantaging of public health nursing in COVID-19 policy and planning (Caxaj et al., 2021; Lefebre et al., 2020). As the world faces increasing political instability and extremism, global pandemics, environmental challenges, aging populations, and a shrinking health care workforce, building knowledge and capacity for nursing leadership is a critical part of meeting the health needs of humanity. The context of nursing leadership is therefore not merely local but global, set within the dynamic context of a rapidly changing world (see Chapter 11).

The Canadian Association of Schools of Nursing's (CASN) *National Nursing Education Framework* (CASN, 2022) identifies leadership as an essential component of baccalaureate education. Leadership opportunities prepare students to coordinate nursing care and influence and advocate for change in nursing and health programs for health equity and social justice. As a nursing student, you will have opportunities to develop insights and awareness for change and influence that will lead to a more just and equitable world. As a nursing student, you have opportunities to provide leadership for practice and nursing education by bringing your vision to the challenges we face today. Box 13.1 presents a case study demonstrating how nurse leaders can influence policy and social justice action by applying nursing knowledge to complex health systems issues.

As you take on your identity as a nurse and begin your nursing practice, your knowledge of leadership roles in nursing will take shape and evolve. As you develop the knowledge and skills to enter the nursing workforce, you will also learn how to become a leader among colleagues and within interprofessional teams. Phrases such as "from the bedside to the boardroom" (Institute of Medicine, 2011) and "leadership in every moment of practice" (Doane & Varcoe, 2021, p. 402) indicate the centrality of leadership in all nursing practice settings and the expansive space for leadership growth in the discipline of nursing.

As the list of competencies required of entry-level nurses illustrate (Box 13.2), leadership begins with a strong professional identity grounded in nursing knowledge and rooted in the relational and ethical practice that is the hallmark of nursing as a profession. Nurse leaders are needed today more than ever to lead the design and delivery of excellent care, and to grow the skills required for managing and leading best practices. Leaders use and create vision, values, strategies, and relationships to achieve health-related goals through a wide range of activities.

BOX 13.1 CASE STUDY

The Application of Nursing Knowledge to Policy Leadership: Addressing Indigenous-Specific Racism in Health Care

On June 19, 2020, allegations of Indigenous-specific racism in health care in British Columbia (BC) went public when the Minister of Health announced the launch of an independent investigation (Government of British Columbia, 2020). The investigation initially focused on reports of a racist game being played in emergency departments. It was then expanded to broadly encompass reports and experiences of racism in health care from both Indigenous peoples and non-Indigenous people. Led by Mary Ellen Turpel-Lafond, the investigation resulted in the publication of the *In Plain Sight* report (Turpel-Lafond, 2020). In it, Turpel-Lafond documents the stories of Indigenous peoples who have faced racism and discrimination in the health care system and makes recommendations for action to address Indigenous-specific racism.

In Plain Sight is the most recent of many such reports on Indigenous-specific racism and the resilience of Indigenous peoples experiencing genocide, discrimination, and the ongoing impacts of colonialism. Reports by the Truth and Reconciliation Commission of Canada (2015), the National Inquiry Into Missing and Murdered Indigenous Women and Girls (Buller, 2019), and the Public Inquiry Commission on Relations Between Indigenous Peoples and Certain Public Services in Québec (Viens, 2019) are all examples of the intersecting testimonies and recommendations now guiding anti-racism work in health care. As BC health organizations attempted to respond to the recommendations in the *In Plain Sight* report, the need for a systematic analysis of the diverse recommendations emerged to guide decision makers in effectively enacting anti-racism work.

In response to this need, two nurse leaders in a regional health authority were commissioned to undertake a systematic analysis of recommendations from six intersecting reports, using the *In Plain Sight* report as the reference point. Initial analysis identified for decision makers the ways in which recommendations aligned and diverged between reports. In charting the full landscape for potential policy action, this analysis enabled decision makers, including Indigenous nurse executives, to make meaning out of the recommendations within each report and to make decisions on key areas for immediate action. Secondary analysis, including the development of a logic model, matched recommendations to governance layers, drawing clear lines of accountability and responsibility among interlocking parts of the health system. For example, recommendations that had legislative requirements were aligned to the provincial government's task force rather than to a health authority. This has prevented duplication of effort and supported decision makers in communicating clearly to staff and communities what expectations and responsibilities are within their areas of authority.

As a further measure of its success, the analysis supported the rapid development of an anti-racism strategy for the provincial health authorities and was escalated to the Ministry of Health as a knowledge resource. Critically, the work of these two nurse leaders enabled a major change in the BC health system: instead of asking Indigenous peoples what colonial health systems should do to provide better patient care, health system leaders began to align with and respond to what Indigenous peoples had named for decades. This work has not only supported project coordination, but also cultivated a sense of possibility and strengthened relationships that are the foundation for truth and reconciliation.

BOX 13.2 Entry-Level Registered Nurse Competencies Related to Nursing Leadership Roles

Recently developed national **entry-level competencies** for registered nurses in Canada relate specifically to the roles of collaborator, coordinator, and leader (British Columbia College of Nurses and Midwives [BCCNM], 2020). The role of coordinator of care is becoming increasingly complex as nurses provide leadership at the point of care, ensuring that people receive the right care or service from the provider. Nurses in coordinator roles navigate people's experiences of health and illness transitions across institutional and community-based sectors of care, a role that involves complex consultations and information exchanges (BCCNM, 2020). This role also requires the enactment of competencies related to collaboration, as it involves leading and supporting teams (MacKinnon et al., 2018). Other roles for which nursing students must develop competencies include the role of collaborator and advocate, whereby nurses work with others to advocate and support health equity for all and human rights (BCCNM, 2020). Specific competencies associated with the role of leader appear below.

Leader

Registered nurses are leaders who influence and inspire others to achieve optimal health outcomes for all.

Competencies:
6.1 Acquires knowledge of the Calls to Action of the Truth and Reconciliation Commission of Canada.
6.2 Integrates continuous quality improvement principles and activities into nursing practice.
6.3 Participates in innovative client-centred care models.
6.4 Recognizes the impact of organizational culture and acts to enhance the quality of a professional and safe practice environment.
6.5 Participates in creating and maintaining a healthy, respectful, and psychologically safe workplace.
6.6 Demonstrates self-awareness through reflective practice and solicitation of feedback.
6.7 Takes action to support culturally safe practice environments.
6.8 Uses and allocates resources wisely.
6.9 Provides constructive feedback to promote professional growth of other members of the health care team.
6.10 Demonstrates knowledge of the health care system and its impact on client care and professional practice.
6.11 Adapts practice to meet client care needs within a continually changing health care system.

Adapted from British Columbia College of Nurses and Midwives (BCCNM). (2020). *Entry-level competencies for registered nurses* (pp. 10–11). https://www.bccnm.ca/Documents/competencies_requisite_skills/RN_entry_level_competencies_375.pdf

Historically, nursing leadership often meant clinical operational *management*, where nurses held responsibility for the day-to-day delivery of patient care, upholding standards of professional practice, and stewarding health care resources through financial management (Hibberd et al., 2006). Today, **nursing leadership** also refers to management in clinical operations, but it extends much further to include leadership in knowledge creation through research, policy advocacy and development in governance contexts, executive leadership in executive teams and boards of directors, health care quality leadership in quality improvement and assurance, education as nurse educators and professors, and so much more (Marcellus et al., 2018). To meet the needs of communities and populations, nurse leaders in every domain must demonstrate leadership practices that honour the importance of relationships, values, and ethics and the unique contribution of nursing knowledge to how we think about health and health systems (Doane & Varcoe, 2021; Institute of Medicine, 2011; Wong, 2015). Nursing leadership is needed at every level, and nurse leaders must work across professional roles to improve health systems with other providers and sectors of society (Institute of Medicine, 2011). Figure 13.1 provides a conceptual model of leadership that has been identified as contributing to health outcomes.

A healthy work environment enables nurses to provide high-quality care and supports nurses in being well at work. A psychologically safe workplace is essential for the promotion of human rights and anti-racist practice, as well as the ability to work with difference and to resolve conflicts. For nursing students, as with all nurses, this begins with self-awareness and knowing oneself in terms of one's own values, biases, and aspirations. Developing as a leader also requires a high level of reflection on the purpose of leadership, as well as observations of how others enact leadership and to what ends (Doane & Varcoe, 2021).

Researchers note that transformational and relational models of leadership best contribute to healthy work environments for nurses, including nurse retention and recruitment needed for quality patient care (Cummings et al., 2010; Wong & Laschinger, 2013). At the staff and patient level, this translates, for instance, into registered nurses working collaboratively with other members of the nursing team, with providers from other disciplines, and with patients and families.

Healthy work environments and wellness at work takes many forms. Federal employment standards and provincial/territorial workplace safety organizations set the standards for physical workplace safety that govern health care workplaces. Nurse leaders are responsible for ensuring that workplaces meet these standards and that they comply with healthy workplace legislation, regulations, and rules. However, wellness at work also includes psychological well-being and the need for mental, emotional, and cultural safety at work. In 2013, the Mental Health Commission of Canada created the National Standard of Canada for Psychological Health and Safety in the Workplace. This standard provides a unifying approach to reducing psychological harm and increasing mental well-being at work (Mental Health Commission of Canada, 2013), which is particularly important for those who work in complex environments like health care. Nurse leaders use tools such as legislation and standards to ensure the wellness of health care teams and to enable the delivery of quality care.

While nurses represent the largest group of health care providers on the planet (WHO, 2020), nurses work in diverse teams. Nurse leaders must therefore be well versed in collaborative practice, which is defined as working together toward mutually identified goals while valuing the different perspectives and accountabilities of individual team members (Canadian Interprofessional Health Collaborative, 2010; Canadian Nurses Association [CNA], 2011; Health Professions Network Nursing and Midwifery Office, 2010; Healthcare Excellence Canada, 2012; Jacobson, 2012; Orchard et al., 2017a, 2017b; Virani, 2012). This chapter therefore focuses on current thinking on nursing leadership, including definitions, roles, and relationships, all within the context of collaborative practice models where nurse leaders work with others to create healthy practice environments (Doane & Varcoe, 2021). The ideas and examples included in this chapter apply to the multitude of different practice settings in which nurses work: in homes, in institutions, and in communities.

Leaders support people in being well and in achieving necessary outcomes, often during intense periods of transformation and change

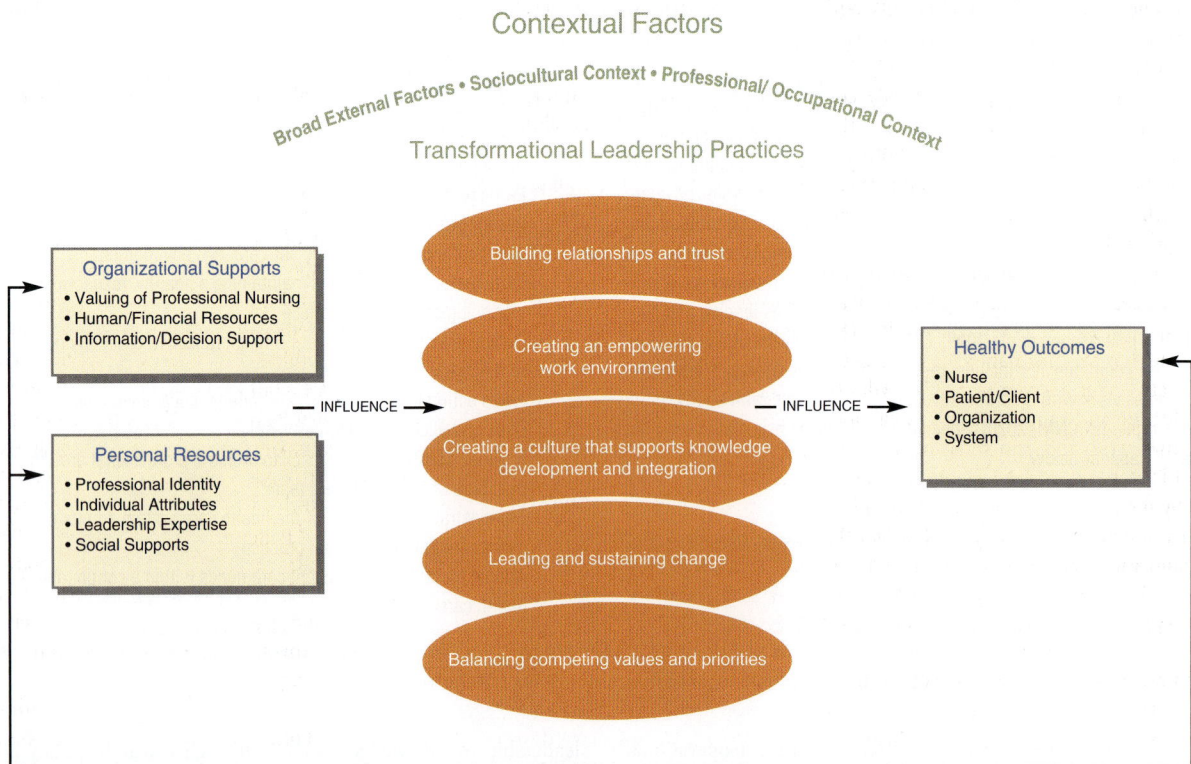

FIGURE 13.1 Conceptual model for developing and sustaining leadership. This model organizes and guides the discussion of the Registered Nurses' Association of Ontario (RNAO) recommendations. It provides a framework for understanding the leadership practices needed to achieve healthy work environments and the organizational supports and personal resources that enable effective leadership practices. (From Registered Nurses' Association of Ontario. [2013]. *The healthy work environments quick reference guide for nurses* [p. 23].)

(Public Health Agency of Canada, 2018). In the current global context, this imperative requires nurse leaders to be active in working toward social justice, equity, and **anti-racism**, which is defined as dismantling the institutions, policies, and social constructs that perpetuate white supremacy, colonialism, and oppression.

It is especially critical that nurses lead the way in addressing Indigenous-specific racism in health care. This starts with cultivating a deep understanding of the history of the lands colonially known as Canada. It also requires a commitment to reading and understanding the decades of testimony from Indigenous peoples set out in reports prepared by the Truth and Reconciliation Commission of Canada (2015), the National Inquiry Into Missing and Murdered Indigenous Women and Girls (Buller, 2019), the Public Inquiry Commission on Relations Between Indigenous Peoples and Certain Public Services in Québec (Viens, 2019), and the Addressing Racism Review in British Columbia (Turpel-Lafond, 2020). Nurse leaders must also be well-acquainted with the legislative and practice implications of the United Nations Declaration on the Rights of Indigenous Peoples and other frameworks for guiding anti-racism action (see Chapter 12, Indigenous Health). The Joyce Echaquan inquiry into nurses' expression of racism toward an Indigenous woman has also prompted the need for critical reflection, inquiry, and action within the nursing profession. Ensuring cultural humility and cultural safety in the health care system requires every nurse to invest in learning and self-reflection on the biases, stigmatizing beliefs, and structural racism that exist within us and within the health care structures we work in.

LEADERSHIP THEORIES

Nurses draw on multiple views and theories of leadership that come from a variety of disciplines, including sociology, psychology, and management science. There is also an emerging body of research on nursing leadership that illuminates critical issues for nursing and nurses (Cummings et al., 2010; Wong et al., 2013). **Theoretical perspectives on leadership** support nurses in critically considering the kinds of leadership practices they wish to adopt and the ways in which different leadership practices impact others. Students may become familiar with one or more leadership theories and reflect on how these theories resonate with their own values and aspirations to make a difference through leadership.

One theory that has resonated with nurses is **transformational leadership**, an approach emphasizing that a leader with vision and values can inspire others in a certain direction (Kouzes & Posner, 2017). Closely related to transformational theory is the idea of the emotionally intelligent leader, a leader who "leads with their heart" and engages in self-reflection and supportive and collaborative relationships while sharing power with those in their organization (Smith et al., 2009). Relational leaders can inspire others by building on what is working well and by focusing on the strengths and identities of nurses instead of on issues and problems (Gottlieb et al. 2012). Leading change in this era will require leaders to develop competencies that are closely aligned with the relational and ethical values of nursing, as well as the ability to think at a systems level, inspire innovation, and collaborate for shared power.

Recent analyses of nursing systems indicate that nursing leadership is needed at all organizational levels, and that more attention needs to be paid to leadership that inspires and supports nurses and nursing at the point of care. Therefore, nurses who are in formal leadership positions, such as at executive and managerial levels, must enable leadership at every level of health organizations, including at the point of care (Duncan et al., 2014). Box 13.3 presents a global case study that illustrates the need to work together across

| BOX 13.3 | **Global Allyship to Advance Nursing Leadership Theories** |

The conditions to encourage leadership in nursing are often hindered by considerations of nursing as a workforce only, the gendered nature of the nursing profession, and the absence of nursing leaders in local and national governments (Cassiani et al., 2019). Following the launch of the global Nursing Now campaign in 2018, nursing leaders across the globe fielded questions about why nursing leadership matters and why a global focus on nursing was needed. In response to these questions, a group of nursing leaders from across the WHO Pan American Health Organization (PAHO) region came together to release a letter to the editor that was published in the *Pan American Journal of Public Health*.

This bold letter stated that "to address shortages, strategies often call for producing more nurses to meet the demand, but those new professionals are frequently not adequately prepared to function and lead in an increasingly complex, strained workplace" (Cassiani et al., 2019, p. 1). Going even further, the authors noted that "the demands and complexity of health systems require professionals capable of mobilizing cognitive and material resources to propose and formulate policies . . . professionals capable of working interprofessionally, and making fundamental decisions that will improve working conditions, expand universal access and coverage, and promote societal well-being." (Cassiani et al., 2019, p. 1). The authors then set out the Strategic Direction for Nursing in the Region of the Americas, which proposes three priority areas of action for nursing: leadership, working conditions, and quality nursing education.

The publication of this letter and the subsequent launch of a WHO region-wide strategy for nursing speaks to what is possible when nurses work collaboratively to address global challenges. Working as allies to speak up and stand strong for the value of nursing, the authors took back the narrative about nursing and named the value of nursing leadership in advancing global health goals.

interprofessional and national boundaries in order to advance leadership in health care.

LEADERSHIP ROLES FOR NURSES

Nurses assume a wide variety of leadership roles in health care organizations, always centring on the health, well-being, and safety of individuals, families, and communities. A primary and essential nursing leadership role is to nurture environments where nurses can practise according to their codes of ethics; this is made possible when nurses and other team members are encouraged to come together in reflection and dialogue over pressing everyday ethical tensions that are pervasive in health care settings (Austin, 2007; CNA, 2017). Nursing leadership can ensure that nursing practice takes place in environments that nurture moral communities, knowledge-informed care, and excellence in standards of practice, care, and patient safety (Aiken, 2008; Aiken et al., 2014; Duncan et al., 2014; CNA, 2017; Estabrooks et al., 2005; Health Canada, 2002; Wong et al., 2013). A high-quality practice environment is also a healthy work environment, defined as on in which "nurses experience respect and are involved in decision-making" (CNA & Canadian Federation of Nursing Unions, 2015, p. 1).

A **healthy practice environment** begins with the senior nurse leader in the organization, who most often holds the title of Chief Nurse Executive, Chief Nursing Officer, or Director or Vice-President of Nursing or of Patient Care (Health Canada, 2002). These positions are key to ensuring that nurses influence the policy directions that governments take to provide high-quality health care for Canadians. As a student, you will learn the skills required to advocate successfully in health and

Nursing Leadership in Primary Health Care

Nursing as a profession has taken a strong leadership role in implementing primary health care throughout the world. Since 1978, the International Council of Nurses (ICN), the Canadian Nurses Association (CNA), and other national, provincial, and territorial nursing associations have been instrumental in lobbying for inclusion of primary health care principles and programs in health care professional education, in service planning and delivery, and in research and evaluation. The CNA (2009b) actively promotes initiatives to incorporate primary health care into nursing practice and policy. Enshrining primary health care principles in policy is the way to promote health for all people and is based on a social justice model and related values (Reutter & Ogilvie, 2011). Nursing advocacy for primary health care as the foundation of health care is required of leaders at all levels of practice and organizations (Reutter & Kushner, 2010; Smith, 2014).

If nurses are to have the influence that is needed to transform health systems, they must develop the vision, knowledge, and skills for primary health care. Nurses learn to influence systems through their work in organizations and, most importantly, by working collectively in nursing and other types of associations. Nursing associations play a pivotal role in ensuring that the voice and influence of nurses is expressed and reflects their status as the largest group of health professionals worldwide.

The ICN and its member national nurses associations (NNAs) promote and support all efforts to improve the preparation of nurses for management, leadership, and policy development. The preparation should be broad and must include the development of knowledge and skills for influencing change, engaging in the political process, social marketing, forming coalitions, working with the media, and other means of exerting influence (Smith, 2014).

In 2015, Dr. Becky Palmer assumed her position as the first Chief Nursing Officer of the First Nations Health Authority in British Columbia. Dr. Palmer is a passionate nursing leader in nursing and health care with a vision for transforming nursing services within First Nations communities. Dr. Palmer's leadership contributes to the health and care of First Nations as she supports Indigenous, trauma-informed, and culturally safe models of care. Dr. Palmer works collaboratively with many nursing and health organizations to influence ways of thinking and being that contribute to cultural safety and humility and to broad understandings of Indigenous health and healing that benefit all.

From Canadian Nurses Foundation. (2021). *Award recipient—Becky Palmer*. https://cnf-fiic.ca/becky-palmer/. Reprinted with permission from Dr. Becky Palmer.

policy environments and will assume the role of advocate to promote the health of people. This includes the important function of shaping **clinical governance**, which is defined as "a systematic approach used by organizations to oversee, shape, manage, and continuously improve clinical health and social services" (Health Standards Organization, 2021). It also includes policy instruments such as policies, procedures, protocols, best practice guidelines, and decision support tools. Nurses today "stand on the shoulders of giants"; the nurse leaders of the past held a powerful vision for the development of nursing as a profession and advocated tirelessly to bring this vision to fruition ("A century of progress," 2005) (Box 13.4). Examples of Canadian nurse leaders are Dr. Becky Palmer, the first Chief Nursing Officer for the First Nations Health Authority in British Columbia (Box 13.5); and Dr. Leigh Chapman, appointed in September 2022 as the new Chief Nursing Officer of Canada.

Health Care Models, Collaborative Practice, and Health Care Teams

As in the past, a strong nurse leader at the senior level of the organization unites the strategic direction of the organization with the values and goals of nursing. Nurse executives must also build teams of leaders who will work across the organization to implement best practices and develop high-quality work environments in which excellent patient care can flourish. Although it takes a strong senior nursing leader to amplify the work of nurses and consistently champion the value of nursing knowledge, the role and responsibility of every nurse is to make a difference through leadership by displaying attributes such as articulating a vision, enabling others to act, encouraging others, and taking initiative (CNA, 2009a). The leader and nursing staff must share a philosophy of care that integrates purpose, best practices, and

concern for relationships, including how staff will work together and with patients and families (Box 13.6).

Integral to the philosophy of care is the selection of a care delivery model and a management structure that support professional nursing practice. A *nursing care delivery model* is a system for organizing and delivering nursing care to patients and their families that represents the structural and contextual elements of nursing practice (Fowler et al., 2006, as cited in CNA et al., 2012). Key factors that contribute to the successful implementation of a nursing care delivery model are strong nursing leadership, decision-making authority for nurses who provide direct care, and effective and respectful communications with colleagues, physicians, and other health care providers (Health Canada, 2002; Healthcare Excellence Canada, 2020).

Nursing care delivery models are designs that determine how nurses provide care. The choice of a nursing care delivery model is influenced by patient, provider, and organizational factors (Harris & McGillis Hall, 2012). Continuity of care is an extremely important concept in determining the choice of a nursing care delivery model. **Continuity of care** is defined as "a seamless continuous implementation of a plan of care that is reviewed and revised to meet the changing needs of the client" (Registered Nurses' Association of Ontario [RNAO], 2010, p. 61)—where the client is a person, a family, or a population. It refers to continuity of information or knowledge, continuity of relationships between a patient and one or more health care providers over time, and continuity of management of care across organizational boundaries (Smith et al., 2006). In the choice of nursing care delivery models, it is important to consider how nurses ensure that a patient's plan of care is as consistent as possible. For instance, evidence shows that the presence and knowledge of the registered nurse is a key factor in determining quality patient care outcomes (Aiken et al., 2014; Wong, 2015).

As changes occur in health care delivery and nursing practice, new care delivery models are evolving. In the current context, a patient care model known as the *collaborative practice model*, or the **team-based care** model, is emerging. This model depends on strong

What Is the Nursing Unit's Purpose or Mission?
- Articulating why it exists
- Ensuring that nursing services are based on primary health care principles
- Knowing the background of health needs and perspectives of patients and population (internal and external)
- Knowing the background of its collaborative team members: their professional preparation, identity, and unique contributions
- Demonstrating how it accomplishes organizational goals or vision

How Will Nurses Engage and Practice With Persons, Families, and Communities?
- By placing person, family, and community needs first with a participatory approach
- By involving care recipients and community members as members of a collaborative practice team
- By making relational practice and communication priorities

What Are the Standards of the Work Unit?
- Nurses adhere to professional accountability practice according to standards of practice and codes of ethics.
- Nurses practise within a culture of safety.
- The work unit integrates evidence-informed best practices.
- Nurses work collaboratively with all members of the health care team.

What Are the Key Values?
- Creating and maintaining a healthy practice environment
- Enacting anti-racist practices and promoting cultural safety
- Promoting principles of equity, inclusion, and human rights
- Enacting the principles of primary health care
- Recognizing social justice issues
- Providing culturally safe care and responding to the Truth and Reconciliation Commission of Canada (TRC) Calls to Action
- Supporting relational practice and the upholding of the CNA *Code of Ethics*
- Being self-aware, motivated, and accountable
- Supporting a learning environment

professional identities and working relationships between nurses at all levels and with patients, other health care providers, and community members. The care delivery models of today involve a wide range of health care team members, including multiple nursing designations, allied health professionals, and health team members that have historically been known as unregulated care providers (UCPs). These diverse teams support patients in many settings of practice, including home care, institutional acute care, and residential long-term care.

The health team members whose practice is unregulated provide personal and delegated care to increasing numbers of patients across different health care settings in Canada. The title of the roles for health team members differs from province to province, as does the requirement for training or educational programs. In British Columbia, for example, these roles may be referred to as health care assistants (HCAs), and individuals are prepared for practice following completion of a 6- to 8-month certification program offered in public and private postsecondary educational institutions.

Nurses that lead diverse teams need to be intimately familiar with the scopes of practice for each role within the team, including their own role, in order to ensure safe patient care, appropriate delegation, and strong, safe collaborative practice.

Models of Care

The terms used to describe **models of care** over the past century include *functional nursing*, *team nursing*, and *primary nursing*. These models have existed primarily in institutional settings, and elements of them may be seen in practice today. Functional nursing became popular during World War II in response to a nursing shortage, where nurses focused on tasks instead of assuming responsibilities for a group of patients. The disadvantages of functional nursing lie in problems with continuity of care, the absence of a holistic view of patients, and the possibility that care will become mechanical and fragmented (Sportsman & MacMillan, 2015). Despite the critique of functional nursing, aspects of this model are still evident today—for example, when a nurse performs a "medication run," assuming sole responsibility for dispensing and administering medications to all patients in a long-term care setting.

Team nursing developed in response to the nursing shortage after World War II (Sportsman & MacMillan, 2015). It involves the coordinated delivery of nursing care by various staff members. A registered nurse (RN) leads a team of other RNs, registered psychiatric nurses (RPNs), licensed practical nurses (LPNs), health team members, or a combination of these professionals. The task orientation of the model in the past and the fact that nurses do not always interact with the same patients each day can result in a lack of continuity of care. An advantage of team nursing is its collaborative style, which encourages each member of the team to help the other members. Elements of this former team nursing model may be present in emerging models of collaborative practice that are evolving to feature more participatory relationships with other members of the intraprofessional nursing team and the broader interprofessional team. For nursing teams to work effectively, it is most important that RNs and LPNs have a strong identity with respect to their roles and unique contributions to practice—often referred to as *scope of practice*. RNs in particular have responsibilities for leading and supporting teams in diverse practice settings, and LPNs work in teams and provide leadership to others in settings such as residential and long-term care.

The **case management** model is one that emphasizes the coordination of an array of health services and links them to patients and their families while streamlining costs and maintaining quality (Dadich, 2003). Case managers can be nurses, but not all are. The term *case manager* has been criticized as impersonal because patients and families are not "cases" to be managed (Smith et al., 2006). Case management, as it has evolved, is "a collaborative process which assesses, plans, implements, coordinates, monitors, and evaluates the options and services required to meet an individual's health needs, using communications and available resources to promote quality, cost-effective outcomes" (Case Management Society of America, 2016). Clinicians, as individuals or in teams, care for patients with specific conditions and associated care needs (e.g., patients with complex nursing and medical problems) and are usually held accountable for quality and cost management. Many case managers use critical pathways, or "care maps," which are multidisciplinary treatment plans for patients with specific case types (see Chapter 14).

The roles of case managers vary across health care settings, including long-term care, home care, community mental health, and acute care institutions, and these professionals increasingly coordinate and integrate care across settings. The roles and responsibilities of case managers across settings include clinical expert, advocate, educator, facilitator, negotiator, manager, and researcher (Smith et al., 2006).

Collaborative Models of Care. Emerging models of care emphasize the ways in which the system of nursing operates to provide continuity of care to patients across settings. Another goal of emerging models of care is to emphasize and acknowledge that the skills and knowledge of RNs are needed at the point of care, as well as for providing coordination and management of teams. In British Columbia, the provincial government is funding the implementation of nurse-led primary care clinics with the goal of establishing team-based care among RNs, including nurse practitioners and other team members.

The collaborative practice model is increasingly used by **intraprofessional teams** (teams whose members provide nursing care) and by other health care providers who are members of **interprofessional teams**. All health professional education programs, including nursing, are called upon to prepare graduates to practise and lead collaborative team approaches to care (CNA, 2011; Health Professions Network Nursing and Midwifery Office, 2010). A call for collaborative practice development has been sounded across Canada because this model is viewed as the way to ensure that all professionals and providers can practise to the full potential of their role and competencies. Collaborative practice is therefore also the best way to ensure that health human resources are used most effectively during a time of shortage in the achievement of quality care and population health outcomes.

Students in nursing and other professional health care programs ought to learn the competencies associated with collaborative practice by focusing on relationships with nurses and others in diverse settings of care. Students and entry-level nurses need to acquire competencies that promote collaboration among teams of nurses and others to ensure that optimal care is provided. Indeed, collaboration as an entry-level competency is an expectation of all members of the nursing team, including LPNs, RNs, and RPNs. The student nurse is an integral member of both nursing and interprofessional teams that cross health care settings, including acute care, mental health care, community and home care, and public and population health care. One of the first and most important responsibilities is to articulate the role and contribution of nurses to care, and then to be able to learn about and relate to the roles and responsibilities of other team members. Central to the collaborative practice model are the patient, family, and population as full participants in care or service delivery.

The RNAO has developed evidence-informed **Best Practice Guidelines** for intraprofessional collaborative practice among nurses (RNAO, 2016) and interprofessional health teams among health professionals (RNAO, 2013). These guidelines show how teamwork and collaborative practice can be supported at individual, team, organizational, and system levels of nursing practice. The guidelines are comprehensive and indicate the need for transformational leadership to support a culture of teamwork and collaboration. One Best Practice Guideline that supports collaborative practice focuses on developing the ability to share power (Box 13.7; RNAO, 2013).

Nurses are well situated to provide leadership for collaborative practice in many health care settings. One example may be found in the home care setting. In this setting, nurses work closely with the broader health care team, the members of which provide a large amount of the continuous day-to-day care for patients who have been discharged from hospitals after undergoing surgery or who have chronic illnesses and disabilities. Health care team members must have opportunities to meet and communicate regularly with all those involved in the care of these patients to ensure that they understand the patient situation and receive support for the challenges they face in providing care. Nurses can also aid health team members by providing education and other supports so that they are able to contribute to best practices in important areas such as safety, emotional support, and wound healing. In this way, all members of the health care team are recognized and valued for their roles, and the continuity of care to a single patient or family is supported by all. Nurses working in long-term or residential care settings may also provide leadership for collaborative practice by creating opportunities for communication and learning among professionals involved in teams or systems of care.

Home care delivery also often includes social workers, physicians, nutritionists, physiotherapists, and other health care providers, as well as nurses and health care team members, a situation requiring even more collaborative practice. According to the Health Professions Network Nursing and Midwifery Office (2010), "collaborative practice in health care occurs when multiple health workers from different professional back grounds provide comprehensive services by working with patients, families, and carers and communities to deliver the highest quality of care across settings" (p. 13). Implementing collaborative practice among professionals requires that no one professional group dominates, leadership is shared, and differences in knowledge and contributions are understood and respected. Educators and practice leaders in the health professions are working to envision and develop education strategies to prepare students to graduate with the interprofessional competencies needed to carry out collaborative practice. iPANEL is an example of an initiative where nurse researchers work collaboratively with nurses in practice, patients and families, and other care providers to collect evidence that addresses the most pressing challenges of palliative care (Box 13.8).

Health care in the twenty-first century will require nurses to work with other members of the health care team and collaborate with other

---

BOX 13.7   RNAO Best Practice Guideline Recommendation 12: Power and Hierarchy in Teams

12.1 Team members demonstrate their willingness to share power by:
  a. Building a collaborative environment through recognizing and understanding power and its influence on everyone involved;
  b. Creating balanced power relationships through shared leadership, decision making, authority, and responsibility;
  c. Including diverse voices for decision making;
  d. Sharing knowledge with each other, openly; and
  e. Working collaboratively with patients/clients and their families to plan and deliver care.

From Registered Nurses' Association of Ontario (RNAO). (2013). *Developing and Sustaining Interprofessional Health Care: Optimizing patient, organizational and system outcomes* (p. 44). https://rnao.ca/sites/rnao-ca/files/DevelopingAndSustainingBPG.pdf

---

BOX 13.8   The iPANEL Collaboration

The Initiative for a Palliative Approach in Nursing: Evidence and Leadership (iPANEL) is an example of strong leadership and collaboration among nurse researchers, practising nurses, and other professionals. iPANEL, a project that ran between 2011 and 2018, aimed to provide research and evidence to promote the best care for people with chronic and life-limiting illnesses. Palliative care is vital to promoting quality of life during illnesses that are life limiting. Nurses are on the forefront of providing palliative care, and they require the most up-to-date knowledge to direct all aspects of their care.

iPANEL was a unique collaboration because it valued and answered the kinds of questions and challenges that nurses face every day, including:
• "What should I say?"
• "Can't we do better when she is so short of breath?"
• "What does she want for her future care? Is it my role to talk with her about this?"

Adapted from Palliative Approaches to Care in Aging and Community Health. (n.d.). *Initiative for a Palliative Approach in Nursing: Evidence and Leadership*. https://www.uvic.ca/research/groups/palliative/projects/current/ipanel.php

community members, agencies, and organizations outside the health sector. Intersectoral collaboration is a principle of primary health care, requiring nurses and others to develop skills in engaging with others to influence health in the broadest way possible. This ability to collaborate across professions and organizations requires the development of competencies in communication and conflict resolution, team functioning, and collaborative leadership. This process starts with a deep understanding of one's own professional role and contribution, as well as the appreciation of others' contributions (Orchard et al., 2017a, 2017b) (see Chapter 19 for further information about interprofessional practice).

Nursing Influence and Shared Governance

One of the most important recommendations for achieving healthy practice environments is to involve nurses, including those at the point of care, in making decisions about nursing practice. In addition, it is imperative to value and amplify the voices and perspectives of the nurses who are providing care at every table where health care and health systems decisions are made. Likewise, the executive level of a health organization must include nursing roles explicitly responsible for escalating nursing practice issues, championing nursing needs, and demonstrating the unique contributions of nursing knowledge to health care governance. The nurse executive may or may not have operational responsibility, but when such responsibility exists, the nurse executive supports operational leaders, managers, and staff by enabling a governance structure that both achieves organizational goals and provides support for participatory decision making and collaborative practice models. The nurse executive must also establish and communicate a vision for nursing within the organization and must motivate and engage nurses and others across the system to share and advance that vision. However, having a nurse at the table is not enough. A critical perspective on this change is required in order to determine the ability of nurse executive leaders to engage nurses and influence the quality of nursing practice.

The concept of trauma-informed leadership has become highly relevant following nurses' experiences of supporting care and populations during the COVID-19 pandemic. Further exacerbating this health care crisis are the associated societal and relational challenges that have led to increasing violence in the workplace and within the community. Trauma-informed leadership builds the conditions for resilience while acknowledging the pervasive nature of trauma. **Trauma-informed leadership** aims to create safety, build trust through transparency, build collaboration in the context of mutually affirming relationships, empower voice and choice, and critically examine the institutions and systems that perpetuate harm (Wignall, 2021).

Every nurse in every position can be a leader. In addition to leadership approach and orientation, nurses must develop core competencies to realize the potential for leadership that nursing has across all domains of health care and beyond (Table 13.1). This includes a recognition that leadership is a shared responsibility (CNA, 2018) that involves a commitment to taking action on issues of equity and social justice, enabling quality care environments, and mentoring others. Growing one's leadership competencies is a key part of every nurse's journey, from student nurse to chief nurse.

Nurse leaders must enable decision making by the professionals who are most involved in patient care. They must also encourage respect for the unique contributions made by team members whose practice touches the patient journey. Leaders of today are making crucial decisions about the nursing care delivery models and staff mix that will best meet patient needs and promote optimal health outcomes. Three national nursing groups, representing RNs, LPNs, and RPNs, have worked with leading nurse researchers, including Dr. Linda McGillis

TABLE 13.1	Position Statement: Nursing Leadership

Key Competencies for Nursing Leadership

- Ability to act courageously and think critically
- Advocacy skills
- Visionary and innovative
- Willingness to be visible in a nursing leadership practice
- Ability to view nursing as more than a series of tasks or acts
- Commitment to ethics
- Connected to research and able to translate research knowledge into practice
- Policy skills, including policy analysis, interpretation, and development
- Commitment to building excellent learning and practice environments
- Ability to influence and participate in the creation of the interlocking legislative, regulatory, and policy controls that shape health care
- A strong understanding of how to enact nursing practice in political, administrative, leadership, governance, and management contexts

Adapted from Canadian Nurses Association. (2009). *Position statement: Nursing leadership.* https://www.cna-aiic.ca/en/policy-advocacy/policy-support-tools/position-statements

BOX 13.9	Five Guiding Principles for Staff Mix Decision Making

- Decisions concerning staff mix respond to clients' health care needs and enable the delivery of safe, competent, ethical, quality, evidence-informed care in the context of professional standards and staff competencies.
- Decision making regarding staff mix is guided by nursing care delivery models based on the best evidence related to (1) client, staff, and organizational factors influencing quality care and work environments, and (2) client, staff, and organizational outcomes.
- Staff mix decision making is supported by the organizational structure, mission, and vision and by all levels of leadership in the organization.
- Direct care nursing staff and nursing management are engaged in decision making about the staff mix.
- Information and knowledge management systems support effective staff mix decision making.

From Canadian Nurses Association, Canadian Council for Practical Nurse Regulators, & Registered Psychiatric Nurses of Canada. (2012). *Joint position statement: Staff mix decision-making framework for quality nursing care.* Canadian Nurses Association. https://www.cna-aiic.ca/en/policy-advocacy/policy-support-tools/position-statements

Hall, to identify evidence-informed guiding principles for making staff mix decisions for quality care (Box 13.9). These principles can only be realized through collaborative nursing leadership, with values of inclusiveness and evidence-informed decisions about nursing care delivery models.

Responsibility refers to the duties and activities that an individual nurse is employed to perform. A nurse's responsibilities in a given role are outlined in the position description, which details the nurse's duties in patient care and participation as a member of the nursing team. Managers must ensure that staff members understand their responsibilities, particularly during change. For example, when hospitals are restructured and patient care delivery models are changed, the manager must clearly define the nurse's role within the new patient care delivery model. All nurses are responsible for knowing which competencies they need to develop in their role.

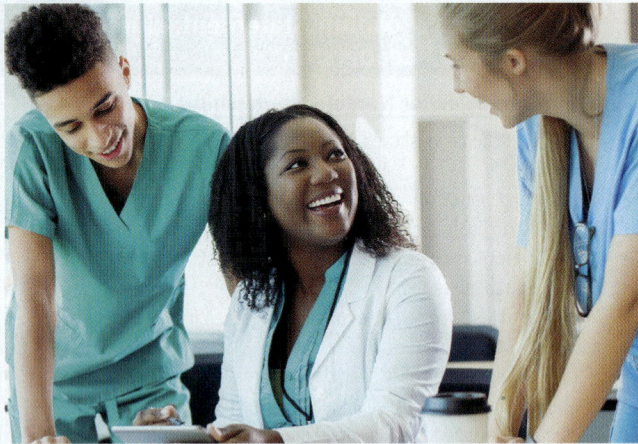

FIGURE 13.2 Students in nursing and other health care provider programs learning about their roles and contributions to collaborative practice. (iStockphoto/Steve Debenport.)

Autonomy in nursing practice means having the authority to make decisions and the freedom to act in accordance with one's professional knowledge base. Innovation by nurses, increased productivity, higher employer retention of nurses, and greater patient satisfaction are the results of autonomy in nursing practice (Keeley et al., 2015).

Authority to act is the right to act in areas in which a nurse has and accepts responsibility according to legislation, standards, and the code of ethics governing the professional practice of nursing. Nurses have authority to act and to question actions concerning the practice of other professionals in relation to this scope of responsibility. The nurse as case manager has accepted responsibility for the care of a group of patients and therefore has final authority in selecting the best course of action for the patient's care while collaborating with others to ensure quality outcomes.

Accountability means being answerable for one's actions. A nurse is accountable to meet the standards of nursing practice and for patient's health outcomes. In the example just described, the nurse as case manager is accountable for the patient's health outcomes by ensuring a continuity of care across hospitalization and home care.

A nursing unit works collaboratively to realize the four elements of decision making: responsibility, autonomy, authority, and accountability. The staff must meet routinely to discuss how to maintain equality and balance in these elements (Figure 13.2). Individuals should be comfortable in expressing differences of opinion and challenging the status quo while at the same time understanding their own responsibility, autonomy, authority, and accountability.

Establishment of Nursing Practice or Professional Shared Governance Councils. Chaired by senior clinical staff, these councils are empowered to maintain care standards for nursing practice (Gokenbach, 2007) and bring voice and influence to address nursing practice issues at the most senior levels of organizations. The councils review and establish standards of care, develop clinical policy and procedures, resolve patient satisfaction issues, or develop new documentation tools. Mechanisms are established to empower all staff to contribute their input on practice issues. The types of work in the nursing unit are what determine council membership. Professionals from other disciplines (e.g., pharmacy, respiratory therapy, social work, medicine, or clinical nutrition) might participate on these councils. Professional practice councils can advocate for the resources and conditions necessary for healthy practice environments and patient safety.

Interprofessional and Intraprofessional Collaboration. As previously described, collaborative practice among professionals from different disciplines and across nursing roles is essential (Canadian Interprofessional Health Collaborative, 2010; CNA, 2011; Healthcare Excellence Canada, 2012; Jacobson, 2012; Orchard et al., 2017a, 2017b; Virani, 2012) (see Chapter 19 for further information about interprofessional collaboration). Whenever systems or programs are redesigned, interprofessional involvement is crucial because most health care processes involve more than one discipline. Nurses must recognize the importance of prompt referrals and timely communication with other care providers. Inclusion of professionals from various disciplines in practice projects, in-service programs, conferences, and staff meetings fosters improvement in health outcomes. Learning the skills and knowledge for interprofessional and intraprofessional practice begins in nursing education. Student nurses are therefore encouraged to seek practicums and other opportunities that allow them to work collaboratively.

Communication and Information Technology. Communication is one of the greatest challenges leaders face, especially in a large work group in which change is constant. It is vital that all staff members and partners receive the correct messages. In the current health care environment, staff quickly become uneasy and distrusting if they fail to hear about planned changes in their work unit that often include the introduction of new information technology such as electronic health records and standardized nomenclatures for patient care (CASN, 2012) (see Chapter 16 for more information about documentation). Social media has radically altered patterns of communications in the workplace, resulting in the need for nurses to develop new competencies and ethical awareness of privacy and confidentiality considerations. As technology continues to evolve as a dominant mode of communication, nurse leaders can find exciting ways to enable relationships virtually and to extend nursing presence, influence, and contributions across traditional boundaries.

Developing a Learning Culture. In this era of unprecedented change, leaders and managers are challenged to develop the conditions in which learning will flourish; such conditions create what has been described as a *learning organization* (Senge, 2006). In learning organizations, many forms of knowledge are shared. Leadership strategies are needed to help nurses incorporate evidence-informed best practice guidelines into their nursing practice. These strategies include "support, role-modelling commitment to best practices, and reinforcing organizational policies and goals consistent with evidence-based care" (Gifford et al., 2006, p. 73). Technology such as web-based applications and social media will continue to transform how we learn and communicate in organizations as well as the power of the media to influence change in systems (Risling, 2016). Learning health systems also leverage data systems—including electronic health records, patient experience surveys, complaints data, learning analytics, and service utilization data—to drive quality, improve care, and identify trends.

Practice Coordination

As a nursing student, you develop the skills necessary to ensure timely and effective nursing practice. Care coordination includes decision making, priority setting, use of organizational skills and resources, and evaluation. Eventually, you will also lead teams responsible for not only delivering care but also designing care.

Decision Making. Leadership and decision-making skills are critical as the nurse engages in the complexity of health care. Nursing students learn to value and practise patient-centredness in every interaction, putting the patient at the centre of every decision, conversation, and interaction. They also learn to adopt a critical thinking approach that questions the status quo and advances change through collaboration (see Chapter 7 for more information about critical thinking and clinical reasoning). Decision making as a core nursing practice transcends designation and underpins the work of LPNs, RNs, and registered psychiatric nurses as the foundational piece of the discipline of nursing.

Priority Setting. Nurses must establish priorities to meet the needs of those they serve. This is particularly important in caring for groups of patients that have health challenges involving immediate needs and actions to be taken. Setting priorities requires that nurses take time to understand the needs of each patient; assess each patient and involve them in the plan for care; and address needs in a timely manner through collaborative practice in interprofessional teams. As a nurse, you will find that prioritization is not a single action but rather a constant part of your work. You will learn to prioritize and reprioritize within the complex context of health care.

Evaluation. Evaluation is an important and ongoing process that provides focus and direction for each phase of nursing care. As a nurse, once you begin to provide care, you should also learn to immediately evaluate its effectiveness in terms of the quality of care and health outcomes. In the evaluation process, you compare expected health outcomes with actual outcomes. For example, a Chief Nursing Officer might evaluate the impact of a new policy on involuntary admission of a patient under the *Mental Health Act*, conducting a chart audit to identify stigmatizing language and behaviours. Upon evaluation, the nurse might realize that additional anti-stigma learning is required to safely care for these unique patients. Focusing on the evaluation of an intervention gives nurses an opportunity to change direction and improve the quality and efficacy of care.

Delegation. Changes in staff mix have resulted in a wider range of health care team members delivering care to patients (Harris & McGillis Hall, 2012). In the new working environment, a nurse must understand the evolving role of nursing and delegated care responsibilities in order to ensure the safety and quality of patient care. **Delegation** is "an active process whereby the responsibility for performance of an intervention is transferred to an individual (delegate) whose scope of practice or employment does not authorize the performance of that intervention" (Nova Scotia College of Nursing, 2019, p. 3). An important point here is that the person delegating the function remains accountable for the practice, while the delegate is responsible for performing it safely (Nova Scotia College of Nursing, 2019; Peebles & Nguyen, 2013).

As a student, you will work as part of interprofessional teams in many health care settings, including home care, residential care, community health care, acute care, and executive leadership. As you develop in your role, it is important to understand the roles and scopes of practice of all health team members in your practice setting. Nurses must also know how their role relates to the roles of others and how the principles of delegation are applied in practice. Students and nurses also have access to valuable resources such as nursing practice consultants and practice guidelines to assist them in making complex decisions about delegation.

Provincial regulations define the scope of a nurse's practice, including activities that are limited to each individual nursing designation. While most provinces and territories identify the delegation and supervision of work as an RN's responsibility, each jurisdiction addresses the specifics of delegation differently. In Ontario, British Columbia, and Alberta, for example, legislation that applies to all regulated health care providers identifies specific tasks or activities that can be performed by only certain providers. In British Columbia, these authorized tasks are known as *reserved acts*; in Ontario, they are called *controlled acts*; and in Alberta, they are known as *restricted activities*. Health team members that are UCPs are not allowed to perform actions authorized for nurses unless those actions have been delegated to them by a nurse, are within the health team member's job description, and are in line with employer policy.

An institution's policies, procedures, and job descriptions for health team members provide specific guidelines regarding which tasks or activities can be delegated. The job description should specify any required education and the types of tasks health team members can perform, either independently or under a nurse's direct supervision. Institutional policy helps in defining the amount of training required of health team members while they are employed. Procedures specify who is qualified to perform a given nursing procedure, whether supervision is necessary, and the type of reporting required.

Effective delegation requires trust between the nurse and other members of the health care team. It also requires constant communication—sending clear messages and listening carefully so that all participants understand expectations regarding patient care. A nurse should provide clear instructions when delegating tasks. These instructions may initially focus on the procedure itself and the unique needs of the patient. As the nurse becomes more familiar with a staff member's scope of practice, trust builds and fewer instructions may be needed, but clarification of patients' specific needs is always necessary.

A key step in delegation is the evaluation of a staff member's performance and patient outcomes. A health team member may fail to meet expectations because of inadequate training or the assignment of too many tasks. The nurse must work together with team members, taking time to ensure that the work is well understood and that each team member has the training and education needed to meet best practice guidelines. All staff should discuss delegation on their unit collaboratively so that all team members can work to the top of their scope of practice in a safe and supported way. The Nova Scotia College of Nursing (2019) has developed guidelines for what a nurse must consider and do when assigning or delegating care (Box 13.10).

QUALITY CARE AND PATIENT SAFETY

As discussed throughout this chapter, safe and high-quality care is delivered when leadership, staffing models, and collaborative practice are in place to support it. Studies show that high-quality practice environments produce better patient outcomes and more satisfied patients and staff (Aiken et al., 2014; CNA, 2014).

Accreditation Canada (2017) engages at an organizational level "to improve client outcomes and health system performance" (see https://www.accreditation.ca). The organization engages people at all levels of the organization and the public to determine whether organizations meet standards. Accredited organizations have achieved a standard of safety and quality in all aspects of the care provided, including leadership, infection control, safe medication management, and other areas. Influential nurse leaders, including the CNA's past president Dr. Karima Velji, Vice-Chair of the Board of Directors at Accreditation Canada, can ensure that organizations set and achieve the highest standards of safety and quality care.

BOX 13.10 Summary of Points to Consider in Assignment and Delegation

Assignment = client and/or interventions—**within** individual scope of practice

Delegation = responsibility for client interventions is transferred to a delegatee—**outside** authorized individual scope of practice

Supervision = an active process of directing, assigning, delegating, guiding, and monitoring the provision of care by an individual nurse, student, other health professional or provider

Supervision is essential in both the assignment and delegation of client care. Nurses may provide supervision of unregulated care providers (UCPs) in the case of delegation or supervision of colleagues who are assigned new care processes or procedures with which they are unfamiliar. Nurses may also supervise the practice of a student or a UCP.

Nurses do not delegate responsibilities to other nurses, including licensed practical nurses.

Education and supervision of a delegatee is always required. It is a collaborative process involving self-assessment of competency and ongoing evaluation of competency and safety by the delegator and delegatee.

Nurses must always retain accountability for monitoring and evaluating the client care and safety outcomes of a delegated care process or intervention.

Eligibility Criteria for Delegation

An intervention may be appropriate for delegation if it meets the following criteria:

- Falls within the nursing scope of practice
- Occurs frequently in daily care for a specific client
- Is part of a well-established plan of care for a specific client
- There is a standard process based on evidence for the delegation
- Has a readily predictable outcome
- Does not require ongoing assessment, interpretation, or decision making
- Aligns with the client's plan of care, and
- Is at low risk of endangering the client.

Adapted from Nova Scotia College of Nursing. (2019). *Assignment and delegation: Guideline for nurses.* https://cdn3.nscn.ca/sites/default/files/documents/resources/Assignment_Delegation.pdf

Quality in Nursing Practice

Quality Defined. Standards or guidelines define the meaning of quality. For example, in order to judge whether rehabilitation has been delayed, there must be a standard indicating when rehabilitation should begin. Quality of care in nursing practice is not arbitrarily defined. A definition of quality begins with the mission, vision, philosophy, and values of the nursing department. These statements define how all nurses within an organization are to perform and which services must be provided. Written values give direction for professional standards and care guidelines that lead to positive patient outcomes.

Professional Standards. Professional standards are authoritative statements that a profession uses to describe the responsibilities for which its practitioners are accountable (Kilty, 2005; Peters, 1995). They include the policies and position descriptions that identify performance expectations within an organization. Standards are an organization's interpretation of the professional's competency. The adherence to professional standards is measured through professional outcomes.

Care and Best Practice Guidelines. Best practice guidelines are evidence-informed resources that assist nurses in providing the best care possible (Folse & Wong, 2015). Guidelines can be developed by single disciplines or be interprofessional in focus. Examples of nursing

practice guidelines are found in the literature encompassing some of the examples referred to in this chapter, including wound care and prevention of falls. The effectiveness of nursing practice is measured through patient outcomes and the accumulation of evidence (Graham & Harrison, 2008).

Nurse-Sensitive Outcomes. *Outcomes* are conditions to be achieved as a result of care. The outcomes selected to measure the effectiveness of nursing care should be related to the work nurses do. A **nurse-sensitive outcome** reveals whether interventions are effective, whether patients progress, how well standards are being met, and whether changes are necessary. Examples of outcomes related to the implementation of best practice guidelines may include incidence of pressure sores, falls in elderly patients, and hypertension control measures.

To judge whether standards of care are being met, processes and outcomes are measured. For example, a staff team measures its success in implementing a new process of diabetes instruction and then measures the outcome: Can patients administer insulin correctly? When selecting quality indicators, teams should consider processes and related outcomes that are most likely to improve nursing practice. Processes to improve may include the following:

- A weak process that is causing problems (e.g., poor pain management for patients with cancer who are at home)
- A stable process that is adequate but can be improved (e.g., access to education and support for people with diabetes in rural communities)
- A process linked to negative outcomes (e.g., care of intravenous access sites with the occurrence of phlebitis).

Building a Culture of Safety

Quality care to ensure patient safety has been recognized as a crucial component of health care delivery. **Patient safety** is "the reduction of risk of unnecessary harm associated with health care to an acceptable minimum" (Healthcare Excellence Canada & Canadian Institute for Health Information, 2016, p. 7). The Health Quality Matrix developed by the British Columbia Patient Safety and Quality Council (2020) identifies seven dimensions of quality that enable high-quality care and reduce patient harm: respect, safety, accessibility, appropriateness, effectiveness, equity, and efficiency. Quality has moved away from focusing solely on reporting adverse events and toward a more complete understanding of how care impacts the whole person in the context of relational care (British Columbia Patient Safety and Quality Council, 2020). Issues such as staff shortages, new technology, and other demands on health care systems have prompted a re-examination of how errors and adverse events affecting patients can be prevented. Increasingly, the emphasis is on enabling a culture of safety where care providers are collectively invested in learning to improve the quality of care and the safety of patients. This shift is reflected in nursing education, where nurses and other health care students are supported in viewing mistakes as learning, knowing and preventing the system and practice conditions that lead to patient risk and harm, and developing the **competencies for safe practice** (CASN, 2018; Davidson et al., 2006). Healthcare Excellence Canada (2020) has identified six core safety competencies for all health care providers, including their contributions to developing a culture of patient safety as the foundation (Box 13.11).

Coming Full Circle: Leadership for a High-Quality Work Life and High-Quality Health Care. Leaders at all levels of health care organizations must do what they can to improve the quality of work life for health care providers to ensure patient safety and quality health care; evidence and awareness of this need are growing. For example, nurse fatigue has been identified as a current factor in patient safety

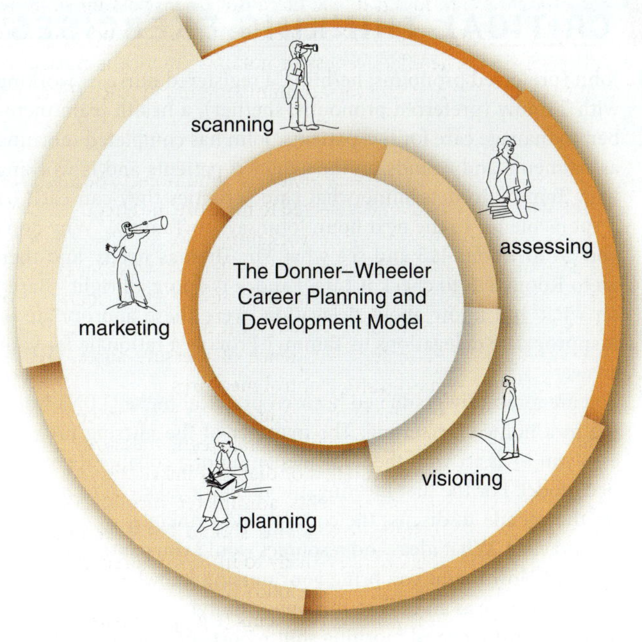

FIGURE 13.3 The Donner–Wheeler career planning and development model. (From Waddell, J., Donner, G. J., & Wheeler, M. M. [2009]. *Building your nursing career: A guide for students* [3rd ed., p. 2]. Elsevier Canada.)

BOX 13.11 | Canadian Safety Competencies for Health Care Providers

Domain 1: Patient Safety Culture

Patient safety culture is "an integrated pattern of individual and organizational actions and behaviours based on shared beliefs and values" (Healthcare Excellence Canada, 2020, p. 14). A safety culture rests on psychological safety, where every team member can name problems without fear of blame or reprisal. The ability to take accountability and speak up about safety is the cornerstone of a just culture where patient safety is the collective goal.

Key and enabling competencies for a just culture of patient safety include the following:

- Contribute to the establishment and maintenance of a just culture
- Advocate for improved patient safety culture, and
- Contribute to the continuous improvement of safety culture.

Each competency calls on care providers to understand the knowledge, skills, and attitudes required to practice within and co-create a culture of safety.

From Healthcare Excellence Canada. (2020). *The safety competencies* (2nd ed.). https://www.patientsafetyinstitute.ca/en/toolsResources/safetyCompetencies/Documents/CPSI-SafetyCompetencies_EN_Digital.pdf

---

that requires the attention of governments, organizations, and individual nurses (CNA & RNAO, 2010). One recommended solution backed by research is to give nurse managers responsibility for instituting fatigue management policies and programs. These measures require significant changes in the workplace and collaboration with nursing unions and nursing education programs. Measures to be considered include rest and sleep policies, as well as reform of scheduling practices (CNA & RNAO, 2010). Nurse managers have significant responsibilities in implementing these solutions, and they provide leadership in this area to make a difference in both the quality of nurses' work lives and patient safety outcomes.

LEADERSHIP SKILLS FOR NURSING STUDENTS

Nursing students lead within their cohorts and prepare for the leadership roles they will enact upon graduation. This does not mean that you as a student need to quickly learn how to lead a team; rather, you must first learn to become an accountable and competent health care provider. Leadership development is ongoing throughout a career, and individual leadership styles are influenced from a variety of sources, including theories, best practices, mentors, role models, and experiences. You learn leadership by considering your own values and beliefs, making decisions, advocating for public health and quality care, learning from mistakes, seeking guidance, engaging in collaborative practice with nursing teams and other professionals, seeking mentors, and reflecting on your practice in each patient interaction. Recent research in Canada indicates that mentorship components of new graduate transition programs are key to helping new graduate nurses become part of the nursing workforce (Baumann et al., 2011; Brewer et al., 2016). Your nursing education program provides you with the opportunity to develop leadership competencies: advocacy, conflict management, collaborative practice, person-centredness, delegation, and evidence-informed decision making.

Career Development and Mentoring for Nursing Students

Nursing students can begin to envision their preferred career paths early in their nursing education. In fact, the earlier students begin planning their careers or "course of life work," the more likely they will achieve their goals and develop personal and professional strengths that enable future career satisfaction and success (Waddell et al., 2009). As you develop a career vision, you may identify opportunities that can further your **career development** as a nurse leader, such as attending meetings of professional associations, presenting your work at student conferences, and finding a career coach or mentor (Cooper & Wheeler, 2010; Mata et al., 2010). Waddell and colleagues (2009) have developed the Career Planning and Development Model for students to use during their nursing education program (Figure 13.3). The model includes stages of planning that engage the student in learning about nursing realities and trends, developing a self-assessment, and creating a career vision and marketing approach. These authors contend that having a career vision is "perhaps the most forceful motivator for using your nursing practice placement and classroom experiences and your summer and part-time work opportunities to the fullest" (Waddell et al., 2009, p. 7).

Nursing leadership is needed to shift the current culture of health care to achieve the vision of health care providers delivering high-quality health care, adopted by collaborators. This means that nurses and other professionals that work directly with patients and mid-level managers have key roles to play in leading change. They must be inspired and supported through **mentoring** and by the implementation of leadership best practice guidelines and collaborative practice. Senior leaders must ensure adequate staffing and support for the culture of a healthy workplace. The way forward is to inspire lifelong learning at all levels of the organization and provide access and resources to education that enables staff to work with the patient and the patient's family at the centre of health care delivery and decision making.

Nurses working at all levels of organizations can contribute by making a commitment to this vision and being part of the change that is required to transform Canadian health care. Indeed, the CNA in its centenary year inspired the theme of leadership for a transformed Canadian health care system and has called for Canadian nurses to "be the change" required to sustain quality health care for all. As a student and as a qualified nurse, you have the opportunity and the challenge to effect positive change in nursing practice and health care in Canada.

KEY CONCEPTS

- A leader must set a vision or philosophy for a work unit, ensure appropriate staffing, mobilize staff and institutional resources to achieve objectives, motivate staff members to carry out their work, set standards of performance, and make the right decisions to achieve objectives.
- Leadership theories and perspectives are evolving and informed by nursing research.
- Nursing's ethics and relational competencies are the foundation of leadership.
- Management and leadership are related processes; both are essential to nursing practice and health care delivery.
- Healthy practice environments are essential to quality nursing and patient care outcomes.
- Transformational leadership that emphasizes relationships, trust, and vision plays a key role in ensuring healthy practice environments. Trauma-informed leadership can extend transformation into justice and equity.
- Empowered nursing staff have decision-making authority to change how they practice.
- Nursing care delivery models vary by the responsibility of the registered nurse in coordinating care delivery and the roles other staff members play in assisting with care.
- Continuity of nursing care can be compromised in total patient care delivery, functional nursing practice, and team nursing.
- Best practice guidelines are evidence informed and contain recommendations for developing and sustaining collaborative practice models and leadership.
- For decentralized decision making to succeed, staff members must be aware that they have the responsibility, authority, autonomy, and accountability for the care they give and the decisions they make.
- A nurse manager can foster decentralized decision making by establishing nursing practice committees, supporting collaborative practice, implementing quality improvement plans, and maintaining timely staff communication.
- Clinical care coordination involves accurate clinical decision making, establishing priorities, efficient organizational skills, appropriate use of resources and time management skills, and ongoing evaluation of care activities.
- To promote an enriching professional environment, each member of a nursing work team is responsible for open, professional communication.
- Delegation involves transferring responsibility for performing an activity while retaining accountability for the outcome.
- When accomplished correctly, delegation can improve job efficiency and job enrichment.
- An important responsibility for the nurse who delegates nursing care is evaluation of the staff member's performance and patient outcomes.
- In a quality improvement–oriented environment, every staff member becomes involved in finding ways to improve or change work processes in order to promote patient safety and quality care outcomes.
- Nurses' career development involves planning and opportunities for mentorship.

CRITICAL THINKING EXERCISES

1. John (preferred pronouns: he/him), a registered nurse, is working with Tammy (preferred pronouns: she/her), a health team member, to manage care for five patients. John has completed morning assessments and rounds on the assigned patients and is working with Tammy to determine what care activities they can each be responsible for in the next hour. John says to Tammy, "Why don't you go to Room 415 and see what Mr. Thomas needs, and then go to Room 418 to check if Mrs. Landry is doing all right." Based on what you know about delegation, were these appropriate or inappropriate delegations to Tammy? Provide a rationale for your answer.

2. You are a recently graduated licensed practical nurse (LPN) working in a home care setting. The manager of the nursing program asks you to assist with the implementation of a collaborative practice model. For the first meeting, the manager asks you to help her set the agenda to discuss the concept and principles of collaborative practice. What ideas and resources would you contribute to the agenda? How might you bring your nursing knowledge and practice experience as an LPN to this opportunity?

3. You have just received morning shift reports on your patients. You have been assigned the following patients:
- A 52-year-old patient (preferred pronouns: he/him) who was admitted yesterday with a diagnosis of angina. The patient is schedule for a cardiac stress test at 0900.
- A 60-year-old patient (preferred pronouns: she/her) who was transferred out of intensive care at 0630 today. The patient underwent uncomplicated coronary bypass surgery yesterday.
- A 45-year-old patient (preferred pronouns: he/him) who experienced a myocardial infarction 3 days ago and is complaining of chest pain, which he rates 5 on a scale of 0 to 10.
- A 76-year-old patient (preferred pronouns: she/her) who had a permanent pacemaker inserted yesterday and is complaining of incision pain, which she rates as 7 on a scale of 0 to 10.

Which of these patients do you need to see first? Explain your answer.

🌐 *Answers to Critical Thinking Exercises appear on the Evolve website.*

REVIEW QUESTIONS

Review Questions 1 to 10 relate to the case study at the beginning of the chapter.

1. A.B. invited K.H. to expand her leadership practice by taking part in creating a new approach to falls prevention. A.B. recognized that K.H. had an interest in falls prevention and emerging skills in collaborative leadership. A.B.'s approach to enabling emerging leaders is a good example of which characteristic of leadership?
   a. Creating an environment of trust and mutual respect where team members can grow
   b. Delegating tasks to other members of the team to optimize existing resources
   c. Capitalizing on the personal traits and interests of team members to drive change
   d. Engaging team members to deliver on her vision for change

2. K.H. chooses to build a working group that includes nurses and diverse members of the health care team. She invites each member to bring their unique skills, experiences, and ideas to the table to build the best possible solution for residents. Which style of leadership is K.H. demonstrating?
   a. Collaborative leadership
   b. Executive leadership
   c. Participatory leadership
   d. Transformational leadership
3. The learning community includes residents, family members, and members of the care team. This approach to creating solutions is best described by which of the following terms?
   a. Informing, where those impacted by the change are made aware of what is changing
   b. Consulting, where feedback is sought to improve solutions and decisions
   c. Co-creating, where what is implemented is decided on together
   d. Involving, where concerns and ideas are understood and considered as changes are made
4. Evaluation of the process K.H. led indicates that staff, residents, and families feel engaged and satisfied. What type of evaluation metric captures this kind of result?
   a. Engagement and buy-in
   b. Impact
   c. Change readiness
   d. Quality improvement
5. In considering what needs to change to improve patient safety, K.H. and the learning group might consider which tools of clinical governance? (*Select all that apply.*)
   a. Policies
   b. Participation
   c. Best practice guidelines
   d. Medication reconciliation tools
   e. Opinions
6. Nurses practising in a small rural hospital are challenged to adjust roles and responsibilities within a nursing team that includes advanced practice nurses, registered nurses, practical nurses, and health care aides. They are particularly interested in increasing their understanding of roles and ways of working together. You are to consider those concepts and resources that the nursing team should initially undertake. For each resource/process listed in the following table, insert an "X" in the row to indicate whether it would be considered *essential* to their learning, *not initially helpful* to their learning, or *possibly irrelevant* to their learning. (*Select only one response option per row.*)

Resources and Processes	Essential to Learning	Not Initially Helpful	Possibly Irrelevant
a. Circulate documents on delegation based on regulatory standards			
b. Bring in an expert from the Human Resources department			
c. Develop a case study to demonstrate how workers in other sectors create teams and work effectively			
d. Create opportunities to learn about each of the nursing roles on the unit and their contributions			
e. Engage nursing leadership processes to support learning			

Answers: 1. a; **2.** a; **3.** c; **4.** a; **5.** a, b, c; **6.** Essential to learning: d, e; Not initially helpful to learning: a, b; Possibly irrelevant to learning: c.

🌐 *Rationales for the Review Questions appear on the Evolve website.*

RECOMMENDED WEBSITES

Accreditation Canada. https://www.accreditation.ca.
Accreditation Canada, formerly known as the Canadian Council on Health Services Accreditation, is a national, not-for-profit, independent organization whose role is to help health services organizations, across Canada and internationally, examine and improve the quality of care and service they provide to their patients.
British Columbia College of Nurses and Midwives (BCCNM): https://www.bccnm.ca
The BCCNM is a health regulator that has the legal obligation to protect the public through the regulation of licensed practical nurses, midwives, nurse practitioners, registered nurses, and registered psychiatric nurses by ensuring that the care they provide is safe, competent, ethical, and meets the standards set out by the college.
Canadian Academy of Nursing: https://www.cna-aiic.ca/en/academy

The Canadian Academy of Nursing is housed within the Canadian Nurses Association (CNA) and aims to educate, empower, and support nursing leadership and influence public policy.
Canadian Association of Schools of Nursing (CASN): https://www.casn.ca
The CASN is the national voice for nursing education, research, and scholarship and represents baccalaureate and graduate nursing programs across Canada.
Canadian Interprofessional Health Collaborative (CIHC): http://www.cihc-cpis.com
The CIHC is made up of health organizations, health educators, researchers, health professionals, and students across Canada. This collaborative group shares best practices and advances knowledge in interprofessional practice and collaborative practice.
Canadian Nurses Association (CNA): https://www.cna-aiic.ca/en

The CNA is a federation of 11 provincial and territorial nursing associations representing more than 120 000 RNs. Its mission is to advance the quality of nursing in the interest of the public.

Canadian Nursing Students Association (CNSA): https://www.cnsa.ca

The CNSA is the national voice of nursing students in Canada. For more than 30 years, the CNSA has represented the interests of nursing students to federal, provincial, and international governments and to other nursing and health care organizations.

Donnerwheeler: http://www.donnerwheeler.com

This website includes information and resources for career development and mentoring, developed by Canadian nurse leaders Gail Donner and Mary Wheeler.

Healthcare Excellence Canada: https://www.healthcareexcellence.ca

Healthcare Excellence Canada works with partners to spread innovations, build capability, and catalyze policy changes so that everyone in Canada has access to safe and high-quality health care. The organization formed in 2021 from the amalgamation of the Canadian Foundation for Healthcare Improvement and the Canadian Patient Safety Institute.

International Council of Nurses (ICN): https://www.icn.ch

The ICN is a federation of national nurses' associations representing nurses in more than 120 countries. Operated by nurses for nurses, ICN works to ensure quality nursing care for all patients, sound health policies globally, and the advancement of nursing knowledge.

Nurse and Nurse Practitioners of British Columbia (NNPBC): https://www.nnpbc.com

This website offers examples of nursing leadership in policy advocacy including policy blogs as well as examples of nursing family collaboration across nursing designations.

Registered Nurses' Association of Ontario (RNAO): https://rnao.ca

This website offers a complete and up-to-date inventory of Best Practice Guidelines, including implementation and evaluation.

Truth and Reconciliation Commission of Canada (TRC): https://nctr.ca/about/history-of-the-trc/trc-website

This website includes all the archived and up-to-date proceedings of the TRC, including the document containing all the Calls to Action. This resource is essential reading that helps nurses to provide leadership for understanding the meaning, shared responsibilities, and opportunities inherent in reconciliation.

REFERENCES

A full reference list is available on the website for this book at
http://evolve.elsevier.com/Canada/Potter/fundamentals/

14

Nursing Assessment, Diagnosis, and Planning

Canadian content written by Shawna M. Ryan, RN, BN, OHN, MN, and Marnie L. Kramer, RN, MEd, PhD, with original chapter contributions by Patricia A. Potter, RN, MSN, PhD, FAAN

OBJECTIVES

Mastery of content in this chapter will enable you to:

- Define the key terms listed.
- Identify and discuss the steps and importance of nursing assessment.
- Explain the relationship of critical thinking to assessment, diagnosis, and planning.
- Differentiate between subjective and objective data.
- Explain the purposes of a patient interview and the use of interview techniques in obtaining a health history.
- Describe the components of a nursing history.
- Describe the relationship between data collection and data analysis.
- Explain the relationship between data interpretation, validation, and clustering.
- Differentiate between a nursing diagnosis, medical diagnosis, and collaborative problem.
- Describe the steps of the nursing diagnostic process.
- Explain the benefit of using the NANDA International nursing diagnoses in practice.
- Describe sources of diagnostic errors.
- Identify nursing diagnoses from a nursing assessment.
- Describe criteria used in a priority setting.
- Describe goal setting and discuss the difference between a goal and an expected outcome.
- Develop a plan of care from a nursing assessment.

KEY TERMS

Actual nursing diagnosis
Assessment
Clinical criteria
Closed-ended questions
Collaborative problem
Concept map
Consultation
Critical pathways
Cue
Data analysis
Database
Defining characteristics
Diagnosis
Diagnostic label
Etiology

Evaluation
Expected outcomes
Goals
Health promotion nursing diagnosis
Implementation
Inference
Interview
Kardex
Long-term goal
Medical diagnosis
NANDA International
Nursing care plan
Nursing diagnosis
Nursing health history
Nursing process

Nursing-sensitive patient outcome
Objective data
Open-ended questions
Person-centred goal
Person-centred plan of care
Planning
Priority setting
Related factor
Review of systems
Risk nursing diagnosis
Short-term goal
Standards
Subjective data
Validation
Wellness nursing diagnosis

🌐 WEBSITE

http://evolve.elsevier.com/Canada/Potter/fundamentals/

CASE STUDY

Mr. Fletcher (preferred pronouns: he/him) is a 56-year-old patient who has been experiencing headaches and dizziness for the past 2 months. He lives in a rural community and works 12-hour shifts as a haul truck operator in an open-pit coal mine. Mr. Fletcher is 23 kg overweight and has a sedentary lifestyle. He has been married for 25 years and has two grown children who no longer live at home. Mr. Fletcher recently attended a blood pressure clinic where he was told he had "high blood pressure." He has been referred to his local general practitioner for follow-up, and the primary health care nurse is preparing to complete his initial health history and assessment. Mr. Fletcher has brought his wife with him for his clinic visit.

Think about this case study as you read this chapter. There are Review Questions at the end of the chapter about this case study.

When providing nursing care, nurses engage in an intellectual process of reasoning—the **nursing process** (The University of British Columbia, 2017). It is a cognitive framework through which the nurse aims to identify, diagnose, and treat actual and potential health issues and challenges of patients from a holistic perspective. As a nursing student, you will begin by learning the steps of the nursing process: assessment, analysis, planning, implementation, and evaluation. As you gain familiarity with the nursing process, you will learn that it is not a linear approach; rather, the steps of the nursing process are unified and continuously relate to each other (Moghadas & Sedaghati Kesbakhi, 2020) (Figure 14.1). The nursing process guides clinical judgement, decision making, and reflective nursing practice when used in a manner that encourages critical thinking in each of the steps (Basit & Korkmaz, 2021; Ead, 2019).

The nursing process begins with the first step, **assessment**, which is the collection of data pertinent to the patient's health status or situation. While the patient may come to the nurse with one problem in mind, the nurse spends time collecting a variety of different types of data in order to fully understand the patient's priority needs. It is imperative to complete "holistic and comprehensive assessment of diverse patients, to plan and provide competent, ethical, safe compassionate nursing care" (Canadian Association of Schools of Nursing [CASN], 2022, competency 3.1). In the next step, **diagnosis**, the nurse analyzes the assessment data to determine key issues and make clinical judgements in the form of a *nursing diagnosis*. This step is important because it directs the plan of care for the patient. In this process, the nurse will *identify outcomes* for the patient that are individualized to the patient and their current situation. The next step is **planning**, which involves the creation of a formal plan that prescribes strategies and alternatives to attain the expected outcomes. The nurse then carries out **implementation** of the plan. This may occur by coordinating care delivery, providing health teaching and health promotion activities to the patient, consulting with other health care providers, or providing medications or other therapies within the scope of practice of the registered nurse. Finally, the nurse conducts an **evaluation** of the patient's response to the selected interventions and determines whether the interventions were effective. Consider the case scenario about Mr. Fletcher presented at the beginning of the chapter.

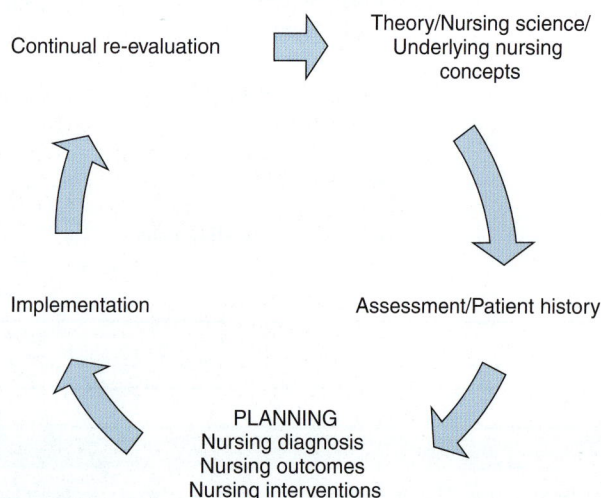

FIGURE 14.1 The modified nursing process. (From T. Heather Herdman / Shigemi Kamitsuru / Camila Takáo Lopes [Eds.], NANDA International, Inc.: *Nursing diagnoses: Definitions and classification 2021–2023*, 12th ed. © 2021 NANDA International, ISBN 978-1-68420-454-0. Used by arrangement with the Thieme Group, Stuttgart / New York.)

CRITICAL THINKING APPROACH TO ASSESSMENT

Assessment is the deliberate and systematic collection of data to determine a patient's current and past health and functional status and to determine the patient's present and past coping patterns (Carpenito, 2017). Nursing assessment consists of the following steps:

- Collection and verification of data from a primary source (the patient) and secondary sources (e.g., caregivers, health care providers, and patient record), and
- The analysis of all data as a basis for developing nursing diagnoses, identifying collaborative problems, and developing a plan of individualized care.

The purpose of assessment is to establish an individualized database about the patient's health status that includes their perceived needs, health challenges, and problems and responds to these challenges or problems (Carpenito, 2017).

Nurses observe a patient's behaviour, ask questions about the nature of the problem, listen to the cues that the patient provides, and conduct a physical examination (see Chapter 33 for further information about conducting a health assessment). Sometimes they also interview caregivers who are familiar with the patient's health problem and review any existing medical record data. It is important that nurses understand that the "coordination of patient care in collaboration with individuals, families and other members of the health care team" is completed in all phases of the nursing process (CASN, 2022, competency 3.10). All of the data collected will form different sets or patterns of information that point to a diagnostic conclusion. Similarly, once a nurse understands the nature and source of a patient's health problems, the nurse is able to provide patient-focused interventions that will restore, maintain, or improve the patient's health.

Critical thinking is foundational to a comprehensive and accurate nursing assessment (see Chapter 7 for further information about critical thinking). Critical thinking enables the nurse to have a broader perspective from which to form conclusions and make decisions about a patient's health condition. While gathering data about a patient, the nurse synthesizes relevant knowledge, recalls prior clinical experiences, applies critical thinking **standards** and available evidence, and uses standards of practice that direct assessment in a meaningful and purposeful way (Figure 14.2). A nurse's knowledge of the physical, biological, and social sciences enables them to ask relevant questions and collect history and physical assessment data relevant to the patient's presenting health care needs.

Figure 14.2 highlights how critical thinking impacts the assessment process. Assessment requires more than collecting data on a patient; it also involves collecting the right data in a way that elicits openness from the patient and integrates the nurse's knowledge base and experience. Nurses use provincial and national standards to guide their care and ensure best practice in order to maintain safe, quality care, upholding confidentiality during all aspects of this process. Most importantly, nurses who have strong assessment skills demonstrate an ability to be focused, detailed, and creative in their approach to assessment.

◆ ASSESSMENT

Nurses begin their assessment by documenting a comprehensive **nursing health history**, a detailed **database** that allows them to plan and carry out nursing care to meet patients' needs. Box 14.1 presents guidelines for documenting a comprehensive history. The goal of the health history is to focus on the patient's strengths and available supports while also highlighting pressing or potential health challenges. As a nurse begins the patient assessment, they need to think critically about what to assess. On the basis of the nurse's clinical knowledge and experience

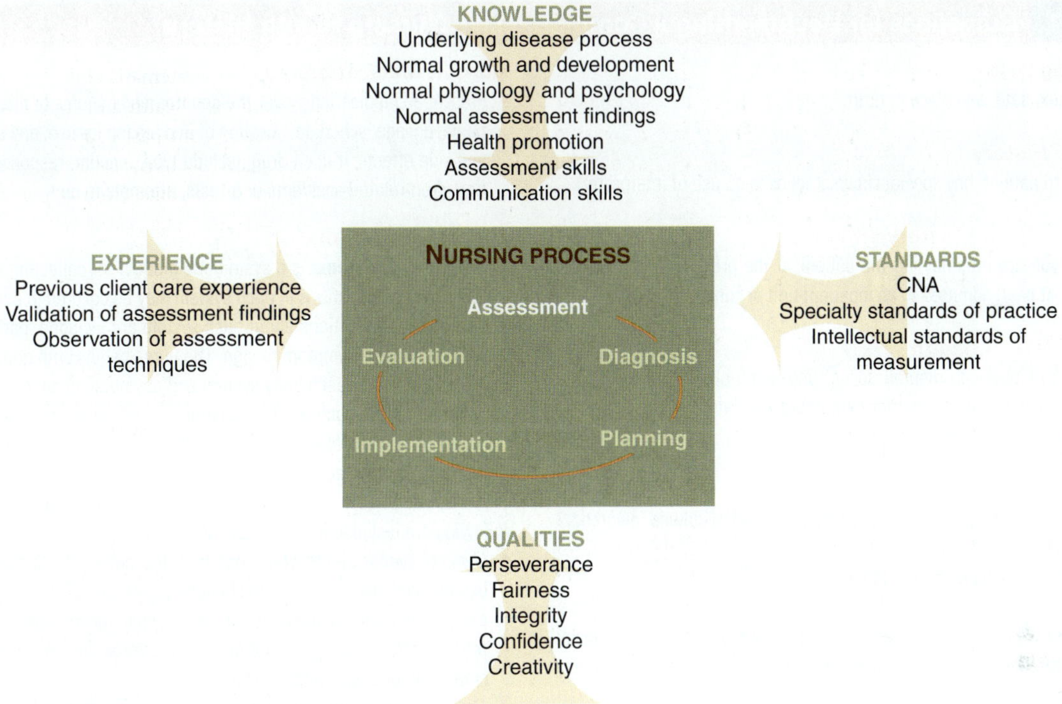

KNOWLEDGE
Underlying disease process
Normal growth and development
Normal physiology and psychology
Normal assessment findings
Health promotion
Assessment skills
Communication skills

EXPERIENCE
Previous client care experience
Validation of assessment findings
Observation of assessment
techniques

NURSING PROCESS
Assessment
Evaluation   Diagnosis
Implementation   Planning

STANDARDS
CNA
Specialty standards of practice
Intellectual standards of
measurement

QUALITIES
Perseverance
Fairness
Integrity
Confidence
Creativity

FIGURE 14.2 Critical thinking and the assessment process. *CNA,* Canadian Nurses Association.

and the patient's health history and responses, the nurse will determine what questions or measurements are appropriate. When a nurse first meets a patient, the nurse makes a quick observational overview or screening. Usually, an overview is based on a treatment situation. For example, a community health nurse assesses the neighbourhood and the community of the patient; an emergency department nurse uses the circulation–airway–breathing (CAB) sequence; and an oncology nurse focuses on the patient's symptoms from disease and treatment and on the grief response (Heart and Stroke Foundation of Canada, 2015).

Nurses learn to differentiate important data from the total data collected (Byermoen et al., 2021). A **cue** is information that a nurse obtains through use of the senses. An **inference** is one's judgement or interpretation of those cues. For example, a patient's crying is a cue that can imply fear or sadness. The nurse asks the patient about any concerns and makes known any nonverbal expressions noticed in an effort to direct the patient to share their feelings. It is possible to miss important cues when a nurse conducts an initial overview. However, with creativity, flexibility, inquisitiveness, intuition, and open-mindedness, the nurse can become aware of unusual or unexpected cues (Chodzaza et al., 2018).

As nurses collect data, they begin to categorize cues, make inferences, and identify emerging patterns, potential problem areas, and solutions. To do this well, nurses critically anticipate patterns, problems, and solutions, staying a step ahead in their assessment. Once the nurse asks a patient a question or makes an observation, the information "branches" to an additional series of questions or observations (Figure 14.3). It is key that nurses anticipate assessment questions, otherwise the overall assessment may be incomplete or the nurse may miss relevant problem areas. Nurses learn to hone these skills and anticipate which questions to ask as they become more experienced in their practice.

Types of Data

Patient data can be categorized in two ways: subjective and objective. **Subjective data** are patients' verbal descriptions of their health concerns. Subjective data are obtained through the health history and the

nurse's questions and the explanation the patient provides (Jarvis et al., 2018). Only patients provide subjective data. Subjective data usually include feelings, perceptions, and self-report of symptoms. Although only patients provide subjective data relevant to their health condition, the data sometimes reflect physiological changes, which nurses further explore through objective data collection. For example, a patient may state they feel nauseous. The nurse will then collect further data to support this symptom.

Objective data are observations or measurements of a patient's health status. Inspection of the condition of a wound, description of an observed behaviour, and measurement of blood pressure are examples of objective data. The measurement of objective data is based on an accepted standard, such as the Celsius measure on a thermometer, centimetres on a measuring tape, or known characteristics of behaviours (e.g., anxiety or fear). Objective data may be considered a normal or abnormal finding. When nurses collect objective data, they apply critical thinking standards (e.g., whether the data are clear, precise, and consistent) to help interpret their findings. In the previous example about the subjective symptom of nausea, vomiting (emesis) would be a piece of objective data that would support this symptom.

Sources of Data

Nurses obtain data from a variety of sources. Each source of data provides information about the patient's level of wellness, strengths, anticipated prognosis, risk factors, health practices and goals, and patterns of health and illness. Sources of data include primary, secondary, and tertiary sources (Nugent & Vitale, 2020) (Box 14.2). The only *primary source* of data is the patient, while *secondary sources* include information from someplace other than the patient, such as caregivers and the patient's medical records. *Tertiary sources* provide information outside the specific patient's frame of reference and are a result of the nurse's or other health care team member's response to care. Sources include textbooks, a nurse's experience, and patterns noticed in other patients with similar presentations and conditions (Nugent & Vitale, 2020, pp. 67–68).

BOX 14.1   Guidelines for Documenting a Comprehensive Nursing Health History

A. Identifying Data
- Name, age, sex, date, and place of birth

B. Source of History
- Relationship to patient, any special circumstances (e.g., use of interpreter)

C. Reason for Health History Interview
- Explain why you are interviewing the patient at the present time (e.g., the patient has just been admitted to an inpatient unit or clinic).

D. Current State of Health
- General state of physical, mental, social, and spiritual health, and health goals. If an illness is present, gather data about the nature of the illness by conducting a symptom analysis (see Chapter 33).

E. Developmental Variables
- Relationship status: single, married, partner, separated, widowed, divorced
- Number of children
- Developmental stage (see Chapter 22)
- Current occupation
- Significant life experiences (e.g., education, previous occupations, financial situations, retirement, coping or stress tolerance, and measures normally used to reduce stress)
- Safety hazards (e.g., biological, chemical, ergonomic, physical, psychosocial, reproductive)
- Housing, environmental hazards (e.g., type of housing, location, living arrangements; specific hazards in the home or community)
- Safety measures (e.g., use of seat belts, helmets, presence of smoke detectors and fire extinguishers, and other measures related to specific hazards of work, community, and home)

F. Psychological Variables
- Mental processes, relationships, support systems, statements regarding patient's feelings about self

G. Spiritual Variables
- Rituals, religious practices, beliefs about life, patient's source of guidance in acting on beliefs, and the relationship with family in exercising faith (see Chapter 29 for further information about spiritual health)

H. Sociocultural Variables
- Culture: values, beliefs, and practices related to health and illness
- Primary language and other languages spoken
- Recreation (exercise, hobbies, socializing, use of leisure time)
- Family and significant others, such as authorized representative (i.e., enduring power of attorney). Include family composition, relationships, special problems experienced by family, patient's and family's response to stress, roles, and support systems. The family history provides information about family structure, interaction, and function that may be useful in planning care. For example, a cohesive, supportive family can help a patient adjust to an illness or disability and should be incorporated into the plan of care. However, if the patient's family members are not supportive, it may be better not to involve them in care.
- Outline a family tree (genogram; see Chapter 20 for further information about how to construct a genogram) to determine whether the patient is at risk for genetic illnesses and to identify areas of health promotion and illness prevention.

I. Physiological Variables (Body Structure and Function)
History of Past Illnesses and Injuries
- Include dates

Current Medications
- Prescribed medications, over-the-counter medications, or illicit drugs. Include name, dosage, schedule, duration of and reason for use, and expected effects and side effects; if illicit drug, include type, amount, response, adverse reaction, drug-related accidents or arrests, attempts to quit.

Review of Systems
The review of systems is a systematic method for collecting data on all body systems. Not all questions in each system may be covered in every history. Nevertheless, some questions about each system are included, particularly when a patient mentions a symptom or sign. The nurse begins with questions about the usual functioning of each body system and any noted changes and follows with specific questions, such as the questions noted for each system. Nurses also focus on measures taken by the patient to promote and maintain health and those to prevent illness or injury. Therefore, after a set of questions is asked, the nurse will always follow up with a review of health promotion activities. The following are included in the review of systems:
- *General overall health state:* Ask how the patient feels overall ("Have you experienced any recent health changes or symptoms?"), fever, chills, malaise, pain, sleep patterns and disturbances, fatigue, recent alterations in weight
- *Integumentary:* itching, colour or texture change, lesions, dryness and use of creams or lotions, changes in hair or nails
- *Ocular:* visual acuity, blurring, eye pain, recent change in vision, discharge, excessive tearing, date of last examination
- *Auditory:* hearing loss, pain, discharge, dizziness, perception of ringing in ears, wax
- *Upper respiratory:* nosebleeds, nasal discharge, nasal allergies, sinus problems, frequency of colds and usual method of treatment, sore throat and usual type of home remedy, hoarseness or voice changes
- *Lower respiratory:* use of tobacco (amount and number of years of smoking; exposure to tobacco smoke; if smoker, attempts to stop smoking), exposure to airborne pollutants, cough, sputum, wheezing, shortness of breath, tuberculosis test and results, date of last chest X-ray examination
- *Breasts and axillae:* rashes, lumps, discharge, pain, breast self-examination practices
- *Lymphatic:* pain, swelling
- *Cardiovascular:* chest pain or distress, precipitating causes, timing and duration, relieving factors, dyspnea, orthopnea, edema, hypertension, exercise tolerance, circulatory problems, varicose veins
- *Gastrointestinal:* appetite, digestion, food intolerance, dysphagia, heartburn, abdominal pain, nausea or vomiting, bowel regularity, use of laxatives, change in stool colour or contents, constipation or diarrhea, flatulence, hemorrhoids, rectal examinations
  - *Dietary pattern:* assess overall nutritional well-being and eating habits, using *Canada's Food Guide* (Health Canada, 2022) for serving size (see Chapter 43 for further information about nutrition); restrictions to food choice; special diets; use of salt; calculate adequacy of fluid intake (should be 30 to 40 mL of fluid per kilogram of body weight); indicate sources of calcium and amounts per day; alcohol use (average number of ounces per week, recent changes in pattern of consumption)
- *Urinary:* painful urination; blood, stones, or pus in urine; bladder or kidney infections; difficulty stopping urinary stream; dribbling or hesitancy; sudden feeling of need to urinate; frequent urination; nocturia (having to get up to void during the night); incontinence (see Chapter 44 for further information about urinary elimination)
- *Genital and reproductive:*
  - *Patients with male genitalia:* puberty onset, difficulty with erections, emissions, testicular pain, libido, infertility, urethral discharge, genital lesions, exposure to and history of sexually transmitted infections, testicular

Continued

BOX 14.1 Guidelines for Documenting a Comprehensive Nursing Health History—cont'd

self-examinations, testicular lump or pain, hernias, sexual preference, birth control method, safer sex practices used
- *Patients with female genitalia:* menses (onset, duration, regularity, flow, discomfort, date of most recent menstrual period), age at menopause (occurrence of hot flashes, night sweats, vaginal discharge), date of last Pap smear, pregnancies (number, miscarriages, abortions), exposure to and history of sexually transmitted infections, sexual preference, birth control method, safer sex practices used
- *Musculoskeletal:* pain, joint stiffness or swelling, restricted motion, muscle wasting, weakness, general mobility, use of mobility aids, ability to perform activities of daily living

- *Neurological:* injury, headaches, dizziness, fainting, abnormalities of sensation or coordination, tremors, seizures
- *Endocrine:* excessive sweating, thirst, hunger, or urination; intolerance of heat or cold; changes in distribution of facial hair; thyroid enlargement or tenderness; unexplained weight change; change in glove or shoe size
- *Hematological:* anemia, bruise or bleed easily, transfusions
- *Psychiatric:* depression, mood changes, difficulty concentrating, nervousness, anxiety, suicidal thoughts, irritability
- *Immunological:* communicable diseases (indicate disease and age at or year of onset), immunization status (indicate year of most recent immunization), allergies (known allergens and reactions; MedicAlert identification worn)

Adapted from Jarvis, C., Browne, A. J., MacDonald-Jenkins, J., & Luctkar-Flude, M. (2018). *Physical examination and health assessment* (3rd Canadian ed., pp. 62–69). Elsevier.

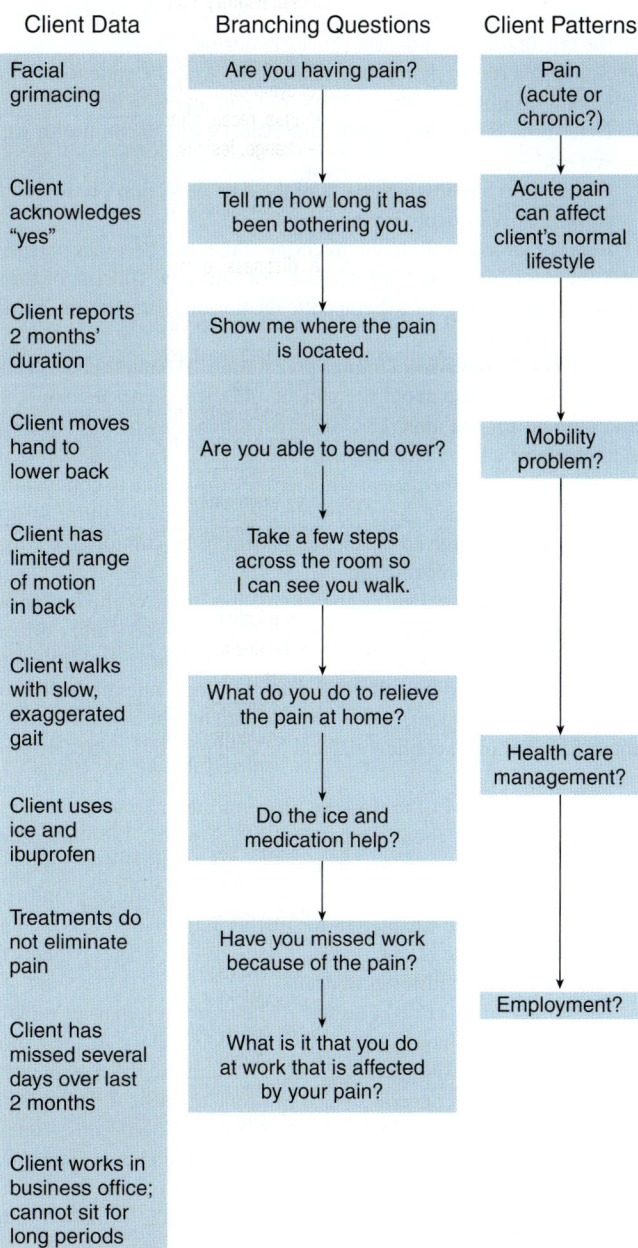

FIGURE 14.3 Example of branching logic for selecting assessment questions.

BOX 14.2 Sources of Data

Primary Sources
- Patient
  Example: Patient's description of the presenting problem and medical history, narratives of health experiences

Secondary Sources
Sources Outside the Patient
- Patient chart
  Examples: nursing notes/charting, health care provider progress notes, medication administration record, diagnostic and laboratory tests, interdisciplinary team notes. It is important to note that the patient is dynamic and changing—chart data show the patient's history and may not reflect the current health status of the patient.
- Caregivers/significant others

Tertiary Sources
Provide information to patient's frame of reference (e.g., illness conditions)
- Relevant literature
- Nurse's experience (e.g. accepted commonalities among patients with similar physical and emotional responses) (Nugent & Vitale, 2020)

Primary Sources

Patient. A patient is usually the nurse's best source of information. Patients who are conscious, alert, and able to answer questions correctly provide the most accurate information about their health care needs, lifestyle patterns, current and past illnesses, perception of symptoms, and changes in activities of daily living. Nurses always need to consider the setting for their assessment. It is important that the patient has privacy and feels safe in disclosing health information. The nurse must also take the current situation into account when taking a health history. For example, a patient experiencing acute symptoms in an emergency department will not offer as much information as one who comes to an outpatient clinic for a routine check-up. It is imperative that the nurse demonstrate a caring presence by actively listening to the patient's concerns and engaging in caring behaviours while completing an assessment (see Chapter 18 for further information about communication skills). In some instances, the use of a translator may be indicated when gathering primary data from the patient. The nurse must ensure that they complete an accurate history and attend when a translator assists the patient.

Secondary Sources

Family and Caregivers. Caregivers and significant others can be the most knowledgeable sources of information for infants or children, critically ill adults, adults with developmental disabilities, and patients who are disoriented or unconscious. In cases of severe illness or emergency situations, families are sometimes the only available sources of information for nurses and the patients' health care providers. The family and significant others are important secondary sources of information. They confirm findings that a patient provides (e.g., whether a patient takes medications regularly at home or how well the patient sleeps or eats). In cases where a language barrier exists, families can often assist in gathering information from the patient in immediate situations. However, the nurse should include the family only when appropriate. A patient may not always want the nurse to question the family or may not wish to reveal certain information in front of family members. The nurse should ask the patient privately if they would like the family present during a health history, and always ask the patient's permission to have family or other health care providers in the room while conducting a physical assessment.

Spouses or close friends often sit in during an assessment and provide their view of the patient's health problems or needs. They not only supply information about the patient's current health status but are also able to tell when changes in the patient's status occurred. Family members are often well informed because of their experiences living with the patient and observing how health problems affect daily living activities. Family and friends make important observations about the patient's needs that can affect the way care is delivered (e.g., how a patient eats a meal or how a patient makes choices). Note that there is a difference between using the family as a source of data and family nursing. Family nursing is a comprehensive primary care approach to the health of the entire family (see Chapter 20) that extends beyond collecting additional data about the patient.

Health Care Team.
Nurses frequently communicate with other health care team members when gathering information about patients. In the acute care setting, the change-of-shift report is a way for nurses from one shift to communicate information to nurses on the next shift (see Chapter 16 for further information about documentation). When nurses, health care providers, physiotherapists, social workers, or other staff consult about a patient's condition, they typically have information about the patient. This information may include how the patient is interacting within the health care environment, the patient's physical or emotional reactions to treatment, the result of diagnostic procedures or therapies, and how the patient responds to visitors. Every member of the health care team is a source of information for identifying and verifying information about the patient.

Medical Records.
The medical record is a source of the patient's medical history, laboratory and diagnostic test results, current physical findings, and the medical treatment plan. Data in the records offer baseline and ongoing information about the patient's response to illness and progress to date. Information in a patient's record is confidential. The medical record is a valuable tool for checking the consistency and similarities of personal observations.

Tertiary Sources

Literature.
Nurses complete the assessment database by reviewing nursing, medical, and pharmacological literature about a patient's present health status. This review increases their knowledge about the patient's diagnosed problems, expected symptoms, treatment, prognosis, and established standards of therapeutic practice. A knowledgeable nurse obtains relevant, accurate, and complete information for the assessment database.

Nurse's Experience.
Manetti (2019) supports the integration of evidence-informed knowledge and good clinical reasoning as essential for eliciting and processing information that will lead the nurse to deliver relevant therapeutic interventions. A nurse's expertise develops after testing and refining propositions, questions, and principle- or standard-based expectations. Practical experience and the opportunity to make clinical decisions strengthen a nurse's critical thinking.

Methods of Data Collection

Nurses use the patient interview, nursing health history, physical examination findings, and results of laboratory and diagnostic tests to establish an assessment database for a patient.

Interview. The first step in establishing a database is to collect subjective information by interviewing the patient. An **interview** is an organized conversation with the patient. The initial formal interview involves obtaining the patient's health history and information about the current illness. During the initial interview, the nurse can do the following:

- Introduce themselves to the patient, explain their role, and explain the role of other health care providers during care.
- Establish a caring therapeutic relationship with the patient.
- Obtain insight about the patient's concerns and worries.
- Determine the patient's goals and expectations of the health care system.
- Obtain cues about which parts of the data collection phase necessitate further in-depth investigation.

Rather than controlling the interview, the nurse becomes partners with the patient during the interview. An interview consists of three phases, similar to that of a therapeutic relationship: orientation, working, and termination.

A successful interview requires preparation. The nurse collects any available information about the patient and then creates a favourable environment for the interview. An environment in which the patient is comfortable and relaxed helps the nurse conduct a good interview. The nurse must ask the patient whether they would like to conduct the interview alone or have caregivers join them. Finally, the nurse selects a place private enough to enable the patient to be comfortable when providing personal information.

Orientation Phase. During the orientation phase of the interview, the nurse introduces themselves, describes their position, and explains the purpose of the interview. It is imperative that the nurse explain to the patient why they are collecting data (e.g., for a nursing history or for a focused assessment) and assure the patient that any information obtained will remain confidential and be used only by health care providers.

Working Phase. In the working phase of the interview, the nurse gathers information about the patient's health status. The nurse does this through focused questioning and other communication strategies such as active listening, paraphrasing, and summarizing to promote a clear interaction (see Chapter 18 for further information about communicating). The use of open-ended questions encourages patients to describe their health histories in detail.

Nurses use **open-ended questions** whenever they want to explore broader issues and have patients describe their history in their own words. Open-ended questions can help to determine the patient's priorities and primary concerns, which can sometimes be different from what the nurse initially thinks the concern is. **Closed-ended questions** can all be answered by stating yes or no (or a choice of answers that the nurse provides); close-ended questions should be limited to issues for which the nurse does not need additional information from the patient (Box 14.3). Both types of questioning can help advance patient care. While open-ended questions can elicit more information about a patient's history and perceptions of their health, closed-ended

BOX 14.3 Examples of Open- and Closed-Ended Questions

Open-Ended Questions

Tell me how you are feeling.

Your discomfort affects your ability to get around in what way?

Describe how your spouse or partner has been helping you.

Give me an example of how you get relief from your pain at home.

Closed-Ended Questions

Do you feel as if the medication is helping you?

Who is the person who helps you at home?

Do you understand why you are having the X-ray examination?

Has the warm compress given you relief from your back pain?

Are you having pain now?

On a scale of 0 to 10, with 0 being no pain at all and 10 being the worst possible pain, how would you rate your pain?

questions can help a patient who is in acute pain or distress identify their emergent or priority needs.

During the working phase, the nurse obtains a nursing health history by exploring the patient's current illness, health history, and expectations of care. The objective for collecting a health history is to identify patterns of health and illness, risk factors for physical and behavioural health problems, changes from normal function, and available resources for adaptation. The initial interview is normally the most extensive. Ongoing interviews, which occur each time a nurse interacts with the patient, do not need to be as extensive; their purpose is to update the patient's status and focus more on changes in previously identified problems and to identify new problems.

Termination Phase. As in the other phases of the interview, termination requires skill on the part of the interviewer. The nurse provides the patient with clues that the interview is coming to an end. For example, the nurse may say, "I want to ask just two more questions" or "We'll be finished in about 2 minutes." This helps the patient maintain direct attention without being distracted by wondering when the interview will end. This approach also gives the patient an opportunity to ask questions. When concluding an interview, the nurse summarizes the important points and asks the patient whether the summary was accurate. The nurse should end the interview in a friendly manner, such as by telling the patient when the nurse will return to provide care.

A skillful interviewer adapts interview strategies based on the patient's responses. Nurses successfully gather relevant health data when they are prepared for the interview and able to carry out each interview phase with minimal interruption.

Cultural Considerations in Assessment

Cultural assessments, combined with critical thinking skills, provide the knowledge necessary for nursing care. It is important that nurses conduct any assessment with cultural competence and cultural safety (see Chapter 12). This involves a conscientious understanding of the patient's culture so that the nurse can offer better care within differing value systems and act with respect and understanding without imposition of the nurse's own attitudes and beliefs (Ball et al., 2019). Good communication techniques are important when assessing a patient whose culture is different from the nurse's own. Communication and culture are interrelated in the way feelings are expressed verbally and nonverbally.

When nurses interact to assess any specific patient, they must first know their own cultural self. Cultural awareness can be achieved by engaging in self-reflection on biases and feelings (see Chapter 12 for more information about cultural awareness). Nurses need to avoid forming conclusions about their sense of a patient based on their prior knowledge of the patient's culture. Doing so may not only affect the quality of patient care but also cause harm to the patient if the person is stereotyped or if assumptions are made about their health practices. The nurse needs to ask questions in a constructive and probing way to establish a comprehensive understanding of the patient with regard to the patient's priorities, beliefs about health, and health concerns.

Approaches to Indigenous Health Assessment

Nurses require skills-based training in intercultural competency, conflict resolution, human rights, and anti-racism (Truth and Reconciliation Commission of Canada [TRC], 2015, Call to Action 24) in order to provide safe and culturally competent care to Indigenous patients. This includes taking courses that address Indigenous health issues, including the history and legacy of residential schools, the United Nations Declaration on the Rights of Indigenous Peoples (United Nations, 2007), treaties and Indigenous rights, and Indigenous teaching and practices (TRC, 2015, Call to Action 24). In consultation with Indigenous communities, nurses should also advocate for policy change at the federal level by requesting that the government publish annual progress reports and assess long-term trends impacting the health of Indigenous communities in Canada. Furthermore, nurses need to understand the value of Indigenous healing practices, assess patients for the use of these practices, and use these practices for the treatment of Indigenous patients in collaboration with Indigenous healers and Elders, when requested (TRC, 2015, Call to Action 22). Significant repercussions from the residential school system persist that may affect the health of Indigenous survivors of this system, their families, and future generations. However, it is imperative that nurses remember that assessing for any type of transgenerational or collective trauma should be conducted by nurses with expertise in this area of assessment. Beginning nurses should focus their efforts on general health assessment and building trusting and therapeutic relationships with their patients by coming to know about them as individuals, their experiences, and their primary health concerns (see Chapter 12, Indigenous Health).

Nursing Health History

Nurses conduct a nursing health history during either their initial contact or an early contact with a patient. The history is a major component of assessment. Although many health history forms are structured, nurses learn to use the questions as starting points. A good assessor learns to refine and broaden questions as needed to correctly assess the patient's unique needs. Time and patient priorities determine how complete a history is. The nurse can identify patterns of information about a patient's health and illness by collecting data about all health dimensions (see Box 14.1). By incorporating data from all dimensions, the nurse can develop a complete plan of care.

Family History

The purpose of collecting the family history is to obtain data about immediate and blood relatives. The objectives are to determine whether the patient is at risk for illnesses of a genetic or familial nature and to identify areas of health promotion and illness prevention (see Chapter 21 for further information about patient education). The family history also provides information about family structure, interaction, and function that is often useful in planning care (see Chapter 20 for further information about assessing the family). For example, a close, supportive family will help a patient adjust to an illness or disability. If the patient's family is not supportive, it is better not to involve family members in their care. Stressful family relationships are sometimes a significant barrier when nurses try to help patients with problems involving loss, self-concept, spiritual health, and personal relationships.

Documentation of History Findings

As nurses conduct the nursing health history, they need to record their assessment in a clear, concise manner using appropriate terminology. Standardized forms make it easy to enter data as the patient responds to questions. In settings that have computerized documentation, entry of assessment data is easy. A clear, concise record is necessary for use by other health care providers (see Chapter 16 for further information about documentation). Regardless of the model used in a documentation system, nurses provide a thorough database inclusive of historical and current information about the patient's health. This information then becomes the baseline against which nurses and the health care team evaluate any future changes.

Physical Examination

A *physical examination* is an investigation of the body to determine its state of health. A physical examination involves use of the techniques of inspection, palpation, percussion, auscultation, and smell (see Chapter 33 for further information about conducting a health assessment). A complete examination includes measurements of a patient's height, weight, and vital signs and a head-to-toe examination of all body systems. By performing actual hands-on physical assessment, nurses gather valuable objective information that helps in forming accurate diagnostic conclusions. It is important for the nurse to conduct an examination with sensitivity and competence to prevent the patient from becoming anxious.

Observation of Patient Behaviour. Throughout an interview and physical examination, it is important for nurses to observe a patient's verbal and nonverbal behaviours closely to enhance their objective database. Nurses learn to determine whether data obtained by observation matches what the patient verbally communicates. For example, if a patient expresses no concern about an upcoming diagnostic test but shows poor eye contact, shakiness, and restlessness, all of which are suggestive of anxiety, then verbal and nonverbal data conflict. Observations direct the nurse to gather additional objective data to form accurate conclusions about the patient's condition. An important aspect of observation includes a patient's level of function: the physical, developmental, psychological, and social aspects of everyday living. Observation of the level of function differs from observations made during an interview. Observation of level of function involves watching what a patient does, such as eating or decision making about preparing a medication, rather than what the patient tells the nurse what they can do. Observation of function can occur in the home or in a health care setting during a return visit.

Diagnostic and Laboratory Data. The results of diagnostic and laboratory tests reveal or clarify alterations questioned or identified during the nursing health history and physical examination. For example, during the history documentation, the patient reports having had a bad cold for 6 days, and the patient currently has a productive cough with brown sputum and mild shortness of breath. On physical examination, the nurse notices an elevated temperature, increased respirations, and decreased breath sounds in the right lower lobe. The nurse reviews the results of a complete blood cell count and notes that the white blood cell count is elevated (indicating an infection). In addition, the radiologist's report of a chest X-ray examination shows the presence of a right lower lobe infiltrate. Such findings combined are suggestive of the medical diagnosis of pneumonia and the associated nursing diagnosis of impaired gas exchange.

Some patients collect and monitor laboratory data in the home. For example, patients with diabetes mellitus often perform daily blood glucose monitoring. The nurse would then ask patients about their routine results to determine their responses to illness and elicit information about the effects of treatment measures. The nurse also compares laboratory data with the established norms for a particular test result, age group, and gender.

Interpreting Assessment Data and Making Nursing Judgements. The successful analysis and interpretation of assessment data requires critical thinking. When nurses correctly analyze data, they recognize patterns that lead them to make necessary clinical decisions about a patient's care. These decisions are in the form of either nursing diagnoses or collaborative problems that require treatment from several disciplines (Carpenito, 2017). When nurses critically think about interpreting assessment information, they determine the presence of abnormal findings, what further observations they need to clarify information, and the patient's health problems.

Data Validation. Before nurses begin analyzing and interpreting data, they need to validate the collected information they have in order to avoid making incorrect inferences (Carpenito, 2017). Validation of assessment data is the comparison of data with another source to determine data accuracy. For example, a nurse observes a patient crying and logically infers that this is related to hospitalization or a medical diagnosis. Making such an initial inference is not wrong, but problems can result if the nurse does not validate the inference with the patient. In this case, the nurse may state, "I notice that you have been crying. Can you tell me about it?" By questioning the patient, the nurse will discover the real reason for the crying behaviour. To validate the information obtained during an interview and history, the nurse relies on the patient to confirm it. The nurse also validates findings from the physical examination and observation of patient behaviour by comparing data in the medical record and consulting with other nurses or health care team members. Often, family or friends are able to validate assessment information. Validation opens the door for gathering more assessment data because it involves clarifying vague or unclear data. On occasion, the nurse may reassess previously covered areas of the nursing history or gather further physical examination data. It is important to continually analyze and think about a patient's database in order to make concise, accurate, and meaningful interpretations. Critical thinking applied to assessment enables the nurse to fully understand the patient's problems, to judge the extent of the problems carefully, and to discover possible relationships between the problems.

Analysis and Interpretation. After the nurse collects extensive information about a patient, the nurse analyzes and interprets the data. The nurse begins analysis by organizing the information into meaningful and usable clusters, keeping in mind the patient's response to illness. A *data cluster* is a set of signs or symptoms that are grouped together in a logical way. During data clustering, the nurse will organize data and focus attention on patient functions to determine which support or assistance for recovery is needed. Data analysis involves recognizing patterns or trends in the clustered data, comparing them with standards, and then establishing a reasoned conclusion about the patient's responses to a health problem. Patterns of meaning begin to form, enabling the nurse to make inferences about patient problems.

Through reasoning and judgement, the nurse decides what information explains the patient's health status. At times, additional information is required to clarify the nurse's interpretation. The ability to cluster or group data during analysis will help the nurse at becoming proficient in identifying individualized nursing diagnoses and identifying collaborative problems (see Figure 14.6).

During clustering, a cue or an individual sign, symptom, or finding will alert the nurse more than others do. Such cues are especially helpful in identifying nursing diagnoses.

Data Documentation

Data documentation is the last part of a complete assessment. The timely, thorough, and accurate documentation of facts is necessary when a patients' data are recorded. Not only does documentation guide patient care, it is also a legal and professional responsibility to record the patient's status. If the nurse does not record an assessment finding or problem interpretation, that information is lost and unavailable to anyone else caring for the patient. If the nurse does not record detailed and specific data, the person reading the report is left with only general impressions. The basic rule is to record all observations. Anything heard, seen, felt, or smelled should be reported exactly. It is important to record objective information in accurate terminology (e.g., "weighs 77.3 kg," "abdomen is soft and nontender to palpation"). Subjective information from a patient is recorded in quotation marks. When entering data, the nurse should not generalize or form judgements through written communication. Conclusions about such data become nursing diagnoses and must be accurate. As nurses become more proficient at identifying data clusters and patterns of signs and symptoms, they are better able to conclude the existence of a correct problem (see Chapter 16).

Concept Mapping

A **concept map** is a visual representation that show the connections between a patient's health problems. It fosters a holistic view of the patient and identifies linkages between the multiple variables affecting the patient's health. Constructing concept maps demonstrates and promotes critical thinking through the use of reflection, creativity, and insight (Aein & Aliakbari, 2017; Doenges et al., 2019). The visual image of patients as holistic, multidimensional, and complex serves as a starting point for the development of a comprehensive, individualized care plan (Aein & Aliakbari, 2017). Figure 14.4 summarizes the primary assessment findings from Mr. Fletcher's case scenario, introduced at the start of this chapter. Review these findings and write out any additional questions you may have about these findings or any additional questions you would ask the patient at this time. It is helpful to address this case scenario as a large group as an in-class exercise. To demonstrate how critical thinking is integrated into assessment, Figure 14.2 is applied here to this case scenario:

Irene (preferred pronouns: she/her) is the local primary health nurse assessing Mr. Fletcher. Irene has practised as a registered

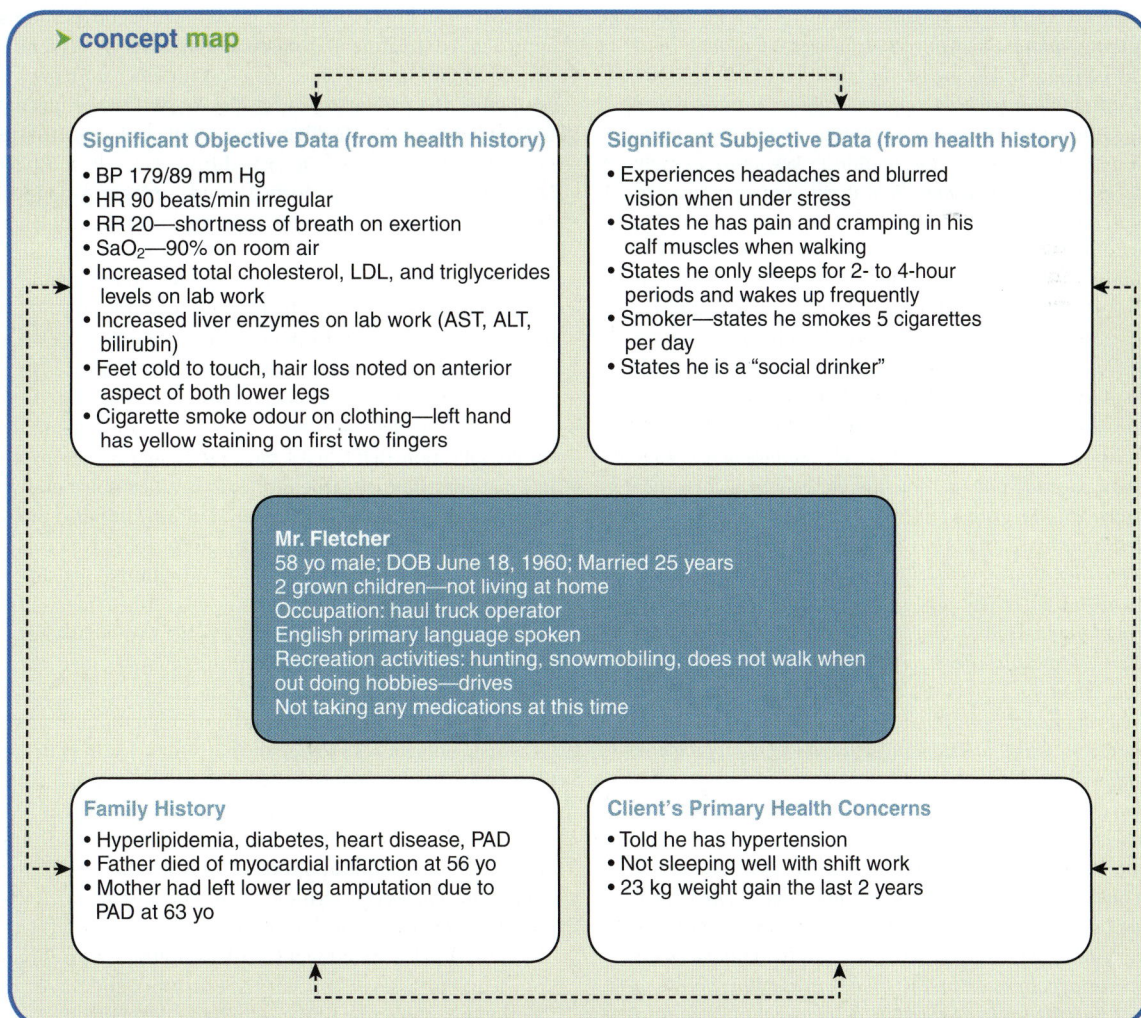

FIGURE 14.4 Concept map for Mr. Fletcher's assessment findings. *ALT,* Alanine aminotransferase; *AST,* aspartate aminotransferase; *BP,* blood pressure; *DOB,* date of birth; *HR,* heart rate; *LDL,* low-density lipoprotein; *PAD,* peripheral arterial disease; *RR,* respiratory rate; *SaO₂,* oxygen saturation; *yo,* years old.

nurse for 25 years in this small mountain community. She is familiar with the daily routines and stresses of a haul truck operator because her husband also works at the coal mine as a heavy-duty mechanic. Irene's practice experience has been in acute care and community health.

Knowledge: Irene is concerned about Mr. Fletcher's high blood pressure and his identification of subjective symptoms such as headache and blurred vision because these are symptoms of advanced disease. She is aware that Mr. Fletcher may have had high blood pressure for years and not been aware of it because high blood pressure can be hidden in a patient who does not take their blood pressure regularly. She is concerned because prolonged hypertension can cause kidney failure, loss of vision, and cardiovascular and peripheral vascular disease. Irene also notes on Mr. Fletcher's laboratory results that he has hyperlipidemia; this condition can worsen vascular disease when paired with uncontrolled hypertension. Irene suspects that Mr. Fletcher is also experiencing peripheral arterial disease owing to the poor circulation in his feet, hair loss on his lower legs, and pain in his calf muscles when walking. Mr. Fletcher has a positive family history for heart disease, vascular disorders, and diabetes—all of these conditions can be genetically linked to future occurrences. She suspects that Mr. Fletcher may be smoking more than five cigarettes per day because he has hypertension, symptoms of vascular disease, a strong odour on his clothing, and stained fingers. However, there may be a reason why he is not disclosing this information to her, so Irene has decided to build a trusting rapport with him before further questioning him about his smoking patterns. At this time, Irene is focused on gathering more information in key areas, namely Mr. Fletcher's hypertension, high lipid levels, and symptoms of vascular disease.

Standards: Irene draws from various resources to help guide her assessment and questioning. For example, Hypertension Canada outlines the standards for the diagnosis and clinical pathways for the diagnosis of hypertension. The organization also provides comprehensive best practice guidelines for the treatment of hypertension that address both medical and nursing management (Rabi et al., 2020). Irene is using both medical knowledge (e.g., pathophysiology, pharmacology, disease management) and nursing knowledge to guide her questioning; she is aware of her scope of practice as a registered nurse.

Qualities: Irene reflects on the assessment interview, her rapport with Mr. Fletcher, and her creativity in collecting information. She listens in the interview process to both what is being said and information that is not pointed out or is being avoided in the conversation. She conducts her interview in a therapeutic manner, ensuring that she is treating Mr. Fletcher fairly and with respect. She does not comment directly on his health practices at this time. Rather, she assesses his understanding, reasoning, and approaches to his health.

Experience: Irene's experience as a nurse in this region informs her approaches to her assessment and the questions that she asks the patient. Irene is familiar with the position of a haul truck operator. She is aware that they work long shifts, often have sleep issues due to shift work, and perform tasks that are mostly stationary (sitting for long periods). She is also familiar with risk factors for hypertension and vascular disease. Therefore, she knows what type of direct questions to ask and what to look for in her assessment. She is confident and proficient in her assessment techniques and knows how to cluster data to gain an understanding of emerging issues.

◆ NURSING DIAGNOSIS

After a patient is assessed thoroughly to compile a database, the next step of the nursing process is to form diagnostic conclusions that determine the nursing care that a patient will receive (Figure 14.5). Figure 14.6 outlines these specific steps to a nursing diagnosis and summarizes key phases of assessment. Some of the conclusions lead to a specific nursing diagnoses, whereas others do not. It is helpful to equate a diagnosis with a health problem or health issue. The diagnostic process is a complex, patient-centred, collaborative activity that involves the health care team as well as information gathering and clinical reasoning to determine the goals of care for a patient's major health problems (Balogh & Miller, 2015). Diagnostic conclusions include problems treated primarily by nurses (nursing diagnoses) and problems necessitating treatment by several disciplines (collaborative problems). More recently, the term "analysis" is often adopted (instead of *diagnosis*) to describe this stage of the nursing process, because nursing diagnoses are not universally used as standardized language (Ignatavicius & Silvestri, 2021). However, diagnosis will remain the central focus of this stage of the nursing process within this chapter in order to help differentiate nursing scope of practice and link assessment findings to patients' relevant health issues or health problems.

When health care providers refer to commonly accepted medical diagnoses, such as myocardial infarction, diabetes mellitus, or osteoarthritis, they all know the meaning of these diagnoses and the standard approaches to treatment. A **medical diagnosis** is the identification of a disease condition on the basis of a specific evaluation of physical signs, symptoms, the patient's medical history, and the results of diagnostic tests and procedures. Health care providers are licensed to treat diseases or pathological processes described in medical diagnostic statements. Nurses have a similar diagnostic language. **Nursing diagnosis**, the second step of the nursing process, determines health problems within the domain of nursing. The term *diagnose* means "distinguish" or "know." A nursing diagnosis is a clinical judgement about individual, family, or community responses to actual and potential health problems or life processes that is within the domain of nursing (NANDA International, 2021). Box 14.4 shows examples of nursing diagnoses to consider in relation to the case scenario regarding Mr. Fletcher.

A **collaborative problem** is an actual or potential physiological complication that nurses monitor to detect the onset of changes in a patient's status (Carpenito, 2017). When collaborative problems develop, nurses intervene in collaboration with personnel from other health care disciplines. Nurses manage collaborative problems such as hemorrhage, infection, and cardiac dysrhythmia by using both health care provider–prescribed and nursing-prescribed interventions to minimize complications. For example, a patient who has a surgical wound is at risk of developing an infection, and thus a health care provider prescribes antibiotics. The nurse monitors the patient for fever and other signs of infection and implements appropriate wound care measures.

Nursing diagnoses provide the basis for selecting nursing interventions to achieve outcomes for which nurses are accountable (NANDA International, 2021). A nursing diagnosis focuses on a patient's actual or potential response to a health problem rather than on the physiological event, complication, or disease. In the case of the diagnosis *inadequate knowledge regarding postoperative routines*, collaborative problems occur or probably will occur in association with a specific disease, trauma, or treatment (Carpenito, 2017). Nurses require expert knowledge to assess a patient's specific risk for these problems, to identify the problems early, and then to take preventive action (Figure 14.7). Critical thinking is necessary in identifying nursing diagnoses and collaborative problems so that nurses individualize care appropriately for their patients.

KNOWLEDGE
Underlying disease process
Normal growth and development
Normal psychology
Normal assessment findings
Health promotion

EXPERIENCE
Previous client care experience
Validation of assessment findings
Observation of assessment
techniques

NURSING PROCESS

Assessment

Evaluation   Diagnosis

Implementation   Planning

STANDARDS
CNA
Intellectual standards
of measurement
Client-centred care

QUALITIES
Perseverance
Responsibility
Fairness
Integrity
Confidence

FIGURE 14.5 Critical thinking and the nursing diagnostic process. *CNA,* Canadian Nurses Association.

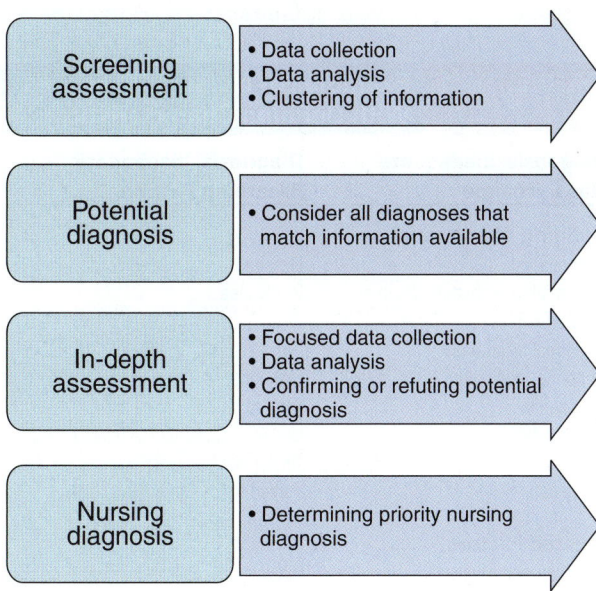

Screening assessment
• Data collection
• Data analysis
• Clustering of information

Potential diagnosis
• Consider all diagnoses that match information available

In-depth assessment
• Focused data collection
• Data analysis
• Confirming or refuting potential diagnosis

Nursing diagnosis
• Determining priority nursing diagnosis

FIGURE 14.6 Steps in moving from assessment to diagnosis. (*From* T. Heather Herdman / Shigemi Kamitsuru / Camila Takáo Lopes [Eds.], NANDA International, Inc.: *Nursing diagnoses: Definitions and classification 2021–2023*, 12th ed. © 2021 NANDA International, ISBN 978-1-68420-454-0. Used by arrangement with the Thieme Group, Stuttgart / New York.)

BOX 14.4	Examples of Nursing Diagnoses Related to the Case Scenario

Acute pain
Altered health maintenance
Lack of compliance
Decreased tissue perfusion
Reduced stamina
Risk for reduced stamina
Anxiety
Risk-prone health behaviour
Activity intolerance
Potential for altered body image
Decreased cardiac output
Defensive coping
Impaired family coping
Impaired coping
Potential for compromised human dignity
Knowledge deficit
Potential for falls

Nursing diagnosis is recognized in Canada as an innovative means of translating nursing observations and assessments into standard conclusions in a common nomenclature. Although nursing diagnosis is part of basic nursing preparation in Canada, it has not yet been incorporated into provincial and territorial nursing practice standards or legislation.

Standard formal nursing diagnostic statements (see Box 14.4) serve several purposes:
1. They provide a precise definition that gives all members of the health care team a common language for understanding the patient's needs.
2. They enable nurses to communicate their actions among themselves, to other health care providers, and to the public.
3. They distinguish the nurse's role from that of the health care provider or other health care providers.
4. They help nurses focus on the scope of nursing practice.
5. They foster the development of nursing knowledge.

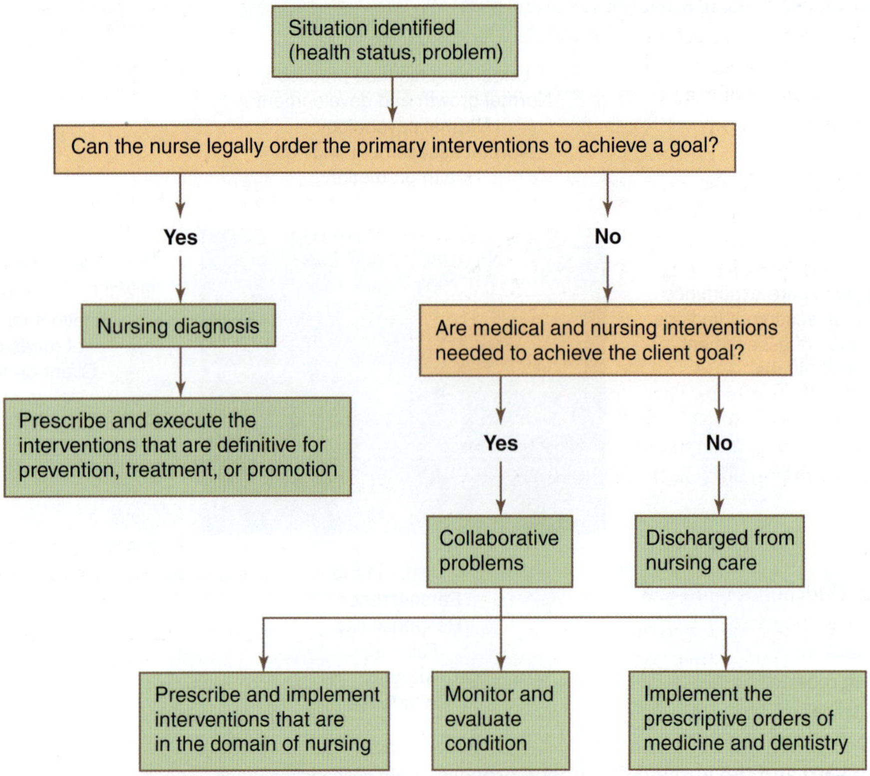

FIGURE 14.7 Differentiating nursing diagnoses from collaborative problems. (Copyright © 1990, 1988, 1985, by Lynda Juall Carpenito. Redrawn from Carpenito, L. J. [1995]. *Nursing diagnosis: Application to clinical practice* [6th ed.]. J. B. Lippincott.)

CRITICAL THINKING AND NURSING DIAGNOSTIC PROCESS

Diagnostic reasoning is a process of using assessment data about a patient to logically explain a clinical judgement—in this case, a nursing diagnosis. The diagnostic process flows from the assessment process and includes decision-making steps. These steps include data clustering, identifying patient needs, and formulating the diagnosis or problem.

Clusters and patterns of data often contain **defining characteristics**—the clinical criteria or assessment findings that help confirm an actual nursing diagnosis. **Clinical criteria** are objective or subjective signs and symptoms, clusters of signs and symptoms, or risk factors that lead to a diagnostic conclusion. A specific set of defining characteristics helps to confirm the identification of each **NANDA International**–approved nursing diagnosis (NANDA International, 2021). Nurses learn to recognize patterns of defining characteristics and then readily select the corresponding diagnosis.

Table 14.1 shows two examples of possible nursing diagnoses and their associated defining characteristics. As nurses analyze clusters of data, they begin to consider various diagnoses that might apply to the patient. For example, the diagnoses of *inadequate gas exchange* and *inadequate breathing pattern* have similar defining characteristics, including dyspnea, abnormal respiratory rate, and abnormal depth of breathing. As the nurse determines a diagnosis, it is important to remember that the absence of certain defining characteristics suggests the rejection of a diagnosis under consideration. Thus, in the same example, if a patient uses accessory muscles to breathe and demonstrates pursed-lip breathing, the correct diagnosis is not *inadequate gas exchange* but *inadequate breathing pattern*. It is important to examine the defining characteristics in the database carefully to confirm or

TABLE 14.1	Examples of Nursing Diagnoses With Defining Characteristics
Diagnosis: Inadequate Gas Exchange	**Diagnosis: Inadequate Breathing Pattern**
Defining Characteristics	
Dyspnea	Dyspnea
Abnormal rate, rhythm, depth of breathing	Bradypnea
Abnormal arterial pH	Decreased vital capacity
Abnormal skin colour (pale, dusky)	Orthopnea
Hypoxemia	Altered chest excursion
Hypercarbia	Use of accessory muscles to breathe
Hypoxia	Tachypnea
Confusion	Pursed-lip breathing
Related Factors	
Ventilation–perfusion	Hyperventilation
Alveolar–capillary membrane changes	Pain
	Chest wall deformity
	Anxiety
	Musculoskeletal impairment
	Body position

eliminate a nursing diagnosis. To be more accurate, review all characteristics, eliminate irrelevant ones, and confirm the relevant ones.

While focusing on patterns of defining characteristics, the nurse compares a patient's pattern of data with data that are consistent with normal, healthy patterns. The nurse uses accepted norms as the basis for comparison and judgement. These norms include laboratory and diagnostic test values, professional standards, and normal anatomical or physiological limits. When comparing patterns, the nurse judges whether the grouped signs and symptoms are normal for the patient and whether they are within the range of healthy responses, then isolates any defining characteristics not within healthy norms in order to identify a problem.

Before finalizing a nursing diagnosis, the nurse needs to review the patient's general health care needs or problems. Identifying patient needs enables the nurse to individualize nursing diagnoses by considering all assessment data and focusing on the more relevant data. NANDA International (2021) has two nursing diagnoses that apply to knowledge: *insufficient knowledge* and *potential for enhanced knowledge*. It is crucial to select the correct diagnostic label for a patient's need. Usually from assessment to diagnosis, the information gathered progresses from general to specific. It helps to think of the problem identification phase in terms of the general health care problem and to think of the formulation of the nursing diagnosis in terms of the specific health problem.

Formulation of the Nursing Diagnosis

NANDA International (2021) identifies four types of nursing diagnoses: actual diagnoses, risk diagnoses, health promotion diagnoses, and wellness diagnoses. An **actual nursing diagnosis** describes responses to health conditions or life processes that exist in an individual, family, or community. Defining characteristics (manifestations, signs, and symptoms) that cluster in patterns of related cues or inferences support this diagnostic judgement (NANDA International, 2021). The selection of an actual diagnosis indicates that sufficient assessment data are available to establish the nursing diagnosis. *Acute pain* is an actual nursing diagnosis. Prioritizing established nursing diagnoses is an important component of the nursing process.

A **risk nursing diagnosis** describes human responses to health conditions or life processes that will possibly develop in a vulnerable individual, family, or community (NANDA International, 2021). Such data include physiological, psychosocial, familial, lifestyle, and environmental factors that increase the patient's vulnerability to, or likelihood of, developing the condition.

A **health promotion nursing diagnosis** is a clinical judgement of a person's, family's, or community's motivation and desire to increase well-being and actualize human health potential, as expressed in their readiness to enhance specific health behaviours, such as those related to nutrition and exercise. Health promotion diagnoses can be used in any health state; they do not reflect current levels of wellness (NANDA International, 2021).

A **wellness nursing diagnosis** describes levels of wellness in an individual, family, or community that can be enhanced (NANDA International, 2021). It is a clinical judgement about an individual, group, or community in transition from a specific level of wellness to a higher level of wellness. Nurses select this type of diagnosis when the patient wishes to or has achieved an optimal level of health. For example, *readiness for enhanced coping related to successful cancer treatment* is a wellness diagnosis, and the nurse and the family unit work together to adapt to the stressors associated with cancer survivorship. In doing so, the nurse incorporates the patient's strengths and resources into a plan of care, with the outcome directed at improving the level of coping.

Components of a Nursing Diagnosis

The nursing diagnosis results from the assessment and diagnostic process. Throughout this text, nursing diagnoses are presented in a two-part format: the diagnostic label followed by the statement of a related factor. It is this two-part format that provides a diagnosis with meaning and relevance for a particular patient. In addition, all NANDA

TABLE 14.2	Comparison of Interventions for Nursing Diagnoses With Different Etiologies
Nursing Diagnoses	**Interventions**
Patient A	
Anxiety related to uncertainty over surgery	Provide detailed instructions about the surgical procedure, recovery process, and postoperative care activities. Plan formal time for patient to ask questions.
Deficient physical mobility related to acute pain	Administer analgesics 30 minutes before planned exercise. Instruct patient in technique to splint painful site during activity.
Patient B	
Anxiety related to loss of job	Consult with social work to arrange for job consulting. Encourage patient to continue health promotion activities (e.g., exercise, routine social activities).
Deficient physical mobility related to musculoskeletal injury	Have patient perform active range-of-motion exercises to affected extremity every 2 hours. Instruct patient on use of three-point crutch gait.

International–approved diagnoses have a definition. Risk factors are a component of all risk nursing diagnoses.

Diagnostic Label. The **diagnostic label** is the name of the nursing diagnosis as approved by NANDA International (2021). It describes the essence of a patient's response to health conditions in as few words as possible. Diagnostic labels include descriptors used to give additional meaning to the diagnosis. For example, the diagnosis *impaired physical mobility* includes the descriptor *impaired* to describe the nature or change in mobility that best describes the patient's response (Table 14.2). Examples of other descriptors are *compromised, decreased, deficient, delayed, effective, imbalanced, impaired,* and *increased*.

Related Factors. The **related factor** is a condition or **etiology** identified from the patient's assessment data. It is associated with the patient's actual or potential response to the health problem and can be changed through the use of nursing interventions. The inclusion of the "related to" phrase requires the nurse to use critical thinking skills to individualize the nursing diagnosis and then select nursing interventions (Figure 14.8). The origin or cause of the nursing diagnosis is always within the domain of nursing practice and a condition that responds to nursing interventions.

Sometimes health care providers record medical diagnoses as the etiology in the nursing diagnosis. This is incorrect. Nursing interventions do not change a medical diagnosis. However, nurses direct nursing interventions at behaviours or conditions that nurses are able to treat or manage. For example, the nursing diagnosis *acute pain related to herniated disc* is incorrect; nursing actions do not affect the medical diagnosis of a herniated disc. Instead, a diagnosis of *acute pain related to pressure on spinal nerves* results in nursing interventions directed at reducing stress on the vertebrae, improving body alignment, and offering nonpharmacological comfort measures.

Table 14.3 displays the association between a nurse's assessment of a patient, the clustering of defining characteristics, and the formulation

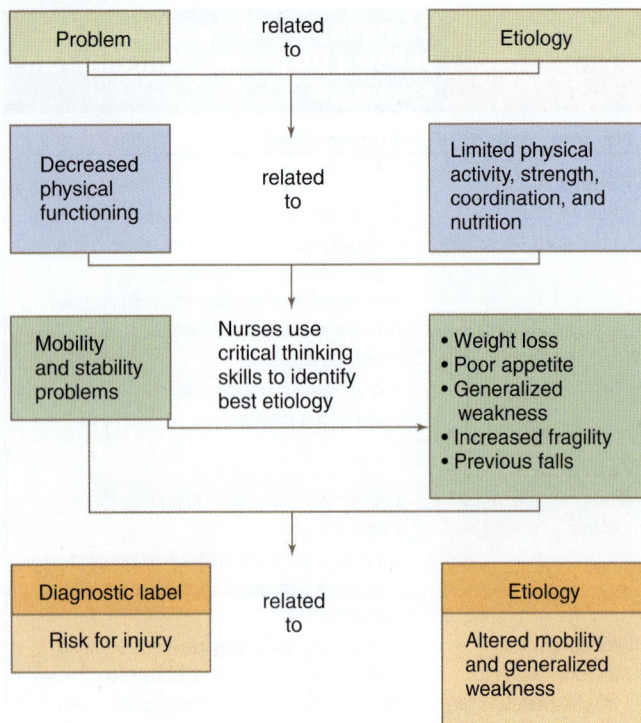

FIGURE 14.8 Relationship between a diagnostic label and an etiology (related factor). (Redrawn from Hickey, P. [1990]. *Nursing process handbook.* Mosby.)

of nursing diagnoses. The diagnostic process results in the formation of a total diagnostic label that enables a nurse to develop an appropriate **person-centred plan of care**. The defining characteristics and relevant etiologies are from NANDA International (2021).

Definition. NANDA International (2021) has approved a definition for each diagnosis that follows clinical use and testing. The definition describes the characteristics of the human response identified. For example, the definition of the diagnostic label *deficient physical mobility* is the "limitation in independent, purposeful physical movement of the body or of one or more extremities" (NANDA International, 2021). Nurses refer to definitions of nursing diagnoses to assist in identifying a patient's correct diagnosis.

Risk Factors. *Risk factors* are environmental, physiological, psychological, genetic, or chemical elements that increase the vulnerability of an individual, family, or community to an unhealthful event (NANDA International, 2021). They are a component of all risk nursing diagnoses. The risk factors are cues to indicate that a risk nursing diagnosis is applicable to a patient's condition. Examples of risk factors for the nursing diagnosis *risk for infection* include invasive procedures, trauma, malnutrition, immunosuppression, and insufficient knowledge to avoid exposure to pathogens. The risk factors help nurses select the correct risk diagnosis, similar to the manner in which defining characteristics help nurses formulate actual nursing diagnoses. In addition, risk factors are valuable in planning preventive nursing interventions.

Support of the Diagnostic Statement. Nursing assessment data must support the diagnostic label, and the related factors must be included in these data. To collect complete, relevant, and correct assessment data, it helps to identify assessment activities that produce specific kinds of data. For example, asking the patient about the quality and perception of pain elicits subjective data. However, if palpating an area elicits a facial grimace, that grimace is objective information. Likewise, asking a patient to describe the perception of an irregular heartbeat elicits subjective information, and using auscultation to obtain a pulse elicits an objective measurement of heart rate and rhythm. As nurses review assessment data, they look for clusters of defining characteristics and consider whether they have probed and assessed the patient accurately and thoroughly to gather a complete database.

CONCEPT MAPPING FOR NURSING DIAGNOSES

Figure 14.9 demonstrates a method for concept mapping a patient's nursing diagnosis using the case study presented at the start of this chapter. While this specific concept map demonstrates nursing diagnosis, it is also important to review other medical and collaborative problems that may influence patient care. Laboratory values and diagnostic testing for patient care may support both medical and nursing diagnosis that will be used in care planning. In the following example of how nurses engage critical thinking in the diagnostic process, Figure 14.5 is used as a template:

After assessing Mr. Fletcher, Irene, the registered nurse, recognizes that there are several areas for diagnosis coming forward for

TABLE 14.3   Defining Characteristics and Etiologies to Confirm Nursing Diagnoses

Assessment Activities	Defining Characteristics (Clustering Cues)	Nursing Diagnosis	Etiology ("Related to")
Ask patient to rate severity of pain on a scale of 0 to 10.	Patient verbally reports pain at a level of 8 or 9 when it becomes sharp.	Acute pain	Physical pressure on spinal nerves
Observe patient's positioning in bed.	Patient bends knees while on back to lessen pain.		
Ask whether patient has difficulty falling asleep or awakens at night from pain.	Patient reports feeling tired, awakens easily.	Acute pain	Physical pressure on spinal nerves
Observe for any nonverbal signs of discomfort.	Patient moans and sighs when attempting to find comfortable position in bed.		
Observe patient's eye contact when patient is talking.	Patient has poor eye contact when discussing surgery. Patient is restless.	Anxiety	Threat to health status as a result of surgery
Observe patient's body language.	Patient is uncertain about what to expect after surgery and the outcome of surgery.		
Ask patient to describe feelings about surgery.			
Give instruction on topic of interest, and return in 15 minutes to measure retention.	Patient forgets details of explanation.	Anxiety	Threat to health status as a result of surgery

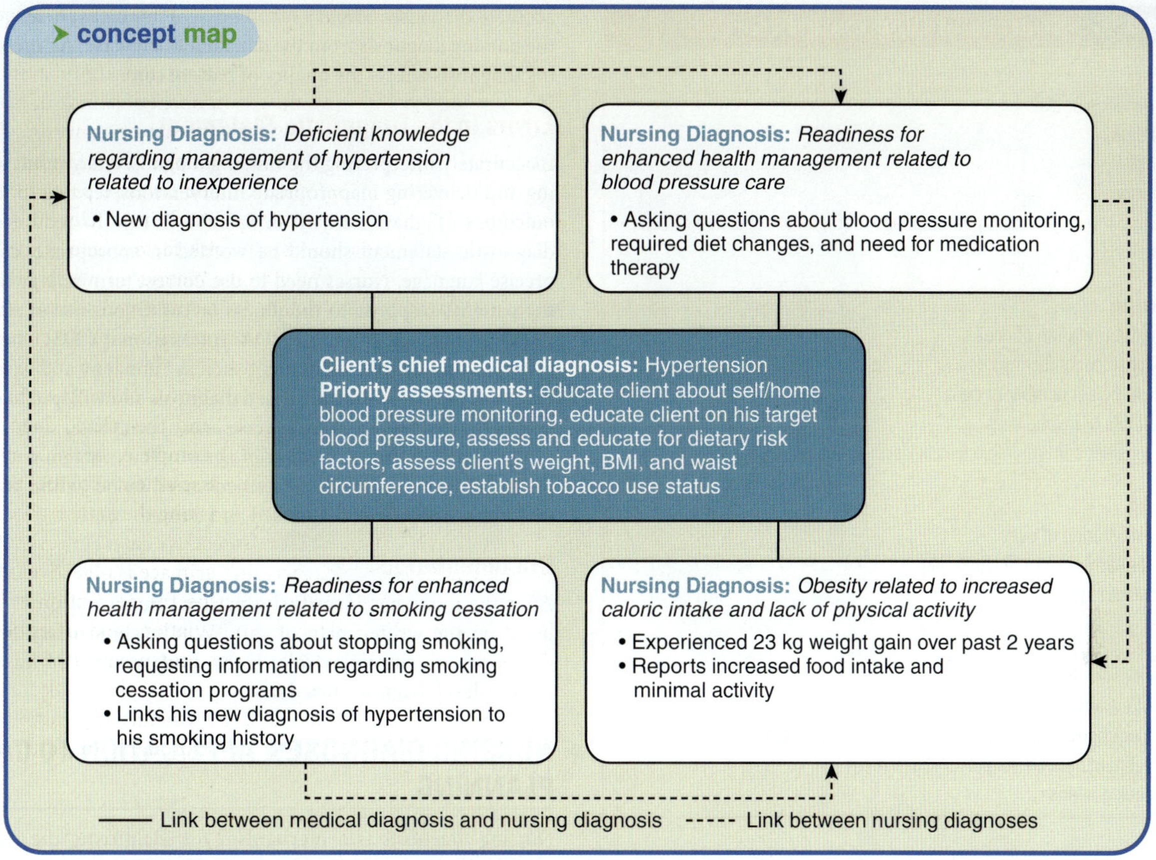

> concept map

Nursing Diagnosis: *Deficient knowledge regarding management of hypertension related to inexperience*

• New diagnosis of hypertension

Nursing Diagnosis: *Readiness for enhanced health management related to blood pressure care*

• Asking questions about blood pressure monitoring, required diet changes, and need for medication therapy

Client's chief medical diagnosis: Hypertension
Priority assessments: educate client about self/home blood pressure monitoring, educate client on his target blood pressure, assess and educate for dietary risk factors, assess client's weight, BMI, and waist circumference, establish tobacco use status

Nursing Diagnosis: *Readiness for enhanced health management related to smoking cessation*

• Asking questions about stopping smoking, requesting information regarding smoking cessation programs
• Links his new diagnosis of hypertension to his smoking history

Nursing Diagnosis: *Obesity related to increased caloric intake and lack of physical activity*

• Experienced 23 kg weight gain over past 2 years
• Reports increased food intake and minimal activity

——— Link between medical diagnosis and nursing diagnosis   ----- Link between nursing diagnoses

FIGURE 14.9 Concept map for Mr. Fletcher's nursing diagnoses. *BMI,* Body mass index.

the patient within both collaborative and nursing diagnostic frameworks. At this time, Irene decides to defer the potential signs of peripheral arterial disease to the health care provider or nurse practitioner and notes it as a collaborative concern on the patient record. She turns her attention to the nursing diagnosis related to Mr. Fletcher's primary concern of hypertension.

Knowledge: Mr. Fletcher's blood pressure is considered high according to clinical guidelines. While is it not in Irene's scope of practice to prescribe medications for the management of hypertension (she notes this as a priority for the health care provider), she continues her assessment to further outline how Mr. Fletcher's lifestyle, weight, diet, exercise, alcohol intake, smoking, and stress may be leading to his hypertension.

Standards: Irene accesses Hypertension Canada's "2020 Comprehensive Guidelines for the Prevention, Diagnosis, Risk Assessment, and Treatment of Hypertension in Adults and Children" (Rabi et al., 2020) to guide her assessment and formulation of the nursing diagnosis. These guidelines provide useful processes to focus her questioning and help direct her plan of nursing care. She also realizes that it would be helpful to follow a self-management framework with Mr. Fletcher because hypertension is considered a chronic health condition.

Qualities: Irene uses therapeutic techniques to ascertain more assessment information from Mr. Fletcher. She actively listens to his responses and focuses her questions on areas that require more information. She does not judge Mr. Fletcher for his weight gain or smoking. Instead, Irene assists him in linking these behaviours to his hypertension and seeks to understand how other social determinants of health or coping practices may be influencing these specific behaviours.

Experience: Irene has learned that the initial interview is of primary importance for helping the patient. It has allowed her to assess Mr. Fletcher's readiness for health behaviour change. It has also enabled her to connect Mr. Fletcher to important community resources that will help him learn more about his hypertension and develop successful strategies for self-care.

SOURCES OF DIAGNOSTIC ERRORS

Errors occur in the nursing diagnostic process during data collection, interpretation and analysis, and clustering, and in the statement of the diagnosis. Nurses must apply methodical critical thinking so that the nursing diagnostic process is accurate.

Errors in Data Collection

To avoid errors in data collection, nurses should be knowledgeable and skilled in all assessment techniques (Box 14.5). It is vital to check for inaccurate or missing data and to collect data in an organized way. The following practice tips are essential for nursing students to learn in order to avoid data collection errors:

• Review your level of comfort and competence with interview and physical assessment skills before you begin data collection.
• Approach assessment in steps. Focus on completing a patient interview before starting a physical examination. Perhaps focus on only one body system in order to learn how to gather a complete assessment. Then move to a more complex head-to-toe examination.
• Review your clinical assessments in clinical or classroom settings. They will provide you with a constructive learning opportunity to determine how to revise an assessment or to gather additional information.

BOX 14.5   Sources of Diagnostic Error

Collecting

Lack of knowledge or skill

Inaccurate data

Missing data

Disorganization

Stereotyping patients or making assumptions that lead to collection of selective data

Interpreting

Inaccurate interpretation of cues

Failure to consider conflicting cues

Using an insufficient number of cues

Using unreliable or invalid cues

Failure to consider cultural influences or developmental stage

Clustering

Insufficient clustering of cues

Premature or early closure of clustering

Incorrect clustering

Labelling

Wrong diagnostic label selected

Existence of evidence that another diagnosis is more likely

Condition incorrectly overlooked as a collaborative problem

Failure to validate nursing diagnosis with patient

Failure to seek guidance

- Determine the accuracy of your data. For example, when you auscultate abnormal lung sounds for the first time, be sure of what you hear through the stethoscope. To minimize the risk of inaccuracy, have a more experienced co-worker validate your findings or explain why they are incorrect. Validate your assessment data by double-checking and verifying them.
- Be organized in any examination. Have the appropriate forms and examination equipment ready to use. Be sure the environment is private, quiet, and comfortable for the patient.

Errors in Interpretation and Analysis of Data

After data collection, nurses will review the database to decide whether it is accurate and complete. Data are reviewed to confirm that measurable, objective physical findings support subjective data. For example, when a patient reports "difficulty breathing," the nurse listens to lung sounds, assesses respiratory rate and oxygen saturation, and measures the patient's chest excursion. The nurse needs to consider any conflicting cues or decide whether cues are insufficient for formulating a diagnosis. Factors such as a patient's developmental stage, for example, may influence how the nurse interprets the meaning of cues.

Errors in Data Clustering

Errors in data clustering occur when data are clustered prematurely or incorrectly or are not clustered at all. Premature closure of clustering occurs when nurses make the nursing diagnosis before grouping all data. For example, the nurse learns that a patient has had urinary incontinence and complains of urgency and nocturia. The available data are clustered, and *ineffective urinary elimination* is considered a probable diagnosis. However, incorrect clustering occurs when nurses try to make the nursing diagnosis fit the signs and symptoms obtained. In this example, further assessment reveals the patient has bladder distension and dribbling, and the condition is probably overflow incontinence. As a result of these findings, the nurse is able to make a more accurate diagnosis: *urinary retention.* It is important to always identify the nursing diagnosis from the data, not the reverse. An incorrect nursing diagnosis affects the quality of patient care.

Errors in the Diagnostic Statement

Inaccurately interpreting the nursing diagnosis may result in developing and delivering inappropriate interventions, leading to undesirable outcomes (Taghavi Larijani & Saatchi, 2019). To reduce errors, the diagnostic statement should be worded in appropriate, concise, and precise language. Nurses need to use correct terminology that reflects the patient's response to the illness or condition. Use of standardized nursing language from NANDA International (2021) helps ensure accuracy. A diagnostic statement such as "unhappy and worried about health" is not a scientifically based diagnosis and will lead to errors. The language needs to be more precise and appropriate, such as *impaired coping related to fear of medical diagnosis.* The problem and etiological portions of the diagnostic statement need to be within the scope of nursing in order to be diagnosed and treated.

Documentation

After the nurse has identified a patient's nursing diagnoses, they are listed on the written plan of care. Within clinical facilities, nursing diagnoses are chronologically listed as they are identified, with the highest-level diagnosis listed first.

◆ NURSING DIAGNOSES: APPLICATION TO CARE PLANNING

Nursing diagnosis is a mechanism for identifying the nursing care needed to address patients' health problems. Diagnoses provide direction for the planning process and the selection of nursing interventions to achieve desired outcomes for patients. Just as the medical diagnosis of *diabetes* guides a health care provider to prescribe a low-carbohydrate diet and medication for blood glucose control, the nursing diagnosis of *reduced skin integrity* directs a nurse to apply certain support surfaces to a patient's bed and to initiate a turning schedule. In the next section, which focuses on the planning phase of the nursing process, you will learn how to unify the language of NANDA International with the Nursing Interventions Classification (NIC) and Nursing Outcomes Classification (NOC) to help facilitate the process of matching nursing diagnoses with accurate and appropriate interventions and outcomes. The care plan is a map for nursing care and demonstrates the nurse's accountability for patient care. Accurate nursing diagnosis will assist in communicating to other health care providers the patient's health care issues and will help to guide the planning of relevant and appropriate nursing interventions.

◆ PLANNING

After a nurse identifies a patient's nursing diagnoses and strengths, the nurse, in consultation with the patient and health care team, will begin planning nursing care. Planning is a category of nursing behaviour in which a nurse sets person-centered goals, outlines expected outcomes, plans nursing interventions, and prioritizes and selects interventions that will resolve the patient's problems and achieve the goals and outcomes. Planning requires critical thinking, applied through deliberate decision making and problem solving, to set priorities for a patient. Many patients have multiple diagnoses and a number of health concerns. Successful planning requires the nurse to collaborate with the patient and caregivers, consult with other members of the health care team, and review related literature. This literature includes available evidence related to the patient's health problems and concerns. A plan of care is dynamic and will change once the patient's needs are met or new needs are identified.

ESTABLISHING PRIORITIES

Priority setting is the ranking of nursing diagnoses or patient problems, using principles such as urgency or importance, to establish a preferential order for nursing actions (Doenges et al., 2019; Figure 14.10). By ranking nursing diagnoses in order of importance, nurses attend to the patient's most important needs first. Priorities help the nurse to anticipate and sequence nursing interventions for a patient who has multiple nursing diagnoses and health problems. When feasible, nurses and patients select mutually agreed-upon priorities based on the urgency of the problems, safety, the nature of the treatment indicated, and the relationship among the diagnoses.

Establishing priorities or determining the urgency of the identified health problems is done on the basis of their severity or physiological importance (Lewis et al., 2019). Nursing diagnoses of conditions that, if left untreated, will result in harm to the patient or others have the highest priorities. For example, *risk for other-directed violence, impaired gas exchange*, and *decreased cardiac output* are typically high-priority nursing diagnoses that raise issues of safety, adequate oxygenation, and adequate circulation. *High priorities* are sometimes both physiological and psychological and may address other basic human needs. *Intermediate priority* nursing diagnoses involve the nonemergency, non–life-threatening needs of the patient. *Low-priority* nursing diagnoses are not always directly related to a specific illness or prognosis but affect the patient's future well-being. Many low-priority diagnoses focus on the patient's long-term health care needs. The order of priorities changes as a patient's condition changes, sometimes within a matter of minutes. Ongoing patient assessment is essential for determining the priority of the patient's nursing diagnoses.

Nurses prioritize the specific interventions or strategies used in order to help a patient achieve desired goals and outcomes. It is important to involve the patient in priority setting whenever possible; in some situations, the nurse and the patient have different priorities.

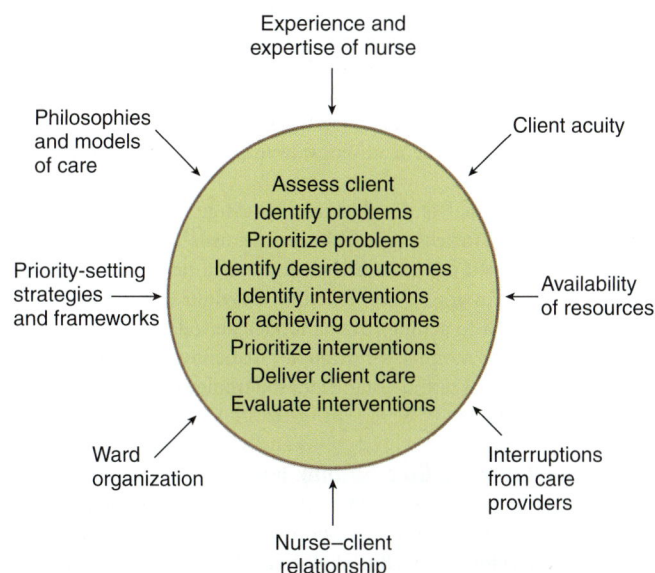

FIGURE 14.10 A model for priority setting. (Adapted from Hendry, C., & Walker, A. [2004]. Priority setting in clinical nursing practice. *Journal of Advanced Nursing, 47*[4], 427–436.)

CRITICAL THINKING IN ESTABLISHING GOALS AND EXPECTED OUTCOMES

Goals and expected outcomes are specific patient behaviours or physiological responses that nurses set to achieve through nursing diagnosis or collaborative problem resolution. They provide a clear focus for the type of interventions necessary to care for the patient.

Planning nursing care requires critical thinking (Figure 14.11). Nurses need to carefully evaluate the identified nursing diagnoses, the urgency of the problems, and the resources of the patient and the health care delivery system. They apply knowledge from the nursing, medical, and sociobehavioural sciences to plan patient care. To select goals, expected outcomes, and interventions, nurses must consider their previous experience with similar patient problems, as well as any established standards for nursing practice.

The diagram in Figure 14.12 illustrates the relationships between nursing diagnoses, goals, expected outcomes, and nursing interventions. To help you understand the role of critical thinking in establishing goals and expected outcomes, we return to Mr. Fletcher's case scenario and outline how the nurse uses this process in the planning of care:

Irene begins planning with Mr. Fletcher how to control and improve his hypertension. Knowing that hypertension is a chronic disease condition, Irene recognizes that Mr. Fletcher will need to be involved in his care and that he needs to help set the expected outcomes for his care.

Knowledge: *Irene needs to educate Mr. Fletcher on the following key aspects related to his hypertension: (1) how to recognize hypertension using clinical parameters, (2) how to monitor his blood pressure, (3) how to identify potential modifiable risk factors, and (4) how to recognize complications. Irene is aware that Mr. Fletcher is dealing with a new diagnosis and that she will need to prioritize and simplify the information given to him. It is likely that the health care provider will prescribe antihypertensive medication to Mr. Fletcher. In this case, Irene will work collaboratively to set goals for patient outcomes resulting from medication therapy.*

Standards: *Irene uses the Hypertension Canada 2020 guidelines (Rabi et al., 2020) to help formulate her teaching plan. She decides to focus on educating Mr. Fletcher about self and home blood pressure monitoring techniques and the appropriate equipment to use to assist in monitoring his hypertension. She will also use these guidelines to plan her educational strategies to guide Mr. Fletcher in optimizing a target blood pressure. She will work with him to identify lifestyle factors that may be contributing to his hypertension.*

Qualities: *Irene takes a person-centred approach in planning nursing care. She has developed a therapeutic relationship with Mr. Fletcher and will use both direct and indirect nursing interventions, accessing collaborative supports as required in her care planning.*

Experience: *For previous patients with newly diagnosed hypertension, Irene has found it helpful to teach them to take their blood pressure at home and to keep a log. This enables patients to see trends in their blood pressure throughout the day and to keep track of any symptoms that may be occurring for them. Irene has also found that including the patient's partner or spouse and/or family in this education has led to increased understanding and practise of the proposed strategies. Irene will set person-centred goals that are both short and long term.*

Goals of Care

A person-centred goal is a specific and measurable behavioural response that reflects a patient's highest possible level of wellness and

KNOWLEDGE
Client's database and selected nursing diagnoses
Anatomy and physiology
Pathophysiology
Normal growth and development
Evidence-informed nursing interventions
Role of other health care disciplines
Community resources
Family dynamics
Teaching and learning process
Delegation principles
Priority-setting principles

EXPERIENCE
Previous client care experience
Personal experience in
organizing activities

NURSING PROCESS
Assessment
Evaluation   Diagnosis
Implementation   Planning

STANDARDS
CNA
Specialty standards of practice
Client-centred goals and outcomes
Intellectual standards

QUALITIES
Creativity
Responsibility
Perseverance
Discipline

FIGURE 14.11 Critical thinking and the process of planning care. *CNA,* Canadian Nurses Association.

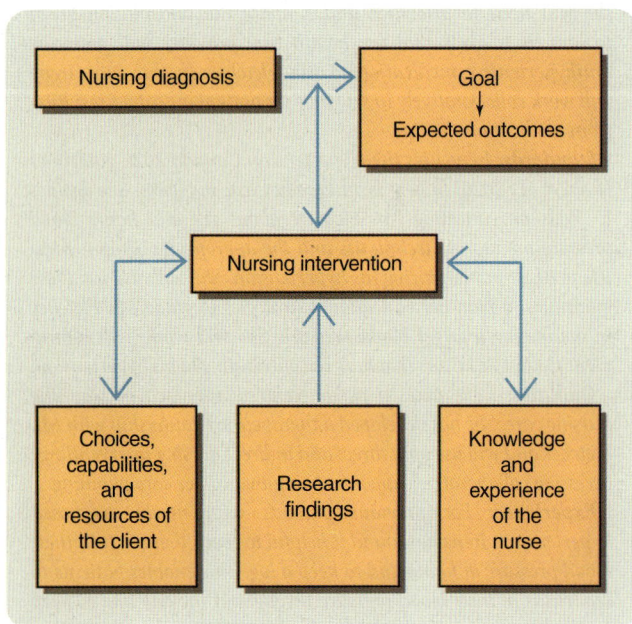

FIGURE 14.12 From diagnosis to outcome. (Revised and redrawn from Gordon, M. [1994]. *Nursing diagnosis: Process and application* [3rd ed.]. Mosby.)

independence in function. Examples are "Patient will perform self-care hygiene independently" and "Patient will remain free of infection." A goal is realistic and based on patient needs and resources. A patient goal represents predicted resolution of a nursing diagnosis or health problem, proof of progress toward resolution, enhanced improved health status, or continued maintenance of optimal health (Carpenito, 2017). A goal involves only one behaviour or response. The example "Patient will administer a self-injection and demonstrate infection control measures" is incorrect because the statement includes two different behaviours: "administer" and "demonstrate." Instead, the goal should be worded as follows: "Patient will administer a self-injection." The specific criteria you use to measure the success of the goal are the expected outcomes: for example, "Patient will prepare medication dose correctly" and "Patient uses aseptic technique when preparing injection site." Each goal is time limited so that the health care team has a common time frame for problem resolution. The time frame depends on the nature of the problem, etiology, overall condition of the patient, and treatment setting.

A **short-term goal** is an objective behaviour or response that a patient is expected to achieve in a short time, usually less than a week. In an acute care setting, goals are set for over a period of just a few hours. A **long-term goal** is an objective behaviour or response that a patient is expected to achieve over a longer period, usually over several days, weeks, or months: for example, "Patient will be tobacco-free within 60 days." Goal setting establishes the framework for the nursing care plan (Table 14.4).

Role of the Patient in Goal Setting. It is important to work closely with patients in setting goals. Mutual goal setting is an activity that includes patients and families in prioritizing the goals of care and in developing plans for action (Bulechek et al., 2019). Patients need to be able to engage in problem solving and decision making to participate effectively in goal setting. Goals that are determined with the patient and have a clear action plan are more likely to be successful.

TABLE 14.4	Examples of Goal Setting With Expected Outcomes	
Nursing Diagnosis	**Goal**	**Expected Outcomes**
Acute pain related to pressure on spinal nerves	Patient's level of comfort will improve before surgery.	Patient will be able to turn without reported discomfort in 2 hours. Patient's self-report of pain will be 3 or less on a scale of 0 to 10 by the time of scheduled surgery.
Anxiety related to uncertainty over surgery	Patient will accept plan for surgical care before scheduled surgery.	Patient will express less uneasiness about surgical experience in next 4 hours.
Deficient knowledge regarding postoperative activities related to inexperience	Patient will understand treatment procedures planned postoperatively within 4 hours.	Patient will describe purpose of postoperative exercises prior to scheduled surgery. Patient will demonstrate use of incentive spirometer and deep breathing and coughing prior to scheduled surgery. Patient will explain purpose of postoperative nursing care prior to scheduled surgery.
Impaired physical mobility related to acute back pain	Patient will move independently in bed before surgery.	Patient will initiate turning without additional discomfort within 2 hours. Patient will position self for care procedures within 2 hours.

Expected Outcomes

An *expected outcome* is a specific measurable change in a patient's status that is expected in response to nursing care. Expected outcomes provide a focus or direction for nursing care because they are the desired physiological, psychological, social, developmental, or spiritual responses that indicate resolution of patients' health problems. Derived from both short- and long-term goals, outcomes determine when a specific person-centred goal has been met.

Usually, several expected outcomes for each nursing diagnosis and goal are listed. The reason for the multiple expected outcomes is that sometimes one nursing action is not enough to resolve a specific problem. In addition, the listing of the step-by-step expected outcomes assists in planning interventions. The nurse should write expected outcomes sequentially, specifying time frames for each. Time frames provide progressive steps to recovery and assist in ranking nursing interventions. In addition, time frames set limits for problem resolution.

The nurse should also write expected outcome statements in measurable terms. This enables the nurse to note the specific behaviour or physiological response expected for resolution of the problem. For example, "Patient will have less pain" is an inaccurate outcome statement because the phrase "less pain" is nonspecific. The statement "Patient will report pain acuity of less than 3 on a scale of 0 to 10" is accurate.

Nursing Outcomes Classification (NOC). In the current health care environment, considerable attention is paid to measuring outcomes sensitive to nursing interventions. Many health care administrators focus on outcomes in determining staffing and other resources in health care settings. The Iowa Intervention Project published the NOC and has linked the outcomes to the NANDA International (2021) nursing diagnoses (University of Iowa College of Nursing, 2021). The Iowa researchers defined a nursing-sensitive patient outcome as an individual, family, or community behaviour or perception that is measurable along a continuum in response to a nursing intervention. For any given NANDA International nursing diagnosis, multiple outcomes are suggested in the NOC. These outcomes provide descriptions of the focus of nursing care and include indicators for measuring success with interventions (Table 14.5).

Combining Goals and Outcome Statements

Nurses within health care settings may refer to the terms, goals, and outcomes interchangeably. This is acceptable as long as the criteria for writing goals and outcomes are met. For example, the statement "Patient will achieve pain control as evidenced by reporting pain acuity of less than 3 on a scale of 0 to 10 within 24 hours" is an acceptable statement. The goal portion of the statement broadly describes the

TABLE 14.5	Examples of NANDA International Nursing Diagnoses and Suggested NOC Linkages	
Nursing Diagnosis	**Suggested NOC-Based Outcomes (Examples)**	**Outcome Indicators (Examples)**
Deficient knowledge	Knowledge: treatment procedures	Description of treatment procedure Description of steps in procedure
	Patient satisfaction: teaching	Explanations provided in understandable terms Explanation of activity restrictions
Activity intolerance	Activity tolerance	Oxygen saturation with activity Pulse rate with activity Respiratory rate with activity
	Self-care status	Bathes self Dresses self Prepares food and fluid for eating

NOC, Nursing Outcomes Classification.

desired patient status ("achieve pain control"), and the outcome portion of the statement contains the observable criterion ("3 on a [pain] scale") needed to measure success.

Guidelines for Writing Goals and Expected Outcomes

There are seven guidelines for writing goals and expected outcomes: patient centred, singular, observable, measurable, time limited, mutual, and realistic.

Patient-Centred Goal or Outcome. Outcomes and goals reflect patient responses that are expected after nursing interventions. The nurse should write a goal to reflect patient behaviour, not to reflect the nurse's goals or interventions. A correct outcome statement is "Patient will ambulate in the hall three times a day." A common error is to write "Ambulate patient in the hall three times a day."

Singular Goal or Outcome. The nurse should be precise in evaluating a patient response to a nursing action. Each goal and outcome addresses only one behaviour or response.

Observable Goal or Outcome. Nurses need to be able to observe whether change in a patient's status occurs. Changes in physiological findings and in the patient's knowledge, perceptions, and behaviour are observable. Nurses observe outcomes by directly asking patients about their condition and by using assessment skills. For the outcome "Chest sounds will be clear on auscultation by 8/31," the nurse would auscultate the patient's chest routinely after therapy (e.g., inhalation, percussion). The outcome statement "Patient will appear less anxious" is not a correct statement because no specific behaviour for "will appear" is observable.

Measurable Goal or Outcome. It is imperative to learn to write goals and expected outcomes that set standards against which to measure the patient's response to nursing care. Examples such as "Body temperature will remain between the normal range of 36.5 and 37.5°C" and "Apical pulse will remain between 60 and 100 beats per minute" enable the nurse to objectively measure changes in the patient's status.

Time-Limited Goal or Outcome. The time frame for each goal and expected outcome indicates when the expected response should occur. Time frames assist in determining progress toward goals and outcomes.

Mutual Goal or Outcome. Mutually set goals and expected outcomes ensure that the patient and nurse agree on the direction and time limits of care. Mutual goal setting increases patients' motivation and cooperation.

Realistic Goal or Outcome. It is important to set goals and expected outcomes that are achievable. Patients are then more likely to feel a sense of empowerment, which increases their motivation and cooperation. In order to establish realistic goals, the nurse needs to assess the resources of the patient, the family, the health care facility, and the community. The nurse should also be aware of the patient's physiological, emotional, cognitive, and sociocultural influences and take into consideration the patient's determinants of health.

WRITTEN PLANS OF CARE

In any health care setting, a nurse is responsible for developing a written plan of care for patients. The written plan of care may take several forms (e.g., a nursing card-filing system, standardized care plans, or computerized plans). In general, a written **nursing care plan** includes nursing diagnoses; goals; expected outcomes, or both; and specific nursing interventions. This format allows any nurse to quickly identify a patient's clinical needs and situation. In hospitals and community-based settings, the patient often receives care from more than one nurse, health care provider, or allied health provider. A written nursing care plan makes possible continuity and coordination of nursing care and consultation by a number of health care providers.

Written care plans organize information exchanged by nurses in change-of-shift reports (see Chapter 17 for further information about nursing informatics). Nurses learn to focus their reports on the nursing care, treatments, and expected outcomes documented in their care plans, and the end-of-shift report allows for discussion of care plans and the overall progress with the next caregiver.

Institutional Care Plans

Institutional care plans become part of a patient's legal medical record. Many hospitals still use a written Kardex nursing care plan. The **Kardex** card-filing system allows quick reference to the needs of the patient for certain aspects of nursing care (see Chapter 16 for further information about documentation). The care plan section of a Kardex system

varies by employer and focuses on planned interventions to meet the needs of the patient and family and prepare the patient for discharge from the hospital. The focus of a nursing care plan differs by setting and the evolving patient situation. For example, nursing care plans developed for patients returning home are usually based solely on long-term health needs. Nursing care plans for same-day surgeries are usually focused on patients' short-term needs (e.g., immediate recovery from surgery and instructions for self-care at home). In a long-term care facility, plans of care focus on patients' long-term rehabilitation needs.

Computerized Care Plans. A majority of health care facilities now have some type of electronic health record (EHR) and documentation system (Canada Health Infoway, 2021). Software programs are available for nursing care plans. In many facilities, standardized care plans have a list of generalized nursing diagnoses, goals, outcome criteria, and interventions for specific patients. The nurse adds or deletes information by making selections from menus on the standardized form to tailor it to a patient's needs. Computerized and standardized nursing care plans organize and enhance care planning. Their design incorporates current evidence-informed practice guidelines to achieve the desired patient outcomes for a specific group of patients.

Care Plans for Community-Based Settings. Planning care for patients in community-based settings—for example, clinics, community centres, or patients' homes—involves using the same principles of nursing practice. In these settings, however, nurses need to complete a more comprehensive community, home, and family assessment. The patient or family unit must be able to provide the majority of health care independently or with the help of external resources provided to meet care demands (see Chapter 4 for further information about community health).

Critical Pathways. **Critical pathways** are interprofessional treatment plans that outline the treatments or interventions that patients may require for treatment of a condition. Most pathways are based on medical rather than nursing diagnoses, but they incorporate related nursing diagnoses and associated nursing interventions. A critical pathway maps out, day to day or even hour to hour, the recommended interventions and expected outcomes. For example, a pathway for a surgical procedure such as a bowel resection will recommend on a day-by-day basis the patient's activities, procedures, and discharge planning activities. A critical pathway improves continuity of care because it clearly maps out the responsibility of each health discipline and can be used to monitor a patient's progress. Well-developed pathways incorporate current evidence in caring for patients with a specific condition. When critical pathways are used to plan care, some forms of documentation are eliminated (e.g., the nursing care plan, flow sheets, and nurses' notes) because all of the pertinent components are included in the pathway.

CONSULTING OTHER HEALTH CARE PROVIDERS

Planning involves consultation with members of the health care team. Although consultation can occur at any step in the nursing process, it occurs most often during planning and implementation, when problems necessitating additional knowledge, skills, or resources arise. A **consultation** involves seeking the expertise of a specialist, such as a nurse educator, registered nurse, or clinical nurse specialist, to identify ways of approaching and managing the planning and implementation of therapies.

Nurse consultants frequently offer advice about difficult clinical problems. For example, a nursing student will consult with the registered nurse assigned to the same patient about ways to individualize interventions, with a clinical specialist for wound care techniques, or with an educator for useful teaching resources. Nurses are consulted for their clinical expertise, patient education skills, or staff education skills. Nurses also consult with other members of the health care team, such as physiotherapists, dietitians, and social workers.

SUMMARY

This chapter has outlined how the nurse approaches assessment, diagnosis, and planning within the nursing process. It is important to remember that nursing practice is complex, dynamic, and at times unpredictable; nurses must be able to prioritize, predict changes in patients' health status, and adapt to new situations as necessary. While nurses use models of care, such as the nursing process, as a beginning structure for approaching, organizing, implementing, and evaluating care, it is their critical thinking and holistic approaches to patient care that help to provide safe, informed, and comprehensive patient care. The next chapter approaches care planning in more detail and discusses the intervention and evaluation stages of the nursing process.

USING THE NURSING PROCESS TO ENHANCE TEST-TAKING SKILLS IN NURSING PROGRAMS

The nursing process is an essential model for helping nursing students understand how nursing care unfolds. It is also a valuable tool to use when learning how to study for and take nursing exams. By understanding the nursing process in full, a nursing student can quickly determine what an exam question is asking and what the most logical answer or next step will be. It is important to speak to the role of the nursing process in exam-taking because nursing students will be evaluated in their nursing programs through exams and on graduation by writing a registration exam for nursing licensure.

The nursing process can be used to organize your studying approach to nursing exams. In Chapter 15 (Implementing and Evaluating Nursing Care), a comprehensive approach to studying using the nursing process is described. In that chapter, we speak to how the nursing process is used in examinations. The focus in this chapter is the assessment, diagnosis (often referred to as *analysis* in exam frameworks), and planning stages of the nursing process. The implementation and evaluation stages of the nursing process will be identified in Chapter 15.

The purpose of nursing exams is to test your ability to recall information, apply information to nursing-specific situations, and learn to think critically using multiple sources of knowledge. Nursing practice requires problem solving that uses critical thinking and decision-making processes—often referred collectively as *clinical judgement* (National Council of State Boards of Nursing, 2021). Many nursing students rely on study strategies that emphasize the memorization of nursing knowledge instead of learning how to apply knowledge to practice situations. *How* you study nursing content is just as important as *what* you are studying.

The nursing process can also be used to help guide your thinking while taking nursing exams. It is important to determine which phase of the nursing process is being tested in each exam question and to understand what the question is asking you to do with the information provided in the question stem. There are several ways that a nursing student can determine this information. You can begin by reflecting on common words that are often present in the stem of the question when you are being asked about the different parts of the nursing process (Nugent & Vitale, 2020). This will help you understand exactly which part of the nursing process (assessment, diagnosis, planning, intervention, or evaluation) the question is speaking to (Table 14.6). When you approach an exam question, engage in the following steps (Kramer-Kile, 2016):

TABLE 14.6 Using the Nursing Process to Help Answer Exam Questions

Nursing Process	Questions in This Stage of the Nursing Process Often Ask You to:	Common Words in the Question Stem Identifying This Area
Assessment	• Perform an assessment technique • Obtain vital signs • Recognize normal and abnormal findings or values • Take a health history • Explore patient feelings • Review diagnostic tests • Review or access a consultation from another health care provider	Inspect, identify, verify, observe, determine, notify, check, inform, question, communicate, verbal and nonverbal, signs and symptoms, stressors, adaptations, sources, perceptions, and assess
Diagnosis	• Clustering data • Determine priorities in data collection • Identifying further data that need to be examined • Interpreting data in the context of illness	Organize, categorize, re-examine, pattern, formulate, nursing diagnosis, reflect, relate, problem, interpret, contribute, related, decision, significant, deduction, statement, analysis
Planning	• Involve the patient in the planning process • Set goals • Establish expected outcomes against which results of care can be compared for the purpose of evaluation • Plan appropriate interventions based on their effects • Establish priorities of nursing interventions • Anticipate patient needs • Collaborate with others • Coordinate planned care with other disciplines • Recognize that plans must be flexible and modified on the basis of changing patient needs	Achieve, desired, plan, effective, desired result, goal, priority, develop, formulate, establish, design, prevent, strategy, select, determine, anticipate, modify, collaborate, arrange, coordinate, expect, outcome

From Kramer-Kile, M. L. (2016). *Transitioning to the NCLEX-RN®: A study guide for Canadian-educated graduates* (2nd ed.). Kramer-Kile Nurse Education Consultants Ltd. Registration No. 1122832. Reprinted with permission.

Step 1: Identify which phase of the nursing process is being addressed in the question stem. You can do this by isolating the verbs in the question stem and determining what the question is asking the nurse to do (see Table 14.6).

Step 2: Determine what the question is asking. Are you being asked to explore a part of the nursing process or to go to the next step? Are you supposed to prioritize among answers that are all correct? Or are you choosing the best answer, knowing that other answers may be incorrect?

Step 3: Link the potential answers back to the question stem and information provided. Are they appropriate with respect to the information you have been given? Are they compatible with the stage of the nursing process that you have identified?

The following are examples of multiple-choice questions focused on assessment, diagnosis, and planning.

Example: The nurse identifies that a patient's heart rate is 48 beats per minute per radial pulse. What is an appropriate next step for the nurse to take in this situation?

1. Call the health care provider immediately.
2. Take a blood pressure.
3. Auscultate the apical pulse.
4. Determine whether the patient is on beta-blocker therapy.

The correct answer is 3. In this question, the nurse is in the assessment phase of the nursing process. The nurse has collected data and is now moving toward the next step, data verification. To verify that the low radial pulse is 48 beats per minute, the nurse takes an apical pulse to confirm the rate. Calling the health care provider at this time is not appropriate because they would ask the nurse to verify the data. Determining whether the patient is on beta-blocker therapy would help the nurse to interpret potential assessment findings, but again, the question already states that the pulse was collected using the radial site. Again, the patient's actual heart rate needs to be verified through a more specific assessment, which is auscultating the patient's apical pulse.

Example: A patient with Alzheimer's disease is admitted to the hospital pale, lethargic, and unable to stand unassisted. His wife states he is refusing to eat or drink. Which of the following nursing diagnoses is the highest priority for this patient?

1. Adult failure to thrive
2. Risk for activity intolerance
3. Risk for caregiver strain
4. Interrupted family processes

The correct answer is 1. In this question, the patient is exhibiting assessment findings associated with failure to thrive. Although family processes, caregiver strain, and activity intolerance are also valid

diagnoses to make, these all stem from the larger problem of failure to thrive. Remember that questions on nursing diagnosis will ask you to analyze the assessment information provided to you. When you are studying nursing diagnosis, instead of attempting to memorize approved diagnoses, think about how each diagnosis would present in a patient case. This will help you to further understand the role of diagnosis (i.e., analysis) in nursing care.

Example: A 60-year-old female patient with 7/10 pain is scheduled for a lumbar laminectomy in 2 hours owing to a ruptured disc. What is an appropriate goal for the nurse to set for the patient?

1. The patient will learn deep breathing and coughing exercises before the surgery.
2. The patient will repeat the purpose of their surgery to the nurse.
3. The patient will achieve improved pain control before the surgery.
4. The patient will tolerate repositioning to their side.

The correct answer is 3. This question is testing the planning phase of the nursing process. When thinking about the *planning phase* in the context of exam questions, always read the information provided in the question stem carefully. Think about whether a long- or short-term goal is required for the patient; then ensure that the potential answers are focused on the specific patient outcomes that are directly related to their care.

Recently, the National Council of State Boards of Nursing (NCSBN), the regulatory body that develops the NCLEX-RN® exam, has created the NCSBN Clinical Judgment Measurement Model (NCJMM) to guide future test plans. The purpose of this model is to build on and expand the nursing process. Learning clinical judgement in nursing practice was originally conceptualized by Tanner's clinical judgement model (Tanner, 2006). Chapter 19 introduces Tanner's clinical judgement model and explains its stages of *noticing, interpreting, responding,* and *reflecting* in more detail. However, nursing exams continue to evolve in order to test more complex aspects of clinical judgement and reasoning. The NCJMM outlines the following six cognitive skills needed demonstrate clinical judgement within an examination:

1. Recognize Cues
2. Analyze Cues
3. Prioritize Hypotheses
4. Generate Solutions
5. Take Action
6. Evaluate Outcomes

These six skills mirror the phases of the nursing process (Table 14.7). However, the NCJMM outlines more specific aspects of clinical judgement. This framework is helpful for learning how to recognize and analyze cues, prioritize what might be happening with the patient,

TABLE 14.7	Understanding How the NCSBN Clinical Judgment Measurement Model (NCJMM) Is Used for Test-Taking/Exams	
Nursing Process	**NCJMM Cognitive Skill Category**	**Cognitive Skill Being Tested with NCJMM Model**
Assessment	Recognize Cues	The ability to recognize whether the patient's findings are normal or abnormal.
Diagnosis/Analysis	Analyze Cues	Understanding the possible complications or medical conditions the patient may be experiencing. The nurse reviews relevant patient data and determines what the data mean. For example, the nurse links the data to a health problem or health issue. Or the nurse may identify potential complications the patient is at risk for based on the assessment data.
Diagnosis/Analysis	Prioritize Hypotheses	The nurse determines the most likely cause of the client's issues.
Planning	Generate Solutions	The nurse identifies possible solutions to address the client's needs and issues.
Implementation	Take Action	The nurse identifies the appropriate action to take. This may include performing an action, which could be an intervention or an assessment. For example, a patient has 8/10 postoperative pain. The nurse may complete a focused assessment to find the source of the pain. While this action is an assessment, it is also an action or intervention.
Evaluation	Evaluate Outcomes	The nurse outlines the parameters to monitor once interventions have been implemented.

generate solutions, take action, and evaluate outcomes. As you review your growing nursing knowledge, think about which cognitive skills within the NCJMM are being tested and how they apply to your future nursing practice.

Chapter 15 revisits the test-taking strategies addressed in this chapter and applies them to the last two steps of the nursing process: implementation and evaluation.

KEY CONCEPTS

- The nursing process employs critical thinking to identify, diagnose, and treat patients' responses to health and illness.
- Nursing assessment involves the collection and verification of data and the analysis of all data to establish a database about a patient's perceived needs, health problems, and responses to those problems.
- By interpreting the meaning of cues, the nurse forms an inference, which then enables the nurse to identify meaningful clusters of information.
- To conduct a comprehensive assessment, nurses use a structured database format or a problem-oriented approach.
- The interview is an organized conversation with a patient that begins by establishing a therapeutic relationship with the patient and aids in the investigation and discussion of the patient's health care needs.
- Open-ended questions encourage patients to describe their health histories in detail, whereas closed-ended questions present a list of possible choices for the patient.
- An interview includes three phases: orientation, working, and termination.
- Once a patient provides subjective data, the nurse considers exploring the findings further by collecting objective data.
- During assessment, nurses critically anticipate and use an appropriate branching set of questions or observations to collect data, and cues of assessment information are clustered to identify emerging patterns and problems.
- Written data statements are descriptive, to the point, and complete and do not include inferences or interpretative statements.
- Caregivers and friends sometimes offer observations about the patient's needs; these observations will affect the way the nurse delivers care.
- During assessment, nurses encourage patients to describe their histories of illnesses or health care problems.
- To form a nursing judgement, nurses critically assess a patient, validate the data, interpret the information gathered, and look for diagnostic cues that will lead them to identify the patient's problems.
- NANDA International has developed a common language that enables all members of the health care team to understand a patient's needs.
- The analysis and interpretation of data require nurses to validate data, recognize patterns or trends, compare data with healthful standards, and then form diagnostic conclusions.
- The absence of defining characteristics suggests that the nurse reject a proposed diagnosis.
- Four types of nursing diagnoses exist: actual, at risk, wellness, and health promotion.
- A nursing diagnosis is written in a two-part format: a diagnostic label and an etiological or related factor.
- The "related to" factor of the diagnostic statement enables nurses to individualize a patient's nursing diagnoses and directs nurses to select appropriate interventions.
- Risk factors serve as cues to indicate that a risk nursing diagnosis applies to a patient's condition.

- Concept mapping is a visual representation of a patient's care and the relationships between assessment, diagnosis, planning, intervention, and evaluation.
- Nursing diagnostic errors occur through errors in data collection, in interpretation and analysis of data, in clustering of data, or in the diagnostic statement.
- Nursing diagnoses improve communication between nurses and other health care providers.
- During planning, nurses determine person-centred goals, set priorities, develop expected outcomes of nursing care, and develop a nursing care plan.
- Priority setting helps nurses anticipate and sequence nursing interventions when a patient has multiple nursing diagnoses and collaborative problems.
- Multiple factors in the nursing care environment influence priority setting.
- Goals and expected outcomes provide clear direction for the selection and use of nursing interventions and provide focus for evaluation of the effectiveness of the interventions.
- In setting goals, the time frame depends on the nature of the problem, etiology, overall condition of the patient, and treatment setting.
- A person-centred goal is singular, observable, measurable, time limited, mutual, and realistic.
- An expected outcome is an objective criterion for goal achievement.
- Care plans and critical pathways increase communication among nurses and facilitate the continuity of care from one nurse to another and from one health care setting to another.

CRITICAL THINKING EXERCISES

Case scenario: Mr. Fletcher returns to the clinic 1 month later. He has been taking a new medication for hypertension and an antilipemic for high cholesterol. The nurse completes Mr. Fletcher's assessment and documents the following findings:

- Temperature = 37.8°C
- Heart rate = 80 beats per minute (bpm) and regular
- Respirations = 20 breaths per minute
- Blood pressure = 132/78 mm Hg
- Left foot is cold to the touch
- Pain and cramping in left calf muscle when walking

1. Place a checkmark next to the assessment findings that require follow-up by the nurse:
   ___ Temperature = 37.8°C
   ___ Heart rate = 80 beats per minute (bpm) and regular
   ___ Respirations = 20 breaths per minute
   ___ Blood pressure = 132/78 mm Hg
   ___ Left foot is cold to the touch
   ___ Pain and cramping in left calf muscle when walking
2. Choose the correct answers (from the list of options provided) for the information missing in the following statement about Mr. Fletcher:

The nurse recognizes that the (1)_____ and (2)_____ are symptoms linked to peripheral arterial disease.

Answer options:
blood pressure
cold left foot
heart rate
pain and cramping in leg
temperature

3. Mr. Fletcher is taking enalapril 7.5 mg daily to manage his hypertension. During the nursing assessment, the following findings are identified:

For each of the nursing assessment findings in the following table, use an "X" to indicate that the assessment finding is directly related to side effects of the medication, is a risk factor for a patient taking this medication, or is not a concern regarding the medication therapy. (*Select only one response option per row.*)

(To assist you with answering this question, consult Chapter 35: Medication Administration.)

Nursing Assessment Finding	Directly Related to the Medication Therapy	Increases the Patient's Risk While on Medication Therapy	Not a Concern for a Patient Taking This Medication Therapy
Patient has a dry and persistent cough			
Patient's blood pressure is 110/60 mm Hg 1 hour after medication administration			
Patient's creatinine and urea levels are elevated			
Patient has decreased capillary refill to their left foot			
Patient is scheduled a nonsteroidal anti-inflammatory medication at the same time as the enalapril			

🌐 *Answers to Critical Thinking Exercises appear on the Evolve website.*

REVIEW QUESTIONS

Review Questions 1 to 9 relate to the case study at the beginning of the chapter.

1. The nurse completes a nursing health history with Mr. Fletcher. What step should the nurse take to avoid incorrect inferences and ensure that the data from Mr. Fletcher's assessment are accurate?
   a. Analyze and interpret the data.
   b. Document the data.
   c. Validate data with the patient.
   d. Share the data with other health care providers.
2. When clustering Mr. Fletcher's data, the nurse should:
   a. Provide documentation of nursing care.
   b. Review data with other health care providers.
   c. Make inferences about patterns of information.
   d. Organize cues into patterns that enable the nurse to identify nursing diagnoses.
3. The nurse is creating nursing diagnoses for Mr. Fletcher. Which of the following statements BEST describes a *nursing diagnosis*?
   a. The diagnosis and treatment of human responses to health and illness
   b. The advancement of the development, testing, and refinement of a common nursing language
   c. A clinical judgement about individual, family, or community responses to actual and potential health problems or life processes
   d. The identification of a disease condition on the basis of a specific evaluation of physical signs, symptoms, the patient's medical history, and the results of diagnostic tests
4. Why would the nurse choose to use a standard formal nursing diagnostic statement for Mr. Fletcher?
   a. To evaluate nursing care
   b. To gather information on patient data

   c. To help nurses focus on the role of nursing in patient care
   d. To facilitate understanding of patient problems among health care providers

5. The nurse determines that Mr. Fletcher has *readiness for enhanced communication*. What type of nursing diagnosis is this an example of?
   a. A risk nursing diagnosis
   b. An actual nursing diagnosis
   c. A potential nursing diagnosis
   d. A wellness nursing diagnosis
6. The word *impaired* in the diagnosis *impaired physical mobility* is an example of:
   a. A descriptor
   b. A risk factor
   c. A related factor
   d. A nursing diagnosis
7. Nurses use a variety of assessment techniques for data collection. When assessing Mr. Fletcher, what is the first appropriate assessment technique for data collection?
   a. Review his medical record.
   b. Interview him.
   c. Consult with the health care team.
   d. Review the literature on hypertension.
8. Mr. Fletcher is advised by the nurse to change his diet. Which of the following are defining characteristics for the nursing diagnosis *impaired nutrition (more than body requirements)*? (*Select all that apply.*)
   a. Patient's weight is 10 to 20% more than his ideal height and frame
   b. Patient reports dysfunctional eating patterns
   c. Patient demonstrates a knowledge deficit related to hypertension diagnosis

d. Patient smokes one pack of cigarettes per day
e. Patient becomes dizzy when he rises from a sitting position
f. Patient expresses feeling anxious and depressed
9. The nurse is completing care planning for Mr. Fletcher and has agreed to see him again in 2 weeks' time. Which of the following would be considered a realistic short-term goal for Mr. Fletcher to achieve prior to the next visit?
   a. To stop smoking

b. To remove two foods that are high in cholesterol from his diet
c. To have his systolic blood pressure decrease by 20 mm Hg by the next clinic visit
d. To ask him to start running 3 days a week

Answers: 1. c; 2. d; 3. c; 4. d; 5. d; 6. a; 7. b; 8. a, b; 9. b.

🌐 *Rationales for the Review Questions appear on the Evolve website.*

RECOMMENDED WEBSITES

Center for Nursing Classification and Clinical Effectiveness: https://nursing.uiowa.edu/center-for-nursing-classification-and-clinical-effectiveness
The University of Iowa's Center for Nursing Classification and Clinical Effectiveness was established to facilitate ongoing research of the Nursing Interventions Classification (NIC) and Nursing Outcomes Classification (NOC). This site provides an overview of the NIC and NOC and offers information about new classification material and publications.
NANDA International: https://www.nanda.org
Through this website, NANDA International (formerly the North American Nursing Diagnosis Association) provides current information on nursing diagnosis research, publications, links, and Internet resources.

National Council of State Boards of Nursing (NCSBN): NCLEX-RN Test Plans: https://www.ncsbn.org/exams/testplans.page
This website outlines the latest NCLEX-RN test plan. This is the registration exam used by the Canadian Council of Registered Nurse Regulators (CCRNR) and provincial regulatory bodies for registration in all the provinces and territories, except Quebec, since January 2015.
Registered Nurses' Association of Ontario (RNAO)—Nursing Best Practice Guidelines: https://rnao.ca/bpg
The RNAO has developed an extensive process to develop Best Practices Guidelines in a variety of areas of clinical nursing. They have received federal and provincial funding for this process, and their work has been made available to all Canadian nurses through this website, which lists all current guidelines that have been developed.

🌐 REFERENCES

A full reference list is available on the website for this book at http://evolve.elsevier.com/Canada/Potter/fundamentals/

Implementing and Evaluating Nursing Care

*Canadian content written by Marnie L. Kramer, RN, MEd, PhD,
Jennifer Girvin, RN, MN, and Candis Spiers, RN, MN,
with original chapter contributions by Patricia A. Potter, RN, MSN, PhD, FAAN*

OBJECTIVES

Mastery of content in this chapter will enable you to:

- Describe the differences between nurse-initiated, physician-initiated, and collaborative interventions.
- Explain the process of selecting nursing interventions.
- Describe the purposes of a written nursing care plan.
- Explain the relationship between implementation and the nursing diagnostic process.
- Explain the differences between protocols and medical directives or standing orders.
- Describe the association between critical thinking and selecting nursing interventions.
- Explain the steps taken to revise a plan of care before implementation.
- Describe and compare direct and indirect nursing interventions.
- Select appropriate interventions for an assigned patient.
- Describe the relationship between critical thinking and evaluation.
- Identify the five elements of the evaluation process.
- Explain the relationship between goals of care, expected outcomes, and evaluative measures in evaluating nursing care.
- Give an example of evaluative measures for determining patients' progress toward an outcome.
- Describe how evaluation leads to discontinuation, review, or modification of a plan of care.

KEY TERMS

Activities of daily living (ADLs)
Adverse reaction
Collaborative interventions
Consultation
Counselling
Dependent nursing interventions
Direct care

Evaluative measures
Independent nursing interventions
Indirect care
Instrumental activities of daily living (IADLs)
Life-saving measure
Medical directive

Nursing intervention
Outcome
Person-centred goals
Preventive nursing actions
Scientific rationale
Standard of care
Standing order

WEBSITE

http://evolve.elsevier.com/Canada/Potter/fundamentals/

CASE STUDY

Mr. Fletcher (preferred pronouns: he/him) is a 56-year-old patient who has been experiencing headaches and dizziness for the past 2 months. He lives in a rural community and works 12-hour shifts as a haul truck operator in an open-pit coal mine. Mr. Fletcher is 23 kg overweight and leads a sedentary lifestyle. He has been married for 25 years and has two grown children who no longer live at home. Mr. Fletcher recently attended a blood pressure clinic where he was told he had high blood pressure. He has been referred to his local general practitioner for follow-up, and the primary health care nurse is preparing to complete his initial health history and assessment. Mr. Fletcher has brought his wife with him for his clinic visit.

The primary nurse has engaged the assessment, diagnosis, and planning phases of the nursing process for Mr. Fletcher's care (Chapter 14).

Based on Mr. Fletcher's assessment, the primary nurse determined that the patient's primary concern is uncontrolled hypertension. He requires a medical intervention to adjust his antihypertensive therapy. Nursing priorities include patient teaching regarding self-care, risk factor modification strategies, and improved supports. The primary nurse is now determining which nursing interventions to implement and outlining how to evaluate Mr. Fletcher's care. (Box 15.1 outlines the care plan constructed for Mr. Fletcher.)

Think about this case study as you read this chapter. There are Review Questions at the end of the chapter about this case study.

◎ BOX 15.1 NURSING CARE PLAN
Hypertension

ASSESSMENT

Mr. Fletcher (preferred pronouns: he/him) is a 56-year-old patient who presented to the clinic with headaches and dizziness over the last 2 months. Current blood pressure is 179/89 mm Hg, HR is 90 beats per minute, and respiration is 20 breaths per minute.

It is noted on his lab work that he has increased levels of total cholesterol, low-density lipoprotein (LDL), and triglycerides. The nurse notes that she detects the odour of cigarette smoke on his clothing and sees yellow staining on his first two fingers.

Assessment Activities	*Finding and Defining Characteristics*
Assess patient's weight, body mass index (BMI), and waist circumference.	Patient weighs 115 kg, 183 cm tall. BMI is 33.9. BMI of 30 or greater is considered a clinical indicator of obesity. Waist circumference of 102 cm (40 inches) is considered a clinical indicator of obesity.
Assess patient's current activity level.	Patient states he hunts, rides a snowmobile, does not walk far when out doing hobbies. Watches 4 hours of television per day.
Establish patient's tobacco use status.	Patient states he has smoked one pack of cigarettes per day for the last 20 years.
Assess patient's dietary patterns and average daily caloric intake.	Patient states that he eats what he feels like eating, and that he snacks often at work. Wife cooks all the meals in the home.

NURSING DIAGNOSIS: Deficient knowledge regarding management of hypertension related to inexperience

PLANNING

Goal (Nursing Outcomes Classification)*	*Expected Outcomes*
Management of Hypertension	*Knowledge of Hypertension Risk Factors*
Patient will identify three lifestyle risk factors associated with the development of hypertension.	Patient will identify the target range for his blood pressure. Patient will link diet to the development of hypertension. Patient will increase physical activity. Patient will decrease tobacco consumption by 25% and work toward cessation.

*Outcome classification labels from Moorhead, S., Swanson, E., Johnson, M., & Maas, M. L. (Eds.). (2018). *Nursing outcomes classification (NOC)* (6th ed.). Mosby/Elsevier.

INTERVENTIONS (NURSING INTERVENTIONS CLASSIFICATION)†

Self-Care Facilitation	*Rationale*
Work with patient to achieve a collaborative goal regarding smoking cessation from a self-care model.	Smoking cessation provides an opportunity for the patient to work toward a goal within a self-care framework. The nurse is supportive in this process, but the patient must take ownership of his goal to quit smoking.
Activity and Exercise Management	Begin the activity plan with a simple activity. Walking 30 minutes per day, 5 times a week, will help the patient to start a pattern of physical activity that can be modified in the future. Intensity-dynamic exercise for 30 to 60 minutes will help to treat hypertension. (The *Canadian 24-Hour Movement Guidelines* state that individuals should exercise 150 minutes a week in bouts of 10 minutes or more [Canadian Society for Exercise Physiology, 2020].)
Patient implements plan to walk for 30 minutes per day, 5 times a week.	
Nutrition Support	The DASH diet will aid the patient in managing his hypertension and introduce him to the basic nutritional principles behind the management of hypertension.
Patient implements the DASH (Dietary Approaches to Stop Hypertension) diet in collaboration with dietitians and other members of the health care team.	

†Intervention classification labels from Butcher, H. K., Bulechek, G. M., McCloskey Dochterman, J. M., & Wagner, C. (Eds.). (2019). *Nursing interventions classification (NIC)* (7th ed.). Mosby/Elsevier.

EVALUATION

Nursing Actions	*Patient Response and Finding*	*Achievement of Outcome*
Ask patient to state three ways to lower his hypertension.	Patient identifies that smoking increases blood pressure. Patient states he will start smoking only half a pack per day. Patient and his wife state they are enjoying walking 30 minutes per day, 5 times a week. Patient identifies that high-salt, high-calorie diets increase BMI and risk for hypertension.	Role of smoking in hypertension is recognized as a contributing factor. Patient is working toward a plan to stop smoking. Patient has initiated an activity plan, and the patient's wife has joined him, leading to increased opportunities for success in the intervention. Patient recognizes the role of diet in the management of hypertension and is beginning to take steps to change and monitor his diet plan.

In the previous chapter, we explored how assessment, diagnosis, and planning inform the nursing process. In this chapter, we discuss the last two steps of the nursing process—implementation and evaluation. This chapter also outlines the important elements to consider when implementing and evaluating nursing care. The case study at the start of this chapter (introduced in Chapter 14) is used to discuss concepts related to implementation and evaluation in the nursing process. Box 15.1 provides an example of a nurse's care plan for Mr. Fletcher.

IMPLEMENTATION

The *implementation* step of the nursing process initiates or completes planned actions or nursing interventions. This step may include organizing and managing planned care, aiding with activities of daily living (ADLs), counselling or teaching the patient and family, providing care, or delegating care to others (Nugent & Vitale, 2020). The nurse aims to implement safe patient care that is designed to achieve planned goals and expected outcomes.

A variety of different interventions may be initiated to ensure comprehensive patient care. With a care plan based on clear and relevant nursing diagnoses, the nurse initiates interventions that are most likely to achieve the goals and expected outcomes needed to support or improve the patient's health status. A **nursing intervention** is any treatment, based on clinical judgement and knowledge, that enhances patient outcomes (Butcher et al., 2019). Ideally, interventions are evidence informed (see Chapter 8 for further information about evidence-informed research), provide the most current, up-to-date, and effective approaches to address patients' health problems, and include both direct and indirect care measures.

Direct care interventions are treatments performed through interactions with patients. Examples of direct care measures include medication administration, insertion of an intravenous infusion, or counselling during a time of grief. **Indirect care** interventions are treatments performed away from the patient but on behalf of the patient or a group of patients (Butcher et al., 2019). Indirect care measures include actions to manage the patient's environment (e.g., safety and infection control), documentation, and interdisciplinary collaboration. Both direct and indirect care measures can be nurse initiated, physician initiated, or collaborative interventions. For example, patient teaching is a direct nurse-initiated intervention. **Consultation**, another type of indirect intervention, is a collaborative intervention.

Each intervention is rendered within the context of a patient's unique situation. This may include the patient's particular situation, how the patient perceives the proposed interventions, and how the nurse can best support the patient as they intervene.

TYPES OF NURSING INTERVENTIONS

Nursing interventions belong to three categories: nurse initiated, physician initiated, and collaborative. Interventions are based on patient needs. Some patients require all three categories of interventions, whereas others need only nurse- and physician-initiated interventions.

Nurse-initiated interventions are **independent nursing interventions**, actions that do not require direction or orders from other health care providers (Nugent & Vitale, 2020). As a nurse, you act independently for patients. Nurses' actions are grounded in evidence-informed decision making. Examples include elevating an edematous extremity, instructing patients about adverse effects of medications, or directing a patient how to splint an incision during coughing.

In contrast to nurse-initiated interventions, physician-initiated interventions are **dependent nursing interventions**, actions that do require orders or directions from physicians (Nugent & Vitale, 2020). These interventions are directed at treating or managing a medical diagnosis. Nurse practitioners working under collaborative agreements with physicians or licensed through provincial or territorial nursing legislation are also able to provide such orders or directions for care. Nurses intervene by carrying out these written or verbal orders in the case of emergency situations. Administering a medication and changing a dressing are examples of written physician-initiated interventions.

Each physician-initiated intervention requires specific nursing responsibilities that are based on nursing knowledge. For example, when administering medications, you are responsible for knowing the classification of the drug, its physiological action, the normal dosage, adverse effects, and nursing interventions related to its action or adverse effects (see Chapter 35 for further information about medications).

Interdependent nursing interventions, or **collaborative interventions**, are therapies that require the combined knowledge, skill, and expertise of numerous health care providers. Typically, when a nurse plans care for a patient, the nurse reviews the necessary interventions and determines whether the collaboration is necessary. An interdisciplinary health care team conference about a patient's care is useful in determining interdependent nursing interventions.

Nurses are required to have the appropriate and specific evidence-informed knowledge, skills, and abilities to be able to recognize and question errors and thus competently care for assigned patient populations (Table 15.1). A nurse is responsible for recognizing incorrect orders or therapies before implementing any order or therapy. Errors may occur in writing or transcribing orders. Clarifying an order is competent nursing practice and protects patients from harm. Nurses who carry out an incorrect or inappropriate intervention have made an error in judgement and are thus legally responsible for any complications

TABLE 15.1	Frequent Errors in Writing Nursing Interventions	
Type of Error	**Incorrectly Stated Nursing Intervention**	**Correctly Stated Nursing Intervention**
Failure to precisely or completely indicate nursing actions	Turn patient every 2 hours	Turn patient every 2 hours, using the following schedule: 0800: supine 1000: left side 1200: prone 1400: right side (repeat this routine beginning at 1600 and 2400)
Failure to indicate frequency	Perform blood glucose measurements	Measure blood glucose before each meal: 0700, 1100, and 1600
Failure to indicate quantity	Irrigate wound once a shift: 0800, 1600, and 2400	Irrigate wound with 100 mL normal saline until clear: 0800, 1600, and 2400
Failure to indicate method	Change patient's dressing once a shift: 0800, 1600, and 2400	Replace patient's dressing with Neosporin ointment to wound and two dry 4 × 4 dressings secured with hypoallergenic tape, once a shift: 0800, 1600, and 2400

resulting from the error (see Chapter 10 for further information about legal implications).

SELECTION OF INTERVENTIONS

Interventions are not selected at random. Patients diagnosed with *anxiety*, for example, may require a variety of interventions. Nurses treat anxiety related to the uncertainty of an impending surgery very differently than anxiety related to a possible loss of family role function. When choosing interventions, the nurse considers six factors: (1) the nursing diagnosis, (2) goals and expected outcomes, (3) the evidence base (e.g., research or proven practice guidelines), (4) feasibility, (5) acceptability to the patient, and (6) the nurse's competence (Butcher et al., 2019) (Box 15.2). During deliberation, the nurse reviews key resources, such as the nursing literature, standard protocols or guidelines, the Nursing Interventions Classification (NIC), critical pathways, policy or procedure manuals, and textbooks. To ensure the best potential for achieving expected patient outcomes, it is important for the nurse to collaborate with other professionals, review a patient's needs and priorities, and allow for previous experiences to factor into the selection of nursing interventions for expected outcomes.

Nursing Interventions Classification

The Iowa Intervention Project (1993) developed the Nursing Interventions Classification (NIC), a set of nursing interventions that nurses perform, providing a level of standardization that enhances communication of nursing care across all health care settings and enables health care providers to compare outcomes (Butcher et al., 2019). The purpose of the NIC model is outlined in Box 15.3. The NIC model has three levels for ease of use: domains, classes, and interventions. The domains are the highest level (level 1) of the model, worded in broad terms (e.g., "safety" and "physiological: basic") to organize the more specific classes and interventions (Table 15.2). The second level of the model includes 30 classes, which offer useful clinical categories for reference in selecting interventions. The third level of the model includes the 514 interventions, defined as any treatment, based on clinical judgement and knowledge, that a nurse performs to enhance the condition of a patient presenting with an alteration within the class (Butcher et al., 2019). Each intervention can be performed with a variety of nursing activities (Box 15.4). Nursing activities are those commonly used in a plan of care. NIC-based interventions are also linked with NANDA International (2021) nursing diagnoses for ease of use. For example,

---

BOX 15.3   Purposes of the Nursing Interventions Classification (NIC)

1. Standardization of the nomenclature (e.g., labelling, describing) of nursing interventions. Standardizes the language nurses use to describe sets of actions in delivering patient care.
2. Expansion of nursing knowledge about connections between nursing diagnoses, treatments, and outcomes. These connections will be determined through the study of actual patient care using a database that the classification will generate.
3. Development of nursing and health care information systems.
4. Teaching decision making to nursing students. Defining and classifying nursing interventions helps to teach beginning nurses how to determine a patient's need for care and to respond appropriately.
5. Determination of the cost of services provided by nurses.
6. Planning for resources needed in all types of nursing practice settings.
7. Language to communicate the unique functions of nursing.
8. Link with the classification systems of other health care providers.

Adapted from Butcher, H. K., Bulechek, G. M., McCloskey Dochterman, J. M., & Wagner, C. (Eds.). (2019). *Nursing interventions classification (NIC)* (7th ed.). Mosby/Elsevier.

BOX 15.2   Choosing Nursing Interventions

Characteristics of a Nursing Diagnosis
Interventions should alter the etiological ("related to") factor or signs and symptoms associated with the diagnostic label.
- When an etiological factor cannot change, direct the interventions toward treating the signs and symptoms (e.g., NANDA International [2021] defining characteristics).
- For potential or high-risk diagnoses, direct interventions at altering or eliminating risk factors for the diagnosis.

Expected Outcomes
Because nurses state outcomes in terms used to evaluate the effect of an intervention, this language assists in selecting the intervention. The Nursing Interventions Classification (NIC) is designed to show the link to the Nursing Outcomes Classification (NOC) (University of Iowa College of Nursing, 2018).

Evidence-Informed Practice
Research evidence in support of a nursing intervention indicates the effectiveness of the intervention in certain types of patients.
- Refer to the evidence (e.g., research articles, evidence-informed decision making, or evidence-informed nursing practice protocols that describe the use of the evidence in similar clinical situations and settings).
- When research is not available, use scientific principles (e.g., infection control) or consult a clinical expert about your patient population.

Feasibility
A specific intervention has the potential to interact with other interventions.
- Be knowledgeable about the total plan of care.
- Consider cost: Is the intervention clinically effective and cost efficient?
- Consider time: Are time and personnel resources available?

Acceptability to the Patient
A treatment plan needs to be acceptable to the patient and/or family and must match the patient's goals, health care values, and culture.
- Promote informed choice; help a patient understand how to participate in and anticipate the effect of interventions.

Capability of the Nurse
The nurse needs to have current knowledge of the intervention, its scientific basis, and considerations for implementation.
- Be prepared to carry out the intervention.
- Know the scientific rationale for the intervention.
- Have the necessary psychosocial and psychomotor skills to complete the intervention.
- Function within the specific setting and use health care resources effectively and efficiently.

Adapted from Butcher, H. K., Bulechek, G. M., McCloskey Dochterman, J. M., & Wagner, C. (Eds.). (2019). *Nursing interventions classification (NIC)* (7th ed.). Mosby/Elsevier.

TABLE 15.2	Nursing Interventions Classification (NIC) Taxonomy					
Domain 1	Domain 2	Domain 3	Domain 4	Domain 5	Domain 6	Domain 7
Level 1 Domains						
1. Physiological: Basic Care that supports physical functioning	2. Physiological: Complex Care that supports homeostatic regulation	3. Behavioural Care that supports psychosocial functioning and facilitates lifestyle changes	4. Safety Care that supports protection against harm	5. Family Care that supports the family	6. Health System Care that supports effective use of the health care delivery system	7. Community Care that supports the health of the community
Level 2 Classes						
A. *Activity and Exercise Management:* Interventions to organize or assist with physical activity and energy conservation and expenditure	G. *Electrolyte and Acid–Base Management:* Interventions to regulate electrolyte/acid–base balance and prevent complications	O. *Behaviour Therapy:* Interventions to reinforce or promote desirable behaviours or alter undesirable behaviours	U. *Crisis Management:* Interventions to provide immediate short-term help in both psychological and physiological crises	W. *Childbearing Care:* Interventions to assist in understanding and coping with the psychological and physiological changes during the childbearing period	Z. *Health System Mediation:* Interventions to facilitate the interface between patient/family and the health care system	c. *Community Health Promotion:* Interventions that promote the health of the whole community
B. *Elimination Management:* Interventions to establish and maintain regular bowel and urinary elimination patterns and manage complications due to altered patterns	H. *Drug Management:* Interventions to facilitate desired effects of pharmacological agents	P. *Cognitive Therapy:* Interventions to reinforce or promote desirable cognitive functioning or alter undesirable cognitive functioning	V. *Risk Management:* Interventions to initiate risk-reduction activities and continue monitoring risks over time	X. *Childrearing Care:* Interventions to assist in rearing children	a. *Health System Management:* Interventions to provide and enhance support services for the delivery of care	d. *Community Risk Management:* Interventions that assist in detecting or preventing health risks to the whole community
C. *Immobility Management:* Interventions to manage restricted body movement and the sequelae	I. *Neurological Management:* Interventions to optimize neurological functions	Q. *Communication Enhancement:* Interventions to facilitate delivering and receiving verbal and nonverbal messages		Y. *Lifespan Care:* Interventions to facilitate family unit functioning and promote the health and welfare of family members throughout the lifespan	b. *Information Management:* Interventions to facilitate communication among health care providers	
D. *Nutrition Support:* Interventions to modify or maintain nutritional status	J. *Perioperative Care:* Interventions to provide care before, during, and after surgery	R. *Coping Assistance:* Interventions to assist another to build on own strength, to adapt to a change in function, or to achieve a higher level of function				
E. *Physical Comfort Promotion:* Interventions to promote comfort using physical techniques	K. *Respiratory Management:* Interventions to provide care before, during, and immediately after surgery	S. *Patient Education:* Interventions to facilitate learning				

Continued

TABLE 15.2 Nursing Interventions Classification (NIC) Taxonomy—cont'd

Domain 1	Domain 2	Domain 3	Domain 4	Domain 5	Domain 6	Domain 7
F. *Self-Care Facilitation:* Interventions to provide or assist with routine activities of daily living	L. *Skin/Wound Management:* Interventions to maintain or restore tissue integrity	T. *Psychological Comfort Promotion:* Interventions to promote comfort using psychological techniques				
	M. *Thermoregulation:* Interventions to maintain body temperature within a normal range					
	N. *Tissue Perfusion Management:* Interventions to optimize circulation of blood and fluids to the tissue					

From Butcher, H. K., Bulechek, G. M., McCloskey Dochterman, J. M., & Wagner, C. (Eds.). (2019). *Nursing interventions classification (NIC)* (7th ed.). Mosby/Elsevier.

BOX 15.4 Examples of Interventions and Associated Nursing Activities

Class: Physical Comfort Promotion Intervention–Environmental Management
Examples of Activities
- Create a safe environment for patient
- Provide a clean, comfortable bed and environment
- Avoid unnecessary exposure, drafts, overheating, or chilling
- Provide music of choice
- Limit visitors
- Manipulate lighting for therapeutic benefit
- Bring familiar objects from home
- Allow family or significant other to stay with patient

From Butcher, H. K., Bulechek, G. M., McCloskey Dochterman, J. M., & Wagner, C. (Eds.). (2019). *Nursing interventions classification (NIC)* (7th ed.). Mosby/Elsevier.

if a patient has a nursing diagnosis of *acute pain*, 21 recommended interventions, including pain management, cutaneous stimulation, and anxiety reduction, may be used. A variety of nursing care activities are presented with each of the recommended interventions.

CRITICAL THINKING IN IMPLEMENTATION

The selection of nursing interventions involves complex decision making and is based on critical thinking to ensure that an intervention is correct and appropriate for the clinical situation. Even when nurses have planned interventions for a patient, good judgement, decision making, and reassessment are needed before each intervention is performed with the understanding that patients' conditions sometimes change rapidly. Some points to consider when working with patients to meet their needs are as follows:

- Review the set of all possible nursing interventions for the patient's problem
- Review all possible consequences associated with each possible nursing action

- Determine the probability of all possible consequences, and
- Determine the effect of the intervention on the patient.

The selection and performance of nursing interventions for a patient is part of clinical decision making. The critical thinking model described in Chapter 7 provides a framework for making decisions about nursing care. As you proceed with an intervention, you should consider the purpose of the intervention, the steps in performing the intervention correctly, and the patient's health status (Figure 15.1). It is essential to know the clinical standards of practice of each agency because procedures and standards of practice vary considerably. The standards of practice are guidelines for nursing practice and sanction principles to provide safe and competent care. To demonstrate the process of critical thinking in the implementation stage (Figure 15.2) for nursing diagnosis and interventions, we return to Mr. Fletcher's case study:

The primary nurse has decided to focus on education as a primary direct nursing intervention for Mr. Fletcher. The nurse will be focusing their efforts on a self-care framework to empower Mr. Fletcher to learn how to manage his hypertension.

Knowledge: *The primary nurse approaches smoking cessation, exercise, and nutrition support as direct nursing interventions for the management of hypertension. The primary nurse also knows that teaching is needed so that Mr. Fletcher can monitor his blood pressure at home. These are areas of education that the primary nurse can address within their nursing scope of practice. If the physician or nurse practitioner orders antihypertensive medications for the patient, the primary nurse will add this area of teaching to the care plan. The primary nurse will be assessing the patient's readiness to learn and apply the most appropriate learning styles to best support the patient's learning.*

Standards: *The primary nurse will aim to help the patient decrease his blood pressure below 140/80 mm Hg as per Best Practice Guidelines. The primary nurse will help the patient to determine a target range for his blood pressure and identify strategies to help the patient understand the links between diet, exercise, and smoking in the development of hypertension. The primary nurse understands that diet and lifestyle modification is*

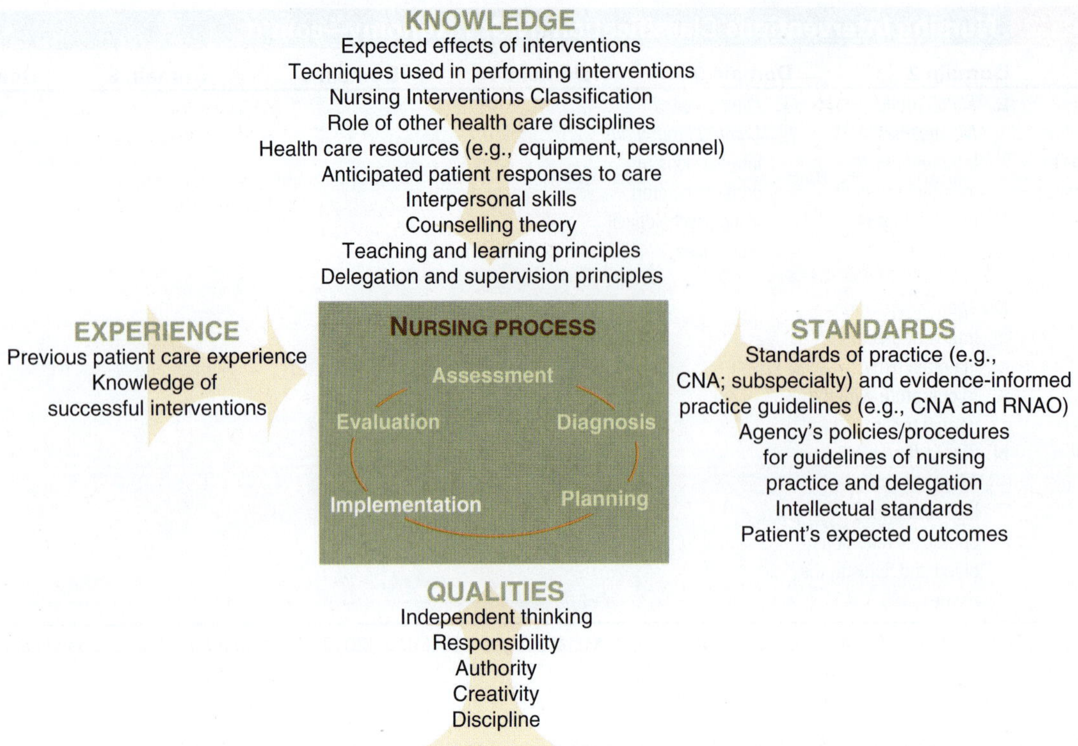

KNOWLEDGE
Expected effects of interventions
Techniques used in performing interventions
Nursing Interventions Classification
Role of other health care disciplines
Health care resources (e.g., equipment, personnel)
Anticipated patient responses to care
Interpersonal skills
Counselling theory
Teaching and learning principles
Delegation and supervision principles

EXPERIENCE
Previous patient care experience
Knowledge of
successful interventions

NURSING PROCESS
Assessment
Evaluation   Diagnosis
Implementation   Planning

STANDARDS
Standards of practice (e.g.,
CNA; subspecialty) and evidence-informed
practice guidelines (e.g., CNA and RNAO)
Agency's policies/procedures
for guidelines of nursing
practice and delegation
Intellectual standards
Patient's expected outcomes

QUALITIES
Independent thinking
Responsibility
Authority
Creativity
Discipline

FIGURE 15.1 Critical thinking and the process of implementing care. *CNA,* Canadian Nurses Association; *RNAO,* Registered Nurses' Association of Ontario.

a first step; if this is unsuccessful in lowering the patient's blood pressure, then the patient may require medication therapy.

Qualities: The primary nurse recognizes that healthy behaviour changes are challenging. Therefore, the nurse sets reasonable short-term goals that will help to build the patient's confidence in managing his condition. The primary nurse starts by helping Mr. Fletcher gain access to a home blood pressure monitor. The primary nurse then teaches the patient and his wife to take their blood pressures at breakfast and before bed. The primary nurse also finds two apps for the patients to download on their smartphones, one to help them both keep track of their diets and another to help Mr. Fletcher track his cigarette consumption.

Experience: In the past, the primary health nurse has found that it is helpful for patients to log their blood pressure and to follow an organized approach when modifying health behaviours. Once the patient has learned to take his blood pressure, the primary nurse will let the patient decide what behaviour he would like to modify next: diet, exercise, or smoking. This will help the patient to stay focused on one task and not be overwhelmed by too many changes at once. The primary nurse has found that with smoking cessation, it is helpful to access the support of a physician or nurse practitioner and to slowly cut back on cigarettes while establishing new habits to replace smoking.

STANDARD NURSING INTERVENTIONS

To facilitate good care planning, systems of standard nursing interventions are available to help the nurse. These are based on common health care problems for which standard interventions can serve as a reference point in determining what is necessary. Of more importance, if the standards are informed by evidence, interventions are more likely to improve patient outcomes (see Chapter 8).

Standard interventions, both nurse initiated and physician initiated, are available in the form of clinical guidelines or protocols, preprinted medical directives or standing orders, and NIC-based interventions.

Clinical Practice Guidelines and Protocols

A clinical guideline or protocol is a document that guides decisions and interventions for specific health care problems. The guideline or protocol is developed through an authoritative examination of current scientific evidence, and assists nurses, physicians, and other health care providers in making decisions about appropriate health care for specific clinical circumstances. Clinicians within a health care agency sometimes choose to review the scientific literature and their own standard of practice to develop guidelines and protocols that improve their standard of care. For example, a hospital may develop a rapid assessment protocol to improve the identification and early treatment of patients suspected of having a stroke. Clinical practice guidelines can also assist you in providing the best possible care. The Best Practice Guidelines, developed by the Registered Nurses' Association of Ontario (RNAO) (http://rnao.ca/bpg), is an excellent example of such guidelines. The Best Practice Guidelines have been critiqued for being difficult to implement into nursing practice. In response, the RNAO developed BPG Order Sets to make it easier for nurses to translate evidence into nursing practice by providing clear, concise, and actionable evidence-informed intervention statements. These BPG Order Sets are available at https://bpgorderset.rnao.ca.

Medical Directives or Standing Orders

A **medical directive** or **standing order** is a statement of orders for the conduct of routine therapies, monitoring guidelines, or diagnostic procedures, or a combination of these, for specific patients with identified clinical problems. These statements direct patient care in various clinical

> concept map

Nursing diagnosis: Deficient knowledge regarding management of hypertension related to inexperience
• New diagnosis of hypertension

Interventions
• Identify normal blood pressure range and targeted range for therapy
• Teach how to take blood pressure on home machine
• Educate regarding treatment for hypertension (diet, medications, activity)

Nursing diagnosis: Readiness for enhanced health management related to blood pressure care
• Asking questions about blood pressure monitoring, required diet changes, and need for medication therapy

Interventions
• Use RNAO 5 A's of self-care management to initiate self-management sessions for blood pressure care
• Have patient list top three priorities for managing his hypertension

Patient s chief medical diagnosis: Hypertension
Priority assessments: educate patient about self/home blood pressure monitoring; educate patient on their target blood pressure; assess and educate for dietary risk factors; assess patient s weight, BMI, and waist circumference; establish tobacco use status

Nursing diagnosis: Readiness for enhanced health management related to smoking cessation
• Asking questions about stopping smoking, requesting information regarding smoking cessation programs
• Links his new diagnosis of hypertension to his smoking history

Interventions
• Complete patient teaching about the relationship between smoking and the risk for cardiovascular disease
• Identify various smoking cessation interventions available

Nursing diagnosis: Obesity related to increased caloric intake and lack of physical activity
• Experienced 23 kg weight gain over past 2 years
• Reports increased food intake and minimal activity
• BMI over 30

Interventions
• Teach patient about the DASH diet
• Implement activity plan of walking 30 minutes 5× per week

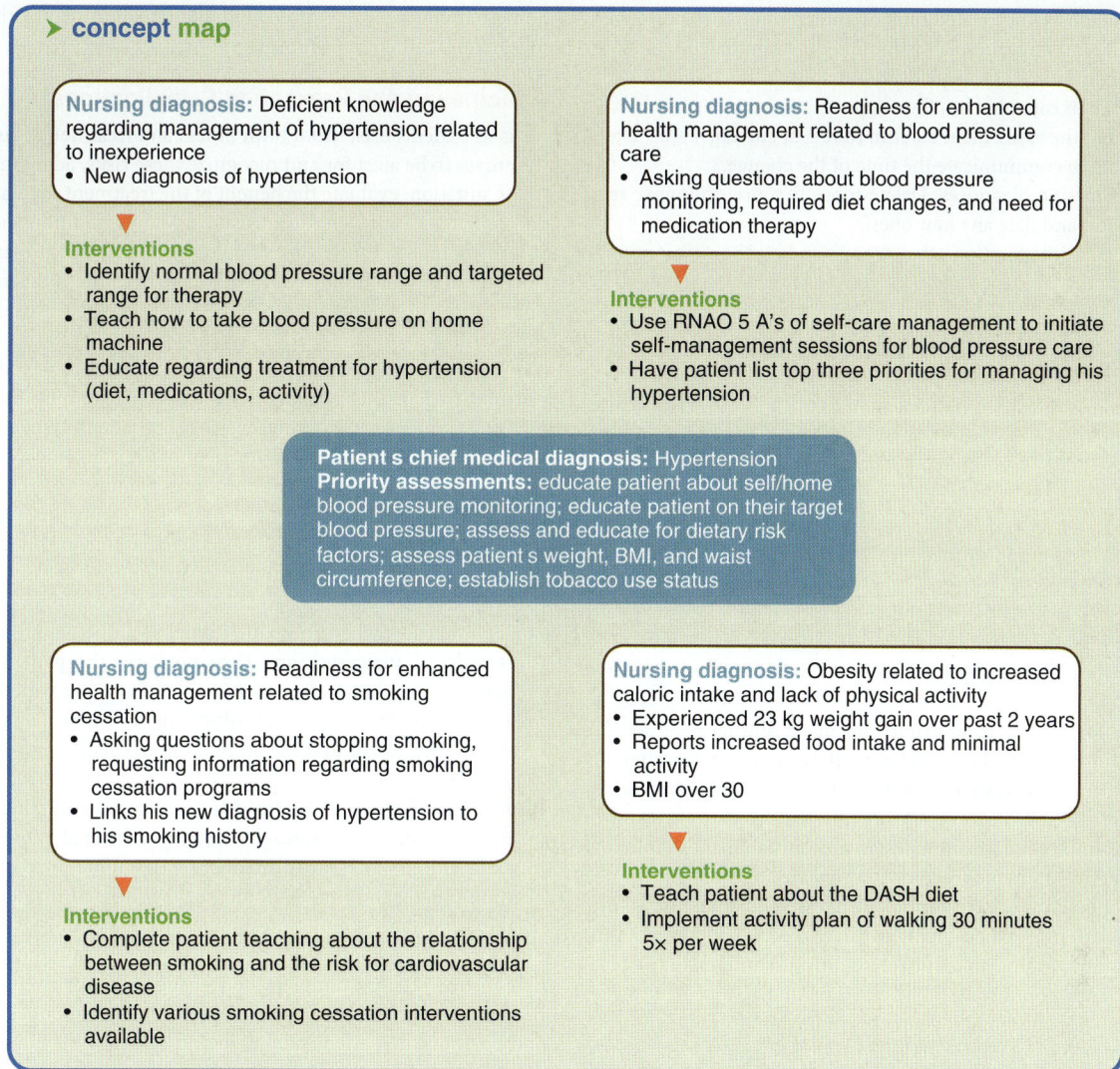

FIGURE 15.2 Concept map for planning Mr. Fletcher's nursing care. *BMI,* Body mass index; *RNAO,* Registered Nurses' Association of Ontario.

settings and must be approved and signed by the prescribing health care provider. Medical directives or standing orders are common in critical care settings and other specialized practice settings in which patients' needs change rapidly and require immediate attention. Examples include those for preoperative blood tests, those for postoperative exercises and positioning, and those for certain medications (such as heparin) for blood coagulation. When these statements are in place, the critical care nurse may administer the specified medication or conduct the specified action without first notifying the physician. Medical directives or standing orders are also common in community health settings in which physicians are not immediately available for consultation. Medical directives, standing orders, and clinical protocols give the nurse legal protection to intervene appropriately in the patient's best interest.

IMPLEMENTATION PROCESS

Preparation for implementation ensures efficient, safe, and effective nursing care. Preparatory activities include reassessing the patient, reviewing and revising the existing nursing care plan, organizing resources and care delivery, anticipating and preventing complications, and implementing nursing interventions.

Reassessing the Patient

Assessment is a continuous process that occurs each time the nurse interacts with a patient. As new data are collected and patient needs change or resolve, nurses modify the plan of care. During the initial phase of planning nursing care, the preliminary assessment may focus on one dimension of the patient, such as level of comfort, or on one system, such as the cardiovascular system. Reassessment helps the nurse decide whether the proposed nursing action continues to be appropriate for the patient's level of wellness. As outlined by the Canadian Association of Schools of Nursing's (CASN) *National Nursing Education Framework*, "theoretically-based and evidence-informed safe, competent, ethical, and culturally respectful nursing care across the lifespan and in diverse contexts through experiential learning opportunities" is essential in any assessment framework (Canadian Association of Schools of Nursing [CASN], 2022, p. 13).

Reviewing and Revising the Existing Nursing Care Plan

After reassessing a patient, the nurse reviews the care plan, compares assessment data in order to validate the nursing diagnoses, and determines whether the nursing interventions remain the most appropriate ones for the patient's situation. If the patient's status has changed and the nursing diagnosis and related nursing interventions are no longer appropriate, the nursing care plan is modified. An outdated or incorrect care plan compromises the quality of nursing care. Modification of the existing written care plan has four steps:

1. Revise data in the assessment column to reflect current status. Date any new data to communicate the time of the change.
2. Revise the nursing diagnoses. Delete those that are no longer relevant and add and date any new ones.
3. Revise specific interventions that correspond to the new nursing diagnoses and goals.
4. Determine the method of evaluation for any outcomes achieved.

Organizing Resources and Care Delivery

A facility's resources include equipment and skilled personnel. Organization of equipment and personnel makes timely, efficient, and skilled patient care possible. Preparation for giving care involves preparing the environment as well as the patient.

Equipment. Most nursing procedures require some equipment or supplies. Nurses must identify which supplies are required for an intervention, determine whether they are available, and ensure that equipment is in working order. It is also imperative that nurses are aware of how to operate equipment safely.

Personnel. Nurses are responsible for determining whether to perform an intervention or to delegate it to another member of the nursing team. Assessment of a patient directs delegation decisions. (Chapter 13 focuses on the principles of delegation in more detail.) For example, practical nurses are accountable and liable for their own practice and able to competently care for stable and predictable patients. If a registered nurse learns in the change-of-shift report that a patient is experiencing cardiac irregularities, changing the patient's status to unstable, the nurse must assume primary care until the patient's condition stabilizes (Canadian Nurses Association [CNA], 2003). Nursing judgement is important for determining the health status of the patient and identifying the appropriate care provider.

Environment. A care environment needs to be safe and conducive to the implementation of therapies. Patient safety is a primary concern. Nurses must anticipate circumstances that place patients at risk, and they must create a culture of patient safety (Healthcare Excellence Canada, 2020). If the patient has sensory deficits, a physical disability, or an alteration in level of consciousness, the environment should be arranged to prevent injury. Privacy should be ensured during procedures that may require some body exposure. Also, lighting should be adequate for performing procedures correctly (see Chapter 38).

Patient. Before providing care, the nurse needs to ensure that the patient is as physically and psychologically comfortable as possible. The patient needs to be comfortable during interventions. The nurse should control environmental factors at the outset, taking care of physical needs (e.g., elimination), minimizing the potential for interruptions, and positioning the patient correctly. The patient's strength and endurance need to be considered, and the nurse should plan only the level of activity that the patient is able to tolerate comfortably. Awareness of the patient's psychosocial needs helps the nurse create a favourable emotional climate.

Some patients feel reassured by having a significant other present for encouragement and moral support.

Anticipating and Preventing Complications

Risks to patients arise from both illness and treatment. It is important for nurses to be alert for and recognize these risks, adapt interventions to the situation, evaluate the benefit of the treatment in relation to risk, and initiate risk-prevention measures. Many conditions heighten the risk for complications. For example, a patient with pre-existing left-sided paralysis that followed a stroke 2 years earlier is at risk of developing a pressure injury after orthopedic surgery because postoperative care entails traction and bed rest.

A nurse's knowledge of pathophysiology and their experience with previous patients help to identify the risk for complications. A thorough assessment reveals the level of the patient's current risk. The scientific rationale, which concerns how certain interventions (e.g., pressure-relief devices, repositioning, or wound care) prevent or minimize complications, helps the nurse select the most useful preventive measures. For example, if an obese patient has uncontrolled postoperative pain, the risk of developing a pressure injury increases because the patient may be unwilling or unable to change position frequently. The nurse anticipates when the patient's pain will be aggravated, administers ordered analgesics, and then positions the patient to remove pressure on the skin and underlying tissues. If the patient continues to have difficulty turning or repositioning, the nurse may then select a pressure-relief device to place on the patient's bed.

Identifying Areas of Assistance. In certain nursing situations, nurses must obtain assistance by seeking additional knowledge, nursing skills, unregulated care providers, or a combination of these. Before beginning care, the nurse should review the plan to determine the need for assistance. Sometimes nurses need assistance with performing a procedure, comforting a patient, or preparing the patient for a diagnostic test. For example, when caring for an overweight, immobilized patient, the nurse may require additional personnel to help turn and position the patient safely. The nurse consults with other health care team members to determine the number of additional personnel required to carry out the intervention. When nurses are less familiar with a situation, they prepare for it by seeking the necessary knowledge and requesting assistance from more experienced nurses.

Implementation Skills

Nursing practice includes cognitive, interpersonal, and psychomotor (technical) skills to implement direct and indirect nursing interventions. Nurses are responsible for knowing which skill is needed in a given situation and for having the necessary knowledge and ability to perform each skill.

Cognitive Skills. Cognitive skills involve the application of critical thinking in the nursing process. To perform any intervention, nurses use good judgement and make sound clinical decisions. No nursing intervention is automatic or routine. Nurses critically think and anticipate to individualize patient care and ensure the safety of patients in their care.

Interpersonal Skills. Interpersonal skills are essential for effective nursing action. The nurse needs to develop a trusting relationship, express a caring attitude, and communicate clearly with the patient and family (see Chapter 18 for further information about relational communication). Good interpersonal communication is crucial for keeping patients informed, providing individualized patient teaching, and effectively supporting patients with challenging emotional needs.

Psychomotor Skills. Psychomotor skills require the integration of cognitive and motor activities. For example, when giving an injection, nurses need to understand anatomy, physiology, and pharmacology (cognitive skills) and use good coordination and precision to administer the injection correctly (motor skills). Nurses are responsible for acquiring the necessary psychomotor skills in a variety of ways: through experience in the nursing laboratory during their nursing education, in practice while learning a new skill, through interactive instructional technology, or through actual hands-on care of patients. Before performing a new skill, nurses always assess their level of competency and obtain the necessary resources to ensure that the patient receives safe treatment.

DIRECT CARE

Nurses provide a wide variety of direct care measures. How a nurse interacts affects the success of any direct care activity, and thus a caring approach is essential. Nurses need to always be sensitive to a patient's clinical condition, values and beliefs, expectations, and cultural views. All direct care measures require safe and competent practice. It is important to note that there are similar direct care activities within the scope of practice of registered nurses (RNs) and licensed practical nurses (LPNs)/registered practical nurses (RPNs). In these cases, teamwork and delegation of direct care activities is essential for the implementation of comprehensive nursing care. However, while scope of practice may overlap at times between RNs, LPNs, and RPNs, there may also be indications where the RN and LPN/RPN roles differ in approach. For example, a patient who is newly diagnosed with a chronic disease or condition may require extensive patient teaching from the RN, while the LPN/RPN may focus on completing teaching from an established care plan for a patient who is being discharged. The following section outlines different types of direct care measures from a general perspective that affects all nurses.

Activities of Daily Living

Activities of daily living (ADLs) are activities usually performed during the course of a normal day, including ambulation, eating, dressing, bathing, brushing the teeth, and grooming (see Chapter 39 for further information about hygiene). A patient's need for assistance with ADLs may be temporary, permanent, or rehabilitative. A patient with impaired mobility because of bilateral arm casts has a temporary need for assistance. A patient with an irreversible injury to the cervical spinal cord is paralyzed and thus has a permanent need for assistance. Occupational therapists and physiotherapists play key roles in rehabilitation to restore ADL function.

When an assessment reveals that a patient is experiencing fatigue, a limitation in mobility, confusion, and pain, the patient needs assistance with ADLs. For example, a patient who experiences shortness of breath avoids eating because of the associated fatigue. The nurse assists the patient by setting up meals, offering to cut up food, and planning for small and frequent meals to maintain nutrition. It is important to determine the patient's preferences when assisting with ADLs and to let the patient participate as much as possible. Involving the patient in planning the timing and types of interventions enhances the patient's self-esteem and willingness to assume more independence.

Instrumental Activities of Daily Living

Illness or disability sometimes alters a patient's ability to be independent in society. **Instrumental activities of daily living (IADLs)** include skills such as shopping, preparing meals, writing cheques, and taking medications. Nurses within home care and community health care settings frequently assist patients in finding ways to accomplish IADLs. Often, family and friends are excellent resources for assisting patients. In acute care, it is important to anticipate how illness will affect the patient's ability to perform IADLs and to involve other health care team members such as occupational therapists or social workers.

Physical Care Techniques

Nurses routinely perform a variety of physical care techniques when caring for a patient. Examples include turning and positioning, changing dressings, administering medications, and providing comfort measures. Considerations in providing physical care include protecting the nurse and the patient from injury, using infection control practices, following applicable practice guidelines, and staying organized. To carry out a procedure, nurses need to be knowledgeable about the procedure, how to perform it, and what the expected outcomes are.

Controlling for Adverse Reactions

An **adverse reaction** is a harmful effect of a medication, diagnostic test, or therapeutic intervention. Nurses are responsible for knowing the potential adverse reactions associated with nursing interventions as they provide patient care.

Nursing actions that control for adverse reactions reduce or counteract the reaction. For example, when applying a moist heat compress, a nurse must take steps to prevent burning the patient's skin. First, the nurse assesses the area where the compress is to be applied. Then, the nurse inspects the area every 5 minutes for any adverse reaction, such as excessive reddening of the skin from the heat or skin maceration from the moisture of the compress. When completing a physician-initiated intervention, such as medication administration, nurses need to know about the potential adverse effects and reactions of the medication. After administration of the medication, the nurse evaluates the patient for the expected outcomes and any adverse effects or reactions.

Nurses need to be knowledgeable about medications that counteract the adverse effects of certain medications or that have adverse reactions themselves. For example, a patient who has an unknown hypersensitivity to penicillin develops hives after three doses. The nurse records the reaction, stops further administration of penicillin, and consults with the physician. Part of this process also includes anticipating an order for diphenhydramine (Benadryl), an antihistamine and antipruritic medication, to reduce the adverse reaction or allergic response and to relieve itching. The nurse recalls how to access and administer this information in advance to help ensure patient safety during this acute event.

Life-Saving Measures

A **life-saving measure** is a physical care technique performed when a patient's physiological or psychological state is threatened (see Chapter 40 for further information about cardiopulmonary functioning). The purpose of life-saving measures is to restore physiological or psychological equilibrium. Such measures include administering emergency medications, instituting cardiopulmonary resuscitation, intervening to protect a confused or violent patient, and providing a safe environment for a patient experiencing a mental health crisis.

Counselling

Counselling is a direct care method that helps the patient use a problem-solving process to recognize and manage stress and to facilitate interpersonal relationships. Nurses may engage in providing emotional, intellectual, spiritual, and psychological support to the patient. "Provide care to individuals with multiple comorbidities and complex health needs, including chronic disease management" is an essential skill of the nurse (CASN, 2022, Competency 3.2.12, p. 15). A patient and family who need nursing counselling may be upset or frustrated, but they are not necessarily disabled psychologically. Family caregivers need assistance in adjusting to the physical and emotional demands of caregiving. Likewise, the recipient of care also needs assistance in adjusting to the disability. Patients with psychiatric diagnoses require therapy provided by psychiatric nurses or by social workers, psychiatrists, or psychologists.

Many counselling techniques foster cognitive, behavioural, developmental, experiential, and emotional growth in patients. Counselling can be used to encourage individuals to examine available alternatives and decide which choices are useful and appropriate.

Teaching

Teaching is an important nursing responsibility and is related to counselling. Both involve the use of communication skills to create a change in the patient. However, in counselling, the focus is on the development of new attitudes and feelings, whereas in teaching, the focus is on intellectual growth or the acquisition of new knowledge or psychomotor skills (Redman, 2007).

The purpose of health teaching is to help patients learn about their health status, ways of promoting health, and ways of caring for themselves. Some common examples of teaching by nurses are related to medication administration, activity restrictions, health promotion activities (e.g., diet, exercise, or smoking cessation), and knowledge about disease and related implications. The nurse's role includes assessment of patients' learning needs and readiness to learn. It is important to know the patient and to be aware of cultural and social factors that influence a patient's willingness and ability to learn. It is also important to know the patient's health literacy levels, that is, whether the patient can read directions or make calculations, which is sometimes necessary with self-care skills. The teaching–learning process is an interaction between the nurse and the patient in which specific learning objectives are addressed (see Chapter 21 for further information about patient education).

Preventive Measures

Preventive nursing actions promote health and prevent illness to avoid the need for acute or rehabilitative health care. Prevention includes assessment and promotion of the patient's health potential, carrying out prescribed measures (e.g., immunizations), health teaching, and identification of risk factors for illness, trauma, or both (see Chapter 1 for further information about health promotion).

INDIRECT CARE

Indirect care measures are actions that support the effectiveness of direct care interventions (Butcher et al., 2019). Nurses spend a good amount of time in indirect care activities (Box 15.5). Communication of information about patients (e.g., change-of-shift report and consultation) is essential to ensure that direct care activities are planned, coordinated, and performed with the proper resources.

Communicating Nursing Interventions

Any intervention provided for a patient will be communicated in writing, verbally, or both. Written interventions are part of both the nursing care plan and the permanent medical record. In a nursing care plan, there are collaborative interventions that represent the contributions of all health care team members involved in caring for a patient.

After completing nursing interventions, the nurse documents the treatment and patient's response in the appropriate record (see

BOX 15.5	Examples of Indirect Care Activities

- Documentation
- Delegation of care activities to unregulated care providers
- Medical order transcription
- Infection control (e.g., proper handling and storage of supplies, use of protective isolation)
- Environmental safety management (e.g., make patient rooms safe, strategically assign patients in geographic proximity to a single nurse)
- Computer data entry
- Telephone consultations with physicians and other health care providers
- Change-of-shift report
- Collecting, labelling, and transporting laboratory specimens
- Transporting patients to procedural areas and other nursing units

Adapted from Butcher, H. K., Bulechek, G. M., McCloskey Dochterman, J. M., & Wagner, C. (Eds.). (2019). *Nursing interventions classification (NIC)* (7th ed.). Mosby/Elsevier.

Chapter 16 for further information about documentation). The entry usually includes a brief description of pertinent assessment findings, the specific procedure, the time and details of the procedure, and the patient's response. The nurse also communicates nursing interventions verbally to other health care providers. Unless communication is clear, concise, accurate, and timely, caregivers may be uninformed, interventions may be needlessly duplicated, procedures may be delayed, and tasks may be left undone.

Delegating, Supervising, and Evaluating the Work of Other Staff Members

Depending on the staffing system, not all the nursing interventions may be performed by the nurse who develops the care plan. Some activities are delegated to other members of the health care team. Interventions such as skin care, ambulation, grooming, measuring vital signs in stable patients, and hygiene measures are examples of care activities that may be assigned to unregulated care providers. When a nurse delegates aspects of a patient's care to another staff member, the nurse assigning the tasks is responsible for ensuring that each task is appropriately assigned and completed.

ACHIEVING PERSON-CENTRED GOALS

Nursing care is implemented to meet **person-centred goals** and outcomes. In most clinical situations, multiple interventions are necessary to achieve the desired outcomes. Because patients' conditions may change rapidly, it is important to apply the principles of care coordination, such as good time management, organizational skills, and appropriate use of resources, to ensure that nurses deliver interventions effectively and that patients achieve the desired outcomes. Therefore, the nurse must demonstrate an ability to "optimize health outcomes by responding effectively in rapidly changing or deteriorating health conditions" (CASN, 2022, Competency 3.2.5, p. 14). Priority setting and time management are also crucial in successful implementation because they help the nurse to anticipate and sequence nursing interventions when a patient has multiple nursing diagnoses and collaborative problems. Another way to achieve person-centred goals is to encourage and assist patients in following their treatment plans. Consultation and collaboration are critical to achieving the patient's goals and expected outcomes.

Effective discharge planning and teaching for patients and families require individualized care that is consistent with culture and health beliefs. The process should be initiated at the outset of care. Adequate and timely discharge planning and education of the patient and family are the first steps in promoting a smooth transition from one health care setting to another or to home. To be effective with discharge planning and education, the nurse needs to individualize care and consider the various factors that influence a patient's health beliefs.

EVALUATION

Evaluation is the final step of the nursing process. Evaluation involves two components: (1) an examination of a condition or situation and (2) a judgement as to whether change has occurred. Ideally, after an intervention takes place, evaluation will reveal an improvement. The nurse uses critical thinking skills throughout the nursing process, from gathering patient data to form nursing diagnoses to developing and implementing a plan of care. At the end of this process, during evaluation, the nurse reviews the expected outcomes for the patient and judges whether the planned goals have been successful. Evaluation ensures that nursing care helped the patient; if it did not, the nurse re-enters the nursing process in order to modify and continue working toward improving the patient's condition or well-being.

CRITICAL THINKING AND EVALUATION

Evaluation is an ongoing process whenever a nurse has contact with a patient. Collaboration is a key component of the evaluation process and is found to be an overarching theme in person-centred care. Nurses gather subjective data from the patient as well as objective data from the family and health care team members prior to and following an intervention; this process ensures that all facets of the patient's health, including past medical history, are considered. Nurses also review knowledge on the patient's current condition, treatment, resources available for recovery, and expected outcomes. In referring to previous experiences caring for similar patients, nurses are in a better position to know how to evaluate their patient's needs.

As in all steps of the nursing process, critical thinking remains a key component in the evaluation process. Critical thinking is a complex phenomenon that can be defined as a process and as a set of skills. Knowledge and reasoning are used to make accurate clinical judgements and decisions (see Chapter 7). Critical thinking also involves using standards of care to determine whether expected outcomes are achieved. Critical thinking fosters analysis of the findings in an evaluation to ensure that a patient's health needs or goals have been met or that the patient is able to improve or meet their health goals in a reasonable amount of time. Critical thinking also enables the identification of internal or external factors that may prevent recovery or the meeting of health goals.

During evaluation, nurses make clinical decisions and continually evaluate nursing care. This involves the nurse's ability to "apply clinical reasoning and clinical judgement when providing care to individuals, families (biological or chosen), communities, and populations" (CASN, 2022, Competency 3.2.6, p. 14). Positive evaluations occur when desired outcomes are met. Unmet or undesirable outcomes, such as the continuation of severe pain, indicate that interventions are not effective in minimizing or resolving the actual problem or in avoiding the risk of a problem. Outcomes need to be realistic and adjusted based on the patient's current prognosis, health goals, and nursing diagnoses. An unmet outcome indicates that the patient has not responded to interventions as planned. As a result, the nurse needs to change the plan of care by trying different healing initiatives or changing the frequency or approach of existing healing initiatives. As a nurse, reflecting on the success or failure of previous interventions will enhance your

clinical expertise when choosing relevant evidence-informed options for future patients.

This sequence of critically evaluating and revising therapies continues until the nurse and the patient successfully and appropriately resolve the health issues, as defined by the nursing diagnoses and the patient's goals. Remember that evaluation is dynamic and ever-changing, depending on the patient's nursing diagnoses, health goals, and condition. As problems change, so will expectations of outcomes. A patient whose health status continuously changes requires more frequent evaluation. In addition, nurses evaluate high-priority diagnoses first; in patient centred-care, the priority will be that set by the patient in collaboration with the nurse.

To highlight the role of critical thinking in evaluation (Figure 15.3), we return to the case study presented in this chapter. The primary nurse is preparing to evaluate their implemented nursing activities for Mr. Fletcher. The primary nurse uses a critical thinking approach to frame the evaluation process (see Figure 15.3), and revisits the nursing care plan to engage in the evaluation process (see Box 15.1).

Knowledge: The primary nurse meets with Mr. Fletcher, who recognizes that smoking influences his blood pressure. While keeping his blood pressure log, he developed an interest in taking his blood pressure before and after having a cigarette. In response, he has decided to decrease his cigarette intake and try to stop smoking. He has also started walking 30 minutes per day, 5 times a week, with his wife. The primary knows that having outside support will help Mr. Fletcher to maintain this practice. His wife has also changed her cooking to include low-salt, low-fat foods and a lower daily caloric intake. The primary nurse plans to seek collaborative support from the nurse practitioner because Mr. Fletcher's blood pressure is still 150/99 mm Hg despite his recent lifestyle changes. He will most likely require an antihypertensive medication to help support his lifestyle modification and decrease his cardiac risk.

Standards: Mr. Fletcher's blood pressure is still high according to clinical guidelines. While he is making significant strides in adopting a self-care approach, he may require extra support or new goals to decrease his overall blood pressure and prevent complications.

Qualities: The primary nurse takes a supportive approach, commending Mr. Fletcher on his changes in health behaviour. The primary nurse helps him to interpret the data he has been collecting and talks about what is working and what he is still having difficulty with. The primary nurse continues to work with Mr. Fletcher to manage his hypertension.

Experience: The primary nurse notes that Mr. Fletcher is making a significant effort to improve his health. His self-care management may become more complicated as he integrates these new behaviours into different social settings. The next step in his care will include the introduction of collaborative approaches to the management of hypertension, including referral to a dietitian to further his education on healthy eating.

The nurse in this scenario developed a comprehensive care plan, but her outcomes were only partially met because the patient remains hypertensive. To understand the evaluation process, think about any additional evaluative data that you would like to ask about or obtain regarding this case study as you read through the rest of this chapter.

EVALUATION PROCESS

The purpose of nursing care is to assist the patient in resolving actual health problems, preventing the occurrence of potential problems, and maintaining a healthy state as defined by the patient. The evaluation

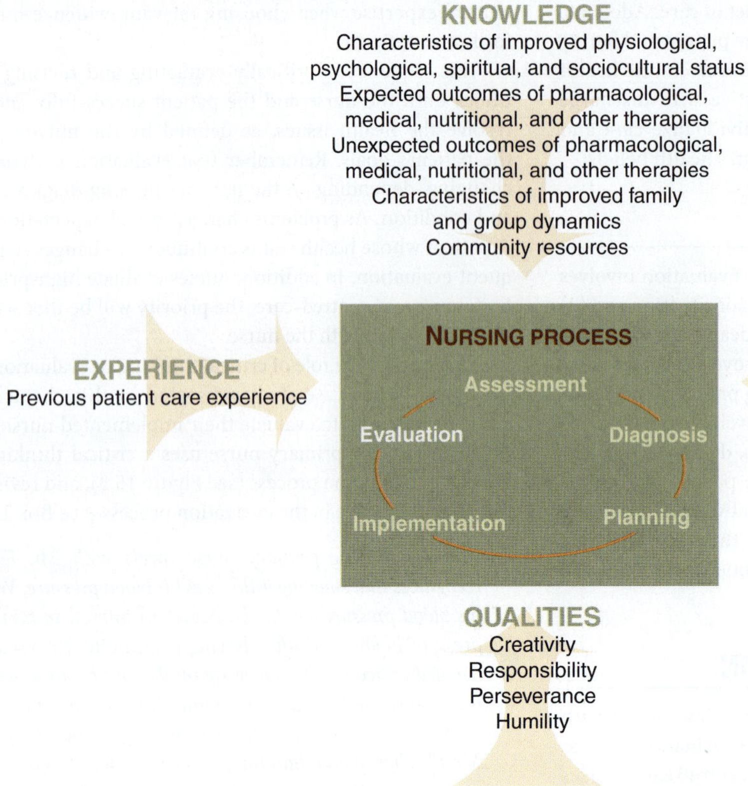

KNOWLEDGE
Characteristics of improved physiological,
psychological, spiritual, and sociocultural status
Expected outcomes of pharmacological,
medical, nutritional, and other therapies
Unexpected outcomes of pharmacological,
medical, nutritional, and other therapies
Characteristics of improved family
and group dynamics
Community resources

EXPERIENCE
Previous patient care experience

NURSING PROCESS
Assessment
Evaluation
Diagnosis
Implementation
Planning

STANDARDS
Expected outcomes of care
Specialty standards of practice
(e.g., Canadian Pain Society)
Intellectual standards

QUALITIES
Creativity
Responsibility
Perseverance
Humility

FIGURE 15.3 Critical thinking and evaluation.

process, which determines the effectiveness of nursing care, consists of five elements: (1) identifying evaluative criteria and standards; (2) collecting data to determine whether the criteria or standards have been met; (3) interpreting and summarizing findings; (4) documenting findings and any clinical judgement; and (5) terminating, continuing, or revising the care plan.

Identifying Criteria and Standards

Nursing care is evaluated by critically analyzing the attainment of the patient's identified goals and expected outcomes. A patient's goals and expected outcomes are the objective criteria by which to judge a patient's response to care. This person-centred approach to care plans falls directly in line with the CNA's *Code of Ethics*, which states, "In health-care decision-making, in treatment and in care, nurses work with persons receiving care to take into account their values, customs and spiritual beliefs, as well as their social and economic circumstances without judgement or bias." (CNA, 2017, p. 12).

Goals. A *goal* is the expected behaviour or response that indicates resolution of a nursing diagnosis or maintenance of a healthy state. It is a summary statement of what will be accomplished when the patient has met all expected outcomes. Successful achievement of this goal depends on the success of interventions, chosen from the NIC, which states that "the classification includes the interventions that nurses do on behalf of patients, both independent and collaborative interventions, both direct and indirect care" (Butcher et al., 2019, p. 2). Goals are also often based on standards of care or guidelines established for minimal safe practice.

The evaluation of interventions considers two factors: the appropriateness of the interventions selected and the correct application of the intervention. The appropriateness of an intervention is based on the standard of care for a patient's health problem. A **standard of care** is

the minimum level of care acceptable to ensure a high quality of care. Standards of care define the types of therapies typically administered to patients with defined problems or needs. If a patient who is receiving chemotherapy for leukemia has a specific nursing diagnosis, such as *nausea related to pharyngeal irritation*, the standard of care established by a nursing department for this problem includes pain control measures for pharyngeal irritation, mouth care guidelines, and diet therapy. The nurse reviews the standard of care to determine whether the right interventions have been chosen or whether additional ones are required. Increasing or decreasing the frequency of interventions is another approach for ensuring appropriate application of an intervention. Nurses adjust interventions based on the patient's actual response to therapy as well as previous experience with similar patients. For example, if a patient continues to have congested lung sounds, the nurse counsels the patient to increase the frequency of coughing and deep breathing exercises to remove secretions.

During evaluation, it is often found that some planned interventions are designed for an inappropriate level of nursing care. In this case, the level of care is changed by substituting a different action verb, such as *assist* in place of *provide* or *demonstrate* in place of *instruct*, in the revised care plan. For example, to assist a patient in walking, a nurse must be at the patient's side during ambulation, whereas providing an assistive device helps the patient ambulate more independently. Also, demonstrating a skill requires that the nurse show a patient how a skill is performed rather than simply telling the patient how to perform it. Sometimes the level of care is appropriate, but the interventions are unsuitable because of a change in the expected outcome. In this case, the current interventions are discontinued and new ones are planned.

Any changes in the plan of care need to be made according to the nature of the patient's unfavourable response. As a beginning nurse, it is good to consult with other nurses to obtain suggestions for improving the approach to care delivery. Senior nurses are often excellent resources because of their experience. Simply changing the care plan is not enough, however. The nurse needs to implement the new plan and re-evaluate the patient's response to the nursing actions, keeping in mind that evaluation is a continuous process.

The nursing process is a systematic problem-solving approach to individualized patient care, but many factors affect each patient with health care problems. Patients who have the same health care problem are not necessarily treated the same way. As a result, nurses will sometimes make errors in judgement. The systematic use of evaluation provides a way to catch these errors. Consistently incorporating evaluation into nursing practice will minimize errors and ensure that the patient's plan of care is appropriate and relevant.

Expected Outcomes. Outcomes have been broadly defined in the health care literature. *Outcomes* refer to the changes that have occurred in response to nursing care (Harris & McGillis Hall, 2012). When a patient enters the health care system (in any care setting) and begins a therapeutic relationship with a nurse, the nursing process steps are set in motion (Doenges et al., 2019). In collaboration with the patient, the nurse collects data, identifies patient needs, establishes goals, creates measurable outcomes, and selects nursing interventions to assist the patient in achieving these outcomes and health-related goals (Doenges et al., 2019). Examples of nursing-sensitive outcomes are reductions in pain severity, incidence of pressure injuries, nosocomial infections (e.g., *Clostridium difficile*), and incidence of falls. By comparison, outcomes influenced largely by medical interventions include patient mortality, hospital readmissions, and length of stay. Outcomes are statements of progressive, step-by-step responses or behaviours that must be achieved in order to accomplish the goals of care. An outcome defines the effectiveness, efficiency, and measurement of the results of nursing interventions. When patient outcomes are achieved, the related factors for a nursing diagnosis usually no longer exist. During the planning phase (see Chapter 14 for more information about the planning process), the nurse needs to select an observable patient state, behaviour, or self-reported perception that will reflect goal achievement.

Nursing-sensitive outcomes (Nursing Outcomes Classification [NOC]) were developed after NICs once nurses realized that NOCs also needed a classification system to aid in documenting a nurse–patient encounter. NOCs are designed to provide the language for the evaluation step of the nursing process. The purposes of the NOC are (1) to identify, label, validate, and classify nursing-sensitive patient outcomes; (2) to field test and validate the classification; and (3) to define and test measurement procedures for the outcomes and indicators using clinical data. The NOC system offers nursing-sensitive outcomes for NANDA International nursing diagnoses (Table 15.3). For each outcome, the NOC system specifies recommended evaluation indicators, that is, the patient behaviours or responses that are measures of outcome achievement. These nursing diagnoses are applied in a meaningful way to provide informed, patient-centred care decisions (NANDA International, 2021).

Collecting Evaluative Data

Proper evaluation enables the nurse to determine the patient's response to nursing care and whether the therapy was effective in improving the patient's physical or emotional health. It is important to evaluate whether each patient reaches a level of wellness or recovery that the health care team and patient established in the goals of care. In addition, the nurse must determine whether they have met the patient's expectations of care. Nurses will ask patients questions about their perceptions of care, such as "Did your pain score out of 10, with 10 being the worst pain you have ever experienced and 0 being no pain, improve after the analgesic was administered?" and "Do you feel that your pain

TABLE 15.3	Linkages Between Nursing Outcomes Classification (NOC) and Nursing Diagnoses	
Nursing Diagnosis	**Suggested Outcomes**	**Indicators (Examples)**
Pain	Comfort level	Reported physical well-being
		Reported satisfaction with symptom control
		Expressed satisfaction with pain control
	Pain control	Recognition of pain onset
		Appropriate use of analgesics
		Control of reported pain
	Pain level	Reported pain severity
		Frequency of pain
		Muscle tension
Deficient knowledge	Knowledge: Treatment procedures	Description of treatment procedures
	Knowledge: Illness care	Description of disease process
		Description of prescribed activity

Adapted from Moorhead, S., Swanson, E., Johnson, M., & Maas, M. (2018). *Nursing outcomes classification (NOC)* (6th ed.). Mosby/Elsevier.

will be appropriately managed when you are discharged from the hospital today?" This level of evaluation is important for determining the patient's satisfaction with care and for strengthening the partnering between the nurse and the patient. Evaluating a patient's response to nursing care requires the use of evaluative measures, which are simply assessment skills and techniques (e.g., auscultation of lung sounds, observation of a patient's skill performance, discussion of the patient's feelings, and inspection of the skin) (Figure 15.4). In fact, evaluative measures are the same as assessment measures, but nurses perform them when making decisions about the patient's status and progress.

The intent of assessment is to identify any problems that exist. The intent of evaluation is to determine whether the known problems have remained the same, improved, worsened, or otherwise changed. In many clinical situations, it is important to collect evaluative measures over time to determine whether a pattern of improvement or change exists. A one-time observation of a pressure injury is insufficient to determine that the injury is healing. Consistent change must be noted. For example, over a period of 2 days, you can observe whether the pressure injury is gradually decreasing in size, whether the amount of drainage is declining, and whether the redness of inflammation is resolving. Recognizing a pattern of improvement or deterioration enables the nurse to reason and decide whether the patient's problems are resolved. The primary source of data for evaluation is the patient. However, nurses also use input from the family and other caregivers. Nursing colleagues may also serve as a source of evaluation when they are consulted regarding how a patient responded to a nursing intervention during a previous shift.

Interpreting and Summarizing Findings

During an acute illness, a patient's clinical condition changes, often minute by minute. In contrast, chronic illness results in slow, subtle changes. When nurses evaluate the effect of interventions, they are essentially performing another nursing assessment whereby they learn to recognize relevant evidence about a patient's condition, even evidence that sometimes does not match clinical expectations. By applying clinical knowledge and life experiences, nurses learn to recognize complications or adverse responses to illness and treatment in addition to expected outcomes. Using evidence, they make judgements about a patient's condition. To develop clinical judgement, nurses learn to match the results of evaluative measures with expected outcomes to determine whether a patient's status is improving. When interpreting findings, the nurse, in conjunction with the patient, compares the patient's behavioural responses and the physiological signs and symptoms expected with the patient's condition. By comparing expected and actual findings, the nurse can interpret and judge the patient's condition and whether predicted changes have occurred (Table 15.4).

To objectively evaluate the degree of success in achieving outcomes of care, use the following steps:

1. Examine the outcome criteria to identify the exact desired patient behaviour or response.
2. Assess the patient's actual behaviour or response.
3. Compare the established outcome criteria with the actual behaviour or response.
4. Judge the degree of agreement between outcome criteria and the actual behaviour or response.
5. If the outcome criteria are not in agreement or are only in partial agreement with the actual behaviour or response, what are the barriers to agreement? Why was agreement not complete?

Evaluation is easier to perform after a nurse has cared for a patient over a long period. The nurse is then able to make subtle comparisons of patient responses and behaviours. When nurses have not had the chance to care for a patient over an extended time, they improve evaluation by referring to previous experiences or asking colleagues who are familiar with the patient to confirm evaluation findings. In short-term stay settings, a plan of care with clearly defined short- and long-term goals provides a framework to guide future care. The accuracy of any evaluation improves when nurses are familiar with the patient's behaviour and physiological status or have cared for more than one patient with a similar problem.

A central part of evaluation is to determine whether each expected outcome was achieved and what its place is in the sequence of care. This aids the nurse in revising and redirecting the plan of care if outcomes are not met. Once a patient achieves an outcome, the nurse either continues the plan of care to reinforce the continuation of the outcome or discontinues the interventions because the goal has been met. If the expected outcome was only partially achieved or not achieved at all, the care plan is reassessed and revised. It is important to note that if progress is not made, the goal or outcome cannot be met. At any time during treatment, the patient may choose to withdraw treatment, regardless of whether or not the goals have been met; in addition, goals may change depending on the patient's desires (Table 15.5).

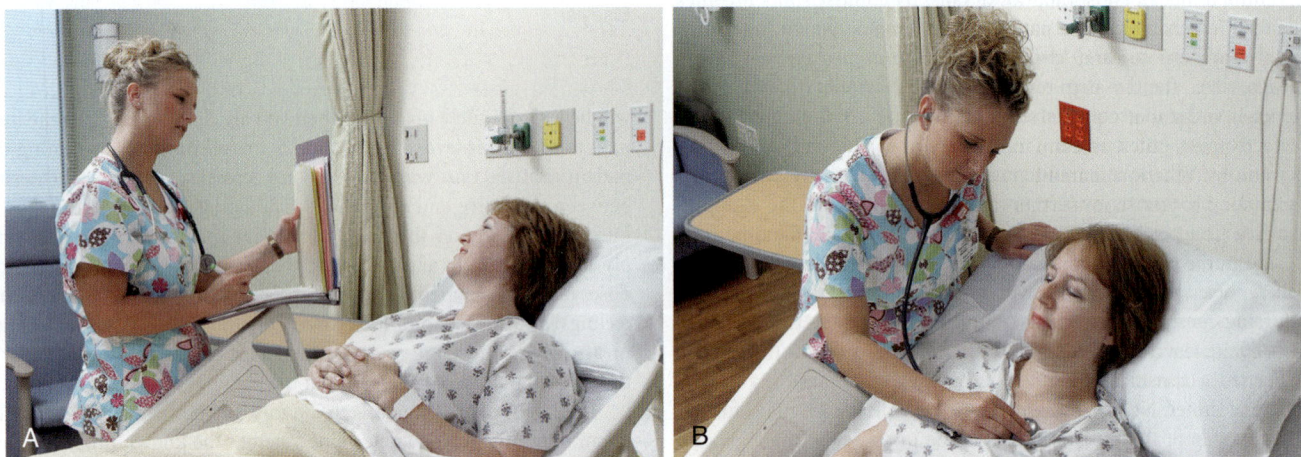

FIGURE 15.4 Evaluative measures. **A,** Nurse confirms patient's medical history. **B,** Nurse evaluates patient's lung sounds.

TABLE 15.4	Evaluative Measures to Determine the Success of Goals and Expected Outcomes	
Goals	**Evaluative Measures**	**Expected Outcomes**
Patient's stage 2 pressure ulcer will heal within 10 days.	Inspect colour, condition, and location of pressure ulcer. Measure and record diameter and depth of ulcer daily. Note odour and colour of drainage from ulcer.	Erythema will be reduced in 2 days. Diameter of ulcer will decrease in 5 days. Ulcer will have no drainage in 2 days. Patient will have increased protein intake for wound healing. Skin overlying ulcer will be closed in 7 days.
Patient will tolerate ambulation to end of hall by 11/20.	Palpate patient's radial pulse before exercise. Palpate patient's radial pulse 10 minutes after exercise. Assess respiratory rate during exercise. Observe patient for dyspnea or breathlessness during exercise.	Pulse will remain below 110 beats per minute during exercise. Respiratory rate will remain within two breaths of patient's baseline rate. Patient will deny feeling of breathlessness.
Patient will have improved grief resolution by 1/15.	Ask patient about frequency of periods of crying, sadness. Review patient's sleeping log. Review patient's dietary intake.	Patient reports decreased frequency of crying and sadness in 2 months. Patient has periods of 6 to 7 hours of sleep without interruption within 10 days. Patient has no weight loss in 1 month.

TABLE 15.5	Examples of Objective Evaluation of Goal Achievement		
Goals	**Outcome Criteria**	**Patient Response**	**Evaluation Findings**
Patient will self-administer insulin by 12/18.	Patient prepares insulin dosage in syringe by 12/17. Patient demonstrates self-injection by 12/18.	Patient prepared accurate dosage in syringe on 12/17. Patient administered morning insulin dosage and performed self-injection correctly on 12/18.	Patient has progressed and achieved desired behaviour.
Patient's lungs will be free of secretions by 11/30.	Coughing will be nonproductive by 11/29. Lungs will be clear to auscultation by 11/30. Respirations will be 20 per minute by 11/30.	Patient coughed frequently and productively on 11/29. Lungs were clear to auscultation on 11/30. Respirations were 18 per minute on 11/29.	Patient will require continued therapy. Condition is improving.
Patient will be able to perform self-care measures without discomfort in 2 days.	Patient will rate pain as 3 on a scale of 0–10 within 2 days. Patient will initiate bathing within 2 days.	Patient rates severe right-sided abdominal pain as 5 on a scale of 0–10 while attempting bathing on day 2.	Patient's condition still indicates a problem. Patient requires continued therapy with possibly new care measures.

Documenting Findings

Documentation and reporting are an important part of evaluation and a legal necessity for nurses to complete. For nurses to make ongoing clinical decisions, a patient's medical record must contain accurate information. Therefore, when documenting a patient's response to interventions, the nurse should always describe the same evaluative measures. For example, "the patient was given 2.5 mg of IV (intravenous) morphine for 8/10 chest pain; after administration the pain level was 0/10." The aim is to present a clear description, informed by the evaluative data, of a patient's progress or lack of progress. Written nursing progress notes, assessment flow sheets, clinical pathways, care maps, and information shared between nurses during change-of-shift reports (see Chapter 16 for further information about documentation) communicate a patient's progress toward meeting expected outcomes and goals in the nursing plan of care.

Care Plan Revision

Nurses evaluate expected outcomes and determine whether the goals of care have been met. They then decide whether the plan of care needs to be adjusted. If goals are successfully met, that portion of the care plan can be discontinued. If goals are unmet or partially met, the intervention continues. After the nurse evaluates a patient, the nurse may want to modify or add nursing diagnoses with appropriate goals and expected outcomes and establish interventions. It is also important to redefine priorities. This is an important step in critical thinking: knowing how the patient is progressing and how problems either resolve or worsen. With chronic conditions, care plans are still used and require revisions based on the progression of the chronic health issue. Care plans help patients with chronic health issues become more proactive in responding to their health needs (Jansen et al., 2015).

Careful monitoring and early detection of problems are a patient's first line of defence. Nurses must make nursing judgements pertaining to observations of what is occurring with a specific patient and not merely of what happens to patients in general. Frequently, changes are not obvious. Evaluations are patient specific, based on a close familiarity with each patient's behaviour, physical status, and reaction to caregivers. Critical thinking skills and life experiences enhance accurate evaluation, which enables appropriate revision of ineffective care plans and discontinuation of therapy that has successfully resolved a problem.

Discontinuing a Care Plan

After a nurse determines that expected outcomes and goals have been met, they confirm this finding with the patient, when possible. If the

nurse and the patient agree, then that portion of the care plan is discontinued. Documentation of a discontinued plan ensures that other nurses will not unnecessarily continue interventions for that portion of the plan of care. Continuity of care ensures that care provided to patients is relevant and timely. In situations of chronic illness, care plans are still used and beneficial; expected outcomes in chronic conditions should aim to improve the quality of the chronic illness. This in turn leads to a better quality of life for patients, improved health outcomes, and decreased health care utilization (Jansen et al., 2015).

Modifying a Care Plan

When goals are not met, nurses identify the factors that interfere with goal achievement. A change in the patient's condition, needs, or abilities usually necessitates changes in the care plan. For example, when teaching self-administration of insulin, a nurse discovers that the patient has developed a new problem, a tremor associated with an adverse effect of a medication. The patient is unable to draw medication from a syringe or inject the needle safely. As a result, the original outcomes "Patient will correctly prepare insulin in a syringe" and "Patient will administer insulin injection independently" cannot be met. The nurse introduces new interventions (instructing a family member in insulin preparation and administration or introducing an alternative method of insulin administration, such as an insulin pen) and revises outcomes to meet the goal of care.

At times, a lack of goal achievement results from an error in nursing judgement or failure to follow each step of the nursing process. Patients often have multiple and complex problems. When a goal is not achieved, no matter the reason, the entire nursing process sequence should be repeated for that nursing diagnosis to determine what changes need to be made in the plan. The patient is then reassessed, the accuracy of the nursing diagnosis is determined, new goals and expected outcomes are established, and new interventions are selected while adhering to national and provincial/territorial nursing standards.

A complete reassessment of all patient factors relating to the nursing diagnosis and etiology is necessary when nurses modify a plan. Reassessment requires critical thinking as new data are compared with previously assessed information.

Knowledge acquired from previous experiences helps to direct the reassessment process. Caring for patients and families who have had similar health problems gives the nurse a strong background of knowledge to use for anticipating patient needs and knowing what to assess. As a nurse's experience increases so too does their knowledge base from which to draw. Reassessment reveals "missing links" (i.e., critical pieces of new information that were overlooked and thus interfered with goal achievement). Nurses sort, validate, and cluster all new data to analyze and interpret differences from the original database. They also document reassessment data to alert other nursing staff to the patient's status and communicate them to the patient. After reassessment, the nurse determines what nursing diagnoses are accurate for the situation and revises the problem list to reflect the patient's changed status and/or goals.

Sometimes a new diagnosis is formed. As the patient's condition changes, the diagnoses also change. For example, the nursing diagnosis *deficient knowledge related to inexperience* for a patient with newly diagnosed diabetes was previously used in the care plan. The original plan was to instruct the patient in how to self-administer insulin. After observing that the patient has difficulty self-administering insulin because of a tremor associated with an adverse effect of a medication, the nurse reassesses the situation and finds that a family member is available as a resource. To develop a plan designed to educate a caregiver about the administration of insulin, the nurse then establishes a new diagnosis: *ineffective health maintenance related to impaired dexterity*.

Goals and Expected Outcomes

When revising care plans, it is imperative to collaboratively review with the patient the goals and expected outcomes for needed changes. Nurses also need to examine the appropriateness of goals for unchanged nursing diagnoses because a change in one problem sometimes affects other problems. Determining that each goal and expected outcome is realistic for the problem, etiology, and time frame is particularly important. Unrealistic expected outcomes and time frames hamper goal achievement. It is important to clearly document goals and expected outcomes for new or revised nursing diagnoses so that all team members are aware of the revised care plan. When the goal is still appropriate but has not yet been met, the nurse can try changing the evaluation data to allow more time. The nurse may also decide to change interventions. For example, when a patient's pressure ulcer does not show signs of healing, the nurse may choose to use a different support surface or a different type of wound cleanser. All goals and expected outcomes are patient-centred, with realistic expectations for patient achievement.

SUMMARY

The evaluation of nursing care is a professional responsibility and a crucial component of nursing care. Evaluation that focuses on a single patient's plan of care enables the nurse to know the effectiveness of interventions and whether expected outcomes are met. At a system or institutional level, evaluation involves quality improvement and performance improvement activities that focus on the delivery of care provided by an agency or a specific nursing division within an agency. Through the continuous evaluation of care, nurses play a key role in the ongoing improvement of patient care.

USING THE NURSING PROCESS TO ENHANCE TEST-TAKING SKILLS IN NURSING PROGRAMS

The nursing process is a useful model for guiding the development of your future nursing practice. It is also an essential tool that will aid in organizing the vast amount of information you will be exposed to in your nursing program. If used in the right way, the nursing process can be an excellent tool to help you to frame your preparation for the registration exam you will write upon graduation from your nursing program. In Chapter 14, the use of the nursing process for test-taking was introduced. The remainder of this chapter will address how to identify test-taking and study strategies focused on the implementation or evaluation stage of the nursing process.

In Chapter 14, common words used in test questions were identified for the nursing process stages of assessment, diagnosis, and planning (Nugent & Vitale, 2020). Table 15.6 identifies common words in test questions for the nursing process stages of implementation and evaluation.

The following questions are examples of how the implementation and evaluation stages of the nursing process can be tested.

Example: A patient (preferred pronouns: he/him) describes having severe abdominal discomfort. On assessment, it is found that the patient's abdomen is distended and the patient has not passed flatus since his bowel resection surgery 24 hours earlier. Which of the following is a priority nursing action at this time?

1. Insert a nasogastric tube per health care provider order.
2. Offer the patient ice chips.
3. Gather more assessment data.
4. Reassess the patient in 15 minutes to see if the discomfort resolves.

The correct answer to this question is 1. In this question, it is made clear that the patient is having abdominal discomfort due to decreased peristalsis of the bowel after a surgical procedure. This can turn into an emergent situation if it is not addressed immediately. Assessment data provided are that the patient had surgery 24 hours earlier and that he has not passed flatus. The question asks, "Which of the following is

TABLE 15.6	Using the Nursing Process to Help Answer Exam Questions	
Nursing Process	**Questions in This Stage of the Nursing Process Often Ask You to:**	**Common Words in the Question Stem Identifying This Area**
Implementation	• Complete nursing actions based on goals established • Prioritize care • Delegate care as appropriate • Advocate for the patient • Document all nursing interventions to therapeutic modalities	Change, assist, counsel, teach, give, supervise, perform, method, procedure, treatment, instruct, strategy, facilitate, provide, inform, refer, technique, motivate, delegate, implement
Evaluation	• Compare actual outcomes with expected outcomes • Communicate findings to health care team • Document and measure goal attainment • Review and modify nursing care plan • Reprioritize care plan based on evaluation	Expected, met, desired, compared, succeeded, failed, achieved, modified, reassess, ineffective, effective, response and evaluate

From Kramer-Kile, M. L. (2016). *Transitioning to the NCLEX-RN®: A study guide for Canadian-educated graduates* (2nd ed.). Kramer-Kile Nurse Education Consultants Ltd. Registration No. 1122832. Reprinted with permission.

a priority nursing action at this time?" The term *action* is associated with the implementation stage of the nursing process—it is focused on what the nurse can do within their scope of practice. The first step in answering this question is to focus on answers that are clearly nursing interventions meant to resolve the identified problem.

Answer 1 (Correct): This is clearly a nursing action focused on alleviating the build-up of gas in the bowel. The insertion of a nasogastric tube is within a nurse's scope of practice; however, it must be under a health care provider's order or directive.

Answer 2 (Incorrect): Offering the patient ice chips will not help to relieve the discomfort and may make the discomfort in the patient's abdomen worse.

Answer 3 (Incorrect): Gathering more assessment data is not an appropriate action at this time. The question stem has provided enough information to determine that this patient is at risk. The nurse needs to move from the assessment phase to the implementation phase of the nursing process.

Answer 4 (Incorrect): This is clearly within the evaluation phase of the nursing process. However, what is the nurse evaluating if they have not performed any nursing interventions?

Example: The nurse inserts a nasogastric tube in a patient who is diagnosed with a paralytic ileus. Which of the following findings indicates the patient's condition has stabilized?

1. The patient is able to eat a full meal.
2. The patient has regular bowel sounds in all four abdominal quadrants.
3. The patient has an increase in their oxygen saturation levels.
4. The patient has their gag reflex return.

The correct answer to this question is 2. You are being asked to evaluate whether the patient's nasogastric tube insertion has relieved the symptoms associated with a paralytic ileus. Therefore, the answer you choose should demonstrate that you understand how to determine that this condition has resolved.

Answer 1 (Incorrect): The patient would not be eating a full meal while a nasogastric tube is in situ. They would be advanced to a full diet once the tube is removed.

Answer 2 (Correct): A common symptom of a paralytic ileus is absence of bowel sounds. Auscultating for the return of bowel sounds would evaluate whether the paralytic ileus has resolved.

Answer 3 (Incorrect): Oxygen saturation levels would not be a way to evaluate the resolution of a paralytic ileus.

Answer 4 (Incorrect): While a gag reflex is essential for protecting the patient's airway, it is not a finding associated with the resolution of a paralytic ileus.

❖ THE NURSING PROCESS AND STUDYING DISEASE MANAGEMENT

While there are many facets to nursing practice, including individual, community, and population approaches to health (which require complex approaches to care), the nursing process is most easily applied to disease management frameworks. Patients may be living with a variety of disease conditions within acute, chronic, or palliative contexts. The nursing process can be used to map out what a plan of care would look like in these instances. For example, if a patient has been diagnosed with a condition such as acute glomerulonephritis, the nurse would need to know what to assess with this condition, how it is diagnosed and what the related nursing diagnoses are, how to plan care, the selected nursing and medical interventions for the patient, and how to evaluate whether these interventions have been successful. Students can begin "mapping" out different disease conditions early in their nursing programs as a way to learn this information and provide a framework for studying for in-class exams and the NCLEX-RN® (Kramer-Kile, 2016). Figure 15.5 outlines a framework for organizing key information regarding disease management using the nursing process as a guide.

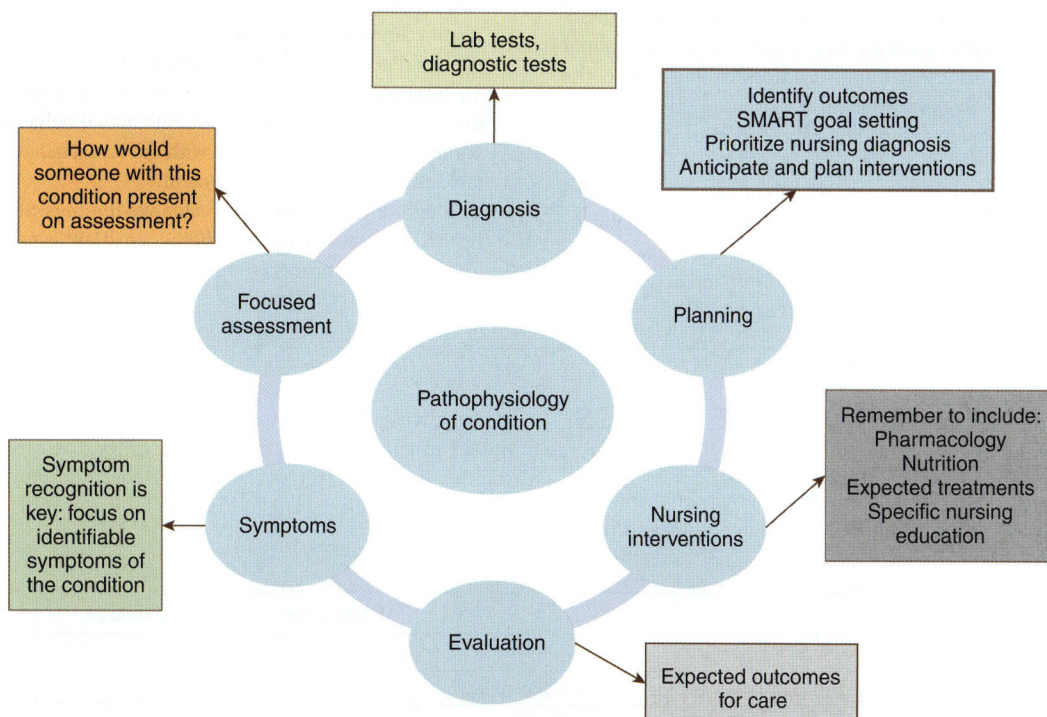

FIGURE 15.5 Using the nursing process to study disease and illness conditions. (From Kramer-Kile, M. L. [2016]. *Transitioning to the NCLEX-RN®: A study guide for Canadian-educated graduates* [2nd ed.]. Kramer-Kile Nurse Education Consultants Ltd. Registration No. 1122832. Reprinted with permission.)

We recommend that you build these study maps while taking your pathophysiology course and moving into acute care practice. While these maps are excellent tools for your clinical practice and for studying, it is important to remember that real patients who are living with these conditions are individuals who may experience their symptoms, understanding, and acceptance of these conditions in differing ways that may directly impact their care. Therefore, the nursing process involves more than listing which activities should be directed through nursing care. It also becomes a tool for learning how to critically think about the provision of holistic and comprehensive nursing care that treats more than the disease process—it is a recognition of the patient and their role in managing their own health.

These maps can serve as a guide for basic content. As you become more comfortable with the topic area, you can begin to add to the maps. For example, it is helpful to attach relevant drug cards to the maps to help you learn the pharmacological treatment of a disease process. Some students also write case studies related to the disease condition on the backs of their maps. This helps them to process the information they have learned. These maps are extremely useful when you are studying for the NCLEX-RN. If you build the maps throughout the program and save them for when it comes time to study, then you will have already organized your study approach so that you can study in the detail needed for the exam; simply reading through your textbooks at the end is far less effective than building maps as you go. It is also extremely helpful to form study groups and to complete the maps together. A list of common diseases to map and a detailed description of the study mapping exercises are provided on the Evolve website.

KEY CONCEPTS

- The Nursing Interventions Classification (NIC) taxonomy provides a standardization to assist nurses in selecting suitable interventions for patients' problems.
- Correctly written nursing interventions include actions, frequency, quantity, and method, and they specify the person to perform them.
- Consultation and collaboration increase a nurse's knowledge about a patient's problem and help nurses learn skills and obtain the resources needed to solve the problem.
- Implementation is the step of the nursing process in which the nurse provides direct and indirect nursing care interventions to patients.
- Clinical guidelines or protocols are evidence-informed documents that guide decisions and interventions for specific health care problems.
- During the initial phase of implementation, the nurse reassesses the patient to determine whether the proposed nursing action is still appropriate for the patient's level of wellness.

- To anticipate and prevent complications, the nurse identifies risks to the patient, adapts interventions to the situation, evaluates the benefit of a treatment in relation to the risk, and initiates risk-prevention measures to create a culture of patient safety.
- Successful implementation of nursing interventions requires the nurse to use appropriate cognitive, interpersonal, and psychomotor skills.
- Counselling is a direct care method that helps patients use problem solving to recognize and manage stress and to facilitate interpersonal relationships.
- Preventive nursing actions include assessment and promotion of the patient's health potential, application of prescribed measures (e.g., immunizations), health teaching, and identification of risk factors for illness, trauma, or both.
- A concept map provides a visual way to understand the relationship between a patient's nursing diagnoses and interventions.
- Evaluation is a step of the nursing process that allows nurses to determine whether nursing interventions are successful in improving a patient's condition or well-being.
- During evaluation, the appropriateness of the intervention should be assessed, as should the outcome.
- Evaluation involves two components: an examination of a condition or situation and a judgement as to whether change has occurred.
- During evaluation, nurses apply critical thinking to make nursing decisions and redirect nursing care to best meet patients' needs.
- Evaluation findings are positive when desired outcomes are met; this enables nurses to conclude that their interventions were effective.
- When the patient's actual response (e.g., behaviours and physiological signs and symptoms) to nursing interventions are compared with expected outcomes established during planning, the nurse determines whether goals of care have been met. At this time, the nurse should also determine whether the goals, outcomes, or both were realistic.
- Evaluative measures are assessment skills or techniques that nurses use to collect data for evaluation.
- It sometimes becomes necessary to collect evaluative measures over time to determine whether a pattern of change exists.
- To interpret evaluative findings, the nurse needs to examine the outcome criteria, assess the patient's actual behaviour or response, compare the outcome criteria with the actual behaviour or response, and judge the degree of agreement.
- Through documentation of evaluative findings, all members of the health care team can know whether a patient is progressing.
- The evaluation process may change a patient's nursing diagnoses, priorities, and interventions.

CRITICAL THINKING EXERCISES

1. The primary nurse is working with Mr. Fletcher to address his modifiable risk factors. These include obesity, inactivity, and smoking. After the session has been completed, Mr. Fletcher makes the following statements.

For each statement, insert an "X" to indicate whether the primary nurse's teaching was *effective* (demonstrates that Mr. Fletcher understands), *ineffective* (shows that Mr. Fletcher does not understand), or *unrelated* (is not relevant to his education regarding modifiable risk factors).

Patient Statement	Effective	Ineffective	Unrelated
"I will walk for 30 minutes per day, 3 times a week."			
"I will do my best to cut down on the number of cigarettes I smoke daily."			
"Some people just have difficulty losing weight."			
"I can use medication to help me stop smoking."			
"I will need to assess my blood pressure before taking my medication."			

2. The primary nurse has finished teaching Mr. Fletcher about the complications of hypertension.

Indicate which nursing action (from the list of actions) is appropriate for each of the three potential complications related to Mr. Fletcher. Note that not all nursing actions will be used.

List of Possible Nursing Actions	Potential Complication	Appropriate Nursing Action for Complication
1. Monitor creatinine and BUN levels	Renal impairment Visual changes Stroke	
2. Teach FAST assessment to the patient and their family		
3. Administer long-term antibiotic therapy		
4. Assess fasting blood glucose levels		
5. Report a severe headache to the health care provider immediately		

🌐 *Answers to Critical Thinking Exercises appear on the Evolve website.*

REVIEW QUESTIONS

Review Questions 1 to 9 relate to the case study at the beginning of the chapter.

1. The primary nurse is watching Mr. Fletcher take his own blood pressure with an automatic blood pressure machine. Which of the following patient actions should the nurse correct first?
   a. Mr. Fletcher has wrapped the blood pressure cuff too loosely.
   b. Mr. Fletcher is moving around during the blood pressure reading.
   c. Mr. Fletcher smokes a cigarette after taking his blood pressure reading.
   d. Mr. Fletcher rests for 5 minutes before taking his first blood pressure reading.

2. Which of the following are examples of dependent nursing interventions? (*Select all that apply.*)
   a. Refer the patient to Best Practice Guidelines for the management of hypertension.
   b. Obtain an order for new antihypertensive medication from the nurse practitioner.
   c. Teach the client to increase their daily activity to 30 minutes a day, three times per week.
   d. Observe the patient for signs of impaired renal function.
   e. Complete a chest X-ray to look for signs of heart failure.

3. The primary nurse writes an expected outcome statement for Mr. Fletcher in measurable terms. An example is:
   a. Patient will be normotensive.
   b. Patient will have decreased blood pressure.
   c. Patient will take his blood pressure daily.
   d. Patient will take his blood pressure daily and report systolic pressures over 140 mm Hg.

4. The primary nurse is exploring a *collaborative intervention* to help assess Mr. Fletcher for peripheral arterial disease. Collaborative interventions are therapies that require:
   a. Nurse and patient intervention
   b. Physician and nurse intervention
   c. Patient and physician intervention
   d. Multiple health care providers

5. When completing an individualized written care plan for Mr. Fletcher, what should the primary nurse prioritize?
   a. Using a critical pathway to provide a strict plan of care
   b. Completing a concept map to comprehensively manage one problem at a time
   c. Collaborating with the patient and family in the development of the plan

   d. Understanding that nursing care plans are the same despite different settings and patient situations

6. Different types of nursing interventions may be incorporated into the plan of care. Which of the following interventions is an example of a specific life-saving measure that the primary nurse may implement?
   a. Administering antihypertensive therapy
   b. Recognizing the signs of stroke in a patient
   c. Initiating stress-reduction therapy
   d. Teaching a patient how to take their blood pressure

7. The primary nurse teaches Mr. Fletcher how to take an antilipemic medication (cholesterol-reducing medication). Which of the following actions would the nurse use to evaluate the long-term impacts of this intervention?
   a. Ask Mr. Fletcher to explain, in his own words, why the medication has been prescribed.
   b. Assess Mr. Fletcher's understanding of why the medication is taken in the evening.
   c. Ensure that Mr. Fletcher is scheduled for blood work that includes a fasting lipid panel monthly.
   d. Track Mr. Fletcher's blood pressure daily over a 3-month period.

8. The primary nurse is evaluating the care provided to Mr. Fletcher. Which of the following objective evaluative criteria would the nurse use to judge the patient's response to the care provided?
   a. Goals and expected outcomes outlined in the care plan
   b. Patient states, "I am feeling better."
   c. Nursing diagnosis chosen for the patient
   d. Patient's satisfaction with the care provided

9. Mr. Fletcher returns to the clinic 2 weeks after starting a new antihypertensive medication. He remains hypertensive, even though he is taking the medication as prescribed. What should be the primary nurse's initial action?
   a. Ask Mr. Fletcher's wife whether he is really taking his medication daily.
   b. Notify the health care provider.
   c. Ask Mr. Fletcher whether he is taking other medications such as NSAID therapy.
   d. Make an appointment for Mr. Fletcher to see a dietitian.

Answers 1. a; **2.** b, e; **3.** d; **4.** d; **5.** c; **6.** b; **7.** c; **8.** a; **9.** c.

🌐 *Rationales for the Review Questions appear on the Evolve website.*

RECOMMENDED WEBSITES

Canadian Nurses Association (CNA): https://www.cna-aiic.ca/en/home
This expansive nursing website provides comprehensive information regarding many nursing issues such as nursing care delivery models and standards and best practices. The CNA's *Code of Ethics for Registered Nurses* is an example of the type of documents available on this site.

Center for Nursing Classification and Clinical Effectiveness:
https://nursing.uiowa.edu/center-for-nursing-classification-and-clinical-effectiveness
The University of Iowa's Center for Nursing Classification and Clinical Effectiveness was established to facilitate ongoing research of the Nursing Interventions Classification (NIC) and Nursing Outcomes Classification (NOC). This website provides an overview of the NIC and NOC and offers information about new classification material and publications.

NANDA International: https://www.nanda.org
Through this website, NANDA International provides current information on nursing diagnosis research, publications, support resources, and Internet resources.

Registered Nurses' Association of Ontario (RNAO)—Best Practice Guidelines: http://rnao.ca/bpg
The RNAO has an extensive process for developing Best Practice Guidelines in a variety of areas of clinical nursing. They have received federal and provincial funding for this process, and the results of their work have been made available to all Canadian nurses through this website, which lists all current guidelines that have been developed.

REFERENCES

A full reference list is available on the website for this book at http://evolve.elsevier.com/Canada/Potter/fundamentals/

16

Documenting and Reporting

Canadian content written by Sarah L. Johnston, RN, MN, with original chapter contributions by Noël Marie Kerr, PhD

OBJECTIVES

Mastery of content in this chapter will enable you to:

- Identify the purpose of a health care record.
- Describe the legal guidelines for documentation.
- Identify ways to maintain the confidentiality of electronic and written records.
- Describe six quality guidelines for documentation and reporting.
- Describe the different methods used in record keeping.
- Explain the advantages of standardized documentation forms.
- Identify elements to include when documenting a patient discharge plan.
- Describe the role of critical pathways in interdisciplinary documentation.
- Identify the important aspects of home care and long-term care documentation.
- Explain how to verify verbal and telephone orders.
- Describe the purpose and content of a change-of-shift report.
- Describe the use of electronic health records in documentation.
- Describe the advantages of clinical information systems.

KEY TERMS

Acuity ratings

Case management

Change-of-shift report

Charting by exception (CBE)

Clinical decision support system (CDSS)

Clinical information system (CIS)

Computerized provider order entry (CPOE)

Consultations

Critical pathways

Data–action–response (DAR) notes

Documentation

Electronic health record (EHR)

Electronic medical record (EMR)

Firewall

Flow sheets

Focus charting

Health informatics

Identification–situation–background–assessment–recommendation–repeat back (I-SBAR-R) technique

Incident (occurrence) report

Information technology (IT)

Kardex

Nursing clinical information system (NCIS)

Patient record

Personal Information Protection and Electronic Documents Act (PIPEDA)

Problem–intervention–evaluation (PIE)

Problem-oriented medical record (POMR)

Referrals

Reports

Situation–background–assessment–recommendation (SBAR) technique

Source record

Standardized care plans

Subjective–objective–assessment–plan (SOAP) note

Subjective–objective–assessment–plan–intervention–evaluation (SOAPIE) note

Transfer of accountability (TOA)

Transfer report

Variance

🌐 WEBSITE

http://evolve.elsevier.com/Canada/Potter/fundamentals/

CASE STUDY

Joseph (preferred pronouns: he/him), who is 80 years old, lives at home with his wife of 52 years. He is seen in the emergency department (ED) for complaints of fatigue and a frequent productive cough. On presentation to the ED, the nursing staffed note a temperature of 39°C and an oxygen saturation of 90%. A medical diagnosis of bacterial pneumonia is confirmed, and Joseph begins receiving supplemental oxygen and antibiotics as a result. Joseph is admitted directly to the inpatient medicine unit for treatment. After reviewing the results of the tests in Joseph's electronic medical record, the health care provider uses the computerized provider order entry (CPOE) feature to write prescriptions for Joseph.

On the inpatient unit, Joseph will be admitted and cared for by Shara (preferred pronouns: she/her), a senior-year nursing student who is starting her final clinical practicum on the unit with a nursing preceptor. She has had a brief orientation to the unit and the documentation system. Shara receives a telephone report from the ED nurse before Joseph is transferred to the unit.

On arrival to the unit, Joseph's vital signs are as follows: blood pressure 150/90 mm Hg; pulse rate 92 beats per minute; respiration rate 22 breaths per minute; and temperature 38.5°C. He states, "It hurts in my chest when I cough." Joseph and his wife have many questions about his admission, and they are worried that he will be sent home without proper support in place.

Think about this case study as you read this chapter. There are Review Questions at the end of the chapter about this case study.

Documentation is a nursing action defined as "the process of documenting nursing information about nursing care in health records" (De Groot et al., 2020). Documentation within a patient health care record is a vital aspect of nursing practice. According to Yen and colleagues (2018), approximately 25% of nursing practice time is concerned with documentation. Nursing documentation needs to be accurate and comprehensive. Nursing documentation systems need to be flexible enough to retrieve clinical data, facilitate continuity of care, track patient outcomes, and reflect current standards of nursing practice. Information in a patient record provides a detailed account of the level of quality of care delivered. The quality of care, the standards of regulatory agencies and nursing practice, and legal guidelines make documentation and reporting an extremely important nursing responsibility.

Effective documentation can positively affect the quality of life and health outcomes for patients and minimize the risk of errors. Accrediting agencies such as Accreditation Canada offer guidelines for documentation. However, documentation and reporting practices differ among institutions and jurisdictions and are influenced by ethical, legal, medical, and agency guidelines.

As a member of the health care team, the nurse needs to communicate information about patients in an accurate, timely, and effective manner. The quality of patient care depends largely on the ability of health care providers to communicate with one another. All care providers require accurate information about patients in order to devise an organized, comprehensive care plan. If the care plan is not communicated to all members of the health care team, care may be fragmented, tasks repeated, and therapies delayed or omitted. Data recorded, reported, or communicated to other health care providers are confidential, and the confidentiality of these data must be protected.

PURPOSE OF MEDICAL RECORDS

A patient's medical record (also known as a patient record or health record) is a valuable source of data for all members of the health care team. Data entered into the medical record facilitate interdisciplinary communication and care planning; provide a legal record of care provided; facilitate funding and resource management; and allow for auditing, monitoring, and evaluation of the care provided. Medical records also serve as sources of research data and as learning resources for nursing and health care education.

Communication and Care Planning

A patient's medical record is one way that health care team members communicate about patient needs and progress responses to care, individual therapies, the content of conferences, patient education, and discharge planning. The plan of care needs to be clear to everyone reading the chart. The record should be the most current and accurate source of information about a patient's health care status.

In the medical record, the nurse must always communicate the manner in which they conduct the nursing process with a patient. The admitting nursing history and physical assessment are comprehensive and provide baseline data about the patient's health status on admission to the facility. These data usually include biographical information (e.g., age and marital status), method of admission, reason for admission, code status, a brief medical-surgical history (e.g., previous surgeries or illnesses), allergies, current medication (prescribed and over the counter), the patient's perceptions about illness or hospitalization, and a review of health risk factors. The results of a health assessment and physical examination of all body systems are either documented in the nursing history or included on a separate form (see Chapter 33 for further information about physical assessment).

The medical record provides data that the nurse uses to identify and support nursing diagnoses, establish expected outcomes of care, and plan and evaluate interventions. Information from the record adds to the nurse's observations and assessment. The nurse does not need to collect information that is already available. If there is reason to believe that the information is inaccurate, the nurse should verify the information and make the appropriate changes to the patient record.

Legal Documentation

Accurate documentation is one of the best defenses against legal claims associated with nursing care (see Chapter 10 for further information about legal implications). From a legal perspective, the purpose of documentation is to provide proof of the health care provided. Documentation should accurately and fully document patient care as well as the patient's response to that care. The medical record is vital evidence in negligent practice lawsuits and is often considered to be the most reliable evidence during legal proceedings (Canadian Nurses Protective Society, 2021). To limit nursing liability, the nurse must clearly document that individualized, goal-directed nursing care, based on the nursing assessment, was provided to a patient and that the nurse continues to monitor for, document, and report deterioration. The record must describe exactly what happened to a patient. Charting should be performed immediately after care is provided. When a chart is reviewed in court, it must show that the patient received the best and most appropriate care possible. In the health care record, the nurse needs to indicate all assessments, interventions, patient responses, instructions, and referrals. It is important to complete all documentation on appropriate forms and to be sure that patient-identifying information (patient's name and identification number) is on every page of documentation.

Seven common charting mistakes have been identified that can result in malpractice: (1) failing to record pertinent health or drug information, (2) failing to record nursing actions, (3) failing to record that medications have been given, (4) recording on the wrong chart, (5) failing to document a discontinued medication, (6) failing to record drug reactions or changes in the patient's condition, and (7) transcribing orders improperly or transcribing improper orders (Nurses Service Organization, 2021). Table 16.1 lists guidelines for maintaining legally sound documentation.

Funding and Resource Management

The patient record reflects the ways in which health care agencies have used their financial resources. Various tools help to monitor the timing and reasons for health care team–patient interactions. These data are then compared with documented entries on the chart to demonstrate the need for and the efficacy of health care resources. In some workload assignment systems, health care interactions and tasks are assigned to specified points in relation to time spent with each patient.

Auditing and Monitoring

A regular review of information in patient records helps the nurse evaluate the quality and appropriateness of care. This audit may involve either a review of care received by discharged patients or an evaluation of care currently being given. Most Canadian health care agencies have continuous quality improvement programs and teams to monitor and improve the delivery of health care services. These teams often consist of members from across the organization, and they normally perform the self-assessment requirements of Accreditation Canada (see Chapter 13). Nurses or interdisciplinary members of a committee monitor or review records throughout the year to determine the degree to which quality improvement standards are

TABLE 16.1	Legal Guidelines for Documentation	
Guidelines for Documentation	**Rationale**	**Correct Action**
Guidelines for Electronic and Written Documentation		
Do not document retaliatory or critical comments about a patient or care provided by another health care provider. Do not enter personal opinions.	Statements can be used as evidence for nonprofessional behaviour or poor quality of care.	Enter only objective and factual descriptions of a patient's behaviour or the actions of another health care provider. Quote all patient statements.
Correct all errors promptly.	Errors in recording can lead to errors in treatment or may imply an attempt to mislead or hide evidence.	Avoid rushing to complete documentation; be sure that information is accurate and complete.
Record all facts.	Record must be accurate, factual, and objective.	Be certain entry is factual and thorough. A person reading your documentation needs to be able to determine that a patient received adequate care.
Document as close as prudently possible to the time of the event.	Most accurate method of recalling details. Details can be lost and discrepancies can arise the longer the wait to the documentation of the event.	Document as soon after the event as possible to ensure accuracy.
If an order is questioned, record that clarification was sought.	If you perform an order known to be incorrect, you are just as liable for prosecution as the prescriber is.	Do not record "physician made error"; instead, chart that "Dr. Wong was called to clarify order for analgesic." Include the date and time of phone call, whom you spoke with, and the outcome.
Document only for yourself.	You are accountable for information you enter into a patient record.	Never enter documentation for someone else. Check agency policy for circumstances when a third party may document for another nurse (e.g., the designated recorder role during a resuscitation).
Avoid using generalized, empty phrases such as "status unchanged" or "had good day."	This type of documentation is subjective and does not reflect patient assessment.	Use complete, concise descriptions of assessments and care so that documentation is objective and factual.
Begin each entry with the date and time and end with your signature and credentials.	Ensures that the correct sequence of events is recorded; signature documents who is accountable for care delivered.	Do not wait until end of shift to record important changes that occurred several hours earlier; sign each entry according to agency policy (e.g., Mei Lin, LPN).
Do not "prechart" (documenting an entry before performing a treatment or an assessment or before giving a medication).	Invites error and thus endangers the health and safety of the patient; it is also illegal and can constitute falsification of health care records.	Document during or immediately after giving care or after administering a medication.
Protect the security of your password for computer documentation.	Maintains security and confidentiality.	Once you are logged into a computer, do not leave the computer screen unattended. Log out when you leave the computer. Make sure the computer screen is not accessible for public viewing.
Guidelines Specific to Written Documentation Only		
Do not erase, apply correction fluid to, or scratch out errors made while recording.	Charting becomes illegible. It may appear as if you were attempting to hide information or deface the record.	Draw a single line through error; write "error" above it, and sign your name or initials and date it. Then record note correctly.
Do not leave blank spaces or lines in a written nurse's progress notes.	Allows another person to add incorrect information in open space.	Chart consecutively, line by line; if space is left, draw a line horizontally through it and place your signature and credentials at the end.
Record all entries legibly and in black ink. Do not use felt-tip pens or erasable ink.	Illegible entries can be misinterpreted, thereby causing errors and lawsuits; ink from felt-tip pens can smudge or run when wet and may destroy documentation; erasures are not permitted in clinical documentation; black ink is more legible when records are photocopied or scanned.	Never use pencil to document in a written clinical record. Never erase entries or use correction fluid. To indicate an error in written documentation, place a single line through the inaccurate information and write your signature with credentials at the end of the text that has been crossed out.

met. Deficiencies are explained to the nursing staff so that corrections in policy or practice can be made.

Research

Statistical data relating to the frequency of clinical disorders, complications, use of specific medical and nursing therapies, recovery from illness, and deaths can be gathered from patient records. For example, as part of a quality improvement program for patients receiving intravenous therapy, a nurse manager reviews patient records to investigate the incidence of infection in patients with a specific type of intravenous catheter. This review reveals that the infection rate is increased, and the

nurse manager and staff nurses design a new method for intravenous catheter care. Once this new intervention is implemented, the manager again reviews patient records to determine whether the infection rate decreases.

A nurse may use patient records during a clinical research study to investigate a new nursing intervention. For example, a nurse wants to compare a new method of pain control with a standard pain protocol by using two groups of patients. The patient records provide data on the two types of interventions: the new method and the standard pain control. The nurse researcher collects data from the patient records that describe the types and doses of analgesic medications used, objective assessment data, and patients' subjective reports of pain relief. The researcher then compares the findings to determine whether the new method was more effective.

Some data collection activities may be part of the quality improvement practices at an agency, whereas other activities may be actual clinical research studies. Different types of permission must be secured before a researcher can review patient records for any type of research study or data analysis. The researcher must be sure that the data collection and analysis adhere to provincial/territorial and agency policies.

Education

One way to learn the nature of an illness and an individual's response to it is to read a patient record. A patient record contains a variety of information, including diagnoses, signs and symptoms of disease, successful and unsuccessful therapies, diagnostic findings, and patient behaviours. No two patients have identical records, but in the course of clinical training, nursing and other health care students review records of patients who have similar health problems to identify patterns of information and anticipate the type of care required for a patient.

THE SHIFT TO ELECTRONIC DOCUMENTATION

Traditionally, health care providers have documented patient information on paper medical records. Paper records are episode oriented, with a separate record created for each patient visit to a health care agency. Key information such as patient allergies, current medications, and complications from treatment are sometimes lost from one episode of care (e.g., hospitalization or clinic visit) to the next, jeopardizing a patient's safety (Hebda et al., 2019).

To enhance communication among health care providers, and thus patient safety, Canadian Health Infoway was given the mandate to partner with multiple jurisdictions to develop and implement an electronic health record to support effective health care delivery for Canadians. In a survey of Canadian nurses conducted in 2020, it was reported that 86% of nurses providing direct patient care were using electronic health records (Canada Health Infoway, 2020a). According to Canada Health Infoway (2020b), 86% of primary care physicians were using an electronic medical record in 2019 (up from 73% in 2015).

Although the terms electronic health record (EHR) and electronic medical record (EMR) are often used interchangeably in practice, there are differences between them. An EHR is a digital version of patient data that is found in traditional paper records. The term *EHR* is used increasingly to refer to a longitudinal (lifetime) record of all health care encounters for an individual patient (Hebda et al., 2019). An EMR is the legal record that describes a single encounter or visit by a patient to a hospital or outpatient health care setting and is the source of data for the EHR (Hebda et al., 2019).

The functionality of an EHR versus a paper chart is increased with the capabilities of multiple health care providers to have concurrent access, the ability to manage orders, access laboratory and diagnostic tests results, access to the medication administration record and/or barcode administration of medication, and access links to external clinical resources as well as clinical decision support (to be discussed later in the chapter) (Hebda et al., 2019).

The general benefits of an EHR include the following (Hebda et al., 2019):
- Improvements in the readability, organization, and accuracy of documentation
- Increased ability to make timely clinical decisions with easier access to data
- Improvements in the quality of care provided, and
- Increase satisfaction among caregivers.

Additional clinical advantages of the EHR include their positive impact on the quality of patient care and improvements in patient safety through reduction of medical errors (Boothe et al., 2020). The EHR provides access to a patient's health record information at the time and place that clinicians need it. A unique feature of an EHR is its ability to integrate all patient information into one record, regardless of the number of times a patient enters a health care system. An EHR also includes the results of diagnostic studies, which may include diagnostic images (e.g., X-ray film or ultrasound images) and decision support software programs. Because an unlimited number of patient records potentially can be stored within an EHR system, health care providers can access clinical data to identify quality issues, link interventions with positive outcomes, and make evidence-informed decisions. For example, of how an EHR works: A patient with a complex medical history sees multiple specialists to manage their health, including an endocrinologist to address diabetes, a pulmonologist to manage emphysema, and a cardiologist to manage heart failure and atrial fibrillation. Each of these providers is able to access patient data from the EMR at the same time.

Members of the health care team use EHRs to improve continuity of health care from one episode of illness to another. A clinician accesses relevant and timely information about a patient and focuses on the priority problems to make timely, well-informed clinical decisions. An EHR includes tools to guide and critique medication administration (see Chapter 35) and basic decision-support tools such as physician order sets and interdisciplinary treatment plans. An EHR gives nurses a way to compare current clinical data about a patient with data from previous health care encounters, and a way to maintain an ongoing record of health education provided to a patient as well as the patient's response to that information.

INTERPROFESSIONAL COMMUNICATION WITHIN THE MEDICAL RECORD

The quality of patient care depends on the nurse's ability to communicate with other members of the health care team. Regardless of whether documentation is entered electronically or on paper, each member of the health care team needs to document patient information in an accurate, timely, concise, and effective manner to develop and maintain an effective, organized, and comprehensive plan of care. When a plan is not communicated to all members of the health care team, care becomes fragmented, tasks are repeated, and delays or omissions in care often occur.

The health care environment creates many challenges for accurately documenting and reporting the care delivered to patients.

CONFIDENTIALITY

Regardless of how patient information is transferred—be it through verbal reports, written documents, or electronic transfer—nurses must follow certain principles to maintain the confidentiality of information. Nurses are legally and ethically obligated to keep information about patients confidential. Under the domain of professionalism in the *National Nursing Education Framework*, the Canadian Association of Schools of Nursing (CASN, 2022, p. 19) lists "maintain confidentiality and privacy of personal health information both at work and outside of work" as an essential component of baccalaureate nursing education. Only members of the health care team who are directly involved in a patient's care have authorized access to the medical record. Thus, the nurse may discuss a patient's diagnosis, treatment, assessment, and any personal conversations only with members of the health care team involved in that patient's care. The nurse must not share information with other patients or health care team members who are not caring for a patient. Patients have the right to request copies of their medical records and read the information contained therein. Each institution has policies that describe how medical records are shared with patients or other people who request them. In most situations, patients are required to give written permission for release of medical information.

Sometimes nurses use health care records for data gathering, research, or continuing education. As long as a nurse uses a record as specified and permission has been granted, this access is permitted. Nursing students in a clinical setting must follow the confidentiality and compliance requirements detailed in the *Personal Information Protection and Electronic Documents Act* (PIPEDA) as part of professional practice (see Chapter 17). Nurses may review patient medical records only when the information is needed to provide safe and effective patient care. For example, when a nurse is assigned to care for a patient, they need to review the patient's medical record and plan of care. A nursing student cannot share this information with classmates (except for clinical conferences) and cannot access the medical records of other patients on the unit. Access to EHRs is traceable through user log-in information. Not only is it unethical to view the medical records of other patients, but it is also breach of confidentiality that can lead to disciplinary action by employers and dismissal from work or nursing school. To protect patient confidentiality, nursing students must ensure that written or electronic materials used in student clinical practice do not include patient identifiers (e.g., room number, date of birth, demographic information), and information from an EHR should never be printed for personal use.

Before the beginning of clinical placements, students and instructors may be required to sign confidentiality agreements with the agencies in question. Students need to understand the practice standards and laws concerning confidentiality. A breach of confidentiality is often a careless rather than deliberate act. Students need to make sure that patient-identifiable information (e.g., files, stickers, information in notebooks, worksheets) is not taken home and that it is disposed of correctly in a secure bin for shredding. Examples of breaches of confidentiality include accessing information not related to one's duties; discussing patient information in an inappropriate area, such as in an elevator or on public transport; revealing confidential patient or co-worker details to a caller; emailing patient information through a public network such as the Internet; and leaving confidential material in a public area. Even after their placement at an agency has been completed, the nursing student is obligated to maintain the confidentiality of patients and co-workers at that agency.

Privacy, Confidentiality, and Security Mechanisms

Electronic documentation has legal risks. It is possible for anyone to access a computer station within a health care agency and obtain information about almost any patient. Therefore, protection of information and computer systems is a top priority. As described in Chapter 17, Canada has both provincial/territorial and national privacy legislation to protect personal health information in electronic and other forms. Under PIPEDA, ensuring appropriate access to and confidentiality of personal health information (PHI) is the responsibility of everyone working in health care. PHI includes individually identifiable health information such as demographic data; facts that relate to an individual's past, present, or future physical or mental health condition; provision of care; and payment for the provision of care that identifies the individual (Hebda et al., 2019).

The *Personal Information Protection and Electronic Documents Act* (PIPEDA) is federal legislation that protects personal information, including health information. PIPEDA delineates how private-sector organizations may collect, use, or disclose personal information while carrying out commercial activities. Individuals also have the right to access and request the correction of any personal information collected about them. PIPEDA applies to all organizations engaged in commercial activities, unless the federal government has exempted an organization or activity in a province with similar legislation. PIPEDA is discussed in more detail in Chapter 17.

Most security mechanisms for computerized information systems use a combination of logical and physical restrictions to protect information. For example, an automatic sign-off is a safety mechanism that logs a user off a computer system after a specified period of inactivity (Hebda et al., 2019). Other security measures include firewalls and the installation of antivirus and spyware-detection software. A **firewall** is a combination of hardware and software that protects private network resources (e.g., the information system of the hospital) from outside hackers, network damage, and theft or misuse of information.

Physical security measures include placing computers or file servers in restricted areas or using privacy filters on computer screens visible to visitors or others without access. This form of security has limited benefit, especially if an organization uses mobile wireless devices such as laptop computers, tablets, and smartphones. These devices are easily misplaced or lost and can therefore fall into the wrong hands. Some organizations use motion detectors or alarms on these devices to help prevent theft.

Access or log-in codes along with passwords are frequently used for authenticating authorized access to electronic records. A *password* is a collection of alphanumeric characters that a user types into a computer before accessing a program after the entry and acceptance of an access code or username. Strong passwords use combinations of letters, numbers, and symbols that are difficult to guess. When using a health care agency computer system, it is essential not to share one's computer password with anyone under any circumstances. A good system requires frequent, random changes in personal passwords to prevent unauthorized people from tampering with records. A password does not appear on the computer screen when it is typed, nor should it be known to anyone but the user and information system administrators (Hebda et al., 2019). In addition, most health care personnel are only given access to patients in their work area. Some staff (e.g., administrators or risk managers) have authority to access all patient records. To protect patient privacy, health care agencies track who accesses patient records and when they access them. Disciplinary action, including loss of employment, occurs when nurses or other health care personnel inappropriately access patient information.

Handling and Disposing of Information

Maintaining the confidentiality of medical records is an essential responsibility of all members of the health care team. It is equally important to safeguard any information that is printed from the medical record or extracted for report purposes. For example, a nurse may print a copy of a nursing activities work list to use as a day planner while providing patient care. The nurse refers to information on the list and writes notes to enter later into the computer. Information on the list is PHI; the nurse cannot leave it out where it may be viewed by unauthorized people. The nurse must destroy (e.g., shred) anything that is printed when the information is no longer needed. Nursing students must write down patient data needed for clinical paperwork directly from a patient's medical record on the computer screen or the physical chart. When writing patient data onto forms or when including it in papers written for nursing courses, you need to de-identify all patient data. Do not remove patient information that is printed out from a clinical agency. If you need to remove printed information from a clinical setting, de-identify all PHI, keep the documents secure, and destroy documents by shredding or disposing of them in a locked receptacle as soon as possible.

Historically, the primary sources for inadvertent, unauthorized disclosure of PHI occurred when information was printed from a patient record or faxed to other health care providers. Thus, nurses need to destroy all papers containing PHI (e.g., social insurance number, date of birth or age, patient's name or address) immediately after using or faxing them. Most agencies have shredders or locked receptacles for shredding and incineration. Some nurses work in settings where they are responsible for erasing files from a computer hard drive that contain calendars, surgery or diagnostic procedure schedules, shift reports, or other daily records that contain PHI (Hebda et al., 2019). It is important to know and follow the disposal policies for records in the institution where you work.

Hebda et al. (2019) have noted key considerations around the security of electronic transmission of patient information, as well as mobile computing. If there is a need for health information to be sent electronically through email, it should be encrypted. Consider, too, the importance of vigilance when accessing patient data on mobile devices. An advantage to mobile access includes the ease with which it can be accessed at the point of care, but this can be complicated by the potential for loss or theft of the devices if they are left unattended. Use care with these technologies. Be aware of, and ensure that you are consistent with, policies regarding their use within the settings in which you practise.

INTERPROFESSIONAL COMMUNICATION WITHIN THE HEALTH CARE TEAM

Patient care requires effective communication among members of the health care team. Communication takes place through the patient record or chart and reports.

A **patient record** (also known as a *medical record*, *health record*, or *chart*), is a confidential, permanent legal document of information relevant to a patient's health care. Information about the patient's health care is recorded after each contact with the patient. The record is a continuing account of the patient's health care status and is available to all members of the health care team. All patient records contain the following information:

- Patient identification and demographic data
- Informed consent for treatment and procedures
- Advance directives
- Admission nursing history
- Nursing diagnoses or problems and the nursing or interdisciplinary care plan
- Record of nursing care treatment and evaluation
- Medical history
- Medical diagnosis
- Therapeutic orders
- Progress notes for various health care providers
- Reports of physical examinations
- Reports of diagnostic studies
- Record of patient and family education
- Summary of operative procedures, and
- Discharge plan and summary.

Reports are oral, written, or audio-recorded exchanges of information between caregivers. Reports commonly compiled by nurses include change-of-shift reports, telephone reports, transfer reports, and incident or occurrence reports (discussed later in this chapter). A physician or nurse practitioner may call a nursing unit to receive a verbal report on a patient's condition and progress. A laboratory submits a written report about the results of diagnostic tests.

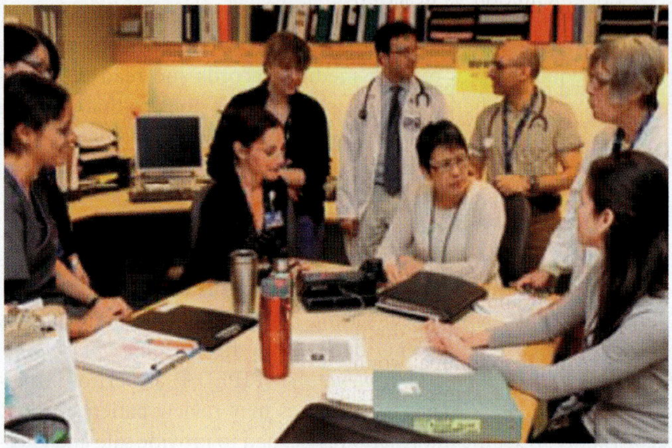

FIGURE 16.1 Staff communicate information about their patients during an interprofessional team conference. (From Registered Nurses' Association of Ontario [RNAO]. [2013]. *Developing and sustaining interprofessional health care: Optimizing patient, organizational and system outcomes.* https://rnao.ca/bpg/guidelines/interprofessional-team-work-healthcare)

Team members communicate information through discussions or conferences (Figure 16.1). For example, a discharge planning conference often involves members of several disciplines (e.g., nursing, social work, dietary, medicine, and physiotherapy) who meet to discuss the patient's progress toward established discharge goals. **Consultations** are another form of discussion whereby one professional caregiver gives formal advice about the care of a patient to another caregiver. For example, a nurse caring for a patient with a chronic wound may need a consultation with a wound care specialist. **Referrals** (an arrangement for services by another care provider), consultations, and conferences must be documented in a patient's permanent record so that all caregivers can plan care accordingly.

GUIDELINES FOR QUALITY DOCUMENTATION AND REPORTING

High-quality documentation enhances efficient, individualized patient care and has the potential to improve patient outcomes. According to Jefferies et al. (2010), nursing documentation too often consists of a list of tasks performed, suggesting that the production of quality documentation can be a challenge for nurses. Quality documentation has six important characteristics: it is factual, accurate, complete, current, and organized, and it complies with the standards set by Accreditation Canada and by provincial or territorial regulatory bodies. It is easier to maintain these characteristics if you continually seek to express ideas clearly and succinctly.

Factual

A factual record contains descriptive, objective information about what a nurse sees, hears, feels, and smells. Avoid vague terms such as *appears*, *seems*, or *apparently*. These words suggest that you are stating an opinion; they do not communicate facts accurately and do not inform another caregiver of details regarding the behaviours exhibited by the patient. Objective data are obtained through direct observation and measurement (e.g., "BP 80/50, patient diaphoretic, heart rate 102 and regular"). Objective documentation includes the observations of the patient's behaviours. The only subjective data that you include in the record is what the patient says. When recording subjective data, you document the patient's exact words within quotation marks wherever possible. Include objective data to support subjective data to make your documentation as descriptive as possible. For example, instead of documenting "the patient seems anxious," provide objective signs of anxiety and document the patient's statement about the feeling(s) experienced (e.g., "the patient's pulse rate is 110/beats/min, respiratory rate is slightly laboured at 22 breaths/min, and the patient states 'I feel very nervous'").

Accurate

The use of exact measurements establishes accuracy and helps the nurse determine whether a patient's condition has changed in a positive or negative way. For example, a description such as "intake, 360 mL of water" is more accurate than "Patient drank an adequate amount of fluid." Documenting that an abdominal wound is "5 cm in length without redness, drainage, or edema" is more descriptive than "large wound healing well." Documentation of concise data should be clear and easy to understand. Avoid the use of unnecessary words and irrelevant detail. For example, the fact that the patient is watching TV is only necessary when this activity is significant to the patient's status and plan of care.

Most health care institutions develop a list of standard abbreviations, symbols, and acronyms to be used by all members of the health care team in documenting or communicating patient care and treatment. Approved abbreviations and acronyms vary depending on the type of facility (i.e., long-term versus acute care facility). Use of an institution's accepted abbreviations, symbols, and system of measures (e.g., metric) ensures that all staff members use the same language in their reports and records. Always use abbreviations carefully to avoid misinterpretation. For example, "od" (every day) can be misinterpreted to mean "O.D." (right eye). If abbreviations are confusing, then you should spell terms out in their entirety to minimize errors.

The Institute for Safe Medication Practices Canada (ISMP Canada, 2021) has published an extensive list of error-prone abbreviations, symbols, and dose designations that health care institutions need to consider adding to their "Do Not Use" lists (see Chapter 35 for further information about abbreviations). Suggestions include writing "unit" instead of "U," always using a zero before a decimal point in a decimal fraction (e.g., "0.25 mg"), and not writing a zero alone after a decimal point (e.g., writing "5 mg," not "5.0 mg").

Correct spelling demonstrates a level of competency and attention to detail. Many terms can easily be misinterpreted (e.g., *dysphagia* and *dysphasia*). Some spelling errors can also result in serious treatment errors (e.g., certain look-alike, sound-alike medications, such as *morphine* and *hydromorphone*, have similar names and package labelling). Transcribe medication names carefully to ensure that patients receive the correct medication.

Patient record entries must be dated, and a method for identifying the authors of entries must be in place. Each entry in a patient record ends with the caregiver's full name or initials and credentials/title/role, such as "Holly Lee, LPN." If initials are used in a signature, the full name and credentials/title/role of the individual need to be documented at least once in the medical record to allow others to readily identify the individual. As a nursing student, you should enter your full name and student nurse (SN) abbreviation, such as "Henri Gauthier, SN." The abbreviation for student nurse varies between SN/SPN (student nurse/student practical nurse) and NS/PNS (nursing student/practical nursing student). Include your educational institution when required by agency policy.

Patient records must reflect accountability during the time frame of the entry. Accountability is best accomplished when you chart only your own observations and actions. Your signature holds you accountable for the information recorded.

You should refer to agency policy before making late entries, correcting errors, or completing an omission. Late entries are often documented by writing the current date and time in the next available space as close to the late entry as possible and writing "late entry for [date and shift]." For adding information to an existing entry, it is good practice to use the current date and time in the next space and add "addendum to note of [date and time of prior note]."

Complete

The information within a recorded entry or a report must be complete and contain appropriate and essential information. Criteria for thorough communication exist for certain health problems or nursing activities (Table 16.2). It is important to document all nursing interventions, such as education and psychosocial support, as this information

TABLE 16.2	Examples of Criteria for Documentation and Reporting
Topic	**Criteria to Report or Record**
Subjective assessment data	Patient's description of episode in quotation marks; for example, "I feel as if I have an elephant sitting on my chest, and I can't catch my breath."
	Describe in patient's own words the onset, location, description of condition (severity, duration, frequency; precipitating, aggravating, and relieving factors) (e.g., "The pain in my left knee started last week after I knelt on the ground. Every time I bend my knee, I have a shooting pain on the inside of my knee.")
Objective assessment data (e.g., rash, tenderness, breath sounds or descriptions of patient behaviour [e.g., anxiety, confusion, hostility])	Onset, location, description of condition (e.g., 1100 hrs: 2-cm raised pale red area noted on back of left hand).
	Onset, precipitating factors, behaviours exhibited (e.g., pacing in room, avoiding eye contact with nurse), patient statements (e.g., repeatedly stating, "I have to go home now.")
Nursing interventions, treatments and evaluation (e.g., enema, bath, dressing change)	Time administered, equipment used (if appropriate), patient's response (objective and subjective changes) compared to previous treatment (e.g., denied incisional pain during abdominal dressing change, ambulated 100 metres in hallway without assistance).
Medication administration	At time of administration when using a computerized barcode medication administration program (or immediately after administration), document time medication given, medication name, dose, route, preliminary assessment (e.g., pain level, vital signs), patient response, or effect of medication. For example:
	1500 hrs: Reports "throbbing headache all over my head." Rates pain at 6 (scale 0 to 10). Tylenol 650 mg given PO.
	1530 hrs: Patient reports pain level 2 (scale 0 to 10) and states, "The throbbing has stopped."
Patient and/or family teaching	Information presented; method of instruction (e.g., discussion, demonstration, video, booklet); and patient response, including questions and evidence of understanding such as return demonstration or change in behaviour.
Discharge planning	Measurable patient goals or expected outcomes, progress toward goals, need for referrals.

and the outcomes of these interventions are not often recorded in nursing documentation (Jefferies et al., 2010). An example of a thorough nurse's note is as follows:

> *1915 hrs: Patient verbalizes sharp, throbbing pain localized along lateral side of right ankle, beginning approximately 15 minutes after twisting his foot on the stairs at 1700. Patient rates pain as 8 on a scale of 0–10. Pain increased with movement, slightly relieved with elevation. Pedal pulses equal bilaterally. Right ankle circumference 1 cm larger than left. Bilateral lower extremities warm, pale pink, skin intact, responds to tactile stimulation, capillary refill less than 3 seconds. Ice applied. Percocet 2 tabs (PO) given for pain. Patient states pain somewhat relieved with ice, rates pain as 6 on a scale of 0–10. Dr. P. Yoshida notified. Lee Turno, RN.*
>
> *1945 hrs: States pain was somewhat relieved with ice and now rates pain as a 3 on a scale of 0–10. States, "The pain medication really helped." Lee Turno, RN*

You will frequently use flow sheets or graphic records to document routine activities such as daily hygiene care, vital signs, and pain assessments. Describe these data in greater detail when they are relevant, such as when a change in functional ability or status occurs. For example, if your patient's blood pressure, pulse, and respirations are elevated above expected values following a walk down the hall, document an additional description that notes the patient's status and response to the walk in the appropriate place in the medical record (e.g., nurses' notes).

Current

Timely entries are essential to the patient's ongoing care. Documentation should occur during or as soon as possible after the incident or intervention, and events should be described chronologically to reflect a clear record of exactly what happened. To increase accuracy and decrease unnecessary duplication, many health care agencies keep records or computers near the patient's bedside to facilitate immediate documentation of information as it is collected.

Flow sheets (described later in this chapter) are a means of entering current information quickly. Portable electronic workstations or secure wall cabinets in patient rooms help ensure that patient confidentiality is maintained. Nurses often keep notes on a worksheet when caring for several patients, making notes as the care occurs to ensure that entries recorded later in the record are accurate. The following activities and findings should be communicated at the time of occurrence:

- Vital signs
- Pain assessment
- Administration of medications and treatments
- Preparation for diagnostic tests or surgery, including preoperative checklist
- Change in patient's status and who was notified (e.g., nurse practitioner, physician, manager, patient's family)
- Admission, transfer, discharge, or death of a patient
- Treatment for a sudden change in patient's status, and
- Patient's response to treatment or intervention.

Most health care agencies use military time, a 24-hour system that avoids misinterpretation of "a.m." and "p.m." times (Figure 16.2). Instead of two 12-hour cycles in standard time, the military clock is one 24-hour time cycle. The military clock ends at midnight (2400) and begins 1 minute after midnight (0001). For example, 10:22 a.m. is 1022 military time; 1:00 p.m. is 1300 military time.

Organized

As a nurse, you want to communicate information in a logical order. For example, an organized note describes the patient's pain, the nurse's

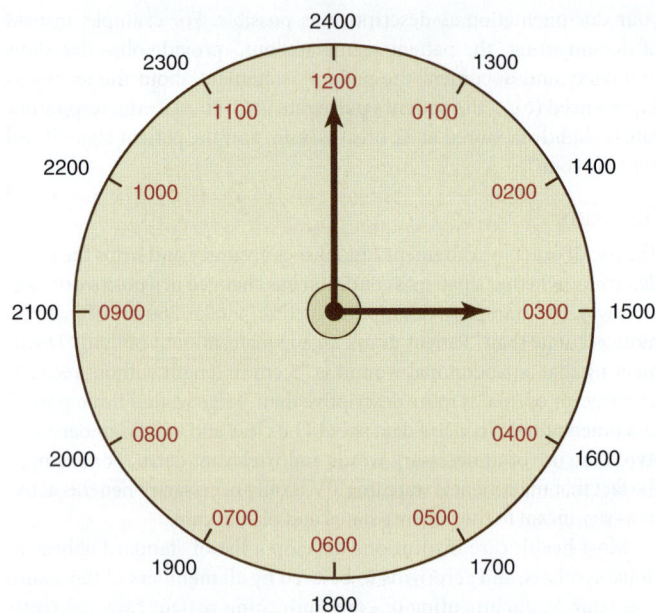

FIGURE 16.2 Comparison of 24-hour military time with the hourly positions for civilian time on the clock face.

assessment and interventions, and the patient's response. To write notes about complex situations in an organized manner, think about the situation and make notes of what is to be included before you begin to write in the permanent legal record.

Compliant With Standards

Documentation needs to follow standards set by Accreditation Canada and by provincial or territorial regulatory bodies in order to maintain institutional accreditation and decrease the risk of liability. Current standards require that all patients who are admitted to a health care institution undergo physical, psychosocial, environmental, and self-care assessments; receive patient education; and be provided discharge planning. In addition, criteria for standards stress the importance of evaluating patient outcomes, including the patient's response to treatments, teaching, or preventive care.

The nursing service department of each health care agency selects a method of documenting patient care. The method reflects the philosophy of the nursing department and incorporates the standards of care. Because the nursing process shapes a nurse's approach and direction of care, effective documentation also reflects the nursing process.

METHODS OF DOCUMENTATION

There are several documentation methods for recording patient assessment data and progress notes. Regardless of whether documentation is entered electronically or on paper, each health care agency selects a documentation system that reflects its philosophy of nursing. The same system is used throughout a specific agency and is sometimes used throughout a health care system as well.

Narrative Documentation

Narrative documentation is the method traditionally used to record patient assessment and nursing care provided. It is simply the use of a story-like format to document information. In an electronic nursing information system, this is accomplished through the use of free text entry or menu selections (Hebda et al., 2019). Narrative documentation tends to be time consuming and repetitive. It requires the reader to sort through a lot of information to locate the desired data. However, in certain situations, this method provides better detail on individual patient assessment findings and complex patient situations (Wilbanks & Moss, 2018). One of the limitations of electronic documentation is the limited use of narrative documentation. Some areas of the EMR are designed to use multiple checkboxes or drop-down lists; however, they might not adequately convey the details of significant events that lead to a change in a patient's condition and thus would require supplementation with a narrative note. EMRs that incorporate options for narrative descriptions in a format that is easily retrieved and reviewed may enhance clinician communication and interdisciplinary understanding for patient care.

Problem-Oriented Medical Records or Health Care Records

The problem-oriented medical record (POMR) is a system for organizing documentation that places the primary focus on patients' individual problems. Data are organized by problem or diagnosis. Ideally, each member of the health care team contributes to a single list of identified patient problems. This assists in coordinating a common plan of care. The POMR has the following major sections: database, problem list, care plan, and progress notes.

Database. The database section contains all available assessment information pertaining to the patient (e.g., history and physical examination, nursing admission history and ongoing assessment, physiotherapist's assessment, laboratory reports, and radiological test results). The database provides the foundation for identifying patient problems and planning care. As new data become available, the database is revised. It accompanies patients through successive hospitalizations or clinic visits.

Problem List. After analyzing the data, health care team members identify problems and make a single problem list. The problem list includes a patient's physiological, psychological, social, cultural, spiritual, developmental, and environmental needs. Team members list the problems in chronological order and file the list at the front of the patient record to serve as an organizing guide for patient care. Team members add and date new problems as they arise. When a problem has been resolved, the text of that problem is highlighted, or lined out, and the date is recorded.

Care Plan. Team members from each discipline involved in a patient's care develop a care plan or plan of care for each problem (see Chapter 14 for further information about the plan of care for patients). Nurses document the plan of care in a variety of formats; generally, all of these formats include nursing diagnoses, expected outcomes, and interventions.

Progress Notes. Health care team members monitor and record the progress made toward resolving a patient's problems in progress notes. Health care providers write progress notes in one of several formats or structured notes within a POMR (Box 16.1).

One method is the subjective–objective–assessment–plan (SOAP) note. The acronym SOAP stands for Subjective data (verbalizations of the patient), Objective data (that which is measured and observed), Assessment (diagnosis based on the data), and Plan (what the caregiver plans to do). In some institutions, an "I" and an "E" are added, for Intervention and Evaluation, respectively, to spell SOAPIE (subjective–objective–assessment–plan–intervention–evaluation). The logic of the SOAPIE note format is similar to that of the nursing process. The nurse collects data about a patient's problems, draws conclusions, develops a plan of care, and then evaluates the outcome(s). Each SOAP note is numbered and titled according to the problem on the list that it addresses.

A second progress note method is the problem–intervention–evaluation (PIE) format (see Box 16.1). It is similar to SOAP charting in its problem-oriented nature. However, it differs from the SOAP method in that PIE charting originated in nursing practice, whereas SOAP charting originated from medical records. The PIE format simplifies documentation by unifying the care plan and progress notes. PIE notes differ from SOAP notes in that the narrative does not include assessment information. A nurse's daily assessment data appear on flow sheets, preventing the duplication of data. The narrative note includes

---

BOX 16.1 Examples of a Nursing Progress Note Written in Different Formats

Narrative Note

Patient stated, "I'm worried about the surgery. Last time I had a lot of pain when I got out of bed." Discussed importance of postoperative ambulation and demonstrated turning, coughing, deep-breathing (TCDB) exercises. Patient set postoperative pain-rating goal at 4 on scale of 0 to 10. Discussed analgesic plan of care and reassured that analgesics will be offered around the clock as ordered. Encouraged to tell nursing staff as soon as possible if pain is not relieved. Provided with teaching booklet on postoperative care. Stated, "I feel less anxious about my pain now." Verbalized understanding of the importance of postoperative ambulation and confidence in the plan of care.

SOAP (Subjective–Objective–Assessment–Plan) Note

S: "I'm worried about the surgery. Last time I had a lot of pain when I got out of bed."

O: Asking multiple questions about how postoperative pain will be addressed.

A: Anxiety related to perceived threat of postoperative pain as evidenced by statement of prior experience with uncontrolled postoperative pain.

P: Explain routine postoperative analgesic plan of care. Encourage to inform nursing staff as soon as possible if pain is not relieved. Explain rationale for early postoperative ambulation and demonstrate TCDB exercises. Provide teaching booklet on postoperative nursing care.

PIE (Problem–Intervention–Evaluation) Note

P: Anxiety related to perceived threat of postoperative pain as evidenced by statement of prior experience with uncontrolled postoperative pain.

I: Explained importance of postoperative ambulation and demonstrated TCDB exercises. Described analgesic plan of care. Encouraged to inform nursing staff as soon as possible if pain is not relieved. Provided teaching booklet on postoperative nursing care.

E: Stated, "I feel less anxious about postoperative pain now," and performed return demonstration of TCDB exercises correctly.

Focus Charting DAR (Data–Action–Response) Note

D: Patient stated, "I'm worried about the surgery. Last time I had a lot of pain when I got out of bed." Asked frequent questions about postoperative pain management.

A: Discussed importance of postoperative ambulation and demonstrated TCDB exercises. Described postoperative analgesic plan of care that is in place. Provided teaching booklet on postoperative nursing care.

R: Demonstrated TCDB exercises correctly. States, "I feel better knowing how my pain will be treated."

the problem, the intervention, and the evaluation. PIE notes are numbered or labelled according to the patient's problems. Resolved problems are dropped from daily documentation after the nurse's review. Continuing problems are documented daily.

The third format used for notes within a POMR is **focus charting**. It involves the use of **data–action–response (DAR) notes**, which include **D**ata (both subjective and objective), **A**ction or nursing intervention, and **R**esponse of the patient (i.e., evaluation of effectiveness). A DAR note addresses patient concerns such as a sign or symptom, condition, nursing diagnosis, behaviour, significant event, or change in a patient's condition (see Box 16.1). Documentation in this format also follows the nursing process. This format enables nurses to broaden their thinking to include any patient concerns, not just problem areas. Focus charting incorporates all aspects of the nursing process, highlights a patient's concerns, and can be integrated into any clinical setting.

Source Records

In a **source record**, the patient's chart is organized so that each discipline (e.g., nursing, medicine, social work, respiratory therapy) has a separate section in which to record data. One advantage of a source record is that caregivers can easily locate the proper section of the record in which to make entries. Table 16.3 lists the components of a source record.

A disadvantage of the source record is that details about a specific problem may be distributed throughout the record. For example, in the case of a patient with bowel obstruction, the nurse describes in the nurses' notes the character of abdominal pain and the use of relaxation therapy and analgesic medication. In a separate section of the record, the physician's notes describe the progress of the patient's condition and the plan for surgery. The findings of X-ray examinations that reveal the location of the bowel obstruction are in the test results section of the record.

The nursing notes or interdisciplinary progress notes section is where nurses enter a narrative description of nursing care and the patient's response (Box 16.2). It is also a section for documenting care that is provided by the physician or nurse practitioner in the nurse's presence. The nurse may record key diagnostic test results from other sections of the record in the nurses' notes if they are of major importance in the care of the patient.

Charting by Exception

The philosophy behind **charting by exception (CBE)** is that a patient meets all standards unless otherwise documented. The method was introduced in the early 1980s. Although the philosophy behind the method has consistently raised professional concern (Brous, 2020), many computerized nursing documentation systems use a CBE design. Exception-based documentation systems incorporate standards of care, evidence-informed interventions, and clearly defined criteria for nursing assessment and documentation of "normal" findings. The predefined statements used to document nursing assessment of body systems are called *within defined limits (WDL)* or *within normal limits (WNL)* definitions. They consist of written criteria for a "normal" assessment for each body system. Automated documentation within a computerized documentation system allows nurses to select a WDL statement or to choose other statements from a drop-down menu, which then enables the description of any assessment findings that deviate from the WDL definition or are unexpected (Elliott et al., 2018). The nurse writes a progress note only when a patient's assessment does not meet the standardized criteria for "normal" in one or more body systems. When changes in a patient's condition develop, the nurse needs to include a thorough and precise description of the effects of the change(s) on the patient and the actions taken to address the change(s) in the progress note.

BOX 16.2   Sample Narrative Note

May 24, 2021

1100 hrs: Patient states, "I'm having a hard time catching my breath." R [Respirations], laboured at 32/min; P [pulse] 120; BP 112/70. Oxygen saturation 90% on room air. Patient alert and oriented. Patient using intercostal muscles during inspiration. Wheezes noted on inspiration in both lower lobes on auscultation of the posterior chest wall. Chest excursion equal bilaterally. Elevated head of bed to Fowler's position. Obtained arterial blood gas (ABG) sample at 1045. O_2 (oxygen) started at 2 L/min per nasal prongs as ordered. Remained at bedside to calm patient. Pam Haske, RN

1130 hrs: Results of ABGs reported to Dr. Stein are pH 7.34; PCO_2 [partial pressure of carbon dioxide] 44 mm Hg; PO_2 [partial pressure of oxygen] 80 mm Hg. Patient states, "It is easier to breathe now." R 24/min; P 96; BP 110/72. Oxygen saturation 97% on O_2 at 2 L/min per nasal prongs, lips pale pink; capillary refill less than 3 seconds. Inspirational wheezing still audible on auscultation to lower lobes. Patient remains in high Fowler's position. Pam Haske, RN

TABLE 16.3   Organization of Traditional Source Record

Sections	Contents
Admission sheet	Specific demographic data about patient: legal name, identification number, sex, age, birth date, marital status, occupation and employer, health card number, nearest relative to notify in an emergency, religious affiliation, name of attending physician, date and time of admission
Order sheet	Record of prescriber's orders for treatment and medications, with date, time, and prescriber's signature
Nurse's admission assessment	Summary of nursing history and physical examination
Graphic sheet and flow sheet	Record of repeated observations and measurements such as vital signs, daily weights, and intake and output
Medical history and examination	Results of initial examination performed by physician, including findings, family history, confirmed diagnoses, and medical plan of care
Medication administration record (MAR)	Accurate documentation of all medications administered to patient: date, time, dose, route, and nurse's signature
Progress notes	Ongoing record of patient's progress and response to therapy completed by all members of the health care team. Included in this section is a narrative record of the nursing process written by nurses: assessment, nursing diagnosis, planning, implementation, and evaluation of care
Health care disciplines' records	Entries made into record by all health care–related disciplines: radiology, social work, laboratories, physiotherapy, and so forth
Discharge summary	Summary of patient's condition, progress, prognosis, rehabilitation, and teaching needs at time of dismissal from hospital or health care agency

Case Management and Use of Critical Pathways

The case management model of delivering care (see Chapter 13 for management models) incorporates an interdisciplinary approach to documenting patient care. In many organizations, the standardized plan of care is summarized into critical pathways for a specific disease or condition. Critical pathways (also known as clinical pathways, practice guidelines, or CareMap tools) are interprofessional care plans that integrate best evidence for the treatment of a condition along a detailed pathway, with expected outcomes noted within an established time frame (Kuntz, 2019). The document facilitates the integration of care because all health care team members use the same critical pathway to monitor a patient's progress. Many organizations summarize the standardized plan of care into critical pathways for a specific disease or condition such as breast cancer. Evidence-informed critical pathways improve patient outcomes. For example, critical pathways to manage hip fractures have been shown to significantly improve health-related quality of life and physical function for patients when compared with usual care (Talevski et al., 2019).

Critical pathways eliminate the need for nurses' notes, flow sheets, and nursing care plans because the pathway document integrates all relevant information. Unexpected occurrences, unmet goals, and interventions not specified within the clinical pathway time frame are called *variances*. A variance is present when the activities on the clinical pathway are not completed as predicted or the patient does not meet the expected outcomes. An example of a negative variance is when a patient postoperatively develops pulmonary complications necessitating oxygen therapy and monitoring with pulse oximetry. An example of a positive variance is when a patient progresses more rapidly than expected (e.g., use of a Foley catheter may be discontinued a day early). A variance analysis is necessary to review the data for trends and for developing and implementing an action plan to respond to the identified patient problems (Box 16.3). In addition, variances may result from changes in the patient's health or because of other health complications not associated with the primary reason why the patient requires care. Once a variance has been identified, the nurse modifies the patient's care to meet the needs associated with the variance.

COMMON RECORD-KEEPING FORMS

Nurses use a variety of electronic or paper forms for the type of information routinely documented. The categories or data fields within a form are usually derived from institutional standards of practice or guidelines established by accrediting agencies.

Admission Nursing History Form

A nursing history form is completed when a patient is admitted to a nursing care unit. The history form guides the nurse through a complete assessment to identify relevant nursing diagnoses or problems (see Chapter 14). Data on history forms provide baselines that can be compared with changes in the patient's condition.

Flow Sheets and Graphic Records

Acute and critical care nurses commonly use flow sheets and graphic records to document physiological data and routine care. Within a computerized documentation system, these forms allow the nurse to quickly and easily enter assessment data about a patient, such as vital signs, admission and daily weights, intake and output, and percentage of meals eaten. They also facilitate the documentation of the provision of routine, repetitive care, such as hygiene measures, ambulation, and safety and restraint checks. These documents provide current patient information accessible to all members of the health care team and help team members quickly see patient trends over time (Box 16.4). Any occurrence on a flow sheet that is unusual or represents a significant change in a patient's condition is explained in detail in a progress note. For example, if a patient's blood pressure becomes dangerously high, the nurse first completes and records a focused assessment and then documents the action taken in a progress note.

Patient Care Summary or Kardex

Many agencies now have computerized systems that provide basic summative information in the form of a patient care summary. This is printed out for each patient during each shift. This summary is continually updated and provides the nurse with a current detailed list of orders, treatment, and diagnostic testing. In some settings, a Kardex system, a portable "flip-over" file or binder, is kept at the nurses' station. Most Kardex forms have an activity and treatment section and a nursing care plan section that organize information for quick reference as nurses give change-of-shift reports or make walking rounds. An updated Kardex form eliminates the need for repeated referral to the chart or computer record for routine information throughout the day. Information commonly found on the patient care summary or Kardex form includes the following:

- Basic demographic data (e.g., age, sex, gender identity [see Chapter 28], religious affiliation)
- Hospital identification number
- Physician's name
- Primary medical diagnosis
- Medical and surgical history
- Current prescriber's treatment orders to be carried out by the nurse (e.g., dressing changes, ambulation, glucose monitoring)
- Nursing care plan
- Nursing orders (e.g., education sessions, symptom relief measures, counselling)

BOX 16.3 Example of Variance Documentation

You are using a critical pathway for "routine postoperative care" for a 56-year-old patient (preferred pronouns: he/him) who had abdominal surgery yesterday. One of the expected outcomes for postoperative day 1 on the critical pathway document is "Afebrile with lungs clear bilaterally." This patient has an elevated temperature, his breath sounds are decreased bilaterally in the bases of both lungs, and he is slightly confused.

The following is an example of how you would document this variance on the pathway:

Breath sounds diminished bilaterally at the bases. T 37.8°C; P 92; R 28/min; oxygen saturation 84% on room air. Family member (she/her) states the patient is "confused" and did not recognize her when she arrived a few minutes ago. Oxygen started at 2 L/min via nasal prongs. Head of bed elevated. Oxygen saturation improved to 92% after 5 minutes. Dr. P. Yoshida (she/her) notified of change in status. The family member remains at bedside.

BOX 16.4 Benefits of Using a Flow Sheet

- Information is accessible to all members of the health care team.
- Time spent on writing a narrative note is decreased.
- Information is current.
- Errors resulting from transfer of information are decreased.
- Team members can quickly see trends over time.

- Scheduled tests and procedures
- Safety precautions to be used in the patient's care
- Factors related to activities of daily living
- Contact information about nearest relative or guardian or person to contact in an emergency
- Emergency code status, and
- Allergies.

Standardized Care Plans

Some institutions use standardized care plans to make documentation easier for nurses. The plans, based on the institution's standards of nursing practice, are preprinted, established guidelines that are used to care for patients who have similar health problems. After a nursing assessment is completed, the staff nurse identifies the standard care plans that are appropriate for the patient. The care plans are placed in the patient's health care record. The standardized plans can be modified (with changes noted in ink) to individualize the therapies. Most standardized care plans also allow the nurse to write in the specific goals or desired outcomes of care and the dates by which these outcomes should be achieved.

One advantage of standardized care plans is establishment of clinically sound standards of care for similar groups of patients. These standards can be useful when quality improvement audits are conducted. These care plans can help nurses recognize the accepted requirements of care for patients and also improve continuity of care.

The use of standardized care plans is controversial. The major disadvantage is the risk that the standardized plans prevent nurses from providing unique, individualized therapies for patients. Standardized care plans cannot replace the nurse's professional judgement and decision making. In addition, care plans need to be updated on a regular basis to ensure that content is current and appropriate.

Discharge Summary Forms

It is important to prepare patients for an efficient, timely discharge from a health care facility. A patient's discharge should also result in desirable outcomes. Interdisciplinary involvement in discharge planning helps ensure that a patient leaves the hospital in a timely manner with the necessary resources in place (Box 16.5).

Ideally, discharge planning begins at admission. The nurse needs to revise the care plan as the patient's condition changes. The patient and family members need to be involved in the discharge planning process so that they have the information needed to return the patient home. Discharge information and instructions should include the following:

BOX 16.5 Discharge Summary Information

- Use clear, concise descriptions in the patient's own language.
- Provide step-by-step instructions for how to perform any procedure that the patient or family member will be doing independently (e.g., emptying a urinary catheter or self-administration of an injectable medication). Reinforce explanation with printed instructions.
- Identify precautions to follow when performing self-care or administering medications.
- Review signs and symptoms of complications that a patient or family member needs to report to a health care practitioner.
- List names and phone numbers of health care providers and community resources that the patient or family member can contact.
- Identify any unresolved problem, including plans for follow-up and continuous treatment.
- List actual time of discharge, mode of transportation, and who accompanied the patient.

- Instruction about potential food–drug interactions, nutrition intervention, and modified diets
- Rehabilitation techniques to support adaptation to, or functional independence in, the environment, or both
- Access to available community resources
- Circumstances in which patients should obtain further treatment or follow-up care
- Methods of obtaining follow-up care as well as any scheduled follow-up appointments
- The patient's and family's responsibilities in the patient's care, and
- Medication instructions, including the times and reasons to take each medication, the dose, the route, precautions, possible adverse reactions, and information about when and how to get prescriptions refilled.

Furthermore, a common standard in nursing practice is to educate patients about the nature of their disease process, its likely progress, and the signs and symptoms of complications.

All of this information is included in a discharge summary that is printed out and given to the patient or family or to the home care, rehabilitation, or long-term care agency on discharge. This information also remains in the EHR as a record of the discharge teaching that was provided (see Box 16.5). Discharge summary forms help make the summary concise and instructive. A summary form emphasizes previous learning by the patient and family and the care that should be continued in any restorative care setting. When given directly to patients, the form may be attached to pamphlets or teaching brochures.

ACUITY RATING SYSTEMS

Nurses use acuity ratings to determine the hours of care and number of staff required for a given group of patients every shift or every 24 hours. A patient's acuity level, usually determined by assessment data entered into a computer program by a registered nurse, is based on the type and number of nursing interventions (e.g., intravenous [IV] therapy, wound care, or ambulation assistance) required by a patient over a 24-hour period. Although acuity ratings are not part of a patient's medical record, nursing documentation within the medical record provides evidence to support the assessment of an acuity rating for an individual patient.

The acuity level is a classification used to compare one or more patients to another group of patients. For example, an acuity system classifies bathing patients from 1 (independent in all but one or two aspects of care; almost ready for discharge) to 5 (totally dependent in all aspects of care; requiring intensive care). Using this system, for example, a postsurgical patient requiring frequent monitoring and extensive care has an acuity level of 3, while another patient awaiting discharge after a successful recovery from surgery has an acuity level of 1. Accurate acuity ratings justify the number and qualifications of staff needed to safely care for patients. The patient-to-staff ratios established for a unit depend on a composite gathering of 24-hour acuity data for all patients receiving care.

DOCUMENTATION IN THE HOME HEALTH CARE SETTING

Home health care is expanding owing to shorter hospitalizations and the larger numbers of older persons needing home care services. Because patients are leaving acute care settings earlier, an increasing number of home care patients are presenting in the community setting with more acuity (i.e., sicker). The focus in home health care is on family-centred care and forming a partnership or collaboration with the patient and the family to help the patient regain health, to help the family take over the patient's care, or to help accomplish both. Documentation in the home health care system has different implications

The usual forms used to document home care include the following:

- Assessment forms
- Referral source information or intake form
- Discipline-specific care plans
- Physician's plan of treatment
- Professional order form (e.g., physician, speech language pathologist, specialty nurses)
- Medication administration record
- Clinical progress notes
- Miscellaneous (case conference notes, professional communication forms, private billing forms, insurance company forms)
- Discharge summary

BOX 16.7	Components of Documentation in Long-Term Care

Section 1: The Health Care Record
The health care record includes the resident's name and medical number; date and time of admission; change in resident's condition; informed consent; note or discharge summary; incident reporting; monthly summary charting; and type of therapy and treatment time.

Section 2: Resident Assessments and Related Documents
This section consists of the admission record; preadmission assessment; admission assessment; assessment of risk for falls; skin assessment; bowel and bladder assessment; physical restraint assessment; record of self-administration of medication; nutrition assessment; and activities, recreation, or leisure interests.

Section 3: Other Records
Other records include drug therapy records, medication or treatment records, flow sheets or other graphic records, laboratory and special reports, consent forms, acknowledgements and notices, advance directives, and discharge or transfer records.

BOX 16.8	Guidelines for Telephone Orders and Verbal Orders

- Clearly determine the patient's name, room number, and diagnosis.
- Repeat any prescribed orders back to the physician or health care provider.
- Use clarification questions to avoid misunderstandings.
- Write telephone order ("TO") or verbal order ("VO"), including date and time, name of patient, and the complete order; sign the names of the physician or other health care provider and nurse.
- Follow agency policies; some institutions require telephone (and verbal) orders to be reviewed and signed by two nurses.
- The physician must co-sign the order within the time frame required by the institution (usually 24 hours).

than in other areas of nursing. Two primary differences are that the majority of the care is performed by the patient and family and that the nurse is often teaching and helping the patient and family achieve greater independence. Nurses must have astute assessment skills to gather the needed information about changes in the patient's health care status. In addition, documentation systems need to provide the entire health care team with the information needed for the nurse, patient, and family to work together effectively (Box 16.6).

In the home care setting, the patient is the guardian of the health care record. A hard copy of the health care record is kept in the patient's home, and the patient is responsible for its safekeeping. Communication is crucial when providing in-home care because much of the interaction between health care providers is conducted virtually by phone or fax over password-protected voice mail or secure fax lines. With the increasing availability of smartphones, laptop computers, or tablets, home health care records can be available in multiple locations, improving accessibility to information and facilitating interprofessional collaboration.

DOCUMENTATION IN THE LONG-TERM HEALTH CARE SETTING

An increasing number of older persons require care in long-term care or residential facilities. Many individuals live in this setting for the rest of their lives and are therefore referred to as *residents* rather than as *patients*. In long-term care settings, nursing personnel face challenges much different from those in acute care settings. Residents' health is often stable, and daily documentation can be completed on flow sheets. Assessments performed several times a day in acute care settings are required only weekly or monthly in long-term care settings.

Governmental agencies and provincial and territorial laws are instrumental in determining the standards and policies for documentation. Documentation is used to review the levels of care given to and needed by residents in long-term care facilities. Although most long-term care facilities have different documentation systems, these systems are based on the need for a concise, nonduplicating method of documentation and on the importance of nursing documentation in support of evidence-informed practice (Box 16.7).

DOCUMENTING COMMUNICATION WITH PROVIDERS AND UNIQUE EVENTS

Telephone Calls Made to a Health Care Provider

Document every phone call you make to a health care provider. Your documentation includes when the call was made, who made it (if you

did not make the call), who was called, to whom information was given, what information was given, and what information was received. An example is as follows: "May 20, 2017 (2030 hrs): Called Dr. Morgan's office. Spoke with Sam Thomas, RN (he/him), who will inform Dr. Morgan (they) that Mr. Wade's (he/him) potassium level drawn at 2000 hrs was 5.9 mEq/dL. Informed that Dr. Morgan will call back after they are finished seeing their current patient. Carla Skala, RN."

Telephone and Verbal Orders

Telephone orders (often written "TO") occur when a health care provider gives therapeutic orders over the phone to a registered nurse or other health care provider. Verbal orders (often written "VO") occur when a health care provider gives therapeutic orders to another health provider while they are standing in proximity to each other. TOs and VOs usually occur at night or during emergencies; they should be used only when absolutely necessary and not for the sake of convenience. In some situations, it is prudent to have a second person listen to TOs. Practitioners and students that can accept a TO or VO may vary by institution. Check agency policy. Box 16.8 lists guidelines that promote accuracy when receiving TOs or VOs.

The health care provider receiving a TO or VO enters the complete order into the computer using the computerized provider order entry (CPOE) software or writes it out on a physician's order sheet for entry in the computer as soon as possible. After taking the order, the health care provider reads it back using the "read-back" process, and documents that they did this as evidence that the information received (e.g., call-back instructions and/or therapeutic orders) was verified with the provider. An example follows: "March 4, 2017 (0815 hrs): Change IV fluid to Lactated Ringer's with potassium 20 mEq/L to run at 125 mL/hour. TO: Dr. Knight/J. Woods, RN, repeat back." The health care provider later verifies the TO or VO legally by signing it within a set time (e.g., 24 hours), as set by hospital policy.

Change-of-Shift Reports

At the end of each shift, nurses report information about their assigned patients to the nurses working on the next shift. While there is an increasing awareness that high-quality handover practices such as standardized methods of providing report (Bukoh & Siah, 2019) are critical to ensuring patient safety, as of yet there has been no gold standard identified in the literature for this component of patient care (Bressan et al., 2019). Various terms are used to describe this exchange of information, such as *change-of-shift reports*, *patient care handover*, *transfer of accountability (TOA)*, *handoffs*, *bedside reporting*, and *shift handover*.

Nurses give a change-of-shift report in one of several ways: orally in person, by audio recording, by writing information on a summary report sheet, or by standing at the patient's bedside. Oral reports can be given in conference rooms, with staff members from both shifts participating, but this is no longer as common as it used to be. Oral reports most often take the form of one-to-one reports—for example, a report given by the night nurse to the day nurse (Figure 16.3). An advantage of oral reports is that they allow staff members to ask questions or clarify explanations. The nurses can see the patient together to perform needed assessments, evaluate progress, and discuss the interventions best suited to the patient's needs. An audio-recorded report is given by the nurse who has completed care for the patient; this type of report is left for the nurse on the next shift to review. However, it is essential to schedule an opportunity for the incoming nurses to ask questions for clarification after they listen to the recorded report. Ineffective communication during handover can have negative consequences for patient outcomes (Hada & Coyer, 2021). Several Canadian hospitals have implemented standardized bedside safe patient handoffs using transfer of accountability (TOA) practice guidelines developed by their institution. The process provides an opportunity for the outgoing nurse and the incoming nurse to engage in a verbal report and to complete a patient safety checklist at the bedside.

Because nurses have many responsibilities, it is important to compile a change-of-shift report quickly and efficiently (Table 16.4). An effective report describes patients' health status and tells staff on the next shift exactly what kind of care patients require. A change-of-shift report should *not* simply be a reading of documented information. Instead, significant facts about patients are reviewed (e.g., condition of wounds, episodes of chest pain) to provide a baseline for comparison during the next shift. Data about patients need to be objective, current, and concise.

An organized report follows a logical sequence. The following is an example of a change-of-shift report:

Background information: Cy Tolan (preferred pronouns: he/him) in bed 4, a 32-year-old patient of Dr. Lang (they), is scheduled for a colon resection this morning at 0800 hrs. He has had ulcerative colitis for 2 years with recent bouts of frank bleeding in his stools. He was admitted at 0600 hrs this morning with slight abdominal discomfort. This is his first experience with surgery. He knows he may require a colostomy. He has been NPO (had nothing by mouth) since midnight at home.

FIGURE 16.3 One-to-one change-of-shift report at a nursing station. (From Registered Nurses' Association of Ontario [RNAO]. [2013]. *Developing and sustaining interprofessional health care: Optimizing patient, organizational and system outcomes* [p. 8]. https://rnao.ca/bpg/guidelines/interprofessional-team-work-healthcare)

TABLE 16.4	Change-of-Shift Reports: Dos and Don'ts
Dos	**Don'ts**
Do provide only essential background information about patient (i.e., name, sex, gender identity [see Chapter 28], age, physician's diagnosis, and medical history).	Don't review all routine care procedures or tasks (e.g., bathing, scheduled changes).
Do identify patient's nursing diagnoses or health care problems and their related causes.	Don't review all biographical information already available in written form.
Do describe objective measurements or observations about patient's condition and response to health problem, and emphasize recent changes.	Don't use critical comments about patient's behaviour, such as "Mrs. Wills is so demanding."
Do share significant information about family members as it relates to patient's problems.	Don't make assumptions about relationships between family members.
Do continuously review ongoing discharge plan (e.g., need for resources, patient's level of preparation to go home).	Don't wait until near discharge to discuss the plan.
Do relay to staff significant changes in the way therapies are given (e.g., different position for pain relief, new medication).	Don't describe basic steps of a procedure.
Do describe instructions given in teaching plan and patient's response.	Don't explain detailed content unless staff members ask for clarification.
Do evaluate results of nursing or medical care measures (e.g., effect of back rub or analgesic administration), and describe results specifically.	Don't simply describe results as "good" or "poor."
Do be clear about priorities to which incoming staff must attend.	Don't force incoming staff to guess what to do first.

Assessment: Mr. Tolan mentioned that he was unable to sleep last night. He had many questions about surgery on admission this morning.

Nursing diagnosis: His chief nursing care problems are anxiety related to inexperience with surgery and risk for body image disturbance.

Teaching plan: I talked to him about postoperative routines and answered all his questions. He attended the preoperative admission clinic 2 weeks ago, but he did not have as many concerns at that time. He stated that he felt less anxious now that he knows what to expect.

Treatments: I started an intravenous infusion of normal saline in his left arm at 0645 hrs and it is running at 125 mL/hr.

Family information: His spouse came with him this morning and will wait in the surgical waiting room till his surgery is complete.

Discharge plan: Mr. Tolan is a very active person and participates in strenuous sports such as swimming. His spouse is concerned about how he might react to a colostomy. I suggest making a referral to the enterostomal therapist early, if the colostomy is performed.

Priority needs: Right now, Mr. Tolan is relaxing in his room. All preoperative procedures have been completed except for his preoperative antibiotic, due on call to the operating room.

A professional demeanour is essential when giving a report about patients or family members. It is often necessary to describe the interactions among patients, nurses, and family members in behavioural terms. Nurses must avoid using judgemental language such as *uncooperative*, *difficult*, or *bad* when describing such behaviours.

In many settings, unregulated care providers (UCPs) are involved in the change-of-shift report. UCPs are part of the health care team and can contribute more when they also know a patient's condition and the nursing team's priorities in care. The nurse can use the report to emphasize to UCPs the tasks that need to be accomplished.

Transfer Reports

Patients may transfer from one unit to another to receive different levels of care. For example, patients are transferred from a critical care unit or the recovery room to general nursing units when they no longer require intense monitoring. To promote continuity of care, the nurse may give a **transfer report** by phone or in person. The components to include in a transfer report are listed Box 16.9. After completion of the transfer report, the receiving nurse needs an opportunity to ask questions about the patient's status. In some cases, written documentation must include a record of the information reported.

Using SBAR or I-SBAR-R for Communication

Nurses communicate information about patients so that all team members can make appropriate decisions about the care of patients. Any verbal report must be timely, accurate, and relevant. Many Canadian hospitals use the **situation–background–assessment–recommendation (SBAR) technique** or **identification–situation–background–assessment–recommendation–repeat back (I-SBAR-R) technique** (Box 16.10) to share important patient information in an effective and efficient way and to help standardize communication (Institute for Healthcare Improvement, 2017). The SBAR/I-SBAR-R technique is a situational briefing system that fosters a culture of patient safety. This technique (see Box 16.10) can be incorporated into a variety of reports (e.g., a nurse's report to a physician about a critically ill patient, change-of-shift reports about individual patients) and can be adapted for use with or by other health care providers.

Incident or Occurrence Reports

An *incident* or *occurrence* is any event that is not consistent with the routine, expected care of a patient or the standard procedures in place

---

BOX 16.9 Components of a Transfer Report

- Patient's name, age, name of primary physician, and medical diagnosis
- Summary of progress up to the time of transfer
- Patient's current health status (physical and psychosocial)
- Patient's allergies
- Patient's emergency code status
- Patient's family support (e.g., spouse or partner, children, parents)
- Patient's current nursing diagnoses or problem and care plan
- Any critical assessments or interventions to be completed shortly after transfer (helps receiving nurse to establish priorities of care)
- Need for any special equipment, such as isolation equipment, suction equipment, or traction

---

BOX 16.10 The Identification–Situation–Background–Assessment–Recommendation–Repeat Back (I-SBAR-R) Technique

When calling the physician, follow the I-SBAR-R process as follows:

Identification: Who is calling and who are you calling about?
- Identify yourself and your role
- Identify the unit, the patient, and the room number

Situation: What is the situation you are calling about?
- Briefly state the problem: What it is, when it started, and the severity

Background: Provide background information as necessary related to the situation, including the following:
- The admitting diagnosis, date of admission, and pertinent medical history
- List of current medications, allergies, intravenous fluids, and laboratory tests
- Laboratory results (date and time each test was performed and results of previous tests for comparison)
- Other clinical information
- Code status

Assessment: What is your assessment of the situation?
Examples include the following:
- Most recent vital signs
- Changes in vital signs or assessment from previous assessments

Recommendations: What is your recommendation, or what do you think needs to be done?
Examples include the following:
- Patient to be admitted or transferred
- New medication or further tests
- Patient to be seen now
- Orders to be changed

Repeat Back:
- Repeat back orders that have been given
- Clarify any questions

Adapted from Joint Commission on Accreditation of Healthcare Organizations. (2005, February). The SBAR technique: Improves communication, enhances patient safety. *Joint Commission Perspectives on Patient Safety, 5*(2), 2; Enlow, M., Shanks, L., Guhde, J., & Perkins, M. (2010). Incorporating interprofessional communication skills (ISBARR) into an undergraduate nursing curriculum. *Nurse Educator, 35*(4), 176–180; Grbach, W., Struth, D., & Vincent, I. (2008, July 17). *Reformulating SBAR to "I-SBAR-R."* Quality and Safety Education for Nurses. http://qsen.org/reformulating-sbar-to-i-sbar-r

on a health care unit. Examples include patient falls, needle-stick injuries, a visit by someone who has symptoms of illness, medication administration errors, accidental omission of ordered therapies, and circumstances that led to injury or risk for patient injury. An **incident (occurrence) report** (or safety learning report) is completed whenever an incident occurs. Incident reports are an important part of the quality improvement program of a unit (see Chapter 13). A *near miss* (or *close call*) is defined as "an event that could have resulted in unwanted consequences, but did not because either by chance or through timely intervention the event did not reach the patient" (ISMP Canada, n.d.).

When an incident occurs, as the nurse, you should document an objective description of what happened; what you observed; and the follow-up actions taken, including notification of the patient's health care provider in the patient's medical record. Remember to evaluate and document the patient's response to the incident.

Incident or occurrence reports contain confidential information; distribution of the report is limited to those responsible for reviewing the forms. It is important to follow agency policy when making an incident report and to file the report with the risk management department of your agency. Analysis of incident reports helps identify trends in an organization that provide justification for changes in policies and procedures or for in-service programs. Do not include any reference to an incident in the medical record. A notation about an incident report in a patient's medical record makes it easier for a lawyer to argue that the reference makes the incident report part of the medical record and therefore subject to attorney review.

INFORMATION MANAGEMENT IN HEALTH CARE

Information technology (IT) refers to the management and processing of information, generally with the assistance of computers. **Health informatics** (see Chapter 17) is defined as follows (Wan & Gurupur, 2020, p. 2):

> *A transdisciplinary study of the data flow and processing into more abstract forms such as information, knowledge, and wisdom along with the associated systems needed to synthesize or develop decision support systems for the purpose of helping the healthcare management processes achieve better outcomes in healthcare delivery.*

A health care information system (HIS) is a group of systems used within a health care organization to support and enhance health care. An HIS consists of two major types of information systems: clinical information systems and administrative information systems. Together the two systems operate to make the entry and communication of data and information more efficient. Any single health care agency uses one or several of these systems.

Nursing competence in health care informatics is becoming a priority as health care providers and facilities across Canada implement electronic documentation. Nurses need informatics competencies to deliver safer and more efficient care, to add to the nursing professional knowledge base, and to facilitate the growth of evidence-informed practice. Professional organizations recommend that all nurses acquire a minimal level of awareness and competence in informatics and use of IT. Under the domain of communication and collaboration in the *National Nursing Education Framework* (CASN, 2022), the CASN lists "communicate clearly and accurately with members of the intraprofessional and interprofessional health care team, verbally and in writing, to improve efficiency and to reduce errors" as an essential component of baccalaureate nursing education (p. 17). The *Nursing Informatics Entry-to-Practice Competencies for Registered Nurses* (CASN, 2012) outlines three entry-to-practice competencies related to nursing informatics: (1) use of relevant information

and knowledge to support the delivery of evidence-informed patient care; (2) use of information and communication technologies (ICTs) in accordance with professional and regulatory standards and workplace policies; and (3) use of ICTs in the delivery of patient/client care. These nursing informatics competencies are considered the minimum knowledge and skills that new graduate nurses require in order to practise.

Competence in informatics is not the same as computer competency. To become competent in informatics, nurses need to be able to use evolving methods of discovering, retrieving, and using information in practice (Hebda et al., 2019). This means that, as a nurse, you learn to recognize when information is needed and have the skills to find, evaluate, and use that information effectively. You also need to know how to use clinical databases within your institution and apply the information so that you can deliver high-quality, appropriate patient care.

Clinical Information Systems

All members of the interprofessional health care team, including nurses, physicians, pharmacists, social workers, and therapists, use programs available on a **clinical information system (CIS)**. These programs include monitoring systems; order entry systems; and laboratory, radiology, and pharmacy systems. A monitoring system includes devices that automatically monitor and record biometric measurements (e.g., vital signs, oxygen saturation, cardiac index, and stroke volume) in acute care, critical care, and specialty areas. The devices electronically send measurements directly to the nursing documentation system.

Order-entry systems allow nurses to order supplies and services from another department. An example is a computer program that provides the ability to order sterile supplies from the central supply department. This eliminates the use of written order forms and expedites the delivery of needed supplies to a nursing unit. **Computerized provider order entry (CPOE)** systems allow health care providers to directly enter orders for patient care into the hospital information system. In advanced systems, CPOE systems have built-in reminders and alerts that help a health care provider select the most appropriate medication or diagnostic test. The direct entry of orders eliminates issues related to illegible handwriting and transcription errors. In addition, a CPOE system potentially speeds the implementation of ordered diagnostic tests and treatments, which improves staff productivity and saves money because the unit secretary no longer transcribes a written order onto a nursing order form (Hebda et al., 2019). Orders made through a CPOE are integrated within the record and sent to the appropriate departments (e.g., pharmacy or radiology).

A **clinical decision support system (CDSS)** is a computerized program used within a health care setting to aid and support clinical decision making. When used to support nursing decisions it is called a *nursing CDSS* (Figure 16.4). An *advanced* CDSS is a tool that makes patient-specific recommendations based on available data (Wasylewicz & Scheepers-Hoeks, 2018). The CDSS will generate tailored recommendations for individual patients, which are presented to nurses as alerts, warnings, or other information for consideration For example, an effective CDSS notifies health care providers of patient allergies before ordering a medication, which enhances patient safety during the medication ordering process. CDSSs also improve nursing care. When patient assessment data are combined with patient care guidelines, nurses are better able to implement evidence-informed nursing care (Box 16.11).

Nursing Clinical Information Systems

A well-designed **nursing clinical information system (NCIS)** incorporates the principles of nursing informatics to support the work that nurses do by facilitating the documentation of nursing process

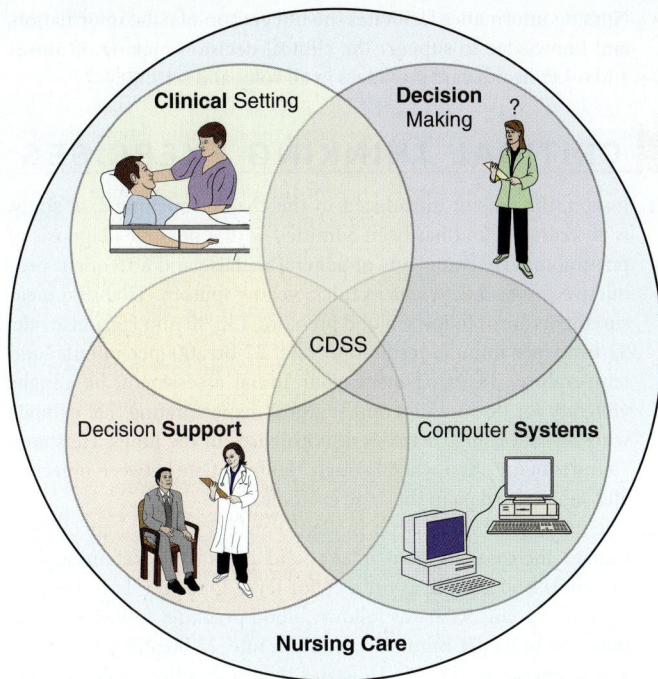

FIGURE 16.4 Model of a nursing clinical decision support system (CDSS).

activities and offering resources for managing nursing care delivery. As a nurse, you need to access a computer program easily, review a patient's medical history and health care provider's orders, and then go to the patient's bedside to conduct a comprehensive assessment. Once you complete an assessment, you will enter data into the computer terminal at the patient's bedside and develop a plan of care from the information gathered. This allows you to quickly share the plan of care with your patient. You will need to periodically return to the computer to check on laboratory test results and document the care you deliver. The computer screens and optional pop-up windows make it easy to locate information, enter and compare data, and make changes.

NCISs have two designs. The nursing process design is the most traditional. It organizes documentation within well-established formats, such as admission and postoperative assessment problem lists, care plans, intervention lists or notes, and discharge planning instructions. The nursing process design facilitates the following:

- Generation of a nursing work list that outlines routine scheduled activities related to the care of each patient
- Documentation of routine aspects of patient care such as hygiene, positioning, fluid intake and output, wound care measures, and blood glucose measurements
- Progress note entries using narrative notes, charting by exception, and flow sheets, and
- Documentation of medication administration (see Chapter 35).

More advanced systems incorporate standardized nursing languages such as the North American Nursing Diagnosis Association (NANDA) International nursing diagnoses, the Nursing Interventions Classification (NIC), and the Nursing Outcomes Classification (NOC) into the software.

The other model for an NCIS is the protocol or critical pathway design (Hebda et al., 2019). This design facilitates interdisciplinary management of information because all health care providers use evidenced-informed protocols or critical pathways to document the care they provide. The information system allows a user to select one or more appropriate protocols for a patient. An advanced system merges

BOX 16.11 EVIDENCE-INFORMED PRACTICE

Effect of Clinical Decision Support Systems on Patient Outcomes

PICO* Question: Do nurses who work at health care agencies that use clinical decision support systems (CDSSs) provide safer and more effective patient care when compared with nurses who work at agencies that do not use CDSSs?

Evidence Summary

Nurses who provide evidence-informed care at the bedside provide safe and effective care. However, one barrier to implementing evidence-informed practice is getting information to nurses at the bedside when they need it. Several studies have investigated the effect of the CDSS on patient outcomes. Huang and colleagues (2020) evaluated the effect of a nursing CDSS on the documentation of risk of pressure ulcer development and incidence of hospital-acquired pressure injury (HAPI). Data collected 4 months before and after the implementation of the CDSS were significant in the reduction of HAPI as well as increases in risk assessment documentation. Additional evidence shows that the use of a nursing CDSS improves adherence to hypoglycemia protocols in in-patient settings (Gibbs et al., 2020) and improves adherence to venous thromboembolism prophylaxis protocols in hospitalized patients (Titi et al., 2021). These studies contribute to the evidence that CDSSs that provide automatic decision support at the time and place clinicians need it enhance the quality and safety of patient care. CDSSs also help nurses initiate evidence-informed care faster and with more accuracy, improving patient outcomes.

Application to Nursing Practice

- CDSSs enhance the implementation of evidence-informed practice into nursing care because they remind nurses which interventions need to be implemented for specific patients at the time the care is needed.
- Nurses need to be involved in the design and selection of CDSSs to ensure that they provide clinical decision support effectively and efficiently.
- Nurses need to evaluate patient outcomes when CDSSs are used. They also need to be involved in developing solutions to improve the effectiveness of CDSSs when opportunities for improvement are identified.

*See Chapter 8 for a description of PICO.

multiple protocols, using a master protocol or path to direct patient care activities. Standard health care provider order sets are included in the protocols and automatically processed. The system integrates appropriate information into the medication delivery process to enhance patient safety. In addition, the system identifies variances of the anticipated outcomes on the protocols as documentation is entered. This provides all caregivers with the ability to analyze variances and offers an accurate clinical picture of a patient's progress.

Advantages of a Nursing Clinical Information System. Anecdotal reports and descriptive studies suggest that NCISs offer important advantages to nurses in practice. According to Hebda and colleagues (2019), some specific advantages include the following:

- Better access to information
- Enhanced quality of documentation through prompts
- Reduced errors of omission
- Reduced hospital costs
- Increased nurse job satisfaction
- Compliance with requirements of accrediting agencies
- Development of a common clinical database, and
- Enhanced ability to track records.

Many NCISs include content-importing technologies that allow the use of templates, macros, and automated data points as well as the ability to copy forward either parts of or entire nursing shift assessments, enabling nurses to quickly document their assessment or the care provided. These features have benefits and risks associated with their use. When allergy and current medication lists are automatically imported into nursing admission documentation from a previous hospital encounter, the nurse needs to meticulously review this information for accuracy and update it as needed to avoid documentation errors and patient safety concerns. When nursing shift assessment data are copied forward from a previous shift or day, the data must be updated so that they accurately reflect a patient's current clinical status (Jacquemard et al., 2021).

KEY CONCEPTS

- The electronic (or paper-based) medical record is a legal document that contains information describing the care delivered to a patient.
- All information contained in the medical record is confidential; access to patient records is limited to individuals involved in the care of the patient.
- Interdisciplinary communication arising among members of the health care team is essential, and the medical record is one tool that supports and facilitates that communication.
- Accurate record keeping requires an objective interpretation of data with precise measurements, correct spelling, and proper use of abbreviations.
- A nurse's electronic or handwritten signature on an entry in a record designates accountability for the contents of that entry.
- To keep medical records accurate, any change in a patient's condition warrants immediate documentation about the event and the action that was taken to address the change.
- Protecting the confidentiality of patient health information and maintaining the security of computer systems is paramount and is achieved through log-in processes, audit trails, firewalls, data-recovery processes, and policies for data handling and disposal.
- Problem-oriented medical records (POMRs) are organized by the patient's health care problems.
- Subjective–objective–assessment–plan (SOAP), subjective–objective–assessment–plan–intervention–evaluation (SOAPIE), problem–intervention–evaluation (PIE), and data–action–response (DAR) charting formats organize entries in the progress notes according to the nursing process.
- Home care documentation is accessible to a variety of caregivers in the home.
- Long-term care documentation is interdisciplinary. Assessments performed several times a day in the acute care setting are required only weekly or monthly in long-term care.
- Patient care information communicated to providers through telephone orders must always be verified by using and documenting use of the "repeat-back" process.
- Incident or occurrence reports objectively describe any event that is not consistent with the routine care of a patient.
- The major purpose of the change-of-shift report is to maintain continuity of care.
- A hospital information system consists of two major types of information systems: a clinical information system and an administrative information system.
- Computerized information systems provide information about patients in an organized and easily accessible fashion.
- Protection of the confidentiality of patient health information and the security of computer systems should be a top priority.
- Nursing informatics facilitates the integration of data, information, and knowledge to support the clinical decision making of nurses and other health care providers in all roles and settings.

CRITICAL THINKING EXERCISES

1. Joseph, the patient introduced in the chapter-opening case study, is 80 years old and has been admitted with a possible diagnosis of pneumonia. He complains of general malaise and a frequent productive cough that produces thick, yellow sputum. Vital sign measurements are as follows: blood pressure, 150/90 mm Hg; pulse rate, 92 beats per minute; respiration rate, 22 breaths per minute; and temperature, 38.5°C. During your initial assessment, he coughs violently for 40 to 45 seconds without expectorating. He exhibits wheezes and coarse crackles at both bases of the lungs. He states, "It hurts in my chest when I cough." Differentiate between objective and subjective data in this case example.

2. The nurse positions Joseph in semi-Fowler's position, encourages him to increase his fluid intake, and gives him acetaminophen (Tylenol), 650 mg PO, as ordered for fever. One hour later, his vital sign measurements are as follows: blood pressure, 130/86 mm Hg; pulse, 86 beats per minute; respiration rate, 22 breaths per minute; and temperature, 37.7°C. He states that he has been able to sleep. His fluid intake over the past hour has been 200 mL of water. Use the given information to write a nurse's progress note using the PIE format.

3. Near the end of the shift, *fluid volume deficit* is identified as a nursing diagnosis for Joseph. Since his admission, he has had a fluid intake of about 600 mL, and his urine output was 300 mL of dark, concentrated urine. His temperature is back up to 38.4°C, his mucous membranes are dry, and he states that he feels very weak. List what should be included in the change-of-shift report.

4. Several days later, after treatment with intravenous antibiotics, Joseph is feeling much better, and preparations are being made for discharge. He is to take cephalexin (Keflex) 500 mg every 6 hours for the next 10 days; continue to drink extra fluids; and get extra rest. Although he is generally cooperative, he does not like drinking water or taking pills. He is to make an appointment with his physician for 1 week from today and should call the physician if symptoms recur. Write a discharge summary that is concise and instructive.

🌐 *Answers to Critical Thinking Exercises appear on the Evolve website.*

REVIEW QUESTIONS

Review Questions 1 to 8 relate to the case study at the beginning of the chapter.

1. Shara, the student nurse caring for Joseph, receives a telephone report for Joseph from the ED nurse. When documenting the content of the call, the ED nurse would include which pieces of information? *(Select all that apply.)*
   a. Joseph is 80 years old.
   b. Joseph's medical diagnosis is pneumonia.
   c. That the receiving nurse was advised the patient's wife is "needy."
   d. Joseph has no allergies to medication.
   e. Joseph is "on the call bell nonstop; good luck."
   f. Joseph is currently receiving oxygen by nasal cannula at 2 L/min.

2. As part of the admission to the inpatient unit, Shara will be documenting her initial assessment for Joseph using an electronic medical record (EMR) on a computer. The computers are located in the hallway of the unit. Shara considers how she will maintain the confidentiality of the patient record. Which of the following actions would require intervention by her preceptor because they do not adequately protect patient confidentiality and the care record? *(Select all that apply.)*
   a. Shara leaves a slip of paper with her username and password in the patient's room.
   b. Shara shares her password with another nursing student who needs to document during a patient emergency.
   c. Shara shreds her patient care worksheet at the end of each shift.
   d. Shara logs out of the electronic medical record when leaving the work station.
   e. Shara allows Joseph's son to view the nursing notes on the computer.
   f. Shara checks her pockets for any paper containing health information before leaving the unit.

3. In the following documentation example, highlight the *subjective data*:
   The patient stated, "I can't get warm no matter how many blankets I have." The patient is diaphoretic, shivering, and has a tympanic temperature of 38.5°C. The patient is experiencing fever related to bacterial lung infection. Covered with a light sheet, acetaminophen 650 mg given and fluids encouraged. S. Coughlin, SN

4. When the nurse is preparing to administer Joseph's first dose of antibiotic, the electronic medication administration record (MAR) flashes an alert to confirm medication allergies because this field is blank in the EMR. By selecting from the list of answer options provided, choose the *most likely* options for the information missing from the following statement:
   Shara recognizes that _____1_____ are computerized programs that create tailored _____2_____ to improve patient safety.
   Answer options for 1 and 2:
   acuity scales
   assessments
   clinical decision support systems
   order sets
   recommendations
   telephone orders

5. Joseph's care provider has used the computerized provider order entry (CPOE) function in the EMR to enter the prescriptions. Shara knows that a CPOE has the following advantages: *(Select all that apply.)*
   a. Reduces transcription errors.
   b. Reduces the time needed for health care providers to write orders.
   c. Eliminates the need for verbal and telephone orders from health care providers.
   d. Reduces the time nurses use to communicate with health care providers.
   e. Keeps track of the hours required for patient care to be provided.
   f. May increase the speed of implementation of ordered tests and procedures.

6. When the nurse enters Joseph's room to administer the antibiotics, Joseph says, "I do not know what is going on; I cannot get an explanation from my doctor about the results of the tests. I want

something done about this." For each of the documentation statements in the following chart, use an "X" to indicate whether the statement represents *appropriate* or *inappropriate* documentation of Joseph's emotional status.

Documentation Statement	Appropriate	Inappropriate
a. The patient has a defiant attitude and demands his test results.		
b. The patient is refusing medications until he speaks to his health care provider.		
c. The patient is demanding and complains frequently.		
d. The patient states that he is frustrated by the lack of information about his test results.		
e. The patient appears to be upset with his health care provider about his test results.		
f. The patient states "I don't know what is going on."		

7. Shara's preceptor is providing feedback on her documentation in the patient record. Indicate which of the following preceptor responses in the following table is *most appropriate* for each entry that Shara has completed. Answer options may be used more than once.

Nursing Student Documentation	Appropriate Preceptor Response No.
a. Patient appears anxious.	
b. Patient complained of chills 4 hours ago on admission to unit—resolved.	
c. Voiding a reasonable amount in bathroom.	
d. Wife is difficult; asks a lot of questions.	
e. Fluid intake is inadequate.	
f. The patient's health care provider was too busy in ED to see patient and address concerns.	

Answer options for preceptor responses:
1. Document as close to the time the assessment occurred as possible.
2. Use exact measurements, where possible, to increase accuracy.
3. Avoid vague statements.
4. Avoid making critical comments about another care provider.

8. At the end of shift, Shara is preparing to give a report to the oncoming nurse. In the following excerpt, highlight phrases

that could be *omitted or reworded* to improve the quality of the report:

> *Joseph is an 80-year-old man that was admitted today with a diagnosis of pneumonia. His spouse is with him in his room. They have been married for 49 years and they live together in an apartment downtown. On admission, his oxygen saturation was 94% on supplemental oxygen and it is now 97% on 2 L/min via nasal cannula. He had a fever but it's getting better. The plan is to send him home with home care if his O2sat continue to improve, but I wouldn't want to be the one doing that, as he can get super-rude when he doesn't think his questions are being answered. Next antibiotics are due at 2200.*

Answers: 1. a, b, d, f; **2.** a, b, e; **3.** Subjective data: "I can't get warm no matter how many blankets I have"; **4.** clinical decision support systems, recommendations; **5.** a, f; **6.** Appropriate statements: d, f; Inappropriate statements: a, b, c, e; **7.** a-3, b-1, c-2, d-3, e-2, f-4, **8.** The following phrases could be omitted or reworded to improve the report: "They have been married for 49 years and they live together in an apartment downtown"; "He had a fever but it's getting better"; "... I wouldn't want to be the one doing that, as he can get super-rude when he doesn't think his questions are being answered."

🌐 *Rationales for the Review Questions appear on the Evolve website.*

RECOMMENDED WEBSITES

Accreditation Canada: https://www.accreditation.ca
Accreditation Canada is a national, not-for-profit, nongovernmental organization that helps health and social service organizations, across Canada and internationally, examine and improve the quality of care and service they provide to their patients through voluntary external peer review.

Canada Health Infoway: https://www.infoway-inforoute.ca
Canada Health Infoway (Infoway) is a federally funded, independent, not-for-profit organization. Members include the 14 federal, provincial, and territorial deputy ministers of health. Infoway has a mandate to improve the health of Canadians by accelerating the development, adoption, and effective use of innovative digital health solutions.

Canadian Nurses Association (CNA): Provincial and Territorial Regulatory Bodies: https://www.cna-aiic.ca/en/nursing/regulated-nursing-in-canada/regulatory-bodies

This part of the CNA website provides links to each provincial and territorial nursing association or college. Most regulatory bodies provide information about documentation standards and requirements in their province or territory.

Canadian Nursing Informatics Association (CNIA): https://cnia.ca
The CNIA is affiliated with the CNA and is the voice for health informatics in Canada. Its aim is to positively impacting health outcomes by advancing nursing informatics leadership.

The Personal Information Protection and Electronic Documents Act (PIPEDA): https://www.priv.gc.ca/en/privacy-topics/privacy-laws-in-canada/the-personal-information-protection-and-electronic-documents-act-pipeda
PIPEDA is the federal privacy law for private-sector organizations. It sets out the ground rules for how organizations must handle the collection, use, and disclosure of individuals' personal information.

🌐 REFERENCES

A full reference list is available on the website for this book at http://evolve.elsevier.com/Canada/Potter/fundamentals/

17

Nursing Informatics and Canadian Nursing Practice

Written by Margaret Ann Kennedy, RN, PhD, CPHIMS-CA, FCAN, and Kathryn J. Hannah, CM, MScN, PhD, DSc(HC)

OBJECTIVES

Mastery of content in this chapter will enable you to:

- Define the key terms listed.
- Describe how nursing informatics differs from routine use of technologies in nursing practice.
- Identify key Canadian issues and challenges in managing nursing data.
- Compare Canadian strategies for identifying and documenting key nursing data.
- Describe how health information data standards influence Canadian nursing practice.
- Explain why using standardized nursing data is important for acknowledging the professional contributions of nursing to health outcomes for Canadians.
- Develop a beginning understanding of the scope of nursing informatics concepts and the ways in which nurses can be involved in nursing informatics.
- Describe the relationship between federal privacy legislation and nursing practice in the context of a digital practice environment.

KEY TERMS

American Medical Informatics Association (AMIA)

Analytics

Australasian Institute of Digital Health (AIDHAU)

Big data

Canada Health Infoway

Canadian Institute for Health Information (CIHI)

Canadian Nursing Informatics Association (CNIA)

C-HOBIC (Canadian Health Outcomes for Better Information and Care) project

Connected health care

Consumer health

Digital health

Digital Health Canada

Discharge Abstract Database (DAD)

eHealth

Electronic health record (EHR)

Health Information: Nursing Components (HI:NC)

International Classification for Nursing Practice® (ICNP®)

International Council of Nurses (ICN)

International Medical Informatics Association (IMIA)

International Medical Informatics Association Special Interest Group in Nursing Informatics (IMIA-SIGNI)

mHealth

Nursing data science

Nursing informatics (NI)

Personal Information Protection and Electronic Documents Act (PIPEDA)

SNOMED CT® (Systematized Nomenclature of Medicine Clinical Terms®)

Standards

uHealth

🌐 WEBSITE

https://evolve.elsevier.com/Canada/Potter/fundamentals/

CASE STUDY

B.S. (preferred pronouns: she/her) is a 46-year-old working professional in human resources (HR) for a large financial consulting firm. Because of the COVID-19 pandemic, B.S. is one among those in many sectors of the workforce who have had to work from home to minimize potential exposure to the virus. She takes Metformin to manage her type II diabetes and supports it through a regular program of blood glucose monitoring at home. Over the past 3 months, B.S. has persistently had a blood glucose well above her recommended levels and was recently placed on insulin injections to control her blood sugar levels.

The pandemic has caused physician offices to remain closed except in the most urgent cases, and most patients are being supported using telehealth. After a telephone consultation with her doctor to review her blood glucose levels, B.S. was referred to the diabetes clinic for additional support. The diabetes clinic uses a videoconferencing program to connect with patients, perform teaching, and track progress. B.S. registers at the diabetes clinic for videoconferencing and is scheduled for biweekly sessions. The diabetes clinic nurses have started a local electronic health record for B.S. Her personal information has been populated by the provincial client registry, and the nurses have completed an

CASE STUDY

intake assessment and clinical assessment. B.S.'s progress is then documented biweekly.

It is now a month later, and B.S. is having home care dressings for a leg wound. The home care nurse wants to access her diabetic record to help inform care and risk assessment associated with the healing of her leg wound. The home

care nurse accesses B.S.'s electronic health record and reviews the relevant information from the diabetic clinic.

Think about this case study as you read this chapter. There are Review Questions at the end of the chapter about this case study.

As health care systems respond to an increasingly complex technological environment and the progression of location-independent health care available through digital technologies (or *connected health care*), long-standing routines and tools are being superseded by strategic, adaptive, and evidence-informed practices that demand high-quality, timely health information. In an era when complex health care is delivered by dynamic interprofessional teams in increasingly diverse locations and using diverse methodologies, effective nursing documentation is critical to support clinical judgement and decision making, as well as to support aggregation of patient-centred documentation from other nurses and clinical disciplines to support optimal patient outcomes (Hussey & Kennedy, 2016). Current information needs in health care challenge nurses to identify the elements of their practice that are most critical to use in nursing decision making. Nursing informatics (NI) is a specialty area of nursing practice dedicated to effective use of information and communication technology (ICT) to support professional nursing practice and enable optimal patient outcomes. NI has been developed to respond to information challenges and to support the effective use and documentation of information in nursing practice. The International Medical Informatics Association (IMIA) Special Interest Group in Nursing Informatics (SIGNI) declared that "Nursing informatics science and practice integrates nursing, its information and knowledge and their management with information and communication technologies to promote the health of people, families and communities worldwide" (IMIA, 2009).

Since the introduction of ICT in the health care sector, nursing has recognized the value of ICT for informing effective practice, fostered technological development in support of patient care, and established core competencies related to ICT and nursing practice (Hussey & Hannah, 2021). Well-established ICT applications in health care include patient scheduling and transfer, billing and financial management, diagnostic imaging, lab reporting, order-entry applications, pharmacy, patient documentation systems, clinical support tools, remote consultation and triage, and resource management applications. Innovative and explosive development of digital tools supporting health information management for both clinicians and consumers have pushed the boundaries of traditional conceptualizations of health care. Terms such as eHealth (electronic health care), mHealth (mobile health care), uHealth (health care available through ubiquitous technologies), connected health care (health care delivered across settings by digital means), and digital health (health care facilitated by digital technologies) have become fully embedded in the daily language of clinicians and consumers. These are collectively included in the term digital health, which the World Health Organization defines as follows:

The field of knowledge and practice associated with the development and use of digital technologies to improve health. Digital health expands the concept of eHealth to include digital consumers, with a wider range of smart-devices and connected equipment. It also encompasses other uses of digital technologies for health such as the Internet of things, artificial intelligence, big data, and robotics.

(World Health Organization, 2021, p. 19)

Such digital information can be generated in acute care facilities, physician practices, or people using apps and wearing sensing devices. Importantly, digital health also includes the administration and data required to coordinate care and processes within the health care system.

Developers of health care software solutions offer integrated suites of applications that incorporate multiple tools for health care facilities or regions, and many health care institutions customize software to meet specific needs. Efforts are underway in every Canadian province and territory to implement a jurisdictional electronic health record (EHR)—a longitudinal record of an individual's health status (including diagnosed morbid conditions), diagnostic tests, treatments, and results—that will be interoperable with a pan-Canadian EHR. This movement toward provincial and federal EHRs requires that developers or vendors design and build interoperability into their information systems. Interoperability allows information to flow freely between other vendors' systems and provides the ability for patient information to be communicated along with the patients as they move across all sectors of the regional, provincial, or federal health care delivery system.

However, despite the vast array of technologies currently available in health care, nurses must continue to contextualize technology within the scope of their professional practice. Leaders such as Kheirkhahan et al. (2019) have advocated that care must be value based, particularly in digital environments where real-time data on the validity and impact of interventions can be provided to clinicians via diverse devices such as smartwatches. Nurses and nurse leaders must therefore recognize that future health care delivery systems relying on digital health will necessarily include informatics competencies and require a shift in practice to incorporate such competencies seamlessly across all practice domains (Hussey & Hannah, 2021). The joint position statement on NI by the Canadian Nurses Association (CNA) and Canadian Nursing Informatics Association (CNIA) (2017) extends this concept further and links practice to NI understanding, stating, "Just as ICT and digitally connected health are becoming integral to nursing practice, nursing informatics knowledge will be integral to evolving models of care . . . in digitally connected health environments that maintain the caring core of nursing" (p. 4).

NURSING INFORMATICS AND THE CANADIAN HEALTH CARE SYSTEM

The term *nursing informatics* was introduced initially by Dr. Marion Ball at the 1983 IMIA Conference in Amsterdam (Hannah et al., 2006a). Since the publication of the first text devoted to NI by Ball and Hannah in 1984, journals and texts have proliferated across Canada and internationally, with both traditional and online resources reflecting discipline-specific informatics (e.g., nursing, medicine, health) and broader, more collaborative topics in informatics and innovation.

Hannah et al. (2006a) have argued that despite the escalation of technology in health care and the recognition of NI, the persistent absence of universally accepted methods for defining and coding nursing contributions to health outcomes has been a significant obstacle to the collection of nursing data and has spurred accelerated innovation. Initiatives designed to capture, document, and share nursing

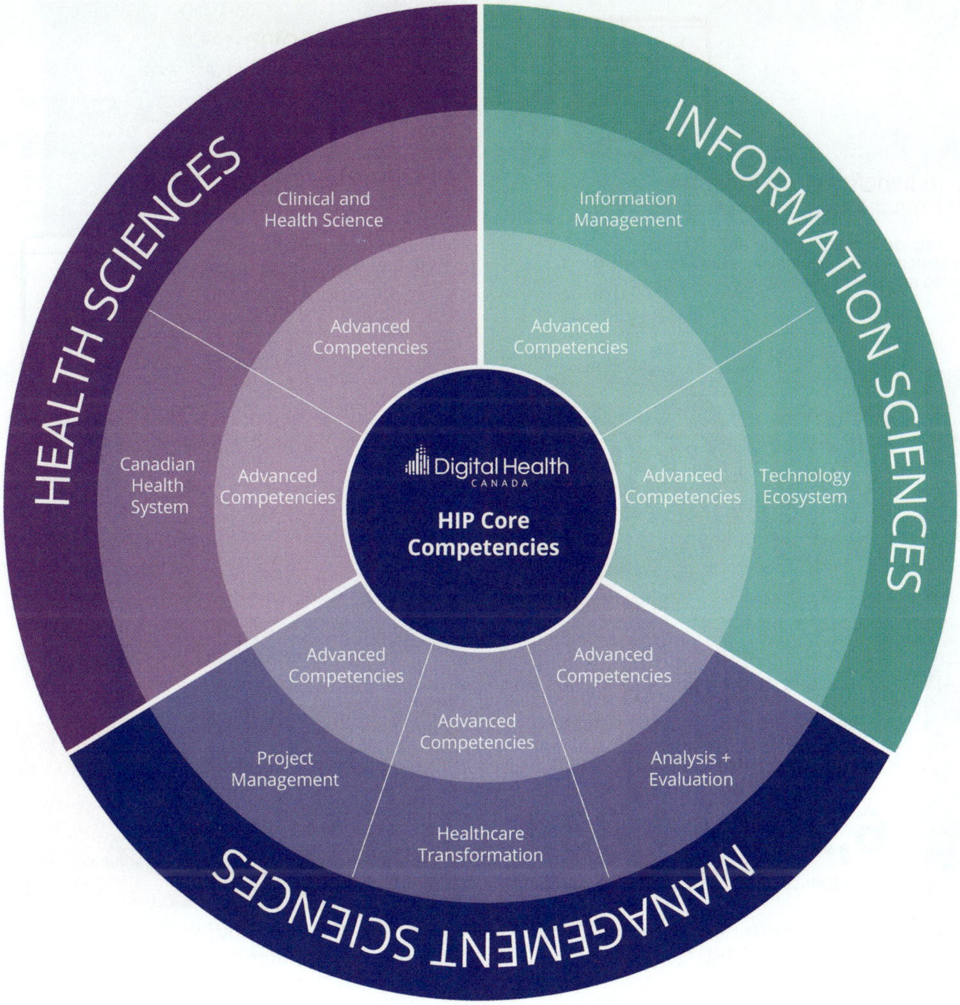

FIGURE 17.1 Digital Health Canada Health Information Professional (HIP) Competency Framework. (From Digital Health Canada. [2018]. *Health Informatics Professional Core Competencies*. Reprinted with permission from Digital Health Canada, copyright 2017. HIP is a registered trademark of Digital Health Canada. HIP Core Competencies is a copyright of Digital Health Canada.)

contributions through tools such as the **C-HOBIC (Canadian Health Outcomes for Better Information and Care) project**, nursing dashboards, and standardized assessment and documentation tools that standardize nursing data are evidence of a new perspective on nursing data and a commitment to articulating how interventions impact patient outcomes. These initiatives will be discussed later throughout this chapter.

Informatics in the Canadian Health Care System

National attention regarding the need for timely, secure, and appropriate health information access is now a given in Canada. Multiple health care and standards development organizations operate to coordinate broad documentation of health information and monitoring of the Canadian health care system. It is essential that nurses have both an awareness and understanding of the roles and relevance of each of these entities in relation to nursing practice.

Health informatics encompasses all health care disciplines, and the unique application of informatics knowledge and skills reflects specialties such as medical informatics, NI, and dental informatics. **Digital Health Canada**, Canada's health informatics association, defines health informatics as "the intersection of clinical, IM/IT (Information Management/Information Technology) and management practices to achieve better health" (Canadian Organization for Advancement of Computers in Health [COACH], 2013, p. 8). The recognition and growth of health informatics has occurred over many years as the result of dedicated efforts by many professionals, and it clearly acknowledges

the dependency on clinical expertise, as reflected in the Health Information Professional (HIP) Competency Framework illustrated in Figure 17.1 (Digital Health Canada, 2019). Although this chapter recognizes the existence of other types of informatics practice in the health sector, the focus will remain on NI.

The **Canadian Institute for Health Information (CIHI)** is the national, independent, and not-for-profit body that records, analyzes, and disseminates essential data and analysis on Canada's health system and the health of Canadians (Canadian Institute for Health Information [CIHI], 2021). Although not initially attentive to nursing data, CIHI later became more important in the context of several issues directly influencing nursing, including nursing workforce recruitment and retention.

Canada Health Infoway (Infoway), incorporated in 2001, was a key outcome of the federal, provincial, and territorial partnership (Canada Health Infoway, 2021a). Infoway has a national mandate to work with provincial and industry partners to accelerate the development, adoption, and use of digital health tools to improve the health of Canadians (Canada Health Infoway, 2021a). Infoway fulfilled this mandate in the past by partnering with jurisdictions as a "strategic investor" to share costs of implementing health information management projects and to provide additional project benefits analysis. Billions of dollars have been invested with partners to develop and implement the EHR in Canada. Six core components make up the pan-Canadian EHR (Canada Health Infoway, 2019):

- Patient registry
- Provider registry

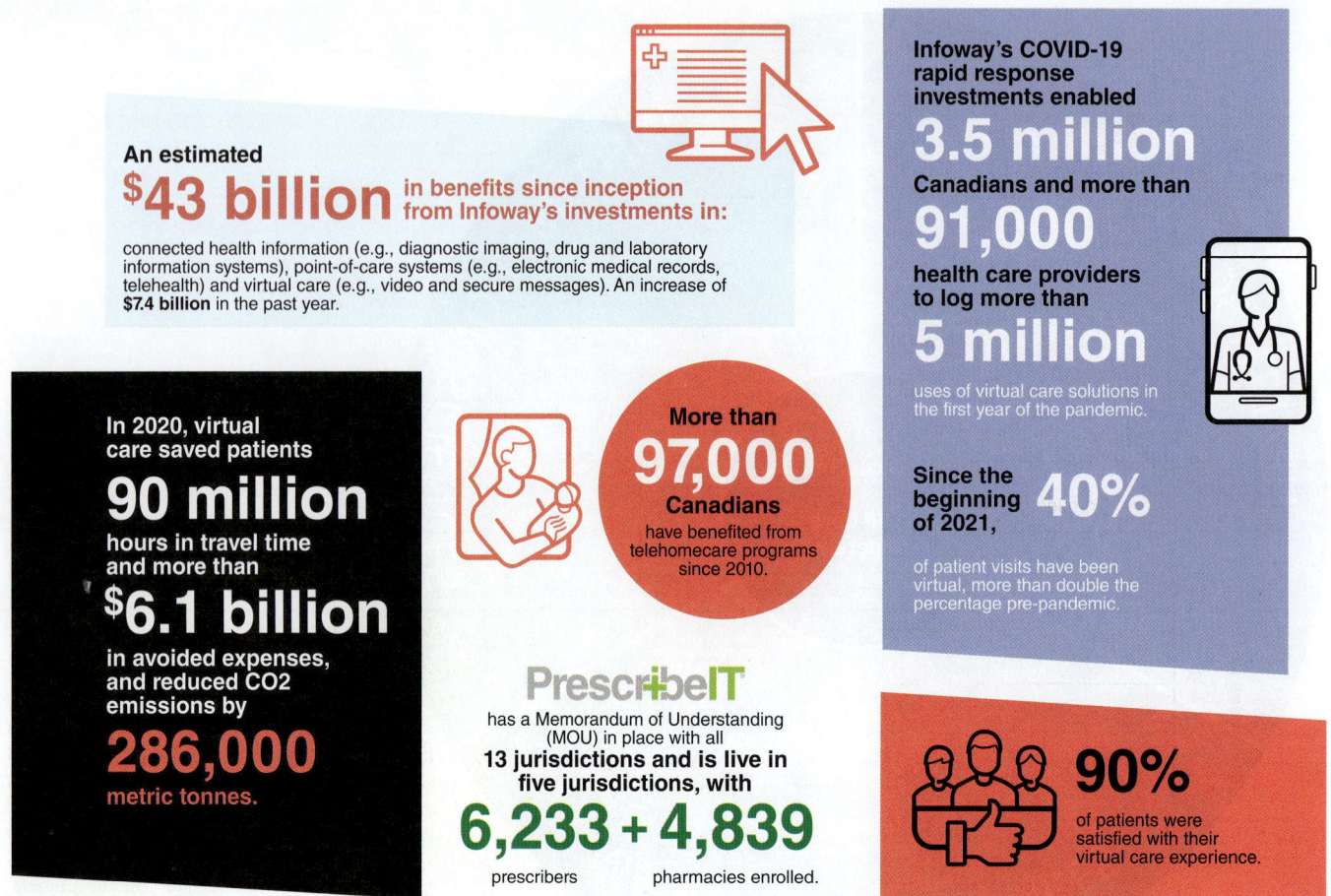

An estimated
$43 billion in benefits since inception from Infoway's investments in:

connected health information (e.g., diagnostic imaging, drug and laboratory information systems), point-of-care systems (e.g., electronic medical records, telehealth) and virtual care (e.g., video and secure messages). An increase of **$7.4 billion** in the past year.

In 2020, virtual care saved patients
90 million hours in travel time and more than
$6.1 billion in avoided expenses, and reduced CO2 emissions by
286,000 metric tonnes.

More than
97,000 Canadians have benefited from telehomecare programs since 2010.

Infoway's COVID-19 rapid response investments enabled
3.5 million Canadians and more than
91,000 health care providers to log more than
5 million uses of virtual care solutions in the first year of the pandemic.

Since the beginning of 2021, **40%** of patient visits have been virtual, more than double the percentage pre-pandemic.

PrescribeIT
has a Memorandum of Understanding (MOU) in place with all **13 jurisdictions** and is live in **five jurisdictions, with**
6,233 + 4,839
prescribers   pharmacies enrolled.

90% of patients were satisfied with their virtual care experience.

FIGURE 17.2 By the numbers. (From Canada Health Infoway. [2019]. *Annual report 2018–2019* [p. 12]. https://www.infoway-inforoute.ca/en/component/edocman/3726-annual-report-2018-2019/view-document?Itemid=101)

- Diagnostic images
- Laboratory results
- Drugs dispensed, and
- Clinical reports/immunization.

Infoway-funded projects have varied in nature—telehealth, registries, picture archiving and communication systems (PACS), and lab and drug information systems—all enabling a faster response time between assessment and treatment (Figure 17.2). And while provinces and territories in Canada have largely completed implementation of EHRs with investment from Infoway, attention has shifted from getting projects started to quantifying the value and benefit of these systems and projects and beyond.

In 2019, Infoway shifted from its role as a strategic investor to that of a service provider (Canada Health Infoway, 2019). PrescribeIT (Figure 17.3) is Infoway's ePrescribing service that is designed to be interoperable across prescribers, pharmacists, hospitals, and community pharmacies in Canada. In the future, this will be extended to community prescribers, community pharmacies, ambulatory clinics, emergency departments, and dentists' offices (Canada Health Infoway, 2019). Initially implemented in limited rollouts in Ontario and Alberta, PrescribeIT has since been launched in New Brunswick, Newfoundland and Labrador, and Saskatchewan (Canada Health Infoway, 2021a).

Consumer Health Informatics in Canada

Canadians are interested in health care technology, particularly if it helps make health care more convenient or puts them in control of their health (Figure 17.4). To support the concept of empowered health care consumers, a variety of self-management tools have been developed over the last few years. Consumers are increasingly using fitness tracking programs along with innovative devices, scheduling apps, and programs such as Google Health to exercise more control over their health and health information. The creation of tools and applications to support consumer self-management of health care is referred to as **consumer health**.

Health care organizations have also developed tools to support consumer health, particularly in the form of patient portals. Gheorghiu and Hagens (2017) have defined the patient portal as a "web-based application that combines an EHR system and a patient portal, not only for patients to interact with their health care providers, but also to access their own medical records and medical exam results." Maloney and Hagens (2021) have noted that the primary drivers of the development of patient portals in many countries are citizen demand and the belief in the empowered and engaged patient. While Gheorghiu and Hagens further noted that some portals provide enhanced functionality, such as secure messaging with health care providers and prescription renewals, Maloney and Hagens point out that the impact of patient portals has not been established or well documented to date.

In Canada, many provinces have patient portals associated with health authorities. One example of a patient portal is MyHealth, developed by Alberta Health Services (Figure 17.5). Patient portals offer access to providers and a variety of digital services. The security of personal health data on MyHealth, for example, is maintained through an authenticated login process, and users can access their health care information in an easy-to-use interface on the website or through a mobile app.

Innovation in care provision has been occurring for quite some time across Canada (Table 17.1). For example, Goodwin and colleagues

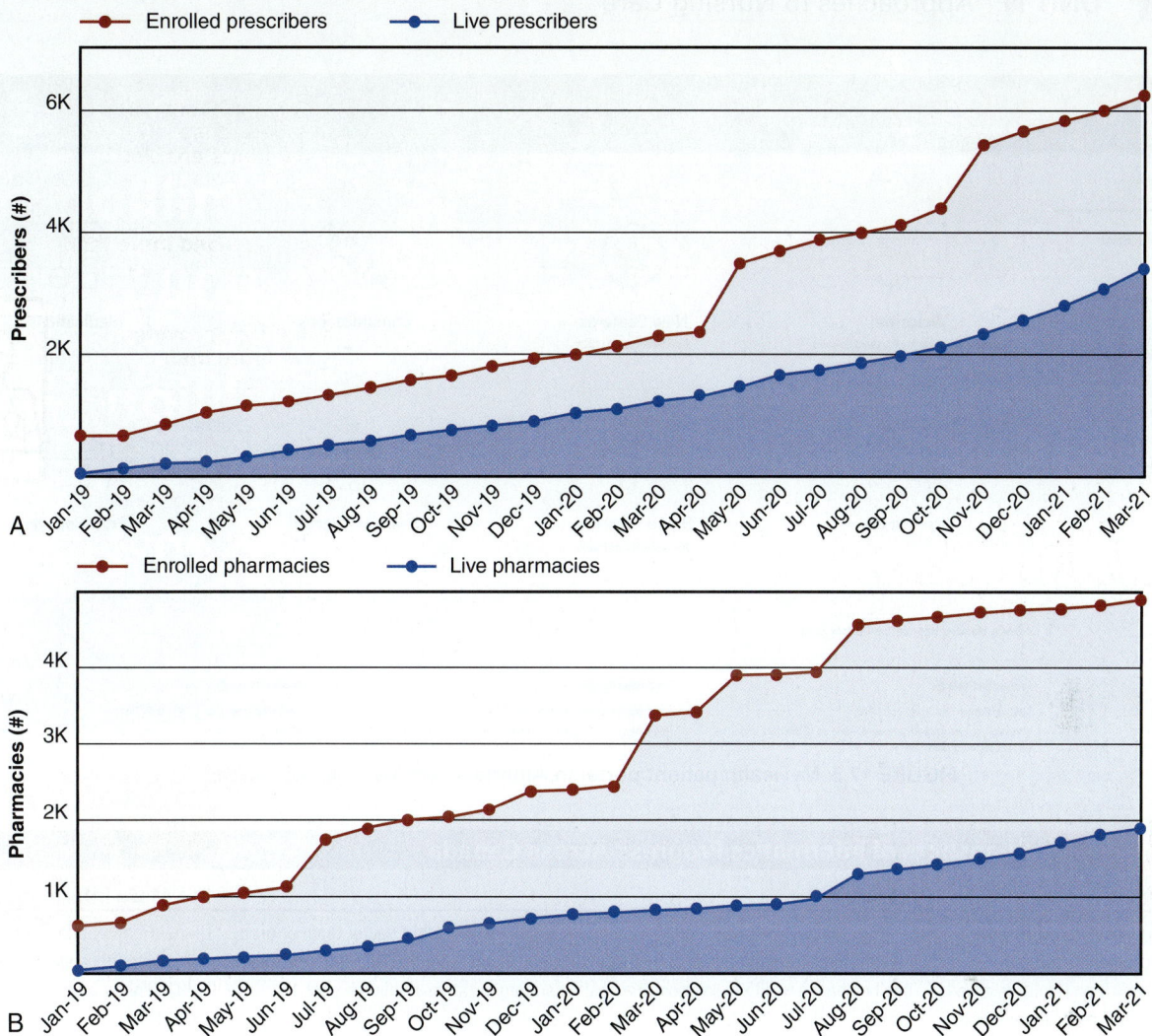

FIGURE 17.3 PrescribeIT implementations across Canada. (From Canada Health Infoway. [2019]. *Annual report 2018–2019* [p. 6]. https://www.infoway-inforoute.ca/en/component/edocman/3726-annual-report-2018-2019/view-document?Itemid=101)

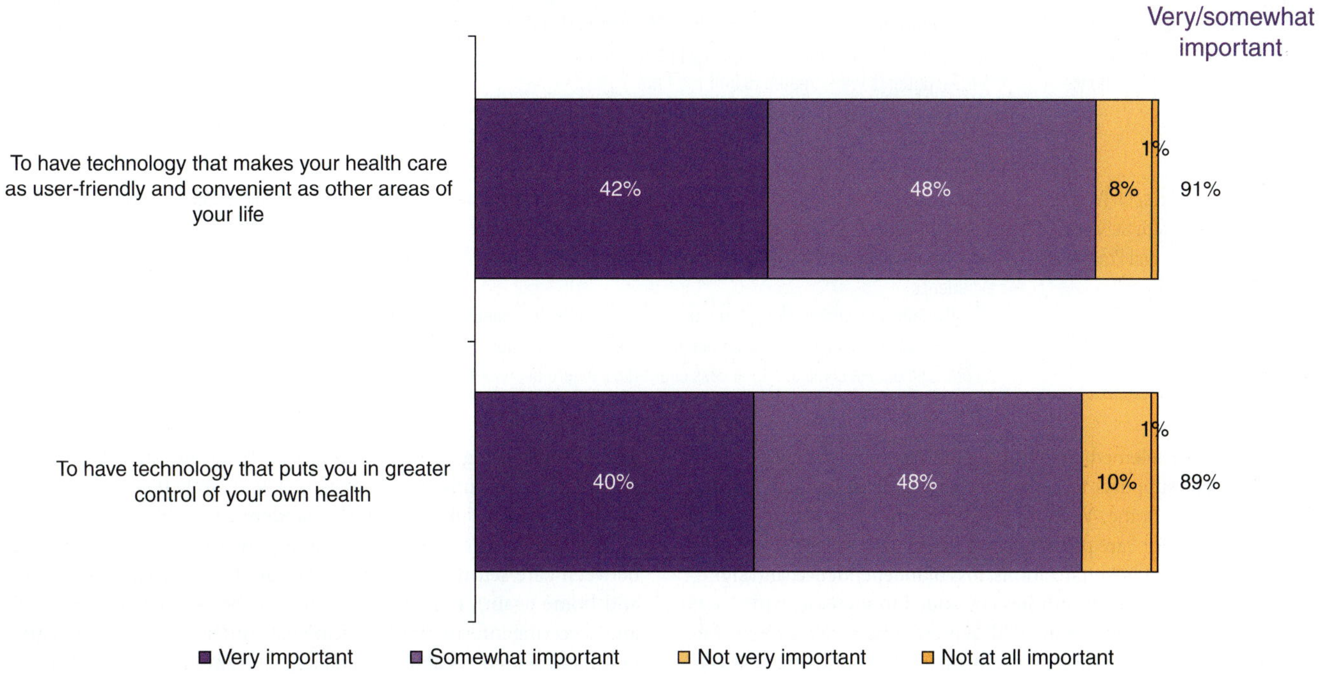

FIGURE 17.4 Outcomes of digital health that are important to Canadians. (Canada Health Infoway. [2020, January]. *Technology use among Canadians.*)

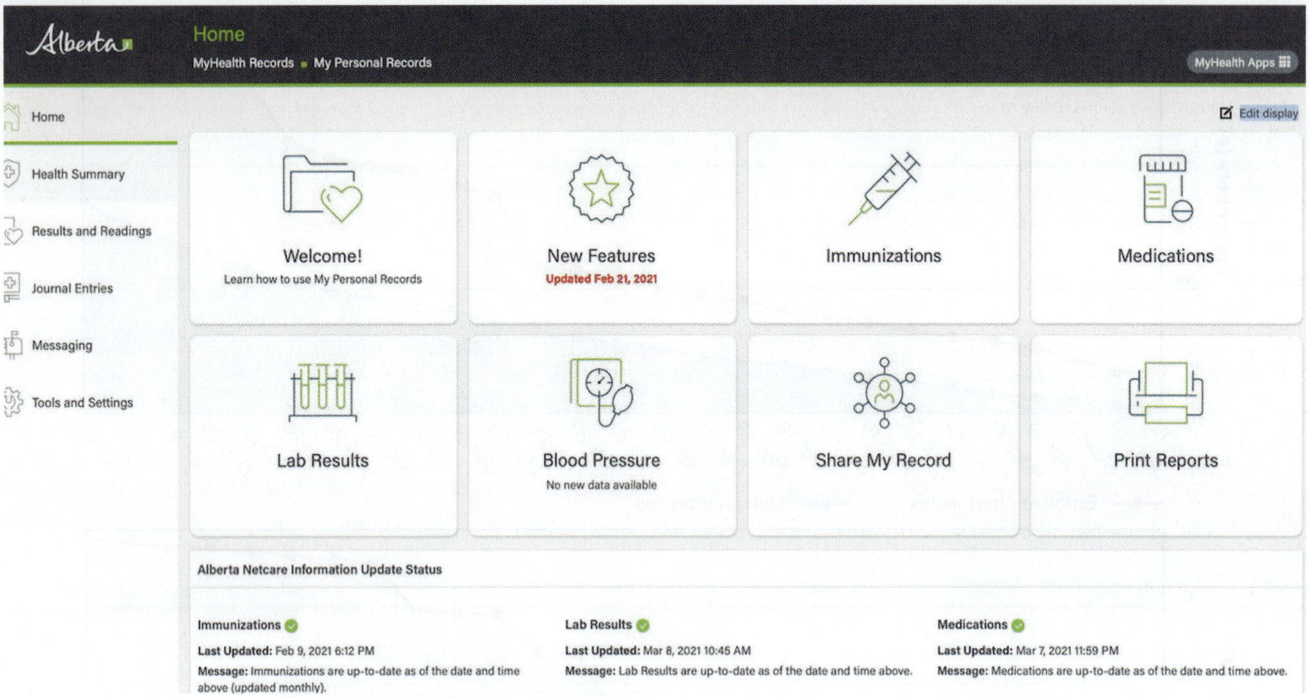

FIGURE 17.5 MyHealth patient portal in Alberta. (From MyHealth.Alberta.ca.)

TABLE 17.1	Snapshots of Informatics Progress Across Canada	
Initiative	**Overview**	**For More Information**
The Newfoundland and Labrador Centre for Health Information (NLCHI) and Orion Health received the 2020 Project Implementation of the Year Award from the Canadian Health Informatics Awards (CHIA)	The Project Implementation Team Award honours private and public sector team effort by recognizing a for-profit health care IT company and client team that have successfully implemented a health IT solution at a health care organization within the past 12 months. The first of its kind in Canada, eOrder is part of the provincial EHR, HEALTHe NL. The solution is an eOrdering referral process that streamlines scheduling and speeds up patient testing in the province's vascular imaging laboratory.	Digital Health Canada (https://digitalhealthcanada.com/news/2020-chiaw-award-winner-eorder)
Mackenzie Health has achieved comprehensive informatics advancement and received the prestigious 2019 HIMSS Nicholas E. Davies Award of Excellence	The Davies Award of Excellence recognized Mackenzie Health for "thoughtful application of health information and technology to substantially improve clinical care delivery, patient outcomes and population health." Mackenzie Health was evaluated on three clinical case studies with the following patient outcomes: • Stroke patients were treated in half the time • Patients with chronic obstructive pulmonary disease (COPD) were discharged home sooner, and • Hospital-acquired infections were reduced.	Canadian Healthcare Technology (https://www.canhealth.com/2019/09/11/mackenzie-health-receives-prestigious-davies-award)
Vancouver Coastal Health (VCH), the Provincial Health Services Authority (PHSA), and Providence Health Care (PHC)	Clinical and Systems Transformation (CST) is one of the largest and most complex projects in Canada. It is designed to transform health care delivery systems and processes to improve the quality and consistency of the patient and caregiver experience. CST will establish common clinical and process standards, including workflows, order sets, clinical guidelines, integrated plans of care, and a common electronic health record, and enable clinicians to access client data where and when needed.	Clinical and Systems Transformation (http://cstproject.ca/about-cst)

(2008) combined telemedicine and telemonitoring with patient education and peer supports in assisting chronically ill patients in rural Ontario to stay at home. Without this program, these patients would have had to travel for care provision and would have potentially experienced more frequent hospitalizations, loss of independence, and significantly less self-care. Telehealth has continued to increase, with 1 045 398 virtual events occurring in 2020, representing a 36% growth rate over the previous year (Ontario Telemedicine Network, 2021). Moreover, the COVID-19 pandemic prompted health care providers across the country to increase their use of telemedicine in the form of virtual assessments (using such tools as Zoom, Doxy.me, and other meeting platforms) to optimize access to care. It is unlikely that this reliance on telemedicine will subside after the pandemic is resolved.

As connected care progresses and patients continue to transition between care settings (from primary care to home care to acute care and home again), nurses are required to be competent in providing and accessing information, ensuring data quality, and using an agreed-upon and shared vocabulary such as that found in the C-HOBIC data set (see Box 17.5 for more information on C-HOBIC). Care provision will become increasingly interprofessional, and nurses must be able to

BOX 17.1	The 5 Vs of "Big Data"

Volume—The sheer scale of data generated by a variety of sources. This is considered by many to be the key hallmark of big data.

Velocity—The unparalleled speed of proliferation and the decreasing amount of time in which information is multiplying.

Variety—The range of different data sources such as electronic health records, electronic medical records, wearables, medical devices, telehealth, and more.

Veracity—The degree of uncertainty of data elements and whether the data are fit for secondary analysis.

Value—The perceived contribution of the data to supporting the organizational mission and objectives.

Adapted from Gu, D., Li, J., Li, X., & Liang, C. (2017). Visualizing the knowledge structure and evolution of big data research in healthcare informatics. *International Journal of Medical Informatics, 98*, 22–32. https://doi.org/10.1016/j.ijmedinf.2016.11.006; Westra, B. L., Sylvia, M., Weinfurter, E. F., et al. (2017). Big data science: A literature review of nursing research exemplars. *Nursing Outlook, 65*(5), 549–561. https://doi.org/10.1016/j.outlook.2016.11.021; Topaz, M., & Pruinelli, L. (2017). Big data and nursing: Implications for the future. *Forecasting Informatics Competencies for Nurses in the Future of Connected Health, 232*, 165–171. https://doi.org/10.3233/978-1-61499-738-2-165

provide leadership on the most important issues and challenges facing the profession.

Analytics in Health Care

The proliferation of digital technologies into everyday life has meant that they are increasingly considered essential tools—whether for personal or professional purposes—and are generating data every minute they consumers use them. As technologies are successfully implemented, the focus shifts from implementation to creating understanding and extracting meaning from the data generated. These data sets are so immense that they require new methodologies to manage them and new ways to interpret their meaning.

The sheer immensity of data being generated has led researchers to characterize data using the "5 Vs" (Box 17.1). The massive *volume* of information being generated is beyond what ordinary research and management programs can manage. SeedScientific (2021) has estimated that by 2025, 175 zettabytes (one zettabyte is 1 000 bytes to the seventh power) will be in the global datasphere. *Velocity*, or the speed of proliferation, is expected to continue rising and is a function of faster computing. The increasing *variety* of data available reflects the ever-expanding diversity of sources of information resulting from continuing integration, interoperability, and convergence of new technologies. SeedScientific recorded that in the first half of 2020, 71.5 billion apps were downloaded by over 4.8 billion Internet users. SeedScientific also found that Google performs 1.2 trillion searches every year. By 2025, 463 exabytes (1 exabyte is 1 000 bytes to the sixth power) of global data will be generated each day from data sources (SeedScientific, 2021). *Veracity* reflects the level of uncertainty—or, conversely, accuracy—of the data or its elements. *Value* reflects the expected worth of the data or its aggregated information to an organization or individual. SeedScientific has noted that Google, Amazon, Microsoft, and Facebook store 1200 petabytes of information, leading to the recognition that information has high value to these companies.

Knowing how to strategically leverage data to make decisions is a key competency regardless of practice domain or role. The prominence of "**big data**" or, more properly, **data science**, is the recognition that the volumes of data created daily in all parts of the health care system can be subjected to sophisticated **analytics** that then inform decisions in all areas of health care delivery and management. Within the domain of nursing,

BOX 17.2	The ISO Standards Life Cycle

The International Organization for Standardization (ISO) standards life cycle has seven phases, each with key events, as follows:

1. *Proposal:* Key stakeholders are identified to help clarify the need for, scope, and purpose of a standard or to determine whether there is a pre-existing standard. At the conclusion of this phase, a decision will be made to *adopt* the pre-existing standard, *adapt* the pre-existing standard, or *develop* an entirely new standard.
2. *Preparatory stage:* A working group of at least five international experts is assembled to create a working draft of the standard. When they are satisfied, the document goes as a Committee Draft to the larger working group and Technical Committee.
3. *Committee stage:* The Committee Draft is registered and distributing for feedback and voting until consensus is reached on the technical content. Once consensus is achieved, the document is packaged as a Draft International Standard (DIS) and distributed to member countries for feedback and voting. A highly structured method (balloting) is used to record feedback, and every comment (e.g., editorial comments or technical comments on the actual content) is addressed.
4. *Enquiry stage:* The DIS is circulated to all ISO members for feedback and voting. It will be approved as a Final Draft International Standard (FDIS) by a two-thirds majority of support.
5. *Approval and publication:* The FDIS is again circulated to all member countries and requires a final yes or no vote. A two-thirds majority is required to pass the FDIS as an international standard.
6. *Implementation:* Countries, including Canada, determine how they will use an international standard. The standard may either be adopted as is or adapted to fit the local context.
7. *Review:* Standards are reviewed every 5 years, at which time decisions are made about whether to confirm, revise, or withdraw.

Adapted from Hussey, P., & Kennedy, M. A. (2021). Health informatics standards. In P. Hussey & M. A. Kennedy (Eds.), *Introduction to nursing informatics* (5th ed.; pp. 139–174). Springer. https://doi.org/10.1007/978-3-030-58740-6_6

"data science" is termed **nursing data science,** where analyses focus on topics of the greatest importance to the profession. Topaz & Pruinelli (2017) define data science as an interprofessional scholarly approach to working with data. They recommend that researchers be trained to apply appropriate analytical methods, such as data mining, artificial intelligence, natural language processing, and visualization. Courses on analytics for leaders, administrators, and clinicians are routinely offered by universities and specialized institutes, supporting the need for informed use of analytical methodologies to manage the vast and largely untapped data sets that are available and continue to be generated.

This burgeoning topic will continue driving change and opportunity in health care and nursing practice. A clear understanding of how nurses can use all types of data to support practice and patient outcomes is imperative. It is also critical that nurses be capable of generating meaning through data aggregation and analytics such as data science. Data standards are essential to data aggregation and digital computation, ensuring not only that the physical management of information is consistent, but also that the understanding of terms is consistent.

STANDARDS AND CLINICAL INTEROPERABILITY

Standards in health care data management refer to a nationally or internationally agreed-upon protocol for representing all types of health information, including types of care provided, location of care provision, pharmaceutical ordering and dispensing, and billing messages. The International Organization for Standardization (ISO) defines an international standard as "a document established by consensus of experts from many countries and is approved and published by a recognized body. It comprises rules, guidelines, processes, or characteristics that allow users to achieve the same outcome time and time again" (International Electrotechnical Commission, 2020).

Standards ensure that data are consistently represented and exchanged between health information systems and thus consistently understood by clinicians. Interoperability between health care systems is critical to ensuring consistent clinical understanding and to measuring the level of conformance (or compliance) to a standard (Box 17.2). This consistent understanding and interpretation of health data contributes to the provision of quality care as well as increasing patient safety.

In their previous mandate for standards development and adoption, Canada Health Infoway (2016) noted that standards ensure interoperability by supporting information exchange. In addition, they identified standards as a critical foundation for the interoperable electronic health record (iEHR). Canada Health Infoway (2016) demonstrated how "standards support integrated, patient-centric health records enabling a longitudinal view of an individual's key health history and care . . . and that this critical information can be updated, managed, shared and interpreted in a meaningful secure way, when and where required" (p. 5).

There are many ways in which standards shape health care data. Standards support both *technical needs*, to ensure consistent communication or transmission of health data in system messages, and *business needs*, for actual clinical work processes and clinical content of messages. For example, a gap may be identified where clinicians need to consistently describe a particular condition or clinical situation and exchange patient data to deliver optimal care. Clinical terminology standards such as **SNOMED CT®**, LOINC (Laboratory Observation Identifiers Names and Codes), and others influence how clinical practice is documented, while technical standards such as HL7 FHIR (Health Level 7 International Fast Healthcare Interoperability Resources) support transmission and exchange across the health care system.

Infoway's commitment to standards development, formerly through structures such as the Standards Collaborative, helped develop and support Canadian adoption of relevant international health information standards, such as SNOMED CT, HL7, and numerous ISO standards. As standards development initiatives matured across Canada, Infoway's focus shifted from development to the practical use and implementation of standards. To this end, Canada Health Infoway (2021b) has assembled all pan-Canadian standards in use across Canada in a single community platform called InfoCentral to ensure easy access (Canada Health Infoway, 2021b) (Box 17.3). Interested Canadians can go to the InfoCentral website to download and learn about the specific standard they are interested in, participate in communities, access implementation guides, and more.

Standardizing Nursing Language

A long-standing perception among many nurses is that nursing, as a professional practice, is generally considered invisible to formal and tangible recognition (Clark, 1999; Clark & Lang, 1992; CNA, 2000; Hannah et al., 2006a). Clark (1999, p. 42) observed that, despite representing the largest group of health care clinicians worldwide, nursing was invisible in health policy decisions, in descriptions of health care, in contracts, and in service specifications. In Canada, health care system performance analyses have historically focused on the financial summaries and analyses evaluating care outcomes, such as hospital discharge summaries; however, analyses were restricted to physician-driven data and contained no clinical nursing data elements. Hannah et al. (2006a, p. 89) made the point that "noteworthy, again, is the

---

BOX 17.3   Canadian Standards for Electronic Health Information

- Canadian Clinical Drug Data Set—Terminology for use in digital health solutions, including pharmacy and electronic prescribing.
- DICOM—Standard for storing, printing, and transmitting medical imaging information.
- HL7 FHIR—A standards framework that enables rapid development of systems to solve real-world clinical and administrative problems.
- HL7 Version 3, CDA—Exchange of information from one system to another using HL7 standards and terminology.
- IHE—Coordinated use of standards to address specific clinical needs.
- ISO—Standardization of health care information to enable and support all aspects of the health care system.
- Nursing Data Standards—The Canadian Nurses Association has endorsed adoption of standardized clinical reference terminologies (C-HOBIC, ICNP, SNOMED CT).
- pCLOCD/LOINC—A comprehensive terminology for sharing laboratory data and clinical documents.
- PHC EMR MDS—The Primary Health Care Electronic Medical Record Minimum Data Set (PHC EMR MDS) increases the availability of structured coded data in EMRs and supports performance measurement for clinical and health system use.
- SNOMED CT CA/SNOMED CT—A comprehensive clinical terminology to capture and exchange clinical data.

Adapted from Canada Health Infoway. (2021). *Canadian standards*. https://infocentral.infoway-inforoute.ca/en/standards/canadian

---

total absence of clinical nursing data." Clark and Lang (1992, p. 109) famously declared in their assessment of the invisibility of nursing, "If we cannot name it, we cannot control it, finance it, teach it, research it, or put it into public policy." Numerous pioneering nurse informaticists supported this position, including Graves and Corcoran (1989), Werley (1988), Ball et al. (2000), and others, arguing that nursing visibility will be gained by developing a standardized language that reflects what nursing is and what nursing does. To accomplish this, significant effort and numerous incremental initiatives would be necessary to distinguish specific components of nursing data and identify key concepts, data sets, and outcomes of care.

Health Information: Nursing Components

Before a standardized nursing language is adopted, it is necessary to identify the most important data elements required for effective nursing decision making and evaluation. The minimum number of essential nursing data elements is referred to as a *nursing minimum data set (NMDS)*. The nursing components of health information, the Canadian version of an NMDS, is known as **Health Information: Nursing Components (HI:NC)**. Since 1992, there has been consensus among Canadian nurses that HI:NC comprises five categories of elements: patient status, nursing interventions, patient outcomes, nursing resource intensity, and primary nurse identifier (AARN, 1994). The CNA describes HI:NC as the "most important pieces of data about the nursing care provided to the client during a health care episode" (CNA, 2000, p. 5). Table 17.2 presents the HI:NC definitions.

In addition to the foundational work on HI:NC, ongoing efforts are being invested into articulating nursing requirements in the EHR. The Nursing Reference Group, hosted by Canada Health Infoway and co-chaired jointly by Infoway and the CNA, sponsored a working group in 2012 that developed the *Pan-Canadian Nursing EHR Business and Functional Elements Supporting Clinical Practice* document. This reference document provides guidance on how nursing data

TABLE 17.2	Health Information: Nursing Components
Nursing Component	**Definition**
Patient status	A label for the set of indicators that reflects the phenomena for which nurses provide care, relative to the health status of patients (McGee, 1993). Although patient status is similar to nursing diagnosis, the term *patient status* is preferred because it represents a broader spectrum of health and illness. The common label *patient status* is inclusive of input from all disciplines. The summative statements referring to the phenomena for which nurses provide care (i.e., nursing diagnosis, similar to medical diagnosis) are merely one aspect of patient status at a point in time.
Nursing interventions	Purposeful and deliberate health-affecting interventions (direct and indirect), based on assessment of patient status, which are designed to bring about results that benefit patients (Alberta Association of Registered Nurses, 1994).
Patient outcome	The "clients' status at a defined point(s) following health care [affecting] intervention" (Marek & Lang, 1993). It is influenced to varying degrees by the interventions of all care providers.
Nursing intensity	"Refers to the amount and type of nursing resource used to [provide] care" (O'Brien-Pallas & Giovannetti, 1993).
Primary nurse identifier	A unique lifetime identification number for each nurse in Canada. This identifier is independent of geographic location (province or territory), practice area (e.g., acute care, community care, public health), and employer.

From Hannah, K. J. (2005). Health informatics and nursing in Canada. *Healthcare Information Management and Communications, 19*(3), 49. Reprinted by permission of Healthcare Computing and Communications Canada, Inc.

should be incorporated into EHRs and covers such topics as privacy and security, safety, data sources, usability, clinical decision support, collaborative practice, communications, information use, and data access.

In 2016, the inaugural National Nursing Data Standards Symposium was held at the University of Toronto, with sponsorship from the CNA, CIHI, Canada Health Infoway, the CNIA, and numerous health informatics industry vendors. Sixty nurse leaders, representatives from the host organizations, and industry vendors from across Canada met to collaborate on a national strategy to "represent, teach, capture, and report nursing practice in Canada" (Nagle & White, 2016). With focused streams of discussion on clinical practice, education, research, and policy, the outcomes of the symposium included a commitment to establishing a national taskforce that would ultimately develop and evaluate a framework for nursing data standards for use across Canada. This work continues through a symposium held annually to advance the objective of ensuring that nursing is represented using standardized data within and across practice domains. In 2017, more than 100 nurse leaders, nurse informaticians, and vendors convened to further this activity. Since 2019, the event has been held virtually.

An overview of computerized nursing documentation is provided in Chapter 16. Some clinical information systems incorporate the HI:NC and nursing functional requirements into the architecture or design of the nursing component of the clinical documentation system,

thereby capturing the most significant data reflective of the nursing contribution to patient care. Many versions of computerized nursing documentation systems continue to evolve, relying on the underlying philosophy of documentation to support design. For example, many systems do not encourage narrative documentation; instead, they provide checklists of common activities and encourage exception charting (see Chapter 16 for additional discussion of this issue).

International Classification for Nursing Practice

The **International Classification for Nursing Practice® (ICNP®)** is a formal terminology developed by the **International Council of Nurses (ICN)** (ICN, 2018b) in response to concerns about the visibility of nursing contributions in health care and calls to standardize nursing data for comparability, analysis, and evidence-informed practice. The ICN's goals were to capture nursing practice across practice settings, cultures or languages, and geographic settings while simultaneously ensuring that professionals who used this new terminology could communicate using the numerous existing nursing terminologies. Initially endorsed for development in 1989 by a resolution at the ICN Nineteenth Quadrennial Conference, the ICNP has evolved through multiple iterations and is currently updated and released biannually to coincide with the ICN Congress (ICN, 2018b).

The standardized terminology for nursing practice in the ICNP is built using the Web Ontology Language (OWL) (ICN, 2018b). This enables the ICNP to function both as a reference terminology (within the system) and as an interface terminology (facing users in a system interface). The ICNP has a seven-axis model, which includes Focus, Judgement, Action, Means, Location, Client, and Time (ICN, n.d.-a). In addition to viewing the ICNP by the axes, users can also view the terminology by hierarchy or in a simple list (see Figure 17.6). The ICN also reports that as ICNP implementations have advanced, some users have experienced success with the seven-axis model; however, the dominant trend has been to use precoordinated concepts or expressions that are accessible through the Diagnosis and Outcome axis or the Intervention axis (ICN, 2018b).

The ICNP is used to generate statements of nursing diagnoses, nursing actions, and nursing outcomes, using terms arranged in a hierarchical order and in catalogues (or subsets) of precombined terms. As of 2021, nine individual catalogues were available to users, with additional catalogues in development (ICN, n.d.-b; Box 17.4). As the ICNP continues to evolve internationally, these numbers will continue to grow over time.

The ICN is working closely with other health care organizations to harmonize nursing terminologies. For instance, the ICN is working with SabaCare to harmonize the Clinical Care Classification (CCC) with the ICNP (ICN, 2018a). Working with teams from the ICN and SabaCare, some of the results include a table of equivalencies that pairs 165 nursing diagnoses from SabaCare's CCC system to the corresponding ICNP concept and a table of 521 ICNP Nursing Diagnoses categorized according to the CCC Care Components (ICN, 2018a). Further work on this mapping initiative continues.

The ICN is also working with SNOMED International to harmonize the ICNP and SNOMED CT to ensure that nursing is adequately represented in interprofessional health information systems. One of the potential risks of a nursing-specific focus, as the ICN has noted, is that "nursing will be somehow disconnected from the larger health information landscape" (ICN, 2018c).

A formal agreement was established to create equivalencies and foster alignment between the ICNP and SNOMED CT. Teams from the ICN and SNOMED International are working to create equivalencies in diagnostic and interventional statements between the ICNP and SNOMED CT to reflect nursing practice and priorities.

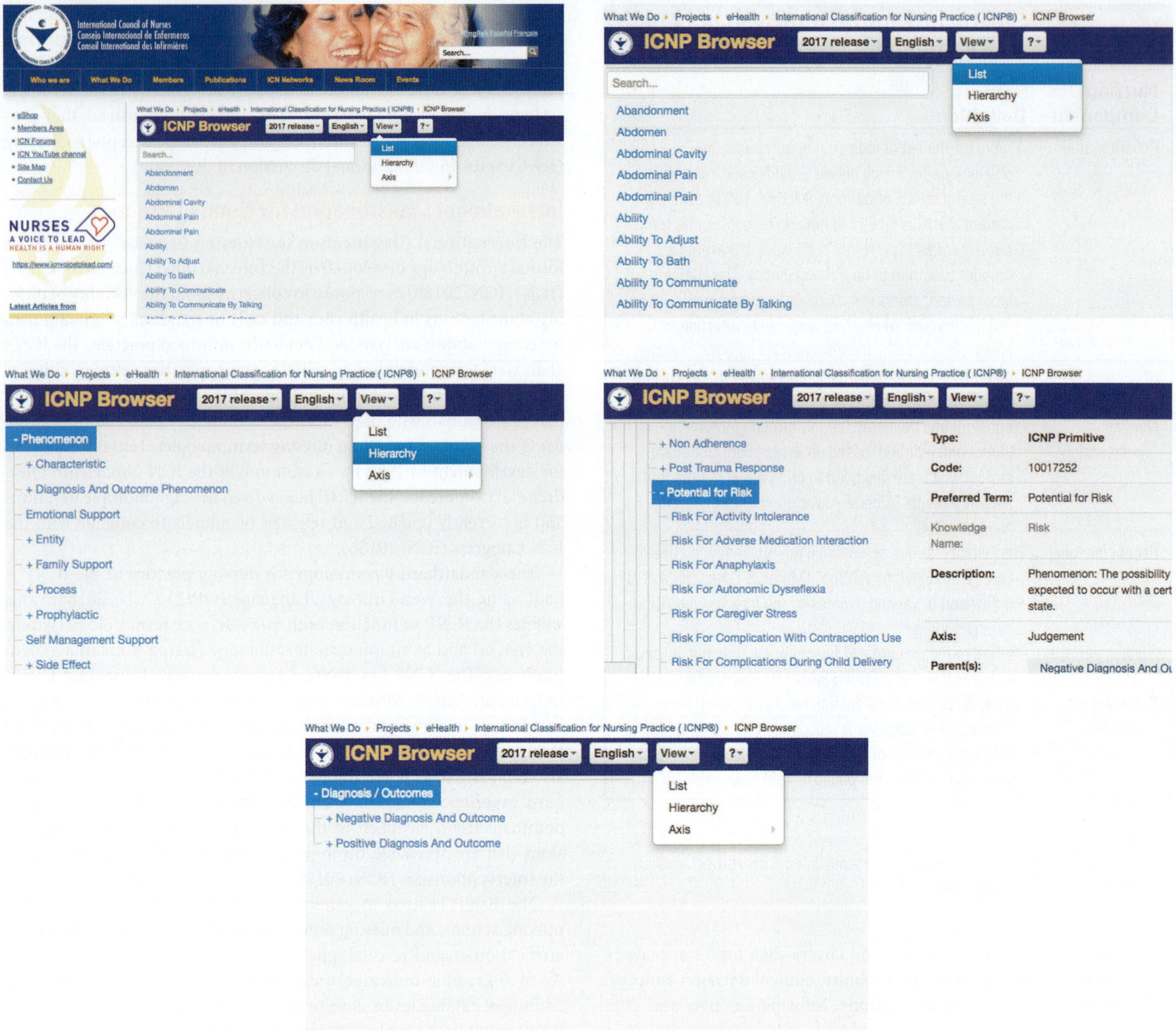

FIGURE 17.6 International Classification for Nursing Practice (ICNP) browser views. (International Council of Nurses. [2021]. *ICNP browser*. https://www.icn.ch/what-we-do/projects/ehealth-icnptm/icnp-browser. Reprinted with permission.)

BOX 17.4   ICNP Catalogues

ICNP Pre-Coordinated Nursing Diagnosis/Outcomes and Interventions
ICNP Diagnosis/Outcomes
ICNP Interventions

ICNP Catalogues Currently Available
Community Nursing
Dementia Care
Disaster Nursing
Nursing Care of Children With HIV and AIDS
Nursing Outcome Indicators
Paediatric Pain Management
Palliative Care
Partnering With Individuals and Families to Promote Adherence to Treatment
Prenatal Nursing Care

ICNP Catalogues in Development
Hospitalized Adult Mental Health Client
Hospitalized Paediatric Client
Post-Surgical Total Hip Replacement
Pressure Ulcer Prevention
Special Care Nursery

Equivalency Tables
ICNP to SNOMED CT Equivalency Table for Diagnosis and Outcome Statements
ICNP to Clinical Care Classification (CCC) Equivalency Table for Nursing Diagnoses

These equivalency tables can be accessed through either SNOMED CT or the ICNP.

The ICNP catalogues are made up of nursing data subsets of diagnoses, actions, and outcomes specific to various practice areas or specialties (such as wound care) and continue to be developed. To begin catalogue development, nurses select a health care topic based on the needs of patients. The organization of the catalogue content is determined by the nurses as associated ICNP diagnoses, outcomes, and interventions are identified. ICN (2021b) has noted that the catalogues can fill a practical need in building health information systems with all the benefits of being part of a unified nursing language.

Box 17.5 discusses the CNA's use of the ICNP to collect information on patient outcomes through the C-HOBIC project.

CANADIAN PRIVACY LEGISLATION

Although both provincial standards of practice and the CNA (2017) *Code of Ethics* address confidentiality, nurses also need to be aware of Canadian privacy legislation affecting nursing practice and the protection of patient data. As a nurse, even as you fulfill the standards of practice, it is possible to violate privacy legislation. Canadians recognize this risk of privacy violation. Among those surveyed, "the vast majority (92%) expressed some level of concern about the protection of their privacy" (Office of the Privacy Commissioner of Canada [OPCC], 2019). Furthermore, approximately 80% of those Canadians surveyed are concerned about the collection and use of the body as information (such as DNA for genetic testing and data from wearable devices such as fitness monitors and smartwatches) (OPCC, 2019). Although

---

BOX 17.5   The C-HOBIC Initiative*

In 2007, the Canadian Nurses Association (CNA) launched a multi-province project, with financial investment by Canada Health Infoway, to introduce the collection of standardized evidence-informed nursing-sensitive patient outcomes (CNA, 2008). The C-HOBIC initiative addresses gaps in health information related to nursing's contribution to patient care and delivers on the need for standardized clinical data for inclusion in electronic health records (EHRs) (CNA, 2021).

Drawing on the work of the original Health Outcomes for Better Information and Care (HOBIC) project, C-HOBIC introduces the standardized collection of the following items into admission and discharge assessments: functional status, symptoms (pain, nausea, fatigue, dyspnea), falls, pressure ulcers, and therapeutic self-care. These items have a concept definition, a valid and reliable measure, and empirical evidence linking them to nursing inputs or nursing interventions (Doran, 2012).

A major component of this project is the systematic approach to gathering nursing content that employs a standardized clinical terminology coded in a format suitable for inclusion in the EHRs. The C-HOBIC concepts were mapped to the International Classification for Nursing Practice (ICNP) terminology, giving Canadian nurses the opportunity to make substantive contributions to the ongoing development of the ICNP. In this case, Canadian nurses proposed multiple new terms that are uniquely Canadian for inclusion in the ICNP catalogues. The initial mapping to ICNP version 1.0 was validated at a national forum (Kennedy, 2008; Kennedy et al., 2008). The final results of this work were used to create the *ICNP Nursing Outcomes Indicators Catalogue* (ICN, 2011). On January 11, 2012, Canada Health Infoway endorsed the C-HOBIC/ICNP Data Set as a Canadian Approved Standard (CAS) (Canada Health Infoway, 2017). This is the first nursing data standard approved as a CAS, and Canada is the first country in the world to approve an ICNP catalogue as a national standard.

The C-HOBIC work has continued to evolve. It was used to create the *Nursing Outcomes Indicators Catalogue* in the ICNP in 2013. C-HOBIC has also been mapped to SNOMED CT and validated through international consensus at SNOMED International (https://www.snomed.org).

In 2017, a demonstration project was undertaken with the Canadian Institute of Health Information (CIHI) to facilitate inclusion of the C-HOBIC data in the

Discharge Abstract Database (DAD) (Figure 17.7). This initiative marked the first time that nursing data was included in DAD submissions. There is value in being able to link this data set with other data sets housed at CIHI, such as the home care and long-term care home data sets, to understand clinical outcomes across the continuum of care and to answer the question "How well is the system doing in improving outcomes for people within the system?"

Early research using this data set in Ontario supported the link between these items and nursing practice (McGillis Hall et al., 2013), the value of the functional status assessment in predicting length of stay and discharge disposition (Jeffs et al., 2013), and the relationship between both symptom status and therapeutic self-care scores on readmission rates to acute care (Wodchis et al., 2012). Furthermore, improvements in therapeutic self-care on discharge from acute care resulted in reduced adverse events in home care clients and reduced readmissions to acute care (Sun & Doran, 2014).

The C-HOBIC data set is designed to assist nurses and other health care providers with planning and evaluating patient care and improving patient outcomes. One Canadian acute care site has created a *patient outcome measures report* (admission and discharge comparison) that allows for nursing staff to monitor the percentage of improvements for the C-HOBIC items between admission and discharge over time, as well as the percentage of patients that came in with an issue and left with the same issue unresolved. They found that monitoring therapeutic self-care assessment allows nurses to determine the care, supports, and education needed to prepare a patient for successful discharge from hospital.

As the largest group of health care providers in Canada, it is important that nursing's contribution to patient care be made visible in EHRs. The inclusion of this standardized data set provides real-time information to nurses about how patients are benefiting from clinical care. Nursing leaders can link the data from real-time reports to staffing, financial, and other data such as length of stay and readmission rates to understand how well their organization is doing in improving clinical outcomes and preparing patients for discharge. Standardized aggregate data will allow for research to support an examination of how well the system is performing, that is, meeting the health care needs of people in Canada.

*Written by section contributor Peggy White, Director, C-HOBIC project.

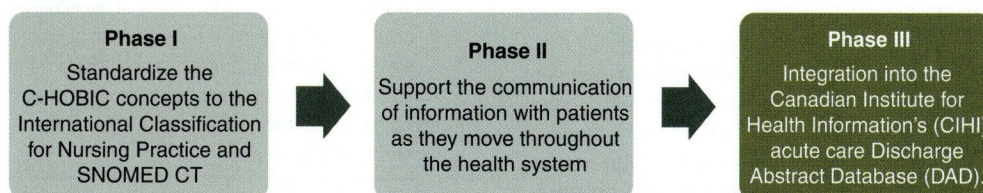

Phase I	Phase II	Phase III
Standardize the C-HOBIC concepts to the International Classification for Nursing Practice and SNOMED CT	Support the communication of information with patients as they move throughout the health system	Integration into the Canadian Institute for Health Information's (CIHI) acute care Discharge Abstract Database (DAD).

FIGURE 17.7 C-HOBIC (Canadian Health Outcomes for Better Information and Care) project phases.

Distinguishing Types of Protected Information

The *Personal Information Protection and Electronic Documents Act* (PIPEDA) distinguishes "personal information" from "personal health information" and provides specific definitions for both as follows:

"*Personal health information,*" with respect to an individual, whether living or deceased, means

(a) Information concerning the physical or mental health of the individual

(b) Information concerning any health service provided to the individual

(c) Information concerning the donation by the individual of any body part or any bodily substance of the individual or information derived from the testing or examination of a body part or bodily substance of the individual

(d) Information that is collected in the course of providing health services to the individual, or

(e) Information that is collected incidentally to the provision of health services to the individual.

"*Personal information*" means information about an identifiable individual, but it does not include the name, title, or business address or telephone number of an employee of an organization.

From *Personal Information Protection and Electronic Documents Act*, SC 2000, c. 5. http://laws-lois.justice.gc.ca/eng/acts/P-8.6/page-1.html#h-3.

BOX 17.7 **Principles of Privacy**

Many pieces of legislation and policies on personal health information (PHI) contribute to best practices in the protection of privacy. The 1996 *Model Code for the Protection of Personal Information* by the Canadian Standards Association is one such example in Canada. It represents a significant foundation to privacy work in Canada by highlighting 10 core principles of data protection:

1. **Accountability for information:** Organizations that collect, use, or disclose PHI are accountable for the protection of such data in their custody.

2. **Identifying purposes for collection, use, and disclosure of information:** Purposes of collection, use, and disclosure must be defined so patients can make informed decisions about whether to provide PHI.

3. **Consent:** Organizations must demonstrate compliance with laws and that patients are reasonably informed and knowledgeable about the purposes of collection, use, and disclosure.

4. **Limiting data collection:** Organizations must limit data collection to only that which is necessary for the defined purposes.

5. **Limiting use, disclosure, and retention:** Upon collection, organizations should only use, disclose, and retain information for the same defined purposes as for collection.

6. **Accuracy:** PHI must be reasonably accurate, up-to-date, and complete.

7. **Safeguards:** Organizations must implement security safeguards to prevent unauthorized access, use, or disclosure of PHI.

8. **Openness:** It should be possible for patients to know the purposes of why information about them is collected, used, and disclosed.

9. **Individual access:** Patients should have the right to access their own PHI so they can validate its accuracy and correct or amend inaccurate information.

10. **Challenging compliance:** Patients have the right to submit a privacy complaint against an organization if they believe their privacy has been violated.

Adapted from Fraser, R. (2021). Data privacy and security. In P. Hussey & M. A. Kennedy (Eds.), *Introduction to nursing informatics* (5th ed.; pp. 267–293). Springer. https://doi.org/10.1007/978-3-030-58740-6_10

privacy legislation varies among provinces, nurses must develop a working knowledge of the relevant provincial and federal legislation supporting the protection of health information.

Two federal legislative acts address the protection of personal information. These are the *Privacy Act* (1985) and the *Personal Information Protection and Electronic Documents Act* (2000). Both acts identify specific limitations to the disclosure of personal information—whether in electronic or other forms. Regardless of the practice setting or mode, you are professionally, ethically, and legally obligated to protect all the personal information of patients in your care (Box 17.6). Knowledge of these two pieces of federal privacy legislation can help you uphold the standards of practice and the *Code of Ethics* (Box 17.7 and Box 17.8).

According to section 8.1 of the *Privacy Act*, "personal information under the control of a government institution shall not, without the consent of the individual to whom it relates, be disclosed by the institution" (*Privacy Act*, 1985). PIPEDA is federal legislation that governs the disclosure of personal health information in any electronic environment. This act extends the *Privacy Act* by addressing specific risks associated with electronic data collection, storage, retrieval, and communication. The purpose of PIPEDA is to "establish, in an era in which technology increasingly facilitates the circulation and exchange of information, rules to govern the collection, use and disclosure of personal information in a manner that recognizes the right of privacy of individuals with respect to their personal information and the need of organizations to collect, use, or disclose personal information for purposes that a reasonable person would consider appropriate in the circumstances" (*Personal Information Protection and Electronic Documents Act*, 2000). Furthermore, PIPEDA restricts the disclosure of personal information under only the most stringent of conditions, such as law enforcement requirements.

PIPEDA was initially applicable only to personal information collected or used in commercial activities by private-sector entities regulated by the federal government. However, the act has been extended over time to cover the retail sector, publishing companies, the service industry, manufacturers, and other provincially regulated organizations, as well as sector-specific data such as health information.

PIPEDA applies to Canadian jurisdictions unless the federal government acknowledges an exemption based on provincial legislation

BOX 17.8 **What's in Your Privacy Policy?**

An organization's privacy policy is an important document that nurses should be familiar with. Posted in a public place in the organization (often in waiting areas or the lobby), the privacy policy informs the public about how their personal health information (PHI) is protected. While there are no standardized rules about what should be contained in the privacy policy, there *are* best practices, and most, if not all, of the following should be in the privacy policy that your organization follows:

- A broad description of the types of personal information held
- A description of the purposes for which data is collected, used, and disclosed
- A statement about how information is used
- A commitment to maintain the privacy of the information
- A nontechnical description of the security in place to protect PHI
- A description of when information will be disclosed to third parties
- A description of situations when data is depersonalized or aggregated
- Contact information and procedures to follow if the person has questions or wishes to lodge a complaint.

Adapted from Fraser, R. (2021). Data privacy and security. In P. Hussey & M. A. Kennedy (Eds.), *Introduction to nursing informatics* (5th ed.; pp. 267–293). Springer. https://doi.org/10.1007/978-3-030-58740-6_10

that is substantially similar. British Columbia, Alberta, and Quebec are considered to have legislation equivalent to PIPEDA, while New Brunswick, Newfoundland, Nova Scotia, and Ontario all have legislation that is substantially similar to PIPEDA (OPCC, 2018). Although provincial/territorial acts take precedence within the provinces/territories, federal legislation continues to govern the transmission of personal information across and between provincial/territorial boundaries.

In addition to domestic legislation, other factors also affect the privacy of the EHR. Infoway's privacy mandate is to support private, secure, and protected information in the EHR. In the course of doing so, Infoway and their partners leverage applicable international standards (for example, from the ISO) that operate in alignment with Canadian legislation and further support the privacy and security of health data in electronic health care systems.

Despite the complex nature of privacy legislation and the standards that support privacy activities, as a nurse you must exercise diligence in examining and applying these pieces of legislation to your professional nursing practice. The privacy legislation in each province and territory can be viewed online (OPCC, 2018) (refer to Chapter 16 to explore how PIPEDA relates to specific nursing documentation).

INFORMATICS COMPETENCIES

As a nursing student, just as you have a responsibility to develop competencies in performing a variety of patient care tasks, such as assessments and treatments, you are likewise responsible for developing and maintaining competencies in technological applications that support information management in professional practice.

In 2014, the Canadian Association of Schools of Nursing (CASN) convened several working groups to identify and establish entry-level informatics competencies for registered nurses. Through this initiative, the CASN, with investment from Infoway, provided a clear path for faculty and nursing students to be equipped with the necessary knowledge, tools, and support to teach, learn, and practise in technology-enabled practice settings. Three primary competencies contribute to a single overarching competency, namely that the nurse "uses information and communication technologies to support information synthesis in accordance with professional and regulatory standards in the delivery of patient/client care" (CASN, 2015). The three component competencies are as follows:

- Uses relevant information and knowledge to support the delivery of evidence-informed patient care
- Uses ICTs in accordance with professional and regulatory standards and workplace policies, and
- Uses information and communication technologies in the delivery of patient/client care.

Each competency is further supported with knowledge and performance indicators, which are defined as assessable and observable examples of various aspects of the required competency (CASN, 2015). This enables clinicians and evaluators to easily identify the specific type of behaviours and knowledge that are required to meet the respective competency statements.

As part of their ongoing commitment to nursing faculty development, the CASN also developed a *Nursing Informatics Teaching Toolkit*, which supports faculty to integrate core NI competencies into curricula. Additionally, through the efforts of the CASN Digital Health Nursing Faculty Peer Network, a second faculty resource, *Consumer Health Solutions: A Teaching and Learning Resource for Nursing Education*, was developed, ensuring that faculty across Canada have access to key NI content to mentor nursing students. Furthermore, the CASN has established peer support workshops for faculty to facilitate development of NI expertise among faculty. Box 17.9 highlights

---

BOX 17.9 RESEARCH HIGHLIGHT

*Informatics Competencies for Nurse Leaders**

Research Focus

The environment in which nurses work and will continue to work in the future is increasingly technology laden. Many nurses document their assessments and care in electronic health record systems, some of which have additional features that support clinical decision making, medication administration, and beyond. Other forms of technology that support virtual assessments and care delivery are increasingly common within the clinical workplace as well. As such, there has been an increasing focus on ensuring that direct care nurses

tise in this technological context.

To support this development, numerous entry-to-practice nursing programs have integrated informatics topics into their curriculum (e.g., use of standardized nursing terminology such as ICNP catalogues in clinical courses and practicums). Thus, nurses entering the workforce today are arriving at work better prepared to deal with technology in their clinical roles. While this approach and level of focus is important in ensuring the adequate use of technologies for clinical care purposes at the direct-care level, important decisions related to technology selection, implementation and support often occur at a senior level. Nurse leaders in these roles would need to possess a different set of competencies to be effective in their roles. At the present time, there is a general feeling that many nurse leaders do not hold the requisite informatics competencies to be effective in technologically supported decision making or decisions about technology acquisition. As a result, direct care nurses may be working with technologies that do not fit within their current workflows or interfere with patient care activities. Direct care nurses may also experience the unintended consequences of technology implementation.

Methods

Strudwick et al. (2019) conducted this research to identify informatics competencies that would be relevant to nurse leaders working in senior management roles in Canada. A review of the literature was completed to identify a list of potential competencies that may be relevant to this population. Nurse leaders in senior roles from across the country were then asked to review this list of competencies and to determine whether they were relevant to the Canadian context.

Findings

After three rounds of consultation with senior nurse leaders, a total of 24 competency statements were agreed upon. These competency statements were related to informatics knowledge and skills and covered a wide range of topics, including ethics, privacy, legislation, change management, interoperability, and other important areas.

Identifying core nurse leader informatics competencies is the first step in supporting the acquisition of appropriate knowledge, skills, and judgement as they relate to technology decision making among nurse leaders in senior roles. The development of nursing informatics competencies in senior nurse leaders should result in fewer unintended negative consequences for nurses and increasing benefits in how technology supports clinical care processes.

*Written by section contributor Gillian Strudwick, RN, PhD, FAMIA, Chief Nursing Executive (Interim) and Independent Scientist, Centre for Addiction and Mental Health, Toronto, ON, Canada.
From Strudwick, G., Nagle, L. M., Morgan, A., et al. (2019). Adapting and validating informatics competencies for senior nurse leaders in the Canadian context: Results of a Delphi study. *International Journal of Nursing Informatics, 129*, 211–218. https://doi.org/10.1016/j.ijmedinf.2019.06.012

current research into nursing leadership competencies and NI, and Box 17.10 discusses health safety technology in nursing.

Schools of nursing have continued to develop curricula that incorporate NI fundamentals. However, few programs have dedicated streams that are devoted solely to NI competencies. Box 17.11 describes an innovative program that is setting the stage across Canada for the development of graduate-level competencies in NI.

The CNA website is a key professional resource for practising nurses. It enables all regulated nurses in Canada, including nursing students and retired nurses, to become CNA members. The site supports competency development and provides members with access to the following services:

- Professional practice (resources with clinical or professional orientation)
- Professional development (including resources for continuing competence, online and continuing education, and career development)
- Certification—details on the 22 nursing specialties available through the CNA

- Policy and advocacy—access to policy statements and advocacy activities
- Academy—access to the Canadian Academy of Nursing, the "first pan-Canadian organization dedicated to identifying, educating, supporting, and celebrating nursing leaders across all the regulated categories and all domains of practice."

Site members can also track current news and nursing information, receive updates and alerts on items of interest, access educational opportunities, and search for practice support. This site continues to develop over time and provides a centralized professional nursing forum for Canadian nurses.

SIMULATION AND VIRTUAL LEARNING

Technology-enhanced learning (TEL), or eLearning, is the use of technology to facilitate and enrich the education experience. As a nursing student, it is important that you have access to the range of technologies you will encounter in clinical practice and to have a broad

---

BOX 17.10   CASE STUDY
Health Technology Safety and Nursing*

Nurses use a variety of health technologies in their everyday practice. Some commonly used technologies in hospital settings and in the community include electronic health records, mobile health applications, blood pressure monitors, digital thermometers, and heart rate monitors. These technologies and others help nurses to monitor a client's health status and support client wellness (Hannah et al., 2015). The types of technologies used by nurses are expanding to include a range of devices and information technology systems. Nurses are increasingly using different types of medical devices and software in the context of health technology systems of care. These technologies are also being used to provide virtual care and remote monitoring of clients' health status in the home and in acute care settings (Seto et al., 2010). This trend is expected to continue in response to consumer demands. For instance, more people may prefer to stay at home in order to protect themselves or vulnerable family members from COVID-19 and other diseases that may be present in the community. Nursing informatics researchers are currently focused on understanding how these technologies (e.g., features and functions) may affect patient care, patient outcomes, nurse clinical decision making, nursing practice, and health care team coordination (Mieronkoski et al., 2017; Tuden et al., 2017, 2019).

Health technologies, such as provider order entry and clinical documentation, can improve patient outcomes and patient safety (Dowding et al., 2012). Health technologies can also lead to unintended consequences, such as introducing new types of errors (i.e., technology-induced errors). "Technology-induced errors arise from the design, development, customization and/or implementation of a technology as well as interactions between a technology and work processes associated with a technology's use" (Borycki, 2013; Borycki & Kushniruk, 2008, p. 150; Borycki et al., 2012). "Mistakes are errors which are not observed or corrected by a user" (Borycki, 2013, p. 70), whereas slips are errors that the "user notices and corrects"; for example, when a system auto-populates a text field with a number and the user, observing this to be an incorrect number, corrects the number in the system (Borycki et al., 2017, p. 70). Nurses need to understand these technologies and exercise nursing judgement when using a technology. If there is a safety issue or the perception that an issue may arise with the technology's use (e.g., if a nurse identifies a technology-induced error, be it a slip or mistake, and reports the safety issue according to the organization's policy), the nurse has a duty to use their best clinical judgement and report this to their manager or leader (Borycki, 2013; CASN, 2015; Nagle et al., 2014).

Nurse researchers have led the way in health technology safety research, developing theories and methods that can be used to improve the safety of technologies and technology systems before they are implemented in real-world settings. They have also developed and extended existing theories, tools, and methods to improve the designs of technology user interfaces (Table 17.3) and configurations of technology systems before their implementation to ensure the safety of these systems (Dhillon-Chattha et al., 2018). Health technology safety theories developed and extended by nurses (such as those listed in Table 17.3) help us to understand where such errors come from and how we can address these sources of error in technology systems to prevent future errors. Health technology safety methods help nurses to identify and diagnose technology errors with the aim of preventing future errors. These tools provide organizations with mechanisms to prioritize fixes (e.g., working with software vendors to update the technology or educating staff nurses about the potential issue so they can prevent it through training) and to prevent errors (see Table 17.3). Lastly, nurse researchers have developed tools that can be applied throughout all phases of the technology design, development, implementation, and maintenance cycle to improve technology systems safety over time.

As a nursing student, you should be aware of the benefits and limitations of the technologies you are using. Seek out your organization's help desk when you identify a potential technology issue that prevents you from providing safe patient care. When your organization is selecting or implementing a technology system, consider participating in that process (Borycki et al., 2012; CASN, 2015; Hannah et al., 2006b). Health care organizations encourage nurse participation in such activities so that the technologies that are being purchased for the organization meet the practice needs of nurses. If you have an interest in health technology design, development, implementation, maintenance, and research, consider studying nursing or health informatics (CASN, 2015; Canadian Nursing Informatics Association [CNIA], 2021). In Canada, there are graduate programs that help nurses to acquire competencies in the areas of health technology design, human factors in health care, project management to support technology implementation, database design, and data science analytic approaches to support patient care (Borycki et al., 2011). Nurses who complete these graduate programs are innovators and leaders in the health care field across Canada.

*Written by section contributor E.M. Borycki, RN, PhD, FACMI, FCAHS, FIAHSI; Professor, School of Health Information Science, University of Victoria, Victoria, BC, Canada; Clinician Scientist, Michael Smith Foundation for Health Research, Vancouver, BC, Canada.

TABLE 17.3	Nursing Theories, Tools, and Methods to Improve the Design of Technology User Interfaces		
Theory, Tool, or Method	Description	Use	Reference
A framework for diagnosing and identifying the source of technology-induced errors	This framework provides an overview of how errors may propagate through a health care system.	Supports investigation and reasoning about technology-induced errors.	Borycki et al., 2009a
A framework for integrating clinical and computer-based simulations	This framework links clinical and computer-based simulations.	Supports decision making and prioritizing decisions about user interface and workflow issues.	Borycki et al., 2009b
Safety heuristics	Safety guidelines enable evaluation of the safety features and functions of a user interface.	Evaluation of the safety of the technology user interface and associated workflows.	Borycki & Keay, 2010
Usability testing	Testing the safety of user interface design features, functions, and workflows.	Testing of technology user interface features, functions, and workflows.	Borycki et al., 2010
Clinical simulations	Testing the safety of technologies under simulated conditions representative of real-world practice and stresses.	Testing of technology under representative real-world conditions in a laboratory setting.	Borycki & Keay, 2010
Clinical plus computer-based simulations	A combination of methods that includes clinical simulations whose outcome data is inputted into a computer-based simulation to forecast future events.	Testing of technology under real-world conditions in a laboratory setting. Data from clinical simulations is used as an input into computer-based simulations.	Borycki & Keay, 2010
Ethnographic studies	The study of the human process of using technology in real-world health care settings.	After the technology has been implemented, evaluators observe users to identify safety issues.	Borycki & Keay, 2010
Case studies	The intensive study of a safety event for the purpose of organizational learning to prevent future events.	After an error has occurred, case studies employ several methods to investigate the contributing factors and causes of an error involving technology.	Borycki & Keay, 2010

BOX 17.11 Program Profile: Double Degree Master's Program in Nursing Informatics*

Nursing informatics as an area of research, education, and practice has grown considerably over the past decade in Canada. The Canadian Association of Schools of Nursing (CASN) has developed entry-to-practice nursing informatics competencies for undergraduate nurses that can be integrated into nursing courses. These competencies are threaded throughout undergraduate nursing programs across Canada. They help students who are learning about nursing develop knowledge, skills, and judgement around using health technologies in their practice to support client care (CASN, 2015).

Several nursing pioneers developed nursing informatics competencies and introduced graduate-level nursing informatics courses into nursing programs across Canada (e.g., Borycki et al., 2017; Hannah et al., 2006b, 2015; Nagle et al., 2014). The intent of this early educational work was to support the development of future nurse educators and researchers as they began learning more about how technology could be used to support nurses caring for clients in hospital, in long-term care, at home, and in the community, as well as to support nurse leadership decision making. Since this early pioneering curriculum research and work, we have seen the introduction of additional nursing informatics courses at the graduate level and joint graduate programs in nursing and health informatics. These courses and programs allow for the development of graduate-level competencies in both nursing and health informatics and at the intersection of competencies in both areas (Borycki et al., 2011). In addition, the nursing and joint nursing – health informatics programs provide students with opportunities for clinical practicums with a focus on informatics and experiential learning opportunities. These opportunities can include co-op placements, where nurse informaticists work in regional health authorities, governments, or private sector organizations such as electronic health record vendors to design, develop, implement, and maintain technologies used in nursing practice.

Canada is a major leader in nursing informatics education and research. Early pioneers in nursing informatics in Canada defined the field internationally (see Hannah et al., 2006b, 2015; Nagle et al., 2014). Canada has led the way in developing and supporting the integration of nursing informatics into undergraduate nursing informatics competencies. More recently, Canada has provided graduate education for nurses who become directors of clinical informatics, chief nursing informatics officers, and vice presidents of technology innovation in health care organizations.

*Written by section contributor E.M. Borycki, RN, PhD, FACMI, FCAHS, FIAHSI; Professor, School of Health Information Science, University of Victoria, Victoria, BC, Canada; Clinician Scientist, Michael Smith Foundation for Health Research, Vancouver, BC, Canada.

understanding of how these digital tools relate to both current and future practice.

A variety of modalities exist for TEL, ranging from simple to sophisticated. Simulations have been carried out for decades using simulation mannequins (Resusci-Annie is one traditional example, but newer high-fidelity simulators provide vital signs and other physiological responses) (Box 17.12) and standardized clients (actors who portray patients in real-life clinical interviews and assessments) (Skiba, 2021). Simulations are increasingly computer-based, involving virtual patients in real-life clinical scenarios (Box 17.13), using avatars and virtual environments. More immersive virtual simulations enable students to interact with avatars, which can be patients, family members, and other health care providers, as they progress through a clinical scenario (Skiba, 2021). Virtual reality devices can also immerse students in the actual environment and allow them to interact with avatars.

Nursing programs have increasingly used these tools to create safe learning environments during the COVID-19 pandemic and when clinical placements are unavailable for a variety of reasons. In some situations, simulations have been used to replace up to 50% of lost clinical

BOX 17.12 CASE STUDY

Simulations and Supporting Student Learning*

Throughout the years, nurse educators have used a variety of teaching strategies to teach nursing students. Teaching strategies are often directed toward cognitive, affective, or psychomotor learning. However, simulation offers the opportunity to address multiple types of learning while using one teaching strategy.

In our nursing program at the University of Saskatchewan, novice nursing students often struggled to learn psychomotor skills and develop communication skills. Historically, low-fidelity simulation was used teach these skills separately. Task trainers were used to teach IV insertions, wound care, and physical assessments, while role playing was used to develop communication skills. Once the student learned these skills, they had little opportunity to integrate these skills before their first clinical experience. Consequently, to support the integration of these skills, a new simulation-based experience was developed.

The INACSL Standards of Best Practice in Simulation Design (INACSL Standards Committee, 2016) guided the development of the simulation-based experience. The first step in the process was to determine the purpose of the simulation—the goal was to provide a standardized experience that promoted readiness for clinical practice in novice nursing students. Next, the learning objectives were developed—the students should be capable of performing critical assessments, interpreting assessment findings, implementing appropriate nursing interventions, and communicating therapeutically with the patient. Once the learning objectives were identified, a backstory and scenario were developed to provide context for the simulation-based experience. Accordingly, the backstory introduced a female patient who had been experiencing multiple episodes of vomiting and diarrhea and was admitted to address her fluid-volume deficit. The scenario was organized into three 15-minute segments and advanced in response to the students' actions. Understanding that enhancing realism helps students buy into the simulation, the physical environment was arranged to mimic an acute care hospital room, the facilitator was the active voice of the high-fidelity mannequin, and all required supplies and equipment were available for use. Lastly, to ensure that the students were prepared, pre-simulation activities

were assigned. These included reviewing lecture content, attending associated practice labs for IV administration, measuring vital signs, and assessing the gastrointestinal, genitourinary, and integument systems.

The simulation-based experience began with a pre-brief session. To ensure consistency, a pre-brief script was shared with all the facilitators. Subsequently, all students were welcomed, expectations were identified, confidentiality was stressed, and a fiction contract was established. Moving forward, nursing and observer roles were assigned, learning objectives were shared, and time allotments were specified. At the end of the pre-brief, students were provided with an orientation to the environment, equipment, and mannequin.

The scenario began with an I-SBAR-R hand-off report to the incoming nursing students. During each segment, nursing students worked together to assess the patient, interpret their findings, and implement appropriate nursing interventions while communicating with each other and the patient.

A 30-minute debrief followed each 15-minute segment. The facilitator used the PEARLS framework (Bajaj et al., 2018) to guide each debrief. The aim of the debrief was to provide formative feedback and to allow students to discuss and reflect on the simulation experience. During the debrief, the students were able to provide a rationale for their actions and receive feedback from the facilitator and their peers that clarified misconceptions or revealed new knowledge.

Overall, the students' responses to the simulation were positive. The majority of students shared that the identification of the expectations and learning objectives during the pre-brief was beneficial to their learning. The opportunity to participate in the scenario, for most students, led to a better understanding of the pathophysiology of the patient's condition and increased their confidence in their assessment skills and their ability to communicate with their patient. Few students appreciated verbalizing their feelings and reflecting on their performance during the debrief. Although the simulation experience was not as fruitful as anticipated, it will be further evaluated and altered to support meeting the learning needs of novice nursing students.

*Written by section contributor Tania Kristoff, RN, PhD, College of Nursing, University of Saskatchewan, Prince Albert, SK, Canada.

BOX 17.13 CASE STUDY

Open-Source Electronic Health Records*

Electronic health record (EHR) systems are being widely adopted in Canada and around the world. Students graduating in the health sciences will be frontline users of these technologies, and their acceptance of, attitudes toward, and proficiency with these systems will be a key factor in their readiness and safety to practise. Moreover, there is a widespread recognition in health care education of the need for interprofessional education to prepare students for interprofessional collaboration in practice.

An open-source educational EHR (EdEHR) has been developed through a collaboration with postsecondary schools and local health authorities in British Columbia (BC). This platform also incorporates interprofessional health case studies that have been specifically developed by the Health Sciences faculty at the BC Institute of Technology for integration into the EdEHR. These case studies, coupled with the EdEHR, have the potential to support interprofessional education and improve advanced communication skills across the health care professions, leading to better patient safety and quality of care.

This platform provides students and faculty with the opportunity to learn and understand the impact of digitized patient health data through experiential learning in a simulated environment. Learning will thus not be limited to training in the navigation of an EHR; it will also provide opportunities to explore and develop knowledge around the impact of EHRs on the patient experience, the clinician experience, interprofessional collaboration, and workflow.

The EdEHR is a server-deployed software tool designed for health education programs that seek a Canadian system focused on the student experience.

The EdEHR is suitable for all health care programs including, but not limited to, nursing, medicine, pharmacy, physiotherapy, and more. The EdEHR is a key learning tool for health care students because it prepares them for employment in ever-evolving digital and technological health care practice environments. The EdEHR has the potential to reduce faculty workload by gathering curricular content, imaging, and laboratory data in one central repository that is easily updated and shared.

The EdEHR is designed to connect to many different learning management systems via LTI (Learning Tools Interoperability). LTI provides access control, authorization, and interconnectivity across different server systems. The software is designed using modules that can be customized to meet the educational needs of its user and enable the sharing of resources with other institutions. The programming languages used to create the EdEHR include HTML5, Python, and JavaScript. The EdEHR data can be edited through JSON files.

Laying the groundwork for education about EHR use by letting students access, and interaction with, an educational EHR in class or laboratory settings will subsequently allow students to quickly learn a "live" system upon their arrival at their clinical placement. It will also give students an enhanced understanding of the benefits of, potential pitfalls in, and rationale for EHR use. Using a tool that spans all health care professions to promote interprofessional collaboration and leverage knowledge has the potential for improved safety and quality of care, greater efficiency, and fewer errors.

For more information on this EdEHR, please see https://edehr.org.

*Written by section contributor Glynda Rees, RN, MSN, Faculty of Nursing, British Columbia Institute of Technology; Past President, Canadian Nursing Informatics Association.

time. Contemporary learning is safely delivered using virtual simulation (VSIM) of a clinical situation and client(s). High-stakes testing can also be conducted using the same virtual environments.

Online or virtual learning is now a common method of delivering and accessing education. Contemporary models of online education no longer consist of just text-based asynchronous delivery—they also incorporate tools to foster communication, teamwork and collaboration, data visualization, knowledge creation, social interactions, and animation. This makes online learning more of a dynamic, active, and enriching experience.

CLINICIAN ENGAGEMENT AND INFORMATICS COMMUNITIES

There are many Canadian and international health informatics communities that offer exciting opportunities to participate in supporting roles, educational programs, and networking. Most importantly, these communities are always welcoming to new members who are interested in advancing informatics. As noted throughout this chapter, involving clinicians in the selection, design, and revision of technology is critically important. Many informatics organizations have specific strategies to foster clinician engagement; despite its historical scarcity, clinician engagement is increasingly recognized as essential to effective design, adoption, and evaluation.

As a professional, you have both an obligation and a right to be involved in issues that affect your professional practice and your work environment. The CNA, the national professional body that represents Canadian nurses, has a mandate to support professional nursing practice, which includes supporting the integration of NI in Canada. The CNA has issued many position statements and professional guidelines to support all nurses as technology has become increasingly integrated into Canadian practice environments. The CNA website provides an excellent starting point from which you can explore NI in Canada.

The **Canadian Nursing Informatics Association (CNIA)** is the national special interest group dedicated to the advancement of NI in Canada (Box 17.14) and is designated as a group affiliated with the CNA. Also affiliated with Digital Health Canada, the CNIA is the Canadian nursing representative to the **International Medical Informatics Association Special Interest Group in Nursing Informatics (IMIA-SIGNI)** (IMIA, n.d.). Originally functioning as a special interest group within Digital Health Canada, this group disbanded in 2000 and reorganized as the CNIA. Since being founded, the CNIA has hosted successful national NI conferences, provided educational offerings, and advocated for the advancement of NI in Canada. The CNIA continues to evolve, producing an online newsletter and offering new initiatives that support continuing education opportunities for nurses.

As noted earlier in this chapter, Digital Health Canada (formerly known as COACH) is another organization dedicated to promoting health informatics within the Canadian health environment through education, information, networking, and communication. Digital Health Canada was formed in 1975 by software developers and health care clinicians (Digital Health Canada, 2022). The original focus was to support effective use of information technology and systems among Canadian health care institutions by sharing ideas and efforts. This focus has expanded to include the effective use of health information for decision making.

Digital Health Canada's interprofessional membership encompasses more than 1 300 individuals, including health care executives, physicians, nurses and allied health providers, researchers and educators, chief information officers, information managers, technical experts, consultants, and information technology vendors (Digital Health Canada, 2022). Member organizations include health care delivery services, government and nongovernment agencies, consulting firms,

BOX 17.14	**Getting to Know Your Canadian Nursing Informatics Association**

The mission of the Canadian Nursing Informatics Association (CNIA) is to "positively impact health outcomes by advancing nursing informatics leadership". The goals of this national organization are as follows:
1. Influence and advance the use of nursing informatics and nursing data standards.
2. Connect nurses and health providers across the country for the purpose of improving best practice.
3. Maintain and grow a diverse and inclusive membership that demonstrates openness, fairness, accountability, and integrity.
4. Support nurses in practice and education by providing resources for the advancement of nursing informatics competencies via education, tool kits, standards, and communities of practice.
5. Establish best practices in clinical information technology and information management.
6. Seek out collaborative opportunities or collaborate with relevant stakeholders to advance common goals and expertise that will improve health outcomes.

Membership offers benefits such as access to a network of national nursing informatics experts and communication forums, valuable educational opportunities and conference events, and the ability to contribute to national discussions shaping the nursing informatics space. Find out more about the CNIA at https://cnia.ca.

From Canadian Nursing Informatics Association. (2020). *2020–2023 Strategic plan.*

commercial providers of information and telecommunications technologies, and educational institutions.

In addition to the groups discussed here, you can contribute your clinician perspective to the various communities of practice and working groups sponsored by Canada Health Infoway. In keeping with the priority of clinical interoperability, Infoway welcomes and encourages clinicians to participate and contribute their expertise on health care and informatics initiatives. Participating in these communities of practice and working groups not only supports your professional practice but also offers you professional development and mentoring opportunities. While many experienced nurses are currently involved in Infoway advisory groups, the communities and working groups consistently need and solicit clinician engagement. Working groups typically focus on a specific challenge, whereas communities may address multiple issues that support both specific and broader issues. The working groups can be accessed at https://ic.infoway-inforoute.ca/en/collaboration/wg, and the communities at https://ic.infoway-inforoute.ca/en/collaboration/communities.

You may also choose to participate in a variety of international informatics organizations. These include the **American Medical Informatics Association (AMIA)**, the **International Medical Informatics Association (IMIA)**, and the **Australasian Institute of Digital Health (AIDH)**, all of which host special interest groups in NI. You can be involved at every level of information management in health care. Your challenge and opportunity is to determine your interests and decide where your energy can best be used.

In addition to the formal organizations that you may consider joining, numerous informal communities are devoted to NI and to creating dialogue among nurses. You may decide to explore a variety of informal communities or social entities, including the following:
- *Blogs:* These are websites that are most often sponsored by an individual or a small group; they are occasionally interactive, but typically present the thoughts and opinions of the blog's sponsor in an informal or conversational style.

- *Wikis:* These are interactive websites that allow multiple subscribers to modify or contribute to the content. Subscribers can use any web browser. Wikis also allow users to incorporate hyperlinks and use a simplified language to rapidly create new pages and linkages.
- *Listservs and discussion groups:* These are email distribution lists. NI sites allow and encourage users to subscribe to the listserv or discussion groups so that users can receive regular updates regarding content, activities, or networking opportunities. These tools also allow participants to ask questions, post messages, and network with colleagues.
- *Social media:* Communities such as Facebook, Twitter, LinkedIn, YouTube, Instagram, and others allow subscribers to join or follow individuals or groups with shared interests. Subscribers may communicate with one another in a variety of ways, including chat, messaging, email, blogs, video, voice chat, file sharing, discussion groups, and message boards. Interest groups and organizations regularly use these types of social media tools to create communities of practice and share experiences. Nurses who use these tools must do so in a fashion consistent with the ethical practice of nursing and privacy legislation.

The value of informal networking cannot be underestimated; however, you should not depend solely on these types of forums for consistent, professional, and credible health informatics information. Some sites may offer highly professional informatics advice or information; unfortunately, no standards exist for either content or process. Many sites offer only personal or anecdotal commentary and may provide misleading information, which can create liability if used in professional practice. Consequently, you must critically evaluate the content of these informal sites and groups to determine the validity of the content, the credibility of the organization or group, and the intent of the networking tool. The most effective way to obtain reliable and authoritative information is through formalized organizations that are committed to the professional advancement of informatics.

CRITICAL THINKING EXERCISES

1. You have been assigned to lead a team tasked with implementing a standardized nursing terminology for your hospital. What critical topics would you assign your team to review? What groups would you connect with to initiate discussions on best practices? What would be the top four activities necessary to proceed with this task?
2. While documenting an admission assessment, you note that your patient has had a previous admission to a psychiatric unit. One of your colleagues is a neighbour of the patient and asks you to confirm whether this patient has a psychiatric history. Your colleague is not providing care to the patient. How do you respond to this inquiry? What pieces of legislation do you consider in helping you come to a decision?
3. Your organization is reviewing its nursing admission assessment forms. You sit on the committee charged with this responsibility. The committee has discovered that across the organization there are 11 units (Internal Medicine, Cardiology, Respiratory, Neurology, General Surgery, Orthopedics, Neurosurgery, Gynecology, Obstetrics, Pediatrics). Each unit has a different nursing admission assessment. The Chief Nursing Officer wants the number of nursing admission assessments reduced and standardized. How should the committee proceed?

Answers to Critical Thinking Exercises appear on the Evolve website.

REVIEW QUESTIONS

Review Questions 1 to 5 relate to the case study at the beginning of the chapter.

1. B.S.'s electronic health record consists of which of the following?
   a. Digital health, analytics, patient registry, diabetic clinic notes, drugs dispensed, and computerized order entry
   b. Patient registry, provider registry, lab results, drugs dispensed, analytics, and a patient portal
   c. Patient registry, provider registry, lab results, drugs dispensed, diagnostic imaging, and clinical reports/immunizations
   d. Patient record, provider notes, lab results, and drugs dispensed
2. The factors behind the need for standardized nursing documentation—regardless of practice domain—include which of the following? *(Select all that apply.)*
   a. To facilitate aggregation of nursing data
   b. To support data analysis
   c. To enhance communication among nurses
   d. To improve representation regarding nursing contributions
3. Which of the following standardized nursing terminology could be used in B.S.'s health care record to document her self-care readiness at the diabetic clinic and at home?
   a. interRAI
   b. ICNP
   c. SNOMED CT
   d. C-HOBIC
4. B.S.'s diabetic clinic nurses want to find information regarding her glucose levels. They will use which of the following forms of clinical documentation?
   a. Lab results
   b. Patient registry
   c. Clinical notes
   d. Clinical reports/immunizations
5. Which of the following enables nurses from both the diabetic clinic and home care to access B.S.'s laboratory records?
   a. Data standards
   b. Patient portal
   c. Big data
   d. Privacy legislation

Answers: 1. c; 2. a, b, c, d; 3. d; 4. a; 5. a.

Rationales for the Review Questions appear on the Evolve website.

RECOMMENDED WEBSITES

American Medical Informatics Association (AMIA): https://www.amia.org
The AMIA is a national association in the United States dedicated to the adoption and advancement of technology in health care.

American Medical Informatics Association (AMIA) Nursing Informatics Community: https://amia.org/communities/nursing-informatics
The nursing informatics community is a special interest group within the AMIA. This group focuses on the advancement of informatics as it relates to American professional nursing practice.

Australasian Institute of Digital Health (AIDH): https://digitalhealth.org.au
The AIDH is the national not-for-profit institute responsible for advancing informatics in Australia (formed from the merger of the Health Informatics Society of Australia [HISA] and the Australasian College of Health Informatics [ACHI]).

Australasian Institute of Digital Health (AIDH) Nursing–Midwifery Community of Practice: https://digitalhealth.org.au/communities-of-practice/nursing-and-midwifery
This AIDH special interest group consists of nursing and midwifery informaticians who are advancing the digital transformation of health care in Australia as it relates to nursing and midwifery informatics priorities.

Canada Health Infoway: https://www.infoway-inforoute.ca/en
Canada Health Infoway is Canada's national not-for-profit organization that generates consensus on health information standards, drives the national agenda for creating an EHR, and acts as the liaison with international standards development organizations.

Canadian Association of Schools of Nursing (CASN) Digital Health in Nursing Education: https://www.casn.ca/education/digital-healthnursing-informatics-casn-infoway-nurses-training-project

The CASN inventory includes a variety of events and resources on the integration of nursing informatics into nursing practice across Canada.

Canadian Nursing Informatics Association (CNIA): https://cnia.ca
The CNIA is a national organization whose mission is to advance nursing informatics in Canada.

Digital Health Canada: https://digitalhealthcanada.com
Digital Health Canada is a member-supported not-for-profit professional organization that connects, inspires, and empowers the digital health professionals who are creating the future of health care in Canada. The organization fosters network growth and connection; brings together ideas from multiple segments for incubation and advocacy; and supports members through professional development at the individual and organizational level.

International Medical Informatics Association (IMIA): https://imia-medinfo.org/wp
The IMIA is an international not-for-profit association dedicated to the adoption and advancement of technology in health care.

International Medical Informatics Association Special Interest Group in Nursing Informatics (IMIA-SIGNI): https://imia-medinfo.org/wp/signi-nursing-informatics
The IMIA-SIGNI is a special interest group within the IMIA. This group is focused on the advancement of nursing informatics in member countries and worldwide.

Office of the Privacy Commissioner of Canada: https://www.priv.gc.ca/en
This site provides access to a range of privacy-related materials, including information on the *Privacy Act* and the *Personal Information Protection and Electronic Documents Act* (PIPEDA).

REFERENCES

A full reference list is available on the website for this book at http://evolve.elsevier.com/Canada/Potter/fundamentals/

18

Communication and Relational Practice

Written by Sonya L. Jakubec, RN, BHScN, MN, PhD, and Barbara J. Astle, RN, PhD, FCAN

OBJECTIVES

Mastery of content in this chapter will enable you to:

- Define the key terms listed.
- Describe aspects of critical thinking that are important to the communication process.
- Describe the five levels of communication and their uses in nursing.
- Describe the basic elements of the communication process.
- Explain the role of communication in relational practice.
- Identify the practices that are important for relational inquiry.
- Identify significant features and therapeutic outcomes of nurse–patient helping relationships.

- List nursing focus areas within the four phases of a nurse–patient helping relationship.
- Describe qualities, behaviours, and approaches that affect interprofessional communication.
- Describe effective approaches to communicating with patients at various developmental levels.
- Identify patient health states and conditions that contribute to impaired communication.
- Describe nursing care measures for patients with special communication needs.

KEY TERMS

Active listening
Aphasia
Assertive
Attention
Authenticity
Autonomy
Channels
Collaborative communication
Communication
Elderspeak
Empathy
Environment
Expressive aphasia
Feedback
Global aphasia

Initiative
Intention
Interpersonal communication
Interpersonal variables
Intrapersonal communication
Message
Metacommunication
Mutuality
Narrative interactions
Nonverbal communication
Perception
Perceptual biases
Public communication
Questioning beyond the surface
Receiver

Receptive aphasia
Referent
Reflexivity
Relational communication
Relational inquiry
Relational practice
Seeking contextual knowledge
Sender
Small group communication
Spiritual inquiry
Symbolic communication
Sympathy
Therapeutic communication techniques
Transpersonal communication
Verbal communication

🌐 WEBSITE

http://evolve.elsevier.com/Canada/Potter/fundamentals/

CASE STUDY

Marie-France (preferred pronouns: she/her), a nurse working in a rural community in Quebec, has been assigned to do the assessment and care planning for Guy (preferred pronouns: he/him), a new home care patient. Guy is 80 years old and lives with his adult child, who participates in a day program for adults with developmental disabilities.

Guy is experiencing aphasia, struggling at times to find words, along with some progressive memory changes and vision loss from macular degeneration. The nurse first aims to understand how to communicate with Guy in order to

engage in a complete home care assessment. The nurse has been told by the program manager that Guy is not resisting the home care referral made by the family physician, but he has expressed concern and suspicion about having people from outside agencies in the house. Communication will be key during each step of the assessment and planning process.

Think about this case study as you read this chapter. There are Review Questions at the end of the chapter about this case study.

Communication involves the exchange of information between individuals, groups, or organizations. For nurses, effective communication is highly consequential to effective patient care and health outcomes. Nurses are intimately involved with patients and their families throughout the lifespan, and they must communicate effectively with people who are experiencing some of the most stressful of life's circumstances. Nurses function as patient advocates and as members of interprofessional teams where other members may have different priorities for patient-centred care. Nurses must also communicate their own needs to avoid burnout and to continue providing effective care (Balzer Riley, 2019). Despite the competing demands on nurses' time and increasing technological complexity, it is the intimate nurse–patient connection that makes the difference in the quality of care and in the meaning of the illness experience for both (Balzer Riley, 2019). Therefore, competency in a variety of communication opportunities supports nurses' ability to develop and maintain therapeutic relationships as well as respect for the profession.

The importance of communication and collaboration is identified as a key domain of nursing education in Canada (Canadian Association of Schools of Nursing, 2022). Effective communication promotes interprofessional collaboration with others on the health care team, helps ensure that ethical and legal responsibilities and professional practice standards are met, earns the public's respect and trust, and contributes to positive patient outcomes (College of Registered Nurses of Alberta [CRNA], 2021; Registered Nurses' Association of Ontario [RNAO], 2013; Slusser et al., 2019) (see Chapter 19 for further information on interprofessional practice). Ineffective communication may lead to poor patient outcomes, increases in adverse incidents, and decreases in professional credibility. The Conference Board of Canada considers communication and interpersonal relationship skills to be crucial for successful employment and the establishment of healthy work environments (Devito et al., 2015). The capacity to communicate effectively evolves over a lifetime.

The qualities, behaviours, and therapeutic communication techniques described in this chapter characterize professionalism in helping relationships. Although the term *patient* is often used, the same principles can be applied in communicating with any person, group, or population in any nursing situation.

COMMUNICATION AND INTERPERSONAL RELATIONSHIPS

At the core of nursing care are therapeutic interpersonal relationships based on caring, mutual respect, and dignity. Communication is the means to establishing these helping–healing relationships. As all behaviour communicates a message, and all communication influences behaviour, nurses must become experts in communication if they are to provide effective care.

Relational practice is "guided by conscious participation with clients using a number of relational skills including listening, questioning, empathy, mutuality, reciprocity, and self-observation, reflection, and a sensitivity to emotional contexts" (College of Nurses of Ontario, 2019, p. 11). The nurse's capacity to be in relation with other people—to take initiative in establishing and maintaining a relationship, to be authentic and responsive to the other person—is a crucial aspect of interpersonal communication. The will and active intention of nurses to join people where they are is what is meant by initiative in relational communication. Reaching out and listening are parts of taking initiative. Being spontaneous and genuine, remaining aware of the patient's and one's own in-the-moment experiences, are aspects of authenticity. Authenticity is often one of the characteristics of nurses that cultivates the public's trust. Effective interpersonal communication also requires

a sense of mutuality and being in a mutual relation. Being "in sync" in this way is based on a belief that the nurse–patient relationship is a partnership and that both partners are equal participants. Mutuality requires that both participants respect each other's autonomy and value system and are committed to the patient's well-being (Arnold & Boggs, 2020).

In their work, nurses honour the fact that people are complex and ambiguous beings. Often, more is communicated than is initially apparent, and patient responses are not always what you might expect. Questioning beyond the surface is an approach to inquiry that nurses employ to facilitate relational practice within complex circumstances of health and illness. Donner and Wiklund Gustin (2020) have found that even when patients are largely silent, nurses communicate effectively through a combination of compassion, willingness to engage, and preparedness to remain in the uncertainty of not knowing. This capacity relies on the balancing of good intentions with the management of fear, through reflection during encounters with patients and on the activities and actions that may be unspoken. Nonverbal interactions provide rich and important joint narratives. Much can be communicated when uncertainty is valued and purposefully brought to interactions. Nurses are further able to engage with complexity and uncertainty and expand their capacity to communicate by focusing on the following specific relational capacities (Hartrick Doane & Varcoe, 2021):

- Collaboration
- Commitment
- Compassion
- Competence
- Leadership
- Orienting
- Scrutinizing

In addition, Hartrick Doane and Varcoe (2021) have proposed the importance of developing a relational orientation that "goes beyond the interpersonal level . . . and includes an examination of the intrapersonal, interpersonal, and contextual dimensions" (p. 2). They detail relational inquiry as an approach to competence in its fullest sense in nursing practice (see Chapter 12 for further information about a relational inquiry approach to nursing competence).

Therapeutic communication occurs within a healing environment between a nurse and a patient (Arnold & Boggs, 2020). Nurses know that attitudes and emotions are easily transmitted and can be communicated intentionally or unintentionally. Every nuance of posture, every small expression and gesture, every word chosen, every attitude held—all have the potential to hurt or heal. Because thought patterns (positive or negative), intention, and behaviour directly influence human energy fields and therefore health, nurses have a tremendous ethical responsibility to pay careful attention to their communication with patients. (Attention is taking notice of someone and regarding them as interesting and important.)

Complementary perspectives of communication and relationships draw upon notions of a collective sense of relationality within a complex interplay of physical, emotional, mental, spiritual, geographical, and historical factors (Van Bewer et al., 2020) as aspects of communication that permeate and connect all beings. Although this approach of balance and nature in communication and healing is a relatively new concept in Western cultures, it has long existed in Indigenous, African, and Eastern cultures. Most nurses embrace the profession's view of people as holistic beings and have experienced synergy in human interactions. All communication must be respected for its potential power and not carelessly misused to hurt, manipulate, or coerce patients. A relational orientation empowers patients and enables them to know themselves and make their own choices within more fulsome contexts and relationships, which is an essential aspect of the healing process. Centring communication on relationships in this way supports the sharing of aspects of culture known only through relationships (McKivett et al., 2018). Nurses have the opportunity to create helping relationships and positive outcomes for themselves, patients, and colleagues through therapeutic communication.

DEVELOPING COMMUNICATION SKILLS

Gaining expertise in communication requires an understanding of the communication process, commitment to an evolving capacity to be in relation to others, and in-depth reflection about personal communication experiences (Balzer Riley, 2019). In addition, the qualities of good critical thinking and problem solving are important to the communication process. Curiosity, perseverance, creativity, self-confidence, independence, fairness, integrity, and humility are useful in approaching a problem (see Chapter 7 for further information on critical thinking).

Interpersonal communication may be challenging because it is based on an individual's perception of received information and is therefore subject to misinterpretation. **Perception** is based on information acquired through the five senses of sight, hearing, taste, touch, and smell (Beauchamp & Baran, 2019). It is a process of mentally organizing and interpreting sensory information to arrive at a meaningful conclusion. An individual's culture, education, and personal background also influence perception (see Chapter 12). Critical thinking and self-reflection can help nurses overcome **perceptual biases**, which are human tendencies that interfere with accurately perceiving and interpreting messages, attitudes, and values from other people. People often assume that others will think, feel, act, react, and behave as they themselves would in similar circumstances. People tend to distort or ignore information that goes against their expectations, preconceptions, or stereotypes (Beebe et al., 2021). By thinking critically about personal communication habits, you will gain awareness of these tendencies and become more responsive to your patients and your goals of therapeutic communication.

As communication skills develop, competence in the nursing process grows. Integration of communication skills throughout the nursing process facilitates collaboration with patients and members of the interprofessional team (Box 18.1). Communication skills are used to gather, analyze, and transmit information and to accomplish the work of each step of the nursing process—assessment, diagnosis, planning, implementation, and evaluation all depend on effective communication among nurse, patient, family, and interprofessional colleagues. Although the nursing process is a reliable framework for patient-centred care, it does not work well unless you master the art of effective interpersonal communication and relational inquiry.

The nature of the communication process requires nurses to constantly make decisions about what, when, where, why, and how to convey messages to other people. Decision making is always contextual; the unique features of any situation influence the nature of the decisions made. For example, the importance of following a prescribed diet will be explained differently to a patient with a newly diagnosed medical condition than to a patient who has repeatedly chosen not to follow dietary restrictions. In nursing communication, **seeking contextual knowledge** is the building block to providing context-based and relevant care (Hartrick Doane & Varcoe, 2021). Effective communication skills such as "seeking contextual knowledge" are easy to learn, but their application is more difficult and nuanced. Deciding which approach is most responsive to each unique nursing situation is challenging and requires tremendous self-awareness and reflexivity. **Reflexivity** is being aware of your own patterns of communication and response to communication, as well as the responses you are evoking in others. When considering self-awareness, imagine how communication

---

BOX 18.1　Communication Throughout the Nursing Process

Assessment

Gathering subjective and objective data through:

Verbal interviewing and history taking

Visual and intuitive observation of nonverbal behaviours and general appearance

Documentation of visual, tactile, and auditory data during physical examination

Written medical records, diagnostic test results, and literature review

Nursing Diagnosis

Intrapersonal analysis of assessment findings

Validation of health care needs and priorities through verbal discussion with patient

Handwritten or electronic documentation of nursing diagnosis

Planning

Interpersonal or small group planning sessions with health care team

Interpersonal collaboration with patient and family to determine implementation methods

Written documentation of expected outcomes

Written or verbal referral to members of the health care team

Implementation

Delegation and verbal discussion with health care team

Verbal, visual, auditory, and tactile health teaching activities

Provision of support through therapeutic communication techniques

Contact with other health care resources and the interprofessional collaboration team

Written documentation of patient's progress in medical record

Communicating targeted, effective public and population health messages

Evaluation

Acquisition of verbal and nonverbal feedback

Comparison of actual and expected outcomes

Identification of factors affecting outcomes

Modification and update of care plan

Verbal or written explanation, or both, of revisions of care plan to patient

Receiving and responding to feedback about one's own nursing care

---

about specific diagnoses such as cancer or end-of-life conditions and dealing with patient and family emotions might be challenging to you. Some nurses do indeed struggle to cope with their own reactions and emotions when communicating difficult news to families and patients (Bumb et al., 2017).

Throughout this chapter, brief clinical examples will guide you in approaches for effective communication. Because the best way to acquire a skill is through practice, it is useful for you to know yourself and your own habits, as well as your typical responses to situations. Discussing and role playing these scenarios before experiencing them at the point of care may be helpful (Slusser et al., 2019).

LEVELS OF COMMUNICATION

Nurses use different levels of communication in their professional role: intrapersonal, interpersonal, transpersonal, small group, and public.

Intrapersonal Communication

Intrapersonal communication, exemplified in one's thinking, is also known as *self-talk* or *inner thought*. It is a powerful form of communication that occurs *within* an individual and relates to personal qualities and values, yet is also highly consequential to interpersonal communication and collaborative practice (Valaitis et al., 2018). Nurses and patients both use intrapersonal communication to develop self-awareness and a positive self-concept that can facilitate self-expression and improve health and self-esteem by supporting reflection and self-awareness practices. Intrapersonal communication can be built upon for a productive and supportive influence on practice.

Interpersonal Communication

Interpersonal communication is the one-to-one interaction between the nurse and patient that often occurs face to face. It is the level most frequently used in nursing practice. It takes place within a social context and includes all the symbols and cues used to give and receive meaning (Valaitis et al., 2018).

Sometimes messages are received differently than the messenger intended. Nurses work with people who have different opinions, experiences, values, and belief systems; therefore, meaning must be validated or mutually negotiated between participants.

Transpersonal Communication. **Transpersonal communication** occurs within a person's spiritual domain. Nurses communicate and relate to their patients within this domain (see Chapter 29). **Spiritual inquiry** is an approach to communication whereby nurses can join with their patients to create a road map of what is meaningful, significant, and important for the patient in their unique context. This inquiry illuminates the patient's contexts, understandings, experiences, and hopes. It is through such dialogue that nurses can communicate with patients in times of deeper, often complex, conflicted, and ambiguous situations (Hartrick Doane & Varcoe, 2021).

Small Group Communication

Small group communication is interaction that occurs when a small number of people meet together for a common purpose. This type of communication is usually goal directed and requires an understanding of group dynamics. When nurses work on committees, lead patient support groups, form research teams, or participate in patient-centred care conferences, they are using the small group communication process. For small groups to function effectively, members must feel accepted, comfortable with sharing their ideas and thoughts openly and honestly, and able to actively listen to other group members and consider possible alternative viewpoints (Arnold & Boggs, 2020).

Public Communication

Public communication is interaction with an audience. Nurses have opportunities to speak with groups of consumers about health-related topics, present scholarly work to colleagues at conferences, lead classroom discussions with peers or students, and engage in public advocacy and media (including social media) activities. Public communication requires special adaptations in eye contact, gestures, and voice inflection and the use of media materials to communicate messages effectively. The purpose of public communication by nurses is to increase audience knowledge about health-related topics, health care issues, and other issues important to the nursing profession. Guidelines are available to support social media and digital communication (CRNA, 2021; RNAO, n.d.).

BASIC ELEMENTS OF THE COMMUNICATION PROCESS

Communication is an ongoing, dynamic, and multidimensional process. Its basic elements are illustrated in Figure 18.1 and described in this section. This simple model represents what is, in practice, a very

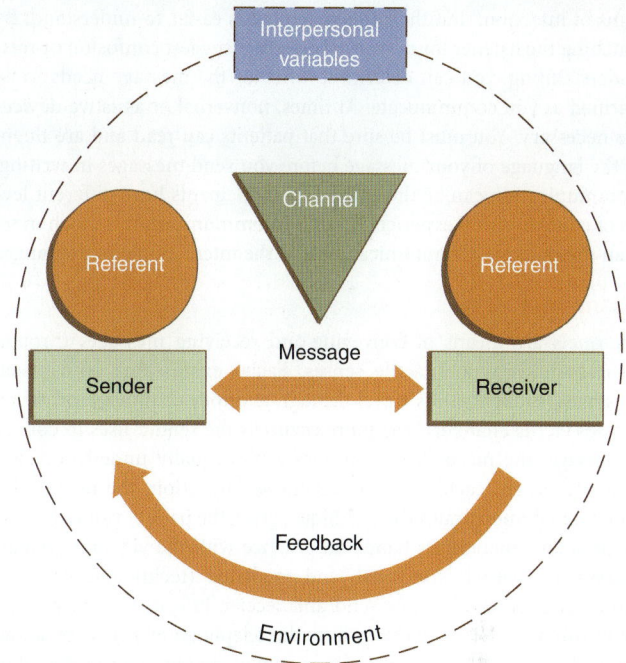

FIGURE 18.1 Communication is an active process between sender and receiver.

complex process. The model helps to identify the essential components of communication.

Referent

The **referent** motivates one person to communicate with another. In a health care setting, sights, sounds, odours, time schedules, messages, objects, emotions, sensations, perceptions, ideas, and other cues trigger communication. When a nurse knows the stimulus that triggered communication, they can develop and organize messages for effective communication.

Sender and Receiver

The **sender** is the person who encodes and delivers the message, and the **receiver** is the person who receives and decodes the message. The sender puts ideas or feelings into a form that can be transmitted and is responsible for accuracy and emotional tone. The sender's message acts as a referent for the receiver, who is responsible for attending to, decoding, and responding to the sender's message. Sender and receiver roles are fluid and change back and forth as people interact; sometimes sending and receiving even occur simultaneously. The more the sender and receiver have in common and the closer their relationship, the more likely they will accurately perceive one another's meaning and respond accordingly.

Messages

The **message** is the content of the communication. It contains verbal, nonverbal, and symbolic expressions of thoughts or feelings that are transmitted from the sender to the receiver (Arnold & Boggs, 2020). Personal perceptions sometimes distort the receiver's interpretation of the message. Two nurses can provide the same information and yet convey very different messages according to their personal communication styles. One nurse can send the same message to two people and be understood differently by each. You can send effective messages by expressing yourself clearly, directly, and in a manner familiar to the receiver. "Your incision is well approximated without purulent drainage" is the same message as "Your wound edges are together, with no signs of infection," but the latter statement is easier to understand. By watching the listener for nonverbal cues that suggest confusion or misunderstanding, you can determine whether the message needs to be clarified as you communicate. At times, nonverbal or assistive devices are necessary. You must be sure that patients can read and are fluent in the language of your message before you send messages in writing. Communication can be difficult when participants have different levels of education and experience, but the communication is much more than the message. Communication is in the interaction and exchange.

Channels

Channels are means of conveying and receiving messages through visual, auditory, and tactile senses. Facial expressions send visual messages, spoken words travel through auditory channels, and touch crosses tactile channels. The more channels the sender uses to convey a message, the more clearly the message is usually understood. For example, when teaching about insulin self-injection, the nurse talks about and demonstrates the technique, gives the patient printed information, and encourages hands-on practice with the vial and syringe. Nurses use verbal, nonverbal, and mediated (technological) communication channels. They send and receive information in person; by informal or formal writing; over the telephone or pager; by audio and video recording; and through fax, email, and interactive digital or social networking media.

Feedback

Feedback is the message returned by the receiver. It indicates whether the intended meaning of the sender's message was understood by the receiver. Senders need to seek verbal and nonverbal feedback to ensure that clear communication has occurred. To be effective, the sender and receiver must be sensitive and open to each other's messages, clarify the messages, and modify behaviour accordingly. In a social relationship, both participants assume equal responsibility for seeking openness and clarification, but in the nurse–patient relationship, this responsibility is primarily the nurse's. The nurse can ask directly for feedback, for example, by asking, "What stands out from the information I have just shared with you?"

Interpersonal Variables

Interpersonal variables are characteristics within both the sender and the receiver that influence communication. People perceive events differently (Austin et al., 2019). A nurse might say, "You have been very quiet since your family left. Is something on your mind?" One patient might perceive the nurse's question as showing caring and concern; another might perceive the nurse as being intrusive. It is the responsibility of the nurse to seek out the variables and contexts that will communicate sensitively and effectively. Other interpersonal variables include educational and developmental levels, sociocultural backgrounds, values and beliefs, emotions, gender, physical health status, and roles and relationships. Variables associated with illness, such as pain, anxiety, and medication effects, can also affect nurse–patient communication and should all be considered in communication choices (West & Turner, 2019).

Environment

The environment is the setting for sender–receiver interaction. For effective communication, the environment should meet nurse and patient needs for physical and emotional comfort and safety. Noise, temperature extremes, distractions, and lack of privacy or space create confusion, tension, and discomfort. Environmental distractions are common in health care settings and interfere with messages sent between people. Establishing as comfortable an environment as possible to create favourable conditions for effective communication is a role of the nurse.

FORMS OF COMMUNICATION

Messages are conveyed verbally, nonverbally, concretely, and symbolically. As people communicate, they express themselves through words, movements, voice inflection, facial expressions, and use of space. These elements work in harmony to enhance a message and can also conflict with one another to contradict or confuse the message.

Verbal Communication

Verbal communication entails the use of spoken or written words. Verbal language is a code that conveys specific meaning through a combination of words. The most important aspects of verbal communication are discussed next.

Vocabulary. Communication is unsuccessful if senders and receivers cannot decode each other's words and phrases. When a nurse cares for a patient who speaks another language, the services of an interpreter may be necessary. Even those who speak the same language use subcultural variations of certain words: *dinner* may mean a noon meal to one person and the last meal of the day to another. Medical jargon (technical terminology used by the interprofessional collaborative practice team) may sound like a foreign language to patients and should be used only with other practitioners of interprofessional collaboration. Children have more limited vocabularies than do adults and may use special words to describe bodily functions or a favourite blanket or toy. Teenagers often use words in unique ways that are unfamiliar to adults.

Denotative and Connotative Meaning. A single word can have several meanings. Individuals who use a common language share the denotative meaning: *baseball* has the same meaning for everyone who speaks English, but *code* specifically denotes cardiac arrest to health care providers, in contrast to other meanings of the word. The connotative meaning is the interpretation of a word's meaning influenced by the thoughts, feelings, or ideas that people have about the word. When families are told that a loved one is "in serious condition," they may believe that death is near, but to the nurse *serious* may simply describe the nature of the condition. As a nurse, you need to select words carefully, avoiding terms that can be easily misinterpreted, especially when explaining a patient's medical condition or therapy. Even a much-used phrase such as "I'm going to take your vital signs" can be unfamiliar to an adult or frightening to a child.

Pacing. Messages are conveyed more successfully when sent at an appropriate speed or pace. It is important to speak slowly enough to enunciate clearly. Talking rapidly, using awkward pauses, or speaking slowly and deliberately can convey an unintended message. Long pauses and rapid shifts to another topic may be unsettling for a patient. Pacing is improved by thinking before speaking and by developing awareness of the cadence of your speech.

Intonation. Tone of voice dramatically affects the meaning of a message. Depending on intonation, even a simple question or statement can express enthusiasm, anger, concern, or indifference. To avoid sending unintended messages, be aware of your tone of voice. For example, patients may interpret a nurse's tone of voice as condescending, which may inhibit further communication. A patient's tone of voice is also highly relevant to communication and may provide information about their emotional state or energy level.

Clarity and Brevity. Effective communication is simple, brief, and direct. Fewer words result in less confusion. You can achieve clarity by speaking slowly, enunciating clearly, and using examples to make explanations easier to understand. Repeating important parts of a message also clarifies communication. Phrases such as "you know" or "okay?" at the end of every sentence detract from clarity as well as professionalism. Brevity is achieved by using short sentences and words that express an idea simply and directly. "Where is your pain?" is much better than "I would like you to describe for me the location of your discomfort."

Timing and Relevance. Timing is critical in communication. Even though a message is clear, poor timing can limit its effectiveness. For example, you should not begin routine teaching when a patient is in severe pain, in emotional distress, or distracted by pressing matters. Often the best time for interaction is when a patient expresses an interest in communicating. If messages are relevant or important to the situation at hand, communication is more effective. For example, when a patient is facing emergency surgery, discussing the risks of smoking is less relevant than explaining preoperative procedures.

Nonverbal Communication

Nonverbal communication makes use of all five senses and refers to transmission of messages that do not involve the spoken or written word. Researchers have estimated that approximately 7% of meaning is transmitted by words, 38% by vocal cues, and 55% by nonverbal body cues. Nonverbal communication serves to accent, complement, contradict, regulate, repeat, or substitute for verbal messages (Devito et al., 2015). Nonverbal communication is unconsciously motivated and thus reflects a person's intended meaning more accurately than spoken words (Austin et al., 2019). When verbal and nonverbal communication are incongruous, the receiver usually "hears" the nonverbal message as the true message.

All kinds of nonverbal communication are important, but interpreting them is often difficult. Sociocultural background is a major influence on the meaning of nonverbal behaviour. Nonverbal messages between people of different cultures are easily misinterpreted. Because the interpretation of nonverbal behaviour is subjective, it is important to check its perceived meaning (Adler & Proctor, 2016). Assessing nonverbal messages is an important communication skill that is highly consequential to patient assessment and nursing care (Austin et al., 2019). Communication through nonverbal means is also important for understanding patient preferences for evidence-informed decision making, which draws on scientific research, best practices, and patient preferences, as discussed in the evidence-informed practice tools in Box 18.2 (Den Hertog & Niessen, 2019).

General Appearance. General appearance includes physical characteristics, facial expression, manner of dress and grooming, and adornments. These factors help communicate physical well-being, personality, social status, occupation, religion, culture, and self-concept. First impressions are largely based on appearance. Nurses learn to develop a general impression of patient health and emotional status through aspects of a patient's appearance, and patients develop a general impression of the nurse's professionalism and caring in the same way.

Posture and Gait. Posture and gait are forms of self-expression. The ways that people sit, stand, and move reflect attitudes, emotions, self-concept, and health status. For example, an erect posture and a quick, purposeful gait communicate a sense of well-being and confidence. Leaning forward conveys attention. A slumped posture and a slow, shuffling gait may be indicative of depression, illness, discomfort, or fatigue.

BOX 18.2 EVIDENCE-INFORMED PRACTICE
Excellent Nurses' Communication Tools

A set of implicit and intuitive communication tools has been identified by Den Hertog and Neissen (2019) to attune professional nursing care to patient preferences for evidence-informed decision making. The use of these tools leads to individual tailored nursing care and appears to be part of nurses' practical wisdom.

The tools include the following: (1) creating a "click," (2) monitoring with "antennae," and (3) framing empathetic questions. Aligned with relational inquiry (Hartrick Doane & Varcoe, 2021) approaches, these tools seek to understand what is said, not said, and under the surface in patient–nurse communication. These tools work together such that when a click is made, it is easy for nurses to monitor whether patients feel safe and confident, allowing nurses to respond to patients' behaviours or needs.

The "click" is the interactive connection with the patient that nurses actively engage in with patients, regardless of patients' verbal communication capacities. The "click" is often highly sensory or intuitively experienced. In part because of the click, nurses experience a unique access to the experiences, thoughts, and feelings of patients—a kind of "antennae." In addition, working with antennae requires constant communication and coordination because the incoming signals need to be checked and action may be required. The empathetic questions are mainly about how the patient is feeling and how they also assess the situation, often with a uniquely shared frankness and honesty.

From Den Hertog, R., & Niessen, T. (2019). The role of patient preferences in nursing decision-making in evidence-based practice: Excellent nurses' communication tools. *Journal of Advanced Nursing, 75*(9), 1987–1995. https://doi.org/10.1111/jan.14083

Facial Expression. The face is the most expressive part of the body. Facial expressions convey emotions such as surprise, fear, anger, happiness, and sadness. Some people have an expressionless face, or flat affect, which reveals little about what they are thinking or feeling. An incongruent affect is a facial expression that does not match the content of a verbal message—for example, smiling when describing a sad situation. People are sometimes unaware of the messages their expressions convey. For example, a nurse may frown in concentration while doing a procedure, and the patient may interpret this as anger or disapproval. Patients closely observe nurses. Consider the impact a nurse's facial expression might have on a person who asks, "Am I going to die?" The slightest change in the eyes, lips, or facial muscles will reveal the nurse's feelings. Although it is hard to control all facial expression, the nurse should try to avoid showing shock, disgust, dismay, or other distressing reactions in the patient's presence. Confidence can be instilled through a well-timed nod or glance, and self-awareness and the careful attention and intention of relational practice during the presentation of self when communicating with another person (Hartrick Doane & Varcoe, 2021).

Eye Contact. People signal readiness to communicate through eye contact. Eye contact also allows people to closely observe one another. Eye movements can also communicate feelings and emotions. Standing above a person (looking downward) conveys authority, whereas interacting at the same eye level indicates equality in the relationship. Rising to the same eye level as an angry person communicates self-assertion. Lack of eye contact may indicate anxiety, defensiveness, discomfort, or lack of confidence in communicating. For some people, maintaining eye contact during conversation shows respect and willingness to listen. For other people, eye contact may be considered intrusive, threatening, or harmful. As with all communication, what is important is to understand the perspective of those you are caring for and working with—and to convey your genuine interest in understanding their needs and concerns. To gain that confidence and understanding, the nurse needs to inquire with the knowledge that a wide array of differences is expected and that communication through eye contact varies in expression that is neither right nor wrong.

Gestures. Gestures emphasize, punctuate, and clarify the spoken word, and they may communicate volumes when speech is not possible. Gestures alone carry specific meanings and create messages. A finger pointed toward a person may communicate several meanings, but when accompanied by a frown and stern voice, the gesture conveys an accusation or a threat. Pointing to an area of pain may be more accurate than verbally describing the location.

Sounds. Sounds such as sighs, moans, groans, or sobs also communicate feelings and thoughts. When combined with other nonverbal communication, sounds help send messages. Sounds can be interpreted in several ways: sighing often suggests boredom or anxiety, moaning may convey pleasure or suffering, and crying may communicate happiness, sadness, or anger. As a nurse, you need to validate such nonverbal messages with the patient in order to interpret them accurately. Simply noticing the sound, such as stating, "I hear you sighing so strongly," can impart concern and signal that you are listening to what is not spoken.

Personal Space. Personal space is the need to gain, maintain, and defend one's right to their space. Personal space is important because it provides people with a sense of identity, security, and control. Personal space can be distinguished and made visible to other people, as with a fence around a yard or a curtain around a bed in a hospital room. Personal space, however, is invisible and individual, connoting boundaries beyond the physical territory. Boundaries such as physical or emotional space can be defended just like another sort of fence or barrier. Some people choose when to open the gate of a fence, and others simply leave the boundary wide open, taking whatever comes through. When personal space becomes threatened, people respond defensively and communicate less effectively. Specific contexts may dictate whether the physical or emotional distance between nurse and patient is appropriate. Because of the nature of caregiving, nurses often must move into a patient's personal space, even entering a more vulnerable zone in that personal space. For instance, when conducting an in-depth patient assessment or performing an intervention such as wound care, there is necessarily close personal and emotional contact between nurse and patient. Before entering a patient's personal space, it is essential that you prepare both your patient and the environment. By explaining to your patient what you will do and preparing the environment for nursing interventions, your patient will recognize a shift toward the establishment of a therapeutic interaction. You need to convey confidence, gentleness, and respect for privacy, especially when your actions will require intimate contact or involve a patient's vulnerable zone. For example, while social distancing was required during the COVID-19 pandemic, this required a different discussion of physical space when providing some care to patients (Newcomb et al., 2021). Box 18.3 provides examples of nursing actions within zones of personal space (Austin et al., 2019) and zones of touch.

Symbolic Communication

Good communication requires awareness of symbolic communication, the verbal and nonverbal symbolism used to convey meaning. Art and music are forms of symbolic communication that nurses use to enhance understanding and promote healing. Morrison and colleagues (2021) found that creative expressions such as art, music, and dance

---

BOX 18.3   Zones of Personal Space and Touch

Zones of Personal Space
Intimate Zone (0 to 45 cm)
Holding a crying infant
Performing physical assessment
Bathing, grooming, dressing, feeding, and toileting a patient
Changing a patient's dressing

Personal Zone (45 cm to 1 m)
Sitting at a patient's bedside
Taking a patient's health history
Teaching an individual patient
Exchanging information with health care staff at change of shift

Social Zone (1 to 4 m)
Participating in patient-centred care rounds
Sitting at the head of a conference table
Teaching a class for patients with a specific disease
Conducting a family support group session

Public Zone (4 m and Greater)
Speaking at a community forum
Testifying at a legislative hearing
Lecturing to a class of students

Zones of Touch
Social Zone (Assess for Permission to Touch)
Hands, arms, shoulders, back

Consent Zone (Consent Needed)
Mouth, wrists, feet

Vulnerable Zone (Consent and Special Care Needed)
Face, neck, front of body

Intimate Zone (Consent and Great Sensitivity Needed)
Genitalia, rectum

---

have a healing effect on patients. Patients reported decreased pain and greater joy and hope and were often more open to communication when creative expression was part of therapeutic communication.

Metacommunication

Metacommunication is a broad term that refers to all factors influencing how a message is perceived by other people (Arnold & Boggs, 2020). It is communication *about* communication that reflects the relational aspects of messages (Adler & Proctor, 2016) and helps people better understand what has been communicated. For example, a nurse observes a young patient holding his body rigidly, and his voice is sharp as he says, "Going to surgery is no big deal." The nurse replies, "You say having surgery doesn't bother you, but you look and sound tense. I'd like to help." Awareness of the tone of the verbal response and the nonverbal behaviour may result in further exploration of the patient's feelings and concerns.

PROFESSIONAL NURSING RELATIONSHIPS

The nurse's application of knowledge, understanding of human behaviour and communication, and commitment to ethical behaviour all contribute to the formation of professional relationships. The intention to promote caring and respect for other people will help you be more successful in establishing professional relationships.

Nurse–Patient Helping Relationships

Helping relationships are the foundation of clinical nursing practice. In such relationships, the nurse assumes the role of professional helper and comes to know the patient as an individual who has unique health care needs, human responses, and patterns of living. The relationship is therapeutic, promoting a psychological climate that facilitates positive change and growth. Therapeutic communication allows patients to achieve their health care–related goals and attain optimal personal growth (Arnold & Boggs, 2020). It includes an explicit time frame and a goal-directed approach, and confidentiality is an expected feature. The nurse establishes, directs, and takes responsibility for the interaction, and the patient's needs take priority over the nurse's needs. The relationship is also characterized by the nurse's nonjudgemental acceptance of the patient. Acceptance conveys a willingness to hear a message or to acknowledge feelings. It does not mean you always agree with the patient or approve of the patient's decisions or actions. A helping relationship between nurse and patient does not just happen; you create it through care, skill, and the development of trust.

The nurse–patient helping relationship is characterized by a natural progression of four goal-directed phases: preinteraction, orientation, working, and termination (Box 18.4). These phases often begin before the nurse meets the patient and continue until the caregiving relationship ends. Even a brief interaction can exhibit an abbreviated version of these four phases. For example, the student nurse gathers patient information to prepare in advance for caregiving, meets the patient and establishes trust, accomplishes health care–related goals through use of the nursing care process, and says goodbye at the end of the shift or when the patient leaves the unit.

Socializing is an important initial component of interpersonal communication. It helps people get to know one another and relax. It is easy, superficial, and not deeply personal, whereas therapeutic interactions are often more difficult, intense, and uncomfortable. A nurse often uses social conversation to lay a foundation for a closer relationship. For example, a nurse may greet a patient by saying, "Hi, Mr. Simpson. I hear it's your birthday today. Happy birthday!" A friendly, informal, and warm communication style helps establish trust, but nurses must get beyond social conversation to talk about issues or concerns affecting the patient's health. During social conversation, patients may ask personal questions about the nurse's family, place of residence, and so forth. Students often wonder whether it is appropriate to reveal such information. The skillful nurse uses judgement about what to share and provides minimal information or deflects such questions with gentle humour and refocuses conversation back to the patient.

Creating a therapeutic environment depends on your ability to communicate, comfort, and help patients meet their needs. Comfort is crucial in the practice of nursing. Therapeutic interactions increase feelings of personal control by helping patients feel secure, informed, and valued. Optimizing personal control facilitates emotional comfort, which minimizes physical discomfort and promotes recovery. Creating an emotionally comfortable interaction is something that can be learned. Without supporting physical and emotional comfort, the communication of information may not be received, and a standard patient history may elicit only short answers.

In a therapeutic relationship, nurses often encourage patients to share personal stories, which are called **narrative interactions**. Through narrative interactions, such as reminiscing with patients, you begin to understand the context of patients' lives and learn what is meaningful from their perspective (Shattell & Hogan, 2005). For example, a nurse asked a patient to share a story about a time in his life when he had to make a difficult decision. The patient related the following story:

"When I was a young man, I worked on the family farm. An uncle died and left me some money. All of a sudden, I could afford to go to university, but Dad didn't want me to go because he needed me there. I had to decide whether to stay or go, and it was real hard

---

BOX 18.4 Phases of the Helping Relationship

Preinteraction Phase
Before meeting the patient, the nurse accomplishes the following tasks:
- Reviews available data, including the medical and nursing history
- Talks to other caregivers who may have information about the patient
- Anticipates health care concerns or issues that may arise
- Identifies a location and setting that will foster comfortable, private interaction with the patient
- Plans enough time for the initial interaction

Orientation Phase
When the nurse and patient meet and get to know one another, the nurse accomplishes the following tasks:
- Sets the tone for the relationship by adopting a warm, empathetic, caring manner
- Recognizes that the initial relationship may be superficial, uncertain, and tentative
- Expects the patient to test the nurse's competence and commitment
- Closely observes the patient and expects to be closely observed by the patient
- Begins to make inferences and form judgements about patient messages and behaviours
- Assesses the patient's health status
- Prioritizes the patient's problems and identifies the patient's goals
- Clarifies the patient's and nurse's roles

- Negotiates a contract with the patient that specifies who will do what
- Lets the patient know when to expect the relationship to be terminated

Working Phase
When the nurse and patient work together to solve problems and achieve goals, the nurse accomplishes the following tasks:
- Encourages and helps the patient to express feelings about their health
- Encourages and helps the patient to explore their own feelings and thoughts
- Provides information that the patient needs to understand and to change behaviour
- Encourages and helps the patient to set goals
- Takes actions to meet the goals set with the patient
- Uses therapeutic communication skills to facilitate successful interactions
- Uses appropriate self-disclosure and confrontation

Termination Phase
During the ending of the relationship, the nurse accomplishes the following tasks:
- Reminds the patient that relationship termination is near
- Evaluates goal achievement with the patient
- Reminisces about the relationship with the patient
- Separates from the patient by relinquishing responsibility for their care
- Facilitates a smooth transition for the patient to other caregivers as needed

because at first I just wanted to get away. I talked to our pastor, and he said it was up to me, to pray about it and do what my heart told me to. So I stayed. Oh, I've thought from time to time what I might have made of myself, but I never regretted it. I had a good life in farming."

Collaboration between nurses and patients builds relationships and is based on principles of mutual gain and respect. It reflects a desire to satisfy the needs of both parties (Dubrin & Geerinck, 2014). Collaborative communication promotes personal responsibility, enables self-expression, and strengthens the patient's problem-solving ability. In addition to communicating with patients, nurses also communicate collaboratively with the interprofessional team. These skills are highly consequential to patient outcomes (Gottlieb et al., 2019).

Nurse–Family Relationships

Many nursing situations, especially those in the community, require the nurse to form helping relationships with entire families. The same principles that guide one-to-one helping relationships also apply when the patient is a family unit. However, communication within families requires additional understanding of the complexities of family dynamics, needs, and relationships (see Chapter 20).

Interprofessional Collaborative Practice (ICP) Relationships

Nurses function in roles that require interaction with interprofessional teams (see Chapter 19 for further information on interprofessional practice). Many elements of the nurse–patient helping relationship also apply to collegial relationships, which focus on accomplishing the work and goals at the point of care. Communication in such relationships may be geared toward team building, facilitating group process, collaboration, consultation, delegation, supervision, leadership, and management (see Chapter 13). Nurses need a variety of communication skills, including presentational speaking, persuasion, group problem solving, providing performance reviews, and writing business reports.

Social and therapeutic interactions are needed between the nurse and members of the interprofessional team to build morale and strengthen relationships within the work setting. Within the interprofessional team, all members need friendship, support, guidance, and encouragement from one another to cope with the many stressors imposed by the demands of the health care context (Gottlieb et al., 2019).

Nurse–Community Relationships

Many nurses form relationships with community groups by participating in local organizations, volunteering for community service, or becoming politically active. In a community-based practice, nurses establish relationships with their community (MacDonald & Jakubec, 2021) (see Chapter 4 for more information about communication in community practice). Communication in the nurse–community relationship includes neighbourhood newsletters, public bulletin boards, newspapers, radio, television, websites, and social media, whereby community and professional practice health information is shared.

ELEMENTS OF PROFESSIONAL COMMUNICATION

Professional appearance, demeanour, and behaviour are important in establishing your trustworthiness and competence as a nurse. They communicate the impression that you have assumed the professional helping role, are clinically skilled, and are focused on the patient.

Professional behaviour should communicate warmth, friendliness, confidence, knowledge, skill, and competence. Professionals speak in a clear, well-modulated voice, use good grammar, listen to other people, help and support colleagues, and communicate effectively. Being punctual, organized, well prepared, and equipped for the responsibilities of the nursing role also communicate respect and trust for patients and colleagues, building trust in the profession as a whole. This expression of trustworthiness and professionalism is also important in electronic and social media communication. Referred to as e-professionalism, any communication on digital platforms must preserve the integrity of the client, person, employer, another health care provider, colleague, or organization, and nurses must carefully consider the potential impact of their communication (CRNA, 2021; RNAO, n.d.). Certainly, the COVID-19 pandemic and the rampant spread of misinformation and disinformation on social media shone the light on the role of nurses in not merely refraining from the exchange of misinformation but also in actively challenging false information and the infodemic (Ritter et al., 2021).

Courtesy

Common courtesy is part of professional communication. To practise courtesy, always greet and say goodbye to patients and knock on doors before entering. A courteous nurse will also state their purpose, address people by name, say "please" and "thank you" to members of the interprofessional team, and apologize for inadvertently causing distress. When a nurse is discourteous, they are perceived as rude or insensitive. Such behaviour sets up barriers between nurse and patient and causes friction among members of the interprofessional team.

Use of Names

Self-introduction is important. Failure to give a name, indicate status (e.g., student nurse, registered nurse, or licensed practical nurse), or acknowledge the patient creates uncertainty about the interaction and conveys a lack of commitment or caring. Making eye contact with and smiling at people communicates recognition. Addressing other people by name conveys respect for human dignity and uniqueness. Asking how to pronounce someone's name and taking the initiative to say the name correctly lays the groundwork for communication. Because using last names is respectful in most cultures, nurses normally use the patient's last name in the initial interaction, but they may use the first name in subsequent interactions at the patient's request.

It is important to ask other people how they would like to be addressed and to honour their preferences and identities. Using first names is appropriate for infants, young children, confused or unconscious patients, and close colleagues. Terms of endearment such as "honey," "dear," "sweetie," or "sweetheart" are inappropriate; they may be perceived as disrespectful and unprofessional. Cultural practices may differ in terms of what is viewed as being respectful or disrespectful (Clucas et al., 2019; Dexter et al., 2016). For example, the term "Auntie" may symbolize respect in some cultural groups, while in others it would be considered disrespectful. Make it a habit to always ask, and never assume what is desired by the patient or what will convey respect. The use of plural pronouns such as "we" when referring to patients is disrespectful, implies a loss of independence, and may be interpreted as condescending. Communication of the possessive, such as "our residents," "our LPNs," or "our Indigenous peoples," suggests ownership and communicates authority and disrespect for the autonomy of others. Referring to a patient by diagnosis, room number, or another attribute is demeaning and implies that you do not care enough to know the patient as an individual.

Trustworthiness

Trust entails relying on someone without doubt or question. Being trustworthy means following through on what you say you are going to do. To foster trust, you need to communicate warmth and demonstrate consistency, reliability, honesty, integrity, competence, and respect. Sometimes it is not easy for a patient to ask for help. Trusting another person involves risk and vulnerability, but it also fosters open, therapeutic communication and enhances the expression of feelings, thoughts, and needs. Without trust, a nurse–patient relationship rarely progresses beyond social interaction and superficial care. Knowingly withholding key information, lying, or distorting the truth violates both legal and ethical standards of practice. Maintaining confidentiality and protecting a patient's privacy are also important aspects of communicating a trustworthy professional relationship. Sharing personal information or gossiping about other people communicates the message that you cannot be trusted, and it damages interpersonal relationships.

Truthfulness in the content of nursing communication plays a pivotal role in establishing trust and respect. The harms of misinformation during the COVID-19 pandemic brought these concerns to light for nurses and all health care providers. Both what and how nurses communicate are highly consequential to patient outcomes. The truth, based on scientific evidence and not on personal ideology, must guide nursing communication (Guest & Villeneuve, 2021). What you say, including your online presence, matters a great deal to health outcomes and professional credibility.

Autonomy and Responsibility

Autonomy is the ability to be self-directed and independent in accomplishing goals and advocating for other people. Nurses make choices and accept responsibility for the outcomes of their actions (Pollard & Jakubec, 2019). They take initiative in solving problems and communicate in a manner that reflects the importance and purpose of the therapeutic interaction (Arnold & Boggs, 2020). Recognizing the patient's autonomy is important to effective communication.

Assertiveness

Assertive communication allows individuals to act in their own best interests without infringing on or denying the rights of others. Assertiveness conveys self-assurance and respect for others (Austin et al., 2019).

Nurses teach assertiveness skills to other people as a means of promoting personal health. Assertive people express feelings and emotions confidently, spontaneously, and honestly. They make decisions and control their lives more effectively than do nonassertive individuals. They can deal with criticism and manipulation by other people and learn to say no, set limits, and resist other people's efforts to impose guilt. For instance, a nurse, when being asked to complete multiple tasks, may set limits by stating, "I will be able to get to that task, but only later today. Will that still work for you?"

Assertive responses are characterized by feelings of security, competence, power, optimism, and professionalism. They are good tools for dealing with criticism, change, negative conditions in one's personal or professional life, and conflict or stress in relationships. Assertive responses often contain "I" messages, such as "I want," "I need," "I think," and "I feel."

❖ COMMUNICATION WITHIN THE NURSING PROCESS

In the following sections, the focus of the nursing process is on providing care for patients who need special assistance with communication.

The section on implementation, to follow, contains examples of therapeutic communication techniques that are appropriate strategies for use in any interpersonal nursing situation.

◆ Assessment

Assessment of a patient's ability to communicate includes gathering data about the many contextual factors that influence communication. The word *context* refers to all the parts of a situation that help determine its meaning. A context includes all the environmental factors that influence the nature of communication and interpersonal relationships. This includes the participants' internal factors and characteristics, the nature of their relationship, the situation prompting communication, the environment, and the sociocultural elements present (Beebe et al., 2021). Box 18.5 lists the contextual factors that influence communication. Understanding these contextual factors helps you make sound decisions during the communication process.

Physical and Emotional Factors. Assessing the psychophysiological factors that influence communication is especially important. Many altered health states and human responses limit communication. People with hearing or visual impairments have fewer channels through which to receive messages (see Chapter 48). Facial trauma, laryngeal cancer, tracheostomy, or endotracheal intubation often prevent movement of air past vocal cords or mobility of the tongue, which results in an inability to articulate words. An extremely breathless person must use oxygen to breathe rather than speak. People with aphasia after a stroke or with late-stage Alzheimer's disease often cannot understand or form words. People with delirium cannot focus attentively, and those with dementia often cannot make sense of what is being said. Certain mental illnesses such as psychoses or depression cause patients to demonstrate flight of ideas (words do not keep up to rapidly changing thoughts), constant verbalization of the same words or phrases, a loose association of ideas, or slowed speech pattern. People who are highly anxious are sometimes unable to perceive environmental stimuli or hear explanations. Unresponsive or heavily sedated people cannot send or respond to verbal messages.

Review of the patient's medical record helps provide relevant information about the patient's ability to communicate. Through the health history and physical examination, the nurse documents physical barriers to speech, neurological deficits, and pathophysiological conditions that affect hearing or vision. Reviewing the patient's medication record is also important. For example, opiates, antidepressants, neuroleptics, hypnotics, or sedatives may cause a patient to slur words or use incomplete sentences. The nursing progress notes may reveal other factors that contribute to communication difficulties, such as the absence of family members who could provide more information about a patient experiencing confusion.

Assessment should include direct communication with patients to determine their ability to attend to, interpret, and respond to stimuli. If patients have difficulty communicating, it is important to assess the effects of the problem. Patients who cannot communicate effectively will often have difficulty expressing their needs and responding appropriately to the environment, perhaps demonstrating frustration or withdrawal. In this way, a patient who is unable to speak is at risk for injury unless the nurse identifies an alternative communication method. Assistive communication tools and devices may support the nurse in assessment and communication more generally, as well as providing relief and comfort to the patient. Some of these aids and tools involve assistive technologies, whereas others may be far simpler, including nonverbal techniques such as simple sign language, lip reading, and so on (Finke et al., 2008). Barriers to the use of these tools may also exist, as was the case when masking was required during the

BOX 18.5   Contextual Factors That Influence Communication

Psychophysiological Context
This refers to the internal factors that influence communication:
- Physiological status (e.g., pain, hunger, weakness, dyspnea)
- Emotional status (e.g., anxiety, anger, hopelessness, euphoria)
- Growth and development status (e.g., age, developmental tasks)
- Unmet needs (e.g., safety or security; love or belonging)
- Attitudes, values, and beliefs (e.g., meaning of illness experience)
- Perceptions and personality (e.g., optimistic or pessimistic, introverted or extroverted)
- Self-concept and self-esteem (e.g., positive or negative)

Relational Context
This refers to the nature of the relationship between the participants:
- Social, helping, or working relationship
- Level of trust between participants
- Level of caring expressed
- Level of self-disclosure between participants
- Shared history of participants
- Balance of power and control

Situational Context
This refers to the reason for the communication:
- Information exchange
- Goal achievement
- Problem resolution
- Expression of feelings

Environmental Context
This refers to the physical surroundings in which communication takes place:
- Privacy level
- Noise level
- Comfort and safety level
- Distraction level

Cultural Context
This refers to the sociocultural elements that affect the interaction:
- Educational level of participants
- Language and self-expression patterns
- Customs and expectations
- Media influences

COVID-19 pandemic (Homans & Vroegop, 2021). These barriers may make it difficult to communicate directly with the patient, which may warrant communicating indirectly with the patient using a mindful and calm approach with clear messaging, as well as reaching out to family or friends to gather collateral information about the patient's communication patterns and abilities and for general assessment (Schlögl & Jones, 2020).

Developmental Factors. Aspects of a patient's growth and development also influence nurse–patient communication. For example, an infant's self-expression is limited to crying, body movement, and facial expression, whereas most older children express their needs more directly, through speech and specific actions such as pointing. Nurses adapt communication techniques to the developmental needs of infants and children (see Chapters 22 and 23 for further discussion of communication with children). Communication with children and their parents requires special considerations. It is important to include the parents, child, or both as sources of information about the child's health, depending on the child's age.

Advancing age may also affect communication abilities. According to Statistics Canada, older persons represent the fasting growing sector of the population, of which 6 to 12% will experience speech, language, or voice difficulties (Speech-Language and Audiology Canada, 2021). Although some older persons have varied communication barriers, nurses need to avoid the patronizing tone of what is referred to as "**elderspeak**," or condescending baby talk. Instead, nurses should communicate simply, clearly, and with respect in order to provide humanistic care that meets the unique needs of their older patients (Shaw & Gordon, 2021). Box 18.6 highlights tips for communicating with older persons who have communication needs and barriers. These tips can be applied to all patients with communication difficulties.

Sociocultural Factors. Culture, like communication more broadly, is a process that is experienced between people in a relationship. Awareness of the relational process of culture, beginning with an appreciation of one's own individual perspective, power, and privilege, can facilitate

BOX 18.6   FOCUS ON OLDER PERSONS

Tips for Improved Communication With Older Persons Who Have Communication Needs or Barriers

- Capture the patient's attention before speaking.
- Check for hearing aids and glasses.
- Introduce yourself.
- Choose a quiet, well-lit environment, and minimize visual and auditory distractions.
- Face the patient, and use facial expressions and gestures as needed.
- Amplify your voice if necessary, but do not shout because it distorts sound and your facial expression could be misinterpreted. Speak clearly at a moderate rate.
- Allow time for the patient to respond. Do not assume the patient is being uncooperative if the patient makes no response or a delayed response.
- Give patients time to ask questions and clarify responses.
- Whenever possible, ask a family member or caregiver to join you and the patient in the room. Such people are usually most familiar with the patient's communication patterns and can assist in the communication process.

---

communication and understanding between nurses and their patients (see Chapter 12). Nurses can communicate in what is considered culturally safe **relational inquiry** (Hartrick Doane & Varcoe, 2021) by responding to their patients and families, following their lead, appreciating their unique contexts, acknowledging difference, and engaging with the relational capacities mentioned earlier.

Make a conscious effort to avoid interpreting messages from your own cultural perspective and to consider communication within the context of the patient's background.

◆ Nursing Diagnosis

Most individuals experience difficulties with some aspect of communication. People who are free of illness or disability may lack skills in attending, listening, responding, and self-expression. Often, nurses will direct care toward individuals who experience more serious communication impairments, though support for everyone's communication regardless of abilities is part of the nursing process.

The primary nursing diagnostic label used to describe the patient with limited or no ability to communicate verbally is *impaired verbal communication*. This is the state in which the ability to receive, process, transmit, and use symbols is decreased or absent (Doenges et al., 2019). Defining characteristics include the inability to articulate words, inappropriate verbalization, difficulty forming words, and difficulty in comprehending, all of which the nurse clusters together to form the diagnosis. This diagnosis is useful for a wide variety of patients with special problems and needs related to communication, such as impaired perception, reception, and articulation. Although a patient's primary problem may be impaired verbal communication, the associated difficulty in self-expression or altered communication patterns may also contribute to other nursing diagnoses as follows:

- Anxiety
- Social isolation
- Ineffective coping
- Compromised family coping
- Powerlessness, and
- Impaired social interaction.

Contributing and contextual factors for a nursing diagnosis focus on the origins of the communication disorder. In the case of impaired verbal communication, these are physiological, mechanical, anatomical, psychological, social/cultural, or developmental in nature. Accuracy in the identification of related factors is necessary to selecting interventions that can effectively resolve the problem. For example, the diagnosis of *impaired verbal communication related to cultural diversity* would be managed very differently than the diagnosis of *impaired verbal communication related to deafness*.

◆ Planning

Once you have identified the origins and context of the patient's communication impairment, you must consider several factors as you design a responsive approach and nursing care plan. Motivation is a factor in improving communication; patients often must be encouraged to try different approaches. It is especially important to involve the patient and family in decisions about the plan of nursing care to determine whether the suggested methods are acceptable. Patients and families must be patient with themselves and each other when learning new skills if communication is to be effective. When the focus is on practising communication, in some instances arranging for a quiet and private place that is free of distractions may be helpful. Communication aids, such as a writing board for a patient with a tracheostomy, an electronic communication device for a patient with autism, or a special call system for a patient with paralysis, may enhance communication.

Goals and Outcomes. The primary goal of nursing interventions is to facilitate the development of trust between the patient and members of the health care team. It is important to identify expected outcomes for all patients, particularly when impaired communication is a concern. Outcomes are specific and measurable and provide the means to determine whether the broader goal is met. For example, outcomes for the patient might be as follows:

- The patient initiates conversation about a diagnosis or health care problem.
- The patient is able to attend to appropriate stimuli.
- The patient conveys clear and understandable messages with family members and members of the health care team.
- The patient expresses increased satisfaction with the communication process.

At times, you will care for well patients whose difficulty in sending, receiving, and interpreting messages interferes with healthy interpersonal relationships. In this case, impaired communication may be contributing to other nursing diagnoses such as *impaired social interaction* or *ineffective coping*. In such cases, you need to plan interventions to help your patients improve their communication skills. For example, you could model effective communication techniques and provide feedback regarding the patient's communication. Role playing helps patients rehearse situations in which they have difficulty communicating. Expected outcomes for a patient in this situation might include demonstrating the ability to appropriately express needs, feelings, and concerns; communicating thoughts and feelings more clearly; engaging in appropriate social conversation with peers and staff; and increasing feelings of autonomy and assertiveness.

Setting of Priorities. It is essential for the nurse to be available for communication with some immediacy so that the patient is able to express any pressing needs or problems. This may involve an intervention as simple as keeping a call light within reach for a patient restricted to bed or providing a communication augmentative device for the patient to use (e.g., message board, Braille keyboard). When you plan to have lengthy interactions with a patient, it is important to address physical care priorities (i.e., pain or elimination needs) first so that the patient is comfortable and the discussion is uninterrupted.

Continuity of Care. To ensure an effective care plan, you may need to collaborate with other members of the interprofessional team who have expertise in communication strategies. Speech therapists help patients with aphasia; interpreters may be of use for communicating with patients in a variety of languages; and psychiatric nurse specialists support communication with patients in crisis or those who may be experiencing altered moods, behaviours, anxiety states, or disordered thoughts and perceptions (Austin et al., 2019).

◆ Implementation

In carrying out any care plan, nurses use communication techniques that are appropriate for the patient's individual needs. Before learning how to adapt communication methods to help patients with serious communication impairments, it is necessary to learn the communication skills and approaches that serve as the foundation for professional communication. It is also important to understand approaches that create barriers to effective interaction (Devito et al., 2015).

Therapeutic Communication Techniques. Therapeutic communication techniques are specific responses that encourage the expression of feelings and ideas and convey acceptance and respect. By learning these techniques, you develop awareness of the variety of nursing responses available for use in different situations. Although some of the techniques seem artificial at first, skill and comfort in using them do increase with practice. Tremendous satisfaction will result from the development of therapeutic relationships and achievement of desired patient outcomes.

Active Listening. Active listening means being attentive to what the patient is saying both verbally and nonverbally. It enhances trust and facilitates patient communication because it demonstrates acceptance and respect for the patient. Several nonverbal skills facilitate active listening. They can be identified by the acronym SOLER (Townsend & Morgan, 2018):

S: *Sit* facing the patient. This posture indicates that you are there to listen and are interested in what the patient is saying.

O: Keep an *open* posture (i.e., keep arms and legs uncrossed). This posture suggests that you are receptive ("open") to what the patient has to say. A "closed" position may convey a defensive attitude, possibly invoking a similar response in the patient.

L: *Lean* toward the patient. This posture indicates that you are involved and interested in the interaction.

E: Establish and maintain intermittent *eye contact*. This behaviour conveys your involvement in and willingness to listen to what the patient is saying. Absence of eye contact or shifting of the eyes indicates that you are not interested in what the patient is saying.

R: *Relax.* It is important to communicate a sense of being relaxed and comfortable with the patient. Restlessness communicates a lack of interest and also conveys a sense of discomfort that may extend to the patient.

Sharing Observations. Nurses make observations by commenting on how the patient looks, sounds, or acts. Stating observations often helps the patient communicate without the need for extensive questioning, focusing, or clarification. This technique helps start a conversation with quiet or withdrawn people. Do not state observations that might anger, embarrass, or upset the patient, such as telling someone, "You look like a mess!" Even if such an observation is made with humour, the patient may be offended or feel belittled.

Sharing observations differs from making assumptions, which means drawing unwarranted conclusions about the patient without validating them. Making assumptions puts the patient in the position of having to contradict the nurse. Examples might include the nurse interpreting fatigue as depression or assuming that untouched food indicates lack of interest in meeting nutritional goals. Sharing observations is a gentler approach that involves simply witnessing without making a judgement about what might be happening: "You look tired" is very different from "You look tired. Were you up all night?," which has a judgement attached. "You seem different today" is different from "You seem much better today". Simply stating "I see you are wearing lipstick today" conveys something quite distinct from "You look very beautiful."

Sharing Empathy. Empathy is the ability to emotionally and intellectually understand another person's reality, to accurately perceive unspoken feelings, and to communicate this understanding to the other person (Devito et al., 2015). Empathy is expressed when you seek to explore the perspective of another person. Cultivating the ability to empathize requires patience, a sense of curiosity, and a willingness to understand a patient's context and viewpoint. This requires a relational approach that starts with the willingness to open the relational space and take action. Empathy can also be expressed in relational communication through clear intention, or a consciousness of the purpose and intention of one's communication, and *reflexivity*, which involves paying attention to one's responses and feelings as they influence communication and decision making (Hartrick Doane & Varcoe, 2021). Such empathetic understanding requires you to be self-aware, sensitive, and imaginative, especially if you have not had similar experiences. Statements reflecting empathy are highly effective because they indicate you heard the emotional content, as well as the factual content, of the communication. Empathetic statements are neutral and nonjudgemental and help to validate the patient and establish a trusting relationship. For example, to an angry patient who has limited mobility after a stroke, you might say, "It must be very frustrating to know what you want to do and not be able to do it."

Sharing Hope. Hope is essential for healing, and thus nurses need to learn to communicate a "sense of possibility" to other people. Appropriate encouragement and positive feedback—without minimizing the reality of an illness or instilling false hope—are important in fostering hope and self-confidence. This approach can encourage people to take the steps necessary to reach their goals. As a nurse, you can instill hope by commenting on the positive aspects of the other person's behaviour,

performance, or response. Sharing a vision of the future is a way to reimagine their situation, which can foster hopefulness and creativity through communication. Reminding patients of their internal resources and coping abilities also conveys a sense of hope as a way to establish action and build relationships. You can also reassure patients that many kinds of hope exist, and that meaning and personal growth can arise from illness experiences. For example, you might say the following to a patient discouraged about progressive changes in mobility: "I have seen your courage and creativity in the past and am curious about how you might be preparing for the changes in your abilities now."

Sharing Humour. Humour is an important but underused and under-researched resource in nursing communication that is particularly useful for gaining rapport and building therapeutic alliance and connection (McCreaddie & Wiggins, 2008; Old, 2012). Research suggests that humour is a useful coping strategy for patients, health care providers, and families, and an essential communication tool for nurses, as it can strengthen the helping relationship (Navarro-Carrillo et al., 2020). Humour has been shown to have positive effects on a person's emotional state and physiological state, and it links to many professional nursing values—empathy in particular (Old, 2012; Scheel & Gockel, 2017).

Humour is not without potential communication challenges. It is common for nurses to care for patients from diverse cultures. When nurses interact with patients who communicate in languages other than their own, it is important to acknowledge that nuances of jokes and humour can be misunderstood. Similarly, when either a nurse or a patient attempts to communicate humour while speaking in a language other than that most familiar to them, mistakes and misunderstandings may also occur. Regardless of culture or background, what is humorous to one person may simply be not funny to another.

Health care providers sometimes use negative humour to deal with extreme tension and stress in the workplace, but this can be problematic. What is referred to as "self-defeating" humour constitutes behaviours such as teasing, practical jokes, and sarcasm. "Aggressive" humour speaks to a more grim or dark style of humour, often used in very difficult situations to relieve anxiety or release anger in order to transform negative feelings into something lighter in mood. This humour frequently includes topics such as body fluids, body parts, physical or slapstick humour, and so on (Navarro-Carrillo et al., 2020). This style of humour has a high likelihood of being perceived as tasteless and lacking in caring by people uninvolved in the situation, though it may release stress temporarily for the nurses who use this type of humour. When nurses use dark humour within earshot of patients or their loved ones, great emotional distress can result. When nurses use humour judiciously and carefully, however, in communication with patients, it can be a highly therapeutic strategy.

Sharing Feelings. Emotions are subjective feelings that result from thoughts and perceptions. Feelings are not right, wrong, good, or bad, although they may be experienced as pleasant or unpleasant. Even though withholding feelings can increase stress and exacerbate illness, people may do so in an attempt to ward off unpleasant feelings or adhere to expectations of others or societal norms. Nurses can gently help patients express their emotions by making observations, acknowledging feelings, encouraging communication, giving them permission to express "negative" feelings, and modelling healthy emotional self-expression. At times, patients may direct anger or frustration prompted by their illness toward nurses, who should not take such expressions personally. Acknowledging patients' feelings demonstrates empathy and communicates that you have listened to and understood the emotional aspects of their situation.

When you care for patients, you must be aware of your own emotions because strong feelings may be difficult to hide. Students may wonder whether it is helpful for nurses to share their feelings with patients. Sharing one's feelings makes nurses seem more human and often brings people closer. It is appropriate to share feelings of caring, or even cry with other people, as long as you are in control of the expression of those feelings and do so in a way that does not burden the patient or break confidentiality. Patients are perceptive and can sense nurses' emotions. It is usually inappropriate and may interfere with assessing and caring for patients to discuss one's negative personal emotions, such as anger or sadness, with patients. A social support system of colleagues is helpful, as are strategies for supervision and debriefing; employee assistance programs, peer group meetings, and the use of interprofessional teams such as social work and pastoral care may provide avenues for nurses to safely express feelings away from patients.

Using Touch. Many patients experience feelings of isolation related to their personal and social contexts, as well as the increasing technological features of society more generally. Thus, more than ever, nurses are required to communicate a human connection to their patients. Touch is an important element of communication that conveys many messages, such as affection, emotional support, encouragement, tenderness, and personal attention. People have unique perspectives on touch based on their past experiences and health conditions. For instance, patients in psychosis may misinterpret touch as threatening; patients who have experienced abusive or violent contact from others may be fearful of even well-intentioned touch from a nurse. Touch may also be misinterpreted by some patients as sexual or romantic (Rovers et al., 2018). In response to the patient's lead, holding a hand or offering a gentle touch on the shoulder may, however, be an expression of comfort, reassurance, and care for some, and may convey empathy in situations when words are insufficient (Arnold & Boggs, 2020) (Figure 18.2). Asking for permission or extending touch with consent may be helpful; for example, the nurse may do so by simply stating, "Reach for my arm as we walk, if you like."

Students may initially find that giving intimate care is stressful, especially when caring for patients that are of a similar age to themselves, for example, or perhaps the age of a parent or even someone they may find attractive. Students learn to cope with intimate contact in these circumstances by reflecting on their perception of the situation, remaining directed by patient needs and the required care. Because much of what nurses do involves touch, you must learn to be sensitive to people's reactions to touch and communicate effectively when touch is required. Touch should be as gentle or as firm as needed and delivered in a comforting, nonthreatening manner. In certain situations, you will need to withhold touch, such as when interacting with highly suspicious or angry people who may respond negatively or even violently to being touched.

Using Silence. It takes time and experience to become comfortable with silence. Most people have a natural tendency to fill silences with words, but sometimes silences serve the need to give the nurse and patient time to observe one another, to really *listen*, to sort out their feelings, to think about how to say things, and to consider what has been communicated. Silence is an important skill in the capacity to relate with curiosity, to live with *complexity and uncertainty*, and to relate with the vulnerability of not knowing it all (Hartrick Doane & Varcoe, 2021, p. 141). Silence may provide sufficient space for some patients to talk freely without the constraint of relying on particular patterns of question and answer. Silence allows patients to think and gain insight into their situation, which is crucial to *reimagining* and hope. In general, you should allow the patient to initiate when the silence is to be broken (Austin et al., 2019).

Silence is particularly useful when people are confronted with decisions that require much thought. For example, silence may help a patient gain the confidence needed to share the decision to refuse medical treatment. Silence also allows the nurse to attend to nonverbal messages, such as worried expressions or loss of eye contact. Reflecting or commenting on the silence can relay the nurses' attention and intention for understanding and communicating (Hartrick Doane & Varcoe, 2021). Remaining silent demonstrates the nurse's patience and responsiveness to the patient who may be unable to reply quickly. For example, recall the introductory case study concerning Guy's home care nursing assessment. Silence may be especially therapeutic during times of profound sadness or grief (Bassett et al., 2018) (Box 18.7).

Providing Information. Providing relevant information that the patient needs or wants to know empowers the patient to make informed decisions, experience less anxiety, and feel safe and secure. It is also an integral aspect of health teaching. Hiding information from patients is not usually helpful, particularly when they are seeking it. If a physician withholds information, you need to clarify the reason with the physician. Patients have a right to know about their health status and what is happening in their environment. Information of a distressing

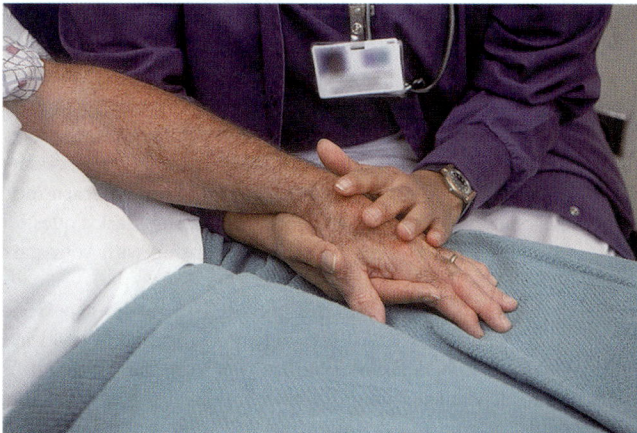

FIGURE 18.2 The nurse uses touch to communicate.

BOX 18.7 CASE STUDY

Communication With a Patient at End of Life

A third-year nursing student (preferred pronouns: she/her) who was assigned to care for a patient at the end of life came to me, as her nursing instructor, to discuss her assignment. The student nurse appeared to be anxious and distraught and was tearful. She requested a change of assignment. When I asked why she felt she needed to be moved, she stated, "I just don't know what I'm supposed to be *doing* with her. She is asking for her family, but they aren't there. She's dying and I just don't know what to do to *help* her." I asked the student what she was doing while she was in the room and she said, "I'm just sitting there holding her hand and listening to her when she's awake. She really isn't talking much, and she drifts off to sleep a lot, but she's afraid of being left alone, so I'm just holding her hand and letting her know I'm there, even when she's sleeping; that way she'll know she's not alone whenever she wakes up. I make sure she's comfortable but I don't know what else she needs. I'm just not *doing* anything." As I looked into her tear-filled eyes, I simply asked her, "So, what makes you think you aren't doing anything?" Communication involves so much more than dialogue. In this case, communication involved very little verbal interaction; it involved active listening, shared empathy, comfort care, gentle touch, silence, presence, and "being with," as the student compassionately accompanied the patient through her final stage of life and assisted with her transition into death.

nature needs to be communicated with sensitivity, at a pace appropriate to what the patient can absorb, and in general terms at first. For example, the nurse may say, "Majid, your heart sounds have changed from earlier today, and so has your blood pressure. I'll let your doctor know." It is important to provide information that enables patients and family members to understand what is happening and what to expect: "Mrs. Ghaed, Majid is getting an echocardiogram right now. This test uses painless sound waves to create a moving picture of Majid's heart structures and valves and should tell us what is causing the murmur."

Clarifying. To check whether understanding is accurate, you should restate an unclear or ambiguous message to clarify the sender's meaning or ask the other person to rephrase it, explain further, or give an example of what they mean. Without clarification, you may make invalid assumptions and miss valuable information. Despite efforts at paraphrasing, you sometimes will still not understand the patient's message and should let the patient know that this is the case. For example, you may say, "I'm not sure I understand what you mean by 'sicker than usual.' What is different now?"

Focusing. Focusing centres on key elements or concepts of a message. If the conversation is vague or rambling or if patients begin to repeat themselves, focusing is a useful technique. Do not use focusing if it interrupts patients while they are discussing an important issue. Rather, use focusing to guide the direction of conversation to important areas: "We've talked a lot about your medications, but let's look more closely at the trouble you're having in taking them on time."

Paraphrasing. Paraphrasing is restating another person's message more briefly in your own words. Through paraphrasing, you let the patient know you are actively involved in the search for understanding. Practice is required to paraphrase accurately. If the meaning of a message is changed or distorted through paraphrasing, communication becomes ineffective. For example, a patient may say, "I've been overweight all my life and never had any problems. I can't understand why I need to be on a diet." Paraphrasing this statement by saying, "You don't care if you're overweight or not," is incorrect and places intentions and ideas that may not be accurate. It would be more accurate to say, "I hear you saying that you're not convinced you need a diet because you've stayed healthy."

Asking Relevant Questions. Nurses ask relevant questions to seek the information needed for decision making. Nurses should ask only one question at a time and fully explore one topic before moving to another area. During patient assessment, questions should follow a logical sequence and proceed from general to more specific. Open-ended questions allow the patient to take the conversational lead and introduce pertinent information about a topic (e.g., "What's your biggest concern now?") Focused questions are used when more specific information is needed in an area (e.g., "How has your pain affected your life at home?") Patients should be allowed to fully respond to an open-ended question before the nurse asks more focused questions. Closed-ended questions elicit yes, no, or one-word responses, such as the question "How many times a day are you taking pain medication?" Although closed-ended questions are helpful during assessment, they are generally less useful during therapeutic exchanges.

Asking too many questions is sometimes dehumanizing. Seeking primarily factual information does not allow you or your patient to establish a meaningful relationship or deal with important emotional issues. It is a way to ignore uncomfortable areas in favour of more comfortable, neutral topics. A useful exercise is to try conversing with another person without asking a single question. By giving general leads ("Tell me about it"), making observations, paraphrasing, focusing, providing information, and so forth, you may discover important information that would have remained hidden if communication were limited primarily to questions.

Summarizing. Summarizing is a concise review of key aspects of an interaction. Summarizing brings a sense of satisfaction and closure to an individual conversation and is especially helpful during the termination phase of a nurse–patient relationship. By reviewing a conversation, participants focus on key issues and add relevant information as needed. Beginning a new interaction by summarizing a previous one helps the patient recall topics discussed and shows the patient that the nurse has analyzed the communication. Summarizing also clarifies expectations, as in the following example of a nurse manager who has been working with a dissatisfied employee: "You've told me a lot of reasons about why you don't like this job and how unhappy you've been. We've also come up with some possible ways to make the situation better, and you've agreed to try some and let me know if any of them help."

Self-Disclosure. Self-disclosures are subjectively true personal experiences about the self that are intentionally revealed to another person. This is not therapy for the nurse; rather, it shows patients that the nurse understands and that their experiences are not unique. You may choose to share experiences or feelings similar to those of the patient and emphasize both the similarities and the differences. This kind of self-disclosure is indicative of the closeness of the nurse–patient relationship and involves a particular kind of respect for the patient. It is offered as an expression of genuineness and honesty and is an aspect of empathy. Self-disclosure should be relevant and appropriate and made to benefit the patient. Self-disclosure should be used sparingly so that the patient remains the focus of the interaction (Steuber & Pollard, 2018). For example, in response to a patient who has suffered a loss, the nurse might say, "That happened to me once, too. I was devastated . . . I went for counselling, and it really helped. What are your thoughts about seeing a counsellor?"

Confrontation. To confront someone in a therapeutic way, you help the other person become more aware of inconsistencies in their feelings, attitudes, beliefs, and behaviours (Moeseneder et al., 2019). Use of this technique improves patient self-awareness and helps the patient recognize growth and deal with important issues. Confrontation should be used only after you have established a trusting relationship with the patient, and it requires gentleness and sensitivity. Asking permission to share an observation can facilitate a confrontation. For example, the nurse might say to a patient who has chronic pain and has decided to forego surgery, "You say you've already decided what to do, but you're still talking a lot about your options."

Nontherapeutic Communication Techniques.

Certain communication techniques hinder or damage professional relationships. These particular techniques are referred to as *nontherapeutic* or *blocking* and will often cause recipients to activate defences to avoid being hurt or negatively affected. Nontherapeutic techniques tend to discourage further expression of feelings and ideas and may engender negative responses or behaviours in other people.

Asking Personal Questions. Asking personal questions that are not relevant to the situation but simply satisfy one's curiosity (e.g., "Why don't you and your partner get married?") is not appropriate professional communication. Such questions are invasive and unnecessary. If patients wish to share private information, they will. To learn more about the patient's interpersonal roles and relationships, ask a question such as "How would you describe your relationship with your partner?"

Giving Personal Opinions. When the nurse provides a personal opinion (e.g., "If I were you, I'd put your dependent adult child in a group home"), it takes decision making away from the patient. It inhibits spontaneity, stalls problem solving, and creates doubt. Personal opinions differ from professional advice. At times, patients need suggestions and help to make choices. Suggestions should be presented to patients as options because the final decision rests with the patient. Remember that the problem and its solution belong to the patient. A much better response is saying, "Let's talk about what options are available for your older child's care as well as yours."

Changing the Subject. When another person is trying to communicate something important, changing the subject (e.g., "Let's not talk about your problems with your job. It's time for your walk") is rude and shows a lack of empathy and mutuality. It tends to block further communication, and the sender then withholds important messages or fails to openly express feelings. Thoughts and spontaneity are interrupted, ideas become tangled, and information provided may be inadequate. In some instances, changing the subject serves as a face-saving manoeuvre. If this happens, reassure the patient that you will return to their concerns: "After your walk, let's talk some more about what's going on with your job."

Automatic Responses. Stereotypes (e.g., "Older persons are always confused" or "Administration doesn't care about the staff") and labels are generalized beliefs held about people. A cliché is a generalizing comment such as "You can't win them all" that tends to dismiss the other person's feelings and minimize the importance of their message. These automatic responses communicate that you are not taking concerns seriously or responding thoughtfully. Another kind of automatic response is parroting, repeating what the other person has said, word for word. Parroting is easily overused and is not as effective as paraphrasing. Automatic remarks about other people lead to assumptions and closed communication, which reflect poor nursing judgement and may well threaten nurse–patient or nurse–team relationships. Nurses may get in the habit of making these automatic remarks as a defence mechanism or to compartmentalize and organize their work. Observation of one's habitual techniques and approaches is key to self-awareness and communication with others (Beauchamp & Baran, 2019).

A nurse who is excessively task oriented automatically makes the task or procedure the central focus of interaction with patients, missing opportunities to communicate with patients as individuals and meet their needs. When you first perform technical tasks, you may have difficulty integrating therapeutic communication because of your need to focus on the procedure. In time, you will learn to integrate communication with high-visibility tasks and accomplish several goals—including relational inquiry—simultaneously.

False Reassurance. When a patient is seriously ill or distressed, you may be tempted to offer hope to the patient with statements such as "Don't worry, everything will be all right," "You'll be fine," or "You have nothing to worry about." When a patient is reaching for understanding, false reassurance discourages open communication. Offering reassurance that is not supported by facts or based in reality typically does more harm than good. Although you may be attempting to be kind, such reassurance has the secondary effect of helping you avoid the patient's distress, tends to block conversation, and discourages further expression of feelings. A more relational nursing response is saying, "It must be difficult not to know what the surgeon will find. What might be helpful to you at this time?"

Sympathy. **Sympathy** is a feeling of concern, sorrow, sadness, or pity for the patient generated by personal identification with the patient's needs (Sinclair et al., 2018). Sympathy is a subjective vision of another person's viewpoint that prevents a clear perspective of the issues confronting that person. If you overidentify with the patient (e.g., "I'm so sorry about your mastectomy; it must be terrible to lose a breast"), then you will lose objectivity and be unable to effectively help the patient work through their situation (Arnold & Boggs, 2020). Although sympathy is a compassionate response to another's situation, it may not be as responsive and therapeutic as empathy (Sinclair et al., 2018). A more empathetic approach is saying, "The loss of a breast is a major change. How do you think it will affect your life?"

Asking for Explanations. You may be tempted to ask your patient to explain why they believe, feel, or have acted in a certain way (e.g., "Why are you so anxious?"). Patients frequently interpret "why" questions as accusations or think you already know the reason and are simply testing them. "Why" questions tend to interrupt patients' descriptions of their feelings and experience and cause them to refocus their energy on providing intellectual or defensive responses (Shattell & Hogan, 2005). Regardless of your motivation, "why" questions can cause resentment, insecurity, and mistrust. If you require additional information, it is best to phrase questions to avoid using "why." For example, saying, "You seem upset. What's on your mind?" or "Tell me about how you are feeling today compared with yesterday," is more likely to help the anxious patient communicate.

Approval or Disapproval. Avoid imposing your personal attitudes, values, beliefs, and moral standards on other people while in the professional helping role (e.g., "You shouldn't even think about assisted suicide; it's not right"). Other people have the right to speak their minds and make their own decisions. Judgemental responses often contain terms such as *should, ought, good, bad, right,* and *wrong.* Agreeing or disagreeing conveys the subtle message that you are making value judgements about the patient's decisions. Approving implies that the behaviour being praised is the only acceptable one. Often the patient shares a decision not to seek approval but rather to provide a means to discuss feelings. On the other hand, disapproving implies that the patient needs to meet your expectations or standards. Instead, help patients explore their own beliefs and decisions.

Defensive Responses. Becoming defensive in response to criticism (e.g., "No one here would intentionally lie to you") implies that the other person has no right to an opinion. The sender's concerns are ignored when you focus on the need for self-defence, defence of the health care team, or defence of other people. When patients express criticism, it is important to listen to what they have to say. Listening does not imply agreement. To discover reasons for a patient's anger or dissatisfaction, you must listen without defensiveness, judgement, or criticism. By avoiding defensiveness, you can defuse anger and uncover deeper concerns: "It sounds as if you believe people have been dishonest with you. That must make it difficult for you to trust anyone."

Passive or Aggressive Responses. Passive responses (e.g., "Things are bad, and I can't do anything about it") serve to avoid conflict or sidestep issues. They reflect feelings of sadness, depression, anxiety, powerlessness, and hopelessness. Aggressive responses (e.g., "Things are bad, and it's all your fault") provoke confrontation at the other person's expense and reflect feelings of anger, frustration, resentment, and stress. When nurses lack assertiveness skills, they may also use triangulation, complaining to a third party rather than confronting the problem or expressing concerns directly to the source. This lowers team morale and draws other people into the conflict situation. Assertive communication establishes boundaries and expectations without the blame or judgement implied in passive and aggressive responses. An assertive approach imparts intention and action that will support the ongoing professional therapeutic relationship.

Arguing. Challenging or arguing against perceptions (e.g., "How can you say you didn't sleep a wink when I heard you snoring all night long?") denies that they are real and valid to the other person. They imply that the other person is lying, misinformed, or uneducated. Skillful nurses give information or present reality in a way that avoids argument: "You feel as if you didn't get any rest at all last night, even though I thought you slept well because you seemed peaceful when I checked your room during the night."

Adapting Communication Techniques for Patients With Special Needs.
The temporary or permanent loss of the ability to speak is

extremely traumatic to an individual. It is important to assess a patient's alternative communication method and whether it causes anxiety in the patient. Patients who have undergone laryngectomies often write notes, use communication boards or laptop computers, speak with mechanical vibrators, or use esophageal speech. Patients with endotracheal or tracheostomy tubes have a temporary loss of speech. Most use a notepad to write their questions and requests. However, the patient may become incapacitated and unable to write messages. You need to determine whether the patient has developed a sign language or system of symbols to communicate needs. If not, you may need to assist the patient in developing a meaningful method during a new or temporary loss of communication.

Interacting effectively with patients who have conditions that impair communication requires special thought, sensitivity, creativity, and responsiveness. Such patients benefit greatly when you adapt communication techniques to their unique circumstances or developmental level. For example, if you are caring for a patient with impaired verbal communication related to mechanical ventilation, you can provide a visual table or construct a coded hand signal to exchange necessary communication. You and the patient can use such tools to help communicate for assessment and interventions. Similar techniques can be used with patients suffering with aphasia or some dementias.

Patients experiencing aphasia may be unable to produce or understand language. Expressive aphasia, a motor type of aphasia, is the inability to name common objects or to express simple ideas in words or writing. For example, a patient may understand a question but be unable to express an answer. Sensory or receptive aphasia is the inability to understand written or spoken language. The patient may be able to express words but is unable to understand the questions or comments of others. Global aphasia is the inability to understand language or communicate orally.

When caring for patients with special needs regarding communication, you need to direct nursing actions toward meeting the goals and expected outcomes identified in the plan of care, addressing both the communication impairment and its contributing factors. Box 18.8 lists many methods available to encourage, enhance, restore, or substitute for verbal communication. You must be sure that the patient is physically able to use the chosen method and that it does not cause frustration by being too complicated or difficult.

◆ Evaluation

To determine whether the plan of care has been successful, both the nurse and patient evaluate the patient's communication outcomes. You

---

BOX 18.8   Communicating With Patients Who Have Special Needs

Patients Who Cannot Speak Clearly (Aphasia, Dysarthria, Muteness)
- Listen attentively, be patient, and do not interrupt.
- Ask simple questions that require yes or no answers.
- Allow time for understanding and response.
- Use visual cues (e.g., words, pictures, and objects) when possible.
- Allow only one person to speak at a time.
- Do not shout or speak too loudly.
- Encourage the patient to converse.
- If you have not understood the patient, let them know.
- Collaborate with a speech therapist as needed.
- Use communication aids:
  - Pad and felt-tipped pen or Magic Slate
  - Communication board with commonly used words, letters, or pictures denoting basic needs
  - Call bells or alarms
  - Sign language
  - Use of eye blinks or movement of fingers for simple responses ("yes" or "no")

Patients Who Are Cognitively Impaired
- Reduce environmental distractions while conversing.
- Capture the patient's attention before you speak.
- Use simple sentences and avoid long explanations.
- Ask one question at a time.
- Allow time for the patient to respond.
- Be an attentive listener.
- Include family and friends in conversations, especially on topics known to the patient.

Patients Who Are Hearing Impaired
- Check for the presence of hearing aids.
- Reduce environmental noise.
- Get the patient's attention before you speak.
- Face the patient so that your mouth is visible.
- Do not chew gum.

- Speak at normal volume; do not shout.
- Rephrase rather than repeat, if your message is misunderstood.
- Provide a sign language interpreter if this is indicated.

Patients Who Are Visually Impaired
- Check for use of glasses or contact lenses.
- Identify yourself when you enter the room and notify the patient when you leave the room.
- Speak in a normal tone of voice.
- Do not rely on gestures or nonverbal communication to convey messages.
- Use indirect lighting, avoiding glare.
- Use an appropriate font size for the impairment (i.e., at least 14-point print).

Patients Who Are Unresponsive
- Call the patient by name during interactions.
- Communicate both verbally and by touch.
- Speak to the patient as though they can hear.
- Explain all procedures and expected sensations.
- Provide orientation to person, place, and time.
- Avoid talking about the patient to other people in their presence.
- Avoid saying things that the patient should not hear (e.g., gossip or speculations about patient's condition).
- Always assume that patients can hear and understand everything said at their bedside.

Patients Who Do Not Speak English
- Speak to the patient in a normal tone of voice (shouting may be interpreted as anger).
- Establish a method for the patient to signal a desire to communicate (call light or bell).
- Provide an interpreter (translator) as needed.
- Develop communication board, pictures, or cards.
- Translate words from the English list into the patient's preferred language for the patient to make basic requests.
- Ensure that a dictionary (English–French, English–Blackfoot, and so forth) is available if the patient can read.

BOX 18.9 Sample Communication Analysis

NURSE: Good morning, to patient. [Smiles and approaches bed, holding clipboard]
- Social greeting to begin conversation

PATIENT: What's good about it? [Arms crossed over chest, frowning, with a direct stare]
- Nonverbal signs of anger

NURSE: You sound unhappy. [Pulls up chair and sits at bedside]
- Sharing observation, nonverbal communication of availability

PATIENT: You'd be unhappy, too, if nobody would answer your questions. [Angry tone of voice, challenging expression]
- Further expression of feelings, facilitated by nurse's accurate observation

NURSE: This hospital has a fine staff. I'm sure no one would intentionally keep information from you.
- Feeling threatened and being defensive: a nontherapeutic technique

PATIENT: All right, then: Why wouldn't that technician tell me what my blood sugar was?

NURSE: I'm not sure. If I were you, I'd forget about it and get a fresh start.
- Giving advice and using cliché, which is nontherapeutic; would have been better to acknowledge that the patient had a right to know the information

NURSE: I'm going to test your blood sugar levels in a minute, and I'll tell you the results. [Performs test] Your blood sugar level was 20.
- Providing information, demonstrating trustworthiness

PATIENT: That's up pretty high, isn't it? [Worried facial expression]
- Feeling very concerned about test results

NURSE: [Nods; long pause]
- Nonverbal affirmation, use of silence to allow patient time to absorb information and gather thoughts

PATIENT: I'm so afraid complications will set in because my blood sugar is high. [Stares out window]
- Feeling free to express deeper concerns, which are hard to face

NURSE: What kinds of things are you worried about?
- Open-ended question to elicit information

PATIENT: I could lose a leg, like one of my parents did. Or go blind. Or have to live hooked up to a kidney machine for the rest of my life.

NURSE: You've been thinking about all kinds of things that could go wrong, and it adds to your worry not to be told what your blood sugar is.
- Summarizing to let patient "hear" what he has communicated

PATIENT: I always think the worst. [Shakes head in exasperation]
- Expressing insight into his "inner dialogue"

NURSE: I'll pass along to the technician that it's okay to tell you your blood sugar levels. And later this afternoon, I'd like us to talk more about some things you can do to help avoid these complications and set some goals for controlling your blood sugar. [Stands up, keeps looking at patient]
- Providing information, encouraging collaboration and goal setting; giving nonverbal cue that conversation is nearing end

PATIENT: Okay, I'll see you later.

---

need to evaluate nursing interventions to determine what strategies or interventions were effective and what changes in the patient's situation resulted because of the interventions. For example, if using pen and paper proves frustrating for a nonverbal patient whose handwriting is shaky, you need to revise the care plan to include use of a picture board instead. If expected outcomes are not met or progress is not satisfactory, you need to determine what factors influenced the outcomes and then modify the plan.

You can evaluate the effectiveness of your own communication by videotaping practice sessions with peers, making recordings, and analyzing written records of your verbal and nonverbal interactions with patients. Process recording analysis reveals faults in personal communication techniques, enabling you to improve your communication effectiveness. Box 18.9 contains a sample communication analysis of such a record. Analyzing a process recording enables you to evaluate the following:
- Determine whether the nurse encouraged openness and allowed the patient to "tell their story," expressing both thoughts and feelings
- Identify any missed verbal or nonverbal cues or conversational themes
- Examine whether nursing responses blocked or facilitated the patient's efforts to communicate
- Determine whether nursing responses were positive and supportive or superficial and judgemental
- Examine the type and number of questions that were asked
- Determine the type and number of therapeutic communication techniques used, and
- Discover any missed opportunities to use humour, silence, or touch.
Evaluation of the communication process helps you gain confidence and competence in interpersonal skills. Becoming an effective communicator greatly increases your professional satisfaction and success. No skill is more basic, and no tool more powerful, than communication.

KEY CONCEPTS

- Communication is a powerful therapeutic tool and an essential nursing skill used to influence other people and achieve positive health care outcomes.
- Relational inquiry depends on approaches to communication that enhance the nurse's capacity to be in relation to patients in their unique contexts and often highly uncertain and difficult circumstances.
- Communication involves the entire human being: body, mind, emotions, and spirit.
- Critical thinking facilitates communication through creative inquiry, focused self-awareness, reflexivity, empathy, and awareness of other people, as well as the intentionality of purposeful analysis and control of perceptual biases.
- Nurses consider many of the contexts and factors influencing communication when making decisions about what, when, where, how, why, and with whom to communicate.
- Nurses use intrapersonal, interpersonal, transpersonal, small group, and public interaction to achieve positive change and health goals.
- Communication is most effective when the receiver and sender accurately perceive the meaning of each other's messages.
- Message transmission is influenced by the sender's and receiver's physical and developmental status, perceptions, values, emotions, knowledge, sociocultural background, roles, and environment.
- Effective verbal communication requires appropriate vocabulary, intonation, clear and concise phrasing, proper pacing of statements, and proper timing and relevance of a message.
- Nonverbal communication often conveys the true meaning of a message more accurately than verbal communication.

- Helping relationships are strengthened when the nurse demonstrates caring by establishing trust, empathy, autonomy, confidentiality, and professional competence.
- Effective communication skills are facilitative and tend to encourage the other person to openly express ideas, feelings, or concerns.
- Ineffective communication techniques are inhibitive and tend to block the other person's willingness to openly express ideas, feelings, or concerns.
- The nurse must blend social and informational interactions with therapeutic communication skills so that other people can explore feelings and manage health issues.
- Older persons with sensory, motor, or cognitive impairments require the adaptation of communication techniques to compensate for their loss of function and special needs.
- Patients with impaired verbal communication require special consideration and alterations in communication techniques to facilitate the sending, receiving, and interpreting of messages.
- Desired outcomes for patients with impaired verbal communication include increased satisfaction with interpersonal interactions, the ability to send and receive clear messages, and attention to and accurate interpretation of verbal and nonverbal cues.

CRITICAL THINKING EXERCISES

1. An Indigenous Elder (preferred pronouns: she/her) who is a member of the Haida community of Atewaas must learn how to manage her diabetes mellitus and self-administer insulin injections. Considering the elements of critical thinking for communication, what communication approaches and skills could you use to help her?

2. A nurse colleague (preferred pronouns: she/her) of yours is having difficulty interacting assertively with Dr. Fielding (they), a physician who has an abrupt, intimidating communication style. The nurse frequently complains of tension headaches, pent-up anger, and crying easily. What can you do to help your colleague?

3. A patient (preferred pronouns: he/him) with Parkinson's disease who is living at a long-term care facility has a stiff, expressionless face from this disease. The patient sits slumped in a recliner chair all day and seems lost in his own world, rarely looking at or interacting with anyone. When he does talk, he mumbles in a soft voice, and his words are difficult to understand. What communication skills would support the nurse's relational inquiry with this patient?

4. A member (preferred pronouns: she/her) of a Hutterite colony in Western Canada is considering whether she should have her two young children immunized before they begin attending school. What communication skills could the nurse use to help her make this decision, and what traps does the nurse need to avoid in communication about information and decision making?

5. A patient (preferred pronouns: he/him) who is receiving palliative care confides in you that he feels overwhelmed by the number of issues he must attend to now that he's facing the possibility of death. He says, "My thoughts are all over the place. I don't know where to start." What communication skills, based on the critical thinking model, can the nurse use to help the patient at this point?

🌐 *Answers to Critical Thinking Exercises appear on the Evolve website.*

REVIEW QUESTIONS

Review Questions 1 to 10 relate to the case study at the beginning of the chapter.

1. Which of the following statements best explains how communication is not about the message intended by Marie-France in her home care assessment, but rather about the message received by Guy?
   a. Clear communication ensures that Guy will receive the message intended.
   b. Authenticity in communication is the responsibility of Marie-France and Guy.
   c. Attention to personal space (physically and emotionally) can minimize Guy's misinterpretation of Marie-France's communication.
   d. Contextual factors, such as Marie-France's attitudes, values, beliefs, and self-concept, influence relational capacity and communication.

2. Marie-France can demonstrate active listening by:
   a. Agreeing with Guy
   b. Repeating everything Guy says in order to clarify
   c. Assuming a relaxed posture, establishing eye contact, and leaning toward Guy in conversation
   d. Smiling and nodding continuously throughout the interview

3. During the orientation phase of the helping relationship, nurse Marie-France:
   a. Discusses the garden and woodwork projects in Guy's yard and home
   b. Works together with Guy to establish goals
   c. Reviews Guy's history to identify possible home care needs
   d. Uses therapeutic communication to manage Guy's memory loss

4. It would be most helpful for a nurse working with a patient who has expressive aphasia to:
   a. Ask open-ended questions
   b. Speak loudly and use simple sentences
   c. Allow extra time for the patient to respond
   d. Encourage a family member to answer for the patient

5. Communication for Guy's (the patient's) plan of care requires that Marie-France:
   a. Collaborate with other interprofessional colleagues and Guy's family to provide combined expertise in planning care
   b. Consult Guy's family physician for direction in establishing goals for the patient
   c. Depend on the latest literature to complete an excellent plan of care for patients with aphasia
   d. Work independently to plan and deliver care without depending on other staff for assistance

6. Marie-France asks Guy, "When you talk about your vision changes, I'm not sure I understand what you mean by 'more difficult than usual.' What is different now?" This reflects the therapeutic technique of:
   a. Paraphrasing
   b. Providing information
   c. Clarifying
   d. Focusing

7. During her communication with Guy, Marie-France says, "We've talked a lot about your immediate home care needs, but let's look more closely at the longer-term care plans for you and for your dependent adult child." This example demonstrates the therapeutic communication skill of:
   a. Paraphrasing
   b. Providing information

c. Clarifying
d. Focusing

8. Marie-France supports herself and her challenging community nursing practice with positive messages about her capacities. This demonstrates communication at the _____ level.
   a. Public
   b. Intrapersonal
   c. Interpersonal
   d. Transpersonal

9. As a nurse working in the community with older persons, Marie-France is advised to avoid:
   a. Touching an agitated patient
   b. Shifting from subject to subject

c. Allowing the patient to reminisce
d. Asking the patient how they feel

10. When completing the patient's health history, Marie-France should acknowledge the appropriate zone of personal space and touch as being:
    a. 0 to 45 cm from the patient
    b. 45 cm to 1 m from the patient
    c. 1 to 4 m from the patient
    d. 4 m or farther from the patient

Answers: 1. d; **2.** c; **3.** a; **4.** c; **5.** a; **6.** c; **7.** d; **8.** b; **9.** b; **10.** b.

Rationales for the Review Questions appear on the Evolve website.

RECOMMENDED WEBSITES

Canadian Hearing Services: https://www.chs.ca/accessibility
This webpage links to services to support effective communication for the Deaf and hearing impaired in Canada, including interpreting services, captioning services, communication devices, and deafblind services.

Communicative Disorders Assistant Association of Canada: https://cdaac.ca/external-resources
This website provides links to various Canadian and international resources for people with conditions that affect communication.

Medscape: https://www.medscape.com
Medscape is a resource for physicians and nurses that requires a one-time registration (free of charge) and offers links to current literature on numerous health care topics. Enter "Communication" in the search frame, and the site will list current articles on communication in health care.

Registered Nurses' Association of Ontario (RNAO)—Establishing Therapeutic Relationships Best Practice Guideline: https://rnao.ca/bpg/guidelines/establishing-therapeutic-relationships
This RNAO Best Practice Guideline addresses the therapeutic relationship and its central importance to nursing practice.

Signing Savvy—American Sign Language Dictionary: https://www.signingsavvy.com/search
This website provides an English and manual alphabet and dictionary, articles about deafness, and one-on-one tutoring.

REFERENCES

A full reference list is available on the website for this book at http://evolve.elsevier.com/Canada/Potter/fundamentals/

19

Client-Centred Care: Interprofessional Collaborative Practice

Written by Carole Orchard, BSN, MEd, EdD

OBJECTIVES

Mastery of content in this chapter will enable you to:

- Define the key terms listed.
- Challenge your existing values and understand how these relate to nursing professional values.
- Explore how knowledge is gained and used.
- Understand how personal and professional ways of knowing shape how you approach and provide nursing care.
- Explore how to integrate your growing nursing professional identity with that of an interprofessional identity.
- Explore your personal ways of knowing and how integrating them supports you in learning how to be a professional nurse and provide care to clients.
- Understand the frameworks that guide what nursing professional practice entails.
- Begin developing skills in client-centred practice using a judgement framework within the context of a case study.
- Explore how to work within interprofessional teams as a new professional nurse.
- Reflect on how your values, knowledge, skills, and judgements have evolved through your learning in this chapter.

KEY TERMS

Action
Aesthetic knowing
Analytic interpreting
Antecedents
Assessment
Behaviourism
Client-centred care
Clinical decision-making process
Collaborative leadership
Constructed knowing
Context
Empirical knowing
Entry-to-practice competencies
Ethical knowing
Evaluation
Feeling

Interprofessional client-centred collaborative practice
Interprofessional communication
Interprofessional team conflict resolution
Intervention
Intuitive interpreting
Narrative interpreting
Norms
Noticing
Nursing process
Patterns of knowing
Perception
Personal knowing
Planning
Procedural knowing
Received knowing

Reflection
Reflection-in-action
Reflection-on-action
Responding
Role clarification
Silence
Situation–background–assessment–recommendation (SBAR) technique
Social contact theory
Socialization
Subjective knowing
Team conflict
Team functioning
Thought
Values
Ways of knowing

WEBSITE

http://evolve.elsevier.com/Canada/Potter/fundamentals/

This chapter uses the term "client-centred" throughout. In the interprofessional field of study, it is always a conundrum as to which term to use to describe recipients of care. The use of "patient" is preferred by medicine, pharmacy, and nursing in acute care areas, while "client" is preferred by social work, occupational health, and physiotherapy; "client" is also preferred by nursing when it is practised in a community setting. Individuals who are the recipients of our care often see themselves as "patients." However, when discussing interprofessional practice, often both the client and a family member or caregiver may be involved in the care. Therefore, using the term "persons" seems more appropriate, but it is still not the norm among health care providers. Therefore, throughout this chapter, we use the term "client."

It would be remiss for a chapter titled "Client-Centred Care" not to begin with the story of a client*—in this case, Jane Black and her

---

* In this chapter, the term "client" is used to denote the persons who are the recipients of nursing care. Other terms often used in the literature include patient, service user, and, at times, consumer.

family. Nurses need to understand clients' stories, or the reasons why clients are seeking nursing help in their care. These stories must be rich enough for nurses to gain an appreciation for the complex health and social issues many clients are faced with. The failure to learn a client's full story may interfere with the effectiveness of nursing care and with a client's capacity to reach health outcomes that are realistic for their situation. Here you will meet Mrs. Black and her family. Through her story, you will learn how to make your nursing care truly client and family centred.

CASE STUDY

Jane Black (preferred pronouns: she/her) is a 32-year-old parent of three who has just been admitted to the hospital unit that you are working on today. She is 22 weeks pregnant and has been diagnosed with diabetes. Mrs. Black was found at home by her partner after she became drowsy and was having difficulty focusing. She has an intravenous line (IV) of 5% dextrose in water (D5W) running and was given a loading dose of insulin. Since she is a newly diagnosed diabetic who is also pregnant, she has been hospitalized by Dr. Johansen. Mrs. Black's three children (aged 3, 5, and 7) have come to the hospital with her and her partner because there is no one at home to take care of them. Mr. Black is a long-distance truck driver who is frequently on the road. He is next scheduled to leave in 2 days. Mrs. Black is a stay-at-home parent who is devoted to her children.

The family lives in a three-bedroom apartment that they rent. In talking to Mr. Black, you learn that his daughter (the 7-year-old; preferred pronouns: she/her) has cystic fibrosis (CF). Mr. Black says that Mrs. Black spends a great deal of time ensuring that their daughter's lungs remain as clear as possible. Mr. Black asks if there is anywhere to smoke. You notice that he has tobacco-stained fingers. He also is somewhat overweight. Mr. Black expresses his concern to you about how he will manage the children's care with Mrs. Black in the hospital, and he wonders how quickly Mrs. Black can be discharged home.

Mrs. Black informs you that she has weakness on the right side of her body because of a previous "small stroke" she had about 5 years ago. She tells you she is worried about whether she has to take insulin by injection because she is right-handed and has not had full use of her right hand since the stroke. Mrs. Black goes on to share that she is often incredibly thirsty and has had urinary frequency (having to void often) for a while but thought it was related to her pregnancy. She also tells you that her mother is a diabetic. She shares that her mother has had many problems with her eyesight and that her mother's doctor recently told her mother that her kidneys were starting to fail.

Think about this case study as you read this chapter. There are Review Questions at the end of the chapter about this case study.

Adapted from Interprofessional Health Education and Research. (2014). *Case of Jane Black*. Western University. From a webpage formerly available at http://www.ipe.uwo.ca/Administration/CaseScenarios/Case%20of%20Jane%20Black.pdf. Reprinted with permission.

In the case study of Mrs. Black, you can see that the complex interplay of the family and their social issues are affected by environmental factors, including housing, finances, parenting, and child-rearing needs. By focusing only on the immediate needs of Mrs. Black, you as the nurse would be neglecting the many other factors that are affecting this family because of Mrs. Black's illness. Therefore, when nurses provide client-centred care, they must integrate multiple dimensions into their practice. As you move through this chapter, you will explore how you can prepare yourself to be able to address stories such as Mrs. Black's. This story is woven throughout the chapter as a way of assisting you to understand how nursing care decisions are made to be client centred.

KNOWING

As you progress in shaping your nursing practice, you will use both your *personal ways of knowing* (Belenky et al., 1986) as well as your *professional patterns of knowing* (Carper, 1978). Each of these terms is discussed in detail the following sections.

Ways of Knowing

Becoming a professional nurse requires that you first look deeply within yourself because the values you bring with you into your nursing studies influence will your future nursing practice. The way you "know" what you know is influenced by how you look at issues and address them. Belenky et al. (1986) carried out a study of women's approaches to how they develop their self, voice, and mind. The authors determined that there are five **ways of knowing**: silence, received knowing, subjective knowing, procedural knowing, and constructed knowing.

Through **silence**, people "feel passive, reactive, and dependent, they see authorities as being all-powerful, if not overpowering" (Belenky et al., 1986, p. 27). For instance, if Mrs. Black used silence, she would listen to whatever you as her nurse told her and would do as you wished. However, she would not question why because she would see you as an authority that she must obey. Therefore, it would be difficult for her to enter into a relationship with you that is client centred, unless you were able to encourage her to participate in her care with you. In order to provide Mrs. Black with client-centred care, you would need to establish a partnership between the two of you in a way that allowed you to learn from one other.

Nurses whose knowing relates to **received knowing** believe what they know based on what they hear, and thus they learn through listening. For example, when you take notes in a class and only memorize those notes and then repeat the notes back in your reflections, you are practising received knowing. If you asked Mrs. Black to repeat the instruction you provided to her and she was able to do this but did not question why this was important to her care, she might be using received knowing. Again, this would not be the true partnership that is needed for client-centred care to occur. In order to establish a true partnership, you would need to encourage Mrs. Black to share how her life situation will affect her ability to do what you are guiding her to do.

If you as a nurse listen to what others say and then internalize it to assess its meaning to you, then you are practising **subjective knowing**. For example, if Mrs. Black shared that she was wondering how she might be able to care for herself at home, she might be demonstrating subjective knowing. Mrs. Black would therefore be more likely to be able to participate with you in making decisions about her care, allowing for a partnership to be created. When this internalization becomes an internal debate as to the personal meaning of what you heard, then you are beginning to use your **procedural knowing**. For example, if Mrs. Black then debated the importance of being at home to care for her daughter with CF, while also realizing that this new diagnosis of diabetes means she could not fulfill this role herself—leading her to explore who might be able to provide her daughter's care at home—she might be demonstrating procedural knowing. In this form of knowing, you are beginning to identify what your assumptions are and how these relate to your own values. If Mrs. Black were using procedural knowing, then a partnership between the two of you would be a likely way of working together.

Finally, when you are able to compare what you have heard against your own beliefs and challenge your own assumptions and those of others, you have moved into **constructed knowing**. If Mrs. Black were using constructed knowing, she might identify which aspects of her daughter's care could be provided by different family members at home. She could then develop in her mind a plan for discussing their respective roles to achieve the total care that needs to be provided to her daughter while she is incapacitated. Again, a partnership between you can be achieved without modifying your interaction with the client. When the more active forms of knowing (received, procedural, and constructive) provide the means for a nurse–client partnership to be established, this allows for client-centred care to occur.

While nursing professional practice requires nurses to use their procedural and constructed knowing, it is important to remember that clients are not always operating using the same ways of knowing. The success of nursing care with such clients requires that nurses explore with them the story that brought them to the hospital in order to gain insight into how the client arrived at the decision to seek help. This will allow you as a nurse to determine how you might develop a relationship with your client and create a client-centred partnership.

In summary, knowing by *receiving knowledge* means deferring to an "authority figure" and accepting without debate what that person tells you. Knowing by *procedural knowing* means receiving knowledge from others but also considering how this knowledge relates to your own understanding. Knowing by *constructing knowledge* means experiencing something and then considering its meaning not only to you but also to others; you also listen to others and consider their perspectives, then assess this in relation to yourself.

In applying these ways of knowing to your own nursing practice, you might consider reflecting on the following questions:

- How do you currently know? By being silent, by receiving knowledge, by perceiving knowledge, or by constructing knowledge?
- What action might you need to take to move yourself into a deeper way of knowing?
- What way of knowing does Mrs. Black present in her story? What impact could it have on how you partner with her?

Professional Patterns of Knowing

As you develop into the nurse you wish to be, you will expand your ways of knowing beyond those just identified. Carper (1978) identified four **patterns of knowing** that are essential to nursing knowledge development: empirical knowing, or "the science of nursing"; aesthetic knowing, or "the art of nursing"; personal knowing; and ethical knowing, or "moral knowledge in nursing" (p. 14).

Empirical Knowing. As you learn about the theories and findings of the research studies that underpin nursing practice, your understanding of how you can implement client-centred nursing practice will expand. When the knowledge you apply to your practice arises from the findings of exploratory, descriptive, or inferential studies that have influenced nursing practice, you will be generating knowledge to guide your **clinical decision-making process** around a pattern of knowing referred to as **empirical knowing**.

However, as Carper and others remind us, this is but one pattern of knowing that nurses use. It does align with much of the research evidence applied in evidence-informed practice, but it also may be limited when it does not include the complex health and social aspects of families that influence how a client responds to such approaches. This does not mean that empirical knowing is not valuable to nursing practice. Rather, it is only one aspect of nursing patterns of knowing.

Aesthetic Knowing. The way we begin to shape our approaches to nursing care using empirical knowing allows us to reflect on our comfort levels. This is where our personalities and approaches to creating relationships with others come into play. Returning to Mrs. Black and her family, you might approach her daughter with CF who is visiting her mother, squat down to her eye level, and ask her how she is doing and how her breathing is today. Then you might ask her daughter what

she has been able to do on her own to help with her breathing. You do this because you know from working with children that they like to participate in adult conversations and share what they are doing rather than be told what to do. This scenario illustrates how to integrate empirical knowledge about the impact of CF on lung capacity with an aesthetic pattern of knowing how to approach children. Another nurse might like to use drawing, and so they encourage the daughter to draw a picture of how she is feeling today. This action may result in different information being gained. Hence, there is no single way to use an aesthetic pattern of knowing. When you are able to use your own comfort level to develop relationships with your clients and their families, you are more likely to be seen as genuine. Genuineness forms the basis for trust. Hence, **aesthetic knowing** relates to how you, as a unique individual, choose to respond in a client situation. It is a unique reflection of your personality and your creativity.

Personal Knowing. How we use our aesthetic pattern of knowing is also based on our pattern of **personal knowing**. Our personal pattern reflects the knowledge that we bring into our nursing understanding that has been accumulated thus far from our lived experiences. Our means of interacting with others, our body movements, our expressions of emotions, the values that influence the way we view our nursing practice, and our interactions with clients, families, and other health care providers create our personal pattern of knowing. Carper (1978) states that, in essence, personal knowing "involves interactions, relationships and transactions between the nurse and the patient–client" (p. 18). Whether practising at the procedural or constructed level of knowing, using empirical and aesthetic patterns of knowing, we are influenced by our personal pattern of knowing.

Ethical Knowing. How we select from our empirical, aesthetic, and personal patterns of knowing is also influenced by our pattern of **ethical knowing**, which is initially shaped by our own values. **Values** are ideals that have significant meaning or importance to you as a person, to your family, or to your community (Keatings & Smith, 2009, p. 16). They arise from a person's cultural, societal, or family norms and shape an individual's morality—that is, what one knows to be right or wrong. In the nursing profession, all members need to have a similar set of nursing professional values. These values form the basis of the nursing profession's code of ethics. One of the characteristics of a profession is having a code of ethics. The Canadian Nurses Association (CNA) *Code of Ethics* (Canadian Nurses Association, 2017, p. 3) includes the following values:

- Providing safe, compassionate, competent, and ethical care
- Promoting health and well-being
- Promoting and respecting informed decision making
- Honouring dignity
- Maintaining privacy and confidentiality
- Promoting justice, and
- Being accountable.

You will need to integrate these values into your own personal values as you socialize yourself to being a professional nurse. These values begin to shape how you approach the care of your clients. You will also need to consider whether any of your own personal values are at odds with nursing professional values, then spend time trying to understand this disjuncture and how you will set aside your own contrary values to ensure that when you practise as a professional nurse, you are not neglecting any of the nursing *Code of Ethics* values in caring for clients.

Now let's go back to our client, Mrs. Black, and your initial "judgement" of the family and their situation. After considering your nursing values, have you changed any of your initial judgements about Mrs. Black and her family? If so, which of the nursing values does this shift in judgement relate to? How will you ensure that the judgement you

TABLE 19.1	Nursing Practice Standards
Standard	**Statement of Standard**
1. Accountability	Each nurse is accountable to the public and responsible for ensuring that their practice and conduct meets legislative requirements and the standards of the profession.
2. Continuing competence	Each nurse maintains and continuously improves their competence by participating in the College of Nurses of Ontario's (CNO's) Quality Assurance Program.
3. Ethics	Each nurse understands, upholds, and promotes the values and beliefs described in the CNO ethics practice standard.
4. Knowledge	Each nurse possesses, through basic education and continuing learning, knowledge relevant to their professional practice.
5. Knowledge application	Each nurse continually improves the application of professional knowledge.
6. Leadership	Each nurse demonstrates leadership by providing, facilitating, and promoting the best possible care to the public.
7. Relationships	Each nurse establishes and maintains respectful, collaborative, therapeutic, and professional relationships.
7.1 Therapeutic nurse–client relationships	Each nurse keeps the client's needs as the focus of the relationship, which is based on trust, respect, intimacy, and the appropriate use of power.
7.2 Professional relationships	Each nurse enters into professional relationships based on trust and respect that result in improved client care.

This content is adapted from the College of Nurses of Ontario; the original work is available at https://cno.org.

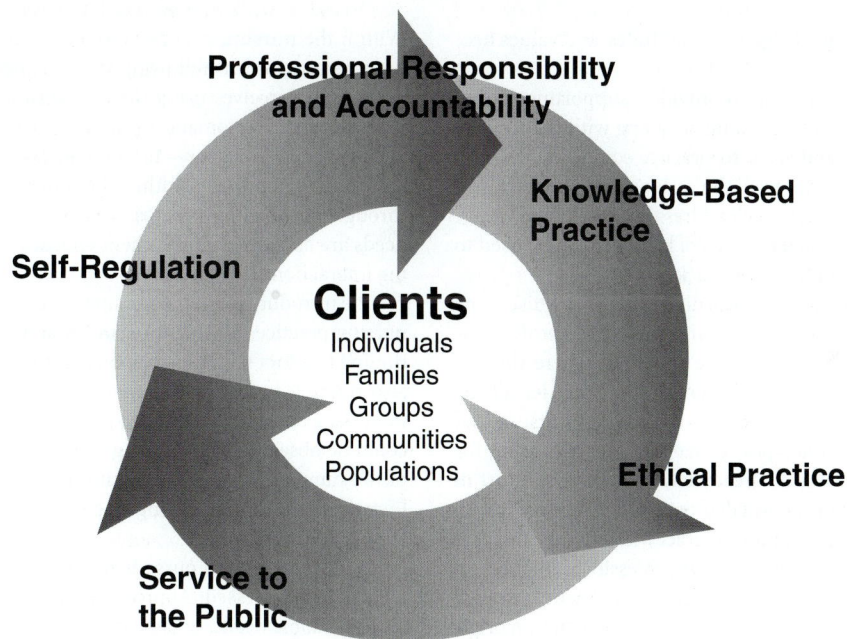

FIGURE 19.1 Canadian Council of Registered Nurses Regulators' framework for entry-to-practice competencies for registered nurses.

initially made of Mrs. Black and her family will not interfere with your enactment of these professional nursing values?

The CNA *Code of Ethics* provides a foundation for how professional nurses practise in Canada. Provincial regulators then use the *Code of Ethics* in generating sets of practice standards that reflect the nursing act in each province and territory. These standards of practice help nurses understand how they can integrate the various patterns of knowing into decision making and the enactment of care into their practice. Therefore, the standards of practice become the norms that nurses use in their professional practice.

Table 19.1 presents one set of nursing practice standards for nurses who practise in Ontario. Your provincial or territorial regulator of nursing practice will have their own set of nursing practice standards. You are encouraged to seek these out through your regulator's website (many of which are listed in the "Recommended Websites" section at the end of this chapter).

These standards are designed to be applied across all settings and situations that nurses find themselves in. But they can be difficult to carry out fully as you are learning to become a professional nurse. Your program faculty will assist you in learning your nursing practice so that you will be able to implement the entry-to-practice competencies. The Canadian nursing **entry-to-practice competencies** (Figure 19.1) comprise a common framework of nursing competencies in Canada. All nursing programs are approved by their provincial or territorial regulators according to how well their graduates are prepared to meet the competencies for entering practice.

These competencies are organized around five categories: (1) professional responsibility and accountability, (2) knowledge-based practice (incorporating both specialized body of knowledge and competent application of knowledge), (3) ethical practice, (4) service to the public, and (5) self-regulation. Practice standards and competencies will assist both you (the aspiring nurse) and your learning facilitators with

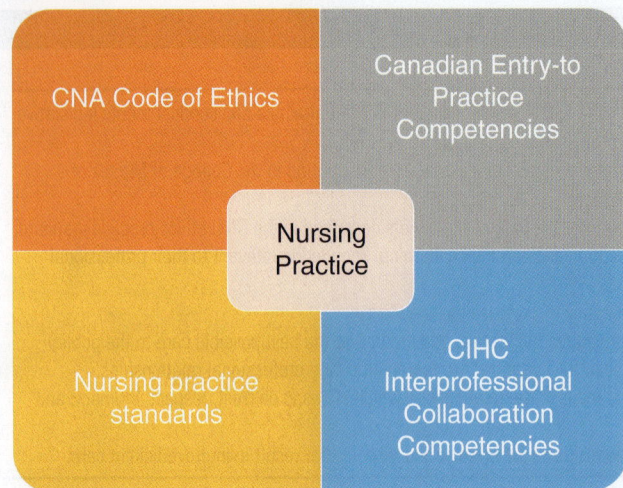

FIGURE 19.2 Foundation of nursing practice. *CIHC,* Canadian Interprofessional Health Collaborative; *CNA,* Canadian Nurses Association.

ensuring that you learn the knowledge, skills, attitudes, and values necessary to practise nursing.

The four patterns of knowing help to provide a supporting framework for your professional practice as a nurse, along with the *Code of Ethics,* standards of practice, and entry-to-practice competencies (Figure 19.2). Now that we have explored all the various ways in which you develop and use your knowledge, we will address how your own way of knowing and evolving professional patterns of knowing can be used to create a plan of care for a client like Mrs. Black.

Keep in mind that restricting one's learning only to the discipline of nursing creates difficulties when practising with other professionals; you will rarely find yourself in practice situations where there is only a professional nurse involved in a client's care. Consider all the other health care providers who need to be involved (e.g., nurse, social worker, physician, and physiotherapist, to name a few) in caring for Mrs. Black and her family. You will already have a level of comfort in using your developing nursing knowledge with other nurses. But in today's health care system, you also must interact with other health care providers. To help you begin to develop your professional interaction with other health care providers for your practice experience, we will explore some useful tips from **social contact theory**, which was originally theorized by Gordon Allport.

When groups (such as your nursing class) study together, they establish strong in-group cohesiveness and loyalty to the group. Consequently, all others outside the in-group (i.e., the other professionals) are seen as out-group members, while those in the in-group feel a level of distrust toward them regarding their understanding of the care needs of clients such as Mrs. Black. This leads to problems of trust and compromises the ability to work collaboratively with other health care providers. It is helpful to be able to explain your role and your current level of competence in your nursing practice to the other health care providers involved in a client's care, particularly in the context of a question you have or the help you are seeking from them. Working with other health care providers is discussed in the context of interprofessional collaborative practice later in this chapter.

THINKING

In the knowing section of this chapter, we explored what can be termed the **antecedents** used to bring us to the point of being able to provide nursing care for Mrs. Black (from our case study). Now we will begin to look at how you can bring the knowledge you are gaining from all your nursing courses to create a plan of care. This is the type of thinking you will use to develop insight into some options that you may share with Mrs. Black that might be of help to her.

There are two common approaches that can be used in this thinking process: the nursing process and the clinical judgement model. First, we will briefly explore how the nursing process evolved and what it comprises, and then we will explore the clinical judgement model. To align with this chapter's focus on the client-centred collaborative process, the integration of Mrs. Black's case will use the latter approach.

❖ NURSING PROCESS

In 1950, Ida Jean Orlando Pelletier put forward her view that nursing would not receive its just rewards until there was a deliberative formulation, later termed the nursing process, guiding nurses' approaches to clients and their care (Sampoornam, 2015; Schmieding, 1983). Orlando theorized that nursing is about clients coming to seek help from nurses, and the role of nurses is to find out what help clients need from nurses and then explore how nurses can meet their needs.

Orlando's work transformed the way nurses practised nursing. Within the **nursing process**, Orlando believed that nurses needed to use a sequence of the following steps: (1) **perception**—finding out how the person perceives using the five senses; (2) **thought**—this perception stimulates automatic thinking; (3) **feeling**—thinking stimulates feelings; and (4) **action**—the person takes action. The processing of these four components within the nurse–client encounter takes place through the nursing process. The process continues until all unmet needs are addressed or the client chooses to withdraw from the ongoing interaction with the nurse.

The introduction of the nursing process created a significant shift in nursing practice. This shift occurred at a time when society was continuing to adopt stimulus–response approaches to learning and action, also referred to as **behaviourism**. Previously, the measure of success in nursing care had been related to which changes in client behaviours could be observed. The nursing profession adopted Orlando's concept of the nursing process and institutionalized its application through a linear set of problem-solving stages: **assessment**, **planning**, **intervention**, and **evaluation**.

In assessment, the nurse is provided with a set of guidelines as to what is to be assessed. Approaches vary depending on the health care agency—some health organizations develop forms related to a specific nursing theory, whereas others may use a "head-to-toe" check system. The criticism of the current approaches relates to how well these approaches assist nurses in linking all the components of nursing care. Others suggest that the centrality of listening to the client's story about why they are seeking help is often missed (Sahlsten et al., 2005). During planning, a set document is provided that provides the means to enter data collected against set goals for each identified problem or nursing diagnosis. The limitation of the nursing process is in its failure to allow for the thinking processes that shape nurses' decision making for client care outcomes. An alternative approach that overcomes this limitation is the clinical judgement model formulated by Tanner (2006).

CLINICAL JUDGEMENT MODEL

Tanner (2006) provided an innovative model for pulling all learning together, the *model of clinical judgement* (Figure 19.3). In this model, Tanner suggests there are four aspects needed to bring all pieces of information together: *noticing, interpreting, responding,* and *reflecting.* All four aspects are influenced by the **context**, or the situation where the client–nurse encounter occurs, the background of all persons involved, and the relationships that develop between the nurse, client,

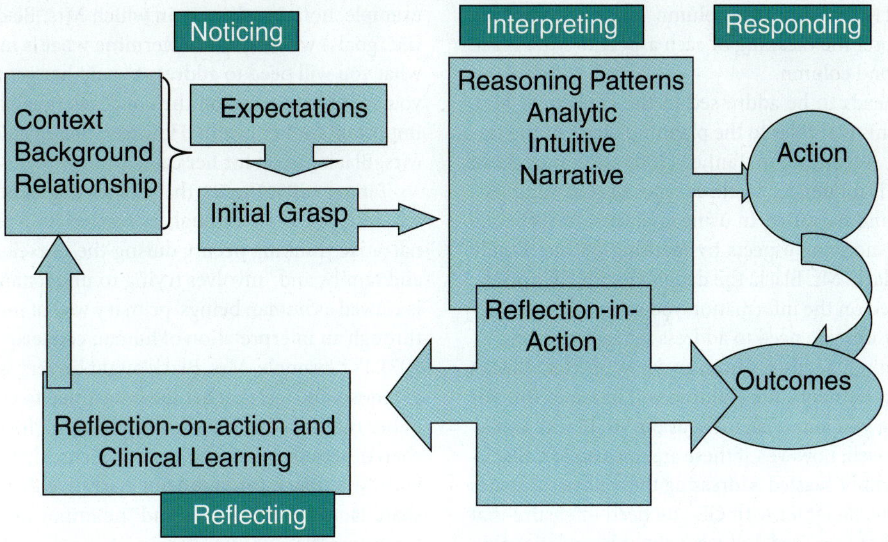

FIGURE 19.3 Tanner's clinical judgement model. (From Tanner, C. [2006]. Thinking like a nurse: A research-based model of clinical judgment in nursing. *Journal of Nursing Education, 45*[6]:208.)

and family. Here, we will bring together all the pieces of information about Mrs. Black and her family.

Noticing

Noticing equates to *assessment* in the traditional nursing process, but it also relates to Orlando's *perception*, *thought*, and *feeling* steps, which are likely to evolve through your use of Carper's patterns of knowing as well. Recalling the case of the Black family, in this process you as the nurse need to notice what key aspects are being presented to more fully understand how each relates to actual observable signs and statements from Mrs. Black. A client's story is not always told in a clear, chronological order, and not all the pieces fit together neatly when the story is first presented. Often, there are pieces in the story that are missing. These missing pieces are critical for you to form a complete picture of the situation that the Black family currently finds themselves in. First, take the key points presented in the case. Then, consider what more you need to learn in order to be able to fully understand the situation and how you might be able to develop a plan to address these needs for the family. In a real situation, you would go back and ask the family members for more information. A critical piece of information to ask is, What does the client want your help with? These pieces of information will then help you to shape, together with the client, their specific goals for care.

Today's fast-paced system of health care prevents a full exploration of all the needs a client may have. Hence, both you and the client need to come to a clear understanding of which of their care needs take priority. Specifically, what is key to care from your nursing professional assessment of the situation? Focusing on what a client's goals are helps you and the client to create a plan of care that is realistic and achievable. Adult education research supports the use of an approach in which the client sets the goal because adults are very problem focused. Moving beyond why a client is seeking your professional help is therefore not likely to be of importance to the client. A further understanding of why such an approach is important relates to the findings of Klein (2008) in *Naturalistic Decision Making*.

In a large study of North Americans, Klein (2008) found that when people faced a problem, they addressed it by focusing on patterns they had used previously to address similar problems. In many cases, when the problem required only a minor adjustment, the change often occurred at an unconscious, reactive level. Consider your own life: Have you ever noticed yourself adjusting to an encountered problem

in the moment or did you notice the adjustment only after you focused on what change you made and why? Klein then reported that when a problem could not be solved unconsciously, a person focused consciously and considered previous ways they had chosen to overcome it. A person might trial that approach and continue making further adjustments until none are found to solve the problem. Finally, a person may move beyond an individual approach and seek someone else's help to overcome the problem. That is, the person is seeking to use a new pattern to resolve the problem.

In many cases, you will be meeting with a client in this situation. Klein's naturalistic decision making further supports your need as an aspiring nurse to explore with clients what prompted them to seek help from you (Klein, 2008). That health-seeking behaviour is very goal directed. It also requires the nurse to find out what approaches have been tried to resolve the problem. This then provides the nurse with a means to build onto the client's norm of problem resolution to enhance the additional approach offered by the nurse. There is therefore a greater chance that such a "scaffolding" of new approaches to the client's past efforts will be accepted and followed through on by clients. Some new approaches may require interventions that the client and you as the nurse might not discover unless you undertake this exploration of the client's problem solving. As an aspiring nurse, focusing on a client's goals for care and what approaches they have already tried can help to create efficient ways to enact your role. Saving time by developing your planning around the client's goals is an important way to achieve this efficiency in practice. Goals also help you to think about what nursing knowledge you would need to help this family. Once you have completed the noticing phase, you are ready to move into the interpreting or planning phase of the nursing process.

Interpreting

Interpreting means translating the information obtained from collecting a client's health history into meaningful nursing actions. As you review the client's set goal(s) as well as all the aspects identified in your noticing, you then identify evidence you have collected and interpret its meaning according to your growing knowledge from theory learning, reading on your own, or previous experience.

To help you see how all aspects identified in your noticing are being addressed, take a piece of paper and draw four columns. Title the first column "Noticing" and the second column "Interpreting." Then, enter all your "noticing" aspects into the first column and start thinking about how you can interpret the meaning of each aspect to Mrs. Black and her family in the second column.

Now consider what needs to be addressed in the context of Mrs. Black's presented goals. This is similar to the planning phase of the traditional nursing process. According to Tanner (2006), the process of interpreting information is influenced by three types of reasoning patterns: analytic, intuitive, and narrative. In using analytic interpreting, you can expand on your noticing aspects by focusing on one family member at a time: Jane Black, Mr. Black, the daughter with CF, and the other children. Then, based on the information you gained from noticing, decide what health issues you need to address for each person.

For Mr. Black, you might focus on how, in view of Mrs. Black's absence and his work requirements, the children will be cared for. For health promotion reasons, you may wish to focus on Mr. Black's smoking and weight control as well; however, if these are not also Mr. Black's goals, then your time might be wasted addressing these physical issues at this time. For the Blacks' daughter with CF, you need to ensure that her breathing capacity is not impaired. But what about her relationship with her parent who will be absent for a few days? These are some of the key needs for this family.

In determining which health issues should be attended to, you will need to consider the family's expressed goals, but you can also present alternatives related to those goals. You will use all the data you have obtained from the Black family and then add your knowledge of the physiology, anatomy, and pathophysiology of diabetes, smoking, CF, obesity, and pregnancy. This is an extensive list but knowing about these elements is key to the analytic reasoning pattern you will use in developing a plan of interaction with the Black family. Further considerations include the following: What would be the genetic impacts of diabetes on Mrs. Black and the children? What care will Mrs. Black require in order to manage herself postdelivery? What are the concerns of other family members about Mrs. Black and the new baby?

Tanner (2006) suggests that you consider which treatments and/or actions will be required to achieve the goals, and then explore with Mrs. Black which alternative approaches to achieving these goals might also be possible. In client-centred care, you first discuss with the client the initial goals that you worked to establish for them. To ensure a successful outcome, you then tailor these initial goals to align with the client's stated goals (not just your goals for them). In a real clinical situation, you will combine all the information that you collected with real clinical data (i.e., tests, blood work, and physical assessment data) to determine how likely it is that the client will achieve their goals. This is the set of analytic processes that you would use in interpreting for a client such as Mrs. Black and her family.

Tanner (2006) identifies another pattern of reasoning that nurses use: intuitive interpreting. She states that "intuition is characterized by immediate apprehension of a clinical situation and is a function of experience with similar situations" (p. 207). Depending on the nursing practice experience you have had up to this point, you will bring learning forward as you consider how you will approach the family and their care. McCutcheon and Pincombe (2001) suggest that intuition "is the result of a complex interaction of attributes, including experience, expertise, and knowledge, along with personality, environment, acceptance of intuition as a valid 'behaviour' and the presence of a nurse/client relationship" (p. 344). Even though you are just at the beginning of your nursing studies, you will also bring to it your own experiential learning (personal knowing) that was gained before you entered nursing. This experiential learning evolved from the environment you grew up in, your personality, and your evolving nursing knowledge and practice (aesthetic knowing). These components will help you shape how you develop your nurse–client relationships in practice. For

example, noticing the way in which Mrs. Black expresses her concerns (i.e., goals) will help you determine what is most important to her, and what you will need to address to help her get past her concerns, so that you are able to work on the concerns (goals) that you feel are equally important for her health. However, these goals need to fit into the goals Mrs. Black has set for her care.

Tanner (2006) notes that nurses augment their analytic and intuitive interpretation through narrative interpreting. She suggests that narrative thinking occurs during the nurse's interactions with a client and family, and "involves trying to understand the particular case and is viewed as human beings' primary way of making sense of experience, through an interpretation of human concerns, intents, and motives" (p. 207). For example, Mrs. Black might be very worried about the diabetes diagnosis and feel that her life is destined to end in renal failure because of her mother's experience with diabetes. It is this type of information, shared because of unspoken concerns, that you will need to explore with Mrs. Black through your narrative thinking. It will allow you to share facts about diabetes and the importance of blood sugar control, for example.

Another point to consider is that this is Mrs. Black's fourth pregnancy. Was it planned? If not, what is the impact on the family of another child? The family lives in an apartment: Will it be large enough for the growing family? Is this an issue of concern to the family? Mr. Black is on the road much of the time. What impact does this have on Mrs. Black? How will Mrs. Black be able to care for the new baby while managing their daughter with CF? What physical, mental, and social costs to her own health will the added pressures of child care have on her? What about their income—will they need assistance to manage? How can you structure your relationship with the family so that it is professional, yet allows trust to develop so that you can explore these questions with the family? How will you determine the right time to approach these issues with the Blacks? All these factors should come to your attention and will require you to use your narrative thinking to ensure that you gain an understanding of which of these issues are the most important to Mrs. Black and her family. You might also consider what resources are available to the family. If you are unfamiliar with such resources, you could approach a social worker or your own instructor or faculty member for examples. Knowing such information enables you to intervene with facts and supports. Each success in Mrs. Black's care is dependent on what goals are important to her.

Consider what further knowledge you need to check on and what information you feel is missing at this time. Then do your research on these missing pieces of needed knowledge. Consider which of Mrs. Black's goals—the ones she has agreed to—you feel confident in working on. See which of these aspects may be out of your depth of understanding and may require you to request assistance from other health care providers.

Responding

Responding means developing actions and planning implementation to address a client's identified health and social issues. Discuss with Mrs. Black what planned interventions you are proposing, and seek her agreement on which of these she can support. Then consider the evidence that is needed for you and Mrs. Black to determine whether each goal has been reached.

As you can see, client-centred care requires ongoing interaction and negotiation with the client and may at times necessitate an adaptation of your plan to fit with the client's capacity to manage. Remember, successful outcomes for the client depend on how well their goals are achieved. Hence, you need to discuss and carry out the plan of care with Mrs. Black and determine how both you and she will know when her goals have been reached. Shaping your care plan around what

Mrs. Black is able and willing to do to achieve her chosen goals is key to effective client-centred care.

Reflecting

Reflection is the process of assessing a client's responses to care at two levels: during provision of care and then again following completion of care when you are evaluating your work. Reflection fits within the evaluation stage in the nursing process. Good nursing care requires that nurses frequently reflect on what has occurred with their care. Citing the work of Schön, Tanner (2006) suggests that two types of reflection are required: **reflection-in-action** and **reflection-on-action**. In *reflection-in-action*, you consider what impact your planned interventions are having in moving the client (i.e., Mrs. Black) toward achieving the desired outcome, as well as how the client (Mrs. Black) feels they are responding to the planned actions. By coming to an agreement with the client about what actions you and they will focus on in order to achieve mutually established goals, you are preparing yourself and the client to reflect on how well the client is progressing toward the goals. This agreement also allows you to look back later at what you and the client have done to achieve the goals (*reflection-on-action*). This is an iterative rather than linear process. Sometimes there is movement in only one goal and not in others. In the case of Mrs. Black, if she is not making satisfactory progress toward achieving a goal, you might have to renegotiate with her to help her adjust the interventions; renegotiating may in turn help Mrs. Black move forward toward achieving her goals in other areas.

An Assessment Rubric for Tanner's Model

At this point you may be thinking, "Well, it's fine for the author to say that this will all come together, but how will I know if what I am doing is moving me toward this level of understanding?" Several approaches have been created to help you assess how well you are using noticing, interpreting, responding, and reflecting. Initially, Lasater (2007) developed what she called an "assessment rubric" for Tanner's model, while Gerdeman et al. (2013) suggested the application of concept mapping to the rubric. Later, Lasater and Neilsen (2009) advocated using reflective journalling. Since reflective journalling is often a part of Canadian nursing professional practice development, an example of how to develop a reflective journal of this case study is provided in Table 19.2.

Journalling using Tanner's clinical judgement model flows through noticing, interpreting, responding, and reflection (both *in action* and *on action*). In this approach, the journalling consists of a set of headings, including a short description of the situation you have found yourself in and the background to your previous experiences. Hence, the use of SBAR elements is also suggested (discussed later in this chapter; see Interprofessional Communication). You then expand on this initial information by discussing what you noticed in the situation and adding to this by interpreting what you saw or experienced. The next step is to reflect on how you responded (e.g., by helping Mrs. Black set her goals for care). As you progress in your care with Mrs. Black, you do further journalling about your reflection-in-action on how the plan for care is moving Mrs. Black toward her goals. At the end of your experience caring for Mrs. Black, you complete your journalling by adding your reflection-on-action about what you learned from the experiences and what the outcome was of your care for Mrs. Black (see Table 19.2).

In nursing care, there are frequently many options available to us. When we ground our practice in a client-centred philosophy, it is up to the client and family to decide which of the goals they wish to work on. Therefore, until you interact with the client and family, you will not be able to finalize any plan you intend to develop.

Returning to the earlier discussion about Orlando and others' conception of the nursing process, the nursing focus is the client and what the client wishes to have help with. This perspective clearly places the control of the interaction in the hands of the client. But in the quest for professional respect, nursing has often veered toward defending professional expertise. This has created a power differential between the client and the nurse. If we reconceptualize health care to have a client-centred focus rather than a system-centred focus (as currently exists), then the expertise of clients, based on their lived experience with their health issues, becomes a critical focus of care. Clients are the experts in their management of illness—they are their own "drivers of their care." The nurse's role is very episodic in that the nurse encounters the client and family only at key points—when they desire nursing assistance. Hence, nurses need to see themselves as partners. Partnering with clients does not mean nurses are totally responsible for a client's care. Today, because of the complex health and social issues that many clients experience, no single health care provider has sufficient knowledge, skills, and expertise to meet all the needs of clients. Hence,

TABLE 19.2 Reflective Journalling With Application of Tanner's (2006) Clinical Judgement Model
SITUATION
Points to consider: Describe your initial encounter with the client and family using Carper's (1978) patterns of nursing.
BACKGROUND
Points to consider: What were your personal and professional experiences that prepared you for this encounter, and what was missing?
Noticing
Points to consider: What did you hear and observe about the client using your five senses? What did you learn from the client about the client's health needs? What patterns were emerging about her desired goals? What might you have missed or failed to consider?
Interpreting
Points to consider: How well did you make sense of the interrelationship between your identified patterns and relationships? What further data did you search for and what additional knowledge did you gain to help you with Mrs. Black and her family's care? What sources did you explore? Were they sufficient? What might have been missed?
Responding
Points to consider: What goals and assessment approach did you develop in your interactions with Mrs. Black and her family? How did you determine with Mrs. Black how to assess for her goal achievement?
Reflecting-in-action
Points to consider: How effective was your planned care for Mrs. Black each day? What were her responses to your care, and what progress did she make toward achieving her goals? How did you and Mrs. Black feel about each of these experiences? What have you learned from each experience?
Reflecting-on-action
Points to consider: What was the outcome of the care you provided for Mrs. Black? What were Mrs. Black's responses to your care? Consider all five—What did you learn from the experience?

while nurses are held accountable for the nursing knowledge, skills, and expertise provided to clients, this is but a part of the totality of care. Addressing the totality of care requires that you learn to practise within your developing professional role. It also requires that you learn how to practise as a member of an interprofessional client-centred collaborative team.

As a segway into our discussion of interprofessional client-centred collaborative practice, you may review all the issues that the Black family is facing. Which other health care providers may need to assist you and the family in addressing all their health and social issues? How would you get their input in care planning in a health care institution? Does the health care institution use a team concept for meeting the complex care needs of clients and their families? If it does not, how would you suggest that other health care providers be consulted to ensure that the best care is provided?

As you learn about the role of a professional nurse, you will begin socialization into the profession. **Socialization** is the development of behaviours and attitudes deemed necessary to fit into a cultural group; in this case, the *nursing culture*. In fact, you started this socialization process long before you began your nursing studies. Your socialization was shaped by the people you talked to about nursing and by the media (both textual and visual), leading you to believe certain things about what a nurse is and what a nurse does. In order to make this career choice, you also explored what other health care providers do. Both sets of beliefs contain truths and myths. While your nursing program will help you to shape your professionalism, it will also cause you to cast off these myths about nursing that are based on information you learned before you came into your program. However, if you do not also attend to learning about the knowledge and roles of other health care providers, your internalized myths about other health professionals will persist well into your practice. This is another component to address from an interprofessional perspective and is referred to as role clarification. **Role clarification** means that you are able to explain to another person what a professional nurse's role is and what knowledge and skills you as a nurse bring to your client-centred care (read the activity outlined in Box 19.1).

INTERACTING

The process of nurses interacting with other health care providers requires artistry. The art of nursing is often an interplay of balancing what the nurse can provide to the care process while interfacing with the way others see the care needs of clients. Varying aesthetic patterns across disciplines can lead to perceived power disputes among professionals, as well as to disputes between professionals and clients. **Interprofessional collaborative practice** is about learning to respect the knowledge, skills, and expertise that are brought into the care process

---

BOX 19.1   Learning Activity: Role Clarification

Reflect for a moment on what thoughts came to mind as you read the case about Mrs. Black and her family at the start of this chapter. Which values do you hold that influence the way you assessed the members of Mrs. Black's family and their current situation? Take a minute to write these down.

Thinking back to your exploration of the nursing role, prepare a written presentation about how you will discuss your nursing role, knowledge, and skill with another student in a health care profession outside of nursing. Then, try it out on a friend in another health-related professional program.

Being able to explain what a nurse's role entails can help clients such as Mrs. Black, as well as other health care providers, appreciate how they can work with you in an interprofessional team.

---

by all health care providers and identifying who is the most appropriate provider to support clients' care needs at key times in their care. When power imbalances occur, these are counterproductive to both effective nursing and effective client-centred care.

Being a member of such a team requires that the nurse understand how the nursing professional role fits in collaboration with the client and the interprofessional team. **Interprofessional client-centred collaborative practice** "involve[s] a partnership between a team of health [care] professionals and a client in a participatory, collaborative and coordinated approach to shared decision-making around health and social issues" (Orchard et al., 2005). This definition has been chosen as the goal within the Canadian Interprofessional Health Collaborative (CIHC) National Interprofessional Competency Framework (Figure 19.4; Canadian Interprofessional Health Collaborative [CIHC], 2010). This framework provides health care providers with a means to understand which competencies they need to enact in order to practise collaboratively within a client's health care team.

In reality, *team* is an amorphous term. In health care, consistency in the composition of teams is often fragmentary owing to the varying needs of clients. But the concepts within a team may be more important to focus on in order to gain an understanding of what it means to function within a team or group. The composition of the health care team changes with each client, and team members often come and go during the course of care. Hence, the approach nurses use to work within collaborative teams has to be adapted to address the realities of health care. The CIHC competency framework attempts to do just this. First, the framework focuses on how the team functions together—how the team achieves being an intact social unit with its "members" working together. In working together, the team members demonstrate the sharing of responsibilities and the use of their interdependencies in managing relationships across the boundaries of each team member's professional competencies.

Together, then, an interprofessional client-centred collaborative team provides care to and with their clients around agreed-upon shared goals. What, then, makes a team collaborative in their practice? Collaboration can be viewed in two ways—as *an outcome of a team working together with a client* or as *a process used by team members working together with a client*—to make shared judgements about care in order to achieve the best outcomes for a client. Hence, the CIHC competency framework focuses on the judgements made within a group of team members who are working interdependently with each other with a shared set of decisions to reach shared goals that have been established in partnership with their clients. In interprofessional client-centred collaborative practice, the client is a full member of the health care team.

Collaborative practice in health care teams is not a constant. Each experience is unique and thus requires ongoing reflection about the team's effectiveness in making judgements with each client. The competencies are interdependent: they overlap and cannot be separated because all are needed to achieve this form of practice. Therefore, the competency framework is viewed as an oval that includes six competency domains. It begins with patient- or client-centred care, as well as family- and community-centred care, which ensures that the focus of all care includes the clients' participation in the care, no matter where clients are located. Client-centred care is achieved through **interprofessional communication**, which entails verbal and nonverbal interactions between health care providers. These interactions include communicating with clients and family members during team-based meetings. Such communication is based on understanding each other's roles through *role clarification*, which allows team members to work together through a set of team norms to enact team functioning, using an interprofessional collaborative leadership approach, and to address

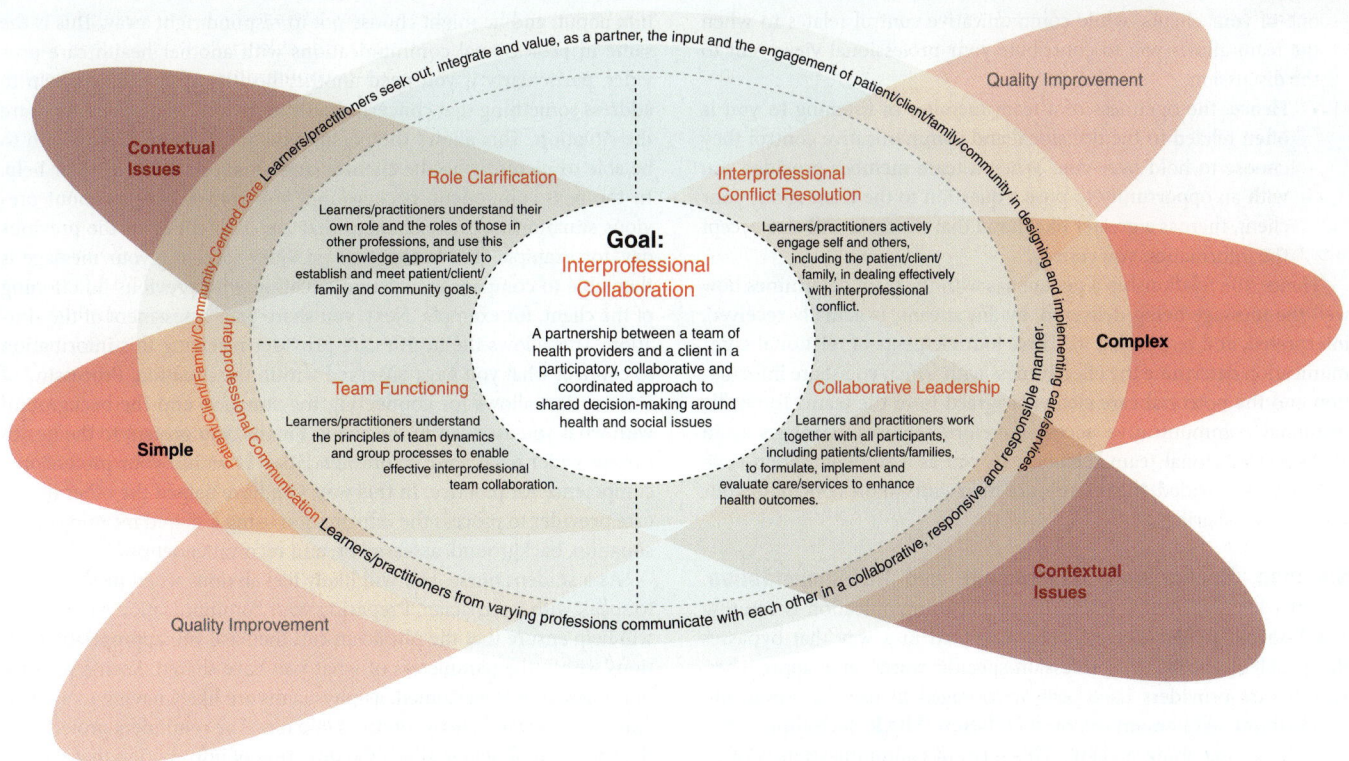

FIGURE 19.4 Canadian Interprofessional Health Collaborative's National Interprofessional Competency Framework. (From Canadian Interprofessional Health Collaborative. [2010]. A National Interprofessional Competency Framework [p. 17]. https://www.cihc.ca/files/CIHC_IPCompetencies_Feb1210.pdf. Reprinted with permission from the Canadian Association of Schools of Nursing, Copyright 2015. This illustration is used with permission of the Canadian Interprofessional Health Collaborative.)

and resolve interprofessional team conflicts or disagreements as they occur (see Figure 19.4).

Throughout this chapter, we have discussed the first competency domain, that of patient-, client-, family-, and community-centred care. It is described as care in which learners "seek out, integrate, and value … the engagement of the patient/client/family/community in designing and implementing care/services" (CIHC, 2010, p. 13). Additional support for focusing on both communication and collaboration for nurses can be found in the Canadian Association of Schools of Nursing's (2022) *National Nursing Education Framework*, which emphasizes the importance of the ability to "communicate and collaborate effectively with clients, families (biological or chosen), intraprofessional and interprofessional health team members, and intersectoral health care partners" (Domain 4: Communication and Collaboration; p. 16).

We will now take each of these remaining competency domains in turn and discuss some key aspects for you to focus on as you gain practice experiences in your program and learn how to work interprofessionally with others, including clients and their family members.

Interprofessional Communication

You have likely already studied communication in your program (and in Chapter 18). Now we will build on that learning by focusing on key aspects that are affected when you work with other health care providers.

When working with other health care providers, it is important to enter into *interactions* with others and create a shared understanding through an exchange of knowledge, skills, and expertise within a moral/ethical framework of practice (Hindmarsh & Pilnick, 2002). In essence, when you come to work with other health care providers, you are using communication that consists of unique nursing language and meanings, nursing-specific communication patterns, and nursing professional

ethical values. Thus, in trying to reach a shared meaning in the message you convey to your non-nursing health care colleagues, there is a greater likelihood of not being fully heard, understood, or both. Interestingly, Adler and colleagues (2008) remind us that whenever we communicate with someone else, we focus on the *content* of our message; however, in reality, our *relationship* with the other person is equally important: "relational [communication] . . . refer[s] to how the parties feel [and respond] toward one another" (Adler et al., 2008, p. 20).

Within any relationship, four aspects will influence how another person receives your message. These are affinity, immediacy, respect, and control, as outlined here:

- *Affinity* refers to how strong a team member's positive feelings are toward you and how much they value your contributions within discussions leading to shared decision making
- *Immediacy* refers to how well another team member pays attention to the content of the message you are delivering as well as the body language you have used to convey that message
- *Respect* refers to your own social need to be viewed as a competent and valued person by other team members
  - Gaining respect from the team is always a difficult task when you are a student who comes into the unit, perhaps only 1 or 2 days a week, and when you are working under the guidance of the nurse who is responsible for your client's care. If that nurse opens the communication with the team by asking you to pose the question, then this support can help the team listen to your message about that client.
- *Control* refers to the *persuasive power* some members in the team may exert over you. This control can take two forms: decisional and communicative. Decisional control reflects how open other team members are to allowing you to lead a point of discussion about

one of your clients, while communicative control relates to when the team allows you to contribute your professional viewpoint to the discussion.

- Hence, the openness of a team member in listening to you is often related to the decisional and communicative control they choose to hold over you. When a team member provides you with an opportunity to pose a question to the team about your client, there is a greater likelihood that the team will also accept the information you convey.

Hence, the relationship a person has with the team determines how well the message being delivered, by any means, is actually received, interpreted, and responded to. These four elements of relational communication determine the effectiveness with which you share information and the potential care elements agreed to in the team. To enable relational communicative access therefore requires openness from all interprofessional team members to you as a student. When such openness is provided, the importance then shifts to the content of your information sharing.

Situation, Background, Assessment, and Recommendation.
Another key to effective interprofessional communication is creating a well-formulated message that is presented in a way that bypasses the problems posed by profession-specific words and approaches. Health care providers have been encouraged to use the situation–background–assessment–recommendation (SBAR) technique when communicating about a client. This form of communication is often needed when a telephone interaction is occurring between two health care providers. The SBAR technique was developed by the US military to improve communications and was later adopted by the health care sector (see https://www.ihi.org/resources/Pages/Tools/SBARToolkit.aspx). Studies have shown SBAR to be effective in improving the clarity of communication within teams (Andreoli et al., 2010; Enlow et al., 2010; Marshall et al., 2009).

Why does SBAR work so well? If we consider communication theory and how we process information, SBAR makes good sense in that it creates shared meanings in interprofessional care. Think about sending a message to a friend: If you would like to find out whether your friend wants to go to a movie with you tomorrow evening, how would you communicate this information? Let's try to formulate your SBAR message:

Communication Element	Message
Situation	Hi, John. Have you heard about the movie *La La Land*? It's playing at the cinema in the local mall. The comments on Facebook says it's really good.
Background	I remember that you love this kind of movie.
Assessment	I know you don't have a car, so I could pick you up if you like. I was thinking of going on Thursday, to the early show at 5 p.m., right after our last class that day.
Recommendations	So, please let me know if you would like to come on Thursday, and if you would like me to drive you. If you want to come, I will go online and buy the tickets.

In this example, if John (preferred pronouns: he/him) didn't know why you were texting him, he would not know what you are contacting him about, and he might choose not to respond right away. This is the same in professional communications with another health care provider, particularly if you need another health care provider's help to address something that concerns you about your client. You first share the situation. This allows the person you are communicating with to be able to picture who the client is and which issue needs their help. In the next component, background, you convey aspects about previous situations, or new changes that are different from the previous day, for example. The health care provider receiving your message is then able to compare the current situation with previous functioning of the client, for example. Next, you share your assessment of the situation. This allows the health care provider receiving this information to connect what you have observed within the situation. Processing of information allows for connecting the situation and the background with what you assessed in the client. Finally, you present to the health care provider what your recommendation is within your professional competence for practice. In this way, you have helped the other health care provider to process the information using a shared meaning of the situation, background, assessment, and recommendation.

As a student nurse, you will likely feel anxious when making a call to speak with a physician. Preparing your communication using SBAR will help ensure that the physician can then ask you appropriate questions within the parameters of what you have shared. Such a package of information is welcomed, as physicians are likely having to address issues with several clients on the same day. The reminders provided in the background help to shape the direction of information that you are likely to receive. Physicians will then learn to respect you, even if you are a student nurse.

To help you create an SBAR communication, we will refer back to the case involving Mrs. Black. You check her glucometer reading at 11 a.m. and note that it is 10. You are concerned and discuss your worry with her assigned nurse. You both agree that the physician needs to be contacted. Try to create your own SBAR for the physician managing Mrs. Black's diabetes, using the following chart:

Communication Element	Message to Be Communicated
Situation	
Background	
Assessment	
Recommendation	

Role Clarification.
The role nurses play within a team often constitutes more than a single role. Earlier in this chapter, we discussed the characteristics of a registered nurse and how standards of practice and entry-to-practice competencies guide you in your practice as a professional nurse. This presentation of your professional role as a nurse is termed a "generic role"—that is, how you are being prepared to be able to practise in any setting. However, when you work with a client such as Mrs. Black in a team environment, you will need to adjust your knowledge, skills, and expertise to the situation that the client and her family present. Hence, nurses do not use all their nursing knowledge and skills with every client. Within an interprofessional collaborative team, the nursing knowledge, skills, and expertise used with a specific client is referred to as the nurse's "focal role." It is a subset of components from within the nurse's entire set of knowledge, skills, and expertise that is needed at a specific time.

In addition, all team members need to understand how they can participate within their team. The role that the nurse uses in the team is then termed a "functional role." While many health professionals learn to work together within their profession and also with their clients, rarely do they learn how to effectively work in a team. We will discuss this role more fully under Team Functioning.

Role clarification has been shown to be a critical element for working collaboratively in teams. This means that not only must you know and be able to articulate your nursing knowledge, skills, and expertise but other members of your team must be able to do so as well.

Most nursing programs in Canada now address this learning as part of the program. If this is not the case in your program, you can learn about other health care providers and their roles at Western University's Office of Interprofessional Education and Practice (https://uwo.ca/fhs//education/ipe/index.html).

A key area that is beginning to be researched is the role of the client and family (or chosen caregiver) within the team. Their role in the team is equally as important as the role of each health care provider. Pettigrew and Tropp (2008) studied the "mediators" of intergroup contact theory. The authors found that three mediators are key to effective role assumptions and must be applied in a particular sequence: (1) decreasing anxiety in joining the team, (2) being shown respect by the team, and (3) having a well-described role within the team. This sequence can also be applied when you join a new group: How do you feel? Are you anxious in joining the team and wondering how they are going to treat you? This is a normal response. It is not likely that you will fully participate in the team unless team members help you to feel like a part of their group. There are many ways this can be accomplished. For example, others may ask you about your background or share their names, roles, and backgrounds. Once you are feeling welcomed, you may also

want to feel respected within the group. This can be achieved by offering your input about something the team is discussing, for example. This allows you to feel valued by the team. Finally, you want to have a team-specified role. In health care teams, any health professional will have unique knowledge, skills, and expertise. It is these capacities that can enhance team practice and the care provided to clients. Challenges to each other's roles, even when the person is a nurse practitioner, registered nurse, or licensed practical nurse, are equally important for the moderators to attend to. Without valuing the role that each team member contributes, collaborative practice cannot occur, and clients may not receive the best care from the team.

These three mediators are also key to making clients feel like full team members involved in shaping and evaluating their care outcomes. Therefore, for clients to be treated as equals in an interprofessional collaborative team, the team must focus on these three mediators. The role of the client in a team is just beginning to be studied. You may review some of the potential roles that a client can have in an interprofessional collaborative team in Box 19.2. You might also wish to review a recently published paper by Metersky and colleagues (2021) that discusses the roles of clients in primary care teams.

Team Functioning. In order for a team to function collaboratively, its members need to develop norms to ensure consistency when working together. **Norms** are standards that are created and shared by team

---

BOX 19.2	Roles of a Patient/Client

Who Is a Patient/Client?
An individual who seeks help to manage a health or social issue that is interfering with their desired capacity to fully participate in their family and community.

What Can the Patient/Client Do in a Team?
The patient/client expresses their lived experience of illness and injury and conveys what their own values and priorities are. This "story" is critical to building the team's understanding of the patient/client and to developing appropriate goals and a care plan. The patient/client brings shares with the health/social care team how their daily life is impacted by their health or social issue (and vice versa) and how the team's suggested treatments or actions can be adapted (or not) into their activities of daily living.

How Does the Patient/Client Fit Into the Team?
The patient/client becomes a true member of the interprofessional patient- or client-centred collaborative team. The patient/client retains control over their care and is provided with the knowledge, skills, and expertise of the health/social care providers so that, between them, they are able to negotiate a plan of care within existing resources.

Education and Preparation
The patient/client brings their understanding of their health/social needs, ensuring that these are recognized within their own frame of reference in the interaction with health/social care providers and help to shape a plan that will address, monitor, and reduce or resolve the identified issues.

As a patient/client, you seek to learn how to prepare yourself to be involved as a team member in your care (e.g., access the patient orientation module: TEAMc Module #6: https://teamc.ca/).

As a caregiver, you seek to learn from the patient/client/legal guardian the role they would like you to serve in the health/social care team.

Patient Associations
Patients/clients can also belong to supportive organizations that provide the means for them to have a voice of influence on the health/social care system. In Canada, these organizations include the following:

Canadian Arthritis Patient Alliance: https://arthritispatient.ca
Patients Canada: https://www.facebook.com/patientscanada

Patient/Client Connecting to a Team
Patients/clients can seek to have a voice in their care and supportive services through three levels of influence.

Policy Level
Serve as a member of the public. Patients/clients may serve on governing boards of hospitals, community agencies (e.g., in Ontario, on a Local Integrated Health Unit [LIHN], and disease-specific organizations (e.g., the Kidney Foundation of Canada or the Canadian Diabetes Association) to influence policy making that supports a patient's/client's voice.

Program Level
Serve as a member of a health organization focusing on quality improvement. In Ontario, the *Excellent Care for All Act* requires that health organizations involve patients in influencing the decisions made about their case.

Health Care Team Level
As a patient/client, you may request that:
- All needed health/social care providers meet with you at the same time to coordinate your care
- Health/social care providers give you, as the patient/client, an equal voice in discussions around your care
- Health/social care providers be willing to negotiate care with you to fit in with what is feasible in your life, and to support a reduction/resolution of your health/social issues
- The community providers necessary to continue to support your care be part of the team, and know the needs and plan developed between you and all the health/social care providers to ensure continuance of the plan through a seamless transition from one level of care to another (e.g., hospital to home).

members to set a tone for teamwork. These are often referred to as the dynamic of **team functioning**. Cohen and Bailey (1997) state that a team is ". . . a collection of individuals who are *interdependent* in their tasks, who *share responsibility* for outcomes, who see themselves and are seen by others as an *intact social entity* embedded in one or more larger social systems and who *manage their relationships* across organizational boundaries." Therefore, norms for collaborative health care team functioning relate to *interdependencies* within a team, how the members *share responsibility* for the care outcomes of their clients, and how these members work together around a set of *shared goals* within the overall organization in which they work (Gittell et al., 2013; van Schaik et al., 2014).

To appreciate team interdependencies, we look at the sharing of knowledge, skills, and expertise to start the process of learning where specific areas of expertise exist and can be used. Also, knowing about each other's roles as professionals helps the health care team members learn where there are shared areas of knowledge, skills, and expertise. In this process, there is a clarification of *role boundaries*. Knowing about shared areas relieves the potential problem of one health care provider trying to limit another's practice because they believe that they are the only provider who can perform in a specific area of care.

Developing collaborative team functioning necessitates creating trust in the team. Trust is essential for effective collaborative practice. Research by McAllister (1995) and further developed by Costa (2003) has identified a two-phase process for developing trust in team members toward one another. First, a team member's *competence* is assessed. This supports the importance of a team member's outright sharing of their knowledge, skills, and expertise. This allows other team members to take this information and assess the key areas identified rather than searching through all the first team member's performance aspects to determine whether they will trust that person. In the second phase, one's ability to work within the team is assessed. This consists of a team member's willingness to *assume responsibility and accountability* for aspects of care that reflect their professional knowledge and skills, as well as their willingness to assist in the team's functioning (Costa, 2003).

One of the areas where a functioning role might be demonstrated is during team meetings. Team meetings need to have a structure and guidelines for attending to meeting processes. These need to be agreed to by the collaborative team and are part of a team's norms. The roles include chair, recorder, summarizer, and re-director. The role of *chair* can rotate within the team membership to ensure the same person is not always required to assume this role. The *summarizer* is the person who assists both the chair and the team to periodically remind team members about what they have discussed and agreed to. The *recorder* takes notes as the meeting progresses. Finally, the *re-director* helps the team refocus if the discussion deviates away from the central topic. Guidelines around the use of these roles should be set by the team. In an effective collaborative team, these guidelines are consistently applied to the team's work. To get acquainted with these roles, try assuming one in your next small-group learning session. Doing so will allow you to gain an appreciation for the value of your role in moving discussion forward and reaching decisions for actions.

Guidelines are also needed to direct how collaborative team members will share information. The SBAR technique discussed earlier in the chapter is used to attend to *what* needs to be communicated (the content), but these additional communication guidelines relate to the *means* (or mechanisms) that will be used within the team (e.g., text messaging, email, paging, etc.). Guidelines are also needed to determine *when* (needed timing) communications are required and *who* needs to provide the communications. When these guidelines are created and used within a collaborative team, there is a greater likelihood

that interdependencies and shared responsibilities within the team can be achieved. A dynamic team is then able to establish *complementary relationships* that result in a cohesive and shared plan of care with the client and team members.

When a team is dynamic, it has a *cohesiveness* that reflects how its members are *committed to a common task* (in our case, client care) and subsequently are *motivated to stay* in the team. Motivation to remain is dependent on the rewards that members see for this teamwork. Hence, rewards should not be individually allocated but rather be team based according to the outcomes of the teamwork. When equivalent reward structures are in place, members are more willing to contribute to the outcomes of the team's work.

Think back to a positive team experience. Why was it so positive? Which of the norms discussed were present? Now consider a negative team experience. What was negative about it? Which of the norms discussed here were not present?

Interprofessional Collaborative Leadership. **Collaborative leadership** "occurs when all members of a team, including the client/family, symbiotically accept their capacity to lead the group by demonstrating mindfulness of the value in working together, and using their shared assets to assist the clients to reach achievable and desired health outcomes" (Orchard et al., 2019, p. 21). Unlike traditional leaders who have formal role assignment and perform a director and monitoring role in interprofessional teams, in collaborative leadership, all the team members work together to reach a shared judgement related to the needs of the client. Hence, the leader of the team can move around the team, functioning in more of a coordinating than directing role. There is a leader or, as discussed earlier, the person in the chair role who assumes a coordinating function to ensure that the work agreed to by team members is moving ahead to achieve the team's shared goals as planned. This leader can also bring the group together in the event that some agreed-upon aspects of the work need to be renegotiated because of unanticipated factors. The coordinator may also move around the team in collaborative leadership so that everyone has the opportunity to learn to lead in the team. All team members hold the team responsible for meeting planned outcomes.

Orchard and Rykoff (2015) developed a theoretical model of a complementary relationship between a formal or vertical leader, as defined by Pearce and Sims, Jr. (2004). They suggest that for the vertical leader to be successful, the leader must enact a role that reflects transformative leadership, interactive leadership, and empowering leadership, all of which complement the collaborative leadership occurring within teams. In the theorized model, the vertical leader and the collaborative leadership in teams are brought together through what Gittel et al. (2013) have termed *relational communication*. For relational communication to be effective, both leadership forms need to emulate the elements of leadership proposed by Kouzes and Posner (2006). While Kouzes and Posner addressed the vertical leader elements, Orchard and Rykhoff (2015) transformed these to also relate to collaborative team leadership, as shown in Table 19.3.

The next time you are in a group learning situation, try using these elements of collaborative leadership to see how they work.

Interprofessional Team Conflict Resolution. Traditionally, conflict in health care was seen as negatively affecting the performance of professionals. Until more recently, the focus was directed at managers and their skills in resolving conflicts that generally occurred between two parties. However, within teams in health care, conflicts are reported as being frequent and can lead to high stress and burnout among health care providers. **Interprofessional team conflict resolution** is defined as "conflict . . . comprised of *substantive, procedural* and

TABLE 19.3	Comparison of Transformative Leadership Elements for a Leader and an Interprofessional Team	
Leadership Element (Kouzes & Posner, 2006)	**Role of a Transformative Leader**	**Interprofessional Client-Centred Collaborative Team**
Inspire a shared vision	Helps the group to see a desired future	Members focus on client-specified goals; when the team considers how to get there, members help each other to bring their ideas together in an agreed-upon plan with the client
Enable others to act	Seeks opportunities to innovate and take risks	Members help to guide the team in promoting respect for all members and in arriving at shared goals with clients and team members; encourage other members to take on the leadership role and support clients in their decision making with the team
Challenge the process	Seeks opportunities to innovate and take risks	Collaborative leader in the team carries out ongoing reflection on how the team is working together with the client and, based on feedback, makes needed changes; thinks about their provider roles within an interprofessional client-centred context
Encourage the heart	Recognizes contributions of others	Collaborative leader in the team recognizes the positive work of all team members, including the client, toward meeting client-set goals for care; helps team members with the client, celebrates achievement of steps toward client-set goals of care and well-being

From Orchard, C., & Rykhoff, M. (2015). Collaborative leadership within interprofessional practice. In D. Forman, M. Jones, & J. Thistlethwaite (Eds.), *Leadership and collaboration: Further developments for interprofessional education* (p. 83). Palgrave Macmillan.

psychological dimensions that participants in conflict respond to on the basis of their perceptions of a particular situation" (Johansen, 2012, p. 50). Jehn has suggested that team conflicts consist of three types of conflict: relationship, task, and process (Jehn, 1995; Jehn et al., 2008). *Relational team conflicts* arise from "interpersonal animosity, tension, or annoyance among members to disagreements on non-work-related issues such as personal or social issues" (Tekleab et al., 2009, p. 152). *Task team conflicts* arise from "disagreements among team members about the content of the tasks being performed, including in differences in viewpoints, ideas, and opinions" (Tekleab et al., 2009, p. 173). And *process team conflicts* "involve incompatibilities regarding how to carry out the work, such as logistical issues and the distribution of task responsibilities" (Jehn & Bendersky, 2003, p. 240).

In further studies, O'Neill and McLarnon (2018) found that when relationship and process conflicts are held in "check," task conflict can be a beneficial form of disagreement. Furthermore, when teams meet three conditions—they deal with nonroutine complex tasks, necessitate a high level of interdependency, and need shared input to reach effective decisions—the beneficial value of task conflict resolution is shown during planning processes (van den Berg et al., 2014). Health care interprofessional teams surely meet all three of these conditions. The nature of client care planning to achieve effective outcomes necessitates a group of different health providers using their shared knowledge, skills, and expertise to arrive at a shared approach to a client's care. To derive the benefit from team task conflict resolution, however, requires that the team adopt a team conflict resolution process. The following six-step process is recommended (Orchard et al., n.d.):

- Step 1: Recognize the disagreement in the team.
- Step 2: Listen to varying points of view.
- Step 3: Consider what is valuable in each viewpoint.
- Step 4: Present reasons for disagreeing with each dissenting viewpoint.
- Step 5: Discuss the importance of each dissenting viewpoint.
- Step 6: Come to a cooperative team decision to resolve disagreement.

These steps reflect the application of Johnson and colleagues' constructive controversy approach to a health care team disagreement (Johnson et al., 2006). The most difficult part of being a team member

is speaking up when a disagreement occurs. Therefore, for all members to feel comfortable addressing a disagreement, there must be trust in the team among all members and agreement that each team member has a responsibility to speak up when a disagreement exists. Think about a recent experience you had when there was a disagreement in the group. How did you feel? What action did you take or not take, and why? Consider the above six recommended steps for conflict resolution—were any of them used?

For a team to be able to effectively deal with disagreements, all the other CIHC dimensions of interprofessional client-centred collaborative practice must be present. For example, when all team members have shared their knowledge, skills, and expertise with each other and the team has teamwork roles for how they operationalize their meetings, then the likelihood of relationship conflicts will be lessened. Process conflicts are also less likely to occur when there are guidelines for meetings; techniques such as SBAR are applied to shape the content of messages; attention is paid to the relational aspects of how messages are communicated; and teams use a conflict resolution process. This allows for the resolution of disagreements to be addressed within the team and allows for a variety of perspectives to be considered when planning clients' care.

In summary, professional nurses integrate their personal, professional, and ethical values with standards of practice to guide their competence to enact nursing founded on patterns of knowing demonstrated through an organizing framework such as the clinical judgement model or nursing process. Nurses apply their nursing lens in care discussions about their clients when relationships with other health care providers within interprofessional client-centred practice are guided by the CIHC competency framework.

KEY CONCEPTS

- Client-centred care is at the heart of nursing professional practice.
- Interprofessional client-centred collaborative practice begins with an understanding of one's personal knowing within the context of ways of knowing.
- Five ways of knowing include silence, received knowing, subjective knowing, procedural knowing, and constructed knowing.

- Nursing professional patterns of knowing include empirical, aesthetic, personal, and ethical.
- A nurse's knowing is then applied to how the nurse thinks about their reasoning process in nursing practice.
- Two approaches used in a nurse's thinking process are the nursing process and the clinical judgement model.
- The nursing process involves perception, thought, feeling, and action.
- The clinical judgement model involves noticing, interpreting, responding, and reflecting.
- Tanner's judgement model of practice is useful for fitting nursing practice within both a nursing team and an interprofessional collaborative team.
- Identifying the nurse's role when working within interprofessional teams of health care providers can enhance competence in such teamwork.

CRITICAL THINKING EXERCISES

1. *Explore your own way of knowing:* It is important to understand how your own ways of knowing shape your interpretation of the information you receive during an encounter with a client. (You may wish to review Belenky et al.'s [1986] ways of knowing before answering these questions.) Recalling your client Mrs. Black, answer the following questions:
   a. Which of the ways of knowing do you use in your learning? What might be Mrs. Black's way of knowing?
   b. Is there *a match* between your way of knowing and Mrs. Black's way of knowing? How can you determine whether there is?
   c. If you perceive that there is a mismatch, how might you adjust the way you communicate with Mrs. Black to help ensure that the communication has meaning for her?

2. *Explore the client's decision-making processes:* Consider how you would determine the decision-making process that Mrs. Black or one of her family members might have used to decide to bring Mrs. Black to the hospital. (Mrs. Black likely felt a change in the normal functioning of her body.) You may wish to review Klein's naturalistic decision-making patterns. These patterns are important to apply as you consider how to gather more information from Mrs. Black in order to shape an effective care plan. Review the patterns that Klein reports are part of a person's naturalistic decision-making process, then answer the following:
   a. What inquiry would you make with the Blacks to determine their initial response to Mrs. Black's reason for seeking professional help?
   b. What inquiry would you make to explore with Mrs. Black the various actions she might have initially taken to address this change in her body's functioning?
   c. What inquiry would you make to explore with Mrs. Black or her family what finally caused them to come to the hospital for professional help?

3. *Setting goal(s) for Mrs. Black's care:* In the first three critical thinking questions, you focused on starting to collect information. Now, identify with Mrs. Black what is/are her goal(s) for her care in the hospital. What might be Mrs. Black's goal(s) for her care?

4. *Challenge your existing personal and professional values within the following scenario:* You are a student nurse working with Mrs. Black. This is the second week you have been in this placement. During morning report, Mrs. Black is scheduled for transition from hospital to home that same day. Her gestational diabetes is under control, and she has received her diabetes education to be able to take care of herself. You enter her room and ask her if she is looking forward to being able to go home today. She seems shocked by this information. You realize that perhaps no one has informed Mrs. Black about this transition today. You ask her about her shocked response. She starts to cry, saying that she did not know she would be going home today and that she is still having trouble giving herself insulin injections. You explore with her what difficulties she is still having with administering the insulin. She explains that she previously had a stroke that left her with some weakness in her dominant hand. She finds it almost impossible to hold the bottle of insulin and to withdraw the required amount into the syringe. You explore further by asking Mrs. Black how she was shown to give herself the insulin. You then ask her whether an occupational therapist came to help her overcome her challenges with the insulin withdrawal process, and she replies no.
   a. What concerns were expressed by Mrs. Black in this scenario?
   b. What are the key issues that Mrs. Black is facing?
   c. What actions could you take to support these values?
   d. What additional information do you need to seek from Mrs. Black and your clinical instructor to fully understand this situation, and what services are likely needed to resolve it?
   e. Which of your personal and professional values were challenged that may have caused these feelings?

5. *Reflection-in-action related to this scenario:*
   a. What surprised you about yourself?
   b. Were the feelings and values that emerged unique to your personal values?
   c. Were these values also consistent with the CNA *Code of Ethics*?

6. *Social determinants of health:* What may appear to be a straightforward health issue for Mrs. Black is really buried in several social determinants of health (SDHs). In the following table, in column 1, list the SDHs that are being challenged within the Black family. In column 2, explore what further information about each SDH you will need to gather from the Black family in order to effectively address the SDHs that are most important to them, according to what you know from this scenario.

SDHs Affecting the Black Family	Additional Information Needed to Address the Black Family's SDHs

7. *Reflect-on-action:* Consider the thoughts that came to mind as you read the case study about the Black family.
   a. What personal values do you hold that influenced the way you judged the members of this family and their current situation?
   b. Which nursing professional values are related to the Black family case study?
   c. Did any of your initial judgements about the Black family change upon reaching the end of this chapter?
   d. What did you learn from this chapter and the Black family case study that you will use in future client situations?

8. *Integration of nursing professional and interprofessional identities:*
   a. What abilities do you need to develop to effectively participate in interprofessional client-centred collaborative practice?
   b. What actions will you take to gain exposure to interprofessional learning with, from, and about other health care providers?
   c. How will you apply your nursing code of ethics in practice situations to ensure that the client's voice is heard and considered as part of care planning?

d. What actions will you take to gain both an understanding of and practice in developing collaborative teamwork skills?

e. What process will you use to address team conflicts or disagreements that may arise during your teamwork?

f. What actions will you take to assume accountability for agreed-upon care interventions that reside within the nursing standards of practice in completing assigned activities?

g. How will you evaluate your own performance with the team and revise your future interactions based on your reflection?

🌐 *Answers to Critical Thinking Exercises appear on the Evolve website.*

REVIEW QUESTIONS

Review Questions 1 to 4 relate to the case study at the beginning of the chapter.

Part 1: You are in your practice setting. You are on a coffee break with other colleagues on the unit. You hear one of the staff members talking about your client, Mrs. Black, and how frustrated she is with her inability to give herself insulin. Others comment that Mrs. Black does not seem to want to go home. You listen to them and wonder whether you should comment on the problems Mrs. Black is experiencing. You then realize that this discussion is a breach of Mrs. Black's privacy, but you are unsure about what to do in this situation.

After the break, you find time to discuss this breach with the staff member. You explain that you overheard the discussion and felt that this was a breach of Mrs. Black's confidentiality, but you wondered whether the other staff member felt the same way. At first, the staff member is angry with you. You explain that you are in a learning situation and are trying to understand when such a discussion about a client does or does not constitute such a breach. The staff member then seems to calm down and comments that you have brought up a very good point and that they will be more careful in the future.

1. Which of the following ethical values are demonstrated in this situation? *(Select all that apply.)*
   a. Providing safe, compassionate, competent, and ethical care
   b. Promoting and respecting informed decision making
   c. Preserving dignity
   d. Promoting justice
   e. Being accountable

2. Which of the following aspects of Tanner's clinical judgement model are demonstrated in the scenario described? *(Select all that apply.)*
   a. Noticing
   b. Interpreting
   c. Responding
   d. Reflection-in-action
   e. Reflection-on-action

Part 2: As a soon-to-graduate registered nurse (RN), you learned to practise as a "real" nurse through your program's practice experiences. However, you are starting to worry about how you will be able to assume your RN role when you encounter other clients like Mrs. Black and her family, and how you will interact with other health care providers who have so much more experience than you do. You recently participated in an interprofessional education workshop at your university that focused on communicating within teams. Yesterday, when you were caring for Mrs. Black in the practice setting, her physician confronted you and questioned whether Mrs. Black had been taken for her prescribed ultrasound yet, since it was ordered for early yesterday morning. You were taken aback by this confrontation with the physician and

were left speechless. You knew that Mrs. Black had not been for her ultrasound, but worried about how the physician would respond if you told them this information. There was a very good reason that Mrs. Black had not yet received the ultrasound—the machine was not working, and the unit staff had called to cancel all tests for that day.

3. Communication consists of content and the relational aspect associated with how the content is received. Which of the following relational aspects were at play in this scenario that likely resulted in your not being able to respond to the physician? *(Select all that apply.)*
   a. Affinity
   b. Immediacy
   c. Respect
   d. Control

Part 3: You are working in a primary care setting within a largely Indigenous population. Mrs. Black comes in to visit the team with her new baby. When you reintroduce yourself to Mrs. Black and comment on her new baby, she is pleased to remember that you had helped her manage her insulin injections. You had not previously realized that Mrs. Black identified as Indigenous. She shares with you that she had left her reservation when she married Mr. Black, who is not Indigenous. This is the first time she has come into the clinic after delivering her new son. She tells you that she no longer has diabetes but worries that it might come back in a few years. She further shares that it is wonderful not to have to take insulin anymore. You ask about her son, and she tells you she was very relieved that he did not have cystic fibrosis. You then ask her how she has been managing her expanded family. She shares that they live in a two-bedroom rented apartment and the space is very tight for all of them. Mr. Black continues to drive long-distance trucks, so they have been able to maintain a steady income during the pandemic. She further shares that Mr. Black is against any of them getting the COVID-19 vaccinations. You begin exploring with her the reasons for Mr. Black's opposition to the vaccine. Mrs. Black shares that her husband believes it was developed too fast and has not been adequately tested yet. Mr. Black wants Mrs. Black to wait until they feel it is safe for all of them to have the vaccine. However, Mrs. Black states that she wants all of them to get vaccinated because three of her relatives have already died from complications of COVID-19.

4. Which actions would you take to assist Mrs. Black in her conflict with Mr. Black about getting vaccinated? *(Select all that apply.)*
   a. Share accurate information about the development and testing of the COVID-19 vaccines.
   b. Explore Mr. Black's views on the other vaccines that the children have already received.
   c. Help Mrs. Black learn an approach that she can use to resolve the conflict between them.
   d. Take no action because you have not heard Mr. Black's viewpoint on COVID-19 vaccines.
   e. Encourage Mrs. Black to bring Mr. Black to the clinic for an appointment, where the team can discuss with Mr. Black his concerns about the vaccine.
   f. Help set up a shared meeting between Mr. and Mrs. Black to allow them to work through this conflict while guiding them through the steps of a conflict resolution process.
   g. Provide Mrs. Black and her children with access to COVID-19 vaccinations at the clinic.

Answers: 1. a, c; **2.** a, b, c; **3.** c, d; **4.** a, e, f.

🌐 *Rationales for the Review Questions appear on the Evolve website.*

RECOMMENDED WEBSITES

British Columbia College of Nurses and Midwives: https://www.bccnm.ca
This website features dropdown menus containing links to practice standards (including Indigenous cultural safety, cultural humility, and antiracism), entry-to-practice competencies, and other important information for nurses and midwives in British Columbia.

Canadian Nurses Association *Code of Ethics for Registered Nurses:* https://cna-aiic.ca/en/on-the-issues/best-nursing/nursing-ethics
This web page links to the *Code of Ethics* that all Canadian nurses must adhere to. While this is a national code, because of the provincial responsibility for health care, some provinces also have their own code of ethics.

College of Nurses of Ontario: Standards and Guidelines: https://www.cno.org/en/learn-about-standards-guidelines/standards-and-guidelines
In Ontario, there are separate ethical standards for nurses practising in this province in addition to the CNA's *Code of Ethics*. This web page links to various standards and guidelines.

College of Nurses of Ontario: Ethical Practice for Nurses: https://www.cno.org/en/learn-about-standards-guidelines/educational-tools/learning-modules/ethics
This web page presents a learning module on ethics, including a video explaining ethical practice for nurses in Ontario.

College of Registered Nurses of Alberta: https://nurses.ab.ca/protect-the-public/standards-for-rns-and-nps/standards
This web page contains links to the practice standards, scope of practice, and entry-to-practice competencies for nurses practising in Alberta.

College of Registered Nurses of Manitoba: https://www.crnm.mb.ca/resource/entry-level-competencies-elcs-for-the-practice-of-registered-nurses
This web page features the entry-to-practice competencies for registered nurses in Manitoba.

College of Registered Nurses of Newfoundland and Labrador: https://crnnl.ca/site/uploads/2021/09/standards-of-practice-for-rns-and-nps.pdf
This document describes the standards of practice for nurses in Newfoundland and Labrador.

College of Registered Nurses of Prince Edward Island: https://crnpei.ca/professional-practice/standards
This web page lists standards for practice and entry-to-practice competencies for nurses who are licensed to practise in Prince Edward Island.

Free Apps for Nurses and Nursing Students: https://www.berxi.com/resources/articles/best-free-nursing-apps
This web page lists a variety of free apps designed for use on smartphones and other mobile devices. Note that the apps have been developed for US practitioners.

Nova Scotia College of Nursing: https://www.nscn.ca/professional-practice/practice-standards/entry-level-competencies
This web page presents the entry-level competencies for each nursing designation in Nova Scotia.

Nurses Association of New Brunswick: http://www.nanb.nb.ca/practice/standards
This web page lists the nursing standards of practice, entry-level competencies, and the code of ethics for nurses in New Brunswick.

Online Journal of Nursing Informatics: https://www.himss.org/resources/online-journal-nursing-informatics
This peer-reviewed journal is published three times a year and covers a wide variety of topics in the field of nursing informatics. There is a separate category for student publications.

Ordre des infirmières et infirmiers auxiliaires du Québec: https://www.oiiaq.org/ordre/systeme-professionnel
This web page links to the Quebec Professional Code, which applies to all regulated professionals, including nurses.

Registered Nurses Association of the Northwest Territories and Nunavut: https://rnantnu.ca/professional-practice
This web page features professional practice information, including the entry-to-practice competencies expected of any nurses wishing to practise in the Northwest Territories and Nunavut.

Saskatchewan Registered Nurses Association: https://www.crns.ca/about-us/what-is-an-rn
On this web page, there is a comprehensive description of what a registered nurse is, along with other important for practising nurses.

Yukon Registered Nurses Association: https://www.yrna.ca/standards
This web page lists the standards of practice for nurses in Yukon, including a recently adopted cultural safety practice standard (based on the cultural safety standard for BC nurses and midwives).

🌐 REFERENCES

A full reference list is available on the website for this book at http://evolve.elsevier.com/Canada/Potter/fundamentals/

20

Family Nursing

Written by Christina H. West, RN, PhD, and Sonya L. Jakubec, RN, BHScN, MN, PhD

OBJECTIVES

Mastery of content in this chapter will enable you to:

- Define the key terms listed.
- Explain the various definitions of family.
- Examine current trends in the Canadian family.
- Describe how family members influence one another's health.
- Compare family as context, family as patient, and family in context, explaining how these different perspectives influence nursing practice with families.
- State the three major categories of the Calgary Family Assessment Model (CFAM) and understand the subcategories to consider in a family assessment.

- Describe key concepts of the Calgary Family Intervention Model (CFIM).
- Explain family nursing as relational inquiry.
- Describe key concepts and approaches to relational inquiry–based practices for family nursing.
- Ask assessment questions to learn relevant information about family functioning in the context of health or illness.
- Describe the relational approaches and practices needed to conduct a family interview and effectively intervene with the family in nursing practice.

KEY TERMS

Alliances and coalitions

Beliefs

Calgary Family Assessment Model (CFAM)

Calgary Family Intervention Model (CFIM)

Circular communication

Circular questions

Commendation

Context (family as context, family in context, family as patient)

Ecomap

Emotional communication

Empowerment

Family

Family centred-care

Family forms

Family nursing

Gender identity

Genogram

Illness narrative

Influence

Linear questions

Nonverbal communication

Problem solving

Relational inquiry

Resiliency

Roles

Two-Spirit

Verbal communication

🌐 WEBSITE

http://evolve.elsevier.com/Canada/Potter/fundamentals/

CASE STUDY

Nuni (preferred pronouns: she/her) is a 75-year-old Oji-Cree Elder and grandmother who has breast cancer. Nuni has recovered from mastectomy surgery and is about to begin chemotherapy treatment in an outpatient clinic 90 minutes from her community, which values Nuni's contributions as an advisor and Elder. Currently, Nuni lives with extended family in an intergenerational household, which includes an adult child, Ramona (60 years of age), who is a single parent of two children, Kiri (42 years old) and Nootau (44 years old), along with three grandchildren. Four adopted grandchildren (step-children from Kiri and Nootau's new and prior partners) spend time with the family on occasion. Nuni's family and community are impacted by this illness experience.

Think about this case study as you read this chapter. There are Review Questions at the end of the chapter about this case study.

The role of the family in health care has evolved significantly throughout Canada's colonial history. In the early twentieth century, visiting public health nurses and private duty nurses worked closely with family members, providing home-based care. After World War II, with the development of a national health care system, there was a significant shift of nursing services into hospital settings. With these historical changes in health care, families and community members were largely excluded from care, while physicians and nurses came to be seen as holding expertise in health care provision (Elliott et al., 2009). Although tensions between the role of professionals and family members continue to persist (Rankin, 2015), families and nurses have increasingly forged more collaborative relationships. Family nursing is a highly contextual, relational, and skill-based practice (International Family Nursing Association, 2015; Shajani & Snell, 2019) that is further complicated by the intensity and complexity of contemporary practice contexts (Hartrick Doane & Varcoe, 2021). The role of family caregivers as essential partners and the challenges of recognizing and consistently integrating family caregivers into health care were also highlighted during the COVID-19 pandemic (Canadian Foundation for Healthcare Improvement, 2020; Chu et al., 2020).

Within family nursing practice, nurses simultaneously attend to the needs of multiple family members in the context of a complex health care environment (Registered Nurses' Association of Ontario [RNAO], 2015). As an example of the complexity faced in contemporary nursing practice, nurses provide support to and education for unpaid family caregivers, who in turn provide essential emotional and physical support to family members during illness, disability, or age-related need (Parmar et al., 2021; Statistics Canada, 2020). The location of a patient's care may create significant challenges for the family in relation to travel, employment, and finances. Other examples include frail older persons isolated from extended family and friends, or recently immigrated families who face illness in the context of significant language, cultural, and economic barriers.

It is within these diverse and challenging contexts that nurses strive to provide family-centred care, an approach characterized by dignity and respect, information sharing, patient and family participation, and family–professional collaboration (RNAO, 2015). Despite the growing adoption of family-centred care within modern health care settings, implementation has been challenging (Thirsk et al., 2021), and differing conceptual understandings persist internationally (Al-Motlaq et al., 2019). Furthermore, Rankin (2015) reported that patient- and family-centred care is "organized to be empty rhetoric" (p. 533), acting to socially organize nurses' work to meet the efficiency-based priorities of the health care system rather than the needs of family members. A lack of research, shared language, relational ethics, and collaborative practice approaches have posed significant challenges to family-centred care implementation (Al-Motlaq et al., 2019; Clay & Parsh, 2016; Tomaselli et al., 2020).

Family nursing is based on the assumption that every person, regardless of age, is a member of some type of family form and carries with them family experiences that profoundly influence their lives and health care encounters (Shajani & Snell, 2019). Also central is the presumption that individuals are best understood within a family context. A change in one family member, such as illness, affects all other family members, and family strengths need to be supported in generalist family nursing practice (International Family Nursing Association, 2015). Family nursing promotes, supports, and provides for the well-being and health of the family and individual family members (Shajani & Snell, 2019). Nurses need to understand the relational contexts as well as the unique strengths and needs of each family encountered in practice. It is also critical that nurses work to understand the historical and contextual influences that shape each family's life experience so that comprehensive, upstream family care is facilitated. Nurses need to be sensitive and attuned to the complex systemic forces that influence health, illness, and family life (Hartrick Doane & Varcoe, 2021).

Through relational inquiry, and the use of family assessment and intervention frameworks, nurses can effectively collaborate with families to enhance the unique strengths and resources they possess while simultaneously working to address the structural influences that shape family members' health experiences (Gottlieb & Gottlieb, 2017; Hartrick Doane & Varcoe, 2021; Shajani & Snell, 2019). Nurses are encouraged to move beyond understanding family as an entity or as the recipient of nursing intervention. Rather, the aim of family nursing is to create a collaborative and respectful nurse–family relationship as well as to support the relationships between family members. Family nursing supports families in achieving and maintaining optimal health throughout the course of an illness and beyond.

WHAT IS A FAMILY?

Defining *family* within complex relational and clinical contexts is not a simple task. Different definitions have resulted in heated debates among social scientists and legislators and have historically excluded Indigenous values and views of relationality and kinship with extended human and more-than-human relations (Campbell et al., 2020). Formal definitions have included understandings of family as a biological or legal entity and as social networks complete with personally or institutionally organized values and ideologies. In addition to the traditional nuclear or extended family, the definition of family has come to include a variety of other family structures: lone-parent families, stepfamilies, same-sex couples with or without children, foster families, formally or informally adoptive families, friends, neighbours, and street family for people who are experiencing homelessness. Pets or other nonhuman beings may also be important members of the family (International Federation on Ageing, 2020).

In the unique and diverse constructs of people's lives, family, simply put, refers to "two or more individuals who depend on one another for emotional, physical, and economic support. The members of the family are self-defined" (Kaakinen, 2018a, p. 5). Shajani and Snell (2019) state, "The family is who they say they are" (p. 55). Based on these contexts and definitions, a family is a group of two or more people whose membership is defined by the family itself. Therefore, it is critical that nurses working with families ask family members who they consider to be their family and then include those members in care provision.

Families are as diverse as the individuals that compose them; patients, as well as health care providers, hold deeply ingrained beliefs and values about family. It is important that nurses intentionally explore these values and beliefs within their nursing practice with families (Shajani & Snell, 2019). As a nurse, your personal beliefs do not have to coincide with those of the patient, but in order to provide responsive, individualized, and compassionate care, it is essential to be aware of your own history, values, and beliefs and to seek to understand the family and their unique needs (Sinclair et al., 2016). Families have their own strengths, resources, challenges, and historical and cultural contexts (Hartrick Doane & Varcoe, 2021; Shajani & Snell, 2019). Families nonetheless share some general characteristics that include future obligations and caregiving functions, such as protection, nourishment, and socialization of family members (McGoldrick et al., 2016).

CURRENT TRENDS IN THE CANADIAN FAMILY

Although the institution of the family remains strong, the form and structure of the family itself has changed. Nurses in Canada will encounter every type of family. In addition to traditionally defined families (i.e., nuclear and extended families), our communities are made up of blended families, cohabiting heterosexual or same-sex partners, sibling-led households, foster families, and, more recently, couples living apart or commuter families, as well as grandparent-led families (grandparents parenting grandchildren) as well as friends and community members functioning as family. Nurses need to be aware of current trends and social factors that affect the structure and function of the family. The following information about current family trends is based on comparative data from Statistics Canada's 2016 Census of Population (Statistics Canada, 2017a, 2022a), alongside provisional and final 2021 census data (Statistics Canada, 2022b), and other sources of demographic data.

Family Forms

Family forms are patterns of people considered by family members to be included in the family (Box 20.1). Although all families have some

BOX 20.1	Family Forms

Blended Family
Formed when both parents bring children from previous relationships into a new, joint living situation or when children from the current union and children from previous unions are living together

Extended Family
Includes the nuclear family and other relatives (perhaps grandparents, aunts, uncles, cousins)

Lone-Parent Family
Consists of one parent and one or more children. The lone-parent family is formed when one parent leaves the nuclear family because of death, divorce, or desertion or when a single person decides to have or adopt a child.

Stepfamily
Formed when at least one child in a household is from a previous relationship of one of the parents

Traditional Nuclear Family
Consists of a mother and father (married or common law) and their children

Family Forms—Increasing Diversity
Family forms and family relationships within Canada have become increasingly diverse. They include married and common-law couples without children, families in which grandparents provide care for their grandchildren, adults living alone, and same-sex couples (with or without children). The proportion of traditional families (two married parents and children living together) in Canada is declining, while the proportion of common-law and lone-parent families is increasing. Today, the average Canadian household consists of 2.9 people, with more one-person households (28.2%) (based on the 2021 census; Statistics Canada, 2022a) than ever with am ever decreasing number of married couple households with children (40.6%) (Statistics Canada, 2022a). These changes hold significant societal implications. For instance, smaller families and more people living alone have led to an increasing need for federal support of affordable child care in Canada. Furthermore, the care and support of young children or older Canadians is now spread among a decreasing number of family members.

common characteristics, each family form has unique challenges and strengths. Nurses should maintain an open mind about what each family sees as their needs so that potential resources and concerns are not overlooked.

The 2021 Census of Population (Statistics Canada, 2022a) reported major changes and some notable stability in the Canadian family in three aspects: structural, functional, and affective. Some of the changes, based on Canadian census data, are as follows:

- The number of adults who are in a couple has been remarkably stable from 1921 (58%) to 2021 (57%). Non-binary and transgender people are less likely to live in a couple arrangement than cisgender people.
- As a long-term pattern, 4.4 million people in Canada lived alone, up from 1.7 million in 1981, representing 15% of all adults.
- 77% of couples in Canada are married (down from 83% in 1981)
  - 22.7% are living as common-law couples (more than triple since 1981).
  - 16.4% are lone-parent families—diverse family structures that are continuously evolving—up from 11% in 1981, though relatively unchanged since 2001.
- Unchanged since 2011, 1 in 10 children lived in step-family households.
- In 2016, there were 72 880 same-sex couple families in Canada, 12% of which were raising children (up from 8.6% in 2001); in 2021, the number of same-sex couples grew to 127 640, 15% of which were raising children.
- In 2016, there were nearly 404 000 multigenerational households in Canada—the *fastest growing household type*, with 442 000 multigenerational households in 2021, a 50% increase over the previous 20 years.
- In 2016, nearly 33 000 children in Canada aged 0 to 14 lived in grand-family households, that is, children living with grandparent(s) with no middle (i.e., parent) generation present; 36 860 children lived solely with grandparents in 2021.

Statistics and historical changes over time require context, conceptual analysis, and critical examination. For instance, family data in the most recent Canadian census may not have data that can be compared on particular family forms over time. For an expanded understanding and more detailed discussion of family diversities and their inherent inequities, refer to the Vanier Institute's *Family Diversities Framework* (https://vanierinstitute.ca/family-diversities-framework).

Lesbian, gay, bisexual, transgender, queer, and Two-Spirit (LGBTQ2) individuals are connected to family through membership in their families of origin, as well as in the families they have chosen to create both within and outside the context of legal marriage (McGoldrick et al., 2016). These individuals, couples, children, and others in the extended family may face discrimination and challenges within the family life cycle, including difficulties with identity development, the process of coming out, coupling, parenting, and transitions in later life.

Canadian society has witnessed a significant shift in how many and which caregivers stay at home—outside of the formal workforce—to care for children. The COVID-19 pandemic radically altered work and domestic arrangements in ways that will continue to unfold. Still, while the majority of stay-at-home parents are women, men are increasingly taking on the caregiver role. In 2017, men represented 1 in 10 stay-at-home parents in Canada (Statistics Canada, 2018). Grandparents have also increasingly taken responsibility for raising their grandchildren. In 2021, nearly 1 in 10 children (9.3%, or 553 855 children) were living in the same household as at least one of their grandparents, unchanged from 2016 but up from 7% in 2001 (Statistics Canada, 2022a). Sharing a home with one's grandchildren, or providing primary care to one's grandchildren, is influenced by numerous factors, including culture, sociodemographics, health, and economic characteristics (Martin et al., 2021).

Family Changes and Challenges: Understanding the Influence of Sociocultural Contexts

Sociocultural and economic changes are significantly increasing challenges to family health. The COVID-19 pandemic glaringly illuminated the many ways in which the social determinants of health (e.g., economic stability and social/community context) profoundly impact family health and well-being. Many families find themselves unable to respond effectively to complex social and health experiences (e.g., poverty, violence, illness, learning disabilities, cognitive decline and/or dementia). These situations can undermine existing relationships of care, leaving family members more vulnerable and socially isolated during times when support is most needed (Reiter, 2019). Cultural influences on family well-being are numerous. For example, culture influences the expectation of contact and time spent between adult children and parents, as well as the expectations that immigrant families have about integration into Canadian society (Kalmijn, 2019). These changes and challenges are crucial to recognize as part of family nursing assessment and intervention.

Domestic Roles and Responsibilities

Domestic roles have become increasingly complex as more and more families consist of two wage earners or single-person households (Statistics Canada, 2021b). Balancing employment and domestic responsibilities creates challenges in child and elder care as well as household work. Maternal well-being and family functioning research provides evidence that maternal life satisfaction and parent–child activities support child development and prosocial behaviour (Richter et al., 2018). However, finding high-quality child care and managing domestic tasks can be a major challenge. Management of domestic tasks and parenting responsibilities varies substantially from family to family. In addition, Indigenous, European, African, Asian, and South Asian communities have historically valued and maintained extended family involvement in family caregiving (Campbell et al., 2020; Hokanson et al., 2018; Hsieh et al., 2017; Lindstrom et al., 2016) (see Chapter 11 for further information on the diversity of the Canadian population).

Economic Status

Families in Canada have experienced profound economic instability as a result of COVID-19. This economic strain has highlighted the powerful influence of the social determinants of health on family well-being. In 2019, the median annual income of Canadian families (including unattached individuals under 65 years of age, singles or couples with children, as well as older persons) was $62 900. The median after-tax income for couples with children was $105 500, while the median annual income for female lone-parent households was $52 500 (Statistics Canada, 2021a). Distribution of wealth greatly affects the capacity to maintain health. Low educational preparation, poverty, and decreased amounts of support all magnify the impact of illness on the family and increase the amount of illness in the family. According to the market basket measure, which was adopted as Canada's official poverty line in June 2019, a family is considered to be living in poverty if it does not have enough income to purchase a basic collection of goods and services in its community. In 2019, in Canada, 3.7 million people, or 10.1% of the population, were living in poverty (Statistics Canada, 2021a).

Indigenous Families

Social and health inequities and disparities have profound impacts on Indigenous individuals, families, and communities in Canada (Browne et al., 2016) and thus need to be comprehensively addressed in family nursing practice. Indigenous families with children younger than 24 years are the fastest growing population in Canada (see Chapter 12). Indigenous families tend to be larger, have younger family members, and contain greater diversity in family members than do non-Indigenous families (Hokanson et al., 2018; Hsieh et al., 2017). Each community of Indigenous peoples has its own traditions, rituals, relationships, and functions that need to be respected and honoured in nursing care. Indigenous families have multigenerational kinship structures that often consist of a network of grandparents, parents, children, aunts, uncles, and cousins. Each member has obligations to the family and all relations human and non-human (Campbell et al., 2020). Traditionally, women and grandmothers held a sacred and central role within Indigenous families, carrying responsibility for nurturing community members, particularly children (Anderson, 2011). Children are held in high esteem within Indigenous communities, and there is an expectation that they be treated gently and protected from harm (Muir & Bohr, 2014).

The colonization and cultural genocide of Indigenous peoples has led to decades of cultural disruption and trauma, including the disruption and loss of traditional Indigenous family values and intergenerational family and parenting patterns; these impacts are felt by Indigenous communities to this day. Forced assimilation of Indigenous peoples was founded on the colonial belief that Indigenous values were inferior to those of the dominant culture (Muir & Bohr, 2014). In the era of truth and reconciliation, traditional values and Indigenous voices are being reclaimed and re-examined, including family values (Lindstrom et al., 2016). The Calgary Family Assessment and Intervention Models (Shajani & Snell, 2019), as well as Hartrick Doane and Varcoe's (2021) approach to relational inquiry with families, can assist nurses in creating sensitivity, cultural safety, and attentiveness to the strengths and knowledge of Indigenous families as well as the challenges they face.

Family Caregivers

Persons 80 years of age and older are Canada's fastest growing age group. One out of every seven Canadians is an older person. Average life expectancy in 2020 was 81.7 years, with women (84.3 years) living slightly longer than men (80.2 years) (Statistics Canada, 2022b). The aging population has affected the family life cycle, especially the middle generation, as many family members serve as informal caregivers for older persons, children, and persons with disabilities. Most of these caregivers are older women, and they frequently provide 10 hours or more of unpaid assistance per week (Arriagada, 2020; Parmar et al., 2021; Statistics Canada, 2020). Family caregiving involves the routine provision of services and personal care activities for a family member by friends, partners, spouses, siblings, or children, all of whom experience their own transitions and needs in this informal but essential work (Duggleby et al., 2017). Caregiving activities include personal and illness care, instrumental activities of daily living (shopping or housekeeping), and ongoing emotional support. The respite needs of family caregivers, which involves the temporary and scheduled relief of caregiving responsibilities, represent an important aspect of family nursing assessment and intervention.

Although family caregivers often find that providing care has many rewards, this group must often balance caring for a family member with many other ongoing demands (e.g., raising children, working full time). As a result, they may suffer physical and emotional health challenges related to these competing demands (Arriagada, 2020; McGoldrick et al., 2016; Parmar et al., 2021). Box 20.2 provides a list of family caregiving concerns in the context of caring for older persons.

THE FAMILY AND HEALTH

The family is the primary context in which health promotion and disease prevention take place (Box 20.3). The health of the family is influenced by many factors such as biology, social status, economic resources, politics, violence, and geographic and environmental contexts. Each family's beliefs, values, and practices also strongly influence the health-promoting behaviours of its members (Hartrick Doane & Varcoe, 2021). The health status of each individual influences how the family unit functions and its ability to achieve its goals. When the family meets its goals, members tend to feel positive about themselves and their family. Conversely, when they do not meet goals, families may view themselves as ineffective.

Family Strengths and Resiliency

Researchers have focused on resiliency as mediating factors for long-term health (Hadfield & Ungar, 2018). Family resiliency is the ability to cope with expected and unexpected stressors: role changes,

- Nurses need to carefully consider caregiver strain; caregivers are typically older persons whose own physical stamina may be declining or middle-aged adult children who often have other responsibilities.
- Older families have a different social network than younger families; friends and same-generation family members may have died or been ill themselves. Family caregivers may experience significant social isolation. Nurses need to look for social support within the community and family's social network.

- Physical health impairments increase the risk of depression in older persons.
- As in other stages of life, members of older families need to work on developmental tasks (see Chapter 25 for further information about older persons).
- Abuse of older persons occurs across all social classes and settings, with family members and family caregivers being the most frequent perpetrators; this situation sadly grew worse during the COVID-19 pandemic (World Health Organization, 2022). Distress, financial changes, unexplained bruises, and skin or other trauma should not be ignored by health care providers.

BOX 20.3 **FOCUS ON PRIMARY HEALTH CARE**

Family practice nurses focus on active collaboration with individual members and the family unit with the goal of supporting their efforts to reach optimal levels of health and well-being. Nurses working in advanced practice roles in primary health care meet families in a wide variety of settings. The goal of this work is often to improve access to primary health care for people in communities, with assessment, treatment, and care planning follow-up all initiated by family practice nurses (typically those with nurse practitioner designations or other advanced practice education and experience). Nursing practices in family health promotion include, but are not limited to, neonatal assessments, palliative and grief care, school health care, occupational health care, mental health and substance use programs, infusion clinics, and home care. Research has shown that these nursing interventions have a positive impact on the health outcomes of families and communities (Lukewich et al., 2018).

developmental milestones, and crises. The goal of the family is not only to survive the challenge but also to thrive and grow from the knowledge acquired by facing the challenge.

Walsh (2016) defined *family resiliency* as successful coping under conditions of stress and adversity that enables individuals and the family unit to flourish with support. Factors influencing family resiliency include positive outlook; spirituality; flexibility; cohesiveness; clear communication; financial management; shared family involvement in recreation, routines, and rituals; and support networks. Resiliency models consider family strengths as a family such as Nuni's (from the chapter-opening case study) copes with a changed and challenging illness situation, attempting to maintain family functioning (Hadfield & Ungar, 2018). Communication is particularly crucial to resilience and general family functioning. It enables individuals within a family unit to express needs, wants, and concerns to one another. Through communication, family members are able to resolve everyday challenges, promote health of all members, and develop resilience for extraordinary challenges (Walsh, 2016).

Health promotion programs, psychosocial supports, and family counselling or therapy aimed at enhancing communication and other resiliency attributes are available for families and children in many communities. Nurses need to make themselves aware of family-oriented community resources so that families can be referred as needed.

FAMILY NURSING CARE

The Canadian Association of Schools of Nursing (2022) has developed a national nursing education framework that emphasizes family nursing in a number of key competency domains, including knowledge of relational practice to affect health outcomes of individuals, families and communities; collaborative practice with families; and family health promotion. This collaborative family nursing practice must be based on mutual respect and trust. Nurses should examine family patterns, relationships, and interactions when they consider how a health challenge or illness affects a family and, conversely, how a family affects a health challenge or illness (Shajani & Snell, 2019). Nurses are uniquely positioned in work with families to address health inequities, and the nurse's relationship with the family can have a significant influence on

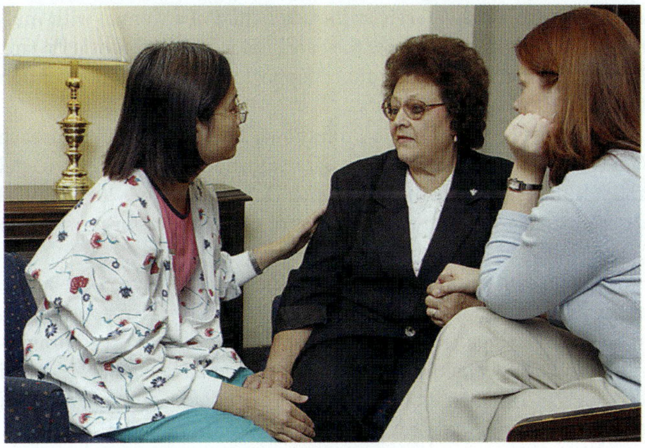

FIGURE 20.1 Nurse (*left*) and family members.

patient and family functioning and health outcomes (Hartrick Doane & Varcoe, 2015; Shajani & Snell, 2021) (Figure 20.1).

Although health care systems in the past tended to emphasize the individual, a family focus is now needed to be able to safely discharge patients to the care of the family or community settings. There is also a pressing need to address within nursing practice the challenges faced by multiple family members, the patient, and the family unit. To begin your nursing practice with families, you must have scientific knowledge of family theory and family nursing. Family nursing care focuses on family as context, family as patient, and understanding families in context. The approach used depends on the care situation and the abilities of the nurse.

Family as Context

When considering the **family as context**, the nurse focuses either on the individual patient within the context of their family or on the family with the individual as context (RNAO, 2015). An example of the first approach is a situation in which a nurse interviews a patient with heart disease, asking the patient's spouse about the family's diet and possible family stressors. The spouse's ability to support their partner's efforts in changing eating patterns and using stress management techniques are also assessed. The focus is the health of the patient within the environment of the family. When patients are unable to communicate, families provide important information about the patient and indicate the patient's wishes. Nurses need to be competent at considering the family as context. Even if there is no opportunity to involve the family directly, the patient is still considered a member of a family.

Family as Patient

When approaching the **family as patient**, the nurse focuses on the entire family—its processes and relationships (e.g., parenting, impacts of the marital relationship, or family caregiving). Family patterns and interactions among family members are the focus rather than individual characteristics. The nursing process concentrates on how these patterns and processes are consistent with achieving and maintaining family and individual health. Nursing practice that focuses on family as patient is also known as *family systems nursing* and requires in-depth knowledge of family dynamics and family systems theory (Shajani & Snell, 2019). Therefore, nurses who specialize in family systems nursing often have advanced skills and training. Specific generalist and advanced practice competencies for family nursing practice have been identified by the International Family Nursing Association (https://internationalfamilynursing.org).

An example of the second approach is a situation in which a community health nurse interviews the adult child of a woman with multiple sclerosis, discussing how they are coping with her mother's care. Family members may need direct support and nursing intervention themselves.

Additionally, using an interprofessional and health equity approach is helpful because family systems are embedded in complex societal and health system structures (Hartrick Doane & Varcoe, 2021). Social determinants of health raise questions of social justice for nurses who are engaged with families (Deatrick, 2017).

In your own nursing practice, it is important that you are aware of the limits of nursing practice and make referrals when appropriate. When considering the family as patient, you aim to support communication and healthy family functioning among family members (Shajani & Snell, 2019). Often, you must support conflict resolution between family members so that each member can confront and resolve challenges in a healthy way. You also may link family members to external and internal resources as necessary.

Understanding Family in Context: Relational Inquiry With Individuals and Families

Family nursing as relational inquiry invites nurses to consider the ways in which families and nurses are embedded within diverse and complex life contexts; this is **family in context**. Hartrick Doane and Varcoe (2021) articulate the importance of critically attending to the social, political, economic, and geographic contexts that influence both family members and nurses who care for them. Nurses need to continually explore how personal and professional definitions of health and family may shape, and possibly constrain, their nursing practice with families. A nurse's perceptions, values, and beliefs about the meaning of family can greatly influence the quality of the therapeutic relationship, the health of patients and families, and the quality of work life experienced by nurses. In a **relational inquiry** approach, nurses intend and act to expand their contextual knowledge of families, developing a more in-depth and comprehensive consideration of the historical, economic, political, social, environmental, and geographic influences at play when families encounter illness or other difficulties related to life transitions.

The nurse's awareness of their own values and beliefs, as well as a critical, reflective consideration of different understandings of health

---

BOX 20.4   **The Five Ws of Relating: An Intentional and Conscious Approach to Family Nursing Inquiry**

You can improve how you relate to family members—aligning your intentions and actions to become more responsive to family health and well-being—by exploring the five Ws of relating: what, who, why, when, and where.

What are you relating to?
On what are you focusing your attention? What are you identifying as priorities? What are you privileging or ignoring? What are you valuing or not valuing?

Who are you relating to?
As you relate to family members, who are you including and who are you leaving out?

Why are you relating?
How do particular purposes and goals guide you in your practice with families?

When are you relating?
When is it that you reach out or distance yourself as you relate to families? How does time and timing shape the way you relate to family members?

Where are you relating?
Consider how context is shaping your experience relating to family members and families.

Adapted from Hartrick Doane, G., & Varcoe, C. (2021). *How to nurse: Relational inquiry in action* (2nd ed., p. 95). Wolters Kluwer.

---

and family, will enhance the nurse's ability to hear the unique stories of family members' lives. Nurses must explore the potential biases they may hold, how those biases may influence the questions they ask, and their ability or inability to listen for and to the experiences of family members.

This practice is guided by several relational capacities that have been described by Hartrick Doane and Varcoe (2021) (also see Chapter 18 for further information about relational practice in communicating). This approach highlights working across differences and acknowledging that power and differences are important, but often invisible, features of relationships. Relational inquiry begins with the five Cs: "being compassionate, curious, committed, competent and corresponding" (Hartrick Doane & Varcoe, 2021, p. 124). Aligning your nursing intentions and values with your approach to inquiry and action in practice takes courage, honesty, and a willingness to look at how you are relating to families. In looking at what you are privileging and what you are ignoring, you can find the gaps between what you intend to do and what you actually do. You can then readjust to relate to patients in ways that are more responsive to family health and well-being. Within your own practice, consider how you might look beyond the surface of patients and families. You can enter your practice with an intentional and conscious approach to inquiry by drawing on the five Ws of relating described in Box 20.4.

ASSESSING THE CHALLENGES, STRENGTHS, AND NEEDS OF THE FAMILY: THE CALGARY FAMILY ASSESSMENT MODEL

Family assessment skills are essential in providing responsive, compassionate, and respectful family care and support. To help families adjust to acute and chronic illness, nurses need to understand the relationships that family members share, what the illness means to family members, how the illness has influenced family functioning, how the family has been affected by the illness, and the support that the family needs most (Shajani & Snell, 2019). Box 20.5 lists the characteristics of families that would most benefit from a family assessment. During such an assessment, the nurse, patient, and family engage relationally and collaboratively in conversation to share information with each other and explore family members' experiences of illness. The nurse will also guide family members to reflect on issues important to the patient and family's well-being.

BOX 20.5 Features of Families: Who Should Be Considered for a Family Assessment?

Families that would most benefit from a family assessment include:

- Families who are experiencing emotional, physical, or spiritual distress or disruption because of a family crisis (e.g., acute, chronic, or life-threatening illness, injury, death, substance use disorder, and/or suspected family violence).
- Families who are experiencing emotional, physical, or spiritual distress or disruption in response to a developmental milestone (e.g., birth, marriage, child leaving home).
- Those who define a problem or illness as a family issue (e.g., the impact of chronic illness on the family).
- Families who have a child or adolescent whom they identify as having difficulties (e.g., cyberbullying at school, fear of cancer treatment, mental health challenges due to COVID-19 social isolation).
- Families who are experiencing issues that are serious enough to threaten family relationships (e.g., terminal illness, abuse, addictions).
- Those who have a family member (adult or child) who is about to be admitted to the hospital.

Adapted from Shajani, Z., & Snell, D. (2019). *Wright and Leahey's nurses and families: A guide to family assessment and intervention* (7th ed., p. 7). F. A. Davis Company.

The **Calgary Family Assessment Model(CFAM)** is a relational, strengths-focused practice model that guides nurses in the completion of comprehensive family assessment (Shajani & Snell, 2019). The CFAM has received international recognition and been adopted by schools of nursing around the world. The CFAM focuses on three key dimensions of family life: structural, developmental, and functional. Each category has several subcategories; however, not all subcategories will be relevant to every family (Figure 20.2). Nurses must decide, on a family-by-family basis, which subcategories are most relevant. Using too many subcategories may result in an overwhelming amount of data and questions for family members; using too few may yield insufficient data, which can distort a family's strengths or challenges. The model can be consulted during discussions about family issues.

Structural Assessment

The structural dimension of the family assessment includes the following:

- *Internal structure:* the people who are included in the family and how they are relationally connected to one another
- *External structure:* the relationships the family shares with people and institutions outside the family unit
- *Context:* the whole situation or background relevant to the family.

Internal Structure. The internal structure of the family—the composition and the relationships among family members—can be further divided into six subcategories: family composition, gender, sexual orientation, rank order, subsystems, and boundaries.

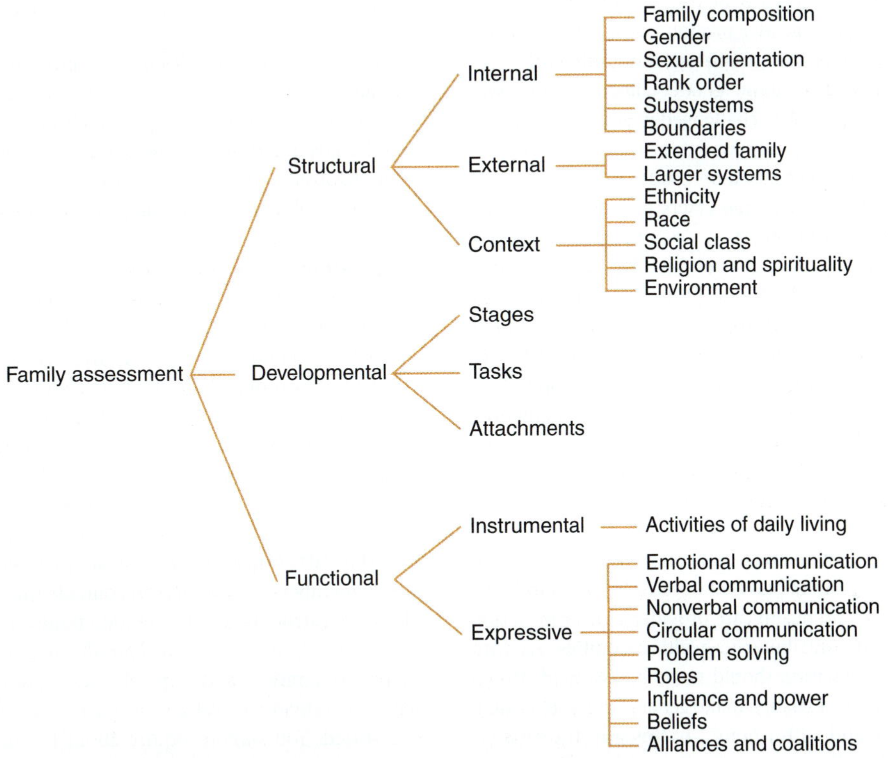

FIGURE 20.2 Branching diagram of the Calgary Family Assessment Model (CFAM). (From Zahra Shajani, Diana Snell. [2019]. *Wright and Leahey's nurses and families: A guide to family assessment and intervention* [7th ed.]. F. A. Davis Company, Philadelphia, PA, with permission.)

Family Composition. *Family composition* refers to the individual members who form the family. The family composition is not limited to the traditional nuclear family; it may include any of the family forms discussed previously (see Box 20.1). It is important to note whether the family composition has changed through additions or losses.

Questions to ask the family
- Who is in your family?
- Does anyone else live with you (e.g., grandparents, boarders, etc.)?
- Has anyone recently moved out of your household, gotten married, or died?
- Can you think of anyone else who is like a family member but is not biologically related?

Gender Identity. *Gender* refers to a person's identity and social classifications, which are often based on masculine or feminine qualities and traits. These identities are fundamental to intimate relationships and are influenced by culture, religion, family, socioeconomic factors, and sexual orientation. Gender identity refers to one's sense of self as male or female. Gender identity can be classified as cisgender (aligned with the gender assigned at birth), transgender (incongruence in a person's gender identity with the gender assigned at birth), gender nonconforming (not conforming to the traditional roles of male or female), and non-binary (identifying as no gender, as a gender other than male or female, or as more than one gender). The term Two-Spirit, which is used by some Indigenous peoples to describe their gender, sexual, or spiritual identity, refers to a person who embodies both a male spirit and a female spirit. The Two-Spirit identity encompasses Indigenous views of gender roles, including the sexual and gender diversity in Indigenous communities (Trans Care BC, 2017). To ensure culturally safe communication and work with an Indigenous family, it is important to understand the gender identify of all family members, how family gender roles and expectations have shaped relationships, and the pronouns they use (Alberta Health Services, 2019; Chang et al., 2018).

Questions to ask the family
- What name would you like me to use for you in our work together? Would you like to share your gender pronouns? (If yes, ask which pronouns the family member prefers you use, if not offered.)
- How have your family's ideas about gender affected your own? Have your ideas about gender been challenged in any way since you became parents?
- Is the division of labour at home based on gender roles?

Sexual Orientation. *Sexual orientation* refers to "a person's emotional and/or sexual attraction to others . . . For many, their sexual orientation can be fluid and may change over time. Sexual orientation may, or may not, reflect sexual behaviours" (Alberta Health Services, 2019, p. 8). Family members may identify as being attracted to people of the opposite sex (heterosexual), the same sex (gay or lesbian), both sexes (bisexual), or all sexes and genders (pansexual, Two-Spirit). In addition, family members may have a sexual orientation or gender identity that differs from the normative binary definition of gender and sexuality (queer), or they may not experience sexual attraction to anyone (asexual) (see Chapter 28 for further information about sexual orientation).

Heterosexism, the belief that heterosexual pairing is the only legitimate sexual orientation, is a form of bias that negatively affects individuals, families, communities, and health care providers. Discrimination based on sexual orientation contributes to health inequities. As with gender, a person's sexual orientation should never be assumed. When asking about sexual activity or sexuality, make general statements such as "Are you sexually active and with whom?" In this way, the nurse is opening the door for further discussion and is letting the patient know that sexuality is diversely understood, and that they can feel comfortable having these conversations.

Questions to ask the family
- When Marti came out to you as lesbian, what did you say? How did you feel?
- When Kiri first told you they were Two-Spirit, what did you say?
- How has your intimacy as partners been most impacted by this illness?
- Who in your family do you feel most comfortable talking to about being bisexual?

Rank Order. The position of children by age is called rank order. The birth order, gender, and distance in age between siblings are important considerations because they may influence expectations, roles, and behaviours.

Questions to ask the family
- How many children are there in your family? What are their ages?
- Do you have different expectations for the older versus the younger children?
- Within your social and cultural community, how are children typically cared for? What is expected at different ages and phases? How do you understand their role in your family?

Subsystems. *Subsystems* are smaller groups of relationships (i.e., based on generation, interests, skills, or gender) within a family. For example, a family could have a sibling subsystem, a spouse subsystem, a parent–child subsystem, or a brother–sister subsystem. Each family member usually belongs to several subsystems, and in each subsystem they play a different role, use different skills, and have a different level of power (i.e., a teenager behaves differently with a younger sibling than with a grandparent or caregiver). Adapting to the demands of different subsystems is a necessary skill for each family member.

Questions to ask the family
- What family members share particularly close relationships in your family?
- Are there times when disagreements occur among and between different groups of people in your family?
- Ramona, who in your family do you talk to when you are worried about your mom going to the hospital for chemotherapy treatment?

Boundaries. Boundaries define family subsystems and distinguish one subsystem from another. They influence how members participate in each subsystem. For example, a child in a parent–child subsystem may be given certain responsibilities and power but is not expected to be involved with family decision making. Boundaries can be weak, rigid, or flexible, and they change over time as family members age or are gained or lost.

Questions to ask the family
- Who do you talk with when you feel happy? Who do you talk to when you feel sad?
- Does the family have any "unwritten" rules about topics never to be discussed outside of the household? For instance, do you avoid certain topics with the stepchildren who visit occasionally?
- Would you be open to having a community worker or nurse come into your home to help you care for Nuni while she is in treatment and recovery? Who would you prefer to play that role?

External Structure. *External structure* refers to the connections that family members have to persons outside the family. Two subcategories of external structure exist: extended family and larger systems.

Extended Family. *Extended family* includes the family of origin, the current generation, and step-relatives. How each member sees themselves as individuals, yet also as part of the family, should be critically assessed. You should inquire about the nature of the relationships shared with extended family members and explore any cultural influences on the value and role of extended family members in family life and experiences of illness.

Questions to ask the family

- In your social and cultural community, how are extended family members involved in your family? Your day-to-day life as a family? What is the role they will play during your chemotherapy?
- Which family members do you see or speak with regularly? Who in your extended family are you the closest to?

Larger Systems. *Larger systems* are groups with whom the family has meaningful contact. Groups include health care organizations, work, religious affiliations, school, friends, and social agencies such as public welfare, child welfare, foster care, and courts. Usually, contact with such larger systems is helpful. However, some families have difficult relationships with individuals from these groups, which can create stress for the family.

Questions to ask the family

- What supports do you have within your social and cultural community to support you during your illness?
- What agency professionals are involved with your family? How have they been helpful or not helpful to your family? How are you hoping I might support you differently than other professionals involved in your family's care?

Context. *Context* refers to the situation or background relevant to the family. A family can be viewed in the context of ethnicity, race, social class, religion/spirituality, and environment.

Cultural Background. A family's cultural, historical, geographic, linguistic, and ethnic background can greatly influence family interaction. Ethnicity may influence a family's functioning, structure, perspectives, values, health beliefs, and philosophies. Cultural influences can affect, for example, religious practices, child-rearing practices, recreational activities, and nutrition. Individually focused assessment is important, as different members of the same cultural group may subscribe to a variety of beliefs, traditions, and restrictions, even within the same generation.

Questions to ask the family

- What aspects of your cultural and historical background are most important for me to understand? What role do you hope they will play in your illness experience?
- How has your cultural background most impacted your experience in the health care system?
- Could you tell me about cultural traditions, rituals, or ceremonies you practice? How would you most like to stay connected to these traditions as you go through chemotherapy treatment?

Race. Family members' interactions among themselves and with health care providers are influenced by racism, white supremacy, racial attitudes, stereotypes, and discrimination. If ignored, and even if expressed unconsciously, these influences may constrain the nurse's relationship with the family. Experiences of structural racism, intergenerational trauma, and colonialism need to be carefully explored with families (Hartrick Doane & Varcoe, 2021).

Questions to ask the family

- Have you ever experienced racism when receiving health care?
- What can I do to counter racism as we begin to work together?

Social Status. *Social status* is shaped by education, income, and occupation, which encodes certain values, lifestyles, and behaviours that influence family interactions and health care practices.

Questions to ask the family

- Are you employed outside the home? What kind of work do you do? How many hours a week do you work? How does this affect family life?
- Does anyone in the family work shifts? How does that influence your family life?
- What education or training have you completed for your work?

- How has COVID-19 impacted your family's finances? Does your family have any financial challenges? Are you experiencing any challenges in managing this illness?

Religion and Spirituality. Family members' spiritual or religious beliefs, rituals, and practices can influence their ability to cope with or manage an illness or health concern (Timmins & Caldeira, 2019; Wright, 2021). Spirituality is often an underused resource in family nursing (see Chapter 29 for further information about spiritual health). Increasingly, families choose to explore the spiritual beliefs and practices that best fit their multifaith lives, beliefs about spirituality, and relationships. Spiritual assessment and support will therefore be highly individualized within an inquiry-oriented approach (Timmins & Caldeira, 2019).

Questions to ask the family

- What spiritual practices or ceremonies are important to your family? Have your family's spiritual beliefs changed or been challenged in any way during this illness?
- What is most important for me to understand about your role as an Elder in your community?
- How do you most want to include your Indigenous healing practices (ceremonies) in Nuni's care? What can I do to support your grandparent?
- Do you consider your spiritual beliefs a resource? A source of stress?

Environment. The family *environment* refers to the larger community, neighbourhood, and home contexts. Environmental factors that may affect family functioning include availability or lack of adequate space, as well as access to schools, day care, recreation, and public transportation.

Questions to ask the family

- What do you most value about living in the community/neighbourhood you are a part of?
- What community services and support does your family use?
- What community services would you like to learn more about within your community? Outside your community?

Structural Assessment Tools. The CFAM encourages you to work with family members to create genograms and ecomaps to facilitate documentation and understanding of the family structure and its contact with outside individuals and organizations. A **genogram** is a sketch of the family structure and relevant information about family members (Figure 20.3). Some agencies have genogram forms, but genograms can also be sketched on other forms, such as admission forms and records. The genogram becomes part of the documentation about the patient and family. An **ecomap** is a sketch of the family's relationships with persons and groups outside the family (Figure 20.4). The family members who share the household are depicted in the centre of the ecomap, and various important extended family members or larger systems are sketched in to show their relationship to the family.

Nurses are encouraged to draw genograms and ecomaps for the families with which they will be involved for more than one day. Information for brief genograms and ecograms can be gleaned from family members during the initial assessment of the family structure. The most essential information for genograms includes data about ages, occupation or schooling, religion, ethnicity, and current health status of family members. For a brief genogram, the focus is only on information relevant to the family and the health problem. The shared creation of a genogram by a nurse and family can be an important time for the nurse to engage with the family, leading to a relational connection between family members and the nurse. Engagement can be facilitated through humour, curiosity, and invitations for family members to describe the strengths they see in one another. For example, the nurse might ask an 8-year-old child, "What do you most like about your grandparent?"

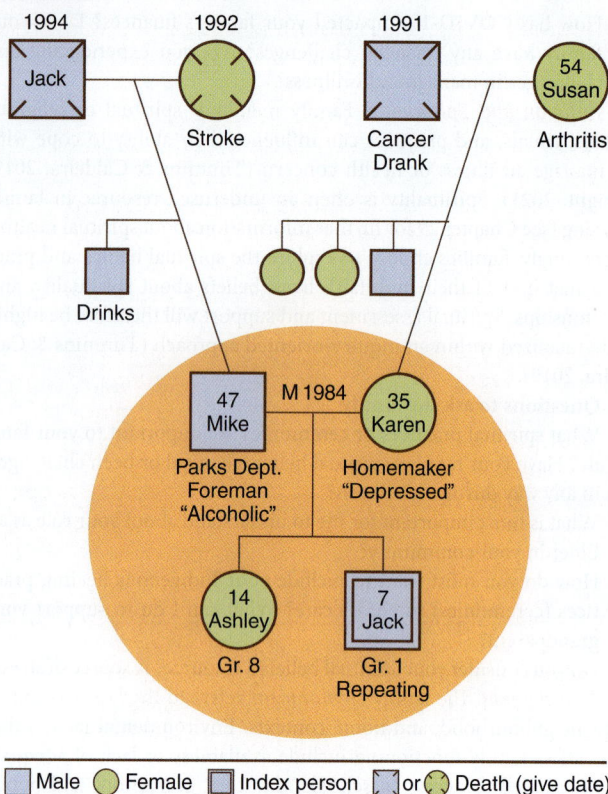

FIGURE 20.3 A sample family genogram. (From Zahra Shajani, Diana Snell. [2019]. *Wright and Leahey's nurses and families: A guide to family assessment and intervention* [7th ed.]. F. A. Davis Company, Philadelphia, PA, with permission.)

Developmental Assessment

Families, like individuals, change and grow over time. Although each family is unique, many families tend to go through certain stages that require family members to adjust, adapt, and change roles. Each developmental stage presents challenges and includes tasks that need to be completed before the family can successfully move on to the next stage. Family development is more than the concurrent development of children and adults. It is the interaction between an individual's development and the phase of the family developmental life cycle, which can be significant for family functioning. Therefore, in addition to understanding family structure, nurses need to understand the developmental life cycle of each family.

In their articulation of the expanded family life cycle, McGoldrick and colleagues (2016) described the emotional process of life cycle transition, as well as the family development tasks for different stages. The family life cycle stages they describe include emerging young adults, couple formation: the joining of families, families with young children, families with adolescents, launching children and moving on at midlife, families in late middle age, and families nearing the end of life (McGoldrick et al., 2016, pp. 24–25). They also discuss the unique challenges faced by lone-parent, lesbian, gay, bisexual, and transgender families, as well as those facing transitions related to divorce. Understanding family development theory can help nurses to promote health during expected family life cycle transitions and experiences of illness. For further information, please see *The Expanding Family Life Cycle: Individual, Family, and Social Perspectives* (McGoldrick et al., 2016).

Functional Assessment

A *functional assessment* focuses on how family members interact and behave toward each other. Nurses assess family functioning by closely

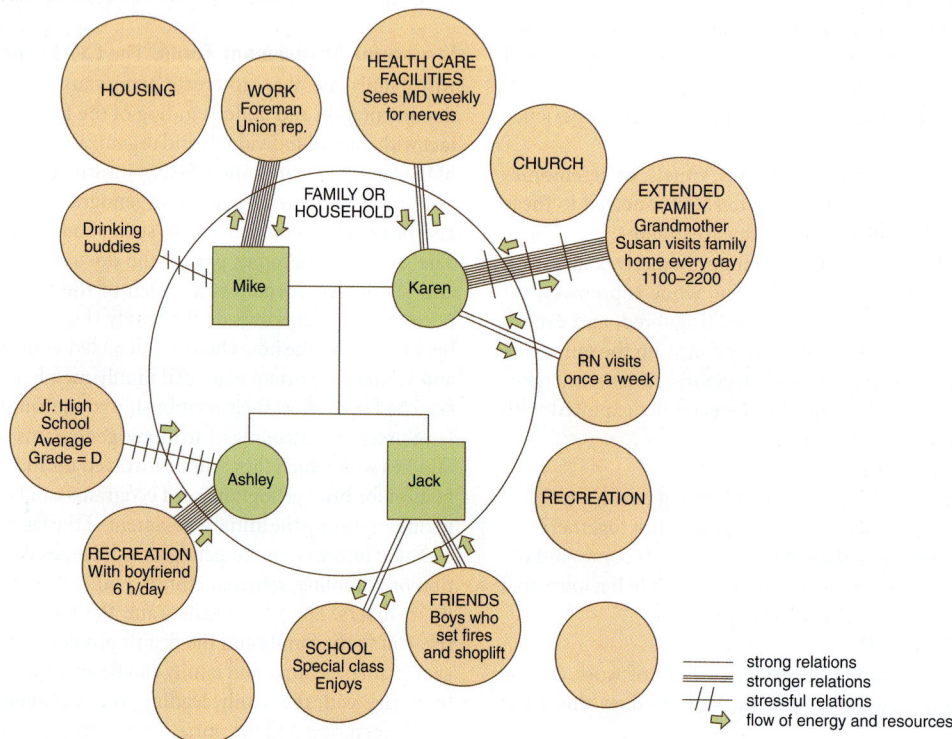

FIGURE 20.4 A sample family ecomap. (From Zahra Shajani, Diana Snell. [2019]. *Wright and Leahey's nurses and families: A guide to family assessment and intervention* [7th ed.]. F. A. Davis Company, Philadelphia, PA, with permission.)

observing the interactions of family members in two subcategories: instrumental and expressive functioning.

Instrumental Functioning.
Instrumental functioning refers to the normal activities of daily living, such as preparing meals, eating, sleeping, and attending to health needs. For families with health problems, these activities often become a challenge. Roles may change as family members cope with a relative's illness or disability. Within the context of illness, nurses and other health care providers play an important role in accessing practical and financial resources to support family members' instrumental needs (e.g., financial resources for medical supplies that parents need to care for an ill child at home).

Questions to ask the family
- Who is usually responsible for housekeeping and child care in your family?
- Do other family members help with these tasks?
- Does anyone in the family require help with activities of daily living?
- Who will be involved in bringing Nuni to the cancer centre, and who will be supporting her care at home?

Expressive Functioning.
Expressive functioning refers to the ways in which people communicate. The significance of communication within the family cannot be emphasized enough, for it has a profound impact on a family's adjustment to illness and their resiliency in the face of developmental and illness-related challenges. Illness and disability often challenge and alter expressive functioning within the family. A diagnosis may cause intense feelings of anxiety or grief, both within the person being diagnosed and within other family members. Nurses should encourage families to explore their understanding of illness and how it affects their lives. Depending on the emotional intensity of the situation, nurses may need to assist family members with having these difficult conversations (Box 20.6). Expressive functioning has 10 subcategories: emotional, verbal, nonverbal, and circular communication; problem solving; roles; influence and power; beliefs; and alliances and coalitions.

Emotional Communication.
Emotional communication encompasses the range and types of feelings that are expressed by the family. Most families express a wide range of feelings. Families with problems may have rigid patterns and narrower ranges of emotional expression (e.g., a family coping with a parent's cancer diagnosis may be anxious and unable to express optimism or hope for the future). Family roles and gender may affect emotional expression.

Questions to ask the family
- How can you tell when each member of your family is happy, sad, or under stress?
- Kiri, when you are sad or worried, who in the family do you most like to spend time with or talk to about that?
- Are there ways, other than talking with each other, that help your family to express or share emotion? (For an Indigenous family, sharing in ceremony might be included.)

Verbal Communication.
Nurses should observe a family's **verbal communication**, focusing on the meaning of the words in terms of the relationship. Is communication among family members clear and direct or vague and indirect? It is useful to ask family members about how well the family communicates.

Questions to ask the family
- Which family member is most able to share what they are thinking and feeling?
- How might you like your family to communicate with each other differently than you do now or have in the past?
- Families sometimes find it helpful to talk with one of the nurses about their life at home after learning about an illness. Other families prefer to talk to friends or community members that they feel close to. What would your family find most helpful?

Nonverbal Communication.
Nonverbal communication consists of messages conveyed without words, including body language, eye contact, gesturing, crying, and tone of voice. An example of a nonverbal communication is a child's body language in response to their grandparent's absence during chemotherapy treatment at the hospital.

Questions to ask the family
- How do you think Nuni feels when your child runs to her for a hug when she has returned from cancer treatment?
- Who shows the most distress when talking about your mother's illness? What are some of the nonverbal signals that indicate your child is distressed when talking about Nuni's illness?

Circular Communication.
Circular communication refers to reciprocal communication between family members; that is, each person

---

⟳ BOX 20.6 RESEARCH HIGHLIGHT

Brief Family Health Conversations Following a Diagnosis of Breast Cancer

Research Focus
When people are diagnosed with breast cancer, they and their families experience physical, emotional, and spiritual distress. Families have described the sadness and fear they live with and the difficulty they experience in talking about cancer. Holst-Hansson et al. (2020) conducted a qualitative family nursing intervention study that analyzed family experiences of participating in three Brief Family Health Conversations (BFamHC) during the outpatient radiation therapy period. Family members were invited to share their stories of illness, and to listen to other family members' experiences. The first BFamHC included interventive questions (Shajani & Snell, 2019, as cited in Holst-Hansson et al., 2020), and family members prioritized topics to focus on. A genogram and ecomap were also constructed. The second BFamHC focused on beliefs and topics raised during the first conversation. The third BFamHC focused on family strengths and resources.

Findings
The 9 families (29 family members, parents, and children) who participated felt the BFamHCs gave them an opportunity to express their feelings and talk about their illness experiences in a safe context. Family members also found it helpful to hear other family members' experiences, which meant they "no longer needed to guess and interpret or protect" each other (Holst-Hansson et al., 2020, p. 331). Participants felt supported as a family and as individuals. One family member expressed their experience in the following way: "It felt safe to have a person one could talk to, to ask questions . . . and to get the time to sit down together as a family" (Holst-Hansson et al., 2020, p. 331). Families came to believe they could get through a difficult experience. This led to their experiencing increased strength as a family. Furthermore, the advice and information offered by the nurse was appreciated: reflections from the nurse "confirmed their feelings and thoughts as "normal" and that there were multiple ways of experiencing a situation" (Holst-Hansson et al., 2020, p. 331). Finally, families experienced new insights. For example, they realized their conversations as a family had tended to focus on practical issues rather than the difficult emotions they were experiencing.

From Holst-Hansson, A., Vejzovic, V., Idvall, E., & Wennick, A. (2020). The usefulness of Brief Family Health Conversations offered to families following the diagnosis of breast cancer. *Journal of Family Nursing, 26*(4), 327–336. https://doi.org/10.1177/1074840720966759

influences the behaviour of the other. Circular communication can be adaptive or create difficulties in family life. For example, an adaptive communication pattern occurs when a parent comforts a child when the child cries. Because the parent responds to the child, the child feels safe and secure. An example of a challenging communication pattern is when a parent criticizes a teenager for not phoning home. The teenager is angry for being criticized and avoids the parent, and then the parent becomes angrier and criticizes more.

Questions to ask the family
- You mentioned that your daughter has been struggling at school since Nuni has been receiving chemotherapy treatment. What have you done to help her with this difficulty?
- Since you have made time to spend more time with your grandchild, what changes have you noticed in them? In their schoolwork?

Problem Solving. **Problem solving** refers to how a family thinks about actions to take to resolve difficult situations.

Questions to ask the family
- Who first notices problems? How does your family tend to handle problems?
- Who in your family "takes the lead" in helping the family manage the problems you face?
- Are there other extended family members or community members who play an important role in helping your family manage difficulties?

Roles. **Roles** are established patterns of behaviour for family members, often developed through interactions with others. Formal roles include those of parent/caregiver, spouse/partner, friend, and so forth. Informal roles may include "the softy," "the angel," "the rock," or "the scapegoat," for example. In the context of illness, family members must often take on new roles, such as medical caregiver.

Question to ask the family:
- Who is the "good listener" in your family? Who is "the rock"?
- Who in the family tends to take on the role of caregiver when someone is ill?

Influence and Power. **Influence** refers to behaviours used by a family member to *influence* or affect another person's behaviour. Influence may be instrumental (e.g., rewards for behaviour such as the promise of candy, computer time), psychological (communication to influence behaviour such as praise, criticism), or physical (the use of body contact, such as hugging, hitting). *Power* focuses on the level of hierarchy, dominance, and equality within family relationships, as well as family–nurse relationships.

Questions to ask the family
- How does Nootau get the grandchildren to go to bed?
- How have the routines and practices of people in the health care system impacted your breast cancer experience? How have they supported or challenged your efforts to integrate traditional Indigenous healing practices into your breast cancer experience?

Beliefs. **Beliefs** are individual- and family-held fundamental ideas, values, opinions, and assumptions (Wright & Bell, 2021). Understanding the core beliefs (Wright & Bell, 2021) of family members is central to understanding their suffering and to facilitating healing in the context of illness (Wright & Bell, 2021; Wright et al., 1996). Beliefs influence behaviours and how the family adapts to illness. For example, if a family believes that traditional Indigenous healing practices and ceremonies are central to Nuni's healing, the family may question continuing with chemotherapy treatment if those ceremonies are not honoured and integrated into her care provision. Beliefs may also influence how a family responds to other family members during illness.

Questions to ask the family
- What do you believe will bring healing to Nuni?
- What do you believe the future holds for Nuni and for your family?

Alliances and Coalitions. **Alliances and coalitions** involve the directionality, balance, and intensity of relationships among family members or between families and nurses.

Questions to ask the family
- If Nuni was sad and struggling with her treatment, is there someone at home she would tend to reach out to? Or would she talk to another extended family member or another Elder in your community?
- Is there anything that you were hoping we would talk about today that we haven't spoken about?

FAMILY INTERVENTION: THE CALGARY FAMILY INTERVENTION MODEL

After assessment, nurses intervene to help families meet their needs, face challenges, and appreciate their strengths. A range of family nursing interventions can be offered to families in the context of a therapeutic relationship. Some, such as parent education and caregiver support, are general; others are specific and require therapeutic communication and family interviewing skills. The ultimate goal is to help family members discover alternative solutions that may lessen or alleviate emotional, physical, and spiritual suffering. Whether caring for a patient with the family as context or directing care to the family as patient, the aim of nursing interventions is to enhance family members' abilities in certain areas, remove barriers to health care, and perform actions that the family cannot perform for itself. Nurses guide the family in problem solving, provide practical services, and convey a sense of acceptance and caring by listening carefully to family members' experiences, concerns, suggestions, and questions.

Interventions for each family must be individualized and focus on particular areas of family functioning (cognitive, affective, behavioural) (Shajani & Snell, 2019). Nurses can only *offer* interventions and must not instruct or insist on a particular kind of change or way of family functioning. Nurses need to sensitively attend to ideas or interventions that the family perceives as being most helpful (Shajani & Snell, 2019).

The **Calgary Family Intervention Model (CFIM)** is a companion to the CFAM and can be used as a guide for nursing intervention with the family (Shajani & Snell, 2019). The CFIM focuses on promoting and improving family functioning in three domains: cognitive, affective, and behavioural. Interventions may affect functioning in any or all of the three domains. For example, when a clinic nurse informs the partner of a patient living with amyotrophic lateral sclerosis that the patient is still capable of large gross motor movement, the nurse can suggest that the patient can help with chores in the house, such as bringing the laundry upstairs. This intervention may challenge the partner's thinking about their spouse's abilities and physical capacities.

The CFIM recommends many relational nursing practices that promote family health and functioning, including asking interventive questions, offering commendations, providing information, validating emotional responses, encouraging illness narratives, supporting family caregivers, and encouraging respite. Central to this interventional practice is the nurse's engagement with family members in a thoughtful, purposeful relation (Box 20.7). Within CFAM and CFIM, as well as in the Illness Beliefs Model (Wright & Bell, 2021; Wright et al., 1996), nurses are guided to continually attend to the cultivation of a relationship that is collaborative, responsive, and nonhierarchical. Within this relationship, there is a privileging of family expertise and a commitment to listening deeply to the concerns, suffering, and questions of family members.

The guidance provided by Hartrick Doane and Varcoe (2021) in their discussion of relational inquiry (and the five Ws of relating in Box 20.4) is another helpful resource for your relational engagement with the families you encounter in your practice.

Asking Interventive Questions

One of the most effective ways that nurses can help families is by engaging in therapeutic conversations with families and asking them questions. Questions lead the family to reflect on their situation, clarify opinions and ideas, and understand how they are affected by their family member's illness or condition. By hearing their own responses to questions, as well as the responses of others, family members can better understand themselves and each other and perhaps discover new possibilities for health and healing. Interventive questions also elicit information important to the nurse.

There are two types of interventive questions: linear and circular (Tomm, 1987, 1988). **Linear questions** elicit information about a patient or family. They explore a family member's descriptions or perceptions of an illness or life challenge. For example, linear questions may be used when exploring a couple's perceptions of their child's anorexia nervosa: "When did you notice that your child had changed their eating habits?" "Have they been hospitalized in the past for this problem?" These questions inform the nurse of the child's eating patterns and illuminate family perceptions or beliefs about eating patterns.

Circular questions help determine possible changes for a patient's or family's life. They help the nurse understand relationships between individuals, beliefs, and events and elicit valuable information to help create change. In this way, circular questions often help patients make new cognitive connections, paving the way for changes in family behaviours. For example, with the same family, the nurse could ask, "Who is most worried about Cheyenne's anorexia?" or "How does Ellen show worry or stress the most?"

Linear questions may imply that you know what is best for the family because they tend to target specific yes or no answers, thereby limiting options for the family. By contrast, circular questions facilitate change by inviting the family to discover their own answers. For example, compare how a family might respond to "Have you tried time out to discipline your 3-year-old?" (a linear question) versus "Which type of discipline seems to work best for your child?" (a circular question). Several types of circular questions exist; each can affect the cognitive, affective, and behavioural domains of family functioning. These types include difference questions, behavioural effect questions, hypothetical or future-oriented questions, and triadic questions (Shajani & Snell, 2019; Tomm, 1987, 1988) (Table 20.1).

Offering Commendations

Families do not always view themselves as having inherent strength and resilience. As their nurse, you can help the family become aware of and communicate their unique strengths, thus increasing their

---

BOX 20.7 Family Intervention Principles

- Interventions (held in partnership and conversation) are the core of clinical work with families.
- Interventions are offered in the context of collaborative, therapeutic conversations as the nurse supports the family to devise solutions to their health challenge together, addressing what might lead or contribute to that challenge. In this way, there can be potential for solutions that fit the family context and circumstances.
- Interventions must be approached within the training, skill, and capacity of the nurse; additional training and supervision should be accessed to continually build capacity.
- Interventions must be devised with respect for the family's values and cultural background in a way to support cultural safety.
- Interventions are not *done to* families; they can only be *offered for* families. The nurse cannot direct change but can create a context for family deliberation, decisions, and actions where change can occur.
- The nurse should make inquiries to the family with an open mind and avoid giving advice while respectfully providing information and correcting any misinformation.
- The nurse should receive feedback without becoming defensive, and offer feedback with respect and permission, avoiding any blaming of self or the family.

From Broekema, S., Paans, W., Roodbol, P. F., & Luttik, M. L. A. (2020). Nurses' application of the components of family nursing conversations in home health care: A qualitative content analysis. *Scandinavian Journal of Caring Sciences, 34*(2), 322–331. https://doi.org/10.1111/scs.12731; Shajani, Z., & Snell, D. (2019). *Wright and Leahey's nurses and families: A guide to family assessment and intervention* (7th ed.). F. A. Davis Company.

TABLE 20.1 Three Types of Circular Questions

	EXAMPLES TO ELICIT CHANGE		
Purpose of Question	**Cognitive Domain**	**Affective Domain**	**Behavioural Domain**
Difference Question Explores differences between people, relationships, time, ideas, or beliefs	What is the best advice you have received about supporting Nuni during breast cancer treatment? What is the worst advice?	Who in the family is most worried about what the future holds for Nuni?	Which family member is best at comforting the children at home when Nuni goes to the cancer centre?
Behavioural Effect Question Explores connections between how one family member's behaviour affects other members	What do you know about the effect of life-threatening illness on children?	How does your child show that he is worried about Nuni being sick?	What could you do to show your son that you understand his fears?
Hypothetical/Future-Oriented Question Explores family options and alternative actions or meanings in the future	What do you think/believe the future holds for Nuni?	If Nuni's treatment is not successful, who do you think will be most distressed?	When you think about the months of treatment ahead, what ceremonies or Indigenous traditions are most important to have integrated into your care?

Adapted from Shajani, Z., & Snell, D. (2019). *Wright and Leahey's nurses and families: A guide to family assessment and intervention* (7th ed., p. 146). F. A. Davis Company.

potential and capabilities. A **commendation** is a conversational statement emphasizing family strengths and abilities. While spending time with the family, you may observe many instances where the family displays its strengths. It is important to acknowledge these moments with the family so that they can recognize and appreciate their capabilities. By commending a family's strengths and capacities, you are not sharing compliments but instead offering family members a new view of themselves, and this may invite a change in how they view their health challenges. Look for patterns of behaviour to commend rather than a single occurrence. For example, you might say, "Your family has shown courage living with your partner's cancer for 5 years. As we have worked together, I have noticed how you have held on to hope for their survival while at the same time being realistic and committing to spending as much time as possible together as a family." Families coping with chronic, life-threatening, or psychosocial problems frequently feel hopeless in their efforts to overcome or live with the illness. Therefore, you should offer as many truthful, genuine commendations as possible.

In the midst of an illness experience, the nurse can observe the family's many strengths. These may include clear communication, adaptability, healthy boundaries, support and nurturing among family members, and the use of crisis for growth. You can help the family focus on these strengths rather than on problems or weaknesses. This practice encourages and reinforces what is working well for the family rather than what might not be working well. This focus on strengths also serves to empower the family to embrace change and to act from their strength. **Empowerment** is a process that nurses use to promote and protect the health of families, encourage autonomy, and provide families with information to actively involve them so that they can make informed choices about their health (Murdaugh et al., 2018).

Providing Information

Families need information from health care providers about developmental issues, health promotion, and illness management, especially if the illness is complex (Shajani & Snell, 2019). Accurate, timely information is essential for the family to make decisions and cope with difficult situations. Health education is a process by which information is exchanged between the nurse, patient, and family. Family and patient needs for information may be elicited through direct questioning but are often far more subtle. In this role of educator, you may recognize, for example, that a new parent is fearful of cleaning their newborn's umbilical cord stump or that an older person is not using their cane safely. Respectful communication is required. Nurses often share information subtly: "I notice you are trying not to touch the umbilical cord stump; I see that a lot with other new parents" or "You use the cane the way I did before I was shown a way to keep from falling or tripping over it; do you mind if I show you?" When you assume a humble, caring position instead of coming across as an authority on the subject, this attitude often decreases the patient's defenses and invites the family to listen without feeling embarrassed.

Validating or Normalizing Emotional Responses

Validating intense emotions can alleviate a family's feelings of isolation and loneliness and help family members make the connection between a family member's illness and their own emotional response. For example, after a diagnosis of a life-shortening illness, families frequently feel powerless or frightened. It is important to validate these strong emotions as normal and reassure families that they will adjust and learn new ways to cope. You may do this by sharing experiences you have had with other families who have faced a similar situation.

Encouraging Illness Narratives

Too often, patients and family members are encouraged to talk only about the medical aspects of their illness rather than the emotional aspects. An **illness narrative** is the person's story of how the illness affects their whole being, including emotional, intellectual, social, and spiritual dimensions (Kleinman, 1988; Wright & Bell, 2021). Hearing the person's illness narrative will help you understand the person's and family's strengths and challenges, and the beliefs they hold about their illness experience. This information enables you to offer commendations to the family. Many people also find that telling their story helps them to better understand themselves, their experience, and their family's experience. Families also benefit from listening to one another's illness narratives. Prior to meeting with their nurse, families may not have had the opportunity to hear and understand how other family members have suffered in living with illness.

Communicating what it is like to live with individual, separate experiences, particularly the experience of illness, is a powerful human need (Wright, 2021). Nurses often believe that listening entails an obligation to "fix" whatever concerns or problems are raised. However, showing compassion through deep listening and offering commendations is usually more therapeutic or helpful than offering solutions to problems (Wright & Bell, 2021).

It is important to frame the family illness narrative solely in terms of problem solving. Otherwise, family members may be overcome with a sense of hopelessness because they view the health concerns as being too overwhelming or because family members may have a fear of failure (Kaakinen, 2018b). By giving commendations, the nurse can help the family identify its strengths, which can make the family feel empowered and hopeful, thus promoting recovery (Halm, 2019).

Encouraging Family Support

Family functioning is enhanced when the nurse encourages and assists family members with listening to each other's concerns and feelings. This assistance can be particularly useful if a family member is embracing some constraining beliefs when a loved one is dying or has died (RNAO, 2015; Wright, 2021; Wright & Bell, 2009). For example, a family may believe that talking with the ill person about death and dying would hasten the person's death.

Supporting Family Caregivers

Family members are often afraid of becoming involved in the care of an ill member without the support of health care providers. One way the nurse can best provide care is through supporting family caregivers. Without preparation and support, caregiving can be stressful, causing a decline in the health of the caregiver and care receiver or the development of abusive relationships. Despite its demands, caregiving—be it one spouse caring for the other or a child caring for a parent—can be a positive and rewarding experience (Parmar et al., 2021). The interpersonal dynamics between family members, along with other variables such as a caregiver's age and own health needs, can greatly influence the family's experiences and, ultimately, the quality of caregiving (Arriagada, 2020).

Nurses can play a key role in helping family members develop better communication and the problem-solving skills needed for caregiving. Support for family caregivers is provided across the lifespan and across diverse contexts of marginalization and privilege. For example, nurses could extend this support to young children experiencing structural vulnerabilities (Wagner et al., 2021), new immigrant families seeking health information (Mason et al., 2021), or caregivers making decisions about the care of older persons (Li & Lee, 2020).

Recently, a competency framework for training health care providers was developed using a multilevel stakeholder co-design approach. Key domains for caregiver-centred care included recognizing the caregiver role; communicating, partnering with and fostering resilience in family caregivers; navigating health and social systems/accessing

---

BOX 20.8 EVIDENCE-INFORMED PRACTICE

Family-Centred Interventions by Primary Health Care Services for Indigenous Early Childhood Well-Being

Primary health care services in Australia, Canada, New Zealand, and the United States have embraced the concept of family-centred care as a promising approach to supporting and caring for the health of young Indigenous children and their families. McCalman and colleagues' (2017) review of evidence-informed programs identified aims, strategies, enablers, and outcomes of family-centred care. Eighteen studies (most published between 2012 and 2015) highlighted the following six family-supporting strategies: support for family behaviours and self-care, increasing maternal knowledge, strengthening links with the clinic, building the Indigenous workforce, promoting cultural/community connectedness, and advocating for social determinants of health. Four enablers of family-supportedness were also identified: competent and compassionate program deliverers, flexibility of access, continuity and integration of health care, and culturally supportive care. Health outcomes were reported for Indigenous children (nutritional status; emotional/behavioural; and prevention of injury and illness); parents/caregivers (depression and substance use disorder; and parenting knowledge, confidence, and skills); health services (satisfaction; access, utilization, and cost); and community/cultural revitalization. These facilitators for family-centred practice show promise for generating diverse health care outcomes for Indigenous children and their parents/caregivers, as well as satisfaction from those using health services.

From McCalman, J., Heyeres, M., Campbell, S., et al. (2017). Family-centred interventions by primary healthcare services for Indigenous early childhood wellbeing in Australia, Canada, New Zealand and the United States: A systematic scoping review. *BMC Pregnancy and Childbirth, 17*(1), 71–71. https://doi.org/10.1186/s12884-017-1247-2

---

resources; and enhancing culture and context of health care (Parmar et al., 2021). Innovative family- and culture-centred care designs are promising to transform health services and outcomes. For example, involving Indigenous Elders as part of routine primary care has been found to significantly improve depressive symptoms and suicidal ideation in Indigenous patients (Tu et al., 2019). Box 20.8 further highlights international research focused on facilitators of family-centred care for Indigenous children.

Encouraging Respite

Nurses should encourage respite for caregivers, who may feel guilty about or not even recognize their need to withdraw, even temporarily, from caregiving tasks. Sometimes an ill person may be encouraged to accept another person's temporary assistance so that family members can take a break. Whatever the situation, the nurse should remember that each family's need for respite varies.

Providing care and support for family caregivers often involves using available family and community resources for respite. Caregiving burden can be lessened by using a schedule to coordinate the participation of multiple family members; sharing any financial burdens posed by caregiving; and communicating support from extended family members who live at a distance. However, it is important to understand the relationship between potential caregivers and care recipients. If the relationship is not a supportive one, community services may be a resource for both the patient and family.

Services that may be beneficial to families include caregiver respite, caregiver support groups, housing and transportation services, food and nutrition services, housecleaning, legal and financial services, home care, hospice, and mental health resources. Before referring a family to a community resource, it is crucial that nurses are aware of the community services themselves, understand the family's dynamics, and know whether such support is desired or welcomed. A family caregiver may resist help, feeling obligated to be the sole source of support to the care recipient. Nurses must be sensitive to family relationships and help normalize the demands of caregiving and the need for respite.

INTERVIEWING THE FAMILY

With a clear conceptual framework for assessment and intervention, you can begin to learn the competencies and skills needed to conduct family interviews. Family interviews follow the same basic principles as any patient interview (see Chapter 14 for further information about interviewing patients). However, family interviews have the complexity of more people and multiple relationships. You must develop keen perceptual, conceptual, and executive skills. *Perceptual skills* refer to the ability to make relevant observations. In family interviewing, you must observe multiple interactions and relationships simultaneously. *Conceptual skills* constitute the ability to formulate observations of the entire family and give meaning to those observations. Remember that observations and subsequent judgements are subjective and not conclusive. *Executive skills* are the actual therapeutic interventions you offer in the context of a family interview. These therapeutic interventions elicit responses from family members and are the basis for further observations and conceptualizations.

During an interview, observe and listen for responses from a patient and family to formulate further therapeutic interventions. The type of intervention that you offer depends on your clinical expertise and experience in working with families, as well as the unique challenges and strengths of the family members you are working with. The four stages of a family interview are engagement, assessment, intervention, and termination. Each of these stages will include specific perceptual and executive skills. For more information on the skills and stages of conducting a family interview, see *Nurses and Families: A Guide to Family Assessment and Intervention* (Shajani & Snell, 2019). With these skills you can assess, explore, and identify strengths and problems in the familiar process of engagement, assessment, intervention, and termination (see Chapter 18 for further information about communication skills). You can also decide to intervene or to refer the family to another health care provider. These skills should not necessarily be applied to all families. You should tailor the interview to each family's individual context.

Not all family interviews are formal, lengthy processes. Even if you do not have the time for a formal family interview, you can still engage the family in therapeutic conversations. Every conversation between you and the patient or family members can improve communication and understanding. Therapeutic conversations can be as short as one sentence or as long as time allows. All therapeutic conversations, regardless of their length, have the potential to assist the family. Even brief interviews or conversations have tremendous healing potential because they offer families the opportunity to acknowledge and affirm their problems and seek solutions (Shajani & Snell, 2019; Svavarsdottir & Gisladottir, 2019).

The integration of task-oriented patient care with interactive, purposeful conversation makes for a time-effective interview (taking less than 15 minutes). Providing information and involving the family in decision making are integral parts of the therapeutic process. You should search for opportunities to engage in purposeful conversations with a family, which may include the following:

- Routinely inviting the family to accompany the patient to the unit, clinic, or hospital
- Routinely including the family's participation in the admission procedure
- Routinely inviting family members to ask questions
- Acknowledging the patient and family's expertise in managing the health problem at home, and
- Routinely consulting the patient and family about their ideas regarding treatment and discharge.

KEY CONCEPTS

- Family members influence one another's health beliefs, practices, and status.
- The concept of family is highly individual; thus, nurses should base care on the patient's definition of family rather than on an inflexible definition of family.
- Family nursing care requires that nurses continually examine the current trends in the Canadian family and their health care implications.
- A healthy, resilient family is one that can integrate the need for stability with the need for growth and change. The family can be viewed as context, where the nurse focuses either on the individual patient within the context of their family or on the family with the individual as context. The family also can be viewed as patient (family systems nursing), where the nurse focuses on family interactions.
- The Calgary Family Assessment Model (CFAM) is a conceptual framework that guides nurses in assessing the structural, developmental, and functional aspects of the family.
- Genograms and ecomaps are structural assessment tools that provide a pictorial image of the family's structure and relation to outside influences.
- Family members that take the caregiver role are often spouses, who may be older persons themselves, or adult children trying to work full time, care for aging parents, and enable children to move out of the home (launch children) successfully.
- Illness and disability often alter expressive functioning and communication within the family.
- Relational inquiry with families is concerned with understanding the family in context (interpersonal, social, geopolitical, historical, environmental context).
- Key components of family nursing as relational inquiry include relational capacities that support being in relation with families in a mode of inquiry that balances letting be and emancipatory action.
- The Calgary Family Intervention Model (CFIM) is a companion to the CFAM that guides nurses in implementing family interventions; it is focused on improving family functioning in three domains: cognitive (thinking), affective (feeling), and behavioural (doing).
- One of the simplest and most effective ways that nurses can help families is by asking them circular questions.
- Offering commendations is important because it encourages the family to recognize their strengths and competencies.
- Other nursing interventions to help the family include providing information, validating emotional responses, encouraging patients to provide illness narratives, supporting family caregivers, and encouraging respite for family caregivers.
- Family caregiving is an interactional process that occurs within the context of the relationships among family members.

- Family interviews require nurses to have perceptual, conceptual, and executive skills; interviews may be formal and lengthy or casual and brief.

CRITICAL THINKING EXERCISES

1. Kathy (preferred pronouns: she/her) is a palliative care nurse working with a family of four: Melinda, a 45-year-old single parent who identifies as female and uses the pronouns she/her; her adolescent children, Etan and Matthew; and Heng, her 76-year-old mother, who is in the last stages of terminal breast cancer. The family has lived together for 10 years, ever since they immigrated to Canada from Hong Kong. Heng helped Melinda to parent Etan and Matthew, and supported Melinda when her husband (the children's father) died 5 years ago. Melinda has decided to care for her mother in the family's home until Heng dies. Kathy will assist this family in achieving their goals. Kathy has just had in-service training in using the Calgary Family Assessment Model (CFAM).
   a. What parts of the CFAM should Kathy use when assessing the family's needs?
   b. How can Kathy help the family achieve their goal of caring for their aging family member at home?
   c. How can Kathy determine this family's strengths, challenges, and resources?
   d. What cultural aspects are important to consider for a family who has immigrated to Canada and is now facing the death of a loved one?
   e. What self-awareness and reflection will support a relational inquiry approach to the assessment and interventions?

2. Dan (preferred pronouns: he/him) and Kim (preferred pronouns: she/her) divorced 7 years ago, and neither has remarried. They have three children, aged 10, 12, and 14 years. At the time of the divorce, Dan was HIV positive and has remained so for 5 years. Kim has had repeated tests and remains HIV negative. Dan is responding to therapy slowly. Kim and Dan share parenting responsibilities and have a friendly relationship. They have decided it would be easier for the family to live together again so that Dan can actively participate in the children's lives without placing caregiver demands on Kim when the extended family visits overnight. Kim also wants to care for Dan, despite their divorced status.
   a. What family development tasks are important to assess for this family as the members attempt to reunite?
   b. How should the nurse determine what support services the family needs?
   c. What assessment questions would be useful to ask in order to assess how the illness is affecting this family? Do family members have any signs of emotional, physical, or spiritual distress?

3. Gilles Leduc (preferred pronouns he/him) and Xavier Bothe (preferred pronouns he/him), both in their early 50s, are the youngest members of large families. They work full time and have two teenage children. Both Gilles's parents and Xavier's parents are in their 80s and have chronic health problems. All their siblings live farther away.
   a. How can the nurse help Gilles and Xavier access resources to aid in caring for their parents and maintain the responsibilities of their own family unit?
   b. What developmental tasks does this family have?
   c. What kinds of questions can you ask to assess the family's emotional and verbal communication (found in CFAM's functional assessment category)?

Answers to Critical Thinking Exercises appear on the Evolve website.

REVIEW QUESTIONS

Review Questions 1 to 11 relate to the case study at the beginning of the chapter.

1. Considering the case of Nuni, who should a nurse consider as Nuni's family?
   a. Nuni's children and grandchildren
   b. People related to Nuni by marriage, birth, or adoption
   c. The nuclear family and aunts, uncles, grandparents, and cousins
   d. A set of relationships that Nuni identifies as family

2. One of Nuni's children, Kiri, has remarried, and the new spouse was also previously married. One child from Kiri's previous marriage lives in Nuni's family household. The new spouse's children from the previous marriage also visit some weeks and on alternate weekends. This is an example of which family configuration?
   a. A nuclear family
   b. A blended family
   c. An extended family
   d. An alternative family

3. What primary social location are the nurses who work with Nuni working at for health promotion and disease prevention?
   a. At educational institutions
   b. With friends and colleagues
   c. With physicians and nurses
   d. In the family, which can include extended family and community members

4. What are two factors that contribute to the long-term health of Nuni's family?
   a. Structure and function
   b. Caregiving and reciprocity
   c. Strength and resiliency
   d. Context and system

5. What does the nurse focus on when viewing Nuni's family as patient?
   a. Nuni's health and development existing within a specific environment
   b. Family process and relationships
   c. Family relational and transactional concepts
   d. Family within a system

6. What is the nurse assessing when asking Nuni the following questions: "Who is in your family? Is there anyone who lives outside of your home who you consider part of your family?"?

a. Internal structure
b. External structure
c. Context
d. Instrumental functioning

7. What is one of the goals of approaching Nuni's family from a relational inquiry perspective?
   a. Professional collaboration
   b. Systematic problem solving
   c. Inquiry to understand the family in context
   d. Circular questions

8. Which two components of relational inquiry are important for the care of Nuni's family?
   a. Using both open-ended and closed-ended questions
   b. Applying both a strict assessment format and corresponding interventions
   c. Incorporating both letting be and emancipatory action
   d. Assessing the presenting problem and the history of the presenting problem

9. The nurse's support of emotional communication in Nuni's family belongs to which CFAM subcategory?
   a. Instrumental functioning
   b. Development
   c. Internal structure
   d. Expressive functioning

10. "Kiri, what is your greatest worry about Nuni starting chemotherapy treatment?" is an example of a circular question. What can asking the family circular questions accomplish?
    a. Facilitating change by inviting the family to discover their own answers
    b. Encouraging family members to be caregivers
    c. Validating their emotional responses
    d. Targeting specific yes or no answers

11. Which intervention can the nurse accomplish during an interview with Nuni's family?
    a. Educate Nuni's family
    b. Enforce change in the family
    c. Engage Nuni's family to assess, explore, and identify strengths and problems
    d. Establish roles within the family

Answers: 1.d; 2.b; 3.d; 4.c; 5.b; 6.a; 7.c; 8.c; 9.d; 10.a; 11.c.

🌐 *Rationales for the Review Questions appear on the Evolve website.*

RECOMMENDED WEBSITES

Family Nursing Resources: http://www.familynursingresources.com
Family nursing videos, books, DVDs, and family genographs are available on this website.

International Family Nursing Association: https://internationalfamilynursing.org
Resources for family nursing practice, education, and research. An online community that promotes connection with family nurses globally.

Journal of Family Nursing: https://journals.sagepub.com/home/jfn
The *Journal of Family Nursing* (JFN) is a peer-reviewed journal publishing scholarly work on nursing research, practice, education, and policy issues related to families in health and illness. The journal seeks to represent cultural diversity and families across the life cycle and encourages interprofessional and collaborative perspectives.

Sexual Orientation and Gender Identity (SOGI) Nursing: https://soginursing.ca
Sponsored by the Canadian Institutes of Health Research and the Canadian Alliance of Nurse Educators Using Simulation, the SOGI nursing website provides a toolkit for nursing students, nurse educators, and nurses in practice who are committed to supportive LGBTQ2 health care.

Vanier Institute of the Family: https://www.vanierinstitute.ca
The Vanier Institute of the Family aims to create awareness of, and to provide leadership on, the importance and strengths of families in Canada and the challenges they face in their structural, demographic, economic, cultural, and social diversity. This website highlights news articles, research, publications, policies, and networks that focus on the family.

🌐 REFERENCES

A full reference list is available on the website for this book at http://evolve.elsevier.com/Canada/Potter/fundamentals/

21

Patient Education

*Canadian content written by Nancy A. Edgecombe, RN-NP, BN, MN, PhD,
with original chapter contributions by Emily McKenna, APN, CNS*

OBJECTIVES

Mastery of content in this chapter will enable you to:

- Define the key terms listed.
- Identify appropriate topics that address a patient's health education needs.
- Explain the role of the nurse in patient education.
- Describe the purposes of patient education.
- Determine appropriate communication principles when providing patient education.
- Describe the domains of learning.

- Identify basic learning principles.
- Explain how to integrate health education into patient-centred care.
- Differentiate factors that determine readiness to learn from those that determine the ability to learn.
- Compare and contrast the nursing process and teaching process.
- Write learning objectives for a teaching plan.
- Establish an environment that promotes learning.
- Include patient teaching while performing routine nursing care.
- Use appropriate methods to evaluate learning.

KEY TERMS

Affective learning

Analogies

Cognitive learning

Health literacy

Learning

Learning objectives

Motivation

Patient-centred approach

Patient-centred care

Patient education

Psychomotor learning

Reinforcement

Return demonstration

Social learning theory

Teaching

🌐 WEBSITE

http://evolve.elsevier.com/Canada/Potter/fundamentals/

CASE STUDY

Susie (preferred pronouns: she/her) has been a community health nurse for 10 years. During the COVID-19 pandemic, she has worked as part of the response team for her community. Community health nurses played an important role in educating the public, counselling individual patients, and spearheading the public health response to the pandemic through screening and prevention, including immunization.

Susie knows that SARS-CoV-2, the virus that causes COVID-19, is highly infectious and results in a range of responses, from mild to severe life-threating symptoms. The mortality rate is significantly higher than from other similar viruses. It has placed considerable stress on the health care system and society in general over the past 3 years. To limit the spread of the disease, several public health measures were implemented at the beginning of the pandemic. Travel and large social gatherings were curtailed, masks and physical distancing

were mandatory in public spaces, and the government periodically imposed total lockdowns of communities.

Susie is aware that there is an abundance of misinformation circulating about COVID-19, especially through social media. This misinformation has led people to question the existence of the pandemic, the cause of the virus, death rates, the need for preventative measures, effective treatment, and potential harm of the vaccines.

In dealing with patients, community health nurses like Susie provide evidence-informed information and must be able to address misinformation to facilitate patient education for informed decision making.

Think about this case study as you read this chapter. There are Review Questions at the end of the chapter about this case study.

PATIENT EDUCATION

Patient education is the process of imparting knowledge to patients and their caregivers about their health. In primary health care settings, nurses are often the main source of information about health promotion, illness prevention, and palliative care (see Chapter 1 for further information about health promotion and Chapter 26 for palliative care). Patient education is a significant part of a nurse's role in any health care setting. Patients and caregivers need health education so that they can make informed decisions about their health care and lifestyles. High-quality patient education has become even more important amid the current trend toward shorter hospital stays, increased demands on nurses' time, and an increasing number of patients with acute or chronic illness. Initial patient education often takes place during acute illness or during management of chronic disease when patients are in the highly stressful stage of their illness, with education taking place over time in a variety of formats. Nurses, both in the hospital setting and out in the community, are not only the primary source of information for people adjusting to health problems but also often in the role of clarifying information provided by physicians, other health care providers, and other sources, including the Internet and social media. By taking a patient-centred approach to patient education, nurses help patients actively participate in their education and better self-manage their needs and care with the support of health care providers across health care settings (Box 21.1).

In order for nurses to be effective patient educators, they require competence in essential domains of nursing education; these include knowledge, critical inquiry, communication and collaboration, professionalism, and leadership (Canadian Association of Schools of Nursing [CASN], 2022). Nurses use both the art and science of nursing to provide professional care to their patients, be they individuals, families, or groups. Providing patient education requires the use of critical thinking skills and the best evidence available. Nurses regularly communicate and collaborate with other members of the health care team to provide patient-centred education to a diverse patient population. Their relationships with patients and their position within the health care team mean that nurses often assume a leadership role in health education.

Over the past couple of decades, the public has become more assertive in seeking knowledge about health and wellness. They have access to more resources via social media and the Internet, and are more actively involved in finding resources available within the health care system. Nurses need to assist patients in navigating the various types of information available to them in all forms of media. The Internet and other forms of technology (telehealth, eHealth) provide nurses and patients with vast amounts of information, some reliable and some not. Patients need guidance regarding the selection of current and reliable resources. Nurses must be able to discuss with patients the criteria for evaluating the validity and reliability of information sources. Nurses educate patients on the use of social media and technology as a medium for obtaining health information related to health promotion and illness prevention, and they facilitate the self-management of individual health needs. The teaching material provided by nurses must honour the copyright rules and must reference both written information and illustrations that are used to support patient learning.

As a nurse providing patient education, you will need to be mindful of the increasing emphasis on scientific evidence and the diminished focus on other kinds of evidence for the efficacy or effectiveness of therapeutic interventions. You should also have a broad perspective on what constitutes meaningful evidence to support the significance of testimonials, lived experiences, and other ways of knowing. Because critical thinking is essential in nursing care, you need to remember that knowledge is limited, beliefs change, and conclusions are temporary. Nonetheless, a well-designed, comprehensive teaching plan that meets a learner's needs can improve quality of care, help patients gain optimal wellness, increase their independence, and reduce health care costs (Bastable, 2019).

BASIC LEARNING PRINCIPLES

Before nurses can teach, they must understand how people learn. Learning depends on the learning environment and on the individual's ability to learn, learning style, and motivation to learn. Learning takes place both in formal learning sessions, which involve planned learning

BOX 21.1 CHRONIC ILLNESS

Self-Management of Chronic Disease

The incidence of chronic illness is increasing across the lifespan, especially in the growing population of persons aged 60 and older. Effective self-management of chronic illness and disease entails a significant educational component, wherein patient teaching focuses on knowledge of the chronic disease, understanding of the health care system, and self-management skills.

Self-managed care requires a patient-centred approach that involves patient participation and a flexible health care interaction, including patient education. The focus of self-management education is to provide patients and their families with the necessary information and knowledge to help them understand the chronic disease, as well as the skills for medical management and living with the chronic disease. A person-centred approach is supported by evidence that patient outcomes improve when patients not only understand their illness, but also develop the knowledge and skills necessary to actively participate in the program, manage symptoms, and engage in interventions to maintain physical functions and activities of daily living (Luhr et al., 2018). While self-management patient education can be offered in a variety of settings and using a variety of methods, research has identified factors that, according to patients, influenced their active participation in self-management.

In a research study by Luhr and colleagues (2018), patients indicated that participation in self-management occurred when they were listened to, considered equal partners, and taken seriously. Active participation in self-management improved when their self-management program provided them with the opportunity to influence the program, to share their knowledge and experiences with others, to learn from others, and to give feedback. Participants indicated that being treated as respected equal members of their self-management program and sharing with others in an open and nonjudgemental environment allowed them to assimilate knowledge, skills, and insights. This in turn improved their self-management and gave them a more positive and hopeful attitude about their chronic disease.

By incorporating a person-centred approach to patient education on self-management, nurses can facilitate patients' understanding of their chronic disease and how to live with it. This leads to patients' having increased confidence in their ability to adapt their lives to their chronic disease and navigate the health care system, which in turn improves quality of life. When patients learn with and from other people living with chronic disease at other stages, they gain peer and social supports, which reduces their isolation and provides them with real-life experiences on how to manage their chronic disease. As a result, patients experience increased hope and optimism about their disease, improved quality of life, and enhanced ability to manage their illness and use the health care system.

From Luhr, K., Holmefur, M., Theander, K., & Eldh, A. C. (2018). Patient participation during and after a self-management programme in primary healthcare—The experience of patients with chronic obstructive pulmonary disease or chronic heart failure. *Patient Education and Counseling, 101*(6), 113–1142. https://doi.org/10.1015/j.pec.2017.12.020

activities, and in teachable moments, which allow nurses to spontaneously take advantage of teaching opportunities as they occur in day-to-day contact with patients.

Learning Environment

Patient education takes place in a variety of settings: the patient's home, community locations, classrooms, and hospital rooms. Specialty clinics in the community (e.g., diabetic, sexual health, prenatal, well child) spend a significant amount of time on patient education related to health promotion and illness prevention. There is a trend toward delivering patient education digitally, including via telehealth, blogs, discussion boards, and self-directed learning modules. The ideal environment for learning is a well-lit, well-ventilated room with appropriate furniture and a comfortable temperature. A quiet setting with few distractions and interruptions can help a person to concentrate. Nurses can provide privacy, even in a busy hospital, by closing cubicle curtains or taking the patient to a quiet spot. In the home, a bedroom might separate the patient from household activities. If the patient desires, caregivers or significant others may join the discussions. However, some patients may be reluctant to discuss their illness when other people, even close caregivers, are in the room. However, an ideal environment is not always achievable. In that case, rather than miss a teachable moment, nurses can adapt the environment as much as possible to provide privacy and minimize distractions.

Ability to Learn

A person's ability to learn depends on their emotional, intellectual, and physical capabilities and on developmental stage. If a patient's learning ability is impaired, the nurse should modify or postpone teaching activities. Learning ability is also impacted by the social determinants of health (see Chapter 1)

Emotional Capability. Emotions can aid or prevent learning. Mild anxiety may help a person focus. However, stronger levels of anxiety can be incapacitating, creating an inability to attend to anything other than the relief of anxiety. The prospect of change makes many people anxious. Seriously ill people, who are faced with multiple losses, may be extremely anxious and distressed. Nurses must be sensitive to a patient's level of anxiety. If a person is incapacitated by anxiety, the nurse needs to find a way to alleviate it. This may mean teaching relaxation techniques before attempting to teach a task or a procedure.

Intellectual Capability. Patients have different levels of intellectual ability. Nurses must assess a patient's knowledge and intellectual level before beginning a teaching plan. For example, measuring liquid or solid food portions requires the ability to perform mathematical calculations. Reading a medication label or discharge instructions requires reading and comprehension skills. Following directions when performing self-care in accordance with limitations requires comprehension and application skills.

Physical Capability. The ability to learn often depends on physical health. To learn psychomotor skills, a patient must possess the necessary strength, coordination, and sensory acuity. Nurses should not overestimate a patient's physical ability. The following physical attributes are necessary for learning psychomotor skills:

- Size (height and weight adequate for performing the task or using the equipment, such as crutch walking)
- Strength (ability of the patient to follow a strenuous exercise program)
- Coordination (dexterity needed for complicated motor skills, such as using utensils, changing a bandage, or opening a medication container)
- Sensory acuity (visual, auditory, tactile, gustatory, and olfactory resources needed to receive and respond to messages taught)

Any physical condition (e.g., pain, fatigue, hunger) that depletes energy also impairs the ability to learn. For example, a patient in a weakened state who has just spent hours undergoing diagnostic tests is likely to be too fatigued to learn. Nurses need to assess the patient's energy level by noting the patient's willingness to communicate, the degree of activity initiated, and the patient's responsiveness to questions. Teaching may be halted if the patient needs rest.

BOX 21.2 Teaching Methods Based on Patient's Developmental Capacity

Infant
Maintain consistent routines (e.g., feeding, bathing).
Hold infant firmly while smiling and speaking softly to convey sense of trust.
Have infant touch different textures (e.g., soft fabric, hard plastic).

Toddler
Use play to teach procedure or activity (e.g., handling examination equipment, applying bandage to doll).
Offer picture books that describe a story of children in a hospital or clinic.
Use simple words such as "cut" instead of "laceration" to promote understanding.

Preschooler
Use role playing, imitation, and play to make learning fun.
Encourage questions and offer explanations; use simple explanations and demonstrations.
Encourage several children to learn together through pictures and short stories about how to perform hygiene.
Use electronic and online age-appropriate teaching tools and games.

School-Age Child
Teach necessary psychomotor skills. (Complicated skills, such as learning to use a syringe, may take considerable practice.)
Offer opportunities to discuss health problems and answer questions.
Offer opportunities to use electronic and online age-appropriate health information sources and tools.

Adolescent
Help adolescent learn about feelings and need for self-expression.
Collaborate with adolescent on teaching activities.
Let adolescent make decisions about health and health promotion (safety, sex education, substance use).
Use problem solving to help adolescent make choices.
Offer opportunity to evaluate and use electronic sources of health information and tools.

Young or Middle-Aged Adult
Encourage participation in teaching plan by setting mutual goals.
Encourage independent learning.
Offer information so that adult can understand effects of health problem.
Offer information so that adult can evaluate electronic sources of information.

Older Person
Teach when patient is alert and rested.
Involve adult in discussion or activity.
Focus on wellness and the person's strengths.
Involve adult in identifying electronic resources to facilitate their health and quality of life.
Use approaches that enhance sensorially impaired patients' reception of stimuli (see Chapter 48).
Keep teaching sessions short.

Developmental Stage. Age and stage of development affect the ability to learn (Box 21.2). Without proper biological, motor, language, and personal–social development, many types of learning cannot take place.

Social Determinants of Health. The ability to learning and access educational resources is influenced by the social determinants of health of the patient, their family, and their community (see Chapter 1). What

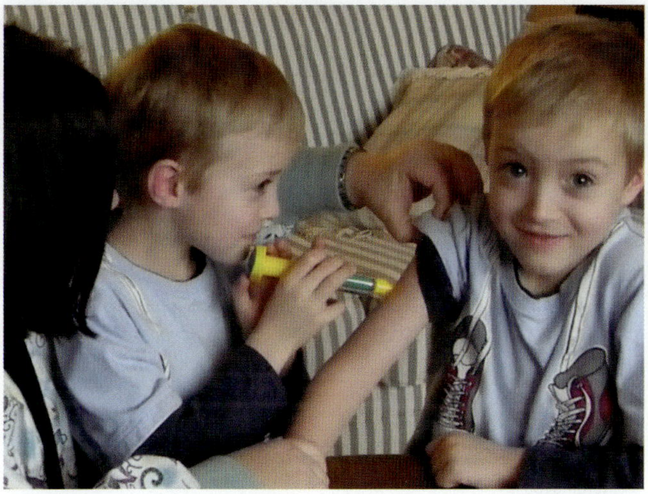

FIGURE 21.1 Teaching aids for children. The nurse uses a developmentally appropriate toy syringe to teach school-aged children about vaccines and immunization.

services and resources are available? Can they be accessed? Are there barriers to participating? These are several of the many factors that need to be considered.

Learning in Children. As a child matures, intellectual growth progresses from concrete to abstract thinking. Therefore, the information presented to children should be understandable, and the expected outcomes should be realistic and based on the child's developmental stage. Developmentally appropriate teaching aids should also be used (Figure 21.1).

Adult Learning. Many adults are independent, self-directed learners. However, they may become dependent in new learning situations. Adults typically learn more successfully when they are encouraged to use past experiences to solve problems. When teaching adult patients, nurses need to collaborate with them on educational topics and goals. Needs or issues that are important to the adult should be addressed early in the teaching–learning process. Ultimately, adults must accept responsibility for changing their own behaviours. Assessing what the adult patient currently knows, teaching what the patient wants to know, and setting mutual goals will improve the outcomes of care and education (Bastable, 2019; Miller & Stoeckel, 2019).

Learning Style and Preference

People have different learning styles. Everyone processes information differently by seeing and hearing, reflecting and acting, reasoning logically and intuitively, and analyzing and visualizing. These styles are not mutually inclusive, and the style(s) used will be influenced by the setting, content, and focus of the learning activity. Some people are visual learners; they learn best by watching. Audiovisual presentations and visual demonstrations often work best for this type of learner. Other people are kinesthetic learners; they learn best when they can manipulate tools and find out how they work. Some people learn by taking detailed notes; others prefer to only listen. Some people need to be engaged in activities and discussion to learn effectively. Others may be too shy to enjoy this type of learning and prefer to learn from an orderly, structured presentation.

Environmental, social, emotional, psychological, and physical stimuli affect people differently. Some people prefer complete silence in the learning environment, whereas others prefer background sounds. Some prefer to learn in a group; others, on their own. Different people prefer different times of the day for learning experiences.

When developing teaching plans, you should assess the favoured learning style and preferences of the patient. With groups, it may not be possible to address every patient's preferences. However, including a combination of approaches to meet multiple learning styles can ensure that most people's learning preferences are met (Bastable, 2019). When the patient is having difficulty with learning, you should consider a change to accommodate a different learning style.

Motivation to Learn

Motivation is a person's desire or willingness to learn. This desire is influenced by four key motivators: the severity of the threat to health, the vulnerability to the threat, the effectiveness of the response in reducing the threat, and the ability of the individual to execute the change in behaviour (Murdaugh et al., 2019; Rosenstock, 1974). If a person is not ready or does not want to learn, learning is unlikely to occur. The stimuli for motivation vary between individuals and may relate to social, task mastery, or physical motives. *Social motives* reflect a need for connection, social approval, or self-esteem. For example, the motivation to exercise may be linked to the social aspects of the exercise activities (Valenzuela et al., 2021). *Task mastery motives* are driven by desire for achievement. For example, a high school student with diabetes begins to test their blood glucose levels and determine insulin dosages before moving away from home and establishing independence. The desire to live independently and manage the disease provides the motivation to master the task or skill. After succeeding at a task, a person is usually motivated to achieve more. *Physical motives* come from a desire to maintain and improve health. Patients motivated by the need to survive or overcome hardship are often more motivated than those who wish merely to improve their health (Murdaugh et al., 2019; Rosenstock, 1974). For example, a patient who has undergone a leg amputation may be extremely motivated to learn to use assistive devices, whereas a patient who is overweight but otherwise healthy may not be motivated to exercise.

Many people do not adopt new health behaviours or change unhealthy behaviours unless they perceive a disease as a threat, overcome barriers to changing health practices, and see the benefits of such changes (Murdaugh et al., 2019; Rosenstock, 1974). Thus, a patient with lung disease may continue to smoke, and an obese patient may worsen their heart condition by refusing to follow a low-fat diet.

Motivation and Social Learning Theory. Health education often involves changing people's attitudes and values. Change can occur only when education plans and interventions are based on sound learning theories. Several theories address the complex patient education process (Bastable, 2019). One of these is social learning theory, which helps educators understand learners and develop interventions that enhance motivation and learning (Bandura, 2001; Bastable, 2019).

When people believe that they can execute a particular behaviour, they are more likely to perform the behaviour consistently and correctly (Bandura, 1997). *Self-efficacy*, a social learning theory concept, is a person's perceived ability to successfully complete a task. Beliefs about self-efficacy arise from four sources: verbal persuasion, vicarious experiences, enactive mastery experiences, and physiological and affective states (Bandura, 1997). Understanding these sources enables nurses to develop appropriate interventions. For example, a nurse teaching a child with asthma to use an inhaler expresses positive reinforcement (verbal persuasion) by encouraging them to use the inhaler on their own. The nurse then demonstrates to the child how to use the inhaler (vicarious experience). The child successfully uses the inhaler alone (enactive mastery experience). As the child begins to control their asthma using the inhaler, the nurse gives the child positive feedback, which further enhances the child's confidence to use the inhaler (physiological and affective states). Interventions such as these enhance perceived self-efficacy, which in turn improves the achievement of desired outcomes.

Motivation and Transtheoretical Model of Change. Health education may involve changes in behaviour, and for many people, behavioural change is often challenging and difficult. It involves a process that occurs over time through a series of stages. By identifying a patient's stage of change and focusing learning activities to match the patient's stage, the nurse can facilitate the learner's motivation to change and their transition from one stage to the next.

Behavioural change involves five stages. These stages have been used in weight management activities, for example (de Freitas et al., 2020; Prochaska & DiClemente, 1992):

- Precontemplation: The person is unaware of the need for change and has no intention of changing their behaviour.
- Contemplation: The person is aware of the need for change and intends to change their behaviour sometime in the future.
- Preparation: The person alters their behaviour in minor ways with the intention of making substantive changes in the immediate future.
- Action: The person modifies their behaviour and experiences in order to make sustainable change.
- Maintenance: The person focuses on not reverting to their previous behaviour and on solidifying the new behaviours.

A Patient-Centred Approach to Patient Education. Patient-centred care is a standard of care that positions the patient as the focus of care delivery and as a partner in the delivery of care (Ortiz, 2018). To engage in a patient-centred approach to patient education, nurses must use both social learning theory and the nursing process. The L.E.A.R.N.S. model, developed by the Registered Nurses' Association of Ontario (RNAO, 2012), consists of a nursing process framework that incorporates social learning theory and a patient-centred approach. The L.E.A.R.N.S. model consists of the following elements (RNAO, 2012, p. 20):

- **Listen** to patient needs.
- **Establish** therapeutic partnership relationships.
- **Adopt** an intentional approach to every learning encounter.
- **Reinforce** health literacy.
- **Name** new knowledge via teach-back.
- **Strengthen** self-management via links to community resources.

Using this approach, the patient is involved as a partner in the learning process.

GOALS OF PATIENT EDUCATION

The goal of patient education is to assist individuals, families, or communities in achieving optimal health (Edelman & Kudzma 2018). Education is an important component of primary health care. It helps individuals, families, and communities to develop the knowledge, understanding, and skills necessary to maintain, improve, and manage their health; reduces hardship; helps contains health care costs; and enables people to take control of and manage their own health (Andrews-Cooper & Kozachik, 2020). Patient education has the following three overall goals (Box 21.3):

- Maintaining and promoting health and preventing illness
- Restoring health, and
- Optimizing quality of life with impaired functioning.

Maintaining and Promoting Health and Preventing Illness

In the home, clinic, or other community health care settings, nurses provide information and skills that people need to prevent disease and maintain, manage, and improve their health (see Box 21.3; see Chapter 4). For example, in prenatal classes, nurses teach expectant parents about fetal development and the physical and psychological

---

BOX 21.3   Topics for Health Education

Health Maintenance and Promotion and Illness Prevention

Educate patients about the following:

First aid

Health resources (e.g., Internet)

Avoidance of risk factors (e.g., smoking, alcoholism, obesity)

Stress management

Typical growth and development patterns

Proper hygiene

Immunizations (e.g., recommendations, risks and benefits)

Prenatal care and normal child-bearing

Nutrition

Exercise

Safety (at home and in health care settings)

Screening for common conditions (e.g., blood pressure, poor vision, cholesterol level)

Behaviour modification to change risky behaviours (e.g., smoking cessation, treatment for substance use disorder)

Restoration of Health

Educate patients about the following:

Patient's disease or condition

Anatomy and physiology of body system affected by disease or condition

Cause of disease

Origin of symptoms

Expected effects on other body systems

Prognosis

Limitations on function

Rationale for treatment

Medications

Alternative therapies (evidence regarding risks and benefits)

Tests and therapies

Nursing measures

Surgical intervention

Expected duration of care

Hospital or clinic environment

Hospital or clinic staff

Long-term care implications

Methods for patient's participation in care

Limitations imposed by disease or surgery

Optimizing Quality of Life When Functions Are Impaired

Educate patients about the following:

Home care

Medications

Intravenous therapy

Diet

Activity

Self-help devices

Rehabilitation of remaining function

Allied health services (e.g., physiotherapy, occupational therapy, speech therapy)

Prevention of complications

Knowledge of risk factors

Implications of nonadherence with therapy

Environmental alterations

Self-help and support groups

---

changes that occur during pregnancy. They also teach about the importance of healthy food choices, exercise, and avoiding substances that might harm the fetus. Greater knowledge can result in better health. When patients become more health conscious, they are more likely to effectively manage their health and seek early diagnosis of health problems (Giese, 2018). With the growth and development of Internet access and health-related websites, patients have been able to access more health information and resources directly. The use of social media, interactive health information sites, and smartphone applications has the potential to enhance health education and patient self-management (Halldorsdottir et al., 2020).

Restoring Health

Many patients seek information and skills that will help them manage, regain, or maintain their health (see Box 21.3). However, patients who find it difficult to adapt to illness may be more passive in their approach. As a student nurse, you will learn to identify barriers to learning, to recognize patients' willingness to learn, and to help motivate their interest in learning (Blevins, 2018).

The family can be a vital part of a patient's return to health, and they may need to know as much as the patient about the patient's recovery. If the nurse excludes the family from a teaching plan, conflicts regarding the patient's care may arise. For example, if the family does not understand a patient's need to regain independent function, their efforts may encourage dependency and thus slow the patient's recovery. It is also important for the nurse to assess the patient–family relationship before involving the family in a teaching plan (see Chapter 20).

Coping With Impaired Functioning

Some patients must learn to cope with permanent health alterations. For example, a patient who loses the ability to speak after surgery of the larynx must learn new ways to communicate. A patient with severe heart disease must learn to modify risk factors that might cause further heart damage. After the patient's needs are identified and the family has expressed their willingness to help, the nurse teaches family members to assist the patient with health care management (e.g., giving medications through gastric tubes and performing passive range-of-motion exercises).

TEACHING AND LEARNING

Teaching is an interactive process that promotes learning. Teaching and learning generally begin when a person identifies a need to know or acquire the ability to do something. A nurse educator provides information that prompts the patient to engage in activities that lead to the desired change (Box 21.4). Teaching is most effective when it addresses the learner's needs, learning style, and capacity. The teacher assesses these needs by asking questions, observing the patient, and determining the patient's interests. With successful teaching, patients can learn new skills or change existing attitudes (Bastable, 2019).

Role of the Nurse in Teaching and Learning

The role of the nurse in patient education is multifaceted. It involves creating or adapting the environment to facilitate learning, using a patient-centred approach in assessing the learning needs of the patient, and using the most appropriate educational strategy (Blevins, 2018). Nurses have an ethical responsibility to teach their patients and enable them to self-manage their health (Miller & Stoeckel, 2019). The Canadian Nurses Association's (2017) *Code of Ethics* states that patients have the right to make informed decisions about their care. The information that patients need to make such decisions must be accurate, complete, and relevant to their needs. Nurses should anticipate patients' needs for information based on their overall condition (physical, mental, emotional, spiritual), identified risks, and interprofessional treatment plans. Nurses often clarify the information provided by physicians

---

BOX 21.4 RESEARCH HIGHLIGHT

Digital Self-Care Intervention in Adults With Chronic Obstructive Pulmonary Disease

Research Focus

This pilot study focused on the development, feasibility, and acceptability of a digital intervention for adults with chronic obstructive pulmonary disease (COPD), as well as evaluating the effects of the intervention.

Research Abstract

Bugajski and colleagues (2020) developed digital self-care modules as an intervention and determined whether the modules affected self-care and symptoms. The study used a quasi-experimental repeated-measures design. The study lasted 21 consecutive days.

Methods

Participants were assessed at the start of the study, 2 weeks into the study, and at the end of the study. Assessment consisted of measurement of self-care ability, anxiety, depression, perceived self-care adherence, and information needs. Digital education modules were developed for seven self-care categories: nutrition/diet, physical activity, medications, breathing control, mental health, environmental modification, and exacerbation planning. Modules consisted of written content, pictures, and videos about self-care behaviours and how to incorporate the behaviours into daily living. Modules and data collection tools were hosted on a website. Participants ($N = 20$) were provided with a tablet computer and received training on using the tablet and the website. In addition, they received a daily text message reminding them to access the website.

Results

Findings indicated that the digital educational web-based intervention significantly improved self-care adherence and self-care knowledge. However, the intervention did not significantly affect perceived self-care ability, anxiety, or depression. The authors suggested that the lack of change in perceived self-care ability may have been related to the short duration of the study and the limited opportunity to practise self-care behaviours. Participant baseline evaluations did not identify the presence of anxiety or depression and may explain the lack of change following the intervention.

Implications for Practice

- Digital web-based educational interventions are an effective method to deliver health education to patients with COPD.
- Digital educational modules significantly improved self-care adherence and self-care knowledge. Perceived self-care ability was not significantly affected by the digital interventions during the 21 days of the study. This may be related to the short time frame and the limited opportunity to practise self-care behaviours.

From Bugajski, A., Frazer, S. K., Cousin, L., et al. (2020). Effects of a digital self-care intervention in adults with COPD: A pilot study. *Western Journal of Nursing Research, 42*(9), 736–746. https://doi.org/10.1177/0193945919892282

---

and other health care providers and may become the patient's primary source of information for adjusting to health problems (Bastable, 2019; Miller & Stoeckel, 2019).

Patients and their families often ask nurses for health information, and it is easy to identify the need for teaching when patients request information. However, in some cases, the need for information may be less apparent. Nurses need to observe and listen carefully to determine patients' needs for information and learning. When nurses value education and ensure that patients learn the necessary information, patients are better prepared to assume health care responsibilities. To be an effective nurse educator, you must do more than just pass on facts; you must determine what patients need to know, find time when they are ready to learn, and evaluate the impact of patient education on patient outcomes (Bastable, 2019; Miller & Stoeckel, 2019).

Teaching as Communication

Effective teaching depends on effective communication (see Chapter 18). To be a good teacher, you must listen empathetically, observe astutely, and speak clearly. Many intrapersonal variables—including attitudes, values, culture, emotions, and knowledge—influence both the nurse's and the patient's styles and approaches. Both you and the patient are also affected by the patient's motivation and ability to learn, which depends on physical and psychological health, education, developmental stage, and previous knowledge.

DOMAINS OF LEARNING

Learning occurs in three domains: cognitive (understanding), affective (attitudes), and psychomotor (motor skills) (Bastable, 2019; Bloom, 1956). Any topic to be learned may involve one domain, all domains, or any combination of the three. For example, patients with diabetes must learn how diabetes affects the body and how to control blood glucose levels for better health (cognitive domain). They must also learn to accept the chronic nature of diabetes by learning positive coping mechanisms (affective domain). Finally, many patients with diabetes must learn to test their blood glucose levels at home. This requires learning how to use a glucose meter (psychomotor domain). By understanding each learning domain, nurses can select appropriate teaching methods (Box 21.5). Learning increasingly involves the use of technology to enhance accessibility and utilization of learning opportunities.

Cognitive Learning

Cognitive learning includes all intellectual behaviours and requires thinking (Alslaity & Tran, 2018). In the hierarchy of cognitive behaviours, the simplest behaviour is remembering, whereas the most complex is creating. Cognitive learning includes the following:

- Remembering: the ability to learn new information and to retrieve knowledge from long-term memory
- Understanding: the ability to construct the meaning of learned material
- Applying: the use of abstract, newly learned ideas in a practical situation
- Analyzing: breaking down information into organized parts and determining how the parts relate to one another
- Evaluating: making judgements based on criteria and standards
- Creating: combining elements to form a coherent and functional whole

---

BOX 21.5   Appropriate Teaching Methods Based on Domains of Learning

Cognitive

Discussion (One-on-One or Group)
May involve nurse and one patient or nurse with several patients
Promotes active participation and focuses on topics of interest to patient
Facilitates peer support
Enhances application and analysis of new information
Can be adapted for online discussion groups or video conferencing

Storytelling
Can involve individual or group
Facilitates cultural relevance and safety
Enhances application of new information to a familiar context
Can use blogs, discussion groups, and video conferencing

Lecture
Is more formal method of instruction because it is teacher controlled
Helps learner acquire new knowledge and gain comprehension
Can be adapted for synchronous or asynchronous online delivery or self-directed learning

Question-and-Answer Session
Is designed to address patient's specific concerns
Assists patient in applying knowledge
May use email or online discussion groups

Role Play and Discovery
Encourages patient to actively apply knowledge in controlled situation
Promotes synthesis of information and problem solving
May use interactive simulations

Independent Projects (e.g., Computer-Assisted Instruction) and Field Experience
Assists patient with assuming responsibility for learning at own pace
Promotes analysis, synthesis, and evaluation of new information and skills

Teach-Back
Allows patient to demonstrate their understanding of material covered
Provides opportunity to identify areas requiring clarification or additional instruction

Affective

Role Play
Debriefing encourages expression of values, feelings, and attitudes

Discussion (Group)
Enables patient to acquire support from other people in group
Encourages patient to learn from other people's experiences
Promotes responding, valuing, and organizing

Discussion (One-on-One)
Facilitates discussion of personal, sensitive topics of interest or concern

Psychomotor

Demonstration
Provides presentation of procedures or skills by nurse in person, through video, or online
Encourages patient to model nurse's behaviour
Allows nurse to control questioning during demonstration

Practice
Enables patient to perform skills by using equipment in a controlled setting
Allows repetition

Return Demonstrations
Enables patient to perform skill as nurse observes
Provides excellent source of feedback and reinforcement

Independent Projects and Games
Require teaching method that promotes adaptation and initiation of psychomotor learning
Enable learner to use new skills

Affective Learning

Affective learning concerns expressions of feelings and acceptance of attitudes, opinions, or values. Values clarification (see Chapter 9) is an example of affective learning. The simplest behaviour in the affective learning hierarchy is receiving, and the most complex is characterizing (Krathwohl et al., 1964; Nelson et al., 2020).

- Receiving: the willingness to attend to another person's words
- Responding: active participation through listening and reacting verbally and nonverbally
- Valuing: attachment of worth to an object, concept, or behaviour, demonstrated by the learner's actions
- Organizing: development of a value system by identifying and organizing values and resolving conflicts
- Characterizing: action and response with a consistent value system

Psychomotor Learning

Psychomotor learning requires the integration of mental and muscular activity in order to acquire a skill, such as the ability to walk or to use an eating utensil. The simplest behaviour in the hierarchy is perception, and the most complex is origination (Muzyk et al., 2018).

- Perception: awareness of objects or qualities through sense organs
- Set: a readiness (mental, physical, or emotional) to take a particular action
- Guided response: the performance of an act under the guidance of an instructor, involving imitation of a demonstrated act
- Mechanism: a higher level of behaviour by which a person gains confidence and skill in performing a behaviour that is more complex or involves several more steps than does a guided response
- Complex overt response: the smooth and accurate performance of a motor skill that requires a complex movement pattern
- Adaptation: the ability to change motor response when unexpected problems occur
- Origination: use of existing psychomotor skills and abilities to perform a highly complex motor act that involves creating new movement patterns

❖ INTEGRATING THE NURSING PROCESS AND TEACHING PROCESS

The nursing process and teaching process are related and usually take place concurrently. Like the nursing process, the teaching process requires assessment, nursing diagnosis, planning, implementation, and evaluation. However, the nursing process is broader than the teaching process. For example, determining a patient's health needs requires an assessment of all data sources. The teaching process is focused on those data sources that reveal the patient's learning needs, willingness and ability to learn, and available teaching resources. The teaching process is especially useful for teaching large groups, where individual learning needs and styles may vary. Table 21.1 compares the teaching process and nursing process.

The teaching process requires assessment. The patient's ability to learn, motivation, and needs should be assessed and analyzed. A diagnostic statement specifies the information or skills that the patient requires. The nurse sets specific **learning objectives** (i.e., what the learner will be able to do after successful instruction), then implements the teaching plan by using teaching and learning principles to ensure that the patient acquires knowledge and skills. Finally, the teaching process requires an evaluation of learning based on the learning objectives.

◆ Assessment

During assessment, the nurse works with the patient to determine the patient's health care needs (see Chapter 14). The patient may indicate a need for health care information, or the nurse may identify a need for education. Learning needs identified by both the patient and the nurse determine the content to be learned. By performing an effective assessment, nurses can individualize instruction for each patient. Nurses need to ask specific questions to assess a patient's unique learning needs (Box 21.6).

Learning Needs. Most patients can identify at least some of their own learning needs. Effective questioning and assessment tools help nurses determine a patient's perceived learning needs. By listening carefully and using open-ended and closed-ended questions (see Chapter 18), nurses can often find out what a patient's needs are. Because a patient's health status is dynamic, assessment is an ongoing activity. Nurses should assess for the following:

- Information or skills that the patient needs to be able to perform self-care and to understand the implications of a health issue (e.g., teaching an adolescent boy to perform a testicular self-exam)
- Experiences that have influenced the patient's need to learn, and
- Information that caregivers or significant others require in order to support the patient's needs; the amount of information needed depends on the extent of the caregiving role.

TABLE 21.1	Comparison of the Nursing Process and Teaching Process	
Basic Steps	**Nursing Process**	**Teaching Process**
Assessment	Collect data about patient's physical, psychological, social, cultural, developmental, and spiritual needs from patient, family, diagnostic tests, medical record, health history, learning style, and literature.	Gather data about patient's learning needs, motivation, ability to learn, and teaching resources from patient, family, learning environment, medical record, health history, and literature.
Analysis	Identify appropriate health concern based on assessment findings, including deficits.	Identify patient's learning needs in the three domains of learning.
Planning	Develop individualized care plan.	Establish learning objectives, stated in behavioural terms.
	Set diagnosis priorities according to patient's immediate needs.	Prioritize learning needs.
	Collaborate with patient on care plan.	Collaborate with patient on teaching plan.
		Identify type of teaching method to use.
Implementation	Perform nursing care therapies.	Implement teaching methods.
	Include patient as active participant in care.	Actively involve patient in learning activities.
	Involve family or significant other in care as appropriate.	Include family or significant other in learning activities as appropriate.
Evaluation	Identify success in meeting desired outcomes and goals of nursing care.	Determine outcomes of teaching–learning process.
	Alter interventions as needed when goals are not met.	Measure patient's ability to achieve learning objectives.
		Reinforce information as needed.

Ability to Learn. The ability to learn can be impaired by many factors, including body temperature, electrolyte levels, oxygenation status, and blood glucose level. Several factors may influence a patient at one time. The nurse assesses the patient's ability to learn by considering the following:

- Physical strength, movement, dexterity, and coordination (the nurse determines the patient's ability to perform skills)
- Sensory deficits that may affect the ability to understand or follow instruction (see Chapter 48)
- Reading level (This can be difficult to assess because functional illiteracy is often easy to conceal; one way to assess a patient's reading level and level of understanding is to ask the patient to read instructions from a teaching brochure and then explain its meaning.)
- Developmental level (influences teaching approaches; see Box 21.2)
- Cognitive function (i.e., memory, knowledge, association, and judgement).

Motivation to Learn. To identify a patient's motivation level, nurses can ask questions that will help them determine readiness to learn (i.e., whether a patient is prepared and willing to learn). The patient's motivation is assessed by studying the following:

- Behaviour (e.g., attention span, tendency to ask questions, memory, and ability to concentrate during the teaching session)
- Health beliefs and perception of a health problem and the benefits and barriers to treatment (For example, asking a patient with coronary artery disease, "How will heart disease affect you over time? What is the value of eating a low-fat diet?")
- Perceived ability to complete a required healthy behaviour
- Desire to learn
- Attitudes about health care providers (exploring the roles of the patient and nurse in making health decisions; e.g., asking the patient, "In what way can I best help you?")

BOX 21.6   Nursing Assessment Questions

Ask Patients

What do you want to know?

What do you know about your illness and your treatment plan?

How does (or will) your illness affect your current lifestyle?

What barriers currently exist that are preventing you from managing your illness the way you would like to manage it?

What cultural or spiritual beliefs do you have regarding your illness and the prescribed treatment?

What experiences have you had that are similar to what you are experiencing now?

Together we can choose the best way for you to learn about your disease. How can I best help you?

What role do you believe your health care provider should take in helping you manage your illness or maintain health?

When you learn new information, do you prefer to have the information given to you in pictures or written down in words?

When you give someone directions to your house, do you tell the person how to get there, write out the instructions, draw a map, or just give the person the address to enter in a smartphone for directions?

How involved do you want your family to be in the management of your illness?

Ask Caregivers

When are you available to help, and how do you plan to help your loved one?

Your spouse needs some help. How do you feel about learning how to assist them?

- Knowledge of information to be learned (The patient must play an active role in seeking health-related information.)
- Pain, fatigue, anxiety, or other physical symptoms that can interfere with the ability to maintain attention and participate (In acute care settings, a patient's physical condition can easily detract from learning.)
- Sociocultural background (A patient's beliefs and values about health and various therapies may be influenced by sociocultural norms or tradition [see Chapter 11]; educational efforts can be especially challenging when patients and educators do not speak the same language.)
- Learning style preference (Patients who learn better by seeing and hearing may benefit from a video; patients who learn best by reasoning logically and intuitively may learn better if presented with written material that they can analyze and discuss with others.)

Teaching Environment. Nurses need to assess the following factors when choosing a teaching environment:

- Distractions or persistent noise (A quiet area should be set aside for teaching.)
- Comfort of the room, including ventilation, temperature, lighting, and furniture, and
- Room facilities and available equipment.

Resources for Learning. Assessment of resources includes a review of available teaching tools and guidelines (RNAO, 2012). If a patient requires family support, the nurse should evaluate the readiness and ability of family and friends to learn to care for the patient and review resources in the home. The nurse needs to assess the following:

- The patient's willingness to have caregivers involved in the teaching plan and care (Information about the patient's health care is confidential unless the patient chooses to share it.)
- Caregivers' perceptions and understanding of the patient's illness and its implications (Caregivers' and patient's perceptions should match; otherwise, conflicts may arise in the teaching plan.)
- Family's willingness and ability to participate in care (Caregivers must be responsible, willing, and able to assist in performing care activities, such as bathing or administering medications.)
- Resources in the home (These resources include health care equipment, access to technology, and a suitable rearrangement of rooms.)
- Teaching tools, including brochures, audiovisual materials, or posters. (Printed material should present current and easy-to-understand information that matches the patient's reading level.)

◆ **Nursing Diagnosis**

After assessing the patient's ability and need to learn, the nurse interprets data to form an accurate health focus. This focus ensures that teaching will be goal directed and individualized. If a patient has several learning needs, the nursing foci guide priority setting. By classifying diagnoses according to the three learning domains, the nurse can focus on subject matter and teaching methods. Examples of nursing foci that indicate a need for education include the following:

- Health maintenance
- Health-seeking behaviours
- Health self-management
- Mastery of a health-related skill, and
- Deficient knowledge.

When health care problems can be managed through education, the foci of patient education are *knowledge* and *skills*. For example, an older person may be unable to manage a medication regimen because of the number of medications that must be taken at different times of day. Education may improve the patient's ability to schedule and take the medications.

Some nursing foci also indicate that teaching is inappropriate. You may identify conditions that hinder learning (e.g., nursing focus of pain or activity intolerance). In these cases, you should delay teaching until the nursing focus is resolved or the health problem is controlled.

◆ Planning

After identifying a patient's learning needs and a nursing focus, the nurse develops a teaching plan, sets goals and expected outcomes, and works with the patient to select a teaching method (Box 21.7). Expected outcomes or learning objectives determine which teaching strategies and approaches are appropriate. Patient participation is essential.

Developing Learning Objectives. Learning objectives identify the expected outcome of instruction and establish learning priorities. Objectives help nurses manage time and resources.

Objectives are either short term or long term. Short-term objectives meet the patient's immediate learning needs, such as needing knowledge about an upcoming test. Long-term objectives, which are often broader, help a patient adapt to a long-term challenge. Learning objectives will guide the teaching plan. SMART objectives provide the following framework for defining objectives:

- Specific—Describes a specific action, behaviour, outcome, or achievement that is observable

BOX 21.7 NURSING CARE PLAN
Learning Needs

ASSESSMENT

A nurse in a surgeon's office is preparing a patient for a colon resection, which is scheduled in 1 week. The patient, aged 75, has recently received a diagnosis of colorectal cancer. The nurse's assessment focuses on the patient's readiness to learn, available resources, and factors that might affect their ability to understand the procedure and related postoperative care.

Assessment Activities	Findings and Defining Characteristics
Assess the patient's readiness to learn and ask what the surgeon has already told them about the surgery.	The patient responds, "I can't remember what the doctor told me at my last appointment. My surgery is scheduled for next week."
Ask the patient to explain postoperative care, including performing a return demonstration of deep breathing and coughing.	The patient is unable to describe postoperative care or provide a return demonstration of deep breathing and coughing.
Assess the patient's visual acuity.	The patient says they have difficulty reading small print.

NURSING FOCUS: Lack of recall and exposure to information

PLANNING

Goals (Nursing Outcomes Classification)*	Expected Outcomes*
	Knowledge: Treatment Regimen
The patient will describe the surgery and the risks.	The patient will verbalize their understanding of the surgical procedure and the related risk factors.
The patient will participate in postoperative care during hospitalization.	The patient will demonstrate deep breathing and coughing; they will advance their level of activity after their surgery.

*Outcome classification labels from Moorhead, S., Swanson, E., Johnson, M., & Maas, M. L. (Eds.). (2018). *Nursing outcomes classification (NOC)* (6th ed.). Mosby/Elsevier.

INTERVENTIONS

Interventions (Nursing Interventions Classification)†	Rationale
Learning Readiness Enhancement	
Determine readiness to learn and what the patient perceives as important to know.	Adult patients' learning is enhanced when they are ready to learn and information is perceived as important (Bastable, 2019).
Learning Facilitation	
Give patient large-print brochure describing preoperative and postoperative care during educational session.	Providing patients with educational methods that use multiple senses is effective in educating older persons. Large fonts with contrasting colours are easier for older persons to see (Miller & Stoeckel, 2019).
Provide patient with Website address associated with clinic to enable access to patient information and instructional video clips.	
Explain postoperative care, demonstrate deep breathing and coughing, and have patient perform return demonstration.	Improving self-efficacy by using role modelling and by having the patient perform behaviours enhances the successful adoption of healthy behaviours (Bandura, 1997).

†Intervention classification labels from Butcher, H. K., Bulechek, G. M., McCloskey Dochterman, J. M., & Wagner, C. (Eds.). (2019). *Nursing interventions classification (NIC)* (7th ed.). Mosby.

EVALUATION

Nursing Actions	Patient Response and Finding	Achievement of Outcome
Ask the patient what they can expect before and after surgery.	The patient is able to state their understanding of preoperative and postoperative care.	The patient's anxiety level has decreased, and they report that they are ready for surgery.
Observe patient as they demonstrate deep breathing and coughing and advance their activity postoperatively.	The patient is able to cough and breathe deeply postoperatively, but they are hesitant to advance their activity level after surgery.	Outcome of advancing activity postoperatively has not been totally achieved. Address and manage barriers inhibiting attainment of this outcome (e.g., pain), and continue to encourage and educate patient.

- **M**easurable—Quantifiable with associated indicators that can be measured
- **A**chievable/**A**ttainable—Objective can be achieved with the available resources
- **R**ealistic—Achievable with the available resources, and
- **T**ime-bound—State a time frame within which the objective will be achieved. (MacDonald & Jakubec, 2022)

Each objective focuses on a single behaviour that will determine the patient's ability to meet health care outcomes. A behavioural objective contains a verb describing what action the learner will perform after the objective is met (e.g., "*will administer* an injection"). Behavioural objectives are achievable, measurable, and observable and indicate how learning will be evidenced (e.g., "will perform *three-point crutch gait*"). The objective describes precise behaviours and content. Nurses should avoid vague or nonspecific objectives that do not explain what the learner is to do.

An objective is more precise when it describes the conditions or timing under which the behaviour occurs. Conditions and time frames should be realistic and designed for the learner's needs (e.g., "will identify the side effects of medication by discharge"). It also helps to consider the conditions under which the patient or family will perform the behaviour (e.g., "will walk from bedroom to bathroom using crutches"). Nurses set criteria for acceptable performance according to the desired level of accuracy, success, or satisfaction. For example, "a patient undergoing therapy for a fractured leg will walk on crutches to the end of the hall within three days." Criteria are more acceptable when the teacher and learner establish them mutually. However, the nurse serves as a resource in setting the minimum criteria for success.

After formulating the learning objectives, the nurse and patient establish a teaching plan. It is the nurse's responsibility to integrate basic teaching principles and to develop a well-timed and organized teaching plan.

Setting Priorities. The teaching plan is prioritized according to the patient's immediate needs, nursing diagnoses, learning objectives, main concerns, anxiety level, and the time available to teach. Patients set priorities based on the importance they assign to a particular aspect of their health experience. They are influenced by (1) internal factors such as control, preferences, and sociocultural values, (2) attitudes to recommended treatment, and (3) functional ability (Liu et al., 2019).

Timing. When is the right time to teach? During a wellness check? In a specialty clinic, before a patient is hospitalized? When a patient enters a clinic or a long-term care facility? At discharge? At home? All of these times are correct because patients continue to have learning needs and opportunities as long as they stay in the health care system. As the nurse, you should plan to teach when a patient is most attentive, receptive, and alert. However, timing can be difficult, particularly in an acute care setting, where the focus is on an early discharge. By the time the patient is ready to learn, discharge may already have been scheduled. Therefore, you need to anticipate a patient's educational needs.

The length of teaching sessions also influences learning. Concentration is difficult to sustain in a prolonged session. You can assess a patient's level of concentration by observing nonverbal cues such as poor eye contact or a slumped posture. Teaching sessions should be held often enough to document the patient's learning progress. The frequency of sessions depends on the learner's abilities and the complexity of the material. For example, a child who has been newly diagnosed with diabetes will require more visits to an outpatient centre than an older person who has been managing diabetes for 15 years. Intervals between teaching sessions should not be so long that the patient might forget information.

Organizing Teaching Material. An outline helps to organize information into a logical sequence. Material should progress from simple to complex. A person needs to learn simple facts and concepts before learning associations or complex concepts.

Essential content should be taught first because people are more likely to remember information that is taught early. Repetition reinforces learning. Summarizing key points helps the learner remember important information (Bastable, 2019).

Maintaining Attention and Promoting Participation. Active participation is key to learning. People learn better when more than one of the body's senses is stimulated. Nurses should engage the patient's interest by changing the tone and intensity of their voice, making eye contact, using gestures, asking questions, and encouraging participation with activities such as role playing.

Building on Existing Knowledge. An effective teacher presents information that builds on a learner's existing knowledge. For example, a patient who has had multiple sclerosis must begin a new medication that is given subcutaneously. On assessment, the nurse asks the patient about experience with injections. The patient explains that they gave their father insulin injections for many years. The nurse can then individualize the teaching plan by building on the patient's previous knowledge and experience with insulin injections.

Selecting Teaching Methods. A teaching method is the way that a teacher delivers information. It is based on the patient's learning needs. More than one method may be used for instruction. For example, a patient who learns best in the psychomotor domain will benefit from demonstrations and supervised practice. The patient masters new skills by manipulating equipment and practising manual skills. Discussions, question-and-answer sessions, and formal lectures can all be effective methods, depending on the patient's needs and learning style. When choosing appropriate teaching methods, nurses should encourage patients to offer suggestions (Box 21.8).

Selecting Resources. Nurses are responsible for ensuring that patients' educational needs are met. Sometimes patients' needs are highly complex. In these cases, nurses need to identify appropriate health education resources within the health care system or the community. Examples of resources for patient education are diabetes education clinics, cardiac rehabilitation programs, prenatal classes, and support groups. Nurses should obtain a referral if necessary, encourage patients to attend these sessions, and reinforce information taught.

Writing Teaching Plans. In all health care settings, nurses develop written teaching plans for use by colleagues. The nurse responsible for developing the teaching plan incorporates all pertinent information into the plan, including topics for instruction, resources (e.g., equipment, teaching booklets, and referrals to education programs), recommendations for involving family, and objectives of the teaching plan. A plan may be detailed or presented in outline form.

In an acute care setting, plans are concise and focused on the primary learning needs of the patient because time for teaching is limited. A care in the community teaching plan or outpatient clinic plan may be more comprehensive because nurses may have more time to instruct patients, and patients are often less anxious in outpatient settings.

A plan should provide continuity of instruction, particularly when several nurses are involved in a patient's care. The more specific the plan is, the easier it is to follow.

BOX 21.8 PATIENT TEACHING

Teaching Strategies

- Establish trust with the patient before beginning the teaching–learning session.
- Limit teaching objectives.
- Use simple terminology to enhance the patient's understanding.
- Avoid medical jargon. If necessary, explain medical terms by using basic one- or two-syllable words.
- Schedule short teaching sessions at frequent intervals; minimize distractions during teaching sessions.
- Begin and end each teaching session with the most important information.
- Present information slowly, pacing the session to provide ample time for the patient to understand the material.
- Repeat important information.
- Provide many examples that have meaning to the patient; for example, relate new material to a previous life experience.
- Build on existing knowledge.
- Use visual cues and simple analogies when appropriate.
- Ask the patient for frequent feedback to determine whether the patient comprehends the information.
- Demonstrate procedures such as measuring dosages; ask for return demonstrations (which provide opportunities to clarify instructions and time to review procedures).
- Provide teaching materials that reflect the reading level of the patient; provide material that uses short words and sentences, large type, and simple format (in general, information written at a Grade 5 reading level is recommended for adult learners).
- Provide teaching materials that reflect the health literacy of the patient; use material that avoids jargon, acronyms, and unnecessary medical terminology and that defines only the necessary medical terms.
- Model appropriate behaviour and use role playing to help patient learn how to ask questions and ask for help effectively.
- Pace the delivery of material so that patients can progress at their own speed.
- Include caregivers or other caregivers in the education process.

From Bastable, S. (2019). *Nurse as educator: Principles of teaching and learning for nursing practice* (5th ed.). Jones & Bartlett Learning; Miller, M. A., & Stoeckel, P. R. (2019). *Client education: Theory and practice* (3rd ed.). Jones & Bartlett Learning.

BOX 21.9 Example of Nursing Interventions Based on Patient's Learning Needs

Assessment Data

A patient, aged 67, has a 15-year history of type 2 diabetes. They are in the hospital because of an infected foot ulcer that requires frequent dressing changes. The patient used to take oral hypoglycemic medications to control their blood glucose levels. However, they now need to start home insulin injections because of the infection and wound. They must also learn how to change their dressings. The patient is anxious about being discharged and requests information about a local diabetes support group and Internet resources. The case manager indicates that the patient will be discharged soon.

Cognitive Interventions

- Ask the patient about what they believe they need to know before they are discharged.
- Encourage the patient to help establish learning outcomes and goals.
- Provide the patient with teaching materials regarding insulin preparation and administration, and how to recognize and manage hypoglycemia and hyperglycemia.
- During teaching sessions, give the patient examples of what problems they might experience at home and ask them how they would respond to the situations (e.g., "If the wound's drainage increases and it looks like there is pus, what would you do?").
- Provide the patient with the website address for Diabetes Canada.

Affective Interventions

- Encourage the patient to attend a support group meeting, if possible, to facilitate learning from others' experiences.
- Encourage the patient to verbalize their feelings and fears about this change in their health status.
- Have the patient role play how they will respond to friends who ask about the patient's health status.
- As they acquire new skills and behaviours, provide the patient with feedback and positive reinforcement.

Psychomotor Interventions

- Demonstrate insulin preparation and injection techniques.
- Demonstrate use of the blood glucose meter and recording of blood glucose measurements.
- Demonstrate dressing changes.
- Ask the patient to perform return demonstrations of insulin preparation and injection, blood glucose testing, and dressing changes.

◆ Implementation

Implementing a teaching plan depends on a nurse's ability to analyze assessment data when identifying learning needs and developing the teaching plan (see Box 21.7). The nurse needs to evaluate the learning objectives and determine the best teaching and learning methods to help the patient meet expected goals and outcomes. A diversified approach can be used to create an active learning environment (Box 21.9).

Teaching Approaches. A *teaching approach* is different from a *teaching method*. Because a learner's needs and motives can change over time, nurses must be ready to modify teaching approaches.

Telling. The telling approach is useful when limited information will be taught (e.g., preparing a patient for an emergency diagnostic procedure). The nurse outlines the task to be done and the patient's role and gives instructions—for example, explaining the insertion of an intravenous line and the need for the patient to remain still. This method provides no opportunity for feedback.

Selling. The selling approach entails two-way communication. The nurse needs to pace instruction according to the patient's response.

Specific feedback is given to the patient who learns successfully. For example, when the patient learns a step-by-step procedure for changing a dressing, first the patient learns to remove the old dressing, then to clean the wound, and finally to apply a new dressing.

Participating. Participating involves setting objectives and becoming involved in the learning process together. The patient helps to decide on content, and the nurse guides and counsels the patient with pertinent information. Opportunities are provided for discussion, feedback, mutual goal setting, and revision of the teaching plan. For example, a patient may request information from the nurse about improving their physical fitness. That leads to a discussion in which the nurse identifies the patient's key areas of interest, such as weight loss and improving cardiovascular fitness. Together with the patient, the nurse identifies goals and learning strategies.

Entrusting. The entrusting approach provides the patient with the opportunity to manage self-care. The nurse observes the patient's progress and remains available to assist without introducing more new information. For example, a patient with metabolic syndrome has decided to make lifestyle changes (e.g., improve diet and exercise) to improve their health. The nurse provides resources and recommends other sources of information. The nurse then meets with the patient on a regular basis to check progress and provide additional information.

Reinforcing. Reinforcement is the use of a stimulus that increases the probability of a response. A person who receives positive reinforcement before or after learning a desired behaviour is likely to repeat the behaviour. People usually respond better to positive reinforcement (Bastable, 2019). Negative reinforcement, such as criticizing, can decrease an undesired response, but its effects are less predictable and often undesirable. Feedback is a common form of reinforcement.

There are three types of reinforcers: social, material, and activity. Most nurses use social reinforcers (e.g., encouraging words) to acknowledge a learned behaviour. Examples of material reinforcers are food, toys, and music. These reinforcers work best with young children. Activity reinforcers are based on the principle that people are motivated to engage in an activity if, after its completion, they are able to engage in a more desirable activity. For example, patients with dementia may be more willing to bathe if they can go for a walk with the nurse afterward. Activity reinforces work when a patient is self-motivated. Choosing an appropriate reinforcer requires attention to individual preferences. Observing behaviour often helps reveal the best reinforcer to use. Reinforcers should never be used as threats and are not effective with every patient.

Incorporating Teaching Into Nursing Care. Many nurses teach effectively while delivering nursing care. This is taking advantage of teachable moments (Reynolds et al., 2020). This activity becomes easier as you gain confidence in clinical skills. For example, while hanging a blood bag, you explain to the patient why the blood is needed, and you describe the symptoms of transfusion reactions that should be reported immediately. When you follow a teaching plan informally, the patient feels less pressure to perform, and learning becomes more of a shared activity. Teaching during routine care is efficient and cost effective (Figure 21.2).

Implementing Teaching Methods. The nurse's choice of teaching methods depends on the patient's learning needs, the time available for teaching, the environment, the resources, and the nurse's own comfort level with teaching. Skilled teachers are flexible in altering teaching methods according to the learner's responses and in using teaching tools that work best with a particular method. Various teaching tools are detailed in Table 21.2.

One-on-One Discussion. In a one-on-one discussion, the nurse presents information informally, providing the patient with the opportunity to ask questions or share concerns. During the discussion, the nurse can use various teaching aids such as models or diagrams, depending on the patient's learning needs. Discussions can be done in person or online.

Group Instruction. Groups are an economical way to teach several patients at once. Patients interact and learn from other's experiences. Groups can also foster positive attitudes that help patients meet learning objectives (Andersson et al., 2019). Video conferencing can be used and may increase access.

Group instruction often involves lecture, activities, and discussion. Lectures are highly structured and help patients learn standard content.

Preparatory Instruction. Patients are often anxious about unfamiliar tests or procedures. By providing information about procedures, nurses help patients anticipate what will happen. Guidelines for giving preparatory explanations are as follows:

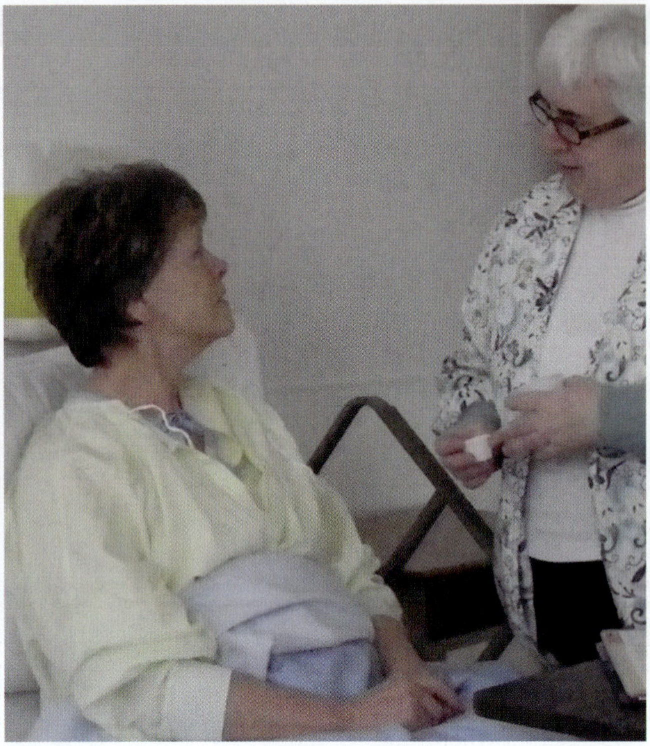

FIGURE 21.2 Teaching during routine care. The nurse uses administration of medication to assess a patient's knowledge about medications and provides additional information as needed.

- Describe physical sensations during the procedure, but do not evaluate them. For example, when you draw a blood specimen, explain to the patient that they will feel a sticking sensation as the needle punctures the skin.
- Describe the cause of the sensation to prevent misinterpretation of the experience. For example, explain that a needle stick burns because the alcohol used to cleanse the skin enters the puncture site.
- Prepare patients only for aspects of the experience that are common to other patients. For example, explain that it is normal for a tight tourniquet to cause a person's hand to tingle and feel numb.

Demonstrations. Demonstrations are used to teach psychomotor skills, such as preparing a syringe, bathing an infant, walking with a crutch, or measuring a pulse. Patients need to observe a skill before practising it. Demonstrations are most effective when patients first observe the nurse doing the skill and then perform a return demonstration to practise the skill. A demonstration should be combined with discussion to clarify concepts and feelings. An effective demonstration requires advanced planning as follows:

- Position the patient to provide a clear view of the demonstration.
- Review the rationale and steps of the procedure.
- Assemble and organize equipment. Make sure it works.
- Perform each step in sequence while analyzing the knowledge and skills involved.
- Determine when to give explanations, considering the patient's learning needs.
- Adjust speed and timing of the demonstration according to the patient's abilities and anxiety level.

The nurse should demonstrate the steps of a procedure in the same order in which the patient will perform them. The demonstration involves the following steps:

- Performing each step slowly and accurately
- Encouraging the patient to ask questions to ensure that each step is understood

TABLE 21.2 Teaching Tools for Instruction

Description of Tool	Implications for Learning
Printed Material Written teaching tools such as pamphlets, booklets, and brochures	Material must be easily readable for learner. Information must be accurate and current. Method is ideal for understanding complex concepts and relationships.
Programmed Instruction Written sequential presentation of learning steps requiring that learners answer questions and that teachers tell them whether their answers are right or wrong	Instruction is primarily verbal, but teacher may use pictures or diagrams. Method requires active learning, giving immediate feedback, correcting wrong answers, and reinforcing right answers. Learner works at own pace.
Computer Resources *Computer Programs* Programmed instruction format in which computers store response patterns for learners and select further lessons based on these patterns (programs can be individualized)	Method requires reading comprehension, psychomotor skills, and familiarity with computer.
Internet Resources Provides access to instructional resources that might not be available locally and that may be interactive, including demonstrations, video clips, self-directed modules, and web-based learning	Method requires access to the Internet, psychomotor skills, and familiarity with computers.
Audiovisual Materials *Diagrams* Illustrations that show interrelationships by means of lines and symbols	Method demonstrates key ideas and summarizes and clarifies key concept.
Graphs (Bar, Circle, or Line) Visual presentations of numerical data	Graphs help learner to grasp information quickly about single concept.
Charts Highly condensed visual summaries of ideas and facts that may highlight series of ideas, steps, or events	Charts demonstrate relationship of several ideas or concepts. Method helps learners know what to do.
Pictures Photographs or drawings used to teach concepts in which the third dimension of shape and space is not important	Photographs are more desirable than diagrams because they more accurately portray the details of the real item. Drawings are pertinent for removing the superfluous detail present in real objects.
Physical Objects Use of actual equipment, objects, models, or simulation to teach concepts or skills	Models are useful when real objects are too small, large, or complicated or unavailable. Learners can manipulate objects that are to be used later in skill development.
Other Audiovisual Materials, Technology Slides, audiotapes, television, and DVDs used with printed material or discussion Social media, websites, electronic games, self-directed modules, blogs, discussion groups	Materials are useful for patients with reading comprehension problems and visual deficits. Allows patient to work at their own speed.

- Explaining the rationale for each step
- Allowing the patient to observe each step, and
- Providing the patient with the opportunity to handle equipment and practise the procedure under supervision.

The patient demonstrates the procedure to ensure that learning has occurred. The demonstration should occur under the same conditions that will be experienced at home or in the place where the procedure is to be performed. For example, for a patient learning to walk with crutches, the nurse needs to simulate the home environment. If short, narrow steps lead to the patient's bedroom, the patient should learn to climb similar stairs in the hospital.

Analogies. Learning occurs when a teacher translates complex language or ideas into words or concepts that the patient understands.

Analogies aid learning by supplementing verbal instruction with familiar images that make complex information simpler and understandable. For example, to explain arterial blood pressure, an analogy is the flow of water through a hose. To use analogies, follow these general principles:

- Be familiar with the concept.
- Know the patient's background, experience, and culture.
- Keep the analogy simple and clear.

Role Playing. Role playing can be used to teach new ideas and attitudes. During role play, patients play themselves or someone else and rehearse a desired behaviour. For example, you can teach a parent to respond to a child's behaviour by pretending to be a child having a temper tantrum. This role playing provides the parent with the opportunity to practise responding in this situation. You then evaluate the parent's response and determine whether an alternative approach would be more appropriate. Role playing helps patients learn skills and feel confident in their ability to perform them independently.

Simulation. Simulation can be used to teach problem solving, application, and independent thinking. During individual or group discussion, a nurse poses a problem or situation for patients to solve. For example, patients with heart disease are asked to plan a low-fat meal. The nurse will then ask the patients to present their diet, providing an opportunity to identify mistakes and reinforce correct information.

Paying Attention to Learning Barriers. Many situations or conditions present a barrier to learning. For example, the patient may have a low reading level (functionally illiterate), a learning disability, a sensory alteration, or depression; may be suffering the effects of prescribed medications or adjusting to life changes or transitions; or may have a poor memory. Patients understand fewer medical words than health care providers predict. Unfortunately, health care providers often use medical terminology and jargon, which prevents patients from understanding the written health information they are given. Nurses should pay special attention to the learning needs of patients who have reading problems, learning disabilities, sensory alterations, or difficulty understanding English or French.

Illiteracy and Learning Disabilities. A recent survey on literacy rates in Canada indicated that about 12.6% of Canadian adults fall within the lowest level of literacy. These people have only rudimentary reading and writing skills; for example, they are not able to read and understand a label on a medicine container. An additional 31.7% of Canadians may read only material that is simple and familiar (Conference Board of Canada, 2022). Therefore, a substantial number of Canadians have problems with reading materials encountered in everyday life. To compound this problem, the readability of printed material ranges from elementary school level to college level. Researchers have found that printed educational material is consistently written above most patients' reading level (Szmuda et al., 2020). Health care providers need to screen materials for readability and clarity.

Some people have learning disabilities, which are disorders that may impair the ability to acquire, organize, remember, understand, or apply information (Learning Disabilities Association of Canada, 2021). The ability to learn or use oral or written language, mathematics, or both may be poor. Teaching strategies need to be adapted to accommodate the learning needs of patients with a learning disability. For example, patients with attention-deficit/hyperactivity disorder (ADHD) may have difficulty recalling information and staying focused during educational sessions; they may also have a low threshold of frustration (Bastable, 2019). Teaching activities should be kept short and delivered in an environment with minimal competing stimuli.

Health Literacy. Health literacy refers to a patient's ability to find, access, read, and understand reliable health information and to use that information to make informed decisions about their health. Many patients have difficulty accessing and understanding health information (Parker & Ratzan, 2019; Simpson et al., 2020). Important aspects of health literacy are the ability to identify, access, and use reliable information. Patients no longer receive health information solely from their health care providers. They are bombarded with health-related advertisements and may seek information on the Internet and social media, some of which is incomplete or inaccurate. They can be either well informed about their health or misinformed about their health, depending on their health literacy. Patient information needs to be presented clearly, avoiding medical terminology, jargon, and acronyms that the patient may not be familiar with.

Sensory Alteration and Other Barriers. Some patients, including many older persons, have sensory deficits (see Chapter 48). Sensory changes such as visual and hearing deficits necessitate teaching methods that enhance functioning. For example, you need to face a patient with hearing problems and speak in a low tone of voice during discussions (lower tones are easier to hear than higher tones). Clearly written materials should be provided. Patients with visual problems can benefit from large-print materials. Patients with slower cognitive function and reduced short-term memory (as in some older persons and patients who have had strokes) learn and remember effectively if the learning is paced properly and the material is relevant to the learner's needs and abilities.

Language. The diverse backgrounds of Canadians can challenge nurses to provide culturally safe care (see Chapters 11 and 12 for further information about cultural safety). Patients may not understand instructions that are not in their native language (see Chapters 11 and 18 for further information about communication). As a nurse, you need to ascertain a patient's fluency in English or French before you choose teaching methods or tools. If possible, instruction should be done collaboratively with an interpreter (Gil-Salmerón et al., 2019).

Cultural Diversity. Nurses need to have knowledge of patients' cultural background, values, and beliefs (see Chapters 11 and 12 for further information about cultural diversity), as well as the patient's ability to understand both verbal and written material (Gil-Salmerón et al., 2019). When educating patients from cultural groups different from your own, you need to be aware of the distinctive aspects of their cultures and develop teaching strategies that are respectful of cultural beliefs, values, and behaviours.

Needs of Patients With Severe Illness. Adapting to serious illness or disability is difficult for most people. Often, people need to grieve the resulting losses. The grieving process gives them time to adapt psychologically to the emotional and physical implications of illness. People experience grief (see Chapter 26) at different rates and in different sequences, depending on their self-concept before illness, the severity of the illness, and the changes and losses caused by the illness. Sensitivity is required to educate patients while they are grieving and adjusting to their illness.

Readiness to learn is related to the grieving stage (Table 21.3). Patients cannot learn when they are unwilling or unable to accept the reality of illness. However, properly timed teaching can help a patient to adjust to illness or disability. The nurse can identify the patient's stage of grieving based on the patient's behaviours. When the patient enters the stage of acceptance—the stage compatible with learning—the nurse can then introduce a teaching plan. Continuous assessment of the patient's behaviours is used to determine the stages of grieving.

◆ Evaluation

Patient education is not complete until outcomes of the teaching–learning process have been evaluated (see Box 21.7). Nurses need to determine whether patients have learned the material. Evaluation reinforces correct behaviour, helps learners realize how they should change incorrect behaviour, and helps the nurse determine the adequacy of the teaching (Bastable, 2019). Success depends on the patient's ability to meet the established outcome and goals, and these in turn are used by the nurse to evaluate success. The following checklist helps to evaluate patient education:

- Were educational goals set mutually between the nurse and the patient?
- Were the patient's goals or outcomes realistic and observable?
- Is the patient able to demonstrate the behaviour or skill on multiple occasions?
- How well is the patient able to answer questions about the topic?

TABLE 21.3	Relationship Between Learning and Psychosocial Adaptation to Illness		
Stage	**Patient's Behaviour**	**Nursing Activities**	**Rationale**
Denial or disbelief	Patient avoids discussion of illness ("Nothing is wrong with me"), withdraws from others, and disregards physical restrictions. Patient suppresses and distorts information that has not been presented clearly.	Provide support, empathy, and careful explanations of all procedures while they are being done. Let patient know you are available for conversation. Explain situation to family or significant other if appropriate. Teach in present tense (e.g., explain what patient needs to know to be discharged).	Patient is not prepared to deal with problem; attempts to teach patient will result in further anger or withdrawal. Provide only information that patient pursues or requires.
Anger	Patient blames and complains and often directs anger toward nurse or others.	Do not argue with patient but listen to concerns. Teach in present tense. Reassure family of the normality of patient's behaviour.	Patient needs opportunity to express feelings and anger. Patient is still not prepared to face future.
Bargaining	Patient offers to live better life in exchange for promise of better health (e.g., "If God lets me live, I promise to manage my disease better").	Continue to introduce only reality and teaching in present tense.	Patient is still unwilling to accept limitations.
Resolution	Patient begins to express emotions openly, realizes that illness has created changes, and begins to ask questions.	Encourage expression of feelings. Begin to share information needed for future, and set aside formal times for discussion.	Patient begins to perceive need for assistance and is ready to accept responsibility for learning.
Acceptance	Patient recognizes reality of condition, actively pursues information, and strives for independence.	Focus on future skills and knowledge required. Continue to teach in present tense. Involve family in planning and teaching for discharge.	Patient is more easily motivated to learn. Acceptance of illness reflects willingness to deal with its implications.

- Does the patient continue to have difficulty in understanding the information or performing a skill? If so, what changes in interventions should be made to enhance skill attainment?

Measurement Methods. Under direct observation, the patient should demonstrate the behaviours described in the learning objectives. If the evaluation process indicates a deficit in knowledge or skill, the nurse must repeat or modify the teaching plan. By watching patients demonstrate behaviours, nurses can see whether correct techniques are being used. However, a patient may behave differently later. Therefore, observation works best in real-life situations.

Oral and written questioning are other useful evaluation methods. Questions are best used for behaviours that are not easily demonstrated. The nurse should phrase questions to ensure that the learner understands them and that objectives are truly measured.

Another form of evaluation includes self-reports (oral and written) and self-monitoring (written). An example is a patient's written log of the foods eaten in a specific time frame, in comparison with a new diet. Nurses rely on patients' honesty and memory in self-reporting.

Patient Expectations. Evaluations of nursing care and teaching sessions help determine whether a patient's needs and expectations have been met. At the end of the session, the nurse asks the patient whether they have questions; in this way, the nurse can identify information that was missing and should have been covered. Patients may also fill out written evaluations of a teaching session or course. Anonymous written evaluations may be more truthful than face-to-face evaluations.

Evaluation may reveal new learning needs or new factors that are interfering with learning, in which case the nurse should try alternative teaching methods. When a patient has difficulty in an acute care setting, the nurse may make a referral to resources, such as care in the community or an outpatient clinic, for further education and evaluation.

Documentation. Because patient teaching often occurs informally, it is difficult to document it consistently. Nurses are legally responsible for providing accurate, timely information that promotes continuity of care; therefore, it is essential to document the outcomes of teaching. The following aspects of patient education should be documented (see Chapter 16):

- *Assessment data and reassessment of learning needs.* Such data and evaluation provide important information for when the teaching plan is developed.
- *Nursing analysis, patient needs, and educational priorities.* These provide support for goals and outcomes that are established.
- *Interventions planned.* A specific plan, including the methods to be used in instruction, enhances continuity of care. When planned interventions are provided, the nurse can determine what information needs to be provided to the patient.
- *Interventions provided.* Specifically describing the subject matter enables other nurses to follow up and reinforce teaching (e.g., "Explained side effects of Inderal" or "Demonstrated umbilical cord care"). Note the date, time, and specific patient or patients taught. Avoid generalizations (e.g., "medications taught"). Resources used, such as pamphlets or audiovisual materials, are documented in the patient's record.
- *Patient's response and outcomes of care.* In documenting evidence of learning (e.g., a return demonstration or the ability to verbalize the purpose and adverse effects of a medication), the nurse is informing staff about the patient's progress and identifying information that must still be taught.
- *Ability of patient, family, or both to manage needs after discharge.* An evaluation of remaining educational needs on discharge helps with identifying the need for outpatient or home health care follow-up. If referrals are appropriate, the patient, family, or both are often able to meet their needs.

KEY CONCEPTS

- The nurse ensures that patients, families, and communities receive information needed to maintain optimal health.
- Health education is aimed at the promotion, restoration, and maintenance of health.
- Teaching is most effective when it is responsive to the learner's needs.
- Teaching is a form of interpersonal communication, with the teacher and student actively involved in a process that increases the student's knowledge and skills.
- The ability to learn depends on a person's physical and cognitive attributes.
- The ability to attend to the learning process depends on physical comfort and anxiety levels and on the presence of environmental distraction.
- A person's health beliefs influence the willingness to gain knowledge and skills necessary to maintain health.
- Teaching must be timed to coincide with the patient's readiness to learn.

- Teaching strategies need to be tailored to a patient's age and developmental capabilities.
- The patient should be an active participant in a teaching plan: agreeing to the plan, helping choose instructional methods, and recommending times for instruction.
- Learning objectives describe what a person is to learn in behavioural terms.
- A combination of teaching methods improves the learner's attentiveness and involvement.
- A teacher is more effective when presenting information that builds on a learner's existing knowledge.
- Nurses should assess which learning materials, methods, and approaches will be most effective for each patient based on their individual abilities and challenges.
- A nurse evaluates a patient's learning by observing performance of expected learning behaviours under desired conditions.
- Effective documentation describes the entire process of patient education, promotes continuity of care, and demonstrates that educational standards have been met.

CRITICAL THINKING EXERCISES

1. Rupinder (pronouns: she/her), the community health nurse, meets with John (pronouns: he/him) to talk about COVID-19 immunization. John has just become eligible to receive the vaccine. Several of his friends have indicated to Rupinder that they have made appointments to get the vaccine and are encouraging him to do the same. John has heard that the vaccine he is eligible for is 70% effective and that blood clots sometimes occur following vaccination. He wants to learn more about the effectiveness and side effects of the vaccine. What should Rupinder's priorities be for patient education? What strategies might she use, and why?

2. You have been asked to train pharmacy technicians who have never administered COVID-19 vaccines. How would you proceed in developing a teaching module?
3. You have been asked by a business to speak to a community group using ZOOM™ about the importance of public health measures to prevent the spread of COVID-19. The employer has indicated that several employees have expressed the belief that COVID-19 is no worse than the common flu and that these public health measures are political. What will you do to prepare for the speaking session?

Answers to Critical Thinking Exercises appear on the Evolve website.

REVIEW QUESTIONS

Review Questions 1 to 12 relate to the case study at the beginning of the chapter.

1. One of Susie's patients must learn to use a face mask properly. Acquisition of this skill will require learning in which domain?
   a. Cognitive
   b. Affective
   c. Psychomotor
   d. Attentional
2. Susie is planning to teach a patient in the community who tested positive for COVID-19 about the importance of following isolation protocols. What is the best time for teaching to occur?
   a. When the patient is in the waiting room of the clinic
   b. When the patient indicates that they are symptom free
   c. Just as the patient is preparing to leave and getting their belongings together
   d. When the patient is talking about current stressors in their life
3. A patient who is newly recovered from COVID-19 is preparing to go home. The patient is avoiding discussion of their illness and discharge orders. In teaching the patient about discharge instructions, the nurse should:
   a. Teach the patient's spouse
   b. Focus on knowledge the patient will need in a few weeks
   c. Provide only the information the patient needs to go home
   d. Convince the patient that learning about her health is necessary

4. Susie is about to teach a Grade 12 health class about infectious disease. To achieve the best learning outcomes, she should do which of the following? *(Select all that apply.)*
   a. Provide information by using a lecture.
   b. Use simple words to promote understanding.
   c. Complete an extensive literature search focusing on COVID-19.
   d. Develop topics that include activities and problem solving.
   e. Explore with students their understanding of infectious disease to determine educational needs.
5. Susie is organizing an illness prevention program for a specific cultural group. To effectively meet the needs of this group, Susie will do which of the following? *(Select all that apply.)*
   a. Assess the needs of the community in general.
   b. Involve those affected by the problem in the planning process.
   c. Use educational materials that are simplified and have many pictures.
   d. Assess commonly held health beliefs among the cultural group.
   e. Educate the group about the Western concepts of health and illness.
   f. Include cultural practices that are relevant to this community.
6. A patient who is having severe respiratory distress is about to be intubated. Which of the following is the most appropriate teaching approach in this situation?
   a. Telling
   b. Selling
   c. Entrusting
   d. Participating

7. Susie is teaching a group of public service employees about strategies to deal with members of the public who are resistant to following COVID-19 precautions. They are asked to respond to several scenarios. This is an example of:
   a. A simulation
   b. An analogy
   c. Role playing
   d. A demonstration

8. A patient with a learning disability is asking Susie about COVID-19 vaccination. In teaching the patient about vaccination, the nurse should do which of the following? *(Select all that apply.)*
   a. Encourage the patient to ask questions.
   b. Provide written material only.
   c. Present the information several times.
   d. Expect the patient to understand the information quickly.

9. Susie has been discussing with a patient the use of social media as a source of information about infectious disease. Susie knows that the patient understands the issues surrounding social media as an information source when the following occurs:
   a. The patient indicates that they will rely on the most popular sites for their information.
   b. The patient indicates that they will verify information from social media with official health information sites.
   c. The patient indicates that they use sites recommended by their friends.
   d. The patient indicates that they are not sure how to evaluate sites for validity of the information provided.

10. A volunteer has just been hired to do COVID-19 screening at a pop-up screening site. They need to learn how to take nasal swabs.

Which of the following would be the best teaching method(s) for this volunteer? *(Select all that apply.)*
   a. Demonstration
   b. Group instruction
   c. One-on-one discussion
   d. Simulation
   e. Step-by-step instructional video

11. Susie is teaching a patient who is required to self-isolate for 14 days in accordance with public health protocols for COVID-19. Susie knows they understand self-isolation when they acknowledge the following: *(Select all that apply.)*
   a. They must not leave their home for 14 days.
   b. One family member can visit at a time.
   c. Food and other items can be delivered to their home if the patient and delivery person wear masks and maintain physical distancing recommendations.
   d. They can go shopping as long as they wear a face mask and practise physical distancing measures.

12. Susie is teaching a group of nurse educators about the different levels of public health infectious disease protocols and how to determine what they should do in various situations. This type of activity addresses learning in the cognitive domain at the level of _____.

Answers: 1. c; **2.** b; **3.** c; **4.** d; **5.** b; **6.** a; **7.** a; **8.** a, c; **9.** b; **10.** a, d, e; **11.** a, c; **12.** Application.

🌐 *Rationales for the Review Questions appear on the Evolve website.*

RECOMMENDED WEBSITES

Canadian Public Health Association: https://www.cpha.ca
This website provides both national and international information and resources on public health issues and services.

Health Canada: https://www.hc-sc.gc.ca
The Health Canada website provides resources to the public about a variety of health issues and topics about maintaining and improving health.

National Institutes of Health: https://health.nih.gov
The National Institutes of Health in the United States provides resources about enhancing health, living longer, and reducing illness and disability.

Public Health Agency of Canada (PHAC): https://www.canada.ca/en/public-health.html
This website provides information and resources on a variety of public health issues and topics, including health promotion, healthy living, diseases, and injury prevention.

Registered Nurses' Association of Ontario (RNAO): https://rnao.ca/bpg/guidelines/facilating-client-centred-learning
This website provides RNAO Best Practice Guidelines and other resources related to patient education.

🌐 REFERENCES

A full reference list is available on the website for this book at http://evolve.elsevier.com/Canada/Potter/fundamentals/

22

Developmental Theories

Canadian content written by Nicole Letourneau, RN, PhD, FCAHS, FCAN, FAAN, with original chapter contributions by Tara Hulsey, BSN, MSN, PhD

OBJECTIVES

Mastery of content in this chapter will enable you to:

- Define the key terms listed.
- Identify basic principles of growth and development.
- Describe factors influencing growth and development.
- Identify five major traditions that underlie modern developmental theories.

- Name and describe the major developmental theories associated with each tradition.
- Describe and compare the mechanisms that underlie the major developmental theories.
- Identify nursing implications associated with the application of developmental principles to patient care.

KEY TERMS

Accommodation
Adverse childhood experiences (ACEs)
Ainsworth's operationalization of attachment theory
Assimilation
Attachment
Autonomous stage
Biophysical developmental theories
Bowlby's attachment and separation theory
Bronfenbrenner's bioecological theory
Cognitive developmental theories
Contextual tradition
Conventional stage
Developmental health
Dialectical tradition
Differentiation
Disorganized attachment
Dynamic maturational model of attachment
Ego

Epigenesis
Epigenetics
Erikson's theory of eight stages of life
Exosystem
Freud's psychoanalytic model of personality development
Gilligan's theory of moral development
Havighurst's developmental tasks
Id
Individuation
Insecure and disorganized parent-infant attachment
Kohlberg's theory of moral development
Libido
Lifespan developmental perspectives
Macrosystem
Maturation
Mechanisms of development
Mechanistic tradition

Mesosystem
Microsystem
Moral developmental theories
Organicism
Parent–child interaction quality
Piaget's theory of cognitive development
Piaget's theory of moral development
Population health approach
Premoral stage
Protective processes
Psychoanalytic and psychosocial tradition
Resilience
Secure parent-infant attachment
Separation
Superego
Temperament
Vulnerability processes
Zone of proximal development

WEBSITE

http://evolve.elsevier.com/Canada/Potter/fundamentals/

CASE STUDY

You are a nurse practitioner working in an interprofessional primary care setting in a large urban centre. Your responsibility is to manage the care of expectant new mothers. Today, you have your monthly appointment with Pritma (preferred pronouns: she/her), a married 23-year-old who is expecting her first child. Having learned a little of Pritma's past since she began her prenatal visits with you 4 months ago, you have grown to respect her sense of duty, intelligence, and tenacity.

Seven years ago, a 16-year-old Pritma immigrated to Canada with her parents and four younger siblings. Her parents went on to have two more children after arriving in Canada. Her siblings now range in age from 4 to 18 years. Prior to immigration, her family spent months in an immigrant camp before finally finding refuge in Canada, far away from the political upheaval in their home country. As the oldest child who could also speak English (thanks to tutoring in the camp), much family responsibility fell to Pritma. She managed to finish high school and then studied information technology (IT) at community college, all the while working to support her family. Her parents struggled to find and maintain employment in Canada owing to their limited proficiency in both English and French. However, at community college, Pritma met her sweetheart, Ahmed (preferred pronouns: he/him). Pritma's Muslim family welcomed Ahmed, and the two married right after graduation. Pritma and Ahmed started their own IT business and shortly after that, Pritma found out she was pregnant.

Today, however, at 7 months pregnant, Pritma does not seem like herself. She has dark circles under her eyes and seems listless as she completes the usual weighing and measuring. Normally careful about her appearance, today Pritma's hair is dishevelled and looks like it has been unwashed for several days. She is wearing a stretchy track suit instead of her usual business maternity wear. Her usual excited chatter about the baby is also subdued. You ask her how she is doing, and she says "fine" and smiles with a tired expression. You also wonder where Ahmed is, because he is usually hovering around Pritma, ensuring her comfort and treating her with such kindness. With growing concern, you examine her measurements to discover she has not gained weight this month. But, you note gratefully, her fundal height is appropriate, the fetal heart rate is

strong, and her urine glucose is normal. Before you begin to discuss your findings with Pritma as usual, you ask her to complete one more test—the Edinburgh Depression Scale (Bergink et al., 2011)—only to find that Pritma scores 14, indicating that she is likely depressed.

As you share your findings with Pritma, you focus in on her lack of weight gain and her depression score. Pritma tells you that her family has had to rely on her more than usual this month because her father has been out of work. To help make ends meet, she and Ahmed have been taking on extra business, working 60 to 70 hours or more per week. She has often missed meals and needed rest due to overwork. "That's where Ahmed is now," she says, "at home, working to catch up. We don't even have time to decorate the baby's room. But who else can help my brothers and sisters?"

Her voice trails off as she sniffles and wipes at the tears that begin to flow. With some additional prodding, it becomes clear that the stress of taking on extra work to help support her parents and siblings is taking its toll on Pritma and her growing fetus.

Think about this case study as you read this chapter. There are Review Questions at the end of the chapter about this case study.

All people progress through phases of growth and development, from the simple to the complex, at a highly individualized rate. Understanding typical growth and development helps nurses to predict, prevent, and detect any changes from patients' expected patterns and to develop approaches and programs that can further enhance the developmental well-being of individuals (Berk, 2018; Bukatko, 2012). Theories from the natural and biomedical sciences, as well as the behavioural and social sciences, help to explain the influence of early childhood experiences on lifespan development. Drawing on these theories enables nurses to care for their patients and provides a foundation from which nurses can advocate for appropriate developmental care for vulnerable children, adults, caregivers, and families (Canadian Association of Schools of Nursing [CASN], 2022).

Knowledge of human developmental processes is crucial to optimal nursing education (CASN, 2022), as it helps nurses to assess and treat a patient's response to an illness and plan appropriate individualized care. Historically, growth and development have been described as orderly, predictable processes that begin with conception and continue until death. However, this view is increasingly recognized as overlooking differences in gender, sexuality, culture, life experiences that influence development, and lifespan perspectives (Baltes, 1987; Green & Piel, 2016). Today, it is no longer assumed that all people progress linearly through universal phases of growth and development. Human growth and development are understood as processes in which sociocultural, biological, and psychological forces interact with the individual over time (Berk, 2018), and lifespan approaches (lifespan developmental perspectives) consider development from conception to old age (Baltes et al., 2007). As a result, theorists have shifted their focus from describing growth and development to explaining it: How do humans develop? What are the mechanisms, or explanatory components, that underlie human growth and development?

In this chapter, five broad traditions of human development are introduced, and the mechanisms of development espoused by key theorists are outlined. Examples are offered to analyze the implications for the nursing process that follow from these mechanisms (see Chapters 23, 24, and 25 for further information about human development).

GROWTH AND DEVELOPMENT

Growth and development are synchronous processes that are interdependent in the healthy individual. Growth and development depend on a sequence of endocrine, genetic, constitutional, environmental, and nutritional influences (Dames et al., 2021).

Physical Growth

Growth is the quantitative, or measurable, aspect of an individual's increase in physical measurements. Measurable growth indicators include changes in height, weight, teeth, skeletal structures, and sexual characteristics. For example, children generally double their birth weight by 5 months of age and their birth height by 36 months. Physical growth is not only genetically determined; it is also affected by other contextual factors such as socioeconomic status.

Development

Development is a progressive and continuous process of change leading to increased skill and capacity to function. Development is the result of complex interactions between biological and environmental influences (Green & Piel, 2016). These changes are qualitative in nature and difficult to measure in exact units. Developmental changes have certain predictable characteristics: they proceed from simple to complex, from general to specific, from head to toe (cephalocaudal), and from trunk to extremities (proximodistal). For example, a child's progressions from rolling over to crawling to walking are developmental changes.

Factors Influencing Growth and Development

Three major categories of factors influence human growth and development: (1) genetic or natural forces within the person, (2) the environment in which the person lives, and (3) the interaction that takes place between these two groups of factors (Table 22.1). Nurses apply their knowledge of these factors when selecting approaches to promote typical growth and developmental progression. For example, as part of planning for a patient's pregnancy, nurses need to consider the patient's genetic endowment, age, socioeconomic status, culture (Box 22.1), available support system, and preconception health.

TRADITIONS OF DEVELOPMENTAL THEORIES

A theory is an organized, often observable, logical set of statements about a subject. Human developmental theories are models intended to account for how and why people develop as they do (Green & Piel, 2016). All theories of development discussed in this chapter make

TABLE 22.1	Major Factors That Influence Growth and Development
Categories	**Implications**
Genetic or Natural Factors	
Heredity	Genetic endowment determines sex, skin, hair, and eye colour, physical growth, stature, and, to some extent, psychological uniqueness.
Temperament	Temperament is the characteristic psychological disposition with which the child is born, typically ranging from difficult to flexible. It influences interactions between an individual and the environment.
Environmental Factors	
Family	The purpose of family is to protect, teach, and nurture its members.
	The functions of family include means for survival, security, promotion of healthy emotional and social development, assistance with maintenance of relationships, instruction about society and the world, and assistance in learning roles and behaviours.
	Family influences values, beliefs, customs, and specific patterns of interaction and communication.
Peer group	The peer group provides a new and different learning environment from the that of the family, with different patterns and structures of interaction and communication, necessitating a different style of behaviour.
	The functions of the peer group include allowing the individual to learn about success and failure; to validate and challenge thoughts, feelings, and concepts; to receive acceptance, support, and rejection as a unique person apart from family; and to achieve group purposes by meeting demands, pressures, and expectations.
Health environment	The level of health affects an individual's responsiveness to the environment and responsiveness of others to the individual.
	It determines availability and accessibility of resources to support health.
Nutrition	Growth is regulated by dietary factors.
	Adequacy of nutrients influences whether and how physiological needs, as well as subsequent growth and development needs, are met.
	The availability of quality nutrients also affects growth.
Rest, sleep, and exercise	Balance between rest, sleep, and exercise is essential for rejuvenating the body; disturbances diminish growth, while equilibrium reinforces physiological and psychological health.
Living environment	Factors affecting growth and development include season, climate, community life, socioeconomic status, quality of the physical environment (e.g., air, water, land) and the presence or absence of ACEs (e.g., abuse, neglect, low income).
	An embryo may be exposed to teratogenic substances (e.g., alcohol, chemicals, or radiation) that cause abnormal development.
	An embryo may also be exposed to the biological substrate of maternal distress that can affect development.
Political and policy environment	Municipal, provincial, and federal policies directly affect the health and well-being of individuals, families, and communities.
Interacting Factors	
Life experiences	Individuals develop by applying what has been learned through experience to their current situation.
	Experiences emerge from both biological and environmental sources.
	The individual deduces meaning from these experiences and bases further actions on them.
	ACEs (e.g., abuse, neglect, low income) are linked to a host of poor health and developmental outcomes.
	The epigenome—genetic expression—changes in response to experience.
Prenatal health	Biological and maturational factors (genetics; maternal age; medical problems) and environmental factors (maternal health; stress and distress; nutrition; use of tobacco, drugs, and alcohol; use of prenatal services) together affect fetal growth and development.
State of health	Health is a product of both intrinsic (biology) and extrinsic (quality of environment, availability of resources for health) factors.
	Changes to health status such as illness or injury may cause inability to cope with and respond to underlying processes and demands of development.

ACEs, Adverse childhood experiences.

different contributions to our understanding of the developmental process.

To help you understand the various developmental theories, this chapter has been grouped into five traditions of (or ways of thinking about) human growth and development: organicism, psychoanalytic and psychosocial, mechanistic, contextualism, and dialectical (see Chapters 21 and 29 for further information about learning and spiritual development, respectively).

Each tradition of developmental theory emphasizes different underlying developmental mechanisms. **Mechanisms of development** are the explanatory components of each theory, or the means by which developmental tasks are achieved. They underlie the developmental process within each theory and enable developmental progression.

These underlying mechanisms are proposed to be universal and to function across the lifespan (not just in childhood) and cultures. Although developmental theories are often presented within a framework of stage-like progressions, what the stages actually represent are the outcomes produced by these mechanisms at each specific age.

ORGANICISM

Organicism refers to a theoretical focus on the organism itself. According to theories in this tradition, development is the result of biologically driven behaviour and the person's adaptation to the environment. Biophysical and cognitive–moral theories of development are included in this tradition.

BOX 22.1 CULTURAL ASPECTS OF CARE

Indigenous Peoples

Nurses need to assess the cultural background of each patient and be prepared to change their practice so that it is congruent with the patient's beliefs and values concerning growth and development. For example, within many Indigenous cultures, the concept of a circle or cycle is a fundamental theme and can be applied to human development and health issues (Douglas, 2013; Greenwood et al., 2018). The human life cycle is symbolized by the Medicine Wheel, which is often depicted as a circle with four equal-sized sections (see Chapter 12). The four sections are linked to the stages of life (birth, youth, adulthood, death), the four aspects of human life (spiritual, emotional, intellectual, physical), or even the four seasons. Its basic symbolism represents a holistic relationship between health, community, and the natural world (plants, animals, and humans) over time (Douglas, 2013). All aspects of human development are viewed as being in harmony with the cycle of life in nature. As in nature, each part of the cycle needs to be balanced with the other parts. Roles and expectations related to developmental age reflect traditional values of respect, honour, balance, and harmony.

Biophysical Developmental Theories

Biophysical developmental theories describe and explain how the physical body grows and changes. The changes that occur as a person grows from fetus, to neonate, to child, to adolescent, and finally to adult can be quantified and compared against established norms; however, regional and cultural differences may exist, as may differences related to the availability of resources in the environment for adequate growth.

How does the physical body age? What are the triggers that change the body's physical characteristics from childhood through adolescence to adulthood? Biological influences on development include many factors, such as genetics and exposure to teratogens (e.g., maternal diseases, drugs, X-rays, or other hazardous substances that interfere with the normal development of the fetus). All biophysical developmental theories give some credence to the roles of nature (genetics) and nurture (caregiving environment and resources). However, the theories differ in how much influence individual and environmental forces have on development.

Gesell's Theory of Maturational Development.
Arnold Gesell (1880–1961) was a psychologist who obtained his medical degree to help him explain the physiological processes he observed in the behaviour of children. Through extensive observations in the 1940s, he developed behavioural norms that today serve as a primary source of information for childhood development.

Fundamental to Gesell's theory of development is the notion that the pattern of growth and development is directed by the activity of genes, although the genetic mechanism was unknown to him at that time. Gesell believed that environmental factors could support, change, and modify the pattern but did not generate the progressions of development (Gesell, 1948). He proposed that the pattern of maturation follows a fixed developmental sequence in all humans and that critical periods exist in which the presence or absence of particular experiences makes a biological system functional or nonfunctional (Weizmann & Harris, 2012). Gesell based some of his observations on the visual system (Gesell et al., 1949). He noted that visual defects not identified until the start of school may be associated with underdeveloped brain pathways that impair long-term vision. New research on child neglect shows a similar pattern: if a child is neglected physically and emotionally early in life, their brain development is affected, with long-term reductions in brain volume observed in neglected children compared with that in non-neglected peers (National Scientific Council on the Developing Child, 2012; Nelson & Gabard-Durnam, 2020).

While Gesell pointed out that the environment does play a part in the development of the child, it does not have any part in the sequence of development. Researchers continue to use Gesell's theories today, probing for gene–environment interactions that affect human development, especially behaviour and mental health (Assary et al., 2020; Letourneau et al., 2019).

Mechanisms of Maturational Development. **Maturation** is the biological internal regulatory mechanism that governs the emergence of all new skills and abilities that appear with advancing age (Beckett & Taylor, 2019). Maturation involves an individual's biological ability, physiological condition, and desire to learn more mature behaviour. To mature, the individual may have to relinquish previous behaviour and learning, integrate new patterns into existing behaviour, or both. Maturation influences the sequence and timing of the changes associated with growth and development. For example, the child relinquishes crawling for walking because walking permits greater investigation of the environment and more learning. However, the child cannot walk until the biological ability and structures to perform the action (i.e., increased muscle cells and tone) have developed.

Differentiation is the process by which cells and structures become modified and refine their characteristics. Development of activities and functions progresses from simple to complex. Embryonic cells begin as vague and undifferentiated and develop into complex, highly diversified cells, tissues, and organs.

Nursing Implications of Maturational Development. As a nurse working with expectant parents, you must consider the sequential development of the fetus and critical periods when you counsel expectant birth parents about prenatal nutrition, environmental teratogens, and protecting their mental health. You need to consider maturational development in your care planning when you help parents or caregivers sequence child play activities appropriate for learning to sit, roll, creep, crawl, and walk. One way to support development during critical periods is to develop or implement evidence-informed early intervention programs for expectant and new parents.

Chess and Thomas's Theory of Temperament Development.
Temperament is a physical and emotional response style that affects a child's interactions with others (Hockenberry & Wilson, 2021). It is the way a person adjusts to life experiences, and it is thought to originate from the person's genetic makeup. A child's temperament influences how others respond to the child and to their needs. Knowledge of temperament helps parents to have a clearer perspective on their child, and enables health care providers to guide parents appropriately (Hockenberry & Wilson, 2021).

Psychiatrists Stella Chess (1914–2007) and Alexander Thomas (1915–2003) conducted a landmark 20-year longitudinal study of development that included children from a range of populations, including children of middle-income parents and intellectually disabled children of lower-income parents. The breadth of the data allowed them to look at people's behaviour from childhood to early adulthood as they interacted with their environment. Their work defined the concept of temperament (Chess & Thomas, 1995), and they proposed that temperament is biologically derived.

Chess and Thomas (1995) described three common categories of temperament, although because of individual variation, approximately 30% of children cannot be classified in any of these groups:

- The *easy child* is easygoing and even-tempered, regular, and predictable in their habits, as well as open-minded, flexible, and adaptable to change. Mood expressions are mild to moderately intense and typically positive.

- The *difficult child* is highly active, irritable, and irregular in habits. Negativity in interactions and withdrawal from other people is typical, and the child requires a highly structured environment. They adapt slowly to new routines, new people, and new situations. Mood expressions are usually intense and primarily negative.
- The *slow-to-warm-up child* typically reacts negatively and with mild intensity to new stimuli. They adapt slowly with repeated contact unless pressured, and respond with mild but passive resistance to novelty or changes in routine.

Mechanisms of Temperament Development. According to temperament theory, biologically derived temperament characteristics drive children's interactions with the environment. Chess and Thomas (1995) proposed that "goodness of fit" between the individual and the immediate environment modulates human development. This assigns significant responsibility for child development outcomes to the family. For instance, the difficult child who has trouble making the transition from one activity or environment to a new one functions best in a family that maintains routines and has a slow, easy attitude toward the introduction of change. The same child in a family that has few routines has much more difficulty moving from one activity (such as play) to the next activity (such as sleep). The first scenario is an example of good fit between the temperament of the child and the family environment. However, recent research has suggested that temperament may be a function of fetal exposures to excessive maternal stress hormones during pregnancy or birth complications, for example (Howland et al., 2020; Takegata et al., 2021).

Nursing Implications of Temperament Development. Nurses can help families identify the unique characteristics of their infants and children. For instance, the Parent–Child Relationship Programs at the University of Washington (Seattle, Washington, USA) offers numerous parenting education programs for nurses and allied health professionals to employ. One such program enables health care providers to become certified to administer the Parent–Child Interaction Teaching Scale (PCITS). The PCITS assesses the qualities of the parent–child relationship linked to children's temperamental characteristics and other health outcomes, such as cognitive and behavioural development (Oxford & Finlay, 2013; see Tryphonopoulos & Letourneau, 2020, for an example of use). This tool was created by pioneering nurse-scientist Kathryn Barnard. Becoming trained to use the PCITS to assess **parent–child interaction quality** requires several days of in-person or online training and passing a test. Once certified, health care providers can use the tool in their practice by videorecording consenting parents as they teach their child a simple age-appropriate task (e.g., shake rattle, stack blocks). Review of the video can reveal many parent and infant behaviours that could explain development or be a focus for intervention. Specifically, the quality of the infant's ability to give clear cues (e.g., smiling, reaching) and respond appropriately to their parent (e.g., soothing when picked up) both underlie temperament and contribute to overall parent–child relationship quality. Currently, many public health nurses in Ontario employ this assessment tool to support parents to engage in sensitive, responsive interactions with their growing infants (Letourneau et al., 2018; McManaman, 2017).

Cognitive Developmental Theories

Cognitive developmental theories focus on reasoning and thinking processes, including the changes in how people perform intellectual operations. These operations are related to the ways people learn to understand the world in which they live. Mental processes, including perceiving, reasoning, remembering, and believing, affect certain types of emotional behaviour. For example, a typical child will have a different emotional reaction to the death of a grandparent than to the death of an older sibling or a parent.

Unlike biophysical developmental theories, cognitive developmental theories emphasize that although the developmental process originates from within the person, it is greatly influenced by interactions between the person and the environment. Therefore, theories of cognitive development emphasize the active role that the individual plays in the developmental process. Cognitive theories are considered to be within the organicism tradition because development is still viewed as originating from within the organism.

Piaget's Theory of Cognitive Development. Jean Piaget (1896–1980), a Swiss biologist and philosopher, studied how people come to know their world. **Piaget's theory of cognitive development** addresses the development of children's intellectual organization and how they think, reason, perceive, and make meaning of the physical world. His theory includes four periods, each of which subsumes several stages (Table 22.2). He recognized that people move through these specific periods at different rates but in the same sequence or order (Piaget, 2000). Piaget also theorized that this would be true in all cultures. He acknowledged that biological maturation plays a role in this developmental theory but believed that rates of development depend on the intellectual stimulation and challenge in the person's environment. Piaget found that children acquire knowledge through acting on the environment. In other words, the individual plays an active role in their own development (Berk 2013; Green & Piel, 2016).

Mechanisms of Cognitive Development. Although it is helpful to be aware of the stages, the importance of Piaget's theory is that development is considered a spontaneous process in which individuals play an active role. Environmental challenges are internalized through the mechanisms of assimilation and accommodation. **Assimilation** is the process of making sense of new information in comparison to what is already known. **Accommodation** is the process of adapting existing ways of thinking to a new experience or new information. Together, these processes reflect adaptation to new information or experience (Feldman, 2019). In a health care situation, a person who has a headache can evaluate it as an everyday or common experience. In this process, the person is assimilating their headache to what they know already as the experience of their body; that is, the person occasionally has headaches. When headaches become extreme or constant, then the person needs to understand the headache pain differently in the experience of their body. For instance, the person may learn to see themselves as someone who has chronic migraines or as a someone with a brain tumour who requires surgery.

The mechanisms of cognitive development apply across the lifespan and to all patient situations. Thus, they also apply to the moral theories and theories of adult development that are described in the following sections.

Nursing Implications of Cognitive Development. Most patients need to know about new ways of adjusting to or behaving with regard to their health. Assimilation and accommodation represent adaptation of the patient to new health challenges. Nurses need to support this process by providing information and support as patients come to terms with new health situations. Nurses must also offer positive feedback when patients successfully adapt to their challenges.

Moral Developmental Theories

Moral developmental theories are a subset of cognitive theories and describe the development of moral reasoning. *Moral reasoning* is how people think about the rules of ethical or moral conduct, but it does not predict what a person would do in each situation. *Moral development* is the ability of an individual to distinguish right from wrong and to develop ethical values on which to base their actions (Berk,

TABLE 22.2 — Piaget's Theory of Cognitive Development

Stage	Description	Nursing Implications
Period 1: Sensorimotor (birth to 2 years of age)	The infant develops the schema or action pattern for dealing with the environment (Berk, 2013; Piaget, 2000). These schemas may include mouthing, looking, vocalizing, grasping, or hitting (Figure 22.1). Schemas become self-initiated activities; for example, the infant who learns that mouthing or sucking achieves a pleasing result generalizes the action to suck fingers, blankets, or clothing. Successful achievement leads to greater exploration. In the second year, children can form primitive mental images as they acquire object permanence. Before this, they do not realize that objects out of sight exist. When a 6-month-old is shown a toy before it is hidden, they will not search for it. At 18 months, the child can understand that even if the object cannot be seen it still exists, so they will search for it.	Educate parents about the need to promote infants' exploration of the environment. Such education supports development of action patterns that help the children achieve motor and cognitive skills. Observe parents during interactions with their infants. Reinforce parents' sensitivity and responsiveness to infant behaviours.
Period 2: Preoperational (2–7 years of age)	Children learn to think with the use of symbols and mental images. Still egocentric, the child sees objects and people from only one point of view: the child's own. Play is the initial method of nonlanguage use of symbols. This is a time of parallel play. Parallel play can be observed as children engage in activities side by side without a common goal. Imitation and make-believe play are ways to represent experience (Berk, 2013; Piaget, 2000). Later, language develops and broadens possibilities for thinking about the past or the future. Children can now communicate about events with others. As the language fits into a logical form, it mirrors the thinking process at the time.	Recognize the use of play as the way the child understands events that are taking place. Parents can be assisted in the use of play materials such as toy thermometers and stethoscopes to encourage children to communicate feelings about health care procedures. Parents can also be encouraged to read and use rich language with their children to promote literacy and language development.
Period 3: Concrete operations (7–11 years of age)	Children achieve the ability to perform mental operations. For example, the child can think about an action that before was performed physically. At the earlier stage, the child could count to 10; at this stage, they can count and understand what each number represents. Children can describe a process without actually performing it. At this stage, they are able to coordinate two perspectives. In other words, they can appreciate the difference between their perspective and that of a friend. Reversibility is the primary characteristic of concrete operational thought. Children can mentally reverse the direction of their thoughts. Children can mentally classify objects according to their quantitative dimensions, known as seriation. Another major accomplishment of this stage is conservation, or the ability to see objects or quantities as remaining the same despite a change in their physical appearance (Berk, 2013; Piaget, 2000). Children can begin to cooperate and share new information about the acts they perform.	Encourage parents to guide the child to perform helpful activities within the home, such as doing chores in exchange for privileges (television or computer time, play with friends). Parents can encourage children to take another person's perspective or to plan ahead in schoolwork deadlines.
Period 4: Formal operations (11 years of age to adulthood)	The individual's thinking moves to abstract and theoretical subjects. Thinking can venture into such subjects as achieving world peace, finding justice, and seeking meaning in life. Adolescents can organize their thoughts in their minds. They have the capacity to reason with regard to possibilities. New cognitive powers allow the adolescent to achieve more far-reaching problem solving. Their thinking matures, and their depth of understanding increases with experience.	Include the adolescent in decision making about their own health care that is based on their ability to think abstractly.

2013). Although various theorists have addressed moral development, Piaget and Kohlberg proposed the most comprehensive theories of moral development. These theories are within the organicism tradition because they are grounded in cognitive developmental theory and development is seen as originating from within the individual. In the context of nursing interventions, the mechanisms of cognitive development also apply to the moral development theories because they both emerged from the original work of Piaget.

Piaget's Theory of Moral Development. Piaget believed that moral development goes through a series of successive stages, just as cognition and learning do. Piaget's theory of moral development presents three stages of morality: the premoral stage, the conventional stage, and the autonomous stage (Feldman, 2019; Green & Piel, 2016). In the premoral stage, the child feels no obligation to follow rules. In the conventional stage, children follow the rules set up by people in authority, such as their parents, teachers, clergy, or police. When a person reaches the stage of autonomous morality, moral judgements are based on mutual respect for the rules. A person also considers the consequences of a moral decision. In making moral judgements that involve others, the person at this stage starts to consider information related to the subjective intent (Patanella, 2011).

Piaget believed that children initially follow the rules without understanding them. Children see these rules as fixed and handed down by adults or by a higher authority (e.g., God) and therefore think they cannot change them. Young children base their moral decisions on the extent of the consequences to the action, not necessarily on the action itself. For example, a young child may refrain from eating a cookie before supper not because the mother said not to but because the child is afraid of the punishment that would result if they did. Around 10 or 11 years of age, children's cognitive ability matures, and the rules they follow are begun to be understood within the context of community life. Children understand that the rules can be modified "by legal channels" if everyone agrees to change the rules (Patanella, 2011). Moral maturity is the internalization of principles—that is, the desire to weigh all relationships and circumstances before making a decision.

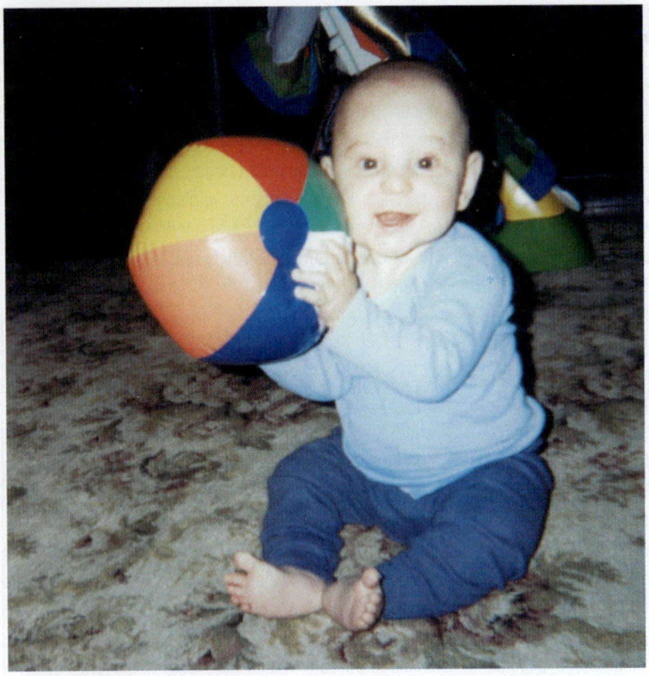

FIGURE 22.1 Piaget's theory of cognitive development, senso-rimotor stage. Successfully achieving action patterns, such as grasping, leads to learning and more exploration.

Kohlberg's Theory of Moral Development. Lawrence Kohlberg (1927–1987) expanded on Piaget's moral developmental theory. From a series of moral dilemmas presented to boys aged 10, 13, and 16 years, he identified six stages of moral development occurring at three levels (Kohlberg, 1981; Table 22.3). Kohlberg found a link between moral development and Piaget's cognitive developmental theory. He theorized that a child's moral development does not advance if the child's cognitive development does not also mature. In this way, **Kohlberg's theory of moral development** follows Piaget's cognitive developmental theory. According to Kohlberg, levels and stages do not occur at specific ages, and people attain different levels of moral development.

Kohlberg's Critics. Although Kohlberg is recognized as a leader in moral developmental theory, critics have questioned the applicability of his theory beyond the study population of adolescents boys of the Western (e.g., North American and European) philosophical traditions. Researchers attempting to support Kohlberg's (1981) theory by studying people raised in the traditions of the Eastern (e.g., East Asian and South Asian) philosophies found that those study participants never proceeded beyond stage 3 or 4 of Kohlberg's model. This cannot mean that Eastern and South Asian people have not reached as high a level of moral development as most Europeans. It is apparent that Kohlberg's research design did not allow for a way to measure moral development in people raised within different cultures. Thus, his theory may be an example of WEIRD (Western, educated, industrialized, rich, and democratic) science (Barrett, 2020).

TABLE 22.3	Kohlberg's Moral Development Theory	
Level/Stage	**Description**	**Nursing Implications**
Level I: Preconventional	The person reflects on moral reasoning based on personal gain. The person's moral reason for acting, the "why," relates to the consequences that the person believes will occur. These consequences can occur in the form of punishment or reward. Therefore, children may view illness as a punishment for fighting with their siblings or disobeying their parents.	Nurses should be aware of this thinking and reinforce teaching that the child cannot become ill because of wrongdoing.
Stage 1: Punishment and obedience orientation	Response to a moral dilemma is in terms of absolute obedience to authority and rules. Avoidance of punishment or the unquestioning deference to authority is characteristic behaviour. The child will do something because an authority figure tells the child to do it.	
Stage 2: Instrumental relativist orientation	The person recognizes that more than one view may be correct. The decision to do something morally correct is based on satisfying one's own needs and occasionally the needs of others.	
Level II: Conventional	The person sees moral reasoning based on their own personal internalization of societal and others' expectations. A person wants to fulfill the expectations of the family, group, or nation; develop loyalty to the dominant order; and actively maintain, support, and justify the order. Moral decision making at this level moves from "What's in it for me?" to "How will it affect my relationships with others?"	Nurses may observe this level of moral development when family members make end-of-life decisions for their loved ones. Grief support will involve an understanding of the level of moral decision making of each family member (see Chapter 26).
Stage 3: Good boy–nice girl orientation	The individual wants to please others and win approval by "being nice," which means having good motives, showing concern for others, and keeping mutual relationships through trust, loyalty, respect, and gratitude.	
Stage 4: Society-maintaining orientation	Focus expands from relationships with others to societal concerns. Correct behaviour is doing one's duty, showing respect for authority, and maintaining the social order. Adolescents at this stage may choose not to attend a party where drugs will be used, not because they are afraid of getting caught but because they know that using drugs is not healthy.	
Level III: Postconventional	The person finds a balance between basic human rights and obligations and societal rules and regulations. Individuals reject moral decisions based on authority or conformity to groups in favour of defining their own moral values and principles. Individuals at this stage start to envision an ideal society.	Focus not only on your individual practice but also on social determinants that affect the well-being of a community, such as poverty and homelessness.
Stage 5: Social contract orientation*	An individual follows the laws but recognizes the possibility of changing the law to improve society. The individual also recognizes that different social groups may have different values but believe in basic rights, such as liberty and life.	
Stage 6: Universal ethical principle orientation	"Right" is defined by the decision of conscience in accord with self-chosen ethical principles. These principles, such as the Golden Rule, are abstract and appeal to logical comprehensiveness, universality, and consistency (Kohlberg, 1981). Whereas stage 5 emphasizes the basic rights and the democratic process, stage 6 defines the principles by which agreements will be most just.	

Kohlberg's (1981) study has also been criticized for age and gender biases. Carol Gilligan was one important critic. As Kohlberg's contemporary, she concentrated on how Kohlberg's findings may have been biased by a narrow focus on only boys. According to Gilligan (1993), all developmental theories are subject to gender bias, and only since the 1990s have scholars researched and recognized the differences between men and women in the way they think and how they have been raised to make decisions.

Gilligan's Theory of Moral Development. Carol Gilligan (1936–present) proposed that Kohlberg's (1981) theory is biased in favour of men. She believes that men and women develop in parallel ways, with one not being superior to the other. In **Gilligan's theory of moral development**, she argues that the developmental difference between women and men lies in relationships and issues of dependency (Gilligan, 1993). Separation and individuation are critically tied to male development. **Separation** refers to a boy's recognition of biological distinctness and is based on his emergence from a dependent relationship with his mother. This separation from the mother is essential for a boy's development of masculinity. Girls do not need to separate from their mothers to achieve feminine identity; it is through this relationship with their mothers that their identity is formed. In most developmental theories, the achievement of increasing separation is a developmental norm. When women are measured against this norm as it relates to their need to maintain relationships, they are seen as failures or as less evolved developmentally. **Individuation** is based on the child's awareness of differences in will, viewpoint, and needs. This process enables the individual to gradually assume a more independent role and identity. In summary, Gilligan argues that while the moral development of boys may focus on logic, justice, and social organization, the moral development of girls focuses on interpersonal relationships.

Nursing Implication of Gilligan's Theory. Gilligan's theory makes a distinction between men and women and how women consider, value, and respect relationships in their health care decision making.

PSYCHOANALYTIC AND PSYCHOSOCIAL TRADITION

Theories in the **psychoanalytic and psychosocial tradition** describe the development of personality, thinking, behaviour, emotions, and mental health. This development is thought to occur with varying degrees of influence from internal biological forces and external societal and cultural forces.

Sigmund Freud

The first scholar to provide a formal structured theory of personality development was Sigmund Freud (1856–1939). His goal was to promote successful participation in society through the development of balance between pleasure-seeking drives and societal pressures. In **Freud's psychoanalytic model of personality development**, he asserted that mature adults should have a strong sense of conscience that allows for the experience of pleasure within the boundaries of society. He believed that two internal biological forces essentially drive psychological change in the child: sexual energy (**libido**) and aggressive energy. Behaviour is motivated by the desire to achieve pleasure and avoid pain created by these forces. These forces come into conflict with the reality of the world as maturational changes occur.

Freud's theory accounts for five psychosexual developmental stages, each associated with different pleasurable zones that serve as the foci for gratification and bodily pleasure (Berk, 2013; Feldman, 2019; Kliegman et al., 2020; Table 22.4). Freud's theory has been soundly criticized

TABLE 22.4	Freud's Five Stages of Psychosexual Development	
Stage	**Description**	**Nursing Implications**
Stage 1: Oral (birth to age 12–18 months)	Initially, sucking and oral satisfaction is not only necessary for living but also extremely pleasurable in its own right. Late in this stage, the infant begins to realize that the mother or parent is something separate from self. Disruption in the physical or emotional availability of the parent (e.g., inadequate bonding or chronic illness) could have an impact on the infant's development.	For an infant, feeding and sucking produces pleasure and comfort and promotes self-regulation. Teach parents/caregivers that feedings should be offered whenever the infant requires them. As well, encourage parents/caregivers to help their infant self-soothe by making the infant's hands available for sucking.
Stage 2: Anal (ages 12–18 months to 3 years)	The focus of pleasure changes to the anal zone. Children become increasingly aware of the pleasurable sensations of this body region with interest in the products of their effort. Through the toilet-training process, the child is asked to delay gratification in order to meet parental and societal expectations.	Teach parents/caregivers that toilet training should be as positive an experience as possible. Praise helps the child achieve a sense of control. Development is not always a smooth, uninterrupted process of moving forward to more advanced stages. Teach parents/caregivers to understand that successes are often accompanied by failures in the normal progression of development.
Stage 3: Phallic or Oedipal (ages 3–6 years)	The genital organs become the focus of pleasure. The boy becomes interested in the penis; the girl becomes aware of the absence of the penis, known as *penis envy*. This is the time of exploration and imagination as the child fantasizes about the parent of the opposite sex as their first love interest, known as the *Oedipus complex* (in boys) or the *Electra complex* (in girls). By the end of this stage, the child attempts to reduce this conflict by identifying with the parent of the same sex in a way to win recognition and acceptance.	Assure parents/caregivers that a child's identifying with the parent of the same sex is a normal developmental phase.
Stage 4: Latency (ages 6–12 years)	Sexual urges from the earlier Oedipal stage are repressed and channelled into productive activities that are socially acceptable. Within the educational and social worlds of the child, much is to be learned and accomplished. The child places energy and effort into these worlds.	Encourage the child to pursue physical and intellectual challenges that will provide opportunities to explore and develop abilities and competencies.
Stage 5: Genital (puberty through adulthood)	This is a time of turbulence when earlier sexual urges reawaken and are directed toward an individual outside the family circle. Unresolved prior conflicts surface during adolescence. Once conflicts are resolved, the individual is then capable of having a mature adult sexual relationship.	Educate parents/caregivers that the child needs to be encouraged to be independent and make their own decisions, within safe limits. Help parents/caregivers to empathize and identify with their growing adolescent. As parent/caregiver–child conflicts associated with increasing adolescent independence arise, empathy will help the parent/caregiver to understand the adolescent's point of view.

for gender and cultural biases and for an extreme focus on sexuality in development. Freud's critics contend that people are more influenced by their life experiences than by their sexual energies. Despite these criticisms, Freud's work provided a basis for observation of emotion, behaviour, and sexuality that has been very influential in the development of many other psychoanalytic theories. Indeed, many agree that development is an ongoing process of resolving conflict between issues of biological maturation and societal expectations.

Mechanisms of Freud's Theory. Components of personality emerge through Freud's developmental stages. The mechanisms of Freud's personality development theory are the id, the ego, and the superego. Freud believed that the functions of these mechanisms regulate behaviour. The **id**—basic instinctual impulses and drives to achieve pleasure—is the most primitive part of the personality and originates in the infant. The **ego** represents the reality mechanism mediating conflicts between the environment and the forces of the id. The ego helps us judge reality accurately, regulate impulses, and make good decisions. The third mechanism, the **superego**, performs regulating, restraining, and prohibiting actions. Often referred to as the *conscience*, the superego is influenced by the standards of outside social forces (parents, teachers).

Nursing Implications of Freud's Theory. The functions of the id, ego, and superego form the historical basis of many, if not all, subsequent theories of personality and social–emotional development. It is important to remember that according to Freudian theory, the mature human personality is the product of conflict between instinctual drives to achieve pleasure and the restraints of adaptive human society. When activities associated with basic pleasure (e.g., eating, sexual activity, and elimination) are altered by illness or disability, knowledgeable and empathetic nursing care is required.

Erikson's Theory of Eight Stages of Life

Erik Erikson (1902–1994) expanded Freud's psychoanalytic stages into a psychosocial model that covered the whole lifespan, not just childhood and adolescence (Erikson, 1993, 1997; Kliegman et al., 2020). He broadened the factors responsible for influencing development to include socialization.

According to **Erikson's theory of eight stages of life**, each person goes through eight stages of development (Table 22.5). In each stage, the person needs to accomplish a particular task before moving on to the next stage. Each task is framed with opposing conflicts that the person must balance. For example, an adolescent needs to develop a sense of personal identity despite many conflicting societal choices (stage 5, identity versus role confusion). Each stage builds upon the successful resolution of the previous developmental conflict. Readiness for the task is necessary for success. Once mastered, tasks are challenged and tested during new situations or at times of conflict (Hockenberry & Wilson, 2021). For example, the infant's trust is built through consistent, reliable caregiving, and the concept of trust is tested when an infant is hospitalized or after the birth of a new sibling.

Mechanisms of Erikson's Theory. *Maturation* and *ego* activity are the primary mechanisms of development in Erikson's theory of eight stages of life. The ego mediates the conflicts between biological needs and societal norms, and maturation establishes the timeline of this mediation. The developmental result of these mechanisms is described as an **epigenesis** (successive gradual change). If the process is adaptive, then a person has successive positive outcomes.

Nursing Implications of Erikson's Theory. The theory of the eight stages of life implies that the quality of early developmental experience is important. For instance, children who live in environments in which violence is common and trust has not been attained are at greater risk of experiencing poor intimate relationships. The mechanism of epigenesis implies that the original required trust elements cannot be retrieved; at best, such a person merely learns to live with the fear and anger associated with this mistrust. Nurses therefore need to practise within the health promotion model to build the familial, community, and societal supports necessary for supporting vulnerable children to achieve successful transitions at each stage (e.g., trust, autonomy, initiative).

John Bowlby

John Bowlby (1907–1990) was a child psychiatrist interested in children's mental health. Much of his theory was developed during his work in the 1930s with maladjusted English adolescents who, he observed, had often been subjected to maternal deprivation in early life (Bretherton, 1992). According to **Bowlby's attachment and separation theory**, the conflict between attachment and separation needs to be resolved to produce healthy social–emotional and mental developmental outcomes across the lifespan. **Attachment** refers to the security (or insecurity) of the emotional tie or relationship between an individual and another person, such as a parent or caregiver. A basic premise of Bowlby's theory is that the quality of attachment relationships stems from interactions between infants and caregivers. A **secure parent-infant attachment** is defined as when infants can rely on their caregivers to meet their emotional and cognitive needs, specifically to provide proximity and companionship, a safe haven in the presence of threat or anxiety, and a secure base from which to explore. **Insecure and disorganized parent-infant attachment** is defined as when infants are less able or unable, respectively, to rely on their caregivers to meet their emotional and/or cognitive needs. In attachment theory, behavioural and psychiatric developmental disorders are considered within the context of family attachment relationships. Empirical research has shown that early attachment patterns predict developmental health (e.g., work, friendships, and intimate relationships), mental health (e.g., anxiety), and physical health (e.g., inflammatory diseases) over the lifespan (Boldt et al., 2020; Madigan et al., 2013; Puig et al., 2013; Sroufe, 2005).

Mechanisms of Bowlby's Theory. Early in life, two complementary behavioural systems, attachment and caregiving, combine into a self-regulating system that supports people in their healthy attachments to and separations from others. The child's experiences within this self-regulating system cause the child to develop a cognitive working model (or "map") of self, other, and the relationship between them. The ability to regulate emotion and behaviour (Box 22.2) is influenced by this working model at each developmental stage throughout life.

Extensions to Bowlby's Theory of Attachment and Separation

Mary Ainsworth (1913–1999) was an American-Canadian psychologist known for operationalizing the measurement of attachment as conceptualized by Bowlby. **Ainsworth's operationalization of attachment theory** (Ainsworth, 1979) categorized child–parent relationships into one of three organized patterns—securely attached (Type B), insecure avoidant (Type A), and insecure ambivalent/resistant (Type C)—based on how 9- to 20-month-old children reacted to a series of separations and reunions from their parents, also known as primary attachment figures. The Type A pattern is dominated by "cognitive" (or unemotional) strategies and Type C by "affective" (emotional) strategies that help maintain the proximity of the caregiver to the child. Type B represents a balance between both extremes and was theorized to be optimal for development (Ainsworth, 1979). Patricia Crittenden

TABLE 22.5 Erikson's Theory of Eight Stages of Life

Stage	Description	Nursing Implications
1. Trust versus mistrust (infancy: birth to 1 year)	The infant learns to trust others. Trust is achieved when the infant will let the caregiver out of sight without undue distress. Key to this stage is consistent caregiving. The question answered at this stage is "Can I trust the world?"	The parent's struggle with building competence can be assisted by the nurse's use of anticipatory guidance and other educative interventions. The parent may need guidance to understand the importance of a safe, nurturing environment when meeting the child's needs.
2. Autonomy versus sense of shame and doubt (toddler years: ages 1–3 years)	The toddler learns to be independent and develops self-confidence. Not learning independence creates feelings of shame and self-doubt. Independence is accomplished through self-care activities, including walking, feeding, and toileting. Toddlers also develop autonomy by making choices. The question answered at this stage is "Can I control my own behaviour?"	Nurses can use empathetic guidance to offer support for and understanding of the challenges at this stage. Parents can be taught to use nonviolent disciplinary methods with their children that promote safety yet discipline. Teach parents to offer children a limited number of choices so as not to overwhelm them; choice promotes children's developing sense of self-efficacy and competence.
3. Initiative versus guilt (preschool years: ages 3–6 years)	The child learns to initiate their activities. Accomplishing this task teaches the child to seek challenges in later life. Children use fantasy and imagination to explore their environment. Conflicts often arise between the child's desire to explore and the limits placed on their behaviour. These conflicts may lead to feelings of frustration and guilt. The question answered during this stage is "Can I become independent of my parents and explore my limits?"	Teaching impulse control and cooperative behaviours to the child is necessary at this stage. Children can be shown appreciation for independent behaviours that demonstrate prosocial skills, such as sharing, kindness to others, and helping with household chores.
4. Industry versus inferiority (middle childhood: ages 6–11 years)	The child develops a sense of competence in physical, cognitive, and social areas. Not learning new skills may lead to a sense of inadequacy and inferiority. Successfully achieving this task leads to positive attitudes toward work in adulthood (Erikson, 1993). The question answered at this stage is "Can I master the skills necessary to survive and adapt?"	Encourage parents to offer the child many opportunities to pursue new interests and challenges in extracurricular activities, such as sports, music, and art.
5. Identity versus role confusion (adolescence: ages 12–18 years)	The task of adolescence is to try out several roles and form a unique identity. Dramatic physiological changes associated with sexual maturation also mark this stage. Acquiring a sense of identity is essential for making later adult decisions such as vocation or marriage partner. New social demands, opportunities, and conflicts arise in relation to the emergent identity and separation from family. The question answered at this stage is "Who am I, and what are my beliefs, feelings, and attitudes?"	Provide education and anticipatory guidance for the parent about the changes in and challenges to the adolescent. Also assist hospitalized adolescents in dealing with their illness by giving them enough information to allow them to make decisions about their treatment plan.
6. Intimacy versus isolation (young adulthood: ages 18–35 years)	The primary task of young adulthood is to form close personal relationships. This is the time to become fully active in the community. If young adults have not achieved a sense of personal identity, they may be unable to form meaningful attachments and will experience feelings of isolation. The question answered during this stage is "Can I give of myself fully to another?"	Understand that during hospitalization, young adults may benefit from the support of their partners/caregivers or significant others because this support helps fulfill their need for intimacy.
7. Generativity versus self-absorption and stagnation (middle adulthood: ages 35–65 years)	The task of middle adulthood is to help younger people. The ability to expand one's personal and social involvement is crucial for this stage of development. Middle-aged adults should be able to see beyond their needs and accomplishments and view the needs of society. Dissatisfaction with one's achievements often leads to self-absorption and stagnation. The question answered during this stage is "What can I offer succeeding generations?"	Assist adults in choosing creative ways to foster social development. Middle-aged people may find a sense of fulfillment from volunteering some time in a local school, hospital, community centre, or place of worship.
8. Integrity versus despair (old age: age 65 years and older)	Older persons reflect on their life and feel satisfaction or disappointment. By suffering physical and social losses, such as those through retirement or illness, the person may also suffer loss of status and function. The person may also have internal struggles, such as the search for meaning in life. Meeting these challenges creates the potential for growth and wisdom (Figure 22.2). The question answered during this stage is "Has my life been worthwhile?"	Nurses can contribute to the valuing of people at all ages and stages in their communities. For example, by promoting older persons' involvement in volunteer activities, such as youth mentoring, you display value for the skills and experience of older people. Such mentoring also helps the younger generation feel important.

Adapted from Erikson, E. (1993). *Childhood and society*. W.W. Norton; Erikson, E. (1997). *The lifecycle completed*. W.W. Norton.

(1945–present) was Ainsworth's student and was heavily influenced by the work of both Bowlby and Ainsworth (1979) in developing her dynamic maturational model of attachment (Crittenden, 2008; Crittenden & Claussen, 2003). Mary Main (1943–present), another of Ainsworth's students, also added to Bowlby's theory by identifying the concept of disorganized attachment (Main & Solomon, 1986; described in the next section).

Mechanisms of the Dynamic Maturational Model of Attachment. The interaction between brain development and experiences

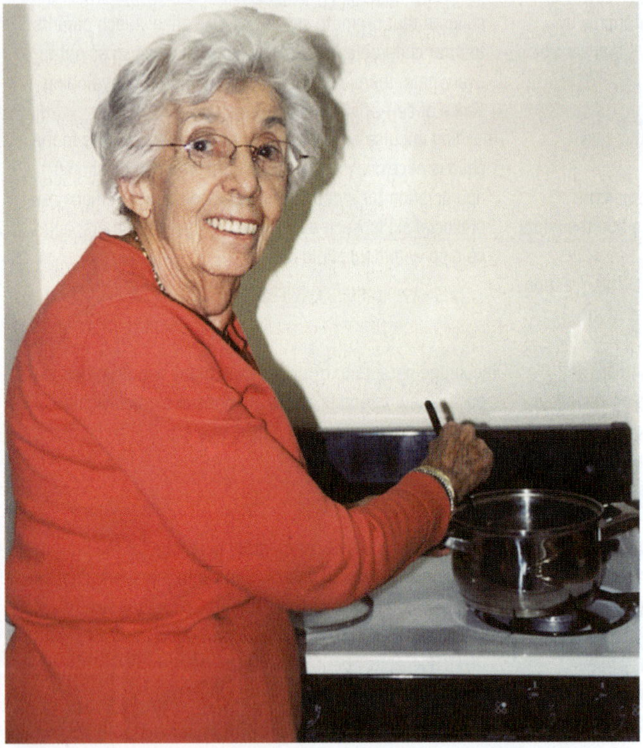

FIGURE 22.2 Maintaining independence is important to a person's self-esteem.

with caregivers is central in the development of self-protective attachment strategies that individuals use over their lifespan (Box 22.3). These attachment strategies are employed to promote safety and security in relationships (Crittenden & Claussen, 2003; Crittenden & Landini, 2011). Unlike the work of other attachment theorists, the dynamic maturational model considers the impact of intimate relationships at different life stages, including preschool, school-age, adolescence, and adulthood, in addition to infancy. People with Type A patterns tend to minimize awareness of negative feelings, compulsively perform what they expect will be reinforced, and avoid doing what will be punished (Crittenden & DiLalla, 1988). People with Type C patterns rely on feelings as guides to behaviour because they lack confidence in what will happen next. When familial relationships fail to protect the child (or adult parent), Type A and Type C coping strategies become more extreme. For example, a child reared by an unresponsive caregiver may learn that "acting out" elicits a needed response from the caregiver. As the child grows and becomes an adult, they may seek attention through extreme emotional outbursts, acting coercively or aggressively in other adult relationships (Type C) (Crittenden & Kulbotten, 2007).

Mechanisms of Disorganized Attachment. Disorganized attachment, also called Type D attachment, is more often seen in maltreated infants and young children but does not necessarily indicate maltreatment. It is often linked to a history of adverse childhood experiences (ACEs). Type D attachment may also be assessed by observing a series of separations and reunions with parents or other attachment figures and represents the child's difficulty in establishing an organized attachment pattern with their parent (Granqvist et al., 2017). Of the four patterns of attachment, Type D is most often linked to behavioural and mental health issues, including hyperactivity and conduct disorder (Fearon et al., 2010; Groh et al., 2012).

Nursing Implications of the Dynamic Maturational Model of Attachment. As a nurse, you will need to design approaches that address both the quality of the attachment system and the caregiving system. Crittenden (2008) asserted that recognizing patients' attachment strategies is crucial to providing helpful treatments and reducing the risk of inappropriate treatment. For instance, in caring for a young hospitalized child, you would need to consider the security of

---

BOX 22.2   CASE STUDY

Jonathan is 5 years old. His father (preferred pronouns: he/him) has brought him to the pediatrician at the advice of his kindergarten teacher. You are the clinic nurse and have been charged with taking Jonathan's history. His father takes time to locate crayons and paper for Jonathan during the office visit. However, Jonathan does not settle for long. As you begin your assessment, you observe Jonny, as his father calls him, spend a minute with the crayons before breaking one and then moving on to examine the stethoscope and then the next item in the office that intrigues him more. Jonny goes back to the crayons and rips the paper, and his father offers him another piece to draw on. Jonny smiles broadly at his dad and you, seeming content to move chaotically about in the office.

As you proceed through your assessment, you learn that Jonny accomplished typical milestones (walking, talking, toilet training) on time and had a few ear infections but no other physical health problems. His weight and height are normal. He gets along well with the other children, except for the occasional skirmish over a toy. His father notes that Jonny does not sit still for very long and that since he and his partner (she/her) separated, Jonny has been more difficult to manage. He has difficulty sitting still in synagogue and fares better in the supervised playroom during service. He adds that his kids miss their

mom, but still see her every week. As he begins to talk about Jonny's mom, Jonny climbs into his father's lap then leaps off and returns quickly with a book held out to his dad. "He loves to read," says Jonny's dad, who opens the book to page 1, points to a rabbit, and pauses his conversation with you to say, "B for bunny," to Jonny. Jonny smiles broadly, then snaps the book shut and begins to play with a car.

The father turns back to you and, laying the book aside, tells you the teacher's concern about his activity level, inability to hold a pencil properly, and failure to pay attention to learning tasks in class. The father relays the teacher's concern that Jonny may have attention-deficit/hyperactivity disorder. You wonder whether Jonny's activity level has anything to do with his parents' separation, an adverse childhood experience. You also wonder whether Jonny's mom was his primary attachment figure, and whether her absence is the reason why Jonny may be reacting with separation anxiety from the loss of his secure base.

Jonny zips back across the office, sprawls out briefly on his dad's lap, hugging his upper legs. As you further observe the father gently tousling his young son's hair, he asks you your opinion on whether medication would help Jonny have an easier time in kindergarten and synagogue.

BOX 22.3 RESEARCH HIGHLIGHT

Toxic Stress, Adverse Childhood Experiences, and Development

In response to stressors such as difficult and challenging experiences, the human body physiologically responds by increasing our capacity to think and act. Energy stores are mobilized, and heart rate and blood pressure are increased, enabling more attention, awareness, and responsiveness to the environment. When stress is controllable, short lived, and predictable, it can help us learn to be adaptive and resilient. This is a "good" form of stress. Some forms of stress are tolerable even though they challenge our abilities to cope. The death of a loved one or moving to a new city are examples of adverse events that are made tolerable by support from our social network and by the fact that many other people have faced similar experiences. But what if the challenges we face are uncontrollable, unpredictable, and pervasive? This is referred to as "toxic" stress.

Toxic stress is a form of stress that results from chronic activation of the biological stress response system, with harmful consequences for child development. Experiences that are chronically disruptive, abusive, neglectful, or unpredictable flood the brain with chemicals that, in large and persistent doses, impair neuronal growth and ultimately make it harder for the brain to form healthy connections. In this way, toxic stress leaves a lasting biological fingerprint of damage on brain structure and function.

For example, parents or caregivers dealing with mental illness, substance use issues, or intimate partner violence are less able to respond sensitively to their infants to meet their needs, placing the infants at risk for unpredictable, neglectful, or abusive parenting. As infants are completely reliant on their parents to have their basic needs met, these situations chronically activate infants' stress response systems and produce changes to the structure and function of some brain regions.

Adverse childhood experiences (ACEs) are stressors that happen before the age of 18 years and include abuse, neglect, and household dysfunction. The more ACEs experienced during childhood, the greater the likelihood of health problems in adulthood (Felitti et al., 2019). The mechanisms of action are likely the same as for toxic stress, in that lack of support to manage the stressors may explain their toxicity. Two major brain regions that are known to be affected by toxic stress and ACEs are the hippocampus and the prefrontal cortex. These brain regions are particularly important to the development of memory and self-regulation—the foundations of school and social success. Over time, the effects of toxic stress and ACEs on brain structure and function can lead to shifts in patterns of behaviour from more organized to more habitual, with the result that children become more rigid and less capable of independent problem solving.

The effects of toxic stress and ACEs are particularly worrisome in early childhood because the brain is exquisitely sensitive to experience during this phase of rapid brain development. As well, children's future brain development builds upon current and past brain development. Thus, changes in brain structure and function due to toxic stress produce cumulative changes—affecting not only current aspects of development for a given stage, but also the next stage that builds upon previous growth. To summarize, it seems that the common adage "what doesn't kill you makes you stronger" is true of good stress, but when it comes to toxic stress and ACEs, "what doesn't kill you now may kill you later."

Adapted from Shonkoff, J. P., Slopen, N., & Williams, D. R. (2021). Early childhood adversity, toxic stress, and the impacts of racism on the foundations of health. *Annual Review of Public Health, 42*, 115–134. https://doi.org/10.1146/annurev-publhealth-090419-101940

the child and provide high-quality substitute care, including by making developmentally appropriate efforts to keep the child attached to their primary caregiver (e.g., using pictures, phone calls, liberal visiting hours, parent rooming-in). If you are working in mental health care, you need to recognize that patients' apparently maladaptive coping strategies (e.g., obsessive–compulsive disorder, anxiety) may be strategies developed to cope with adverse relationships with attachment figures. Alternatively, in working with parents in impoverished environments, you need to support the caregivers through the provision of material, social, and educational resources that will promote the safety and security of adults and children alike. Nurses need to advocate for appropriate support resources for families in which caregiving may be compromised as a result of the stress associated with parental poverty, mental illness, or lack of education (Francis et al., 2018).

Havighurst's Developmental Tasks

Robert Havighurst (1900–1991) was influenced by Erikson's work and observations of the developmental tasks crucial for healthy development. Havighurst defined a series of age-specific essential tasks, such as learning to walk, getting ready to read, learning social and gender roles, developing independence, selecting a mate, rearing children, and, finally, adjusting to decreasing physical strength and health. The essential tasks arise from predictable internal and external pressures, such as increasing physical maturity, the cultural pressure of society, and the individual's personal goals and aspirations (Havighurst, 1972).

According to Havighurst's developmental tasks, several sources of pressure may be present at the same time. Increasing physical maturity is associated with the development of skills such as walking, talking, or eating. Cultural pressure creates the conditions necessary to learn social behaviours and ethical norms. An adolescent girl may be physically able to bear a child, but the preparation and timing for the onset of parenthood can also be considered from the perspective of pressure from both the youth and adult cultures (Havighurst, 1972).

Havighurst believed that at certain critical periods, the individual is most receptive to the learning necessary to achieve success in performing these tasks. Effective learning and achievement of tasks during one period leads to happiness and success with later tasks. Failure leads to unhappiness, disapproval from society, and difficulty with later tasks. An example is the struggle that adolescents might experience in preparing for a work career after having failed to develop fundamental skills in reading and math (Havighurst, 1972; Seiffge-Krenke & Gelhaar, 2008).

Critics argue that Havighurst's theory is limited in its cultural application because it describes developmental milestones from the perspective of middle-class norms in the United States. It would be difficult to fit all cultural or ethnic mores within this theoretical framework (Klaczynski, 1990).

Mechanisms and Nursing Implications of Havighurst's Theory.
Havighurst's work built on that of Freud and Erikson. Therefore, the mechanisms and nursing implications from Freud and Erikson also apply to Havighurst's developmental tasks (Table 22.6).

MECHANISTIC TRADITION

According to the mechanistic tradition, the organism is similar to a machine. Development depends on the level of stimulation, the kind of stimulation, and the history of stimulation from the environment. The environment is responsible for activating human development (Bornstein & Lamb, 2015), and behaviour is seen as responsive to environmental forces rather than driven only by internal causes such as

TABLE 22.6	Developmental Theorists for Adult Stages	
Adult Stages	**Erikson's Description**	**Havighurst's Description**
Early-early adult (ages 16–22 years)	Intimacy versus isolation	Early adulthood stage
Middle-early adult (ages 22–28 years)	Ability to form intimate relationships	Selecting a mate
		Learning to live with a partner
		Starting a family
		Rearing children
		Getting started in an occupation
		Taking on civic responsibilities
		Finding a congenial social group
Early-middle adult (ages 28–45 years)	Generativity versus self-absorption and stagnation	Middle age
	Ability to expand personal and social involvement	Assisting teenage children to become responsible adults
		Achieving adult social and civic responsibility
		Reaching and maintaining satisfactory performance in one's occupation
		Developing adult leisure-time activities
		Relating to one's partner as a person
		Accepting and adjusting to the physiological changes of middle age
		Adjusting to aging of parents
Late adult–old age (age 45 years and older)	Integrity versus despair	Later maturity
	Ability to adapt to changes in lifestyle, functional level, and family structure	Adjusting to decreasing physical strength and health
		Adjusting to retirement and reduced income
		Adjusting to death of a partner
		Establishing an affiliation with one's age group
		Adopting and adapting social roles in a flexible way
		Satisfactory physical living space

maturation. Social learning theory follows from this tradition and is presented in Chapter 21.

CONTEXTUALISM

The way that human development is described and explained is increasingly tied to our understanding of environment and context. Developmental theories within the contextual tradition focus on the relationship between the individual and their social context. Within this tradition, the individual and the environment are viewed as mutually influential, acting on one another in dynamic interaction (Bornstein & Lamb, 2015). Human development is the process of continuously adapting to changing environments.

Bioecological Theory

Urie Bronfenbrenner (1917–2005), a developmental psychologist at Cornell University, developed a theory that stresses the importance of the interaction between the developing individual and their surrounding social environments. Bronfenbrenner's bioecological theory considers multiple "layers" of the environment as follows:

- The microsystem consists of the immediate settings, activities, and personal relationships of the individual. Examples are family, classroom, workplace, and recreation group.
- The mesosystem is made up of the relationships between the different settings in which the person spends time. Examples are relationships between families and schools, between workplaces and schools, between families and spiritual organizations (church parish, mosque, temple), and between spiritual organizations and schools.
- The exosystem is a set of specific social structures that do not directly contain the individual but exert direct and indirect influence on individual development. Examples are the health care system, the education system, the justice system, and religious institutions.

- The macrosystem consists of all the elements contained in the individual's microsystem, mesosystem, and exosystem, as well as the general underlying philosophy, cultural orientation, and values by which the person lives (Bronfenbrenner, 2009). Examples are overarching dimensions such as political orientation, economic model, and cultural values.

Mechanisms of the Bioecological Theory. Lev Semenovich Vygotsky (1896–1934) introduced a concept called the zone of proximal development, which is the key developmental mechanism of ecological theories. This zone is the space between the individual's potential and their actual developmental status (Green & Piel, 2016). For instance, a toddler may have a 10-word vocabulary but could potentially have a repertoire of hundreds of words. Activity that links those two states promotes development. For instance, parents who use joint referencing (looking at things that their toddlers are looking at and naming them) promote toddler vocabulary development within the zone of proximal development.

Bronfenbrenner's modern conception of developmental processes expands upon Vygotsky's idea of the zone of proximal development. In language acquisition, developmental support processes occur at all levels of the system. At the macrosystem level, a process supporting language development in young children would be the adoption of a national child care policy to support working parents. Such a policy would inform regulations concerning issues such as the education level of child care workers, ratio of children to workers in child care centres, and space requirements per child.

Nursing Implications of the Bioecological Theory. An appropriate goal of nursing practice is to influence wellness by promoting health in all layers of the bioecological system. The ecological model applies to nursing practice beyond the individual level of health

BOX 22.4   FOCUS ON PRIMARY HEALTH CARE
Bronfenbrenner's Ecological Theory and Primary Health Care

Three principles of primary health care are to (1) foster public participation, (2) educate the patient to promote health and prevent illness, and (3) foster intersectoral collaboration. Bronfenbrenner's ecological model of human development fits well with these principles. Nurses can initiate actions to promote health at each of the following environmental layers:

- *Microsystem*, which includes the individual and their immediate setting (e.g., family, school, workplace, neighbourhood). As a nurse, you can help the individual develop personal skills, healthy lifestyles and activities, and supportive environments. For example, you can help teach family members caring for an elderly parent how to balance family care and self-care to keep themselves healthy.
- *Mesosystem*, which consists of relations among the individual's various immediate settings. To strengthen the mesosystem, you can work toward strengthening community action. You can link the family to community supports such as adult respite services and older persons' activity groups.

- *Exosystem*, which comprises relations among structures, sectors, services, and policies. The exosystem is strengthened when nurses promote healthy public policy. You are practising at this level when you help develop links between typically separate services such as the health care system and the social service system. For example, you can volunteer to be on planning committees and other decision-making bodies.
- *Macrosystem*, which consists of societal values. To promote optimum health at the macrosystem level, the nurse can be an advocate for social change. For example, if you believe that more value should be placed on older persons in society, you may advocate for higher standards and staff-to-resident ratios in long-term care facilities. Such advocacy might include writing letters to the editor, joining community or national advocacy groups, and lobbying politicians.

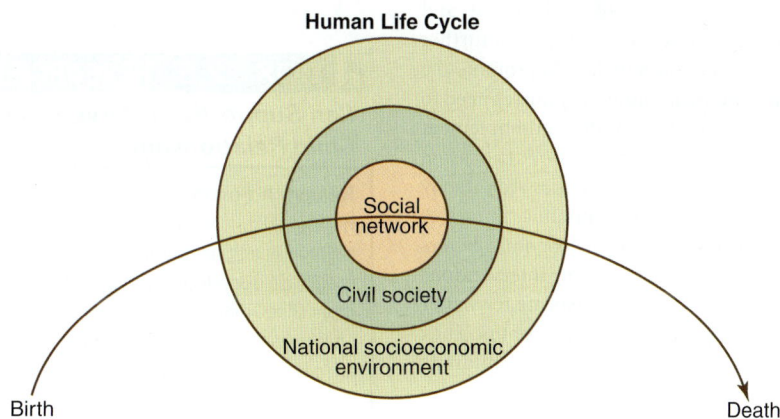

FIGURE 22.3 Framework for human development and the social determinants of health. (Redrawn from Keating, D. P., & Hertzman, C. [Eds.]. [1999]. *Developmental health and the wealth of nations: Social, biological and educational dynamics* [p. 30]. Guilford Press.)

promotion to include higher levels of the social context. Therefore, Bronfenbrenner's theory fits well with the current emphasis on primary health care (Box 22.4).

DIALECTICISM

In the **dialectical tradition**, all developmental theories are considered mutually interactive (Sameroff, 2010). Developmental theorists are increasingly proposing that change or development can occur within the framework of multiple theories. A key element of the dialectic tradition is the ability to incorporate multiple contexts. An example of a dialectical approach from the natural and biomedical sciences is the theory of gene expression or epigenetics. **Epigenetics** links genetics, the environment, and their influences on human development and disease (Cavalli & Heard, 2019). In the behavioural and social sciences, examples of dialectical thinking include the growing awareness of the effect of the economic environment on human development at the population level. Resilience theory is an approach in which the interaction between two processes, previously studied separately, is examined.

Keating and Hertzman's Population Health Theory

Human development has historically been considered an individual characteristic. According to the **population health approach** of Daniel

P. Keating (1949–present) and Clyde Hertzman (1953–2013), human development is a population phenomenon Keating and Hertzman (1999). These Canadian developmental theorists referred to the strong association between the health of a population, developmental outcomes, and the social and economic forces affecting the larger society. They based their developmental theory on epidemiological evidence that improved literacy (one marker of human development) is related to improvements in family economic status, school community economic status, and national economic status (Hertzman, 2011). Hertzman theorized that socioeconomic status created gradients in developmental health, a process he called "biological embedding" (Hertzman & Boyce, 2010).

Keating and Hertzman (1999) proposed that health, behaviour, and cognitive functions are largely set in early life and are then influenced further by succeeding events in the socioeconomic environment. **Developmental health** is defined as the physical and mental health, well-being, coping, and competence of human populations. Developmental health is primarily a function of the overall quality of the social environment, including the national socioeconomic environment, civil society, and social network. Keating and Hertzman's population approach to human development is outlined in Figure 22.3.

Mechanisms of the Population Health Theory. Keating and Hertzman (1999) proposed three interrelated regulatory systems as the mechanisms underlying human population development: emotional regulation, attention regulation, and social regulation. Each regulatory system develops in interaction between the individual's biological processes and their multiple socioeconomic environments. *Emotional regulation*, which involves the modulation of emotional reactions, plays an important role in competent social functioning. *Attention regulation*, which involves regulation of arousal and reactivity of the brain, contributes to the ability to pursue goals and to respond to challenges encountered while pursuing those goals. *Social regulation* involves regulation of social interactions, including aspects such as mutual affection and warmth, particularly in nurturing relationships. Together, these three regulatory systems are thought to influence later competence as individuals interact reciprocally with their socioeconomic environments. Extensions of the work show that early developmental adversity actually affects gene expression or an individual's epigenetic profile and is linked to later heath and developmental outcomes (Barker et al., 2018).

Community Nursing Care Implications of the Population Health Theory.

Community nurses have typically focused on the health and well-being of patients in a community context (see Chapter 4 for further information on caring for patients in the community). To promote the well-being of individuals over their lifespan, community nurses need to understand how socioeconomic context affects health and implement practices that consider socioeconomic impacts (Stanhope & Lancaster, 2019). The ecological levels of health promotion activities are directly applicable to the population health approach for community nurses. A population health approach helps identify these socioeconomic factors and provides direction for designing community nursing interventions that address them. Community health nurses can advocate for better environments for children affected by low socioeconomic status. They can also work with families to help address risks to their children's development that can have lifelong consequences.

Resilience Theory

Resilience is defined as the maintenance of positive adjustment under challenging life conditions (Masten & Barnes, 2018). This approach arose in the field of child psychiatry when clinicians observed that some children and adolescents were able to thrive in severely adverse conditions (e.g., poverty, maternal depression, and paternal criminality), whereas others faltered (Luthar, 2003).

Mechanisms of Resilience.

Resilience theory focuses on the interaction between protective processes and vulnerability processes. **Vulnerability processes** (physical illness, psychological stresses, social risk) and **protective processes** (self-efficacy, good parenting and problem solving, social support acquisition and maintenance) are examined together to understand and explain human growth and development. Individual factors found to promote resilience include self-efficacy, positive attitude, literacy, social competence, and a history of success. Family-level processes that protect from adversity include coherent response to crisis, social supports, stability, flexibility, effective parenting, and responsibilities outside the home (Rutter, 2005). Community-level processes that promote resilience include control over policy, collaborative and cooperative organization, widespread citizen participation in the community, and volunteerism.

Resilience and family adaptation theory has been used to design interventions to support children and families at risk by focusing on protective processes within the context of key risk situations, usually defined by factors such as poverty, chronic illness, and civil conflict. This emphasis is a progression from the previous emphasis on only pathological processes, but the challenge is to design research that

enables scholars to study both protective processes and vulnerability processes as they occur together.

Nursing Implications of Resilience.

The focus of nursing practice is directly on the individual, family, and community factors that promote health. Nursing practice is usually used in situations that are stressful and challenging for individuals and families, such as illness and loss. Resilience theorists acknowledge the complexity of these moments and ask what nurses can use from these challenging situations that will help the family succeed (Box 22.5). For example, a young single woman dealing with the birth of her first child will benefit from nursing interventions that focus both on protective processes (linking to support group, learning parenting skills) and on vulnerability processes (ensuring adequate health care, arranging for financial support).

DEVELOPMENTAL THEORIES AND NURSING

The diverse set of theories included in this chapter suggests that human behaviour is truly complex. No single theory successfully describes

---

BOX 22.5 RESEARCH HIGHLIGHT

Can Supportive Intervention Improve Parent–Child Relationships?

Research Focus

Healthy child development has been identified as one of the key determinants of health and resiliency in adulthood. Attachment security promotes healthy child development. In a systematic review by Letourneau et al. (2015), researchers examined interventions aimed at improving the parent–child attachment security among children from a variety of groups, including those affected by maternal depression, financial stress, or marital problems.

Research Abstract

Early secure maternal–child attachment relationships lay the foundation for children's healthy social and mental development. Interventions targeting maternal sensitivity during the first year of infant life may be the key to promoting secure attachment. Letourneau et al. (2015) conducted a narrative systematic review and meta-analysis to examine the effectiveness of interventions aimed at promoting maternal sensitivity on maternal–child attachment security. Studies included mothers and their infants followed up to 36 months postpartum.

Methods and Results

Ten trials, involving 1 628 mother–infant pairs, were included. Examination of the trials showed that interventions designed to promote maternal sensitivity worked to improve maternal–child attachment security. The authors concluded that interventions aimed at improving maternal sensitivity alone or in combination with maternal reflection, implemented in the first year of infants' lives, are effective in promoting secure maternal–child attachments. Intervention aimed at highest-risk families produced the most beneficial effects.

Implications for Practice

- Helping parents become more sensitive and responsive to their infants to improve the quality of parent–child relationships is an important support mechanism for families at risk.
- Parent training and support have the potential to positively alter the style of interaction between parents and children.

From Letourneau, N., Tryphonopoulos, P., Giesbrecht, G., et al. (2015). Narrative and meta-analytic review of interventions aiming to improve maternal–child attachment security. *Infant Mental Health Journal, 36*(4), 366–387. https://doi.org/10.1002/imhj.21525

human growth and development in all its complexity. Theorists demonstrate their own values and beliefs in their focus and the subjects chosen for their work, and they work within specific cultural and historical perspectives. The theories described in this chapter are meant to provide the basis for meaningful thought and observation of an individual's pattern of growth and development and the role of environments in it. This observation and reflection provide you with a framework within which you can predict human responses to health and illness and recognize deviations from the norm.

Patterns of growth and development help determine future patterns of adjustment to life (Dames et al., 2021). A clear understanding of these patterns and of the contexts within which they occur can assist you in planning questions for health screening and health history and in health teaching for patients of all ages. Nurses need to consider an individual's development within the context of their family, social relationships, community, and the larger society.

Developmental theories help you as a nurse use critical thinking skills when you consider how and why people respond as they do. Your assessment of a patient requires a thorough analysis and interpretation of data to form accurate conclusions about a patient's developmental needs. To accurately identify patients' needs, you need the ability to consider developmental theory in data analysis. Observed developmental behaviours are compared with those projected by the developmental theory.

KEY CONCEPTS

- Nurses provide care for individuals and families throughout their lives. Developmental theories provide a basis for nurses to assess, interpret, and understand the responses seen in their patients.
- Development continues throughout life.
- Individuals have unique patterns of growth and development within broad limits.
- Development is not just a series of distinct linear tasks; it is also a process that varies across and within individuals.
- Three major categories of factors influence human growth and development: (1) genetic or natural forces within the person, (2) the environment in which the person lives, and (3) the interaction that takes place between these two.
- Theories within the organic tradition explore how individuals develop when mostly biological components are believed to stimulate developmental progress.
- Theories in the psychoanalytic and psychosocial tradition describe development of the human personality with regard to conflict resolution between internal biological forces and external societal and cultural forces.
- According to the mechanistic approach, human development and behaviour are responses to environmental forces rather than driven by internal causes such as maturation.
- Within the contextual tradition, the individual and the environment are viewed as mutually influential, acting on one another in dynamic interaction.
- In the dialectical tradition, the complete complexity of development is acknowledged. Theorists who work in this tradition strive to combine divergent ways of viewing human development.

CRITICAL THINKING EXERCISES

1. A 50-year-old parent (preferred pronouns: she/her) is anxious because her children, 20 and 23 years of age, are no longer living at home. Her partner is still working full time but planning to retire in 2 years. She is concerned that she is not needed and is feeling bored with her life. Identify the developmental task of Erikson's theory that best fits her situation. How will you assist this patient in changing her lifestyle while understanding her developmental tasks?

2. A community nurse conducting a routine assessment of an 18-month-old is concerned about the child being underweight for his age. Upon further discussion, the parent (preferred pronouns: he/him) reveals that he is not working at present and that the family is having financial troubles. Using your knowledge of Bronfenbrenner's bioecological theory, what approach and subsequent strategies would be helpful for these parents?

3. Two 11-year-old children (preferred pronouns: she/her) are spending the day together at the mall. As they exit one store, one of the girls shows her friend a small purse that she stole from the store. Her friend is upset and wonders how she should respond. Use Kohlberg's moral developmental theory to discuss this issue.

4. A patient (preferred pronouns: she/her) visits her nurse practitioner at her local health clinic. The patient is struggling with depression and seeking to increase her medication dosage. She also reveals that she is struggling to cope with her 8-year-old child's (he/him) problem behaviours, such as refusing to do homework and having tantrums when he fails to get his way. Using the dynamic maturational model of attachment, discuss how her mental health state could be influencing her child's behaviour.

Answers to Critical Thinking Exercises appear on the Evolve website.

REVIEW QUESTIONS

Review Questions 1 to 8 relate to the case study at the beginning of the chapter.

1. Today, you have your monthly appointment with Pritma, 23 years old, who is 7 months pregnant with her first child. Normally she arrives at the clinic on time and is careful about her appearance. You document the following findings as part of your assessment:
   a. ____ She reports oversleeping from fatigue.
   b. ____ Her urine glucose is high.
   c. ____ The fetal heart rate is normal.
   d. ____ She has not gained weight this month.
   e. ____ Her hair is dishevelled.
   f. ____ Her clothes look slept in.
   g. ____ She smiles throughout the whole clinic visit.
   h. ____ She says, "Everything at home is great."
   Place a checkmark next to the observations suggesting that Pritma may be depressed and require more detailed follow-up assessment.

2. Based on your assessment findings during your prenatal visit with Pritma, you decide to administer a measure of perinatal depression. You find that she scores high, for likely depressed. As you share your findings with Pritma, you focus on problem solving with her to identify solutions to address her symptoms of depression and potential impacts on her unborn child. Which of the following solutions would you discuss with Pritma? (*Select all that apply.*)
   a. Discuss ways to obtain more rest.
   b. Discuss return-to-work options for after her child is born.
   c. Discuss how to engage her support network (e.g., husband, family, friends) for help.
   d. Discuss possibility of medication therapy.
   e. Discuss referral for counselling or psychotherapy.
   f. Discuss how to reduce stress.
   g. Discuss how to attain nutritional needs.
   h. Discuss breastfeeding plans.

3. Recalling some of the details you know about Pritma's journey to Canada, you decide to administer Felitti and Anda's Adverse Childhood Experiences Questionnaire (an inventory of childhood abuse, neglect, and family dysfunction before the age of 18 years). Pritma scores a 5. Upon review of the items, you learn that Pritma experienced childhood sexual and physical abuse and emotional and physical neglect while living at the immigration facility. You also learn that Pritma's mother has been depressed off and on for as long as Pritma can remember, which meant that the care of the younger siblings often fell to Pritma. After immigration, her father was often absent, working two jobs to feed and house his family, so Pritma assumed the role of head of household from a young age.

Choose the most likely options (from the list of options provided) for the information missing from the following statement:

The nurse recognizes that the patient's (1)_____ symptoms of depression may be due to childhood (2)_____, specifically (3)_____, _____ , the experience of her mother's (5)_____, and stress from family (6)_____ before she was 18 years of age.

Answer options:
abuse
depression
dysfunction
elevated
neglect
trauma

4. Today at your monthly appointment with 23-year-old Pritma, who is 7 months pregnant, she flinches when you support her to lay down on the examination table. You document the following findings as part of your assessment:
   a. ___ Bruising on her upper back
   b. ___ When asked what happened to her back and face, she tells you she slipped on the ice.
   c. ___ Makeup that appears to cover a healing bruise or blemish on her face
   d. ___ Her mother-in-law insists on remaining with her throughout the examination.
   e. ___ When asked for details of her fall on the ice, Pritma's mother-in-law answers, and Pritma remains silent.

   Place a checkmark next to the observations suggesting that Pritma may be a victim of family violence and that she requires sensitive follow-up.

5. In her prenatal visit, Pritma is presenting in your office with depressive symptoms. She describes her overwhelming financial responsibilities to her siblings, since her father cannot work and the family relies on her for support.

Choose the most likely options (from the list of options provided) for the information missing from the following statement:

The nurse recognizes that the patient's (1)_____ symptoms may be due to lack of (2)_____ and excessive (3)_____ in the (4)_____. Finding solutions in the social (5)_____ of the (6)_____ may help to reduce burden and promote (7)_____.

Answer options:
burden
depression
mental health
mesosystem
microsystem
network
stress
support

6. At Pritma's first well-baby check and immunization appointment when her infant is 3 months of age, you administer a measure of postnatal depression as part of routine care in your public health unit. You observe two things: first, that Pritma's score is very high, indicating probable depression, and second, that she also scored positively on an item indicating suicidal ideation and possible postpartum psychosis.

For each of the nursing actions in the following table, use an "X" to indicate that the nursing action is *indicated* (appropriate or necessary), *contraindicated* (could be harmful), or *nonessential* (make no difference or not necessary) for the patient's care at this time. (Select only one response option per row.)

Nursing Action	Indi- cated	Contrain- dicated	Non- essential
a. Refer the patient to a mental health professional.			
b. Assess risk for suicidality.			
c. Attribute the mother's symptoms to the baby blues, which are experienced by 80% of new mothers.			
d. Request a prescription for an antipsychotic medication.			
e. Speak to the mother about treatment options for postpartum depression.			
f. Speak to the mother about how her symptoms of depression may impact her relationship with her child and child's development.			
g. Ask the mother whether she is on antidepressants.			
h. Ask the mother whether she is breastfeeding.			
i. Discuss/problem solve ways to enhance the mother's personal and professional social support resources.			

7. After a routine well-child visit with 24-year-old Pritma and her 6-month-old Ana (she/her), you referred the pair to a developmental pediatrics clinic for urgent assessment of failure-to-thrive in Ana. At the appointment, Ana presented as listless, lacking weight gain, and failing to meet developmental milestones. From Ana's chart, you are aware that Pritma was diagnosed with postpartum

depression (DSM-5 major depressive disorder with postpartum onset) when Ana was 4 months old. Pritma was also experiencing symptoms of suicidal ideation at that time. Now, at the 12-month follow-up well-child visit in your public health clinic, you learn that Pritma has been taking an antidepressant (selective serotonin reuptake inhibitor, SSRI) for 6 months. The medication has provided Pritma with some symptom relief, eliminating her suicidal ideation, but she is still experiencing some more moderate symptoms, such as fatigue and anxiety. You also learn that she has attended multiple sessions with her daughter at the developmental pediatrics clinic over the last 6 months.

For each of the assessment findings in the following table, use an "X" to indicate that the intervention was *effective* (helped to meet expected outcomes), *ineffective* (did not help to meet expected outcomes), or *unrelated* (not related to the expected outcomes). *(Select only one response option per row.)*

Assessment Finding	Effective	Ineffective	Unrelated
a. Ana meets developmental milestones.			
b. Ana is at a weight appropriate for her age.			
c. Pritma has decided not to return to work after her 1-year maternity leave.			
d. Pritma has become pregnant again.			
e. Pritma does not respond to her child's requests to play a game or hug during office visit.			
f. Ana does not react positively to being reunited with her mother on brief separation.			
g. Ana reaches out to the nurse for comfort after her needle-stick from immunization.			
h. Ana is comforted by her mother and rapidly returns to play after being upset by the needle-stick from immunization.			

8. At Pritma's 18-month well-child immunization visit, you learn that Pritma's child, Ana, has been receiving early intervention through the public health nursing office. This was indicated by Pritma's postpartum depression and observations of her child's developmental delay in the motor and cognitive domains at 12 months of age. For 6 months, they have been receiving biweekly home visits from early child development specialists, overseen by a public health nurse case manager.

For each of the assessment findings in the following table, use an "X" to indicate that the intervention was *effective* (helped to meet expected outcomes), *ineffective* (did not help to meet expected outcomes), or *unrelated* (not related to the expected outcomes). *(Select only one response option per row.)*

Assessment Finding	Effective	Ineffective	Unrelated
a. Ana does not cry from the immunization.			
b. Pritma is no longer depressed.			
c. Pritma reports a satisfying marriage with her husband.			
d. Ana's language development is at developmental level for her age.			
e. Ana does not walk, preferring to crawl around the office.			
f. Ana is in day care while her parents work.			
g. When Pritma asks Ana if she would like to read her favourite story book, Ana replies yes and recites much of the simple rhymes with her mother.			
h. Ana does not pick up finger foods; her mother has to feed them to her.			

Answers: 1. a, e, f, g; **2.** a, c, d, e, f, g; **3.** (1) elevated, (2) trauma, (3) abuse, (4) neglect, (5) depression, (6) dysfunction; **4.** a, b, c, d, e; **5.** (1) depression, (2) support, (3) stress, (4) microsystem, (5) network, (6) mesosystem, (7) mental health; **6.** Indicated nursing actions: a, b, e, f, g, i; Contraindicated nursing actions: c; Nonessential actions: d, h; **7.** Effective interventions: a, b, h; Ineffective interventions: e, f, g; Unrelated interventions: c, d; **8.** Effective interventions: d, g; Ineffective interventions: a, b, c, f.

🌐 *Rationales for the Review Questions appear on the Evolve website.*

RECOMMENDED WEBSITES

Alberta Family Wellness Initiative: https://www.albertafamilywellness.org
The Alberta Family Wellness Initiative began in Alberta, but the organization's work is used across Canada and the globe to support community and clinical agencies to understand how early experiences and genetics influence child development and health over the lifespan. Their free online resources include the Brain Story Toolkit, information about ACEs, resilience, parent–child interaction quality, and the Brain Story Certification, which enables learners to understand brain development from leading experts.

Centre for Health Promotion: https://www.canada.ca/en/public-health/services/health-promotion/centre-health-promotion.html
Part of the Public Health Agency of Canada, the Centre for Health Promotion uses a life stages approach and is responsible for implementing policies and programs that enhance the conditions conducive to healthy development. The centre addresses the determinants of health and facilitates successful movement through the life stages. Its programs address healthy child development, families, aging and lifestyles, public information, and education, as well as issues related to rural health and support of the voluntary sector.

Centre of Excellence for Early Childhood Development—Encyclopedia on Early Childhood Development: https://www.child-encyclopedia.com
The mandate of the Centre of Excellence for Early Childhood Development at the Université de Montréal is to foster the dissemination of scientific knowledge about the social and emotional development of young children and about the policies and services that influence this development. The centre also formulates recommendations for the services needed to ensure optimum early childhood development. The Encyclopedia on Early Childhood Development is one of the centre's projects. It covers a wide variety of issues and behaviours common to children from conception to age 5, with links to up-to-date scientific content written by leading researchers in the field.

Infant and Early Mental Health Promotion: https://www.imhpromotion.ca
The Infant and Early Mental Health Promotion program, housed at the Hospital for Sick Children in Toronto, is a coalition of professionals representing service agencies across Canada dedicated to promoting optimal outcomes for infants and preschoolers, in collaboration with families and other caregivers. Programs and advocacy initiatives are rooted in sound knowledge of the origins of healthy development in children, based on attachment theory, theories of social–emotional development, and emerging neuroscience. The program provides graduate certificates in infant and early child mental health and publishes a quarterly newsletter, among other initiatives.

Parent–Child Relationships Programs: https://www.pcrprograms.org
Based at the University of Washington, Seattle, this organization aims to give health professionals, parents, and other caregivers the knowledge and skills to provide nurturing environments for young children. PCRP disseminates and develops research-informed products and training programs for practitioners and researchers in many disciplines and settings, which can be used with typically developing children, with those at risk for developmental delays, and with those in whom special health care needs have been identified.

🌐 REFERENCES

A full reference list is available on the website for this book at http://evolve.elsevier.com/Canada/Potter/fundamentals/

23

Conception Through Adolescence

Canadian content written by Heather Meyerhoff, MSN, RN, and Sarah Liva, RN, PhD, with original chapter contributions by Bronwyn Doyle, RN, PhD, CNE

OBJECTIVES

Mastery of content in this chapter will enable you to:

- Define the key terms listed.
- Identify physiological and psychosocial health concerns during the transition of the child from intrauterine to extrauterine life.
- Describe characteristics of physical growth of the fetus and the child from birth to adolescence.
- Describe cognitive and psychosocial development from birth to adolescence.
- Describe the interactions that occur between parent and child.
- Explain the role of play in the development of the child.
- Identify factors that contribute to self-esteem in youth.
- Describe the influence of the school environment on the development of the child.
- Plan appropriate health promotion activities for children of all backgrounds.
- Describe ways in which you can help parents meet their children's developmental needs and promote health.

KEY TERMS

Adolescence
Animism
Apgar score
Artificialism
Blastocyst
Bonding
Circumcision
Classification
Concrete operations
Differentiation
Embryo
Estrogen
Fertilization
Fetus
Fontanels

Formal operations
Hyperbilirubinemia
Immanent justice
Implantation
Inborn errors of metabolism
Infancy
Lanugo
Menarche
Morula
Moulding
Naegele's rule
Neonatal period
Object permanence
Organogenesis
Placenta

Prematurity
Preoperational thought
Preschool period
Preterm labour
Puberty
Quickening
School-age
Sensorimotor period
Sexually transmitted infections (STIs)
Teratogens
Testosterone
Toddlerhood
Vernix caseosa
Zygote

WEBSITE

http://evolve.elsevier.com/Canada/Potter/fundamentals/

CASE STUDY

You are paired to work with Angele (preferred pronouns: they/them), a public health nurse in your community health clinical placement. Angele is scheduled to do follow-up assessments on newly discharged parents and infants in the morning and an immunization clinic in the afternoon.

It is morning; Angele is calling on Rochelle (preferred pronouns: she/her), a 32-year-old first-time parent who is 48 hours postpartum. Newborn Isolde is

healthy, delivered at term, weighs 3 200 grams, and has Apgar scores of 9 and 9. Rochelle is breastfeeding and concerned about milk coming in because Isolde is fussy and feeding frequently. Angele assesses Rochelle's feeding and arranges a follow-up home visit.

Think about this case study as you read this chapter. There are Review Questions at the end of the chapter about this case study.

It is imperative for nurses to have a foundational knowledge of human development and functioning (Canadian Association of Schools of Nursing [CASN], 2022). Human growth and development are continuous, intricate, complex processes that are divided into stages organized by age group. This arbitrary chronological division is used because it coincides with the timing and sequence of maturational changes that allow children to progress through a series of developmental stages and associated tasks (Box 23.1). This chapter focuses on the various physical, psychosocial, and cognitive changes that occur between conception and adolescence. It also focuses on health risks and concerns that may arise during the various stages of growth and development (see Chapter 22 for further information about developmental theories).

SELECTING A DEVELOPMENTAL FRAMEWORK FOR NURSING

Providing developmentally appropriate nursing care is easier when the care plan is based on a theoretical framework (see Chapter 22 for further information about theoretical frameworks). An organized, systematic approach ensures that children's needs are assessed and met by the plan. In a developmental approach, organized care is directed at an individual child's current level of functioning to motivate self-direction and health promotion; for example, the nurse might instruct parents to encourage toddlers to feed themselves in order to advance their developing independence and promote their sense of autonomy. Understanding an adolescent's need to be independent should prompt the nurse to negotiate with the adolescent to establish a contract about the care plan and its implementation. Also, parents may choose to have midwives, who provide developmentally appropriate individualized care, in their child-bearing experiences. In planning care, it is important for nurses to recognize that complex intersecting aspects of social identity (e.g., gender, sexuality, ethnicity) affect growth and development and health experiences (Etherington & Baker, 2018). Patient care needs will be diverse and uniquely shaped by intersecting social characteristics. All care planning should promote culturally safe (see Chapter 11), ethical (see Chapter 9), legal (see Chapter 10), and evidence-informed (see Chapter 8) care.

Conception

From the moment of conception, human growth proceeds at a predictable and rapid rate. During the prenatal period, the embryo grows from a single cell to a complex physiological being. All major organ systems develop in utero, and most function before birth.

Intrauterine Life

Intrauterine life that reaches full term usually lasts approximately 9 calendar months, or 40 weeks. The length of pregnancy is computed according to Naegele's rule, whereby you count back 3 months from the first day of the pregnant person's last menstrual period and then add 7 days. Fertilization occurs when a sperm penetrates the ovum and the material from both cell nuclei unites. The newly formed organism, known as a zygote, has its full genetic complement (1 pair of sex chromosomes and 22 pairs of autosomal chromosomes). The ovum and the sperm each contribute one chromosome to each pair of chromosomes. Through this mechanism, genetically determined characteristics (such as eye colour) are transmitted from parent to child and genetic conditions (such as Down syndrome) may result.

The zygote moves through the fallopian tube to the uterus within 3 to 4 days. During this time, the zygote continues to divide. Within 3 days, a solid ball of cells, the morula, has formed. The morula continues to develop and forms a central cavity, or blastocyst. Even at this early stage of development, cells begin to differentiate in structure and function. Cells at one end of the blastocyst develop into the embryo, and

those at the opposite end form the placenta. Between days 6 and 10, some of the cells secrete enzymes that allow the blastocyst to burrow into the endometrium and become completely covered; this process is known as implantation. Chorionic villi—fingerlike projections that emerge from the outer sac surrounding the embryo—obtain oxygen

BOX 23.1   Developmental Age Periods

Prenatal Period: Conception to Birth
Germinal: Conception to approximately 2 weeks
Embryonic: 2 to 8 weeks
Fetal: 8 to 40 weeks (birth)

Because of the rapid growth rate and total dependency of the embryo and fetus, this is one of the most mutable and vulnerable periods in the developmental process. The relationship between maternal health and certain manifestations of abnormalities in the newborn emphasizes the importance of adequate prenatal care to the health and well-being of the infant.

Infancy Period: Birth to Approximately 12 to 18 Months
Neonatal: Birth to 28 days
Infancy: 1 month to approximately 12 to 18 months

The infancy period is one of rapid motor, cognitive, and social development. Through bonding with the parent or other caregiver, the infant establishes a basic trust in the world and the foundation for future interpersonal relationships. The critical first month of life, termed the neonatal period, although part of infancy, is often differentiated from the remainder of infancy because it is characterized by major physical adjustments to extrauterine existence and by the psychosocial adjustment of the parents to their new roles.

Early Childhood: 1 to 6 Years
Toddler: 1 to 3 years
Preschooler: 3 to 6 years

This period, which extends from the time children begin walking until they start school, is characterized by intense activity and discovery. It is a time of marked physical and psychosocial development. Motor development advances steadily. Children at this age acquire language and wider social relationships, learn role standards, gain self-control and skill mastery, develop increasing awareness of dependence and independence, and begin to develop a self-concept.

Middle Childhood: 6 to 12 Years
Frequently referred to as the *school age*, this period of development is one in which children expand relationships outside the family group and activities revolve around peer relationships. The child's physical, cognitive, and psychosocial development advances steadily, with emphasis on developing skill competencies. Social cooperation and early moral development take on more importance, with relevance for later life stages. This is a critical period in the development of a self-concept.

Adolescence: 12 to Approximately 19 Years
The period of rapid maturation and change known as adolescence is considered to be a transitional period that begins at the onset of puberty and extends to the point of entry into the adult world—in Canada, high school graduation usually signals the beginning of adulthood. Biological and psychological maturation are accompanied by physical changes and emotional turmoil, and the self-concept is redefined. In the late adolescent period, children begin to internalize all previously learned values and to focus on an individual, rather than a group, identity.

Adapted from Hockenberry, M. J., Wilson, D., & Rodgers, C. C. (2019). *Wong's nursing care of infants and children* (11th ed.). Mosby.

and nutrition from the maternal blood supply and dispose of carbon dioxide and waste products.

The placenta produces essential hormones that maintain the pregnancy. It also provides nutrients to the developing fetus and removes wastes. Because the placenta is porous, noxious materials such as viruses and drugs can pass from parent to child. The effect of noxious agents on the fetus depends on the developmental stage in which exposure takes place; the embryonic stage (2 to 8 weeks after conception) is critical because the organ systems and the main external features are developing. The period of gestation is divided equally into three periods called trimesters.

First Trimester: 0 to 13 weeks. During the first trimester, the first 3 calendar months, fetal cells continue to differentiate and develop into essential organ systems. As cellular change (**differentiation**) and rapid organ growth (**organogenesis**) occur, each organ is vulnerable to conditions in the environment. Interference with growth can cause the congenital absence of an organ system or extensive structural or functional alterations. Because several organ systems develop at the same time, disruption of one system often occurs with disruption of others. Toward the end of the first trimester, it is possible to detect fetal heart sounds by fetoscopy or ultrasonography.

Second Trimester: 14 to 26 weeks. During the second trimester, from the end of the third month to the end of the sixth month, the height of the parent's uterus above the symphysis pubis is an indicator of fetal growth and approximate gestational age. Between 16 and 20 weeks, the parent begins to feel fetal movement. This feeling of life is referred to as **quickening**.

By the end of the sixth month, most of the fetal organ systems are complete and can function. The **fetus** is therefore considered viable, or capable of life outside the uterus, if given intensive environmental support. Fingers and toes are differentiated, rudimentary kidneys function, and the genitalia are defined. The fetus is covered with **vernix caseosa**, a cheese-like substance coating the skin. **Lanugo**, or fine hair, covers most of the body. These substances protect the thin, fragile skin and decrease in amount as the pregnancy nears its completion; thus, infants born before 38 weeks' gestation have more of these protective coverings than do full-term infants.

Third Trimester: 27 to 40 weeks. During the last 3 months of gestation, the fetus grows to approximately 50 cm in length. Subcutaneous fat is stored, and weight increases to between 3.2 and 3.4 kg. The skin thickens, lanugo begins to disappear, and the fetal body becomes rounder and fuller.

A tremendous spurt in brain growth begins during this trimester and lasts well into the first few years of life. The central nervous system has established its total number of neurons and connections between neurons, and myelination of nerve fibres progresses at a rapid rate.

At the end of the third trimester, the normal fetus is physically able to make the transition from intrauterine to extrauterine life. The circulatory system, which bypasses the right side of the heart (which, in turn, supplies the lungs with oxygen), can change its circulation to include the lungs. The lungs are capable of maintaining the inflated state for gas exchange. The primitive temperature maintenance systems, reflexes, and sensory organs are ready for use.

Health Promotion

As a nurse, you can address many topics with a patient during pregnancy to protect their health and that of the fetus. Such topics will vary according to the stage of pregnancy. Box 23.2 lists some of the topics to discuss with people and their partners during pregnancy.

TRANSITION FROM INTRAUTERINE TO EXTRAUTERINE LIFE

The transition from intrauterine to extrauterine life requires rapid changes in the newborn. As the nurse, you need to assess the newborn's ability to make these changes, and you should begin to plan before the birth for appropriate nursing interventions (Murray & McKinney, 2019). Circulatory, pulmonary, and thermal changes all contribute to the infant's adaptation to neonatal life. Gestational age and development, exposure to depressant drugs before or during labour, and the newborn's own behavioural style also influence the adjustment to the external environment. Therefore, initial assessment encompasses a variety of physical and psychosocial elements. You can also provide early opportunities for the parents and infant to develop close emotional bonds.

Physical Changes

The most extreme physiological change occurs when the newborn leaves the in utero circulation and assumes independent respiratory functioning. Nursing care is directed at maintaining an open airway, stabilizing and maintaining body temperature, and protecting the newborn from infection. The most widely used assessment tool, the **Apgar score**, rates heart rate, respiratory effort, muscle tone, reflex irritability, and colour in order to determine overall status. The Apgar assessment is generally conducted between 1 and 5 minutes after birth and may be repeated until the newborn's condition stabilizes. Table 23.1 outlines the scoring criteria of physiological functioning. A total score of 0 to 3 signifies severe distress, a score of 4 to 6 represents moderate difficulty, and a score of 7 to 10 indicates little difficulty in adjusting to extrauterine life. Nurses can use the Apgar score to determine areas requiring further assessment and careful observation. In addition, nurses need to monitor and record the newborn's early elimination patterns (i.e., voiding and passage of meconium), as well as body temperature and other vital signs.

Psychosocial Changes

After conducting a physical evaluation, it is important to promote the parents' and newborn's need for close physical contact. Early parent–child interaction encourages parent–child attachment or bonding. Physical factors (e.g., fatigue, hunger, and health) and emotional factors (e.g., needs for affection and touch) are assessed.

Merely placing the family together does not promote closeness. The parents and newborn must be willing and able to respond to each other. Most healthy newborns are awake and alert for the first half-hour after birth. This is a good time for parent–child interaction to begin. Close body contact, often including skin-to-skin

TABLE 23.1	Apgar Scoring		
Sign	**Score 0**	**Score 1**	**Score 2**
Heart rate	Absent	Slow, <100 bpm	>100 bpm
Respiratory effort	Absent	Irregular, slow, weak cry	Strong cry
Muscle tone	Limp	Some flexion of extremities	Strong flexion of extremities
Reflex irritability	No response	Grimace	Cry, sneeze
Colour	Blue, pale	Body pink, extremities blue	Completely pink

bpm, Beats per minute.
Adapted from Hockenberry, M. J., Wilson, D., & Rodgers, C.C. (2019). *Wong's nursing care of infants and children* (11th ed.). Mosby.

♥ BOX 23.2 FOCUS ON PRIMARY HEALTH CARE
Health Promotion Topics for the Patient During Pregnancy

First-Trimester Health Concerns
Nutrition

People with good nutritional practices have fewer complications during pregnancy and childbirth and bear healthier babies than do people with poor nutritional intake (Murray & McKinney, 2019). Inadequate prenatal nutrition has been associated with lower birth weight (Ahmed et al., 2018), and infants with low birth weight have an increased risk for learning disorders, temperament problems, neurological and motor impairment, and developmental delays. Folic acid (vitamin B9) intake must be adequate before and during pregnancy; the recommended daily dose is 0.4 mg. During pregnancy, people should eat foods rich in folic acid, such as leafy green vegetables, liver, lentils, and asparagus. Folic acid intake is believed to be responsible for decreasing the incidence of neural tube defects (Government of Canada, 2018). See Chapter 43 for more information on nutritional needs during pregnancy.

Teratogens

Agents capable of producing functional or structural damage to the developing fetus are called **teratogens**. Nurses need to educate the parent about avoiding exposure to teratogenic agents. One such teratogen is the rubella virus, which can cause stillbirth or congenital anomalies, primarily when exposure occurs in the first trimester. Many drugs are teratogenic during the first trimester. The nurse should assess the person's past and current use of home remedies, medications (prescription and over the counter), and illegal drugs. The benefits of any prescription medication needed to maintain the person's health during pregnancy must be weighed against potential harm to the fetus.

Cigarette smoke and alcohol are also teratogens. Smoking during pregnancy has been shown to reduce birth weight and increase the incidence of premature birth, fetal death, and neonatal death (Murray & McKinney, 2019). It is also considered a risk factor for impaired growth and development among young children (Guille & Aujla, 2019; Soesanti et al., 2019). Alcohol consumed during pregnancy is known to cause fetal alcohol syndrome, fetal alcohol effects, and alcohol-related birth defects. During pregnancy, people must be educated about the risks of cigarette smoke and alcohol to the developing fetus.

Second-Trimester Health Concerns
Preterm Labour

Preterm labour is labour that begins before the thirty-seventh week of pregnancy. With technological advances, it is possible for 500 g babies of 24 to 26 weeks' gestation to survive; however, the risk of morbidity and disability is significant. Causes of preterm labour are poorly understood and may be the result of maternal or fetal problems. Risk factors include physiological stresses such as renal and cardiovascular disease, diabetes mellitus, and uterine and cervical abnormalities. Urinary tract infections greatly increase the risk of preterm labour. Because of dramatic changes occurring in the renal system during pregnancy, it is possible for a person to have an asymptomatic urinary tract infection. Voiding habits should be discussed with the person during this time. People living in poverty, smokers, and those receiving poor prenatal care are at higher risk for preterm labour (Kliegman & St. Geme, 2020). The presence of multiple fetuses and fetal infections are two of the potential fetal factors for preterm labour. Interventions to prevent preterm labour include medications, intravenous fluids, and bed rest.

Third-Trimester Health Concerns
Choices of Birth Setting

In Canada, beginning in the early 1920s, childbirth gradually moved into hospital settings; by 1950, approximately 76% of births were taking place in hospitals (Mitchinson, 2002) because emergency backup was available in case of birth complications. Many hospitals have taken a family-centred approach to childbirth.

In some areas of the country, birthing centres are available for people who prefer a more homelike setting. People delivering in this setting are required to attend childbirth classes, and the pregnancy must be considered low risk. Physicians and midwives with hospital privileges may attend births in these facilities. Patients must understand that they may be transferred to a hospital if the conditions warrant.

A growing number of people choose to deliver at home when professional midwifery services are available. Control over the birth process and the desire for a more natural birth are common reasons why some people choose home births. Another reason is that it allows the entire family or other people close to the family to be part of the birth. Nurses can support the parent by offering information and resources to help them choose the birth setting.

---

contact and breastfeeding, is a satisfying way for most families to start. If immediate contact is not possible, it should be incorporated into the care plan as early as possible, which may mean bringing the newborn to an ill parent or bringing the parents to an ill or premature child.

Bonding occurs when parents and newborn elicit reciprocal and complementary behaviour. Parental bonding behaviours include attentiveness and physical contact. Newborn bonding behaviour involves maintenance of physical contact with the parent. Preterm newborns, ill newborns, and ill parents may have difficulty forming this bond if separation is prolonged; they need to be carefully assessed for any problems with attachment. The bonding process is further complicated if parents are unable to care for the infant. Nurses should give the parents support throughout the early bonding process, particularly if the newborn or parent is ill or if the newborn is separated from the parents.

Wiping excess nasopharyngeal and oropharyngeal secretions away with a towel ensures airway patency. Newborns are susceptible to heat loss and cold stress (Kliegman & St. Geme, 2020). Because hypothermia increases oxygen needs, the newborn's body temperature must be

stabilized and maintained. The newborn may be placed skin-to-skin (directly on the parent's abdomen and covered in warm blankets); dried and wrapped in warm blankets, with the head well covered; or dried and placed unclothed in an infant warmer with a temperature probe in place. The practice of immediately placing the infant skin-to-skin is recommended for healthy newborns because of its many benefits, including temperature regulation, breastfeeding, and parental–newborn bonding (Bigelow & Power, 2020; Breastfeeding Committee of Canada, 2021). For newborns unable to sustain adequate body temperature, isolettes and incubators, which supply radiant heat, are preferred.

Prevention of infection is a major concern in the care of the newborn, whose immune system is immature. Good hand hygiene technique is the most important factor in protecting the newborn and the nurse from infection. Other standard precautions include wearing gloves when touching mucous membranes or skin that is not intact (e.g., as a result of surgery or injury) and when drawing blood (e.g., heel stick).

The most commonly used prophylactic treatment against ophthalmic conjunctivitis is erythromycin (0.5%) because it prevents infections with *Neisseria gonorrhoeae* and other organisms, which can be transmitted during passage through an infected vaginal canal. This treatment should be applied during the newborn's initial assessment with parental consent.

Vitamin K is most commonly administered in a single intramuscular injection shortly after birth. Vitamin K is important for the synthesis of prothrombin, a protein necessary for clotting. Normally, the intestinal flora synthesize vitamin K, and by about the third day the infant should have enough intestinal flora to start to synthesize its own vitamin K.

The stump of the moist umbilical cord is an excellent medium for bacterial growth. The cord should be cleansed with soap and water and dried at each diaper change. Until the stump dries and falls off, the diaper should be folded below the umbilicus to prevent accumulation of moisture.

NEWBORN

The neonatal period is the first month of life. During this stage, the newborn's physical functioning is mostly reflexive, and stabilization of the major organ systems is the body's primary task. Behaviour greatly influences interaction between the newborn and the environment and caregivers. For example, the average 2-week-old newborn may smile and is able to regard the parent's face. The effect of these reflexive behaviours is generally a surge of feelings of love that prompt the parent to cuddle the baby.

Nurses can apply their knowledge of this stage of growth and development to promote neonatal and parental health. If the nurse understands, for example, that the newborn's cry is usually a response to an unmet need (such as hunger), the nurse can assist parents in identifying ways to meet those needs, such as counselling the parents to feed their baby on demand rather than on a rigid schedule.

Physical Changes

A comprehensive nursing assessment is usually performed as soon as the newborn's physiological functioning is stable, generally within a few hours after birth. The infant's height, weight, head circumference, temperature, pulse, and respirations should be measured, and general appearance, body functions, sensory capabilities, reflexes, and responsiveness observed.

The average newborn weighs 3 400 g, is 50 cm in length, and has a head circumference of 35 cm. Up to 10% of birth weight is lost in the first few days after birth, primarily owing to fluid losses through respiration, urination, defecation, and low fluid intake. Birth weight is usually regained by the second week after birth, and a gradual pattern of increase in weight, height, and head circumference is evident. During the first month, weekly increases average 226 to 455 g in weight, 0.6 to 2.5 cm in length, and 2 cm in head circumference.

The newborn's heart rate ranges from 120 to 160 beats per minute. The average blood pressure is 85/54 mm Hg. The newborn's respiratory movements are primarily abdominal and vary in rate and rhythm, with an average rate of 30 to 60 breaths per minute. The axillary temperature ranges from 36°C to 37.5°C and generally stabilizes within 24 hours after birth.

Normal physical characteristics include the continued presence of lanugo on the skin of the back; cyanosis of the hands and feet for the first 24 hours; and a soft, protuberant abdomen. Skin colour varies according to racial and genetic heritage and gradually changes during infancy. **Moulding**, or overlapping of the soft skull bones, allows the fetal head to adjust to various diameters of the maternal pelvis and is a common occurrence with vaginal births. The bones readjust within a

few days, producing a rounded appearance. The sutures and **fontanels** are usually palpable at birth. Figure 23.1 shows the diamond shape of the anterior fontanel and the triangular shape of the posterior fontanel between the unfused bones of the skull.

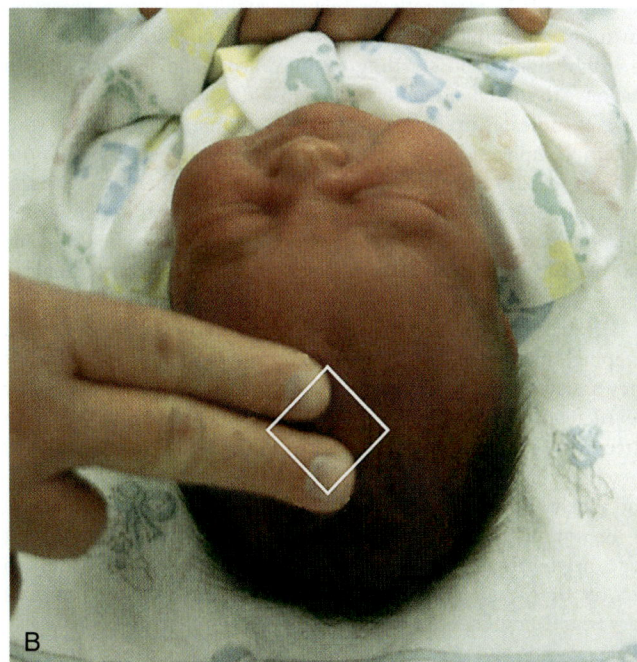

FIGURE 23.1 Fontanels and suture lines. (Adapted from Hockenberry, M. J., Wilson, D., & Rodgers, C. C. [2019]. *Wong's nursing care of infants and children* [11th ed.]. Mosby.)

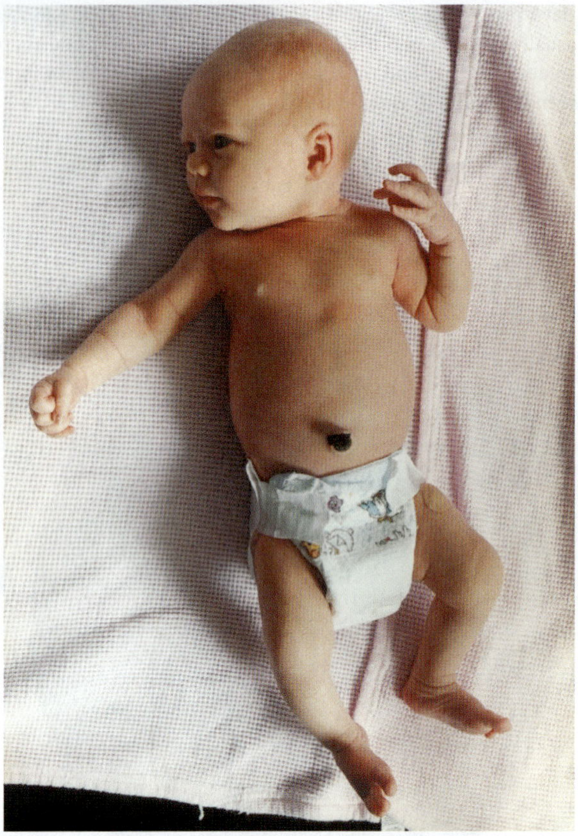

nipple (rooting) and learn that crying results in feeding, diapering, and cuddling by the parent.

Sensory functions contribute to cognitive development in the newborn. At birth, children can fixate on moving objects about 20 to 25 cm from their faces (Hockenberry et al., 2019). A preference for the human face is apparent. Auditory and vestibular (i.e., equilibrium) systems function from birth. These sensory capabilities allow newborns to elicit stimuli rather than simply receive them. Parents should be taught the importance of providing sensory stimulation, such as talking to their newborns and holding them to see their faces. This allows infants to seek or take in stimuli, thereby enhancing learning and cognitive development.

Psychosocial Changes

During the first month of life, parents and newborns normally develop a strong bond that grows into a deep attachment. Interactions during routine care enhance or detract from the attachment process. The processes of feeding, changing, bathing, and comforting an infant promote interaction and provide a foundation for deep attachments. Early on, older siblings should have the opportunity to be involved with the newborn. Family involvement helps support growth and development and promotes nurturing.

If parents or newborns experience health complications after birth, bonding may be compromised. Infants' behavioural cues may be weak or absent, and caregiving may be less mutually satisfying. Tired or ill parents have difficulty interpreting and responding to their infants' cues. Children who have congenital anomalies are often too weak to be responsive to parental cues and require special supportive nursing care. For example, infants born with heart defects may tire easily during feedings. They may rest frequently after several bursts of sucking. They may awaken frequently, crying because they are hungry again. People may think that they are inadequate as parents or that the infants are being fussy. Both infants and parents may feel frustrated. In this case, bonding is not enhanced and may even be reduced unless nursing intervention breaks the sequence of events.

For newborns, crying is a means of communication and provides cues to parents (Lowdermilk et al., 2020). Although it can be a sign of distress, such as from pain, crying is an adaptive response to extrauterine life. Babies may cry because their diapers are wet, they are hungry, they want to be held, or they need a change in position or activity. Between 2 weeks and 3 to 4 months of age, it is normal for infants to cry for several hours a day (Perinatal Services British Columbia, 2019). Infants may be difficult to soothe at times and crying can be unexpected, which can frustrate parents if no cause is apparent (HealthLink BC, 2021). Nurses can support parents by normalizing and suggesting strategies to safely manage crying (National Centre on Shaken Baby Syndrome, n.d.). With help, parents can learn to recognize infants' cues and cry patterns and take appropriate action when necessary, including seeking help when needed (Lowdermilk et al., 2020).

Health Risks

Hyperbilirubinemia is a condition caused by the excessive accumulation of bilirubin in the blood, resulting in yellowish skin, or jaundice (Lowdermilk et al., 2020). The accumulation occurs when the infant's immature liver is unable to balance the destruction of red blood cells with the use or excretion of byproducts (Lowdermilk et al., 2020). The balance can be further upset by prematurity, inadequate intake during breastfeeding, excess production of bilirubin, certain disease states, or a disturbance in the liver. Bilirubin at high levels is highly toxic to neurons, and affected newborns are at risk for brain injury (Canadian Paediatric Society, 2018). Phototherapy is used to help break down the bilirubin for easier excretion. During phototherapy, the infant's eyes

FIGURE 23.2 Tonic neck reflex. Newborns assume this position while supine. (From Hockenberry, M. J., Wilson, D., & Rodgers, C. C. [2019]. *Wong's nursing care of infants and children* [11th ed.]. Mosby. Courtesy Paul Vincent Kuntz, Texas Children's Hospital.)

To assess neurological function, the newborn's level of activity, alertness, irritability, responsiveness to stimuli, and reflexes should be observed. Normal reflexes include sucking, rooting, grasping, yawning, coughing, sneezing, hiccupping, blinking in response to bright lights, and startling (pulling arms and legs inward) in response to sudden, loud noises. An absence of any of these or other reflexes indicates **prematurity**, possible trauma, or central nervous system complications. Because the newborn depends largely on reflexes for survival and response to its environment, it is necessary to assess them. Figure 23.2 shows the tonic neck reflex: When newborns are lying supine, they reflexively turn the head to one side, extend the arm and leg on that side, and flex the opposite arm and leg.

Normal newborn behaviours include periods of sucking, crying, sleeping, and wakefulness. Movements are generally sporadic, but they are symmetrical and involve all four extremities. The relatively flexed fetal position of intrauterine life continues as the newborn attempts to maintain an enclosed, secure feeling. Newborns respond to sensory stimuli, particularly the primary caregiver's face, voice, and touch.

Except for the first hour after birth, when they are in a quiet alert state, newborns sleep almost continuously for the first 2 to 3 days to recover from the exhausting birth process. Thereafter, sleep periods vary from 20 minutes to 6 hours with little day–night differentiation.

Cognitive Changes

Early cognitive development begins with innate behaviour, reflexes, and sensory functions. Newborns initiate reflex activities and learn behaviours and desires. For example, newborns reflexively turn to the

must be shielded because they can be damaged by the light. Because excretion of the extra bilirubin can cause watery stools, adequate fluid balance in the infant must be maintained.

Health Concerns

Feeding Alternatives. Supplying essential nutrients to the infant is an important goal for parents. Nurses can support the parents' choice of feeding methods and facilitate a successful feeding process (Box 23.3). Since promotion of breastfeeding can contribute to maternal guilt, nurses need to develop a respectful, collaborative partnership with parents when discussing feeding choices in order to minimize feelings of guilt (Grant et al., 2018). Breastfeeding is considered the most complete nutritional source until the infant is about 6 months of age. Parents are encouraged to continue breastfeeding for up to 2 years or even longer, if both the parent and child want to continue (Canadian Paediatric Society, 2020a). Breastmilk contains protein, fats, and carbohydrates, as well as immunoglobulins that bolster the infant's ability to resist infection. Breastfeeding has been associated with enhanced cognitive development and parent–child bonding and a decreased frequency of respiratory tract illnesses, sudden infant death syndrome, type 1 and type 2 diabetes, childhood leukemia, obesity, gastroenteritis, necrotizing enterocolitis, otitis media, atopic dermatitis, food allergies, and childhood internalizing behaviour problems (Hockenberry et al., 2019; Kliegman & St. Geme, 2020).

Screening. Screening tests and other laboratory tests should be coordinated as needed. Blood tests can determine **inborn errors of metabolism** (Hockenberry et al., 2019). This term applies to genetic disorders caused by the absence or deficiency of a substance, usually an enzyme, essential to cellular metabolism that results in abnormal protein, carbohydrate, or fat metabolism. Although inborn errors of metabolism are rare, they account for a significant proportion of health problems in children. Neonatal screening can detect phenylketonuria (PKU), hypothyroidism, and galactosemia and thus allow appropriate treatment in order to prevent permanent intellectual disability and other health problems. Routine screening of newborns for PKU is recommended (Kliegman & St. Geme, 2020). Other screening (e.g., for cystic fibrosis or hemophilia) may be necessary, depending on the family history.

Circumcision. **Circumcision** is the removal of the foreskin (prepuce) of the penis (Lowdermilk et al., 2020, p. 516). It is controversial in Canada and is not recommended as a routine procedure by the Canadian Paediatric Society (2021a). The controversy surrounds the risks and benefits of the procedure, especially with regard to pain control. Risks have been identified as hemorrhage, infection, adhesions, and meatal stenosis. Benefits include prevention of penile cancer, prevention of urinary tract infections, and preservation of male body image to be consistent with that of peers when circumcision is part of the culture (Hockenberry et al., 2019). Parents must give informed consent before the procedure. Care of the circumcised site depends on the type of method used for the procedure. Circumcised newborns should be checked frequently for evidence of swelling, oozing, excessive bleeding, and the ability to void.

INFANT

Infancy, the period from 1 month to 1 year of age, is characterized by dramatic physical growth and change. Psychosocial development advances, and interactions between infants and the environment are greater and more meaningful.

BOX 23.3 RESEARCH HIGHLIGHT
Breastfeeding

Research Focus

Nongestational partners in same-sex female relationships may induce lactation in order to co-nurse with the gestational partner. Nurses can support families' perceptions of respect and inclusiveness through education and awareness of diversity in feeding practices.

Research Abstract

Juntreal and Spatz (2020) explored the breastfeeding experiences of birthing partners in same-sex female relationships. The qualitative study was performed with a small sample of birth partners ($n = 18$) in the United States and the United Kingdom. The researchers found that birth partners wanted health care providers to view nongestational partners as essential and equivalent to them in parenthood. Participants wanted ways to share feeding experiences with their partners and desired more clinically competent health care providers who were knowledgeable about induced lactation and the unique needs of co-nursing parents. The researchers concluded that health care providers need to incorporate more inclusive language and seek education about the diverse needs of breastfeeding parents.

Implications for Practice

Assess breastfeeding expectations and desires with birth parents and non-gestational partners.

Provide education about induced lactation and co-nursing to same-sex female couples to support feeding decision making.

Seek ways to involve the nongestational parents in breastfeeding experiences.

Advocate for inclusive language in breastfeeding policies.

From Juntreal, N., & Spatz, D. (2020). Breastfeeding experiences of same-sex mothers, *Birth*, *47*(1), 21–28. https://doi.org/10.1111/birt.12470

Physical Changes

Steady and proportional growth of the infant is more important than absolute growth values. The infant's growth can be compared with charts of normal age- and gender-related growth measurements. Using growth charts, nurses can also evaluate an infant's growth patterns by recording weight, length, and head circumference at selected intervals. Measurements recorded over time are the best way to monitor growth and identify problems. An infant with a growth problem may have measurements generally below the expected norms at all intervals or may experience an acute, brief interference with growth. An infant with a feeding problem or a genetic condition such as cystic fibrosis may have a weight below the expected norm.

Size increases rapidly during the first year; birth weight doubles by approximately 5 months of age and triples by 12 months. On average, weight gain is 680 g during the first 5 months and 340 g for months 7 to 12. Height increases an average of 2.5 cm during each of the first 6 months and 3.8 cm for the next 6 months. This 50% increase in birth height occurs primarily in the trunk, with the chest diameter approximating that of the head by the first birthday (Hockenberry et al., 2019). The fontanels become smaller; the posterior fontanel closes at about 2 months.

Physiological functioning stabilizes. By the end of the first year, the heart rate is 90 to 140 beats per minute, the blood pressure averages 95/65 mm Hg, and the respiratory rate is 30 to 35 breaths per minute. Patterns of body function also stabilize as evidenced by predictable sleep, elimination, and feeding routines. Motor development proceeds steadily in a cephalocaudal direction (from the head toward the feet).

Cognitive Changes

The infant learns by experiencing and manipulating the environment. Developing motor skills and increasing mobility expand an infant's environment and, with developing visual and auditory skills, enhance cognitive development. For these reasons, Piaget (1952) named his first stage of cognitive development, which extends until around the third birthday, the sensorimotor period (see Chapter 22 for further information about developmental theories). Before the acquisition of language, the extraordinary development of the mind occurs through children's developing senses and motor abilities. Improved visual acuity and eye–hand coordination allow grasping and exploration of objects. In addition, rudimentary colour vision begins by age 2 months and improves throughout the first year, making the environment more interesting to see and explore. Infants' hearing also improves, allowing localization and discrimination of sounds.

Infants need opportunities to develop and use their senses. It is important to evaluate the appropriateness and adequacy of these opportunities. For example, ill or hospitalized infants may lack the energy to interact with their environments, and thus their cognitive development may be slowed. Infants need to be stimulated according to their temperament, energy, and age. Stimulation strategies can be used that maximize development of infants while conserving their energy and orientation. An example of this approach is talking to an infant and encouraging them to suck on a pacifier while administering a tube feeding.

Language. Speech is an important aspect of cognition that develops during the first year. Infants proceed from crying, cooing, and laughing to imitating sounds, comprehending the meaning of simple commands, and repeating words with knowledge of their meaning (Hockenberry et al., 2019). One-year-old children can recognize their own names and have two- or three-word vocabularies, usually including "Da-Da," "Ma-Ma," and "no." Nurses can promote language development by encouraging parents to name objects on which their infants' attention is focused.

Psychosocial Changes

Separation. During their first year, infants begin to differentiate themselves from other people, understanding that they are separate beings capable of acting on their own. Initially, infants are unaware of the boundaries of self, but through repeated experiences with the environment, they learn where the self ends and the external world begins. As infants determine their physical boundaries, they begin to respond to others.

At 2 or 3 months of age, infants begin to smile responsively rather than reflexively (Hockenberry et al., 2019). Similarly, they can recognize differences in people when their sensory and cognitive capabilities improve. By 8 months, most infants can differentiate a stranger from a familiar person and respond differently to the two (Hockenberry et al., 2019). Close attachment to the primary caregivers, most often parents, is usually established by this age. Infants seek out these people for support and comfort during times of stress. The ability to distinguish self from others allows children to interact and socialize within their environments. By 9 months of age, for example, children play simple social games, such as patty-cake and peekaboo (Hockenberry et al., 2019). More complex interactive games, such as hide-and-seek and play involving objects, are possible by time a child is 1 year old (Hockenberry et al., 2019). Erikson (1963) described the psychosocial developmental crisis for the infant as trust versus mistrust. If the infant's physical and emotional needs are met, then the infant begins to develop a sense of security (see Chapter 22 for further information about developmental theories).

Nurses should assess the availability and appropriateness of experiences that contribute to psychosocial development. Hospitalized infants may have difficulty establishing physical boundaries because of repeated bodily intrusions and painful sensations. Limiting these negative experiences and providing pleasurable sensations are interventions that support early psychosocial development. Extended separations from parents complicate the bonding process and increase the number of caregivers with whom the infant must interact. Ideally, the parents should provide the majority of care during hospitalization. When parents are not present, an attempt should be made to limit the number of caregivers who have contact with the infant and to follow the parents' directions for care. These interventions will foster the infant's continuing development of trust.

Play. Play is a meaningful set of activities through which individuals interact with their environment and relate to others. Play provides opportunities for the infant to develop many motor skills (Hockenberry et al., 2019). Much of infant play is exploratory, inasmuch as infants use their senses to observe and examine their own bodies and objects of interest in their surroundings. For example, placing their toes in their mouths provides infants with pleasure and information about their own body and helps form their early self-concept. Play becomes manipulative as children learn control of the hands. Adults can facilitate infant learning by planning activities that promote the development of milestones and by providing toys that are safe for infants to explore with the mouth and manipulate with the hands, such as rattles, blocks, stacking rings, and washable stuffed animals. Infants most frequently engage in solitary (one-sided) play, but they do enjoy watching others, particularly siblings. Infants need to be played with and stimulated through interactions with others.

Health Risks

Sudden Infant Death Syndrome. Sudden infant death syndrome (SIDS) is the sudden and unexpected death of an apparently healthy infant. SIDS is rare before 1 month of age, but its incidence peaks among infants between 2 and 4 months of age, and it can occur in infants up to a year old. Other terms for SIDS include sudden unexplained infant death (SUID) and sudden unexpected death in infancy (SUDI). SIDS is the second leading cause of death among infants aged 1 month to 1 year old (Public Health Agency of Canada [PHAC], 2021a). The cause of SIDS is complex and not well understood, but PHAC (2021b) recommends taking the following precautions:

- Infants should sleep alone on their backs on a firm, flat surface alone (i.e., sharing any sleeping surface with another person is hazardous to the infant).
- A smoke-free environment should be provided before and after birth.
- For every sleep, infants should sleep in a crib, cradle, or bassinet that meets current Canadian regulations.
- The crib should be placed next to the adult's bed for the first 6 months.
- A baby's crib must be free of clutter such as toys, bumper pads, pillows, blankets, and other loose bedding. Babies do not need blankets when they sleep. If desired, a well-fitting sleep sack may be used.
- The infant should sleep in a room at room temperature in one-piece fitted sleepwear.
- Infants should be breastfed if possible.

In research studies, the following maternal and antenatal risk factors were associated with a higher risk of SIDS: smoking, alcohol and illicit drug use, inadequate prenatal care, nutritional deficiency, low socioeconomic status, younger age, lower education, single marital status, shorter interpregnancy interval, intrauterine hypoxia, fetal growth restriction, and elevated second-trimester serum α-fetoprotein (Blair et al., 2018; Kliegman & St. Geme, 2020; PHAC, 2021b). Infant risk factors have included age (peak 2 to 4 months), male sex, race and ethnicity (Black, Indigenous, and other minorities), growth failure, no breastfeeding, no pacifier use, prematurity, prone and side sleep position, recent febrile illness, inadequate immunizations, smoking exposure, soft sleeping surface or bedding, bed sharing, thermal stress, overheating, colder season, and no central heating (Blair et al., 2018; Kliegman & St. Geme, 2020).

Accidental Injury. Injury is a major cause of death in children 6 to 12 months old. An understanding of the major developmental accomplishments during this period helps nurses plan for injury prevention. Box 23.4 lists the main types of injuries that occur in this age group and possible prevention strategies.

Child Maltreatment. Nurses need to be aware that child maltreatment may occur during any stage of a child's life, including during infancy. *Child maltreatment* refers to violence, emotional or sexual mistreatment, or neglect of a child or adolescent. More children suffer from neglect than from any other type of maltreatment. Many suffer from more than one type of child maltreatment. In infancy, abusive head trauma that results from vigorous infant shaking is the most common form of maltreatment (HealthLink BC, 2021). Up to 25% of infants who are shaken die, and 80% have permanent brain damage (HealthLink BC, 2021). For this reason, nurses must emphasize to parents that they should never shake their baby in response to crying or frustration. Nurses need to be knowledgeable about the impacts of early childhood maltreatment, relevant legislation, and prevention and intervention strategies to fulfill professional responsibilities (British Columbia College of Nurses and Midwives, 2021; Government of British Columbia, 2017). Research on adverse childhood experiences (ACEs) over the past few decades has provided strong evidence about the significant impact of early childhood experiences on long-term health (Centers for Disease Control and Prevention [CDC], 2021; Felitti et al., 1998). Exposure to abuse, neglect, or household dysfunction in childhood affects development and is linked with lasting negative occupational, relational, and health effects (CDC, 2021). Box 23.5 highlights the initial landmark ACEs study findings that provided foundational evidence for current clinical understandings of early childhood and long-term health.

In Ontario, the incidence of child abuse and neglect is 16 confirmed cases for every 1 000 children (Canadian Child Welfare Research Portal, 2020). Protection of children from maltreatment comes under the jurisdiction of a province or territory. If you suspect any type of maltreatment of children, you are legally required to report it. Document the location and a detailed description of all injuries, and include diagrams and photographs of the injuries using a measurement tool (Hockenberry et al., 2019). Box 23.6 includes possible signs and symptoms of child maltreatment. These indications apply to children from infancy through adolescence.

A combination of signs and symptoms or a pattern of injury should arouse suspicion. It is important to be aware of certain birthmarks (e.g., Mongolian spots, which are flat, dark birthmarks that may look like bruises) and cultural practices (e.g., coining, in which the skin is rubbed or scratched with a coin to improve circulation or restore balance) that may mimic signs of maltreatment.

Health Concerns
Nutrition. The quality and quantity of nutrition influence the infant's growth and development. Nurses need to help parents select a nutritionally adequate diet for their infant. Nutrition is affected by many variables (e.g., culture, food preferences, slow eating, or food allergies), and no single diet will be effective for all children in an age group.

If breastfeeding is not possible or not desired by the parent, parents can feed their infant commercially prepared formula that is fortified with iron. Formulas contain standard ingredients and are fortified with vitamins and minerals. Cow's milk and imitation milks are not recommended in the first year because infants are not able to properly digest the contained fat. If parents introduce cow's milk, they are advised to wait until at least 9 months and to limit intake to less than 750 mL per day (Canadian Paediatric Society, 2020a). Cow's milk also contains more sodium and protein and less iron and essential nutrients than does formula (Hockenberry et al., 2019). Because cow's milk has low levels of iron and high levels of calcium and phosphorus, absorption of iron may be decreased, causing anemia.

The average 1-month-old infant takes in approximately 540 to 630 mL of breast milk or formula per day. This amount increases slightly during the first 6 months and decreases when solid foods are introduced. The amount of formula per feeding and the number of feedings vary among infants.

Developmentally, infants are not ready for solid food until 6 months of age. Before 6 months, the infant's gastrointestinal tract cannot handle the complex nutrients in solid food, and the extrusion reflex causes food to be pushed out of the mouth. Also, early introduction to solid foods may cause food allergies.

Cereals and well-cooked puréed fruits, vegetables, and meats eaten during the second 6 months of life provide iron and additional sources of vitamins. These nutrients become especially important when infants stop consuming breast milk or formula and begin drinking whole cow's milk after the first birthday. Iron-rich meat, meat alternatives, and iron-fortified cereals are recommended as the first foods to introduce (Canadian Paediatric Society, 2020a). It is recommended to introduce lumpy textures no later than 9 months of age and to progress to a variety of textures before the end of the first year (Canadian Paediatric Society, 2020a). Because the amount and frequency of feedings vary among infants, it is important to discuss differing feeding patterns with parents.

Honey has been used to sweeten water and coat pacifiers. However, honey should not be given to infants younger than 1 year because of the potential for infant botulism poisoning (Kliegman & St. Geme, 2020).

Supplementation. The need for dietary vitamin and mineral supplements depends on the infant's diet. Full-term infants are born with some iron stores. The breastfed infant absorbs adequate iron from breast milk during the first 4 to 6 months of life. After 6 months of age, iron-fortified cereal is generally considered an adequate supplemental source. Because the iron in formula is less readily absorbed than that in breast milk, formula-fed infants should receive iron-fortified formula throughout the first year. All Canadian infants who are breastfed need to receive a daily 400 IU vitamin D supplement to prevent rickets (PHAC, 2020a).

Adequate concentrations of fluoride to protect against dental caries are not available in human milk, so fluoridated water or supplemental fluoride is generally recommended. The presence of fluoride in formula depends on the type of formula and the source of water used in preparing the concentrated forms. Fluoride supplementation may be necessary.

Infant Overfeeding and Obesity. The association between overfeeding, infant obesity, and later adult obesity is controversial. However, early feeding experiences can influence later eating habits. Nurses can support the development of healthy dietary habits through educating parents about hunger and satiety cues, emphasizing balanced nutrition and the importance of mutually satisfying feeding experiences. Perceptions about eating and weight can be influenced by the family's

BOX 23.4 | Injury Prevention During Infancy

Age: Birth to 4 Months
Major Developmental Accomplishments

Involuntary reflexes, such as the crawling reflex, may propel the infant forward or backward, and the startle reflex may cause the body to jerk.

The infant may roll over.

Eye–hand coordination improves, and the voluntary grasp reflex increases.

Injury Prevention
Aspiration

Aspiration is not as great a danger in this age group as in others, but caregivers should begin to practise safeguarding early (see "Age: 4 to 7 Months" section in Box 23.4).

Hold the infant for bottle feeding; do not prop the bottle.

Know emergency procedures for choking.

Use pacifiers with one-piece construction and loop handle.

Suffocation and Drowning

Keep all plastic bags stored out of the infant's reach; discard large plastic garment bags after tying them in a knot.

Do not cover the infant's mattress with plastic.

Use a firm mattress; do not use pillows or loose bedding.

Make sure crib design follows federal regulations and the mattress fits snugly; crib slats should be no farther than 6 cm apart. Do not use a drop-side crib.

Position the crib away from other furniture and away from radiators.

Do not tie a pacifier on a string around the infant's neck.

Remove bibs at bedtime.

Never leave the infant alone in a bath.

If the infant is younger than 12 months, do not leave them alone on an adult- or youth-sized mattress or on "beanbag"-type pillows.

Falls

Use a crib with fixed, raised rails.

Never leave the infant on a raised, unguarded surface.

When in doubt as to where to place the child, use the floor.

Restrain the child in an infant seat, and never leave them unattended while the seat is resting on a raised surface.

Avoid using a high chair until the child can sit well with support.

Poisoning

Poisoning is not as great a danger in this age group as in others, but caregivers should begin to practise safeguards early (see "Age: 4 to 7 Months" section in Box 23.4).

Burns

Install smoke detectors in the home.

Avoid warming formula in a microwave oven; always check temperature of liquid before feeding.

Check bath water temperature.

Do not pour hot liquids when the infant is close by (e.g., sitting on lap).

Do not smoke cigarettes around the child.

Do not leave infant in the sun for more than a few minutes; keep exposed areas covered.

Wash flame-retardant clothes according to label directions.

Use cool-mist (rather than hot-mist) vaporizers.

Do not leave the child in a parked car.

Check the surface heat of the car restraint before placing the child in it.

Motor Vehicles

Transport the infant in a federally approved rear-facing infant car seat that has been secured in the back seat.*

Never place infant on seat of car or in lap while driving.

Never place an infant seat in the front passenger seat with an air bag.*

Do not place infant in a carriage or stroller behind a parked car.

Do not leave infant in a vehicle on a warm day.

Bodily Damage

Keep sharp, jagged objects out of infant's reach.

Keep diaper pins closed and away from infant.

Never shake a baby (which can cause shaken baby syndrome); advise caregivers to seek help if they feel irritated or overwhelmed by a baby's crying.

Age: 4 to 7 Months
Major Developmental Accomplishments

The infant rolls over.

The infant sits momentarily.

The infant grasps and manipulates small objects.

The infant picks up a dropped object.

The infant has well-developed eye–hand coordination.

The infant can focus on and locate very small objects.

The infant's tendency to put objects in their mouth is prominent.

The infant can push up on hands and knees.

The infant crawls backward.

Injury Prevention
Aspiration

Keep buttons, beads, syringe caps, and other small objects out of the infant's reach.

Keep the floor free of any small objects.

Do not feed the infant hard candy, nuts, food with pits or seeds, or whole or circular pieces of hot dog.

Exercise caution when giving the infant teething biscuits because large chunks may be broken off and aspirated.

Do not feed the infant while they are lying down.

Inspect toys for removable parts.

Suffocation

Keep all latex balloons out of the child's reach.

Remove all crib toys that are strung across the crib or playpen when the infant begins to push up on hands or knees or is 5 months old.

Use only cribs with well-secured crib sides; do not use drop-side cribs.

Falls

Restrain the infant in a high chair.

Do not use baby walkers (baby walkers are no longer sold in or imported to Canada because of the high rate of injuries that they cause).

Poisoning

Make sure that paint for furniture or toys does not contain lead.

Hang plants or place them on high surfaces rather than on the floor.

Store coin-like batteries and any toxic substances, such as cleaning fluid, paints, and pesticides, out of the reach of babies, either on a high shelf or in a locked cabinet.

Discard used containers of poisonous substances.

Do not store toxic substances in food containers.

Store medication in a locked cabinet, and keep cosmetics and personal care products out of the child's reach.

BOX 23.4 Injury Prevention During Infancy—cont'd

Know the telephone number of the local poison control centre (usually listed in the beginning of telephone directories) and add it to list of contacts on mobile phone.

Burns
Keep faucets out of reach.
Place hot objects (candles, incense) on high surfaces.
Limit the child's exposure to sun; apply sunscreen after 6 months of age.

Motor Vehicles
See "Age: Birth to 4 Months" section in Box 23.4.

Bodily Damage
Give the child toys that are smooth and rounded, preferably made of natural wood or plastic.
Avoid long, pointed objects as toys.
Avoid toys that are excessively loud.
Keep sharp objects out of the infant's reach.
See also the "Age: Birth to 4 Months" section in Box 23.4.

Age: 8 to 12 Months
Major Developmental Accomplishments
The child crawls and creeps.
The child stands, holding on to furniture.
The child stands alone.
The child cruises around furniture.
The child walks.
The child climbs.
The child pulls on objects.
The child throws objects.
The child is able to pick up small objects and has pincer grasp.
The child explores objects by putting them in their mouth.
The child dislikes being restrained.
The child explores away from parents.
The child's understanding of simple commands and phrases increases.

Injury Prevention
Aspiration
Keep lint and small objects off the floor, off furniture, and out of reach of children.

Take care to give very small pieces when feeding solid table food.
Do not use beanbag toys or allow the child to play with dried beans.
See also the "Age: 4 to 7 Months" section in Box 23.4.

Suffocation and Drowning
Keep doors of appliances (ovens, dishwashers, refrigerators, coolers, and front-loading washers and dryers) closed at all times.
If storing an unused appliance, such as a refrigerator, remove the door.
Supervise contact with inflated balloons; immediately discard popped balloons, and keep uninflated balloons out of children's reach.
Fence in swimming pools.
Always supervise the child when near any source of water, such as baths, cleaning buckets, drainage areas, and toilets.
Keep bathroom doors closed.
Eliminate unnecessary pools of water.
When swimming, keep child within arm's reach at all times.
Keep one hand on the child at all times when they are in the tub.

Falls
Gate the stairways at the top and bottom if the child has access to either end.
Dress the child in safe shoes (soles that do not "catch" on the floor, tied shoelaces) and clothing (pant legs that do not touch the floor).
Ensure that furniture is sturdy enough for the child to hold while they pull themselves to a standing position and while cruising.

Poisoning
Never call medications "candy."
Avoid use of over-the-counter cough and cold preparations for infants.
Do not administer medications unless they are prescribed by a practitioner.
Put away medications and poisons immediately after use; put child-resistant caps on properly.
Keep phone number for poison control centre readily available.

Burns
Place guards in front of or around any heating appliance, fireplace, or furnace.
Keep electrical wires hidden or out of the child's reach.
Place plastic guards over electrical outlets; place furniture in front of outlets.
Keep hanging tablecloths out of reach (the child may pull down hot liquids or heavy or sharp objects).

*Further information is available from Caring for Kids (2020b), Transport Canada (2019), and Canadian Paediatric Society (2020b).
Adapted from Hockenberry, M. J., Wilson, D., & Rodgers, C. C. (2019). *Wong's nursing care of infants and children* (11th ed.). Mosby.

sociocultural background. For example, in some cultures, there may be beliefs that it is normal for infants to be overweight because it reflects health and status (Cheng et al., 2020). Nurses need to assess patients' beliefs about infant feeding in order to develop effective nursing interventions.

Dentition. The average age at which the first tooth erupts is 7 months, but considerable variation exists among infants because of their genetic endowment. Occasionally, an infant is born with a tooth, whereas others remain toothless at 1 year. The order of tooth eruption is fairly predictable: the lower central incisors are first to appear, closely followed by the upper central incisors. Most 1-year-olds have six teeth.

Teething may result in considerable discomfort for some infants and little or none for others. The inflammation of the gums before the tooth emerges may result in a low-grade fever and irritability. Some infants exhibit increased drooling, biting, or finger sucking. Biting on a frozen teething ring or ice cube wrapped in a washcloth may be soothing. Appropriate doses of acetaminophen are helpful when the infant is irritable and has difficulty eating or sleeping.

Most dentists recommend that parents cleanse their infant's teeth after each feeding. The parent can place a clean, wet washcloth or piece of gauze over a finger and use it to wipe the infant's teeth. Once teeth come in, parents can begin brushing the child's teeth twice a day. Several strategies are recommended to reduce the risk of developing dental caries (Health Canada, 2018). Prolonged breast- or bottle-feeding is discouraged, especially just before the infant goes to sleep because the infant is likely to leave milk in the mouth and around the teeth. The infant should never go to bed with a bottle of juice or milk (Kliegman & St. Geme, 2020). By age 1, it is recommended to use open-lid cups instead of bottles and to visit a dentist.

Immunizations. Widespread immunization since the 1950s has resulted in the dramatic decline of infectious diseases and is therefore an important factor in health promotion during childhood. Although most vaccines can be given to people of any age, the Canadian government recommends that the administration of the primary series begin soon after birth and be completed during early childhood (PHAC,

BOX 23.5   RESEARCH HIGHLIGHT
Adverse Childhood Experiences

Research Focus

Adverse childhood experiences (ACEs), including neglect, abuse, and household dysfunction, increase the risk of premature death and health conditions in adulthood. The greater the exposure to ACEs, the more at risk individuals are to negative health outcomes.

Research Abstract

In one of the largest studies ever conducted on childhood abuse and health outcomes, Felitti et al. (1998) surveyed 13 494 adults about their current health and childhood exposure to abuse, neglect, and household dysfunction. More than half of participants reported at least one adverse childhood exposure, while less than 10% were exposed to four or more adverse experiences. The more ACEs participants reported, the greater their risk of health risk factors and chronic health conditions, such as cancer and liver, heart, and lung disease.

Results

Participants exposed to four or more ACEs had the most prevalent and severe negative health outcomes, including greater than a ten-fold increased risk of suicide attempt and substance use. The authors conclude that the high prevalence of ACEs and their strong relationships to long-term health outcomes warrant significant health care investments in prevention efforts.

Implications for Practice

Be aware that it is common for patients to have been exposed to abuse, neglect, or household dysfunction at least once in their childhood.

Seek further knowledge about ACEs, their negative effects, and signs/symptoms of exposure.

Reflect on personal ACEs and their potential impacts on nursing care.

From Felitti, V. J., Anda, R. F., Nordenberg, D., et al. (1998). Relationship of childhood abuse and household dysfunction to many of the leading causes of death in adults. The Adverse Childhood Experiences (ACE) Study. *American Journal of Preventive Medicine, 14*(4), 245–258. https://doi.org/10.1016/s0749-3797(98)00017-8

2020b). The Canadian national immunization guidelines for infants and children are available online (PHAC, 2018). Publicly funded immunization schedules also vary from province to province or territory. Therefore, nurses must know the specific immunization schedule for their jurisdiction. PHAC maintains an online tool where parents can create a personal immunization schedule for their child based on age and provincial or territorial residence (PHAC, 2018). Parents must receive instructions regarding the potential adverse effects of vaccines. Minor adverse effects may occur, but serious reactions are rare. High fever and extreme irritability should be reported to the health care provider.

Most caregivers in Canada ensure that their children receive the recommended vaccines in a timely manner; however, a worldwide barrier is vaccine hesitancy, which results in delays in, or refusal of, immunization (Canadian Paediatric Society, 2022). As a nurse, one of your roles is to discuss the importance of vaccination for infants and children, provide up-to-date information to parents, and encourage them to make an informed decision for their children. General contraindications to vaccination include moderate illness; allergic response to a previous dose of a particular vaccine; and, with live vaccines only, pregnancy, immunosuppression, and taking high doses of corticosteroids. The Canadian Paediatric Society (2022) recommends using a five-step approach to discussing immunizations and addressing vaccine hesitancy (Figure 23.3).

Sleep. Sleep patterns vary among infants, with many having their days and nights "mixed up" until 3 to 4 months of age. By that age, most infants sleep between 9 and 11 hours a night. Total daily sleep averages 15 hours. Most infants take one or two naps a day by the end of the first year. Sleep disturbances with a physiological basis are rare, with the possible exception of colic. Behavioural sleep problems (such as frequent waking at night, difficulty falling asleep, bedtime resistance) persist beyond infancy in 20 to 30% of children and can negatively affect functioning, cognition, and development (Paavonen et al., 2020). Parents' perceptions about sleep problems and infant sleeping environments are influenced by multiple factors, including family and cultural expectations (Sadler et al., 2020). The Canadian Paediatric Society does not endorse bed sharing (PHAC, 2021b), although globally, bed sharing is the most common sleeping arrangement. In Canada, 33% of parents report regularly bed sharing with their infants (Gilmour et al., 2019). Nurses can strategize family-centred approaches to promote sleep health and safety (described in Table 23.2) through assessment of parental perceptions, sleep environments, and infant sleeping patterns.

TODDLER

Toddlerhood lasts from 12 to 36 months of age. Toddlers have increasing independence, physical mobility, and cognitive abilities. Toddlers become aware of their abilities to control their environments and are pleased with successful efforts. This success leads them to continue attempting to control their environments. Unsuccessful attempts at control may result in the toddler refusing to do something, saying no frequently, or engaging in temper tantrums.

Physical Changes

The rapid development of motor skills allows toddlers to participate in self-care activities, such as feeding, dressing, and toileting. Initially, toddlers walk with a broad stance and gait, protuberant abdomen, and arms out to the sides for balance. Soon they begin to navigate stairs, using a rail or the wall to maintain balance. Locomotion skills eventually include running, jumping, standing on one foot for several seconds, and kicking a ball. Most toddlers can ride tricycles, climb ladders, and run well by their third birthday.

Fine motor capabilities move from scribbling spontaneously to drawing circles and crosses accurately. By 3 years, children draw simple stick people and can usually stack a tower of small blocks (Hockenberry et al., 2019). Increased locomotion skills, the ability to undress, and development of sphincter control allow toilet training if a toddler has developed the necessary language and cognitive abilities. Parents often consult nurses for an assessment of readiness for toilet training. A child's recognition of the urge to urinate and defecate is a crucial component of the child's mental readiness. At this stage, children usually show a willingness to please parents and take pride in their accomplishments (Santrock et al., 2021). Nurses must remind parents that patience, consistency, and a nonjudgemental attitude, in addition to child readiness, are essential to successful toilet training.

The cardiopulmonary system becomes stable in the toddler years. The heart and respiratory rates slow to an average of 110 beats and 25 breaths per minute, respectively, and the blood pressure varies slightly from infancy. The average blood pressure in toddlers is 90/50 mm Hg.

The anterior fontanel closes between 12 and 18 months of age, ending the period of the most rapid growth of the skull and brain. However,

BOX 23.6	Clinical Manifestations of Potential Child Maltreatment

Physical Neglect
Suggestive Physical Findings

Failure to thrive (infants), signs of malnutrition (e.g., unhealthy looking skin and hair, sunken eyes or cheeks), evidence of poor health care (e.g., delayed immunization)

Poor personal hygiene, especially of teeth; unclean or inappropriate dress

Frequent injuries resulting from lack of supervision

Suggestive Behaviours

Dull and inactive (infants)

Self-stimulatory behaviours, such as finger sucking or rocking

Begging or stealing food, vandalism, or shoplifting

Absenteeism from school

Substance use in older children

Emotional Maltreatment and Neglect
Suggestive Physical Findings

Failure to thrive

Feeding disorders, such as rumination

Enuresis (bedwetting after toilet training has been established)

Sleep disorders

Suggestive Behaviours

Self-stimulatory behaviours such as biting, rocking, sucking

Stranger anxiety and lack of social smile (infants)

Withdrawal and unusual fearfulness

Antisocial behaviour, such as destructiveness, stealing, cruelty

Extremes of behaviour, such as overcompliance, passivity, aggressiveness, or being demanding

Lags in emotional and intellectual development, especially language

Suicide attempts

Physical Maltreatment
Suggestive Physical Findings

Bruises and welts on face, lips, mouth, back, buttocks, thighs, or areas of torso

Regular patterns on skin that are descriptive of certain objects, such as belt buckle; hand; wire hanger; chain; wooden spoon; squeeze or pinch marks; round cigar or cigarette burns; burns in the shape of an iron, radiator, or electric stove burner

Burns, injuries, fractures, lacerations, or bruises in various stages of healing on soles of feet, palms of hands, back, or buttocks

Presence of symmetrical burns in the absence of "splash" marks

Unusual symptoms, such as abdominal swelling, pain, and vomiting from punching

Marks such as those resembling human bites, or pulling out of hair

Unexplained repeated poisoning or unexplained sudden illness

Suggestive Behaviours

Wariness of physical contact with adults

Apparent fear of parents or of going home

Lying very still while surveying environment, lack of reaction to frightening events

Inappropriate reaction to injury, such as failure to cry from pain

Apprehensiveness when hearing other children cry

Indiscriminate friendliness and displays of affection, superficial relationships

Acting-out behaviour, attention-seeking behaviours

Withdrawn behaviour

Sexual Maltreatment
Suggestive Physical Findings

Bruises, bleeding, lacerations, or irritation of external genitalia, anus, mouth, or throat

Torn, stained, or bloody underclothing

Pain on urination or pain, swelling, and itching of genital area; penile discharge; unusual odour in the genital area

Sexually transmitted infection, nonspecific vaginitis, venereal warts, or presence of sperm

Difficulty in walking or sitting

Recurrent urinary tract infections

Pregnancy in a young adolescent

Suggestive Behaviours

Sudden emergence of sexually related problems, including excessive or public masturbation, age-inappropriate sexual play, promiscuity, or overtly seductive behaviour

Withdrawn behaviour, excessive daydreaming, preoccupation with fantasies, especially in play

Poor relationships with peers

Sudden changes, such as anxiety, weight loss or gain, clinging behaviour

In incestuous relationships, a child's excessive anger at one parent for not protecting the child from the other parent

Regressive behaviour, such as bedwetting or thumb-sucking

Sudden onset of phobias or fears, particularly fears of the dark, men, strangers, or particular settings or situations (e.g., undue fear of leaving the house, of staying at the day care centre, or of staying at the babysitter's house)

Running away from home

Substance use, particularly of alcohol or mood-elevating drugs

Profound and rapid personality changes, especially extreme depression, hostility, and aggression (often accompanied by social withdrawal)

Rapidly declining school performance

Suicide attempts or suicidal ideation

Adapted from Hockenberry, M. J., Wilson, D., & Rodgers, C. C. (2019). *Wong's nursing care of infants and children* (11th ed.). Mosby.

head circumference should be measured routinely until a toddler is 3 years of age.

The rate of increase in a toddler's weight and length slows. By 2.5 years, children's weights are four times their birth weight. The average weight of a 2-year-old is 12 kg. Height during the toddler years increases by approximately 7.5 cm a year, mainly as a result of increases in leg length. The average height of 2-year-olds is 85 cm. Slowed growth rates are accompanied by decreased caloric need, and reduced food intake leads some parents to worry about the adequacy of dietary intake. Parents need encouragement to offer appropriate servings of food, as recommended in *Healthy Eating for Parents and Children* (Health Canada, 2022), and should avoid force-feeding or allowing children to fill up on

foods that have high levels of fat and sugar. Nurses can reassure parents that a child's nutrition is adequate by demonstrating the child's satisfactory status on a growth chart.

Cognitive Changes

Toddlers' completion of the development of **object permanence**, their ability to remember events, and their beginning ability to put thoughts into words at about 2 years of age signal their transition to Piaget's (1952) **preoperational thought** stage of cognitive development (see Chapter 22 for further information about development). Toddlers recognize that they are separate beings from their parents, but they are unable to assume another person's point of view. They use symbols to

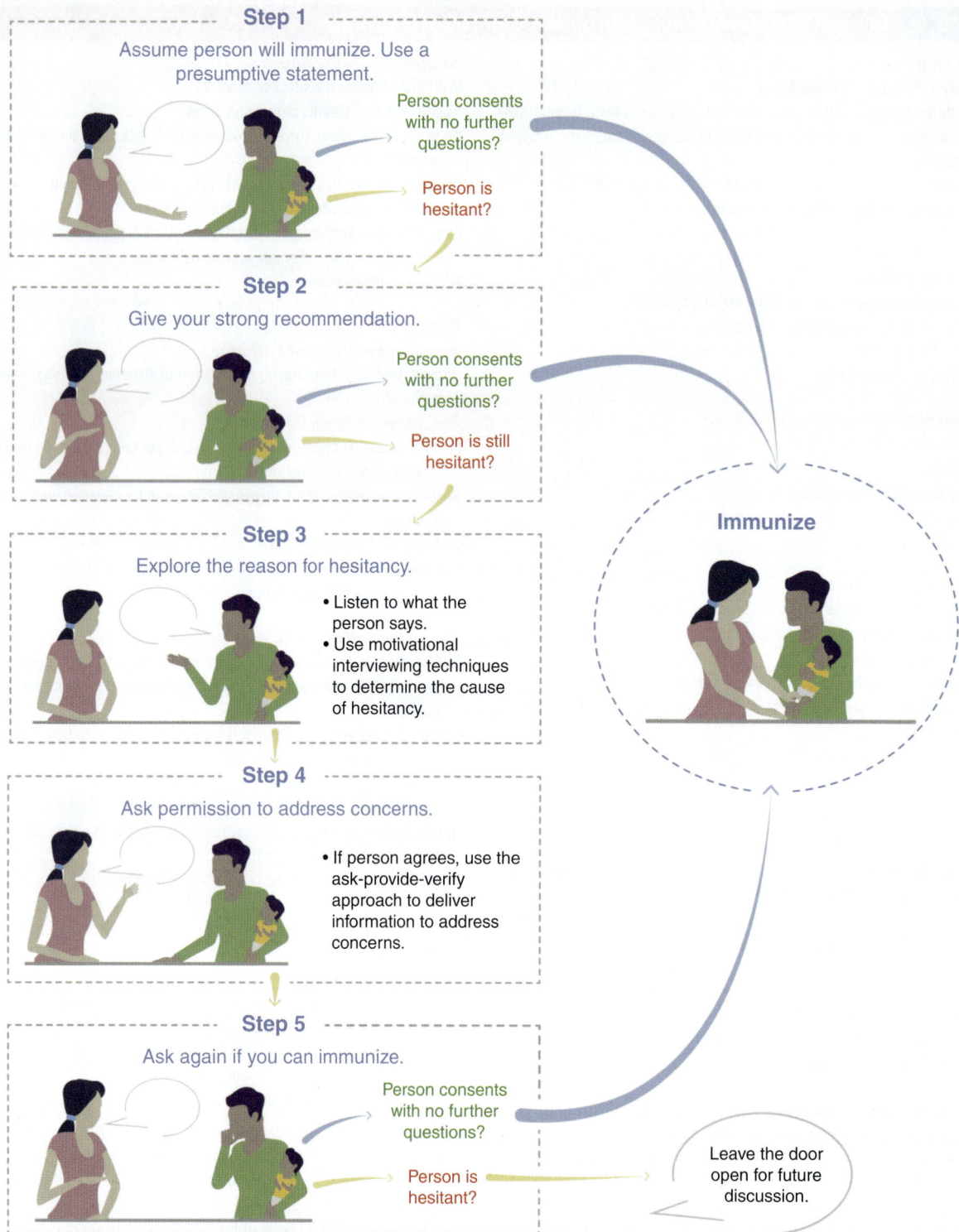

FIGURE 23.3 A 5-step approach to discussing immunizations and addressing vaccine hesitancy. (From BC Centre for Disease Control. [2021]. *A 5-step approach to discussing vaccines and addressing vaccine hesitancy.* http://www.bccdc.ca/resource-gallery/Documents/Guidelines%20and%20Forms/Guidelines%20and%20Manuals/Immunization/Vaccine%20Safety/bccdc-vh-5-steps.pdf. Adapted from *Moving to Acceptance: How to address vaccine hesitancy in your busy practice,* with permission from the Canadian Paediatric Society.)

represent objects, places, and people. This function is demonstrated when children imitate the behaviour of another person that they viewed earlier (e.g., pretend to shave like daddy), pretend one object is another (e.g., pretend that a doll is a baby), and use language to stand for absent objects (e.g., request a bottle).

Language. An 18-month-old child uses approximately 50 words (Santrock et al., 2021). A 24-month-old child has a vocabulary of up to 200 words and is generally able to speak in two-word sentences. "Who's that?" and "What's that?" typify questions asked during this period. First-person expressions such as "Me do it" and "That's mine"

TABLE 23.2	Selected Nursing Approaches to Promote Infant Sleep Health and Safety
Goal	**Nursing Approaches**
Early identification of sleep problems and appropriate management	• Assess infant sleep history and parents' perceptions, including assessment of parental concerns/expectations about sleep, bedtime routines, characteristics of nighttime wakings, sleep environment, differences between weekends and weekdays, different caregivers, infant settling strategies, and daytime functioning and sleep patterns (i.e., daytime naps). • Assess need and provide education to support parental understanding about normal infant sleep patterns and sleep cycles (e.g., frequent infant nighttime wakings are developmentally appropriate for infants) • Refer parents to their health care provider to rule out physiological reasons for sleep problems • Advise parents to wait at least 6 months before engaging in any form of behavioural sleep intervention to allow for circadian rhythms to develop
Parents will make informed sleep environment decisions	• Assess parental beliefs about infant sleep environments • Provide information about safe sleep evidence and recommendations (e.g., placing the infant on their back to sleep, room sharing) • Provide information about strategies to reduce bed sharing risks. Strategies include the following: tying long hair back; not allowing bed sharing with siblings, pets, or parents who are overly drowsy from fatigue, licit or illicit drugs, or alcohol; putting the mattress on the floor; not swaddling the infant; keeping the infant away from heavy blankets/duvets; having the infant sleep on the outside of the bed, not between the parents; ensuring both parents are aware that the infant is in the bed
Parent-identified sleep problems are addressed in ways that work for individual families to maximize sleep health and well-being	• Assess for parental concerns about infant sleep behaviours and effects on family well-being. • Refer to health care provider as needed to rule out physiological causes for sleep problems. • Discuss various strategies to manage parent-identified sleep problems once infant is at least 6 months old and physiological problems are ruled out. Common evidence-informed approaches to manage sleep problems include promoting increased sleep consistency and developmentally appropriate infant self-settling. • Some strategies to promote sleep consistency include having consistent bedtimes/daytime naps and calming sleep routines ("bath, book, bed"). • Some strategies to promote infant self-settling include settling babies into their cribs while they are drowsy but still awake; putting infant to bed without a bottle; avoiding overstimulation during nighttime feeds or diaper changes; waiting a few minutes to see if infant settles to sleep on their own at bedtime or with nighttime wakings • Parents may need referral to a health care provider who specializes in infant sleep problems for advisement on more complex withdrawal or behaviour modification strategies such as gradual parental withdrawal at bedtime (by lying near but not interacting with children until they fall asleep, leaving the room and not returning for 2–5 minutes before responding to crying, then lengthening that interval), differential reinforcement, and controlled comforting • Collaboratively select sleep management approaches that fit parents' values and preferences. • Reassess effectiveness of strategies and ongoing need for parental support or referral to a health care provider who specializes in infant sleep.

Adapted from Canadian Paediatric Society. (2019). *Relationships matter: How clinicians can support positive parenting in the early years.* https://www.cps.ca/en/documents/position/positive-parenting; HealthLink BC. (n.d.). *Safer sleep for my baby.* https://www.healthlinkbc.ca/pregnancy-parenting/parenting-babies-0-12-months/baby-safety/safer-sleep-my-baby

demonstrate 2-year-old children's use of pronouns and desire for independence and control. Despite the expanded vocabulary of older toddlers, the word they use most often is *no* until well into the third year. Offering choices to toddlers helps reduce their sense of frustration and builds their sense of independence (Santrock et al., 2021).

Because children's moral development is closely associated with their cognitive abilities, the moral development of toddlers is only beginning and is also egocentric. Toddlers do not understand concepts of right and wrong. However, they understand that some behaviours bring pleasant results and others elicit unpleasant results. Therefore, until toddlers achieve a higher level of cognitive function, they behave simply to avoid the unpleasant and seek out the pleasant (Hockenberry et al., 2019).

Psychosocial Changes

According to Erikson (1963), a sense of autonomy emerges during the toddler years (see Chapter 22 for developmental stages). Children strive for independence by using their developing muscles to do everything for themselves and to control their bodily functions. Their strong wills are frequently exhibited in negative behaviour when caregivers attempt to direct their actions; for example, temper tantrums may result when toddlers are frustrated by parental restrictions. Parents need to provide

toddlers with graded independence, allowing them to do things that do not result in harm to themselves or others. This strategy prevents them from doubting their abilities or feeling a sense of shame for what they have done. Firm and consistent limits, patience, and support allow toddlers to develop socially acceptable behaviour and cope with the frustration of learning self-control (Santrock et al. 2021).

Socially, toddlers remain strongly attached to their parents and fear separation from them. In their parents' presence, toddlers feel safe, and their curiosity is evident in their exploration of the environment. Children continue to engage in solitary play during toddlerhood, but also begin to participate in parallel play, which is playing beside rather than with another child. Toddlers who are just learning what belongs to them are often possessive of their toys. They learn the joy of sharing when they offer parents or caregivers toys to hold and the parents or caregivers express pleasure.

Health Risks

Their newly developed locomotion abilities and insatiable curiosity put toddlers at risk for injury. Toddlers need close supervision at all times, particularly when they are in environments that have not been childproofed (Figure 23.4). Creating a safe, childproof environment in the home is essential for preventing accidental injuries.

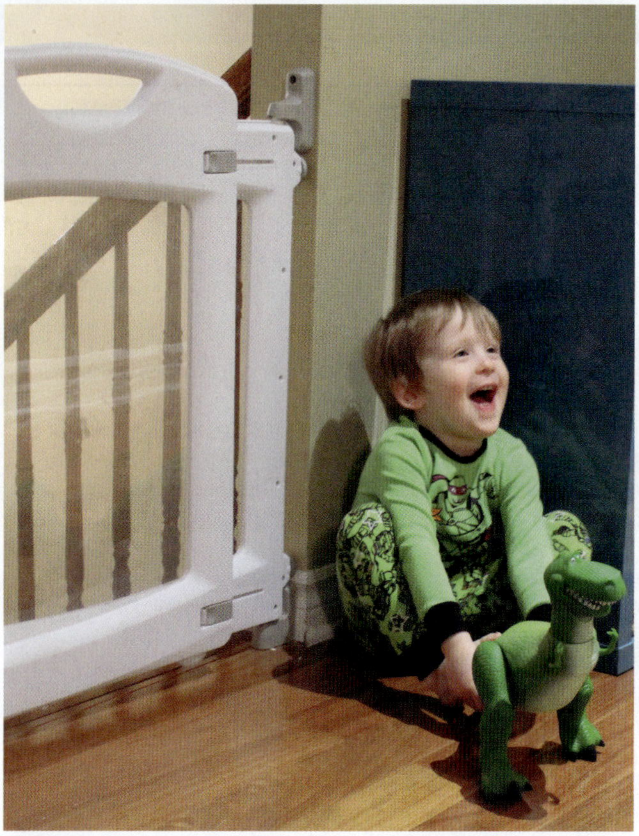

FIGURE 23.4 Creating a safe environment for toddlers. Safety precautions (such as child safety gates) should be provided for toddlers. (Courtesy Cynthia Murray, BN, MN, PhD.)

Poisonings occur frequently in children nearing 2 years of age because they are interested in placing any object or substance in their mouths to learn about it. Parents must remove or lock up all possible poisons, including plants, cleaning materials, and medications. Lead poisoning can pose a health hazard for younger children (Hockenberry et al., 2019). Health care providers need to educate families living in older homes about the risks, screening, and treatment of lead poisoning.

Because of toddlers' lack of awareness regarding the danger of water and their newly developed walking skills, drowning is a major cause of accidental death in this age group. Toddlers can easily become separated from a parent because they often wander away. It is important that parents closely supervise toddlers, especially in an open public space. Setting limits is extremely important for toddlers' safety.

In automobiles, toddlers must remain in car seats. Under Canadian law, infants up to 9 kg must ride in rear-facing car seats, but it is safer for children to remain in this position until they grow out of these seats (Transport Canada, 2019). Rear-facing car seats are required for all children under the age of 2 (Caring for Kids, 2020a). Children often learn to release the car restraints, and parents must be firm in their resolve not to drive unless their children are securely restrained. Toddlers depend completely on their parents for physical safety. Health care providers must educate parents on proper use of child passenger restraints.

Table 23.3 identifies developmental abilities acquired during this stage along with injury prevention strategies.

Health Concerns

Nutrition. Most toddlers stop drinking breastmilk or formula and begin drinking cow's milk. Nutritional requirements are increasingly met by solid foods. Because the consumption of more than 1 L of milk per day usually decreases children's appetite for these essential solid foods and results in inadequate iron intake, nurses should advise parents to limit milk intake to between 500 and 750 mL (two to three servings) per day (Canadian Paediatric Society, 2020a). Children should not drink low-fat or skim milk until 2 years of age because they need the fat in whole milk for physical and intellectual growth. Nutritional needs can be met with diverse diets (Canadian Paediatric Society, 2020a). By age 1, children should generally follow Canada's Food Guide recommendations, which include eating a variety of vegetables and fruit, protein foods, and whole grains and a regular schedule of meals and snacks (Canadian Paediatric Society, 2020a) (see Chapter 43 for further information about nutrition). Nurses can provide information to parents about the recommended "plate method" (foods on the plate are one-quarter protein, one-quarter whole grains, and one-quarter vegetables and fruit) to help support healthy serving sizes and intake of a variety of foods (SickKids, 2021).

Mealtime has psychosocial and physical significance. If the parents struggle to control toddlers' dietary intake, problematic behaviour and conflicts may result. Toddlers often develop "food jags," or the desire to eat one food repeatedly. Rather than becoming disturbed by this behaviour, parents should be encouraged to offer a variety of nutritious foods at meals and to provide only nutritious snacks between meals. Serving finger foods to toddlers allows them to eat by themselves and to satisfy their need for independence and control. Small, reasonable servings enable toddlers to eat their entire meal.

PRESCHOOLER

The **preschool period** applies to children between the ages of 3 and 5 years. Children refine the mastery of their bodies and often are eager to begin school. Many people consider these the most intriguing years of parenting because children exhibit positive emotions and can more effectively share their thoughts, interact, and communicate. Physical development occurs at a slower pace than does cognitive and psychosocial development.

Physical Changes

Physical development continues in the preschool years. Heart and respiratory rates range from 60 to 100 beats and 23 to 25 breaths per minute, respectively. Blood pressure rises slightly to an average of 92/56 mm Hg. Children gain about 2.27 kg per year; the average weight is 14.5 kg at 3 years, 16.8 kg at 4 years, and about 18.6 kg at 5 years. Preschoolers grow 6 to 7.5 cm per year, double their birth length at about 4 years of age, and stand an average of 1 m tall by their fifth birthday. The elongation of the legs results in a more slender appearance. Little difference exists between boys and girls, although boys are slightly larger with more muscle and less fatty tissue.

Large and fine muscle coordination improves. Preschoolers run well, walk up and down steps with ease, and learn to hop. By age 5, they can usually skip on alternate feet, can jump rope, and begin to skate and swim. Improvements in fine motor skills allow intricate manipulations. Children learn to copy crosses and squares. Triangles and diamonds are usually mastered between 5 and 6 years of age. Scribbling and drawing help children develop the fine muscle skills and eye–hand coordination needed for printing letters and numbers.

Children need opportunities to learn and practise new physical skills. Early intervention programs are helpful in developing these skills, especially among disadvantaged children. Nursing care of both healthy and ill children includes assessment of the availability of these opportunities. Although children with acute illnesses benefit from rest and exclusion from usual daily activities, children who have chronic

TABLE 23.3   Injury Prevention for Toddlers and Preschoolers

Developmental Abilities Related to Risk of Injury	Injury Prevention
	Motor Vehicles
• Walks, runs, and climbs • Able to open doors and gates • Can ride tricycle • Can throw ball and other objects	• Continue to use federally approved car restraint. Children should ride in rear-facing car seats until they weigh at least 10 kg. Children weighing up to 18 kg should be placed in a forward-facing child seat that is anchored to the vehicle frame with a tether strap. A child weighing 18–36 kg should be seated in a booster seat. Each province and territory may have its own age, height, and weight restrictions (Transport Canada, 2019). • Supervise child while they are playing outside to prevent them from entering street. • Do not allow child to play on curb or behind a parked car. • Do not permit child to play in pile of leaves, snow, or anywhere that they are not visible. • Supervise tricycle riding. • Supervise child playing outside. • Teach children to obey pedestrian safety rules. • Supervise child when near traffic.
	Drowning
• Has great curiosity • Helpless in water; unaware of its danger at any depth	• Supervise closely when child is near any source of water, including buckets. • Keep bathroom doors and lid on toilet closed. • Have fence around swimming pool, and lock gate. • Teach the child swimming and water safety (and continue to protect them from injury).
	Burns
• Able to reach heights by climbing, stretching, standing on toes, and using objects as a ladder • Pulls objects • Explores any holes or openings • Can open drawers and closets • Unaware of potential sources of heat or fire • Plays with mechanical objects	• Turn pot handles toward back of stove. • Place electric appliances, such as coffeemaker or frying pan, toward back of counter. • Place guard rails in front of radiators, fireplaces, and heating appliances. • Store matches and cigarette lighters in locked or inaccessible area; discard carefully. • Place burning candles, incense, hot foods, ashes, embers, and cigarettes out of reach. • Do not let tablecloth hang within child's reach. • Do not let electric cord from iron or other appliance hang within child's reach. • Cover electrical outlets with protective devices. • Keep electrical wires hidden or out of reach. • Do not allow child to play with electrical appliance, wires, or lighters. • Stress danger of open flames; teach child what "hot" means. • Always check bath water temperature; adjust hot-water heater temperature to 49°C or lower; do not allow child to play with faucets. • Apply a sunscreen with SPF 30 or higher when child is exposed to sunlight.
	Poisoning
• Explores by putting objects in mouth • Can open drawers, closets, and most containers • Climbs • Cannot understand warning labels	• Place all potentially toxic agents (including plants) in a locked cabinet or out of reach. • Put away medications and poisonous substances immediately after use; position (and tighten) child-resistant caps properly. • Refer to medications as "drugs," not "candy." • Do not store large amounts of toxic agents. • Promptly discard empty poison containers; never reuse such containers to store a food item or other poison. • Teach child not to play in trash containers. • Never remove labels from containers of toxic substances. • Know number and location of nearest poison control centre (usually listed at beginning of telephone directories); add phone number to list of contacts on mobile phone.
	Falls
• Able to open doors and some windows • Goes up and down stairs • Has unrefined depth perception	• Keep screen in window, nail securely, and install guard rail. • Place gates at top and bottom of stairs. • Keep doors locked or use child-resistant doorknob covers at entry to stairs, high porch, or other elevated area such as laundry chute. • Remove unsecured or scatter rugs. • Apply nonskid mat in bathtub or shower. • Use a crib with fixed, raised rails. Keep mattress at lowest level. • Place carpeting under crib and in bathroom. • Keep large toys and bumper pads out of crib or playpen (child can use these as "stairs" to climb out). • Move child to youth bed when they are able to climb out of crib. • Dress child in safe clothing (soles that do not "catch" on floor, tied shoelaces, pant legs that do not hang on floor). • Never leave child unattended in shopping cart or stroller. • Supervise child at playgrounds; select play areas with soft ground cover and safe equipment.

Continued

TABLE 23.3	Injury Prevention for Toddlers and Preschoolers—cont'd	
Developmental Abilities Related to Risk of Injury	**Injury Prevention**
	Choking and Suffocation
• Puts things in mouth • May swallow hard or nonedible pieces of food	• Do not give child large, round chunks of meat, such as whole hot dogs (instead, slice into thin pieces). • Do not give child fruit with pits, fish with bones, dried beans, hard candy, chewing gum, nuts, popcorn, grapes, or marshmallows. • Choose large, sturdy toys without sharp edges or small removable parts. • Discard unused refrigerators, unused ovens, and other unused appliances; if storing old appliance, remove doors. • Keep automatic garage door opener in inaccessible place. • Select safe toy boxes or chests without heavy, hinged lids. • Keep window blind strings out of child's reach. • Remove drawstrings from clothing.
	Bodily Damage
• Still clumsy in many activities • Easily distracted from tasks • Unaware of potential danger from strangers or other people	• Avoid giving child sharp or pointed objects—such as knives, scissors, or toothpicks—especially when child is walking or running. • Do not allow lollipops or similar objects in the child's mouth when they are walking or running. • Teach safety precautions (e.g., to hold fork or scissors with pointed end away from face). • Store all dangerous tools, garden equipment, and firearms in locked cabinet. • Be alert to danger of animals, including household pets. • Use safety glass and decals on large glass areas, such as sliding glass doors. • Teach personal safety. • Teach child their name, address, and phone number; also teach them to ask for help from appropriate people (cashier, security guard, police officer) if lost; have identification on child (sewn in clothes, inside shoe). • Avoid dressing child in personalized clothing in public places. • Teach child to never go anywhere with a stranger. • Teach child to tell parents if anyone makes child feel uncomfortable in any way. • Always listen to child's concerns regarding others' behaviour. • Teach child to say no when confronted with uncomfortable situations.

Adapted from Hockenberry, M. J., Wilson, D. & Rodgers, C. C. (2019). *Wong's nursing care of infants and children* (11th ed.). Mosby.

conditions or have been hospitalized for long periods need ongoing exposure to developmental opportunities. With the parents, the nurse can weave these opportunities into the children's daily experiences depending on their abilities, needs, and energy level.

Cognitive Changes

Preschoolers continue to master the preoperational stage of cognition. The first phase of this period, known as *preconceptual thought* (2 to 4 years), is characterized by perception-bound thinking, in that children judge people, objects, and events by their outward appearance or what seems to be true (Piaget, 1952). For example, a child may think that a 240 mL glass full of fluid contains more than a 300 mL glass that also contains 240 mL of fluid because the smaller glass appears fuller. Even if they watch the fluid from the smaller glass being poured into the larger glass and the smaller glass refilled, they still assert that the full, smaller glass contains more.

Children's thinking is hindered by their limited attention and attending skills. Artificialism, the misconception that everything in the world has been created by humanity, may result in children's asking questions such as "Who built the mountains?" Another misconception of preschool thinking, animism, the attribution of sentience to inanimate objects, often results in statements such as "Trees cry when their branches are broken." A third misconception is a type of reasoning called immanent justice, the notion that if a built-in code of law and order is broken, punishment will occur immediately (Santrock et al., 2021). For example, a child might think that he became sick because he lied to his parent.

At about the age of 4, the intuitive phase of preoperational thought develops. Children's ability to think more complex thoughts is demonstrated by their ability to classify objects according to size or colour and by questions such as "Why do they call it the thirty-first day of the month instead of the thirty last?" Egocentricity persists, but during these 3 years it begins to be replaced with social interaction; for example, a 5-year-old child offers a bandage to a child with a cut finger. Children become aware of cause-and-effect relationships, as illustrated by the statement "The sun sets because people want to go to bed." Early causal thinking is also evident in preschoolers' transductive thoughts (reasoning occurs from one particular to another). If two events are related in time or space, children link them in a causal manner. A hospitalized child, for example, may reason, "I cried last night, and that's why the nurse gave me the shot." As children near the age of 5 years, they begin to use, or can be taught to use, rules to understand causation. They then begin to reason from the general to the particular. This development forms the basis for more formal logical thought. The hospitalized child now reasons, "I get a shot twice a day, and that's why I got one last night."

Preschoolers' knowledge of the world remains closely linked to concrete (perceived by the senses) experiences. Even their rich fantasy life is grounded in the perception of reality. The mixing of the two aspects can lead to many childhood fears, and adults may misinterpret children's stories as lying when children are actually presenting reality from their perspective.

The greatest fear of this age group appears to be that of bodily harm, and it can be seen in children's fear of the dark, thunderstorms, and medical personnel. This fear often makes children unwilling to allow nursing interventions such as measurement of vital signs. Preschoolers may cooperate if they are allowed to help the nurse measure the blood pressure of a doll or teddy bear or if they are allowed to handle the equipment the nurse will use.

Preschoolers' moral development expands to include a beginning understanding of behaviours considered socially right or wrong. Children continue to be motivated, however, by the wish to avoid punishment and the desire to obtain a reward. The primary difference between this stage of moral development and that of toddlers is that preschoolers are better able to identify behaviours that elicit rewards or punishment and begin to label these behaviours as right or wrong.

Language. Preschoolers' vocabularies continue to increase rapidly. By the age of 6, children know more than 2 100 words and can construct sentences containing 5 to 6 words (Hockenberry et al., 2019). Language is more social, and questions expand to "Why?" and "How come?" Phonetically similar words such as "die" and "dye" or "wood" and "would" might cause confusion in preschool children. Nurses should avoid such words when preparing children for procedures and assess their comprehension of explanations.

Psychosocial Changes

The world of preschoolers expands beyond the family into the neighbourhood, where children meet other children and adults. Their curiosity and developing initiative lead to the active exploration of the environment, the development of new skills, and the making of new friends. Preschoolers have much energy, which enables them to plan and attempt many activities that may be beyond their capabilities, such as pouring milk into their cereal bowls. Guilt arises within children when they overstep the limits of their abilities and feel they have not behaved correctly (Hockenberry et al., 2019). For example, a child who, in a moment of anger, wishes that their sibling were dead will experience guilt if that sibling then becomes ill. Children need to be taught that "wishing" for something to happen does not make it occur. Parents should allow preschoolers to perform tasks on their own but must set firm limits and provide guidance.

During times of stress or illness, preschoolers may revert to bedwetting or thumb-sucking and want the parents to feed, dress, and hold them (Hockenberry et al., 2019). These dependent behaviours are often confusing and embarrassing to parents, who can benefit from a nurse's reassurance that they are the children's normal coping behaviours. Nurses should provide experiences that these children can master. Such successes help children return to their prior level of independent functioning. As language skills develop, children should be encouraged to talk about their feelings. Play is also an excellent way for preschoolers to vent frustration or anger and is a socially acceptable way to deal with stress.

Play. Children become more social after their third birthday as they shift from parallel to associative play (Hockenberry et al., 2019). Children playing together engage in similar, if not identical, activity; however, no division of labour or rigid organization or rules exist. Most 3-year-old children are able to play with one other child in a cooperative manner in which they make something or play designated roles, such as parent and baby. By the age of 4 years, children play in groups of two or three, and by 5 years, the group has a temporary leader for each activity (Hockenberry et al., 2019).

In many play activities, preschoolers display awareness of social context. Gender-role identification is strengthening, and children most often assume roles of people of their own gender. Children frequently mimic or repeat social experiences. This tendency is especially significant in hospitalized children. Through play, children may express questions, fears, anger, and misunderstanding about their illnesses and care. It is important to be alert to such clues and ensure that children can play within energy limits. Play can provide a healthy outlet for frustration, especially when children have been subjected to painful or restrictive experiences against their will.

Imaginative play depends on children's memory of things they have seen or heard. This sociodramatic play involving other children occupies about a third of 5-year-old children's playtime. Pretending allows children to learn to understand others' points of view, develop skills in solving social problems, and become more creative. Some children have imaginary playmates, which are a sign of creativity and healthy development.

Health Risks

As fine and gross motor skills develop, children become more coordinated with better balance; nevertheless, falls and other accidents remain a leading cause of injury. Guidelines for injury prevention in toddlers also apply to preschoolers (see Table 23.3). Nurses should alert parents of children in this age group to the risks of poisoning and pedestrian–motor vehicle accidents. In Canada, the leading cause of death in children is unintentional injury (PHAC, 2022). All these injuries are preventable. Children should be taught about safety in the home, and this teaching should be reinforced early in elementary school.

Health Concerns

Nutrition. Nutrition requirements for preschoolers vary little from those for toddlers. Parents may nonetheless worry about the amount of food their child is consuming. In most situations, however, the quality of the food is more important than quantity. Preschoolers consume about half of the average adult portions. Finicky eating habits are characteristic of 4-year-olds; in contrast, 5-year-olds are more interested in trying new foods. Parents should provide healthy food on a regular daily schedule of three meals and two snacks, while allowing the child to decide the amount to eat (Kliegman & St Geme, 2020).

Sleep. Preschoolers average 12 hours of sleep a night and take infrequent naps. Sleep disturbances are common during these years. Disturbances may range from trouble getting to sleep, to night terrors and nightmares, to a prolonged bedtime due to extensive rituals. Many preschoolers have had an overabundance of activity and stimulation during the day. Having children follow a set routine before bedtime helps them prepare for sleep.

Vision. Preschoolers should routinely be screened for vision problems. One of the common problems in the preschool period is amblyopia (blindness from disuse of an eye if a child has untreated strabismus). Early detection and treatment can improve vision for most children (Hockenberry et al., 2019).

SCHOOL-AGE CHILDREN AND ADOLESCENTS

School-age children and adolescents lead demanding, challenging lives. The changes that occur between 6 and 19 years of age are diverse and span all areas of growth and development. Physical, psychosocial, cognitive, and moral skills are developed, expanded, refined, and synchronized. The environment in which the individual develops skills also expands and diversifies. Instead of only family and close friends, the environment may now include the school, their community, and a religious institution. Because of expectations for development, increasing skill and knowledge base, and environmental expansion, the individual experiences new difficulties and dilemmas. With age-specific assessment, nurses should review the appropriate developmental expectations for each age group. For example, before assessing risk-taking behaviours, recognize that adolescents normally strive to achieve a sense of identity while developing a moral code compatible with society.

Nurses can direct school-age children and adolescents toward normal developmental behaviours, assisting them in improving their abilities and using them to cope. Table 23.4 provides an overview of developmental behaviours typical of school-age children and adolescents. Nurses must also increasingly involve children or adolescents in charting a developmental course. Not only can they describe their feelings about the changes, but they also can think through these changes. Problem solving becomes more purposeful and sophisticated and results in the achievement of the outcomes they desire. This paced, active participation may initiate a style of involvement in lifelong self-care.

School-age children and adolescents must cope with many changes, and these can be a source of stress for children. For example, 6-year-old children beginning school are confronted with new authority figures, teachers, and rules and restrictions. They need to work and play cooperatively with a large group of children of various cultural backgrounds.

School-age children must meet the challenge of developing cognitive skills that enhance their reasoning and allow them to learn to read, write, and manipulate numbers. Because of the stress of these changes, children may develop physical and psychosocial health problems (e.g., increased susceptibility to upper respiratory infections, inadequate peer relationships, or poor performance in school). It is important to design health promotion interventions that are based on an individual child's developmental stage.

SCHOOL-AGE CHILD

During these "middle years" of childhood, the foundation for adult roles in work, recreation, and social interaction is laid. In industrialized countries, this period begins when children start formal schooling, at about the age of 5. Puberty, which occurs at around 12 years of age, signals the end of middle childhood (Hockenberry et al., 2019). Great developmental strides are made during these years as children develop competencies in physical, cognitive, and psychosocial skills.

The school or educational experience expands children's worlds and is a transition from a life of relatively free play to a life of structured play, learning, and work (Hockenberry et al., 2019). The school and

TABLE 23.4	Developmental Behaviours of School-Age Children and Adolescents
School-Age Children	**Adolescents**
Relationships With Parents Children gradually learn that parents are less than perfect; children can become disillusioned with parents and wish that friends' parents were their own. They still rely on parents for unconditional love, security, guidance, and nurturing.	Adolescents desire increasing independence and autonomy, and yet continue needing some dependence and limit setting by parents; this conflict places strain on the parent–child relationship. Effective communication and democratic parenting are the best tools for meeting this challenge.
Relationships With Siblings Siblings seem to be at odds with one another at home, and yet they tend to be each other's best defenders away from home. Younger children often idolize older siblings, and this frequently leads to competition. Older children may envy the attention that younger siblings require.	Younger siblings rarely understand their adolescent siblings' need for privacy. Adolescents often enjoy interacting with and guiding younger siblings when the timing is convenient for them and they can remain in control.
Relationships With Peers During primary grades (6–7 years), children of all genders play together, depending on who is available and interested. Around age 8, children form social groupings with peers of the same gender. These groups allow children to declare their independence from parental rules and establish their own rules of membership and behaviour. Preadolescent (ages 10–12 years) friendships are characterized by having a best friend of the same gender. These relationships may be transient, but they are intense and allow discussion of all areas of life. Childhood "crushes" are common.	The peer group is of critical influence on adolescents, who increasingly need recognition and acceptance. Companionship offered by peer groups provides a secure environment for individuals to try out new ideas and share similar feelings and attitudes. Adolescents often form cliques with peers who have similar interests and are from the same socioeconomic group. Cliques, which are highly exclusive, help their members develop their identities.
Self-Concept Children's feelings of competence regarding mastery of tasks are key elements in forming self-esteem. Children need to receive positive feedback regarding their efforts. It is important for children to develop skills in at least one area, such as reading, music, or swimming.	Formal and informal peer groups are a primary force in shaping self-concept of group members. Popularity and recognition within the peer group enhance self-esteem and reinforce self-concept. Total immersion in the peer group may make it appear that adolescents have no original thoughts and are incapable of making decisions. Adolescents who withdraw from peers into isolation struggle with developing identity.
Fears Fears related to body safety decline. Fears of supernatural beings, such as ghosts and witches, persist and decline slowly. New fears related to school and family occur. Children fear ridicule from teachers and friends and disapproval of and rejection by parents. They also become frightened about death and events that they hear on the news, such as war and destruction of the environment.	Fears in this age group centre on peer group acceptance, body changes, loss of self-control, and emerging sexual urges. Adolescents constantly examine their bodies for changes and signs of imperfection. Any defect, real or imagined, is the cause of endless worry.

TABLE 23.4	Developmental Behaviours of School-Age Children and Adolescents—cont'd
School-Age Children	**Adolescents**

Coping Patterns

To deal with stress, school-age children use problem solving and defence mechanisms such as denial and aggression. Several categories of coping behaviours of hospitalized school-aged children are inactivity (total silence, lack of activity, and apathy), orientation or precoping (looking and listening, walking around and exploring, and asking questions), cooperation (compliance with care), resistance (attempt to get away from the situation by turning away or making physical or verbal attacks), and controlling (assuming responsibility for self-care and suggesting how things could be done).

Coping behaviours expand with experiences adolescents have gained from life and from developing cognitive maturity. By age 15, most adolescents use a full range of defence mechanisms, including rationalization and intellectualization. Adolescents' problem-solving abilities have matured, and they can reason through philosophical discussions and complex situations that require abstract thinking and proposition of hypotheses. Some adolescents use avoidance coping strategies in which a problem is denied or repressed, and an attempt is made to reduce tension by engaging in substance abuse or avoiding people.

Morals

Children learn rules from parents, but their understanding of rules or the reasons for them is limited until about age 10. Before that, they are concerned with their own needs first and may cheat to win games. After 10 years of age, they advocate for justice and believe that the punishment should fit the crime (e.g., if children break something, they should pay to have it fixed).

According to Kohlberg (1964), as youths approach adolescence, they reach the *conventional level*, where internalization of expectations of their family and society begins. Initially, youths exhibit considerable conformity to rules to win praise or approval from others and to avoid social disapproval or rejection; later, they seek to avoid criticism from authority figures in institutions.

Diversional Activities

School-age children play cooperatively in group activities, such as sports and jumping rope. Play becomes competitive, and children often have difficulty learning to accept losing. Teasing, insults, dares, superstitions, and increased sensitivity are characteristics of this age.

Many teenagers develop special interests in certain sports and concentrate on developing maximal skills in them. Recreational activities are often determined by what is popular with peers and what can provide independence from parents (e.g., computers, cars).

Nutrition

Children have definite likes and dislikes. Few nutritional deficiencies occur in this age group. Children have voracious appetites after school and need quality snacks, such as fruit and sandwiches, to avoid empty-calorie foods such as chips and candy.

Total nutritional needs become greater during adolescence. Girls' caloric needs decrease and their need for protein increases slightly. Adolescents need to increase their consumption of iron-rich foods, and growth spurts increase calcium demand.

home influence growth and development, necessitating adjustment by parents and children. Children must learn to cope with rules and expectations presented by the school and peers. Parents must learn to allow their children to make decisions, accept responsibility, and learn from life's experiences.

Physical Changes

The rate of growth during these early school years is slower than at any time since birth, but continues steadily. A particular child may not follow the pattern precisely. School-age children appear slimmer than preschoolers as a result of changes in fat distribution and thickness (Dames et al., 2021). Growth accelerates at different times for different children. The average increase in height is 5 cm per year, while weight, which is more variable, increases by 2 to 3 kg per year. An average 6-year-old is 116 cm tall and weighs 21 kg; the average 12-year-old is 150 cm tall and weighs 40 kg. Many children double their weight during these middle childhood years (Hockenberry et al., 2019).

School provides children with the opportunity to compare themselves with other children of the same age. The physical examination is an excellent opportunity to discuss with a child and their parents the influences of genetic endowment, nutrition, and exercise on height and weight. Annual measurement of height and weight may reveal alterations in growth that are symptoms of the onset of a variety of childhood diseases (Hockenberry et al., 2019).

Boys are slightly taller and heavier than girls during these early school years. Approximately 2 years before puberty, children experience a rapid acceleration in skeletal growth. Girls, who generally reach

puberty first, begin to surpass boys in height and weight, which causes embarrassment to both genders. In North America, puberty occurs between the ages of 9 and 13 years in girls and 11 and 14 years in boys (Hockenberry et al., 2019).

Cardiovascular functioning is refined and stabilized during the school years. The heart rate averages 75 to 100 beats per minute, the blood pressure normalizes to approximately 110/65 mm Hg, and the respiratory rate stabilizes to 20 to 30 breaths per minute. Lung growth is minimal, and respirations become slower, deeper, and more regular. However, by the end of this period, the heart is six times the size it was at birth and has generally reached its adult size (Hockenberry et al., 2019)

School-age children become more graceful during the school years because their large-muscle coordination improves and their strength doubles. Most children practise the basic gross motor skills of running, jumping, balancing, throwing, and catching during play, which results in refinement of neuromuscular function and skills. Fine motor skills improve, and control is gained over fingers and wrists. Children become proficient in a wide range of activities, although much individual difference exists in the rate and degree of proficiency (Hockenberry et al., 2019).

Most 6-year-olds can hold a pencil adeptly and print letters and words. By age 12, children can make detailed drawings and write sentences in script. Activities such as painting, drawing, playing computer games, and making models allow children to practise and improve newly refined skills. Parents should encourage children to pursue these activities. Table 23.5 describes specific gross motor and fine motor skills and their use in self-care activities.

TABLE 23.5	Average Motor Development in School-Age Children	
Ages 6–7 Years	**Ages 8–10 Years**	**Ages 11–12 Years**
Fine Motor Skills		
• Uses knife to butter bread and learns to cut tender meat	• Uses knife and fork simultaneously	• Learns to peel apples and potatoes
• Cuts, folds, and pastes paper	• Learns to thread needle and tie knot	• Sews simple garments on machine
• Prints with pencil	• Uses hammer, saw, and screwdriver	• Builds simple objects like birdhouse
• Draws person with 12–16 details	• Becomes proficient at cursive writing	• Enjoys writing in decorative script
• Copies triangle at age 6 and diamond by age 7	• Uses symbols in drawing (e.g., bird, star)	• Begins to use creative and artistic talents
• Colours within lines of picture	• Builds simple models of cars and planes and does simple handicrafts	• Builds complex models of cars and planes and does complex handicrafts
• Needs assistance to clean teeth thoroughly	• Can learn to floss teeth effectively and be independent in tooth care	• Learns to play musical instrument
		• Becomes proficient in caring for teeth with braces and other appliances
Gross Motor Skills		
• Remains in constant motion when awake	• Catches, throws, and hits a baseball	• Can perform standing broad jump of 1.5 m
• Moves more cautiously at age 7 than at age 6	• Engages in alternate rhythmic hopping	• Can perform standing high jump of 1 m
• Hops and jumps into small squares	• Engages in complex styles of skipping rope while reciting verbal jingles	• Engages in sports involving simultaneous use of two or more complex motor skills, such as ice skating, skateboarding, or playing hockey
• Learns to roller skate, skip rope, ride a bicycle, and swim		
Self-Care		
• Takes bath without supervision	• Learns to clean bathroom after bath	• Dusts, vacuums, and straightens own room
• Often returns to finger feeding	• Enjoys fixing own snacks and sack lunch	• Learns to cook simply prepared foods
• Learns to brush and comb hair in acceptable manner without help	• Learns to part hair and insert barrettes	• Washes, dries, and fixes own hair
• Puts on most clothes, but may need assistance with final adjustments	• Dresses self completely and can help younger siblings with clothes	• Learns to sort, wash, dry, and press own clothing
	• Can make own bed	• Learns to care for fingernails and toenails

The improved fine motor capabilities of school-age children allow them to become independent in bathing, dressing, and taking care of other personal needs. They develop strong personal preferences in the way these needs are met. Illness and hospitalization threaten children's control in these areas; therefore, it is important to allow them to participate in care and maintain as much independence as possible. For example, children whose care mandates restriction of fluids cannot be allowed to decide the volume of fluids they will drink in 24 hours, but they can help to decide the type of fluids and keep a record of their intake.

Assessment of neurological development is often based on fine motor coordination. This assessment may include penmanship, stacking ability, and performance of sequential, rapid, alternating movements, such as touching the finger to the nose and then to the examiner's finger (smooth movement without tremors is the normal response). Fine motor coordination is crucial for academic success because children must be able to hold pencils and crayons, use scissors and rulers, and develop computer skills. The opportunity to practise these skills through schoolwork and play is essential for the acquisition of coordinated, complex behaviours.

Other physical changes take place during the school years. Steady skeletal growth in the trunk and extremities occurs, and small- and long-bone ossification is present, but not complete, by age 12 years. Dental growth is prominent during the school years. The first permanent or secondary teeth begin to erupt at approximately 6 years of age. Development of the permanent teeth has, however, been occurring for some time before eruption. The root of a primary tooth is absorbed, leaving the crown, which causes the tooth to become loose and fall out, making room for the permanent tooth. Eruption of secondary teeth usually begins with the 6-year molars, and the others follow the same order as with the primary teeth. By 12 years, all primary teeth have been shed, and the majority of permanent teeth have erupted. Infrequent or inadequate dental care remains a persistent problem for many children.

As skeletal growth progresses, body appearance and posture change. Earlier posture, which was characterized by a stoop-shouldered, slight lordosis and prominent abdomen, changes to a more erect posture. It is essential that children, especially girls after the age of 12 years, be evaluated for scoliosis, the lateral curvature of the spine.

Eye shape alters because of skeletal growth. This improves visual acuity, and normal adult 20/20 vision is achievable. Screening for vision and hearing problems is easier, and results are more reliable because school-age children can more fully understand and cooperate with the test directions. The community health nurse typically assesses the dental, visual, and auditory status of school-age children and refers those with possible deviations to their family practitioner or pediatrician.

Cognitive Changes

Cognitive changes provide school-age children with the ability to think in a logical manner and to understand the relationship between things and ideas (Hockenberry et al., 2019). The thoughts of school-age children are no longer dominated by their perceptions, and thus their ability to understand the world greatly expands. At about 7 years of age, children enter Piaget's (1952) third stage of cognitive development, known as concrete operations, in which they are able to use symbols to carry out operations (mental activities) in thought rather than in action. They begin to use logical thought processes with concrete materials (people, events, and objects they can touch and see).

Children in the concrete operational stage are considerably less egocentric than are younger children and develop the ability to concentrate on more than one aspect of a situation. School-age children now have the ability to recognize that the amount or quantity of a substance remains the same even when its shape or appearance changes. For instance, they can understand that two balls of clay of equal size retain the same amount of clay even when one is flattened and the other remains in the shape of a ball.

The mental process of classification becomes more complex during the school years. Younger children can separate objects into groups according to shape or colour, whereas school-age children understand that the same element can exist in two classes at the same time. School-age children are becoming "thinkers" and are more capable of understanding another person's views and feelings (Santrock et al., 2021).

In middle childhood, youngsters can use their newly developed cognitive skills to solve problems. Some individuals are better than others at problem solving because of intelligence level, education, and experience, but all children can improve these skills. Children who are good problem solvers demonstrate the following characteristics: a positive attitude that the problem can be solved with persistence, a concern for accuracy, the ability to divide the problem into parts for study, and the ability to avoid guessing while searching for facts. Adults can help children improve their problem-solving strategies by helping them define the problem, plan a solution, and then evaluate their solution. Nurses can use these strategies to help hospitalized school-age children understand their illness and assume responsibility for their general health.

Language Development. Language growth is so rapid during middle childhood that these ages cannot be matched with language achievements. Children improve their use of language and expand their structural knowledge. They become more aware of the rules for linking words into phrases and sentences. They can also identify generalizations and exceptions to rules. They accept language as a means of representing the world in a subjective manner and realize that words have arbitrary, rather than absolute, meanings. They can use different words for the same object or concept, and they understand that a single word may have many meanings. Like younger children, school-age children watch parents and other adults to obtain clues about how to understand events (Santrock et al., 2021). Many school-age children use "bad language" to gain peer status and to shock adults. It often begins with bathroom language and progresses to sexual or genital words. Children begin to think about language, which enables them to appreciate jokes and riddles. Language acquisition is nurtured by social interactions with their parents and caretakers.

Psychosocial Changes

Erikson (1963) identified the developmental task for school-age children as industry versus inferiority (see Chapter 22 for further information about developmental theories). During this time, children strive to acquire the competence and skills necessary for them to function as adults. School-age children who are positively recognized for success feel a sense of worth. Those faced with failure can feel a sense of unworthiness, which may result in withdrawal from school activities and peers (Hockenberry et al., 2019).

Moral Development. The need for a moral code and social rules becomes more evident as school-age children's cognitive abilities and social experiences increase. For example, 12-year-old children are able to consider what society would be like without rules because of their ability to reason logically and their experiences with group play. They view rules as necessary principles of life, not just dictates from authorities. In the early school years, children strictly interpret and adhere to rules. As they grow older, their judgements become more flexible and they can evaluate rules for applicability to a given situation. School-age children consider motivations and behaviour when

making judgements about the way their behaviours affect themselves and others. The abilities to be flexible when applying rules and to take the perspective of other people are essential in developing moral judgements. These abilities are present at times in earlier years, but are more consistently displayed in later school years (Hockenberry et al., 2019).

Peer Relationships. Group and personal achievements are important to school-age children. Success is important in physical and cognitive activities. Play involves peers and the pursuit of group goals. Although solitary activities are not eliminated, they are overshadowed by group play. Learning to contribute, collaborate, and work cooperatively toward a common goal becomes a measure of success.

For the most part, school-age children prefer same-gender peers to opposite-gender peers. In general, girls and boys view the opposite gender negatively. Peer influence becomes diverse during this stage of development. Conformity is evidenced in mannerisms, clothing styles, and speech patterns, which are reinforced and influenced by contact with peers. During this period, clubs and peer groups become prominent. Group identity increases as school-age children approach adolescence. Also, during the "tween" years (i.e., ages 8 to 12), children are increasingly exposed to digital media. To help tweens and teens safely navigate the digital social world, the Canadian Paediatric Society Digital Health Task Force (Ponti, 2019) recommends the following 4 "M" approach for parents:

- *MANAGE* use of screen time:
  - Be present and engaged during screen use.
  - Discourage multitasking of media, particularly while doing homework.
  - Set appropriate time limits.
  - Use parental controls and ensure that privacy settings are appropriate.
  - Discuss appropriate online behaviour (e.g., discourage gossiping, spreading rumours, and bullying).
- Encourage *MEANINGFUL* screen use:
  - Encourage face-to-face contact, sleep, and physical activity rather than screen time.
  - Encourage educational, active, or social screen activities.
  - Participate with tweens and adolescents by joining them in video game play.
- *MODEL* healthy screen use:
  - Review own social media habits.
  - Encourage daily "screen-free" times.
  - Avoid use of screens before bedtime.
  - Do not text or use headphones while walking, biking, or driving.
- *MONITOR* for signs of problematic screen use:
  - Screen time that interferes with physical activity, face-to-face time, schoolwork, or sleep
  - Being unhappy or bored when social media is not available
  - Negative emotions after interactions online or playing video games.

Bullying is a significant problem for school-age children and adolescents. In Canada, 47% of parents have at least one child who has experienced bullying, and one-third of Canadians have experienced bullying as children (Public Safety Canada, n.d.). Approximately 15% and 18% of girls and boys, respectively, reported being bullied at least twice in previous months (PREVNet, n.d.-a). Bullied children have higher rates of academic, physical, and mental health problems, including depression, anxiety, and suicide (PREVNet, n.d.-a). There are four types of bullying: physical (e.g., hitting and pushing); verbal (e.g., insults and taunts); social (e.g., spreading rumours and social exclusion); and cyber (e.g., sending mean or threatening text messages). In addition, bullying may target a person because of their ethnicity, religion, sexual orientation, or disability (PREVNet, n.d.-c). Nurses can work with other professionals to develop bullying prevention programs and strategies, recognize signs of bullying, and offer early intervention (PREVNet, n.d.-a). Interventions include encouraging children to report bullying to a trusted adult, teaching children how to be assertive and step in when someone they know is being bullied, and promoting healthy relationships (PREVNet, n.d.-b).

Sexuality. Sigmund Freud described middle childhood as the latency period because he believed that children had little interest in their sexuality at this age. Today, many researchers believe that school-age children have a great deal of curiosity about their sexuality. Some may experiment, but this play is usually temporary. Children's curiosity about adult magazines or the meanings of sexually explicit words is another example of their sexual interest. This is the time for children to have exposure to sex education, including information on sexual maturation, reproduction, and relationships (Dames et al., 2021) (see Chapter 28).

Health Risks

Accidents and injuries are major health problems affecting school-age children. Motor vehicle accidents and accidents related to recreational activities or equipment are the leading causes of death or injury from the age of 1 year onward (Dames et al., 2021). Nurses play an essential role in injury prevention initiatives. Also, nurses must respond competently and ethically to rapidly changing conditions (CASN, 2022) when accidents and injuries occur. Unintentional injuries account for nearly half of all childhood deaths, many of which can be prevented through the use of precautionary measures (Table 23.6).

Although falls account for 45% of pediatric unintentional injury–related hospital admissions, they account for less than 5% of pediatric deaths resulting from unintentional injuries (Parachute, 2016). Even though an accident may not result in death, it still can be a major cause of disability in children.

"On road" injuries account for nearly 50% of all unintentional injury–related deaths among Canadian children (Parachute, 2016). This includes children who are motor vehicle occupants, cyclists, and pedestrians. The rates of injury and death have decreased since the introduction of legislation requiring the use of car/booster seats and helmets.

School-age children are also significantly affected by respiratory illnesses, especially asthma, cancer, and heart disease (Hockenberry et al., 2019). In this age group, these problems have a relatively low mortality rate but a high morbidity rate in comparison with accidents. Cancers are the second leading cause of death in children aged 5 to 14 years (Hockenberry et al., 2019). Leukemia is the most frequent type, and brain tumours and lymphoma are the second and third most common, respectively.

Infections account for the majority of all childhood illnesses; respiratory infections are the most prevalent. The common cold remains the chief illness of childhood. Children living in poverty are more prone to disease and disability. Intellectual disabilities, learning disorders, sensory impairments, emotional difficulties, behavioural problems, and malnutrition are far more prevalent among children living in poverty (Campaign 2000, 2021). Of particular concern is the high rate of poverty among First Nations, Inuit, and Métis children (53% on reserve, 41% off reserve) compared with the overall rate of childhood poverty in Canada (18.6%) (Campaign 2000, 2021).

Poverty and the prevalence of illness are highly correlated, probably because access to health promotion and preventive health care activities are minimal for children living in poverty. Poor nutrition and limited access to early intervention programs continue to be major health concerns for impoverished families. Education, social and health care reform, and environmental change are necessary to positively influence the health of children.

Children's developing cognitive and psychomotor skills make it possible for them to become more involved in health promotion and the management of chronic illness.

Health Concerns

During the school years, identity and self-concept become stronger and more individualized. School-age children are aware of their bodies and are sensitive about body privacy. In providing nursing care, it is important to ensure their privacy and to offer explanations of common procedures. This approach helps to foster children's self-esteem and lessens their fear of pain and intrusion (Hockenberry et al., 2019).

Health Education

The school years are crucial for the acquisition of behaviours and health practices for a healthy adult life. Because cognition is advancing during this period, effective health education must be developmentally appropriate. Promotion of good health practices is a nursing responsibility. Comprehensive school health is an internationally recognized approach that is based on the World Health Organization's (1986) *Ottawa Charter for Health Promotion* (see Chapter 1 for more information about health promotion). It considers the social and physical environment, teaching and learning, partnerships and services, and policy to enable children and youth to reach their full potential as healthy, productive members of society (Pan-Canadian Joint Consortium for School Health, n.d.; Box 23.7).

School-age children should receive age-appropriate education about sexuality (Hockenberry et al., 2019). Other topics for elementary health education curricula include the promotion of adequate nutrition, oral hygiene, physical activity, and injury prevention. School-age children should also be educated about prevention of tobacco, drug, and alcohol use (Hockenberry et al., 2019).

Nurses can instruct parents in health promotion that is appropriate for school-age children. Parents need to recognize the importance of annual checkups for immunizations, screenings, and dental care. When school-age children reach 10 years of age, it is recommended that their parents talk to them about upcoming pubertal changes (Hockenberry et al., 2019). Topics should include introductory information regarding menstruation, sexual intercourse, and reproduction. Nurses can provide age-appropriate written materials to aid parents in their efforts. The settings in which health promotion activities can occur are varied: the classroom, a school-based clinic, a community-based clinic, or community settings such as a public library or community centre.

BOX 23.7   Comprehensive School Health

The comprehensive school health approach supports student learning as part of health promotion in the following ways:
- Recognizes that healthy students learn better and achieve more
- Understands that schools can directly influence students' health and behaviours
- Encourages healthy lifestyle choices and promotes students' health and well-being
- Incorporates health into all aspects of school and learning
- Links health and education issues and systems
- Needs the participation and support of families and the community at large

From Pan-Canadian Joint Consortium for School Health. (n.d.). *Comprehensive school health framework.* http://www.jcsh-cces.ca/en/concepts/comprehensive-school-health

TABLE 23.6   Injury Prevention for School-Age Children

Developmental Abilities Related to Risk of Injury	Injury Prevention
	Motor Vehicles
• Is increasingly involved in activities away from home • Is excited by speed and motion • Can be reasoned with • Does not always perceive injury risk • Is easily distracted by environment	• Educate child regarding proper use of seat belts while a passenger in a vehicle. • Maintain discipline while a passenger in a vehicle (e.g., keep arms inside, do not lean against doors, do not interfere with driver). • Remind parents and children that no one should ride in the bed of a pickup truck. • Emphasize safe pedestrian behaviour. • Insist that child wear safety apparel (e.g., helmet) when applicable, such as when riding a bicycle or using a skateboard, all-terrain vehicle, or snowmobile.
	Drowning
• Is apt to overdo activities • May work hard to perfect a skill • Is cautious but not fearful	• Teach child to swim. • Teach basic rules of water safety. • Select safe and supervised places to swim. • Check sufficient water depth for diving. • Insist that child swim with a companion. • Use an approved flotation device in water or boat. • Learn cardiopulmonary resuscitation (CPR).
	Burns
• Demonstrates increasing independence • Is adventurous • Enjoys trying new things	• Make sure working smoke detectors are in homes. Set water heaters to 48.9°C to avoid scald burns. • Instruct child in behaviour in areas involving contact with potential burn hazards (e.g., gasoline, matches, bonfires or barbecues, lighter fluid, firecrackers, cigarette lighters, cooking utensils, chemistry sets). • Instruct child to avoid climbing or flying kites around high-tension wires. • Instruct child in proper behaviour in the event of fire (e.g., fire drills at home and school). • Teach child safe cooking (use low heat; avoid any frying; be careful of steam burns, scalds, or exploding foods, especially from microwaving). • Teach children about the danger of fire and instruct them that if their clothing is on fire, they should "stop," "drop," and "roll."
	Substance Use and Poisoning
• May be easily influenced by peers • Adheres to group rules • Has strong allegiance to friends	• Educate child regarding hazards of taking nonprescription drugs and chemicals, including tobacco and alcohol. • Teach child to say no if they are offered illegal or dangerous drugs or alcohol. • Keep potentially dangerous products in properly labelled receptacles, preferably locked and out of child's reach.
	Bodily Damage
• Demonstrates increased physical skills • Needs strenuous physical activity • Is interested in acquiring new skills and perfecting attained skills • Is daring and adventurous, especially with peers • Frequently plays in hazardous places • Confidence often exceeds physical capacity • Desires group loyalty and has strong need for friends' approval • Attempts hazardous feats • Accompanies friends to potentially hazardous facilities • Delights in physical activity • Is likely to overdo activity • Has growth in height that exceeds muscular growth and coordination	• Help provide facilities for supervised activities. • Encourage playing in safe places. • Keep firearms safely locked up. • Teach proper care of, use of, and respect for devices with potential danger (e.g., power tools). • Teach children not to tease or surprise dogs, invade their territory, take dogs' toys, or interfere with dogs' feeding. • Stress use of eye, ear, or mouth protection when using potentially hazardous objects or devices or when engaged in potentially hazardous sports. • Do not permit use of trampolines except as part of supervised training. • Teach safety regarding use of corrective devices (glasses); if child wears contact lenses, monitor duration of wear to prevent corneal damage. • Stress careful selection, use, and maintenance of sports and recreation equipment such as skateboards and inline skates. • Emphasize proper conditioning, safe practices, and use of safety equipment for sports or recreational activities. • Caution against engaging in hazardous sports, such as those involving trampolines. • Use safety glass and decals on large areas of glass, such as sliding glass doors. • Use window guards to prevent falls. • Teach name, address, and phone number, and emphasize that child should ask for help from appropriate people (e.g., cashier, security guard, police) if lost; have identification on child (e.g., sewn in clothes, inside shoe). • Teach safety and stranger awareness. • Avoid personalized clothing in public places. • Caution child to never go anywhere with a stranger. • Have child tell parents if anyone makes child feel uncomfortable in any way. • Always listen to child's concerns regarding others' behaviour. • Teach child to say no when confronted with uncomfortable situations. • Help child avoid carrying more than 5–10% of body weight in a backpack, and teach child to always put backpack on in a way that evenly distributes weight; a lightweight backpack with wide shoulder straps, a waist strap, a padded back, and multiple compartments should be used.

Adapted from Hockenberry, M. J., Wilson, D., & Rodgers, C. C. (2019). *Wong's nursing care of infants and children* (11th ed., p. 488). Mosby; National Safety Council. (2021). *Backpack safety: It's time to lighten the load.* https://www.nsc.org/home-safety/safety-topics/child-safety/backpacks

Table 23.7 presents a list of possible health promotion interventions for school-age children.

Safety. Because accidents are the leading cause of death and injury in school-age children, safety is a priority health teaching consideration. Nurses can contribute to the general health of children by educating them about safety measures to prevent accidents. At this age, children should be encouraged to take responsibility for their own safety.

Nutrition. Nurses can contribute to the promotion of children's healthy lifestyle habits, including nutrition. School-age children should participate in educational programs that enable them to plan, select, and prepare healthy meals and snacks. These foods should be consistent with the recommendations in *Canada's Food Guide* (Health Canada, 2019a), which include eating plenty of fruits and vegetables, whole grain foods, and plant-based protein foods; limiting highly processed foods; making water the drink of choice; and being aware of how food marketing influences our food choices. Box 23.8 outlines several learning activities appropriate for this age group. In addition, it is important to encourage daily physical activity for all children.

Growth may slow down during the school years in comparison with infancy and adolescence. Obesity is the most common nutritional problem during childhood, with rates among children and youth having tripled in the last 30 years (Health Canada, 2016). Obesity increases the risk for hypertension, type 2 diabetes, coronary heart disease, sleep apnea, abnormal menstruation, and emotional health problems; some children with obesity have low self-esteem, poor body image, depression, and reduced quality of life and interpersonal relationships (Health Canada, 2016). Obesity may occur because children often rush into the home after school or play and eat the most easily obtainable and appealing foods. Unfortunately, these foods are often high in calories and low in nutrition. Providing nutritious snacks is often the best way for a parent to ensure good nutritional intake. Caregivers should follow *Canada's Food Guide* and provide ready access to fresh fruit, raw vegetables, cheese, popcorn, and high-protein snacks such as skim-milk pudding and hot chocolate. When planning successful eating interventions, nurses need to consider cultural, economic, and social issues (Health Canada, 2016, 2019a).

Nurses can help families and children prevent obesity by recommending proper nutrition and physical activity. Many families often eat in fast-food restaurants, where the food is high in fat, calories, and salt. Nurses should encourage healthy food choices in these situations. Selections should include meats that are not breaded and are broiled, shakes that are made with low-fat yogurt or skim milk, and fruits and vegetables that are fresh or prepared in a low-calorie manner. Children and teens should participate in at least 60 minutes of physical activity each day (Canadian Society for Exercise Physiology, 2020; see Box 37.11).

ADOLESCENCE

Adolescence is the period of development between childhood and adulthood, usually between 12 and 19 years of age (Hockenberry et al., 2019). The term *adolescent* usually refers to psychological maturation of the individual, whereas *puberty* refers to the point at which reproduction becomes possible. The hormonal changes of puberty result in physical changes in the young person's appearance, most notably in the primary sexual characteristics (maturation of the reproductive organs) and secondary sexual characteristics (such as the development of pubic hair and breasts). Mental development during puberty results in the ability to hypothesize and deal with abstractions. In addition, adolescents become much more social,

TABLE 23.7	Health Promotion for School-Age Children
School-Age Health Concerns	**Health Promotion Interventions**
Nutrition	• Provide nutrition education that promotes healthy lifestyle; for example, eat plenty of fruits and vegetables, eat protein foods, choose whole-grain foods, and make water your drink of choice (Health Canada, 2019a).
Oral hygiene	• Provide examples of low-cariogenic snacks. • Review mechanics of dental hygiene: brushing, flossing. • Stress importance of regular dental checkups.
Infections	• Provide immunization information and follow-up. • Teach infection prevention practices (hand hygiene, care of minor skin injuries). • Teach concepts of viral and bacterial illness. • Promote hand hygiene and regular bathing.
Tobacco, alcohol, and drug use	• Provide programs in preventing tobacco use. • Provide information regarding the hazards of alcohol and drug use.
Human sexuality	• Provide information about sex, gender identity, sexual orientation, intimacy, sexual maturation, and reproduction in age-appropriate manner. • Encourage parents to view their children's sexual curiosity as part of the developmental process. • Discuss with parents the learning needs of their children regarding sexuality. Provide age-appropriate education about sexuality.

BOX 23.8	Interventions to Promote Education About Nutrition

• Include healthy eating as part of education programs at school.
• Make healthy foods available in school vending machines and at school sporting or other events.
• Encourage nutritious and nonfood items for school fundraising projects and classroom rewards or prizes.
• Use positive messages to reinforce healthy eating and physical activity.
• Have teachers and school personnel model healthy eating habits.
• Limit access to unhealthy foods and beverages.
• Provide positive reinforcement for healthy food choices.
• Create a healthy food environment.
• Celebrate birthdays and special events with healthy food choices.
• Promote safe food handling practices.
• Involve parents and the community in promoting healthy eating in schools.

Adapted from Knowledge Network. (n.d.). *Making it happen: Healthy eating at school.* http://healthyeatingatschool.ca; Health Canada. (2020). *Healthy eating at school.* https://food-guide.canada.ca/en/tips-for-healthy-eating/school

and their behavioural patterns far less predictable. Adjustments and adaptations are needed to cope with these simultaneous changes and the adolescent's attempt to establish a mature sense of identity. Many people refer to adolescence as a stormy and stressful period filled with inner turmoil, but it is recognized that most teenagers successfully meet the challenges of this period. These challenges may cause adolescents to be moody and difficult. Within adolescence, three subphases exist: early adolescence, including puberty (ages 11 to 14 years), middle adolescence (ages 15 to 17 years), and late adolescence (ages 18 to 20 years). Opportunities, challenges, changes, skills, pressures, and physical, cognitive, and psychosocial development vary widely among the subphases (Table 23.8).

As a nurse, your understanding of development offers teenagers and parents a unique perspective that can help them anticipate and cope with the stresses of adolescence. Primary health care activities, particularly education, can promote healthy development. These activities occur in a variety of settings and can be directed at adolescents, parents, or both. For example, a nurse can conduct seminars in a high school to provide practical suggestions for solving problems of concern to a large group of students, such as treating acne or making responsible decisions about drugs or alcohol use. Similarly, a group education program for parents about how to cope with teenagers would promote parental understanding of adolescent development. These programs can be held in the school, clinic, private office, or community centre. To learn more about specific topics or problems, it is important to identify teenagers' needs and desires. Involvement produces more active and interested learners.

Physical Changes

Physical changes occur rapidly in adolescence. Sexual maturation occurs with the development of primary and secondary sexual characteristics. The four main focuses of these physical changes are as follows:

- Increased growth rate of the skeleton, muscles, and viscera
- Sex-specific changes, such as changes in shoulder and hip width
- Alteration in distribution of muscle and fat
- Development of the reproductive system and secondary sexual characteristics

The timing of physical changes associated with puberty varies. Individuals (patients) with female genitalia tend to begin their physical changes earlier than individuals (patients) with male genitalia. The sequence of pubertal growth changes is the same in most individuals (Table 23.9).

Changes are created by hormonal fluctuations within the body when the hypothalamus begins to produce gonadotropin-releasing hormones. This change sends the pituitary gland a signal to secrete gonadotropic hormones. Gonadotropic hormones stimulate ovarian cells to produce **estrogen** and testicular cells to produce **testosterone**. These hormones contribute to the development of secondary sexual characteristics, such as hair growth and voice changes, and play an essential role in reproduction. The changing concentrations of these hormones are also linked to acne and body odour. Understanding these hormonal changes enables nurses to reassure adolescents and educate them about body care needs.

Boys who mature early have been shown by some researchers to be more poised, relaxed, good natured, skilled in athletic activities, and likely to be school leaders than boys who mature late. In contrast, girls who mature early have been found to be less sociable and more shy and introverted, perhaps as a result of feeling conspicuous (Dames et al., 2021). Such girls are more conscious of the physical changes of puberty, such as breast development, and thus stand out from many of their peers.

Being like their peers is extremely important for adolescents. Nurses need to stress that normal sexual changes are quite variable. As with increases in height and weight, the pattern of sexual changes is more significant than their time of onset. Large deviations from normal patterns necessitate investigation.

Any deviation in the timing of the physical changes can be extremely difficult for adolescents to accept. It is important to provide emotional support for those undergoing early or delayed puberty. Even adolescents whose physical changes are occurring at the normal times may seek reassurance about their normality.

Height and weight usually increase during the prepubertal growth spurt. The growth spurt for girls generally begins between 8 and 14 years of age. Height increases by 5 to 20 cm, and weight increases by 7 to 25 kg. The growth spurt in boys usually occurs between 10 and 16 years of age. Height increases by approximately 10 to 30 cm, and weight increases by 7 to 30 kg. In both sexes, the final 20 to 25% of adult height and 50% of adult weight are attained during this time (Hockenberry et al., 2019).

Girls attain 90 to 95% of their adult height by **menarche** (the onset of menstruation) and reach their full height by 16 to 17 years of age, whereas boys continue to grow taller until 18 to 20 years of age. Fat is redistributed into adult proportions as height and weight increase, and gradually the adolescent torso takes on an adult appearance. Despite individual and biological sex differences, growth follows a similar pattern for both sexes. Growth in the length of the extremities occurs earliest, making the hands and feet appear very large and the legs very long; the individual often appears awkward and clumsy. At the same time, the lower jaw and nose become longer and the forehead higher and wider as the baby face of childhood disappears. Next, the thighs widen; then the shoulders broaden, and growth of the trunk proceeds. The female hips widen and the male shoulders broaden throughout adolescence.

Personal growth curves can help a nurse in assessing physical development. The individual's sustained progression along the curve, however, is more important than a comparison of measurements with the norm. To evaluate changes, the nurse should chart growth measurements during routine health assessments.

Adolescents are sensitive about physical changes that make them different from peers. For this reason, they are generally interested in the normal pattern of growth and in their personal growth curves. Therefore, nurses should share this information to reassure adolescents that their own patterns are normal.

Cognitive Changes

According to Piaget (1952), the changes that occur within the mind and the widening social environment of adolescents result in the highest level of intellectual development, known as **formal operations** (see Chapter 22 for further information on development). However, without an appropriate educational environment, some people may not attain this stage. Those who are guided toward developing rational thinking may reach this stage early.

Adolescents develop the ability to determine possibilities, rank options, solve problems, and make decisions through logical operations. The teenager can deal effectively with hypothetical problems. When confronted with a problem, the teenager is able to consider an infinite variety of causes and solutions. Adolescents can move beyond the physical or concrete properties of a situation and use reasoning powers to understand the abstract. School-age children think about what is, whereas adolescents can imagine what might be. These newly developed abilities allow the individual to have more insight and skill when playing video games, computer games, and board games that require abstract thinking and deductive reasoning about many possible strategies. A teenager can solve problems by simultaneously manipulating several abstract concepts.

Development of the ability to reason abstractly is important in the pursuit of an identity. For example, newly acquired cognitive skills enable the teenager to define appropriate, effective, and comfortable gender-role behaviours and consider their impact on peers, family, and society. The ability to think logically about these behaviours and their outcomes helps adolescents to develop personal thoughts about

TABLE 23.8   Growth and Development During Adolescence

Early Adolescence (11–14 Years)	Middle Adolescence (15–17 Years)	Late Adolescence (18–20 Years)
Growth		
Rapidly accelerating growth reaches peak velocity. Secondary sexual characteristics appear.	Growth decelerates in girls. Stature reaches 95% of adult height. Secondary sexual characteristics are well advanced.	The body is physically mature. Structural and reproductive growth are almost complete.
Cognition		
The person explores newfound ability for limited abstract thought. Clumsy groping for new values and energies occurs. One's "normality" is compared with that of peers of same gender.	Capacity for abstract thinking develops. Intellectual powers, often in idealistic terms, are increased. Concerns with philosophical, political, and social problems arise.	Abstract thought is established. The person can perceive and act on long-range options. The person is able to view problems comprehensively. Intellectual and functional identity are established.
Identity		
The person is preoccupied with rapid body changes. The person tries out various roles. Attractiveness is measured by acceptance or rejection by peers. Conformity to group norms is typical. Self-esteem declines.	Body image is modified. The person is very self-centred; narcissism is increased. A tendency toward inner experience and self-discovery develops. Fantasy life is rich. The person becomes idealistic. The person is able to perceive future implications of current behaviour and decisions, with variable application.	Body image and gender-role definition are nearly secured. Gender identity is mature. Identity is consolidated. Self-esteem increases. The person is comfortable with physical growth. Social roles are defined and articulated.
Relationships With Parents		
Independence–dependence boundaries are defined. The person has a strong desire to remain dependent on parents while trying to detach from them. No major conflicts over parental control occur.	Major conflicts over independence and control occur. This is the low point in the parent–child relationship. The person makes the greatest push for emancipation and disengagement. Emotional detachment from parents is final and irreversible; mourning occurs.	Emotional and physical separation from parents is completed. Independence is achieved from family with less conflict. Emancipation is nearly secured.
Relationships With Peers		
The person seeks peer affiliations to counter instability generated by rapid change. The person experiences an upsurge of close, idealized friendships with members of the same gender. Struggle for mastery takes place within the peer group.	The person has a strong need for identity to affirm self-image. Behavioural standards are set by peer group. Acceptance by peers is extremely important; rejection is feared. The person explores the ability to attract a sexual partner.	The peer group recedes in importance in favour of individual friendship. Male–female and same-gender relationships are tested against the possibility of permanent alliance. Relationships are characterized by giving and sharing.
Sexuality		
Self-exploration and evaluation occur. Dating is limited; the person usually socializes with a group. Intimacy is limited.	Multiple plural relationships are characteristic. "Self-appeal" is explored. Feeling of "being in love" is common. Relationships are tentatively established.	The person forms stable relationships and attachment to another person. The capacity for mutuality and reciprocity grows. Dating is common. The person may publicly identify as lesbian, gay, transgender, queer, or Two-Spirit (LGBTQ2). Intimacy involves commitment rather than exploration and romanticism.
Psychological Health		
Wide mood swings occur. Intense daydreaming is characteristic. Anger is outwardly expressed with moodiness, temper outbursts, verbal insults, and name-calling.	A tendency toward inner experiences is exhibited; the person becomes more introspective. The person tends to withdraw when upset or when feelings are hurt. Emotions vacillate in time and range. Feelings of inadequacy are common; asking for help is difficult.	The person experiences more constancy of emotion. Anger is more apt to be concealed.

Adapted from Hockenberry, M. J., Wilson, D., & Rodgers, C. C. (2019). *Wong's nursing care of infants and children* (11th ed.). Mosby.

TABLE 23.9	Average Sequences of Physiological Changes in Adolescence	

	AGE RANGE (YEARS)	
Characteristics	**Girls**	**Boys**
Beginning of skeletal growth spurt	8–14.5 (peak: 12)	10.5–16 (peak: 14)
Beginning of breast development	8–13	—
Enlargement of testes and scrotal sac	—	10–13.5
Appearance of straight, pigmented pubic hair, which gradually becomes curly	8–14	10–15
Early voice changes (cracks)	—	11–14.5
Enlargement of penis and prostate gland	—	11–14.5
Menarche	10–18 (average: 12.25)	—
Spermatogenesis (ejaculation of sperm)	—	11–17 (average: 13.5)
Ovulation and completion of breast development	14–18 (average: 15.52)	—
Appearance of downy facial hair	—	12–17
Appearance of axillary (underarm) hair and increased output of oil and sweat-producing glands, which may lead to acne	10–16	12–17
Widening and deepening of pelvis, with deposition of subcutaneous fat that gives rounded appearance to body	10–18	—
Increase in shoulder width	—	11–21
Deepening of voice; appearance of coarse and pigmented facial hair; appearance of chest and axillary hair; other body hair also becomes more prominent, such as that on forearms and legs	—	16–21

the capability to think as logically as adults, they do not yet have experiences from which to gain perspective. It is common for teenagers to view their parents as too narrow minded or too materialistic. This perception can result in conflicts between teenagers and parents. Cognitive abilities and performance vary greatly among adolescents. In fact, an adolescent may perform at different levels in different situations on the basis of past experiences, formal education, and motivation in the use of logic and effective deductive reasoning.

Language Skills. Language development is fairly complete by adolescence, although vocabulary continues to expand. The primary focus becomes practising communication skills that can be used effectively in various situations. Adolescents need to communicate thoughts, feelings, and facts to others. The skills used in communication situations are varied. Adolescents must select the person with whom to communicate, decide on the message, and choose the way to transmit the message. For example, the way teenagers tell parents about failing grades is not the same as the way they tell friends. Adolescents develop different skills and styles of communication and learn how and when to use them most effectively. These diverse communication skills are used and refined throughout life (Santrock et al., 2021). Good communication skills are crucial for overcoming peer pressure and unhealthy behaviours. The following are some hints for communicating with adolescents:

- Do not avoid discussing sensitive issues. Asking questions about sexuality, drugs, and school demonstrates your interest in their well-being and may open the channels for further discussion.
- Ask open-ended questions.
- Try to discern the meaning behind their words or actions.
- Be alert to clues to their emotional state.
- Involve other individuals and resources when necessary.

Psychosocial Changes

The search for personal identity is the major characteristic of adolescent psychosocial development. Teenagers must establish close peer relationships or risk remaining socially isolated. Erikson (1963) viewed identity (or role) confusion as the prime danger of this stage, and suggested that the cliquishness and intolerance of differences seen in adolescent behaviour are defences against identity confusion (Erikson, 1968). Adolescents work at becoming emotionally independent from their parents while retaining family ties. In addition, they need to develop their own ethical systems that are based on personal values. Choices about vocation, future education, and lifestyle must be made. The various components of identity evolve from these stages and compose a total adult personal identity that is unique to the individual. Indecisiveness and the inability to make an occupational choice are behaviours indicating the lack of resolution to certain developmental tasks.

Gender Identity. Achievement of gender identity is enhanced by the physical changes of puberty. According to Freud, these physiological changes of puberty stimulate the libido, the energy source that fuels the sex drive (see Chapter 22 for further information on development). Transgender adolescents have gender identities that are different from their biological sex, and they may transition to their affirmed gender (Arrington Sanders & Fields, 2021). Nurses should be aware of resources to assist transgender youth (see Recommended Websites at end of the chapter).

Group Identity. Adolescents seek a group identity because they need esteem and acceptance (Figure 23.5). Similarity in dress, speech, or both is common in teenage groups. Popularity is a major concern for

and the means of expressing gender identity. In addition, because their level of cognitive functioning is higher, adolescents are receptive to more detailed and diverse information about sexuality and sexual behaviours.

By middle adolescence, an introspective quality emerges. At this time, adolescents believe that they are unique. They also may believe, because of their new physical skills, that they are invulnerable, and so they engage in risk-taking behaviours; many state that they "can drive fast and not get into an accident." Other typical adolescent behaviours include self-consciousness and the desire for privacy.

The complex development of thought during this period leads adolescents to question society and its values. Although adolescents have

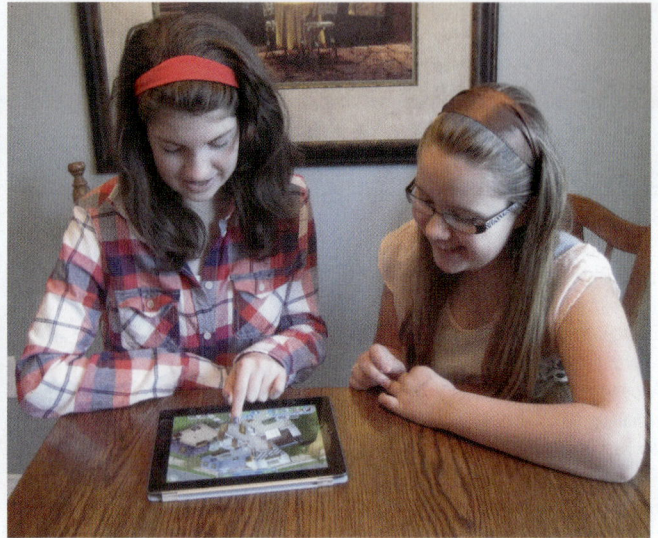

FIGURE 23.5 Social interactions strengthen a teenager's group identity. (Courtesy Cynthia Murray, BN, MN, PhD.)

teenagers. Peer groups provide adolescents with a sense of belonging, approval, and the opportunity to learn acceptable behaviour. Popularity with peers is important. The strong need for group identity seems to conflict at times with the search for personal identity. It is as though adolescents require close bonds with peers so that they can later achieve a sense of individuality.

Family Identity. The movement toward stronger peer relationships contrasts with adolescents' movements away from parents. Although financial independence for adolescents is not the norm in Canadian society, many adolescents work part-time, using their income to bolster independence. When adolescents cannot have a part-time job because of studies, school-related activities, and other factors, parents can provide allowances for clothing and incidentals, which encourage adolescents to develop decision-making and budgeting skills.

Some adolescents and families have more difficulty during these years than others. Adolescents need to make choices, act independently, and experience the consequences of their actions. This testing, however, is best done against the background of firm family support. The family needs to allow independence while providing a haven in which adolescents can contemplate actions. Families unable to provide this support complicate movement toward identity formation. Health care support of a family and an adolescent may be essential to their success.

Nurses can assist families in considering ways that are appropriate for them to foster the independence of their adolescent while maintaining the family structure. Many of these discussions involve curfews, jobs, and participation in family chores. Emancipation from the immediate family is most successful when accomplished gradually and when it results in a balance between independence and family ties.

Vocational Identity. Selecting an occupation or a vocational direction in life is a goal for adolescents. Because of society's changing needs, adolescents must be future oriented when making these choices. However, adolescents do not know which jobs will be available and rewarding 10 or 20 years in the future, and selecting a career is thus a complicated task. Nurses need to be supportive to the family during

this process and help adolescents select courses of action that promote self-satisfaction, identity, and continued opportunity for growth.

Moral Identity. The development of moral judgement depends heavily on cognitive and communication skills and peer interaction. Although moral development begins in early childhood, it is consolidated in adolescence because of the presence of certain skills. Adolescents learn that rules are cooperative agreements that can be modified to fit the situation rather than being absolutes. Adolescents learn to use their own judgement rather than following the rules to avoid punishment as in earlier years. Kohlberg (1964) explained moral development in terms of stages (see Chapter 22 for further information on development). At the highest level, morality is derived from individual principles of conscience. Adolescents judge themselves by internalized ideals; such judgement often leads to conflict between personal and group values. Group values become less significant in later adolescence.

Not all adolescents attain the same level of moral development; however, they generally advance through the stages of moral development, and the sequence of the stages is similar for all individuals, even though the time at achievement varies. Kohlberg's (1964) moral development theory focuses on justice based on reciprocity and equal respect. Adolescent girls have been found to be more likely to give caring responses to moral problems, whereas adolescent boys have been found to give more justice-oriented responses (Gilligan, 1982).

Health Identity. Healthy adolescents evaluate their own health according to feelings of well-being, ability to function normally, and absence of symptoms (Hockenberry et al., 2019). Interventions to improve health perception might, therefore, concentrate on the adolescent period. The rapid changes during this period make primary health care programs especially crucial. Adolescents try new roles, begin to stabilize their identity, and acquire values and behaviours from which their adult lifestyle will evolve.

Health Risks

Injuries. Unintentional injuries and suicide are the leading causes of death in Canadian youth aged 15 to 19 (Statistics Canada, 2020). Feelings of being indestructible can lead to risk-taking behaviour. Many injuries are preceded by the use of alcohol (Hockenberry et al., 2019).

Nurses can play an important role in planning, implementing, and evaluating injury prevention strategies (CASN, 2014). For example, in partnership with community members and other stakeholders, a nurse might identify alcohol-related motor vehicle accidents among adolescents as a community health need and assist in the development, delivery, and evaluation of preventive programs and healthy public policies aimed at addressing the need.

Mental Health. One in five Canadians live with mental illness, and more than 70% of these people first experienced symptoms before the age of 18 (Mental Health Commission of Canada, 2021). During the COVID-19 pandemic, 20% fewer youth reported excellent or good mental health, while the number of interactions with Kids Help Phone doubled compared with 2019 (Canadian Institute for Health Information [CIHI], 2022). The most common mental health conditions seen in children and youth are anxiety disorders; other conditions include depression, schizophrenia, attention-deficit/hyperactivity disorder, and conduct disorders (Hockenberry et al., 2019). Nurses play an important role in early detection of symptoms and referral to mental health services. As adolescents transition to adulthood, they must be taught how to manage and live with their condition. Through the principles of hope, empowerment, self-determination, and responsibility, adolescents can learn to manage their condition as they transition to adulthood (Mental Health Commission of Canada, 2016).

Suicide. Suicide is increasing as a cause of death in adolescents aged 15 to 19. Depression and social isolation commonly precede a suicide attempt, but suicidal thoughts probably result from a combination of several factors (Box 23.9).

A nurse must be able to identify the factors associated with adolescent suicide risk and precipitating events. In addition, the nurse should be alert to the following warning signs, which often occur for at least a month before suicide is attempted:

- Deterioration in school performance
- Social withdrawal
- Loss of initiative
- Loneliness, sadness, and crying
- Appetite and sleep disturbances
- Verbalization of suicidal thought

Immediate referrals to mental health providers are needed when assessment findings suggest that adolescents may be considering suicide. Guidance can help them focus on the positive aspects of life and strengthen coping abilities.

Substance Use. Adolescents may believe that mood-altering substances create a sense of well-being or improve performance. All adolescents are at risk for experimental or recreational substance use, but those with dysfunctional families are more at risk for chronic use and physical dependency. Some adolescents believe that substance use makes them more mature. They further believe they will look and feel better with drug usage. From 2017 to 2018, 5% of all hospital stays among youth aged 10 to 24 were related to the adverse effects of substances, with cannabis being the most common followed by alcohol (CIHI, 2019). Of growing concern is the use of cannabis edibles. An ongoing study by the Canadian Paediatric Surveillance Program (Canadian Paediatric Society, 2021b) has found that unintentional consumption of cannabis in gummies, candies, and chocolate has led to an increased rate of hospitalization for the adverse effects of cannabis. Rates of opioid use and overdose are increasing in Canada, with the fastest rate of growth in hospitalizations for opioid poisoning occurring in adolescents and youth aged 15 to 24 (Health Canada, 2019b). The use of substances before age 14 increases the likelihood of lifelong

dependence (CIHI, 2019). Tobacco use, although decreasing, continues to be a problem among adolescents.

Eating Disorders. Weight extremes resulting from excessive or inadequate caloric intake are common during the adolescent years. The number of eating disorders is on the rise in adolescents, particularly among girls. If an adolescent's growth deviates radically from the usual pattern, further assessment is necessary to identify the cause. Items to include in the assessment are past and present diet history, food records, eating habits, attitudes, health beliefs, and socioeconomic and psychosocial factors (Hockenberry et al., 2019). Knowledge of growth progression may be a way to discourage radical weight reduction activities. Allowing an adolescent to see when and how the weight curve changed can be a first step in identifying the problem and implementing dietary changes.

BOX 23.9 **Factors Associated With Suicide**

History
Previous suicide attempt
Suicide attempt by family member or friend
History of child maltreatment
Past psychiatric hospitalization
Death of a parent when child was young

Individual Factors
Hopelessness
Marked, persistent depression
Alcohol or drug use
Impulsiveness
Difficulty tolerating frustration
Feelings of self-hatred, excessive guilt, or humiliation
Thinking disorder (wishes to join a deceased person, hears voices saying to kill self)
Physical, behavioural, developmental, or body image problems (delayed puberty, chronic illness, disability, attention-deficit/hyperactivity disorder, learning disorders)
Gender identity or sexual orientation concerns; being LGBTQ2 in an unsupportive environment
Seeing self as totally helpless, a victim of fate
Perfectionistic tendencies

Family Factors
Difficult home situation: long, bitter parent–child conflict
Hostile parents
Overt rejection by one or both parents
Divorce or separation of parents
Recent or impending move
Family breakup or loss of parent
Stress of unrealistically high parental expectations
Parental indifference with very low expectations

Social and Environmental Factors
Firearms in the home
Incarceration
Lack of effective social support system
Isolation
Suicide of someone known
Few social, vocational, or educational opportunities

Adapted from Hockenberry, M. J., Wilson, D., & Rodgers, C. C. (2019). *Wong's nursing care of infants and children* (11th ed.). Mosby.

Although anorexia nervosa and bulimia are classified as separate eating disorders, manifestations of the two overlap. Anorexia nervosa is considered a clinical syndrome with both physical and psychosocial components. The majority of patients are adolescents and young women. Attending a highly competitive high school and being from an upper-middle-class family of professionals increase the risk for this disorder. People with anorexia nervosa have an intense fear of gaining weight and refuse to maintain body weight at the normal minimum for their age and height (Hockenberry et al., 2019).

Bulimia nervosa is most identified with binge eating and behaviours to prevent weight gain, including self-induced vomiting, misuse of laxatives and other medications, fasting, and excessive exercise (Hockenberry et al., 2019). Because adolescents rarely volunteer information about behaviours to prevent weight gain, it is important to take a thorough dietary history. Society's expectations for thinness may have a strong influence on the development of these disorders. While eating disorders tend to be more common among girls, boys may also suffer from these disorders. Causes of eating disorders are the same for girls and boys.

Obesity and Physical Inactivity. Overweight and obesity, together with a decrease in physical activity, are becoming serious public health problems in Canada. Over the last 30 years, obesity rates have nearly tripled among Canadian children and adolescents (Health Canada, 2016). A contributing factor is a lack of physical activity; children and adolescents spend more time watching television and using computers, especially for playing computer games. Parents and other people working with adolescents must encourage them to participate in more physical activity, monitor their computer use, and promote healthy nutrition.

Sexual Exploration. Sexual exploration is common among adolescents. Peer pressure, physiological and emotional changes, and societal expectations contribute to early heterosexual and same-sex relations. Two prominent consequences of adolescent sexual activity are sexually transmitted infections and pregnancy (Hockenberry et al., 2019).

Sexually Transmitted Infections. The incidence of sexually transmitted infections (STIs) is highest among Canadians who are 25 years of age or younger (PHAC, 2020c). Therefore, sexually active adolescents must be screened for STIs, even when they have no symptoms, because STIs can be asymptomatic. The annual physical examination of a sexually active adolescent should include a thorough sexual and genitourinary history and a careful examination of the genitalia so that genital warts, herpes, and other STIs are not missed. Recommended tests for women include Papanicolaou (Pap) smears, cervical cultures for gonorrhea and *Chlamydia* species, and syphilis tests; for men, urethral cultures for gonorrhea and *Chlamydia* species and syphilis tests are recommended. If men have participated in same-sex activities, rectal and pharyngeal cultures also need to be taken to check for gonorrhea. Because the human papillomavirus (HPV) is a common STI, all Canadian provinces and territories have HPV vaccine programs; the vaccine is effective against some HPV viruses associated with cervical cancer (PHAC, 2020d). The vaccine is given to both boys and girls. Health care providers can be proactive by using the patient interview process to identify risk factors in adolescents. Once risk factors are identified, corresponding strategies for prevention should be carried out.

The human immunodeficiency virus (HIV), which causes acquired immune deficiency syndrome (AIDS), is transmitted through unprotected sexual intercourse, the use of shared needles for injecting drugs, and infected blood products (see Chapter 28 for further information about HIV). Therefore, the risk-taking behaviours of sexual activity and drug use make adolescents vulnerable to the threat of AIDS and other STIs. Adolescents who have placed themselves at risk for AIDS should be tested for HIV infection. All adolescents need thorough and up-to-date knowledge about HIV and AIDS.

Pregnancy. Adolescent pregnancy occurs across socioeconomic classes, in public and private schools, among all ethnic and religious backgrounds, and in all parts of the country. Adolescent pregnancy with early prenatal supervision is considered less physically harmful to both the parent and child than earlier believed. Pregnant teenagers need special education about nutrition, as well as health supervision and psychological support.

Health Concerns

Adolescents need to form healthy habits of daily living. Nurses should emphasize the importance of exercise, sleep, nutrition, and stress reduction and identify ways to convey these needs to each adolescent. To do this, the nurse must assess the individual's positive and negative habits and attitudes about health. Extensive and long-term follow-up is required if individualized interventions are to succeed. Nurses must be aware of the prevalence of health problems and make assessments accordingly.

Health Education. Community and school-based health programs for adolescents focus on health promotion and illness prevention. Nurses can become involved in these programs by providing screening and teaching for adolescents (Table 23.10). Developing and implementing programs to respond to adolescents' needs is another important strategy that nurses can be involved in. Helping adolescents make decisions about their health care strengthens their autonomy and promotes healthy behaviours. However, remember that adolescents first need to feel comfortable and respected as individuals before they will reveal

TABLE 23.10	Health Promotion for Adolescents	
Adolescent Health Concerns	**Health Promotion Intervention**	
Unintentional injuries	Advise the adolescent to take a driver's education course and to wear a seat belt.	
	Inform the adolescent of risks associated with drinking and driving and use of drugs.	
	Promote helmet use by adolescents who ride bicycles, motorcycles, all-terrain vehicles, and snowmobiles.	
	Ensure the adolescent receives proper orientation in the use of all sports equipment.	
	Encourage the adolescent to swim with a "buddy."	
Firearm use and violence	Teach conflict resolution skills.	
	Implement gang-prevention strategies.	
Tobacco, alcohol, and drug use	Screen for tobacco (including smokeless), vaping, alcohol, and drug use, and inform the adolescent of risks of use.	
Suicide	Offer suicide prevention information.	
	Teach methods of dealing with a suicidal peer.	
	Promote alternatives to suicide.	
Sexually transmitted infections	Provide the adolescent with information regarding disease, mode of transmission, and related symptoms.	
	Encourage safer sexual practices, including abstinence from sexual activity or the use of condoms.	
	Provide accurate information about the consequences of sexual activity.	

intimate information about their risk-taking behaviours. Discussions with adolescents must therefore be private and confidential.

A nurse can play an important role in preventing injuries and accidental deaths by taking part in activities such as injury prevention programs; working with organizations that promote responsible behaviour, including Mothers Against Drunk Driving (MADD) and Drug Abuse Resistance Education (DARE); and encouraging students to participate in organizations such as Students Against Drunk Driving (SADD). By engaging adolescents in a discussion of the alternatives to driving when under the influence of drugs or alcohol, you can prepare them to consider the alternatives when such an occasion arises. It is also important to identify adolescents at risk for substance use, provide education to prevent accidents related to substance use, and provide counselling to patients in rehabilitation programs.

The nurse can also play a strategic role in an antismoking movement, such as participating in a smoking prevention program initiated in a school. Education should also include information about the risks of vaping, which can cause lung damage and altered brain development from nicotine (Government of Canada, 2020).

Regardless of health setting, nurses need to provide sex education and counselling and can play a key role in counselling teenagers on ways to avoid pregnancy. Nurses can also assist adolescents in making decisions about pregnancies that do occur (e.g., becoming a parent, adoption, or abortion). Some schools have instituted day care programs so that adolescent parents can continue their schooling after their babies are born. Whatever choice an adolescent makes, it is important that they receive appropriate health care, including counselling.

Extensive educational efforts to prevent the spread of AIDS and other STIs in this age group are a nursing responsibility. Formal or informal education, in a one-on-one or group setting, may be provided in the school or community. Speakers and organizations can be used to help in the educational process.

Adolescents in Rural Communities. Approximately 18% of Canadians lived in rural areas and small towns in 2020 (Trading Economics, 2022); however, this percentage varies by province and territory. Although adolescents living in these areas have many of the same health needs as their urban counterparts, they also have some unique risks. For example, those living on farms are at increased risk for accidents because of exposure to heavy equipment, chemicals, huge vehicles, and large animals. Safety days and education programs for children are provided by organizations such as the Canadian Agricultural Safety Association (2019). Other concerns for adolescents living in rural areas and small towns are the limited availability of recreational facilities and limited access to specialized services.

Nurses can play an important role in improving the health of adolescents who live in rural areas by acting to decrease barriers to care, providing health promotion education, developing coping strategies for these adolescents, and assessing their health beliefs.

Indigenous Adolescents. Health status and the factors affecting it are generally worse for Indigenous adolescents than for any other adolescent populations in Canada (Kumar & Tjepkema, 2019) (see Chapter 12: Indigenous Health). In Canada, suicide rates are 2 to 9 times higher for Indigenous peoples, with suicide rates being highest among 15- to 24-year-olds (Kumar & Tjepkema, 2019). Among First Nation boys under the age of 15, suicide rates are 4 time higher than rates for non-Indigenous boys and 10 times higher for boys who live on reserve. Factors that contribute to the high suicide rates among Indigenous peoples include the effects of colonization, a history of mental health conditions, a family history of suicide and violence, intergenerational trauma, and difficulty accessing health care services. In contrast, several factors have been identified that increase the resilience of Indigenous youth and decrease the rates of suicide. These include communities with 50% or more people with knowledge of the Indigenous language, Indigenous title to traditional lands, self-government, and cultural facilities (Kumar & Tjepkema, 2019).

When working with Indigenous adolescents, nurses need to be aware of the unique factors that may affect these young people's health. First, nurses need to be aware that health beliefs and practices, as well as health problems, vary among Indigenous populations and communities. Nurses must be sensitive to culturally appropriate interventions. Many Indigenous communities take responsibility for their own health and well-being, develop their own health services, and include traditional methods of healing to improve well-being.

LGBTQ2 Adolescents. Although research on lesbian, gay, bisexual, transgender, queer, and Two-Spirit (LGBTQ2) youth is limited, special consideration must be given to the developmental and health challenges that may result from nonheterosexual orientations and societal attitudes toward those orientations (Hockenberry et al., 2019). It may be difficult for adolescents to discuss some of these challenges because of the stigma associated with being LGBTQ2. As a consequence, LGBTQ2 youth could be at greater risk for emotional distress, depression, suicide, and alcohol or other drug use. LGBTQ2 youth may need assistance with disclosing their sexual orientation; before coming out, they may also need help developing a plan for dealing with the negative and sometimes violent reactions from others who are nonaccepting of them, including family members. It is important to respond to these individuals in a sensitive and nonjudgemental way (see Chapter 24: Young to Middle Adulthood).

KEY CONCEPTS

- A developmental perspective helps the nurse understand commonalities and variations in each stage and the impact they have on the patient's health.
- During the intrauterine period, while the embryo and fetus grow and develop, genetic factors and environmental factors (teratogens) may cause impairments in any body system.
- Physiological, cognitive, and psychosocial development continue from conception through adolescence, and nurses must be familiar with normal parameters to determine potential problems and to promote normal development.
- Physical growth during the school years is slow and steady until the skeletal growth spurt just before puberty.
- The major psychosocial developmental task of school-age children is the development of a sense of competence.
- Cognitive development in young school-age children involves developing the ability to think in a logical manner.
- The prepubertal growth spurt usually occurs 2 years earlier in girls than in boys.
- Adolescents move forward to the last stage of cognitive development, formal operations, in which they begin to think in an abstract manner, reflect on thought processes, and plan for the future.
- Adolescence begins with puberty, which manifests as changes in the primary sexual characteristics (maturation of the reproductive organs) and the secondary sexual characteristics (such as the development of pubic hair and female breasts).
- Adolescents are able to solve complex mental problems by using deductive reasoning.
- Adolescents' rapid change in physical appearance heightens self-consciousness and concerns about body image.

- Accidents are the major cause of death in all age groups up to adulthood.
- Motor vehicle accidents are the major cause of accidental death in adolescence.
- Adolescents begin the long process of emancipation from their parents and need parental support to accomplish this task in a timely manner.

CRITICAL THINKING EXERCISES

1. Alana (preferred pronouns: she/her), who is in her first trimester of pregnancy, is attending the antepartum clinic for the first visit. What are the main health promotion topics you need to explore with her at this stage of her pregnancy?
2. The parents of 2-year-old Mark (preferred pronouns: he/him) are concerned because his language does not seem to be at the same level as that of their neighbour's 2-year-old daughter. How would you reassure these parents and help them with language development?
3. Eight-year-old Lisa (preferred pronouns: she/her) sometimes tells her parents that she feels "like a failure." According to Erickson's task for this stage of development, what measures can her parents and teacher use to help negate these feelings and help her meet this stage of development?
4. Twelve-year-old Maya (preferred pronouns: she/her) is brought to the pediatric clinic for a physical examination. Maya is concerned about her lack of physical development in comparison with her peers. Discuss ways to educate Maya about puberty and the variations that occur.
5. Fifteen-year-old Ricardo (preferred pronouns: he/him) wants very much to belong and to be accepted by his peers. He expresses concern when his peers begin to plan a party with alcohol and drugs. What should be discussed to help support his feelings and need to belong?

🌐 *Answers to Critical Thinking Exercises appear on the Evolve website.*

REVIEW QUESTIONS

Review Questions 1 to 9 relate to the case study at the beginning of the chapter.

1. Nurse Angele (preferred pronouns: they/them) does a home visit with Rochelle (preferred pronouns: she/her) and newborn Isolde. Rochelle is concerned because Isolde is crying more frequently than expected. Isolde is currently fussy and displaying infant feeding cues. What nursing actions should Angele take? *(Select all that apply.)*
   a. Assess Rochelle's knowledge about feeding cues and infant crying.
   b. Provide client-centred education based on Rochelle's needs.
   c. Suggest to Rochelle that she feed Isolde.
   d. Explain the risks of infant crying.
2. Nurse Angele weighs baby Isolde the day following birth and finds that 5% of the infant's birthweight has been lost. What action should the nurse take?
   a. Inform the parent that the infant's weight is normal.
   b. Notify the doctor about the infant's weight loss.
   c. Instruct the parent to breastfeed the infant more frequently.
   d. Instruct the parent to supplement breastfeeding with formula.
3. According to Piaget's theory of development, at about 2 years of age, toddlers transition to preoperational thought. Which of the

following would indicate that Isolde, your 3-year-old patient, has reached this cognitive milestone? *(Select all that apply.)*
   a. The child can understand your point of view.
   b. The child likes to play pretend.
   c. The child understands object permanence.
   d. The child can logically reason why something is happening to them.
4. You are caring for preschooler Isolde, who is now 4 years old and talking well. Which of the following would be cognitively and behaviourally appropriate nursing interventions when caring for a preschooler? *(Select all that apply.)*
   a. Allow the child to handle equipment you will use in assessment.
   b. Encourage play and talking about feelings to vent frustration or anger.
   c. Avoid using phonetically similar words when explaining procedures.
   d. Provide experiences the child can master to support return to prior level of functioning.
5. Rochelle is concerned about the amount of time Isolde is spending on digital media. What findings may indicate that Isolde's screen use is problematic? *(Select all that apply.)*
   a. Isolde appears upset during or after screen time.
   b. Isolde occasionally enjoys playing online games with friends.
   c. Isolde is not completing assigned homework.
   d. Isolde uses a cell phone in the evenings and has difficulty falling asleep.
   e. Isolde complains of being bored when away from Internet access.
6. During a wellness check in Grade 9, Isolde (preferred pronouns: they/them) discloses that they are being bullied at school. The nurse should assess for which warning signs of suicide? *(Select all that apply.)*
   a. Loneliness, sadness, and crying
   b. Stable school performance
   c. Social withdrawal
   d. An increase in appetite
   e. A decrease in appetite
   f. Verbalization of suicidal thought
7. Isolde is now 12 years old. Isolde tells the school nurse that they are concerned because, unlike their friends, they have not started menstruating, although they have had some breast development. Which is the most likely reason for the client's concern?
   a. The client has a gynecological condition that is impeding menstruation.
   b. The client is in prepuberty.
   c. The client has an eating disorder that is impeding menstruation.
   d. The client is undergoing puberty at a normal rate.
8. The nurse gives a presentation to a group of parents at Isolde's school on health risks for Canadian adolescents. Which parental statement indicates the need for more teaching about the health risks? *(Select all that apply.)*
   a. "The leading cause of death in adolescence is substance use."
   b. "The leading cause of death in adolescence is injuries."
   c. "Eating disorders are only a concern for parents with daughters."
   d. "The number of adolescents smoking cigarettes is increasing."
9. The local public health office is offering COVID-19 vaccines to high school students. Isolde feels mildly ill with seasonal allergies and is worried about the safety of the vaccine. What approach should the public health nurse use? *(Select all that apply.)*

a. Provide up-to-date information about the vaccine.
b. Acknowledge vaccine hesitancy and address concerns.
c. Discuss the importance of vaccines in reducing the severity of COVID-19.
d. Delay administration of the vaccine until Isolde is feeling better.

Answers: 1. a, b, c; 2. a; 3. b; c 4. a, b, c, d; 5. a, c, d; 6. a, c, d, e, f; 7. d; 8. a, c d 9. a, b, c.

Rationales for the Review Questions appear on the Evolve website.

RECOMMENDED WEBSITES

BC Children's Hospital—Gender Resources:
http://www.bcchildrens.ca/health-info/coping-support/gender-resources
This website provides information for families, children, youth, and health care providers.

Campaign 2000: https://campaign2000.ca
Campaign 2000 is a nonpartisan, cross-Canada coalition of more than 120 national, provincial, and community organizations committed to working together to end child and family poverty in Canada.

Canadian Paediatric Society—Position Statements and Practice Points:
https://www.cps.ca/en/documents
This website includes the Canadian Paediatric Society's position statements on a variety of child health issues. Updated information is released on an ongoing basis.

Immunize Canada: https://immunize.ca
Immunize Canada (formerly the Canadian Coalition for Immunization Awareness and Promotion) is a partnership of national nongovernmental, professional, health, consumer, government, and private-sector organizations focused on promoting the understanding and use of vaccines recommended by the National Advisory Committee on Immunization. This website provides evidence-informed resources on immunization for parents and health care providers.

Parachute: https://parachutecanada.org
Parachute is Canada's national charity dedicated to injury prevention in the home, at play, or on the move.

REFERENCES

A full reference list is available on the website for this book at http://evolve.elsevier.com/Canada/Potter/fundamentals/

24

Young to Middle Adulthood

Canadian content written by J. Craig Phillips, RN, PhD, LLM, ACRN, FAAN, FCAN, with original chapter contributions by Anne Griffin Perry, RN, MSN, EdD, FAAN

OBJECTIVES

Mastery of content in this chapter will enable you to:

- Define the key terms listed.
- Describe the major life events and developmental tasks of young and middle-aged adults.
- Explain the significance of family in the life of the adult.
- Describe normal physiological changes in young and middle adulthood, including pregnancy.
- Explain the cognitive and psychosocial changes that occur during the adult years.
- Describe the health concerns of young and middle-aged adults.
- Apply clinical decision making to administering care to young and middle-aged adults.

KEY TERMS

Braxton-Hicks contractions

Breastfeeding

Computer-mediated communication

Erasure

Gender expression

Gender identity

Health literacy

Heteronormativity

Infertility

Lesbian, gay, bisexual, transgender, queer, and Two-Spirit (LGBTQ2)

Menopause

Nesting

Peer support worker

Perimenopause

Prenatal care

Puerperium

Sandwich generation

🌐 WEBSITE

http://evolve.elsevier.com/Canada/Potter/fundamentals/

CASE STUDY

Transgender-Affirming Care

Justine is a 40-year-old Two-Spirit transgender woman (preferred pronouns: she/her) who has been brought to the emergency department by the police because she was found wandering around a local park. She is disoriented, emaciated, and agitated.

Psychosocial history: *Justine is known to hospital staff and has been treated by them many times over the years. She was forcibly removed from her birth family at 3 years of age and spent 5 years in the child welfare system. She was adopted at 8 years of age. Justine is estranged from her adoptive family, as they do not accept her "lifestyle choices." Justine smokes and has used alcohol and drugs in the past.*

Medical history: *Diagnosed with human immunodeficiency virus (HIV) at age 23. No known drug allergies.*

Current medications: *Cross-sex hormone therapy, antiretroviral therapy, and selective-serotonin reuptake inhibitor (SSRI; anti-depressant).*

Think about this case study as you read this chapter. There are Review Questions at the end of the chapter about this case study.

Young to middle adulthood is a life stage marked by challenges, rewards, and crises. Challenges may include the demands of working and raising a family; rewards may include career, family, and personal successes; and crises may include job loss and caring for children or adolescents in crisis in addition to caring for aging parents. At the time of writing this chapter, the world was in its third year of navigating the worst pandemic in more than a century. We have all been learning to live with COVID-19, an emerging pathogen that affects all humans across the lifespan. Sadly, the pandemic has caused over 6.3 million deaths worldwide (https://covid19.who.int/) and revealed persistent health inequities.

Adult developmental changes are unique to each person and are influenced by the social and ecological contexts in which we live. These changes are based on characteristics that originate in childhood and subsequent behaviours that people develop to adapt to these characteristics, environments, and new experiences. Young adulthood is the period from about 20 to 35 years of age (American Psychological Association [APA], 2020). In 2020, young adults between 20 and 34 years of age constituted approximately 20.5% of the Canadian population (Statistics Canada, 2021a). During young adulthood, people move away from their families of origin, establish career goals, and decide whether to marry and begin families or to remain single.

Middle age is the period between the mid- to late 30s and the mid-60s (APA, 2020). During this period, people become aware of changes in reproductive and physical abilities and may reassess life goals. In 2020, the median age of the Canadian population was 40.9 years of age; this age group continues to grow because fertility rates have declined and life expectancy has increased (Statistics Canada, 2021a).

Developmental theories provide nurses with a basis for understanding the life events and developmental tasks of young and middle-aged adults. Developmental theorists Erikson (1963, 1982), Havighurst (1972), and Gilligan (1993) have described the phases of adulthood and related developmental tasks (see Chapter 22). The Canadian Association of Schools of Nursing's *National Nursing Education Framework* provides a competency framework to guide nurses in acquiring relevant knowledge and skills (Canadian Association of Schools of Nursing [CASN], 2022). This chapter provides foundational knowledge of human development and functioning across the lifespan, drawing from secondary education, natural and life sciences, and behavioural and social sciences. This foundational knowledge will help you develop "the ability to recognize and respond safely, competently and ethically to rapidly changing client-conditions and context" (CASN, 2022).

You may be a young or middle-aged adult yourself, coping with the demands of your own developmental period. As a nurse, you must be careful to recognize and respect the needs of your patients even if you are not experiencing the same challenges and events. You can help young and middle-aged adults achieve their potential by offering support and providing information and appropriate referrals.

YOUNG ADULTHOOD

Physical Changes

Most young adults have completed physical growth by 20 years of age. Young adults are usually quite active, experience fewer severe illnesses than those in older age groups, tend to ignore physical symptoms of illness, and often postpone seeking health care. The physical characteristics of young adults begin to change as middle age approaches.

Individuals in this developmental stage may benefit from a personal lifestyle assessment to identify habits that increase the risk for cardiac, malignant, pulmonary, renal, or other chronic diseases. A personal lifestyle assessment of the young adult includes assessment of general life satisfaction; hobbies and interests; habits (e.g., diet, sleep, exercise, sexual practices, use of caffeine, alcohol, and illicit drugs); home conditions (e.g., housing, finances); and occupational environment (e.g., type of work, exposure to hazardous substances, physical or mental strain).

Cognitive Changes

Cognitive changes are variations in reasoning and thinking. Critical thinking habits increase steadily through the young and middle-adult years. Formal and informal education, life experiences, and work opportunities increase people's conceptual and problem-solving skills. Young adults that use flexible decision-making processes cope most effectively by continually evolving and adjusting to changes and challenges in their home, workplace, and personal lives.

Choosing an occupation is a major task of young adults. It requires knowledge of one's skills, talents, and personality characteristics. Occupational choices for many young adults are limited by the lack of resources or support systems for pursuing higher education.

By addressing health literacy issues (Box 24.1) and understanding how adults learn, nurses can develop relevant patient teaching plans (see Chapter 21 for further information about patient education).

BOX 24.1 Health Literacy

Health literacy is an important health determinant for many health outcomes. Health literacy requires the patient to be able to access information, process that information to understand it, and act on that information to make good health decisions. People who are health literate can find the information they need; read, interpret, and understand the message conveyed; weigh their treatment options; navigate the available health services to determine which ones are appropriate; and understand instructions that health care providers give them.

Strategies that you as a nurse can use to increase health literacy include the teach-back technique. In this process you provide an initial teaching or explanation, followed by a summary of key information in manageable chunks. Then, you check the person's understanding and clarify any of their questions or concerns. When you seek to enhance someone's health literacy, encourage questions by using body language that invites questions (e.g., position yourself at the person's level), solicit questions (e.g., "Let me know when you have questions"), help the person form questions, take time for questions, and check that teaching is complete (e.g., "Have all your questions been answered?").

Comprehending medical information is challenging. Assessing health literacy and taking steps to ensure that people understand the information presented to them and can make informed decisions can improve health outcomes. Helping people develop health literacy will become a rewarding part of your nursing practice.

Adapted from McCall, J., & Wilson, C. (2015). Promoting health literacy in an HIV-infected population: Creating staff awareness. *Journal of the Association of Nurses in AIDS Care, 26*(4), 498–502. https://doi.org/10.1016/j.jana.2014.11.003

Adults enter learning situations already having a background of unique life experiences, including illness. Therefore, nurses should always view each adult as a unique individual. When determining the amount of information that a person needs in order to make decisions about a prescribed course of therapy, nurses should consider the range of factors that may affect the person's adherence to the regimen, including educational level, sociocultural factors, social context, motivation (Etowa et al., 2021a), and desire to learn.

Psychosocial Changes

The emotional health of young adults is related to their ability to address and resolve personal and social tasks. Young adults often want to prolong adolescence and yet assume adult commitments. Between the ages of 23 and 28 years, people usually refine self-perception and capacity for intimacy. From 29 to 34 years of age, people usually focus on achieving personal and occupational goals and improving their socioeconomic status. For many young adults, a dual-income family is needed to achieve and maintain middle-class status. Career and personal counselling can help people identify career choices and set realistic goals.

Ethnicity and gender issues influence an adult's life and can pose challenges for nursing care, as each person holds culture-bound definitions of health and illness. An understanding of ethnicity, race, and gender differences enables nurses to provide individualized care (see Chapter 11 for further information about culture and context).

Traditional gender roles have changed in recent decades, resulting in changes to traditional family structures. Since the 1970s, women have been entering the workforce and pursuing careers outside the home in high numbers. In 2021, about 78.5% of Canadian women aged 25 to 54 years were employed (Statistics Canada, 2021b). Women contribute significantly to their families' incomes and tend to bear primary caregiving responsibilities. As a result, many women deal with the stresses of being a partner, a parent, a caregiver to aging parents, and an employee. Some men choose to put their careers on hold to be stay-at-home parents.

Career. Young people hope to have fulfilling careers. They may formulate short- and long-term career goals. Successful employment ensures economic security and promotes friendships, social activities, support, and self-respect.

In many two-career relationships, the benefits experienced (e.g., improved finances) may outweigh potential stressors (e.g., child care demands; household needs; increased physical, mental, or emotional demands). To reduce stress in a two-career family, neither partner should assume all household responsibilities. For some families, one solution is to hire a housekeeper. Others may set up an equal division of household and child care duties. During the COVID-19 pandemic, women assumed more homeschooling responsibilities than men, and it is unclear whether women or men were assuming more caregiving and household responsibilities (Statistics Canada, 2020a).

Sexuality. Young adults usually have the emotional maturity necessary to establish intimacy and develop fulfilling sexual relationships. Young adults who have failed to achieve the developmental tasks of adolescence may develop superficial relationships (Austin et al., 2018).

For most young adults, the emotional aspect of sexual activity is as important as its type or frequency. Understanding the differences between sexual desire (i.e., responses to physical and mental stimuli during or in anticipation of sexual activity), sexual behaviour (i.e., how humans experience and express their sexuality), and sexual identity (i.e., how a person identifies their sexuality) will facilitate your work as a nurse with young adults. Recognizing the distinct differences between each of these categories and how they are influenced by internal and external factors will facilitate open dialogue and collaborative approaches to patient teaching about sexual health. This open dialogue has the capacity to reduce potential sexual health risks, including human immunodeficiency virus (HIV) and other sexually transmitted infections (Phillips et al., 2021). Adults should be encouraged to explore various aspects of their sexuality and be aware that their sexual needs and concerns evolve (see Chapter 28).

Nurses should be aware of how the social determinants of health impact individuals who identify as **lesbian, gay, bisexual, transgender, queer, and Two-Spirit (LGBTQ2).** For example, despite the lack of fundamental health differences between the LGBTQ2 and heterosexual populations, there are health disparities between the two groups (Henriquez et al., 2019). Within the LGBTQ2 population, health disparities and risks also differ among subgroups (Phillips et al., 2021).

Gender Identity and Expression. **Gender identity** is a person's inner sense of their gender (e.g., cisgender man, cisgender woman, transgender, bigender, non-binary, Two-Spirit), which may or may not align with their biological sex (Aisner et al., 2020). **Gender expression** is how people outwardly express their gender (e.g., masculine, feminine, androgynous, neutral), usually through physical appearance or behaviours (Aisner et al., 2020). Challenges may arise for young adults who do not conform to traditional gender presentation. LGBTQ2 individuals may face challenges in navigating the health care system and social context because of **heteronormativity**—the exclusionary belief that heterosexuality and the gender binary of male–female are the norm— which in turn limits their ability to lead happy and healthy lives (Burton et al., 2021; Phillips et al., 2021; Unger, 2016; Ziegler et al., 2020).

For transgender persons, navigating the world may be particularly challenging owing to "erasure," the social process through which transsexuality is managed in cultures and institutions as being ultimately impossible (Bauer et al., 2009). **Erasure** describes the way in which a heteronormative society systematically "erases" sexual minority identities by allowing only gender binary designations (male–female) on health records and other documents (Bauer et al., 2009). The 2021 Census of Population in Canada was recently expanded to rectify this problem (Statistics Canada, 2020b, 2020c).

For other sexual minorities, the common use of the epidemiological categories of *men who have sex with men* (MSM) and *women who have sex with women* (WSW) serves to "erase" the existence of gay and lesbian communities (Phillips et al., 2021). Governmental apologies, such as the one delivered by Prime Minister Justin Trudeau on November 28, 2017 (Harris, 2017), acknowledge the structural challenges faced by LGBTQ2 individuals and offer hope to members of these groups. This apology requires nurses to be vigilant in promoting equity in health care delivery in order to address the health disparities experienced by LGBTQ2 individuals living in Canada (Harris, 2017).

Two-Spirit is a term used by some Indigenous peoples to describe a person whose gender identity, sexual orientation, or spiritual identity does not align with the gender binary and heteronormativity (LGBTQ2 Secretariat, 2022). Two-Spirit individuals assume cross-gender or multiple gender roles, attributes, dress, and attitudes for personal, spiritual, cultural, ceremonial, or social reasons. These roles are defined by each Indigenous cultural group and can be fluid over a person's lifetime. Some Indigenous people also use terms such as *gay, lesbian, bisexual, transgender, transsexual,* or *intersex* (exclusively or in combination with Two-Spirit) to define who they are (Lezard et al., 2021).

Singlehood. Social pressure to get married is not as great as it once was. Family structures and living arrangements continue to diversify. Young adults who choose to remain single and maintain independence may consider siblings and parents as their family. However, close friends and associates may also be viewed as the person's "chosen family." Some single people choose to become parents, either biologically or through adoption.

The population of single people is increasing partly because women have greater career opportunities than before and partly because single people often choose to live together and share housing costs rather than marry. In addition, many adults become single again after a marriage ends.

Marriage. In the latest Census of Population, married and common-law families accounted for 47.6% of all families, and the number of lone-parent families continued to increase (Statistics Canada, 2021c). The 2011 census cycle was the first full cycle in which all areas of Canada recognized same-sex marriage, and the number of same-sex marriages increased by 42% between 2006 and 2011 (Statistics Canada, 2012). The number of same-sex marriages across Canada increased by 16% between 2011 and 2016 (Statistics Canada, 2017) and by 61% between 2016 and 2021 (Statistics Canada, 2022).

Every married couple's relationship is unique, regardless of the gender makeup of the couple. Although no rules can guarantee a successful marriage, there are some useful guidelines for building a happy marriage. Before getting married, a couple ideally should (1) ensure that their emotions are based on love rather than physical attraction alone, (2) explore their motivations for marriage, (3) develop clear communication, (4) accept that behaviour and habits are unlikely to change after marriage, and (5) determine their compatibility in important beliefs and values.

When establishing a household and family, the married couple must work as a team. People require maturity and self-esteem to accomplish the following major tasks of marriage: establishing an intimate relationship; deciding on and working toward mutual goals; establishing guidelines for decision making; setting boundaries and standards for social interactions; and choosing morals, values, and ideologies acceptable to both. Accomplishing these tasks sets the foundation for a stable relationship.

Marriage also requires the couple to learn patterns of sexual expression, establish roles, and practise effective conflict resolution and decision-making skills. Each partner may experience a sense of loss of their individuality in the transition from being single to being married.

Child-Bearing Cycle. Conception, pregnancy, birth, and the puerperium (postpartum period) are phases of the child-bearing cycle. The changes during these phases are complex. Childbirth education classes can prepare the pregnant person, their partner, and other supportive people to participate in the birthing process. Pregnant people and their families may benefit from having a peer support worker.

Breastfeeding offers many advantages to both the child-bearing parent and their baby (see Chapter 43). However, for the inexperienced parent, breastfeeding may cause anxiety and frustration. Child-bearing parents who have had no previous contact with newborns and other child-bearing parents who breastfeed may require assistance to breastfeed successfully. Nurses must be alert for signs that the parent needs information and assistance. By observing the parent while they breastfeed, the nurse may catch problems such as improper positioning or ineffective sucking by the infant (Registered Nurses' Association of Ontario, 2018).

As a nurse, you will need to be sensitive to the diverse needs of child-bearing parents who seek guidance about breastfeeding and other options for feeding their infants, including parents living with HIV and transmasculine gestational parents. For example, a parent living with HIV may desire to breastfeed; however, nurses need to know that this practice is counter to current infant-feeding guidelines in Canada and may pose challenges for child-bearing parents from other parts of the world (Etowa et al., 2021a, 2021b). In the case of a transmasculine parent who wishes to breastfeed, nurses need to be knowledgeable about lactation and chest care as well as sensitive to their gender identity and gender expression experiences (MacDonald et al., 2016).

The personal and social changes that occur in parents' lives after the birth of a baby cannot be overstated. Nursing assessment of a parent's response to the birthing experience and parent–child attachment are discussed later in this chapter.

Parenthood. Contraception allows couples or individuals to decide when and whether to start a family. One factor influencing this decision is the reason for wanting a child. Social pressures may encourage a couple to have a child or may influence them to limit the number of children they have. Economic considerations frequently enter the discussion because raising children is expensive. Because couples are getting married later and are postponing pregnancies, general health status and age may influence whether a couple decides to have children. To overcome the economic challenges to parenthood, Canada offers 15 weeks of maternity benefits for child-bearing parents; 35 weeks of parental benefits for either parent; and, as of 2019, 5 weeks of paternity benefits for the father or second parent (UNICEF Canada, 2019).

Parenting roles must be defined and practised. The nurturing and socialization needs of children and adolescents can put pressure on a couple's relationship. In addition, parents' images of the "perfect parent" may conflict with reality. For example, parents may be blamed for parental failures when an adolescent engages in substance misuse. A qualitative literature synthesis highlighted mothers' experiences of parenting adolescents who misused substances and the complex social and familial factors that intersect with adolescent substance misuse (Katouziyan et al., 2018).

Alternative Family Structures and Parenting. Norms and values about family life in Canada are evolving continuously, as demonstrated

by judicial rulings on same-sex marriage since 2000. More infants are being born to cohabiting (common-law) couples (see Chapter 20). Families may take the form of a single parent and children, same-sex couples with or without children, or a blended family consisting of children from previous relationships. Parents living in alternative family structures may perceive a lack of support and bias from the health care system (Malmquist & Nieminen, 2021). Same-sex parents and their children may need support for adoption of children and the parenting role.

Hallmarks of Emotional Health

Most young adults have the physical and emotional resources and support systems to meet their challenges, tasks, and responsibilities. During psychosocial assessment of young adults, nurses can assess for 10 hallmarks of emotional health that indicate successful maturation in this developmental stage (Box 24.2). If one or more of these hallmarks are not attained, further assessment and action may be required.

Social Support in Health and Illness

A current trend in health care is the use of a peer support worker (or peer navigator) to facilitate well-being (Figure 24.1). This trend is evident in states of health when a family uses the services of a peer support worker to help a child-bearing person and their family to navigate the challenges of pregnancy. In chronic disease states such as cancer, mental illness, and HIV, peer navigators can help people

BOX 24.2	10 Hallmarks of Emotional Health

- A sense of meaning and direction in life
- Successful negotiation through transitions
- Absence of feelings of being cheated or disappointed by life
- Attainment of several long-term goals
- Satisfaction with personal growth and development
- When married, feelings of love for partner; when single, satisfaction with social interactions
- Satisfaction with friendships
- Generally cheerful attitude
- Acceptance of constructive criticism
- No unrealistic fears

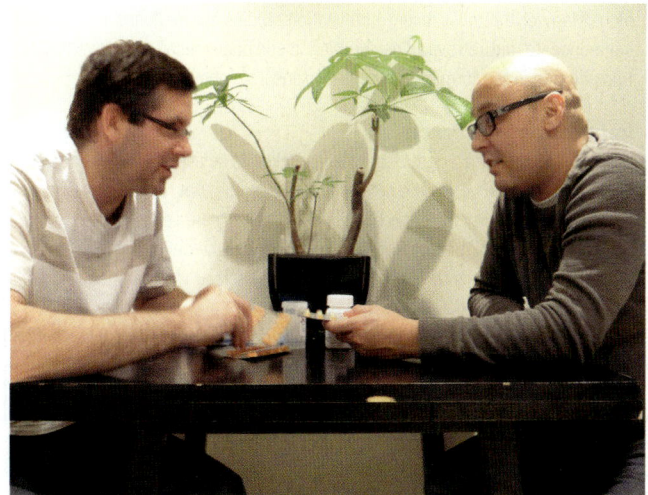

FIGURE 24.1 A peer navigator and person discuss medication adherence strategies.

navigate the complexities of the health care system and therapeutic regimens (Box 24.3).

Health Risks

Health risk factors for a young adult originate in lifestyle patterns, family history, and their environment and occupation.

Lifestyle. Lifestyle habits such as poor food choices, smoking, stress, high-risk sexual behaviour, substance use, and inactivity increase the risk of illness. For example, prolonged stress can cause ulcers, emotional disorders, and infections (see Chapter 30 for further information about stress and adaptation). Smoking and second-hand smoke can cause lung cancer and pulmonary, cardiac, and vascular diseases. **Computer-mediated communication** (e.g., Internet dating, "sexting") can lead to high-risk sexual encounters and adverse health outcomes (Phillips et al., 2021). Your role as a nurse in health promotion is to identify lifestyle risk factors and provide education and support to reduce unhealthy behaviours.

Family History. A family history of a disease may put a young adult at risk for developing that disease in middle age or later. For example, a family history of certain cancers or cardiovascular, renal, endocrine, or neoplastic disease increases the family member's risk of developing the disease.

Accidental Death and Injury. Accidents are the leading causes of injury and death in young adults (Statistics Canada, 2021d). Death and injury can result from motor vehicle or other accidents, physical assaults, and suicide attempts. In 2018, 24% of driver fatalities were among drivers between 20 and 34 years of age (Transport Canada, 2021).

Physical assault and violence also lead to injury and death. Police-reported crimes increased between 2018 and 2019 but remained lower than they were in 2009 (Allen, 2022). Firearm-related and gang-related violent crime, including homicide, accidental death, and suicide, remain a significant public health and social issue (Allen, 2022). The homicide rate for Indigenous peoples was approximately 6.5 times higher than that for the non-Indigenous population (Statistics Canada, 2020d). Risk factors for violence include poverty, breakdown of family relations, child abuse and neglect, and access to firearms. To detect personal and environmental risk factors for violence, nurses need to perform a thorough psychosocial assessment, including assessment of behavioural patterns, history of physical violence and substance use, education, work history, and social support systems.

Substance Misuse. Substance misuse directly or indirectly contributes to mortality and morbidity in young adults. Regular heavy drinking (five or more drinks on one occasion) is most common among Canadians aged 20 to 34 years, and more men than women in this age group drink. Regular heavy drinking appears to be decreasing among both sexes, although more slowly in women compared to men in this age group (Statistics Canada, 2021e). Intoxication is often a factor in motor vehicle accidents.

Rates of opioid use are on the rise in the population and have reached epidemic proportions across North America. Dependence on stimulants ("uppers") puts stress on the cardiovascular and nervous systems and can thus cause overdose and death. Use of depressants ("downers") can lead to accidental or intentional overdose and death. Nurses can provide counselling and support for people seeking treatment for substance misuse.

Substance use disorder cannot always be diagnosed, particularly in its early stages. Nonjudgemental questions about the use of legal drugs (prescription medications, over-the-counter medications, tobacco, alcohol, and cannabis [which became legalized in Canada in 2020]) and illegal drugs (cocaine, heroin) should be a routine part of any physical assessment and psychosocial history. Important information may be obtained by making specific inquiries about past medical problems, changes in food intake or sleep patterns, or issues with emotional lability. A record of arrests for impaired driving, domestic or child abuse, or disorderly conduct should alert the nurse to the possibility of substance use disorder.

Unplanned Pregnancies. Unplanned pregnancies, although more common among adolescents, also occur in young and middle-aged adults of child-bearing age. Unplanned pregnancies are a source of

---

🔰 BOX 24.3 RESEARCH HIGHLIGHT

Expanding Nurses' Knowledge to Achieve Equity and a Right to Health With LBGTQ2 People

Research Focus

Building nursing workforce capacity to achieve equity and the human right to health for LGBTQ2 people requires ongoing action by all nurses to eliminate stigma and discrimination. To understand how nurses have contributed to this goal, Phillips and colleagues (2021) systematically reviewed all HIV nursing literature that addressed the health of LGBTQ2 people living with HIV over the first 40 years of the HIV pandemic.

Research Abstract

The research team members had diverse ancestry and were gender diverse. They applied an inclusive approach by using a literature review and the 15 health-related Yogyakarta Principles plus 10 (International Commission of Jurists, 2017, as cited in Phillips et al., 2021) to identify specific actions that nurses can take with LGBTQ2 people to realize those principles.

Methods and Results

The search strategy identified 1 109 articles after duplicates were removed. Data were extracted from 68 articles; these were categorized as practice guidance articles (n = 44) or intervention studies (n = 24). Evidence-informed recommendations to improve the health of LGBTQ2 people's health were categorized as those that are applicable to all LGBTQ2 people, LGBTQ2 adolescents, lesbian women and women who have sex with women (WSW), transgender people, and gay men and men who have sex with men (MSM).

The authors found that HIV nurses have engaged in and led intervention studies by, with, or for LGBTQ2 people at the individual, family, and structural levels. Most of the intervention studies have been conducted with gay men. Many of the most recent intervention studies are designed to improve adherence to antiretroviral prescription medications used to prevent HIV transmission in the form of pre- or post-exposure prophylaxis.

Implications for Practice

- International human rights legal frameworks can be used to guide nurses to develop approaches to the care of LGBTQ2 people that reduces the stigma and discrimination they may experience in health care settings.
- Including LGBTQ2 people and their loved ones in the development of interventions to address their health conditions may lead to greater success of interventions.
- Nurses are well positioned in the health care system to improve health outcomes for LGBTQ2 people and to advocate for policy changes to improve health equity.

From Phillips, J. C., Hidayat, J., Clark, K., et al. (2021). A review of the state of HIV nursing science with sexual orientation, gender identity/expression (SOGI) peoples. *Journal of the Association of Nurses in AIDS Care, 32*(3), 225–252. https://doi.org/10.1097/jnc.0000000000000250

stress that can result in adverse health outcomes for the child-bearing parent, infant, and family. Many young adults have educational and career goals that take precedence over family development. Interference with these goals can affect future relationships and later parent–child relationships. When assessing the child-bearing parent faced with an unplanned pregnancy, nurses should determine the situational factors that will affect pregnancy outcome. These include exploring issues such as family support systems; potential parenting disorders; depression; coping mechanisms; and possible financial, career, or housing problems.

Sexually Transmitted Infections. Sexually transmitted infections (STIs) are a major health issue in young adults. STIs include syphilis, chlamydia, gonorrhea, genital herpes, human papilloma virus (HPV) infection, and HIV (see Chapter 28 for further information about STIs). STIs have immediate physical effects such as discharge and discomfort. STIs also can lead to chronic conditions (from genital herpes), infertility (from gonorrhea), or death. Many people have an STI without experiencing symptoms. Young adults need information about transmission, prevention, symptoms, and management of STIs.

Many young adults have misconceptions regarding the transmission and treatment of STIs. Partners should be encouraged to know one another's sexual history and sexual practices. Nurses should be alert for STIs when people come to clinics with complaints of urological or gynecological problems (see Chapter 33). Young adults should be assessed for their knowledge and use of safer sex practices and genital self-examinations.

Environmental or Occupational Factors. A common environmental or occupational risk factor is exposure to work-related hazards or agents. Diseases observed in workplaces include silicosis from inhalation of talcum and silicon dust, emphysema from inhalation of smoke, and hearing loss from noise exposure. Cancers resulting from occupational exposures may involve the lungs, liver, brain, blood, or skin. Environmental exposures through leisure activities include outdoor exposure to mosquitoes (which may transmit West Nile virus) and ticks (which may transmit Lyme disease). Questions regarding environmental and occupational exposures should be a routine part of nursing assessment.

Health Concerns

Infertility. Infertility refers to a lack of conception after a reasonable period of sexual intercourse without contraception. Infertility affects as many as one in eight couples. For many couples, the use of infertility clinics can facilitate pregnancy. There are many causes of infertility, including female reproductive factors, such as ovulatory dysfunction or a pelvic factor, and male reproductive factors, such as sperm and semen abnormalities. Couples who delay conception until their mid-thirties may experience fertility problems (Public Health Agency of Canada, 2019). For some infertile couples, a nurse may be the first resource contacted. Nursing assessment of infertile couples should include comprehensive histories of both partners to determine factors that may affect fertility, as well as pertinent physical findings.

Exercise. Exercise patterns can affect health status. Adults between 18 and 64 years of age should engage in activity of moderate to vigorous intensity, in bouts of 10 minutes or more, for at least 150 minutes per week (Canadian Society for Exercise Physiology, 2020). Exercise improves cardiopulmonary function by decreasing blood pressure and heart rate. In addition, exercise decreases fatigue, insomnia, tension, and irritability. When assessing a person's health status, nurses should

conduct a thorough musculoskeletal assessment, including evaluations of joint mobility and muscle tone, and a psychosocial assessment for improved tolerance of stress to determine the effects of exercise.

Routine Health Screening. Routine screening examinations enable early detection of an illness and thus lower the risk of illnesses becoming severe. People should be encouraged to perform monthly skin, breast, or testicular self-examination (see Chapter 33). In Canada, cancer is the leading cause of death; more than half of all cases are prostate, breast, lung, or colorectal cancers. While the highest incidence of cancer is among persons over the age of 50, cancer contributes to illness and death in young and middle-aged adults. Breast and genital cancers continue to be considerable issues in Canada (Brenner et al., 2020). Therefore, as a nurse, you have an extremely important role in educating people about breast self-examination and the current breast screening recommendations, and you must provide male patients with information about testicular self-examination and prostate cancer screening.

In adolescence and early adulthood, prolonged exposure to ultraviolet rays from the sun or in tanning salons can increase the risk of developing skin cancer. People should be encouraged to undergo routine assessment of the skin for changes in colour or presence of lesions and changes in their appearance. Persons living with chronic conditions such as cancer, diabetes mellitus, or HIV may require specific condition-related screenings on a routine basis (Figure 24.2).

Job Stress. Job stress can be a daily occurrence or periodic. Most young adults can handle day-to-day crises. Situational job stress may occur when a new boss enters the workplace, a deadline is approaching, or new responsibilities are assigned. Corporate restructuring may lead to layoffs and increased responsibilities for remaining employees and is a major source of stress. Job dissatisfaction is another source of job stress. Because people perceive jobs differently, the types of job stressors vary from person to person. Your assessment of the young or middle-aged adult should include a description of their work, including conditions and hours, duration of employment, changes in sleep or eating habits, and evidence of increased irritability or nervousness.

Family Stress. Family stressors can arise at any time in family life. Family life is a dynamic process that includes times when everyone in the family works together and times when everyone appears to pull

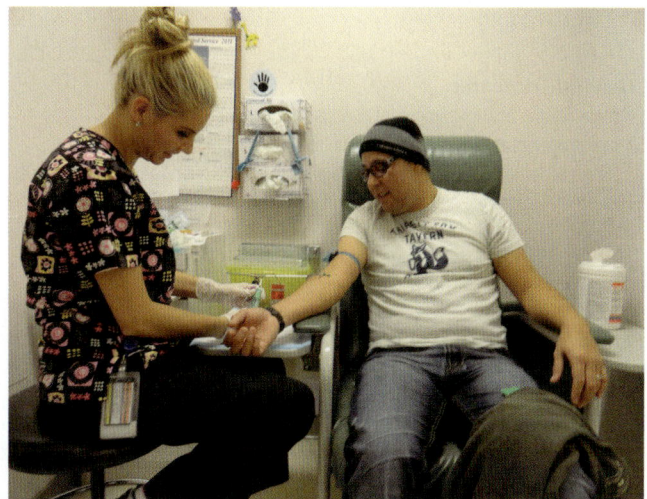

FIGURE 24.2 Routine health screening for persons living with chronic conditions.

apart. Situational stressors occur during major life events such as birth, death, illness, marriage, divorce, and job loss. Because of changing relationships and structures in the emerging young adult family, stress levels are frequently high and may be related to a number of variables that can lead to family dysfunction. Stress and the possible resulting family dysfunction may account for high divorce rates during the first 3 to 5 years of marriage for young adult couples. When a patient seeks health care and exhibits stress-related symptoms, the nurse should ask whether the person has recently experienced a life-changing event.

Each family has certain predictable roles or jobs for members. These roles enable the family to function and be an effective part of society. One necessary role is the family leader. In most families, one parent is the leader or both parents act as co-leaders. In lone-parent families, the parent or, on occasion, a member of the extended family is the family leader. When this role changes because of illness, a situational crisis may occur. Nurses should assess environmental and familial factors, including support systems and coping mechanisms, commonly used by family members.

Pregnancy. Although the physiological changes associated with pregnancy and childbirth occur only in the pregnant person, cognitive and psychosocial changes and health concerns affect the child-bearing person's entire family. The entire family, therefore, needs education about pregnancy, labour, delivery, breastfeeding, and integration of the newborn into the family structure.

Child-bearing parents who are anticipating pregnancy benefit from learning good health practices before conception, including the importance of eating a balanced diet, exercising, attending regular dental checkups, and avoiding alcohol, drugs, and smoking. Child-bearing parents trying to become pregnant should not follow weight-reduction diets.

Prenatal Care. Prenatal care includes routine assessment of the pregnant person by a nurse, family physician, obstetrician, nurse practitioner, or midwife. Health promotion interventions are important during the prenatal period and can improve the well-being of the pregnant person and fetus. Prenatal care includes a thorough physical assessment of the pregnant person during regularly scheduled intervals; provision of information regarding STIs, vaginal infections, and urinary infections that could adversely affect the fetus; and counselling about exercise patterns, diet, and child care. Regular prenatal care can address health concerns that arise during pregnancy.

Physiological Changes. The physiological changes and needs of the pregnant person vary with each trimester (Table 24.1). Temporary changes in visual and hearing acuity, taste, and smell also occur. Nurses must be familiar with these physiological changes, their causes, and helpful interventions. All child-bearing persons experience some physiological changes in the first trimester, but some changes affect only certain child-bearing persons. During the second trimester, growth of the uterus and fetus results in some of the physical signs of pregnancy, and the pregnant person will see a growing abdomen and feel fetal movements. During the third trimester, irregular, short contractions (Braxton-Hicks contractions), fatigue, and urinary frequency may occur. Close to the onset of labour, the person may experience a burst of energy during preparation for the baby's arrival, a period called nesting.

The puerperium is the period of about 6 weeks after childbirth. During this time, the person's body reverts to its prepregnant physical status. Nurses should assess the person's knowledge of and ability to care for themselves and their newborn. Assistance with infant feeding and care and assessment of parenting skills and child-bearing parent–infant interactions are important. During this period, nurses should assess for postpartum depression, symptoms of which may include

TABLE 24.1	Major Physiological Changes During Pregnancy	
Signs and Symptoms	**Causes**
First Trimester	
Amenorrhea	Fertilization and implantation of egg
	Increases in hormone levels
"Morning sickness" (nausea, sometimes vomiting)	Increased serum hormone levels
Breast changes: enlargement, tenderness, darkened and enlarged nipples	Increased estrogen levels
Urinary frequency	Pressure of uterus on bladder
Fatigue	Increased nutritional demands
	Decreased nutritional intake resulting from morning sickness
Second Trimester	
Integumentary changes: pigment changes in nipple and breast, hyperpigmentation of abdominal line (linea nigra), mottling of cheeks or forehead (chloasma, or "mask of pregnancy"), localized or generalized pruritis	Increased levels of melanocyte-stimulating hormone
Hypertrophy of gums, causing gingival swelling and bleeding	Proliferation of interdental papillary blood vessels, caused by increased estrogen levels
Increasing height of uterine fundus	Growth of fetus
Sensation of movement or of abdominal gas (quickening)	Fetal movement
Third Trimester	
Braxton-Hicks contractions	Expansion and preparation of uterus for labour
Increased colostrum	Hormonal influence; preparation of breasts for lactation
Increased urinary frequency	Pressure on bladder from enlarged fetus
Shortness of breath	Pressure on diaphragm from enlarged uterus
Supine hypertension	Uterine pressure on inferior vena cava
Heartburn	Slower gastric emptying and esophageal reflux

Data from Perry, S. E., Hockenberry, M. J., Lowdermilk, D. L., et al. (2017). *Maternal child nursing care in Canada* (2nd ed.). Elsevier Canada.

TABLE 24.2	Major Psychosocial Changes During Pregnancy
Type of Change	**Implications for Nursing Intervention**
Body image	Morning sickness and fatigue may contribute to poor body image. Increase in breast size may make the pregnant person feel more feminine and sexually appealing but may also be uncomfortable.
	The pregnant person begins to "show" during the second trimester. The pregnant person may experience a general feeling of well-being, feel the baby move, and hear the baby's heartbeat.
Role changes	Both partners think about impending role changes and can have feelings of uncertainty about them.
	Both partners may have feelings of ambivalence about becoming parents and concern about their ability to be parents.
Sexuality	Partners need reassurance that sexual activity will not harm the fetus.
	Desire for sexual activity may be influenced by body image.
	Partners may desire cuddling and holding rather than sexual intercourse.
Coping mechanisms	Partners need reassurance that childbirth and child-rearing are natural and positive experiences but can also be stressful.
	Partners should be provided guidance in preparation for childbirth and encouraged to participate in childbirth classes.
Stresses during puerperium	Partners may return home from the hospital fatigued and unfamiliar with infant care.
	Partners may experience physical discomfort or feelings of anxiety. The pregnant person may have to return to work soon after delivery, with subsequent feelings of guilt, anxiety, or, possibly, a sense of freedom or relief.
Postpartum anxiety and depression (often called postpartum blues)	Postpartum blues symptoms include transient emotional or mood disturbances such as weepiness, insomnia, anxiety, and poor concentration about 3 to 6 days after birth.
	Postpartum depression symptoms include extreme anxiety, a sense of failure, feelings of guilt, sleep disturbances, appetite disorders, excessive concerns about the baby, and suicidal ideation. Interventions include medication, therapy, counselling, and support.
Postpartum psychosis	Symptoms of postpartum psychosis may include delusions or strange beliefs, visual or auditory hallucinations (seeing or hearing things that are not there), feelings of irritability, hyperactivity, decreased need for sleep or insomnia, paranoia and suspiciousness, rapid mood swings, or difficulty communicating at times.
	Risk factors for postpartum psychosis include history of bipolar disorder, history of postpartum psychosis in a previous pregnancy, history of schizoaffective disorder or schizophrenia, family history of postpartum psychosis or bipolar disorder, first pregnancy, discontinuation of psychiatric medications for pregnancy.
	Interventions include medication, therapy, counselling, and support.

maladaptive coping strategies and ineffective bonding interactions between the child-bearing parent and newborn. Postpartum anxiety and psychosis may also occur during this period, and the nurse should assess for signs and symptoms of these conditions.

Psychosocial Changes. Like the physiological changes of pregnancy, psychosocial changes may occur at various times during pregnancy and in the puerperium. Table 24.2 summarizes the major categories of psychosocial changes and implications for nursing intervention.

Acute Care. The young adult years are generally a time of good physical and emotional health. Potential health hazards may be related to lifestyle. Acute care for young adults is frequently related to accidents, substance use, exposure to environmental and occupational hazards, stress-related illnesses, respiratory infections, gastroenteritis, influenza, urinary tract infections, and minor surgery.

Major mental illnesses such as anxiety, depression, and schizophrenia are often diagnosed during the young adult years and can persist across the lifespan. Anxiety disorder often arises during the young adult years. There are 11 "types" of anxiety and related disorders, and adults may experience more than one anxiety or related disorder at the same time. Anxiety symptoms usually manifest in one of four categories: physical responses, thoughts, emotions, or behaviours (Anxiety Canada, n.d.). Interventions for anxiety and related disorders include behavioural, biomedical, and psychosocial approaches to enhance coping and manage symptoms.

Depression "is a complex mood disorder caused by various factors, including genetic predisposition, personality, stress and brain chemistry" (Centre for Addiction and Mental Health [CAMH], n.d.-a). The main symptom of depression is a sad and despairing mood that is present most days and lasts most of the day for more than 2 weeks, and impairs the

person's ability to function at work, school, play, home, or social relationships. Additional symptoms of depression may include changes in appetite and weight; sleep disturbances; loss of interest in work, hobbies, people, or sex; withdrawal from family members and friends; feeling useless, hopeless, excessively guilty, or pessimistic or having low self-esteem; agitation or feeling slowed down; irritability; fatigue; trouble concentrating, remembering, or making decisions; crying easily, or feeling like crying but being unable to cry; thoughts of suicide (which should always be taken seriously); a loss of touch with reality, hearing voices (hallucinations), or having strange ideas (delusions) (CAMH, n.d.-a). Interventions for depression include behavioural, biomedical, and psychosocial approaches to enhance coping and manage symptoms.

Schizophrenia "is a complex mental illness that affects how a person thinks, feels, behaves and relates to others" (CAMH, n.d.-b). Schizophrenia is slightly more common in men, but also occurs in women. The first episode of schizophrenia typically occurs in the late teens to early twenties—usually earlier in men than in women. People can also develop schizophrenia later in life. Schizophrenia includes cognitive symptoms and "positive" and "negative" symptoms of psychosis. Cognitive symptoms include difficulties with attention, concentration, and memory. Positive symptoms of psychosis are those that add to or distort the person's normal functioning. Negative symptoms involve lost or reduced normal functioning (CAMH, n.d.-b). Interventions for schizophrenia include behavioural, biomedical, and psychosocial approaches to enhance coping and manage symptoms.

An acute, minor illness can disrupt the life activities of a young adult and increase stress in an already hectic lifestyle. Dependency and limitations posed by treatment regimens can also increase their frustration. To give young adults control of their health care choices, it is important for nurses to keep them informed about their health status and involve them in health care decisions. Acute phases of chronic illnesses may pose challenges for young adults.

Restorative and Continuing Care. Chronic conditions in young adulthood, although not common, do occur. Chronic illnesses such as hypertension, coronary artery disease, and diabetes may have their onset in young adulthood and remain unknown to the person until later in life. Causes of chronic illness and disability in a young adult can include accidents, multiple sclerosis, rheumatoid arthritis, HIV, and cancer. Chronic illness and disability can affect the accomplishment of important developmental tasks in young adulthood. They can reduce a young adult's independence and require the person to change personal, family, and career goals. Young adults with chronic illness or disability may experience developmental problems related to their sense of identity. They may need support to establish independence, reorganize intimate relationships and family structure, and start a chosen career.

MIDDLE ADULTHOOD

The middle adult years begin around the mid- to late thirties and last through the mid-sixties (APA, 2020). Personal and career achievements have often already been experienced. Many middle-aged adults enjoy assisting their children and other young people to become productive and responsible adults. Middle-aged adults may also begin to help aging parents. Using leisure time in satisfying and creative ways is a challenge that, if met satisfactorily, enables middle-aged adults to prepare for retirement. Socioeconomic instability brought on by corporate restructuring and economic realities, however, may leave many middle-aged adults either jobless or forced to accept lower-paying jobs.

People must adjust to inevitable biological changes. Middle-aged adults need to adapt self-concept and body image to physiological realities and changes in physical appearance. Exercising, eating well, getting enough sleep, and practising good hygiene promote good health and a positive attitude toward physiological changes.

Physical Changes

Major physiological changes occur between the ages of 40 and 65 years. Table 24.3 summarizes normal developmental changes that are important to consider when conducting a physical examination. The most visible changes are greying of the hair, wrinkling of the skin, and thickening of the waist. Decreases in hearing and visual acuity are often noted during this period. These physiological changes may affect the person's self-concept and body image. For individuals with female genitalia, the most significant physiological change during middle age is menopause. Individuals with male genitalia may also notice several sexual changes as androgen levels decrease, such as weaker erections and less frequent ejaculation (see Chapter 28). However, many middle-aged individuals with male genitalia are still capable of producing fertile sperm and causing a pregnancy.

Perimenopause and Menopause. Menstruation and ovulation occur in a cyclical rhythm in women from adolescence into middle adulthood. **Perimenopause** is the period during which ovarian function declines, resulting in a diminishing number of ova and irregular menstrual cycles. During perimenopause, however, individuals with female genitalia can still become pregnant. **Menopause** is the permanent cessation of menstruation. It occurs primarily because the ovaries stop producing the hormones estrogen and progesterone. Menopause typically occurs between 45 and 60 years of age and includes symptoms such as hot flashes and insomnia. Experiences of menopause can range from asymptomatic and mild to severe enough to interfere with activities of daily living.

TABLE 24.3	Physical Assessment Findings in the Middle-Aged Adult
Body System	**Expected Findings**
Integument	Intact condition
	Appropriate distribution of pigmentation
	Slow, progressive decrease in skin turgor
	Greying and loss of hair (baldness patterns in men are established by age 55; hair loss after this time might have other causes)
Head and neck	Symmetry of scalp, skull, and face
Eyes	Normal accessory organs of vision
	Visual acuity (according to Snellen chart) that is less than 20/50
	Normal pupillary reaction to light and accommodation
	Normal visual fields and extraocular movements
	Normal retinal structures
Ears	Normal auditory structures and acuity
Nose, sinuses, and throat	Patent nares and intact sinuses, mouth, and pharynx
	Location of trachea at midline
	Nonpalpable lateral thyroid lobes
Thorax and lungs	Increased anteroposterior diameter
	Respiratory rate: 12–20 breaths per minute and regular
	Ratio of respiratory rate to heart rate: 1:4
	Normal tactile fremitus, resonance, and breath sounds
Heart and vascular system	Normal heart sounds
	Systole: first heart sound loudest at apex
	Diastole: first heart sound loudest at base
	Point of maximal impulse: at fifth intercostal space in midclavicular line and 2 cm or less in diameter
	Temperature: 36.1–37.6°C
	Pulse: 60–100 bpm (50 bpm in a conditioned athlete)
	Blood pressure: 130 mm Hg systolic, 85 mm Hg diastolic
	All pulses palpable
Breasts	Decreased size resulting from decreased muscle mass
	Normal nipples
Abdomen	No tenderness or organomegaly
	Decreased strength of abdominal muscles
Female reproductive system	Change in menstrual cycle and in duration and quality of menstrual flow to cessation of menses
	"Hot flashes"
Male reproductive system	Normal penis and scrotum
	Prostatic enlargement in some individuals
Musculoskeletal system	Decreased muscle mass
	Decreased range of joint motion
Neurological system	Appropriate affect, appearance, and behaviour
	Lucidity and appropriate level of cognitive ability
	Intact cranial nerves
	Adequate motor responses
	Responsive sensory system

bpm, Beats per minute.

Cognitive Changes

Changes in the cognitive function of middle-aged adults are rare except in the case of illness or trauma. The middle-aged adult can learn new skills and information. Some middle-aged adults enter educational or vocational programs to prepare themselves for entering the job market or changing jobs.

Psychosocial Changes

The psychosocial changes in middle-aged adults may involve expected events, such as children moving away from home, or unexpected events, such as a marital separation or the death of a loved one. Many middle-aged adults may find themselves in the so-called **sandwich generation**, simultaneously having the responsibilities of raising their own children and caring for aging parents. These changes may result in stress that can affect middle-aged adults' overall health. During middle age, the person examines their life goals and relationships. Self-reflection often results in a "midlife crisis," whereby the person feels turmoil or anxiety about the course of their life and desires change. As a result, the person may change relationships, lifestyle, or occupation.

In assessing for psychosocial changes, nurses should assess the major life changes occurring in the middle-aged adult and the impact that the changes have on that person's state of health. The assessment should also include individual psychosocial factors such as coping mechanisms and sources of social support.

In the middle adult years, as children depart from the household, the family enters the postparental family stage. Time and financial demands on the parents decrease, and the couple faces the task of redefining their relationship. If grandchildren are born, grandparenting styles must be chosen. Many middle-aged adults begin to adopt a healthier lifestyle. Health promotion needs for the middle-aged adult include adequate rest, leisure activities, regular exercise, good nutrition, reduction or cessation in the use of tobacco or alcohol, and regular screening examinations. A middle-aged adult's social environment is also important, including relationship concerns; communication and relationships with children, grandchildren, and aging parents; and caregiver concerns with their own aging or disabled parents.

According to Erikson's (1968, 1982) developmental theory, the primary developmental task of the middle adult years is to achieve generativity (see Chapter 22). *Generativity* is the willingness to care for and guide others. Middle-aged adults can achieve generativity with their own children or other younger people. If middle-aged adults fail to achieve generativity, stagnation occurs, which may manifest as excessive concern with themselves or destructive behaviour toward their children and the community. For some Indigenous peoples, the Medicine Wheel teachings are also important for understanding their life stages (see Chapter 12 for information about the Medicine Wheel).

Career Transition. Career changes may occur by choice or because of changes in the workplace or society. Middle-aged adults change occupations for a variety of reasons, including limited upward mobility, decreasing availability of jobs, and desire for a more challenging occupation. In some cases, technological advances or other changes force middle-aged adults to seek new jobs. Some middle-aged adults choose not to retire and continue working if they are able to. Such changes, particularly when unanticipated, may result in stress that can affect health, family relationships, self-concept, and other dimensions. Assessing levels of coping and adaptation to work-related stress and changes is an essential part of the nurse's role.

Sexuality. After the departure of their last child, many couples rejuvenate their relationship and find increased marital and sexual satisfaction during middle age. Onset of menopause can affect the sexual health of the middle-aged woman. A woman may desire increased sexual activity because pregnancy is no longer possible. Menopausal women may also experience vaginal dryness and dyspareunia or pain during sexual intercourse (see Chapter 28). A middle-aged man may notice changes in the strength of his erection and a decrease in his ability to experience repeated orgasms. This may result in the use of erectile function–enhancing agents (e.g., sildenafil citrate, tadalafil). Other factors influencing sexuality during this period include work stress, diminished health of one or both partners, and the use of prescription medications with adverse effects that may influence sexual desire or functioning (e.g., antihypertensive agents). Both partners may experience stresses related to sexual changes or a conflict between their sexual needs and self-perceptions and social attitudes or expectations. Assessing sexual functioning contributes to identification of potential risks for STIs and adverse health outcomes that can result from erectile function–enhancing agents.

Family Types. Psychosocial factors involving the family may include the stresses of singlehood, marital changes, family transition as children leave home, and the care of aging parents.

Singlehood. Many adults older than 35 years have never been married. Many of them have chosen to delay marriage and parenthood. Some single middle-aged adults, however, have chosen to become parents, either biologically or through adoption. Many single middle-aged adults may have no relatives but share a family type of relationship with close friends or work associates. Consequently, some single middle-aged adults may feel isolated during traditional "family" holidays. In times of illness, single adults may have to rely on relatives or friends. The nursing assessment of single middle-aged adults should include a thorough assessment of psychosocial factors, including the individual's definition of family and available support systems.

Marital Changes. Marital changes that may occur during middle age include death of a spouse, separation, divorce, and the choice to remarry or remain single. If a single middle-aged adult decides to marry, the stressors of marriage are similar to those for the young adult. A widowed, separated, or divorced person goes through a period of grief and loss in which it is necessary to adapt to the change in marital status. Normal grieving progresses through a series of phases, and the resolution of grief may take a year or more. Nurses should assess middle-aged adults' coping with the grief and loss associated with life changes (see Chapter 26).

Family Transitions. Departure of the last child from the home may be a stressor. Many parents welcome freedom from child-rearing responsibilities, whereas others feel lonely or without direction because of "empty-nest syndrome." Eventually, parents must reassess their marriage, resolve conflicts, and plan for the future. On occasion, this readjustment phase may lead to marital conflicts, separation, and divorce.

Care of Aging Parents. Increasing lifespans have led to more older persons in the population. Therefore, more middle-aged adults must address the personal and social issues confronting their aging parents, including becoming caregivers for their older parents.

Traditional social expectations between generations in families have changed because of housing, employment, health, and economic realities. Conflicts may arise between middle-aged adults and their older parents, who may strive to remain independent. Negotiations and compromises help in defining and resolving problems. As a nurse, you may encounter middle-aged and older persons in the community, in long-term care facilities, and in hospitals. You can help identify the health needs of both groups, as well as assist multigenerational families to determine the health and community resources available to them as they make decisions and plans. You will need to assess family relationships to determine family members' perceptions of responsibility and loyalty in relation to caring for older family members. Nurses also help to assess the environmental resources (e.g., number of rooms in the house, stair rails, handrails in bathrooms) needed by adults to care for their older parents.

When working with adults who are caring for older parents, the nurse should monitor for signs of caregiver role strain, which can include feelings of overwhelm or constant worry; frequent tiredness;

sleep disturbances; weight changes; irritability or anger; loss of interest in enjoyable activities; sadness; frequent headaches, bodily pain, or other physical problems; or misuse of alcohol or prescription medications.

Health Concerns

Physiological concerns for middle-aged adults include stress, level of wellness, obesity, and the formation of positive health habits. When adults seek health care, the nurse's focus includes evaluating their health behaviours, lifestyle, and environment to help them achieve their wellness goals. Health can be undermined by modifiable factors such as stress, obesity, tobacco use, excessive alcohol consumption, poor nutrition, and unsafe sexual practices. Drug use and misuse may also occur. Attention to these risk factors can increase quality of life and add years to it.

Stress and Stress Reduction.
Middle-aged adults' perceptions of health and health behaviours are often important factors in maintaining health. People in this life stage are prone to stress-related illnesses such as heart attacks, hypertension, migraine headaches, ulcers, colitis, autoimmune disease, backache, arthritis, and cancer. Stress levels may also increase as the middle-aged adult tries to balance responsibilities related to employment, family life, care of children, and care of aging parents.

People are exposed to many stressors throughout life (see Chapter 30). After these stressors are identified through an assessment, the nurse and patient can work together to intervene and modify the stress response. Stress can be reduced in three ways. First, the frequency of stress-producing situations can be minimized. Together, the nurse and patient should identify approaches to prevent stressful situations, such as habituation, change avoidance, time blocking, time management, and environmental modification. Second, stress resistance can be increased by psychophysiological preparation, such as increasing self-esteem, improving assertiveness, redirecting goal alternatives, and reorienting cognitive appraisal. Third, the physiological response to stress can be avoided. Nurses can teach people relaxation techniques and introduce stress-reduction strategies to recondition their response to stress. Chapter 36 explains these general interventions in greater detail.

Levels of Wellness.
Nurses need to be able to assess the health status of the middle-aged adult. Such assessment offers direction for planning nursing care and is useful in evaluating the effectiveness of nursing interventions. Nurses should use standard assessment techniques as guides for physical assessment (see Table 24.3 for the expected physical assessment findings of the middle-aged adult; also see Chapter 33).

Obesity.
Obesity, defined as having a body mass index of 30 or more, peaks in middle age and is thus a health concern for many middle-aged adults. Among Canadian adults aged 35 to 64 years, nearly 70% are overweight or obese, and more men than women are overweight or obese (Statistics Canada, 2019). Health conditions associated with obesity include high blood pressure, high blood cholesterol levels, type 2 (noninsulin-dependent) diabetes mellitus, coronary heart disease, osteoarthritis, and obstructive sleep apnea. Continued focus on the goal of wellness can assist people in evaluating health behaviours and lifestyle that contribute to obesity during the middle adult years. Counselling related to physical activity and nutrition is an important component of the plan of care for overweight and obese people.

Forming Positive Health Habits.
A *habit* is a person's usual practice or manner of behaviour. This behavioural pattern is reinforced by frequent repetition until it becomes the person's customary way of behaving. Some habits support health, such as exercise, eating a balanced diet, participating in routine screening and diagnostic tests (e.g., laboratory work for cholesterol, mammography), reducing stress, and daily brushing and flossing of teeth. Other habits involve behaviours harmful to health, such as smoking, consuming excessive alcohol, using illegal drugs, or eating foods with little or no nutritional value.

During assessment, nurses frequently obtain data about people's positive and negative health behaviours. In the planning, implementation, and evaluation phases, nurses can help people maintain habits that protect health and offer healthier alternatives to poor habits.

Health teaching and health counselling are often directed at improving health habits (Box 24.4). The more fully you as a nurse understand the dynamics of behaviour and habits, the more likely your interventions will help the person to achieve or reinforce health-promoting behaviours. Motivational interviewing techniques can be used to build the person's capacity to achieve their health goals (motivational interviewing is described in Chapter 18).

As a nurse, you can coach people about forming positive health habits and improve their health literacy. By providing information about how the body functions and how habits are formed and changed, you raise people's understanding of the impact of behaviour on health. You cannot change people's habits—people have control of and are responsible for their own behaviours. But you can explain the psychological principles of changing habits and offer information about health risks. Ultimately, however, the person decides which behaviours will become habits of daily living.

Barriers to change exist (Box 24.5), and unless these barriers are minimized or eliminated, it is futile to encourage the person to take actions that are going to be blocked. Internal and external barriers may require providing support or motivational interviewing techniques to

---

BOX 24.4 PATIENT TEACHING

Encouraging Positive Health Habits

Objective
- Establish a collaborative relationship with the patient, using reflective listening to build trust and mutual respect, to support their goal of walking 2 km three times per week to lose weight and improve cardiopulmonary function.

Teaching and Evaluation Strategies
- Use open questions to:
  - Review patient's daily work schedule and identify potential times for exercise.
  - Determine patient's knowledge about how to calculate target heart rate and assess pulse correctly; then develop strategies with them to acquire those skills if needed.
  - Explore patient's knowledge of warm-up and cool-down exercises; then devise a plan to carry out those activities with them.
  - Determine patient's understanding of the importance of support shoes for walking, and develop a strategy for accessing and acquiring them if needed.
- Affirm the effect of the patient's exercise efforts on weight control and improved cardiac function, then re-evaluate strategies, as needed, to help keep them motivated to achieve their health goals.
- End conversations with patients by using summarizing questions or statements, such as "Here is what I have heard; have I missed anything?"
- Document teaching interventions and patients' response. Determine with patient the need for further interventions and strategies to overcome challenges.

BOX 24.5 Barriers to Health Literacy

External Barriers	Internal Barriers
Lack of facilities	Lack of knowledge
Lack of materials	Lack of motivation
Lack of social supports	Insufficient skills to effect change in health habits
	Undefined short- and long-term goals

BOX 24.6 CULTURAL ASPECTS OF CARE

Cultural safety is a concept that has been proposed as an approach to address health inequities. Cultural safety was originally developed by Indigenous nurse-scholars and educators to provide more respectful care to Indigenous peoples. Cultural safety extends beyond cultural sensitivity and cultural competence to address the power imbalances, institutional discrimination, and inequitable positioning of certain groups (Pauly et al., 2015).

Implications for Practice

- Recognize that some people may choose to delay or avoid accessing health care because of perceived or actual adverse health encounters that they or their friends, family, or community members have experienced.
- Be aware of cultural influences that may affect the experiences of people from vulnerable populations who seek the assistance of health care providers.
- Educational materials that combine Western remedies with traditional approaches may be more easily accepted and utilized.
- Nurses should critically reflect on how health issues are framed in health care and how that influences people's ability to access culturally safe health care.

From Pauly, B., McCall, J., Browne, A. J., et al. (2015). Toward cultural safety: Nurse and patient perceptions of illicit substance use in a hospitalized setting. *Advances in Nursing Science, 38*(2), 121–135. https://doi.org/10.1097/ans.0000000000000070

identify strategies to overcome them. In some cases, the person may require referral for more intense therapeutic intervention.

As with adolescents and young adults, nurses need to continue educating middle-aged adults about STIs, substance use, and accident/injury prevention.

Anxiety. Adults often experience anxiety in response to the physiological and psychosocial changes of middle age. Such anxiety can motivate the adult to rethink life goals and can stimulate their productivity. For some adults, anxiety precipitates psychosomatic illness and preoccupation with death. Some middle-aged adults may view life as being half (or more) over and think in terms of the time left to live.

Clearly, a life-threatening illness, marital transition, or job stressor increases the anxiety of the person and their family. Nurses may need to use crisis intervention or stress management techniques to help the person adapt to a new diagnosis or the changes that span the adult years (see Chapter 30).

Depression. Risk factors for depression include being female; disappointments or losses at work, at school, or in family relationships; departure of the last child from the home; and family history. The incidence of depression in women is higher than in men.

People experiencing mild depression may feel sad, "blue," downcast, "down in the dumps," and tearful. Other symptoms include changes in the amount of sleep (not sleeping [insomnia], sleeping too much [hypersomnia]) or quality of sleep (multiple awakenings), irritability, feelings of social disinterest, and decreased alertness. Physical changes such as weight loss or weight gain, headaches, or feelings of fatigue regardless of the amount of rest may also be depressive symptoms. Depression that occurs during the middle years is commonly characterized by moderate to high anxiety and physical complaints. Mood changes and depression are common phenomena during menopause. Depression may be worsened by the use of alcohol or other substances.

Nursing assessment of a depressed middle-aged adult includes focused data collection regarding individual and family history of depression, mood changes, cognitive changes, behavioural and social changes, and physical changes. Assessment data should be collected from both the patient and their family. Family data may be particularly important, depending on the level of depression being experienced by the middle-aged adult.

Primary Health Care Programs. Primary health care programs for young and middle-aged adults are designed to prevent illness, promote health, and detect disease in the early stages. Nurses can make valuable contributions to community health by taking an active part in the planning of screening programs, teaching programs, and support groups for young and middle-aged adults.

Family planning, birthing, and parenting skills are program topics in which adults might be interested. Health screening for diabetes, hypertension, eye disease, and cancer is a good opportunity for nurses to perform assessments and provide health teaching and health counselling.

Health education programs can promote changes in behaviour and lifestyle. As a health teacher, the nurse can offer information that enables the patient to make decisions about health practices and that increases their health literacy (see Box 24.1), or the ability to access, comprehend, evaluate, and communicate health information as a way to promote, maintain, and improve health. Educational programs must be culturally appropriate (Box 24.6) (refer to Chapter 11 for information about cultural humility). Encouraging young to middle-aged adults to adopt more positive health practices during young and middle adulthood may lead to fewer or less complicated health problems during older adulthood. During health counselling, the patient and nurse should design a plan of action that addresses the patient's health and well-being. Through objective problem solving, the nurse can support the patient to grow and change.

Acute Care. Acute illnesses and conditions experienced in middle adulthood may be similar to those experienced in young adulthood. Injuries and acute illnesses in middle adulthood, however, may require a longer recovery period because recuperative processes slow with aging. In addition, acute illnesses and injuries experienced in middle adulthood are more likely to become chronic conditions.

HIV infection affects all age groups and is a consideration for middle-aged adults as well. Although HIV is typically thought of as a health concern of young adults, middle-aged adults should be assessed for risk factors and given information to help prevent HIV transmission.

Restorative and Continuing Care. Chronic illnesses such as diabetes mellitus, hypertension, rheumatoid arthritis, chronic obstructive pulmonary disease, and multiple sclerosis may affect the roles and responsibilities assumed by the middle-aged adult. Chronic illness may lead to strained family relationships, modifications in family activities, increased health care tasks, increased financial stress, the need for housing adaptation, social isolation, medical concerns, and grieving. The degree of disability and the person's perception of both the illness and the disability determine the extent to which lifestyle changes will occur. A few examples of the challenges experienced by people who develop debilitating chronic illness during adulthood include role reversal, changes in sexual behaviour, and altered self-image.

Nursing assessment of the chronically ill middle-aged adult includes assessment of their emotional, physical, social, and spiritual health status and the knowledge base of both the person and their family. This assessment should include the medical course of the illness and the prognosis for the person. In addition, it is important to determine the coping mechanisms of the person and their family, their adherence to treatment and rehabilitation regimens, and the need for community and social services, along with appropriate referrals.

KEY CONCEPTS

- Adult development involves orderly and sequential changes over time.
- Young adults are generally in a stable period of physical development, except for pregnancy-related changes.
- Cognitive development continues throughout the young and middle-adult years.
- LGBTQ2 individuals encounter worse health outcomes than other Canadians, primarily owing to their collective experiences with stigma and discrimination, which are rooted in historical social processes that persist in some segments of Canadian society.

- Increased health literacy among young and middle-aged adults can promote positive health outcomes for people in this stage of life.
- The emotional health of young adults is correlated with their ability to address and resolve personal and social problems.
- Young adults must choose a career and decide whether to remain single or marry and begin a family.
- Pregnant people need to understand the physiological changes that occur during each trimester.
- Psychosocial changes and health concerns during pregnancy and the puerperium period affect the child-bearing parent and the rest of the family.
- Health promotion interventions are important during the prenatal period and can improve the well-being of the child-bearing person and fetus.
- Midlife transition begins when a person becomes aware that physiological and psychosocial changes signify passage to another stage in life.
- Two significant physiological changes in the middle adulthood are menopause in women and changes in sexual response in men.
- Cognitive changes are rare in middle age except in cases of illness or physical trauma.
- Psychosocial changes for middle-aged adults may be related to career transition, sexuality, marital changes, family transition, and care of aging parents.
- Health goals of middle-aged adults commonly involve preventing stress-related illnesses, participating in health assessments, and adopting positive health habits.

CRITICAL THINKING EXERCISES

1. Daoud (preferred pronouns: he/him) is a 24-year-old gay man who smokes two packs of cigarettes per day. He began smoking when he was 14 years old. When Daoud arrives at the clinic, he tells you, "I just can't seem to kick the habit, no matter how hard I try." What information do you need to know to assist Daoud in quitting smoking?

2. Ray-Jean (preferred pronouns: she/her) is 48 years old, divorced, and the mother of two sons, ages 13 and 16. She has recently had to assume the responsibility of caring for her 78-year-old father after he suffered a stroke. Describe your role in assisting Ray-Jean to care for her father.

🌐 *Answers to Critical Thinking Exercises appear on the Evolve website.*

REVIEW QUESTIONS

Review Questions 1 to 10 relate to the case study at the beginning of the chapter.

1. Justine is being seen by the triage nurse in the emergency department. She is accompanied by the police because she was found wandering around a local park and is disoriented, emaciated, and agitated. Which actions does the nurse take to determine the plan of care for this patient? *(Select all that apply.)*
   a. Assess level of consciousness
   b. Obtain or access patient's medical record
   c. Ask the patient about their sexuality
   d. Determine education level
   e. Determine the patient's health literacy
   f. Assess motivation and desire to learn

2. The triage nurse is caring for Justine in the emergency department. The triage nurse's assessment of the patient includes the following data:
   - Temperature = 38.9°C (102°F)
   - Heart rate = 100 bpm
   - Respirations = 20 per minute
   - Oxygen saturation = 98% (on room air)
   - Pain = 2/10 on a 0–10 pain scale
   - Oriented to name only
   - Conscious and aware of surroundings
   - Responds appropriately to directions and answers questions when asked
   - Agitated, but responds to directions and is not currently a danger to self or others

   Choose the *MOST LIKELY* options for the information missing from the following statements by selecting from the list of options provided:

   The triage nurse recognizes that a(n) _____(1)_____ temperature and _____(2)_____ are factors that can influence a patient's emotional states and behaviours. The triage nurse suspects that these symptoms are related to a(n) _____(3)_____ interaction.

   Answer options:
   agitated
   calm
   drug–drug
   elevated
   police
   subnormal

3. When monitoring the prescribed course of cross-sex hormone therapy, the triage nurse considers which of the following factors that may affect Justine's adherence to the regimen? *(Select all that apply.)*
   a. Gender identity
   b. Lifestyle
   c. Sexuality
   d. Education level
   e. Health literacy
   f. Motivation and desire to learn

4. The triage nurse assesses that Justine is agitated and oriented to name only. The triage nurse recognizes her from previous visits to the emergency department.

For each nursing action in the following table, use an "X" to indicate that the action is *anticipated* (appropriate or necessary), *contraindicated* (could be harmful), or *nonessential* (makes no difference or not necessary) for the patient's care at this time. *(Select only one response option per row.)*

Nursing Action	Anticipated	Contraindicated	Nonessential
a. Review current medications.			
b. Determine symptoms of possible drug–drug interactions.			
c. Confirm whether the patient is taking medications as directed.			
d. Refer the patient to a mental health professional.			
e. Place the patient in the least restrictive restraints.			
f. Assess whether the patient is a danger to themselves or others.			
g. Make eye contact with the patient if culturally appropriate.			

5. The triage nurse notes from Justine's electronic medical record that she is an Indigenous survivor of the child welfare system.

For each nursing action in the following table, use an "X" to indicate that the action is *anticipated* (appropriate or necessary), *contraindicated* (could be harmful), or *nonessential* (makes no difference or not necessary) for the patient's care at this time. *(Select only one response option per row.)*

Nursing Action	Anticipated	Contraindicated	Nonessential
a. Employ cultural humility when interacting with the patient.			
b. Provide care that is informed by cultural safety.			
c. Confirm whether the patient is taking medications as directed.			
d. Refer the patient to a mental health professional.			
e. Place the patient in the least restrictive restraints.			
f. Assess whether the patient is a danger to themselves or others.			
g. Make eye contact with the patient if culturally appropriate.			

6. The triage nurse assesses that Justine is agitated and oriented to name only. The triage nurse receives orders from the attending physician to admit the patient for further observation and treatment.

For each of the nursing actions in the following table, use an "X" to indicate that the action is *anticipated* (appropriate or necessary), *contraindicated* (could be harmful), or *nonessential* (makes no difference or not necessary) for the patient's care at this time. *(Select only one response option per row.)*

Nursing Action	Anticipated	Contraindicated	Nonessential
a. Initiate discharge planning.			
b. Notify the admitting office that the patient will be admitted and request a bed assignment.			
c. Place the patient in the least restrictive restraints.			
d. Assess whether the patient is a danger to themselves or others.			
e. Notify police that the patient will be admitted.			
f. Notify social work to mobilize post-discharge services.			

7. Justine is admitted to the medical unit from the emergency department. The admitting nurse receives a report indicating that the patient was accompanied by the police and is disoriented, emaciated, and agitated. Which actions does the nurse take to determine the plan of care for this patient? *(Select all that apply.)*
   a. Assess the patient's level of consciousness
   b. Determine the patient's capacity to engage in the care planning process
   c. Obtain or access patient's medical record
   d. Obtain the patient's medical and psychosocial history from the electronic medical record
   e. Ask the patient about her family medical history
   f. Use motivational interviewing techniques to facilitate medication adherence

8. As part of the care planning process for Justine, the nurse is planning for discharge from the hospital.

For each nursing action listed in the following table, use an "X" to indicate that the action is *anticipated* (appropriate or necessary), *contraindicated* (could be harmful), or *nonessential* (makes no difference or not necessary) for the patient's care at this time. *(Select only one response option per row.)*

Nursing Action	Anticipated	Contrain-dicated	Non-essential
a. Engage the patient in discharge planning.			
b. Notify admitting office that the patient will be admitted and request a bed assignment.			
c. Determine the patient's housing situation (e.g., stably housed versus homeless).			

Nursing Action	Anticipated	Contrain-dicated	Non-essential
d. Assess whether the patient is a danger to themselves or others.			
e. Notify police that the patient will be discharged.			
f. Notify social work to mobilize post-discharge services.			

9. The licensed/registered practical nurse is discharging Justine from the medical unit. Which actions does the nurse take to determine the plan of care for this patient? *(Select all that apply.)*
   a. Assess the patient's level of consciousness.
   b. Determine the patient's capacity to engage in the discharge process.
   c. Ensure the patient has referrals for follow-up appointments.
   d. Give the patient prescriptions for medications at discharge.
   e. Ask the patient about their family medical history.
   f. Use motivational interviewing techniques to facilitate medication adherence.

Answers: 1. a, b; **2.** (1) elevated; (2) agitated; (3) drug–drug; **3.** a, b, d, e, f. **4.** Anticipated: a, b, c, f; g; Contraindicated: e; Nonessential: d; **5.** Anticipated: a, b, g; Contraindicated: e; Nonessential: c, f; **6.** Anticipated: a, b, d, f; Contraindicated: c; Nonessential: e; **7.** a, b, c, d; **8.** Anticipated: a, c, d, f; Contraindicated b; Nonessential: e; **9.** a, b, c, d, f.

🌐 *Rationales for the Review Questions appear on the Evolve website.*

RECOMMENDED WEBSITES

Breastfeeding Committee for Canada: https://www.breastfeedingcanada.ca/en
The Breastfeeding Committee for Canada was established in 1991 as a Health Canada initiative dedicated to the protection, promotion, and support of breastfeeding. This website provides videos and other educational resources that address breastfeeding issues.
Canadian AIDS Treatment Information Exchange (CATIE): https://www.catie.ca
This website provides information about the treatment, management, and prevention of HIV and hepatitis C.
Canadian Cancer Society: https://cancer.ca/en
This website provides information on specific cancers, clinical trials, support services, and ways to get involved.
Canadian Foundation for Women's Health: https://cfwh.org
The Canadian Foundation for Women's Health is a not-for-profit fundraising foundation focused on research, education, and advocacy in obstetrics and gynecology.
Institute of Indigenous Peoples' Health: https://cihr-irsc.gc.ca/e/8668.html
The Institute of Indigenous Peoples' Health fosters the advancement of a national health research agenda to improve and promote the health of

First Nations, Inuit, and Métis peoples in Canada through research, knowledge translation, and capacity building.
La Leche League Canada: https://www.lllc.ca
La Leche League Canada encourages, promotes, and provides mother-to-mother/parent-to-parent/peer breastfeeding support and educational opportunities, thus contributing to the health of children, families, and society.
Movember Foundation: https://ca.movember.com
The Movember Foundation is the leading global organization for improving men's health.
Public Health Agency of Canada (PHAC): https://www.canada.ca/en/public-health.html
The PHAC website has links to topics concerning health issues affecting Canadians, including information on chronic diseases, infectious diseases, and healthy living.
World Professional Association for Transgender Health (WPATH): https://www.wpath.org
WPATH is a world leader in advancing the health of transgender people. This website features information and resources to help improve the care of transgender people globally.

🌐 **REFERENCES**

A full reference list is available on the website for this book at https://evolve.elsevier.com/Canada/Potter/fundamentals/

25

Older Persons

Canadian content written by Sherry Dahlke, RN, PhD, GCN(c), and Robin Coatsworth-Puspoky, RN, PhD, with original chapter contributions by Shari Kist, RN, PhD, CNE

OBJECTIVES

Mastery of content in this chapter will enable you to:

- Define the key terms listed.
- Describe demographic trends related to older persons in Canada.
- Identify common myths and stereotypes about older persons.
- List the types of community-based and institutional health care services available to older persons.
- Describe the concept of quality of life.
- Describe common developmental tasks of older persons.
- Describe common physiological changes associated with aging.
- Differentiate among delirium, dementia, and depression.
- Describe issues related to psychosocial changes connected with aging.
- Describe selected health concerns of older persons.
- Identify nursing interventions related to the physiological, cognitive, and psychosocial changes of aging.

KEY TERMS

Age-friendly community
Ageism
Alzheimer's disease
Cognitive stimulation
Delirium

Dementia
Depression
Elder abuse
Functional status
Long-term care

Palliative care
Personal care home
Polypharmacy
Reminiscence
Restorative care

WEBSITE

http://evolve.elsevier.com/Canada/Potter/fundamentals/

CASE STUDY

Mrs. Jones, a 74-year-old individual (preferred pronouns: she/her), came to the clinic for help with recent health problems related to memory and dizziness. The patient shared that she had three adult children who lived in neighbouring towns, is a retired public school teacher, and up until 2 years ago tutored children in her home. Two years ago, Mrs. Jones' husband was diagnosed with terminal cancer and Mrs. Jones became a caregiver. Becoming a caregiver ended the tutoring business and outings with friends. Six weeks ago, her husband passed away.

To minimize the burden on their children, Mrs. Jones has been preparing to sell the family home. Mrs. Jones tells the nurse that she is not ready for a long-term care facility but would like to move closer to her children and to a smaller, more affordable place where she could meet new friends. Since her husband's death, Mrs. Jones has felt overwhelmed with grief and with the caretaking of the family home. She confides that she has felt isolated and lonely in the large family home. Recently, Mrs. Jones has experienced periods of dizziness, along with the feeling like she was going to fall. Mrs. Jones has also missed or was often late for appointments because she forgot them.

Think about this case study as you read this chapter. There are review questions at the end of the chapter that relate to the case study.

The identification of 65 years of age as the start of older adulthood dates back to social reform in Germany in the nineteenth century. The age of 65 years continues to be used as the lower boundary to define older adulthood in demographics and social policy, although many older persons consider themselves to be "middle-aged" well into their 70s (Bartlett & Smith Fowler, 2019). The term *older person* is the most appropriate term for persons over the age of 65 years. Sometimes the older age group is broken down into groups of youngest old, old, and oldest old, with oldest old comprising people over 85; however, how people age is diverse, because an 80-year-old could have the physical and mental capacities of many 20-year-olds (Bartlett & Smith Fowler, 2019; World Health Organization [WHO], 2021a). All people age in their own way according to their own schedules and life histories. Even though generalizations are made in this chapter about the aging process and its effect on individuals, every older person is unique and must be treated by nurses as a unique individual.

The number of older persons in Canada is growing, both absolutely and as a proportion of the total population. In 2019, 17.5% of the overall population in Canada were older persons (Public Health Agency of Canada [PHAC], 2021a). Geographical variations in the aging population exist across Canada; the largest numbers of older people are estimated to live in the Atlantic provinces and the far north

(PHAC, 2021a; Statistics Canada, 2021a). Older Canadians are living an additional 21 years longer (19.5 years longer for men and 22.3 years longer for women) than they did in the past (PHAC, 2021a). Two other factors contribute to the projected increase in the number of older persons: the aging of the baby-boom generation, and advances in health care practices to manage chronic diseases. The *baby boomers* are the large cohort of people born between 1946 and 1964. In 2011, the oldest baby boomers reached the age of 65 years and represented the fastest growing age group in Canada. By 2031, all baby boomers will have reached the age of 65 and will comprise of 23% of older persons in Canada. The baby boomers are often still working; 53% of men and 38.8% of women are working after the age of 65 (Yssaad & Fields, 2018). As baby boomers age, social and health care programs will need to expand to meet their needs, as well as the needs of the second fastest growing group of persons, those aged 100 years and older (Jackson et al., 2017; PHAC, 2021a). The numbers of centenarians have increased from 8 643 in 2016 to an estimated 11 517 in 2019 (Statistics Canada, 2021b).

The diversity of the population older than 65 years is also projected to increase, as future cohorts of older persons will be born outside of Canada. It is estimated that by 2036, between 24.5 and 30% of the Canadian population will have been born outside of Canada (Yssaad & Fields, 2018). Although many of these people immigrated when they were young, others immigrated when they were older, often accompanied by their younger family members (Yssaad & Fields, 2018). In 2016, 31% of older persons in Canada were immigrants, with 24% of them having immigrated as older persons (Kei et al., 2019). In caring for older persons from these groups, nurses must account for diversity in cultures, values, and languages. Examples of culturally safe nursing approaches to older persons include respect for preferences in food, music, and religion; attentive listening; use of physical assessment norms appropriate for diverse groups; and asking about personal health practices, family customs, lifestyle preferences, and spiritual resources (Touhy et al., 2019). Chapter 9 provides further information on culturally safe care. Before the 1950s, when the specialties of gerontology and geriatrics emerged, there was little differentiation between general principles of nursing care and nursing care for older people (Dahlke, 2011). The Canadian Gerontological Nurses Association (CGNA) has demonstrated strong support for nursing care of older people through their establishment of Gerontological Nursing Competencies and Standards of Practice (CGNA, 2020).

VARIABILITY AMONG OLDER PERSONS

The nursing care of older persons poses special challenges because of the great variation in their physiological, cognitive, and psychosocial health. Levels of functional ability also vary widely among older persons. The majority of older persons are active and involved members of their communities. A smaller number have lost the ability to care for themselves, have cognitive impairment, are withdrawn, are unable to make decisions concerning their needs, or have a combination of these factors. Most older persons (92%) live in private homes; even at 85 years of age and over 69.9% of older persons are living in private homes, with only 6.8% residing in institutions such as nursing homes (Bartlett & Smith Fowler, 2019). Age influences living arrangements: the proportion of older persons living with a spouse decreases with age, and the proportion living alone or living in an institution increases with age, with women being more likely than men to live in a communal setting (Bartlett & Smith Fowler, 2019).

Aging does not inevitably lead to disability and dependence. Most older people remain functionally independent despite the increasing prevalence of chronic disease. Nursing assessment, a complex and challenging process, can provide valuable clues to the effect a disease

or illness is having on a patient's functional status. Chronic conditions add to the complexity of assessment and care of the older person. Approximately 73% of older persons report one or more chronic conditions; hypertension, periodontal disease, osteoarthritis, ischemic heart disease, diabetes, osteoporosis, cancer, chronic obstructive pulmonary disease, asthma, and mood and anxiety disorders are the most common conditions in noninstitutionalized older persons (PHAC, 2021a); 30% of all Canadian older persons have two or more chronic diseases. About 37% of older persons living in private dwellings and 41% living in institutions with multiple chronic conditions report persistent pain. These chronic conditions impose limitations on activities: slightly more than 22% of persons 65 to 74 years of age and nearly 50% of those 85 years or older report some limitations in activities.

The physical, cognitive, and psychosocial aspects of aging are closely related. For the older person, a reduced ability to respond to stress, the experience of multiple losses, and the physical changes associated with normal aging may combine to increase the risk for illness and functional deterioration. Although the interaction of these physical and psychosocial factors can be serious, nurses should not assume that all older persons have signs, symptoms, or behaviours representing disease and decline or that these are the only items to be assessed. An older person's strengths and abilities must also be identified during the assessment.

MYTHS AND STEREOTYPES

Despite ongoing research in the field of gerontology, false beliefs and myths about older persons persist. These stereotypes include beliefs about the physical and psychosocial characteristics and the lifestyles of older persons. Sometimes negative perceptions about older people are perpetuated through jokes, with up to half of jokes about getting old portraying a negative attitude toward aging and old people, or by speaking in a manner that suggests a negative perspective toward older people (Touhy et al., 2019). Despite the diversity among older persons, it is estimated that 63% have experienced ageism, which is discrimination due to age (Bartlett & Smith Fowler, 2019). These negative perceptions about older people, in combination with the projected increases in numbers of older people, has led to concerns about older people using too many of our limited health care resources. However, increased costs in health care are often associated with the cost of health care technology rather than the age of the health care consumer (WHO, 2015). Negative stereotypes may adversely affect access to and the quality of care provided to older patients (WHO, 2021b). Nurses, although personally susceptible to the myths and stereotypes held by society, have the responsibility to dispel the myths and replace the stereotypes with accurate information.

Older persons are sometimes stereotyped as ill and disabled. However, although many experience chronic conditions or have at least one disability that limits performance of activities of daily living (ADLs), only 23% of older persons describe their health as poor or fair (PHAC, 2021a). Despite increased incidence of chronic diseases with age, 80% of older people are able to live independently, and 72% of older Canadians rate their mental health as very good or excellent (PHAC, 2021a). Other common misconceptions are that older persons are generally not interested in sex and that any interest in sexual activities is abnormal and should be discouraged. However, many older persons report continued enjoyment of sexual relationships. Another common misconception is that older persons are unable to use computers. Yet, over 68% of older Canadians use the Internet (Davidson & Schimmele, 2019) (Figure 25.1).

Some people believe that older persons are forgetful, confused, rigid, bored, unfriendly, and unable to understand and learn new

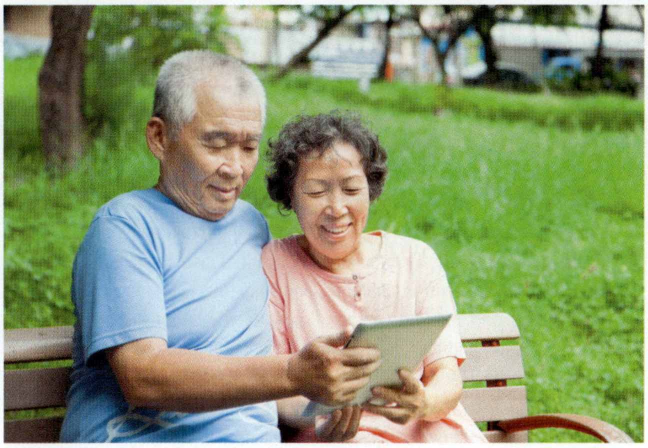

FIGURE 25.1 Most Canadian older persons use the Internet. (© tomwang/CanStock Photo Inc.)

BOX 25.1 FOCUS ON OLDER PERSONS

Strategies for Communicating Effectively With Older Persons

- Try to find a quiet room with minimal outside noises for communication.
- Sit facing the patient so that they can watch your lip movements and facial expressions.
- If masks must be worn for safety, consider how to maintain an interaction that is warm, open, and demonstrates interest in what the older person is saying.
- If needed, make sure that glasses and hearing aids are being worn.
- Speak slowly and clearly (do not speak loudly).
- Keep your tone of voice low; older persons can hear low-frequency sounds better than high-frequency sounds.
- Periodically summarize what has been said to clarify that you have understood what the older person was saying, and repeat key points.
- Ask the older person to explain what they understood and invite questions to clarify information. There may also be cultural aspects related to communication. (Please refer to Chapter 18 for more information.)
- Emphasize and integrate emotional and personal values in the acquisition of skills and ideas.

Adapted from Harper, L., & Dobbs, L. (2018). *Adult development and aging: The Canadian experience.* Nelson.

---

information. However, centenarians, the oldest of the old, are described as having an optimistic outlook on life, good memories, broad social contacts and interests, and tolerance for others (Touhy et al., 2019). Although the process of learning may be affected by age-related changes in vision or hearing or by reduced energy and endurance, older persons are lifelong learners. When communicating with older persons, nurses should use techniques that compensate for sensory changes, provide additional time for remembering and responding, and present concrete rather than abstract material to older persons. Effective teaching techniques draw from older persons' past experiences and correspond to their identified interests rather than to the content areas believed important by the health care provider. Box 25.1 presents communication strategies that nurses can use to address the learning needs of older persons.

In a society that values attractiveness, energy, and youth, these myths and stereotypes lead to the undervaluing of older persons. Some people believe that older persons are unattractive and become worthless to society after they leave the workforce. Others consider the knowledge and experience of older persons to be too old-fashioned

---

BOX 25.2 Developmental Tasks for Older Persons

- Adjusting to decreasing health and physical strength
- Adjusting to retirement and reduced or fixed income
- Adjusting to the death of a spouse
- Accepting oneself as an aging person
- Maintaining satisfactory living arrangements
- Redefining relationships with adult children
- Finding ways to maintain quality of life

Adapted from Erikson, E. H., Erikson, J. M., & Kivnick, H. Q. (1986). *Vital involvement in old age: The experience of old age in our time.* W. W. Norton.

---

to have any current value. These notions underlie the concept of age-ism, which is discrimination against people because of increasing age, just as racism and sexism are discrimination based on skin colour and gender, respectively. Ageism has the potential to undermine the self-confidence of older persons, limit their access to care, and distort caregivers' understanding of the uniqueness of each older person (Harper & Dobbs, 2018; WHO, 2021b). By contrast, a society that values the contribution and wisdom of older people helps them to maintain decision making and function to their greatest ability.

NURSES' ATTITUDES TOWARD OLDER PERSONS

It is important for you as a nurse to assess your attitudes toward older persons, your own aging, and the aging of your family and friends. Your attitudes toward older persons result partly from your personal experiences with older persons, your education and employment experiences, attitudes of co-workers and employers, and your own age. Cultivation of positive attitudes toward older persons and specialized knowledge about aging and the health care needs of older persons are priorities for nurses.

Positive attitudes regarding older persons are based in part on a realistic portrayal of the characteristics and health care needs of older persons. Health care providers, under the influence of negative attitudes toward older persons, often lack respect for older persons and ignore the opportunity to actively involve them in care decisions and activities. At times, health care providers in hospitals and long-term care facilities have treated older persons as objects to be acted on rather than as independent, dignified persons (Dahlke et al., 2020; McCloskey et al., 2020). All nurses need to recognize and address ageism by questioning prevailing negative attitudes and stereotypes about older persons and advocating for them in all care settings.

Developmental Tasks for Older Persons

Although no two individuals age in the same way, either biologically or psychosocially, frameworks outlining developmentally appropriate tasks for older persons have been developed. Seven developmental tasks of older persons are listed in Box 25.2.

These developmental tasks are common to many older persons and are associated with varying degrees of change and loss. The more common losses involve health, significant others, a sense of being useful, socialization, income, and independent living. The ways that older persons adjust to the changes of aging are highly individualized. For some, adaptation and adjustment are relatively easy. For others, coping with the changes caused by aging may require the assistance of family, friends, and health care providers. As a nurse, you must be sensitive to the effect of such losses on older persons and their families and be prepared to offer support.

Older persons must also adjust to the physical changes that accompany aging. The extent and timing of these changes vary from individual to individual, but as body systems age, changes occur in appearance and functioning. These changes are not associated with a disease but are normal changes. The presence of disease may alter the timing of the changes or their impact on daily life. Structural and functional changes associated with aging are described in "Physiological Changes" later in the chapter.

QUALITY OF LIFE

There is debate among gerontologists regarding what it means to experience a good old age. More recently, resilience to adversity and a perception of physical and psychological wellness have been found to be connected to the older person's perception of quality of life (Fullen et al., 2018). Interdependence and relationships are important aspects of quality of life for older persons (Nosraty et al., 2019). However, the definition of quality of life varies from person to person. As a nurse you must listen to what an older person considers most important, rather than making assumptions about that individual's priorities. Together, you and the older person may set objectives for maintaining quality of life, whether quality of life is defined as maintenance of social relationships, continuing to live alone, or continuing activities such as driving or gardening or dancing.

COMMUNITY-BASED AND INSTITUTIONAL HEALTH CARE SERVICES

As a nurse, you may encounter older persons in a wide variety of community-based and institutional health care settings. Outside the acute care hospital setting, you and other nurses may care for older persons in private homes and apartments, adult day care centres, home care, assisted-living facilities (also known as *supportive housing*), long-term care facilities, and hospices. Nursing care in older persons' homes can be provided by Canadian home care services and private-duty nursing. A **personal care home** is a private business that provides accommodation, meals, and supervision or assistance with personal care in a family-like atmosphere. In some provinces, personal care homes are offered as a type of assisted-living facility. *Assisted-living facilities* are designed for residents who need only minimal to moderate care. Residents live independently in their own apartments and are provided with support services such as homemaking or personal care. Some assisted-living facilities are small group homes where residents share common eating and living areas. Nursing services are not usually included in assisted-living facilities. **Long-term care** facilities provide accommodations, 24-hour nursing care, and support services for people who cannot care for themselves at home but do not need hospital care. *Palliative care facilities* such as hospices focus on providing care for persons who are dying. They can be publicly or privately funded.

Canadian older persons, because of their changing health status, will need different types of care options during their life. These include health care and social services that can support them to stay in their own home (Box 25.3). Nurses can assist older persons and their families by providing information and answering questions as they make choices among care options. During the decision-making period, the actual move from a private home to an assisted-living or long-term care facility, and the time after the move, the nurse's role is to support the older person and their family. Nurses can provide information about the selection of a good assisted-living or long-term care facility (Harper & Dobbs, 2018).

BOX 25.3 **FOCUS ON OLDER PERSONS**

Community Resources for Older Persons

- *Information and referral:* Local programs within communities offer an "info line" that provides information about agencies and services. Health Link is also a Canadian resource.
- *Senior centres:* Community-based centres provide services such as meals, limited transportation, and social and educational programming.
- *Home-delivered meals:* Programs that deliver hot meals to older person are run by community centres, churches, and hospitals.
- *Companions and friendly visitors:* Programs that offer socially focused home visitation and accompaniment for appointments are run by seniors centres, churches, and not-for-profit organizations.
- *Telephone reassurance:* Service providers make scheduled telephone calls to older people to provide support and reminders.
- *Personal emergency response systems:* An emergency response system that involves wearing a "call button" in a necklace or bracelet will initiate a phone call to designated support people when assistance is needed.
- *Energy assistance programs:* Provincial and territorial programs offer financial assistance to older people with limited income for paying utility bills.
- *Financial support:* National programs exist to support older persons' ability to subsidize their income, as well as support community engagement.

From Government of Canada. (n.d.). *Programs and services for seniors.* https://www.canada.ca/en/employment-social-development/campaigns/seniors.html

---

ASSESSING THE NEEDS OF OLDER PERSONS

Gerontological nursing offers creative approaches for maximizing the potential of older persons. The standards of practice of the CGNA (2020) were developed to define the uniqueness and scope of gerontological nursing practice, which includes functions such as assessment. With comprehensive assessment information regarding an older person's strengths, resources, and limitations, the nurse and the older person can identify needs and problems and select interventions that maintain the older person's physical abilities and create an environment for psychosocial and spiritual well-being. To conduct a thorough assessment, nurses need to actively engage older persons and provide them with enough time to share important information about their health. Nurses should assess for changes in physiology, cognition, and psychosocial behaviour (please refer to Chapter 14 on nursing assessment and diagnosis for more information).

Nursing assessment must take into account five key points to ensure an age-specific approach: 1) the interrelation between physical and psychosocial aspects of aging, 2) the effects of disease and disability on functional status, 3) the decreased efficiency of homeostatic mechanisms, 4) the lack of standards for health and illness norms, and 5) altered manifestations of and responses to specific disease (Touhy et al., 2019). Obtaining a comprehensive assessment of an older person often takes more time than does an assessment of a younger person because of the longer life and medical history and the potential complexity of that history. By planning to spend extra time with the assessment, the nurse and older person are less likely to feel rushed. During the physical examination, the nurse may find it necessary to allow rest periods or to conduct the assessment in several sessions because of the reduced energy and limited endurance experienced by some frail older persons.

Sensory changes may also affect data gathering. The choice of communication techniques is influenced by any visual or hearing impairment experienced by the older person. If older persons are unable to understand the nurse's visual or auditory cues, assessment data may be inaccurate or misleading. For example, if an older person has difficulty hearing the nurse's questions, their responses may be inappropriate, and the nurse may wrongly believe that the older person is confused.

Memory deficits, if present, will affect the accuracy and completeness of the data collected. Information contributed by a family member or other caregiver, such as a history of allergies and documentation of immunizations, may be necessary to supplement the older person's recollection of past medical events and information. Nurses must use tact when involving another adult in the assessment interview with an older person. The additional adult supplements the answers of the older person with their consent, but the older person remains the focus of the interview.

Interpreters or cultural brokers must be present when an older person does not speak the nurse's language. The spoken word must be interpreted within the context of the older person's culture. To ensure culturally safe means of communication during assessment, it is important to 1) identify how the older person wishes to be addressed (use culturally appropriate titles); 2) assess the health-related beliefs and practices of the older person; and 3) know the beliefs and practices of the older person's culture group with regard to spatial requirements, eye contact, and touch, and use them to establish rapport. (See Chapter 11 for more information on providing culturally safe care.)

In older patients, signs and symptoms of diseases and laboratory values may be different from those in younger persons; the classic signs and symptoms of diseases may be absent, blunted, or atypical in older persons (Touhy et al., 2019). These differences may result from age-related changes in organ systems and homeostatic mechanisms, from progressive loss of physiological and functional reserves, or from coexisting acute or chronic conditions. As a result, an older person with a urinary tract infection may present with confusion, loss of appetite, weakness, dizziness, or fatigue instead of fever, dysuria, frequency, or urgency. An older person with pneumonia may have tachycardia, tachypnea, and confusion without the more common symptoms of fever and productive cough. And instead of substernal chest pain and diaphoresis, an older person with a myocardial infarction may experience epigastric discomfort, restlessness, hypotension, confusion, or referred or no pain. Variations from the usual norms for laboratory values may result from age-related changes in cardiac, pulmonary, renal, and metabolic function (Schuff-Werner, 2018). Examples of laboratory values that may be increased by these changes include, but are not limited to, levels of alkaline phosphatase, serum cholesterol, triglycerides, serum glucose (postprandial), and serum uric acid. Examples of laboratory values that may be decreased by the aging process include, but are not limited to, levels of serum calcium and serum creatine kinase, as well as creatinine clearance.

It is important to recognize the early indicators of acute illness in older persons: change in mental status, falls, dehydration, decrease in appetite, loss of function, dizziness, and incontinence (Hao et al., 2019). Two key principles of providing age-appropriate nursing care are timely detection of these cardinal signs of illness and a focus on finding underlying causes so that treatment can begin (Box 25.4). Attention is often not paid to underlying causes because of mistaken assumptions about normal aging (Touhy et al., 2019). Many health challenges can coexist, which adds to the difficulty in isolating the causes of symptoms. Mental status commonly changes as a result of disease and psychological issues, but more often in relation to drug toxicity or adverse drug events. A fall is a complex event, and careful investigation is necessary to find out whether it has environmental causes or is the symptom of a new-onset illness; such illnesses include cardiac, respiratory, musculoskeletal, neurological, urological, and sensory disorders. Dehydration is common in older persons because the thirst response is

| BOX 25.4 | Examples of Atypical Presentation of Illness |

- Delirium (acute confusion) with an acute illness is considered a medical emergency.
- Depression without sadness
- Infectious disease without fever or tachycardia
- Myocardial infarction without chest pain
- Nondyspneic pulmonary edema
- Abdominal pain is absent or vague.
- Confusion is not inevitable. Look for neurological events, new medication, or the presence of risk factors for delirium.
- Many hospitalized older persons suffer from chronic dehydration accelerated by acute illness.
- Not all older persons have fevers with infection; most common are respiratory or urinary tract infections. Symptoms may include increased respiratory rate, falls, incontinence, or confusion.

Adapted from Vonnes, C., & El-Rady, R. (2020). When you hear hoof beats, look for the zebras: Atypical presentation of illness in the older adults. *Journal for Nurse Practitioners, 17*(4), 1555–4155. https://doi.org/10.1016/j.nurpra.2020.10.017

reduced, which results in less water intake, and because less free water is available as a consequence of decreased muscle mass. Vomiting and diarrhea can accompany the onset of an acute illness, and older persons are then at risk for further dehydration. Decrease in appetite is a common symptom with the onset of pneumonia, heart failure, and urinary tract infection. Loss of functional ability occurs either in a subtle manner over time or suddenly, depending on the underlying cause. Thyroid disease, infection, cardiac or pulmonary conditions, metabolic disturbances, and anemia are common causes of functional decline, so nurses need to identify them early and notify health care providers so that proper treatment can be initiated. Dizziness is a common sign of various acute illnesses, including anemia, arrhythmia, infection, myocardial infarction, stroke, and brain tumour. New-onset urinary incontinence in an older person is often associated with a urinary tract infection, but it can also be a symptom of an electrolyte abnormality or adverse drug event.

Physiological Changes

Perception of well-being can define quality of life. Understanding a patient's perceptions about health status is essential for the accurate assessment and development of clinically relevant interventions. Older persons' concepts of health generally depend on personal perceptions of functional ability. Therefore, older persons engaged in ADLs usually consider themselves healthy, whereas those whose activities are limited by physical, emotional, or social impairments may perceive themselves as ill.

Many observed physiological changes in older persons are called "normal." Finding such changes during an assessment is not unexpected. These physiological changes are not always pathological processes, but they may make older persons more vulnerable to some common clinical conditions and diseases. Some older persons experience all of these physiological changes, and others experience only a few. The body changes continuously with age, and specific effects on particular older persons depend on health, lifestyle, stressors, and environmental conditions. As a nurse, you should know about these commonly experienced changes in order to provide appropriate care for older persons and to assist with adaptation to the changes. Common physiological changes are summarized in Table 25.1.

TABLE 25.1	Common Physiological Changes With Aging
System	**Common Changes**
Integumentary	Loss of skin elasticity with fat loss in extremities; pigmentation changes; glandular atrophy (oil, moisture, sweat glands); thinning hair, with hair turning grey-white (facial hair: decreased in men, increased in women); slower nail growth; atrophy of epidermal arterioles
Respiratory	Decreased cough reflex; decreased cilia; increased anterior–posterior chest diameter; increased chest wall rigidity; fewer alveoli, increased airway resistance; increased risk of respiratory infections
Cardiovascular	Thickening of blood vessel walls, narrowing of vessel lumen, loss of vessel elasticity, lower cardiac output, decreased number of heart muscle fibres, decreased elasticity and calcification of heart valves, decreased baroreceptor sensitivity, decreased efficiency of venous valves, increased pulmonary vascular tension, increased systolic blood pressure, decreased peripheral circulation
Gastrointestinal	Periodontal disease; decrease in saliva, gastric secretions, and pancreatic enzymes; smooth-muscle changes with decreased peristalsis and small intestinal motility; gastric atrophy; decreased production of intrinsic factor; increased stomach pH; loss of smooth muscle in the stomach; hemorrhoids; rectal prolapse; impaired rectal sensation
Musculoskeletal	Decreased muscle mass and strength, decalcification of bones, degenerative joint changes, dehydration of intervertebral disks, fat tissue increases, with loss of muscular-skeletal integrity postural kyphosis may occur
Neurological	Degeneration of nerve cells, decrease in neurotransmitters, decrease in rate of conduction of impulses
Sensory	
Eyes	Decrease in accommodation to near/far vision (presbyopia), difficulty adjusting to changes from light to dark, yellowing of the lens, altered colour perception, increased sensitivity to glare, smaller pupils
Ears	Loss of acuity for high-frequency tones (presbycusis), thickening of tympanic membrane, sclerosis of inner ear, buildup of earwax (cerumen)
Taste	Often diminished; often fewer taste buds
Smell	Often diminished
Touch	Decreased skin receptors
Proprioception	Decreased awareness of body positioning in space
Genitourinary	Fewer nephrons, 50% decrease in renal blood flow by age 80, decreased bladder capacity
	Male—enlargement of prostate
	Female—reduced sphincter tone
Reproductive	Male—sperm count diminished, smaller testes, erections less firm and slow to develop
	Female—decreased estrogen production, degeneration of ovaries, atrophy of vagina, uterus, and breasts
Endocrine	General—alterations in hormone production with decreased ability to respond to stress
	Thyroid—diminished secretions
	Cortisol, glucocorticoids—increased anti-inflammatory hormone
	Pancreas—increased fibrosis, decreased secretion of enzymes and hormones, decreased sensitivity to insulin
Immune system	Thymus decreases in size and volume
	T-cell function decreases
	Core temperature elevation is lowered

Modified from Touhy, T. A., Jett, K. F., Boscart, V., et al. (2019). *Ebersole and Hess' gerontological nursing and healthy aging* (2nd Canadian ed). Elsevier.

General Survey. The general survey occurs during the initial encounter with an older person and includes a quick, but careful, head-to-toe scan of the client, which the nurse should document in a concise description. An initial inspection of an older person might reveal whether eye contact and facial expression are appropriate to the situation, as well as common aging changes such as facial wrinkles, grey hair, loss of body mass in the extremities, and an increase of body mass in the trunk.

Functional Changes

Optimizing functional ability is also an important part of healthy aging and is influenced by older persons' intrinsic capacity and the environments in which they live (WHO, 2021c). Declines in physical, psychological, cognitive, and social function that can occur with aging are usually linked to illness or disease and its degree of chronicity. However, the complex relationship among all of these areas ultimately influences an older person's functional abilities and overall well-being. It is difficult for older persons to accept the changes that occur in all the areas of their lives, which in turn have a profound effect on function. Some older people deny the changes and continue to expect the same performance from themselves regardless of age. Conversely, some overemphasize these changes and prematurely limit their activities and involvement in life. Also, the fear of becoming dependent can be overwhelming for an older person who is experiencing functional decline as a result of aging.

Nurses need to educate older persons to promote understanding of age-related changes, appropriate lifestyle adjustments, and effective coping. Factors that promote the highest level of function in all areas include a healthy, well-balanced diet; paced and appropriate activity; regularly scheduled visits with a health care provider; regular participation in meaningful activities; use of stress management techniques; and avoidance of use of alcohol, tobacco, and illicit drugs. **Functional status** in older persons ordinarily refers to the capacity and safe performance of ADLs and is a sensitive indicator of health or illness in older persons. ADLs are essential to independent living; therefore, nurses must carefully assess whether an older person has changed the way in which they complete these tasks. In fact, a sudden change in function, as evidenced by a decline or change in an older person's ability to perform any one or combination of ADLs, is often a sign of the onset of an acute illness, pain, or worsening of a chronic condition (Vonnes & El-Rady, 2021). Pneumonia, urinary tract infection, dehydration, electrolyte disturbances, and delirium are examples of acute illnesses that may manifest as a change in function. Worsening of chronic conditions such as diabetes, cardiovascular disease, and chronic lung disease can also manifest as a change in function.

Various health care providers in a range of different settings are able to perform a functional assessment. Several standardized functional assessment tools are widely available; an online collection of tools is available at http://www.consultgeri.org. Some examples include FAN-CAPES, a functional assessment that will assist health care providers in identifying areas where help is needed (Touhy et al., 2019). FANCAPES includes the following:

1. **F**luids—assessing hydration and functional capacity to obtain fluids
2. **A**eration—assessing oxygen exchange, respiratory rate at rest and during activities, and auscultating breath sounds
3. **N**utrition—assessing ability to eat, which includes diet and oral health
4. **C**ommunication—assessing hearing, vision, and comprehension
5. **A**ctivity—assessing the capacity to toilet, groom, ambulate, and balance
6. **P**ain—assessing for physical, psychological, or spiritual pain
7. **E**limination—Assessing for bowel and bladder functioning and challenges
8. **S**ocialization and social skills—assessing the ability to navigate relationships

When a decline in function is identified, nursing interventions should be focused on maintaining, restoring, and maximizing the older person's functional status so that they can maintain independence while preserving dignity.

Cognitive Changes

A common misconception about aging is that cognitive impairments are widespread among older persons. Forgetfulness is not an expected consequence of aging. Older persons often fear that they are, or soon will be, cognitively impaired. Younger persons often assume that older persons are confused and no longer able to handle their affairs. Structural and physiological changes within the brain—such as reduction in the number of cells, deposition of lipofuscin and amyloid in cells, and change in neurotransmitter levels—are normal with aging and are observed in older persons whether they do or do not have cognitive impairment. Symptoms of cognitive impairment such as disorientation, loss of language skills, loss of the ability to calculate, and poor judgement are not normal aging changes. When nurses identify these changes during the assessment, they must further investigate the underlying causes.

The three common conditions affecting cognition are delirium, dementia, and depression (Table 25.2). As a nurse, you may find that distinguishing among these three conditions is challenging, but it is essential for selecting appropriate nursing interventions.

Delirium. **Delirium**, or acute confusional state, is a potentially reversible cognitive impairment that often has a physiological cause. Physiological causes of delirium include, but are not limited to, too many medications, dehydration, malnutrition, infection, pain, and stress (Casey, 2019). Delirium in older persons sometimes accompanies systemic infections and may be the presenting symptom for pneumonia or urinary tract infection. Delirium may also have environmental causes (e.g., sensory deprivation, unfamiliarity with surroundings) or psychosocial causes (e.g., emotional distress, pain). Although delirium may occur in any setting, an older person in the acute care setting is especially at risk because of predisposing factors (physiological, psychosocial, and environmental) in combination with the medical condition that led to the hospital admission. Older people with dementia are at increased risk of experiencing delirium.

The onset of delirium is typically sudden, and symptoms and severity fluctuate rapidly. Since delirium can fluctuate throughout the 24-hour period, it is important that nurses conduct frequent assessments. The presence of delirium necessitates prompt assessment and intervention. The cognitive impairment secondary to delirium is usually reversed once the cause of delirium is identified and treatment is started, unless permanent brain injury has occurred. The three main types of delirium are *hypoactive, hyperactive,* and *mixed delirium;* there is also a *subsyndromal delirium* in which the person presents with only some of the features of delirium. Scholars have also described a *persistent delirium,* which lasts longer than days and is associated with poor outcomes, such as increases in cognitive impairment and decreased functional ability (Casey, 2019). Treatment of delirium is focused on determining causative factors; however, prevention of delirium is also important. To prevent delirium and maintain a patient's functioning, nurses must address the causative factors, which may be multidimensional.

Casey (2019) recommends that nurses establish and maintain person-centred and family-centred relationships with older patients in any setting. If the older person is experiencing cognitive changes, the family can be a resource in explaining whether or not this is a new onset of confusion and, thus, delirium and if a new medication was started. The family can also provide other nuances of the client's health history that can aid in determining the cause of the delirium.

Dementia. **Dementia** is an umbrella term for a variety of diseases that cause irreversible changes in the brain. The Alzheimer Society of Canada (2022) classifies five major types of dementia: Alzheimer's disease, diffuse Lewy body disease, frontotemporal dementia, Creutzfeldt-Jacob dementia, and vascular dementia. The symptoms of dementia include loss of memory, judgement, and reasoning and changes in mood, behaviour, and communication abilities. Deterioration of cognitive function leads to a decline in the ability to perform basic and instrumental ADLs. Unlike delirium, dementia is characterized by progressive, irreversible cerebral dysfunction. Because of the close resemblance of delirium to dementia, the presence of delirium must be ruled out whenever dementia is suspected. The most common form of dementia is Alzheimer's disease. In Canada, 6.9% of older persons are living with dementia, with the incidence of dementia being higher among those over the age of 85 (PHAC, 2021b).

The cause of **Alzheimer's disease** is not known, and although several theories are being studied, none is definitive. Cholinesterase-inhibiting medications—memantine (Ebixa), donepezil (Aricept), rivastigmine (Exelon), and galantamine (Reminyl)—are currently prescribed to slow progression of symptoms. These medications prevent breakdown of the neurotransmitter acetylcholine by the enzyme cholinesterase (Hsu et al., 2018). It is hypothesized that by increasing the amount of acetylcholine available to transmit impulses among neurons, cognition in some older persons with Alzheimer's disease will improve.

The characteristic progressive symptoms of Alzheimer's disease are loss of memory (amnesia), loss of the ability to recognize objects and people (agnosia), loss of the ability to perform familiar tasks (apraxia), and loss of language skills (aphasia). As Alzheimer's disease progresses, the affected person becomes more dependent on caregivers for assistance with ADLs. Safety issues must be addressed as the disease progresses and the ability to judge risks diminishes.

Like Alzheimer's disease, diffuse Lewy body disease is progressive. The features of diffuse Lewy body disease include dementia, fluctuating cognition, visual or auditory hallucinations (or both), exhaustion, and the motor features of parkinsonism.

Frontotemporal dementia has an insidious onset and progresses slowly. Early symptoms include poor hygiene, lack of social tact, hyperorality, and sexual disinhibition. Incontinence is also an early symptom in frontotemporal dementia, whereas it is a late symptom in Alzheimer's disease. Repetitive behaviours (wandering, clapping, singing, picking up objects) are frequently observed. Safety and behaviour management are major concerns for caregivers.

TABLE 25.2   Comparison of Clinical Features of Delirium, Dementia, and Depression

	Delirium	Dementia	Depression
Definition	Delirium is a medical emergency. It is characterized by acute and fluctuating onset of confusion, disturbances in attention, disorganized thinking, and/or decline in consciousness. It can coexist with dementia. Older people with dementia have a higher risk of delirium.	Dementia is a gradual and progressive decline in mental processing ability that affects short-term memory, language, judgement, reasoning, and abstract thinking. It eventually affects long-term memory and the ability to perform familiar tasks. Some types of dementia are associated with changes in mood and behaviour.	*Depression* is a term used to describe presence of a cluster of depressive symptoms on most days, most of the time, for at least 2 weeks, and when the intensity of the symptoms is out of the ordinary for that person. It is a biologically based illness that affects a person's thoughts, feelings, behaviour, and even their physical health.
Onset and course	Sudden onset—it lasts hours to days. Often it is reversible with treatment of the underlying cause. Often it fluctuates over a 24-hour period and can be worse at night.	Gradual deterioration occurs over months to years. It has slow, chronic progression and is irreversible.	Recent unexplained changes in mood persist for at least 2 weeks. Usually, it is reversible with treatment. Often it is worse in the morning.
Thinking	Fluctuations in alertness, cognition, perceptions, and thinking occur. The person may have misperceptions and delusions.	Cognitive decline with problems in memory occurs plus one or more of the following: apraxia, agnosia, and/or executive functioning. The person may have paranoia and delusions of theft, and some types of dementia include hallucinations.	Reduced memory, concentration, and thinking occur, along with low self-esteem. The person may have delusions of poverty, feel guilt, and complain of somatic symptoms.
Mood	Fluctuations in emotions occur, with outbursts, anger, crying, and/or feeling fearful. Sleep may be disturbed, but there is no set pattern.	The person is depressed, especially in early stages. Apathy occurs. Sleep may be disturbed, with a pattern in the disturbance.	The person has depressed mood with decreased interest in or experiences of pleasure. Changes in appetite occur, with possible suicidal ideation and/or feelings of hopelessness. Sleep is disturbed, with early morning waking.
Psychomotor activities	Hyperactive: agitation, restlessness, hallucinations Hypoactive: unarousable, very sleepy Mixed: combinations of hyper- and hypoactive manifestations	Wandering with exit seeking Agitation The person is withdrawn (which may be related to an existing depression).	Hyperactive: agitated Hypoactive: withdrawn, decreased motivation and interest
Screening tools	Confusion Assessment Method (CAM) If the person has features 1 and 2 plus either 3 or 4 they are positive for delirium. 1. Presence of acute onset and fluctuating course and 2. Inattention and either 3. Disorganized thinking or 4. Altered level of consciousness	Folstein's Mini Mental Status Exam measures cognitive functioning. A score of 23 or lower is indicative of cognitive impairment.	Geriatric Depression Scale (GDS) Interpretation of the 15 GDS screen: Less than or equal to 4 = no depression 5–7 = borderline depression Greater than 7 = probable depression
Next steps	Notify the physician—delirium is considered a medical emergency. Determine and treat the underlying cause of the delirium (e.g., urinary tract infection, reaction to medication).	Management of behaviours should focus on nonpharmaceutical interventions.	Refer patient to a physician if there is suicidal risk. Refer to geriatric outreach teams.

Adapted from Casey, G. (2019). Delirium—too often overlooked. *Kai Tiaki Nursing New Zealand, 25*(10), 20–24.

A sudden onset of memory loss, behavioural changes, or difficulties with speech and movement occur with Creutzfeldt-Jakob disease (CJD). CJD is a rare, rapid, and fatal form of dementia caused by infectious agents called *prions*. Two types of CJD exist. *Classical CJD* (also called *sporadic CJD*) occurs at random. *Variant CJD* (vCJD) is a disease linked to eating beef products from cattle with bovine spongiform encephalopathy, also called "mad cow disease."

The cause of vascular dementia is interruption of blood supply to areas of the brain by thromboembolism, hemorrhage, or ischemia (Wolters & Ikram, 2019). Symptoms of vascular dementia vary according to the areas of the brain affected. Progression of vascular dementia may be either stepwise, with repeated episodes of damage to the brain over time, or steadily progressive. Management of vascular dementia parallels the recommendations for cerebrovascular disease (i.e., reduction of risk factors by treatment of hypertension, hyperlipidemia, carotid disease, arrhythmias, diabetes mellitus, and polycythemia vera). Because the use of nicotine has been linked with vascular disease, older persons with vascular dementia should stop or reduce their use of tobacco products. If an older person has a cardiac arrhythmia such as atrial fibrillation, anticoagulant therapy may be indicated to reduce the risk of thromboembolism.

In the nursing management of older persons with any form of dementia, nurses must consider the needs of the patient and the needs of the family. Those needs change because the progressive nature of dementia leads to increased cognitive deterioration. In addition to the patient's physical needs, their safety needs and psychosocial needs must be considered. The patient's family requires information and support. Nursing care objectives are promotion of the use of remaining functional abilities and behavioural interventions to decrease the incidence of responsive behaviours.

The Alzheimer Society of Canada (2019) has compiled suggestions for care of persons with dementia. The most challenging behaviours are those that include verbal and physical aggression. Often, these behaviours are a response to an unmet need, such as the need to go to the toilet, or hunger. When caring for patients with dementia, nurses should be calm and reassuring, look for an immediate cause, try distracting the patient, and, if safety is an issue, leave the situation and get assistance. Gentle Persuasive Approaches in Dementia Care (GPA®) is a geriatric program to teach caregivers positive strategies to use for their interactions with persons experiencing dementia (Geriatric Certificate Program, 2022). Restraints cause physical harm and are not an efficacious alternative. Minimal restraint (policy of least restraint) for the shortest period of time should be used only as the last resort when safety is an issue. Unfortunately, older persons are more likely to be restrained than are younger people, often because of the older person's "confusion," which could be dementia, delirium, or dementia (Thomann et al., 2021). Before resorting to restraints, nurses should try nonpharmacological methods to meet the older person's needs. These include walking the person (if they are able), providing a distracting activity, asking family to sit and visit with the older person, or using a one-to-one nurse.

Depression.
Late-life **depression** may be experienced by older persons. However, the incidence of depression in later life is lower than it is in earlier life (Harper & Dobbs, 2018). Depression reduces happiness and well-being, contributes to physical and social limitations, complicates the treatment of concomitant medical conditions, and increases the risk of suicide. The manifestation of depression in older persons differs from that in younger persons. Older persons are more likely to talk about being "blue" or "down in the dumps" and may express feelings of diminished life satisfaction (Touhy et al., 2019).

Delirium and depression, both reversible disorders, are often mistaken for irreversible dementia in older persons because cerebral dysfunction and cognitive impairment occur with these conditions, as well as with dementia. Careful and thorough assessment of older persons with cognitive impairment is essential to distinguish among delirium, dementia, and depression. People with dementia and depression have a higher risk of developing delirium (Touhy et al., 2019). As a beginning nurse, you may choose to consult with a clinical nurse specialist in gerontology. Accurate assessment is necessary to select appropriate nursing interventions.

Psychosocial Changes
The psychosocial changes that occur with aging involve changes in roles and relationships. Roles and relationships within the family change as parents become grandparents, as adult children become caregivers for aging parents, or as spouses become widows or widowers. Group membership roles and relationships change as older persons retire from work, move from a familiar neighbourhood, or stop attending social activities because of declining health status.

In an assessment, nurses should assess both the nature of the psychosocial changes facing an older person and the adaptation to those changes. It is important to ask the older person how they feel about themselves, in relation to self and others and as an aging person. Areas to be addressed during the assessment include the family, intimate relationships, past and current occupation, finances, housing, social

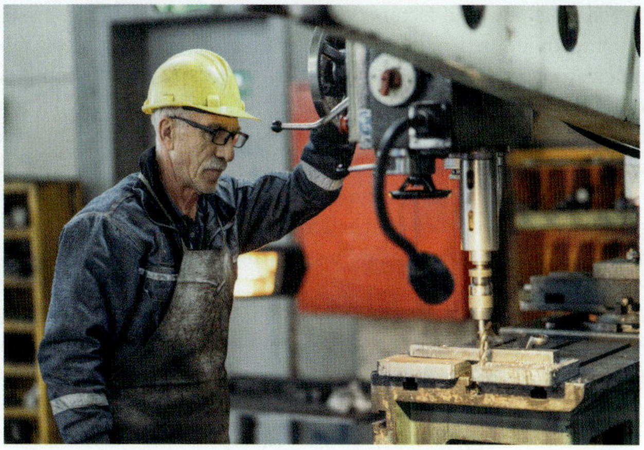

FIGURE 25.2 This older person works part-time at a machine shop. (iStockphoto.com/RainStar)

networks, activities, and spirituality. Specific topics related to these areas include retirement, housing and environment, social isolation, abuse, sexuality, and death.

Retirement.
The great majority of Canadian older people are retired; 13.4% of them are employed outside the home (Milan & Ouelett-Leveille, 2022). Some older people return to work after retirement for financial reasons, others prefer to work part-time hours, still others return to work for social reasons (Figure 25.2). Older workers often face negative stereotypes about aging, such as older persons being more difficult to train (Harper & Dobbs, 2018).

Retirement is a stage of life characterized by transitions and role changes. The psychosocial stresses of retirement may be related to role changes within the partner relationship or within the family and to loss of role. Problems may also arise in relation to social isolation and finances. Retirement, which may be mandatory or voluntary, occurs at a variety of ages. Regardless of the age at retirement, it is one of the major turning points in life.

Planning for retirement is an important, advisable task for middle-aged individuals. People who plan in advance for retirement generally have a smoother transition into that stage of life. Planning begins with consideration of the "style" of retirement desired and includes an inventory of interests, current skills, and general health. Meaningful retirement planning is critical because retirement can last for 30 years or more.

Retirement has an impact on other individuals besides the retired person. Partners, adult children, and grandchildren are all affected. When the partner is still working, the retired older person faces time alone. Friction may develop when the plans of the retired person conflict with the work responsibilities of the working partner. The working partner's expectations of the retired person must be clarified. For couples, adjustment to retirement is affected by the quality of communication with each other, their process of decision making about issues such as money or activities, their adherence to either traditional or shared role orientations, and their level of affection and intimacy (Harper & Dobbs, 2018). Adult children may expect the retired person to become an automatic babysitter for grandchildren.

Loss of the work role has a major impact on some retired people. Personal identity may be rooted in the work role and work relationships; with retirement, a new identity must be constructed. This is similar to Erickson's final stage of integrity versus despair (see Chapter 22). Life review is a strategy that might assist the person with construction of a new identity.

The most powerful factors that influence the retired person's satisfaction with life are health status, the option to continue working, and sufficient income (Harper & Dobbs, 2018). Positive expectations also contribute to satisfaction in retirement. Nurses can help an older person and family prepare for retirement by discussing several key areas, including relationships with partner and children, meaningful activities to replace the work role, adjusting or rebuilding social networks, issues related to the promotion and maintenance of income and health, and long-range planning, including wills and advance directives.

Social Isolation. Social isolation and loneliness are significant issues for older persons regardless of gender and geographical location (Petersen et al., 2020). *Social isolation* is defined as the lack of a sense of belonging, social engagement, and quality relationships, whereas *loneliness* is a feeling of dissatisfaction with the level of social contact. Isolation exists in two forms: it may be a choice to not interact with others, or it may be a response to conditions that inhibit the ability or the opportunity to interact with others, such as has happened during the pandemic (Brooke & Jackson, 2021). Geographical dispersion of families also leads to decreased opportunities for interaction among family members. Regardless of whether isolation is a choice for older persons, they are vulnerable to its consequences.

Living alone and having multiple chronic illnesses are factors contributing to social isolation and loneliness (Harper & Dobbs, 2018). Some older persons may isolate themselves because of cognitive issues or concerns about incontinence or decreased mobility (Touhy et al., 2019). Social isolation is prevalent in immigrant communities, in part because of language and cultural differences (Walsh et al., 2017). Nurses can assist lonely older persons to rebuild social networks and reverse patterns of isolation (Touhy et al., 2019). Many communities have outreach programs designed to make contact with isolated older persons. Outreach programs, such as Meals on Wheels, may help meet nutritional needs; daily telephone calls by volunteers may help meet socialization needs; and outings may help meet needs for activities. Social service agencies in most communities welcome older persons as volunteers and provide them with the opportunity to serve and to be served. Other organizations within communities such as religious institutions, colleges, and libraries offer a variety of programs for older persons that increase the opportunity to meet people with similar activities, interests, and needs.

Abuse. **Elder abuse** is the mistreatment of an older person by other people who are in a position of trust or power or who are responsible for the adult's care. Neglect is commonly associated with abuse. For example, elder abuse includes not performing an action (inaction) that a caretaker has a duty to perform, such as not providing medications to an older person who needs them (McDonald, 2018). Types of abuse are as follows:

- Physical abuse: use of physical force that may result in bodily injury, physical pain, or impairment
- Sexual abuse: nonconsensual sexual contact of any kind, which includes sexual contact with any person incapable of giving consent
- Psychological or emotional abuse: infliction of anguish, emotional pain, or distress through verbal or nonverbal acts
- Material abuse (financial abuse): illegal or improper exploitation of an older person's funds, property, or assets
- Neglect: the intentional or unintentional harmful behaviour on the part of an informal or formal caregiver in whom the older person has placed their trust
- Self-neglect: behaviour by an older person that threatens their health and safety, such as not eating

In most provinces in Canada, elder abuse must be reported. As a nurse, you play an important role in assessment, recognition, and reporting of elder abuse, as well as its prevention, through education and resources for families.

Nurses often must put together clues to determine if elder abuse has occurred. By its nature, it is a hidden problem, and assessment begins with a suspicion that abuse may be occurring.

Sexuality. Sexuality is increasingly recognized as an important factor in the lives of older persons. All older persons, whether healthy or frail, need to express sexual feelings. Sexuality involves love, warmth, sharing, and touching, not just the act of intercourse. Sexuality is linked with identity and validates the belief that people can give of themselves to others and have the gift appreciated.

Maintaining sexual health requires integration of somatic, emotional, intellectual, and social aspects of the sexual being. To help an older person achieve or maintain sexual health, nurses need to understand the physical changes in sexual response (see Chapter 28). They should provide privacy for any discussion of sexuality and should maintain a nonjudgemental attitude. Open-ended questions inviting the patient to explain sexual activities or concerns may elicit more information than closed-ended questions about specific activities or symptoms. Older persons may appreciate information about the typical age-related changes in sexuality. Information about the prevention of sexually transmitted infections should be included when appropriate. The libido does not decrease in older persons, although frequency of sexual activity may decline. An older person who does not understand physical changes affecting sexual activity—such as when they discover a change in the firmness of their erection, a decreased need for ejaculation with each orgasm, or a longer recovery period between episodes of intercourse—may be concerned that their sex life is nearly over.

In addition to the physical changes that affect sexual functioning, many older persons use prescription medications that depress libido, such as antihypertensives, antidepressants, sedatives, and hypnotics. Some drugs increase libido in older persons. For example, phenothiazines increase sexual desire in women, and levodopa has a similar effect in men.

While considering an older person's need for sexual expression, nurses must not ignore the important need to touch and be touched. Touch is an overt expression with many meanings and is an important part of sexuality in some cultures. Before using touch, nurses should respect the fact that it may not be appropriate for some older persons because of culturally associated meanings.

Experience in caring for older persons, in combination with the ability to establish therapeutic connection, will enable you as a nurse to learn how to explore patients' sexual concerns. Knowing an older person's sexual needs can help you incorporate this information into the nursing care plan. In addition, improving communication and creating open and supportive environments of care will promote successful, healthy sexual expression.

The sexual preferences of older persons are as diverse as those of younger persons. Not all older persons are heterosexual. Although little is known about aging as a lesbian, gay, bisexual, or transsexual (LGBTQ2) person, some scholars suggest that the LGBTQ2 community has increased physical and mental health concerns, with exposure to violence and loneliness due to inequities in social care environments (Kneale et al., 2019). To be effective caregivers for older LGBTQ2 persons, nurses need to be aware of their own beliefs about sexuality and the potential impact of those beliefs on their ability to provide care.

You may find that you are called on to advise older persons and help other health care providers understand the sexual needs of older persons. You may feel uncomfortable counselling older persons about sexual health and need not feel obligated to do so. But you should be prepared to refer older persons to appropriate professional counsellors.

Housing and Environment. Most Canadians want to stay in their communities as long as possible (Boucher et al., 2019). However, housing choices are strongly determined by an older person's ability to live independently. Changes in social roles, family responsibilities, health status, retirement, and income influence this ability. For example, physical impairments may necessitate relocation to a smaller, single-level home. Because of health problems, an older person may need to live with relatives or friends or move to an assisted-living or long-term care facility. A change in living arrangements may require an extended period of adjustment during which assistance and support from health care providers, friends, and family members are needed.

Some older persons choose to live with family members. Others prefer their own homes or apartments near their families. Leisure or retirement communities provide older people with living and social opportunities in a one-generation setting. Federally subsidized housing, where available, offers apartments with communal, social, and, in some cases, food service arrangements. There are Canadians, however, who because of poverty are unable to find adequate housing (Harper & Dobbs, 2018; Woo, 2018). When assisting older persons with housing needs, nurses should assess activity level, financial status, availability of access to public transportation and community activities, environmental hazards, and support systems. Housing choices should also account for anticipated future needs of older persons. For instance, a housing unit with only one floor and without exterior steps may be a prudent choice for an older person with severe arthritis who has already had some lower extremity joint replacement surgeries and anticipates the need for future surgeries.

Housing and environment have a major impact on the health of older persons. **Age-friendly community** is a concept that is spreading across Canada; it focuses on transportation, lighting, sidewalks, community centres, and supports that promote older people's ability to live independently (Harper & Dobbs, 2018). The environment can support or hinder physical and social functioning, can enhance or drain energy, and can complement or tax existing physical changes such as vision and hearing. For example, older persons can most easily see the colours red, orange, and yellow; in contrast, they have difficulty distinguishing between green and blue and among pastel shades. To help older persons in health care settings find their rooms, pictures or other decorations near their doors can be used as landmarks. To improve perception of the boundaries of halls and rooms, door frames and baseboards should be painted in a colour that contrasts with the colour of the wall. Glare from highly polished floors, metallic fixtures, and windows is poorly tolerated.

Furniture should be comfortable and designed for the musculoskeletal changes of older persons. Older persons should examine furniture carefully for size, comfort, and function before purchasing it. Furniture should be easy to get into and out of and should provide back support. Dining room chairs should be tested for comfort during meals and height in relation to the table. Older persons may prefer transferring out of a wheelchair to another chair for meals because some styles of wheelchairs prevent sitting close enough to the table to eat comfortably. Raising the table to clear the wheelchair arms may bring the table closer to the adult but make it too high for comfortable use. To make getting out of bed easier and safer, the height of the bed should allow the adult's feet to be flat on the floor when the adult is sitting on the side of the bed.

The goal of nursing assessment of the environment is the promotion of independence and functional ability. Assessment of safety, a major component of an older person's environment, includes determining risks within the environment and the adult's ability to recognize and respond to the risks (see Chapter 38). Risks include factors leading to injury within the home (such as water heaters set at excessively hot temperatures or throw rugs that could cause a fall) and factors outside the home (such as deteriorating sidewalks and steps or a high incidence of street crime).

Death. Part of the life history of an older person is the experience of the death of family members and friends (see Chapter 26). As persons age, friends gradually die. The majority of older persons are faced with the death of a spouse. Some older persons must also cope with the death of children and grandchildren. All experience the deaths of friends. These deaths represent both losses and reminders of personal mortality. Nurses should not, however, assume that older persons are comfortable with the idea of death. Coming to terms with death is often difficult. As a nurse, you can play a key role in assisting older persons through the grieving process.

Older people have a wide variety of attitudes and beliefs about death. To support a patient at the end of life, you can use the Dignity in Care Toolkit (Manitoba Palliative Care Research Unit, 2016). This toolkit includes an assessment tool to assess a person's sense of dignity, as well as strategies to improve their dignity at the end of life. Another model of care that is available is a Living with Hope program (Duggleby, 2019), which can be used to foster a patient's hope and improve quality of life. Such strategies to improve end-of-life care can be easily incorporated into everyday nursing practice. Nurses are often the one person to whom the older person and family members or friends turn for assistance in coping with death and loss. It is critical that you understand the grieving process, have excellent communication skills, understand the legal issues, are familiar with community resources, and are aware of your own feelings, limitations, and strengths as they relate to the care of older persons confronting death.

ADDRESSING THE HEALTH CONCERNS OF OLDER PERSONS

The two most common causes of death in Canadian older persons are cancer and heart disease. Other frequently reported causes of death are respiratory diseases, stroke, accidents or falls, diabetes, kidney disease, and liver disease (PHAC, 2021a). For all these causes of death, preventive measures exist that could potentially reduce the frequency of these conditions and delay disability, death, or both.

Nursing interventions for older persons are directed toward improving or maintaining their health needs and concerns. Although various interventions cross all three levels of care—health promotion, acute care, and restorative care—approaches to each level are unique. When planning interventions, it is important to incorporate a patient's routines or rituals when possible because patients feel more secure when routines are continued. In general, the interventions are aimed at promoting independence and supporting self-care abilities. Box 25.5 describes a study aimed at understanding older men's experiences with exercise to promote their health. Box 25.6 outlines guidelines for prevention and health promotion interventions for older persons.

Health Promotion and Maintenance: Physiological Health Concerns

Older persons, like persons of any age, vary in their desire to participate in health promotion activities; therefore, nurses should use an individualized approach, taking into account the person's beliefs about the importance of staying healthy and fit and remaining independent. Researchers have not fully identified the factors that lead to good health in advanced age, but four factors seem to be important:

BOX 25.5   **EVIDENCE-INFORMED PRACTICE**

Engaging Older Men in Physical Activity: Implications for Health Promotion Practice

In this qualitative study by Thandi and colleagues (2018), four men over the age of 65 participated in a semi-structured interview, three walk-along interviews, and a photovoice project to understand their perceptions about exercise. The research question was "How can older men's day-to-day experiences with physical activity inform the development of targeted physical activity programs?" Using an interpretive descriptive approach to data analysis, three key themes related to men's experiences with exercise were found: (a) "the things I've always done"; (b) "out and about"; and (c) "you do need the group atmosphere at times." Health promotion activities for older men that focus on social connection could engage men in physical activity and their community.

Reference: Thandi, M. K. G., Phinney, A., Oliffe, J. L., et al. (2018). Engaging older men in physical activity: Implications for health promotion practice. *American Journal of Men's Health, 12*(6), 2064–2075. https://doi.org/10.1177/1557988218792158

genetics, chance, good health habits, and preventive measures. As a nurse, you cannot alter an older person's genetic heritage or the chance occurrence of disease or injury, but you can promote health habits by establishing health maintenance programs, and you can recommend preventive measures. Health maintenance programs have been found to have a positive impact on the physical, mental, and social health of older persons. Community centres, houses of worship, schools, shopping malls, libraries, and hospital lobbies can be used as settings to conduct screening tests and present information on health topics. Using creative approaches, nurses can include health promotion activities for older persons in all health care settings.

Approximately 80% of older persons living at home have at least one chronic health condition. The most common conditions are arthritis, high blood pressure, back problems, chronic heart problems, cataracts, and diabetes (PHAC, 2021a). The effect of chronic conditions on the lives of older persons varies widely, but, in general, chronic conditions diminish well-being and threaten independence of older persons. This is particularly the case when an older person has more than one chronic condition. Box 25.7 describes the impact on older persons returning home from the hospital.

Nursing interventions are often directed at the management of these conditions, but interventions can also focus on prevention. Nurses can recommend the following general preventive measures:

- Regular exercise (150 minutes per week)
- Weight reduction if the older person is overweight
- Management of hypertension
- Smoking cessation
- Immunization for influenza, pneumococcal pneumonia, tetanus, and COVID-19

Approximately 18 per 100 000 people died from influenza in 2019, more than in previous years (Statista, 2021). As of this writing, the COVID-19 pandemic has resulted in over 41 000 deaths in Canada (10 times the usual yearly amount), most of which were among people over the age of 70 (Government of Canada, 2022). These deaths highlight the importance of COVID-19 vaccination and boosters, as well as annual immunization against influenza for all older persons, especially residents of long-term care facilities and persons of any age with chronic cardiovascular, pulmonary, and metabolic disorders. Vaccination against pneumococcal pneumonia is recommended for all persons older than 65 years. Influenza vaccine is needed every year, whereas pneumococcal pneumonia vaccine is given only once (although some authorities recommend a booster vaccination 10 years after the initial

BOX 25.6   **Guidelines for Prevention and Health Promotion Interventions for Older Persons**

Screening for Healthy Older Persons
- Blood pressure checks at least annually
- Risk assessment for lipid screening every 5 years
- Fecal occult blood test or fecal immunochemical test (FIT) every 2 years, or flexible sigmoidoscopy every 10 years after the age of 50 to screen for cancer
- Screen for osteoporosis
- Visual acuity and glaucoma screening every year
- Monthly breast self-examination for both individuals with male and female genitalia and annual breast examination by primary care practitioner
- Individuals with female genitalia should have a Pap smear and pelvic examination annually until three consecutive negative examinations, then every 3 years until age 69; after age 70 they may stop after three consecutive negative examinations. They should also have a mammogram every 2 years, and stop at age 75.
- Men should have a digital rectal examination annually.

Screening for Older Persons With Risk Factors
- Blood glucose level
- Thyroid function
- Bone density
- Heart function
- Screening for dementia, depression, and substance use
- Fall assessment
- Medication review for drug interactions
- Functional assessment
- Individuals with male genitalia should have prostate-specific antigen blood test.
- Gonorrhea and chlamydia, VDRL, HIV, and HBV if high risk

Health Promotional Counselling (for All Older Persons, Unless Contraindicated)
- Exercise 150 minutes a week
- Healthy food and nutritious intake that includes vitamins and minerals
- Dental care every 6 months
- Protective measures:
  - Use sunscreen and seatbelts
  - Avoid tobacco use
  - Light to moderate alcohol use
  - Get 7–8 hours of sleep a night

HBV, hepatitis B virus; *HIV,* human immunodeficiency virus; *VDRL,* Venereal Disease Research Laboratory.
Adapted from Public Health Agency of Canada. (2020). *Aging and chronic diseases: A profile of Canadian seniors.* https://www.canada.ca/en/public-health/services/publications/diseases-conditions/aging-chronic-diseases-profile-canadian-seniors-report.html; *Canada preventative screening guidelines—Objective health.* (2018). https://objectivehealth.ca/screening/

vaccination). For tetanus immunization, booster injections every 10 years are recommended for persons who have received the primary series for tetanus immunization. However, not all older persons are up to date with their booster injections, and some have never received the primary series of injections. During assessment, nurses should ask older persons about the current status of all three types of immunizations, provide information about the immunizations, and make arrangements for the older person to receive the immunizations as

BOX 25.7 RESEARCH HIGHLIGHT

Warning Signs Intervention for Rural Older Persons Returning Home After Hospitalization

Research Focus

When patients are unprepared to manage their care and recovery after discharge from hospital, they may not know the warning signs that indicate their health conditions are worsening. A lack of preparation may cause some patients to wait too long to get medical help, causing their health conditions to get worse. For patients in rural communities, who usually do not live close to medical services, knowing the signs that their health conditions are worsening and what to do about them is especially important. In a previous study, older rural patients and their families were asked in what was important to them postdischarge from hospital. They indicated that their most pressing unmet need is how to detect and respond to signs of worsening health conditions. To meet this need, a health care service called the *warning signs intervention* was designed to prepare patients to detect and respond to the warning signs of worsening health conditions.

Research Abstract

This study's aims were to determine the perceived acceptability of evidence-informed interventions to patients, families, and nurses and then adapt the interventions to fit patients' and families' needs in the rural nursing practice context.

Methods

Telephone interviews were conducted with patients who had been recently discharged from hospital. They were asked their perceptions about the warning signs intervention and to rate the acceptability of the intervention. Descriptive statistics were used to describe participants' average standing on preparedness for managing postdischarge care.

Results

Patients who received the intervention had more knowledge and confidence in managing changes in their health conditions at home; they had fewer emergency room visits and hospital readmissions than patients who did not receive the intervention.

Implications for Nursing Practice

Another project is planned with health care providers to understand what they think about the intervention and what they need in order to provide it in rural communities. The results will guide in developing a plan to help health care providers give the intervention to older rural patients and their families.

Reference: Fox, M. T., Sidani, S., Butler, J. I., et al. (2019). Protocol of a multimethod descriptive study: Adapting hospital-to-home transitional care interventions to the rural healthcare context in Ontario, Canada. *BMJ Open, 9*, 1–9. https://doi.org/10.1136/bmjopen-2018-028050

needed. Older persons should also be referred for screening for the early detection of cancer and depression.

Most older persons are interested in their health and are capable of taking charge of their lives. They want to remain independent and to prevent disability. Initial screenings establish baseline data that can be used to determine wellness, identify health needs, and design health maintenance programs. After initial screening sessions, nurses can share information on nutrition, exercise, medications, and safety precautions with older persons. They may also provide information about specific conditions, such as hypertension or arthritis, or about self-care procedures, such as foot and skin care. By providing information about health promotion and self-care, nurses can significantly improve the health and well-being of older persons.

Cancer. Malignant neoplasms are the most common cause of death among older persons (PHAC, 2021a). Nurses may participate in programs designed to educate older persons about early detection, treatment, and risk factors. Examples include smoking cessation programs, teaching breast self-examination (see Chapter 4), and encouraging all older persons to have screening for fecal occult blood or have a fecal immunochemical test (FIT) every 2 years. It is also important to educate older persons about the signs of cancer and to encourage prompt reporting of nonhealing skin lesions, unexpected bleeding, change in bowel habits, and unexplained weight loss. Detection is complicated when cancer symptoms are mistakenly identified by patients and health care providers as part of the normal aging process, thus it is important to carefully distinguish between normal aging and pathological conditions.

Heart Disease. Heart disease is the second leading cause of death in older persons. Common cardiovascular disorders are hypertension and coronary artery disease. Hypertension is diagnosed when repeated diastolic blood pressure measurements are 90 mm Hg or greater and systolic measurements are 140 mm Hg or greater. Over 27% of older persons in Canada have been diagnosed with heart disease (PHAC, 2021a). Research on treatment threshold in people older than 80 is limited; it is nonetheless suggested that blood pressure be 139/89 or lower (Touhy et al., 2019). In coronary artery disease, partial or complete blockage of one or more coronary arteries leads to myocardial ischemia and myocardial infarction. Risk factors for both hypertension and coronary artery disease include smoking, obesity, lack of exercise, and stress. Additional risk factors for coronary artery disease include hypertension, hyperlipidemia, and diabetes mellitus. Nursing interventions for hypertension and coronary artery disease address weight reduction, exercise, dietary changes to limit salt and fat, stress management, and smoking cessation. Patient education includes information about medications, blood pressure monitoring, nutrition, stress reduction techniques, and the symptoms that indicate the need for emergency care.

Smoking. Tobacco use has been recognized as the major preventable cause of death and disease in Canada (PHAC, 2021a). Smoking cessation is a health promotion strategy as much for older persons as for younger persons. Older persons who smoke can benefit from smoking cessation. In addition to reducing risk, smoking cessation may help stabilize existing conditions, such as chronic obstructive pulmonary disease. Smoking cessation may even contribute to the extension of life or of independent functioning. Use of the stages-of-change model has had success in smoking cessation (Martinasek et al., 2021). The first stage in this model is *pre-contemplation*—when the person has not yet made a change but might be willing to read some information about their condition and how to improve it. The second stage is *contemplation*—the person is beginning to think about making some positive changes. In the third stage, *preparation*, the person is making an active plan about improving their health. Next the person puts the plan into action—the *action* stage. Finally, in the *maintenance* stage, the person is developing strategies to maintain healthy behaviours.

Substance Use. In 2017 in Canada, the numbers of older persons exceeding low-risk drinking recommendations was 9%, with men 1.2 times more likely than women to have engaged in heavy drinking (PHAC, 2021a). *Heavy drinking* is defined as five or more drinks for men and four or more drinks for women on one occasion at least once a month. Studies of alcohol addiction in older persons have revealed two patterns: a lifelong pattern of frequent heavy drinking and a late-onset pattern in which heavy drinking begins late in life. Frequently cited causes of excessive alcohol use are depression, loneliness, and lack of social support. Problematic use of alcohol may be underidentified in older people (Touhy et al., 2019).

Substance use, one of which is alcohol, is often associated with a chronic health challenge. Some older people initially use alcohol as a means to address pain. Signs of alcohol dependence are subtle, and the assessment may be complicated by coexisting dementia or depression. Alcohol dependence should be suspected when the older person has a history of repeated falls and accidents, exhibits a change in behaviour or personality, is socially isolated, has recurring episodes of memory loss and confusion, has a history of skipping meals or medications, and has difficulty managing household tasks and finances. When problematic use of alcohol is suspected, treatment includes age-specific approaches in which the health care provider acknowledges the stresses experienced by the older person and encourages involvement in activities that match the person's interests and boost feelings of self-worth. The identification and treatment of coexisting depression is also important.

Older persons may also be using cannabis to manage a health challenge (Baumbusch & Sloan Yip, 2020). Older persons may be obtaining cannabis without consulting their primary health care provider and might be reticent to volunteer their use of cannabis, for fear of stigmatization. It is important that nurses ask older persons if they are using substances such as cannabis or alcohol to manage their health concerns.

Nutrition. Lifelong eating habits and situational factors influence how older persons meet their needs for good nutrition. Such habits are based in tradition, ethnicity, and religion and influence choices of what foods are eaten and how those foods are prepared. Situational factors affecting nutrition include availability of access to food stores, finances, the physical and cognitive capability for food preparation, and a place to store food and prepare meals. Almost one fifth of older persons are at nutritional risk due to eating fewer than two fruits and vegetables a day (PHAC, 2021a).

Nutritional needs of older persons are affected by levels of activity and by clinical conditions. Level of activity has implications for the total amount of calories: more sedentary older persons usually need fewer calories than more active older persons. However, caloric requirements are not determined solely by activity. Additional calories may be required in clinical situations such as recovery from surgery, whereas calories may be restricted when the patient is diabetic or overweight. Beyond caloric requirements, therapeutic diets may restrict fat, sodium, or simple sugars or may increase fibre or foods with high levels of calcium, iron, vitamin A, or vitamin C.

Good nutrition for older persons includes appropriate caloric intake and limited intake of fat, salt, refined sugars, and alcohol. Although the nutritional guidelines displayed in *Canada's Food Guide* (Health Canada, 2022) are the basic recommendations for nutrition in older persons (see Chapter 43), some older persons do not follow these guidelines. Protein intake may be lower than recommended if people have reduced financial resources or limited access to grocery stores. Difficulty chewing meat may also limit protein intake. Fat intake may be higher than recommended because fast-food restaurant meals may be substituted for meals prepared at home or because methods of cooking may feature fried foods and sauces made with butter and cream. Extra salt and sugar may be used in cooking or at the table to compensate for a diminished sense of taste. Vitamin intake may be reduced if the adult has difficulty shopping for fresh fruits and vegetables. As a nurse, you should assess the nutritional status of older persons in all settings and identify interventions to improve their nutritional status (Touhy et al., 2019).

Older persons with dementia have special nutritional needs. As memory and functional skills decline, they lose the ability to remember when to eat, how to prepare food, and, eventually, how to feed themselves. At the same time, caloric needs may increase because of the energy expended in pacing and wandering activities. Nurses and other caregivers of older persons with dementia should routinely monitor weight and food intake, serve food that is easy to eat, provide assistance with eating, and offer food supplements as needed to maintain weight (Fetherstonhaugh et al., 2019). Mealtime interventions for older persons with dementia provide opportunities for socialization and practice with functional skills.

Oral Health. Oral health is very important for older persons, as dental problems are common in older persons and include conditions involving natural teeth and dentures. Dental caries, gingivitis, broken or missing teeth, and ill-fitting or missing dentures may affect nutritional adequacy, cause pain, and lead to infection. Nurses can help prevent dental and gum disease through education about routine dental care (see Chapter 39). Nurses can also help older persons find dental services that offer reduced rates and that are accessible to patients with impaired mobility.

Exercise. Older persons should be encouraged to maintain physical exercise and activity. The primary benefits of exercise include maintaining and strengthening functional ability and promoting a sense of enhanced well-being. Mobility is important to older persons for maintaining their physical and psychological health (Langhammer et al., 2018). An exercise such as walking builds endurance, increases muscle tone, improves joint flexibility, strengthens bones, reduces stress, and contributes to weight loss. Other benefits of an exercise program include improvement of cardiovascular function, improved plasma lipoprotein profiles, increased metabolic rate, increased gastrointestinal transit time, and improved quality of sleep.

An exercise program should meet physical needs while allowing for physical impairments, and nurses should encourage the older person to persevere with the program. Willingness to participate in and persevere with an exercise program is influenced by general beliefs about exercise, specific benefits from exercise, past experiences with exercise, personal goals, personality, and any unpleasant sensations associated with exercise. Walking is the preferred exercise of many older persons (Figure 25.3).

Walking and other low-impact exercises such as riding an exercise (stationary) bicycle or exercises in a swimming pool protect the

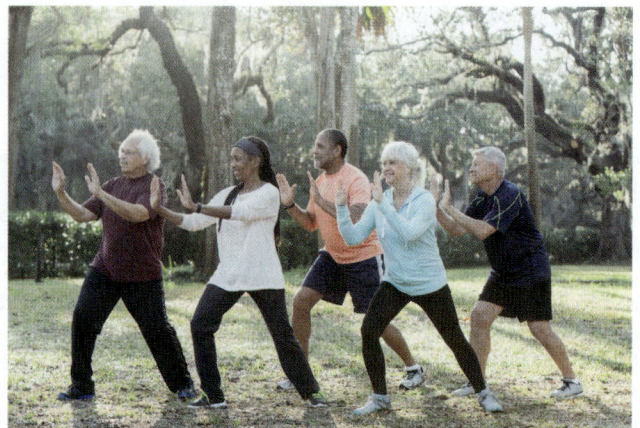

FIGURE 25.3 A group of five multi-ethnic older persons taking an exercise class in the park. They are practicing tai chi, standing with their hands raised. (iStockphoto/kali9)

musculoskeletal system and joints. Other exercises can be incorporated into an older person's ADLs. For example, the adult can perform arm and leg circles while watching television. However, before beginning an exercise program, the older person should have a physical examination. Exercise programs for sedentary older persons who have not been exercising regularly should begin conservatively and progress slowly. Safety considerations include wearing appropriate shoes and clothing, drinking water before and after exercising, avoiding outdoor exercise when the weather is very warm or very cold, and exercising with one or more partners. The older person should be instructed to stop exercising and seek help if they experience tightness or pain in the chest, shortness of breath, dizziness or lightheadedness, or palpitations during exercise.

Arthritis. Arthritis is common in older persons, especially women. The degree to which the mobility of older persons is impaired depends on the extent of disease and which joints are affected. Changes in joint range of motion and stability, combined with the amount of pain experienced, affect quality of life. Arthritis has no cure, but pharmacological agents can decrease pain and swelling and therefore increase joint motion. Nursing interventions are aimed at promoting comfort, functional ability, and safety. Education on self-care techniques, joint protection, and exercises for flexibility and strength is also important.

Falls. Falls are the leading cause of injuries among Canadians 65 years and over, with up to 30% of community-dwelling Canadian older persons experiencing a fall (PHAC, 2021a). Falls are a safety concern and one of the most common causes of functional dependence among older persons. They may lead to fear of additional falls, withdrawal from usual activities, and loss of independence (see Chapter 37). Hospitalization and placement in a long-term care facility may be required. Older persons who are hospitalized from a fall stay in the hospital 7 days longer than a hospitalization for another cause (PHAC, 2021a). Falls are more frequent and have more serious consequences among persons older than 85 years.

Falls are caused by a combination of individual and environmental factors (PHAC, 2021a). Individual factors include impaired vision; cardiovascular conditions, such as postural hypotension or syncope; conditions affecting mobility, such as arthritis, muscle weakness, and foot problems; conditions affecting balance; alterations in bladder function, such as frequency or incontinence; cognitive impairment; and adverse medication reactions. Medications can also have an impact on fall risk. Medications such as benzodiazepines and other hypnotics can impair an older person's central nervous system and affect gait. Environmental factors include, but are not limited to, poor lighting, slippery or wet floors, stairs or sidewalks in poor repair, shoes in poor repair or with slippery soles, and household items that could be tripped over, such as throw rugs, foot stools, and electric extension cords.

Multifactor falls-prevention programs such as sit-to-stand activity have been found to significantly reduce falls among community-dwelling older people (Winsnesky et al., 2020). Nurses can encourage older persons to perform exercises aimed at increasing leg strength and balance, which also reduce the risk of falls. Simple interventions in the home, such as rearranging furniture to provide a clear pathway to the bathroom and providing a night light in the bathroom, can reduce falls related to nighttime trips to the toilet. Removing throw rugs and other items on the floor helps reduce slipping and tripping. Nurses can also instruct older persons in the safe use of assistive devices such as canes, walkers, and wheelchairs. Older persons taking medications that may have adverse effects such as postural hypotension, dizziness, or sedation can be instructed to be aware of these potential effects and to take precautions, such as changing position slowly or holding onto sturdy

---

BOX 25.8 EVIDENCE-INFORMED PRACTICE

Effect of the Sit-to-Stand Activity on Mobility Outcomes Among Canadian Continuing-Care Residents With and Without Dementia

Evidence Summary

After an admission to a long-term care facility, the mobility of older residents declines because of sedentary behaviour and limited mobility. In this study by Slaughter and colleagues (2018), care staff received education on the importance of promoting function and independence in older people, as well as instructions on how to safely conduct the sit-to-stand activity. The time to complete the sit-to-stand activity was 30 seconds to 5 minutes. The aim of this study was to examine the effect of the sit-to-stand activity delivered by health care assistants on mobility outcomes in older persons who were living in supportive and long-term care settings. The study method was a hybrid type 3 cluster randomized controlled trial to evaluate the frequency and intensity of reminder implementation strategies and to evaluate the effect on older persons.

Results

Older people's mobility, function, and quality of life were measured before the intervention and then at 3 and 6 months during the intervention. Older people receiving the sit-to-stand activity over 6 months had less decline in their mobility and functional outcomes than did the control group. Moreover, the quality of life for the sit-to-stand group improved.

Application to Nursing Practice
- Nurses should assess older persons in long-term care facilities for functional decline.
- Promoting functional ability in older persons in long-term care facilities also increases their feelings of well-being.
- Nurses can use the sit-to-stand intervention when providing care to older persons.

Reference: Slaughter, S., Ickert, C., Jones, C. A., et al. (2018). Effect of a sit-to-stand activity on mobility outcomes among Canadian continuing care residents with and without dementia. *Journal of Aging and Long-Term Care, 1*(2), 65–72. https://doi.org/10.5505/jaltc.2018.52724

---

furniture if they are unsteady. Other health conditions such as ear infections can also contribute to falls. Box 25.8 describes a physical intervention to prevent falls among older people living in long-term care settings.

Sensory Impairments. Most older persons have changes in vision, hearing, taste, and smell as a result of normal aging. Chapter 48 describes in detail the nursing interventions used to maintain and improve sensory function.

Pain. National statistics reveal that one in four Canadians live with persistent pain, and since pain is often associated with chronic diseases, older persons are at a higher risk of living with pain (Health Canada, 2020). Causes of pain in older persons include acute and chronic conditions (e.g., trauma, infection, neuropathies). Consequences of persistent pain include depression, sleep difficulties, changes in gait and mobility, and decreased socialization. Older persons are most at risk of having their pain inadequately assessed and treated. Many factors influence the management of pain, including cultural influences on the meaning and expression of pain in older persons, fears related to the use of analgesic medications, and the difficulty of pain assessment with cognitively impaired older persons.

In caring for older persons, nurses must advocate for appropriate and effective pain management and for the use of standardized pain tools in assessing pain (see Chapter 32). The goal of nursing management of pain in older persons is to maximize function and improve quality of life.

Medication Use. Because older people tend to have more than one chronic health problem, they may receive multiple prescriptions, or they may combine prescription drugs with over-the-counter products or with natural remedies. The combinations can cancel the benefits of any or all medications and produce adverse reactions, such as memory loss, sleepiness, agitation, and confusion. These effects have been associated with falls and other injuries (PHAC, 2021a). The medications most commonly used are cardiovascular drugs, antihypertensives, analgesics, sedatives, tranquilizers, laxatives, and antacids. **Polypharmacy** (the concurrent use of many medications) increases the risk for adverse reactions. Although polypharmacy may reflect inappropriate prescribing, the concurrent use of multiple medications may be necessary if the older person has multiple acute and chronic conditions. However, a periodic and thorough review of all medications being used is important in helping older persons use the fewest necessary medications. The nurse's role with an older person is to ensure that the medications achieve the greatest therapeutic benefit with the least amount of harm. A good resource is *10 Tips for Safe Medication Management for Seniors* (Daily Caring, 2020).

Older persons are at risk for adverse reactions because of age-related changes in the absorption, distribution, metabolism, and excretion of drugs (see Chapter 35). Medications may interact with one another; one medication may augment or negate the effect of another. Medications may also cause confusion; affect balance and mobility; cause dizziness, nausea, and vomiting; or lead to constipation, urinary frequency, or incontinence. Because of these effects, some older persons are unwilling to take medications, and others do not adhere to the prescribed dosing schedule.

Managing medications is a very important component of maintaining and promoting good health in old age. For some older persons taking large numbers of medications, safely managing medications can be a complex activity that can easily become overwhelming. Nurses can provide valuable assistance to these older persons as they carry out this important self-care activity.

As a nurse, you need to work collaboratively with an older person to ensure safe and appropriate use of prescribed and over-the-counter medications. The older person should be taught the names of all drugs being taken, when and how to take them, and the desirable and undesirable effects of the drugs. You should also teach how to avoid adverse effects and interactions of drugs and how to establish and follow an appropriate self-administration pattern. To reduce the risk for an adverse medication reaction, you should review the medications at each visit; examine for potential interactions with food or other drugs; simplify and individualize the drug regimen; take every opportunity to inform the older person and their family about all aspects of medication use; and encourage them to question the physician, advanced practice nurse, pharmacist, or all three about all prescribed and over-the-counter drugs.

When medications are used in the management of confusion, special care is necessary. The sedatives and tranquilizers sometimes prescribed for acutely confused older persons may themselves cause or exacerbate confusion. These medications should be carefully administered; age-related changes in body systems can affect the pharmacokinetic activity. When confusion has a physiological cause (such as an infection), the cause, rather than the confused behaviour, should be specifically treated. When confusion varies by time of day or is related to environmental factors, creative, nonpharmacological measures can be used, such as changing the environment to include things that are familiar to the older person, providing adequate light, encouraging use of assistive devices (glasses, hearing aids), or even encouraging the older person to make telephone calls to friends or family members to hear reassuring voices (Touhy et al., 2019).

Health Promotion and Maintenance: Psychosocial Health Concerns

Interventions supporting psychosocial health of older persons resemble those for other age groups. However, some interventions are more crucial for older persons experiencing social isolation, cognitive impairment, or stresses related to retirement, relocation, or approaching death. These interventions include therapeutic communication, touch, cognitive stimulation, reminiscence, and measures to improve body image. Social isolation can cause loneliness for older persons (O'Rourke et al., 2018).

Therapeutic Communication. With therapeutic communication, the nurse perceives and respects the older person's uniqueness and meets their expectations. Older persons expect nurses to be attentive, caring, and knowledgeable. Being attentive means providing care in a timely manner and meeting the older person's expressed or unexpressed needs. As a caring nurse, you convey concern, kindness, and compassion. To show that you are knowledgeable, you need to demonstrate procedural competence and be adept at recognizing needs and relaying information. Older persons also expect others to respect their individuality. When you meet expectations and communicate effectively, they will accept you as someone who has a genuine concern for their welfare. However, you cannot simply enter an older person's environment and immediately establish a therapeutic relationship; you must first be knowledgeable and skilled in communication techniques (see Chapter 18).

Touch. Throughout life, touch tells people about their environment and the people around them. Gentle touch conveys affection and friendliness. A firm hand clasp may convey security. Although human touch is important, researchers have been exploring the use of social robots in the care of older persons, for tasks such as lifting and carrying (Parviainen et al., 2019). Robots could be useful in many ways, but they cannot replace human touch (Hung et al., 2019). Touch can provide sensory stimulation, induce relaxation, provide physical and emotional comfort, orient the adult to reality, convey warmth, and communicate interest. It is a powerful physical expression of a relationship.

Older persons may be deprived of touching when separated from family or friends. An older person who is isolated, dependent, or ill; fears death; or lacks self-esteem has a greater need for touch. You may recognize touch deprivation by behaviours as simple as an older person reaching for your hand or standing close to you. When you use touch, you must be aware of cultural variations and individual preferences (see Chapter 11). Touch should convey respect and sensitivity; it should not be used in a condescending way, such as patting an older person on the head.

Cognitive Stimulation. With **cognitive stimulation**, persons engage in physical activity and also benefit from improved cognitive function (Falch et al., 2019). Lobbia and colleagues (2019) reviewed research related to cognitive stimulation programs in people with mild to moderate dementia. These programs provided moderate improvements in general cognition, specifically language. The improvement enhanced the older persons' quality of life and their interactions with caregivers. Atypical types of cognitive stimulation include the use of current information; topics of general interest; historical events; attention, memory, and visuospatial exercises; and clocks and calendars. Some older persons may benefit more from cognitive stimulation than others; however, this pattern still remains unknown. Until more information is available, nurses should be sensitive to individuals' responses. As a nurse, you should always be respectful, patient, and calm, and in communicating, you should answer questions simply, honestly, and with sensitivity.

Reminiscence. **Reminiscence** is recalling the past. Many older persons find enjoyment in sharing past experiences. In reminiscence as therapy, the recollection of the past is used to find meaning and understanding of the present and to resolve current conflicts. Remembering positive resolutions to problems reminds older persons of previous coping strategies used successfully. Reminiscing is also a way to express personal identity. Reflection on past achievements supports self-esteem. For some older persons, the process of remembering past events uncovers new meanings for those events and has been found to decrease depression (Park et al., 2019). Researchers demonstrated that computer software can be used to aid older people to get in touch with their past and to engage in conversations with younger people (Welsh et al., 2018). The software enables older people to talk to other people and plays music and movies from decades past.

During the assessment process, nurses may use reminiscence to assess self-esteem, cognitive function, emotional stability, unresolved conflicts, coping ability, and expectations for the future. Reminiscence also occurs during direct care activities. Taking time to ask the older person questions about their experiences and listening attentively conveys to an older person an attitude of respect and concern.

Although reminiscence is often useful in a one-on-one situation with older persons, reminiscence can also be useful in group therapy for cognitively impaired or depressed older persons. A community nurse, for instance, can organize the group and select strategies to start a conversation (e.g., ask the group to discuss families or childhood memories). The group's size, structure, process, goals, and activities are then adapted to meet its members' needs.

Body-Image Interventions. The way that older persons present themselves influences body image and, potentially, feelings of isolation. Some physical characteristics of aging, such as distinguished-looking grey hair, may be socially desirable. Other features, such as a lined face that displays character or wrinkled hands that convey a lifetime of hard work, may also be impressive. Consequences of illness and aging that threaten the older person's body image include invasive diagnostic procedures, pain, surgery, loss of sensation in a body part, skin changes, loss of scalp hair, and incontinence. Body image is also affected by the use of devices such as dentures, hearing aids, artificial limbs, indwelling catheters, ostomy devices, and enteral feeding tubes.

The importance to the older person of presenting a socially acceptable image must be considered. When older persons have acute or chronic illnesses, the related physical dependence can make it difficult for them to maintain a healthy body image. Nurses can influence the older person's appearance by assisting with grooming and hygiene, such as combing hair, cleaning dentures, shaving, or changing clothing. Nurses should also be sensitive to odours in the environment. Odours may be created by urine and some illnesses. By controlling odours, nurses may encourage visitors to stay longer or visit more often.

OLDER PERSONS AND THE ACUTE CARE SETTING

Older persons in the acute care setting need special attention to help them adjust to the acute care environment and to meet their basic needs for comfort, safety, nutrition, hydration, and skin integrity. The acute care setting poses increased risk for older persons who have geriatric syndromes (such as cognitive impairment, malnutrition, incontinence, and fall risk). Older persons with geriatric syndromes on admission to acute care have increased incidence of adverse events such as delirium, dehydration, malnutrition, nosocomial infections (often respiratory or urinary tract infections), urinary incontinence, and falls (Van Seben et al., 2019).

The risk for delirium is increased when hospitalized older persons experience immobilization, infection, dehydration, pain, and hypoxia. Multiple medications and multiple medical diagnoses, infections, and dementia are also risk factors (Gual et al., 2018). Nonmedical causes include placement in unfamiliar surroundings, separation from supportive family members, and stress. Impaired vision or hearing contributes to confusion and interferes with nurses' attempts to reorient the patient. When prevention of delirium fails, the basis of nursing management is identification and treatment of the cause of delirium. Supportive interventions include encouraging family visits, providing memory cues (e.g., clocks, calendars, name tags), and compensating for sensory deficits. Reality orientation techniques may be useful.

Older persons are at greater risk for dehydration and malnutrition during hospitalization because of standard procedures such as limiting food and fluids in preparation for diagnostic tests. The risk for dehydration and malnutrition is also increased when older persons are unable to reach beverages or to feed themselves while in bed or connected to medical equipment. Interventions include getting the patient out of bed, providing beverages and snacks frequently, and including favourite foods and beverages in the diet plan.

The risk for health care–associated infections in older persons is increased by age-related reductions in immune system response. Of all health care agency–acquired infections, urinary tract infection is the most common in older people because of age-related changes; urinary catheter-related bacteriuria in older persons is the most common infection (Gbinigie et al., 2018). Other health care–associated infections include surgical site infection, pneumonia, and bloodstream infections. Prevention begins with hand hygiene and measures to minimize the risk of infection from procedures (see Chapter 34). Prevention also includes measures to increase the older person's resistance to infection.

Older persons in acute care settings are also at risk for acquiring urinary incontinence (transient incontinence). Causes of transient urinary incontinence include delirium, untreated urinary tract infection, excessive urine production, medications, restricted mobility, and constipation or impaction. Interventions for transient urinary incontinence should be geared toward correcting contributing factors. The interventions may include an individualized plan to provide voiding opportunities and modification of the environment to improve access to the toilet. In-dwelling urinary catheters should be avoided if possible. Skin breakdown should be prevented.

The risk for skin breakdown and the development of pressure injury is increased by changes in aging skin and situations that arise in the acute care setting, such as immobility, incontinence, and malnutrition. To prevent skin breakdown in older persons, nurses must avoid pressure on the skin, reduce shear forces and friction, provide skin care and moisture management, and provide nutritional support (see Chapter 43).

Older persons in the acute care setting are at risk for falling and sustaining injuries. This could occur because they get out of bed without assistance, or because they have received sedating medications. Medications causing orthostatic hypotension may also increase the risk for falls because the blood pressure drops when the patient arises from a bed or chair. Diuretics increase the risk for falling because the adult must get out of bed often to void. Attempts to get out of bed when physically restrained may lead to injury if the patient becomes entangled in the restraint. Equipment such as wires from monitors, intravenous tubing, urinary catheters, and other medical devices become obstacles to safe ambulation. Impaired vision may prevent the patient from seeing tripping hazards such as garbage cans. Interventions to reduce the risk for falling include assistance with ambulation, strengthening exercises, medication monitoring, assistance with toileting, and removal of tripping hazards and having friends or family at the bedside (see Chapter 38). Falls may be reduced by minimizing fall risk factors; through staff, patient, and family education; and through individualized fall-reduction interventions. The goal is to minimize the risk of falling without compromising mobility and functional independence.

Since the 1980s, many hospitals in Canada have established hospital acute care for elderly (ACE) units to provide specialized care for older people who have complex health care needs and to prevent functional decline (Flood et al., 2018). Key elements of ACE units are patient-centred care, interprofessional team management, medical review, discharge planning, and assessments and interventions for common geriatric syndromes such as falls, incontinence, confusion, and skin integrity. The ACE principles can be applied to older patients regardless of which unit they are on, to promote best care practices.

When caring for older persons in acute care, it is important for nurses to identify their pre-hospitalization level of functioning, which includes cognition, mobility, continence, and their living circumstances. This information is important for discharge planning, which should begin on admission. While in hospital, nurses must work with the interprofessional team to assist older persons to restore or maintain their function by walking them to the toilet, frequently orientating them to who the nurse is, as well as encouraging them to mobilize. This will facilitate older persons' ability to return home. When this is not possible and another type of living accommodation (such as a rehabilitation unit, assisted living, or long-term care) is required, nurses must work with the interprofessional team and the older person's family in assessing the older person's care needs and living preferences.

OLDER PERSONS AND RESTORATIVE CARE

Restorative care consists of two types of ongoing care: (1) continuing the convalescence from acute illness or surgery that began in the acute care setting and (2) addressing chronic conditions that affect day-to-day functioning. Both types of care take place in private homes and long-term care settings.

Interventions during convalescence from acute illness or surgery are directed toward regaining or improving the prior level of independence in ADLs. Interventions that began in the acute care setting should be continued and later modified as convalescence progresses. To achieve this continuation, the acute care setting's discharge information should describe the ongoing interventions (e.g., exercise routines, wound care routines, medication schedules, vital sign monitoring, and blood glucose monitoring). To ensure that all the patient's needs are addressed, a team approach to discharge planning is important. Interventions should also address the restoration of interpersonal relationships and activities either at their previous level or at the level desired by the patient.

When restorative care addresses chronic conditions, the goals of care include stabilizing the chronic condition, promoting health, and promoting independence in ADLs. Interventions to stabilize the chronic condition may focus on regulation or prevention. An example of a regulatory intervention is the monitoring of blood glucose levels in diabetes. An example of promoting health is a smoking cessation program for older persons with chronic obstructive pulmonary disease.

Health promotion interventions for older persons, as addressed in this chapter, should occur in all health care settings. For example, nurse-directed programs in long-term care settings improve ambulation, reverse urinary incontinence, and reduce confusion.

Interventions to promote independence in ADLs address physical ability, cognitive ability, and safety. The physical ability to perform ADLs requires strength, flexibility, and balance. Impairments of vision, hearing, and touch must be accommodated. The cognitive ability to perform ADLs requires the ability to recognize, judge, and remember. Cognitive impairments, such as Alzheimer's disease, may interfere with the safe performance of ADLs, although the affected patient is still physically capable of the activities. Interventions to promote independence in ADLs adapt these requirements to the needs and lifestyle of the older person. Safety is always an important consideration. An older person should be able to perform the ADLs with the least amount of risk.

Beyond the basic ADLs, the older person's ability to perform instrumental ADLs must be assessed and appropriate interventions implemented. Instrumental ADLs are tasks such as using a telephone, preparing meals, shopping, doing laundry, cleaning the home, and driving an automobile. To remain independent at home or in assisted-living residences, older persons must be able to perform instrumental ADLs, be able to purchase services by outside workers, or have a supportive network of family and friends who assist with these tasks.

Restorative care measures focus on activities to prevent, improve, reduce, or eliminate problems. Priorities of care are established, patient goals and expected outcomes are determined, and appropriate interventions are selected. These are done with the patient's participation so that interventions are understood and conflicts in approaches or priorities can be avoided. An older person's lifetime experiences, values, and sociocultural background are the bases for planning individual care. When deterioration of the patient's cognitive status prevents participation in care decisions, family or significant others must be consulted. Family and friends are rich sources of data because they knew the patient before the impairment. Frequently they can provide explanations for the older person's behaviours and suggest methods of management. Thoughtful assessment and planning involve consideration of the influence of normal aging changes, facilitating an optimal level of comfort and coping, and promoting independence in self-care activities.

OLDER PERSONS AND PALLIATIVE CARE

As the proportion of older persons in Canada increases, so too will the number of deaths. Although older persons are living longer and in better health than before, there is an increased incidence of chronic conditions with age (PHAC, 2021a). Thus, many individuals will require some form of assistance during their final years. The WHO (2020) describes the purpose of palliative care as improving overall quality of life for persons with life-limiting illness and for their families. It includes good symptom management and interprofessional collaboration, with a focus on fostering patient and family hopes, and achieving their goals and expectations for illness management over time. Often, this is viewed as happening in the last months, weeks, or days of life under the care of palliative care specialists. However, with the rising numbers of older persons worldwide, the WHO suggests a public health approach to meet a person's and family's full range of needs at all stages of frailty or chronic illness, not just at the end of life (Callaway et al., 2018). A palliative approach to care incorporates the ideals of palliative care for all patients with chronic conditions and their families, early on in the chronic disease trajectory as well as at the end of life, and is part of generalist health care practice in all settings (Sawatzky et al., 2018). As a nurse, you will be using the principles of the palliative approach for all of your patients who have chronic conditions.

KEY CONCEPTS

- The number of older persons in Canada, especially the number of older persons older than 85 years, is increasing.
- Because the nurse's attitudes toward older persons influence the quality of care, those attitudes should be based on accurate information about older persons, rather than on myths and stereotypes.
- Biological and psychosocial theories of aging offer possible explanations for the changes seen in aging, but every older person is a unique individual who ages in a unique way.
- The physical changes that accompany aging are considered normal, not pathological, although they may predispose older persons to disease.
- Cognitive impairment is not normal in older persons, and it necessitates assessment and intervention.
- Cognitive impairment includes acute, potentially reversible disorders (delirium) and chronic, irreversible, progressive disorders (dementia).
- Issues and events involving psychosocial changes related to aging include retirement, social isolation, change in housing, death of friends and family, sense of own mortality, and sexuality.
- Nursing interventions for psychosocial concerns include therapeutic communication, touch, cognitive stimulation, reminiscence, and interventions to improve body image.
- The leading causes of death in the older population are cancer, heart disease, stroke, lung disease, accidents and falls, diabetes, kidney disease, and liver disease.
- Health promotion recommendations for older persons include good nutrition, regular exercise, smoking cessation, measures to reduce the risk for falls, and measures to reduce adverse medication reactions.
- Acute care settings increase older persons' risk for delirium, dehydration, malnutrition, health care–associated infections, urinary incontinence, and falls.
- Restorative nursing interventions, whether accomplished in the older person's home or in long-term care facilities, stabilize chronic conditions, promote health, and promote independence in basic and instrumental ADLs.

CRITICAL THINKING EXERCISES

Critical Thinking Exercises 1 to 3 relate to the case study at the beginning of the chapter.

1. What are some possible questions to ask Mrs. Jones to begin to differentiate between delirium, depression, and dementia?
2. What are some of the cues that explain Mrs. Jones's feelings of social isolation and loneliness?
3. Identify some health promotion recommendations for Mrs. Jones.

Answers to Critical Thinking Exercises appear on the Evolve website.

REVIEW QUESTIONS

Review Questions 1 to 8 relate to the case study at the beginning of the chapter.

1. Identify and prioritize the three most urgent assessments that the nurse should focus on with Mrs. Jones. Highlight or place an X beside the assessments that the nurse should focus on.
   a. Assess the patient's dizziness and falls
   b. Rule out delirium and assess memory problems
   c. Assess grief and loneliness associated with husband's death
   d. Isolation from family and loss of friends and friendships
   e. Paranoia related to the loss of her husband and living alone
   f. Loss of her tutoring business and income
   g. Discuss potential living options and arranging a moving truck
   h. Create a budget and plan for her to stay in her own home
   i. Arrange for the installation of home security system
   j. Educate patient about peer support program in the area

2. In the table below, identify whether each of the listed screening tools or nursing actions would be indicated, contraindicated, or nonessential in assessing Mrs. Jones for delirium, dementia, and depression.

Nursing Action	Indicated	Contraindicated	Nonessential
a. Confusion Assessment Method (CAM)			
b. Geriatric Depression Scale (GDS)			
c. Folstein Mini-Mental Status Exam (MMSE)			
d. Falls Assessment			
e. Blood pressure assessment			
f. Elder abuse assessment			
g. Sexuality assessment			
h. Housing and environment assessment			
i. Palliative care			
j. Blood glucose screening			
k. Incontinence assessment			
l. Skin assessment			

3. Which care options would the nurse discuss with Mrs. Jones? *(Select all that apply.)*
   a. Personal care home
   b. Private home
   c. Private apartment
   d. Assisted living facilitates
   e. Long-term care
   f. Palliative care
   g. Restorative care
   h. Acute care

4. A. What type of support might the nurse suggest if Mrs. Jones decides to remain in her own home? *(Select all that apply.)*
   i. Homemaking
   ii. Personal care
   iii. Day-care centres
   iv. Information and referral
   v. Seniors' centres
   vi. Home-delivered meals

vii. Companions and friendly visitors
viii. Telephone reassurance
ix. Personal emergency response systems
x. Energy assistance programs

B. What type of support might the nurse suggest if Mrs. Jones chooses to move? (Select all that apply.)
  i. Homemaking
  ii. Personal care
  iii. Day-care centres
  iv. Information and referral

v. Seniors' centres
vi. Home-delivered meals
vii. Companions and friendly visitors
viii. Telephone reassurance
ix. Personal emergency response systems
x. Energy assistance programs

5. For each nursing intervention listed in the table below, highlight or place an X in the correct category column for each assessment to identify whether it would be indicated, contraindicated, or nonessential to address Mrs. Jones's dizziness and fear of falling.

Nursing Intervention	Indicated	Contraindicated	Nonessential
a. Contact physician for assessment			
b. Evaluate the need to involve other members of the health care team for assessment of balance and gait			
c. Explore patient's understanding of prescribed and over-the-counter medications, paying attention to benzodiazepines and hypnotics			
d. Assess patient's vision and hearing			
e. Assess patient's blood pressure			
f. Advocate for nonpharmacological and pharmacological agents to decrease pain and swelling of joints			
g. Assess living environment (indoors and outdoors) for lighting and clear pathways			
h. Encourage patient to wear nonskid footwear			
i. Educate about exercises to increase leg strength and balance, precautions to take to reduce chances of falling, such as changing positions slowly			
j. Refer to real estate agent			
k. Assess ability to perform ADLs and instrumental ADLs			
l. Explore past strategies for managing dizziness and feeling like they were falling			

6. When Mrs. Jones tells the nurse that she is afraid she has dementia because she was not able to remember her appointment, how should the nurse respond?
  a. "Don't worry, not remembering happens to everyone, and you are probably just overwhelmed."
  b. "I have some strategies that I can share with you to cue your memory. Would you like to go over those now?"
  c. "I understand you are afraid you have dementia. Tell me more about your concerns."
  d. "Dementia is reversible and is sometimes misdiagnosed. I am sure you are fine."

7. Choose the most likely options for the information missing from the statements below by selecting from the list of options provided.

Completing a comprehensive assessment with an older person may take longer than with a younger person because an older person has a longer and more complex _____ and may require _____ as a result of decreased energy and endurance or additional time to _____. This may be related to changes in understanding the nurse's _____, to _____, or to the older person being not able to accurately recall _____.

Answer Options:
Life history
Rest periods
Respond to questions
Visual or auditory cues
Memory deficits
Past medical events and information

8. To ensure cultural safety during a comprehensive assessment with an older person, which of the following should the nurse implement? (Select all that apply.)
  a. Identify how the older person wishes to be addressed
  b. Assess and uphold the health-related beliefs and practices of the older person
  c. Establish rapport using the cultural beliefs and practices about spatial requirements, eye contact, and touch
  d. Always use an interpreter or cultural broker with assessments with older persons

Rationales for the Review Questions appear on the Evolve website.

events and information. 8. a, b, c
or to the older person not being able to accurately recall past *medical*
understanding the nurse's *visual or auditory cues*, to *memory deficits*,
time to *respond to questions*. This may be related to changes in
periods as a result of decreased energy and endurance or additional
has a longer and more complex *life history* and may require *rest*
may take longer than with a younger person because an older person
c; 7. Completing a comprehensive assessment with an older person
Contraindicated interventions: k; 6.
ix, x; 5. *Indicated nursing interventions:* a, b, c, d, e, f, g, h, i, l;
a, b, c, d; 4. **A:** i, iii, iv, v, vii, viii, ix, x; **B:** i, iii, iv, v, vi, vii, viii,
j; *Contraindicated actions:* i, k, l; *Nonessential actions:* f, g; 3.
Answers: 1. a, b, c; 2. *Indicated nursing actions:* a, b, c, d, e, h,

RECOMMENDED WEBSITES

Alzheimer Society of Canada: https://www.alzheimer.ca
The Alzheimer Society of Canada provides current information about Alzheimer's disease, related dementias, caregiving, support, research, treatment, and programs and services.

Canadian Coalition for Seniors' Mental Health: https://ccsmh.ca
This website provides information on national guidelines, tools, and resources about older persons' mental health issues.

Canadian Gerontological Nursing Association: https://www.cgna.net
This website provides information about gerontological nursing practice in Canada, including current standards of practice.

Canadian Network for the Prevention of Elder Abuse: https://www.cnpea.ca
This website provides information about elder abuse in Canada and Best Practice Guidelines for the prevention of elder abuse.

Hartford Institute for Geriatric Nursing: https://hign.org
This website provides continually updated evidence-informed protocols and assessment tools for nurses to use with older persons.

Public Health Agency of Canada, Division of Aging and Seniors:
https://www.phac-aspc.gc.ca/seniors-aines/
This federal website provides links to new services, publications, and news releases on issues relevant to aging.

REFERENCES

A full reference list is available on the website for this book at http://evolve.elsevier.com/Canada/Potter/fundamentals/

26

The Experience of Loss, Death, and Grief

Canadian content written by Lorraine Holtslander, RN, MN, PhD, CHPCN(c), with original chapter contributions by Emily McClung, MSN, RN, PhD

OBJECTIVES

Mastery of content in this chapter will enable you to:

- Define the key terms listed.
- Identify your role in assisting patients and families experiencing loss, death, and grief.
- Describe and compare various theories and models of grieving.
- List and describe categories of loss and grief and types of death.
- Describe the characteristics of a person experiencing grief.
- Describe variables that influence a person's response to grief, loss, and death, including cultural aspects.
- Explain eligibility criteria and the nurse's role in medical assistance in dying (MAiD).

- Develop a nursing care plan for a patient or family experiencing loss and grief.
- Describe principles of hospice and palliative care.
- Describe how to involve family members in palliative care.
- Describe the procedure for care of the body after death.
- Reflect on your own experience of loss when caring for dying patients.
- Consider ways to improve palliative care for Indigenous people.
- Explore resources available to families and nurses regarding death, loss, and grief.

KEY TERMS

Actual loss
Advance care planning
Anticipatory grief
Bereavement
Complicated grief
Disenfranchised grief
Disorganization, hopelessness, and despair
Grief
Health care proxy

Hope
Hospice
Maturational loss
Meaning-making approach
Medical assistance in dying (MAiD)
Necessary losses
Neurological death
Numbness
Palliative approach to care

Perceived loss
Postmortem care
Prolonged grief
Prolonged grief disorder (PGD)
Reorganization
Situational loss
Specialist palliative care
Substitute decision-maker
Yearning and protest

WEBSITE

http://evolve.elsevier.com/Canada/Potter/fundamentals/

CASE STUDY

As a community nurse, you are asked to visit, assess, and support Mrs. Long (preferred pronouns: she/her) with her medication management. Mrs. Long is an 86-year-old woman who is currently living alone after the death of her husband 13 months ago. The referral states that her family doctor has requested a community nurse to assist with her medications because she has been missing important doses and her health is deteriorating. As you complete your assessment, you realize that her main concern relates to the loss of her husband of 60 years. Mrs. Long describes how she provided 24-hour physical and emotional care for her husband for over 5 years and is still quite exhausted. She expresses feeling very sad and lonely, and says that living without her husband feels like "someone has chopped one of my arms off." She has three adult children who

are supportive, but they are also busy with their own families and dealing with the death of their father after his lengthy illness.

After a month of weekly visits to monitor Mrs. Long's ability to self-administer her medications after they were placed in "bubble packaging" and to assess her general physical and emotional health, you realize that Mrs. Long is losing weight, taking extra naps, and has increasing pain in her back. After some tests and referrals organized by her family doctor, you learn that Mrs. Long has been diagnosed with both prolonged grief and lung cancer. Mrs. Long and her children are in shock and are not sure what to do next.

Think about this case study as you read this chapter. There are review questions at the end of the chapter that relate to the case study.

Loss, death, and grief are experiences that affect not only patients and their families but also the nurses who care for them. Palliative, hospice, and end-of-life care programs and practices continue to develop in health care and gain acceptance, even though most Canadians deny the possibility of death, even when their health may be significantly deteriorating. Loss and death are an inevitable part of life, offering nurses important opportunities to promote quality of life for patients and families and to improve the outcomes of grief, which is a response to any type of loss.

Grief affects survivors physically, psychologically, socially, and spiritually because of actual, situational, and perceived losses. The death of a patient may leave family, friends, and caregivers feeling sad and uncertain. Most nurses enter the profession with the intent of helping patients recover from illness, adjust to illness-related changes in lifestyle, and move toward restoration of health. However, the reality is that loss, grief, and death will be encountered in every area of nursing practice.

The nurse's role in facilitating the grief process includes providing emotional, physical, and psychosocial support for survivors to move forward in their own unique ways. To be effective, nurses must acknowledge the loss, its significance and meaning to the patient and family, and how it affects their ability to carry on. Providing care for patients in crisis from loss or at the end of life requires knowledge, caring, and compassion to help bring comfort to patients and families. Helping patients to experience a peaceful, dignified death is an important aspect of nursing care. Although working with dying patients can be emotionally challenging, many nurses also find it to be a valuable and truly transformative experience (Parola et al., 2018).

SCIENTIFIC KNOWLEDGE BASE

Loss

Throughout their lives, as social beings, people form attachments that result in many types of loss. They develop independence from their parents, start and leave school, change friends, begin careers, and form and end relationships. The growing-up process is natural and positive, and yet as people's lives unfold, they suffer these necessary losses, an integral part of each person's life. People expect their losses to be replaced by something different or better, but some losses have long-lasting and devastating effects (Pohlkamp et al., 2019). Losses such as the death of a child, losses that come with a divorce, or a loss of independence due to an accident are significant and can have long-term effects on physical and psychological health. Loss comes in many forms, depending on the values and priorities learned within a person's sphere of influence, made up of family, friends, society, and culture. A person experiences

loss in the absence of an object, person, pet, body part or function, emotion, or idea that was formerly present (Table 26.1). Losses may be actual or perceived. An actual loss is any loss of a person or object that can no longer be felt, heard, known, or experienced by the individual. Examples are the loss of a body part, a child, a relationship, or a role at work. Lost objects that have been valued by a patient could be any possession that is worn out, misplaced, stolen, or ruined. For example, a child may grieve over the loss of a favourite toy. A perceived loss is any loss that is defined uniquely by the grieving patient. It may be less obvious to others. An example is the loss of confidence or prestige. Perceived losses are easily overlooked or misunderstood, and yet the process of grief may be very similar to actual losses. Individual interpretation makes a difference in how the perceived loss is uniquely valued and the response that a person will have during grieving.

Losses may also be maturational, situational, or both. A maturational loss is any change in the developmental process that is normally expected during a lifetime. One example would be a parent's feeling of loss as a child goes to school for the first time. Events associated with maturational loss are part of normal life transitions, but the feelings of loss may persist, and grieving helps a person cope with the change. Situational loss is any sudden, unpredictable external event. Often this type of loss includes multiple losses rather than a single loss; for example, an automobile accident may leave a driver paralyzed, unable to return to work, and grieving over the death of a passenger in the accident.

The type of loss and the perception of the loss influence the depth and duration of grief that a person experiences. Each individual responds to loss differently. It is incorrect to assume that the loss of an object does not generate the same level of grieving as the loss of a loved one. The value an individual places on the lost item, or attachment to the person or object, determines the emotional response to the loss. As a nurse, you must assess the special meaning that a loss has for a patient and validate its effect on the patient's health and well-being.

Hospitalization, chronic illness, and disability are circumstances associated with multiple losses. When patients enter a hospital, they lose their privacy, control over their daily routines, and any illusions that they may have about their personal indestructibility. In addition, modesty and control over bodily functions may be compromised. A chronic illness or disability often engenders concern over financial security. Furthermore, long-term illness may necessitate a job change, threaten independence, and force alterations in lifestyle. Even a brief illness or hospitalization necessitates temporary shifts in family role functioning. Chronic or debilitating illness may pose a major threat to the stability of relationships.

TABLE 26.1 Types of Loss	
Definition	**Implications of Loss**
Loss of external objects (e.g., loss, misplacement, deterioration, theft, fire, or destruction by natural causes)	Extent of grieving depends on object's value, sentiment attached to it, and its usefulness.
Loss of known environment (e.g., moving from a neighbourhood, hospitalization, leaving or losing a job, moving into a long-term care or a residential setting)	Loss occurs through maturational or situational events and through injury or illness. Loneliness or newness of an unfamiliar setting threatens self-esteem and makes grieving difficult.
Loss of a significant other (e.g., through being promoted, moving, or running away; loss of a family member, friend, trusted nurse, acquaintance, animal companion or pet)	Significant other typically fulfills another person's need for psychological safety, love and belonging, and self-esteem.
Loss of an aspect of self (e.g., body part, psychological function, or physiological function)	Illness, injury, and developmental changes result in loss of an aspect of the self that causes grief and permanent changes in body image and self-concept.
Loss of life (e.g., death of family members, friend, or acquaintance; own death)	Loss of life creates grief for the survivors. The person facing death often fears pain, loss of control, and dependency on others.

Death is the ultimate loss, resulting in a period known as *bereavement* for the survivors. Although death is part of the continuum of life and a universal and inevitable part of being human, it is also a mystical event that generates anxiety and fear. Death ends relationships and separates people. Even with a strong spiritual and emotional grounding, facing death is often difficult for the dying person, as well as for the person's family, friends, and caregivers. A person's terminal illness reminds close friends and associates of their own mortality. A person with an advanced, progressive, ultimately fatal illness, such as chronic renal failure, end-stage heart failure, amyotrophic lateral sclerosis (ALS), or metastatic cancer, faces many—often progressive—levels of suffering.

The way a person approaches death and dying is influenced by personal fundamental beliefs and values, past experiences with death, culture, spirituality, and the quality of the emotional support available. More and more often, many Canadians are choosing to die at home, with the support and involvement of their family. This goal can be enabled and accomplished by implementing a person-centred palliative approach to care, facilitating choice, and supporting family caregivers in the community (Hammond & Baxter, 2019).

Grief

Each individual will experience grief and grieving in unique ways (Lundorff et al., 2020). Differences are based on individual experience, previously established coping strategies, cultural expectations, and spiritual beliefs (see Chapters 11, 12, and 29) and involve the process of mourning and adapting to a loss. Most people will find the support and develop the coping strategies they need to remain resilient through grief, while a smaller but significant number will experience prolonged or complicated grief that requires intervention and professional support (Lundorff et al., 2020). Table 26.2 offers a comparison of several theories of the grief process.

Bereavement is the state of having lost a significant other to death, resulting in grief and mourning. The bereavement process is not linear, nor does it proceed through sequential stages that can be precisely predicted, which may imply passivity on the part of the bereaved person. Although it is often not possible to just "get over" a loss, an individual can heal and develop the ability to cope with grief (Harrop et al., 2020). Over time, many researchers have explored the processes of grief and identified stages, phases, and tasks that may describe how people work through bereavement and adapt to life with a loss. It is important not to "impose" these models on individuals, recognizing the uniqueness and complexity of each situation.

Theories of Grief. The work of Kübler-Ross (1969) is seminal, although controversial and often misinterpreted since it was based on her research with dying patients. She described five stages in the process of coming to terms with a terminal illness as denial, anger,

bargaining, depression, and acceptance. The work of Kübler-Ross provides an explanation that is often applied to other losses and to the bereaved as well, which may or may not be helpful, but may show some of the ways in which people cope with grief.

Bowlby's (1980) important contribution is theories of attachment, exploring the essential need for attachment of babies to their parents, and then to other significant people. Being social, humans require these attachments, and when they end through separation such as death, there is grief. Bowlby and Parkes (1970) built on attachment theory by describing four stages of grief as follows: **numbness**, characterized by shock and denial, then **yearning and protest** with waves of grief, guilt, blame, tension, physical symptoms, and difficulty thinking. In the phase of **disorganization, hopelessness, and despair**, an individual may constantly examine how and why the loss occurred. During the final phase of **reorganization**, attachments begin to change and new relationships are built.

In a **meaning-making approach** to grief (Neimeyer, 2006) the death of a significant person can lead to great difficulty in finding meaning in the loss and in life. Meaning reconstruction, through a narrative (telling of the story) approach, can enable a more positive adaptation to the loss. Survivors of a death that was tragic or violent, for example from suicide or homicide, are particularly vulnerable to negative outcomes and may be unable to make sense of their loss (Zakarian et al., 2019) without resources and therapy to support the meaning-making process (Neimeyer, 2019).

Stroebe and Schut's (1999) dual process model (DPM) does not define stages but rather depicts grief as an oscillation or a process of going in and out of grief work. Individuals are both dealing with the daily stressors of "loss-oriented (LO) coping," or ruminating on the loss, and "restoration-oriented (RO) coping," or finding a new identity. The movement between LO and RO coping indicates a moving forward, including adapting to new roles while also spending necessary time with difficult emotions. A Finding Balance Intervention that is based on the DPM has shown promise to increase RO coping (Holtslander, 2019), and the DPM has remained a realistic framework that is often used to illustrate the bereavement experience (Fiore, 2019).

Continuing Bonds (Klass, 2006) is based on attachment theory. When someone we are attached to dies, the bond may continue in memories, dreams, and at many significant points in future events, such as anniversaries. Persons who are bereaved aren't required to "move on" and reach acceptance or complete the "work" but rather are encouraged to maintain a bond with the deceased that may enable coping. For example, visits to the cemetery demonstrate a physical bond with the deceased. Research with bereaved parents has described how promoting an internalized continuing bond with the deceased child predicted post-traumatic growth and improved coping (Albuquerque et al., 2018).

TABLE 26.2	Theories of the Grief Process			
Kübler-Ross's (1969) Stages of the Dying Process	Bowlby's (1980) Attachment Theory; (Bowlby & Parkes, 1970) Phases of Mourning	Dual-Process Model (Stroebe & Schut, 1999)	Meaning-Making (Neimeyer, 2006)	Continuing Bonds (Klass, 2006)
A person with a terminal diagnosis may experience the following: • Denial • Anger • Bargaining • Depression • Acceptance	Attachment as a human need that, when broken, results in phases of grief/mourning: Numbness Yearning and protest Disorganization, hopelessness, and despair Reorganization	Grief as a process of oscillation between loss-oriented and restoration-oriented coping	The meaning of the loss will affect outcomes; need for meaning reconstruction, through a narrative approach	Continuing a connection with the deceased has benefit toward processing the loss

Types of Grief. Grief can be a normal process, but some people will have great difficulties and for them it can become **complicated grief** or **prolonged grief**, defined as grief that is chronic and unmanageable. Knowledge of types of grief, which are based on characteristics or signs and symptoms of grief, enables you as a nurse to respond with appropriate bereavement support and interventions.

Normal Grief. Normal or uncomplicated grief consists of the feelings, behaviours, thoughts, and reactions to a loss, including resentment, sorrow, anger, crying, loneliness, and temporary withdrawal from activities. Most people in bereavement will follow a "resilient" trajectory, with symptoms of grief they can manage based on their abilities to maintain mental health and optimism for the future (Lundorff et al., 2020), resulting in the development of adaptive coping strategies on which the person can rely in the future.

Anticipatory Grief. Faced with many losses often encountered during the terminal phase of an illness, death may become anticipated in a phenomenon called **anticipatory grief** (Coelho et al., 2020). In the study by Coelho and colleagues, caregivers of a person with terminal cancer experienced traumatic distress, uncertainty, images of suffering, and a very challenging caregiving experience, leading to an anticipation of the care recipient's death in order to escape the burden of caregiving.

Anticipatory grief is commonly experienced by caregivers of persons with dementia because the trajectory of dementia is experienced as a series of losses pre-death (Cheung et al., 2018), including loss of a companion, of freedom, and of social roles. These caregivers may begin preliminary bereavement before the physical death of the person with dementia in anticipation of their loss (Liew et al., 2018). By seeking and receiving social support, those who "proactively cope" may experience positive outcomes during anticipatory grief, even through the traumatic experience of caregiving for a person at the end of life (Rogalla, 2020).

Anticipatory grieving entails some risks. For example, in a study of caregivers of patients admitted to the Critical Care Unit (CCU), levels of anticipatory grief were high and associated with anxiety, depression, and difficulty making important decisions on behalf of the patient (Glick et al., 2018). Anticipatory grief may also contribute to complicated or prolonged grief; thus, assessment of coping, type of grief, and available support is very important.

Complicated or Prolonged Grief. Most individuals will have the coping skills and support they need to move forward in their grief without professional intervention. However, a significant minority will experience intense, prolonged, and disabling symptoms of grief, also known as "complicated grief" (Iglewicz et al., 2020). Complicated grief encompasses debilitating feelings of loss that do not improve after a significant amount of time has passed (Oates & Maani-Fogelman, 2020). When a person has difficulty progressing through the "normal" phases or stages of grieving, grief may present as chronic and disabling, requiring detection and formal intervention. There is a lack of agreement on these terms and the time frames, but they indicate that grief has become overwhelming and intervention is usually required.

Prolonged grief disorder (PGD) is a mental disorder described in the *Diagnostic and Statistical Manual of Mental Disorders*, 5th edition, text revision (*DSM-5-TR*). PGD is characterized by distressing, disabling yearning and difficulties engaging in life activities that persist for a year or more after the loss (Prigerson et al., 2021). Following a natural death, approximately 1 out of 10 bereaved individuals will experience impairing and pervasive grief symptoms requiring intervention and treatment (Lundorff et al., 2020); however, PGD can be predicted by poor physical and mental well-being prior to the loss. In one study, when the experience of the death was unnatural (for example suicide, homicide, accidental, or death of a child), the rate of PDG increased to

50% of individuals (Djelantik et al., 2020). A diagnosis of PGD is also made when there is persistent separation distress that impairs daily functioning for more than 6 months after the loss (Pohlkamp et al., 2019). In Pohlkamp et al.'s study, for some parents whose child had died of cancer, grief symptoms persisted for the 5 years of the study. Strong attachments form between parents and children and even more so when children become ill.

Disenfranchised Grief. **Disenfranchised grief** is defined as the experience of grief that is not openly acknowledged, publicly mourned, or socially supported. This sense of isolation can make grief difficult to express, and it may become complicated grief because societal rules exist regarding who has a right to grieve, when and how they should grieve, for whom, and for how long (Doka, 1999). Individuals who experience disenfranchised grief may struggle with emotional expression and deny themselves support (Albuquerque et al., 2021). Examples are the loss of a partner from an accidental drug overdose, divorce, the health care provider who experiences the loss or multiple losses of patients, or the loss of a pet (Spain et al., 2019). In the context of attachment theory, any significant emotional bond that is lost can be overwhelming and distressing when grief cannot be expressed or is not socially accepted. Limitations imposed during the COVID-19 pandemic have also led to disenfranchised grief, due to limitations on attending funerals and burials, as well as restricted hospital and care home visits at the end of life (Albuquerque et al., 2021).

Application of Grief Theory to Other Types of Loss. Although grief theories apply mainly to the way that individuals cope with the death of a loved one, they also apply to other losses. The theories are relevant to the way people respond to a loss of body function, as in the case of joint replacement or heart attack, and to disability, such as amputation or paralysis. Grief theory applies to individuals who mourn for lost independence, body integrity, and a change in body image. These individuals experience genuine emotional pain as they progress through the grieving process and may face similar complications such as prolonged grief.

Death

Types of Death. Death is an event that could be categorized into types such as biological/physiological, social, psychological, and theological (Table 26.3). *Biological death* is the clinical definition of death, when the body dies due to a lack of oxygen, which can be subcategorized into two types: *circulatory death* and *neurological death* (Gardiner et al., 2020). **Neurological death** is a medical determination in which there is irreversible cessation of all functions of the entire brain, including the brainstem (de Tantillo et al., 2019). *Circulatory death* is declared after cardiorespiratory arrest, when the entire body is subjected to ischemia due to the cessation of blood flow. However,

TABLE 26.3	Types of Death
Types of Death	**Definition**
Biological death	Cells cease to function due to lack of oxygen
Neurological	Irreversible cessation of all functions of the brain, including the brainstem
Circulatory	Declared after the circulatory system stops, resulting in cardiorespiratory arrest
Social death	When an individual is no longer accepted as an active agent within their relationships
Psychological death	An individual's acceptance of their impending death
Theological death	The body, mind, and soul cease to act as one, and the soul leaves the body.

BOX 26.1 A Dying Person's Bill of Rights

I have the right to be in control.

I have the right to be treated as a living human being until I die.

I have the right to have a sense of purpose.

I have the right to be cared for by those who can maintain a sense of hopefulness.

I have the right to express my feelings and emotions about my approaching death in my own way.

I have the right to have a respected spirituality.

I have the right to participate in decisions about my care.

I have the right to expect continuing medical and nursing attention even though "cure" goals must be changed to "comfort" goals.

I have the right not to die alone.

I have the right to be comfortable.

I have the right to have my questions answered honestly.

I have the right not to be deceived.

I have the right to have help from and for my family in accepting my death.

I have the right to die in peace and dignity.

I have the right to laugh and to be angry and sad.

I have the right to retain my individuality and not be judged for my decisions that may be contrary to beliefs of others.

I have the right to be cared for by caring, sensitive, knowledgeable people who will try to understand my needs and will be able to gain some satisfaction in helping me face my death.

Adapted from Barbus, A. J. (1975). The dying person's bill of rights. *American Journal of Nursing, 75,* 99; and from Hospice RN. (2003). *Patient's bill of rights.*

neurological death is often considered to be equivalent to circulatory death, because the brain is required to maintain the functioning of the organism as a whole and without the brain, circulatory death is certain to occur (Truog, 2020).

The term *social death* is relevant when the individual is not yet deceased but is no longer an active being in social relationships and in a social context (Gatti & Blanes, 2020). Social death can occur when an individual becomes advancingly ill; for example, persons with dementia may become ostracized and no longer recognized and responded to as active participants within their relationships (Watson, 2019). *Psychological death* involves an individual's acceptance of their impending death (Philipp et al., 2019). Individuals may begin to withdraw from relationships and social activities while experiencing this type of death (Secinti et al., 2019). *Theological death* occurs when there is an irreversible loss of a being's capacity to function as a whole, where "wholeness" is the integration of body, mind, and soul (Veatch, 2019). In other words, theological death is when the soul leaves the body.

Another term, a "good death," has been described from the patient's perspective as one where pain and symptoms are controlled, there is a feeling of closure and preparedness, and the patient feels they are seen as a person who is able give back to others (Krikorian et al., 2020). The elements of a good death are shaped by culture, society, religion and spirituality, and age and life circumstances. A good death can vary greatly within cultural groups and depends on the disease and the trajectory of dying. The concept of a good death is highly individualized and changes depending on circumstances.

The nurse needs to respect the values and wishes of dying patients, while exploring their own expectations and experiences of death, to avoid imposing an ideal image on each patient and family's situation at the end of life. Box 26.1 describes a bill of rights for a dying person that reflects individuality in the dying process and offers ways to provide end-of-life care that is meaningful to the patient, the family, and their care providers.

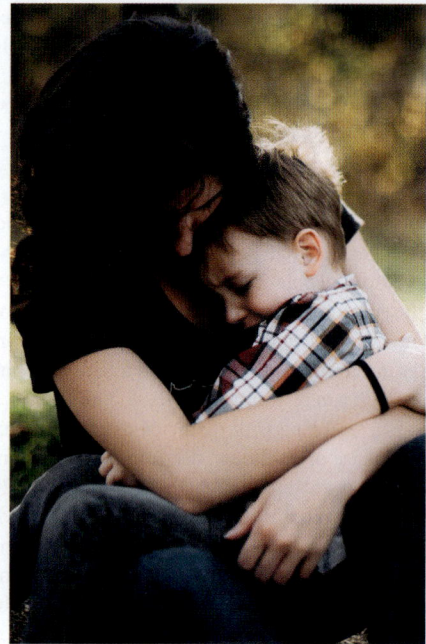

FIGURE 26.1 Children need support through the emotions of loss. (Jordan Whitt/Unsplash)

NURSING KNOWLEDGE BASE

Nursing knowledge has traditionally focused on the acute care setting, in which losses may seem mainly physical in nature. As nurses enter home and community settings, the types of loss are more apparent, comprehensive, and in some ways different. As a nurse you must develop assessment skills and interventions for each unique patient, family, and community situation.

Factors Influencing Loss and Grief

The way that an individual perceives a loss and responds to it during bereavement is influenced by many factors.

Human Developmental Stage. People of differing ages and stages of development display different and unique symptoms of grief. For example, toddlers are unable to understand the permanence of loss or death, but they feel great anxiety over the loss of objects and separation from parents. School-aged children experience grief over the loss of a pet, friend, sibling, parent, or grandparent through death, divorce, changing schools, or moving. Children are not able to process loss as well as adults because of the disruption in their developmental progress, lack of coping skills, lack of supports and relationships, and misperceptions that result in them feeling they are to blame for what happened (Ferow, 2019). As Ferow explains, these risk factors that are specific to children need to be recognized. Children can be helped to face grief and loss through open and honest communication and by being provided a safe place for them to express how they feel. When a parent is dying, parents and children need to spend quality time together, create positive and lasting memories, maximize networks of support, and strengthen relationships with open communication (Hanna et al., 2019) (Figure 26.1). Children need a safe place to express their feelings about a loss.

Middle-aged and older persons may experience anticipatory grief because of changes associated with aging and the possible loss of self-care abilities. Aging is frequently associated with multiple losses, such as physical changes, loss of employment, loss of social respect, loss of relationships, and threats to a sense of fulfillment and contributions

Excerpted from Goveas, J. S., & Shear, M. K. (2020). Grief and the COVID-19 pandemic in older adults. *American Journal of Geriatric Psychiatry, 28*(10), 1119–1125. https://doi.org/10.1016/j.jagp.2020.06.021

BOX 26.2 FOCUS ON OLDER PERSONS

Grief and the COVID-19 Pandemic

- Grief is a normal response to bereavement and is intensely painful and disruptive, yet most older people will adapt even while facing secondary losses, such as loss of physical and emotional support and independence.
- Most older persons restore meaning and purpose, but when grief is stalled, the result might be prolonged grief, characterized by persistent yearning, distress, and impairment in daily functioning.
- Risk factors for prolonged grief include previous depression or anxiety, previous trauma, loss through a sudden death, and secondary losses, such as loss of a caregiver or partner.
- Risk factors related to death during COVID-19 include sudden and unexpected deaths, family members dying alone, restrictions on visiting in hospital, disruption and delay of rituals such as funerals, fear of the disease, and ongoing social isolation and loneliness.
- Nurses can help older persons through active listening, reflecting on emotions, and talking to older persons about their experiences of death and their ongoing concerns.
- It is important to recognize the risk factors and symptoms of prolonged grief because they are associated with physical health changes, impaired coping, increased risk of suicide, and overall increased mortality. Immediate action is needed, such as a referral for professional support of a mental health clinician, especially for older persons who are often isolated.

made in life. Older persons have many coping skills and are often resilient in responding to grief. However, the COVID-19 pandemic has presented major challenges for older persons facing grief (Goveas & Shear, 2020) (Box 26.2).

Psychosocial Perspectives of Loss and Grief. Loss and death are life experiences that each person faces, even more so in nursing practice settings. Culture can have a significant influence on people's views of death and how the dying person should be cared for. As a nurse you may share some of your patients' biases or perspectives gained during your childhood and sociological development. Exploring your own experiences of loss, personal beliefs, and experiences of death and grief will help you be self-aware in supporting patients and families who have beliefs that are different from your own (Schreiner & Bordonaro, 2019).

An individual's expression of grief evolves as the person matures. Personal experiences shape the coping mechanisms that an individual uses to deal with stressors. As psychologists explain, the coping mechanisms that were effective in the past are repeated as a first response to the pain of a loss. When older coping strategies are unsuccessful, new coping mechanisms are attempted (see Chapter 30). When faced with a loss, a patient or family member learns what is needed for their own coping through repetition that is based on the successes and failures of different coping mechanisms. Sometimes the number or depths of losses become overwhelming, and familiar coping styles are not successful. For example, in the case of disenfranchised grief, routine coping strategies such as expressing emotions and seeking support are not available to the person or sanctioned by society. Professional support may be required to help the individual or family move forward through the pain associated with the loss.

Socioeconomic Status. Socioeconomic status influences a person's ability to obtain options and use support mechanisms when coping with loss. In general, people feel greater burden from a loss when financial, educational, or occupational resources are lacking. For example, a patient with limited finances may not be able to access mental health resources or may not be able to purchase necessary medications or supplies to manage a newly diagnosed disease. These patients require referral to community social support agencies that can provide access to needed resources.

Personal Relationships. The quality and meaning of the relationship is critical in understanding a survivor's grief experience. It has been said that to lose parents is to lose the past, to lose a spouse is to lose the present, and to lose a child is to lose the future. When a relationship between two individuals has been very close, the one left behind can have great difficulty coping, as explained by the complexity of attachment theory (Smigelsky et al., 2020). Support from family and friends is based, in part, on the person's relationships with members of a social network and the manner and circumstances of the loss. People who do not easily receive support and compassion from others may have difficulty grieving.

Nature of the Loss. The ability to manage grief depends on the meaning of the loss and the situation surrounding the loss. The visibility of a loss influences the support a person receives. For example, the loss of one's home from a fire prompts support from the community, whereas a private loss of an important possession may prompt less support from others. Some losses are not highly visible, such as reproductive loss (e.g., miscarriage, stillbirth, abortion, giving up a child for adoption, infertility). The suddenness of a loss can delay resolution from grief. For example, a sudden and unexpected death is generally more difficult for a family to accept than death after a long-term chronic illness.

Culture and Ethnicity. A person's cultural background strongly influences their ways of coping with loss and beliefs about life-sustaining treatments during terminal illness. For example, in a CCU setting, when the patient has limited English proficiency, communication and relationships with clinicians can be significantly impaired and may result in difficulty understanding and accepting treatment options such as palliative care (Barwise et al., 2019). Barwise and colleagues (2019) recommend the use of cultural humility, interpreters, and refraining from generalizing and stereotyping each patients' specific culture.

Culture affects how patients, and their support systems or families, respond to loss (see Chapters 11 and 12). For example, in the Western hemisphere, the grieving process is usually personal and private; individuals tend to show restrained emotion. However, the ceremonies surrounding a person's death offer time for grief resolution and reminiscing. In Eastern hemisphere nations, such as the Philippines, respect for the dead is shown by wailing and physically demonstrating grief for a specified period. Despite these trends, members of the same ethnocultural background will respond to loss and death differently. Nurses must acquire an understanding and appreciation of each individual patient's and family's cultural values as they apply to the experience of loss, death, and grieving.

Canada is a multicultural society, and as a nurse, you can anticipate many cultural contexts and responses to loss, death, grief, and bereavement. You must be able to support and guide patients and families through the end-of-life process in a culturally informed and acceptable manner. Indigenous people in Canada face inequitable access to health care—including palliative care—due to racism, discrimination, stigma, sexism, and bias that prevents Indigenous people from accessing health services. Providing culturally safe care involves building trust, conveying respect, and ensuring a partnership in which the patient and family determine whether cultural safety is achieved (Bourassa, 2018).

⊕ BOX 26.3   CULTURAL ASPECTS OF CARE

Improving the Cancer Journey for Indigenous People in Canada

Cancer survival rates in Canada are lower for Indigenous Canadians as a result of many factors, including racism and a lack of respectful, trusting relationships with health care providers.

- Loss of culture, ceremony, and language and the subsequent trauma as a result of colonialism and residential schools have negatively impacted equitable access to health resources and services for Indigenous people.
- Historical trauma, ongoing racism, and discrimination are social determinants of health that have resulted in the statistic that First Nations people are 35% less likely to survive lung cancer (Canadian Partnership Against Cancer, 2020).
- Reconciliation, cultural safety, and humility among health care providers are necessary and expected, which can result in improved utilization of health care services and improved outcomes.
- Cultural safety and humility involve a process of self-reflection for health care providers to understand personal and systemic biases.
- Creating relationships of trust will engage Indigenous people in partnerships to improve equity in access to health services.

From Caron N, Linn, K., Spinelli, JJ, Johnson, H. (2018). Improving First Nations cancer journeys: Current policy perspectives and approaches in British Columbia, Canada. *Cancer Health Disparities, 2*, e1–e8. https://doi:10.9777/chd.2018.10012

Incorporating cultural safety and humility could improve the care and outcomes for Indigenous people within the health care system (Caron et al., 2018), as detailed in Box 26.3.

At the end of life, rituals, mourning practices, and specific expressions of grief are necessary for participants of all cultures in order to have a sense of acceptance and inner peace. These rites and rituals provide an opportunity to express emotions, share grief with others, and recognize the value and importance of who has died, enabling a healthier response and grief journey. The COVID-19 pandemic has greatly affected gatherings and connection and resulted in the loss of many important farewell rituals (Cardoso et al., 2020), predisposing many individuals to complicated grief.

Spiritual Beliefs. Individuals' spirituality significantly influences their ability to cope with loss. Some of the spiritual resources on which patients may depend during a loss include faith in a higher power or influence, their community of fellowship with friends, their sources of hope and meaning in life, and their use of religious rituals and practices. Loss can sometimes cause internal conflicts about spiritual values and the meaning of life. Patients who have a strong spiritual interconnectedness may be able to face death with relatively minimal discomfort (see Chapter 29). Alternatively, patients faced with a life-threatening or terminal illness may begin to question their faith and wonder why this would be allowed to happen to them.

Coping With Grief and Loss

In order to support patients and families during loss, nurses must understand how people usually cope with grief and loss. Nursing interventions involve reinforcing the patient's successful coping mechanisms and introducing new coping approaches, such as protecting and promoting hope. Chapter 30 summarizes the nursing care principles for assisting patients to cope with stressful situations.

Hope. Hope enables us to achieve goals and to cope with life's challenges, offering ways to stay positive about the future while giving meaning to the present (Callina et al., 2018). Hope, or similarly, optimism, is often about future expectations, but hope can also be centred in the present, especially when linked to agency and trust. Hope enhances coping skills by giving inner strength when hopes are changing, such as during a terminal illness. The nurse can promote hope during difficult times by exploring the meaning of events, building trust, and offering ways to maintain a sense of control during challenging circumstances.

Bally and colleagues (2021) developed a "Keeping Hope Possible" (KHP) toolkit for parents of children with life-limiting and life-threatening conditions. Parents face many challenges while caregiving, including significant life disruption and feelings of a total loss of control. The KHP toolkit offers activities and information to foster hope and self-efficacy while reducing uncertainty and distress. The toolkit encourages journalling, self-reflection, and ways to find support and information. Nurses and other health care providers can offer personal connectedness that is essential to hope. Nurses can help patients and families to identify their emotions, to remember to care for themselves, and to live in the moment. Chapter 29 discusses the conceptual components of hope and related nursing care implications.

CRITICAL THINKING

Successful critical thinking involved in caring for patients who have experienced losses requires a synthesis of knowledge, previous experience with loss and grief, and information gathered from patients and families. To provide appropriate and responsive nursing care, nurses must apply both critical thinking qualities and intellectual and professional standards.

During assessment, nurses must analyze all sources of information in order to select appropriate nursing diagnoses (Figure 26.2). To understand the process of grief and its effect on the patient and family, the nurse integrates knowledge from nursing and other disciplines and from previous experiences in caring for patients suffering loss. Knowledge of the processes of grief, for example, enables the nurse to better empathize with a patient and family and to understand their reactions. Critical thinking qualities and standards of care then help the nurse apply this information in a relevant and therapeutic way for the patient's and family's benefit. For example, as a nurse you need the critical thinking quality of perseverance so that you can learn as much as possible about the type of grief a patient is experiencing, in order to ultimately select the most appropriate nursing interventions.

❖ THE NURSING PROCESS AND GRIEF

◆ Assessment

For a patient who has experienced or is facing a loss, nursing assessment includes the patient, family, significant others, and the psychosocial context. Grief assessment is ongoing throughout the course of an illness for the patient and family and for the bereavement period after the death for the survivors (Holtslander et al., 2017). As a nurse you should not assume how or whether the patient or family experiences grief. You should also avoid assuming that a particular behaviour indicates grief; rather, you should allow patients to share what is happening in their own way. An effective nurse encourages patients to tell their stories. This requires the nurse to establish trust with patients and to evoke a caring presence. It is helpful to have patients and families find a time and place to express their grief and describe their experiences (Figure 26.3). A thorough and comprehensive approach to the assessment of grief will result in a well-designed plan of care that will facilitate patients' and families' abilities to work through grief.

Knowledge
- Grief process
- Pathophysiology of related illness threatening a loss
- Therapeutic communications principles
- Cultural perspectives on the meaning of loss or death
- Family dynamics in offering social support
- Concepts of caring
- Concepts of stress and coping

Experience
- Caring for a patient who experienced a physical or emotional loss
- Caring for a patient who died
- Personal experience with loss or death of a significant other

Assessment
- Assess meaning of loss for this patient
- Observe behaviours and other symptoms indicative of grief response
- Note quality and extent of patient's family support

Standards
- Apply principles outlined in professional and clinical standards
- Demonstrate the ethical principles of health care
- Apply intellectual standards of significance; know what is important to the patient

Qualities
- Take risks if necessary to develop a close relationship with the patient to understand loss

FIGURE 26.2 Critical thinking model for loss, death, and grieving assessment.

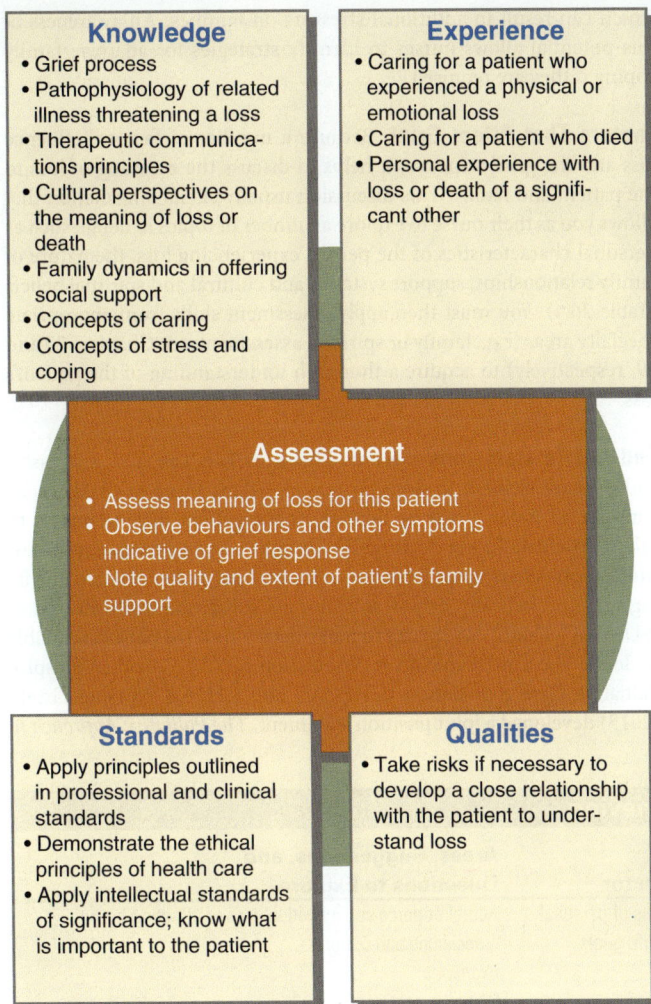

FIGURE 26.3 Nurse meeting with a family caregiver. (© CanStockphoto/obencem)

Assessment begins by interviewing, using honest and open communication to build trust. Listening carefully and observing their responses and behaviours is important. The nurse should assume a neutral perspective and remain alert for nonverbal cues such as affect, facial expressions, voice tones, and topics that are avoided. While gathering data, the nurse summarizes and validates any impressions formed

with the patient and family so that appropriate nursing diagnoses can be made. Information from other health care workers, such as social workers, and providers of pastoral care, will contribute to the database.

Type and Stage of Grief. It is important to assess how a patient *is reacting* rather than how the patient *should be reacting*. The sequencing of stages or behaviours of grief may occur in order, they may be skipped, or they may recur. A single behaviour can be representative of any number of types of grief. Therefore, the identification of the type and stage of grief should be used only to guide the assessment and not to judge the outcomes of the grieving process. By understanding the processes of grief, nurses can begin to assess a situation. For example, if a patient is complaining of loneliness and difficulty falling asleep, all factors surrounding the loss need to be considered. When did the loss occur? What type of loss occurred? The patient may be experiencing a normal grief reaction, or, if the loss occurred 2 years ago, the patient may be experiencing prolonged or complicated grief.

As a nurse assessing grief, ask the patient to describe their loss and how it has affected them: "Tell me how your diagnosis of heart disease makes you feel." You can anticipate characteristics or responses during a phase of grieving, but you should allow patients to describe their feelings as thoroughly as possible: "How has this change in your life affected you today?" "Tell me more." Then probe and validate feelings expressed in the patient's emotions: "You seem angry; tell me more . . .," "You seem sad; tell me . . .," "What are your feelings about . . .?" Avoid premature assumptions about the type of grief that a patient might be experiencing, so that you do not terminate the assessment too early.

Grief Reactions. Nurses use psychological and physical assessment skills to compile a complete database about the patient, family, or both. Although no two people grieve exactly the same way, most people who grieve have at least some outward signs and symptoms (Box 26.4). Clinical reasoning is needed to analyze the data and cues collected and to determine the appropriate related cause. For example, a patient who is experiencing complicated grieving may have a changing affect, lowered activity level, somatic symptoms such as headache or upset stomach, and alterations in sleep patterns, memory, and concentration. These symptoms might be associated with any number of health problems, such as anxiety, gastrointestinal disturbances, or even impaired memory. However, the focus is to assess the patient's symptoms in context. What are the meaning and significance of the loss, and how are they affecting the patient in physical, social, emotional and behavioural ways? With what does the patient associate the symptoms? In what ways are the symptoms related to one another when they occur? What symptoms are observed when the patient openly expresses grief? Over what time period have the symptoms been present—before the loss or during the loss? Careful analysis refines the nurse's ability to make judgements about the patient's condition.

A loss takes place in a social context. When the primary provider in a family has a terminal illness, the family begins to reorganize itself as soon as the patient is no longer able to fulfill the same number and types of roles. When a person is disabled, the patient and family undergo similar reorganization, realigning roles and responsibilities to meet demands. During this time, patients and families can experience a variety of physical and psychological symptoms. Nurses need to assess the entire family's response to loss, recognizing that family members may be dealing with aspects of grief different from those of the patient. Good interviewing and physical assessment skills guide nurses in planning appropriate nursing care. It is important to assess for changes in family relationships or interactions during a patient's illness. Terminal illness may bring distant family members together,

BOX 26.4	Symptoms of Normal Grief

Feelings
Sadness
Anger
Guilt or self-reproach
Anxiety
Loneliness
Fatigue
Helplessness
Shock or numbness (lack of feeling)
Yearning
Feeling of emancipation or relief

Cognitions (Thought Patterns)
Disbelief
Confusion
Preoccupation about the deceased
Sense of the presence of the deceased
Auditory hallucinations
Perceptual disturbances
Hopelessness ("I'll never be okay again")

Physical Sensations
Hollowness in the stomach
Tightness in the chest
Tightness in the throat
Oversensitivity to noise
Depersonalization ("Nothing seems real")
Shortness of breath
Muscle weakness
Lack of energy
Dry mouth
Headache
Abdominal pain

Behaviours
Sleep pattern changes
Appetite disturbances
Absent-minded behaviour
Dreams about the deceased
Sighing
Emotional lability
Carrying objects that belonged to the deceased

which can result in additional stressors on families. An awareness of this potential allows nurses to identify strategies for adaptive family coping if they are required.

Factors That Affect Grief. Because a number of factors influence loss and the grief response, it helps to discuss the meaning of loss to the patient and family. This discussion usually elicits information that allows you as their nurse to explore a number of topics in detail, such as personal characteristics of the person experiencing loss, the nature of family relationships, support systems, and cultural and spiritual beliefs (Table 26.4). You must then apply assessment skills from appropriate specialty areas (e.g., family or spiritual assessment; see Chapters 20 and 29, respectively) to acquire a thorough understanding of the patient's loss.

End-of-Life Decisions. Serious illness or loss can add a stressful and difficult element to decision making. Time to make decisions or consider all options may be limited, or the patient may be unable to fully participate in the decision-making process. Advance care planning involves having earlier conversations about end-of-life care, revising them periodically, as well as naming a substitute decision-maker (SDM) or a health care proxy to make decisions if the patient is unable to do so. The Canadian Nurses Association (CNA), Canadian Hospice Palliative Care Association (CHPCA), and CHPCA Nursing Group (2015) developed a joint position statement, *The Palliative Approach to*

TABLE 26.4	Assessment of Factors That Influence Grieving		
Factor	**Areas, Suggestions, and Questions to Explore**	**Factor**	**Areas, Suggestions, and Questions to Explore**
Nature of relationships	Functions of the family, community, and society *Examples:* "How long have you known your friend?" "What role has your mother played in your family?" "What is your relationship? Will it change?" "How will family relationships change as a result of the loss?"	Loss of personal life goals	Actual or perceived individual losses affecting future decisions and options *Examples:* "What is your goal in life?" "How has this goal changed as a result of your diagnosis?" "How will your role change your personal goals?" "What planning have you and your family made for your own life?"
Social support system	Availability of family, friends, health care providers *Examples:* Who is present? Absent? Supportive? Not supportive? What do family and friends do that is most meaningful? Are family and friends available when needed? Are health care providers accepting and exploring ways to preserve the patient's dignity and lifestyle?	Family's grief	Relationships, involvement with the dying process *Examples:* Observe patient and family's level of grief, patterns of behaviour, rank of leadership or power. What has helped family members deal with problems in the past? What was not helpful? What are the family's strengths and weaknesses?
Nature of loss	Actual versus perceived; death issues; impact on roles *Examples:* "Tell me what the loss means to you." "What factors help you to grieve?" "What factors interfere with grieving?" "What past experiences or outcomes have you had with loss?"	Survivor risk factors	High risk, such as sudden death, violent death, loss of a child, multiple losses, as well as previous and current mental and physical health concerns. *Examples:* "Describe your feelings and thoughts at this time." "Let's talk about why you think you could have prevented this. Are you feeling guilty because . . .?" "What are the unresolved issues or perceptions toward others?" "What other losses are you currently dealing with?"
Cultural and spiritual beliefs	Values, cultural norms, spirituality, customs, attitudes *Examples:* "What is your belief about death? About the meaning of life?" "What customs do you value at the time of death?" "How is this loss viewed by other people of your culture or religious group?" "Do medical treatments interfere with religious practices?" "Who has the right to say yes or no to life-sustaining measures?"	Hope	Goals, worth, adaptation to future changes *Examples:* "Tell me what you think about your treatment plan." "What are you hoping will happen to you?" "How does this illness affect your hopes and goals in life?" "What are you hoping for after your surgery?"

Care and the Role of the Nurse, which includes a statement on advance care planning. This document states: "Nurses should encourage all people to reflect on, communicate and document their values (i.e., personal, cultural, religious and those that constitute a legacy for enduring and sustaining life), in addition to health and personal care wishes that include end-of-life care" (p. 5). An advance care plan documents a person's preferences regarding life-sustaining treatment and communicates these preferences if the person becomes incapable of doing so for themselves (CNA et al., 2015). This upholds the nursing professional value of autonomy. As a nurse, you must be aware of the legal status of advance care plans or instructional directives, as well as the specific terms used (agent, representative, proxy, SDM) in your province or territory. You also need to know the laws regarding a person's competence to consent to treatment, as well as legislation regarding the selection and responsibilities of the SDM or a health care proxy (see Chapter 10).

When a person has a terminal illness, family members must face end-of-life decisions that have ethical, legal, and practical implications. Families may experience higher levels of stress, discomfort, or even guilt when deciding whether to initiate or withdraw life-sustaining treatments. Some treatments may offer symptom relief but simultaneously prolong life, which creates conflict or dilemmas for families and caregivers. Although some patients may have advance care plans or directives, it is important for family members to know in advance a patient's wishes in regard to life-sustaining measures. At times, family members may disagree with each other about treatment plans, or the values of the family may be in conflict with those of the health care provider. Situations such as these often result in ethical dilemmas for families, nurses, or other care providers. Decision making related to ethical situations should consider the primary nursing values from the CNA (2017a) *Code of Ethics for Registered Nurses.* Ethicists and ethical decision-making models may be used if agreement on treatment is not possible.

The *Code of Ethics for Registered Nurses* (CNA, 2017a) identifies three values that are pertinent to nurses assisting individuals in end-of-life decision making:

1. *Promoting health and well-being:* Nurses must ensure that an individual's wishes as stated in an advance directive are respected and that continuing care and support are provided.
2. *Promoting and respecting informed decision making:* Nurses must respect and promote the autonomy of individuals, help patients express their needs and values, and help patients obtain appropriate care.
3. *Preserving dignity:* Nurses must advocate on the patient's behalf and examine biological, psychological, social, cultural, and spiritual factors that affect end-of-life treatment decisions.

Responsibility statements associated with each value in the code give more direction to nurses in upholding the values. For example, the value "health and well-being" includes this responsibility statement:

> *When a person receiving care is terminally ill or dying, nurses foster comfort, alleviate suffering, advocate for adequate relief of discomfort and pain, and assist people in meeting their goals of culturally and spiritually appropriate care. This includes providing a palliative approach to care for the people they interact with across the lifespan and the continuum of care, support for the family during and following the death, and care of the person's body after death (CNA, 2017a, p. 13).*

Palliative Approach to Care. The **palliative approach to care**, as supported by the CNA, CHPCA, and the CHPCA-NG (2015), is focused on helping people to live well until death, across the lifespan and in all settings. Nurses have a central role in implementing a palliative approach to care for patients and families faced with diagnoses of illnesses that are life-threatening. Person-centred care is the foundation, honouring people's values, promoting autonomy, dignity, control, and shared decision-making. Nurses work with interprofessional colleagues, employers, and governments to support high-quality palliative and end-of-life care that is accessible and available in any setting of care. A palliative approach may include treating the illness at the same time as comfort and supportive care. The aim of the palliative approach is to reduce hospitalizations and inappropriate medical treatments, with goals of better symptom management, reduced suffering, and better bereavement outcomes for families. For example, research shows that early introduction of a palliative approach to care for persons with Parkinson's spectrum disorders would improve quality of life, focus on support for family caregivers, and include person-centered advance care planning (Katz, 2020). The introduction of a palliative approach to care would greatly improve quality of life for many Canadians (Hammond & Baxter, 2019), as well as the outcomes of grief and bereavement for family caregivers. The conversation needs to be open and ongoing to ensure the patient and family have their wishes and values upheld and that the goal of a comfortable and peaceful death is achieved.

Medical Assistance in Dying (MAiD). Residents of Canada may voluntarily request medical assistance (or **medical assistance in dying [MAiD]**) to hasten their death following a process which became legal in 2016 under Bill C-14 of the *Criminal Code.* Criteria for MAiD include being older than 18 years of age and being mentally competent, suffering from a grievous and irremediable medical condition, and being in an advanced state of illness that cannot be reversed. Additional criteria for MAiD were included in Bill C-7, which received royal assent on March 17, 2021. These changes removed the requirement that the person's natural death be "reasonably foreseeable" and allowed eligible persons to waive final consent if they are at risk of losing capacity.

Canadians cannot include MAiD in their advance care plans. Both medical doctors and nurse practitioners are able to provide MAiD to patients, either through direct administration or prescription of medications, based on a voluntary written and witnessed patient request and assessments by two independent practitioners. Nurses have the right to conscientiously object or refuse to participate in MAiD, based on moral or religious beliefs, but they must respect patient decisions, discuss all treatment options, and not impede access; nor may they counsel someone to choose MAiD (CNA, 2017b; Pesut et al., 2020a, 2020b). Each nurse should check with their own provincial regulatory body about limits and conditions regarding their own involvement with MAiD.

The MAiD decision is complex, and consideration for grief and bereavement is important. The patient's family may face unique challenges after a MAiD death, such as disenfranchised grief if the circumstances are not openly shared, and complicated grief if there was family conflict over the decision. The journey through MaiD includes the grief and bereavement process; support and information are available through organizations such as Dying with Dignity Canada and Bridge C-14. More information can be found in the Recommended Websites at the end of the chapter.

Nurses' Experience With Grief. When caring for grieving patients, nurses must assess their own emotional well-being. Self-reflection, which is a part of critical thinking, is a valuable tool in assessing whether a person's sadness is related to the patient, to unresolved personal experiences from the past, or to a combination of both. It is normal to have personal feelings and emotions about certain illnesses and death. However, as a nurse it is inappropriate to emphasize your personal family situations and values over those of the patient. Talking

BOX 26.5   NURSING DIAGNOSTIC PROCESS

Assessment Activities	Defining Characteristics	Nursing Diagnosis
Ask patient to discuss future goals and plans.	Patient sighs and says, "I have no future; I don't want to face life alone."	*Hopelessness related to grief and failing physical condition*
Observe patient's nonverbal behaviour.	Patient becomes passive with little affect and turns away from speaker.	*Ineffective individual coping related to low mood, and inability to manage loss*
Offer patient choices and observe responses.	Patient shrugs and says, "What does it matter?"	*Powerlessness related to perceived poor outcomes*
Assess activity level.	Patient refuses to eat. Patient sleeps all the time, keeping blinds closed and lights out. Patient refuses to participate in care.	*Self-care deficit related to inability to perform activities of daily living* *Social isolation related to inability to cope with loss*

with friends and professional colleagues may help you resolve conflicts about caring for dying patients. Some nurses choose to work in a specialty area in which deaths are usual. Close bonds between nurses and patients often develop in these situations. Part of being a professional involves knowing oneself and when to move away from a situation. Nurses who choose to work in palliative care settings often obtain support and feedback from their peers, as well as from interprofessional team debriefings. A safe environment in which to express concerning behaviours, thoughts, and feelings is an important aspect of self-care through taking time for reflection and relaxed moments (Parola et al., 2018).

Nursing Diagnosis

From data collected during the assessment, the nurse can identify a nursing diagnosis that accurately reflects the needs of the patient or family experiencing the loss. Critical thinking skills are used to apply concepts of assessment, clustering of cues, and drawing a conclusion of the actual or perceived needs of the patient. The nurse clusters defining characteristics and identifies the nursing diagnosis applicable to the patient's situation (Box 26.5). Clustering of patient or family behaviours, actual or potential losses, the patient's attempts at coping, and data involving the nature and meaning of the loss will lead to individualized nursing diagnoses, such as the following:

- *Anticipatory grieving*
- *Anxiety*
- *Caregiver role strain*
- *Compromised family coping*
- *Dysfunctional grieving*
- *Fear*
- *Hopelessness*
- *Ineffective coping*
- *Ineffective denial*
- *Powerlessness*
- *Readiness for enhanced spiritual well-being*
- *Social isolation*
- *Spiritual distress*

The presence of one or two defining characteristics is usually insufficient for an accurate diagnosis. As a nurse you must carefully review the data to consider whether competing diagnoses exist. For example, if a dying person cries, displays anger, and reports nightmares, this could signal several possible nursing diagnoses, as these characteristics are common to more than one diagnosis. Possibilities include *pain, ineffective coping,* and *spiritual distress.* It is important to examine all available data and inquire about and observe for the presence of other behaviours and symptoms until you can identify an accurate diagnosis.

Part of the diagnostic process is to identify the appropriate related factor for each diagnosis. For example, *dysfunctional grieving related to the loss of the ability to walk from paralysis* necessitates different interventions than does *dysfunctional grieving related to the loss of a spouse.*

In order to promote a holistic approach to care, wellness-oriented diagnoses need to be included, such as *readiness for enhanced spiritual well-being.* These diagnoses allow for recognizing and drawing from patient strengths. In addition, the nursing diagnostic process is continual because the patient situation will change.

When identifying nursing diagnoses for the dying patient, other conditions are identified separately according to specific standards of care. Other nursing diagnoses can include *disturbed body image, impaired physical mobility,* or *ineffective role performance.* More physical nursing diagnoses are identified when the patient begins to experience physical changes accompanying the progression of illness, including *impaired urinary elimination and/or bowel incontinence, acute pain, nausea, disturbed sensory perception,* and *ineffective breathing pattern.* The comfort of dying patients, including specialized pain control and acceptance of the dying process by the family, is a realistic expectation. With terminal illness, physical assessment of the dying process is ongoing so that nurses can adapt or validate the actual nursing diagnoses with the patient's changing condition.

Planning

Grieving is the natural response to loss and thus has therapeutic value. The focus in planning nursing care is to support the patient physically, emotionally, developmentally, and spiritually in the expression of grief. Figure 26.4 illustrates the interrelatedness of critical thinking factors during the planning phase of the nursing process. Through critical thinking, nurses ensure a well-designed plan in which they support a patient's personhood, self-esteem, and autonomy by including the patient in making decisions about the plan of care. When caring for the dying patient, it is important to devise a plan that helps a patient die with dignity and offers family members the assurance that their loved one is being cared for compassionately (Box 26.6). The care planning process is highly individual to the patient and family, and when possible, both must be included as active participants in a nurse's planning, goal setting, and development of realistic interventions and timelines.

Goals and Outcomes. Realistic goals and expected outcomes are established on the basis of a patient's nursing diagnoses. Patient resources such as physical energy and activity tolerance, supportive family members, spiritual faith, and methods for coping are integrated into the plan of care. For example, if a patient with a life-threatening illness has the diagnosis *powerlessness related to planned cancer therapy,* a goal of "Patient will be able to discuss expected course of disease" is realistic if the patient is able to remain attentive and participate in educational discussions without becoming fatigued. In contrast, the expected outcome "Patient will participate in series of mini, planned teaching discussions about disease" accounts for the patient's need for teaching sessions to be short to avoid exhaustion.

Goals of care for a patient dealing with loss might be long or short term, depending on the nature of the loss, the patient's phase of grieving,

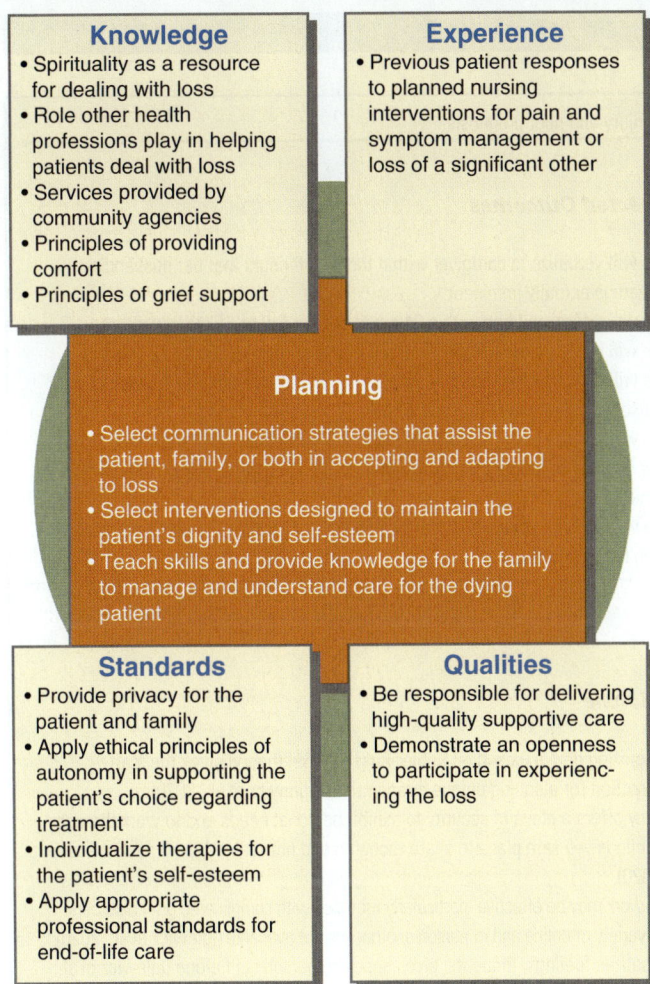

Knowledge
- Spirituality as a resource for dealing with loss
- Role other health professions play in helping patients deal with loss
- Services provided by community agencies
- Principles of providing comfort
- Principles of grief support

Experience
- Previous patient responses to planned nursing interventions for pain and symptom management or loss of a significant other

Planning
- Select communication strategies that assist the patient, family, or both in accepting and adapting to loss
- Select interventions designed to maintain the patient's dignity and self-esteem
- Teach skills and provide knowledge for the family to manage and understand care for the dying patient

Standards
- Provide privacy for the patient and family
- Apply ethical principles of autonomy in supporting the patient's choice regarding treatment
- Individualize therapies for the patient's self-esteem
- Apply appropriate professional standards for end-of-life care

Qualities
- Be responsible for delivering high-quality supportive care
- Demonstrate an openness to participate in experiencing the loss

FIGURE 26.4 Critical thinking model for loss, death, and grief planning.

and the nature of the illness. Many terminally ill patients experience plateaus (periods of relatively stable health) interspersed with periods of exacerbation of symptoms. Because a patient may move back and forth between coping with grief, nurses may need to revise goals and outcomes to ensure that they remain relevant. Help from the patient's partner in deciding which goals are relevant is important. General nursing care goals for patients with a loss include accommodating grief, accepting the reality of a loss, and renewing regular relationships. When a patient has a terminal illness, controlling pain and symptoms, maintaining autonomy, and achieving spiritual comfort are important goals. For the goal "achieving a sense of dignity for a parent diagnosed with cancer," expected outcomes might include the following:

- Patient will be able to continue parental responsibilities in care of toddler.
- Patient will express hopefulness that cancer treatment will control symptoms.
- Patient will engage in playing chess with friends on a weekly basis.

Setting Priorities. When a patient has multiple nursing diagnoses, the problems cannot be addressed simultaneously. At any given time, two or three issues dominate the nurse's attention. Figure 26.5 is a concept map developed for a patient with a medical diagnosis of depression after the death of his wife 6 months previously. As a result of the patient's medical condition, associated health problems include the nursing diagnoses *dysfunctional grieving, disturbed sleep pattern,* and *imbalanced nutrition: less than body requirements.* The nurse must determine which of the three diagnoses necessitates greater attention. The prolonged grief experienced by the patient might be the focus. Until the patient is able to accept his loss and begin moving forward through his grief, he may be unable to attend to interventions that will improve his nutritional intake and sleep status.

Patients' conditions always change. In the ongoing assessment of a patient's condition, nurses can quickly discover a new problem. The nurse must always consider which of the patient's most urgent physical or psychological needs require immediate intervention.

BOX 26.6 NURSING CARE PLAN

Ineffective Coping

ASSESSMENT

Jan Runyon is the nurse who admits Mr. Miller, a 48-year-old man, from the emergency department to the Critical Care Unit (CCU) after traumatic brain injury incurred in a motor vehicle accident. Mr. Miller is a successful business executive who has a wife and two sons. The intensivist has explained to the family that Mr. Miller's prognosis is poor. Tests are underway to determine the extent of brain injury. Mrs. Miller and the children are in the CCU waiting area, waiting on word about Mr. Miller.

Assessment Activities

Jan asks Mrs. Miller, "Tell me how you are feeling about your discussion with the intensivist."
Jan observes Mrs. Miller's interaction with her children.

Jan overhears Mrs. Miller on the phone in the waiting area.

Jan accompanies the transplant coordinator, who asks Mrs. Miller if the family has ever discussed organ donation.

Findings and Defining Characteristics

"I know they are doing everything they can. He is going to be okay, I just know he is. He has never been sick a day in his life."
Mrs. Miller has difficulty problem solving. The family has posed several questions to her as to what she plans to say to Mr. Miller's employees. Mrs. Miller is unable to decide what to say at this time.
Mrs. Miller states over the phone, "Don't worry, he's having some tests right now. I know Bill; he'll be back in the office before you know it. Tell the staff everything will be okay."
Mrs. Miller responds, "Bill will be fine. That's not important right now!"

Continued

◎ BOX 26.6   NURSING CARE PLAN

Ineffective Coping—cont'd

NURSING DIAGNOSIS: Ineffective coping related to husband's traumatic brain injury and poor prognosis

PLANNING

Goal (Nursing Outcomes Classification)*

Grief Resolution

Wife will accept the fact that the patient will probably die within 48 hours.

Wife will demonstrate effective expression of grief within the next 48 hours.

Expected Outcomes

Wife will verbalize to caregiver within the next 6 hours that her husband's death is actually imminent.

Wife will inform children within 24 hours of their father's likely death.

Wife will make a decision about organ donation within the next 12 hours.

Wife will discuss immediate lifestyle changes that will occur as a result of her husband's death over the next 48 hours.

Wife will discuss with her children their concerns about what they need to do as a family to prepare for their father's impending death within the next 48 hours.

Wife will discuss effects that loss has on her personally with caregiver within the next 48 hours.

*Outcomes classification label from Moorhead, S., Swanson, E., Johnson, M., et al. (2018). *Nursing outcomes classification (NOC)* (6th ed.). Elsevier Health Sciences.

INTERVENTIONS

Interventions (Nursing Interventions Classification)†

Presence

Display interest in wife's situation and accept her behaviours of denial.

Establish trust and a positive regard by creating an atmosphere of sharing. Offer privacy and security.

Grief Work Facilitation

Offer wife encouragement to explore and verbalize feelings of grief.

Identify personal coping strategies used in the past; assess their effectiveness and promote them when appropriate.

Determine wife's acceptance of available community resources and initiate as appropriate: significant other (business partner), children, clergy, or other health care providers.

Rationale

Recognizing denial (based on Kübler-Ross's [1969] theory) gives the staff direction for planning unique interventions (Iglewicz et al., 2020).

Privacy offers a place of security to exhibit personal needs and to work through feelings—a safe place to share thoughts and not feel judged (Iglewicz et al., 2020).

Grief work may be effective, particularly for those with complicated grief disorders. A variety of online and in-person approaches are available (Iglewicz et al., 2020).

Normalizes feelings, thoughts; gives hope the person isn't alone (Iglewicz et al., 2020).

Previously successful coping strategies are the first to be used when a person is under stress (Chapter 30).

Assesses effectiveness of the available support network (Iglewicz et al., 2020).

†Intervention classification labels from Butcher, H. K., Bulechek, G. M., McCloskey Dochterman, J. M., et al. (2018). *Nursing interventions classification (NIC)* (7th ed.). Elsevier Health Sciences.

EVALUATION

Nursing Actions	Patient Response and Finding	Achievement of Outcome
Say to patient's wife, "This has been a difficult time. Your husband's injury has been so sudden." Ask, "Tell me how you are feeling now."	Wife responds, "I still cannot believe it. The doctors do not believe he will live through the night." Wife explains, "I am worried about my kids. Both boys are close to their dad. I feel this unbelievable sadness."	Wife begins to acknowledge patient's impending death. Wife is able to express normal grieving feelings, thoughts, and behaviours.
Observe wife's behaviour when with children. Wife discusses decisions that must be made.	Wife discusses decisions that must be made because of impending death of her husband. She allows the children to express their sadness.	Wife is able to express grief with family; maintains role as supportive mother.

The patient's expectations and preferences also need to be taken into account when determining the priorities of care. If a terminally ill patient's priorities include controlling pain and maintaining self-esteem, pain control is the priority when analgesics become ineffective and the patient experiences acute distress. If the patient is progressing as desired, the nurse may refocus priorities to address unmet needs. For example, the patient suffering prolonged grief after his wife's death also has problems of imbalanced nutrition and disturbed sleep pattern. If the patient reports improved appetite and has shown weight stabilization since the last clinic visit, the nurse can focus more attention on the sleep pattern disturbance. If a terminally ill patient places more emphasis on spiritual support than on other priorities, such as learning about planned treatments, the nurse must attend to the patient's priorities. Meeting patient priorities may allow the nurse to then address other needs more effectively with less effort.

> concept map

Dysfunctional grieving
- Sadness
- Crying
- Avoidance of social contacts
- Unable to express feelings about loss
- Altered sleep pattern

Disturbed sleep pattern
- Reports unable to fall asleep easily at night
- Awakens frequently during night, thinks about wife
- Reports feeling very tired

Patient's chief medical diagnosis: Depression
Priority assessments: Behaviour, activities of daily living, patient's self-perceptions

Imbalanced nutrition
- Consumes less than body requirements
- Has reduced appetite
- Stops eating shortly after starting a meal, "feels full"
- Lost 1 kg during last 2 weeks

—— Link between medical diagnosis and nursing diagnosis

----- Link between nursing diagnoses

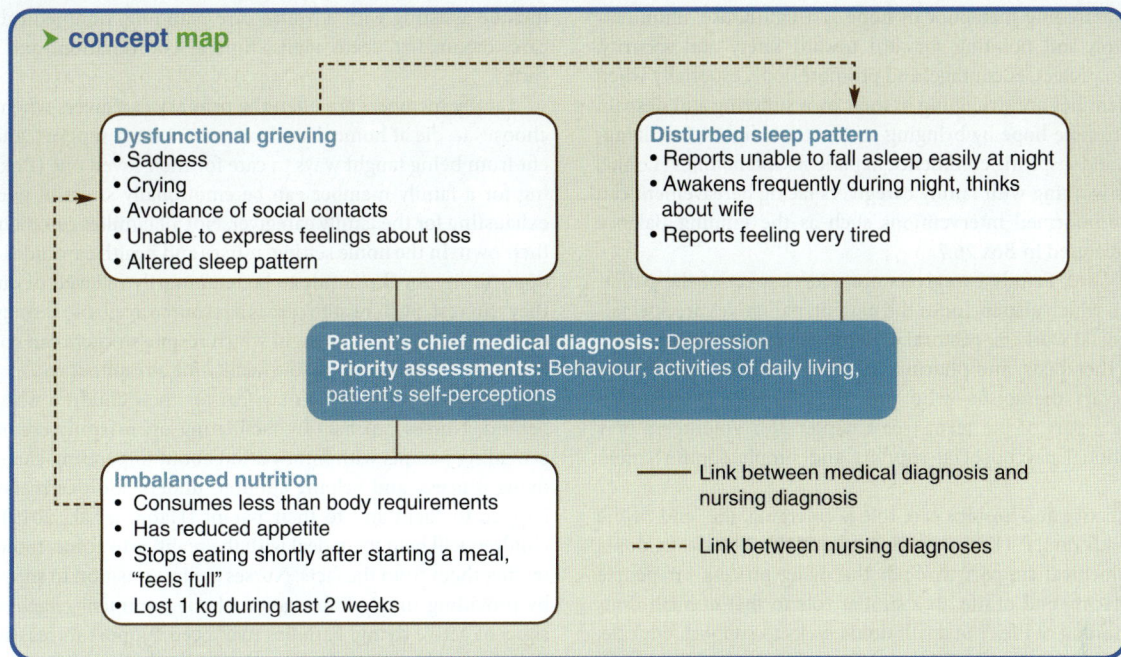

FIGURE 26.5 Concept map for a patient with prolonged grief after the death of his wife.

Continuity of Care. Interprofessional teams work to help identify and meet the needs of people who experience losses. Dietitians, clergy, social workers, physiotherapists, psychologists, chaplains, and other specialty health care providers can assist a patient and family in their grief. A coordinated team approach to managing a patient's needs results in a well-managed care plan. When a patient of yours dies, the loss that you and your colleagues experience can be shared within the interprofessional group. Support is needed to promote healing for all who worked with the dying patient and the family. Conflicts and differences can be discussed openly and solutions found in a healthy manner with the patient and family as the primary focus. For example, ethical conflicts may have arisen related to proposed or performed medical treatments or interventions. Through working together, the sharing of feelings, alternatives, and solutions becomes the basis for learning from challenging experiences.

Many terminally ill patients return home and require continued intensive nursing care. Community nurses collaborate closely with family members to meet the patient's ongoing needs. Important interventions to include in planning a return home are arranging for main-floor access, arranging appropriate medical equipment, and providing sufficient family respite. For example, judicious application of orthotic devices, along with physiotherapy and occupational therapy, can often bolster a patient's functional capacity and maintain safety for both the patient and the caregivers. Essential elements for a successful palliative home care program involve an integrated team approach, careful and holistic symptom management, and preparing the patient and family for what lies ahead in the end-of-life trajectory (Seow & Bainbridge, 2018).

◆ **Implementation**
Health Promotion. Although a return to full function is not an expected outcome for a terminally ill patient or even for a patient who has significant disability, optimal physical and emotional functioning is a realistic goal. The goal of nursing care is to help patients and families cope with the stressors in their lives and to achieve healthy grief outcomes. Nurses help patients and families in dealing with loss, making decisions about the patient's health care, and adjusting to any disappointment, frustration, and anxiety created by their loss.

Therapeutic Communication. Nursing care of the grieving patient and family begins with establishing a caring presence and determining the significance of their loss. This is difficult if the patient is unwilling or unable to express feelings or if the family is experiencing numbing or denial. Therapeutic communication strategies can be used that enable patients and families to discuss their loss and find ways to work through it. A nurse's presence, attentive listening, and use of open-ended questions enable open communication of thoughts, emotions, and concerns. The nurse will gain their trust by showing a desire to enter into a caring, therapeutic relationship.

Some patients will not discuss feelings about their loss, or sometimes a patient does not want to discuss loss, symptoms, or impending death. In this case, as their nurse you must observe for expressions of anger, denial, depression, or guilt. You must also know your own feelings before encouraging patients to express their anger. Individuals may express anger toward family or health care providers. Patients can also become demanding and accusing. Nurses must remain supportive by letting patients and family members know that feelings such as anger are normal. For example, you might say, "You are obviously upset. I just want you to know I am here to talk with you if you want." You must avoid barriers to communication such as denying the patient's grief, providing false reassurance, or avoiding discussion of sensitive issues (see Chapter 18).

Promoting Hope. When faced with loss, grief, and uncertainty, hope is a source of courage and inner strength (Lohne, 2022). Lohne compared the types of hope found in different clinical contexts and described the following dimensions and metaphors of hope:
- In acute and critical care, hope meant change and transformation, a creative, flexible process that was indispensable and continually in mind. Hope meant possibilities.
- In long-term care and rehabilitation, hope was represented as an inner flame, increasing the capacity to endure. Hope was related to faith, daily struggling, and never giving up.
- In the context of health promotion, expanding hope pushed the limit toward becoming a better person. Hope was for safety and meant vitality and freedom.

Lohne's overarching metaphor of hope is a lighthouse, illuminating the horizon and pointing forward toward safety and security. Nurses need to protect, encourage, and promote hope, especially when patients and families are struggling in their own suffering and despair. Nurses can promote hope by bringing comfort and light in challenging situations and inspiring confidence in patients and families (Lohne, 2022). Nurses working with family caregivers facing bereavement can offer evidence-informed interventions such as the Finding Balance Intervention featured in Box 26.7.

Palliative Care. Family caregivers are a key aspect of the palliative care team, which also includes the patient, palliative care specialists, nurses, social workers, pastoral care providers, physiotherapists, occupational therapists, and pharmacists. Massage therapists, music therapists, or art therapists—who provide alternative therapies—might also be a part of the team (see Chapter 36). Volunteers may provide additional psychosocial support and simple comfort measures.

A new palliative and hospice care role is emerging: the "end-of-life doula" or "death doula" (Krawczyk & Rush, 2020). The death doula provides nonmedical support through the dying process for people and families facing end of life, in a similar role to that of birth doulas at the beginning of life. The death doula seeks to support, educate, and empower individuals, families, and the public by building death literacy and contributing to societal change that would involve returning death care to the family and community. Roles for a death doula

include assisting with advance care planning, nonmedical supportive care, organizing death vigils, funeral coordination, and after-death care.

Family members are often the primary caregivers when the patient chooses to die at home. Family members need support, and they benefit from being taught ways to care for their loved one (Box 26.8). Caring for a family member can be emotionally stressful and physically exhausting for the family caregiver. Not all families can manage care on their own. In the home setting, nurses and health care aides provide the opportunity for the family to be temporarily relieved of duties so that they can rest. Such respite care is a resource available through palliative care and hospice programs, in which respite workers can come into the home, or a patient can go to a facility for a respite stay.

Parents who are dying may fear for their children who will be left behind. Nurses can help by facilitating open family communication, providing parents with information about impending changes and the dying process, and helping children understand death and what may happen to them and to their parent (Hanna et al., 2019). Preparing children will help them deal with the realities to come, rather than protecting them from the facts. Nurses are in a position to support families by providing timely information about imminent changes, including signs of active dying. Families may need support to reassure children that they will be cared for after the death of a parent.

Family caregivers may enter bereavement with many painful emotions such as sadness, emptiness, guilt, and regret, and even anger and

---

BOX 26.7 RESEARCH HIGHLIGHT

A Finding Balance Intervention for Bereaved Caregivers

Research Focus

Holtslander and colleagues (2016) conducted a multimethod pilot study employing a randomized trial design to test the feasibility, acceptability, and potential of a self-administered writing intervention for older persons who were bereaved after caregiving, to increase hope, coping, and oscillation balance.

Research Abstract

Family caregivers provide an immense amount of care and support to patients at the end of life yet receive very little attention or support during bereavement. A theory-based writing intervention, called the Finding Balance Intervention, was developed on the basis of the dual process model (Stroebe & Schut, 1999). It was tested using both qualitative and quantitative approaches with two groups of older persons to evaluate the effectiveness of this intervention.

Methods

Nineteen older persons were randomized into either the intervention group or the control group. The intervention group received the Finding Balance Intervention and a follow-up visit from an RN research assistant. The control group received the intervention at a second visit. Data were collected at baseline and at a follow-up visit for each group, including measures of hope (using the Herth Hope Index), grief (using the Hogan Grief Reaction Checklist), and the oscillation balance of restoration- and loss-oriented approaches to coping (using the Inventory of Daily Widowed Life). Quantitative data were analyzed with a paired samples t-test and qualitative data were analyzed with content analysis.

Following are the components of the Finding Balance Intervention:

- *Deep grieving:* Write down a list of your emotions while also identifying ways to take a "time out" from these difficult emotions, such as calling a friend or going for a walk.

- *Walking a fine line:* Write out a list of activities that take you back to grieving and also involve moving forward, such as creating a memory book, planting a tree, or planning a memorial or family event.

- *Moving forward:* Write down your thoughts as you reflect on your caregiving story. Think about what you have learned while caregiving and how these lessons might be of help to others. Write out a plan for the day and ways to reach out to others in need.

Results

The participants found the Finding Balance Intervention to be very positive, acceptable, and easy to use. There was a statistically significant increase in restoration-oriented coping and oscillation balance for the intervention group, indicating that the intervention group was spending more time thinking about, and giving more attention to, their grief journey. According to the dual-process model of grief (Stroebe & Schut, 1999), oscillating between activities focused on loss and activities focused on restoration after loss improved grief outcomes by enabling individuals to find unique ways to move forward in grief.

Implications for Practice

Writing itself has been shown to have a therapeutic benefit in grief (Holtslander, 2019). This writing tool could be given to family caregivers in palliative and hospice care and could also be used in grief support groups so that individuals could share their writing if they wished. Nurses can provide much-needed support through offering information, tools, and resources while monitoring for signs of complicated or prolonged grief and providing appropriate referrals.

References: Holtslander, L., Duggleby, W., Teucher, U., et al. (2016). Developing and pilot-testing a Finding Balance Intervention for older adult bereaved family caregivers: A randomized feasibility trial. *European Journal of Oncology Nursing, 21,* 66–74. https://doi.org/10.1016/j.ejon.2016.01.003; Holtslander, L. (2019). Finding balance through a writing intervention. In L. Holtslander, S. Peacock, & J. Bally (Eds.), *Hospice palliative home care and bereavement support* (pp. 137–142). Springer. https://doi.org/10.1007/978-3-030-19535-9_5

BOX 26.8   PATIENT TEACHING

Preparing the Dying Patient's Family

Objectives
- Improve the family's ability to provide appropriate physical care for the dying patient.
- Improve the family's ability to provide appropriate psychological support to the dying patient.

Teaching Strategies
- Describe and demonstrate feeding techniques and selection of foods to facilitate the patient's ease of chewing and swallowing.
- Demonstrate bathing, mouth care, and other hygiene measures, and allow the family to perform return demonstration.
- Show the family a video on simple transfer techniques to prevent injury to themselves and the patient; help the family practice these techniques.
- Instruct the family on the need to take rest periods.
- Teach the family to recognize signs and symptoms to expect as the patient's condition worsens and provide information on whom to call in an emergency.
- Discuss ways to support the dying patient and listen to needs and fears.
- Solicit questions from the family and provide information as needed.

Evaluation
- Ask the family members to demonstrate physical care techniques (e.g., turning, feeding, mouth care).
- Ask the family members to describe how they vary approaches to care when the patient has symptoms such as pain or fatigue.
- Ask the family to discuss how they feel about their ability to support the patient.

---

resentment (Holtslander et al., 2017), while some will experience relief and a feeling of accomplishment. The latter is more likely when a caregiver has strong support networks and positive coping strategies. Caregivers have also described the support they have received as lacking or unhelpful. Sometimes caregivers experience pressure to "move on" and feel alienated from family, friends, and formal supports. Research shows that family caregivers who had a positive experience of the death, with an opportunity to say goodbye, were left with positive memories that supported the grief process. Key messages from a metasummary of research on bereaved caregivers were as follows: a) the caregiver's experiences while caregiving will affect them in bereavement; b) each caregiver's situation is unique; and c) many kinds of support are required during grief and bereavement, depending on the situation and the needs of each person and family (Holtslander et al., 2017).

Families also need to be informed of palliative and hospice care options, including care in the community, so they can choose among the resources available. There are many online resources to help families meet the needs of terminally ill patients, including the Canadian Virtual Hospice (see Recommended Websites listed at the end of the chapter). Each province and health region has varying support programs and resources; therefore, nurses are required to know what is available to them in the individual family's jurisdiction. In some cases, families may need assistance and support in making the decision about placement in a health care facility.

Nurses must keep the family informed so that they can anticipate the type of symptoms the patient will probably experience and the implications for care. Family members should be encouraged to express their grief openly with the patient and to give the patient the opportunity to discuss any remaining concerns or requests. The family also needs personal time to share their concerns with nursing staff and

to ask questions about treatment options, the course of the patient's disease, and the meaning of the patient's behaviours. It is wise for nurses to communicate news of the patient's impending death when the family is together, if possible, as family members can provide support for one another. The nurse should convey the news in a private area and be willing to remain with the family as needed. In some situations, in which families are large or cannot all be together, it may be beneficial to have a designated family spokesperson or representative through whom information can be relayed.

It is also important to educate the family regarding the signs of impending death. Tissue perfusion becomes impaired, which results in cool and clammy skin. Alterations in heart rate or rhythms, hypotension, and pooling of blood in dependent areas may occur. The extremities often have a mottled appearance. Breathing patterns may be impaired. Patients may exhibit shortness of breath or increased secretions. Later signs include increasingly longer and more frequent periods of apnea, alternating with hyperpnea; this pattern is known as *Cheyne-Stokes respirations*. Patients may exhibit alterations in level of consciousness and changes in behaviour; for example, disorientation and restlessness may occur. Urine output decreases, and incontinence may occur. In addition, periods of sleep increase, and eventually some patients may become unconscious as death nears.

In the hospital setting, nurses assist in planning a visitation schedule for family members to keep the patient and family from excessive fatigue. Young children should visit dying parents. During the final moments of a patient's life, the nurse can help the family to stay in communication with the patient through their frequent visits, caring silence, attentive listening, touch, and telling the patient of their love. After the patient's death, the family should be encouraged to remain with the deceased for as long as they feel they need to. Nurses are required to provide support and assist the family with decision making, such as notification of the death, contacting the funeral home, transportation of additional family members, and collection of the patient's belongings.

Hospice Care. In Canada, the terms *palliative* and *hospice* care are used interchangeably, although the term *hospice care* may be used to describe care in the community rather than in a hospital. Hospice services may be available in the home, stand-alone facilities, and long-term care settings. Availability and accessibility vary across Canada. Hospice programs include the following components:
Patient and family as the unit of care
Coordinated community care with access to beds in available inpatient and long-term care facilities
Control of symptoms (physical, sociological, psychological, and spiritual)
An interprofessional team to provide specialist palliative care, which is defined as experts in palliative care who support a patient's primary care team to meet complex patient care needs during serious illness
Availability of medical and nursing services at all times
Bereavement follow-up after a patient's death
Use of trained volunteers for frequent visitation and respite support

Canada's first hospice was established in Toronto in 1979. Casey House in Toronto and the John Gordon home in London, Ontario, provide hospice care for people dying from HIV/AIDS. Canuck Place, in Vancouver, was the first freestanding children's hospice in North America and provides a continuum of care that comprises three components: respite, palliative, and bereavement.

Nurses need to support a patient's choice in maintaining comfort and dignity. Whether the patient ultimately dies at home or in a facility, the patient's wishes are followed as much as possible. One or more bereavement visits are often made by the staff of the hospice team to the family after the death of the patient, to support the family through the grieving process.

It is important to know the patient's preference regarding where their death should take place. Many patients prefer to die at home in a familiar setting, whereas others, who require support and symptom management, choose to die in a hospice, hospital, or long-term care facility. Some families are ill-prepared or unable to care for a patient at home, and some patients suffer distressing physical ailments that prevent them from being cared for at home.

A patient receiving palliative care may be hospitalized because of a change in condition or exacerbation of symptoms, and the health care team coordinates care between the home and inpatient setting. An effort is always made to keep patients at home for as long as possible (or as long as they desire). The family provides basic supportive care. However, if the family cannot meet all of the patient's needs, a nurse is available to coordinate and administer symptom management therapies. The goal of the interprofessional team is 24-hour accessibility as needed. As a patient's death becomes imminent, members of the team are available to give support to the patient and family.

Care After Death. When a patient dies in a home, facility, or hospital setting, nurses provide **postmortem care**. Nurses are responsible for coordination of all aspects of care surrounding a patient's death. Box 26.9 summarizes the nurse's responsibilities for care of the body after death. Nurses need to be familiar with policies and procedures that are established for postmortem care. Many of these practices also depend on the individual and family's unique experiences, culture, religion, and personal preferences. In all cases, it is most important to care for the patient's body with dignity and sensitivity and in a manner consistent with the patient's religious or cultural beliefs.

Patients' and families' cultural beliefs are very important in postmortem care. Maintaining the integrity of rituals and mourning practices helps families acknowledge the patient's death and achieve inner peace. The ethical decisions that surround a patient's death are based on the values of a culture. Health care providers must determine the makeup of a family network and which members should be involved in decisions such as organ and tissue donation and end-of-life care.

Hospitals are required to formulate policies and procedures that are based on current provincial and territorial laws to validate death, identify potential organ or tissue donors, and provide postmortem care. For transplantation of organs, the patient must be maintained in a CCU on ventilatory and circulatory support until vital organs are harvested. The family must clearly understand that the patient is neurologically dead or "brain dead" and that the equipment (i.e., ventilator and vasopressor medications) is not keeping the patient alive but keeping the physical body in a state so that the organs will not be damaged before being harvested.

Support of the family is crucial at the time of the patient's death. If family members are not present at that time, the assigned nurse (or another staff member who knows the family) makes contact with the family. If you are the assigned nurse, you inform the family of the death and respond to any immediate questions from the family. It is important that you find out from the family whether they will come to the facility to view the deceased and to collect any personal belongings. Make a note of which family members will come and when. In some situations, family members may be too distraught to safely drive themselves and need to be encouraged to have someone else drive or to take alternative transportation. After a death, it is acceptable to lower the head of the bead, to straighten the body, and attempt to gently close the eyes and mouth. Once the family has arrived to view the deceased, it is beneficial, before they view the body, for the nurse to explain to the family what they may expect to see. Typically, a deceased person has a peaceful expression (as facial muscles have relaxed); however, the body

---

BOX 26.9   PROCEDURAL GUIDELINE   ◖

Care of the Body After Death

Delegation Considerations

Care of the body after death can be delegated to unregulated care providers except in cases of organ or tissue donation. Check employer policy for which staff member is authorized to remove any invasive tubes or catheters.

Equipment

Bath towels, washcloths, wash basin, scissors, shroud kit with name tags, bed linen, documentation forms

Procedure

1. Legislated health care providers must complete the medical certificate of death: cause of death, time when death was pronounced, therapy used, and actions taken. In some provinces, such as Saskatchewan and British Columbia, nurses may pronounce the death if it was from natural causes. (This may not be the policy in all agencies. Follow your employer's policy.)

2. An autopsy may be requested, especially for deaths that have occurred under unusual circumstances.

3. Trained staff members offer survivors the option of donating the organs or tissue of the deceased; personal, religious, and cultural needs should be included during this process.

4. Nurses work with sensitivity to preserve the patient's and family's dignity.
   a. Check orders for any specimens or special orders.
   b. Ask if the family wish to be involved in after-death care, such as washing the body.
   c. Remove all equipment, tubes, supplies, and dirty linens according to employer protocol. Exceptions to this process include organ donation (leave support systems in place) and sudden or unexpected deaths that necessitate coroner involvement or investigation (leave tubing and lines in situ but cut them near the body and clamp them).
   d. Cleanse the body.
   e. Brush and comb the patient's hair.
   f. Position according to protocol: The eyes should be closed by gently holding the patient's eyelids closed for a few minutes; dentures should be in the patient's mouth to maintain facial alignment.
   g. Cover the body with a clean sheet up to the chin with arms outside covers if possible.
   h. Encourage the family to say goodbye through both touch and talk. Do not rush the goodbye process; this is an important time for coming to terms with the loss.
   i. Clarify which personal belongings should stay with the body and who will take personal items; documentation requires both a descriptor of the objects (i.e., rings, jewellery, electronics) and the name of each person who received them, with the time and date.
   j. Do not discard items found after the family is gone; call the family and tell them what was found and ask who might pick it up. Descriptions of the articles help the patient's family make decisions accordingly.
   k. Apply name tags according to protocol, such as on the wrist, on the right big toe, or outside a shroud.
   l. Complete documentation in the nursing notes. Documents vary, depending on the employer (see Box 26.10).
   m. In most cases, the funeral home/transfer company will arrive to pick up the body. Remain sensitive to other hospitalized patients or visitors when transporting the body, such as covering the body with a clean sheet, temporarily and gently closing doors to patients' rooms, and watching to avoid visitors when moving the body to another part of the hospital or to the exit for the funeral home.
   n. Follow all protocol and policies to meet all legal requirements in caring for the body.

BOX 26.10	Documentation of End-of-Life Care

The following items must be documented at the end of a patient's life:

- Time of death and actions taken to prevent death, or cardiac arrest record, if applicable
- The name of the person who pronounced the patient's death
- Any special preparation and type of donation, including time, staff, and company
- The name of the family member or friend who was called and who came to the hospital: donor organization, morgue, funeral home, chaplain, and individual family members making any decisions
- Personal articles left on the body and taped to skin, or tubes left in
- Personal items given to the family: specific names and descriptors of items
- Time of discharge and destination of the body
- Location of name tags on the body
- Special requests made by the family
- Any other statements that might be needed to clarify the situation

feels cool to touch and appears greyish-white. Within several hours, the body begins to stiffen as rigor mortis sets in. The body may have areas of pooled blood that appear bruised. The eyes and mouth may be partially open, but mucous membranes will appear dry. This appearance may be difficult for some family members to observe.

Nurses can be very helpful in supporting families through the organ and tissue request process. It is important to provide a private area in which to discuss all issues with the family. The staff member designated to make a request, such as a formal transplant coordinator, a social worker, chaplain, or nurse, must offer the family clarification of what defines brain death because support systems must remain in place even after the patient is pronounced "dead" (see Table 26.3) for vital organ retrieval (i.e., heart, lungs, kidneys, and liver). Nurses reinforce explanations throughout the organ retrieval process. The family must know who legally can give final consent, the options for organ or tissue donation, any associated costs, and how donation will affect burial or cremation. Nonvital tissues such as corneas, skin, long bones, and middle ear bones can be harvested when the patient is proclaimed dead, without artificially maintaining vital functions. If the patient did not make specific documented requests before death, the family must agree on organ and tissue donation. Nurses should review the organ retrieval laws in the family's province or territory, as well as the institution's policy and procedure regarding the formal consent process.

Another topic that can create tension or anxiety is autopsy. It is very difficult to approach a grieving family with such a request; ideally, the topics of autopsy and donation are discussed before the patient's death. The value of an autopsy is that it may improve knowledge in the field of medicine or bring answers or clarification for the family. To help the living, the autopsy can lead to new therapies or new understanding of diseases. The more reasons nurses can think of to support organ donation, tissue donation, or autopsy, the more the family will be helped to realize the good that can be accomplished by either donation or research autopsy.

The family becomes the primary patient when the actual death has occurred, and the shift of concern moves from the deceased patient to the living family. At this time, it is important to appropriately use the resources that are available. For example, pastoral care staff can be a helpful resource to assist the family even before the actual death, if no bereavement team is available. However, it is important to know whether the family chooses to have spiritual counsellors present. Some families prefer to grieve alone, whereas others may desire the support of other people. Social workers and counsellors can also offer assistance.

Documentation of all the events surrounding a patient's death is important for avoiding misunderstandings and clarifying final events in a patient's life. Each facility's policies and procedures support legal guidelines that must be followed and accurately documented. Box 26.10 lists the content to be documented about end-of-life care. Documentation validates the success of meeting goals identified for the patient or provides a justification for failure to meet any goals. Complete and accurate documentation offers a summary of activities that can become the focus for risk management or legal investigations.

In cases of legal matters, the family expects a clear, concise description of what occurred in the care of the patient at the time of death. Opinions must be avoided, and facts are stated in a nonjudgemental, objective manner. Provincial and territorial guidelines direct the type of information that is to be charted and when it is to be charted. Patients have the right to access their health records. Copies of parts of the chart can be given to family members upon written request and the approval of the hospital (see your employer's guidelines). Nurses must understand and uphold the legal guidelines of documentation at all times (see Chapter 16).

The Grieving Nurse. When nurses have cared for a patient for a period of time, it is possible to have deep personal feelings of loss and sadness when the patient dies. It is common for nurses to want to hold the hand of the patient who is dying. By being present at the time of the patient's death, nurses are able to "let go." You, as a nurse, can attempt in many ways to cope with the loss of a dying patient. Attending the funeral is one way to say goodbye. Writing a letter of sympathy to the family can prove helpful. Some agencies routinely send out sympathy cards from the interprofessional team, in which you can write an individual note. It is natural for you to go through the grieving process. When you work in an area in which multiple losses occur, it is easy for bereavement overload to develop unless you have ways to process grief. You might feel frustration, anger, guilt, sadness, or anxiety. Often nurses seek out other nurses or health care providers to discuss their own grief (Figure 26.6). It is important for you to develop your own support systems that allow time away from the care setting and provide opportunities to share personal feelings. The process of debriefing with colleagues after a death allows nurses to talk about their experiences, share thoughts, information, and advice and provide emotional support to one another (Zheng et al., 2018). Debriefing, reflection, and expressing emotions are beneficial for mental health and increase knowledge and confidence when dealing with the deaths of future patients.

Stress management techniques (see Chapter 30) can help restore a nurse's energy and continued enjoyment in caring for patients. Your self-care is crucial for your survival and recovery from loss, not only for your sake but also for the sake of future patients. Interprofessional team debriefings regarding complex or ethical issues are valuable in helping nurses cope with loss. Nurse managers and administrators have a responsibility to ensure nurses have opportunities to obtain support from a team within the work environment (Parola et al., 2018).

◆ Evaluation

Patient Care. Nurses care for patients and families at every phase of the grief process. This requires nurses to remain aware of signs and symptoms of grief, even when patients are not specifically seeking care directly related to a loss. These signs and symptoms help in evaluation of whether a patient is able to deal with a loss and move forward in the grief process. Critical thinking ensures that the evaluation process is thorough and relevant to the patient's situation (Figure 26.7).

In order for nurses to determine the effectiveness of nursing interventions, they must refer to the goals and expected outcomes established in the plan of care. By comparing actual patient behaviours with expected outcomes, nurses evaluate the patient's health status and

FIGURE 26.6 Nurses need support within the team for their own grief. (© istockphoto/Juanmonino)

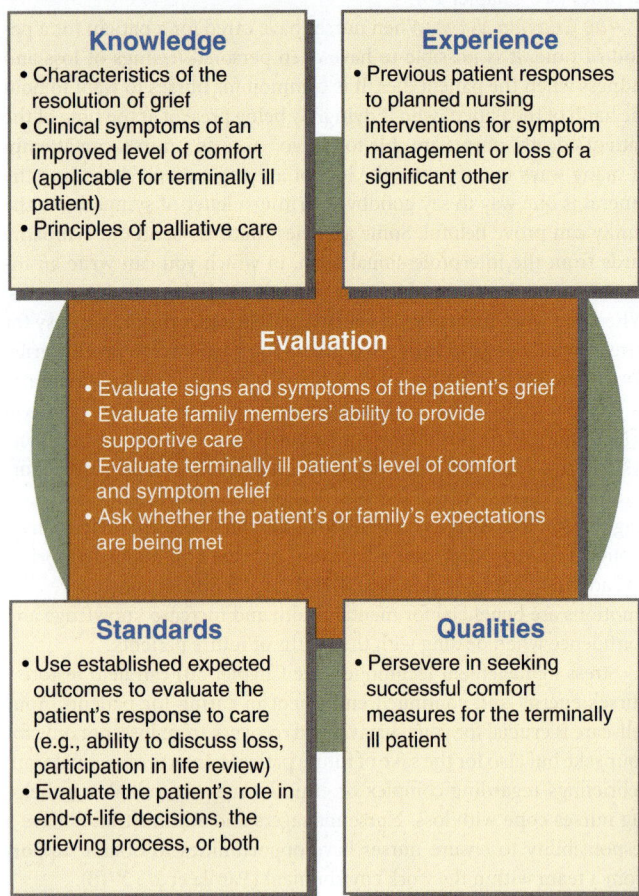

Knowledge
- Characteristics of the resolution of grief
- Clinical symptoms of an improved level of comfort (applicable for terminally ill patient)
- Principles of palliative care

Experience
- Previous patient responses to planned nursing interventions for symptom management or loss of a significant other

Evaluation
- Evaluate signs and symptoms of the patient's grief
- Evaluate family members' ability to provide supportive care
- Evaluate terminally ill patient's level of comfort and symptom relief
- Ask whether the patient's or family's expectations are being met

Standards
- Use established expected outcomes to evaluate the patient's response to care (e.g., ability to discuss loss, participation in life review)
- Evaluate the patient's role in end-of-life decisions, the grieving process, or both

Qualities
- Persevere in seeking successful comfort measures for the terminally ill patient

FIGURE 26.7 Critical thinking model for loss, death, and grieving evaluation.

whether the plan needs to be revised. For example, if the goal is to have the patient communicate a sense of hope with family members, the nurse evaluates the verbal and nonverbal communication process for cues related to hope. The patient's responses indicate whether new therapies are needed or whether existing therapies should be revised. The nurse would continue to evaluate the progress of the patient, the effectiveness of interventions, and the interactions between the family and patient. It is important for the patient and family to share experiences and be active participants in the evaluation process.

Patient Expectations. Patients expect individualized care, including relief of symptoms, preservation of dignity, and support of the family to maximize quality of life. The success of the evaluation depends partially on the bond that the nurse forms with the patient. If the patient does not trust you as the nurse, they are not likely to share personal expectations or desires with you. It thus becomes important for you to take the time to talk with the patient and learn whether expectations are being met. The following are examples of questions that will validate whether patient expectations have been achieved:

- "Am I helping you in the way you have hoped?"
- "Would you like me to assist you in a different way?"
- "Do you have a specific request that I have not yet met?"
- "What is most important for us to do for you at this time?"
- "Are we dealing with your problems in a timely manner?"

Through communication and evaluation, you can continue to determine whether outcome criteria were met to support the goals of patient and family-centred care.

KEY CONCEPTS

- When caring for patients who have experienced a loss, nurses facilitate the grieving process by recognizing the loss and listening with compassion to their experiences and stories.
- Loss comes in many forms and is to be expected throughout life, depending on the values and priorities learned from family, friends, society, and culture.
- The type of loss and the meaning and perception of the loss influence the grief that a person experiences.
- Death is a challenging—yet meaningful—journey for the dying person, as well as for the person's family, friends, and caregivers.
- Survivors move through a time of bereavement that is not linear; rather, a grieving individual will move back and forth through various processes, stages, or phases lasting an unknown length of time.
- Several theorists have attempted to describe stages of the grieving process and how a person begins to adapt to life with a loss.
- Nurses' knowledge of the types of grief enables them to offer appropriate bereavement supports and interventions.
- The way an individual perceives and responds to a loss is influenced by development, psychosocial perspectives, socioeconomic status, personal relationships, the nature and meaning of the loss, culture, spiritual beliefs, and the type and degree of attachment.
- Nursing interventions involve reinforcing patients' successful coping mechanisms and introducing new coping approaches, such as the promotion of hope.
- When assessing patients in grief, nurses must not assume how or whether patients experience grief or whether a particular behaviour indicates grief; rather, they allow patients to share in their own way what is happening.
- Nurses must assess the terminally ill patient and family's wishes for end-of-life care, including the preferred place for death, the type and level of life-sustaining measures to use, and expectations regarding pain and symptom management.
- A plan of care is developed by integrating patients' resources such as physical energy and activity tolerance, supportive family members, spiritual faith, and methods for coping.
- Nurses need to establish a caring presence and use therapeutic communication strategies that enable patients to discuss their loss as they find ways to manage it.
- A palliative approach to care enables patients and families to make more informed choices, better alleviate symptoms, and have more opportunity to manage unfinished business.

- Nurses can promote a patient's self-esteem and dignity by conveying respect for the patient as a whole person.
- Hospice palliative care is a specialized approach for patient- and family-centred care designed for providing comfort, dignity, and quality of life for the patient and family facing the challenges of advanced illness and end of life.

CRITICAL THINKING EXERCISES

Critical Thinking Exercises 1 and 2 refer to the case study at the beginning of the chapter.

1. Mrs. Long says, "I don't know what's wrong with me. I lost my husband more than a year ago and I still miss him and really wish I could bring him back from the funeral home to sit in his old chair so I could talk to him. I am quite angry that he left me this way." How could you respond to Mrs. Long? What might be your next steps in addressing her concerns related to her grief journey?

2. Mrs. Long is admitted to hospital with shortness of breath and pain in her chest due to her stage IV lung cancer. What are some questions you could ask together with her family, once she is comfortable? Is she a candidate for palliative care? How is palliative care different from a palliative approach?

3. A nursing colleague is discussing her patient with you. She says, "My patient is a 48-year-old man with a degenerative neurological disease. The disease is progressive. He is having trouble walking and taking care of his daily needs. The only thing I can do is assist him with bathing, feeding, and walking. He is requesting information about MAiD; but I'm not sure how I feel about that." How might you respond to your colleague?

🌐 *Answers to Critical Thinking Exercises appear on the Evolve website.*

REVIEW QUESTIONS

Review Questions 1 to 3 relate to the case study at the beginning of the chapter.

1. Mrs. Long is reporting chest pain and shortness of breath and is asking to see her husband, who died more than a year ago. What is your priority response in this situation?
   a. Reorient Mrs. Long to time, place, and person.
   b. Give prn analgesia and reassess symptoms in 1 hour.
   c. Assess Mrs. Long for air entry, apply oxygen as ordered, and call for assistance.
   d. Reassure Mrs. Long that her husband died and cannot return.

2. A conversation with the family reveals that they are uncertain about who is the health care proxy for Mrs. Long. The nurse refers to an advance care plan that was placed on the chart in order to clarify Mrs. Long's wishes. The nurse reassures the family that: *(Select all that apply.)*
   a. The advance care plan indicates that her youngest child is her health care proxy; however, legally the oldest child would be the person the nurse would call for a decision if needed.
   b. Since Mrs. Long's named health care proxy is the youngest child, this person will be called to make health care decisions if Mrs. Long is unable to do so.
   c. The next step is to call the hospital ethicist to meet with the family.
   d. Since Mrs. Long is becoming more confused each day, the advance care plan is going to be integrated into her care as much as possible.

3. Mrs. Long returns home on the palliative care program, with the support of her children. As the community nurse, your priorities include: *(Select all that apply.)*
   a. Describing to the family not to call "911" if Mrs. Long dies expectedly from her lung cancer at home, but rather to call the palliative home care nurse who is on call.
   b. Reassuring Mrs. Long and her family that all her needs will be met at home.
   c. Drawing up vials of morphine for pain and shortness of breath.
   d. Assessment of the family dynamics and assisting the family to develop a plan to arrange a schedule for caregiving.

Review Questions 4 to 5 relate to Jonathan, a patient seen in a community health clinic.

4. Jonathan's father died 6 months ago in the hospital during the COVID-19 pandemic, and he was unable to visit to say goodbye at the time because of visitor restrictions. Jonathan states, "Without being able to say goodbye, or even have a funeral, I feel as though I'm trapped in my bed every morning. I feel like I'm not allowed to be sad." What kind of grief is Jonathan experiencing?
   a. Anticipatory grief
   b. Disenfranchised grief
   c. Prolonged grief
   d. Normal grief

5. What is the best response to Jonathan's expressions of grief?
   a. "I can't imagine how difficult this must be for you. Can I get you a cup of tea?"
   b. "I think this is a conversation to best be had with your counsellor."
   c. "Let me get you some contact information for a grief counsellor."
   d. "Expressing these feelings is important. Do you have any support people in your life?"

Review Questions 6 to 8 relate to Sylvie, a patient on a medical unit.

6. Sylvie has advanced dementia and is experiencing complications related to end-of-life care. She is on the palliative care program, admitted to your medicine ward to receive "comfort measures only" (no vital signs, no formal head-to-toe assessments). Sylvie has her daughter, who is her substitute decision maker and power of attorney, at the bedside. You are assigned to be Sylvie's primary nurse for the day. Sylvie's daughter approaches the nursing station and is very upset. She yells loudly, "My mom is in pain and you guys are doing nothing for her!" What would be the most appropriate response to Sylvie's daughter?
   a. "I need to ask you to stop yelling, please; let's go talk somewhere in private."
   b. "Let me get your mother some pain medication."
   c. "If you don't stop yelling, I will call security."
   d. "Let's go see your mother together and figure out what's going on."

7. You enter the room to assess Sylvie and she is visibly in pain. You return a few minutes later with hydromorphone and midazolam to help alleviate her symptoms, but she is restless and refuses to let you administer the medications. What is your next nursing action?
   a. Administer the medication anyway because the daughter is telling you to.
   b. Offer to bring warm blankets, a face cloth, and a moist oral sponge instead.
   c. Leave the patient and come back in a while to see if she is calm enough to receive the medication.
   d. Call the charge nurse and ask for assistance in dealing with Sylvie's daughter.

8. Your patient, Sylvie, is gradually changing her breathing patterns with periods of apnea, and her extremities are cool and mottled. You speak with her daughter to explain options for the next few hours. What should you say?

    a. Ask Sylvie's daughter if she would like to step away from the unit and take a coffee break.

    b. Explain to Sylvie's daughter that her mother's death is imminent and ask if anyone else should be called at this point.

    c. Prepare to administer Sylvie's prn medication because she appears to be in distress.

    d. Sit Sylvie up in bed to assist with her breathing and apply oxygen for dyspnea.

9. A 16-year-old patient has been admitted to the Critical Care Unit after suffering a closed-head injury. The patient is soon declared brain dead. The intensivist and nurse are preparing to approach the family to consider donation of the patient's heart and lungs. When working with families in this situation, it is important to explain that:

    a. The ventilator is being used to prevent brain death.

    b. The ventilator maintains organ perfusion until time for harvesting.

    c. Tissues such as corneas can be harvested only if the patient remains ventilated.

    d. Organ donation can occur only if the patient has made a request to donate organs in the past.

10. Following the death of a child who had been a patient on the pediatric unit for many months, several nurses are planning to attend the funeral, based on permission from their manager. What should the manager realize about this situation: *(Select all that apply.)*

    a. Attending the patient's funeral may cause even more burnout among the nurses.

    b. Attending the patient's funeral expresses support for the family to help them in their own grief journey.

    c. Attending the patient's funeral provides an opportunity for the nurses to express their grief more openly.

    d. Attending the patient's funeral takes time away from other patients and is mainly a ritual that is focused on the family.

Answers: 1. c; **2.** b; **3.** a, d; **4.** b; **5.** d; **6.** a; **7.** b; **8.** b; **9.** b; **10.** b, c.

🌐 *Rationales for the Review Questions appear on the Evolve website.*

RECOMMENDED WEBSITES

Advance Care Planning in Canada: https://www.advancecareplanning.ca
This website provides resources, tools, and guides to develop your own advance care plan and campaign to raise awareness. Speak Up is spearheaded by the CHPCA.

Bridge C-14: https://www.bridgec-14.org
This organization provides compassionate support to families throughout their journey with medical assistance in dying (MAiD).

Canadian Hospice Palliative Care Association (CHPCA): https://www.chpca.ca
The Canadian Hospice Palliative Care Association is a national organization that promotes excellence in care for people approaching death. One of its goals is to advocate for improved hospice palliative care policy, resource allocation, and supports for caregivers.

Canadian Virtual Hospice: https://www.virtualhospice.ca
The Canadian Virtual Hospice is the most comprehensive online centre in the world on palliative and end-of-life care, loss, and grief. It provides information and support to people living with a life-limiting illness and to their families, health providers, educators, and researchers. Canadian Virtual Hospice operates many other excellent websites, including: LivingMyCulture.ca, LivingOutLoud.life.ca for teens and young adults

with advanced illnesses, and Methadone4Pain.ca for clinical training for analgesia in palliative care.

Dying With Dignity Canada: https://www.dyingwithdignity.ca
Dying With Dignity Canada is the national human-rights charity committed to helping Canadians avoid unwanted suffering, advocating for MAiD, and advocating for the importance of advance care planning.

End of Life Doula Association of Canada: https://endoflifedoulaassociation.org
This association provides information and support for end-of-life doulas, to help promote the provision of high-quality end-of-life care in a holistic, person-centred way.

Government of Canada, End of Life Care: https://www.hc-sc.gc.ca/hcs-sss/palliat/index-eng.php
This federal government website includes information on the involvement of the federal government in palliative care and contains links to publications, supportive programs, and other related resources.

KidsGrief.ca: https://kidsgrief.ca
Developed by the Canadian Virtual Hospice, KidsGrief.ca can help you understand how children (ages 0 to 18 years) grieve and how to support them as they face the life-limiting illness, dying, and death of someone important to them.

🌐 REFERENCES

A full reference list is available on the website for this book at http://evolve.elsevier.com/Canada/Potter/fundamentals/

27

Self-Concept

Canadian content written by Judee E. Onyskiw, RN, MN, PhD, with original chapter contributions by Victoria N. Folse, PhD, APRN, PMHCNS-BC, LCPC

OBJECTIVES

Mastery of content in this chapter will enable you to:

- Define the key terms listed.
- Describe factors that influence the following components of self-concept: identity, body image, and role performance.
- Identify stressors that affect self-concept and self-esteem.
- Describe the components of self-concept as related to psychosocial and cognitive developmental stages.

- Analyze ways in which a nurse's self-concept and nursing actions can affect a patient's self-concept and self-esteem.
- Incorporate research findings to promote evidence-informed practice for addressing identity confusion, disturbed body image, low self-esteem, and role conflict.
- Examine cultural considerations that affect self-concept.
- Apply the nursing process to promote a patient's self-concept.

KEY TERMS

Body image
Identity
Identity confusion
Role ambiguity

Role conflict
Role overload
Role performance
Role strain

Self-concept
Self-esteem
Sick role

WEBSITE

http://evolve.elsevier.co /Canada/Potter/fundamentals/

CASE STUDY

Amil (preferred pronouns: he/him) is a 48-year-old married individual and father of two teenagers who has always thought of himself as an active, healthy person—until yesterday, when at work he had a sudden, unexpected stroke. This morning, he woke up in the hospital to find that he cannot move his right hand. He is unable to get out of bed himself to use the bathroom alone or to sit in a chair. His speech is slurred and people keep asking him to repeat himself. His physician tells him that he was fortunate to get to the hospital when he did and receive acute stroke care interventions, but he is frightened and worried about his future.

Everything in his life has changed so suddenly. Amil used to think of himself as someone who is physically strong; he now feels weak and helpless. He is concerned about his family's welfare. Although his partner works, he is the primary financial provider for his family. They plan to help their children with

their university education, which requires both incomes. If his condition does not improve, his role as the primary financial provider will drastically change.

Amil's recovery and rehabilitation progress slowly. His self-concept has changed from thinking of himself as someone who is self-sufficient and independent to someone who must rely on others. Although he is able to leave the hospital and now attends rehabilitation as an outpatient, Amil is not able to perform most basic household tasks and must wait until someone comes home to help him with any activities that require strength. He is barely able to care for his own needs with bathing and eating. He feels fortunate to be alive, but his adaptation capabilities are stretched to the maximum. His identity is not clear to him anymore. His body image has been radically altered, his self-esteem is low, and his role in the family has changed.

Think about this case study as you read this chapter. There are review questions at the end of the chapter that relate to this case study.

Self-concept is the mental image that a person has of themselves. It is a subjective and complex mixture of conscious and unconscious thoughts, attitudes, and perceptions that a person has about their own identity. *Self-concept and self-esteem* are two independent but related terms that are often used interchangeably; however, there is a difference in these terms. *Self-concept* is considered the cognitive aspect of self,

whereas *self-esteem* refers to subjective feelings of self-acceptance and self-respect. Self-esteem refers to the extent to which we like, accept, approve of, or value ourselves. In other words, reflecting on the question "Who am I?" relates to self-concept, whereas reflecting on "Am I worthy?" relates to self-esteem. Self-esteem is subjective and does not necessarily reflect a person's objective characteristics and competencies

455

or how a person is evaluated by others. High self-esteem is characterized by feelings of self-acceptance and self-respect, whereas low self-esteem involves self-doubts and feelings of being a failure.

Self-concept comprises several domains: social, emotional, physical, and academic. Self-concept affects how people adapt to health challenges, difficult situations, and relationships. Individuals with a positive self-concept and self-esteem are better able to cope with illness and stressful life challenges and events. They are also more likely to choose healthy behaviours and participate in activities that promote their health and prevent illness (Orth & Robins, 2019).

Nurses care for patients with a variety of health problems that can threaten patients' self-concept and self-esteem. The loss of a bodily function, a decline in activity tolerance, and difficulty managing a chronic illness are all situations that can potentially affect patients' self-concept. Nurses need to assess patients to determine if they have a healthy self-concept and to develop nursing strategies to meet their patients' needs. Nurses who are sensitive to their patients' expressions of self-concept can use each nurse–patient interaction to enhance their patient's sense of self, assist their patients to adjust to alterations in self-concept, and support components of self-concept that enable patients to address life's challenges and cope more adaptively with difficulties. Nurses also facilitate communication and ensure that the nursing care plan is individualized to meet each patient's needs when the terms *self-concept* and *self-esteem* are used appropriately.

SCIENTIFIC KNOWLEDGE BASE

An individual is not born with a self-concept. Self-concept is considered to be a social creation that develops as a result of interacting with others. Developing self-concept and self-esteem is a lifelong process that begins in early childhood and continues across the lifespan. In general, self-concept and self-esteem levels are high in childhood, decrease in adolescence, rise gradually throughout adulthood, peak at age 60 years, then decline in old age (Orth & Robins, 2019; Orth et al., 2021). In infancy, the development of self-concept is largely influenced by children's interactions with their primary caregivers. As children grow and develop and have relationships with other people such as extended family, friends, teachers, and coaches, those individuals also influence their self-concept. Other factors that influence self-concept are the child's gender, developmental stage, socioeconomic status, culture, and social environment. Young children start out with reasonably high levels of self-concept (Orth & Robins, 2019). In childhood, children tend to rate themselves higher on measures of self-concept than they rate other children, which is perhaps a reflection of their egocentric view of the world (Figure 27.1). The biological, social, and cognitive changes of late childhood take a toll on children's positive view of themselves. Self-concept begins to decline by adolescence and gender differences appear. Adolescence is a particularly critical time when many factors affect self-concept. Research has shown that the adolescent experience appears to adversely affect girls slightly more than boys (Bleidorn et al., 2016). For girls, adolescence brings overt physical changes, such as the development of breasts, a gain in body fat, and the onset of menarche with its associated symptoms. As a result, adolescent girls may be more sensitive to their appearance and how others view them. For boys, there are no sudden physical changes to indicate puberty. Maturational changes are generally regarded as more positive.

Self-esteem generally increases from adolescence to middle adulthood. A large number of studies using different samples and assessments of self-esteem provide evidence that both men and women show age-related increases in self-concept and self-esteem from late adolescence to middle adulthood. While earlier studies showed clear gender differences, with men reporting higher levels of self-esteem

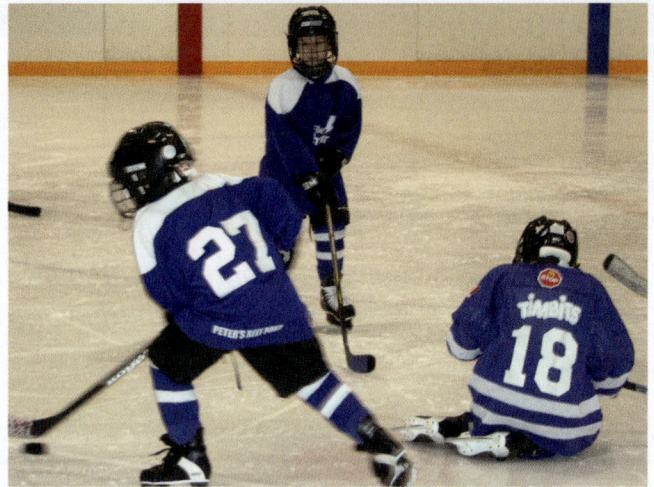

FIGURE 27.1 Participating in group activities can foster children's self-esteem. (From https://morguefile.com/search/morguefile/3/hockey/pop.)

than women, more recent studies using large samples, as well as meta-analyses that synthesize findings from numerous studies using nationally representative samples, found fewer gender differences (Orth et al., 2018, 2021).

A growing body of scientific evidence does suggest that self-esteem affects individuals' lives and well-being in many diverse domains. Self-esteem has been linked to both emotional and physical health and well-being, positive social relationships, school and academic achievements, as well as satisfaction with employment (Möller et al., 2020; Orth et al., 2018, 2021).

Self-esteem remains relatively stable during adulthood, peaks at about 60 years of age, and then declines slightly in older persons (Orth, 2019; Orth et al., 2018; Orth & Robins, 2019). The sense of self may be negatively affected by declines in health, cognitive abilities, and socioeconomic status associated with aging. When older persons develop health problems or lose their spouses or partners, for example, they may experience negative changes in independence or social interaction, which may alter their perceptions of themselves.

Ethnic and cultural differences in self-concept and self-esteem have also been demonstrated. Findings from cross-cultural research show age and gender differences in self-concept and self-esteem (Cicero, 2018). For example, across all nations, males consistently reported slightly higher levels of self-esteem than females, and all genders' self-esteem increased from late adolescence to middle adulthood. Despite these broad cross-cultural similarities, the cultures differed significantly in the magnitude of the age and gender differences. These differences were associated with cultural differences in socioeconomic, sociodemographic, gender-equality, and cultural-value indicators (Bleidorn et al., 2016). Nurses must be sensitive to factors that affect self-concept and self-esteem in the diverse cultures that make up the multicultural fabric of Canadian society, in order to ensure an individualized and patient-centred approach to nursing care.

Individuals' perceptions of themselves and of their health are closely related. Patients' beliefs about their personal health can enhance their self-concept. Statements such as "I'll beat this" or "I've never been sick a day in my life" indicate that a person's thoughts about personal health are positive. Self-concept is also affected by illness, hospitalization, and surgery. Chronic illness may affect the ability to provide financial support, thereby affecting an individual's self-esteem and perceived roles within the family. Negative perceptions regarding health status may be reflected in such statements as "It's not worth it anymore" or "I'm just a burden to my family." Chronic illness can affect identity and body image. This is reflected in statements such as "I'll never get any better" or "I can't stand to look at myself this way."

What individuals think and how they feel about themselves affects the way they care for themselves physically and emotionally and the way they care for others. How a person behaves is generally consistent with both self-concept and self-esteem. Individuals who have poor self-concept and poor self-esteem often do not feel in control of situations and may not feel worthy of care, which can influence decisions regarding health care. Nurses' knowledge of factors that affect both self-concept and self-esteem is critical to provide effective nursing interventions.

NURSING KNOWLEDGE BASE

Knowledge developed from medical and social sciences, humanities, and psychology, as well as knowledge from nursing research and clinical practice, is used to provide patients with evidence-informed practice. This broad knowledge base enables nurses to have a holistic view of patients, which promotes quality patient care that best meets the self-concept needs of patients.

Development of Self-Concept

Self-concept begins in infancy and continues throughout the lifespan. Erik Erikson's psychosocial theory of development (1963) helps us understand key tasks that individuals face at various stages of development from infancy to late adulthood. The eight stages of psychosocial development are discussed in a previous chapter (see Chapter 22). Each stage builds on the tasks of the previous stage, and successful mastery of each stage leads to a positive sense of self. Most individuals master each stage; however, individuals can regress during times of major stressful life events, illness, significant trauma, or other life-changing experiences. Nurses need to recognize when individuals fail to achieve an age-appropriate developmental stage or regress to an earlier stage in a period of crisis, in order to be able to individualize care and determine appropriate nursing interventions to support healthy adaptation.

Self-concept is always changing and is based on the following:
- Sense of competency and mastery of prior and new experiences
- Perceived reactions of other people to one's body
- Ongoing perceptions and interpretations of other people's thoughts and feelings
- Personal and professional relationships
- Collective beliefs and images one holds about oneself
- Academic and employment-related identity
- Ability to cope with and resolve problems
- Racial and ethnic identity
- Gender and sexual identity
- Personality structure
- Perceptions of events that have an impact on the self
- Personal appearance and physical attractiveness
- Current feelings about the physical, emotional, and social self
- Self-expectations

Components and Interrelated Terms of Self-Concept

A positive self-concept provides a sense of meaning, wholeness, and clarity. A healthy self-concept has a high degree of stability, generates positive feelings toward the self, and helps individuals adapt positively to stressors. There are many components of self-concept. Social scientists refer to a bundle of interrelated concepts when referring to self-concept. Those particularly relevant to nurses are identity, body image, and role performance.

Identity. Identity involves the internal sense of individuality, wholeness, and consistency of a person over time and in various circumstances. Our identity distinguishes us from others. Identity is influenced by age, gender, sexuality, social class, ethnicity, and culture. Establishing an individual identity is an important developmental task from childhood to adolescence to young adulthood. Identity develops over time and ends in the "uniqueness" of each individual. A child learns culturally and socially accepted values, behaviours, and roles through observing other people and modelling their behaviour. Identity is often gained from self-observation and from what individuals are told about themselves (Austin et al., 2019). A child first identifies with parental figures and later with teachers, peers, and role models. To form an identity, a child must be able to integrate learned behaviours and expectations into a coherent, consistent, and unique whole (Erikson, 1963, 1997).

Achieving one's identity is necessary for developing intimate relationships, because individuals express identity in relationships with others (Austin et al., 2019; McIntyre et al., 2017). Sexuality is part of one's identity. Gender identity is a person's internal psychological sense of being male or female, or not identifying with either male or female, and includes a person's sexual orientation. It is one of the most central aspects of self-concept (Rathus et al., 2019). This image and its meaning depend on culturally determined values of gender-appropriate behaviour that are affected by socialization (see Chapter 23). Gender identity is a complex concept that is based partly on a person's anatomy (i.e., sexual organs) and partly on the psychology of the individual, which is influenced by culture and tradition.

Traditionally, children have been raised to have a female or male gender identity in accordance with their assigned genital anatomy. This rigidity in how society classifies gender is referred to as *gender binary*, a classification system that assumes either a male or female gender identity and ignores the fact that there are variations in gender identification (Rathus et al., 2019). Instead, advocates encourage gender to be viewed on a continuum. While most people identify with the sexual anatomy they were born with, some do not and struggle to find an expression of their gender identity that is comfortable for them. The internal conflict between a person's assigned gender and the gender they identify with is referred to as *gender dysphoria*. Some individuals may be uncomfortable with their assigned gender because of the expected roles assigned to that gender, or as a consequence of biological processes that result in a variation of gender development (D'Angelo, 2020). However, not all individuals who do not identify with their assigned gender at birth experience distress or are uncomfortable with their expression of gender. *Transgender* is the term used to describe individuals whose gender identity, expression, or behaviour differs from those typically associated with their assigned sex at birth (Rathus et al., 2019).

Religious faith also may foster identity formation through participation in traditions and rituals. Associating with others in a religious community provides strong identity experiences that influence an individual's sense of self. Adopting, adapting, or alternately even rejecting religious traditions is a prominent way in which young people may confirm or challenge societal expectations and help individuals express and define *who they are* (Gareau et al., 2019).

Race and ethnicity are other factors which can influence the formation of identify. Racial-ethnic or cultural identity is a sense of commitment or belonging to an identified racial or ethnic group, as well as participation and pride in its cultural traditions. Racial or cultural identity develops from identification and socialization within an established group, as well as through the experience of integrating the response of individuals outside the cultural or racial group into a person's sense of self. Differences in ethnic identity (e.g., Polish Canadian, Lebanese Canadian) exist through participation in traditions, customs, and rituals. The evolution of cultural identity may be challenging for some individuals. For example, the children of Chinese immigrants who were born in Canada may experience two different environments on a daily basis—a traditional Chinese home and a largely Euro-Canadian school environment.

Indigenous people recognize the pivotal role of personal and cultural identity and the losses suffered from governmental policies that forced assimilation with the Euro-Canadian culture, such as removing children from their parents and communities to attend residential schools. Children's forced assimilation with the dominant Euro-Canadian culture resulted in the loss of traditional spiritual practices and loss of Indigenous languages, cultural practices, and traditions and affected gender roles, child-rearing, and family relationships. The loss of cultural identity has had deleterious effects on Indigenous people's physical, mental, and emotional health, not only among residential school attendees but in the generation following them (Wilk et al., 2017). Indigenous people have engaged in strategies to reclaim their culture by revitalizing their language, history, customs, and the traditional practices that support their identity (see Chapter 12 for further discussion of Indigenous identity). For people of diverse cultures, a strong racial-cultural identity generally buffers against the effects of prejudice and discrimination and is positively related to self-concept, self-esteem, as well as psychological health and well-being and engaging in positive health practices (Box 27.1).

BOX 27.1   CULTURAL ASPECTS OF CARE
Racial and Cultural Background

Racial and cultural identity are important components of a person's self-concept. Early in growth and development, an individual develops racial and cultural identity within the family context. As the individual grows, the cultural aspects of their self-concept may be reinforced through family, social, cultural, or religious experiences. An individual's self-concept may be strengthened or challenged through political, social, or cultural influences experienced in school or work environments. Positive or negative cultural role modelling and past experiences also influence self-concept.

Implications for Practice
- To improve patients' self-concept, develop an open, nonrestrictive attitude when assessing for and encouraging cultural or religious practices.
- Ask patients what they think is important to help them feel better or gain a stronger sense of self.
- Encourage cultural identity by individualizing self-care practices, dietary choices, and clothing to meet each patient's self-concept needs.
- Facilitate culturally sensitive health promotion activities identified through evidence-informed practice that address at-risk behaviors (such as smoking, problematic substance use, premature sexual experiences).

From Orth, U. (2018). The family environment in early childhood has a long-term effect on self-esteem: A longitudinal study from birth to age 27 years. *Journal of Personality and Social Psychology, 114*(4), 637–655. https://doi.org/10.1037/pspp0000143; Orth, U. (2019). Self-esteem. In D. Gu & M. E. Dupre (Eds.), *Encyclopedia of gerontology and population aging.* Springer; Orth, U., Erol, R. Y., & Luciano, E. C. (2018). Development of self-esteem from age 4 to 94 years: A meta-analysis of longitudinal studies. *Psychological Bulletin, 144*(10), 1045–1080. https://doi.org/10.1037/bul0000161; Orth, U., & Robins R. W. (2019). Development of self-esteem across the lifespan. In D. P. McAdams, R. L. Shiner, & J. L. Tackett (Eds.), *Handbook of personality development* (pp. 328–344). Guilford.

Body Image. Body image is the perception we have of our bodies, including size, appearance, and functioning. This perception or mental image is affected by both conscious and subconscious thought. Feelings about body image include those related to femininity and masculinity, youthfulness, sexuality, health, and vitality. These perceptions are not always consistent with a person's actual physical structure or appearance. Sometimes, an individual's mental image can be different from how other people perceive them. Some body-image distortions have psychological origins, such as those that occur in an eating disorder (e.g., anorexia nervosa). Other alterations occur as a result of situational events, such as an amputation of a limb as a result of trauma, a scar due to surgery, or disfigurement from a caustic burn.

Most individuals experience some degree of body dissatisfaction, which can affect body image and overall self-concept. Disturbances in body image can be exaggerated when a change in health status occurs. The way other people view a person's body and the feedback offered are also influential. For example, a controlling, violent husband might tell his wife that she is ugly and that no one else would want her. Over time, with repeated humiliation and degradation, she may incorporate this devalued image into her self-concept. Likewise, a patient who has suffered disfiguring burns has to cope with their own psychological reaction to their altered body, as well as with how other people react to them (Dekel & van Niekerk, 2018).

Body image is affected by cognitive growth and physical development and by normal developmental transitions such as puberty or menopause. Hormonal changes during adolescence affect body image. The development of secondary sex characteristics and changes in body fat distribution affect adolescents' self-concept. In older persons, changes associated with aging, such as decreasing visual acuity and hearing or loss of physical strength and stamina also can affect body image.

Cultural and societal attitudes and values influence body image. Culture and society dictate accepted social norms for body image that can influence a person's attitudes (Figure 27.2). Values such as ideal body weight and shape, as well as attitudes toward body markings, piercings, and tattoos, are culturally based. In North American culture, people have been socialized to value youth and fear the aging process. Youth, beauty, and vitality are emphasized in actors who appear in television programs, movies, and advertisements and on social media. The media play a dominant role in creating and perpetuating unrealistic standards of thinness, youth, and physical attractiveness that are difficult or impossible for individuals to attain. Exposure to societal messages that reflect the sociocultural norm has been shown to have a negative impact on both females and males even as early as late childhood (Salomon & Brown, 2019). Having a positive body image is a

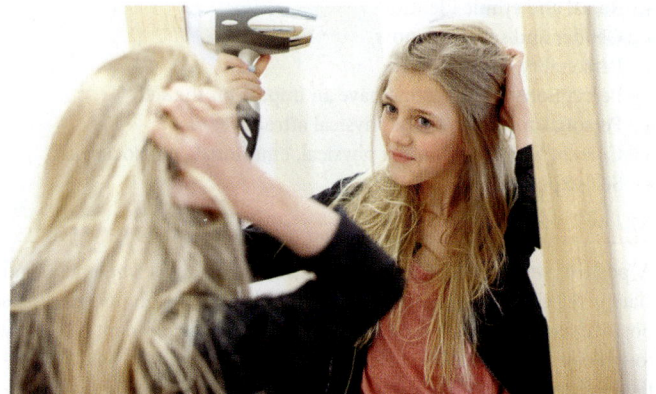

FIGURE 27.2 An individual's appearance influences self-concept. (iStockphoto/stocknroll.)

protective factor for self-concept clarity and psychological health and well-being.

Body image depends only partly on reality. When physical changes occur, individuals may or may not incorporate these changes into their body image. For example, people who have experienced significant weight loss may not perceive themselves as thin and thus may have a distorted body image. Body-image issues are often associated with impaired self-concept and self-esteem. In recent years, a body-positive movement has emerged on social media to challenge mainstream notions of beauty and to encourage people to both accept and appreciate their own bodies. There is also research showing that viewing positive messages on social media can positively influence people's appreciation and acceptance of their bodies and emotional well-being (Cohen et al., 2019; Stevens & Griffiths, 2020).

Role Performance. **Role performance** is the way in which individuals perceive their ability to carry out significant roles. Common roles include parent, child, spouse, employee, and student. Some roles are temporary (e.g., student or patient role) while others are permanent (e.g., child or parent). An individual's perception of competency in a role may or may not match other people's evaluation. Roles that individuals follow in given situations involve socialization to expectations or standards of behaviour. Individuals learn behaviours that are approved by society through the following processes:

- *Reinforcement-extinction:* Certain behaviours become common or are avoided, depending on whether they are approved and reinforced or are discouraged and punished.
- *Inhibition:* An individual learns to refrain from certain behaviours, even when tempted to engage in them.
- *Substitution:* An individual replaces one behaviour with another, which provides the same personal gratification.
- *Imitation:* An individual acquires skills or behaviours by observing and then imitating the skills and behaviours of other members of the family or other social or cultural groups.
- *Identification:* An individual internalizes the beliefs, behaviours, and values of role models into a personal, unique expression of self.

Ideal societal role behaviours are often hard to achieve in real life. Individuals have multiple roles and personal needs that often conflict. For example, an individual may be a mother of small children, a daughter of older parents, a student, and an employee. Each role involves meeting certain expectations. To function effectively in multiple roles, a person must know the expected behaviour and values, desire to conform to them, and be able to meet the role requirements. Successful adults learn to distinguish between ideal role expectations and realistic possibilities. Fulfillment of these expectations leads to an enhanced sense of self. Difficulty or failure in meeting role expectations leads to deficits in the sense of self and often contributes to decreased self-esteem or altered self-concept.

Self-Esteem. **Self-esteem** is an individual's overall sense of self-worth or the emotional appraisal of self-concept. It represents the overall judgement of personal worth or value. It is a subjective feeling and does not always reflect how people are evaluated by others. Self-esteem is positive when a person feels capable, worthwhile, and competent. Self-esteem is shaped by individuals' appraisals of how they are perceived by significant others.

There are both genetic and environmental factors that influence the development of self-esteem, but environmental factors play the major role in the formation of self-esteem (Lodi-Smith & Crocetti, 2018; Orth, 2018; Orth & Robbins, 2019). Children's self-esteem is shaped by early experiences in important interpersonal relationships, most importantly by the parent–child relationship. The impressions of our early caregivers serve as a "looking glass," reflecting back an image of ourselves that is then internalized and serves as the basis for self-esteem (Cooley, 1902). Parental warmth, parental support, and support of children's autonomy help children develop greater self-esteem. Other significant family relationships (e.g., siblings, grandparents) also help children form beliefs about their self-worth. These early experiences with social relationships help children develop a strong sense of self and self-worth. Later, other significant people's evaluation, such as that of teachers and peers, also has a profound influence on children's self-esteem. While this perspective suggests that self-esteem is co-constructed through relational processes that first emerge in childhood, they also persist across the lifespan (Harris et al., 2017; von Soest et al., 2018).

In early and middle adolescence, self-esteem remains relatively constant. Several factors have been shown to be positively associated with self-esteem in adolescents—for example, parental support, family cohesion, greater number of siblings, and social and emotional support from other adult role models (Orth, 2018; Orth & Robins, 2019). Supportive and caring relationships will help foster self-esteem in adolescents. Other factors related to greater self-esteem include family income above the poverty level, safe and nurturing environments, and religious community. Participating in physical activity that is developmentally appropriate and enjoyable can lead to positive self-esteem in adolescents (Fernández-Bustos et. al., 2019).

Self-esteem levels rise gradually during adulthood until approximately middle-age and then decline slightly in old age (Orth & Robins, 2019). In general, this pattern holds true across gender, socioeconomic status, and ethnicity. Erikson's (1963) emphasis on the generativity stage (see Chapter 22) may explain the increase in self-esteem and self-concept in adulthood. The individual is focused on being increasingly productive and creative at work, while at the same time promoting and guiding the next generation. Other than childhood, the mid-60s represents the highest level of self-esteem across the lifespan. At around 70 years of age, self-esteem declines slightly, which, according to Erikson's theory of psychosocial development (1963), reflects a diminished need for self-promotion and a shift in self-concept to a more modest and balanced view of the self.

> **SAFETY ALERT** Adolescence marks a time when youth begin to experiment with risky behaviours, such as engaging in substance use, premature sexual activity, and unprotected sex. These risks threaten adolescents' health and have implications for health care interventions. A decline in self-esteem is often associated with an increased need for attention, which may be demonstrated by engaging in risky behaviours. In addition, the influence of peers is strong during adolescence. Research has shown, however, that adolescents with a strong sense of identity are not as susceptible to the influence of peers and are not as likely to engage in risky behaviours compared to adolescents with a weaker sense of identity.

To better understand self-esteem, consider the relationship between a person's self-concept and the ideal self. The *ideal self* is a representation of the attributes the person would like to have—an image of the person ideally. The ideal self acts as a motivator that gives the individual an incentive for future behaviour—providing an image of what they want to be or not be. The ideal self is also used as a standard to evaluate the actual self. The ideal self originates in the preschool years and develops throughout life. Early in life, parents set ideals for their children, to have certain attributes, such as honesty, intelligence, and success. Through socialization practices, children often internalize their parents' ideals. The ideal self is also influenced by other factors,

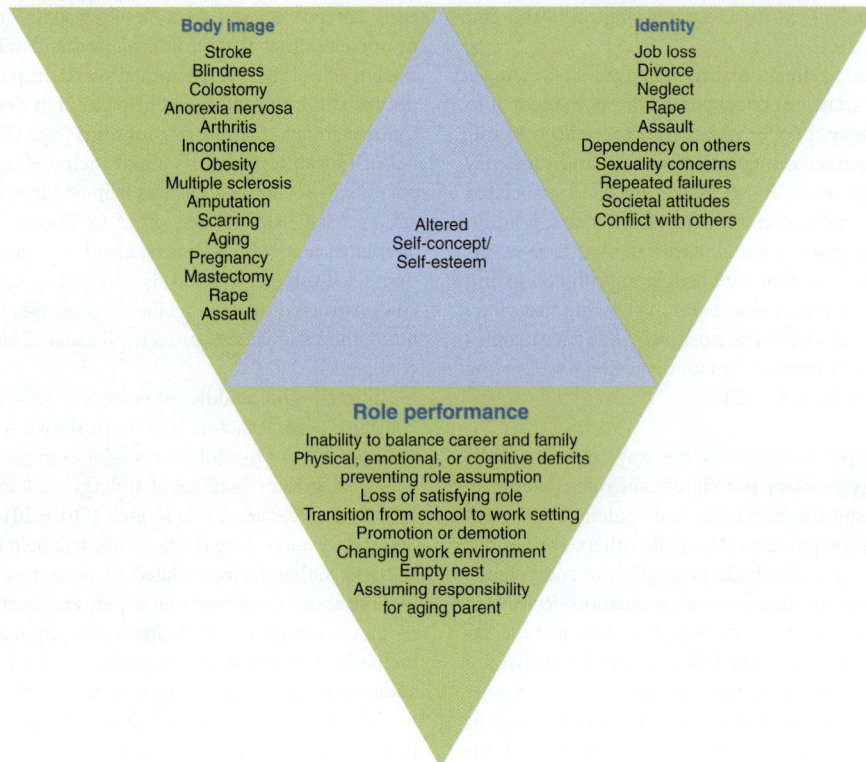

FIGURE 27.3 Common stressors that influence self-concept.

such as school, peer relations, and the media. Self-evaluation is an ongoing mental process. In general, a person whose self-concept comes close to matching the ideal self has high self-esteem, whereas a person whose self-concept varies widely from the ideal self tends to have low self-esteem.

A positive sense of self-esteem is an important variable in determining how an individual functions in the world. A person's ability to contribute to society in a meaningful way often affects self-concept and self-esteem. Once established, basic feelings about the self tend to be relatively stable, although they may fluctuate somewhat. A situational crisis may temporarily affect one's self-esteem. Individuals who are sick and unable to be involved in society may feel worthless. Accepting a patient as an individual with worth and dignity can help maintain and improve the patient's self-esteem.

Stressors Affecting Self-Concept

A *self-concept stressor* is any real or perceived change that threatens identity, body image, or role performance (Figure 27.3). A stressor challenges a person's adaptive capacities. The most important factor in determining an individual's response is the individual's perception of the stressor. The ability to re-establish balance is related to numerous factors, including the number, intensity, and duration of the stressors; the individual's health status; and their coping mechanisms (see Chapter 30). The normal process of maturation and development itself is a stressor. Changes that occur in physical, spiritual, emotional, sexual, familial, and sociocultural health can affect self-concept. Being able to adapt to stressors is likely to lead to a positive sense of self, whereas failure to adapt may lead to a negative sense of self.

Any change in health can be a stressor that potentially affects self-concept. A physical change can alter body image, thereby affecting identity and self-esteem. Chronic illnesses often alter role performance, which may affect identity and self-esteem. An essential process

in adjusting to loss is the development of a new self-concept. The case study at the beginning of this chapter about Amil, who suffered a sudden and unexpected stroke, illustrates the interrelationships among the various components of self-concept. As a result of the stroke, Amil's self-concept was dramatically affected. His body image changed radically from seeing himself as someone who was strong and independent to someone who was dependent on others for his activities of daily living. While he was once the main provider for his family, now his role as the primary provider changed too. His self-esteem was negatively affected as he experienced a loss of self-worth.

Try to put yourself in Amil's place. How would you cope with these changes? What if this happened to a relative who was the same age as your patient? How would these changes affect them? As Amil's nurse, ask some questions to help you gain an understanding of the experience from the patient's perspective and point of view. Consider asking Amil to describe his experience in his own words.

More broadly, give the patient the opportunity to express their feelings. How has this sudden alteration in health affected their life, their image of themselves, and ability to lead the lifestyle they were used to before their stoke?

Ask the patient about other health challenges or major obstacles in their life that they have had in the past. Can they identify strengths and capabilities they have used previously to help in their present situation?

These questions will help you as a nurse understand the impact of this major health event on Amil's self-concept and help you plan strategies to assist him to adapt positively to these changes. If necessary, referral for in-depth assessment by other health care providers with expertise in mental health may be useful to ensure Amil's optimal long-term recovery (Lanctôt et al., 2020).

Crisis occurs when people cannot overcome obstacles with their usual methods of problem solving and adaptation. Any crisis potentially threatens self-concept and self-esteem. Some crises, such as the one described in the case study, directly affect all components of self-concept. The stressors created by a crisis—identity confusion, disturbed body image, low self-esteem, role conflict, role strain, role ambiguity, and role overload—may result in illness. During self-concept crises, supportive and educative resources can help people learn new ways of coping and responding to the stressful event or situation.

Identity Stressors. Developmental markers such as puberty, menopause, child-bearing, and retirement may affect identity. Identity, like body image, is closely related to appearance and abilities. An individual's identity is affected by stressors throughout life, but it is particularly vulnerable during adolescence, a time characterized by physical, emotional, and mental changes of increasing maturity, which can result in insecurity and anxiety. It is also a time when adolescents are developing psychosocial competence, including coping strategies (see Chapter 30). A positive self-concept in adolescence enhances psychological and physical health in young adulthood.

Adults generally have a more stable identity and thus a more firmly developed self-concept than younger people. Cultural and social stressors, rather than personal stressors, may have more effect on an adult's identity. For example, an adult may have to balance career and family or make choices regarding religious or cultural traditions. Retirement may mean the loss of an important means of achievement and the loss of social connections. People at retirement may begin to re-evaluate their identities and accomplishments. Also, when individuals lose their significant other this can lead the surviving individual to re-examine aspects of their identity.

Identity confusion results when people do not maintain a clear, consistent, and continuous consciousness of personal identity. It may occur at any stage of life if a person is unable to adapt to identity stressors. Under extreme stress, an individual may experience disturbed personal identity, a state in which differences between the self and others cannot be determined. One example of identity confusion is when an adolescent realizes that some of their feelings and behaviours are focused on individuals of the same sex. A period of anxiety and confusion may begin regarding sexuality and gender expectations. The person needs to adjust and accept this new identity of the self.

Body Image Stressors. Changes in appearance, structure, or function of a body part require an adjustment in body image. An individual's perception of the change and the relative importance placed on body image affects the significance of the loss of function or change in appearance. For example, if a woman's body image incorporates reproductive functions as the ideal, a hysterectomy to treat uterine cancer may be a significant alteration and may result in a perceived loss of femininity or wholeness. Changes in body appearance, such as an amputation, facial disfigurement, or scars from burns or surgery, are physically obvious stressors affecting body image. Mastectomy and colostomy are surgical procedures that alter body appearance and function; although these changes are usually undetected by other people, they nonetheless can have a significant effect on the individual. Even elective changes such as breast augmentation or reduction can affect body image. Chronic illnesses such as heart and renal disease affect body image because the body no longer functions at an optimal level. Anticipated body changes resulting from developmental processes can also affect body image. The effects of pregnancy, significant weight gain or loss, pharmacological management of illness, or radiation therapy can change body image and lead to adverse health outcomes. Stressors are not always the result of physical health problems. Sometimes, psychological health challenges also can affect body image (Box 27.2). Social media has also been found to have a negative effect on adolescent body image for all genders (Spurr et al., 2013).

BOX 27.2   RESEARCH HIGHLIGHT

Visible and Invisible Disabilities, Self-Concept, and Body Image

Research Focus

Individuals with visible differences often face stigma and discrimination. Some visible differences are those caused by congenital conditions (e.g., cleft lip, birthmarks, Down syndrome) while other visible differences are caused by accidents such as traumatic injuries (e.g., loss of a limb). Even minor differences that affect individuals' mobility and require them to use a cane or walker can influence other people's reactions (e.g., staring, startled reactions) and as a result may lead to negative thoughts and feelings ultimately influencing a person's self-concept and body image. While research has focused on the way people with visible disabilities think about themselves, less is known about the impact of invisible disabilities on self-concept and body image. Some disabilities, such as cognitive disabilities due to head injuries or psychiatric illnesses, are not observable to others but may still have negative impacts on individuals' self-concept and body image.

Research Abstract

In a unique study, Shpigelman and HaGani (2019) examined the impact of the type of disability on self-concept and body image in 119 adults with disabilities who were diagnosed at birth or during childhood or adolescence. They compared adults with a visible physical (or motor) impairment such as cerebral palsy or muscular dystrophy to adults with a mental illness such as an affective disorder or schizophrenia.

Results

Results showed that individuals with invisible psychiatric disabilities reported lower levels of self-concept and body image than individuals with visible physical disabilities. Gender, family status, and the severity of the disability were also found to be associated with self-concept and body image. Women reported lower levels of body image than men. Single or divorced individuals reported lower levels of self-concept than married participants, and individuals with severe disabilities reported lower levels of self-concept and body image than participants with mild or moderate disabilities.

Implications for Practice

- Nurses need to enhance the self-concept and body image of individuals who have invisible disabilities.
- Nurses should assist individuals to identify strategies that will help them cope with their disability.
- Nurses should examine their attitudes about caring for individuals with disabilities since it may have an impact on individuals' well-being.
- Family members may benefit from support to help the individual with a disability cope.

From Shpigelman, C., & HaGani, N. (2019). The impact of disability type and visibility on self-concept and body image: Implications for mental health nursing. *Journal of Psychiatry and Mental Health Nursing, 26*, 77–86. https://doi.org/10.1111/jpm.12513

Many people associate success with a specific body part or function. For example, athletes may consider their bodies and physical activities to be the focus of personal success. Adaptation and rehabilitation may be affected if they can never again participate in athletics as they know it because of an accident or injury. To surgeons, an amputation of a finger would significantly alter their ability to perform surgery. This change may affect their perception of their self-worth. Body image changes necessitate the revision of long-accepted self-perceptions, as well as alterations in lifestyle. To regain a positive self-concept and self-esteem, each person must adapt to their body image stressors.

Society's response to an individual's physical changes may be affected by the conditions surrounding the alteration. For example, individuals may be treated as heroes and praised for self-sacrifice when paralysis was the result of military duty, whereas individuals who were paralyzed as a result of driving intoxicated may elicit different responses.

Role Performance Stressors. Throughout life, a person undergoes numerous role changes. Normal changes associated with growth and maturation result in developmental transitions. Situational transitions occur when parents, spouses, children, or friends die or when people move, marry, divorce, or change jobs. A *health–illness transition* is changing from a state of health or well-being to one of illness. A shift along the continuum from illness to wellness is as stressful as a shift from wellness to illness. Any transition may lead to role conflict, role ambiguity, role strain, or role overload.

Role conflict results when a person simultaneously assumes two or more roles that are inconsistent, contradictory, or mutually exclusive. For example, when a middle-aged woman with teenage children assumes responsibility for caring for her older parents, conflicts may arise in relation to being both the adult child and the parents' caregiver. Role conflicts can occur when trying to balance time and energy between her children and parents. The perceived importance of each conflicting role influences the degree of conflict experienced. The sick role involves the expectations of other people and society about how a person should behave when sick. Role conflict may occur when general societal expectations ("Take care of yourself so you will get better") conflict with the expectations of co-workers ("The job needs to get done"). The conflict of taking care of oneself while getting everything done can be a major challenge.

Role ambiguity involves unclear role expectations. When expectations are unclear, people may be unsure about what to do or how to behave. Such situations are often stressful and confusing. Role ambiguity is common in adolescence. Parents, peers, and the media pressure adolescents to assume adultlike roles, but many adolescents may still lack the resources to move beyond the role of dependent children. Role ambiguity can occur in employment situations. Employees may become unsure about job expectations in complex, rapidly changing, or highly specialized organizations.

Role strain is the stress or frustration experienced by individuals when behaviours, expectations, or obligations associated with a single social role are incompatible. Individuals who feel inadequate or unsuited for a new social role may experience role strain. For example, individuals who marry someone with children often feel unprepared to suddenly assume a parental role.

Role overload involves having more roles or responsibilities within a role than are manageable. It is frequently reflected in unsuccessful attempts to meet the demands of work and family while still having some personal time. During periods of illness or change, the people involved, either as the person who is ill or as a significant other, often find themselves in role overload.

Self-Esteem Stressors. Individuals with high self-esteem are generally more resilient and are better able to cope with demands and stressors than are those with low self-esteem. High self-esteem is associated with more optimal mental and physical health, greater control over circumstances, and greater adaptation and productivity in adulthood (Orth & Robins, 2019). Low self-worth can contribute to feeling unfulfilled and isolated and can result in depression and unremitting uneasiness or anxiety. Illness, surgery, or accidents that change life patterns can also influence feelings of self-worth. Chronic illnesses such as diabetes, arthritis, and cardiac dysfunction necessitate changes in

accepted and long-assumed behavioural patterns. The more the illness interferes with the ability to engage in activities contributing to feelings of worth or success, the more it affects self-esteem.

Self-esteem stressors vary with developmental stages. Perceived inability to meet parental expectations, lack of parental warmth, harsh criticism, and inconsistent discipline may reduce children's sense of self-worth and self-esteem. Children with low self-esteem and self-worth are more likely to experience internalizing disorders such as fear, anxiety, and depression. They are also more likely to bully other children and are more likely to be bullied (Box 27.3). In adolescence, low self-esteem is one of the strongest predictors of depression, risk-taking behaviors, and psychopathology. In older persons, self-concept stressors include health problems, reduced functional ability, and stressful life events and circumstances. Longitudinal studies have found that self-esteem prospectively predicts better health. Thus, having high self-esteem may be an important resource in older adulthood when health problems become more prevalent (Lodi-Smith & Crocetti, 2018; Orth, 2019) (Box 27.4).

The Family's Effect on the Development of Self-Concept

The family plays a key role in creating and maintaining each family member's self-concept. Children develop a basic sense of who they are from their caregivers. Bowlby's (1982) attachment theory suggests that the quality of the attachment that children develop with their caregivers influences the development of a set of expectations about the self, their interpretations of the actions of other people, and ideas about how to respond to them. Attachment theory suggests that children who experience sensitive and supportive caring will develop expectations that they are worthy of other people's love and that other people are supportive. The quality of parenting interactions also influences children's development. Parents who respond in a firm, consistent, and warm manner promote positive self-esteem in their children. Parents who are harsh, behave inconsistently, or have low self-esteem themselves may foster negative self-concepts in their children. Even well-meaning parents can cultivate negative self-concepts in children. To assist patients in developing a positive self-concept, it is important to assess the family's style of relating (see Chapter 20).

The Nurse's Effect on the Patient's Self-Concept

As a nurse, your acceptance of a patient with an altered self-concept helps promote positive change. When a patient's physical appearance has changed, likely both the patient and the family will observe your verbal and nonverbal responses and reactions. You need to be aware of your own feelings, ideas, values, expectations, and judgements. Self-awareness is critical in initially understanding and accepting others. Nurses who are secure in their own identities more readily accept and thus reinforce patients' identities (Box 27.5). It is important to assess and clarify the following self-concept issues:

- Thoughts and feelings about lifestyle, health, and illness
- Awareness of how nonverbal communication may affect patients and families
- Personal values and expectations and how they affect patients
- Ability to convey a nonjudgemental attitude toward patients
- Preconceived attitudes toward cultural differences in self-concept and self-esteem

Some patients with a change in body appearance or function are very sensitive to health care providers' verbal and nonverbal responses. A positive and matter-of-fact approach to care can provide a model for the patient and family to follow. As their nurse, you can have a positive effect by conveying genuine interest and acceptance. By recognizing and including self-concept issues in planning and delivering care, you can positively influence patient outcomes. By building a trusting

BOX 27.3   **RESEARCH HIGHLIGHT**

Bullying and Self-Concept

Research Focus

Bullying is defined as physical, psychological, or verbal intimidation or attack, or a combination of these meant to cause distress, harm, or both to an intended victim. School-aged children report being bullied in the classroom, schoolyard, or playground, as well as on social media and the Internet (i.e., cyberbullying). Bullying is a serious problem both for the victims and for the children who bully others.

Bullying has always been a concern among parents, educators, and health care providers because of the serious impact on children's health and well-being. Public concern in Canada increased dramatically after the tragic death of Reena Virk, a teen who was bullied by her peers and then murdered, and the tragic deaths of two teens (Amanda Todd and Rehtaeh Parsons) who committed suicide after being bullied. Participation in bullying also increases the risk of suicidal ideation in youth. In the school context, bullying is the most common form of violence among children and youth and has both short- and long-term deleterious effects on children's physical and psychological health and well-being.

Results

Menesini and Salmivalli (2017) conducted a review of research to better understand the complexity of bullying among youth and to focus on effective interventions. Although rates of bullying varied across studies, 9 to 25% of students reported victimization by peers, and 4 to 9% reported bullying others. While all children are at risk, bullying presents heightened risks for vulnerable children, such as children with disabilities, children affected by migration, children who belong to minority groups, or children who simply differ from their peers. The rate of bullying increased to 61% for those who identified as a sexual minority (i.e., lesbian, gay, bisexual, transgender, or queer) (Menesini & Salmivalli, 2017).

Both boys and girls engage in bullying; however, there are some gender differences. The most consistent finding was boys' greater involvement in physical bullying and girls' greater use of relational or verbal aggression and cyberbullying. Children can simultaneously be victims of bullies and bullies of other children, such as their younger siblings. Bullying peaks during middle school years (i.e., 12 to 15 years) and tends to decrease by the end of high school (Hymel & Swearer, 2015).

Bullying has been linked with a host of negative mental health outcomes for both bullies and victims, such as internalizing problems (e.g., depression, anxiety, low-self-esteem and suicidal ideation), as well as having a negative influence on social relationships (e.g., low peer acceptance, having no or few friends, negative friendship quality) and academic functioning (e.g., increased absenteeism, poorer academic achievement) (Menesini & Salmivalli, 2017). Further, there are negative long-term adjustment difficulties in adulthood for individuals who were victimized in their youth (McDougall & Vaillancourt, 2015).

Although the reasons why children bully other children are complex and multifaceted, one explanation focuses on self-concept. Studies have shown that children with a positive self-concept are less likely to be bullied, less likely to bully other children, and less likely to engage in delinquent behaviour or be instigators of peer conflict (Hymel & Swearer, 2015).

Implications for Practice

- Encouraging children's self-concept is an important strategy to prevent bullying behaviour in children and to prevent children from being victimized by a bully.
- Parents must be helped to understand how children are affected by parenting behaviour in particular, and by the family environment.
- It is important to involve the entire family system in the intervention process when children are identified as victims or bullies.
- Youth are reluctant to report bullying. Positive relationships between parents and their children may enhance the likelihood that children report bullying.
- Referral to other health care providers may be necessary to assist vulnerable children and families.

Note: The articles by Hymel and Swearer (2015) and McDougall and Vaillancourt (2015) are two of six in the 2015 special issue (May-June) of *American Psychologist*, "School Bullying and Victimization."
From Hymel, S., & Swearer, S. M. (2015). Four decades of research on school bullying: An introduction. *American Psychologist*, 70(4), 293–299. https://doi.org/10.1037/a0038928; McDougall, P., & Vaillancourt, T. (2015). Long-term adult outcomes of peer victimization in childhood and adolescence: Pathways to adjustment and maladjustment. *American Psychologist*, 70(4), 300–310. https://doi.org/10.1037/a0039174; Menesini, E., & Salmivalli, C. (2017). Bullying in schools: The state of knowledge and effective interventions. *Psychology, Health & Medicine, 22*(Suppl. 1), 240–253. https://doi.org/10.1080/13548506.2017.1279740; Shemesh, D. O., & Heiman, T. (2021). Resilience and self-concept as mediating factors in the relationship between bullying victimization and sense of well-being among adolescents. *International Journal of Adolescence and Youth, 26*(1), 158–171. https://doi.org/10.1080/02673843.2021.1899946

BOX 27.4   **FOCUS ON OLDER PERSONS**

Promoting a Positive Self-Concept

Promoting a positive self-concept in older persons is essential, but it is especially important for those experiencing disability, frailty, or reduced functional capacity.

- Examples of activities to help older persons feel a sense of self-worth while providing a legacy for younger family members include conducting a life review or participating in a reminiscence group, recording an oral history, or making a photo scrapbook of meaningful life events (Eliopoulos, 2018).
- Potential threats to an older person's self-esteem may arise from the institutional environments where they receive care. These threats can include dependence, devaluation, depersonalization, functional impairments, and lack of control over one's environment. Nursing interventions directed toward reducing or eliminating these threats can improve an older person's quality of life.

- Self-concept may be negatively affected in older adulthood by a number of life changes, including health problems, reduced functional ability, lower income or socioeconomic status, spousal loss or bereavement, loss of social support, and decline in achievement experiences after retirement.
- Health care providers should be alert to an older person's preoccupation with physical complaints. They should conduct a comprehensive assessment and encourage patients to verbalize needs, feelings, and emotions such as fear, insecurity, and loneliness (Austin et al., 2019).
- By actively listening and accepting the person's feelings; being respectful; praising health-seeking behaviours; and recognizing, acknowledging, and praising accomplishments, health care providers convey respect for an older person's worth.

BOX 27.5   RESEARCH HIGHLIGHT
Professional Identity and Nursing

Research Focus

Individuals' professional identity is a component of their overall identity. It is a sense of self that is derived and perceived from the role we take on in the careers, occupations, or work we choose to do. A positive and healthy professional identity is critical for nurses to function skillfully and competently, and it ultimately benefits patients and families. Nurses feeling positively about themselves can support patient care in a positive health care environment and enhance job satisfaction and retention rates in nursing.

The formation of a professional identity is the result of socialization into the nursing profession, a process in which individuals learn and internalize nursing knowledge, values, and norms of the profession in addition to the knowledge, skills, and competencies needed for safe, competent, and ethical nursing practice (Rose et al., 2018). Although a professional identity is separate from self-concept, it is inextricably linked to self-concept. Several researchers explored the factors that influence professional identity in nurses.

Key Findings

- Nurses' professional identities start prior to entering their formal nursing education, as potential students have some preconceived values and beliefs about the profession.
- Nurses' professional identities develop throughout the years of educational preparation and continue to develop in their nursing careers.

- The education period is a critical time for nursing students because during this time, students gain the knowledge and skills to gain entry into the profession and to self-identify with the profession.
- The different educational contexts all play a vital role in constructing a professional identity. While nurse educators are a key influence, clinical preceptors in clinical learning environments have significant influence in helping students develop a professional identity.
- Professional identity is a key issue in transitioning from being a student to a practising nurse. Students need to feel comfortable and confident as they assume their new positions after graduation.
- Professional identity continually evolves. Nurses undergo constant reshaping of professional identity throughout their careers, with frequent advances occurring in nursing, health, and medical knowledge, as well as changes in technology, roles, and patient expectations.
- Values of trust, respect, recognition, advocacy, accountability, responsibility, knowledge, and caring are seen as core to professional identity.
- Perceptions of professional identity are also related to external factors. For example, the environment where nurses work affects their professional identity. A good team environment where nurses feel valued positively influence professional identity, whereas an environment constrained by a lack of system resources negatively impacts professional identity.
- Obtaining advanced education in nursing through certifications, specialization, and graduate education in nursing further enhances professional identity.

From Karanikola, M., Doulougeri, K., Koutrouba, A., et al. (2018). A phenomenological investigation of the interplay among professional worth appraisal, self-esteem and self-perception in nurses: The revelation of an internal and external criteria system. *Frontiers in Psychology, 9.* https://doi.org/10.3389/fpsyg.2018.01805; Landis, T. T., Severtsen, B. M., Shaw, M. R., et al. (2020). Professional identity and hospital-based registered nurses: A phenomenological study. *Nursing Forum, 55,* 389–394. https://doi-org.ezproxy.macewan.ca/10.1111/nuf.12440; Rasmussen, P., Henderson, A., McCallum, J., et al. (2021). Professional identity in nursing: A mixed method research study. *Nurse Education in Practice, 52,* 1–7. https://doi.org/10.1016/j.nepr.2021.103039; Rose, T., Nies, M. A., & Reid, J. (2018). The internalization of professional nursing values in baccalaureate nursing students. *Journal of Professional Nursing, 34,* 25–30. https://doi.org/10.1016/j.profnurs.2017.06.004

nurse–patient relationship and appropriately involving the patient and family in decision making, you can enhance self-concept. An individualized approach may highlight a patient's unique needs, including incorporating alternative health care practices or methods of personal and spiritual expression.

You also can significantly influence a patient's body image. For example, for a woman who has undergone a mastectomy, you can positively affect her body image by showing acceptance of the mastectomy scar. Patients closely watch other people's reactions to their wounds and scars. A facial expression of shock or disgust can contribute to the patient developing a negative body image. It is important to monitor your responses. Statements such as "Your wound is healing nicely" or "The tissue looks healthy" will be affirming to the patient. Nonverbal behaviours help to convey caring for the patient and can affect self-esteem (Figure 27.4). For example, the self-concept of an incontinent patient can be threatened by the perception that the caregivers find the situation unpleasant. A good practice is to anticipate personal reactions, acknowledge them, and focus on the patient instead of on the unpleasant task or situation. Imagining yourself in the patient's position will help you find strategies to ease your patient's embarrassment, frustration, and anger.

Preventive measures, early identification, and appropriate treatment can minimize the intensity of self-esteem stressors and the potential effects on the patient and family. Learn to design specific self-concept interventions to fit a patient's profile of risk factors. Assess the patient's perception of a problem and work collaboratively with the patient and with other members of the health care team to resolve issues related to self-concept (Box 27.6).

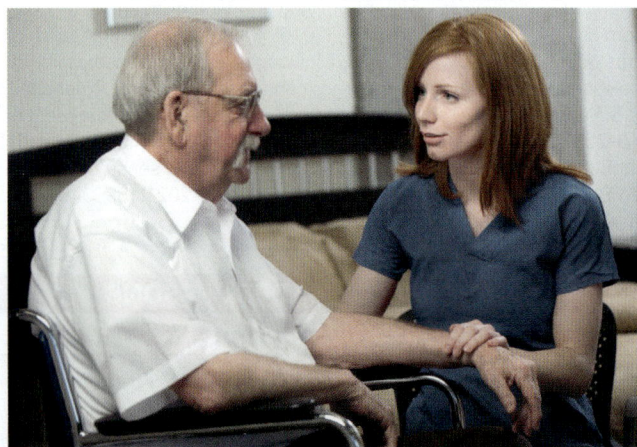

FIGURE 27.4 Nurses can use touch and eye contact to enhance a patient's self-esteem.

CRITICAL THINKING

Self-concept profoundly influences a person's response to illness. Because of this, a critical thinking approach to nursing care is essential. This approach requires synthesis of knowledge, experience, information gathered from patients and families, critical thinking abilities, and knowing and adhering to professional standards. Solid clinical judgement requires anticipating the required information, collecting

BOX 27.6	Behaviours Suggestive of Altered Self-Concept

- Avoidance of eye contact
- Slumped posture
- Unkempt appearance
- Being overly apologetic
- Hesitant speech
- Being overly critical or angry
- Frequent or inappropriate crying
- Negative self-evaluation
- Being excessively dependent
- Hesitancy in expressing views or opinions
- Lack of interest in what is happening
- Passive attitude
- Difficulty in making decisions

and analyzing the data, and making appropriate decisions regarding patient care.

It is essential to integrate knowledge from nursing and other disciplines, including self-concept theory and communication principles, and to consider cultural and developmental factors. Previous experience in caring for patients with alterations in self-concept can assist the nurse to individualize care for each patient. The nursing process continues until the patient's self-concept is improved, restored, or maintained.

❖ SELF-CONCEPT AND THE NURSING PROCESS

◆ Assessment

In assessing self-concept, nurses must focus on the various components of self-concept: identity, body image, role performance, and self-esteem. Assessment should include observing behaviours suggestive of an altered self-concept (see Box 27.6), actual and potential self-concept stressors (see the earlier case study), and coping patterns. Nurses need to be sensitive to the effect that cultural influences have on the patient's behaviours and needs. Some behaviours suggestive of an altered self-concept for someone in one culture may be normal for individuals in other cultures. For example, in many Indigenous and Asian cultures, eye contact is a sign of disrespect. In order to gather comprehensive assessment, information from multiple sources must be synthesized critically (Figure 27.5).

At appropriate times, the nurse will need to ask specific questions to assess the patient's self-concept, paying close attention to their responses (Table 27.1). It is important to closely observe nonverbal behaviour. Note the manner in which patients talk about significant people in their lives. This can provide clues to both stressful and supportive relationships, as well as to key roles that the patient assumes. Using knowledge of developmental stages to determine what areas are likely to be important to the patient, the nurse can inquire about these aspects of the person's life. For example, older patients should be asked about their lives and what has been important to them. At this stage of development, individuals are examining their lives and considering the effects they have had in the world. The conversation will probably provide data relating to role performance, identity, self-esteem, stressors, and coping patterns.

Coping Behaviours.
Nursing assessment should also include consideration of previous coping behaviours; the nature, number, and intensity of the stressors; and the patient's internal and external resources. Knowledge of how patients have handled past stressors can provide

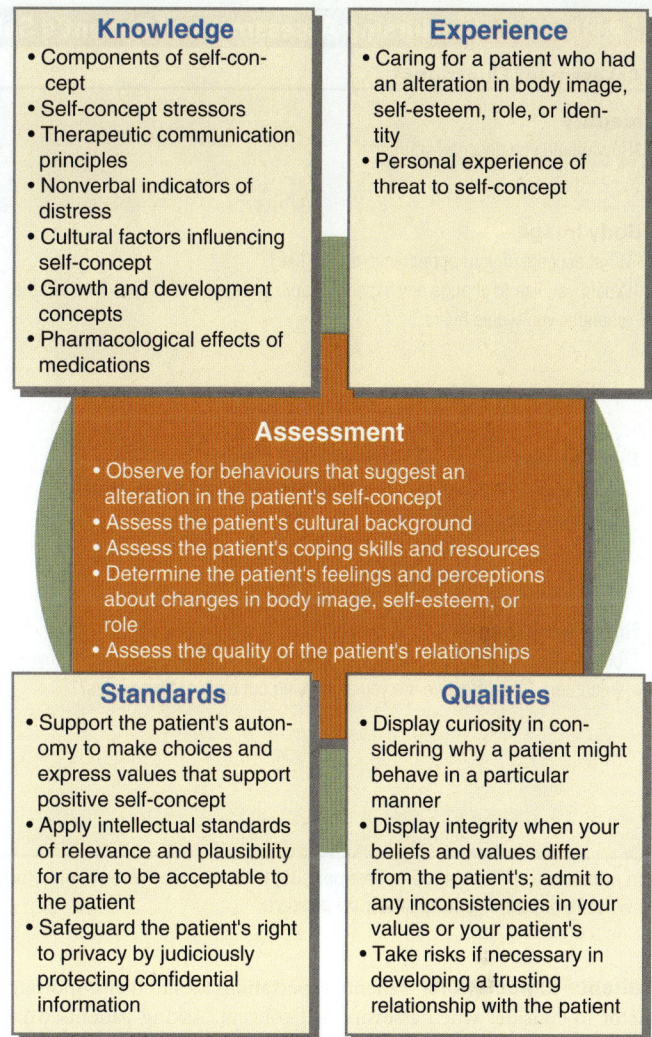

Knowledge
- Components of self-concept
- Self-concept stressors
- Therapeutic communication principles
- Nonverbal indicators of distress
- Cultural factors influencing self-concept
- Growth and development concepts
- Pharmacological effects of medications

Experience
- Caring for a patient who had an alteration in body image, self-esteem, role, or identity
- Personal experience of threat to self-concept

Assessment
- Observe for behaviours that suggest an alteration in the patient's self-concept
- Assess the patient's cultural background
- Assess the patient's coping skills and resources
- Determine the patient's feelings and perceptions about changes in body image, self-esteem, or role
- Assess the quality of the patient's relationships

Standards
- Support the patient's autonomy to make choices and express values that support positive self-concept
- Apply intellectual standards of relevance and plausibility for care to be acceptable to the patient
- Safeguard the patient's right to privacy by judiciously protecting confidential information

Qualities
- Display curiosity in considering why a patient might behave in a particular manner
- Display integrity when your beliefs and values differ from the patient's; admit to any inconsistencies in your values or your patient's
- Take risks if necessary in developing a trusting relationship with the patient

FIGURE 27.5 Critical thinking model to assess self-concept.

insight into the patient's style of coping. People do not address all issues in the same way, but they often use a familiar coping pattern for newly encountered stressors. As previous coping patterns are identified, it is useful to determine whether these patterns have contributed to healthy functioning or created more problems. For example, abused women sometimes use alcohol or drugs to cope with the abuse, but use of these harmful substances only creates additional stressors (see Chapter 30).

Exploring resources and strengths, such as the availability of significant others or prior use of community resources, can be important when developing a realistic and effective plan. It is also critical to understand how patients view their situation. For example, older women may be more accustomed to changes in their health status because of the aging process in general, and experiencing heart disease may be one more aspect of growing older. On the other hand, a cardiac event occurring in middle age may be less expected and more problematic for women because of family and career responsibilities and may thus elicit greater anxiety.

Significant Others. A patient's family or friends can help identify changes in a patient's behaviour that may suggest alterations in self-concept. These individuals may have insights into the patient's way of dealing with stressors or knowledge about what is important to the patient's self-concept. The way a family member or friend talks about the patient and the person's nonverbal behaviours may provide information about what kind of support is available for the patient.

TABLE 27.1	Nursing Assessment of Patient's Self-Concept
Assessment Questions*	**Responses Reflecting Difficulties With Self-Concept**
Identity "How would you describe yourself?"	Derogatory answers (e.g., "I don't know; not too much is worth mentioning") should raise concern.
Body Image "What aspects of your appearance do you like?" "Would you like to change any aspects of your appearance? If yes, describe the changes you would make."	Most people can identify something positive about their appearance (e.g., "I have nice eyes"). If a person cannot identify any positive characteristic, this may suggest a negative body image and poor self-esteem. Most people have something that they would like to change (e.g., "My nose is too big" or "My hips are too large"), but a long list of problem areas may suggest difficulties with self-concept.
Self-Esteem "Tell me about the things you do that make you feel good about yourself." "How do you feel about yourself?"	Statements about not having any strengths or being able to do anything well should raise concern. Statements that are very negative about the patient should raise concern (e.g., "I am hopeless" or "I have never felt good about myself").
Role Performance "Tell me about your primary roles (e.g., partner, parent, friend, sister, employee, volunteer). How effective are you at carrying out each of these roles?"	Listen for the different roles identified. A large number of primary roles increases the risk for role conflict and role overload. As with previous questions, if the patient indicates that they do not believe that these roles are adequately covered, the patient may be experiencing alterations in self-concept. Most people carry out several roles and often feel as though some of them are not adequately addressed; listen for the patient's perception about their overall role competency.

*In addition to patients' verbal responses, note any nonverbal behaviours. A negative self-concept is suggested by hesitant speech, lack of interest in what is happening, and slumped posture.

Patients' Expectations. Patients' expectations are another important factor to consider when assessing self-concept. Asking patients what they think you as their nurse can do to help is important. Collaborating with patients is essential so that interventions are acceptable to them. Asking patients how they think the interventions will make a difference elicits useful information regarding their expectations and provides an opportunity to discuss their goals. For example, while working with patients who are experiencing anxiety related to upcoming diagnostic tests, you might ask about the relaxation exercise that they have been practising. Patients' responses provide valuable information about their beliefs and attitudes regarding the efficacy of the intervention, as well as the potential need to modify the nursing approach.

◆ **Nursing Diagnosis**

Nurses need to carefully consider the assessment data to identify patients' actual or potential problem areas. Nurses should rely on knowledge and experience, apply appropriate professional standards, and observe for clusters of defining characteristics that indicate a nursing diagnosis. Although multiple nursing diagnostic labels exist for altered self-concept, the following list (Herdman & Kamitsuru, 2021) provides examples of self-concept–related nursing diagnoses:

- *Disturbed body image*
- *Caregiver role strain*
- *Disturbed personal identity*
- *Ineffective role performance*
- *Chronic low self-esteem*
- *Situational low self-esteem*
- *Risk for situational low self-esteem*
- *Readiness for enhanced self-concept*

Making nursing diagnoses about self-concept is complex. Often, isolated data could be the defining characteristics for more than one nursing diagnosis (Box 27.7). For example, a patient might express feelings of uncertainty and inadequacy. These are defining characteristics for both anxiety and situational low self-esteem. If the patient is demonstrating defining characteristics for more than one nursing diagnosis, then the nurse needs to gather specific data to validate and differentiate the underlying problem. To further assess the possibility of anxiety as the nursing diagnosis, the nurse might consider whether the patient has any of the following defining characteristics: Is the person experiencing increased muscle tension, shakiness, a sense of being "rattled," or restlessness? These symptoms may suggest anxiety rather than low self-esteem. On the other hand, if the person expresses a predominantly negative self-appraisal, including inability to handle situations or events and difficulty making decisions, then situational low self-esteem may be the more appropriate nursing diagnosis. To further aid in differentiating between the two diagnoses, information regarding recent events in the person's life and how the person has viewed themselves in the past provides insight into the most appropriate nursing diagnosis. As additional data are gathered, usually the priority nursing diagnosis becomes evident.

To validate critical thinking regarding a nursing diagnosis, it is important to share observations and allow the patient to provide input and verify perceptions. This approach often encourages the patient to provide additional data, which further clarifies the situation. In the example in Box 27.7, if you were to say, "I notice you haven't eaten very much lunch today," the response to this statement, coupled with the patient's nonverbal communication, could facilitate further discussion. An alternative approach may be to state, "I notice you jumped when I

BOX 27.7 NURSING DIAGNOSTIC PROCESS

Assessment Activities	Defining Characteristics	Nursing Diagnosis
Observe patient's behaviour during conversation.	Patient demonstrates restlessness, inability to maintain eye contact, facial tension, increased perspiration, and self-preoccupation.	Anxiety related to accidental injury, pain, uncertainty of outcome of upcoming surgery
Empathically communicate, "Tell me how you are coping" or "How are you feeling about tomorrow's procedure?"	Patient replies, "I'm scared. They may amputate my leg tomorrow. I don't know how I'll manage. I was awake all night. I just kept thinking about everything."	

Knowledge
- Principles of caring to establish trust
- Nursing interventions to promote self-awareness and facilitate change in self-concept
- Family dynamics
- Available services offered by health care providers and community agencies

Experience
- Establishing rapport with diverse patients
- Previous client responses to planned nursing interventions to enhance or support a patient's self-concept

Planning
- Select therapies that strengthen or maintain the patient's coping skills
- Involve the patient to ensure that realistic therapies are chosen
- Refer to community services as appropriate
- Minimize stressors affecting the patient's self-concept

Standards
- Maintain the patient's dignity and identity
- Demonstrate the ethics of care

Qualities
- Think independently; explore various approaches to address the issue or problem
- Be creative; be willing to try unique interventions
- Exhibit perseverance because changes in self-concept often happen slowly; continue to support the vision that change is possible

FIGURE 27.6 Critical thinking model for self-concept planning.

walked up behind you. Are you feeling uneasy today?" This statement allows the patient to verify whether they are in fact anxious and to discuss any concerns.

◆ Planning

Planning involves synthesizing knowledge, experience, critical thinking qualities, and standards (Figure 27.6). Critical thinking ensures that the nursing care plan integrates all that the nurse knows about the individual, as well as key critical thinking elements (Box 27.8). Professional standards are important to consider when developing a plan of care. These standards often establish ethical or evidence-informed practice guidelines for selecting effective nursing interventions.

A concept map is another method used to help plan nursing care. The concept map illustrated in Figure 27.7 shows the relationship between a medical diagnosis, postoperative reconstruction of severe facial scars, and the four nursing diagnoses. The concept map also links the nursing diagnoses and shows how they are interrelated. In this example, disturbed body image is related to situational low self-esteem. As the patient's facial scars improve, she should begin to feel better about her appearance.

Goals and Outcomes. In collaboration with the patient, the nurse needs to develop a plan of care for each nursing diagnosis. Goals should be established that are individualized, are realistic, and have measurable outcomes. The nurse consults with the patient to determine if the goals are perceived as realistic. By consulting with the patient and with significant others, mental health clinicians, and community resources, the nurse can design a more comprehensive and workable plan. Once a goal has been formulated, the nurse should consider how the data that illustrated the problem would change if the problem were diminished. These changes should be reflected in the outcome criteria. For example, a patient receives a diagnosis of *situational low self-esteem related to a recent job layoff*. The nurse and the patient establish a goal: "Patient's self-esteem and self-concept should begin to improve in 2 weeks." Examples of expected outcomes include the following:

- The patient will discuss a minimum of three areas of their life in which they are functioning well.
- The patient will be able to voice the recognition that losing the job is not reflective of their worth as a person.
- The patient attends a support group for unemployed individuals.

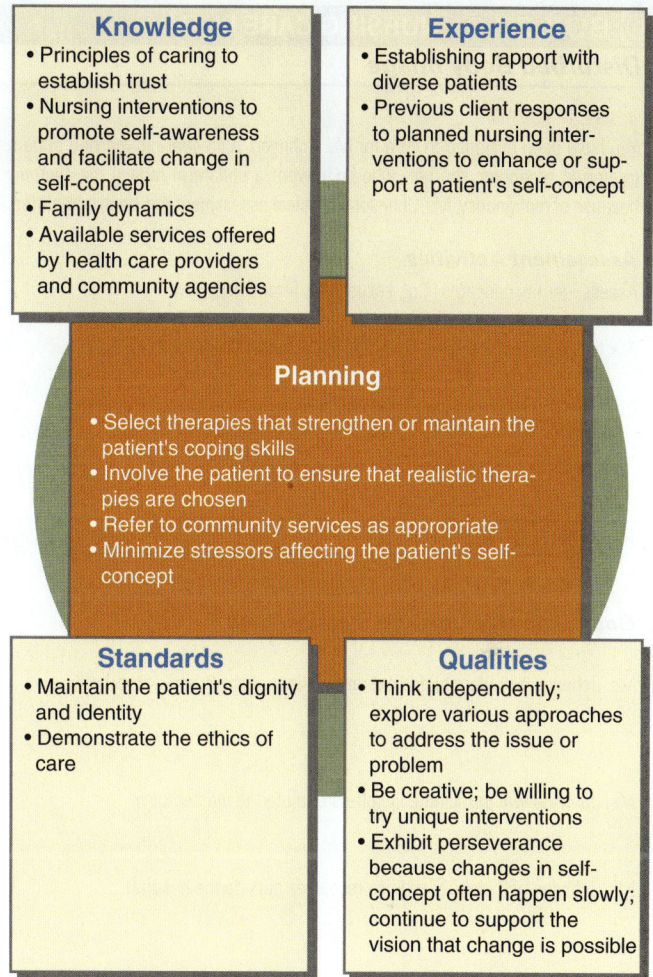

Setting Priorities. The care plan lists the goals, expected outcomes, and interventions for a patient with an alteration in self-concept. Interventions focus on helping the patient adapt and cope with the stressors that led to the disturbance in self-concept. A patient may perceive a situation as overwhelming and may feel hopeless about returning to the previous level of functioning. The patient may need time to adapt to physical changes.

Establishing priorities may include therapeutic communication to address self-concept issues to ensure that the patient's ability to address physical needs is maximized. The nurse should assess for strengths in both the patient and their family and provide resources and education to assist the patient in changing limitations into strengths. Patient teaching creates an understanding of the normality of certain situations (e.g., the nature of a chronic disease, change in a relationship, or the effect of a loss). Often, once this is understood, the sense of hopelessness and helplessness decreases.

Continuity of Care. The perceptions of significant others must be incorporated into the plan of care. Patients who have experienced deficits in self-concept before the current episode of treatment may have established a system of support that includes mental health clinicians, clergy, and other community resources. Before involving the family, the nurse must consider the patient's desires for their involvement and cultural norms regarding who most frequently makes decisions in the family.

◎ BOX 27.8 NURSING CARE PLAN
Disturbed Body Image

ASSESSMENT

You have been assigned to care for Ms. Johnson, a 45-year-old married patient (preferred pronouns: she/her) who underwent a unilateral radical mastectomy because of malignancy. Ms. Johnson's physical assessment has been completed, and she has received adequate medication for pain. You sit down to discuss how the mastectomy has affected her self-concept.

Assessment Activities	Findings and Defining Characteristics
Assess identity concerns (e.g., sexual role, femininity).	Ms. Johnson looks away, shakes her head, and states, "I don't feel feminine. My husband says it won't affect how he feels about me, but I'm sure it will."
Ask Ms. Johnson how the mastectomy is affecting her sense of self.	Intermittent eye contact, frequent crying when alone, pulling hospital gown tightly across chest
Observe Ms. Johnson's mood and interactions with others, including family members.	Has superficial conversations with staff and family members
Determine Ms. Johnson's participation in self-care activities.	Avoids looking in mirror and touching or looking at the dressing; ignoring basic hygiene (e.g., bathing, combing hair, or brushing teeth)

NURSING DIAGNOSIS: Disturbed body image related to negative thoughts and feelings to actual change in body

PLANNING

Goal (Nursing Outcomes Classification)*	Expected Outcomes
	Body Image
Ms. Johnson will identify and express feelings verbally and nonverbally.	Ms. Johnson will discuss disturbed body image with staff members and significant others within 3 days. Ms. Johnson will consider exploring support groups by the time of discharge.
	Acceptance and Health Status
Ms. Johnson will participate in self-care related to mastectomy.	Ms. Johnson will look at tissue surrounding surgical site within 2 days.
	Ms. Johnson will begin to attend to basic hygiene needs within 2 days.
	Social Involvement
Ms. Johnson will identify and use resources outside the hospital.	Ms. Johnson will verbalize commitment to participating in community resources (e.g., mastectomy support group) by the time of discharge.
	By postoperative visit, Ms. Johnson will determine whether she wishes to attend support group.

*Outcome classification labels from Moorhead, S., Swanson, E., Johnson, M., et al. (Eds.). (2018). *Nursing outcomes classification (NOC)* (6th ed.). Mosby.

INTERVENTIONS

Interventions (Nursing Interventions Classification)†	Rationale
Initially assign the same staff members to work with Ms. Johnson.	Continuity in care will facilitate the establishment of a therapeutic relationship; familiarity and trust will enhance communication.
Approach Ms. Johnson and initiate conversation; use silence and active listening to promote communication.	Ms. Johnson's ability to initially find the words for what she is experiencing may be limited.
Remain aware of your own feelings regarding Ms. Johnson's bodily changes and physical appearance.	Inadvertently communicating your own discomfort or negativity will interfere with Ms. Johnson's ability to openly communicate her feelings.
Have Ms. Johnson spend time alone and with supportive family members for crying, recording in her journal, reflection, or prayer.	This use of time encourages expression of thoughts and feelings, including depression, grief, resentment, and fear of rejection. Family involvement is an essential element of comprehensive care.
Facilitate evaluation of overall self-concept.	The effect on body image may influence other aspects of self-concept and self-esteem, including perception of identity and role performance.
Involve Ms. Johnson's husband in discussion of uncomfortable issues, such as sexual concerns.	Sexuality is a basic need and concern for both men and women, and yet it can be one of the most difficult discussions for patients to initiate.
Assist Ms. Johnson in identifying and using appropriate support systems outside the hospital, including home health care.	Support can assist the patient in feeling normal again and in integrating a new body image into her self-concept.

†Intervention classification labels from Butcher, H. K., Bulechek, G. M., McCloskey Dochterman, J. M., et al. (Eds.). (2019). *Nursing interventions classification (NIC)* (7th ed.). Elsevier.

Continued

◎ BOX 27.8 NURSING CARE PLAN—cont'd

EVALUATION

Nursing Actions	*Patient Response and Finding*	*Achievement of Outcome*
Ask Ms. Johnson how effective she feels in her ability to identify and express feelings verbally and nonverbally.	Ms. Johnson responds, "It's hard for me to talk about myself, but I have really made an effort to talk about what the loss of my breast means to me."	Ms. Johnson reports improvement in communication skills and success with discussing disturbed body image with her primary nurse and husband.
Observe Ms. Johnson's participation in self-care related to mastectomy.	Ms. Johnson assumes responsibility for basic hygiene immediately after establishing the goal and has used a mirror to examine her mastectomy scar.	Ms. Johnson has increased her independence and has begun to integrate body image change into her self-concept.
Assist Ms. Johnson in identifying resources outside the hospital; secure a commitment to use resources.	Ms. Johnson verbalizes commitment to participating in community resources (e.g., mastectomy support group).	Outcome has not been completely achieved; Ms. Johnson has expressed hesitancy in attending a support group but is receptive to care in the community. The home care nurse will ensure that the goal is re-evaluated and addressed as appropriate.

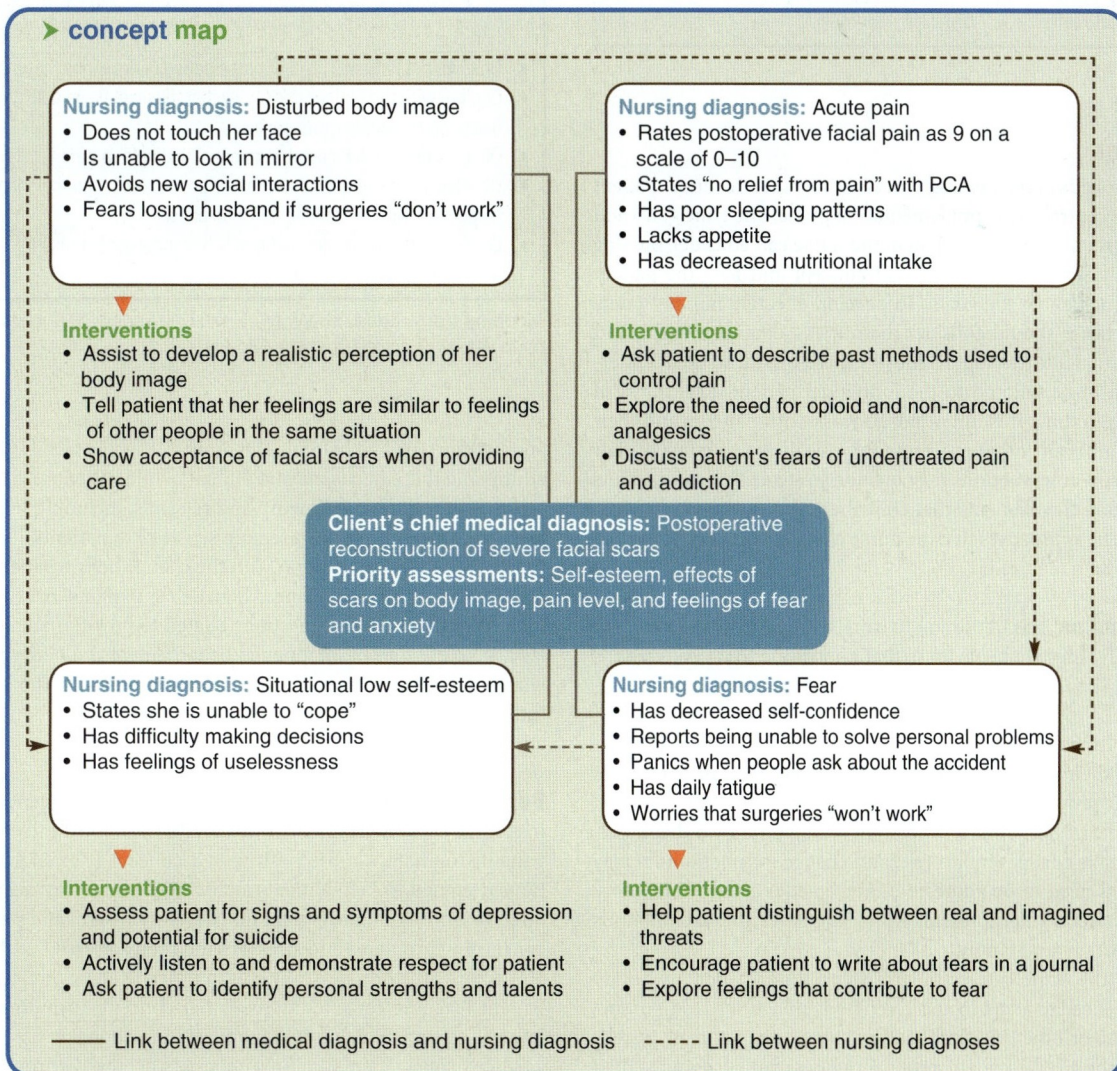

➤ concept map

Nursing diagnosis: Disturbed body image
- Does not touch her face
- Is unable to look in mirror
- Avoids new social interactions
- Fears losing husband if surgeries "don't work"

Nursing diagnosis: Acute pain
- Rates postoperative facial pain as 9 on a scale of 0–10
- States "no relief from pain" with PCA
- Has poor sleeping patterns
- Lacks appetite
- Has decreased nutritional intake

Interventions
- Assist to develop a realistic perception of her body image
- Tell patient that her feelings are similar to feelings of other people in the same situation
- Show acceptance of facial scars when providing care

Interventions
- Ask patient to describe past methods used to control pain
- Explore the need for opioid and non-narcotic analgesics
- Discuss patient's fears of undertreated pain and addiction

Client's chief medical diagnosis: Postoperative reconstruction of severe facial scars
Priority assessments: Self-esteem, effects of scars on body image, pain level, and feelings of fear and anxiety

Nursing diagnosis: Situational low self-esteem
- States she is unable to "cope"
- Has difficulty making decisions
- Has feelings of uselessness

Nursing diagnosis: Fear
- Has decreased self-confidence
- Reports being unable to solve personal problems
- Panics when people ask about the accident
- Has daily fatigue
- Worries that surgeries "won't work"

Interventions
- Assess patient for signs and symptoms of depression and potential for suicide
- Actively listen to and demonstrate respect for patient
- Ask patient to identify personal strengths and talents

Interventions
- Help patient distinguish between real and imagined threats
- Encourage patient to write about fears in a journal
- Explore feelings that contribute to fear

—— Link between medical diagnosis and nursing diagnosis   - - - - - Link between nursing diagnoses

FIGURE 27.7 Concept map for patient after surgical reconstruction of severe facial scars. *PCA,* Patient-controlled analgesia.

♥ BOX 27.9 FOCUS ON PRIMARY HEALTH CARE
Promoting Patients' Self-Concept

The focus of primary health care is to promote health and prevent illness by stressing patient education and self-care. Measures that contribute to a healthy self-concept and therefore promote health and well-being include those that support adaptation to stress, such as proper nutrition and regular exercise within the patient's capabilities; those that facilitate adequate sleep and rest; and those that reduce stress.

Nurses are in a unique position to identify lifestyle practices that put a patient's self-concept at risk or are suggestive of an altered self-concept. For example, a young adult visits a clinic with complaints of being unable to sleep and experiencing anxiety attacks. As the nurse gathering the health history, you may learn of lifestyle practices such as excessive use of alcohol or nonprescription medications, too little rest, or a large number of life changes occurring simultaneously. These data, when taken together, may suggest actual or potential self-concept disturbances. In this situation, you determine how the patient views the various lifestyle elements so that you can facilitate the patient's insight into behaviours. If necessary, you provide needed health teaching or make appropriate referrals to other community services. Patients who are experiencing threats to or alterations in self-concept often benefit from mental health and community resources to promote increased awareness. Knowledge of available community resources enables you to make appropriate referrals.

◆ Implementation

As with all the steps of the nursing process, a therapeutic nurse–patient relationship is central to the implementation phase. Once the goals and outcome criteria have been developed, the nurse can consider nursing interventions to promote a healthy self-concept and help the patient move toward achieving the goals. To develop effective nursing interventions, the nurse should consider the nursing diagnosis and broad interventions that address the diagnosis. These broad, standard interventions need to be tailored to the individual patient. Regardless of the health care setting, it is important to work with patients and their families or significant others to promote a healthy self-concept. For example, nursing interventions may include strategies to help patients regain or restore the elements that contribute to a strong and secure sense of self. The approaches that the nurse chooses will vary according to the level of care required.

Health Promotion. It is important to work with patients to help them develop healthy lifestyle behaviours that contribute to a positive self-concept (Box 27.9).

Acute Care. In the acute care setting, some patients experience potential threats to their self-concept because of the nature of the treatment and diagnostic procedures. Threats to a person's self-concept can result in anxiety or fear. Numerous stressors, including unknown diagnoses, the need to make changes in lifestyle, and change in functioning, may be present and need to be addressed. In the acute care setting, more than one stressor is often present, which increases the overall stress level for the patient and family.

Nurses in the acute care setting also encounter patients who are faced with the need to adapt to an altered body image as a result of surgery, accidents, or other physical changes. Sometimes, threats to self-concept and the need to adapt result in aggressive behaviour. Often a visit by someone who has experienced similar changes and adapted to them (e.g., someone who has undergone a mastectomy or an

BOX 27.10 PATIENT TEACHING
Alterations in Self-Concept

Objective
- Risks for situational low self-esteem will be reduced in the home care setting.

Teaching Strategies
- Reinforce the patient's expression of thoughts and feelings; clarify meaning of verbal and nonverbal communication.
- Encourage opportunities for self-care.
- Elicit the patient's perceptions of strengths and weaknesses.
- Convey verbally and behaviourally that the patient is responsible for their own behaviour.
- Identify relevant stressors with the patient and ask for the patient's appraisal of these stressors.
- Explore the patient's adaptive and maladaptive coping responses to problems.
- Collaboratively identify alternative solutions; encourage the patient to use alternatives not previously tried.
- Continue to reinforce the patient's strengths and successes.

Evaluation
- Confirm the patient's perception of and actual use of improved communication skills.
- Observe the patient's level of participation in decisions that affect care.
- Confirm with the patient and family that the increase in activities and tasks has been a positive experience.
- Observe the patient's establishment of a simple routine.
- Observe the patient take necessary action to change maladaptive coping responses and maintain adaptive responses.
- Confirm with the patient and family how new coping resources can be applied to continued change.

Modified from Stuart, G. W. M. T. (2013). *Principles and practice of psychiatric nursing* (10th ed.). Mosby.

amputation) may be helpful. The timing of such a visit is vital. Because addressing these needs may be difficult while patients are in acute care settings, appropriate follow-up and referrals, including home care, are essential. It is important to remain sensitive to patients' level of acceptance. Forcing confrontation with the change before patients are ready could delay their acceptance. Signs that patients may be receptive include patients asking questions related to how to manage a particular aspect of what has happened or looking at the body part that has changed. As patients express readiness to integrate the body change into their self-concept, the nurse can let them know about groups that are available and make the initial contact.

Restorative Care. Often, in a long-term nurse–patient relationship in a home care environment, nurses have the opportunity to work with patients to attain a more positive self-concept (Box 27.10). Interventions designed to help patients attain a positive self-concept are based on the premise that the patient first develops insight and self-awareness concerning problems and stressors and then acts to solve the problems and cope with the stressors. This approach can be incorporated into patient teaching for alterations in self-concept, including situational low self-esteem, which might manifest in the home care setting.

Increasing patients' self-awareness is achieved through establishing a trusting nurse–patient relationship that allows patients to openly explore their thoughts and feelings. A priority nursing intervention is the expert use of communication skills to clarify patient and family expectations. Open exploration can make the situation less threatening and encourages behaviours that expand self-awareness. The nurse can encourage patients' self-exploration by accepting their thoughts and feelings, by helping them clarify interactions with others, and by being empathetic. Self-expression should be encouraged and patients' self-responsibility stressed. To promote patients' self-evaluation, patients should be helped to define problems clearly and to identify positive and negative coping mechanisms. The nurse needs to work closely with patients to help analyze adaptive and maladaptive responses, contrast different alternative responses, and discuss outcomes.

Collaborating with patients to establish realistic goals involves helping patients to identify alternative solutions and develop realistic goals based on them. This collaboration facilitates real change and encourages further goal-setting behaviours. The nurse can design opportunities that result in success, reinforce patients' skills and strengths, and help the patient to obtain needed assistance. To assist the patient in becoming committed to decisions and actions to achieve goals, the nurse needs to help the patient to develop successful coping strategies. Supporting attempts that are health promoting is essential, because with each success, another attempt can be made. Supporting adaptive, flexible coping is crucial to helping a patient with an altered self-concept.

Establishing a therapeutic environment and a therapeutic relationship (see Chapter 18) and increasing self-awareness are also critical to successfully helping patients who have alterations in self-concept, whether care is focused on health promotion, dealing with an acute process, or addressing restorative care. To support patients in developing a positive self-concept, nurses must convey genuine caring (see Chapter 19) and establish partnerships with their patients to address underlying problems.

◆ **Evaluation**

Patient Care. Critical thinking is needed to evaluate success in meeting patients' goals and the established expected outcomes (Figure 27.8). Frequent evaluation of patient progress is recommended so that changes can be instituted if necessary. The nurse needs to use knowledge of behaviours and characteristics of a healthy self-concept when reviewing patients' behaviours. This method determines whether outcomes have been met.

Expected outcomes for patients with a self-concept disturbance may include nonverbal behaviours indicating a positive self-concept, statements of self-acceptance, and acceptance of change in appearance or function. Nonverbal behaviours can be key indicators of patients' self-concept. For example, patients who have had difficulty making eye contact may demonstrate a more positive self-concept by making more frequent eye contact. Social interaction, adequate self-care, acceptance of the use of prosthetic devices, and statements indicating understanding of teaching all indicate progress. A positive attitude toward rehabilitation and increased movement toward independence facilitate a return to pre-existing roles at work or at home. Patterns of interacting can also reflect changes in self-concept. For example, patients who have been hesitant to express their views may more readily offer opinions and ideas as self-esteem increases. The goals of care may be unrealistic or inappropriate as patients' condition changes. The plan may need to be revised, to reflect on successful experiences with other patients. Patient adaptation to major changes may take a year or longer, but such length is not suggestive of problems with adaptation. The nurse needs to look for signs that patients have reduced some stressors and that some behaviours have become more adaptive. Changes in self-concept take time. For some patients, the sense of hopelessness and helplessness may persist and referral to other mental health specialists may be necessary.

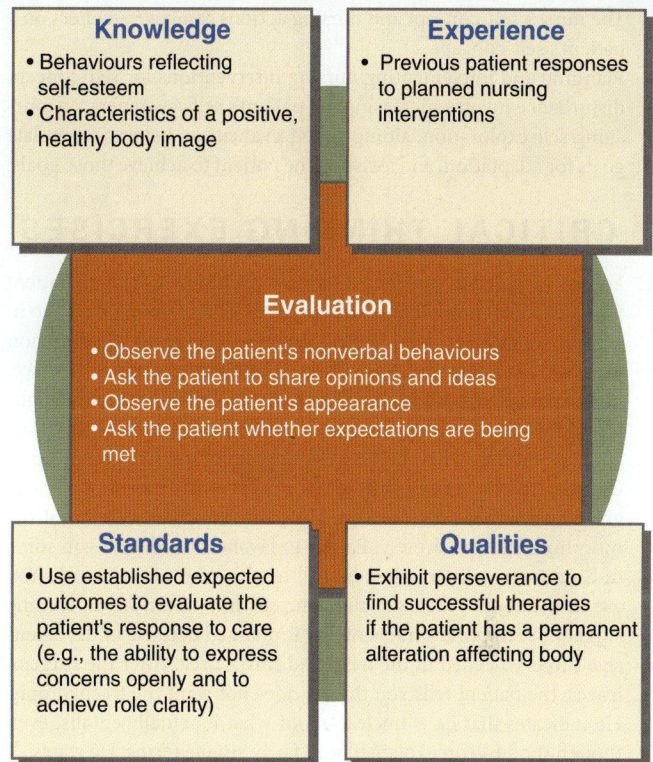

FIGURE 27.8 Critical thinking model for self-concept evaluation.

Patient Expectations. If nurses have a good rapport with their patients, patients may be able to share how things are going from their perspective. The nurse may be able to facilitate this sharing by initiating a review of what has happened over time. This offers the opportunity to share perceptions and encourages patients to consider and voice how they have conceptualized any changes.

KEY CONCEPTS

- Self-concept is an integrated set of conscious and unconscious attitudes and perceptions about the self.
- Components of self-concept are identity, body image, and role performance.
- Each developmental stage involves factors that are important to developing a healthy, positive self-concept.
- Identity is particularly vulnerable during adolescence.
- Body image is the mental picture of one's own body and is not necessarily consistent with a person's actual body structure or appearance.
- Body image stressors include changes in physical appearance, structure, or functioning that are caused by normal developmental changes or illness.
- Self-esteem is the emotional appraisal of self-concept and reflects the overall sense of being capable, worthwhile, and competent.
- Self-esteem stressors include developmental and relationship changes, illness (particularly chronic illness involving changes in what were once normal activities), surgery, accidents, and the responses of other individuals to changes resulting from these events.
- Role stressors, including role conflict, role ambiguity, and role strain, may originate in unclear or conflicting role expectations and may be aggravated by illness.

- The nurse's self-concept and nursing actions can have an effect on a patient's self-concept.
- Planning and implementing nursing interventions for self-concept disturbance involve increasing the patient's self-awareness, encouraging self-exploration, aiding in self-evaluation, helping formulate goals for adaptation, and assisting the patient to achieve those goals.

CRITICAL THINKING EXERCISES

1. You are assigned to care for a 23-year-old Chinese Canadian patient who sustained multiple fractures to his face and femur 4 days ago in a motor vehicle accident. He had surgery the evening of admission to repair his femur but was admitted to await surgery to his face. The patient lives with his girlfriend and their 7-month-old daughter and works as a custodian in the local university. He left China with his mother when he was a young child and has grown up in Canada. You have been with him for most of the morning. He was given an analgesic for his pain. His pain rating decreased, but the morphine left him drowsy. Earlier today, he shared with you some of his concerns about when he will be able to return to work. You are in the room when the surgeon tells him about his upcoming surgery. A temporary tracheotomy is planned because of the extensive surgery needed in the nasal and throat area. After the surgeon leaves, the patient tells you that he does not want the tracheotomy. He indicates that he is unclear about what it actually entails, even though the surgeon explained it in fairly simple terms. He states, "I just want to get back to normal." How would you address this comment and his lack of understanding regarding the tracheotomy?

2. A 16-year-old (preferred pronouns: she/her) is preparing for discharge from the hospital after giving birth a day earlier. She is unmarried, is uninvolved with the baby's father, and has minimal support from her family to help her care for her newborn. Before admission, she arranged to give the baby up for adoption. She reaffirms this as a good decision because she will be able to return to school and still graduate with her peers. The patient confides in you that her biggest concerns right now are how she feels about herself and how she looks. Taking into account the developmental needs of this adolescent, how will you collaborate with her to establish priority interventions to address her self-concept difficulties?

3. As a part of your community health experience, you are assigned to visit a 75-year-old patient who has gone to live with her daughter after being hospitalized for agitation and aggression secondary to Alzheimer's disease. When you go to their home, you find the 55-year-old daughter tearful. She says, "I just don't know if I can do this. She is so confused. She calls me two or three times a night but often doesn't recognize me when I come to her. I've been missing a lot of work. Even when I'm there, I'm not as productive because I'm so tired." What additional assessment data would be important to gather? What provisional nursing diagnosis could be made for the daughter?

🌐 *Answers to Critical Thinking Exercises appear on the Evolve website.*

REVIEW QUESTIONS

Review Questions 1 to 3 relate to the case study at the beginning of the chapter.

1. What are nurses assessing for when they ask Amil, "How do you feel about yourself?"
   a. Identity
   b. Body image
   c. Self-esteem
   d. Role performance

2. Which of the following questions would be appropriate to ask to assess the Amil's satisfaction and dissatisfaction associated with role responsibilities and relationships? *(Select all that apply.)*
   a. How do you feel about yourself?
   b. What are your responsibilities in your family?
   c. Are you comfortable discussing your stroke?
   d. What are your relationships like with your relatives?
   e. What changes in your body are you expecting after your stroke?

3. Which of the following would help increase Amil's self-awareness?
   a. Establishing a trusting nurse–patient relationship that allows him to explore his thoughts and feelings
   b. Accepting the patient's thoughts and feelings
   c. Helping the patient to define his problems clearly
   d. Having the patient identify his positive and negative coping mechanisms

4. When a nurse is caring for a patient after a mastectomy, interventions to promote physiological stability and pain control are necessary. What other nursing interventions would the nurse need to develop?
   a. Interventions to improve the patient's mobility
   b. Interventions to improve the patient's self-concept
   c. Interventions to improve the patient's activity tolerance
   d. Interventions to improve the patient's ability to perform self-care activities

5. Adolescents are at risk for body image disturbance. Which of the following is an accurate statement about body image?
   a. Body image is not influenced by the opinions of others.
   b. Body image refers to the external features of a person.
   c. Body image includes actual and perceived perceptions of one's body.
   d. Physical changes during adolescence are quickly incorporated into the person's body image.

6. What age group is particularly vulnerable to stressors that can affect an individual's identity because it is a time of great change?
   a. Infants
   b. Children
   c. Adolescents
   d. Adults

7. What is the possible outcome when a person does not maintain a clear, consistent, and continuous consciousness of personal identity?
   a. Identity confusion
   b. Low self-esteem
   c. Low self-concept
   d. Body image difficulties

8. Which of the following findings from a nursing assessment suggest a negative self-concept? *(Select all that apply.)*
   a. The patient avoids eye contact.
   b. The patient has a stooped or slumped posture.
   c. The patient shows independence in self-care.
   d. The patient has an untidy or unkempt appearance.
   e. The patient requests a visit from the hospital chaplain.

9. The nurse is caring for a patient after back surgery. He states, "I'm a construction worker. I won't be able to work and provide for my family." Which component of self-concept does this statement address?
   a. Identity
   b. Body image
   c. Self-esteem
   d. Role performance

10. The nurse is assessing a 16-year-old who has been diagnosed with a sexually transmitted infection. Which of the following may be associated with risk-taking behaviours such as unprotected sex?
    a. Peer pressure
    b. Poor self-esteem
    c. Social expectation
    d. Lack of information

Rationales for the Review Questions appear on the Evolve website.

RECOMMENDED WEBSITES

Canadian Centre for Gender + Sexual Diversity: https://ccgsd-ccdgs.org
This website promotes diversity in gender identity and gender expression and provides resources for education, health, and advocacy.
Canadian Mental Health Association: Children and Self-Esteem: https://reddeer.cmha.ca/wp-content/uploads/2017/04/ChildrenAndSelfEsteem.pdf
This web page offers advice about how to promote a positive self-esteem in children.
Canadian Paediatric Society: How to Foster Your Child's Self-Esteem: https://caringforkids.cps.ca/handouts/behavior-and-development/foster_self_esteem

The website provides a resource for how to foster self-esteem in children, including how to identify low and high levels of self-esteem, strategies for promoting self-esteem, and when to contact a health care provider.
Media Smarts: Canada's Centre for Digital and Media Literacy: Body Image: https://mediasmarts.ca/digital-media-literacy/media-issues/body-image
This website provides resources about how body image is represented in different media for boys and girls.
Public Agency of Canada: Parents: Feeling Good About Yourself: https://publications.gc.ca/site/eng/9.801373/publication.html
The site is a resource to help parents with strategies to feel confident and secure in their own parenting practices and to help them develop self-esteem in their children.

REFERENCES

A full reference list is available on the website for this book at http://evolve.elsevier.com/Canada/Potter/fundamentals/

28

Sex, Gender, and Sexuality

Written by Carla T. Hilario, RN, PhD, and Elizabeth Saewyc, RN, PhD, FSAHM, FCAHS, FAAN, FCAN

OBJECTIVES

Mastery of content in this chapter will enable you to:

- Define the key terms listed.
- Understand key concepts related to sex, gender, and sexuality across the lifespan.
- Describe aspects of sexual development in relation to sexual health.
- Describe a nurse's role in maintaining or enhancing a patient's sexual health.
- Assess a patient's sexual health.
- Identify risk factors in the area of sexual health.
- Compare types and causes of sexual dysfunction.
- Identify common sexually transmitted infections.
- Formulate appropriate nursing diagnoses for patients with alterations in sexual health.
- Apply critical thinking and clinical judgement to assist patients in meeting their sexual health needs.
- Select appropriate nursing interventions using clinical judgement to improve sexual health outcomes of patients.
- Evaluate patient outcomes related to sexual health needs.

KEY TERMS

Asexual

Biphobia

Bisexual

Cisgender

Cissexism

Consent

Contraception

Dyspareunia

Gender

Gender expression

Gender identity

Heterosexism

Heterosexual orientation

Homophobia

Homosexual orientation

Infertility

Intersex

LGBTQ2

Non-binary

Pansexual

Queer

Safer sex

Sex

Sexual assault

Sexual dysfunction

Sexual health

Sexual orientation

Sexual response cycle

Sexual violence

Sexuality

Sexually transmitted infections (STIs)

Transgender

Transphobia

Two-spirit

Vasocongestion

🌐 WEBSITE

http://evolve.elsevier.com/Canada/Potter/fundamentals/

CASE STUDY

Alex (preferred pronouns: they/them) is a new nurse at an ambulatory care clinic for patients with alterations in cardiac functioning. They are conducting a follow-up assessment with a patient they are meeting for the first time. The patient, Elliott, is 65 years old and had a myocardial infarction (MI) 4 weeks ago. Elliott has hypertension, which is treated with propranolol. The patient is married and currently lives with their partner, who was unable to join them for their follow-up appointment.

Alex takes the patient's blood pressure and asks if the patient has noticed any new changes since their last visit. The patient responds, "Not really. I have been taking my medications and I'm trying to exercise and eat healthy. But things have been a little difficult for my partner . . ." Alex recognizes an opening to ask the patient about their sexual health needs and says, "A common adverse effect of blood pressure medications is that it can affect sexual function. Changes in health status can also often result in stressors that can affect one's sexuality. Is this a concern right now for you?" Alex plans to begin caring for Elliott by using their clinical judgement to identify current stressors affecting the patient and their partner. Alex will select tailored nursing interventions that support the patient's adaptation to this change in sexual health status and evaluate the outcomes of those interventions. At the end of the visit, Alex provides Elliott with resources, including evidence-informed patient education materials about sexual dysfunction related to medications, suggests referrals to other health care providers, and creates a care plan to structure their next visits at the clinic.

Think about this case study as you read this chapter. There are review questions at the end of the chapter that relate to the case study.

Sexuality and its expression are vital elements to the wholeness we feel as human beings. **Sexuality** can be defined as "a central aspect of being human throughout life [and] encompasses sex, gender identities and roles, sexual orientation, eroticism, pleasure, intimacy, and reproduction" (World Health Organization [WHO], 2021). Sexuality can be expressed and experienced through thoughts, beliefs, fantasies, behaviours, practices, and relationships with others. People's view of themselves and others as sexual beings is influenced by social, cultural, legal, and historical factors, as well as religious and spiritual beliefs and practices. Sexual functioning is seen as what people *do* as sexual beings and their satisfaction with their sexual practices. Sexual dysfunction could be defined as alteration in sexual functioning that causes dissatisfaction or distress for the patient and possibly their partner.

The World Health Organization (WHO) defines **sexual health** as "a state of physical, emotional, mental and social well-being related to sexuality; it is not merely the absence of disease, dysfunction or infirmity. Sexual health requires a positive and respectful approach to sexuality and sexual relationships, as well as to the possibility of having pleasurable and safe sexual experiences, free of coercion, discrimination and violence. For sexual health to be attained and maintained, the sexual rights of all persons must be respected, protected and fulfilled" (WHO, 2021, paragraph 4). Sexual health is linked to diverse sexualities and is influenced by gender norms, roles, and power dynamics.

Nurses have a role in the promotion of positive sexuality and sexual health across the life course. Nurses can also educate patients and can provide care in response to sexual health and related outcomes, including unintended pregnancy, **sexually transmitted infections (STIs)**, sexual dysfunction, and other sequelae from sexual violence. Religious teachings, culturally prescribed gender roles, beliefs about sexual orientation, and social and environmental climates influence both the patient's and the health care provider's value systems. As a nurse, you need to explore your own beliefs, values, and assumptions and strive to develop a nonjudgmental, caring and respectful approach that integrates sexual health care into your everyday practice.

SCIENTIFIC KNOWLEDGE BASE

To assist patients in meeting their sexual needs, nurses must have a sound scientific knowledge base about sex, gender, and sexuality, including sexual orientation, sexual development, the sexual response cycle, safer sex behaviours, STIs, contraception, and abortion. As a nurse, it is also important to continue to read widely and to ask your patients about the language and terminology they would use to identify themselves. Listen to your patients for the words they would choose, what these mean to them, and how they understand their experiences. This is a key practice in providing safe and competent patient-centred care.

Sex and Gender

Sex refers to biological attributes in humans, including chromosomes, gene expression, hormone levels and function, and reproductive/sexual anatomy, that are usually categorized as female or male (Canadian Institutes of Health Research [CIHR], 2020). **Intersex** refers to "individuals whose physical sex characteristics, such as their reproductive or sexual anatomy or chromosome patterns, do not conform with typical notions of female or male sex. These patterns may become apparent at birth, may develop later (at puberty or in adulthood), or may remain unrecognized" (Government of Canada, 2020a). While previously defined as "disorders of sex development" (for example, Turner's syndrome, Klinefelter's syndrome), these patterns are more common than previously thought and are identified in an estimated 1 to 2% of births (Blackless et al., 2000). Variations in genitalia, chromosomes,

hormone levels, or pubertal development that are divergent from the commonly recognized binary of female/male sex are increasingly being recognized as normal variations in sex development (Saewyc, 2017).

Gender refers to "the socially constructed roles, behaviours, expressions and identities of girls, women, boys, men, and gender diverse people. It influences how people perceive themselves and each other, how they act and interact, and the distribution of power and resources in society" (CIHR, 2020). "**Gender identity** is not confined to a binary (girl/woman, boy/man) nor is it static; it exists along a continuum and can change over time. There is considerable diversity in how individuals and groups understand, experience and express gender through the roles they take on, the expectations placed on them, relations with others and the complex ways that gender is institutionalized in society" (CIHR, 2020). Understanding others' and one's own gender identity begins in early childhood as the child becomes aware of the sexes (female, male, intersex) and the roles within their culture around different genders.

Gender identity is most commonly consistent with physical sex at birth, which is also referred to as **cisgender**. For **transgender** and non-binary people, their physical body may not be aligned with their gender identity. Transgender people experience their gender identity differently from the gender and sex they were assigned at birth, whereas the gender identity of cisgender individuals aligns with the sex they were assigned at birth (Meggetto et al., 2019; Puechl et al., 2019). About 75 000 Canadians identify as transgender (Statistics Canada, 2020). Some people may identify as **non-binary** or as *genderqueer,* which refers to individuals whose gender identity does not align with binary notions of gender (man/woman) and may be androgynous, multiple, fluid, no gender, or a different gender (Government of Canada, 2020b).

Individuals who identify as transgender, non-binary, or genderqueer may experience barriers to accessing health care, in addition to experiences of discrimination (Puechl et al., 2019). Transgender patients have reported stigmatization, being mis-gendered, and health care provider insensitivity and incompetency as factors that contribute to poorer access and utilization of health care (Kiran et al., 2019; Puechl et al., 2019). Gender-affirming care, including hormone therapy and surgeries, involves a variety of procedures that help alter the body to better align with one's gender identity (Trans Care BC, 2021). The types of surgeries that are performed and associated costs covered in each province vary, though most provinces cover some or all of the costs for these surgeries.

Gender expression (e.g., feminine, masculine, androgynous, neutral) refers to the ways in which a person presents themselves through their outward appearance (e.g., dress, hair, makeup) and behaviours (body language, mannerisms, gait, and voice), which may be associated with gender (Government of Canada, 2020a). In many cultures, gender is organized into categories with rules about how people of different sex or genders should appear and behave, including how particular presentations are perceived to be masculine, feminine, neutral, etc. However, gender expressions are contextually and culturally bound, and some appearances may not signal the same gender. While dresses and skirts are categorized as being feminine in some cultures, for example, they are also worn by boys and men in other cultures and parts of the world, such as Saudi Arabia and Scotland. The ways that gender is expressed varies widely and may change for each individual throughout their lifetime. A person's chosen pronoun and name are also ways of expressing gender.

Sexual Orientation

Sexual orientation describes "a person's physical, romantic and/or emotional attraction to, and/or intimate relations with, individuals of a different gender, the same gender, no gender, or more than one gender"

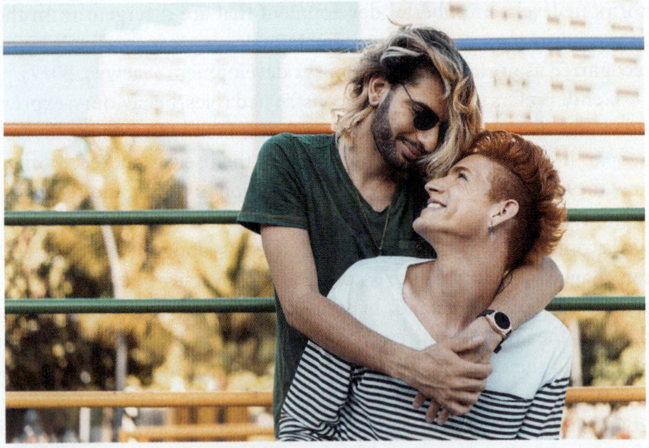

FIGURE 28.1 Gender identity and sexual orientation are fluid, changing over time. (iStockphoto/Pollyana Ventura.)

(Government of Canada, 2020a). A person's understanding of their sexual orientation may change (Figure 28.1). **Heterosexual orientation** refers to emotional, romantic, and/or sexual attraction to, and/or intimate relations with, individuals of a different gender. **Homosexual orientation** refers to attraction and/or intimate relations toward individuals of the same gender; however, the term *homosexual* can be perceived as negative in LGBTQ2 communities, and people with this orientation in Canada commonly identify as gay or lesbian (Saewyc, 2019). **Bisexual** individuals are emotionally, romantically, and/or sexually attracted to more than one gender. Some bisexual individuals may also identify as **pansexual**, who may feel physical, romantic, and/or emotional attraction to individuals regardless of their gender or sex. Some people may identify as **asexual**, which refers to individuals who do not experience sexual attraction or have interest in sexuality, although they may still have sexual and/or romantic partners (Government of Canada, 2020a).

As a nurse, you should not assume that you know your patients' gender identity or sexual orientation. You may offer to share your own pronouns (they/them, she/her, and/or he/him) when you introduce yourself if you are comfortable with doing that, and this can be an invitation for the patient to share their pronouns as well. If you learn a patient's sexual orientation, you should not assume that you may tell anyone else or include it in the medical record without the patient's knowledge. Some people might want to keep their sexual orientation confidential.

Two-spirit is "an Indigenous-defined pan-Native North American term that refers to a diversity of Indigenous LGBTQ identities, as well as culturally specific non-binary expressions of gender" (Hunt, 2018, p. 27). The term was coined by Indigenous lesbian, gay, bisexual, transgender, queer, and/or non-heterosexual (LGBTQ2) leaders at the Third Annual Intertribal Native American/First Nations Gay and Lesbian Conference in Winnipeg in 1994 (Thomas, 1997). Two-spirit is a way for Indigenous people to describe themselves in terms of embodying diverse sexualities, gender identities, roles, and/or expressions (Pruden & Salway, 2020). Two-spirit can refer to sexual orientation or gender, as well as cultural and spiritual roles within Indigenous communities, depending on the individual and the context, while at the same time challenging Western binary notions of gender and sexual orientation (Pruden & Salway, 2020).

LGBTQ2 is a term that is frequently used to refer to people who identify as lesbian, gay, bisexual, transgender, queer, questioning, or two-spirit. The term is used to help bring awareness to the needs and experiences of people who identify with LGBTQ2 communities. It refers to a number of different communities and groups of people who hold diverse and fluid sexual orientations and identities. (University of Toronto, Centre for Addiction and Mental Health, 2022). **Queer**, while seen as bearing negative and offensive connotations, is used by some sexual minority people as a label for a nonheterosexual orientation (Saewyc, 2019). Generally, however, people outside the LGBTQ2 communities should be cautious about using this term.

There are many variations of sexual orientation. Earlier thinking about sexual orientation led to the assumption that heterosexuality was normal and mentally healthy and that all other orientations were abnormal or signs of a psychological disorder. Today, this theory is rejected; scientists agree that there are normal variations in sexual orientation, and these are not associated with mental illness or abnormal psychological functioning. Those earlier views about sexual orientation reflect the perspective of **heterosexism**, which assumes that heterosexuality is the norm and that everyone is heterosexual by default, or should be. A related concept is **cissexism**, which privileges cisgender bodies and identities over transgender bodies and identities (Saewyc, 2019).

Nevertheless, prejudice and negative attitudes toward LGBTQ2 groups still exist, which can affect the extent to which these individuals choose to disclose or limit disclosure about their sexual orientation. **Homophobia** refers to "the fear, hatred, or aversion of people who experience same-sex attraction" (Government of Canada, 2020a). It is usually based on assumptions and is expressed through derogatory language, jokes, and discriminatory treatment toward individuals perceived to be gay or lesbian (Saewyc, 2019). **Biphobia** is a type of prejudice toward bisexual people, and **transphobia** refers to prejudice and hatred toward transgender individuals (Government of Canada, 2020a). These prejudices can be demonstrated through verbal harassment, discrimination, and, in extreme cases, violence toward individuals perceived to be LGBTQ2 (Saewyc, 2019).

LGBTQ2 terminology is continuously evolving, and it is important to view definitions as a starting point for learning. To help foster inclusivity, the use of gender-neutral terms can help reduce bias. For example, instead of using *husband* or *wife*, use *spouse* or *partner*, or use the term *their* instead of *him* or *her*. Organizations like the Canadian Centre for Diversity and Inclusion (CCDI) have worked to build more inclusive environments and equity for members of the LGBTQ2 communities. Issues around pay equity, spousal benefits, and job promotion have been areas where members of LGBTQ2 communities have faced discrimination in the past.

Sexual Development

As a person grows and develops, so does their sexuality. Each stage of development brings changes in sexual functioning and in the role of sexuality in relationships.

Infancy and Childhood. Beginning at early ages, young children start to explore their sexuality through various means (Balter et al., 2018; Bragg, 2020). They are socialized into cultural, societal, and familial norms through interactions with parents, caregivers, and peers. Sexual development can be influenced by the ease with which parents and caregivers are able to communicate with children in terms of their sexuality. This can include exploring their bodies and emotions, the naming of genital parts, learning about safe behaviours, and learning about gender and sex through play (such as learning about the body parts of other sexes).

Puberty and Adolescence. This is a developmental period in which social and emotional changes are also significant. Peer group attachments are strong; sexual attraction to other people is common (Figure 28.2). Often, peer groups can encourage or reinforce adolescents'

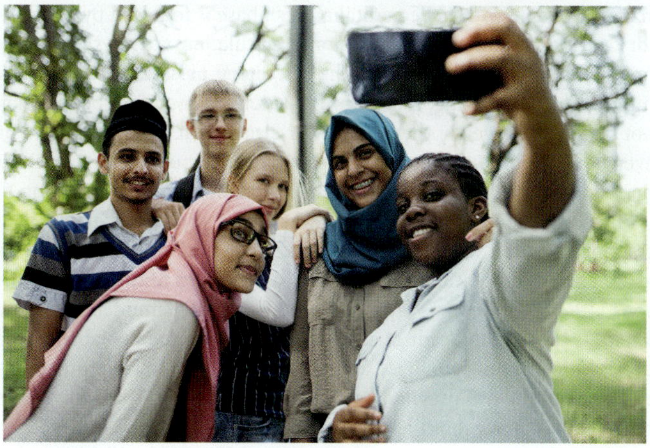

FIGURE 28.2 Adolescents with peers. Adolescents function within a network of peers as they explore their sexual orientation and gender identity. (iStockphoto/Rawpixel.)

decisions about whether or not to engage in sexual activity. Decisions about sexual activity can also be influenced as the adolescent moves from thinking concretely (where only the here and now is important) to thinking abstractly (often considering the future). Promoting safe, healthy group interactions (such as watching movies or listening to music) with adolescents of all genders as they develop can help promote healthy intimate relationships (Koch, 2020; Zani & Cicognani, 2020). Many adolescents who engage in sexual activity are influenced by the amount of sexual activity they perceive their peers to partake in, and they perceive their activities to be low risk in nature. Adolescents are often surprised to learn that far fewer of their peers are sexually active than they think and that the rates have actually been declining slightly over the past 20 years. In the British Columbia Adolescent Health Survey, for example, a large representative school-based survey of adolescent students aged 12–18 that is conducted every 5 years, fewer than one in four adolescents reported ever having sex—23% in 1998, declining to 20% in 2018 (Smith et al., 2019). Older adolescents were more likely to be sexually experienced than younger teens, with only about 2% of 12-year-olds, 16% of 15-year-olds, and 44% of 18-year-olds reporting they had ever had sex, but that is still fewer than half of 18-year-olds. A national study of 15-year-olds from the Health Behaviour of School-Age Children Survey found 22% of boys and 21% of girls in 2014 reported ever having sexual intercourse (Havaei et al., 2019), which is slightly higher than among 15-year-olds in British Columbia in 2018 (Smith et al., 2019).

Support for adolescents who have questions or concerns around their sexual health should be safe and developmentally appropriate and provide them with evidence-informed knowledge so that they can make informed choices for preventing negative health outcomes. Interventions should match the adolescent's cognitive development, address the effects of peer pressure and common misconceptions regarding sexuality, and emphasize the importance of family, friends, and extended family in building healthy relationships (Koch, 2020). Sex education is an important component of sexual health promotion by nurses. Delivering comprehensive sex education in school settings is one strategy for ensuring that adolescents have access to accurate information; however, it can be controversial in some school settings, where educators and parents mistakenly worry that sex education might encourage adolescents to become sexually active early. At the request of the Public Health Agency of Canada, the Sex Information and Education Council of Canada (SIECCAN) has recently updated national guidelines on the principles and key components of comprehensive

sex education for adolescents (SIECCAN, 2019), providing access to existing curriculum and lesson plans on their online portal. SIECCAN also provides research-based responses to questions and concerns that parents and educators might have about offering comprehensive sex education in school settings (SIECCAN, 2020).

Adulthood. While adults have matured physically, they continue to explore and define emotional maturation in relationships. Intimacy and sexuality are issues for all adults of all sexual orientations, whether they are in a sexual relationship, choose to abstain from sex, are single, are widowed, or are divorced—whatever circumstances arise. People can be sexually healthy in numerous ways.

Through middle adulthood, physical changes can affect sexual functioning. Decreasing levels of estrogen during perimenopause (during the years leading up to menopause) and menopause (after menstruation has ceased) may result in diminished vaginal lubrication and decreased vaginal elasticity. Both of these changes may lead to **dyspareunia**, which is painful intercourse. Declining levels of testosterone result in decreased desire for sexual activity. Suggestions such as using vaginal lubrication and creating time for foreplay, caressing, and tenderness can help patients adjust to normal changes related to aging. Aging can also lead to physiological changes in people with male genitalia, such as an increase in the post-ejaculatory refractory period, delayed ejaculation, and erectile dysfunction. Advising patients of these normal changes related to aging can ease concerns regarding functioning. Aging adults may also need to adjust to the effects of chronic illness, medications, aches, pains, and other health concerns that affect sexuality.

Older Adulthood. As people age, sexual practices and desires may change. For some older persons, there may be a shift in preference from genital sex to other activities that promote affection, romance, intimacy, and companionship (Figure 28.3). Many older persons continue to experience interest in sex. However, older people are often hesitant to disclose sexual concerns or to seek health care for sexual difficulties because of barriers such as cultural views about sexuality and aging, stigma, embarrassment, and discrimination (Ezhova et al., 2020). Often nurses are reluctant to initiate conversations about sexual health and sexuality with older persons, which is related to the lack of education and training of health care providers (Chen et al., 2020). Many health care providers avoid discussing issues around sex with older persons unless the issue is obvious. As well, many clinical trials around STIs do not include people from this age group. However, many issues can and should be addressed with sexually active older persons, including body image, erectile dysfunction, and STIs. Studies have shown that a number of misconceptions exist in regard to sexuality of older persons (Gianotten, 2020). At the same time, people are remaining sexually active for longer periods of time, and rates of STIs have been increasing in this population (Choudhri et al., 2018a, 2018b).

Sexual Response Cycle. The sexual response cycle in humans includes several phases or stages. Kaplan (1979) developed a three-phase model that includes the independent phases of desire, excitement, and orgasm. In Kaplan's model, emotion and cognition, which lead to the subjective feeling of desire, are an important part of sexual response. According to this model, it is possible to experience excitement without having experienced desire first. Excitement and orgasm in this model are as described in Masters and Johnson's (1966) model (discussed below).

Masters and Johnson (1966) developed a four-stage model explaining the human **sexual response cycle**. The four stages of the model are excitement, plateau, orgasm, and resolution, and they represent

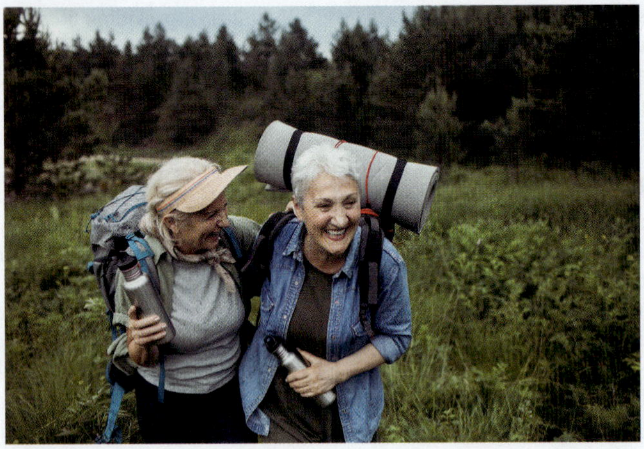

FIGURE 28.3 Intimacy and affection are important to older persons. (iStockphoto/Geber86.)

episodes of **vasocongestion** (swelling of tissues) and muscle contractions. Physical and psychological stimulation can contribute to arousal and the sexual response.

In the *excitement* stage, the heart rate and blood pressure increase, and blood flows into the sexual organs. Breasts enlarge in size, and a reddish flush may be seen over the upper torso. The nipples become more erect. Increased blood flow to the genitalia results in a variety of changes such as enlargement of the clitoris; engorgement of the labia majora, which flatten and spread outward; and swelling of the labia minora. The upper two-thirds of the vagina enlarge, and the vaginal walls thicken. The vaginal walls also secrete a fluid that allows for penetration. The penis becomes erect as blood flows into the spongy tissues. The skin of the scrotum thickens, and the testicles swell; the scrotum elevates, and the testicles move in toward the body.

The *plateau* phase is a state of advanced arousal. Blood pressure and heart rate continue to increase, and breathing may become rapid. The lower third of the vagina (at the entry to the vagina) swells. The upper vagina continues to expand, and the uterus moves into an upright position. The labia minora become more engorged with blood and become a darker colour. The clitoris shortens and withdraws below the clitoral hood. The breasts continue to increase in size. The testicles continue to enlarge. The head or glans of the penis changes to a deeper colour.

Orgasm is the phase of significant muscular contractions. During this phase, respiration and heart rates peak, and subjective feelings of intense pleasure radiate through the body. Most of the major muscles in the body contract and may go into spasm. Oxytocin is released. The pelvic muscles contract between 3 and 15 times and the muscles of the anal sphincter contract. In people with female genitalia, the vaginal walls and the uterus itself contract. These contractions are accompanied by subjective feelings of intense pleasure. In people with male genitalia, an orgasm occurs when seminal fluid is forced into the bulb of the penis by contractions of the vas deferens, the two seminal vesicles, the ejaculatory ducts, and the prostate gland. The bladder neck closes off to prevent urine from mixing with the semen. The muscles around the urethra contract, and fluid is propelled along the urethra and out of the urethral meatus. These contractions are also accompanied by subjective feelings of intense pleasure.

In the *resolution* phase, vasocongestion diminishes, and the rest of the body returns to its normal state: muscle tension is reduced within minutes, and heart rate, blood pressure, and respiration rate return to normal. During this phase, blood flow to the pelvic organs is reduced. Breasts return to their normal size and flushing of the skin disappears. The penis loses its rigidity, and the testicles and scrotum shrink in

size. For people with male genitalia, this phase is followed by a refractory period during which orgasm and ejaculation are physiologically impossible. In younger people, the refractory period may last a few minutes, but with aging, this period lasts longer, and older people may not be able to have another orgasm or ejaculation for many hours or even days. People with female genitalia may not experience a refractory period; they may have multiple orgasms with continued stimulation.

Basson (2005) described an alternative model of the sexual response cycle. It accounts for interpersonal and contextual factors, as well as physiological and biological factors as in Masters and Johnson's (1966) and Kaplan's (1979) models. In Basson's model, desire (or *libido*) is thought to occur at a variety of points in the sexual response cycle, which is conceptualized as a circular rather than linear process as described in the two previous models. Basson suggests that individuals rely on different reasons to be receptive to or instigators of sexual activity; rewards such as emotional intimacy, feelings of well-being, and lack of negative feelings resulting from avoiding sex are all factors that may cause one to feel desire. With varied motivations for sexual activity, one responds to sexual stimuli from a partner. When stimuli are received, they are processed psychologically and physically; this may then lead to subjective feelings of arousal and a responsive feeling of desire. Basson (2005) reasoned that satisfaction does not necessarily mean orgasm and suggests that for many individuals, feelings of closeness and intimacy and the partner's satisfaction may be sufficient for sexual fulfilment.

The sexual response cycle, as described in Masters and Johnson's (1966) and Kaplan's (1979) models, are limited in terms of accounting for dimensions of desire, pleasure, and sexual intimacy. Basson's (2005) model recognizes that sexual fulfillment and satisfaction can be achieved regardless of an orgasm or a particular physiological sexual response. Some people who are asexual (i.e., they do not have sexual arousal or interest) may still experience romantic attraction and intimacy.

Sexual Behaviour

Sexual behaviour typically comprises the broad array of sexual activities people participate in, such as masturbation, touching, kissing, manual stimulation of a partner, vaginal or anal intercourse or penetration, oral–genital stimulation, oral–anal stimulation, sexual excitement while looking at erotica, and telephone sex or cybersex (Society of Obstetricians and Gynaecologists of Canada [SOGC], 2021a). Wide variation in terms of sexual behaviour and practices exists between cultures and at different times in society. An inclusive attitude is that whatever people find pleasurable is "normal" as long as it occurs between consenting adults and youth, who engage in sexual behaviour by choice, in a safe environment where rules and boundaries are negotiated and respected (Box 28.1).

Safer Sexual Behaviour. Safer sex refers to sexual activities that present minimal or reduced risk for disease transmission or unintended pregnancy. The risks of sexual activities can vary. Because body fluids can be transferred between partners, unprotected sex can result in the transmission of STIs and in unintended pregnancy. It is important to understand risk based on the particular type of risk that is of concern, for example, STIs, physical injury, or unintended pregnancy.

Less safe sex refers to activities through which risk for infection, unintended pregnancy, or injury is increased. Less safe sex may include anal–penile or vaginal–penile intercourse without a condom; however, this is not always the case. For example, for people in long-term monogamous relationships who have been tested for STIs and for whom preventing pregnancy is not a concern, anal– or vaginal–penile sex without a condom may not be less safe.

BOX 28.1   RESEARCH HIGHLIGHT

A Qualitative Study of Sexuality Education for Sexual- and Gender-Minority Youth

Research Focus
This study examined contextual factors that shape sexual violence victimization and perpetration against sexual- and gender-minority youths, with a focus on the role of schools.

Research Abstract
MacAulay and colleagues (2022) conducted interviews with 50 young people aged 14–26 years who participated in the Growing up with Media survey and who reported sexual violence perpetration. Sexual violence included sexual acts without consent, sexual harassment, sexual assault, and rape. The interviewers asked the young people about thoughts and opinions about sexual violence, their sources of information, and ideas about reducing sexual violence. The study found that sexuality education in schools often did not include education about sexual violence and that if it was included, it was infrequent, incomplete, and based on binary and heteronormative assumptions regarding sex and gender that excluded sexual- and gender-minority youth. The study also found that schools struggle when it comes to intervening in sexual misconduct in learning environments, using sexist generalizations to excuse sexual harassment and often trivializing sexual violence between students.

Evidence-Informed Practice
- Schools contribute to sexual violence perpetration by not fully addressing sexual violence, especially in relation to gender and sexuality.
- When sexual- and gender-minority young people do learn about sexual violence in formal education settings, they rarely see their identities and their lives reflected in that content.
- The exclusion of sexual- and gender-minority youths in sexuality education content leaves them less prepared to navigate sexual situations.
- Being aware of binary thinking about sex and gender, homophobia, and transphobia, and being open to communicate about how these may shape the sexual health of sexual- and gender-minority young people can be an important aspect of the nurse–patient relationship and can provide some valuable assessment data.

From MacAulay, M., Ybarra, M. L., Saewyc, E. M., et al. (2022). 'They talked completely about straight couples only': schooling, sexual violence and sexual and gender minority youth. *Sex Education, 22*(3), 275–288. https://doi.org/10.1080/14681811.2021.1924142

Sexually Transmitted Infections

A number of STIs are of concern to public health and are reportable by law, including chlamydia, gonorrhea, and syphilis (Government of Canada, 2021a). There is some variance between provinces in terms of which STIs are reported and how they are reported. Nurses need to be aware of the mandatory reporting requirements in their province.

A major problem in dealing with STIs is finding and treating the people who have them. Because symptoms may be absent or go unnoticed, some people may not even know that they are infected. Sexual behaviour may include the whole body rather than just the genitalia; therefore, many parts of the body are potential sites for an STI. The mouth, tongue, and throat are commonly used for sexual pleasure. The vagina, perineum, anus, and rectum are also frequently included in sexual activity. Furthermore, any contact with another person's body fluids near an open lesion on the skin, anus, or genitalia can result in transmission of an STI.

Sometimes people do not seek treatment because they are embarrassed to discuss sexual symptoms or concerns. They may also hesitate to talk about their sexual behaviour if they believe that it is not "normal." This hesitation to seek help often hinders the detection of an STI.

Human Papillomavirus. Human papillomavirus (HPV) is the most common STI in the world according to the Society of Obstetrics and Gynaecologists of Canada (SOGC, 2021b). HPV may be manifested as external genital warts that occur on the penis, scrotum, perineum, vulva, and perianal area; they usually appear as small, hard, painless bumps. These warts can also occur in the vagina, on the cervix, inside the urethra, and inside the anus. If untreated, they may grow and develop a fleshy, cauliflowerlike appearance. Because they are caused by a virus, genital warts cannot be cured. They are treated with a topical drug (applied to the skin), by freezing, or, if they recur, with injections of medication. If the warts are very large, they can be removed surgically.

HPV is strongly linked with cervical cancer and is the leading cause of oropharyngeal cancers. HPV subtype 16 causes 90% of oral cancers, and the virus is readily spread through mucosal contact. Men have a higher incidence of oral HPV infection and HPV-related oropharyngeal cancer than women, with peaks in incidence between the ages 25–30 years and 55–60 years (Kreimer et al., 2020). HPV vaccines have been approved for the prevention of cervical cancer and adenocarcinoma in situ. In Canada, HPV vaccines are recommended for all healthy individuals who are 9 years of age and older, as well as for immunocompromised and immunocompetent HIV-infected individuals (Government of Canada, 2021b).

Chlamydia. Chlamydia is one of the most common of all bacterial STIs (SOGC, 2021a). Chlamydial infection may cause an abnormal genital discharge and burning with urination; however, it is often asymptomatic. It is treated by an antibiotic.

Chlamydia produces many serious complications in females. If undetected and thus untreated, it can progress to pelvic inflammatory disease (PID), a very painful and sometimes debilitating disease that is linked to infertility. An untreated chlamydial infection may cause scarring of the uterine tubes, which increases the risk for ectopic pregnancy and infertility. Research findings suggest that chlamydial infection can also cause another form of STI called *lymphogranuloma venerum*, also known as LGV, or venereal disease. It may also lead to miscarriage, preterm birth, and an infant's low birth weight for women who are pregnant (SOGC, 2021a).

Syphilis. Syphilis, a bacterial infection, can be transmitted through oral, vaginal–penile, or anal sex with an infected person. A pregnant person with syphilis can pass it on to their baby, which can lead to birth defects or death in the baby. Syphilis also can be transmitted through injection drug use or through broken skin or sores, although transmission by these routes is not common. Syphilis can be diagnosed with a simple blood test and is easily treated with antibiotics. If it is not treated, syphilis can affect the brain, blood vessels, heart, and bones. It can also cause death. Males older than 30 years account for the majority of syphilis cases in Canada (SOGC, 2021a), and local outbreaks are reported periodically across the country.

Gonorrhea. Gonorrhea is easily transmitted during vaginal–penile intercourse, anal–penile intercourse, and oral sex (SOGC, 2021a). Infection rates are on the rise in Canada; it is currently the second most common STI and is often found as a co-infection with chlamydia. It can affect the penis, cervix, rectum or anus, throat, and eyes. Pain during sex or during urination, or unusual discharge, may be indications of a gonorrheal infection. Gonorrhea must be treated with antibiotics.

If left untreated, it may cause serious health problems, including infertility. It can also cause blood, joint, and eye infections in a baby born to an infected individual.

Genital Herpes. Genital herpes, caused by the herpes simplex virus, is the most common manifestation of genital ulceration and is transmitted by people who have no visible or symptomatic lesions in up to 70% of cases (SOGC, 2021a). Genital herpes can cause extensive ulceration (painful blisters or open sores) with severe pain. The infection can be passed on from parent to baby during birth and can cause lesions and possibly life-threatening infections of the central nervous system for the baby. Without treatment, episodes can last for 3 or more weeks, and many people with herpes have recurrent episodes. At present, the viral infection is incurable; antiviral drugs can only control the symptoms and suppress transmission.

Human Immunodeficiency Virus Infection. In the vast majority of people living with human immunodeficiency virus (HIV) and who have access to treatment, the infection is well managed and is a chronic health condition. HIV is the virus that causes acquired immune deficiency syndrome (AIDS). The HIV virus destroys the body's ability to defend against infection. Many people do not have symptoms when they first are infected with HIV, although some may have a flulike illness within 1 to 2 weeks after exposure. More persistent or severe symptoms may not appear for 10 years or more after infection. During the asymptomatic period, however, the virus is actively multiplying, infecting, and killing cells of the immune system. As the immune system weakens, various complications occur (SOGC, 2021a).

AIDS represents the most advanced stage of HIV infection. The syndrome can result in many infections that do not usually affect healthy people. In people with AIDS, these infections are often severe and sometimes fatal. People with AIDS are particularly prone to developing cancers, especially those caused by viruses (such as Kaposi's sarcoma or cervical cancer) and those of the immune system (such as lymphomas).

In an infected and untreated person, HIV is present in the majority of body fluids. For transmission to occur, therefore, some exchange of body fluid, particularly blood, must occur. Primary routes of transmission include contaminated intravenous needles, unprotected sexual activity (anal intercourse, vaginal intercourse, and oral–genital sex), and transfusion of blood and blood products. HIV can also be spread from infected parents to their babies during pregnancy, at birth, or during breastfeeding. HIV has not been proved to be transmitted through sweat, tears, saliva, or urine.

The number of people living with HIV continues to rise in Canada. HIV affects an estimated 62 050 people in Canada, according to 2018 estimates (Government of Canada, 2020c). Approximately 20% of people who have HIV are unaware that they are infected (SOGC, 2021a). For people who are knowingly going to have sex with an HIV-positive partner or otherwise be exposed to body fluids, pre-exposure prophylaxis may be available. Post-exposure prophylaxis is also available (i.e., for needlestick injuries) but must be started within 72 hours to be most effective. In HIV-positive individuals who take antiretroviral therapy (or ART) as prescribed, this treatment can reduce the amount of HIV in their body to an undetectable viral load (200 copies of HIV per millilitre of blood) and can prevent transmission to others (Centers for Disease Control and Prevention, 2021).

Prevention of Sexually Transmitted Infections. People most likely to be infected with an STI are those who have unprotected sex. Exposure to multiple partners, or to sexual partners who have multiple partners, increases the risk of acquiring an STI. Injection drug use can also increase the risk of STI transmission when needles are shared between users who are affected by HIV. Primary prevention of STIs starts with changing the sexual behaviour that heightens the risk for infection. STIs often occur together, and screening is usually performed for all STIs at the same time. Health promotion must emphasize education and counselling regarding safer sexual behaviour.

Safer Sex and STIs. Safer sex practices and behaviour can reduce the risk of contracting and transmitting STIs, especially HIV. These practices include reducing one's number of sex partners, mutual monogamy, and using condoms and/or oral dams. When a partner is infected and untreated, or when the infection status of a partner is not known, it is crucial to practice safer sex. For vaginal–penile and penile–anal intercourse, the correct use of male latex condoms is effective for reducing STI transmission. Safer sex practices are also necessary for oral sex; if one of the partners has a vagina, a female or vaginal condom, an oral latex dental dam, or a male condom cut open to form a flat piece of latex should be placed between the other partner's mouth and the vulva before any oral contact is made. Penises should be covered with a condom before any oral contact is made (SOGC, 2021a).

Using Condoms. Condoms were originally sold to promote birth control. However, when used correctly, they also provide protection against STIs. A condom acts as a barrier to keep blood, semen, and vaginal fluids from passing from one person to another. In Canada, condoms are free at many public health clinics and readily available from drugstores and supermarkets. Condoms can be made from latex, polyurethane, or natural membranes such as sheepskin or lambskin. Latex and polyurethane condoms reduce the risk of most STIs (including HIV) and help protect against pregnancy. Natural membrane condoms do not protect against STIs because some bacteria and viruses can pass through small pores in the material (Healthwise Staff, 2021).

The female or vaginal condom is a strong, soft, seamless nitrile polymer sheath with two flexible rings at either end (SOGC, 2021a). One end covers the cervix and the other end covers part of the external genitalia. It is placed inside the vagina (up to 8 hours) before sex and prevents sperm from entering the vagina. A new condom must be used for each act of sexual intercourse. Female condoms protect against STIs, including HIV, and pregnancy, and can be purchased without a prescription.

Contraception

Contraception is a crucial facet of sexual health to avoid unintended pregnancies. Some forms of contraception require a health care provider's intervention: hormonal contraceptives (e.g., birth control pills or patch, injectable contraceptives), intrauterine devices (IUDs), the diaphragm, the vaginal contraceptive ring, and the cervical cap. Surgical procedures that provide permanent contraception are also available, such as vasectomies and tubal ligation. Other forms of contraception do not require a prescription or intervention from a health care provider: condoms, contraceptive sponges, vaginal spermicides, and fertility awareness methods (i.e., timing of intercourse in relation to the menstrual cycle). Table 28.1 summarizes some of the contraceptive choices available.

Effective contraception involves factors relating to the sexually active couple, the method of contraception, the couple's understanding of the contraceptive method, the consistency of contraceptive use, and the adherence to the requirements of the chosen method. Personal characteristics that have been identified as positively influencing contraceptive use include motivation to avoid unplanned pregnancy, ability to plan, comfort with sexuality, and previous contraceptive use (Running & Berndt, 2003). Cultural and religious background may also influence the choices people make with regard to the use of contraception.

TABLE 28.1	Available Contraceptives and Effectiveness for Birth Control	
Type	**Effectiveness**	**Description**
Penile condom	82–98%	A thin, skin-tight sheath placed on an erect penis to stop sperm from entering a partner's body. Water-based lubricants can make them more comfortable, increase sensation, and reduce the risk of breakage.
Vaginal condom	79–95%	A lubricated pouch that is placed in the vagina before penile insertion; it stops sperm from entering the vagina. It may break or slip, and some people may have difficulty placing it correctly.
Birth control pills	91–99%	Pills taken every day that contain a low dose of hormones (estrogen and progestin or progestin alone). The ovaries are prevented from releasing an egg for fertilization, eggs are prevented from implanting, and the mucus around the cervix is thickened, which makes entry of the sperm more difficult. They are available only by prescription.
Cervical cap	Previous childbirth: 68–74% No previous vaginal childbirth: 84–91%	A small, flexible cup that is inserted into the vagina before penile insertion. It covers the cervix and prevents sperm from entering the uterus. The caps are available in different sizes; proper fitting by a trained health care provider is required.
Intrauterine device (IUD) (both hormonal and copper IUD)	99.2–99.9%	A small piece of plastic or copper that is inserted into the uterus by a health care provider. Sperm is prevented from fertilizing an egg, or, if an egg is fertilized, the egg is prevented from implanting in the uterus. Some IUDs also release hormones to prevent pregnancy. IUDs can stay in place for 1–8 years.
Birth control patch	91–99%	A thin, 2 cm × 2 cm patch that can be worn on the lower abdomen, buttock, upper arm, or upper torso. The patch is applied once a week for 3 consecutive weeks; the fourth week is patch-free. The mechanism of action is the same as that of oral contraceptives.
Injectable contraceptive	94–99%	Progestin is injected into the arm or buttocks once every 12 weeks. The hormone prevents the ovaries from releasing eggs. A health care provider administers the injections.
Vaginal contraceptive ring	91–99%	A soft, flexible, transparent ring that is self-inserted into the vagina and delivers hormones over 3 weeks, after which time the ring is removed for 1 week. A new ring is then inserted.
Contraceptive sponge	Previous childbirth: 68–80% No previous childbirth: 84–91%	A soft sponge that is filled with spermicide and placed in the vagina before vaginal–penile intercourse. It is effective for 24 hours after placement. The sponge must be kept in place for 6 hours after intercourse.
Vaginal spermicides	72–82%	Gels, films, and suppositories, which contain a spermicidal agent, that are inserted into the vagina before vaginal–penile intercourse. The agent kills sperm and acts as a physical barrier to prevent any surviving sperm cells from entering the cervix. This approach may be used by individuals who are at low risk for STIs and whose partners are at low risk.
Fertility awareness method	76–95%	A female can monitor their fertility patterns and know, on the basis of daily observations of body temperature and cervical mucus, when they are most likely and least likely to conceive. They must abstain from vaginal–penile intercourse when they are most likely to conceive. This method can also be used to achieve pregnancy.
Tubal ligation	99%	A surgical procedure in which the uterine tubes are tied into a loop and then cut. This procedure is performed under general anaesthesia, and its effects should be considered permanent.
Vasectomy	99%	A minor surgical procedure in which the vas deferens that carry the sperm are cut, "tied," cauterized, or otherwise interrupted. The semen no longer contains sperm after the tubes are cut, and conception cannot occur. The procedure can be performed in a health care provider's office with a local anaesthetic. The results of this procedure should be considered permanent.

Adapted from HealthWise Staff. (2021). *Birth control.* MyHealth.Alberta. https://myhealth.alberta.ca/Pages/default.aspx

Emergency Contraception. There are two types of emergency contraception currently available in Canada: "the morning after pills" and the copper IUD (SOGC, 2021a). Commonly referred to as "the morning after pill" or Plan B, this medication is similar to regular hormonal contraception pills but taken in higher doses. The medication is available in two forms. The first is LNG-EC pills, which are available without a prescription from a pharmacy and are most effective within 24 hours of unprotected intercourse but can be taken up to 5 days after. A body mass index (BMI) of greater than 25 may decrease their effectiveness (SOGC, 2021a). The second form is UPA-EC, which remains more effective for a longer period of time (5 days) and appears to be equally effective for those who have a higher BMI. The most effective type of emergency contraception is the copper IUD, which is inserted by a physician within 7 days of unprotected intercourse. This method also provides ongoing secure birth control.

Emergency contraception is intended for use in the following situations: contraception was not used; the condom slipped or broke; missed birth control pill, patch, or injection; and in the case of nonconsensual sexual intercourse (sexual assault). It is available for free or at minimum cost at many sexual health clinics, birth control clinics, university health services, Planned Parenthood clinics, and women's health clinics. Parental consent is not required to obtain emergency contraception, and medical examination is not required.

Abortion

Since 1988, Canada has been one of the few countries without any legal restrictions on abortion. Canada has no requirements for waiting periods, parental or spousal consent, gestational limits, or restrictions on types of elective abortion. Some provinces fully fund all elective abortions; others fund only those performed in hospitals. In Prince Edward

Island, abortions became available in 2017. However, access to abortion services can be a challenge for individuals who live outside major cities. Abortion rates have been declining in Canada since 2011, with a total rate of 83 576 in 2019 (24 852 occurring in hospital and 58 724 in clinics) (Abortion Rights Coalition of Canada, 2022).

Abortion is a safe procedure, especially if performed within the first trimester of pregnancy. Couples faced with an unwanted pregnancy may consider an elective abortion. As a nurse, you can provide an environment in which the issue of abortion can be discussed openly and various options with an unwanted pregnancy can be explored. You should discuss religious, social, and personal issues in a non-judgemental manner with patients. Reasons for choosing an elective abortion vary and may include terminating an unwanted pregnancy or aborting a fetus known to have abnormalities. When abortion is chosen as a way of dealing with an unwanted pregnancy, the expecting individual, and often their partner, may experience a sense of loss, grief, or guilt or a combination of these. Guilt may surface immediately, or it may be more covert and manifest as sexual dysfunction.

Nurses must reflect on their own personal beliefs and attitudes related to abortion. The health care provider should not engage in care or in procedures that are contrary to their beliefs and values. Nurses should choose specialties or places of work that align with their beliefs and attitudes, so that the care and health outcomes of a patient are not compromised.

NURSING KNOWLEDGE BASE

In planning to help patients address sexual needs, nurses should use critical thinking skills and basic nursing knowledge. Nurses may draw from the following areas of nursing knowledge: sociocultural dimensions of sexuality; how to discuss sexual issues; alterations in sexual health (sexual dysfunction, sexual abuse, infertility); and conditions that create sexual health concerns (pregnancy, surgery, illness, disability).

Sociocultural Dimensions of Sexuality

Sexuality is influenced by cultural norms and expectations that determine acceptable behaviour and practices within a culture. Society plays a powerful role in shaping sexual values and attitudes and in supporting specific expression of sexuality in its members. Each cultural and social group has its own set of rules and norms that guide the behaviour of its members. These rules become an integral part of an individual's thinking and underlie sexual behaviour; they include, for example, how people find partners, their choices of partners, how they relate to one another, how often they have sex, and what they do when they have sex.

It is widely suggested that nurses include information about sexual health and the implications for sexuality when they care for patients. Nurses should also routinely ask patients whether they have any sexual concerns related to their condition or treatments. However, this question is frequently omitted, and a valuable opportunity to be proactive and holistic in the care provided is thus missed (Fennell & Grant, 2019). Moreover, missing this aspect of health can lead to negative health outcomes. Some nurses may not be engaging in conversations about sexual health with patients because of lack of knowledge about and discomfort with discussing sexual health, or because of attitudes among nurses that sexual health care is a private issue (Fennell & Grant, 2019). Some nurses may feel that asking about sexuality might make patients feel uncomfortable, or they may believe that it is another health care provider's responsibility (Åling et al., 2021). Beliefs and attitudes toward age, gender, and sexual identity can also be a barrier for discussions around sexuality and sexual health. Some nurses continue to consider older patients as uninterested in sex and find it more challenging to have these discussions with patients of different genders and sexual orientations (Åling et al., 2021). Some nurses may presume that because of the seriousness of the patient's disease or because of the patient's stage of life, sexuality is not an important issue for them. As a result, sexual health issues may not be assessed in a timely way, leading to missed opportunities for early intervention and appropriate care.

Discussing Sexual Issues

Sexuality is a significant part of each person's being; however, as stated earlier, sexual assessment and interventions are not always included in health care. The area of sexuality can be emotionally charged for nurses as well as for patients. Discomfort with talking about sexual issues, lack of information, and differences between a patient's values and the nurse's values may prevent the nurse from discussing issues of sexuality with patients. The most valuable tool that nurses can develop for providing care in areas of sexuality is effective, nonjudgemental communication. If you as a nurse have difficulty discussing topics related to sexuality, you should understand why, and you should develop a plan for addressing your discomfort.

Discussing matters of a sexual nature can also be embarrassing for patients. Often, patients do not mention sexual health issues; they may worry about looking stupid, using incorrect words, or being offensive, or they may simply have no way of describing their concerns. It is crucial that nurses be comfortable in asking questions about sexuality and in responding to issues that arise from such questioning. By using a perceptive and educated approach to talking about sexuality, nurses can offer the support that many patients require.

Effective communication about sexuality requires caring, sensitivity, tact, compassion, the use of appropriate language, and nondiscriminatory attitudes. When talking with patients about sexuality, it is important not to have preconceived notions about their sexual orientation or sexual activities. LGBTQ2 people may not receive adequate health care if health care providers assume patients have a heterosexual orientation and fail to obtain complete sexual histories. Older persons' sexual health may also be overlooked if health care providers stereotype these patients as asexual.

When talking with patients about sexuality nurses also need to take into account consent. **Consent** is described as the voluntary agreement to engage in sexual activity and can be demonstrated verbally or by a person's conduct without undue pressure; the person must be capable of consent. In Canada, the legal age of consent to sexual activity is 16 years old. A person who is under 16 years of age cannot consent to sexual activities with someone 5 or more years older than them; if under 14 years of age, the person is unable to consent to sexual activity with someone who is 2 or more years older than they are (Department of Justice, 2017).

Alterations in Sexual Health

Sexual Violence. Sexual violence is defined as an "act committed against someone's sexual integrity without that person's freely given consent. It can be physical or non-contact, affects all ages and genders, and the person committing the act may be known or a stranger" (Government of Alberta, 2022). Sexual violence is a widespread health problem and includes, but is not limited to, sexual abuse, sexual assault, rape, incest, childhood sexual abuse, sexual harassment, stalking, cyber-harassment, trafficking, and sexual exploitation (Government of Ontario Ministry of Children, Community and Social Services, 2021). In Canada, about one in three women and one in eight men experience sexual violence (Government of Ontario Ministry of Children, Community and Social Services, 2021). Most often, this abuse is perpetrated by a former intimate partner or by a family member.

Sexual Abuse. Sexual abuse has far-ranging effects on physical and psychological functioning (Sabella, 2016). Increasingly, sexual abuse is occurring through the Internet: sexual predators recruit victims on social networking sites and then arrange to meet the victims, after which the abuse begins. In Canada, nurses are required by law to report suspected child abuse to child protection authorities (Smith et al., 2020).

Evidence of sexual abuse in children may be uncovered during history taking or physical examination (see Chapter 33). Symptoms that should raise suspicion of sexual abuse include a child showing an early, exaggerated awareness of sex or exhibiting seductive behaviour toward adults; swelling or bruising of the external genitalia, anus, breasts, or buttocks; lacerations of or a foreign substance in the vagina or anus; and an STI in a child younger than 15 years. Signs and symptoms of sexual abuse are listed in Box 28.2.

When sexual abuse is recognized, support needs to be mobilized for the victim and the family. All family members may require therapy, particularly in situations of incest, to address issues of safety and recovery for the victim and the family members. Rape victims may need to address the mental and emotional impacts of the trauma before feeling comfortable with intimate interactions or relationships. The victim's partner may need support in understanding this process and ways to assist the victim. Children who have been sexually abused need to understand that they are not at fault for the incident. The parents must understand that their response is critical to how the child reacts and adapts. As a nurse, you may come in contact with patients confronting these stressors. You can use your position to assess occurrences of sexual violence and to educate individuals about community services. You should be aware of resources for referral and support in the community where you work.

Sexual assault occurs when a person is touched in a sexual nature *without consent*, and it may involve physical force or a position of authority against another person (Royal Canadian Mounted Police [RCMP], 2021). Sexual assault can involve unwanted sexual activity (including penetration or attempted penetration of the mouth, vagina, or anus) touching, and kissing. Consent refers to a freely given agreement from all persons involved to take part in a sexual activity and it must be given every single time for the activity to be consensual (RCMP, 2021). In Canada, the legal age of consent is 16 years of age.

According to the Department of Justice Canada (2019), the majority (83%) of sexual assaults are not reported to police, with only 5% reported and fewer than half of reported cases resulting in a finding of guilt. Women experience a higher rate of victimization, especially in the 15- to 24-year age group. In over half of sexual assault incidents, the assailant was known to the victim (Department of Justice Canada, 2019).

In the digital era, sexting (*sex + texting*) has emerged has a component of intimate and sexual interactions. *Sexting* refers to the sharing of sexually suggestive or explicit messages, photographs, or videos, including nude or nearly nude images, through electronic devices. An estimated one in four emerging adults (18 to 29 years old) engage in sexting, which indicates that it is a common behaviour, particularly in young adulthood (Mori et al., 2020). In youth younger than 18 years old, the average prevalence for sending and receiving sexts have been found to be 15% and 27%, respectively, and 12% (or one in eight youth) have reported forwarding a sext without consent (Madigan et al., 2018). While many who participate in sexting view it as being satisfying (i.e., providing immediate gratification) and safer than sex (no chance of developing an STI or getting pregnant), there are potential health implications. Among youth, engaging in sexting (either sending or receiving) has been linked to higher levels of mental health issues (Kim et al., 2020) as well as in substance use and sexual behaviours

> **BOX 28.2 Signs and Symptoms That May Indicate Current or Previous Sexual Abuse**
>
> - Trauma or injury (such bruises, scars, chafing, or bite marks) to the genital or anal areas
> - Pain to breasts, genital, or anal areas
> - Vaginal discharge or bleeding
> - Rectal discharge or bleeding
> - Anal tears or dilation
> - Trauma to mouth and throat, including petechiae of the oral cavity
> - Symptoms of a sexually transmitted infections
> - Pregnancy
> - Post-traumatic stress, depression, anxiety, and other mental health conditions
>
> Adapted from Healthwise Staff. (2019). *Sexual abuse: Signs and symptoms.* MyHealth.Alberta https://myhealth.alberta.ca/Health/Pages/conditions.aspx?hwid=not34212

(i.e., sexual activity, multiple sexual partners, lack of contraception use) (Mori et al., 2019). Educational campaigns have focused on increasing awareness around safety, security, and potential harm in the digital era of interpersonal communication.

Sexual Dysfunction. **Sexual dysfunction** is a common, complex condition that arises because of biological, psychological, and social factors and can be categorized using *Diagnostic and Statistical Manual of Mental Disorders*, 5th edition, text revision *(DSM-5-TR)* classifications (Table 28.2). Although sexual dysfunction is prevalent, affecting an estimated 30 to 40% of the general population, these conditions are frequently under-recognized and under-diagnosed in clinical settings (Avasthi et al., 2017). Sexual difficulties and dysfunction have been associated with heart disease, diabetes, cancer, and mental illness.

For most people, sexual dysfunction can have a significant impact on their sexual and mental health, as well as on their relationships. Sexual dysfunction can usually be treated with either medical interventions (mostly pharmacological) or psychological interventions (e.g., cognitive and behaviour change methods). A symptom-based approach, for example, can be used to organize the assessment and care of women experiencing sexual dysfunction with the aim of providing care to address sexual pain, low desire, low arousal, and orgasmic dysfunction, which are also aligned with the *DSM-5* classifications of female sexual dysfunction (Krakowsky & Grober, 2018).

Low desire is the most common sexual difficulty reported, particularly among people with female genitalia (Quinn-Nilas et al., 2018). Despite considerable research, sexual desire is poorly understood. Medical conditions including depression, stress, and fatigue affect sexual desire. Painful intercourse is another common sexual dysfunction. Sexual pain disorders have been linked to anxiety and depression and disturbed body image, a sense of isolation, and lower arousal and frequency of intercourse and sexual dissatisfaction (Lakshmi & Khan, 2019). An estimated 40% of reproductive age females are affected by sexual dysfunction (McCool et al., 2016), including sexual interest/arousal disorder, female orgasmic disorder, and genitopelvic pain/penetration disorder according to the diagnostic criteria of the *DSM-5* (American Psychiatric Association, 2013). Consistent risk factors for female sexual dysfunction include poor physical health, poor mental health, genitourinary conditions, sexual abuse, and religious concerns, while protective factors include physical activity, positive body image, sex education, and older age at marriage (McCool et al., 2018).

TABLE 28.2 Types of Sexual Dysfunction

Category	Type*	Definition
Sexual desire disorders	Hypoactive sexual desire disorder	Persistent or recurrent deficiency or absence of sexual fantasies and desire for sexual activity
	Sexual aversion disorder	Persistent or recurrent extreme aversion to, and avoidance of, all or almost all genital sexual contact with a sexual partner
Sexual arousal disorders	Female sexual arousal disorder	Failure to attain or maintain the lubrication-swelling response or to experience a subjective sense of sexual excitement and pleasure during sexual activity
Male erectile dysfunction		Persistent or recurrent inability to attain an adequate erection or to maintain an adequate erection until completion of the sexual activity
Orgasmic disorders	Female orgasmic disorder (anorgasmia)	The recurrent and persistent inhibition of the female orgasm, as manifested by the absence or delay of orgasm after a period of sexual excitement the clinician judges adequate in intensity and duration to produce such a response
	Male orgasmic disorder (retarded ejaculation)	Persistent or recurrent delay in, or absence of, orgasm after a normal sexual excitement phase during sexual activity that the clinician, taking into account the age of the patient, judges to be adequate in focus, intensity, and duration
	Male orgasmic disorder (premature ejaculation)	Persistent or recurrent ejaculation with minimal sexual stimulation before, upon, or shortly after penetration and before the individual wishes it
Sexual pain disorders	Dyspareunia	Recurrent or persistent genital pain before, during, or after sexual intercourse that is not associated with vaginismus or with lack of lubrication
	Vaginismus	An involuntary constriction of the outer third of the vagina that prevents penile insertion and intercourse
Sexual dysfunction resulting from drug use or diseases		Sexual dysfunction judged to be caused by the direct physiological effects of a general medical condition or use of a substance

*According to American Psychiatric Association. (2013). *Diagnostic and statistical manual of mental disorders* (5th ed.). Author.

For people with male genitalia, one of the most common types of sexual dysfunction is erectile dysfunction. Erectile dysfunction, which is the repeated inability to achieve or maintain an erection, affects between 3 and 77% of the population worldwide and is associated with increasing age and with health conditions such as cardiovascular disease, benign prostatic hyperplasia, and dementia (Kessler et al., 2019) and with unhealthy lifestyle (Allen & Walter, 2019). Erectile dysfunction itself might be a warning sign of undiagnosed cardiovascular disease.

Infertility. Infertility is the inability of a couple to conceive after 1 year of unprotected intercourse; it affects one in six couples. Generally, infertility is caused by either hormonal or structural causes, including fallopian tube damage and sperm dysfunction. Primary care nurses often provide support and education around obesity management, smoking cessation, and alcohol and drug use, all of which can affect fertility. Treatment for infertility depends on the cause and may include medication, surgery, assisted reproductive technology, or a combination of these (Cunningham, 2017).

Choices for the infertile couple include medical assistance with fertilization, adoption, or exploring the possibility of remaining childless. Nurses can give emotional support and refer couples to infertility support groups that can provide couples with further emotional and educational help.

Patients With Particular Sexual Health Concerns

Pregnant and Postpartum Individuals. Sexual interest tends to fluctuate during pregnancy; it increases during the second trimester and often decreases during the first and third trimesters. The decrease in libido during the first trimester may be caused by nausea, fatigue, and breast tenderness. During the second trimester, blood flow to the pelvic area is increased to supply the placenta, and sexual enjoyment and libido accordingly increase. During the third trimester, increased abdominal size may make finding a comfortable position difficult.

Sexual health concerns are common during pregnancy, with sexual distress affecting about 40% of pregnant people (Vannier & Rosen, 2017). Some pregnant people refrain from sex because they are worried it could harm their pregnancy, and this fear is associated with greater sexual distress (Beveridge et al., 2018). In a healthy pregnancy, sexual activity is not associated with harm to a fetus, including miscarriage, except among individuals with a history of preterm labour or placenta problems (Public Health Agency of Canada, 2022). Most couples resume sexual activities within the first year of their baby's life.

Patients Recovering From Surgery. Surgeries that result in disfigurement, especially of the face, breasts, genitalia, and reproductive organs, can affect a patient's self-image and sexuality. The effects of surgery, whether temporary or permanent, are often not fully anticipated and may not be fully manifested until after discharge from the hospital. Patients' partners might also have adjustments to make and may find it difficult to resume sexual activity. Coping with anxiety, fear, or depression about the surgery is essential. Health care providers need to be prepared to discuss sexual health concerns with patients in providing pre- and postsurgical care (Marsh et al., 2020). Patients who have had ileostomies, colostomies, or urostomies are particularly concerned about possible loss of control, unpleasant smells or sounds, seepage or broken bags, and their partners' responses (see Chapter 45). Peri- and postoperative counselling and support are essential for these patients.

Patients With Illness or Disabilities. Illness and disability often affect sexuality and sexual health. During periods of illness, individuals may experience major physical changes, the effects of medications or treatments, the emotional stress of a prognosis, concern about future functioning, and separation from significant others. Situational stressors could include a heart attack (myocardial infarction), cancer diagnosis and treatment, or chronic disease such as diabetes, multiple sclerosis, or Parkinson's disease. In some instances, patients may wrongly believe that their condition prohibits sexual activity, or they may need some guidance to promote satisfactory sexual functioning. Nurses should not assume that sexuality and sexual functioning is not a health concern for individuals who are living with illness (O'Connor et al., 2019).

Many myths are prevalent about people living with a disability or different abilities, including the idea that they are asexual or somehow different (Addlakha et al., 2017; Loeser et al., 2018). Long-term disability can have profound effects on a person's sense of sexuality and sexual function. Congenital or birth impairments commonly affect sexual development; for example, for people with disabilities who require assistance in activities of daily living, the resulting lack of privacy and independence may affect their ability to engage in sexual activities. Acquired disabilities may have different implications: impairments sustained in youth may bring about low social and sexual confidence, and people who sustain disabilities as adults may be far more aware of what they have lost. It is important that health care providers validate sexuality in individuals with disabilities. Nurses can do this by sensitively initiating conversations about sexual function and safer sex practices.

CRITICAL THINKING

Successful critical thinking requires synthesis of knowledge, experience, information gathered from patients, critical thinking qualities, and intellectual and professional standards. Clinical judgement requires nurses to anticipate the information necessary, analyze the data, and make appropriate decisions regarding patient care. Figure 28.4 depicts numerous critical thinking elements, as well as patient assessment data, that contribute to appropriate nursing diagnoses regarding sexuality.

In the case of sexuality, nurses need to integrate knowledge from nursing and other disciplines. Nurses must have a good understanding, for example, of the human sexual response cycle, safer sex practices, and sexual health concerns, as well as solutions to these, to anticipate how to assess a patient and then how to interpret findings. Previous experience in caring for patients whose sexuality becomes threatened can help nurses approach the next patient in a more reflective and helpful way. Patients may have customs and values different from those of the nurse. Professional standards require that nurses respect each patient as an individual.

❖ SEXUALITY AND THE NURSING PROCESS

As stated earlier, a person's sexuality has physical, psychological, social, and cultural elements. Nurses must assess all relevant elements to determine a patient's sexual well-being. Nurses should build a sound knowledge base and be willing to explore personal issues regarding sexuality. The nursing role in addressing sexual concerns can range from ongoing assessment to providing information to counselling to referral.

◆ Assessment
Factors Affecting Sexuality. In gathering a sexual history, nurses should consider physical, functional, relationship, lifestyle, and self-esteem factors that may influence sexual functioning.

Sexual Health History. When taking a health history, it is good to include a few questions related to sexual functioning to determine whether the patient has any sexual concerns (Fennell & Grant, 2019). Nurses can incorporate these questions in the review of systems and address them in a routine, matter-of-fact manner. Any mention a patient makes of sexual activity offers a good opportunity to open a discussion about this topic. The nurse should use language that is appropriate to the age and educational level of the patient and that is

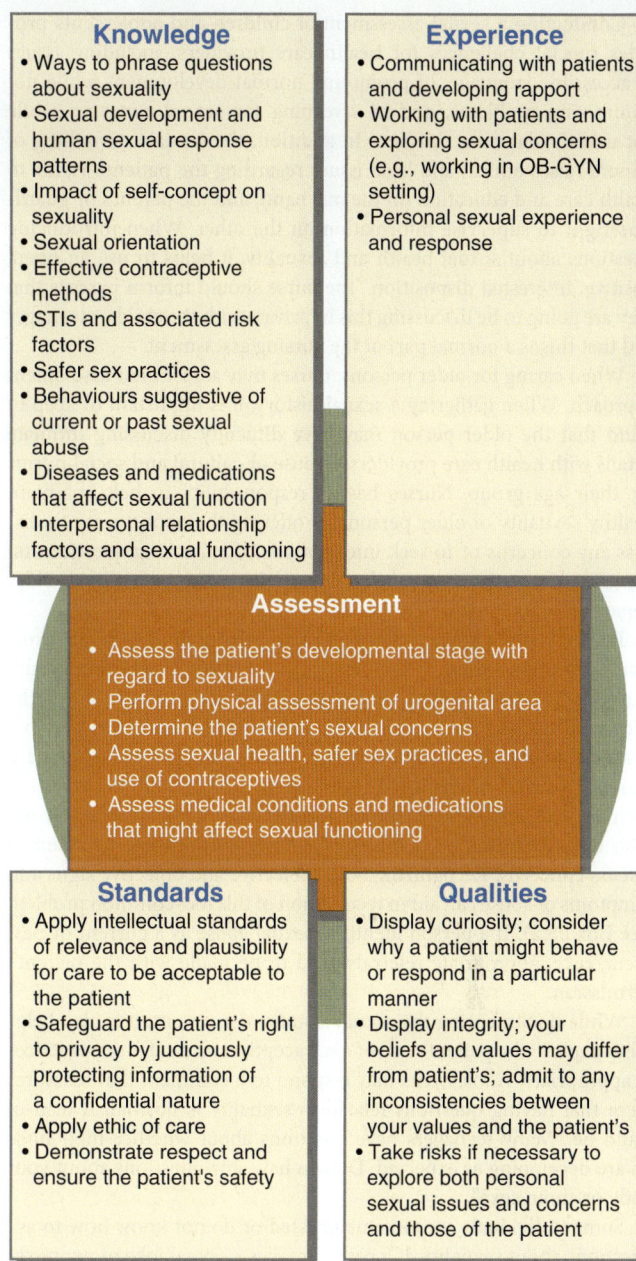

Knowledge
- Ways to phrase questions about sexuality
- Sexual development and human sexual response patterns
- Impact of self-concept on sexuality
- Sexual orientation
- Effective contraceptive methods
- STIs and associated risk factors
- Safer sex practices
- Behaviours suggestive of current or past sexual abuse
- Diseases and medications that affect sexual function
- Interpersonal relationship factors and sexual functioning

Experience
- Communicating with patients and developing rapport
- Working with patients and exploring sexual concerns (e.g., working in OB-GYN setting)
- Personal sexual experience and response

Assessment
- Assess the patient's developmental stage with regard to sexuality
- Perform physical assessment of urogenital area
- Determine the patient's sexual concerns
- Assess sexual health, safer sex practices, and use of contraceptives
- Assess medical conditions and medications that might affect sexual functioning

Standards
- Apply intellectual standards of relevance and plausibility for care to be acceptable to the patient
- Safeguard the patient's right to privacy by judiciously protecting information of a confidential nature
- Apply ethic of care
- Demonstrate respect and ensure the patient's safety

Qualities
- Display curiosity; consider why a patient might behave or respond in a particular manner
- Display integrity; your beliefs and values may differ from patient's; admit to any inconsistencies between your values and the patient's
- Take risks if necessary to explore both personal sexual issues and concerns and those of the patient

FIGURE 28.4 Critical thinking model for sexuality assessment. *OB-GYN,* Obstetrical-gynecological; *STIs,* sexually transmitted infections.

culturally safe, as the patient may be hesitant to talk to a nurse who is much older or younger than the patient, is of a different gender, or from a different cultural or ethnic background. Asking open-ended questions will help encourage patients to ask questions and use words they are comfortable with. Nurses need to let patients know that they are about to ask a few questions to obtain a sexual health history and that these questions are asked of all patients, as this can assure patients that the questions are routine.

When taking a sexual health history, it is beneficial to think of the five Ps:
- **P**artners
- **P**ractices
- **P**rotection from STIs
- **P**ast history of STIs
- **P**revention of pregnancy

Conducting a sexual assessment of children and adolescents provides special challenges for health care providers, including issues of accessible language, of promoting normal development while not minimizing problems, and of screening for sexual concerns while not unduly alarming children. In addition, the sexual counselling of minors raises ethical and legal issues regarding the patient's rights to health care and education on the one hand, and the parent's or guardian's right to supervise information on the other. When introducing questions about sexual health and sexuality, it helps to use an open, positive, interested disposition. The nurse should inform parents that they are going to be discussing this in private with the child or teenager and that this is a normal part of the nursing assessment.

When caring for older persons, nurses may adjust their assessment approach. When gathering a sexual history, it is important to keep in mind that the older person may have difficulty discussing intimate details with health care providers because of cultural and social norms for their age group. Nurses have a responsibility to help maintain healthy sexuality of older persons by offering the opportunity to discuss any concerns or to seek information. Often, asking questions on the topic of sexuality in a comfortable, relaxed manner facilitates older persons' discussion of their sexual needs.

Because of the prevalence of intimate partner violence and sexual abuse, questions relating to abusive relationships can be important. Questions that address intimate partner violence or abuse should be addressed to the patient in private. A question such as "Are you in a relationship in which someone is hurting you?" may encourage a patient to reveal current or previous abuse. An additional question such as "Has anyone ever forced you to have sex when you did not wish to participate?" may more specifically encourage the patient to discuss concerns. Recognizing both subjective and objective signs and symptoms of abuse can aid in recognition of this too-common problem (see Box 28.2). If a person identifies sexual abuse as a current or past occurrence, appropriate referrals need to be made with the patient's permission.

While documenting the sexual history of a patient, it is also helpful to explore the patient's use of contraceptives and safer sex practices as appropriate. Adolescents may respond to a comment that reassures them that having questions related to sexuality is normal. A lead-in could be "Many teenagers have questions about whether their bodies are developing as expected. Do you have any questions about your body or about sex?"

Some individuals are too embarrassed or do not know how to ask questions about sexuality. If a patient makes a sexual joke or expresses concern about relations with a partner, they may have questions. Observing for and listening to concerns about sexuality takes practice. With experience, you will develop skill in clarifying and paraphrasing to help patients express their sexual concerns. By including sexuality in the health history, you are acknowledging that sexuality is an important part of health and creating an opportunity for the patient to discuss sexual concerns.

Physical Assessment. The physical examination is important in evaluating the cause of sexual concerns or problems; however, this is beyond the scope of the generalist nurse and more appropriate for the advanced practice nurse or physician. Talking about sexuality at the time of the genital examination is not appropriate and can be misconstrued by the patient and may make them feel uncomfortable. Discussions about sexuality are best held when the patient is fully clothed and sitting comfortably in a private room.

Patient Expectations. As in the case of any patient assessment, it is important to understand the patient's expectations regarding their

BOX 28.3 NURSING DIAGNOSTIC PROCESS

Assessment Activities	Defining Characteristics	Possible Nursing Diagnosis
Observe readiness to discuss sexual concerns through verbalization (e.g., "When can I return to life as normal?" or "There goes my love life") or behaviour (e.g., exhibitionism).	Patient verbalizes concern that sexual activity may cause another myocardial infarction or death.	Ineffective sexuality patterns related to fear of recurrent myocardial infarction
Ask patient and spouse about previous level and method of sexual expression (e.g., frequency, initiator).		Ineffective relationship related to reported sexual dissatisfaction between partners
Observe for affectionate behaviour (e.g., touching, hand holding, kissing).	Patient's spouse exhibits reluctance to touch patient.	Ineffective relationship related to reported sexual dissatisfaction between partners
In privacy, ask spouse about perceptions of patient's recovery and return to full functioning.	Spouse verbalizes concern that patient will need continuous care, attention, and protection.	Anxiety
Observe for facial expressions and gestures that may indicate anxiety (e.g., hand wringing).	Patient maintains eye contact, shifts position frequently.	Anxiety

care. Questions such as "What would you like to have happen in regard to [expressed concern]?" and "What initial steps might you take?" can help the person identify desired outcomes. It is important for the nurse to set aside personal views and not assume what a patient's expectations might be.

Nursing Diagnosis

After completing an assessment and applying critical thought to the diagnostic process (Box 28.3), the nurse selects diagnoses applicable to the patient's needs. Possible nursing diagnoses related to sexual functioning (Ackley et al., 2020) are as follows:

- *Sexual dysfunction* related to insufficient knowledge about sexual function
- *Sexual dysfunction* related to altered body function
- *Sexual dysfunction* related to altered body structure, tissue trauma
- *Sexual dysfunction* related to painful intercourse
- *Ineffective relationship* related to reported sexual dissatisfaction between partners
- *Anxiety*
- *Chronic sorrow* related to loss of ideal sexual experience, altered relationships
- *Risk for situational low self-esteem*: Risk factor: alteration in body function
- *Ineffective sexuality pattern*

Clues that may signal risk or an actual nursing diagnosis related to sexuality include a history of surgery involving the reproductive organs, changes in appearance, past or current physical or sexual abuse, chronic illness, and developmental milestones such as puberty or menopause. Before making nursing diagnoses related to sexual dysfunction, the nurse must first assess anatomical, physiological, sociocultural, and situational issues thoroughly.

When making a nursing diagnosis regarding sexuality, the nurse must clarify with the patient that the defining characteristics do in fact exist and that the patient perceives a concern with regard to sexuality. Determining the etiological or contributing factors is important in order to focus effective planning and to select appropriate nursing interventions. For example, the nursing interventions appropriate for the nursing diagnosis *low self-esteem* would be different from those appropriate for other etiological factors. For *self-esteem disturbance related to chronic, recurring herpes infection*, the appropriate interventions include counselling and education on how to maintain safer sexual practices. In contrast, *self-esteem disturbance related to sexual abuse* would necessitate counselling and referral to community resources (e.g., crisis services or a sexual abuse support group).

◆ **Planning**

Goals and Outcomes. During planning, nurses again synthesize information from multiple resources (Figure 28.5). Critical thinking skills are used to integrate professional standards and knowledge about the patient's sexuality as it relates to their health into the care plan. It is especially important to maintain a patient's dignity and identity when developing the care plan. For example, nurses can convey respect for a LGBTQ2 patient by including the help of their partner in the plan to the degree that the partner can assist the patient in maintaining their identity and dignity.

Nurses develop an individualized care plan for each nursing diagnosis (Box 28.4). Together, the nurse and the patient set realistic goals for care. Expected outcomes must be individualized and realistic. For example, for a patient with a nursing diagnosis of *sexual dysfunction related to dyspareunia*, the nurse and the patient would develop a goal to be free from pain or discomfort during sexual intercourse. Expected outcomes for this goal may be as follows:

- The patient will report decreased anxiety and greater satisfaction with sexual activity.
- The patient will consistently use a water-soluble lubricant with sexual intercourse.
- The patient will avoid the use of hygiene products that destroy the natural flora and secretions of the vaginal walls.

A concept map is useful for organizing patient care (Figure 28.6). A concept map shows the relationship of a medical diagnosis (e.g., decreased libido and depression) with the four nursing diagnoses identified from the patient assessment data. The map also shows links and relationship with the nursing diagnosis. For example, ineffective coping affects and contributes to social isolation; as long as the patient has ineffective coping, social isolation continues or perhaps worsens.

Continuity of Care. Planning in the area of sexuality may include referrals to community resources (Box 28.5). Sexual violence in relationships or trauma related to sexual abuse or incest may necessitate intensive treatment with a mental health care provider. For individuals experiencing intimate partner violence, most communities have shelters that provide counselling and serve as a safe haven while they plan for their future.

◆ **Implementation**

Health Promotion. Because of their education, clinical expertise, and wellness orientation, nurses are among the health care providers best

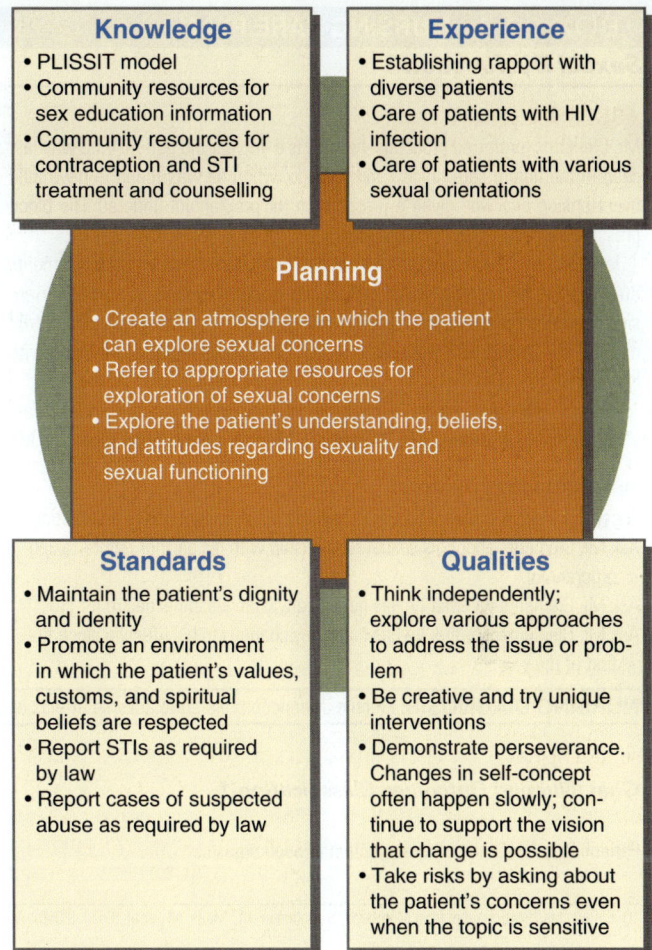

Knowledge
- PLISSIT model
- Community resources for sex education information
- Community resources for contraception and STI treatment and counselling

Experience
- Establishing rapport with diverse patients
- Care of patients with HIV infection
- Care of patients with various sexual orientations

Planning
- Create an atmosphere in which the patient can explore sexual concerns
- Refer to appropriate resources for exploration of sexual concerns
- Explore the patient's understanding, beliefs, and attitudes regarding sexuality and sexual functioning

Standards
- Maintain the patient's dignity and identity
- Promote an environment in which the patient's values, customs, and spiritual beliefs are respected
- Report STIs as required by law
- Report cases of suspected abuse as required by law

Qualities
- Think independently; explore various approaches to address the issue or problem
- Be creative and try unique interventions
- Demonstrate perseverance. Changes in self-concept often happen slowly; continue to support the vision that change is possible
- Take risks by asking about the patient's concerns even when the topic is sensitive

FIGURE 28.5 Critical thinking model for sexuality planning. *HIV,* Human immunodeficiency virus; *PLISSIT,* permission giving, limited information, specific suggestions, and intensive therapy; *STI,* sexually transmitted infection.

situated to develop and implement sexual health initiatives. Nurses can promote sexual health by identifying patients at increased risk, providing appropriate information, helping individuals gain insight into their problems, and exploring methods to deal with problems effectively. A health promotion perspective ought to guide nurses in designing a number of programs: informal educational opportunities, continuing education, peer learning activities for adolescents, community and political initiatives, and health care provider education (Begley et al., 2022). Topics for education vary, depending on the nursing diagnosis (Box 28.6).

Acute Care. In general, nursing interventions that address alterations in sexuality are aimed at raising awareness, assisting in clarification of issues or concerns, providing information, or performing a combination of these. Nurses who have pursued specialized education in sexual functioning and counselling may provide more intensive sex therapy. Nurses should recognize when an individual's needs exceed the nurses' expertise, in which case they should provide an appropriate referral.

In the initial intervention, the nurse often explores current sexual practices of the patient. The patient should be encouraged to investigate and acknowledge social and ethical values and consider the role of sexuality in their self-concept. When significant discrepancy exists between values and past or current practices, the patient may need referral for more intensive counselling.

⊚ BOX 28.4   NURSING CARE PLAN
Sexual Dysfunction

ASSESSMENT

Mr. Clements (preferred pronouns: he/him) is a 46-year-old patient who was last seen in the health care office 2 months ago, when he was found to have mild hypertension and was given a prescription for propranolol (Inderal). His blood pressure today is 122/82 mm Hg.

Jack (preferred pronouns: he/him), a nursing student, talks with Mr. Clements after reading his records, which include the recent diagnosis of mild hypertension, the order for propranolol, and the current blood pressure reading of 122/82 mm Hg. The record also indicates that Mr. Clements is married and living with his partner.

Jack tells Mr. Clements of the improvement in his blood pressure since his last visit. He inquires whether Mr. Clements is taking his medication regularly. Mr.

Clements reports that he has been taking his medication regularly. He relates that it scared him when his blood pressure was up because both his parents had died of strokes. Jack then inquires whether Mr. Clements has noted any adverse effects from the medicine. Mr. Clements says that he has not, except that he may be a little more tired than he used to be. Jack then states, "Some people find that certain blood pressure medications affect their sexual performance. Have you noticed any changes in sexual functioning since you began your medication?" Mr. Clements replies that he has had some problems achieving an erection since starting the medication.

Assessment Activities

Ascertain when Mr. Clements began noticing his inability to have an erection.
Ask Mr. Clements about his sexual relationship with his partner before taking propranolol.
Ask Mr. Clements whether he has noticed any changes in his desire for sex.
Ask Mr. Clements whether he has made any changes to his lifestyle since the first of the year.

Findings and Defining Characteristics

He responds that it was at about the same time he started taking propranolol.
He states that he and his partner used to have intercourse one to three times per week.
He states that he has the same level of interest as before.
He denies any changes.

NURSING DIAGNOSIS: Erectile dysfunction related to adverse effects of antihypertensive medication

PLANNING
Goal (Nursing Outcomes Classification)*

Patient sustains penile/clitoral erection through orgasm.

Expected Outcomes
Sexual Functioning

Patient will talk to their health care provider about this goal, and a change of medication may be warranted.

*Outcome classification label from Moorhead, S., Johnson, M., Maas, M., et al. (Eds.). (2018). *Nursing outcomes classification* (6th ed.). Elsevier.

INTERVENTIONS
Interventions (Nursing Interventions Classification)†
Sexual Counselling

Establish trust and respect with patient. Offer privacy during conversations.

Discuss possible effects of antihypertensive medication on sexual functioning and encourage patient to discuss sexual concerns with their health care provider.
Encourage patient to discuss concerns with their partner. Role-play so that the patient can practise ways to approach concerns.
Anxiety Reduction
Assure patient that other blood pressure medications are available to maintain blood pressure control that do not negatively affect sexual function.

Rationale

Conveys sense of caring, increasing likelihood of patient's ability to express concerns fully
Helps patient understand possible cause for sexual difficulties and gives patient important options to review with the health care provider

Many of the sexual difficulties in relationships involve poor communication

Anxiety and embarrassment can be difficult and can interfere with adult-to-adult relationships. Knowing that options exist and that blood pressure can continue to be safely managed gives patient a sense of control.

†Intervention classification labels from Bulechek, G. M., Butcher, H. K., & McCloskey Dochterman, J. M. (2018). *Nursing interventions classification (NIC)* (7th ed.). Elsevier.

EVALUATION
Nursing Actions
At his next visit, ask Mr. Clements whether his problems have been resolved.

Patient Response and Finding
He responds that since he has been on new medication, he has had no trouble having an erection.

Achievement of Outcome
Mr. Clements reports sexual function with the new medication.

Major developmental milestones (e.g., puberty or menopause) should prompt education about potential effects on sexuality. Situational crises such as a life change with pregnancy, illness, extreme financial stress, placement of a spouse in a long-term care facility, or loss and grief affect sexuality. Effects may last for days, months, or years and can generate performance anxieties that lead to continued sexual

dysfunction. If an individual is prepared for possible changes in sexual functioning, performance anxieties may be minimized.

When concerns are assessed and identified, they can be addressed in the context of the patient's value system. In response to identified concerns, the nurse may initiate discussion in pertinent areas. It may be appropriate to discuss sexual practices such as oral–genital sex or

▶ concept map

Sexual dysfunction
- Patient has decreased interaction with partner
- Patient blames partner for dysfunction
- Patient states that they do not enjoy sex
- Patient is unwilling to have nonsexual intimacy
- Dysfunction began within 4 months after diagnosis of depression

Ineffective coping
- Patient neglects partner and their relationship
- Patient exhibits withdrawal from job, friends, and children
- Patient blames family for problem
- Patient will not seek out medical treatment for sexual dysfunction

Patient's chief medical diagnosis: Decreased libido and depression
Priority assessments: Coping, sexual activity, and socialization

Fear
- Patient verbalizes fear that condition is permanent
- Patient exhibits lack of appetite/weight loss
- Patient fears that partner will leave
- Dysfunction began after prostate surgery

Social isolation
- Patient refuses to go out with couples group
- Patient seeks out solitary hobbies away from family
- Patient avoids interaction with co-workers

—— Link between medical diagnosis and nursing diagnosis   - - - - Link between nursing diagnoses

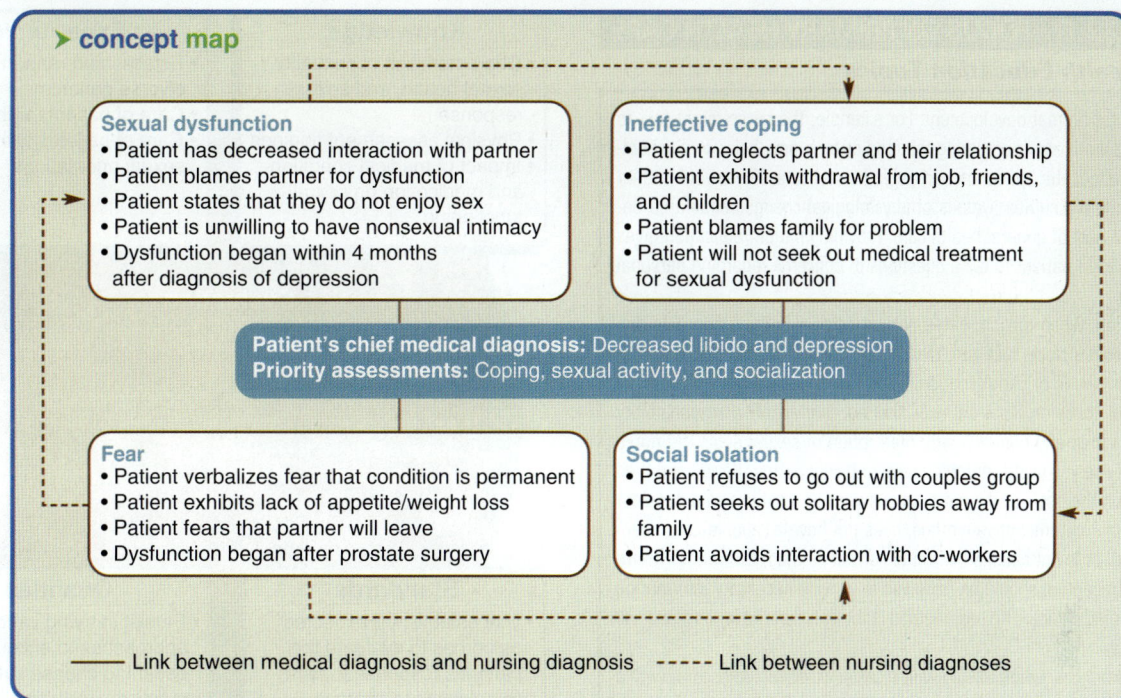

FIGURE 28.6 Concept map for patient with decreased libido and depression.

BOX 28.5	Community Resources Relating to Sexuality

Planned Parenthood
Sex therapists
Clinical psychologists
Social workers
Health department (often for both family planning and treatment of STIs)
Groups that provide education and services for those with particular conditions include the following:
   Diabetes Canada
   Heart and Stroke Foundation of Canada
   Muscular Dystrophy Canada
   Sexual abuse support groups
   Women's shelters (for those who have been physically abused, sexually abused, or both)
   Hotlines for help (which have lists of community support resources)

mutual masturbation as methods of expressing intimate affection when vaginal–penile intercourse is contraindicated. Often, if a partner's abilities (physical or mental) change, dealing with sexuality needs to be addressed with both partners. Dealing with issues of fatigue, a change in sensory perceptions, pain, and limited motion may require a change in positioning, touch, and so on. Often, counselling is needed to deal with these kinds of changes.

Restorative Care. In the patient's home, the nurse can help create an environment that is comfortable for sexual activity. This may involve recommending ways to arrange the bedroom to accommodate an individual's limitations. For example, a patient using a wheelchair may prefer to move the chair close to the side of the bed at an angle that allows for more ease in touching and caressing. Suggestions regarding how to accommodate barriers such as Foley catheters or drainage tubes can contribute to enhanced sexual activity.

In the long-term care setting, there is often a lack of policies and education to guide staff in navigating the sexual activities and sexual expressions of the residents. This can be particularly salient when at least one of the residents has a cognitive impairment. It is important to explore possibilities for dealing with such issues, including the possibility of having a semi-private room that provides for both visual and auditory privacy, should the need arise.

◆ Evaluation

Patient Care. To determine whether patient goals and outcome criteria have been met, nurses review patients' responses to interventions (Figure 28.7). Using critical thinking, nurses apply what they know about sexuality and the patient's unique situation.

In follow-up discussions with the patient and partner, the nurse determines whether goals and outcomes have been achieved. Patients can be asked to relate risk factors, verbalize concerns, share stories of their experiences, and clarify their level of satisfaction. Nurses can also observe behavioural cues, such as eye contact, posture, and extraneous hand movements, that indicate comfort or are suggestive of continued anxiety or concern as topics are addressed. As outcomes are evaluated, the nurse, the patient, and the partner may need to modify expectations or establish time frames in which to achieve the target goals. All involved may need to be reminded of the individual nature of sexuality and the multiple factors that affect perceptions and responses. Sexual wellness is not an absolute. An individual must define what is acceptable and satisfying. The partner's level of sexual satisfaction must also be considered. Sexual performance is seldom the exclusive focus of sexual satisfaction. Open communication and positive self-esteem are essential factors in effectively resolving concerns.

Patient Expectations. In evaluating the outcomes of interventions related to sexuality, the nurse must consult with the patient. Resolution of sexual concerns must meet the patient's perceptions of improvement. A patient must define what is acceptable and satisfying. In considering

❤ BOX 28.6 FOCUS ON PRIMARY HEALTH CARE
Sexual Health Education Topics

- Guidelines for normal development: For example, the nurse might talk to a toddler's parent about preparing the toddler for a new baby, to a school-aged child about the appearance of pubic hair, or to a 60-year-old patient about erectile difficulties. Details of physiological changes should be described as a part of general health care. Providing patient education gives permission for a patient to raise questions or concerns regarding personal functioning.
- Contraception, when talking with a patient of child-bearing age: The discussion should include such topics as the desire for children, usual sexual practices, methods of contraception, frequency of sexual activity, comfort with genital touching, comfort with sharing contraceptive responsibility with the partner, and comfort with interruption of sexual acts. The nurse might ask, "Are you using contraceptives with your partner now?" and then follow up, on the basis of the patient's answer. For a patient who does not have a regular contraceptive method, does not have a reliable contraceptive method, or is not satisfied with the current method, the various methods of contraception should be reviewed to provide necessary information for an informed choice. The best method is the one that the patient will use consistently.
- Safer sex practices, when talking with a sexually active adolescent, with a patient who has more than one sex partner, or with a patient whose partner has multiple sexual partners: The nurse should provide information regarding STI symptoms and transmission, use of condoms, and less safe sexual activities (e.g., trauma from penile–anal sex). An important topic in discussing sexuality and sex is consent. Role-play can be a useful educational tool for helping a person learn to say no or negotiate with a partner to use a condom.
- The need for regular physical examinations: Regular health examinations are important for maintaining sexual health. The annual health examination also provides an easy opportunity to discuss contraception and safer sex practices. Regular clinical breast examinations, mammography, and Papanicolaou (Pap) smears are important for individuals with female genitalia, as are testicular self-examinations for individuals with male genitalia.

the status of sexual health, the patient's partner's perceptions of sexual satisfaction are also significant.

KEY CONCEPTS

- Sexuality is related to all dimensions of health; therefore, as a part of nursing care, sexual concerns or problems should be addressed.
- Sexuality is a part of each individual's identity and is linked to sex, gender, and sexual orientation.
- Attitudes toward sexuality vary widely and are influenced by societal values, cultural norms, religious beliefs, the family, and other factors.
- Nurses' attitudes toward sexuality also vary and may differ from those of patients; nurses should be sensitive to patients' sexual health needs.
- Sexual development is a process beginning in infancy and involves some level of sexual behaviour or growth in all developmental stages.
- The physiological sexual response changes with aging, but aging does not lead to diminished sexuality.
- Sexual health involves physical and psychosocial aspects and contributes to an individual's sense of self-worth and positive interpersonal relationships.

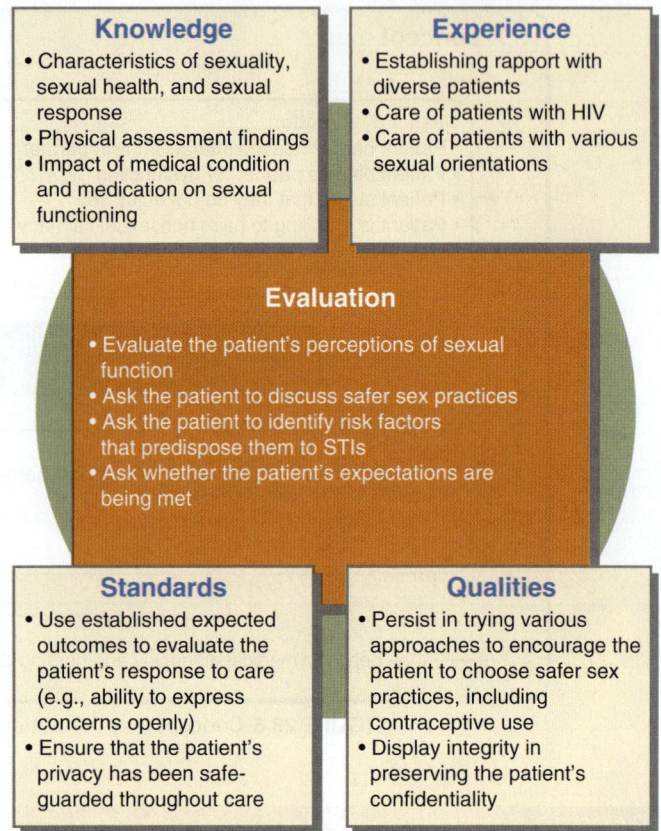

FIGURE 28.7 Critical thinking model for sexuality evaluation. *HIV*, Human immunodeficiency virus; *STI*, sexually transmitted infection.

- Sexual dysfunction can have an easily identified cause or varied and complex causes.
- Interventions for sexual dysfunctions depend on the condition and the patient; interventions may include giving information, teaching specific exercises, improving communication between partners, and referral to a specialized care provider.
- Choice and use of contraceptive methods are affected by desire for children, usual sexual practices, acceptable methods of contraception, frequency of sexual activity, comfort with genital touching, comfort with sharing contraceptive responsibility with the partner, and comfort with interruption of sexual acts.
- A brief review of sexuality should be included in every nursing assessment of a patient's level of wellness.
- Most nursing interventions to enhance a patient's sexual health involve providing information and education.

CRITICAL THINKING EXERCISES

1. Your current clinical experience is in a community health care setting. You are conducting the initial interview with a 48-year-old patient who started taking antihypertensive medications 2 weeks ago. You take their blood pressure and find it to be 136/74 mm Hg. You ask them how they have been doing since their last visit. They look down at the floor and say, "Oh, okay, I guess. Seems like I'm just getting old now." What kind of follow-up would be indicated on the basis of this information?

2. You are assigned to care for a 15-year-old patient who was admitted after a motor vehicle accident. Yesterday they underwent internal fixation of a fractured ankle. In gathering their nursing history,

you explore sexuality and learn that they have just recently become sexually active with their partner of 3 months. When you ask about safer sex and the use of birth control, they tell you that they know that they do not have to worry about STIs with their partner because they are just not the type. In regard to birth control, they say that their partner has reassured them that because they are pulling out before ejaculation, there is no risk of becoming pregnant. How would you proceed?

3. You are working on a rehabilitation unit and caring for a 67-year-old patient who had a stroke 3 weeks ago. They share a room with a patient of the same sex and who is recovering from a stroke. Your patient has been progressing in their self-care skills and is now able to get around with a cane, feed themselves, and perform most of their bathing. Their partner is in fairly good health, and the plan is for the patient to return home within the next 1 to 2 weeks. As you work with the patient one morning, they say to you, "You know, one of the things that is hardest about being here is not being able to sleep in the same bed as Greta [their partner]. I miss her so much. Even though she visits every day, it is just not the same." How would you explore their comment, and what planning would you consider?

🌐 *Answers to Critical Thinking Exercises appear on the Evolve website.*

REVIEW QUESTIONS

Review Questions 1 to 8 relate to the case study at the beginning of the chapter.

1. In the case study at the beginning of this chapter, Alex is a nurse conducting a follow-up assessment with a patient (Elliott) who had an MI. Alex knows that sexual health issues are common after an MI but is unsure about how to best bring up the topic. What is the best way for Alex to handle this situation? *(Select all that apply.)*
   a. Wait for the patient to bring up the topic.
   b. Instruct the patient to discuss any sexual concerns with their partner.
   c. Ask a more experienced nurse to cover this with the patient and learn from observing their approach.
   d. Plan to obtain training on how to discuss sexual health issues.
   e. Encourage the patient to discuss their sexual health concerns with the cardiologist.

2. Alex is concerned about Elliot's sexual health. Sexual health refers to:
   a. Having no STIs
   b. Awareness of and positive attitudes toward sexual functioning
   c. Using contraception all the time
   d. Frequent sexual activity
   e. Abstinence from sexual activity

3. Elliott is concerned about sexual functioning. Inability or difficulty in sexual functioning caused by numerous factors is called:

   a. Sexual behaviour
   b. Sexual response
   c. Sexual identity
   d. Sexual orientation
   e. Sexual dysfunction

4. In the case study, the patient (Elliott) is experiencing erectile dysfunction. Erectile dysfunction is a common adverse effect of which of the following? *(Select all that apply.)*
   a. Antihypertensive medications
   b. Heart disease
   c. Depression
   d. Exercise
   e. Diet

5. Gender identity is the individual's:
   a. Sexual behaviour
   b. Sexual orientation
   c. Sense of being a woman, man, non-binary, or gender-fluid
   d. Sense of preferring one gender over another
   e. Sexual identity

6. The most valuable tool that the nurse can use when providing sexual health care is:
   a. Knowledge of right and wrong sexual behaviours
   b. Effective, nonjudgemental communication
   c. Nursing diagnoses
   d. Firm personal convictions about what constitutes normal sexual behaviour
   e. Referral to a physician

7. When Alex is gathering a sexual history from an older person (Elliott), they must keep in mind that: *(Select all that apply.)*
   a. Older persons do not usually participate in sexual activity.
   b. Older individuals with male genitalia always lose fertility.
   c. Older persons may have difficulty discussing intimate matters.
   d. Nurses may hold assumptions and biases about older people's sexuality.
   e. Both older individuals with male and female genitalia are sexually dysfunctional.

8. A nurse is providing education about changes in sexual response with age. Which statement made by the patient indicates the need for further information?
   a. "Health conditions such as diabetes and hypertension have little effect on sexual functioning and desire."
   b. "It usually takes longer to reach an orgasm."
   c. "Many medications can interfere with sexual function."
   d. "Most of the normal changes in function are related to alterations in circulation and hormone levels."
   e. "As people age, sexual function and desires may change."

Answers: 1. c, d; **2.** b; **3.** e; **4.** a, b, c; **5.** c; **6.** b; **7.** c, d; **8.** a

🌐 *Rationales for the Review Questions appear on the Evolve website.*

🌐 REFERENCES

A full reference list is available on the website for this book at
http://evolve.elsevier.com/Canada/Potter/fundamentals/

RECOMMENDED WEBSITES

Online Training Modules: Integrating Sex & Gender in Health Research: https://cihr-irsc.gc.ca/e/49347.html

Developed by the Canadian Institutes of Health Research (CIHR) Institute of Gender and Health, these learning modules were designed to help researchers account for sex and gender in health research. The modules contain helpful information about concepts and issues related to sex, gender, and health.

Project Implicit: https://www.projectimplicit.net

Developed by researchers at Harvard University, University of Virginia, and University of Washington, this resource is designed to educate the public about bias. The website contains a range of implicit bias tests, including tests about sexuality and transgender people (https://implicit.harvard.edu/implicit/selectatest.html).

Public Health Agency of Canada: Sexual Health and Sexually Transmitted Infections: http://www.phac-aspc.gc.ca/index-eng.php

The Public Health Agency of Canada works with provinces, nongovernmental organizations, and health care providers to improve and maintain the sexual health and well-being of Canadians. This website offers links to sexual health and STI information, publications, and resources.

Sexual Education Resource Centre MB: http://www.serc.mb.ca

SERC Manitoba is a community-based organization that promotes sexual health through education to both health care providers and the general public.

Women's Health Matters: Sexual Health: http://www.womenshealthmatters.ca/health-centres/sexual-health

Developed by Sunnybrook and Women's College Health Sciences Centre and the Centre for Research in Women's Health, this website provides information about women's sexual matters, including sexual expression, how female bodies work, pregnancy, birth control, abortion, and safer sex.

29

Spirituality in Health and Health Care

Written by Sheryl Reimer-Kirkham, RN, PhD, FCAN, Savitri Singh-Carlson, RN, PhD, FAAN, and Harjit Kaur, RCC, PhD

OBJECTIVES

Mastery of content in this chapter will enable you to:

- Define the key terms listed.
- Compare and contrast the concepts of religion and spirituality.
- Describe the historical influences of spirituality and religion on nursing.
- Describe spiritual and religious diversity in Canada and the implications for nursing practice.
- Describe research findings that suggest a relationship between spiritual practices and patients' health status.
- Describe how spirituality may facilitate coping during times of illness or suffering
- Recognize how spirituality and spiritual care may vary in different clinical contexts.
- Describe the relational attributes that facilitate spiritual nursing care.
- Describe the competencies, process, and qualities of spiritual nursing care.
- Describe an ethical approach to spiritual nursing care.
- Describe the role of the nurse in providing spiritual nursing care.
- Describe a process for understanding patients' spirituality.
- Explain appropriate ways to facilitate patients' spiritual practices.
- Describe when it is necessary to involve a spiritual leader or make a referral to a spiritual care provider.
- Describe spiritual practices that can support the nurse's spiritual well-being.

KEY TERMS

Compassion

Faith

Holism

Person-centred approach

Religion

Spiritual care

Spiritual care competencies

Spiritual practices

Spiritual support

Spiritual well-being

Spirituality

Suffering

Transcendence

WEBSITE

http://evolve.elsevier.com/Canada/Potter/fundamentals/

CASE STUDY

Understanding the Spirituality of Someone Who Is Spiritual but Not Religious

Blair Williams (preferred pronouns: he/him) is a 65-year-old person receiving home health care for metastatic cancer. He refers to himself as "a very spiritual person, but I just don't believe in God. I believe the divine is in nature all around." He describes his custom of having a morning coffee on his deck, appreciating the silence and the rising sun. When asked about where he finds strength and meaning, he speaks of sitting by the river "for tranquility and wholeness," connecting back to childhood hours spent by the river where he was away from an abusive family situation: "I was alone there; I didn't have to worry about things."

When the home health nurse, Amy, asks how they might support him, Blair emphasizes a blend of compassion and professionalism as a "partner in my healing, to come with the intention to co-manage my care." As his condition deteriorates, he values the consistency of having the same nurse assigned to his care. Amy is intentional using a holistic approach to care that integrates spirituality. This involves communicating dignity and nonjudgement in caring for Blair's ileostomy. Because Amy has learned about the comfort he experiences from nature, Amy ensures that he is able to see out the window and also places a device with the sound of running water near his bedside.

Think about this case study as you read this chapter. There are review questions at the end of the chapter that relate to the case study.

The word *spirituality* is derived from the Latin word *spiritus*, which refers to breath or wind. The spirit gives life to, or animates, a person. **Spirituality** is described as a way of being in the world in which a person feels a sense of connectedness to self, others, and/or a higher power or nature; a sense of meaning in life; and transcendence beyond self, everyday living, and suffering (Weathers, 2019). Spirituality is expressed through beliefs, values, traditions, and practices and can help individuals achieve the balance needed to maintain health and well-being and to cope with illness. Caring for a patient's spiritual needs means caring for the whole person, accepting their beliefs and experiences, and helping with issues concerning meaning and hope.

Many people use the terms *religion* and *spirituality* interchangeably. Although closely associated, these terms are not synonymous. **Religion** is an organized system of beliefs concerning the cause, nature, and purpose of the universe, especially belief in or the worship of a God or gods, and is typically practised in a faith community (Balboni & Peteet, 2017). A person might describe themselves as spiritual but not religious, as both spiritual and religious, or as neither spiritual nor religious. Although nursing defines spirituality and religion differently, these differences may be less clear in practice. Individuals who describe themselves as spiritual but not religious may draw on religious ideas and practices as they grow in their spiritual journey. As a result, nurses need to know how to give skillful spiritual and religious care.

Another common term individuals use to express their spirituality is **faith**. Faith is often used in two ways: in the context of a cultural or institutional religion, such as Judaism, Buddhism, Islam, Hinduism, or Christianity, and as a relationship with a divinity, a higher power, an authority, or a spirit. Faith may involve a sense of **transcendence**—an awareness of something beyond oneself that gives a wider perspective and meaning in life's experience. It is mystical in nature, although the experience does not necessarily need to be understood in relation to God—it may be in relation to the universe, nature, or humanity (Lalani, 2020).

HISTORICAL PERSPECTIVES

Nursing has deep historical ties to spirituality, building on centuries of caring traditions and sacred texts (Alshmemri & Ramaiah, 2021). Florence Nightingale's model of nursing, rooted in Christianity, was spread around the world during the colonial era. Canadian missionary nurses were among those who brought Nightingale's ideas of modern nursing methods to China, India, Japan, and Korea during the first half of the twentieth century (Grypma, 2021). In Canada, the earliest nurses belonged to Roman Catholic orders devoted to care of the sick—most notably, the Sisters of Charity of Montreal (Grey Nuns), an order founded by Marie Marguerite d'Youville in 1737 (Nelson & Paul, 2020). During the late nineteenth and early twentieth centuries, confidence in religion was replaced by confidence in medical science. Religious aspects of care became less visible. However, many nurses became dissatisfied with a medical approach to care that neglected spirituality, in part because a purely scientific approach could not answer the existential questions raised by patients. The last decades have seen a renewed interest in spirituality, reflected by an increase in nursing literature on spirituality, as well as a growing interest in parish nursing as a way for faith communities to reclaim their healing mission (LeBlanc-Kwaw et al., 2021).

Canadian nursing scholarship has made important contributions to this renewed interest by emphasizing the relationships between spirituality, religion, culture, and health. Reimer-Kirkham and colleagues have used a social justice lens to explore how religious and spiritual diversity is negotiated in Canadian health care (e.g., Reimer-Kirkham, 2019). Likewise, Canadian research by Etowa and colleagues regarding Black Canadians (Bernard et al., 2020), Singh-Carlson and colleagues regarding South Asian Canadians (Singh-Carlson et al., 2013), and Bourque Bearskin and colleagues regarding Indigenous people (Bourque Bearskin et al., 2020) highlight the intersections between spirituality, religion, culture, and health. Just as nurses must understand cultural influences in health and illness, they must also recognize the need for sensitive, safe, and ethical nursing care in which patients' spiritual needs and resources are recognized and supported.

SPIRITUALITY AND RELIGION IN CANADA

Canada's landscape is characterized by a "new diversity" (Beaman, 2017) of secularism and fading majoritarian religions, newcomer and diasporic religions, Indigenous histories and spiritualities, and those who identify as "nones." This diversity requires the nurse to be conversant with and responsive to a range of spiritual and religious identities. There are regional variations that impact nursing care, such as the high levels of non-religion on the West Coast, the larger numbers of newcomers representing diasporic religions in urban settings, and variations in government policies regarding religious symbols in public institutions.

Although declining in numbers, just over sixty-five percent (65.4%) of Canadians report having a religious affiliation (Statistics Canada, 2022). Within this affiliation, there is considerable diversity, including Christianity (53.3%), Muslim (4.9%), Hinduism (2.3%), Sikhism (2.1%), Buddhism (1.4%), Judaism (1%), and other traditions (1.3%). There has been a steady decline in the numbers of affiliates and the social influence of these religions on social life in Canada over the last decades. At the same time, increasing numbers of Canadians (34.6%) indicate "no religion" on census surveys (Statistics Canada, 2022). Also referred to as "nones," this is a broad category that includes emergent spiritualities not tied to formal religions, as well as agnostics, atheists, and people who do not view themselves as spiritual. Many Canadians refer to themselves as spiritual but not religious. The case study in the chapter introduction portrays how a nurse can provide care to someone who positions themselves this way.

Diasporic minority religions are on the rise, in step with patterns of immigration to Canada. Immigration from Asia, South Asia, the Middle East, and Africa has created ever-growing Buddhist, Hindu, Muslim, and Sikh communities, collectively representing 10.3% of Canada's population (Statistics Canada, 2022). With our diverse Canadian citizenry, and the rising evidence of religion and spirituality as social determinants of health (Reimer-Kirkham, 2019), nurses' knowledge of spirituality in health care must include consideration of the beliefs and practices of diasporic religions. In this regard, Canadian health care services have received scrutiny of the degree to which religious and spiritual diversity is accommodated (Taher, 2020)—all the more so in the era of emerging stories of racialized religions, including Islamophobia (Reimer-Kirkham, 2019; Samari et al., 2020). The case study in Box 29.1 describes the care of a South Asian person who is receiving care at a cancer clinic.

Also reshaping the Canadian landscape is the young and growing Indigenous population and an overdue movement to acknowledge and reconcile the long-standing government history of land dispossession and colonial oppression, much of which was operationalized by the church through residential schools and Native Indian hospitals (see Chapter 12). Reconciliation involves acknowledgement of the immeasurable damage wrought by residential schools, together with appreciation for the resilience of Indigenous spiritualities with the view that the sacred is embedded in all aspects of Indigenous life. As Canadian institutions—including higher education and health care—take up the Truth and Reconciliation Commission of Canada's Calls to Action

BOX 29.1 CASE STUDY

Diasporic Religion and Spiritual Support (See also Chapter 12)

Mrs. Singh (preferred pronouns: she/her) is a married 49-year-old South Asian woman who lives with her husband, children, and one grandchild from her eldest married son. She was diagnosed with breast cancer 2 years ago and was given a culturally specific survivorship care plan called HOUNSLA (translated to hope, faith, and trust; Singh-Carlson et al., 2013) after completing her first chemotherapy treatments. Her cancer has progressed to stage IV with metastasis to her bones, and she is receiving palliative treatment of radiation and chemotherapy treatments. Today she is at the cancer clinic for her post-treatment follow-up appointment.

The chart does not include information about her community support, affiliation with a religious group or faith, or notes on discussions for initiating an advance care plan. You read that the oncologist is concerned with her lack of engagement in discussions about her prognosis; she has turned down referrals with patient and family counselling for social support, although she shows concerning signs of sadness and distress. She communicates through an interpreter for medically related appointments and is usually accompanied by family members. She is dressed in a traditional South Asian outfit with a scarf over her head and is accompanied by her eldest son, who is on the phone when you enter the room.

Reflection Questions for the Nurse:
- What personal biases are important for the nurse to be aware of given Mrs. Singh's physical appearance, her quiet appearance, and her accompanying family member who is on the phone?
- How would the nurse engage with Mrs. Singh in order to retrieve the missing information regarding her community support, any religious affiliation, or her faith?

BOX 29.2 CASE STUDY

Indigenous Spiritualities and Healing (see also Chapter 13)

Perry Monture (preferred pronouns: she/her) is a 50-year-old Indigenous person who is hospitalized for diabetes and renal failure. She lives in an urban setting, some distance away from her nation. She has experienced housing insecurity, ongoing intravenous drug use, and chronic hepatitis C infection. In the hospital, she is quiet and withdrawn. A nurse asks Perry if she would like to be visited by someone from the Indigenous Wellness Team (Hadjipavlou et al., 2018). An Elder-in-Residence comes to her bedside to provide a traditional healing service with drumming, prayer, and cedar brushing and does so daily during her hospitalization. Perry explains how the Elder has brought healing: "They come from the same background as I do, the residential school, the breaking of families, of loss of tradition and language. I can talk to and trust them. It is hard for an Indigenous person to be open, to trust. The ceremony brought comfort and soothing to heal my soul. Having this Elder support is life-changing in connecting to my people and our ways."

Reflection Questions for the Nurse:
- What assumptions do you bring to your care for Perry? Do you see her as having made poor life choices or experiencing structural vulnerability? Do you see the spiritual dimensions of her health?
- How can nurses support Indigenous patients through interpersonal encounters and program changes?

(Truth and Reconciliation Commission, 2015) in the spirit of decolonization, we see a way forward that can contribute to healthier relations and better health outcomes. The case study in Box 29.2 portrays the experience of an Indigenous patient who is hospitalized.

A **person-centred approach** to spirituality involves respect for diversity, regardless of how someone identifies. Part of respecting diversity is recognizing that some individuals might be offended by the claim often made in nursing literature that all individuals are spiritual (Pesut et al., 2009). Other people affiliated with diasporic religions may not find a generic spirituality, intended to be inclusive, as being representative of their views. Along with a person-centred approach, an equity orientation is needed, where the nurse understands that some people may be disadvantaged on account of their religious affiliation or spiritual beliefs and practices, as in situations of Indigenous-specific racism and racialized religion

EMPIRICAL EVIDENCE ABOUT SPIRITUALITY AND HEALTH EXPERIENCES

Spirituality, Health, and Illness

The Canadian Nurses Association (CNA) recognizes spirituality as an essential dimension of overall health (CNA, 2010). Evidence from thousands of studies shows that religion and spirituality are largely associated with positive health outcomes (Litalien et al., 2022; Shattuck & Muehlenbein, 2020). There are, however, also some negative correlations, such that nurses must strive to maintain a person-centred approach in understanding individual experiences.

Taylor (2020) summarizes three mechanisms by which spirituality, health, and illness are interrelated and affect health outcomes: religious/spiritual beliefs, behaviours or practices, and a sense of belonging. Religious/spiritual beliefs affect how individuals view health and the meaning they make of illness and suffering. For example, many faith traditions emphasize that health is holistic, requiring balancing of mind, body, and soul. Research demonstrates that beliefs may impact adjustment to stress and illness. Roberto et al. (2020), in their study of women's resilience and coping during the COVID-19 pandemic, found that participants' faith and spirituality aided them in coping with the day-to-day experiences of living during a pandemic as well as with having hope for the future. Singh-Carlson et al.'s (2013) study of South Asian (Indian ethnicity) women with breast cancer identified their state of "quiet acceptance" as derived from a combination of their faith and inner strength, their beliefs about *karma* and fate, *hounsla* (hope, faith, and trust), and their family and community social network.

Evidence shows that religious/spiritual behaviours and practices such as meditation, yoga, prayer, fasting, and attending religious services result in positive health outcomes (Taylor, 2020). In a mixed-methods study that explored racism-related experiences of 50 African-heritage women in Nova Scotia, Bernard et al. (2020) found that spirituality served as a sustaining life force, providing a key coping mechanism for racism-related stress; elements of coping included prayer, guidance, and meaning-making. For some women, spiritual belief provided a means of cognitive reinterpretation, allowing them to make sense of racism and other life challenges, recasting these as tests and trials that they were capable of surmounting with God's blessing and protection.

The mechanism of religious/spiritual belonging includes informal caregiving and venues for health promotion. For example, Salami et al. (2019), in their study with immigrant service providers in Alberta, found that religious communities serve as an important point of community belonging and social support for recent immigrants. The substantial body of evidence on health outcomes of religious and spiritual belief, behaviour, and belonging indicates the need for nurses to provide timely, culturally responsive, and person-centred spiritual support to patients.

Spirituality, Suffering, and Loss

As we encounter illness, we are entering the domains of spirituality and suffering. Canadian nurse scholar Wright (2017), in her book *Suffering and Spirituality: The Path to Illness Healing*, defines suffering as the experience of physical, emotional, or spiritual anguish, pain, or distress. Few individuals experience life's journey without facing an unexpected or chronic illness or injury resulting in suffering and loss. Spiritual beliefs can shape how suffering is interpreted. An unhealthy view of suffering can see it as a form of punishment from God, stemming from wrong choices or not being "good enough" (Westera, 2016). Others may accept a cancer diagnosis and its treatments as their fate and part of their individual *karma* on account of wrong-doing in past lives. A healthy view of suffering sees suffering as part of the human condition and that one can draw on spiritual resources to deal with suffering. A compassionate, relational approach can help nurses inquire about a patient's narrative of suffering. Articulating and reformulating an illness narrative can provide a way to withstand suffering. For the nurse, this requires deep listening, attending to, and being present, rather than providing answers.

Suffering and illness can lead to both spiritual challenges and transformation. Spiritual dimensions of the illness experience may include reconsidering beliefs about life; maintaining spiritual or religious practices; connecting with God and significant others; and finding balance, courage, and growth. In the face of suffering, individuals may feel alone or even abandoned by a higher power. They may question their spiritual values and beliefs, raising questions about their way of life and purpose for living. Anger is not uncommon, and patients may express anger toward God, their families, themselves, or health care providers. People also look for ways to remain faithful to their beliefs during their suffering. They may pray, attend religious services, or reflect on the positive aspects of their lives.

Spirituality, Life Journey, and Clinical Context

Spirituality and the need for spiritual support can vary by life journey, health challenge, and clinical context. Research is increasingly providing guidance as to best practices for various populations and settings.

Children and Youth. Nurses are often not comfortable discussing spirituality with children and families and may consider a child's young age to be a barrier to providing spiritual care. In a study with pediatric Critical Care Unit (CCU) nurses, Nascimento et al. (2016) found that nurses were more likely to consider spirituality of the parents of a sick child, because they were unclear about the spiritual dimension as expressed by a child. O'Brien (2022) notes that perhaps no therapeutic intervention calls on the nurse's creative skills as much as that of providing spiritual care to a child. This creativity might involve using pictures or stories to encourage children to talk about aspects of their spirituality, such as the meaning they assigned to their illness and connectivity to others and the sacred (Alvarenga et al., 2021).

Maternity Nursing. In many cultures, childbirth is seen as a deeply spiritual event, marked by ritual and celebration. Yet, as birth has become increasingly medicalized, existential and spiritual aspects are, for the most part, left unspoken and even hidden within dominant professional discourses around safety and risk (Crowther et al., 2021). Spirituality can emerge not only from the unordinary or difficult situations that can arise during childbirth but also from any childbirth as an "intensification of the human experience" (Belanger-Levesque, et al.,

2016). Nurses' responses can include questions about offering spiritual support and affirmation of the emotions, meaningfulness, and mystery of childbirth.

Mental Health Nursing. Spirituality and religion can have a dual nature in the context of mental health. Saiz and colleagues (2021) report that some people find religion to encourage hope, purpose, and meaning in their lives, whereas for others it induces spiritual despair. In their systematic review on experiences of spirituality among adults with mental health difficulties, Milner et al. (2019) indicate that being spiritual and being diagnosed with a mental illness can serve as a double stigma, but that spiritual themes such as meaning-making, spiritual identity, and coping were aspects of holistic mental health care. A person-centred approach is vital in helping the nurse to understand the role of spirituality for some people with mental illness and to offer spiritual support, including nonjudgemental listening and facilitating those spiritual practices that someone has found to be helpful. Referring back to the case study of Perry (see Box 29.2), the nurse understands the importance of connecting her to the Elder, who performs traditional ceremony that can reconnect her to her Indigenous identity.

Community-Based Nursing. Providing nursing care in someone's home or in other community-based settings can shift the dynamics of spiritual care. In a project on spiritual diversity in home health settings, Reimer-Kirkham et al. (2017) found that patients were often the ones making a deliberate effort to create an interpersonal space that would diminish the awkwardness of the personal care they were requiring. For some, this connection came through shared religious affiliations. Mrs. Singh (see Box 29.1) appreciates the South Asian nurse who understands the importance of prayer to her spirituality, along with genuine respect (*ijiat*) for her humanity. Referring to the case study of Blair at the beginning of the chapter, the home health nurse scanned the home for cues regarding spiritual practices and noticed the presence of several water features. As the nurse inquired about these, Blair shared the strength he derived from water and the connotations of safety based on his childhood experiences. Fewer resources for spiritual care tend to exist in community-based care, which means that rather than making a referral to a spiritual care provider, the nurse may need to connect to community-based faith leaders.

Long-Term Care. For individuals living with dementia, spirituality can provide a means of finding peace, affirmation, home, meaning, and linkage with the past, present, and future. Faith practices and the social support of faith communities are also identified in the literature as important (Daly et al., 2019). Discerning what would be meaningful in relation to spiritual care occurs through relationship over time, but also through spiritual and social assessments completed at the time of admission to a long-term care facility. These assessments are foundational to person-centredness and spiritual care. Indoor and outdoor spaces dedicated to spiritual care that are available and accessible can facilitate religious and spiritual practices that are important to the identity of older persons.

End-of-Life and Palliative Care Nursing. Terminal illness marks the end of the life journey and brings with it unique struggles. As the physical body is in the process of dying, individuals are confronted with questions about the meaning of their life and what comes after life. Fears of physical pain, isolation, and losing control are common, both for oneself and for one's family. Spiritual beliefs and practices often provide a source of comfort and strength, and individuals may experience the end of life as a time of positive spiritual transformation. Advance care planning, during which wishes for future care and treatment are

Domain	Competence
Awareness and use of self	1. Attitude toward the patient's spirituality: The nurse's handling of their own values, convictions, and feelings in their professional relationships with patients of different beliefs and religions
	2. Communication: Addressing the subject of spirituality with patients from a range of backgrounds, in a caring manner
Spiritual dimensions of the nursing process	3. Assessment and implementation of spiritual care: The nurse collects information about the patient's spiritualty and identifies the patient's need
	4. Personal support and patient counselling: Discussing with the patient and team members how spiritual care is planned, provided, and evaluated
	5. Referral to professionals
Assurance of quality and expertise	6. Contributing to quality assurance and improving expertise in spiritual care in the organization

TABLE 29.1 Profile of Spiritual Care Competencies

From van Leeuwen, R. (2020). Providing spiritual care: An exploration of required spiritual care competencies in healthcare and their impact on healthcare provision. In F. Timmins & S. Caldeira (Eds.), *Spirituality in healthcare: Perspectives for innovative practice* (p. 99). Springer.

discussed and recorded, is a culturally and spiritually imbued process that must be approached through a person-centred lens (de Vries et al., 2019).

NURSING AND SPIRITUAL CARE

Keeping in view the meanings associated with spirituality and religion, how they are represented in the history of nursing and in Canadian society, and how they are connected to health, illness, and suffering, it is appropriate to explore nurses' response to spirituality and their provision of spiritual care. The nursing commitment to holism and holistic care recognizes the unity and balance of the mind, body, and spirit and the social dimensions and interrelatedness of these dimensions (Westera, 2016). Incorporating spirituality into nursing practice is an enactment of this commitment to holistic care. Spiritual care should be considered a natural part of compassionate care, not a discrete set of actions. To provide holistic, person-centred, spiritual care, nurses require competencies that encompass the nurse's self-awareness and attitude, spiritual dimensions of the nursing process, and workplace resources and health care policy (van Leeuwen, 2020) (Table 29.1). Nursing education programs vary in Canada in how students are prepared for spiritual caregiving, and these spiritual care competencies provide guidance regarding the knowledge, skills, and attitudes that nurses require.

The Professional Role of Nurses—Awareness and Use of Self

The starting point of awareness and use of self involves nurses examining their own spirituality and examining ethical boundaries to the use of self. Spirituality can be a source of well-being and resilience for the nurse, a topic we return to later in the chapter. The *Code of Ethics for Registered Nurses* (CNA, 2017a) requires nurses to treat all patients with dignity and respect. In providing nursing care, the nurse must not discriminate on the basis of spiritual beliefs, age, ethnicity, marital status, gender, race, sexual orientation, health status, or disability.

However, for many, discrimination is not a conscious process but rather an unchallenged set of biases that cause us to react to others in less than caring ways. Therefore, an important part of ethical spiritual care is constantly working to be aware of one's own potential biases as a nurse. This is commonly known as *reflective practice*. In the process of delivering care, the nurse remains open to internal dialogues and feelings that have the potential to violate patients' dignity or respect. Once the nurse identifies those internal feelings, they can do the hard work of trying to understand the origins of those feelings so that engagement with patients can grow ethically. This is particularly important in the context of religion and spirituality, as society tends to polarize over religious beliefs. For instance, if you are a "believer," do you judge harshly the "unbeliever"? If you are agnostic or atheist, do you dismiss the believer? Box 29.3 provides some questions that can be useful for you as a nurse to reflect on.

Beyond a foundational approach of respect, there are two important ethical issues when nurses engage in spiritual care. The first is understanding and respecting appropriate nurse–patient boundaries. The second is ensuring that the nurse is competent to engage in spiritual care and knowing when they are beyond their competency, so that they can refer to a spiritual care provider or social worker. Spiritual care requires an interdisciplinary approach. Nursing is a relational process, so it is not always easy to discern where the professional boundaries lie. This is particularly relevant in spiritual care. When we establish a relationship with patients and we discern that they want to share the more intimate aspects of their spiritual lives with us, it is not always easy to know what is appropriate to do. Here is where questions arise for the nurse, such as the following:

- Is it appropriate to share my own beliefs with patients, whether they are the same or different from theirs?
- Is there a role for proselytizing in nursing, or what do I do if patients try to proselytize to me?
- Should I participate in religious practices like prayer if patients request it of me, regardless of the patient's own religion?
- How do I respond to what I perceive to be unhelpful spiritual beliefs (e.g., when individuals feel that they are being punished by God or resist health care treatment because they believe they will be divinely healed)?

The answers to these questions are complex, and the responses will vary according to the context. The *Code of Ethics for Registered Nurses* (CNA, 2017a) provides some important guidelines:

- Nurses provide care directed first and foremost toward the health and well-being of persons receiving care, recognizing and using the values and principles of primary health care (p. 16).
- Nurses are sensitive to the inherent power differentials between care providers and persons receiving care. They do not misuse that power to influence decision making (p. 17).
- Nurses provide education to support the informed decision making of capable persons. They respect the decisions a person makes, including choice of lifestyles or treatment that are not conducive to good health, and continue to provide care in a nonjudgemental manner (p. 17).
- In health care decision making, in treatment and in care, nurses work with persons receiving care to take into account their values, customs, and spiritual beliefs, as well as their social and economic circumstances without judgement or bias (p. 17).
- If nursing care is requested that is in conflict with the nurse's moral beliefs and values but in keeping with professional practice, the nurse provides safe, compassionate, competent, and ethical care until alternative care arrangements are in place to meet the person's needs or desires (p. 23).

BOX 29.3 Nursing Care Reflective Exercises

Take a few moments to reflect on the following questions:

- Do you believe that there is a God or an ultimate authority in the universe? If so, how does that belief influence your behaviour and, ultimately, your nursing care?
- How do you feel about religion? Should religious beliefs be accounted for in the context of nursing care?
- How do you feel about spirituality? Should spiritual beliefs be accounted for in the context of nursing care?
- Why does suffering happen in the world? How should individuals respond to suffering such as incest, sexual assault, violence, abandonment, terminal illness, or dying?
- What behaviours, practices, or lifestyles do you consider immoral or wrong? What patients might you look after who would exhibit those behaviours, and how might your beliefs influence your ability to give care?
- Do you come from a religious background, and does that background encourage you to share your beliefs and possibly to convert others to those beliefs? How might that influence your practice? Should patients be allowed to try to convert you to their beliefs?
- How comfortable do you feel asking about your patient's religious or spiritual practices and the individual meanings of their illness in relation to their beliefs? How comfortable are you with patients from diverse ethnic and age groups?
- How would you approach the conversation of spirituality or religion with non-English-speaking patients?
- What happens to a person after they die?
- How do you approach patients on preparing an advance care plan for themselves?

Although these may seem like questions unrelated to nursing practice, understanding more about what you believe will help you to deal more authentically with the beliefs of others. It will also help you to think through issues that will ultimately arise in the context of your practice. It is also important to know that nursing practice itself might challenge you to rethink and reframe your beliefs. That is an important part of growing as a person.

BOX 29.4 RESEARCH HIGHLIGHT
Medical Assistance in Dying

Canada's legalization of medical assistance in dying (MAiD) in 2016 has important implications for nurses. Nurses perform a central role in negotiating initial inquiries about assisted death and provide "wrap-around" supportive care for patients and their families. Pesut et al. (2020) found among nurses a range of moral responses and uncertainty about MAiD. For a variety of reasons, including religious views and differences in philosophy (e.g., tensions between palliative care and MAiD), some nurses may abstain from being involved in MAiD. The Canadian Nurses Association's (2017b) *National Nursing Framework on Medical Assistance in Dying in Canada* provides clear guidance to the nurse in this situation, stating if nurses can anticipate a conscientious objection to MAiD, they have an obligation to notify their employer as soon as possible and are required to "take all reasonable steps to ensure that the quality and continuity of care for clients are not compromised" (p. 12).

Implications for Practice
- Nurses may have a range of moral responses to MAiD and require education and support to assist them with moral decision making when choosing to participate in MAiD.
- Nurses have care responsibilities to the patient requesting MAiD and their family, to preserve dignity and respect their values.
- Nurses who anticipate conscientious objection to MAiD must inform their employers so that a safe, continuous, and respectful transfer of care can be ensured.

From Pesut, B., Thorne, S., & Greig, M. (2020). Shades of gray: Conscientious objection in medical assistance in dying. *Nursing Inquiry, 27*(1), e12308. https://doi.org/10.1111/nin.12308.

As you study these guidelines, you can see that there are some important principles to adopt in relation to boundaries and spiritual care. First, it is always the patient's best interest that should be foremost. In the case of sharing your own values and beliefs, the first question should be, whose interests does this serve, yours or the patient's? Second, patients have a right to make decisions about their health care on the basis of spiritual and religious beliefs that we as nurses may not agree with. Our role is to inform them of the best evidence in relation to their decision. They have the right to choose. Third, as a nurse, you, too, have the right to abstain from health care situations that violate your religious or spiritual beliefs, provided you ensure that alternative arrangements can be made. Supporting care for the person who chooses medical assistance in dying (MAiD) may be one such a situation (Box 29.4).

Spiritual Dimensions of the Nursing Process—Understanding Patients' Spirituality

Understanding patients' spirituality is different from the physical aspects of care. Spirituality contains an element of mystery that cannot be assessed and treated in the same way that one might treat a physical problem, such as a pressure injury. Diagnosing and intervening in a patient's spirituality could be considered disrespectful and intrusive. Instead, nurses should think about *understanding* rather than assessing patients' spirituality. It could be thought of as a series of conversations whereby nurses seek to understand what is important and meaningful

to individuals. The depth of that conversation will rest largely on the circumstances the patient is facing and the extent of relational development. But even more important, the nurse should discover those values and beliefs that are important to take into account in health care. Does the patient have beliefs that will influence important health care decisions? Are there religious rituals or restrictions that should inform care? Without knowing these details, the nurse risks harming the patient. For example, a nurse who removes sacramental garb or provides food that is prohibited may actually be contributing to the breaking of religious law and thus be seen to be harming that individual's spirit.

In these conversations, the nurse is not the expert but rather a co-learner in the mysteries of life. This kind of work generally consists of quiet conversations, effective listening, and communication through presence and touch. In many cases, nurses would say that they are the learners in such conversations. Patients teach them about life as they share their stories of transition and suffering. An example of two simple questions that can open conversation are offered by the Ross & McSherry 2 Question Spiritual/Holistic Assessment Model (2Q-SAM) (McSherry et al., 2020): What's most important to you right now? How can we help? Applying the 2Q-SAM to the case of Mrs. Singh in Box 29.1, her nurse learns the importance of including her son in the process of establishing trust and rapport. Her son is an advocate and source of information, and his inclusion in the provision of care can lend support to reducing stress for Mrs. Singh while creating a safe environment to understand her spirituality. The process of learning about a patient's spirituality should be grounded in an understanding of **compassion**, which is defined as "a virtuous response that seeks to address the suffering and needs of a person through relational understanding and action" (Sinclair et al., 2018, p. 2). To practise compassion, a nurse requires virtues (such as honesty, kindness, helpfulness, and nonjudgement), relational skills, and a commitment to responding with action to the spiritual concerns that arise (Sinclair et al., 2018).

Even though understanding is a relational and evolving process, it is still important that the nurse have some form of systematic approach to ensure that critical information is obtained. When patients enter the health care system, it is essential to obtain information about their religious and spiritual beliefs and practices. This has been referred to as a *spiritual screening* and has the aim of discerning whether spirituality and religion are important to the individual and, if so, what beliefs or practices are most important to take into account in the context of care.

Numerous tools are available to enable nurses to gain a deeper understanding of patients' spirituality. Canadian nurse scholar Karen Scott Barss (2012) has developed the T.R.U.S.T. Model for Spiritual Assessment and Care as an inclusive approach, to prompt spiritual reflection and holistic health promotion on the part of the nurse and to offer spiritual care and promote healing. The acronym reminds the nurse of how important trust is to healing and guides the nurse in five topics for exploration:

1) **T**raditions (What healing traditions are meaningful for the patient?)
2) **R**econciliation (What unresolved issues or trauma might be reconciled?)
3) **U**nderstandings (What patient beliefs influence their health?)
4) **S**earching (How is the patient making meaning of their illness and suffering?)
5) **T**eachers (What resources or referrals would be helpful?) (Barss, 2012)

Applying the T.R.U.S.T. model to the case of Perry Monture (see Box 29.2), the nurse learns that the traditions of drumming, prayer, and cedar brushing are meaningful for the patient. The nurse also keeps in mind that *reconciliation* means that Perry may be experiencing intergenerational trauma stemming from the colonial history of Indian residential schools. Considering *understandings*, Perry is disconnected from her community and traditional lands and yet carries a sense of interconnectedness to them. An assessment of *searching* leads the nurse to understand that Perry seeks respect for her Indigenous identity. For *teachers*, time spent with an Elder brings Perry this sense of identity and much comfort.

Another helpful tool for clinical practice is the FICA Spiritual History Tool, developed by Puchalski and Romer (2000) (see Box 29.5 for a systematic process of understanding a patient's spirituality). Applying the FICA Spiritual History Tool to the chapter-opening case of Blair Williams, the nurse learns that Blair does not affiliate with a religion but does consider himself to be spiritual (*faith and belief*). As the nurse asks about the influence of spirituality in his life, they learn that Blair finds peace and a sense of well-being when out in nature, especially when near the river (*importance*). Blair does not consider himself to belong to a spiritual community (*community*) but likes to have nature incorporated into his care, through views out the window and the sound of running water (*address in care*).

It is important to think about how and when the information will be gathered and recorded. Numerous nurses are involved in one patient's care, and having all of these nurses using spiritual assessment tools to inquire about a patient's spirituality is not appropriate. For each nursing context, it is important to ask the following questions and to create policies and procedures that address these questions:

- Who should be collecting this data?
- How extensive should the assessment be in light of the clinical context?
- At what point in the care trajectory should this information be obtained?

BOX 29.5 PROCEDURAL GUIDELINE

Understanding a Patient's Spirituality: Applying the FICA Spiritual History Tool

F—Faith and Belief

"Do you consider yourself spiritual or religious?" or "Is spirituality something important to you?" or "Do you have spiritual beliefs that help you cope with stress and difficult times?" (Contextualize to reason for visit if it is not the routine history.) If the patient responds "No," the health care provider might ask, "What gives your life meaning?" Sometimes patients respond with answers such as family, career, or nature. (The question of meaning should also be asked even if people answer "Yes" to spirituality.)

I—Importance

"What importance does your spirituality have in your life? Has your spirituality influenced how you take care of yourself and your health? Does your spirituality influence you in your health care decision making (e.g., advance directives, treatment, etc.)?"

C—Community

"Are you part of a spiritual community?" Communities such as churches, temples, and mosques or a group of like-minded friends, family, or yoga can serve as strong support systems for some patients. This can be explored further: "Is this of support to you? How? Is there a group of people you really love or who are important to you?"

A—Address in Care

"How would you like me, your health care provider, to address these issues in your health care?" (With the newer models including diagnosis of spiritual distress, *A* also refers to the assessment and plan of patient spiritual distress or issues within a treatment or care plan.)

From The George Washington Institute for Spirituality and Health. *FICA Spirituality History Tool.* https://smhs.gwu.edu/gwish/clinical/fica/spiritual-history-tool © Copyright, Christina M. Puchalski, MD, 1996.

- Which responses should be documented so that the information is available to all health care providers, and which responses should be held in confidence?

Pondering and answering these questions in the health care context is part of expert nursing thinking and critical judgement.

Spiritual Dimensions of the Nursing Process—Offering Spiritual Support

What do patients expect from nurses in terms of spiritual care? Although nurses are not typically seen as being primary spiritual care providers, patients do appreciate having nurses know about their spirituality and show concern in this regard. This is most often the case if spirituality is important to the patient, in the context of life-threatening illness, and if there is a relationship between the patient and nurse (Taylor, 2019). As nurses establish a healing relationship through presence and compassion, they gain insight into a patient's spiritual resources and needs. In a study set in Quebec, patients with advanced cancer indicated that they did not expect help from the hospital in handling spiritual issues per se, but wished for their spiritual dimension to be recognized as part of their identity and dignity (Pujol et al., 2016).

Facilitating spiritual practices is an aspect of a nurse's spiritual care competencies. Research suggests that spiritual and religious practices may do more than just provide a comforting effect. Prayer, meditation, contemplation, sacraments, rituals, and other practices that support spiritual and religious expression may indeed reduce stress and support health and healing. Many spiritual practices are integrated

BOX 29.6	Examples of Spiritual Practices

Meditation
Contemplation
Prayer
Gratitude
Presence
Mantra
Yoga
Tai chi
Qi gong
Reflection
Ritual participation
Sacred readings
Incense use
Active listening, guidance
Journalling
Service
Exercise
Listening to music
Worship
Affirmations
Solitude
Study
Fasting
Simplicity
Confession

The spiritual practice of prayer is a part of most faith traditions. The practices of prayer may vary, but the common thread is communion with a higher power. This communion occurs through reciting memorized prayer, chanting, singing, dancing, meditation, supplication, stream-of-consciousness, or silence. Reimer-Kirkham et al. (2020) drew on research to explore the ways that prayer is enacted in health care contexts. They suggest that prayer can be used to support or challenge dominant religious and health care views. Prayer can also provide an important way to bridge religious differences. This is important for nurses to think about, as patients may ask nurses to pray with or for them.

From Reimer-Kirkham, S., Sharma, S., Brown, R., et al. (2020). *Prayer as transgression? The social relations of prayer in healthcare*. McGill-Queens University Press.

throughout a person's daily activities and do not necessarily take place in a church or mosque or formal setting. What is considered spiritual practice varies greatly from person to person, even for people of the same spiritual or religious tradition. These may be as varied as practices or sacraments associated with a person's religion, such as prayer, daily readings, or communion, and informal practices, such as enjoying a sense of connectedness with others or enjoying the beauty of nature (Box 29.6 provides examples of spiritual practices). Along with rituals, personal clothing or garments, such as veils for women or turbans for men, and personal items, such as crosses, jewellery, or a rosary, that bring meaning of spiritual connectedness are to be respected by the nurse for patients of all ethnic, religious or spiritual, and age groups.

Food and nutrition are important aspects of patient care and often are a significant component of religious observances. Nurses can consult with a dietitian to integrate the patient's dietary preferences into daily care. In the event that an agency cannot prepare food in the preferred way, the family may be asked to bring meals that accommodate dietary restrictions. Personal care of the patient should be planned to allow time for spiritual readings, visits by spiritual advisors, or attendance at religious services.

Some churches and synagogues offer audio recordings of their services for those members who cannot attend in person. Family members can plan a prayer session or an organized reading of spiritual material on a regular basis. Arrangements may need to be made with spiritual care staff for the patient and family to receive the sacraments. Clergy will routinely offer to make home visits for people unable to attend religious services. Recorded meditations, classical or spiritual music, and televised spiritual services are other options. Nurses should be respectful of icons, medals, prayer rugs, or crosses that patients bring to a health care setting and ensure that items are not accidentally lost, damaged, or misplaced.

Nurses may be uncertain about providing care across diverse religious and spiritual traditions. This is a valid concern in light of the risk for harm if nurses fail to take into account these beliefs. For example, taking off the sacred garb of a baptized Sikh has important religious implications. Although doing so is often unavoidable in health care, it requires sensitivity to the implications and assistance (if necessary) with reconnecting the patient with their religious community for restoration of their baptized state. This is just one of many examples of religious implications for care. Unfortunately, many of these situations have been downplayed in nursing because of the desire to recognize spirituality apart from religion and to not stereotype individuals within religious traditions. These certainly are valid concerns. However, it is possible to recognize the validity of spirituality and religion and to understand the possible implications of religious traditions without stereotyping.

Table 29.2 provides *possible* care considerations for some of the most common religious traditions. Naturally, it is important to remember that this is just a starting point. While the information presented in the table enables nurses to enter the caregiving situation with some background knowledge, it is essential to clarify with each individual the practices they follow within their tradition. There is great variability among religions, and individuals will pick and choose the practices they adhere to within that religion. Nurses need not be afraid to ask, because by not asking, they may be doing more harm. Many religious individuals will gladly talk about their faith and practices if the nurse is open and genuine. It is important to take the time to be present, practise attentive listening, and be curious. Think of yourself as an explorer among the mystery of sacred stories and commitments that characterizes persons' lives (Pesut, 2016).

The Interprofessional Team and Making Referrals

One of the most important competencies for nurses is knowing when to refer to a spiritual care provider (the term *spiritual care provider* refers here to both health care chaplains and spiritual leaders from the community who provide spiritual oversight to a group). Although nurses can provide a caring context for patients' spirituality, this should not in any way be misconstrued to suggest that nurses have expertise in spiritual care (unless they have additional education in this field). Part of excellent care is understanding when patients require expert assistance, either from a spiritual leader from their tradition or from a psychologist, counsellor, or social worker if they do not adhere to a religious tradition. It is critical that the nurse check with the patient if they would like to see a spiritual care provider (or faith leader) prior to making a referral. See Box 29.7 for reasons to make a referral to a spiritual care provider.

Sinclair and Chochinov's (2012) model of the levels of spiritual care (Figure 29.1) provides clarity about the interprofessional provision of spiritual care. Nurses are involved in the first level, primary spiritual care, which consists of basic communication with patients' spiritual issues through explicit or implicit means. Self-awareness, assessing patients' spirituality, compassionate presence, referring for additional

TABLE 29.2   Religious Beliefs About Health

Religious or Cultural Background	Possible Health Care Beliefs and Practices	Nursing Implications
Hinduism	Modern medical science is accepted. Illness is caused by past sins. Holy days are celebrated with fasting, prayer, and feasting. Autopsies and organ donations may be discouraged as interfering with *karma* and reincarnation.	Privacy is needed for prayer and meditation. Modesty in clothing is important, and hospital gowns may be considered indecent; same-sex caregivers may be preferred. Important sacraments are associated with birth, naming, puberty, and death. Religious symbols should not be removed.
Sikhism	Modern medical science is accepted. Baptized and nonbaptized Sikhs have different religious requirements.	Prayers are said twice a day; privacy is preferred. Modesty in clothing is important, and hospital gowns may be considered indecent; same-sex caregivers may be preferred. Religious symbols include uncut hair, comb, steel bracelet, symbolic dagger, undershorts, and turban; these should not be removed. Cleanliness during eating and prayers is important.
Buddhism	Modern medical science is accepted. Understanding, rather than belief, is emphasized. *Dharma*, the law of nature, teaches that life is impermanent and all people have to age and die. Death is usually accepted as the last stage of life, and withdrawal of life support may be permitted. Buddhists may believe in rebirth after death.	Treatment may be refused on holy days. Prayers may occur five times daily. Privacy is needed for meditation. The dying process is encouraged to be calm, meditative, and reflective to facilitate an auspicious rebirth and communicate beliefs about impermanence. The patient may want a Buddhist monk or teacher in attendance for spiritual support.
Islam	Muslims must be able to practise the Five Pillars of Islam. Muslims may have a fatalistic view of health. Faith healing is used. Withdrawal of life support may be permitted. Autopsies are generally forbidden.	Prayers are said five times per day, facing toward Mecca. Privacy is important. Fasting may occur on holy days. Modesty in clothing is important, and hospital gowns are considered indecent; same-sex caregivers may be required. Family may request turning the bed so that the head faces Mecca at the time of death.
Judaism	Jews believe in the sanctity of life. God and medicine must have a balance. Observance of the Sabbath is important.	Prayers are said three times per day; men may wear prayer shawl and skull cap. Treatment may be refused on the Sabbath.
Christianity	Modern medical science is accepted. Prayer and faith healing are used; some Christians use laying on of hands. Most believe in an afterlife that involves spiritual restoration for believers.	Times of prayer vary between individuals; privacy is preferred. Sacraments of Holy Communion and the Anointing of the Sick may be practised. Religious symbols may include cross and prayer beads.
Hutterian	Modern science is accepted. About 80% of Hutterites seek alternative therapies. All things are shared communally. Hutterites live on colonies to help avoid earthly distractions that impede spiritual practice and devotion. Praying for good health is not appropriate; rather, prayers may be for wisdom to live a healthy life or bear suffering without complaint. Created order is God over man, man above woman, older person above younger person, and parent over child.	Education about health is appreciated. Straightforward discussions are preferred. Health care providers are respected. Families expect to be involved in health care discussions. Decision-making processes about what health concerns are important for the colony are made by the leaders. Individual decisions regarding medical treatment may be made in consultation with other members of the colony.
Indigenous (e.g., Anishinaabe)	Central value is that everything belongs to everyone in extended family. Health is having spiritual, emotional, mental, and physical balance. Connecting with the land, one's traditional territory and community, and traditional medicines and healing practices are critical factors in being healthy. Disease and illness may be caused by soul loss or spiritual intrusion.	Families generally want to be involved in health care decisions and may wish to stay with the ill individual. They desire to get to know the nurse before sharing problems. They may use Western medicine blended with traditional healing practices.

support, and dialogue (SACR-D) are key components of communication at this level. The second level, supportive spiritual care, is offered by team members who have additional training or experience in addressing spiritual issues and may involve counselling, peer support, and administration of religious rites. The third level, specialized spiritual care, is concerned with treating spiritual issues from a patient-centred approach, involving the assessment and treatment of spiritual distress and emotional distress, and is provided by those with professional training, such as spiritual care providers or faith leaders. Nurses need to exercise caution when addressing spiritual issues, as guided in the Safety Alert below.

Organizational Resources to Support Spiritual Care and Staff Well-Being

Despite the links between spirituality and health and the professional guidance for nurses to provide spiritual care, it is often overlooked in the provision of nursing care. Some barriers to nurses offering spiritual care are time constraints, lack of privacy, inadequate training, and role

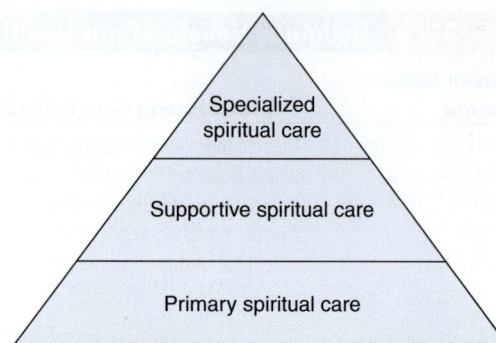

FIGURE 29.1 Levels of spiritual care. (From Shane Sinclair & Harvey Max Chochinov [2012]. Communicating with patients about existential and spiritual issues: SACR-D work. *Progress in Palliative Care*, *20*[2], 72–78. https://doi.org/10.1179/1743291X12Y.0000000015)

confusion (Neathery et al., 2020). Support from organizational leadership is also important in communicating the value of spiritual care. A study in Vancouver and London, England showed that nurses looked for permission to provide spiritual support from their organizations (Reimer-Kirkham et al., 2020). Such permission could be communicated through mission statements (e.g., with references to person-centredness), resource allocation, and policy statements about spiritual care. Nurses, patients, and families in this study often availed themselves of the designated sacred spaces (e.g., chapels, multifaith rooms) to participate in spiritual practices such as prayer and meditation.

Along with providing spiritual care to patients, spiritual care providers are increasingly involved in supporting the **spiritual well-being** of staff. Drake et al. (in press) report on how a health care team consisting of a spiritual care provider, manager, nurse educator, and nurse researchers developed a Compassion Cart intervention with a debriefing script and a grounding exercise to support nurses following a Code Blue. During the COVID-19 pandemic at one community health site in Metro Vancouver, a spiritual care provider created a Lavender Room (Gregory, 2021) for staff for meditation and respite, to help offset fatigue and stress.

DEVELOPING AND MAINTAINING SPIRITUALITY AS A NURSE

Understanding one's own spirituality is a lifelong process. It shifts and evolves with life experiences and with meanings derived from these experiences. Maintaining and increasing our understanding of spirituality is a contemplative and reflective process. Learning to recognize what gives one's life meaning and purpose and cultivating opportunities to experience this feeling of purpose are ways to develop one's own spirituality. Consider for a moment the things that bring the greatest meaning to your life, the times when you feel peace, joy, and purpose. What were you doing right before you experienced these feelings? Did you pause for a moment and take a breath? Did you recognize the beauty of the garden outside your window? Did you feel gratitude for the meal before you? Did you recognize the humanity in a face before you? Did you comfort your colleague with kindness and compassion because they just lost a patient? These are all spiritual experiences and can be nurtured and grown once they are brought to awareness. Through this awareness, one can choose to consciously connect and be fully present in the moment. Being fully present in the moment, or "presence," facilitates spiritual care.

Spiritual practices like reflective journalling; paying attention to our thoughts, emotions, and sensations; noticing when we feel most connected to those around us; and reflecting on what was occurring for us in that moment can help us understand our spirituality. In addition, it is useful to take time for contemplation on life's big questions—spend time in meditation, join a spiritual community, ask questions, be curious. Look for new ways to experience the feeling of transcendence, spend time in nature, and then practise what works for you. If you feel a sense of peace from meditation, then meditate. If moving the body with fluidity in yoga gives you a feeling of peace, then move the body in union with the self. If a walk in nature creates a sense of connection, then walk in nature. If quiet contemplation or prayer provides a feeling of transcendence, then pray. Each person will have a unique experience of spirituality and of learning to recognize when they are most connected to all things around them. Seeking out these opportunities will expand and deepen your understanding of spirituality and enhance your ability to understand the spiritual needs of your patients and will provide space to connect with them. It is important to nurture this awareness, as nurses who have a spiritual base or identity are more likely to facilitate spiritual practices and provide spiritual care in practice (Oxhandler & Parrish, 2018).

Mindfulness

Mindfulness can be an important strategy for developing spiritual practice, both for yourself and for others (see Chapter 36). Mindfulness is "awareness, cultivated by paying attention in a sustained and particular way: on purpose, in the present moment, and non-judgmentally" (Kabat-Zinn, 2013, p. 1). There are seven attitudinal factors at the foundation of mindfulness practice (Kabat-Zinn, 2013):

- An attitude of nonjudgement
- An attitude of patience (both with yourself and the process), allowing things to unfold at their own pace
- An attitude of open curiosity, approaching each moment as if encountering everything for the first time
- An attitude of trust in ourselves
- An attitude of nonstriving, relinquishing the tendency to strive toward a goal in exchange for a willingness to pay attention to whatever arises in each moment
- An attitude of acceptance—an acceptance of the present moment as it is, accepting what we notice without trying to make it different
- An attitude of letting go or nonattachment; we let things be as they are in the present moment, without grasping or pushing away

Adopting these attitudes of mindfulness helps create an environment that is safe for patients to express their spirituality.

Research examining the effectiveness of mindfulness programs with university students demonstrated that it is beneficial for stress reduction and improves quality of life. Students who learned mindfulness had an increased nonjudgemental and nonreactive stance toward feelings, thoughts, and emotions; thus, mindfulness can be an effective intervention to support mental health (Canby et al., 2015). Research with health care providers who have received mindfulness training has found that levels of burnout and stress were reduced, mental well-being improved, and patient satisfaction increased (Suleiman-Martos et al., 2020).

REFLECTING ON NURSES' SPIRITUAL CARE

Personal growth along the journey of spirituality is a lifelong pursuit and one that is not easily evaluated by others. Particularly during times of illness and suffering, patients need to clarify values, reshape philosophies, strengthen relationships, and live experiences that help to shape their purpose in life. It is not normally within the nursing role to "evaluate" whether patients achieve connectedness, meaning, peace, hope, or other indicators of spirituality. Meaning-making during suffering is often a mysterious, highly personal experience. As nurses,

we can always be present for patients in their suffering and we can do everything within our power to alleviate distress. We should aggressively treat pain and other symptoms. We should provide a hospitable climate for those who are most important in patients' lives. We should put great effort into ensuring that patients can continue with their religious and spiritual practices. We should know the values and beliefs that are important to take into account as part of the overall picture of care. These are all spiritual "interventions." But we need to be cautious about entering into the areas of mystery, particularly if we are sensing our own need to explain or control patients' suffering.

In this aspect of nursing care, it is appropriate to reflect on your own contributions to a healing relationship. Were patients' spiritual practices respected? Was the relationship characterized by caring, respect, and support? Does the patient express trust and confidence in you? Is the patient able to discuss important issues or topics? Is the patient comfortable expressing spiritual needs to you? That sense of rapport that develops within a nurse–patient relationship is often the best indicator that you have helped to provide a safe context within which patients can live their spiritual journey.

KEY CONCEPTS

- Spirituality is personal and unique to each individual, while influenced by sociocultural meanings and relationships.
- Nurses must be aware of their own spirituality in order to recognize the spirituality of others.
- Religion is a system of organized beliefs and worship that a person practises to outwardly express spirituality.
- Faith is a relationship with God or a higher power or authority that enables action and gives purpose and meaning to an individual's life.
- Canadian nursing practice has a rich spiritual heritage that has influenced contemporary practice.
- Canada represents a wide range of religious and spiritual diversity, requiring nurses to have an understanding of various traditions.
- Spirituality may have beneficial health outcomes.
- When patients experience acute or chronic illness or a terminal disease, spiritual resources may help a person recover.
- Faith communities can be a vital source of social support, connectedness, and healing practices.
- Spirituality is a lifelong journey that may reflect the age and life experiences of the patient, as well as their current context.
- Spiritual concerns can vary by life events, illnesses, and clinical contexts.
- Spiritual practices are varied and may include private worship, prayer, meditation, sacraments, singing, use of a rosary or prayer beads, and reading religious texts.
- Nurses require spiritual care competencies that encompass the nurse's self-awareness and attitude, spiritual dimensions of the nursing process, and workplace resources and health care policy.
- Critical thinking in spiritual care includes an understanding of the unique perspective of the patient.
- A spiritual assessment is most successful when nurses attempt to understand rather than assess patients' spirituality, allowing the development of the relationship.
- Spiritual assessment tools should be flexible, and the depth of the assessment must be sensitive to the circumstances.
- The personal nature of spirituality requires open communication and the establishment of trust between nurse and patient.
- Ethical care includes respecting appropriate nurse–patient boundaries and knowing when patients should be referred to a spiritual care provider or to a social worker.

- Certain religions may have dietary restrictions or beliefs and practices of health care that may have implications for nursing practice.
- Spiritual care is an expression of self; how nurses learn to be with patients and the qualities that nurses bring are important to nursing care.
- Spiritual practices may be an effective coping resource for physical and psychological symptoms.
- Spiritual practices can be effective forms of self-care for nurses.
- Spiritual care cannot be evaluated like other aspects of nursing practice. Rather, nurses should focus on being present for patients while seeking to alleviate suffering.

CRITICAL THINKING EXERCISES

1. Renee (pronouns: they them) is a 40-year-old business owner with more than 100 employees. A 12-hour workday is not unusual for them. Renee is married, has four teenage children, and is solely responsible for providing financially for the family. Last evening, Renee was admitted to the cardiac care unit with severe chest pain resulting from a myocardial infarction (heart attack). They are now stabilized but frequently ask about their diagnostic tests and what to do to go home. Renee tells the nurse, "My doctor tells me I will need surgery once I am more stable. I hope they can do that soon. I just can't believe this is happening. I worry about what will happen to my business while I am gone and to my family if I can't keep my business going." Renee asks, "Could I die from this?" You notice that Renee has devotional literature at the bedside. How might you go about conducting a spiritual health assessment for Renee?
2. Tejal is a new graduate nurse caring for Clare for the first time. Clare, who is 27 years old, has recently received a diagnosis of renal cancer and is scheduled for a nephrectomy. Tejal notices from the patient chart that Clare has identified as Jewish. What factors might be important to consider in relation to Clare's spirituality or religion for the plan of care? How might Tejal determine which factors are relevant for the patient?
3. Critical thinking is an ongoing process. When you learn that you are assigned to care for Fangzhou Lin, you note that the Kardex information includes their religion (Buddhist) and place of birth (Hong Kong). A colleague tells you Fangzhou can speak some English. The patient is 80 years old and reportedly has a hearing deficit. What knowledge might you wish to reflect on critically before beginning a spiritual assessment of this patient?

Answers to Critical Thinking Exercises appear on the Evolve website.

REVIEW QUESTIONS

Review Questions 1 to 10 relate to the case study at the beginning of the chapter.

1. Which of the following answers *best* demonstrates caring for a patient's spiritual needs?
   a. Having the same beliefs as the patient
   b. Praying for the patient
   c. Accepting the patient's beliefs and experiences
   d. Calling for a religious leader if the nurse determines a need
2. In the case of Blair, what is the FICA Tool helpful for?
   a. Understanding a patient's spirituality
   b. Making referrals to community resources
   c. Planning spiritual assessment and care
   d. Guiding spiritual intervention

3. In caring for Blair, Amy, the home health nurse, decides to compete a spiritual assessment using the FICA tool. Referring to the FICA Tool, match the criteria in the left column with the appropriate assessment question in the right column.

   _____ 1. **F** – Faith
   _____ 2. **I** – Importance of spirituality
   _____ 3. **C** – Community
   _____ 4. **A** – Interventions to address spiritual needs

   a. Do you have a higher power or authority that helps you act on your values or beliefs?
   b. Are there activities that give you comfort spiritually?
   c. To whom do you go for support in times of difficulty?
   d. Is spirituality an important aspect of who you are?

4. Which statements are *true* when considering the spiritual practices of the patient? *(Select all that apply.)*
   a. They have no place in the health care setting.
   b. They provide structure and support for the patient.
   c. They can be a barrier to providing nursing care.
   d. There are many different types.
   e. They are dependent on religious beliefs.
5. Which of the following statements *best* describes establishing presence with a patient?
   a. Offering a closeness—physically, psychologically, and spiritually
   b. Offering touch
   c. The nurse sharing their own spiritual beliefs
   d. Performing procedures
6. Which of the following *best* describes spirituality?
   a. A structured search for God
   b. A different word to describe religion
   c. An appropriate term to describe atheists
   d. Commonly identified as meaning, purpose, and connectedness
7. Based on research findings, which of the following interventions by the nurse might be appreciated by Blair? *(Select all that apply.)*
   a. Intimate interventions like meditation and journalling
   b. Support of the patient's spiritual practices
   c. Sharing of the nurse's personal beliefs and practices
   d. An attitude of open curiosity regarding the patient's spiritual beliefs and spiritual concerns
   e. Sharing of the nurse's religious beliefs
8. Which of the following may be *most* beneficial to a patient like Blair who is experiencing a terminal illness?
   a. Grief work
   b. Diet therapy
   c. Acupuncture
   d. Values clarification
9. Which of the following *best* describes spiritual assessment?
   a. It is structured and follows a specific process.
   b. It can only be done by a spiritual care provider.
   c. It should be flexible, and the depth of the assessment is dependent on the circumstances.
   d. It is the first component of the nursing assessment.

10. Which of the following *best* describe relational practice? *(Select all that apply.)*
    a. Creates the environment for spiritual care
    b. Allows the nurse to create clear boundaries
    c. Is unlikely if the patient and nurse hold different spiritual beliefs
    d. Is not a component of spiritual care
    e. Is respectful, compassionate, and authentic inquiry into the experience of another

🌐 *Rationales for the Review Questions appear on the Evolve website.*

RECOMMENDED WEBSITES

Canadian Association for Parish Nursing Ministry: https://www.capnm.ca
The Canadian Association for Parish Nursing Ministry is committed to the development of parish nursing as a health and ministry resource within Canada.

Canadian Multifaith Federation: http://omc.ca
The Canadian Multifaith Federation provides services and advocates on spiritual and religious matters for Canadians.

Center for Spirituality and Healing: https://www.csh.umn.edu
Established in 1995 at the University of Minnesota in the United States, the Center for Spirituality and Healing provides education about integrative medicine, combining biomedical, complementary, cross-cultural, and spiritual care.

Center for Spirituality, Theology and Health: https://spiritualityandhealth.duke.edu
The purpose of this Center, which is part of Duke University in the United States, is to conduct research on the effects of spirituality on physical and mental health.

Global Network for Spirituality and Health: https://smhs.gwu.edu/gwish/global-network
This network provides a way for members to work together internationally toward high-quality comprehensive and compassionate spiritual care.

Institute for the Bio-Cultural Study of Religion: http://www.ibcsr.org/index.php/irr-basicinfo/ibcsr-research-review
This organization produces a regular annotated bibliography of the recent research in the field.

Nurses Christian Fellowship: https://ncf-jcn.org
Nurses Christian Fellowship, a US institution, is a Christian organization with the goal of connecting Christian faith with nursing. This website contains information about the scope and trend of research related to spiritual care. The Canadian chapter of Nurses Christian Fellowship can be found at https://www.ncfcanada.ca

Spirituality in Health-Care Network: https://www.spiritualityinhealthcare.net/links.html
This Canadian site provides links to a number of resources.

🌐 REFERENCES

A full reference list is available on the website for this book at http://evolve.elsevier.com/Canada/Potter/fundamentals/

30

Stress and Adaptation

Canadian content written by Tanya Park, RN, PhD, with original chapter contributions by Carla Armstead Harmon, PhD (Curriculum & Instruction), MSN, BSN

OBJECTIVES

Mastery of content in this chapter will enable you to:

- Define the key terms listed.
- Describe how stress is conceptualized.
- Define the key biological systems involved in stress responses.
- Describe how overwhelming stress or chronic stress can affect health.
- Differentiate acute stress disorder and post-traumatic stress disorder.
- Describe the integration of stress theory with nursing theories.
- Formulate nursing diagnoses from assessment data.
- Describe stress management techniques beneficial for coping with stress.
- Describe the process of crisis intervention.
- Develop a care plan for patients experiencing stress.
- Explain how stress in the workplace can affect health care providers.

KEY TERMS

Acute stress disorder
Adaptation
Alarm reaction
Appraisal
Burnout
Coping
Crisis
Crisis intervention
Developmental crises

Distress
Endorphins
Eustress
Exhaustion stage
Fight-or-flight response
Flashbacks
General adaptation syndrome
Homeostasis
Post-traumatic growth

Post-traumatic stress disorder (PTSD)
Primary appraisal
Resistance stage
Secondary appraisal
Situational crises
Stress
Stressor
Trauma

🌐 WEBSITE

http://evolve.elsevier.com/Canada/Potter/fundamentals/

CASE STUDY

Missing What Is Important

I was so keen! I wanted to be such a good nurse. In the second year of my nursing program, I began my first day on an assessment unit within our provincial psychiatric hospital with eager anticipation of testing my newly learned communication techniques, mixed with some curiosity and anxiety about how I would react to patients.

As it turned out, what I was stressed about was so far off the mark! I was so concerned about how I would react to patients that I did not consider how patients would react to me. We were to complete verbatim reports regarding our interactions with our patients. However, my assigned patient was a middle-aged person with paranoid schizophrenia who apparently was suspicious of new people. It was suggested that I "hang around" the unit for a few days, so that my patient could get used to seeing me before I actually approached them. But what about those verbatim reports? How could I initiate the first conversation? Maybe discreet observations could fill in for the time being. I was caught up in my role as an unobtrusive staff member. On the second day, the patient abruptly approached me and in an angry tone stated, "You have been following me and watching me

for 2 days!" So much for my discretion. In focusing only on my own perceptions and needs, I had thought little about how perception, like communication, can be different for the participants. My spontaneous response was, "You're right, I have. I just didn't know how to approach you." The patient's anger dissolved into a laugh at my awkwardness. That clear, honest response was the start of a very rewarding nurse–patient relationship that spanned the entire 2-month rotation. They taught me so much about mental health nursing: how perceptions about potential stressors affect our interactions, how spontaneity can be powerful in interactions, and how our own self-perceptions need to be checked against the perceptions of our patients, regardless of diagnosis.

I subsequently enjoyed mental health nursing as a career choice, which spanned more than 30 years. I worked with many different clinical populations over the years, but I still remember my stress and distress over my first patient assignment and how it made me blind to what was really going on.

Think about this case study as you read this chapter. There are review questions at the end of the chapter that relate to the case study.

Stress: Everyone has experienced it, but the term **stress** is difficult to define and is often loosely used. It has been used to describe a stimulus, a process, a response, and a state, which often leads to confusion and ambiguity. In this chapter, the term **stressor** is used to describe an event that activates stress response systems—that is, it acts as a stimulus. This activation of multiple biological systems and psychological schemas has a collective goal of maintaining a state of dynamic equilibrium. Stressors can arise in the external environment and range from motivational prompts, such as taking a school examination, to devastating personal events, such as a life-threatening illness, a motor vehicle crash, a sexual assault, or a natural disaster (e.g., an earthquake or a tornado). Internal stressors, such as hunger or infection, can also activate stress response systems. Behavioural responses to stressors presumably reflect the activation of numerous biological systems. Behavioural responses can change over time, inasmuch as previous stressful experiences and individual contextual factors can produce **adaptation** in stress response systems. Among animals, biological systems help alert the animal to some type of threat in the environment and prepare it to mount a defence. These systems also turn off when the threat is past. For humans, in addition to acute threats to body integrity, psychological well-being and sense of self-worth can be threatened. Physical and psychological health can be severely affected by serious or chronic stressors, and these effects can be long-standing and pervasive. It is important for health care providers to understand conceptual frameworks that have been developed to explain the relationship between stress (overwhelming or chronic) and health.

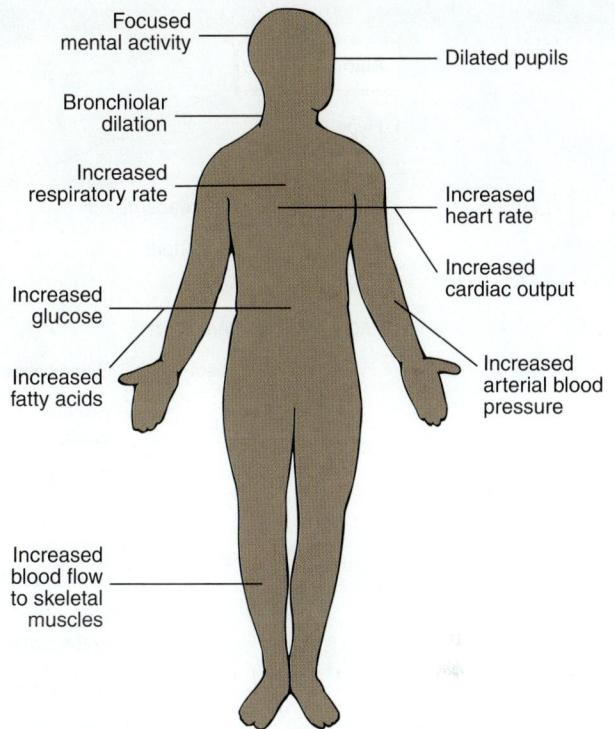

FIGURE 30.1 Fight-or-flight response.

Labels: Focused mental activity; Bronchiolar dilation; Increased respiratory rate; Increased glucose; Increased fatty acids; Increased blood flow to skeletal muscles; Dilated pupils; Increased heart rate; Increased cardiac output; Increased arterial blood pressure.

CONCEPTUALIZATIONS OF STRESS

Physiological Conceptualizations

Walter Cannon was one of the pioneers of the early twentieth century who laid the groundwork for regulatory physiology and concepts of adaptation. Cannon demonstrated that the sympathetic–adrenal–medullary (SAM) system acted to maintain homeostasis of the internal environment. Cannon first coined the term **fight-or-flight response**, in 1915, to describe an animal's response to threats through the activation of the SAM system (Figure 30.1; Le Moal, 2007). Hans Selye, another pioneer, focused on maladaptation and the pathology of stress. Selye demonstrated the existence of a biological stress syndrome, called the **general adaptation syndrome** (Selye, 1974; Figure 30.2). This three-stage syndrome occurs in response to serious stressors. The first stage is the **alarm reaction**, analogous to Cannon's fight-or-flight response to stress. In this stage, complex physiological changes help the organism mobilize energy and react to the stressor. The second stage of the general adaptation syndrome is the **resistance stage**. During resistance, the organism maintains arousal while the body works to defend against and adapt to the stressor and maintain homeostasis. Should the stressors continue for an extended period, organisms use up their finite ability to adapt, and they enter a third stage of the adaptation syndrome, called the **exhaustion stage**. This is a pathological state in which organisms start showing diverse health consequences, which may eventually result in death. Selye was also the first to emphasize the role of the pituitary–adrenal axis in the pathological processes of stress.

At this point, two systems for stress were proposed: (1) the SAM system for behavioural fight-or-flight responses to stress and immediate adaptation and (2) the pituitary–adrenal axis for maintaining homeostasis. The concept of the pituitary–adrenal axis was expanded to the hypothalamic–pituitary–adrenal (HPA) axis; this axis is thought to mediate a bidirectional brain–body communication during physiological and psychological stress and is activated to promote homeostasis and to adapt to threatening or stressful situations (Herman et al., 2016). The concept of **homeostasis** is the return of systems to a

stable set point; *allostasis* is the term used to describe how cumulative stressors can change physiological set points through adaptation (Fava et al., 2019). In this way, organisms are readied to respond and adapt to future stressors, but maintaining this state of readiness has an energy cost. This cost is termed *allostatic load*, which refers to the physiological burden of repeated stressors and enduring a heightened stress response system. When this load becomes too great, stress responses change from adaptation to health problems and stress-related disorders.

Psychological Conceptualizations

In addition to physiological models of stress and stress responses, cognitive approaches to stress were also studied. The general adaptation syndrome and fight-or-flight responses to stress did not explicitly take into account perceptions and appraisals of stress in humans. Researchers began to look at the relationship between the person and the environment. The roles of perception and appraisal in stress responses are integral in the framework of stress proposed by Richard Lazarus. Lazarus (1999) maintained that a person is under stress only if the person evaluates the event or circumstance as personally significant. **Appraisal** of an event or circumstance is an ongoing perceptual process (Aguilera, 1998). Evaluating an event for its personal meaning is called **primary appraisal**. If as a result of primary appraisal the person identifies the event or circumstance as a harm, loss, threat, or challenge, the person experiences stress. If stress is present, **secondary appraisal** then focuses on possible coping strategies. **Coping** is the active process of managing circumstances, expending effort to solve personal and interpersonal problems, and seeking to master, minimize, reduce, or tolerate stress or conflict. Balancing factors contribute to restoring equilibrium.

If previous ways of coping are not effective, a **crisis** may occur, in which the person faces a turning point in life and the person must change. Caplan (1981) distinguished two types of crises: those associated with changing developmental levels, or **developmental crises**, and **situational crises**. Examples of developmental crises could be related to mastering developmental tasks as an individual (independence in adolescence) or as a family (children leaving home, caregiving to older

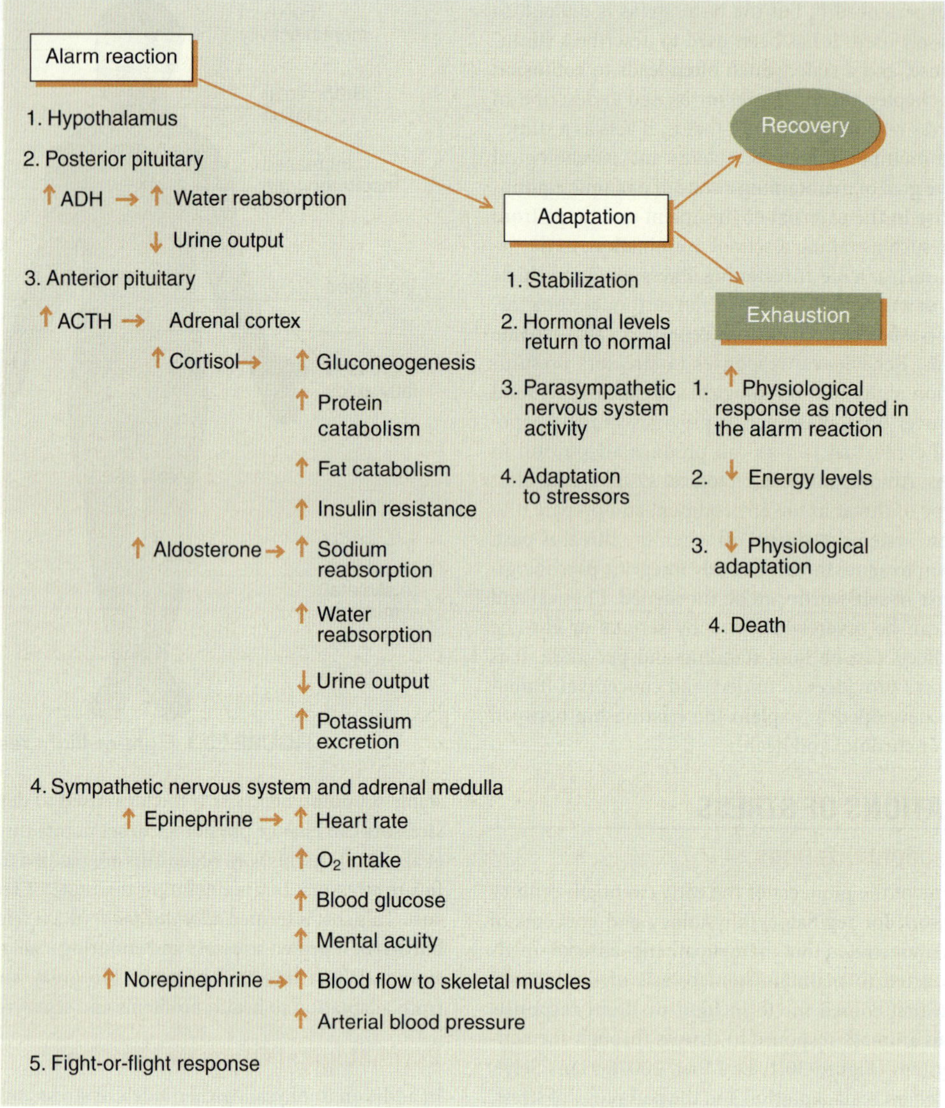

FIGURE 30.2 General adaptation syndrome. *ACTH,* Adrenocorticotropic hormone; *ADH,* antidiuretic hormone.

parents). Examples of situational crises could include natural disasters like floods or famine, the end of an intimate relationship, or loss of work transportation through a motor vehicle crash. The frame of reference for a crisis is the viewpoint of the person experiencing the crisis. According to Aguilera's (1998) crisis theory, the vital questions for a person in crisis are "What does this mean to you?" and "How is it going to affect your life?" A basic assumption of crisis theory is that a person can either advance or regress as a result of a crisis, depending on how the crisis is managed. Feedback cues lead to ongoing reappraisals of original perceptions. Therefore, coping behaviours constantly change as new information is perceived.

Later work in the important role of appraisal and perception focused on the contribution of age and gender to responses to stressful events. Coping strategies, meaning attached to events, and responses to stressors change with age. Gender differences may be conceptualized as an interaction between biologically based sex differences and an individual's social context. People may perceive a stressor differently, may attach different meanings to that stressor, and thus may have different responses and reactions (Mélendez et al., 2012). Interestingly, Mélendez and colleagues (2012) found that gender and age affected

overt emotional expression and the development of coping strategies across the lifespan.

In summary, individual differences in response to stressors can be affected by previous vulnerabilities and experiences, coexisting health problems, age, gender, allostatic load, and coping resources. Psychological and biological conceptualizations are not mutually exclusive. Indeed, the integration of the various frameworks helps explain the complexity of the relationship between stress and health.

STRESS RESPONSE SYSTEMS

Sympathetic–Adrenal–Medullary System

Activation of the SAM system results in increased heart rate, diversion of blood from the intestines to the brain and skeletal muscles, increased blood pressure, bronchodilation and increased respiratory rate, and increases in blood glucose levels (Chrousos et al., 1988; Selye, 1991). All these changes are meant to prepare for fight-or-flight responses. A stressor activates specific cells in the brainstem that release norepinephrine into the bloodstream. Norepinephrine stimulates the adrenal medulla to release epinephrine. Epinephrine produces the cardiovascular, respiratory, and metabolic changes and the heightened awareness or alertness. Chronic stimulation brings about a chronic arousal state, with sleep disturbance, edginess and irritability, gastrointestinal upset, and increased startle responses. Brain areas that are involved in this stress response system include the following:

- *Reticular formation:* This is a small, integrative cluster of neurons in the brainstem and spinal cord that continuously monitor the physiological status of the body through connections with sensory and motor tracts. For example, certain cells within the reticular formation can cause a sleeping person to regain consciousness or increase the level of consciousness when a need arises.
- *Limbic system:* This is another integrative cluster of neurons that interconnect several parts of the brain and are involved in processing strong emotional experiences. Fear and perceived threat will cause increased activity within this system.
- *Midbrain and pons:* The midbrain joins the lower part of the brainstem and the spinal cord with the higher part of the brain and acts as a reflex centre for certain auditory, visual, and postural stimuli. The pons mainly relays impulses to and from the medulla oblongata to other parts of the brain and the peripheral nervous system, and it also controls the rate and depth of breathing.
- *Medulla oblongata:* This brain region controls vital functions necessary for survival, including heart rate, blood pressure, and respiration. Impulses travelling to and from the medulla oblongata can increase or decrease these vital functions. For example, heart rate is regulated by sympathetic or parasympathetic nervous system impulses travelling from the medulla oblongata to the heart. The rate increases in response to pulses from sympathetic fibres and decreases with impulses from parasympathetic fibres.

Hypothalamic–Pituitary–Adrenal Axis

Activation of the HPA axis results in the release of a cascade of hormones. A stressor activates the hypothalamus to release a corticotrophin-releasing hormone (CRH). This hormone activates receptors in the anterior pituitary, which in turn signal the release of adrenocorticotropic hormone (ACTH) into the bloodstream. ACTH interacts with its receptors in the adrenal cortex to release glucocorticoids. In humans, the major glucocorticoid is cortisol. Cortisol has effects similar to those of epinephrine, contributing to the increase in heart rate and blood pressure, causing shunting of blood to skeletal muscles, and increasing the availability of glucose in the bloodstream. This stress response system is tightly controlled by negative feedback, whereby rising cortisol levels activate receptors in the hypothalamus and the pituitary gland, shutting off further release of CRH and ACTH (Takahashi et al., 2018). Other brain chemicals, such as β-endorphin arginine vasopressin and oxytocin, are also involved in the regulation of the HPA axis.

This part of the endocrine system interacts with other parts that regulate sex hormone levels, thyroid hormones, electrolyte and fluid balance, and insulin release. Therefore, overwhelming or chronic stressors can have diverse and complex impacts on health. The following brain areas are involved in this stress response system:

- *Hypothalamus:* This region of the brain is involved with many basic physiological processes, including appetite, sexual drive, sleeping, motor activity, and mood states (all of which are affected by stress). The hypothalamus is highly interconnected with many other areas of the brain. Dysregulation of the hypothalamus is thought to be involved in depression.
- *Pituitary gland:* This small gland, attached to the hypothalamus, produces and releases hormones that control vital functions. It is divided into the anterior and posterior portions. The anterior pituitary releases stress-, thyroid-, growth-, and reproduction-related

hormones, whereas the posterior pituitary releases hormones related to electrolyte and water balance, as well as oxytocin. Both the pituitary gland and the hypothalamus can produce endorphins. Endorphins are hormones that produce a sense of well-being and reduce pain (Lazarus, 1999).

- *Adrenal glands:* One of these glands rests atop each kidney, and they are fundamental to stress responses. Each is composed of two very different regions. The outer region, or cortex, is where glucocorticoids such as cortisol are produced and released, and the inner region, or medulla, is where epinephrine is produced and released.

STRESS AND THE IMMUNE SYSTEM

Physiological responses to stress also include immunological responses, although the mechanisms through which stress affects the immune system are not fully understood (Takahashi et al., 2018; Box 30.1). The immune system differentiates between self and non-self material, so that, under normal conditions, one's own cells are not treated as threats in the way that bacteria, viruses, parasites, or toxins are treated. An antigen on the surface of bacteria cells identifies them as invaders. After being exposed to a particular antigen, the immune system remembers how to respond to that antigen and is prepared to respond with antibodies when the same antigen appears at a later time. Autoimmune illnesses such as multiple sclerosis, fibromyalgia, or insulin resistance can occur when the immune system misinterprets the body's own cells as foreign. Glucocorticoids are powerful anti-inflammatory agents and play a role in the cascade of homeostatic immune responses that are activated by infection or inflammation and clinical depression. Dysregulation or chronic activation of the SAM system and the HPA axis may increase the risk of stress-related mental illnesses, as well as cardiovascular disease, insulin resistance (which in turn can increase risk for type 2 diabetes), metabolic syndromes, and autoimmune illnesses.

THE RELATIONSHIP BETWEEN TYPE OF STRESSOR AND HEALTH

Selye (1974) identified two types of stress: distress, or damaging stress, and eustress, or stress that protects health. Eustress is stress that is

---

BOX 30.1	Factors Influencing the Response to Stressors

Aspects of a Stressor That Influence the Stress Response
Intensity
Scope
Duration
Number and nature of other stressors
Past exposure to serious stressors
Predictability

Individual Characteristics That May Influence the Stress Response
Age
Gender
Perception of personal control or inescapability
Availability of social supports
Feelings of competence
Cognitive appraisal

experienced due to a positive event. Eustress often leads to feelings of happiness and hopefulness. Eustress is a positive, healthy adaptation to stressors in daily life. In reference to this concept, Selye (1974) wrote the book *Stress Without Distress.* However, Aldwin (2007) wrote that the idea of healthy stress is controversial because it is difficult to tell whether a person has benefited from stress or is coping by denying the stress in some way.

Distressing events can be categorized in many ways, including work stressors, family stressors, chronic stressors, acute stressors, daily hassles, trauma, and crisis: "Work and family stress interact, family being the background for work stress, and work the background for family stress" (Lazarus, 1999). Parents who have preschool children, for example, may experience full-time work as stressful when their child cannot go to day care because the child is ill and their spouse's job involves extended periods away from home. It is difficult to categorize some events, such as the COVID-19 pandemic. The loss of life and changes like changing work sites—working from home or loss of work—were experienced throughout the world as a result of the pandemic, and it is difficult to predict what long-term health implications will result. Chronic stress can arise also from stressful roles, such as being a caregiver for a spouse with Alzheimer's disease, or persistent physical or psychological conflict. Another example of chronic stress is living with a long-term illness. Conversely, acute stress is provoked by time-limited events that are threatening for a relatively brief period. In the context of chronic or acute stress, daily life activities, such as commuting to work, maintaining a home, social and personal interactions, and managing money, can become more difficult to manage. Trauma can refer to any physical damage to the body or, in psychological terms, can refer to feelings of fear, threat, and persistent reliving after witnessing or experiencing an emotionally painful, distressful, or shocking event or series of events. Severe stressors such as natural disasters or interpersonal events such as family violence or child maltreatment are often considered traumatic events; however, as in other types of stressors, perception plays a major role in the individual's response to such events. Indeed, for some people, serious stressors can lead to positive change or personal growth, leading in turn to greater self-knowledge, improved coping skills, stronger social ties, and positive changes in values and perspectives called post-traumatic growth. The COVID-19 pandemic has led to increased trauma and stress for nurses and can be an opportunity for nurses to experience post-traumatic growth (Chen et al., 2021).

Stress-Related Disorders

Prolonged exposure to a serious stressor or an acute stressor that overwhelms the ability to cope can lead to stress-related disorders (Box 30.2). However, even if an individual's stress-related symptoms do not meet full criteria for a stress disorder, it is important to recognize that those symptoms may have a significant impact on the individual's functioning and relationships with others. If interventions are not implemented, these symptoms can decrease quality of life and increase the risk of developing the full disorder. Early emerging stress-related symptoms include poor sleep, tension and jitteriness, and inability to concentrate, to a degree that day-to-day activities are affected.

Although stress-related psychiatric disturbances are usually considered to be acute stress disorder and post-traumatic stress disorder (PTSD), these are only two potential health outcomes. It is important to recognize the diversity of health effects from serious stressors. Indeed, clinical depression, chronic pain syndromes, somatization disorder, and irritable bowel syndrome have all been linked to chronic stress (Kivimaki & Steptoe, 2018). Health providers need to perform thorough, multifaceted assessments to identify the full range of health effects.

BOX 30.2   RESEARCH HIGHLIGHT
COVID-19, Critical Care Nurses, and Stress

Research Focus

In early 2020, the world came to know about a virus that was causing widespread infection: a novel coronavirus called SARS-CoV-2. The global COVID-19 pandemic we have experienced since that time has caused health care systems to rapidly require changes like increased and mandatory use of personal protective equipment. During the pandemic, nurses were often the only person with whom patients interacted while in hospital, due to strict public health rules implemented to stop the spread of the virus. Nurses often work in high-stress, rapidly changing work environments; however, the COVID-19 pandemic significantly affected many nurses' work. The project reported by Crowe et al. (2021) highlights the increased potential for mental health disorders due to the high stress experienced during the pandemic.

Research Abstract & Methods

This article presents the findings from a study aimed at examining the mental health of Critical Care Registered Nurses (CCRN) providing direct patient care during the initial phase of the COVID-19 pandemic in Canada: 109 CCRNs participated in two self-reported validated surveys (the Impact of Events Scale-Revised, and the Depression, Anxiety and Stress Scale), and 15 CCRNs participated in an interview.

Results

The results from the surveys showed that symptoms of post-traumatic stress disorder (PTSD) were experienced by 50% of participants, as well as significant experiences of depression, anxiety, and stress symptoms for many participants. The interview participants all described feelings of anxiety, worry, distress, and fear. Challenges that were identified included rapidly changing policy, communication, meeting patient care needs, and managing personal commitments. The authors concluded that CCRNs have experienced significant psychological distress related to the COVID-19 pandemic.

Implications for Practice

- Regardless of age, sex, marital status, or years in health care, similar findings of increased psychological distress were experienced by CCRNs.
- Trust and clear communication are needed by CCRNs to support their work during rapidly changing health care information.
- Health care workplaces urgently need to implement evidence-informed strategies to strengthen resilience and coping strategies for their employees.

From Crowe, S., Howard, F. A., Vanderspank-Wright, B., et al. (2021). The effect of COVID-19 pandemic on the mental health of Canadian critical care nurses providing patient care during the early phase pandemic: A mixed method study. *Intensive & Critical Care Nursing, 63,* 102999. https://doi.org/10.1016/j.iccn.2020.102999

Acute Stress Disorder. Acute stress disorder is caused by exposure to one or more traumatic events and lasts at least 3 days to 1 month after experiencing, witnessing, or being confronted with a traumatic event; the reaction is one of intense fear, helplessness, or horror (American Psychiatric Association, 2013). Other criteria of acute stress disorder are the presence of the following symptoms: (1) the patient displays acute dissociative symptoms; (2) the patient has at least one recurring symptom (intense memories, flashbacks [recurring, intensely vivid mental images of a past traumatic experience], or distressing dreams); (3) the patient displays marked avoidance of stimuli that arouse memories of the trauma; (4) the patient shows marked hyperarousal; and (5) the patient experiences arousal symptoms such as sleep disturbance, irritable behaviour, and angry outbursts. These symptoms must have a significant effect on the individual's occupational, social, or personal functioning to meet full criteria for acute stress disorder. Examples of traumatic events that lead to acute stress disorder are motor vehicle crashes, natural disasters, violent personal assault, emergency service work experiences, and military combat. Nurses are also not immune to acute stress disorder. Treatment usually focuses on symptoms, to aid in sleeping and to relieve the jitteriness and irritability. If the trauma-related symptoms persist longer than 1 month, the individual will likely meet the criteria for PTSD.

Post-Traumatic Stress Disorder. Symptoms of post-traumatic stress disorder (PTSD) are more persistent, having endured for at least 1 month (American Psychiatric Association, 2013). The symptom clusters are similar to those of acute stress disorder, with less emphasis on dissociative symptoms. The diagnosis of PTSD was formulated from research with men returning from the Vietnam War and was first thought to be quite rare. Recognizing the extensive impact on people and their families, in June 2018 the Government of Canada enacted the *Federal Framework on Post-Traumatic Stress Disorder Act,* followed closely by the development of a federal framework. This Act has three priority areas: improving tracking of PTSD rates, establishing guidelines for the treatment and management of PTSD, and the creation of standardized educational materials (Public Health Agency of Canada, 2020).

NURSING KNOWLEDGE BASE

Nurses have proposed theories related to stress and coping. Because stress plays a role in vulnerability to disease, symptoms of stress often necessitate nursing intervention.

Nursing Theory and the Role of Stress

Neuman's (1995) systems model is based on the concepts of stress and reaction to stress. Nurses are responsible for developing interventions to prevent or reduce stressors on the patient or to make them more bearable for the patient (Neuman, 1995). Because Neuman's model is a systems model, it is applied to understand not only patients' individual responses to stressors but also families' and communities' responses. All systems experience multiple stressors, each of which has a differing potential to disturb the person's, family's, or community's dynamic balance. Every person has developed a set of responses to stress that constitute the "normal line of defence" (Neuman, 1995). This line of defence helps maintain health and wellness. However, when "physiological, psychological, sociocultural, developmental, or spiritual influences" are unable to buffer stress, the normal line of defence is broken, and disease can result. Neuman's systems model coincides with Selye's (1974) general adaptation syndrome and the concept of allostatic load.

Neuman's (1995) systems model stresses the importance of accuracy in assessment and interventions that promote optimal wellness through the use of primary, secondary, and tertiary prevention strategies. According to Neuman's theory, the goal of primary prevention is to promote patient wellness by stress prevention and reduction of risk factors. Secondary prevention occurs after symptoms appear. The nurse helps the patient determine the meaning of the illness and stress and finds resources available to handle them. Tertiary prevention begins when the patient is becoming more stable and recovering. At the tertiary level of prevention, the nurse supports rehabilitation processes involved in healing, moving the patient back to wellness, and the primary level of disease prevention.

In their health promotion model, Pender and colleagues (2002) proposed that health promotion is directed toward increasing the level of well-being of an individual or group. Conversely, primary, secondary, and tertiary types of prevention (health protection) focus on avoiding negative events. Pender and colleagues considered stress reduction strategies important to reducing threats to well-being, helping people fulfill their potential, and shaping and maintaining health behaviours. To change behaviour, the patient must initiate the change and behave differently in interactions. On the basis of core assumptions regarding the capability and desire of people to be healthy, Pender and colleagues suggested strategies for stress prevention and for health promotion related to stress management.

Situational, Maturational, and Sociocultural Factors

Multiple factors affect the types of potential stressors and coping mechanisms. Age is one; for example, adolescence, adulthood, and old age bring different stressors (Mélendez et al., 2012). Appraisal of stressors, amount and type of social support, and coping strategies are other factors that affect appraisal of stressors, as are previous life experiences (Mélendez et al., 2012).

Situational Factors. Situational stress can arise from a person's current circumstances, such as moving, changing jobs (stressful job changes include promotions, transfers, downsizing, restructuring, and changes in supervisors and responsibilities), and adjusting to a chronic illness or condition. Common diseases and conditions that can be exacerbated by stress are obesity, hypertension, diabetes, depression, asthma, and coronary artery disease. Being a family caregiver may also cause situational stress, although the source of stress may be not necessarily the caregiving but other factors in the caregiver's life, such as work, finances, or lack of respite (Rao et al., 2020). Spouses and other family members also experience stress when a loved one is ill.

Maturational Factors. Stressors vary with life stage and are not necessarily related to negative events. Important individual and family developmental milestones can be anticipated with excitement but can nonetheless be stressful. Preadolescents may experience stress related to self-esteem issues, changes in family structure as a result of divorce or death of a parent, or hospitalizations. As adolescents search for their identity with peer groups and separate from their families, they may view these developmental tasks as stressors. In addition, they must make decisions about using mind-altering substances, peer pressure, sexuality, jobs, school, and career choices; the decision-making process may also be viewed as stressful. Stress for adults can arise from major changes in individual and family life circumstances (Aguilera, 1998). These changes include the many milestones of beginning a family and a career, losing parents, helping children leave home, and accepting physical aging. In old age, stressors include the loss of autonomy and mastery, as a result of general frailty or health problems that limit mobility, stamina, and strength, and the loss of a spouse, close friends, and family that provided social support over the years (Box 30.3).

Social Determinants of Health. The social determinants of health are the conditions in which people are born, grow, work, and live that influence their life. Disparities in the social determinants of health affect quality of life, health status, and life expectancy (Lathrop, 2020). For example, poverty, food insecurity, abuse, and racism can lead to chronic stress (Lathrop, 2020). Nurses can positively influence the social determinants of health by understanding the impact of disparities on individuals and advocating for systemic and policy changes that prioritize health equity (Lathrop, 2020).

A person's cultural background can also influence their perception of and reaction to stress (Aldwin, 2007). Cultural context must be integrated into any assessment. Differences are observed from culturally distinct groups within the general population, such as Indigenous cultures, as well as from immigrant populations. It is important to recognize that

BOX 30.3 FOCUS ON OLDER PERSONS

Stress

- Older persons are incorrectly presumed to be more vulnerable to the psychosocial effect of stressors (Nwachukwu et al., 2020). With age, the diurnal pattern of hypothalamic–pituitary–adrenal (HPA) axis activity changes, with higher evening levels of cortisol (Lanfear et al., 2020). As a result, sleep patterns may be altered, memory may be impaired (Sivertsen et al., 2021), and immune system functioning may be blunted (Lanfear et al., 2020). These changes can lead to increasing physical and mental frailty (Liu et al., 2020).
- A study of stress and coping in people in their 70s found that chronic stressors including physical, economic, and interpersonal stressors were experienced (Murayama et al., 2020). This study found that women used coping strategies such as support-seeking more than men did.
- The timing of stress-inducing events can significantly influence older persons' ability to cope. Many older people experience several stressful events (e.g., loss of a spouse and new medical diagnosis) within a brief time frame, which may result in reduced coping ability.
- Older people with strong spiritual beliefs effectively use religious coping in response to medical illness and disasters (Lima et al., 2020).
- Major depressive disorder and anxiety disorders are the most prevalent mental health disorders in later life (Murayama et al., 2020).

BOX 30.4 CULTURAL ASPECTS OF CARE

Intergenerational Trauma, Residential Schools, and Family

Understanding the consequences of intergenerational trauma is important for nurses who work with diverse cultural groups. *Intergenerational trauma* is described as trauma that occurs as a result of historical occurrences, such as colonization, and that has an impact on health for many generations after the original events took place. Maladaptive patterns of usually destructive behaviour (e.g., addictions, suicide, violence) developed in response to the original trauma and are absorbed into the culture and transmitted as learned behaviour from generation to generation. Coping strategies are influenced by culture. Cultures vary in their emotion-focused and problem-focused coping strategies. For example, according to some cultures, emotions should be controlled; according to others, they should be expressed.

Implications for Practice

- Realize that intergenerational stress can affect health and stress-related illness for many generations.
- Use introspection to examine your own experiences and perceptions of stress and coping.
- Assess the influence of culture on a patient's appraisal of stress.
- Determine the available resources within a patient's culture that may facilitate coping.

From Cowan, K. (2020). How residential schools led to intergenerational trauma in the Canadian Indigenous population to influence parenting styles and family structures over generations. *Canadian Journal of Family and Youth, 12*(2), 2. https://doi.org/10.2917 3/cjfy29511

Indigenous culture is not singular. Indeed, potential stressors vary by geographic region (e.g., urban, rural, or remote parts of Canada) and by historical events, such as colonization and residential schooling. Although stressors related to the social determinants of health have been described, ongoing stressors also may influence the health of families for generations, or intergenerational stress. Initial stressors can include career and financial issues related to underemployment, loss of extended family supports, language barriers, and unfamiliarity regarding accessing health services (Bowers & Yehuda, 2016). Later stressors can be related to raising children in a dual context (between cultural norms of the country of origin and the current environment) (Bowers & Yehuda, 2016). An example of intergenerational stress and how this may influence mental health is discussed in Box 30.4.

CRITICAL THINKING

When caring for a patient who is experiencing stress, the nurse needs to integrate knowledge from nursing and other disciplines, previous experiences, and information gathered from the patient to understand the particular stressor, its meaning for the patient and family, and current and past events that influence their responses to this stressor. Nurses must know the neurophysiological changes that occur in response to overwhelming or chronic stress. Nurses must also be able to determine the patient's perception of the situation and help the patient identify and use coping strategies that have helped in the past. If the patient's usual coping skills are unsuccessful or support systems are inadequate, the nurse must implement crisis intervention counselling (see "Crisis Intervention" section in this chapter).

As a nurse, you should be confident in the belief that you can help the patient manage the current situation effectively. Patients who are overwhelmed and perceive events as being beyond their capacity to cope rely on you as their guide to action. Through a nurse's expert advice and counsel, many patients gain confidence in their own ability to manage the consequences of the recent event. Standards of practice can help nurses make an accurate assessment of the level of a patient's stress, previously successful coping mechanisms, and available support systems before intervening.

❖ NURSING PROCESS

◆ Assessment

When assessing a patient's stress level and coping resources, the nurse must ask the patient to share personal and sensitive information. Therefore, the nurse must first establish a trusting nurse–patient relationship. By asking open-ended questions, listening carefully, observing the patient's nonverbal behaviour, and observing the patient's environment, the nurse can learn about the patient's stress. Nurses use critical thinking skills to synthesize and analyze information (Figure 30.3). Often patients have difficulty expressing what is troubling them until they have the opportunity to talk with someone who has time to listen.

Subjective Findings. When assessing a patient's level of stress and coping resources, it is important to ensure that the environment is nonthreatening. The nurse needs to assume the same height as the patient, arranging the interview environment so that eye contact can be comfortably maintained or avoided. Placing chairs at a 90-degree angle or side by side can help reduce the intensity of the interaction. The interview is used to determine the patient's view of the stress, past successful coping resources, any possible maladaptive coping, and adherence to prescribed medical recommendations, such as medication or diet (Table 30.1). If the patient is using denial as a coping mechanism, the nurse must be alert to whether the patient is overlooking necessary information. Other patients may state that they feel overwhelmed and unable to cope, but with help, they can reduce their multiple interacting stressors to manageable pieces. As in all patient interactions, nurses must respect the confidentiality and sensitivity of the information shared.

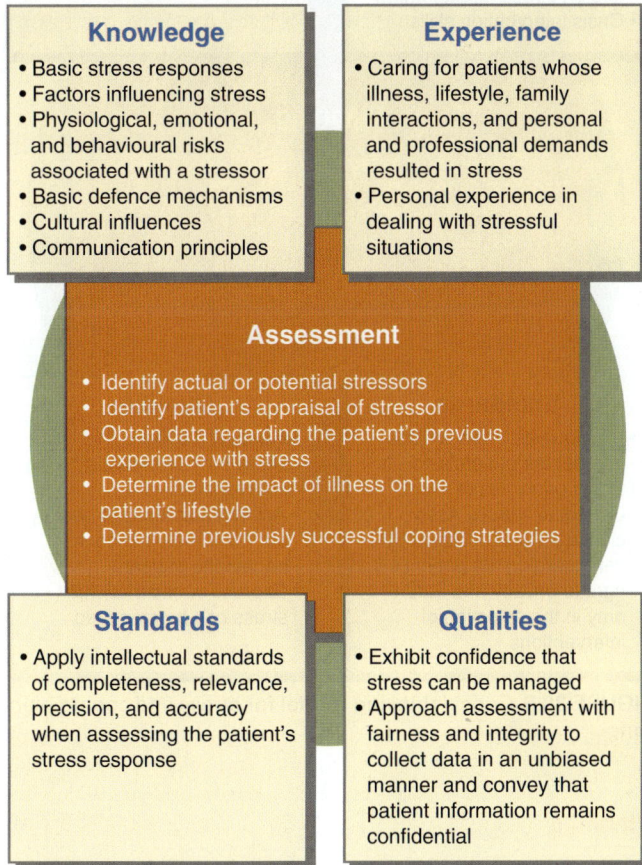

Objective Findings. Nurses obtain further findings about stress and coping by observing the patient's appearance and nonverbal behaviour during the interview, including grooming and hygiene, handshake and gait, body language, speech quality, eye contact, and attitude. However, it is important to consider that someone who is experiencing stress may not be behaving as "usual" when meeting a health care provider for the first time, so care should be exercised in making judgements at this time. During the assessment, depending on the patient's anxiety level, the nurse takes basic vital signs to assess for physiological signs of stress, such as elevated blood pressure, heart rate, or respiratory rate (Figure 30.4).

Patient Expectations. It is crucial that nurses understand the meaning the patient attaches to the precipitating event and how stress responses are affecting the patient's life. Nurses must allow the patient time to express priorities for coping. For example, if a woman has just been told that a breast mass was identified on a routine mammogram, the nurse must discern what the patient wants and needs most from the nurse. Some patients identify an immediate need for information about biopsy or mastectomy; others need guidance and support on how to share the news with family members. In some cases, when nothing can be done to change or improve the situation, just being with the patient can be helpful. Once the nurse understands patient expectations, it is important to support the patient in meeting their identified needs.

◆ Nursing Diagnosis

Nurses cluster data that indicate a potential or actual stressor and the patient's response. Keeping in mind previous knowledge and experiences with patients under stress, nurses then make individualized nursing diagnoses (Box 30.5).

Nursing diagnoses for people experiencing stress generally focus on coping. Major defining characteristics of *ineffective coping* include verbalization of both an inability to cope and an inability to ask for help. Defining characteristics are identified by asking patients what currently concerns them most and allowing them sufficient time to answer. The nurse observes for nonverbal signs of anxiety, fear, anger, irritability, and tension. Other defining characteristics include the presence of life stressors, an inability to meet role expectations and basic needs, alteration in societal participation, self-destructive behaviour, change in usual communication patterns, high rate of accidents, excessive food and alcohol intake, smoking, and sleep

Knowledge
- Basic stress responses
- Factors influencing stress
- Physiological, emotional, and behavioural risks associated with a stressor
- Basic defence mechanisms
- Cultural influences
- Communication principles

Experience
- Caring for patients whose illness, lifestyle, family interactions, and personal and professional demands resulted in stress
- Personal experience in dealing with stressful situations

Assessment
- Identify actual or potential stressors
- Identify patient's appraisal of stressor
- Obtain data regarding the patient's previous experience with stress
- Determine the impact of illness on the patient's lifestyle
- Determine previously successful coping strategies

Standards
- Apply intellectual standards of completeness, relevance, precision, and accuracy when assessing the patient's stress response

Qualities
- Exhibit confidence that stress can be managed
- Approach assessment with fairness and integrity to collect data in an unbiased manner and convey that patient information remains confidential

FIGURE 30.3 Critical thinking model for stress and coping assessment.

TABLE 30.1	**Focused Assessment Interview**	
Factors to Assess	**Questions and Approaches**	**Physical Assessment Strategies**
Perception of stressor	Ask the patient what is of most concern at this time. Ask the patient about problems sleeping, eating, working, and concentrating. Ask whether the patient has had accidents in the home, in the car, or on the job. Ask about previous stressors that are influencing current appraisals.	Observe nonverbal behaviour and expressions of feelings that indicate anxiety, fear, anger, irritability, or tension.
Available coping resources	Ask the patient about current friendships and contacts with family members. Ask what the patient has done in the past to cope with similar problems or stress. Ask how the patient spends leisure time. Ask the patient to describe any specific stress management techniques.	Observe whether the patient is alone or with others. Observe grooming and hygiene. Observe the patient's communication skills. Determine whether the patient is able to ask for help. Observe developmental level and sociocultural circumstances.
Maladaptive coping used	Assess current and past patterns of use of tobacco, alcohol, prescription or over-the-counter drugs, and caffeine.	Observe for effects of heavy use of tobacco, alcohol, illegal drugs, and caffeine.
Adherence to healthy practices	Ask whether the patient visits a health care provider regularly for checkups. Ask about nutritional habits, exercise, use of seat belts, helmets (if applicable), and safer sexual practices.	Monitor pulse, blood pressure, weight. Observe nonverbal behaviour.

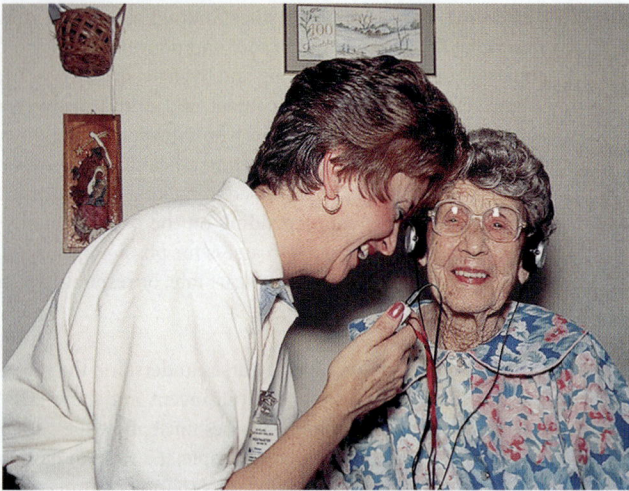

FIGURE 30.4 Sharing a joke or laughing with patients can reduce stress and support a therapeutic relationship.

BOX 30.5 NURSING DIAGNOSTIC PROCESS

Assessment Activities	Defining Characteristics	Nursing Diagnosis
Ask patient about change in sleeping patterns.	Sleep disturbance; difficulty falling asleep at night or staying asleep Nightmares or disturbing dreams Sighing	Anxiety
Ask patient to complete a sleep diary for 2 weeks.	Excessive sleeping	Sleep disturbance
Observe patient's behaviour and response to questions during assessment.	Fatigue Inability to concentrate Inaccurate response to questions Inappropriate laughing or crying	Ineffective coping
Observe patient's appearance.	Poor grooming Self-harm	Ineffective coping
Ask patient about changes in eating patterns.	Weight gain or loss Lack of interest in food	Nutritional imbalance

Knowledge
- Role of community resources in assisting patient and family adaptation
- Role of health care providers in stress management
- Impact of diet, exercise, medication, and other health promotion indicators on stress management
- Crisis intervention skills

Experience
- Previous patient responses to planned nursing interventions for improving patient's adaptation to stress
- Previous experience in partnering with patient in goal setting

Planning
- Select nursing interventions to promote adaptation to stress
- Consult with mental health providers
- Involve the patient and family
- Identify community resources accessible to the patient

Standards
- Individualize interventions to meet the patient's needs
- Apply principles of the Canadian Nurses Association's *Code of Ethics* by safeguarding the patient's right to privacy and autonomy in the selection of interventions

Qualities
- Respect the patient's lifestyle when creating interventions
- Act independently to seek out resources that could benefit the patient
- Express confidence that stress can be managed

FIGURE 30.5 Critical thinking model for stress and coping planning.

disturbances. Stress can result in multiple nursing diagnoses, such as the following:
- *Anxiety*
- *Caregiver role strain*
- *Chronic pain*
- *PTSD*
- *Powerlessness*

Crises differ from stressors in the degree of severity, although stressors and crises have many similarities. A patient who perceives a situation as stressful, who is unable to cope in ways that have worked before, and who has insufficient support is experiencing a crisis. A crisis can be devastating and requires the nurse to help mobilize all resources available.

Planning

Goals and Outcomes. Desirable outcomes for people experiencing stress are the development of behavioural and cognitive coping strategies. Coping strategies may include self-control, seeking support, acceptance, avoidance, and problem solving (Martinez et al., 2020). Nurses may select interventions for stress and improved coping such as coping enhancement or crisis intervention, which are in the *Nursing Interventions Classification (NIC)* (Butcher et al., 2018). In addition, nurses select individualized interventions after considering the nursing diagnosis, the resources available to the patient, and the goals identified by the patient and nurse (Figure 30.5).

Nursing interventions may be designed within the framework of primary, secondary, and tertiary prevention (Heard et al., 2020). At the primary level of prevention, individuals and populations who may be at risk for stress are identified. At the secondary level, nursing actions are directed at symptoms, such as decreasing the frequency or intensity of specific symptoms. At the tertiary level, nursing interventions assist the patient in readapting and might include relaxation training and time management training (Box 30.6). Another method of planning care involves using a concept map (Figure 30.6). The nurse creates the map after identifying relevant nursing diagnoses from the assessment database. In this example, the nursing diagnoses are linked to

◎ BOX 30.6 NURSING CARE PLAN

Caregiver Role Strain

ASSESSMENT

When the professional nurse first goes to Carl's house, the nurse finds the home to be in slight disarray. The lawn is overgrown, dirty dishes are in the sink, and an empty can of soup is sitting on the kitchen counter. Carl is standing in the living room, folding clothes from a laundry basket, and Evelyn, Carl's wife, is sitting in a chair watching TV. Evelyn recently received a diagnosis of Alzheimer's disease.

Assessment Activities	*Findings and Defining Characteristics*
Ask Carl about recent stressors and coping strategies.	Carl continues to fold clothes during the visit, stating, "There's so much to do that I don't even know where to begin." Carl describes being awakened three to four times per night to find Evelyn wandering in the house. Carl is not participating in any outside activities, and their children live in other provinces. Carl does have several close friends who live nearby but does not know of community resources.
Observe Carl's grooming and hygiene.	Carl is unshaven and appears dishevelled.
Ask Carl about sleep and nutrition patterns.	Carl has lost 9 kg in the past 6 months and has a poor appetite.
Assess Carl's mood and affect.	Carl states, "I feel very tired. Everything feels overwhelming."
Assess Carl's suicide potential.	Carl denies being suicidal.
Assess health status and health care status.	Carl has not seen a health care provider for a health check in over a year.

NURSING DIAGNOSIS: Caregiver role strain related to recent diagnosis of wife's Alzheimer's disease

PLANNING

Goal (Nursing Outcomes Classification)*	*Expected Outcomes*
	Caregiver's Physical Health
Patient will appear rested in 1 month.	Patient will report waking up less frequently during the night within 1 week.
	Patient will verbalize approaches used to involve other people in caregiving activities within 2 weeks.
Patient will maintain a stable weight over next 4 weeks.	Patient will re-establish normal eating pattern within 1 week.
	Patient will report improved appetite.
	Caregiver's Lifestyle Disruption
Patient will state that they have resumed one outside activity within 1 month.	Patient will report within 1 week an improvement in a balanced routine that incorporates time for own rest or relaxation.

*Outcome classification labels from Moorhead, S., Swanson, E., Johnson, M., et al. (Eds.). (2018). *Nursing outcomes classification (NOC)* (6th ed.). Elsevier.

INTERVENTIONS

Interventions (Nursing Interventions Classification)†	*Rationale*
Caregiver Support	
Assist patient in establishing a consistent care routine.	Routines can help tasks be simplified and more time efficient.
Discuss ways that patient agrees will simplify care routine, such as hiring someone to mow the lawn, buying frozen meals, having groceries delivered, and having a cleaning service.	Caregivers experience stress outside of their caregiving roles. Frequently, providing ways to assist the caregiver with home maintenance, meal planning, and shopping assists caregivers with stress management.
Identify sources of respite care.	Caregiving can be stressful when there is only one caregiver.
	The caregiver may be hesitant to ask for help.
Explore community resources such as care in the community, adult day care, and Meals on Wheels with patient.	Feelings of burden have been found to be lower among caregivers with social supports.
Teach patient stress-management techniques.	Stress, especially long-term stress, can precipitate physical illness.
Set up monthly health checks for patient that include vital sign and weight measurements.	Teaching the caregiver health maintenance strategies is important for sustaining his own physical and mental health.

†Intervention classification labels from Butcher, H. K., Bulechek, G. M., McCloskey Dochterman, J. M., et al. (Eds.). (2018). *Nursing interventions classification (NIC)* (7th ed.). Elsevier.

EVALUATION

Nursing Actions	*Patient Response and Finding*	*Achievement of Outcome*
Observe for signs of fatigue.	Carl states he feels more rested and less depressed.	Carl is able to sleep for 6 hours during night and takes a 30-minute nap in the afternoon.
Review new care routines. Ask patient what other modifications may need to be made.	Carl buys frozen meals to use when he is busy with other caregiving responsibilities.	Carl has reduced his personal expectation that he must cook every meal.

Continued

◎ BOX 30.6   NURSING CARE PLAN—cont'd

Nursing Actions	*Patient Response and Finding*	*Achievement of Outcome*
Ask patient about how community and additional family support is helping to relieve stress.	Meals on Wheels delivers lunch 5 days per week. A neighbour mows the lawn for Carl.	Carl is mobilizing community resources.
Ask patient to compare past and current energy levels.	Carl reports having more energy and smiles spontaneously.	Carl has improved balance between their routines.
Weigh patient regularly.	Carl reports gaining 2 kg in 1 month.	Carl has resumed a normal eating pattern.
Ask patient about recent food intake.	Carl reports having eaten lunch with Evelyn on the day of the visit.	Carl has been able to sustain reasonable food intake recently.

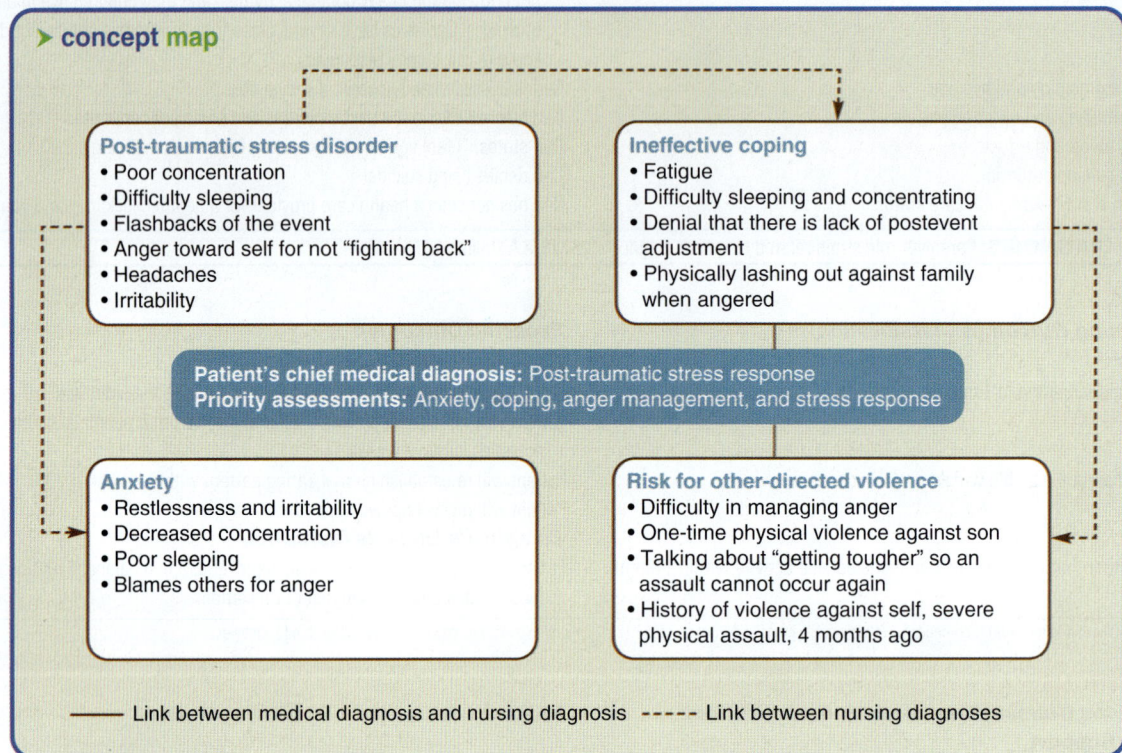

> **concept map**

Post-traumatic stress disorder
- Poor concentration
- Difficulty sleeping
- Flashbacks of the event
- Anger toward self for not "fighting back"
- Headaches
- Irritability

Ineffective coping
- Fatigue
- Difficulty sleeping and concentrating
- Denial that there is lack of postevent adjustment
- Physically lashing out against family when angered

Patient's chief medical diagnosis: Post-traumatic stress response
Priority assessments: Anxiety, coping, anger management, and stress response

Anxiety
- Restlessness and irritability
- Decreased concentration
- Poor sleeping
- Blames others for anger

Risk for other-directed violence
- Difficulty in managing anger
- One-time physical violence against son
- Talking about "getting tougher" so an assault cannot occur again
- History of violence against self, severe physical assault, 4 months ago

—— Link between medical diagnosis and nursing diagnosis   - - - - Link between nursing diagnoses

FIGURE 30.6 Concept map for patient with PTSD after experiencing a severe physical assault 4 months ago.

the patient's medical diagnosis of PTSD. The concept map shows the relationships with the nursing diagnoses: PTSD, *ineffective coping, anxiety, and risk for outward-focused violence.* In this approach, nurses use critical thinking skills to organize patient data and plan for patient-centred care.

Just as the nursing assessment of stress and coping depends on patient perception of the problem and coping resources, interventions focus on a partnership of the nurse with the patient and support system, usually the family. In the case of a family or community stressor and impaired family or community coping, the view of the situation and resources is broader.

Setting Priorities. When nurses prioritize needs for a person experiencing stress or a crisis, the first question to be answered is "What is happening in your life that you needed to come in today?" or "What happened in your life that is *different*?" This question requires the patient to focus. The nurse should then assess the patient's perception of the event, situational supports, and what the patient usually does when faced with a problem As in all areas of nursing, safety of the patient and family is the first priority.

SAFETY ALERT Direct questions help to determine whether a person is suicidal or homicidal. The nurse might ask, "Have you thought that life is not worth living? Are those thoughts with you most of the day?" "Have you thought your problems would be solved if that other person were not around anymore?" If the patient answers "yes" to any of these questions, the nurse should calmly determine whether the patient has a plan and determine how lethal the means are. If suicide or homicide is not an issue, the nurse should consider other threats to the safety of people who are under the patient's care and provide for their temporary care or supervision if necessary. When immediate assessment is completed and safety is ensured, the problem-solving process should begin.

Continuity of Care. Sometimes the scope of nursing practice is insufficient to meet all of the patient's needs. For patients experiencing stress from medical conditions or psychiatric disorders, nurses must consult with advanced practice mental health nurses, psychiatrists, psychologists, psychiatric social workers, or other mental health experts. An interprofessional approach to care is often most effective in addressing the holistic needs of the patient and should be included in the planning

BOX 30.7 FOCUS ON PRIMARY HEALTH CARE

Preventing Stress

Nurses address their patients' stress or potential stress in many different primary health care settings. In a community setting, the nurse might work with a group of teenage mothers on how to care for their newborns and themselves. The goal is to improve the health and safety of the babies and mothers and to prevent stress, health breakdown, and crises in their lives. In a home setting, the nurse might help the family of a patient who has cancer to recognize and deal with symptoms of stress in their lives. At a community clinic, the nurse might assess the stress in the life of a patient with sleep problems and plan interventions with the patient to help improve their sleep. Nurse practitioners who work in primary health care settings can provide a range of services related to family health and ongoing management of chronic health conditions.

BOX 30.8 PATIENT TEACHING

Stress Management Strategies

Objective
- Improved coping with daily hassles in the workplace (such as a depending on others for transportation to work, chronically late co-worker, multiple competing work demands, intense work demands at specific times)

Teaching Strategies
- Teach the patient how to break down hassles into specific aspects in order to begin coping with them.
- Advise the patient to avoid impulsive changes in lifestyle when stressed.
- Assist the patient with time management skills and setting priorities.
- Assist the patient in examining lifestyle issues that may serve as stress relievers, such as walking.
- Assist the patient in examining dietary sources of increased tension, such as excessive caffeine intake (e.g., coffee, tea, chocolate).
- Assist the patient in building a network of social support.
- Teach the patient relaxation techniques, such as rhythmic breathing.

Evaluation
- Observe the patient for signs of active coping strategies.
- Ask the patient to keep a record of hours of sleep.
- Ask the patient to list activities that are soothing or enjoyable.

Data from Pender, N. J., Murdaugh, C., & Parsons, M. A. (2002). *Health promotion in nursing practice* (4th ed.). Haworth Press.

of care. The nurse's role is to recognize the need for collaboration and consultation, inform the patient about potential resources, and make arrangements for interventions, such as consultations, group sessions, or therapy as needed.

❖ **Implementation**

Health Promotion. Pender's health promotion model focuses on three areas; individuals' characteristics, behaviours, and outcomes of behaviour (Pouresmali et al., 2021). Nurses can use this model to guide their practice in health promotion. Nurses are in a position to educate patients and families about the importance of health promotion (Boxes 30.7 and 30.8). Several strategies help increase resistance to stress and reduce response to stress.

Regular Exercise. A regular exercise program improves muscle tone and posture, controls weight, reduces tension, and promotes relaxation. In addition, exercise improves mood and immune system and cardiopulmonary functioning (Karatas & Polat, 2020). Patients who have a history of a chronic illness, who are at risk for developing an illness, or who are older than 35 years should begin a physical exercise program only after discussing the plan with a health care provider. In general, for a fitness program to have positive physical effects, a person should exercise three to four times per week for at least 20 to 30 minutes (Figure 30.7).

Support Systems. A support system of family, friends, and colleagues who listen, offer advice, and provide emotional support may be of benefit to patients experiencing stress. Many support groups are available to individuals, such as those sponsored by the Heart and Stroke Foundation of Canada, the Canadian Cancer Society, local hospitals and churches, and mental health organizations.

Time Management. Time management techniques include developing lists of tasks to be performed in order of priority—for example, tasks that require immediate attention, those that are important but can be delayed, and those that are routine and can be accomplished when time becomes available. In many cases, setting priorities helps individuals identify tasks that are not necessary or perhaps can even be delegated to someone else.

Guided Imagery and Visualization. The concept of guided imagery is based on the belief that a person can significantly reduce stress with imagination (see Chapter 36). Guided imagery is a relaxed state in which a person actively uses imagination to visualize a soothing, peaceful setting. The image created or suggested typically evokes many sensory words to engage the mind and offer distraction and relaxation.

Progressive Muscle Relaxation. In the presence of anxiety-provoking thoughts and events, a common physiological symptom is muscle tension. Physiological tension is diminished through a

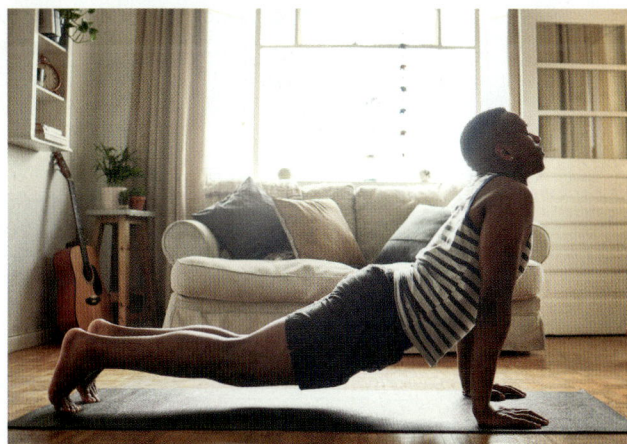

FIGURE 30.7 Regular exercise assists in coping with stress. (iStockphoto/PeopleImages.)

systematic approach to releasing tension in major muscle groups. A relaxed state is achieved typically through deep chest breathing, and then the patient is directed to alternately tighten and relax muscles in specific groupings (see Chapter 36).

Assertiveness Training. Assertiveness comprises skills that help individuals communicate their needs and desires effectively. The ability to resolve conflict through assertiveness training is important for reducing stress. When assertiveness is taught in a group setting, benefits of the experience are increased.

Journal Writing. For many people, keeping a private, personal journal provides a therapeutic outlet for stress. Nurses can suggest this activity to patients and assist by providing space and privacy to enable time for contemplation and reflection. In a private journal, patients can express a full range of emotions, venting their feelings honestly without hurting anyone's feelings and without concern for how they might appear to others. The writings can help individuals by increasing their awareness of situations through self-reflection. Journal entries can also be shared with health care providers to help plan interventions.

Stress Management in the Workplace. Rapid changes in health care technology, diversity in the workforce, organizational restructuring, and changing work systems can place stress on nurses (Lee & Kim, 2020). Additional causes of job stress include particular job assignments, challenging schedules, such as two different work shifts within a short period of time, working predominantly night shifts, fear of failure, and inadequate support services (Lee & Kim, 2020). **Burnout** is an occupational phenomenon resulting from chronic work stress and is characterized by three domains: emotional exhaustion, depersonalization, and a diminished sense of accomplishment (Woo et al., 2020). This can be reflected in high rates of sick leave, irritability with co-workers, increased risk of errors at work, and increased home stress. Nurses are not immune to maladaptive coping, such as use of alcohol, in response to chronic stress or burnout.

Primary prevention is essential to addressing risk for burnout and is important for all health care providers. Personal stress management strategies need to be a part of professional practice; they can include working on crafts, scheduled social outings with friends, participation in a team sport or an individual recreational or physical activity, limiting amount of overtime worked, taking an art class, or reading for pleasure.

If nurses recognize feelings of burnout, they can engage in some of the same strategies that help patients: increase their own self-reflections regarding potential sources of stress, use daily journal writing to increase recognition of contextual factors, seek a colleague or mentor to help with their reflections, create an inventory of available personal and support resources, and devise a plan for addressing the various stressors in a manageable and positive manner. An important step is identifying the limits and scope of responsibilities at work (Woo et al., 2020). It is essential that nurses recognize the areas over which they have control and can change and those for which they do not have responsibility.

Acute Care

Crisis Intervention. When stress overwhelms a person's usual coping mechanisms and all available resources must be mobilized, the situation becomes a crisis. A crisis creates a turning point in a person's life because it changes the direction of a person's life in some way. According to Aguilera (1998), the precipitating event usually occurs 1 to 2 weeks before the individual seeks help, but it may have occurred within the past 24 hours. In general, a crisis is resolved in some way within approximately 6 weeks. The aim of crisis intervention is to return the person to a pre-crisis level of functioning and to promote growth (Figure 30.8). The use of unfamiliar strategies can result either

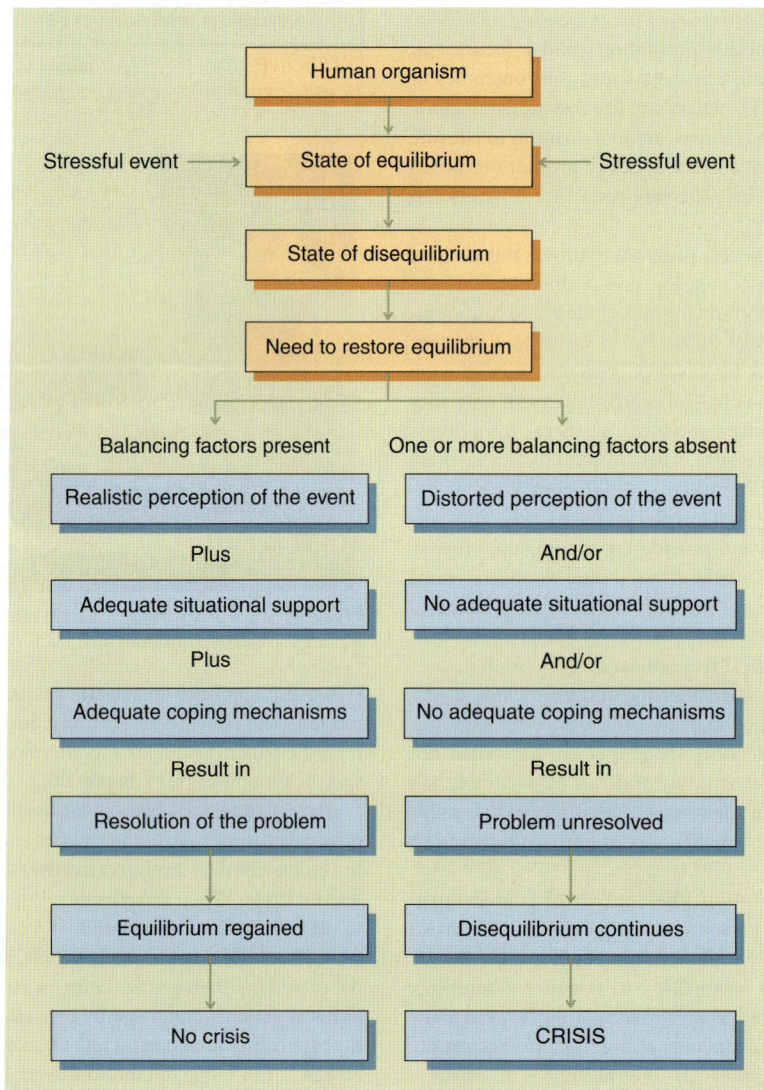

FIGURE 30.8 Crisis intervention model. (Redrawn from Aguilera, D. C. [1998]. *Crisis intervention: Theory and methodology* [8th ed.]. Mosby.)

in a heightened awareness of previously unrecognized strengths and resources or in deterioration in functioning. Thus, a crisis is often referred to as a situation of both danger and opportunity. Some people or families emerge from a crisis state functioning more effectively, whereas others are weakened, and still others are rendered completely dysfunctional. There are a variety of crisis intervention models. Figure 30.8 presents an example of a crisis intervention model that is widely and currently used.

Crisis intervention is a specific type of brief psychotherapy with prescribed steps. Crisis intervention is more directive than traditional psychotherapy or counselling and can be used by any member of the health care team who has been trained in its techniques. The basic approach is problem solving, and the focus is on only the problem presented by the crisis.

When using a crisis intervention approach, the nurse helps the patient make the mental connection between the stressful event and the patient's reaction to it. This is crucial because the patient may be unable to envision the whole situation clearly. The nurse can help the patient become aware of current feelings, such as anger, grief, or guilt, in order to reduce tension. The nurse can also assist the patient in exploring coping mechanisms, perhaps identifying ways of coping that the patient had not thought of. Finally, the nurse may help increase the patient's social contacts if the patient has been internally focused and isolated.

Restorative and Continuing Care. A person under stress recovers when the stress is removed or coping strategies are successful; however, a person who has experienced a crisis has changed, and the effects may last for years or for the rest of the person's life. The final stage of adapting to a crisis is acknowledgement of the long-term implications of the crisis.

◆ Evaluation

Patient Care. By evaluating the goals and expected outcomes of care, the nurse knows whether the nursing interventions were effective and whether the patient is coping with the identified stress. The nurse needs to review the measurable goals and assess whether the patient has met the criteria for success as stated in the outcomes. If the nursing interventions have not been effective in helping the patient achieve targeted goals, the nurse must re-evaluate the strategies implemented and revise the care plan in light of the patient's current health status (Figure 30.9).

To evaluate whether goals and outcomes of care have been achieved, nurses should observe patient behaviours and interactions between the patient and family, if appropriate. If the nurse's contact with a patient ends before goals have been achieved, the patient should be referred to appropriate resources so that progress is not delayed or interrupted.

Patient Expectations. It is crucial to maintain ongoing communication with patients in regard to the care plan. Patients under severe stress or trauma often feel powerless and vulnerable. Nurses can help reduce these feelings by actively involving patients and families in assessment, prioritizing, goal setting, and evaluation. Being involved enables patients to direct their energy positively and encourages them to take responsibility for their health. It also facilitates open communication, which makes it easier for the patient to report on interventions that are successful and helps nurses better understand why some interventions fail to meet the patient's goals.

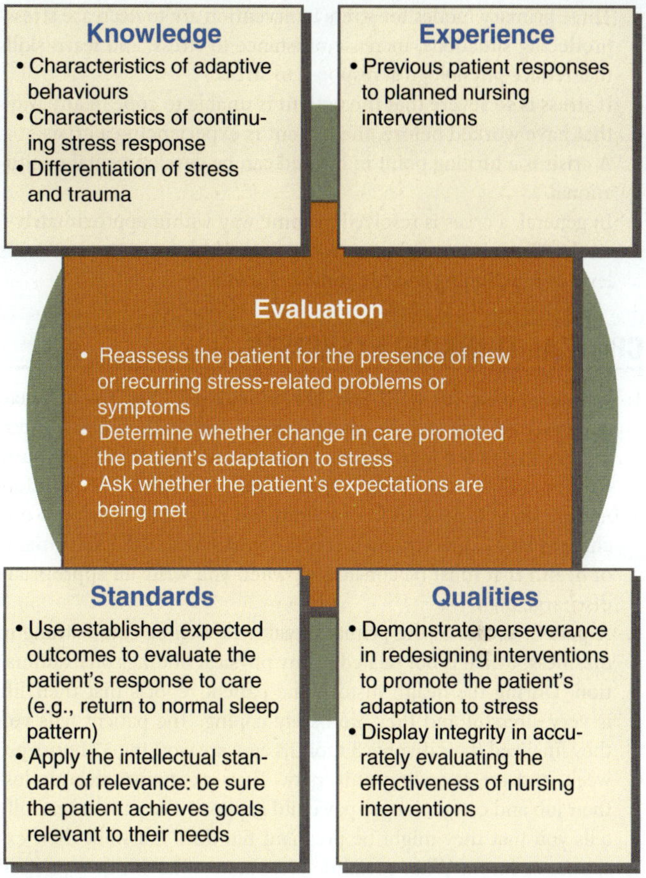

FIGURE 30.9 Critical thinking model for stress and coping evaluation.

KEY CONCEPTS

- Physiological and psychological frameworks have been developed to describe how stress affects biological systems and psychological well-being.
- Overwhelming or chronic stress can increase the risks of (1) serious and long-standing physical and mental health problems; (2) choosing coping strategies that are unhealthy, such as isolating oneself, not getting enough rest or a proper diet, or using tobacco, alcohol, or caffeine; (3) ignoring warning signs of illness; and (4) neglecting to take prescribed medicines or treatments.
- A person is under psychological stress only if the person evaluates the event or circumstance as personally significant. Such an evaluation of an event for its personal meaning is called *primary appraisal.*
- Several types of stressors are work stressors, family stressors, chronic stressors, acute stressors, daily hassles, traumatic events, and crisis.
- Rapid changes in health care technology, diversity in the workforce, organizational redesign, and changing work systems can place nurses at risk for stress-related symptoms and burnout.
- Potential stressors and coping mechanisms vary across the lifespan: from childhood through adolescence, adulthood, and old age.
- Coping is a means of managing psychological stress and reflects a dynamic process in response to the current situation, past experiences, and available resources.

- Three primary modes for stress intervention are to decrease stress-producing situations, increase resistance to stress, and learn skills that reduce physiological response to stress.
- If stress is so severe that the patient is unable to cope in any ways that have worked before, the patient is experiencing a crisis.
- A crisis is a turning point in life and can be developmental or situational.
- In general, a crisis is resolved in some way within approximately 6 weeks. Crisis intervention aims to return the person to a pre-crisis level of functioning and to promote growth.

CRITICAL THINKING EXERCISES

1. You are caring for a 30-year-old patient who has recently had surgery as a first step in treatment for metastatic breast cancer. The patient is the lone parent and sole provider for three young children (all younger than 7 years of age). What additional information do you need to know about the patient to develop a discharge plan? Consider and discuss the various social determinants of health that must be considered when you write an appropriate discharge plan.

2. A patient comes to the primary health care clinic complaining of dizziness, which is not related to any physical findings on examination. During the health history, the patient reports that their life is very stressful and they are barely coping. The patient tells you they finalized their divorce 3 months ago, are working 32 hours per week, and are attending university. Their ex-spouse recently lost their job and can no longer pay child support. The patient tearfully tells you that they might be pregnant but does not want their ex-spouse to know. What social determinants of health do you need to consider in order to develop a plan of care? What short-term and long-term coping strategies could you consider to support the patient to cope with their life events?

3. An older person is admitted to the hospital with a fractured hip. Before this injury, they lived with their partner, who has advancing Alzheimer's disease. While the person is hospitalized, their partner is staying with a niece who lives 50 km away, but this cannot be a permanent situation because their niece is also in frail health. The patient has no other family who can help when they return home. They are concerned about who will care for their partner after discharge and while rehabilitating. What approach would be the best to take in establishing goals for treatment?

Answers to Critical Thinking Exercises appear on the Evolve website.

▐ REVIEW QUESTIONS

Review Questions 1 to 9 relate to the case study at the beginning of the chapter.

1. When the patient says to the nurse, "You have been following me and watching me for 2 days!" the patient is likely feeling stressed with changes in their heart rate, blood pressure, and respiration. What controls this physiological response?
   a. Medulla oblongata
   b. Reticular formation
   c. Pituitary gland
   d. Limbic system

2. The nurse in the case study describes feeling stressed to another student nurse. The student nurse notices their respirations have increased and knows that which of the following physiological changes that the nurse is experiencing are also due to stress?
   a. Heart rate increases.
   b. Blood volume is unstable.
   c. Vital signs return to normal.
   d. Blood glucose level is fluctuating.

3. The nurse says, "But I still remember my stress and distress over my first patient assignment." If the nurse also said that they have vivid images of this interaction and that their heart rate increased every time a patient approaches them on the unit, even 30 years later, these reactions would be considered flashbacks, which are symptoms of:
   a. Social phobia
   b. Acute anxiety
   c. Post-traumatic stress disorder
   d. Borderline personality disorder

4. When the patient said, "You have been following me and watching me for 2 days," and the nurse turned and ran out of the unit, the nurse would have been experiencing which stage of the general adaptation syndrome response to stress?
   a. Flight adaptation
   b. Resistance stage
   c. Alarm reaction
   d. Exhaustion stage

5. The nurse is describing the incident with the patient to a group of new nurses. The nurse tells the students that after this experience, they have developed many new ways of working in new situations. What the nurse is describing reflects that:
   a. Individual stresses are personal.
   b. Coping strategies develop across the lifespan.
   c. This incident has nothing to do with stress.
   d. The nurse has a personality disorder.

6. The nurse describes feeling stressed. Which of the following actions is most important for the clinical educator to consider first?
   a. Help the nurse realize that they haven't got what it takes to be a nurse.
   b. Tell the nurse they are experiencing a stress response and should take some time off to relax.
   c. Ask the nurse to describe their day and how they are feeling.
   d. Tell the nurse it's okay to be stressed and that it's a normal part of nursing work.

7. The nurse in the case study described feeling stressed about how they would react to meeting new patients. This stressor could be described as which type of stressor?
   a. External stressor
   b. Internal stressor
   c. Behavioural stressor
   d. Personal stressor

8. Burnout occurs as a result of chronic stress. If you were the clinical educator supporting the nurse in the case study, what strategies would you introduce to ensure that chronic stress doesn't develop in this situation?
   a. Primary prevention—Tell the nurse to write in their journal at the end of each day.
   b. Primary prevention—Ask the nurse to share what strategies they already use to manage stress.
   c. Primary prevention—Tell the nurse to put it all behind them and start again tomorrow.
   d. Primary prevention—Discuss how you are feeling sad that they are not happy being a nurse.

9. In the case study, the nurse describes their perception and appraisal of their experience. How do individual perception and appraisal influence a person's stress and coping responses?

   a. Discussing a stressful situation increases the stress response and leads to burnout.

   b. Evaluating an event for its personal meaning influences the response to the event.

   c. Coping strategies are developed only when experiencing stress.

   d. Observing others' experiences of a stress experience leads to developing coping responses.

Answers: 1. a; **2.** d; **3.** c; **4.** c; **5.** b; **6.** c; **7.** a; **8.** b; **9.** b.

Rationales for the Review Questions appear on the Evolve web site.

RECOMMENDED WEBSITES

Health Canada: Mental Health—Coping With Stress: https://www.hc-sc.gc.ca/hl-vs/iyh-vsv/life-vie/stress-eng.php
This website provides links to taking care of mental health by identifying symptoms of stress and strategies to decrease its effect on health.

Heart & Stroke Foundation: Healthy Living/Reduce Stress: https://www.heartandstroke.ca/healthy-living/reduce-stress
This website provides information and resources related to coping with stress.

REFERENCES

A full reference list is available on the website for this book at http://evolve.elsevier.com/Canada/Potter/fundamentals/

31

Vital Signs

Written by Tracy Stephen, RN, MN, and Mi-Yeon Kim, RN, PhD

OBJECTIVES

Mastery of content in this chapter will enable you to:

- Define the key terms listed.
- Explain the principles and mechanisms of thermoregulation.
- Describe nursing measures that promote heat loss and heat conservation.
- Describe physiological changes associated with fever.
- Accurately assess temperature via multiple routes: tympanic, oral, temporal, rectal, and axillary.
- Accurately assess pulse, respirations, oxygen saturation, and blood pressure.
- Explain the physiology of normal regulation of blood pressure, pulse, oxygen saturation, and respirations.
- Describe factors that cause variations in body temperature, pulse, oxygen saturation, respirations, and blood pressure.
- Describe ethnic variations in blood pressure.
- Identify ranges of acceptable vital sign values for an infant, a child, and an adult.
- Explain variations in technique used to assess an infant's, a child's, and an adult's vital signs.
- Describe the benefits and precautions involving self-measurement of blood pressure.
- Identify when vital signs should be measured.
- Accurately record and report vital sign measurements.
- Appropriately delegate vital sign measurement to unregulated care providers.

KEY TERMS

Afebrile
Antipyretics
Auscultatory gap
Basal metabolic rate (BMR)
Blood pressure
Bradycardia
Cardiac output
Celsius
Conduction
Convection
Core temperature
Diaphoresis
Diastolic (blood pressure)
Diffusion
Dysrhythmia
Eupnea
Evaporation
Febrile

Fever
Fever of unknown origin
Frostbite
Heat exhaustion
Heatstroke
Hematocrit
Hypertension
Hyperthermia
Hypotension
Hypothalamus
Hypothermia
Hypoxemia
Malignant hyperthermia
Masked hypertension
Nonshivering thermogenesis
Orthostatic hypotension
Perfusion
Postural hypotension

Pulse
Pulse deficit
Pulse oximeter
Pulse pressure
Pyrexia
Pyrogens
Radial pulse
Radiation
Shivering
Sphygmomanometer
Stroke volume
Systolic (blood pressure)
Tachycardia
Thermoregulation
Tidal volume
Ventilation
Vital signs (VS)
White coat hypertension

WEBSITE

http://evolve.elsevier.com/Canada/Potter/fundamentals/

CASE STUDY

Johnathan (preferred pronouns: he/him) is a 58-year-old who works as a manager at a large warehouse that distributes essential goods to grocery stores in the city. With the COVID-19 pandemic period persisting, his employer laid off staff members, and since that time Johnathan has been feeling pressured to pitch in to help as well as to manage his own work responsibilities. The increased workload has added to his stress, which has worsened his high blood pressure.

He was diagnosed with hypertension 7 years ago and is currently on antihypertensive medication, which he occasionally forgets to take. Lately, he has been feeling excessively fatigued and short of breath when he gets home from work, but he has simply attributed it to the stress of his job. Yesterday, his dyspnea gradually worsened while at work and he also began to cough frequently. By the time he reached home after work, he was feeling feverish and could hardly walk around the house because he was severely short of breath. Johnathan's spouse became very alarmed about his deteriorating condition and despite his protest drove Jonathan to a local emergency department (ED).

Following are his vital signs taken in the ED:
- Temperature: 38.2°C
- Blood pressure: 150/86 mm Hg

- Heart rate: 102 beats per minute
- Respiratory rate: 28 breaths per minute
- SpO_2 90% on room air
- Johnathan was also tested for COVID-19 and the result was positive.

Think about this case study as you read this chapter. There are review questions at the end of the chapter that relate to the case study.

The most frequent measurements obtained by health care providers are those of temperature, pulse, blood pressure, respiratory rate, and oxygen saturation. These measurements indicate the effectiveness of circulatory, respiratory, neural, and endocrine body functions. Because of their importance, they are referred to as *vital signs (VS)*. Many factors, such as environmental temperature, physical state, activities, or illness, can cause vital signs to change, sometimes to values outside an acceptable range. Recently, pain has been referred to as the "fifth vital sign," demonstrating the importance of its assessment not only as a factor that influences the standard vital signs but as an indicator of the necessity to ensure the inclusion of its assessment as part of baseline data (see Chapter 32 for further information about pain assessment).

Vital signs provide important data to determine the usual state of health (baseline data). A change in vital signs indicates a change in physiological function, which may signal the need for medical or nursing intervention. Measuring vital signs is a quick and efficient way of monitoring a patient's condition, identifying health problems, or evaluating responses to interventions. With knowledge of the physiological variables influencing vital signs and recognition of the relationship of vital signs changes to other physical assessment findings, precise determinations of health are made. Inspection, palpation, and auscultation are used to determine vital signs. These simple skills should not be taken for granted. Careful measurement techniques ensure accurate and consistent findings. When measuring vital signs, it is important to remember that they are often interconnected; for example, with an increase in temperature you will often see an increase in the respiratory rate and an increase in pulse. Blood pressure and pulse will often rise and fall together; however, in cases of hypovolemic shock or severe infection, the blood pressure often falls as the pulse increases. Vital signs and other physiological measurements are the basis for clinical problem solving.

GUIDELINES FOR MEASURING VITAL SIGNS

Vital signs are an important part of all assessments. Data are obtained during a complete physical assessment (see Chapter 33 for further information about conducting a physical assessment) and as needed to assess a patient's condition. Vital sign measurements during a routine physical examination provide a baseline for future assessments. The patient's needs and condition determine when, where, how, and by whom vital signs are measured. The nurse must measure vital signs correctly or delegate their measurement appropriately. Vital sign values must be understood, and knowledge of the person's developmental stage and functioning over the lifespan are crucial to correct interpretation (Canadian Association of Schools of Nursing [CASN], 2022). Then findings must be communicated appropriately and interventions begun as needed. Often the prioritization of interventions can be determined in part by vital signs, using the acronym *ABC*, which stands for

| BOX 31.1 | Vital Signs: Acceptable Readings for Adults |

Temperature Range: 36°C to 38°C*
Average oral/tympanic/temporal: 37°C
Average rectal: 37.5°C
Average axillary: 36.5°C

Pulse
60–100 beats per minute

Respirations
12–20 breaths per minute

Blood Pressure
Systolic: 120–139 mm Hg
Diastolic: 80–89 mm Hg
Pulse pressure: 30–50 mm Hg

Oxygen Saturation
95–100%

*Geneva, I., Cuzzo, B., Tasaduq, F., et al. (2019). Normal body temperature: A systemic review. *Open Forum Infectious Diseases, 6*(4).

airway, breathing, and circulation. Box 31.1 lists acceptable adult values for vital signs.

Use the following guidelines to incorporate vital sign measurement into your nursing practice:
- Unregulated care providers (UCPs) may measure selected vital signs (i.e., in stable patients), and then the nurse responsible for the patient may interpret and act on these measurements.
- Use equipment that is functional and appropriate for the size and age of the patient to ensure accurate findings (e.g., an oral thermometer is not appropriate for use in an infant).
- Select equipment on the basis of the patient's condition and characteristics (e.g., an adult-size blood pressure cuff should not be used for a child).
- Minimize environmental factors that may affect vital signs (e.g., assessing the patient's temperature in a warm, humid room may yield a value that is not a true indicator of the patient's condition).
- Use an organized, step-by-step approach to ensure accuracy.
- Approach the patient in a calm, caring manner while demonstrating proficiency in handling supplies needed for vital sign measurement. The manner of approach can alter vital signs.
- Follow guidelines cited in Box 31.2 to decide frequency of vital sign assessment. Increase the frequency of vital sign assessment if the patient's condition warrants it (i.e., frequency of vital signs ordered

| BOX 31.2 | When to Measure Vital Signs |

Upon admission to a health care facility

During a care-in-the-community visit

According to the health care provider's order or the health facility's standards of practice

Before, during, and after a surgical procedure or an invasive diagnostic procedure

Before, during, and after the administration of blood products

Before, during, and after administration of medications that affect cardiovascular, respiratory, and temperature-control function

When a patient's general physical condition changes (e.g., loss of consciousness or increased pain)

Before and after nursing interventions that affect a vital sign (e.g., before a patient previously on bed rest ambulates or before a patient performs range-of-motion exercises)

When a patient reports nonspecific symptoms of physical distress (e.g., feeling "funny" or "different")

Before a patient is sent home on a day or weekend pass and when the person returns to the floor

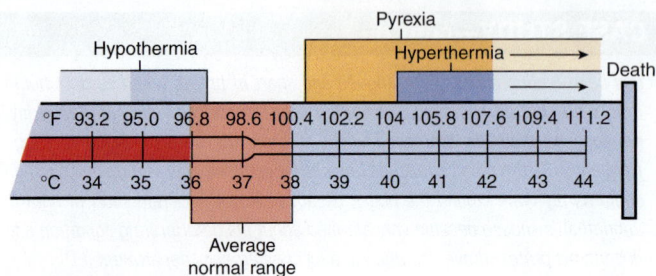

FIGURE 31.1 Ranges of normal temperature values and physiological consequences of abnormal body temperature.

| BOX 31.3 | Sites of Measurement of Core and Surface Temperature |

Core Temperature
Rectum
Tympanic membrane
Temporal artery
Esophagus
Pulmonary artery
Urinary bladder
Nasopharynx

Surface Temperature
Skin
Mouth
Axillae

by the health care provider is the *minimum* number of times that they should be checked).

- Use vital sign measurements to determine indications for prescribed medication administration (e.g., certain cardiac medications are given only if pulse or blood pressure values are in a certain range; antipyretics are administered only when temperature is elevated outside the acceptable range for the patient).
- Analyze the results of vital sign measurement by considering the patient's usual baseline values, medical history, therapies, and prescribed medications. A patient's baseline values may differ from the acceptable range for that age or physical state; for example, long-distance runners often have a lower resting heart rate. Some illnesses or treatments cause predictable changes in vital signs; for example, patients with chronic obstructive pulmonary disease (COPD) typically have a lower oxygen saturation level. Some medications affect one or more vital signs. The nurse is often in the best position to assess all clinical findings about a patient and must be knowledgeable of related physical signs or symptoms and the patient's ongoing health status.
- Baseline measurements allow the identification of changes in vital signs. When vital signs appear abnormal, it is useful to have another nurse repeat the measurement. Verify, document, and communicate significant changes in vital signs to the health care provider or nurse in charge.
- Involve the patient, caregiver, or both in vital sign assessment and the significance of findings through implementation of teaching plans as necessary.

BODY TEMPERATURE

Physiology

Body temperature is the difference between the amount of heat produced by body processes and the amount lost to the external environment. Despite extremes in environmental conditions and physical activity, temperature-control mechanisms keep the body's *core temperature* (temperature of structures deep within the body) relatively constant (Figure 31.1), whereas body surface temperature fluctuates, depending on blood flow to the skin and the amount of heat lost to the external environment. Because of these surface temperature fluctuations, acceptable body temperature ranges from 36°C to 38°C, a narrow range in which the body's tissues and cells function best.

The measurement of body temperature is aimed at obtaining an average temperature of core body tissues, such as the internal organs

deep within the body. Sites reflecting core temperatures (i.e., rectal or temporal) are more reliable indicators of body temperature than are sites reflecting surface temperatures of the skin (i.e., oral or axillae) (Box 31.3). The temperature value obtained may also differ between one measurement site and another. In clinical practice, nurses learn the temperature range of individual patients, recognizing that no single temperature reading is normal for all people.

Regulation. The balance between heat lost and heat produced, or *thermoregulation*, is precisely regulated by physiological and behavioural mechanisms. For body temperature to stay constant and within an acceptable range, the relationship between heat production and heat loss must be closely maintained. This relationship is regulated by neurological and cardiovascular mechanisms. To regulate patients' temperatures, knowledge of temperature-control mechanisms is applied.

Neural and Vascular Control. The *hypothalamus*, located between the cerebral hemispheres, controls body temperature the same way that a thermostat works in a building. A comfortable temperature is the *set point* at which a heating system operates. In the building, a decrease in environmental temperature activates the furnace, whereas a rise in temperature shuts the system down. The hypothalamus is like the building's furnace; it senses minor changes in body temperature. The anterior hypothalamus controls heat loss, and the posterior hypothalamus controls heat production.

When nerve cells in the anterior hypothalamus become heated above the set point, impulses are sent to reduce body temperature. Mechanisms of heat loss include sweating, vasodilation (widening) of blood vessels, and inhibition of heat production. Blood is redistributed to surface vessels to promote heat loss. If the posterior hypothalamus senses that the body's temperature is lower than the set point, heat conservation mechanisms are instituted: vasoconstriction (narrowing) of blood vessels reduces blood flow to the skin and extremities.

Compensatory heat is produced through voluntary muscle contraction and muscle shivering. When vasoconstriction is ineffective in preventing additional heat loss, shivering begins. Disease or trauma to the hypothalamus or to the spinal cord, which carries hypothalamic messages, can cause serious alterations in temperature control.

Heat Production. Thermoregulation depends on the normal function of heat production processes. Heat is produced in the body as a by-product of metabolism, the chemical reaction in all body cells. Food is the primary fuel source for metabolism. Activities requiring additional chemical reactions increase metabolic rate. As metabolism increases, additional heat is produced. When metabolism decreases, less heat is produced. Heat production occurs during rest, voluntary movements, involuntary shivering, and nonshivering thermogenesis.

Basal metabolism accounts for the heat produced by the body at absolute rest. The average *basal metabolic rate (BMR)* depends on the body surface area. Thyroid hormones also affect the BMR. By promoting the breakdown of body glucose and fat, thyroid hormones increase the rate of chemical reactions in almost all cells of the body. When large amounts of thyroid hormones are secreted, the BMR can increase 100% above normal. Absence of thyroid hormones can reduce the BMR by half, causing a decrease in heat production. The male sex hormone testosterone increases BMR. Men have a higher BMR than do women. Voluntary movements such as muscular activity during exercise require additional energy. Metabolic rates can increase up to 2 000 times normal during exercise. Heat production can increase up to 50 times normal.

Shivering is an involuntary body response to temperature differences in the body. The skeletal muscle movement during shivering requires significant energy. In vulnerable patients, shivering can seriously deplete energy sources, which results in further physiological deterioration. Shivering can increase heat production four to five times greater than normal. The heat produced assists in equalizing body temperature, and shivering ceases. Newborns and older persons are less able to generate heat by shivering or preserve heat by vasoconstriction, putting them at an increased risk for hypothermia (Cheshire, 2016, p. 97).

Nonshivering thermogenesis (NST) occurs primarily in newborns and is the main source of heat generation due to their inability to shiver. Sympathetic nerve endings secrete norepinephrine in response to chilling, which stimulates fat metabolism in the richly vascularized brown adipose tissue to produce internal heat that is conducted to surface tissues through the blood (Hockenberry & Wilson, 2019, p. 275).

Heat Loss. Heat loss and heat production occur simultaneously. The skin's structure and exposure to the environment result in constant, normal heat loss through radiation, conduction, convection, and evaporation.

Radiation is the transfer of heat from the surface of one object to the surface of another without direct contact between the two. Up to 85% of the human body's surface area radiates heat to the environment. Peripheral vasodilation increases blood flow from internal organs to the skin to increase radiant heat loss. Peripheral vasoconstriction minimizes radiant heat loss. Radiation increases as the temperature difference between the objects increases. If the environment is warmer than the skin, the body absorbs heat through radiation.

Heat loss is increased through radiation by removing clothing or blankets. The patient's position enhances radiation heat loss (e.g., standing exposes a greater radiating surface area, and lying in a fetal position minimizes heat radiation). Covering the body with dark, closely woven clothing also reduces the amount of heat lost from radiation.

Conduction is the transfer of heat from one object to another through direct contact. Heat is conducted through contact with solids, liquids, and gases. When warm skin touches a cooler object, heat is lost. Conduction normally accounts for a small amount of heat loss. Interventions such as applying a cool cloth increase conductive heat loss. Applying several layers of clothing reduces conductive loss. The body gains heat by conduction when contact is made with materials warmer than skin temperature (e.g., application of an aquathermia pad).

Convection is the transfer of heat away from the body by air movement. A fan promotes heat loss through convection. Convective heat loss increases when moistened skin comes into contact with slightly moving air.

Evaporation is the transfer of heat energy when a liquid is changed to a gas. The body continuously loses heat by evaporation. About 600 to 900 mL per day evaporates from the skin and lungs, resulting in water and heat loss. By regulating perspiration (sweating), the body promotes additional evaporative heat loss. Millions of sweat glands located in the dermis of the skin secrete sweat through tiny ducts on the skin's surface. When body temperature rises, the anterior hypothalamus signals the sweat glands to release sweat. Sweat evaporates from the skin surface, which results in heat loss. During exercise and emotional or mental stress, sweating is one way to lose excessive heat produced by the increased metabolic rate.

Diaphoresis is visible perspiration, which occurs primarily on the forehead and upper thorax, although it can be seen elsewhere on the body. Excessive evaporation can cause skin scaling and itching, as well as drying of the nares and pharynx. Lowered body temperature inhibits sweat gland secretion. People who have a congenital absence of sweat glands or a serious skin disease that impairs sweating are unable to tolerate warm temperatures because they cannot cool themselves adequately.

Skin in Temperature Regulation. The skin regulates temperature through insulation of the body, vasoconstriction (which affects the amount of blood flow and heat loss to the skin), and temperature sensation. The skin, subcutaneous tissue, and fat keep heat inside the body. When blood flow between skin layers is reduced, the skin alone is an excellent insulator. People with more body fat have more natural insulation than do slim and muscular people.

In the human body, the internal organs produce heat. During exercise or increased sympathetic stimulation, the amount of heat produced is greater than the usual core temperature. Blood flows from the internal organs, carrying heat to the body surface. The skin is well supplied with blood vessels, especially the areas of the hands, feet, and ears. Blood flow through these vascular areas of skin may vary from minimal flow to as much as 30% of the blood ejected from the heart. Heat transfers from the blood through vessel walls to the skin's surface and is lost to the environment through the heat-loss mechanisms. The body's core temperature remains within safe limits.

The degree of vasoconstriction determines the amount of blood flow and heat loss to the skin. If the core temperature is too high, the hypothalamus inhibits vasoconstriction. As a result, blood vessels dilate, and more blood reaches the skin's surface. On a hot, humid day, the blood vessels in the hands are dilated and easily visible. In contrast, if the core temperature becomes too low, the hypothalamus initiates vasoconstriction and blood flow to the skin lessens, thus conserving body heat.

Behavioural Control. Healthy individuals voluntarily act to maintain a comfortable body temperature when exposed to temperature extremes. A person's ability to control body temperature depends on (1) the degree of temperature extreme, (2) the person's ability to sense feeling comfortable or uncomfortable, (3) thought processes or emotions, and (4) the person's mobility or ability to remove or add clothes. Body temperature control is difficult if any of these abilities is absent. Infants can sense uncomfortably warm conditions but cannot change their environment. Older persons and people with spinal cord injuries may need assistance in detecting cold environments and minimizing heat loss. Illness, altered levels of consciousness, or impaired thought processes result in an inability to recognize the need to change behaviour for temperature control. In extreme temperatures, health-promoting behaviours, such as removing or adding clothing, have a limited effect on controlling temperature. It is important for the nurse to assess for factors that place patients at high risk for ineffective thermoregulation.

Factors Affecting Body Temperature

Many factors affect body temperature. Changes in body temperature within an acceptable range occur when the relationship between heat production and heat loss is altered by physiological or behavioural variables. Nurses need to be aware of these factors when assessing temperature variations and evaluating deviations from normal.

Age. At birth, the newborn leaves a warm, relatively constant environment and enters one in which temperatures fluctuate widely. Temperature-control mechanisms are immature. An infant's temperature may respond dramatically to changes in the environment, requiring extra care to protect the newborn. Body coverings must be adequate, and exposure to temperature extremes must be avoided. A newborn loses up to 30% of body heat through the head and thus needs to wear a cap to prevent heat loss. When protected from environmental extremes, the newborn's core and peripheral body temperature can be normally maintained between 36.5°C and 37.6°C.

Temperature regulation is unstable until children reach puberty. The normal temperature range gradually drops as individuals approach older adulthood. Older persons have a lower and narrower range of body temperatures than do younger adults. An oral temperature of 35°C is not unusual for older persons in cold weather. However, the average body temperature of older persons is approximately 36°C. Older persons are particularly sensitive to temperature extremes because of deterioration in control mechanisms, particularly poor vasomotor control (control of vasoconstriction and vasodilation), reduced amounts of subcutaneous tissue, reduced sweat gland activity, and reduced metabolism.

Exercise. Muscle activity requires increases in blood supply and in carbohydrate and fat breakdown. This increased metabolism causes an increase in heat production. Any form of exercise can increase heat production and thus body temperature. Prolonged strenuous exercise, such as long-distance running, can temporarily raise body temperatures up to 41°C.

Hormone Level. Women generally experience greater fluctuations in body temperature than men. Hormonal variations in progesterone during the menstrual cycle cause body temperature fluctuations. When progesterone levels are low, the body temperature is a few tenths of a degree below the baseline level. This lower temperature persists until ovulation occurs. During ovulation, greater amounts of progesterone enter the circulatory system and raise the body temperature to previous baseline levels or higher. These temperature variations can be used to predict a woman's most fertile time to achieve pregnancy.

Body temperature changes also occur during menopause (cessation of menstruation). Menopausal women may experience times of intense body heat and sweating, lasting anywhere from 30 seconds to 5 minutes. Skin temperature may increase intermittently by up to 4°C, which is known as a *hot flash*. These increases in temperature result from the instability of the vasomotor controls for vasodilation and vasoconstriction.

Circadian Rhythm. Body temperature normally changes 0.5°C to 1°C during a 24-hour period. In persons who are awake during the day and sleep during the night, the temperature is usually lowest between 0100 and 0400 hours (Figure 31.2). During the day, body temperature rises

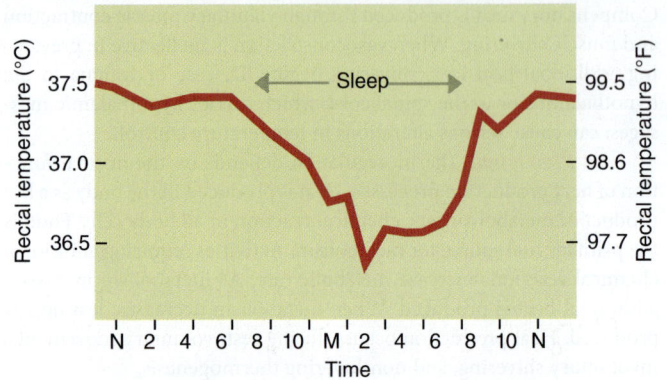

FIGURE 31.2 Temperature cycle for 24 hours.

steadily, until a maximum temperature value is reached at about 1800 hours, and then declines back down to early morning levels. It takes 1 to 3 weeks for temperature patterns to reverse in people who work at night and sleep during the day. In general, the circadian temperature rhythm does not change with age.

Stress. Physical and emotional stress increases body temperature through hormonal and neural stimulation. These physiological changes increase metabolism, which increases heat production. The patient who is anxious about entering a hospital or undergoing a procedure may register a higher normal temperature.

Environment. Environment influences body temperature. If body temperature is measured in a very warm room, a patient may be unable to regulate body temperature by heat-loss mechanisms, resulting in the elevation of body temperature. If the patient has just been outside in the cold without warm clothing, body temperature may be low because of extensive radiant and conductive heat loss. Infants, older persons, and those with spinal cord injuries are most likely to be affected by environmental temperatures, because their temperature-regulating mechanisms are less efficient. Body temperature often adjusts to the environmental temperature in people with spinal cord injuries; this is called *poikilothermia* (Krassioukov et al., 2020).

Temperature Alterations. Body temperatures outside the usual range affect the hypothalamic set point. Such changes can be related to excess heat production, excessive heat loss, minimal heat production, minimal heat loss, or any combination of these alterations. The nature of the change affects the type of clinical problems experienced.

Fever. Pyrexia, or *fever*, occurs because heat-loss mechanisms are unable to keep pace with excess heat production; as a result, body temperature rises to an abnormal level. A fever is usually not harmful if it stays below 39°C, and a single temperature reading may not indicate a fever. In addition to physical signs and symptoms of infection, determination of fever is based on several temperature readings at different times of the day that are compared with the usual value for that person at those times.

A true fever results from an alteration in the hypothalamic set point. *Pyrogens* such as bacteria and viruses cause a rise in body temperature. Pyrogens act as antigens, triggering immune system responses. The hypothalamus reacts to raise the set point, and the body responds by producing and conserving heat. Several hours may pass before the body temperature reaches the new set point. During this period, the person experiences chills, shivers, and feels cold, even though the body temperature is rising (Figure 31.3). The chill phase resolves when the new set point, a higher temperature, is achieved. During the next

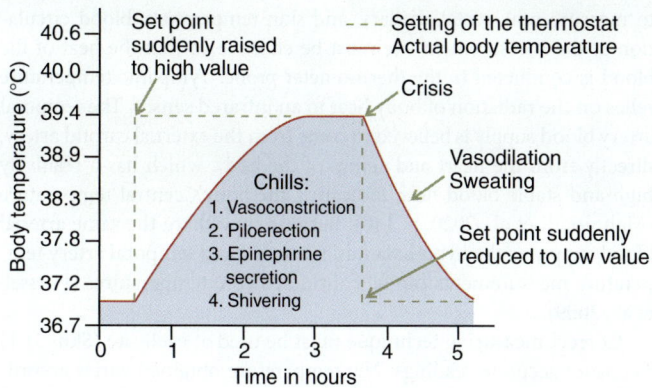

FIGURE 31.3 Effect of changing the set point of the hypothalamic temperature control during a fever. (Adapted from Hall, J. E. [2011]. *Guyton & Hall textbook of medical physiology* [12th ed., p. 876]. W. B. Saunders.)

TABLE 31.1	Classification of Hypothermia
Description	**Temperature (°C)**
Mild	34–36
Moderate	30–34
Severe	<30

phase, the plateau, the chills subside, and the person feels warm and dry. If the new set point is "overshot" or the pyrogens are removed (e.g., destruction of bacteria by antibiotics), the third phase of a febrile episode occurs. The hypothalamus set point drops, initiating heat loss responses. The skin becomes warm and flushed because of vasodilation. Diaphoresis assists in evaporative heat loss. When the fever "breaks," the person becomes *afebrile*.

Fever is an important defence mechanism. Temperature elevations up to 38°C enhance the body's immune system. During a *febrile* episode, white blood cell production is stimulated. Increased temperature reduces the concentration of iron in the blood plasma, suppressing the growth of bacteria. Fever also fights viral infections by stimulating production of interferon, the body's natural virus-fighting substance.

By analyzing a fever pattern, health care providers can make diagnoses. Fever patterns differ, depending on the causative pyrogen. The increase or decrease in pyrogen activity results in fever spikes and declines at different times of the day. The duration and degree of fever depend on the strength of the pyrogen and the ability of the individual to respond. The term *fever of unknown origin* refers to a fever that does not have a determined cause.

During a fever, cellular metabolism increases and oxygen consumption rises. Heart and respiratory rates increase to meet the increased metabolic needs of the body for nutrients. The increased metabolism entails the use of energy that produces additional heat. If the patient has a cardiac or respiratory problem, the stress of a fever can be great. A prolonged fever can weaken a person by exhausting energy stores. Increased metabolism requires additional oxygen. If the demand for additional oxygen cannot be met, cellular hypoxia (inadequate oxygenation) occurs. Myocardial hypoxia produces angina (chest pain); cerebral hypoxia produces confusion. Interventions during a fever may include oxygen therapy. Water loss through increased respiration and diaphoresis can be excessive, placing a patient at risk for fluid volume deficit. Dehydration is a serious concern for older persons and for children with low body weight. Maintaining optimum fluid volume status is an important nursing intervention (see Chapter 41 for further information about fluids and electrolytes).

Hyperthermia. *Hyperthermia* is body temperature that is elevated as a result of the body's inability to promote heat loss or reduce heat production. Whereas fever is an upward shift in the set point, hyperthermia results from an overload of the body's thermoregulatory mechanisms. Any disease or trauma to the hypothalamus can impair heat-loss mechanisms. *Malignant hyperthermia* is a life-threatening disorder of the skeletal muscle in people with a pharmacogenetic predisposition. It is characterized by muscle contractions and a severe hypermetabolic crisis, in response to the use of volatile anaesthetics or the neuromuscular blocking agent succinylcholine (Ortiz et al., 2020).

Heatstroke. Prolonged exposure to the sun or high environmental temperatures can overwhelm the body's heat-loss mechanisms. Heat also depresses hypothalamic function. These conditions cause *heatstroke*, a dangerous heat emergency with a high mortality rate. Patients at risk include the very young, older persons, and those who have cardiovascular disease, hypothyroidism, diabetes, spinal cord injury, or alcoholism. Also at risk are patients who take medications that decrease the body's ability to lose heat (e.g., phenothiazines, anticholinergics, diuretics, amphetamines, and β-adrenergic receptor antagonists) and those who exercise or engage in strenuous physical labour (e.g., athletes, construction workers, and farmers).

Signs and symptoms of heatstroke include confusion, delirium, excess thirst, nausea, muscle cramps, visual disturbances, giddiness, and incontinence. The most important sign is hot, dry skin. Patients with heatstroke do not sweat because of severe electrolyte loss and hypothalamic malfunction. Vital signs reveal a body temperature sometimes as high as 45°C, with an increase in heart rate and lowering of blood pressure. If the condition progresses, loss of consciousness can occur. Permanent neurological damage may result unless cooling measures are rapidly started.

Heat Exhaustion. *Heat exhaustion* occurs when profuse diaphoresis results in excessive water and electrolyte loss. The patient exhibits signs and symptoms of fluid volume deficit (see Chapter 41 for further information about fluids and electrolytes). Treatment includes transporting the patient to a cooler environment and restoring fluid and electrolyte balance.

Hypothermia. Heat loss during prolonged exposure to cold overwhelms the body's ability to produce heat, causing hypothermia. *Hypothermia* is classified by core temperature measurements (Table 31.1). It can be unintentionally induced (e.g., by falling through the ice of a frozen lake) or intentionally induced (e.g., during specific surgical procedures) to reduce metabolic demand and the body's need for oxygen. Accidental hypothermia usually develops gradually and may go unnoticed for several hours. When body temperature drops to 35°C, uncontrolled shivering, loss of memory, depression, and poor judgement occur. As the body temperature falls below 34.4°C, heart rate, respiratory rate, and blood pressure fall and the skin becomes cyanotic. If hypothermia progresses, cardiac dysrhythmias, loss of consciousness, and unresponsiveness to painful stimuli occur. In cases of severe hypothermia, clinical signs similar to death (e.g., lack of response to stimuli and extremely slow respirations and pulse) are demonstrated. The assessment of core temperature is critical when hypothermia is suspected. A special thermometer that displays low readings may be required because most standard devices do not register below 35°C.

Frostbite occurs when the body is exposed to subnormal temperatures. Ice crystals forming inside cells can result in permanent circulatory and tissue damage. Areas on the body particularly susceptible to frostbite are the earlobes, tip of the nose, fingers, and toes. The injured area becomes white, waxy, and firm to the touch and loss of sensation occurs in the affected area. Intervention includes gradual warming measures, analgesia, and protection of the injured tissue.

❖ NURSING PROCESS AND THERMOREGULATION

Knowledge of the physiology of body temperature regulation is essential for assessing and evaluating the patient's response to temperature alterations and for intervening safely. Independent measures can be implemented to increase or minimize heat loss, promote heat conservation, and increase comfort. These measures complement the effects of medically ordered therapies. Many measures can be taught to caregivers and parents of children.

◆ Assessment

Sites. Core and surface body temperature may be measured at several sites. The core temperatures of the pulmonary artery, esophagus, nasopharynx, and urinary bladder are measured in critical care settings. These measurements require the use of invasive devices placed in body cavities or organs that continuously display readings on an electronic monitor.

Intermittent temperature measurements are obtained invasively from the sites of the mouth, rectum, and tympanic membrane or non-invasively from the axilla and temporal artery sites. Chemically prepared thermometer patches can also be applied to the skin. In order to measure oral, rectal, axillary, and skin temperature, blood circulation at the measurement site must be effective so that the heat of the blood is conducted to the thermometer probe. Tympanic temperature relies on the radiation of body heat to an infrared sensor. The temporal artery blood supply is believed to come from the external carotid artery, directly from the heart and centre of the body, which has a relatively high and stable blood flow, indicating the body's central temperature (Mahmoudi et al., 2020, p. 148). Because they share the same arterial blood supply as the hypothalamus, tympanic and temporal artery temperature measurements can be considered core temperatures (Purssell et al., 2009).

Correct measuring technique must be used at each site (Skill 31.1) to ensure accurate readings. The temperature obtained varies according to the site used but should remain between 36.0°C and 38.0°C. Rectal temperatures are usually 0.5°C higher than oral temperatures, and axillary temperatures are usually 0.5°C lower than oral temperatures. Each measurement site has advantages and disadvantages (Box 31.4). The rectal site was traditionally chosen because of the close replication of core body temperature but is now less routinely measured given the availability of less invasive and accurate alternative measurement devices such as the temporal thermometer. The safest and most

---

SKILL 31.1	MEASURING BODY TEMPERATURE

Delegation Considerations

The task of measuring temperature can be delegated to unregulated care providers (UCPs). The nurse is responsible for assessing the impact of changes in body temperature; therefore, when the task of measuring temperature is delegated, it is important to *inform the UCP* about the following:

- The appropriate route and device to measure temperature
- Patient-specific factors that can falsely raise or lower temperature
- Appropriate precautions when positioning the patient
- Frequency of temperature measurement for the patient
- Usual values for patient
- Abnormalities that should be reported to the health care provider

Equipment

- Appropriate thermometer
- Soft tissue or wipe
- Alcohol swabs
- Lubricant (for rectal measurements only)
- Pen and either vital sign flow sheet or documentation form
- Disposable gloves
- Plastic thermometer sleeve or disposable probe cover

PROCEDURE

STEPS	RATIONALE
1. Identify patient using at least two person specifics (e.g., name and date of birth or name and medical record number) according to employer policy.	• Ensures correct patient. Complies with Accreditation Canada's standards and improves patient safety (Accreditation Canada, 2020).
2. Assess for signs and symptoms of temperature alterations and for factors that influence body temperature.	• Physical signs and symptoms may indicate abnormal temperature. You can accurately assess the nature of variations.
3. Determine previous activity that would interfere with accuracy of temperature measurement. Wait before measuring oral temperature in the following situations: 2 minutes after patient has smoked, 5 minutes after patient has chewed gum, and 20 minutes after patient has ingested hot or cold liquids or foods.	• The oral temperature can be affected by the temperature of the smoke, liquids, or food.
4. Determine appropriate temperature site and device for patient.	• This choice is based on advantages and disadvantages of each site (see Box 31.4) Use a disposable, single-use thermometer for a patient who has isolation precautions.
5. Explain to patient the route by which temperature will be measured and the importance of maintaining the proper position until the reading is complete.	• Patients are often curious about measurements and should be cautioned against prematurely removing the thermometer to read results.
6. Perform hand hygiene.	• Hand hygiene reduces transmission of microorganisms between the patient and the nurse.
7. Obtain temperature reading.	

Continued

SKILL 31.1 MEASURING BODY TEMPERATURE—cont'd

STEPS	RATIONALE

A. Oral temperature measurement with electronic thermometer

(1) Put on disposable gloves (optional).

- Use of oral probe cover, removed without physical contact, minimizes the need to wear gloves.

(2) Remove thermometer pack from charging unit. Attach oral probe (blue tip) to thermometer unit. Grasp top of probe stem, being careful not to press the ejection button.

- Charging provides battery power. Removal of hand-held unit from base prepares it to measure temperature. Pressing ejection button releases plastic probe cover from tip.

(3) Slide disposable plastic probe cover over thermometer probe until cover locks in place (see Step 7A[3] illustration).

- The soft plastic cover will not break in the patient's mouth, and it prevents transmission of microorganisms between patients.

STEP 7A(3) Inserting thermometer stem into plastic probe cover.

(4) Have patient sit or lie in bed. Ask patient to open their mouth; gently place thermometer probe under the patient's tongue in posterior sublingual pocket lateral to centre of lower jaw (see Step 7A[4] illustration).

- Heat from superficial blood vessels in the sublingual pocket produces temperature reading. Temperatures in right and left posterior sublingual pockets are significantly higher than in area under front of tongue.

STEP 7A(4) Probe under tongue in posterior sublingual pocket. (iStockphoto/YinYang.)

(5) Ask patient to hold thermometer probe with lips closed.

- Holding the probe this way helps maintain proper position of thermometer during recording.

(6) Leave thermometer probe in place until the audible signal sounds and the patient's temperature appears on the digital display; remove thermometer probe from under the patient's tongue.

- The probe must stay in place until the signal occurs, to ensure accurate reading.

(7) Push ejection button on thermometer stem to discard plastic probe cover into appropriate receptacle.

- Discarding probe cover reduces transmission of microorganisms between patients.

(8) Return thermometer stem to storage well of recording unit.

- Proper storage protects the probe from damage. Returning the probe automatically causes digital reading to disappear.

(9) If gloves were worn, remove and dispose in appropriate receptacle. Perform hand hygiene.

- Glove disposal and hand hygiene reduce transmission of microorganisms between patients.

(10) Return thermometer to charger.

- Charging provides battery power.

B. Rectal temperature measurement with electronic thermometer

(1) Prepare patient for procedure.

(a) Draw curtain around patient's bed or close room door, or do both.

(b) Assist patient in a side-lying or modified left lateral recumbent position with upper leg flexed.

- Provides appropriate access for insertion of rectal probe.

(c) Move aside bed linen to expose only anal area. Keep patient's upper body and lower extremities covered with a sheet or blanket.

- These actions maintain patient's privacy, minimize embarrassment, and promote comfort. Anal area is exposed for correct thermometer placement.

(d) Remind patient to remain in position until the procedure is complete.

SKILL 31.1   MEASURING BODY TEMPERATURE—cont'd

STEPS	RATIONALE
(2) Put on disposable gloves.	• Gloves help maintain standard precautions during exposure to items soiled with body fluids (e.g., feces).
(3) Remove thermometer pack from charging unit. Attach rectal probe (red tip) to thermometer unit. Grasp top of probe stem, being careful not to press the ejection button.	• Charging provides battery power. Removal of hand-held unit from base prepares it to measure temperature. Pressing the ejection button releases the plastic probe cover from the tip.
(4) Slide disposable plastic probe cover over thermometer probe until cover locks in place.	• Probe cover prevents transmission of microorganisms between patients.
(5) Squeeze a liberal portion of lubricant on a tissue. Dip thermometer's blunt end into lubricant, covering 2.5–3.5 cm for an adult patient or 1.2–2.5 cm for an infant or a child.	• Lubrication minimizes trauma to rectal mucosa during thermometer insertion. Use of tissue avoids contamination of remaining lubricant in container.
(6) With nondominant hand, separate patient's buttocks to expose anus. Ask patient to breathe slowly and relax.	• Separating buttocks fully exposes anus for thermometer insertion. Relaxing anal sphincter facilitates thermometer insertion.
(7) Gently insert thermometer into patient's anus in direction of umbilicus, 3.5 cm for an adult patient. Do not force thermometer.	• Insertion in this direction ensures adequate exposure against blood vessels in the rectal wall.
(8) If resistance is felt during insertion, withdraw thermometer.	• This action prevents trauma to mucosa.

CRITICAL DECISION POINT: *If thermometer cannot be adequately inserted into the rectum, remove thermometer and consider an alternative method for obtaining temperature.*

---

(9) Once positioned, thermometer probe should be left in place (see Step 7B[9] illustration) until an audible signal sounds and the patient's temperature appears on digital display; remove thermometer probe from anus.	• Probe must stay in place until signal occurs, to ensure accurate reading.

STEP 7B(9) Probe positioned in anus.

(10) Push ejection button on thermometer stem to discard plastic probe cover into appropriate receptacle. Wipe probe adequately with an alcohol swab, paying particular attention to ridges where probe cover is connected to the probe.	• Discarding probe cover reduces transmission of microorganisms between patients.
(11) Return thermometer stem to storage well of recording unit.	• Proper storage protects the probe from damage. Returning probe automatically causes digital reading to disappear.
(12) Wipe patient's anal area with a soft tissue to remove lubricant or feces, and discard tissue. Assist patient to assume a comfortable position and be sufficiently covered with linens.	• These actions provide for comfort and hygiene.
(13) Remove and dispose of gloves in an appropriate receptacle. Perform hand hygiene.	• Glove disposal and hand hygiene reduce transmission of microorganisms between the patient and the nurse.
(14) Return thermometer unit to charger. Verify that charger and probes are wiped with alcohol daily (in isolation areas, they are wiped whenever they are removed from the room).	• Charging provides battery power. Wiping with alcohol reduces transmission of microorganisms between the patient and the nurse.
C. Axillary temperature measurement with electronic thermometer	
(1) Prepare patient for procedure.	
(a) Draw curtain around patient's bed or close room door, or do both.	• These actions maintain patient's privacy, minimize embarrassment, and promote comfort.
(b) Assist patient to a supine or sitting position.	• These positions enable easy access to axilla.
(c) Move clothing or gown away from patient's shoulder and arm.	• This action exposes axilla for correct thermometer probe placement.
(2) Remove thermometer pack from charging unit. Ensure oral probe (blue tip) is attached to thermometer unit. Grasp top of probe stem, being careful not to press the ejection button.	• Charging provides battery power. Removal of hand-held unit from base prepares it to measure temperature. Pressing ejection button releases plastic cover from probe.
(3) Slide disposable plastic probe cover over thermometer probe until cover locks in place.	• The soft plastic cover prevents transmission of microorganisms between patients.

Continued

SKILL 31.1 MEASURING BODY TEMPERATURE—cont'd

STEPS	RATIONALE
(4) Raise patient's arm away from torso; inspect for skin lesions and excessive perspiration. Insert probe into centre of patient's axilla, lower patient's arm over probe (see Step 7C[4] illustration).	• Maintains proper position of probe against blood vessels in axilla.

STEP 7C(4) Proper placement of thermometer tip in patient's axilla. (Courtesy Barbara J. Astle, RN, PhD.)

CRITICAL DECISION POINT: *Do not use axilla if skin lesions are present, because local temperature may be altered and area may be painful to touch. Wipe off excessive perspiration.*

STEPS	RATIONALE
(5) Hold probe in place until an audible signal sounds and temperature appears on digital display.	• Probe must stay in place until signal occurs, to ensure accurate reading.
(6) Remove probe from patient's axilla.	
(7) Push ejection button on thermometer stem to discard plastic probe cover into appropriate receptacle.	• Discarding probe cover reduces transmission of microorganisms between the patient and the nurse.
(8) Return thermometer stem to storage well of recording unit.	• Proper storage protects probe from damage. Returning probe automatically causes digital reading to disappear.
(9) Assist patient to assume a comfortable position and move linen or gown back over patient's shoulder.	• These actions restore comfort and promote privacy.
(10) Perform hand hygiene.	• Hand hygiene reduces transmission of microorganisms between the patient and the nurse.
(11) Return thermometer to charger.	• Charging provides battery power.
D. Tympanic membrane temperature measurement with electronic thermometer	
(1) Assist patient in assuming a comfortable position with head turned to the side, away from the nurse. Right-handed caregivers should obtain temperature from the patient's right ear. Left-handed caregivers should obtain temperature from the patient's left ear.	• This positioning ensures comfort and exposes the auditory canal for accurate temperature measurement. The less acute the angle of approach, the better the probe seal.
(2) Check for the presence of obvious cerumen in the patient's ear canal.	• To ensure a clear optical pathway, the lens cover of the speculum must not be impeded by cerumen. Switch to the other ear or select an alternative measurement site if necessary.
(3) Remove thermometer hand-held unit from charging base, being careful not to press the ejection button.	• Charging provides battery power. Removal of hand-held unit from base prepares it to measure temperature. Pressing ejection button releases plastic probe cover from tip.
(4) Slide clean disposable speculum cover over otoscope-like lens tip until it locks into place; be careful not to touch the lens cover.	• The lens cover must be clear of dust, fingerprints, and cerumen to ensure a clear optical pathway.
(5) Insert speculum into the patient's ear canal in accordance with manufacturer's instructions for tympanic probe positioning:	• Correct positioning of the probe with regard to the ear canal ensures accurate readings. Operator errors cause false readings.
(a) Pull patient's pinna backward, up, and out. For children younger than 3 years, pull pinna down and back.	• The speculum does not get a panoramic view of the ear canal unless it is straightened, because the canal is curved (Hockenberry & Wilson, 2019, p. 118).

SKILL 31.1   MEASURING BODY TEMPERATURE—cont'd

STEPS	RATIONALE
(b) Fit otoscope probe snugly into ear canal and do not move (see Step 7D[5][b] illustration).	• Gentle pressure seals the ear canal from ambient temperature, which can alter readings as much as 2.8°C.

STEP 7D(5)(b) Tympanic thermometer with probe cover inserted into auditory canal.

STEPS	RATIONALE
(c) Point speculum tip toward patient's nose.	
(6) When probe is in place, press scan button on hand-held unit. Leave thermometer probe in place until an audible signal sounds and the patient's temperature appears on digital display.	• When scan button is pressed, the probe detects infrared energy. The otoscope tip must stay in place until signal occurs, to ensure accurate reading.
(7) Carefully remove speculum from auditory canal.	• Careful removal prevents rubbing of sensitive outer ear lining.
(8) Push ejection button on hand-held unit to discard plastic probe cover into an appropriate receptacle.	• Discarding probe cover reduces transmission of microorganisms between the patient and the nurse and automatically causes digital reading to disappear.
(9) If a second reading is necessary, replace probe lens cover and wait 2 to 3 minutes before inserting probe tip.	• The lens cover must be free of cerumen to maintain an optical path. Time allows the auditory canal to regain its usual temperature.
(10) Return hand-held unit to charging base.	• Proper storage protects probe from damage.
(11) Assist patient to assume a comfortable position.	• This action restores comfort and a sense of well-being.
(12) Perform hand hygiene.	• Hand hygiene reduces transmission of microorganisms between the patient and the nurse.
8. Discuss findings with patient as needed.	• Such discussion promotes patient's participation in care and understanding of their health status.
9. If patient's temperature is being assessed for the first time and is within normal range, document temperature as baseline.	• Baseline is used to compare future temperature measurements.
10. Compare current temperature reading with patient's previous baseline and with acceptable temperature range for patient's age group.	• Normal body temperature fluctuates within a narrow range; comparison helps reveal presence of abnormality. Improper placement or movement of thermometer causes inaccuracies. A second measurement confirms initial findings of abnormal body temperature.

UNEXPECTED OUTCOMES	RELATED INTERVENTIONS
Temperature 1°C above usual range	• Assess possible sites (e.g., central line catheter, wounds) for localized infection and for related data suggestive of a systemic infection. • Implement appropriate nursing measures (see Box 31.9).
Persistent fever	• Notify appropriate health care provider and administer antipyretic and antibiotics as prescribed.
Temperature 1°C below usual range	• Remove any drafts, wet clothing, or damp linens. • Apply extra blankets, and, unless contraindicated, offer warm liquids.

RECORDING AND REPORTING

• Record temperature on vital sign flow sheet. Document temperature after administration of specific therapies in nurses' narrative notes.
• Report abnormal findings to nurse in charge or to health care provider.

CARE IN THE COMMUNITY CONSIDERATIONS

• Assess temperature and ventilation of the patient's environment to determine existence of any environmental condition that may influence outcome of patient's temperature.
• In the home, patients may continue to use mercury-in-glass thermometers. Educate patient and caregiver about mercury hazards and encourage replacement with an electronic thermometer.

BOX 31.4	Advantages and Disadvantages of Select Temperature Measurement Sites

Temperature Site	Advantages	Disadvantages
Tympanic membrane	• Site is easily accessible; minimal patient repositioning is required. Temperature reading can be obtained without disturbing or waking patient. • Device provides core reading, as the eardrum is close to the hypothalamus. • Measurement is very rapid (2 to 5 seconds). • Measurement is unaffected by oral intake of food or fluids or by smoking. • Device can be used for tachypneic patients without affecting breathing. • Device can be used in newborns to reduce handling of infants and subsequent heat loss.	• Measurement is more variable with this device than with other core temperature devices. • Hearing aids must be removed before measurement. • Site cannot be used in patients following surgery of the ear or tympanic membrane. • Readings are altered by cerumen impaction and otitis media. • Disposable probe cover comes in only one size. • Device does not accurately measure core temperature changes during and after exercise. • Accuracy of results is influenced by size of the probe (most are 8 mm). This may be a problem in young children, due to the small diameter of their ear canal (Hockenberry & Wilson, 2019, p. 210). • Inaccuracies can result from incorrect technique with temperature differences as much as 2.8°C between the opening of the ear canal and the tympanic membrane (Jevon & Joshi 2019, p.4) • Obtaining continuous measurement is not possible. • Temperature readings are affected by ambient temperature devices such as incubators, radiant warmers, and fans.
Rectum	• Site is argued to be more reliable when oral temperature cannot be obtained.	• Measurement at this site lags behind those at sites of core temperature during rapid temperature changes. • Site should not be used in patients with diarrhea, rectal surgery, a rectal disorder, or bleeding tendencies. • Site should not be used for routine measurement of vital signs in newborns. • Given the invasiveness of this approach and the positioning that is required, this may be a source of patient discomfort, embarrassment, and anxiety. • Impacted stool alters readings. • Measurement at this site carries risk of exposure to body fluids. • Lubrication is required.
Mouth	• Site is accessible and no position change is required. • Measurement is comfortable for patients. • Measurement provides accurate reading of surface temperature. • Measurement reflects rapid change in core temperature.	• Readings are affected by ingestion of fluids or foods, smoking, and oxygen delivery. • Site is not suitable for patients who have had oral surgery, have suffered trauma, have a history of epilepsy, or have shaking chills. • Site should not be used for infants and small children or in confused, unconscious, or uncooperative patients. • Measurement at this site carries risk of exposure to body fluids.
Axilla	• Site is safe and noninvasive. • Site is appropriate for use in newborns and in uncooperative or unconscious patients.	• Measurement time is long. • Measurement at this site necessitates continuous positioning by the nurse. • Measurement time lags behind those at sites of core temperature during rapid temperature changes. • Site requires exposure of thorax, which can result in temperature loss, especially in newborns. • Readings are affected by exposure to the environment during device placement. • Site is not recommended for detecting fever in infants and young children.
Skin	• Continuous reading can be obtained. • Site is safe and noninvasive. • Site requires minimal disturbance to patient. • It is appropriate site for newborn measurement.	• Measurement time lags behind those at other sites during temperature changes, especially during hyperthermia. • Adhesion of the thermometer can be impaired by diaphoresis or sweat. • Measurement at this site can be affected by environmental temperature. • Site cannot be used for patients who have an allergy to adhesive.
Temporal artery	• Site provides a considerable reduction in nursing time required to measure (Mahmoudi et al., 2020, p. 150). • Measurement reflects rapid change in core temperature. • Site is easy to access without changing the patient's position. • Measurement is comfortable and eliminates the need to remove clothing. • Measurement is useful in premature infants, newborns, and children.	• Measurement is not effective through head covering (e.g., dressing) or hair. • Results are affected by diaphoresis or sweating. • Continuous measurement is not possible. • Measurement at this site fails to detect fever at the two critical temperature points of 38°C or greater, and 39°C in children younger than 36 months (Hoffman et al., 2013).

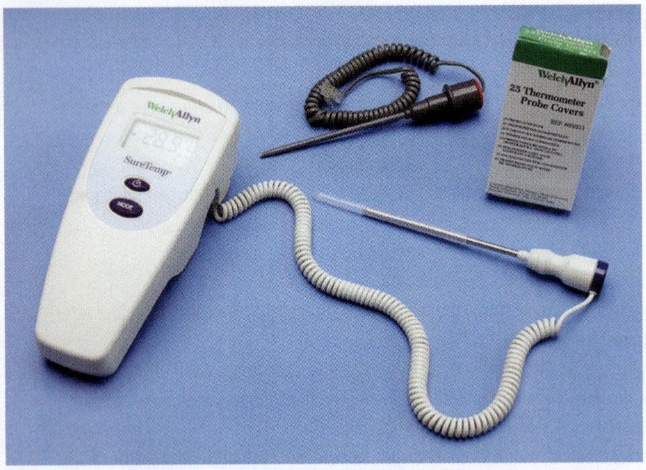

FIGURE 31.4 Electronic thermometer. The blue probe is for oral or axillary use. The red probe is for rectal use.

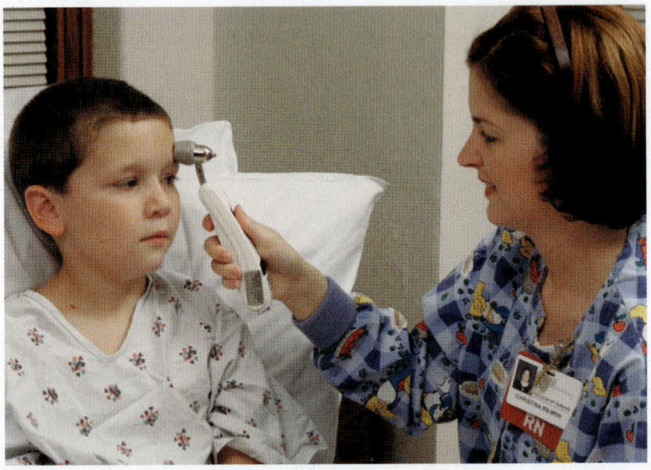

FIGURE 31.5 Temporal artery thermometer scanning the child's forehead.

effective site should be chosen for each patient. When possible, the same site should be used when measurements must be repeated.

Thermometers. Two types of thermometers are commonly available for measuring body temperature: electronic and disposable. A third type, the mercury-in-glass thermometer, was once the standard device for the clinical setting. Most municipalities have now prohibited the sale or use of mercury-containing medical devices because of potential toxins associated with mercury spills, in addition to the potential hazards associated with glass breakage during temperature measurement.

Temperature is recorded according to the *Celsius* scale. Electronic thermometers allow conversion to alternative scales by activating a switch.

Recently, because of the coronavirus pandemic and similar to previous epidemics, infrared thermography (IRI) is now being utilized. IRI is a noninvasive, low-cost technology that measures the radiation from a body. It provides information on the superficial temperature without requiring contact or any dosage of radiation, making this technique completely safe. Its use is particularly encouraged in mass screening in places like health care and transport hubs such as airports because of its contactless features (Perpetuini et al., 2021).

Electronic Thermometer. The electronic thermometer consists of a rechargeable battery-powered display unit, a thin wire cord, and a temperature-processing probe covered by a disposable plastic cover (Figure 31.4). Separate unbreakable probes are available for oral and rectal use. The oral probe can also be used for axillary temperature measurement. Electronic thermometers provide two modes of operation: a 4-second predictive temperature and a 3-minute standard temperature. When the first mode is used, a reading appears on the display unit within 20 to 50 seconds of insertion depending on the device used; please refer to the user's manual. A signal is sounded when the peak temperature reading has been measured.

Another form of electronic thermometer is used exclusively for tympanic temperature. An otoscope-like speculum with an infrared sensor tip detects heat radiated from the tympanic membrane. Within seconds after the speculum is placed in the auditory canal, a reading appears on the display unit. A signal sounds when the peak temperature reading has been measured.

Newer to the market is an electronic thermometer that measures the temperature of the superficial temporal artery. A hand-held scanner with an infrared sensor tip detects the temperature of cutaneous blood flow: the sensor is swept across the forehead and just behind the ear (Figure 31.5). Once scanning is complete, a reading appears on the display. Temporal artery temperature is a reliable and noninvasive measure of core temperature and has become an institutional standard in many health care settings (Box 31.5).

The greatest advantages of electronic thermometers are that they can be used immediately and read easily within seconds. The plastic sheath is unbreakable, making these devices ideal for use with children. Their expense is a major disadvantage. Maintaining cleanliness of the probes is important: for example, if a rectal probe is not properly cleaned between patients, contamination of the rectal probe by gastrointestinal disease organisms can be a vector of disease transmission. The thermometer must be wiped frequently with alcohol, and the thermometer probe must be wiped with an alcohol swab after each use. Particular attention must be paid to the probe hub, which has ridges, where the probe cover is secured to the probe.

Chemical Strip Thermometers. Single-use or reusable chemical strip (or dot) thermometers are thin strips of plastic containing a temperature sensor at one end. The sensor consists of chemically impregnated dots that change colour at different temperatures in increments of 0.1°C between 35.5°C and 40.4°C (Figure 31.6). Most of these devices are intended for single use, but the dots on reusable strips return to their original colour in seconds. The devices are used for measuring oral or axillary temperatures, particularly in children, and may be used rectally in a special sheath. The thermometer is removed after 60 seconds and read after another wait of 10 seconds to ensure that the temperature reading has stabilized. Research has shown that disposable single-use thermometers tend to overestimate or underestimate true temperature readings. The device is recommended only for screening purposes. When an abnormal temperature is suspected, the temperature should be confirmed with an electronic thermometer. Chemical strip thermometers are useful in caring for patients with isolation precautions (see Chapter 34 for further information about infection control), to avoid the need to take electronic instruments into these patients' rooms.

Another type of disposable thermometer is a temperature-sensitive patch or tape. Applied to the forehead or abdomen, the patch changes colour at different temperatures. These thermometers are also useful for screening patients, especially infants, for altered temperature. If an abnormal temperature is suspected, the temperature must be confirmed with an electronic temperature device. Disposable thermometers are not appropriate for monitoring temperature therapies.

Glass Thermometers. The traditional glass thermometer is a glass tube sealed at one end and with a mercury—or more recently, due to safety

BOX 31.5 PROCEDURAL GUIDELINE ▶

Measurement of Temporal Artery Temperature

Delegation Considerations

The measurement of temporal artery temperature can be delegated to unregulated care providers (UCPs). The nurse is responsible for assessing the impact of changes on body temperature; therefore, when measurement of temporal artery temperature is delegated, it is important to *inform the UCP* about the following:

- Frequency of temperature measurement
- Factors that falsely raise or lower temperature readings
- Reporting abnormalities to the nurse for further assessment

Equipment

- Temporal artery thermometer, alcohol wipes or probe cover (optional)

Procedure

1. Perform hand hygiene.
2. Ensure that the patient's forehead is dry; wipe it with a towel if it is moist.
3. Place the probe flush on the patient's forehead to avoid measuring ambient temperature.
4. Press the red scan button with your thumb. Scanning for the highest temperature will be continuous until you release the scan button.
5. Slowly slide the thermometer straight across the patient's forehead while keeping the probe flush on the patient's skin.
6. Keeping scan button pressed, lift the probe from the patient's forehead, and touch the probe to the patient's neck just behind the earlobe (the area where perfume is typically applied).
7. While the probe is scanning, a clicking sound occurs; this sound stops when peak temperature is scanned.
8. Release the scan button; read and record the temperature. Reading remains on the screen for 15 seconds after the button is released.
9. Clean the probe with an alcohol wipe, or, if a probe cover was used, remove and dispose of the probe cover.

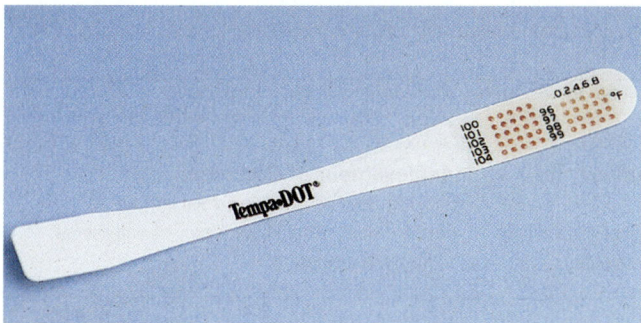

FIGURE 31.6 Disposable, single-use thermometer strip.

BOX 31.6 NURSING DIAGNOSTIC PROCESS

Assessment Activities	Defining Characteristics	Nursing Diagnosis
Measure vital signs, including temperature, pulse, respirations, and pulse oximetry (SpO₂).	Increased body temperature above usual range	*Ineffective thermoregulation related to aging and inability to adapt to environmental temperature*
Palpate skin.	Tachycardia	
Observe patient's appearance and behaviour while talking and resting.	Tachypnea	
Review medical history.	Hypoxemia	
	Warm, dry skin	
	Restlessness	
	Confusion	
	Flushed appearance	
	Location (e.g., found in unventilated apartment during heat wave) and other patient characteristics (e.g., 85 years old with history of dementia)	

recommends phasing out use of mercury-containing thermometers and all other nonessential mercury-containing products and implementing safe use and disposal of these products. However, mercury-in-glass thermometers can sometimes still be found in patients' homes or being used in developing countries (Oncel et al., 2013, p. 193).

◆ Nursing Diagnosis

Nurses identify assessment findings and cluster defining characteristics to form a nursing diagnosis. Nursing diagnoses for patients with body temperature alterations include the following:

- *Risk for imbalanced body temperature*
- *Hyperthermia*
- *Hypothermia*
- *Ineffective thermoregulation*

For example, an increase in body temperature, flushed skin, skin warm to touch, and tachycardia are indicative of the diagnosis *hyperthermia.* The nursing diagnosis is stated as either an at-risk or an actual temperature alteration. If the patient has risk factors for temperature alterations, the nurse should minimize or eliminate them.

Once the diagnosis is established, the nurse accurately determines the related factor or cause (Box 31.6). The related factor directs the selection of appropriate nursing interventions. In the example of hyperthermia, a related factor of vigorous activity will result in interventions much different from those for a related factor of decreased ability to perspire.

◆ Planning

During planning, nurses integrate knowledge gathered from assessment and patient history to develop and modify a person-centred plan of care (CASN, 2022) (Box 31.7). It is important to match a patient's needs with interventions that are supported and recommended in the clinical research literature.

Goals and Outcomes. The care plan for a patient with alteration in temperature must include realistic and individualized goals along with relevant outcomes. The nurse needs to collaborate closely with the patient in setting goals and outcomes and choosing nursing

factors, an alcohol-filled—bulb at the other end of the device. Exposure of the bulb to heat causes the internal fluid to expand and rise in the enclosed tube. The length of the thermometer is marked with centigrade (Celsius) calibrations from which the temperature reading is obtained. The thermometer must be positioned properly at the oral, rectal, or axillary site and must be maintained for the appropriate length of time to obtain an accurate reading. There are many disadvantages to using this type of device. In addition to the time delay (approximately 3 minutes with the device held in place), the mercury-in-glass device is easily breakable and, when broken, releases the contents, which may include hazardous mercury. With the potent toxicities associated with mercury spills, in addition to injuries from the use of glass thermometers, most health care agencies no longer supply these devices. The World Health Organization (2017)

◎ BOX 31.7 NURSING CARE PLAN

Hyperthermia

ASSESSMENT

Mr. Coburn is a 45-year-old teacher (preferred pronouns: he/him) who arrives at the outpatient clinic complaining of malaise. His medical history includes a past urinary tract infection. Several of his students have had colds lately. He has been feeling unwell for the past 3 days.

Assessment Activities	**Findings and Defining Characteristics**
Palpate skin.	Skin is warm and dry to touch
Observe patient's behaviour when talking and resting.	Breathing appears laboured; face is flushed
Measure vital signs.	Blood pressure: right arm, 116/62 mm Hg; left arm, 114/64 mm Hg
	Right radial pulse: 128 beats per minute, regular and bounding
	Respiratory rate regular at 26 breaths per minute
	SpO$_2$: 98% on room air
	Oral temperature: 39.2°C
Review medical history.	Smokes one pack of cigarettes per day and recently began expectorating yellow-green sputum
	Tired for past 3 days and dizzy upon rising in the morning

NURSING DIAGNOSIS: Hyperthermia related to infectious process

PLANNING

Patient Outcomes*	**Expected Outcomes**
Thermoregulation	
Patient will maintain core body temperatures within adaptive levels (less than 40°Celsius) in the next 24 hours.	Body temperature will decline at least 1°C within the next 8 hours.
Patient will remain free of dehydration in the next 24 hours.	Patient will verbalize increased satisfaction with rest and sleep pattern.
	Patient will verbalize signs and symptoms of dehydration and necessary fluid intake to prevent this.

*Patient outcomes from Ackley, B.J., Ladewig, G.B., Makic, M.B., et al. (2020). *Nursing diagnosis handbook: An evidence guide to planning care* (12th ed.). Elsevier.

INTERVENTIONS

Interventions (Nursing Interventions Classification)†	**Rationale**
	Fever Treatment
Instruct patient to reduce external coverings and keep clothing and bed linen dry.	Heat loss is promoted through conduction and convection.
Instruct patient to monitor temperature at home frequently and take acetaminophen every 4 hours as ordered for temperature higher than 38°C.	Antipyretics reduce set point.
Instruct patient to limit physical activity and increase frequency of rest periods over next 2 days.	Activity and stress increase metabolic rate, contributing to heat production.

†Intervention classification label from Bulechek, G.M., Butcher, H.K., McCloskey Dochterman, J.M., et al. (Eds.). (2018). *Nursing interventions classifications (NIC)* (7th ed.). Mosby.

EVALUATION

Nursing Actions	**Patient Response and Finding**	**Achievement of Outcome**
Obtain body temperature measurement.	Body temperature: 37.8°C	Body temperature is within normal limits.
Ask Mr. Coburn whether his energy level has changed since the last visit.	He responds, "I am sleeping much better and have returned to work with a lot more energy."	Rest and sleep pattern have improved, and energy level has increased.

---

interventions. Expected outcomes are established to gauge progress toward returning the body temperature to an acceptable range. Goals may be short term, such as regaining normal range of body temperature in 24 hours, or long term, such as helping the patient modify the environment (e.g., obtaining appropriate clothing to wear in cold weather). Outcomes must be related to what is learned about the patient.

Setting Priorities

The severity of temperature alteration and its effects, together with the patient's general health status, influence care priorities. Safety is a top priority. In many cases, other medical problems complicate the care plan. For instance, alterations in body temperature affect the body's requirements for fluids. Patients with cardiac disease may have difficulty tolerating required fluid replacement therapy.

Continuity of Care. Patients at high risk for alterations in body temperature require an individualized care plan directed at maintaining normothermia (normal body temperature) and reducing risk factors. For example, the outcome of care may be that the patient can explain actions to take during a heat wave. The nurse should teach the patient and caregiver the importance of thermoregulation and actions to take during very hot weather. Education is particularly important for parents who need to know how to take action at home when an infant or child develops temperature alteration.

Implementation

Health Promotion. Health promotion for patients at risk for altered body temperature is directed toward promoting balance between heat production and heat loss. Patient activity, temperature of the environment, and clothing are all considered. In the prevention of hyperthermia, nurses teach patients to avoid strenuous exercise in hot, humid weather; to drink fluids such as water or clear fruit juices before, during, and after exercise; to wear light, loose-fitting, light-coloured clothes; to avoid exercising in areas with poor ventilation; to wear a protective covering over the head when outdoors; and, when entering hot climates, to expose themselves to the heat gradually.

Prevention is key for patients at risk for hypothermia and involves educating not only patients but also their caregivers and friends. Patients most at risk are at the extremes of age—very young, very old—and people debilitated by trauma, spinal cord injury, stroke, diabetes, drug or alcohol intoxication, sepsis, and Raynaud's disease. Mentally ill and disabled patients may acquire hypothermia because they are unaware of the dangers of cold conditions. People without adequate home heating, shelter, diet, or clothing are also at risk. Fatigue, skin colour (dark-skinned patients are more susceptible), malnutrition, hypoxemia, and body piercing can contribute to the risk of frostbite.

Acute Care

Fever. When body temperature is elevated, it is important to initiate interventions to treat fever. The objective of therapy is to increase heat loss, reduce heat production, and prevent complications.

The procedures used to intervene and treat the temperature depend on the cause; any adverse effects; and the strength, intensity, and duration of the elevation. The nurse plays a key role in assessing and implementing temperature-reducing strategies (Box 31.8). The health care provider may try to determine the cause of the elevated temperature by isolating the causative pyrogen. Necessary culture specimens for laboratory analysis, such as urine, blood, sputum, and tissue from wound sites (see Chapter 34 for further information about infection control), may need to be obtained. After the cultures have been sent, the prescribing health care provider orders administration of antibiotic medications, to destroy pyrogenic bacteria and eliminate the cause of the elevated temperature.

In children, most fevers are caused by viruses, last only briefly, and have limited effects. Children still have immature temperature-control mechanisms so temperatures can rise rapidly. Dehydration and febrile seizures can occur while temperatures are rising in children between 6 months and 6 years of age. Febrile seizures are unusual in children older than 6 years. The actual temperature, often exceeding 38.8°C, seems to be more important than the rapidity of the temperature increase. Children are at particular risk for fluid volume deficit because they can quickly lose large amounts of fluids in proportion to their body weight. It is important to maintain accurate intake and output records and encourage fluid consumption.

A fever may also indicate a hypersensitivity response to a medication. Drug fevers can be accompanied by other symptoms of allergy, such as rash or pruritus. Treatment involves withdrawing the particular medication.

Antipyretics are medications that reduce fever. Nonsteroidals such as acetaminophen, salicylates, indomethacin, and ketorolac reduce fever by increasing heat loss. Corticosteroids reduce heat production by interfering with the immune system and can mask signs of infection. Corticosteroids are not used to treat a fever. However, it is important to be aware of their effect on suppressing the patient's ability to develop a fever in response to a pyrogen.

Nonpharmacological therapy for fever involves methods that increase heat loss by evaporation, conduction, convection, or radiation.

BOX 31.8 Nursing Measures for Patients With a Fever

Assessment
- Obtain core temperature during each phase of a febrile episode.
- Assess for contributing factors such as dehydration, infection, and environmental temperature.
- Identify physiological response to temperature.
- Measure all vital signs.
- Observe skin colour.
- Assess skin temperature.
- Observe for shivering and diaphoresis.
- Assess the patient's comfort and well-being.
- Determine phase of fever: chill, plateau, or fever break.

Interventions (Unless Contraindicated)
- Obtain blood cultures when ordered: Blood specimens are obtained to coincide with temperature spikes when the antigen-producing organism is most pervasive.
- Minimize heat production: Reduce frequency of activities that increase oxygen demand, such as excessive turning in bed; allow rest periods; and limit physical activity.
- Maximize heat loss: Reduce external covering on patient's body to promote heat loss through radiation and conduction without inducing shivering; keep clothing and bed linen dry to increase heat loss through conduction and convection.
- Meet requirements for increased metabolic rate: Provide oxygen as ordered to improve oxygen delivery to body cells; provide measures to stimulate appetite; offer well-balanced meals; provide fluids (3 L per day for patient with normal cardiac and renal function) to replace fluids lost through insensible water loss and sweating.
- Promote patient comfort: Encourage the patient to practise oral hygiene for dry oral mucous membranes; control environmental temperature without inducing shivering (between 21°C and 27°C).
- Identify febrile episode phases: Examine previous temperature measurements to identify trends.
- Initiate health teaching as indicated.

Blankets cooled by circulating water delivered by motorized units increase conductive heat loss. The manufacturer's instructions for applying these hypothermia blankets must be followed because of risk for skin breakdown and "freeze burns." Placing a bath blanket between the patient and the hypothermia blanket and wrapping distal extremities (fingers, toes, and genitalia) are recommended to reduce the risk of injury to the skin and tissue from hypothermia therapy. Traditional methods such as tepid sponge baths, bathing with alcohol water solutions, applying ice packs to axillae and groin areas, and cooling fans should be used cautiously because they lead to shivering. These methods have no demonstrated advantage over antipyretic medications. Nursing measures used to enhance body cooling must avoid stimulating shivering. Shivering is counterproductive and increases energy expenditure up to 400%. Wrapping the patient's extremities has been recommended to reduce the incidence and intensity of shivering.

Heatstroke. Heatstroke is an emergency. Treatment for heatstroke includes moving the patient to a cooler environment; reducing clothing covering the body; placing cool, wet towels over the skin; and using oscillating fans to increase convective heat loss. Emergency medical treatment may include intravenous fluids and irrigation of the stomach and lower bowel with cool solutions, in addition to use of cooling blankets.

Hypothermia. The priority of treatment for hypothermia is to prevent a further decrease in body temperature. Removing wet clothes and replacing with dry clothes and wrapping the patient in blankets are key interventions. In health care settings, forced-air warming blankets can actively rewarm hypothermic patients. Away from a health care setting, the patient should be laid under blankets next to a warm person. A conscious patient should drink hot liquids (e.g., soup) and avoid alcohol and caffeine. It is important to keep the patient's head covered, place the patient near a fire or in a warm room, or place heating pads next to areas of the patient's body (head and neck) that lose heat most rapidly.

Restorative and Continuing Care. A patient who has been febrile should be educated about the importance of taking and continuing antibiotics as directed until the course of treatment is completed. Children and older persons are at risk for fluid volume deficit because they can quickly lose large amounts of fluids in proportion to their body weight. Intake of preferred fluids should be encouraged.

◆ Evaluation

All nursing interventions are evaluated by comparing the patient's actual response with the expected outcomes of the care plan. This evaluation reveals whether goals of care have been met or whether the plan must be revised. After any intervention, the nurse should measure the patient's temperature to evaluate for change. Other evaluative measures such as palpation of the skin and assessment of pulse and respirations can be used. If therapies are effective, body temperature will return to an acceptable range, other vital sign measurements will stabilize, and the patient will report a sense of comfort.

PULSE

The pulse is the bounding of arterial blood flow that is palpable at various points on the body. Blood flows through the body in a continuous circuit. The pulse is an important indicator of the status of the circulatory system.

Physiology and Regulation

Pulse is the palpable high pressure created by blood that occurs as a result of alternate actions of expansion and recoil of an artery. Two elements contribute to the existence of pulse: 1) intermittent ejection of blood from the heart into the aorta that causes alternate increase and decrease of pressure in the artery, and 2) the ability of the arterial wall to stretch with each injection of blood, which is then followed by the recoil. As one of the most commonly performed physical assessments, palpation of pulse yields information about pulse rate, rhythm, strength, and equality that can be used to identify different types of pathology.

Pulse, commonly known as *heart rate,* is regulated by two branches of the autonomic nervous system: the sympathetic nervous system and parasympathetic nervous system. Stimulation of the sympathetic nervous system releases epinephrine and norepinephrine, which leads to an increase in heart rate, whereas stimulation of the parasympathetic nervous system releases acetylcholine, which leads to a decrease in heart rate.

Electrical impulses originating from the sinoatrial node travel through heart muscle to stimulate cardiac contraction. Approximately 60 to 70 mL of blood enters the aorta with each ventricular contraction (*stroke volume*). With each stroke volume ejection (blood pushed out of the heart), the walls of the aorta distend, creating a pulse wave that travels rapidly toward the distal ends of the arteries. When a pulse wave reaches a peripheral artery, it can be felt by palpating the artery lightly against underlying bone or muscle. The number of pulsing sensations occurring in 1 minute is the *pulse rate.*

The volume of blood pumped by the heart during 1 minute is the *cardiac output*: the product of heart rate and ventricular stroke volume. In an adult, the heart pumps about 5000 mL of blood per minute (e.g., if heart rate is 70 beats per minute and stroke volume is 70 mL, the cardiac output is 4900 mL per minute). A change in heart rate or stroke volume does not always change the heart's output or the amount of blood in the arteries. Mechanical, neural, and chemical factors regulate the strength of heart contractions and its stroke volume. When these factors are unable to alter stroke volume, the heart rate changes to subsequently adjust blood pressure. As heart rate increases, the heart has less time to fill. Without a change in stroke volume, blood pressure decreases. As the heart rate decreases, filling time is increased, and blood pressure increases. The inability of blood pressure to respond to increases or decreases in heart rate may indicate a health deviation and must be reported to the health care provider. An abnormally slow, rapid, or irregular pulse alters cardiac output. It is important to be able to assess the ability of the patient's heart to meet the demands of the body tissues for nutrients by palpating a peripheral pulse or by using a stethoscope to listen to heart sounds (apical rate).

Assessment of Pulse

All arteries have a pulse, but it is most easily felt at points where the vessel approaches the surface of the body. Although any artery can be assessed for pulse rate, the radial artery is commonly used because it is easily palpated. When a patient's condition suddenly worsens, the carotid artery is the recommended site for quickly finding a pulse. The heart will continue delivering blood through the carotid artery to the brain as long as possible. When cardiac output declines significantly, peripheral pulses weaken and are difficult to palpate. Nurses most commonly assess the radial and apical pulses in adult patients, but people who are learning to monitor their own heart rates use the radial or carotid pulse (e.g., athletes, patients taking medications for cardiac disease, and patients starting a prescribed exercise regimen). If the *radial pulse* at the wrist is abnormal or intermittent, or if it is inaccessible because of a dressing or cast, the apical pulse should be assessed. When a patient takes medication that affects the heart rate, the apical pulse provides a more accurate assessment of cardiac function. In infants or young children, it is best to assess the brachial or apical pulse because other peripheral pulses are deep and difficult to palpate accurately.

Assessment of other peripheral pulse sites, such as the popliteal or femoral, is unnecessary in routine measurement of vital signs. These alternative peripheral pulses are assessed during a complete physical examination, when surgery or treatment has impaired blood flow to a body part, or when a patient has clinical indications of impaired peripheral blood flow (see Chapter 33). Table 31.2 summarizes pulse sites and criteria for measurement. Skill 31.2 outlines heart rate assessment. Table 31.3 lists acceptable heart rate ranges.

Use of a Stethoscope. A stethoscope is used to assess the apical rate (Figure 31.7). The five major parts of the stethoscope are the earpieces, binaurals, tubing, bell chest piece, and diaphragm chest piece.

The plastic or rubber earpieces fit snugly and comfortably in the ears. The binaurals are angled and strong enough so that the earpieces stay firmly in the ears without causing discomfort. To ensure the best reception of sound, the earpieces follow the contour of the ear canal, pointing toward the face when the stethoscope is in place. Stethoscopes can have single or dual tubes. The tubing has thick walls and is flexible yet moderately rigid to eliminate transmission of environmental noise and to prevent the tubing from kinking. Tubing that is longer than 30 to 40 cm decreases the transmission of sound waves, making it more difficult to accurately auscultate sounds.

TABLE 31.2	Pulse Sites	
Site (Artery)	**Location**	**Use and Assessment Criteria**
Temporal	Over temporal bone of head, above and lateral to eye	Of significance in the diagnosis of temporal arteritis
Carotid	Along medial edge of sternocleidomastoid muscle in neck	During physiological shock or cardiac arrest, when other sites are not palpable
Apical	Fourth to fifth intercostal space at left midclavicular line	Auscultation is performed to obtain apical pulse
Brachial	Groove between biceps and triceps muscles at antecubital fossa	Provides status of circulation to lower arm; to auscultate blood pressure
Radial	Radial or thumb side of forearm at wrist	Common site to assess peripheral pulse and status of circulation to hand
Ulnar	Ulnar side of forearm at wrist	Assess status of circulation to hand; also to perform Allen's test (test for patency of radial artery)
Femoral	Below inguinal ligament, midway between symphysis pubis and anterior superior iliac spine	Appropriate location to assess pulse during physiological shock or cardiac arrest when other pulses are not palpable; to assess status of circulation to leg
Popliteal	Behind knee in popliteal fossa	Assess status of circulation to lower leg
Posterior tibial	Inner side of ankle, below medial malleolus	Assess status of circulation to foot
Dorsalis pedis	Along top of foot, between extension tendons of the great toe and next toe	Assess status of circulation to foot

SKILL 31.2   ASSESSING THE RADIAL AND APICAL PULSES

Delegation Considerations

The task of pulse measurement can be delegated to unregulated care providers (UCPs). The nurse is responsible for assessing changes in pulse; therefore, when the task of pulse measurement is delegated, it is important to *inform the UCP* about the following:

- Patient's history or risk for irregular pulse
- Frequency of pulse measurement in patient
- Patient's usual pulse values
- Abnormalities that should be reported to the health care provider

Equipment

- Stethoscope (for measurement of apical pulse only)
- Watch or clock with second hand or digital display
- Pen and either vital sign flow sheet or documentation record
- Alcohol swab

PROCEDURE

STEPS	RATIONALE
1. Identify patient using at least two person specifics (e.g., name and date of birth or name and medical record number) according to employer policy.	• Ensures correct patient. Complies with Accreditation Canada's standards and improves patient safety (Accreditation Canada, 2020).
2. Determine need to assess radial or apical pulse.	• Use clinical judgement to determine need for assessment.
A. Note risk factors for alterations in apical pulse.	• Certain conditions heighten risk for pulse alterations (e.g., cardiac disease, cardiac dysrhythmias, sudden chest pain or acute pain from any site, invasive cardiovascular diagnostic tests, surgery, sudden infusion of large volume of intravenous fluid, hemorrhage, administration of medications that alter cardiac function).
B. Assess for signs and symptoms of altered stroke volume and cardiac output, such as dyspnea, fatigue, chest pain, orthopnea, syncope, palpitations (unpleasant awareness of heartbeat), jugular venous distension, edema of dependent body parts, and cyanosis or pallor of skin.	• Physical signs and symptoms may indicate alteration in cardiac function.
3. Assess for factors that normally influence heart rate and rhythm: age, exercise, position changes, fluid balance, medications, temperature, sympathetic nervous system stimulation.	• These assessments enable you to accurately evaluate the presence and significance of pulse alterations. Acceptable range of heart rate changes with age (see Table 31.3).
4. Determine previous baseline apical rate (if available) from patient's record. Otherwise, note baseline radial rate.	• By comparing rates you can assess for change in the patient's condition and evaluate future apical pulse measurements.
5. Explain to patient that pulse or heart rate is to be assessed. If patient was active, wait 5–10 minutes before taking their pulse. Encourage patient to relax and not to speak.	• Activity and anxiety elevate heart rate. The patient's voice interferes with your ability to hear sound when you measure apical pulse. Measuring heart rates at rest allows for objective comparison of values.
6. Perform hand hygiene.	• Hand hygiene reduces transmission of microorganisms between the patient and the nurse.
7. If necessary, draw curtain around the patient's bed or close room door, or do both.	• These actions maintain the patient's privacy, minimize embarrassment, and promote comfort.

STEPS	RATIONALE

8. Obtain pulse measurement.

   A. Radial pulse

      (1) Assist patient to assume a supine or sitting position.

      (2) If patient is supine, place patient's forearm straight alongside their body, across the lower chest, or across the upper abdomen with wrist extended straight (see Step 8A[2] illustration). If patient is sitting, bend patient's elbow 90 degrees and support their lower arm on a chair or on your arm. Slightly flex patient's wrist with palm down (see Step 8A[3] illustration).

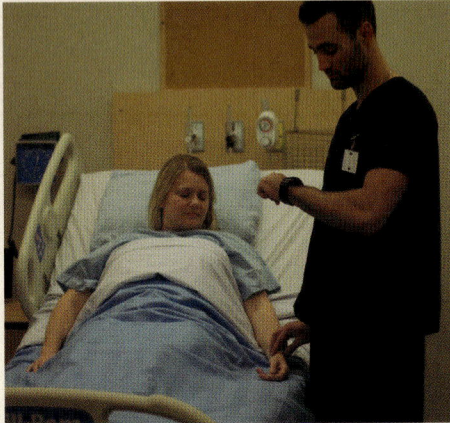

- These positions enable easy access to pulse sites.
- Relaxed position of lower arm and slight flexion of wrist promotes exposure of artery to palpation without restriction.

STEP 8A(2) Pulse check with patient's forearm at side with wrist extended. (Courtesy Barbara J. Astle, RN, PhD.)

STEP 8A(3) Hand placement for pulse checking radial pulse. (Courtesy Barbara J. Astle, RN, PhD.)

      (3) Place tips of your first two or middle three fingers over groove along radial or thumb side of patient's inner wrist (see Step 8A[3] illustration).

- Fingertips are the most sensitive parts of the hand to palpate arterial pulsation. The thumb has pulsations that may interfere with accuracy.

      (4) Lightly compress your fingertips against the patient's radius, obliterate pulse initially, and then relax pressure so that pulse becomes easily palpable.

- Pulse is more accurately assessed with moderate pressure. Too much pressure occludes pulse and impairs blood flow.

      (5) Determine strength of pulse. Note whether thrust of vessel against your fingertips is bounding (+4), strong (+3), weak (+2), thready (+1), or absent (0).

- Strength reflects volume of blood ejected against the arterial wall with each heart contraction. Accurate description of strength improves communication among health care providers, although keep in mind this is subjective data.

      (6) After you can feel a regular pulse, look at your watch and begin to count heart rate when the second hand reaches a number on the watch dial; start counting pulse with "one," then "two," and so on.

- You can determine heart rate accurately only after you can palpate the pulse. Count of "one" is the first beat palpated after you begin timing.

      (7) If pulse is regular, count rate for 30 seconds and multiply total by 2.

- A 30-second count is accurate for rapid, slow, or regular heart rates.

      (8) If pulse is irregular, count rate for 1 minute (60 seconds). Assess frequency and pattern of irregularity. Compare bilateral radial pulses.

- Inefficient contraction of the heart fails to transmit pulse wave, interfering with cardiac output, resulting in irregular pulse. Longer measurement time ensures accurate count.

CRITICAL DECISION POINT: *If pulse is irregular, assess apical or radial pulse to detect a pulse deficit. Count apical heart rate while a colleague counts radial heart rate. Begin apical pulse count out loud to simultaneously assess pulses. If pulse count differs by more than two, a pulse deficit exists; this can indicate altered cardiac output.*

   B. Apical pulse

      (1) Perform hand hygiene; clean earpieces and diaphragm of stethoscope with alcohol swab.

- These actions reduce transmission of microorganisms between patients and when stethoscopes are shared.

      (2) Draw curtain around the patient's bed or close room door, or do both.

- These actions maintain patient's privacy, minimize embarrassment, and promote comfort.

      (3) Assist patient to supine or sitting position. Move aside bed linen and gown to expose sternum and left side of chest.

- Expose portion of patient's chest wall to select auscultatory site.

Continued

SKILL 31.2   ASSESSING THE RADIAL AND APICAL PULSES—cont'd

STEPS	RATIONALE

(4) Locate anatomical landmarks to identify the *point of maximal impulse* (PMI), also called the *apical impulse* (see Steps 8B[4][a]–8B[4][d]; illustrations). The heart is located behind and to the left of the sternum with base at top and apex at bottom. Find angle of Louis just below the suprasternal notch between the sternal body and manubrium; it can be palpated as a bony prominence (see Step 8B[4][a] illustration). Slip your fingers down each side of angle to find second intercostal space (ICS; see Step 8B[4][b] illustration). Carefully move fingers down left side of sternum to fifth ICS (see Step 8B[4][c] illustration) and laterally to the left midclavicular line (MCL; see Step 8B[4][d] illustration). A light tap felt in an area within 1 to 2 cm of the PMI is reflected from the apex of the heart.

- Use of anatomical landmarks allows correct placement of stethoscope over apex of the heart, enhancing ability to hear heart sounds clearly. In a patient with large breasts, ask the patient to move the breast aside so that you can access the PMI site. If you are unable to palpate the PMI, reposition patient on their left side. In the presence of severe cardiac disease, the PMI may be located to the left of the MCL or at the sixth ICS.

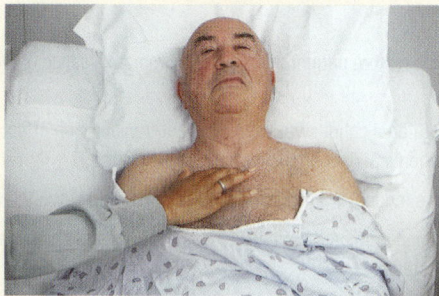

STEP 8B(4)(a) Locating the angle of Louis.

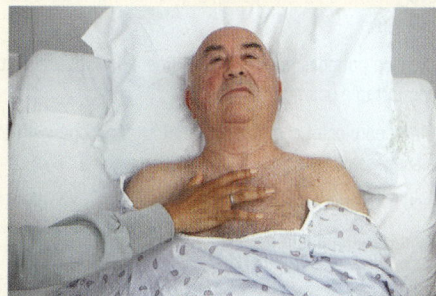

STEP 8B(4)(b) Locating the second intercostal space.

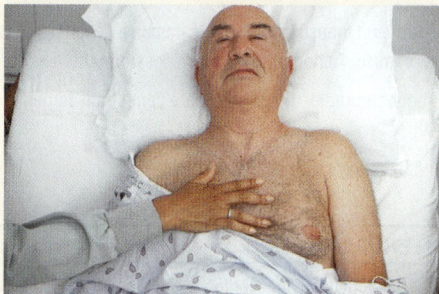

STEP 8B(4)(c) Locating the fifth intercostal space.

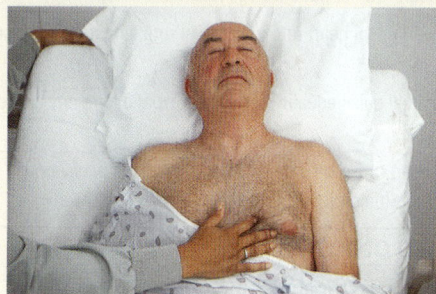

STEP 8B(4)(d) Identifying the midclavicular line.

(5) Place diaphragm of stethoscope in palm of your hand for 5–10 seconds.

- By warming metal or plastic diaphragm, you avoid startling patient and promote patient's comfort.

(6) Place diaphragm of stethoscope over PMI at the fifth ICS, at left MCL, and auscultate for normal S_1 and S_2 heart sounds (heard as "lub-dub" see Step 8B[6] illustrations).

- Allow stethoscope tubing to extend straight without kinks that would distort sound transmission. Normally, S_1 and S_2 heart sounds are high-pitched and best heard with the diaphragm.

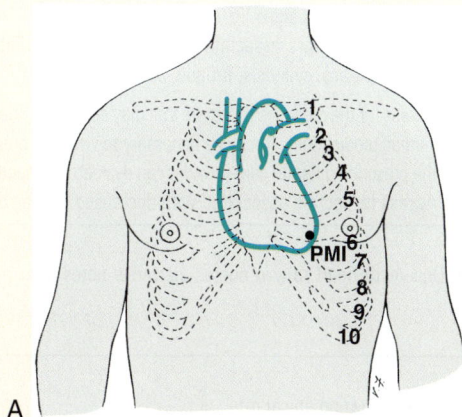

STEP 8B(6) A, Location of point of maximal impulse (PMI) in adult. **B,** Stethoscope placement over PMI.

SKILL 31.2	ASSESSING THE RADIAL AND APICAL PULSES—cont'd
STEPS	**RATIONALE**

STEPS	RATIONALE
(7) When S₁ and S₂ are heard with regularity, look at your watch and begin to count rate: when second hand reaches a number on the watch dial, start counting with "one," then "two," and so on.	• You can accurately determine apical rate only after you can auscultate sounds clearly. Count of "one" is first sound auscultated after timing begins.
(8) If apical rate is regular, count for 30 seconds and multiply by 2.	• Regular apical rate can be assessed within 30 seconds.

CRITICAL DECISION POINT: *If heart rate is irregular or if patient is receiving cardiac medication, count for 1 minute (60 seconds). An irregular heart rate is more accurately assessed when measured over a longer interval.*

STEPS	RATIONALE
(9) If heart rate is irregular, or patient is receiving certain cardiovascular medications, for example, digoxin, count for a full 1 minute (60 seconds) and describe pattern of irregularity (S₁ and S₂ occurring early or later after previous sequence of sounds; e.g., every third or every fourth beat is skipped). Digoxin is held if the apical rate is less than 60.	• Regular occurrence of dysrhythmia within 1 minute may indicate inefficient contraction of heart and alteration in cardiac output.
(10) Replace patient's gown and bed linen; assist patient to return to a comfortable position.	• These actions restore patient's comfort and promote a sense of well-being.
(11) Clean earpieces and diaphragm of stethoscope with alcohol swab as necessary.	• Cleaning with an alcohol swab helps prevent transmission of microorganisms between patients and when the stethoscope is shared.
9. Perform hand hygiene.	• Hand hygiene reduces transmission of microorganisms between patients.
10. Discuss findings with patient as needed.	• Such discussion promotes patient's participation in care and understanding of their health status.
11. Compare current readings with previous baseline measurement or acceptable range of heart rate for patient's age (see Table 31.3).	• Evaluate for change in condition and alterations.
12. Compare peripheral heart rate with apical rate, and note any discrepancy.	• Differences between measurements indicate pulse deficit and possibly cardiovascular compromise. Abnormalities may necessitate therapy.
13. Compare radial pulse equality between arms and note any discrepancy.	• Differences between radial arteries indicate compromised peripheral vascular system.
14. Correlate heart rate with data obtained from blood pressure and related signs and symptoms (palpitations, dizziness).	• Heart rate and blood pressure are interrelated.

UNEXPECTED OUTCOMES	RELATED INTERVENTIONS
Radial pulse is weak or thready	• Assess both radial pulses and compare findings. Local obstruction to one extremity (e.g., clot, edema) may decrease peripheral blood flow. • Perform complete assessment of all pulses (see Chapter 33). • Observe for symptoms associated with decreased tissue perfusion, such as pallor and cool skin temperature of tissue distal to the weak pulse. • Measure apical and radial pulse simultaneously to determine presence of pulse deficit.
Apical pulse is greater than 100 beats per minute (tachycardia)	• Assess for presence of fever, anxiety, pain, recent exercise, hypotension, decreased oxygenation, or dehydration, all of which can elevate pulse. • Measure all vital signs. • Assess for factors associated with decreased cardiac output, such as chest pain, dizziness, cyanosis, fatigue, and orthopnea.
Apical pulse is less than 60 beats per minute (bradycardia)	• Assess for the presence of factors that may alter heart rate, such as digoxin or other cardiac medications. It may be necessary to withhold prescribed medications until the prescribing health care provider can evaluate the need to adjust dosage. • Assess for factors associated with decreased cardiac output.

RECORDING AND REPORTING
• Record heart rate with assessment site in nurses' notes or vital signs flow sheet. Document heart rate in nurses' narrative notes after administration of specific therapies.
• *Report abnormal findings* to nurse in charge or health care provider.

CARE IN THE COMMUNITY CONSIDERATIONS
• Assess home environment to determine which room will afford a quiet environment for auscultating apical rate.

TABLE 31.3	Normal Heart Rates Across Age Groups
Age	Heart Rate (Beats per Minute)
0–28 days	104–162
1–3 months	104–162
4–11 months	109–159
1–3 years	89–139
4–6 years	71–128
7–11 years	60–114
>12 years	50–104

From Child Health BC. (2018). *BC PEWS vital sign, assessment & documentation guidelines.* https://www.childhealthbc.ca/sites/default/files/bc_pews_vital_sign_assessment_and_documentation_guidelines_1.pdf

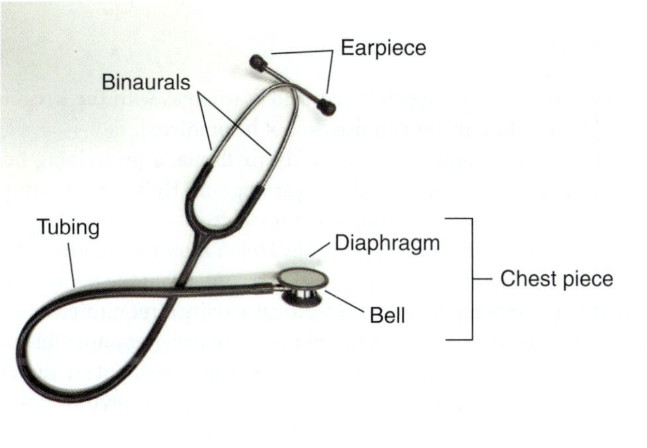

FIGURE 31.7 Parts of a stethoscope. (Image courtesy of Mi-Yeon Kim, RN, PhD.)

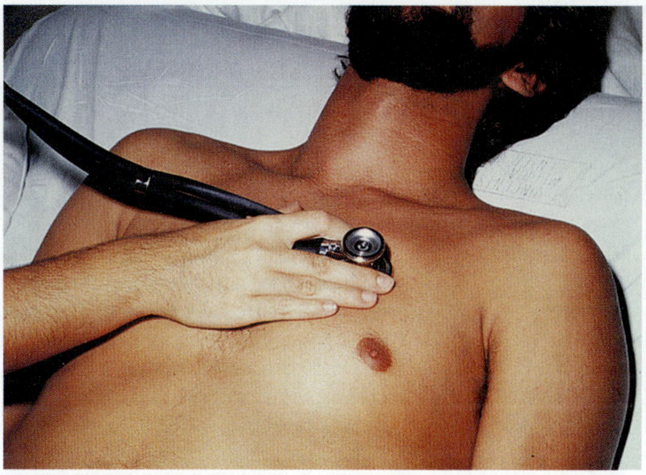

FIGURE 31.8 Positioning the diaphragm of the stethoscope firmly and securely when high-pitched heart sounds are auscultated.

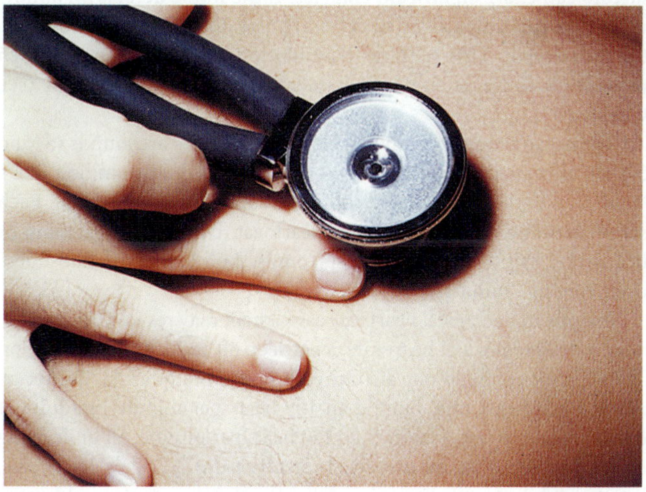

FIGURE 31.9 Positioning the bell of the stethoscope lightly on the skin to hear low-pitched heart sounds.

The chest piece consists of a bell and a diaphragm that are typically rotated from one to the other into position. The diaphragm or bell must be in proper position to hear sounds through the stethoscope. The position of the chest piece can be tested by tapping lightly on the diaphragm to determine which side is functioning. The diaphragm is the circular, flat portion of the chest piece and is covered by a thin plastic disk. It transmits high-pitched sounds created by the high-velocity movement of air and blood. Lung, heart, and bowel sounds are best auscultated by using the diaphragm. The diaphragm is positioned to make a tight seal against the patient's skin (Figure 31.8).

The bell is the bowl-shaped chest piece usually surrounded by a rubber ring. The ring prevents chilling the patient with cold metal when the chest piece is placed on the skin. The bell transmits low-pitched sounds created by the low-velocity movement of blood. Heart and vascular sounds are auscultated through the bell. The nurse should apply the bell lightly, resting the chest piece on the patient's skin (Figure 31.9). Compressing the bell against the skin reduces low-pitched sound amplification and creates a "diaphragm of skin." Some stethoscopes have just one chest piece that combines the features of the bell and diaphragm. With the use of light pressure, the chest piece acts as a bell; with more pressure, it acts as a diaphragm.

The stethoscope is a delicate instrument and requires proper care for optimal function. The earpieces should be removed regularly and cleaned (to remove cerumen) according to the manufacturer's instructions. The bell and diaphragm need to be cleaned (to remove dust, lint, and body oils) routinely with alcohol to help prevent transmission of microorganisms. The tubing can be cleaned with mild soap and water. Nurses are encouraged to have their own stethoscope. If several nurses use the same stethoscope, the earpieces should be cleansed with an antiseptic prior to each use.

Character of the Pulse

Assessment of the radial pulse includes measurement of the rate, rhythm, strength, and bilateral equality. When auscultating an apical pulse, the nurse assesses rate and rhythm only.

Rate. Before measuring a pulse, the patient's baseline rate should be reviewed for comparison (see Table 31.3). Some practitioners make baseline measurements of the heart rate with the patient sitting, standing, and lying. Changes in posture cause changes in heart rate because of alterations in blood volume and sympathetic nervous system activity. The heart rate temporarily increases when a person changes from a lying to a sitting or standing position.

It is important to always consider the variety of factors influencing the heart rate (Table 31.4). A single factor or a combination of

TABLE 31.4	Factors Influencing Heart Rates	
Factor	**Increases Heart Rate**	**Decreases Heart Rate**
Exercise	Short-term exercise	Long-term exercise, which conditions the heart and results in a lower resting pulse and a quicker return to resting level after exercise
Temperature	Fever and heat	Hypothermia
Emotions	Anxiety increases sympathetic stimulation, affecting heart rate	Relaxation
Pain	Acute pain, which increases sympathetic stimulation and thereby increases heart rate; the effect of chronic pain on heart rate varies	Unrelieved severe pain, which increases parasympathetic stimulation and thereby affects heart rate
Medications	Positive chronotropic medications such as epinephrine. Cholinergic blocking agents (anticholinergics), such as atropine	Negative chronotropic medications such as digitalis, β-adrenergic blockers, and calcium channel blockers
Hemorrhage	Loss of blood increases sympathetic stimulation	
Postural changes	Standing up from a sitting position	Lying down
Pulmonary conditions	Diseases causing poor oxygenation, such as asthma and chronic obstructive pulmonary disease (COPD)	

factors can cause significant changes. If the nurse detects an abnormal rate while palpating a peripheral pulse, the next step is to assess the apical rate. This requires auscultation of heart sounds, which provides a more accurate assessment of cardiac contraction (see Chapter 33).

The nurse should identify the first and second heart sounds (S_1 and S_2). At normal slow rates, S_1 is low-pitched and dull, sounding like a "lub." S_2 is higher pitched and shorter, creating the sound "dub." Each set of "lub-dub" is counted as one heartbeat. Using the diaphragm or bell of the stethoscope, the nurse counts the number of "lub-dubs" occurring in 1 minute.

Peripheral and apical heart rate assessment may reveal variations in heart rate. The normal heart rate is between 60 and 100. Two common abnormalities in heart rate are tachycardia and bradycardia. *Tachycardia* is a fast heart rate, more than 100 beats per minute in adults. If the heart rate at rest is faster than 120 beats per minute, an underlying health problem may be suspected. *Bradycardia* is a slow heart rate, less than 60 beats per minute in adults. The slow heart rate could occur from heart block or the use of medications such as β-blockers. Often, the slow resting heart rate can be observed in athletes.

An inefficient contraction of the heart that fails to transmit a pulse wave to the peripheral pulse site creates a *pulse deficit*. Two people are required to detect a pulse deficit—one to assess either the radial or apical rate, and the second to simultaneously assess the other rate. Then the two rates are compared. The difference between the apical and radial pulse rates is the pulse deficit. For example, if the apical rate is 92 beats per minute and the radial rate is 78 beats per minute, the pulse deficit is 14 beats per minute. Pulse deficits are frequently associated with abnormal rhythms.

Rhythm. Normally, a regular interval occurs between each pulse or heartbeat. In other words, the pulse should be regular under the normal circumstance. An interval interrupted by an early or late beat or a missed beat indicates an abnormal rhythm, or *dysrhythmia*. Dysrhythmia threatens the heart's ability to provide adequate cardiac output, particularly if it occurs repetitively. Dysrhythmia is identified by palpating an interruption in successive pulse waves or auscultating an interruption between heart sounds. If dysrhythmia is present, the nurse should assess the regularity of its occurrence and auscultate the apical rate for one full minute (see Chapter 33 for further information about conducting a health assessment). Dysrhythmias are described as "regularly irregular" or "irregularly irregular." With the regularly irregular

rhythm, the next pulse can be predicted, whereas with the irregularly irregular rhythm, the next pulse cannot be predicted.

To document and investigate a dysrhythmia, a prescribing health care provider may order an electrocardiogram, Holter monitoring, or telemetry. In an electrocardiogram, the electrical activity of the heart is recorded for a 12-second interval. The Holter monitor records 24 hours of electrical activity in a small portable recorder that the patient wears. In cardiac telemetry, the heart's electrical activity is monitored continuously, and the data are transmitted to a stationary monitor. Telemetry enables observation of heart rhythm during all the patient's daily activities and thus allows for immediate treatment if the rhythm becomes erratic or the patient's condition becomes unstable.

Strength. The strength of a pulse reflects both the volume of blood ejected against the arterial wall with each heart contraction and the condition of the arterial vascular system leading to the pulse site. The simplest way to describe pulses is absent, present, and bounding. One of the common approaches to express the strength of pulses is by using a grading scale of 0 to 4: absent (0), diminished (1+), normal (2+), moderate increased (3+), and markedly increased (4+). It is included during assessment of the vascular system (see Chapter 33 for further information about conducting a health assessment).

Equality. Pulses on both sides of the body should be assessed to compare their characteristics. A pulse in one extremity may be unequal to the pulse in the other extremity in strength, or it may be absent in many disease states (e.g., thrombus [clot] formation). All symmetrical pulses can be assessed simultaneously except for the carotid pulses, which should never be measured simultaneously because excessive pressure may occlude blood supply to the brain or trigger carotid reflexes that may result in altered cardiac output.

❖ NURSING PROCESS AND PULSE DETERMINATION

Pulse assessment helps to determine the general state of cardiovascular health and the body's response to other system imbalances. Tachycardia, bradycardia, and dysrhythmia are defining characteristics of many nursing diagnoses, including the following:

- *Activity intolerance*
- *Anxiety*
- *Decreased cardiac output*
- *Deficient/excess fluid volume*

- *Impaired gas exchange*
- *Hyperthermia*
- *Hypothermia*
- *Acute pain*
- *Ineffective tissue perfusion*

The nursing care plan includes interventions specific for the nursing diagnosis identified and its related factors. For example, the defining characteristics of an abnormal heart rate, exertional dyspnea, and a patient's verbal report of fatigue lead to a diagnosis of *activity intolerance*. When the related factor is "inactivity after a prolonged illness," interventions focus on increasing the patient's daily exercises. Patient outcomes are evaluated by assessing the heart rate, rhythm, strength, and equality after each intervention.

RESPIRATION

Human survival depends on the ability of oxygen (O_2) to reach body cells and of carbon dioxide (CO_2) to be removed from the cells. *Respiration* is the mechanism that the body uses to exchange gases between the atmosphere and the blood and between the blood and the cells. Respiration involves *ventilation* (the movement of gases in and out of the lungs), *diffusion* (the movement of oxygen and carbon dioxide between the alveoli and the red blood cells), and *perfusion* (the distribution of red blood cells to and from the pulmonary capillaries). To analyze respiratory efficiency, assessment data must be integrated from all three processes. Ventilation is assessed by determining respiratory rate, respiratory depth, and respiratory rhythm. Diffusion and perfusion are assessed by determining oxygen saturation.

Physiological Control

Breathing is generally a passive process; a person thinks little about it. The respiratory centre in the brainstem regulates the involuntary control of respirations. Adults normally breathe in a smooth, uninterrupted pattern, 12 to 20 times a minute.

Ventilation is regulated by levels of CO_2, O_2, and hydrogen ion concentration (pH) in the arterial blood. The most important factor is the level of CO_2 in the arterial blood. An elevation in the CO_2 level causes the respiratory control system in the brain to increase the rate and depth of breathing. The increased ventilatory effort removes excess CO_2 (which is the state of hypercarbia) by increasing exhalation. However, patients with chronic lung disease have ongoing hypercarbia. For them, chemoreceptors in the carotid artery and aorta become sensitive to *hypoxemia*, or low levels of arterial O_2. If arterial O_2 levels fall, these receptors signal the brain to increase the rate and depth of ventilation. Hypoxemia helps control ventilation in patients with chronic lung disease. Because low levels of arterial O_2 provide the stimulus that allows the patient to breathe, administration of high oxygen levels can be dangerous for these patients.

Mechanics of Breathing

Although breathing is normally passive, muscular work is involved in moving the lungs and chest wall. Inspiration is an active process. During inspiration, the respiratory centre sends impulses along the phrenic nerve, causing the diaphragm to contract. Abdominal organs move downward and forward, increasing the length of the chest cavity to move air into the lungs. The diaphragm moves approximately 1 cm, and the ribs retract upward from the body's midline approximately 1.2 to 2.5 cm. During a normal, relaxed breath, a person inhales 500 mL of air. This amount is referred to as the *tidal volume*. During expiration, the diaphragm relaxes and the abdominal organs return to their original positions. The lung and chest wall return to a relaxed position (Figure 31.10). In contrast to inhalation, expiration is a passive process.

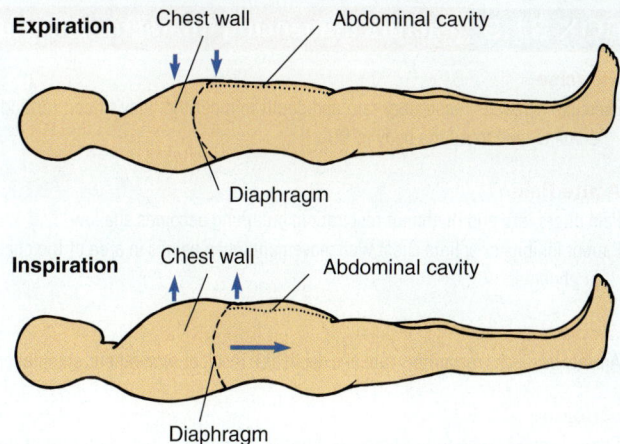

FIGURE 31.10 Illustration of diaphragmatic and chest wall movement during inspiration and expiration.

The normal rate and depth of ventilation, *eupnea*, is interrupted by sighing. The *sigh*, a prolonged deeper breath, is a protective physiological mechanism for expanding small airways and alveoli not ventilated during a normal breath.

The accurate assessment of respiration depends on the recognition of normal thoracic and abdominal movements. During quiet breathing, the chest wall gently rises and falls. Contraction of the accessory muscles of breathing (i.e., the intercostal muscles between the ribs and the muscles in the neck and shoulders) is not visible. During normal quiet breathing, diaphragmatic movement causes the abdominal cavity to rise and fall slowly.

Assessment of Ventilation

Special equipment is not needed to measure respirations, but measurement must not be haphazard. Accurate measurement requires observation and palpation of chest wall movement.

A sudden change in the character of respirations is important to note. Because respiration is tied to the function of numerous body systems, all variables need to be considered when changes occur (Box 31.9). For example, abdominal trauma may injure the phrenic nerve, which is responsible for diaphragmatic contraction. The extent of the injury and the implications for the respiratory system are important to understand.

In a nursing assessment, you should try to not let the patient know that you are assessing their respiration. A patient aware of your intentions may consciously alter the rate and depth of breathing. The best time to measure respiration is immediately after measuring the pulse while your hand remains on the patient's wrist as it rests over the chest or abdomen. When assessing, keep in mind the patient's usual ventilatory rate and pattern, the influence any disease or illness has on respiratory function, the relationship between respiratory and cardiovascular function, and the influence of therapies on respiration. The objective measurements in assessing respiratory status include the rate and depth of breathing and the rhythm of ventilatory movements (Skill 31.3).

Respiratory Rate. The nurse should observe both inspiration and expiration when counting ventilation or respiration rate. The respiratory rate varies with age (Table 31.5) and usually decreases with age.

An *apnea monitor* is a respiratory monitoring device that aids in respiratory assessment. Leads that sense movement are attached to the patient's chest wall. Absence of chest wall movement triggers the apnea

BOX 31.9   Factors Influencing Character of Respiration

Exercise

Exercise increases respiratory rate and depth to meet the body's need for additional O_2 and to rid the body of CO_2.

Acute Pain

Pain alters rate and rhythm of respiration; breathing becomes shallow.

Patient inhibits or splints chest wall movement when pain is in area of the chest or abdomen.

Anxiety

Anxiety increases respiratory rate and depth as a result of sympathetic stimulation.

Smoking

Chronic smoking changes pulmonary airways, resulting in increased rate of respirations at rest when the person is not smoking.

Body Position

A straight, erect posture promotes full chest expansion.

A stooped or slumped position impairs ventilatory movement.

Lying flat prevents full chest expansion.

Medications

Opioids, general anaesthetics, and sedative hypnotics depress respiratory rate and depth.

Amphetamines and cocaine may increase respiratory rate and depth.

Bronchodilators slow respiratory rate by causing airway dilation.

Neurological Injury

Injury to the brainstem impairs the respiratory centre and alters respiratory rate and rhythm.

Hemoglobin Function

In the state of anemia, decreased hemoglobin levels reduce O_2-carrying capacity of the blood, which results in increases in respiratory rate.

Increased altitude lowers the amount of saturated hemoglobin, which increases respiratory rate and depth.

Abnormalities in blood cell function (e.g., sickle cell disease) reduce ability of red blood cells to carry oxygen, which results in increases in respiratory rate and depth.

SKILL 31.3   ASSESSING RESPIRATIONS

Delegation Considerations

The task of measuring respiration can be delegated to unregulated care providers (UCPs). The nurse is responsible for assessing for change in respiration rate, rhythm, and depth; therefore, when the task of measuring respiration is delegated, it is important to *inform the UCP* about the following:

- The patient's history or risk for abnormal respiratory status
- The frequency of respiration measurement for a specific patient
- Abnormalities that should be reported to the health care provider

Equipment

- Watch with a second hand or digital display
- Pen and either vital sign flow sheet or record form

PROCEDURE

STEPS	RATIONALE
1. Identify patient using at least two person specifics (e.g., name and date of birth or name and medical record number) according to employer policy.	• Ensures correct patient. Complies with Accreditation Canada's standards and improves patient safety (Accreditation Canada, 2020).
2. Determine need to assess patient's respiration.	• Use clinical judgement to determine need for assessment.
A. Note presence of risk factors for respiratory alterations.	• Conditions that heighten risk for alterations in ventilation—detected by changes in respiratory rate, depth, and rhythm—include fever, pain, anxiety, diseases of chest muscles, constrictive chest or abdominal dressings, gastric distension, chronic pulmonary diseases, traumatic chest injury, presence of a chest tube, respiratory infection, pulmonary edema and emboli, anemia, and head injury with damage to the brainstem.
B. Assess for signs and symptoms of respiratory alterations, such as bluish (cyanotic) appearance of nail beds, lips, mucous membranes, and skin; restlessness, irritability, confusion, and reduced level of consciousness; pain during inspiration; laboured or difficult breathing; adventitious breath sounds (see Chapter 33 for further information about conducting a health assessment), inability to breathe spontaneously; thick, frothy, blood-tinged, or copious sputum produced on coughing.	• Physical signs and symptoms indicate alterations in respiratory status related to ventilation.
3. Assess pertinent laboratory values.	

A. **Arterial blood gases** (normal values may vary slightly between institutions):
    pH: 7.35–7.45 mm Hg
    PaCO2: 35–45 mm Hg
    PaO$_2$: 80–100 mm Hg
    HCO$_3$: 22–26 mEq/L
    SaO$_2$: 95–100%
	• Arterial blood gases measure arterial blood pH, partial pressure of O_2 (PaO_2) and CO_2 (PaCO_2), and arterial O_2 saturation (SaO_2), which reflects patient's oxygenation status.

Continued

SKILL 31.3   ASSESSING RESPIRATIONS—cont'd

STEPS	RATIONALE
B. Pulse oximetry (SpO₂): Normal levels are 95–100%; 85–89% may be acceptable for certain chronic disease conditions: less then 85% is abnormal (see Skill 31.4).	• Although 95% is considered normal, 90% can be considered acceptable in patients with disorders such as sleep apnea. SpO_2 less than 85% is often accompanied by changes in respiratory rate, depth, and rhythm.
C. Specific tests of the complete blood cell count (CBC): (normal values for adults may vary between institutions and references consulted): *Hemoglobin:* 140–180 g/L in patients with male genitalia; 120–160 g/L in patients with female genitalia *Hematocrit:* 0.42–0.54 in patients with male genitalia; 0.37–0.47 in patients with female genitalia *Red blood cell count:* $4.7–6.2 \times 10^{12}$/L in male patients; $4.2–5.4 \times 10^{12}$/L in patients with female genitalia (Pike-MacDonald et al., 2019).	• Hemoglobin, hematocrit, and red blood cell count (three of several CBC tests) measure the concentration of hemoglobin volume of red blood cells, and red blood cell count, all of which reflect the patient's capacity to carry O_2.
4. Determine previous baseline respiratory rate (if available) from patient's record.	• This enables nurses to assess for changes in the patient's condition and provides comparison with future respiratory measurements.
5. Perform hand hygiene.	• Hand hygiene reduces transmission of microorganisms between the patient and the nurse.
6. Draw curtain around the patient's bed or close room door, or do both.	• Drawing the curtain and closing the room door maintains patient's privacy, minimizes embarrassment, and promotes comfort.

CRITICAL DECISION POINT: *Patients with difficulty breathing (dyspnea), such as those with heart failure, with abdominal ascites, or in late stages of pregnancy, should be assessed in the position of greatest comfort. Repositioning may increase the work of breathing, which increases respiratory rate.*

---

7. Ensure patient is in a comfortable position, preferably sitting or lying with the head of the bed elevated 45 to 60 degrees. Move bed linen or gown to be sure patient's chest is visible.	• Sitting erect promotes full ventilatory movement. A clear view of the chest wall and abdominal movements is needed for assessment.
8. Place patient's arm in a relaxed position across their abdomen or lower chest, or place your hand directly over the patient's upper abdomen (see Step 8 illustration).	• A similar position used during pulse assessment allows you to assess respiratory rate inconspicuously. The patient's hand or your hand rises and falls during respiratory cycle.

STEP 8 Nurse's hand over patient's abdomen to check respiration. (Courtesy Ouni Liao.)

9. Observe complete respiratory cycle (one inspiration and one expiration).	• You can determine rate accurately only after you have viewed the patient's respiratory cycle.
10. After observing the cycle, look at the watch's second hand. When the second hand reaches a number on the watch dial, begin counting respiratory cycles, starting with "one" for the first full cycle, then "two," and so on.	• Timing begins with count of one. Respirations occur more slowly than pulse.
11. If rhythm is regular, count number of respiratory cycles in 30 seconds and multiply by 2. If rhythm is irregular, slower than 12 per minute, or faster than 20 per minute, count for 1 full minute.	• Respiratory rate is equivalent to number of respiratory cycles per minute. Suspected irregularities necessitate assessment for at least 1 minute.

Continued

SKILL 31.3 ASSESSING RESPIRATIONS—cont'd

STEPS	RATIONALE
12. Note depth of respirations, which you subjectively assess by observing the degree of chest wall movement while counting respiratory rate. You can also objectively assess respiratory depth by palpating the patient's chest wall excursion or auscultating the posterior thorax after respiratory rate has been counted (see Chapter 33). Depth is described as "shallow," "normal," or "deep."	• Character of ventilatory movement may reveal specific disease state restricting volume of air from moving into and out of the lungs.
13. Note rhythm of ventilatory cycle. Normal breathing is regular and uninterrupted. Sighing should not be confused with abnormal rhythm.	• Character of ventilations can reveal specific types of alterations. Without being aware of it, people periodically take single deep breaths or sigh to expand small airways prone to collapse.

CRITICAL DECISION POINT: *Any irregular respiratory pattern or period of apnea (the cessation of respiration for several seconds) in an adult is a symptom of underlying disease and must be reported to the health care provider or nurse in charge. Further assessment may be required (see Chapter 33), and immediate intervention may be needed. An irregular respiratory rate and short apneic spells are normal only in newborns.*

STEPS	RATIONALE
14. Move back bed linen and patient's gown.	• This action restores patient's comfort and promotes sense of well-being.
15. Perform hand hygiene.	• Hand hygiene reduces transmission of microorganisms between patients.
16. Discuss findings with patient as needed.	• Such discussion promotes patient's participation in care and understanding of their health status.
17. If patient's respiration is assessed for the first time, document rate, rhythm, and depth as baseline values.	• These data are used for comparing data from future respiratory assessments.
18. Compare respiration data with patient's previous baseline values and with normal values for rate, rhythm, and depth.	• These data allow you to assess for changes in patient's condition and for presence of respiratory alterations.

UNEXPECTED OUTCOMES	RELATED INTERVENTIONS
Patient's respiratory rate is less than 12 (bradypnea) or more than 20 (tachypnea) breaths per minute, depth is increased or decreased, rhythm is irregular, or patient feels "short of breath"	• Observe for related factors, including obstructed airway, abnormal breath sounds, productive cough, restlessness, irritability, anxiety, and confusion. • Position patient in a supported sitting position (semi-Fowler's or high Fowler's), unless contraindicated. • Provide oxygen as ordered. • When possible, remove respiratory irritants from the environment, such as second-hand smoke and perfumes.

RECORDING AND REPORTING
- Record respiratory rate and character in nurses' notes or vital sign flow sheet. Indicate type and amount of oxygen therapy if it was used by the patient during assessment. Document respiratory rate in nurses' narrative notes after administration of specific therapies.
- Report abnormal findings to nurse in charge or to health care provider.

CARE IN THE COMMUNITY CONSIDERATIONS
- Assess for environmental factors in the home that may influence patient's respiration, such as second-hand smoke, poor ventilation, or gas fumes.

TABLE 31.5	Acceptable Ranges of Respiratory Rates by Age
Age	**Rate (Breaths per Minute)**
Premature	40–70
0–3 months	35–55
3–6 months	30–45
6–12 months	22–38
1–3 years	22–30
3–6 years	20–24
6–12 years	16–22
Greater than 12 years	12–20
Adult	12–20

Data from United Medical Education. (2021). *PALS algorithms 2020 (pediatric advanced life support)*. https://www.acls-pals-bls.com/algorithms/pals/

alarm. Apnea monitoring is used frequently with infants in hospitals and at home to observe for prolonged apneic events.

Ventilatory Depth. Depth of respiration is assessed by observing the degree of excursion or movement in the patient's chest wall. Ventilatory movements can be described as "deep," "normal," or "shallow." A deep respiration involves full expansion of the lungs with full exhalation. Respirations are shallow when only a small quantity of air passes through the lungs and ventilatory movement is difficult to see. Objective techniques are used if chest excursion is unusually shallow (see Chapter 33). Table 31.6 summarizes breathing pattern alterations.

Ventilatory Rhythm. Breathing pattern can be determined by observing the chest or the abdomen. Diaphragmatic breathing results from the contraction and relaxation of the diaphragm and is best observed by

TABLE 31.6 Alterations in Breathing Pattern

Alteration	Description
Bradypnea	Rate of breathing is regular but abnormally slow (<12 breaths per minute).
Tachypnea	Rate of breathing is regular but abnormally rapid (>20 breaths per minute).
Hyperpnea	Respirations are laboured, increased in depth, and increased in rate (>20 breaths per minute). This occurs normally during exercise.
Apnea	Respirations cease for several seconds and then resume. Persistent cessation results in respiratory arrest.
Hyperventilation	Rate and depth of respirations increase. Hypocarbia may occur.
Hypoventilation	Respiratory rate is abnormally low, and depth of ventilation may be depressed. Hypercarbia may occur.
Cheyne-Stokes respiration	Respiratory rate and depth are irregular, characterized by alternating periods of apnea and hyperventilation. Respiratory cycle begins with slow, shallow breaths that gradually increase to abnormal rate and depth. The pattern reverses, breathing slows and becomes shallow, climaxing in apnea before respiration resumes.
Kussmaul respirations	Respirations are abnormally deep, regular, and increased in rate.
Biot's respiration	Respirations are abnormally shallow for two to three breaths, followed by irregular periods of apnea.

watching abdominal movements. Healthy men and children usually demonstrate diaphragmatic breathing. Women tend to use thoracic muscles to breathe; therefore, movements are best observed in the upper chest. Laboured respirations involve use of the accessory muscles of respiration visible in the neck. When a foreign body interferes with the movement of air in and out of the lungs, the intercostal spaces in the rib cage retract during inspiration, indicating increased respiratory effort. A longer expiration phase is evident when the outward flow of air is obstructed (e.g., as in asthma). In infants, additional indicators of respiratory distress are nasal flaring, grunting, and wheezing, making it important to look, listen, and feel when assessing breathing patterns in this population.

With normal breathing, a regular interval occurs after each respiratory cycle. Infants tend to breathe less regularly. The young child may breathe slowly for a few seconds and then suddenly breathe more rapidly. In assessment, the nurse should estimate the time interval after each respiratory cycle. Respiration is regular or irregular in rhythm.

Assessment of Diffusion and Perfusion

To evaluate the respiratory processes of diffusion and perfusion, the oxygen saturation of the blood is measured. Blood flow through the pulmonary capillaries contains red blood cells for oxygen attachment. After oxygen diffuses from the alveoli into the pulmonary blood, most of the oxygen attaches to hemoglobin molecules in red blood cells. The red blood cells then carry the oxygenated hemoglobin molecules through the left side of the heart and out to the peripheral capillaries, where the oxygen detaches, depending on the needs of the tissues.

The percentage of hemoglobin that is bound with oxygen in the arteries is the percentage of saturation of hemoglobin (SaO_2). This value is usually between 95 and 100%. SaO_2 is affected by factors that interfere with ventilation, perfusion, or diffusion (see Chapter 40). The saturation of venous blood (SvO_2) is lower because the tissues have removed some of the oxygen from the hemoglobin molecules. A normal value for SvO_2 is 70%. SvO_2 is affected by factors that interfere with or increase the tissue's need for oxygen.

Measurement of Arterial Oxygen Saturation. A *pulse oximeter* enables the indirect measurement of oxygen saturation (Skill 31.4). This device contains a probe with a light-emitting diode (LED) and photo detector connected by cable to an oximeter (Figures 31.11 and 31.12). The LED emits light wavelengths that are absorbed differently by oxygenated and deoxygenated hemoglobin molecules. The photo detector detects the amount of oxygen bound to hemoglobin molecules; the oximeter calculates the pulse saturation (SpO_2).

The photo detector is in the oximeter probe. The appropriate probe should be selected to reduce measurement error. Digit probes are spring-loaded and conform to various sizes. Earlobe probes have greater accuracy at lower saturations and are least affected by peripheral vasoconstriction. Disposable sensor pads can be applied to a variety of sites, even the bridge of an adult's nose or the sole of an infant's foot. Factors that affect light transmission or peripheral arterial pulsations also affect the ability of the photo detector to measure SpO_2 (Box 31.10). Control of these factors allows accurate interpretation of abnormal SpO_2 measurements.

❖ NURSING PROCESS AND RESPIRATORY VITAL SIGNS

Measurements of respiratory rate, pattern, and depth, along with SpO_2, enable the assessment of ventilation, diffusion, and perfusion. Other assessments also involve respiratory status (see Chapter 33). Each measurement provides clues in determining the nature of a patient's health problem. Respiratory assessment data are defining characteristics of many nursing diagnoses, including the following:

- *Activity intolerance*
- *Ineffective airway clearance*
- *Anxiety*
- *Ineffective breathing pattern*
- *Impaired gas exchange*
- *Acute pain*
- *Ineffective tissue perfusion*
- *Dysfunctional ventilatory weaning response*

The nursing care plan includes interventions specific for the nursing diagnosis identified and the related factors (Box 31.11). For example, the defining characteristics of tachypnea, changes in depth of respirations, use of accessory muscles, cyanosis, and a decline in SpO_2 lead to a diagnosis of *impaired gas exchange*. Related factors may include lung surgery, history of chronic obstructive lung disease, and history of heavy smoking. Patient outcomes are evaluated by assessing the respiratory rate, ventilatory depth, rhythm, and SpO_2 after each intervention.

BLOOD PRESSURE

Blood pressure is the force exerted on the walls of an artery by the pulsing blood under pressure from the heart. Blood flows throughout the circulatory system because of pressure changes. It moves from an area of high pressure to an area of low pressure. Systemic or arterial blood pressure (the blood pressure in the system of arteries in the body) is a good indicator of cardiovascular health. The heart's contraction forces blood under high pressure into the aorta. The peak of maximum pressure when ejection occurs is the *systolic* blood pressure. When the ventricles relax, the blood remaining in the arteries exerts *diastolic* blood pressure, which is the minimal pressure exerted against the arterial walls at any time.

The standard unit for measuring blood pressure is millimetres of mercury (mm Hg). The measurement indicates the height to which the blood pressure can raise a column of mercury. It is recorded as the systolic reading over the diastolic reading (e.g., 120/80). The difference

| SKILL 31.4 | MEASURING OXYGEN SATURATION (PULSE OXIMETRY) |

Delegation Considerations

The task of measuring oxygen saturation can be delegated to unregulated care providers (UCPs). The nurse is responsible for assessing the effect of changes in oxygen saturation; therefore, when the task of measuring oxygen saturation is delegated, it is important to *inform the UCP* about the following:

- The importance of notifying the nurse immediately of any reading lower than SpO_2 of 90%
- How to select and appropriate sensor site and probe for measurement of oxygen saturation
- The frequency of oxygen saturation measurements for the patient
- Factors that can falsely lower SpO_2 (see Box 31.10)

Equipment

- Oximeter
- Oximeter probe appropriate for patient and recommended by manufacturer
- Acetone or nail polish remover, if needed
- Pen and either vital sign flow sheet or documentation form

PROCEDURE

STEPS	RATIONALE
1. Identify patient using at least two person specifics (e.g., name and date of birth or name and medical record number) according to employer policy.	• Ensures correct patient. Complies with Accreditation Canada's standards and improves patient safety (Accreditation Canada, 2020).
2. Determine need to measure patient's oxygen saturation.	• Clinical judgement is used to determine need for assessment.
A. Note risk factors, including acute or chronic compromised respiratory function; recovery from general anaesthesia or monitored sedation; traumatic injury to chest; ventilator dependence; activity intolerance; and changes in supplemental oxygen therapy.	• Certain conditions heighten risk for decreased oxygen saturation.
B. Assess for signs and symptoms such as altered respiratory rate, depth, or rhythm; adventitious breath sounds (see Chapter 33 for further information about conducting a health assessment); cyanotic appearance of nail beds, lips, mucous membranes, and skin; restlessness, irritability, or confusion; reduced level of consciousness; and laboured or difficult breathing.	• Physical signs and symptoms may be indicative of abnormal oxygen saturation.
3. Assess for factors that normally influence measurement of SpO_2 (see Box 31.10), such as oxygen therapy, hemoglobin level, temperature, and medications (e.g., bronchodilators).	• This assessment enables you to accurately assess oxygen saturation variations. Peripheral vasoconstriction related to hypothermia can interfere with SpO_2 determination.
4. Review patient's medical record for pulse oximetry order, or consult agency policy or procedure manual for standard of care for measurement.	• A medical order may be needed to assess oxygen saturation.
5. Determine site most appropriate for sensor probe placement (e.g., digit, earlobe) by assessing capillary refill (see Chapter 33 for further information about conducting a health assessment) and skin condition. If capillary refill is less than 3 seconds, choose another site.	• The sensor requires a pulsating vascular bed to identify hemoglobin molecules that absorb emitted light. Changes in SpO_2 are reflected in the circulation of the finger capillary bed within 30 seconds and the capillary bed of earlobe within 5–10 seconds.
A. Site needs to have adequate circulation and be free of moisture.	• Moisture prevents the sensor from detecting SpO_2 levels.
B. If a peripheral digit is selected, it must be free of polish or artificial nail.	• Artificial nails and nail polish interferes with accuracy of readings. Opaque coatings decrease light transmission; nail polish containing blue pigment can absorb light emissions and falsely alter saturation measurement.
C. If tremors are present, use earlobe as site.	• Motion artifact is the most common cause of a false reading.
D. If patient has obesity, a clip-on probe may not fit; obtain a single-use tape-on probe.	
6. Determine previous baseline SpO_2 (if available) from patient's record.	• Baseline information provides basis for comparison and assists in assessment of current status and evaluation of interventions.
7. Explain purpose of procedure to patient and how oxygen saturation will be measured.	• Explaining procedures promotes patient's cooperation and increases adherence.
8. Perform hand hygiene.	• Hand hygiene reduces transmission of microorganisms between the patient and the nurse.
9. Position patient comfortably. If finger is chosen as monitoring site, support patient's lower arm.	• This positioning enables probe positioning and decreases motion artifact that interferes with SpO_2 determination.

Continued

SKILL 31.4	**MEASURING OXYGEN SATURATION (PULSE OXIMETRY)—cont'd**
STEPS	**RATIONALE**

10. Use acetone to remove any fingernail polish from digit to be assessed.
   - Nail polish can interfere with accuracy of readings. Opaque coatings decrease light transmission; polish containing blue pigment can absorb light emissions and falsely alter oximetry measurements.

11. Instruct patient to breathe normally.
   - Normal breathing prevents large fluctuations in respiratory rate and depth and prevents possible errors in SpO_2 reading.

12. Attach sensor probe to monitoring site. Inform patient that clip-on probe feels like a clothespin on the finger but will not hurt.
   - To avoid startling patient, prepare patient to feel pressure of sensor probe's spring tension on a peripheral digit or earlobe.

CRITICAL DECISION POINT: *Do not attach probe to a finger, an ear, or bridge of the nose if area is edematous or skin integrity is compromised. Do not attach probe to hypothermic fingers. Select ear or bridge of nose if adult patient has history of peripheral vascular disease. Do not use sensors on an earlobe and bridge of nose in infants and toddlers because of skin fragility. Do not use disposable adhesive probes if patient has latex allergy. Do not place probe on the same extremity as used for electronic blood pressure cuff because blood flow to finger is temporarily interrupted when the cuff inflates; this results in inaccurate readings that trigger alarms.*

13. Once sensor is in place, turn on oximeter. Observe pulse waveform and intensity display, and listen for an audible beep. Correlate oximeter heart rate with patient's radial pulse. Oximeter pulse rate and patient's radial pulse should be the same. If differences are present, re-evaluate oximeter probe placement, and reassess pulse rates.
   - Pulse waveform and intensity display enables detection of valid pulse to SpO_2 value. Double-checking heart rate ensures oximeter accuracy.

14. Leave probe in place until oximeter readout reaches constant value and pulse display reaches full strength during each cardiac cycle. Inform patient that oximeter alarm will sound if probe falls off or if patient moves probe. Read SpO_2 on digital display.
   - Reading takes 10 to 30 seconds, depending on site selected.

15. If SpO_2 monitoring is to be continuous, verify SpO_2 alarm limits and alarm volume, which are preset by the manufacturer at a minimum of 85% and a maximum of 100%. Determine limits for SpO_2 and heart rate alarms on the basis of each patient's condition. Verify that alarms are functional. Assess skin integrity under sensor probe every 2 hours. Relocate sensor probe at least every 4 hours and more frequently if skin integrity is altered or tissue perfusion compromised.
   - Alarms must be set at appropriate limits and volumes to avoid frightening patients and visitors.
   - Spring tension of sensor probe or sensitivity to disposable sensor probe adhesive can cause skin irritation and lead to disruption of skin integrity.

16. Assist patient to return to a comfortable position.
   - This action restores patient's comfort and promotes a sense of well-being.

17. Perform hand hygiene.
   - Hand hygiene reduces transmission of microorganisms between the patient and the nurse.

18. Discuss findings with patient as needed.
   - Such discussion promotes patient's participation in care and understanding of their health status.

19. If SpO_2 measurements are intermittent or spot-checked, remove probe and turn oximeter power off between measurements. Store probe in an appropriate location.
   - Batteries will be depleted if oximeter is left on. Sensor probes are expensive and vulnerable to damage.

20. Compare SpO_2 readings with patient's baseline and acceptable values.
   - Comparison reveals presence of abnormality.

21. Correlate SpO_2 with SaO_2 obtained from arterial blood gas measurements (see Chapter 41) if available.
   - Reliability of noninvasive assessments is documented.

22. Correlate SpO_2 reading with data obtained from assessment of respiratory rate, depth, and rhythm (see Skill 31.3).
   - Measurements of ventilation, perfusion, and diffusion are interrelated.

UNEXPECTED OUTCOMES	**RELATED INTERVENTIONS**

SpO_2 is less than 90%
   - Verify that oximeter probe is intact and that outside light transmission does not influence measurement.
   - Observe for signs associated with decreased oxygenation (e.g., anxiety, restlessness, tachycardia, cyanosis) (see Box 31.11).
   - Verify that supplemental oxygen delivery system is delivered as ordered and is functioning properly.
   - Minimize factors that alter SpO_2 (e.g., lung secretions, increased activity, hyperthermia).
   - Position patient to promote optimal ventilation (e.g., high Fowler's position for patient with obesity).
   - Recheck SpO_2 after interventions and notify physician if still below 90%.

SKILL 31.4   MEASURING OXYGEN SATURATION (PULSE OXIMETRY)—cont'd

STEPS	RATIONALE
Heart rate indicated on oximeter is lower than patient's radial or apical pulse	• Reposition sensor probe to alternative site with increased blood flow. • Assess patient for signs of altered cardiac output (e.g., decreased blood pressure, cool skin, confusion).

RECORDING AND REPORTING
- Record SpO_2 value on nurses' notes or vital sign flow sheet, indicating type and amount of oxygen therapy used by patient during assessment. Record any signs and symptoms of oxygen desaturation in nurses' narrative notes. Report abnormal findings to nurse in charge or health care provider.
- Document SpO_2 in nurses' narrative notes after administration of specific therapies.
- Record in nurses' notes the patient's use of continuous or intermittent pulse oximetry.

CARE IN THE COMMUNITY CONSIDERATIONS
- Pulse oximetry is used in community care to noninvasively monitor oxygen therapy or changes in oxygen therapy.
- Instruct caregivers to examine oximeter site before applying sensor.
- Instruct caregivers on procedure to implement when oxygen saturation is not within acceptable values.

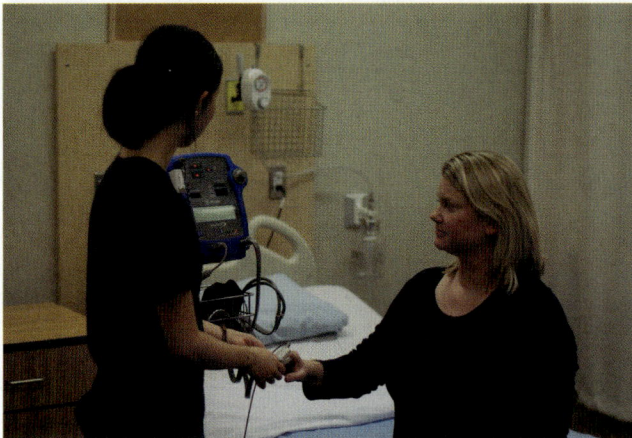

FIGURE 31.11 Portable pulse oximeter. (Courtesy Barbara J. Astle, RN, PhD.)

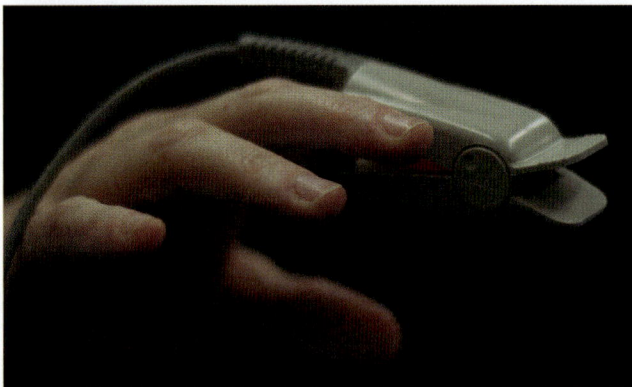

FIGURE 31.12 Spring tension oximeter probe. (Courtesy Barbara J. Astle, RN, PhD.)

between systolic and diastolic pressure is the *pulse pressure*. For a blood pressure of 120/80, the pulse pressure is 40. This parameter has been recently considered a potential indicator of cardiovascular disease, given its relationship to compliance or stiffening of the arteries.

Physiology of Arterial Blood Pressure

Blood pressure reflects the interrelationships of cardiac output, peripheral vascular resistance, blood volume, blood viscosity, and artery elasticity. Knowledge of these hemodynamic variables helps in the assessment of blood pressure alterations.

BOX 31.10   Factors Affecting Determination of Pulse Oxygen Saturation (SpO_2)

Interference With Light Transmission

Outside light sources interfere with the oximeter's ability to process reflected light.

Carbon monoxide (caused by smoke inhalation or poisoning) artificially elevates SpO_2 by absorbing light in a way similar to oxygen.

Patient motion interferes with the oximeter's ability to process reflected light.

Jaundice interferes with the oximeter's ability to process reflected light.

Intravascular dyes (e.g., methylene blue) absorb light in a way similar to deoxyhemoglobin and artificially lower saturation.

Nail polish, artificial nails, and metal studs in nails interfere with light absorption and the ability of the oximeter to process reflected light.

Dark skin pigment sometimes results in signal loss or overestimation of saturation.

Reduction of Arterial Pulsations

Peripheral vascular disease (atherosclerosis) reduces pulse volume.

Hypothermia at assessment site decreases peripheral blood flow.

Pharmacological vasoconstrictors (epinephrine, dopamine) decrease peripheral pulse volume.

Low cardiac output and hypotension decrease blood flow to peripheral arteries.

Peripheral edema obscures arterial pulsation.

A tight probe records venous pulsations in the finger that compete with arterial pulsations.

Cardiac Output. Blood pressure depends on cardiac output. When volume increases in an enclosed space, such as a blood vessel, the pressure in that space rises. As cardiac output increases, more blood is pumped against arterial walls, causing the blood pressure to rise. Cardiac output increases as a result of an increase in heart rate, greater heart muscle contractility, or an increase in blood volume. Changes in heart rate can occur faster than changes in heart muscle contractility or blood volume. A rapid or significant increase in heart rate decreases the heart's ability to fill, resulting in blood pressure decreasing.

Peripheral Resistance. Blood pressure depends on peripheral vascular resistance. Blood circulates through a network of arteries, arterioles, capillaries, venules, and veins. Arteries and arterioles are surrounded by smooth muscle that contracts or relaxes to change the size of the lumen. Normally, arteries and arterioles remain partially constricted to maintain a constant flow of blood. The size of arteries and arterioles changes to adjust blood flow to the needs of local tissues.

For example, when a major organ requires more blood, the peripheral arteries constrict, decreasing their supply of blood. More blood then becomes available to the major organ because of the resistance change in the periphery. Peripheral vascular resistance is the resistance to blood flow determined by the tone of the vascular musculature and diameter of blood vessels. The smaller the lumen of a vessel, the greater the resistance to blood flow. As resistance rises, arterial blood pressure rises. As vessels dilate and resistance falls, blood pressure subsequently decreases.

Blood Volume. The volume of blood circulating within the vascular system affects blood pressure. Most adults have a circulating blood volume of approximately 5 000 mL. Normally, this blood volume remains constant. However, if volume increases, more pressure is exerted against arterial walls. For example, the rapid, uncontrolled infusion of intravenous fluids would typically increase blood pressure. When circulating blood volume decreases, as with hemorrhage or dehydration, blood pressure would subsequently decrease.

Viscosity. The thickness or viscosity of blood affects the ease with which blood flows through the small vessels. The *hematocrit*, or percentage of red blood cells in the blood, determines blood viscosity. When the hematocrit rises and blood flow slows, the heart must contract more forcefully to move the viscous blood through the circulatory system. This results in arterial blood pressure increasing.

Elasticity. Normally, the walls of an artery are elastic and easily distensible. As pressure within the arteries increases, the diameter of the vessel walls increases to accommodate the rising pressure change. Arterial distensibility prevents wide fluctuations in blood pressure. However, in certain diseases, such as arteriosclerosis, vessel walls lose their elasticity and are replaced by fibrous tissue that cannot stretch as well. With reduced elasticity, resistance to blood flow is greater. As a result, when the left ventricle ejects its stroke volume, the vessels no longer yield to pressure. Instead, a given volume of blood is forced through the rigid arterial walls, and systemic pressure rises. Systolic pressure is more significantly elevated than diastolic pressure as a result of reduced arterial elasticity.

Most importantly, each hemodynamic factor significantly affects the others. For example, as arterial elasticity declines, peripheral vascular resistance increases. The complex control of the cardiovascular system normally prevents any single factor from permanently changing the blood pressure. For example, if the blood volume falls, the body compensates with increased vascular resistance.

Factors Influencing Blood Pressure

Blood pressure is not constant; it is continually influenced by many factors. One measurement cannot adequately reflect a patient's blood pressure. Blood pressure changes from heartbeat to heartbeat. Blood pressure trends, not individual measurements, guide nursing interventions. By understanding these factors, nurses can more accurately interpret blood pressure readings.

Age. Normal blood pressure levels vary throughout life. Blood pressure increases during childhood. The level of a child's or adolescent's blood pressure is assessed with regard to body size and age. The systolic blood pressure of a child 6 to 12 months old ranges from 80 to 100, and the diastolic pressure ranges from 55 to 65. The normal systolic blood pressure for a 3- to 6-year-old is 95 to 110, and the normal diastolic pressure is 60 to 75 (United Medical Education, 2021). Larger children (heavier and/or taller) have higher blood pressures than do smaller children of the same age. During adolescence, blood pressure continues to vary according to body size.

An adult's blood pressure tends to increase with advancing age. Canadian guidelines indicate that blood pressure should be assessed at all appropriate health care visits. In most people, including those with nondiabetic chronic kidney disease, blood pressure should be treated to lower than 140/90 mm Hg. In those people with diabetes, blood pressure should be treated to below 130/80 mm Hg (Table 31.7). Individuals with high normal blood pressure should be followed up annually to assess for risk of early-onset hypertension (Rabi et al., 2020). Older persons may have a rise in systolic pressure and increased pulse pressure related to higher arterial stiffness (Sapra et al., 2022).

Stress. Anxiety, fear, pain, and other emotional stress result in stimulation of the sympathetic nervous system, which increases heart rate, cardiac output, and peripheral vascular resistance. These alterations, in turn, increase blood pressure. Anxiety can raise blood pressure by as much as 30 mm Hg.

Gender. Patients with male genitalia and those with female genitalia do not have clinically significant differences in blood pressure levels. After puberty, children with male genitalia tend to have higher blood pressure readings. Factors such as pregnancy, birth control, and menopause can increase the risk of hypertension in persons with female genitalia throughout the lifespan. After the age of 65, individuals with female genitalia are more likely to have higher levels of blood pressure than individuals with male genitalia (Heart and Stroke Foundation of Canada, 2022).

Daily Variation. A daily peak and trough, the diurnal rhythm, occurs in blood pressure. Blood pressure undergoes a steep increase in the morning, peaking in late afternoon, then decreasing at night during rest (Douma, & Gumz, 2018).

Medications. During blood pressure assessment, it is important to determine if the patient is on any type of medications, as some can directly or indirectly affect blood pressure. Antihypertensive or other

TABLE 31.7	Blood Pressure Thresholds for Initiation of Antihypertensive Therapy and Treatment Targets in Adults	
Patient Population	BP Threshold (mm Hg) for Initiation of Antihypertensive Therapy	BP Target (mm Hg) for Treatment
Low risk (no target organ damage or cardiovascular risk factors)	SBP ≥ 160 DBP ≥ 100	SBP < 140 DBP < 90
High risk of cardiovascular disease	SBP ≥ 130	SBP < 120
Diabetes mellitus	SBP ≥ 130 DBP ≥ 80	SBP < 130 DBP < 80
All others	SBP ≥ 140 DBP ≥ 90	SBP < 140 DBP < 90

BP, Blood pressure; DBP, diastolic blood pressure; SBP, systolic blood pressure.
From Rabi, D., McBrien, K., Sapir-Pichhadze R., et al. (2020). Hypertension Canada's 2020 comprehensive guidelines for the prevention of, diagnosis, risk assessment and treatment of hypertension in adults and children. *Canadian Journal of Cardiology 36*(5), 596–694 (Table 5, p. 606).

TABLE 31.8	Antihypertensive Medications	
Medication Type	Names	Action
Diuretics	Hydrochlorothiazide (Microzide), furosemide (Lasix), spironolactone (Aldactone), metolazone (Zaroxolyn), triamterene (Dyazide)	Reduce kidneys' reabsorption of sodium and water, thus lowering circulating fluid volume
β-Adrenergic blockers	Atenolol (Tenormin), nadolol (Corgard), propranolol (Inderal), metoprolol (Lopressor)	Combine with β-adrenergic receptors in the heart, arteries, and arterioles to block response to sympathetic nerve impulses; this results in reduced heart rate and thus cardiac output
Vasodilators	Hydralazine (Apresoline), minoxidil (Loniten)	Act on arteriolar smooth muscle to cause relaxation and reduce peripheral vascular resistance
Calcium channel blockers	Diltiazem (Cardizem, Dilacor XR), verapamil hydrochloride (Calan SR), nifedipine (Procardia)	Reduce peripheral vascular resistance by systemic vasodilation
Angiotensin-converting enzyme (ACE) inhibitors	Ramipril (Altace), captopril (Capoten), enalapril (Vasotec), lisinopril (Prinivil, Zestril), benazepril (Lotensin)	Block the conversion of angiotensin I to angiotensin II, which prevents vasoconstriction; also reduces aldosterone production and fluid retention, thereby lowering circulating fluid volume
Angiotensin II receptor blockers	Losartan (Cozaar), olmesartan (Benicar)	Block the binding of angiotensin II, which prevents vasoconstriction

cardiac medications may lower blood pressure (Table 31.8). Opioid analgesics can lower blood pressure. Vasoconstrictors and an excess of intravenous fluids can increase blood pressure. It is therefore critical to always assess blood pressure before administering any of these medications.

Activity, Weight, and Smoking. Blood pressure can be reduced for several hours after a period of exercise. Older persons often experience a 5- to 10-mm Hg fall in blood pressure about 1 hour after eating. Increases in oxygen demanded by the body during activity leads to increases in blood pressure. Obesity is a factor in hypertension. Smoking results in vasoconstriction. Blood pressure rises when a person is smoking, and it returns to baseline 15 minutes after smoking ceases.

Hypertension

The most common alteration in blood pressure is *hypertension*. Hypertension is often asymptomatic. Hypertension is associated with thickening and loss of elasticity in the arterial walls. Peripheral vascular resistance increases within thick, inelastic vessels. The heart must continually pump against greater resistance. As a result, blood flow to vital organs such as the heart, brain, and kidney decreases.

According to Rabi et al. (2020), patients who exhibit features of a hypertensive urgency or emergency should be diagnosed as hypertensive and treated immediately. Hypertension is also diagnosed with the following criteria:

1. Mean blood pressure (MBP), obtained either by office blood pressure measurement (OBPM) or automated office blood pressure (AOBP), is systolic blood pressure (SBP) ≥180 mm Hg or diastolic blood pressure (DBP) ≥110 mm Hg,

2. First reading of SBP measured by AOBP is between 135 and 179 mm Hg, or DBP is between 85 and 109 mmHg, or

3. SBP measured by OBPM is between 140 and 179 mmHg, or DBP is between 90 and 109 mmHg.

To rule out *white coat syndrome*, out-of-office blood pressure measurement should be taken prior to the second visit with the recommended ambulatory blood pressure monitoring (APBM). The diagnosis of hypertension using APBM is established if:

1. Mean SBP is ≥135 mm Hg, or DBP is ≥85 mm Hg, or

2. 24-hr mean SBP is ≥130 mm Hg or DBP is ≥80 mm Hg.

Home blood pressure measurement (HBPM) is used if ABPM is not tolerated or readily available and should consist of two readings taken each morning and evening for 7 days (28 days total). The first day's readings should be discarded and the last 6 days should be averaged. If the mean of the readings SBP is ≥135 mm Hg, or DBP is ≥85 mm Hg, then a diagnosis of hypertension is made. If out-of-office measurements cannot be performed, the patient can be diagnosed as hypertensive using serial office visits under certain conditions (Figure 31.13). Nurses need to incorporate these blood pressure measurement recommendations into practice in order to correctly interpret blood pressure and minimize error. Box 31.12 describes a nursing example of such practice.

Home measurement of blood pressure is an important facet in the diagnosis of white coat hypertension and masked hypertension. In *white coat hypertension*, blood pressure is elevated during a visit to a

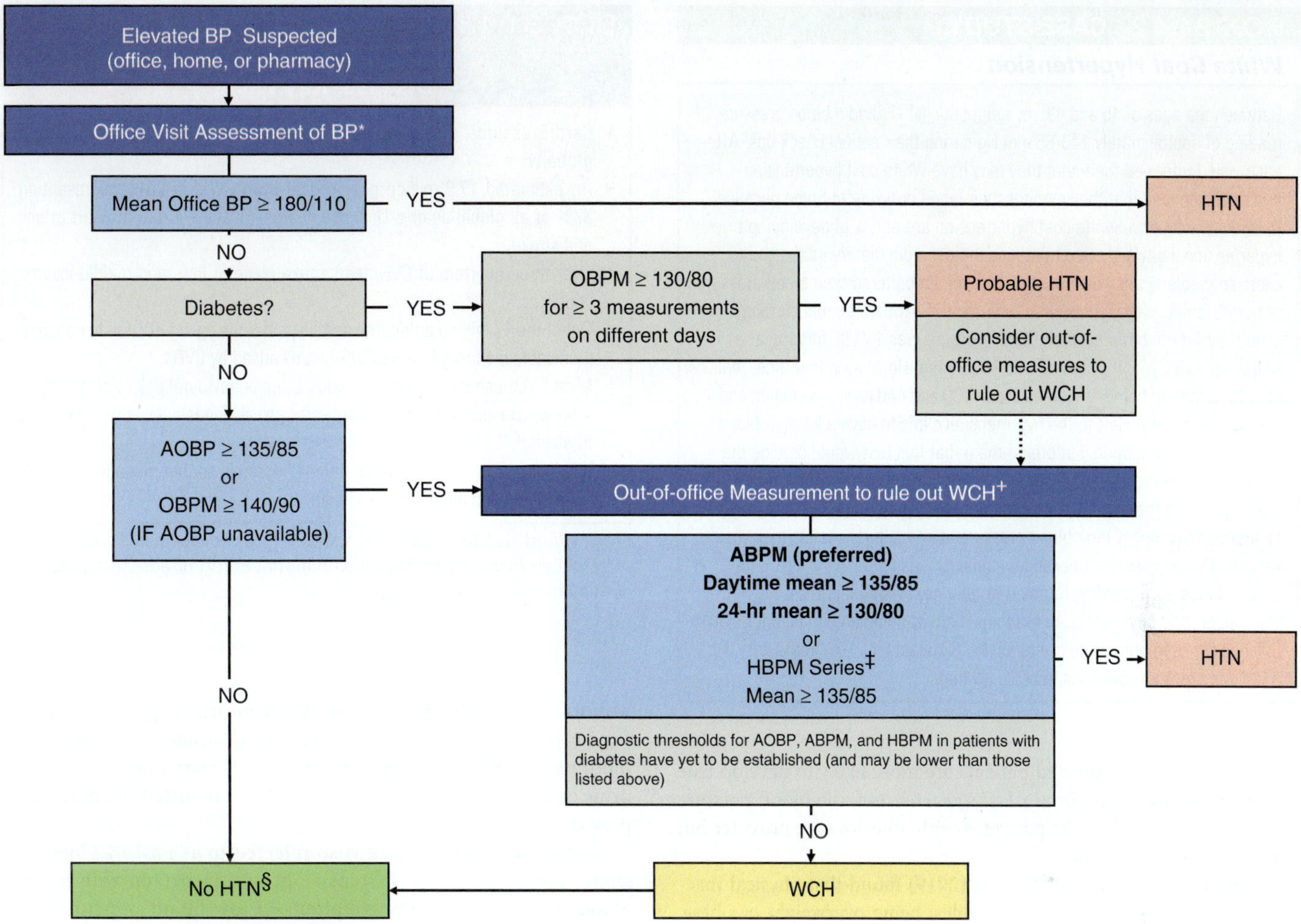

FIGURE 31.13 Hypertension diagnostic algorithm for adults. The diagnostic algorithm has been revised for the 2020 guidelines. In 2017 and 2018, diabetes was included in the diagnostic algorithm to provide a comprehensive overview of the diagnosis of hypertension. However, this created several challenges: the OBPM diagnostic threshold is different in patients with diabetes; evidence for defining AOBP and out-of-office (ABPM and HBPM) diagnostic thresholds is lacking; and the potential prognostic value of out-of-office measurements in patients with diabetes, including the identification of white coat hypertension or masked hypertension, exists, but definitions are not established. The committee elected to revise the 2018 algorithm to include the recommendation that a series of three to five office measurements can be used to establish a diagnosis of hypertension in diabetes. Although it is plausible that an AOBP threshold could be lower, there is currently no published evidence to guide a specific AOBP threshold. There are no studies to date that have established ABPM or HBPM thresholds in patients with diabetes. Other guideline bodies have elected to estimate corresponding values for HBPM and ABPM on the basis of the established thresholds for the general population; however, the evidence is not clear and these are not validated for diabetes. With respect to identifying white coat hypertension in patients with diabetes, there are currently no evidence-based definitions. However, a comprehensive review of the published evidence is required to establish thresholds on which diagnostic and treatment decisions can be based. *ABPM*, Ambulatory blood pressure measurement; *AOBP*, automated office blood pressure (performed with the patient unattended in a private room); *BP*, blood pressure; *HBPM*, home blood pressure measurement; *HTN*, hypertension; *OBPM*, office blood pressure measurement (measurements are performed in the office using an electronic upper arm device with a provider in the room); *WCH*, white coat hypertension. *If AOBP is used, use the mean calculated and displayed by the device. If OBPM is used, take at least three readings, discard the first, and calculate the mean of the remaining measurements. A history and physical examination should be performed, and diagnostic tests ordered. †Serial office measurements over three to five visits can be used if ABPM or HBPM are not available. ‡Home BP Series: Two readings taken each morning and evening for 7 days (28 total). Discard first-day readings and average the last 6 days. §In a patient with suspected masked hypertension, ABPM or HBPM could be considered to rule out masked hypertension. (Reprinted with permission from Rabi, D., McBrien, K., Woo, V., et al. [2020]. Hypertension Canada's 2020 comprehensive guidelines for prevention, diagnosis, risk assessment, and treatment for hypertension in adults and children. *Canadian Journal of Cardiology, 36*[5], 596–624. https://www.onlinecjc.ca/action/showPdf?pii=S0828-282X%2820%2930191-4)

BOX 31.12 CASE STUDY

White Coat Hypertension

Between the ages of 45 and 49, my neighbour, M. J., had a blood pressure reading of approximately 140/85 mm Hg during their annual check-ups. After each visit, I informed them that they may have white coat hypertension and recommended that they monitor their blood pressure at home because individuals who have white coat hypertension are at risk of developing true hypertension. I advised them to reduce their sodium dietary intake and to exercise regularly; they did not drink alcohol. I monitored their blood pressure at home; results were all below 135/85 mm Hg. At their annual checkup after their fiftieth birthday, their blood pressure was 140/86 mm Hg; at a follow-up visit 2 months later, it was 142/88 mm Hg. During that time, their blood pressure at home ranged between 136 and 140 (systolic) and 82 and 86 (diastolic). They went to the hypertension clinic to have a 24-hour blood pressure monitor applied. I informed them that this test would provide the physician with information to make treatment decisions. Because of high readings during the test, Dyazide (triamterene), 25 mg daily, was prescribed. I continued to monitor their blood pressure at home, but because their results remained in the hypertensive range, enalapril (Vasotec) 2.5 mg was added to their blood pressure drug regimen at their next visit 4 months later. Since then, all of their blood pressure readings, both at home and in the physician's office, have been below 126 (systolic) and 82 (diastolic). Four years later, M. J.'s blood pressure continues to be controlled.

BOX 31.13 Cardiovascular Disease (CVD)—A Noncommunicable Disease: Key Facts

- Cardiovascular diseases (CVDs) are the leading cause of death globally.
- An estimated 17.9 million people died from CVDs in 2019, representing 32% of all global deaths. Of these deaths, 85% were due to heart attack and stroke.
- Over three-quarters of CVD deaths take place in low- and middle-income countries.
- Out of the 17 million premature deaths (under the age of 70) due to noncommunicable diseases in 2019, 38% were caused by CVDs.
- Most CVDs can be prevented by addressing behavioural risk factors such as tobacco use, unhealthy diet and obesity, physical inactivity, and harmful use of alcohol.
- It is important to detect CVD as early as possible so that management with counselling and medicines can begin.

From World Health Organization. (2021). *Cardiovascular diseases (CVDs) key facts*. https://www.who.int/news-room/fact-sheets/detail/cardiovascular-diseases-(cvds)

health care provider. Affected patients are more likely to develop true hypertension over time. In *masked hypertension*, the blood pressure reading is normal while the patient is with a health care provider but becomes elevated at home.

A study by Leung and colleagues (2019) found that physical inactivity, a diet low in fruits and vegetables, being overweight or obese, the presence of diabetes, and chronic kidney disease were strong, often modifiable, risk factors for hypertension. This is why health behaviour strategies have proven to effectively lower blood pressure. The following actions should be recommended as a first-line intervention to individuals in both the prevention and treatment of hypertension (Hypertension Canada, 2022):

- Becoming more physically active
- Weight reduction
- Moderation in alcohol intake
- Eating healthier
- Relaxation therapies
- Smoking cessation

Hypertension is also a major risk factor for cardiovascular disease and the number one risk factor for stroke (Heart and Stroke Foundation of Canada, 2022). People with a family history of hypertension are at significant risk for developing hypertension and cardiovascular disease. Cardiovascular disease is a noncommunicable disease (NCD) that accounts for most NCD deaths—17.9 million people died in 2019. (World Health Organization, 2021) (Box 31.13).

Hypotension

Hypotension is considered present when the systolic blood pressure decreases to 90 mm Hg or lower. Some adults may have a low blood pressure normally; however, for the majority of people, low blood pressure is an abnormal finding associated with illness.

Hypotension occurs because of the dilation of the arteries in the vascular bed, the loss of a substantial amount of blood volume (e.g.,

hemorrhage), or the failure of the heart muscle to pump adequately (e.g., myocardial infarction). Hypotension associated with pallor, skin mottling, clamminess, confusion, increased heart rate, or decreased urine output is life-threatening and should be reported to a health care provider immediately.

Orthostatic hypotension, also referred to as *postural hypotension*, occurs when a normotensive person (a person with normal blood pressure) develops symptoms of low blood pressure when rising to an upright position. When a healthy individual changes from lying down to a sitting or standing position, the peripheral blood vessels in the legs constrict. Vasoconstriction in the lower extremities during standing prevents the pooling of blood in the legs caused by gravity. Thus, no symptoms are normally felt when standing. In contrast, when patients have a decreased blood volume, their blood vessels are already constricted. When a volume-depleted patient stands, blood pressure drops significantly, and heart rate increases to compensate for the drop in cardiac output. Patients who are dehydrated, are anemic, or have experienced prolonged bed rest or recent blood loss are at risk for orthostatic hypotension.

To assess for orthostatic hypotension, during vital sign measurements, blood pressure and pulse are obtained with the patient supine, sitting, and standing. The readings are obtained 1 to 3 minutes after the patient changes position. In most cases, orthostatic hypotension is detected within a minute of standing up. If it occurs, the nurse needs to assist the patient to a lying position and notify the health care provider or nurse in charge. While obtaining orthostatic measurements, it is important to observe for other symptoms of hypotension, such as fainting, weakness, or light-headedness. When recording orthostatic blood pressure measurements, the nurse records the patient's position, in addition to the blood pressure measurement—for example, "140/80 supine, 132/72 sitting, 108/60 standing." Because the skill of orthostatic measurements requires advanced reasoning and ongoing nursing judgement, the nurse *should not delegate this procedure* to unregulated care providers.

Measurement of Blood Pressure

Arterial blood pressure may be measured either directly (invasively) or indirectly (noninvasively). The direct method requires the insertion of a thin catheter into an artery. Tubing connects the catheter to electronic monitoring equipment. The monitor displays a constant arterial pressure waveform and reading. Because of the risk of sudden blood loss from an artery, invasive blood pressure monitoring is used only in critical care settings. For noninvasive blood pressure measurement, Hypertension Canada's *2020 Guidelines* (Rabi et al., 2020) continue to recommend that validated oscillometric upper arm measurements are preferred over auscultation, with AOPB being the preferred method for in-office measurement, and out-of-office measurements are essential in ruling out white coat hypertension and diagnosing masked hypertension. Despite this recommendation, the auscultatory method is still often being utilized. According to a survey of Canadian family physicians, 52% of them still use aneroid or mercury devices with auscultation to manually measure blood pressure instead of following the current Canadian guidelines (Kaczorowski et al., 2017). A literature review by Elias and Goodell (2021) states that although many experts have suggested that the auscultation method is a more complex skill that increases human error, the introduction of automated blood pressure monitoring devices has not completely eliminated human error. Electronic measurement of blood pressure should be encouraged; however, it is important for nurses to know the proper technique for both auscultation and automated measurement (Skill 31.5).

SKILL 31.5	MEASURING BLOOD PRESSURE

Delegation Considerations

In most provinces and territories, the task of measuring blood pressure can be delegated to unregulated care providers (UCPs). The nurse is responsible for assessing changes in blood pressure; therefore, when the task of measuring blood pressure is delegated, it is important to *inform the UCP* about the following:

- Selection of appropriate limb for blood pressure measurement—typically the arm, but can also be measured on leg
- Selection of appropriate-size blood pressure cuff for designated extremity
- Frequency of blood pressure measurement for patient
- Patient's usual values
- Abnormalities that should be reported to the health care provider

Equipment

- Aneroid sphygmomanometer
- Cloth or disposable vinyl pressure cuff of appropriate size for patient's extremity
- Stethoscope
- Alcohol swab
- Pen and either vital sign flow sheet or documentation form

PROCEDURE

STEPS	RATIONALE
1. Identify patient using at least two person specifics (e.g., name and date of birth or name and medical record number) according to employer policy.	• Ensures correct patient. Complies with Accreditation Canada's standards and improves patient safety (Accreditation Canada, 2020).
2. Determine need to assess patient's blood pressure.	• Use clinical judgement to determine need for assessment.
A. Note risk factors for alteration in blood pressure, including cardiovascular disease, renal disease, diabetes, circulatory shock, acute or chronic pain, rapid intravenous infusion of fluids or blood products, increased intracranial pressure, postoperative conditions, and toxemia of pregnancy.	• Certain conditions heighten risk for blood pressure alteration.
B. Observe for signs and symptoms of blood pressure alterations.	• Physical signs and symptoms may indicate alterations in blood pressure.
(1) High blood pressure (hypertension): headache (usually occipital), flushing of face, nosebleed, and fatigue (older persons); often asymptomatic until pressure is very high	
(2) Low blood pressure (hypotension): dizziness, mental confusion; restlessness; pale, dusky, or cyanotic skin and mucous membranes; and cool, mottled skin over extremities	
3. Determine best site for blood pressure assessment. Avoid applying cuff to extremity where intravenous fluids are infusing; where an arteriovenous shunt or fistula is present; on the side where breast or axillary surgery has been performed; and when extremity has been traumatized, is diseased, or requires a cast or bulky bandage (Box 31.14). Use lower extremities when the brachial arteries are inaccessible.	• Inappropriate site selection results in poor amplification of sounds, causing inaccurate readings. Application of pressure from inflated cuff bladder temporarily impairs blood flow and can exacerbate existing impairment of circulation in extremity.
4. Determine previous baseline blood pressure (if available) from patient's record.	• Baseline measurement enables assessment of change in patient's condition and provides comparison with future blood pressure measurements.
5. Identify factors likely to interfere with accuracy of blood pressure measurement (e.g., acute anxiety, stress, pain). Encourage patient to avoid using caffeine and tobacco for 30 minutes before blood pressure is assessed, and rest quietly for 5 minutes beforehand (Hypertension Canada, 2022).	• Exercise and smoking cause false elevations in blood pressure. Smoking increases blood pressure immediately, with the effect lasting up to 15 minutes. Caffeine (e.g., in coffee) increases blood pressure for up to 3 hours.

STEPS	RATIONALE
6. Explain to patient that blood pressure is to be assessed, and have patient rest at least 5 minutes before blood pressure is measured in sitting or lying position; wait 1 minute if patient is standing. Ask patient not to speak when blood pressure is being measured.	• These preparations allow patients to relax and help avoid falsely elevated readings. Blood pressure readings taken at different times can be objectively compared with readings taken with the patient at rest.
7. Select appropriate cuff size.	• Improper cuff size results in inaccurate readings. If cuff is too small or comes loose when inflated, this may result in falsely high readings. A cuff that is too large may produce falsely low readings.
8. Ensure proper functioning of cuff components: the release valve should be clean and freely movable in either direction; the inflation bulb and tubing should be intact and free of leaks.	• Improper functionality results in difficulty with regulation of cuff inflation and deflation.
9. Perform hand hygiene.	• Hand hygiene reduces transmission of microorganisms between the patient and the nurse.
10. Have patient assume sitting or lying position. Be sure the room is warm, quiet, and relaxing.	• These actions maintain patient's comfort during measurement. The patient's perceptions that the physical or interpersonal environment is stressful affect the blood pressure measurement.
11. With patient sitting or lying, position patient's forearm at heart-level position with patient's thigh flat (provide support as needed). To measure at patient's arm, turn palm up (see Step 11 illustration); to measure at patient's thigh, position with knee slightly flexed. If patient is sitting, the legs should not be crossed and feet should be touching the floor.	• If extremity is unsupported, patient may perform isometric exercise that increases diastolic blood pressure. Leg crossing falsely elevates blood pressure (Peters et al., 1999).

STEP 11 Patient's forearm supported in bed.

STEPS	RATIONALE
12. Expose patient's extremity arm, or the leg in certain medical situations, by fully removing constricting clothing.	• Exposure ensures proper cuff application.
13. Palpate patient's brachial artery (arm; see Step 13A illustration) or popliteal artery (leg). With cuff fully deflated, apply bladder of cuff above artery by centring cuff over artery. If no centre arrows appear on the cuff, estimate the centre of the bladder and place this centre over artery. Position cuff 2.5 cm above site of pulsation (antecubital or popliteal space). Wrap cuff evenly and snugly around extremity (see Step 13B illustrations). Do not place blood pressure cuff over clothing.	• Inflating bladder directly over artery ensures that proper pressure is applied during inflation. A loose-fitting cuff causes false high readings.

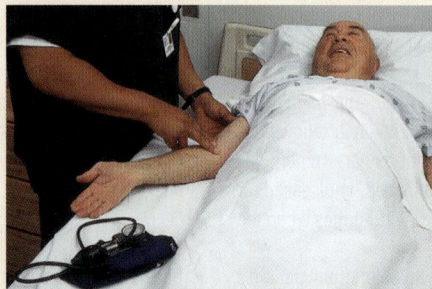

STEP 13A Palpating patient's brachial or popliteal artery.

Continued

SKILL 31.5

SKILL 31.5   **MEASURING BLOOD PRESSURE—cont'd**

STEPS   **RATIONALE**

STEP 13B *Left,* Bladder of cuff centred above artery. *Right,* Blood pressure cuff wrapped around upper arm.

14. Position aneroid manometer gauge no further than 1 metre away.
15. Measure blood pressure.
    A. Two-step method

    (1) Relocate patient's brachial or popliteal pulse. Palpate the artery distal to the cuff with fingertips of nondominant hand while inflating cuff rapidly to pressure 30 mm Hg above the point at which the pulse disappears. Slowly deflate cuff, and note reading when the pulse reappears. Deflate cuff fully and wait 1 minute.
    (2) Place stethoscope earpieces in your ears, and be sure sounds are clear, not muffled.
    (3) Relocate patient's brachial or popliteal pulse and place bell or diaphragm chest piece of stethoscope over it. Do not allow chest piece to touch cuff or clothing (see Step 15A[3] illustration).

- Gauge indicates correct readings.

- Provides estimate of systolic pressure, which assists in level of cuff inflation, particularly when baseline blood pressure is unknown.
- Relocating prevents false low readings. Maximal inflation point for accurate reading can be determined by palpation. If you are unable to palpate artery because of weakened pulse, an ultrasonic stethoscope can be used (see Chapter 33). Completely deflating the cuff prevents venous congestion and false high readings.
- Each earpiece should follow angle of ear canal to facilitate hearing.

- Proper stethoscope placement ensures optimal sound reception. An improperly positioned stethoscope causes muffled sounds that often result in false low systolic readings and false high diastolic readings.

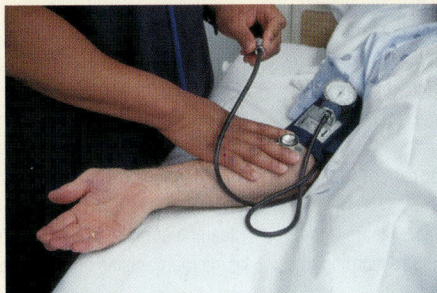

STEP 15A(3) Stethoscope over brachial artery to measure blood pressure.

    (4) Close valve of pressure bulb clockwise until it is tight.
    (5) Rapidly inflate cuff to 30 mm Hg above previously palpated systolic pressure (patient's estimated systolic pressure; see Step 15A[5] illustration).

- Tightening of valve prevents air leak during inflation.
- Rapid inflation ensures accurate measurement of systolic pressure.

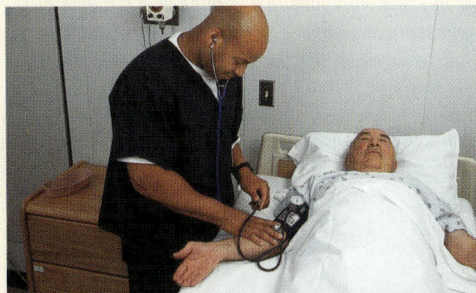

STEP 15A(5) Inflating blood pressure cuff.

    (6) Slowly release pressure bulb valve, and allow needle of manometer gauge to fall at rate of 2–3 mm Hg/second. Make sure no extraneous sounds are audible.

- Too rapid or slow a decline in pressure can cause inaccurate readings. Noise interferes with precise determination of Korotkoff phases.

STEPS	RATIONALE
(7) Note point on manometer when first clear sound is heard. The sound will slowly increase in intensity.	• First Korotkoff sound indicates systolic pressure.
(8) Continue to deflate cuff, noting point at which sound becomes muffled or dampened.	• Fourth Korotkoff sound is distinctly muffled and is indication of diastolic pressure in children.
(9) Continue to deflate cuff gradually, noting point at which sound disappears in adults. Listen for 10–20 mm Hg after the last sound, and then allow remaining air to escape quickly.	• Beginning of the fifth Korotkoff sound is indication of diastolic pressure in adults. Cuff is deflated as soon as possible because continuous cuff inflation causes arterial occlusion, resulting in numbness and a tingling sensation in patient's arm.
B. One-step method	• Used for frequent measurements and when there is previous awareness of systolic inflation level.
(1) Place stethoscope earpieces in your ears, and be sure sounds are clear, not muffled.	• Each earpiece should follow angle of ear canal to facilitate hearing.
(2) Relocate patient's brachial or popliteal artery, and place bell or diaphragm chest piece of stethoscope over it. Do not allow chest piece to touch cuff or clothing.	• Proper stethoscope placement ensures optimal sound reception. Improper positioning of stethoscope causes muffled sounds that often result in false low systolic readings and false high diastolic readings.
(3) Close valve of pressure bulb clockwise until tight. Quickly inflate cuff to 30 mm Hg above palpated systolic pressure.	• Tightening of valve prevents air leak during inflation. Inflation above systolic level ensures accurate measurement of systolic pressure.
(4) Slowly release pressure bulb valve, and allow needle of manometer gauge to fall at rate of 2–3 mm Hg/second.	• Too rapid or slow a decline in pressure can cause inaccurate readings.
(5) Note point on manometer when first clear sound is heard (first Korotkoff sound). The sound will slowly increase in intensity.	• First Korotkoff sound indicates systolic pressure.
(6) Continue to deflate cuff, noting point at which sound becomes muffled or dampened (fourth Korotkoff sound).	• Fourth Korotkoff sound is distinctly muffled and indicates diastolic pressure in children.
(7) Continue to deflate cuff gradually, noting point at which the sound disappears (fifth Korotkoff sound) in adults. Listen for 10–20 mm Hg after the last sound, and then allow remaining air to escape quickly.	• Beginning of the fifth Korotkoff sound is indication of diastolic pressure in adults. Cuff is deflated as soon as possible because continuous cuff inflation causes arterial occlusion, resulting in numbness and a tingling sensation in patient's arm.
16. Hypertension Canada (Rabi et al., 2020) recommends that for auscultation, at least three measurements should be taken in the same arm with the patient in the same position. The first reading should be discarded, and the latter two averaged.	• Multiple readings increase accuracy of blood pressure measurement.
17. Remove cuff from extremity unless measurement must be repeated. If patient's blood pressure is being assessed for the first time, repeat blood pressure assessment on other extremity.	• By comparing blood pressure in both extremities, circulation problems can be detected. (Difference of 5–10 mm Hg between extremities is normal.)
18. Assist patient to return to a comfortable position, and cover patient's upper arm if it was previously clothed.	• These actions restore patient's comfort and promote a sense of well-being.
19. Wipe the blood pressure cuff with disinfectant or, if disposable, keep in the patient's room until no longer needed; then dispose of the cuff according to agency policy.	• Cleaning or disposing of the blood pressure cuff helps reduce the transmission of microorganisms between patients.
20. Discuss findings with patient as needed.	• Such discussion promotes patient's participation in care and understanding of their health status.
21. Perform hand hygiene.	• Hand hygiene reduces transmission of microorganisms between the patient and the nurse.
22. Compare reading with previous baseline value, acceptable value of blood pressure for patient's age, or both.	• Evaluate for change in condition and alterations.

CRITICAL DECISION POINT: *In some situations (e.g., critically ill patients or those with peripheral vascular disease), it is often necessary to compare blood pressure readings in both arms, both legs, or all four extremities. If using upper extremities, use the arm with the higher pressure for subsequent assessments, unless this is contraindicated.*

23. Correlate blood pressure with data obtained from pulse assessment and other related cardiovascular signs and symptoms.	• Blood pressure and heart rate are interrelated.

Continued

SKILL 31.5	MEASURING BLOOD PRESSURE—cont'd
STEPS	RATIONALE

UNEXPECTED OUTCOMES	RELATED INTERVENTIONS
Blood pressure reading cannot be obtained	• Determine whether any immediate crisis is present by measuring pulse and respiratory rate. • Assess for signs of decreased cardiac output (e.g., weak or thready pulse, confusion, pallor, or cyanosis). If any sign is present, notify the nurse in charge or health care provider immediately. • Use alternative sites or procedures to obtain blood pressure. Auscultate blood pressure in lower extremity; use a Doppler ultrasonic instrument or a palpation method to obtain systolic measurement. • Repeat blood pressure measurement with sphygmomanometer. Electronic blood pressure devices are less accurate in conditions of low blood flow.
Blood pressure is not sufficient for adequate perfusion and oxygenation of tissues	• Compare blood pressure value with baseline value. A systolic reading of 90 mm Hg is an acceptable value for some patients. • Position patient in supine position to enhance circulation, and restrict activity if this is the cause of blood pressure to decrease. • Assess for signs of decreased cardiac output (e.g., weak or thready pulse, confusion, pallor, or cyanosis). If any sign is present, notify the nurse in charge or health care provider immediately. • Increase rate of intravenous infusion, or administer vasoconstrictor medications if ordered.
Blood pressure is elevated above acceptable range	• Repeat measurement in patient's other arm and compare findings. Verify correct size and placement of cuff. • Ask a colleague to repeat measurement in 2 minutes. • Observe for related symptoms (e.g., headache, confusion), although symptoms are sometimes not apparent until blood pressure is extremely elevated. • Report elevated blood pressure to the nurse in charge or health care provider immediately. • Administer antihypertensive medications as ordered.

RECORDING AND REPORTING
- Inform patient of value and need for periodic reassessment of blood pressure.
- Record blood pressure in nurses' notes or vital sign flow sheet. Document blood pressure in nurses' narrative notes after administration of specific therapies.
- Report abnormal findings to the nurse in charge or health care provider.

CARE IN THE COMMUNITY CONSIDERATIONS
- Assess home noise level to determine which room will provide the quietest environment for assessing blood pressure.
- Consider using an electronic blood pressure cuff in the home if patient has hearing difficulties, adequate financial resources, and adequate dexterity.

BOX 31.14 CASE STUDY

Blood Pressure Measurement in Patients With Mastectomies

I was assessing vital signs during my morning rotation as a student nurse and was just about to measure a patient's (preferred pronouns she/her) vital signs when I noted a sign above her bed that said "no blood pressure on arms, please." This puzzled me and made me nervous as to what I should do. I had never been faced with this situation before, and so far, I had only been taught how to take blood pressure on the arm. Thankfully, I found an experienced registered nurse (RN) and, despite the fact that I felt like it was a silly question, asked how I was supposed to measure this patient's blood pressure and why it could not be done on her arms. I then took her blood pressure on her thigh as the RN instructed. Prior to this, the thought had actually occurred to me that it probably wouldn't hurt the patient to take her blood pressure on her arm, but I discovered later that this is not true, and that the pressure of the cuff on her arm could possibly lead to lymphedema. When lymph nodes are removed from the axilla, as often happens with mastectomies, it can cause the lymph fluid to build up in the soft tissue of the arm instead of flowing normally through lymph vessels of the body; this buildup is called *lymphedema*. Lymphedema can cause swelling, a feeling of puffiness or heaviness, an aching or burning feeling, trouble moving the joint in the affected limb, and many other complications (Canadian Cancer Society, 2022). The National Lymphedema Network (NLN Medical Advisory Committee, 2012) recommends that, to reduce the risk of lymphedema, patients should avoid excessive or prolonged constriction of the at-risk body part. This tightening or squeezing could restrict lymph flow through that area or cause tissue trauma, and blood pressure cuffs used improperly or with extreme pressure may excessively constrict tissues in the affected arm. Although newer studies may dispute these facts and report that medical procedures like blood pressure measurement do not result in lymphedema initiation or worsening in breast cancer survivors, there are still case reports of harmful effects of, hesitation in, and cautions toward using most of these procedures in daily practice (Sheikhi-Mobarakeh et al., 2021).

FIGURE 31.14 Parts of a blood pressure cuff. (Image courtesy of Mi-Yeon Kim, RN, PhD.)

FIGURE 31.15 Wall-mounted aneroid sphygmomanometer.

FIGURE 31.16 Guidelines for proper blood pressure cuff size. Bladder length should cover 80 to 100% of arm circumference, and bladder width should be close to 40% of arm circumference (Hypertension Canada, 2022).

Blood Pressure Equipment. Before assessing blood pressure, make sure that you know how to use a sphygmomanometer and stethoscope. A *sphygmomanometer* includes a pressure manometer, an occlusive cloth or vinyl cuff that encloses an inflatable rubber bladder, and a pressure bulb with a release valve that inflates the bladder (Figure 31.14). Manometers are of two types: aneroid (Figure 31.15) and mercury. Aneroid manometers have the advantages of being safe, lightweight, portable, and compact. The aneroid manometer contains a glass-enclosed circular gauge with a needle that registers millimetre calibrations.

Mercury manometers, once the gold standard, are less commonly used because they contain mercury, a hazardous substance. As stated earlier, most municipalities have prohibited the sale or use of mercury-containing devices because of potential hazards. Pressure created by the inflation of the cuff moves the column of mercury upward against the force of gravity. Millimetre calibrations mark the height of the mercury column. To ensure accurate readings, the mercury column should fall freely as pressure is released and always remain at zero when the cuff is deflated. Measure at the meniscus of the mercury at eye level; looking up or down results in distorted readings.

Cloth or disposable vinyl compression cuffs contain an inflatable bladder and come in several sizes. The size selected is proportional to the circumference of the limb being assessed (Figure 31.16). Ideally, the bladder width of the cuff should be 40% of the circumference of the upper arm and the length should cover 80 to 100% of the arm's circumference. The lower edge of the cuff should be positioned 3 cm above the patient's antecubital fossa, allowing room for placement of the stethoscope bell or diaphragm. Many adults require a large-sized cuff. Using the forearm when a large cuff is not available is not recommended. Blood pressure measurements are not accurate unless the correct size cuff is applied appropriately (Table 31.9).

The release valve of the aneroid or mercury sphygmomanometer should be clean and freely movable in either direction. The valve, when closed, holds the pressure constant. A sticky valve makes pressure cuff deflation hard to regulate. The pressure bulb should be free of leaks.

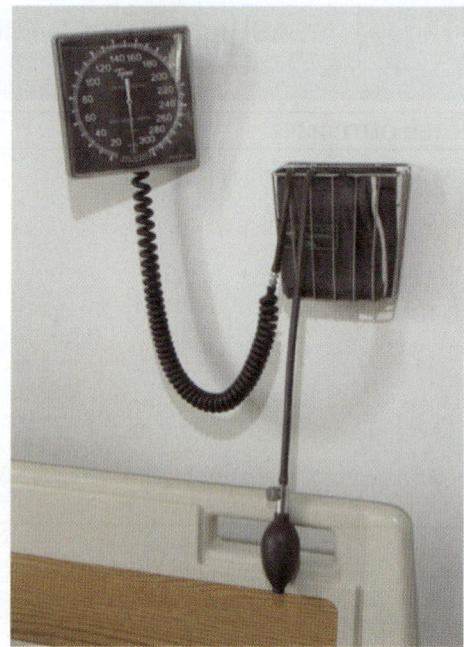

Auscultation. The best environment for blood pressure measurement by auscultation is a quiet room at a comfortable temperature. Although the patient may lie or stand, sitting is the preferred position. In most patients, blood pressure readings obtained in the supine, sitting, and standing positions are similar.

Patient position should be consistent during routine blood pressure measurements to enable meaningful comparison of values. Before measuring blood pressure, attempt to control factors responsible for artificially high readings, such as pain, anxiety, or exertion. It is important to minimize the patient's perceptions that the physical or interpersonal environment is stressful in order to reduce any effect on blood pressure measurement.

TABLE 31.9	Common Mistakes in Blood Pressure Assessment
Error	**Effect**
Bladder or cuff too wide	False low reading
Bladder or cuff too narrow or too short	False high reading
Cuff wrapped too loosely or unevenly	False high reading
Deflating cuff too slowly	False high diastolic reading
Deflating cuff too quickly	False low systolic reading and false high diastolic reading
Arm below heart level	False high reading
Arm above heart level	False low reading
Arm not supported	False high reading
Stethoscope fits poorly or impairment of the examiner's hearing, causing sounds to be muffled	False low systolic reading and false high diastolic reading
Stethoscope applied too firmly against antecubital fossa	False low diastolic reading
Cuff inflating too slowly	False high diastolic reading
Repeating assessments too quickly	False high systolic reading
Inadequate inflation level	False low systolic reading
Multiple examiners using different Korotkoff sounds for diastolic readings	False high systolic reading and low diastolic reading

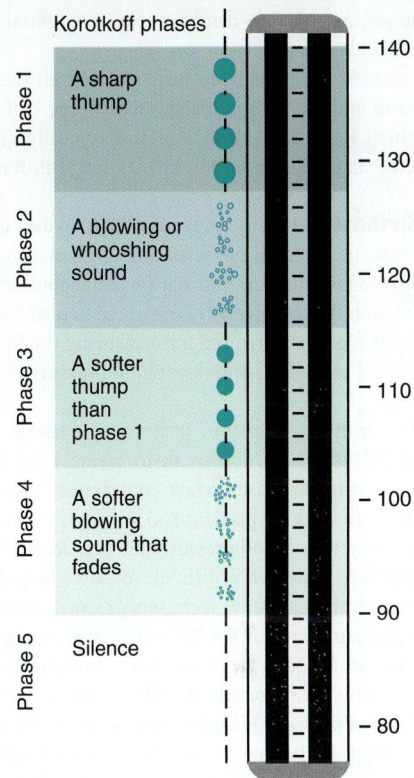

FIGURE 31.17 The sounds auscultated during blood pressure measurement can be differentiated into five Korotkoff phases. In this example, blood pressure is 140/90 mm Hg.

During the initial assessment, measure and record the blood pressure in both arms. Normally, pressures in the arms differ by 5 to 10 mm Hg. In subsequent assessments, the blood pressure in the arm with the higher pressure is measured. Pressure differences greater than 10 mm Hg indicate vascular problems and should be reported to the health care provider or nurse in charge.

The patient should be asked to state their usual blood pressure. If the patient does not know, inform the patient of their blood pressure reading after measuring and recording the blood pressure. It is important to educate the patient about optimal values of blood pressure, the risk factors for developing hypertension, and the dangers of hypertension.

Indirect measurement of arterial blood pressure works on a basic principle of pressure: blood flows freely through an artery until an inflated cuff applies pressure to tissues and causes the artery to collapse. After the cuff pressure is released, the point at which blood flow returns and sound appears through auscultation is the systolic pressure.

In 1905, Nikolai Korotkoff, a Russian surgeon, first described the sounds heard over an artery distal to the blood pressure cuff. The first Korotkoff sound is a clear rhythmical tapping that corresponds to the heart rate and gradually increases in intensity. Onset of the sound corresponds to the systolic pressure. A blowing or swishing sound occurs as the cuff continues to deflate; this is the second Korotkoff sound. As the artery distends, blood flow becomes turbulent. The third Korotkoff sound is a crisper and more intense tapping. The fourth Korotkoff sound is muffled and low-pitched as the cuff is further deflated. At this point, the cuff pressure has fallen below the pressure within the vessel walls; this sound is the diastolic pressure in infants and children. The fifth Korotkoff "sound" is actually the disappearance of sound. In adolescents and adults, the fifth sound corresponds to the diastolic pressure (Figure 31.17). In some patients, the sounds are clear and distinct. In other patients, only the beginning and ending sounds are clear. When recording numbers for blood pressure measurement,

note the point on the manometer when the first sound is heard (systolic reading), and the point on the manometer when the fifth sound is heard (diastolic reading). Some institutions recommend recording the point when the fourth sound is heard as well, especially for patients with hypertension. The numbers are presented by slashed lines (e.g., "120/80" or "120/100/80"). The arm used to measure the blood pressure (e.g., "right arm [RA] 130/70") and the patient's position (e.g., "sitting") should be noted.

Blood pressure findings prompt many medical decisions and nursing interventions concerning a patient's health care. Obtaining an accurate blood pressure measurement is essential. Error can arise from several sources (see Table 31.9). When unsure of a reading, it is good to ask a colleague to reassess the blood pressure.

Assessment in Children. All children 3 years of age through adolescence should have blood pressure measured regularly; presently, the auscultatory method is the gold standard (Rabi et al., 2020). Blood pressure in children changes with growth and development. Nurses can help parents understand the importance of this routine screening in children who may be at risk for hypertension.

The measurement of blood pressure in infants and children is difficult for several reasons:
- Different arm sizes necessitate careful selection of an appropriate cuff size. Do not choose a cuff on the basis of the name of the cuff; for example, an "infant" cuff may be too small for some infants.
- Readings are difficult to obtain in restless or anxious infants and children. Allow a delay of at least 15 minutes for patients to recover from recent activities and apprehension.
- Preparing the child for the blood pressure cuff's unusual sensation can increase cooperation. Most children understand the analogy of a "tight hug on your arm."

- Placing the stethoscope too firmly on the antecubital fossa causes errors in auscultation.
- Korotkoff sounds are difficult to hear in children because of low frequency and amplitude. A pediatric stethoscope bell can be helpful. The fourth Korotkoff sound, which is typically quite muffled, represents the diastolic pressure in infants and children.

Ultrasonic Stethoscope. If the nurse is unable to auscultate sounds because of a weakened arterial pulse, an ultrasonic stethoscope can be used (see Chapter 33 for further information about conducting a health assessment). This stethoscope enables the nurse to hear low-frequency systolic sounds. It is commonly used for measuring the blood pressure of infants, children, and adults with low blood pressure.

Palpation. The indirect palpation technique is useful for patients whose arterial pulsations are too weak to create Korotkoff sounds. Severe blood loss and decreased heart contractility are examples of conditions that result in blood pressure too low to auscultate accurately. In these cases, the systolic blood pressure can be assessed by palpation; the diastolic pressure, however, is difficult to assess by palpation (Box 31.15). When using the palpation technique, record the systolic value and how it was measured (e.g., "RA 90/—, palpated, supine").

The palpation technique can be used with auscultation. In some hypertensive patients, the sounds usually heard over the brachial artery when the cuff pressure is high disappear as pressure is reduced, and then they reappear at a lower level. This temporary disappearance of sound is the *auscultatory gap*. It typically occurs between the first and second Korotkoff sounds. The gap in sound may cover a range of 40 mm Hg and the failure to recognize this gap may cause nurses to underestimate systolic pressure or overestimate diastolic pressure. It is important to inflate the cuff high enough to hear the true systolic pressure before the auscultatory gap. Palpation of the radial artery helps in determining how high to inflate the cuff. Inflate the cuff to 30 mm Hg above the pressure at which the radial pulse disappeared and rapidly

deflate the cuff. While it is deflating, take note of the levels of pressure when the radial pulse disappeared and then reappeared—this is the auscultatory gap. Record the range of pressures in which the auscultatory gap occurs (e.g., "blood pressure RA 180/94 with an auscultatory gap from 180 to 160, sitting").

Lower Extremity Blood Pressure. Dressings, casts, intravenous catheters, arteriovenous fistulas, or shunts can render the upper extremities inaccessible for blood pressure measurement. In such cases, blood pressure is measured in the lower extremities. Comparing upper extremity blood pressure with that in the legs is also necessary for patients with certain cardiac or blood pressure abnormalities. The popliteal artery, palpable behind the knee in the popliteal space, is the site for auscultation. The cuff must be wide and long enough to allow for the larger girth of the thigh. Placing the patient in a prone position is best. If such a position is impossible, ask the patient to flex the knee slightly for easier access to the artery. Position the cuff 2.5 cm above the patient's popliteal artery with the bladder over the posterior aspect of the midthigh (Figure 31.18). The procedure is identical to that for brachial artery auscultation. Systolic pressure in the legs is usually 10 to 40 mm Hg higher than in the brachial artery, but the diastolic pressure should be the same.

Automatic Blood Pressure Devices. Many styles of electronic devices are available to determine an automatic blood pressure assessment rather than a manual one (Figure 31.19). For example, some devices rely on an electronic sensor to detect the vibrations caused by the rush of blood through an artery. When the cuff deflates, the sensor determines the initial burst of vibrations and translates the information into a systolic pressure reading. When the vibrations are lowest, just before they stop, the diastolic pressure is determined.

Rabi and colleagues (2020) recommend the use of automated blood pressure measurement over manual measurement, and AOBP measurement is the preferred in-office method as it provides a more standardized assessment of blood pressure. The AOBP method has multiple preprogrammed measurements, each administered at 1- to 2-minute intervals. The first measurement is taken by the nurse to verify cuff position and validity of measurement. The rest of the measurements should be taken while the patient is alone in a quiet room. The average blood pressure displayed on the electronic device, heart rate, arm used, and whether the patient was supine, sitting, or standing should all be recorded. The use of AOPB measurement reduces the risk of white coat hypertension and lowers the prevalence of masked hypertension (Box 31.16).

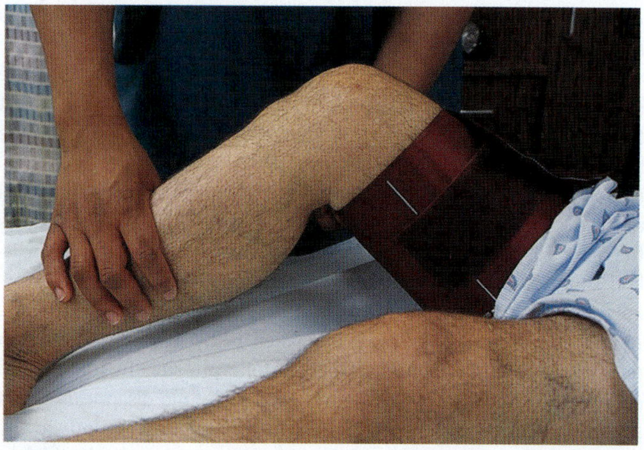

BOX 31.15 PROCEDURAL GUIDELINE
Palpating the Systolic Blood Pressure

Delegation Considerations
The skill of palpation of blood pressure *may not be delegated* to unregulated care providers.

Equipment
- Sphygmomanometer

Procedure
1. Perform hand hygiene.
2. Apply the blood pressure cuff to the patient's extremity selected for measurement.
3. Continually palpate the pulse of the patient's brachial, radial, or popliteal artery with fingertips of one of your hands.
4. Rapidly inflate the blood pressure cuff 30 mm Hg above the point at which the patient's pulse cannot be palpated.
5. Slowly release the valve and deflate the cuff at a rate of 2 to 3 mm Hg per second.
6. Note the manometer reading when the pulse is again palpable; this is the systolic blood pressure.
7. Deflate the cuff rapidly and completely. Remove the cuff from the patient's extremity unless repeat measurement is needed.
8. Perform hand hygiene. Record pressure as "[systolic]/—" and palpated (e.g., "blood pressure 108/—, palpated").

FIGURE 31.18 A lower extremity blood pressure cuff is positioned above the popliteal artery at midthigh with the knee flexed. (Courtesy St. Mary's Health Center. St. Louis, MO.)

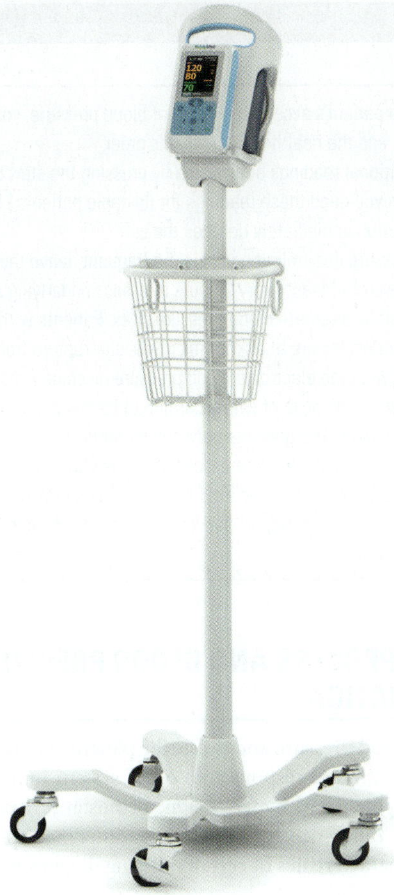

FIGURE 31.19 Automatic blood pressure monitor. (Photo courtesy Welch Allyn, http://www.welchallyn.com)

Automatic devices are easy to use and efficient, and knowledge about how to use a stethoscope is not required. The automated device enables assessment of blood pressure during interpersonal interactions (Figure 31.20). AOBP measurement limits interaction because the patient is alone while the measurements are being taken. The AOBP method can thus decrease the risk of nursing error related to blood pressure measurement.

Self-Measurement of Blood Pressure. More people are measuring their own blood pressure because of improved technology in home-monitoring devices and a greater interest in health promotion. Portable home devices include aneroid sphygmomanometers and the now recommended electronic digital readout devices that do not require use of a stethoscope. The electronic devices inflate and deflate cuffs with the push of a button, and their use minimizes or eliminates many auscultation-induced errors.

Stationary automatic blood pressure devices can be found in public places such as grocery stores, drug stores, fitness clubs, airports, and worksites. Users rest their arm within the machine's inflatable cuff, which contains a pressure sensor. The cuff fits over clothing. A visual display tells users their blood pressure within 60 to 90 seconds. The reliability of the stationary machines is limited. Blood pressure values (both systolic and diastolic) may vary by 5 to 10 mm Hg or more in comparison with values measured by a manual sphygmomanometer.

Self-measurement of blood pressure has several benefits. Elevated blood pressure may be detected in people previously unaware of a health problem. People with high normal blood pressure can provide information about the pattern of blood pressure values. Patients with hypertension can benefit from actively participating in their treatment through self-monitoring, which may subsequently enhance adherence to treatment. Self-monitoring also helps to confirm elevated blood pressure readings related to white coat hypertension (Rabi et al., 2020). The

---

BOX 31.16 PROCEDURAL GUIDELINE

Electronic Blood Pressure Measurement

Delegation Considerations

The task of obtaining an electronic blood pressure measurement can be delegated to an unregulated care provider (UCP) unless the patient is considered unstable or needs close monitoring. The nurse is responsible for assessing the impact of changes in blood pressure; therefore, when the task of obtaining an electronic blood pressure measurement is delegated, it is important to *ensure that the UCP* performs the following tasks:

- Selects appropriate limb for measurement
- Selects appropriate-size cuff for designated limb
- Selects blood pressure cuff recommended by the manufacturer
- Obtains blood pressure measurement for patient with ordered frequency
- Reports abnormalities

Equipment

- Electronic blood pressure machine and blood pressure cuff of appropriate size as recommended by manufacturer

Procedure

1. Determine the appropriateness of using electronic blood pressure measurement. This device is not suitable for use in patients with irregular heart rates, peripheral vascular disease, seizures, tremors, or shivering.

2. Determine the best site for cuff placement. Validated wrist devices can be used on patients with large arm circumferences, in situations where standard arm cuffs cannot be used (Rabi et al., 2020) (see Skill 31.5, Step 2).

3. Select the appropriate cuff size for the patient's extremity and appropriate cuff for machine. The electronic blood pressure cuff and machine are matched by the manufacturer and are not interchangeable.

4. Assist patient to a comfortable position, either lying or sitting. Plug in the device and place it near the patient, ensuring that the connector hose between the cuff and machine will reach the patient.

5. Prepare blood pressure cuff by manually squeezing all air out of the cuff and connecting the cuff to the connector hose.

6. Turn on the machine to enable the device to perform a self-test on internal computer systems.

7. Expose the patient's extremity for measurement by removing restrictive clothing, to ensure proper cuff application. Do not place blood pressure cuff over clothing.

8. Wrap flattened cuff snugly around the patient's extremity, verifying that only one finger fits between the cuff and the patient's skin. Make sure the "artery" arrow marked on the outside of the cuff is correctly placed.

Electronic Blood Pressure Measurement

9. Verify that the connector hose between the cuff and machine is not kinked. Kinking prevents proper inflation and deflation of the cuff.
10. In accordance with manufacturer's directions, set the frequency control to automatic or manual, and then press "start" button. The first blood pressure measurement will pump the cuff to a pressure of about 180 mm Hg. After this pressure is reached, the machine begins a deflation sequence that helps measure the blood pressure. The first reading is the peak pressure inflation for additional measurements.
11. When deflation is complete, the digital display provides the most recent values and flashes time (in minutes) that has elapsed since measurement occurred (see Figure 31.20).
12. Set the frequency of blood pressure measurements and upper and lower alarm limits for systolic, diastolic, and mean blood pressure readings. Intervals between blood pressure measurements can be set from 1 to 90 minutes. Determine measurement frequency and alarm limits on the basis of the patient's acceptable range of blood pressure, your nursing judgement, and the health care provider's order.
13. Obtain additional readings at any time by pressing the start button. (Sometimes you need these readings for unstable patients.) Pressing the "cancel" button immediately deflates the cuff.
14. If blood pressure determinations must be frequent, leave the cuff in place. Remove the cuff at least every 2 hours to assess underlying skin integrity, and, if possible, alternate blood pressure sites. Patients with abnormal bleeding tendencies are at risk for microvascular rupture from repeated inflations. When the electronic blood pressure machine is no longer needed, clean or dispose of cuff according to facility policy, to reduce transmission of microorganisms between patients.
15. Record blood pressure and site assessed on the vital sign flow sheet or in nurses' notes. Record associated signs of blood pressure alterations in nurses' progress notes. Report abnormal findings to the nurse in charge or health care provider.

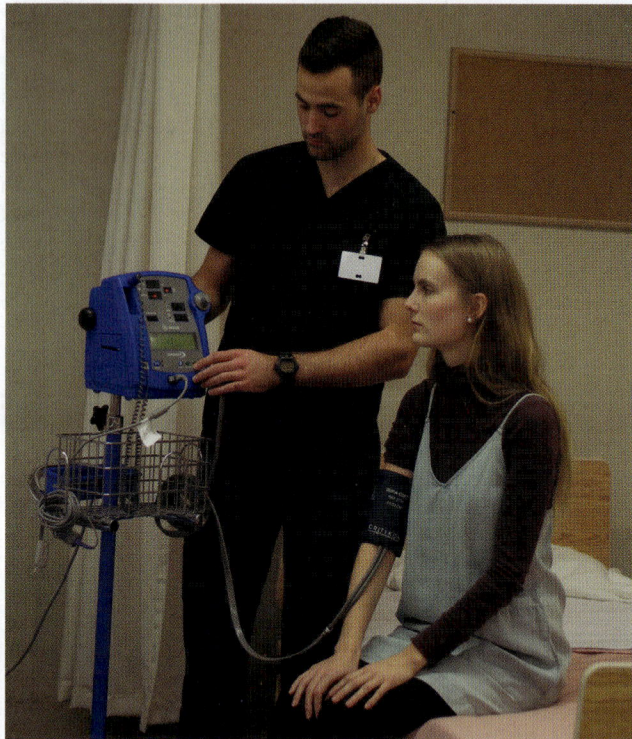

FIGURE 31.20 Taking an electronic blood pressure measurement. (Courtesy Barbara J. Astle, RN, PhD.)

disadvantages of self-measurement include improper use of the device and inaccurate readings. A patient may be needlessly alarmed by one elevated reading. Patients with hypertension may become overly conscious of their blood pressure and inappropriately adjust medication intake.

Patients can learn to use self-measurement devices if they have the information needed to perform the procedure correctly and know when to seek medical attention. Patients should be advised that because of possible inaccuracies in the blood pressure devices, they must not adjust their medication regimens without consulting the health care provider. It is important to teach patients the meaning and implications of readings and ensure understanding of proper measurement techniques.

NURSING PROCESS AND BLOOD PRESSURE DETERMINATION

In assessing blood pressure and pulse, the patient's general state of cardiovascular health and responses to other system imbalances can be evaluated. Hypotension, hypertension, orthostatic hypotension, and narrow (small difference) or wide (large difference) pulse pressures are defining characteristics of certain nursing diagnoses, including the following:

- *Activity intolerance*
- *Anxiety*
- *Decreased cardiac output*
- *Deficient/excess fluid volume*
- *Risk for injury*
- *Acute pain*
- *Ineffective tissue perfusion*

The nursing care plan includes interventions specific for the nursing diagnosis identified and the related factors. For example, the defining characteristics of hypotension, dizziness, pulse deficit, and dysrhythmia lead to a diagnosis of *decreased cardiac output*. Related factors may include poor oral intake, excessive heat exposure, and a history of valvular heart disease. The related factor guides the choice of nursing interventions. The nurse evaluates patient outcomes by assessing the blood pressure after each intervention.

HEALTH PROMOTION AND VITAL SIGNS

The emphasis on health promotion and health maintenance, as well as early discharge from hospital settings, has resulted in an increased need for patients and their families to monitor vital signs in the home. The CASN (2022) also underlines the importance of health teaching in its statement that baccalaureate nursing graduates should have "the ability to counsel and educate patients to promote health, symptom and disease management" (p. 13). Therefore, teaching regarding all vital sign measurements in order to promote and maintain health should be incorporated within the patient's plan of care (Box 31.17). In addition, when teaching patients and their families about vital sign measurements, caregivers must be aware of changes that are unique to older persons. Box 31.18 identifies some of these variations.

BOX 31.17 ♥ FOCUS ON PRIMARY HEALTH CARE

Health Promotion and Vital Signs

Temperature
- Identify the patient's ability to initiate preventive health care and recognize alteration in body temperature. Educate the patient and caregiver about ways to prevent body temperature alterations.
- Teach the patient risk factors for hypothermia and frostbite: fatigue; malnutrition; hypoxemia; cold, wet clothing; and alcohol intoxication.
- Teach the patient risk factors for heat stroke: strenuous exercise in hot, humid weather; sudden exposure to hot climates; insufficient fluid intake before, during, and after exercise.
- Teach the patient the importance of taking and continuing to take antibiotics as directed until the course of treatment is completed (e.g., to decrease chance of resurgence of infection or the development of antibiotic-resistant organisms).

Pulse Rate
- Patients taking certain cardiac medications need to learn to assess their own pulse rates to detect adverse effects.
- Patients undergoing cardiac rehabilitation need to learn to assess their own pulse rates to determine their response to exercise.

Blood Pressure
- Patients with a family history of hypertension are at significant risk for hypertension. Teach risk factors for hypertension: obesity, cigarette smoking, heavy alcohol consumption, high blood cholesterol and triglyceride levels, and continued exposure to stress.
- Patients with hypertension need to learn about their blood pressure values, long-term follow-up care and therapy, the lack of obvious symptoms indicative of high blood pressure, the ability of therapy to control but not cure hypertension, and benefits of consistently following the treatment plan.

- Teach patient the importance of using an appropriate-sized blood pressure cuff and recommend electronic measurement for home use.
- Instruct the patient or primary caregiver to measure blood pressure at the same time each day and after the patient has had a brief rest. Patients should measure blood pressure while sitting or lying down, and they should use the same position and arm each time they measure pressure.
- Recommend electronic measurement of blood pressure, but if auscultation is all that is available, instruct the patient or primary caregiver that if it is difficult to hear the pressure, the cuff may be too loose, not big enough, or too narrow; the stethoscope is not over the arterial pulse; the cuff was deflated too quickly or too slowly; or the cuff was not pumped high enough for systolic readings.

Respirations
- Patients who demonstrate decreased ventilation benefit from learning deep-breathing and coughing exercises (see Chapter 49 for further information about care of surgical patients).
- Instruct the patient or caregiver to contact the community care nurse or health care provider if unusual fluctuations in respiratory rate occur.
- Teach the patient signs and symptoms of hypoxemia: headache, somnolence, confusion, dusky colour of skin and mucous membranes, shortness of breath, and dyspnea.
- Teach patient the effect of high-risk behaviours on respiratory function, such as cigarette smoking and environmental pollutants.
- When considering how to teach patients and their families about vital sign measurements and their importance and significance, the patient's age is an important factor (see Box 31.18 for factors to consider in measuring and interpreting vital signs in older persons).

BOX 31.18 FOCUS ON OLDER PERSONS

Vital Signs

Temperature
- Normal body temperature ranges from 36°C to 36.8°C orally and 36.6°C to 37.2°C rectally. Temperatures considered to be within normal range sometimes reflect a fever in an older person.
- Because of sensorineural changes in thermoregulation, older persons have a diminished awareness of temperature changes, which may impair their behavioural and thermoregulatory responses to dangerously or low environmental temperatures and put them at greater risk for hyperthermia and hypothermia (Touhy et al., 2019, p. 195).
- Sweat gland reactivity decreases in older persons; as a result, sweating may not occur until temperatures are very high, leading to hyperthermia and heatstroke.
- Loss of subcutaneous fat reduces the insulating capacity of the skin; older men are at especially high risk for hypothermia.
- For older persons, the nurse must be especially attentive to subtle temperature changes and other manifestations of fever, such as tachypnea, anorexia, falls, delirium, and decline in overall function.

Pulse Rate
- If it is difficult to palpate the pulse of an older person or a patient with obesity, a Doppler device provides a more accurate reading.
- In older persons, it takes longer for the pulse rate to rise to meet sudden increased demands that result from stress, illness, or excitement. Once elevated, the pulse rate of an older person takes longer to return to normal resting rate (Touhy et al., 2019, p. 75).
- Heart sounds are sometimes muffled or difficult to hear in older persons because of an increase in air space in the lungs.

Blood Pressure
- In older persons with decreased upper arm mass, blood pressure cuff size must be selected especially carefully.

- Blood pressure measurement is more variable and fluctuates more in response to other factors, such as postural changes, making accurate assessment difficult (Miller, 2019).
- Owing to a combination of age-related changes and risk factors, orthostatic hypertension and postprandial hypotension are conditions that often happen in older persons. *Postprandial hypotension* is defined as a drop of 20 mm Hg in systolic blood pressure after eating. Assessing for these conditions will help to reduce the incidence of syncope, falls, strokes, and other complications (Millar, 2019).
- Instruct older persons to change position slowly and wait after each change before beginning activity, to avoid orthostatic hypotension and to prevent injuries.

Respirations
- Aging causes ossification of costal cartilage and causes the ribs to slant downward, which results in more rigidity of the rib cage, which in turn reduces chest wall expansion. Kyphosis and scoliosis that can occur in older persons restrict chest expansion and decrease tidal volume.
- Older persons depend more on accessory abdominal muscles during respiration than on weaker thoracic muscles.
- The respiratory system matures by the time a person reaches the age of 20 and then begins to decline. Despite this decline, older persons are able to perform customary life activities with little or no effort under usual conditions. Sudden events that increase demand for oxygen (e.g., stress, exercise, illness) may cause a respiratory deficit to become evident in the older person (Touhy et al., 2019, p. 76).
- Identifying an acceptable site for the pulse oximeter probe may be difficult in older persons because of the likelihood of peripheral vascular disease, decreased cardiac output, cold-induced vasoconstriction, and anemia.

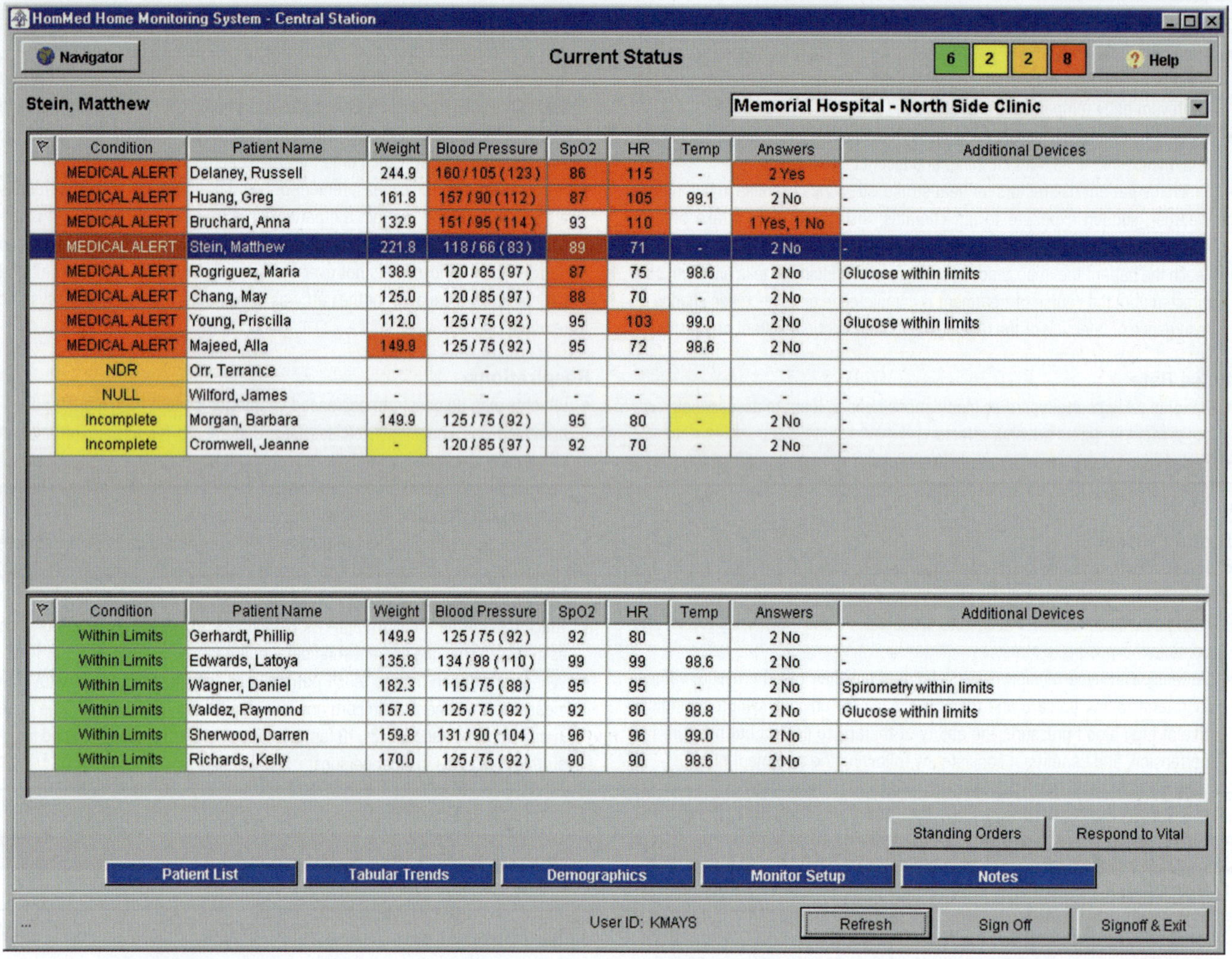

HomMed Home Monitoring System - Central Station

Navigator | Current Status | 6 | 2 | 2 | 8 | Help

Stein, Matthew | Memorial Hospital - North Side Clinic

Condition	Patient Name	Weight	Blood Pressure	SpO2	HR	Temp	Answers	Additional Devices
MEDICAL ALERT	Delaney, Russell	244.9	160 / 105 (123)	86	115	-	2 Yes	-
MEDICAL ALERT	Huang, Greg	161.8	157 / 90 (112)	87	105	99.1	2 No	-
MEDICAL ALERT	Bruchard, Anna	132.9	151 / 95 (114)	93	110	-	1 Yes, 1 No	-
MEDICAL ALERT	Stein, Matthew	221.8	118 / 66 (83)	89	71	-	2 No	-
MEDICAL ALERT	Rogriguez, Maria	138.9	120 / 85 (97)	87	75	98.6	2 No	Glucose within limits
MEDICAL ALERT	Chang, May	125.0	120 / 85 (97)	88	70	-	2 No	-
MEDICAL ALERT	Young, Priscilla	112.0	125 / 75 (92)	95	103	99.0	2 No	Glucose within limits
MEDICAL ALERT	Majeed, Alla	149.9	125 / 75 (92)	95	72	98.6	2 No	-
NDR	Orr, Terrance	-	-	-	-	-	-	-
NULL	Wilford, James	-	-	-	-	-	-	-
Incomplete	Morgan, Barbara	149.9	125 / 75 (92)	95	80	-	2 No	-
Incomplete	Cromwell, Jeanne	-	120 / 85 (97)	92	70	-	2 No	-

Condition	Patient Name	Weight	Blood Pressure	SpO2	HR	Temp	Answers	Additional Devices
Within Limits	Gerhardt, Phillip	149.9	125 / 75 (92)	92	80	-	2 No	-
Within Limits	Edwards, Latoya	135.8	134 / 98 (110)	99	99	98.6	2 No	-
Within Limits	Wagner, Daniel	182.3	115 / 75 (88)	95	95	-	2 No	Spirometry within limits
Within Limits	Valdez, Raymond	157.8	125 / 75 (92)	92	80	98.8	2 No	Glucose within limits
Within Limits	Sherwood, Darren	159.8	131 / 90 (104)	96	96	99.0	2 No	-
Within Limits	Richards, Kelly	170.0	125 / 75 (92)	90	90	98.6	2 No	-

Standing Orders | Respond to Vital

Patient List | Tabular Trends | Demographics | Monitor Setup | Notes

User ID: KMAYS | Refresh | Sign Off | Signoff & Exit

FIGURE 31.21 Image of an electronic medical record of vital signs. (From http://www.aaronnursing.com/Telehealth.asp)

Recording Vital Signs

Measurements of vital signs can be recorded on graphic flow sheets (and/or in progress notes) or, in some institutions, using electronic medical records (EMR) (Figure 31.21). Improved patient safety and decreased medication errors in practice have been noted with the use of information systems such as the EMR (Gardner & Jones, 2012). It is important to identify institutional procedures for documenting and to remember that timely documentation is critical. In one study, nurses who memorized the vital signs because they did not have time to document them in the patient's electronic or paper record or interim paper notes created additional errors, compromised the data, and potentially jeopardized the safety of the patient (Yeung et al., 2012). In addition to the actual vital sign values, it is important to record in the progress notes any accompanying or precipitating symptoms, such as chest pain and dizziness with abnormal blood pressure, shortness of breath with abnormal respiration, cyanosis with hypoxemia, or flushing and diaphoresis with elevated temperature. Any interventions initiated as a result of abnormal vital sign measurements should be documented, such as administration of oxygen therapy or an antihypertensive medication.

For patients for whom critical paths or care maps are used, vital sign values may be listed as outcomes (see Chapter 14 for further information about nursing assessments). If a vital sign value is higher or lower than the anticipated outcomes, a variance note should be written to explain the nature of the variance and the nurse's course of action. For example, a care map for a patient who has undergone a thoracotomy may list a postoperative outcome of "afebrile." If the patient has a fever, the nurse's variance note addresses possible sources of fever (e.g., retained pulmonary secretions) and nursing interventions (e.g., increased suctioning, postural drainage, or hydration).

KEY CONCEPTS

- Vital sign measurement includes the physiological measurement of temperature, pulse, blood pressure, respiration, and oxygen saturation.
- Vital signs are measured as part of either a complete physical examination or a review of a patient's condition.
- Changes in vital signs are evaluated with other physical assessment findings; a critical decision point is used to determine frequency of measurement.
- Knowledge of the factors influencing vital signs assists in determining and evaluating abnormal values.
- Vital signs provide a basis for evaluating the response to nursing and medical interventions.

- Vital signs should be measured when the patient is inactive and the environment is controlled for comfort.
- Patients should be assisted in maintaining body temperature by interventions that promote heat loss, production, or conservation.
- A fever is one of the body's normal defence mechanisms.
- Measurement of temperature with the temporal artery is the least invasive, most accurate method of obtaining core temperature.
- Respiratory assessment includes determining the effectiveness of ventilation, perfusion, and diffusion.
- Assessment of respiration involves observing ventilatory movements through the respiratory cycle.
- Variables affecting ventilation, perfusion, and diffusion influence oxygen saturation.
- Heart rate and rhythm, measured at the radial or apical pulses, are documented to assess cardiac function. Hypertension is diagnosed immediately if the mean of electronic measurement is systolic blood pressure ≥180 mm Hg and/or diastolic blood pressure ≥110 mm Hg; however, if the electronic measurement mean is lower than these but is still considered high, additional out-of-office measurements are required for diagnosis (Rabi et al., 2020).
- Hypertension Canada (Rabi et al., 2020) encourages the use of validated electronic digital oscillometric devices over auscultation for blood pressure measurement.
- Improperly selecting the blood pressure cuff size and improperly applying the blood pressure cuff results in measurement errors.
- Changes in one vital sign often influence characteristics of the other vital signs.

CRITICAL THINKING EXERCISES

1. A 74-year-old patient living in a long-term residential care facility has had an in-dwelling urinary catheter inserted for the past week to help pass urine. When an unregulated care provider (UCP) was emptying the urine collection bag, they noticed the urine was cloudy with sediment and had a foul odour. The resident also reported "I feel chills" to the UCP. The UCP reported these findings to the nurse in charge.
   a. As the nurse in charge, what would be the appropriate course of action?
   b. The resident's vital signs are as follows: temperature 38.0°C (oral), blood pressure 100/74 mm Hg, heart rate 88 beats per minute, and SpO$_2$ is 95% on room air. Based on the resident's current vital signs and their physical signs and symptoms, should the nurse be concerned?
   c. What would be the next appropriate nursing action?
2. A patient is visiting the health clinic for a routine physical examination by the nurse practitioner. The unregulated care provider obtains the following vital sign measurements: tympanic temperature, 36.9°C; right radial heart rate, 96 beats per minute and irregular; blood pressure, sitting, right arm, 162/82 mm Hg, and left arm, 150/70 mm Hg; SpO$_2$, 95% on room air; respiratory rate, 22 breaths per minute.
   a. As the admitting nurse, what questions would you ask this patient to evaluate their risk for hypertension?
   b. On the basis of these vital sign measurements, what actions should you take?
3. A parent brings their child into the care centre and notes that the child has been fussy, has not had much of an appetite, and is "not their active self." The child is crying and struggling to get out of the parent's lap during the interview. You note that the child is small for their age but their physical development appears normal.
   a. Describe the sequence you would use for obtaining vital signs.

   b. When you select the appropriate equipment for measuring the vital signs, what, if any, special considerations are needed?
   c. The unregulated care provider reports they have obtained a temperature reading of 37.7°C. What additional information do you request from the unregulated care provider?
4. A patient is admitted to the medical unit for chronic dyspnea and discomfort in their left chest with deep breathing and coughing. The patient has been smoking for 35 years and has a 20-year history of emphysema. Over the past 4 months, the patient has lost 4.5 kg and currently weighs 50 kg.
   a. When delegating the measurement of vital signs to an unregulated care provider, what information and directions should you provide?
   b. The blood pressure and heart rate are within acceptable ranges. The temperature is 37.5°C, obtained with an oral electronic thermometer; the respiratory rate is 32 breaths per minute and shallow; and the SpO$_2$ is 89%. On the basis of these results, list your actions in priority order.
5. A woman arrives at the prenatal clinic for her first visit. She is 8 months pregnant. The unregulated care provider assesses her vital signs, height, and weight. The patient weighs 104 kg and is 160 cm tall; blood pressure in her right arm is 210/92 mm Hg; her heart rate is 104 beats per minute; her respiratory rate is 24 breaths per minute; her tympanic temperature is 37.1°C. You are concerned about the patient's blood pressure. In repeating the measurement, you obtain 148/86 mm Hg in the right arm and 144/84 mm Hg in the left arm.
   a. What blood pressure measurement should be recorded? Provide some possible explanations for the difference between your measurements.
   b. What explanation about the abnormal vital signs will you share with the patient?
   c. What will be included in your discharge teaching?

🌐 *Answers to Critical Thinking Exercises appear on the Evolve website.*

REVIEW QUESTIONS

Review Questions 1 to 6 relate to the case study presented at the beginning of the chapter. Review Questions 7 to 11 are vital signs review questions.

1. In the case study, Johnathan's heart rhythm is referred to as:
   a. Dysrhythmia
   b. Tachycardia
   c. Bradycardia
   d. Regularly irregular rhythm
2. Choose the most likely options for the information missing from the statements below by selecting from the list of options provided. The ED nurse recognizes that Johnathan's _____1_____ and _____1_____ are symptoms that would require an immediate attention. The most likely cause of these symptoms is _____2_____.

Answer Options for 1
a. Temperature
b. Blood pressure
c. Heart rate
d. Respiratory rate
e. SpO$_2$ level
f. Spouse's worry and agitation
g. Johnathan's difficulty with ambulation

Answer Options for 2
a. Hypertension
b. Johnathan's anxiety
c. COVID-19 virus (SARS-CoV-2)
d. Stress at work
e. Temperature
f. SpO$_2$ level

3. Given Johnathan's presenting conditions to ED, which of the following nursing actions would be the priority? *(Select all that apply.)*
   a. Auscultate his lungs
   b. Administer supplemental oxygen as per prescription of health care provider or according to the institution's protocol on oxygen therapy.
   c. Provide verbal assurance.
   d. Ask Johnathan to slow down his respiratory rate.
   e. Continue to monitor Johnathan's SpO$_2$ level
   f. Administer a β-blocker.
   g. Administer antihypertensive medication.

4. Should the nurse be concerned about Johnathan's temperature of 38.2°C? Use an X for the nursing actions listed below to indicate which ones are indicated (appropriate or necessary), which ones are contraindicated (could be harmful), or which ones are nonessential (makes no difference or not necessary) for Johnathan's care at this time.

Nursing Action	Indicated	Contra-indicated	Non-essential
a. Check the health care provider's order for the prescription of antipyretics.			
b. Immediately administer an antipyretic before blood culture is collected.			
c. Administer an antipyretic after blood culture has been collected, if ordered.			
d. Apply a cold cloth to Johnathan's forehead.			
e. Monitor Johnathan's temperature following the administration of an antipyretic.			

5. The contributing factors for Johnathan's heart rate on presentation to the ED would include _____, _____, and _____.
   Answer options:
   a. Antihypertensive medication he took earlier in the day
   b. Anxiety related to dyspnea
   c. Dyspnea
   d. Fever
   e. Pain

6. SARS-CoV-2 is a type of coronavirus (commonly known as COVID-19) that is responsible for the onset of the pandemic in 2019. Which of the following factors associated with SARS-CoV-2 would contribute to the clinical picture of the disease? *(Select all that apply.)*
   a. SARS-CoV-2 virus is transmitted only from touching parts of human body.

b. SARS-CoV-2 virus is transmitted by person-to-person close contact.
c. The primary mode of transmission is via respiratory droplets.
d. SARS-CoV-2 causes pathological changes in the lung and contribute to severe pneumonia.
e. All individuals infected with SARS-CoV-2 have fever.

7. During a nursing assessment the nurse notes that the patient has a pulse deficit. A pulse deficit is the difference between the _____ and _____. Choose from the options below.
   Answer options:
   a. Apical pulse and systolic pressure
   b. Radial and apical pulses
   c. Radial and ulnar pulses
   d. Systolic and diastolic pressures

8. The nurse has decided to hold the scheduled metoprolol to an adult patient after the morning assessment that is documented below. Place a check mark by the assessment that would have led to the decision. *(Select all that apply.)*
   _____ a. Heart rate 54 beats per minute
   _____ b. Respiratory rate 18 breaths per minute
   _____ c. Blood pressure 98/56 mmHg
   _____ d. Patient reported, "I'm feeling a little dizzy this morning."

9. A 55-year-old patient returns from the post-anaesthesia care unit after a left total hip replacement. During surgery they had an epidural and regional anaesthesia. The nurse takes the patient's vital signs and documents the following.
   ___ a. Temperature: 36.3ºC
   ___ b. Heart rate: 120 beats per minute
   ___ c. Blood pressure: 96/52 mmHg
   ___ d. Respiratory rate: 24 beats per minute
   ___ e. SpO$_2$ 95%
   Highlight or put a check mark beside the vital signs that require follow-up, either in the form of an ongoing assessment of this vital sign, or with the physician.

10. Which of the following conditions could increase a respiratory rate? *(Select all that apply.)*
    a. Opioids
    b. Brainstem injury
    c. Smoking
    d. Anxiety
    e. Pain
    f. A low hemoglobin

11. When measuring oxygen saturation, the nurse recalls that some of the following factors can influence the measurement and lead to inaccurate results. Which of the following assessments would have led to the erroneous measurement? *(Select all that apply.)*
    a. Rapid heart rate
    b. Reduced circulation to extremities
    c. Nail polish, artificial fingernails
    d. Decreased respiratory depth and effort
    e. Bright light near the measurement site

Answers: 1. b; **2.** Option 1—d, e; Option 2—c; **3.** a, b, c, e; **4.** Indicated: a, c, e; Contraindicated: b; Nonessential: d; **5.** b, c, d; **6.** b, c, d; **7.** b; **8.** a, d; **9.** b, c, d; **10.** c, d, e, f; **11.** a, b, c, e.

🌐 *Rationales for the Review Questions appear on the Evolve website.*

RECOMMENDED WEBSITES

British Columbia Ministry of Health Services, Guidelines and Protocols Advisory Committee (GPAC): Hypertension—Detection and Management: https://www2.gov.bc.ca/gov/content/health/practitioner-professional-resources/bc-guidelines/hypertension?keyword=hypertension

Part of the British Columbia Ministry of Health Services, the Guidelines and Protocols Advisory Committee developed several documents to recommend proper blood pressure management, including the recommended technique for measuring blood pressure. Other topics are home blood pressure monitoring, dietary approaches, and a patient guide.

Government of Canada: Heart Diseases and Conditions: https://www.canada.ca/en/public-health/services/publications/diseases-conditions/heart-disease-canada.html

This web page, part of the website of the Public Health Agency of Canada, provides links to a variety of Canadian resources on cardiovascular health, including the Canadian Association of Cardiovascular Prevention and Rehabilitation, the Canadian Stroke Strategy, Heart and Stroke Foundation of Canada, and the Canadian Stroke Network.

Heart & Stroke Foundation of Canada: https://www.heartandstroke.ca
This website provides information about stroke and heart disease.

Hypertension Canada: https://hypertension.ca
This website offers information on hypertension to health care providers and the public. The mission of Hypertension Canada is to advance health through the prevention and control of high blood pressure and its complications. Hypertension Canada is a volunteer, nonprofit hypertension education program that provides annually updated, relevant, evidence-informed hypertension guidance. All sites provide educational tools.

REFERENCES

A full reference list is available on the website for this book at http://evolve.elsevier.com/Canada/Potter/fundamentals/

32

Pain Assessment and Management

Canadian content written by Monakshi Sawhney, NP (Adult), BScN, MN, PhD, and Brenda L. Martelli, RN(EC), BScN, BEd, MEd, with original chapter contributions by Angela Renee Starkweather, PhD, ACNP-BC, FAAN

OBJECTIVES

Mastery of content in this chapter will enable you to:

- Define the key terms listed.
- Describe common misconceptions about pain.
- Describe the physiology of pain.
- Identify components of the pain experience.
- Explain how the physiology of pain relates to selecting interventions for pain relief.
- Describe the components of pain assessment.
- Perform an assessment of a patient experiencing pain.
- Explain how cultural factors influence the pain experience.
- Describe the appropriate nursing diagnoses, outcomes, and interventions for a patient with pain.
- Describe guidelines for selecting and individualizing pain interventions.
- Explain the various pharmacological approaches to treating pain.
- Describe applications of nonpharmacological pain interventions.
- Describe nursing implications for administering analgesics.
- Identify barriers to effective pain management.
- Evaluate a patient's response to pain interventions.

KEY TERMS

Acupuncture
Acute pain
Addiction
Adjuvants
Anaesthetics
Analgesics
Biofeedback
Breakthrough pain
Chordotomy
Chronic pain
Cutaneous stimulation
Dorsal rhizotomy
Drug tolerance

Epidural analgesia
Epidural space
Guided imagery
Local anaesthesia
Modulation
Nociception
Nociplastic pain
Opioids
Pain
Pain threshold
Pain tolerance level
Patient-controlled analgesia (PCA)
Perception

Persistent postoperative pain (PPP)
Physical dependence
Placebo
Regional anaesthesia
Reiki
Relaxation
Therapeutic touch
Transcutaneous electrical nerve stimulation (TENS)
Transduction
Transmission

🌐 WEBSITE

http://evolve.elsevier.com/Canada/Potter/fundamentals/

CASE STUDY

As a nurse, your patient assignment includes a 6-kg ex-premature infant, Sam, who is now 47 weeks corrected age. Sam has undergone a laparotomy for a bowel anastomosis. How would you optimally manage their pain?

The anaesthesiologist and pain service have opted for nurse-controlled analgesia (NCA) with a basal infusion of morphine 20 mcg/kg/hr, with the ability to offer breakthrough doses of 0.04 mg/kg/dose every 20 minutes as needed. This is beneficial because the breakthrough dose is available immediately at the bedside and can be timed to manage a potentially painful intervention. For instance, if Sam needed to be repositioned or if the parents wanted to hold their infant, an NCA dose

could be administered pre-emptively prior to the infant's movement. Nonsteroidal anti-inflammatory drugs are contraindicated with this patient; however, Tylenol IV can be used on a scheduled basis × 48 hours with reassessment. Adjuncts such as acetaminophen will be opioid-sparing in this case.

Although interprofessional care is optimal for pain assessment and management, nurses (RNs, LPNs, and RPNs) play an integral role because they provide care around the clock.

Think about this case study as you read this chapter. There are review questions at the end of the chapter that relate to the case study.

Pain assessment and management is a process that is multidimensional in nature. Pain assessment can be challenging because of the inconsistent use of validated pain tools, leading to suboptimal pain management in some cases. Also, despite being a commonly occurring symptom that is experienced even by premature infants, pain is not well understood and is inconsistently and inadequately addressed. Given the complex and dynamic nature of pain, it is imperative to utilize a systematic approach for both assessment and management of pain (Brand & Al-Rais, 2019). The above case study provides a framework for further discussion and application, taking into consideration the unique specifications for the pediatric population.

Pain is a common reason why people seek health care. In 2020, the International Association for the Study of Pain (IASP) defined **pain** as "an unpleasant sensory and emotional experience associated with, or resembling that associated with, actual or potential tissue damage" (Raja et al., 2020). The updated definition is supported by six additional key concepts:

1. Pain is a personal experience and is influenced by biological, psychological, and social factors.
2. Pain is more than a neurological response (i.e., experienced through the activity of sensory neurons).
3. An individual's understanding of pain changes over the lifespan.
4. Clinicians need to respect the individual's experience of pain and be cognizant of patient's cultural and linguistic diversities (Bostick et al., 2021).
5. Pain can be a catalyst for adaptation, but it can also have negative effects on function and social and psychological well-being.
6. There are many ways to express pain (verbal and behavioural) (Raja et al., 2020).

Using this new definition, health care providers need to expand how they assess and manage pain to include individualized physiological and psychological interventions. Pain is a highly subjective experience; hence it is best described by the person experiencing it. This concept has endured for more than 40 years, when McCaffery first coined the "self-report" concept. Self-report is the preferred measurement for pain (Birnie et al., 2019).

Almost all acute and cancer pain can be relieved, and most patients with chronic noncancer pain achieve pain control. Treatment of pain is deemed to be a basic human right (Canadian Pain Society, 2020). The Canadian Pain Coalition (2002) has further delineated patients' rights regarding pain to include the right to have one's pain reports taken seriously, to receive compassionate care, and to be allowed to actively participate in one's own treatment. Furthermore, patients should have timely access to care, have follow-up with reassessment of their pain, and be provided information that allows them to give consent to appropriate treatments. Yet, in Canada, acute pain in hospitalized infants, children, and adults continues to be undermanaged.

Nurses are ethically responsible for promoting the health and well-being of individuals, families, and communities in their care; this includes assessing and managing pain through the use of appropriate, evidence-informed measures in order to improve patient outcomes (Canadian Nurses Association, 2017). Responsive, evidence-informed pain management can reduce pain and improve quality of life. Effective pain management promotes earlier mobilization and return to work and school, resulting in fewer hospital and clinic visits, shortened hospital stays, and reduced overall health care costs.

SCIENTIFIC KNOWLEDGE BASE

Pain is part of the human experience and, as noted above, is one of the most common reasons for individuals seeking medical care (Alles & Smith, 2018). In the past, pain was viewed simply as a symptom of an illness or condition. Pain is now understood to be complex and affected by physical, psychological, biological, and social factors. Moreover, while chronic pain can develop from an injury or disease process, it is no longer thought to be strictly a symptom but is a disease process within itself (Mills et al., 2019). The Canadian Pain Task Force (2021) has deemed chronic pain to be a disease, and it has now been listed in by the World Health Organization (WHO) as a diagnostic classification in the *International Classification of Diseases* (11th revision) (WHO, 2019).

Nature of Pain

Pain is more than a physical sensation caused by a specific stimulus. An individual's perception of pain includes affective (emotional), cognitive, behavioural, and sensory components that are shaped by past experience, culture, and situational factors. The nature of the stimulus for pain can be physical, psychological, or a combination of both.

Physiology of Pain

Pain is a multifaceted experience that involves both the peripheral and central nervous systems. Pain can be classified by its inferred pathophysiology: nociceptive (physiological) pain or neuropathic pain. *Nociceptive pain* is the experience of pain that represents a fundamental physiological process that signals actual or potential tissue damage (Alles & Smith, 2018). It involves the neural processing of noxious stimuli that occurs when nociceptors (pain-sensing nerves) are activated by tissue damage or inflammation (Beck et al., 2019). *Neuropathic pain* involves the abnormal processing of stimuli due to a lesion or disease of the somatosensory nervous system (Alles & Smith, 2018). This processing can cause alterations in the normal sensory signalling at the level of the periphery, spinal cord, and brain.

Nociception has four specific processes: transduction, transmission, perception, and modulation (Ringkamp et al., 2018). Patients in pain cannot discriminate among these four processes. However, understanding them will help you as a nurse to recognize factors that can cause pain, symptoms that accompany pain, and the rationale and actions of a selected treatment plan.

The first process involved in nociception is **transduction**. When tissue cells are damaged by either thermal stimuli (e.g., burn), mechanical stimuli (e.g., cut), or chemical stimuli (e.g., chemotherapy), the damaged cells release pain-sensitizing and inflammatory substances, including prostaglandins, bradykinin, histamine, prostaglandins, serotonin, and substance P (Box 32.1). These substances activate nociceptors, resulting in transduction, or the generation of electrical activity in peripheral terminals (an action potential) (Ringkamp et al., 2018).

In the second process, **transmission**, these pain-sensitizing and inflammatory substances surround the pain nerve fibres in the extracellular fluid, creating the spread of the pain message via the afferent peripheral nerve fibres to the dorsal horn of the spinal cord. Within the dorsal horn of the spinal cord, a synaptic transmission from the *afferent* (sensory) peripheral nerve to the spinothalamic tract nerves occurs through a complex neurophysiological and neurochemical mechanism, resulting in the relay of the signal to various higher brain centres (Figure 32.1) (Ringkamp et al., 2018).

Two types of afferent peripheral nerve fibres conduct painful stimuli: the fast, myelinated A-delta fibres, and the very small, slow, unmyelinated C fibres. The A fibres send sharp, localized, and distinct sensations that focus the source of the pain and detect its intensity. The C fibres relay impulses that are poorly localized, burning, and persistent. For example, after stepping on a nail, a person initially feels a sharp, localized pain, which is a result of A-fibre transmission. Within a few seconds, the pain becomes more diffuse and widespread, until the whole foot aches, as a result of C-fibre innervation.

BOX 32.1 Neurophysiology of Pain: Neuroregulators

Neurotransmitters (Excitatory)
Substance P
Found in the pain neurons of the dorsal horn (excitatory peptide)
Needed to transmit pain impulses from the periphery to the higher brain centre
Causes vasodilation and edema

Serotonin
Released from the brainstem and dorsal horn to inhibit pain transmission

Prostaglandins
Generated from the breakdown of phospholipids in cell membranes
Believed to increase sensitivity to pain

Neuromodulators (Inhibitory)
Endorphins and Dynorphins
Function as the body's natural supply of morphine-like substances
Activated by stress and pain
Located within the brain, spinal cord, and gastrointestinal tract
Cause analgesia when they attach to opiate receptors in the brain
Present in higher levels in people who have less pain than others with a similar injury

Bradykinin
Released from plasma that leaks from surrounding blood vessels at the site of tissue injury
Binds to receptors on peripheral nerves, increasing pain stimuli
Binds to cells that cause the chain reaction–producing prostaglandins

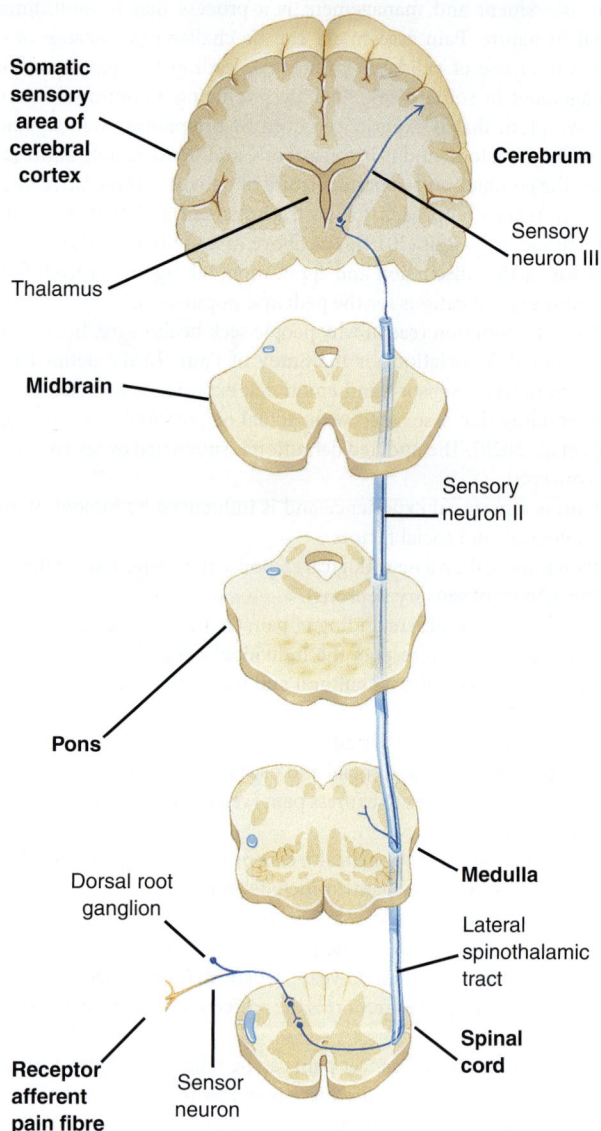

FIGURE 32.2 Spinothalamic pathway that conducts pain stimuli to the brain.

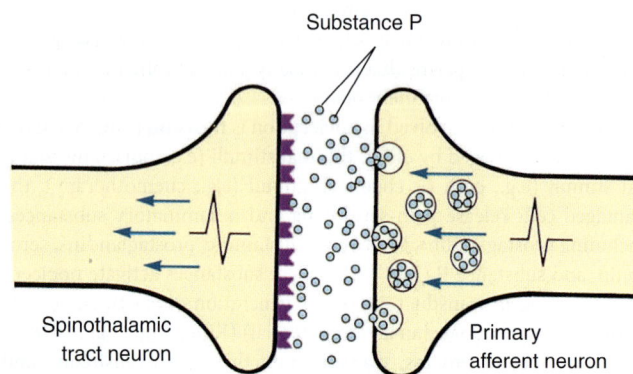

FIGURE 32.1 Substance P and other neurotransmitters are released from primary afferent fibres that terminate in the dorsal horn of the spinal cord. (From Paice, J. A. [1991]. Unraveling the mystery of pain. *Oncology Nursing Forum, 18*[5], 843.)

Pain stimuli continue to travel through nerve fibres in the spinothalamic tracts that cross to the opposite side of the spinal cord. Pain impulses then travel up the spinal cord. Figure 32.2 shows the normal pain reception pathway. After the pain impulse ascends the spinal cord, information is quickly transmitted by the thalamus to higher centres in the brain. These centres include the reticular formation, limbic system, somatosensory cortex, and association cortex. It only takes microseconds for the pain signal to be transmitted from the site of injury to the brain.

Perception, the third nociceptive process, is the conscious awareness of pain. Once a pain stimulus reaches the cerebral cortex, the brain interprets the intensity, quality, and character of the pain, as well as information from past experiences. Psychological, social, spiritual, and cultural associations are also involved in processing the perception of the pain. The somatosensory cortex identifies the location and intensity of the pain, and the association cortex determines how we feel about the pain. Cells within the limbic system are believed to control emotion, particularly anxiety. Thus, the limbic system may play an active role in processing the emotional reaction to pain and the memory of the pain experience. However, the human ability to experience and remember pain does not depend on *cognitive ability* (explicit memory). The experience of pain is remembered by even the youngest of infants, including those born prematurely.

As a person becomes aware of pain, a complex reaction unfolds. Psychological and cognitive factors interact with neurophysiological factors in the perception of pain. Perception gives awareness and meaning to pain so that a person can then react. The reaction to pain comprises the physiological and behavioural responses that occur after pain is perceived.

Modulation of pain is the final nociceptive phase and refers to the increase or decrease in pain signal intensity that can occur before,

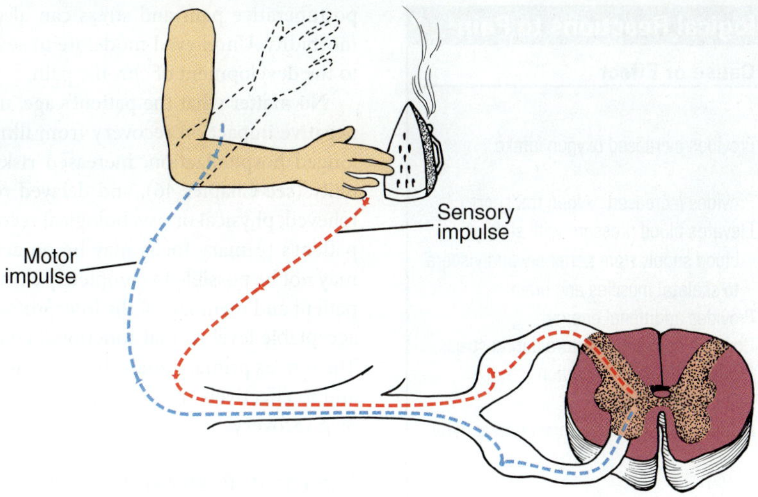

FIGURE 32.3 Protective reflex to pain stimulus.

during, and after pain is perceived. For example, once the brain perceives the pain, inhibitory neurotransmitters are released (see Box 32.1); these include endogenous opioids (endorphins and enkephalins), serotonin, norepinephrine, and gamma aminobutyric acid, which work to hinder the transmission of pain and help produce an analgesic effect.

A protective reflex response may also occur with pain reception (Figure 32.3). A-delta fibres send sensory impulses to the spinal cord, where they synapse with spinal motor neurons. The motor impulses travel via a reflex arc along *efferent* (motor) nerve fibres back to a peripheral muscle near the site of stimulation, thus bypassing the brain. Contraction of the muscle leads to a protective withdrawal from the source of pain. For example, when a person touches a hot iron, a burning sensation is felt, but the hand also reflexively withdraws from the iron's surface. When superficial fibres in the skin are stimulated, a person moves away from the pain source. If internal tissues such as muscle or mucous membranes become stimulated, tightening and guarding of muscles occur. This reflex is usually absent below the injury in patients with spinal cord injuries. However, patients with spinal cord injuries can still experience pain above the level of injury.

Theory of Pain. The gate-control theory, first coined by Melzack and Wall in 1965, introduced the concept that, in addition to the physical sensation of pain, there exist emotional and cognitive dimensions of pain. It was proposed that pain can be transmitted via pain impulses and regulated or even blocked by gating mechanisms located along the central nervous system. The theory suggests that pain impulses pass through when a gate is open and that impulses are blocked when a gate is closed. Closing the gate is the basis for pain-relief interventions. Gating mechanisms can be found in substantia gelatinosa cells within the dorsal horn of the spinal cord, thalamus, and limbic system. Understanding what physiological, emotional, and cognitive processes can influence these gates will help guide your approach as a nurse to pain management. For example, stress, exercise, and other factors increase the release of endorphins, raising an individual's **pain threshold**, or the minimal intensity of a stimulus that is perceived as painful (IASP, 2017). Knowing that the amount of modulating substances varies with each person will help you to understand why pain intensity varies among patients, even for comparable stimuli, and why individuals exhibit different responses to pain.

More recently, researchers have identified neuronal modifiability, or "plasticity," of the nervous system. This refers to the nervous system's

ability to create adaptive changes in response to varied internal and external stimuli (Sasmita et al., 2018). In response to repeated noxious stimuli, or unrelieved pain, neurons develop a memory of the pain. This leads to changes in pain mechanisms in the peripheral and central nervous system, called *peripheral* and *central sensitization*. With central sensitization, dorsal horn spinal cord neurons may become increasingly sensitive and responsive to all stimuli, leading to chronic pain. Thus unrelieved acute pain can lead to chronic pain.

Physiological Responses. As pain impulses ascend the spinal cord toward the brainstem and thalamus, the autonomic nervous system (ANS) becomes stimulated, as part of the stress response (see Chapter 30). Stimulation of the sympathetic branch of the ANS results in physiological responses (Table 32.1). If the pain is continuous, severe, or deep, typically involving the visceral organs (e.g., with a myocardial infarction or colic from gallbladder or renal stones), the parasympathetic nervous system goes into action. Sustained physiological responses to pain could cause serious harm to an individual, such as an altered immune response. However, most people reach a level of adaptation in which physical signs return to normal. Therefore, patients in pain will *not* always have changes in their vital signs. Although nurses need to consider a person's physiological responses to pain, they should avoid using them as a primary indicator of pain.

Behavioural Responses. Once pain is perceived, if it is not managed effectively, a cycle of events begins that can significantly diminish the meaning and quality of a person's life. Pain—especially intense acute pain or chronic pain—is physically and emotionally exhausting and can interfere, short or long term, with the ability to function and engage with others. Anxiety is a common initial response to pain, while depression, irritability, and chronic fatigue often accompany persistent pain. These responses to pain help explain why pain management can be so multifactorial and challenging.

Unrelieved pain affects physical, psychological, social, and spiritual well-being. Patient factors may contribute to unrelieved pain. For example, some patients will endure severe pain without asking for assistance, whereas others may not report pain if they believe their pain may inconvenience others or signals a loss of self-control. To ensure optimal health outcomes and minimize the impact on activities of daily living, it is important to discuss the benefits of using effective pain-management strategies.

TABLE 32.1 Physiological Reactions to Pain

Response	Cause or Effect
Sympathetic Stimulation*	
Dilation of bronchial tubes and increased respiratory rate	Provides increased oxygen intake
Increased heart rate	Provides increased oxygen transport
Peripheral vasoconstriction (pallor, elevation in blood pressure)	Elevates blood pressure with shift of blood supply from periphery and viscera to skeletal muscles and brain
Increased blood glucose level	Provides additional energy
Diaphoresis	Controls body temperature during stress
Increased muscle tension	Prepares muscles for action
Dilation of pupils	Affords better vision
Decreased gastrointestinal motility (nausea, vomiting)	Frees energy for more immediate activity
Parasympathetic Stimulation†	
Pallor	Causes blood supply to shift away from periphery
Muscle tension	Results from fatigue
Decreased heart rate and blood pressure	Results from vagal stimulation
Rapid, irregular breathing	Causes body defences to fail under prolonged stress of pain
Weakness or exhaustion	Results from expenditure of physical energy

*Superficial pain and pain of low to moderate intensity.
†Severe or deep pain.

Nonverbal or behavioural indicators of pain may include body movements, facial expressions, and vocalizations. Bracing, splinting, or protecting the painful part, rocking, body stiffening, jaw clenching, grimacing, frowning, crying, moaning, or screaming may indicate that pain is present. Affective responses can include social withdrawal, changes in eating or sleep patterns, stoicism, fear, anxiety, anger, or feelings of hopelessness. Valid and reliable tools exist to assist in the assessment of pain in people who are unable to self-report their pain. Lack of pain expression does not necessarily mean that a person has no pain. For example, premature and full-term infants sometimes do not cry in response to painful stimuli and they may exhibit few motor movements, especially after excessive and repeated exposure to pain. Similarly, opioids can blunt the behavioural expression of pain by sedating the patient. Yet, the patient who is sedated or sleeping can still be in pain.

Types of Pain

Pain may be categorized by its duration, such as acute and chronic pain; by its pathology, such as cancer pain and noncancer pain (e.g., pain associated with arthritis, diabetic neuropathy, low back pain, and headache); or by the process of action (nociceptive or neuropathic).

Acute Pain. Acute pain usually has an identifiable cause—either somatic, visceral, or nociceptive—and is of short duration (usually less than 3 months). Acute pain has a predictable ending (healing) and an identifiable cause. Eventually it resolves with or without treatment after a damaged area heals. Evidence suggests, however, that unrelieved acute pain may have developmental and age-related consequences. For instance, significant and repeated exposure to acute pain during epochs of rapid early infant brain development may alter an infant's pain response. Untreated or poorly treated intraoperative and postoperative pain and stress can also increase infant mortality and morbidity. Unrelieved moderate to severe postoperative pain can lead to the development of chronic pain.

No matter what the patient's age, unrelieved acute pain can have a negative impact on recovery from illness or surgery, resulting in prolonged hospitalization, increased risk of complications from immobility (see Chapter 46), and delayed rehabilitation. When pain is not relieved, physical or psychological recovery can be delayed because the patient's primary focus may be on achieving pain relief. Although it may not be possible to completely eliminate the pain, working with the patient and members of the interprofessional team to reduce pain to an acceptable level so that functional goals can be met is a realistic goal. The nurse's primary goals should be to prevent pain whenever possible and to effectively manage pain so that patients can participate in their own recovery.

Persistent Postoperative Pain. Persistent postoperative pain (PPP) is defined as pain that persists beyond 2 to 3 months after a surgical procedure, with other pain causes excluded, which may include pre-existing pain or postoperative infection (Wang et al., 2018). PPP can be somatic, visceral, or neuropathic in origin. PPP occurs frequently, with incidences reported between 5 and 50%, and can be challenging to manage effectively, so prevention is paramount. PPP can be debilitating for the patient and can impact health care costs. Studies are underway to evaluate the efficacy of the role that regional anaesthesia plays in reducing the incidence of PPP (Weinstein et al., 2019).

Chronic Pain. Chronic pain is defined as pain that persists longer than 3 months and is associated with actual or potential tissue damage (IASP, 2017). It is estimated that one in four Canadians, or 25% of the population over 15 years of age, lives with chronic pain (Canadian Pain Task Force, 2021). It is distinctly different from acute pain. Chronic pain can be intermittent (occurs in a pattern) or persistent (lasting more than 12 hours daily), experienced at any point in life, including early childhood, and lead to great personal suffering. Chronic pain may be nonmalignant or related to cancer. Chronic noncancer pain is usually not life-threatening. However, patients with chronic noncancer pain are often frustrated because they cannot predict how they will feel from day to day, and the pain they experience may be unrelenting. The pain may result from an injured area that healed long ago but continues to be nonresponsive to treatment. Chronic noncancer pain may be experienced along with other symptoms such as sleep disturbances, depression, anxiety, and anger. This type of pain may be a major cause of psychological and physical disability, leading to issues such as job loss, school absenteeism, the inability to perform simple daily activities, sleep disturbances, sexual dysfunction, and social isolation.

Despite the fact that Canadians are among the largest opioid users per capita in the world, undertreated chronic noncancer pain is a challenge faced by patients and health care providers alike. Now, more than ever, health care providers may be reluctant to treat chronic noncancer pain with opioids. To help break the cycle of poor pain management, nurses should inform patients about concerns raised when they seek help from multiple health care providers and refer the patient to a pain team or chronic pain clinic, if available. The current Canadian guideline for chronic noncancer pain addresses the challenges with assessment and management of chronic noncancer pain and provides recommendations and tools for safe and responsible selection, prescription, titration, and monitoring of opioids.

For Canadian pain clinics, managing chronic pain during a pandemic has been increasingly challenging and approaches to care have pivoted. For pediatric patients with chronic pain (incidence 20%), access to interprofessional care was shifted from in-person appointments to virtual visits through a program provided by Hospital for Sick Children in Toronto during the COVID-19 pandemic. This program provided continued access to care while reducing risk of exposure and transmission (D'Alessandro et al., 2020).

The coping strategies used by individuals with chronic pain, as well as their personal beliefs, may determine how they will function with and adjust to pain. When managing pain, a comprehensive approach that includes both nonpharmacological and pharmacological strategies should be utilized. Furthermore, the treatment for chronic pain needs to be based on a triad of therapies using the following 3-P approach: **p**hysical, **p**sychological, and **p**harmacological (Canadian Pain Task Force, 2021). Other methods, such as interventional pain management (IPM) strategies—which include peripheral nerve blocks, neuroaxial injections, and radiofrequency treatments that serve as target-specific interventions—can be used effectively to treat chronic pain. The IPM strategies further compliment the 3-P approach (Shanthanna et al., 2020). The use of evidence-informed adaptive coping strategies is encouraged, such as cognitive-behavioural therapy (CBT), relaxation techniques, positive thinking, visual imagery, and distraction.

Cancer Pain. Pain in a patient with cancer may be acute, chronic, or both. The pain may also be nociceptive, neuropathic, or both. Cancer pain may be caused by tumour progression and its related pathological process, invasive procedures, toxicities of treatment, infection, and physical limitations. It can be sensed at the actual site of the tumour or distant to the site. When pain is sensed at a site that is distant to the area of tissue damage it is called *referred pain*. For example, a patient who has pancreatic cancer may sense the pain from a pancreatic tumour in the lower back. Referred pain can occur in patients experiencing cancer pain or noncancer pain.

Any new report of pain by a patient with existing pain needs to be investigated. Although the need for treatment of cancer pain has become increasingly evident, the issue of undertreatment continues. Many individuals with cancer pain live at home in their community and pain is managed by themselves, by their families, or both. Research findings suggest that accessing community resources when pain is not well managed may be difficult for these families and that the stress of caring for a loved one with cancer pain can affect the health of family caregivers. The importance of establishing an organized, systematic,

and comprehensive approach to pain assessment and treatment, as well as communicating with and supporting patients' families, cannot be overemphasized; nurses have the potential to play pivotal roles in these endeavours.

Pain by Inferred Pathology Process. Identifying the cause of pain is one of the first steps in successfully managing pain. Nociceptive pain is pain caused by tissue damage and is subdivided into *somatic* (musculoskeletal) and *visceral* (internal organ) pain. Neuropathic pain arises from abnormal or impaired pain nerves (Table 32.2). Each of these pathological processes has distinct pain characteristics that are discussed later, under "Assessment" in the "Nursing Process and Pain" section.

Although nociceptive and neuropathic pain have historically been classified by nociceptor activation or lesions of the somatosensory system, the classification system has a gap in areas that do not specifically meet these criteria, namely complex regional pain syndrome (CRPS), fibromyalgia, and nonspecific low back pain. Subsequently, a new classification to capture these gaps is *nociplastic pain* (IASP, 2017). **Nociplastic pain** has been defined as "pain that arises from altered nociception despite no clear evidence of actual or threatened tissue damage causing the activation of peripheral nociceptors or evidence for disease or lesion of the somatosensory system causing the pain" (Trouvin & Perrot, 2019, p. 3).

Finally, the concept of mixed pain is emerging as well. Mixed pain can be a complex overlap of the nociceptive, neuropathic, or nociplastic pain types and can be acute or chronic in nature (Trouvin & Perrot, 2019).

Breakthrough Pain. Some patients experience occasional, transitory exacerbations of their baseline pain, called **breakthrough pain**—so called because the pain "breaks through" the regular pain medication or treatment that adequately controls the baseline pain. Research has shown that breakthrough pain is not routinely recognized, evaluated, or treated. When breakthrough pain is brief and precipitated by an activity-related action, such as movement, sneezing, or coughing, it is referred to as *incident pain*. *Idiopathic pain*, another subtype of breakthrough pain, is not associated with an identifiable cause and has a longer duration than that of incident pain (Box 32.2). Breakthrough pain

TABLE 32.2 **Classification of Pain by Inferred Pathology: Two Major Types of Pain**	
I. Nociceptive pain: Normal processing of stimuli that damages normal tissues or has the potential to do so if prolonged; usually responsive to nonopioids, opioids, or both	**II. Neuropathic pain:** Abnormal processing of sensory input by the peripheral or central nervous system; treatment usually includes adjuvant analgesics. Typically, it is not responsive to opioids.
A. Somatic pain: Arises from bone, joint, muscle, skin, or connective tissue. It is usually aching or throbbing in quality and is well localized.	**A. Centrally generated pain**
	1. Deafferentation pain. Injury to either the peripheral or central nervous system. Examples: Phantom pain may reflect injury to the peripheral nervous system; burning pain below the level of a spinal cord lesion reflects injury to the central nervous system
	2. Sympathetically maintained pain. Associated with dysregulation of the autonomic nervous system. Examples: May include some of the pain associated with complex regional pain syndrome (CRPS—type I, type II)
B. Visceral pain: Arises from visceral organs, such as the gastrointestinal tract and pancreas. This source may be subdivided:	**B. Peripherally generated pain**
1. Tumour involvement of the organ capsule, which causes aching and fairly well-localized pain	1. Painful polyneuropathies. Pain is felt along the distribution of many peripheral nerves. Examples: Diabetic neuropathy, alcohol-nutritional neuropathy, and those associated with Guillain-Barré syndrome
2. Obstruction of hollow viscus, which causes intermittent cramping and poorly localized pain	2. Painful mononeuropathies. Usually associated with a known peripheral nerve injury, and pain is felt at least partly along the distribution of the damaged nerve. Examples: Nerve root compression, nerve entrapment, trigeminal neuralgia

CRPS, Complex regional pain syndrome.

can occur spontaneously as a result of predictable or unpredictable triggers and can occur despite stable and well-controlled background or baseline pain (Gonella et al., 2019).

NURSING KNOWLEDGE BASE

Nurses have a long history of dealing with the effects of pain on patients, dating back to the days of Florence Nightingale. In this section, factors that influence pain are explored.

Knowledge, Attitudes, and Beliefs

Pain assessment and management may be influenced by the nurse's or members of the interprofessional team's personal beliefs, attitudes, or pain-related myths. There are many factors that influence clinicians' belief in patients' reports of pain. It is important to acknowledge that the knowledge, attitudes, and preferences of health care providers, including your own, will influence pain care decision making.

Health care provider bias can affect care and can negatively affect patient care, through inadequate patient assessment, treatment, and follow-up (Narayan, 2019). Biases can be unconscious, when we categorize or assign judgement (favourable or prejudiced) to different groups of people based on their cultural background, gender, or physical characteristics (Deska & Hoffman, 2018). Negative bias and stereotypes can impact treatment and create disparities in access to effective pain management (Hoffman et al., 2016; Mack et al., 2018).

A patient's tolerance to pain and response to pain may influence the nurse's perception of the patient's degree of discomfort. **Pain tolerance level** is the greatest level of pain an individual is prepared to endure in a given situation and is strictly a patient's subjective expression (IASP, 2017). Patients with a low pain tolerance level may be perceived to be complainers. To avoid making judgements about another's pain, it is important for you as a nurse to acknowledge your own beliefs about pain. Consider the immediate context in which a patient is experiencing pain, as well as their past pain experiences. Base your pain assessment and pain care decision making on a variety of sources and observations, such as the patient's self-report, information from family and significant others, the patient's behaviour, and internal and external environmental factors.

Studies on how clinicians judge the pain of others have indicated that, when compared with patients' self-reports, health care providers tend to underestimate or, on occasion, overestimate the patient's pain (Alotaibi et al., 2018; Drake & de C Williams, 2017; Keen et al., 2017). For example, it has been demonstrated that nurses tend to overestimate pain when patients report no pain and underestimate pain when patients report mild to intense pain or when they are told that patients might be faking pain to obtain opioids. Differences in pain ratings may

also result from the type of tool used for pain assessment. Nurses are often unaware of the process of inferring pain in others, yet nurses' judgements guide their actions. For example, a nurse's personal opinion about the patient's report of pain may affect the type of analgesia chosen or the titration of opioid doses.

Making assumptions about patients in pain may seriously limit a nurse's ability to offer effective pain relief. Too often, nurses allow misconceptions about pain (Box 32.3) to affect their willingness to intervene. Some even avoid acknowledging a patient's pain because of their own fear and denial. Nurses have their personal beliefs; however, they must accept the patient's report of pain and act according to professional guidelines, standards, position statements, policies and procedures, and evidence-informed research findings. Moreover, nurses have an ethical obligation not only to treat all patients for pain but also to do so in an unbiased manner (Sturdivant et al., 2020). Most importantly, pain treatment should be equitable, regardless of a patient's ethnicity, gender, sexual orientation, or underlying medical conditions such as opioid abuse.

Factors Influencing Pain

As stated earlier, pain is complex and involves physiological, social, spiritual, psychological, and cultural influences. Each individual's pain experience is different. Nurses need to consider all factors that affect the patient in pain.

Physiological Factors

Age. Age is an important variable that influences pain, particularly in infants, children, and older people. Developmental differences among these age groups influence how children and older people perceive and react to pain. Young children have difficulty understanding the procedures that nurses perform that may cause pain. Cognitively, toddlers and preschoolers are often unable to recall explanations about pain, or they associate pain with experiences that can occur in various situations. They may also have difficulty expressing their pain or may use verbal descriptors that differ from those used by older individuals. When assessing pain in a child, consider adapting your approaches (including what to ask and the behaviours to observe). Help prepare the child for a painful procedure and consider consulting a child life specialist, if available. Ask the child and parents about the terms most often used by the child to describe the pain experience and pain treatment, and then use those terms when communicating about pain with the child. For instance, children have developed words for pain by the age of 18 months and may describe pain as an "ache" or "hurt." As cognitive development matures, so does the ability for a toddler to report the degree of pain, such as it hurts a lot or a little. School-age children and adolescents are capable of seriation, hence can better rate their pain intensity using validated pain tools, such as the numerical rating scale (Health Quality Ontario, 2020).

Frail older persons and obese older persons are more likely to report experiencing chronic pain than are normal-weight, healthy older persons (Chen et al., 2019). Older patients may experience cognitive impairment, confusion, or memory loss, either from pathology or medication, which can be compounded by sight and hearing impairment. Mobility, activities of daily living (ADLs), social activities outside the home, and activity tolerance may all be reduced among older persons (Chen et al., 2019). Therefore, pain in an older person requires careful, comprehensive assessment, diagnosis, and management (Schofield, 2018) (Box 32.4). The ability of older patients to interpret pain can be complicated by the presence of multiple diseases with vague symptoms that affect similar parts of the body. Nurses need to undertake a detailed pain history and conduct a thorough physical assessment when a patient has more than one source of pain. Older patients who experience multiple sites of musculoskeletal pain are more prone to disability and are at risk for falls (Thapa et al., 2019). The manifestations of different diseases can cause atypical presentations of painful conditions. Different diseases can also cause similar symptoms. For example, chest pain does not always indicate a heart attack; it may be a symptom of arthritis of the spine or of an abdominal disorder. And while not all older people experience cognitive impairment, when older persons are confused, they may not be able to recall and explain details of pain experiences.

BOX 32.4 FOCUS ON OLDER PERSONS

Factors Influencing Pain

With aging, muscle mass decreases, body fat increases, and the percentage of body water decreases. These changes result in the potential for an increased concentration of water-soluble medications, such as morphine. Also, the volume of distribution for fat-soluble medications, such as fentanyl, increases.

Older persons frequently eat poorly, resulting in them having low serum albumin levels. Many medications are highly protein bound. In the presence of low serum albumin, more of the active form of a medication remains unbound, which increases the risk for adverse effects, toxic effects, or both (Maher et al., 2020):

- Decline of hepatic and renal function is a natural occurrence with aging and results in reduced metabolism and excretion of medications. Hence, older people often experience a greater peak effect and longer duration of analgesics (Maher et al., 2020).
- Age-related changes in the skin, such as thinning and loss of elasticity, could affect the absorption rate of topical analgesics. However, transdermal analgesics have been proven beneficial for older patients and are particularly suitable for those with impaired gastrointestinal function (Maher et al., 2020).
- Patient-controlled analgesia (PCA) and regional analgesia are not contraindicated in older persons, but frequent assessment for pain and the adverse effects of analgesics and of cognition are necessary to ensure the efficacy of these interventions (Cornelius et al., 2017).
- The loss of the efficiency of homeostatic mechanisms puts older persons at risk for falls or delirium after the administration of sedative medications or regional anaesthesia.

Older individuals may not only have age-related physiological changes but may also have other comorbidities and polypharmacy, which can affect the treatment plan. Therefore, the goal would be to use a multimodal plan consisting of both nonpharmacological and pharmacological approaches (Horgas, 2017).

Misconceptions about pain management in the very young and in older persons may seriously hamper effective pain management for these populations (Tables 32.3 and 32.4).

Sleep. Sleep disturbances, including insomnia and sleep interruption, can heighten pain perception, increase pain intensity, and decrease coping abilities. Sleep disturbance and fatigue are common challenges for patients with long-term illnesses or as a result of treatment. Acute or chronic pain can affect a patient's sleep, often leading to poor-quality or fragmented sleep, which can further exacerbate pain (Andersen et al., 2018; Chun & Lee, 2019). It is important to ask patients if pain interferes with their ability to sleep, if it awakens them, or if it keeps them awake (see Chapter 42). Nonpharmacological or pharmacological pain management interventions may be needed to aid sleep (Nijs et al., 2018).

Pharmacogenetics. Increasingly, research has provided evidence that genetic information can influence the ability to metabolize pain medicine, pain threshold, pain tolerance, and susceptibility to develop chronic pain (Aroke & Kittelsrud, 2020).

Neurological Function. A patient's neurological function can influence the pain experience. Any factor that interrupts or influences normal pain reception or perception affects the patient's awareness of and response to pain. For example, patients who have a spinal cord injury, peripheral neuropathy (e.g., from diabetes mellitus), or a neurological disease (e.g., multiple sclerosis) experience altered pain sensation. Certain pharmacological medications influence pain perception and response. Analgesics (medications that relieve pain), sedatives, and anaesthetics (medications that cause temporary loss of sensation) depress functions of the central nervous system. Because patients at risk for pain insensitivity could suffer injury, they require preventive nursing care that includes neurological assessment (see Chapter 33).

Social Factors

Distraction. The degree to which a patient focuses on pain can influence pain perception. Distraction has been associated with a decreased pain response. Innovations such as virtual reality are one effective adjunct pain therapy, for both children and adults, that uses distraction (Ahmadpour et al., 2019). However, there are many ways to use distraction that nurses can implement. By focusing a patient's attention and concentration on other stimuli, the person's awareness of pain temporarily declines.

Previous Experience. Prior painful experiences may shape how a patient responds to subsequent painful events. If a person has had frequent episodes of pain or severe pain without relief, pain-related anxiety or fear may occur. In contrast, if a person has had repeated experiences with the same type of pain but the pain has been successfully relieved, it becomes easier to interpret the pain sensation, and the patient is better prepared to take actions to relieve the pain.

When patients have no prior exposure to a particular pain-inducing event, they may be unprepared to manage their pain, and this may impair their coping abilities. For example, incisional pain is common after abdominal surgery. When a patient is not informed to expect pain, they may view the incisional pain as a serious complication of surgery. As a result, they may tense up, exhibit more shallow breaths, and become anxious. It is important to inform patients of the type of pain that might be anticipated, based on the type of surgery or procedure performed, or pain that may be attributed to a particular illness.

Family and Social Support. People in pain often depend on family or friends for support, assistance, or protection. A loved one can help minimize loneliness and fear. An absence of support can make the pain experience more stressful. The presence of parents is especially important for children with pain. Nurses should explain to parents that children typically want their parents with them during a pain event,

TABLE 32.3 Pain in Infants

Misconception	Correction
Infants cannot feel pain or are less sensitive to pain because of an immature nervous system.	Infants can feel pain. Their immature inhibitory capacities can enhance the pain experience. Complete myelination is not required in order for infants to feel pain.
Infants are incapable of expressing pain.	Behavioural cues, such as facial expression and motor movements, along with responses such as crying and physiological cues such as vagal tone can be indicators of pain and have led to the development of validated pain assessment tools for infants.Infants can react to pain via afferent/efferent pathways but cannot cognitively modulate the pain.
Infants must learn about pain from previous painful experiences.	Emotional processing and cognitive abilities are maturational in nature and can influence the expression of pain and the ability to cope with pain.
Pain cannot be accurately assessed in infants.	Behavioural responses, primarily facial expressions, can be reliably and validly assessed. Specific facial expressions are acknowledged as being the most specific indicator of pain in response to acute noxious stimuli. Numerous behavioural validated pain-assessment tools have been developed to use with infants.
Because infants cannot demonstrate cognitive awareness, they are insensible and lack memory for pain.	Early and repeated exposure to noxious stimuli can affect the infant's future responses to painful events.
Analgesics and anaesthetics cannot be safely given to infants and newborns because of their immature capacity to metabolize and eliminate medications, as well as their sensitivity to opioid-induced respiratory depression.	Infants older than 1 month of age metabolize medications in the same manner as older infants and children. Careful selection of the medication, dosage, administration route, and time; frequent monitoring for desired and undesired effects; and medication titration and weaning can minimize the adverse effects of opioids and nonopioids for pain management in newborns.

TABLE 32.4 Pain in Older Persons

Misconception	Correction
Pain is a natural outcome of growing old.	Older persons are at greater risk than younger adults for many painful conditions; however, in the absence of disease, pain is not a normal part of aging.
Pain perception, or sensitivity, decreases with age.	Some studies suggest that greater age brings a higher threshold for painful electrical, thermal, and mechanical stimuli to the skin, while others have reported that older patients have alterations in the sensorineural apparatus, thus diminishing the perception of pain (Domenichiello & Ramsden, 2019).
If the older patient does not report pain, they do not have pain.	Older patients commonly underreport pain. Reasons include expecting to have pain with increasing age; not wanting to alarm loved ones; being fearful of losing independence; not wanting to distract, anger, or bother caregivers; and believing that caregivers know that the older patient has pain and are doing all that can be done to relieve it. The absence of a report of pain does not mean the absence of pain.
If an older patient appears to be occupied, asleep, or otherwise distracted from pain, they do not have pain.	Older patients often believe it is unacceptable to show pain and have learned to use a variety of ways to cope with it instead (e.g., many patients use distraction successfully for short periods of time). Sleeping may be a coping strategy or may indicate exhaustion, not pain relief. Assumptions about the presence or absence of pain cannot be made solely on the basis of a patient's behaviour.
The potential adverse effects of opioids make them too dangerous to use to relieve pain in older persons.	Opioids may be used safely in older persons. Although the opioid-naïve older person may be more sensitive to opioids, this does not justify withholding their use in pain management for this population. Potentially dangerous opioid-induced adverse effects can be prevented with slow titration; regular, frequent monitoring and assessment of the patient's response; and adjustment of dose and interval between doses when adverse effects are detected. If necessary, clinically significant respiratory depression can be reversed by an opioid antagonist medication.
Patients with Alzheimer's disease and other cognitive impairments do not feel pain, and their reports of pain are most likely invalid.	No evidence exists that cognitively impaired older persons experience less pain or that their reports of pain are less valid than those of individuals with intact cognitive function. It is probable that patients with dementia or other deficits of cognition suffer significant unrelieved pain and discomfort. Assessment of pain in these patients is challenging, but possible. The best approach is to accept the patient's report of pain and treat the pain as it would be treated in an individual with intact cognitive function (Domenichiello & Ramsden, 2019).

but warn them that a parent's own anxiety and responses may influence how the child experiences and responds to pain. Parents should be provided with information about the procedure, and the nurse should involve them by explaining how they can use pain-related distraction strategies with their child during the painful procedure. For example, skin-to-skin contact or kangaroo care is a useful strategy to use with preterm infants experiencing procedural pain. Also, breastfeeding should be encouraged as a means of pain reduction for procedural pain in infants (Harrison et al., 2016).

Psychological Factors

Anxiety. The relationship between pain and anxiety is complicated. Anxiety is associated with many types of pain; however, the cause-and-effect relationship has not been established. Pain often causes anxiety, but it is not clear that anxiety increases the intensity of pain. However, pain-related anxiety can result in the avoidance of activities that a patient fears may cause pain. When anxiety goes unnoticed, it may be difficult to manage pain effectively. The management of anxiety through the use of nonpharmacological and

TABLE 32.5	Classification of Pain by Location		
Location	**Characteristics**	**Examples of Causes**	**Examples of Common Medications**
Superficial or Cutaneous			
Pain resulting from stimulation of skin	Pain is localized and of short duration. It is usually a sharp sensation.	Needle-stick; small cut or laceration	Topical analgesics and anaesthetics (e.g., Ametop or EMLA for infants >37 weeks gestational age or Pain Ease topical spray for children >3 years of age given prior to painful procedures such as venipuncture or intravenous initiation) Lidoderm patch for cutaneous neuropathic pain in adults
Deep or Visceral			
Pain resulting from stimulation of internal organs	Pain is diffuse and may radiate in several directions. Duration varies, but it usually lasts longer than superficial pain. Pain may be sharp, dull, or unique to the organ involved.	Crushing sensation (e.g., angina pectoris); burning sensation (e.g., gastric ulcer)	Opioids such as morphine, hydromorphone
Referred			
Common phenomenon in visceral pain because many organs themselves have no pain receptors; entrance of sensory neurons from affected organ into same spinal cord segment as neurons from areas where pain is felt; perception of pain is in unaffected areas	Pain is felt in a part of the body separate from the source of pain and may assume any characteristic.	Myocardial infarction (MI), which may cause referred pain to the jaw, left arm, and left shoulder; kidney stones, which may refer pain to groin	Opioids for acute MI
Radiating			
Sensation of pain extending from initial site of injury to another body part	Pain feels as though it travels down or along the body part. It may be intermittent or constant.	Low back pain from ruptured intravertebral disc, accompanied by pain radiating down leg from sciatic nerve irritation	Temporary treatment with one-time epidural injection of a steroid; injections of anaesthetics (e.g., xylocaine or bupivacaine)
Neuropathic			
Arises from abnormal or damaged pain nerves as a result of prior injury or disease; certain nerves may continue to send pain messages to the brain even though no ongoing tissue damage is present (see Table 31.2)	Pain is usually described as burning, shooting, numbing, or electric-like.	Consequence of disease or prior injury to either the peripheral or central nervous system CRPS type I, type II, stroke, spinal cord injury, multiple sclerosis; diabetic neuropathy, alcohol-nutritional neuropathy, and those associated with Guillain-Barré syndrome; nerve root compression, nerve entrapment, trigeminal neuralgia; post-thoracotomy, herniorrhaphy, mastectomy; herpes zoster	Opioids, tricyclic antidepressants (e.g., nortriptyline/amitriptyline), anticonvulsants (e.g., gabapentin/pregabalin), and topical lidocaine

CRPS, Complex regional pain syndrome.

pharmacological approaches is appropriate. However, anxiolytic medications should not be used as a substitute for good analgesia, nor used long term.

Meaning of Pain. The meaning of pain affects the experience of pain and how one adapts to it. A person will perceive pain differently if it suggests a threat, loss, punishment, or challenge. For example, a woman in labour may perceive pain differently than a woman with a history of cancer who experiences new pain and fears recurrence.

Spiritual Factors. Religion and/or spirituality can help individuals become part of a community or feel connected with nature or the universe. In some traditions, pain is viewed as punishment from God, or as an opportunity to demonstrate the strength of character that will be rewarded after death. Prayer, hope, and seeking spiritual support, such as through attendance at church, have been linked to less suffering associated with pain (Barbato, 2017). However, severe or prolonged pain can permeate the very essence of the person, often challenging established beliefs and values, which may result in increased pain. Similarly, for those who view humans as irreducible energy fields in continual interaction with universal sources of energy, pain may be intensified or lessened as a result of changes in energy patterns.

Health care providers should explore religious and spiritual coping strategies with patients, such as meaning-making, distraction, spiritual supports, and relaxation techniques. For example, for patients whose faith or spirituality is based in a religious tradition, nurses can suggest a visit from a clergyperson. Other strategies include supporting the choice of meditation, therapeutic touch, Reiki, or acupuncture as restorative modalities designed to improve energy-flow patterns. Providing interventions designed to holistically heal can be an essential component of pain management.

Cultural Factors. Culture shapes individuals' responses to, attitudes toward, and meaning of pain and how they react to and cope with pain (Van Looveren et al., 2018). It is important to understand that pain has different meanings for different cultures. Effective pain management requires that each patient be viewed as an individual with many characteristics, including a particular cultural background.

In some cultures people are demonstrative about pain; in others, people are introverted. Health care providers should recognize that some people adapt or assimilate to the culture into which they migrate. Health care providers should not assume that every person affiliated with a specific cultural group will display the pain behaviours of that cultural group. For example, if several generations of an Asian patient's family have lived in Canada, the influence of their Asian culture may be more limited. In contrast, a recent immigrant to Canada may have different beliefs from those of the larger Canadian population. As a nurse caring for a patient in pain, explore the impact of cultural differences on the patient's pain experience and adjust the plan of care (Box 32.5). Work with the patient and family to facilitate communication about the assessment and management of pain. Find a culturally appropriate assessment tool and communicate the use of that tool to other health care providers.

CRITICAL THINKING

Critical thinking requires synthesizing knowledge, experience, patient information, critical thinking attitudes, and professional standards. Clinical judgement requires that nurses anticipate the information needed, analyze the data, and make decisions about patient care. A patient's condition or situation is always changing; thus, it is essential during pain assessments for nurses to consider all critical elements that will enable them to make a nursing diagnosis.

Assessing Pain

Culture affects behavioural responses to pain and treatment preferences. The way people define and express pain is influenced by their culture and is similar to how their family members respond to pain. For example, patients of Chinese descent may be reluctant to express pain because they feel that revealing and admitting to pain is a sign of weakness. As a result, they may endure the pain and not report it until the pain becomes unbearable. In order to provide quality care, nurses need to acquire cultural competence regarding the cultural and linguistic diversity of patients (Kaihlanen et al., 2019). With the acquisition of cultural competence, nurses can further develop cultural sensitivity and awareness by seeking additional information from each patient and family about their specific beliefs (Givler et al., 2020).

Implications for Practice
- Emotional and cognitive responses to pain (overt, stoic) vary between and within cultures.
- Words used to express pain vary among cultures (*hurt, ache, discomfort*).
- Personal and social meanings of pain and past pain experiences affect pain perception.
- The meaning of pain may influence the perception of pain intensity.
- Health care providers' beliefs and expectations regarding pain expression influence the use of pain management strategies.
- Therapeutic goals of pain management are influenced by cultural beliefs.
- It is important to be aware of perceived causal factors of pain (fate, lifestyle, punishment).
- Believe patients' reports about their perceived pain; do not act on your own beliefs about a patient's pain.

Successful pain management does not necessarily mean pain elimination, but rather the attainment of mutually agreed-upon pain-relief goals that allow patients to manage their pain and maintain function and quality of life.

NURSING PROCESS AND PAIN

The nursing process provides nurses with a systematic approach to understanding and treating a patient's pain. An important aspect of effective pain management is establishing a trusting relationship with the patient and family. Pain management extends beyond pain relief; it encompasses the patient's quality of life and their ability to work and play productively and to function within the family and society (Health Quality Ontario, 2020).

The nurse's application of the nursing process can be optimized by framing it around readily available clinical pain guidelines, which are based on best evidence and are continuously updated (see the Recommended Websites at the end of this chapter).

Assessment

Pain assessment is the basis of all pain management (Busse et al., 2017; Health Quality Ontario, 2018a, 2020). The patient's pain should be consistently monitored along with other assessments, such as vital signs, especially if the pain is not well controlled. Establishing a nursing diagnosis, deciding on appropriate interventions, and evaluating the patient's response to the interventions are contingent on a timely and accurate pain assessment (Figure 32.4). Effective and unbiased pain assessment is best achieved by using a validated pain assessment tool appropriate to the patient.

Factors to consider when choosing an assessment tool include the age and developmental stage of the patient, patient condition, type of

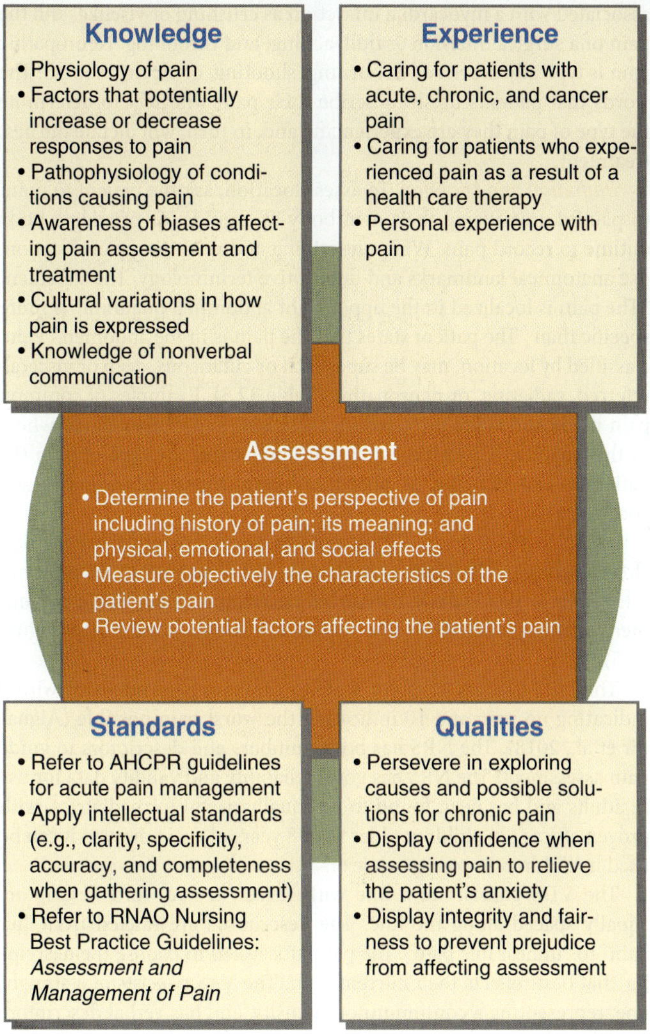

Knowledge

- Physiology of pain
- Factors that potentially increase or decrease responses to pain
- Pathophysiology of conditions causing pain
- Awareness of biases affecting pain assessment and treatment
- Cultural variations in how pain is expressed
- Knowledge of nonverbal communication

Experience

- Caring for patients with acute, chronic, and cancer pain
- Caring for patients who experienced pain as a result of a health care therapy
- Personal experience with pain

Assessment

- Determine the patient's perspective of pain including history of pain; its meaning; and physical, emotional, and social effects
- Measure objectively the characteristics of the patient's pain
- Review potential factors affecting the patient's pain

Standards

- Refer to AHCPR guidelines for acute pain management
- Apply intellectual standards (e.g., clarity, specificity, accuracy, and completeness when gathering assessment)
- Refer to RNAO Nursing Best Practice Guidelines: *Assessment and Management of Pain*

Qualities

- Persevere in exploring causes and possible solutions for chronic pain
- Display confidence when assessing pain to relieve the patient's anxiety
- Display integrity and fairness to prevent prejudice from affecting assessment

FIGURE 32.4 Critical thinking model for pain and comfort assessment. *AHCPR,* Agency for Health Care Policy and Research; *RNAO,* Registered Nurses' Association of Ontario.

BOX 32.6 Pain Assessment OPQRSTUV Mnemonic

O = Onset / Origin: When and where did it start?

P = Palliation / Provocation: What makes the pain better? What makes it worse?

Q = Quality: What does the pain feel like (i.e., descriptors—sharp, dull, continuous, intermittent)?

R = Region / Radiation: Where is your pain, and does it radiate?

S = Severity: Score pain using a validated pain tool, such as 4/10 on 0–10 scale, using a numerical rating scale. Obtain pain assessment at rest and with activity and note current pain, worst pain, and average pain.

T = Timing / Treatment: When did the pain begin or end and how long did it last? What time of the day is the pain better and worse? What nonpharmacological and pharmacological treatments are effective?

U = Understanding: What do you believe is causing this symptom? How is this symptom affecting you, your family, or both?

V = Value: Are there any other views or feelings about this symptom that are important to you or your family? (This may include cultural and religious values.). What is your comfort goal or acceptable level with respect to this symptom (0 = none, 10 = worst possible)?

Adapted from Fraser Health Authority. (2018). *Symptom assessment acronym.* https://www.fraserhealth.ca/-/media/Project/FraserHealth/FraserHealth/Health-Professionals/Professionals-Resources/Hospice-palliative-care/SymptomAssessmentRevised_Sept09.pdf

---

BOX 32.7 Sources of Error When Assessing Pain

- Bias, which causes nurses to consistently overestimate or underestimate their patients' pain
- Unclear assessment questions, which lead to unreliable assessment data (see OPQRSTUV mnemonic in Box 32.6 to optimize pain history and symptom assessment)
- Use of pain assessment tools that have no established reliability or validity
- Expecting self-reports of pain from individuals who cannot rate their pain using a pain scale or who cannot provide a complete verbal account of their pain
- Not considering the pain context and the trajectory or change in an individual's expression of pain over time

---

pain, culture, cognitive ability, preference, and ease of use for both the patient and health care provider. Specific tools are available that are appropriate for patients across the lifespan, from preterm infants to cognitively impaired persons. Pain assessment should include obtaining a pain history, determining the pain severity and intensity and its location, and noting the pain descriptors. Assessing how pain is impacting a person's function and mood is critical.

Establishing a pain management goal with the patient enables nurses to interpret the pain assessment data collected. Pain management goals should be patient-led and "SMART"—**S**pecific, **M**easurable, **A**chievable, **R**ealistic, and have a **T**ime frame associated with them (Health Quality Ontario, 2020). When a SMART pain management goal is established, the nurse can help support the patient in achieving this goal. For patients with chronic or complex pain conditions, thorough assessment of pain should include affective, cognitive, and behavioural dimensions of the pain experience as well as a pain history. The nurse's assessment of chronic noncancer complex pain should focus on the relationship between pain, function, quality of life, and treatment adverse effects because complete pain relief may not be possible or realistic. In the home setting, family members may assist with pain assessment. The mnemonic *OPQRSTUV* can be used to guide the pain assessment process (Box 32.6).

Failure of clinicians to assess a patient's pain, accept the findings, and treat the report of pain is a common cause of unrelieved pain and suffering. Nurses need to use the right tools and methods to avoid errors in managing a patient's pain and to choose the best pain interventions. It is important to become aware of possible errors in pain assessment (Box 32.7).

Expression of Pain. A patient's self-report of pain is considered the gold standard and, as such, is the single most reliable indicator of the existence and intensity of pain. Many patients fail to report or discuss pain; at the same time, many nurses believe that patients will report pain. If patients sense that the nurse doubts their pain, they may share little about pain or minimize their report of pain. It is important to establish a caring, therapeutic, trusting relationship that enables open communication about pain.

Patients having difficulty communicating their pain because of their age, medical condition, language requirements, or cognitive disability require special consideration throughout the pain assessment and treatment process. A self-report or behavioural observation pain assessment tool should be selected that is appropriate for age, language, and condition of the patient (Beltramini et al., 2017; Herr et al., 2019). The nurse should assess and document pain and comfort behaviours before and after pain management interventions to gauge the effectiveness of treatments.

Cognitively impaired patients might require simple assessment approaches involving close observation of behaviour changes, especially with movement. The Pain Assessment in Advanced Dementia (PAINAD) provides a clinically relevant and easy-to-use pain assessment tool for individuals with advanced dementia. Adults in a critical care setting who may not be able to self-report their pain can be assessed using the Critical Care Pain Observation Tool (CPOT) (Gélinas et al., 2021). The r-FLACC tool is validated for cognitively impaired children, as they cannot report or quantify the severity of their pain, and takes parental input into consideration (Crellin et al., 2018).

Characteristics of Pain. Assessment of common pain characteristics will help you as a nurse to understand the type and pattern of pain and will aid in choosing interventions. When you assess pain and when you ask the patient for their self-report of pain, it is important to remember that using instruments to quantify the intensity and characteristics of pain depends on having a good fit between the needs of the patient and the attributes of the assessment tool. Developmental level, cognitive ability, language, and culture are a few factors to consider when assessing pain characteristics.

Onset, Duration, and Sequence of Pain. Ask questions to determine the onset, duration, and sequence of pain. When did the pain begin? How long has it lasted? Does it occur at the same time each day? How often does it recur? Is there frequent breakthrough pain or prolonged pain recovery? Understanding the pattern and cycles of pain will enable you to intervene before the pain occurs or worsens (refer to the OPQRSTUV mnemonic presented earlier in this chapter; see Box 32.6).

Provocation and Pain Pattern. Various factors affect the pain pattern. It is important to assess for factors that precipitate or aggravate pain. Ask the patient to describe activities that cause or increase pain—for example, specific actions such as turning or bending. The low back pain and radiation down the leg associated with a ruptured intravertebral disc are usually aggravated by bending or lifting. Similarly, swallowing and talking typically aggravate the pain of pharyngitis. Asking the patient if the pain is worse at certain times of day, or if it is intermittent, constant, or a combination of both, will help you to plan effective interventions.

Palliation and Relief Measures. Ask the patient what pain-relief measures they use and which measures are found to be most effective. Patients with chronic, complex pain often have a number of pharmacological and nonpharmacological measures that help relieve pain. Physical and cognitive modalities such as heat or cold, exercise, gentle stretching, massage, acupuncture, imagery, relaxation, distraction, or music are components of a tool kit of pain-relief measures. You should also note practitioners whose services the patient has used for pain management (e.g., orthopedist, acupuncturist, chiropractor, massage therapist, or naturopath).

Quality. Another subjective characteristic of pain is its quality; the descriptors that patients use will vary according to their habits, culture, age, and preference. For example, some patients may use "hurt" and "ache" for mild pain but reserve the word "pain" for severe discomfort. The patient may describe the pain as crushing, throbbing, sharp, or dull. Certain pain descriptors are typically associated with certain conditions or injuries. For example, patients will often describe pain

associated with a myocardial infarction as crushing or viselike, and the pain of a surgical incision as dull, aching, and throbbing. Neuropathic pain is typically described as burning, shooting, or electric shocks. The words that patients use to describe their pain will help to determine the type of pain they are experiencing and, in turn, will dictate the best treatment.

Radiation and Location. To assess location, ask the patient to point to painful areas using their own body as a guide, or provide a body outline to record pain. When describing and recording pain location, use anatomical landmarks and descriptive terminology. The statement "The pain is localized in the upper right abdominal quadrant" is more specific than "The patient states that the pain is in the abdomen." Pain, classified by location, may be superficial or cutaneous, deep or visceral, referred, radiating, or neuropathic (Table 32.5). Examples of common pain medications are provided in Table 32.5 and explained elsewhere in this chapter. It is critical that you understand the type of pain the patient is experiencing, as pharmacological treatments will vary accordingly.

Severity and Intensity. Tools used to assess pain intensity fall into two categories, self-report and behavioural observation. Examples of self-report scales include the verbal descriptor scale (VDS), the numerical rating scale (NRS), and the visual analogue scale (VAS) (Figure 32.5).

The NRS uses an 11-point scale to measure pain intensity, with 0 indicating no pain and 10 indicating the worst pain possible (Alghadir et al., 2018). The NRS has both numbers and descriptors to guide pain assessment. The NRS has good reliability and validity data for use in adults and has been found to be equally useful for pediatrics, with proven efficacy in children older than 8 years of age; however, it can be used in children as young as age 6.

The VDS consists of a line with three- to five-word descriptors equally spaced along the line. The descriptors are ranked from "no pain" to "unbearable pain." The patient is asked to choose the descriptor that best reflects their current pain. The VAS consists of a straight line, representing a continuum of intensity, and has verbal descriptors at each end.

Faces scales are validated self-report scales that can be used by children as young as 3 or 4 years of age. In addition, these scales are often well understood and acceptable to cognitively impaired persons. The

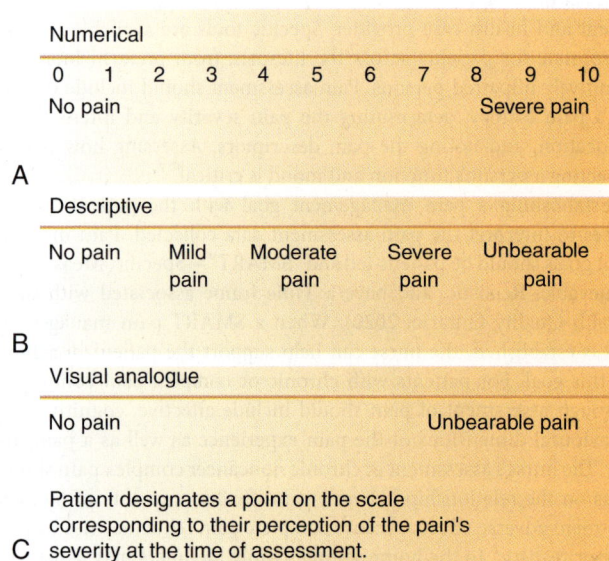

Numerical

0	1	2	3	4	5	6	7	8	9	10
No pain										Severe pain

A

Descriptive

No pain	Mild pain	Moderate pain	Severe pain	Unbearable pain

B

Visual analogue

No pain	Unbearable pain

Patient designates a point on the scale corresponding to their perception of the pain's severity at the time of assessment.

C

FIGURE 32.5 Sample pain scales. **A,** Numerical rating scale. **B,** Verbal descriptive scale. **C,** Visual analogue scale.

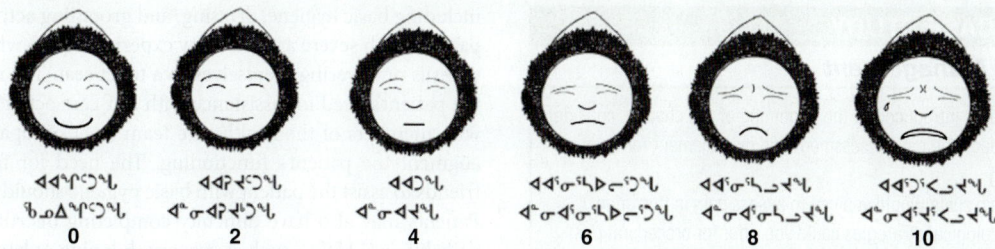

FIGURE 32.6 Northern Pain Scale. Brief word instructions: Point to each face using words to describe the pain intensity. Ask the child to choose the face that describes their own pain and record the appropriate number. (From Ellis, J., Ootoova, A., Blouin, R., et al. [2011]. Establishing the psychometric properties and preferences for the Northern Pain Scale. *International Journal of Circumpolar Health*, 70[3], 274–285. Ellis/Ootoova is an adapted version of the Wong/Baker FACES Pain Rating Scale from Hockenberry, M. J., & Wilson, D. [2006]. *Wong's nursing care of infants and children* [8th ed., p. 1876]. Elsevier/Mosby.)

Wong-Baker FACES scale consists of six faces with verbal descriptors depicting increasing amounts of pain. The FACES scale was adapted to provide a culturally sensitive pain assessment tool in Inuktitut for use with Indigenous children and adults and is referred to as the Northern Pain Scale (Ellis et al., 2011) (Figure 32.6). The Faces Pain Scale–Revised (FPS-R) is another commonly used self-report scale that can be utilized in patients 4–12 years of age, but it also has proven validity for use with older children, with strong psychometric properties for use with children up to 17 years of age (Le May et al., 2018). The FPS-R is composed of six visual analogue pain scales that are intended to measure pain intensity using a 0–10 metric scale. The FPS-R has good clinical utility, can be downloaded for free, and is available in many languages (https://www.iasp-pain.org/Education/Content.aspx?ItemNumber=1519).

If the patient cannot provide a self-reported pain rating, a validated behavioural observation tool can be used. Although subjective input from parents is warranted with respect to pain assessment, their observations alone cannot be solely relied on because there is a tendency to either overestimate or underestimate their child's pain because of contextual influences (Birnie et al., 2019). Focus should be placed on using validated observational tools. These tools prompt the nurse to observe the patient and score typical pain behaviours that provide a total pain intensity score. The Neonatal Infant Pain Scale (NIPS) and the Premature Infant Pain Profile–Revised (PIPP-R) specifically focus on the pain behaviours of premature and term babies. The PIPP-R is a validated measure for infant pain assessment, and an e-learning tool has been developed by researchers at The Hospital for Sick Children to promote standardization of the training (Bueno et al., 2021). The FLACC tool is a validated tool primarily aimed at assessing pain in children 2 months to 18 years of age and can be used for patients who have cognitive impairment and developmental delay who are unable to self-report their pain. The FLACC tool consists of five categories of behaviour, each of which is scored accordingly: **f**acial expression (F), **l**eg movement (L), **a**ctivity (A), **c**ry (C), and **c**onsolability (C). An e-learning educational tool was developed by clinicians at the Children's Hospitals of Eastern Ontario to assist nurses in uptake of the tool, using a case-based approach aimed at improving the clinical utility of the tool (Choueiry et al., 2020).

A pain scale should be easy for the patient to use and easy for the nurse to document. The nurse should use the same scale for the same patient consistently. A pain scale should be used before and after an intervention to gauge the effectiveness of the intervention. A rating of greater than 4 on a 0-to-10 scale indicates moderate pain and requires immediate attention. However, a pain intensity score is only one component of best practice pain care. Box 32.8 describes one nurse's effective solutions in caring for the young patient from the case study at the beginning of the chapter who underwent a laparotomy for a bowel anastomosis.

Contributing Symptoms. Symptoms such as depression, anxiety, fatigue, nausea, anorexia, sleep disruption, spiritual distress, or guilt may increase suffering and aggravate pain. It is important to assess for pain-associated symptoms and evaluate their effects on the patient's pain perception and pain tolerance. Monitoring and treating these symptoms contributes to effective pain management and improved quality of life. A referral to psychology or psychiatry may be warranted for workup of depression and anxiety or for pain coping strategies, as well as to physiotherapy to optimize function and address any deconditioning.

Effects of Pain. Pain is a physiological, psychological, and psychosocial stressor that negatively affects all aspects of a patient's life. Unrelieved acute pain prolongs hospital stays, delays healing, and may lead to chronic pain. Poorly controlled procedural pain—for example, from needle-sticks that lead to "needle phobia—can set the stage for treatment refusal or delay. Chronic and complex pain can severely challenge a patient's ability to function in all domains of their life.

Behavioural effects and nonverbal indicators. When a patient has pain, the nurse needs to assess verbalization, vocal response, facial and body movements, and social interaction. For patients who cannot provide a verbal report of pain (e.g., infants; unconscious patients; disoriented, confused, aphasic patients; and patients who speak a foreign language), it is important to assess behaviours that are indicative of pain. Grimacing, moaning, crying, inability to settle and rest, poor appetite, and negative emotions such as anger, fear, and anxiety are cues that the patient may be experiencing pain. Also, the patient may exhibit behaviours when in pain that may not be an intuitive pain behaviour; hence, it is important to consult with the parents or caregivers, if available, to ascertain typical pain behaviours for that patient (e.g., a cognitively impaired child may rub their ear continuously when in pain) (Box 32.9). For patients who are unable to speak either French or English, an interpreter should be used to translate the patient's pain assessment and to enable health care providers to outline the treatment plan.

Some nonverbal expressions characterize sources of pain. A person with chest pain often grabs or holds the chest. A person with severe abdominal pain often assumes a fetal position. The nonverbal expression of pain may support or contradict other information about pain. If a person in labour reports that that their labour pains are occurring more frequently and begins to massage their abdomen more frequently, their report is confirmed. If a patient complains of severe abdominal pain but grasps the chest, a more detailed assessment may be necessary, including an assessment for referred pain. For some patients, vocalizations are culturally acceptable ways to communicate and do not necessarily indicate a higher severity of pain or reduced pain tolerance.

Premature and full-term infants in pain often display behavioural characteristics as part of their pain expression. The preterm infant undergoes up to 16 painful diagnostic or therapeutic procedures per day, with many procedures (up to 31%) being repeated if they have been unsuccessful (Karimi et al., 2019). As noted earlier, the PIPP is a validated pain tool for premature infant pain assessment and has undergone rigorous psychometric testing. The scale was recently revised (PIPP-R) to increase

BOX 32.8   CASE STUDY
Pediatric Pain Management

Based on the case study introduced at the beginning of the chapter, consider how you would approach the pain assessment and management for Sam. Check your learning:
1. What validated pain scale would you use to assess pain in this infant?
2. What nonpharmacological strategies could you offer for procedural pain during blood work for this infant?
3. Why is nurse-controlled analgesia (NCA) a good modality for this patient?

Responses:
1. The Neonatal Infant Pain Scale (NIPS) or FLACC scale could be used to measure pain.
2. Kangaroo care, breastfeeding, and sucrose are nonpharmacological approaches that can be used to address procedural pain.
3. NCA allows for a basal infusion with stable opioid levels and can be used to provide nurse-initiated breakthrough doses at the point of care and pre-emptive doses before performance of painful procedures such as turning and positioning.

BOX 32.9   Behavioural and Nonverbal Indicators of Pain

Vocalizations
Moaning
Crying
Gasping
Grunting

Facial Expressions
Grimacing
Clenched teeth
Wrinkled forehead
Tightly closed or widely opened eyes
Lip biting

Body Movement
Restlessness
Immobilization
Muscle tension
Increased hand and finger movements
Pacing activities
Rhythmic or rubbing motions
Protective movement of body parts

Social Interaction
Avoidance of conversation
Focused only on activities for pain relief
Avoidance of social contacts
Reduced attention span
Withdrawn
Despondent—failure to interact purposefully and meaningfully with immediate environment

its clinical reliability. PIPP-R is a multidimensional, seven-item measure used to assess acute pain. It includes behavioural, physiological, and contextual indicators of pain (Bueno et al., 2019).

Influence on activities of daily living. The primary goal of pain management should be to improve the patient's function. Depending on the location of the pain, the patient may have difficulty performing ADLs,

including basic hygiene, dressing, and grooming activities. For example, patients with severe arthritis may experience pain when grasping eating utensils or lowering themselves to a toilet seat. The nurse should assess the patient's need for assistance with self-care activities and collaborate with members of the health care team (e.g., occupational therapist) to augment the patient's functioning. The need for family members or friends to assist the patient with basic hygiene should also be considered. Patients may also have difficulty completing instrumental activities of daily living (IADLs), such as grocery shopping or banking.

Pain can also affect sexual activity. Fear of worsening pain, arousal, confidence, performance, difficulty finding a comfortable position, and relationship issues are frequently reported pain-related problems. Prolonged use of opioids for chronic pain or cancer pain may affect sexual function and libido, as can the use of some adjuvant analgesics such as antidepressants (Healy, 2020). Nurses need to explore with the patient pain-related sexual issues and determine the patient's preference for information and for individual or group discussion to address these concerns. It is important to convey a willingness to have a discussion regarding pain and sexual health regardless of the patient's sexual orientation.

Pain also affects the ability of a patient to work or for children and adolescents to perform and attend school. The more physical activity required in a job, the greater the risk of discomfort when the pain is associated with musculoskeletal and certain visceral alterations. Pain may increase if the job is stressful. The nurse should inquire about the patient's work and assess whether pain affects their ability to function in their job, including performance of any household duties. Nurses should also assess whether it is necessary for patients to stop activity occasionally because of pain, and then help patients select ways of minimizing or controlling the pain so that they are able to remain productive.

It is also important to include an assessment of the effect of pain on social activities. The pain may be so debilitating that the patient becomes too exhausted to socialize. The nurse should identify the patient's normal social activities, the extent to which they have been disrupted, and the patient's desire to participate in them. Grief over lost goals or unfilled desires may augment pain. For an adolescent with pain, the nurse can explore options such as having a peer over to watch a movie, rather than participating in a group activity such as a volleyball game that may exacerbate the adolescent's pain.

Navigating a global pandemic, such as COVID-19, has led to further isolation and loneliness for many individuals. The need for connectivity then becomes even greater, along with access to platforms that facilitate social interactions and support. Technological advancements in platforms like Zoom™ provide such a network, as does the availability of smartphones that facilitate the use of different apps, from pain apps to mindfulness apps (Tolley et al., 2020).

Patient Expectations. Patients who seek health care assistance with pain as a major symptom may have experienced the pain for many hours or days or even months. Hospitalized patients may expect and even accept some pain. Asking patients to describe an acceptable pain level is a first step in encouraging them to take control of their pain. Assessing previous pain experiences and effective home interventions provides a treatment care foundation on which the nurse can build. Patients expect that nurses will believe their reports of pain and act on meeting their comfort needs.

◆ Nursing Diagnosis

Nurses should not diagnose pain simply because they assume that a patient will have discomfort. The nurse can make an accurate diagnosis only after having performed a complete assessment. The development of an accurate nursing diagnosis of pain results from thorough data collection and analysis (Box 32.10). Careful assessment, which should include examination of the patient's history for recent procedures or pre-existing painful conditions, will reveal the presence of or potential for pain.

BOX 32.10 NURSING DIAGNOSTIC PROCESS
Utilize OPQRSTUV Mnemonic

Assessment Activities	Defining Characteristics	Nursing Diagnosis
Have patient describe pain intensity.	Pain is constant; 5 out of 10	*Potential chronic pain related to chronic physical disability*
Assess onset and location of pain.	Present for 7 months in lower lumbar area	
Observe patient behaviours.	Grimaces and grunts with movement, rubs flanks frequently; reduced movement with sitting and standing	
Assess effect of pain on activities of daily living (ADLs).	Appetite poor; gets little sleep; difficulty bathing and dressing	
Review medical history and history of pain management treatments.	Previous trauma	
	Previous analgesic trials including opioids and nonopioids and note their effectiveness.	
	Determine previous nonpharmacological treatment trials including physiotherapy, acupuncture, massage therapy or chiropractic services and note their effectiveness.	

The nursing diagnosis focuses on the nature of the pain so that the nurse can identify the best interventions for relieving pain and minimizing its effect on function. Accurate identification of related factors ensures that appropriate nursing interventions will be chosen. For example, *acute pain related to physical trauma* versus *acute pain related to natural low-risk childbirth processes* each requires very different nursing interventions, such as "monitoring of vital signs for possible shock" versus "controlled breathing techniques." Examples of other diagnoses that may be applicable to patients at risk for pain are the following:

- *Anxiety*
- *Ineffective coping*
- *Fatigue*
- *Fear*
- *Hopelessness*
- *Impaired physical mobility*
- *Imbalanced nutrition: less than body requirements*
- *Acute pain*
- *Chronic pain*
- *Powerlessness*
- *Ineffective role performance*
- *Self-care deficit*
- *Chronic low self-esteem*
- *Situational low self-esteem*
- *Risk for situational low self-esteem*
- *Sexual dysfunction*
- *Disturbed sleep pattern*
- *Impaired social interaction*
- *Spiritual distress*

◆ Planning

The care plan integrates key patient information, critical thinking elements (Figure 32.7), and professional standards, which provide the best evidence for selecting nursing interventions (Box 32.11). Professional standards of care regarding pain management are available as agency policies or through professional organizations such as the Registered Nurses' Association of Ontario (RNAO) or the Canadian Pain Society and its affiliated special interest groups. See the "Recommended Websites" section at the end of this chapter.

A concept map can help with care planning. Patients in pain frequently have interrelated health problems. As one problem worsens, others also change. The concept map shows how nursing diagnoses link to one another and to medical diagnoses. For example, when planning care for the patient with arthritis, the nurse notes the relationships between *acute pain, impaired physical mobility, self-care,* and *fatigue*

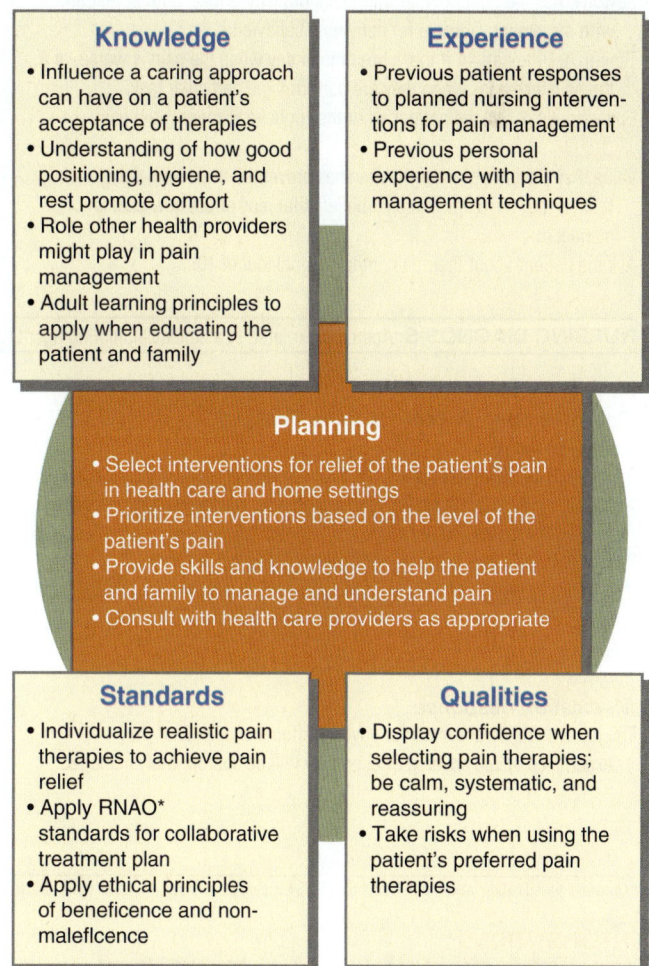

Knowledge
- Influence a caring approach can have on a patient's acceptance of therapies
- Understanding of how good positioning, hygiene, and rest promote comfort
- Role other health providers might play in pain management
- Adult learning principles to apply when educating the patient and family

Experience
- Previous patient responses to planned nursing interventions for pain management
- Previous personal experience with pain management techniques

Planning
- Select interventions for relief of the patient's pain in health care and home settings
- Prioritize interventions based on the level of the patient's pain
- Provide skills and knowledge to help the patient and family to manage and understand pain
- Consult with health care providers as appropriate

Standards
- Individualize realistic pain therapies to achieve pain relief
- Apply RNAO* standards for collaborative treatment plan
- Apply ethical principles of beneficence and non-maleficence

Qualities
- Display confidence when selecting pain therapies; be calm, systematic, and reassuring
- Take risks when using the patient's preferred pain therapies

FIGURE 32.7 Critical thinking model for comfort planning. *The Registered Nurses' Association of Ontario (RNAO) has developed evidence-informed practice guidelines specifically with regard to pain. See https://rnao.ca/bpg/guidelines/assessment-and-management-pain

(Figure 32.8). Understanding these relationships helps the nurse to develop a holistic and patient-centred care plan.

Goals and Outcomes. Pain management goals enable the patient to function to the best possible extent. The nurse should determine with the

◎ BOX 32.11 NURSING CARE PLAN

Acute Pain

ASSESSMENT

A 40-year-old patient was diagnosed with a cancerous tumour in their left lung 8 months ago. After treatment, they were taking oral analgesics on an as-needed basis. The patient can no longer tolerate taking medications orally and is now hospitalized with uncontrollable chest pain and possible pneumonia. The patient's spouse is with them. A patient-controlled analgesia (PCA) of morphine 0.5 mg on-demand dose with a 10-minute lockout is begun.

Assessment Activities	*Findings and Defining Characteristics*
Onset: Ask the patient when the pain began. Review their past medical and nursing history.	The pain started 6 months ago but has gotten worse over the last 2 weeks. The patient's past history of illness includes a cancer diagnosis and the subsequent treatments that they received over the past 8 months.
Palliative/Provoking factors: Ask the patient what they did at home to control the pain. Ask them what makes the pain worse.	The pain escalated from a 3 to a 10, so they doubled the medication and went to bed. This did not help. Lying flat and coughing make the pain worse.
Quality: Ask the patient what the pain feels like.	They describe the pain as constant and dull. It becomes sharp when they cough.
Radiating: Ask the patient where the pain is located and if it travels anywhere.	The pain is in the left-side thoracic area. They state it radiates to their upper back when they cough.
Severity: Ask the patient what their pain intensity is now, both at rest and with movement. Observe for nonverbal behaviours.	On a scale of 0 to 10, currently they report a 9 at rest and >10/10 with movement. They are restless and unfocused during the history-taking.
Timing: Ask the patient if there is a time of day when the pain is worse, or if the pain increases when they are performing a particular task.	The patient reports that the pain is worse at night when they are lying down.
Understanding: Ask the patient what they believe is causing the pain.	The patient believes that they have a recurrent tumour in the left lung that is causing the pain.
Value: Ask the patient what the pain has prevented them from doing. Ask them if they have any personal beliefs that may affect how pain is managed.	The patient responds that they are unable to complete their own hygiene activities and sleep is poor. They explain that they have been taught to not complain about pain and to be stoic.
Ask the patient about their pain intensity goal (out of 10).	They report that a pain intensity of 5 out of 10 would help them function better. A goal of 3 would be preferred.

NURSING DIAGNOSIS: Acute pain related to a biological injuring agent (tumour).

PLANNING

Goals (Nursing Outcomes Classification) *	*Expected Outcomes*
Pain Control	
Patient will obtain an acceptable level of comfort as soon as possible.	Patient will report pain at stated goal or below prior to discharge.
The spouse will assist in restoring the patient to a more comfortable state.	The spouse will provide selected comfort measures to the patient before bedtime.
Pain: Disruptive Effects	
Patient will actively participate in ADLs.	The patient will report sleeping for 5 to 6 hours without interruption from pain. Perhaps a sleep aid can be initiated while in the hospital if disrupted sleep persists.
	They will complete their own hygiene with minimal assistance.
	They will walk the hallway with their spouse every 4 hours for 15 minutes.
Medication Response	
The patient will be assessed for adverse effects of opioids. If they experience opioid adverse effects, they will be appropriately managed.	The patient will be assessed for nausea, pruritus, constipation, and sedation. Their bowel pattern will be maintained and they will have a normal bowel movement as per their baseline routine. Consideration will be given for starting a bowel agent before discharge for the period of time they are taking opioids. Any adverse effects will be managed with the appropriate treatment options.

*Outcome classification labels form Moorhead, S., Swanson, E., Johnson, M., et al. (Eds). (2018). *Nursing outcomes classification (NOC)* (6th ed.). Mosby/Elsevier.

INTERVENTIONS

Interventions (Nursing Interventions Classification)†	*Rationale*
Pain Management	
Begin PCA at the prescribed dose. Explain to the patient and spouse how to use the PCA. Emphasize the importance of only the patient pushing the button; they know best when they are having pain and they can pre-emptively activate the button prior to mobilization.	The patient is experiencing an acute episode of their cancer pain. Confirming that only the patient should activate the button will minimize potential over sedating effects of the opioid because the patient must be awake to activate it in response to pain.
Monitor PCA opioid use. Explain to patient and spouse the action of the medication, potential adverse effects, and the importance of reporting if the pain is not relieved.	Pain is easier to prevent than to treat. Provide patient and spouse with written instructions regarding the use of the PCA pump. Instruct the spouse to inform staff of unrelieved pain or unmanageable adverse effects.

Continued

BOX 32.11 NURSING CARE PLAN—cont'd
Acute Pain

Interventions (Nursing Interventions Classification)†	Rationale
Administer nonopioid analgesics as prescribed.	Nonopioid analgesics can effectively assist in the management of pain and can be opioid sparing.
Have the patient select nonpharmacological interventions that have relieved pain in the past (e.g., distraction, music, simple relaxation therapy or massage).	Personal control allows a patient to shape immediate circumstances through their own actions. Nonpharmacological interventions augment pharmacological strategies but should not be used in place of analgesics.

†Intervention classification labels from Bulechek, G. M., Butcher, H. K., McCloskey Dochterman, J. M., et al. (Eds.). (2019). *Nursing interventions classification (NIC)* (7th ed.). Mosby/Elsevier.

EVALUATION

Nursing Actions	Patient Response and Finding	Achievement of Outcome
Ask the patient if they attained their pain-relief goal most of the time.	They respond, "My pain usually runs around a 3, which is my goal, except when I start walking."	The patient reports an acceptable level of comfort, which is a change from the level that indicated unacceptable pain. Instruct them to push their button pre-emptively about 5 minutes before ambulating to further assist with pain at movement.
Observe the patient's ability to perform ADLs, walk, and sleep.	They are dressed for breakfast and are walking the hallway every 4 hours with their spouse. The handover report indicates the patient slept through the night.	Ability to perform ADLs and to sleep has improved. Continue to monitor.
Ask the patient's spouse if they were able to offer a massage.	They reported that the patient did not want a massage but preferred to have their feet rubbed, which the spouse was happy to perform.	A nonpharmacological intervention was successful and the nursing care plan was updated.
Ask the patient the about the timing and consistency of their last bowel movement.	They had not had a bowel movement in 3 days and typically they do so every 2 days.	Assess the patient's abdomen for bowel sounds and distension. Inquire about passing flatus. As constipation is one of the most common opioid adverse effect, consult with the health care provider about starting a stool softener and mild peristaltic stimulant. It is recommended to start these agents as soon as possible.

patient what the pain has prevented the patient from doing and decide on a realistic and acceptable level of pain that will allow a return of function. Success is determined through attainment of goals and positive outcomes. For example, if the goal is "the patient will achieve a satisfactory level of pain relief within 24 hours," the following are possible outcomes:

- Reporting that pain is a 3 or less on a scale of 0 to 10, or does not interfere with ADLs
- Identifying factors that intensify pain, and modifying behaviour accordingly
- Using pain-relief measures safely, both pharmacotherapies and nonpharmacological supports

Setting Priorities. When setting priorities in pain management, the nurse needs to consider the type of pain the patient is experiencing and the effects the pain has on various body functions. The nurse should discuss with the patient the selected interventions appropriate for the nature and effects of the pain. For example, if a patient has had acute pain but an analgesic has brought relief, attention is focused on how the pain is influencing activity, appetite, and sleep. In contrast, when a patient's pain continues to be severe, immediate pain relief is the obvious priority. Nursing priorities will change as the patient's pain experience changes. Plans should take into account expected occurrences of pain.

Collaborative Pain Care. A comprehensive plan includes a variety of resources and all members of the interprofessional team to work

together toward pain control. This approach includes staff nurses, advanced practice nurses and nurse practitioners, pharmacists, physiotherapists, occupational therapists, psychologists, social workers, and pastoral and spiritual care. For children, child life specialists can also assist with pain management. Pharmacists are knowledgeable about the effects, interactions, and adverse effects of multiple medication regimens often required to treat pain. Physiotherapists can plan exercises that strengthen muscle groups and lessen pain in affected areas. Occupational therapists can devise splints to support painful body parts. Child life specialists can plan social and play activities that reflect the developmental needs of the child. Psychologists can assist with augmenting coping behaviours for chronic pain or for patients with chronic pain and an acute exacerbation. The family should also be involved in the care within the hospital because they may need to administer or assist with care at home after discharge. The home care instructions should be both verbal and written. If the pain management plan is not successful, the nurse should discuss the need for a change in treatment plan with the most responsible health care provider, consult a pain service, or both. Nurse practitioners working on pain management teams can be instrumental in providing holistic care by adjusting modalities or managing unbearable adverse effects during the trajectory of the patient's hospitalization. Nurse practitioners within various pain teams can work in the perioperative areas managing acute pain, in outpatient chronic pain clinics, and with patients with complex pain and patients with opioid misuse and addictions (Katz et al., 2019).

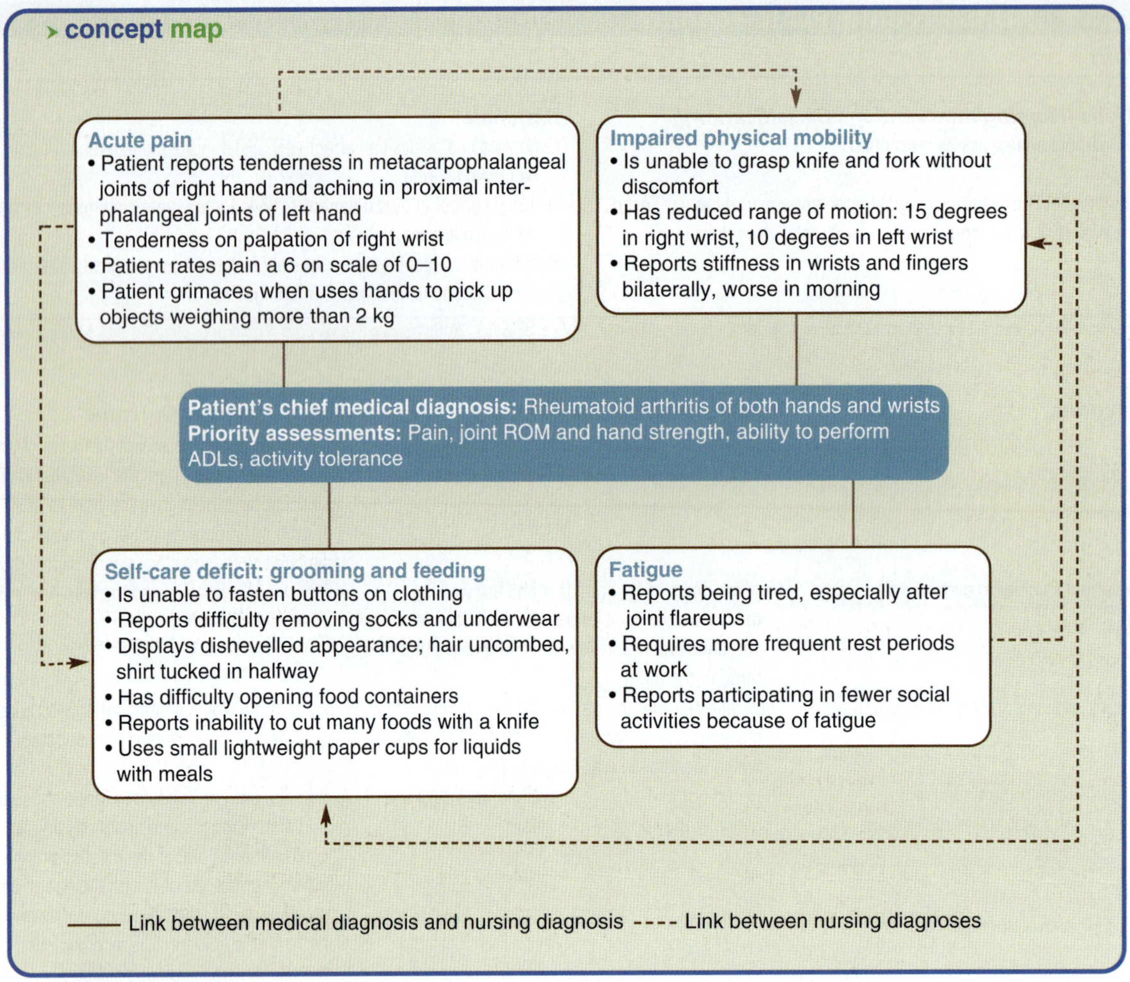

> concept map

Acute pain
- Patient reports tenderness in metacarpophalangeal joints of right hand and aching in proximal interphalangeal joints of left hand
- Tenderness on palpation of right wrist
- Patient rates pain a 6 on scale of 0–10
- Patient grimaces when uses hands to pick up objects weighing more than 2 kg

Impaired physical mobility
- Is unable to grasp knife and fork without discomfort
- Has reduced range of motion: 15 degrees in right wrist, 10 degrees in left wrist
- Reports stiffness in wrists and fingers bilaterally, worse in morning

Patient's chief medical diagnosis: Rheumatoid arthritis of both hands and wrists
Priority assessments: Pain, joint ROM and hand strength, ability to perform ADLs, activity tolerance

Self-care deficit: grooming and feeding
- Is unable to fasten buttons on clothing
- Reports difficulty removing socks and underwear
- Displays dishevelled appearance; hair uncombed, shirt tucked in halfway
- Has difficulty opening food containers
- Reports inability to cut many foods with a knife
- Uses small lightweight paper cups for liquids with meals

Fatigue
- Reports being tired, especially after joint flareups
- Requires more frequent rest periods at work
- Reports participating in fewer social activities because of fatigue

—— Link between medical diagnosis and nursing diagnosis   - - - - Link between nursing diagnoses

FIGURE 32.8 Concept map for patient with pain related to rheumatoid arthritis. *ADLs,* Activities of daily living; *ROM,* range of motion.

◆ Implementation

The nature of the pain and how much it affects well-being determines the choice of interventions. Pain therapy requires an individualized approach, perhaps more so than any other patient health challenge. The nurse, the patient, and the family must be partners in using pain-control measures. While nurses administer and monitor pain treatments ordered by a health care provider, they should also consider using other complementary comfort measures. Patient remedies are often successful, especially when the patient has already had experience with pain. Generally, the least invasive and safest therapy should be tried first.

Health Promotion. *Health promotion* is the process of enabling individuals to gain control over and improve their health, with the ultimate goal of equity in health for all. Chronic pain and suffering diminish quality of life; thus, relieving pain and promoting self-control are important. Once pain is controlled to an acceptable level, patients and their families need to be provided with education and information about pain so that they can participate in the pain care decision-making process. This will help reduce anxiety and increase a patient's sense of control. For example, patients who are in the hospital for the first time may know that they require tests but do not understand the rationale for such tests. They may also not be able to decipher the results. Consequently, they may become anxious and fearful, which can increase the pain threshold.

Nonpharmacological Pain-Relief Interventions. Several nonpharmacological interventions do not need a prescriber's order but are initiated by nurses. These approaches are used in addition to, not in place of, pharmacological measures (Health Quality Ontario, 2018a, 2020). Nonpharmacological interventions include cognitive-behavioural and physical approaches.

The goals of cognitive-behavioural interventions, such as relaxation and guided imagery, are to change pain perceptions, alter pain behaviour, and provide a greater sense of control (Vitoula et al., 2018). The aim of physical agents is to provide comfort, correct physical dysfunction, alter physiological responses, and reduce fears associated with pain-related immobility. Complementary and alternative medicine (CAM) therapies, such as herbal supplements, energy therapies, and manipulation or body-based therapies, are also available. The National Center for Complementary and Integrative Health (NCCIH) and the Canadian Health Network, a health promotion service operated by the Public Health Agency of Canada, offer up-to-date information on their websites to assist health care providers in answering their patients' questions, in a nonjudgemental manner, about the use of these methods. Most hospitals support complementary therapies, as long as they serve to augment the primary therapy.

Relaxation and guided imagery. Relaxation is mental and physical freedom from tension or stress. Relaxation techniques provide patients with self-control and can be used at any phase of health or

BOX 32.12 Body Positions for Relaxation

Sitting
Sit with the entire back resting against the back of the chair.
Place feet flat on the floor.
Keep legs separated.
Hang arms at the side or rest on chair arms.
Keep head aligned with the spine.

Lying
Keep legs separated with toes pointed slightly outward.
Rest arms at sides without touching sides of the body.
Keep head aligned with the spine.
Use a thin, small pillow under the head.

illness. Relaxation techniques include meditation, yoga, guided imagery, and progressive relaxation exercises (see Chapter 36).

For effective relaxation, patients must be in a state that will enable them to participate. Relaxation is difficult to teach to patients who are in severe pain, because they may not be able to focus and concentrate. The environment should be quiet and free of stimuli. The patient may sit in a comfortable chair or lie in bed (Box 32.12). A light sheet or blanket may help the patient feel more comfortable. Guided imagery and relaxation exercises may be done together or separately.

Progressive relaxation of the entire body takes about 15 minutes. The patient pays attention to the body, noting areas of tension. Warmth and relaxation replace tension in these areas. Some patients relax better with their eyes closed. Soft background music can help in this process.

Progressive relaxation exercises involve controlled breathing exercises and a series of contractions and relaxation of muscle groups. The patient begins by breathing slowly and diaphragmatically, allowing the abdomen to rise slowly and the chest to expand fully. When the patient establishes a regular breathing pattern, the nurse can coach the patient to locate any area of muscular tension, to think about how it feels, to tense muscles fully, and then to relax them completely. This creates the sensation of removing all discomfort and stress. Gradually the patient can relax the muscles without first tensing them. When full relaxation is achieved, pain perception may be lowered and anxiety about pain may decrease. Chapter 36 offers several relaxation exercise approaches.

If a patient becomes agitated or uncomfortable, it is best to stop the exercise. If the patient has difficulty relaxing any part of the body, it is best to slow the progression of the exercise and concentrate on the tensed body part. The patient must know that the exercise can be stopped at any time. With practice, the patient can soon perform relaxation exercises independently.

In **guided imagery**, the patient creates an image in their mind, concentrates on that image, and gradually becomes less aware of pain. The nurse coaches the patient in forming the image and concentrating on the sensory experience. Initially, the patient is asked to think of a pleasant scene or experience that promotes the use of all of the senses. The patient may describe the image, which the nurse may record for use during later exercises. The nurse should use the information the patient provides and not change the patient's image. The following is an example of part of a guided imagery exercise:

Imagine you are lying on a cool bed of grass with the sounds of rushing water from a nearby stream. It's a balmy day. You turn to see a patch of blue wildflowers in bloom and can smell their fragrance.

The nurse should sit close enough to be heard and speak in a calm, soft voice. While relaxing, the patient focuses on the image, and it will become unnecessary for the nurse to speak continuously. If the patient shows signs of agitation, restlessness, or discomfort, the exercise is stopped and then tried again when the patient is more at ease.

Distraction. The reticular activating system inhibits painful stimuli if a person receives sufficient or excessive sensory input. Boredom or isolation may cause patients to focus on their pain and thus perceive it more acutely. Pleasurable stimuli cause the release of endorphins that help a person ignore or become unaware of pain. Distraction, particularly effective for young children, directs attention to something else, thus reducing pain awareness and increasing tolerance. It works best for short, intense pain lasting a few minutes, such as during a needle-stick or intravenous insertion. Examples are praying, describing photos or pictures aloud, listening to music, using therapeutic humour, and playing games, some involving the use of virtual reality technology. Most distractions can be used in a hospital, home, or long-term care facility.

Music. Music can promote relaxation and decrease physiological pain, stress, and anxiety by diverting attention away from pain (Lin et al., 2020). Music can be chosen by either the patient or health care provider. The nurse can help create a relaxing setting so that music can be listened to uninterrupted. The use of earbuds or noise-cancelling headphones may assist with concentration and block out ambient noise. Although some benefits can be achieved with music therapy as a means of distraction, the evidence is weak to moderate regarding the effects of music therapy on reducing acute pain.

Biofeedback. **Biofeedback** is a behavioural therapy that involves educating patients about how to alter their physiological activity in order to improve both health and performance. Specific instrumentation can measure physiological activity such as brain oscillations, heart rate, breathing, muscle activity, and skin temperature. The instrument then provides "feedback" of the information to the patient, and this information, combined with changes in one's thinking, emotions, and behaviour, can elicit a targeted physiological response. Biofeedback allows the patient to have control over their perceptions, mood, and sensations. It is often combined with cognitive-behavioural therapy (CBT) to treat chronic pain. CBT has been shown to be efficacious in treating patients with chronic pain and has been demonstrated in multiple randomized controlled trials (Fukui et al., 2020). (Chapter 36 describes the benefits and limitations of biofeedback.) A referral to a psychologist will be warranted to initiate biofeedback within the hospital.

Acupuncture. **Acupuncture**, traditionally embedded in naturalistic theories and in Chinese medicine dating back 2 500 years, may help reduce chronic and acute pain and, if properly performed, is a safe procedure. Acupuncture involves the insertion of acupuncture needles into specific "acupuncture points" (acupoints) on the patient's body, followed by the twisting of the needle up and down by hand. Evidence from numerous systematic reviews indicates that acupuncture is potentially effective for emesis developing after surgery or chemotherapy in adults, for nausea associated with pregnancy, and for relieving dental pain. There is also evidence for the use of acupuncture to treat low back pain (Li et al., 2020). During the last decades, our understanding of how acupuncture analgesia works has undergone considerable development. Acupuncture activates endogenous opioid mechanisms and may stimulate gene expression of neuropeptides. The training of practitioners and the provision of acupuncture care in Canada are rapidly expanding. Chapter 36 describes the benefits and limitations of acupuncture.

Cutaneous stimulation. **Cutaneous stimulation**, also referred to as *touch healing* (TH) therapies, is the stimulation of the skin to relieve pain. A massage, warm bath, ice bag, and transcutaneous electrical nerve stimulation are simple ways to reduce pain perception. How

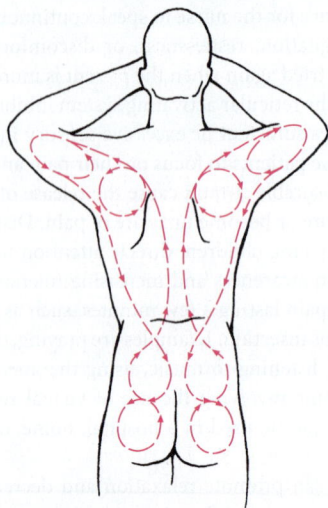

FIGURE 32.9 Back massage pattern.

methods of cutaneous stimulation work is unclear. It has been suggested that TH therapies involve mechanisms of neural plasticity in somatosensory maps, thus resulting in sensory reorganization.

An advantage to cutaneous stimulation is that the measures can be used in the home, giving patients and families some control over pain symptoms and treatment. With the proper use of cutaneous stimulation, pain perception can be reduced, as well as muscle tension that might otherwise increase pain. The practitioner first helps the patient get into a comfortable position and explains the purpose of the therapy. Cutaneous stimulation should not be used directly on sensitive skin areas (e.g., burns, bruises, skin rashes, inflammation, underlying bone fractures).

Massage is a safe and effective way to reduce anxiety and minimize tension (Figure 32.9). Massage involves the manipulation of the soft tissues by either mechanical or physical means. Recent literature suggests that hand and foot massage can be an option for reducing pain, along with back or body massage.

Tactile stimulation such as rubbing or stroking using moderate intensity can be used just prior to and during the vaccination of children over 4 years of age. This method works within the framework of the gate control theory whereby touch competes with pain in routing the message to the brain, thereby reducing pain.

Therapeutic touch (TT) and **Reiki** are classified as alternate or complementary treatments. With Reiki, the universe is understood to consist of energy, which includes the human body, and alteration of this energy can lead to disease (Dogan, 2018). Practitioners of Reiki use subtle energy fields in and around the body for positive health effects. TT and Reiki both involve the practitioner's use of hands to help strengthen the body's ability to heal. Reiki is an ancient practice believed to have originated thousands of years ago. In recent years, nursing has been instrumental in exploring the benefits of energy work. Reiki is an effective complementary therapy aimed at reducing pain; however, sample sizes in randomized controlled trials have been small, necessitating further research regarding the effectiveness of this approach. Energy work has been endorsed as a valid modality for nursing intervention by a number of nursing groups across Canada, such as the Canadian Holistic Nurses Association and the RNAO's Complementary Therapies Nurses' Interest Group. Please see Chapter 36 for additional information.

Cold and heat applications have been shown to relieve pain and promote healing. The choice of heat or cold varies with patients' condition and preference. Use of either method may require a prescriber's order. Moist heat can help relieve pain from a tension headache, and cold applications can reduce acute pain from inflamed joints. To avoid injury, it is important to check the temperature and avoid direct application of cold or heat to the skin. Patients at most risk for injury include those with spinal cord or other neurological injury, older people, and patients with confusion.

Application of cold packs may be effective for pain relief in certain conditions. Cold is particularly effective for dental pain and has been used to relieve pain associated with coughing and breathing in postcardiac surgery. Following orthopedic surgery, ice packs or cooling devices can help relieve postoperative pain (Kunkle et al., 2021). Cold applications are also useful before needle-stick procedures. Cold may be placed either near or distal to the pain site. The cold should be applied for 20 minutes to achieve maximum effect. Placement of a cold pack near the actual site of pain tends to provide the most relief.

Heat application is another option for relieving pain. Heating pads or hot water bottles may be used, as can commercial heated pillows that can contour to the body. These methods are ideal at home; disposable heat and warmth solutions are used in the hospital as an infection prevention and control measure.

Although heat and cold applications are methods to consider when promoting comfort, few studies have been published addressing their impact on pain or functional qualities. Refer to Cobbett and colleagues' (2020) textbook *Canadian Clinical Nursing Skills and Techniques* for further guidance on the application of warm and cold therapy and the necessary safety precautions for use.

Another form of cutaneous stimulation, sometimes called *counterstimulation*, is **transcutaneous electrical nerve stimulation (TENS)**. TENS involves stimulation of the skin with a mild electrical current passed through external electrodes. This therapy requires a prescriber's order. The TENS unit consists of a battery-powered transmitter, lead wires, and electrodes. The electrodes are placed directly over or near the pain site. TENS works by providing electrical stimulation via the skin and can be used with acute and chronic pain conditions. The frequency, intensity, and duration can be adjusted to meet the needs of the patient. However, a recent Cochrane Review reported that given the low quality of the evidence reviewed, researchers could not conclusively state the efficacy of TENS for chronic pain and suggested that future studies of this approach are warranted (Gibson et al., 2019). Physiotherapy should be consulted for TENS assessment and application.

Herbal supplements. Herbal supplements have not been sufficiently studied to be recommended for pain relief; however, many patients self-medicate using supplements such as echinacea, ginseng, ginkgo biloba, and garlic supplements. Some herbal products may interact with prescribed analgesics—in particular, ginkgo biloba may decrease the ability of blood to clot after surgery. The patient should be asked to report all supplements taken to relieve pain, and this should be part of the medication reconciliation while the patient is in hospital (see Chapter 36). Patients may support using complementary and alternative methods, such as following a special dietary plan (Atkins, macrobiotic, or vegan diets) or consuming herbal or non-vitamin supplements, because of the perceived benefits of these methods being a natural treatment that focuses on the whole person. Studies of the use of rosa damascena (damask rose—a rose hybrid) to treat pain have shown promising safety and evidence, but the results need to be interpreted with caution, and more studies are required (Arruda et al., 2019).

Reducing pain perception. One simple way to promote comfort is to remove or prevent painful stimuli. As a nurse you can take steps to reduce patients' pain by paying attention to the way you perform procedures. This is especially important for patients who are immobilized or have difficulty expressing themselves. Consider a patient's condition and the aspects of the procedure that are uncomfortable.

Use techniques to avoid pain-producing situations. For example, in a patient with severe arthritic knee pain, know that extreme flexion of the knee can cause pain. Before walking the patient to the bathroom, make sure that an elevated toilet seat is available. The patient can then be seated and can rise with minimal discomfort.

Acute Pain Management. Some patients have acute pain from invasive procedures (e.g., surgery or endoscopy), trauma, or cancer. The key to successful pain relief is ongoing evaluation of interventions. In caring for the patient, the nurse needs to ask the following questions: Is relief obtained? Do the medications cause any unacceptable adverse effects? It is the responsibility of the health care team to collaborate in order to find the combination of therapy that works best for the patient.

Pharmacological Pain-Relief Interventions. While the ideal analgesic has yet to be developed, many opioid and nonopioid pain-relieving medications are available. Most require a physician's or nurse practitioner's prescription.

> **SAFETY ALERT** As a nurse, your critical thinking and judgement in the selection and administration of analgesics helps to ensure safe and effective pain relief.
> - Be cognizant of the pain diagnosis or nature of the patient's pain, the patient's physical characteristics (e.g., age), and severity of their illness; know that some analgesics will be contraindicated.
> - Employ the 10 rights (person, medication, dose, route, time, documentation, reason, evaluation, patient education, and right to refuse) of medication administration.
> - When dispensing opioids, be sure to check the dose and medication type, as the names of some common medications sound alike. Some institutions employ an independent double-check policy for high-alert medications, including opioids.
> - Administer all opioids using standardized guidelines.
> - Evaluate analgesic effectiveness, and report and document any adverse effects.

Analgesics. Analgesics are a common and effective method of pain relief. Although analgesics can effectively relieve pain, nurses and physicians still tend to undertreat patient's pain.

Three types of analgesics exist: (1) acetaminophen and nonsteroidal anti-inflammatory drugs (NSAIDs) and nonopioids, (2) **opioids**, and (3) co-analgesics, a variety of medications that enhance analgesics or have analgesic properties.

Acetaminophen (Tylenol®) has no anti-inflammatory effects and works peripherally and centrally; its action is unknown. Its major adverse effect is hepatotoxicity. It is in a variety of over-the-counter (OTC) cold, flu, and allergy remedies. The maximum 24-hour dose for an adult is 4 g (the same dose limitation as Aspirin) and is weight-dependent for infants and children. Pediatric patients who weigh over 50 kg receive dosing parameters similar to those for adults. Acetaminophen does not affect platelet function and has minimal impact on the gastrointestinal tract. For postoperative or moderate to severe pain, it is often combined with opioids (e.g., hydromorphone, morphine, oxycodone) because it is opioid sparing and part of multimodal therapy (Baichoo et al., 2019). Intravenous acetaminophen was approved for use by Health Canada in 2018. It is becoming more available for use via hospital formularies, under restricted use by certain teams such as the pain services. It has been somewhat cost-prohibitive (it is approximately 300 times more expensive than the same oral dose); however, it has been proven to be beneficial for patients who are NPO and is used for short periods, typically 72 hours or until oral doses can be tolerated (Richebe, 2020). More studies are required in pediatrics to

provide further evidence about whether the intravenous formulation provides superior analgesia to the oral version (Ulrich et al., 2021). An overdose of acetaminophen can be fatal, and toxicity can have hepatotoxic and nephrotoxic sequelae. The usual treatment for overdose is N-acetylcysteine or Mucomyst®, which can be administered via intravenous, inhalation, or oral routes (Hendrickson, 2019).

Nonselective NSAIDs, such as Aspirin, ibuprofen (OTC), and dicofenac available by prescription, and selective NSAIDS, such as celecoxib (Celebrex®) available by prescription, provide relief for mild to moderate acute pain resulting from trauma or an inflammatory process. NSAIDs act directly by inhibiting the synthesis of cyclooxygenase (COX) enzymes. Two types of COX enzymes exist, COX-1 and COX-2. COX-1 acts directly on homeostasis functions whereas COX-2 is mostly expressed via an inflammatory response (Capuano et al., 2020). Nonselective NSAIDs have been found to be safe when taken for short periods. Selective NSAIDs are at times preferred for longer use because they do not interfere with platelets and cause less gastric irritation. Celecoxib is a selective COX-2 inhibitor and should not be used in patients with a sulfa allergy. Most NSAIDs act on peripheral nerve receptors to reduce transmission of pain stimuli. Unlike opioids, NSAIDs do not depress the central nervous system, nor do they interfere with bowel or bladder function.

Use of salicylates or Aspirin is typically avoided in pediatrics because of the associated development of Reye's syndrome with salicylate use. Reye's syndrome can manifest as neurological compromise, acute hepatitis, and cerebral edema. Given cases studies that have identified a strong correlation between Reye's syndrome and aspirin use, its use has decreased in pediatric practice. In fact, use of Aspirin® should be avoided in all children less than 18 years of age who are recovering from chickenpox or a viral-type illness, because of its association with Reye's syndrome, which can manifest early with behavioural changes and nausea and vomiting (Noor & Gradidge, 2018) .

Chronic NSAID use in older patients is associated with more frequent adverse effects (e.g., gastrointestinal bleeding and renal insufficiency) and should be avoided (Capuano et al., 2020). Taking NSAIDs with food reduces the likelihood of gastrointestinal upset.

Opioids are also used to help manage pain, and there are many opioids that are available. Opioid or opioid-like analgesics are generally prescribed for moderate to severe pain. These analgesics act by binding with opiate receptors, namely mu, delta, and kappa, to modify the perception of pain (Machelska & Celik, 2018).

Codeine is a weak opioid used for moderate to severe pain. Although codeine has been widely prescribed for pain relief, recent advances in our understanding of the pharmacogenetics of codeine have forced more investigation of its properties and adverse effects, particularly in the pediatric age group. Codeine is a prodrug. A *prodrug* is a drug that must undergo chemical and enzymatic conversion to morphine to have an analgesic effect. Codeine's pharmacokinetics are variable and, in some patients, unpredictable. Because codeine is a prodrug, it has pharmacokinetic properties that vary between individuals, owing to genetic variations of CYP2D6 and CYP3A4 genes. This affects how codeine converts to morphine and is highly depended on CYP2D6 functionality. In poor metabolizers, codeine may not be expressed at all, leading to poor or no pain control, whereas other patients may be ultra-rapid metabolizers, resulting in rapid conversion of codeine to morphine, even despite recommended dosing (Sobczak & Gorynski, 2020). This places high metabolizers at risk for oversedation and respiratory depression that could result in death. As a result of several pediatric deaths secondary to codeine ingestion, most pediatric hospitals have removed it from their formulary. Health Canada has issued a recommendation that codeine-containing cough medications should not be administered to children under 13 years of age because of rare, yet fatal, adverse effects. Codeine-containing OTC products can be misused, as they may cause euphoria, relaxation, and a warm feeling with pleasurable sensations and can thus serve as a substitute for illicit drug use (Sobczak & Gorynski, 2020).

Opioid overdose is a potentially fatal adverse effect of opioids. People are at increased risk of an opioid overdose if they consume opioids with sedatives or if they consume opioids with alcohol. Signs of an overdose include pin-point pupils plus oversedation (somnolent and unable to wake) and respiratory depression (respiration rate of less than 10 breaths per minute). Opioid-induced respiratory depression can be prevented through careful titration of opioids, close monitoring of sedation scores, and a thorough respiratory assessment that includes the depth, quality, and regularity of respirations (Government of Canada, 2021; Jungquist et al., 2020). In pediatric settings, protocols exist for monitoring requirements (nurse in room or constant observation) for children under 1 year of age with basal infusions or opioid-containing epidural infusions, as they are at greater risk of respiratory depression.

If a patient experiences respiratory depression, an opioid antagonist such as naloxone (Narcan®) can be administered. The dose must be titrated carefully and given as per health care provider prescription. Administering naloxone too quickly or administering too much can reverse the analgesic effect and produce severe pain that may be difficult to control. In addition, rapid administration can increase the sympathetic response and the patient may experience tachycardia, dysrhythmias, hypertension, pulmonary edema, and even cardiac arrest. Nurses need to carefully assess and reassess patients every 15 minutes for 2 hours after medication administration because of the risk of renarcotization and the return of respiratory depression. Naloxone is also used in smaller doses (0.25–2 mcg/kg/hour by continuous infusion) for the treatment of opioid adverse effects such as pruritus and nausea without reversing the opioid.

Opioid receptors can also mediate adverse effects. Common adverse effects of opioids include nausea, vomiting, pruritus, constipation, sedation, and confusion. Less common effects include urinary retention, dry mouth, sweating, orthostatic hypotension, and seizures. Most adverse effects are dose related; hence, a reduction in the opioid dose may eliminate the adverse effect or allow it to be more tolerable. If intolerable adverse effects persist, sometimes an opioid rotation will reduce the adverse effects such that intractable nausea with morphine patient-controlled analgesia (PCA) may be minimized or eliminated with a rotation to hydromorphone PCA.

Around-the-clock (ATC) dosing of pain medications should be considered when pain exists for 12 of 24 hours. The benefits of ATC dosing include prevention in delay of timely medication administration and more stable blood levels of opioids to prevent the peaks and valleys of pain.

Pro re nata or PRN dosing can be used to treat breakthrough pain; however, this method requires the patient's participation since they need to request analgesia. Undertreatment of pain can occur if PRN dosing is used for continuous pain. As-needed or rescue dosing is most useful when initiating opioid therapy to treat moderate to severe escalating pain or when pain is diminishing.

The proper use of analgesics requires careful assessment and critical thinking in the application of pharmacological principles. A patient's response to an analgesic is highly individualized. An NSAID can be as effective as or more effective than an opioid for some patients if the pain is caused by inflammation. An orally administered analgesic usually has a longer onset and duration of action than an injectable form. In addition, controlled- or extended-release opioid formulations (MS Contin, H Contin, OxyContin, Kadian, Avinza, and methadone) are available for administration every 8 to 12 hours ATC with short-acting breakthrough dosing ordered. Health care providers should not prescribe these long-acting formulations on an as-needed basis. Typically, the long-acting opioids are calculated on the basis of the previous 24-hour requirements and are adjusted according to the amount of breakthrough doses required. Prescribers wishing to prescribe methadone no longer have regulatory constraints, and exemptions no longer are required from Health Canada to prescribe or administer methadone (Government of Canada 2017). Effective May 19, 2018, nurse practitioners gained the authority to prescribe methadone, which can be used for pain and to treat opioid use disorder (Government of Canada, 2017).

It is essential that nurses know the comparative potencies of analgesics in both oral and injectable forms. It is equally important to know the route of administration most effective for a patient so that pain relief can be achieved. *Equianalgesic charts* are charts that convert one opioid to another (e.g., morphine to hydromorphone) or parenteral forms of opioids to oral forms (or vice versa). They are available online or by contacting pharmacy team members. To see an example of an equianalgesic chart, refer to the *Oral Opioids Analgesic Conversion Table* (Machealth, 2019). An application of this is noted in the following example: morphine 20–30 mg orally is equivalent to morphine 10 mg parenterally (refer to switching opioids using equivalency tables at *Switching Opioids Using Equivalency Tables* [MedSask, 2012] from the University of Saskatchewan).

Before administering opioids, it is important to consider the patient's situation, including current treatments, comorbidities, and kidney and liver function. Opioid doses often need adjusting according to patient circumstances. Patients requiring special consideration include opioid-naïve patients, breastfeeding patients, patients on dialysis, persons with neurological or respiratory conditions, and patients at either end of the age spectrum, including pediatric and geriatric populations. Pharmacists are instrumental in assisting with specific dosing requirements in special circumstances, such as renal impairment. Furthermore, pharmacists play a key role in pain management by advising providers about dosing, determining interactions with other medications, and assisting in the review of adverse reactions. This collaborative practice undoubtedly improves patient outcomes and supports the mandate of Canadian pharmacists (Canadian Pharmacists Association, 2021).

Adjuvants, or co-analgesics, are medications that were originally developed to treat conditions other than pain but have been shown to have analgesic properties (Chin et al., 2020). Adjuvants used for acute or chronic pain can be employed as foundational analgesia or as a primary therapy for some specific painful conditions. Classes of medications considered adjuvant therapy or nonopioid analgesics include the following: anticonvulsants, such as gabapentin and pregabalin for neuropathic pain; antidepressants, such as amitriptyline for neuropathic pain; corticosteroids; α_2-adrenergic agonists, such as clonidine; cannabinoids; and topical analgesic agents.

Patient-controlled analgesia. Patients benefit from having control over their own pain therapy because they are the ones experiencing the pain. When patients depend on nurses for analgesia, an erratic cycle of alternating pain and analgesia often occurs. The patient feels pain and asks for medication, but the nurse must first assess the patient and then prepare the medication, which can cause a delay in timely administration. Within an hour, analgesia finally occurs, but adequate pain relief may last only 30 to 60 minutes. The patient's discomfort then gradually escalates, and the cycle is repeated.

A medication delivery system called **patient-controlled analgesia (PCA)** is a safe method for pain management that allows patients to self-administer opioid doses (e.g., morphine, hydromorphone, fentanyl) on demand with minimal risk of overdose. PCA can be

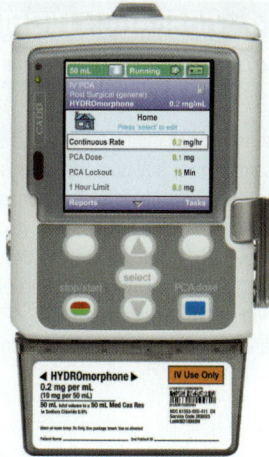

FIGURE 32.10 Ambulatory patient-controlled analgesia (PCA) pump. (*Smiths Medical: CADD Solis Ambulatory PCA Pump:* https://www.smiths-medical.com/brands/cadd)

administered with a continuous or basal infusion with demand-mode capabilities or demand mode only. PCA demand mode allows patients to control when they request analgesia and avoids the delay in waiting for pain relief as the patient can time the dose to a painful stimulus, such as coughing, turning, and positioning. The goal is to maintain a constant plasma level of analgesic so that the problems of rescue dosing are avoided. Systemic PCA typically pertains to intravenous administration, but PCA devices can be used to deliver pain medication via subcutaneous, epidural, intrathecal, and transdermal routes. PCA devices are portable computerized infusion pumps containing a chamber for a syringe, cassette (Figure 32.10), or bag that delivers a small, preset dose of medication. To receive a bolus dose, the patient activates a button attached to the PCA pump. To minimize overdoses, the system is designed with a preset "lockout" or delay interval, typically 6–8 minutes, based on the pharmacotherapies of the medication. The system is designed to deliver a specified number of doses every hour as required and demanded by the patient. PCA dosing is based strictly on weight, and dosing for any pediatric patient over 50 kg is based on adult dosing. Pediatric patients typically need to be older than 6 years of age to use PCA so that they have the comprehension to use it. For patients under 6 years of age or those with cognitive or developmental impairment, a nurse-controlled analgesia (NCA) modality can be administered using the same principles of weight-based dosing as for PCA, with the option of a basal infusion. The advantage of NCA includes pre-emptive analgesia timed to a painful procedure or for use for breakthrough pain. The pump can be activated by the nurse and be titrated on an individualized patient basis depending on the patient's unique needs. Furthermore, it avoids delays in providing breakthrough dosing because it is readily available (Donado et al., 2019).

SAFETY ALERT *Independent Double-Checks*

Remember to perform an independent double-check with a nurse colleague to ensure that the medication and the pump settings (e.g., basal rate, bolus dose, lockout interval, and total hourly dose) are congruent with the orders and that the appropriate documentation is provided within the medication administration record.

PCA is beneficial in many ways. The patient gains control over their pain, and pain relief does not depend on nurse availability. Patients can also access medication when they need it. This can decrease patient anxiety and lead to decreased medication use. Small doses of

BOX 32.13 Preparation for Patient-Controlled Analgesia

Objectives
- Patient will be able to explain the purpose of patient-controlled analgesia (PCA) in managing pain.
- Patient will demonstrate the correct use of the PCA device.
- Patient will achieve effective pain control.

Teaching Strategies
Some institutions employ both written and verbal instructions with PCA and offer instructions in advance for using PCA with elective surgery so that the patient is not learning this modality in the post–anaesthetic care unit for the first time. The Children's Hospital of Eastern Ontario (CHEO) created an instructional video in both English and French for the use of PCA that can be accessed via YouTube. It is posted on their website for patients to view preoperatively before the surgery and postoperatively as required to reinforce concepts. The video script was vetted via the youth forum for feedback and suggestions prior to final production.
- Teach the use of PCA before it is needed so that the patient can understand how to use it after awakening from anaesthesia or sedation. Reinforce teaching as needed.
- Instruct patient on the purpose of PCA, emphasizing that the patient controls the medication delivery.
- Explain that the lockout or delay interval prevents the risk of overdose.
- Tell family members or friends that they should not operate the PCA device for the patient.
- Ask the patient to demonstrate use of the PCA delivery button.

Evaluation
- Ask patient to tell you the purpose of the PCA device.
- Observe the patient administering a dose.
- Evaluate the severity of the patient's pain, both at rest and with movement, with PCA and determine if the patient's preset pain goal has been achieved.
- Evaluate and treat any adverse effects.

medications are delivered at short intervals, stabilizing serum medication concentrations for sustained pain relief.

Patients who may not be appropriate candidates for PCA are those who have cognitive impairment or who have short-term memory loss or states of confusion that make comprehension of the technology more difficult. Patient suitability, preparation, and teaching are critical to the safe and effective use of PCA devices (Box 32.13). It is important to teach patients how to use the technology and determine if they are physically able to locate and activate the button to deliver the dose. Family members need to be reminded that they must not press the button for patients, as this is deemed unauthorized administration of a dose by another person, referred to as *PCA by proxy*. Nurses need to check to ensure that their institution has established a policy that provides safeguards for PCA by proxy.

The intravenous line and PCA device need to be checked regularly to ensure proper functioning. Errors in pump programming can occur, placing the patient at risk for an overdose, resulting in oversedation and respiratory depression. In addition, opioid-naïve patients should be monitored carefully for both of these adverse effects with PCA therapy.

Local analgesic infusion pump. Postoperatively following cardiac, general, or orthopedic surgery, an infusion of a local anaesthetic into the operative site may be effective for pain management and help to avoid systemic adverse effects of oral or intravenous analgesics. A catheter from the wound, placed during surgery, is connected to a pump containing a local anaesthetic, such as bupivacaine (Marcaine) or ropivacaine. The infusion is usually left in place for 48 hours and may be set to either demand or continuous modes. Oral analgesics may still be needed by the patient, but the total dose is often reduced. Either single-shot nerve blocks or continuous nerve blocks can be used in pediatrics. Some pediatric patients who qualify can be discharged home on an ambulatory nerve block pump (On-Q pump) that is discontinued by the patient or family within 48 hours of discharge. Daily phone follow-ups are conducted by the Department of Anaesthesiology and Pain Medicine until the catheter is discontinued, and parents have emergency contact numbers for queries. Patient satisfaction scores are high, and pain is well controlled with nerve blocks. The block can reduce opioid requirements and reduce length of hospital stay. Many hospitals in Canada now use ambulatory pumps for pain management. Children's Hospital of Eastern Ontario (CHEO) has an outpatient program and has developed a teaching video that provides an overview of the pump, troubleshooting, and removal instructions (refer to https://www.cheo.on.ca/en/Video-Outpatient-Catheter-Therapy).

Topical analgesics and anaesthetics. Topical local analgesics such as Maxilene, Ametop, and EMLA (eutectic mixture of local anaesthetic containing lidocaine and prilocaine) are available for both children and adults. The topical agents are used for intravenous cannulation, lumbar puncture, and immunizations in pediatrics (Trottier et al., 2019). Some agents such as Ametop have the advantage of earlier onset of action than that of EMLA. Other topical medications are available for pain relief using a transdermal drug delivery system (TDDS), whereby the medication enters the systemic circulation via the skin and capillaries (Ma et al., 2021). Transdermal routes are advantageous in that they are simple to administer, avoid indirect interaction of medications with food or other drugs in the gastrointestinal tract, and assist in controlling drug delivery while reducing frequency of dosing. An example of a transdermal NSAID is ketoprofen. Transdermal applications can include ointment, gel, gel paste, or patch. Furthermore, transdermal opioids such as a fentanyl patch can be used to treat chronic pain, whereas capsaicin and lidocaine transdermal patches are used to treat neuropathic pain (Leppert et al., 2018; Ma et al., 2021).

Sucrose. Oral sucrose is an effective strategy to reduce procedural pain in infants (Mangat et al., 2018) (Box 32.14). Sweet taste is thought to trigger a release of endogenous opioids. Small volumes of sucrose (weight-based) are administered 2 minutes prior to the procedure and continue in small aliquots throughout the duration of the procedure. Non-nutritive sucking, as with use of a pacifier, may further assist with the uptake of sucrose. The efficacy of sucrose has been well demonstrated in infants undergoing painful procedures such as immunizations, venipunctures, and intravenous cannulation.

Local and regional anaesthetics and analgesics. Local anaesthesia is the infiltration of a local anaesthetic medication to induce loss of sensation to a localized body part. Physicians use local anaesthesia during brief surgical procedures, such as the removal of a skin lesion or suturing a wound. The local anaesthetic is topically applied on skin and mucous membranes or injected subcutaneously or intradermally to anaesthetize a body part. The medications produce temporary loss of sensation by inhibiting nerve conduction. Local anaesthetics can also block motor and autonomic functions, depending on the amount used and the location and depth of an injection. Smaller sensory nerve fibres are more sensitive to local anaesthetics than are large motor fibres. As a result, the patient loses sensation before losing motor function and, conversely, motor activity returns before sensation.

Local anaesthetics can cause adverse effects, depending on their absorption into the circulation. Itching or burning of the skin or a localized rash is common after topical applications. Application to vascular mucous membranes increases the chance of systemic effects, such as a change in heart rate.

BOX 32.14 RESEARCH HIGHLIGHT
Sucrose for Reducing Pain in Infants

Research Focus

Infants undergo painful procedures during their first year of life. Even healthy infants require blood sampling for newborn screening and receive injections for scheduled childhood immunization. Effective management of pain during these procedures is vital for the well-being of the developing infant. Canadian researchers have contributed substantially to the development of effective pain-management strategies for infants and have demonstrated analgesic effects of sweet-tasting solutions, such as sucrose 24%, in infants up to 18 months of age who were undergoing a painful procedure (DeBernardo et al., 2019).

Research Abstract

A randomized double-blind pilot study was conducted from February to September 2017 in a neonatal intensive care unit in Naples, Italy. The inclusion criteria included infants 37–42 weeks of gestational age, weighing 2 500–4 500 g, able to feed orally, and greater than 1 week of age at the time of the intervention. Newborns were randomly assigned to receive oral sucrose and non-nutritive sucking (NNS). Previous research findings indicated that the combination of sucrose and nonpharmacological approaches, such as NNS, seemed to be more effective in managing pain than when sucrose is used alone. This study supports the efficacy of sucrose for reducing pain prior to and during a single painful procedure beyond the first week of life (DeBernardo et al., 2019).

Evidence-Informed Practice

- Effective management of pain during painful procedures is critical for the well-being of infants. Poorly controlled pain can affect neurodevelopment (DeBernardo et al., 2019).
- Small volumes or aliquots of sucrose significantly reduce pain during procedures in infants up to 12–18 months of age, with the initial dose administered 2 minutes prior to the procedure and during the procedure.
- Other pain-management strategies can be used in conjunction with sucrose, such as topical anaesthetic agents. Sucrose does not replace providing appropriate analgesia.
- Mothers should be supported to help their infants during immunization. For example, sucrose can be offered, and mothers can be encouraged to breast-feed during the immunization and to provide kangaroo care.

From DeBernardo, G., Riccitelli, M., Sordino, D., et al. (2019). Oral 24% sucrose associated with nonnutritive sucking for pain control in healthy term newborns receiving venipuncture beyond the first week of life. *Journal of Pain Research, 12,* 299–305. https://doi.org/10.2147/jpr.s184504

Regional anaesthesia is the injection of a local anaesthetic to block a group of sensory nerve fibres. Tissues are anaesthetized layer by layer as the surgeon or anaesthesiologist introduces the agent into deeper structures of the body. Some types of regional anaesthesia are epidural anaesthesia, nerve blocks, and spinal anaesthesia.

Whereas epidural anaesthesia induces temporary loss of sensation, **epidural analgesia** permits control or reduction of severe pain without the sedative effects of parenteral or oral opioids. Epidural analgesia is commonly used for the treatment of acute postoperative pain, labour and delivery pain, and chronic pain, especially when associated with cancer (Galligan, 2020).

Epidural catheters can be placed via the caudal, lumbar, or thoracic region. However, intraspinal opioids can produce the same adverse effects of nausea, mental clouding, and sedation because they are absorbed via the cerebrospinal fluid into the circulation of the

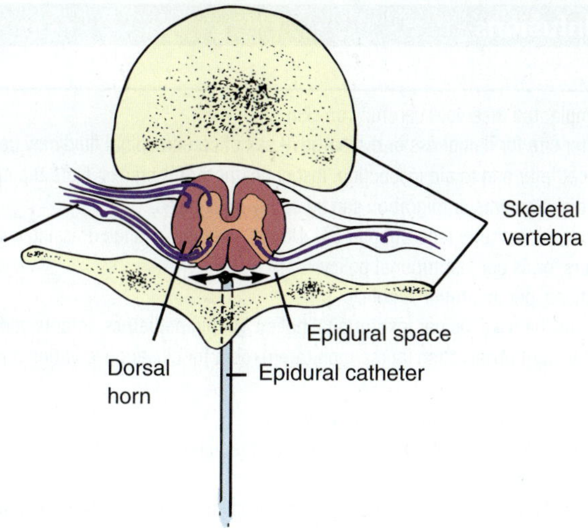

FIGURE 32.11 Anatomical drawing of epidural space.

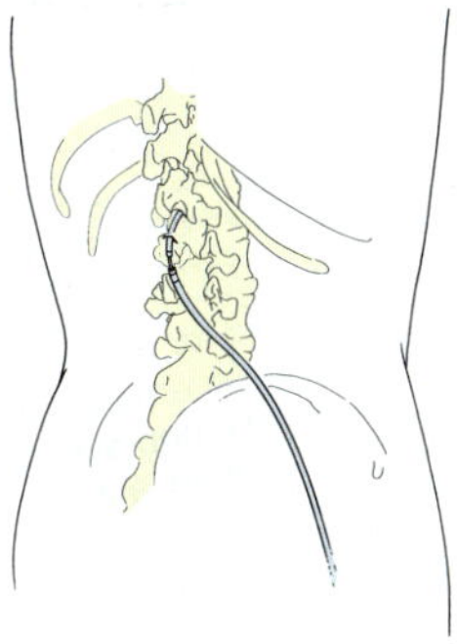

FIGURE 32.12 Epidural catheter taped in place.

epidural vascular plexus. Epidural analgesia can be short or long term, depending on the patient's condition and life expectancy. Short-term therapy is used for pain after intrathoracic, abdominal, and orthopedic surgery. Long-term therapy is particularly useful for intractable cancer pain.

Epidural analgesia is administered into the **epidural space**, which lies between the dura mater and the vertebrae (Figure 32.11) (Galligan, 2020). The physician inserts a needle into the level of the vertebral interspace nearest to the dermatomal area requiring analgesia. When the needle reaches the space, preservative-free local anaesthetic and opioids may be injected and a small catheter may be passed into the space. Once a catheter is advanced into the epidural space and the needle is removed, the remainder of the catheter is secured with a dressing and taped along the back of the patient (Figure 32.12). If the catheter is only temporary, it is connected to tubing positioned along the spine and over the patient's shoulder. The end of the catheter can then be placed on the patient's chest for easy access. Patients may also be given control of the demand dose, which is known as patient-controlled epidural analgesia (PCEA). When PCEA is used, the basal rate is intended to meet the patient's analgesic requirements and the PCEA bolus doses are intended to control periods of breakthrough pain. Infants may benefit from a single caudal block whereby a one-time dose of local anaesthetic is administered to manage surgical pain, specifically with procedures below the level of the umbilicus. When local anaesthetic agents are administered via any route, observation for adverse effects is critical. Local anaesthetic systemic toxicity (LAST) is a life-threatening adverse event that is characterized by peri-oral paresthesia, confusion, visual disturbances, agitation, and reduced level of consciousness and

may progress to dysrhythmias, conduction disturbances, and, eventually, cardiac arrest. Health care organizations will have a standardized management strategy for LAST, including rescue kits that contain intravenous lipid emulsion therapy, which is used as first-line therapy (El-Boghdadly et al., 2018).

Nursing implications. Nurses can provide emotional support to patients receiving local or regional anaesthesia by explaining the procedure to them and informing them that they will temporarily lose sensory function. Patients commonly fear paralysis because epidural and spinal injections come close to the spinal cord. To reassure the patient, the nurse should explain that numbness, tingling, and coldness are common.

After administration of a local anaesthetic, the patient should be protected from injury until full sensory and motor function return. Patients are at risk for injuring the anaesthetized body part without knowing it. For example, after an injection into a joint, the nurse needs to inform the patient to avoid using the joint until function returns (Galligan, 2020). For patients with topical anaesthesia, heat or cold should not be applied to numb areas. After spinal anaesthesia, the patient should be instructed to stay in bed until sensory and motor function return. The nurse needs to assist the patient during the first attempt at mobilizing and ensure that the patient is wearing proper footwear to prevent falls and to optimize stability.

When managing epidural infusions, the nurse connects the catheter to an infusion pump, a port, or a reservoir or caps it off for bolus injections. To reduce the risk of accidental epidural injection of medications intended for intravenous use, the catheter should be clearly labelled an "epidural catheter." The nurse should always administer continuous infusions through dedicated electronic infusion devices for proper control. Because of the catheter location, surgical asepsis is used to prevent a serious and potentially fatal infection. The nurse must notify the health care provider immediately of any signs or symptoms of infection or pain at the insertion site. Nursing implications for managing epidural analgesia are summarized in Table 32.6.

Supplemental doses of opioids or sedatives (hypnotics) are avoided because they have additive effects that can be detrimental to the central nervous system. Monitoring of medication adverse effects differs, depending on whether infusions are intermittent or continuous. If opioids are to be administered, mu-agonist opioids, such as morphine, fentanyl, and hydromorphone, are the most common choices. Adverse reactions can be related to the opioid or the local anaesthetic agent. Nurses should refer to their specific institutional protocols for monitoring standards.

Patients should be instructed about the action of the medication, advantages and disadvantages of the epidural route of medication, and potential adverse effects. They should be instructed to notify a health care provider if they develop any adverse effects. If the patient requires a long-term epidural, a tunnelled catheter can be placed, which exits at the patient's side. Nurses need to provide education about long-term therapy, including how to safely administer infusions. For these patients, home care will likely be required.

Invasive Interventions for Pain Relief. When pain is severe, invasive interventions may give relief when more conservative treatment is neither tolerated nor effective. These interventions include intrathecal implantable pumps or injections, spinal cord stimulators, deep brain stimulation, neuroablative procedures (e.g., **chordotomy**, **dorsal rhizotomy**, thalamotomy), trigger point injections, radiofrequency ablation, cryoablation, intradiscal electrothermal (IDET) annuloplasty, vertebroplasty, or intraspinal medications (e.g., opioids, steroids, local anaesthetics, alpha agonists) (Corallo et al., 2020; Deer et al., 2017). Patients with pain that is unresponsive to traditional therapies require consultation with a pain expert or an interprofessional pain team.

TABLE 32.6 Nursing Care for Patients With Epidural Infusions

Goal	Actions
Prevent catheter displacement	Secure catheter (if not connected to implanted reservoir) carefully on skin.
Maintain catheter function	Check external dressing around catheter site for dampness or discharge. (Leak of cerebrospinal fluid may develop.) Use transparent dressing to secure catheter and to aid inspection. Inspect catheter for breaks. Note the epidural catheter marking at the skin so any dislodgments or migration can be easily recognized.
Prevent infection	Use strict aseptic technique when caring for catheter (see Chapter 34). Do not routinely change dressing over site. Change infusion tubing every 24 hours, or as per institutional policy.
Monitor for respiratory depression	Monitor vital signs, especially respirations, per institutional policy. Pulse oximetry and apnea monitoring may be used, as per institutional policy. Within pediatrics, infants under 1 year of age are often placed in a constant observation (nurse-monitored) room for closer observation and monitoring.
Prevent and treat complications	Assess for potential adverse effects, such as pruritus, nausea, and vomiting. Administer appropriate treatments to manage adverse effects as ordered and required.
Maintain urinary and bowel function	Monitor intake and output. Assess for bladder and bowel distension. Protect lumbar epidural catheters from soilage with infants who are diapered or patients who are incontinent to avoid contamination of the catheter. Assess for discomfort, frequency, and urgency. Some institutions will place a urinary catheter with lumbar epidurals, which remains until the epidural is discontinued.

Procedure Pain Management. Many of the following procedures can evoke pain:

- Turning
- Wound drain removal
- Tracheal suctioning
- Femoral catheter removal
- Placement of central line
- Changing of wound dressings

Premedicating patients before painful procedures may assist them in cooperating during the procedure and may help to reduce the experience of pain. This is also true for patients who present in the emergency department with pain.

Cancer Pain Management. Cancer pain may be chronic or acute or a combination of the two. A number of key organizations across Canada, such as Cancer Care Ontario's Cancer-Related Pain Management Guideline Panel and the Canadian Pain Society, have released evidence-informed clinical practice guidelines for the management of cancer pain. These guidelines are designed to treat cancer pain in a more comprehensive and aggressive manner and to provide patients and families with options for pain relief. The choice of treatment may change as the patient's condition and the characteristics of pain change. Effective pain management is best achieved when pharmacological and nonpharmacological pain interventions are used together and is part of an interprofessional approach to care.

Various medications and routes of administration provide relief for patients with cancer pain. Long-acting or controlled-release medications have been successful in managing all types of chronic pain. These controlled-released medications (e.g., MS Contin©, Hydromorph Contin©) relieve pain for 8 to 12 hours. A 72-hour fentanyl patch is also available. Management of most chronic pain can be achieved with oral or patch medications.

Administering analgesics to treat chronic noncancer and cancer pain requires principles different from those used to treat acute pain. The WHO recommends a three-step approach to managing cancer pain (Figure 32.13). Therapy begins with using NSAIDs, adjuvants, or both and progresses to strong opioids if pain persists. However, when a patient with cancer first experiences pain, it is recommended to begin with a higher dosage than will be needed for continued pain relief.

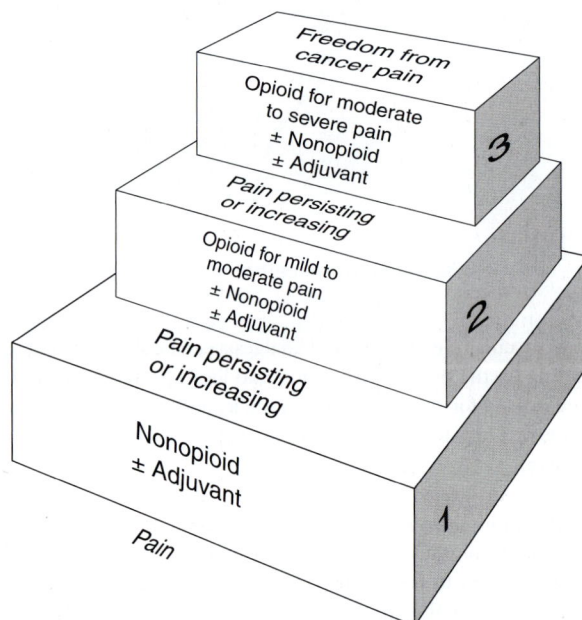

FIGURE 32.13 World Health Organization's pain relief ladder. (*From World Health Organization. [1996]. Cancer pain relief—with a guide to opioid availability [2nd ed.].* http://apps.who.int/iris/bitstream/10665/37896/1/9241544821.pdf. *Figure also available at* http://www.who.int/cancer/palliative/painladder/en/)

The dosing can then be decreased accordingly to the patient's needs. Adverse effects of analgesia, such as nausea, pruritus, and constipation, can be aggressively treated so that analgesia can be continued. Patients may become tolerant to the adverse effects of nausea, but not to the constipating effects of analgesics. Stimulant laxatives should be routinely administered to both prevent and treat constipation.

The WHO pain relief ladder (see Figure 32.13) was first developed in 1986 as a simple guide to pain management using pharmacotherapies to treat pain in cancer patients. The ladder has since been adopted as a tool for managing pain in acute, chronic, and noncancer conditions as well (Anekar & Cascella, 2020). The analgesic ladder utilizes a three-step approach to pain management that is primarily focused on pharmacological agents only; recently, some researchers have added an additional step, before strong opioids, that would include minimally invasive interventional procedures such as nerve blocks, radiofrequency, spinal cord stimulation, intrathecal administration of local anaesthetic agents, and epidural analgesia. This additional step would also encompass other nonpharmacological treatments such as yoga and would be aimed at strengthening the patient's quality of life. The philosophy is that this step should be considered with patients who have acute pain (pain <3 months), chronic pain (pain >3 months), and cancer pain where trials of weak opioids and nonopioids have failed to control the pain (Yang et al., 2020).

Patients with persistent pain requiring prolonged opioid administration sometimes develop an opioid tolerance. As a result, higher doses of opioids are required to attain pain relief. The higher opioid dose is not lethal because patients also develop a tolerance to the medication. For patients with chronic pain, it is necessary to give required analgesics on a regular, ATC basis, even when the pain subsides. Prescribing analgesics on an as-needed basis for chronic pain is likely to be ineffective and result in more pain and dysfunction. Regular administration maintains therapeutic medication blood levels for ongoing pain control. Helping patients to understand this principle will help prevent breakthrough pain and loss of pain control.

The transdermal route is useful when patients are unable to take medications orally. Patients find these systems easy to use, and they allow for continuous opioid administration without needles or pumps. Self-adhesive patches release the medication slowly over time, achieving effective analgesia. Transdermal medication systems administer fentanyl at predetermined doses for up to 48 to 72 hours. Fentanyl is about 100 times more potent than morphine. The nurse needs to exercise caution when administering transdermal patches to adult patients who weigh less than 45 kg (too little subcutaneous tissue for absorption) or who are hyperthermic. Hyperthermia causes more rapid medication absorption. The patch should never be cut or folded as this alters the medication-releasing mechanism. The patch remains in place for 48 to 72 hours, and sites should be rotated with each change. The transdermal patch is generally applied to the back, flank, chest, or upper arm and is deemed to be safe for long-term therapy. Care providers should wear plastic gloves while manipulating the patches so as to avoid inadvertent absorption of the fentanyl. Medication disposal procedures should be followed within institutions and proper disposal in the home environment to avoid the potential for misuse or diversion by other persons and to minimize environmental contamination.

> **SAFETY ALERT** Fentanyl should be used only in patients who are opioid tolerant and is not used for acute pain.

A transmucosal fentanyl "unit" (it resembles a lozenge on a handle) has been developed to treat breakthrough pain—a transient flare of moderate to severe pain superimposed on continuous or persistent pain—in opioid-tolerant patients. The unit is placed in the mouth and swabbed over the buccal mucosa and lower gums. The unit must remain intact to dissolve in the mouth, allowing 15 minutes for absorption. No more than two units per breakthrough pain episode should be used. If the patient's pain is not relieved after two units, the nurse should notify the health care provider.

Analgesics may be given rectally when patients have nausea and vomiting or are fasting before or after surgery. This route is contraindicated if patients have diarrhea or if cancerous lesions involve the anus or rectum. Morphine, hydromorphone, and oxymorphone are available as suppositories.

Another way to treat severe cancer pain in the home or acute care setting is with continuous infusions or a basal rate on a PCA device. This provides improved, uniform pain control with fewer peaks and valleys in plasma concentration, more effective medication action, and lower medication dosages overall. Candidates for continuous infusions include patients with severe pain for whom oral and injectable medications provide minimal relief, patients with severe nausea and vomiting, and patients unable to swallow oral medications. The intramuscular route should not be used for controlling cancer pain because the injection itself is painful and absorption of the medication is inconsistent and erratic.

When a patient is first given continuous morphine infusion, it is essential that the intravenous access be patent and without complications (see Chapter 41). A central-line catheter such as a Groshong or Hickman catheter, an implanted venous access port, or a peripherally inserted central catheter (PICC) is usually best suited for long-term intravenous therapy. When intravenous access is poor, the subcutaneous route with a concentrated dose is possible.

The Opioid Epidemic and Stewardship.
The opioid misuse and abuse epidemic is a public safety crisis that is affecting all Canadians in all provinces. *Prescription drug misuse* is defined as the use of any prescription opioid in a way that is not directed by the prescriber. It includes use without a prescription (e.g., using another person's opioid); use in greater amounts, more often or longer than instructed to take the opioid; or use in any other way than that instructed by the prescriber (National Institute on Drug Abuse, 2020).

The challenge associated with prescription drug misuse is that opioids have a role in the management of pain that needs to be considered. Opioids are recommended to be used in combination with nonopioid analgesics to manage acute pain following surgery on a short-term basis (Busse et al., 2017; Chou et al., 2016; Health Quality Ontario, 2018a). Long-term and high-dose opioid prescription rates have escalated, placing Canadians at risk of developing an opioid use disorder, overdose, and death. Canada ranks third in the world for opioid prescription use per capita (Tilli et al., 2020). Therefore, the recommended watchful (maximum) daily dose of an opioid is 60 mg oral morphine equivalents (Busse et al., 2017).

Another strategy implemented to help curtail the opioid misuse crisis in many hospitals and community pharmacies is an opioid stewardship program (Tilli et al., 2020). Opioid stewardship programs are aimed at reducing the total amount of opioid prescriptions, reducing the duration of days for opioids prescription to 3–5 days. In addition, the continued use of multimodal therapies using nonopioids is championed by hospitals as a risk-reduction strategy, in addition to providing education to patients and families about pain management using alternate strategies. Opioid Wisely is a resource for patients and families, developed by Choosing Wisely Canada, that is intended to provide a framework for discussion about harm reduction with respect to opioid prescribing. The document *Opioids—When You Need Them and When You Don't* (Choosing Wisely Canada, n.d.) is a good resource as it outlines other pain treatments that are effective, along with associated risks.

Unfortunately, *medication diversion* (defined as prescription medications that are either obtained or used illegally) can occur within hospitals or within homes. Medications commonly diverted are opioids and benzodiazepines (Chant, 2019). To reduce the risk of medication diversion within the community, it is important to discuss with and help patients plan the safe storage of opioids in their home. Also, pharmacies have a take-back program whereby one can return any prescription medications, OTC medications, and natural health products (unused and expired) to any pharmacy in Canada on any day of the year for disposal (Government of Canada, 2014).

Cannabinoids. Cannabis was legalized in Canada in 2018, and with reduced stigma related to usage, it has also continued to gain popularity in the medical field (Allan et al., 2018). Cannabinoids are found in the human body as part of the endogenous cannabinoid system, as a plant form, or as a synthetic form (Markovic et al., 2017). There is evidence that cannabinoids improve chemotherapy-induced nausea and vomiting, reduce spasms, and reduce neuropathic pain (Allan et al., 2018; Darkovska-Serafimovska et al., 2018). The most common adverse effects of cannabinoids include dizziness, sedation, and dissociation or "feeling high" (Allan et al., 2018). There is conflicting evidence about the efficacy of cannabis for the management of pain; therefore, more research is needed to support the use of cannabis as a treatment option in pain management. If patients are suffering with chronic or oncological pain and have failed first- and second-line therapies, the use of a cannabis trial may be a next step. With the inclusion of cannabinoids as part of the arsenal of treatment options, a discussion about risks and benefits needs to occur between the health care provider and patient.

One downside of legalizing cannabis is the unintended consequences seen within the pediatric sector. The pediatric population is at greater risk via prenatal exposure and unintentional ingestion of edibles containing cannabis that look, taste, and smell like regular food products. Furthermore, a single gummy candy, brownie, or cookie can contain 5–100 mg of tetrahydrocannabinol (THC), placing the child at risk of significant harm (Wang, 2017). Cannabis abuse can be exhibited during adolescence through alternative methods such as vaping and ingestion of edibles. Youth may have misconceptions that these methods of use are safer. Overall, there is concern about negative cognitive effects and academic performance associated with cannabis use in adolescents as reported in some cohort studies (Wang, 2017). Cannabidiol (CBD) has been used to treat seizures in pediatrics with some benefit. With the latter form, more rigorous clinical trials need to be performed before a true evaluation of efficacy can be determined.

Barriers to Effective Pain Management. Barriers to effective pain management are complex and can involve the patient, health care provider, and health care system (Box 32.15). A concern shared by health care providers and patients is the fear of addiction when long-term opioid use is prescribed to manage pain. Health care providers should be careful with their terminology when assessing someone who has a substance use disorder. Using stigmatizing terms, such as "substance abuse" can negatively impact quality of care (Saitz et al., 2021). Differences exist between **physical dependence**, **addiction**, and **drug tolerance** (Box 32.16). Experiencing a physical dependency does not imply addiction, and drug tolerance in and of itself does not constitute addiction. Nurses and other health care providers should avoid labelling patients as "drug seeking" because this term may negatively affect their care, without justification. If the nurse is concerned that a patient is misusing opioids, they should screen for addictive issues and engage in a discussion with the patient (Health Quality Ontario, 2018b).

Some of the characteristics that put individuals at a higher risk for opioid use disorder and that suggest they may be candidates for screening include having a history of involvement with the criminal justice system; receiving care in a mental health setting; being prescribed long-term opioid therapy for chronic pain; seeking health care for symptoms that suggest the possibility of opioid use disorder (for example, medical complications related to injection drug use); having alcohol use disorder; having a diagnosis of substance use disorder; and having a history of psychological trauma or adverse childhood experiences, including intergenerational trauma (Health Quality Ontario, 2018b). If the nurse suspects that a person has an opioid use disorder, the nurse should notify the primary health care provider, explaining the characteristics identified. The nurse and the health care team could

---

BOX 32.15 Barriers to Effective Pain Management

Barriers for Patients

Previous experience with poorly controlled pain
Fear of addiction
Worry about adverse effects
Fear of tolerance (medication will not continue to work when needed)
Concern about taking an abundance of pills already
Fear of injections
Concern about not being a "good" patient
Not wanting to worry family and friends
More tests may be needed
Belief that one needs to suffer to be cured
Belief that pain is punishment for past indiscretions
Inadequate education
Reluctance to discuss pain
Belief that pain is inevitable
Belief that pain is part of aging
Fear of disease progression
Belief that health care team members are already doing all that they can
Fear that patient will forget to take analgesics
Fear of distracting health care providers from treating illness
Belief that health care providers have more important or more ill patients to see
Belief that suffering in silence is noble and expected

Barriers for Health Care Providers

Concern that patient did not receive adequate pain assessment
Concern about addiction
Opiophobia (fear of opioids)
Fear of legal repercussions
No visible cause of pain exists
Belief that patients must learn to live with pain
Reluctance to deal with adverse effects of analgesics
Not believing patient's report of pain
Fear of giving a dose that will kill the patient
Time constraints
Belief that opioids may "mask" symptoms
Belief that pain is part of aging or disease progression
Overestimation of risks of respiratory depression
Not viewed as ethical obligation to properly treat pain

Barriers for the Health Care System

Concern with creating "addicts" or a substance use problem
Ability to fill prescriptions
Extensive documentation requirements
Poor pain policies and procedures regarding pain management
Lack of resources and education
Inadequate access to pain clinics; long waiting lists for chronic pain clinics, for both pediatric and adult patients
Poor understanding of economic impact of unrelieved pain

---

consider using an opioid contract—a written agreement between a sole prescribing health care provider and the patient—that outlines key points regarding opioid therapy or daily dispensing with a maximum number of pills allotted per day (Busse et al., 2017).

Individuals with an active opioid use disorder or a history of substance misuse are at increased risk of poorly managed pain because of clinicians' negative attitudes toward and inadequate knowledge about addiction, and their fears of exacerbating addiction by administering

BOX 32.16 Definitions Related to the Use of Opioids for Pain Treatment

Physical Dependence

A state of adaptation that is manifested by a class-specific drug withdrawal syndrome that can be produced by abrupt cessation, rapid dose reduction, decreasing blood level of the drug, or administration of an antagonist. An individual has a subjective sense of need for a specific psychoactive substance, to benefit from its positive effects, or to avoid negative effects associated with not consuming the substance (American Society of Addiction Medicine, 2019). It is not the same as addiction; it is a pharmacological effect (Saitz et al., 2021).

Drug Tolerance

A state of adaptation in which exposure to a drug induces changes that result in a diminution of one or more of the drug's effects over time. It is not the same as addiction.

Addiction

A neurobiological disease that has genetic, psychosocial, and environmental factors influencing its development and manifestations. It is characterized by behaviours that include one or more of the following: impaired control over drug use, compulsive use, continued use despite harm, and craving.

Addiction is a treatable, chronic medical disease involving complex interactions among brain circuits, genetics, the environment, and an individual's life experiences. People with addiction use substances or engage in behaviours that become compulsive and often continue despite harmful consequences (American Society of Addiction Medicine, 2019). Refer to the Centre for Addiction and Mental Health for additional information: http://www.camh.ca/en/hospital/health_information/a_z_mental_health_and_addiction_information/drug-use-addiction/Pages/addiction.aspx

---

opioids. Poorly managed pain in these populations results in increased length of hospital stays and more frequent readmissions and outpatient and emergency department visits. The rate of addiction to opioids and alcohol among patients with pain is approximately the same as it is in the general population, ranging from 6 to 10%.

In contrast to medications used to treat pain, a **placebo** is any treatment thought not to have a specific effect. Placebos may be appropriately used as controls in randomized controlled medication trials. However, the use of placebos, without patient consent, to treat pain is considered unethical and sets up an adversarial relationship between the health care providers and the patient and their family. If a placebo is prescribed, the nurse should question the prescription and ask "Why?" Many health care agencies have policies that limit placebo use only to research.

Restorative and Continuing Care

Pain Clinics, Palliative Care, and Hospices. In recent years, health care providers have recognized pain as a significant health problem and, as a result, a number of programs and pain clinics have been developed. A comprehensive pain centre can treat patients on an inpatient or outpatient basis, conduct research into new treatments, and train professionals. Clinicians from various health disciplines, such as pharmacists, nurses and nurse practitioners, physicians, physiotherapists, psychologists, spiritual care workers, nutritionists, and social workers, work with patients to discover effective pain-relief measures from a holistic perspective. Many hospitals have palliative care teams to assist patients and families in managing their chronic or end-of-life pain and symptoms from diseases. Learning to live life fully with an incurable condition is one goal of palliative care (see Chapter 26).

Patients and their families need ongoing assistance in managing the patient's pain at home. Some palliative care programs have a pain and symptom management team that may be consulted for complex pain and symptom management.

In Canada, palliative care and end-of-life care continue to be recognized as a necessary part of the continuum of care. A hospice or palliative care unit provides specialized end-of-life care in the patient's home or at a facility (see Chapter 26), helping patients with life-limiting illnesses to continue to live in comfort and privacy, with effective pain control as one of the priorities. Under the guidance of hospice nurses, families learn to monitor patients' symptoms and become the patients' primary caregivers. A hospice patient may become hospitalized in the event of a brief, acute care crisis or family challenge. The Canadian Virtual Hospice is an online resource for patients, families, and health care providers.

Medical assistance in dying (MAiD) was legalized in Canada with the passing of Bill C-14, which outlines requirements that patients must meet in order to be eligible for MAiD. Under the auspices of this program, physicians or nurse practitioners can provide a substance to a person upon their request, and the person can self-administer the substance that will lead to their death. Some of the eligibility criteria include the following: the patient must be over 18 years of age, have capacity to make their own decisions pertaining to health care, and have a grievous or irremediable medical condition (patient has a serious or incurable disease or disability); the patient is in an advanced state of irreversible decline in capabilities; and the patient is enduring physical or psychological suffering, or their natural death is reasonably foreseeable. Refer to the federal legislation for specifics regarding the amended MAiD legislation (Government of Canada, 2022). For an example of provincial MAiD legislation information, refer to the Ontario Ministry of Health and Long-Term Care (2022).

◆ Evaluation

Patient Care. Evaluating pain is one of many nursing responsibilities that require critical thinking (Figure 32.14). The patient's behavioural responses to pain-relief interventions are not always obvious. Evaluating the effectiveness of a pain intervention requires that the nurse be an intent observer and know what responses to anticipate on the basis of the type of pain, the type of intervention, the timing of the intervention, the physiological nature of the injury or disease, the pharmacotherapies used, and the patient's previous responses. The nurse's input should be extracted from the three Ps or domains of pain management: **p**hysiotherapies, **p**sychological therapies and support, and **p**harmacotherapies.

If a patient continues to have discomfort after an intervention, the nurse can try a different approach. For example, if an analgesic provides only partial relief, relaxation or guided-imagery exercises might be added. The nurse should consult with the health care provider about increasing the dosage, decreasing the interval between doses, or trying different analgesics. The nurse should also evaluate tolerance to therapy and the overall relief obtained. If an intervention aggravates discomfort, it should be stopped immediately and an alternative sought. Time and patience are necessary to maximize the effectiveness of pain management. Nurses need to evaluate the entire pain experience to determine the most effective interventions and times for medication administration.

Patient Perceptions. The patient, if able, is the best resource for evaluating the effectiveness of pain-relief measures. Nurses must regularly assess whether the character of the patient's pain changes. The family or caregiver can be a valuable resource, particularly if the patient is unable

Knowledge
- Characteristics of an improved level of comfort for a patient

Experience
- Previous patient responses to pain relief measures

Evaluation
- Reassess signs and symptoms of the patient's pain response (the severity and characteristics of pain, the patient's self-report)
- Evaluate the family and friends' observations of the patient's response to therapies

Standards
- Use established expected outcomes to evaluate the patient's response to care (e.g., reduced pain severity)
- Apply RNAO* guidelines for chronic pain evaluation
- Determine if the patient's expectations are met

Qualities
- Demonstrate humility; rethink your approach; if pain continues, confer with other clinicians
- Be responsible and accountable when care is ineffective and the patient's rights must be maintained

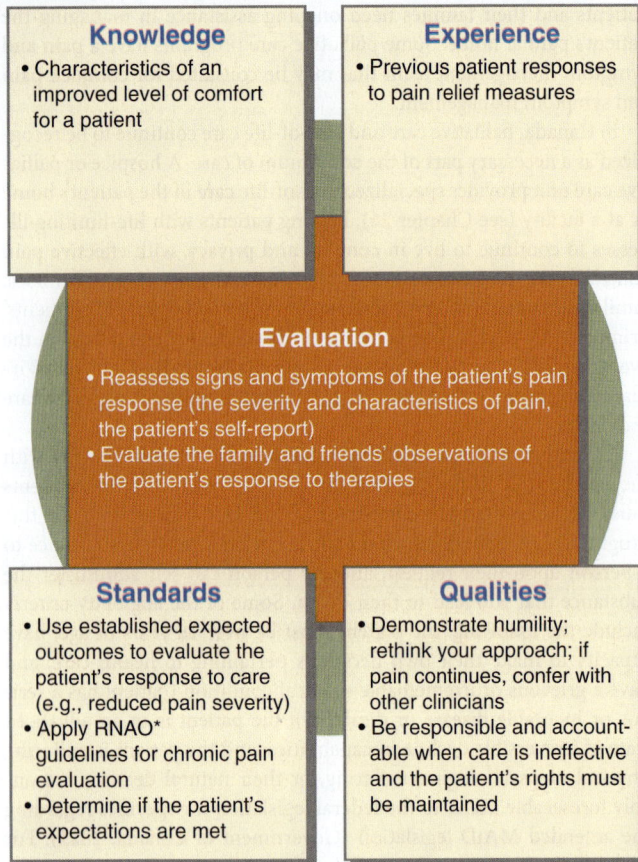

FIGURE 32.14 Critical thinking model for pain relief evaluation. *The Registered Nurses' Association of Ontario (RNAO) has developed evidence-informed practice guidelines specifically with regard to pain. See https://rnao.ca/bpg/guidelines/assessment-and-management-pain

to self-report their pain (Herr et al., 2019). Pain treatment is successful when the patient's expectations of pain relief are assessed and met. However, some patients may unnecessarily experience uncontrolled pain because they lack knowledge of available pain-relief interventions.

Pain assessment and responses to intervention should be accurately documented so that they can be communicated to the health care team. Communication occurs from nurse to nurse, shift to shift, and nurse to other health care providers. The nurse caring for the patient is responsible for reporting and documenting what has been effective for managing pain. Various bedside tools, such as validated pain tools and a pain management flow sheet, help centralize information about pain management. Patients expect the nurse to be sensitive to their pain and to be diligent in managing that pain. Because pain relief is a team effort, it is vital to communicate effectively with all members, including the patients' family and significant others, seek a collaborative approach, and determine optimal treatment goals (Box 32.17).

KEY CONCEPTS

- Pain is a subjective physical and psychosocial experience.
- A nurse's misconceptions about pain may result in doubt about the degree of the patient's suffering and in unwillingness to provide relief.
- Knowledge of the pathophysiology of pain—transmission, transduction, perception, and modulation—provides the nurse with guidelines for determining pain-relief measures.

BOX 32.17 **Establishing a Collaborative Team Approach to Pain Management**

1. Establish common goals for pain relief and optimal functioning.
2. Use common language regarding pain assessment and management.
3. Use validated pain-rating scales.
4. Secure a common knowledge base and encourage the use of clinical practice guidelines.
5. Optimize regular team communication opportunities for direct communication and problem solving.
6. Assess patient and caregiver expectations regarding pain control.

Data from Health Quality Ontario. (2020). *Chronic pain: Care for adults, adolescents and children, quality standard.* Queen's Printer for Ontario. https://www.hqontario.ca/evidence-to-improve-care/quality-standards/view-all-quality-standards/chronic-pain

- An interaction of psychological and cognitive factors affects pain perception.
- A person's cultural background influences the meaning of pain and how it is expressed.
- It is common for older patients not to report pain.
- Patients who have chronic pain are unlikely to show behavioural changes.
- An in-depth pain history should not be collected when the patient is experiencing discomfort.
- Pain can cause physical signs and symptoms similar to the signs and symptoms of other diseases.
- The nurse individualizes pain interventions by collaborating closely with the patient, using assessment findings, and trying a variety of multimodal interventions.
- Eliminating sources of painful stimuli is a basic nursing measure for promoting comfort.
- A regular schedule should be used for analgesic administration for persistent pain, as this is more effective than an as-needed schedule in controlling pain.
- A patient-controlled analgesic device gives patients control over their pain management with low risk of overdose.
- While caring for a patient who receives local anaesthesia, the nurse should protect the affected limb from injury.
- When administering epidural analgesia, the nurse needs to take steps to prevent infection and monitor closely for respiratory depression.
- The nurse's primary goal in pain management is to anticipate and prevent pain, rather than to treat it.
- In evaluating the effectiveness of a pain intervention, the nurse needs to consider the changing character of pain, the patient's response to the intervention, and the patient's perceptions of a therapy's effectiveness.
- Nurses must report any unexpected change in analgesia usage, or in the site, severity, or character of the pain.

CRITICAL THINKING EXERCISES

1. Do you have a friend or family member who lives with cancer and is willing to talk about it? If so, ask the individual to tell you about different painful experiences they may have had and what they would recommend to help nurses provide better care during these painful events.
2. A 40-year-old patient is newly diagnosed with fibromyalgia. The patient is married and has a daughter and son who are 2 and 5 years

old, respectively. Their spouse travels frequently and is often home only on weekends. The patient informs the nurse: "The pain is so bad at night that I only get 3 or 4 hours of sleep. I have no opportunity to rest during the day because I'm busy caring for my children. I am so tired that I don't know how I am going to cope with this pain long term." Identify two follow-up care plan components that would be important when considering the patient's concerns regarding the management of their pain.

3. Alexis is a 3-year-old patient admitted to the pediatric unit for a third-degree burn to their right lower extremity. How would you proceed in assessing this child's pain?

4. An older patient with metastatic breast cancer to the bone has been receiving intravenous morphine for a week for severe back and leg pain. The frequently increased infusion of morphine is not reducing their pain to an acceptable level, and they are becoming increasingly sedated. What other pharmacological interventions might be considered?

🌐 *Answers to Critical Thinking Exercises appear on the Evolve website.*

▮ REVIEW QUESTIONS

Review Questions 1 to 10 relate to the case study at the beginning of the chapter.

1. Sam's nurse uses gentle touch to soothe him after his physical examination. The intent of gentle massage is to provide comfort. What is this nonpharmacological pain intervention known as?
   a. Recall
   b. Distraction
   c. Imagery
   d. Relaxation technique

2. Sam has pain along the incision as noted during the examination. An infant expressing pain at the surgical site is indicative of which type of pain?
   a. Transient pain
   b. Superficial pain
   c. Phantom pain
   d. Referred pain

3. Sam has undergone a laparoscopic bowel anastomosis. Which of the following validated pain assessment tools would be most appropriate for the nurse to use to assess this infant's pain?
   a. FLACC
   b. Numerical rating scale
   c. The Northern Pain Scale
   d. Wong-Baker FACES Scale

4. Which one of the following responses would the nurse expect to be good corroborative data with respect to Sam experiencing moderate pain?
   a. Restlessness or inconsolability
   b. Decreased heart rate
   c. Decreased blood pressure

   d. Low FLACC scores

5. Sam is starting to take oral feeds. What would the nurse expect as the next steps with Sam's nurse-controlled analgesia (NCA)?
   a. Stop the basal infusion and allow NCA boluses for breakthrough pain
   b. Only administer acetaminophen for pain
   c. Stop the NCA
   d. Only administer pain medications if the parents request this

6. Sam receives an NCA breakthrough dose prior to turning and positioning. Afterward, he settles, with a FLACC score of 0/10. Which one of the following interpretations about the dosage of pain medications is the most appropriate?
   a. Adequate
   b. Excessive
   c. Insufficient
   d. Unnecessary

7. Which one of the following nursing actions is most appropriate when Sam is scheduled to have a painful procedure?
   a. Discuss analgesic options with the physician
   b. Inform the parents that the discomfort will be minimal
   c. Teach about the procedure and its associated discomfort
   d. Provide education about the procedure and the need to consider offering a breakthrough dose prior to the procedure

8. Sam requires that bloodwork be drawn after his laparoscopic bowel anastomosis. Which nonpharmacological approaches are the best options for pain management?
   a. Physical interventions such as sucrose and non-nutritive sucking
   b. Support for parents
   c. Request to the health care provider to delay bloodwork
   d. Holding the infant so that the phlebotomist can perform the venipuncture

9. The assessment of infant pain can be challenging, as infants cannot self-report. In addition to obtaining a pain score using a validated tool, it is important to do the following:
   a. Check that the patient is on a monitor.
   b. Determine if they need bloodwork to check electrolytes.
   c. Assess other sources of discomfort, such as hunger.
   d. Only offer nonpharmacological approaches.

10. NCA is often used for postoperative pain management for infants, for which one of the following reasons?
    a. To improve pain control by allowing pre-emptive use by the nurse at the point of care
    b. To promote sustained pain relief, with the patient in control
    c. To enable family members to administer the medication dosage
    d. To decrease the quantity of opioid medication use

Answers: 1. d; **2.** b; **3.** a; **4.** a; **5.** a; **6.** a; **7.** d; **8.** a; **9.** c; **10.** a.

🌐 *Rationales for the Review Questions appear on the Evolve website.*

RECOMMENDED WEBSITES

Canadian Cancer Society: https://www.cancer.ca

This site is an educational resource to help cancer patients and their caregivers. It has the most up-to-date knowledge and tools available related to cancer prevention, diagnosis, treatments, and supports and services. It also features a number of pain-management publications, which include information on traditional and complementary therapies.

Canadian Hospice Palliative Care Association: https://chpca.ca

This site is intended as an educational resource for professional and informal caregivers and interest groups. It includes an extensive listing of online resources for those interested in palliative and end-of-life care, including cancer, clinical, and research sites.

Canadian Pain Society: https://www.canadianpainsociety.ca

The Canadian Pain Society (CPS) is an association whose members include physicians, nurses, and other clinicians involved with the management of pain. Its aim is to foster and encourage research on pain, to promote education and training in the field of pain, and to improve the management of patients with acute and chronic pain.

Canadian Virtual Hospice: https://www.virtualhospice.ca/en_US/Main+Site+Navigation/Home.aspx

This site is a resource for patients, families, caregivers, and health care providers who would like more information on palliative care or end-of-life care.

Choosing Wisely Canada—Opioid Wisely: https://choosingwiselycanada.org/campaign/opioid-wisely

Choosing Wisely provides a framework and resources for safe options for managing pain that can be used for discussions between prescribers and patients. The ultimate aim is to reduce harm associated with opioid prescribing.

College of Nurses of Ontario (CNO): https://www.cno.org

CNO is the governing body of registered nurses (RNs), registered practical nurses (RPNs), and nurse practitioners (NPs) in Ontario. NPs (Registered Nurse, Extended Class RN-EC) can prescribe controlled substances, including methadone. (For information on NPs and Prescribing Controlled Substances, see https://www.cno.org/en/trending-topics/nps-and-prescribing-controlled-substances.)

Health Canada: https://www.canada.ca/en/health-canada.html

Health Canada provides an extensive listing of clinical guidelines for nurses in primary care. It provides the public, clinicians, and researchers with information on pain and other public health concerns. The following URL provides a document outlining questions, issues, and research surrounding neuropathic pain: https://www.collectionscanada.gc.ca/obj/thesescanada/vol2/OKQ/TC-OKQ-1762.pdf

International Association for the Study of Pain (IASP): https://www.iasp-pain.org

The IASP is the leading professional forum for science, practice, and education in the field of pain. IASP brings together scientists, clinicians, health care providers, and policymakers to stimulate and support the study of pain and to use that knowledge for improved pain relief worldwide.

Pain BC: https://painbc.ca

This site is a noncommercial resource for health care providers and their patients, providing open access to clinical news, information, research, and education for a better understanding of evidence-informed pain-management practices.

Registered Nurses' Association of Ontario: Assessment and Management of Pain: https://rnao.ca/bpg/guidelines/assessment-and-management-pain.

The Registered Nurses' Association of Ontario's website is specific to nursing and is available in English and French. It features a number of Best Practice Guidelines, including those for the assessment and management of pain.

University of Toronto Centre for the Study of Pain: http://sites.utoronto.ca/pain

The University of Toronto Centre for the Study of Pain is a partnership involving the faculties of dentistry, medicine, nursing, and pharmacy. The mission of the centre is to lead, both nationally and internationally, in pain research, education, knowledge translation, networking, and sustainability.

🌐 REFERENCES

A full reference list is available on the website for this book at http://evolve.elsevier.com/Canada/Potter/fundamentals/

33

Health Assessment and Physical Examination

*Canadian content written by Janet Luimes, NP, MScN, and Mary Ellen Labrecque, NP, PhD,
with original chapter contributions by Angela McConachie, FNP, DNP*

OBJECTIVES

Mastery of content in this chapter will enable you to:

- Explain the purposes of physical assessment.
- Describe cultural diversity, cultural competency, and cultural safety as these relate to the provision of culturally competent health and physical assessment and improved patient health outcomes.
- Identify data to collect from the nursing history before a physical examination.
- Describe environmental preparations necessary prior to a physical examination.
- List techniques used to prepare a patient physically and psychologically before and during an examination.
- Demonstrate the techniques used with each physical assessment skill.

- Describe physical measurements made in assessing each body system.
- Describe normal physical findings in young, middle-aged, and older persons.
- Identify preventive screenings and the appropriate age(s) for each screening to occur.
- Identify self-screening examinations commonly performed by patients.
- Describe ways to incorporate health promotion and health teaching into the examination.
- Identify how nurses use physical assessment skills during routine nursing care and care provided using telehealth or virtual patient care.

KEY TERMS

Acromegaly
Adventitious sounds
Alopecia
Aneurysm
Aphasia
Apical impulse
Arcus senilis
Atherosclerosis
Atrophy
Basal cell carcinoma
Benign (fibrocystic) breast disease
Borborygmi
Bronchophony
Bruit
Capillary refill
Caries
Cerumen
Chancre
Cherry angiomas
Cholecystitis
Cirrhosis
Clubbing
Conjunctivitis
Cyanosis
Dermatitis
Distension
Dysrhythmia
Ectropion
Eczema

Edema
Entropion
Erythema
Excoriation
Exophthalmos
Exostosis
Hemorrhoids
Hepatitis B
Hernia
Hirsutism
Hydrocephalus
Hypertonicity
Hypotonicity
Indurated
Integument
Jaundice
Kyphosis
Leukoplakia
Lordosis
Melanoma
Metastasize
Murmurs
Nystagmus
Occlusion
Ophthalmoscope
Orthopnea
Osteoporosis
Otoscope
Ototoxicity

Palpation
Pancreatitis
Papanicolaou (Pap) smear
Paralytic ileus
Peristalsis
Peritonitis
PERRLA
Petechiae
Phlebitis
Pigmentation
Point of maximal impulse (PMI)
Polyps
Ptosis
Pulse deficit
Scoliosis
Senile keratosis
Squamous cell carcinoma
Stenosis
Strabismus
Striae
Syncope
Tactile fremitus
Telehealth
Thrill
Turgor
Varicosities
Ventricular gallop
Vocal fremitus
Whispered pectoriloquy

⊕ **WEBSITE**

http://evolve.elsevier.com/Canada/Potter/fundamentals/

CASE STUDY

Mrs. Smith is a 76-year-old patient (preferred pronouns: she/her) who has just been admitted to the medical unit where you are working as a student nurse. You have been asked to perform an admission history for and physical examination of this patient. The following information is provided in the notes from the emergency department (ED):

Admitted to the ED 2 hours ago.

Admission history: Patient states that she feels "unable to catch her breath" and has been coughing up thick green phlegm for the past 2 days. She does not think that she has had a fever or chills, but does state that she has been "mostly sleeping for the past 2 days" and is "very tired."

Vital signs on admission to ED:

T: 38.3º C, Pulse: 94 bpm, Resp: 25/min, BP: 142/90, SaO$_2$: 88% on room air

- *Admission diagnosis: Chronic obstructive pulmonary disease—exacerbation*
- *Patient chart notes indicate that the patient was placed on O$_2$ at 15 mL/min using a non-rebreather mask. After 5 minutes her vitals were as follows: SaO$_2$ increased to 97%, Resp: 22/min, Pulse: 86 bpm, BP: 132/86.*

The patient's vital signs have remained stable on oxygen as you begin your history and physical examination of this patient.

As you read each section in this chapter, reflect back on the information about this patient and identify the following:

1. *Which of the vital signs are concerning to you? What will you continue to monitor?*
2. *What history information would be important to collect that focuses on her diagnosis?*
3. *What physiological systems will you complete in the physical assessment of this patient?*

In answering the questions, it might be helpful to begin by reviewing anatomical and physiological information about chronic obstructive pulmonary disease:

- *How the disease develops*
- *Relevant lifestyle elements that contribute to the disease process*
- *Anatomical and physiological changes in the body systems to look for when performing a history and physical assessment*

Think about this case study as you read this chapter. There are related review questions at the end of the chapter that refer to the case study.

A holistic assessment of a patient's health status involves the collection of a broad range of data regarding the emotional, intellectual, physical, psychosocial, spiritual (see Chapter 14), and cultural dimensions of the patient's life (see Chapter 11). The process of collecting data about a patient includes a thorough health history and the physical examination. The physical exam, although primarily focused on physiological function, may also include assessment of cognition, mood, and functional status.

Nurses are often the first persons that patients come in contact with when they are provided health care services. It is thus extremely important that nurses be able to detect changes in a patient's condition. Whether the nurse is conducting health assessments in a primary care clinic, in acute care agencies, or in a patient's home, nurses continually seek information about patients' health status. For this reason, the ability to think critically and interpret the meaning of a patient's behaviour and physiological status is an important skill in professional nursing practice.

The skills of physical assessment and examination provide powerful tools for detecting subtle, as well as obvious, changes in a patient's health. Physical assessment enables the nurse to assess patterns reflecting health problems and to evaluate the patient's progress following therapy. Health screenings may focus on a specific physical condition or assess cognition, mood, and functional status. For example, nurses perform blood pressure screenings to detect the risk for high blood pressure. If screening determines that a patient has a risk for hypertension, the nurse refers the patient for a more complete physical examination.

A complete health assessment involves a nursing history (see Chapter 14), behavioural and physical examination, and cultural assessment (see Chapter 11). The focus of this chapter is to introduce the skills necessary to perform a physical examination. For more information on physical examination and health assessment, nursing students and health care providers should consult comprehensive textbooks such as those by Ball et al. (2019) and Jarvis et al. (2019).

A complete physical examination is a head-to-toe review of each body system that offers objective information about the patient. This enables the nurse to make clinical judgements and develop the plan for nursing care. The patient's condition and response affect the extent of the examination. The accuracy of the physical assessment will influence the choice of therapies a patient receives and the evaluation of the response to those therapies. Continuity in health care improves when the nurse makes an ongoing, objective, and comprehensive assessment.

SOCIAL AND CULTURAL CONSIDERATIONS

Culturally competent health and physical assessment requires the nurse to be culturally aware and sensitive (see Chapter 11). The nurse demonstrates cultural competence, in part, by respecting patient preference when completing an examination. It is important to remember that social or cultural background may influence a patient's behaviour and beliefs about health. Integrating cultural assessment with health and physical assessment for every patient provides the nurse with the background data needed to facilitate a culturally competent physical examination. Assessment data about gender identity, the use of complementary and alternative therapies, dietary preferences, caregiver relationships, and past experiences with health care offer the nurse important clues to performing a physical assessment in ways that are respectful to the patient and help build relational practice. Ethnohistorical, biocultural, and socioeconomic assessment data may provide important information about potential health risks.

Cultural assessment data are used to inform a culturally safe physical assessment; such data help the nurse think critically about the political, social, and economic contexts of patients' lives and how inequities in power and access to resources for health care can influence the health of individuals (see Chapter 11; Jarvis et al., 2019, pp. 28–45). Applying a cultural safety lens will help the nurse avoid stereotyping patients on the basis of gender or ethnicity. Nurses need to learn to recognize common biocultural variations of what is considered normal or healthy, as well as disorders that may be more common in certain populations in the community. For example, infants of Indigenous, Asian, or Black descent may exhibit congenital dermal melanocytosis, which is a common variation of hyperpigmentation seen in newborns (Jarvis et al., 2019, p. 241).

Canadians of Indigenous, Black, or South Asian ancestry may be more likely to exhibit the signs and symptoms of high blood pressure or diabetes. Providing culturally competent care leads to greater patient satisfaction and improved clinical outcomes (Brunett & Shingles, 2021).

Purposes of Physical Examination

Examinations are designed to address the patient's needs. In an acutely ill patient, the nurse assesses only the involved body system or systems. When a patient with asthma is having an acute episode with difficulty breathing, the nurse initially focuses on assessing the pulmonary and cardiac systems. Then a more comprehensive examination about the patient's total health status is completed when the patient is physiologically more stable. A complete physical examination is often performed as part of a periodic health examination to promote wellness behaviours and preventive health care measures (Canadian Task Force on Preventative Health Care, 2017). Additionally, a complete medical examination is often required to determine eligibility for extended health insurance, military service, or a specialized driver's license; as a pre-employment medical exam for a new job; with initiating care by a new practitioner; for a presurgical assessment; and for the admission process to a hospital or long-term care facility.

A complete physical examination provides valuable information for all members of the patient's interprofessional health care team. Thorough examination and documentation contribute to the following essential elements for comprehensive evidence-informed care:

- Gather baseline data about the patient's health history, present status, and health concerns
- Supplement, confirm, or refute data obtained in the history
- Confirm and identify nursing diagnoses
- Make clinical judgements about a patient's changing health status and management
- Evaluate the outcomes of care

While a complete physical examination has many benefits, it is important to have a reason for performing a complete examination. Annual physical examination of asymptomatic adults is no longer recommended because repeated research shows they do not improve health status and can result in false-positive test results. These false-positive test results often cause anxiety for patients and lead to unnecessary follow-up tests and treatment, creating more possible harm than benefit (Canadian Task Force on Preventative Health Care, 2017; College of Family Physicians of Canada, 2020).

To assist in learning about the physical assessment of body systems, it is helpful to review anatomy and physiology. There are many anatomy and physiology textbooks available that will assist you in the identification of the structures and functions of the human body and interconnectedness of the physiological systems. For example, to conduct an assessment of cranial nerves, it is important to develop an understanding of the function of each nerve and the motor and sensory pathways innervated by these nerves.

Gathering a Health History

The main objective of interacting with patients is to find out what their concerns are and to help them find solutions. As a nurse you must pay close attention to a patient's concerns. Direct the interview and examination so that you can create a clear picture of the patient's condition. The collection of health history and physical examination data requires patience and a dedication to comprehensiveness and detail. Conducting a successful interview and physical examination is based on several principles, relational practice being foremost (see Chapters 11, 14, and 18). The interview allows for the formation of a partnership with the patient. Orient the interview to the patient, not to a disease. For example, a patient is not a "diabetic"; rather, the patient should be referred

to as "a person who has diabetes." Make sure you know your own idiosyncrasies (e.g., wanting to be liked, fear of catching a disease) so that you are able to prevent these feelings from affecting your therapeutic relationship with the patient.

Developing Nursing Diagnoses and a Care Plan

After gathering information about the patient's health from the health history, a subsequent physical assessment can reveal information that refutes, confirms, or supplements the history. As a nurse you need to think critically about the information the patient provides, apply knowledge from previous clinical care, and methodically conduct the examination to create a clear picture of the patient's health status. For example, if a patient reports back pain, ask the patient several questions to clarify the nature of the pain. During the examination, look carefully for the source of the pain (e.g., discomfort when changing position or a bruise across the patient's back) to rule out a variety of potential conditions (e.g., back strain, contusions, trauma, scoliosis). It is important to remember that one assessment finding (e.g., back pain) does not conclusively reveal the nature of an abnormality. A complete assessment is necessary to form a definitive nursing or medical diagnosis. Grouping significant findings into clusters of data assists in revealing actual or "risk for" nursing diagnoses (see Chapter 14). In addition, each abnormal finding suggests the need to gather additional information.

Information gathered during the initial history and physical assessment provides a baseline for the patient's health status and functional abilities. This baseline assessment is a record of findings identified when the patient was first assessed that can be used as a comparison for future assessment findings. The comprehensiveness and attention to detail in the documentation of the initial assessment enables the nurse and other health care providers to determine changes in a patient's condition during subsequent assessments.

The accuracy of the database of assessment information allows for the development of an individualized nursing diagnosis. Physical assessment findings determine the etiology of the diagnosis so that the selection of interventions is appropriate for the care plan. It is important to view physical assessment as an ongoing process; thus, the care plan changes as health conditions resolve or deteriorate, and when new health problems arise. Ongoing monitoring of the patient's progress and responses to therapies and treatments necessitates a review of the nursing diagnoses and plan of care.

Managing Patient Problems

When caring for patients, the nurse assesses and performs a variety of interventions. Yet the nurse's success in providing care depends on the ability to recognize a change in status and to modify interventions so that patients gain the most desirable outcomes. Physical assessment skills enable nurses to judge the status of patients' health and direct the management of care. For example, the nurse inspects the skin during a routine bath and finds it excessively dry. The nurse does not use soap and applies body lotion to the skin. The nurse revises the written care plan so that other nurses know the type of skin care to provide and instructs the patient about skin care. Performing the mechanics of physical assessment is relatively simple. The challenge lies in applying critical thinking skills to interpret assessment findings and make care decisions.

Evaluating Nursing Care

Nurses demonstrate accountability for their nursing care through evaluating the results of nursing interventions. Physical assessment skills enhance the evaluation of nursing measures through monitoring physiological and behavioural outcomes of care. Nurses use physical assessment skills to assess a condition (e.g., palpation of the patient's pulse) and evaluate a patient's response to care (e.g., an evaluation of a patient's tolerance to an exercise plan). Accurate, detailed, objective documentation of measurements through physical assessment assists in determining whether the expected outcomes of care are met.

SKILLS OF PHYSICAL ASSESSMENT

A comprehensive physical examination involves the use of four skills: inspection, palpation, percussion, and auscultation. Olfaction (use of one's sense of smell) is also an element in the assessment of patients during care, as hygiene, infections, and physiological processes can have unique odours. All interactions with patients require health care providers to thoroughly clean their hands and check patient identification.

Inspection

Inspection is the use of vision and hearing to distinguish normal from abnormal findings. It is important to know what to consider normal or healthy for patients of different age groups. Nurses need experience to recognize common healthy variations among patients. Inspection is a simple technique that can provide valuable clues about a patient's health status. The quality of an inspection depends on the nurse's willingness to spend time doing a thorough job. To inspect body parts accurately, the principles should be followed:

- Make sure adequate lighting is available.
- Position and expose body parts so all surfaces can be viewed.
- Inspect each area for size, shape, colour, symmetry, position, drainage, and abnormalities.
- When possible, compare each area inspected with the same area on the opposite side of the body.
- Use additional light (e.g., a penlight) to inspect body cavities.
- Do not hurry inspection. Pay attention to detail.

Findings from inspection of a body part sometimes indicate the need for further examination. Palpation should be used with or after visual inspection.

Palpation

Palpation involves the use of the hands to touch body parts to make sensitive assessments. Palpation is used to examine all accessible parts of the body. For example, the skin is palpated for temperature, moisture, texture, turgor, tenderness, and thickness. The abdomen is palpated for tenderness, **distension** (swelling), or masses. Different parts of the hand are touched to detect characteristics such as texture, temperature, and perception of movement (Table 33.1).

Palpation is conducted as follows: Before palpation, help the patient relax and be comfortable because muscle tension during palpation impairs effective assessment. To promote relaxation, have the patient take slow, deep breaths and place their arms along the side of their body. *Palpate tender areas last.* Be sure to ask the patient to point out the more sensitive areas. Watch the patient's facial expressions and body movements and note any nonverbal signs of discomfort.

Palpation requires warm, clean hands, short fingernails, and a gentle approach. Perform palpation slowly, gently, and deliberately. Light, intermittent pressure is best when palpating; heavy, prolonged pressure causes a loss of sensitivity in the hand. To avoid injuring a patient, do not attempt deep palpation without clinical supervision; caution is the rule. Use the most sensitive parts of the hand, the palmar surface of the fingers and finger pads, to determine position, texture, size, consistency, masses, fluid, and crepitus. Measure temperature using the dorsal surface or back of the hand. The ulnar surface of the hand and finger is more sensitive to vibration. Measure position, consistency, and turgor by lightly grasping the body part with the fingertips.

TABLE 33.1	Examples of Characteristics Measured by Palpation	
Area Examined	**Criteria Measured**	**Portion of Hand to Use**
Skin	Temperature	Dorsum of hand/fingers
	Moisture	Palmar surface
	Texture	Palmar surface/pads of fingertips
	Turgor and elasticity	Grasping with fingertips
	Tenderness	Palmar surface/pads of fingertips
	Thickness	Palmar surface/pads of fingertips
Organs (e.g., liver and intestine)	Size	Entire palmar surface of hand or palmar surface of fingers
	Shape	Palmar surface/pads of fingertips
	Tenderness	Entire palmar surface of hand or palmar surface of fingers
	Absence of masses	Palmar surface/pads of fingertips
Glands (e.g., thyroid and lymph)	Swelling	Pads of fingers
	Symmetry and mobility	Palmar surface/pads of fingertips
Blood vessels (e.g., carotid or femoral artery)	Pulse amplitude Elasticity Rate Rhythm	Palmar surface/pads of fingertips
Thorax	Excursion	Palmar surface
	Tenderness	Finger pads/palmar surface of fingers
	Fremitus	Palmar or ulnar surface of entire hand

Do not palpate without considering the patient's condition. For example, if the patient has a fractured rib, use extra care to locate the painful area. Do not palpate a vital artery with pressure that obstructs blood flow. Also consider the body area being palpated, as well as the reason for using palpation.

Percussion

Percussion involves tapping the body with the fingertips to produce a vibration that travels through body tissues. The character of the sound determines the location, size, and density of underlying structures to verify abnormalities assessed by palpation and auscultation. This vibration is transmitted through body tissues, and the character of the sound heard depends on the density of the underlying tissue. By knowing the way various densities influence sound, the nurse can locate organs or masses, map their boundaries, and determine their size. An abnormal sound suggests a mass or substance such as air or fluid within an organ or body cavity. The skill of percussion requires dexterity and is usually used by advanced practitioners.

Auscultation

Auscultation involves listening to sounds the body makes to detect variations from normal. Some sounds can be heard without assistance, but most will require a stethoscope.

First, learn the normal sounds created by the cardiovascular, respiratory, and gastrointestinal (GI) systems, such as the passage of blood through an artery. Recognize abnormal sounds after learning normal variations. To become more proficient in auscultation one needs to know the types of sounds each body structure makes and the location in which the sounds are heard best. Also, it is good to learn which areas do not normally emit sounds.

To auscultate correctly, the nurse needs to hear well, have a good stethoscope, and know how to use it properly. For those with a hearing disorder, a stethoscope with greater sound amplification should be used. The stethoscope is always placed directly on the skin because clothing obscures sound. Chapter 31 describes the parts of the stethoscope and general use. The bell is best for low-pitched sounds, such as vascular and certain heart sounds, and the diaphragm is best for high-pitched sounds, such as bowel and lung sounds.

Be familiar with the stethoscope before attempting to use it. Practise using the stethoscope. Extraneous sounds created by movement of the tubing or chest piece interfere with auscultation of body organ sounds. By deliberately producing these sounds, learn to recognize and disregard them during the actual examination.

Learn to recognize the following characteristics of sounds:

- *Frequency*, or the number of sound wave cycles generated per second by a vibrating object. The higher the frequency, the higher the pitch of a sound, and vice versa.
- *Loudness*, or the amplitude of a sound wave. Auscultated sounds are loud or soft.
- *Quality*, or sounds of similar frequency and loudness from different sources. Terms such as *blowing* or *gurgling* describe the quality of sound.
- *Duration*, or the length of time that sound vibrations last. The duration of sound is short, medium, or long. Layers of soft tissue dampen the duration of sounds from deep internal organs.

Auscultation requires concentration and practice. Always consider the part of the body auscultated and the cause of the sound. For example, closure of the mitral valve causes the first heart sound. Learn where to hear the sounds best. Typically, the first heart sound is heard best when auscultated at the left fifth intercostal space along the midclavicular line. It is also important to learn the characteristics of normal sounds. The first heart sound has the quality of a loud "lub," whereas the second sound is a "dub." After understanding the cause and character of normal auscultated sounds, it becomes easier to recognize abnormal sounds and their origins.

Olfaction

While assessing a patient, it is good to become familiar with the nature and source of body odours (Table 33.2). Olfaction helps in detecting abnormalities that cannot be recognized by any other means. For example, if a patient's cast has a sweet, heavy, thick odour, this indicates an underlying infection. Findings from olfaction and other assessment skills should prompt the nurse to investigate the origin of the odour, as it may indicate abnormalities.

PREPARATION FOR EXAMINATION

Proper preparation of the environment, equipment, and patient ensures a smooth physical examination with few interruptions. A disorganized approach when preparing for a physical examination will cause errors and incomplete findings.

Infection Control

During an examination, some patients will present with open skin lesions or weeping wounds. Use standard precautions and routine practices throughout the examination (see Chapter 34) as appropriate. It is necessary to wear gloves during palpation and percussion of patients presenting with open skin lesions or weeping wounds to reduce contact with microorganisms (see Chapter 47). If a patient has excessive drainage or risk of spray from a wound, wear a gown and other personal protective equipment as needed. Always practise hand hygiene before initiating and after completing a physical assessment.

TABLE 33.2	Assessment of Characteristic Odours	
Odour	**Site or Source**	**Potential Causes**
Alcohol	Oral cavity	Ingestion of alcohol, diabetes
Ammonia	Urine	Urinary tract infection, renal failure
Body odour	Skin, particularly in areas where body parts rub together (e.g., underarms and under breasts)	Poor hygiene, excess perspiration (hyperhidrosis), foul-smelling perspiration (bromhidrosis)
	Wound site	Wound abscess
	Vomitus	Abdominal irritation, contaminated food
Feces	Vomitus/oral cavity (fecal odour)	Bowel obstruction
	Rectal area	Bowel incontinence
Foul-smelling stools in infant	Stool	Malabsorption syndrome
Halitosis	Oral cavity	Poor dental and oral hygiene, gum disease
Sweet, fruity ketones	Oral cavity	Diabetic acidosis
Stale urine	Skin	Uremic acidosis
Sweet, heavy, thick odour	Draining wound	*Pseudomonas* (bacterial) infection
Musty odour	Casted body part	Infection inside cast
Fetid, sweet odour	Tracheostomy or mucous secretions	Infection of bronchial tree (*Pseudomonas* bacteria)

Environment

A physical examination requires privacy. A well-equipped examination room is preferable, but often the examination occurs in the patient's hospital or tertiary care room. In the home, nurses will often perform an examination in the patient's bedroom. Any examination room needs to be well equipped for all necessary procedures. Adequate lighting is necessary for proper illumination of body parts. Ideally, an examination room is soundproof so that patients feel comfortable discussing their conditions. Eliminate sources of noise, take precautions to prevent interruptions from others, and make sure the room is warm enough to maintain comfort.

Sometimes it is difficult to perform a complete examination when the patient is in a bed or on a stretcher. Special examination tables make patients easily accessible and help them assume positions conducive to examination. Patients need to be carefully assisted so that they do not fall while getting on and off the examination table. A confused, combative, or uncooperative patient should not be left unsupervised on an examination table.

Examination tables are often hard and uncomfortable. When the patient lies supine, raise the head of the table about 30 degrees and give the patient a small pillow to use. When examining a patient in bed, the bed should be raised to reach the patient's body parts more easily. Remember to use proper body mechanics to ensure your physical safety and the safety of the patient while performing an exam (see Chapter 46).

Equipment

Before equipment preparation and the examination, perform thorough hand hygiene. Set up equipment so it is readily accessible and check that it is functioning properly. Box 33.1 lists typical assessment equipment used to perform a complete physical examination.

BOX 33.1   Equipment and Supplies for Physical Assessment

- Cervical brush, broom, or spatula devices (if needed)
- Cotton applicators
- Disposable pad/paper towels
- Drapes
- Eye chart (e.g., Snellen chart)
- Flashlight and spotlight
- Forms (e.g., physical, laboratory)
- Gloves (sterile and clean)
- Gown for patient
- Ophthalmoscope
- Otoscope
- Papanicolaou (Pap) slides (labelled with patient information) and cytological fixative (if needed), or liquid cytology
- Percussion (reflex) hammer
- Pulse oximeter
- Ruler
- Scale with height measurement rod
- Specimen containers (e.g., tissue or urine samples)
- Sphygmomanometer and cuff
- Sterile swabs (e.g., for culture or viral collection)
- Stethoscope
- Tape measure
- Thermometer
- Tissues
- Tongue depressors
- Tuning fork
- Vaginal speculum (if needed)
- Water-soluble lubricant
- Wristwatch with second hand or digital display

Physical Preparation of the Patient

The patient's physical comfort is vital for an accurate examination. Before starting, ask if the patient needs to use the washroom. An empty bladder and bowel facilitate examination of the abdomen, genitalia, and rectum. Collection of urine or stool specimens occurs at this time, if needed. Be sure to explain the proper method for collecting specimens and label each specimen properly according to the policies of the receiving laboratory.

Physical preparation involves being sure the patient is dressed and draped properly. The patient in the hospital will likely be wearing a gown. In an outpatient setting, a patient may need to undress and put on a gown to allow proper examination of underlying body systems. The patient should be given privacy and plenty of time during undressing. Walking into the room as the patient undresses can cause embarrassment. After the patient has undressed and put on a gown, they sit or lie down on the examination table with a drape over their lap or lower trunk. Make sure the patient stays warm, by eliminating drafts, controlling room temperature, and providing warm blankets. Routinely ask the patient if they are comfortable.

Positioning. During the examination, ask the patient to assume positions so that body parts are accessible and the patient stays comfortable. Table 33.3 lists the preferred positions for each part of the examination and contains figures illustrating these positions. Patients' abilities to assume positions will depend on their physical strength, mobility, ease of breathing, age, and degree of wellness. Explain the positions and assist patients in assuming them. Adjust the drapes so that the area being examined is accessible, making sure not to unnecessarily expose

a body part. To decrease the number of times the patient changes positions, organize the examination so that all techniques requiring a sitting position are performed first, then perform those that require a supine position next, and so forth. It is important to use extra care when positioning an older person, because they are more prone to having disabilities and postural limitation.

Psychological Preparation of the Patient

Many patients find an examination stressful or tiring, or they experience anxiety about possible findings. A thorough explanation of the purpose and steps of each assessment lets patients know what to expect and what to do so that they can cooperate. Explanations should be kept simple and in understandable terms. As the examiner, you can help patients feel free to ask questions and to mention any discomfort. As each body system is examined, give a more detailed explanation. Convey an open, professional approach while remaining relaxed (see Chapter 18).

When the patient and nurse are of opposite gender, it helps to have a third person or chaperone present during physical examination. A chaperone can provide protection and reassurance to both the patients and health care provider. This person is also a witness to the examiner's and the patient's conduct.

During the examination, watch the patient's emotional responses. Observe whether the patient's facial expression shows fear or concern and if body movements show anxiety. Remain calm and explain each step clearly. It is sometimes necessary to stop the examination and ask the patient how they feel. Do not force the patient to continue with the examination. Postponing the examination is advantageous because the findings may be more accurate when the patient can cooperate and relax. If the patient's fears result from misconceptions, clarify the purpose of the examination and prior to performing each element of the exam, verbalize what you will be assessing and ask for the patient's consent.

Assessment of Age Groups

Different interview styles and approaches to physical examination are used for patients of different age groups. When assessing children, the nurse must be sensitive and anticipate the child's reaction to the examination as a strange and unfamiliar experience. Routine pediatric examinations focus on assessment of developmental milestones, growth, weight, health promotion, and illness prevention (Rourke et al., 2020). Children with acute or chronic health conditions also require health care visits to address these concerns. When examining children, the following tips assist in data collection:

- Gather all or part of the histories on infants and children from parents or guardians.
- Perform the examination in a nonthreatening area; provide time for play to become acquainted.
- Because parents sometimes think the examiner is testing them, offer support during the examination and do not pass judgement.
- Call children by their first name, and address the parents as "Mr.," "Mrs.," or "Ms." rather than by their first names.
- Use open-ended questions to allow parents to share more information and describe more of the child's health issues. This practice also enables observation of parent–child interactions. Interview older children, who often provide details about their health history and severity of symptoms.
- Treat adolescents as adults because they tend to respond best when treated as such.
- Remember that adolescents have the right to confidentiality. After talking with parents about health history, make an opportunity to speak alone with adolescents.

TABLE 33.3 Positions for Examination

Position	Areas Assessed	Rationale	Limitations
Sitting	Head and neck, back, anterior and posterior thorax and lungs, breasts, axillae, heart, vital signs, and upper extremities	Sitting upright provides full expansion of lungs and provides better visualization of symmetry of upper body parts.	A physically weakened patient is sometimes unable to sit. Use the supine position with the head of the bed elevated instead.
Supine	Head and neck, anterior thorax and lungs, breasts, axillae, heart, abdomen, extremities, pulses	This is the most normally relaxed position. It provides easy access to pulse sites.	If the patient becomes short of breath easily, raise the head of the bed.
Dorsal recumbent	Head and neck, anterior thorax and lungs, breasts, axillae, heart, abdomen	This position is for abdominal assessment because it promotes relaxation of abdominal muscles.	Patients with painful disorders are more comfortable with knees flexed.
Lithotomy*	Female genitalia and genital tract	This position provides maximal exposure of genitalia and facilitates insertion of a vaginal speculum.	Lithotomy position can be embarrassing and uncomfortable, so the examiner should minimize time that the patient spends in it. The patient should be kept well draped.
Modified left lateral recumbent	Rectum and vagina	Flexion of hip and knee improves exposure of rectal area.	Joint deformities hinder the patient's ability to bend their hip and knee.
Prone	Musculoskeletal system	This position is only for assessing extension of the hip joint, skin, and buttocks.	Patients with respiratory difficulties do not tolerate this position well.
Left lateral recumbent	Heart	This position aids in detecting murmurs.	Patients with respiratory difficulties do not tolerate this position well.
Knee–chest*	Rectum	This position provides maximal exposure of rectal area.	This position can be embarrassing and uncomfortable.

*Some patients with arthritis or other joint deformities are unable to assume this position.

Pediatric (Box 33.2) and geriatric (Box 33.3) assessment tools are used to document and evaluate changes in health status. The Rourke Baby Record (Rourke et al., 2020) assists in the examination of normal growth and development in children from birth to the age of 5 years. In the geriatric population, a functional assessment of activities of daily living might help determine the need for assistance in the home.

ORGANIZATION OF THE EXAMINATION

The complete physical examination is made up of assessments for each body system. Patients with specific symptoms or returning for follow-up care typically require a focused examination of specific body systems. For example, a patient who comes to a clinic with symptoms of a severe chest cold requires a focused assessment of the ears, nose,

BOX 33.2 Developmental Assessment of Infants and Children

A good Canadian resource for the assessment of children is the Rourke Baby Record (Rourke et al., 2020). This tool provides information about growth and developmental milestones for children from birth to the age of 5 years. The tool combines helpful information on nutrition, child safety, and the childhood immunization schedule. A Rourke Baby Record can be downloaded free from https://www.rourkebabyrecord.ca/. Information about the tool development and associated evidence is also accessible from this website. Additionally, infant and child growth charts for Canada can be accessed from the Canadian Paediatric Society website, with additional information for the use of these tools: http://www.cps.ca/tools-outils/who-growth-charts.

BOX 33.3 Assessment Tools for Older Persons

A number of assessment tools are used to help assess the health of older persons. These tools help identify the functional, cognitive, and affective status of older persons, as well as health risks such as falls, polypharmacy, and elder abuse (see Chapter 25).

Functional independence is the ability to perform basic personal care and activities that support independent living (activities of daily living [ADLs] and instrumental ADLs [IADLs]). Most often, functional assessment tools are used to assess older persons; however, these tools can also be used for younger individuals who have functional limitations through such injuries as spinal cord or traumatic brain injuries (TBI). Functional status assessment tools help nurses assess a person's independence in the home or their level of functioning on return home from the hospital. The Katz Index (Katz et al., 1963), although published a number of years ago, is a common and simple screening tool used to assess independence with ADLs. The Lawton-Brody Instrumental Activities of Daily Living (IADL) scale is a common tool for assessing tasks that are necessary for independent functioning in the community. Other examples of functional assessment tools include the Functional Analysis Screening Tool (FAST), Global Assessment of Functioning (GAF) Scale, and Barthel Index. Access to many of these tools is free from online sources.

Screening for elder abuse is also an important consideration when working with older persons. Several tools have been developed to screen older persons for maltreatment, such as the Elder Abuse Suspicion Index (EASI), Hwalek-Sengstock Elder Abuse Screening Test (H-S/EAST), and the Vulnerability to Abuse Screening Scale (VASS) (Gallione et al., 2017). A good online resource for assessment tools in older persons is the Hartford Institute for Geriatric Nursing (https://hign.org/consultgeri/resources).

throat, and respiratory and cardiovascular systems but will not routinely require a neurological assessment. When a patient is admitted to the hospital, a complete examination is performed. A patient who is receiving a routine health promotion examination undergoes specific preventive screenings, depending on the patient's age or health risk (Table 33.4). Nurses need to use judgement to ensure that an examination involves assessment of relevant body systems and that the correct observations are documented.

The performance of a complete health assessment follows the format of the nursing history interview review of body systems. The nurse should obtain information from the history to focus attention on specific parts of the examination. Findings from the history generally reveal a pattern of related signs and symptoms. The physical examination supplements information from the history to confirm or refute the data.

Nurses need to be systematic and well organized about the examination so that they do not miss important assessment findings. A head-to-toe approach includes all body systems and helps in anticipating each step. In an adult, the examination begins by assessing the head and neck structures, including hair and skin, and progressing methodically down the body to incorporate all body systems. The following tips help keep an examination well organized:

- Compare both sides of the body for symmetry. A degree of asymmetry is normal (e.g., the biceps muscles in the dominant arm are sometimes more developed than the same muscles in the nondominant arm).
- If a patient is seriously ill, first assess the systems of the body more at risk for being abnormal. For example, a patient with chest pain first undergoes a cardiovascular assessment.
- If a patient becomes fatigued, offer rest periods between assessments.
- Perform painful procedures near the end of the examination.

TABLE 33.4 Recommended Preventive Screenings

Screening Measure	Ages 19–49	Ages 50–64	Ages 65+
Blood pressure (BP)	Measure BP at each appropriate visit. Automated office BP is preferred.	Measure BP at each appropriate visit. Automated office BP is preferred.	Measure BP at each appropriate visit. Automated office BP is preferred (Rabi et al., 2021).
Breast cancer	Screening may be considered in high-risk individuals (e.g., first-degree relative with *BRCA* gene).	Mammogram every 2–3 years	Mammogram every 2–3 years until age 75 years
Cervical cancer	Sexually active women age 25 years and older: Papanicolaou (Pap) test every 3 years if results are normal	Pap test every 3 years if results are normal	Pap test every 3 years if results are normal; stop at age 69 if there are three normal results in last 10 years
Colon/rectal cancer	Screening may be considered in individuals at high risk (e.g., first-degree relative with colon/rectal cancer prior to age 50).	Fecal immunochemical test (FIT) or fecal occult blood test (FOBT) every 2 years or flexible sigmoidoscopy every 10 years	FIT or FOBT every 2 years or flexible sigmoidoscopy every 10 years until 75 years
Dental	Dental exam every 6 months	Dental exam every 6 months	Dental exam every 6 months
Diabetes	Fasting blood glucose (FBG) and/or A1c every 3 years in all individuals age 40 and older. Screen earlier and/or more frequently (q 6–12 months) in people with high risk for diabetes.	FBG and/or A1c every 3 years. Screen individuals at high risk more frequently (q 6–12 months).	FBG and/or A1c every 3 years. Screen individuals at high risk more frequently (q 6–12 months) (Diabetes Canada Clinical Practice Guidelines Expert Committee, 2018).
Intimate partner violence (IPV)	Screen all patients, especially women of child-bearing age, for intimate partner violence and offer referral to intervention services if they screen positive.		

Continued

TABLE 33.4	Recommended Preventive Screenings—cont'd		
Screening Measure	**Ages 19–49**	**Ages 50–64**	**Ages 65+**
Lipid disorders/ cardiovascular risk	Ages 19–39: Screen based on risk assessment with lipid profile (blood test) Ages 40–49: Screen men and postmenopausal woman with lipid profile and cardiovascular risk assessment (e.g., Framingham Risk Score) every 5 years.	Screen with lipid profile and cardiovascular risk assessment (e.g., Framingham Risk Score) every 5 years.	Screen with lipid profile and cardiovascular risk assessment (e.g., Framingham Risk Score) every 5 years up to age 75 (Pearson et al., 2021).
Obesity	Height, weight, body mass index (BMI), and waist circumference at each appropriate visit. Use Edmonton Obesity Staging System to evaluate obesity.	Height, weight, BMI, and waist circumference at each appropriate visit. Use Edmonton Obesity Staging System to evaluate obesity.	Height, weight, BMI, and waist circumference at each appropriate visit. Use Edmonton Obesity Staging System to evaluate obesity (Obesity Canada and the Canadian Association of Bariatric Physicians and Surgeons, 2020).
Osteoporosis		Screen patients with risk of fracture using clinical risk assessment tool (e.g., FRAXX or CAROC). Screen patients with recent hip or fragility fracture using bone mineral density (BMD).	Screen women and men aged 65 years and older at risk of fracture using clinical risk assessment tool (e.g., FRAXX or CAROC). Screen patients with recent hip or fragility fracture using BMD (Papaioannou et al., 2010).
Prostate cancer	Consider prostate-specific antigen (PSA) screening for individual 45 years and older with increased risk of prostate cancer, after discussing strengths and limits of available screening with patient and using shared decision-making approach. Frequency of screening is based on PSA level (e.g., repeat q 2 years if PSA 1–3 ng/mL).	Consider for individuals with at least a 10-year life expectancy, after discussing strengths and limits of available screening with patient and using shared decision-making approach. Frequency of screening is based on PSA level (e.g., repeat q 2 years if PSA 1–3 ng/mL).	Consider for individuals age 65–70 with at least a 10-year life expectancy, after discussing strengths and limits of available screening with patient and using shared decision-making approach. Frequency of screening is based on PSA level (e.g., repeat q 2 years if PSA 1–3 ng/mL) (Rendon et al., 2017).
Sexually transmitted infections (STIs)	Annual chlamydia and gonorrhea screening for sexually active individuals under 30 years at average risk; more frequent screening for high-risk groups (e.g., serial monogamy, men who have sex with men [MSM], injection drug user). Hepatitis C and HIV screening for adolescents and adults at risk of infection. (Public Health Agency of Canada, 2021a).		
Skin cancer	Routine self-exam and annual health care provider exam for those at high risk	Routine self-exam and annual health care provider exam for those at high risk	Routine self-exam and annual health care provider exam for those at high risk
Substance use	Ask all individuals 18 years and older about substance use, including alcohol, marijuana, tobacco, and illicit drugs		
Vision	Every 2–5 years	Every 2–3 years	Every year

Based on Bouchard, B. (2021). *Canadian preventative screening guidelines.* https://objectivehealth.ca/screening/; Canadian Task Force on Preventative Health Care. (2021). *Published guidelines.* https://canadiantaskforce.ca/guidelines/published-guidelines/

- Record assessments in specific terms on a physical assessment form or in the nurses' notes.
- Use common and accepted medical abbreviations to keep notes brief and concise.
- Record quick notes during the examination to avoid keeping the patient waiting. Complete any observations at the end of the examination.
- A physical assessment form allows the nurse to record information in the same sequence as it was gathered.

A guide for performance of a complete physical assessment can be found in the textbook by Jarvis et al. (2019, pp. 819–840), Chapter 28, The Complete Health Assessment: Putting It All Together.

GENERAL SURVEY

Assessment begins when the nurse first meets the patient and observes their behaviour, appearance, and mobility. This forms the beginning of the general survey, the first step in physical examination of the patient. The survey provides information about characteristics of an illness, a patient's hygiene and body image, emotional state, recent changes in weight, and developmental status. If there are abnormalities or health problems, the nurse needs to closely assess the affected body system later during the physical examination of that system.

General Appearance and Behaviour

Assess appearance and behaviour while interacting with the patient. The review of general appearance and behaviour includes the following:

- *Age and gender:* A person's gender and age affect the type of examination performed and the manner in which the assessments are made. Physical characteristics offer clues that help guide the examination. Certain conditions are more likely to affect individuals of a specific gender or who have certain physical characteristics; for example, breast cancer is more common in women than men, and the incidence of skin cancer is higher in individuals who have fair complexions.
- *Signs of distress:* There are sometimes obvious signs or symptoms indicating pain (grimacing, splinting painful area) or difficulty in breathing (shortness of breath, sternal retractions) or anxiety (fidgeting, pacing). These signs establish priorities regarding what to examine first.
- *Body type:* Observe if a patient appears trim and muscular, obese, or excessively thin. Body type reflects the level of health, age, and lifestyle.
- *Posture:* Normal standing posture is an upright stance with parallel alignment of the hips and shoulders. Normal sitting posture involves some degree of rounding of the shoulders. Observe whether the patient has a slumped, erect, or bent posture. Posture often reflects mood or pain. Older persons may assume a stooped, forward-bent posture, with the hips and knees somewhat flexed and arms bent at the elbows, raising the level of the arms.
- *Gait:* Observe the patient walking into the room or at the bedside (if the patient is ambulatory). Note whether movements are coordinated or uncoordinated. A person normally walks with arms swinging freely at their sides, with their head and face leading the body.
- *Body movements:* Observe whether movements are purposeful, and note if there are any tremors involving the extremities. Determine if any body parts are immobile.
- *Hygiene and grooming:* Note the patient's level of cleanliness by observing the appearance of the hair, skin, and fingernails. Note if the patient's clothes are clean. Grooming depends on the activities being performed just before the examination, as well as the patient's occupation. Also note the amount and type of cosmetics used.
- *Dress:* Culture, lifestyle, socioeconomic level, and personal preference affect the type of clothes worn. Note if the type of clothing worn is appropriate for the temperature and weather conditions. Depressed or cognitively impaired individuals are often unable to choose proper clothing. An older person tends to wear extra clothing because of the sensitivity to cold.
- *Body odour:* An unpleasant body odour often results from physical exercise, poor hygiene, or certain disease states.
- *Affect and mood:* Affect is a person's feelings as they appear to others. Patients express mood or emotional state verbally and nonverbally. Note if verbal expressions match nonverbal behaviour. Observe if mood is appropriate for the situation. Observe facial expressions while asking questions.
- *Speech:* Normal speech is understandable and moderately paced. It shows an association with the person's thoughts. Note if the patient speaks rapidly or slowly. Emotions or neurological impairment sometimes causes an abnormal pace. Observe whether the patient speaks in a normal tone with clear inflection of words.

- *Victims of violence:* Physical and verbal intimidation and violence toward children, women, and older persons is a growing health concern. Obvious physical injury or neglect are signs of possible physical intimidation and violence (e.g., evidence of malnutrition or presence of bruising on the extremities or trunk). Assess for the patient's fear of the spouse or partner, caregiver, parent, or adult child. Note if the partner or caregiver has a history of violence, alcoholism, or drug abuse. Is the person unemployed, ill, or frustrated at caring for the patient? Most provinces mandate a report to social service if a health care provider suspects violence or neglect (Box 33.4). During an assessment, if you suspect the patient is experiencing physical and/or verbal intimidation and violence, interview the patient in private. It is difficult to detect physical and verbal intimidation and violence because victims often will not complain or report that they are in an abusive situation (Jarvis et al., 2019, pp. 124–140). Patients are more likely to reveal intimidation or abuse when the suspected abuser is absent from the room.

> **SAFETY ALERT** The risk for further violence is high once the victim has reported the event or tries to leave the situation. Provide counselling options for these individuals.

- *Substance use and misuse:* Substance use and misuse affects all socioeconomic groups. A single visit to a clinic does not always reveal the problem. Several visits often reveal behaviours that nurses can confirm with a well-focused history and physical examination. The patient should be approached in a caring and nonjudgemental way, as issues of problematic substance use involve both emotional and lifestyle issues. Box 33.5 lists characteristics of patients that may raise suspicion of substance use and misuse. When substance misuse is suspected, ask the patient the following CAGE questions (CAGE is an acronym for the following):
  - Have you ever felt the need to **C**ut down on your drinking or drug use?
  - Have people **A**nnoyed you by criticizing your drinking or drug use?
  - Have you ever felt bad or **G**uilty about your drinking or drug use?
  - Have you ever used or had a drink first thing in the morning as an **E**ye-opener to steady your nerves or feel normal?

Vital Signs

Assessment of vital signs (see Chapter 31) is the first part of the physical examination.

Height and Weight

Height and weight reflect a person's general level of health. Weight is a routine measure during health screenings and clinical visits. Both measures are routine when patients are admitted to a health care setting. Health care providers measure an infant or child's height and weight to assess growth and development. In older persons, height and weight are usually coupled with a nutritional assessment by a dietitian in order to determine possible causes of chronic diseases or contributions to treatment, or to help identify the older person who has difficulty with eating and other functional activities.

It is important to look for overall trends in height and weight, as changes can be indicative of health problems. A patient's weight will normally vary daily because of fluid loss or retention. A downward trend in a frail older person indicates serious reduction in nutritional reserves. The nursing history helps to focus on possible causes for a

BOX 33.4	Clinical Indicators of Abuse

Physical Findings	Behavioural Findings
Child Sexual Abuse	
Vaginal or penile discharge	Difficulty in sleeping or eating
Blood on underclothing	Fear of certain people or places
Pain, itching, or unusual odour in genital area	Play activities recreate the abuse situation
Genital injuries	Regressed behaviour
Difficulty sitting or walking	Sexual acting out
Pain while urinating; recurrent urinary tract infections	Knowledge of explicit sexual matters
Foreign bodies in rectum, urethra, or vagina	Preoccupation with others' or own genitals
Sexually transmitted infections	Profound and rapid personality changes
Pregnancy in a young adolescent	Rapidly declining school performance
	Poor relationship with peers
Intimate Partner Violence	
Injuries and trauma are inconsistent with reported cause	Attempted suicide
Multiple injuries involving head, face, neck, breasts, abdomen, and genitalia (black eyes, orbital fractures, broken nose, fractured skull, lip lacerations, broken teeth, strangulation marks)	Eating or sleeping disorders
	Anxiety
	Panic attacks
	Pattern of problematic substance use (follows physical abuse)
	Low self-esteem
X-ray films show old and new fractures in different stages of healing	Depression
	Sense of helplessness
	Guilt
Abrasions, lacerations, bruises/welts	Increased forgetfulness
	Stress-related symptoms (headache, anxiety)
Burns	
Human bites	
Elder Abuse	
Injuries and trauma are inconsistent with reported cause (cigarette burn, scratch, bruise, or bite)	Dependent on caregiver
	Physically or cognitively impaired, or both
Hematomas	Combative
Bruises at various stages of resolution	Wandering
	Verbally aggressive
Bruises, chafing, excoriation on wrist or legs (restraints)	Minimal social supporProlonged interval between injury and medical treatment
Burns	
Fractures inconsistent with cause described	
Dried blood	

Data from Perry, S. E., Hockenberry, M. J., Lowdermilk, D. L., et al. (Eds.). (2017). *Maternal child nursing care in Canada* (2nd ed.). Mosby; Jarvis, C., Browne, A., MacDonald-Jenkins, J., et al. (Eds.), (2019). *Physical examination and health assessment* (3rd Canadian ed., pp. 110–123). Elsevier Canada.

BOX 33.5	Red Flags for Suspicion of Substance Use and Misuse

- Patients who frequently miss appointments
- Patients who frequently request written excuses for absence from work
- Patients who have chief complaints of insomnia, "bad nerves," or pain that does not fit a particular pattern
- Patients who often report lost prescriptions (e.g., tranquilizers or pain medications) or ask for frequent refills
- Patients who make frequent emergency department (ED) visits
- Patients who have a history of changing health care providers or who bring in medication bottles prescribed by several different providers
- Patients with a history of gastrointestinal bleeds, peptic ulcers, pancreatitis, cellulitis, or frequent pulmonary infections
- Patients with frequent sexually transmitted infections (STIs), complicated pregnancies, multiple abortions, or sexual dysfunction
- Patients who experience chest pains or palpitations or who have a history of admissions to rule out myocardial infarctions
- Patients who give histories of activities that place them at risk for human immunodeficiency virus (HIV) infection (multiple partners, multiple rapes)
- Patients with a family history of addiction; history of childhood sexual, physical, or emotional abuse; or social and financial or marital problems
- If two or more of the CAGE questions are positive, strongly suspect substance use disorder and consider how to motivate the patient to seek treatment.

Data from American Psychiatric Association. (2013). *Diagnostic and statistical manual of mental disorders* (5th ed.). Miller, S. C., Fiellin, D. A., Rosenthal, R. N., et al. (Eds.). (2019). *The ASAM principles of addiction medicine* (6th ed.). Lippincott Williams & Wilkins.

Body mass index (BMI) tables are used to help determine the normal expected weight range for a patient at a given height (Figure 33.1). With the BMI, waist circumference of adults is used to measure the health risk associated with obesity. A patient's waist is measured midway between the costal margin and the iliac crest. Measurement should be taken to the nearest 0.5 cm at the end of expiration. The tape measure should fit snugly but should not compress soft tissue. Locating the intersection of the patient's height and weight on the BMI table will indicate the patient's BMI. The risk for health problems based on this value can be assessed using the BMI categories. Patients at high risk should be encouraged to seek the care of a health care provider for weight loss, dietary changes, and exercise programs.

Patients should always be weighed at the same time of day, on the same scale, and in the same clothes to allow an objective comparison of subsequent weights. Accuracy of weight measurement is important because health care providers will base medical and nursing decisions (e.g., drug dosage determinations, lifting, and positioning) on changes. Electronic scales are the most reliable and commonly used form of scales. They are automatically calibrated each time they are used and display the weight within seconds.

Stretcher and chair scales are available for patients unable to bear weight. After the patient is transferred to the scale, a hydraulic device lifts the patient above the bed and measures their weight on a balance beam or digital display. Caution is required when transferring patients to and from the scales.

Infants should always be weighed in baskets or on platform scales. To weigh the infant, remove the infant's clothing, and weigh the infant in dry, disposable diapers. Adjust the measurement later for the weight of the diaper, ensuring an accurate reading. Keep the room warm to

change in weight (Table 33.5). When measuring a patient's height and weight, first ask the patient their current height and weight. Also assess for weight gains or losses. A weight gain of 2.3 kg (5 lb) in a day indicates problems with fluid retention. If the patient has lost more than 5% of body weight in a month or 10% in 6 months, the loss is considered significant.

TABLE 33.5	Nursing History for Weight Assessment
Assessment Category	**Rationale**
Ask about total weight lost or gained; compare with usual weight; note time period for loss (e.g., gradual, sudden, desired, or undesired).	Determines severity of issue and reveals if weight change is related to disease process, change in eating pattern, or pregnancy
If weight loss is desired, ask about eating habits, diet plan followed, food preparation, calorie intake, appetite, exercise pattern, support group participation, and weight goal.	Aids in determining appropriateness of diet plan followed
If weight loss is undesired, ask about anorexia, vomiting, diarrhea, thirst, frequent urination, and change in lifestyle, activity, stress levels, alcohol intake.	Focuses on conditions that cause weight loss (e.g., gastrointestinal conditions)
Assess if patient has noted changes in social aspects of eating: more meals in restaurants, rushing to eat meals, stress at work, or skipping meals.	Lifestyle changes sometimes contribute to weight changes.
Assess if patient takes chemotherapy, diuretics, insulin, fluoxetine, prescription and nonprescription appetite suppressants, laxatives, oral hypoglycemics, and herbal supplements (weight loss); steroids, oral contraceptives, antidepressants, insulin (weight gain).	Weight gain or loss is a side effect of these medications.
Assess for preoccupation with body weight or body shape, never feeling thin enough, unusually strict caloric intake, laxative abuse, induced vomiting, amenorrhea, and excessive exercise.	These are symptoms of a potential eating disorder.

prevent chills. A light cloth or paper placed on the scale's surface prevents cross-infection from urine or feces. When placing infants in baskets or on platforms, hold a hand lightly above to prevent accidental falls. An infant's weight is measured in grams.

To measure the height of weight-bearing patients, have them remove their shoes. A measuring stick or tape is attached vertically to the weight scales or wall. Have the patient stand erect. The platform scale has a metal rod attached to the back of the scale; this swings out and over the crown of the head. When a scale is unavailable, place a measuring stick or flat book on the patient's head. With the rod or stick placed level horizontally at a 90-degree angle to the measuring stick, measure the patient's height in centimetres.

Remove the shoes of a non–weight-bearing patient and position the patient (such as an infant) supine on a firm surface. Portable devices are available that provide a reliable means to measure height. Place the infant on the device, having the parent hold the infant's head against the headboard. With the infant's legs straight at the knees, place the footboard against the bottom of the infant's feet (Figure 33.2). Record the infant's length to the nearest 0.5 cm.

THE INTEGUMENTARY SYSTEM: SKIN, HAIR, AND NAILS

The integument consists of the skin, hair, scalp, and nails. Developing a routine approach to physical assessment helps to ensure the completeness of the examination. The approach to patient assessment might begin with the inspection of all skin surfaces. Alternatively, as your assessment skills develop, you may choose to assess the skin gradually while examining other body systems (e.g., inspecting the skin of the torso while assessing the respiratory, cardiovascular, and abdominal systems). Use the skills of inspection, palpation, and olfaction to assess the integument's function and integrity.

Skin

Assessment of the skin reveals changes in oxygenation, circulation, nutrition, local tissue damage, and hydration. In a hospital setting, the majority of patients are older persons, debilitated patients, or young and seriously ill patients. There are significant risks for skin lesions resulting from trauma to the skin during administration of care, from exposure to pressure during immobilization, or from reaction to various medications used in treatment. Patients at high risk are persons who

are neurologically impaired or chronically ill and orthopedic patients. Others at risk are patients with diminished mental status, poor tissue oxygenation, low cardiac output, or inadequate nutrition. In long-term care and extended-care facilities, patients are often at risk for many of the same skin conditions, depending on their level of mobility and the presence of chronic illness. It is important to routinely assess the skin for development of primary or initial lesions. Without proper care, primary lesions can deteriorate to become secondary lesions that require more extensive nursing care. The development of a pressure injury, for example, will lengthen a hospital stay unless the nurse prevents or discovers it early and treats it properly (see Chapter 47).

Melanoma, an aggressive form of skin cancer, and other cutaneous malignancies are the most common neoplasms seen in patients. It is thus important to incorporate a thorough skin assessment on all patients and to educate them about self-examination (Box 33.6).

Assessing the integrity of a patient's skin can reveal the need for nursing intervention (see Chapter 47). Use assessment findings to determine the type of hygiene measures required to maintain skin integrity (see Chapter 39). Adequate nutrition and hydration are important goals of therapy if an alteration in skin integrity is identified (see Chapter 43).

Appropriate lighting is essential to accurately observe a patient's skin. Natural or halogen lighting provides optimal lighting for assessing most patients, with sunlight being optimal for detecting skin changes in the dark-skinned patient. Fluorescent light is not recommended because it imparts a bluish tone to dark skin (Morgan, 2015). Room temperature also affects skin assessment. A room that is too warm causes superficial vasodilation, resulting in an increased redness of the skin. A cool environment causes the sensitive patient to develop cyanosis (bluish discoloration) around the lips and nail beds.

Use disposable gloves for palpation if open, moist, or draining lesions are present. Although each part of the body is inspected during an examination, it is helpful to make a brief but careful overall visual sweep of the entire body. This provides a good assessment of the distribution and extent of any lesions, as well as the overall symmetry of skin colour. Because all skin surfaces need to be inspected, the patient will assume several positions. Table 33.6 outlines the nursing history for skin assessment. If during an examination you notice abnormalities, palpate the involved areas. Skin odours are usually apparent in the folds of the skin, such as the axillae or under the female patient's breasts.

FIGURE 33.2 Measurement of infant length. (From Ball, J. W., Dains, J. E., Flynn, J. A., et al. [2019]. *Seidel's guide to physical examination* [9th ed.]. Mosby. Courtesy SECA GmbH, Hamburg, Germany.)

A

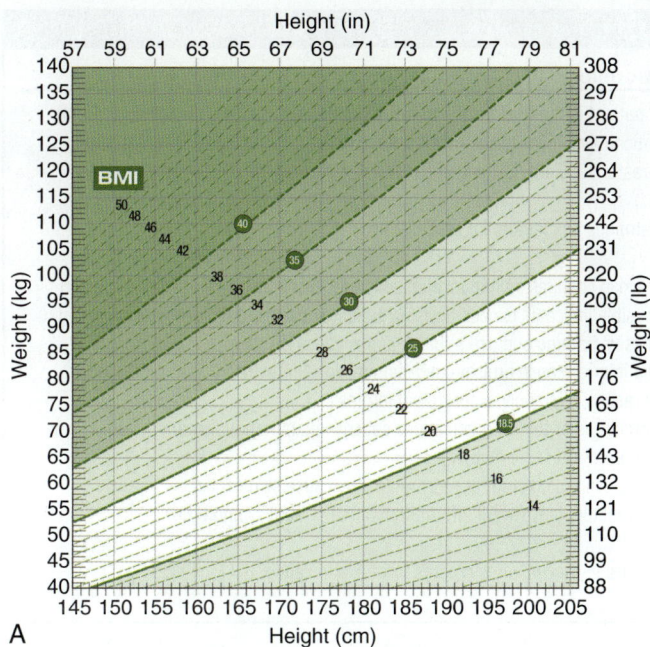

Waist circumference	BMI category		
	Normal 18.5–24.9 kg/m²	Overweight 25–29.9 kg/m²	Obese class I 30–34.9 kg/m²
Men: < 102 cm Women: < 88 cm	Least risk	Increased risk	High risk
Men: ≥ 102 cm Women: ≥ 88 cm	Increased risk	High risk	Very high risk

B

FIGURE 33.1 Height and weight measures: Weights for people over 18 years (excluding pregnant or lactating women).

- Weight and height are required to measure a person's body mass index (BMI), which is calculated by dividing weight (kg) by height squared (m²).
- Weight is measured with the patient wearing light clothing and no footwear and is recorded to the nearest 0.2 kg.
- Height is measured with the person wearing no shoes, standing in an erect position, looking straight ahead with feet together and heels against a wall or measuring board. A horizontal bar or other similar device should be lowered so that it rests flat on top of the person's head. Height is recorded to the nearest 0.5 cm.
- For a quick determination of BMI, use a straight edge to help locate the point on the chart below where height and weight intersect. Read the number on the dashed line closest to this point. For example, a person who weighs 69 kg and is 173 cm tall has a BMI of about 23. NOTE: The BMI cannot be used to distinguish between increased body weight due to adiposity or fluid retention (e.g., peripheral edema), although this distinction should be apparent clinically. The BMI may have limitations in people who are very muscular or very lean, in those who are very tall or very short, in people with long limb lengths relative to trunk size (e.g., those with Marfan syndrome), and in people with short limb lengths relative to trunk size (e.g., those with achondroplasia).

BOX 33.6 PATIENT TEACHING

Skin Assessment

Objectives
- Patient will perform a monthly self-examination of the skin.
- Patient will identify factors that increase the risk of skin cancer.
- Patient will follow hygiene practices aimed at maintaining skin integrity.

Teaching Strategies
- Instruct patient to conduct a complete monthly self-examination of all skin surfaces, noting moles, blemishes, and birthmarks. Cancerous melanomas start as small, molelike growths that increase in size, change colour, become ulcerated, and bleed (see Box 33.8).
- Tell patient to report any change to a skin lesion, a lesion that bleeds or fails to heal, or a sore that does not heal to a health care provider. Especially instruct older persons, who tend to have delayed wound healing.
- To treat excessively dry skin, the patient should avoid using hot water, harsh soaps, and drying agents such as rubbing alcohol. Tell patient to use a superfatted (Dove) soap, and pat rather than rub the skin after bathing.
- Instruct patient to apply moisturizers (mineral oil) to the skin regularly to reduce itching and drying, and to wear cotton clothing (Marks & Miller, 2019).

Evaluation
- Observe patient performing a skin assessment.
- Have the patient describe signs of skin cancer and measures to take to prevent skin cancer.
- Ask the patient to describe methods for keeping the skin lubricated and supple.

Colour. Skin colour varies from body part to body part and from person to person. Despite individual variations, skin colour is usually uniform over the body. Table 33.7 lists common variations. Normal skin **pigmentation** ranges in tone from ivory or light pink to ruddy pink in light skin and from light to deep brown or olive in dark skin. In older persons, pigmentation increases unevenly, causing discoloured skin.

TABLE 33.6	Nursing History for Skin Assessment
Assessment Category	**Rationale**
Ask the patient about history of changes in the skin: dryness, pruritus, sores, rashes, lumps, colour, texture, odour, lesion that does not heal.	The patient is the best source to recognize change. Usually skin cancer is first noticed as a localized change in skin colour.
Consider if the patient has the following history: fair, freckled, ruddy complexion; light-coloured hair or eyes; tendency to burn easily.	Characteristics are risk factors for skin cancer.
Determine whether patient works or spends excessive time outside. If so, ask whether patient wears sunscreen, other protective clothing, or both.	Determines risk factors for skin cancer
Determine whether patient has noted lesions, rashes, or bruises.	Most skin changes do not develop suddenly. A change in character of a lesion possibly indicates cancer. Bruising indicates trauma or bleeding disorder.
Question patient about frequency of bathing and type of soap used.	Excessive bathing and use of harsh soaps cause dry skin.
Ask if patient has had recent trauma to skin.	Some injuries cause bruising and changes in skin texture.
Determine whether patient has a history of allergies.	Skin rashes commonly occur from allergies.
Ask if patient uses topical medications or home remedies on skin.	Incorrect use of topical medications causes inflammation, irritation, and compromised skin integrity.
Ask if patient goes to tanning parlours, uses sun lamps, or takes tanning pills.	Overexposure of skin to these irritants may cause skin cancer.
Ask if patient has family history of serious skin disorders such as skin cancer or psoriasis.	Family history may reveal information about patient's condition.
Determine if patient works with creosote, coal, tar, petroleum products, arsenic compounds, or radium.	Exposure to these agents creates risk for skin cancer.

TABLE 33.7	Skin Colour Variations		
Colour	**Condition**	**Causes**	**Assessment Locations**
Bluish (cyanosis)	Increased amount of deoxygenated hemoglobin (associated with hypoxia)	Heart or lung disease, cold environment	Nail beds, lips, mouth, skin (severe cases)
Pallor (decrease in colour)	Reduced amount of oxyhemoglobin	Anemia	Face, conjunctivae, nail beds, palms of hands
	Reduced visibility of oxyhemoglobin resulting from decreased blood flow	Shock	Skin, nail beds, conjunctivae, lips
Loss of pigmentation	Vitiligo	Congenital or autoimmune condition causing lack of pigment	Patchy areas on skin over face, hands, arms
Yellow-orange (jaundice)	Increased deposit of bilirubin in tissues	Liver disease, destruction of red blood cells	Sclera, mucous membranes, skin
Red (erythema)	Increased visibility of oxyhemoglobin caused by dilation or increased blood flow	Fever, direct trauma, blushing, alcohol intake	Face, area of trauma, sacrum, shoulders, other common sites for pressure injury
Tan-brown	Increased amount of melanin	Suntan, pregnancy	Areas exposed to sun: face, arms, areolae, nipples

While inspecting the skin, be aware that cosmetics or tanning agents sometimes mask colour.

The assessment of colour first involves areas of the skin not exposed to the sun, such as the palms of the hands. Note if the skin is unusually pale or dark. Areas exposed to the sun, such as the face and arms, will be darker. It is more difficult to note changes such as pallor or cyanosis in patients with dark skin tones. Usually, colour hues are seen best in the palms, soles of the feet, lips, tongue, and nail beds. Areas of increased colour (*hyperpigmentation*) and decreased colour (*hypopigmentation*) are common. Skin creases and folds are darker than the rest of the body in the dark-skinned patient.

Inspect sites where abnormalities can be identified more easily. For example, pallor can be seen more easily in the face, buccal (mouth) mucosa, conjunctiva, and nail beds. Observe for cyanosis in the lips, nail beds, palpebral conjunctivae, and palms. In recognizing pallor in the dark-skinned patient, observe that normal brown skin appears to be yellow-brown and normal black skin appears to be ashen grey. Also assess the lips, nail beds, and mucous membranes for generalized pallor; if pallor is present, the mucous membranes will be ashen grey. Assessment of cyanosis in the dark-skinned patient requires observation of areas where pigmentation occurs least (conjunctiva, sclera, buccal mucosa, tongue, lips, nail beds, and palms and soles). In addition, verify these findings with clinical manifestations (Marks & Miller, 2019).

The best site to inspect for jaundice (yellow-orange discoloration) is the patient's sclera. Normal reactive hyperemia, or redness, can be seen most often in regions exposed to pressure, such as the sacrum, heels, and greater trochanter. Inspect for any patches or areas of skin colour variation. Localized skin changes, such as pallor or erythema (red discoloration), indicate circulatory changes. For example, an area of erythema is due to localized vasodilation resulting from a sunburn, inflammation, or fever. It is difficult to observe erythema in the dark-skinned patient, so palpate the area for heat and warmth to note the presence of skin inflammation (Jarvis et al., 2019). An area of an extremity that appears unusually pale results from arterial occlusion or edema. Be sure to ask the patient if they have noticed any changes in skin colouring.

A pattern of skin assessment findings can be indicative of substance use disorder (Table 33.8). For example, a patient who takes repeated intravenous (IV) injections has edematous, reddened, and warm areas

TABLE 33.8	Physical Findings of the Skin Indicative of Substance Use Disorder
Body System	**Commonly Associated Drug**
Diaphoresis	Sedative hypnotic (including alcohol)
Spider angiomas	Alcohol, stimulants
Burns (especially fingers)	Alcohol
Needle marks	Opioids
Contusion, abrasions, cuts, scars	Alcohol, other sedative hypnotics
"Homemade" tattoos	Cocaine, intravenous (IV) opioids (prevents detection of injection sites)
Increased vascularity of face	Alcohol
Red, dry skin	Phencyclidine (PCP)

Data from Miller, S. C., Fiellin, D. A., Rosenthal, R. N., et al. (Eds.). (2019). *The ASAM principles of addiction medicine* (6th ed.). Lippincott Williams & Wilkins.

along the arms and legs suggestive of recent injections. Evidence of old injection sites appears as hyperpigmented and shiny or scarred areas.

Moisture. The hydration of skin and mucous membranes helps to reveal body fluid imbalances, changes in the skin's environment, and regulation of body temperature. *Moisture* refers to wetness and oiliness. The skin is normally smooth and dry. Skin folds such as the axillae are normally moist. Minimal perspiration or oiliness is often present (Jarvis et al., 2019). Increased perspiration is sometimes associated with activity, warm environments, obesity, anxiety, or excitement. Use ungloved fingertips to palpate skin surfaces and observe for dullness, dryness, crusting, and flaking. *Flaking* is the appearance of flakes resembling dandruff when the skin surface is lightly rubbed. *Scaling* involves fishlike scales that are easily rubbed off the skin's surface. Both flaking and scaling indicate abnormally dry skin. Excessively dry skin is common in older persons and in individuals who use excessive amounts of soap during bathing. Other factors causing dry skin include lack of humidity, exposure to sun, smoking, stress, excessive perspiration, and dehydration. Excessive dryness worsens existing skin conditions such as eczema and dermatitis.

Temperature. The temperature of the skin depends on the amount of blood circulating through the dermis. Increased or decreased skin temperature indicates an increase or decrease in blood flow. An increase in skin temperature often accompanies localized erythema or redness of the skin. A reduction in skin temperature reflects a decrease in blood flow. It is important to remember that if an examination room is cold, this will affect the patient's skin temperature and colour.

Accurately assess temperature by palpating the skin with the dorsum, or back of the hand. Compare symmetrical body parts. Normally the skin temperature is warm. Sometimes skin temperature is the same throughout the body, and other times it varies in one area. Always assess skin temperature for patients at risk of having impaired circulation, such as after a cast application or vascular surgery. A stage I pressure injury can be identified early by noting warmth and erythema on an area of the skin (see Chapter 47).

Texture. The character of the skin's surface and the feel of deeper portions are its *texture*. Determine whether the patient's skin is smooth or rough, thin or thick, tight or supple, and indurated (hardened) or soft by stroking it lightly with the fingertips. The texture of the skin is normally smooth, soft, even, and flexible in children and adults. However,

the texture is usually not uniform throughout. The palms of the hand and soles of the feet tend to be thicker. With advancing age, the skin becomes wrinkled and leathery because of a decrease in collagen, subcutaneous fat, and sweat glands.

Localized changes result from trauma, surgical wounds, or lesions. When finding irregularities in texture such as scars or induration, ask the patient if a recent injury to the skin has occurred. Deeper palpation sometimes reveals irregularities such as tenderness or localized areas of induration commonly caused by repeated injections.

Turgor. Turgor is the skin's elasticity. Edema or dehydration diminishes turgor. Normally the skin loses its elasticity with age. To assess the skin turgor, grasp a fold of skin on the back of the forearm or sternal area with the fingertips and release it. Normally the skin lifts easily and snaps back immediately to its resting position. The back of the hand is not the best place to test for turgor, because the skin is normally loose and thin (Jarvis et al., 2019). The skin stays pinched when turgor is poor. Note the ease with which the skin moves and the speed at which it returns to place. Failure of the skin to reassume its normal contour or shape indicates dehydration. The patient with poor skin turgor does not have resilience to the normal wear and tear on the skin. A decrease in turgor predisposes the patient to skin breakdown.

Vascularity. The circulation of the skin affects colour in localized areas and the appearance of superficial blood vessels. With aging, capillaries become fragile. Localized pressure areas, found after a patient has remained in one position, appear reddened, pink, or pale (Jarvis et al., 2019). Petechiae are pinpoint-sized, red or purple spots on the skin caused by small hemorrhages in the skin layers. Petechiae do not blanch but may indicate serious blood-clotting disorders, drug reactions, or liver disease.

Edema. Areas of the skin become swollen or edematous from a buildup of fluid in the tissues. Direct trauma and impairment of venous return are two common causes of edema (Jarvis et al., 2019). Inspect edematous areas for location, colour, and shape. The formation of edema separates the skin's surface from the pigmented and vascular layers, masking skin colour. Edematous skin also appears stretched and shiny. Palpate edematous areas to determine mobility, consistency, and tenderness. When pressure from the examiner's fingers leaves an indentation in the edematous area, it is called *pitting edema*. To assess the degree of pitting edema, press the edematous area firmly with the thumb for several seconds and release. The depth of pitting, recorded in millimetres, determines the degree of edema (Jarvis et al., 2019, p. 552). For example, 1+ edema equals a 2-mm depth, 2+ edema equals a 4-mm depth, 3+ equals 6 mm, and 4+ equals 8 mm (see Figure 33.40).

Lesions. The skin is normally free of lesions, except for common freckles or age-related changes such as skin tags, senile keratosis (thickening of skin), cherry angiomas (ruby-red papules), and atrophic warts. Lesions are primary (occurring as initial spontaneous manifestations of a pathological process), such as an insect bite, or secondary (resulting from later formation or trauma to a primary lesion), such as a pressure injury. When a lesion is detected, inspect it for colour, location, texture, size, shape, type, grouping (clustered or linear), and distribution (localized or generalized). Observe any exudate for colour, odour, amount, and consistency. Measure the size of the lesion by using a small, clear, flexible ruler divided in centimetres. Comparing a lesion with a household measure, such as a coin or eraser, is not reliable (Jarvis et al., 2019, p. 237). Measure lesions in height, width, and depth.

Palpation determines the lesion's mobility, contour (flat, raised, or depressed), and consistency (soft or indurated). Certain types of

BOX 33.7   Types of Primary Skin Lesions

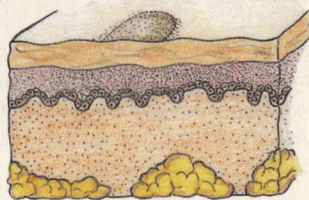

Macule: Flat, nonpalpable change in skin colour, smaller than 1 cm (e.g., freckle, petechiae)

Papule: Palpable, circumscribed, solid elevation in skin, smaller than 1 cm (e.g., elevated nevus)

Nodule: Elevated solid mass, deeper and firmer than papule, 1–2 cm (e.g., wart)

Tumour: Solid mass that extends deep through subcutaneous tissue, larger than 1–2 cm (e.g., epithelioma)

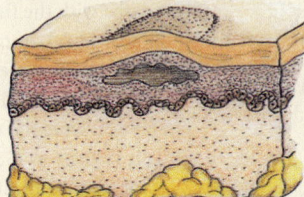

Wheal: Irregularly shaped, elevated area or superficial localized edema; varies in size (e.g., hive, mosquito bite)

Vesicle: Circumscribed elevation of skin filled with serous fluid, smaller than 1 cm (e.g., herpes simplex, chicken pox)

Pustule: Circumscribed elevation of skin similar to vesicle but filled with pus; varies in size (e.g., acne, staphylococcal infection)

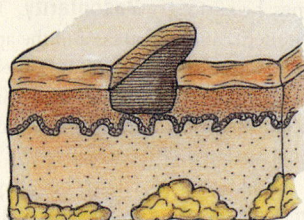

Ulcer: Deep loss of skin surface that extends to dermis and frequently bleeds and scars; varies in size (e.g., venous stasis ulcer)

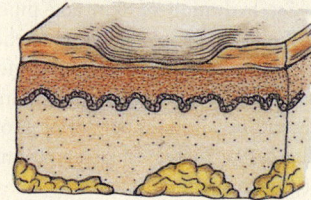

Atrophy: Thinning of skin with loss of normal skin furrow, with skin appearing shiny and translucent; varies in size (e.g., arterial insufficiency)

lesions present a characteristic pattern. For example, a tumour is usually an elevated, solid lesion larger than 1 cm. Primary lesions, such as macules and nodules, come from some stimulus to the skin (Box 33.7). Secondary lesions, such as ulcers, occur as alterations in primary lesions. Upon identifying a lesion, closely inspect it in good lighting. Palpate gently, covering the entire area of the lesion. If the lesion is moist or draining fluid, wear gloves during palpation.

Note if the patient reports tenderness during palpation. Cancerous lesions frequently undergo changes in colour and size (Box 33.8). Basal cell carcinoma is most common in sun-exposed areas and frequently occurs in a background of sun-damaged skin; it almost never spreads to other parts of the body. Squamous cell carcinoma is more serious than basal cell carcinoma and develops on the outer layers of sun-exposed skin; these cells may travel to lymph nodes and throughout the body. Report abnormal lesions to the health care provider for further examination.

Every nurse should be able to perform a complete examination of the skin and recognize abnormalities. Box 33.9 presents patient education that nurses should communicate while performing an examination of the integumentary system and in discussions about health screening.

> **SAFETY ALERT** Individuals exposed to the sun through sunbathing or artificial means increase their risk for development of skin cancer. Provide appropriate teaching to inform patients of ways to decrease their risk (see Boxes 33.6 and 33.9).

Hair and Scalp

The following types of hair cover the body: *terminal hair* (long, coarse, thick hair easily visible on the scalp, axillae, pubic areas, and in the beard in men) and *vellus hair* (small, soft, tiny hairs covering the whole body except for the palms and soles). Inspection of the condition and distribution of hair and the integrity of the scalp requires good lighting.

Inspection. During inspection, explain to the patient that it is necessary to separate parts of the hair to detect abnormalities. If lesions, infectious disease, or pests are probable, wear clean gloves. Table 33.9 describes the nursing history for assessment of the hair and scalp.

First inspect the colour, distribution, quantity, thickness, texture, and lubrication of body hair. Scalp hair is coarse or fine; curly or straight; and should be shiny, smooth, and pliant. While separating sections of scalp hair, observe characteristics of colour and coarseness. Colour varies from very light blond to black to grey and sometimes shows alterations from rinses or dyes. In older persons, the hair becomes dull grey, white, or yellow. The hair also thins over the scalp, axillae, and pubic areas. Older men often lose facial hair, whereas some older women develop hair on the chin and upper lip.

Be aware of the normal distribution of hair growth in a man and a woman. At puberty, a change in the amount and distribution of hair growth occurs. Some patients with hormone disorders experience an unusual distribution and growth. A woman with hirsutism has hair

BOX 33.8 Skin Malignancies

Basal Cell Carcinoma
0.5- to 1.0-cm crusted lesion that is flat or raised and has a rolled, somewhat scaly border.
Frequently there are underlying, widely dilated blood vessels that appear within the lesion.

Basal cell carcinoma

Squamous Cell Carcinoma
Occurs more often on mucosal surfaces and nonexposed areas of skin, compared with basal cell.
0.5- to 1.5-cm scaly lesion is sometimes ulcerated or crusted. Appears frequently and grows more rapidly than basal cell.

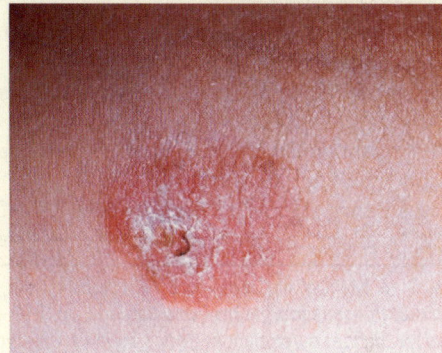

Basal squamous cell carcinoma

Melanoma
0.5- to 1.0-cm brown, flat lesion that appears on sun-exposed or nonexposed skin. Variegated pigmentation, irregular borders, and indistinct marginsUlceration, recent growth, or recent changes in long-standing mole are ominous signs.

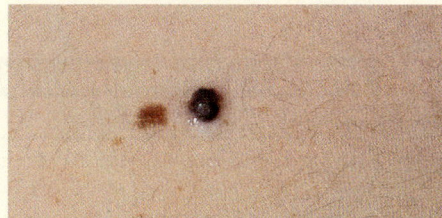

Melanoma

Illustrations from Marks, J., & Miller, J. (Eds.) (2019). *Lookingbill and Mark's principles of dermatology* (6th ed.). Elsevier; *Basal cell:* Fig. 5.14A; *Squamous cell:* Fig. 5.12. *Melanoma:* From Paller, A. S., & Mancini, A. J. (2016). *Hurwitz clinical pediatric dermatology* (5th ed., Fig. 9.18). Elsevier/Saunders.

growth on the upper lip, chin, and cheeks, with vellus hair becoming coarser over the body. For some, a change in hair growth negatively affects body image and emotional well-being.

Some changes occur in the thickness, texture, and lubrication of scalp hair. Disturbances such as a febrile illness or scalp disease sometimes result in hair loss. Conditions such as thyroid disease alter the condition of the hair, making it fine and brittle. Hair loss (**alopecia**) or thinning of the hair is usually related to genetic tendencies and endocrine disorders such as diabetes, thyroiditis, and even menopause. Poor nutrition causes stringy, dull, dry, and thin hair. The oil of sebaceous glands lubricates the hair. Excessively oily hair is associated with androgen hormone stimulation. Dry, brittle hair occurs with aging and with excessive use of chemical agents.

The amount of hair covering the extremities is sometimes reduced as a result of aging. Arterial insufficiency is most common over the lower extremities and results in hair loss.

Inspect the scalp for lesions. The scalp is normally smooth and inelastic, with even coloration. Carefully separating strands of hair, thoroughly examine the scalp for lesions. Note the characteristics of any scalp lesion. If you find lumps or bruises, ask the patient if they have experienced recent head trauma. Moles on the scalp are common. Warn the patient that combing or brushing sometimes causes a mole to bleed. Dandruff or psoriasis frequently causes scaliness or dryness of the scalp.

Careful inspection of hair follicles on the scalp and pubic areas may reveal lice or other parasites. The three types of lice are *Pediculus*

BOX 33.9 EVIDENCE-INFORMED PRACTICE GUIDELINE

Skin Cancer Prevention

Evidence-Informed Guideline Summary

What is cancer? More specifically, what is skin cancer? Cancer is an uncontrolled growth and spread of abnormal cells. Skin cancer is characterized by abnormal skin cells, which can spread and invade other tissues. More importantly, what can we do about skin cancer? As nurses, it becomes our responsibility to assess for and educate patients about all types of skin cancers, especially the most serious form, called *melanoma*. There are several risk factors for melanoma—major factors are positive family history of melanoma, a prior melanoma, and multiple or unusual moles. Other factors include fair complexion or skin that is sensitive to the sun, excessive exposure to the sun (especially before age 18), and the use of tanning beds or booths.

When detected early and treated properly, most forms of skin cancer are highly curable. Therefore, early assessment and intervention are of utmost importance.

Application to Nursing Practice

Nurses have a responsibility to screen for cancer. Promoting and teaching self-screening of skin, hair, and nails to all patients and their caregiver(s) is one way in which nurses can help prevent skin cancer.

- Instruct patients to conduct a complete monthly self-examination of the skin and scalp, noting moles, blemishes, and birthmarks.
  - Perform the examination after a bath or shower, including a head-to-toe check.
  - Use a well-lit room and mirrors to examine all skin surfaces. If necessary, ask a caregiver to aid in the investigation.
  - Remember the warning signs of skin cancer by using the ABCD mnemonic: *A* is for asymmetry—look for uneven shape; *B* is for border

irregularity—look for edges that are blurred, notched, or ragged; *C* is for colour—pigmentation is not uniform; blue, black, brown variegated and areas of pink, white, grey, blue, or red are abnormal; and *D* is for diameter—greater than 6 mm.

- Instruct patients to contact their health care provider if a skin lesion or mole starts to bleed or ooze or feels different (swollen, hard, lumpy, itchy, or tender to the touch). Stress this point to older persons, who tend to have delayed wound healing.
- Inform patients of ways to prevent skin cancer by avoiding overexposure to the sun:
  - Wear wide-brimmed hats and long sleeves.
  - Apply broad-spectrum sunscreens with SPF of 15 or greater to protect against ultraviolet B (UVB) and ultraviolet A (UVA) rays, approximately 15 minutes before going into the sun and after swimming or perspiring.
  - Avoid tanning under the direct sun at midday (11 a.m. to 3 p.m.).
  - Do not use indoor sunlamps, tanning parlours, or tanning lotions.
- Inform patients who are on medications that make the skin more sensitive to the sun (e.g., oral contraceptives, antibiotics, anti-inflammatories, antihypertensives, immunosuppressives) to take extra precautions when spending time in the sun.
- Instruct patients to protect their children from the sun. Severe sunburns in childhood greatly increase melanoma risk later in life.

These interventions will provide the patient with self-screening measures to detect, prevent, and seek early treatment for skin cancer.

Data from Jarvis, C., & MacDonald-Jenkins, J. (2019). Skin, hair, and nails. In C. Jarvis, A. J. Browne, J. MacDonald-Jenkins, et al. (Eds.), *Physical examination and health assessment* (3rd Canadian ed., pp. 219–270). Elsevier Canada; Canadian Cancer Society. (2022). *What is melanoma skin cancer?* https://www.cancer.ca/en/cancer-information/cancer-type/skin-melanoma/melanoma/?region=on; Canadian Cancer Society. (2022). *What is non-melanoma skin cancer?* https://www.cancer.ca/en/cancer-information/cancer-type/skin-non-melanoma/non-melanoma-skin-cancer/?region=on

TABLE 33.9 Nursing History for Hair and Scalp Assessment

Assessment Category	Rationale
Ask patient if they are wearing a wig or hairpiece and, if so, ask them to remove it.	Wigs or hairpieces interfere with inspection of hair and scalp. (Patient sometimes requests to omit this part of examination.)
Determine if patient has noted change in growth or loss of hair; change in texture or colour.	Change often occurs slowly over time.
Identify type of hair care products used for grooming.	Excessive use of chemical agents and burning of hair cause drying and brittleness.
Determine if patient has recently had chemotherapy (medications that cause hair loss) or taken a vasodilator (minoxidil) for hair growth.	Chemotherapeutic medications kill cells that rapidly multiply, such as tumour cells and normal hair cells. Minoxidil causes excessive hair growth.
Has patient noted changes in diet or appetite?	Nutrition influences condition of hair.

humanus capitis (head lice), *Pediculus humanus corporis* (body lice), and *Pediculus pubis* (crab lice). Head and crab lice attach their eggs to hair. The tiny eggs look like oval particles of dandruff. The lice themselves are difficult to see. Head and body lice are very small with greyish white bodies. Crab lice have red legs. Observe for bites or pustular eruptions in the hair follicles and in areas where skin surfaces meet, such as behind the ears and in the groin. The discovery of lice requires immediate treatment (Box 33.10).

Nails

The condition of the nails reflects general health, state of nutrition, a person's occupation, and level of self-care. Nail biting can reveal a person's psychological state. Before assessing the nails, gather a brief

history (Table 33.10). The most visible portion of the nails is the *nail plate*, the transparent layer of epithelial cells covering the nail bed (Figure 33.3). The vascularity of the nail bed creates the nail's underlying colour. The semilunar, whitish area at the base of the nail bed is called the *lunula*, from which the nail plate develops.

Inspection and Palpation. Inspect the nail bed for colour, cleanliness, and length; the thickness and shape of the nail; the texture of the nail; the angle between the nail and the nail bed; and the condition of the lateral and proximal nail folds around the nail. Also palpate the nail base. Inspecting the nails can give the examiner a quick sense about the patient's hygiene practices. The nails are normally transparent, smooth, well rounded, and convex, with a nail bed angle of about 160 degrees.

BOX 33.10 PATIENT TEACHING

Hair and Scalp Assessment

Objective
- Patient and/or caregiver will perform proper hygiene practices for care of the hair and scalp.

Teaching Strategies
- Teach patient and caregiver(s) about basic hygiene practices for care of the hair and scalp (see Chapter 39).
- Inform patient and caregiver(s) about signs and symptoms of lice and how to check for infestations. Dispel myths regarding lice, emphasizing that they are a common occurrence in school-aged children and are not associated with poor hygiene.
- Discuss treatment options for lice. Currently in Canada, there are three different types of pharmacotherapy available for lice: topical insecticides (pyrethrins, permethrins), noninsecticidal agents (isopropyl myristate/ST-cyclomethicone [Resultz], dimethicone solution [NYDA], benzyl alcohol lotion [Ulesfia lotion]), and oral medications (ivermectin). Both topical insecticides and noninsecticides can be purchased over the counter at drug stores and are the preferred treatment options. There is little evidence to support the efficacy of oral medications for head lice treatment, and they require a written prescription.
  - Pyrethrins and permethrins are approved for children 2 months of age and older with confirmed head lice.
  - Demethicone solution is approved for use in children 2 years of age and older.
  - Myristate/ST-cyclomethicone is approved for use in children 4 years of age and older.
  - Benzyl alcohol lotion is approved for use in children 6 months of age and older and is more expensive than other medications.
  - Because of its neurotoxic effects, lindane is no longer recommended for treatment of lice.
  - Household products such as petroleum jelly, oil, mayonnaise, and tea tree oil are NOT recommended for treating lice as their efficacy of killing lice is low or not proven.
- Upon selection of a pharmacological treatment option, instruct patient and caregiver(s) to follow the directions on the product box, as treatment methods vary by product type. A second treatment 7–10 days after initial treatment is recommended for all cases where a live infestation is found (i.e., live lice).
- Inform patient and caregiver(s) that pediculicides can cause scalp itching, rash, and mild burning sensation. This does not indicate reinfestation; reinfestation must be diagnosed by presence of live lice or eggs.
- There is little evidence to support the added benefit of wet combing (removing lice by combing wet hair with a fine-tooth comb) after application of lice products. However, some patients may choose to do wet combing as a precautionary measure, to remove detectable nits and eggs.
- Inform patient and caregiver(s) that lice and nits do not live long away from the skin. Therefore, thorough environmental cleaning and disinfecting after a household infestation may not be necessary. However, items that have been in close contact with the head or body hair of an infested individual should be decontaminated to prevent reinfestation and transmission. Such items can be decontaminated by:
  - Washing items in hot water (≥66°C) and drying them in a hot dryer for 15 minutes.
  - Dry-cleaning, or sealing nonwashable items in a plastic bag for 14 days.
  - Soaking combs, brushes, and hair accessories in lice-killing products for 1 hour or in boiling water for 10 minutes.
- Instruct patient and caregiver(s) about ways to reduce transmission of lice:
  - Do not share personal-care items with others (e.g., brushes, hats, hair bands).
  - Use thorough hand hygiene practices.
  - If lice were sexually transmitted, the patient needs to notify their partner.
  - Avoid close physical contact with infested individuals, especially head-to-head or skin-to-skin contact.
  - Generally, there is no medical rationale to exclude individuals with lice from school, day care, or work. Rather, the Canadian Paediatric Society recommends a full course of treatment and avoiding close head-to-head activities.

Evaluation
- Have patient or parents describe methods used to care for the hair and scalp.
- Have patient or parents explain the steps to take to reduce lice transmission in the home.
- Have patient or parents explain the steps to treat lice infestations in the home.

Data from Canadian Pediatric Society. (2016). *Head lice*. Caring for Kids. https://www.caringforkids.cps.ca/handouts/health-conditions-and-treatments/head_lice; Cummings, C., Finlay, J. C., MacDonald, N. E., & the Canadian Paediatric Society Community Paediatrics Committee. (2018). *Head lice infestations: A clinical update*. https://www.cps.ca/en/documents/position/head-lice

TABLE 33.10 Nursing History for Nail Assessment

Assessment Category	Rationale
Ask if patient has experienced recent trauma or changes in nails (splitting, breaking, discoloration, thickening).	Trauma changes shape and growth of nail. Systemic conditions cause changes in colour, growth, and shape.
Has the patient had other symptoms of pain, swelling, presence of systemic disease with fever, or psychological or physical stress?	Alterations sometimes occur slowly over time.
Question patient's nail care practices. Determine if patient has acrylic nails or silk wraps.	Helps to determine if change in nails is due to a local or systemic problem. Acrylic nails and silk wraps are areas for fungal growth.
	Chemical agents cause drying of nails. Improper care damages nails and cuticles.
Determine if patient has risks for nail or foot conditions (e.g., diabetes, peripheral vascular disease, obesity).	Vascular changes associated with diabetes and peripheral vascular disease reduce blood flow to peripheral tissues; foot lesions and thickened nails are common. Some older persons have trouble performing foot and nail care because of poor vision, incoordination, or inability to bend over. Patients with obesity have difficulty bending over.

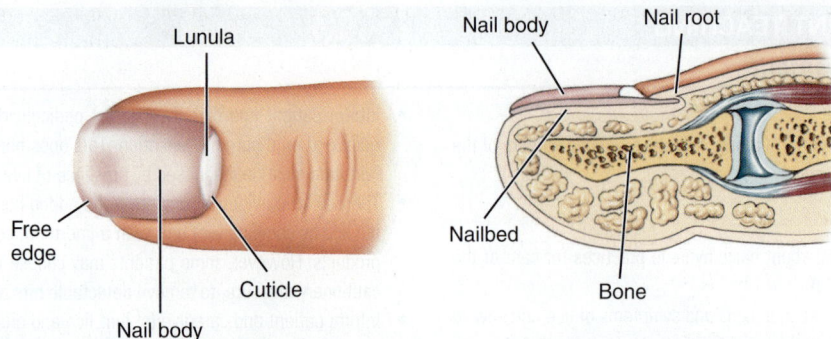

FIGURE 33.3 Components of the nail unit. (From Herlihy, B. [2018]. *The human body in health and illness* [6th ed., Figure 7.3]. Elsevier.)

The surrounding cuticles are smooth, intact, and without inflammation. If the nails are ragged, dirty, and poorly kept, this is a good indication that either the patient practises infrequent nail care or is physically unable to perform care. However, consider the patient's profession, because some individuals have dirty nails as part of their employment (e.g., gardeners, mechanics, coal miners, and farmers) despite excellent nail care. Jagged, bitten, or broken nail edges or cuticles predispose a patient to localized infection. Report any abnormalities such as erythema or swelling.

> **SAFETY ALERT** Patients with impaired circulation are at greater risk for localized infection. It is important to observe the condition of hand and foot nails and nail beds to identify risks for and early signs of infection.

In light-skinned individuals, nail beds are pink with translucent white tips. In dark-skinned patients, nail beds are darkly pigmented with a blue or reddish hue. A brown or black pigmentation is normal with longitudinal streaks. Trauma, cirrhosis, diabetes mellitus, and hypertension cause splinter hemorrhages. Vitamin, protein, and electrolyte changes cause various lines or bands to form on the nail beds.

Nails normally grow at a constant rate, but direct injury or generalized disease impairs growth. With aging, the nails of the fingers and toes become harder and thicker. Longitudinal striations develop, and the rate of nail growth slows. Nails become more brittle, dull, and opaque and turn yellow in older persons because of insufficient calcium. Also with age, the cuticle becomes less thick and wide.

Inspection of the angle between the nail and nail bed normally reveals an angle of 160 degrees (Box 33.11). A larger angle and softening of the nail bed indicate chronic oxygenation problems. Palpate the nail base to determine firmness and the condition of circulation. The nail base is normally firm.

To palpate, gently grasp the patient's finger and observe the colour of the nail bed. Next, apply gentle, firm, quick pressure with the thumb to the nail bed and release and observe capillary refill. As pressure is applied, the nail bed will appear white or blanched; however, the pink colour should return immediately on release of pressure. Capillary refill is measured in seconds; less than 2 seconds is brisk, while greater than 4 seconds is sluggish. Failure of the pinkness to return promptly indicates circulatory insufficiency. An ongoing bluish or purplish cast to the nail bed occurs with cyanosis. A white cast or pallor results from anemia.

Calluses and corns are commonly found on the toes or fingers. A callus is flat and painless, resulting from a thickening of the epidermis. Friction and pressure from shoes cause corns, usually over bony prominences. During the examination, the patient should be instructed in proper nail care (Box 33.12).

BOX 33.11 Abnormalities of the Nail Bed

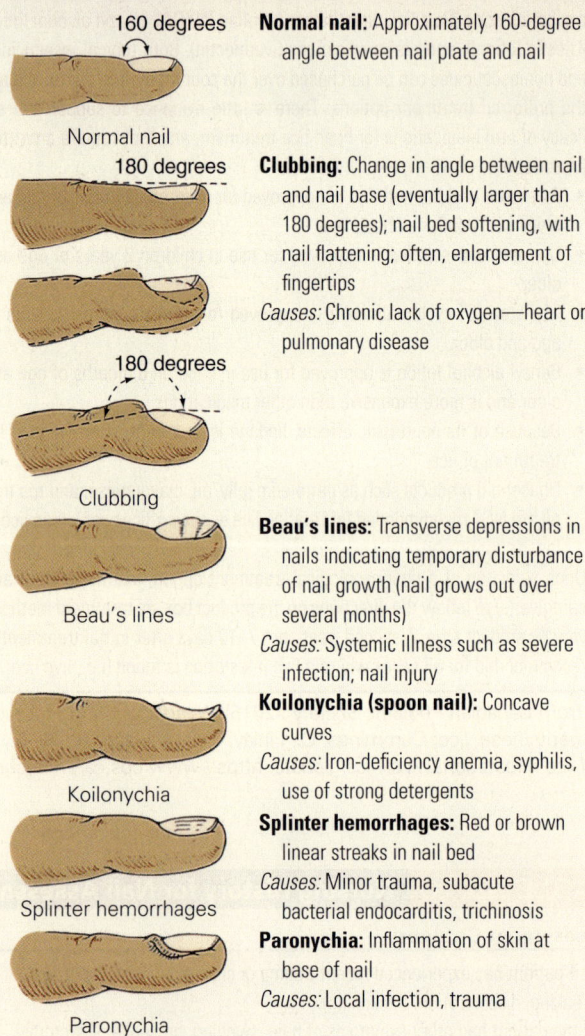

Normal nail: Approximately 160-degree angle between nail plate and nail

Clubbing: Change in angle between nail and nail base (eventually larger than 180 degrees); nail bed softening, with nail flattening; often, enlargement of fingertips
Causes: Chronic lack of oxygen—heart or pulmonary disease

Beau's lines: Transverse depressions in nails indicating temporary disturbance of nail growth (nail grows out over several months)
Causes: Systemic illness such as severe infection; nail injury

Koilonychia (spoon nail): Concave curves
Causes: Iron-deficiency anemia, syphilis, use of strong detergents

Splinter hemorrhages: Red or brown linear streaks in nail bed
Causes: Minor trauma, subacute bacterial endocarditis, trichinosis

Paronychia: Inflammation of skin at base of nail
Causes: Local infection, trauma

HEAD AND NECK

An examination of the head and neck includes assessment of the head, eyes, ears, nose, mouth, pharynx, and neck (lymph nodes, carotid arteries, thyroid gland, and trachea). This assessment is commonly referred to in clinical documentation under *EENT* (eyes, ears, nose, and throat) and includes all of the associated physical structures (e.g., peripheral arteries and carotid arteries). Assessment of the head and neck requires inspection, palpation, and auscultation, with inspection and palpation often done simultaneously.

Head

Inspection and Palpation. The nursing history involves screening for intracranial injury and local or congenital deformities (Table 33.11). This starts with inspecting the patient's head, noting the position, size, shape, and contour. The head is normally held upright and midline to the trunk. The patient holding the head tilted to one side can be an indication of unilateral hearing, visual loss, or musculoskeletal concern. A horizontal jerking or bobbing indicates a tremor or tic.

Note the patient's facial features, looking at the eyelids, eyebrows, nasolabial folds, and mouth for shape and symmetry. It is normal for slight asymmetry to exist. If there is facial asymmetry, note if all features on one side of the face are affected or if only a portion of the face is involved. Various neurological disorders (e.g., facial nerve paralysis) affect different nerves that innervate muscles of the face.

Examine the size, shape, and contour of the skull. The skull is generally round with prominences in the frontal area anteriorly and the occipital area posteriorly. Trauma typically causes local skull deformities. In infants, a large head results from a congenital anomaly or the buildup of cerebrospinal fluid in the ventricles (**hydrocephalus**). Some adults have enlarged jaws and facial bones resulting from **acromegaly**, a disorder caused by excessive secretion of growth hormone. Palpate the skull for nodules or masses. Gently rotate the fingertips down the midline of the scalp and then along the sides of the head to identify abnormalities. Then palpate the temporomandibular joint (TMJ) space bilaterally. Place the fingertips just anterior to the tragus of each ear. The fingertips should slip into the joint space as the patient's mouth opens, to gently palpate the joint spaces. Normally, the movements should be smooth, although it is not unusual to hear or feel a clicking or snapping in the TMJ (Jarvis et al., 2019, pp. 642–643).

Eyes

Examination of the eyes includes inspection of external and internal eye structures and extraocular movement and the assessment of visual acuity and visual fields. Figure 33.4 shows a cross-section of the eye. Through assessment, visual alterations are detected, and the level of assistance that patients require when ambulating or performing self-care activities is determined. Some patients with visual difficulties also need special aids for reading educational materials or instructions (e.g., medication labels). Table 33.12 outlines the nursing history for an eye examination. Box 33.13 describes common types of visual conditions.

BOX 33.12 PATIENT TEACHING

Nail Assessment

Objective
- Patient properly cares for fingernails, feet, and toenails.

Teaching Strategies
- Instruct patient to cut nails only after soaking them about 10 minutes in warm water. (Exception: Diabetic patients are warned against soaking nails because this dries the hands and feet out; dry skin leads to infection.)
- Tell the patient to cut nails straight across and even with the tops of the fingers or toes. If patient has diabetes, tell patient to file rather than cut the nails (see Chapter 39).
- Instruct patient to shape nails with a file or emery board.
- If *patient is diabetic:*
  - Wash feet daily in warm water, and carefully dry them, especially between the toes. Inspect feet each day in good lighting, looking for dry places and cracks in the skin. Soften dry feet by applying a cream or lotion.
  - Do not put lotion between the toes; moisture between the toes allows microorganisms to grow, leading to infections.
  - Caution patient against using sharp objects to poke or dig under the toenail or around the cuticle.
  - Have patient see a podiatrist for treatment of ingrown toenails and nails that are thick or tend to split.

Evaluation
- Inspect nails during subsequent patient interactions.
- Have patient explain steps to take to avoid injury.

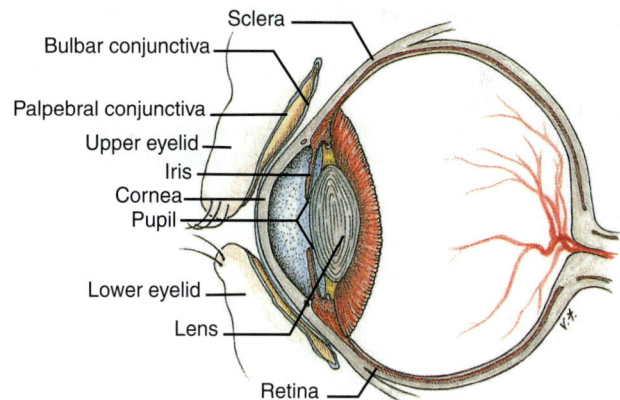

FIGURE 33.4 Cross-section of the eye.

TABLE 33.11 Nursing History for Head Assessment

Assessment Category	Rationale
Determine if patient has experienced recent head trauma. If so, assess state of consciousness after injury (immediately on return and 5 minutes later), duration of unconsciousness, and predisposing factors (e.g., seizure, poor vision, blackout).	Trauma is a major cause of lumps, bumps, cuts, bruises, or deformities of scalp or skull. Loss of consciousness after head injury indicates possible brain injury.
Ask if patient has history of headache; note onset, duration, character, pattern, and associated symptoms.	Character of headache helps in determining causative factors, such as sinus infection, migraine, or neurological disorders.
Determine length of time patient has experienced neurological symptoms.	Duration of signs or symptoms indicates severity of problem.
Review patient's occupational history for use of safety helmets.	Nature of some occupations creates a risk for head injury.
Ask if patient participates in contact sports or higher-risk recreational activities (e.g., motor cross, skiing).	These activities require use of safety helmets.

TABLE 33.12	Nursing History for Eye Assessment
Assessment Category	**Rationale**
Determine if patient has history of eye disease, (e.g., glaucoma, retinopathy, cataracts), eye trauma, diabetes, hypertension, or eye surgery.	Some diseases or trauma cause risk for partial or complete visual loss. Patient may have had surgery for a visual disorder.
Determine symptoms that prompted patient to seek health care. Ask patient about eye pain, photophobia (sensitivity to light), burning or itching, excess tearing or crusting, diplopia (double vision) or blurred vision, awareness of a "film" or "curtain" over field of vision, floaters (small, black spots that seem to float across field of vision), flashing lights, or halos around lights.	Common symptoms of eye disease indicate need for a health care provider.
Determine whether there is family history of eye disorders or diseases.	Certain eye conditions such as glaucoma or retinitis pigmentosa are inherited.
Review patient's occupational history and recreational hobbies; are safety glasses worn?	Performance of close, intricate work causes eye fatigue. Working with computers causes eye strain. Certain occupational tasks (e.g., working with chemicals) and recreational activities (e.g., fencing, motorcycle riding) place people at risk for eye injury unless patients take precautions.
Ask patient if they wear glasses or contacts and if so, how often.	Patients need to wear glasses or contacts during certain portions of the examination for accurate assessment.
Determine when patient last visited an ophthalmologist or optometrist.	Date of last eye examination indicates level of preventive care patient takes.
Assess medications patient is taking, including eye drops or ointment.	Determines need to assess patient's knowledge of medications. Certain medications cause visual symptoms.

BOX 33.13	Common Eye and Visual Conditions

Hyperopia

Hyperopia is farsightedness, a refractive error in which rays of light enter the eye and focus behind the retina. Individuals are able to clearly see distant objects but not close objects.

Myopia

Myopia is nearsightedness, a refractive error in which rays of light enter the eye and focus in front of the retina. Individuals are able to clearly see close objects but not distant objects.

Presbyopia

Presbyopia is impaired near vision in middle-aged and older persons, caused by loss of elasticity of the lens and associated with the aging process.

Retinopathy

Retinopathy is a noninflammatory eye disorder resulting from changes in retinal blood vessels. It is a leading cause of blindness.

Strabismus

Strabismus is a congenital condition in which both eyes do not focus on an object simultaneously; these eyes appear crossed. Impairment of the extraocular muscles or their nerve supply causes strabismus.

Amblyopia

Amblyopia is a congenital condition, commonly referred to as a "lazy eye," which occurs when the nerve pathway in one eye does not develop in early childhood.

This weakness to one eye can result in blurred vision, distortion of depth perception, or progressive vision loss to the affected eye. Early screening and referral of children for amblyopia and strabismus is important to correct and preserve vision.

Cataracts

A cataract is an increased opacity of the lens, which blocks light rays from entering the eye. Cataracts sometimes develop slowly and progressively after age 35 or suddenly after trauma. Cataracts are one of the most common eye disorders. Most older persons (age 65 years and older) have some evidence of visual impairment from cataracts. Protection of the eyes from the sun's rays and trauma through the use of sunglasses and protective eyewear when there is an occupational or recreational risk for eye injury is an important factor in the prevention of cataracts.

Glaucoma

Glaucoma is intraocular structural damage resulting from elevated intraocular pressure. Obstruction of the outflow of aqueous humor causes this. Without treatment, the disorder will lead to blindness.

Macular Degeneration

Macular degeneration is blurred central vision often occurring suddenly, caused by a progressive degeneration of the centre of the retina. It is the most common visual impairment of individuals over age 50 and the most common cause of blindness in older persons. There is no cure.

External Eye Structures. To inspect external eye structures, stand directly in front of the patient at eye level and ask the patient to look at your face.

Position and Alignment. Assess the position of the eyes in relation to one another. Normally, they are parallel to each other. Bulging eyes (exophthalmos) usually indicate hyperthyroidism. The crossing of eyes (strabismus) results from neuromuscular injury or inherited abnormalities. Tumours or inflammation of the orbit often cause abnormal eye protrusion.

For the remainder of the eye examination, have the patient remove their glasses or contact lenses.

Eyebrows. Inspect the eyebrows for size, extension, texture of hair, alignment, and movement. Normally, the eyebrows are symmetrical. Coarseness of hair and failure to extend beyond the temporal canthus possibly reveals hypothyroidism. If the brows are thinned, this may be a result of waxing or plucking. Aging causes loss of the lateral third of the eyebrows. Have the patient raise and lower the eyebrows. The brows normally raise and lower symmetrically. An inability to move the eyebrows indicates a facial nerve paralysis (cranial nerve VII).

Eyelids. Inspect the eyelids for position, colour, condition of the surface, condition and direction of the eyelashes, and the patient's ability to open and close their eyes and blink. When the eyes are open in a normal position, the lids do not cover the pupil and the sclera cannot be seen above the iris. The lids are also close to the eyeball. An abnormal drooping of the lid over the pupil is called **ptosis** (pronounced "toe-sis"), caused by edema or impairment of the third cranial nerve. In the older person, ptosis results from a loss of elasticity that accompanies aging. Observe for defects in the position of the lid margins. An older person frequently has lid margins that turn out (**ectropion**) or in (**entropion**). An entropion sometimes leads to the lashes of the lid irritating the conjunctiva and cornea, increasing the risk of infection. The eyelashes are normally distributed evenly and curved outward away from the eye. An erythematous or yellow lump (hordeolum or stye) on the follicle of an eyelash indicates an acute suppurative inflammation.

To inspect the surface of the upper lids, ask the patient to close their eyes. Then raise both eyebrows gently with the thumb and index finger to stretch the skin. The lids are normally smooth and the same colour as the skin. Redness indicates inflammation or infection. Lid edema is sometimes due to allergies or to heart or kidney failure. Edema of the eyelids prevents them from closing. Inspect lesions for typical characteristics and discomfort or drainage. Wear clean gloves if drainage is present.

The lids normally close symmetrically. Failure of the lids to close exposes the cornea to drying. This condition is common in unconscious patients or in those with facial nerve paralysis. Ask the patient to open the eyes for inspection of the lower lids. Assess the same characteristics noted for the upper lids. Normally, a patient blinks involuntarily and bilaterally up to 20 times a minute. The blink reflex lubricates the cornea. Report absent or infrequent, rapid, or monocular (one-eyed) blinking.

Lacrimal Apparatus. The lacrimal gland (Figure 33.5), located in the upper outer wall of the anterior part of the orbit, is responsible for tear production. Tears flow from the gland across the eye's surface to the lacrimal duct, which is in the nasal corner or inner canthus of the eye. The lacrimal gland is sometimes the site of tumours or infections. Inspect this area for edema and redness. Palpate the gland gently to detect tenderness. Normally the gland cannot be felt.

The nasolacrimal duct sometimes becomes obstructed, blocking the flow of tears. Observe for evidence of edema in the inner canthus. Gentle palpation of the duct at the lower eyelid just inside the lower orbital rim causes a regurgitation of tears.

Conjunctivae and Sclerae. The bulbar conjunctiva covers the exposed surface of the eyeball up to the outer edge of the cornea. Observe the sclera under the bulbar conjunctiva; it normally has the colour of white porcelain in White patients and light yellow in dark-skinned patients. Sclerae become pigmented and appear either yellow or green if liver disease is present.

Take care when inspecting the conjunctivae. For adequate exposure of the bulbar conjunctiva, retract the eyelids without placing pressure directly on the eyeball. Gently retract both lids, with the thumb and index finger pressed against the lower and upper bony orbits. Ask the patient to look up, down, and from side to side. Many patients begin to blink, making the examination difficult. Inspect for colour, texture, and the presence of edema or lesions. Normally, the conjunctivae are free of erythema. The presence of redness indicates an allergic or infectious **conjunctivitis**. Bright red blood in a localized area surrounded by normal-appearing conjunctiva usually indicates subconjunctival hemorrhage. Conjunctivitis is a highly contagious infection. It is easy to spread the crusty drainage that collects on eyelid margins from one eye to the other. Wear clean gloves during the examination. Performing proper hand hygiene is necessary before and after the examination.

Corneas. The cornea is the transparent, colourless portion of the eye covering the pupil and iris. While the patient looks straight ahead, inspect the cornea for clarity and texture while shining a penlight

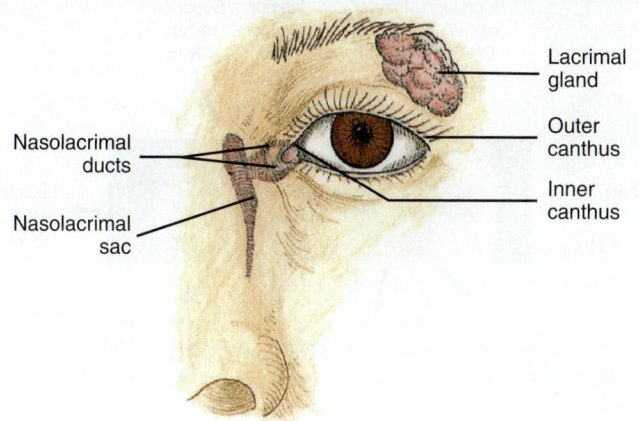

FIGURE 33.5 The lacrimal apparatus secretes and drains tears, which moisten and lubricate eye structures.

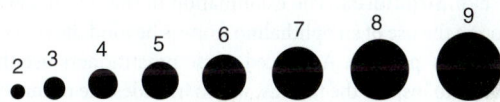

FIGURE 33.6 Chart depicting pupillary size in millimetres.

obliquely across the cornea's entire surface. The cornea is normally shiny, transparent, and smooth. As a result of aging, the cornea loses its lustre. Any irregularity in the surface indicates an abrasion or tear that requires further examination by a health care provider. Both conditions are very painful. Note the colour and details of the underlying iris. The iris becomes faded in an older person. A thin white ring along the margin of the iris, called an **arcus senilis**, is common with aging but is abnormal in anyone under age 40. To test for the corneal blink reflex, see the cranial nerve test section of this chapter.

Pupils and Irises. Observe the pupils for size, shape, equality, accommodation, and reaction to light. The pupils are normally black, round, regular, and equal in size (3 to 7 mm in diameter) (Figure 33.6). The iris should be clearly visible.

Cloudy pupils indicate cataracts. Dilated pupils result from glaucoma, trauma, neurological disorders, eye medications (e.g., atropine), or withdrawal from opioids. Inflammation of the iris or use of medications (e.g., pilocarpine, morphine, or cocaine) causes constricted pupils. Pinpoint pupils are a common sign of opioid intoxication. Shining a beam of light through the pupil and onto the retina stimulates the third cranial nerve and causes the muscles of the iris to constrict. Any abnormality along the nerve pathways from the retina to the iris alters the ability of the pupils to react to light. Changes in intracranial pressure, lesions along the nerve pathways, locally applied ophthalmic medications, and direct trauma to the eye alter pupillary reaction.

Test pupillary reflexes (to light and accommodation) in a dimly lit room. While the patient looks straight ahead, bring a penlight from the side of the patient's face, directing the light onto the pupil. If the patient looks at the light, there will be a false reaction to accommodation. A directly illuminated pupil constricts, and the opposite pupil constricts consensually. Observe the quickness and equality of the reflex. Repeat the examination for the opposite eye.

To test for accommodation, ask the patient to gaze at a distant object (the far wall) and then at a test object (finger or pencil) held approximately 10 cm from the bridge of the patient's nose. The pupils normally converge and accommodate by constricting when looking at close objects. The pupillary responses should be equal. If assessment of pupillary reaction is normal in all tests, record the abbreviation **PERRLA** (**p**upils **e**qual, **r**ound, **r**eactive to **l**ight, and **a**ccommodation).

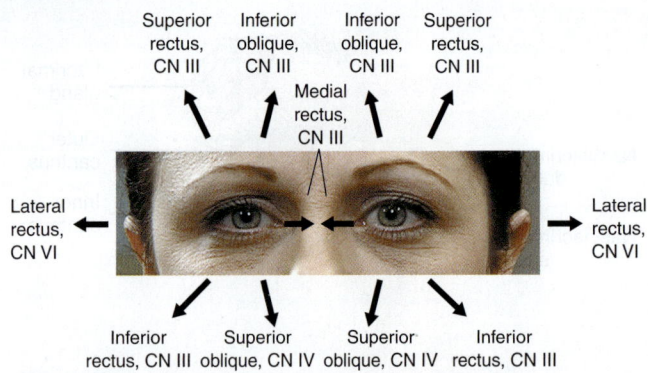

FIGURE 33.7 Six directions of gaze. Direct the patient to follow finger movement through each gaze. *CN,* cranial nerve. (From Ball, J. W., Dains, J. E., Flynn, J. A., et al. [2019]. *Seidel's guide to physical examination* [9th ed.]. Mosby.)

Internal Eye Structures. The examination of the internal eye structures through the use of an ophthalmoscope is beyond the scope of new graduate nurses' practice. Advanced nurse practitioners use the **ophthalmoscope** to inspect the fundus, which includes the retina, choroid, optic nerve disc, macula, fovea centralis, and retinal vessels. Patients in greatest need of an examination are those with diabetes, hypertension, and intracranial disorders.

Extraocular Movements. Six small muscles guide the movement of each eye. Both eyes move parallel to each other in each of the six directions of gaze (Figure 33.7). To assess extraocular movements, have the patient sit or stand 60 cm away, facing you. Hold a finger at a comfortable distance (15 to 30 cm) from the patient's eyes. Have the patient maintain their head in a fixed position facing forward and follow the movement of the finger with their eyes only. Have the patient look to the right, to the left, and diagonally up and down to the left and right. The finger moves smoothly and slowly within the normal field of vision.

As the patient gazes in each direction, observe for parallel eye movement, the position of the upper eyelid in relation to the iris, and the presence of abnormal movements. As the eyes move through each direction of gaze, the upper eyelid covers the iris only slightly. **Nystagmus,** an involuntary, rhythmical oscillation of the eyes, is assessed by periodically stopping movement of the finger. To initiate nystagmus in patients with normal eye movements, have them gaze to the far left or right. Disturbances in eye movement reflect local injury to eye muscles and supporting structures or a disorder of the cranial nerves innervating the muscles.

Visual Fields. As a person looks straight ahead, they are normally able to see all objects in the periphery. To assess visual fields, have the patient stand or sit 60 cm away, facing you at eye level. The patient gently closes or covers one eye (e.g., the left) and looks at your eye directly opposite. Close the opposite eye (in this case, the right) so that the field of vision is superimposed on that of the patient. Move a finger equidistant from you and the patient outside the field of vision, then slowly bring it back into the visual field. Ask the patient to tell when they are able to see the finger. If you see the finger before the patient does, a portion of the patient's visual field is reduced. To test temporal field vision, the object should be slightly behind the patient. (Note: The nurse can see the finger.) Repeat the procedure for each field of vision for the other eye.

SAFETY ALERT Some patients with visual field restrictions are at risk for injury because they cannot see all the objects in front of them. Older persons commonly have loss of peripheral vision caused by changes in the shape of the lens.

Visual Acuity. The assessment of *visual acuity,* the ability to see small details, involves testing central vision. The easiest way to assess near vision is to ask patients to read printed material under adequate lighting. If patients wear glasses or contact lenses, they should wear them during assessment. It is important to determine the language the patient speaks and reading ability. Asking patients to read aloud will help determine literacy. If the patient has difficulty reading, move to the next step.

Assessment of distance vision requires use of a Snellen chart (paper chart or projection screen). The chart should be well lit. Vision without corrective lenses is tested first. Have the patient sit or stand 6.1 m (20 feet) away from the chart and try to read all the letters beginning at any line with both eyes open. Then have the patient read the line with each eye separately (the patient covers the opposite eye with an index card or eye cover). The patient should avoid applying pressure to the eye. Note the smallest line in which the patient is able to read all the letters correctly and record the visual acuity for that line. Repeat the test with the patient wearing corrective lenses. Complete the test rapidly enough so that the patient does not memorize the chart (Jarvis et al., 2019).

If a patient is unable to read, use an *E* chart or one with pictures of familiar objects. Instead of reading letters, patients tell which direction each *E* is pointing or the name of the object. The visual acuity score for each eye and for both eyes is then recorded.

The Snellen chart has standardized numbers at the end of each line of the chart. The numerator is the number 20, or the distance the patient stands from the chart. The denominator is the distance from which the normal eye is able to read the chart. Normal vision is 20/20. The larger the denominator, the poorer the patient's visual acuity. For example, a value of 20/40 means that the patient, standing 6.1 m (20 feet) away, can read a line that a person with normal vision can read from 40 feet away. Visual acuity is recorded as O.D. (right eye) and O.S. (left eye) as well as *sc* (without correction) or *cc* (with correction), depending on whether the patient wears glasses or contact lenses.

If patients cannot read even the largest letters or figures of a Snellen chart, test their ability to count upraised fingers or to distinguish light. Hold a hand 30 cm from the patient's face, and have the patient count the upraised fingers. To check light perception, shine a penlight into the eye and then turn the light off. If the patient notes when the light is turned on or off, light perception is intact.

Near vision is assessed by asking the patient to read a hand-held card containing a vision screening chart. Instruct the patient to hold the card a comfortable distance (5 to 6 cm) from the eyes and read the smallest line possible. This portion of the examination is a good time to discuss the need for routine eye examinations (Box 33.14).

Ears

The three parts of the ear are the external, middle, and inner ear (Figure 33.8). Assessment involves inspecting and palpating external ear structures, inspecting middle ear structures with an otoscope, and testing the inner ear by measuring the patient's hearing acuity. External ear structures consist of the auricle, outer ear canal, and tympanic membrane (eardrum). The ear canal is normally curved and approximately 2.5 cm long in an adult. It is lined with skin containing fine hairs, nerve endings, and glands secreting cerumen. The middle ear is an air-filled cavity containing the three bony ossicles (malleus, incus, and stapes). The eustachian tube connects the middle ear to the nasopharynx. Pressure between the outer atmosphere and the middle ear is stabilized through the eustachian tube. The inner ear contains the cochlea, vestibule, and semicircular canals.

Assessment of the ears helps in determining the integrity of ear structures and the condition of hearing (Box 33.15). Nursing history data (Table 33.13) aid in identifying risks for hearing disorders.

BOX 33.14 PATIENT TEACHING

Eye Assessment

Objectives

- Patient follows recommendations for regular eye examinations.
- Patient recognizes warning signs and symptoms of eye disease.
- Patient takes appropriate safety precautions for visual deficits.

Teaching Strategies

- Inform adult patients that people between ages 19 and 49 need to have a complete eye examination every 2–5 years (or more often if family history reveals risk factors, such as diabetes or hypertension, for eye disorders).
- Inform adult patients that people between ages 50 and 64 need to have an eye examination every 2–3 years, and people over 65 years of age need to have an eye exam annually, to screen for conditions that may develop without symptoms (e.g., glaucoma).
- Inform patient that people with diabetes should have an eye exam every 1–2 years because of increased risk of retinopathy.
- Describe the typical symptoms of eye disease (see Box 33.13).
- Instruct older persons to take the following precautions because of normal visual changes:
  - Avoid or use caution while driving at night.
  - Increase lighting in the home to reduce risk of falls.
  - Paint the first and last steps of a staircase and the edge of each step in between a bright colour to aid depth perception.

Evaluation

- Ask patient or caregiver(s) to report on patient's most recent visit to an ophthalmologist or optometrist.
- Have patient describe when to have an eye examination.
- Ask patient to describe common symptoms of eye disease.
- Observe the home environment of a patient with visual deficits.

Based on Canadian Ophthalmological Society. (2021). *When should you see and ophthalmologist?* https://www.cos-sco.ca/when-should-you-see-an-ophthalmologist/; Diabetes Canada Clinical Practice Guidelines Expert Committee. (2018). Diabetes Canada 2018 clinical practice guidelines for the prevention and management of diabetes in Canada. *Canadian Journal of Diabetes, 42*(Supp 1), S1–S325. http://guidelines.diabetes.ca/cpg

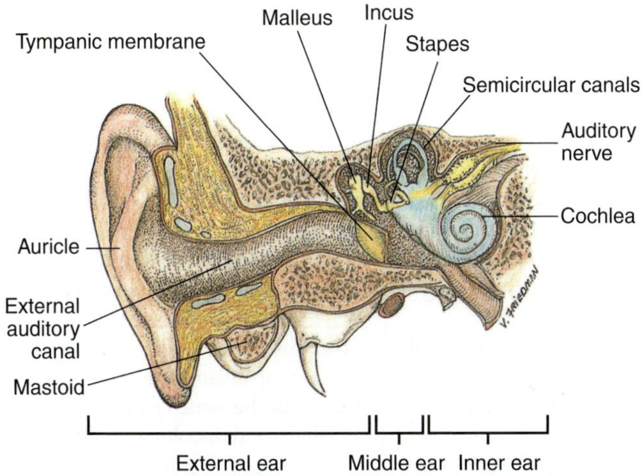

BOX 33.15 PATIENT TEACHING

Ear Assessment

Objectives

- Patient uses proper technique for cleaning the ears.
- Patient follows preventive guidelines for screening of hearing loss.
- Patient with hearing loss communicates effectively.

Teaching Strategies

- Instruct patient in the proper way to clean the outer ear (see Chapter 39), avoiding use of cotton-tipped applicators and sharp objects such as hairpins, which cause impaction of cerumen deep in the ear canal or cause trauma.
- Tell patient to avoid inserting pointed objects into the ear canal.
- Encourage patients over age 65 to have regular hearing checks. Explain that a reduction in hearing is a normal part of aging (see Chapter 25).
- Instruct caregiver(s) of patients with hearing loss to avoid shouting and instead speak in low tones, and to be sure the patient is able to see the speaker's face.

Evaluation

- Ask patient to explain the proper technique for cleaning the ears.
- In a follow-up visit, question patient about frequency of hearing checks.
- Observe patient with hearing loss interacting with caregiver(s).

Understanding the mechanisms for sound transmission helps in identifying the nature of hearing disorders. Sound travels through the ear by air and bone conduction; the following explains the steps of hearing:

1. Sound waves in the air enter the external ear, passing through the outer ear canal.
2. The sound waves reach the tympanic membrane, causing it to vibrate.
3. Vibrations are transmitted through the middle ear by the bony ossicular chain to the oval window at the opening of the inner ear.
4. The cochlea receives the sound vibration.
5. Nerve impulses from the cochlea travel to the auditory (eighth cranial) nerve and to the cerebral cortex.

Disorders of the ear result from several types of problems, including mechanical dysfunction (blockage by earwax or foreign body), trauma (foreign bodies or noise exposure), neurological disorders (auditory nerve damage), acute illnesses (viral infection), and toxic effects of medications.

Auricles. With the patient sitting comfortably, inspect the auricle's size, shape, symmetry, landmarks, position, and colour. The auricles are normally of equal size and level with each other. The upper point of attachment is in a straight line with the lateral canthus, or corner of the eye. The position of the auricle is almost vertical. Ears that are low-set or at an unusual angle are a sign of chromosome abnormality (e.g., Down syndrome) or may indicate the possibility of fetal alcohol affects or syndrome. Ear colour is usually the same as that of the face, without moles, cysts, deformities, or nodules. Redness is a sign of inflammation or fever. Extreme pallor indicates frostbite. Deformities of the ear can be a sign that there may be other organ abnormalities that occurred during fetal development (e.g., kidney).

Palpate the auricles for texture, tenderness, and skin lesions. Auricles are normally smooth and without lesions. If the patient reports pain, gently pull the auricle, press on the tragus, and palpate behind the ear over the mastoid process. If palpating the external ear increases the pain, an external ear infection is likely. If palpation of the auricle and

FIGURE 33.8 Structures of the external, middle, and inner ear.

TABLE 33.13	Nursing History for Ear Assessment
Assessment Category	**Rationale**
Ask if patient has experienced ear pain, itching, discharge, vertigo, tinnitus (ringing in ears), or change in hearing.	These signs and symptoms indicate infection or hearing loss.
Assess risks for hearing impairment.	Risk factors predispose patient to permanent hearing loss.
Infants/children: Hypoxia at birth, meningitis, birth weight less than 1500 g, family history of hearing loss, congenital anomalies of skull or face, nonbacterial intrauterine infections (rubella, herpes), maternal drug use, excessively high bilirubin, head trauma	It is difficult to assess an infant's hearing status with examination only.
Adults: Exposure to industrial or recreational noise, genetic disease (Meniere disease), neurodegenerative disorder	
Determine patient's exposure to loud noises at work and availability of protective devices.	Prolonged noise exposure causes temporary or permanent hearing loss.
Note behaviours indicative of hearing loss, such as failure to respond when spoken to, requests to repeat comments, leaning forward to hear, and child's inattentiveness or use of monotonous voice tone.	Individuals with hearing loss cope with sensory deficit through a variety of behavioural cues.
Assess if patient takes large doses of aspirin or other ototoxic medications (e.g., aminoglycosides, furosemide, streptomycin).	Medications have adverse effects of hearing loss.
Determine whether patient uses hearing aid.	Indicates need to assess ability to care for device and informs nurse to adjust voice tone or pace or to face patient to communicate.
If patient had recent hearing difficulty, note onset, contributing factors, affected ear, and effect on activities of daily living.	Helps determine nature and severity of hearing impairment.
Determine whether patient has repeated history of cerumen buildup in ear.	Cerumen impaction is a common cause for conduction deafness.

tragus does not influence the pain, the patient possibly has a middle ear infection. Tenderness in the mastoid area indicates mastoiditis.

Inspect the opening of the ear canal for size and presence of discharge. If discharge is present, wear clean gloves during the examination. A swollen or occluded meatus is not normal. Cerumen, a yellow, waxy substance, is common. Yellow or green, foul-smelling discharge indicates infection or a foreign body.

Ear Canals and Eardrums. Deeper structures of the external and middle ear are assessed with the use of an otoscope. The examination of the internal ear structures through the use of an otoscope is beyond the scope of new graduate nurses' practice. Advanced nurse practitioners use the otoscope to inspect the ear canal, tympanic membrane, and bony landmarks. Patients in greatest need of an examination are those with a possible foreign body in the ear canal, pain, swelling, discharge, tinnitus, injury, change in hearing, or disorders related to balance. A detailed presentation of an otoscope examination of the inner ear can be found in the textbook by Jarvis et al. (2019, pp. 360–365).

Hearing Acuity. A patient with a hearing loss often fails to respond to conversation. The three types of hearing loss are conduction, sensorineural, and mixed. A conduction loss interrupts sound waves as they travel from the outer ear to the cochlea of the inner ear, because the sound waves are not transmitted through the outer and middle ear structures. Examples of causes of a conduction loss are swelling of the auditory canal or tears in the tympanic membrane. A sensorineural loss involves the inner ear, auditory nerve, or hearing centre of the brain. Sound is conducted through the outer and middle ear structures, but the continued transmission of sound becomes interrupted at some point beyond the bony ossicles. A mixed loss involves a combination of conduction and sensorineural loss.

> **SAFETY ALERT** Patients working or living around loud noises are at risk for hearing loss. In addition, adolescents are at risk for premature hearing loss from continued exposure to loud music in their car or home or at concert events. The use of earbuds also increases the risk for hearing loss in all patients.

Older persons experience an inability to hear high-frequency sounds and consonants (e.g., *S, Z, T,* and *G*). Deterioration of the cochlea and thickening of the tympanic membrane cause older persons to gradually lose hearing acuity. They are especially at risk for hearing loss due to ototoxicity (injury to auditory nerve) resulting from high-maintenance doses of antibiotics (e.g., aminoglycosides).

To conduct a hearing assessment, have the patient remove any hearing aid, if worn. Note the patient's response to questions. Normally, the patient responds without excessive requests to have the questions repeated. If hearing loss is suspected, check the patient's response to the whispered voice. Test one ear at a time while the patient occludes the other ear with a finger. Ask the patient to gently move the finger up and down during the test. While standing 30 to 60 cm from the testing ear, cover the mouth so that the patient is unable to read lips. After exhaling fully, whisper softly toward the unoccluded ear, reciting random numbers with equally accented syllables, such as *nine-four-ten*. If necessary, gradually increase voice intensity until the patient correctly repeats the numbers. Then test the other ear for comparison. Ball and colleagues (2019) reported that patients normally hear numbers clearly when whispered, responding correctly at least 50% of the time. If a hearing loss is present, patients are referred for an audiometric assessment. While there are tests that can be performed using a tuning fork (Weber and Rinne tests), these are a gross screening tool and not as reliable as audiometry.

Nose and Sinuses

The integrity of the nose and sinuses is assessed through inspection and palpation. The patient sits during the examination. Use of a penlight enables gross examination of each naris. A more detailed examination requires use of a nasal speculum to inspect the deeper nasal turbinates. Table 33.14 lists components of the nursing history. Box 33.16 describes teaching guidelines during nose and sinus assessment.

Nose. When inspecting the external nose, observe for shape, size, skin, colour, and the presence of deformity or inflammation. The nose is normally smooth and symmetrical with the same colour as the face. Recent trauma sometimes causes edema and discoloration. If swelling or deformities exist, gently palpate the ridge and soft tissue of the nose by placing one finger on each side of the nasal arch and gently moving

TABLE 33.14	Nursing History for Nose and Sinus Assessment
Assessment Category	**Rationale**
Ask if patient has had trauma to the nose.	Trauma causes septal deviation and asymmetry of external nose.
Ask if patient has a history of allergies, nasal discharge, epistaxis (nosebleeds), or postnasal drip.	History is useful in determining source or nature of nasal and sinus drainage.
If there is history of nasal discharge, assess colour, amount, odour, duration, and associated symptoms (e.g., sneezing, nasal congestion, obstruction, or mouth breathing).	Aids in ruling out presence of infection, allergy, or drug use
Assess for history of nosebleed, including site, frequency, amount of bleeding, treatment, and difficulty stopping bleeding.	Characteristics sometimes reveal trauma, medication use, or excessive dryness as causative factors.
Ask if patient uses nasal spray or drops, including amount, frequency, and duration of use.	Overuse of over-the-counter nasal preparations causes physical change in mucosa.
Ask if patient snores at night or has difficulty breathing.	Difficulty with breathing or snoring indicates septal deviation or obstruction.

BOX 33.16   PATIENT TEACHING

Nose and Sinus Assessment

Objectives
- Patient will safely use over-the-counter nasal sprays.
- Parents will take proper measures to stop a child's nosebleed.
- Older persons will take safety precautions with loss of olfaction.

Teaching Strategies
- Caution patient against overuse of over-the-counter nasal sprays, which leads to "rebound" effect, causing excess nasal congestion.
- Instruct parents in care of a child with nosebleeds: Have child sit up and lean forward to avoid aspiration of blood, apply pressure to the anterior nose with the thumb and forefinger as the child breathes through the mouth, and apply ice or a cold cloth to the bridge of the nose if pressure fails to stop bleeding.
- Instruct all patients to install smoke detectors on each floor of their home.
- Instruct older persons to always check dated labels on food to ensure against spoilage.

Evaluation
- Have patient explain proper use of over-the-counter nasal sprays.
- Have parents demonstrate and describe technique for stopping a nose-bleed.
- Inspect patient's home during visit, and look for smoke detectors. Ask to check some food items in the refrigerator.

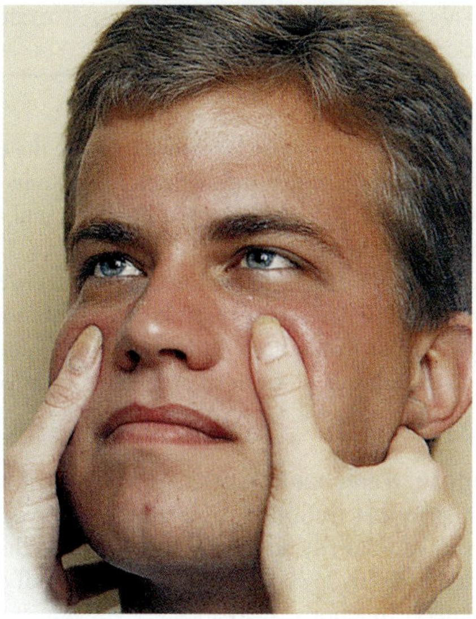

FIGURE 33.9 Palpation of maxillary sinuses.

the fingers from the nasal bridge to the tip. Note any tenderness, masses, or underlying deviations. Nasal structures are usually firm and stable.

Air normally passes freely through the nose when a person breathes. To assess patency of the nares, place a finger on the side of the patient's nose and occlude one naris. Ask the patient to breathe with the mouth closed. Repeat the procedure for the other naris.

While illuminating the anterior nares, inspect the mucosa for colour, lesions, discharge, swelling, and evidence of bleeding. If discharge is present, apply gloves. Normal mucosa is pink and moist without lesions. Pale mucosa with clear discharge indicates allergy. A mucoid discharge indicates rhinitis. A sinus infection results in yellowish or greenish discharge. Habitual use of intranasal cocaine and opioids causes puffiness and increased vascularity of the nasal mucosa. For the patient with a nasogastric tube, routinely check for local skin breakdown (excoriation) of the naris, characterized by redness and skin sloughing.

To view the septum and turbinates, have the patient tip the head back slightly to provide a clear view. Illuminate the septum and observe for alignment, perforation, or bleeding. Normally the septum is close to the midline and thicker anteriorly than posteriorly. The turbinates are covered with mucous membranes that warm and moisten inspired air. Normal mucosa is pink and moist, without lesions. A deviated septum obstructs breathing and interferes with passage of a nasogastric tube. Perforation of the septum often occurs after repeated use of intranasal cocaine. Note any **polyps** (tumour-like growths) or purulent drainage.

Sinuses. Examination of the sinuses involves palpation. In cases of allergies or infection, the interior of the sinuses becomes inflamed and swollen. The most effective way to assess for tenderness is by externally palpating the frontal and maxillary facial areas (Figure 33.9). Palpate the frontal sinus by exerting pressure with the thumb up and under the patient's eyebrow. Gentle, upward pressure elicits tenderness easily if sinus irritation is present. Do not apply pressure to the eyes. If tenderness of sinuses is present, the sinuses may be transilluminated.

Mouth and Pharynx

The mouth and pharynx are assessed to detect signs of overall health, determine oral hygiene needs, and develop therapies for patients with dehydration, restricted intake, oral trauma, or oral airway obstruction. To assess the oral cavity, use a penlight and tongue depressor or a single gauze square. Wear clean gloves during the examination. Have the patient sit or lie down during the examination. The oral cavity can also be assessed while administering oral hygiene (see Chapter 39). Table 33.15 describes the nursing history for assessment of the mouth and pharynx.

TABLE 33.15	Nursing History for Mouth and Pharyngeal Assessment
Assessment Category	**Rationale**
Determine if patient wears dentures or retainers and if they are comfortable.	Patient needs to remove dentures for nurse to visualize and palpate gums. Ill-fitting dentures chronically irritate mucosa and gums.
Determine if patient has had recent change in appetite or weight.	Symptoms result from painful mouth conditions or poor hygiene.
Determine if patient uses tobacco products:	
Smoking of cigarette, cigar, or pipe	Smoking of these products increases risk for lung, oral cavity, larynx, and esophageal cancers.
Smokeless tobacco: use of chewing tobacco and snuff	Smokeless tobacco causes various cancers and noncancerous oral disorders. Long-term snuff users have increased risk for cancer of the gums and cheeks.
Review history for alcohol consumption.	Excessive alcohol consumption appears to put a person at greater risk for oral cavity and pharynx cancer. Effects of alcohol are independent of tobacco use.
Assess dental hygiene practices, including use of fluoride toothpaste, frequency of brushing and flossing, and frequency of dental visits.	Assessment reveals patient's need for education, financial support, or both. Periodontal disease has a higher prevalence among older persons who have a history of high plaque buildup, use tobacco, and visit the dentist infrequently.
Ask if patient has pain from chewing or eating. If so, ask if mouth lesions are present, including duration and associated symptoms.	Pain is often associated with a broken tooth, tooth grinding, or temporomandibular joint problems. Extra care is needed during oral hygiene administration.

Lips. Have patients wearing lipstick remove it before the examination. Inspect the lips for colour, texture, hydration, contour, and lesions. With the patient's mouth closed, view the lips from end to end. Normally they are pink, moist, symmetrical, and smooth. Lip colour in dark-skinned patients varies from pink to plum. Anemia causes pallor of the lips, with cyanosis caused by respiratory or cardiovascular problems. Cherry-coloured lips indicate carbon monoxide poisoning. Any lesions such as nodules or ulcerations are related to infection, irritation, or skin cancer.

Buccal Mucosa, Gums, and Teeth. Ask the patient to clench the teeth and smile so that teeth occlusion can be observed. The upper molars normally rest directly on the lower molars, and the upper incisors slightly override the lower incisors. A symmetrical smile reveals normal facial nerve function.

Inspect the teeth to determine the quality of dental hygiene (Box 33.17). Note the position and alignment of the teeth. To examine the posterior surface of the teeth, have the patient open the mouth with the lips relaxed. Use a tongue depressor to retract the lips and cheeks, especially when viewing the molars. Note the colour of teeth and presence of dental caries (cavities), tartar, and extraction sites. Normal, healthy teeth are smooth, white, and shiny. A chalky white discoloration of the enamel is an early indication of caries formation. Brown or black discolorations indicate the formation of caries. A stained yellow colour is from tobacco use, whereas coffee, tea, and colas cause a brown stain. In the older person, loose or missing teeth are common because bone resorption increases. An older person's teeth often feel rough when tooth enamel calcifies. Yellow or darkened teeth are also common in the older person because of the general wear and tear that exposes the darker, underlying dentin.

To view the mucosa and gums, ask the patient to first remove any dental appliance. View the inner oral mucosa by having the patient open and relax the mouth slightly and then gently retract the patient's lower lip away from the teeth (Figure 33.10). Repeat this process for the upper lip. Inspect the mucosa for colour, hydration, texture, and lesions such as ulcers, abrasions, or cysts. Normally the mucosa is a glistening pink, smooth, and moist. Some common small, yellow-white raised lesions on the buccal mucosa and lips are Fordyce spots, or ectopic sebaceous glands (Ball et al., 2019). If lesions are present, palpate them gently with a gloved hand for tenderness, size, and consistency.

BOX 33.17 PATIENT TEACHING

Mouth and Pharyngeal Assessment

Objectives
- Patient will practise proper oral hygiene measures and dental care.
- Patient will describe warning signs of oral cancer.
- Older patient will maintain normal solid food intake.

Teaching Strategies
- Discuss proper techniques for oral hygiene, including brushing and flossing (see Chapter 39).
- Explain the early warning signs of oral cavity and pharynx cancer: a sore that bleeds easily and does not heal, a lump or thickening, and a red or white patch on the mucosa that persists. Difficulty chewing, swallowing, or moving the tongue or jaw are late symptoms (Canadian Cancer Society, 2022c).
- Encourage regular dental examination every 6 months for children, adults, and older persons.
- Identify older persons who have difficulty chewing and changes in the teeth. Teach patients to eat soft foods and cut food into small pieces.

Evaluation
- Ask patient to demonstrate brushing.
- Have patient identify when to have regular dental checkups.
- Have patient identify the warning signs of oral cavity and pharynx cancer.
- Ask an older person to keep a diet record for 3 days.

To inspect the buccal mucosa, ask the patient to open the mouth, and then gently retract the cheeks with a tongue depressor or gloved finger covered with gauze (Figure 33.11). View the surface of the mucosa from right to left and top to bottom. A penlight illuminates the most posterior portion of the mucosa. Normal mucosa is glistening, pink, soft, moist, and smooth. Varying shades of hyperpigmentation are normal in 10% of light-skinned patients after age 50 and up to 90% of dark-skinned patients by the same age. For patients with normal pigmentation, the buccal mucosa is a good site to inspect for jaundice and pallor. In older persons, the mucosa is normally dry because of reduced salivation. Thick white patches (leukoplakia) are often a precancerous lesion seen in heavy smokers and alcoholics. Palpate for any buccal lesions by placing the index finger within the buccal cavity and the thumb on the outer surface of the cheek.

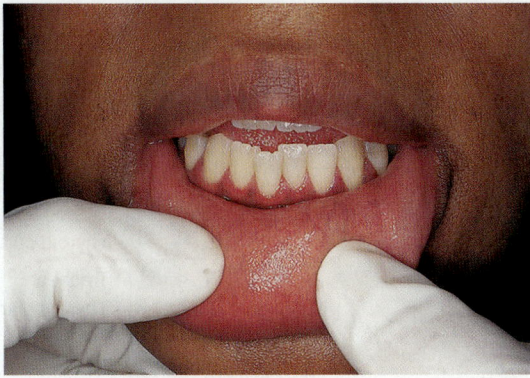

FIGURE 33.10 Inspection of inner oral mucosa of the lower lip.

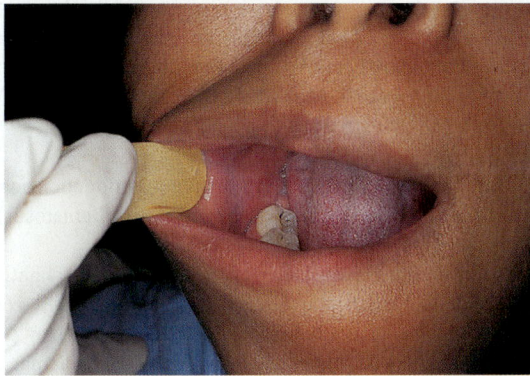

FIGURE 33.11 Retraction of the buccal mucosa allows for clear visualization.

> **SAFETY ALERT** Patients who smoke cigarettes, cigars, or pipes and those who use smokeless tobacco have an increased risk of oral, laryngeal, and esophageal cancer. These individuals may have leukoplakia or other lesions anywhere in their oral cavity (e.g., lips, gums, tongue) at an early age.

Inspect the gums (gingivae) for colour, edema, retraction, bleeding, and lesions while retracting the cheeks. Healthy gums are pink, smooth, and moist and tightly fit around each tooth. Dark-skinned patients often have patchy pigmentation. In older persons, the gums are usually pale. Using clean gloves, palpate the gums to assess for lesions, thickening, or masses. Normally there is no tenderness. Spongy gums that bleed easily indicate periodontal disease and vitamin C deficiency. If the patient has loose or mobile teeth, swollen gums, or pockets containing debris at the tooth margins, suspect periodontal disease or gingivitis.

Tongue and Floor of Mouth. Carefully inspect the tongue on all sides, as well as the floor of the mouth. Have the patient relax the mouth and stick the tongue out halfway. Note any deviation, tremor, or limitation in movement. This tests hypoglossal nerve function. If the patient protrudes the tongue too far, this will elicit the gag reflex. When the tongue protrudes, it lies midline. To test for tongue mobility, ask the patient to raise the tongue up and move it from side to side. The tongue should move freely.

Using a penlight for illumination, examine the tongue for colour, size, position, texture, and coatings or lesions. A normal tongue is medium or dull red in colour, moist, slightly rough on the top surface, and smooth along the lateral margins. The undersurface of the tongue and the floor of the mouth are highly vascular (Figure 33.12). Take extra care to inspect this area, a common site for oral cancer lesions. The patient lifts the tongue by placing its tip on the palate behind the

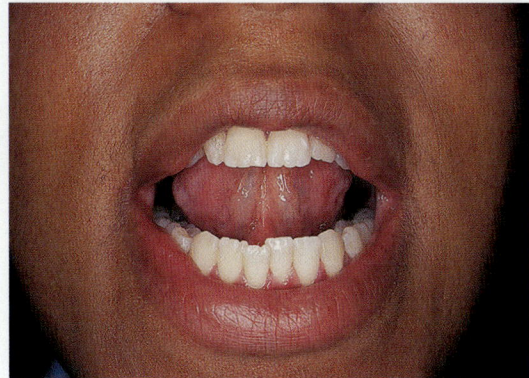

FIGURE 33.12 The undersurface of the tongue is highly vascular.

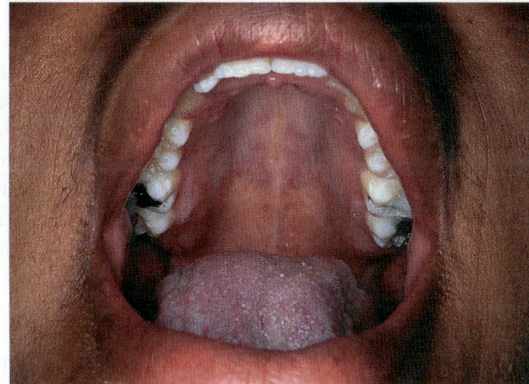

FIGURE 33.13 The hard palate is located anteriorly in the roof of the mouth.

upper incisors. Inspect for colour, swelling, and lesions such as nodules or cysts. The ventral surface of the tongue is pink and smooth, with large veins between the frenulum folds. To palpate the tongue, explain the procedure and ask the patient to protrude the tongue. Grasp the tip with a gauze square and gently pull it to one side. With a gloved hand, palpate the full length of the tongue and the base for any areas of hardening or ulceration. **Varicosities** (swollen, tortuous veins) are common in the older person and rarely cause health problems.

Palate. Have the patient extend the head backward, holding the mouth open, to inspect the hard and soft palates. The hard palate, or roof of the mouth, is located anteriorly. The whitish hard palate is dome shaped. The soft palate extends posteriorly toward the pharynx. It is normally light pink and smooth. Observe the palates for colour, shape, texture, and extra bony prominences or defects (Figure 33.13). A bony growth, or **exostosis**, between the two palates is common.

Pharynx. Perform an examination of pharyngeal structures to rule out infection, inflammation, or lesions. Have the patient tip the head back slightly, open the mouth wide, and say "Ah" while you place the tip of a tongue depressor on the middle third of the tongue. Take care not to press the lower lip against the teeth. By placing the tongue depressor too far anteriorly, the posterior part of the tongue mounds up, obstructing the view. Placing the tongue depressor on the posterior tongue elicits the gag reflex.

With a penlight, first inspect the uvula and soft palate (Figure 33.14). Both structures, which are innervated by the tenth cranial (vagus) nerve, should rise centrally as the patient says "Ah." Examine the anterior and posterior pillars, soft palate, and uvula. View the tonsils in the cavities between the anterior and posterior pillars and note the presence or absence of tissue. The posterior pharynx is behind the pillars.

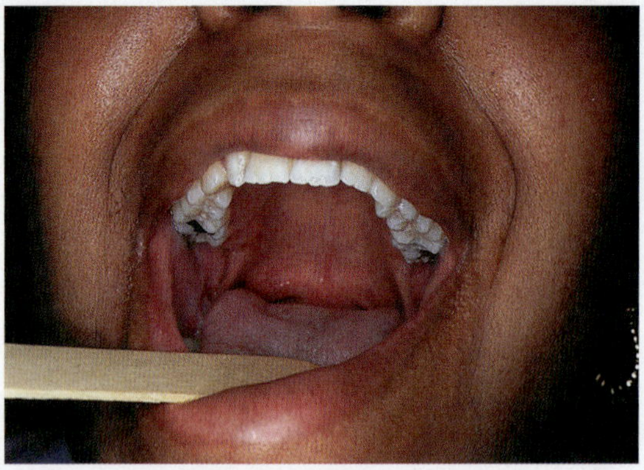

FIGURE 33.14 Use of a penlight and tongue depressor enables visualization of the uvula and posterior soft palate.

Normally, pharyngeal tissues are pink and smooth and well hydrated. Small, irregular spots of lymphatic tissue and small blood vessels are normal. Note edema, petechiae (small hemorrhages), lesions, or exudate. Patients with chronic sinus problems frequently exhibit a clear exudate that drains along the wall of the posterior pharynx. Yellow or green exudate indicates infection. A patient with a typical sore throat has a red and edematous uvula and tonsillar pillars with possible presence of yellow exudate.

Neck

Assessment of the neck includes assessment of the neck muscles, lymph nodes of the head and neck, carotid arteries, jugular veins, thyroid gland, and trachea (Figure 33.15). The examination of the jugular veins and carotid arteries is included under the vascular system assessment. Inspection and palpation of the neck are performed to determine the integrity of the neck structures and to examine the lymphatic system. The lymphatic system is examined region by region during the assessment of body systems (head and neck, breast, genitalia, and extremities). An abnormality of superficial lymph nodes sometimes reveals the presence of an infection or malignancy. Examination of the thyroid gland and trachea also aids in ruling out malignancies. This examination is carried out with the patient sitting. The sternocleidomastoid and trapezius muscles outline the areas of the neck, dividing each side of the neck into two triangles. The anterior triangle contains the trachea, thyroid gland, carotid artery, and anterior cervical lymph nodes. The posterior triangle contains the posterior lymph nodes. Table 33.16 reviews the nursing history for the head and neck examination.

Neck Muscles. The neck is inspected first in the usual anatomical position, with slight hyperextension. Observe for symmetry of the neck muscles. Ask the patient to flex the neck with the chin to the chest, hyperextend the neck backward, and move the head laterally to each side and then sideways with the ear moving toward the shoulder. This tests the sternocleidomastoid and trapezius muscles. The neck normally moves without discomfort. Tests that assess muscle strength and function can be performed during assessment of the head and neck; the description of these tests is included in the assessment of the musculoskeletal system.

Lymph Nodes. An extensive system of lymph nodes collects lymph from the head, ears, nose, cheeks, and lips (Figure 33.16). The immune system protects the body from foreign antigens, removes damaged cells from the circulation, and provides a partial barrier to growth of malignant cells within the body. Assessing the lymph nodes requires competence when caring for patients with suspected immunoincompetence,

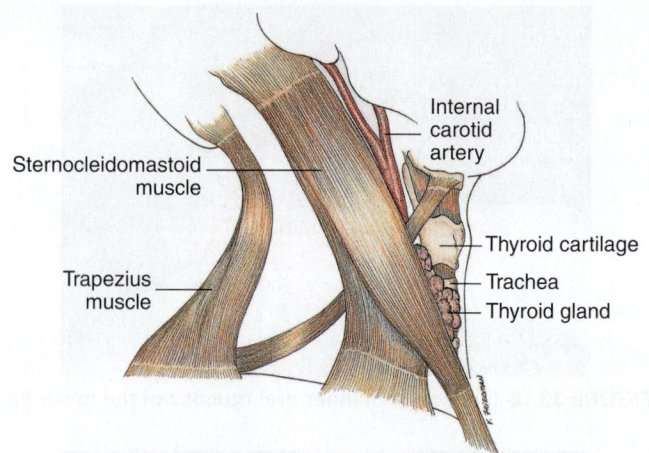

FIGURE 33.15 Anatomical position of the major neck structures. Note the triangles formed by the sternocleidomastoid muscle, lower jaw, and anterior neck anteriorly and by the sternocleidomastoid muscle, trapezius muscle, and lower neck posteriorly.

which is often linked to allergies, human immunodeficiency virus (HIV) infection, autoimmune disease (e.g., lupus erythematosus), lymphomas, or serious infection.

With the patient's chin raised and the head tilted slightly, first inspect the area where lymph nodes are distributed and compare both sides. This position stretches the skin slightly over any possible enlarged nodes. Inspect visible nodes for edema, erythema, or red streaks. Nodes are not normally visible.

Use a methodical approach to palpate the lymph nodes to avoid overlooking any single node or chain. The patient relaxes with the neck flexed slightly forward. Inspect and palpate both sides of the neck for comparison. During palpation, either face or stand to the side of the patient for easy access to all nodes. Using the pads of the middle three fingers of each hand, gently palpate in a rotary motion over the nodes. Check each node methodically in the following sequence: occipital, postauricular nodes, preauricular, retropharyngeal, submandibular, and submental. Try to detect enlargement and note the location, size, shape, surface characteristics, consistency, mobility, tenderness, and warmth of the nodes. If the skin is mobile, move the skin over the area of the nodes. It is important to press underlying tissue in each area and not simply move the fingers over the skin. However, if excessive pressure is applied, it is easy to miss small nodes and destroy palpable nodes.

To palpate supraclavicular nodes, ask the patient to bend the head forward and relax the shoulders. Palpate these nodes by hooking the index and third finger over the clavicle, lateral to the sternocleidomastoid muscle. Palpate the deep cervical nodes only with the fingers hooked around the sternocleidomastoid muscle.

Normally lymph nodes are not easily palpable. However, small, mobile, nontender nodes are common. Lymph nodes that are large, fixed, inflamed, or tender indicate a condition such as local infection, systemic disease, or neoplasm (Jarvis et al., 2019) (Box 33.18). If enlarged nodes are found, explore the adjacent areas and regions drained by the nodes. Tenderness almost always indicates inflammation. An anomaly involving a lymph node of the head and neck means an abnormality in the mouth, throat, abdomen, breasts, thorax, or arms. These are the areas drained by the head and neck nodes.

Thyroid Gland. The thyroid gland lies in the anterior lower neck, in front of and to both sides of the trachea. The gland is fixed to the trachea with the isthmus overlying the trachea and connecting the two irregular, cone-shaped lobes (Figure 33.17). Inspect the lower neck

TABLE 33.16	Nursing History for Neck Assessment
Assessment Category	**Rationale**
Assess for history of recent cold or infection or enlarged lymph nodes, exposure to radiation or toxic chemicals.	Colds or infections (e.g., mononucleosis) cause temporary or permanent lymph node enlargement. Lymph nodes are also enlarged in various diseases such as cancer.
If there is an enlarged lymph node, consider reviewing history of intravenous drug use, hemophilia, sexual contact with people infected with human immunodeficiency virus (HIV), history of blood transfusion, multiple and indiscriminate sexual contacts, or if the patient is male, having sex with other men.	These are risk factors for HIV infection.
Ask if patient has had a history of neck pain with restriction in movement.	This indicates muscle strain, head injury, local nerve injury, or enlarged or swollen lymph node.
Ask if patient has had a change in temperature preference (more or less clothing); swelling in neck; change in texture of hair, skin, or nails; or change in emotional stability.	Symptoms are indicative of thyroid disease.
Ask if patient has a history of hypothyroidism or hyperthyroidism or takes thyroid medication or has a family history of thyroid disease.	Disease or medications influence tissue growth of gland.
Review medical history of pneumothorax (collapsed lung) or bronchial tumour.	Conditions place patient at risk for tracheal displacement or lateral deviation.

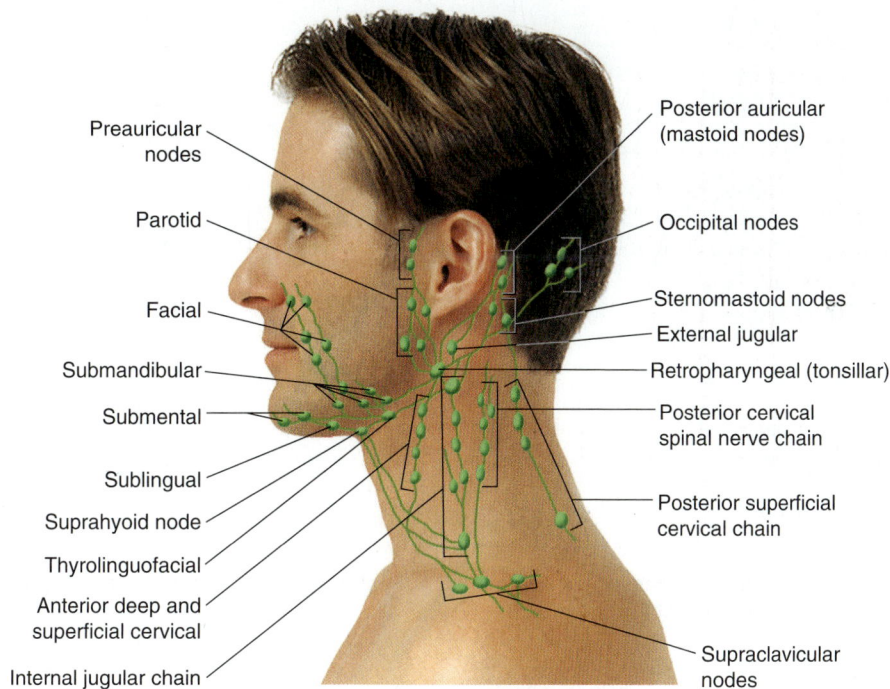

FIGURE 33.16 Palpable lymph nodes in the head and neck. (From Ball, J. W., Dains, J. E., Flynn, J. A., et al. [2019]. *Seidel's guide to physical examination* [9th ed.]. Mosby.)

overlying the thyroid gland for obvious masses, symmetry, and any subtle fullness at the base of the neck. Ask the patient to hyperextend the neck, which helps tighten the skin for better visualization. Offer the patient a glass of water, and, while observing the neck, have the patient swallow. This manoeuvre helps with visualizing an abnormally enlarged thyroid. Normally, the thyroid cannot be visualized.

Carotid Artery and Jugular Vein. This portion of the examination is described under examination of the vascular system (see later section).

Trachea. The trachea is a part of the upper respiratory system that the examiner directly palpates. It is normally located in the midline above the suprasternal notch. Masses in the neck or mediastinum and pulmonary abnormalities cause displacement laterally. Have the patient sit or lie down during palpation. Determine the position of the trachea by palpating at the suprasternal notch, slipping the thumb and index fingers to each side. Note if the finger and thumb shift laterally. Do not apply forceful pressure because this elicits coughing.

THORAX AND LUNGS

Accurate physical assessment of the thorax and lungs requires review of the ventilatory and respiratory functions of the lungs. If disease is affecting the lungs, this will affect other body systems as well. For example, reduced oxygenation causes changes in cognitive functioning and alertness because of the brain's sensitivity to lowered oxygen levels. Data from all body systems are used to determine the nature of pulmonary alterations.

BOX 33.18 PATIENT TEACHING

Neck Assessment

Objective
- Patient takes proper preventive action if they notice a mass in the neck.

Teaching Strategies
- Stress importance of regular adherence to medication schedule to patients with thyroid disease.
- Instruct patient about the lymph nodes and how infection commonly causes node tenderness.
- Instruct patient to call a health care provider when they notice an enlarged lump or mass in the neck.
- Teach patient risk factors for human immunodeficiency virus (HIV) infection and other sexually transmitted infections.

Evaluation
- Have patient explain when to notify a health care provider about a neck mass.

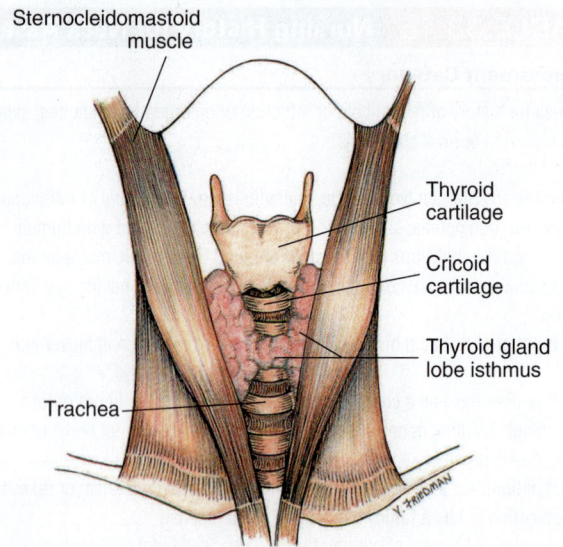

FIGURE 33.17 Anatomical position of the thyroid gland.

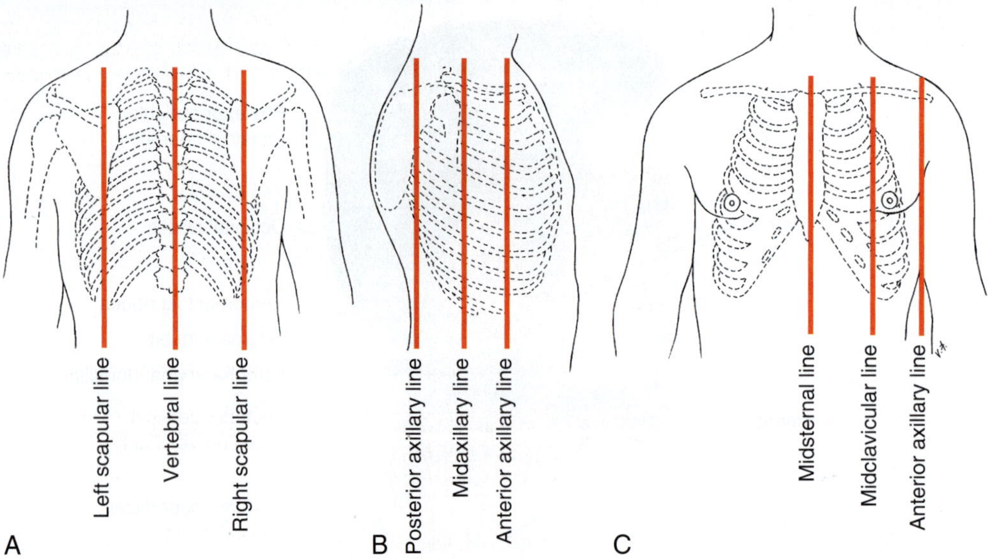

FIGURE 33.18 Anatomical chest wall landmarks. **A,** Posterior chest landmarks. **B,** Lateral chest landmarks. **C,** Anterior chest landmarks.

Before assessing the thorax and lungs, be familiar with the landmarks of the chest (Figure 33.18). These landmarks help in identifying findings and using assessment skills correctly. The patient's nipples, angle of Louis, suprasternal notch, costal angle, clavicles, and vertebrae are key landmarks that provide a series of imaginary lines for sign identification. Keep a mental image of the location of the lobes of the lung and the position of each rib (Figure 33.19). The proper orientation to anatomical structures ensures a thorough assessment of the anterior, lateral, and posterior thorax.

Locating the position of each rib is critical to visualizing the lobe of the lung being assessed. To begin, locate the angle of Louis at the manubriosternal junction. The angle is a visible and palpable angulation of the sternum and is the point at which the second rib articulates with the sternum. Count the ribs and intercostal spaces (between the ribs) from this point. The number of each intercostal space corresponds with that of the rib just above it. The spinous process of the third thoracic vertebra and the fourth, fifth, and sixth ribs helps to locate the lung's lobes laterally. The lower lobes project laterally and anteriorly (Figure 33.20). Posteriorly, the tip or inferior margin of the scapula lies approximately at the level of the seventh rib (Figure 33.21). After

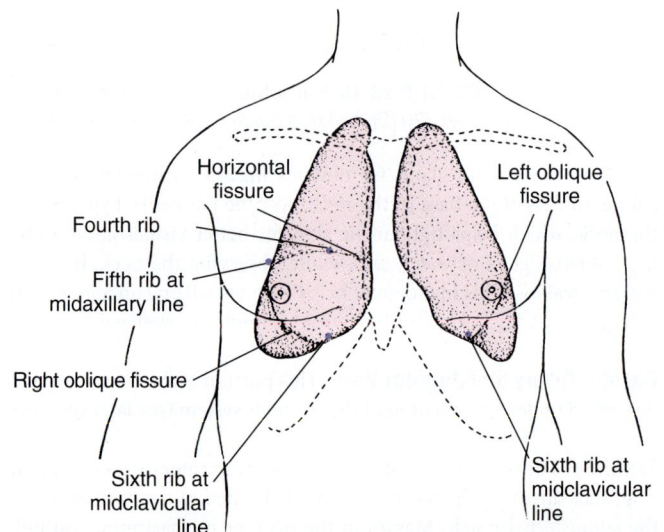

FIGURE 33.19 Anterior position of lung lobes in relation to anatomical landmarks.

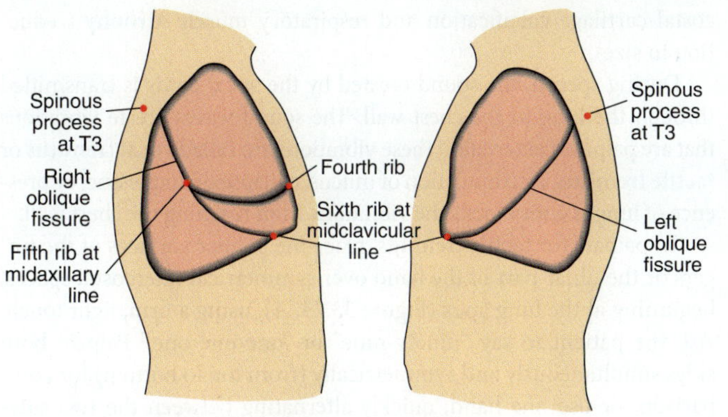

FIGURE 33.20 Lateral position of lung lobes in relation to anatomical landmarks.

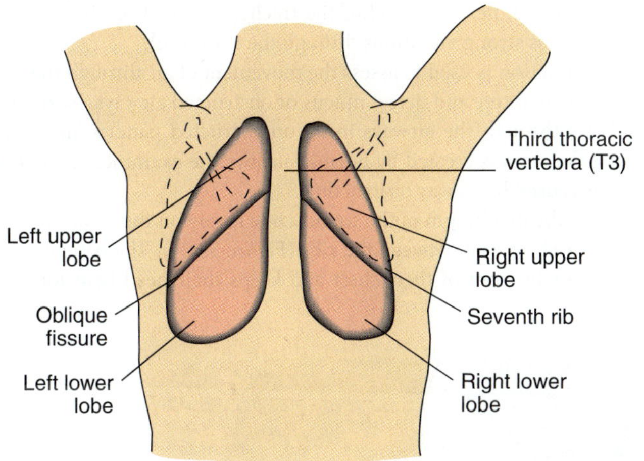

FIGURE 33.21 Posterior position of lung lobes in relation to anatomical landmarks.

identifying the seventh rib, count upward to locate the third thoracic vertebra and align it with the inner borders of the scapula to locate the posterior lobes.

The examination requires the patient to be undressed to the waist, in good lighting. Assess patients at risk for pulmonary conditions, such as the patient confined to bed rest or the patient with chest pain who cannot fully expand the lungs. The examination begins with the patient sitting for assessment of the posterior and lateral chest. Have the patient sit or lie down for assessment of the anterior chest. Table 33.17 reviews the nursing history for lung examination.

Posterior Thorax

Begin examination of the posterior thorax by observing for any signs or symptoms in other body systems that indicate pulmonary conditions. Reduced cognitive impairment or alertness, nasal flaring, somnolence, and cyanosis are examples of signs assessed that indicate difficulties with oxygenation. Inspect the posterior thorax by observing the shape and symmetry of the chest from the patient's back and front. Note the anteroposterior diameter. Body shape or posture significantly impairs ventilatory movement. Normally the chest contour is symmetrical, with the anteroposterior diameter one-third to one-half of the transverse, or side-to-side, diameter. A barrel-shaped chest (anteroposterior diameter equals transverse diameter) characterizes aging and chronic lung disease. Infants have an almost round shape. Congenital and postural alterations cause abnormal contours. Some patients lean over a table or splint the side of the chest because of a breathing difficulty. Splinting or holding the chest wall because of pain causes a patient to bend toward the side affected. This posture impairs ventilatory movement.

Standing at a midline position behind the patient, look for deformities, position of the spine, slope of the ribs, retraction of the intercostal spaces during inspiration, and bulging of the intercostal spaces during expiration. The scapulae are normally symmetrical and closely attached to the thoracic wall. The normal spine is straight without lateral deviation. Posteriorly, the ribs tend to slope across and down. The

TABLE 33.17	Nursing History for Lung Assessment
Assessment Category	**Rationale**
Assess history of tobacco or marijuana use, including type of tobacco, duration and amount (pack-years = number of years smoked × number of packs per day), age started, and efforts to quit and length of time since smoking stopped.	Smoking is a risk factor for lung cancer, heart disease, cerebrovascular disease, emphysema, and chronic bronchitis. Smoking accounts for a significant percentage of all cancer deaths.
Ask if patient has had a *persistent cough* (productive or nonproductive), *sputum streaked with blood, voice change, chest pain*, shortness of breath, **orthopnea**, dyspnea during exertion or at rest, poor activity tolerance, or *recurrent attacks of pneumonia or bronchitis*.	Symptoms of cardiopulmonary alterations help localize objective physical findings. (Warning signals for lung cancer are in italic type.)
Determine if patient works or lives in an environment containing pollutants (e.g., asbestos, arsenic, coal dust) or requiring exposure to radiation. Does patient have exposure to second-hand smoke?	These risk factors increase the chance for various lung diseases.
Review history for known or suspected human immunodeficiency virus (HIV) infection, substance use disorder, or low income, or being a resident or employee of a long-term care facility or shelter, homeless, a recent prison inmate, caregiver of a tuberculosis (TB) patient, or an immigrant to Canada from a country where TB is prevalent.	These are risk factors for HIV.
Ask if patient has a history of persistent cough, hemoptysis, unexplained weight loss, fatigue, night sweats, or fever.	These are risk factors for both TB and HIV infection.
Does patient have a history of chronic hoarseness?	Hoarseness indicates a laryngeal disorder or abuse of cocaine or opioids (sniffing).
Assess history of allergies to pollens, dust, or other airborne irritants and to foods, medications, or chemical substances.	Symptoms such as choking feeling, bronchospasm with respiratory stridor, wheezes on auscultation, and dyspnea are often caused by allergic response.
Review family history for cancer, TB, allergies, or chronic obstructive pulmonary disease.	These conditions place patient at risk for lung disease.
Ask if patient has had a pneumonia or influenza vaccine and a TB test; if not, educate patient on the need to do so.	The very young, the very old, and those with chronic respiratory conditions or with immunosuppressive diseases are at increased risk for respiratory disease.

ribs and intercostal spaces are easier to see in a thin person. Normally, no bulging or active movement occurs within the intercostal spaces during breathing. Bulging indicates that the patient is using great effort to breathe.

Also assess the rate and rhythm of breathing (see Chapter 31). Observe the thorax as a whole. The thorax normally expands and relaxes regularly with equality of movement bilaterally. In healthy adults, the normal respiratory rates vary from 12 to 20 respirations per minute.

The posterior thorax is palpated to assess further characteristics. Palpate the thoracic muscles and skeleton for lumps, masses, pulsations, and unusual movement. If the patient notes pain or tenderness, avoid deep palpation. Fractured rib fragments could be displaced against vital organs. Normally the chest wall is not tender. If there is a suspicious mass or swollen area, lightly palpate it for size, shape, and the typical qualities of a lesion.

To measure chest excursion or depth of breathing, stand behind the patient and place the thumbs along the spinal processes at the tenth rib, with the palms lightly contacting the posterolateral surfaces (Ball et al., 2019). Place thumbs 5 cm apart, pointing toward the spine and fingers pointing laterally (Figure 33.22, *A*). Press the hands toward the spine so that a small skin fold appears between the thumbs. Do not slide the hands over the skin. Instruct the patient to take a deep breath after exhaling. Note movement of the thumbs (see Figure 33.22, *B*). Chest excursion is symmetrical, separating the thumbs 3 to 5 cm. Reduced chest excursions may be caused by pain, postural deformity, or fatigue. In the older person, chest movement normally declines because of

costal cartilage calcification and respiratory muscle **atrophy** (reduction in size).

During speech, the sound created by the vocal cords is transmitted through the lung to the chest wall. The sound waves create vibrations that are palpated externally. These vibrations are called **vocal fremitus** or **tactile fremitus**. Accumulation of mucus, collapse of lung tissue, or presence of lung lesions blocks the vibrations from reaching the chest wall.

To palpate for tactile fremitus, place the palmar surfaces of the fingers or the ulnar part of the hand over symmetrical intercostal spaces, beginning at the lung apex (Figure 33.23, *A*), using a firm, light touch. Ask the patient to say "ninety-nine" or "one-one-one." Palpate both sides simultaneously and symmetrically (from top to bottom) for comparison, or use one hand, quickly alternating between the two sides (Ball et al., 2019). Normally, a faint vibration is present as the patient speaks. If fremitus is faint, ask the patient to speak in a louder or lower tone of voice. Normally, fremitus is symmetrical. Vibrations are strongest at the top, near the level of the tracheal bifurcation. In a crying infant, assess strong vibrations through the chest wall.

Auscultation is used to assess the movement of air through the tracheobronchial tree and detect mucus or obstructed airways. Normally, air flows through the airways in an unobstructed pattern. In recognizing the sounds created by normal airflow, the examiner can detect sounds caused by airway obstruction.

Place the diaphragm of the stethoscope firmly on the skin, over the posterior chest wall between the ribs (Figure 33.24). The patient folds their arms in front of their chest and keeps their head bent forward

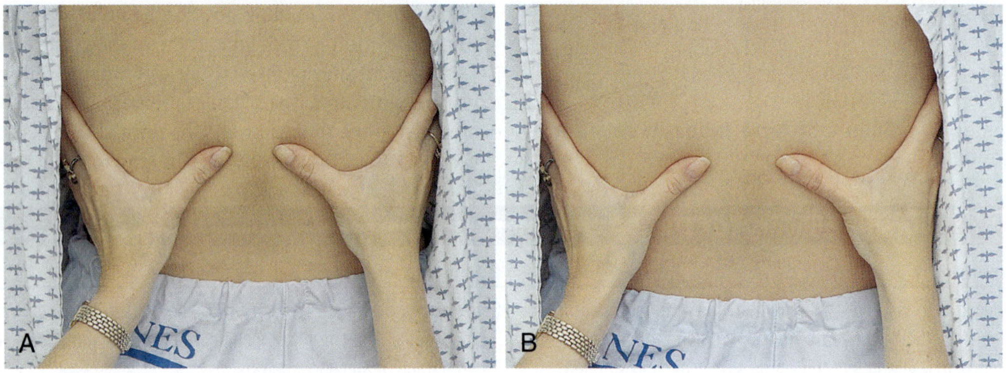

FIGURE 33.22 A, Hand position for palpation of posterior thorax excursion. **B,** As patient inhales, movement of chest excursion separates the thumbs.

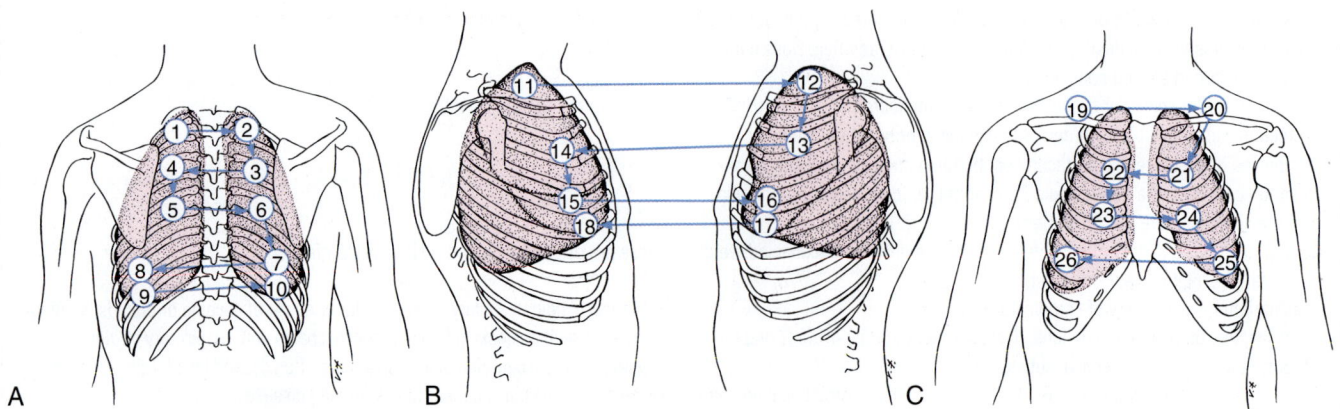

FIGURE 33.23 A–C, A systematic pattern (posterior–lateral–anterior) is followed when palpating and auscultating the thorax. (From Ball, J. W., Dains, J. E., Flynn, J. A., et al. [2019]. *Seidel's guide to physical examination* [9th ed.]. Mosby.)

while taking slow, deep breaths with the mouth slightly open. Listen to an entire inspiration and expiration at each position of the stethoscope. If sounds are faint, as in the patient with obesity, ask the patient to breathe harder and faster temporarily. Breath sounds are much louder in children because of their thin chest walls. In children, the bell, or a pediatric stethoscope, works best because of a child's small chest. Use a systematic pattern comparing lung sounds in one region on one side of the body with sounds in the same region on the opposite side. It is impossible to remember the quality of all sounds noted on one side of the body and then compare them with sounds on the other side (see Figure 33.23, *A*).

Auscultate for normal breath sounds and abnormal or **adventitious sounds**. Normal breath sounds differ in character, depending on the area being auscultated. Normally, bronchovesicular and vesicular sounds are heard over the posterior thorax (Table 33.18).

Abnormal sounds result from air passing through moisture, mucus, or narrowed airways. They also result from alveoli suddenly reinflating or from an inflammation between the pleural linings of the lung.

Adventitious sounds often occur superimposed over normal sounds. The four types of adventitious sounds are crackles, rhonchi, wheezes, and pleural friction rub. A specific entity causes each sound, and each has typical auditory features (Table 33.19). During auscultation, note the location and characteristics of the sounds, and listen for the absence of breath sounds (found in patients with collapsed or surgically removed lobes).

If there are abnormalities in tactile fremitus or auscultation, perform the vocal resonance tests (spoken and whispered voice sounds). Place the stethoscope over the same locations used to assess breath sounds, and have the patient say "ninety-nine" in a normal voice tone. Normally, the sound is muffled. If fluid is compressing the lung, the vibrations from the patient's voice are transmitted to the chest wall and the sound becomes clear (**bronchophony**). Then ask the patient to whisper "ninety-nine." The whispered voice is usually faint and indistinct. Certain lung abnormalities cause the whispered voice to become clear and distinct (**whispered pectoriloquy**). Bronchophony and whispered pectoriloquy can be indicative of lung disorders such as

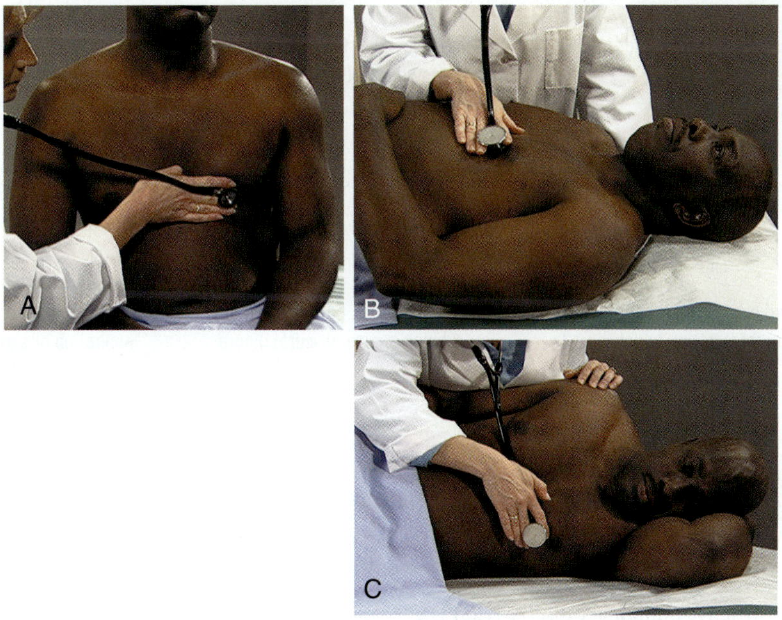

FIGURE 33.24 A–C, Use the diaphragm of the stethoscope to auscultate breath sounds. (From Ball, J. W., Dains, J. E., Flynn, J. A., et al. [2019]. *Seidel's guide to physical examination* [9th ed.]. Mosby.)

TABLE 33.18	**Normal Breath Sounds**	
Description	**Location**	**Origin**
Vesicular		
Vesicular sounds are soft, breezy, and low-pitched. Inspiratory phase is three times longer than expiratory phase.	Best heard over lung's periphery (except over scapula)	Created by air moving through smaller airways
Bronchovesicular		
Bronchovesicular sounds are blowing sounds that are medium-pitched and of medium intensity. Inspiratory phase is equal to expiratory phase.	Best heard posteriorly between scapulae and anteriorly over bronchioles lateral to sternum at first and second intercostal spaces	Created by air moving through large airways
Bronchial		
Bronchial sounds are loud and high-pitched with hollow quality. Expiration lasts longer than inspiration (3:2 ratio).	Heard only over trachea	Created by air moving through trachea close to chest wall

TABLE 33.19	**Adventitious Breath Sounds**		
Sound	**Site Auscultated**	**Cause**	**Character**
Crackles	Most common in dependent lobes: right and left lung bases	Random, sudden reinflation of groups of alveoli; disruptive passage of air through small airways	Fine crackles are high-pitched fine, short, interrupted crackling sounds heard during end of inspiration, usually not cleared with coughing. Medium crackles are lower, more moist sounds heard during middle of inspiration; not cleared with coughing. Coarse crackles are loud, bubbly sounds heard during inspiration; not cleared with coughing.
Rhonchi (sonorous wheeze)	Primarily heard over trachea and bronchi; if loud enough, can be heard over most lung fields	Muscular spasm, fluid, or mucus in larger airways, new growth or external pressure causing turbulence	Loud, low-pitched, rumbling coarse sounds heard most often during inspiration or expiration; sometimes cleared by coughing
Wheezes (sibilant wheeze)	Heard over all lung fields	High-velocity airflow through severely narrowed or obstructed airway	High-pitched, continuous musical sounds like a squeak heard continuously during inspiration or expiration; usually louder on expiration
Pleural friction rub	Heard over anterior lateral lung field (if patient is sitting upright)	Inflamed pleura, parietal pleura rubbing against visceral pleura	Has dry, rubbing, or grating quality heard during inspiration or expiration; does not clear with coughing; heard loudest over lower lateral anterior surface

Data summarized from Ball, J. W., Dains, J. E., Flynn, J. A., et al. (2019). *Seidel's guide to physical examination* (9th ed. p. 299–302). Mosby.

pneumonia, asthma, chronic obstructive pulmonary disease (COPD), and lung tumours and suggest the need for diagnostic assessment (Box 33.19).

Lateral Thorax

Assessment of the posterior thorax is extended to the lateral sides of the chest. The patient sits during examination of the lateral chest. Have the patient raise their arms, to improve access to lateral thoracic structures. Use inspection, palpation, and auscultation skills to examine the lateral thorax (see Figure 33.23, *B*). Do not assess excursion laterally. Normally, the breath sounds heard are vesicular.

Anterior Thorax

The anterior thorax is inspected for the same features as the posterior thorax. The patient sits or lies down with the head elevated. Observe the accessory muscles of breathing: sternocleidomastoid, trapezius, and abdominal muscles. The accessory muscles move little with normal passive breathing. When an adult patient requires effort to breathe as a result of strenuous exercise or disease (e.g., COPD), the accessory muscles and abdominal muscles contract. Some patients produce a grunting sound. In children, an increased effort to breathe can cause an increased use of accessory muscles of the neck and chest, resulting in nasal flaring, tracheal tug (indrawing of the suprasternal area), and chest wall retractions. Children sometimes produce an audible wheeze or barking sounds.

Observe the width of the costal angle; it is usually larger than 90 degrees between the two costal margins. Observe the breathing pattern. Normal breathing is quiet and barely audible near the open mouth. Most often, respiratory rate and rhythm are assessed anteriorly (see Chapter 31). The respirations of patients with male genitalia are usually diaphragmatic, whereas those of patients with female genitalia are more costal. Accurate assessment occurs as a patient breathes passively.

Palpate the anterior thoracic muscles and skeleton for lumps, masses, tenderness, or unusual movement. The sternum and xiphoid are relatively inflexible. Place the thumbs parallel along the costal margin approximately 6 cm apart with the palms touching the anterolateral chest. Push the thumbs toward the midline to create a skin fold. As the patient inhales deeply, the thumbs normally separate approximately 3 to 5 cm, with each side expanding equally.

Assess tactile fremitus over the anterior chest wall. Anterior findings differ from posterior findings because of the heart and female breast tissue. Fremitus is felt next to the sternum at the second intercostal space, at the level of the bronchial bifurcation. It decreases over the heart, lower thorax, and breast tissue.

BOX 33.19 PATIENT TEACHING

Lung Assessment

Objectives
- Patient describes warning signs of lung disease.
- Children receive routine childhood immunizations.
- Older persons receive influenza and pneumonia vaccines annually.
- Patients will verbalize an understanding of air pollutants in the home and the importance of a smoke-free environment at home and in the community.
- Patient with chronic obstructive pulmonary disease (COPD) clears airways more effectively and reports less shortness of breath.

Teaching Strategies
- Explain risk factors for chronic lung disease and lung cancer, including cigarette smoking, history of smoking for over 20 years, exposure to environmental pollution, and radiation exposure from occupational, medical, and environmental sources. Exposure to radon and asbestos also increases risk, especially for cigarette smokers. Other risk factors include certain metals (arsenic, cadmium, chromium), some organic chemicals, and tuberculosis. Exposure to second-hand cigarette smoke increases risk for nonsmokers.
- Share brochures on lung cancer from the Canadian Cancer Society with patient and their caregiver(s).
- Discuss warning signs of lung cancer, such as a persistent cough, sputum streaked with blood, chest pains, and recurrent attacks of pneumonia or bronchitis.
- Counsel parents of young children on benefits from receiving annual influenza and routine childhood vaccinations.
- Counsel older persons on benefits from receiving annual influenza and pneumonia vaccinations because of their greater susceptibility to respiratory infection.
- Instruct patient with COPD in coughing and pursed-lip breathing exercises.
- Refer individuals at risk for tuberculosis to visit clinics or health care centres for skin testing.

Evaluation
- Have patient describe risk factors for lung disease and cancer.
- Ask patient to identify any known risks for cancer.
- Ask patient to name warning signs for cancer.
- In a follow-up visit, review patient's immunization record.
- Observe patient performing breathing exercises and coughing.

Auscultation of the anterior thorax follows a systematic pattern (see Figure 33.23, *C*). Have the patient sit, if possible, to maximize chest expansion. Give special attention to the lower lobes, where mucous secretions commonly gather. Listen for bronchovesicular and vesicular sounds above and below the clavicles and along the lung periphery. Auscultate also for bronchial sounds, which are loud, high-pitched, and hollow sounding, with expiration lasting longer than inspiration (3:2 ratio). Normally, this sound is heard over the trachea.

Use a systematic pattern when comparing the right and left sides (see Figure 33.23). Compare lung sounds in one region on one side of the body with sounds in the same region on the opposite side of the body.

HEART

Findings from the assessment of heart function are compared with findings from the vascular assessment (see later section). Alterations in either system sometimes manifest as changes in the other. Some patients with signs or symptoms of cardiac disorders have a life-threatening condition requiring immediate attention. In this case, it is vital to act quickly and conduct only the portions of the examination that are absolutely necessary. When a patient is more stable, a more thorough assessment can be conducted. The nursing history (Table 33.20) provides data to help interpret physical findings.

Cardiac function is assessed through the anterior thorax. In the adult, the heart is located in the centre of the chest (precordium), behind and to the left of the sternum, with a small section of the right atrium extending to the right of the sternum. The base of the heart is the upper portion, and the apex is the bottom tip. The surface of the right ventricle composes most of the heart's anterior surface. A section of the left ventricle shapes the left anterior side of the apex. The apex actually touches the anterior chest wall at approximately the fourth to fifth intercostal space just medial to the left midclavicular line. This is where the **apical impulse** can be palpated, also referred to as the **point of maximal impulse (PMI)**.

An infant's heart is positioned more horizontally. The apex of the heart is at the third or fourth intercostal space, just to the left of the midclavicular line. By the age of 7 years, a child's PMI is in the same location as the adult's. In tall, slender individuals, the heart hangs more vertically and is positioned more centrally. With increased stockiness and shortness, the heart tends to lie more to the left and horizontally (Jarvis et al., 2019, pp. 512–513).

To assess heart function, a clear understanding of the cardiac cycle and associated physiological events is of utmost importance. The heart normally pumps blood through its four chambers in a methodical, even sequence. Events on the left side occur just before those on the right. As blood flows through each chamber, the valves open and close, the pressures within the chambers rise and fall, and the chambers contract. Each event creates a physiological sign. Both sides of the heart function in a coordinated fashion.

There are two phases to the cardiac cycle: systole and diastole. During *systole*, the ventricles contract and eject blood from the left ventricle into the aorta and from the right ventricle into the pulmonary artery. During *diastole*, the ventricles relax and the atria contract to move blood into the ventricles and fill the coronary arteries.

Heart sounds occur in relation to physiological events in the cardiac cycle. As systole begins, ventricular pressure rises and closes the mitral and tricuspid valves. Valve closure causes the first heart sound (S_1), often described as "lub." The ventricles then contract, and blood flows through the aorta and pulmonary circulation. After the ventricles empty, ventricular pressure falls below that in the aorta and pulmonary artery. This allows the aortic and pulmonic valves to close, causing the second heart sound (S_2), described as "dub." As ventricular pressure continues to fall, it drops below that of the atria. The mitral and tricuspid valves reopen to allow ventricular filling. Rapid ventricular filling creates a third heart sound (S_3), heard more often in children and young adults. An S_3 is also an abnormality in adults over 30 years of age. A fourth heart sound (S_4) occurs when the atria contract to enhance ventricular filling. An S_4 is heard in healthy older persons, children, and athletes, but it is not normal in adults. Because S_4 also indicates an abnormal condition, it needs to be reported to a health care provider.

Inspection and Palpation

Before the examination, ensure that the patient is relaxed and comfortable. Explain the procedure to relieve the patient's anxiety. An anxious or uncomfortable patient will have mild tachycardia, which will lead to inaccurate findings.

Use the skills of inspection and palpation simultaneously. The examination begins with the patient in the supine position or with the upper body elevated 45 degrees because patients with heart disease frequently

TABLE 33.20   Nursing History for Heart Assessment

Assessment Category	Rationale
Determine history of smoking, alcohol intake, caffeine intake, use of prescriptive and recreational drugs, exercise habits, and dietary patterns and intake (including fat and sodium intake).	Smoking, alcohol ingestion, cocaine use, lack of regular exercise, and intake of foods high in carbohydrates, fats, and cholesterol are risk factors for cardiovascular disease. Caffeine can cause heart dysrhythmias.
Determine if patient is taking medications for cardiovascular function (e.g., antidysrhythmics, antihypertensives) and if patient knows their purpose, dosage, and adverse effects.	Knowledge enables nurse to assess adherence to drug therapies. Medications sometimes affect vital sign values.
Assess for chest pain or discomfort, palpitations, excess fatigue, cough, dyspnea, leg pain or cramps, edema of feet, cyanosis, fainting, and orthopnea. Ask if symptoms occur at rest or during exercise.	These are key symptoms of heart disease. Cardiovascular function is sometimes adequate during rest but not during exercise.
If patient reports chest pain, determine if it is cardiac in nature. Angina pain is usually a deep pressure or ache that is substernal and diffuse, radiating to one or both arms, neck, or jaw.	Assessment determines nature of pain and need to initiate care immediately.
Determine whether patient has a stressful lifestyle. What physical demands or emotional stress exists?	Repeated exposure to stress increases risk for heart disease.
Assess family history for heart disease, diabetes, high cholesterol levels, hypertension, stroke, or rheumatic heart disease.	Factors increase risk for heart disease.
Ask patient about history of heart trouble (e.g., heart failure, congenital heart disease, coronary artery disease, dysrhythmias, murmurs).	Knowledge reveals patient's level of understanding of condition. A pre-existing condition influences examination techniques used, as well as findings to expect.
Determine whether patient has pre-existing diabetes, lung disease, obesity, or hypertension.	These disorders alter heart function.

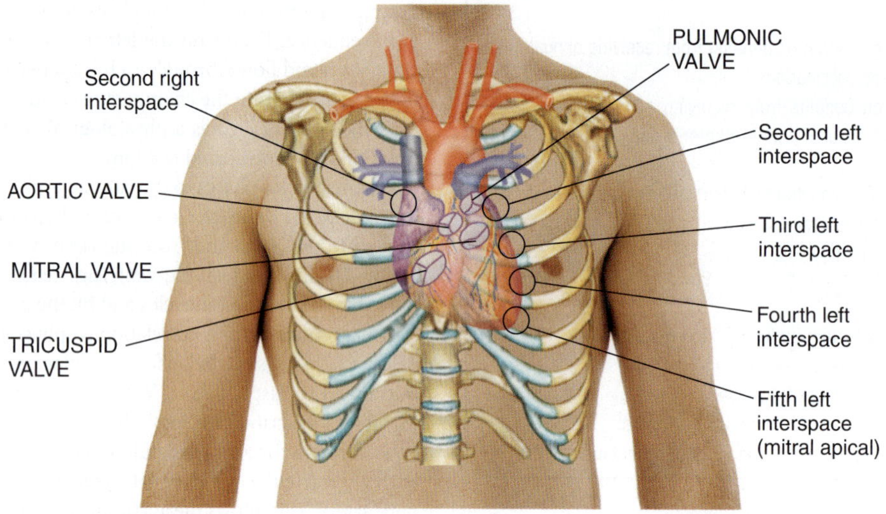

FIGURE 33.25 Areas for auscultation of the heart. (From Ball, J. W., Dains, J. E., Flynn, J. A., et al. [2019]. *Seidel's guide to physical examination* [9th ed.]. Mosby.)

suffer shortness of breath while lying flat. Stand at the patient's right side. Do not let the patient talk, especially when auscultating heart sounds. Good lighting in the room is essential.

During inspection and palpation, look for visible pulsations and exaggerated lifts, and palpate for the apical impulse and any source of vibrations (thrills). Follow an orderly sequence, beginning with assessment of the base of the heart and moving toward the apex. First inspect the angle of Louis, which lies between the sternal body and manubrium, and feel the ridge in the sternum approximately 5 cm below the sternal notch. Slip the fingers along the angle on each side of the sternum to feel adjacent ribs. The intercostal spaces are just below each rib. The second intercostal space allows identification of each of the anatomical landmarks (Figure 33.25). The second intercostal space on the right is the aortic area, and the left second intercostal space is the pulmonic area. Deeper palpation is needed to feel the spaces in obese or heavily muscled patients. After locating the pulmonic area, move the fingers down

the patient's left sternal border to the third intercostal space, called the *second pulmonic area*. The tricuspid area is located at the fourth or fifth intercostal space along the sternum. To find the apical or mitral area, locate the fifth intercostal space just to the left of the sternum and move the fingers laterally, to the left midclavicular line. Locate the apical area with the palm of the hand or the fingertips. Normally, the apical pulse is felt as a light tap in an area 1 to 2 cm in diameter at the apex (Figure 33.26). Another landmark is the epigastric area at the tip of the sternum. Typically, this is used to palpate for aortic abnormalities.

Locate the six anatomical landmarks of the heart and inspect and palpate each area. Look for the appearance of pulsations, viewing each area over the chest at an angle to the side. Normally, pulsations will not be seen, except perhaps at the PMI in thin patients or at the epigastric area as a result of abdominal aorta pulsation. Use the proximal halves of the four fingers together, and then alternate this with the ball of the hand to palpate for pulsations. Touch the areas gently to

FIGURE 33.26 Palpation of apical pulse. (From Ball, J. W., Dains, J. E., Flynn, J. A., et al. [2019]. *Seidel's guide to physical examination* [9th ed.]. Mosby.)

allow movements to lift the hand. Normally, no pulsations or vibrations are felt in the second, third, or fourth intercostal spaces. Loud murmurs cause a vibration. Time palpated pulsations or vibrations and their occurrence in relation to systole or diastole by auscultating heart sounds simultaneously.

The apical impulse or PMI should be felt easily. If it is hard to find, have the patient roll onto their left side, moving the heart closer to the chest wall. Estimate the size of the heart by noting the diameter of the PMI and its position relative to the midclavicular line. In cases of serious heart disease, the cardiac muscle enlarges, with the PMI found to the left of the midclavicular line. The PMI is sometimes difficult to find in an older person because the chest deepens in its anteroposterior diameters. It is also difficult to find in muscular or overweight patients. An infant's PMI is usually found near the third or fourth intercostal space. It is easy to palpate because of the child's thin chest wall.

Auscultation

Auscultation of the heart enables detection of normal heart sounds, extra heart sounds, and murmurs. Concentrate on detecting low-intensity sounds created by valve closures. To begin auscultation, eliminate all sources of room noise and explain the procedure to the patient to reduce their anxiety. Follow a systematic pattern beginning at the aortic area and inching the stethoscope across each of the anatomical sites (Figure 33.27). Listen for the complete cycle ("lub-dub") of heart sounds clearly at each location. Then repeat the sequence using the bell of the stethoscope. Sometimes the patient will assume three different positions during the examination (see Figure 33.27): sitting up and leaning forward (good for all areas and to hear high-pitched murmurs), supine (good for all areas), and left lateral recumbent (good for all areas; best position for hearing low-pitched sounds in diastole).

Learn to identify the first (S_1) and second (S_2) heart sounds. At normal rates, S_1 occurs after the long diastolic pause and preceding the short systolic pause. S_1 is high-pitched, dull in quality, and heard best at the apex. If it is difficult to hear S_1, time it in relation to the carotid pulsation. S_2 follows the short systolic pause and precedes the long diastolic pause; it is best heard at the aortic area.

Auscultate for rate and rhythm after hearing both sounds clearly. Each combination of S_1 and S_2 or "lub-dub" counts as one heartbeat. Count the rate for 1 minute, and listen for the interval between S_1 and S_2, and then the time between S_2 and the next S_1. A regular rhythm

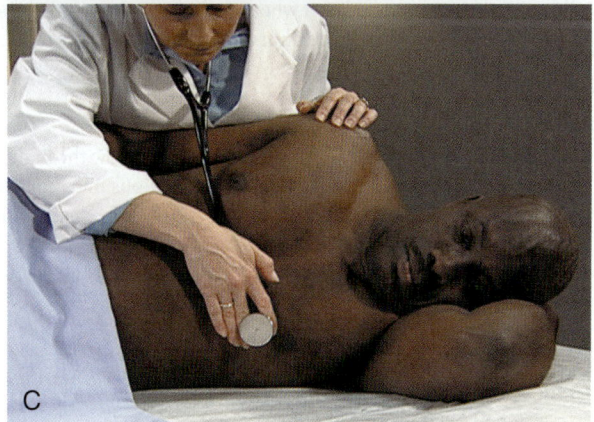

FIGURE 33.27 Sequence of patient positions for heart auscultation. **A,** Sitting. **B,** Supine. **C,** Left lateral recumbent. (From Ball, J. W., Dains, J. E., Flynn, J. A., et al. [2019]. *Seidel's guide to physical examination* [9th ed.]. Mosby.)

involves regular intervals of time between each sequence of beats. There is a distinct silent pause between S_1 and S_2. Failure of the heart to beat at regular successive intervals is a **dysrhythmia**. Some dysrhythmias are life-threatening.

When assessing an irregular heart rhythm, compare apical and radial pulse rates simultaneously to determine if a pulse deficit exists. Auscultate the apical pulse first, and then immediately palpate the radial pulse (one-examiner technique). Assess the apical and radial rates at the same time when two examiners are present. When a patient has a **pulse deficit**, the radial pulse is slower than the apical pulse because ineffective contractions fail to send pulse waves to the periphery. Report a difference in pulse rates to the health care provider immediately.

Assess for extra heart sounds at each auscultatory site. Use the bell of the stethoscope and listen for low-pitched extra heart sounds such as S_3 and S_4 gallops, clicks, and rubs. Auscultate over all anatomical areas. S_3, or a **ventricular gallop**, occurs just after S_2 at the end of ventricular diastole. This is due to a premature rush of blood into a ventricle that is stiff or dilated as a result of heart failure and hypertension. The combination of S_1, S_2, and S_3 sounds like "Ken-tuck'-y."

S_4, or an atrial gallop, occurs just before S_1 or ventricular systole. The sound of an S_4 is similar to that of "Tenn'-es-see." Physiologically, it is due to an atrial contraction pushing against a ventricle that is not accepting blood because of heart failure or other alterations. Extra heart sounds are heard more easily with the patient lying on their left side and the stethoscope at the apical site.

The final portion of the examination includes assessment for heart murmurs. **Murmurs** are sustained swishing or blowing sounds heard at the beginning, middle, or end of the systolic or diastolic phase. They are due to increased blood flow through a normal valve, forward flow through a stenotic valve or into a dilated vessel or heart chamber, or backward flow through a valve that fails to close. A murmur is asymptomatic or a sign of heart disease (Box 33.20). Murmurs are common in children. The following factors should be kept in mind when auscultating to detect murmurs:

- When a murmur is detected, auscultate the mitral, tricuspid, aortic, and pulmonic valve areas for placement in the cardiac cycle (timing), the place it is heard best (location), radiation, loudness, pitch, and quality.
- If a murmur occurs between S_1 and S_2, it is a systolic murmur. If it occurs between S_2 and the next S_1, it is a diastolic murmur.
- The location of a murmur is not necessarily directly over the valves. With experience, you will learn where each type of murmur is best heard. For example, mitral murmurs are heard best at the apex of the heart.
- To assess for radiation, listen over areas beside where it is heard best. Murmurs are also heard over the neck or back.
- Intensity or loudness is related to the rate of blood flow through the heart or the amount of blood regurgitated. In serious murmurs, feel for a thrust or intermittent palpable sensation at the auscultation site. A **thrill** is a continuous palpable sensation like the purring of a cat. Intensity is recorded in the following grades (Ball et al., 2019, p. 313):
  Grade 1: Barely audible in a quiet room
  Grade 2: Clearly audible but quiet
  Grade 3: Moderately loud
  Grade 4: Loud, with associated thrill
  Grade 5: Very loud, thrill easily palpable
  Grade 6: Louder, may be heard without a stethoscope, thrill palpable and visible
- A murmur is low, medium, or high in pitch, depending on the velocity of blood flow through the valves. A low-pitched murmur is heard best with the bell of the stethoscope. If it is heard best with the diaphragm, the murmur is high pitched.

The quality of a murmur refers to its characteristic pattern and sound. A crescendo murmur starts softly and builds in loudness. A decrescendo murmur starts loudly and then becomes less intense.

VASCULAR SYSTEM

Examination of the vascular system includes measuring the blood pressure (see Chapter 31) and assessing the integrity of the peripheral vascular system. Table 33.21 reviews the nursing history data collected before the examination. The skills of inspection, palpation, and auscultation are used to assess the vascular system, and portions of the vascular examination are performed during other body systems assessments.

BOX 33.20 PATIENT TEACHING

Heart Assessment

Objectives
- Patient describes risk factors for cardiovascular disease (CVD) and takes appropriate steps to eliminate risks from lifestyle.
- Patient with risk for CVD will seek support from appropriate caregivers.

Teaching Strategies
- Explain risk factors for CVD, including diabetes, arterial hypertension, chronic kidney disease, obesity, abdominal aortic aneurysm, clinical evidence of atherosclerosis, current smoking, inflammatory bowel disease, human immunodeficiency virus (HIV), hypertensive disorder of pregnancy, erectile dysfunction, chronic obstructive pulmonary disease, high dietary intake of saturated fat or cholesterol, lack of regular aerobic exercise, stressful lifestyle, and family history of premature CVD or dyslipidemia (Pearson et al., 2021).
- Refer patient (if appropriate) to resources available for controlling or reducing risks (e.g., dietitian, exercise class, stress reduction programs).
- Explain that lifestyle interventions play an important role in preventing and reducing risk of CVD. For example, research shows that achieving and maintaining a healthy body weight, healthy diet (e.g., Mediterranean diet, DASH diet), regular physical activity, smoking cessation, moderate alcohol consumption, and sufficient sleep duration are associated with CVD prevention and risk reduction (Pearson et al., 2021).
- Encourage patients with risk factors for CVD and individuals 40 years of age and older to have lipid testing as part of risk assessment for CVD (Pearson et al., 2021).
- Explain the components of lipid testing and results to patient. Common components of lipid testing include low-density lipoprotein (LDL) cholesterol, high-density lipoprotein (HDL) cholesterol, and triglycerides.
  - LDL cholesterol is often referred to as "bad cholesterol" as too much of it can lead to atherosclerotic plaques and CVD. In individuals with moderate to high risk for CVD, target LDL levels are ≤2.0 mmol/L.
  - HDL cholesterol is known as "good" cholesterol because it carries cholesterol from other parts of the body to the liver where it can be broken down and eliminated. Target HDL levels are generally ≥1.2 mmol/L.
  - Triglycerides are a type of fat the body uses. High levels of triglycerides and LDL can increase risk for CVD. Generally, target triglyceride levels are ≤1.7 mmol/L.
- Cardiovascular risk can be assessed using the Framingham Risk Score (calculator accessible at https://myhealth.alberta.ca/alberta/Pages/Heart-Disease-Risk-Calculator-Overview.aspx).
- Advise patient to avoid cigarette smoke because nicotine causes vasoconstriction.
- Advise patient to quit smoking because this lowers the risk for CVD.

Evaluation
- Ask patient to identify risk factors for CVD.
- Have patient develop and implement lifestyle interventions to reduce risk of CVD.
- Monitor patient's cholesterol level during follow-up appointments at the clinic or with a health care provider.

For example, the carotid pulse is checked after palpating the cervical lymph nodes. Signs and symptoms of arterial and venous insufficiency are noted when assessing the skin.

Blood Pressure

Blood pressure readings can vary by as much as 5–10 mm Hg between the arms (Jarvis et al., 2019, p. 163). The higher reading should be recorded. Systolic readings that differ by 10–15 mm Hg or more suggest atherosclerosis or arterial obstruction.

TABLE 33.21	Nursing History for Vascular Assessment
Assessment Category	**Rationale**
Determine if patient experiences leg cramps, numbness or tingling in extremities, sensation of cold hands or feet, pain in legs, or swelling or cyanosis of feet, ankles, or hand.	These signs and symptoms indicate vascular disease.
If patient experiences leg pain or cramping in lower extremities, ask if walking or standing for long periods, or during sleep, aggravates or relieves it.	Relationship of symptoms to exercise will clarify whether condition is vascular or musculoskeletal. Pain caused by a vascular condition tends to increase with activity. Musculoskeletal pain is not usually relieved when exercise ends.
Ask patients if they wear tight-fitting leg wear or hosiery and sit or lie in bed with legs crossed.	Tight hosiery around lower extremities and crossing legs can impair venous return.
Reconsider previous heart risk factors (e.g., smoking, exercise, nutritional problems).	These predispose patient to vascular disease.
Assess medical history for heart disease, hypertension, phlebitis, diabetes, or varicose veins.	Circulatory and vascular disorders influence findings gathered during the examination.

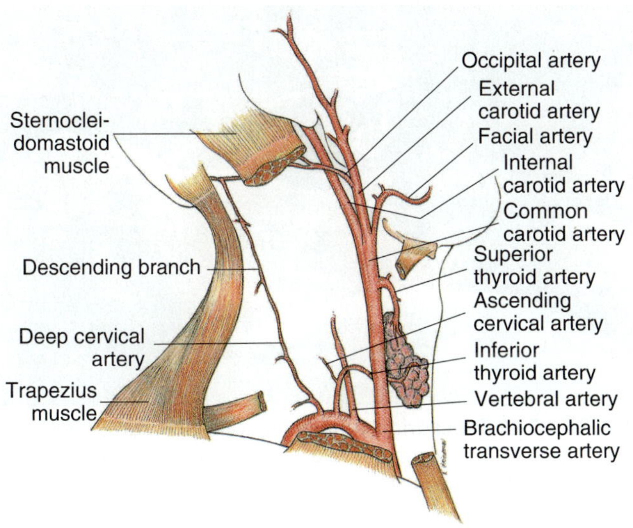

FIGURE 33.28 Anatomical position of the carotid artery.

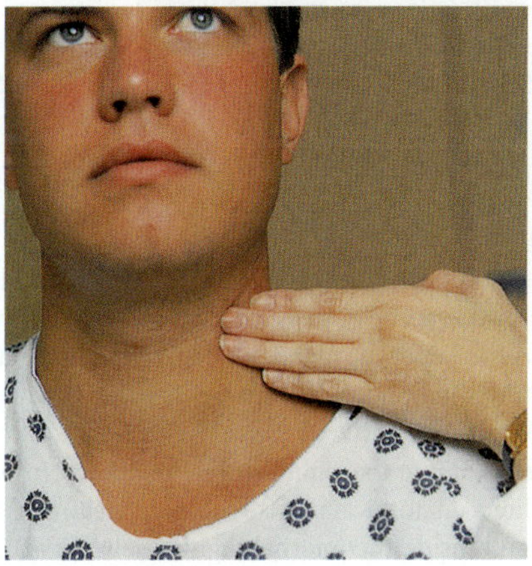

FIGURE 33.29 Palpation of internal carotid artery along the margin of the sternocleidomastoid muscle.

Carotid Arteries

When the left ventricle pumps blood into the aorta, the arterial system transmits pressure waves. The carotid arteries reflect heart function better than peripheral arteries because their pressure correlates with that of the aorta. The carotid artery supplies oxygenated blood to the head and neck (Figure 33.28). The overlying sternocleidomastoid muscle protects the carotid artery.

To examine the carotid arteries, have the patient sit or lie supine with the head of the bed elevated 30 degrees. Examine one carotid artery at a time. If both arteries are simultaneously occluded during palpation, the patient will lose consciousness as a result of inadequate circulation to the brain. The carotid arteries should not be palpated or massaged vigorously because the carotid sinus is located at the bifurcation of the common carotid arteries in the upper third of the neck. This sinus sends impulses along the vagus nerve. Its stimulation causes a reflex drop in heart rate and blood pressure, which causes syncope or circulatory arrest. This is a particular problem for older persons.

Begin inspection of the neck for obvious pulsation of the artery. Have the patient turn their head slightly away from the artery being examined. Sometimes the wave of the pulse is visible. The carotid is the only site for assessing the quality of a pulse wave. An absent pulse wave indicates arterial occlusion (blockage) or stenosis (narrowing).

To palpate the pulse, ask the patient to look straight ahead or turn their head slightly toward the side being examined. Turning relaxes the sternocleidomastoid muscle. Slide the tips of the index and middle fingers around the medial edge of the sternocleidomastoid muscle. Gently palpate to avoid occlusion of circulation (Figure 33.29).

The normal carotid pulse is localized rather than diffuse. As a strong pulse, the carotid has a thrusting quality. As the patient breathes, no change occurs. Rotation of the neck or a shift from a sitting to a supine position does not change the carotid artery's quality. Both carotid arteries are normally equal in pulse rate, rhythm, and strength and are equally elastic. Diminished or unequal carotid pulsations indicate atherosclerosis or other forms of arterial disease.

The carotid is the most commonly auscultated pulse. Auscultation is especially important for a middle-aged or an older person suspected of having cerebrovascular disease. When the lumen of a blood vessel is narrowed, this disturbs blood flow. As blood passes through the narrowed section, this creates turbulence, causing a blowing or swishing sound. The blowing sound is called a bruit (pronounced "brew-ee").

Place the bell of the stethoscope over the carotid artery at the lateral end of the clavicle and the posterior margin of the sternocleidomastoid muscle. Have the patient turn their head slightly away from the side being examined (Figure 33.30). Ask the patient to hold their breath for a moment so that breath sounds do not obscure a bruit. Normally, no sounds are heard during carotid auscultation. Palpate the artery lightly for a thrill (palpable bruit) if a bruit is audible.

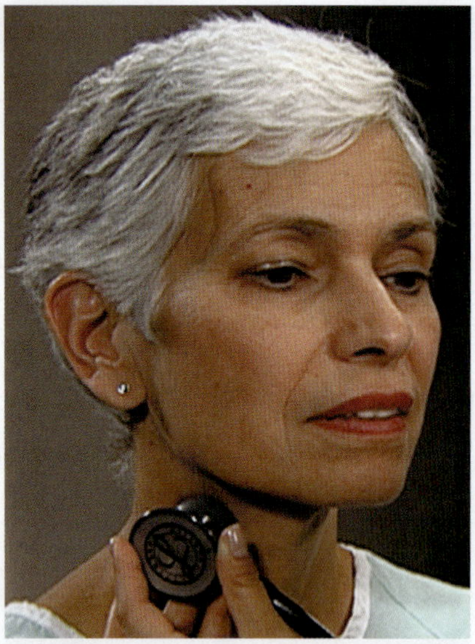

FIGURE 33.30 Auscultation for carotid artery bruit. (From Ball, J. W., Dains, J. E., Flynn, J. A., et al. [2019]. *Seidel's guide to physical examination* [9th ed.]. Mosby.)

Jugular Veins

The most accessible veins for examination are the internal and external jugular veins in the neck. Both veins drain bilaterally from the head and neck into the superior vena cava. The external jugular vein lies superficially and is just above the clavicle. The internal jugular vein lies deeper, along the carotid artery.

It is best to examine the right internal jugular vein because it follows a more direct anatomical path to the right atrium of the heart. The column of blood inside the internal jugular vein serves as a manometer, reflecting pressure in the right atrium. The higher the column, the greater the venous pressure. Raised venous pressure reflects right-sided heart failure.

Normally, when a patient lies in the supine position, the external jugular vein distends and becomes easily visible. In contrast, the jugular veins normally flatten when the patient is in a sitting or standing position. Some patients with heart disease, however, have distended jugular veins when sitting.

To measure venous pressure, inspect the jugular veins. Blood volume, the capacity of the right atrium to receive blood and send it to the right ventricle, and the ability of the right ventricle to contract and force blood into the pulmonary artery all influence venous pressure. Any factor resulting in greater blood volume within the venous system results in elevated venous pressure. Assess venous pressure by using the following steps:

1. Ask the patient to lie supine with the head elevated 30 to 45 degrees (semi-Fowler's position).
2. Expose the neck and upper thorax. Use a pillow to align the head. Avoid neck hyperextension or flexion, to ensure that the vein is not stretched or kinked (Figure 33.31).
3. Usually pulsations are not evident with the patient sitting up. As the patient slowly leans back into a supine position, the level of venous pulsations begins to rise above the level of the manubrium as much as 1 or 2 cm as the patient reaches a 45-degree angle. Measure venous pressure by measuring the vertical distance between the angle of Louis and the highest level of the visible point of the internal jugular vein pulsation.
4. Use two rulers. Line up the bottom edge of a regular ruler with the top of the area of pulsation in the jugular vein. Then take a centimetre ruler and align it perpendicular to the first ruler at the level of

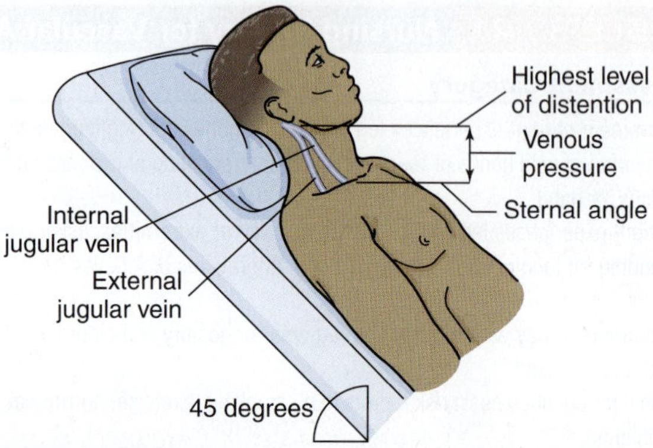

FIGURE 33.31 Position of patient to assess jugular vein distension. (From Ball, J. W., Dains, J. E., Flynn, J. A., et al. [2019]. *Seidel's guide to physical examination* [9th ed.]. Mosby.)

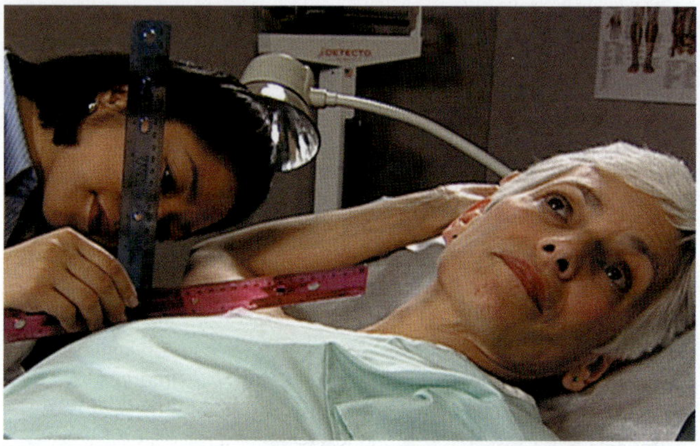

FIGURE 33.32 Measuring jugular venous pressure. (From Ball, J. W., Dains, J. E., Flynn, J. A., et al. [2019]. *Seidel's guide to physical examination* [9th ed.]. Mosby.)

the sternal angle. Measure in centimetres the distance between the second ruler and the sternal angle (Figure 33.32).

5. Repeat the same measurement on the other side. Bilateral pressures higher than 2.5 cm are considered elevated and are a sign of right-sided heart failure. One-sided pressure elevation is due to obstruction.

Peripheral Arteries and Veins

To examine the peripheral vascular system, first assess the adequacy of blood flow to the extremities by measuring arterial pulses and inspecting the condition of the skin and nails. Next assess the integrity of the venous system. Assess the arterial pulses in the extremities to determine sufficiency of the entire arterial circulation.

Factors such as coagulation disorders, local trauma or surgery, constricting casts or bandages, and systemic diseases impair circulation to the extremities (Table 33.22). Discuss risk factors and ways to monitor for circulatory conditions with the patient (Box 33.21).

Peripheral Arteries. Each peripheral artery is examined using the distal pads of the second and third fingers. The thumb helps anchor the brachial and femoral artery. Apply firm pressure but avoid occluding a pulse. When a pulse is difficult to find, it helps to vary pressure and feel all around the pulse site. Be sure not to palpate your own pulse.

Routine vital signs usually include assessment of the rate and rhythm of the radial artery because it is easily accessible. Count the pulse for either 30 seconds or a full minute, depending on the character of the

TABLE 33.22	Indicators for Assessing Local Blood Flow
Indicator	**Rationale**
Systemic diseases (e.g., arteriosclerosis, atherosclerosis, diabetes)	Diseases result in changes in integrity of walls of arteries and smaller blood vessels.
Coagulation disorders (e.g., thrombosis, embolus)	Blood clot causes mechanical obstruction to blood flow.
Local trauma or surgery (e.g., contusion, fracture, vascular surgery)	Direct manipulation of vessels or localized edema impairs blood flow.
Application of constricting devices (e.g., casts, dressings, elastic bandages, restraints)	Constriction causes tourniquet effect, impairing blood flow to areas below site of constriction.

BOX 33.21 PATIENT TEACHING
Vascular Assessment

Objectives
- Patient will know normal blood pressure range for age and compare it with own blood pressure readings to identify normalcy of blood pressure.
- Patient with vascular insufficiency will avoid activities that worsen circulatory status.

Teaching Strategies
- Tell patient the blood pressure reading. Explain the normal reading for the patient's age. Discuss implications of abnormalities.
- Instruct patient with risk or evidence of vascular insufficiency in the lower extremities to avoid wearing tight clothing over the lower body or legs, to avoid sitting or standing for long periods, to walk regularly, and to elevate feet when sitting.
- Advise patient to avoid cigarette smoking because nicotine causes vasoconstriction.
- Identify patients with hypertension; they sometimes benefit from regular monitoring of blood pressure (daily, weekly, or monthly). Teach patients how to use home monitoring kits (see Chapter 31).

Evaluation
- Ask patient to identify if blood pressure reading is within normal limits for age.
- Have patient with vascular insufficiency describe precautions to take to avoid further circulatory deficiency.
- Have patient demonstrate self-monitoring of blood pressure.

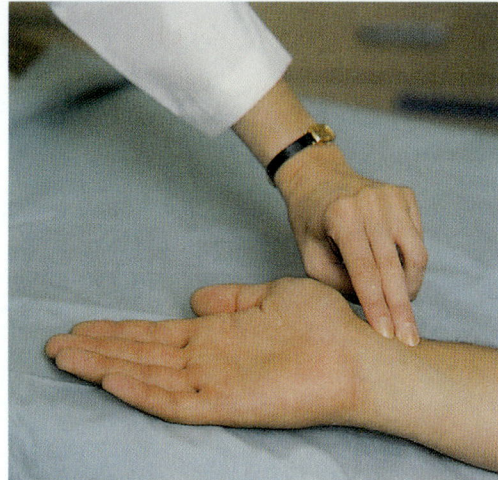
FIGURE 33.33 Palpation of radial pulse.

pulse. Always count an irregular pulse for 60 seconds. With palpation, normally the pulse wave is felt at regular intervals. When an interval is interrupted by an early, late, or missed beat, the pulse rhythm is irregular. In emergencies, health care providers usually assess the carotid artery because it is accessible and most useful in evaluating heart activity. To check local circulatory status of tissues, palpate the peripheral arteries long enough to note that a pulse is present.

Assess each peripheral artery for elasticity of the vessel wall, strength, and equality. The arterial wall is normally elastic, making it easily palpable. After depressing the artery, it will spring back to shape when the pressure is released. An abnormal artery is hard, inelastic, or calcified.

The strength of a pulse is a measurement of the force at which blood is ejected against the arterial wall. Some examiners use a scale rating from 0 to 4+ for the strength of a pulse (Ball et al., 2019, p. 363):

0   Absent, not palpable
1+   Pulse diminished, barely palpable
2+   Expected/normal
3+   Full pulse, increased
4+   Bounding pulse

All peripheral pulses need to be measured for equality and symmetry. Compare the left radial pulse with that of the right, and so on. Lack of symmetry indicates impaired circulation, such as a localized obstruction or an abnormally positioned artery.

In the upper extremities, the brachial artery channels blood to the radial and ulnar arteries of the forearm and hand. If circulation in this artery becomes blocked, the hands will not receive adequate blood flow. If circulation in the radial or ulnar arteries becomes impaired, the hand will still receive adequate perfusion. An interconnection between the radial and ulnar arteries guards against arterial occlusion.

To locate pulses in the arm, have the patient sit or lie down. Find the radial pulse along the radial side of the forearm at the wrist. Thin individuals have a groove lateral to the flexor tendon of the wrist. Feel the radial pulse with light palpation in the groove (Figure 33.33). The ulnar pulse is on the opposite side of the wrist and feels less prominent (Figure 33.34). Palpate the ulnar pulse only when evaluating arterial insufficiency to the hand.

To palpate the brachial pulse, find the groove between the biceps and triceps muscle above the elbow at the antecubital fossa (Figure 33.35). The artery runs along the medial side of the extended arm. Palpate the artery with the fingertips of the first three fingers in the muscle groove.

The femoral artery is the primary artery in the leg, delivering blood to the popliteal, posterior tibial, and dorsalis pedis arteries. An interconnection between the posterior tibial and dorsalis pedis arteries guards against local arterial occlusion.

Find the femoral pulse with the patient lying down with the inguinal area exposed (Figure 33.36). The femoral artery runs below the inguinal ligament, midway between the symphysis pubis and the anterosuperior iliac spine. Sometimes deep palpation is required to feel the pulse. Bimanual palpation is effective in patients with obesity. Place the

FIGURE 33.34 Palpation of ulnar pulse.

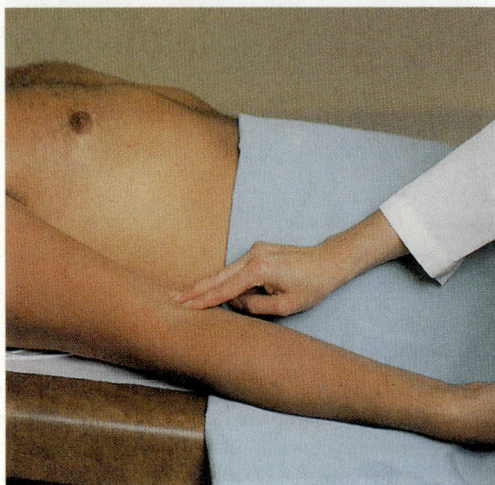

FIGURE 33.37 Palpation of popliteal pulse.

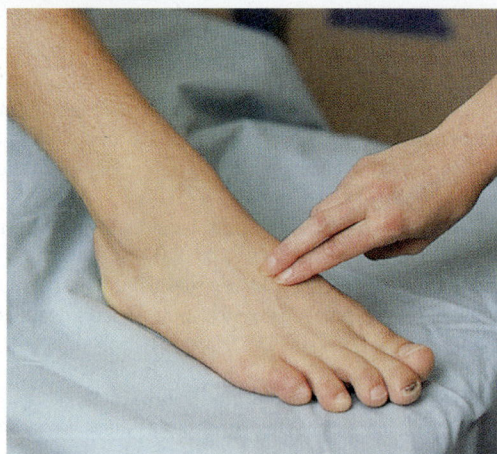

FIGURE 33.35 Palpation of brachial pulse.

FIGURE 33.38 Palpation of dorsalis pedis pulse.

FIGURE 33.36 Palpation of femoral pulse.

With the patient's foot relaxed, locate the dorsalis pedis pulse. The artery runs along the top of the foot in line with the groove between the extensor tendons of the great toe and first toe (Figure 33.38). To find the pulse, place the fingertips between the first and second toes and slowly move up the dorsum of the foot. This pulse is sometimes congenitally absent.

Find the posterior tibial pulse on the inner side of each ankle (Figure 33.39). Place the fingers behind and below the medial malleolus (ankle bone). With the patient's foot relaxed and slightly extended, palpate the artery.

Tissue Perfusion. The condition of the skin, mucosa, and nail beds offers useful data about the status of circulatory blood flow. Examine the face and upper extremities, looking at the colour of the skin, mucosa, and nail beds. The presence of cyanosis requires special attention. Heart disease sometimes causes central cyanosis, which indicates poor arterial oxygenation. Some characteristics of this are a bluish discoloration of the lips, mouth, and conjunctivae. Blue lips, earlobes, and nail beds are signs of peripheral cyanosis, which indicates peripheral vasoconstriction. When cyanosis is present, consult with a health care provider to have laboratory testing of oxygen saturation to determine the severity of the condition. Examination of the nails involves inspection for clubbing, a bulging of the tissues at the nail base. Clubbing is due to insufficient oxygenation at the periphery resulting from conditions such as chronic emphysema and congenital heart disease.

fingertips of both hands on opposite sides of the pulse site. A pulsatile sensation is felt when the arterial pulsation pushes the fingertips apart.

The popliteal pulse runs behind the knee. Have the patient slightly flex the knee, with the foot resting on the examination table, or assume a prone position with the knee slightly flexed (Figure 33.37). Instruct the patient to keep leg muscles relaxed. Palpate with the fingers of both hands deeply into the popliteal fossa, just lateral to the midline. The popliteal pulse is difficult to locate.

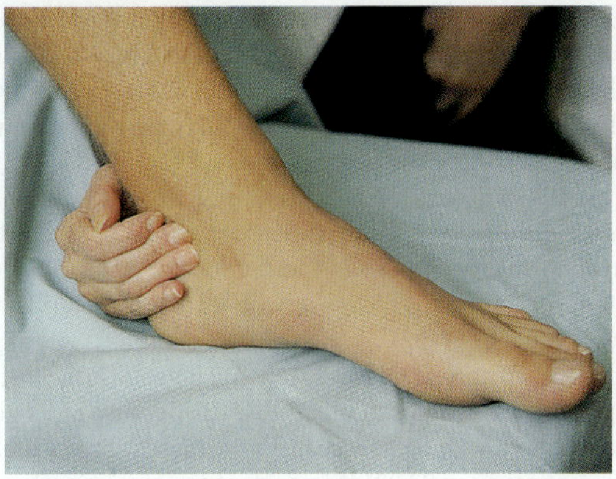

FIGURE 33.39 Palpation of posterior tibial pulse.

TABLE 33.23	**Signs of Venous and Arterial Insufficiency**	
Assessment Criterion	**Venous**	**Arterial**
Colour	Normal or cyanotic	Pale; worsened by elevation of extremity; dusky red when extremity is lowered
Temperature	Normal	Cool (blood flow blocked to extremity)
Pulse	Normal	Decreased or absent
Edema	Often marked	Absent or mild
Skin changes	Brown pigmentation around ankles	Thin, shiny skin; decreased hair growth; thickened nails

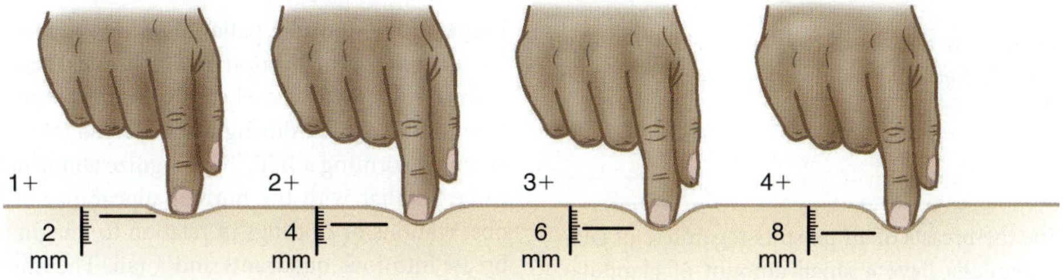

FIGURE 33.40 **Assessing for pitting edema.** (From Ball, J. W., Dains, J. E., Flynn, J. A., et al. [2019]. *Seidel's guide to physical examination* [9th ed.]. Mosby.)

Inspect the lower extremities for changes in colour, temperature, and condition of the skin indicating either arterial or venous alterations (Table 33.23). This is a good time to ask the patient about any history of pain in the legs. If an arterial occlusion is present, the patient has signs resulting from an absence of blood flow. Pain will be distal to the occlusion. The *P*s—pain, pallor, pulselessness, paresthesias, and paralysis—characterize an occlusion. Venous congestion causes tissue changes indicating an inadequate circulatory flow back to the heart.

During examination of the lower extremities, also inspect skin and nail texture; hair distribution on the lower legs, feet, and toes; the venous pattern; and scars, pigmentation, or ulcers. Palpate the legs and feet for colour and temperature. Also assess capillary refill. Measure capillary refill by blanching the nail bed with a substantial pressure for several seconds. Release the pressure, and observe the time elapsed before the nail regains its full colour. An acceptable capillary refill time is less than 2 seconds (Jarvis et al., 2019, p. 240).

The absence of hair growth over the legs indicates circulatory insufficiency. Chronic recurring ulcers of the feet or lower legs are a serious sign of circulatory insufficiency and require a health care provider's intervention.

Peripheral Veins. The status of the peripheral veins is assessed by asking the patient to assume sitting and standing positions. Assessment includes inspection and palpation for varicosities, peripheral edema, and phlebitis. Varicosities are superficial veins that become dilated, especially when the legs are in a dependent position. They are common in older persons because the veins normally fibrose, dilate, and stretch. They are also common in people who stand for prolonged periods. Varicosities in the anterior or medial part of the thigh and the posterolateral part of the calf are abnormal.

Dependent edema around the area of the feet and ankles is a sign of venous insufficiency or right-sided heart failure. Dependent edema

is common in older persons and individuals who spend a lot of time standing (e.g., waitresses, security guards, and nurses). To assess for pitting edema, use the index finger to press firmly for several seconds and then release over the medial malleolus or the shins. A depression left in the skin indicates edema. Grading 1+ through 4+ characterizes the severity of the edema (Figure 33.40).

Phlebitis is an inflammation of a vein that occurs commonly after trauma to the vessel wall, infection, immobilization, and prolonged insertion of IV catheters (see Chapter 40). Phlebitis promotes clot formation, a potentially dangerous situation because a clot within a deep vein of the leg can become dislodged and travel through the heart, causing a pulmonary embolus. To assess for phlebitis, inspect the calves for localized redness, tenderness, and swelling over vein sites. Gentle palpation of calf muscles reveals warmth, tenderness, and firmness of the muscle. Unilateral edema of the affected leg is one of the most reliable findings of phlebitis. Homan sign is not a reliable indicator of phlebitis. Performing the Homan sign test is contraindicated in patients with deep vein thrombosis. If a clot is present, it may become dislodged from its original site during this test, resulting in a pulmonary embolism.

Lymphatic System

Lymphatic drainage of the lower extremities is assessed during examination of the vascular system or during the female or male genital examination. Superficial and deep nodes drain the legs, but only two groups of superficial nodes are palpable. With the patient supine, palpate the area of the superficial inguinal nodes in the groin area (Figure 33.41). Then move the fingertips toward the inner thigh, feeling for any inferior nodes. Use a firm but gentle pressure when palpating over each lymphatic chain. Multiple nodes are not normally palpable, although a few soft, nontender nodes are not unusual. Enlarged, hardened, tender nodes reveal potential sites of infection or metastatic disease.

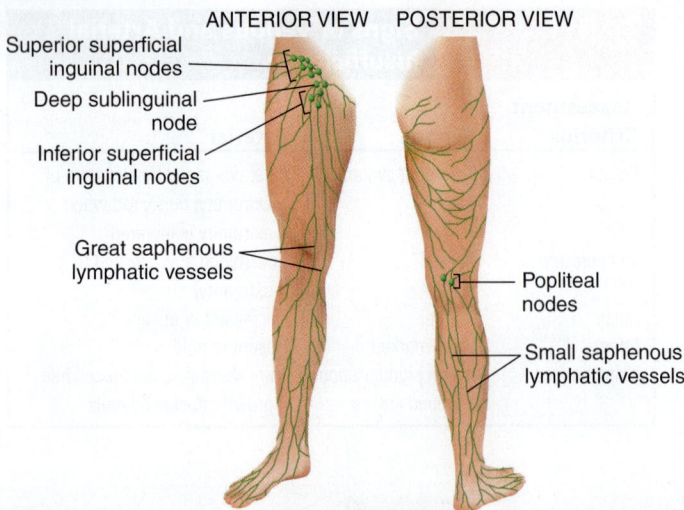

FIGURE 33.41 Inguinal lymph nodes. (From Ball, J. W., Dains, J. E., Flynn, J. A., et al. [2019]. *Seidel's guide to physical examination* [9th ed., Fig. 10.4]. Mosby.)

BREASTS

It is important to examine the breasts of all patients regardless of gender. Patients with male genitalia have a small amount of glandular tissue, a potential site for the growth of cancer cells, in the breast. In contrast, the majority of the female breast is glandular tissue.

Female Breasts

Breast cancer is the most common invasive cancer among Canadian women and is second to lung cancer as the leading cause of death from cancer in women (Canadian Cancer Society, 2022a). Early detection is the key to cure.

Recently published clinical practice guidelines have moved away from routine recommendation of annual clinical breast examinations (CBEs) by health care providers, as research has not proven CBEs to be an effective screening tool. However, CBE may still help in detecting abnormalities in breast tissue (Canadian Cancer Society, 2022a). Women are also encouraged to be aware of what is normal in their own breasts, through use of breast self-examination (BSE), so they can detect an abnormality (American Cancer Society, 2022). For a detailed overview of teaching BSE please see the textbook by Jarvis and colleagues (2014, pp. 421–422).

The patient's history (Table 33.24) should note normal developmental changes, as well as signs of breast disease. Because of its glandular structure, the breast undergoes changes during a woman's life. Knowing these changes (Box 33.22) is important to completing an accurate assessment. Both men and women should be encouraged to observe their breasts for changes.

Inspection. Have the patient remove the top gown or drape to allow simultaneous visualization of both breasts. Have the patient stand or sit with arms hanging loosely at their sides. If possible, place a mirror in front of the patient during inspection so they can see what to look for when performing a BSE. To recognize abnormalities, the patient needs to be familiar with the normal appearance of their breasts. Describe observations or findings in relation to imaginary lines that divide the breast into four quadrants and a tail. The lines cross at the centre of the nipple. Each tail extends outward from the upper outer quadrant (Figure 33.42).

Inspect the breasts for size and symmetry. Normally, the breasts extend from the third to the sixth ribs, with the nipple at the level of the fourth intercostal space. It is common for one breast to be smaller. However, inflammation or a mass causes a difference in size. As the person becomes older, the ligaments supporting the breast tissue weaken, causing the breasts to sag and the nipples to lower.

TABLE 33.24	Nursing History for Breast Assessment	
Assessment Category	**Rationale**	
Determine if woman is over age 50; has a personal or family history of breast cancer or other cancer; has a personal or family history of *BRCA* gene mutations; has dense breasts; is of Ashkenazi Jewish ancestry; has been exposed to ionizing radiation (i.e., cancer treatment); has been on hormone replacement therapy; has atypical hyperplasia; drinks more than one alcoholic beverage per day; is overweight or obese; is of high socioeconomic status; has early-onset menarche (before age 13) or late-age menopause (after age 52); never had children or gave birth to first child after age 30; or has used oral contraceptives.	These are risk factors for breast cancer (Canadian Cancer Society, 2022a).	
Ask if patient (both sexes) has noticed lump, thickening, pain, or tenderness of breast; discharge, distortion, retraction, or scaling of the nipple; or change in size of breast.	Potential signs and symptoms of breast cancer help the nurse to focus on specific areas of the breast during assessment.	
Determine patient's use of medications (oral contraceptives, digitalis, diuretics, steroids, or estrogen). Determine patient's caffeine intake.	Some medications cause nipple discharge. Hormones and caffeine cause fibrocystic changes in the breast.	
Determine patient's level of activity, alcohol intake, and weight.	Breast cancer incidence rates correlate with being overweight or obese (postmenopausal), physical inactivity, use of oral contraceptives, and consumption of one or more alcoholic beverages per day (Canadian Cancer Society, 2022a).	
Ask if patient performs breast self-examination (BSE). If so, determine time of month the patient performs examination in relation to menstrual cycle. Have patient describe or demonstrate method used.	The nurse's role is to educate patient about breast cancer and techniques for BSE.	
If patient reports a breast mass, ask about length of time since patient first noticed the lump. Does the lump come and go, or is it always present? Have there been changes in the lump (e.g., size, relationship to menses), and are there associated symptoms?	Information helps in determining nature of mass (e.g., breast cancer or fibrocystic disease).	

BOX 33.22 Normal Changes in the Breast During a Person's Lifespan

Puberty (8 to 20 Years)

Tanner staging (1–5) is a method of assessment for sexual maturity of adolescents (Jarvis et al., 2019, pp. 120–124; Tanner, 1962). Breasts mature in five stages. One breast may grow more rapidly than the other. The ages at which changes occur and rate of developmental progression vary.

Stage 1 (Preadolescent)

This stage involves elevation of the nipple only.

Stage 2

The breast and nipple elevate as a small mound, and the areolar diameters enlarge.

Stage 3

There is further enlargement and elevation of the breast and areola, with no separation of contour.

Stage 4

The areola and nipple project into the secondary mound above the level of the breast (does not occur in all girls).

Stage 5 (Mature Breast)

Only the nipple projects, and the areola recedes (varies in some individuals with female genitalia).

Young Adulthood (20 to 30 Years)

Breasts reach full (nonpregnant) size. Shape is generally symmetrical. Breasts are sometimes unequal in size.

Pregnancy

Breast size gradually enlarges to two to three times the previous size. Nipples enlarge and become erect. Areolae darken, and diameters increase. Superficial veins become prominent. The nipples expel a yellowish fluid (colostrum).

Menopause

Breasts shrink. Tissue becomes softer, sometimes flabby.

Older Women

Breasts become elongated, pendulous, and flaccid as a result of glandular tissue atrophy. The skin of the breasts tends to wrinkle, appearing loose and flabby. Nipples become smaller and flatter and lose erectile ability. Nipples sometimes invert because of shrinkage and fibrotic changes.

Data from Perry, S. E., Hockenberry, M. J., Lowdermilk, D. L., et al. (Eds.). (2017). *Maternal child nursing care in Canada* (2nd ed.). Mosby; Ball, J. W., Dains, J. E., Flynn, J. A., et al. (2019). *Seidel's guide to physical examination* (9th ed.). Mosby.

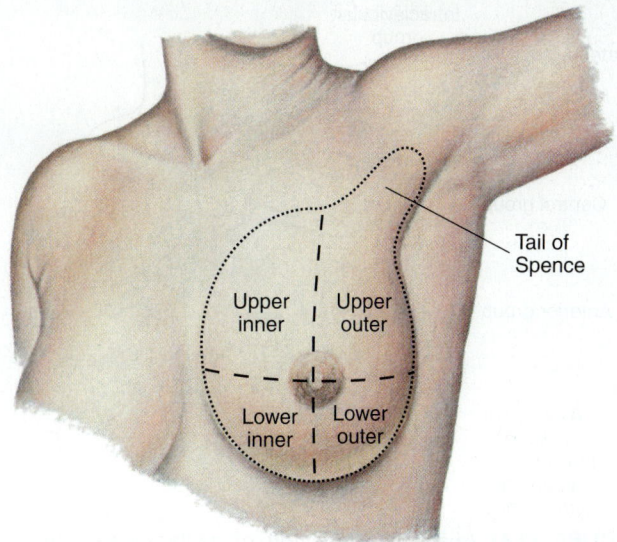

FIGURE 33.42 Quadrants of the left breast and axillary tail of Spence. (From Ball, J. W., Dains, J. E., Flynn, J. A., et al. [2019]. *Seidel's guide to physical examination* [9th ed.]. Mosby.)

Observe the contour or shape of the breasts, and note masses, flattening, retraction, or dimpling. Breasts vary in shape and can be convex, pendulous, or conical. Retraction or dimpling results from invasion of underlying ligaments by tumours. The ligaments fibrose and pull the overlying skin inward toward the tumour. Edema also changes the contour of the breasts. To bring out retraction or changes in the shape of breasts, ask the patient to assume three positions: raise their arms above their head, press their hands against their hips, and extend their arms straight ahead while sitting and leaning forward. Each manoeuvre causes a contraction of the pectoral muscles, which will accentuate the presence of any retraction.

Carefully inspect the skin for colour; venous pattern; and the presence of lesions, edema, or inflammation. Lift each breast when necessary to observe lower and lateral aspects for colour and texture changes. The breasts are the colour of neighbouring skin, and venous patterns are the same bilaterally. Venous patterns are easily visible in thin or pregnant women. Individuals with large breasts often have redness and excoriation of the undersurfaces caused by rubbing of skin surfaces.

Inspect the nipple and areola for size, colour, shape, discharge, and the direction the nipples point (Ball et al., 2019, pp. 378–382). The normal areolae are round or oval and nearly equal bilaterally. Colour ranges from pink to brown. In light-skinned individuals, the areola turns brown during pregnancy and remains dark. In dark-skinned individuals, the areola is brown before pregnancy. Normally, the nipples point in symmetrical directions, are everted, and have no drainage. If the nipples are inverted, ask if this has been a lifetime history. A recent inversion or inward turning of the nipple indicates an underlying growth. Rashes or ulcerations are not normal on the breast or nipples. Note any bleeding or discharge from the nipple. Clear yellow discharge 2 days after childbirth is common. While inspecting the breasts, explain the characteristics you see. Teach the patient the significance of abnormal signs or symptoms.

Palpation. Palpation is used to assess the condition of underlying breast tissue and lymph nodes. Breast tissue consists of glandular tissue, fibrous supportive ligaments, and fat. Glandular tissue is organized into lobes that end in ducts that open onto the nipple's surface. The largest portion of glandular tissue is in the upper outer quadrant and tail of each breast. Suspensory ligaments connect to skin and fascia underlying the breast to support the breast and maintain its upright position. Fatty tissue is located superficially and to the sides of the breast.

A large portion of lymph from the breasts drains into axillary lymph nodes. If cancerous lesions **metastasize** (spread), the nodes commonly become involved. Study the location of supraclavicular, infraclavicular, and axillary nodes (Figure 33.43). The axillary nodes drain lymph from the chest wall, breasts, arms, and hands. A tumour of one breast sometimes involves nodes on the opposite side, as well as those on the same side.

To palpate the lymph nodes, have the patient sit with arms at their sides and muscles relaxed. While facing the patient and standing on

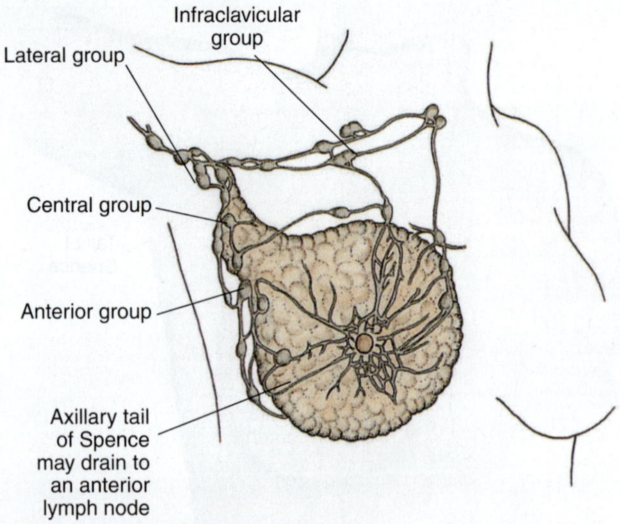

FIGURE 33.43 Anatomical position of axillary and clavicular lymph nodes.

Labels on figure:
Infraclavicular group
Lateral group
Central group
Anterior group
Axillary tail of Spence may drain to an anterior lymph node

the side being examined, support the patient's arm in a flexed position and abduct the arm from the chest wall. Place the free hand against the patient's chest wall and high in the axillary hollow. With the fingertips, press gently down over the surface of the ribs and muscles. Palpate the axillary nodes with the fingertips gently rolling soft tissue. Palpate four areas of the axilla: at the edge of the pectoralis major muscle along the anterior axillary line, the chest wall in the midaxillary area, the upper part of the humerus, and the anterior edge of the latissimus dorsi muscle along the posterior axillary line.

Normally, lymph nodes are not palpable. Carefully assess each area, and note their number, consistency, mobility, and size. The presence of one or two small, soft, nontender palpable nodes is normal. A palpable node feels like a small mass that is hard, tender, and immobile. Also palpate along the upper and lower clavicular ridges. Reverse the procedure for the patient's other side.

It is sometimes difficult for patients to learn to palpate for lymph nodes. Lying down with the arm abducted makes the area more accessible. Instruct the patient to use their left hand for the right axillary and clavicular areas. Take the patient's fingertips and move them in the proper fashion. Then have the patient use their right hand to palpate for nodes on the left side.

With the patient lying supine and one arm behind their head (alternating with each breast), palpate the patient's breast tissue. The supine position allows the breast tissue to flatten evenly against the chest wall. The patient raises their hand and places it behind their neck to further stretch and position breast tissue evenly. Place a small pillow or towel under the patient's shoulder blade to further position breast tissue.

The consistency of normal breast tissue varies widely. The breasts of a young patient are firm and elastic. In an older person, the tissue sometimes feels stringy and nodular. The patient's familiarity with the texture of their own breasts is very important. Patients gain this familiarity through BSE (Box 33.23).

If the patient reports a mass, examine the opposite breast to ensure an objective comparison of normal and abnormal tissue. Use the pads of the first three fingers to compress breast tissue gently against the chest wall, noting tissue consistency. Perform palpation systematically in one of three ways: (1) clockwise or counter-clockwise, forming small circles with the fingers along each quadrant and the tail; (2) using a vertical technique with the fingers moving up and down each quadrant; or (3) palpating from the centre of the breast in a radial fashion, returning to the areola to begin each spoke. Whatever approach used,

---

BOX 33.23   PATIENT TEACHING

Breast Assessment of Individuals With Female Genitalia

Objectives
- Patient will perform breast self-examination (BSE).
- Patient will have screening mammography performed at recommended intervals, beginning at age 50.
- Patient will identify signs and symptoms of breast cancer.
- Patient will identify signs and symptoms of benign (fibrocystic) breast disease.
- Patient will follow a low-fat diet.

Teaching Strategies
- Instruct patient on how to perform BSE
- Have patient perform return demonstration of BSE and offer the opportunity to ask questions.
- Explain recommended frequency of mammography and assessment by a health care provider.
- Discuss signs and symptoms of breast cancer.
- Discuss signs and symptoms of benign (fibrocystic) breast disease.
- Inform patient with obesity or who has a family history of breast cancer that they are at higher risk for the disease (Canadian Cancer Society, 2022a). Encourage dietary changes, including limiting meat consumption to well-trimmed, lean beef, pork, or lamb; removing skin from cooked chicken before eating it; selecting tuna and salmon packed in water and not oil; and using low-fat dairy products.

Evaluation
- Have patient demonstrate BSE.
- During follow-up visit, determine whether patient has had mammography performed.
- Ask patient to explain frequency of mammography.
- Have patient describe signs and symptoms of breast cancer compared with those of benign (fibrocystic) breast disease.

---

be sure to cover the entire breast and tail, directing attention to any areas of tenderness.

When palpating large, pendulous breasts, use a bimanual technique. Support the inferior portion of the breast in one hand while using the other hand to palpate breast tissue against the supporting hand.

During palpation, note the consistency of breast tissue. It normally feels dense, firm, and elastic. With menopause, breast tissue shrinks and becomes softer. The lobular feel of glandular tissue is normal. The lower edge of each breast sometimes feels firm and hard. This is the normal inframammary ridge and not a tumour. It helps to move the patient's hand so that the patient can feel normal tissue variations. Palpate abnormal masses to determine location in relation to quadrants, diameter in centimetres, shape (e.g., round or discoid), consistency (soft, firm, or hard), tenderness, mobility, and discreteness (clear or unclear boundaries).

Cancerous lesions are hard, fixed, nontender, irregular in shape, and usually unilateral. A common benign condition of the breast is **benign (fibrocystic) breast disease**. Bilateral lumpy, painful breasts and sometimes nipple discharge characterize this condition. Symptoms are more apparent during the menstrual period. When palpated, the cysts (lumps) are soft, well differentiated, and movable. Deep cysts feel hard.

Pay special attention when palpating the nipple and areola to assess for nodules, edema, ulceration or discharge. Palpate the entire surface gently. Use the thumb and index finger to compress the nipple, and note any discharge. During the examination of the nipple and areola,

TABLE 33.25	Nursing History for Abdominal Assessment
Assessment Category	**Rationale**
If patient has abdominal or low back pain, assess character of pain in detail (location, onset, frequency, precipitating factors, aggravating factors, type of pain, severity, course).	Pattern of characteristics of pain helps determine its source.
Carefully observe patient's movement and position, including lying still with knees drawn up, moving restlessly to find comfortable position, and lying on one side or sitting with knees drawn to chest.	Positions assumed by patient reveal nature and source of pain, including peritonitis, renal stone, and pancreatitis.
Assess normal bowel habits and stool character; ask if patient uses laxatives.	Data compared with physical findings help in identifying the cause and nature of elimination problems.
Determine if patient has had abdominal surgery, trauma, or diagnostic tests of gastrointestinal (GI) tract.	Surgical or traumatic alterations of abdominal organs cause changes in expected findings (e.g., position of underlying organs). Diagnostic tests change character of stool.
Assess if patient has had recent weight changes or intolerance to diet (e.g., nausea, vomiting, cramping, especially in last 24 hours).	Data possibly indicate alterations in upper GI tract (stomach or gallbladder) or lower colon.
Assess for difficulty in swallowing, belching, flatulence (gas), bloody emesis (hematemesis), black or tarry stools (melena), heartburn, diarrhea, or constipation.	These characteristic signs and symptoms indicate GI alterations.
Ask if patient takes anti-inflammatory medication (e.g., aspirin, ibuprofen, steroids) or antibiotics.	Pharmacological medications cause GI upset or bleeding.
Ask patient to locate tender areas before examination begins.	Assess painful areas last to minimize discomfort and anxiety.
Inquire about family history of cancer, kidney disease, alcoholism, hypertension, or heart disease.	Data possibly reveal risk for alterations identifiable during examination.
Determine if patient with female genitalia is pregnant; note last menstrual period.	Pregnancy causes changes in abdominal shape and contour.
Assess patient's usual intake of alcohol.	Chronic alcohol ingestion causes GI and liver problems.
Review patient's history for the following: health care occupation, hemodialysis, intravenous drug user, household or sexual contact with hepatitis B virus (HBV) carrier, more than one sex partner in previous 6 months, international traveller in area of high HBV infection rate.	These are risk factors for HBV exposure.

the nipple sometimes becomes erect with wrinkling of the areola. These changes are normal.

After completing the examination, have the patient demonstrate self-palpation. Observe the patient's technique and emphasize the importance of a consistent and systematic approach. Urge the patient to see their health care provider if they discover an abnormal mass during self-examination. The patient also needs to know all of the signs and symptoms of breast cancer.

Male Breasts

Examination of the male breast is relatively easy. Inspect the nipple and areola for nodules, edema, and ulceration. An enlarged male breast results from obesity or glandular enlargement. Breast enlargement in young individuals with male genitalia results from steroid use. Fatty tissue feels soft, whereas glandular tissue is firm. Use the same techniques to palpate for masses as those used in examination of the female breast.

> **SAFETY ALERT** Individuals with male genitalia, especially those who have a first-degree relative (e.g., mother, sister) with breast cancer, are at risk for breast cancer and need to palpate their breasts at regular intervals. In discussion with their health care provider, these individuals may also be scheduled for routine mammograms.

ABDOMEN

The abdominal examination is complex because of the number of organs located within and near the abdominal cavity. A thorough nursing history (Table 33.25) helps with interpretation of physical signs.

The examination includes an assessment of structures of the lower GI tract in addition to the liver, stomach, uterus, ovaries, kidneys, and bladder. Abdominal pain is one of the most common symptoms that patients report when seeking medical care. An accurate assessment requires matching patient history data with a careful assessment of the location of physical symptoms.

The organs are assessed anteriorly and posteriorly. A system of landmarks helps map out the abdominal region. The xiphoid process (tip of the sternum) is the upper boundary of the anterior abdominal region. The symphysis pubis marks the lower boundary. Divide the abdomen into four imaginary quadrants (Figure 33.44, A), and refer to assessment findings and record them in relation to each quadrant. Posteriorly, the lower ribs and heavy back muscles protect the kidneys, which are located from the T12 to L3 vertebrae (see Figure 33.44, B). The costovertebral angle formed by the last rib and vertebral column is a landmark used during kidney and liver palpation.

During the abdominal examination, the patient needs to relax. A tightening of abdominal muscles hinders palpation. Ask the patient to void before beginning. Be sure the room is warm, and drape the patient's upper chest and legs. The patient lies supine or in a dorsal recumbent position with arms at their sides and knees slightly bent. Place a pillow beneath the knees. If the patient places their arms under their head, the abdominal muscles tighten. Proceed calmly and slowly, being sure that there is adequate lighting. Expose the abdomen from just above the xiphoid process down to the symphysis pubis. Warm hands and stethoscope further promote relaxation. Ask the patient to report any pain and to point out tender areas. Assess tender areas last.

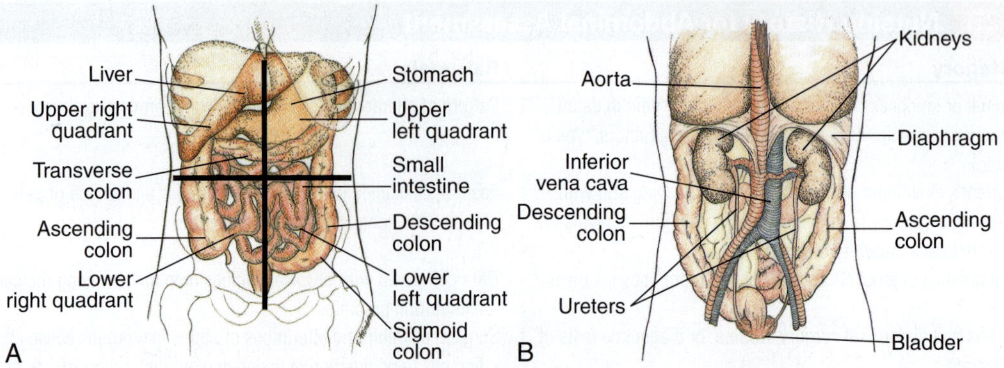

FIGURE 33.44 **A,** Anterior view of abdomen divided by quadrants. **B,** Posterior view of abdominal section.

The order of an abdominal examination differs slightly from previous assessments. Begin with inspection and follow with auscultation. By using auscultation before palpation, there is less chance of altering the frequency and character of bowel sounds. Be sure to have a tape measure and marking pen available during the examination.

Inspection

Make it a habit to observe the patient during routine care activities. Note the patient's posture and look for evidence of abdominal splinting: lying with the knees drawn up or moving restlessly in bed. A patient free from abdominal pain will not guard or splint the abdomen. To inspect the abdomen for abnormal movement or shadows, stand on the patient's right side and inspect from above the abdomen. To assess abdominal contour, sit down to look across the abdomen. Direct the examination light over the abdomen.

Skin. Inspect the skin over the abdomen for colour, scars, venous patterns, lesions, and **striae** (stretch marks). The skin is subject to the same colour variations as the rest of the body. Venous patterns are normally faint, except in thin patients. Striae result from stretching of tissue by obesity or pregnancy. Artificial openings indicate drainage sites resulting from surgery (see Chapter 49) or an ostomy (see Chapter 45). Scars reveal evidence of past trauma or surgery that has created permanent changes in underlying organ anatomy. Bruising indicates accidental injury, physical abuse, or a type of bleeding disorder. Ask the patient about self-administered injections (e.g., low-molecular-weight heparin or insulin). Unexpected findings include generalized colour changes such as jaundice or cyanosis. A glistening, taut (tight) appearance indicates ascites.

Umbilicus. Note the position; shape; colour; and signs of inflammation, discharge, or protruding masses. A normal umbilicus is flat or concave with the colour the same as that of the surrounding skin. Underlying masses cause displacement of the umbilicus. An everted (pouched-out) umbilicus usually indicates distension. A **hernia** (protrusion of abdominal organs through the muscle wall) causes upward protrusion of the umbilicus. Normally, the umbilical area does not emit discharge.

Contour and Symmetry. Inspect for contour, symmetry, and surface motion of the abdomen, noting any masses, bulging, or distension. A flat abdomen forms a horizontal plane from the xiphoid process to the symphysis pubis. A round abdomen protrudes in a convex sphere from the horizontal plane. A concave abdomen appears to sink into the muscular wall. Each of these findings is normal if the abdomen's shape is

symmetrical. In the older person, there is often an overall increased distribution of adipose tissue. The presence of masses on only one side, or asymmetry, possibly indicates an underlying pathological condition.

Intestinal gas, a tumour, or fluid in the abdominal cavity causes distension. When distension is generalized, the entire abdomen protrudes. The skin often appears taut, as if it were stretched over the abdomen. When gas causes distension, the flanks do not bulge. However, if fluid is the source of the problem, the flanks bulge. Ask the patient to roll onto one side. A protuberance forms on the dependent side if fluid is the cause of the distension. Ask the patient if the abdomen feels unusually tight. Be careful not to confuse distension with obesity. In obesity, the abdomen is large, rolls of adipose tissue are often present along the flanks, and the patient does not experience tightness in the abdomen. If abdominal distension is expected, measure the abdomen by placing a tape measure around the abdomen at the level of the umbilicus. Consecutive measurements will show any increase or decrease in distension. Use a marking pen to indicate the location of tape measure.

Enlarged Organs or Masses. Observe the contour of the abdomen while asking the patient to take a deep breath and hold it. Normally, the contour remains smooth and symmetrical. This manoeuvre forces the diaphragm downward and reduces the size of the abdominal cavity. Any enlarged organs in the upper abdominal cavity (e.g., liver or spleen) will descend below the rib cage to cause a bulge. Perform a closer examination with palpation.

To evaluate the abdominal musculature, have the patient raise their head off the examination table. This position causes superficial abdominal wall masses, hernias, and muscle separations to become more apparent.

Movement or Pulsations. Inspect for movement. Normally, men breathe abdominally and women breathe more costally. A patient with severe pain has diminished respiratory movement and tightens the abdominal muscles to guard against the pain. Closely inspect for peristaltic movement and aortic pulsation by looking across the abdomen from the side. These movements are visible in thin patients; otherwise, no movement is present.

Auscultation

During the abdominal assessment, auscultation is performed before palpation because manipulation of the abdomen alters the frequency and intensity of bowel sounds. The patient should be asked not to talk so that the examiner can hear bowel sounds. Patients with GI tubes connected to suction need them temporarily turned off before beginning the examination.

BOX 33.24   PATIENT TEACHING
Abdominal Assessment

Objectives
- Patient will maintain normal bowel elimination.
- Patient will achieve pain relief.
- Patients at high risk for **hepatitis B** virus (HBV) will receive immunization.
- Patient will identify signs and symptoms of colon cancer.

Teaching Strategies
- Explain factors that promote normal bowel elimination, such as diet, regular exercise, limited use of over-the-counter medications causing constipation, establishment of regular elimination schedule, and a good fluid intake (see Chapter 45). Stress importance for older persons.
- Caution patients about dangers of excessive use of laxatives or enemas.
- Instruct patient to have acute abdominal pain evaluated by a health care provider.
- If patient has chronic pain, explain measures used for pain relief (e.g., relaxation exercises, positioning) (see Chapter 32).
- If patient is a health care worker or has contact with blood or fluids of infected persons, encourage patient to receive the series of three HBV vaccine doses.
- Instruct patient about warning signs of colon cancer, including rectal bleeding, cramping pain in lower abdomen, black or tarry stools, blood in stool, and a change in bowel habits (constipation or diarrhea).

Evaluation
- Reassess patient's bowel elimination pattern and stool character after therapies begin.
- Observe patient using pain-relief measures and reassess character of pain.
- During follow-up clinic or office visit, check patient's adherence to HBV vaccine schedule.
- Ask patient to state signs and symptoms of colon cancer.

Bowel Motility. **Peristalsis**, or the movement of contents through the intestines, is a normal function of the small and large intestine. Bowel sounds are the audible passage of air and fluid that peristalsis creates. To perform auscultation, place the warmed diaphragm of the stethoscope lightly over each of the four quadrants. Normally, air and fluid move through the intestines, creating soft gurgling or clicking sounds that occur irregularly 5 to 30 times per minute (Jarvis et al., 2019, p. 580). Sounds usually last from half a second to several seconds. It takes 5 minutes of continuous listening before determining that bowel sounds are absent. Auscultate all four quadrants to be sure not to miss any sounds. The best time to auscultate is between meals. Sounds are generally described as normal, audible, absent, hyperactive, or hypoactive. Absent sounds indicate a lack of peristalsis, possibly due to late-stage bowel obstruction, **paralytic ileus**, or **peritonitis**. Normally, absent or hypoactive bowel sounds occur postoperatively following general anaesthesia. Hyperactive sounds are loud, "growling" sounds called **borborygmi**, which indicate increased GI motility. Inflammation of the bowel, anxiety, diarrhea, bleeding, excessive ingestion of laxatives, and reaction of the intestines to certain foods cause increased motility (Box 33.24).

Vascular Sounds. Bruits indicate narrowing of the major blood vessels and disruption of blood flow. The presence of bruits in the abdominal area will possibly reveal aneurysms or stenotic vessels. Use the bell of the stethoscope to auscultate in the epigastric region and each of the four quadrants. Normally, there are no vascular sounds over the aorta (midline through the abdomen) or femoral arteries (lower quadrants). Renal artery bruits are heard by placing the stethoscope over each upper quadrant anteriorly or over the costovertebral angle posteriorly. If a bruit is detected, report it immediately to a health care provider.

Kidney Tenderness. With the patient sitting or standing erect, use direct or indirect percussion to assess for kidney inflammation. With the ulnar surface of the partially closed fist, percuss posteriorly the costovertebral angle at the scapular line. If the kidneys are inflamed, the patient feels tenderness during percussion (Jarvis et al., 2019, p. 588) (Figure 33.45).

Palpation

Palpation is used primarily to detect areas of abdominal tenderness, distension, or masses. As their skill base increases, nurses learn to palpate for specific organs. Both light and deep palpation are used.

Light palpation is performed over each abdominal quadrant. Initially, areas previously identified as problem spots should be avoided. Lay the palm of the hand with fingers extended and approximated lightly on the abdomen. Explain the manoeuvre to the patient, and then with the palmar surface of the fingers depress approximately 1 cm in a gentle dipping motion (Jarvis et al., 2019, p. 582) (Figure 33.46). Avoid quick jabs, and use smooth, coordinated movements. For ticklish patients, first place the patient's hand on the abdomen with your hand on the patient's; continue this until the patient tolerates palpation.

Use a systematic palpation approach for each quadrant and assess for muscular resistance, distension, tenderness, and superficial organs or masses. Observe the patient's face for signs of discomfort. The abdomen is normally smooth with consistent softness and nontender without masses. The older person often lacks abdominal tone. Guarding or muscle tenseness sometimes occurs while palpating a sensitive area. If tightening remains after the patient relaxes, peritonitis, acute **cholecystitis**, or appendicitis is sometimes the cause. It is easy to detect a distended bladder with light palpation. Normally, the bladder lies below the umbilicus and above the symphysis pubis. Routinely check for a distended bladder if a patient has been unable to void (e.g., because of anaesthesia or sedation) or has been incontinent, or if an in-dwelling urinary catheter is not draining well.

With practice and experience, nurses perform deep palpation to delineate abdominal organs and to detect less obvious masses. For deep palpation, nurses must have short fingernails. It is important for the patient to be relaxed while the hands depress approximately 5 to 8 cm into the abdomen in a similar procedure when performed with light palpation (Jarvis et al., 2019, p. 588). Deep palpation should never be done over a surgical incision or over extremely tender organs. It is also unwise to use deep palpation on abnormal masses. Deep pressure causes tenderness in the healthy patient over the cecum, sigmoid colon, aorta, and the midline near the xiphoid process.

Each quadrant is surveyed systematically. Palpate masses for size, location, shape, consistency, tenderness, pulsation, and mobility. Test for rebound tenderness by pressing a hand slowly and deeply into the involved area and then letting go quickly. The test is positive if the patient feels pain with the release of the hand. Rebound tenderness occurs in patients with peritoneal irritation such as occurs in appendicitis; **pancreatitis**; or any peritoneal injury causing bile, blood, or enzymes to enter the peritoneal cavity.

Aortic Pulsation. To assess aortic pulsation, palpate with the thumb and forefinger of one hand deeply into the upper abdomen, just left of the midline. Normally a pulsation is transmitted forward. If there is enlargement of the aorta from an **aneurysm** (localized dilation of a vessel wall), the pulsation expands laterally. A pulsating abdominal mass should not be palpated. In patients with obesity it is often necessary to palpate with both hands, one on each side of the aorta.

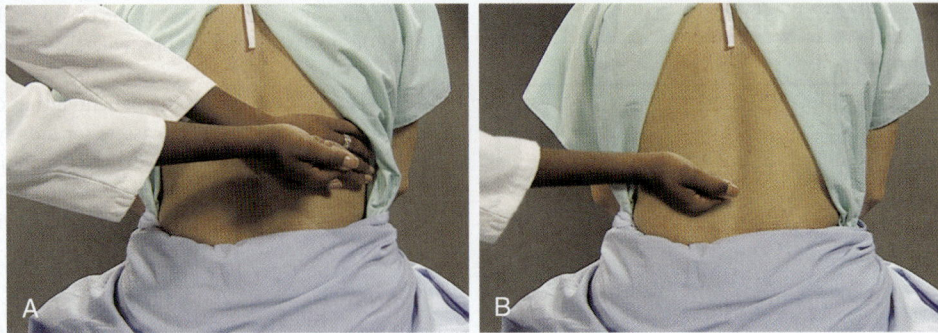

FIGURE 33.45 Costovertebral angle tenderness. **A,** Indirect percussion. **B,** Direct percussion. (From Ball, J. W., Dains, J. E., Flynn, J. A., et al. [2019]. *Seidel's guide to physical examination. An interprofessional approach* [9th ed.]. Mosby.)

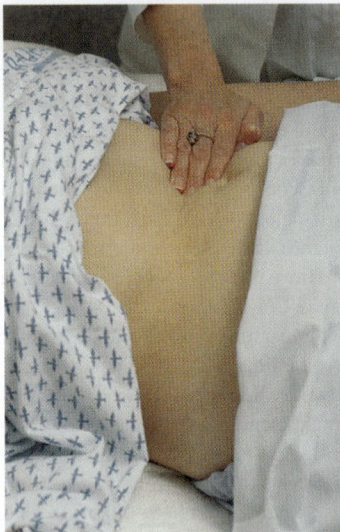

FIGURE 33.46 Light palpation of abdomen.

> **SAFETY ALERT** When enlargement from an aneurysm is present, only someone with advanced education and experience should perform palpation of this area.

GENITALIA EXAMINATION

Sensitive patient examination, including examinations of male and female genitalia, begin with appropriate assessment of gender identity, sexual orientation, and sex assigned at birth. Open and respectful assessment of how patients express sex and gender helps to avoid inaccurate biases and promotes provision of high-quality care (Aisner et al., 2020) (see Chapter 28). Examination of the genitalia of a transgender person must be done with sensitivity and must be relevant to the anatomy present, as sex organs and secondary sex characteristics will vary depending on whether the patient has had sex reassignment surgery or hormone therapy (Jarvis et al., 2019).

FEMALE GENITALIA AND REPRODUCTIVE TRACT

Examination of the female genitalia can be embarrassing to the patient, so the nurse needs to use a calm, relaxed approach. The gynecological examination is also one of the more difficult health care experiences for adolescents. Cultural background can further add to apprehension. In some cultures, women do not expose their bodies to men or even to other women. In other cultures, the examination of genitalia may

be considered offensive. Cultural expression of these values, and the level of emotional or physical comfort with the procedure, needs to be explored prior to any genital exam. The lithotomy position assumed during the examination can be an added source of embarrassment. It is often the nurse's role to provide a thorough explanation for the examination and the procedures that will be used. The nurse can also assess the patient's level of anxiety regarding a genital exam while obtaining the nursing history (Table 33.26). Patient acceptance and comfort can be augmented through correct positioning and draping. Adolescents sometimes choose to have parents present in the examination room.

Sometimes a patient requires a complete examination of the female reproductive organs: assessment of the external genitalia and a vaginal examination. The nurse will examine external genitalia while performing routine hygiene measures or preparing to insert a urinary catheter. An internal examination, to assess for signs of cancer or other disorders, is part of the preventative health care visit for sexually active individuals with female genitalia who are aged 25–69 and as indicated by health history findings (Canadian Task Force on Preventative Health Care, 2021). Genital examination may also be indicated for patients with suspected sexually transmitted infections (STIs).

Preparation of the Patient

As a beginning nurse, your responsibility will be assisting the patient's health care provider with the examination (Jarvis et al., 2019, pp. 789–790). For a complete examination, the following special equipment is needed: examination table with stirrups, vaginal speculum of correct size, adjustable light source, sink, clean disposable gloves, sterile cotton swabs, glass slides, plastic or wooden spatula, cervical brush or broom device, cytological fixative, and culture plates or media.

The equipment needs to be ready before the examination begins. Ask the patient to empty their bladder so that the uterus and ovaries are readily palpable. Often it is necessary to collect a urine specimen. Assist the patient to the lithotomy position, in bed or on an examination table, for the external genitalia assessment. Help the patient place their feet into stirrups for a speculum examination. Have the patient stabilize each foot in a stirrup and then have them slide the buttocks down to the edge of the examining table. Place a hand at the edge of the table and instruct the patient to move until touching the hand. The patient's arms should be at their sides or folded across the chest to prevent tightening of abdominal muscles.

Some patients who suffer from pain or deformity of the joints are unable to assume a lithotomy position. In this situation, the patient need abduct only one leg, or another person can assist in separating the patient's thighs. The side-lying position can also be used, with the patient lying on their left side with the right thigh and knee drawn up to her chest.

TABLE 33.26	Nursing History for Female Genitalia and Reproductive Tract Assessment
Assessment Category	**Rationale**
Determine if patient has had previous illness, including sexually transmitted infections (STIs), or surgery involving reproductive organs.	Illness or surgery influences appearance and position of organs being examined.
Determine if patient has received a human papillomavirus (HPV) vaccine.	HPV vaccine is recommended for immunocompetent patients of all genders (ages 9–26) to prevent HPV infection and potential risks for cancers (Public Health Agency of Canada, 2021b). HPV may also be given after the age of 26, based on risk assessment and potential benefits.
Review menstrual history, including age at menarche, frequency and duration of menstrual cycle, character of flow (e.g., amount, presence of clots), presence of dysmenorrhea (painful menstruation), pelvic pain, dates of last two menstrual periods, and premenstrual symptoms.	This information is useful to determine level of reproductive health, including normalcy of menstrual cycle.
Ask patient to describe obstetrical history, including each pregnancy and history of abortions or miscarriages.	Observed physical findings will vary, depending on patient's history of pregnancy.
Ask patient to describe current and past contraceptive practices and problems encountered. Determine whether patient uses safer sex practices. Discuss risk of STIs and HIV infection.	Use of certain types of contraceptives influences reproductive health (e.g., sensitivity reaction to spermicidal jelly). Sexual history reveals risk for and understanding of STIs.
Assess if patient has signs and symptoms of vaginal discharge, painful or swollen perianal tissues, or genital lesions.	These signs and symptoms may indicate an STI or other pathological condition.
Determine if patient has symptoms or history of genitourinary conditions, including burning during urination, frequency, urgency, nocturia, hematuria, incontinence, or stress incontinence (see Chapter 44).	Urinary problems are associated with gynecological disorders, including STIs.
Ask if patient has had signs of bleeding outside of normal menstrual period or after menopause or has had unusual vaginal discharge.	These are warning signs for cervical and endometrial cancer or vaginal infection.
Determine if patient has history of HPV (condyloma acuminatum, herpes simplex, or cervical dysplasia); has multiple sex partners; smokes cigarettes; has had multiple pregnancies; or was young at first intercourse.	These are risk factors for cervical cancer. Vaccines are available for HPV for individuals with female genitalia who are 9–26 years of age.
Determine if patient is older than 40, has obesity, and has history of ovarian dysfunction, breast or endometrial cancer, irradiation of pelvic organs, or endometriosis; has family history of ovarian, breast, or colon cancer; has history of infertility or nulliparity; or uses estrogen (alone) or as part of hormone replacement therapy.	These are risk factors for ovarian cancer.
Determine if patient is postmenopausal, obese, or infertile; had early menarche; had late menopause; has history of hypertension, diabetes, gallbladder disease, or polycystic ovary disease; has family history of endometrial, breast, or colon cancer; or has a history of estrogen-related exposure (estrogen replacement therapy, tamoxifen use).	These are risk factors for endometrial cancer.

Give the patient a square drape or sheet: The patient holds one corner over their sternum, the adjacent corners fall over each knee, and the fourth corner covers the perineum. After the examination begins, lift the drape over the perineum. A male examiner always needs to have a female attendant present during the examination. A female examiner may prefer to work alone but should have a female attendant present if the patient is particularly anxious or emotionally unstable.

External Genitalia

The perineal area needs to be well illuminated to be examined. The examiner must wear clean gloves on both hands to help prevent contact with infectious organisms. The perineum is extremely sensitive and tender; this area should not be touched suddenly without warning the patient. It is best to touch the neighbouring thigh first before advancing to the perineum.

As the examiner, while the patient is sitting at the end of the examination table or bed, inspect the quantity and distribution of hair growth. Preadolescents have no pubic hair. During adolescence, hair grows along the labia, becoming darker, coarser, and curlier. In an adult, hair grows in a triangle over the female pubis and along the medial surfaces of the thighs. Hair should be free of nits and lice. The underlying skin should be free of inflammation, irritation, or lesions.

A common practice among younger individuals of all genders is the removal of genital hair by means of waxing or shaving. The genital region in these patients should be assessed for abrasion, ingrown hair, irritation from clothing, and signs of infection.

Inspect surface characteristics of the labia majora. The skin of the perineum is smooth, clean, and slightly darker than other skin. The mucous membranes appear dark pink and moist. The labia majora are gaping or closed and appear dry or moist. They are usually symmetrical. After childbirth, the labia majora separate, causing the labia minora to become more prominent. When a woman reaches menopause, the labia majora become thinned. With advancing age, they become atrophied (reduced in size). The labia majora are normally without inflammation, edema, lesions, or lacerations.

To inspect the remaining external structures, use the nondominant hand and gently place the thumb and index finger inside the labia minora and retract the tissues outwardly (Figure 33.47). Be sure to have a firm hold to avoid repeated retraction against the sensitive tissues. Use the other hand to palpate the labia minora between the thumb and second finger. On inspection, the labia minora are normally thinner than the labia majora, and one side is sometimes larger. The tissue feels soft on palpation and without tenderness. The size of the clitoris is variable, but it normally does not exceed 2 cm in length and 0.5 cm in width. Look for atrophy, inflammation, or adhesions. If inflamed, the

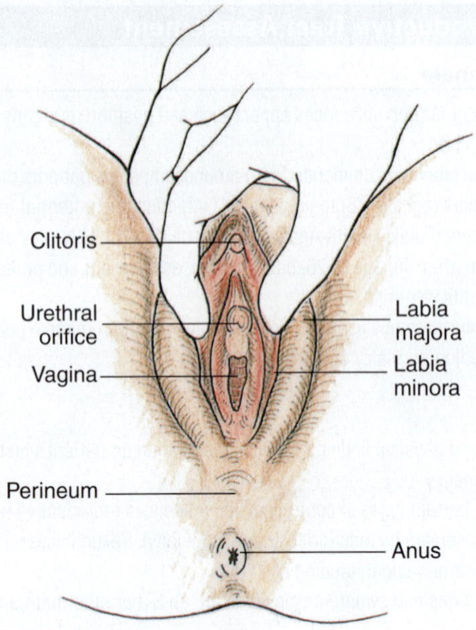

FIGURE 33.47 External female genitalia.

clitoris will be a bright cherry red. In young individuals with female genitalia, it is a common site for syphilitic lesions, or chancres, which appear as small open ulcers that drain serous material. Some older individuals with female genitalia have malignant changes that result in dry, scaly, nodular lesions.

Inspect the urethral orifice carefully for colour and position. It is normally intact without inflammation. The urethral meatus is anterior to the vaginal orifice and is pink. It appears as a small slit or pinhole opening just above the vaginal canal. Note any discharge, polyps, or fistulas.

Inspect the vaginal orifice (introitus) for inflammation, edema, discoloration, discharge, and lesions. Normally the introitus is a thin, vertical slit or a large orifice. The tissue is moist. While inspecting the vaginal orifice, note the condition of the hymen, which is just inside the introitus. In a virgin, the hymen restricts the opening of the vagina. Only remnants of the hymen remain after sexual intercourse.

Inspect the anus, looking for lesions and hemorrhoids. After completion of the external examination, dispose of examination gloves and offer the patient perineal hygiene.

Patients who are at risk for contracting an STI need to learn to perform a genital self-examination (GSE) (Box 33.25). The purpose of the examination is to detect any signs or symptoms of an STI. Many people do not know they have an STI (e.g., chlamydia), and some STIs (e.g., syphilis) remain undetected for years.

Speculum Examination of Internal Genitalia

An examination of the internal genitalia requires skill and practice. Advanced practice nurses and primary care providers will perform this examination. Beginning students will more than likely only observe the procedure or assist the examiner by helping the patient with positioning, handing off specimen supplies, and supporting the patient. A detailed presentation of the internal genital exam can be found in the textbook by Jarvis et al. (2019, pp. 791–804). The examination involves use of a plastic or metal speculum, consisting of two blades and an adjustment device. The examiner inserts the speculum into the vagina to assess the internal genitalia for cancerous lesions and other abnormalities. During the examination, the examiner will collect a specimen for a Papanicolaou (Pap) test for cervical cancer.

BOX 33.25 PATIENT TEACHING

Female Genitalia and Reproductive Tract Assessment

Objectives
- Patient will pursue routine gynecological examinations based on their level of risk for cervical cancer and other gynecological pathology.
- Patient with a sexually transmitted infection (STI) will follow safer sex practices.
- Patient will use measures to prevent acquisition and transmission of STIs.

Teaching Strategies
- Teach patient about purpose and recommended frequency of Papanicolaou (Pap) smears and gynecological examinations. Explain that the Pap smear is relatively painless and needed with a pelvic examination for individuals with female genitalia who are over the age of 25 and sexually active. Pap smear screening is recommended every 3 years when results are normal, and more often when results are abnormal (Canadian Task Force on Preventive Health Care, 2021).
- Counsel patient with an STI about diagnosis and treatment.
- Instruct patient in genital self-examination (GSE): Using a mirror, position self in order to examine the area covered by the pubic hair. Spread the hair apart, looking for bumps, sores, or blisters. Also, look for any warts, which appear as small, bumpy spots and that enlarge to fleshy, cauliflower-like lesions. Next, spread the outer vaginal lips apart and look at the clitoris for bumps, blisters, sores, or warts. Also look at both sides of the inner vaginal lips. Inspect the area around the urinary and vaginal opening for bumps, blisters, sores, or warts.
- Explain warning signs of STIs: pain or burning on urination, pain during sex, pain in pelvic area, bleeding between menstruation, itchy rash around vagina, and abnormal vaginal discharge.
- Teach measures to prevent STIs: use of condoms by partners with male genitalia, restricting number of sexual partners, avoiding sex with individuals who have several other partners, and perineal hygiene measures.
- Tell patients with an STI to inform sexual partners of the need for an examination and treatment.
- Reinforce the importance of performing perineal hygiene (as appropriate).

Evaluation
- Ask patient to explain when they should routinely have a gynecological examination and Pap smear.
- Have patient describe ways to prevent transmission of STIs.
- For patient with an STI, determine during follow-up visit if patient has followed safer sexual practices (use nonthreatening inquiry).

MALE GENITALIA

An examination of the male genitalia is done to assess the integrity of the external genitalia (Figure 33.48), inguinal ring, and canal. Because the incidence of STIs in adolescents and young adults is high, an assessment of the genitalia needs to be a routine part of any health maintenance examination for this age group (Box 33.26). The examination begins by having the patient void. The examination room should be warm. The patient lies supine with the chest, abdomen, and lower legs draped or stands during the examination. The examiner must wear clean gloves.

Using a calm, gentle approach can lessen the patient's anxiety. The position and exposure of the body during the examination is embarrassing for some patients. To minimize the patient's anxiety, it often helps to offer explanations of the steps of examination so the patient can anticipate all actions. The genitalia should be manipulated gently

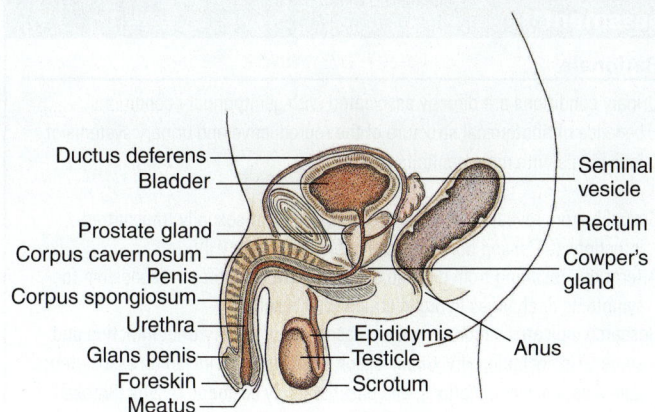

FIGURE 33.48 External and internal male sex organs.

to avoid causing an erection or discomfort. A thorough history (Table 33.27) is obtained before the examination to ensure that the assessment is complete.

Sexual Maturity

First, note the sexual maturity of the patient by observing the size and shape of the penis and testes; the size, colour, and texture of the scrotal skin; and the character and distribution of pubic hair. Use Tanner stages to assess and document sexual maturation (Jarvis et al., 2019, p. 750). In stage 1, the penis and scrotum show no change in size and there is no evidence of pubic hair. In stage 2, the testes first increase in size during preadolescence. At this time, there is little to no pubic hair. At stage 3, the scrotal hair becomes coarse and dark and the penis begins to enlarge. Further growth and coverage of the pubic area occur in stage 4 and the glans penis matures and scrotum darkens. By the end of stage 5, the testes and penis enlarge to adult size and shape and scrotal skin darkens and becomes wrinkled. The penis has no hair, and the scrotum has very little hair. Also inspect the skin covering the genitalia for lice, rashes, excoriations, or lesions. Normally the skin is clear, without lesions.

Penis

To inspect penile surfaces thoroughly, manipulate the genitalia or have the patient assist. Inspect the shaft, corona, prepuce (foreskin), glans, and urethral meatus. The dorsal vein is apparent on inspection. In uncircumcised individuals with male genitalia, retract the foreskin to reveal the glans and urethral meatus. The foreskin usually retracts easily. A small amount of white, thick smegma sometimes collects under this foreskin. Obtain a culture if abnormal discharge is present. The urethral meatus is slitlike and is positioned on the ventral surface just millimetres from the tip of the glans. In some congenital conditions, the meatus is displaced along the penile shaft. The area between the foreskin and glans is a common site for venereal lesions. Gently compress the glans between the thumb and index finger; this opens the urethral meatus for inspection of lesions, edema, and inflammation. Normally the opening is glistening and pink, without discharge. Palpate any lesion gently to note tenderness, size, consistency, and shape. When inspection and palpation of the glans is complete, pull the foreskin down to its original position.

Continue by inspecting the entire shaft of the penis, including the undersurface, looking for lesions, scars, or edema. Palpate the shaft between the thumb and first two fingers to detect localized areas of hardness or tenderness. A patient who has lain in bed for a prolonged period of time sometimes develops dependent edema in the penis shaft.

It is important for any patient with male genitalia to learn to perform a GSE to detect signs or symptoms of STIs. Many people who have an STI do not know it. Self-examination is a routine part of self-care (Box 33.27).

Scrotum

The examiner should be particularly cautious while inspecting and palpating the scrotum because the structures lying within the scrotal sac are very sensitive. The scrotum is divided internally into two halves. Each half contains a testicle, epididymis, and the vas deferens, which travels upward into the inguinal ring. Normally, the left testicle is lower than the right. Inspect the scrotum's size, shape, and symmetry while observing for lesions or edema. Gently lift the scrotum to view the posterior surface. The scrotal skin is usually loose, and the surface is coarse. The scrotal skin is more deeply pigmented than body skin. Tightening, loss, or wrinkling of skin indicates edema. The size of the scrotum normally changes with temperature variations because the dartos muscle contracts in cold and relaxes in warm temperatures. Lumps in the scrotal skin are commonly sebaceous cysts.

The testes are normally sensitive but not tender. The underlying testicles are normally ovoid and approximately 2 to 4 cm in size. Gently palpate the testicles and epididymis between the thumb and first two fingers. The testes feel smooth, rubbery, and free of nodules. The epididymis is resilient. Note the size, shape, and consistency of the organs. The most common symptoms of testicular cancer are a painless enlargement of one testis and the appearance of a palpable, small, hard lump, about the size of a pea, on the front or side of the testicle. In older individuals with male genitalia, the testicles decrease in size and are

TABLE 33.27   Nursing History for Male Genitalia Assessment

Assessment Category	Rationale
Review normal urinary elimination pattern, including frequency of voiding; history of nocturia; character and volume of urine; daily fluid intake; symptoms of burning, urgency, and frequency; difficulty starting stream; and hematuria (see Chapter 44).	Urinary conditions are directly associated with genitourinary conditions because of anatomical structure of the reproductive and urinary systems of individuals with male genitalia.
Assess patient's sexual history and use of safer sex habits (multiple partners, infection in partners, failure to use condom).	Sexual history reveals risk for and understanding of sexually transmitted infections (STIs) and human immunodeficiency virus (HIV).
Determine if patient has had previous surgery or illness involving urinary or reproductive organs, including STI.	Alterations resulting from disease or surgery are sometimes responsible for symptoms or changes in organ structure or function.
Ask if patient is circumcised or uncircumcised.	Research indicates circumcision decreases risk of urinary tract infection and some STIs, including HIV. Circumcision also has risks, including associated pain, surgical complications, and unsatisfactory cosmetic results (Sorokan et al., 2021).
Ask if patient has noted penile pain or swelling, genital lesions, or urethral discharge.	These signs and symptoms may indicate STI.
Determine if patient has noticed heaviness or painless enlargement of testis or irregular lumps.	These signs and symptoms are early warning signs for testicular cancer.
If patient reports an enlargement in inguinal area, assess if it is intermittent or constant, associated with straining or lifting, and painful, and whether pain is affected by coughing, lifting, or straining at stool.	These signs and symptoms reflect potential inguinal hernia.
Ask if patient has difficulty achieving erection or ejaculation; also review whether patient is taking diuretics, sedatives, antihypertensives, or tranquilizers.	These medications influence sexual performance.

BOX 33.27   Male Genital Self-Examination

All individuals with male genitalia who are aged 15 years and older need to perform this examination on a regular basis using the following steps.

Genital Examination

Perform the examination after a warm bath or shower, when the scrotal skin is less thick.

Stand naked in front of a mirror, and hold the penis in your hand and examine the head. Pull back the foreskin if uncircumcised to expose the glans.

Inspect and palpate the entire head of the penis in a clockwise motion, looking carefully for any bumps, sores, or blisters (bumps and blisters may be light coloured or red, resemble pimples) (see illustration). Look also for any genital warts.

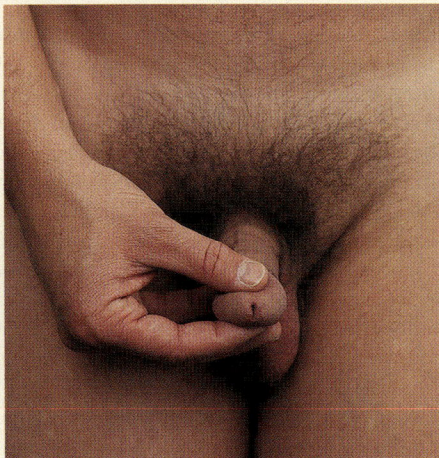

Male genital examination.

Look at the opening (urethral meatus) at the end of the penis for discharge.

Look along the entire shaft of the penis for the same signs.

Be sure to separate pubic hair at the base of the penis and carefully examine the skin underneath.

Testicular Self-Examination

Look for swelling or lumps in the skin of the scrotum while looking in the mirror.

Use both hands, placing the index and middle fingers under the testicles and the thumb on top (see illustration).

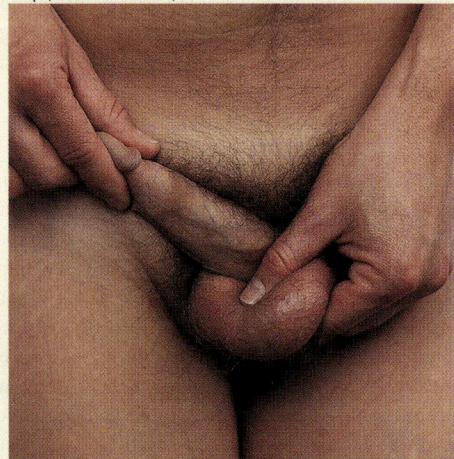

Testicular self-examination.

Gently roll the testicle, feeling for lumps, swelling, soreness, or a change in consistency (hardening).

Find the epididymis (a cordlike structure on the top and back of the testicle; it is not a lump).

Feel for small, pea-sized lumps on the front and side of the testicle. The lumps are usually painless and are abnormal.

Call your health care provider if you are uncertain whether you have detected any abnormal findings.

Photos from Ball, J. W., Dains, J. E., Flynn, J. A., et al. (2019). *Seidel's guide to physical examination. An Interprofessional approach* (9th ed.). Mosby.)

TABLE 33.28	Nursing History for Rectal and Anal Assessment
Assessment Category	**Rationale**
Determine whether patient has experienced bleeding from rectum, black or tarry stools (melena), rectal pain, or change in bowel habits (constipation or diarrhea).	These are warning signs of colorectal cancer* or other gastrointestinal alterations.
Determine whether patient has personal or strong family history of colorectal cancer, polyps, or chronic inflammatory bowel disease. Ask if patient is over age 40.	These are risk factors for colorectal cancer.*
Assess dietary habits, including high fat intake, diet high in processed or red meats, or deficient fibre content (inadequate fruits and vegetables).	Bowel cancer is often linked to dietary intake of fat or insufficient fibre intake.*
Determine if patient has obesity, is physically inactive, smokes, or consumes alcohol.	These are risk factors for colorectal cancer.
Determine whether patient has undergone screening for colorectal cancer (digital examination, fecal immunochemical test [FIT], fecal occult blood test [FOBT], flexible sigmoidoscopy, and colonoscopy).	Undergoing this screening reflects understanding of and adherence to preventive health care measures.
Assess medication history for use of laxatives or cathartic medications.	Repeated use causes diarrhea and eventual loss of intestinal muscle tone.
Assess for use of codeine or iron preparations.	Codeine causes constipation. Iron turns the color of feces black and tarry.
Ask patient with male genitalia if they have experienced weak or interrupted urine flow, inability to urinate, difficulty in starting or stopping urine flow, polyuria, nocturia, hematuria, or dysuria. Does patient have continuing pain in lower back, pelvis, or upper thighs?	These are warning signs of prostatic cancer.* Symptoms also suggest infection or prostate enlargement.

*Data from Canadian Cancer Society (2022b).

less firm during palpation. Continue to palpate the vas deferens separately as it forms the spermatic cord toward the inguinal ring, noting nodules or swelling. It normally feels smooth and discrete.

Testicular cancer is a solid tumour that is common in young men ages 15 to 29 years (Canadian Cancer Society, 2022d). Early detection is critical. Testicular self-examination (TSE) should be explained to the patient while they are being examined. Further details on teaching TSE can be found in the textbook by Jarvis et al. (2019, p. 764).

Inguinal Ring and Canal

The external inguinal ring provides the opening for the spermatic cord to pass into the inguinal canal. The canal forms a passage through the abdominal wall, a potential site for hernia formation. A *hernia* is a protrusion of a portion of intestine through the inguinal wall or canal. Sometimes an intestinal loop enters the scrotum. Often hernias are asymptomatic. However, complications of hernias can be serious, including severe pain and bowel obstruction. Physical examination of inguinal hernias is an advanced practice nursing skill. A detailed overview of this examination can be found in the textbook by Jarvis et al. (2019, p. 776).

RECTUM AND ANUS

The rectal examination is usually performed after the genital examination. It is not commonly performed during the examination in young children or adolescents. A rectal examination may detect colorectal cancer in its early stages. In individuals with male genitalia, the rectal examination is also used to detect prostatic tumours. A thorough history (Table 33.28) is collected to determine the patient's risk for bowel or rectal disease or prostatic disease.

An examination of the rectum and anus requires much skill and practice; advanced nurse practitioners and primary care providers will perform this examination. Beginning students will more than likely only observe the procedure or assist the examiner by helping the patient with positioning, handing off specimen supplies, and comforting the patient. A detailed presentation of the anus, rectum, and prostate examinations can be found in the textbook by Jarvis et al. (2019, pp. 607–616).

The rectal examination is uncomfortable, so explaining all steps to the patient can help the patient relax. A calm, slow-paced, gentle approach should be used during the examination. Patients with female genitalia remain in the dorsal recumbent position following genitalia examination or they assume a modified side-lying position. The best way to examine patients with male genitalia is to have the patient stand and bend over forward with hips flexed and upper body resting across the examination table. A nonambulatory patient is examined in the lateral recumbent position where the person lies on their left side, with their left hip and lower extremity straight and the right hip and knee bent. The examiner must use disposable gloves.

Inspection

Using the nondominant hand, the examiner gently retracts the buttocks to view the perianal and sacrococcygeal areas. Perianal skin is smooth and more pigmented and coarser than skin over the buttocks. Anal tissue is inspected for skin characteristics, lesions, external **hemorrhoids** (dilated veins that appear as reddened protrusions), ulcers, fissures and fistulas, inflammation, rashes, or excoriation. Anal tissues are moist and hairless, and the voluntary external muscle sphincter holds the anus closed. Next, the examiner asks the patient to bear down as though having a bowel movement. Any internal hemorrhoids or fissures will appear at this time. Clock reference (e.g., 3 o'clock, 8 o'clock) is used to describe location of findings. Normally, there is no protrusion of tissue.

Digital Palpation

The anal canal and sphincters are examined with digital palpation, and in patients with male genitalia, the prostate gland is palpated to rule out enlargement (Box 33.28). A detailed presentation of the anus, rectum, and prostate examinations can be found in the textbook by Jarvis et al. (2019, pp. 606–616).

MUSCULOSKELETAL SYSTEM

The musculoskeletal assessment can be conducted as a separate examination or integrated into other portions of the total physical examination. Assessment can be performed during other nursing care measures such as bathing or positioning. The assessment of musculoskeletal function focuses on determining range of joint motion, muscle strength and tone, and joint and muscle condition. The assessment of musculoskeletal integrity is especially important when the patient reports pain

BOX 33.28   PATIENT TEACHING

Rectal and Anal Assessment

Objectives

- Patient will have a regular digital examination performed appropriate to age and symptom presentation.
- Patient will be able to identify symptoms of colorectal and prostatic cancer.
- Patient will follow a nutritiously sound diet.

Teaching Strategies

- Discuss recommendations for early detection of colorectal cancer and preventive health screening methods (Canadian Task Force on Preventative Health Care, 2021).
- Discuss warning signs of colorectal cancer (see Table 33.28).
- Discuss dietary planning and healthy lifestyle choices to maintain or improve colon health.
- Warn patient against health problems caused by overuse of laxatives, cathartic medications, codeine, or enemas.
- Discuss benefits and harms of prostate cancer screening with patients with male genitalia who are 50–70 years of age, using a shared decision-making approach. Potential harms include false-positive results, unnecessary invasive procedures, and anxiety. Benefits include potential for early detection and treatment of prostate cancer (Rendon et al., 2017).
- Inform patients with male genitalia that if they have a first-degree relative diagnosed with prostate cancer, they should consider screening starting at age 45 (Rendon et al., 2017).
- Discuss the warning signs of prostatic cancer.

Evaluation

- During follow-up visits, determine whether patient has had a rectal examination performed.
- Have patient explain warning signs of colorectal and prostatic cancer.
- Ask patient to describe appropriate lifestyle and food choices for a healthy colon.

---

or loss of function in a joint or muscle. Frequently, muscular disorders are the result of neurological disease. For this reason, health care providers often conduct a neurological assessment simultaneously.

While examining the patient's musculoskeletal function, it helps to visualize the anatomy of bone and muscle placement and joint structure (see Chapter 46). Joints vary in their degree of mobility. The spinal vertebrae are examples of slightly movable joints in comparison to the hinge joint movement of the knee or elbow.

For a complete examination, the muscles and joints should be exposed so they are able to move without restriction from clothing and so that they are easy to visualize. The patient assumes a sitting, supine, prone, or standing position while certain muscle groups are assessed. Table 33.29 lists the information gathered in the nursing history.

General Inspection

To begin assessment, observe the patient's gait when they enter the examination room. When a patient is unaware of the nature of the observation, gait is more natural. Later, a more formal test has the patient walk in a straight line away and then return to point of origin. Note how the patient walks, sits, and rises from a sitting position. Normally, patients walk with arms swinging freely at their sides and their head leading the body. Older persons often walk with smaller steps and a wider base of support. Any foot dragging, limping, or shuffling and the position of the trunk in relation to the legs should be noted.

Observe the patient from the side in a standing position. The normal standing posture is upright with parallel alignment of the hips and shoulders. There is an even contour of the shoulders, level scapulae and iliac crests, alignment of the head over the gluteal folds, and symmetry of extremities. Looking sideways at the patient, note the normal cervical, thoracic, and lumbar curves. Holding the head erect is normal. As the patient sits, some degree of rounding of the shoulders is normal. Older persons tend to assume a stooped, forward-bent posture with hips and knees somewhat flexed and arms bent at the elbows, raising the level of their arms.

Common postural abnormalities include lordosis, kyphosis, and scoliosis. **Kyphosis**, or hunchback, is an exaggeration of the posterior curvature of the thoracic spine. This postural abnormality is common in the older person. **Lordosis**, or swayback, is an increased lumbar curvature. A lateral spinal curvature is called **scoliosis**. Loss of height is frequently the first clinical sign of osteoporosis, in which height loss occurs in the trunk as a result of vertebral fracture and collapse. **Osteoporosis** is a metabolic bone disease that causes a decrease in quality and quantity of bone. One in three individuals with female genitalia and one in five individuals with male genitalia will experience an osteoporotic fracture in their lifetime (Public Health Agency of Canada [PHAC], 2020). Osteoporosis affects not only adults; it strikes any age group, including children. Although a small amount of height loss is to be expected with aging, if the amount of loss is great, osteoporosis is likely (Box 33.29). As people age, they are more likely to have osteoporotic fractures of the forearm or wrists, hips, and vertebrae (PHAC, 2020).

During general inspection, the examiner looks at the extremities for overall size, gross deformity, bony enlargement, alignment, and symmetry. Normally, there is bilateral symmetry in length, circumference, alignment, and position and in the number of skin folds. A general review pinpoints areas requiring specialized assessment.

Palpation

During a complete examination, the examiner applies gentle palpation to all bones, joints, and surrounding muscles. In a focused assessment, the involved area and adjacent muscle groups or joints are examined. Any heat, tenderness, edema, or resistance to pressure is noted. The patient should not feel any discomfort upon palpation. Muscles should be firm.

Range of Joint Motion

The examination includes comparison of both active and passive range of motion (ROM); the patient puts each major joint through active and passive full ROM (see Chapter 46). Beginning students need to learn the correct terminology for the movements that the joints are capable of making (Table 33.30) and know how to instruct the patient in how to move through each ROM. ROM should be demonstrated to the patient when possible. To assess ROM passively, ask the patient to relax and then passively move the extremities through their ROM. Compare the same body parts for bilateral equality and symmetry in movement. Figure 33.49 shows an example of ROM positions for the hand and wrist. A joint must not be forced into a painful position. Examiners must know the normal range of each joint and the extent to which they can move the patient's joints. ROM is equal between contralateral joints. Ideally, the patient's normal range should be assessed to determine a baseline for assessing later change.

Joints are typically free from stiffness, instability, swelling, or inflammation. There should be no discomfort when applying pressure to bones and joints. In older persons, joints often become swollen and stiff with reduced ROM resulting from cartilage erosion and fibrosis of synovial membranes (see Chapter 46). If a joint appears swollen and inflamed, it should be palpated for warmth.

TABLE 33.29 Nursing History for Musculoskeletal Assessment

Assessment Category	Rationale
Determine if patient is involved in competitive sports (particularly involving collision and contact), fails to warm up adequately, is in poor physical condition, or has had a rapid growth spurt (adolescents).	These are risk factors for sports injury.
Review patient history for use of alcohol and caffeine; cigarette smoking; constant dieting; calcium intake less than 500 mg daily; thin and light body frame; nulliparous status; menopause before age 45; estrogen deficiency; postmenopause status; family history of osteoporosis; advanced age; history of fractures or falls; sedentary lifestyle; chronic diseases (Cushing's hyperthyroidism and hypothyroidism, malabsorption or malnutrition disorders, neoplasm); long-term use of corticosteroids, methotrexate, phenytoin, aluminum-containing antacids; lack of weight-bearing exercise; lack of exposure to sunlight or inadequate vitamin D intake.	These are risk factors for osteoporosis.
Ask patient to describe history of problems in bone, muscle, or joint function (e.g., recent fall, trauma, lifting of heavy objects, history of bone or joint disease with sudden or gradual onset, location of alteration).	History assists in assessing nature of musculoskeletal problem.
Assess nature and extent of pain, including location, duration, severity, predisposing and aggravating factors, relieving factors, and type.	Pain frequently accompanies alterations in bone, joints, or muscle. This has implications for not only comfort but also ability to perform activities of daily living.
Assess patient's normal activity pattern, including type of exercise routinely performed.	Provides baseline in assessment. Sedentary lifestyle and lack of appropriate exercise increase bone loss and risk of fractures.
Determine how alteration influences the patient's ability to perform activities of daily living (e.g., bathing, feeding, dressing, toileting, ambulating) and social functions (e.g., household chores, work, recreation, sexual activities).	The extent to which the patient is able to perform self-care will determine the level of nursing care. Type and degree of restriction in continuing social activities influence topics for patient education and ability of nurse to identify alternative ways to maintain function.
Assess height loss of individuals with female genitalia over age 50 by subtracting current height from recall of maximum adult height.	Measurement is useful screening tool to predict osteoporosis.

BOX 33.29 PATIENT TEACHING

Musculoskeletal Assessment

Objectives
- Patient will follow measures to prevent or minimize osteoporosis.
- Patient will assume proper body posture.
- Patient will be able to perform self-care measures.

Teaching Strategies
- Instruct patient in correct postural alignment. Consult with physiotherapist to provide patient with exercises for improving posture.
- Recommend to patients age 50 and older that they should undergo routine screening for osteoporosis (Papaioannou et al., 2010).
- To reduce bone demineralization, instruct older persons in a proper exercise program (e.g., weight-bearing, muscle-strengthening, and balance-training exercise) to be followed three or more times a week.
- Encourage intake of calcium to meet the recommended daily allowance. Increased vitamin D will aid calcium absorption.
  - Recommendation for daily calcium intake: age 4 to 8 years (1 000 mg), 9 to 18 years (1 300 mg), 19 to 50 years (1 000 mg), and 50+ years (1 200 mg) (Health Canada, 2020). If supplementing to achieve recommended calcium intake, instruct patient to take no more than 600 mg of calcium at one time.
  - Recommended vitamin D supplementation is 400 to 1 000 IU for low-risk adults and 800 to 2 000 IU for individuals considered at high risk (Health Canada, 2020).

- Explain to patients with low back pain that they will benefit from modification of worker risk factors (e.g., lifting heavy weights, use of protective equipment), regular aerobic exercise, exercises that strengthen the back and increase trunk flexibility, and learning how to lift properly.
- Instruct older persons and those with osteoporosis in proper body mechanics and range-of-motion and moderate weight-bearing exercises (e.g., swimming and walking), to minimize trauma and subsequent fracture of bones.
- Instruct patient in use of assistive devices (e.g., zippers on clothing instead of buttons; elevation of chairs to minimize bending of knees and hips) when patient is unable to perform activities of daily living.
- Instruct an older person to pace activities to compensate for loss in muscle strength and to avoid falls.

Evaluation
- Observe patient's posture.
- Ask patient to describe therapies for preventing osteoporosis.
- Observe patient perform range-of-motion exercises.
- Have patient keep log of regular weight-training exercises.
- Ask patient or caregiver(s) to describe patient's use of self-care aids.

TABLE 33.30	Terminology for Normal Range-of-Motion Positions	
Term	**Range of Motion**	**Examples of Joints**
Flexion	Movement decreasing angle between two adjoining bones; bending of limb	Elbow, fingers, knee
Extension	Movement increasing angle between two adjoining bones	Elbow, knee, fingers
Hyperextension	Movement of body part beyond its normal resting extended position	Head
Pronation	Movement of body part so that front or ventral surface faces downward	Hand, forearm
Supination	Movement of body part so that the front or ventral surface faces upward	Hand, forearm
Abduction	Movement of extremity away from midline of body	Leg, arm, fingers
Adduction	Movement of extremity toward midline of body	Leg, arm, fingers
Internal rotation	Rotation of joint inward	Knee, hip
External rotation	Rotation of joint outward	Knee, hip
Eversion	Turning of body part away from midline	Foot
Inversion	Turning of body part toward midline	Foot
Dorsiflexion	Flexion of toes and foot upward	Foot
Plantar flexion	Bending of toes and foot downward	Foot

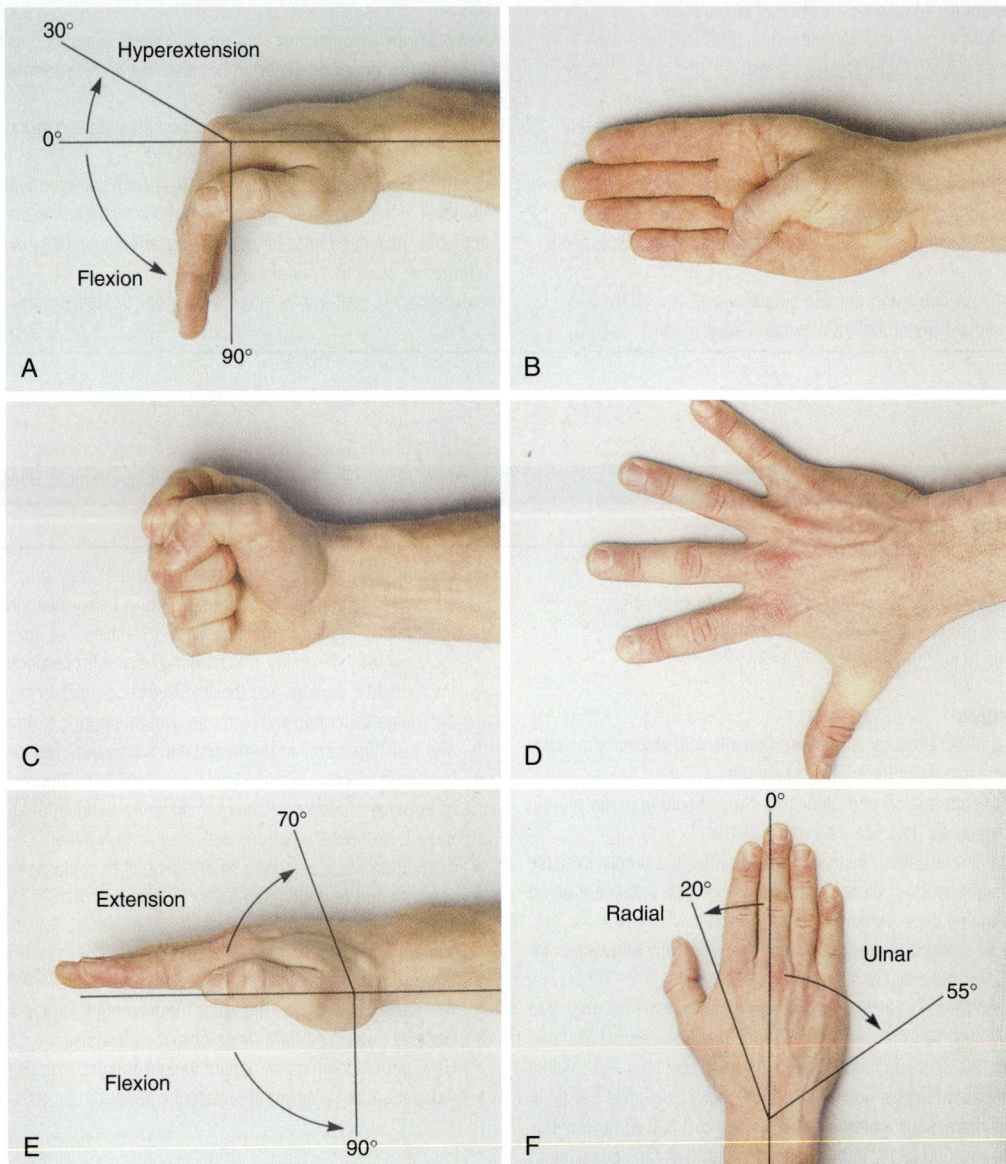

FIGURE 33.49 Range of motion of the hand and wrist. **A,** Metacarpophalangeal flexion and hyperextension. **B,** Finger flexion: thumb to each fingertip and to the base of the little finger. **C,** Finger flexion, fist formation. **D,** Finger abduction. **E,** Wrist flexion and hyperextension. **F,** Wrist radial and ulnar movement. (From Ball, J. W., Dains, J. E., Flynn, J. A., et al. [2019]. *Seidel's guide to physical examination* [9th ed.]. Mosby.)

TABLE 33.31	Manoeuvres to Assess Muscle Strength
Muscle Group	**Manoeuvre**
Neck (sternocleidomastoid)	Place hand firmly against patient's upper jaw. Ask patient to turn head laterally against resistance.
Shoulder (trapezius)	Place hand over midline of patient's shoulder, exerting firm pressure. Have patient raise shoulders against resistance.
Elbow	
Biceps	Pull down on forearm as patient attempts to flex arm.
Triceps	As you flex patient's arm, apply pressure against forearm. Ask patient to straighten arm.
Hip	
Quadriceps	When patient is sitting, apply downward pressure to thigh. Ask patient to raise leg up from table.
Gastrocnemius	Patient sits, while examiner holds shin of flexed leg. Ask patient to straighten leg against resistance.

TABLE 33.32	Assessing Muscle Strength
Muscle Function Level	**Grade**
No evidence of movement	0
Trace of movement	1
Full range of motion, but not against gravity*	2
Full range of motion against gravity, but not against resistance	3
Full range of motion against gravity and some resistance, but weak	4
Full range of motion against gravity, full resistance	5

*Passive movement.
From Ball, J. W., Dains, J. E., Flynn, J. A., et al. (2019). *Seidel's guide to physical examination* (9th ed., Table 22.1). Mosby.

Muscle Tone and Strength

Muscle strength and tone are assessed during ROM measurement. These findings are integrated with those from the neurological assessment. Muscle tone is noted through the slight muscular resistance felt as the examiner moves the relaxed extremity passively through its ROM.

To assess muscle tone, ask the patient to allow an extremity to relax or hang limp. This is often difficult, particularly if the patient feels pain in the extremity. Support the extremity, and grasp each limb, moving it through the normal ROM. Normal tone causes a mild, even resistance to movement through the entire range.

If a muscle has increased tone, or **hypertonicity**, the examiner will meet considerable resistance with any sudden passive movement of a joint. Continued movement eventually causes the muscle to relax. A muscle that has little tone (**hypotonicity**) feels flabby. The involved extremity hangs loosely in a position determined by gravity.

For assessment of muscle strength, the patient assumes a stable position. The patient performs manoeuvres demonstrating strength of major muscle groups (Table 33.31). Symmetrical muscle pairs are compared for strength on the basis of a grading scale of 0 to 5 (Table 33.32). The arm on the dominant side is normally stronger than the arm on the nondominant side. In older persons, a loss of muscle mass causes bilateral weakness, but muscle strength remains greater in the dominant arm or leg.

Each muscle group needs to be examined. To start, ask the patient to first flex the muscle being examined and then to resist when you apply an opposing force against that flexion. It is important to not allow the patient to move the joint. Gradually increase pressure to a muscle group (e.g., elbow extension). Have the patient resist the pressure applied by attempting to move against resistance (e.g., elbow flexion). The patient resists until instructed to stop. Vary the amount of pressure applied, then observe the joint move. If you identify a weakness, compare the size of the muscle with its opposite counterpart by measuring the circumference of the muscle body with a tape measure. A muscle that has atrophied feels soft and boggy when palpated.

NEUROLOGICAL SYSTEM

The neurological system is responsible for many functions, including initiation and coordination of movement, reception and perception of sensory stimuli, organization of thought processes, control of speech, and storage of memory. A close integration exists between the neurological system and all other body systems. For example, urine production relies in part on the adequacy of blood flow to the kidneys, and the size of arterioles supplying the kidneys is under neural control.

An assessment of neurological function alone is quite time consuming. For efficiency, neurological measurements should be integrated with other parts of the physical examination. For example, cranial nerve function is tested during the survey of the head and neck. Cognitive and emotional status is observed during the initial interview.

Many variables need to be considered when deciding the extent of the examination. A patient's level of consciousness influences the ability to follow directions. General physical status influences tolerance to assessment. The patient's chief complaint also helps determine the need for a thorough neurological assessment. If the patient reports headache or a recent loss of function in an extremity, the patient will need a complete neurological review. Table 33.33 reviews the data collected in the nursing history. For a complete examination, the following special equipment is needed:

- Reading material
- Vials containing aromatic substances (e.g., vanilla extract and coffee)
- Opposite tip of cotton swab or tongue blade broken in half
- Snellen eye chart
- Penlight
- Vials containing sugar or salt
- Tongue blade
- Two test tubes, one filled with hot water and the other with cold water
- Cotton balls or cotton-tipped applicators
- Tuning fork
- Reflex hammer

Mental and Emotional Status

Nurses learn a great deal about a patient's mental capacities and emotional state by simply interacting with the patient. They ask questions during an examination to gather data and observe the appropriateness of emotions and thoughts. There are special screening tools designed to assess a patient's mental health status. A widely used tool in the screening for cognitive impairment is the Montreal Cognitive Assessment (MoCA), which is focused on the assessment of mild cognitive impairment (available at https://www.mocatest.org/). The Mini-Mental State Examination (MMSE) is another screening instrument that measures orientation and cognitive function. The MMSE is available online from numerous sources. The maximum score on the MMSE is 30; patients with scores of 21 or less generally have cognitive impairment requiring further evaluation.

To ensure an objective assessment, nurses need to consider the patient's cultural and educational background, values, beliefs, and

TABLE 33.33 Nursing History for Neurological Assessment

Assessment Category	Rationale
Determine if patient uses analgesics, alcohol, sedatives, hypnotics, antipsychotics, antidepressants, nervous system stimulants, or recreational drugs.	These medications alter level of consciousness or cause behavioural changes. Medication misuse sometimes causes tremors, ataxia, and changes in peripheral nerve function.
Determine if patient has recent history of seizures or convulsions: clarify sequence of events (aura, fall to ground, motor activity, loss of consciousness); character of any symptoms; and relationship of seizure to time of day, fatigue, or emotional stress.	Seizure activity often originates from central nervous system alteration. Characteristics of seizure aid in determining its origin.
Screen patient for symptoms of headache, tremors, dizziness, vertigo, numbness or tingling of body part, visual changes, weakness, pain, or changes in speech. Presence of any symptom requires more detailed review (onset, severity, precipitating factors, or sequence of events).	These symptoms frequently originate from alterations in central nervous system or peripheral nervous system function. Identification of specific patterns aids in diagnosis of pathological condition.
Discuss with patient's family any recent changes in patient's behaviour (e.g., increased irritability, mood swings, memory loss, change in energy level).	Behavioural changes sometimes result from intracranial pathological states.
Assess patient for history of change in vision, hearing, smell, taste, or touch.	Major sensory nerves originate from the brainstem. These symptoms help in localizing nature of the problem.
If an older person displays sudden acute confusion (delirium), review history for drug toxicity (anticholinergics, diuretics, digoxin, cimetidine, sedatives, antihypertensives, antiarrhythmics), serious infections, metabolic disturbances, heart failure, and severe anemia.	This is one of the most common mental health disorders in an older person. The condition is always potentially reversible (see Box 33.30).
Review past history for head or spinal cord injury, meningitis, congenital anomalies, neurological disease, or psychiatric counselling.	These factors cause neurological symptoms or behavioural changes to develop, focusing assessment on possible cause.

previous experiences. Such factors influence responses to questions. An alteration in mental or emotional status reflects a disturbance in cerebral functioning. The cerebral cortex controls and integrates intellectual and emotional functioning. Cerebrovascular accidents (CVAs), medication, and metabolic changes are examples of factors that can change cerebral function.

Delirium is an acute mental health disorder characterized by confusion, disorientation, and restlessness. The acute condition is often misdiagnosed as a form of *dementia*, a more progressive, organic mental health disorder such as in Alzheimer's disease. Thus, many health care providers miss the underlying cause of the condition. Delirium is often overlooked in older persons because of a failure to adequately assess cognition and alterations in mental status. Fortunately, the condition often reverses when it is correctly assessed and the underlying cause is treated (central nervous system, metabolic, and cardiopulmonary disorders; systemic illnesses; and sensory deprivation or overload) (Hshieh et al., 2020). Delirium may occur with older persons but also may occur in children having surgery and in hospitalized children (Dechnik & Traube, 2020). It is important to obtain a good history of the patient's behaviour before delirium develops in order to recognize the condition early. Caregivers are usually a good resource in diagnosing delirium. Box 33.30 summarizes clinical criteria for delirium.

Level of Consciousness. A person's level of consciousness exists along a continuum from full awakening, alertness, and cooperation to unresponsiveness to any form of external stimuli. To assess level of consciousness, the nurse talks with the patient, asking questions about events involving the patient or concerns about any health problems. A fully conscious patient responds to questions quickly and expresses ideas logically. With a lowering of the patient's consciousness, the Glasgow Coma Scale (GCS) is used for an objective measurement of consciousness on a numerical scale (Table 33.34). The patient needs to be as alert as possible before testing. One should use caution when using the scale if a patient has sensory losses (e.g., vision, hearing). The GCS enables evaluation of a patient's neurological status over time. The higher the score, the better the patient's neurological function. Short,

BOX 33.30 Clinical Criteria for Delirium

- *Definition:* An acute disturbance of attention (i.e., reduced ability to direct, focus, sustain, and shift attention) and awareness (i.e., reduced orientation to the environment) that is accompanied by a change in cognition. It is not due to a pre-existing or evolving dementia, substance withdrawal or intoxication, exposure to a toxin, or multiple etiologies. Delirium develops over a short period of time, usually hours to days, and tends to fluctuate during the course of the day. It is usually a direct physiological consequence of a general medical condition. It is most common in older persons but occurs occasionally in younger patients.
- There is reduced clarity of awareness of the environment.
- Ability to focus, sustain, or shift attention is impaired (questions must be repeated).
- Irrelevant stimuli easily distract the person.
- There is an accompanying change in cognition (memory impairment, disorientation, or language disturbance).
- Dementia commonly affects recent memory.
- Disorientation usually occurs, with the patient disoriented to time, place, or person.
- Language disturbance involves impaired ability to name objects or ability to write; speech is sometimes rambling.
- Perceptual disturbances include misinterpretations, delusions, or visual and auditory hallucinations. Neurological signs include tremor, unsteady gait, asterixis, or myoclonus.

Modified from American Psychiatric Association. (2013). *Diagnostic and statistical manual of mental disorders* (5th ed.). Stuart, G. (2013). *Principles and practice of psychiatric nursing* (10th ed.). Mosby.

simple questions are asked, such as "What is your name?" "Where are you?" and "What day is this?" The patient is also asked to follow simple commands, such as "Move your toes."

If a patient is not conscious enough to follow commands, the nurse can try to elicit the pain response. To do this, the nurse applies firm pressure with the thumb over the root of the patient's fingernail. The

TABLE 33.34 Glasgow Coma Scale

Action	Response	Score
Eyes open	Spontaneously	4
	To speech	3
	To pain	2
	None	1
Best verbal response	Oriented	5
	Confused	4
	Inappropriate words	3
	Incomprehensible sounds	2
	None	1
Best motor response	Obeys commands	6
	Localized pain	5
	Flexion withdrawal	4
	Abnormal flexion	3
	Abnormal extension	2
	Flaccid	1
	TOTAL SCORE	15

normal response to the painful stimuli is withdrawal of the body part from the stimulus. A patient with serious neurological impairment exhibits abnormal posturing in response to pain. A flaccid response indicates the absence of muscle tone in the extremities and severe injury to brain tissue.

Behaviour and Appearance. Behaviour, moods, hygiene, grooming, and choice of dress reveal pertinent information about mental status. Nurses need to remain perceptive of a patient's mannerisms and actions during the entire physical assessment. Nonverbal and verbal behaviours are noted. Does the patient respond appropriately to directions? Does the patient's mood vary with no apparent cause? Does the patient show concern about appearance? Is the patient's hair clean and neatly groomed, and are the nails trim and clean? The patient should behave in a manner expressing concern and interest in the examination. The patient should make eye contact with the nurse and express appropriate feelings that correspond to the situation. Normally, the patient will show some degree of personal hygiene.

Choice and fit of clothing reflect socioeconomic background or personal taste rather than deficiency in self-concept or self-care. It is important to avoid being judgemental and to focus assessment on the appropriateness of clothing for the weather. Older persons sometimes neglect their appearance because of a lack of energy, finances, mobility, or impaired vision.

Language. Healthy cerebral function enables a person to understand spoken or written words and to express themselves through written words or gestures. Thus, to assess cerebral function, the patient's voice inflection, tone, and manner of speech are assessed. Normally, the patient's voice has inflections, is clear and strong, and increases in volume appropriately. Speech is fluent. When communication is clearly ineffective (e.g., omission or addition of letters and words, misuse of words, or hesitations), the nurse should assess for aphasia, as injury to the cerebral cortex results in aphasia.

The two types of aphasia are sensory (or receptive) and motor (or expressive). With *receptive aphasia,* a person cannot understand written or verbal speech. With *expressive aphasia,* a person understands written and verbal speech but cannot write or speak appropriately when attempting to communicate. A patient sometimes suffers a combination of receptive and expressive aphasia. Language capabilities should

be assessed when it is clear that ineffective communication with the patient exists. Some simple assessment techniques are the following:

- Point to a familiar object and ask the patient to name it.
- Ask the patient to respond to simple verbal and written commands, such as "Stand up" or "Sit down."
- Ask the patient to read simple sentences out loud.

Normally, a patient can name objects correctly, follow commands, and read sentences correctly.

Intellectual Function

Intellectual function includes memory (recent, immediate, and past), knowledge, abstract thinking, association, and judgement. Testing each aspect of function involves a specific technique. However, because cultural and educational background influences the ability to respond to test questions, questions related to concepts or ideas with which the patient is unfamiliar should not be asked.

Memory. To assess memory, immediate recall and recent and remote memory are assessed. Patients demonstrate immediate recall by repeating a series of numbers (e.g., *7, 4, 1*) in the order they are presented or in reverse order. Patients normally recall a series of five to eight digits forward and four to six digits backward.

Assessment begins with the nurse first asking the patient permission to test their memory. Then the nurse states clearly and slowly the name of three unrelated objects. After mentioning all three, the patient is asked to repeat each. The nurse continues until the patient is successful. Then, later in the assessment, the patient is asked to repeat the three words again. The patient should be able to identify the three words. Another test for recent memory involves asking the patient to recall events occurring during the same day (e.g., what was eaten for breakfast). Information can be validated with a caregiver.

To assess past memory, the patient is asked to recall the maiden name of the patient's mother, a birthday, or a special date in history. It is best to ask open-ended questions rather than simple yes/no questions. A patient usually has immediate recall of such information. With an older person, hearing loss should not be interpreted as confusion. Good communication techniques are essential throughout the examination to ensure that the patient clearly understands all directions and testing.

Knowledge. Knowledge is assessed by asking how much the patient knows about their illness or the reason for seeking health care. By assessing a patient's knowledge, the nurse can determine a patient's ability to learn or understand. If there is an opportunity to teach, the patient's mental status can be tested by asking for feedback during a follow-up visit.

Abstract Thinking. Interpreting abstract ideas or concepts reflects the capacity for abstract thinking. An individual requires a higher level of intellectual function to explain phrases that are common to them depending on their primary language and culture, such as "A stitch in time saves nine" or "Don't count your chickens before they're hatched." It is important first to determine the person's primary or most used language and their cultural background. Based on this information the nurse should use the most appropriate phrases. The patient with altered mental status will probably interpret the phrase literally or merely rephrase the words.

Association. Another higher level of intellectual functioning involves finding similarities or associations between concepts: a dog is to a beagle as a cat is to a Siamese. The nurse names related concepts and asks the patient to identify their associations. Questions are appropriate to the patient's level of intelligence. Using simple concepts is sufficient.

Judgement. Judgement requires a comparison and evaluation of facts and ideas to understand their relationships and to form appropriate conclusions. A patient's ability to make logical decisions may be measured using questions such as "Why did you seek health care?" or "What would you do if you became ill at home?" Most often, a patient makes logical decisions.

Cranial Nerve Function

A physical examination can involve the assessment of all 12 cranial nerves or a single nerve or related group of nerves. A dysfunction in one nerve reflects an alteration at some point along the distribution of the cranial nerve. Measurements used to assess the integrity of organs within the head and neck also assess cranial nerve function. A complete assessment involves testing the 12 cranial nerves in order of their numbers. To remember the order of the nerves, use this simple phrase: "On old Olympus' towering tops, a Finn and German viewed some hops." The first letter of each word in the phrase is the same as the first letter of the names of the cranial nerves listed in order (Table 33.35).

Sensory Function

The sensory pathways of the central nervous system conduct sensations of pain, temperature, position, vibration, and crude and finely localized touch. Different nerve pathways relay the sensations. Most patients require only a quick screening of sensory function unless there are symptoms of reduced sensation, motor impairment, or paralysis.

> **SAFETY ALERT** The risk of skin breakdown is greater in a patient with impaired sensation. When assessing decreased sensation, complete a skin and tissue assessment of the area affected by the sensory loss. In addition, teach the patient to avoid pressure, thermal, and chemical trauma to the area.

Normally, a patient has sensory responses to all stimuli that are tested. A patient feels sensations equally on both sides of the body in all areas. To assess the major sensory nerves the nurse must know the sensory dermatome zones (Figure 33.50). Some areas of the skin are innervated by specific dorsal root cutaneous nerves. For example, if assessment reveals reduced sensation when checking for light touch along an area of the skin (e.g., the lower neck), this determines, in general, where a neurological lesion exists (e.g., fourth cervical spinal cord segment).

All sensory testing is done with the patient's eyes closed so that the patient is unable to see when or where a stimulus strikes the skin (Table 33.36). Then stimuli are applied in a random, unpredictable order to maintain the patient's attention and prevent detection of a predictable pattern. The nurse asks the patient to describe when, what, and where the patient feels each stimulus. Symmetrical areas of the body are compared while applying stimuli to the patient's arms, trunk, and legs.

Motor Function

An assessment of motor function includes measurements made during the musculoskeletal examination. In addition, cerebellar function is assessed. The cerebellum coordinates muscular activity, maintains balance and equilibrium, and controls posture.

TABLE 33.35 Cranial Nerve Function and Assessment

Number	Name	Type	Function	Method
I	Olfactory	Sensory	Sense of smell	Ask patient to identify different nonirritating aromas, such as coffee and vanilla.
II	Optic	Sensory	Visual acuity	Use Snellen chart, or ask patient to read printed material while wearing glasses.
III	Oculomotor	Motor	Extraocular eye movement	Assess directions of gaze.
IV	Trochlear	Motor	Pupil constriction and dilation	Measure pupillary reaction to light reflex and accommodation.
			Upward and downward movement of eyeball	Assess directions of gaze.
V	Trigeminal	Sensory and motor	Sensory nerve to skin of face	Lightly touch cornea with wisp of cotton. Assess corneal reflex. Measure sensation of light pain and touch across skin of face.
			Motor nerve to muscles of jaw	Palpate temples as patient clenches teeth.
VI	Abducens	Motor	Lateral movement of eyeballs	Assess directions of gaze.
VII	Facial	Sensory and motor	Facial expression	As patient smiles, frowns, puffs out cheeks, and raises and lowers eyebrows, look for asymmetry.
			Taste	Have patient identify salty or sweet taste on front of tongue.
VIII	Auditory	Sensory	Hearing	Assess ability to hear spoken word.
IX	Glossopharyngeal	Sensory and motor	Taste	Ask patient to identify sour or sweet taste on back of tongue.
			Ability to swallow	Use tongue blade to elicit gag reflex.
X	Vagus	Sensory and motor	Sensation of pharynx	Ask patient to say "ah." Observe movement of palate and pharynx.
			Movement of vocal cords	Assess speech for hoarseness.
XI	Spinal accessory	Motor	Movement of head and shoulders	Ask patient to shrug shoulders and turn head against passive resistance.
XII	Hypoglossal	Motor	Position of tongue	Ask patient to stick out tongue to midline and move it from side to side.

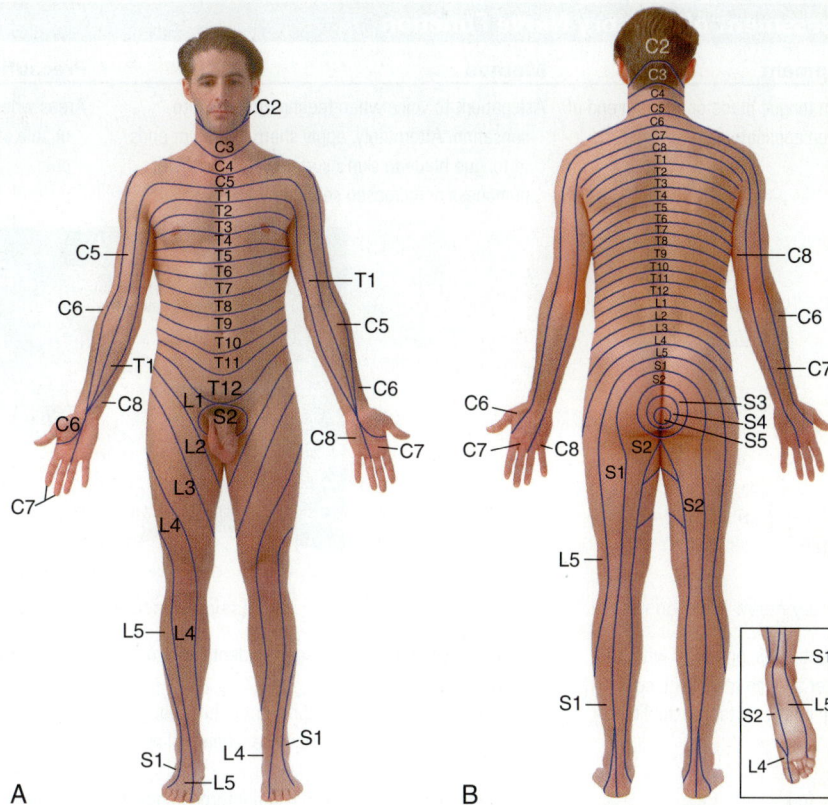

FIGURE 33.50 Dermatomes of the body, the body surface areas innervated by particular spinal nerves. C1 usually has no cutaneous distribution. **A,** Anterior view. **B,** Posterior view. It appears that there is a distinct separation of surface area controlled by each dermatome, but there is almost always overlap between spinal nerves. (From Ball, J. W., Dains, J. E., Flynn, J. A., et al. [2019]. *Seidel's guide to physical examination* [9th ed.]. Mosby.)

Coordination. To avoid confusion, it is good to demonstrate each manoeuvre and then have the patient repeat it, observing for smoothness and balance in the patient's movements (Box 33.31). In older persons, normally slow reaction time causes movements to be less rhythmical.

To assess fine motor function, have the patient extend their arms out to the sides and touch each forefinger alternately to their nose (first with eyes open, then with eyes closed). The patient should be able to alternately touch the nose smoothly. Performing rapid, rhythmical, alternating movements demonstrates coordination in the upper extremities. While sitting, the patient begins by patting the knees with both hands. Then the patient alternately turns up the palm and back of the hands while continuously patting their knees. Normally, patients perform the manoeuvre smoothly and regularly with increasing speed.

An additional manoeuvre for upper extremity coordination involves touching each finger with the thumb of the same hand in rapid sequence. The patient moves from the index finger to the little finger and back, with one hand tested at a time. The patient's dominant hand is slightly less awkward when performing this movement. Movement is smooth and in succession.

To test lower extremity coordination the patient lies supine, legs extended. Place a hand at the ball of the patient's foot. The patient taps the hand with the foot as quickly as possible. Test each foot for speed and smoothness. The feet do not move as rapidly or evenly as the hands.

Balance. Use one or two of the following tests to assess balance and gross motor function:

- Have the patient perform a Romberg test by standing with feet together, arms at their sides, both with eyes open and with eyes closed. Protect the patient's safety by standing at their side, observing for swaying. Expect slight swaying of the body in the Romberg test. A loss of balance (positive Romberg) causes a patient to fall to the side. Normally the patient does not break the stance.
- Have the patient close their eyes, with arms held straight at their sides, and stand on one foot and then the other. Normally patients are able to maintain balance for 5 seconds with slight swaying.
- Ask the patient to walk a straight line by placing the heel of one foot directly in front of the toes of the other foot.

> **SAFETY ALERT** When examining an older person's gait, be aware of the risk for falls. An older person may need assistance with this portion of the examination.

Reflexes

Eliciting reflex reactions provides data about the integrity of sensory and motor pathways of the reflex arc and specific spinal cord segments. Assessment of reflexes does not determine higher neural centre functioning. Figure 33.51 traces the pathway of the reflex arc. Each muscle contains a small sensory unit called a *muscle spindle*, which controls muscle tone and detects changes in the length of muscle fibres. Tapping a tendon with a reflex hammer stretches the muscle and tendon, lengthening the spindle. The spindle sends nerve impulses along afferent nerve pathways to the dorsal horn of the spinal cord segment.

TABLE 33.36	Assessment of Sensory Nerve Function		
Function	**Equipment**	**Method**	**Precautions**
Pain	Broken tongue blade or wooden end of cotton applicator	Ask patient to voice when feeling dull or sharp sensation. Alternately, apply sharp and blunt ends of tongue blade to skin's surface. Note areas of numbness or increased sensitivity.	Areas where skin is thick, such as heel or sole of foot, are less sensitive to pain.

Assessing sensory nerve function in foot.

Assessing sensory nerve function in face.

Function	Equipment	Method	Precautions
Temperature	Two test tubes, one filled with hot water and the other with cold	Touch skin with tube. Ask patient to identify hot or cold sensation.	Omit test if pain sensation is normal.
Light touch	Cotton ball or cotton-tip applicator	Apply light wisp of cotton to different points along skin's surface. Ask patient to voice when feeling a sensation.	Apply at areas where skin is thin or more sensitive (e.g., face, neck, inner aspect of arms, top of feet and hands).
Vibration	Tuning fork	Apply stem of vibrating fork to distal interphalangeal joint of fingers and interphalangeal joint of great toe, elbow, and wrist. Have patient voice when and where vibration is felt.	Be sure patient feels vibration and not merely pressure.
Position		Grasp finger or toe, holding it by its sides with thumb and index finger. Alternate moving finger or toe up and down. Ask patient to state when finger is up or down. Repeat with toes.	Avoid rubbing adjacent appendages as you move finger or toe. Do not move joint laterally; return to neutral position before moving again.
Two-point discrimination	Two broken tongue blades	Lightly apply one or both tongue blade tips simultaneously to the skin's surface. Ask patient whether one or two pricks are felt. Find the distance at which patient can no longer distinguish two points.	Apply blade tips to same anatomical site (e.g., fingertips, palm of hand, or upper arms). Minimum distance at which patient discriminates two points varies (2 to 8 mm on fingertips).

Within milliseconds, the impulses reach the spinal cord and synapse to travel to the efferent motor neuron in the spinal cord. A motor nerve sends the impulses back to the muscle, causing the reflex response.

The two categories of normal reflexes are *deep tendon reflexes*, elicited by mildly stretching a muscle and tapping a tendon, and *cutaneous reflexes*, elicited by stimulating the skin superficially. Table 33.37 summarizes common deep tendon and cutaneous reflexes. Reflexes are graded as follows (Jarvis et al., 2019, p. 713):

0   No response
1+ Sluggish or diminished
2+ Active or expected response
3+ More brisk than expected, slightly hyperactive
4+ Very brisk and hyperactive with intermittent or transient clonus

When assessing reflexes, have the patient relax as much as possible to avoid voluntary movement or tensing of muscles. Position the limbs to slightly stretch the muscle being tested. Hold the reflex hammer loosely between the thumb and fingers so that it is able to swing freely and tap the tendon briskly (Figure 33.52). Compare the responses on corresponding sides. Normally, older persons present with diminished reflexes. Stick figures are sometimes used to record reflexes.

AFTER THE EXAMINATION

Findings from the physical assessment are recorded during the examination or at the end. Special forms are available to record data. It is good to review all findings before assisting the patient with dressing, in case any information needs to be rechecked or additional data gathered. Physical assessment findings should be integrated into the plan of care.

After completing the assessment, give the patient time to dress. The hospitalized patient sometimes needs help with hygiene and returning to bed. When the patient is comfortable, it helps to share a summary of the assessment findings. If the findings have indicated serious abnormalities, such as a mass or highly irregular heart rate, consult the patient's health care provider before revealing any findings. It is the health care provider's responsibility to make definitive medical diagnoses. Explain the type of abnormality found and the need for the health care provider to conduct an additional examination.

When cleaning the examination area, use infection-control practices in removing materials or instruments soiled with potentially infectious wastes into a garbage container. If the patient's bedside was the examination site, clear away soiled items from the bedside table, and make sure that the bed linen is dry and clean. The patient will appreciate a clean gown and the opportunity to wash their face and hands. Afterward, be sure to perform hand hygiene.

Be sure to record a complete assessment. If you delayed entering any items into the assessment form, record them at this time to avoid forgetting any important information. If you made entries periodically during the examination, review them for accuracy and thoroughness. Communicate significant findings to appropriate health care providers, either verbally or in the patient's written care plan.

The patient often needs a number of ancillary examinations, such as X-ray examinations, laboratory tests, or ultrasonography, after a physical examination. The tests provide additional screening information to rule out the presence of abnormalities and help in the diagnosis of specific abnormalities found during the examination. Explain the purpose of these tests and the sensations that the patient will experience.

BOX 33.31 PATIENT TEACHING

Neurological Assessment

Objectives
- Patient's caregiver(s) will understand relationship of patient's behavioural and mental health changes to physical status.
- Patient with sensory or motor impairment will select safety measures for self-care.
- Older person will routinely inspect skin for injuries.

Teaching Strategies
- Explain to caregiver(s) the implications of any behavioural or mental health impairment shown by patient.
- If patient has sensory or motor impairments, explain measures to ensure safety (e.g., use of ambulation aids or safety bars in bathrooms or stairways).
- Teach an older person to plan enough time to complete tasks because reaction time is slow.
- Teach an older person to observe skin surfaces for areas of trauma because perception of pain is reduced.

Evaluation
- Ask caregiver(s) to discuss patient behaviours that result from neurological impairments.
- Have patient explain safety measures used to avoid injury from sensory and motor limitations.
- Have an older person explain the reason for inspecting skin surface routinely.

INTEGRATION OF PHYSICAL ASSESSMENT WITH NURSING CARE

It is important to learn to integrate an examination into routine patient care. For example, the condition of the skin should be assessed during a bed bath, or a patient's gait, ROM, and balance observed as the patient ambulates. Assisting with activities of daily living offers an additional opportunity to obtain cognitive assessment data. This practice makes more efficient use of time and decreases anxiety involved in formal physical assessment examinations.

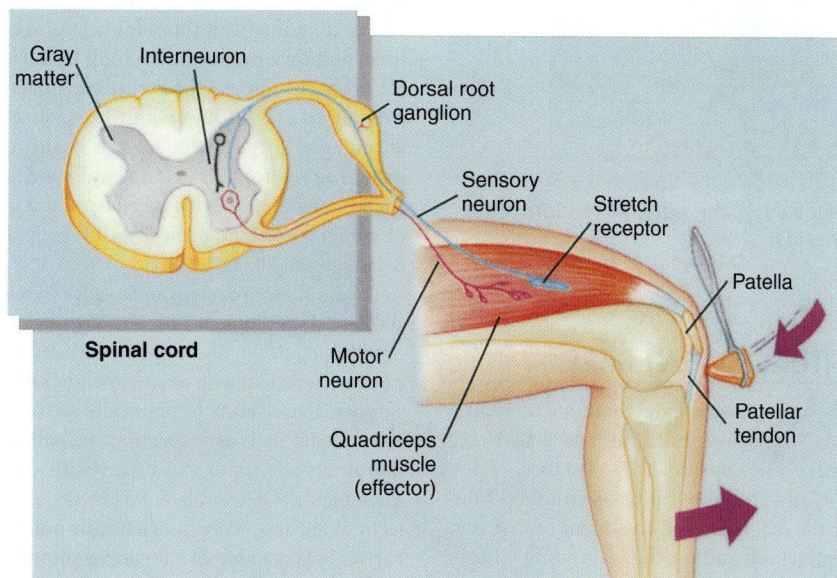

FIGURE 33.51 Pathway of the reflex arc. (From Thibodeau, G. A., & Patton, P. T. [1996]. *Anatomy and physiology* [3rd ed.]. Mosby.)

TABLE 33.37   Assessment of Common Reflexes

Type	Procedure	Normal Reflex
Deep Tendon Reflexes		
Biceps	Flex patient's arm up to 45 degrees at elbow with palms down. Place your thumb in antecubital fossa at base of biceps tendon and your fingers over biceps muscle. Strike triceps tendon with reflex hammer.	Flexion of arm at elbow
Triceps	Flex patient's arm at elbow, holding arm across chest, or hold upper arm horizontally and allow lower arm to go limp. Strike triceps tendon just above elbow.	Extension at elbow
Patellar	Have patient sit with legs hanging freely over side of table or chair, or have patient lie supine and support knee in a flexed 90-degree position. Briskly tap patellar tendon just below patella.	Extension of lower leg
Achilles	Have patient assume same position as for patellar reflex. Slightly dorsiflex patient's ankle by grasping toes in palm of your hand. Strike Achilles tendon just above heel at ankle malleolus.	Plantar flexion of foot
Cutaneous Reflexes		
Plantar	Have patient lie supine with legs straight and feet relaxed. Take handle end of reflex hammer and stroke lateral aspect of sole from heel to ball of foot, curving across ball of foot toward big toe.	Plantar flexion of all toes
Gluteal	Have patient assume side-lying position. Spread buttocks apart and lightly stimulate perineal area with cotton applicator.	Contraction of anal sphincter
Abdominal	Have patient stand or lie supine. Stroke abdominal skin with base of cotton applicator over lateral borders of rectus abdominis muscle toward midline. Repeat test in each abdominal quadrant.	Contraction of rectus abdominis muscle with pulling of umbilicus toward stimulated side

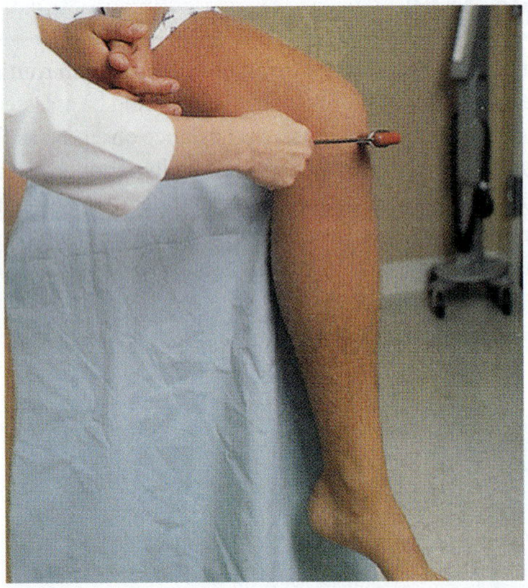

FIGURE 33.52 Position for eliciting the patellar tendon reflex. The lower leg normally extends.

TELEHEALTH AND VIRTUAL PATIENT CARE

Telehealth assessment has become increasingly common in health care. Telehealth is defined as "the delivery of health care services, where patients and providers are separated by distance. Telehealth uses ICT (information and communications technology) for exchange of information for the diagnosis and treatment of diseases and injuries, research and evaluation, and for the continuing education of health professionals" (World Health Organization, 2016, p. 56). Telehealth may also be referred to as telenursing, telemedicine, telepractice, virtual care, and e-health. It includes patient–provider interactions by telephone, email, text messaging, computer chat, video conferencing, remote monitoring, digital devices, and other forms of Internet-based communication (Canadian Nurses Association, 2017).

Telehealth has many advantages. Enhanced accessibility to care is at the forefront of telehealth's benefits. It enables individuals in rural and remote communities, who would otherwise need to travel long distances to seek care, to access a provider in a timely manner. It also reduces barriers to accessing care for individuals with limited mobility, people with young children at home, and individuals who have difficulty taking time off from work. Telehealth has been shown to reduce wait times for access to care, decrease waiting-room time, and save money in the long term (Kaminski, 2021). Telehealth also reduces the risk of spreading infectious disease, allowing sick patients to stay at home and be assessed remotely. There are also advantages to telehealth from a health care provider's perspective, including reduced clinician travel time, enhanced opportunities for timely consultation with specialists, and increased work flexibility, all of which contribute to health care provider satisfaction (Gajarawala & Pelkowski, 2021).

While there are many advantages to telehealth, there are also some shortcomings. Some health concerns cannot be appropriately assessed or managed over a distance and patients need to be seen in person. For example, a patient with acute appendicitis needs to be seen in person for surgery. The inability to physically see or touch the patient to perform assessments such as inspection, palpation, percussion, and auscultation limits telehealth to patients with conditions not requiring these assessments (Gajarawala & Pelkowski, 2021). However, innovations in technology and evolving telehealth practices are helping address this barrier. Use of video conferencing allows for observational assessment (inspection), and remote monitoring devices (e.g., blood pressure and heart rate monitors) allow for vital sign measurements.

Patient-assisted (provider-directed) physical examination is another strategy used to help assess patients by telehealth. In patient-assisted physical examination, the health care provider explains to the patient how to perform a health assessment on themselves (e.g., how to check their own pulse). The patient then reports findings back to the provider, and if video conferencing is being used, the provider can observe the assessment (Benzinger et al., 2021).

When providing telehealth, it is helpful to think of the similarities between in-person and telehealth encounters. Like an in-person visit, the nurse will start with the health history and conduct a general survey using information available to the nurse (e.g., speech and thought process if talking via telephone; appearance and behaviours if using video conferencing). Next, the nurse needs to consider what other assessments are needed for the patient and if these can be done by telehealth. It is important to remember that if the patient cannot be safely assessed using telehealth, an in-person visit should be arranged.

Nurses working in telehealth should further their knowledge of telehealth nursing through resources such as *Fundamentals of Telemedicine and Telehealth* (Gogia, 2020) and the South Central Telehealth Resource Center (https://learntelehealth.org/telehealth-training/courses/). Several online videos are also available to assist in learning virtual physical examination, such as Old Dominion University's (ODU's) (2021) *Telehealth Physical Exam Playlist,* available at https://www.youtube.com/playlist?list=PLM0VF0yZsE6eRiWVQ-RwnkIqruaFzDAON.

KEY CONCEPTS

- Baseline assessment findings reflect the patient's functional abilities and serve as the basis for comparison with subsequent assessment findings.
- Physical assessment of a child or infant requires application of the principles of growth and development.
- The normal process of aging affects physical findings collected from an older person.
- Patient teaching should be integrated throughout the examination to help patients learn about health promotion and disease prevention.
- Inspection requires good lighting, full exposure of the body part, and a careful comparison of the part with its counterpart on the opposite side of the body.
- Palpation involves the use of parts of the hand to detect different types of physical characteristics.
- Auscultation is used to assess the character of sounds created in various body organs.
- A physical examination is performed only after proper preparation of the environment and equipment and after preparing the patient physically and psychologically.
- Throughout the examination, the patient should be kept warm and comfortable and should be informed of each step of the process.
- A competent examiner is systematic while combining assessment of different body systems simultaneously.
- Information from the history helps focus the assessment on body systems likely to be affected.
- When assessing a seriously ill patient, the nurse concentrates on the body systems most likely to be affected.

- Creating a mental image of internal organs in relation to external anatomical landmarks enhances accuracy in assessing the thorax, heart, and abdomen.
- When assessing heart sounds, it helps to imagine events occurring during the cardiac cycle.
- The carotid arteries should never be palpated simultaneously.
- When examining the breasts of a patient with female genitalia, the nurse should explain the techniques for breast self-examination.
- The abdominal assessment differs from other portions of the examination in that auscultation follows inspection.
- During assessment of the genitalia, the technique for genital self-examination should be explained.
- An assessment of musculoskeletal function is conducted when observing the patient ambulate or participate in other active movements.
- Mental health and emotional status are assessed by interacting with the patient throughout the examination.
- At the end of the examination, the nurse provides for the patient's comfort and then documents a detailed summary of physical assessment findings.

CRITICAL THINKING EXERCISES

You are caring for Fallon (preferred pronouns: she/her), a 75-year-old patient of Indigenous ancestry who underwent repair of a right fractured femur attributed to osteoporosis. Fallon was transferred to your hospital from the health centre in her small rural home community. This is her first postoperative day on your clinical unit. The night nurse reported that the patient had an "uneventful" night. The patient has an intravenous line (IV) for fluids and medication, a right hip dressing, a Jackson-Pratt drain, and a Foley (urethral) catheter to gravity and is on bed rest.

1. What body systems would you assess for this patient? Describe the key elements in these assessments.
2. Upon entrance to the room, you observe that Fallon appears agitated and confused. How do you further evaluate the patient's mental health status? What condition may these symptoms indicate?
3. After you reorient Fallon, the patient allows you to continue with your assessment. On auscultation of the patient's posterior lung field bases, you hear a crackling noise on inspiration. What is this sound, and what does it indicate?
4. You next assess the patient's cardiac status. The apical heart rate is 72 beats per minute, rhythm regular. You interpret this finding as
   1. Abnormal
   2. Bradycardia
   3. Normal
   4. Tachycardia
5. You are performing neurovascular checks of the lower extremities. Describe how you would evaluate for capillary refill.
6. How will you demonstrate cultural competency in your care and assessment of Fallon?

🌐 *Answers to Critical Thinking Exercises appear on the Evolve website.*

REVIEW QUESTIONS

Review Questions 1 to 5 refer to the case study at the beginning of the chapter.

1. What assessment information is important to obtain as part of the general survey on Mrs. Smith?
   a. Shortness of breath, posture, moods and affect
   b. Skin colour, moisture, temperature, and turgor
   c. Auscultation of the heart and lungs
   d. Height, weight, and complete vital signs

2. Which of the following assessment findings, as documented in the case study, require follow-up by the nurse? (*Select all that apply.*)
   a. History of coughing up thick green phlegm
   b. No reported history of fever or chills
   c. History of being "very tired"
   d. Blood pressure of 132/86
   e. Respiratory rate of 22 breaths per minute
   f. SaO_2 of 97% on a non-rebreather mask

3. When auscultating Mrs. Smith's lungs, the nurse hears a loud, low-pitched, rumbling, coarse sound during inspiration and expiration. What do these sounds indicate?
   a. Crackles, caused by increased fluid in the airways
   b. Normal breath sounds
   c. Rhonchi, caused by secretions in the bronchial airways
   d. Wheezes, a normal variation in adults with chronic obstructive pulmonary disease

4. The nurse assesses Mrs. Smith's heart, noting a regular rhythm with a distinct silent pause between S1 and S2 and a rate of 86 bpm. What do these finding indicate?
   a. Dysrhythmia
   b. Normal findings
   c. Abnormal heart sounds
   d. Pulse deficit

5. The nurse conducts an assessment of Mrs. Smith's neurological system and documents the following:
   a. Alert and oriented to person and place; incorrect identification of day, month, and year
   b. GCS: 14
   c. Clear and strong voice with inflections
   d. PERRLA
   e. Sensation intact
   f. Reflexes 2+ bilaterally

   Place a checkmark beside findings requiring follow-up by the nurse.

   Review Questions 6 to 12 review general health examination and physical assessment topics.

6. The nurse is teaching the patient to inspect all skin surfaces for abnormal skin pigmentation and lesions. Which of the following abnormalities should the patient be instructed to report to a health care provider? (*Select all that apply.*)
   a. An asymmetrical, flat lesion that is 10 mm × 6 mm diameter
   b. A symmetrical, flat lesion that is uniform in colour
   c. A flat, brown-coloured lesion with irregular borders
   d. A symmetrical, raised lesion that is 8 mm × 8 mm in diameter
   e. A raised lesion with irregular borders that is 3 mm × 4 mm in diameter
   f. A symmetrical, purple-coloured lesion with regular borders

7. A patient has a suspected fracture of the left scaphoid bone. Which pulse is a priority for the nurse to assess?

   a. The dorsalis pedis
   b. The radial
   c. The posterior tibialis
   d. The apical

8. The nurse assesses a patient with abdominal pain. Place in correct order the assessment techniques employed during this examination.
   a. Palpation
   b. Inspection
   c. Percussion
   d. Auscultation

9. The nurse is teaching a patient how to perform a testicular self-examination. What is the correct information to provide the patient?
   a. "The testes are normally round, movable, and have a lumpy consistency."
   b. "Contact your health care provider if you feel a painless pea-sized nodule."
   c. "The best time to do a testicular self-examination is before you bathe or shower."
   d. "Perform a testicular self-examination weekly to detect signs of testicular cancer."

10. When the nurse is assessing range of motion of a patient's knee, what movements are assessed? (*Select all that apply.*)
    a. Flexion
    b. Extension
    c. Abduction
    d. Adduction
    e. Internal rotation
    f. External rotation

11. The nurse is assessing the patient's visual direction of gaze. What cranial nerve(s) does this assessment evaluate? (*Select all that apply.*)
    a. II—Optic
    b. III—Oculomotor
    c. IV—Trochlear
    d. VI—Abducens
    e. VII—Facial
    f. XI—Spinal accessory

12. The nurse recognizes which of the following as common biocultural variations of normal physical exam findings? (*Select all that apply.*)
    a. Darker skin creases on the body of a patient with a dark complexion
    b. Dry, flaky cerumen in the ear canal of a child of Indigenous descent
    c. Elevated blood pressure in an individual of Black ancestry
    d. Dark brown areolae in a fair-complexioned patient aged 45 years

Answers: 1. a; **2.** a, c, e, f; **3.** c; **4.** b; **5.** a, b; **6.** a, c, d, e; **7.** b; **8.** b, d, c, a; **9.** b; **10.** a, b; **11.** b, c, d; **12.** a, b, d.

Rationales for the Review Questions appear on the Evolve website.

RECOMMENDED WEBSITES

Canadian Cancer Society (CCS): https://www.cancer.ca
This website is a source of general information about all types of cancers, including Canadian statistics on the prevalence, mortality, and survival rates for specific cancers. Please note that screening guidelines for cancer vary slightly from region to region. Students are encouraged to consult with the guidelines of their local region and to be aware of national guidelines for cancer screening and prevention.

Canadian Diabetes Association (CDA): https://www.diabetes.ca
The Canadian Diabetes Association website (Diabetes Canada) contains a wealth of resources on diabetes and evidenced-informed guidelines for patient care. The site contains information about risk factors and associated disease processes and conditions.

Canadian Task Force on Preventive Health Care (CTFPHC): http://www.canadiantaskforce.ca
This site provides information on health prevention and evidence-informed recommendations.

Choosing Wisely Canada: https://www.choosingwiselycanada.org
This site provides information for patients and health care providers on unnecessary tests and treatments, with the intent of increasing awareness of effective, high-quality, patient-centred care.

Montreal Cognitive Assessment: https://www.mocatest.org
This site provides access to the Montreal Cognitive Assessment (MoCA) and research on cognitive impairment.

Osteoporosis Canada: https://www.osteoporosis.ca
The Osteoporosis Canada website provides information and support to individuals who have osteoporosis. The site contains links to information on calcium and vitamin D, as well as health promotion and prevention recommendations.

Public Health Agency of Canada (PHAC): https://www.phac-aspc.gc.ca/index-eng.php
The Public Health Agency of Canada is a repository of a wealth of information on infectious and chronic diseases, immunization, food and travel safety, and emergency preparedness. The site also provides daily updates on current concerns (e.g., flu virus tracking) and other health promotion and disease prevention issues.

Rourke Baby Record: https://www.rourkebabyrecord.ca/
The Rourke Baby Record website provides information about children's first 5 years of life. Literature and research that contributed to the development of this tool are linked to the website. This tool and the website offer information about pediatric assessment.

REFERENCES

A full reference list is available on the website for this book at http://evolve.elsevier.com/Canada/Potter/fundamentals/

34

Infection Control

Canadian content written by Colleen M. Astle, RN, BScN, MN, CNeph(C), NP, Deborah Hobbs, BScN, RN, CIC, and Laurence Fernandez, RN, MN, NP(Cand.), with original chapter contributions by Lorri A. Graham, DNP-L, RN

OBJECTIVES

Mastery of content in this chapter will enable you to:

- Define the key terms listed.
- Explain the relationship between the chain of infection and the transmission of infection.
- Identify the body's normal defences against infection.
- Describe the events in the inflammatory response.
- Describe the signs and symptoms of a localized and a systemic infection.
- Identify patients most at risk for infection.
- Explain conditions that promote the transmission of health care–associated infection.

- Explain the difference between medical and surgical asepsis.
- Give an example of preventing infection for each element of the infection chain.
- Perform proper procedures for hand hygiene.
- Explain the rationale and components of routine practices.
- Explain the rationale and practices for additional (isolation) precautions.
- Explain how infection-control measures in the home may differ from those in the hospital.
- Properly don and doff a surgical mask, sterile gown, and sterile gloves.

KEY TERMS

Aerobic
Anaerobic
Asepsis
Broad-spectrum antibiotics
Carriers
Colonizing
Communicable
Disinfection
Edema
Endogenous infection
Epidemiology
Exogenous infection
Exudates
Hand hygiene
Handwashing

Health care–associated infection (HAI)
Immune response
Immunocompromised
Inflammatory response
Invasive
Isolation precautions
Leukocytosis
Localized
Medical asepsis
Microorganisms
Necrotic
Normal flora
Nosocomial infection
Pathogenicity
Pathogens

Phagocytosis
Purulent
Resident microorganism
Routine practices
Sanguineous
Serosanguineous
Serous
Sterile field
Sterilization
Superinfection
Surgical asepsis
Susceptibility
Systemic
Transient microorganism
Virulence

WEBSITE

http://evolve.elsevier.com/Canada/Potter/fundamentals/

CASE STUDY

Susan (preferred pronouns: she/her) is a 48-year-old woman in end-stage renal failure secondary to focal segmental glomerulosclerosis, diagnosed 2 months previously. Susan is dialysis dependent, which required the insertion of a central venous catheter. Susan was admitted to the nephrology service on Friday evening from the emergency department with complaints of chills, headache, fatigue, and a painful maculopapular rash of new onset located across her upper chest and on her abdomen, involving more than two dermatomes. Susan described it as itchy and burning. Susan also stated that she had felt well until the end of her dialysis treatment 2 days earlier.

In this chapter you will learn how to assess Susan, develop a treatment plan, and evaluate this plan.

Think about this case study as you read this chapter. There are review questions at the end of the chapter that relate to the case study.

Good health depends in part on a safe environment. Practices or techniques that control or prevent transmission of infection help to create an environment that protects patients and health care workers from disease. Patients in all health care settings are at risk for acquiring infections because they often have lower resistance to infectious microorganisms and increased exposure to numbers and types of disease-causing microorganisms, and they sometimes undergo **invasive** procedures wherein a body cavity or organ is entered by either puncture or incision. In acute care or ambulatory care facilities, patients can be exposed to pathogens, some of which may be resistant to most antibiotics. By practising infection prevention and control techniques, nurses can avoid spreading microorganisms to patients.

In all settings, patients and their families must be able to recognize sources of infections and be able to institute protective measures. Patient teaching should include information concerning infections, modes of transmission, and methods of prevention.

Health care workers can protect themselves from contact with infectious materials or exposure to communicable diseases by having knowledge of the infectious process and appropriate barrier protections. The spread of diseases such as hepatitis B and C, acquired immune deficiency syndrome (AIDS), sudden acute respiratory syndrome (SARS), tuberculosis (TB), and, more recently, Ebola and Coronavirus/COVID-19 (CoV) has resulted in a greater emphasis on infection-control techniques. Infection control has three purposes: (1) protecting patients from acquiring infections, (2) protecting health care workers from becoming infected, and (3) protecting entire populations from contracting infectious diseases. Many of the techniques used to protect patients or entire populations also provide effective protection for nurses. Nurses must remain constantly vigilant to prevent the spread of infection while providing care.

SCIENTIFIC KNOWLEDGE BASE

Microorganisms are typically a single cell and can only be seen with the aid of a microscope. They include bacteria, protozoa, certain types of algae, and fungi. Microorganisms live and grow on inanimate objects and in air, water, food, soil, plants, and animals. They also live and grow in and on people. Most microorganisms are nonpathogens, meaning that they do not cause a person to be ill; however, some are **pathogens**, meaning that they can cause disease. An *infection* is a disease state resulting from the entry and multiplication of a pathogen in the tissues of a host, causing the body to manifest clinical signs and symptoms. If the infection can be transmitted from one person to another, it is a **communicable** (infectious, contagious) disease. Resident skin microorganisms are usually nonpathogenic. However, they can cause serious infection when surgery or other invasive procedures allow them to enter deep tissues, or when a patient is severely **immunocompromised** (has an impaired immune system).

Chain of Infection

The presence of a pathogen does not mean that an infection will begin. The development of an infection occurs in a cycle that depends on the presence of all the following elements:

- An infectious agent (pathogen)
- A reservoir (source for pathogen growth)
- A portal of exit from the reservoir
- A mode of transmission
- A portal of entry to a host
- A susceptible host

An infection develops if this chain remains intact (Figure 34.1). Nurses need to follow infection prevention and control practices to break the chain so that infections do not develop.

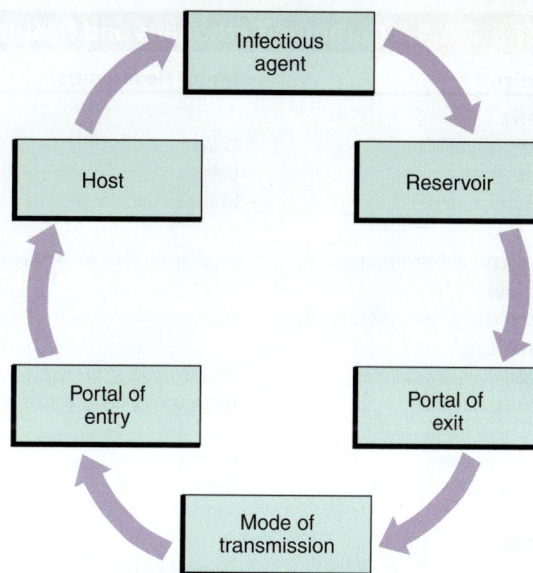

FIGURE 34.1 Chain of infection.

Infectious Agents. As stated earlier, microorganisms include bacteria, viruses, fungi, and protozoa (Table 34.1). Microorganisms on the skin are called *resident* or *transient flora*. **Resident microorganisms** are considered permanent residents of the skin, where they survive and multiply without causing harm. They are not easily removed by handwashing with plain soaps unless considerable friction is used. Resident microorganisms in deep skin layers are usually killed only by performing hand hygiene with products containing antimicrobial ingredients. *Staphylococcus aureus* is a resident microorganism of the skin.

Transient microorganisms attach to the skin when a person has contact with another person or object. For example, when a person touches a bedpan or a contaminated dressing, transient bacteria adhere to their skin. The organisms attach loosely to the skin in dirt and grease and under fingernails. These organisms may be readily transmitted unless removed by proper handwashing or hand hygiene (Hillier, 2020). *Escherichia coli* (*E. coli*) is found in the bowel and is an example of transient bacteria of the skin.

The potential for microorganisms to cause disease depends on the following factors:
- A sufficient number of organisms
- **Virulence**, or the ability to produce disease
- The ability to enter and survive in the host
- The susceptibility of the host

Reservoir. A *reservoir* is a place where a pathogen can survive but may or may not multiply. For example, hepatitis A virus survives in shellfish but does not multiply; *Pseudomonas* organisms can survive and multiply in nebulizer reservoirs used in the care of patients with respiratory conditions. The most common reservoir is the human body. A variety of microorganisms live on the skin and within body cavities, fluids, and discharges. When a pathogen is present on or in the body but does not cause harm, the pathogen is **colonizing** the site. **Carriers** are animals or persons who show no symptoms of illness but who have pathogens on or in their bodies that can be transferred to others. For example, a person can be a carrier of hepatitis B virus without having any signs or symptoms of infection. Animals, food, water, insects, and even inanimate objects can also be reservoirs for infectious organisms. For example, the bacterium *Legionella pneumophila*, which causes Legionnaires' disease, lives in contaminated water and water systems.

TABLE 34.1 Common Pathogens and Resulting Major Infections

Organism	Major Reservoir(s)	Major Infections
Bacteria		
Clostridioides difficile	Colon	Colitis, diarrhea
Escherichia coli	Colon	Gastroenteritis, urinary tract infection
Staphylococcus aureus	Skin, hair, anterior nares	Wound infection, pneumonia, food poisoning, cellulitis, bacteremia, meningitis, osteomyelitis, septic arthritis
Streptococcus (β-hemolytic group A) organisms	Oropharynx, skin, perianal area	"Strep throat," rheumatic fever, scarlet fever, impetigo, wound infection, glomerulonephritis (CDC, 2022)
Streptococcus (β-hemolytic group B) organisms	Adult genitalia	Urinary tract infection, wound infection, postpartum sepsis, neonatal sepsis
Mycobacterium tuberculosis	Droplet nuclei from lungs	Tuberculosis
Neisseria gonorrhoeae	Genitourinary tract, rectum, mouth	Gonorrhea, pelvic inflammatory disease, infectious arthritis, conjunctivitis
Rickettsia rickettsii	Wood tick	Rocky Mountain spotted fever
Staphylococcus epidermidis	Skin	Wound infection, bacteremia
Viruses		
Coronavirus	Respiratory	Pneumonia (Hasöksüz et al., 2020)
COVID-19	Respiratory	Cold
Severe acute respiratory syndrome (SARS)	Respiratory	Pneumonia (CDC, 2017)
Ebola virus	Blood and body fluids	Gastrointestinal bleeding (CDC, 2021a)
Hepatitis A virus	Feces	Hepatitis A
Hepatitis B virus	Blood and body fluids	Hepatitis B
Hepatitis C virus	Blood	Hepatitis C
Herpes simplex virus (type 1)	Lesions of mouth or skin, saliva, genitalia	Cold sores, aseptic meningitis, genital herpes, herpetic whitlow
Human immunodeficiency virus (HIV)	Blood, semen, vaginal secretions, breast milk (has also been isolated in saliva, tears, and urine, but these have not proved to be sources of transmission)	Acquired immune deficiency syndrome (AIDS)
Varicella-zoster virus	Spreads from human to human via respiratory droplets or vesicular fluid	Primary infection chicken pox, reactivation infection shingles, disseminated shingles
Fungi		
Aspergillus organisms	Soil, dust, construction dust, decaying or organic matter	Sinusitis or skin, lung, wound, or central nervous system infection (CDC, 2021b)
Candida albicans	Mouth, skin, colon, genital tract	Candidiasis, pneumonia, sepsis
Protozoan		
Plasmodium falciparum	Blood	Malaria

To thrive, pathogens require a reservoir that provides food, oxygen (or no oxygen, depending on the pathogen), water, an appropriate temperature and pH, and minimal light.

Food. Microorganisms require nourishment. Some, such as *Clostridium perfringens,* the microbe that causes gas gangrene, thrive on organic matter. Others, such as *Escherichia coli,* consume undigested food in the bowel. Carbon dioxide and inorganic materials such as soil provide nourishment for other organisms.

Oxygen. **Aerobic** bacteria require oxygen to survive and to multiply sufficiently to cause disease. Aerobic organisms cause more infections than do **anaerobic** organisms (i.e., organisms that can survive only in the absence of oxygen). Examples of aerobic organisms are *Staphylococcus aureus* and strains of *Streptococcus* organisms.

The gastrointestinal tract is colonized by large numbers of anaerobic bacteria that can cause infections if the bowel is damaged. Infections deep within the pleural cavity, in a joint, or in a deep sinus tract are typically caused by anaerobes. Bacteria that cause tetanus, gas gangrene, and botulism are anaerobes.

Water. Most organisms require water or moisture for survival. For example, microorganisms thrive in the moist drainage from a surgical wound. However, some bacteria assume a form called a *spore.* Spores remain viable even when deprived of water and are resistant to drying. Spore-forming bacteria, such as those that cause anthrax, botulism, and tetanus, can live without water.

Temperature. Microorganisms can live only in certain temperature ranges. The ideal temperature for most pathogens in humans is 35°C to 37°C; however, some can survive temperature extremes that would be fatal to humans (Taylor, 2018). Cold temperatures tend to prevent the growth and reproduction of bacteria.

pH. The acidity of an environment determines the viability of microorganisms. Most microorganisms prefer an environment within a pH range of 5 to 8. Bacteria, in particular, thrive in urine with an alkaline pH. Most organisms cannot survive the acidic environment of the stomach. Acid-reducing medications (e.g., antacids and histamine 2 blockers) can cause an overgrowth of gastrointestinal organisms, which can contribute to development of nosocomial pneumonia (Taylor, 2018).

Minimal Light. Microorganisms thrive in dark environments, such as those under dressings and within body cavities. Ultraviolet light may be effective in killing certain forms of bacteria (e.g., *Mycobacterium tuberculosis*).

Portal of Exit. After microorganisms find a site in which to grow and multiply, they must find a portal of exit if they are to enter another host and cause disease. *A portal of exit* is the path by which the pathogen leaves the reservoir (AusMed, 2020). Exits in the human body include body openings (mouth, nose, rectal, vaginal, and urethral openings; and artificial openings such as those resulting from ostomies), breaks in the skin (a scrape, cut, or other wound), and breaks in the mucous membranes (the skin in the mouth, eyes, nose, vagina, and rectum). Pathogens are carried through portals of exit by blood, body fluids, excretions, and secretions (e.g., urine, stool, vomitus, saliva, mucus, pus, vaginal discharge, semen, wound drainage, bile, and sputum). For example, pathogens that infect the respiratory tract, such as *M. tuberculosis,* can be released from the body through the mouth and nose when an infected person sneezes, coughs, talks, or even breathes. In patients with artificial airways such as tracheostomy or endotracheal tubes (see Chapter 40), organisms easily exit the respiratory tract through these devices. Similarly, when a patient has a urinary tract infection, microorganisms exit during urination or through urinary diversions such as ileal conduits, urostomies, and suprapubic drains (see Chapter 44).

Modes of Transmission. Microorganisms can be transmitted from the reservoir to the host in many ways. Certain infectious diseases tend to be transmitted more commonly by specific modes (Table 34.2). However, a microorganism may be transmitted by more than one mode. For example, human chicken pox virus may be spread by the airborne route or through direct contact.

Indirect contact is a major mode of transmission in health care facilities. The health care worker's hands can easily pick up microbes from one person, place, or thing and then transmit them to other people, places, or things. However, almost any object within the environment (e.g., a stethoscope or thermometer) can be a mode of indirect transmission of pathogens. Some organisms, such as *Clostridioides difficile,* which can produce spores, can live in hospital environments for months. *C. difficile* can be spread by direct or indirect contact. All health care workers providing direct care (e.g., nurses and licensed practical nurses, physiotherapists, and physicians) or performing diagnostic and support services (e.g., laboratory technicians, respiratory therapists, and dietary workers) must follow practices to minimize the spread of infection. Each group follows procedures for handling equipment and supplies used by a patient. For example, respiratory therapists perform hand hygiene before working with each patient and dispose of contaminated therapy equipment in a prescribed manner. Certain medical devices and diagnostic procedures provide avenues for the spread of pathogens. Invasive procedures such as cystoscopy (the

TABLE 34.2 Modes of Transmission	
Mode of Transmission	**Examples of Organisms**
Contact Transmission The transfer of microbes by physical touch; may be by direct contact, indirect contact, or droplet	
Direct Contact Physical skin-to-skin contact between an infected or colonized individual and a susceptible host (e.g., via touching patient)	*Clostridioides difficile, Staphylococcus,* herpes simplex virus, methicillin-resistant *Staphylococcus aureus* (MRSA), vancomycin-resistant enterococci (VRE), carbapenemase-producing organisms (CPO), Ebola (CDC, 2021a)
Indirect Contact Contact between a susceptible host and a contaminated intermediate object (e.g., via touching soiled linen, equipment, or dressings; transferring pathogens to a patient via hands that are not washed between handling patients)	*Clostridioides difficile, Staphylococcus,* respiratory syncytial virus (RSV), *Pseudomonas,* MRSA, VRE, CPO
Droplet Transmission Large particles (droplets) from the respiratory system of an infected source propelled up to 2 m through the air and deposited onto a susceptible host (e.g., droplets produced via coughing, sneezing, or talking)	Influenza virus, rubella virus, RSV, Coronavirus (Jayaweera et al., 2020), *Neisseria meningitis*
Airborne Transmission Small airborne particles (droplet nuclei) containing microbes remain suspended in the air for long periods of time (e.g., droplets and aerosolized airborne particles produced via coughing and sneezing); air currents transmit these particles long distances (>2 m); susceptible host inhales them	*Mycobacterium tuberculosis* (causes tuberculosis), varicella-zoster virus (causes chicken pox), Coronavirus, measles virus
Vehicle Transmission A single contaminated source (e.g., water, medications, intravenous fluid, food, equipment) transmits infection to multiple hosts, possibly resulting in an outbreak	*Pseudomonas* (via water, medications), *Escherichia coli* (via food, water), *Enterobacter cloacae* (via intravenous fluid), *Salmonella* (via food)
Vectorborne Transmission Insects (fleas, mites, ticks, mosquitoes) or pests (e.g., mice) transmit microbes to humans	*Vibrio cholerae, Plasmodium falciparum* (causes malaria), West Nile virus, Lyme disease

Data from Public Health Agency of Canada. (2017). *Routine practices and additional precautions for preventing the transmission of infection in health care settings* (Table 5: Transmission characteristics and precautions by specific etiology). https://www.canada.ca/en/public-health/services/publications/diseases-conditions/routine-practices-precautions-healthcare-associated-infections.html

use of an endoscope to visualize the bladder) facilitate the diagnosis of health problems but also increase the risk of infection transmission. Because so many factors can promote the spread of infection to a patient, all health care workers must be conscientious about using infection-control practices, such as performing proper hand hygiene and ensuring that equipment has been adequately cleaned, disinfected, or sterilized.

Portal of Entry. Organisms can enter the body through the same routes they use to exit (i.e., body openings and breaks in the skin or mucous membranes). For example, organisms enter the body when a needle pierces the skin. As long as the device is in place, more organisms are able to enter the body. In patients with a urinary catheter, any obstruction to the flow of urine allows organisms to travel up the urethra. Factors that reduce the body's defences enhance the chances of pathogens entering the body.

Susceptible Host. Whether a person acquires an infection is related to their susceptibility to an infectious agent—**susceptibility** depends on the individual's degree of resistance to a pathogen. Although everyone is constantly in contact with large numbers of microorganisms, an infection does not develop until an individual becomes susceptible to the strength and numbers of microorganisms capable of producing infection. The more virulent an organism is, the greater the likelihood that a person will be susceptible to it. Organisms with resistance to antibiotics are becoming more common in acute care settings—this is believed to be associated with the frequent and sometimes inappropriate use of antibiotics. A person's resistance to an infectious agent may be enhanced by receiving an appropriate vaccine or actually contracting the disease.

Infectious Process

By understanding the chain of infection, nurses can intervene to prevent infections from developing. If a patient is at risk for acquiring an infection, the nurse should observe for signs and symptoms of infection and take appropriate actions to prevent its spread. Infections follow a progressive course (Box 34.1). The severity of a patient's illness depends on the extent of the infection, the ability of the microorganism to cause disease (**pathogenicity** of the microorganisms), and the susceptibility of the host (patient).

If infection is **localized**, or restricted to a limited area (e.g., a wound infection), proper care controls the spread and minimizes the illness. The patient may experience localized symptoms such as pain and tenderness at the wound site. An infection that affects the entire body instead of just a single organ or part is **systemic** and can be fatal.

The course of an infection influences the level of nursing care provided. Nurses are responsible for properly administering antibiotics and monitoring the response to medication therapy (see Chapter 35). Supportive therapy includes providing adequate nutrition and rest to bolster the patient's defences against the infectious process. The complexity of care depends on body systems affected by the infection.

Regardless of whether an infection is localized or systemic, nurses play a critical role in minimizing its spread. For example, an organism causing a simple wound infection can spread to involve an intravenous needle–insertion site if the nurse uses an improper technique when changing a dressing at this site. Nurses who have breaks in their own skin can also acquire infections from patients if their techniques for controlling infection transmission are inadequate.

Defences Against Infection

The body has several mechanisms that protect it against infection. Normal body flora that live inside and outside the body protect a person

---

BOX 34.1 Course of Infection by Stage

Incubation Period
- Interval between the entrance of the pathogen into the body and the appearance of first symptoms (e.g., in chicken pox, 2 to 3 weeks; in the common cold, 1 to 2 days; in influenza, 1 to 3 days; in mumps, 15 to 18 days)

Prodromal Stage
- Interval from the onset of nonspecific signs and symptoms (malaise, low-grade fever, and fatigue) to more specific symptoms (during this time, microorganisms grow and multiply and the patient may be more capable of spreading disease to others)

Illness Stage
- Interval when the patient manifests signs and symptoms specific to type of infection (e.g., the common cold is manifested by a sore throat, sinus congestion, and rhinitis; mumps is manifested by an earache, a high fever, and parotid and salivary gland swelling)

Convalescence
- Interval when the acute symptoms of infection disappear, and the body tries to replenish its resources and return to a state of homeostasis; the length of recovery depends on the severity of the infection and the patient's general state of health (may take several days to months)

---

from several pathogens. Each organ system has defence mechanisms that fight infectious microorganisms. The **immune response** is a protective reaction that neutralizes pathogens and repairs body cells. The immune system is composed of cells and molecules that help the body resist disease; certain responses of the immune system are nonspecific and protect against microorganisms regardless of prior exposure (e.g., normal flora, body system defences, and inflammation), whereas others are specific defences against particular pathogens. If any of the body's defences fail, an infection can quickly progress to a serious health problem.

Normal Flora. The body normally contains microorganisms that reside on the surface and in deep layers of skin, in the saliva and oral mucosa, and in the gastrointestinal and genitourinary tracts. A person normally excretes trillions of microbes daily through the intestines. The skin also has a large population of resident flora—these **normal flora** do not typically cause disease when residing in their usual area of the body but, instead, participate in maintaining health.

Normal flora of the large intestine exist in great numbers without causing injury. Normal flora may assist in fighting infection and inflammation and maintaining homeostasis. Gut microorganisms change dietary fibre into fatty acids, which are reabsorbed by the large bowel and synthesize vitamins B and K, bile acids, and sterols; this synthesis has a benefit to both the host and the flora. Bile has antibacterial properties as well as fatty acids that stabilize the normal flora populations and prevent invasion of pathogens (Howerton et al., 2018). When the normal flora are disrupted, disease-causing organisms can proliferate. The skin's normal flora exert a protective action by inhibiting the multiplication of organisms landing on the skin. The mouth and pharynx are also protected by flora that impair the growth of invading microbes. The mass of normal flora maintains a sensitive balance with other microorganisms to prevent infection. Any factor that disrupts this balance places a person at increased risk for acquiring an infectious disease. For example, according to studies, when a patient acquires microorganisms within the hospital, the person's resident flora change, which may lead to an infection (Prinzi, 2020).

In addition, the use of broad-spectrum antibiotics for the treatment of infection can lead to a superinfection, which develops when broad-spectrum antibiotics eliminate a wide range of microorganisms, not just those causing infection. Normal bacterial flora are eliminated, reducing the body's defences and thus allowing disease-producing microorganisms to multiply (Lishman et al., 2018). An example is *Clostridioides difficile* (*C. diff*).

Body System Defences. A number of the body's organ systems have unique defences against infection (Table 34.3). The skin, respiratory tract, and gastrointestinal tract are easily accessible to microorganisms: pathogenic organisms easily adhere to the skin's surface, are inhaled into the lungs, or are ingested with food. Each organ system has defence mechanisms physiologically suited to its structure and function. For example, the lungs cannot completely control the entrance of microorganisms; however, the airways are lined with hair-like projections (cilia) that rhythmically beat to move a blanket of mucus and adherent or trapped organisms up to the pharynx to be removed. Conditions that impair an organ's specialized defences increase the person's susceptibility to infection.

Inflammation. *Inflammation* is the body's cellular response to injury or infection. Inflammation is a protective vascular reaction that delivers fluid, blood products, and nutrients to interstitial tissues in an area of injury. The process neutralizes and eliminates pathogens or necrotic (dead) tissues and establishes a means of repairing body cells and tissues. Signs of localized inflammation are swelling, redness, heat, pain or tenderness, and loss of function in the affected body part. When infection becomes systemic, other signs and symptoms develop, including fever, leukocytosis, malaise, anorexia, nausea, vomiting, and lymph node enlargement.

The inflammatory response may be triggered by physical agents, chemical agents, or microorganisms. Mechanical trauma, temperature extremes, and radiation are examples of physical agents. Chemical agents include external and internal irritants, such as harsh poisons and gastric acid.

After tissues are injured, the inflammatory response, a series of well-coordinated events, occurs:
- Vascular and cellular responses
- The formation of inflammatory exudates (fluid and cells that are discharged from cells or blood vessels, e.g., pus or serum)
- Tissue repair

Vascular and Cellular Responses. Acute inflammation is an immediate response to cellular injury. Arterioles supplying the infected or injured area dilate, allowing more blood into the local circulation. The increase in local blood flow causes the characteristic redness of

TABLE 34.3	Normal Defence Mechanisms Against Infection	
Defence Mechanisms	**Action**	**Factors That May Alter Defence**
Skin		
Intact multilayered surface (body's first line of defence against infection)	Provides barrier to microorganisms and antibacterial activity	Cuts, abrasions, wounds, areas of maceration (softening of the skin due to moisture), burns, or penetration by invasive devices
Shedding of outer layer of skin cells	Removes organisms that adhere to skin's outer layers	Failure to bathe regularly
Sebum	Contains fatty acid that kills some bacteria	Excessive bathing
Mouth		
Intact multilayered mucosa	Provides mechanical barrier to microorganisms	Lacerations, trauma, extracted teeth
Saliva	Washes away particles containing microorganisms, contains microbial inhibitors (e.g., lysozyme)	Poor oral hygiene, dehydration
Eye		
Tearing and blinking	Blinking prevents entry of particles containing pathogens, and tearing helps to wash particles away	Injury
Respiratory Tract		
Cilia lining upper airway, coated with mucus	Trap inhaled microbes and sweep them outward in mucus to be expectorated or swallowed	Smoking, high concentration of oxygen and carbon dioxide, decreased humidity, cold air
Macrophages	Engulf and destroy microorganisms that reach the lung's alveoli	Smoking
Urinary Tract		
Flushing action of urine flow	Washes away microorganisms on lining of bladder and urethra	Obstruction to normal flow by urinary catheter placement, obstruction from growth or tumour, delayed micturition
Intact multilayered epithelium	Provides barrier to microorganisms	Introduction of urinary catheter, continual movement of catheter in urethra
Gastrointestinal Tract		
Acidity of gastric secretions	Acids destroy some microorganisms	Administration of antacids to neutralize acids
Increased peristalsis in small intestine	Prevents retention of bacterial contents	Delayed motility resulting from impaction of fecal contents in large bowel or mechanical obstruction by masses
Vagina		
At puberty, normal flora causing vaginal secretions to achieve low pH	Inhibit growth of many microorganisms	Use of antibiotics or oral contraceptives, which disrupt normal flora

inflammation. The symptom of localized warmth results from a greater volume of blood at the inflammatory site. Local vasodilation enables blood and white blood cells (WBCs) to travel to the injured tissues.

Injury causes tissue necrosis, and, as a result, the body releases histamine, bradykinin, prostaglandin, and serotonin. These chemical mediators increase the permeability of small blood vessels, allowing fluid, protein, and cells to enter interstitial spaces. Accumulated fluid appears as localized swelling (edema).

Another symptom of inflammation is pain—the swelling of inflamed tissues increases the pressure on nerve endings, causing pain. Chemical substances such as histamine stimulate nerve endings. As a result of physiological changes occurring with inflammation, the involved body part usually undergoes a temporary loss of function. For example, a localized infection of the hand causes the fingers to become swollen, painful, and discoloured. Joints may become stiff as a result of the swelling, but the function of the fingers returns when inflammation subsides.

The cellular response of inflammation involves WBCs arriving at the site. These cells pass through the blood vessels and into the tissues. Through the process of phagocytosis, specialized WBCs, called *neutrophils* and *monocytes,* ingest and destroy microorganisms and other small particles. As inflammation becomes systemic, other signs and symptoms develop. Leukocytosis, or an increase in the number of circulating WBCs, is the body's response to WBCs leaving blood vessels. A serum WBC count is normally $5000/mm^3$ to $10000/mm^3$ but may rise to $15000/mm^3$ or even higher during inflammation. Fever is caused by the phagocytic release of pyrogens from bacterial cells that cause a rise in the hypothalamic set point (see Chapter 31).

Inflammatory Exudates. The accumulation of fluid, dead tissue cells, and WBCs forms an exudate at the site of inflammation (see Chapter 47). The exudate may be serous (clear, watery plasma), sanguineous (bloody drainage), serosanguineous (thin, watery drainage that is blood tinged), or purulent (thick drainage that contains pus). Eventually, the exudate is cleared away through lymphatic drainage. Platelets and plasma proteins such as fibrinogen form a meshlike matrix at the site of inflammation to prevent the spread of infection.

Tissue Repair. When tissues are injured, healing involves the inflammation, proliferation, and remodelling stages (see Chapter 47). Damaged cells are eventually replaced with healthy new ones, which undergo a gradual maturation until they take on the same structural characteristics and appearance as the previous cells. However, unless a wound is minor, the healed wound does not usually have the tensile strength of the tissue it replaces, and scarring may occur.

Health Care–Associated Infections

Patients in health care settings have an increased risk of acquiring infections. A health care–associated infection (HAI), also known as nosocomial infection or *iatrogenic infection,* is an infection acquired after admission to a health care facility that was not present or incubating at the time of admission. Patients in hospitals are at risk for infections because they may have a high acuity of illness and frequently undergo aggressive treatments, many of which compromise immunity (Public Health Agency of Canada [PHAC], 2020a). Transmission of antibiotic-resistant organisms also can occur in health care facilities because a large population of susceptible people who frequently receive antibiotics are in close proximity to each other.

Clostridioides difficile infection (CDI) is one of the most common and costly HAIs. *C. difficile* is a Gram-positive, spore-forming, anaerobic bacillus that produces two toxins, A and B, which cause diarrhea and colitis in patients whose bacterial flora have been disrupted by prior antibiotic use. Pseudomembranous colitis (PMC) is a more severe form of CDI, in which patients have a colitis characterized by the presence

of pseudomembranes on the colon surface seen during endoscopy. Infection-control measures to prevent transmission of *C. difficile* to patients include placing the patient on contact isolation, good hand hygiene (preferably with soap and water for patients who have diarrhea), gloves and gowns, as well as thorough environmental cleaning (Centers for Disease Control and Prevention [CDC], 2019a). Another important preventative measure is good antibiotic stewardship.

HAIs can result from a diagnostic or therapeutic procedure, such as a urinary tract infection that develops after catheter insertion. The incidence of nosocomial infections can be reduced if nurses use critical thinking when practising aseptic techniques. Nurses should always consider the patient's risks for infection and anticipate how the approach to care may increase or decrease the chances of infection transmission (Box 34.2).

HAIs may be exogenous or endogenous. An exogenous infection arises from microorganisms external to the individual that do not exist as normal flora; examples are *Salmonella* organisms and *Clostridium tetani*. An endogenous infection can occur when some of the patient's flora become altered and overgrowth results. Examples are infections caused by enterococci, yeasts, and streptococci. When sufficient numbers of microorganisms normally found in one body cavity or lining are transferred to another body site, an endogenous infection develops. For example, the transmission of enterococci, normally found in fecal material, from the hands to the skin is a common cause of wound infections. The number of microorganisms needed to cause an infection depends on the virulence of the organism, the host's susceptibility, and the site affected.

A patient's risk for infection is influenced by the number of health care workers having direct contact with the patient, the type and number of invasive procedures the patient has undergone, the therapy received, and the length of hospitalization. Major sites for HAI are surgical and traumatic wounds, urinary and respiratory tracts, and the bloodstream (Box 34.3).

Older persons have an increased susceptibility to HAIs because they are more likely to have a chronic disease and because of the effects of the aging process itself (Box 34.4). Extended stays in health care institutions, increased disability, and prolonged recovery times are all potential outcomes of HAIs. HAIs decrease the patient's quality of life and increase costs to the health care system. Therefore, their prevention is an important part of managed care.

❖ NURSING PROCESS IN INFECTION CONTROL

◆ Assessment

When considering infection prevention, the nurse must assess a patient's defence mechanisms, susceptibility, and knowledge of infections. A review of disease history with the patient and family may reveal an exposure to a communicable disease. A thorough review of the patient's clinical condition may allow the nurse to detect signs and symptoms of an infection or a risk for infection. Information about the patient's defences against infection can be determined by an analysis of laboratory findings. By knowing the factors that increase susceptibility or risk for infection, nurses are better able to plan preventive therapy that includes aseptic techniques. With recognition of early signs and symptoms of infection, nurses can alert others on the health care team to the potential need for therapy and to initiate supportive nursing measures.

Status of Defence Mechanisms

Nurses can determine the status of a patient's normal defence mechanisms against infection through a review of the physical assessment findings and the patient's medical condition. For example, any break in

⊚ BOX 34.2 NURSING CARE PLAN

Infection Control Measures—Preventing the Spread of Infection

ASSESSMENT

Susan Serious (case study) related that she is allergic to co-trimoxazole (Bactrim). Her medication list is composed of amlodipine (Norvasc), ramipril (Altace), furosemide (Lasix), prednisone, calcium carbonate, multivitamins (Replavite), ferrous gluconate, and darbepoetin alpha (Aranesp).

Assessment Activities	Findings and Defining Characteristics
Assess for the presence and location of skin lesions.	Lesions are vesicular, turn yellow in colour, and crust over. They follow the path of dermatomes in bandlike strips.
Assess for secondary infection from scratching due to skin irritation.	Scratching can open the pustules and introduce bacteria.
Review signs and symptoms of localized and systemic infections.	Signs of localized infection include swelling, redness, pain, or tingling.
	Signs and symptoms of systemic infection include fever, chills, headache, and malaise.
Research susceptibility to infection in patients with end-stage renal failure.	The literature shows that infections are a significant cause of morbidity and mortality in patients with end-stage renal failure, in part because of the clinical setting where treatment is received, the type of dialysis access, and the use of immunosuppressive medications (Szarnecka-Sojda et al., 2020). Susan has been taking prednisone 10 mg daily.
Review effects of medications.	Prednisone suppresses the body's response to infection.
Assess the need for additional isolation precautions.	In addition to routine practices, the new onset of a rash may require additional precautions. Some conditions that present with the development of a rash require airborne precautions.
Confirm the diagnosis.	A potential diagnosis of disseminated herpes zoster was made on the basis of the physical examination and Susan's history. Culture specimens of the lesions were obtained and sent to the hospital laboratory to confirm the diagnosis.

NURSING DIAGNOSIS: Risk for infection related to end-stage renal disease, immunosuppressive medications, and new onset of painful burning rash diagnosed as herpes zoster.

PLANNING

Goals	Expected Outcomes
Susan will be treated for the rash and will remain free of future infections.	Follow-up results of cultures with attending nephrologist to diagnose and treat the rash: Provide antiviral medications and initiate intravenous (IV) antibiotics, as ordered, to treat existing secondary infection.
	Provide analgesia to control the pain.
	Contact precautions and airborne isolation precautions are implemented and in use until the risk of transmission has subsided. The use of a single room with negative pressure was provided because Susan is immunocompromised from prednisone usage.
Susan will become knowledgeable of infection risks.	Susan will self-monitor for signs and symptoms of infection, report these to health care providers, and be observed for good aseptic technique by the health care providers.
	Review the use and dosage of prednisone with Susan to increase her understanding of immunosuppressive medications.

INTERVENTIONS

Prevention and Early Detection	Rationale
Monitor Susan's temperature and vital signs, and inspect the rash for evidence of infection.	Interventions are designed to prevent and ensure early detection of infection.
	Increased knowledge will aid in the prevention of infection and manage the discomfort from pain.
	Handwashing reduces bacterial counts on hands (Joint Commission, 2019).
Practise isolation precautions to prevent airborne transmission of disseminated herpes zoster infection.	Isolation precautions prevent the transmission of a communicable disease, such as herpes zoster.
	Negative pressure isolation protects others from airborne infections. Susan is aware that if she has to leave the room for essential reasons, she needs to wear a surgical mask to protect others. *Note: People entering the room also need to wear an N95 mask.*

Continued

◎ BOX 34.2 NURSING CARE PLAN—cont'd
Infection Control Measures—Preventing the Spread of Infection

Prevention and Early Detection

Teach Susan about her medications, indications, adverse effects, and dosages.

Rationale

Increased knowledge will increase adherence to the medication regimen and reporting of any related issues.

EVALUATION

Nursing Actions	Patient Response and Finding	Achievement of Outcome
Compare Susan's temperature, vital signs, and physical findings with baseline data.	Susan remains afebrile, free of signs and symptoms of infection and in control of pain.	Susan has no active infection at this time and is able to manage her pain.
Ask Susan to review knowledge of her rash and its care.	Susan is able to identify signs and symptoms of infections from scratching.	Susan has demonstrated a good knowledge base of secondary infections.
Ask Susan to explain the importance of hand hygiene.	Susan is able to relate that hand hygiene helps to reduce microorganisms that may contribute to infections.	Susan understands the principles and rationale of hand hygiene.
Ask Susan to review isolation precautions used to prevent the transmission of communicable diseases, such as disseminated herpes zoster.	Susan is able to explain why and how isolation precautions are used.	Susan understands the principles of isolation precautions used for disseminated herpes zoster. Additional precautions are discontinued when the lesions are dry and crusted.
Ask Susan to review the medications she is currently using.	Susan is able to list and explain the use of her current medications.	Susan has demonstrated an understanding of her medications regarding their use, effects, and potential concerns.

BOX 34.3 Sites for and Causes of Health Care–Associated Infections

Surgical and Traumatic Wounds

Improper skin preparation (shaving) before surgery
Failure to cleanse skin surface properly
Failure to use aseptic technique during dressing changes
The use of contaminated antiseptic solutions
Improper hand hygiene

Urinary Tract

Inappropriate and unsterile catheterization techniques
Inadequate monitoring of in-dwelling urinary catheters
Obstruction or blockages in tubing
An improper specimen-collection technique
Urine in the catheter or drainage tube being allowed to re-enter bladder (reflux)
Improper hand hygiene

Respiratory Tract

Contaminated respiratory therapy equipment
Failure to use aseptic technique while suctioning airway
Improper disposal of secretions
Improper hand hygiene

Bloodstream

Contamination of intravenous fluids by tubing or needle changes
The insertion of medication additives to intravenous fluid
The addition of a connecting tube or stopcocks to an intravenous system
Improper care of a needle-insertion site
Improper insertion technique
Contaminated needles or catheters
Failure to change the intravenous access site when inflammation first appears
Improper technique during the administration of multiple blood products
Improper care of peritoneal or hemodialysis catheters
Improper hand hygiene

BOX 34.4 FOCUS ON OLDER PERSONS

Immune Function

- An age-related decline in immune system function, termed *immune senescence*, increases the body's susceptibility to infection and lessens the strength of the overall immune response (Azar & Ballas, 2022).
- Age-related changes alter the response to infection, resulting in atypical signs and symptoms.
- Chronic disease, prevalent among older persons, allows infectious agents to readily invade; hospitalization and institutionalization as a result of chronic disease also increase older persons' exposure to pathogens (Yoshikawa, 2020).
- Risks associated with the development of infections in older patients include poor nutrition, unintentional weight loss, and low serum albumin levels (Government of Canada, 2020). Age-related changes in immunity contribute to the increased risk for acquiring pneumonia and influenza in older adulthood, both of which have significant age-related increases in mortality rates (Yoshikawa, 2020).
- Older persons present with an altered response to infection with atypical signs and symptoms such as confusion.

Data from Yoshikawa, T. (2020). Epidemiology and unique aspects pf aging and infectious diseases. *Clinical Infectious Diseases, 30*(6), 931–933.

the skin or mucosa is a potential site for infection. Similarly, a chronic smoker is at greater risk for acquiring a respiratory tract infection after general surgery because the cilia of the lung are less likely to propel retained mucus from the lung's airways. Any reduction in the body's primary or secondary defences against infection places a patient at risk (Box 34.5).

Patient Susceptibility

Many factors influence susceptibility to infection. Nurses need to gather information about each factor through the patient's and family's history.

Age. Throughout the lifespan, susceptibility to infection changes. An infant has immature defences against infection. Born with only the antibodies provided by the mother, the infant's immune system is incapable of producing the necessary immunoglobulins and WBCs to adequately fight some infections. However, breastfed infants have greater immunity than do bottle-fed infants because they receive the mother's antibodies through the breast milk. As the child grows, the immune system matures; however, the child is still susceptible to organisms that

cause the common cold, intestinal infections, and, if the child is not vaccinated, infectious diseases such as mumps and measles.

The young or middle-aged adult has refined defences against infection. Normal flora, body system defences, inflammation, and the immune response provide protection against invading microorganisms. Viruses are the most common cause of infectious illness in young and middle-aged adults.

Defences against infection change with aging (Yoshikawa, 2020). The immune response, particularly cell-mediated immunity, declines. Older persons also undergo alterations in the structure and function of the skin, urinary tract, and lungs. For example, the skin loses its turgor and the epithelium thins; as a result, the skin is more easily abraded or torn. This increases the potential for invasion by pathogens (Table 34.4).

Nutritional Status. When protein intake is inadequate as a result of poor diet or debilitating disease, the rate of protein breakdown exceeds that of tissue synthesis (see Chapter 43). A reduction in the intake of protein and other nutrients such as carbohydrates and fats reduces the body's defences against infection and impairs wound healing (see Chapter 43). Patients with illnesses or conditions that increase protein requirements are at further risk. These conditions include traumatic injury, extensive burns, and conditions causing fever. Patients who have had surgery also require increased protein.

Nurses need to assess patients' dietary intake and ability to tolerate solid foods. Patients who have difficulty swallowing, who experience

---

BOX 34.5 | Risk Factors for Infection

Inadequate Primary Defences
Broken skin or mucosa
Traumatized tissue
Decreased ciliary action
Obstructed urine outflow
Altered peristalsis
A change in the pH of secretions
Decreased mobility

Inadequate Secondary Defences
A reduced hemoglobin level
The suppression of white blood cells (WBCs) (medication or disease related)
A suppressed inflammatory response (medication or disease related)
A low WBC count (leukopenia)

TABLE 34.4 | Assessing the Risk of Infection in Older Persons

Component	Possible Changes With Aging	Possible Outcomes
Skin	Thinner dermal and epidermal layers, decreased collagen strength, decreased skin elasticity, decreased sweating	Pressure injuries
Peripheral nerves	Reduced sensitivity, particularly in patients with a history of alcohol use disorder, vitamin B_{12} deficiency, and diabetes mellitus	Pressure injuries, patients unaware of trauma to skin, leading to infection
Circulation	Heart failure, calcified mitral and aortic valves	Pneumonia, bacterial endocarditis
Peripheral circulation	Loss of elasticity of veins (prone to distension), less effective venous valves, blood pooling in lower extremities	Venous stasis ulcers
Mouth	Dehydration, reduction in saliva production, functional inability to maintain oral hygiene	Parotid gland infection, periodontal disease, localized abscess, bacteremia (i.e., bacteria in the blood)
Gastrointestinal tract	Loss of ability to secrete stomach acid in 30% of persons older than 70 years	*Salmonella* diarrhea
Pulmonary system	Increased colonization of oropharynx, impaired mucociliary clearance, decreased macrophage function, decreased cough reflex	Viral and bacterial pneumonia
Genitourinary tract	Prostatic hypertrophy or hyperplasia, urethral strictures, age-related hormonal changes in vaginal wall, pelvic floor relaxation, ureterocele or cystocele, degeneration of nerves leading to neurogenic bladder, use of tricyclic antidepressants results in urinary retention, dehydration	Asymptomatic bacteriuria (i.e., bacteria in the urine), cystitis, pyelonephritis
Nutrition	Malnutrition, vitamin deficiency (vitamin A, vitamin C, pyridoxine, and riboflavin), protein and caloric deficiencies	Impaired immune response to infection
Medication therapy	Corticosteroid and cytotoxic medications	Impaired immune response to infection in patients already at risk for decline in immune system function
Long-term care residency	Age-related changes are multifactorial and include changes in all systems of the body that contribute to the risk of infection. The increasing use of invasive devices, antimicrobials, and multiple medications contribute to infections in this population. The health care setting may provide a setting that promotes the development and spread of infections. Preventive measures should be instituted, such as increased hand hygiene, reduced use of in-dwelling catheters, increased efforts to reduce aspiration, increased administration of vaccines, and prudent use of antibiotics.	Frequent serious infection, increased risk of pneumonia and urinary tract infections. Increased risk of acquiring a multidrug-resistant organism

From Yoshikawa, T. (2020). Epidemiology and unique aspects of aging and infectious diseases. *Clinical Infectious Diseases 30*(6), 931–933. https://doi.org/10.1086/313792

alterations in digestion, or who are too confused or weak to feed themselves are at risk for inadequate dietary intake. A dietitian may be called in to assess the nutritional adequacy of a patient's diet. When preparing a patient for discharge, the nurse should evaluate the patient's and family's understanding of nutritional needs.

Stress. The general adaptation syndrome is the body's response to emotional or physical stress (see Chapter 30). During the alarm stage, the basal metabolic rate increases as the body uses energy stores. Adrenocorticotropic hormone acts to increase serum glucose levels and decrease unnecessary anti-inflammatory responses through the release of cortisone. If stress continues or becomes intense, elevated cortisone levels result in a decreased resistance to infection. Continued stress leads to exhaustion, wherein energy stores are depleted and the body has no resistance to invading organisms. The same conditions that increase nutritional requirements, such as surgery or trauma, also increase physiological stress. Chronic diseases also increase risk for infections. Examples of chronic diseases and how they are at risk for infection are presented in Box 34.6.

Disease Process. Patients with diseases of the immune system are at particular risk for infection. Leukemia, AIDS, lymphoma, and aplastic anemia are conditions that compromise a host by weakening defences against infectious organisms. Patients with leukemia, for example, are unable to produce normal WBCs to effectively ward off infection.

Patients with chronic diseases such as coronary artery disease (CAD), diabetes mellitus, arthritis, and multiple sclerosis are also more susceptible to infection because of general debilitation and nutritional impairment. Cancer and end-stage renal failure (which alters the immune response), peripheral vascular disease (which reduces blood flow to injured tissues), and diseases that impair body system defences, such as emphysema and bronchitis (chronic obstructive pulmonary disease [COPD]) (which impair ciliary action and thicken mucus), increase susceptibility to infection. Patients with burns have an exceedingly high susceptibility to infection because of the damage to skin surfaces. The greater the depth and extent of the burns, the higher the risk for infection.

Medical Therapy. Some drugs and medical therapies compromise immunity to infection. Nurses need to assess their patients' history to determine whether they take medications at home that increase infection susceptibility. A review of therapies received within the health care setting may further reveal risks. Adrenal corticosteroids, prescribed for several conditions, are anti-inflammatory medications that cause protein breakdown and impair the inflammatory response against bacteria and other pathogens. Cytotoxic or antineoplastic medications attack cancer cells but cause adverse effects such as depression of bone marrow activity and normal cell toxicity. When bone marrow activity is depressed, the body is unable to produce lymphocytes and sufficient WBCs. When normal cells become altered by antineoplastic agents, cellular defences against infection fail. Cyclosporine and other immunosuppressant medications, which decrease the body's immune response, are commonly taken by organ transplant recipients. The immunosuppressants prevent organ and tissue rejection, but they also increase the recipients' susceptibility to infection.

Patients with cancer who are receiving radiotherapy are at risk for infection. The massive doses of radiation that destroy cancerous cells can also depress bone marrow activity and destroy normal cells.

Clinical Appearance

The signs and symptoms of infection may be local or systemic. Localized infections are most common in areas of skin or mucous membrane

---

BOX 34.6	Chronic Diseases and Risks for Infection

Chronic diseases are diseases of slow progression and long duration. They primarily occur at any age but are more prevalent in people over 65 years of age. Individuals with chronic diseases are more at risk for infection for a variety of reasons, including those listed below.

Chronic Diseases: Types	Risk Factors for Infection	Risk Factors for Hospital-Acquired Infections (HAI)
Coronary artery disease (CAD)	Comorbidities: two or more	Long hospitalizations
Cancer	Smoking/alcohol use	Surgical procedures
COPD	Poor nutrition	Procedures: intubation, invasive lines
Diabetes mellitus	Obesity	Antibiotic use
Cardiovascular disease	Age	Wounds, incisions, burns, ulcers
Arthritis	Low economic state	Inadequate hand hygiene by staff and clients
Neurodegenerative disease	Environment	
	Inactivity	
Renal failure	Impaired circulation	Exposure to health care environment
Asthma	Immunosuppressive medications	Immobility
	Compromised host defences (low WBC)	Treatments: dialysis, TPN
	Compromised immune system	
	Stress	

COPD, Chronic obstructive pulmonary disease; *TPN,* total parenteral nutrition; *WBC,* white blood cells.

Data from Canadian Nosocomial Infection Surveillance Program. (2020). *Healthcare-associated infections and antimicrobial resistance in Canadian acute care hospital, 2014–2018. Canadian Communicable Diseases Report, 46*(5), 99–112. https://www.canada.ca/content/dam/phac-aspc/documents/services/reports-publications/canada-communicable-disease-report-ccdr/monthly-issue/2020-46/issue-5-may-7-2020/ccdrv46i05a01-eng.pdf; Centers for Disease Control and Prevention (CDC). (2022). *Chronic diseases: How you can prevent chronic diseases.* https://www.cdc.gov/chronicdisease/about/prevent/; AusMed. (2020). *The relationship between chronic conditions and infections.* https://www.ausmed.com/cpd/articles/chronic-conditions-and-infections; CDC. (2022). *People who are immunocompromised. Know how to protect yourself and what to do if you get sick.* https://www.cdc.gov/coronavirus/2019-ncov/need-extra-precautions/people-who-are-immunocompromised.html

---

breakdown, such as surgical and traumatic wounds, pressure injuries, and mouth lesions. Infections also develop locally in cavities beneath the skin; an example is an abscess.

To assess an area for localized infection, the nurse should first inspect the area for redness and swelling caused by inflammation. Because drainage from open lesions or wounds may occur, nurses must wear disposable gloves. Infected drainage may be yellow, green, or brown, depending on the pathogen. Ask the patient about pain or tenderness around the site. The patient may complain of tightness and pain caused by edema. If the infected area is large enough, movement of a body part may be restricted. Gentle palpation of an infected area usually results in some degree of tenderness.

Systemic infections cause more generalized symptoms than do local infections. Systemic infections usually result in fever, fatigue, and malaise. Lymph nodes that drain the area of infection often become enlarged, swollen, and tender during palpation. For example, an abscess in the peritoneal cavity may cause the enlargement of the lymph nodes in the groin. An infection of the upper respiratory tract may cause cervical lymph node enlargement. If an infection is serious and widespread, all major lymph nodes may enlarge. Systemic infections commonly cause a loss of appetite, nausea, and vomiting.

Systemic infections may develop after treatment for a localized infection has failed. Nurses should be alert for changes in a patient's level of activity and responsiveness. As systemic infections develop, the patient may become lethargic and experience a loss of energy. An elevation in body temperature may lead to episodes of increased heart and respiratory rates and low blood pressure. The involvement of major body systems may produce specific signs. For example, a pulmonary infection may result in a productive cough with purulent sputum. A urinary tract infection may result in cloudy, foul-smelling urine.

In older persons, infection may not present with typical signs and symptoms. Fever, pain, and swelling are often absent in older people because they tend to have lower body temperatures, decreased pain sensation, and less immune response to infection. As a result, in older persons, infection is often advanced before it is identified. Atypical symptoms such as a change in behaviour (e.g., new or increased confusion, incontinence, or agitation) may be the only symptoms of an infectious illness (Yoshikawa, 2020). For example, as many as 20% of older persons with pneumonia do not have the typical signs and symptoms of fever, shaking, chills, and "rusty" productive sputum. The only symptoms present may be an increased heart rate with no apparent reason, confusion, or generalized fatigue.

Laboratory Data

A review of laboratory test results may confirm infection (Table 34.5). However, laboratory values alone are not sufficient to detect infection; other clinical signs must be assessed. Factors other than infection may alter test values. For example, trauma and physical stress can cause an elevation in the number of neutrophils. A culture may show the growth of an organism in the absence of overt signs of infection.

Patients With Infection

A patient with infection may have a variety of health problems. Nurses need to assess ways that the infection affects the patient's and family's needs—these may be physical, psychological, social, or economic. For example, a patient with a chronic disease such as AIDS may experience serious psychological challenges as a result of self-imposed isolation or rejection by family and friends. Using a case-management approach, the nurse can determine the patient's and family's ability to adjust to the disease and the resources available to help them manage health care challenges (Australian College of Nursing, 2019).

◆ Nursing Diagnosis

During assessment, nurses gather objective findings, such as an open incision or a reduced caloric intake, and subjective data, such as a patient's report of tenderness over a surgical wound site (Box 34.7). The nurse then interprets the data carefully, looking for clusters of defining characteristics or risk factors that create a pattern suggesting a specific nursing diagnosis. The following are examples of nursing diagnoses that may apply:

- *Disturbed body image*
- *Risk for infection*
- *Risk for injury*
- *Imbalanced nutrition—less than body requirements*
- *Impaired oral mucous membrane*
- *Risk for impaired skin integrity*
- *Social isolation*
- *Impaired tissue integrity*

TABLE 34.5	Laboratory Tests to Screen for Infection	
Laboratory Value	**Normal (Adult) Values**	**Indication of Infection**
White blood cell (WBC) count	$5–10 \times 10^9$/L	Increased in acute infection, neoplasm, allergy, immunosuppression.
		Decreased in aplastic anemia, and in certain viral or overwhelming infections
Erythrocyte sedimentation rate (ESR) Westergren method	$4.7–6.1 \times 10^{12}$/L Male $4.2–5.4 \times 10^{12}$/L Female	Elevated in presence of inflammatory process, acute and chronic infection, tissue necrosis, infarction, dehydration.
		Decreased in anemia, leukemia, post-hemorrhage
Iron level	14–32 mcmol/L Male 11–29 mcmol/L Female	Increased in hemochromatosis, massive transfusions.
		Decreased in chronic infection, anemia of chronic disease
C-reactive protein	<10 mg/L	An acute-phase reactant protein that is elevated in the presence of an acute inflammatory process
Cultures of urine and blood	Normally sterile, without microorganism growth	Presence of infectious microorganism growth
Cultures and Gram stain of wound, sputum, and throat	No WBCs on Gram stain, possible normal flora	Presence of infectious microorganism growth and WBCs on Gram stain
WBC: Differential Count (Percentage of Each Type of WBC)		
Neutrophils–segmented	62–68%	Increased in bacterial infections, collagen diseases
		Decreased in overwhelming bacterial infection (older persons)
Lymphocytes	20–40%	Increased in chronic bacterial and viral infection
		Decreased in sepsis
Monocytes	2–8%	Increased in protozoal, rickettsia, and tuberculosis infections
Eosinophils	1–4%	Increased in parasitic or allergic infection
		Decreased in steroid therapy
Basophils	0.5–1%	Increased in hypothyroidism, ulcerative colitis
		Normal during infection
		Decreased in hyperthyroidism

Data from Pagana, K. D., Pagana, T. J., & Pike-MacDonald, S. A. (2019). *Mosby's Canadian manual of diagnostics and laboratory tests* (2nd ed.). Elsevier Inc.

It may be necessary for the nurse to validate data (e.g., by inspecting the integrity of a wound more carefully). Likewise, additional data such as laboratory findings may be helpful. The proper selection of appropriate nursing diagnoses depends on the correct analysis and organization of data.

The diagnosis must have the correct etiological factor for a nurse to establish an appropriate and well-thought-out plan. For example, minimizing the risk for infection related to broken skin requires good hygiene measures and wound care; minimizing the risk for infection related to malnutrition requires good nutritional support and fluid balance.

Nurses may diagnose a risk for infection or make diagnoses that result from the effects of infection on the patient's health status. Nurses' success in planning appropriate nursing interventions depends on the accuracy of the diagnosis and their ability to meet the patient's needs.

◆ **Planning**

Goals and Outcomes. The patient's care plan is based on each nursing diagnosis and related factors (Box 34.8). The nurse develops a plan that sets attainable outcomes so that interventions are purposeful and directed. For example, if you are caring for a patient with the nursing diagnosis *risk for infection related to broken skin,* you must implement skin and wound care measures to promote healing. The expected outcomes "reduction in wound size by 1 cm" and "absence of drainage" represent targets for measuring the patient's improvement. Once outcomes are met, the goal of "skin intact and without drainage" can be reached. Interventions are selected in collaboration with the patient, the family, and others on the health care team. Nurses direct the care in the acute care setting; care may also involve other professionals in

BOX 34.7   NURSING DIAGNOSTIC PROCESS

Assessment Activities	Defining Characteristics	Nursing Diagnosis
Check results of laboratory tests.	WBC count 3.9 × 10⁹/L	*Risk for infection related to neutropenia*
Review current medications.	Patient receiving azathioprine (Imuran), an immunosuppressant	
Identify potential sites of infection.	Intravenous catheter in right forearm in place for 3 days	
	Foley catheter draining amber-coloured urine	

WBC, White blood cell.

BOX 34.8   NURSING CARE PLAN

Risk for Infection

ASSESSMENT

Mrs. Spicer (preferred pronouns: she/her) was admitted to the medical nursing unit 3 days ago with a diagnosis of lymphoma. She received her first dose of multiagent chemotherapy yesterday. Jess Ralston (preferred pronouns: he/him) is the student nurse caring for Mrs. Spicer. He begins his shift by conducting a focused assessment.

Assessment Activities

Review patient's chart for laboratory data reflecting immune function.
Ask patient to describe appetite and review food intake for past 24 hours. Weigh patient. Measure height.

Palpate patient's cervical and clavicular lymph nodes.
Review effects of chemotherapy in medication reference.

Findings and Defining Characteristics

Data show a reduction in number of white blood cells (WBCs) (leukopenia).
Mrs. Spicer reports she has not had interest in eating for a couple of weeks. She has lost approximately 2.5 kg. Her current weight is 57 kg, and her height is 170 cm. Her food intake yesterday consisted of a small cup of applesauce, a half bowl of soup, three crackers, and two glasses of juice. Mrs. Spicer states, "I get full easily and lose interest in food."
Lymph nodes are enlarged and painless.
Multiagent chemotherapy causes medication-induced pancytopenia.

NURSING DIAGNOSIS: Risk for infection related to immunosuppression and reduced food intake.

PLANNING

Goals (Nursing Outcomes Classification)*
Risk Detection
Patient will remain free of infection.

Knowledge: Infection Control
Patient will become knowledgeable of infection risks.

Expected Outcomes

Patient will remain afebrile.
Patient will develop no signs or symptoms of local infection (e.g., will remain free of cough, cloudy or foul-smelling urine, and purulent drainage from open wound or normal body opening).

Patient will identify routines to follow in the home that reduce the transmission of microorganisms.
Patient will identify signs and symptoms indicating infection to report to her health care provider.

*Outcome classification labels from Moorhead, S., Swanson, E., Johnson, M., et al. (Eds.). (2018). *Nursing outcomes classification (NOC)* (6th ed.). Mosby.

Continued

◎ BOX 34.8 NURSING CARE PLAN—cont'd

INTERVENTIONS

Interventions (Nursing Intervention Classification)[†]	Rationale
Prevention and Early Detection	
Monitor patient's body temperature routinely, inspect oral cavity for lesions, inspect urethral and vaginal orifices for drainage or discharge, inspect intravenous access site for drainage, and observe patient for evidence of cough.	Interventions are designed to prevent and ensure early detection of infection in a patient at risk (Vera, 2022).
Practise hand hygiene routinely before caring for a patient, between patients, and before any invasive procedures.	Rigorous hand hygiene reduces bacterial counts on the hands (PHAC, 2020a; Vera, 2022).
Teach patient how to perform hand hygiene correctly.	Patient can easily come in contact with infectious agents that can cause infection.
Consult with dietitian about providing a high-calorie, high-protein, low-bacteria diet. Minimize intake of salads, undercooked meat, pepper, paprika, and raw fruits and vegetables. Offer small, frequent meals.	Maintaining calorie and protein intake will prevent weight loss. Foods high in bacteria should be avoided because they increase the risk for gastrointestinal infection (Vera, 2022).
Infection Control	
Instruct patient to report the following to the health care provider: temperature >38°C, persistent cough with or without sputum, pus or foul-smelling drainage from the body site, the presence of an abscess, urine that is cloudy or foul smelling, or burning on urination.	Signs and symptoms are indicative of local or systemic infection.
Teach patient to follow these activities at home:	These measures are designed to prevent infection in patients with impaired immune function (Vera, 2022).
• Avoid crowds and large gatherings of persons.	
• Bathe daily.	
• Do not share personal hygiene items with family members (e.g., toothbrush, washcloth, and deodorant stick).	
• Take your temperature twice daily.	
• Do not drink water that has been standing for >15 minutes.	
• Do not reuse cups or glasses without washing.	

[†]Intervention classification labels from Butcher, H. K., Bulechek, G. M., McCloskey Dochterman, J. M., et al. (Eds.). (2019). *Nursing interventions classification (NIC)* (7th ed.). Mosby; Vera, M., (2022). *Nursing diagnosis guide and list: All you need to know to master diagnosing.* https://nurseslabs.com/nursing-diagnosis/

EVALUATION

Nursing Actions	Patient Response and Finding	Achievement of Outcome
Compare patient's body temperature and other physical findings with baseline data.	Mrs. Spicer remains afebrile and denies having cough or burning on urination. No signs of drainage or discharge from body site are evident.	Mrs. Spicer has no active infection at this time.
Ask patient to describe signs and symptoms to report to health care provider.	Mrs. Spicer is able to identify the temperature range to report. She is able to describe cough. She is unable to identify signs of urinary infection or local discharge.	Mrs. Spicer has a partial understanding of signs and symptoms to report. She will need additional instruction and an information sheet.
Ask patient to explain the measures to take at home to reduce exposure to infectious agents.	Mrs. Spicer is able to discuss the need to avoid sharing personal hygiene articles. She has asked for a list of other precautions and requested that her husband be included in the discussion.	Mrs. Spicer has a partial understanding of restrictions. Nurse will obtain printed guidelines and include her husband in discussion this evening.

assisting with instructions on postdischarge procedures. Common goals of care relating to infection include the following:

- Preventing exposure to infectious organisms
- Controlling or reducing the extent of the infection
- Maintaining resistance to infection
- Educating the patient and family about infection-control techniques

Setting Priorities. In collaboration with the patient, the nurse establishes priorities for the goals of care. For example, for a patient who has an open wound and cancer and cannot tolerate solid foods, the priority of administering therapies that promote wound healing exceeds the goal of educating the patient to assume self-care therapies at home.

When the patient's condition improves, the priorities will change, and patient education will become an essential intervention.

Continuity of Care. The development of a care plan includes infection prevention practices. Nurses may initiate appropriate referrals, such as to a dietitian, infection control professional, or home care nurse, to collaborate in a patient's care. When care is being administered in the home, the nurse should ensure that the environment supports good infection-control practices. For example, if a patient does not have running water, the nurse needs to bring a waterless antimicrobial solution during visits to ensure adequate hand hygiene. Educating patients and families is also an important aspect of prevention.

BOX 34.9 **FOCUS ON PRIMARY HEALTH CARE**

Immunizations

Immunizations are an essential component of disease prevention. Nurses should encourage proper immunization of infants, children, individuals at risk, and older persons. In Canada, most provinces provide free-of-charge immunization to infants against measles, mumps, rubella, diphtheria, tetanus, acellular pertussis, and poliomyelitis. Parents may be required to pay to have their infant or child vaccinated against *Haemophilus influenzae* type b (Hib), human papillomavirus (HPV), varicella, and hepatitis B. The HPV vaccine is available in Canada for both male and female patients 9 to 26 years of age. For maximum benefit, it should be given before the patient becomes sexually active (PHAC, 2021).

Older persons and those who have underlying medical conditions are at risk for influenza and pneumonia and are therefore offered influenza vaccines each year and pneumococcal vaccines as per the recommended schedule, which varies according to the recipient's age (Weinberger et al., 2018). Nurses should remind patients of the importance of having a tetanus–diphtheria booster vaccination every 10 years. Health care workers who care for persons at high risk for complications from influenza should be immunized for influenza yearly as well.

In most provinces and territories, public health nurses or community nurses hold free immunization clinics for patients at risk during an outbreak of a potentially deadly infection such as bacterial meningitis or COVID-19.

From Public Health Agency of Canada. (2021). *Canadian immunization guide* (8th ed.). https://www.canada.ca/en/public-health/services/canadian-immunization-guide.html

◆ Implementation

By recognizing and assessing a patient's risk factors and implementing appropriate measures, nurses can reduce the risk of infection.

Health Promotion. Nurses may prevent an infection from developing or spreading by minimizing the numbers and kinds of organisms transmitted to potential infection sites. Eliminating reservoirs of infection, controlling portals of exit and entry, and avoiding actions that transmit microorganisms prevent pathogens from finding a new site in which to grow. The proper use of sterile supplies, barrier protection, and proper hand hygiene are examples of methods that nurses use to control the spread of microorganisms. A further preventive measure is to strengthen a potential host's defences against infection. Nutritional support, rest, maintenance of physiological protective mechanisms, and receipt of recommended immunizations (Box 34.9) protect a patient from invasion by pathogens.

Being vigilant about infection control helps nurses to apply good medical–surgical aseptic practices at the right time and in the right clinical situation. When a patient develops an infection, the nurse needs to continue preventive care so that health care personnel and other patients are not exposed to the infection. Isolation precautions may be necessary for patients with communicable diseases; the environment is controlled by barriers against the transmission of infection (see "Isolation Guidelines" section).

Communicable Diseases. *Communicable diseases* are infectious diseases that spread disease from one person to another. They are caused by bacteria, fungi, or viruses. The transmission may be direct, indirect, droplet, airborne, or vehicle. Examples include influenza, HIV, salmonella, *E. coli*, TB, malaria, Coronavirus, Ebola, MRSA, meningitis, cholera, chickenpox, West Nile virus, SARS, avian influenza, and H1N1. Prevention against the spread of these diseases includes good hand hygiene, surface cleansing, the use of protective equipment, vaccinations, isolation, and education and training of health care staff.

Many health care centres are already taxed trying to meet the current demand for services, so a pandemic limits their ability to handle a large influx of patients. Communication between centres, the community, and emergency management organizations is of vital importance to deal with an influx of infectious patients. Resources and guidance for infection control and prevention are found at federal, regional, and local levels. They assist in the planning and organization of centres to stop the spread of disease, coordinate resources, and manage care. When a pandemic occurs, there is no time to plan; rather, plans that were previously developed need to be implemented (Joint Commission, 2019).

Acute Care Measures. Treatment of an infectious process includes eliminating the infectious organisms and supporting the patient's defences. To identify the causative organism, nurses may collect specimens of body fluids or drainage from infected body sites for cultures. When the disease process or causative organism has been identified, the prescriber prescribes the treatment that is most effective for the situation. Nurses properly administer antibiotics and other treatments, watch for adverse reactions, and assess the progress of the infection.

Systemic infections necessitate measures to prevent complications of fever (see Chapter 31). Maintaining the patient's intake of fluids prevents dehydration resulting from diaphoresis. Because of the patient's increased metabolic rate, adequate nutritional intake must be ensured. Rest preserves energy for the healing process.

Localized infections often necessitate measures to remove debris to promote healing. Nurses need to apply the principles of wound care to remove any infected drainage from the wound site and support the integrity of healing wounds. Special dressings can be applied to facilitate the removal of infectious drainage and promote healing of wound margins. Drainage tubes may be inserted to remove infected drainage from body cavities. Nurses must use medical and surgical aseptic techniques to manage wounds and ensure correct handling of all drainage or body fluids (see Chapter 47).

During the course of infection, nurses can support the patient's body defence mechanisms. For example, if a patient has infectious diarrhea, the nurse must maintain skin integrity to prevent breakdown and the entrance of microorganisms. Other routine hygiene measures such as bathing and oral care protect the skin and mucous membranes from invasion and overgrowth of microorganisms.

Asepsis

Nurses' efforts to minimize the onset and spread of infection are based on the principles of aseptic technique. **Asepsis** is the process for keeping away disease-producing microorganisms. *Aseptic technique* refers to practices designed to render an area and objects as free from microorganisms as possible. The two types of aseptic technique are medical asepsis and surgical asepsis.

Medical asepsis, or clean technique, includes procedures used to reduce and prevent the spread of microorganisms. Hand hygiene, using clean gloves (i.e., disposable gloves) to prevent direct contact with blood or body fluids, and cleaning the environment routinely are examples of medical asepsis. The principles of medical asepsis are commonly followed in the home, as in washing hands before preparing food.

After an object becomes unsterile or unclean, it is considered *contaminated*. In medical asepsis, an area or object is considered contaminated if it contains or is suspected of containing microorganisms. For example, a used bedpan, the floor, and a used dressing are contaminated.

Nurses need to follow certain principles and procedures, including routine practices, to prevent infection and control its spread (see "Isolation Guidelines" section). During daily routine care, nurses use basic medical aseptic techniques to break the infection chain. Because infections are readily transmitted between patients and caregivers, it may become necessary for the nurse to follow isolation precautions as appropriate (see "Isolation Guidelines" section).

Nurses are responsible for providing the patient with a safe environment. The effectiveness of infection-control practices depends on the nurse and their colleagues' conscientiousness and consistency in using effective aseptic technique. It is easy to forget key procedural steps or, in a hurry, to take shortcuts that break aseptic procedures. However, a nurse's failure to be meticulous places the patient at risk for an infection that can seriously impair recovery or lead to death.

Control or Elimination of Infectious Agents.

Proper cleaning, disinfection, and sterilization of contaminated objects significantly reduce and often eliminate microorganisms. In health care centres, a sterile processing department disinfects and sterilizes reusable supplies. However, nurses also may be required to perform these functions. Many principles of cleaning and disinfection also apply to the home.

Cleaning. Cleaning is the physical removal of foreign material (e.g., dust, soil, and organic material such as blood, secretions, excretions, and microorganisms) from objects and surfaces (Joint Commission, 2019; Provincial Infectious Diseases Advisory Committee [PIDAC], 2018). In general, cleaning involves the use of water and mechanical action with detergents or enzymatic products. When an object comes in contact with infectious or potentially infectious material, the object is contaminated. Reusable objects must be cleaned thoroughly before reuse and then either disinfected or sterilized according to the manufacturer's recommendations.

When cleaning equipment that is soiled by organic material such as blood, fecal matter, mucus, or pus, nurses should take appropriate measures to protect themselves against contamination. These may include wearing a mask and protective eyewear (or a face shield) and waterproof gloves. These barriers provide protection from infectious organisms. A brush and detergent or soap are needed for cleaning.

The following steps ensure that an object is clean:

1. Rinse a contaminated object or article with cold running water to remove organic material. Hot water causes the protein in organic material to coagulate and stick to objects, making removal difficult.
2. After rinsing, wash the object with soap and warm water. Soap or detergent reduces the surface tension of water and emulsifies the dirt or remaining material. Rinse the object thoroughly to remove the emulsified dirt.
3. Use a brush to remove dirt or material in grooves or seams. Friction dislodges the contaminated material for easy removal. Open any hinged items for cleaning.
4. Rinse the object in warm water.
5. Dry the object and prepare it for disinfection or sterilization if indicated by the intended use of the item.
6. The brush, gloves, and sink in which the equipment is cleaned should be considered contaminated and should be cleaned and dried.

Disinfection and Sterilization. **Disinfection** is the elimination of all pathogens except bacterial spores (Joint Commission, 2019; PIDAC, 2018). Disinfectants are used on inanimate objects; antiseptics are used on living tissue. Disinfection usually involves chemicals, heat, or ultraviolet light. An item must be thoroughly cleaned before it is disinfected. Examples of disinfectants are alcohols, chlorines, glutaraldehydes, phenols, and quaternary ammonium compounds. These chemicals can

---

> ## BOX 34.10 Categories for Sterilization, Disinfection, and Cleaning
>
> ### Critical Items
> Critical items are instruments and devices that enter sterile tissue or the vascular system. They present a high risk of infection if the items are contaminated with microorganisms, including bacterial spores. Critical items must be thoroughly cleaned and sterilized. Examples of these items follow:
> - Surgical instruments
> - Intravascular catheters
> - Urinary catheters
> - Needles
> - Respiratory deep suction catheters
>
> ### Semicritical Items
> Semicritical items are devices that come in contact with mucous membranes or nonintact skin but do not penetrate them. These items also present a risk of infection and must be free of all microorganisms (except bacterial spores). Semicritical items must be thoroughly cleaned and disinfected.
>   The following are examples of these items:
> - Electronic thermometers
> - Respiratory therapy equipment
> - Oral suctioning catheters
> - Endotracheal tubes
> - Gastrointestinal endoscopes
> - Vaginal and nasal specula
>
> ### Noncritical Items
> Noncritical items are items that either touch only intact skin but not mucous membranes or do not directly touch the patient. Noncritical items must be cleaned or cleaned and disinfected. Examples of these items follow:
> - Bedpans, urinals, and commodes
> - Blood pressure cuffs
> - Linens
> - Stethoscopes
> - Some eating utensils

---

be caustic and toxic to tissues. Some disinfectants are indicated for use only on noncritical items; nurses should read the label and follow the manufacturer's recommendations for use.

Sterilization is the destruction of all microorganisms, including spores. Steam under pressure, ethylene oxide gas, hydrogen peroxide plasma, and chemicals are the most common sterilizing agents. Items must be cleaned thoroughly before they can be sterilized.

Whether an item is to be simply cleaned, or cleaned and disinfected or sterilized, depends on the intended use of the item. Devices are classified in three categories (Box 34.10). Nurses should be familiar with their agency's policy and procedures for cleaning, handling, and delivering care items for eventual disinfection and sterilization. Workers especially trained in disinfection and sterilization should perform most of the procedures (CDC, 2019b). Efficacy of the disinfecting or sterilizing method is influenced by the following factors:

- *Concentration of solution and duration of contact.* A weakened concentration or shortened exposure time may lessen effectiveness.
- *Type and number of pathogens.* Certain organisms are killed more easily than others by disruption. Higher numbers of pathogens on an object necessitate longer disinfecting time.
- *Surface areas to treat.* All dirty surfaces and areas must be fully exposed to disinfecting and sterilizing agents.
- *Temperature of the environment.* Disinfectants tend to work best at room temperature.

TABLE 34.6	Examples of Disinfection and Sterilization Processes
Characteristics	**Examples of Use**
Moist Heat Steam is moist heat under pressure. When exposed to high pressure, water vapour can attain a temperature above the boiling point to kill pathogens and spores.	An autoclave is used to sterilize surgical instruments and dressings.
Chemicals A number of chemical disinfectants are used in health care, including alcohols, chlorines, formaldehyde, glutaraldehydes, hydrogen peroxide, iodophors, phenolics, and quaternary ammonium compounds. Each product performs in a unique manner and is used for a specific purpose.	Chemicals are used for the disinfection of instruments and equipment such as thermometers and endoscopes. Use the appropriate facility-approved disinfectant in a safe manner (e.g., with gloves, proper ventilation) for the approved purpose (CDC, 2019b).
Ethylene Oxide Gas Ethylene oxide gas destroys spores and microorganisms by altering cells' metabolic processes. Fumes are released within an autoclave-like chamber. This gas is toxic to humans, and aeration time varies with products.	This gas sterilizes some rubber and plastic items.
Boiling Water Boiling is the least expensive method of sterilization for use in the home. Bacterial spores and some viruses resist boiling. It is not used in hospitals.	The items (e.g., glass baby bottles) should be boiled for at least 15 minutes.

- *Presence of soap.* Soap may cause certain disinfectants to be ineffective. Thorough rinsing of an object is necessary before disinfecting.
- *Presence of organic materials.* Disinfectants can become inactivated unless blood, saliva, pus, or body excretions are already washed off.

Table 34.6 lists processes for disinfection and sterilization and their characteristics. Selection of the method for disinfecting or sterilizing an item depends on the intended use and nature of the item (e.g., some delicate instruments cannot tolerate steam and must be sterilized with gas or plasma).

Control or Elimination of Reservoirs. To control or eliminate reservoir sites for infection, nurses need to eliminate or control sources of body fluids, drainage, or solutions that might harbour microorganisms. Nurses must also carefully discard articles that become contaminated with infectious material (Box 34.11). All health care institutions must have guidelines for the disposal of infectious waste according to provincial or territorial laws.

Control of Portals of Exit. Nurses need to follow several measures to minimize or prevent infectious organisms from exiting the body. To control organisms exiting via the respiratory tract, the nurse should wear a mask as needed, avoid talking directly into patients' faces, and never talk, sneeze, or cough directly over surgical wounds or sterile dressing fields. The nurse should cover the mouth or nose when sneezing or coughing. Nurses are also responsible for teaching patients to protect others when they sneeze or cough and for providing patients with disposable wipes or tissues to control the spread of microorganisms.

Nurses who have an upper respiratory tract infection should consider not working; they may be required to remain at home. Nurses who continue to work with patients should wear a mask when working closely with a patient and pay special attention to hand hygiene. Nurses should not be caring for patients who are highly susceptible to infection (e.g., an immunosuppressed patient or a newborn).

Another way of controlling the exit of microorganisms is through the careful handling of blood, body fluids, secretions, or excretions (e.g., urine, feces, vomitus, and exudate). Contaminated fluids can easily splash while being discarded or cleaned up. Nurses should always

---

BOX 34.11	Infection Control to Reduce Reservoir Sites

Bathing
Use soap and water to remove drainage, dried secretions, or excess perspiration.

Dressing Changes
Change dressings that become wet or soiled (see Chapter 47).

Contaminated Articles
Place tissues, soiled dressings, and soiled linen in moisture-resistant bags for proper disposal.

Contaminated Needles
Engage the safety features of all sharp devices and dispose of them in a puncture-proof container. Place syringes, uncapped hypodermic needles, and intravenous needles in puncture-proof containers, which should be located in patient rooms or treatment areas so that exposed, contaminated equipment need not be carried a distance (see Chapter 35). *Do not recap needles* or attempt to break them.

Bedside Unit
Keep table surfaces clean and dry.

Bottled Solutions
Do not leave bottled solutions open for prolonged periods. Keep solutions tightly capped. Date bottles when opened and discard according to the facility's policy.

Surgical Wounds
Keep drainage tubes and collection bags patent to prevent the accumulation of serous fluid under the skin surface.

Drainage Bottles and Bags
Empty and dispose of drainage suction bottles according to the health agency's policy. Empty all drainage systems on each shift unless otherwise ordered by a physician. Never raise a drainage system (e.g., urinary drainage bag) above the level of the site being drained unless the drainage system is clamped off.

wear disposable gloves when handling blood, body fluids, secretions, or excretions. Masks, gowns, and protective eyewear should be worn if splashing or contact with any fluids is possible. Disposable soiled items should be appropriately disposed of in impervious plastic bags. Laboratory specimens from all patients are handled as if they were infectious.

Control of Transmission. Effective control of infection requires nurses to remain aware of the modes of transmission and ways to control them. In the hospital, home, or long-term care facility, a patient should have a personal set of care items. The sharing of bedpans, urinals, bath basins, and eating utensils can easily lead to transmission of infection. Thermometers, even when individually used, warrant special care. Because the patient's own mucus can become a source of microorganism growth, the electronic thermometer is used with a disposable sheath over the probe; the sheath is discarded after each use. Single-use chemical strip thermometers present less risk of infection than do other thermometers. Use of electronic thermometers for rectal temperatures has been associated with nosocomial diarrhea (CDC, 2019a). The organism *C. difficile* is able to survive on inanimate surfaces such as a thermometer probe for weeks to months. In institutions where nosocomial diarrhea occurs, electronic thermometers are not recommended for taking rectal temperatures.

To prevent transmission of microorganisms through indirect contact, soiled items and equipment must not touch the nurse's clothing. A common error is to carry dirty linen in one's arms against the uniform. Fluid-resistant linen bags should be used, or soiled linen should be carried with hands held out from the body. Laundry hampers should be replaced before they are overflowing.

Hand Hygiene. Hand hygiene is the most important and most basic technique in preventing the transmission of infections. Hand hygiene includes using an instant alcohol hand antiseptic before and after providing patient care, handwashing with soap and water when hands are visibly soiled, and performing a surgical scrub when necessary. The components of good handwashing include using an adequate amount of soap, rubbing the hands together to lather the soap and create friction, and rinsing under a stream of water (Infection Prevention and Control [IPAC] Canada, 2020a). The purpose is to remove soil and transient organisms from the hands and to reduce total microbial counts over time.

Contaminated hands are a prime cause of cross-infection. For example, imagine you are caring for a patient who has excessive pulmonary secretions, and you assist the patient in expectorating mucus and disposing of the tissues in a bedside container. The patient's roommate asks you to open containers of food on the meal tray. You then leave the patient's room to pour a dose of medication that is to be taken in 5 minutes. If you fail to perform hand hygiene before opening the containers of food or pouring the medication, organisms from the first patient's mucus can easily be transmitted to the roommate's food and to the medication container. Decreased nosocomial infection rates have been reported with improved hand hygiene adherence (IPAC Canada, 2020b).

The decision of when and what type of hand hygiene should occur depends on the following: the intensity of contact with patients or contaminated objects, the degree or amount of contamination that could occur with that contact, the susceptibility of the patient or the health care worker to infection, and the procedure or activity to be performed (Joint Commission, 2019). For example, after prolonged and direct contact with a patient's wound drainage, the nurse must perform thorough hand hygiene.

It takes 40–60 seconds to clean hands by washing with soap and water (IPAC Canada, 2022). If the hands are visibly soiled, more time may be needed. Routine handwashing may be performed with plain soap. Plain soap with water can physically remove a certain level of microbes, but antiseptic agents are necessary to kill or inhibit microorganisms and reduce the level still further (CDC, 2019c). Skill 34.1 lists the steps for performing hand hygiene.

SKILL 34.1 HAND HYGIENE

Delegation Considerations
- Monitor an unregulated care provider (UCP) to ensure that they are using the proper method of hand hygiene.
- Instruct the UCP to report any skin irritation from soaps or antimicrobials.

Equipment
- Easy-to-reach sink with warm running water
- Antimicrobial or regular soap
- Alcohol-based waterless antiseptic
- Paper towels or air dryer
- Clean plastic nail stick

PROCEDURE

STEPS	RATIONALE
1. Inspect surface of hands for breaks or cuts in skin or cuticles. Report and cover lesions before providing patient care.	• Open cuts or wounds can harbour high concentrations of microorganisms. Agency policy may prevent you from caring for high-risk patients. If dermatitis occurs, additional interventions may be needed.
2. Inspect hands for visible soiling.	• Lengthier handwashing is needed if soiling is heavy.
3. Inspect nails for length and presence of artificial acrylics or chipped nail polish.	• Nails should be short and filed because most microbes on hands come from beneath the fingernails. Nails should be free of artificial applications and chipped or old nail polish (Joint Commission, 2019).
4. Assess patient's risk for, or extent of, infection (e.g., white blood cell [WBC] count, extent of open wounds, known medical diagnosis).	• Use of alcohol-based waterless antiseptic is encouraged if you will be working with patients who are immunosuppressed (CDC, 2019c).
5. Push wristwatch and long uniform sleeves above wrists. Avoid wearing rings. If worn, remove for duration of the procedure.	• Provide complete access to fingers, hands, and wrists. Wearing of rings increases number of microorganisms on the hands (Joint Commission, 2019).

Continued

PROCEDURE

| **STEPS** | **RATIONALE** |

6. If hands are visibly dirty or contaminated with protein-containing material, use water and plain soap or antimicrobial soap for handwashing:

   A. Stand in front of sink, keeping hands and uniform away from sink surface. (If hands touch sink during handwashing, repeat procedure.)

   - Inside of sink is a contaminated area. Reaching over the sink increases the risk of touching the edge, which is contaminated.

   B. Turn on water. Turn faucet on or push knee pedals laterally or press pedals with foot to regulate flow and temperature (see Step 6B illustration).

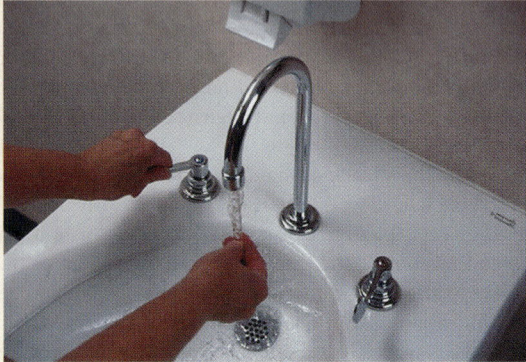

STEP 6B Turn on water.

   C. Avoid splashing water against uniform.

   - Microorganisms travel and grow in moisture.

   D. Regulate flow of water so that temperature is warm.

   - Warm water removes less of the protective oils than does hot water.

   E. Wet hands and wrists thoroughly under running water. Keep hands and forearms lower than elbows during washing.

   - Hands are the most contaminated parts to be washed. Water flows from the least to most contaminated area, rinsing microorganisms into the sink.

   F. Apply a small amount of soap, lathering thoroughly (see Step 6F illustration). Soap granules and leaflet preparations may be used.

   - Antimicrobial soaps used exclusively can be drying to hands and can cause skin irritations. The decision of whether to use an antimicrobial soap or alcohol-based hand antiseptic should depend on the procedure to be performed and the patient's immune status.

STEP 6F Lather hands thoroughly.

   G. Wash hands using plenty of lather and friction for at least 10 to 15 seconds. Interlace fingers and rub palms and back of hands with circular motion at least five times each. Keep fingertips down to facilitate removal of microorganisms. Rub knuckles of one hand into the palm of the other; repeat with the other hand (see Step 6G illustration).

   - Soap cleanses by emulsifying fat and oil and lowering the surface tension of water. Friction and rubbing mechanically loosen and remove dirt and transient bacteria. Interlacing fingers and thumbs and rubbing knuckles ensure that all surfaces are cleansed.

   H. Rub thumb on one hand with the palm of the other hand; repeat with the other hand (see Step 6H illustration).

   - Thumbs are frequently missed areas.

Continued

SKILL 34.1   HAND HYGIENE—cont'd

PROCEDURE

STEPS	RATIONALE

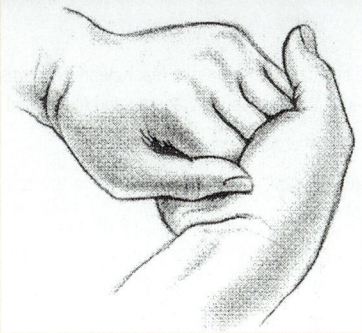

STEP 6G Rub the knuckles of one hand into the palm of the other.

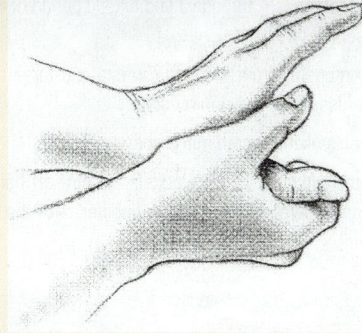

STEP 6H Rub the thumb into the palm of the other hand.

I. Work the fingertips on one hand into the palm of the other. Massage soap into nail spaces; repeat with the other hand (see Step 6I illustration).

- Fingertips are frequently missed areas.

J. Areas under fingernails are often soiled. Clean them with an orangewood stick or fingernails of the other hand and additional soap.

- Areas under the nails can be highly contaminated, which increases the risk of infection.

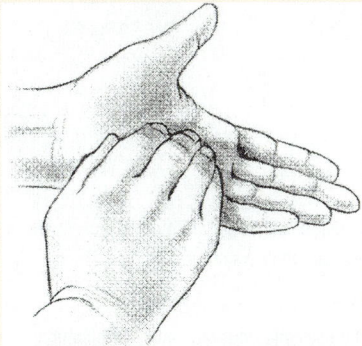

STEP 6I Work the fingertips into the palm of the other hand.

CRITICAL DECISION POINT: *Do not tear or cut skin under or around nail.*

K. Rinse hands and wrists thoroughly, keeping hands down and elbows up (see Step 6K illustration).

- Rinsing mechanically washes away dirt and microorganisms.

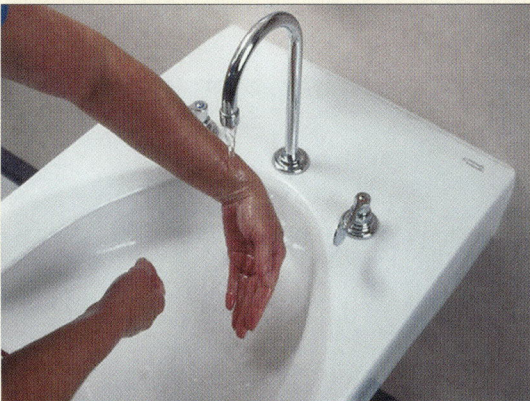

STEP 6K Rinse hands.

Continued

PROCEDURE

STEPS	RATIONALE
L. Optional: Repeat steps A through J and extend period of washing if hands are heavily soiled.	
M. Dry hands thoroughly from fingers to wrists and forearms with a paper towel, single-use cloth, or warm-air dryer.	• Drying from the cleanest (fingertips) to least clean (forearms) area avoids contamination. Drying hands prevents chapping and roughened skin.
N. If paper towel is used, discard it in proper receptacle.	• Prevents transfer of microorganisms.
O. Turn off water with foot or knee pedals. To turn off hand faucet, use a clean, dry paper towel; avoid touching handles with the hands (see Step 6O illustration).	• Faucets are contaminated. Using paper towels to touch the faucet prevents contamination of hands.

STEP 6O Turn off faucet.

P. If hands are dry or chapped, a small amount of lotion or barrier cream can be applied.	• Use an agency-provided container of lotion because many lotions may interfere with antimicrobial action or disintegrate gloves.
Q. Inspect surfaces of hands for obvious signs of soil or other contaminants.	• Determine whether handwashing is adequate.
R. Inspect hands for dermatitis or cracked skin.	• The presence of these conditions indicates complications from excessive handwashing.

7. If hands are not visibly soiled, use an alcohol-based waterless antiseptic for routine decontamination of hands in all clinical situations.

A. Apply an ample amount of product to the palm of one hand (see Step 7A illustration).	• Enough product is needed to thoroughly cover the hands.
B. Rub hands together, covering all surfaces of hands and fingers with antiseptic (see Step 7B illustration).	• Complete coverage of the hands and fingers by using friction ensures antimicrobial effect.

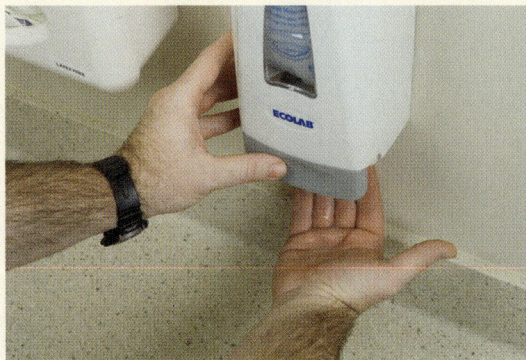

STEP 7A Apply enough waterless antiseptic to the palm of one hand to cover all hand surfaces—usually two to three pumps.

STEP 7B Rub hands thoroughly.

Continued

SKILL 34.1   HAND HYGIENE—cont'd

PROCEDURE

STEPS	RATIONALE
C. Rub hands together for several seconds until alcohol is dry. Allow hands to dry before applying gloves.	• Drying ensures full antiseptic effect (Gammon & Hunt, 2019).
D. If hands are dry or chapped, a small amount of lotion or barrier cream can be applied.	• Use the agency-provided container of lotion, because many lotions may interfere with antimicrobial action or disintegrate gloves.

RECORDING AND REPORTING

- It is not necessary to record or report this procedure.
- Report any dermatitis to employee health or infection control per agency policy.

HOME CARE CONSIDERATIONS

- Evaluate the handwashing facilities in the home to determine the possibility of contamination, the proximity of the facilities to the patient, and available supplies in the area.
- Evaluate the availability of warm running water and soap when conducting home visits, and anticipate the need for alternative handwashing products such as alcohol-based hand rubs and antiseptic wipes.
- Instruct the patient and primary caregiver in the proper techniques and situations for handwashing.

The use of alcohol-based waterless antiseptics is recommended (Joint Commission, 2019) to improve hand hygiene practices, protect health care workers' hands, and reduce the transmission of pathogens to patients and personnel in health care settings. Alcohols have excellent germicidal activity and are more effective than either plain soap or antimicrobial soap and water. Emollients are added to alcohol-based antiseptics to prevent drying of the skin. Researchers have found that these antiseptics may be more effective than water because they are used quickly and are available at the bedside (CDC, 2019c).

The Centers for Disease Control and Prevention (CDC, 2019c) recommends that hands be washed with plain soap when hands are visibly soiled. If the hands are not visibly soiled, an alcohol-based waterless antiseptic agent can be used for routine decontamination of hands in all other clinical situations.

For indications of when to perform hand hygiene in health care settings, IPAC Canada (2022) recommends the following "four moments for hand hygiene":

1. Before initial contact with the patient or the patient's environment
2. Before aseptic procedures
3. After body fluid exposure risk
4. After contact with the patient or patient's environment
   Hands should also be cleaned at the following times:
- Before and after glove use
- When moving from a contaminated body site to a clean body site during patient care
- Before clean procedures such as preparing, handling, or serving food or medications

Alternatively, if alcohol-based hand rub is not available, health care workers may wash hands in all clinical situations (US Food and Drug Administration, 2019). Also, health care workers are advised to wash their hands with soap and water if patient exposure to *C. difficile* is suspected or proven. The physical action of washing and rinsing hands under such circumstances is recommended because alcohol-based hand rub has poor activity against spores (CDC, 2019a).

Nurses need to instruct patients and visitors about the proper technique and times for hand hygiene. Nurses should ensure that patients and visitors understand the importance of cleaning under their nails and that artificial nails should not be worn because they harbour increased numbers of pathogens. Teaching proper hand hygiene is particularly important if health care is to continue at home. Patients should wash their hands before eating or handling food; after handling contaminated equipment, linen, or organic material; and after elimination. Visitors are encouraged to wash their hands before eating or handling food, after coming in contact with infected patients, and after handling contaminated equipment or organic material.

Using gloves does not replace the need for hand hygiene. Hand hygiene must be performed before entering the box of gloves, to prevent contamination of the gloves to be used and the rest of the gloves in the box. Gloves may not be completely free of tears or punctures; therefore, hands must also be cleaned before donning and after doffing gloves.

Control of Portals of Entry. Many measures that control the exit of microorganisms likewise control their entrance. Maintaining the integrity of skin and mucous membranes reduces the chances of microorganisms reaching a host. The patient's skin should be kept well lubricated by using lotion as appropriate. Immobilized and debilitated patients are particularly susceptible to skin breakdown. Patients should not be positioned on tubes or objects that might cause breaks in the skin. Dry, wrinkle-free linen also reduces the chances of skin breakdown. Frequent turning and positioning are needed in order to prevent a patient's skin from becoming reddened. Frequent oral hygiene prevents the drying of mucous membranes. A water-soluble ointment keeps the patient's lips well lubricated.

After elimination, a person with female genitalia should clean the rectum and perineum by wiping from the urinary meatus toward the rectum. Cleansing in a direction from the least to the most contaminated area helps reduce genitourinary infections. Meticulous and frequent perineal care is especially important in persons who wear incontinence pads.

Patients, health care workers, and even housekeepers are at risk for acquiring infections from accidental needle sticks. After administering an injection or inserting an intravenous catheter, the nurse should engage any safety device and carefully dispose of needles in a puncture-resistant box (see Chapter 35). A stray needle lying in the bed linen or carelessly thrown into a wastebasket is a prime source of exposure to bloodborne pathogens. Hepatitis B and C are the infections most commonly transmitted by contaminated needles. A needle stick should be reported immediately. Health care agencies require the victim of a needle stick to complete an injury report and seek appropriate treatment. The Canadian Needle Stick Surveillance Network (PHAC, 2020b) has the mandate to monitor health care workers exposed to needle sticks and the subsequent outcomes of these exposures.

Another cause of microorganism entrance into a host is improper handling and management of urinary catheters and drainage sets (see Chapter 44). The point of connection between a catheter and drainage tube should remain closed and intact. As long as such systems are closed, their contents are considered sterile. Outflow spigots on drainage bags should also remain closed to prevent the entrance of bacteria. Movement of the catheter at the urethra should be minimized by stabilizing the catheter with tape to reduce chances of microorganisms ascending the urethra into the bladder. Urine-measuring containers should not be shared between patients.

Nurses may care for patients with closed drainage systems that collect wound drainage, bile, or other body fluids. In each example, the site from which a drainage tube exits should remain clear of excess moisture and accumulated drainage. All tubing should remain connected throughout use. Drainage receptacles should be opened only when it is necessary to discard or measure the volume of drainage.

At times, nurses will obtain specimens from drainage tubes or intravenous tubing ports. First, the nurse must perform hand hygiene; then tubes and ports are disinfected by wiping the surface outward with alcohol, iodine, or a chlorhexidine alcohol solution before entering the system. Temporarily placing squares of sterile gauze around the ends of an open drainage tube, such as a urinary catheter, adds further protection against bacteria. However, keeping drainage tubes closed and secure is the best practice.

A final method for reducing the entrance of microorganisms is the technique for cleansing wounds (see Chapter 47). A surgical wound is considered to be sterile. To prevent the entrance of microorganisms into the wound, clean outward from a wound site. When applying an antiseptic or cleaning with soap and water, wipe around the wound edge first and then clean outward away from the wound. Clean gauze should be used for each revolution around the wound's circumference.

Protection of the Susceptible Host. Patients' resistance to infection improves as nurses protect patients' normal body defences against infection. Nurses can intervene to maintain the body's normal reparative processes (Box 34.12). Nurses must also protect themselves and others by following their agency's isolation guidelines.

BOX 34.12 Infection Control: Protecting the Susceptible Host

Protecting Normal Defence Mechanisms

Regular bathing removes transient microorganisms from the skin's surface. Lubrication helps keep the skin hydrated and intact.

Regular oral hygiene removes proteins in the saliva that attract microorganisms. Flossing removes tartar and plaque that can cause infection.

Maintenance of adequate fluid intake promotes normal urine formation and a resultant outflow of urine to flush the bladder and urethral lining of microorganisms.

For physically dependent or immobilized patients, nurses should encourage routine coughing and deep breathing to keep patients' lower airways clear of mucus.

Nurses should encourage proper immunization of children and adult patients (see Box 34.9).

Maintaining Healing Processes

Nurses need to encourage the intake of adequate fluids and a well-balanced diet containing essential proteins, vitamins, carbohydrates, and fats. Nurses should also use measures to increase the patient's appetite.

A patient's comfort and sleep need to be promoted, as both are vital to replenishing energy stores on a daily basis.

Nurses can assist a patient in learning techniques to reduce stress.

Isolation Guidelines. The risk of transmitting an HAI or infectious disease among patients is high. When a patient has a suspected or known infection, health care workers are alerted and follow infection control practices. However, sometimes health care workers are not aware that patients have infections. The majority of organisms causing nosocomial infections are found in the colonized body substances of patients regardless of whether a culture has confirmed infection and a diagnosis has been made (CDC, 2019d). Body substances such as feces, saliva, mucus, and wound drainage always contain potentially infectious organisms.

The CDC issued isolation guidelines in 1996 that contain a two-tiered approach (Garner, 1996). These guidelines were updated and expanded in 2007 and have been adopted by most health care agencies. Some health care agencies have adopted Public Health Agency of Canada's (PHAC's) isolation guidelines (2017), which contain a similar two-tiered approach. The PHAC guidelines were written to accommodate acute, long-term, home, and ambulatory care settings, whereas the CDC guidelines were written specifically for acute care settings. Nevertheless, the CDC guidelines and PHAC's guidelines are essentially interchangeable.

The first tier of the isolation guidelines contains practices designed to care for all patients in any setting, regardless of their diagnosis or presumed infectiousness (Table 34.7). In the PHAC's guidelines, it is called *routine practices*. **Routine practices** apply when a health care worker is or potentially may be exposed to (1) blood; (2) all body fluids, secretions, and excretions except sweat; (3) nonintact skin; or (4) mucous membranes. Routine practices include the appropriate use of gowns, gloves, masks, eyewear, and other protective devices or clothing. Barrier protection is indicated for use with all patients because every patient has the potential to transmit infection via blood and body fluids, and the risk for infection transmission can be unknown. Routine practices also include rules on appropriate handwashing, cleaning of equipment, and disposal of contaminated linen and sharps.

The second tier of the isolation guidelines is additional precautions. These precautions are designed to contain pathogens in one area, usually the patient's room; therefore, they are often called **isolation precautions**. Only patients infected or colonized with certain highly transmissible or epidemiologically significant pathogens are placed under isolation precautions. These precautions are followed in addition to routine practices. Isolation precautions are categorized in three ways: airborne, droplet, and contact precautions (see Table 34.7). The precautions used depend on how the pathogen is spread. For example, a patient diagnosed with (or suspected of having) active TB would require the use of airborne precautions, using a special mask and ventilated room, in conjunction with routine practices.

Regardless of the category of isolation precaution (Box 34.13; Box 34.14), nurses must observe the following basic principles:

- Observe thorough hand hygiene before entering and leaving the room of a patient in isolation.
- Dispose of contaminated supplies and equipment in a manner that prevents the spread of microorganisms to other persons as indicated by the mode of transmission of the organism.
- Apply knowledge of a disease process and the mode of infection transmission when using protective barriers.
- Ensure that all persons who might be exposed during transport of a patient outside the isolation room are protected.

Psychological implications of isolation precautions. A patient required to be in isolation in a private room may become lonely because normal social relationships are disrupted. This situation can be psychologically harmful, especially for children (Box 34.15).

Patients' body image may be altered as a result of the infectious process. Patients may feel unclean, rejected, lonely, or guilty. Infection prevention and control practices further intensify these feelings of difference or undesirability. Isolation in a private room limits sensory contact. Unless nurses act to minimize feelings of psychological and physical isolation, patients' emotional state can interfere with their recovery.

Before isolation measures are instituted, a patient and family must understand the nature of the disease or condition, purposes of isolation, and steps for carrying out specific precautions. If they are able to participate in maintaining infection prevention, the chances of reducing the spread of infection are increased. The patient and family should be taught to perform hand hygiene and use barrier protection if appropriate. Each procedure should be demonstrated, and the patient and family should be given an opportunity to practise it. It is also important to explain how infectious organisms can be transmitted so that the patient understands the difference between contaminated and clean objects.

Nurses should take measures to improve the patient's sensory stimulation during isolation. The room environment should be clean and pleasant. Drapes or shades should be opened, and excess supplies and equipment removed. Nurses must listen to the patient's concerns or interests. If the nurse hurries through care or shows a lack of interest, the patient will feel rejected and even more isolated. Mealtime is a particularly good opportunity for conversation. Providing comfort measures such as repositioning, a back massage, or a tepid sponge bath increases physical stimulation. If appropriate for the patient's condition, the nurse should encourage the patient to walk and to sit up in a chair. Recreational activities such as board games or cards may be an option to keep the patient mentally stimulated.

TABLE 34.7	Public Health Agency of Canada Routine Practices and Additional Precautions

Routine Practices

Routine practices and precautions are for the care of all patients; they incorporate previous precautions against bloodborne pathogens (universal precautions) and body substance isolation.

Hand hygiene must be performed before and after direct patient contact; before and after contact with the patient's environment; after contact with blood, body fluids, secretions, and excretions and after contact with equipment or articles contaminated by them; and before gloves are put on and immediately after gloves are removed. (Refer to the agency's policy for use of alcohol-based waterless antiseptics.)

Gloves are worn when touching blood, body fluids, secretions, excretions, nonintact skin, mucous membranes, or contaminated items. Gloves should be removed and hand hygiene performed between care of patients. Gloves should also be changed and hand hygiene performed between procedures on the same patient and after contact with material that may be highly contaminated.

Masks, eye protection, or face shields are worn if patient care activities or procedures may generate splashes or sprays of blood or body fluid or by droplet transmission.

Gowns should be used to protect uncovered skin and prevent soiling of clothing during procedures and patient care activities likely to generate a splash or spray of blood or body fluid.

Reusable patient care equipment is properly cleaned and reprocessed before use in the care of another patient. Single-use items are discarded.

All soiled linen from health care facilities should be handled the same way for all patients. If the bag soaks through, an additional bag should be used.

Used sharp instruments and needles are discarded in a puncture-resistant container, which is located in the area where the item is used.

Generally, a single room is unnecessary for routine patient care. Patients who visibly soil the environment or for whom appropriate hygiene cannot be maintained should be placed in a single room with dedicated toileting facilities.

ADDITIONAL (ISOLATION) PRECAUTIONS (TIER TWO)

Category	Description and Disease	Barrier Protection
Airborne precautions	For known or suspected infections caused by microbes transmitted by airborne droplets; examples: measles, chicken pox (varicella), disseminated zoster, tuberculosis	Private room (room door kept closed), negative-pressure airflow of at least six exchanges per hour, respiratory protection device (e.g., N95 respirator) must be worn when the patient has tuberculosis or when the patient has varicella, disseminated zoster, or measles and the worker is not immune
Droplet precautions	For known or suspected infections caused by microbes transmitted by droplets produced by coughing, sneezing, or talking; examples: diphtheria (pharyngeal), rubella, influenza, pertussis, mumps, meningococcal pneumonia, coronavirus, sepsis	Private room or cohort patients (room door closed unless bed is more than 2 m from the door), mask is worn when within 2 m of the patient
Contact precautions	For known or suspected infections caused by direct or indirect contact; examples: colonization or infection with multidrug-resistant organisms; *C. difficile*; major wound infections; gastrointestinal, respiratory, or skin infections	Private room or cohort patients (door can be open); gloves and gown upon entry into isolation room; limiting patient movement outside isolation room to necessary medical treatments or procedures; cleaning and disinfecting or discarding items before removal from isolation room

Adapted from Canadian Center for Occupational Health and Safety. (2021). *Routine practices.* https://www.ccohs.ca/oshanswers/prevention/universa.html; Canadian Committee on Antibiotic Resistance. (2007). *Infection prevention and control best practices for long term care, home and community care including health care offices and ambulatory clinics.* http://www.designit.ca/ccar/english/pdfs/IPC-BestPractices-June2007.pdf

Nurses must explain to the family the patient's risk for depression or loneliness. Visiting family members should be taught the principles of isolation and encouraged to avoid expressions or actions that convey revulsion, fear, or disgust. Ways to provide meaningful stimulation should also be discussed.

Protective Environment. Private rooms used for isolation may have negative-pressure airflow to prevent infectious particles from flowing out of the room. Special rooms with positive-pressure airflow are used for highly susceptible patients, such as organ transplant recipients. On the door or wall outside the room, the nurse needs to post a card listing the precautions for the isolation category according to the agency's policy. The card is a handy reference for health care workers and visitors, and it alerts anyone who might enter the room that special precautions must be followed.

The isolation room should contain hand hygiene, bathing, and toilet facilities. Soap and water and alcohol-based hand rub must be made available. Personnel and visitors perform hand hygiene before approaching the patient's bedside and again before leaving the room. If toilet facilities are unavailable, special procedures for handling portable commodes, bedpans, or urinals must be followed. Personal protective equipment should be stored in an anteroom between the room and hallway or in a convenient location close to the point of use.

All patient care rooms, including those used for isolation, contain an impervious bag for soiled or contaminated linen as well as a waste receptacle with plastic liners. Impervious receptacles stop the transmission of microorganisms by preventing seepage and soiling of the outside surface. A disposable rigid container should be available in the room for discarding used needles, syringes, and sharp objects.

Nurses should remain aware of infection prevention and control techniques while working with patients in protected environments. Depending on the microorganism and the mode of transmission, the nurse must evaluate what articles or equipment may be taken into an

---

⊚ BOX 34.13   NURSING CARE PLAN

Clostridioides difficile: *Infection Control Measures to Prevent Spread*

ASSESSMENT

Susan has been in the hospital for 7 days when she develops a temperature of 38°C and watery diarrhea. She has three episodes of diarrhea in a 12-hour period. Susan's nurse is concerned about the diarrhea and informs the most responsible health practitioner (MRHP). An order is obtained to send a sample of Susan's stool to the laboratory to test for *Clostridioides difficile*.

Assessment Activities	*Finding and Defining Characteristics*
Review signs and symptoms of *Clostridioides difficile* infection.	Signs and symptoms include watery diarrhea, abdominal pain, cramping, weight loss, and fever.

NURSING DIAGNOSIS: Risk for dehydration and infection related to *C. difficile*.

PLANNING

Goals	*Expected Outcomes*
Susan will recover from *C. difficile* and remain infection free.	Follow up with stool specimens for culture to diagnose and treat infection.
Isolation control practices will be employed to prevent cross-contamination.	Employ the use of isolation precautions: private room with contact precautions, appropriate signage on the door, single-use supplies, use personal protective equipment, and sporicidal agents.

INTERVENTIONS

Interventions (Nursing Intervention Classification)[†]	*Rationale*
Monitor laboratory values, including electrolytes.	Monitoring labs will alert heath care professionals regarding low potassium, which is associated with diarrhea
Monitor daily weights and vital signs (VS).	Monitoring weights and VS will alert health care professionals of dehydration.
Manage diet.	Prevent weight loss and dehydration through IV fluid replacement and diet.
Monitor skin.	Protect skin from breakdown by applying barrier cream.
Review antibiotic coverage and change as required.	Treat infection through the use of antibiotics.
Employ isolation precautions.	Prevent cross-contamination to protect others within the hospital.
Provide analgesia	To manage abdominal discomfort

[†]Intervention classification labels from Butcher, H. K., Bulechek, G. M., McCloskey Dochterman, J. M., et al. (Eds.). (2019). *Nursing interventions classification (NIC)* (7th ed.). Mosby.

EVALUATION

Nursing Actions	*Patient Response and Finding*	*Achievement of Outcome*
Compare laboratory results, vital signs, weights, diet, and condition of skin to baseline.	Susan will remain afebrile, free of signs and symptoms of infection.	Susan has recovered from *C. difficile*.
Ask Susan about the need for isolation and hand hygiene.	Susan is able to explain the need for isolation, including details of contact precautions.	Susan understands the principles and practices of contact isolation.
Contact isolation is used for *C. difficile*.	Susan will recover from *C. difficile* and will not transmit the infection to others.	No other patients are infected as a result of Susan's infection.

BOX 34.14 PROCEDURAL GUIDELINE

Caring for a Patient on Isolation Precautions

Delegation Considerations

Care of a patient in isolation can be delegated to an unregulated care provider (UCP) when necessary procedures are within the UCP's competence.

Equipment

- Barrier protection determined by type of isolation
- Supplies necessary for procedures performed in room

Procedure

1. Assess isolation indications (e.g., current laboratory test results or the patient's history of exposure).
2. Review agency policies and precautions necessary for the specific isolation category, and consider care measures to be performed while in the patient's room.
3. Review nurses' notes or confer with colleagues regarding the patient's emotional state and adjustment to isolation.
4. Perform hand hygiene and prepare all equipment to be taken into the patient's room.
5. Prepare for entrance into isolation room:
   A. Perform hand hygiene.
   B. Apply gown (when needed), making sure it covers you from neck to knees. Pull sleeves down to wrist. Tie securely at neck and waist (see Step 5B illustration).
   C. Apply either surgical mask or respirator around mouth and nose when needed. (Type will depend on type of isolation and facility policy.)
   D. Apply eyewear or goggles snugly and adjust to fit around face and eyes (when needed).
   E. Apply disposable nonsterile gloves for isolation. (NOTE: Unpowdered, latex-free gloves should be worn if the patient or the health care worker has a latex allergy.) If gloves are worn with a gown, bring the glove cuffs over edge of the gown sleeves.

STEP 5B Tie gown at waist.

6. Enter the patient's room. Arrange supplies and equipment. (If equipment will be removed from room for reuse, place it on a clean paper towel.)
7. Explain purpose of isolation and necessary precautions to the patient and family. Offer an opportunity to ask questions. Assess for evidence of emotional issues that may be caused by being in isolation.
8. Assess vital signs:
   A. If patient is infected or colonized with a resistant organism (e.g., methicillin-resistant *Staphylococcus aureus* [MRSA]), the equipment remains in the room. Proceed to assess vital signs. Avoid contact of stethoscope or blood pressure cuff with infectious material.
   B. If stethoscope is to be reused, the entire stethoscope must be thoroughly cleaned after leaving the room. You may use a few alcohol swabs to clean and disinfect the stethoscope. (Ideally, equipment is dedicated for the use of the patient with an antibiotic-resistant organism and remains in the room.) Clean diaphragm or bell with alcohol. Set aside on clean surface.
   C. Individual or disposable thermometers should be used.
9. Administer medications:
   A. Give oral medication in wrapper or cup.
   B. Dispose of wrapper or cup in plastic-lined receptacle.
   C. Administer injection.
   D. Discard syringe and uncapped needle or sheathed needle into special container.
   E. If gloves are not worn and hands contact contaminated article or body fluids, wash hands immediately.
10. Administer hygiene measures, encouraging the patient to discuss questions or concerns about isolation. Informal teaching can be used at this time:
    A. Prevent the gown from becoming wet.
    B. Remove linen from the bed; avoid contact with the gown. Place linen in an impervious bag.
    C. Change gloves and wash your hands if they become excessively soiled and further care is necessary.
11. Collect specimens:
    A. Place specimen containers on a clean paper towel in the patient's bathroom.
    B. Follow procedure for collecting specimen of body fluids.
    C. Transfer specimen to the container without soiling the outside of the container. Place the container in a plastic bag and place a label on the outside of the bag or as per agency policy.
12. Dispose of linen and garbage bags as they become full:
    A. Use sturdy, moisture-resistant single bags to contain soiled articles.
    B. Tie bags securely at the top in a knot (see Step 12B illustration).

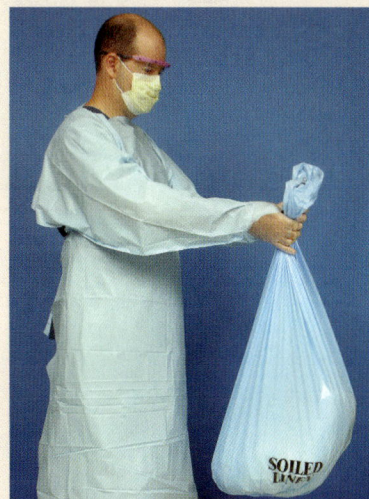

STEP 12B Tie linen bag securely.

Continued

BOX 34.14 PROCEDURAL GUIDELINE—cont'd

Caring for a Patient on Isolation Precautions

13. Resupply room as needed.
14. When leaving isolation room, remove personal protective equipment, except for N95 respirator, inside doorway or in anteroom. Remove N95 respirator after leaving the patient's room and closing the door.
    A. Remove gloves. Remove one glove by grasping the cuff and pulling the glove inside out over the hand. Discard the glove. With the ungloved hand, tuck a finger inside the cuff of the remaining glove and pull it off, inside out (see Step 14A illustration).

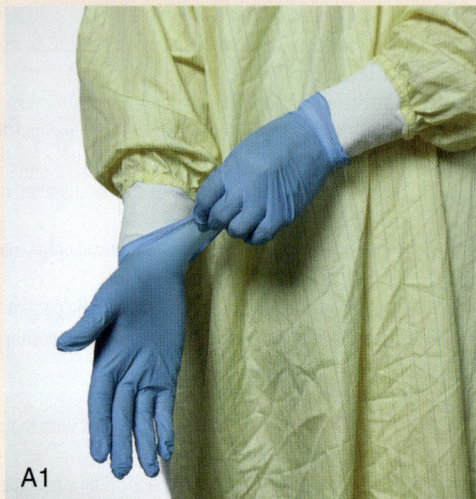

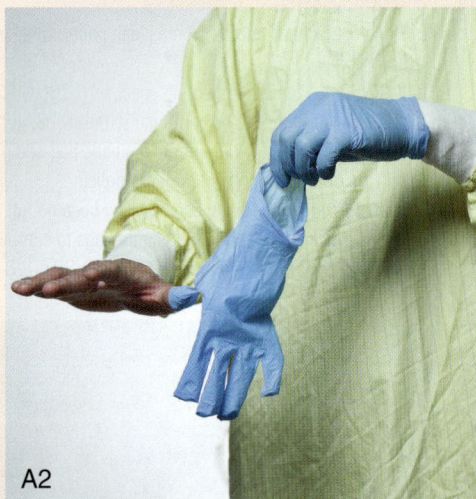

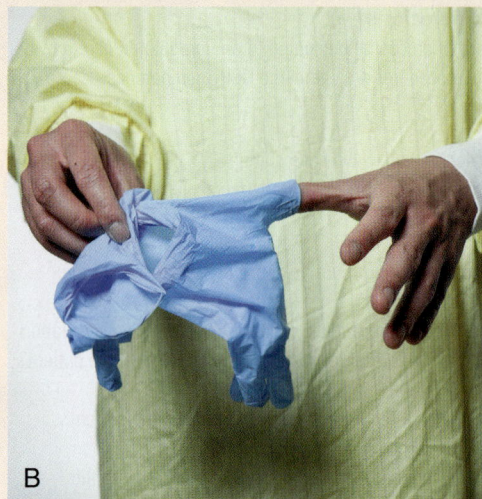

A1

A2

B

C

STEP 14A **Doffing gloves. A,** Grasp the outside edge of the glove near the wrist and peel away from the hand (A1), turning the glove inside out (A2). **B,** Hold the glove in the opposite gloved hand. Slide an ungloved finger or thumb under the wrist of the remaining glove. **C,** Peel the glove off and over the first glove, making a bag for both gloves. Dispose of gloves in the garbage. (Alberta Health Services. [2021]. *Taking off [doffing] personal protective equipment [PPE].* https://www.albertahealthservices.ca/assets/Infofor/hp/if-hp-ipc-doffing-ppe-poster.pdf. Reprinted with permission.)

Continued

BOX 34.14   PROCEDURAL GUIDELINE—cont'd

Caring for a Patient on Isolation Precautions

B. Perform hand hygiene using alcohol-based hand rub unless your hands are visibly soiled or feel dirty, then use soap and water (see Step 14B illustration).

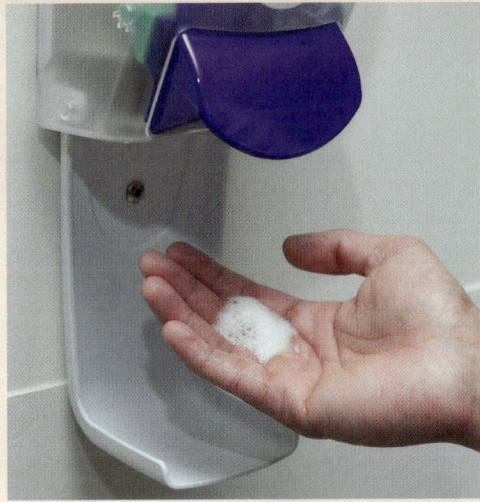

STEP 14B Hand hygiene. 1) Using an alcohol-based hand rub is the preferred way to clean your hand. **2)** If your hands look or feel dirty, soap and water must be used to wash your hands. Clean your hands. Exit the patient room, close the door, and clean your hands again. (Alberta Health Services. [2021]. *Taking off [doffing] personal protective equipment [PPE]*. https://www.albertahealthservices.ca/assets/Infofor/hp/if-hp-ipc-doffing-ppe-poster.pdf. Reprinted with permission.)

Continued

BOX 34.14   PROCEDURAL GUIDELINE—cont'd

Caring for a Patient on Isolation Precautions

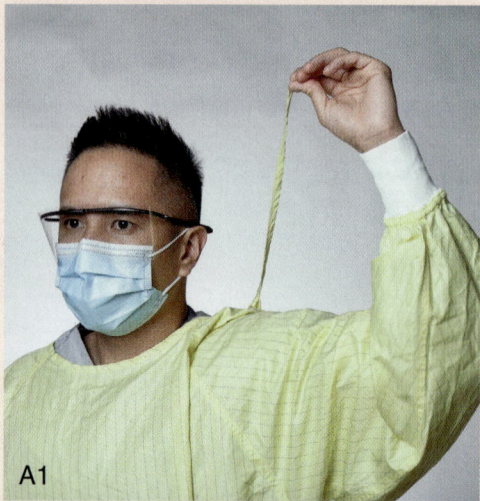

A1

B

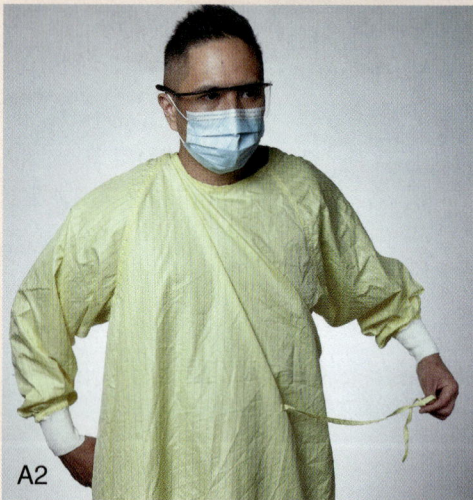

A2

C

STEP 14C **Doffing gown.** Remove hands from sleeves without touching outside of the gown. **A1–A2,** Carefully unfasten ties. **B,** Grasp the outside of the gown at the back of the shoulders and pull the gown down over the arms. **C,** Turn the gown inside out during removal. Put in hamper or, if disposable, put in garbage. (Alberta Health Services. [2021]. *Taking off [doffing] personal protective equipment [PPE].* https://www .albertahealthservices.ca/assets/Infofor/hp/if-hp-ipc-doffing-ppe-poster.pdf. Reprinted with permission.)

    C. Untie waist and neck strings of the gown. Allow the gown to fall from your shoulders. Remove hands from sleeves without touching the outside of the gown (see Step 14C illustration). Hold the gown inside at shoulder seams and fold inside out; discard in laundry bag.

    D. Perform hand hygiene.

    E. Remove eyewear or goggles (see Step 14E illustration).

Continued

BOX 34.14   PROCEDURAL GUIDELINE—cont'd

Caring for a Patient on Isolation Precautions

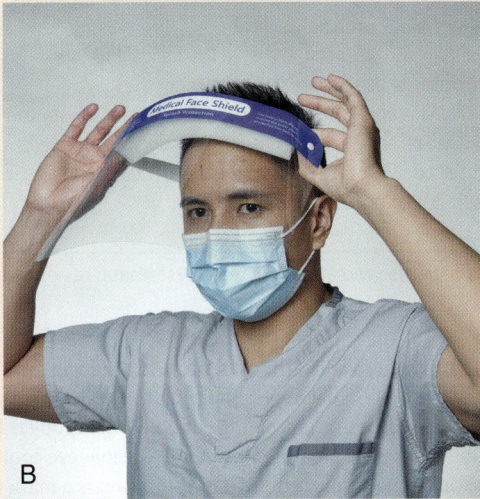

A

B

STEP 14E **Removing eye protection or face shield.** Handle eye protection only by headband (**A**) or ear pieces (**B**). Carefully pull away from face. Put reusable items in appropriate area for cleaning. Put disposable items into garbage. (Alberta Health Services. [2021]. *Taking off [doffing] personal protective equipment [PPE].* https://www.alber tahealthservices.ca/assets/Infofor/hp/if-hp-ipc-doffing-ppe-poster.pdf. Reprinted with permission.)

F. Remove mask away from face. Untie first bottom mask string and then top strings; pull the mask away from your face and drop mask into a waste receptacle (see Step 14F illustration). (Do not touch outer surface of mask.) Note: If patient is on airborne precautions, remove N95 respirator once you have exited the patient room.

G. Perform handwashing and hand hygiene.

H. Explain to the patient when you plan to return to the room. Ask whether the patient requires any personal-care items, books, or magazines.

I. Leave the room and close the door, if necessary. (Door should be closed if airborne precautions are being used.)

J. All contaminated supplies and equipment should be disposed of in a manner that prevents the spread of microorganisms to other individuals (see your agency's policy).

A

B

C

STEP 14F **Doffing mask or N95 respirator.** There are different styles of masks and N95 respirators, but all styles have the same basic steps for doffing. Bend forward slightly and carefully remove the mask from your face by touching only the ties or elastic bands. Start with the bottom tie (**A**), then remove the top tie (**B**). Pull mask away from the face (**C**) and throw mask in the garbage. (Alberta Health Services. [2021]. *Taking off [doffing] personal protective equipment [PPE].* https://www.albertahealthservices.ca/assets/Infofor/hp/if-hp-ipc-doffing-ppe-poster.pdf. Reprinted with permission.)

BOX 34.15   RESEARCH HIGHLIGHT

Adverse Effects of Isolation

Research Focus

Purssell and colleagues (2020) reviewed the impact of isolation due to highly contagious microorganisms, both psychological and nonpsychological outcomes, on adult hospitalized patients and compared the results with those from non-isolated, hospitalized patients.

Methods

The information sources used were Embase, Medline, and PsycINFO, which were searched from inception to December 2018. A total of 3 839 papers were retrieved, of which 38 were assessed for eligibility. Of these studies, 13 provided data suitable for calculation of the risk ratio, 5 giving psychological outcomes and 8 providing data for calculation of standardized mean difference. Outcomes were divided into three categories: quality of care, satisfaction of care, and adverse events. The search items included patient safety or harm, depression, anxiety, adaptation, stress, patient satisfaction, and quality of life.

Results

The results did not indicate significant differences in psychological outcomes; however, when it did make a difference, it was primarily negative. There were significant declines in control and self-esteem and increases in depression and anxiety. No change was noted in the isolated versus non-isolated patients for the development of ulcers or falls. For nonpsychological outcomes, there was a trend

for less time to be spent with patients in isolation compared to non-isolated patients, and more errors occurred. The authors found that older individuals felt more depression and loneliness; women in isolation were more concerned about precautions and transmission; while men were more resigned, rational, and tended to cope better. In conclusion, the study authors found a number of apparently negative aspects to contact precautions or isolation, in particular with regard to psychological effects and a reduction in the quality of some aspects of care. The study was able to quantify the extent of the issues associated with isolation but unable to identify solutions in the literature. The authors suggested that risks and benefits of isolation should be weighed for each individual, and if it is demonstrated that there is a need for isolation, patient harm should be minimized. They also recommended larger longitudinal studies, including older age groups who were underrepresented.

Implications for Practice

- Nurses must be extra vigilant to ensure the standard of care is similar for all patients, including those on isolation precautions.
- Nurses should ensure that both physical and psychological factors are addressed when planning and carrying out care for isolated patients.
- Nurses must be sure to record observations and complete nursing notes for all patients, including those in isolation.

From Purssell, E., Gould, D., & Chudleigh, J. (2020). Impact of isolation on hospitalized patients who are infectious: Systematic review with meta-analysis. *BMJ, 10*(2). https://doi.org/10.1136/bmjopen-2019-030371

isolation room. For example, Ontario's Provincial Infectious Diseases Advisory Committee on Infection Prevention and Control (PIDAC, 2018) recommends the dedicated use of articles such as stethoscopes, sphygmomanometers, and rectal thermometers in the isolation room of a patient infected or colonized with methicillin-resistant *Staphylococcus aureus* (MRSA). These devices should not be used on other patients unless the devices are first adequately cleaned and disinfected. If the nurse brings an article into the room, exposes the article to infected material, and then touches or removes the article, the nurse increases the risk of transmitting infection to other patients or personnel.

Personal protective equipment. Personal protective equipment (gowns, masks, protective eyewear, and gloves) should be readily available. The primary reason for gowning is to prevent the contamination of clothes during contact with the patient. Gowns and cover-ups protect health care workers and visitors from coming in contact with infected material, blood, or body fluid. Gowns may also be required for contact precautions, depending on the expected amount of exposure to infectious material. Gowns used for barrier protection are made of a fluid-resistant material and should be changed immediately if damaged or heavily contaminated.

Isolation gowns usually open at the back and have ties or snaps at the neck and waist to keep the gown closed and secure. They should be long enough to cover all outer garments. Long sleeves with tight-fitting cuffs provide added protection. No special technique is required for applying clean gowns as long as they are fastened securely. However, nurses must be careful when removing a gown to minimize the contamination of their hands and uniform. Isolation gowns are disposable or reusable, depending on the agency's policy.

Full face protection (with eyes, nose, and mouth covered) should be worn when splashing or spraying of blood or body fluid into the face is possible. Masks and eye protection should also be worn when working with a patient placed on droplet precautions; they protect the wearer from inhaling microorganisms from a patient's respiratory tract and prevent the transmission of pathogens from the wearer's respiratory

tract to the patient. Surgical masks protect a wearer from inhaling large-particle aerosols that travel short distances (2 m). Eye protection protects a wearer from receiving large-particle droplets to the eye. Prescription eyeglasses are not considered suitable eye protection. At times, a patient who is susceptible to infection wears a mask to prevent inhalation of pathogens. Patients on droplet or airborne precautions who are transported outside their rooms should wear masks to protect other patients and personnel. According to the PIDAC (2018), masks may prevent the transmission of infection through direct contact with mucous membranes. In addition, masks discourage the wearer from touching their eyes, nose, or mouth.

A properly applied mask fits snugly over the mouth and nose so that pathogens and body fluids cannot enter or escape through the sides (Box 34.16). If a person wears glasses, the top edge of the mask fits below the glasses so that the glasses do not cloud over as the person exhales. Talking should be kept to a minimum while wearing a mask to reduce respiratory airflow—a mask that has become moist may not provide a barrier to microorganisms and should be discarded. A mask should never be reused. Patients and family members should be warned that a mask can cause a sensation of smothering. If family members become uncomfortable wearing a mask, they should leave the room and discard the mask.

Specially fitted respiratory protective devices or N95 masks are required when nurses care for a patient with known or suspected TB or when the patient has varicella, disseminated zoster, measles, or coronavirus, and the worker is not immune. The mask must have a higher filtration rating than the regular surgical mask and be fitted snugly to the wearer's face to prevent leakage around the sides. Nurses should be aware of their agency's policy regarding the type of respiratory protective device required.

Gloves help to prevent the transmission of pathogens by direct and indirect contact. Clean, nonsterile gloves (also called *disposable gloves*) should be worn when contact with blood, body fluid, secretions, excretions, or contaminated items is possible. Clean gloves should be donned just before touching mucous membranes and nonintact skin. Gloves should be changed between tasks and procedures on the same patient

BOX 34.16   PROCEDURAL GUIDELINE
Donning and Removing a Surgical-Type Mask

Procedure

1. Find top edge of the mask (usually has a thin metal strip). The pliable metal fits snugly against the bridge of the nose.
2. Hold the mask by the top two strings or loops. Tie the two top ties at the top of back of the head (see Step 2 illustration), with ties above the ears (alternative: slip loops over each ear).
3. Tie the two lower ties snugly around the neck, with mask well under the chin (see Step 3 illustration).

4. Gently pinch upper metal band around bridge of the nose.
   Note: Mask should be changed if it becomes wet, moist, or contaminated.
5. To remove the mask, grasp the loops and remove away from the face. If there are ties, undo the bottom tie, then the top tie (reverse order for donning a mask), and remove them away from the face. Wash hands for 15 seconds (see Step 5 illustration).

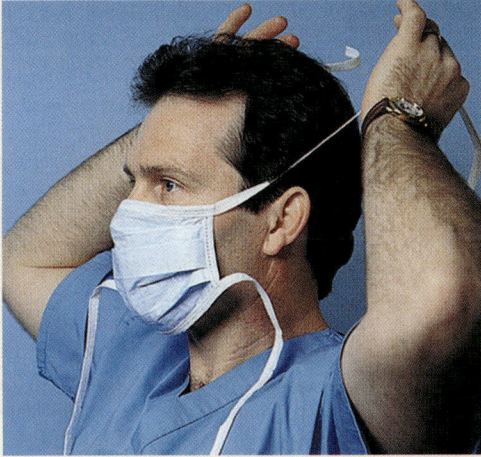

STEP 2 Tie two top ties at top of back of the head.

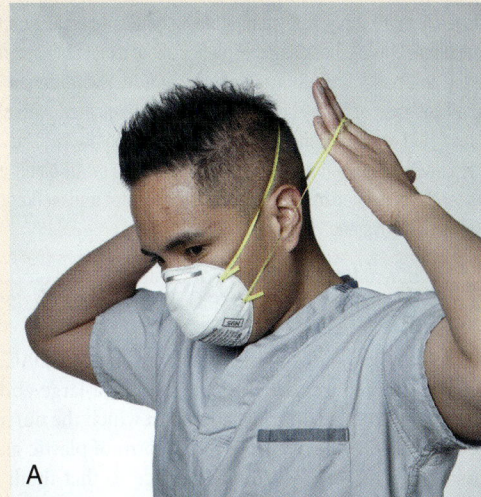

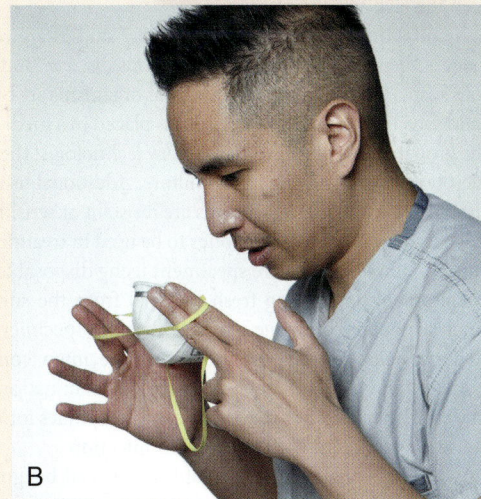

STEP 5 (**A**) Grasp the loops (or if mask has ties, undo bottom and then top tie) and (**B**) remove the mask away from the face.

STEP 3 Tie two lower ties snugly around the neck.

Alberta Health Services. (2021). *Taking off (doffing) personal protective equipment (PPE).* https://www.albertahealthservices.ca/assets/Infofor/hp/if-hp-ipc-doffing-ppe-poster.pdf. Reprinted with permission.

after contact with material that may contain a high concentration of microorganisms. Gloves should be removed promptly after use, before touching noncontaminated items and environmental surfaces, and before going to another patient. Hand hygiene should be performed immediately after removing the gloves to avoid the transfer of microorganisms to other patients and environments. Facilities provide nonlatex gloves for health care staff who are allergic or sensitive to latex. When full protective apparel is needed, the nurse must first perform hand hygiene, apply a mask and eyewear or goggles (as needed), apply a gown, and then put on gloves. Disposable gloves are easily applied and are designed to fit either hand. The glove cuffs should be pulled up over the wrists or

over the cuffs of the gown. The gloves' thin rubber can be easily torn; if a break or tear is detected in a glove while providing care, the nurse should change gloves if care is not completed. If no additional contact with the patient is planned, reapplying gloves is unnecessary.

Family members visiting patients who are in isolation that necessitates the use of gloves must know when and how to apply gloves properly. Nurses need to demonstrate the application of gloves to family members and explain the reason for glove use, placing emphasis on the importance of hand hygiene after the removal of gloves.

When participating in a procedure that may create droplets or splashing or spraying of blood or other body fluids, nurses must

BOX 34.17 Specimen Collection Techniques*

Wound Specimen

Clean the site with sterile water or saline before wound specimen collection. Wear gloves and use a cotton-tipped swab or a syringe to collect as much drainage as possible. Set a clean test tube or culture tube on a clean paper towel close by. After swabbing the healthiest-looking tissue of the wound site, grasp the collection tube by holding it with a paper towel. Carefully insert the swab without touching the outside of the tube. After securing the tube's top, transfer the tube into a bag for transport and then perform hand hygiene.

Blood Specimen

Wearing gloves, use a syringe and culture media bottles to collect up to 10 mL of blood per culture bottle (check agency's policy about exact amounts required). After prepping the patient, perform a venipuncture at two different sites, to decrease the likelihood of both specimens being contaminated with skin flora. Place the blood culture bottles on the bedside table or another surface; swab off the bottle tops with alcohol. Inject the appropriate amount of blood into each bottle. Transfer the specimen into a clean, labelled bag for transport and remove gloves. Perform hand hygiene.

Stool Specimen

Wearing gloves, use a clean cup with sealing top (it does not need to be sterile) and a tongue blade to collect a small amount of stool, approximately the size of a walnut. Place the cup on a clean paper towel in the patient's bathroom; using the tongue blade, collect the needed amount of feces from the patient's bedpan and transfer the feces to the cup without touching the cup's outside surface. Dispose of the tongue blade and place the seal on the cup. Transfer the specimen into a clean bag for transport. Remove gloves and perform hand hygiene.

Urine Specimen

Wearing gloves, use a syringe and sterile cup or tube to collect 1 to 5 mL of urine. Place the cup or tube on a clean towel in the patient's bathroom. If the patient has a urinary catheter, use the syringe to collect the specimen. If the patient is not catheterized, have the patient follow the procedure to obtain a clean, voided specimen (see Chapter 44). Transfer the urine into a sterile container by injecting urine from the syringe or by pouring it from the collection cup. Secure the top of the container and transfer the specimen into a clean, labelled bag for transport. Remove gloves and perform hand hygiene.

*Agency policies may differ on the type of containers and amount of specimen material required.
Data from Pagana, K. D., Pagana, T. J., & Pike-MacDonald, S. A. (2019). *Mosby's Canadian manual of diagnostic and laboratory tests* (2nd ed.). Elsevier Inc.

wear protective eyewear and a mask or a face shield (PIDAC, 2018). Examples of such procedures are the irrigation of a large abdominal wound or the insertion of an arterial catheter in which the nurse assists a physician. Eyewear may be available in the form of plastic glasses or goggles. They should fit snugly around the face so that fluids cannot enter between the face and the glasses.

Specimen collection. Often, many laboratory studies are required when a patient is suspected of having an infectious disease. Body fluids and secretions suspected of containing infectious organisms are collected for culture and sensitivity tests. The specimen is placed in a medium that promotes the growth of organisms. A laboratory technologist then identifies the microorganisms growing in the culture. Additional test results indicate antibiotics to which the organisms are resistant or sensitive, and sensitivity reports determine the antibiotics to be used in treatment.

Nurses need to obtain all culture specimens using disposable gloves and sterile equipment. Collecting fresh material from the site of the infection, such as wound drainage, ensures that the specimen is not contaminated by neighbouring microbes. All specimen containers should be sealed tightly to prevent spillage and contamination of the outside of the container. Box 34.17 describes the techniques for collecting specimens from a patient with a suspected infection.

Bagging waste or linen. Nurses should use special bagging procedures when removing contaminated items from a patient's environment. Bagging contaminated items and ensuring that the outside of the bag is not contaminated prevents accidental exposure of personnel and contamination of the surrounding environment.

The PIDAC (2018) recommends using a single bag for discarding items if the bag is impervious and sturdy and if the article can be placed in the bag without contaminating the outside of the bag. Soiled linen should be placed in an impervious laundry bag in the patient's room. Double bagging is recommended *only* if it is impossible to prevent the contamination of the bag's outer surface. Studies have shown that double bagging is otherwise not necessary to control infection (PIDAC, 2018). The use of one standard-sized linen bag that is not overfilled, is tied securely, and is intact is adequate to prevent infection transmission. The same rule applies to garbage bags.

Transporting patients. Before transferring a patient to a wheelchair or stretcher, the nurse should have the patient perform hand hygiene and give the patient a clean gown and robe. Patients infected

with organisms transmitted by the airborne route should leave their rooms only for essential purposes, such as diagnostic procedures or surgery. These patients must also wear masks. Personnel transporting these patients may also need to wear barrier protection depending on the amount of contact they will be having with the patient.

At times, a patient being transported may drain body fluids onto a stretcher or wheelchair. When this occurs, the nurse must be sure to have the equipment cleaned and, if necessary, disinfected after the patient returns to the room. An extra layer of sheets may be used to cover the stretcher or seat of the wheelchair.

Personnel in diagnostic or procedural areas or the operating room should be notified that the patient is on isolation precautions. Record the type of isolation on the patient's chart. Explain to the patient ways that they can help prevent the transmission of infection during transport. A patient on airborne or droplet isolation is provided with a mask and given tissues and a bag to allow for the proper disposal of secretions.

Role of the Infection Control Professional. Many hospitals employ professionals who are specially trained in infection prevention and control; most of these professionals are nurses. These individuals are responsible for advising hospital personnel regarding infection prevention and control and for monitoring infections within the hospital. Infection Prevention and Control (IPAC) Canada is a voluntary multidisciplinary association of infection-control professionals. Its mission is to promote excellence in the practice of infection prevention and control (IPAC Canada, 2022). The duties of an infection-control professional include the following:

- Provide staff with education on infection prevention and control.
- Develop and review infection prevention and control policies and procedures.
- Recommend appropriate isolation procedures.
- Screen patient records for community-acquired infections that may be reportable to the public health department.
- Consult with employee health departments concerning recommendations to prevent and control the spread of infection among personnel, such as TB testing.
- Gather statistics regarding the **epidemiology** (cause and effect) of HAIs.

- Notify the public health department of incidents of communicable diseases within the facility.
- Confer with all hospital departments to investigate unusual events or clusters of infection.
- Recommend education for patients and families.
- Identify infection-control problems related to equipment.
- Monitor antibiotic-resistant organisms in the institution.
- Monitor construction sites in hospitals to ensure that appropriate dust-containment measures are used.

An infection-control professional can be a valuable resource for nurses in controlling HAIs.

Infection Prevention and Control for Hospital Personnel. Health care workers are continually at risk of exposure to infectious microorganisms. Each agency has protocols in place to advise staff and to monitor infection protocols. Hospitals offer regularly scheduled staff education programs. Each province and territory has rules and procedures to ensure that health care workers are not unnecessarily exposed to pathogens.

Patient Education. Often patients must learn to use infection-control practices at home (Box 34.18). Preventive technique will become almost second nature to you as a nurse if practised daily, but your patients will be less aware of factors that promote the spread of infection and ways to prevent its transmission. The home environment does not always lend itself to infection prevention—often you must help patients adapt according to the resources available to maintain hygienic techniques. However, patients in a home care setting generally have a lower risk of infection than do patients in a hospital because they have less exposure to resistant organisms and undergo fewer invasive procedures.

Surgical Asepsis. Surgical asepsis, or sterile technique, requires precautions different from those of medical asepsis. Surgical asepsis includes procedures used to eliminate all microorganisms, including spores, from an object or area. In surgical asepsis, an area or object is considered contaminated if touched by any object that is not sterile. When nurses are working with a sterile field or with sterile equipment, they must understand that the slightest break in technique results in contamination. Surgical asepsis should be used in the following situations:

- During procedures that require the intentional perforation of the patient's skin (e.g., the insertion of intravenous catheters or administration of injections)
- When the skin's integrity is broken as a result of trauma, surgical incision, or burns
- During procedures that involve the insertion of catheters or surgical instruments into sterile body cavities

Although surgical asepsis is commonly practised in the operating room, labour and delivery area, and major diagnostic areas, nurses may also use surgical aseptic techniques at the patient's bedside—for example, when inserting intravenous or urinary catheters, suctioning the tracheobronchial airway, or reapplying sterile dressings. In an operating room, nurses must follow a series of steps to maintain sterile technique, including applying a mask, protective eyewear, and a cap; performing a surgical hand scrub; and applying a sterile gown and gloves. In contrast, when performing a dressing change at a patient's bedside, nurses may only perform hand hygiene and apply sterile gloves (see "Principles of Surgical Asepsis" section). When using the principles of surgical asepsis, nurses need to remember that they are trying to prevent infections. For more information on infection control, see Box 34.19.

Patient Preparation. Because surgical asepsis necessitates exact techniques, the nurse must have the patient's cooperation. Therefore, the nurse must prepare the patient before any procedure. Some patients may fear moving or touching objects during a sterile procedure, but others may try to assist. Nurses need to explain how a procedure is to be performed and what the patient can do to avoid contaminating sterile items, including the following:

- Avoid sudden movements of body parts covered by sterile drapes.
- Refrain from touching sterile supplies, drapes, or the nurse's gloves and gown.
- Avoid coughing, sneezing, or talking over a sterile area.

BOX 34.18 PATIENT TEACHING

Infection Control

Objective
- Patient will perform self-care using proper infection-control techniques.

Teaching Strategies
- Instruct patient to clean equipment using soap and water and to disinfect it with an appropriate disinfectant.
- Demonstrate proper hand hygiene, explaining that it should be done before and after all treatments and when infected body fluids are contacted.
- Inform patient of the signs and symptoms of wound infection.
- For patients who receive tube feedings at home, explain the importance of following instructions regarding how long formula can be prepared ahead of time and left unrefrigerated. Tell patient that contaminated enteral feedings can cause infections. Teach patient to care for the feeding bag and tubing as per the organization's protocol.
- Instruct patient to place contaminated dressings and other disposable items containing infectious body fluids in impervious plastic bags and to place needles in a puncture-proof and leak-proof container, such as an empty bleach bottle with the opening taped shut or a coffee can with the lid taped closed. Glass containers should not be used. Ensure that the patient knows to contact the local municipality or public health department before disposing of contaminated items (Provincial Infection Control Network of British Columbia [PICNet], 2014).

- Instruct patient (or family) to separate noticeably soiled linen from other laundry, wash it in water that is as hot as the fabric will tolerate, add 250 mL of bleach to detergent, and set the dryer temperature as high as the fabric will allow.

Evaluation
- Ask patient or family member to describe techniques used to reduce the transmission of infection.
- Ask patient to demonstrate select techniques.
- Ask patient to explain the risks for infection, based on the condition.

After patients are at home, nurses need to educate them about infection and techniques to prevent or control its spread, and nurses need to determine patients' adherence to infection-control practices. Family members caring for patients must be involved in the teaching plan: Patients and family members should be taught a common-sense approach to controlling and preventing infection. Topics to address in a teaching session include the following:
- The patient's susceptibility to infection
- The chain of infection, with specific reference to the means of transmission
- Hygienic practices that minimize organism growth and spread; emphasize hand hygiene
- Preventive health care (e.g., proper diet, immunizations, and exercise)
- The proper methods for handling and storage of food
- An awareness of family members who are at risk for acquiring infection

Certain sterile procedures may take an extended period of time. The nurse should assess the patient's needs and anticipate factors that may disrupt a procedure. If a patient is in pain, the nurse should try to administer analgesics no more than half an hour before a sterile procedure begins. The patient should be given the opportunity to void. Often patients must assume uncomfortable positions during sterile procedures; the nurse can help the patient to assume the most comfortable position possible. Finally, the patient's condition may result in actions or events that contaminate a sterile field. For example, a patient with a respiratory infection transmits organisms by coughing or breathing; the nurse needs to anticipate such a situation and offer the patient a mask.

Principles of Surgical Asepsis. When beginning a surgically aseptic procedure, nurses must follow certain principles to ensure the maintenance of asepsis. Failure to follow these principles places patients at risk for infection. The following principles are important:

1. *A sterile object remains sterile only when touched by another sterile object.* This principle guides nurses in the placement of sterile objects and how to handle them.
   A. Sterile objects that touch sterile objects remain sterile; for example, sterile gloves are worn or sterile forceps are used to handle objects on a sterile field.
   B. Sterile objects that touch clean objects become contaminated; for example, if the tip of a syringe or other sterile object touches the surface of a clean disposable glove, the object is contaminated.

BOX 34.19   Surgical Asepsis: Infection Control

Objective
- The goal of surgical asepsis or aseptic technique is to prevent microorganisms from becoming introduced to a susceptible site. It should also prevent transmission of microorganisms to other patients or to staff.

Principles
- Ensure that all required supplies are gathered and that there is a clear and dry field to carry out the procedure.
- Movement within or around a sterile field should be done in a manner that does not contaminate the sterile field.
- Sterile fields should be prepared as close to the time of use as possible; the potential for environmental contamination from dust and particles in the ambient environment that settle on surfaces increases over time.
- Conversation in a sterile field should be kept to a minimum, to reduce contamination by means of respiratory droplets.
- Perform hand hygiene prior to setting up a sterile field.
- Ensure that the sterile barrier covering the supplies is intact, with no punctures or evidence of moisture damage.
- If there is any question of the item's sterility, the item must be considered unsterile.
- Open sterile packs carefully to prevent contamination of the contents of the pack.
- All items in a sterile field must be sterile.
- Once a sterile package is opened, a 2.5-cm border around the edges is considered unsterile.
- Pour solutions into receptacles on the sterile field slowly to avoid splashing. Splashing can cause strike-through or splash-back from nonsterile surfaces to the sterile field.
- An object is considered no longer sterile if it is below a person's waist or if it is out of the range of vision.
- Wear sterile gloves for the procedure to prevent the introduction of microorganisms to the site and to protect the wearer from coming into contact with body fluids.

C. Sterile objects that touch contaminated objects become contaminated; for example, when you touch a sterile object with an ungloved hand, the object is contaminated.
D. Sterile objects that touch questionable objects are considered contaminated; for example, when a tear or break in the covering or packaging of a sterile object is found, the object is discarded regardless of whether the object itself appears untouched.

2. *Only sterile objects may be placed on a sterile field.* All items are properly sterilized before use. Sterile objects are kept in clean, dry storage areas. The package or container holding a sterile object must be intact and dry—a package that is torn, punctured, wet, or open is considered to be contaminated.

3. *A sterile object or field out of the range of vision or an object held below a person's waist is contaminated.* The nurse must never turn their back on a sterile tray or leave it unattended. Contamination can occur accidentally by a dangling piece of clothing, falling hair, or an unknowing patient touching a sterile object. Any object held below waist level is considered contaminated because it cannot be viewed at all times. Sterile objects should be kept in front of the nurse, with hands as close together as possible.

4. *A sterile object or field becomes contaminated by prolonged exposure to air.* Nurses need to avoid activities that may create air currents, such as excessive movements or rearranging linen after a sterile object or field becomes exposed. When sterile packages are being opened, it is important to minimize the number of persons walking into the area. Microorganisms travel by droplets through the air; therefore, no one should talk, laugh, sneeze, or cough over a sterile field or when gathering and using sterile equipment. Microorganisms travelling through the air can fall on sterile items or fields if the nurse reaches over the work area. When opening sterile packages, hold the item or piece of equipment as close as possible to the sterile field without touching the sterile surface. Keeping the movement or rearranging of sterile items to a minimum also reduces contamination by air transmission.

5. When a sterile surface comes in contact with a wet, contaminated surface, the sterile object or field becomes contaminated by capillary action. If moisture seeps through a sterile package's protective covering, microorganisms travel to the sterile object. When stored sterile packages become wet, the objects must be discarded immediately, or the equipment sent for re-sterilization. When working with a sterile field or tray, the nurse may have to pour sterile solutions. Any spill can be a source of contamination unless the object or field rests on a sterile surface that cannot be penetrated by moisture. Urinary catheterization trays contain sterile supplies that rest in a sterile, plastic container. In this example, sterile solutions spilled within the container will not contaminate the catheter or other objects. In contrast, if the nurse places a piece of sterile gauze in its wrapper on a patient's bedside table and the table surface is wet, the gauze is considered contaminated.

6. *Fluid flows in the direction of gravity.* A sterile object becomes contaminated if gravity causes a contaminated liquid to flow over the object's surface. To avoid contamination during a surgical hand scrub, the nurse holds their hands above the elbows. This allows water to flow downward without contaminating the hands and fingers. This is also the reason for drying from the fingers to elbows with hands held up, after the scrub.

7. *The edges of a sterile field or container are considered to be contaminated.* Frequently, sterile objects are placed on a sterile towel or drape (Figure 34.2). Because the edge of the drape touches an unsterile surface, such as a table or bed linen, a 2.5-cm border around the drape is considered contaminated. Objects placed on the sterile field must be inside this border. The edges of sterile

FIGURE 34.2 Placing sterile item on a sterile field.

FIGURE 34.3 Opening a sterile package on a cleaned work area above waist level.

containers become exposed to air after they are open and are thus contaminated. After a sterile needle is removed from its protective cap, or after forceps are removed from a container, the objects must not touch the container's edge. After a sterile needle is removed from its protective cap or after forceps are removed from a container, the objects must not touch the container's edge.

Performing Sterile Procedures. All necessary equipment should be assembled before a procedure is done, to avoid having to leave a sterile area to obtain equipment. A few extra supplies should be available in case objects accidentally become contaminated. Before the sterile procedure, each step should be explained so that the patient can cooperate fully. If an object becomes contaminated during the procedure, it should be discarded immediately.

Donning and removing caps, masks, and eyewear. For sterile procedures on a general nursing division, nurses may wear a surgical mask and eyewear without a cap. Eyewear is worn as a part of standard precautions or routine practices if fluid or blood could splash into the nurse's eyes. For sterile surgical procedures, the nurse must first apply a clean cap that covers all the hair and then put on the surgical mask and eyewear. The mask must fit snugly around the face and nose to prevent contamination by droplet nuclei. After a mask is worn for several hours, the area over the mouth and nose often becomes moist. Because moisture promotes the spread of microorganisms, the mask should be changed if it becomes moist.

Protective glasses or goggles should fit snugly around the forehead and face to fully protect the eyes. Eyewear needs to be worn only for procedures that create the risk of body fluids splashing into the eyes.

Before removing a mask, eyewear, and cap, remove the gloves to prevent contamination of the hair, neck, and facial area. After untying the mask, hold it by the ties and discard it with the cap. Masks should not be worn hanging from the neck after removal from the face. Eyewear is removed and cleaned later for reuse. After removing all protective wear, perform hand hygiene.

Opening sterile packages. Sterile items such as syringes, gauze dressings, and catheters are packaged in paper or plastic containers that are impervious to microorganisms as long as they are dry and intact. Some institutions wrap reusable supplies in a double thickness of paper, linen, or muslin. These packages are permeable to steam and thus allow for steam autoclaving. Sterile items are kept in clean, enclosed storage cabinets and are separated from nonsterile equipment.

Sterile supplies carry chemical tapes indicating that a sterilization process has taken place. The tapes change colour during the sterilization process; if the tapes do not change colour, the item is not sterile. A sterile item should never be used if the integrity of the packaging is compromised. Health care facilities may apply the date processed and a lot number to the item after processing ("event-related expiration"), or they may apply an expiration date ("date-related expiration") to the

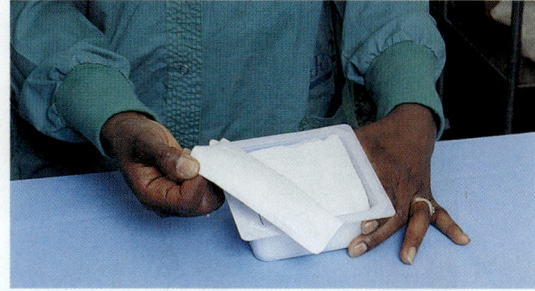

item. With either system, it is important for nurses to check the integrity of the packaging before using an item.

Before opening a sterile item, perform thorough hand hygiene. Inspect the supplies for package integrity and sterility and assemble the supplies in the work area, such as the bedside table or treatment room, before opening the packages. A cleaned bedside table or countertop provides a large, clean working area for opening items. The work area should be above waist level. Sterile supplies should not be opened in a confined space where a dirty object might fall on or strike them.

Opening a sterile item on a flat surface. Sterile packaged items must be opened without contaminating the contents. Commercially packaged items are usually designed so that the user has to tear away or separate only the paper or plastic cover. The item is held in one hand while the wrapper is pulled away with the other hand (Figure 34.3). Take care to keep the inner contents sterile before use. When opening items processed by the facility and packed in paper or linen, observe the following steps:

1. Place the item flat in the centre of the work surface.
2. Remove the sterilization tape or seal.
3. Grasp the outer surface of the tip of the outermost flap.
4. Open the outer flap away from the body, keeping the arm outstretched and away from the sterile field (Figure 34.4, A).
5. Grasp the outside surface of the first side flap.
6. Open the side flap, allowing it to lie flat on the table surface. Keep your arm to the side and not over the sterile surface (see Figure 34.4, B). Do not allow the flaps to spring back over the sterile contents.
7. Grasp the outside surface of the second side flap and allow it to lie flat on the table surface (see Figure 34.4, C).
8. Grasp the outside surface of the last and innermost flap.
9. Stand away from the sterile package and pull the flap back, allowing it to fall flat on the surface (see Figure 34.4, D).
10. Use the inner surface of the package (except for the 2.5-cm border around the edges) as a sterile field to add additional sterile items. The 2.5-cm border can be grasped to manoeuvre the field on the table surface.

If the sterile supplies are not for immediate use, you can close the sterile package. In this case, touch only the wrapper's outside surface. To close a package, the order of unwrapping is reversed, and you should not touch the inside contents or reach over the field.

Opening a sterile item while holding it. To open a small, sterile item, hold the package in your nondominant hand. Using the dominant hand, carefully open the side and top flaps away from the enclosed sterile item in the order previously mentioned. Open the item in a hand so that the item can be handed to a person wearing sterile gloves or transferred to a sterile field.

Preparing a sterile field. When performing sterile procedures, nurses need a sterile work area that provides room for the handling and placing of sterile items. A **sterile field** is an area free of microorganisms

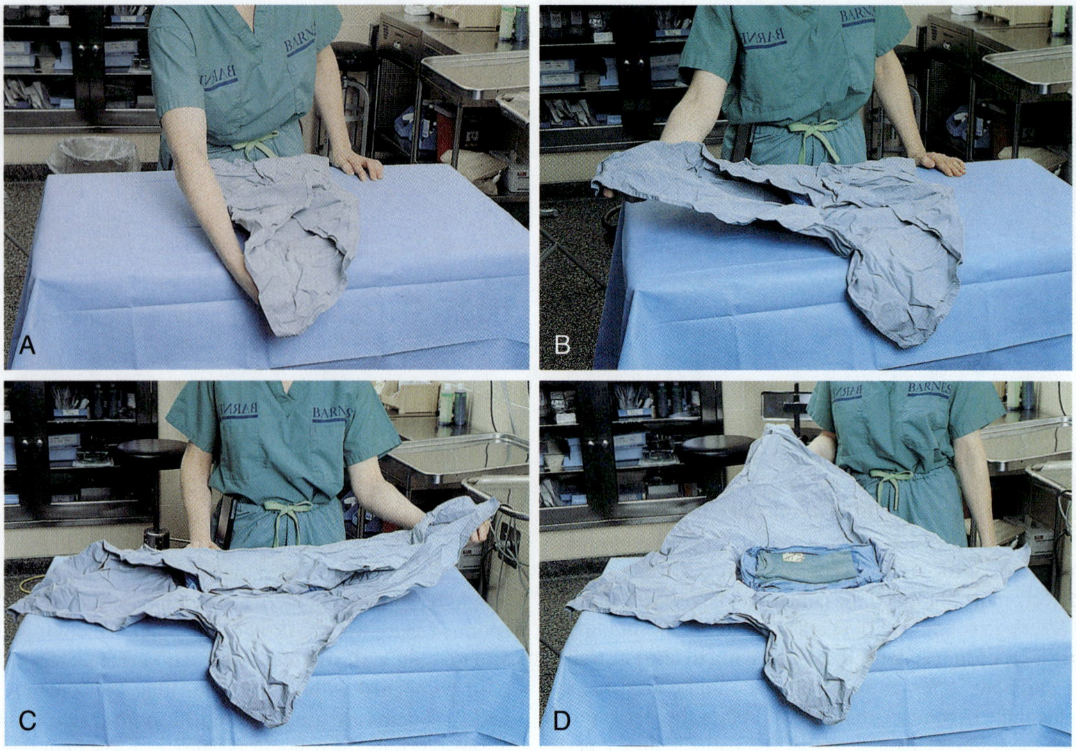

FIGURE 34.4 Opening sterile packaged items on a flat surface. **A**, Open the top flap away from the body. **B**, Keep your arm away from the sterile field while opening the side flap. **C**, Open the second side flap. **D**, Open the back flap.

and prepared to receive sterile items. The field may be prepared by using the inner surface of a sterile wrapper as the work surface or by using a sterile drape or dressing tray. Skill 34.2 describes preparation of a sterile field. After the surface for the field is created, add sterile items by carefully placing them directly on the field or by transferring them with a sterile forceps. A sterile object that comes in contact with the 2.5-cm border must be discarded.

You may choose to wear sterile gloves while preparing items on the field. If this is done, you can touch the entire drape, but sterile items must be handed over by an assistant. Your gloves cannot touch the wrappers of sterile items.

Pouring sterile solutions. Often nurses must pour sterile solutions into sterile containers. A bottle containing a sterile solution is sterile on the inside and contaminated on the outside; the outside neck of the bottle is also contaminated, but the inside of the bottle cap is considered sterile. After the cap or lid is removed, it is held in the hand or placed sterile side (inside) up on a clean surface. This means that the inside of the lid can be seen as it rests on the table surface. A bottle cap or lid should never rest on a sterile surface, even though the inside of the cap is sterile. The outer edge of the cap is unsterile and would contaminate the sterile surface. Likewise, placing a sterile cap down on an unsterile surface increases the chances of the inside of the cap becoming contaminated.

It is important to check the label of the bottle to ensure it is the correct solution. Then hold the bottle with its label in the palm of the hand to prevent the possibility of the solution wetting and fading the label. The edge of the bottle is kept away from the edge or inside of the receiving container. Pour the solution slowly to avoid splashing the underlying drape or field. The bottle should be held outside the edge of the sterile field. Pour medications or sterile solutions from the container once only. Discard the remaining fluids in the container at the end of the procedure (Operating Room Nurses Association of Canada [ORNAC], 2021, 5.7.2).

Surgical hand scrub. Patients undergoing operative procedures are at an increased risk for infection. When working in operating rooms, nurses must decontaminate their hands to decrease and suppress the growth of skin microorganisms in case the glove tears (ORNAC, 2021).

During surgical hand antisepsis before an operation, scrub from the fingertips to the elbows with an antiseptic soap. The optimum duration of the surgical hand scrub is unclear, although research indicates that it may be dependent on the type of antimicrobial product. Either an antimicrobial surgical scrub agent intended for surgical hand antisepsis or an alcohol-based antiseptic surgical hand rub that has persistent or cumulative activity is acceptable to use as a surgical scrub. For a traditional scrub, a 3- to 5-minute scrub should be performed to allow adequate contact time with the product, using the manufacturer's written instructions (Seal et al., 2017). Nurses should follow their agency's policy for length of scrub time. A study by Fry (2019) suggested that the alcohol rub appears to have comparable results to the surgical scrub and is a reasonable alternative for preparation of the hands for surgical procedures.

For maximum elimination of bacteria, all jewellery should be removed, including wristwatches, and the nails should be kept clean and short (Seal et al., 2017). Artificial nails or any fingernail enhancements should not be worn because they may harbour a greater number of bacteria. Similarly, nail polish should be avoided because it conceals soil under the nails and because chipped nail polish may increase the bacterial load (Seal et al., 2017). Nurses who have active skin infections, open lesions or cuts, or respiratory infections should be excluded from the surgical team. Skill 34.3 describes the steps for surgical hand hygiene.

Applying sterile gloves. Sterile gloves are an additional barrier to bacterial transfer. Nurses who work on general nursing divisions use *open gloving* before procedures such as dressing changes and urinary catheter insertions. *Closed gloving,* which is performed after applying

SKILL 34.2	PREPARATION OF A STERILE FIELD

Delegation Considerations

Delegation of the preparation of a sterile field is inappropriate unless you are delegating to an unregulated care provider (UCP) who has received specialized training. Operating room technicians are usually trained for this skill.

Equipment

- Sterile drape
- Assorted sterile supplies

PROCEDURE

STEPS	RATIONALE
1. Prepare sterile field just before planned procedure. Supplies are to be used immediately.	• Prevents exposure of sterile field and supplies to air and contamination.
2. Select clean work surface above waist level.	• A once-sterile object held below the waist is considered contaminated.
3. Assemble necessary equipment.	• Preparation of equipment in advance prevents a break in the technique.
4. Check dates or labels on supplies for sterility of equipment.	• Equipment stored beyond the expiration date is considered unsterile.
5. Perform hand hygiene. Option: Procedure may be performed with gloves on.	• Reduces microbial counts on skin.
6. Place pack containing sterile drape on work surface and open as described in Figure 34.4.	• Ensures sterility of packaged drape.
7. With fingertips of one hand, pick up folded top edge of sterile drape.	• The 2.5-cm border around drape is unsterile and may be touched with fingers or clean gloves.
8. Gently lift drape up from its outer cover and let it unfold by itself without touching any object. Discard outer cover with your other hand.	• If sterile object touches any nonsterile object, it becomes contaminated.
9. With your other hand, grasp adjacent corner of drape and hold it straight up and away from your body (see Step 9 illustration).	• Drape can now be properly placed while using two hands. Drape must be held away from unsterile surfaces.
10. Holding drape, first position and lay bottom half over intended work surface (see Step 10 illustration).	• Prevents reaching over sterile field.
11. Allow top half of drape to be placed over work surface last (see Step 11 illustration).	• Creates flat sterile work surface.

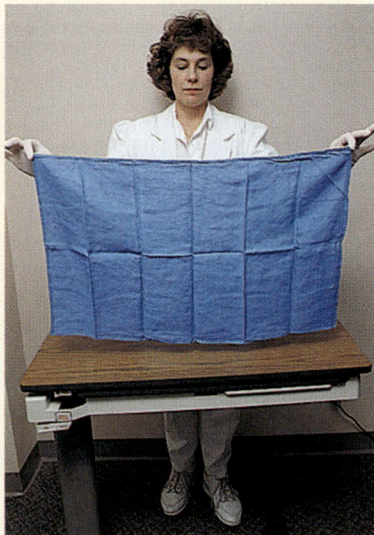

STEP 9 Hold drape straight up and away from body.

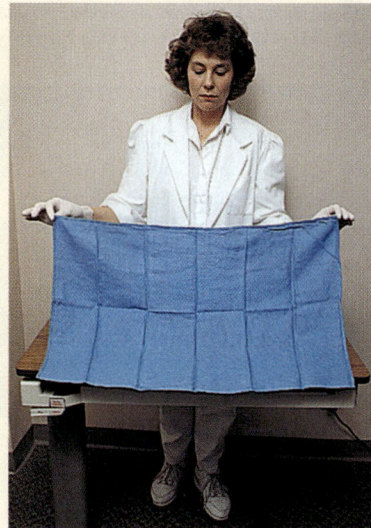

STEP 10 Lay bottom half of drape over work surface.

Continued

SKILL 34.2   PREPARATION OF A STERILE FIELD—cont'd

PROCEDURE

STEPS	RATIONALE

STEP 11 Place top half of drape over work surface.

12. Grasp 2.5-cm border around edge to position as needed.	• Assists in differentiating and organizing the sterile surface.

ADDING STERILE ITEM

13. Open sterile item (according to package directions) while holding outside wrapper in nondominant hand.	• Frees dominant hand for unwrapping outer wrapper.
14. Carefully peel wrapper onto nondominant hand. Do not shake item onto sterile field.	• Item remains sterile.
15. Being sure wrapper does not fall down on sterile field, place item onto field at angle. Do not hold arm over sterile field (see Step 15 illustration).	• Prevents reaching over field and contaminating its surface.

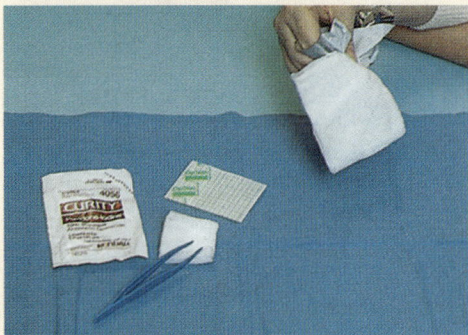

STEP 15 Adding item to sterile field.

16. Dispose of outer wrapper.	• Prevents accidental contamination of sterile field.
17. Perform procedure using sterile technique.	• Prevents transmission of infection to patient.

RECORDING AND REPORTING

• It is not necessary to record or report this procedure.

SKILL 34.3	SURGICAL HAND SCRUB: PREPARING FOR GOWNING

Delegation Considerations

The role of the scrub nurse can be delegated to a surgical technologist or licensed practical nurse. Unregulated care providers (UCPs) can help the registered nurse in the circulating nurse role by opening sterile supplies, setting up sterile fields, and running errands under the direction of the registered nurse.

Equipment

- Deep sink with foot or knee controls for dispensing water and soap (faucets should be high enough for hands and forearms to fit comfortably)
- Antimicrobial surgical scrub agent or alcohol-based waterless antiseptic, according to agency policy (product should be nonirritating, broad spectrum, fast acting, and effective in reducing skin microorganisms and have a residual effect) (Seal et al., 2017)
- Surgical scrub sponge (if using traditional surgical hand scrub) and a disposable nail cleaner
- Paper mask and cap or hood
- Sterile towel
- Proper scrub attire
- Protective eyewear (goggles or face shield)

PROCEDURE

STEPS	RATIONALE
1. Consult your agency's policy regarding required length of scrub time and antiseptic to use for hand antisepsis.	• Guidelines vary regarding ideal time needed and antiseptic to use for surgical scrub.
2. Be sure fingernails are short, clean, and healthy. Artificial nails should be removed. Natural nails should be less than 0.5 cm long.	• Long nails and chipped or old polish increase the number of bacteria residing on nails. Long fingernails can puncture gloves, causing contamination. • Artificial nails are known to harbour Gram-negative microorganisms and fungus.

CRITICAL DECISION POINT: *Remove nail polish if chipped or worn longer than 4 days because it may harbour microorganisms (Seal et al., 2017).*

STEPS	RATIONALE
3. Inspect hands for presence of abrasions, cuts, or open lesions.	• These conditions increase the likelihood of microorganisms residing on skin surfaces.
4. Apply surgical shoe covers, cap or hood, face mask, and protective eyewear.	• The mask prevents escape into the air of microorganisms that can contaminate hands. Other protective wear prevents exposure to blood and body fluid splashes during the procedure.
5. Surgical hand hygiene:	
A. Turn on water-activating sensor or use knee or foot controls.	
B. Wet hands and arms under running water and lather with detergent to 5 cm above elbows. (Hands need to be above elbows at all times.)	• Water runs by gravity from fingertips to elbows, flowing from least to most contaminated areas. Hands become the cleanest part of the upper extremity. • Washing a wide area reduces the risk of contaminating an overlying gown that you later apply.
C. Rinse hands and arms thoroughly under running water. **Remember to keep hands raised above the elbows.**	• Rinsing removes transient bacteria from fingers, hands, and forearms.
D. Under running water, clean under nails of both hands with a nail pick. Discard after use (see Step 5D illustration).	• Removes dirt and organic material that harbour large numbers of microorganisms.
E. Wet clean sponge and apply antimicrobial detergent. Scrub nails of one hand with 15 strokes. Holding sponge perpendicular, scrub palm, each side of thumb and fingers, and posterior side of hand with 10 strokes each. The arm is mentally divided into thirds, and each third is scrubbed 10 times (see Step 5E illustrations). The duration of scrub is determined by the manufacturer's recommendations for the scrub agent used, which is usually 2 to 6 minutes). Rinse sponge and repeat sequence for the other arm. A two-sponge method may be substituted. Check your agency's policy.	• Friction loosens resident bacteria that adhere to skin surfaces. Technique ensures coverage of all surfaces. Scrubbing is performed from the cleanest area (hands) to the marginal area (upper arms).

Continued

SKILL 34.3   SURGICAL HAND SCRUB: PREPARING FOR GOWNING—cont'd

PROCEDURE

STEPS	RATIONALE

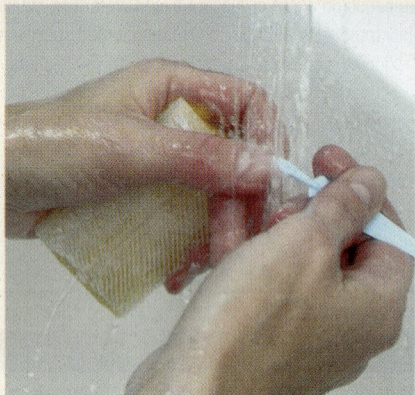

STEP 5D Clean under fingernails.

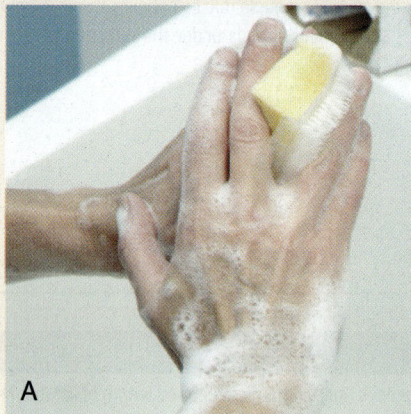

A

B

STEP 5E **A,** Scrub side of fingers. **B,** Scrub forearms.

F. Discard sponge and rinse hands and arms thoroughly (see Step 5F illustration). Turn off water with foot or knee control and back into room entrance with hands elevated in front of and away from the body.

G. Walk up to sterile tray and lean forward slightly to pick up a sterile towel (see Step 5G [A] illustration). Dry one hand thoroughly, moving from fingers to elbow. Dry in a rotating motion. Dry from the cleanest to least clean area (see Step 5G [B] illustration).

• After touching skin, the sponge is considered contaminated. Rinsing removes resident bacteria. Using the foot or knee tap control and backing into the room prevent accidental contamination.

• Drying prevents chapping and facilitates donning of gloves. Leaning forward prevents accidental contact of arms with scrub attire.

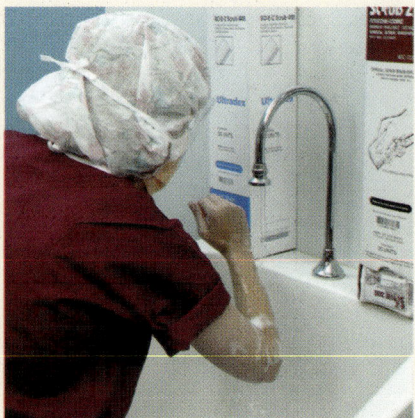

STEP 5F Rinse arms.

Continued

SKILL 34.3   SURGICAL HAND SCRUB: PREPARING FOR GOWNING—cont'd

PROCEDURE

STEPS	RATIONALE

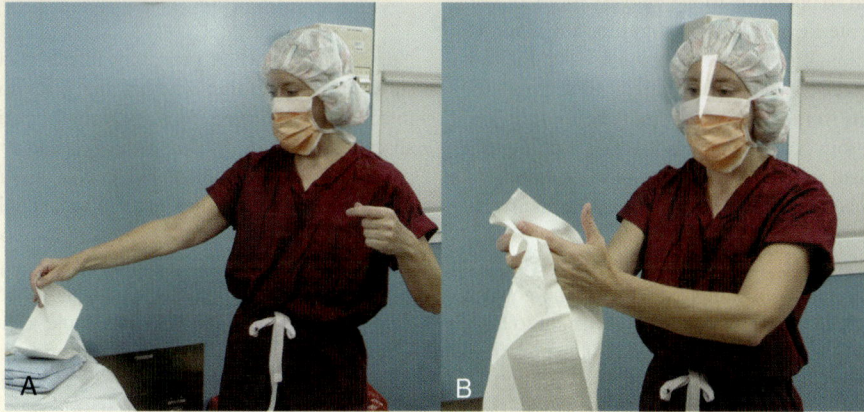

STEP 5G A, Grasping sterile towel. **B,** Drying sequence.

H. Repeat drying method for the other hand by carefully reversing towel or using a new sterile towel.
- Prevents accidental contamination.

I. Discard towel.
- Prevents accidental contamination.

J. Proceed with sterile gowning (see Skill 34.4).

6. Alternative method of surgical hand hygiene using alcohol-based antiseptic:

A. Wash hands with soap and water for at least 15 seconds to remove soil.
- Removes dirt and organic material that harbour large numbers of microorganisms.

B. Under running water, clean under nails of both hands with disposable nail cleaner. Discard after use and dry hands with a paper towel.

C. Apply enough alcohol-based waterless antiseptic to one palm to cover both hands thoroughly (see Step 6C illustration). Spread the antiseptic over all surfaces of the hands and fingernails. Follow product instructions for length of time to rub over hand surfaces. Allow to air-dry.
- Ensures coverage of all surfaces. Air-drying ensures that complete antisepsis is achieved.

D. Repeat the process and allow hands to air-dry before applying sterile gloves.

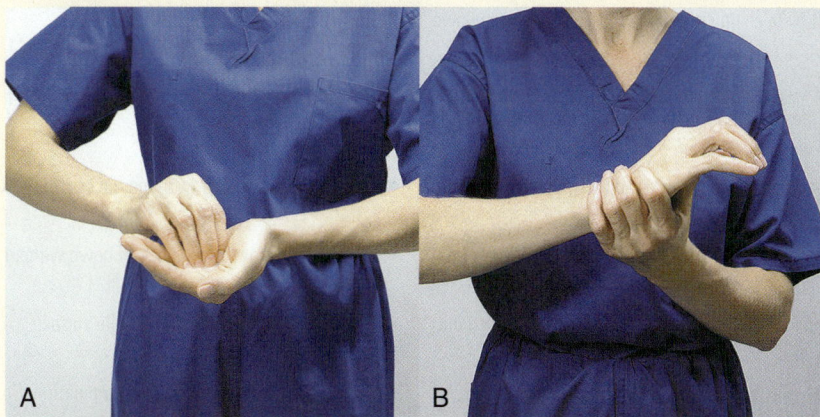

STEP 6C Application of antimicrobial agent for brushless hand scrub. This nurse is using 3M Avagard. (Photo courtesy of 3M Health Care.)

RECORDING AND REPORTING

- It is not necessary to record or report this procedure.
- Report any dermatitis to employee health or infection control per your agency's policy.

sterile gowns, is practised in operating rooms and special treatment areas. The proper glove size should be selected; the glove should not stretch so tightly that it can easily tear, yet it should be tight enough that objects can be picked up easily.

Donning a sterile gown. Nurses must wear a sterile gown when assisting at the sterile field in an operating room, delivery room, or special treatment areas so that sterile objects can be comfortably handled with less risk of contamination. The circulating nurse usually does not wear a sterile gown. The sterile gown acts as a barrier to decrease the shedding of microorganisms from skin surfaces into the air, thus preventing wound contamination. Nurses may also wear a sterile gown if they are caring for a patient with a large open wound or assisting a physician during a major invasive procedure (e.g., inserting an arterial catheter).

After the nurse has applied a mask and surgical cap and performed the surgical hand scrub, the nurse dons a sterile gown. The gown is picked up from a sterile pack, or the nurse can ask an assistant to hand the gown to them. Only a certain portion of the gown—the area from the anterior waist to, but not including, the collar and the anterior surface of the sleeves—is considered sterile. The back of the gown, the area under the arms, the collar, the area below the waist, and the underside of the sleeves are not sterile because the nurse cannot keep these areas in constant view and ensure their sterility. Skill 34.4 reviews the steps for applying a sterile gown and closed gloving, and Skill 34.5 reviews the method of open gloving.

◆ **Evaluation**

Nurses' success when practising infection-control techniques is measured by determining whether the goals for reducing or preventing infection are achieved. By comparing the patient's response, such as the absence of fever or development of wound drainage, with expected outcomes, nurses determine the success of nursing interventions. Similarly, nurses determine whether interventions should be revised or eliminated. Correctly assessing wounds for healing and conducting a physical assessment of body systems (see Chapter 33) are important skills in evaluation. Nurses need to closely monitor patients, especially those at risk, for signs and symptoms of infection. For example, a patient who has undergone a surgical procedure is at risk for infection at the surgical site, as well as at sites of invasive procedures such as a venipuncture or central-line insertion. In addition, the patient is at risk for a respiratory tract infection

---

SKILL 34.4	**APPLYING A STERILE GOWN AND PERFORMING CLOSED GLOVING**

Delegation Considerations

The role of the scrub nurse can be delegated to a surgical technician.

Equipment

- Surgical cap
- Surgical mask
- Eye protection
- Foot covers
- Sterile gown (prepared by circulating nurse)

PROCEDURE

STEPS	**RATIONALE**
1. Before entering the operating room or treatment area, apply cap, face mask, and eyewear. Foot covers are also required in the operating room.	• Prevent hair and air droplet nuclei from contaminating sterile work areas. Eyewear protects mucous membranes of the eye. • Foot covers are paper or cloth and fit over work shoes.
2. Perform thorough surgical hand hygiene (see Skill 34.3).	• Removes transient and resident bacteria from fingers, hands, and forearms.
3. Ask circulating nurse to assist by opening sterile pack containing sterile gown (folded inside out).	• Gown's outer surface remains sterile.
4. Have circulating nurse prepare glove package by peeling outer wrapper open while keeping inner contents sterile. Inner glove package is then placed on the sterile field created by sterile outer wrapper.	• This action keeps gloves sterile and allows the nurse who has scrubbed to handle sterile items.
5. Reach down to sterile gown package; lift folded gown directly upward and step back away from table.	• This action provides a wide margin of safety, avoiding contamination of gown.
6. Holding folded gown, locate the neckband. With both hands, grasp inside front of gown just below the neckband.	• Clean hands may touch inside of gown without contaminating outer surface.
7. Allow gown to unfold, keeping inside of gown toward body. Do not touch outside of gown with bare hands or allow it to touch the floor.	• Outside of gown will remain sterile surface.
8. With hands at shoulder level, slip both arms into armholes simultaneously (see Step 8 illustration). Ask circulating nurse to bring gown over shoulders by reaching inside to arm seams and pulling gown on, leaving sleeves covering hands.	• Careful application prevents contamination. Gown covers hands to prepare for closed gloving.
9. Have circulating nurse securely tie back of gown at neck and waist (see Step 9 illustration). (If gown is a wraparound style, the sterile flap to cover gown is not touched until you have gloved.)	• Gown must completely enclose underlying garments.

Continued

PROCEDURE

STEPS	RATIONALE

STEP 8 Place arms in sleeves.

STEP 9 Circulating nurse ties scrub gown.

10 Closed gloving:

A. With hands covered by gown sleeves, open inner sterile glove package (see Step 10A illustration).

- Hands remain clean. Sterile gown cuff will touch sterile glove surface.

B. With dominant hand inside gown cuff, pick up glove for nondominant hand by grasping folded cuff.

- Sterile gown touches sterile glove.

C. Extend nondominant forearm with palm up and place palm of glove against palm of nondominant hand. Glove fingers will point toward elbow.

- Position glove for application over cuffed hand, keeping glove sterile.

D. Grasp back of glove cuff with covered dominant hand and turn glove cuff over end of nondominant hand and gown cuff (see Step 10D illustration).

- The seal that is created by the glove cuff over gown prevents exit of microorganisms over operative sterile field.

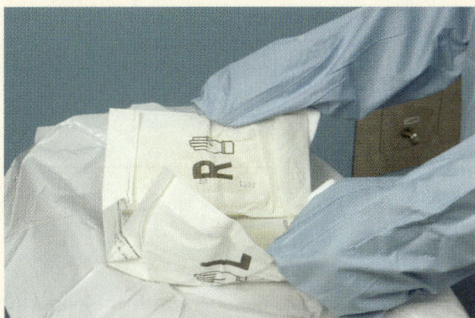

STEP 10A Open glove package.

STEP 10D Apply glove to nondominant hand, keeping dominant hand inside cuff.

Continued

SKILL 34.4   APPLYING A STERILE GOWN AND PERFORMING CLOSED GLOVING—cont'd

PROCEDURE

STEPS	RATIONALE

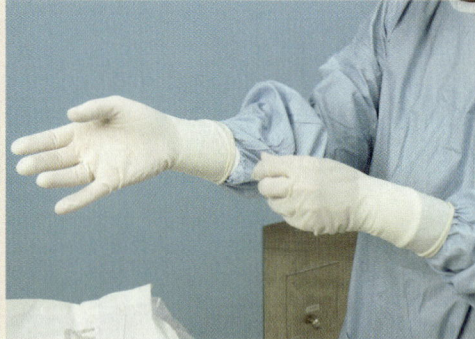

STEP 10F Apply second glove.

E. Grasp top of glove and underlying gown sleeve with covered dominant hand. Carefully extend fingers into glove, being sure the glove's cuff covers the gown's cuff.

F. Glove dominant hand in the same manner, reversing hands (see Step 10F illustration). Use gloved nondominant hand to pull on glove. Keep hand inside sleeve (see Step 10F illustration).

- Sterile object touches sterile object and therefore stays sterile. Touching the sterile sleeve with the sterile gloved hand allows the gloved hands to remain sterile.

G. Be sure fingers are fully extended into both gloves.

- Ensure that you have full dexterity while using gloved hand.

11. For wraparound sterile gowns, take gloved hand and release fastener or ties in front of gown.

- Front of gown is sterile.

12. Hand tie to sterile team member, who stands still (see Step 12 illustration). Allowing margin of safety, turn around to the left, covering back with extended gown flap. Take back tie from team member and secure tie to gown.

- Contact with team member could contaminate gown and gloves. Garments worn under the gown must be enclosed.

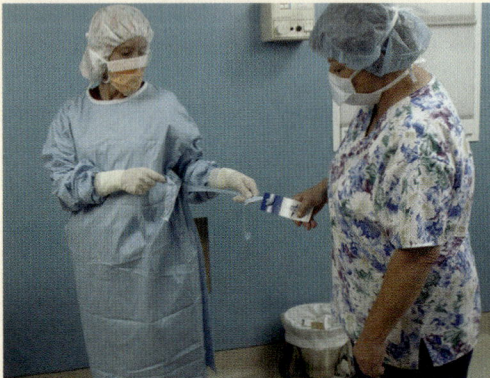

STEP 12 Hand tie to sterile team member.

RECORDING AND REPORTING

- It is not necessary to record or report this procedure.

---

as a result of decreased mobility and for a urinary tract infection if an in-dwelling catheter is present. Nurses must closely monitor all invasive and surgical sites for swelling, erythema, and purulent drainage. Breath sounds are monitored for changes, and sputum character is checked for purulence. Laboratory test results are reviewed for leukocytes in the urine, which may indicate a urinary tract infection. The absence of signs or symptoms of infection is the expected outcome of infection prevention and monitoring activities.

The patient at risk for infection must understand the measures needed to reduce or prevent microorganism growth and spread.

Providing patients or family members with the opportunity to discuss infection-control measures and to demonstrate procedures will increase their ability to adhere to therapy. Nurses may determine that patients require new information or that previously instructed information needs reinforcement.

The nurse needs to document the patient's response to therapies for infection control. A clear description of any signs and symptoms of systemic or local infection is necessary to give all nurses a baseline for comparative evaluation. The efficacy of any intervention in reducing infection must be reported.

SKILL 34.5	OPEN GLOVING

Delegation Considerations

Delegation of open gloving depends on whether an unregulated care provider (UCP) has received special training and is competent to perform the sterile procedure.

Equipment

• Sterile gloves (proper size)

PROCEDURE

STEPS	RATIONALE
1. Perform thorough hand hygiene.	• Removes bacteria from skin surfaces and reduces risk of transmitting infection.
2. Remove outer glove package wrapper by carefully separating and peeling apart sides.	• Prevents inner glove package from accidentally opening and touching contaminated objects.
3. Grasp inner package and lay it on a clean, dry, flat surface just above waist level. Open package, keeping gloves on wrapper's inside surface (see Step 3 illustration).	• Sterile object held below the waist is contaminated. Inner surface of glove package is sterile.

STEP 3 Open package.

4. If gloves are not pre-powdered, take packet of powder and apply lightly to hands over sink or wastebasket.	• Powder allows gloves to slip on easily. (Some staff members do not use powder for fear of promoting growth of microorganisms.)
5. Each glove has a cuff approximately 5 cm wide. Glove dominant hand first.	• Proper identification of gloves prevents contamination by improper fit. Gloving of dominant hand first improves dexterity.
6. With thumb and first two fingers of nondominant hand, grasp edge of cuff of glove for dominant hand. Touch only glove's inside surface.	• Inner edge of cuff will lie against skin and is thus not sterile.
7. Carefully pull glove over dominant hand, being sure cuff does not roll up wrist. Be sure thumb and fingers are in proper spaces (see Step 7 illustration).	• If glove's outer surface touches the hand or wrist, it is contaminated.
8. With gloved dominant hand, slip fingers underneath second glove's cuff (see Step 8 illustration).	• Cuff protects gloved fingers. Sterile surface touching sterile surface prevents glove contamination.

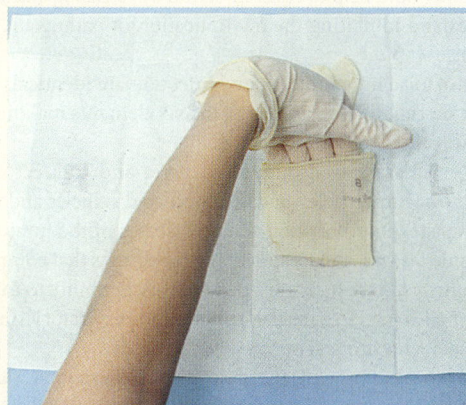

STEP 7 Pull glove over dominant hand.

STEP 8 Slip fingers underneath second glove's cuff.

Continued

SKILL 34.5	OPEN GLOVING—cont'd

PROCEDURE

STEPS	RATIONALE
9. Carefully pull second glove over nondominant hand. Do not allow fingers and thumb of gloved dominant hand to touch any part of exposed nondominant hand. Keep thumb of dominant hand abducted back (see Step 9 illustration).	• Contact of gloved hand with exposed hand results in contamination.

STEP 9 Pull second glove over nondominant hand.

STEP 10 Interlock hands. Gloved hands must be kept above waist level within the visual field at all times or clasped together above elbow level.

10. After second glove is on, interlock hands. The cuffs usually fall down after application. Be sure to touch only sterile sides (see Step 10 illustration).	• Ensure smooth fit over fingers.

GLOVE DISPOSAL

11. Grasp outside of one cuff with other gloved hand; avoid touching wrist.	• Minimize contamination of underlying skin.
12. Pull glove off, turning it inside out. Discard in receptacle.	• Outside of glove does not touch skin surface.
13. Take fingers of bare hand and tuck inside remaining glove cuff. Peel glove off, inside out. Discard in receptacle. Perform hand hygiene.	

RECORDING AND REPORTING

• It is not necessary to record or report this procedure.

KEY CONCEPTS

• Hand hygiene is the most important technique to use in preventing and controlling the transmission of infection.
• The potential for microorganisms to cause disease depends on the number of organisms, their virulence, their ability to enter and survive in a host, and the susceptibility of the host.
• Normal body flora help to resist infection by releasing antibacterial substances and inhibiting the multiplication of pathogenic microorganisms.
• The signs of local inflammation and infection are identical.
• An infection can develop as long as the six elements making up the chain of infection are uninterrupted.
• Microorganisms are transmitted by direct and indirect contact, droplets, airborne particles, and contaminated vehicles and vectors.
• Advancing age, poor nutrition, stress, diseases of the immune system, chronic disease, and treatments or conditions that compromise the immune response increase a person's susceptibility to infection.
• The major sites for HAI are the urinary and respiratory tracts, the bloodstream, and surgical or traumatic wounds.
• The CDC now recommends the use of alcohol-based waterless antiseptics as an alternative to handwashing to more effectively reduce the transmission of microorganisms.
• Invasive procedures, medical therapies, long hospitalization, and contact with health care personnel increase a hospitalized patient's risk for acquiring an HAI.

• Isolation practices may prevent personnel and patients from acquiring infections and may prevent the transmission of microorganisms.
• Standard precautions or routine practices entail the use of generic barrier techniques in the care of all patients.
• Transmission-based (isolation) precautions are used for patients with specific, highly transmissible infections.
• Proper cleansing involves the mechanical removal of soil from an object or area.
• A patient in isolation is subject to sensory deprivation because of the restricted environment.
• An infection-control professional monitors the incidence of infection within an institution and provides educational and consultative services to maintain infection prevention.
• Surgical asepsis necessitates more stringent techniques than does medical asepsis and is directed at eliminating all microorganisms.
• Surgical aseptic practices are followed if the skin is broken or if the nurse performs an invasive procedure in a body cavity that is normally free of microorganisms.

CRITICAL THINKING EXERCISES

1. Your patient had an in-dwelling urethral catheter for 1 week. The catheter has now been out for 24 hours. The patient complains of frequency of and pain on urination. The patient suggests that the catheter be reinserted so that she does not need to get up frequently.

What can frequency of or pain on urination indicate? Should the catheter be reinserted? Why or why not? Describe at least one appropriate assessment measure and independent nursing action for this patient.

2. You are caring for a patient who has a large, open, draining abdominal wound. You notice another health care worker changing the patient's dressing without wearing gloves or using sterile supplies or sterile technique. When you question the health care worker regarding this practice, the person says, "Don't worry, the wound is already infected, and the antibiotics and draining will take care of any contaminants." How would you respond to this comment? What would your next steps be in following up on this incident?

3. Penelope (preferred pronouns: she/her) is 83 years of age and lives alone. She has difficulty walking and relies on a church volunteer group to deliver lunches during the week. Her fixed income limits her ability to buy food. Last week, Penelope's 79-year-old sister died. The two sisters had been very close. Explain the factors that might increase Penelope's risk for infection.

4. A patient (preferred pronouns: he/him) is admitted to your facility with a history of recent weight loss, a cough that has persisted for 2 months, and hemoptysis. His chest X-ray film shows a cavity in one lung, and his physician suspects tuberculosis. What type of isolation precautions would you use for this patient? What protection would you use when providing care? What education would you provide for the patient and his family?

🌐 *Answers to Critical Thinking Exercises appear on the Evolve website.*

REVIEW QUESTIONS

Review Questions 1 to 10 relate to the case study at the beginning of the chapter.

1. Shingles cannot be passed from one person to another. However, the virus (varicella zoster) that causes shingles can be spread from a person with active shingles to another person who has never had chickenpox. If an infection can be transmitted from one person to another, it is a:
   a. Communicable disease
   b. Portal of entry to a host
   c. Portal of exit from a reservoir
   d. Susceptible host

2. The patient, Susan, has been diagnosed with disseminated herpes zoster. The mode of transmission for disseminated herpes zoster is:
   a. Direct and indirect contact
   b. Droplet transmission
   c. Airborne transmission
   d. Airborne, droplet, and contact transmission

3. Disseminated herpes zoster is no longer infectious when:
   a. All lesions are dry and crusted
   b. Fever resolves
   c. Generalized red rash blanches when touched
   d. The patient no longer feels itchy

4. Susan was in the hospital for 7 days when she developed symptoms of *Clostridioides difficile*. The most common symptom of *C. difficile* is:
   a. Bleeding gums
   b. Diarrhea
   c. Maculopapular rash
   d. Headache

5. The most effective way to prevent transmission of microorganisms is hand hygiene. The minimum handwashing time with soap and water necessary to remove most transient microorganisms is:
   a. 1.5 seconds
   b. 15 seconds
   c. 40–60 seconds
   d. 3 minutes

6. Staff entering Susan's room are required to use an N95 mask. Which organism requires the use of an N95 mask?
   a. Methicillin-resistant *Staphylococcus aureus* (MRSA)
   b. Herpes zoster
   c. Influenza viruses
   d. Paramyxoviruses

7. Disseminated herpes zoster is treated by:
   a. Antifungal medication
   b. Antibiotics
   c. Antiviral medication
   d. Antiemetics

8. Susan is placed on airborne and contact precautions. The most appropriate room placement would be:
   a. A four-bed ward with each bed 2 metres apart and shared washroom
   b. A two-bed room with shared washroom
   c. A single room, with dedicated washroom and anteroom
   d. A single room and dedicated washroom

9. Susan is at risk for disseminated herpes zoster because:
   a. She is immunocompromised because she is taking prednisone.
   b. She is in end-stage renal failure.
   c. She has a central venous catheter for dialysis.
   d. She is an inpatient in a hospital.

10. The people involved in direct or indirect patient care needs for Susan need to be concerned about hand hygiene and should be able to perform it correctly and at the right time. When should hand hygiene be performed?
    a. Before entering Susan's room.
    b. Before and after direct contact with the patient or the patient's environment; before an aseptic procedure, after exposure or risk of exposure to blood or body fluids; and following the removal or gloves and before gloves are put on.
    c. After leaving Susan's isolation room.
    d. Before donning a gown and mask.

Answers: 1. a; **2.** d; **3.** a; **4.** b; **5.** c; **6.** b; **7.** c; **8.** c; **9.** a; **10.** b.

🌐 *Rationales for the Review Questions appear on the Evolve website.*

RECOMMENDED WEBSITES

Infection Prevention and Control Canada: https://ipac-canada.org
Infection Prevention and Control Canada (IPAC Canada) is a national,
multidisciplinary, voluntary association of infection-control professionals
committed to improving infection prevention and control.

REFERENCES

A full reference list is available on the website for this book at
http://evolve.elsevier.com/Canada/Potter/fundamentals/

Public Health Agency of Canada: https://www.phac-aspc.gc.ca
This federal government site provides links to documents related to
infection-control practices, including the *Canada Communicable
Disease Report.*

35

Medication Administration and Management

Canadian content written by Pamela Durepos, RN, PhD, with original chapter contributions by Sharon Kaasalainen, RN, PhD

OBJECTIVES

Mastery of content in this chapter will enable you to:

- Define the key terms listed.
- Examine the nurse's role and responsibilities regarding medication administration.
- Describe the physiological mechanisms of medication action, including absorption, distribution, metabolism, and elimination of medications.
- Differentiate among different types of medication actions.
- Explain developmental factors that influence pharmacokinetics.
- Explain factors that influence medication actions.
- Describe methods of educating a patient about prescribed medications.
- Compare and contrast the roles of the physician and nurse practitioner, the pharmacist, the licensed practical nurse, and the registered nurse in medication administration.
- Implement nursing actions to prevent medication incidents.
- Describe factors to consider when choosing routes of medication administration.
- Calculate a prescribed medication dose.
- Describe factors to use when assessing a patient's needs for and response to medication therapy.
- Explain the rights of medication administration.
- Prepare and administer subcutaneous, intramuscular, and intradermal injections; intravenous medications; hypodermoclysis infusions; oral and topical skin preparations; eye, ear, and nose drops; vaginal instillations; rectal suppositories; and inhalants.
- Describe the importance of safe medication techniques.
- Describe the importance of establishing and adhering to employer policies and procedures when administering medications.
- Identify and describe how principles of primary health care are applied to medication administration in nursing practice.

KEY TERMS

Absorption
Adverse effects
Anaphylactic reactions
Automated dispensing cabinet (ADC)
Barcode scanning
Best possible medication history
Biotransformation
Buccal
Close call or near miss
Computers on wheels (COWs)
Computerized physician-order entry (CPOE)
Concentration
Controlled substances or drugs
Culture of safety
Deprescribing
Detoxify
Dispensing
High-alert medications
Hypodermoclysis

Infusions
Inhalation
Injection
Instillation
Intradermal (ID)
Intramuscular (IM)
Intraocular
Intravenous (IV)
Irrigations
Medication allergy
Medication incidents
Medication interaction
Medication nonadherence
Medication reconciliation
Metered-dose inhalers (MDIs)
Metric system
Nebulizer
Ophthalmic
Opioids
Parenteral administration

Peak concentration
Pharmacokinetics
Polypharmacy
Precipitation reaction
Prescribing nurse
Prescription for medication
Serum half-life
SMART outcomes
Solution
Standardized order sets
Subcutaneous (sub-Q)
Sublingual
Synergistic effect
Therapeutic effect
Toxicity
Transdermal disc
Verbal order prescription
Z-track method

WEBSITE

http://evolve.elsevier.com/Canada/Potter/fundamentals/

CASE STUDY

Mr. Blackstock (preferred pronouns: he/him) is an 81-year-old man who resides in a long-term care facility. Mr. Blackstock was transferred to the emergency department and has been diagnosed with pneumonia. He has a history of respiratory conditions and uses a wheelchair. Mr. Blackstock is now admitted to an inpatient medicine ward in the hospital, where you are assigned to be Mr. Blackstock's primary care nurse. On your initial assessment, you note that his temperature is 39.2°C. He is experiencing chills, complaining of nausea, and asks for something to "take away the nausea." Mr. Blackstock is unable to tolerate oral fluids. His medical administration record (MAR) states that he has an environmental allergy to pollen. The prescriptions in his medical record read as follows:

- *0.9% normal saline IV infusion at 75 mL per hour*
- *Amoxicillin 500 mg IV*
- *Acetaminophen 650 mg orally for temperature above 38.5°C q4h PRN*
- *Ondansetron 2–4 mg sublingually q8h PRN*
- *Hydromorphone 0.5–2 mg sub-Q q4h PRN*

Think about the case study as you read this chapter. There are review questions at the end of the chapter that relate to the case study.

A *medication* is a substance used in the prevention, diagnosis, relief, treatment, or cure of health alterations. Medications are a primary treatment that patients associate with restoration and maintenance of health. Nurses play an essential role in preparing and administering medications, teaching patients about medications and self-administration, and evaluating patients' responses to medications across health settings. As a nurse, you are responsible for evaluating the effects of the medications on the patient's health status, teaching patients about their medications and their adverse effects, promoting patient adherence to the medication regimen, and evaluating the patient's technique for all routes of medication delivery. Additionally, you must assess the relationship between a patient's medication regimen and their social determinants of health—for example, income, access to health care, social support, physical environment, and genetics. Nurses can implement interventions to address barriers to effective medication management and wellness.

SCIENTIFIC KNOWLEDGE BASE

Medications are administered to patients to prevent, diagnose, or treat disease and health conditions. To safely and accurately administer medications, nurses must have an understanding of pharmacology, pharmacokinetics (the study of how medications enter, affect, and exit the body), anatomy, pathophysiology, nutrition, stages of growth and development, psychology, cultural considerations, and math. The nursing process provides the framework for nurses to organize their thoughts and actions, and it is the foundation for medication administration.

Pharmacological Concepts

Medication Names. A medication may have as many as three different names: chemical, brand, and generic. Chemical names provide an exact description of the medication's molecular structure and are rarely used in clinical practice. The brand name (i.e., trade or proprietary name) is the name the medication is marketed under by a manufacturer. The generic name is given by the manufacturer that first develops the medication. For example, the chemical name N-acetyl-para-aminophenol is more commonly known by the brand name *Tylenol* and the generic name *acetaminophen*. The medication's generic name is used in official publications, such as the *Compendium of Pharmaceuticals and Specialties (CPS)*. Medication products approved for distribution in Canada also have an eight-digit number drug identification number (DIN) that

is assigned by the Health Protection Branch of the federal government to track medication information across Canada.

Similarities in medication names are a common cause of confusion and medical incidents (i.e., errors). The Institute for Safe Medication Practices (ISMP) publishes a list of medication pairs whose names "look-alike and sound-alike" (LASA), as well as recommendations for how nurses and institutions can prevent incidents related to LASA medication names. Common prescription medications in Canada, with their associated brand and generic names, are listed at https://www.medbroadcast.com/drug.

Classification. Medication classification indicates the effect or action of the medication on a body system. For example, patients with type 2 diabetes often use medications classified as *sulfonylureas* to stimulate insulin secretion. Six different medications, including glyburide and gliclazide, are classified as sulfonylureas (Miller et al., 2018). Some medications belong to more than one class. For example, Aspirin is classified as an *analgesic*, *antipyretic*, and an *anti-inflammatory* medication. Each classification of medication has implications for nursing care (Box 35.1).

Medication Forms. Medications are available in a variety of forms, preparations, or compositions (Figure 35.1). The form of the medication determines its route of administration. The composition of a medication is designed to enhance its absorption and metabolism. Many medications are made in several forms, such as tablets, capsules, elixirs, and suppositories. When administering a medication, the nurse must be certain to use the proper form (Table 35.1).

Medication Legislation and Standards

Canadian Medication Legislation. Regulation of medication standards began in Canada in 1884, when the *Adulteration Act* set the conditions under which a medication could be adulterated. The *Food and Drugs Act* of 1920 replaced this Act and, with amendments in 1950, gave the federal government control of the manufacture and sale of all medications (except opioids), all food, all cosmetics, and certain

BOX 35.1 | Clinical Tip

Medications in the same class often have similar adverse effects, nursing considerations, and required patient teaching. Students and new practitioners are often overwhelmed by the number of medications they need to know. Classifying medications makes it easier to recall information, thus increasing patient safety.

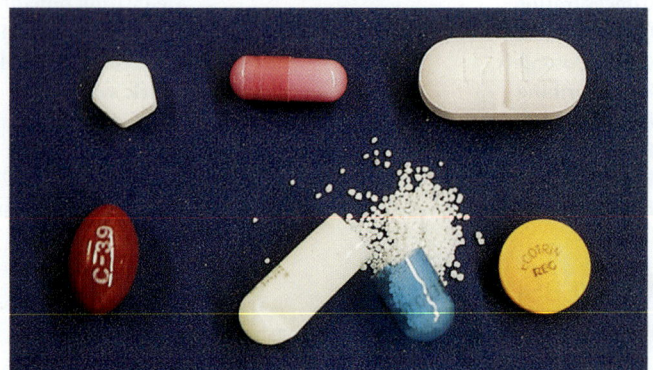

FIGURE 35.1 Forms of oral medications. **Top row:** Uniquely shaped tablet, capsule, scored tablet. **Bottom row:** Gelatin-coated liquid, extended-release capsule, enteric-coated tablet.

TABLE 35.1	Forms of Medication
Form	**Description**

Medication Forms Commonly Prepared for Administration by Oral Route
Solid Forms

Capsule	• Particles or powdered medication • Encased in a gelatin shell/container that opens
Tablet	• Powdered medication compressed into a hard disc or oblong shape (e.g., caplet) • Contains medication, binders (for powder adhesion), disintegrators (for tablet dissolution), lubricants and fillers (for ease of swallowing)
Enteric-coated tablet	• Coated tablet, coating protects against absorption in the stomach • Dissolves and is absorbed in the intestines
Pill	• Generally refers to any solid medication, e.g., tablet, capsule
Sustained release	• Solid tablet or capsule • Contains small, coated medication particles • Dissolves over an extended period of time

Liquid Forms

Elixir	• Clear fluid • Contains medication, water, alcohol, and/or sweetener
Extract	• Syrup or dried medication • Concentrated preparation created by evaporating any nonactive ingredients (e.g., water)
Oral solution	• Medication dissolved in water
Oral suspension	• Fine medication particles dispersed in liquid • Particles settle to the bottom of the container when left standing
Syrup	• Medication dissolved in a concentrated sugar solution
Lozenge (troche)	• Flat, round tablet • Dissolves in the mouth to release medication; not intended for ingestion
Aerosol	• Liquid medication • Sprayed or inhaled; not intended for ingestion • Absorbed in the mouth and upper airway

Medication Forms Commonly Prepared for Administration by Topical Route

Ointment	• Semisolid, moderate consistency • Provides a protective film • Contains medication, hydrocarbons (e.g., mineral oil, petrolatum), no water
Lotion	• Liquid suspension, thin consistency • Moisturizes or cleanses skin • Contains high water content, alcohol, and dissolved medication
Paste	• Semisolid, thick consistency, porous and breathable on skin • Protects and treats skin excoriation • Absorbed slowly, easily confined to one area (e.g., to treat diaper rash) • Contains ointment and powdered medication
Transdermal disc or patch	• Adhesive disc or patch • Contains a medication reservoir and membrane • Provides controlled release of medication (e.g., nicotine) over hours to weeks

Medication Forms Commonly Prepared for Administration by Parenteral Route

| Solution | • Sterile liquid
• Contains water with one or more dissolved medicinal compounds (e.g., sodium chloride) |
| Powder | • Solid sterile particles of medication (e.g., ceftriaxone)
• Dissolved into a sterile liquid (e.g., water or normal saline) for administration |

Medication Forms Commonly Prepared for Instillation Into Body Cavities

Solution	• Liquid medication, dissolved in water or other liquid
Intraocular disc	• Solid small, flexible oval (similar to a contact lens) • Contains two outer layers and one middle layer with medication • Slowly releases medication when moistened by ocular fluid
Suppository	• Solid medicine, shaped into a smooth, narrow tablet • Contains gelatin • Inserted into a body cavity (rectum or vagina); melts at body temperature and releases medication

medical devices. The federal government first began to control opioids in 1908 through the *Opium Act.* In 1961, the *Narcotic Control Act,* which controls the manufacture, distribution, and sale of opioids, was enacted. This Act was repealed in 1996 and replaced by the *Controlled Drugs and Substances Act.* Federal legislation also regulates the manufacture and sale of herbs and other natural health products. This legislation addresses the content of these products as well as the products' packaging, labelling, distribution, and storage.

Medication Standards. Official publications, such as the *Canadian Formulary,* set standards for medication strength, quality, purity, packaging, safety, labelling, and dosage form. Health care providers depend on these standards to ensure that patients receive pure medications in safe and effective dosages. Standards include the following:

- *Purity*: The standard quantity of active substance or drugs in a medication product
- *Potency*: The concentration of the active substance or drug in the medication affects its strength, or potency.
- *Bioavailability*: The ability of the active substance or drug to be released, dissolved, absorbed, and transported by the body to the site of action
- *Efficacy*: Laboratory studies demonstrating medication action and effectiveness
- *Safety*: All medications need to be continually evaluated to determine risk for adverse effects.

Control. Administration of the *Food and Drugs Act* and the *Controlled Drugs and Substances Act* is carried out by the Health Protection Branch (HPB) of the federal government. Before a new medication can be marketed in Canada, it must be intensely tested for safety and effectiveness with humans, and an application for approval must be made to the HPB. If approved, the HPB issues a DIN and Notification of Compliance, which allow the medication to be sold in Canada. Stringent controls are applied to a new medication until sufficient information has been accumulated to ensure its safety and efficacy. Monitoring of the medication is ongoing to report adverse effects, safety concerns, or changes in the indications for use.

Provincial, Territorial, and Local Regulation of Medication. The provincial and territorial governments do not directly regulate the manufacture or sale of medications. However, the provincial and territorial governments have most of the legislative responsibility for health care, which indirectly affects the use and sale of medications. Each province and territory has legislation regarding medical, dental, pharmacy, and nursing practice that dictates each health care provider's role in the prescribing, **dispensing**, and administering of medications. Legislation includes schedules or lists of medications that can be sold with and without prescription. The National Association of Pharmacy Regulatory Authorities facilitates and promotes the harmonization of medication sales across the country.

Health care institutions and employers establish policies that conform to federal and provincial/territorial regulations. The size of an institution, the types of services it provides, and the types of health care providers it employs influence an institution's policies for medication management. Institutional policies are often more restrictive than government controls, to avoid medication-related incidents and promote quality assurance. For example, a common institutional policy is the automatic discontinuation of antibiotic therapy after a predetermined number of days. This policy controls the length of time a medication is prescribed, avoiding unnecessary expenses and prolonged, unwarranted, and potentially harmful therapies.

Medication Regulation and Nursing Practice. In Canada, nurses must be familiar with both the federal and provincial/territorial regulations for medication administration and management by registered nurses and licensed practical nurses in their practice areas. In New Brunswick, for example, licensed practical nurses can administer medications by all routes except for intravenous (IV) push, when supervised and collaborating with a registered nurse (Association of New Brunswick Licensed Practical Nurses, 2022). If a nurse moves to another province, they may discover significant differences in the laws governing medication administration. For example, new legislation surrounding registered nurse prescribing was introduced in British Columbia in February 2021, allowing nurses with additional training to prescribe specific medications. Nursing regulatory bodies each have their own standards for registered and licensed practical nurse medication administration and management to promote safety—for example, the College of Nurses of Ontario's *Practice Standard on Medication* (2019), the College of Licensed Practical Nurses of Alberta's (CLPNA) *Practice Guidelines: Medication Management* (2021), the College of Registered Nurses of Alberta's (CRNA) *Medication Management Standards* (2021), and the Saskatchewan Registered Nurses' Association's *Medication Management Guideline* (2021).

Nurses adhere to additional legal provisions when administering **controlled substances or drugs** (medications that affect the mind or behaviour), such as opioids. Violations of the *Controlled Drugs and Substances Act* are punishable by fines, imprisonment, and loss of nursing license. Health care institutions must meet accreditation standards for medication management, which includes stringent policies for the proper storage, dispensing, and administration of controlled substances like opioids (Box 35.2). **Opioids** are natural, synthetic, or semisynthetic chemicals that reduce the intensity of pain by interacting with nerve cell opioid receptors (Centers for Disease Control and Prevention [CDC], 2022a).

Institutions also have policies for the safe storage and use of **high-alert medications,** which have an increased risk of harm if used inappropriately (Institute for Safe Medication Practices [ISMP], 2018a). Examples of high-alert medications include adrenergic agonists (e.g., epinephrine), anaesthetics (e.g., propofol), antithrombolitics (e.g., heparin), antiarrhythmics (e.g., amiodarone), and insulin. Strategies that enhance safe use of high-alert medications include the following:

1. Standardized processes for prescribing, storing, preparing, administering medications
2. Limiting access
3. Using automated alerts and additional bright-coloured labels
4. Improving access to medication information for health care providers

For a complete list of high-alert medication see the list prepared by the Institute for Safe Medication Practices (ISMP) (2018a).

Pharmacokinetics as the Basis of Medication Actions

For medications to be therapeutic, they must be taken into a patient's body, where they are absorbed and distributed to cells, tissues, or a specific organ, and they must alter physiological functions. **Pharmacokinetics** is the study of how medications enter the body, reach their site of action, metabolize, and exit the body. Nurses must use their knowledge of pharmacokinetics when timing medication administration, selecting the route of administration, considering the patient's risk for alterations in medication action, and evaluating the patient's response.

Absorption. **Absorption** refers to the passage of medication molecules into the blood from the medication's site of administration. Medication absorption is affected by the route of administration, the ability of the medication to dissolve, blood flow to the site of administration, the

BOX 35.2	Guidelines for Safe Storage and Preparation of Controlled Substances

Storage

- Store controlled substances in a locked, secure cabinet or automated (i.e., computerized) medication dispensing cabinet (ADC).
- Maintain an accurate count of controlled substance medication doses in the ADC or locked cabinet in the computer or on a paper inventory flowsheet.
- Count and record the number of doses removed and remaining each time an ADC drawer or cabinet is opened and on a scheduled basis (e.g., nursing shift change).
- Report discrepancies (i.e., differences) between the documented inventory and the actual available doses immediately.
- If you require a partial dose (e.g., half a tablet), a second nurse must witness disposal of the unused portion. Two nurses must document the quantity, volume, and reason for the waste.
- Dispose of medications in a designated medication disposal container or return unopened medications to the pharmacy. Do not dispose of medications in a sharps container, sink, toilet, or garbage can. Persons have obtained substances by reaching into sharps containers, and medications cause environmental harm if improperly disposed of.

Preparation

1. Perform hand hygiene.
2. If using an ADC, log into your institutional account. Select the patient's name and confirm their identity by comparing the patient's name, date of birth, and identification number on the computer screen to information on the medication administration record (MAR). It is easy to select the wrong patient on an ADC.
3. Confirm the last time the patient received the controlled substance according to the patient's MAR, and the last time the medication was

withdrawn for the patient according to the ADC or inventory flowsheet. This ensures doses given have been accurately documented.

4. Select the prescribed medication and dose listed under your patient's profile on the ADC and the required drawer will automatically open. If using a locked cabinet, you will need to access a key and manually locate the medication.
5. Count the quantity of doses of the medication you are collecting in the drawer or cabinet.
6. Collect only the dose you require right now. Do not remove additional doses to be administered at a later time. Controlled substances cannot be stored securely except in the ADC or locked cabinet.
7. Immediately draw up ampoules or vials into a syringe and label the syringe. It is easy to leave vials or ampoules in your pocket where they are not secure.
8. Count the quantity of doses remaining in the drawer or cabinet.
9. Document the quantity removed and remaining in ADC or if using an inventory flowsheet: document your patient's name, the date, time, medication, and dose and route of medication you collected, with your signature.
10. Log off the ADC to ensure other persons cannot use your account to access medication, or securely lock the cabinet and return the key to safe storage.
11. Perform hand hygiene.
12. Complete any required patient assessments (e.g., vital signs) and follow the guidelines for administering medication at the bedside.
13. Monitor your patient's response to the medication, and evaluate and document the medication's effectiveness.

patient's body surface area, and lipid solubility (maximum concentration of a chemical that will dissolve in fatty substances) of medication.

Route of Administration. Absorption rates differ according to the route of medication administration. Medications applied to the skin are absorbed slowly. Medications placed on the mucous membranes and respiratory airways are absorbed quickly because of high blood flow (vascularization) to these tissues. Oral medications have a slow rate of absorption because they must pass through the gastrointestinal (GI) tract. The IV route is the most rapid route of absorption because medications are directly injected into the circulating blood.

Ability of the Medication to Dissolve. The ability of an oral medication to dissolve depends on its form or preparation. For example, liquid medications are absorbed more rapidly than solid tablets or capsules. Acidic medications are absorbed quickly in the stomach, whereas alkalotic medications are not absorbed until they reach the small intestine.

Blood Flow to the Site of Administration. Medication is absorbed as it comes into contact with blood. Therefore, medications administered at sites with more blood supply (i.e., highly vascularized sites) will be distributed and absorbed more rapidly into the bloodstream

Body Surface Area. When a medication is in contact with a large surface area (SA), the medication will be absorbed at a faster rate. For example, most medications are absorbed in the small intestine rather than in the stomach.

Lipid Solubility of a Medication. Cell membranes have a lipid layer that allows highly lipid-soluble medications to easily cross the cell membrane and be absorbed quickly. The absorption of medication is also affected by the presence of food in the stomach. Food can change the structure of a medication and impair its absorption. Therefore, some oral medications must be absorbed more easily when

administered between meals or on an empty stomach. Medications administered at the same time can also interact (i.e., medication–medication interaction) and affect absorption. Nurses should be aware of potential medication–medication interactions listed in the *CPS*, in medication manuals, and on packaging. If medications prescribed at the same time interact, the prescriber must be notified immediately to revise medication administration times.

Safe medication administration requires knowledge of factors that may impair or alter (i.e., increase) the absorption of the prescribed medications. This information is based on an understanding of the medication's pharmacokinetics, the patient's history, dietary patterns, and the physical and diagnostic assessment of the patient (e.g., blood pressure, kidney function values).

Distribution. After a medication is absorbed by the body it enters the bloodstream and is distributed throughout the body tissues and organs to a site of action. The rate and extent of distribution depend on the physical and chemical properties of the medications and the physiology of the person taking the medication.

Circulation. After a medication enters the bloodstream, the speed at which it reaches the site of action (i.e., intended organ or tissue) depends on the vascular content of the patient's tissues and organs. Circulation conditions (i.e., conditions that limit blood flow), such as heart failure, inhibit or slow the distribution of a medication to an intended site of action. The efficacy of medications in patients with circulation challenges can be delayed or altered or increased (if the medication is not distributed and is absorbed at a site that was not intended). For example, a patient with heart failure may have impaired circulation to their feet. If this patient has a fungal infection on their foot and is taking oral antibiotics, the medication may not be distributed or circulated to the foot. The patient may require a prolonged course of antibiotics and additional medications (e.g., ointment) applied directly to the site of infection.

Membrane Permeability. Medications pass through all the organ's tissues and biological membranes to be distributed to the target organ. Some membranes serve as barriers to the passage of medications. For example, the blood–brain barrier allows only fat-soluble medications to pass into the brain and cerebrospinal fluid. Therefore, central nervous system (CNS) infections require treatment with antibiotics that selectively cross the blood–brain barrier. Some older patients experience confusion and other adverse effects when taking medications that cross the blood-brain barrier. The placental membrane has a nonselective barrier that allows both fat and non-fat-soluble medications to cross the placenta, resulting in conditions such as fetal deformities and fetal alcohol syndrome. In contrast, medications that are highly ionized, like heparin and insulin, do not cross the placenta (OpenAnesthesia, 2022).

Protein Binding. The degree to which medications bind to serum proteins (e.g., albumin) affects medication distribution. Most medications bind to proteins and then become inactive. The unbound, or free, medication is the active form of the medication. Patients who have liver disease or malnutrition and older persons have a decrease in albumin circulating in their blood to bind to medication and therefore can experience increased or toxic effects of medication.

Metabolism. After a medication reaches its site of action, it metabolizes into a less active/inactive form that is more easily eliminated. Biotransformation occurs when enzymes detoxify, degrade (break down), and remove the biologically active substance or drug. Most biotransformation occurs within the liver, although the lungs, kidneys, blood, and intestines also metabolize medications. The liver oxidizes and transforms many toxic substances, degrading harmful chemicals before they are distributed to the tissues. Decreases in liver function usually cause medications to be eliminated more slowly and accumulate. Patients with alterations in organs that metabolize medications are at increased risk for medication toxicity. For example, administering anaesthetics such as fentanyl or lorazepam in patients with liver failure can result in stupor or coma.

Elimination. After medications are metabolized, they exit the body through the kidneys, liver, bowel, lungs, or exocrine glands. The chemical makeup of a medication determines the organ of elimination. Gaseous and volatile medications, such as nitrous oxide and alcohol, exit through the lungs. Deep breathing and coughing (see Chapter 49) help the postoperative patient to eliminate anaesthetic gases more rapidly. The exocrine glands (e.g., sweat glands) eliminate lipid-soluble medications, often causing skin irritation. Nurses can assist the patient in good hygiene practices (see Chapter 39) to protect skin integrity. Medications eliminated through the mammary gland place a breastfeeding infant at risk of ingesting the chemicals. Nurses must be aware of what medications pass through the placenta to ensure the newborn is not at risk.

The GI tract is another route for medication elimination. Many medications enter the hepatic circulation where they are broken down by the liver and eliminated into the bile. After medications enter the intestines through the biliary tract, they may be reabsorbed by the intestines. Factors that increase peristalsis (e.g., laxatives and enemas) accelerate medication elimination through the feces, whereas factors that slow peristalsis (e.g., inactivity and improper diet) may prolong a medication's effects.

The kidneys are the main organs for medication elimination. Some medications escape extensive metabolism and exit unchanged in the urine. Other medications must undergo biotransformation in the liver before being eliminated by the kidneys. If renal function declines, a patient is at risk for medication toxicity. If the kidneys cannot effectively eliminate a medication, the dose may need to be reduced. Maintenance of an adequate fluid intake (50 mL/kg/day) promotes proper elimination of medications for the average adult.

Types of Medication Action

Medications vary considerably in the way they act and in their types of action. Factors other than characteristics of the medication also influence medication actions. Patients may respond differently to subsequent doses of a medication, and patients may each respond differently to the same medication.

Therapeutic Effects. The therapeutic effect is the expected or predictable physiological response that a medication causes. Each medication has a desired therapeutic effect, which is the reason it is prescribed. For example, nitroglycerine reduces the body's cardiac workload and increases myocardial oxygen supply. A single medication may have more than one therapeutic effect. For example, Aspirin reduces platelet aggregation (clumping) and is an analgesic, an antipyretic, and an anti-inflammatory medication. Understanding the medication's desired therapeutic effect enables nurses to provide patient education to evaluate the medication's effectiveness.

Adverse Effects. *Side effects* are the unintended, often predictable, secondary effects that a medication causes. Side effects may be harmless or cause injury; when they cause injury they are called *adverse effects*. For example, a common adverse effect of opioids is pruritus; however, a rash might indicate an allergy. Patients often stop taking medications because of adverse effects. The prescriber and patient must always weigh the burden (i.e., discomfort) of a medication's adverse effects with the medication's beneficial effects to decide if the medication is of value. If the burden outweighs the benefits, the prescriber may discontinue the medication. When an adverse effect (an injurious, serious, negative response to medication) occurs (for example, if a patient becomes comatose after ingesting a medication), the prescriber immediately discontinues the medication. Some adverse reactions are effects that were not discovered during medication testing, or rare, unpredicted responses. Health care providers are required to report adverse reactions to the Health Canada Vigilance Program (Health Canada, 2022a). Reporting became mandatory in 2013 with the introduction of *Vanessa's Law,* named after 15-year-old Vanessa Young, who died of a cardiac arrhythmia after being prescribed a medication (Health Canada, 2021, 2022b).

Medication Toxicity. Toxicity develops after prolonged intake of a medication or after a medication accumulates in the blood because of impaired metabolism or impaired elimination. Excess amounts of a medication within the body may have lethal effects, depending on the medication's action. For example, toxic levels of morphine (an opioid) can cause severe respiratory depression and death. Antidotes such as naloxone (for opioid toxicity) are available to treat specific types of medication toxicity.

Allergic Reactions. Allergic reactions are unpredictable responses to a medication. Some patients become immunologically sensitized to the initial dose of a medication. After repeated administration of the medication, the patient develops an allergic response to the medication, its chemical preservatives, or a metabolite. The medication or chemical acts as an antigen, triggering the release of the body's antibodies. A patient's medication allergy symptoms may vary, depending on the individual and the medication (Table 35.2). Among the different classes of medications, antibiotics cause a high incidence of allergic reactions.

Anaphylactic reactions are severe reactions that are life-threatening and are characterized by sudden constriction of bronchial muscles, edema of the pharynx and larynx, severe wheezing, shortness of breath, and circulatory collapse. Immediate use of antihistamines, epinephrine, or bronchodilators is required to treat anaphylactic reactions. Emergency resuscitation measures are sometimes required. A patient with a known history of an allergy to a medication needs to avoid exposure to that medication and must wear a bracelet or medal engraved with emergency medical information, including medication allergies (e.g., a MedicAlert bracelet; Figure 35.2). These bracelets alert health care workers to the patient's medical information, including allergies, if the patient is unable to communicate this information when receiving medical care. Additionally, some patients with allergies leading to anaphylactic reactions carry their own epinephrine pens.

Medication Interactions

When one medication modifies the action of another medication, a **medication interaction** occurs. Medications that do not interact are referred to as *compatible*. Some medications increase or diminish the action of other medications or may alter the way another medication is absorbed, metabolized, or eliminated from the body. When two medications have a **synergistic effect**, the combined effect of the two medications is greater than the effect of the medications when given separately. For example, alcohol acts as a depressant on the CNS and has a synergistic effect (i.e., increases sedation effects of) antihistamines, antidepressants, barbiturates, and opioids.

Some medication interactions are desired; prescribers combine medications to create an interaction that has a beneficial effect. For example, a patient with high blood pressure may be prescribed diuretics and vasodilators, which act together to decrease blood pressure. Nurses need to be aware of reactions that can occur if medications

and other substances (e.g., food, IV fluid solutions) come into contact. In particular, nurses should refer to IV monographs and compatibility charts to ensure medications and IV fluids will not interact if they come into contact. For example, a **precipitation reaction** can occur if phenytoin (an antiseizure medication) is infused with IV solutions containing dextrose. A precipitate reaction causes visible cloudiness or crystals if contact occurs within IV tubing and is harmful to a patient (ISMP, 2017).

Medication Dose Responses

When a medication is prescribed, the goal is to achieve a constant blood level of the medication within a safe therapeutic range. Repeated doses are required to achieve a plateau or therapeutic **concentration** (constant steady state), because although medication accumulates over time, a portion of a medication is continuously being eliminated. The **peak concentration** (highest serum concentration) of a medication occurs when the rate of absorption equals the rate of elimination usually after half of the medication has been absorbed. After peaking, the serum concentration falls progressively. After IV medication **infusions**, the peak concentration occurs quickly, but the serum level also begins to fall immediately (Figure 35.3). The peak concentration takes longer to achieve when a medication is delivered for the first time or in a single dose. Once a therapeutic concentration (steady state) is achieved, the peak concentration will occur more quickly because medication has accumulated and remains in the system (see Figure 35.3). The point at which the lowest amount of medication is detected in the serum is called the *trough concentration*. Some medications doses (e.g., vancomycin) are based on peak and trough serum levels. The trough level is generally drawn 30 minutes before the medication is administered, and the peak level is drawn whenever the medication is expected to reach its peak concentration. The time a medication takes to reach its peak concentration varies depending on the medication's pharmacokinetics (Burchum & Rosenthal, 2019).

A medication's **serum half-life** is the time it takes for the serum medication concentration to be eliminated by half. To maintain a therapeutic concentration or plateau, the patient needs to receive regular, fixed doses. For example, pain medications are most effective when they are given around the clock to maintain a constant level of medication, rather than being given intermittently when a patient complains

TABLE 35.2	Mild Allergic Reactions
Symptom	**Description**
Urticaria	• Raised, irregularly shaped skin eruptions with varying sizes and shapes • Eruptions have reddened margins and pale centre
Rash	• Small, raised vesicles that are usually reddened • Often distributed over entire body
Pruritus	• Itchiness, accompanies most rashes
Rhinitis	• Inflammation of mucous membranes lining nose • Causes swelling and clear, watery discharge

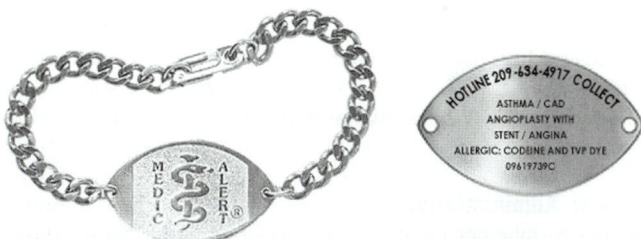

FIGURE 35.2 A MedicAlert bracelet is engraved with a person's emergency medical information, including medication allergies.

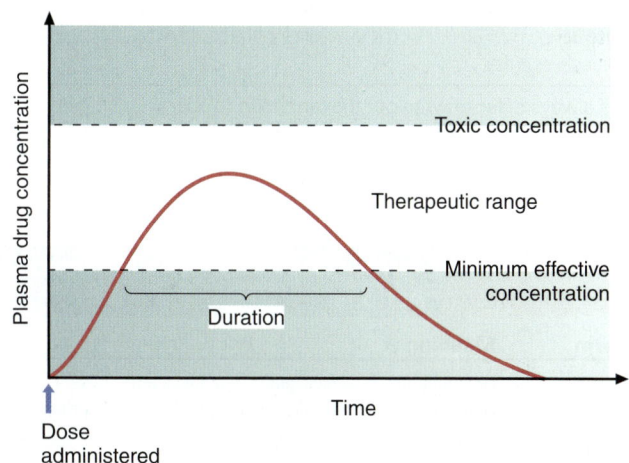

FIGURE 35.3 The therapeutic range of a medication provides maximum efficacy and safety, occurring between the minimum effective concentration and the toxic concentration. (From Burchum J. R., & Rosenthal, L. D. [2019]. *Lehne's pharmacology for nursing care* [10th ed.]. Elsevier.)

of pain. After the initial medication dose, the patient receives each subsequent dose when the previous dose reaches its half-life.

Patients and nurses follow regular dosage schedules and adhere to prescribed doses and dosage intervals (Table 35.3). Some employers set schedules for medication administration. However, nurses can alter this schedule on the basis of knowledge about a medication. For example, at some employers, medications prescribed to be taken once a day are given at 9:00 A.M. However, if a medication causes drowsiness, a nurse may routinely administer the medication at 9 P.M.

It is important to teach patients about dosage schedules and expected effects using plain language. For example, rather than telling a patient to take a medication every 12 hours with food, explain that they should take the medication with breakfast and dinner. Table 35.4 lists common terms associated with medication actions.

Routes of Administration

The route prescribed for administering a medication depends on the medication's properties, the medication's desired effect, the patient's physical and mental condition, and their preferences (Table 35.5).

Oral Routes. The oral route is the easiest, most comfortable, and the most commonly used route of administering medication. Medications are given by mouth and swallowed with fluid. Oral medications

TABLE 35.3	Common Dosage Administration Schedules
Dosage Schedule	**Abbreviation or Notation***
Before meals	AC
Twice a day	BID
At bedtime	HS
After meals	PC
When needed	PRN
Every morning, every A.M.	qam
Every hour	q1hr, q1h
Every 2, 4, 6, 8, 12, or 24 hours	q2h, q4h, q6h, q8h, q12h, q24h
Four times a day	QID
Every 2 days/every other day	q 2 days
Give immediately	STAT
Give now	NOW
Once daily	Once daily (no abbreviation)
Three times a day	TID

*It is always safer to write out the term than to abbreviate it (see Table 35.7). Follow your employer's policy regarding the use of abbreviations. See ISMP website: https://www.ismp.org/recommendations/error-prone-abbreviations-list

TABLE 35.4	Terms Associated With Medication Actions
Term	**Meaning**
Onset	Length of time for a medication to produce a response
Peak	Length of time for a medication to reach its highest effective concentration
Trough	Minimum level of medication blood serum concentration, typically reached just before the next scheduled dose
Duration	Length of time a medication produces a response
Plateau	Therapeutic level of medication blood serum concentration, reached and maintained after repeated doses

have a slower onset of action and a longer effect than parenteral medications.

Sublingual Administration. Sublingual medications are placed under the tongue to dissolve and are readily absorbed (Figure 35.4). A medication given by the sublingual route should not be swallowed because the medication will not have the desired effect. After giving a sublingual medication (e.g., nitroglycerine), the patient should be instructed to avoid liquids until the medication is completely dissolved.

Buccal Administration. Buccal medications are placed in the mouth against the mucous membranes of the cheek where the medication dissolves (Figure 35.5). To avoid mucosal irritation, patients should be instructed to alternate cheeks with each subsequent dose, not to chew or swallow the medication, and not to take liquids with it. A buccal medication acts locally on the mucosa or systemically when it is dissolved in a person's saliva.

Parenteral Routes. Parenteral administration involves injecting a medication into body tissues. The following are the four major sites of injection (i.e., the insertion of liquid into the body with a syringe):
- **Intradermal (ID):** Injection into the dermis just under the epidermis
- **Subcutaneous (sub-Q):** Injection into tissues just below the dermis
- **Intramuscular (IM):** Injection into a muscle
- **Intravenous (IV):** Injection into a vein

Medications are also administered into other body cavities through epidural, intrathecal, intraosseous, intrapleural, and intra-arterial routes. Employer policies dictate which health care providers are able (as well as the training required) to administer medications through different routes.

Epidural Route. Medications are administered through the epidural space via a catheter by an anaesthesiologist. This route is often used for the administration of analgesia both intraoperatively and postoperatively (see Chapter 32). Additional employer training is required to administer medications in bolus form or by continuous infusion via this route. Institutions have policies for the frequency of physical assessment and documentation when patients receive epidural medications.

Intrathecal Route. Medications are administered through an intrathecal catheter that has been placed into the subarachnoid space or into one of the ventricles of the brain. Intrathecal administration is often associated with the administration of medications such as antibiotics directly into the brain.

Intraosseous Route. Medications are infused directly into the bone marrow. Intraosseous routes are most commonly used during emergencies when access is required quickly and for infants and toddlers because their intravascular space (i.e., veins) is difficult to access. Additional training is required for health care providers to insert an intraosseous infusion needle into the bone, usually the tibia.

Intrapleural Route. Medications are injected into the pleural space usually through a chest tube. Chemotherapeutic medications are the most common medications administered by this method.

Intra-Arterial Route. Medications are administered through an indwelling catheter into the arteries. The intra-arterial route is commonly used to deliver tissue plasminogen activators ([tPA], clot busters) to patients who have arterial clots. Patients can experience systemic and GI bleeding related to the administration of tPA and must be monitored closely by nurses.

Topical Administration. Medications applied to the skin and to mucous membranes usually cause a localized effect. Nurses should wear gloves when applying medications, to avoid absorbing the medication through their skin. Topical medications are administered by painting or spreading the medication over the skin, applying moist

TABLE 35.5	Factors Indicating Choice of Administration Routes
Advantages	**Disadvantages or Contraindications**

Oral, Buccal, and Sublingual Routes

Advantages	Disadvantages or Contraindications
• Economical	• Contraindicated if unable to swallow, e.g., patients with neuromuscular disorders, esophageal strictures, mouth lesions, confusion
• Convenient	• Slow absorption
• Comfortable for the patient	• Unpleasant adverse effects, e.g., stomach upset, discoloured teeth, unpleasant taste
• Local or systemic effects	• Contraindicated if alterations in GI function and reduced/increased motility (e.g., nausea, vomiting, GI surgery, anaesthetic, opioid use) inhibit or alter absorption
	• Contraindicated if using gastric suction, unless gastric suction can be held
	• May be contraindicated for medical procedures or diagnostic test

Subcutaneous, Intramuscular (IM), Intravenous (IV), and Intradermal (ID) Routes

Advantages	Disadvantages or Contraindications
• An alternative when oral medications are contraindicated, particularly for critically ill patients	• Risk of introducing infection
• Rapid, increased absorption	• Expensive
• Appropriate for long-term therapy	• Uncomfortable, anxiety-provoking
• IV infusion can maintain therapeutic levels of a medication over time.	• Inconvenient
• IV infusion effectively distributes medication.	• Unpleasant adverse effects, e.g., pain, tissue damage
	• Increased absorption increases risk for adverse reactions
	• Injections contraindicated for alterations in bleeding
	• Risk of needle-stick injuries for nurses

Dermal Route
Topical Medications

Advantages	Disadvantages or Contraindications
• Primarily local effects	• Slow absorption
• Comfortable	• Adverse effects: rash, irritation
• Convenient	• Contraindicated in patients with poor skin integrity and abrasions, can cause rapid, systemic effects
• Minimal adverse effects	

Transdermal Medications

Advantages	Disadvantages or Contraindications
• Prolonged systemic effects	• Expensive
• Convenient	• Leaves oily or pasty residue, may soil clothing
• Comfortable	
• Limited adverse effects	
• Therapeutic medication level can be maintained	
• Useful for long-term therapy	

Mucous Membranes*

Advantages	Disadvantages or Contraindications
• Alterative for some oral medications (e.g., acetaminophen)	• Mucous membranes are highly sensitive
• Local application	• Insertion of rectal and vaginal medications can be uncomfortable, anxiety-provoking.
• Liquid medications have rapid absorption	• Rectal suppositories are contraindicated if patient has rectal surgery or GI bleeding.
• Systemic or local effects	• Ear irrigations are contraindicated if patient has ruptured ear drums.

Inhalation Routes

Advantages	Disadvantages or Contraindications
• Convenient	• Expensive
• Comfortable	• Systemic adverse effects (e.g., hypotension, tachycardia)
• Fast absorption	• Aerosolized medications can be inhaled by nurses.
• Rapid relief of local respiratory problems (e.g., stridor)	• Gaseous medications (e.g., oxygen) must be stored under pressure.
• Rapid delivery of anaesthetic gases	

GI, Gastrointestinal.
*Includes mouth (buccal, sublingual), eyes, ears, nose, vagina, rectum, and ostomy.

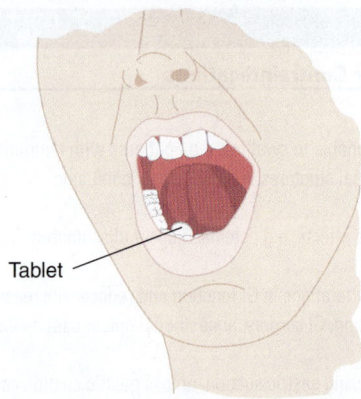

FIGURE 35.4 Sublingual administration of a tablet.

FIGURE 35.5 Buccal administration of a tablet.

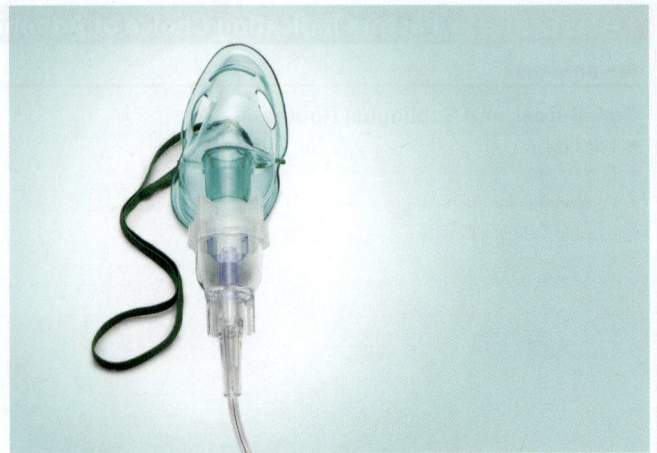

FIGURE 35.6 Face mask with a nebulizer for delivery of inhaled medications and humidified oxygen. (iStockphoto/Bombaert.)

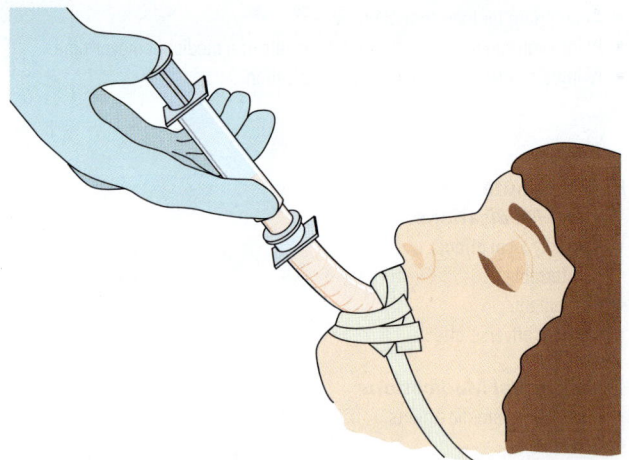

FIGURE 35.7 Medication being instilled through an endotracheal tube.

dressings, soaking body parts in a solution, or giving medicated baths. Systemic effects often occur if a patient's skin is thin or broken down, if the medication concentration is high, or if the medication's contact with the skin is prolonged.

A **transdermal disc** or patch is an adhesive-backed patch that has a medication reservoir and membrane. Medications such as nitroglycerine, nicotine, and fentanyl are released from the reservoir into the skin and cause systemic effects. Transdermal patches are applied for between 12 hours and 7 days.

Medications can be applied to mucous membranes in a variety of ways: 1) by directly applying a liquid or ointment; 2) by inserting a medication into a body cavity (e.g., rectal suppository); 3) by instilling fluid into a body cavity (e.g., ear drops); 4) by irrigating a body cavity (e.g., flushing the bladder and removing the flush fluid); and 5) by spraying.

Inhalation Route. The deeper passages of the respiratory tract provide a large surface area for medication absorption. Medications can be administered through the nasal passages, the oral passage, or endotracheal or tracheostomy tubes. Devices such as **metered-dose inhalers (MDIs)** and **nebulizers** are used to deliver aerosolized (i.e., vaporized) medications (Figure 35.6). Endotracheal tubes are inserted into the patient's mouth and extend to the trachea (Figure 35.7), whereas tracheostomy tubes directly enter the trachea through an incision in the patient's neck. Inhaled medications are absorbed and work rapidly because of the rich blood supply (i.e., vascular alveolar–capillary network) in the pulmonary tissue. Inhaled medications have either local or systemic effects.

Intraocular Route. In **intraocular** medication delivery, a medication in a form similar to a contact lens, is inserted directly into the patient's eye. The eye medication disc has two soft outer layers that enclose the medication. The disc can remain in the patient's eye for up to 1 week. Pilocarpine, a medication used to treat glaucoma, is the most common medication delivered through the intraocular route.

Systems of Medication Measurement

Nurses are responsible for calculating medication doses, measuring medications, and checking the accuracy of the dose before giving a medication to avoid causing harm. The metric, apothecary, and household systems of measurement are used. Canada uses the metric system as the standard of measurement.

Metric System. The **metric system** (Système Internationale d'Unités [SI]) is a decimal system. Metric units can easily be converted and computed through simple arithmetic, such as multiplication and division. Each basic unit of measurement is organized into units of 10. Secondary units are formed by multiplying or dividing by 10. In multiplication, the decimal point moves to the right; in division, the decimal moves to the left. For example:

$$10 \text{ mg} \times 10 = 100 \text{ mg}$$

$$10 \text{ mg}/10 = 1 \text{ mg}$$

When designating a metric dosage, *do not write a zero* alone after a decimal point (e.g., write 5 mg, not 5.0 mg) and always include a zero before the decimal point (e.g., 0.1 mg) to comply with current guidelines (ISMP, 2021a). The basic units of measurement in the metric system are the metre (length), the litre (volume), and the gram (weight). For medication calculations, use only the measurements for volume and weight. In the metric system, the basic units are designated by the use of lowercase or uppercase letters:

Gram = g or Gm

Litre = L or l

Lower-case letters are used for abbreviations for other units:

Milligram = mg

Millilitre = mL

A system of Latin prefixes designates a subdivision of the basic units: *deci-* (1/10 or 0.1), *centi-* (1/100 or 0.01), and *milli-* (1/1 000 or 0.001). Greek prefixes designate multiples of the basic units: *deka-* (10), *ector-* (100), and *kilo-* (1 000). When medication doses are written in metric units, prescribers and nurses use either divisions or multiples of a unit. Convert any fractions to the decimal form.

500 mg or 0.5 g, not 1/2 g

10 mL or 0.01 L, not 1/100 L

Solutions. Solutions of various concentrations are used for injections, **irrigations**, and infusions. A **solution** contains a mass of solid substance dissolved in a known volume of fluid or a given volume of liquid dissolved in a known volume of another fluid. When a solid is dissolved in a fluid, the concentration is expressed in units of mass per units of volume (e.g., g/mL, g/L, mg/mL). A concentration of a solution may also be expressed as a percentage. A 10% solution, for example, is 10 g of solid dissolved in 100 mL of solution. A proportion also expresses concentrations. A 1/1 000 solution represents a solution containing 1 g of solid in 1 000 mL of liquid or 1 mL of liquid mixed with 1 000 mL of another liquid.

Household Measurements. Household measures include drops, teaspoons, tablespoons, cups, pints, and quarts (or litres) for volume, and ounces and pounds (or grams and kilograms) for weight. Although ounces and pounds are considered household measures, they are also used in the apothecary system. The advantage of household measurements is their convenience and familiarity. When the accuracy of a medication dose is not critical, household measures can be safely used. For example, many over-the-counter (OTC) medications can safely be measured by this method. To calculate medications accurately, nurses need to be familiar with the common equivalents of metric and household units (Table 35.6). The disadvantage of household measures is their inaccuracy. Household utensils, such as teaspoons and cups, often vary in size. The scales used to measure pints or quarts are often not well calibrated.

NURSING KNOWLEDGE BASE

Between 2020 and 2021, 72 929 medication and care incidents occurred in Canadian hospitals that caused harm (Canadian Institute for Health Information [CIHI], 2021). To safely administer medications, nurses must calculate medication doses accurately, strictly adhere to employer policy and procedure, and report medication incidents that occur. The nursing process provides the framework for organizing a nurse's thoughts and actions, and it is the foundation for medication

TABLE 35.6 Equivalents of Measurement

Metric Measurement	Household Measurement
1 mL	15 drops (gtt)
4–5 mL	1 teaspoon (tsp)
15 mL	1 tablespoon (tbsp)
30 mL	2 tablespoons (tbsp)
250 mL	1 cup (c)
480 mL (approximately 500 mL)	1 pint (pt)
960 mL (approximately 1 L)	1 quart (qt)
3840 mL (approximately 4 L)	1 gallon (gal)

BOX 35.3 EVIDENCE-INFORMED PRACTICE

Reducing Distractions During Medication Administration

Evidence Summary

Many medication incidents (e.g., missed or incorrect dose, inappropriate medication, incorrect timing or route) occur when nurses are distracted, interrupted, or do not follow standard procedures during medication administration. Effective approaches to reduce distractions include using 1) a separate room for medication preparation; 2) standardized checklists; 3) "Do Not Interrupt" signs; 4) diversion strategies (e.g., designating another nurse to answer phone calls and non-emergency requests); and 5) storage of medications close to the patient (Alrabadi et al., 2021).

Application to Nursing Practice
- Consistently follow a standardized procedure for medication administration.
- Reduce distractions by placing "Do Not Disturb" signs in medication preparation areas.
- Prepare medications in a separate room.

From Alrabadi, N., Shawagfeh, S., Haddad, R., et al. (2021). Medication errors: A focus on nursing practice. *Journal of Pharmaceutical Health Services Research, 12*(1), 78–86. https://doi.org/10.1093/jphsr/rmaa025

administration. Box 35.3 describes ways of reducing distractions that can lead to medication incidents.

Clinical Calculations

Nurses use basic arithmetic to calculate medication doses and mix solutions because medications are not always dispensed in the unit of measure which is prescribed. For example, the prescriber may prescribe or order 20 mg of a medication that is supplied (i.e., on hand/available) in 40-mg vials. Nurses must convert the available units of volume or weight to the prescribed doses.

Conversions within One System. To convert units of measurement in the metric system, divide or multiply. To change milligrams to grams, divide by 1 000, moving the decimal three places to the left.

1000 mg = 1 g

350 mg = 0.35 g

To convert litres to millilitres, multiply by 1 000 or move the decimal three places to the right.

1 L = 1000 mL

0.25 L = 250 mL

To convert units of measurement within the apothecary system or the household system, consult an equivalence table. For example, when converting fluid ounces to quarts, recall that 32 ounces is the equivalent of 1 quart. To convert 8 ounces to a quart measurement, divide 8 by 32 to get the equivalent, which is 0.25 quart.

Dose Calculations. Many formulas can be used to calculate medication doses. Apply the following basic formula when preparing solid or liquid doses of a medication:

$$\text{Dose prescribed} / \text{Dose on hand} \times \text{Amount on hand} = \text{Amount to administer}$$

The dose is the amount or quantity of medication prescribed. The dose on hand is the dose of medication supplied by the pharmacy (e.g., milligrams, units) and is expressed on the medication label as the contents of a tablet or capsule or as the amount of medication dissolved per unit volume of liquid. The amount on hand is the basic unit or quantity of the medication that contains the dose on hand. For solid medications, the amount on hand may be one capsule; the amount of liquid on hand may be a millilitre or litre, depending on the container. For example, a liquid medication comes in the strength of 125 mg per 5 mL. Thus, 125 mg is the dose on hand, whereas 5 mL is the amount on hand. The amount to administer is the actual amount of medication the nurse will administer. Always express the amount to administer in the same unit as the amount on hand.

For example, a patient is prescribed morphine 2 mg IV. Thus, the dose prescribed is 2 mg. The medication is available in a vial containing 10 mg per mL, and the amount on hand is 1 mL. The formula is applied as follows:

$$2 \text{ mg}/10 \text{ mg} \times 1 \text{ mL} = \text{Amount in millilitres to administer}$$

To simplify the 2/10 fraction to decimal form, divide numerator and denominator by 2:

$$1/5 \times 1 \text{ mL} = 1/5 \text{ mL or } 0.2 \text{ mL to administer}$$

Syringes are calibrated only in decimals. After converting the fraction 1/5 to 0.2 mL, prepare the correct dose.

The following is an example of how the formula applies when calculating solid dose forms. Digoxin 0.125 mg orally (PO) is prescribed. The medication is available in tablets containing 0.25 mg of digoxin.

$$0.125 \text{ mg}/0.250 \text{ mg} \times 1 \text{ tablet} = \text{Number of tablets to administer}$$

The fraction 0.125/0.250 equals 1/2, or 0.5. Therefore,

$$0.5 \times 1 \text{ tablet} = 0.5 \text{ or } {}^1\!/_2 \text{ tablet to be administered}$$

Many tablets are manufactured with scores, or indentations, across the centre (Figure 35.8). If half a tablet is required, then the pharmacy will often split the tablet and dispense the prescribed unit-dose of medication for the patient. The majority of hospital pharmacies in Canada use a unit-dose medication management and dispensing system, whereby the pharmacy delivers the exact dose of every prescribed medication in separate packages, at the required time, for each patient (Canadian Society of Hospital Pharmacists, 2021). This reduces the need for nurses to split tablets or calculate dosages, which is associated with medication incidents (Cicero et al., 2021).

Often, liquid medications are manufactured in volumes greater than 1 mL. In applying the formula, be careful to use the correct concentration

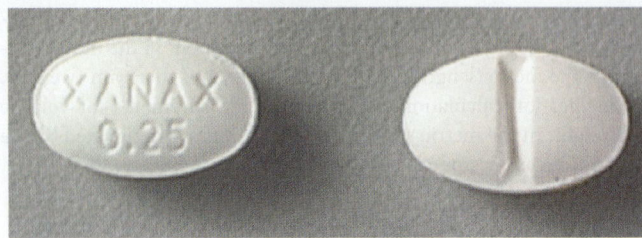

FIGURE 35.8 Scored medication tablet. (Courtesy Sharon Kaasalainen, RN, PhD.)

to avoid a medication incident. For example, a medication prescription is for "erythromycin suspension 250 mg PO." The pharmacy dispenses a 100-mL bottle labelled "erythromycin 125 mg per 5 mL." The concentration is 125 mg in 5 mL. To obtain the correct dose calculate:

$$\text{Dose prescribed} / \text{Dose on hand} \times \text{Amount on hand} = \text{Amount to administer}$$

$$250 \text{ mg}/125 \text{ mg} \times 5 \text{ mL} = \text{Volume to administer}$$

The fraction 250/125 equals 2. Therefore,

$$2 \times 5 \text{ mL} = 10 \text{ mL to administer}$$

Some employers require a nurse to double-check calculations with another nurse before administering the medication, especially when the risk of harm from administering the wrong medication dose is high (e.g., heparin or insulin). Double-check your calculations or confer with another nurse if you are uncertain or your calculation result seems unusual.

Pediatric Doses. Use additional caution when calculating children's medication doses. Children metabolize medications at different rates than adults. Premature and newborn infants are especially vulnerable to adverse effects of medications because the liver and kidneys are not fully functioning. After the newborn period, a child's liver metabolizes some medications more quickly, which means the child may require larger or more frequent doses (Cicero et al., 2021). It is also more difficult to assess the hydration status of a child and to evaluate if a medication has the desired effect in children. The prescriber often calculates the required medication dose for a child and includes this information on the prescription. However, nurses are responsible for knowing the safe dose range (listed on the medication package insert) and for rechecking doses prior to administering medication. Formulas used to calculate the appropriate medication dosages for children often consider the child's age, weight in kilograms, body surface area, and the adult dosage of the medication (Berchum & Rosenthal, 2019). The most accurate method of calculating pediatric doses is based on estimating a child's body surface area (SA) using the West nomogram and Mosteller's formula (Sigurdsson & Lindberg, 2020) (Figure 35.9).

The formula used to calculate a pediatric dose is a ratio of the child's body surface area compared with the body surface area of an average adult, which is 1.7 square metres, or 1.7 m².

$$\text{Child's dose} = \text{Surface area of child}/1.7 \text{ m}^2 \times \text{Normal adult dose}$$

For example, ampicillin is prescribed for a child weighing 12 kg. The normal adult dose for ampicillin is 250 mg. According to the West nomogram (see Figure 35.9), a child weighing 12 kg has a surface area of 0.54 m². Using this information, calculate the appropriate child's dose:

$$\text{Child's dose} = 0.54 \text{ m}^2/1.7 \text{ m}^2 \times 250 \text{ mg}$$

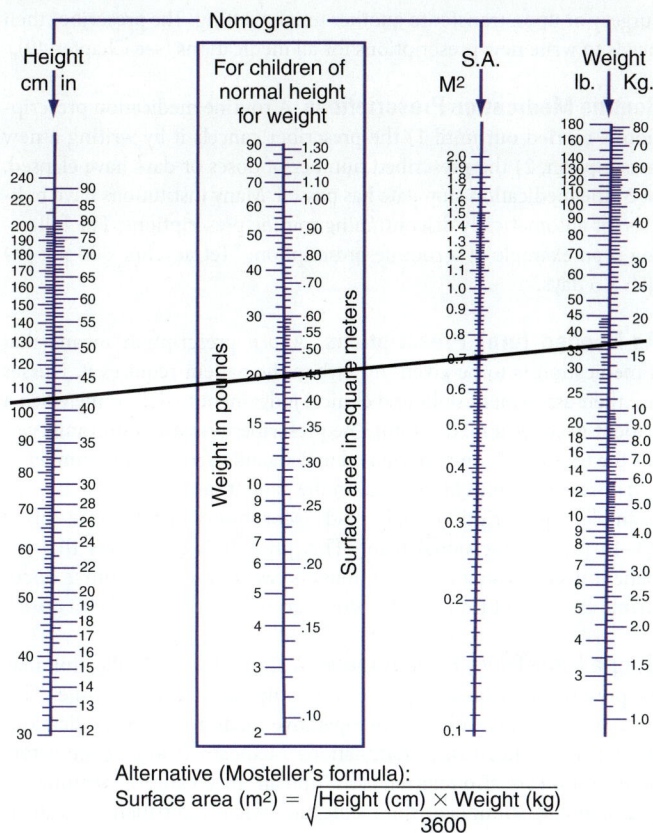

FIGURE 35.9 West nomogram used to estimate the body surface area of children. A straight line is drawn between a child's height and weight. The point where the line crosses the surface area *(S.A.)* column is the child's estimated body surface area. (From Kliegman, R., & St. Geme, J. [2020]. *Nelson textbook of pediatrics* [21st ed.]. Elsevier.)

The m² units are cancelled out.

$$\text{Child's dose} = 0.54/1.7 \times 250 \text{ mg}$$

$$0.54/1.7 = 0.3$$

$$\text{Child's dose} = 0.3 \times 250 \text{ mg} = 75 \text{ mg}$$

An alternative method to determine medication doses for children involves basing the amount of medication to administer (usually in milligrams) on the weight of the child (usually in kilograms). For example, a child weighing 14 kg is prescribed 5 mg/kg. Using this information, calculate the appropriate dosage based on the following calculation:

$$\text{Child's dose} = 5 \text{ mg/kg} \times 14 \text{ kg} = 70 \text{ mg to be delivered}$$

Role of Authorized Prescribers

Prescribing occurs when a health care provider issues an authorization to dispense a specified medication for use by a designated individual (British Columbia College of Nurses and Midwives [BCCNM], 2022). Prescribers in Canada vary according to the province/territory in which they work and include physicians, nurse practitioners, and pharmacists in some provinces. Pharmacists can independently prescribe medications in Alberta and prescribe in collaborative care settings in most provinces (Canadian Pharmacists Association, 2022). Additional

Adapted from Institute for Safe Medication Practices (ISMP). (2020). Strategies for safer telephone and other verbal orders in defined circumstances. *ISMP Canada Safety Bulletin, 20*(4), 2–5. https://www.ismp-canada.org/download/safetyBulletins/2020/ISMPC SB2020-i4-TelephoneOrders.pdf

training, licensing, or supervision is required for health care providers to prescribe some controlled substances such as methadone.

The scope of practice for registered nurses has expanded in some areas of Canada to include nurse prescribing (called a **prescribing nurse**). Beginning in 2021, in accordance with employer policies, registered nurses with additional training in British Columbia could diagnose and prescribe a limited number of medications to treat condition such as anaphylaxis, cardiac dysrhythmias, opiate overdoses, respiratory distress associated with asthma, hypoglycemia, postpartum hemorrhage, and symptoms of influenza (BCCNM, 2022). Standards for registered and licensed practical nurses' dispensing or recommending non-prescription medications and natural health products also vary across Canada. In Nova Scotia, for example, nurses can administer nonprescription medications (e.g., Tylenol) in accordance with employer policies if the medication will treat an existing diagnosis and the nurse has the necessary knowledge, skill, and judgement to dispense the medication (Nova Scotia College of Nursing [NSCN], 2022a).

Prescribing

A prescriber issues a legal authorization for a medication to be dispensed to a designated individual by writing or ordering a **prescription** for medication on a form in the patient's medical record, on a legal prescription pad or electronically through a **computerized-physician order entry system (CPOE)**. The patient's diagnosis, condition, or indication for use is described for each prescription. A health care provider may also prescribe a medication by speaking to the nurse in person or by telephone. This is called a **verbal order prescription**. Strategies to reduce medication incidents when receiving a verbal order prescription (ISMP, 2020a) are outlined in Box 35.4. Nursing students cannot receive verbal order prescriptions and can only give medications after the prescription has been written or entered electronically and verified by two registered nurses.

Abbreviations are used when writing prescriptions to indicate dosage frequencies, times, routes, and special instructions (see Table 35.3). Employers have policies for the use of abbreviations; some shortened forms can lead to confusion and increased risk for medication incidents (Table 35.7). Nurses must not use error-prone abbreviations when documenting medication prescriptions (ISMP, 2021a; Joint Commission, 2022).

Standardized order sets (SOS) or standardized prescription sets include a predefined set of medication prescriptions with recommended dosages for specific conditions. Frequently used in acute care, standardized order sets are computerized and allow the prescriber to select the appropriate medications and desired dosages for a patient on a form with predefined, suggested prescriptions, based on clinical practice guidelines. Prescriptions using standardized order sets have been shown to reduce mortality for persons with ischemic stroke and coronary heart failure, improve symptom management for patients at end of life, and improve the accuracy of antibiotic dosing with vancomycin (Wells & Loshak, 2019).

Types of Medication Prescriptions

Five types of medication prescriptions and orders are common in acute care settings: routine, prn, single (one-time), STAT, and now prescriptions. Medication prescriptions are based on the frequency and the urgency of administration. Some conditions change the status of a patient's medication prescriptions. For example, in some agencies, the patient's preoperative medications are automatically discontinued after

surgery or upon transfer to another unit or setting. The prescriber then needs to write new prescriptions for all medications (see Chapter 49).

Routine Medication Prescriptions. A routine medication prescription is carried out until 1) the prescriber cancels it by writing a new prescription, 2) the prescribed number of doses or days have elapsed, or 3) the medication stop date has passed. Many institutions have policies for automatically discontinuing routine prescriptions. The following is an example of a routine prescription: "Tetracycline 500 mg PO q6h × 5 days."

As-Needed (prn) Prescriptions. A *prn* prescription means that a medication is to be given only when the patient requires it. Nurses use their assessment skills and clinical judgement to determine when a patient needs *prn* medication. The prescriber sets minimum intervals for the time of administration and may include a maximum number of *prn* doses or amount of medication the patient can receive in a day. For example, a prescription might read: "Morphine sulphate 5 mg sub-Q q3–4h prn for incisional pain." This prescription indicates that the patient needs to wait at least 3 hours between doses. The nurse documents assessment findings, *prn* doses given, and the effects of a dose.

Single (One-Time) Prescriptions. A single dose of medication may be prescribed to be given "one time only" at a specified time. This prescription is common for preoperative medications or medications given prior to diagnostic examinations. Medications to be given before an operation are also referred to as "on-call" medications, meaning the nurse should administer the medication when the patient "is called"

TABLE 35.7	Abbreviations, Symbols, and Dose Designations With Potential for Errors in Medication Administration		
Do Not Use Abbreviations	**Meaning**	**Misinterpretation**	**Correction**
U or uu	Unit	• Mistaken for the number 0, causing a 10-fold overdose • Mistaken for "40" or "4u" • Mistaken for "cc" causing the dose to be administered in volume instead of in units	Write out "unit"
IU	International unit	• Mistaken for "IV" or "10"	Write out "international unit"
Q.D., q.d., QD, or qd	Every day	• Mistaken for "q.i.d."	Write out "daily"
Q.O.D., q.o.d., QOD, or qod	Every other day	• Mistaken for "q.d." (daily) or "q.i.d." (four times daily)	Write out "every other day"
MS, MSO$_4$	Morphine sulphate	• Mistaken for magnesium sulphate	Write out the complete medication name
MgSO$_4$	Magnesium sulphate	• Mistaken for morphine sulphate	Write out the complete medication name
μg	Microgram	• Mistaken for "mg" (milligram)	Write the abbreviation "mcg"
hs	At bedtime, hours of sleep (hora somna)	• Mistaken for "half-strength"	Write out "bedtime" or "half-strength"
T.I.W. or tiw	3 times a week	• Mistaken for 3 times a day or twice in a week	Write out "three times weekly"
S.C., S.Q., SC, and SQ	Subcutaneous	• SC mistaken for S.L. (sublingual) • SQ mistaken for the words "5 every" • "q" mistaken for the word "every"	Write the abbreviation "sub-Q" or the term "subcutaneously"
D/C	Discharge patient AND Discontinue medications	• Medications to be prescribed on patient's "discharge" mistaken for medications to be discontinued	Write out "discharge" and "discontinue"
cc	Cubic centimetres	• Mistaken for the letter "u" (units)	Use the abbreviation "mL"

Adapted from The Joint Commission for Accreditation of Health Care. (2021). *2021 National patient safety goals: Medication management.* https://www.jointcommission.org/standards/standard-faqs/#first=10&f:_FacetChapter=[Medication%20Management%20(MM)]; Institute for Safe Medication Practices. (2021) *List of error-prone abbreviations.* https://www.ismp.org/Tools/errorproneabbreviations.pdf

to proceed to the operating room (OR). For example: "Ancef 1 g IV on call to OR."

STAT Prescriptions. A *STAT* prescription signifies that a single dose of a medication is to be given immediately and only once. STAT prescriptions are often written for emergencies when the patient's condition changes suddenly. For example: "Give Apresoline 10 mg IV STAT."

Now Prescriptions. A "now" prescription is used only once, when a patient needs medication quickly but not immediately, as in a STAT emergency prescription. A now prescription needs to be administered within 90 minutes. An example of a now prescription is "Give vancomycin 1 g IV piggyback now."

Prescriptions in Home and Community Settings. Prescribers frequently write prescriptions for medications that are to be self-administered in the community by the patient or a caregiver. The prescription includes additional detailed instructions to ensure the patient understands how to take the medication and when to refill the prescription. The parts of a prescription are illustrated in Figure 35.10. Nurses need to assess the patient's social determinants of health (e.g., access to pharmacies, income and medication coverage benefits, social support) to determine if they need additional support.

Pharmacist's Role

The pharmacist prepares (e.g., selects, mixes, compounds), dispenses, labels, monitors, and evaluates the effects of prescribed medications. In some areas (e.g., Alberta), pharmacists also prescribe or recommend medications and provide patient teaching (e.g., in the community). Pharmacists are valuable team members with advanced knowledge that is integral to the care of patients.

Dispensing Systems

Systems for storing and dispensing medications vary. Institutions conform to regulations and use medication management systems to maintain an accurate inventory and store, prepare, and dispense medications in a safe and secure way. Typically, pharmacists or technicians dispense medications and nurses administer them.

Stock Supply System. In a stock system, medications are available in multidose containers. The stock system is time-consuming because nurses must collect each dose of medication from shared containers for each patient. Repeatedly accessing multidose containers also increases the risk for infection transmission.

Unit-Dose System. The unit-dose system provides each patient with a 24-hour supply of medications in a drawer or tray within a portable cart or medication room. Each drawer is labelled with the name of a patient. Each unit-dose is packaged and includes the exact medication dose the patient is prescribed. Pharmacy technicians refill the patient's medication drawer at a designated time each day (e.g., 0600 and 1800 hours). Limited numbers of prn and stock medications are also provided. Controlled substances are kept separately in a locked cabinet or electronic automated dispensing cabinet. The unit-dose system reduces the number of medication incidents, reduces medication waste, and decreases dispensing and preparation time.

Automated Dispensing Cabinets. Automated dispensing cabinets (ADC) use computerized controls to dispense opioids and unit-dose medications (Figure 35.11). Each nurse accesses the ADC by logging in and entering a security code. All patients have a computerized profile listing their prescribed medications. The nurse selects the patient's profile, confirms their identity, and selects the required medication, the correct dose, and the route from the ADC computer screen. The ADC drawer containing the medication then opens and the nurse collects the medication. The ADC medication system automatically records the transaction. If the nurse is collecting a controlled substance, they physically count the available medications in the drawer and record the new inventory after removing the collected dose (see Box 35.5).

Nurse's Role

When administering medications, as a nurse you are accountable for knowing the following information: 1) what medications are prescribed; 2) the medication purpose; 3) appropriate dosages and routes; 4) therapeutic and adverse effects; 5) assessment and monitoring requirements; 6) patient education needs; and 7) why the patient is taking this medication and if the medication is appropriate for this patient

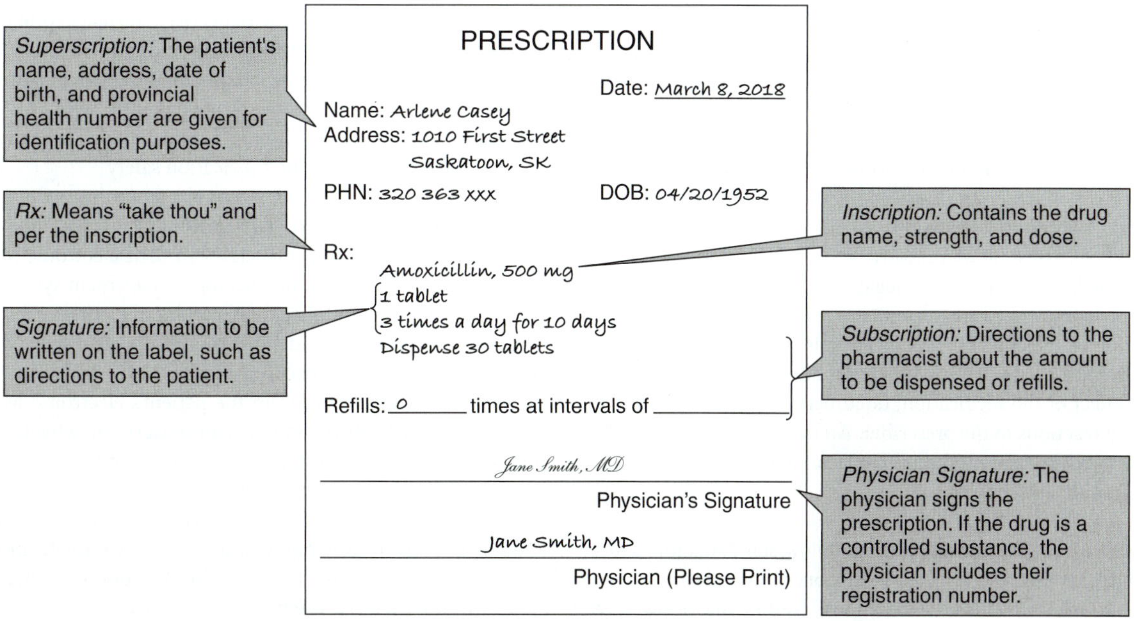

FIGURE 35.10 Sample handwritten medication prescription.

A

B

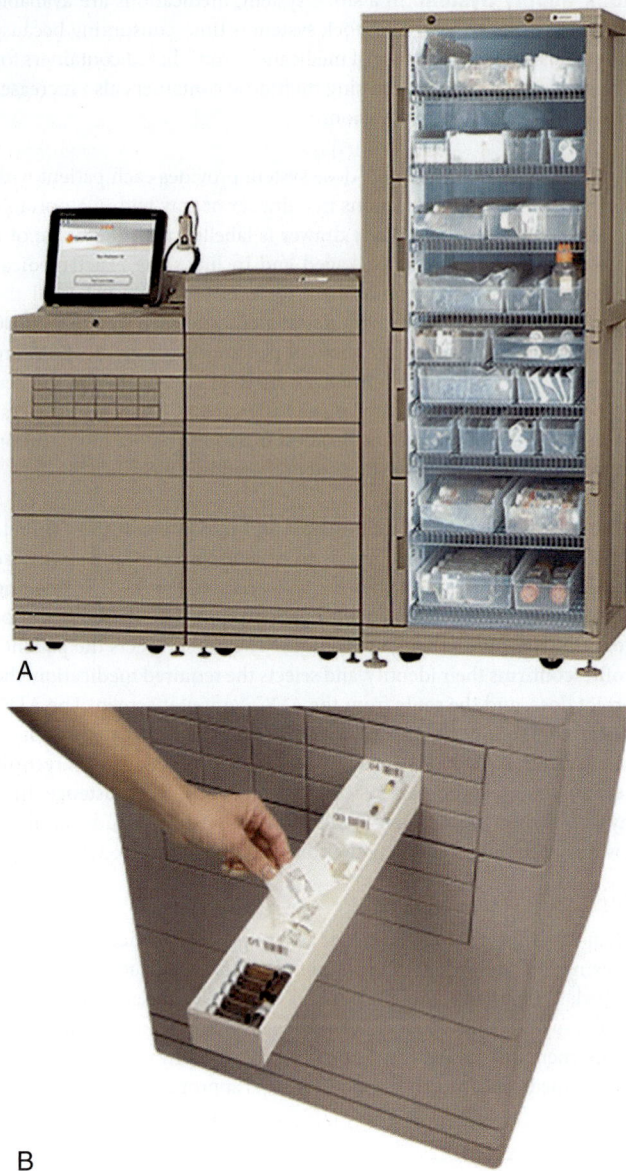

FIGURE 35.11 A, Automated dispensing cabinet. **B,** Drawer access. (Photo of Pyxis Medication Management System courtesy and © Becton, Dickinson and Company.)

at this time. Use the nursing process to integrate medication therapy into nursing care. In order to determine if the medication is safe to administer and is appropriate, you must perform a physical assessment of the patient (e.g., assess blood pressure before administering an anti-hypertensive medication). Do not delegate any part of the medication administration process to unregulated care providers. Based on your assessment, you will decide if the medication is safe to administer and what route is appropriate. After medication administration, you will evaluate the effect of the medication, document any effects observed, and report any reactions to the prescriber. An integral part of your role is also educating the patient and their caregiver about proper medication administration and monitoring.

Safe Medication Management. Nurses follow standards for medication management described by their regulatory body and employer—for example, by checking dose calculations; confirming dosages of medications with a colleague before administration; fulfilling the rights

BOX 35.5 Process for Medication Reconciliation

1. ***Collect:*** Collect the best possible medication history (BPMH). Obtain a current list of the patient's medications, and interview people (e.g., patient, caregivers, health care providers, pharmacist), as necessary, to understand the patient's actual medications used. Document the BPMH, including the accurate medications, dosages, and frequencies.
2. ***Compare:*** Identify discrepancies. Compare the BPMH you documented with new medications recorded in the patient's chart. Document any discrepancies (i.e., differences) for clarification.
3. ***Correct:*** Resolve discrepancies. Correct any discrepancies by communicating with the patient, caregivers, and health care providers.
4. ***Communicate:*** Ensure continuity of medication information. Discuss any medication changes with the patient. Provide the patient and persons involved in their care with a reconciled list of medications.

Adapted from ISMP Canada. (2021). *MedRec process in primary care practice settings.* https://www.ismp-canada.org/primarycaremedrecguide/MedRecProcess.htm

of medication administration (see the section "Standards" for a sample list of common rights); and documenting assessment findings before medication administration (e.g., patient's blood glucose levels or blood pressure). Employers also utilize a system of checks and balances to optimize safe medication management.

The aim of patient safety strategies is to reduce human and system issues and address the core processes of prescribing, dispensing, and administering medications. Examples include 1) having standardized processes for medication reconciliation when patients are transferred; 2) computerizing prescription entry, medication administration records (MARs), and documentation; 3) dispensing medications in unit-dose packages; 4) involving patients in medication checks and medication administration; and 5) implementing medication barcode scanning (CIHI & Healthcare Excellence Canada, 2021; Institute for Healthcare Improvement, 2021).

Medication Reconciliation. The process of assessing and documenting a patient's **best possible medication history** and resolving any discrepancies in the patient's current mediation list is called **medication reconciliation.** Medication incidents (e.g., mistakes) often occur when a patient is transferred between care settings. Therefore, reconciling the list of a patient's medications when a patient is admitted, transferred, or discharged is pivotal to safe patient care (Killin et al., 2021). Medication reconciliation (Box 35.5) may be time-consuming, but it is an essential step for ensuring medication safety.

Barcode Scanning. **Barcode scanning** links a unique barcode on the patient's identification bracelet with their electronic MAR and the institution's computerized medication management system in order to enhance safety. To administer medications, the nurse scans the patient's barcode, scans their own identification badge, and then scans the barcode on the medication package (Figure 35.12). The administration is then automatically recorded in the patient's electronic MAR and the institution's medication system. **Computers on wheels (COWs)** or portable computer workstations also enable nurses to access patient data (e.g., lab values) and medication information (e.g., IV monograph) quickly and easily, thus avoiding medication incidents. Innovations and advances in technology that aim to reduce medication incidents are further described in Box 35.6. Table 35.8 outlines situations associated with student nurse medication incidents and prevention strategies (ISMP, 2007; Asensi-Vicente et al., 2018).

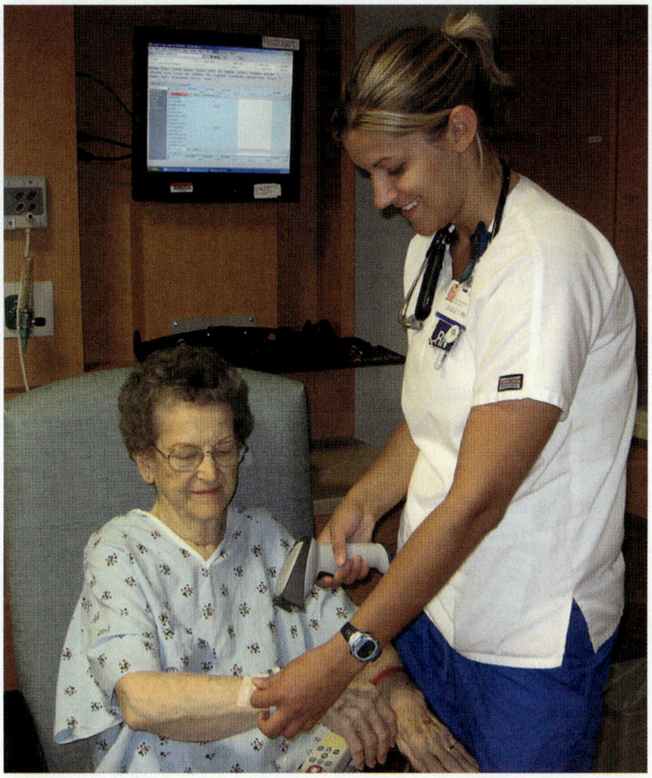

FIGURE 35.12 Nurse using a barcode scanner to identify patient during medication administration.

BOX 35.6 Technology to Enhance Medication Safety

- Electronic medical records (EMR), electronic health records (EHR), and computerized medication administration records (MAR) provide an up-to-date record of the patient's allergies, conditions, prescriptions (past and present), doses administered, and patient responses (Carayon et al., 2021).
- Internet/intranet services, computer applications, and computers on wheels in the workplace enhance access to medication resources (e.g., IV infusion monographs and rates).
- Computerized physician order-entry (CPOE) reduces illegible handwriting and aims to increase efficiency in medication dispensing.
- Automated medication dispensing cabinets (ADC) and medication systems dispense personalized doses, monitor and store controlled medications, and eliminate the need for manual in-person inventory (Zheng et al., 2020)
- Barcode medication administration requires the nurse to scan the medication, the patient's identification bracelet, and the nurse's identification badge to fulfill the rights of medication adherence (Zheng et al., 2020).
- Smart IV infusion pumps have medication libraries and dose error reduction systems (DERS). Nurses must select the medication and solution they are infusing when administering it through an IV pump and confirm that medication guidelines (i.e., guardrails) for dose and rate are being followed.

Application to Nursing Practice
- Participate in the selection, implementation, and evaluation of technology for nursing.
- Be aware of employer policies for when the technology cannot be used (e.g., during power outages).
- Follow the manufacturer's guidelines for care of electronic equipment and report any problems with technology immediately.

Medication Incidents

Medication incidents, previously referred to as *medication errors*, are preventable events or situations that lead to the inappropriate use of medications and/or patient harm while the medication is being managed by a patient or health care provider (ISMP, 2019). A **close call or near miss** is when a potential medication incident is caught and avoided before it occurs and causes harm. Incidents occur through human (e.g., dose miscalculation, illegible handwriting, inappropriate use of abbreviations) and system issues (e.g., similar medication packaging, incorrect labels) during the prescribing, transcribing, dispensing, and administering process.

In 2019 alone, 72 950 medication-related incidents occurred that caused harm to patients in Canada (CIHI, 2021). Medications and health care environment (e.g., wrong medication, pressures) account for 45% of harm-related events in hospital. The medications most frequently associated with incidents include insulin, hydromorphone, and heparin, and the most common reported cause of medication incidents is distractions or interruptions and heavy workload. The most common types of incidents associated with nursing students are errors of medication omission (i.e., missed dose) and improper dose administration caused by distractions or interruptions and lack of knowledge or supervision (Asensi-Vicente, et al., 2018) (see Table 35.8).

Responding to Medication Incidents

When an incident occurs, the patient's safety and well-being is top priority. The nurse needs to assess the patient's condition, notify the prescriber immediately, and take measures to counteract the incident. After the patient is stabilized, the nurse reports the incident to their employer and government monitoring agencies. The nurse is usually responsible for preparing an incident report for their employer within 24 hours. The report does not usually include patient identifying information but describes the location, time, factual description of the incident; factors perceiving as causing the situation; the patient's response; actions taken; and persons notified. The incident report is not a permanent part of the patient's medical record (see Chapter 10). Institutions use incident reports to track patterns and identify areas for quality improvement. Many institutions have procedures in place for disclosing incidents to patients or their caregiver.

All medication incidents, even those that do not cause obvious or immediate harm and near misses, must be reported to the employer and to Health Canada to avoid similar incidents in the future. Creating a **culture of safety** through strategies such as "close call" or "near miss" reporting aims to shift negative perspectives and encourage reporting.

Coping with medication incidents often causes feelings of guilt, shame, loss of confidence, concern for the patient, and fear, all of which lead to under-reporting of incidents (Meulenberg, 2020) (Box 35.7). If you are involved in a medication incident, reflect on how the incident could have been prevented. Evaluate the situation to determine whether you have the necessary resources, environment, and systems for safe medication administration. If repeated medication incidents occur within a work area, identify and analyze the factors that may be contributing to the incidents and take corrective actions. Internationally, employers and health care authorities have introduced nonpunitive strategies to encourage reporting. Nurses must be vigilant in preventing incidents and advocate for work environments that are conducive to safe medication administration.

TABLE 35.8 Situations Associated With Student Nurse Medication Incidents

Situation	Concern	Prevention Strategies
Preparing medications for multiple patients	Leads to administering medications to the wrong patient	Prepare medications for one patient at a time. Apply patient labels to medication cups, syringes, and IV bags. Confirm the patient's identity with two to three unique identifiers.
Nonstandard and uncommon medication times	Leads to dose omissions if uncommon times, single-doses, or new medications are prescribed	Develop a proactive plan with the staff nurse. Clarify who is responsible for administering each medication. Clarify how new prescriptions will be addressed. Instructors and staff nurse monitor the patient's MAR and review potential omissions with the student nurse.
Neglecting to document or review documentation	Leads to dose omissions or extra doses if both a student nurse and staff nurse are administering medications to a patient	Both student nurses and staff nurses use the same MAR. Always take the MAR to the bedside during medication administration. Document administration immediately. Review all sources of documented medication administration, especially for patients who are transferred from a different unit. Include student nurses in all verbal reports to receive information about the patients they are caring for.
MAR is unavailable or not reviewed.	Leads to incidents (e.g., wrong patient, inappropriate medication, dose, route, time) if the MAR is not reviewed for preparing and administering medications	Always review the patient's MAR when preparing and administering medications; worksheets should not be used. Bring the MAR to the patient's bedside for verification before administering medications. Always use two to three unique identifiers to verify the correct patient before administering medications. *The room and bed number are not patient identifiers.*
Permitted types of medication for administration vary.	Leads to dose omissions if the student does not administer all mediation types	Instructors provide a daily report to staff nurses indicating the types of medications the student nurses will and will not be administering. At the beginning of a shift, the student nurse confirms with the staff nurse the types of medications the student nurse will be administering, medications the nurse will be responsible for administering, and when.
Held or discontinued medication processes or policies are unfamiliar.	Leads to extra or inappropriate doses if held or discontinued medications are administered	Employers have a clear, reliable process and accessible policy for holding or discontinuing medications. Instructors and staff nurses explain the process for holding or discontinuing medications and review the MAR with the student to identify medications on hold or for discontinuation.
Assessments and monitoring are not performed.	Leads to adverse reactions if vital signs or lab values are not assessed before administering some medications	Know which medications require vital signs monitoring (e.g., antihypertensive medications) and lab values assessment (e.g., warfarin) before being administered. Schedule and plan required assessments prior to medication administration. Routinely access the computer and assess the patient's most recent lab values. Instructors review the MAR with the student at the beginning of the shift to identify assessments that must be performed prior to medication administrations.
Nonspecific or stock doses dispensed	Leads to excessive doses administered if students assume medications are all in a unit-dose package	Pharmacists dispense packaged unit-doses or include detailed instructions on the MAR and stock bottles. Include the patient-specific dose on the MAR followed by the unit-dose, e.g., "Lopressor 25 mg," followed by "25 mg = 1/2 of a 50-mg tab."
Preparing oral/enteral liquids in parenteral syringes without labels	Leads to administering medication in the wrong route if syringes with oral or enteral solutions are injected IV	Pharmacists dispense all oral liquid products in oral (non-parenteral) syringes. Stock medication areas with oral syringes. Only use oral syringes to prepare oral medications.

MAR, Medication administration record.
Adapted from ISMP. (2007). *Error-prone conditions that lead to student nurse–related errors.* https://www.ismp.org/resources/error-prone-conditions-lead-student-nurse-related-errors

CRITICAL THINKING

Knowledge

Nurses use knowledge they have acquired from many disciplines to administer medications. For example, from physiology, they learn that potassium is a major intracellular ion. When patients do not have enough potassium in their body (hypokalemia), they experience signs and symptoms such as muscle fatigue or weakness. In some cases, severe hypokalemia is fatal because of the dysrhythmias that may occur as a result. To restore the patient's potassium level to normal, medications may be prescribed, which will also relieve the patient's signs and symptoms of hypokalemia. New medications are constantly being manufactured, and evidence for treatments change. As a result, nurses must continuously check resources (e.g., *CPS*, drug guides) to ensure they are administering medications safely.

Experience

Clinical experiences provide nursing students with the opportunity to apply the nursing process to medication administration and practise psychomotor skills. The patient's attitudes, knowledge, physical and mental status, and responses can make medication administration a complex experience.

Cognitive and Behavioural Attributes

Medication administration requires a disciplined attitude and a comprehensive, systematic approach. As a nurse, you are responsible and accountable for your actions. When administering a medication to a patient, do not assume that the prescribed or dispensed medication is appropriate or is the correct dose. You are accountable for administering a medication that is inappropriate, even if it is prescribed for the patient. You are also responsible for ensuring that patients who self-administer medication do so properly. Understand the therapeutic effect, usual dosage, laboratory references, and adverse effects of each medication before you administer it. Conduct a comprehensive physical assessment of the patient and critically analyze the assessment data.

Each institution has policies that define the classes, doses, and routes of medications that nurses can administer in each setting (e.g., critical care, medicine unit, diagnostic imaging). For example, phenytoin (Dilantin), a medication prescribed to treat seizures, may be administered by mouth or by IV push. In large doses, phenytoin can affect the rhythm of the heart. Therefore, when a nursing unit does not have the ability to monitor the patient's heart rate and rhythm, some institutions limit the amount of phenytoin that can be given to a patient. To ensure safe medication administration, nurses must adhere to evidence-informed practice guidelines and employer policy and procedure. Prescribers are sometimes unaware of nurses' scope of practice and may prescribe medications that nurses cannot give. Nurses must be aware, practice within their scope, and communicate any discrepancies.

Standards

Standards are actions that ensure safe nursing practice. In Canada, the activity of medication administration by registered nurses is governed by the Canadian Nurses Association's (CNA) (2017) *Code of Ethics for Registered Nurses* and professional practice standards set by provincial and territorial nursing associations. Nurses are legally and ethically responsible for acquiring the knowledge needed to administer medications and upholding the patient's rights, dignity, and uniqueness in the process. To ensure safe nursing practice, each time a nurse administers a medication, they must be aware of the rights of medication administration. All medication incidents can be linked, in some way, to an inconsistency in adhering to the following rights of medication administration:

1. The right medication
2. The right dose
3. The right patient
4. The right route
5. The right time and frequency
6. The right documentation
7. The right reason
8. The right to refuse
9. The right patient education
10. The right evaluation

Right Medication. A prescription is required for every medication administered to a patient. When medications are first prescribed, compare the MAR with the original handwritten or computerized prescription order entered by the prescriber. Always verify new medication information when new prescriptions are written or when patients transfer from one nursing unit or health care facility to another (ISMP, 2021b; Killin et al., 2021). When preparing medications, compare the label of the medication container with the medication form. Check the label against the medication form three times: (1) before removing the container from the drawer or shelf, (2) when the amount of medication prescribed is removed from the container, and (3) before returning the container to storage. Never prepare medications from unmarked containers or from containers with illegible labels (Joint Commission, 2022). When using unit-dose prepackaged medications, check the label against the MAR when taking medications out of the medication dispensing system. After determining that the information on the patient's MAR is accurate, the record is used to prepare and administer the medications. Verify all medications against the MAR at the patient's bedside before opening the medication packages and delivering the medications to the patient.

Administer only the medications that you prepare. If an incident occurs, the nurse who administers the medication is responsible. If a patient questions the medication, do not ignore the patient's concerns. An alert patient will know whether a medication is different from one previously received. In most cases, the patient's prescription has been changed; however, the patient's questions might reveal an incident. If an incident does occur, withhold the medication and recheck or compare it directly against the most recent prescription.

Patients who self-administer medications should keep the medications in their original labelled containers, separate from other medications, to avoid confusion. Many hospitals request that all medication in the hospital setting be administered by nurses, rather than allowing patients to self-administer; this process ensures that patients do not receive double doses of medication. If a patient refuses a medication, the nurse should discard it; it should not be returned to the original container. Unit-dose packaged medications can be saved if they are unopened. However, because of infection control, some employers require medication to be discarded if it has been taken into a patient's room. If a patient refuses an opioid or other controlled substance, follow the proper hospital procedure of having another nurse witness the wastage of the medication.

Right Dose. The unit-dose system is designed to minimize medication incidents. The chance of incident increases when a medication must be prepared from a larger volume or strength than needed or when the prescriber, in prescribing a medication, uses a system of measurement different from what the pharmacist supplies. When performing a medication calculation or conversion, ensure that another nurse verifies the calculated dose.

After confirming the calculated dose, prepare the medication by using standard measurement devices. Use graduated cups, syringes, and scaled droppers to measure medications accurately. At home, patients should use measuring spoons and cups, not household spoons and cups, which vary in volume.

Only tablets that are scored by the manufacturer should be broken. When a scored tablet needs to be broken, ensure the break is even. A tablet can be cut in half by using a knife or a pill-cutting device. Discard tablets that do not break evenly. Some agencies allow nurses to save the unadministered portion of the scored medication tablet for subsequent doses if the remaining tablet is repackaged and labelled. Nurse should verify with the employer policy before administering a tablet that has been opened, cut, and repackaged. In the community care setting, pill splitting is particularly risky. It is important to determine whether the patient has both the motor dexterity and visual acuity needed to split tablets (Baig et al., 2016). If possible, prescribers need to avoid prescribing medications that require splitting.

Often a nurse prepares a tablet by crushing it so that it can be mixed in food. The crushing device should always be cleaned completely before the tablet is crushed. Remnants of previously crushed medications may increase a medication's concentration or result in the patient receiving a portion of an unprescribed medication. Crushed medications should be mixed with very small amounts of food or liquid but should not be mixed with the patient's favourite foods or liquids because a medication may alter the taste of the food or liquid and thereby decrease the patient's desire for them. This is particularly important when administering crushed medications to pediatric patients.

> **SAFETY ALERT** Not all medications can be crushed. Some medications, such as timed-release or extended-release capsules, are coated with special material to prevent the medication from being absorbed too quickly. Before crushing a medication, refer to a medication manual or another medication reference to ensure that the medication can be safely crushed.

Right Patient. Medication incidents often occur because one patient receives a medication intended for another patient. An important step in administering medications safely is to ensure medications are given to the right patient. Remembering every patient's name and face is difficult. To identify a patient correctly, ask the patient to state their name. Compare the patient's name and another identifier (e.g., hospital identification number) on the MAR against the information on the patient's identification bracelet. Scan the patient's barcode on their identification bracelet, if applicable (see Figure 35.12).

If an identification bracelet is missing or the text is smudged or illegible, acquire a new bracelet for the patient. When asking the patient's name, you should not merely speak the name and assume that the patient's response indicates that they are the right person. Instead, ask the patient to state their full name. To avoid making the patient feel uneasy, simply explain that the question is routine for giving medications.

Right Route. If a prescription does not designate a route of administration, or if the specified route is not the recommended route, always consult with the prescriber.

When administering injections, take precautions to ensure that the medications are given correctly. Prepare injections only from preparations designed for parenteral use. The injection of a liquid designed for oral use can produce local complications, such as a sterile abscess, or

fatal systemic effects. Medication companies label parenteral medications "for injectable use only."

Right Time and Frequency. Nurses must know why a medication is prescribed for certain times of the day and whether the time schedule can be altered. For example, two medications are prescribed: one q8h (every 8 hours) and the other three times a day. Both medications are scheduled three times within a 24-hour period. The prescriber intends the q8h medication to be given around the clock to maintain therapeutic blood levels of the medication. In contrast, the nurse needs to give the three-times-a-day medication during the waking hours. Each institution has a recommended or standard time schedule to guide the administration of medications prescribed for various intervals. Nurses may alter recommended times if necessary or appropriate.

The prescriber often gives specific instructions for the timing of administration of a medication. Medications prescribed to follow an ongoing, consistent, standard dosing schedule are referred to as ROUTINE. As mentioned, when a preoperative medication is to be given ON CALL the nurse needs to administer the medication when notified that the patient can be transferred for surgery by health care providers in the operating room. A medication prescribed pc (after meals) is to be given within half an hour after a meal, when the patient has a full stomach. A STAT medication is to be given immediately. Priority is given to medications that must act at certain times. For example, insulin should be administered at a precise interval before a meal. Antibiotics should be administered on time around the clock to maintain therapeutic blood levels. Medications should be given within 60 minutes of the times for which they are prescribed (i.e., 30 minutes before or after the prescribed time).

Some medications require nurses to use their clinical judgement to determine the proper time for administration. A prn sleeping medication should be administered when the patient is prepared for bed or at another time appropriate for maximum benefit. When administering prn analgesics, nurses need to use their judgement. For example, the nurse may need to obtain a STAT prescription if the patient requires a medication before the prn interval has elapsed. The nurse must always document calls made to the patient's prescriber regarding changes to medication prescriptions.

Before a patient is discharged from the hospital setting, the nurse evaluates the patient's need for care in the community setting, especially if the patient was admitted to the hospital as the result of a problem with medication self-administration. Patients often leave the hospital with a basic knowledge of their medications but are unable to retrieve and implement this knowledge after they return to the community setting. Before discharge, the nurse evaluates whether medications are adequate or are prescribed at therapeutic levels for the patient. At home in the community setting, a patient may need to take several medications throughout the day. Nurses can help patients to plan their schedules on the basis of preferred medication intervals, the medications' pharmacokinetics, and the patients' own daily schedule. For patients who have difficulty remembering when to take medications, a chart can be made that lists the times when each medication is to be taken or a special container prepared to hold each timed dose.

Right Documentation. Nurses and other health care providers use accurate documentation to communicate with each other. Correct documentation is essential to ensure safe medication administration. Because medication incidents may result from inaccurate documentation, it is vital to ensure that the documentation is appropriate before giving the medications. Appropriate documentation includes the patient's name; the name of the prescribed medication written out in full (no medication name abbreviations); the time the medication was administered; and the medication's dose, route, and frequency. Common problems with medication prescriptions are omission of the medication type (e.g., tablet, liquid), frequency, route or dosage, illegible handwriting, and use of inappropriate abbreviations (Suclupe et al., 2020). If any pieces of information are missing, the nurse needs to contact the prescriber to verify the prescription. The prescribing health care provider is responsible for providing accurate, complete, and understandable medication prescriptions.

After administering a medication, the nurse completes the MAR according to employer policy to verify that the medication was administered as prescribed. Nurses are also responsible for documenting any preassessment data regarding the administration of certain medications (e.g., antihypertensive medications, blood glucose–lowering medications, and medications for pain management). Inaccurate documentation of medications, such as failing to document an administered medication or documenting an incorrect dose, can lead to incidents or errors in subsequent decisions about the patient's care. For example, inaccurate documentation about insulin often results in negative patient outcomes. Consider the following situation: a patient receives insulin at breakfast, but the nurse who gave the insulin neglected to document it. The nurse leaves, and a new nurse is assigned to care for the patient. The new nurse notices that the previous nurse did not document the insulin and assumes that the prescribed insulin was not given. Therefore, the new nurse gives the patient another dose of insulin. Two hours later, the patient experiences a low blood glucose level that causes the patient to experience seizures. Timely and accurate documentation would have prevented this situation.

Right Reason.
Nurses are professionally responsible for obtaining the rationale for prescribed medications. If you are unaware of a new medication, you have the professional responsibility to research the medication by using the following sources: the *Compendium of Pharmaceuticals and Specialties (CPS)*, medication manuals, or electronic medication information databases. When retrieving information about a medication, be attentive to nursing implications, including routes of administration, pre-administration physical assessments, expected onset of action, contraindications, and follow-up nursing assessments and evaluation for both adverse effects and desired responses. Nurses are professionally obligated to contact the prescriber for verification in any of the following situations: a health care provider prescribes a medication that the nurse identifies as contraindicated on the basis of either the patient's medical history or the patient's current condition, the prescribed dose exceeds the recommended limits, or the prescribed route is contraindicated for the patient. Being vigilant in critically assessing a patient's medication regimens is essential to maintaining patient safety.

Right to Refuse.
With the emerging focus on patient-centred care and the recognition that patients are not passive recipients of care, more attention has been given to ensuring that the rights of patients are also upheld during the medication administration process (CNA, 2017). Nurses are responsible for ensuring that a patient is aware of the medications being administered to them and that the patient is aware that they can make an informed choice regarding whether to accept or refuse a medication (NSCN, 2022b). Thus, it is important to remember that a patient has the right to refuse a medication. Patients need to be informed that they have this right, but at the same time, they also need to be fully informed about the potential consequences of their refusal. If a patient refuses medication therapy, the nurse should not become defensive and instead recognize that every person of consenting age has the autonomous right to refuse a medication. *Covert medication administration* refers to the administration of medications to a patient

---

> **BOX 35.8   CASE STUDY**
>
> ### *The Right to Refuse Medication*
>
> You have been caring for Ishmael (preferred pronouns: he/him), who lives with schizophrenia, for over 2 years now as a mental health nurse in the community. During one of your visits with him, Ishmael tells you he has stopped taking his antipsychotic medications because he feels he is doing much better now. You worry that Ishmael will develop severe symptoms again and wonder what you should do, although you understand he has the right to refuse medications.
>
> **Thinking Points**
> 1. What should be your immediate response to Ishmael?
> 2. What clinical assessments are needed?
> 3. Who should you communicate this issue to?
> 4. How will this change your visits with Ishmael in the future?

without their knowledge or consent. If a patient has the capacity to make an informed decision and refuses their medication, the medication should not be given, and the prescriber should be notified. If a patient does not have capacity, the patient's substitute decision-maker will make decisions about accepting or refusing medications (NSCN, 2022b) (Box 35.8).

Right Patient Education.
In order for patients to be fully informed about their medication and the consequences of refusing to take it, it is imperative that they receive the right education about their medications and their overall treatment plan. For some patients, education may be required for a caregiver as well, particularly if they are involved in helping patients manage their medications at home in the community setting. Education should include providing information about the medication being given, such as the reason for taking it, its action, and possible adverse effects that the patient might experience while taking it. This information is important for patients and their caregiver to know, to ensure patient safety (Bastable, 2021). Patients and their caregivers need to be involved in the decision-making process about managing and administering medications, and to achieve this, they need the right information.

Right Evaluation.
Patients also need to have the right evaluation at the appropriate times. Before a medication is given, the nurse needs to check to make sure that the prescribed medication is correct or appropriate and that the medication is available and accessible to the patient. Nurses need to follow up with the pharmacy or prescriber if they have any concerns or questions about the medication.

Nurses also need to make sure that any special assessments that are required have been completed, such as taking a pulse or blood pressure or checking important laboratory results that are necessary for a particular medication. If a nurse is working in the community, it is essential to ensure that patients and their caregivers have the necessary equipment and resources that facilitate safe and effective administration of medications. This assessment should include a thorough functional and cognitive assessment since many older people and persons with mental or other disorders are faced with several conditions, such as cognitive impairments and physical limitations, which may affect their ability to manage their medications properly.

Once a medication has been given, careful monitoring of the effectiveness of the medication, its adverse effects, and signs of adverse reactions and medication interactions is necessary. If the medication has not achieved its desired effect, additional follow-up is needed. Within a collaborative model of care, nurses should be working closely with

BOX 35.9   Nursing Assessment Questions

- Do you have a list of medications from your pharmacy?
- What medications (prescription, over-the-counter, herbal) do you actually take, when do you take them, and how do you take them?
- What are your medications for?
- What adverse effects have you experienced?
- Do you have any allergies to medications or foods? What is your reaction to these foods and medications?
- What are your normal eating and drinking patterns?
- How do you pay for your medications?
- How do you remember to take your medications?
- How do you obtain your prescription medications in your community?
- What questions do you have about your medications?

pharmacists and health care providers such as physicians if further follow-up or assessments are necessary (CNA, 2017).

Risk Management: Employer Policy and Procedure. Institutions have policies and procedures to guide nursing practice. Policies and procedures are reviewed on a consistent basis (e.g., annually) and updated to reflect new evidence. Policies describe the types of medications that nurses are permitted to administer, the preparation of medications, the administration of medications, and guidelines for evaluating patients' response to medications. For example, some employers require nurses to complete specialized training to qualify them to safely administer IV chemotherapeutic medications. Furthermore, the administration of certain medications (e.g., IV inotropic medications for regulating a patient's blood pressure) is permitted only by nurses in critical care areas where the patient is on a continuous heart monitor to evaluate the response to medication.

Maintaining Patients' Rights. Because there are risks related to medication administration, patients have the right to the following:

- To be informed of the medication's name, purpose, action, and potential undesired effects
- To refuse a medication regardless of the consequences
- To have qualified health care providers assess their medication history, including allergies and use of herbal therapies (Box 35.9)
- To be advised if a medication is experimental or part of a research study and provide written consent for its use
- To receive labelled medications safely without discomfort in accordance with the rights of medication administration
- To receive appropriate supportive therapy in relation to medication therapy
- To only receive necessary medications
  Nurses need to be aware of these rights and handle all inquiries by patients and their families courteously and professionally.

❖ NURSING PROCESS AND MEDICATION ADMINISTRATION

❖ Assessment

To determine the appropriateness and safety of medications for administration for each patient, nurses must understand the medication (e.g., purpose, contraindications), perform a physical assessment, and explore the patient's medical history.

Information About Medications to Be Administered.. The nurse should review the medications the patient has been prescribed. The nurse must understand each medication's action, purpose, normal dosages, routes, adverse effects, and nursing implications for administration and monitoring to determine if the medication is appropriate and safe for the patient. Common questions to ask include the following: Is the smallest dose possible prescribed? Will the medications interact? How is this medication administered? Valuable resources include the *CPS*, online medication manuals, medication package inserts, the pharmacist, and pharmacology or drug textbooks.

Health History. Review the patient's medical history prior to administering medications. A patient's medical history provides indications and contraindications (i.e., reasons to not administer) medications. For example, a patient who has experienced a thyroidectomy surgery may require levothyroxine (Synthroid) for hormone replacement; therefore, levothyroxine may be indicated. Alternatively, if a patient has a gastric ulcer, taking Aspirin may increase the risk of bleeding, making Aspirin contraindicated.

Allergies. A patient's history of allergies (i.e., environmental, medication or food) needs to be communicated to the health care team. Many medications contain ingredients found in food, and patients with a food allergy may experience an allergic reaction. For example, a patient who is allergic to shellfish may also be sensitive to any product containing iodine, such as povidone iodine (Betadine) or dyes used in radiological testing. To ensure patient safety, when patients are admitted to a hospital, they are issued an identification band that lists the medications they are allergic to. All allergies must be noted on the nurse's admission notes, the medication records, and the health care provider's documentation of the patient's history.

Best Possible Medication History. The nurse must collect or review the patient's best possible medication history, including information about each medication (prescription; OTC; traditional, natural, or herbal) that the patient takes. The nurse must record the length of time the medication has been taken, the current dosage, and whether the patient has experienced any adverse effects. Traditional medications can interact with prescription medications.

Diet History. A diet history reveals the patient's normal eating patterns and food preferences. Nurses can then plan the dosage schedule and advise patients to avoid foods that may interact with their medications. It is important to be aware of patients' cultural preferences for food, and if these foods counteract the effects of medications, nurses should provide the patients and their families with comprehensive, respectful explanations (Young & Guo, 2020).

Patient's Current Condition. Assess the patient's physical or mental status, as this will affect whether a medication is given and how it is administered and provides a baseline to evaluate if the medication is effective. For example, a patient who is nauseated may be unable to swallow a tablet. A patient with low urine output may have impaired kidney function that can increase medication effects. A patient with frequent diarrhea may have decreased intestinal absorption, which can decrease oral medication effects.

Patient's Perception and Coordination Abilities. It is important to assess people's perceptual, fine motor, or coordination skills in order to understand any difficulties a patient may have with self-administering medication. For example, a patient with arthritis who takes insulin to manage blood glucose levels may have difficulty manipulating a syringe. If the patient is unable to self-administer medications, the nurse must determine whether a caregiver will be available to assist the patient, or consult with the health care team and refer the patient to supports in the community setting.

Patient's Attitude and Beliefs About Medications. The patient's attitude and beliefs about medications needs to be assessed because these factors influence a patient's adherence to medication therapy. It

BOX 35.10 CULTURAL ASPECTS OF CARE
Influences on Medication

Administration

Assess a patient's beliefs and preferences before medication administration and do not assume that the patient's beliefs are the same as your own. Health beliefs vary within cultural, ethnic, spiritual, and religious practices and will influence how patients perceive, manage, and respond to medication therapy. For example, some Muslim patients may refuse opioids when dying, in order to be fully conscious and enter the afterlife (Attum et al., 2022). Herbal remedies, traditional or natural medicines, and alternative therapies are also commonly used, and their value to people must be respected. For example, some Indigenous people perform smudging ceremonies with sacred medicines such as sage, sweetgrass, and cedar for healing to combat illnesses and promote healing (Redvers & Blondin, 2020). Previous negative experiences in the health care system and the history of colonialism in Canada may cause patients to distrust nurses and Western medicines. Nurses must practice cultural humility, respect differences in values and beliefs surrounding medication use, and form therapeutic trusting relationships with diverse patients (Young & Guo, 2020).

In addition to the psychosocial aspect of medication therapy, genetics associated with race and ethnicity can influence medication response, metabolism, and adverse effects. Therefore, factors such as the patient's age, culture, ethnicity, race, and sex must be considered when administering medication.

Implications for Practice
- Assess a patient's beliefs about medications—for example, "How do you feel about your medications?"
- Do not assume a persons' beliefs and experiences with medications are the same as your own.
- Assess whether the patient uses any traditional medicines.
- If a patient is not responding to medication therapy as expected, consider whether the person is taking the medication as prescribed and if their genetics (race or ethnicity) is influencing their medication response, metabolism rate, and adverse effects.
- Contact the prescriber regarding changes to the patient's medication regimen if needed.

Adapted from Young, S., & Guo, K. L. (2020). Cultural diversity training: The necessity of cultural competence for health care providers and in nursing practice. *Health Care Manager, 39*(2), 100–108.

is unlikely that a patient will take a medication if they or their caregiver perceives that medication does not align with their cultural beliefs (Box 35.10); will cause harmful adverse effects, addiction, or dependence; will interfere with their identity or role (e.g., medication causing drowsiness will make it difficult to work); or will not be beneficial. In contrast, patients may seek medications even if they cause them harm but have a desired effect (i.e., addiction) or if they have become dependent on them (i.e., experience withdrawal symptoms when medications are stopped) (see Chapter 11).

Health Literacy and Learning Needs. Health literacy refers to the patient's ability to find, understand, and utilize services and information to make health-related decisions, such as taking medication (CDC, 2022b). A patient's level of health literacy, knowledge, and understanding of their medication therapy influences their willingness, motivation, and ability to follow a medication regimen. Adherence is unlikely unless a patient understands the medication's purpose, the importance of regular dosage schedules and proper administration methods, and the medication's possible adverse effects and perceives the medication as valuable to their personal health goals.

The nurse can assess a patient's health literacy, learning needs, and information preferences by asking questions such as "What is your medication for?", "When do you take it?", "How do you obtain your medications?", "Where do you go for information about your health?", "How much information would you like to have about your medications?" and "How do you like to learn about new things?" The nurse needs to provide education that is appropriate to the patient's developmental stage and education level surrounding the medication's purpose, adverse effects, and administration techniques. The nurse should describe tools the patient can use to assist with medication management, such as using a dosette, and demonstrate techniques (e.g., administering injection). The patient's learning is evaluated by asking them questions about their medication or by asking them to demonstrate administering an injection.

◆ Nursing Diagnosis

Assessing and then analyzing the patient's history and physical assessment data will enable the nurse to recognize if the patient has a problem that is influencing medication administration and formulate a nursing diagnosis, if needed. The nursing diagnosis medication nonadherence refers to the intentional or nonintentional overuse, underuse, or incorrect use of medications as prescribed (ISMP, 2022). Nonadherence occurs most often because of uncomfortable adverse effects and expensive costs of medication. Examples of related nursing diagnoses include the following:
- *Anxiety*
- *Deficient knowledge of medications*
- *Medication nonadherence*
- *Disturbed visual sensory perception*
- *Impaired swallowing*
- *Ineffective therapeutic regimen management*

After the patient's diagnosis has been selected, the nurse identifies related factors that guide nursing interventions. For example, if the diagnosis *medication nonadherence* is related to lack of knowledge, an appropriate intervention might be providing patient education about medication.

◆ Planning

Nurses organize care and schedule time to prepare and administer medications according to the prescribed medication times, special instructions (e.g., take with food), and patient preferences (e.g., take when in bed). When preparing and administering medications it is important to minimize distractions and interruptions and avoid rushing (Kavanagh & Donnelly, 2020). Plan sufficient time and multiple sessions for patient education; do not wait to educate patients about their medications and self-administration on the day they are being discharged home from the hospital.

Goals and Outcomes. Setting broad goals and specific, measurable, achievable, relevant, and time-bound, or SMART outcomes will help the nurse to use time wisely during medication administration. Whether the patient, caregiver, or nurse administers the medication, the nurse is responsible for ensuring that the following goals and outcomes are met:
1. The patient understands the medication therapy.
2. The patient gains the therapeutic effect of the prescribed medications without discomfort or complications.
3. The patient experiences no complications related to the route of administration.
4. The patient can safely self-administer the prescribed medications.

For example, the following goal and related outcomes are appropriate for a patient with type 2 diabetes:

Broad goal: The patient will safely administer all prescribed medications before discharge.

SMART Outcomes:

- The patient will describe the desired and adverse medication effects by May 1.
- The patient will explain the signs, symptoms, and treatment of hypoglycemia by May 1.
- The patient will monitor and interpret blood glucose levels and determine medication management or treatment for hypoglycemia by May 3.
- The patient will explain and follow the daily routine, coordinating medications with mealtimes by May 3.

Setting Priorities. The information gathered from the patient assessment and history enables a nurse to prioritize which medication is given first. For example, medication for a life-threatening symptom that is affecting the patient's airway, breathing, or circulation (e.g., low oxygen saturation, extreme tachycardia, low potassium) is given first. If one symptom is causing another (e.g., pain is causing high blood pressure) the primary cause (e.g., pain) is treated before administering medication to treat the related symptom (blood pressure). Similarly, when teaching, the nurse should provide the most important information first. For example, teach patients about *how to administer insulin* and *signs of hypoglycemia* before explaining the complex actions of insulin.

Collaborative Care. Nurses collaborate with a variety of health care providers (e.g., physician, nurse practitioner, pharmacist, dietitian, visiting nurse, case coordinator), the patient, and their caregiver. It is important to develop a therapeutic relationship and collaborate with the patient's caregiver who will support the medication regimen at home. Medical information can be overwhelming, and two listeners are better than one. The nurse should ensure that patients and their caregivers can read the medication labels and educational information provided. In the community, patients frequently require referrals to supportive resources (e.g., visiting nurses, community care) for the administration, monitoring, and evaluation of medication therapy. Patients must be connected to the essential resources prior to being discharged home from hospital or they risk nonadherence and poor health outcomes.

◆ Implementation

Health Promotion. Teaching is an essential component of primary health care, empowers patients in their self-management, and can promote adherence to the medication regimen (Box 35.11). Medication administration is an ideal time to continuously educate patients and caregivers about the conditions the medications are treating, factors influencing their health (e.g., personal health practices, genetics, physical environment), and nonmedicinal strategies that can also improve their health (e.g., diet). It is important to maintain a positive, nonjudgemental attitude and focus on a patient's strengths. The patient's health beliefs and personal, cultural, religious, and spiritual practices must also be considered when creating a schedule for medications with patients, which can improve adherence. Lastly, all patients must be educated about medication safety, which includes the proper storage, administration, and disposal of medications, such as insulin, in the home (Box 35.12).

Acute Care. Patients are often hospitalized for close observation, medication administration, and evaluation. When receiving a medication prescription, several nursing interventions are essential for safe and effective medication administration.

BOX 35.11   FOCUS ON PRIMARY HEALTH CARE

Improving Medication Adherence

When a patient is in the community setting, their ongoing treatment may include regularly taking medications. Medication adherence is especially important for persons with chronic illnesses. Ensure the patient and their caregiver:

- Understand the reason for the medication, administration techniques, adverse effects, and possible consequences of nonadherence.
- Recognize symptoms of medication adverse effects or toxicity (e.g., confusion, sedation).
- Have the cognitive and physical abilities (e.g., memory, coordination, grip strength, eyesight) necessary to safely administer medication by the intended route according to a schedule.
- Have resources (e.g., financial, transportation) and tools to manage medications (e.g., dosette, medication list with pictures, medication schedule, logbook).
- Have ongoing follow-ups and support from the health care team (e.g., visiting community nurses, scheduled reminders from the pharmacy).

BOX 35.12   PATIENT TEACHING

Safe Insulin Administration

Objective

- The patient will correctly administer subcutaneous insulin.

Teaching Strategies

Use discussion, printed information, videos, websites, and demonstration to explain:

- Where the insulin needs to be stored (e.g., refrigerator)
- That the insulin needs to be kept in its original labelled container
- Why and how to rotate sites for injection
- How to check the expiry date on the insulin vial
- How to determine the amount of insulin required (if on a sliding scale) based on the results of capillary glucose monitoring
- How to perform hand hygiene
- How to prepare a syringe with insulin for injection or prepare a prefilled insulin syringe pen
- How to select a site, cleanse the skin, and administer the subcutaneous insulin injection
- How to dispose of needles and supplies in a safe sharps container
- Keeping a daily logbook to record blood glucose results, type and dose of insulin, and injection site

Evaluation

Ask the patient to describe and demonstrate:

- Signs of hypoglycemia and actions to take
- The schedule they will follow for testing their blood and administering insulin
- The reason they are taking insulin
- Where they will store their insulin and supplies
- Reading the label of the insulin vial and the numbers on the syringe aloud (to show visual acuity)
- Performing hand hygiene and testing their capillary blood glucose
- Preparing the required insulin dose (based on the results if on a sliding scale)
- Selecting an injection site, cleansing the skin, and self-administering the insulin injection
- Disposing of needles safely
- Recording information in the logbook

Receiving Medication Prescriptions. A complete medication prescription is necessary for a medication to be administered by a nurse (Box 35.13). The nurse must inform the prescriber if any element is missing and ensure completeness before administering or altering the prescribed medication.

Accurate Transcription and Communication of Prescriptions. Nurses or a unit clerk (depending on the employer policy) transcribe (i.e., write out) the prescriber's complete prescription on the MAR. The transcribed prescription includes the patient's name, identification number, bed number, allergies, medication name, dose, frequency, route, and start and stop dates. If an institution has CPOE, the prescription may be automatically transcribed onto an electronic MAR and a computer printout may be used for medication administration (Figure 35.13). When transcribing prescriptions, the nurse must ensure that names, doses, and symbols are legible, and rewrite any smudged or illegible transcriptions. Each time a medication dose is prepared, the nurse refers to the MAR.

Transcribed prescriptions must be checked against the original prescription for accuracy and confirmed by two nurses. If the original prescription is incorrect, incomplete, or inappropriate, the nurse must consult the prescriber. The nurse is responsible for medication incidents associated with administration.

Accurate Dose Calculation and Measurement. When measuring liquid medications use a standard measuring container (e.g., oral syringe). Calculate each dose when preparing the medication, and avoid interruptions and distractions. Consult with other nurses when calculating a new or unusual dose.

Correct Administration. It is important to use aseptic techniques and proper procedures when handling and giving medications. Verify the patient's identity by using at least two and preferably three patient identifiers (Joint Commission, 2022). Some employers have *barcode medication administration* whereby the nurse scans a barcode on the patient's identification bracelet, their own identification badge, and the barcodes on medication packages to confirm identify. Perform the necessary assessments prior to administration (e.g., assessing heart rate before giving antidysrhythmic medications). Carefully monitor the patient's response to medication, especially when administering the first dose of a new medication. Document the patient's response in the patient's chart or electronic medical record.

Documenting Medication Administration. After administering a medication, document it immediately on the appropriate record form (see Figure 35.13). Some nurses will place a "dot" next to the medication to indicate that they have prepared the medication, but do not sign for a medication until after it is actually administered. Documenting immediately after administration reduces incidents.

Documenting and "signing off" an administered medication includes writing one's signature on the patient's MAR along with the date, name of the medication, dose, route, site, and exact time of administration. Document assessment parameters (e.g., blood glucose level, blood pressure, pain score) in the patient's medical record. If a patient refuses a medication or undergoes tests or procedures that result in a missed dose, the reason the medication was not given must be recorded in both the MAR and in the medical record. Some PRN medications also require the nurse to document if the medication was effective, by charting an "E," or not effective, "NE." This helps health care providers understand if current treatments for symptoms (e.g., morphine administered for pain) have been effective or if a change is needed.

Restorative Care. Medication administration activities vary among the numerous types of restorative care settings (e.g., hospice, long-term care, home). Patients with functional or cognitive limitations may require the nurse to administer medications. In the home setting, patients usually administer their own medications. Nurses are responsible for instructing patients and their families in medication action, administration, and adverse effects, even if the patient is self-administering their medications. The nurse also needs to monitor the patient's medication adherence and evaluate medication effectiveness.

Special Considerations for Administering Medications to Specific Age Groups. Nurses' knowledge of a patient's developmental stage affects the way they administer medication and allows them to anticipate reactions or responses to medication.

Infants and Children. Children vary in age, weight, body surface area, and their ability to absorb, metabolize, and eliminate medications. Medication doses are lower for children than for adults, and caution is needed when preparing children's medications. Medications are usually not packaged in unit-doses for children. Preparing the prescribed dose from an available amount of medication requires careful calculation.

All children need emotional preparation before receiving medications. The child's parents or caregivers are valuable resources for learning the best way to administer medications to their child. Sometimes the child will experience less trauma if a parent or caregiver administers the medication and the nurse supervises.

When administering medication to a child, explain the procedure to the child, using short words and simple language appropriate to the child's level of comprehension. Long explanations may increase the child's anxiety, especially for painful procedures such as an injection. Nurses need to administer medications to children even when they refuse to cooperate or they resist consistently despite explanation and encouragement. Depending on the legislation in a territory or province, children under 16 years of age usually cannot provide consent for medical treatment, and their legal surrogate decision-maker (parent/caregiver) will make decisions about medications, even if the child refuses. Children as young as 5 years old may be able to self-administer oral medications and like to be involved in their own care. This builds the basis for self-management later. If the child is uncooperative, administer the medication to the child quickly and carefully (Alberta Health Services, 2018). Allow children

---

BOX 35.13   Components of Medication Prescriptions

A complete medication prescription includes all the following information:
- *Patient's Full Name:* Distinguishes the patient from other persons with the same last name. Patients with similar names should each have an additional name alert on their medical record. May also include a patient or pharmacy identification number
- *Date and Time:* Clarifies when the medication was initially prescribed
- *Medication Name:* Correct spelling of the generic or brand name to prevent confusion with similar-sounding medications or those with similar spelling
- *Dose:* The amount or strength of the medication
- *Route:* Acceptable routes by which the medication can be given and permitted abbreviations (e.g., PO, IV, PR)
- *Timing, Frequency of Administration, Start and Stop Dates:* Time a medication needs to be initiated, how often it is given, and when the medication should be discontinued. For example: "Prednisone 5 mg PO daily for 7 days starting March 5th and stopping after the dose is administered on March 11th."
- *Special Considerations:* Additional instructions, such as "Take with food" or "Do not take while driving."
- *Prescriber's Signature:* The prescriber's signature makes the prescription a legal request.

Room: 3700-03

Saint Francis Medical Center

MEDICATION ADMINISTRATION RECORD

Patient: PDM, Pharmacy
Birth: 11/30/79 Admit: 01/01/XX
MRN: 2000403 Acct: 900015
Doctor: Jim Smith

Date: 01/18/XX – 01/19/XX

Age: 39 y Ht: 5 ft 2 in Wt: 125.2 lbs
Metric: Ht: 1 m 57 cm Wt: 56.79 kg

ADEs/Nondrug allergies: Latex – Zosyn – Amoxicillin – Insulins – Darvocet – Lugols soln. – Antihi +

	0800	0900	1000	1100	1200	1300	1400	1500	1600	1700	1800	1900	2000	2100	2200	2300	2400	0100	0200	0300	0400	0500	0600	0700
P00014 Bacitracin ointment AKA: Bacitracin ointment Dose: Apply STRGH: 30 gm/tube TID Topical: Right lower leg For external use only Testing			RL 10																					
P00029 Insulin/human regular AKA: Humulin R Dose: 15 units STRGH: 1 ml = 100 units AC Sub-Q	RL 0730																							
P00030 Fexofenadine 60 mg/pseudo 120 mg AKA: Allegra–D Sr Tab Dose: 1 tab STRGH: 60/120/tab BID Oral Auto Sub: 1 Allegra–D Tab bid For Claritin–D 12 hr and 24 hr Per P&T Comm			RL 10																					
P00036 Aspirin AKA: Aspirin 325 mg Tab Dose: 2 tab 650 mg STRGH: 325 mg/tab Q3–4h Oral Testing								RL 1315	RL 1615															
P00039 Haloperidol tablet AKA: Haldol 0.5 mg tab Dose: 1 mg STRGH: 1 mg/tab QHS Oral																								
P00035 Zolpidem AKA: Ambien 5 mg tab Dose: 5 mg STRGH: 5 mg/tab QHS PRN Oral MR × 1 Testing																								

| | 0800 | 0900 | 1000 | 1100 | 1200 | 1300 | 1400 | 1500 | 1600 | 1700 | 1800 | 1900 | 2000 | 2100 | 2200 | 2300 | 2400 | 0100 | 0200 | 0300 | 0400 | 0500 | 0600 | 0700 |

Circle = Dose not given
Initials = Dose given Page: 01 (continued)
Deltoid = R.D., L.D.
Vastus Lateralis = R.V.L., L.V.L.
Lower Abdominal = R.L.A., L.L.A.
Anterior Gluteal = R.A.G., L.A.G.
Posterior Gluteal = R.P.G., L.P.G.

Initials and signature	Initials and signature	Initials and signature
Rita Lassater RL		
Initials and signature	Initials and signature	Initials and signature
Initials and signature	Initials and signature	Initials and signature

FIGURE 35.13 Example of a medication administration record (MAR). *AC,* Active control; *ADEs,* adverse drug/medication events/effects; *AKA,* also known as; *BID,* twice a day; *MR,* medication record; *PRN,* as needed; *Q3–4h,* every 3 to 4 hours; *QHS,* before bed; *STRGH,* strength; *TID,* three times a day.

BOX 35.14 Tips for Administering Medications to Children

Oral Medications
- Use liquid forms whenever possible.
- Use droppers or oral syringes, rather than cups, which spill easily and are less accurate.
- To help them swallow pills, suggest children put the pill in their mouth and then sip liquid through a straw.
- Offer juice, a soft drink, or a frozen juice bar after a medication is swallowed.
- Mix medications with the smallest amount of food (e.g., apple sauce or syrup) if needed so they receive the entire dose.

Injections
- Use caution when selecting intramuscular (IM) injection sites for infants and small children. The deltoid muscle should not be used.
- Children are unpredictable. Ensure that someone (ideally another nurse) is available to help restrain a child if needed.
- Awake a sleeping child before giving an injection.
- Distract the child with conversation, a ringing bell, or a toy to reduce the perception of pain.
- Give the injection quickly and do not argue with the child.
- Apply a local anaesthetic (EMLA) cream to the site before the injection if possible.

BOX 35.15 FOCUS ON OLDER PERSONS
Medication Administration and Adherence
- Simplify the medication therapy plan and schedule, and deprescribe (i.e., reduce) the number of prescription medications when possible.
- Keep instructions clear and simple, and provide written material in large print.
- Assess whether the patient requires physical or cognitive support (e.g., reminders) to take medications.
- Have the patient drink a fluid before taking oral medications, to ease swallowing.
- Ask the patient to sit up straight and to tuck in their chin to decrease risk of aspiration.
- Encourage the patient to drink 1 cup of fluid after taking medications, to ensure hydration.
- Older persons have a greater sensitivity to medications, especially medications that act on the central nervous system. Carefully monitor patients' responses to medications and adverse effects, and anticipate dosage adjustments as needed.
- Ask the prescriber to substitute a liquid medication if the patient has difficulty swallowing a solid form (e.g., tablet).
- Promote healthy activities (e.g., exercise) and diet (e.g., fibre, fruits, vegetables) as alternatives to reduce the need for medications such as laxatives and vitamins.
- On a regular basis, reconcile the patient's medication list.

Adapted from Verloo, H., Chiolero, A., Kiszio, B., et al. (2017). Nurse interventions to improve medication adherence among discharged older adults: A systematic review. *Age and Ageing, 46*(5), 747–754.

to make a simple choice if possible. For example, "It's time to take your medicine now. Do you want it with water or juice?" Do not give the child the option of not taking a medication. After a medication is given, praise the child; offer a simple reward, such as a star or a token, if possible. Tips for administering medications to children are listed in Box 35.14.

Older Persons. Older persons also require consideration during medication administration (Box 35.15), related to physiological changes of aging (Figure 35.14) and other factors. Common administration challenges among older persons include forgetting to take medication doses, taking someone else's medication, and refusing doses in order to avoid adverse effects. Medication nonadherence (i.e., not taking medications as prescribed) can be related to poor eyesight, functional limitations (e.g., difficulty opening packaging), social determinants of health (e.g., lack of access to a pharmacy, lack of social support network, low income), and limited understanding of the importance or purpose of the medication (Lewis et al., 2023).

Polypharmacy. **Polypharmacy** commonly refers to the use of five or more medications by a patient, including prescribed, herbal, and OTC (i.e., nonprescription) medications. In Canada, 66% of persons over 65 years old take five medications or more (ISMP, 2018b). Polypharmacy is common because many older people live with multiple chronic health conditions, self-manage their own symptoms, and see multiple health care providers who prescribe medications and may not communicate with one another (Davies et al., 2020). Patients with polypharmacy are at increased risk of adverse effects (e.g., sedation resulting in falls) and adverse reactions (e.g., delirium) due to medication interactions, medication accumulation, and decreased elimination from the body. Polypharmacy is associated with emergency department visits, hospitalizations, increased length of hospital stay, readmission to hospital, and placement in a long-term care facility (Davies et al., 2020).

Deprescribing is an effective way to reduce polypharmacy among older persons and is being utilized internationally. **Deprescribing** refers to a collaborative, systematic process whereby the patient, caregivers, prescriber(s), and other health care providers (e.g., pharmacist,

nurse) review the patient's medications and identify opportunities to discontinue prescribed medications, inappropriately prescribed medications, or medications associated with adverse effects in older persons (ISMP, 2018b). Deprescribing usually requires the "weaning-off" or slow, reduced titration and discontinuation of one medication at a time. The Canadian Deprescribing Network and Choosing Wisely Canada provide resources to assist patients and health care providers in identifying medications for deprescribing, which typically include the following types: benzodiazepines, antipsychotics, proton pump inhibitors, and anticholinergics (ISMP, 2018b). See Choosing Wisely Canada: https://cshp.ca/choosing-wisely-canada.

◆ Evaluation

Nurses monitor patient responses to medications on an ongoing basis. For each medication, nurses require knowledge of the desired effect, the therapeutic action, and the common adverse effects. A change in a patient's condition can be physiologically related to health status, medications, or both. Nurses must be alert for reactions in a patient who takes several medications. To achieve the goal of safe and effective medication administration, a careful evaluation of both the patient's response to therapy and the patient's ability to assume responsibility for self-care is required.

To evaluate the effectiveness of nursing interventions in meeting established goals of care, nurses use evaluative measures to identify whether patient outcomes were met. Various evaluation measures are applied in the context of medication administration, including direct observation of the patient's behaviour or response, rating scales and checklists, and oral questioning. Physiological measurement is the most common method of evaluation. Examples of physiological measures are blood pressure, heart rate, and visual acuity. Patient statements can also be used as evaluative measures. Table 35.9 gives examples of goals, expected outcomes, and corresponding evaluative measures.

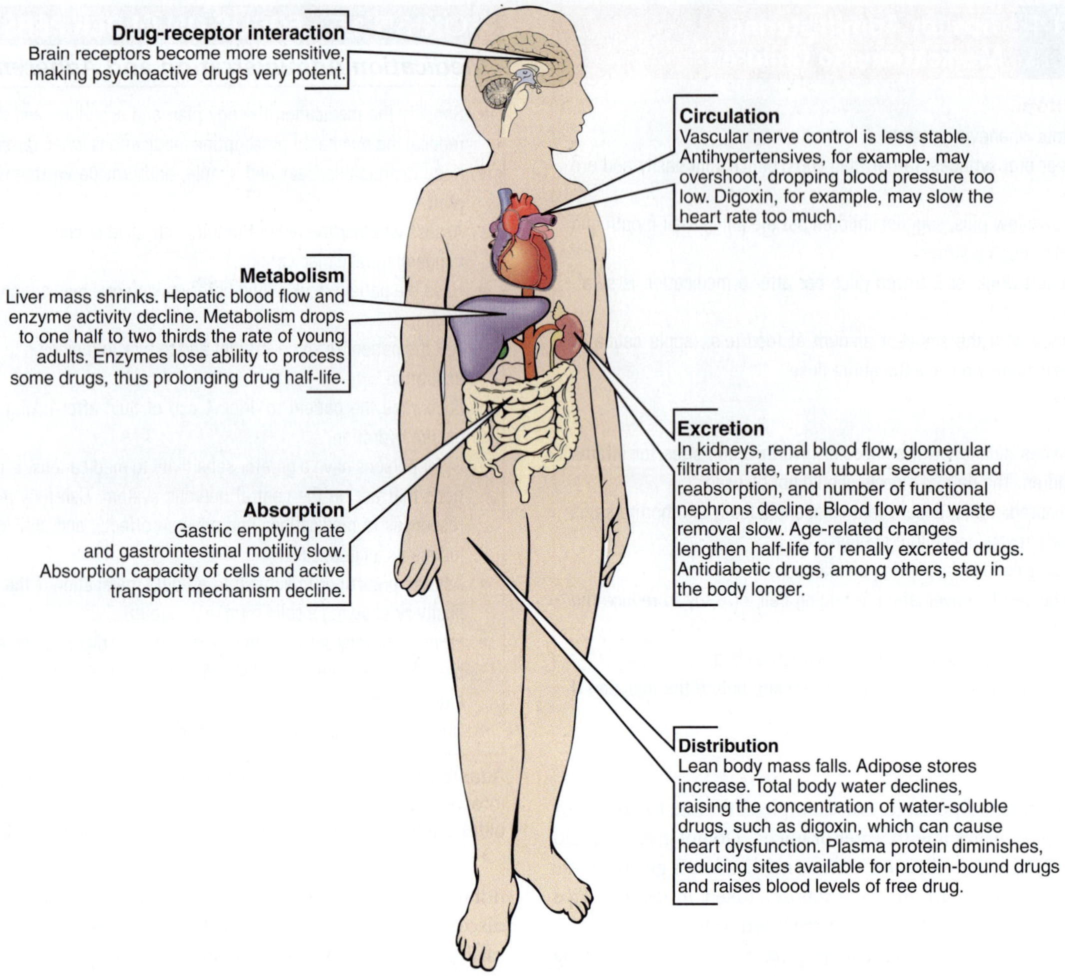

Drug-receptor interaction
Brain receptors become more sensitive, making psychoactive drugs very potent.

Circulation
Vascular nerve control is less stable. Antihypertensives, for example, may overshoot, dropping blood pressure too low. Digoxin, for example, may slow the heart rate too much.

Metabolism
Liver mass shrinks. Hepatic blood flow and enzyme activity decline. Metabolism drops to one half to two thirds the rate of young adults. Enzymes lose ability to process some drugs, thus prolonging drug half-life.

Excretion
In kidneys, renal blood flow, glomerular filtration rate, renal tubular secretion and reabsorption, and number of functional nephrons decline. Blood flow and waste removal slow. Age-related changes lengthen half-life for renally excreted drugs. Antidiabetic drugs, among others, stay in the body longer.

Absorption
Gastric emptying rate and gastrointestinal motility slow. Absorption capacity of cells and active transport mechanism decline.

Distribution
Lean body mass falls. Adipose stores increase. Total body water declines, raising the concentration of water-soluble drugs, such as digoxin, which can cause heart dysfunction. Plasma protein diminishes, reducing sites available for protein-bound drugs and raises blood levels of free drug.

FIGURE 35.14 The aging body and medication use. (From Lewis, S. M., Bucher, L., Heitkemper, M. M., et al. [Eds.]. [2019]. *Medical-surgical nursing in Canada: Assessment and management of clinical problems* [4th ed., Fig. 7.8]. Elsevier.)

TABLE 35.9	Example Evaluation for Patient Goals	
Goals	**Expected Outcomes**	**Evaluation**
The patient and their caregiver understand the patient's medication therapy.	The patient and their caregiver describe information about the medication, its dosage, schedule, purpose, and adverse effects.	Written measurement: Ask the patient to write out the medication schedule for a 24-hour period.
		Oral questioning: Ask the patient to describe the purpose, dosage, and adverse effects of each prescribed medication.
	The patient and their caregiver identify situations that require medical intervention.	Oral questioning: Ask the patient's caregiver to describe what to do if the patient has adverse effects from a medication.
	The patient and their caregiver demonstrate the appropriate administration technique.	Direct observation: Ask the patient to demonstrate the filling of an insulin syringe and self-injection.
The patient safely self-administers medications.	The patient follows a prescribed treatment regimen.	Anecdotal notes: Have the patient's caregiver keep a log of the patient's adherence to therapy for 1 week.
	The patient performs administration techniques correctly.	Direct observation: Observe while the patient instills eye drops.
	The patient identifies available resources for obtaining the necessary medication.	Oral questioning: Ask the patient's caregiver to identify how to contact the local pharmacy or community clinic to obtain the patient's medications.

MEDICATION ADMINISTRATION

Medication administration is an essential part of nursing practice and requires a sound knowledge base in anatomy, physiology, pathophysiology, pharmacology, psychology, and research. The following sections illustrate the steps involved in administering medications through various routes.

Oral Administration

The preferred way to administer medications is by mouth (Skill 35.1). Patients usually are able to ingest or self-administer oral medications with few problems. Most tablets and capsules should be administered and swallowed with approximately 60 to 100 mL of fluid; however, some situations contraindicate administering medications by mouth. The primary contraindications to giving oral medications include swallowing difficulties (i.e., dysphagia), which may impair the patient's ability to swallow medications, and the presence of GI alterations or concurrent use of gastric suction, which may impair or alter absorption.

An important precaution to take when administering any oral preparation is to protect patients from aspiration. Aspiration occurs when food, fluid, or medication intended for GI administration is inadvertently administered into the respiratory tract. Therefore, nurses must assess the patient's ability to manage and swallow oral medications prior to administering medications to protect against aspiration. Many

SKILL 35.1	**ADMINISTERING ORAL MEDICATIONS**

Delegation Considerations

The administration of oral medications cannot be delegated to unregulated care providers (UCPs). Instruct UCPs to report the occurrence of medication adverse effects immediately.

Equipment

- Medication cart or tray
- Disposable medication cups
- Patient identification labels
- Glass of water, juice, or preferred liquid (e.g., thickened)
- Pill-crushing device (if needed)
- Medication administration record (MAR)
- Barcode medication scanner (if applicable)

PROCEDURE

STEPS	RATIONALE
1. Check the accuracy and completeness of the MAR (i.e., patient's name, medication name, dosage, route, time for administration, start and stop dates). If difficult to read, review the original prescription and rewrite the prescription on the MAR.	• Ensures that the patient receives the right medication • Illegible MARs are a source of medication incidents. The original prescription is the most reliable source and only legal record of medications the patient is to receive.
2. Assess the patient's health history, medications, and allergies	• Characteristics (e.g., age) affect how a patient will respond to medications. • Medications should correspond to medical diagnoses. • Certain substances have similar compositions; never administer a substance to which a patient has a known allergy. • Recognize if the patient has any contraindications to oral medications (e.g., difficulty swallowing).
3. Collect the necessary information to administer the medication safely (i.e., action, purpose, adverse effects, normal dose, time of peak onset, whether the medication can be crushed).	• It is necessary to determine if the medication, dose, and route are appropriate, and how to administer it safely; not all medications are safe to crush.
4. Prepare medications:	
A. Organize your medication cart or room and reduce distractions. Move the medication cart to a quiet location near the patient's room or use a separate medication room.	• Saves time, reduces need to leave medications unmonitored • Reduces distractions
B. Access the patient's medicine drawer in the cart, or log in to the medication automated dispensing cabinet (ADC).	• Medications are protected from misuse when kept in a cart in a secure, monitored area or in a locked cabinet.
C. Perform hand hygiene. Prepare medications for one patient at a time. View only one patient's MAR at a time and keep all paper sheets of the MAR together.	• Ensures that the nurse prepares the right medication for the right patient
D. Collect correct medication from the patient's unit-dose medication drawer, the stock supply, or ADC cabinet. Compare the label on the medication package with the MAR at least two times (see Step 4D illustration). Check the medication expiry date.	• *This is the first and second accuracy check.* • Potency increases or decreases when medication expires.

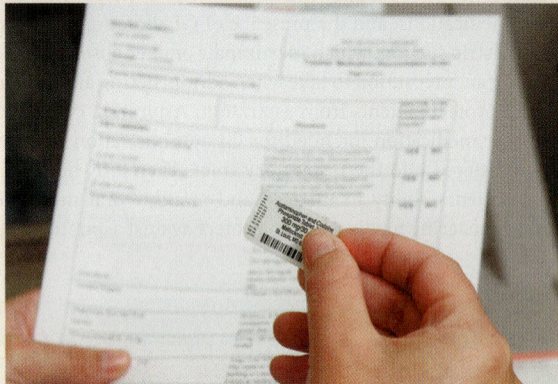

STEP 4D The nurse verifies each medication with the MAR.

E. Calculate the medication dose as necessary. Double-check calculations and verify calculations with another nurse according to your employer policies or if needed.

- Double-checking reduces the risk of calculation errors.

F. If preparing a controlled substance, check the patient's MAR and the controlled substance inventory flowsheet or ADC to determine the last time the medication was administered. Compare the inventory recorded with the actual supply available to identify any discrepancies.

- This reduces the risk of double-dosing if the patient is receiving controlled substances on a prn (as needed) schedule.
- Controlled substance laws require nurses to carefully monitor and count controlled substances such as opioids to avoid incidents and misuse.

G. If preparing tablets or capsules from a multidose stock bottle, pour the required number into an empty medication cup. Do not touch the medication with your fingers. Return extra tablets or capsules to the bottle. If necessary, split scored or unscored medications using a clean a pill-splitter. Identify scored tablets by looking for a line that divides the tablet in half.

- A clean (nonsterile) technique is required of medication administration.
- Cleaning the pill-splitter removes potential contaminants.

H. If preparing unit-dose tablets or capsules, place the packaged tablet or capsule directly into a medicine cup. Do not remove the package (see Step 4H illustration.)

- Packaging maintains the cleanliness of medication and enables the nurse to identify the medication name and dose at the bedside.

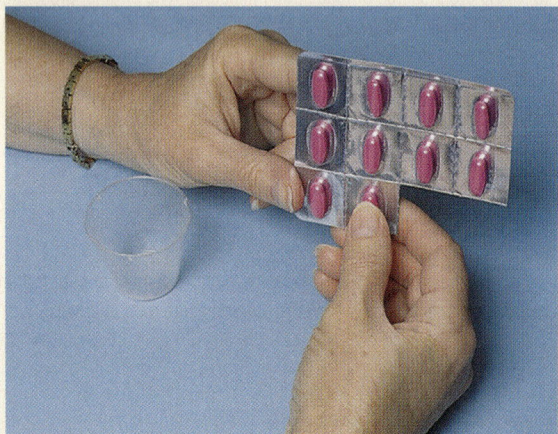

STEP 4H Place tablets or capsules into medicine cup without removing the packaging.

CRITICAL DECISION POINT: *If you are preparing controlled substances, check the controlled substance inventory flowsheet or computerized ADC record for the previous medication count and compare it against the actual stock present. You are responsible for being aware of and upholding laws regarding the use of controlled substances.*

SKILL 35.1   ADMINISTERING ORAL MEDICATIONS—cont'd

STEPS	RATIONALE
I. Place all tablets or capsules to be given to the patient at one time in a single medicine cup in their packaging, with the patient's identification label attached. If a medication requires an assessment prior to administration (e.g., pulse rate or blood pressure), keep this medication separate. Remove the patient's identification label and discard the label in the appropriate confidential garbage can.	• Labelling ensures that the nurse administers the medication to the right patient. • Separating medications that require an assessment before administration makes it easier for the nurse to withhold medications, if needed. • Disposing of the patient's label in a confidential garbage can is necessary to protect patient confidentiality.

> **CRITICAL DECISION POINT:** *Not all medications can be crushed (e.g., capsules and enteric-coated medications). When in doubt whether a medication can be crushed, consult your pharmacist. When pills are crushed, the patient is more likely to experience choking or aspiration of particles of medication or soft food. Please see the ISMP (2020b) document at https://www.ismp.org/tools/donotcrush.pdf for information about crushing pills if the pharmacy is not available or is closed.*

J. If the patient has difficulty swallowing, and liquid medications are not an option, use a pill-crushing device to crush the pills (see Step 4J illustration). Clean a grinder pill crusher before using. If a pill-crushing device is not available, place the tablet inside a medication cup, place another medication cup on top of it, and press on the top cup with a blunt instrument until the pill is crushed. Mix crushed tablets in a small amount of soft, moist food (custard or applesauce).	• Large tablets can be difficult to swallow. A crushed tablet mixed with palatable, moist soft foods such as applesauce is usually easier to swallow. • Cleaning pill-crushing devices ensures contamination of medications does not occur.

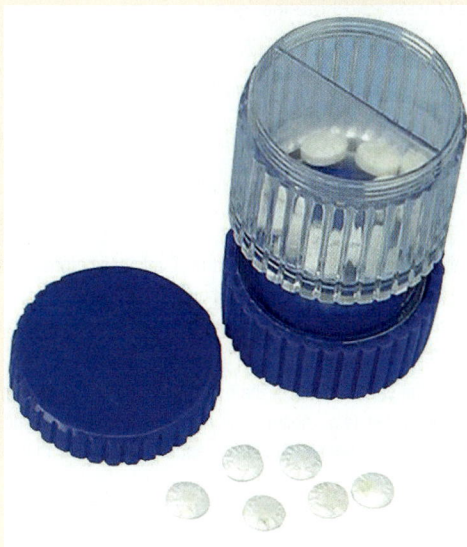

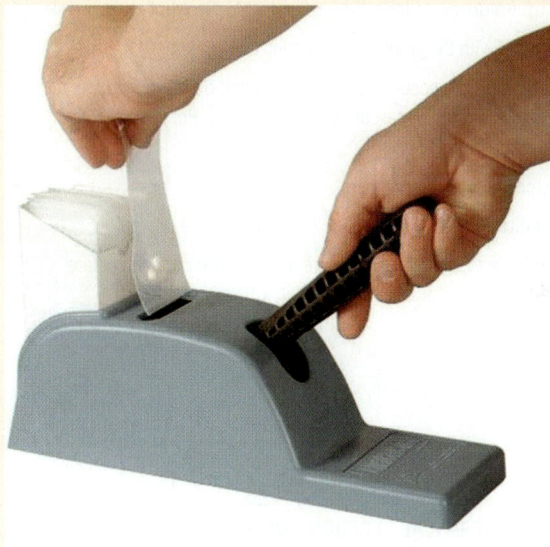

STEP 4J Pill-crushing devices. **A,** Grinder pill crusher. **B,** Pill crusher with medication bags. (Photos reprinted with permission from Ocelco, Inc., 2021.)

K. To prepare liquids:	
(1) Read the directions for each medication, as some may require you to shake the container. Medications in a unit-dose container (e.g., sealed cup or syringe) with the correct amount to administer are ready for use. If preparing medications from a multidose stock bottle, remove the bottle cap and place the cap on its side.	• If directed, shaking the container mixes the medication before administration. • Placing the cap of the bottle on its side avoids contaminating the inside of the cap.
(2) Hold a multidose bottle with the label against the palm of your hand while pouring.	• Holding the bottle with your hand over the label ensures that spilled liquid will not soil or fade the label.
(3) Fill a medication cup to the desired level on the scale and measure at eye level (see Step 4K[3] illustration). The scale should be even with the fluid level at its surface or the base of the meniscus, not at its edges. Draw up volumes of less than 10 mL in a needleless oral syringe (see Step 4K[3] illustration).	• Ensures the right dose is prepared • Oral syringes are more accurate for small doses of medication.

Continued

SKILL 35.1 ADMINISTERING ORAL MEDICATIONS—cont'd

STEPS	RATIONALE

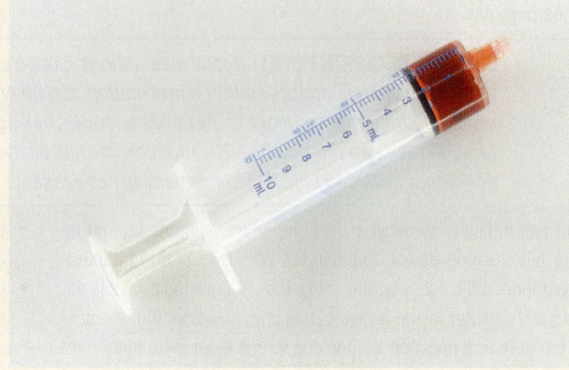

STEP 4K(3) A, Pour the desired volume of liquid so that the base of the meniscus is level with the line on the scale. **B,** Use a needleless oral syringe to draw up volumes of less than 10 mL. (*A,* iStockphoto/mayakova; *B,* © CanStock Photo Inc./georgeburba.)

L. Compare the MAR with the prepared medication and container.	• *This is the second accuracy check.*
M. Return stock containers, unopened and unneeded unit-dose medications to safe storage (e.g., medication cart drawer) immediately. Read the labels of stock bottles again.	• This is an additional *accuracy check* for medication in multiple-dose containers.
N. Do not leave medications unattended.	• Medications must be monitored and secure at all times.
5. Administering medications:	
A. Take medications to the patient at the correct time. Perform hand hygiene.	• Medications are administered within 30 minutes before or after the prescribed time to ensure the intended therapeutic effect. • Give STAT medications immediately or single-time medications at the time prescribed.
B. Identify the patient using two to three patient identifiers.	• Asking the patient to state their name, comparing the patient's name and one other identifier (e.g., hospital ID number) on the MAR and ID bracelet, and scanning the patient's barcode (if applicable) ensure that you have the right patient.

CRITICAL DECISION POINT: *Replace patient identification bracelets (i.e., armbands) that are missing, illegible, or faded.*

C. Assess the patient to determine if oral medications are indicated and safe to administer (e.g., blood pressure is elevated and patient is due for antihypertensive) or contraindicated (e.g., vomiting, drowsy, unable to swallow) to be administered or avoided.	• Impaired swallowing and drowsiness are risks for aspiration. • Alterations in gastrointestinal (GI) function affect medication distribution, absorption, and elimination. • Medications may be removed through GI suction before being absorbed. • Poor liver and kidney functions affect medication metabolism and elimination.

CRITICAL DECISION POINT: *If the patient has any contraindications for receiving oral medications, or if you are in doubt of the patient's ability to swallow, temporarily withhold medication and inform the prescriber.*

D. Explain the purpose and action of each medication to the patient. Assess the patient's understanding and encourage them to ask questions.	• The patient has the right to be informed. • Questions indicate the need for teaching. • Understanding improves medication adherence. • Assessment may reveal problems such as medication adverse effects, cost, access, misuse, or lack of perceived benefit.
E. Assess the patient's preferences for fluids. Maintain fluid restriction when applicable.	• Offering fluids during medication administration increases the patient's fluid intake (unless contraindicated). • Fluids ease swallowing and facilitate absorption from the GI tract.

SKILL 35.1	**ADMINISTERING ORAL MEDICATIONS—cont'd**
STEPS	**RATIONALE**

STEPS	RATIONALE
F. Compare labels of the medications with the MAR at the patient's bedside.	• *This is the third accuracy check.*
G. Assist the patient to a sitting position (or side-lying position if sitting is contraindicated).	• A sitting position prevents aspiration during swallowing (Mandel & Niederman, 2019).
H. Administer medications:	
(1) *For tablets:* The patient may wish to hold solid medications in their hand or in a cup before placing them in their mouth.	• The patient can become familiar by seeing of each of their medications.
(2) Offer water or juice to help the patient swallow the medications. Give cold carbonated water if it is available, not contraindicated, and preferred by the patient.	• Offering a choice of fluids promotes the patient's comfort and can improve fluid intake. Carbonated water helps passage of the tablet through the esophagus.
(3) *For sublingual-administered medications:* Have the patient place the medication under the tongue and allow it to dissolve completely (see Figure 35.4). Caution the patient against swallowing the tablet.	• Medication is absorbed through the blood vessels of the undersurface of the tongue. • If the medication is swallowed, it is destroyed by gastric juices and not delivered.
(4) *For buccal medications:* Have the patient place the medication in the mouth against the mucous membranes of the cheek until it dissolves (see Figure 35.5). Avoid administering liquids until the buccal medication has dissolved.	• Buccal medications act locally on mucosa or systemically as they are swallowed in saliva.
(5) *For powdered medications:* Mix with the directed quantity of liquids at bedside and give to the patient to drink immediately.	• Powdered medications may thicken and harden if mixed far in advance.
(6) Caution the patient against chewing or swallowing lozenges.	• Lozenges are absorbed through the oral mucosa, not gastric mucosa.
(7) Give effervescent powders and tablets immediately after they have dissolved.	• Effervescence improves medication taste and often relieves GI problems.
I. If the patient is unable to hold medications in their hand or in a cup, place the medication cup to the patient's lips and gently introduce each medication into the mouth, one at a time. Do not rush.	• Administering a single tablet or capsule eases swallowing and decreases the risk of aspiration.
J. If a tablet or capsule falls to the floor, discard it and repeat the preparation.	• Medication is contaminated when it touches the floor.
K. Stay at the bedside until the patient has completely swallowed each medication. If you are uncertain whether the medication was swallowed, ask the patient to open their mouth and check their cheeks for "pocketing."	• The nurse is responsible for ensuring that the patient receives the prescribed dose. If left unattended, the patient may discard, save (i.e., stockpile), or divert the medication to someone else, which could be harmful.
L. For highly acidic medications (e.g., aspirin), offer the patient a nonfat snack (e.g., crackers) if not contraindicated.	• A nonfat snack reduces the possible gastric irritation from highly acidic medication.
M. If the patient has received any crushed or liquid medications and they are at risk for aspiration (e.g., older age, problems swallowing), encourage them to complete oral care by swishing and spitting out water, and brushing their tongue and teeth.	• Oral care reduces the risk of aspiration pneumonia related to medication, food, and liquid residue in the mouth.
N. Assist the patient in returning to a comfortable position.	• The patient's comfort is maintained.
O. Clean the work area and restock any materials you have used.	• A clean and organized work area allows for efficient medication preparation.
P. Evaluate the patient's response to medications at times that correlate with the medication's onset, peak, and duration.	• Allows the nurse to evaluate the medication's benefit and elimination (e.g., when the medication effect is wearing off) and notice adverse effects or allergic reactions

UNEXPECTED OUTCOMES	**RELATED INTERVENTIONS**
Adverse effects (e.g., toxic effects, allergic reactions)	• Symptoms such as urticaria, rash, pruritus, rhinitis, and wheezing may indicate an allergic reaction. • Withhold further doses, and add allergy information to the patient's health record. • Notify the prescriber, the pharmacy, and Health Canada if a patient exhibits adverse effects or an adverse reaction.

Continued

SKILL 35.1   ADMINISTERING ORAL MEDICATIONS—cont'd

UNEXPECTED OUTCOMES	RELATED INTERVENTIONS
Patient refuses medication	• Explore reasons why the patient does not want to take the medication. • Provide education to address any misunderstandings of the medication. • Do not force the patient to take the medication; patients have the right to refuse treatment. • If the patient continues to refuse medication after you have provided education, document this on the MAR. Refused medications are usually indicated by circling the dose missed. Record in the medical record why the medication was withheld and notify the prescriber.

DOCUMENTATION AND REPORTING
• Record the administration of oral medications on the MAR immediately after administering the medications.
• Record the reason any medication was withheld, according to employer policies.
• Record the medication's effect in the patient's medical record and/or MAR, and report effects to the prescriber, if indicated (e.g., report urine output following administration of a diuretic if prescribed).

CARE IN THE COMMUNITY CONSIDERATIONS
• To ensure safe medication administration at home in the community, instruct patients on all aspects of medication administration, including dosage, desired effect, when to take the medications, proper storage of the medications, anticipated adverse effects, and whether to take medication with or without food.
• Evaluate the patient's ability to safely self-administer medications. If the patient needs assistance in self-administration, introduce nursing interventions, such as a chart or pillbox. If interventions fail and the patient still is unable to safely administer medications, notify the prescriber.

BOX 35.16   Strategies to Protect Patients From Aspiration

• Assess the patient's swallowing abilities, including their ability to cough, the presence of a gag reflex, and their level of alertness, which may fluctuate.
• Give medications at mealtimes or when the patient is most alert.
• Prepare oral medications in the form that is easiest for the patient to swallow.
• Allow the patient to hold and drink from a cup of water, if possible. Thicken liquids or offer fruit nectar if thin fluids (i.e., water) are not tolerated.
• Avoid using straws, which can increase the risk of aspiration and swallowing of air.
• Position the patient in a side-lying or upright semi-Fowler or high-Fowler position.
• Allow the patient to self-administer medications, if possible.
• If the patient has unilateral weakness, place the medication in the stronger side of the mouth.
• Administer pills one at a time, ensuring that each pill is fully swallowed and not caught in the patient's cheek before administering the next.
• Stop administering medications if the patient starts sputtering or coughing. Consult the prescriber and administer medications through another route or form, if available (e.g., rectal).
• Advise or assist the patient to perform oral hygiene following medication administration.

organizations have standardized processes for nurses to assess patients' safe swallowing at the bedside. A multidisciplinary approach through consults with a speech-language pathologist, dietitian, or occupational therapist is also recommended to help manage swallowing difficulties. Proper positioning is essential in preventing aspiration. The patient should be seated upright and slightly flex their head in a chin-down position when receiving oral medications, unless these positions are contraindicated by the patient's condition (Mandel & Niederman, 2019). Box 35.16 summarizes techniques used to protect the patient from aspirating.

For patients with enteral tubes (i.e., nasogastric, orogastric, gastrostomy, intestinal), liquid medications are preferred, but some tablets can be crushed and some capsules opened to mix in a solution for administration. Buccal, sublingual, enteric-coated, or sustained-release medications cannot be crushed. The nurse must read medication labels carefully before crushing a tablet or opening a capsule. Enteral (i.e., tube) feeding may need to be held for a time before or after a medication is administered. The nurse should check with the medication monograph and the employer policy. Medication times should be consolidated to avoid frequent enteral feeding interruptions. If the desired effect is not achieved following medication administration via the enteral route, there may be a problem with the medication's bioavailability or absorption and a different medication or route may be required. The need for medication administration through an enteral tube should be continuously reassessed because complications can occur. The procedure for administering medications via the enteral route is described in Box 35.17. Figure 35.15 illustrates a patient holding a gastrostomy feeding tube that may be used to administer medications.

Topical Medication Applications
Topical medications are medications that are applied locally, most often to intact skin but also to mucous membranes. They are prepared in many forms, including lotions, pastes, and ointments (see Table 35.1).

Skin Applications. Because many locally applied medications, such as lotions, pastes, oils, and ointments, cause both systemic and local effects, these medications are applied with the use of gloves and applicators. The nurse uses sterile techniques if the patient has an open wound. Skin encrustation and dead tissues harbour microorganisms and block contact of the medications from the tissues to be treated. Before applying medications, the area to be treated is cleaned thoroughly by washing the skin gently with soap and water, soaking an involved site, or locally debriding tissue (see Chapter 47).

Each type of topical medication is applied according to the directions to ensure proper penetration and absorption. When applying ointments or pastes, spread the medication evenly over the involved surface and cover the area well without applying an overly thick layer. Application of a gauze dressing over the medication may be prescribed to prevent soiling of clothes and wiping away of the medication. Lightly

BOX 35.17 PROCEDURAL GUIDELINE
Administering Medications Through an Enteral Tube

Delegation Considerations

The administration of medications through a feeding tube cannot be delegated to an unregulated care provider. Instruct unregulated care providers to recognize and report any adverse effects immediately—for example, pain at the gastrostomy site, tube displacement, patient vomiting or coughing up liquid feeds or medications.

Equipment

- 60-mL syringe (catheter tip for large-bore tubes, Luer-Lok tip for small-bore tubes)
- Graduated container
- Sterile water
- Medications to be administered
- Pill crusher, if medication is in tablet form
- Medication administration record (MAR)
- Clean, disposable gloves
- Barcode scanner (if applicable)

Procedure

1. Check the accuracy and completeness of the MAR (i.e., patient's name, medication name, dosage, route, time of administration, start and stop dates). If it is difficult to read, review the original prescription and rewrite the prescription on the MAR.
2. Assess the patient's health history, medications, and allergies.
3. Collect the necessary information to administer the medication safely (i.e., purpose, normal dose, adverse effects). Determine if medications need to be given on an empty stomach or if they are compatible with the enteral feeding.
4. Verify the confirmed enteral tube placement in the medical record and the prescription to use the tube for medication administration (see Chapter 43).

5. Perform hand hygiene. Prepare the medications in a liquid form (i.e., elixir, suspension, solution). Ensure tablets are crushable before crushing. Check the expiry dates of medications (see Skill 35.1, Steps 5A–H).
6. Check the label of the medication with the MAR two times during preparation. (This is the *first and second accuracy check*.)
7. Take the medication to the patient at the correct time. Perform hand hygiene.
8. Identify the patient using two to three identifiers. Asking the patient to state their name, comparing the patient's name and one other identifier (hospital ID number) on the MAR and the patient's ID bracelet, and scanning the patient's barcode on their ID bracelet ensure that you have the right patient.
9. Compare the labels on the medications against the MAR record one more time at the patient's bedside. This is the *third accuracy check*.
10. Explain the procedure and the medications to the patient. Assess the patient's understanding of their medications.
11. Perform hand hygiene and put on clean, disposable gloves.
12. Dissolve the crushed tablets, powders, and opened capsules in at least 30 mL of sterile water. Do not give solid medications through the tube, and do not add medications to an enteral feed pouch.
13. Assess the patient. Verify the placement of tubes that enter the patient's mouth or nose by attaching the 60-mL syringe to the primary large port on the feeding tube and aspirating gastric contents (see Chapter 43).
14. Draw up 30–60 mL of sterile water in the syringe and flush the enteral tube slowly to ensure it is patent.
15. Draw up the medications and administer them slowly through the enteral tube.
16. Flush the enteral tube with 30–60 mL of sterile water when complete.
17. Remove gloves and perform hand hygiene.
18. Document administration on the MAR.
19. Continually evaluate the patient's response to medication therapy.

Adapted from Morgan, B. (2021). *Standard of care enteral feeding tubes and nutrition.* London Health Science Centre, London, Ontario, Canada. https://www.lhsc.on.ca/critical-care-trauma-centre/standard-of-care-enteral-feeding-tubes-and-nutrition

spread lotions, oils, and creams onto the skin's surface; rubbing often causes irritation. Apply a liniment by rubbing it gently but firmly into the skin. After that, dust a powder lightly to cover the affected area with a thin layer. During any application, assess the skin thoroughly. When recording the administration, note the area where the medication was applied, the name of the medication, and the condition of the skin.

Some topical medications are applied in the form of a transdermal patch that remains in place for an extended period of time (e.g., 12 hours or 7 days). Many patches are clear, which makes them difficult to see. Common transdermal patches exist with fentanyl (for pain control), nicotine (for smoking cessation), and nitrogen (for blood pressure reduction) and for contraception. Nurses and patients may inadvertently leave old transdermal patches in place, which results in the patient receiving an overdose of the medication. Therefore, it is important to carefully assess the patient's skin and ensure that the existing patch is removed before applying a new patch. Do not apply transparent film dressings such as Tegaderm over the top of transdermal patches as this can affect the medication action. The following guidelines are used to ensure safe administration of transdermal or topical medications (Khan & Sharman, 2021):

1. Perform hand hygiene and apply clean, disposable gloves. Transdermal medications can be absorbed through the nurse's skin during administration.

2. Assess if the patient has an old transdermal patch applied. Remove the old patch and document the removal.
3. Rotate the site of the transdermal patch application (e.g., right upper arm for 24 hours followed by left upper arm for 24 hours).
4. Disinfect and clean the skin where the new patch is to be applied.
5. Apply the new patch to the skin. If it is difficult to see, write the date and your initial directly on the patch.
6. Remove gloves and perform hand hygiene.
7. Document on the MAR the name of medication, dose, site where the new patch was applied and your initials.
8. Monitor for effectiveness of the medication.

Nasal Instillation. Patients with nasal sinus alterations may receive medications by spray, drops, or tampons (Box 35.18). The most commonly administered form of nasal instillation (administration of a liquid) is a decongestant spray or drops, which are used to relieve symptoms of sinus congestion and colds. Patients should be cautioned to avoid abuse of medications because overuse can lead to a rebound effect in which the nasal congestion worsens. When excess decongestant solution is swallowed, serious systemic effects can develop, especially in children. Saline drops are safer as a decongestant for children than nasal preparations that contain sympathomimetics (e.g., Afrin or Neo-Synephrine).

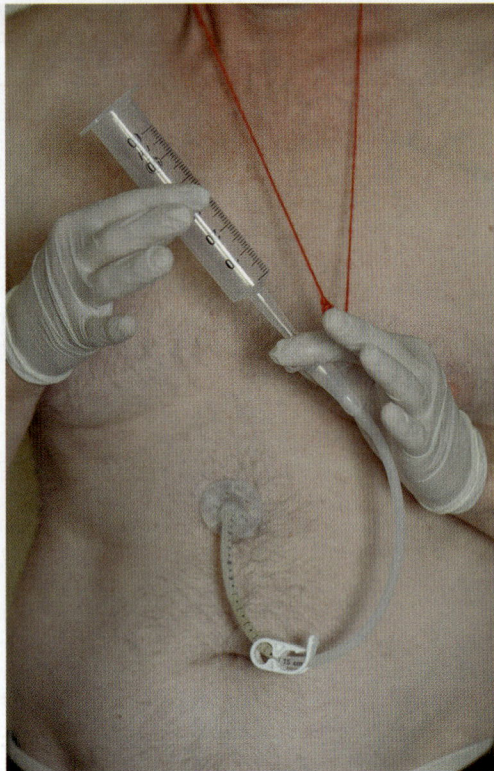

FIGURE 35.15 Patient with a percutaneous gastrostomy tube and 60-mL syringe for medication administration (iStockphoto/Lighthousebay.)

Self-administering sprays is easier because the patient can control the spray and inhale as it enters the nasal passages. For patients who use nasal sprays repeatedly, check the nares for irritation. Position patients to permit the medication to reach the affected sinus.

Eye Instillation. Common eye medications used by patients are eye drops and ointments, including OTC preparations, such as artificial tears and vasoconstrictors (e.g., Visine and Murine). Many patients receive prescribed **ophthalmic** medications for eye conditions, such as glaucoma, and after cataract extraction. In older persons, the ease with which eye medications can be self-administered can be affected by physiological changes, including poor vision, hand tremors, and difficulty grasping or manipulating containers. Patients and their caregivers should be instructed in the proper techniques for administering eye medications (Skill 35.2). Determine the ability of the patient and their caregiver to administer the eye medication by demonstrating the procedure. Showing patients each step of the procedure for instilling eye drops can improve their adherence. Follow these principles when administering eye medications:

- The cornea of the eye is richly supplied with pain fibres and thus is very sensitive to anything applied to it. Avoid instilling any form of eye medication directly onto the cornea.
- The risk of transmitting infection from one eye to the other is high. Avoid touching the eyelids or other eye structures with eyedroppers or ointment tubes.
- Use eye medication only for the patient's affected eye.
- Never allow a patient to use another patient's eye medications.

Intraocular Administration. Some medications are administered intraocularly (see Skill 35.2). Intraocular medications resemble a contact

---

BOX 35.18 PROCEDURAL GUIDELINE

Administering Nasal Instillations

Delegation Consideration

The administration of nasal drops and ointments cannot be delegated. Instruct unregulated care providers to report the occurrence of medication adverse effects immediately.

Equipment

- Prepared medication with a clean dropper or spray container
- Facial tissue
- Small pillow (optional)
- Washcloth (optional)
- Clean, disposable gloves
- Penlight (to inspect nares; if ointment is to be applied to a specific lesion inside the nares)
- Medication administration record (MAR)
- Barcode scanner (if applicable)

Procedure

1. Check the accuracy and completeness of each MAR, including the following: the patient's name and the medication name, dosage, route, time for administration, and start and stop dates. If difficult to read, review the original prescription and rewrite the prescription on the MAR.
2. If nasal drops are to be administered, refer to the medical record to determine which sinus is affected, so that you can position the patient appropriately for medication instillation.
3. Review the patient's health history, medications, and allergies. Medical conditions (e.g., cardiovascular disease, hyperthyroidism) can contraindicate the use of decongestants that stimulate the central nervous system. Adverse effects may occur, such as transient hypertension, tachycardia, palpitations, and headache.

4. Collect the information necessary to administer the medication safely, including the medication's action, purpose, adverse effects, normal dose, time of peak onset, method of delivery, and nursing implications.
5. Perform hand hygiene. Prepare the medication.
6. Ensure that you compare the label of the medication against the MAR at least two times.
7. Take the medication to the patient at the correct time. Perform hand hygiene. Put on clean, disposable gloves.
8. Identify the patient by using two to three identifiers. Asking the patient to state their name, comparing the patient's name and one other identifier (e.g., the hospital ID number) on the MAR and the patient's ID bracelet, and scanning the patient's barcode on their ID bracelet (if applicable) ensure that you have the right patient.
9. Explain the procedure to the patient regarding the positioning and the sensations to expect, such as a burning or stinging of the mucosa, or a choking sensation as the medication trickles into the throat.
10. Assess the patient's knowledge regarding the use of nasal instillations and the technique for instillation, and determine whether the patient is willing to learn self-administration.
11. Using a penlight, inspect the condition of the nose and sinuses. Palpate sinuses for tenderness. Remove gloves and perform hand hygiene.
12. Compare the MAR with the medication labels at the patient's bedside.
13. Perform hand hygiene. Put on clean, disposable gloves.
14. Gently roll or shake the medication container as directed.
15. Instruct the patient to clear or blow the nose gently before you administer the medication, unless contraindicated (e.g., risk of increased intracranial pressure or nosebleeds). Clearing the nose helps to remove mucus and secretions that can block medication distribution.

BOX 35.18 PROCEDURAL GUIDELINE—cont'd

Administering Nasal Instillations

16. Administer nasal drops:
   A. Assist the patient to a supine position and position the head properly to facilitate access to the nasal passages.
      (1). To access the posterior pharynx, tilt the patient's head backward.
      (2). To access the ethmoid and sphenoid sinuses, tilt the head back over the edge of the bed or place a small pillow under the patient's shoulder and tilt the head back (see Step 16A[2] illustration).
      (3). To access the frontal and maxillary sinuses, tilt the head back over the edge of the bed or pillow with the head turned toward the side to be treated (see Step 16A[3] illustration). This position will allow the medication to drain into the affected sinus.

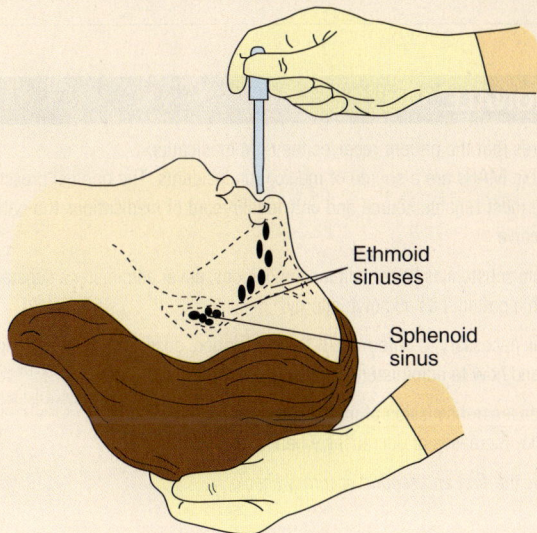

STEP 16A(2) Position for instilling nose drops into the ethmoid and sphenoid sinuses.

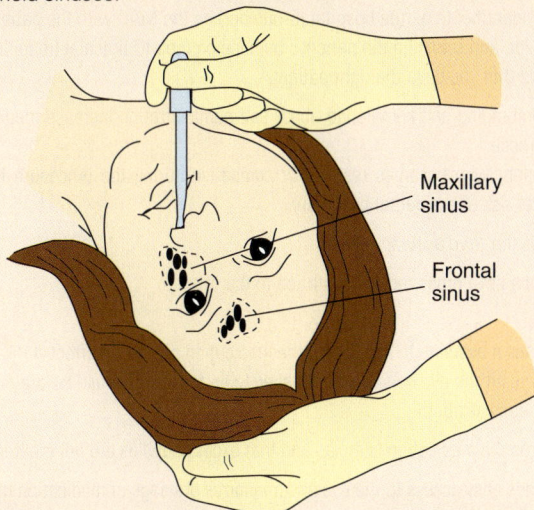

STEP 16A(3) Position for instilling nose drops into the frontal and maxillary sinuses.

   B. Support the patient's head with your nondominant hand to prevent the straining of neck muscles.
   C. Instruct the patient to breathe through the mouth, which reduces the chance of aspirating nasal drops into the trachea and lungs.
   D. Hold the dropper 1 cm above the nares to avoid contamination of the dropper. Instill the prescribed number of drops toward midline of the ethmoid bone to facilitate distribution of medication over the nasal mucosa.
   E. Have the patient remain in a supine position for 5 minutes to prevent premature loss of medication through the nares.
   F. Offer a facial tissue to blot a runny nose, but caution the patient against blowing the nose for several minutes.
17. Assist the patient to a comfortable position after the medication is absorbed.
18. Administering nasal spray:
   A. Assist the patient to a comfortable high Fowler's position or a sitting position.
   B. Administer the nasal spray with the patient's head upright. Tipping the opening of the nasal spray container downward will cause the medication to be administered in a stream, not a spray, and will deliver more medication than the prescribed medication.
   C. Offer a facial tissue to blot a runny nose, but caution the patient against blowing the nose for several minutes.
19. Dispose of soiled supplies in the garbage can, and perform hand hygiene.
20. Document administration on the MAR.
21. Observe the patient for adverse effects for 15 to 30 minutes after administration. Medications absorbed through mucosa can cause a systemic reaction.
22. Assess whether the patient can breathe through the nose, to determine the medication's effectiveness. The patient may need to occlude one nostril at a time and breathe deeply.
23. Evaluate the patient's response to the medications at times that correlate with the medication's onset, peak, and duration. Re-inspect the condition of the nasal passages between the instillations.
24. If possible, have the patient demonstrate self-administration at the next time of medication administration.

SKILL 35.2 ADMINISTERING OPHTHALMIC MEDICATIONS

Delegation Considerations

The administration of eyedrops and ointments cannot be delegated. Instruct unregulated care providers to report the occurrence of medication adverse effects, including the potential for visual difficulty, immediately.

Equipment

- Medication bottle with sterile eyedropper, ointment tube, or medicated intraocular disc
- Cotton ball or tissue
- Washbasin filled with warm water and washcloth if eyes have crust or need drainage
- Eye patch and tape (optional)
- Clean, disposable gloves
- Medication administration record (MAR)
- Barcode scanner (if applicable)

PROCEDURE

STEPS	RATIONALE
1. Check the accuracy and completeness of each MAR, including the following: patient's name, the medication name and dosage (e.g., number of drops), the route and eye to be treated, time of administration, and start and stop dates. If difficult to read, review the original prescription order and rewrite the MAR.	• Ensures that the patient receives the right medication • Illegible MARs are a source of medication incidents. The original prescription is the most reliable source and only legal record of medications the patient is to receive.
2. Assess the patient's health history, medications and allergies, including latex.	• Certain substances have similar compositions; never administer a substance to which a patient has a known allergy.
3. Collect the information necessary to administer the medication safely.	• This is necessary to determine if the medication, dose, and route are appropriate, and how to administer it safely.
4. Perform hand hygiene. Prepare medication (see Skill 35.1, Steps 4A–H): Check the medication expiry date.	• Decreases transmission of microorganisms • Potency increases or decreases when medication expires.
5. Ensure that you check the label of the medication against the MAR at least two times while preparing the medication.	• This is the *first and second accuracy check*.
6. Take the medication to the patient at the correct time. Perform hand hygiene.	
7. Identify the patient by using two to three patient identifiers.	• Asking the patient to state their name, comparing the patient's name and one other identifier (e.g., the hospital ID number) on the MAR with the patient's ID bracelet, and scanning the patient's barcode on their ID bracelet (if applicable) ensure that you have the right patient.
8. Explain the procedure to the patient, including the positioning and sensations to expect, such as burning or stinging. Assess the patient's level of consciousness, knowledge of medication therapy, and ability to manipulate and hold an eye dropper for self-administration.	• Understanding and knowledge about self-administration increase medication adherence. • A patient who becomes restless or combative during the procedure is at a greater risk of accidental eye injury.
9. Compare labels of medications with the MAR.	• This is the *third accuracy check*.
10. If eye drops are stored in the refrigerator, allow them to reach room temperature before instilling them.	• Warming eye drops reduces irritation to the eye.
11. Perform hand hygiene and put on clean disposable gloves. Assess the patient's external eye structures and any symptoms of visual alterations.	• Provides a baseline to evaluate if the medication causes an effect • Indicates if the eye needs to be cleaned (e.g., to remove crust) before medication administration
12. Gently roll the medication container; do not shake.	• Ensures the medication is mixed and that excess bubbles are not created
13. Ask the patient to lie supine or to sit back in a chair with the head slightly hyperextended.	• Provides easy access to the eye and minimizes drainage of medication through the tear duct
14. If crusts or drainage is present along the eyelid margins or the inner canthus, gently wash it away. Soak any crusts that are dried and difficult to remove by applying a damp washcloth or cotton ball over the eye for a few minutes. Always wipe from the inner canthus to the outer canthus.	• Crusts or drainage harbours microorganisms. • Soaking allows easy removal of the crusts and prevents pressure from being applied directly over the eye. • Cleansing from the inner canthus to the outer canthus helps prevent entrance of microorganisms into the lacrimal duct.
15. Hold a cotton ball or clean tissue in your nondominant hand.	• Cotton or tissue absorbs the medication that escapes the eye.

SKILL 35.2	ADMINISTERING OPHTHALMIC MEDICATIONS—cont'd
STEPS	**RATIONALE**

16. With the tissue or cotton resting below the lower lid, gently press downward with your thumb or forefinger against the bony orbit.

- Exposes the lower conjunctival sac. Retraction against the bony orbit prevents pressure and trauma to the eyeball and prevents your fingers from touching the eye.

17. Ask the patient to look at the ceiling and explain the steps to the patient.

- Retracts the sensitive cornea up and away from the conjunctival sac and reduces stimulation of the blink reflex.

A. Instill the eye drops:
  (1) With your dominant hand resting on the patient's forehead, hold the filled medication eyedropper or the ophthalmic solution approximately 1–2 cm above the conjunctival sac (see Step 17A[1] illustration).

- Prevents accidental contact of the eyedropper with eye structures, reducing risk of injury to the eye and transfer of infection to dropper. Ophthalmic medications are sterile.

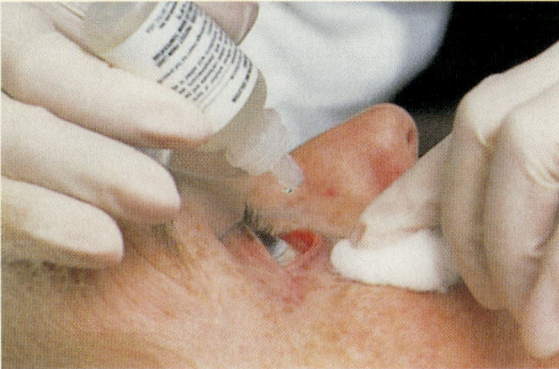

STEP 17A(1) Hold the eyedropper above the conjunctival sac.

  (2) Instill the prescribed number of medication drops into the conjunctival sac.

- The conjunctival sac normally holds one or two drops, which provides even distribution of medication across the eye.

  (3) If the patient blinks or closes their eye, or if the drops land on the outer lid margins, repeat the procedure.

- Medication must enter the conjunctival sac to be effective.

  (4) After instilling the drops, ask the patient to close the eye gently.

- Helps to distribute the medication. Squinting or squeezing of eyelids forces medication from the conjunctival sac (Safe Medication, 2021).

  (5) When administering medications that cause systemic effects, apply gentle pressure with your finger and a clean tissue on the patient's nasolacrimal duct for 30–60 seconds.

- Prevents the overflow of medication into the nasal cavity

B. Instill eye ointment:
  (1) Ask the patient to look at the ceiling.

- Retracts the sensitive cornea up and away from the conjunctival sac and reduces stimulation of the blink reflex

  (2) Holding the ointment applicator above the lower lid margin, apply a thin stream of ointment evenly along the inner edge of the lower eyelid on the conjunctiva (see Step 17B[2] illustration) from the inner canthus to outer canthus.

- Distributes the medication evenly across the eye and lid margin

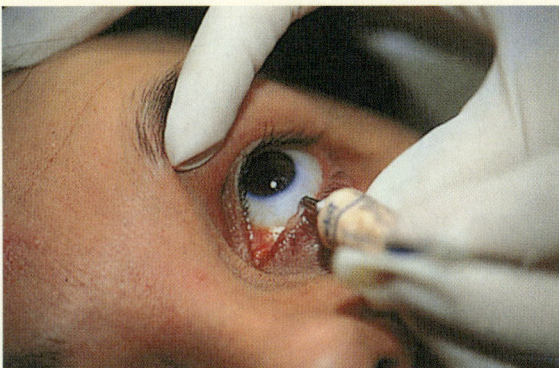

STEP 17B(2) Apply ointment along the lower eyelid.

Continued

SKILL 35.2	ADMINISTERING OPHTHALMIC MEDICATIONS—cont'd
STEPS	**RATIONALE**

(3) Have the patient close the eye and use a cotton ball to rub the lid lightly in a circular motion, if rubbing is not contraindicated.	• Distributes the medication without traumatizing the eye
C. Intraocular disc	
(1) Application:	
(a) Open the package containing the disc. Gently press your fingertip against the disk so that it adheres to your finger. Position the convex side of the disc on your fingertip (see Step 17C[1][a] illustration).	• Enables the nurse to inspect the disc for damage or deformity
(b) With your other hand, gently pull the patient's lower eyelid away from the eye. Ask the patient to look up.	• Prepares the conjunctival sac for receiving the medicated disc
(c) Place the disc in the conjunctival sac, so that it floats on the sclera between the iris and the lower eyelid (see Step 17C[1][c] illustration).	• Ensures accurate delivery of the medication

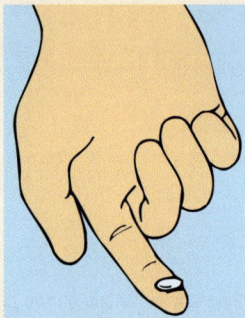

STEP 17C(1)(A) Gently position the convex side of the disc against your fingertips.

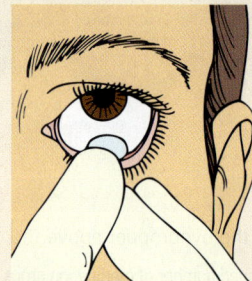

STEP 17C(1)(C) Place the disc in the conjunctival sac between the iris and the lower eyelid.

(d) Pull the patient's lower eyelid out and over the disc (see Step 17C[1][d] illustration).

• Ensures accurate medication delivery

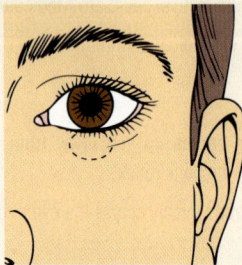

STEP 17C(1)(D) Gently pull the lower eyelid over the disc.

CRITICAL DECISION POINT: *You should not be able to see the disc at this time. If you can see the disc, repeat Step 17C(1)(d).*

---

(2) Removal:

(a) Perform hand hygiene and put on clean, disposable gloves.

(b) Explain the procedure to the patient.

(c) Gently pull on the patient's lower eyelid to expose the intraocular disc.

STEPS	RATIONALE

(d) Using your forefinger and thumb of the opposite hand, pinch the disc and lift it out of the patient's eye (see Step 17C[2][d] illustration).

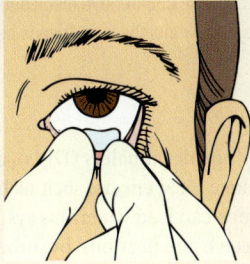

STEP 17C(2)(D) Carefully pinch the disc to remove it from the patient's eye.

18. If excess medication is on the eyelid, gently wipe it from the inner canthus to outer canthus.

- Promotes the patient's comfort and prevents trauma to eye (Safe Medication, 2021)

19. If the patient wears an eye patch, apply a clean patch by placing it over the affected eye so that the entire eye is covered. Tape securely without applying pressure to eye.

- Reduces the chance of infection

CRITICAL DECISION POINT: *If the patient receives more than one eye medication to the same eye at the same time, wait at least 5 minutes before administering the next medication to avoid interaction between medications (Safe Medication, 2021).*

---

20. If the patient receives eye medication to both eyes at the same time, use a different tissue or cotton ball for each eye.

- The use of separate tissues or cotton balls prevents cross-contamination between eyes.

21. Remove gloves, dispose of soiled supplies in proper receptacle, and perform hand hygiene.

22. Note the patient's response to instillation; ask whether the patient felt any discomfort.

- The patient's response determines whether the procedure was performed correctly and safely and whether the patient is experiencing adverse effects of the medication.

23. Observe the patient's response to the medication by assessing any visual changes and noting any adverse effects.

24. Ask the patient to discuss the medication's purpose, action, adverse effects, and the technique of administration.

25. If possible, have the patient demonstrate self-administration of the next dose.

UNEXPECTED OUTCOMES	RELATED INTERVENTIONS

Inability of patient to instill drops without supervision

- Reinforce your teaching and allow the patient to self-administer drops as often as possible to enhance confidence.
- If the patient cannot self-administer drops, teach their caregiver to instill drops into the patient's eye.

Signs of reaction to medication, such as allergic reaction (e.g., tearing, reddened sclera) or systemic response (e.g., bradycardia)

- Follow your employer's policy or guidelines for the reporting of adverse events and allergic reactions to medications.
- Notify the patient's health care provider immediately, and withhold further administration of the medication.
- Add information about the allergy to the patient's medical record, according to employer policy.

Continued

DOCUMENTATION AND REPORTING
- Document on the MAR the medication, concentration, number of drops, time of administration, and the eye (left, right, or both) that received medication.
- Record the appearance of the eye in the nurses' notes.

CARE IN THE COMMUNITY CONSIDERATIONS
- Patients with chronic health care conditions should consult with their health care provider before they use over-the-counter eye medication.
- When they use eye drops at home in the community, patients should not share medications with caregivers, family members, or friends because the risk of infection transmission is high.

lens. Place the medication into the conjunctival sac, where it remains in place for up to 1 week. Medications such as pilocarpine are administered this way. Patients need to be taught about monitoring for adverse reactions to the disc. Patients also need to be taught how to insert and remove the disc.

Ear Instillation. Internal ear structures are very sensitive to temperature extremes. Failure to instill ear drops or irrigating fluid at room temperature may cause vertigo (severe dizziness) or nausea. Although the structures of the outer ear are not sterile, sterile drops and solutions are used in case the eardrum is ruptured. The entrance of nonsterile solutions into middle ear structures can result in infection. If the patient has ear drainage, assess the ear to ensure the patient does not have a ruptured eardrum. Never occlude the ear canal with the dropper or an irrigating syringe. Forcing medication into an occluded ear canal creates pressure that will injure the eardrum. Box 35.19 provides guidelines for administering ear drops and ear irrigations and describes the differences in straightening the ear canal for children and adults.

The external ear structures of children differ from those of adults. When instilling drops or irrigating solutions, first straighten the ear canal. In infants and young children, straighten the cartilaginous canal by grasping the auricle of the ear and pulling it gently down and backward. In adults, the ear canal is longer and composed of underlying bone. The adult ear canal is straightened by pulling the auricle upward and outward. Failure to straighten the canal properly may prevent medicinal solutions from reaching the deeper external ear structures.

Vaginal Instillation. Vaginal medications are available as suppositories, foam, jellies, and creams. Suppositories are individually packaged in foil wrappers and are sometimes stored in a refrigerator to prevent the solid, oval-shaped suppositories from melting. After a suppository is inserted into the vaginal cavity, body temperature causes it to melt and be distributed and absorbed. Foam, jellies, and creams are administered with an applicator inserter (Box 35.20). A suppository is given with a gloved hand in accordance with standard precautions and routine practices (see Box 35.21 for administering rectal suppositories; see also Chapter 34). Patients often prefer administering their own vaginal medications, which requires privacy. After instillation of the medication, a patient may wish to wear a perineal pad to collect the drainage. Because vaginal medications are often given to treat infection, the discharge may be foul smelling. Follow aseptic techniques and offer the patient frequent opportunities to maintain their perineal hygiene (see Chapter 39).

Administering Medications by Inhalation

Medications administered by hand-held inhalers are dispersed through an aerosol spray, mist, or powder that penetrates the lung airways. The alveolocapillary network absorbs medications rapidly. Metered-dose inhalers (MDIs), dry powder inhalers (DPIs), and slow-stream inhaler devices usually produce local effects, such as bronchodilatation; however, some medications can lead to serious systemic adverse effects.

Patients who receive medications by **inhalation** frequently have chronic respiratory disease, such as chronic asthma, emphysema, or bronchitis. Medications given by inhalation provide these patients with control of their airway obstruction. Inhaled medications are often described as "rescue" or "maintenance" medications. *Rescue medications* are short-acting medications that are taken for immediate relief of acute respiratory distress. *Maintenance inhalers* are used on a daily scheduled basis to prevent acute respiratory distress. The effects of maintenance inhalers start within hours of administration and last for a longer period of time than rescue inhalers. Because these patients depend on these medications for disease control, they must learn about the inhalers and how to administer them safely (Skill 35.3). If a patient uses more than one type of inhaler, the bronchodilator is given first.

An MDI delivers a measured dose of medication with each push of the canister. Chemical propellants (e.g., hydrofluorocarbons) push the medication out of the MDI. MDIs are either squeeze-and-breathe inhalers or inhalers activated by the patient's breath. The squeeze-and-breathe MDI requires the application of approximately 2 to 5 kg of pressure to the top of the canister to administer the medication. To use this type of MDI, the patient must have hand strength, which often diminishes as a result of aging or the effects of chronic respiratory disease. Lack of sufficient hand strength can restrict the patient's ability to self-administer medication via MDIs. Breath-activated MDIs release the medication when the patient inhales. Release of the medication is dependent on the strength of the patient's breath on inspiration (Asthma Canada, 2022). The MDI can be used with a spacer to allow the particles of medication to slow down and break into smaller pieces, which improves the medication's absorption in the patient's airway. Spacers are equipped with a face mask when they are used by infants and children younger than 4 years of age. Spacers are especially helpful for patients who have difficulty coordinating the steps involved in self-administering inhaled medications. When patients do not use their inhalers and spacers correctly, they do not receive the full effect of the medication. Therefore, patient education is essential.

DPIs hold dry, powdered medication and create an aerosol when the patient inhales through a reservoir that contains a dose of the medication. DPIs require less manual dexterity than MDIs, and because the device is activated by the patient's breath, the patient does not need to coordinate puffs with inhalation, as required when an MDI is used. DPIs do not require use of a spacer; however, the medication inside the DPI may clump if the DPI is used in a humid climate, and some patients cannot inspire at the speed needed to administer the entire dose of the medication.

One important aspect of patient teaching is to help the patient determine when the MDI or DPI is empty and needs to be replaced.

BOX 35.19 PROCEDURAL GUIDELINE

Administering Ear Medications

Delegation Considerations

The administration of ear medications cannot be delegated. Instruct unregulated care providers about the potential adverse effects of ear medications and the need to report their occurrence immediately.

Equipment

- Medication administration record (MAR)
- Clean, disposable gloves
- Medication bottle with dropper, cotton-tipped applicator, and cotton ball (optional) if ear drops are being administered
- Irrigating syringe, kidney-shaped basin, and towel if ear is to be irrigated
- Barcode scanner (if applicable)

Procedure

1. Check the accuracy and completeness of the MAR, including the following: patient name and medication name, route, dosage, time of administration, and start and stop date. If difficult to read, review the original prescription order and rewrite the MAR.
2. Assess the patient's health history, medications, and allergies.
3. Collect the necessary information to administer the medication safely (i.e., purpose, adverse effects).
4. Prepare the medication. Check expiry dates. Ensure that you compare the label of the medication against the MAR at least two times during the medication preparation.
5. Take the medication to the patient at the correct time. Perform hand hygiene.
6. Identify the patient by using at two to three patient identifiers. Asking the patient to state their name, comparing the patient's name and one other identifier (e.g., the hospital ID number) on the MAR and the patient's ID bracelet, and scanning the barcode on the patient's ID bracelet (if applicable) ensure that it is the right patient.
7. Compare the label on the medication with the MAR one more time at the patient's bedside.
8. Teach the patient about the medication and explain the procedure: positioning, sensations to expect, such as hearing bubbling or feeling water in the ear as medication trickles into the ear.
9. Administer the ear drops:
   A. Have the patient assume a side-lying position (if this position is not contraindicated by patient's condition) with the ear to be treated facing up. Alternatively, the patient may sit in a chair or at the bedside.
   B. Perform hand hygiene. Put on gloves.
   C. Straighten the ear canal by pulling the auricle down and back (for children under 3 years of age) or upward and outward (for adults).

D. Hold the dropper 1 cm above the ear canal and instill the prescribed drops (see Step 9D illustration).

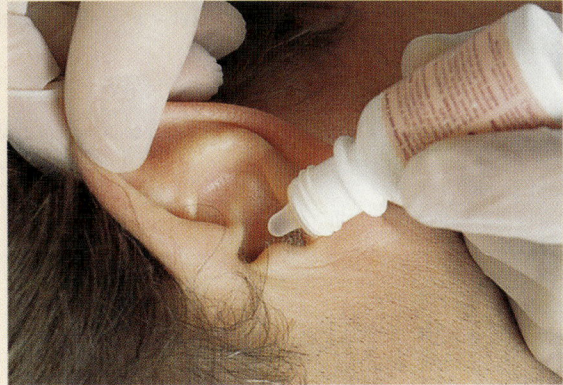

STEP 9D Placing ear drop in ear.

   E. Ask the patient to remain in a side-lying position for 2 to 3 minutes. Apply gentle massage or pressure to the tragus of the ear with your finger unless contraindicated due to pain.
   F. If a cotton ball is needed, place the cotton ball into the outermost part of the ear canal. Do not press cotton deep into the canal. Remove cotton after 15 minutes.
10. Administer ear irrigations:
   A. Assess the tympanic membrane or review the medical record for a history of eardrum perforation, which would contraindicate ear irrigation.
   B. Assist the patient in assuming a sitting or lying position with the head tilted or turned toward the affected ear. Place a towel under the patient's head and shoulder and have the patient hold a kidney-shaped basin under the affected ear.
   C. Perform hand hygiene. Put on clean, disposable gloves.
   D. Fill the irrigating syringe with approximately 50 mL of the solution.
   E. Gently grasp the auricle and straighten the ear canal by pulling it down and back (for children under 3 years of age) or upward and outward (for children 4 years of age and older and adults).
   F. Slowly instill the irrigating solution by holding the tip of the syringe 1 cm above the opening of the ear canal. Allow the fluid to drain out during instillation. Continue until the canal is clean or until all solution is used.
11. Clean the work area and put the medication supplies away.
12. Remove gloves and perform hand hygiene.
13. Document medication administration on the MAR.
14. Evaluate the patient's response to the medication.

Floating the MDI to determine the amount of medication remaining is no longer recommended because extra propellant may cause buoyancy even if no medication remains in the inhaler. Furthermore, MDIs with hydrofluoroalkanes (HFA) should never be immersed (Asthma Canada, 2022). Some DPIs have mechanisms that indicate the number of doses remaining; however, these mechanisms are not always accurate. To calculate how long the medication in an MDI or DPI will last, divide the capacity of the canister by the number of doses the patient takes per day. For example, a patient is to take albuterol, a β-adrenergic agonist bronchodilator. The prescribed dose is two puffs four times a day. The canister has a total of 200 puffs. Complete the following calculations to determine how long the MDI will last:

$$2 \text{ puffs} \times 4 \text{ times a day} = 8 \text{ puffs per day}$$

$$200 \text{ puffs} \div 8 \text{ puffs per day} = 25 \text{ days}$$

The canister in this example will last 25 days. To ensure the patient does not run out of medication, teach the patient to refill the medication prescription at least 7 to 10 days before it is expected to run out (Asthma Canada, 2022).

BOX 35.20 PROCEDURAL GUIDELINE

Administering Vaginal Medications

Delegation Consideration

The administration of medications by the vaginal route cannot be delegated. Instruct unregulated care providers to report new or increased vaginal discharge or bleeding and occurrence of potential adverse effects of the medications immediately.

Equipment

- Vaginal cream, foam, jelly, or suppository, or irrigating solution with applicator (if required)
- Clean, disposable gloves
- Towels, or a washcloth, or both
- Paper towels
- Perineal pad
- Drape or sheet
- Water-soluble lubricating jelly
- Medication administration record (MAR)
- Barcode scanner (if applicable)

Procedure

1. Check the accuracy and completeness of the MAR, including the following: patient name and medication name, route, dosage, form (e.g., ointment, lotion), time of administration, and start and stop date. If difficult to read, review the original prescription order and rewrite the MAR.
2. Assess the patient's health history, medications, and allergies (including latex).
3. Collect the information necessary to administer the medication safely.
4. Perform hand hygiene. Prepare the medication (see Skill 35.1, Steps 4 A–H). Check expiry dates. Compare the label of the medication with the MAR two times while preparing the medication.
5. Take the medication to the patient at the correct time. Perform hand hygiene.
6. Identify the patient by using two to three patient identifiers. Asking the patient to state their name, comparing the patient's name and one other identifier (e.g., the hospital ID number) on the MAR and the patient's ID bracelet, and scanning the barcode on the patient's ID bracelet ensure that you have the right patient.
7. Compare the label on the medication with the MAR one more time at the patient's bedside.
8. Teach the patient about the medication. Explain to the patient the procedure for positioning and the sensations they can expect, such as feelings of moisture or wetness in the vaginal area. Assess the patient's ability to manipulate the applicator or suppository and to position themselves to insert the medication. Explain the procedure to the patient. Especially if the patient plans to self-administer the medication, it is important to be specific in your explanation.
9. Allow the patient to empty or attempt to empty their bladder before administration of vaginal medication. To facilitate adequate absorption, the patient needs to lie quietly for at least 10 minutes.
10. Close the room curtain or door and arrange the supplies at the bedside.
11. Assist the patient in lying in a dorsal recumbent position. This position provides full exposure and easy access to the vaginal canal and allows the suppository to dissolve without escaping through an orifice.
12. Perform hand hygiene. Put on clean, disposable gloves.
13. Keep the abdomen and lower extremities draped.
14. Ensure that the lighting is adequate to visualize the vaginal opening. Inspect the condition of external genitalia and the vaginal canal, noting the appearance of any discharge. Clean the area with a towel or washcloth if necessary.
15. Insert the vaginal suppository:
    A. Remove the suppository from its foil wrapper. Apply a liberal amount of sterile water-based lubricating jelly to the smooth or rounded end of the suppository. Lubricate the gloved index finger of your dominant hand.
    B. With your nondominant gloved hand, expose the vaginal orifice by gently retracting the labial folds.
    C. With your dominant gloved hand, gently insert the rounded end of the suppository along the posterior wall of the vaginal canal for the entire length of your finger (7.5 to 10 cm) to ensure equal distribution of the medication along the walls of the vaginal cavity (see Step 15C illustration).
    D. Withdraw your finger and wipe any remaining lubricant from around the orifice and labia.

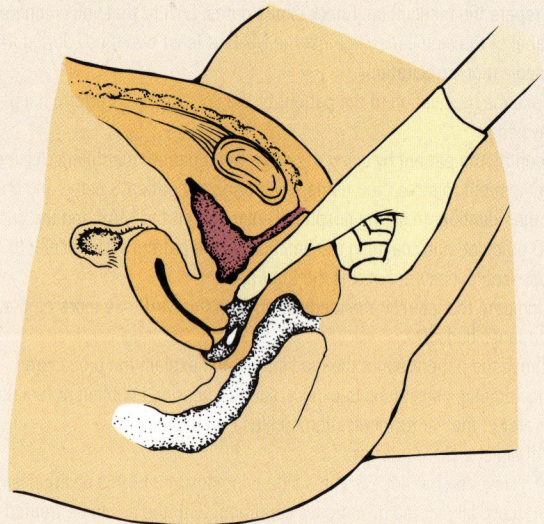

STEP 15C Insertion of a suppository into the vaginal canal.

16. Administer the cream or foam:
    A. Fill the cream or foam applicator, as described on the package directions.
    B. With your nondominant gloved hand, expose the vaginal orifice by gently retracting the labial folds.
    C. With your dominant gloved hand, insert the applicator approximately 5 to 7.5 cm. Push the applicator plunger to deposit the medication into the vagina to allow equal distribution of medication (see Step 16C illustration).
    D. Withdraw the applicator and place it on a paper towel. Wipe residual cream from the labia or vaginal orifice.

BOX 35.20 PROCEDURAL GUIDELINE—cont'd

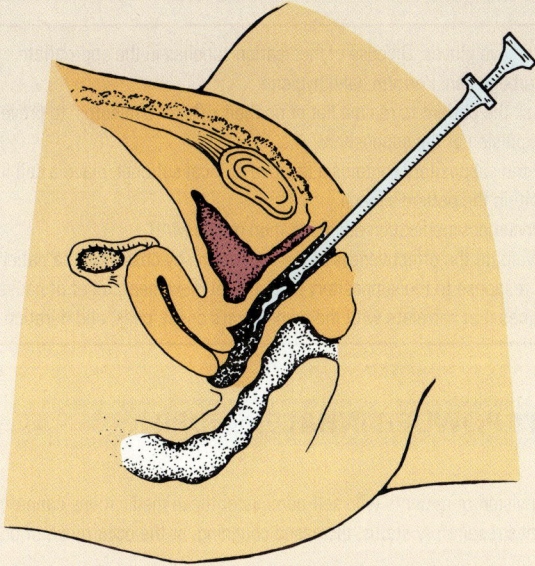

STEP 16C Instillation of medication in the vaginal canal.

17. Dispose of supplies, remove gloves, and perform hand hygiene.
18. Instruct the patient to remain on their back for at least 10 minutes.
19. Document the medication administration on the MAR.
20. Offer the patient a perineal pad when they resume ambulation, to prevent vaginal discharge from spreading to clothing.
21. Inspect the appearance of discharge from the vaginal canal and the condition of external genitalia between applications to evaluate the medication's effectiveness.

BOX 35.21 PROCEDURAL GUIDELINE

Administering Rectal Suppositories

Delegation Considerations
The administration of medications by the rectal route cannot be delegated. Instruct unregulated care providers to expect and report fecal discharge or a bowel movement and to report the occurrence of potential adverse effects or medications immediately.

Equipment
- Rectal suppository
- Water-soluble lubricating jelly
- Clean, disposable gloves (two pairs)
- Drape or sheet
- Tissue
- Medication administration record (MAR)
- Barcode scanner (if applicable)

Procedure
1. Check the accuracy and completeness of the MAR, including the following: patient name and medication name, route, dosage, time of administration, and start and stop date. If difficult to read, review the original prescription order and rewrite the MAR.
2. Assess the patient's health history, medications, and allergies. Previous rectal surgery or bleeding may contraindicate a rectal suppository.
3. Collect the necessary information to administer the medication safely.
4. Perform hand hygiene. Prepare medication (see Skill 35.1, Steps 4A–H). Check the medication expiry date. Compare the label of the medication with the MAR two times during medication preparation.
5. Take the medication to the patient at the correct time.
6. Perform hand hygiene. Identify the patient by using two to three patient identifiers. Asking the patient to state their name, comparing the patient's name and one other identifier (e.g., the hospital ID number) on the MAR and the patient's ID bracelet, and scanning the barcode on the patient's ID bracelet (if applicable) ensure that you have the right patient.
7. Compare the label of the medication with the MAR one more time at the patient's bedside.
8. Teach the patient about the medication. Explain the procedure to the patient regarding the positioning and the sensations to expect, such as feelings of needing to defecate. Ensure that the patient understands the procedure and that they can self-administer the medication.
9. Close the room curtain or door and arrange supplies at the bedside.
10. Perform hand hygiene. Put on clean, disposable gloves.
11. Assist the patient in assuming modified left lateral recumbent position to expose the anus and facilitate relaxation of the external anal sphincter. Keep the patient draped with only the anal area exposed.
12. Ensure the lighting is adequate to visualize the anus. Check for evidence of active rectal bleeding. Examine the condition of the anus externally and palpate the rectal walls to assess for presence of feces, which may interfere with the suppository placement (see Chapter 33). Dispose of gloves in proper garbage can. Perform hand hygiene.
13. Put on a new pair of clean, disposable gloves.
14. Remove the suppository from its package and lubricate the rounded end (see Step 14 illustration) with a sterile water-soluble lubricating jelly to reduce the friction when the suppository enters the rectal canal. Lubricate the index finger of your dominant hand with a water-soluble lubricant.

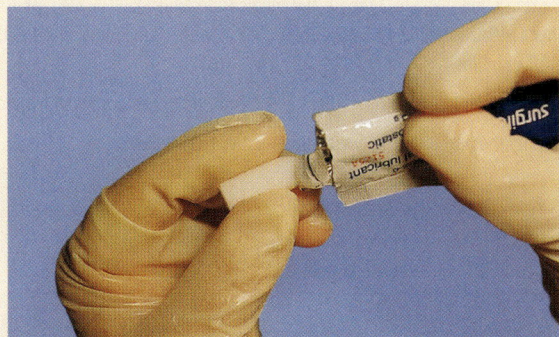

STEP 14 Remove the suppository from its packaging.

Continued

BOX 35.21   PROCEDURAL GUIDELINE—cont'd

Administering Rectal Suppositories

15. Ask the patient to take slow, deep breaths through the mouth and relax the anal sphincter.
16. Retract the buttocks with your nondominant hand. Insert the suppository gently through the anus, past the internal sphincter and against the rectal wall, 10 cm in adults, 5 cm in children and infants. Apply gentle pressure to hold the buttocks together momentarily, if necessary, to keep medication in place and to facilitate medication distribution and absorption.
17. Withdraw your finger and wipe the anal area with tissue.

18. Remove gloves. Dispose of medication supplies in the appropriate garbage can. Perform hand hygiene.
19. Ask the patient to remain flat or on their side for 5 minutes, to prevent expulsion of the suppository.
20. If the suppository contains a laxative or fecal softener, place a call light within the patient's reach.
21. Document medication administration on the MAR.
22. Evaluate the effectiveness of the medication by observing the patient for a response to the suppository (e.g., bowel movement, relief of nausea) at times that correlate with the medication's onset, peak, and duration.

SKILL 35.3   USING METERED-DOSE (MDI) AND DRY POWDER INHALERS (DPI)

Delegation Considerations

The administration of a metered-dose inhaler (MDI) or dry powder inhaler (DPI) and the supervision of patients who self-administer these medications cannot be delegated to unregulated care providers (UCPs). Instruct UCPs to report changes in the patient's respiratory status, increased coughing, or the occurrence of potential adverse effects immediately.

Equipment

- MDI or DPI
- Spacer (i.e., Aerochamber) (optional)
- Washbasin or sink with warm water (to wash a spacer)
- Paper towel
- Oral hygiene supplies (e.g., water, mouthwash)
- Medication administration record (MAR)
- Barcode scanner (if applicable)

PROCEDURE

STEPS	RATIONALE
1. Check the accuracy and completeness of the MAR, including the following: patient name, medication name, route, dosage, time of administration, and start and stop date. If difficult to read, review the original prescription order and rewrite the MAR.	• Ensures that the patient receives the right medication • Illegible MARs are a source of medication incidents. The original prescription is the most reliable source and only legal record of medications the patient is to receive.
2. Assess the patient's health history, medications, and allergies.	• Medications should correspond to medical diagnoses (e.g., chronic obstructive pulmonary disease [COPD] and bronchodilators). • Certain substances have similar compositions; never administer a substance to which a patient has a known allergy.
3. Collect the necessary information to administer the medication safely.	• This is necessary to determine if the medication, dose, and route are appropriate, and how to administer it safely.
4. Perform hand hygiene. Prepare the medication (see Skill 35.1, Steps 4A–H). Check medication expiry dates. Compare the label of the medication with the MAR two times.	
5. Take the medication to the patient at the right time. Perform hand hygiene.	
6. Identify the patient using two to three patient identifiers.	• Asking the patient to state their name, comparing the patient's name and one other identifier (e.g., the hospital ID number) on the MAR and the patient's ID bracelet, and scanning the patient's barcode on their ID bracelet, ensure that you have the right patient.

SKILL 35.3	USING METERED-DOSE (MDI) AND DRY POWDER INHALERS (DPI)—cont'd
STEPS	**RATIONALE**

STEPS	RATIONALE
7. Assess the patient's respiratory status, breath sounds, and strength in inhalation by asking them to exhale and inhale strongly.	• Assessment provides a baseline to compare breath sounds before and after treatment; symptoms may indicate the need for inhaled medications (e.g., wheezes). • DPI and breath-activated MDIs require the patient to forcefully inhale to aerosolize the medication.
8. Compare the label on medications with the MAR one more time at the bedside. If using an MDI see Step 10 or DPI Step 11.	• This is the *third accuracy check.*

CRITICAL DECISION POINT: *If the patient is using an MDI with or without a spacer and the inhaler is new or has not been used for several days, push a "test spray" into the air (Asthma Canada, 2022). A test spray is not needed for a DPI.*

STEPS	RATIONALE
9. If using an MDI with a spacer, teach the patient about the medication and explain the following steps:	• Understanding increases medication adherence.
A. Shake the inhaler vigorously five or six times. Insert the MDI canister into the holder.	• Shaking ensures that fine particles are aerosolized.
B. Remove the MDI and spacer mouthpiece covers. Inspect the spacer for foreign objects. If the spacer has a valve, ensure that the valve is intact. Insert the MDI into the end of the spacer.	• A spacer breaks up and slows down the medication particles, enhancing the amount of medication received by the patient (Asthma Canada, 2022).
C. Instruct the patient to take a deep breath and exhale.	• Exhaling empties the lungs and prepares the airway for medication.
D. The patient closes their mouth around the spacer mouthpiece without covering the exhalation holes (see Step 9D illustration).	• The spacer emits a spray that allows finer particles to be inhaled. • Large droplets are retained in the spacer.

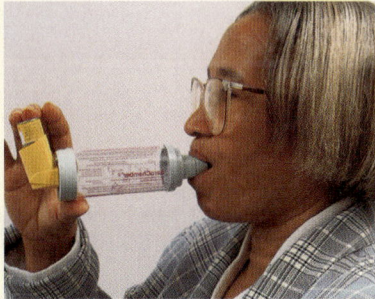

STEP 9D Instruct the patient to place the mouthpiece in their mouth and close their lips, being careful to keep the exhalation slots exposed.

STEPS	RATIONALE
E. The patient depresses the medication canister and sprays one puff into the spacer.	
F. The patient inhales deeply and slowly through their mouth for 3–5 seconds.	• Deep inhalations maximize the amount of medication that enters the lungs.
G. The patient then holds their breath for 10 seconds and removes the spacer from their mouth before exhaling.	• Holding the breath ensures full medication distribution. • Removing the MDI and spacer allows the patient to exhale normally.
H. Note: The steps are the same if the patient uses an MDI without a spacer, except the following: the patient closes their mouth around the MDI with the opening toward the back of the throat (see Step 9H(1) illustration), or holds the inhaler 2–4 cm in front of the mouth (see Step 9H(2) illustration). The patient tilts their head back while inhaling, depresses the canister fully, and exhales through pursed lips.	• Positioning the inhaler directs the medication toward the airways.

Continued

SKILL 35.3	USING METERED-DOSE (MDI) AND DRY POWDER INHALERS (DPI)—cont'd
STEPS	**RATIONALE**

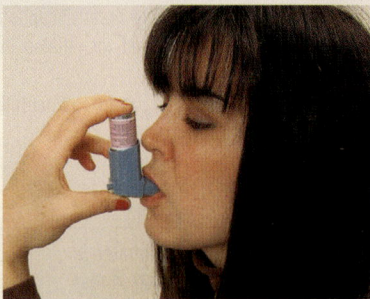

STEP 9H(1) The patient places the inhaler in their mouth with opening toward back of throat.

STEP 9H(2) The patient places the mouthpiece of the inhaler 2 to 4 cm away from their mouth. This placement is considered the best way to deliver the medication.

10. If using a DPI or breath-activated MDI, teach the patient about the medication and explain the following steps:	
A. Remove the cover from the mouthpiece. Do not shake the inhaler.	
B. Prepare the medication as directed by the manufacturer (e.g., hold the inhaler upright and turn the wheel to the right and then to the left until a click is heard, load the medication pellet, etc.).	• Preparing the medication properly primes the inhaler to ensure the medication will be delivered to the patient (Asthma Canada, 2022).
C. Instruct the patient to exhale away from the inhaler before inhalation.	• Exhaling before using the inhaler prevents loss of powder.
D. The patient places the mouthpiece between their lips.	• Properly positioning the mouthpiece prevents the medication from escaping through the mouth.
E. The patient inhales deeply and forcefully through the mouth. There is no canister to depress.	• Deep inhalations create aerosol.
F. The patient holds their breath for 5–10 seconds and then exhales.	• Holding the breath ensures full medication distribution.
11. Instruct the patient to wait at least 20–30 seconds between each inhalation (i.e., puffer).	• Time is needed for each dose to be absorbed.
12. Assist the patient in performing oral hygiene by swishing and spitting out water or mouthwash after taking inhaled medications.	• Inhaled medications can cause patients to develop thrush. • Medications must be inhaled sequentially. The first inhalation opens the airways and reduces inflammation. The second or third inhalation penetrates the deeper airways.

CRITICAL DECISION POINT: *If two medications are to be administered, give the bronchodilator first.*

---

13. After medication administration, assess the patient's respiratory status, including work of breathing, respiratory rate, breath sounds, and oxygenation. Perform hand hygiene.	• Evaluate the patient's response to the medication and respiratory status.
14. Instruct the patient in cleaning the inhaler:	
A. Once a day, rinse the inhaler and its cap in warm running water. Completely dry before use.	• Spray accumulates around the mouthpiece and interferes with proper distribution during use.
B. Twice a week, wash the L-shaped plastic mouthpiece with mild dishwashing soap and warm water. Rinse and dry well before placing the canister back inside the mouthpiece (Asthma Canada, 2022).	• Removes residual medication. Do not place inhalers holding cromolyn, nedocromil, or HFA (hydrofluoroalkane) in water.

SKILL 35.3	USING METERED-DOSE (MDI) AND DRY POWDER INHALERS (DPI)—cont'd
STEPS	**RATIONALE**

STEPS	RATIONALE
15. Educate the patient on their respiratory condition, medications, and self-administration:	• Understanding increases medication adherence.
A. Allow adequate time and use a quiet, comfortable location for teaching. Assemble supplies for demonstration and patient education materials (e.g., pamphlet, videos).	• Patients are more receptive to education if in a comfortable environment (Bastable, 2021).
B. Assess the patient's readiness and ability to learn. For example, does the patient ask questions about the medication, are they fatigued or in respiratory distress?	• Influences the patient's ability to understand information and actively participate (Bastable, 2021)
C. Assess the patient's knowledge and understanding of the disease and the prescribed medications.	• Knowledge of disease is essential for the patient to understand when and why to use the inhaler.
D. Explain what a metered dose is and the prescribed frequency for use. Warn the patient about over- or underusing the inhaler.	• Misusing inhalers can cause harm.
E. Explain the steps and demonstrate how to use an inhaler. Allow the patient to handle the medication cartridge, the inhaler, and devices (e.g., spacer).	• Demonstrating allows the patient to visualize and see a role model.
F. Assess the patient's ability to hold an inhaler, spacer, or DPI and depress a canister or prepare a DPI dose.	• Functional limitations may make it difficult for the patient to effectively self-administer medications.
G. Ask whether the patient has any questions.	• Clarifies patient misconceptions or misunderstandings
H. Ask the patient to explain the medication schedule, adverse effects, and when to call health care providers.	• Allows the nurse to evaluate the patient's understanding and improves adherence
I. Ask the patient to calculate how many days the inhaler will last.	• Helps the patient recognize when to refill or request a new prescription
J. Have the patient explain and demonstrate how to use an inhaler.	• Allows the nurse to evaluate and provide feedback on learning

UNEXPECTED OUTCOMES	RELATED INTERVENTIONS
Need for a bronchodilator more frequently than every 4 hours	• Respiratory conditions are indicated. The type of medication and delivery methods need to be reassessed. Notify the health care provider if respiratory status does not improve.
Cardiac dysrhythmias, especially in patient receiving β–adrenergics	• Withhold doses of medication and notify the prescriber if symptoms with dysrhythmias (e.g., lightheadedness).
Inability of patient to self-administer medication properly	• Explore alternative delivery routes and methods (e.g., caregiver administration).
Paroxysms of coughing	• Aerosolized particles irritate the posterior pharynx. Notify the prescriber; reassess the type of medication or the delivery method.

DOCUMENTATION AND REPORTING
- Document the skills that you taught the patient and the patient's ability to perform these skills.
- Document on the MAR the medication, time of administration, and number of puffs.
- Report any undesirable effects from the medication.

CARE IN THE HOME OR COMMUNITY CONSIDERATIONS
- Remind patients to carry their prescribed inhalers to use immediately in case of an acute asthma attack.

Administering Medications by Irrigations

Some medications irrigate or wash out a body cavity and are delivered through a stream of solution. Irrigations most commonly use sterile water, saline, or antiseptic solutions to irrigate the eye, ear, throat, vagina, or urinary tract. The nurse must use aseptic technique if the patient has a break in the skin or mucosa. When the cavity to be irrigated is not sterile, as in the case of the ear canal (see Box 35.19) or vagina, the nurse uses a clean technique. In health care settings, sterile solutions are usually used. Irrigations are used to clean an area, instill a medication, or apply heat or cold to injured tissue.

Administering Parenteral Medications

Parenteral administration of medications is the administration of medications by injection. Parenteral administration is an invasive procedure that must be performed with aseptic techniques (Box 35.22). After a needle pierces the skin, the patient is at risk of infection. Each type of injection requires the application of specific skills to ensure the medication reaches the proper location. The effects of a parenterally administered medication develop rapidly, depending on the rate of medication absorption. The nurse must always closely observe the patient's response.

- To prevent contamination of the solution, draw the medication from the ampoule or vial quickly. Do not allow it to stand open.
- To prevent needle contamination, avoid letting the needle intended for the injection touch a contaminated surface (e.g., the outer edges of the ampoule or vial, the outer surface of the needle cap, your hands, a countertop, a table surface).
- To prevent syringe contamination, avoid touching the length of the plunger or the inner part of the barrel. Keep the tip of the syringe covered with a cap or needle.
- To prepare the skin, wash skin soiled with dirt, drainage, or feces with soap and water and then dry. Use friction and a circular motion to clean the skin with an antiseptic swab for 30 seconds. Swab from centre of site and move outward in a 5-cm radius. Allow the skin to fully dry before administering the injection and do not blow air on the site to speed up the drying time; this contaminates the surface.

FIGURE 35.17 Various syringe sizes for fluid volume injection. (Courtesy and © Becton, Dickinson and Company.)

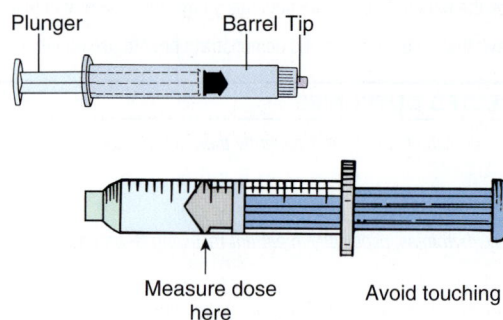

FIGURE 35.16 Types of syringes. **A,** Luer-Lok syringe marked in 0.1 (tenths). **B,** Tuberculin syringe marked in 0.01 (hundredths) for doses of less than 1 mL. **C,** Insulin syringe marked in units (100). **D,** Insulin syringe marked in units (50).

FIGURE 35.18 Parts of a syringe.

Equipment. A variety of syringes and needles are available, each designed to deliver a precise volume of medication to a specific type of tissue. Use nursing judgement when determining the syringe or needle that will be most effective.

Syringes. Syringes consist of a close-fitting plunger and a cylindrical barrel with a tip designed to fit the hub of a hypodermic needle. Syringes, in general, are classified as being Luer-Lok or non–Luer-Lok. This nomenclature is based on the design of the syringe's tip. Luer-Lok syringes (Figure 35.16, A) require special needles, which are twisted onto the tip and lock in place. This design prevents the inadvertent removal of the needle. Non–Luer-Lok syringes (see Figure 35.16, B–D) require needles that slip onto the tip. In clinical settings, all syringes now have safety devices to prevent needle-stick injuries. Various sizes of syringes exist to allow the administration of different fluid volumes (Figure 35.17)

Fill the syringe by aspiration, by pulling the plunger outward while the needle tip remains immersed in the prepared solution. The outside of the syringe barrel and the handle of the plunger may be handled.

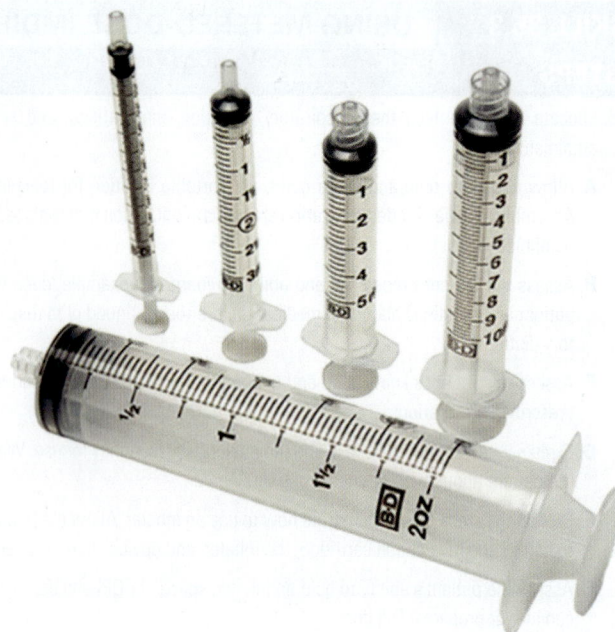

To maintain sterility, avoid letting any unsterile object touch the tip or the inside of the barrel, the hub, the shaft of the plunger, or the needle (Figure 35.18).

Syringes come in numerous sizes, from 0.5 mL to 60 mL. A 1- to 3-mL syringe is usually adequate for a subcutaneous or IM injection. The use of a syringe larger than 5 mL is unusual for an injection. The larger volume creates discomfort. Instead, larger syringes are used to administer certain IV medications, to add medications to IV solutions, and to irrigate wounds or drainage tubes. Syringes may be prepackaged with a needle attached; however, the needle size may be changed depending on the route of administration and the size of the patient.

Insulin syringes (see Figure 35.16, C–D) are available in sizes from 0.3 mL to 1 mL and are calibrated in units. Insulin syringes that hold 0.3 mL are known as *low-dose syringes* (30 units per 0.3 mL). Most insulin syringes are known as *U-100s* and are designed to be used with insulin that has a strength of U-100. Each millilitre of U-100 insulin contains 100 units of insulin.

The tuberculin syringe (see Figure 35.16, B) has a long, thin barrel with a preattached thin needle. The syringe is calibrated in sixteenths of a minim and in hundredths of a millilitre and has a capacity of 1 mL. Use a tuberculin syringe to prepare small amounts of medications

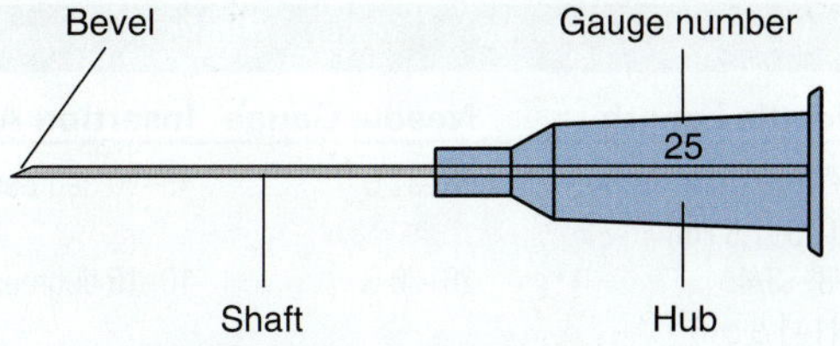

FIGURE 35.19 Parts of the needle.

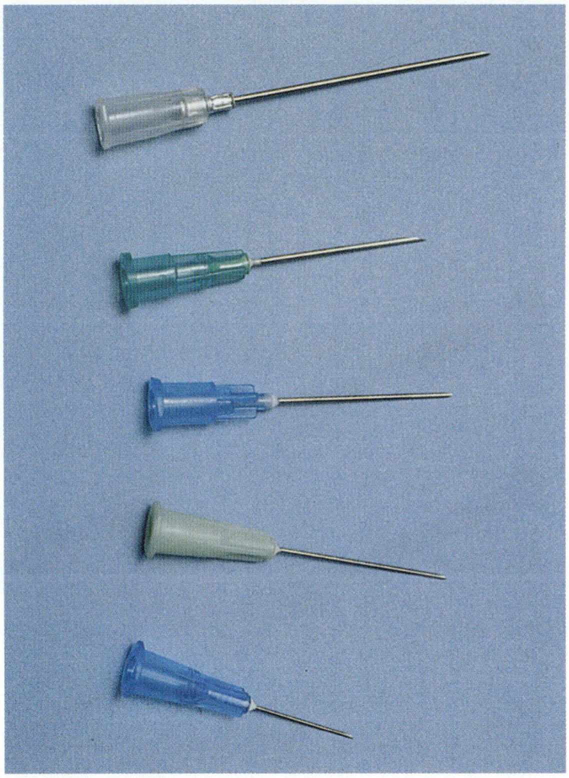

FIGURE 35.20 Needles. **Top to bottom:** 19 gauge, 3.8 cm length; 20 gauge, 2.5 cm length; 21 gauge, 2.5 cm length; 23 gauge, 2.5 cm length; and 25 gauge, 1.6 cm length.

FIGURE 35.21 Blunt filter needle (pink) and blunt fill needle (red). (Courtesy and © Becton, Dickinson and Company.)

(e.g., intradermal or subcutaneous injections). A tuberculin syringe is also useful when preparing small, precise doses for infants or young children.

Needles. Needles are packaged in individual sheaths to allow flexibility in choosing the right needle for a patient. Some needles are pre-attached to standard-sized syringes. Most needles are made of stainless steel and are disposable.

The needle has three parts: the *hub*, which fits onto the tip of a syringe; the *shaft*, which connects to the hub; and the *bevel*, or slanted tip (Figure 35.19). The tip of a needle, or the bevel, is always slanted. The bevel creates a narrow slit when it is injected into tissue.

When the needle is removed, the slit in the skin quickly closes to prevent leakage of medication, blood, or serum. Long, bevelled tips are sharper and narrower to minimize discomfort to the patient when entering tissue used for subcutaneous or IM injections.

Needles vary in length from 0.6 to 7.6 cm (Figure 35.20). Although metric measurement is preferred in Canada, most needles used here come from the United States and likely will not appear in metric sizes. Choose the needle length according to the patient's size and weight and the type of tissue into which the medication is to be injected. In general, a child or slender adult requires a shorter needle. Use longer

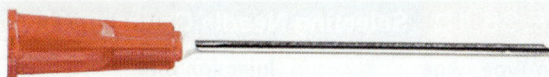

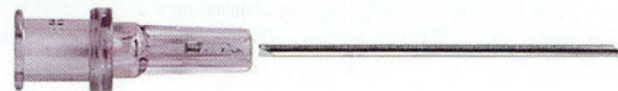

needles (2.5 to 3.8 cm) for IM injections and use a shorter needle (1 to 1.6 cm) for subcutaneous injections.

Blunt needles are frequently used to aspirate medications from vials or ampoules in preparation for injection into a patient or an IV bag of fluid solution. Blunt needles have a dull tip to reduce the risk of needle-stick injuries. Blunt filter needles include a filter inside the needle hub to prevent the aspiration of glass particles from ampoules (Harmon, 2013). Blunt fill needles have no filter and are used to draw up medications from a vial. Prior to injecting a patient, the blunt needle must be removed from the syringe and the appropriate sharp, bevelled needle applied (Figure 35.21).

Needle diameter is measured by gauge. As the gauge becomes smaller, the needle diameter becomes larger (see Figure 35.20). Gauge selection depends on the viscosity of fluid to be injected or infused. An adult IM injection usually requires a 19- to 25-gauge needle, depending on the viscosity of the medication. Subcutaneous injections require small-diameter needles ranging from 29- to 32-gauge for adults. A 26- to 28-gauge needle is used for an adult intradermal injections. Needle length varies depending on the site (i.e., location), type (determines depth required), and the size and age of the patient. The standard length of a needle for IM injections is 3.8 cm (1.5 inches). Table 35.10 summarizes needle lengths, gauges, sites, and angles for injection types.

Retractable needle syringes also exist with a variety of needle gauges and syringe sizes. When the syringe plunger handle is fully depressed at the completion of an injection, the needle automatically retracts into the syringe, reducing the risk of needlestick injury to the health care provider (Figure 35.22) (Reddy et al., 2017; Retractable Technologies Inc., 2021).

Disposable Injection Units. Disposable, single-dose, prefilled syringes are available for some medications. It is important to check the medication and concentration because all prefilled syringes look very similar. When using these syringes, the nurse does not have to prepare medication doses, except perhaps to expel portions of unneeded medications. Anticoagulant medications for injection (such as heparin or dalteparin) are usually supplied in single-dose, prefilled syringes (Figure 35.23).

The Carpuject injection systems (such as the Abboject from Pfizer, Inc.) include 1) an empty syringe shaft and needle and 2) a prefilled, sterile cartridge with medication for emergency use (Figure 35.24). To prepare these systems follow the package directions, which usually describe slipping the cartridge into the syringe shaft and securing the cartridge to the needle and shaft by twisting the cartridge. After the medication is given, safely dispose of the entire unit in a puncture-proof and leakproof receptacle. The design of these injection systems supports efficient and timely administration of medications such as

TABLE 35.10	Selecting Needle Gauge and Length				
Injection Type	Age	Injection Site	Needle Length	Needle Gauge	Insertion Angle
Subcutaneous	<12 mo; 12 mo–18 yr; >18 yr	Anteriolateral thigh, upper outer triceps, upper buttocks, abdomen (>2" from umbilicus)	½"–5/8" (1.3–1.6 cm)	26–31 G	45–90 degrees
Intradermal	<12 mo; 12 mo–18 yr; >18 yr	Anterolateral forearm, upper chest, upper back, upper arm posterior	3/8"–3/4" (1–1.9 cm)	26–28 G	10–15 degrees
Intramuscular	<18 mo	Vastus lateralis (<0.5 mL volume)	7/8"–1" (2.2–2.5 cm)	25–27 G	90 degrees
	12 mo–18 yr	Deltoid, ventrogluteal, dorsogluteal (>3 years), vastus lateralis	7/8"–1 1/4" (2.2–3.2 cm)	22–25 G	
	>18 yr	Deltoid, ventrogluteal, dorsogluteal, vastus lateralis	1"–1 ¼" (2.5–3.2 cm) (large adults 3" maximum)	19–25 G	

Adapted from Becton, Dickinson and Company. (2019). *Chart injection guidelines for needle length and gauge selection.* https://www.bd.com/documents/in-service-materials/syringes-and-needles/MPS_HY_Injection-guidelines-for-needle-length-and-gauge-selection_IM_EN.pdf

FIGURE 35.22 Retractable needle and syringe: Vanishpoint Syringe. (Photo courtesy of Retractable Technologies Inc., 2021.)

FIGURE 35.23 Single-dose, prefilled disposable syringe. (Courtesy and © Becton, Dickinson and Company.)

dextrose, epinephrine, and sodium bicarbonate in an emergency and reduces the risk of needle-stick injuries.

Preparing an Injection From an Ampoule. Ampoules contain single doses of medication in a liquid. Ampoules are available in several sizes, from 1 mL to 10 mL or more (Figure 35.25). An *ampoule* is made of glass with a constricted neck that must be snapped off to access the medication. A coloured ring around the neck indicates where the ampoule is scored to be broken easily. Aspiration of the medication from an ampoule into a syringe (Skill 35.4) often requires the use of a blunt filter needle to prevent small glass fragments from entering the syringe (see Figure 35.21). Change the blunt filter needle to an appropriate-sized sharp needle for the actual injection.

Preparing an Injection From a Vial. A *vial* is a single-dose or multidose container with a rubber seal at the top (see Figure 35.25). A metal

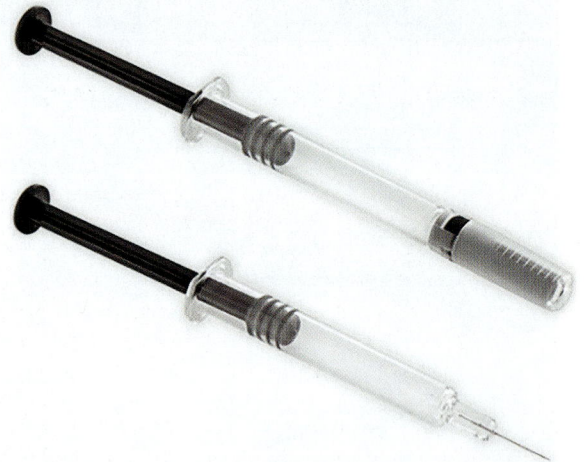

or plastic cap protects the seal until it is ready to be used. Vials contain liquid or dry forms of medications. Medications that are unstable in solution are packaged dry. The vial label specifies the solvent or diluents to be used to dissolve the medication and the amount of diluent needed to prepare a desired medication concentration. Normal saline and sterile distilled water are solutions commonly used to dissolve medications.

Unlike the ampoule, the vial is a closed system, and air must be injected into the vial to permit easy withdrawal of the solution. Failure to inject air creates a vacuum within the vial that makes withdrawal difficult (see Skill 35.4).

To prepare a powdered medication, draw up the amount of diluent or solvent recommended on the vial's label. Inject the diluent into the vial in the same manner used for injecting air into the vial. Most powdered medications dissolve easily, but you may need to withdraw the needle to mix the contents thoroughly. If this step is needed, remove the needle and gently roll the vial between your hands to dissolve the powdered medication, then reinsert the needle to draw up the dissolved medication. After mixing multidose vials, make a label that records the date and time of the mixing and indicates the concentration of medication per millilitre. Multidose vials may require refrigeration after the contents are reconstituted.

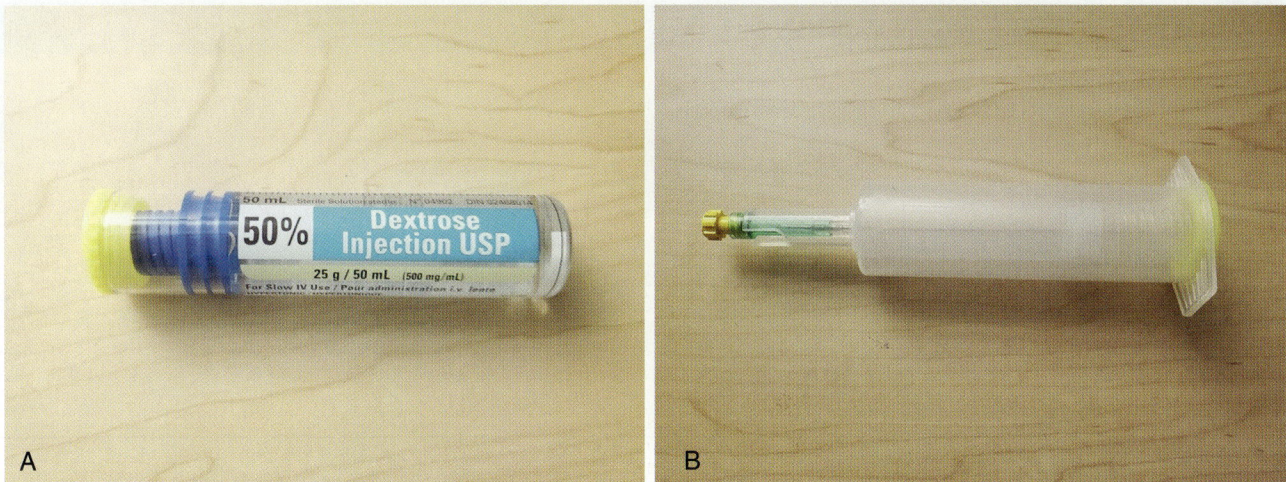

FIGURE 35.24 The Carpuject or Abboject injection system includes a prefilled single-dose 50-mL cartridge and syringe. The syringe is screwed onto the base of the cartridge by the nurse for injection. **A,** Cartridge containing 50% dextrose (25 g/50 mL). **B,** Syringe with Luer-lok tip and protected needle. (Photos courtesy of Steph Auer, RN.)

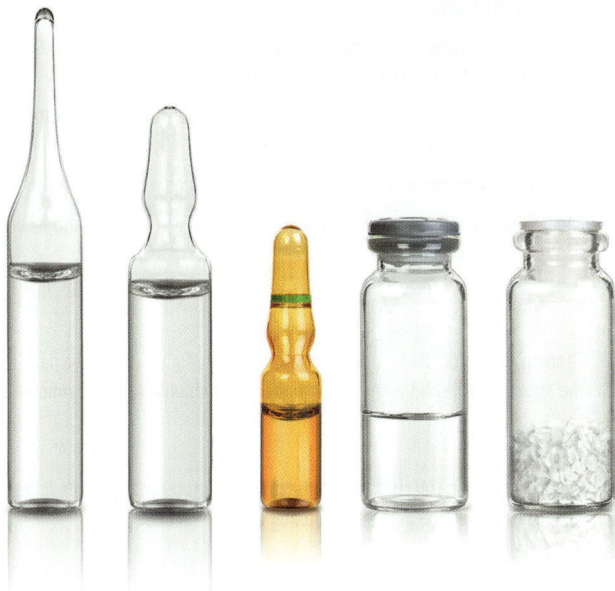

FIGURE 35.25 Medications in ampoules and vials. (iStockphoto/urfinguss)

Mixing Medications. If two medications are compatible, they can be mixed in one injection if the total dose is within accepted limits. When two or more medications are mixed, the patient will not have to receive more than one injection at a time. Most nursing units keep charts that list common compatible medications. If you have any uncertainty about medication compatibilities, consult a pharmacist.

Mixing Medications From Two Vials. Apply the following principles when mixing medications from two vials:
1. Do not contaminate one medication with another.
2. Ensure the final dose is accurate.
3. Maintain an aseptic technique.

To mix medications from two vials, use only one syringe with a needle or use a syringe with a needleless access device attached (Figure 35.26). Aspirate a volume of air equivalent to the first medication's dose

(vial A). Inject the air into vial A, ensuring the needle does not touch the solution. Withdraw the needle and aspirate a volume of air equivalent to the second medication's dose (vial B). Inject the air into vial B. Immediately withdraw the medication from vial B into the syringe, then insert the needle back into vial A, being careful not to push the plunger and expel the medication in the syringe into the vial. Withdraw the desired amount of medication from vial A into the syringe. After withdrawing the necessary amount, withdraw the needle from the syringe. Insert into the syringe a new needle or a needleless access device suitable for injection.

Mixing Medications From One Vial and One Ampoule. When mixing medication from a vial and an ampoule, prepare medication from the vial first and then use the same syringe and filter needle to withdraw medication from the ampoule. Prepare the medication combination in this prescription because air does not need to be added to withdraw medication from an ampoule.

Insulin Preparation. Insulin is the hormone used to treat diabetes in some patients. Although inhaled insulin has recently been approved for use, insulin is most commonly administered by injection. Because insulin is a protein, if it were taken orally, it would break down and be destroyed in the GI tract. Most patients who have diabetes that requires them to take insulin learn to self-administer the injections. In Canada, health care providers usually prescribe insulin in concentrations of 100 units per millilitre of solution, which is called *U-100 insulin*. Make sure to use the correct syringe when preparing insulin. For example, use a 100-unit insulin syringe to prepare U-100 insulin.

Prefilled insulin pens are becoming more commonly used in hospitals to minimize incidents related to dosing and type of insulin administered (Table 35.11). Insulin pens are easy to use but they take more time to inject the insulin compared to a syringe. The insulin pen type must match the insulin brand prescribed.

Insulin is classified by its rate of action: rapid-acting, short-acting, intermediate-acting, or long-acting. Each type has a different onset, peak, and duration of action (Table 35.12). Only regular (short-acting) insulin can be administered intravenously. Prescriptions for insulin injections attempt to imitate the normal pattern of a patient's insulin release from the pancreas. Some insulins come in a stable premixed solution (e.g., 30/70 insulin comprises 30% regular or short-acting insulin to 70% NPH

SKILL 35.4   PREPARING INJECTIONS

Delegation Considerations
The preparation of injections cannot be delegated to unregulated care providers.

Equipment
- Medication administration record (MAR)
- Barcode scanner (if applicable)
- Small gauze pad and alcohol swab
- Syringe and needle for injection
- Medication in an ampoule or vial
- Blunt filter or fill needle
- Medication diluent (e.g., normal saline or sterile water) (if indicated)

PROCEDURE

STEPS	RATIONALE
1. Check the accuracy and completeness of the MAR, including the following: patient name and medication name, route, dosage, time of administration, and start and stop date. If difficult to read, review the original prescription and rewrite the MAR.	• Ensures the patient receives the right medication • Illegible MARs are a source of medication incidents. The original prescription is the most reliable source and only legal record of medications the patient is to receive.
2. Assess the patient's health history, medications, and allergies.	• Certain substances have similar compositions; never administer a substance to which a patient has a known allergy.
3. Collect the necessary information to administer medication safely, including action, purpose, adverse effects, and nursing implications.	• This is necessary to determine if the medication, dose, and route are appropriate, and how to administer it safely.
4. Assess the patient's body build, muscle size, and weight.	• Determines the type and size of the syringe and the needles for injection
5. Perform hand hygiene. Prepare medication (see Skill 35.1, Steps 4A–H): Check the expiry date on medication vials and ampoules. Ensure that you compare the label of the medication with the MAR at least two times while preparing the medication.	• Medication potency may increase or decrease when medications are expired.
A. Ampoule preparation	
(1) Attach the blunt filter needle to the syringe or select the appropriate sharp needle for injection according to employer policy. Tap the top of the ampoule lightly and quickly with your finger until the fluid moves from the neck of the ampoule (see Step 5A[1] illustration).	• Tapping the ampoule dislodges any fluid that collects above the neck of the ampoule. All solution moves into the lower chamber of the ampoule.
(2) Place a small gauze pad or an unopened alcohol swab around the neck of the ampoule (see Step 5A[2] illustration).	• Placing a pad around the neck of the ampoule protects the user's fingers from injury when the glass tip is broken off.

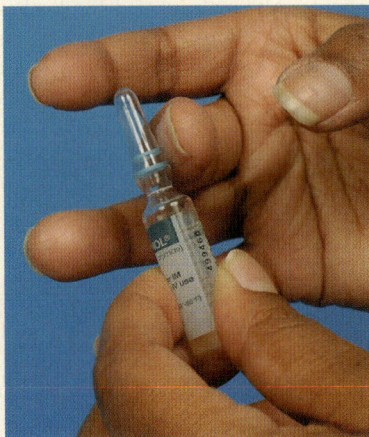

STEP 5A(1) Tapping the ampoule moves the fluid down the neck of the ampoule.

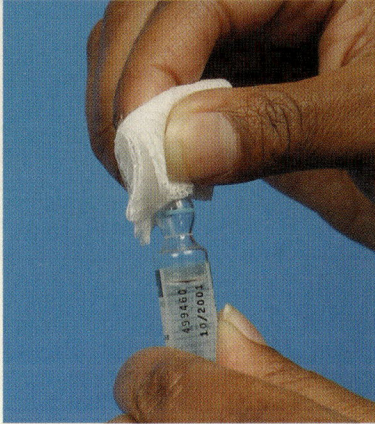

STEP 5A(2) Gauze pad placed around the neck of the ampoule.

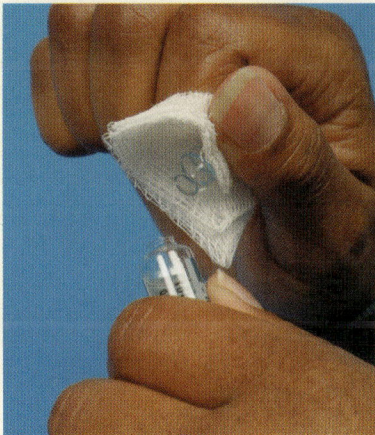

STEP 5A(3) Snapping the neck of the ampoule away from the hands.

(3) Snap the neck of the ampoule quickly and firmly away from the hands (see Step 5A[3] illustration).

- Snapping the neck quickly and firmly protects the user's fingers and face from the shattering glass.

(4) Draw up the medication immediately, using a blunt filter or sharp needle long enough to reach the bottom of the ampoule.

- The injection system is vulnerable to airborne contaminants. The needle must be long enough to access the medication for preparation. Filter needles are used to sift out any fragments of glass (Mitchell, 2020).

(5) Hold the ampoule sideways, inverted, or set it on a flat surface. Insert the needle into the centre of the ampoule opening. Do not allow the needle tip or shaft to touch the rim of the ampoule.

- The broken rim of the ampoule is considered contaminated. When the ampoule is inverted, the solution dribbles out if the needle tip or shaft touches the rim of the ampoule.

(6) Keep the needle tip under the surface of the liquid. Tip the ampoule to bring all fluid within reach of the needle.

- Keeping the needle tip under the surface of the liquid prevents the aspiration of air bubbles.

(7) Aspirate the medication into the syringe by gently pulling back on the plunger (see Step 5A[7] illustrations).

- Withdrawal of the plunger creates negative pressure within the syringe barrel, which pulls the fluid into the syringe.

STEP 5A(7) Aspirate medication from the ampoule using a blunt filter needle. (Courtesy and © Becton, Dickinson and Company.)

Continued

(8) If air bubbles are aspirated, do not expel the air into the ampoule.

- Expelling air into the ampoule may force fluid out of the ampoule, which could lead to loss of the medication.

(9) To expel excess air bubbles, remove the needle from the ampoule. Hold the syringe with the needle pointing up. Tap the side of the syringe to cause the bubbles to rise toward the needle. Draw back slightly on the plunger, then push the plunger upward to eject the air. Do not eject any fluid.

- Withdrawing the plunger too far will remove it from the barrel. Holding the syringe vertically allows fluid to settle in the bottom of the barrel. Pulling back on the plunger allows the fluid within the needle to enter the barrel so that fluid is not expelled. Air at the top of the barrel and within the needle is then expelled.

(10) If the syringe contains excess fluid, dispose of it in the appropriate receptacle. Hold the syringe vertically with the needle tip up and slanted slightly toward the receptacle. Recheck the fluid level in the syringe by holding it vertically. Do not dispose of excess liquids into a sink, toilet, or garbage can.

- The position of the needle allows the medication to be safely expelled without flowing down the needle shaft. Rechecking the fluid level ensures the proper dose.

(11) Recap the blunt filter needle and replace the blunt filter needle with the appropriate sharp needle for injection. If you have drawn up the medication with the appropriate sharp bevelled needle for the patient's size and weight, cover the tip with safety sheath (if applicable).

- Covering the needle prevents contamination of the needle and minimizes needle-stick injuries. Filter needles cannot be used for injection.

B. Vial containing a solution

(1) Attach a blunt fill needle to a syringe or select the appropriate sharp needle for injection based on employer policy (see Step 5B[1] illustration). Remove the cap covering the top of the unused vial to expose the sterile rubber seal. If a multidose vial has been previously used, the cap has already been removed. Firmly and briskly wipe the surface of the rubber seal with an alcohol swab for 30 seconds and allow it to dry.

- The vial comes packaged with a seal that cannot be replaced after the cap has been removed. Not all medication manufacturers guarantee that caps of unused vials are sterile. Therefore, seals must be swabbed with alcohol before preparing the medication. Allowing the alcohol to dry prevents the needle from being coated with alcohol, which could mix with the medication.

(2) Pick up the syringe and remove the needle cap. Draw up air into the syringe equivalent to volume of medication you will be aspirating from the vial (e.g., 2 mL) by pulling back on the plunger.

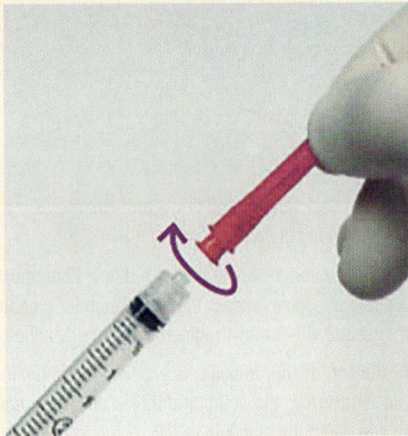

- Inject air into the vial to prevent the buildup of negative pressure in the vial when aspirating medication.

STEP 5B(1) Attach the blunt fill needle to the syringe and draw up air. (Courtesy and © Becton, Dickinson and Company.)

STEP 5B(3) Insert the tip of the needle through the centre of the vial diaphragm (with the vial flat on the table). (Courtesy and © Becton, Dickinson and Company.)

SKILL 35.4 PREPARING INJECTIONS—cont'd

STEPS	RATIONALE

CRITICAL DECISION POINT: *Some medications require that a filter needle be used when preparing medications from a vial. The same policy is required by some institutions. Check the employer policy to determine whether the use of a filter needle is indicated (Mitchell, 2020). If using a filter needle to aspirate the medication, replace the blunt needle with use an appropriately sized sharp needle to administer an injection.*

(3) Hold the vial firmly on a flat surface. Insert the bevelled tip of the needle first, followed by the rest of the needle through the centre of the rubber seal at a 90-degree angle (see Step 5B[3] illustration).

- The centre of the seal is thinner and easier to penetrate than the sides of the seal. Injecting the bevelled tip of the needle first and using firm pressure prevents coring of the rubber seal, which could enter the vial or needle.

(4) Inject the air into the empty airspace in the vial. Hold the plunger with firm pressure so it is not forced backward by air pressure within the vial.

- Injecting air before aspirating the fluid creates a vacuum that is needed to allow the medication to flow into the syringe. Injecting air into the empty airspace in the vial prevents the formation of bubbles, which can lead to an inaccurate dose.

(5) Invert the vial while keeping a firm hold on the syringe and plunger (see Step 5B[5] illustration). Hold the vial between your thumb and the middle fingers of your nondominant hand. Grasp the end of the syringe barrel and plunger with the thumb and forefinger of your dominant hand to counteract pressure in the vial.

- Inverting the vial allows the fluid to settle in the lower half of the container. Correct positioning of your hands prevents forceful movement of the plunger and permits easy manipulation of the syringe.

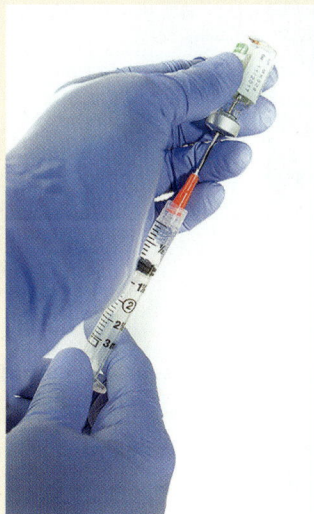

STEP 5B(5) Withdraw fluid with the vial inverted. (iStockphoto/Teresa Otto.)

(6) Keep the tip of the needle below the fluid level.

- Keeping the needle tip under the surface of the liquid prevents the aspiration of air.

(7) Allow air pressure from the vial to fill the syringe gradually with medication. If necessary, pull back slightly on the plunger to obtain the correct amount of solution.

- Positive pressure within the vial forces the fluid into the syringe (unless the vial has been used several times).

(8) When the desired volume of solution is obtained, position the needle into the vial's airspace; tap the side of the syringe barrel carefully to dislodge any air bubbles. Eject any air remaining at the top of the syringe into the vial.

- Forcefully striking the barrel while the needle is inserted in the vial may bend the needle. The accumulation of air displaces the medication and can lead to inappropriate doses.

(9) Remove the needle from the vial by grasping the syringe barrel. Do not pull on the plunger.

- Accidentally pulling the plunger instead of the barrel can cause the plunger to separate from the barrel and spray out the medication.

(10) Hold the syringe at eye level, at a 90-degree angle, to ensure the correct volume has been obtained and no air bubbles are present (see Step 5B[10] illustration). Remove any remaining air by tapping the barrel to dislodge the air bubbles. Draw back slightly on the plunger; then push the plunger upward to eject any air. Do not eject the fluid. Recheck the volume of the medication.

- Holding the syringe vertically allows fluid to settle in the bottom of the barrel. Pulling back on the plunger allows the fluid within the needle to enter the barrel so that fluid is not expelled. Air at the top of the barrel and within the needle is then expelled.

Continued

SKILL 35.4	PREPARING INJECTIONS—cont'd
STEPS	RATIONALE

STEP 5B(10) Hold the syringe upright to check if the correct volume has been obtained. (iStockphoto/pinkomelet.)

STEP 5B(11A) Recap the blunt needle by sliding the needle into the cap lying on a flat surface. (Courtesy and © Becton, Dickinson and Company.)

STEP 5B(11B) Replace the blunt needle with the appropriate sharp needle for injection.

(11) Recap the blunt fill needle (see Step 5B[11a] illustration). Remove the blunt needle and replace it with the appropriate sharp needle for injection (see Step 5B[11b] illustration). If you have drawn up the medication using the appropriate sharp bevelled needle for the patient's size and weight, cover the tip with safety sheath (if applicable).

- Inserting a needle through a rubber stopper may dull the bevelled tip. New needles are sharper. Because no fluid remains along the shaft, the needle will not track medication through the tissues.

STEPS	RATIONALE
(12) If using a multidose vial, make a label that includes the date of opening, the concentration of the medication per millilitre, and your initials.	• Labelling ensures that future doses will be prepared correctly. Some medications are discarded a specific number of days after opening the vial. For example, insulin vials are discarded 30 days after opening.
C. Vial containing a powder (reconstituting medications)	
(1) Remove the cap covering the vial of powdered medication and the cap covering the vial of proper diluent. Firmly wipe both seals with the alcohol swab for 15 seconds and allow to dry for 30 seconds.	• Not all medication manufacturers guarantee that caps of unused vials are sterile. Therefore, seals must be swabbed with alcohol before preparing the medication. Allowing the alcohol to dry prevents the needle from being coated with alcohol, which could mix with the medication.
(2) Draw up diluent into the syringe following Steps 5B(2) through 5B(11).	• Drawing up the diluent prepares the diluent for injection into a vial containing powdered medication.
(3) Insert the tip of the needle through the centre of the rubber seal on the vial of powdered medication. Inject the diluent into the vial. Remove the needle.	• The diluent begins to dissolve and reconstitute medication.
(4) Mix the medication thoroughly. Roll the vial in your palms. Do not shake.	• Rolling ensures proper dispersal of medication throughout the solution. Shaking produces bubbles.
(5) Reconstituted medication in the vial is ready to be drawn into a new syringe. Read the label carefully to determine the dose after reconstitution.	• After the diluent has been added, the concentration of medication (mg/mL) determines the dose to be given.
(6) Prepare medication in syringe following Steps 5B(2) through 5B(11).	

CRITICAL DECISION POINT: *Some institutions may require prepared parenteral medications to be verified for accuracy by another nurse. Check the employer policy before administering medication.*

6. Dispose of all soiled supplies. Place broken ampoule vials, used vials, and used needles in a puncture-proof and leak-proof container. Clean the medication work area and perform hand hygiene.	• Proper disposal of glass and needle prevents accidental injury to staff and controls the transmission of infection.

UNEXPECTED OUTCOMES	RELATED INTERVENTIONS
Air bubbles remaining in syringe	• Expel air from the syringe and add medication to the syringe until the correct dose is prepared.
Incorrect dose prepared	• Discard the prepared dose and prepare the corrected new dose.

TABLE 35.11   Preparing a Preloaded Pen Device

Loading	Please refer to the pen manufacturer's instruction sheets.
Appropriate mixing	NPH and premixed insulins. Roll 10 times, tip 10 times, and visually check that insulin has a consistent milky appearance.
Priming shot	A priming shot is required when changing a cartridge or using a new needle. Typically, it is recommended to use two units to prime the pen; however, please refer to the pen instruction sheets from the manufacturer.
Dialing up dose	Dial-up units of insulin required.
Delivery of insulin	Inject insulin at a 90-degree angle in desired injection site when using a shorter needle (4, 5, or 6 mm). A 45-degree angle may be needed if the person is thin or if a longer needle (>8 mm) is being used. A proper skin lift should also be used in thin individuals or when using longer needles. Hold the injection for 10 seconds to ensure full delivery of dose.

Adapted from Diabetes Canada. (2018). *Clinical practice guidelines: Insulin pen start checklist for healthcare providers.* http://guidelines.diabetes.ca/BloodGlucoseLowering/InsulinChecklist

TABLE 35.12   A Comparison of Insulin Preparations

Type of Insulin	Onset	Peak	Duration
Rapid-Acting and Short-Acting (Clear)			
Insulin glulisine (Apidra)	10–15 minutes	1–2 hours	3–5 hours
Insulin lispro (Humalog)	10–15 minutes	1–2 hours	3.5–4.75 hours
Insulin aspart (NovoRapid)	10–15 minutes	1–1.5 hours	3–5 hours
Regular insulin (short-acting insulin)* (Humulin-R, Novolin ge Toronto)	30 minutes	2–3 hours	6.5 hours
Intermediate-Acting (Cloudy)			
Isophane insulin suspension (Novolin ge NPH insulin, Humulin N)	1–3 hours	5–8 hours	Up to 18 hours
Long-Acting (Clear)			
Insulin glargine (Lantus)†	90 minutes	Plateau	24 hours
Insulin detemir (Levemir)†	90 minutes	"Peakless"	16–24 hours

Continued

TABLE 35.12	A Comparison of Insulin Preparations—cont'd			
Type of Insulin		**Onset**	**Peak**	**Duration**
Premixed Insulins (Cloudy)‡				
Premixed regular insulin—NPH (Humulin 30/70, Novolin ge 30/70, 40/60, 50/50)		30–60 minutes	2–12 hours	18–24 hours
Premixed insulin analogues		30–60 minutes	2–12 hours	18–24 hours
• Biphasic insulin aspart (NovoMix 30)				
• Insulin lispro/lispro protamine (Humalog Mix25 and Mix50)				

*Regular insulin is the only insulin for intravenous use; when administered intravenously, the onset of action is within 10 to 30 minutes and the peak effect is within 20 to 30 minutes.
†Cannot be mixed with other insulins.
‡A single vial or cartridge contains a fixed ratio of insulin (% of rapid-acting or short-acting insulin to % of intermediate-acting insulin).
Based on Diabetes Canada. (2020). *Clinical practice guidelines for the prevention and management of diabetes in Canada.* http://guidelines.diabetes.ca/fullguidelines

BOX 35.23	Example of a Sliding Scale Insulin Prescription According to Capillary Blood Sugars (CBS)

Give Novolin ge Toronto Regular Insulin subcutaneously before meals and at bedtime (0800, 1200, 1700, 2200 hours) according to sliding scale:

CBS	<4.0	Follow hypoglycemia protocol and notify prescriber
CBS	4.1–8.0	No insulin
CBS	10.1–12.0	1 unit
CBS	12.1–14.0	2 units
CBS	14.1–16.0	2 units
CBS	16.1–18	3 units
CBS	18.1–20	4 units
CBS	>20	Notify prescriber

Adapted from Diabetes Canada. (2018). *Insulin orders sets & in-hospital management of diabetes.* https://guidelines.diabetes.ca/docs/resources/in-hospital-management-clinical-order-set-fillable.pdf

[neutral protamine Hagedorn] or intermediate-acting insulin). Patients receiving premixed insulins do not need to mix insulins.

A patient with diabetes may require more than one type of insulin. For example, by receiving both a short-acting insulin and an intermediate-acting insulin, a patient receives a more sustained control of blood glucose levels over 24 hours.

Insulin is prescribed either by a specific dose at select times or by a sliding scale. A sliding scale dictates a certain dose on the basis of the patient's blood glucose level (Box 35.23). Usually, rapid-acting or short-acting insulins are used for sliding scales. Before drawing up the insulin doses, gently roll all cloudy insulin preparations between the palms of the hands (or rotate the vial for at least 1 minute) to resuspend the insulin. Do not shake insulin vials; shaking causes the formation of bubbles, which take up space in the syringe and thereby alter the dose. If more than one type of insulin is required to manage the patient's diabetes, two different types of insulin can be mixed in one syringe *if they are compatible* (Box 35.24), by following the steps demonstrated in Figure 35.26. When two types of insulin are mixed, the single injection minimizes the patient's discomfort that is associated with multiple injections. In hospitals, when taking capillary blood samples for blood glucose monitoring, always swab the patient's anticipated sample site (e.g., the fingertip) with an alcohol swab before taking the sample. Use of an aseptic technique prevents the introduction of microorganisms and protects patients from infection while in the hospital. Although diabetic patients are commonly educated not to use alcohol swabs in the community setting, their use is essential to maintain asepsis and infection-control

standards in hospital settings. Always consult with employer protocol for special care required when treating diabetic patients.

Administering Injections

Each injection route differs depending on the type of tissues the medication enters. The characteristics of the tissues influence the rate of medication absorption and thus the onset of medication action. Before injecting a medication, the nurse must know the volume of the medication to administer, the medication's characteristics and viscosity, and the location of anatomical structures underlying the injection sites (Skill 35.5).

If injections are not administered correctly, negative patient outcomes can result. Failure to select an injection site in relation to anatomical landmarks can result in nerve or bone damage during needle insertion. An inability to maintain stability of the needle and syringe unit can result in pain for the patient and possible tissue damage. It was previously considered best practice to aspirate for 5 to 10 seconds prior to administering intramuscular medications, in order to avoid puncturing a vein or artery. Research on this topic has had inconsistent results, and the practice is still common and recommended by some institutions' policies. However, the World Health Organization and the U.S. Centers for Disease Control and Prevention now both recommend aspirating only if performing an IM in the dorsogluteal location, due to the proximity of the gluteal artery (Thomas et al., 2016). Aspirating is considered more painful and, due to the rapid rate of aspiration that most nurses perform, it is not believed to be effective for ensuring that injury does not occur. A new clinical practice guideline from 2018 is available on the subject (Mraz et al., 2018), although in clinical practice aspirating still remains common.

Many patients, particularly children, fear injections. Patients with serious or chronic illness often are given several injections daily. Nurses may be able to minimize the patient's discomfort in the following ways:

- Using a sharp-bevelled needle in the smallest suitable length and gauge
- Positioning the patient as comfortably as possible, to reduce muscular tension
- Selecting the proper injection site, by using anatomical landmarks
- Diverting the patient's attention from the injection by asking open-ended questions
- Inserting the needle quickly and smoothly to minimize tissue pulling
- Holding the syringe steady while the needle remains in the tissues
- Injecting the medication slowly and steadily

Subcutaneous Injections. Subcutaneous injections involve administering medications into the loose connective tissue under the dermis (see Skill 35.5). Because subcutaneous tissue is not as richly supplied

BOX 35.24 PROCEDURAL GUIDELINE

Mixing Two Kinds of Insulin in One Syringe

Delegation Considerations

The mixing of two kinds of insulin in one syringe cannot be delegated.

Equipment

- Insulin vials
- Insulin syringe
- Alcohol swabs
- Medication administration record (MAR)
- Barcode scanner (if applicable)

Procedure

1. Check the accuracy and completeness of the MAR, including the following: patient name and medication name, route, dosage, time of administration, and start and stop date. If difficult to read, review the original prescription order and rewrite the MAR.
2. Assess the patient's health history, medications, and allergies.
3. Collect the necessary information to administer the medication safely.
4. Perform hand hygiene. Carefully verify the insulin labels; compare the medication labels against the MAR before preparing the dose to ensure that the correct type of insulin is prepared.
5. If the insulin is cloudy, roll the bottle of insulin between your hands to resuspend the insulin preparation.
6. Wipe the tops of both insulin vials with the alcohol swabs for 30 seconds.
7. Verify the insulin dosage against the MAR a second time.
8. If mixing rapid- or short-acting insulin with intermediate- or long-acting insulin, take the insulin syringe and aspirate a volume of air equivalent to the dose of insulin to be withdrawn from the intermediate- or long-acting insulin first. If two intermediate- or long-acting insulins are mixed, either vial can be prepared first.

9. Insert the needle and inject air into the vial of the intermediate- or long-acting insulin. Do not let the tip of the needle touch the insulin.
10. Remove the syringe from the vial of the intermediate- or long-acting insulin without aspirating the insulin.
11. With the same syringe, inject a volume of air that is equivalent to the dose of insulin to be withdrawn into the vial of the rapid- or short-acting insulin. Withdraw the correct dose into the syringe.
12. Remove the syringe from the rapid- or short-acting insulin vial after carefully removing air bubbles in the syringe to ensure the correct dose.
13. After verifying the insulin dosage with the MAR a third time, show the insulin preparation in the syringe to another nurse to verify that the correct dose of insulin was prepared. Determine which point on the syringe scale represents the total of the combined units of insulin by adding the number of units of both insulins together (e.g., 3 units regular insulin + 10 units NPH insulin = 13 units total insulin).
14. Place the needle of the syringe back into the vial of the intermediate- or long-acting insulin. Be careful not to push the plunger, which would inject the insulin in the syringe into the vial.
15. Invert the vial, and carefully withdraw the desired amount of insulin into the syringe.
16. Withdraw the needle and check the fluid level in the syringe. Keep the needle of the prepared syringe sheathed or capped until you are ready to administer the medication. Show the syringe to another nurse to verify the correct dose was prepared.
17. Dispose of soiled medication supplies in the proper receptacle and perform hand hygiene.
18. Because rapid- or short-acting insulin binds with intermediate- or long-acting insulin, which reduces the action of the faster-acting insulin, administer the mixture within 5 minutes of preparing it.

Adapted from Healthwise. (2021). *My Health Alberta: Steps for preparing a mixed dose of insulin.* https://myhealth.alberta.ca/health/Pages/conditions.aspx?hwid=hw39025&lang=en-ca

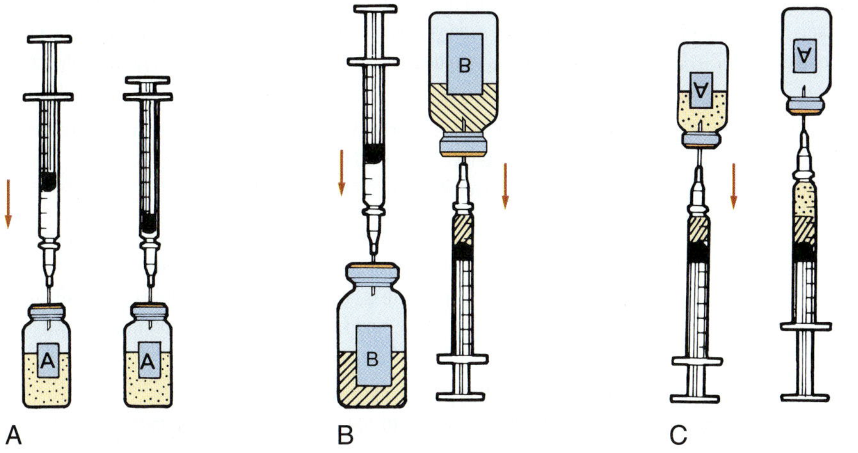

FIGURE 35.26 Mixing medications from two vials. **A,** Injecting air into vial A. **B,** Injecting air into vial B and withdrawing the dose. **C,** Withdrawing medication from vial A; the two medications are now mixed.

SKILL 35.5 ADMINISTERING INJECTIONS

Delegation Considerations

The administration of injections cannot be delegated to an unregulated care provider (UCP). Instruct UCPs to report the occurrence of potential medication adverse effects or any changes in the patient's vital signs or level of consciousness (e.g., sedation) immediately.

Equipment

- Proper size syringe and needle:
  - *Subcutaneous:* Syringe (1–3 mL) and needle (26–31 G, 1.3–1.6 cm length)
  - *Subcutaneous U-100 insulin:* Insulin syringe (0.3, 0.5, or 1 mL) with preattached needle (29–32 G, 0.3–1.3 cm length)
  - *Intramuscular (IM):* Adults: syringe (2–3 mL) and needle (19–25 G, 2.5–3.2 cm length); Children: syringe (0.5–1 mL) and needle (22–25 G; 2.2–3.2 cm length); Infants: syringe (0.5–1 mL) and needle (25–27 G; 2.2–2.5 cm length)
  - Needle length corresponds to the site of injection and the age of the patient (see Table 35.10)
- Small gauze pad, or alcohol swab, or both
- Vial or ampoule of medication
- Clean, disposable gloves
- Medication administration record (MAR)
- Barcode scanner (if applicable)

PROCEDURE

STEPS	RATIONALE
For All Injections	
1. Check the accuracy and completeness of the MAR, including the following: patient name and medication name, route, dosage, time of administration, and start and stop date. If difficult to read, review the original prescription order and rewrite the MAR.	• Ensures that the patient receives the right medication • Illegible MARs are a source of medication incidents. The original prescription is the most reliable source and only legal record of medications the patient is to receive.
2. Assess the patient's health history, medications, and allergies.	• Certain substances have similar compositions; never administer a substance to which a patient has a known allergy.
3. Collect the information necessary to safely administer the medication.	• This is necessary to determine if the medication, dose, and route are appropriate, and how to administer it safely.
4. Perform hand hygiene. Aseptically prepare the correct medication dose from an ampoule or vial (see Skill 35.4). Check the expiry dates on ampoules or vials. Ensure that all air is expelled from the syringe.	• Aseptic preparation ensures that the medication is sterile. Preparation techniques differ for ampoules and vials. • Medication potency may increase or decrease when medications are expired.
5. Check the label of medication against the MAR two times while preparing the medication. Create a removable label that shows the patient's name, the name of the medication, and the dosage. Apply the label to the syringe (not the needle).	• Ensures that the right medication is prepared for the right patient • Labelling the syringe (and not the needle) ensures that the medication in the syringe is recorded and a label on the needle is not moved to another syringe.
6. Take the medication to the patient at the right time. Perform hand hygiene.	• Taking the medication according to schedule ensures that the patient receives the effect of the medication at the right time. • Hand hygiene reduces the transfer of microorganisms.
7. Close the room curtain or door.	• Provides privacy and avoids distractions
8. Identify the patient using two to three patient identifiers.	• Asking the patient to state their name, comparing the patient's name and one other identifier (e.g., the hospital ID number) on the MAR and the patient's ID bracelet, and scanning the barcode on the patient's ID bracelet ensure that you have the right patient.
9. Explain the procedure and observe the patient's verbal and nonverbal responses to receiving the injection. Inform the patient that the injection will cause a slight burning or stinging sensation. Assess the patient's understanding.	• Injections can be painful and anxiety-provoking. • Describing the process to the patient helps to minimize the patient's anxiety. • Understanding increases medication adherence.
10. Assess the patient for contraindications.	

SKILL 35.5 ADMINISTERING INJECTIONS—cont'd

STEPS	RATIONALE
A. *For subcutaneous injections:* Assess the patient for factors such as circulatory shock and reduced local tissue perfusion. Assess the adequacy of the patient's adipose tissue.	• Reduced tissue perfusion interferes with medication absorption and distribution. Physiological changes of aging and the patient's health may affect the amount of the patient's subcutaneous tissue. The amount of subcutaneous tissue influences the methods chosen for administering injections.
B. *For intramuscular injections:* Assess the patient for muscle atrophy, reduced blood flow, and circulatory shock.	• Atrophied muscles absorb medication poorly. Factors that interfere with blood flow to muscles will impair the medication's absorption.

CRITICAL DECISION POINT: *Because of documented adverse effects to intramuscular injections, other routes of medication administration are safer. Verify that an intramuscular injection is necessary and explore alternative medication routes, if possible (Polania Gutierrez & Munakomi, 2021).*

STEPS	RATIONALE
11. Compare the label on the medication with the MAR one more time at the patient's bedside.	• This is the *third accuracy check.*
12. Perform hand hygiene; put on clean, disposable gloves.	• Reduces the transfer of microorganisms
13. Keep a sheet or gown draped over the patient's body parts that do not need to be exposed.	• Respects the dignity of the patient while only the area to be injected is exposed
14. Assess the patient and select an appropriate injection site. Inspect the skin surface over the injection site for bruises, inflammation, and edema.	• Injection sites should be free of abnormalities or hardening that may interfere with medication absorption. Sites used repeatedly can become hardened from lipohypertrophy (increased growth in fatty tissue). Do not inject an area that is bruised or shows signs associated with infection.
A. *Subcutaneous injection:* Palpate the injection site for masses or tenderness. Avoid using these areas. For patients who require daily insulin, rotate the injection site daily. Ensure that the needle is the correct size by grasping a skin fold at the injection site with your thumb and forefinger. Measure across the skin fold. The needle should be one-half the distance across the fold to give it at a 90-degree angle.	• Subcutaneous injections can be inadvertently given in the muscle, especially when the injection site is in the abdomen or thigh. Use of the appropriate size of needle ensures that medication will be injected in the subcutaneous tissue (Polania Gutierrez & Munakomi, 2021).
B. *Intramuscular injection:* Note the integrity and size of the muscle and palpate for tenderness or hardness. Avoid using these areas. If injections are given frequently, rotate the injection sites. Use the ventrogluteal site if possible.	• Unless contraindications exist for this site, the ventrogluteal site is the preferred injection site for adults and children, but for infants the vastus lateralis site should be used (Polania Gutierrez & Munakomi, 2021).
C. *Intradermal injection:* Note any lesions or discolorations of the patient's forearm. Select an injection site three to four fingerwidths below the antecubital space and a handwidth above the wrist. If the forearm cannot be used, inspect the patient's upper back. If necessary, sites for subcutaneous injections may be used.	• An intradermal site should be free from lesions or discolorations so that results of a skin test can be seen and interpreted correctly.
15. Assist the patient to a comfortable position:	
A. *Subcutaneous injection:* Have the patient relax the arm, leg, or abdomen, depending on the site chosen for injection.	• Minimizes the patient's discomfort
B. *Intramuscular injection:* Position the patient depending on the site chosen (e.g., have the patient sit, lie flat, lie on one side, or lie prone).	• Reduces strains on the patient's muscle and minimizes the discomfort of the injection
C. *Intradermal injection:* Have the patient extend their elbow and support the elbow and forearm on a flat surface.	• Stabilizes the injection site for easy accessibility
D. Speak with the patient about a subject of interest. Ask open-ended questions.	• Reduces anxiety

CRITICAL DECISION POINT: *Ensure that the patient's position is not contraindicated by a medical condition.*

STEPS	RATIONALE
16. Relocate the injection site using anatomical landmarks.	• Prevents injury to nerves, bones, and blood vessels
17. Clean the injection site with an antiseptic swab. Touch the swab to the centre of the site and rotate outward in a circular direction about 5 cm for 30 seconds. Air to dry (see Step 17 illustration).	• Removes microorganisms

Continued

STEPS	RATIONALE

STEP 17 Clean the injection site by using a circular motion.

18. Hold the swab or gauze between the third and fourth fingers of your nondominant hand.

19. Remove the needle cap or sheath from the needle by pulling it straight off.

20. Hold the syringe between the thumb and forefinger of your dominant hand.

   A. *Subcutaneous injection:* Hold the syringe as if you were holding a dart, palm down; or hold the syringe across the tops of your fingertips (see Step 20A illustration).

   B. *Intramuscular injection:* Hold the syringe as if you were holding a dart, palm down.

- The gauze or swab is readily accessible when the needle is withdrawn.
- Avoids contaminating the needle

- Quick, smooth injection requires proper manipulation of the syringe parts.

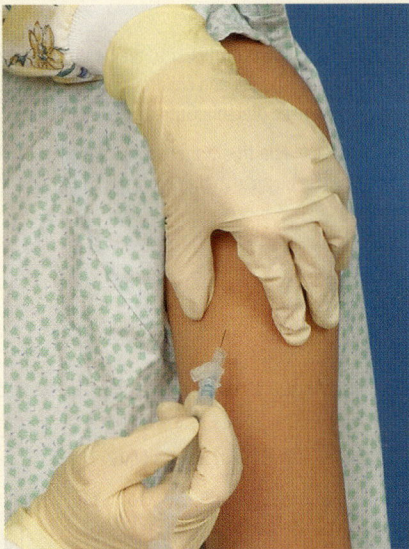

STEP 20A Hold the syringe as if grasping a dart.

   C. *Intradermal injection:* Hold the bevel of the needle pointing up.

21. Administer the injection:

   A. Subcutaneous injection

      (1) For an average-sized patient, spread the skin tightly across the injection site or pinch the skin with your nondominant hand.

- With the bevel pointing up, the medication is less likely to be deposited into tissues below the dermis.

- A needle penetrates tight skin easier than loose skin. Pinching the skin elevates the subcutaneous tissue and may desensitize the area.

SKILL 35.5	ADMINISTERING INJECTIONS—cont'd
STEPS	**RATIONALE**

(2) Inject the needle quickly and firmly at a 45- to 90-degree angle. Hold the skin fold until the needle has been withdrawn from the skin.	• Quick, firm insertion minimizes the patient's discomfort. (Injecting medication into compressed tissue irritates the nerve fibres.) Injecting at the correct angle prevents accidental injection into the muscle. Injecting into a raised skin fold is thought to result in a more diffuse depot of insulin, in contrast to a compact bolus injected without a raised skin fold (Polania Gutierrez & Munakomi, 2021).
(3) For a patient with obesity, pinch the skin at the injection site and insert the needle at a 90-degree angle below the tissue fold.	• Ensure that the injection is given in the subcutaneous adipose tissue rather than intradermally (just under the epidermis) or into the muscle (Polania Gutierrez & Munakomi, 2021).

CRITICAL DECISION POINT: *Piercing a blood vessel during a subcutaneous injection is very rare, so aspiration is not necessary when administering subcutaneous injections.*

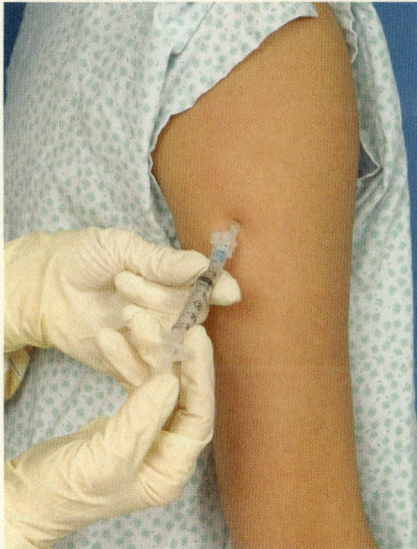

STEP 21A(4) Inject the medication slowly.

(4) Inject the medication slowly (see Step 21A[4] illustration).

B. Intramuscular injection

(1) Position your nondominant hand at the proper anatomical landmarks and pull the skin down approximately 2.5–3.5 cm or laterally with the ulnar side of your hand to administer the injection in a Z-track. Hold this position until the medication is injected. Use your dominant hand to insert the needle quickly at a 90-degree angle into the muscle.	• Creates a zigzag path through the tissues to seal the needle track and avoid tracking of the medication. The Z-track should be used for all intramuscular injections (smaller needles may be needed for smaller muscles) (Polania Gutierrez & Munakomi, 2021).
(2) If the patient's muscle mass is small, grasp a body of muscle between your thumb and fingers.	• Ensures that the medication reaches the muscle mass
(3) After the needle pierces the skin, grasp the lower end of the syringe barrel with your nondominant hand to stabilize the syringe. Continue to hold the skin tightly with your nondominant hand. Move your dominant hand to the end of the plunger. Do not move the syringe.	• Reduces the patient's discomfort from needle movement. The skin must remain pulled until after the medication is injected to ensure Z-track administration.
(4) Pull back on the plunger to aspirate. If no blood appears, slowly inject the medication at 10 mL/second.	• Aspirating rules out potential vascular puncturing (Polania Gutierrez & Munakomi, 2021).

CRITICAL DECISION POINT: *If blood appears in the syringe, remove the needle and dispose of the medication and syringe properly. Prepare another dose of medication for injection.*

(5) Slowly and steadily withdraw the needle and release the skin. Apply gentle pressure over the injected site with dry gauze.	• Allows time for the medication to absorb into the muscle before removal of the syringe (Polania Gutierrez & Munakomi, 2021)

Continued

SKILL 35.5	ADMINISTERING INJECTIONS—cont'd
STEPS	**RATIONALE**

C. Intradermal injection

(1) With your nondominant hand, stretch the skin over the injection site with your forefinger or thumb.

- A needle pierces tight skin more easily than loose skin.

(2) With the needle almost against the patient's skin, insert it slowly with the bevel pointed up at a 5- to 15-degree angle until resistance is felt. Advance the needle through the epidermis to approximately 3 mm below the skin surface. The needle tip can be seen through skin.

- Ensures the needle tip is in the dermis

(3) Inject the medication slowly. Normally, resistance is felt. If resistance is not felt, the needle is in too deep; remove it and begin again. Your nondominant hand can stabilize the needle during the injection.

- Minimizes the discomfort at the injection site. The dermal layer is tight and does not expand easily when the solution is injected. Stabilizing the needle prevents unnecessary movements and decreases the patient's discomfort.

(4) While injecting medication, notice that a small bleb of approximately 6 mm in diameter (resembling a mosquito bite) appears on the skin's surface (see Step 21C[4] illustration). Instruct the patient that this bleb is a normal finding.

- Indicates the medication is deposited in the dermis

STEP 21C(4) The injection creates a small bleb.

22. Withdraw the needle while wiping an alcohol swab or gauze gently over the injection site.

- Minimizes the patient's discomfort during withdrawal of the needle. Dry gauze may minimize the patient's discomfort associated with the use of alcohol on nonintact skin.

23. Apply gentle pressure. Do not massage the injection site. Put on a bandage if needed.

- Massage may cause underlying tissue damage. Massage of the intradermal site may disperse the medication into underlying tissue layers and thereby alter the test results.

24. Assist the patient to a comfortable position.

- Gives the patient a sense of well-being

25. Discard into a puncture- and leak-proof receptacle the uncapped needle or the needle enclosed in safety shield and attached to the syringe. Do *not* recap the needle.

- Prevents needlestick injuries

26. Remove disposable gloves and perform hand hygiene.

- Reduces the transmission of microorganisms

27. Stay with the patient for 3–5 minutes to observe for any allergic reactions.

- Severe anaphylactic reaction is characterized by dyspnea, wheezing, and circulatory collapse and is a life-threatening emergency.

28. Regularly reassess the patient and evaluate whether the patient feels any acute pain, burning, numbness, or tingling at the injection site.

- Continued discomfort may indicate injury to underlying bones or nerves.

29. Inspect the injection site, noting any bruising or induration.

- Bruising or induration indicates a complication associated with the injection. Document your findings and notify the patient's health care provider. Provide a warm compress to the site.

30. Observe the patient's response to medication at times that correlate with the medication's onset, peak, and duration.

- Intramuscular medications are rapidly absorbed. Adverse effects of parenteral medications may develop rapidly. The nurse's observations are to evaluate the efficacy of the medication action.

31. For intradermal injections, use a skin pencil and draw a circle around the perimeter of the injection site. Read the site within an appropriate amount of time, which is determined by the type of medication or skin test administered.

- The pencil mark makes the injection site easy to find. Results of skin testing are read at various times, on the basis of the type of medication used or the type of skin test completed. Refer to the manufacturer's directions to determine when to read the test's results.

SKILL 35.5   ADMINISTERING INJECTIONS—cont'd

UNEXPECTED OUTCOMES	RELATED INTERVENTIONS
Raised, reddened, or hard zone (induration) around intradermal test site	• Notify the patient's health care provider. • Document the patient's sensitivity to the injected allergen or the positive test if tuberculin skin testing was completed.
Hypertrophy of skin, resulting from repeated subcutaneous injections	• Do not use this site for future injections. • Instruct the patient not to use the injection site for 6 months.
Signs and symptoms of allergy or adverse effects	• Follow the institutional policy or guidelines for the appropriate response to medication adverse effects. • Notify the patient's health care provider immediately. • Add allergy information to the patient's medical record.
Complaints of localized pain, numbness, tingling, or burning sensation at injection site, indicating possible injury to nerve or tissues	• Assess the injection site. • Document your findings. • Notify the patient's health care provider.

DOCUMENTATION AND REPORTING
• Chart the medication dose, route, site, time, and date of injection on the MAR immediately after giving medication, as per employer policy.
• Document if the scheduled medication is withheld and record the reason as per employer policy.
• Report any undesirable effects from the medication to the prescriber.
• Record the patient's response to medications in the nurses' notes and report to the prescriber if required.

CARE IN THE COMMUNITY CONSIDERATIONS
• Assess the patient's readiness to learn before instructing them in how to administer self-injections. Some patients are hesitant to administer injections to themselves; relieve any anxiety before teaching this skill to a patient.
• Patients can often purchase or obtain sharps boxes for use in the home or community setting. If this purchase is not feasible, a hard plastic bottle that is nontransparent (e.g., a fabric softener bottle or a detergent bottle) may be used to safely store syringes after use. Disposal of used needles varies in homes and community settings. Check with local authorities to verify how to appropriately dispose of needles.

Adapted from Becton, Dickinson and Company. (2019). *Chart injection guidelines for needle length and gauge.* https://www.bd.com/documents/in-service-materials/syringes-and-needles/MPS_HY_Injection-guidelines-for-needle-length-and-gauge-selection_IM_EN.pdf.

with blood as the muscles, medication given by subcutaneous injection is absorbed more slowly than medication given by IM injections; however, medications injected subcutaneously are absorbed completely if the patient's circulatory status is normal. Because subcutaneous tissue contains pain receptors, the patient may experience some discomfort.

The best subcutaneous injection site and most frequently recommended site is the abdomen from below the costal margins to the iliac crests (i.e., umbilical area) (Li et al., 2020). The lateral sides of the arms and the anterior aspects of the thighs are also commonly used (Figure 35.27). Subcutaneous heparin injections in the abdomen are associated with less bruising and pain (Li et al., 2020) (Figure 35.28). Other acceptable sites are the scapular areas of the upper back and the upper ventral or dorsal gluteal areas. The injection site chosen should be free of skin lesions, bony prominences, and large underlying muscles or nerves.

The administration of low-molecular-weight heparin (LMWH) (e.g., enoxaparin) requires special considerations. The injection site is the right or left side of the abdomen at least 5 cm from the umbilicus. Administer LMWH in its prefilled syringe with the attached needle; do not expel the air bubble in the syringe before giving the medication. The needle should be introduced into a skin fold held between the thumb and forefinger; the skin fold should be held throughout the injection. A slow injection rate of 30 seconds should be used, to reduce bruising and pain (Janini & Akbari Sari, 2017; St. Clair-Jones et al., 2020). Apply light pressure with a cotton gauze for 10 seconds after the injection (Yılmaz et al., 2020). Cold application at the injection site can also decreases bruising and pain (Amaniyan et al., 2020).

When administering insulin from a vial, use U-100 insulin syringes with a preattached 26- to 31-gauge needle 6–8 mm in length (Forum for Injection Technique [FIT] Canada, 2020). This needle length is

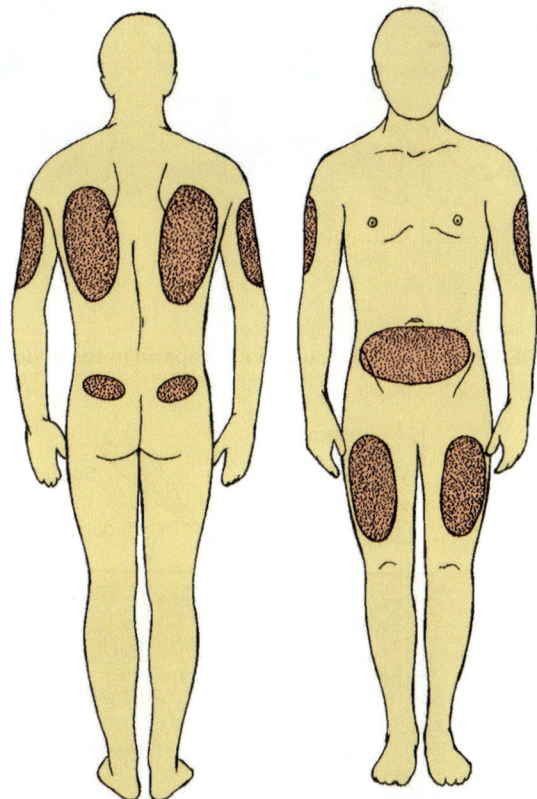

FIGURE 35.27 Sites recommended for subcutaneous injections.

required to pierce the vial, inject air, and withdraw the insulin. Recommended sites for insulin injections include the upper arm and the anterior and lateral portions of the thigh, buttocks, and abdomen. Patients with diabetes who inject insulin should practise intrasite rotation (rotating injection sites within the same body part) to provide greater consistency in the absorption of insulin. For example, if the morning insulin is injected into the patient's arm, then a subsequent injection should also be given in the arm but at least 2.5 cm away from the previous site. No injection site should be used again for at least 1 month. The rate of insulin absorption varies depending on the site: the abdomen has the quickest absorption, followed by the arms, thighs, and buttocks (Miller et al., 2018). If using a 6-mm long needle, the nurse can either insert the needle at a 90-degree angle directly into the flat skin or pinch and lift the skin. If using an 8-mm needle, the nurse must pinch and lift the skin. The nurse then injects the insulin, releases the skin if pinched, and slowly withdraws the needle at the same direction at which it was inserted (FIT Canada, 2020).

Only small doses (0.5 to 1.5 mL) of water-soluble medications should be given subcutaneously because the tissue is sensitive to irritating solutions and large volumes of medications. Medications can collect within the tissues to cause sterile abscesses, which appear as hardened, painful lumps under the skin.

A patient's body weight indicates the depth of the subcutaneous layer. Therefore, choose the needle length and angle of insertion based on the patient's weight and an estimation of the amount of subcutaneous

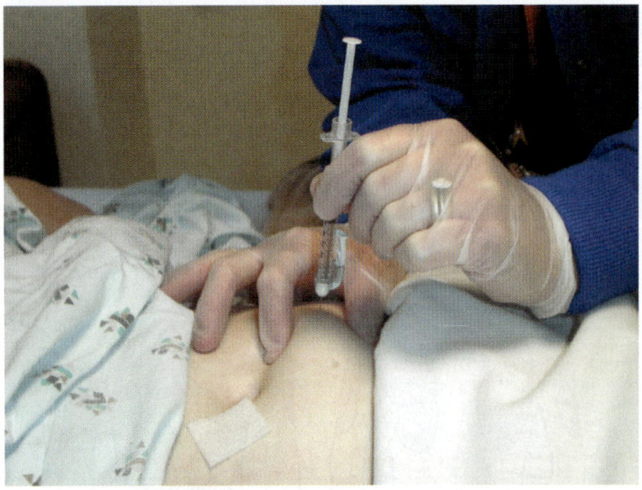

FIGURE 35.28 Giving subcutaneous heparin in the abdomen.

tissue (FIT Canada, 2020). In general, medications can be injected in the subcutaneous tissue of a normal-sized patient using a 25-gauge 1.6-cm needle inserted at a 45-degree angle (Figure 35.29) or a 1.3-cm needle inserted at a 90-degree angle. A child may require only a 1.3-cm needle. If the patient has obesity, pinch the tissue and use a needle long enough to insert through the fatty tissue at the base of the skinfold. The preferred needle length is one-half the width of the skinfold; the angle of insertion may be between 45 and 90 degrees. Thin patients may have insufficient tissue for subcutaneous injections; the upper abdomen is the best injection site for these patients. To ensure that a subcutaneous medication reaches the subcutaneous tissue, follow this rule: if you can grasp 5 cm (or greater than 1 inch) of tissue, insert the needle at a 90-degree angle; if you can grasp 2.5 cm (or less than 1 inch) of tissue, insert the needle at a 45-degree angle (Rushing, 2004).

Intramuscular Injections. The IM route provides faster medication absorption than the subcutaneous route because of a muscle's greater vascularity; however, IM injections are associated with many risks. Therefore, when administering a medication by the IM route, it is important to first verify that the injection is justified (Polania Gutierrez & Munakomi, 2021). In many cases, such as with influenza and pneumonia vaccinations, no alternative routes exist to administer the medication.

A longer and heavier-gauge needle is used to pass through the subcutaneous tissue and penetrate the deep muscle tissue (see Skill 35.5). The patient's body weight and the amount of adipose tissue can influence the selection of a needle size. For example, a patient with obesity may require a needle 7.5 cm long, whereas a thin patient may require a 1.3- to 2.5-cm needle. It is not necessary to aspirate during the administration of an IM injection except if injecting into the dorsogluteal site, to ensure not having punctured the gluteal artery (Polania Gutierrez & Munakomi, 2021).

The angle of insertion for an IM injection is 90 degrees (see Figure 35.29). Muscle is less sensitive to irritating and viscous medications. An average adult patient can tolerate 2–5 mL of medication injected into the ventrogluteal site, or 2 mL into the deltoid muscle, without severe muscle discomfort. A larger volume of medication is unlikely to be absorbed properly. Children over 18 months, older people, and thin patients can tolerate only 2 mL of an IM injection. Do not give more than 0.5 mL to infants under 18 months old and 1 mL to small children (Polania Gutierrez & Munakomi, 2021).

Assess the muscle integrity of the selected site before giving an injection. The muscle should be free of tenderness. Repeated injections in the same muscle can cause severe discomfort. Ensure that the patient is relaxed, then palpate the muscle to rule out any hardened

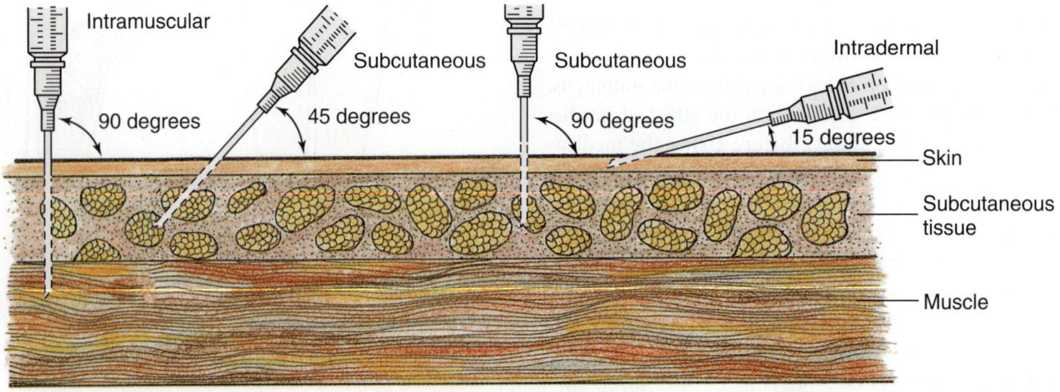

FIGURE 35.29 Comparison of angles of insertion for intramuscular (90 degrees), subcutaneous (45 and 90 degrees), and intradermal (15 degrees) injections.

lesions. Discomfort can be minimized during an injection by helping the patient to assume a position that will help reduce muscle strain. Other interventions, such as distraction and applying pressure to the IM site, may be used to decrease pain during an IM injection.

Sites. When selecting an IM site, consider the following: Is the area free of infection or necrosis? Do local areas show signs of bruising or abrasions? Where is the location of underlying bones, nerves, and major blood vessels? What volume of medication is to be administered? Each site has certain advantages and disadvantages. The characteristics of each IM site and the indications for use of each site are listed in Box 35.25.

> **SAFETY ALERT** Researchers who have investigated complications associated with IM injection sites indicate that the ventrogluteal and deltoid muscle are the preferred sites for IM injections for adults. The vastus lateralis and deltoid are preferred for children, and the dorsogluteal muscle is not recommended for children less than 3 years old. The only IM site recommended for infants less than 18 months old is the vastus lateralis (Polania Gutierrez & Munakomi, 2021).

Ventrogluteal Muscle. The ventrogluteal muscle, which involves the gluteus medius, is situated deep and away from major nerves and blood vessels. It is a safe site for most patients because it is a large muscle that is usually well developed in adults and children, even if they are not yet walking. Complications associated with IM injections—including fibrosis, nerve damage, abscess, tissue necrosis, muscle contraction, gangrene, and pain—have not been associated with the ventrogluteal site, making it the safest perceived site for IM injection (Nakajima et al., 2020).

To locate the ventrogluteal muscle, place the heel of your hand over the greater trochanter of the patient's hip with the wrist perpendicular to the femur. Use your right hand for the left hip, and your left hand for the right hip. Point your thumb toward the patient's groin and point your fingers toward the patient's head; point your index finger to the anterior superior iliac spine, and extend your middle finger back along the iliac crest toward the buttocks. The index finger, the middle finger, and the iliac crest form a V-shaped triangle; the injection site is the centre of the triangle (Figure 35.30). The patient may lie on their side or back. Flexing of the knee and hip helps the patient to relax this muscle.

Vastus Lateralis Muscle. This thick and well-developed muscle is located on the anterior lateral aspect of the thigh and extends in an

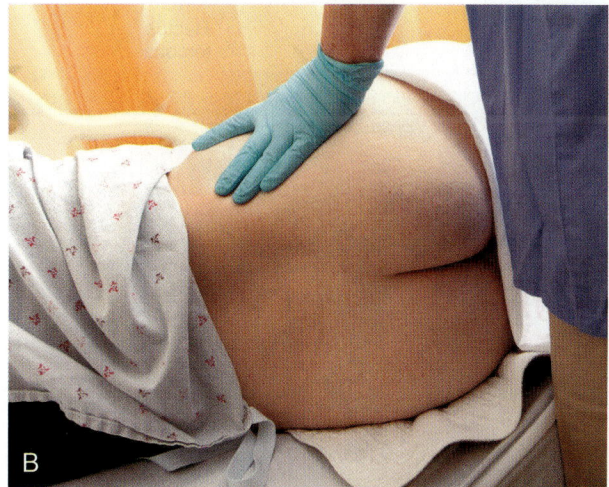

A

B

C

FIGURE 35.30 A, Landmarks for the ventrogluteal site. **B,** Locating ventrogluteal site in patient. **C,** Giving intramuscular injection in ventrogluteal muscle using Z-track method.

BOX 35.25	**Characteristics of Intramuscular Sites and Indications for Usage**

Vastus Lateralis Muscle
- Lacks major nerves and blood vessels
- Facilitates rapid medication absorption
- Used frequently with infants (younger than 18 months old) receiving immunizations
- May also be used in older children and toddlers receiving immunizations

Ventrogluteal Muscle
- Offers a deep site, situated away from major nerves and blood vessels
- Offers less chance of contamination in incontinent patients and infants
- Identified easily by prominent bony landmarks
- Is preferred site for medications (e.g., antibiotics) that are larger in volume, more viscous, and irritating for adults, children, and infants over 18 months

Deltoid Muscle
- Is easily accessible but the muscle is not well developed in most patients
- May be used for small amounts of medications
- Not used in infants under 18 months old or children with underdeveloped muscles
- Use of the muscle involves potential for injury to the brachial artery and to the radial and ulnar nerves
- May be used for immunizations of toddlers over 18 months, older children, and adults
- Recommended site for hepatitis B vaccine and rabies injections

adult from a handbreadth above the knee to a handbreadth below the greater trochanter of the femur (Figure 35.31). Use the middle third of the muscle for injection. The width of the muscle usually extends from the midline of the thigh to the midline of the thigh's outer side. When administering injections to infants under 18 months or cachectic patients, grasp the body of the muscle during injection to ensure the medication is deposited in the muscle tissue. To help relax the muscle, ask the patient to assume a sitting position or to lie flat with leg extended. The vastus lateralis site is often used when infants, toddlers, and children are administered biologicals (e.g., immune globulins, vaccines, or toxoids) (Polania Guiterrez & Monakomi, 2021).

Dorsogluteal muscle. In the past, the dorsogluteal muscle has been a traditional site for IM injections. However, the exact location of the

sciatic nerve varies from one person to another. If a needle hits the sciatic nerve, the patient may experience permanent or partial paralysis of the involved leg. Therefore, do *not* use the dorsogluteal site (Nakajima et al., 2020; Polania Guiterrez & Monakomi, 2021).

Deltoid Muscle. Although the deltoid site is easily accessible, the muscle is not well developed in many patients. A potential for injury exists when using this site because the axillary, radial, brachial, and ulnar nerves and the brachial artery lie within the upper arm along the humerus (Figure 35.32, A). Use this site only for small medication volumes, when giving immunizations, or when other sites are inaccessible because of dressings or casts (Nakajima et al., 2020; Polania Guiterrez & Monakomi, 2021).

To locate the deltoid muscle, fully expose the patient's upper arm and shoulder. Do not roll up a tight-fitting sleeve. Have the patient relax the arm at the side and flex the elbow. The patient may sit, stand, or lie down (see Figure 35.32, B). Palpate the lower edge of the acromion process, which forms the base of a triangle in line with the midpoint of the lateral aspect of the upper arm. The injection site is in the centre of the triangle, approximately 3 to 5 cm below the acromion process (Nakajima et al., 2021). The site can also be located by placing four fingers across the deltoid muscle, with the top finger along the acromion process. The injection site is then three fingerwidths below the acromion process.

Technique for Intramuscular Injections. When administering IM injections, the **Z-track method** is recommended because it minimizes local skin irritation by sealing the medication in the muscle tissue (Zeyrek et al., 2019). Insert a new needle into the syringe after preparing the medication so that no solution remains on the outside of the needle shaft. For the Z-track technique, select an IM site, preferably in a large, deep muscle, such as the ventrogluteal muscle; smaller needles may need to be used for smaller muscles (Nakajima et al., 2021). After preparing the site with an antiseptic swab, pull the overlying skin and subcutaneous tissues approximately 2.5 to 3.5 cm laterally to the side. Holding the skin taut with the nondominant hand, insert the needle deep into the muscle, and slowly inject the medication over 10 seconds (Polania Guiterrez & Monakomi, 2021). The slow injection allows the medication to disperse evenly rather than channelling back up the track of the needle. Then, withdraw the needle and release the skin. This technique leaves a zigzag path that seals the needle track where the tissue planes slide across each other (Figure 35.33). The medication cannot escape from the muscle tissue. Injections using this technique cause less discomfort and fewer lesions at the injection site (Zeyrek et al., 2019).

FIGURE 35.31 A, Landmarks for the vastus lateralis site. **B,** Giving intramuscular injection in the vastus lateralis muscle.

Intradermal Injections. Intradermal injections are commonly performed for skin testing (e.g., tuberculin screening and allergy tests).

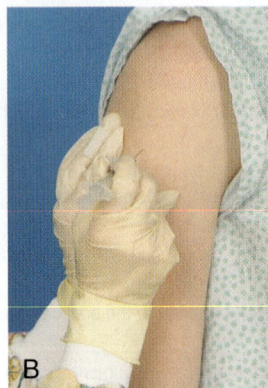

FIGURE 35.32 A, Landmarks for the deltoid site. **B,** Giving intramuscular injection in the deltoid muscle.

Because these medications are potent, they are injected into the dermis, where blood supply is reduced and medication absorption occurs slowly. If the medications enter the circulation too rapidly, a patient may have a severe anaphylactic reaction.

For accurate skin testing, the nurse must be able to see the injection site clearly to detect changes in colour and tissue integrity. Intradermal sites should be lightly pigmented, free of lesions, and relatively hairless. The inner forearm and upper back are ideal locations.

Use a tuberculin or small hypodermic syringe for skin testing. The angle of insertion for an intradermal injection is 5 to 15 degrees (see Figure 35.29), with the bevel of the needle pointed up. As the

medication is injected, a small bleb resembling a mosquito bite should appear on the skin's surface (see Skill 35.5). If a bleb does not appear or if the site bleeds after withdrawal of the needle, the medication may have entered the subcutaneous tissues. In this case, the test results will not be valid.

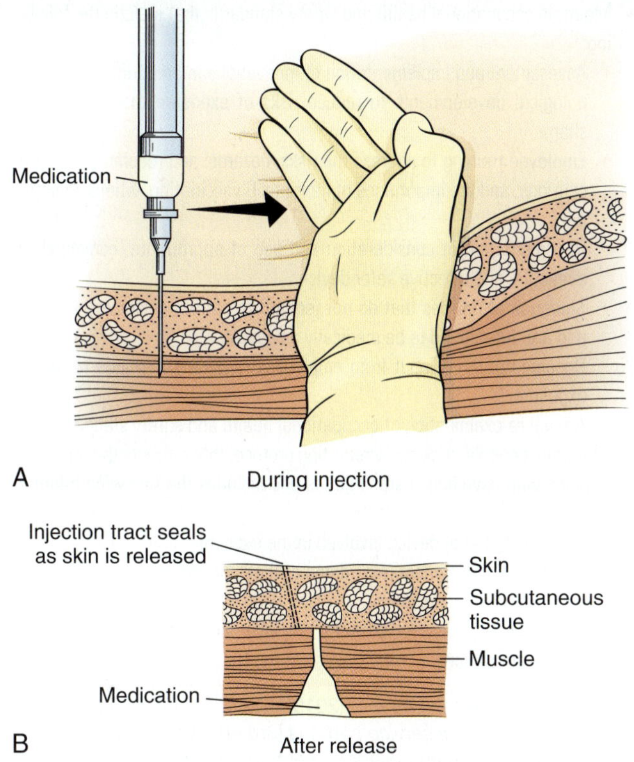

Safety in Administering Medications by Injection

Needleless Devices. Needle-stick injuries occur frequently in all health care settings, with approximately 70 000 occurring in Canadian hospitals each year (Isada et al., 2018). However, because many workers do not report their injuries, the incidence of needle-stick injuries is probably higher. Needle-stick injuries commonly occur when needles are recapped, IV lines and needles are mishandled, or needles are left at a patient's bedside. The risk of exposure of health care workers to bloodborne pathogens has led to the development of "needleless devices" or special needle safety devices.

Special syringes are designed with a sheath or guard that covers the needle after it is withdrawn from the skin (Figure 35.34). The needle is immediately covered to eliminate the possibility of a needle-stick injury, similar to retractable syringes and needles. The syringe and sheath are disposed of together in a receptacle. Needleless devices should be used whenever possible to reduce the risk of injury from needle sticks and sharps (Public Health Ontario, 2019).

Needles and other instruments that are considered "sharps" are always disposed of into clearly marked containers that are puncture-proof and leak-proof (Figure 35.35). A needle should never be forced into a needle disposable receptacle that is full. Nurses should never place used needles and syringes in a garbage can, in their pocket, on a patient's meal tray, or at the patient's bedside. Box 35.26 summarizes recommendations for the prevention of needle-stick injuries.

Intravenous Administration.
Medications are administered intravenously by the following methods:

1. By adding medication to a large volume/primary bag of IV fluids, e.g., Add 20 mEq KCl to 1 L normal saline and infuse over 1 hour.
2. By injecting or "pushing" an IV bolus through an existing IV infusion line or intermittent venous access (i.e., saline lock), e.g., Give 0.5 mg adenosine IV push STAT.
3. By secondary IV set (i.e., piggyback) infusion of the prescribed medication and diluent through an existing IV line, while stopping the primary infusion, e.g., Give 2 mg morphine IV in 25 mL

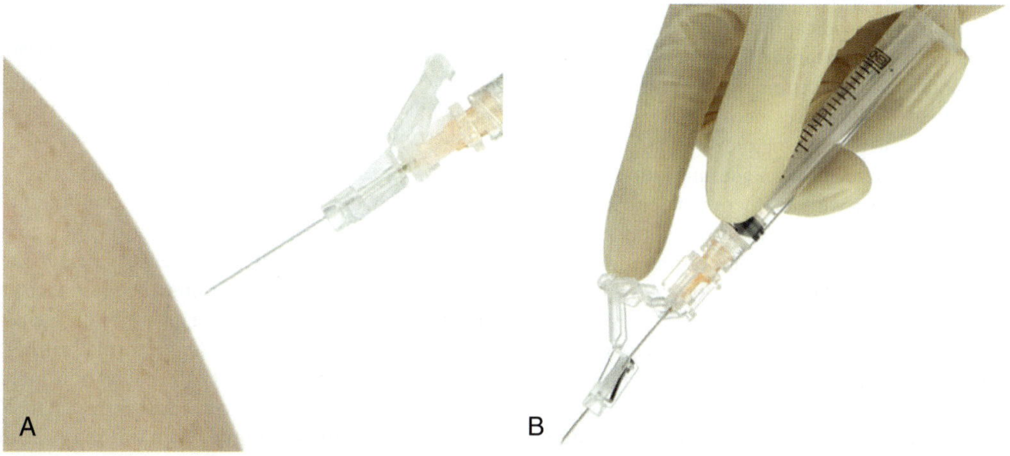

A During injection

B After release

FIGURE 35.33 A, Pulling on the overlying skin during intramuscular injection moves tissue to prevent later tracking. **B,** The Z-track left after injection prevents the deposit of medication through sensitive tissue.

(Figure 35.33 labels: Medication; Injection tract seals as skin is released; Skin; Subcutaneous tissue; Muscle; Medication)

A   **B**

FIGURE 35.34 Needle with plastic guard to prevent needle sticks. **A,** Position of guard before injection. **B,** After injection, the guard locks in place, covering the needle. (BD Safety Glide needle photo courtesy and © Becton, Dickinson and Company.)

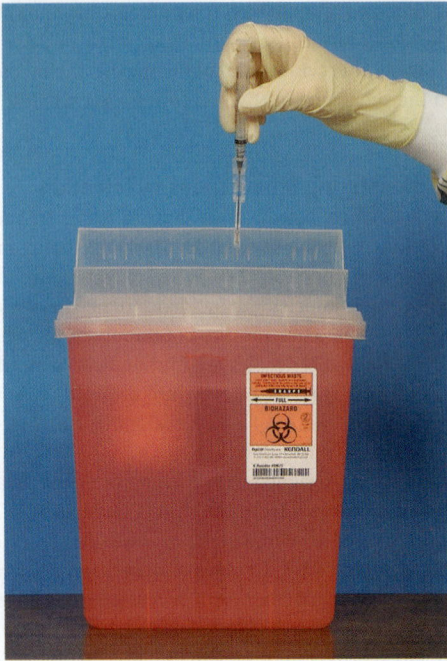

FIGURE 35.35 Sharps disposal using only one hand.

normal saline over 15 minutes (primary infusion automatically shuts off).

4. By tandem or mini-pump IV infusion of the prescribed medication and diluent through an existing IV line, while continuing the primary infusion, e.g., Give 5 g magnesium sulphate in 250 mL normal saline over 5 hours (primary infusion continues).

In all four methods, the patient has either an existing IV infusion line or an IV access site (i.e., saline lock). In most institutions, policies and procedures list the persons who may give IV medications and the situations in which these medications may be given. These policies are based on the medication, capability, and availability of staff and on the type of monitoring equipment available.

Chapter 41 describes the technique for performing venipuncture and establishing continuous IV fluid infusions. Medication administration is only one reason for supplying IV fluids. IV fluid therapy is used primarily for fluid replacement in patients unable to take oral fluids and as a means of supplying the patient with electrolytes and nutrients.

When using any method of IV medication administration, patients should be closely monitored for symptoms of adverse effects. After a medication enters the bloodstream, it begins to act immediately, and its action cannot be stopped. Thus, nurses need to take special care to avoid inappropriate dose calculations or preparation. They must carefully follow the rights of safe medication administration, double-check their medication calculations with another nurse, and know the desired action and adverse effects of every medication administered. If the medication has an antidote, it must be available during administration. When administering potent medications, the patient's vital signs are assessed before, during, and after infusion.

Administering medications by the IV route has advantages. The IV route is used in emergencies when a fast-acting medication must be delivered quickly. The IV route is also preferred when constant therapeutic blood levels need to be established. Some medications are highly alkaline and irritating to the muscle and subcutaneous tissue. These medications cause less discomfort when given intravenously.

SAFETY ALERT Because IV medications are immediately available to the bloodstream after they are administered, verify the prescribed rate of administration with a medication reference manual or a pharmacist before giving any IV medication. This step ensures that the medication is administered safely over the appropriate amount of time. Patients can experience severe adverse effects if IV medications are administered too quickly.

Large-Volume Infusions. Of the four methods of administering IV medications, mixing medications in a compatible fluid (e.g., normal saline, dextrose 5% or sterile water) is the safest and easiest (Skill 35.6). In many institutions, the pharmacist creates the admixture by adding medications (e.g., antibiotics, electrolytes, vitamins) to an IV container of fluid (e.g., normal saline) to ensure asepsis and to reduce the possibility of medication incidents. Because the medication is not in a concentrated form, the risk of adverse effects or fatal reactions is minimal when infused over the prescribed time frame. However, the nurse must be aware of the patient's fluids status to determine if they can safely circulate additional fluid given with medications.

SKILL 35.6   ADDING MEDICATIONS TO INTRAVENOUS FLUID CONTAINERS

Delegation Considerations

Adding medications to IV fluid containers cannot be delegated to unregulated care providers (UCPs). (In some institutions, the pharmacist may add medications to the primary containers of IV solutions to promote safe medication administration and ensure asepsis.)

Equipment

- Medication vial or ampoule
- Syringe of appropriate size (5–20 mL)
- Sterile blunt fill or filter needle
- Sterile, compatible intravenous (IV) fluid container for medication
- Antiseptic swab
- Medication label
- Medication administration record (MAR)
- Barcode scanner (if applicable)

PROCEDURE

STEPS	RATIONALE
1. Check the accuracy and completeness of the MAR, including the following: patient name and medication name, route, dosage, time of administration, and start and stop date. If difficult to read, review the original prescription order and rewrite the MAR.	• Ensures that the patient receives the right medication • Illegible MARs are a source of medication incidents. The original prescription is the most reliable source and only legal record of medications the patient is to receive.
2. Assess the patient's health history, medications, and allergies.	• Medications should correspond with the patient's medical diagnoses. • Certain substances have similar compositions; never administer a substance to which a patient has a known allergy.
3. Collect information necessary to administer the medication safely, including the medication's action, purpose, adverse effects, normal dose, time of peak onset, method of delivery, and nursing implications.	• Some medications contain particles that require an IV filter in the tubing. For example, parenteral nutrition IV tubing must have a 0.22-micron filter. • This is necessary to determine if the medication, dose, and route are appropriate, and how to administer it safely.
4. Assess for medication compatibility with the primary IV solution and other medications infusing.	• Medications may be incompatible when mixed together. • Chemical reactions can result in a precipitate reaction (i.e., clouding or crystallization of IV fluids).
5. Perform hand hygiene. Prepare the prescribed medication (see Skill 35.4); use aseptic techniques. Check the expiry dates on medication vials and ampoules.	• Ensures the medication is sterile • Medication potency increases or decreases when expired.
6. Compare the label of the medication with the MAR two times while preparing the medication, and compare the label of the IV fluid bag or bottle with the MAR two times.	• Ensures it is the right medication • Ensures it is the right diluent for the medication
7. Add the medication to the new IV bag or bottle container (usually in the medication room or at medication cart):	• Avoids distractions and additional microorganisms at the bedside
A. *Solution in a bag or bottle:* Locate the correct medication injection port; a small rubber stopper on an IV bag, or a metal or plastic cap and rubber seal on an IV bottle.	• The injection port self-seals to prevent introduction of microorganisms. • Incorrect injection into the IV bag main port or IV bottle air vent causes leaks.
B. Wipe the port or injection site with alcohol or an antiseptic swab.	• Reduces the risk of introducing bacteria into the port

Continued

SKILL 35.6   ADDING MEDICATIONS TO INTRAVENOUS FLUID CONTAINERS—cont'd

STEPS   **RATIONALE**

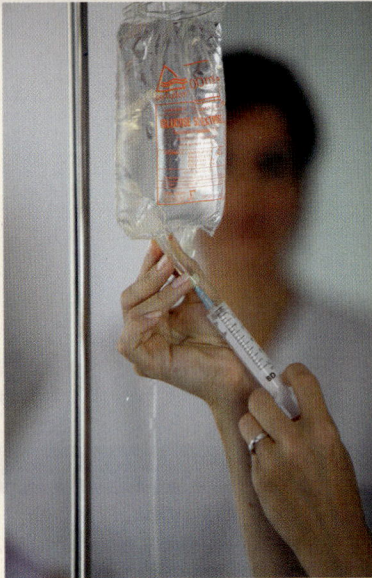

STEP 7C Inject the medication through a rubber port. (© CanStock Photo/photography33.)

C. Insert the blunt syringe needle through the centre of the port and inject the medication (see Step 7C illustration).

- Accidentally piercing the sides of the port causes a leak and contamination.

D. Withdraw the syringe from the bag or bottle.

- The injection port self-seals to prevent the introduction of microorganisms.

E. Mix the medication and the IV solution by holding the bag or bottle and turning it gently end to end.

- Allows even distribution of the medication

F. Complete and affix the medication label to the IV bottle or bag, i.e., medication name, dose, date, time of administration, and your initials. Ensure that important information preprinted on the IV bag or bottle (e.g., fluid name) is still visible.

- The label informs health care providers of the contents of the bag or bottle.
- Concealing important information can lead to medication incidents.

8. Take the IV medication bag or bottle and supplies to the patient's bedside at the right time. Perform hand hygiene.

9. Identify the patient using at two to three patient identifiers.

- Asking the patient to state their name, comparing the patient's name and another identifier (e.g., hospital ID number) on the MAR against information on the patient's ID bracelet, and scanning the patient's barcode (if applicable) ensure that it is the right patient.

10. Perform hand hygiene. Assess the IV insertion site for signs of infiltration or phlebitis (see Chapter 41).

- Ensures medication is infused correctly into the vein, i.e., the IV is not interstitial

11. Assess the patient, including signs of fluid balance: skin hydration, turgor, body weight, pulse, blood pressure, and ratio of fluid intake to urine output.

- Rapid infusions and volume can cause circulatory overload, especially in children and older persons.

12. Explain to the patient that the medication is to be given through an IV line and no discomfort should be felt. Encourage the patient to report symptoms of discomfort.

- IV medications should not cause discomfort when diluted; however, some are irritating (e.g., KCl).
- Pain may be a sign of infiltration.

13. Assess the patient's understanding of the purpose of the medication therapy and possible adverse effects.

- Patient understanding increases medication adherence.

14. Spike the medication container with the IV tubing. Prime (i.e., fill) the tubing and drip chamber ensuring that it is free of air before connecting the tubing to the patient's primary IV line.

- Priming the tubing ensures that air does not cause an air embolus.

15. Manually regulate the infusion using the roller clamp, or secure the tubing inside a SMART IV infusion pump and program the pump using the drug library.

- Prevents rapid infusion of fluid
- Ensures medication is mixed and infused according to the guideline

SKILL 35.6	ADDING MEDICATIONS TO INTRAVENOUS FLUID CONTAINERS—cont'd
STEPS	**RATIONALE**

> **CRITICAL DECISION POINT:** *Some medications (e.g., potassium chloride) can cause serious adverse effects, including fatal cardiac dysrhythmias. These medications should be infused on an IV pump. Check the institutional guidelines or policies indicating which IV medications require administration on an IV pump.*

STEPS	RATIONALE
16. Label IV tubing with the date and time of opening and change date (according to employer policy).	• Most IV tubing is changed every 72 hours but varies based on the solution (e.g., parenteral nutrition is changed daily). • Prevents infection from microorganisms in tubing
17. Dispose of any soiled supplies and perform hand hygiene.	
18. Observe the patient for a medication reaction (e.g., rash) and circulatory overload (e.g., new or worsening chest crackles).	• IV medications can cause rapid effects. • Rapid infusion and volume can cause circulatory overload.
19. Regularly reassess the IV insertion site, rate of infusion, tubing integrity, fluid bag volume, and air bubbles in the tubing.	• Patient movement can cause the IV to become interstitial or disconnect or cause the flow rate to change. • Interstitial medications injure tissues (i.e., extravasation). • Empty IV bags or air bubbles in tubing can cause an air embolus. • Tubing occlusions or leaks prevent the patient from receiving the medication dose.

UNEXPECTED OUTCOMES	RELATED INTERVENTIONS
Adverse effects or allergic reaction to medication	• Follow institutional policy or guidelines for your appropriate response to and reporting of adverse effects or adverse medication reactions. • Notify the patient's health care provider immediately. • Add the allergy information to the patient's medical record.
Signs of fluid volume overload (e.g., abnormal breath sounds, shortness of breath, intake greater than output)	• Assess the patient for compromised circulatory regulation (vital signs, input:output, focused respiratory and cardiac assessments). • Stop the IV infusion. • Notify the patient's health care provider immediately.
Swelling, warmth, redness, and tenderness at IV site, indicating phlebitis (see Chapter 41)	• Stop IV infusion and discontinue IV. • Treat the IV site as indicated by institutional policy. • If continuation of IV therapy is indicated, insert a new IV.
Coolness, pallor, and swelling at IV site, indicating infiltration (see Chapter 41)	• Some IV medications are extremely harmful to the subcutaneous tissue. • Provide IV extravasation wound care as indicated by institutional policy.

DOCUMENTATION AND REPORTING
* Record the medication and IV solution administered on the MAR.
* Document the volume of fluid, rate, and site of infusion in the patient's health record.
* Report any adverse effects to the patient's health care provider, and document adverse effects.

Intravenous Bolus. An IV bolus, or "push," involves the introduction of a concentrated dose of a medication directly into the patient's systemic circulation (Skill 35.7). A bolus has the advantage of requiring only a small amount of fluid to deliver the medication; therefore, the bolus is useful when the patient is on restricted fluids. However, an IV bolus, or "push," is the most dangerous method for administering medications because the nurse has no time to correct or stop an incident. Also, a bolus may cause direct irritation to the lining of the blood vessels. Before administering a bolus, confirm the placement of the IV line by obtaining a blood return through the IV catheter or needle. The inability to obtain a blood return suggests that the needle or catheter is in the patient's tissues or is resting against the vein wall. Never give a medication intravenously if the insertion site appears puffy or edematous or if the IV fluid cannot flow at the proper rate. Accidental injection of a medication into the tissues around a vein can cause pain, sloughing of tissues, and abscesses, depending on the medication's composition.

The rate of administration of an IV bolus medication is determined by the amount of medication that can be given per minute. For example,

if a patient is to receive 4 mL of a medication over 2 minutes, give 2 mL of the IV bolus medication every minute. Research each medication to determine the recommended concentration and rate of administration. When delivering a medication IV push, consider the purpose for which a medication is prescribed and any potential adverse effects related to the rate or route of administration.

Volume-Controlled Infusions. IV medications can also be administered in small amounts (e.g., 25 to 100 mL) of compatible IV fluids. Containers used to precisely control infusion volumes include secondary medication sets, buretrols, and mini-infusers. A second container with a medication solution is connected to the primary IV fluid line using an additional set of IV tubing. The use of volume-controlled infusions has several advantages:
* The risk of rapid-dose infusion by IV push is reduced. Medications are diluted and infused over longer time intervals (e.g., 30 to 60 minutes).
* Medications that are stable for only a limited time in solution (e.g., antibiotics) can be administered.
* IV fluid intake can be controlled.

SKILL 35.7   ADMINISTERING MEDICATIONS BY INTRAVENOUS BOLUS

Delegation Considerations

The administration of medications by intravenous (IV) bolus cannot be delegated to unregulated care providers (UCPs). Instruct UCPs to report immediately any unexpected medication reactions or adverse effects, discomfort at the infusion site, and changes in any required vital signs.

Equipment

- A watch with a second hand
- Medication administration record (MAR)
- Clean, disposable gloves
- Antiseptic swab or new disinfectant cap
- Medication vial or ampoule
- Needleless syringe for medication
- Blunt fill or filter needle
- Two syringes for flushing (prefilled with saline, sterile water, OR for preparation)
- Vial of saline/sterile and blunt needle (if preparing flushes)
- Barcode scanner (if applicable)

PROCEDURE

STEPS	RATIONALE
1. Check the accuracy and completeness of the MAR, including the following: patient name and medication name, route, dosage, time of administration, and start and stop date. If difficult to read, review the original prescription and rewrite the MAR.	• Ensures that the patient receives the right medication • Illegible MARs are a source of medication incidents. The original prescription is the most reliable source and only legal record of medications the patient is to receive.
2. Assess the patient's health history, medications, and allergies.	• IV bolus medications have rapid effects; allergic reactions can be fatal. • Substances have similar compositions; never administer a substance to which a patient has a known allergy.
3. Collect the necessary information to administer the medication safely, including pace (i.e., speed) of administration, appropriate diluents, and filter requirements.	• This is necessary to determine if the medication, dose, and route are appropriate, and how to administer it safely.

CRITICAL DECISION POINT: *Some IV medications can be pushed safely only when the patient is being continuously monitored for dysrhythmias, blood pressure changes, or other adverse effects. Therefore, some medications can be pushed only by nurses (or physicians or nurse practitioners) in specific areas (e.g., cardiac care unit). Confirm employer guidelines regarding requirements for monitoring and verify that these requirements are met before giving medication.*

STEPS	RATIONALE
4. If pushing the medication into an IV line, determine the compatibility of the medication with any IV fluids and medications infusing.	• IV medications are not always compatible with IV solutions and can cause a precipitate reaction. • Some medications require a tubing filter.
5. Perform hand hygiene. Prepare the prescribed medication from the vial or ampoule using aseptic technique (see Skill 35.4). Check the expiry date on medication vials or ampoules.	• Potency increases or decreases when medications are expired.
6. Check the label of the medication carefully with the MAR two times. Apply a removable label to the medication syringe indicating the patient's name and the medication name, dosage, date, and your initials. Do not apply medication labels to syringe needle caps.	• Ensures that you have the right medication • Medication labels applied to needle caps can be easily removed or accidently applied to the wrong syringe.

CRITICAL DECISION POINT: *Some IV medications require dilution before administration. Verify the dilution requirements with the employer policy. If a small amount of medication is given (e.g., less than 1 mL), dilute the medication in 5 to 10 mL of normal saline or sterile water so that the medication does not collect in the "dead spaces" (e.g., the Y-site injection port or IV cap) of the IV delivery system.*

STEPS	RATIONALE
7. Take the medication to the patient at the correct time. Perform hand hygiene.	
8. Identify the patient using two to three patient identifiers.	• Asking the patient to state their name, comparing the patient's name and one other identifier (e.g., the hospital ID number) on the MAR against information on the patient's ID bracelet, and scanning the patient's barcode (if applicable) ensure that you have the right patient.

SKILL 35.7	ADMINISTERING MEDICATIONS BY INTRAVENOUS BOLUS—cont'd

STEPS	RATIONALE
9. Compare the label of the medication with the MAR at the patient's bedside.	• The *third check* of the medication label against the MAR at bedside ensures that you have the right medication.
10. Explain the procedure to the patient. Encourage the patient to report symptoms of discomfort at the IV site. Assess the patient's understanding of the medication.	• Explanation helps identify infiltration early. • Understanding increases medication adherence.
11. Perform hand hygiene. Put on clean, disposable gloves.	• Reduces the transmission of infection and risk of exposure to blood from the IV site
12. Assess the patient, including the IV or saline lock insertion site for signs of infiltration or phlebitis (see Chapter 41).	• Ensures that the medication is infused into the vein (i.e., is not interstitial) • Infiltration causes tissue injury (i.e., extravasation).
13. Administer the medication by IV push through an infusing IV line: A. Select the needleless injection port of the IV tubing closest to the IV insertion site and the patient.	• Needleless injection ports decrease needle-stick injuries. • Injecting the port closest to the insertion site ensures that the medication will reach the patient rapidly.
B. Wipe the injection port with an antiseptic swab for 15 seconds and allow to dry. Or, if the port has a disinfectant cap applied, remove and discard the cap (see Step 13B illustrations). There is no additional need to swab the port.	• Prevents the introduction of microorganisms during needle insertion
C. Connect the tip of the needleless syringe to the centre of the injection port (see Step 13C illustration).	• The port is self-sealing.
D. Occlude the IV line by pinching the tubing just above the injection port (see Step 13D illustration).	• Prevents the medication from flowing backward toward the primary IV bag. This step is the *final check* that the medication is being delivered into the bloodstream.

STEP 13B A, Swab the top of the needle-free connector with alcohol and allow to dry for 30 seconds. **B,** Removing the disinfectant cap. (*A* and *B:* Courtesy and © Becton, Dickinson and Company.)

STEP 13C Connecting the needleless syringe to the IV line port.

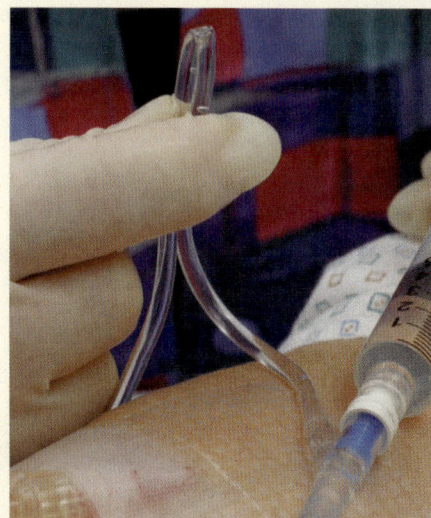

STEP 13D Pinching the IV line above the injection port for medication infusion.

Continued

CRITICAL DECISION POINT: *In some cases, especially with a smaller-gauge IV needle, the blood return may not be aspirated, even if the IV is patent (open and unblocked). If the IV site does not show signs of infiltration, and the IV fluid is infusing without difficulty, proceed with the IV push.*

E. Inject the medication over the prescribed amount of time (e.g., 1–2 minutes) or according to employer policy. Use your watch to time the administration.

- Rapid injection of IV medication can cause adverse effects or fatality.

CRITICAL DECISION POINT: *If the IV medication is incompatible with the primary IV fluid infusing, stop the IV fluids, clamp the IV line, and flush with 10 mL of normal saline or sterile water. Then give the IV bolus over the appropriate amount of time, flush with another 10 mL of normal saline or sterile water at the same rate as the medication was administered, and then restart the IV fluids at the prescribed rate. If the IV that is currently hanging is a medication, disconnect the IV, and administer the IV push as outlined in Step 13. This step avoids giving the patient a sudden bolus of the medication in the existing IV line and avoids creating potential risks associated with IV incompatibilities. Some IV medications and fluids cannot be stopped. Verify the institutional policy regarding the temporary stopping of IV fluids or continuous IV medications. If unable to stop the IV infusion, start a new IV site and administer the medication using the IV lock method.*

F. After injecting the medication, release the pinched tubing and remove the syringe. Wipe the port with an antiseptic swab for 15 seconds or apply a new disinfectant cap.

G. Recheck the fluid infusion rate.

- Injection of the bolus may alter the rate of fluid infusion. Rapid fluid infusion can cause circulatory overload.

14. If administering medications by IV push through a saline lock:

A. Select syringe sizes for flushing according to employer policy (e.g., 5 mL, 10 mL). Prepare two syringes with 3–5 mL of sterile fluid (i.e., saline or sterile water). If using prefilled sterile flushes, eject the air from the syringe and fill the syringe tip with fluid by depressing the plunger (see Step 14A illustration). If using regular syringes, attach a blunt fill needle to each syringe and withdraw 3–5 mL of sterile fluid from a vial. Eject any air bubbles from the syringes.

- Follow employer policies for syringe size when flushing or injecting medications intravenously. Small syringes (e.g., 1 mL or 3 mL) create higher pressure per square inch (PSI) and can damage certain types of IV catheters (e.g., central lines, peripherally inserted central catheter [PICC] lines).
- Most employers require flushes with normal saline because it is effective in keeping IV locks patent and is compatible with most medications.
- Heparin is not routinely used because it places patients at risk for thrombocytopenia.

B. Administer medication:

(1) Wipe the lock's injection port with an antiseptic swab or remove the disinfectant cap if present.

(2) Connect a flush syringe containing sterile flush fluid into the injection port of the IV lock (see Step 14B[2] illustration).

- Wiping the injection port prevents introduction of microorganisms during the needle insertion. Disinfectant caps are antiseptic; therefore, no additional wiping is needed.

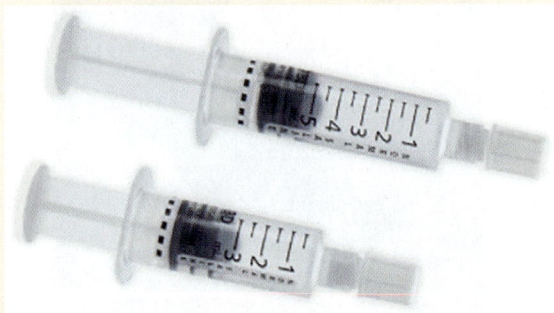

STEP 14A Prefilled saline flush syringe. (Courtesy and © Becton, Dickinson and Company.)

STEP 14B(2) Flushing a saline lock. Attach the saline-filled syringe to the needle-free connector on the saline lock. Use positive pressure to slowly inject (i.e., flush) the catheter. (Courtesy and © Becton, Dickinson and Company.)

SKILL 35.7	**ADMINISTERING MEDICATIONS BY INTRAVENOUS BOLUS—cont'd**
STEPS	**RATIONALE**

(3) Pull back gently on the syringe plunger and look for blood return.
• This step determines whether the IV needle or catheter is positioned in the vein.

CRITICAL DECISION POINT: *Sometimes a saline lock will not yield a blood return even though the lock is patent. If the IV site does not show signs of infiltration, proceed with the IV push.*

(4) Flush the IV lock with sterile fluid by pushing slowly on the plunger.
• Flushing the IV lock clears it of blood.

CRITICAL DECISION POINT: *Observe closely the area of skin above the IV catheter. As the IV lock is flushed, note any puffiness or swelling, which could indicate infiltration into the vein and thereby require removal of the catheter.*

(5) Remove the empty flush syringe.

(6) Connect the syringe containing the prepared medication to the injection port of the IV lock.

(7) Inject the medication within the amount of time prescribed or based on employer policy, timing the administration with your watch (see Step 14B(7) illustration). Observe the patient for effects and the IV site during injection any swelling.
• Rapid injection can cause adverse effects (e.g., hearing loss due to rapid injection of furosemide) or fatality.
• Swelling indicates infiltration into tissues surrounding the vein.

STEP 14B(7) Pushing an IV bolus medication over a specific amount of time. (Courtesy and © Becton, Dickinson and Company.)

(8) After administering the bolus, withdraw the syringe.

(9) Attach the second syringe with sterile flush fluid and inject the fluid.
• Prevents occlusion of the IV access device and ensures all medication is delivered

(10) Clamp the intermittent access device (e.g., saline lock). Wipe the port with an aseptic alcohol swab for 15 seconds and allow it to dry. Or apply a new disinfectant cap.
• Prevents the introduction of microorganisms

15. Dispose of needles and syringes in a puncture-proof and leak-proof container.
• Proper disposal reduces the risk of accidental needle sticks.

16. Remove and dispose of gloves. Perform hand hygiene.
• Proper hygiene reduces the transmission of microorganisms.

17. Observe the patient closely for several minutes to evaluate medication effects and potential adverse effects.
• IV bolus medications cause rapid changes and require careful monitoring (e.g., vasopressors instantly change blood pressure and heart rate).

18. Consult the employer's policy with regard to the frequency and process for routine sterile flushes of intermittent devices (e.g., saline lock).
• Routine flushing is required to keep IV catheters patent. Short-term peripheral IV catheters are usually flushed every 12 hours; central IV catheters are usually flushed every 25 hours.
• Different flushing procedures are required for IV access devices, based on whether they have an internal valve: e.g., "Turbulent flush and positive pressure" means the nurse intermittently flushes, stops, flushes, and stops until an entire saline flush is injected, maintaining a positive pressure inside the IV catheter and preventing introduction of microorganisms.

Continued

SKILL 35.7 ADMINISTERING MEDICATIONS BY INTRAVENOUS BOLUS—cont'd

UNEXPECTED OUTCOMES	RELATED INTERVENTIONS
Adverse effects or adverse reaction to medication	• Stop delivering medication immediately and follow institutional policy or guidelines for the appropriate response and reporting of medication adverse effects. • Notify the patient's health care provider of adverse effects immediately. • Add allergy information to the patient's medical record.
Symptoms of infiltration or phlebitis at IV site	• Immediately discontinue administration of the injection and discontinue use of the site. • Follow institutional guidelines on appropriate extravasation care.

DOCUMENTATION AND REPORTING
• Record the medication, dose, time, and route on the MAR.
• Report adverse effects immediately to the health care provider, because the reactions could be life-threatening. The patient's response may indicate the need for additional therapy.
• Record the patient's response to medication in the nurses' notes and on the MAR.

Volume-Control Administration. Volume-control administration sets are small (50- to 150-mL) containers used to administer precise, small amounts of fluid or medication. A **buretrol** or burette attaches directly below a primary IV solution bag or IV medication bag. Usually, a buretrol is filled with a diluent fluid from a larger primary IV bag above (e.g., normal saline), and medication is injected into the buretrol through a needleless injection port (Figure 35.36). Buretrols are frequently used to dilute and safely deliver medications to children and adults, such as sodium bicarbonate, where only a small, precise volume (e.g., 3 mL to 20 mL per hour) may be prescribed. Follow package directions for priming sets (see Chapter 41).

Secondary IV Medication Set. A secondary IV medication set, or "piggyback" set, is a small (25- to 250-mL) IV bag or bottle of fluid or medication that is connected using a second, short IV tubing set to the upper port of primary IV tubing (Figure 35.37). The secondary IV tubing set is a microdrip or macrodrip system (see Chapter 41). The secondary set is also referred to as a *piggyback* because the small bag or bottle is set higher than the primary IV bag on the IV pole. The difference in height and a back-check valve within the tubing causes the primary IV infusion to stop automatically when the elevated secondary medication or fluid is infusing. After the secondary medication or fluid infusion is complete, gravity causes the primary IV infusion to automatically restart.

Tandem. A tandem setup is an additional IV bag or bottle with its own IV tubing that connects to the lower port (closest to the patient) on the primary IV tubing. The tandem set is placed at the same height as the primary infusion bag or bottle. In the tandem setup, the tandem and the primary IV line infuse simultaneously. This setup is frequently used to infuse a bolus of fluid or medication (e.g., red blood cells, albumin, Ringer's lactate) when the primary infusion also needs to continue. The tandem setup must be monitored closely. If it is not immediately clamped when the medication is infused, the IV solution from the primary line will back up into the tandem line.

Mini-Infusion Pump. The mini-infusion pump is a small, SMART IV infusion pump used to deliver medications from a syringe or small IV bag container in very small amounts (5 to 60 mL). Syringe pumps are frequently used for patient-controlled analgesia (PCA) with opioids like hydromorphone and morphine. The syringe is secured and locked into the infusion pump, and safeguards are in place to prevent the patient from administering extra doses or accessing the medication beyond those prescribed (Figure 35.38). Similarly, continuous epidural infusions, such as bupivacaine with fentanyl solutions, are normally locked inside a mini-infusion pump, programmed, and only accessible to the nurse (Skill 35.8).

Intermittent Venous Access. An intermittent venous access (commonly called a *saline lock*) is an IV catheter attached to a small set of IV tubing with one or multiple needleless access ports (Figure 35.39). Special rubber-seal injection caps accept the needleless safety devices and can be inserted into most IV catheters (see Chapter 41). Advantages to intermittent venous access include the following:
• Reduced risk of the patient developing fluid volume excess
• Increased mobility, safety, and comfort for the patient

Before administering an IV bolus or medication via a secondary IV set, assess the patency and placement of the IV site. After the medication has been administered through an intermittent venous access, the access must be flushed with a solution to keep it patent. Normal saline is an effective flush solution for peripheral catheters. Heparin is used only in specific situations (e.g., for flushing dialysis catheters) because of the risk of thrombocytopenia. Verify and follow the institution's policies regarding the care and maintenance of the IV site.

Administration of IV Therapy in the Community Setting. Sometimes patients are discharged from an acute care setting and continue to receive IV therapy in the community setting (e.g., home or residence). Medications such as antibiotics, chemotherapy, total parenteral

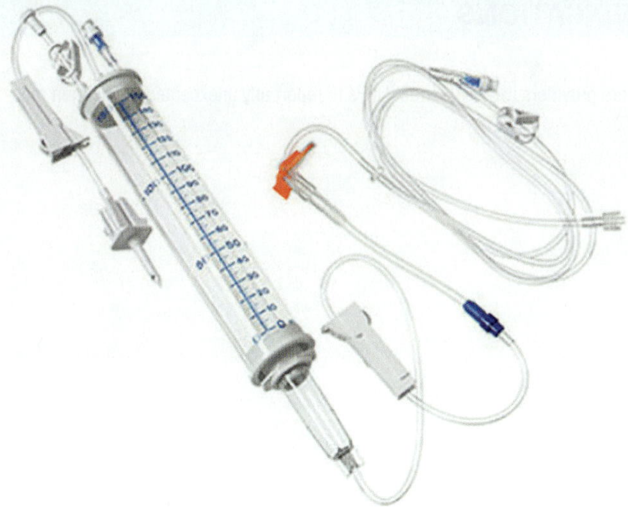

FIGURE 35.36 Buretrol for volume-controlled administration with needleless injection port. (Courtesy and © Becton, Dickinson and Company.)

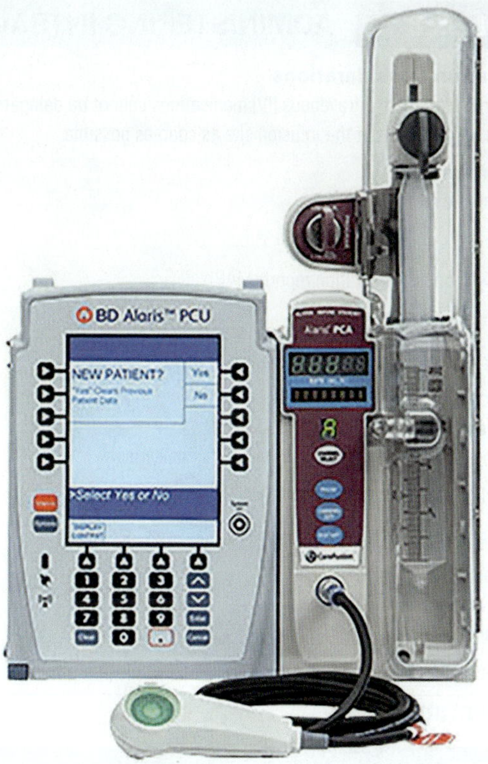

FIGURE 35.38 Mini-infusion pump with patient-controlled analgesia (PCA). (BD Alaris PCA photo courtesy and © Becton, Dickinson and Company.)

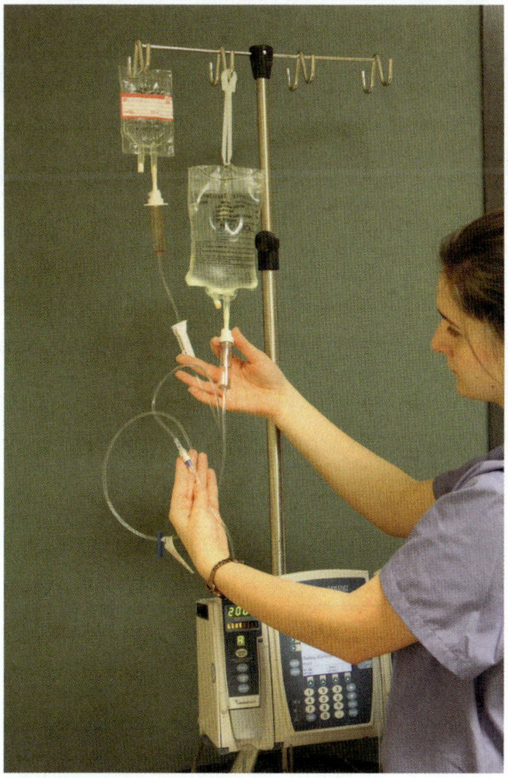

FIGURE 35.37 Secondary IV setup. (Courtesy Sharon Kaasalainen, RN, PhD.)

However, patients and their families need to be carefully assessed for their ability to manage this therapy in their community setting. Instruction on IV care management must be provided while the patient is still in the hospital. Patients and their families need to be taught how to recognize problems and what to do when these problems occur. It is important for the patient and caregiver to recognize signs of infection and complications and to know that when these signs occur, a visiting nurse or health care provider (e.g., physician) must be notified. In addition, patients and their families need information regarding the maintenance of IV administration equipment, including the infusion pump.

Subcutaneous Butterfly Catheters. Subcutaneous butterfly catheters provide a route for both subcutaneous medication administration and hypodermoclysis (Box 35.27). As a route for medication administration, subcutaneous butterfly catheters reduce the frequency of breaking the skin barrier to inject a medication. This route is used for patients requiring longer-term therapy with medication that is administered via subcutaneous injection. Hypodermoclysis is the administration of fluids through a butterfly catheter and is commonly used for patients with limited IV access, palliative care patients, and patients at risk for or with mild dehydration.

A fine-gauge needle (e.g., 24-gauge) is inserted into the patient's subcutaneous tissue. The preferred site for subcutaneous butterfly catheters is the subcutaneous tissue of the abdomen. Other appropriate sites include the subcutaneous tissue of the upper arms, upper back (scapular area), anterior thighs, and the anterior upper chest (avoiding the breast and axilla). A subcutaneous butterfly catheter must not be inserted into tissues that have recently been irradiated or where a rash, bruising, or scar tissue is present. After inserting a subcutaneous

nutrition, pain medications, and blood transfusions may be given in the community setting. Most patients who have IV therapy in the community setting will have a central venous catheter inserted before their discharge (see Chapter 41). In addition, patients who need to receive IV therapy in the community have visiting nurses who assist in the management of the IV therapy.

Delegation Considerations

The administration of intravenous (IV) medications cannot be delegated to unregulated care providers (UCPs). Instruct UCPs to report any unexpected medication reactions or discomfort at the infusion site as soon as possible.

Equipment
- Antiseptic swabs
- IV pole
- Medication administration report (MAR)
- Medication label
- Adhesive tape
- Barcode scanner (if applicable)

Medication preparation:
- Medication in an ampoule, vial, mini-infusion syringe
- Needleless syringe for medication
- Blunt fill or filter needle
- IV bag/bottle of diluent

Medication administration:
- Secondary IV medication set tubing
- Buretrol, IV infusion tubing, or mini-infusion syringe pump tubing

PROCEDURE

STEPS	RATIONALE
1. Check the accuracy and completeness of the MAR, including the following: patient name and medication name, route, dosage, time of administration, and start and stop date. If difficult to read, review the original prescription order and rewrite the MAR	• Ensures that the patient receives the right medication • Illegible MARs are a source of medication incidents. The original prescription is the most reliable source and only legal record of medications the patient is to receive.
2. Check the patient's health history, medications, and allergies.	• Effects from IV infusion are rapid; allergic reactions can be severe. • Substances have similar compositions; never administer a substance to which a patient has a known allergy.
3. Collect the necessary information to administer the medication safely: action, purpose, adverse effects, normal dose, time of peak onset, and nursing implications.	• This is necessary to determine if the medication, dose, and route are appropriate, and how to administer it safely.
4. Assess the compatibility of the medication with the patient's existing primary IV infusion and additives.	• Medications that are incompatible with IV solutions may result in clouding or crystallization of the solution in IV tubing (precipitate reaction), which may harm the patient.

CRITICAL DECISION POINT: *Never administer IV medications through tubing that is infusing blood, blood products, or parenteral nutrition solutions.*

5. Perform hand hygiene. Prepare the prescribed medication. Check the expiry date for medications and IV diluents.	• Potency increases or decreases when medications are expired.
6. Compare the label of the medication with the MAR two times while preparing the medication. Compare the label of the IV bag or bottle diluent with the MAR at least two times.	• Ensures that the right medication is given to the right patient
7. Take the medication and supplies to the patient at the correct time. Perform hand hygiene.	
8. Identify the patient using two or three patient identifiers.	• Asking the patient to state their name, comparing the patient's name and one other identifier (e.g., the hospital ID number) on the MAR against information on the patient's ID bracelet, and scanning the patient's barcode on their ID bracelet (if applicable) ensure that you have the right patient.
9. Compare the medication label with the MAR at the patient's bedside.	• *This is the third accuracy check.*
10. Explain the purpose of the medication and potential adverse effects to the patient.	• Communication with the patient keeps the patient informed of planned therapies.

SKILL 35.8	ADMINISTERING INTRAVENOUS MEDICATIONS—cont'd
STEPS	**RATIONALE**

11. Explain the procedure and that medication will be delivered through the IV equipment. Encourage the patient to report symptoms of discomfort at the IV site. Assess the patient's understanding of the medication.
- Patients who can verbalize pain at the IV site can help detect IV infiltrations early, reducing the possibility of damage to the surrounding tissues.
- Patient understanding influences medication adherence.

12. Perform hand hygiene. Put on clean, disposable gloves.

13. Assess the patient, including the primary IV flow rate and IV insertion site for signs of infiltration or phlebitis: redness, pallor, swelling, or tenderness on palpation.
- Ensures IV is in the vein and not interstitial
- Infiltration causes tissue injury (e.g., extravasation) and prevents medication from being delivered.

CRITICAL DECISION POINT: *If the patient's IV site is saline locked, clean the port with alcohol or remove the disinfectant cap if present. Assess the patency of the IV line by flushing it with 2–3 mL of sterile normal saline. Attach the appropriate IV tubing to the saline lock and administer the medication via secondary IV set, tandem, mini-infusion, or other volume-control administration set (e.g., buretrol). When the infusion is completed, disconnect the tubing, clean the port with alcohol, and flush the IV line with 2–3 mL sterile normal saline. Clean the port with alcohol again, or apply a new disinfectant cap. Maintain sterility of the IV tubing between intermittent infusions.*

14. Administer the infusion:

   A. Secondary IV set or tandem infusion
   1. Hang the tandem infusion at the same level as the primary fluid bag. Hang a secondary IV medication bag or bottle high on the IV pole and move the primary IV bag to a lower hook. Clamp the regulator flow clamp on the new IV tubing set and remove the cap on the end of the tubing. Be careful to keep the end clean (i.e., untouched), hold the tubing, and do not let it touch the floor.
   - Clamping the regulator flow clamps prior to connecting or spiking the IV bag reduces the amount of air drawn into the tubing. The infusion tubing should be filled with solution and be free of air bubbles to prevent an air embolus.

   2. Spike the medication bag or bottle with the IV tubing or connect the mini-syringe pump container to IV tubing (see Chapter 41). Open any roller clamp and prime (i.e., fill) the IV tubing and any drip chamber with fluid. Once the tubing is full, close the roller clamp and recap the end of the tubing, keeping it clean.
   - The height of the fluid bag affects the rate of medication flow to the patient.

   3. Wipe the appropriate port on the primary IV tubing with an aseptic swab, or remove the disinfectant cap if present.
      a) Connect a secondary IV set to the highest port on the primary IV tubing and hang the medication bag higher than the primary IV bag.
      b) Alternatively, in some instances, you may want to infuse the secondary fluid/medication through the port closest to the patient on the primary IV line. This may be desired if you want the primary IV fluid to continue infusing simultaneously with the secondary fluid/medication, or if you are hanging blood products, fluids, or medications that you do not want to pass through the primary IV tubing (e.g., because it requires a special filter or type of tubing or is not compatible with the primary IV fluid). In these instances:
         i) If the secondary fluid/medication is not compatible with the primary IV fluid, flush the IV port closest to the patient on the primary IV line with a syringe containing 3–5 mL of sterile IV fluid compatible with the secondary fluid/medication.
         ii) Connect the primed secondary fluid/medication IV set to the port. Be sure to use an IV tubing set long enough to reach from the port closest to the patient to the top of the IV pole. Hang the secondary fluid/medication bag higher than the primary IV bag if you want only the secondary fluid/medication to infuse and the primary IV fluid infusion to stop.
         iii) Hang the secondary fluid/medication bag at the same height as the primary IV bag if you want both fluids to infuse at the same time.
   - A secondary IV set causes the primary IV infusion to automatically shut off while the medication is infusing and then restart when the medication bag is empty.
   - A tandem IV and mini-infusion pump cause the primary IV infusion to continue infusing while the medication is infusion.

   4. Adjust the flow rate of the medication using the roller clamp, or insert the tubing into the SMART IV pump and program the IV infusion pump using the library.
   - Ensures the medication is infused at the right rate and volume

Continued

SKILL 35.8   **ADMINISTERING INTRAVENOUS MEDICATIONS—cont'd**

STEPS	RATIONALE
(5) After the medication has been infused, recheck the flow rate on the primary infusion. The primary infusion should automatically begin to flow after the secondary IV set with medication is empty and should continue to flow when the tandem solution or mini-infusion pump is empty.	• Ensure that the primary IV fluid container is infusing at the correct rate and does not empty to prevent an air embolus. • The primary IV infusion rate could be altered after a tandem or secondary medication infusion.
(6) Leave the secondary IV bag and tubing in place for future medication administration (according to the employer policy) or discard in appropriate containers.	• Repeatedly accessing an IV access device or IV tubing introduces microorganisms. IV tubing is usually changed every 72 hours or more frequently, depending on the medication; follow employer policies.
B. Buretrol volume-control administration set	• Use of the medication room controls the risk of contaminating the IV solution.
(1) Assemble the supplies in the medication room. Perform hand hygiene.	
(2) Prepare medication from a vial or ampoule (see Skill 35.4).	• Ensures that the medication is sterile
(3) Hang the primary IV bag or medication solution on the IV pole. Clamp the buretrol roller clamps. Remove the cap from the end of the buretrol tubing, being sure to keep it clean by not touching it. Do not let the end touch the floor. Spike the buretrol tubing into the IV bag. Open the upper roller clamp. Allow the buretol to fill with the desired amount of fluid (25–100 mL) (see Step 14B[3] illustration).	• Use of a small volume of fluid dilutes the IV medication and reduces the risk of rapid infusion.

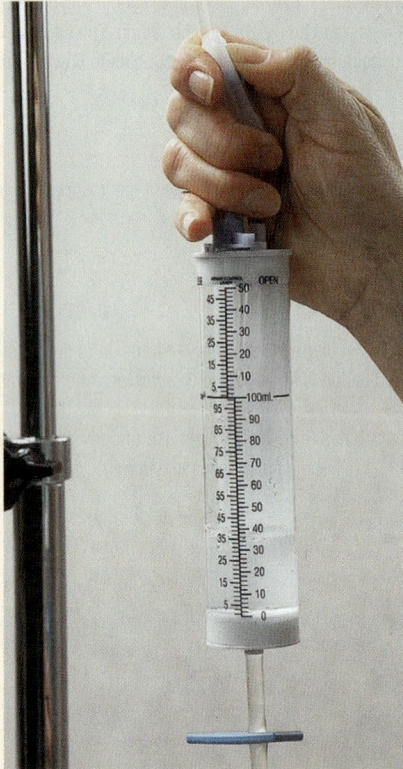

STEP 14B(3) Filling the buretrol volume-control administration device from a primary IV bag of diluent solution.

(4) Close the upper roller clamp and ensure that the clamp on the air vent of the buretrol chamber is open. Remove the cap from the end of tubing and be sure to keep it clean by not touching it. Open the lower clamp and allow the fluid to fill and prime the tubing. Once the tubing is primed (i.e., full), close the lower clamp and replace the cap on the end.	• This prevents air from accumulating in the tubing and reduces risk for air embolus. • Air vent allows fluid in the buretrol to exit at a regulated rate.

SKILL 35.8   **ADMINISTERING INTRAVENOUS MEDICATIONS—cont'd**

STEPS	RATIONALE
(5) Swab the buretrol port with an antiseptic swab for 15 seconds.	• Prevents the introduction of microorganisms
(6) Attach the needleless syringe containing the medication to the buretrol port, then inject the medication (see Figure 35.36). Gently rotate the buretrol between your hands.	• Rotating mixes the medication with the fluid solution in the buretrol to ensure equal distribution.
(7) Label the buretrol with the name of the medication, dose, volume (including the diluent), time of administration, and your initials. See the buretrol setup in Step 14B(7) illustration.	• Proper labelling alerts nurses to medication being infused and prevents other medications from being added to the buretrol.

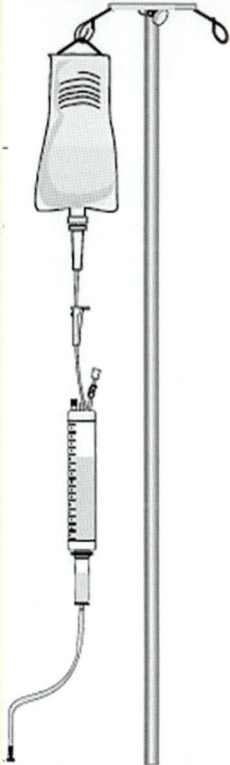

STEP 14B(7) The prepared Buretrol setup. (Courtesy and © Becton, Dickinson and Company.)

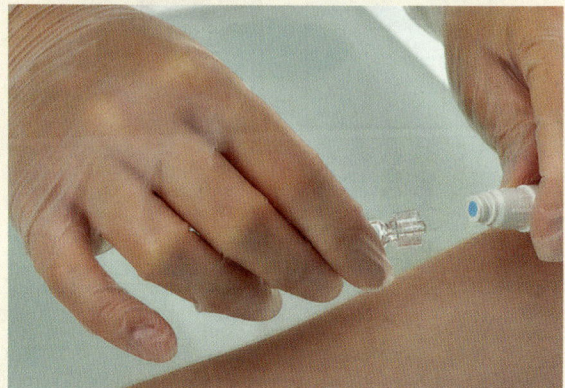

STEP 14B(8) Connecting the Buretrol tubing to the primary IV tubing or IV access device. (Courtesy and © Becton, Dickinson and Company.)

(8) Swab the appropriate port on the primary IV tubing for 15 seconds and allow to dry or remove the disinfectant cap if present. Connect the buretrol tubing to the port. (see Step 14B(8) illustration). Regulate the IV infusion rate by opening the lower clamp and infusing the medication at the prescribed rate, or insert the IV tubing into the SMART IV infusion pump and program the pump.	• Ensures the right rate and volume of medication is infusing
(9) Dispose of soiled supplies in a proper container. Perform hand hygiene.	• Reduces the transmission of microorganisms

SKILL 35.8   **ADMINISTERING INTRAVENOUS MEDICATIONS—cont'd**

STEPS	RATIONALE
C. Mini-infusion administration	
(1) Connect the prefilled syringe container to the mini-infusion tubing.	• The special tubing is designed to fit the syringe to deliver the medication to the main IV line.
(2) Place the syringe into a mini-infusion pump (follow product directions). Ensure that the syringe is secure (see illustration Step 14C[2].)	
(3) Fill and prime the tubing using the mini-infusion automatic priming features. Recap the end of the tubing, keeping it clean.	

STEP 14C(2) The syringe is secure in a mini-infusion pump. (Courtesy and © Becton, Dickinson and Company.)

STEPS	RATIONALE
(4) Select the lowest injection port on the primary IV tubing close to the patient. Swab the port with an antiseptic swab for 15 seconds or remove the disinfectant cap.	
(5) Connect the mini-infusion tubing to the lowest needleless port close to the patient on the primary IV tubing.	
(6) If the mini-infusion pump is for patient-controlled analgesia (PCA), educate the patient in how to administer their medication, and the dose and the frequency available.	• Monitoring a PCA or epidural mini-infusion pump requires teaching, scheduled assessment and documentation of the patient's pain level, doses administered, and doses requested to understand if the patient's pain analgesia is adequate.
(7) Program the pump to deliver the medication with the prescribed dose and frequency. Usually a second nurse is required to confirm the programming if a controlled substance (e.g., fentanyl) is being administered via the mini-infusion pump.	• Medication is delivered at a constant rate or on demand by pressing a button that injects the correct volume into the tubing.
15. Observe the patient for signs of adverse effects, particularly if they are receiving an opioid.	• IV medications act rapidly; adverse effects such as respiratory depression and sedation related to opioids can be harmful.
16. Regularly reassess the infusion rate and the condition of the IV site according to employer policy (e.g., hourly, every 4 hours)	• Ensures the IV is in the vein and not interstitial

SKILL 35.8 ADMINISTERING INTRAVENOUS MEDICATIONS—cont'd

UNEXPECTED OUTCOMES	RELATED INTERVENTIONS
Adverse effects or adverse reactions	• Stop or decrease medication infusion rates or dosages immediately. • Follow institutional policy or guidelines for the appropriate response, assessments, and reporting of medication adverse effects. • Notify the patient's health care provider of adverse effects immediately. • Document evidence of allergies in the patient's medical record.
Medication does not infuse over desired period	• Determine the reason for the lack of infusion (e.g., improper calculation of flow rate, wrong positioning of the IV needle at the insertion site, or infiltration). • Take corrective action as indicated.
Swelling, warmth, reddening, and tenderness at IV site, indicating phlebitis (see Chapter 41)	• Stop IV infusion. • Discontinue IV. • Treat the IV site as indicated by the institutional policy. • Select a new IV site if continuation of therapy is indicated.
Coolness, pallor, and swelling at IV site (see Chapter 41)	• Signs of infiltration are indicated. • Some IV medications are extremely harmful to subcutaneous tissue. • Provide IV extravasation care as indicated by institutional policy; or use a medication reference manual or consult a pharmacist to determine the appropriate follow-up care.

DOCUMENTATION AND REPORTING
• Record the medication, dose, route, and time administered on the MAR.
• Record the patient's intake from the volume of fluid in the medication bag, buretrol, or syringe container and the remaining volume of fluid in the container.
• Report any adverse effects to the nurse in charge or the health care provider.

CARE IN THE COMMUNITY CONSIDERATIONS
• Teach the patient and caregiver to dispose of any supplies in safe containers (e.g., needles in a coffee can).
• Instruct the patient and caregiver about community resources for obtaining supplies.
• Collaborate with the interdisciplinary team to facilitate access to supplies for patients who have barriers (e.g., income, transportation).

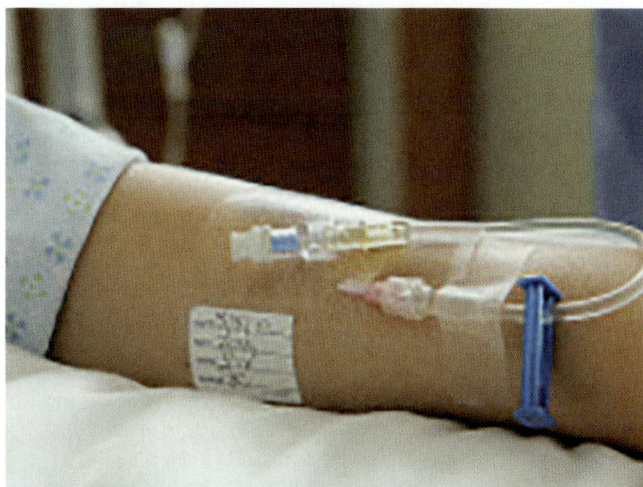

FIGURE 35.39 Intermittent IV access device with needleless Luer-lock port. (Courtesy and © Becton, Dickinson and Company.)

butterfly catheter, only one type of medication can be injected (e.g., morphine).

Contraindications to using the hypodermoclysis route for IV fluid administration include cardiac failure, prerenal or renal failure, low platelet or coagulation disorders, and existing fluid overload or marked

edema (see Chapter 41). If a patient is severely dehydrated, the IV route is preferred for fluid administration.

KEY CONCEPTS

• Learning the medication classifications improves a nurse's understanding of nursing implications for administering medications with similar characteristics.
• Federal medication legislation regulates the production, distribution, prescription, and administration of medications.
• All controlled substances are handled according to strict procedures that account for each medication.
• The nurse applies understanding of the physiology of medication action when physically assessing a patient before medication, timing the administration, selecting routes, initiating actions to promote medication efficacy, and observing responses to medications.
• The older person's body undergoes structural and functional changes that alter medication actions and influence the way in which medication therapy is provided.
• Children's medication doses are computed on the basis of body surface area and weight.
• Medications given parenterally are absorbed more quickly than medications administered by other routes.

BOX 35.27   PROCEDURAL GUIDELINE
Subcutaneous Butterfly Catheters and Hypodermoclysis

Delegation Considerations

The insertion of subcutaneous butterfly catheters cannot be delegated. Instruct unregulated care providers to report the occurrence of adverse effects of medications immediately.

Equipment:
- Butterfly catheter with 24-gauge, 19-mm needle (the smallest and shortest gauge should be used)
- Interline injection site
- Antiseptic swab
- Occlusive dressing (Tegaderm or Opsite)
- Tape
- Clean, disposable gloves
- Barcode scanner (if applicable)

Subcutaneous Medication Administration
- Prescribed medication
- Syringe and needleless access device

Hypodermoclysis
- Prescribed intravenous (IV) fluid
- IV administration set

Procedure:
1. Check the accuracy and completeness of each medication administration record (MAR), including patient name and medication name, route, dosage, time of administration, and start and stop date. If difficult to read, review the original prescription order and rewrite the prescription on the MAR.
2. Assess the patient's health history, medications, and allergies.
3. Collect the necessary information to administer the medication safely.
4. Perform hand hygiene. Remove the butterfly catheter from the package (see Step 4 illustration).

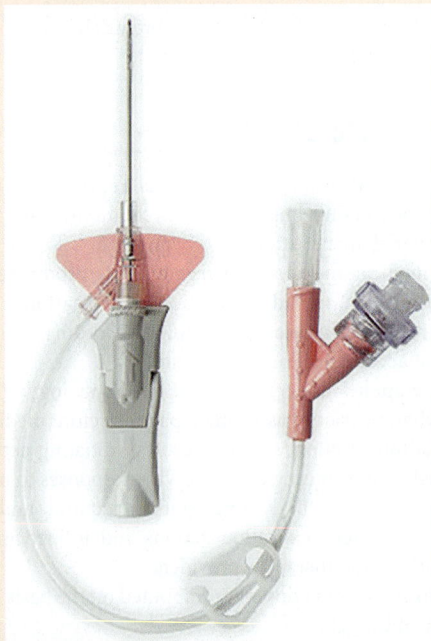

STEP 4 Subcutaneous butterfly catheter for infusion. (Courtesy and © Becton, Dickinson and Company.)

5. Check expiry dates on medication ampoules, vials, or the IV fluid for infusion. Check the label of the medication with the MAR two times while preparing the medication or fluid.
   a) *Subcutaneous medication administration:* Prepare the medication dose from an ampoule or vial (see Skill 35.4). Swab the butterfly connection port with an antiseptic swab for 15 seconds and allow to dry. Remove the blunt needle and connect the syringe to the butterfly tubing. Inject the medication to prime the tubing. Keep the syringe with the medication connected to the butterfly. Apply a medication label to the syringe with the medication name, dose, and date and your initials.
   b) *Hypodermoclysis:* Check the expiry date on the IV fluid for infusion. Attach the IV bag tubing to the butterfly port after the port is swabbed. Prime the IV tubing and the butterfly port.
6. Take the medication to the patient at the right time. Perform hand hygiene.
7. Close the room curtain or door to provide privacy.
8. Identify the patient, using two to three identifiers. Asking the patient to state their name, comparing the patient's name and one other identifier (e.g., the hospital ID number) on the MAR against information on the patient's ID bracelet, and scanning the patient's barcode on their ID bracelet ensure that you have the right patient.
9. Compare the label of the medication with the MAR one more time at the patient's bedside. This is the *third* accuracy check.
10. Explain to the patient the steps of the procedure and the sensations to expect, including a slight burning or stinging when the catheter is inserted. Inform the patient that the catheter will remain and will be used for medication administration of a particular medication.
11. Keep a sheet or gown draped over the body parts not requiring exposure.
12. Perform hand hygiene. Put on clean, disposable gloves.
13. Assess the patient for adequate subcutaneous tissue. Select an appropriate injection site. Inspect the skin surface over the sites for bruises, inflammation, or edema.
14. Palpate the sites for masses or tenderness. Avoid these areas.
15. Assist the patient into a comfortable position; have the patient relax the abdomen, thigh, or upper arm, depending on selected site.
16. Locate the site, using appropriate anatomical landmarks.
17. Clean the site with an antiseptic swab for 30 seconds. Apply the swab at the centre of the site and rotate outward in a circular direction for about 5 cm.
18. Remove the sheath from the catheter needle.
19. Hold the subcutaneous butterfly wings between the thumb and forefinger of your dominant hand with the palm down.
20. Ensure that the bevel of the needle is pointed upward.
21. Using the thumb and index finger of your nondominant hand, gently pinch the patient's skin around the selected injection site to create a roll of skin 1.25 to 2.5 cm in diameter.
22. Insert the full length of the needle through the skin at a 30-degree angle.
23. Assess for blood return into the catheter tubing. If blood return occurs, withdraw the needle and repeat the procedure at a new site.
24. Release the catheter wings and stabilize them on the skin surface with your thumb and index finger.
25. Apply an occlusive dressing (e.g., Tegaderm, Opsite) over the insertion site and some of the tubing. Reinforce the dressing with tape.
26. Apply a label to the occlusive dressing that shows the date and time of administration and your initials.
27. a) *Subcutaneous medication administration:* Inject the medication from the syringe. Remove the syringe and apply a new cap or disinfectant cap.

BOX 35.27 PROCEDURAL GUIDELINE—cont'd

b) *Hypodermoclysis:* Adjust the flow rate of the IV fluid as prescribed manually using the roller clamp or insert the tubing into the SMART IV infusion pump and program the pump using the library.

28. Dispose of supplies into the designated containers. Remove gloves and discard. Perform hand hygiene.

29. Document the procedure, including the site, type, and gauge of subcutaneous butterfly catheter; the date and time of insertion; the patient's response to the insertion; and your initials.

30. If infusing hypodermoclysis, regularly reassess the patient and infusion site until the fluid is complete. When complete, disconnect the tubing and apply a new cap or disinfectant cap to the butterfly.

Courtesy and © Becton, Dickinson and Company.

- Each medication prescription should include the patient's name; the prescription date; the medication name, dosage, route, time of administration, and indication; and the prescriber's signature.
- A medication history reveals allergies, medications that the patient is taking, and the patient's adherence to therapy.
- The nursing process should be used when administering medication.
- The rights of medication administration ensure accurate preparation and administration of medication doses.
- The rights of medication administration are the right medication, right dose, right patient, right route, right time and frequency, right documentation, right reason, right evaluation (or assessment), right patient education, and right to refuse.
- The nurse should administer only the medications that they prepare; prepared medications must never be left unattended.

- The nurse needs to avoid distractions and follow the same routines when preparing medications to reduce the chance of medication incidents.
- To prevent medication incidents, the nurse must document immediately all medications they administer.
- The nurse must use clinical judgement to determine the best time to administer PRN (when needed) medications.
- Medication incidents must be reported immediately.
- When preparing medications, the nurse checks the medication container label against the medication administration record three times.
- The Z-track method for intramuscular injections protects the subcutaneous tissues from irritating parenteral fluids.
- Failure to select injection sites by anatomical landmarks may lead to tissue, bone, or nerve damage.

CRITICAL THINKING EXERCISES

1. A 69-year-old patient has recently experienced a stroke and has right-sided weakness. The nurse practitioner in the neurological care unit wrote a prescription for routinely scheduled oral medications to start today. The prescription reads:
   - Acetaminophen 650 mg, 2 tabs, PO q4h
   - Metoprolol 25 mg PO daily
   - Senna 2 tabs PO qHS
   a) How will you assess if the patient can safely receive their oral medications? What symptoms would you recognize that would make you concerned that the patient cannot swallow?
   b) How would you respond if the patient cannot swallow safely?
   c) What steps would you take to administer the patient's oral medications if the patient can safely swallow?
2. Tega (pronouns: she/her) is a 25-year-old patient who delivered a healthy infant 24 hours ago. Tega has Rh-negative blood and the baby is Rh positive. Tega has a new prescription in her medical record which reads: "Administer WinRho 300 mcg IM × 1 today." (Here is a link to the Medication Package Insert for WinRho: https://www.fda.gov/media/77860/download.)

a) How would you assess if the prescription is appropriate for Tega?
b) Based on the information you have, do you think the medication prescription is appropriate for Tega? Why or why not?
c) How would you administer Tega's IM injection?
3. Mr. Gleason is a 75-year-old retired farmer who has developed a chronic cough and mild shortness of breath. Mr. Gleason is a widower and lives alone in a rural area. The physician at his family health team has prescribed an albuterol inhaler with a spacer, to start. You are the patient educator and will meet with Mr. Gleason about his new medication. You notice that Mr. Gleason has a shuffling walk, uses a cane, and wears thick glasses.
a) What is important to consider and assess when Mr. Gleason starts a new medication?
b) What information would you want to share with Mr. Gleason about his medication?
c) How would you evaluate if Mr. Gleason has the knowledge and skills needed to self-administer his inhaler at home?

🌐 *Answers to Critical Thinking Exercises appear on the Evolve website.*

REVIEW QUESTIONS

Review Questions 1 to 14 relate to the case study at the beginning of the chapter.

1. What symptoms is Mr. Blackstock experiencing that may benefit from medication administration currently?
   a. Chest pain
   b. Confusion

c. Weakness
d. Nausea, fever, and chills

2. Based on your assessment of Mr. Blackstock, what factor will affect your medication administration?
   a. He has an allergy to pollen.
   b. His symptoms are mild.
   c. He is not tolerating oral fluids.
   d. He is refusing medication.

3. What do you think is the best route to administer acetaminophen and treat Mr. Blackstock's fever?
   a. Rectal suppository
   b. Oral liquid
   c. Oral tablet
   d. Intravenous

   New information: Both Mr. Blackstock and another of your patients, Mrs. Young, are requesting medications at the same time. Your medication cart is in the hallway outside of Mr. Blackstock's room and you have both patients' medication administration records (MARs) and medication drawers. The hallway is loud with family members and patients talking, and you are scheduled to monitor your colleague's patients while they are on break.

4. What factors in this situation may interfere with your ability to safely prepare medications? *(Select all that apply.)*
   a. Distractions and interruptions
   b. Time constraints
   c. Preparing medications for multiple patients at the same time
   d. Reviewing two MARs at the same time

5. What medication administration right is most at risk if you prepare medications in this environment?
   a. The right patient
   b. The right documentation
   c. The right reason
   d. The right to refuse

6. What strategies can you use to fulfill the rights of medication administration and avoid incidents? *(Select all that apply.)*
   a. Prepare medications for only one patient at a time.
   b. Check the MAR two times during preparation, once at the bedside, and once after medication administration
   c. Document medication administration at the end of your shift
   d. Ask the patient to state their name, compare the patient's name and identification number on their MAR and identification bracelet, scan the patient's barcode.

7. It is time to deliver Mr. Blackstock's amoxicillin and you are reviewing his MAR. What do you notice about the medication prescription?
   a. The frequency is missing.
   b. The dose is missing.
   c. The route is missing.
   d. It is a single-time dose.

   New information: You consult the prescriber and obtain a complete prescription, which reads as follows: Amoxicillin 500 mg IV q12h starting today for 5 days.

8. What process should be completed prior to administering Mr. Blackstock's medications to ensure the amoxicillin is given at the correct time and will not interact with Mr. Blackstock's other medications?
   a. Medical history
   b. Diet history
   c. Patient education
   d. Medication reconciliation

9. You are unsure about whether or not Mr. Blackstock received a dose of amoxicillin IV in the emergency department before being transferred to the medicine unit. What is the most reliable way to assess this information?

   a. Review the MAR from the emergency department
   b. Ask the patient
   c. Ask the patient's family or friend
   d. Ask your colleague

   New information: The amoxicillin is in a powdered form inside a glass vial. The instructions state:
   - *Add 10 mL of sterile water to vial to reconstitute the medication.*
   - *Dilute in 50 mL of normal saline for IV infusion.*

10. Place the following steps in the correct order to describe how you would prepare the vial of powdered amoxicillin for IV administration.
    a. #___ Dispose of the supplies in the correct waste garbage containers. Perform hand hygiene. The medication is ready for administration.
    b. #___ Remove the blunt fill needle and syringe with medication from the vial. Tap the vial the push air bubbles to the tip. Eject any air bubbles. Confirm you have the desired amount of medication.
    c. #___ Insert the blunt fill needle and syringe with medication into the rubber port on the 50-mL IV bag of normal saline. Inject the medication into the IV bag.
    d. #___ Attach a blunt fill needle to a 10-mL syringe and draw up 10 mL of sterile water diluent from a vial or use a prefilled syringe of 10 mL sterile water.
    e. #___ Perform hand hygiene and check the expiry date on the medication vial.
    f. #___ Insert the blunt fill needle of the syringe containing the diluent into the medication vial at a 90-degree angle and inject the diluent. Remove the blunt fill needle and empty syringe.
    g. #___ Remove the top of the medication vial, swab the rubber cap vigorously for 15 seconds, and allow to dry.
    h. #___ Roll the vial to dissolve the powdered medication in the diluent.
    i. #___ Insert the blunt fill needle of the syringe containing the air into the medication vial at a 90-degree angle and inject the air into the vial's empty airspace.
    j. #___ Withdraw the blunt fill needle and syringe. Mix the medication in the IV bag by turning it upside down multiple times until the medication is dissolved.
    k. #___ Invert the vial, keeping the blunt fill needle under the fluid level. Withdraw the medication into the syringe. Check the level of the medication in the syringe to ensure you have the desired amount.
    l. #___ Swab the rubber injection port on a 50-mL IV bag of normal saline with an antiseptic swab for 15 seconds and allow to dry. Affix a medication additive label to the IV bag stating the name of the medication, the dose, the time, the date, and your signature.
    m. #___ Recap the blunt fill needle of the syringe containing the reconstituted medication.
    n. #___ Draw up the amount of air equal to the amount of reconstituted medication (e.g., 5 mL) into the syringe with the blunt fill needle.

11. How will you recognize if Mr. Blackstock is tolerating the IV medication infusion?
    a. Redness and swelling at the IV site
    b. Hives and rash at the IV site

c. Reported pain and burning at the IV site

d. No changes to skin colour, swelling, pain, or leaking fluid at IV site

New information: Mr. Blackstock is now complaining of pain associated with coughing. The ampoule of hydromorphone contains 1 mg per mL and you want to deliver 0.5 mL of hydromorphone sub-Q injection to Mr. Blackstock.

12. What will the volume of the hydromorphone be that you administer to Mr. Blackstock?

    a. 0.5 mL of medication
    b. 1 mL of medication
    c. 0.25 mL of medication
    d. 1.2 mL of medication

13. How much hydromorphone will need to be discarded and witnessed by two nurses?

    a. 0.8 mg

b. 0.75 mg

c. 0.5 mg

d. 0 mg

New information: You prepare and administer 0.5 mg hydromorphone sub-Q by injection into Mr. Blackstock's abdomen.

14. What signs would indicate that Mr. Blackstock tolerated the hydromorphone injection without adverse effects?

    a. Patient becomes confused and agitated 20 minutes after receiving the hydromorphone.
    b. Patient reports decreased pain severity from 6/10 to 3/10, 20 minutes after receiving the hydromorphone.
    c. Patient's respiratory rate and blood pressure decrease below normal limits 20 minutes after receiving the hydromorphone.
    d. Patient develops a rash at the injection site.

Rationales for the Review Questions appear on the Evolve website.

Answers: 1. d; **2.** c; **3.** a; **4.** a, b, c, d; **5.** a; **6.** a, b, d; **7.** a; **8.** d; **9.** a; **10.** Correct order: E G D F H B I K N M L C J A; **11.** d; **12.** a; **13.** c; **14.** b.

RECOMMENDED WEBSITES

Canadian Nursing Colleges: Each nursing regulatory body for registered and/or licensed practical nurses in Canada has its own medication management standard. Some samples of regulatory guidelines are listed below:

- British Columbia College of Nurses and Midwives: https://www.bccnm.ca/NP/PracticeStandards/General%20Resources/NP_PS_Medication.pdf
- College of Licensed Practical Nurses of Alberta: https://www.clpna.com/wp-content/uploads/2013/02/doc_CCPNR_CLPNA_Standards_of_Practice.pdf
- College of Nurses of Ontario: https://www.cno.org/globalassets/docs/prac/41007_medication.pdf
- College of Registered Nurses of Alberta: Standards of Medication Management: https://www.nurses.ab.ca/media/3lfhdrrq/medication-management-standards-mar-2021.pdf
- College of Registered Nurses of Manitoba: https://www.crnm.mb.ca/uploads/document/document_file_254.pdf?t=1580488652
- College of Registered Nurses of Newfoundland and Labrador: https://crnnl.ca/site/uploads/2021/09/standards-of-practice-for-rns-and-nps.pdf
- College of Registered Nurses of Prince Edward Island: https://crnpei.ca/wp-content/uploads/2021/03/Practice-Directive-Medication-Administration-with-CLPNPEI-2021-02-25.pdf
- Nova Scotia College of Nursing: https://cdn1.nscn.ca/sites/default/files/documents/resources/MedicationGuidelines.pdf
- OIIQ: Ordre des infirmières et infirmiers du Québec: https://www.oiiq.org/
- Registered Nurses Association of the Northwest Territories and Nunavut: https://rnantnu.ca/wp-content/uploads/2019/10/2019-standards-of-practice.pdf
- Saskatchewan Registered Nurses Association: http://www.srna.org/images/stories/Nursing_Practice/Resources/Medication_Management_for_RNs_FINAL_2015_09_03_Rev_2015_09_30_Web.pdf
- Yukon Registered Nurses Association: https://drive.google.com/file/d/1sHLWj49h9yZlr8HG86hMdXiA4r7vMyV-/view

Canadian Council for Practical Nurse Regulators: https://ccpnr.ca

This council promotes best practice and leadership in practical nursing and includes the 2020 Standards of Practice.

Canadian Nurses Protective Society: https://cnps.ca

This society provides advice and information for nurses regarding their legal rights and obligations when providing patient care.

Canadian Pharmacists Association: https://www.pharmacists.ca

The Canadian Pharmacists Association (CPhA) is a national organization of pharmacists. CPhA's website provides links to medication information, patient information, and resources.

Choosing Wisely Canada: https://choosingwiselycanada.org/nursing

Choosing Wisely Canada is a national organization that aims to reduce unnecessary use of medications and treatments. Guidelines for deprescribing and questions for nurses to ask about prescribed medications are provided.

Forum for Injection Technique (FIT) Canada: https://www.fit4diabetes.com/canada-english

The FIT provides recommendations and instructions for safe injection techniques worldwide, with a focus on techniques for persons with diabetes.

Health Canada: Drug Product Database: https://www.hc-sc.gc.ca/dhp-mps/prodpharma/databasdon/index-eng.php

This website provides access to government reports, resources, and programs about the safety and effectiveness of pharmaceutical medications and other therapeutic products.

Health Canada: Pharmaceutical Drugs Directorate: https://www.hc-sc.gc.ca/ahc-asc/branch-dirgen/hpfb-dgpsa/tpd-dpt/index-eng.php

Health Canada's Pharmaceutical Drugs Directorate (formerly the Therapeutic Products Directorate) is the Canadian federal authority that regulates pharmaceutical medications and medical devices for human use. This website provides access to information on reporting adverse effects or adverse reaction information.

Health Canada Vigilance Program: https://www.canada.ca/drug-device-reporting

This website allows consumers (i.e., patients) and health care providers to report side effects and adverse (i.e., harmful) reactions to medications, medical devices, natural health products, and vaccines. It is mandatory for hospitals to report serious adverse effects within 30 days. Reporting both serious and mild side effects allows for safer monitoring of medications and the identification of risks and effects.

Institute for Safe Medication Practices (ISMP) Canada: https://ismpcanada.ca

This website has information about preventing medication incidents, practising medication reconciliation, and managing high-alert medications and controlled substances. Reports, publications, educational opportunities, newsletters, and tip sheets are also provided to optimize patient safety. Practitioners can also report medication incidents and near misses confidentially at https://www.ismp-canada.org/err_ipr.htm through ISMP to help identify opportunities for enhanced medication safety.

University of Saskatchewan: medSask: https://medsask.usask.ca
medSask, operating from the University of Saskatchewan, aims to give health care providers and laypersons access to objective and concise information on medications and medication therapy.

REFERENCES

A full reference list is available on the website for this book at
http://evolve.elsevier.com/Canada/Potter/fundamentals/

36

Integrative Health Care

Written by Deborah Gibson, RN, MSN

OBJECTIVES

Mastery of content in this chapter will enable you to:

- Define the key terms listed.
- Explain the conceptualization and evolution of integrative health care.
- Describe the various treatments associated with integrative medicine.
- Explain the scope of naturopathic and chiropractic medicine.
- Understand how integrative health care assists in health promotion and disease prevention.
- Recognize botanical treatments as an approach to integrative medicine.
- Understand the nurse's role in interprofessional collaboration in relation to integrative health care.

KEY TERMS

Acupoints
Acupuncture
Allopathic medicine
Alternative approaches
Biofeedback
Botanicals
Cannabinoids
Chiropractic medicine
Complementary and alternative medicine (CAM)
Complementary approaches

Energy flow
Healing touch
Holistic health
Imagery
Integrative health care/medicine
Medical use of cannabis
Meditation
Meridians
Mindfulness
Natural health products
Naturopathic medicine

Nutrition
Prayer
Qi
Relaxation
Spiritual nursing care
Stress response
Therapeutic dry needling
Therapeutic touch
Traditional Chinese medicine (TCM)
Yin and yang
Yoga

WEBSITE

https://evolve.elsevier.com/Canada/Potter/fundamentals/

CASE STUDY

A Holistic Approach to Health

As the nurse at an integrative medicine clinic, you are responsible for completing initial assessments, providing counselling, and advising new patients about integrative health care approaches. You meet Mrs. Shari Lorimer (preferred pronouns: she/her), a 48-year-old woman employed full time as a high school teacher. Shari indicates that she has anxiety and is currently taking anti-anxiety medication. Her primary reason for visiting the clinic is to learn about other approaches to treating her anxiety as an alternative to taking additional medication.

Key Points

- Past history: Mrs. Lorimer indicates that her parents immigrated from Ireland before she was born. Her extended family currently lives in Ireland. Her mother has a history of anxiety and depression. Her father recently died. He had been living in a care facility on a dementia unit for the past 2 years.
- Social history: Her relationships with her children and spouse are strong. She attends church regularly and expresses a connection to her faith.
- Medications: She currently takes a selective serotonin reuptake inhibitor (SSRI) medication for her anxiety (as prescribed by her general practitioner).

Mrs. Lorimer's physician has suggested adding another SSRI medication to help her feel better.

- Attitude toward health: She cries during the interview and expresses feelings of loss and sadness about her father's recent death and her perceived inability to control her anxiety. She expresses that her occupation and family activities are stressful, and she feels that she has little time or energy left at the end of the day. She states that she does not want to take additional medication unless it is absolutely necessary.

Critical Thinking Questions

1. What additional health assessment information would be important to ask Mrs. Lorimer?
2. What would you need to consider in order to offer holistic nursing care?
3. What approaches could you offer that are considered nursing interventions?
4. What integrative health approaches may be indicated for Mrs. Lorimer?
5. Which health care provider would you refer Mrs. Lorimer to?

Think about this case study as you read this chapter. There are review questions at the end of the chapter about this case study.

Interest in wellness and integrative health, or other systems of care, continues to gain momentum in Canada, with 75% of Canadians having used at least one integrative health care/medicine or complementary and alternative medicine (CAM) approach for the treatment of cancer, persistent pain, trauma recovery, anxiety, depression, and health promotion (Ashraf et al., 2021; Bolton et al., 2018; Canizares et al., 2017; de Jonge et al., 2018; Esmail, 2017; Mattar & Frewen, 2020; Ng & Sharma, 2020; Pratt et al., 2020; Yang et al., 2019). The current culture of health care delivery is evolving in alignment with values and beliefs toward health and life, trending toward less invasive, more traditional treatments such as nutrition, botanicals, manipulation, meditation, massage, and others that were neglected during the explosion of medical science and technology during the twentieth century. This trend is supported by the World Health Organization's (WHO) statement of health as "a state of complete physical, mental, and social well-being and not merely the absence of disease or infirmity" (Leonardi, 2018, p. 736).

The terminology used to describe the field of integrative medicine has evolved several times. It was called *holistic medicine* in the 1970s, *complementary and alternative medicine* in the 1980s, and *integrative medicine* in the 1990s; since 2020, it has been referred to as *integrative health* (Micozzi, 2019a, 2019b; Rakel & Weil, 2018). However, the philosophy of holistic health itself is not new. "Health is derived from the old English word *hal*, which means whole, soundness or spiritual wellness" (Rakel & Weil, 2018, p. 7). Holistic health addresses all aspects of a person's psychological, physical, spiritual, and social needs to promote the balance and health of the body.

Aristotle first proposed that the body and mind could not be separated and that a healer must observe and reflect upon the total person. Ancient civilizations dating from 5000 BC, including the Egyptians and Chinese, were employing and recording the effects of various herbal and energy healing traditions on the body. Despite the intervening Dark Ages (1493–1541), a period characterized by a loss of interest in science and an increase in magic to explain the world environment, interest in the human condition continued to grow.

The roots of twentieth-century conventional medicine (allopathic medicine) can be traced back to René Descartes (1595–1650), a deeply religious mathematician and philosopher who believed that the mind and body must be separated to protect the "spirit" from scientific inquiry. Consequently, the development of medicine focused exclusively on physical function and a reduction of the larger whole into its smaller parts (Rakel & Weil, 2018). This paradigm is still evident to this day in the many fields of specialization that exist within modern medicine.

Contrary to the popular views of her day, Florence Nightingale (1820–1910), most often remembered as the founder of modern nursing, practised a holistic approach to health. She incorporated various healing modalities along with advocating for cleanliness, sanitation, fresh air, light, and compassionate and spiritual care while providing nursing care to soldiers during the Crimean War.

In the mid-twentieth century, Canada experienced broad cultural shifts and paradigm changes. Social activism grew, and attitudes toward traditional health care delivery systems changed. These social movements coincided with demographic changes, increased cultural diversity, and global mobility. Ultimately, these forces have led consumer interest toward a less invasive, more holistic approach. Integrative health care underscores relational-centred care while combining the best treatment options from both allopathic medicine and integrative medicine for the patient's needs. The goal is to understand the "interplay of mind, body, and spirit and what is needed to restore balance of health of the body" (Rakel & Weil, 2018, p. 9). Today, the public has access to a massive volume of health

---

BOX 36.1	**Characteristics of Integrative Health Care**

- Integrative health care approaches:
  - Work in conjunction with the body's own self-healing mechanisms
  - Are "holistic" (view the whole person as unique with their own inner resources)
  - Focus on disease prevention and well-being.
- Nutrition and natural products are fundamental to maintain tissue and cell growth.
- Each person's body heals itself. The focus is on the healed body instead of the healer.
- Knowledge is shared between the patient and the practitioner. Both are active participants in the interaction.

From Micozzi, M. S., & Cassidy, C. M. (2019). Translation from conventional medicine. In M. S. Micozzi, *Fundamentals of complementary and alternative medicine* (6th ed., pp. 12–22). Elsevier.

information online, including the websites of organizations that promote personal, holistic, and integrative health approaches (e.g., https://www.chna.ca; https://www.cand.ca/; https://www.chiropractic.ca; https://www.cancer.gov/about-cancer/treatment/cam).

INTEGRATIVE HEALTH CARE

Integrative health care complements conventional medicine and includes numerous care approaches based on paradigms of health and healing. Integrative health care primarily focuses on the underlying causes of illness and imbalance in the body instead of on disease symptoms (Micozzi, 2019a). It provides health care consumers with access to both allopathic and integrative health care providers. While integrative approaches such as Indigenous healing, traditional Chinese medicine, chiropractic, naturopathic medicine, massage, and relaxation therapy represent a wide range of complexity in their approaches to health, these approaches all emphasize holistic health and wellness relative to the standards of the mainstream medical model (Micozzi, 2019a). The common characteristics of integrative health approaches are listed in Box 36.1.

Within integrative health care, the terms *complementary medicine* and *alternative medicine* are often used interchangeably and as an "adjunct to, if not a replacement for, biomedicine" (Micozzi & Cassidy, 2019, p. 13). Complementary approaches align with or contribute to and enhance conventional medical treatments, whereas alternative approaches may be used instead of conventional medical treatments (Micozzi, 2019a). Integrative medicine approaches such as naturopathy and chiropractic require diagnostic and therapeutic treatments specific to their respective disciplines, whereas other complementary approaches, such as imagery, do not require diagnostic examination. Nurses should be knowledgeable about the safety and efficacy of the various integrative health approaches in order to educate and support patients in their decision making (Steinhorn et al., 2017).

CAM approaches gained legitimacy because of the growing consumer movement and favourable patient-reported outcomes (Micozzi, 2019a; Rakel & Fortney, 2018). Although the terms CAM and integrative medicine are often used interchangeably, they are not synonymous. Integrative health care/medicine consists of best practices chosen from among conventional, complementary, and alternative approaches (National Center for Complementary and Integrative Health, 2016; Rakel & Weil, 2018). In integrative medicine, healing is facilitated through safe, evidence-informed practice based on medical and biomedical research that simultaneously respects patient choice (Ng, 2020). It is worth noting that both chiropractic and naturopathy are regulated health professions in Canada, and both use evidence-informed integrative health care approaches (Ng, 2020). In some institutions, nurses may practise massage, reiki, and therapeutic touch.

Integrative health approaches are often organized into six categories that researchers find useful (Box 36.2). Some categories and examples of integrative health approaches are presented in Table 36.1. This list is not exhaustive and does not address issues of safety and efficacy. Commonly used approaches include chiropractic and naturopathy, prayer, massage, acupuncture, cupping, botanicals, relaxation techniques, mindfulness, and yoga.

Public Interest in Integrative Health

The popularity of, and demand for, alternative health care services and providers has been growing nationally and globally. Although integrative health care is less expensive and more cost effective for the health care system, individuals (or their private insurance plans) must pay for these services. Despite the cost, a 2016 Canadian survey to determine the prevalence and patterns of CAM use indicated that more than three-quarters (79%) of Canadians had used at least one CAM therapy at some point during their lives (Esmail, 2017; Micozzi, 2019a), and more than 50% of the populations in Europe, North America, and other industrialized regions have sought CAM therapies at least once (Esmail, 2017). The 2016 survey results also indicated that age, income, education, spirituality, and perceived control over health are important predictors of whether or not a person is willing to explore integrative health care (Esmail, 2017). Individuals with cancer, depression, asthma, diabetes, and migraines and those receiving palliative care visit integrative health providers at a significantly higher rate and with more positive outcomes than do individuals within the general population (Alsharif, 2021; Ashraf et al., 2021; Steinhorn et al., 2017).

BOX 36.2 Categories and Examples of Integrative Health Care

Natural Products

Interventions use substances found in nature.

Examples: herbs, (botanicals), vitamins, minerals, dietary supplemental probiotics

Mind–Body–Spirit Interventions

Interventions include a diverse group of therapies to enhance the mind's ability to affect body functions and symptoms.

Examples: relaxation techniques, imagery, meditation, yoga, music therapy, prayer, journalling, hypnotherapy, biofeedback, humour, tai chi, art therapy, acupuncture

Manipulative and Body-Based Methods

Interventions focus on manipulation or movement of one or more parts of the body.

Examples: chiropractic, osteopathy, massage

Energy Therapies

Interventions focus on the use of energy fields, such as magnetic fields and biofields, that are believed to surround and permeate the body.

Examples: healing touch, therapeutic touch, Reiki, external qi gong, magnets

Other Integrative Health Care Approaches

Whole systems of care are built on theory and practice and often evolved apart from and earlier than Western medicine. Each has its own therapies and practices.

Examples: traditional Chinese medicine, Ayurveda, naturopathy, homeopathy

From Lindquist, R., Snyder, M., & Tracy, M. (Eds.). (2018). *Complementary and alternative therapies in nursing* (8th ed.) Springer.

TABLE 36.1 Integrative Health Practices

Types	Mechanism or Philosophy of Action
Whole Medical Systems	
Integrative health care	A health care system augmented by approaches directed toward the underlying causes of disease and preventative measures as opposed to only the symptoms of disease.
Integrative approaches	Health care approaches used in addition to conventional medical treatment that contribute to or enhance overall well-being.
Ayurveda	A traditional system of medicine, rooted in Hinduism, that dates to ancient India. Ayurveda practitioners use a combination of remedies, such as herbs, purgatives, and oils, to treat disease.
Latin American practices	The curanderismo medical system includes a humoral model (used by Hippocrates to explain disease) for classifying food, activity, drugs, illnesses, and a series of folk illnesses.
Traditional Indigenous healing	Traditional wellness is central to improving and transforming First Nations health in Canada. Health practices, approaches, knowledge, and beliefs incorporate First Nations healing and wellness while using ceremonies; plant-, animal-, or mineral-based medicines; energetic therapies; and physical or hands-on techniques (First Nations Health Authority, 2021) (see Chapter 12).
Naturopathic medicine	Naturopathic medicine views disease as a process instead of an entity, recognizing the body's inherent healing abilities. Approaches include botanical medicine, nutrition, hydrotherapy, naturopathic manipulation, traditional Chinese medicine, acupuncture, and cupping.
Traditional Chinese medicine	Traditional and systematic techniques that promote health and treat disease through acupuncture, herbal remedies, massage, acupressure, qigong (balancing energy flow through movement), and moxibustion (the use of heat from burning herbs).
Biologically Based Approaches (Natural Health Products)	
Amino acids, essential fatty acids (EFAs), and antioxidant supplements	These products, packaged as tablets or capsules, reduce the body's inflammatory response and limit oxidative stress within the body.
Botanicals/Plants	Botanicals are used singly or in mixtures, offering a therapeutic benefit. They provide a source of nutrients, essential oils, and energy and have biomedical guidelines for nutrition and disease prevention.

Continued

TABLE 36.1	Integrative Health Practices—cont'd
Types	**Mechanism or Philosophy of Action**
Homeopathic medicines	A system of medicinal treatment based on the theory that certain diseases can be cured with small doses of substances that, in a healthy person, would produce symptoms similar to the symptoms of disease. The prescribed remedies are made from naturally occurring plant, animal, or mineral substances.
Vitamins and minerals (megavitamin therapy)	Megavitamin therapy involves the increased intake of nutrients, such as vitamins B, C, D, and beta-carotene. Treatment focuses on a variety of health concerns, including cancer, schizophrenia, and coronary artery disease.
Traditional medicines (Ayurvedic remedies, traditional Chinese herbal remedies)	Ayurvedic remedies use a combination of herbs, purgatives, and rubbing oils to treat disease. Herbs and medicinal plants, considered the backbone of traditional Chinese medicine, have been studied extensively.
Probiotics	Living microorganisms that are orally administered to confer a protective benefit on the immune system of the small intestine.
Cannabis and cannabinoids for medical use	Cannabis is a dried or fresh plant and oil administered by ingestion or other means and that contains psychoactive chemicals. Cannabis contains many chemicals, including THC (delta-9-tetrahydrocannabinol) and CBD (cannabidiol). THC is the best-understood chemical and is responsible for most of the physical and psychotropic effects of cannabis. CBD is found in lesser amounts in the plant and has fewer psychotropic properties. Canadian licensed producers of cannabis for medical use have manufactured a variety of cannabis forms (with varying levels of THC and CBD for patients with prescriber authorization to access cannabis for medical reasons (Abramovici et al., 2018; Health Canada, 2022a).
Nutrition as Medicine	
Gerson therapy	In this therapy, disease is believed to be caused by the accumulation of toxic substances that disrupt the body's immune system. This therapy advocates a low-salt, high-potassium organic diet of fruit juices, raw vegetables, and nutritional supplements and is primarily used in the treatment of cancer.
Macrobiotic diet	A predominantly vegan diet (white meat, fish, occasional fruits, seeds, and nuts) believed to have anticancer properties. The diet consists of 40–60% whole cereal grain, 20–30% vegetables, and 5–10% beans.
Mediterranean diet	This diet, commonly eaten by people living in the Mediterranean region, is high in whole grains, nuts, fruits, vegetables, and omega-3 essential fatty acids. It produces a protective benefit for cardiac health and various inflammatory diseases.
Manipulative and Body-Based Approaches	
Acupressure	A therapeutic technique wherein digital pressure is applied on designated body points to relieve pain, produce analgesia, or regulate bodily function.
Chiropractic medicine	This practice emphasizes that the body has an inherent recuperative ability to restore and maintain health and well-being through the evaluation and conservative treatment of neuromuscular disorders. Care includes therapeutic adjustments of the spinal column and counselling patients on lifestyle choices (diet, nutrition, exercise, and stress management) (Canadian Chiropractic Association, 2019).
Massage therapy	The manipulation of soft tissue through stroking, rubbing, or kneading increases the body's circulation and improves muscle tone and relaxation.
Simple touch	Touching the patient in appropriate, gentle ways is used to stimulate a connection, display acceptance, and give appreciation.
Tai chi	This technique incorporates breath, movement, and meditation to cleanse, strengthen, and circulate vital energy and blood. Tai chi helps to stimulate the immune system and maintain balance.
Therapeutic dry needling	Dry needling, a treatment often used to improve neck pain, uses thin "filiform needles to penetrate the skin and stimulate myofascial trigger points, muscular and connective tissues for the management of neuromusculoskeletal pain and movement impairments" (Boyce et al., 2020, p. 103). This treatment is different in its application and mechanism from acupuncture and must be performed by a certified health care provider. It is usually provided by physiotherapists; however, some naturopathic doctors have been certified to perform dry needling. Adverse effects (while minor) include mild bleeding, bruising, and pain during the procedure (Fernández-De-Las-Peñas et al., 2021).
Mind–Body Interventions	
Aromatherapy	The use of essential plant oils to promote relaxation or stimulation, thereby enhancing overall well-being.
Art therapy	A form of psychotherapy in which self-expression through visual art is used to reconcile emotional conflicts and foster self-awareness and creativity.
Biofeedback	A mind–body therapy whereby a person receives visual or auditory information about their autonomic physiological body functions, such as muscle tension, skin temperature, and brain wave activity, through an electrical instrument. Biofeedback highlights the relationships between thoughts, feelings, and physiological responses.
Breath work	Using a variety of breathing patterns to relax, invigorate, or open the emotional channels. In yoga, control of the breath (*prana*, or life force energy) is referred to as *pranayama*.
Dance therapy	A form of psychotherapy in which dance and movement are used as a therapeutic intervention to heal social, emotional, cognitive, or physical difficulties.
Hypnotherapy	The induction of trance states and the use of therapeutic suggestion to treat paralysis, headaches, addictions, pain, and phobias.

TABLE 36.1	Integrative Health Practices—cont'd
Types	**Mechanism or Philosophy of Action**
Imagery	A mind–body practice using imagination to evoke emotions for the treatment of acute and chronic illness, stress management, anxiety, relaxation, and enhancement of wellness (Fitzgerald & Langevin, 2018).
Labyrinth meditation	Labyrinths are ancient spiritual symbols found in many religious traditions. Walking the labyrinth is regarded as a spiritual act of meditation, reflection, and prayer and as a pilgrimage.
Meditation	A self-directed practice that relaxes the body and calms the mind through focused awareness on rhythmic breathing.
Mindfulness	Drawing from Buddhist psychology, **mindfulness** helps to build awareness of the present moment with an attitude of openness and equanimity. Mindfulness promotes being in the present moment, on purpose and nonjudgementally (Rakel & Fortney, 2018).
Music therapy	The clinical use of music to stimulate the physical, psychological, cognitive, and spiritual dimensions. Music can "elicit an emotional response associated with dopamine activity in the brain's mesolimbic reward system, physiological processes (BP, temperature, digestion and adrenal hormones" (Chlan & Heiderscheit, 2018, p. 110). It is used to manage pain and improve physical movement, communication, emotional expression, and memory.
Spiritual nursing care and prayer	**Spiritual nursing care**, which is practised through relational care and interconnectedness with patients, is essential to nursing practice (Hawthorne & Gordon, 2020) (see Chapter 29). **Prayer** is a method of communication (verbal or silent, within a group or solitary) that expresses one's desires and needs and is often identified as an important source of help in managing physical and spiritual pain and quality of life (Piasseschi de Bernardin Gonçalves et al., 2017). A variety of techniques are used in a variety of cultures to incorporate caring, compassion, love, and empathy in prayer.
Psychotherapy	The treatment of mental and emotional disorders using psychological techniques.
Yoga	**Yoga** combines physical poses, controlled breathing (*pranayama*), and meditation to cultivate present-moment awareness, resulting in greater physical and mental well-being.
Energy Medicine	
Qigong	Qigong is derived from the ancient Chinese practice of breathing, movement, and meditation and involves the coordination of body postures and movement. This practice promotes strength, balance, and optimal body functioning and is used to treat stress-related conditions, fatigue, and musculoskeletal stiffness.
Reiki therapy	Reiki is derived from ancient Buddhist practices in which a practitioner places a hand on or above the body and transfers "universal life energy" to the patient. The energy from this therapy provides strength, harmony, and balance to treat health issues.
Therapeutic listening	A dynamic and intentional process that requires attention to a patient verbal and nonverbal cues. Active listening is an effective therapeutic technique for nurses and is foundational to building the nurse–patient relationship (Watanuki et al., 2018).
Therapeutic touch	Practitioners direct balance their own energies toward the energies of a patient by laying the hands on or close to a patient's body.

The Canadian Interdisciplinary Network of Complementary Medicine Researchers was launched in 2004 to foster CAM research and disseminate information. Objectives include providing information that reflects a Canadian perspective on the safety and efficacy of various CAM approaches.

Medical Use of Cannabis.
Medical use of cannabis is the use of cannabis (marijuana) and cannabinoids according to a prescriber's orders. There is limited evidence that cannabis and prescription **cannabinoids** (dronabinol, nabilone, and nabiximols) may be useful in alleviating symptoms in palliative care, chemotherapy, multiple sclerosis (e.g., tremors, spasticity, epilepsy, pain, anxiety, and depression [secondary to chronic conditions]), and sleep (associated with chronic conditions). Adverse effects include a potential for carcinogenesis. Evidence from preclinical studies indicates that cannabis smoke contains the same carcinogens as tobacco smoke and thus can have a negative effect on many body systems, including the respiratory tract and the immune, reproductive, cardiovascular, gastrointestinal, cognitive, and psychomotor systems. Cannabis can also potentially cause psychiatric effects, schizophrenia and psychosis, and suicidal ideation.

Nurses should be aware of the complex nature of cannabis and its derivatives:

> Cannabis products and cannabinoids should not be considered equivalent. Cannabis and cannabis products are highly complex materials with hundreds of chemical constituents whereas cannabinoids are typically single molecules. Direct comparisons between cannabis products and cannabinoids must account for route of administration, dosage, individual pharmacological components and their potential interactions, and the different pharmacokinetic and pharmacodynamic properties of these different substances.
>
> **Abramovici et al., 2018**

Integrative Health Care and Holistic Nursing

Integrative medicine and holistic nursing care have similar goals. Holistic nursing values the "awareness of whole-people and whole-system interconnectedness" (Rosa et al., 2019, p. 381) that is foundational to current global health initiatives focused on the improvement of human, animal, and planetary health, and for the essential nature of partnerships in attaining these goals (Rosa et al., 2019). The practice of holistic nursing regards the human health experience as a complicated, dynamic relationship of health, illness, and wellness, acknowledging mind-, body-, spirit-, and relationship-centred care and optimal healing environments. Integrative health care approaches consider the whole person—physical, emotional, mental, and spiritual—with the goal of creating balance for the individual (Canadian Holistic Nurses Association [CHNA], 2020; Snyder & Lindquist, 2018).

A holistic approach to health care is increasingly relevant in Canada owing to how diverse the population is. In addition to Indigenous peoples and cultural practices that were originally present on this land are those who have migrated to Canada from all over the world, bringing with them their own sets of cultural beliefs. A person's cultural beliefs about a chronic condition can impact their continued use of traditional and conventional (i.e., allopathic) healing approaches. While some healing practices can be complementary, Western health care providers must assess for the safety of practices that a patient may wish to use in order to ensure safe care (Snyder & Lindquist, 2018).

Nurses may encounter and use a wide variety of holistic interventions, including relaxation therapy, imagery, music therapy, simple touch, massage, and prayer (Box 36.3). Complementary and integrative health therapies target the whole person as opposed to a specific disease or symptoms (Snyder & Lindquist, 2018), while holistic interventions can augment standard treatments, replace ineffective or debilitating interventions, and promote and maintain health (Blaszko et al., 2020). The CHNA (2020) has developed standards of practice for holistic nursing and promotes holistic nursing practice, education, research, and administration. Furthermore, the Canadian Association of Schools of Nursing (CASN, 2022) released the *National Nursing Education Framework,* a document highlighting nursing competency domains that emphasize the necessary entry-level competencies related to CAM approaches in health care (Table 36.2).

A growing appreciation for the importance of healing the mind, body, and spirit has influenced the development of hospital programs, such as music, art, and recreation therapy. At the University of Alberta Hospital, the Artists on the Wards program connects local artists with individual patients at the bedside, assisting patients in developing their creativity and aiding in physical, spiritual, emotional, and mental healing. The University of Alberta Hospital also offers patients and families both a chapel and a teepee (Figure 36.1). The teepee, built specifically for Indigenous patients and their families, is used for prayer, reflection, and healing ceremonies. A few hospitals have built or are considering the construction of labyrinths on their grounds. Patients and visitors can use these labyrinths for walking, meditation, and prayer (see Table 36.1).

NURSING-ACCESSIBLE APPROACHES

Nurses practise a variety of holistic approaches such as presence, imagery, meditation, support groups, music therapy, journaling, massage, therapeutic listening, and touch with patients who have acute and/or chronic conditions. These techniques are easily learned and provided to patients within independent nursing practice (Blaszko Helming et al., 2020; Snyder & Lindquist, 2018). Presence, through assessment and therapeutic listening, along with a patient's consent, are prerequisites for implementation. There are minimal precautions, however, since some integrative approaches may alter physiological responses, and thus health care provider–prescribed treatments (e.g., medication dosages) may need to be adjusted. All approaches should be chosen according to the patient's diagnosis, functional status, beliefs or religious perspectives, access to health care, and insurance coverage.

These holistic techniques are designed to educate patients about how physical responses to stress and associated symptoms such as muscle tension, gastrointestinal discomfort, pain, and sleep disturbances can be altered through nonpharmaceutical approaches. Key principles include effective communication, collaboration, and client participation in the selection and delivery of the specific approach to facilitate capacity building and positive outcomes.

Relaxation Therapy

People are exposed to stressful situations in everyday life that evoke a **stress response** (see Chapter 30 for further information about stress and adaptation). The biochemical functions of major organ systems are modulated by the mind. Thoughts and feelings influence the production of chemicals (i.e., neurotransmitters, neurohormones, and peptides) that circulate in the body and convey messages to various body systems. Physiologically, the stress response can cause increased heart, respiratory, and metabolic rates; tightened muscles; and a general sense of foreboding, fear, nervousness, irritability, and negative mood. Other physiological responses include elevated blood pressure, dilated pupils, stronger cardiac contractions, and increased blood glucose, serum cholesterol, circulating free fatty acids, and triglycerides. Although these responses effectively prepare a person for a short-term stress response, long-term stress can cause structural damage and chronic illness, such as angina, tension headaches, cardiac arrhythmias, pain, and ulcers (Blaszko Helming et al., 2020). In a meta-analysis of randomized

---

BOX 36.3 | **Focus on Palliative Care**

Palliative care focuses on holistic, human-centred care of the whole person, including spiritual care. Treating the disease may provide relief for the physical symptoms but does not attend to the complexity of the psychological, social, and spiritual concerns (Ferrell et al., 2015; Rathore et al., 2020). End-of-life illnesses can generate a plethora of challenges, including confusion, doubt, and despair, while seeking meaning and purpose in one's life. Spiritual care can be achieved through encouraging meditation, reflective journalling, yoga, breathing practices, prayer, family and friends, support groups, and supportive environments. Interprofessional care is essential for innovative approaches focused on "tending to the spirit" in order to minimize suffering and promote well-being (Rosa et al., 2018). Nurses should invest in learning about holistic and integrative approaches that could promote presence, introspection, joy, and acceptance and reduce fear within a healing environment for their patients and families.

Further research studies on the use of complementary and alternative therapy in palliative care units are warranted.

TABLE 36.2 | **Competency Domains for Integrative Health Care Approaches (CASN National Nursing Education Framework)**

Domain 1: Knowledge	Competency 1.2.2 Integrate foundational knowledge from the health sciences related to illness, pathophysiology, psychopathology, epidemiology, genomics, and pharmacology, across the lifespan (p. 9).
Domain 3: Nursing Practice	Competency 3.2.1 Provide promotive, preventive, curative, and rehabilitative care to individuals across the lifespan, families (biological or chosen), communities, and populations (p. 13).
	Competency 3.2.12 Provide care to individuals with multiple comorbidities and complex health needs, including chronic disease management (p. 15).
Domain 5: Professionalism	Competency 5.2.1 Participate in lifelong learning to remain current in complex and changing health care environments (p. 19).

From Canadian Association of Schools of Nursing (CASN). (2022). *National Nursing Education Framework: Final report.* https://www.casn.ca/wp-content/uploads/2022/12/National-Nursing-Education-Framework_2023_EN_FINAL-002.pdf

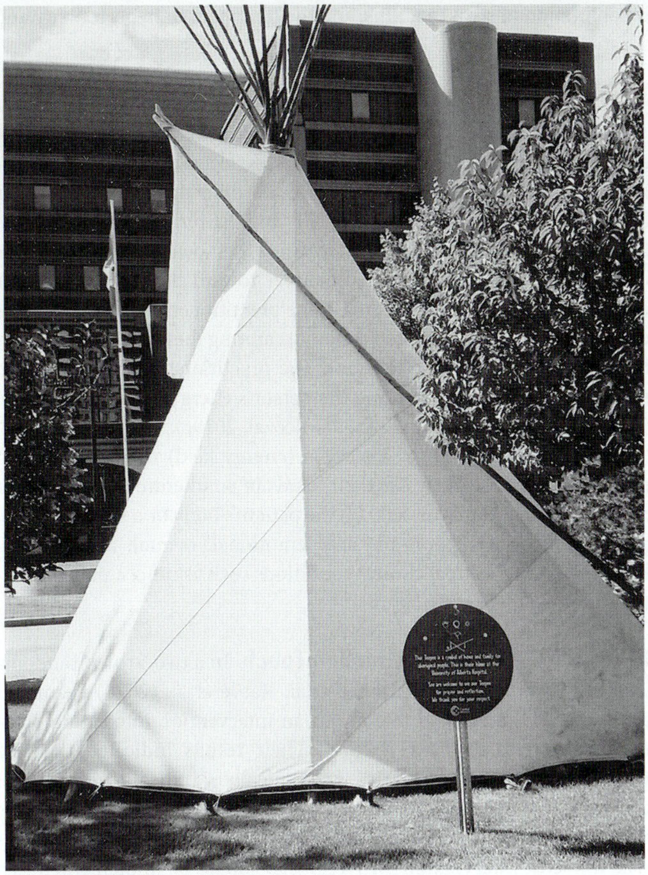

FIGURE 36.1 This teepee outside the university of alberta hospital provides space for prayer and healing. (Courtesy University of Alberta Hospital.)

FIGURE 36.2 Yoga is an ancient mind–body practice that combines physical postures, breathing, and meditation or relaxation. (Courtesy Deborah Gibson, RN, MSN.)

controlled trials, Scott-Sheldon et al. (2022) found that stress management interventions offered an integrative approach to standard treatment in the management of psychological stress associated with chronic heart failure.

Relaxation is a state of overall decreased cognitive, physiological, and behavioural arousal. The process of relaxation reduces neural impulses sent to the brain, thus decreasing the brain's activity. Relaxation is characterized by decreases in heart and respiratory rates, blood pressure, and oxygen consumption and increases in muscle relaxation and alpha-wave brain activity.

Clinical Applications of Relaxation Therapy. Relaxation techniques can lower heart rate and blood pressure, decrease muscle tension, improve perceived well-being, and reduce symptoms of distress in individuals facing a variety of situations, from medical concerns to loss and grief. The type of relaxation intervention should be matched to the individual's functional status, the energy expenditure of the relaxation technique, and the individual's motivation to practise frequently.

Relaxation therapy—either alone or in combination with deep breathing, imagery, yoga (Figure 36.2), biofeedback (also referred to as biofeedback-assisted relaxation [BFAR]), or music—can bring about healthy physiological changes such as reduced pain, decreased anxiety, lower blood pressure and heart rate, and alleviation of tension headaches as well as symptoms of diabetes. Of note is that BFAR has been effective in improving physical symptoms in patients with heart failure (Micozzi, 2019a; Moss, 2020).

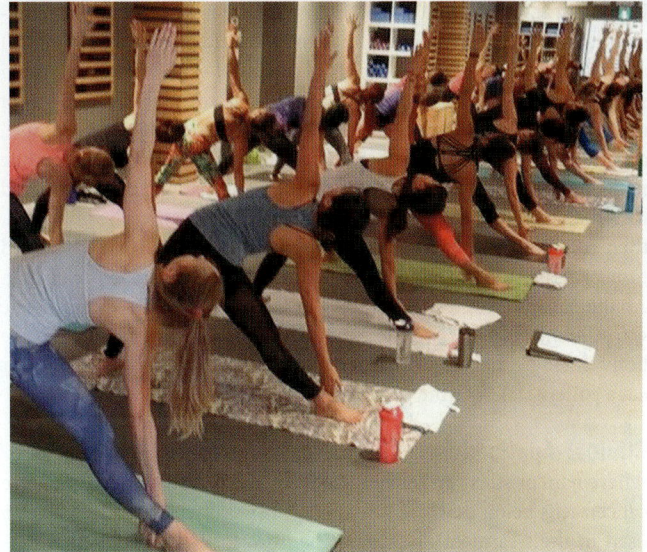

Meditation and Breathing

Meditation is a practice in which a person limits stimulus input to the mind and body by directing their attention and awareness to a single unchanging or repetitive stimulus, a practice that can enhance attention, cognitive ability, and mental health (Fortney, 2018). Meditation encapsulates a range of practices that relax the body and still the mind. The root word of meditation, *meditari*, means "to consider." In 1975, Dr. Herbert Benson's book *The Relaxation Response* drew the attention of Western health care providers to the physical and psychological benefits of relaxation. As Benson (1975) noted, the components of meditation are simple: a quiet space, a comfortable position, a receptive attitude, and a focus of attention. He described meditation as a process that anyone can use to calm down, to cope with stress, and, for those with spiritual inclinations, to feel at one with God or the universe. Most meditation techniques involve slow, relaxed, deep, usually abdominal breathing. Meditation evokes a restful state, lowers oxygen consumption, reduces respiratory and heart rates, and decreases anxiety.

Clinical Applications of Meditation. Meditation has positive effects on mood, cardiac function, blood pressure, muscle tone, and breathing patterns, and assists in managing stress-related illnesses when practised regularly. The effects of mindful meditation are facilitated through the development of nonjudgemental awareness of feelings, thoughts, a sense of gratitude, and balance between the sympathetic and parasympathetic nervous systems (Coeytaux & Mann, 2018). Meditation may be indicated for anxiety, stress, chronic bereavement, chronic fatigue syndrome, chronic pain, substance use, hypertension, low self-esteem, depression, and sleep disorders. Furthermore, meditation in conjunction with yoga has been found to lower diastolic and systolic blood pressure and may be an effective alternative to pharmacotherapy for some patients (Gross et al., 2018; Park & Han, 2017).

Imagery

Imagery or visualization techniques, which are frequently used as part of relaxation training, help a person create mental images in order to stimulate physical, emotional, or spiritual changes, improve perceived well-being, and enhance self-awareness. Imagery can be either self-directed or guided by a practitioner (Blaszko Helming et al., 2020;

Fitzgerald & Langevin, 2018). Active imagery can be an outcome (envisioning a goal) or a process (imagining a strong immune response) and works by eliciting the benefits of a relaxed state of mind by using suggestions and affirmations that enable one to integrate feelings of relaxation into daily living (Fitzgerald & Langevin, 2018). For example, a patient may be directed to begin slow abdominal breathing while focusing on the rhythm of their breath. The patient is then guided to visualize ocean waves washing onto a shore with each inhalation, then receding with each exhalation. Next, the patient is encouraged to notice the smells, sounds, and temperatures they are experiencing. As the session progresses, the patient may be instructed to visualize warmth entering the body during inhalation and tension leaving the body during exhalation. Imagery scenarios can be individualized for each patient or left to the patient to develop.

Clinical Applications of Imagery. Imagery is used to control or relieve pain or stress, to achieve calmness and serenity, and to visualize cancer cells being destroyed by immune system cells. Imagery is also used in the treatment of chronic conditions, such as asthma, hypertension, functional urinary disorders, menstrual and premenstrual syndromes, and rheumatoid arthritis, as well as in the treatment of gastrointestinal disorders, such as irritable bowel syndrome (Blaszko Helming et al., 2020). A recent study measured the impact of cognitive behavioural therapy with relaxation versus imagery on test anxiety in university settings. The results indicated that group treatments along with imagery were an effective method of treating test anxiety (Reiss et al., 2017).

INTEGRATIVE MEDICINE APPROACHES REQUIRING EDUCATION

Integrative medical treatments may be administered by nurses, but only after the completion of a specific course of study. A professional nurse must have a certification, degree, or license beyond their nursing degree to administer most of these holistic approaches, such as biofeedback, therapeutic touch, and massage therapy.

Biofeedback

Biofeedback techniques are frequently used in addition to relaxation interventions to assist individuals with learning how to control specific autonomic nervous system responses. **Biofeedback** is a therapeutic procedure that uses electronic or electromechanical instruments to measure, process, and provide rapid and accurate information about neuromuscular and autonomic nervous system activity. This feedback is provided through pneumography in the form of physical, physiological, auditory, and visual measurements. Biofeedback practitioners help patients to develop awareness of and voluntary control over physiological responses and thereby enable them to change their behaviour or activity to improve health. Moss (2020) has identified that BFAR training is a widely applied protocol and has been found to be effective in clinical studies from 1969 to the present for anxiety disorders, diabetes, and headaches, as well as for other common medical and psychological conditions. In audio biofeedback, patients may hear a sound of their pulse rate or blood pressure increases outside of their therapeutic zone. This approach is helpful because the information is transmitted without the need for visual attention. Biofeedback is considered a complement to Western science–based relaxation programs because it can immediately demonstrate to patients their ability to control some physiological responses.

Clinical Applications of Biofeedback. Biofeedback has numerous applications, including the treatment of migraine headaches,

rehabilitation of stroke victims, and the treatment of hypertonicity and spasticity.

Therapeutic Touch and Healing Touch

Therapeutic touch (TT) is a training-specific therapy that was developed in the 1970s by a nurse, Dr. Dolores Krieger. Although the philosophical and religious assumptions of TT differ from those of other Eastern healing modalities, both TT and Eastern practices involve trained practitioners who attempt to direct their own balanced energies in an intentional and motivated manner toward the patient (Krieger et al., 1979; Micozzi, 2019c). In TT, the practitioner places their hands either on or close to the person's body, scanning the body and diagnosing areas of accumulated tensions. The practitioner then attempts to redirect these energies to bring the person's energy back into balance (Krieger, 1975; Krieger et al., 1979; Micozzi, 2019c).

Healing touch (HT) is a biofield (energy field) therapy in which practitioners consciously use their hands in an intentional way (either by placing their hands directly on the patient's body or a small distance away from it) to support physical, emotional, mental, and spiritual health. It is used to treat clinical conditions such as cancer, pain, arthritis, and movement restriction.

Clinical Applications of Healing Touch. In a two-armed randomized crossover waitlist-controlled trial, Reeve et al. (2020) examined the use of HT, a biofield therapy, as an intervention in treating posttraumatic stress disorder (PTSD). Their results indicated that the reduction in symptom severity was clinically significant for both the test and control groups. While continued research using larger samples is needed, Reeve and colleagues (2020) concluded that HT is a "low-risk, low-cost intervention for PTSD that should be implemented as a treatment option" (p. 897).

Chiropractic Medicine

Chiropractic medicine was developed in the late 1890s and has grown rapidly in popularity, particularly in the treatment of musculoskeletal conditions, becoming the third largest independently practised health profession in the Western world (Micozzi, 2019d; Pratt et al., 2020). Practitioners of chiropractic medicine are regulated in all 10 provinces and are designated to use the title "doctor" after graduating from the extensive 4-year Doctor of Chiropractic Medicine degree program and passing four national board examinations for licensure. These requirements ensure that chiropractors have extensive training in their area of expertise and are able to provide a diagnosis (Malik, 2019). The broad chiropractic model of health care is committed to a holistic approach that focuses on the assessment and treatment of the spine, joints, nervous system, and musculoskeletal system. The basic principles of chiropractic medicine incorporate the idea that human beings have an innate healing potential; harnessing this potential is the goal of this healing profession.

The central tenet of chiropractic treatment is correction of the body's alignment and improvement of function through spinal manipulation (manual or manipulative approaches), postural and exercise education, ergonomic training, nutrition consultation, and ultrasound and laser approaches. This model theorizes that joint dysfunction or subluxation operates as an irritant that lowers the body's ability to resist disease (Micozzi, 2019d). *Manipulation* is defined as a therapeutic movement of the spine or a quick but strong pressure on a joint between two vertebrae of the spine that rotates the joint beyond its normal range of motion. Additional components of chiropractic medicine in patient management and health promotion include dietary modification, nutritional supplementation, physiotherapy, and regular exercise to optimize overall health and body function (Hartvigsen & French, 2020; Micozzi, 2019d).

Clinical Applications of Chiropractic Therapy. In contrast to the musculoskeletal biomedical approach, many chiropractors employ a "vertebral subluxation vitalistic practice approach" (Glucina et al., 2020, p. 1). The basic goals of chiropractic therapy focus on restoring structural and functional imbalances in the body that may result in pain. One of the major structural distortions that chiropractors treat is vertebral subluxation, in which joint mobility is decreased owing to slight changes in the position of the articulating bones. Subluxation exists when joint motion is restricted or malpositioned. Chiropractic interventions treat musculoskeletal abnormalities, headaches, dysmenorrhea, disorders of blood pressure, vertigo, tinnitus, and visual disorders (Micozzi, 2019d).

Traditional Chinese Medicine

Traditional Chinese medicine (TCM), as it has been practised since the mid-twentieth century, blends several healing modalities, including herbal remedies, acupuncture, diet, exercise, and meditation, with scientific theoretical principles. Foods exist in connection with medicines among plant sources (Ergil, 2019). A major concept in TCM is **yin and yang**, which represent opposing, yet complementary, phenomena that exist in a state of dynamic equilibrium. Examples of yin and yang are night and day, hot and cold, and shade and sun. Yin represents shade, cold, and inhibition, whereas yang represents fire, light, and excitement. Yin also represents the inner part of the body, specifically the viscera, liver, heart, spleen, lungs, and kidneys, whereas yang represents the outer part, specifically the bowels, stomach, and bladder. According to TCM, when an imbalance occurs in these paired opposites, disease can emerge (Micozzi & Cassidy, 2019).

Qi (pronounced *chee*) refers to the body's vital energy, which has the qualities of "flow and balance" (Micozzi & Cassidy, 2019, p. 19). In TCM, disease is classified into three major categories: external causes, internal causes, and neither internal nor external causes. Regardless of the cause, when yin and yang are out of balance, the movement of qi is altered. The body has several forms of qi that directly influence its physiological functions and help maintain homeostasis.

Another important aspect of TCM involves the five elements: earth, metal, water, wood, and fire. Various health phenomena are organized according to these elements and interact with each other. In TCM, outward manifestations reflect the internal environment. Two primary areas assessed in TCM are the tongue and various pulses. The colour, shape, and coating of the tongue reflect the general condition of the internal organs. The pulses provide information about the condition and balance of qi, blood, yin and yang, and internal organs (Micozzi & Cassidy, 2019).

Naturopathic Medicine. **Naturopathic medicine** is a popular paradigm for integrative primary health care that combines modern evidence-informed knowledge with traditional and natural forms of medicine (Canadian Association of Naturopathic Doctors [CAND], 2020; Pizzorno et al., 2015). The WHO (2019) considers traditional and complementary medicine and naturopathic medicine to be credible approaches to eliminating health care inequality and achieving sustainable health care as a human right. Naturopathic doctors (NDs) graduate from a 4-year program at a naturopathic school and are required to write national board examinations for licensure. Naturopathic medicine offers a new perspective on safe and effective methods to restore health using a variety of health promotion and preventative treatment approaches. These treatments integrate traditional and natural approaches with modern scientific knowledge and medicines, including botanical (plant) medicine, to stimulate healing and treat underlying causes of diseases (CAND, 2020). Acupuncture, nutritional counselling and supplementation, cupping, and hydrotherapy are also used.

Clinical Applications of Naturopathic Medicine. You and colleagues (2021) evaluated the effectiveness and safety of acupuncture in relieving chronic pain–related depression. The results showed that acupuncture is an effective and safe treatment, and that acupuncture along with drug therapy is a more effective treatment than single-drug therapy.

Acupuncture

Acupuncture is becoming a preferred alternative to treating disease because it does not involve the ingestion of medications (Chen et al., 2018; Michelfelder, 2018). According to TCM, channels of energy run in regular patterns throughout the body and over its surface. These channels, called **meridians**, are like rivers flowing through the body. An obstruction of these meridians functions like a dam, backing up the flow in one part of the body and restricting the flow in other parts, eventually leading to disease. Located along the channels are **acupoints**, or holes through which qi can be influenced by the insertion of needles, a process known as acupuncture.

Acupuncture is the stimulation of certain points (acupoints) on the body through the insertion of special needles to modify the perception of pain, normalize physiological functions, or treat or prevent disease (Figure 36.3). Acupuncture involves inserting thin, firm needles into specific points to "clear blockages, regulate and promote the free flow of a person's qi" (Berger et al., 2021, p. 1; Ergil & Ergil, 2019). According to TCM, acupuncture needles unblock obstructed **energy flow** and reestablish the flow of qi through the meridians, thereby stimulating the skin and underlying muscles, leading to afferent nerve excitement. The sensory information is then transported to the central nervous system, which ultimately affects visceral function. The effects of the acupuncture needles may be enhanced by applying heat or weak electrical currents to the needles. Since acupuncture can produce side effects, Health Canada regulates the needles used to ensure the safety and sterility of the procedure (Health Canada, 2019).

Clinical Applications of Acupuncture. Acupuncture is the primary treatment used by TCM practitioners and naturopathic doctors who have learned TCM theory. Other health care providers must receive additional training for certification in acupuncture.

Acupuncture is used to treat back and neck pain, myofascial pain, headaches, tennis elbow, osteoarthritis, and musculoskeletal sprains.

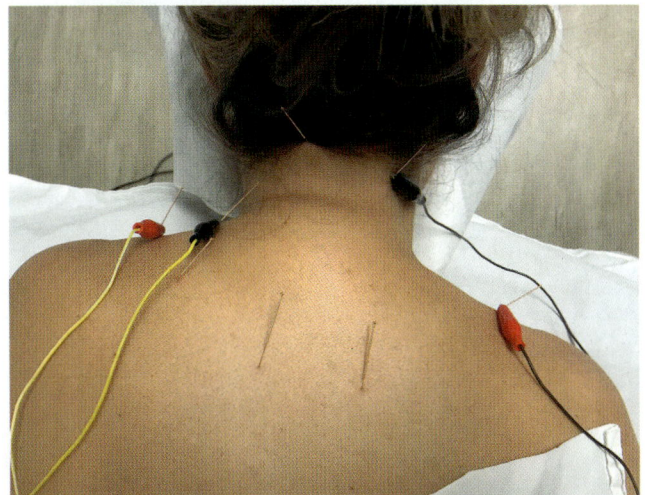

FIGURE 36.3 Acupuncture involves the insertion of special needles to regulate the flow of energy. Electric current connected to the needles enhances energy flow and healing. (Courtesy Deborah Gibson, RN, MSN.)

Other problems that have been successfully treated are sinusitis, gastrointestinal disorders, menstrual symptoms, neurological disorders, chronic pulmonary diseases (including asthma), hypertension, smoking and other addictions, anxiety, and clinical depression (Ergil & Ergil, 2019).

Cupping

Cupping is a therapeutic approach that originated in China and is used in TCM and by naturopathic doctors. Practitioners place a small glass cup on bare skin where the body's acupuncture points are located and then use a vacuum or suction technique to pull skin upward. Cupping stimulates qi and ultimately reduces chronic neck pain, lessens upper or lower back pain, and improves range of motion (Ergil, 2019) (Figure 36.4).

Clinical Applications of Cupping. Patients with chronic low-back pain were enrolled into a randomized control trial to evaluate whether a single cupping session would reduce chronic back pain. Patients were evaluated both immediately and 1 week after the session. The results from the study indicated a significant improvement in pain and sleep and a decrease in disability (Volpato et al., 2019).

Massage Therapy

Practitioners of massage therapy, a regulated health care profession in Canada, offer assessment, treatment, and prevention of pain in soft tissues and joints. Therapists use manipulation and stimulation of pressure receptors to augment physical functioning and promote pain relief (Harris, 2018; Micozzi, 2019e).

Clinical Applications of Massage Therapy. Patient-reported outcomes suggest that massage therapy offers therapeutic benefits for individuals experiencing medical conditions across the lifespan. Da Rocha Rodrigues and colleagues (2021) studied the impacts of touch massage on the experience of patients with chronic pain. Results highlighted that the inclusion of massage in care planning for patients suffering from chronic pain was beneficial and positively impacted patients' physical and psychological dimensions, well-being, and quality of life.

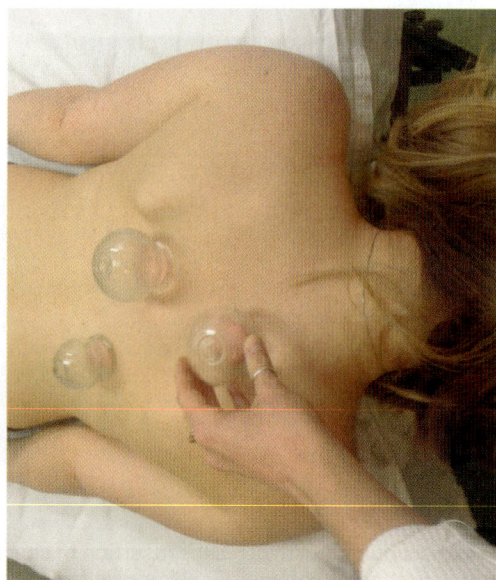

FIGURE 36.4 Cupping is a complementary approach used to stimulate qi and alleviate pain. (Courtesy Dr. Annie Gibson, ND.)

HEALTH PROMOTION: NUTRITION IN DISEASE PREVENTION

A growing body of scientific research has explored the relationship between nutrition and its effects on disease. Substantial evidence from epidemiological studies indicates that nutrition plays a critical role in health and development, and that the relationship between diet, nutrition, diabetes, cancer, and cardiovascular disease is directly linked to lifestyle and nutritional choices (Micozzi, 2019f). Poor nutrition is also a factor in low mood, and improving diet may help to protect the physical and mental health of a population (Firth et al., 2020). The COVID-19 pandemic has greatly disrupted the global food system, resulting in the undernourishment of millions of people, which could in turn impact global illness and disease processes (International Labour Organization et al., 2020).

In nutritional science aimed at prevention of disease, quality, not quantity, of nutritional intake is emphasized, and a shift toward a Mediterranean diet high in nuts, olive oil, fish, fruits, vegetables, yogourt, and whole grains is recommended.

Many practitioners of CAM, including naturopathic and chiropractic physicians, are required to take nutritional science courses as part of their programs of study. Nutritional and dietary interventions are being explored as part of cancer prevention strategies because of speculation that therapeutic or protective nutritional strategies could reduce cancer rates, particularly for aging populations worldwide (Gray et al., 2019). Gray and colleagues found that while early nutrition intervention can improve outcomes, the pathology and current treatment of cancers can result in malnutrition and "that undernutrition or overnutrition can have an impact on either accelerating or reducing cancer risk or tumour burden" (Gray et al., 2020, p. 11). As such, it would be conceivable that nutritional science should be fully integrated into medical school curricula.

A single fruit or vegetable contains many protective compounds and nutrients that cannot be sourced from a supplement alone. These plant compounds, commonly called *phytochemicals* or antioxidants, destroy free radicals, protect cells from damage, and offer defence against disease. The Canadian Cancer Society (2021) addresses key dietary sources of phytochemicals and advises choosing a variety of colourful foods each day. Examples include dark green and orange (carrots, spinach, oranges); red and blue or purple (beets, red peppers, blueberries); and white, brown, and tan (cauliflower, garlic, bananas).

Botanicals/Natural Health Products

An estimated 25 000 plant species are used in medicinal approaches globally. Botanical therapy, the oldest form of medicine, was widespread for thousands of years, but its popularity declined with the development of modern scientific medicine in the early eighteenth century. The philosophy of botanical therapy differs from that of conventional drug therapy in that the former aims to restore balance within the individual by facilitating a person's self-healing ability, while the latter treats a specific disease or symptoms. However, because approximately 80% of the world's population lives in developing countries, herbal medicine remains a prominent form of health care globally. In countries that use predominantly allopathic medicine, an increased interest in herbal medicine has developed from consumer interest in natural foods and growing concern about the complications and limitations of scientific medicine.

Botanicals are extracted from plants, animals, and microorganisms, and the active ingredients are prepared in tinctures or extracts, elixirs, syrups, capsules, pills, tablets, lozenges, powders, ointments, or creams, drops, and suppositories. As with other medications, some herbal substances contain powerful chemicals that can cause harm or adverse effects. As such, botanicals and herbs should be examined for interaction and compatibility with other prescribed or nonprescribed substances. Botanical products are, in general, classified as beneficial, harmful, or neutral, in which case they have no effects on the specific ailment.

Health Canada (2019) establishes standards for the safety and quality of all foods and drugs sold in Canada through the *Food and Drugs Act, 1985*, and associated regulations. Health Canada regulates all over-the-counter **natural health products** (NHPs) and botanicals for safety, effectiveness, and quality, with the most recent amendments due between 2022 and 2024 (Health Canada, 2019, 2022b). NHPs include herbs, probiotics, essential fatty acids, vitamins, minerals, and homeopathic medicines that are used to "diagnose, treat, prevent disease; restore or correct function, maintain or promote health" (Health Canada, 2019). NHP regulations include good manufacturing practices and guidelines for obtaining a product license. Botanicals/NHPs approved for sale under the new regulations are assigned a Drug Identification Number (DIN; DIN-HM for homeopathic medicines) or natural product number (NPN). These numbers certify that the product has passed a review of its formulation, labelling, and instructions for use. Health Canada advises Canadians to use only those health products that carry a DIN, DIN-HM, or NPN on the label.

Clinical Applications of Botanicals/Natural Health Products. Numerous NHPs have been determined to be safe and effective for a variety of conditions (Table 36.3). Milk thistle (*Silybum marianum*), for example, has been used in the treatment of many diseases, particularly liver disorders. Its antioxidant and anti-inflammatory properties are believed to protect and facilitate the regeneration of liver cells, reduce blood cholesterol, and assist in the prevention of liver cancer (Ashie et al., 2021; Valkova et al., 2020). The potential health benefits of fenugreek (*Trigonella foenum-graecum*) include management of blood glucose in type 2 diabetes, reduction of cholesterol, anti-inflammatory and anti-cancer effects, enhancement of milk production in new mothers, and increase of male libido (Gupta et al., 2021). Preparations of St. John's wort with compound derivatives of hyperforin have been found to have antidepressant effects; however, Nicolussi and colleagues (2019) caution that the amount of hyperforin should be clearly identified in medicinal products owing to potential drug interactions.

Limitations of Botanicals/Natural Health Products. Although botanicals are known to provide beneficial effects for a variety of conditions, concerns may exist. Concentrations of active ingredients can vary, and contamination may occur with prescription medication and other herbs or chemicals, including pesticides and heavy metals. Some

TABLE 36.3	Botanicals/Natural Health Products Commonly Used and Considered Safe			
Common Name	**Effects**	**Indications***	**Warnings†**	**Other**
Black cohosh	Estrogen-like effects	Menopausal hot flashes Premenstrual syndrome	Significant estrogenic activity has not been found, but not recommended if patient has a history of breast cancer	Is promising for the relief of moderate hot flashes related to menopause
Chamomile (German or Hungarian)	Topically: Anti-inflammatory Orally: Anti-inflammatory, antiestrogenic effects	Chemotherapy-induced mucositis Dyspepsia Colic Inflammatory conditions Insomnia Menstrual disorders	Contraindicated if allergies to the daisy family May potentiate the effect of anticoagulants and CNS depressants	Avoid confusion with Roman chamomile
Echinacea	Topically: Anaesthetic and anti-inflammatory, wound healing Orally: Stimulates the immune system	Upper respiratory infections Colds Urinary tract infections	Contraindicated in patients receiving cancer treatments and for people with autoimmune diseases, multiple sclerosis, tuberculosis, diabetes, asthma, leukemia, HIV/AIDS, lupus, or allergies to the daisy family Not to be used longer than 8 weeks	Chemical constituents differ among roots, leaves, and flowers
Evening primrose oil	Anti-inflammatory constituents omega-6 and gamma-linoleic fatty acids	Mastalgia Atopic dermatitis Premenstrual syndrome (PMS) Menopausal hot flashes Rheumatoid arthritis	Contraindicated in patients with seizure disorders Large doses may cause loose stools and abdominal pain	Studies have shown positive effects on relieving mastalgia (cyclic breast pain)
Fenugreek (*Trigonella foenum-graecum*)	Management of blood glucose in type 2 diabetics, cholesterol-lowering effect, effect on growth hormone leading to modulation of metabolic syndrome, anti-inflammatory and anticancer effects, enhancement of milk production in new mothers, increase of male libido		Avoid use during pregnancy until embryonic/fetal development has reached a safe stage	Potentially allergenic to persons with known peanut allergy

Continued

TABLE 36.3	Botanicals/Natural Health Products Commonly Used and Considered Safe—cont'd			
Common Name	**Effects**	**Indications***	**Warnings†**	**Other**
Fish oil	Omega-3 essential fatty acids are believed to have anti-inflammatory properties	Rheumatoid arthritis Prevention of cardiovascular disease and cancer	Possible increase of INR with warfarin (Coumadin) Avoid doses greater than 3 g/day to avoid inhibiting blood coagulation Quality of product should be monitored for cancer-causing pollutants, such as dioxins and PCBs	Effective in reducing triglyceride levels The Mediterranean diet, which is rich in fish, has been associated with lower rates of cancers. May improve overall cognitive functioning and behaviour in children with attention deficit–hyperactivity disorder (ADHD).
Garlic	Major constituent allicin reduces oxidative stress and stimulates the immune system Inhibits platelet aggregation	Hypertension Cold and flu prevention Athlete's foot (topically)	May prolong bleeding time Possible interactions with anticoagulants Topical application may cause skin irritation	Supplementation not recommended during pregnancy owing to its effect on bleeding time
Ginger	Antiemetic Antibiotic	Motion/morning sickness Nausea and vomiting Vertigo	May enhance the effects of Coumadin, aspirin, and NSAIDs	Recent studies indicate no fetal harm when used for morning sickness
Ginkgo biloba	Contains flavonoids and organic acids that have anti-inflammatory/antioxidant effects Inhibits platelet-activating factor	Dementia Respiratory and circulatory dysfunctions Poor memory	Ingestion may increase the risk of serious bleeding, especially in patients taking anticoagulants or NSAIDs Can cause contact dermatitis High doses can cause seizures	Potential promise in enhancing cognitive functions in people with dementia and improving peripheral arterial disease
Ginseng (root of *Panax* species)	Restoration of homeostasis	Adaptation to changing circumstances and environment		Adaptation restores energy and sleep
Glucosamine (Hydrochloride/sulphate)	Naturally occurring amino sugar that stimulates the synthesis of proteins responsible for cartilage growth and maintenance	Joint pain Osteoarthritis	May increase the anticoagulant effects of Coumadin	Mounting evidence for pain reduction and disease-modifying effects in osteoarthritis
Liquorice (*Glycyrrhiza glabra*)	Anti-inflammatory, antibacterial, antifungal, antidiabetic, antiviral, antiulcer, antioxidant	Antiviral effect against HIV, herpes simplex virus, hepatitis B, and hepatitis C		
Milk thistle	Silymarin, the active constituent, is a potent inhibitor of tumour necrosis factor (TNF), which reduces toxicity to the liver and reduces inflammation	Chronic hepatitis Cirrhosis, gastrointestinal upset	Reports on significant decrease in fasting blood glucose in diabetics using conventional diabetic therapy	Do not confuse with blessed thistle. Mixed evidence on effectiveness in managing hepatitis or cirrhosis
Saw palmetto	Androgen receptor blocker Anti-inflammatory	Benign prostatic hyperplasia (BPH) Urinary problems	Increased risk of bleeding if on anticoagulants	Evidence suggests mild improvement of urinary problems
St. John's wort	Inhibits reuptake of serotonin, dopamine, and norepinephrine neurotransmitters Wound healing (topical)	Depression Sedative Menopausal symptoms	Not appropriate for severe depression May enhance the effects of SSRIs and other antidepressants Significant interactions with many medications (digoxin, warfarin, antiretrovirals, cyclosporine, oral contraceptive therapy) Photosensitivity with chronic use	Studies support its use in treating mild to moderate depression
Valerian	Valepotriate constituents have sedative–hypnotic and smooth muscle effects	Muscle spasms Sleep disorders Restlessness	May cause headaches or gastrointestinal disturbances Avoid using concurrently with other sedatives	Studies support its use in treating insomnia and improving sleep quality

CNS, Central nervous system; *INR*, international normalized ratio; *NSAIDs*, nonsteroidal anti-inflammatory drugs; *PCBs*, polychlorinated biphenyls; *SSRIs*, selective serotonin reuptake inhibitors.

*Unless otherwise noted, these natural health products have not shown sufficient evidence to rate their effectiveness for all stated indications.

†Data do not support the use of these herbs in infants or children or during pregnancy or lactation.

Adapted from Sharma, A., Keservani, R., & Gautam, S. P. (Eds.). (2021). *Herbal product development: Formulation and applications.* Apple Academic Press Inc.

herbs have been found to contain toxic products associated with cancer. Comfrey, for example, has been used for its wound-healing properties; however, some species of comfrey contain highly carcinogenic pyrrolizidine alkaloids and have caused liver cancer in small animals. Other unsafe botanicals (NHPs) are listed in Table 36.4.

Not all companies follow strict quality-control and manufacturing guidelines that set standards for acceptable levels of pesticides, residual solvents, bacterial, and heavy metals. For this reason, botanicals/NHPs should only be purchased from reputable manufacturers (Box 36.4). In addition, labels on herbal products should include the scientific name of the botanical, the name and address of the manufacturer, the batch or lot number, the date of manufacture, the expiration date, and the DIN-HM or NPN identifying safety and effectiveness.

NURSING ROLE IN INTERPROFESSIONAL COLLABORATION WITH COMPLEMENTARY AND ALTERNATIVE MEDICINE

The integrative medicine approach is consistent with the nursing holistic approach. Indeed, many nurses already practise the use of simple touch, including a variety of modalities designed to promote the health and well-being of the patient. The use of these modalities assumes that nurses are working within their scope of practice, as defined by the provincial or territorial nursing regulatory body, the Canadian Nurses Association (CNA) (2015), and the CHNA (2020). As health care providers, nurses who provide integrative health care approaches must possess the knowledge and skill necessary to provide safe and ethical

TABLE 36.4	Unsafe Botanicals/Natural Health Products	
Common Name	**Claimed Benefits**	**Risks**
Aconite (*Aconitum*, blue monkshood root)	Pain and inflammation (joint pain, gout, etc.)	Nausea, vomiting, weakness, paralysis Contains alkaloids toxic to the heart, lungs, and CNS
Coltsfoot (British tobacco, coughwort)	Cough Bronchitis Asthma Sore throat	Liver damage Contains large number of hepatotoxic pyrrolizidine alkaloids that are carcinogenic
Comfrey (blackwort, slippery root)	Relieves cough, heavy menstrual periods, stomach problems, chest pain May be used to treat cancer	Liver damage Contains large number of toxic hepatotoxic pyrrolizidine alkaloids that can cause cancer
Country mallow (heartleaf, white mallow)	Asthma Colds and nasal congestion	Contains ephedrine, similar to the stimulant ephedra, which can cause heart attack and seizure (unauthorized for sale as a natural health product by Health Canada)
Germander (*Teucrium chamaedrys, Teucrium viscidum*)	Weight loss Alleviates fever, arthritis, gout, stomach problems	Liver damage, hepatitis, and even death
Greater celandine (celandine, *Chelidonii herba*)	Dyspepsia, IBS, gastric cancer	Liver damage
Green tea extract powder (*Camellia sinensis*)	Weight loss	Dizziness, ringing in ears, reduced absorption of iron; exacerbates anemia and glaucoma; elevates blood pressure and heart rate; liver damage
Ephedra (ma huang, herbal Ecstasy)	Weight loss Athletic performance enhancer	Unsafe for people with hypertension, diabetes, or thyroid disease because of stimulant effects Many interactions with herbs and drugs Health Canada (2019) advises against use of any product containing this substance
Kava (Ava pepper, kava kava)	Anxiety and stress; improves insomnia	Hepatotoxicity and liver failure May exacerbate Parkinson's disease and depression Issues related to contaminants in product Health Canada (2019) advises against use
Lobelia (asthma weed, Indian tobacco)	Improves respiratory problems such as asthma, bronchitis; aids smoking cessation	Nausea, vomiting, diarrhea CNS overstimulation may cause tremors, tachycardia, confusion, seizures, coma, and even death
Methylsynephrine (Oxilofrine, *p*-hydroxyephedrine)	Weight loss Increased energy and athletic performance	Causes heart rate and heart rhythm abnormalities, cardiac arrest Risky when taken with other stimulants
Usnic acid (Beard moss)	Weight loss Pain relief	Liver damage
Yohimbe (Johimbi)	Used to treat low libido or impotence, depression, and obesity	Hypertension, tachycardia, headache, seizures, liver and kidney problems, panic attacks, cardiac conduction disorders

CNS, Central nervous system; *IBS*, Irritable bowel syndrome.
Adapted from Consumer Reports. (2019, October 30). *15 supplement ingredients to always avoid.* https://www.consumerreports.org/vitamins-supplements/15-supplement-ingredients-to-always-avoid/

BOX 36.4 FOCUS ON PRIMARY HEALTH CARE

Patient Education: Purchasing Botanicals/NHPs

When purchasing botanicals, individuals may be unaware of the lack of regulation around the manufacture and sale of such products. It is difficult to make informed decisions owing to the vast variety of available products. Botanicals and natural health products (NHPs) should be used only on the advice of a health care provider to prevent medication contraindications, and they should be purchased only from reputable manufacturers to ensure safety and appropriate use..

Patients can be assisted in making informed choices about botanicals/NHPs by offering them the following guidelines:

- Avoid hype: Be wary of supplements that offer a "cure" or a "secret formula."
- All product labels should indicate the following:
  - The scientific name of the botanical; the quantity and concentration; the expiration date and manufacturer's name; the purpose and dosage form; the route of administration; warnings of possible adverse reactions; the names of other key ingredients; and the natural product number (NPN) or Drug Identification Number (DIN-HM) indicating that the formulation has been reviewed by Health Canada
- Ensure that the product is supported by published research. Avoid "multi-ingredient" formulations when possible; otherwise, determining potential reactions with other medicines will be difficult. Consumers often pay more for secondary products that may not be present at established therapeutic levels.
- Look for well-educated service staff who can answer consumers' questions.
- Be cautious about "mega" doses of anything: even excess ingestion of certain vitamins can be toxic.
- Be skeptical about cheap herbal remedies. Consumers must pay for the manufacturer's investments in ensuring product quality and purity. Very inexpensive herbal products are often of inferior quality.

NHPs used for weight loss, body building, sleep problems, and diabetes have become a worldwide problem because of their use with prescription and nonprescription drugs. Purchasing unauthorized NHPs through the Internet may increase patients' risks for unsafe products.

care through continued education and certification courses offered by universities, colleges, and professional associations or through study with expert practitioners. Nurses should understand provincial and territorial legislation regarding complementary approaches, practise within the scope of these laws, and be able to make appropriate recommendations about integrative health care to allopathic primary care providers.

Nursing resources on nursing scope of practice in relation to integrative health care have been developed and are available through a variety of professional associations, including the Canadian Holistic Nurses Association, provincial and territorial nursing regulatory bodies such as the British Columbia College of Nurses and Midwives (2021), the Registered Nurses' Association of Ontario (RNAO), and the CNA (2015). These resources assist nurses in understanding their professional responsibilities, the ethics related to implementation and advisement of integrative health care, and the implications for nurses.

It is important for nurses to remain current on Best Practice Guidelines as well as current research in the field of integrative health care in order to provide accurate information to patients and other health care providers. For example, the Canadian Interdisciplinary Network of Complementary Medicine Researchers has been created to foster excellence in integrative medicine research.

Nurses are well placed to advise patients about the appropriate times to use conventional and integrative approaches. Since patients often

trust nurses to provide sound advice on the use of different approaches, nurses should maintain knowledge of the potential benefits and risks associated with different integrative health care approaches. Furthermore, nurses are in the unique position of being able to become familiar with patients' religious and cultural viewpoints and to determine integrative approaches that would be best suited to individuals' beliefs.

Patients should be reminded to inform their health care providers about the medications and approaches they receive. Complete information about the use of botanicals and NHPs should be added to a patient's medical record to prevent potential interactions between prescribed medications and botanical medicines. See Chapter 19 for further information about interprofessional collaboration.

KEY CONCEPTS

- An increasing number of Canadians are using integrative health care and natural health products to treat illness and promote health.
- Integrative health care approaches are used in conjunction with allopathic medicine, whereas alternative therapy is generally used without the addition of conventional health care methods.
- Integrative medicine uses a multidisciplinary (both allopathic and complementary) treatment approach.
- Stress is an adaptive response that allows individuals to react to demanding situations.
- Chronic stress may be maladaptive, thereby leading to chronic muscle tension and changes in mood and immunity.
- Relaxation is a beneficial state characterized by improved mood, relaxed muscle tension, reduced blood pressure, and slower heart and respiratory rates.
- To promote effectiveness and beneficial outcomes, complementary and alternative medicine approaches require collaboration and active participation with the patient.
- Integrative health care approaches should be chosen according to the patient's functional status, cultural beliefs or religious perspectives, access to health care, and insurance coverage.
- Some integrative approaches may alter physiological responses, thereby requiring changes in routine prescription medication doses.
- Imagery, when used as part of relaxation techniques, is usually visual but can also involve the auditory, gustatory, and olfactory senses.
- Many integrative health approaches are considered effective based on a growing volume of scientific research published in professional nursing and medical journals and the positive outcomes observed in patients who have used these approaches.
- Current research supports various nutritional practices as a form of health promotion and disease prevention.
- Not all natural health products are safe.

CRITICAL THINKING EXERCISES

Margaret is a 76-year-old patient (preferred pronouns: she/her) who has been diagnosed with a slow-growing renal tumour. Surgery is scheduled to take place in 2 weeks, and Margaret is afraid of both the procedure and the outcome. Is it cancer? Will the surgery result in a disability?

1. What nursing-specific integrative health care interventions can you offer Margaret to reduce her anxiety and prepare her for the surgery?
2. After surgery, Margaret becomes depressed. What integrative health care approaches may be appropriate to assist Margaret with her depression?

🌐 *Answers to Critical Thinking Exercises appear on the Evolve website.*

REVIEW QUESTIONS

Questions 1 to 10 relate to the case study at the beginning of the chapter.

1. Despite the success of allopathic medicine (modern Western medicine), many patients find that integrative health care approaches provide relief for a variety of conditions. For which of the following conditions is Mrs. Lorimer (preferred pronouns: she/her) seeking assistance?
   a. Heart disease and pancreatitis
   b. Cancer
   c. Chronic neck and back pain
   d. Anxiety

2. Many integrative health approaches, such as acupuncture and therapeutic dry-needling, have diagnostic and therapeutic methods specific to their field. Which approach can be provided to the patient as part of independent nursing practice?
   a. Massage therapy
   b. Traditional Chinese medicine
   c. Shamanism
   d. Imagery

3. When asked about her reason for requesting an integrative health approach, which of the following statements best describes the patient's reason for attending the clinic?
   a. "Everyone uses complementary and alternative medicine therapy to prevent illness or maintain wellness."
   b. "A few of my colleagues found these approaches helpful."
   c. "Most of my friends and family members have had these complementary and alternative approaches covered through health care coverage."
   d. "Most of my friends are from lower socioeconomic backgrounds."

4. As the clinic nurse, which of the following do you know is representative of holistic nursing care?
   a. Mind, body, and spirit
   b. Disease, spirit, and family
   c. Desires and emotions
   d. Muscles, nerves, and spine disorders

5. After the clinic nurse has completed the initial assessment of the patient, whose permission is required before implementing complementary and alternative medicine therapy?
   a. The physician
   b. The patient
   c. The family
   d. No permission is required.

6. According to the principles of integrative medicine approaches, which of the following statements best describes the patient?
   a. Actively involved in the treatment
   b. A person who adheres to what is being taught
   c. Submissive to the practitioner
   d. Less competent in her own care

7. The patient asks the health care provider about using St. John's wort for her symptoms. Which of the following describes the most effective use of St. John's wort?
   a. Antioxidant
   b. Anti-inflammatory
   c. Mild antidepressant
   d. Vasodilator

8. Meditation may augment the effects of which of the following medications?
   a. Antidepressants
   b. Insulin and vitamins
   c. Prednisone
   d. Cough syrups and aspirin

9. After discussing potential treatment options, the patient decides to try acupuncture. Acupuncture techniques are frequently used to:
   a. Bring the patient's body back into balance through the transfer of energy
   b. Stimulate and activate the body's self-healing abilities
   c. Treat diseases of the spine and joints
   d. Create a state of relaxation through reduction of neural impulses sent to the brain

10. The patient and nurse also discuss the option of therapeutic touch to assist with feelings of anxiety. Therapeutic touch is a specific therapy that was developed by which profession?
    a. Medicine
    b. Physiotherapy
    c. Occupational therapy
    d. Nursing

Answers: 1. d; **2.** d; **3.** c; **4.** a; **5.** d; **6.** a; **7.** c; **8.** a; **9.** b; **10.** d.

Rationales for the Review Questions appear on the Evolve website.

RECOMMENDED WEBSITES

Canadian College of Naturopathic Medicine (CCNM): https://ccnm.edu.
This website provides detailed information about the 4-year full-time program offered by CCNM, a professional college of naturopathic medicine. The site includes a resource centre with links to other websites.

Canadian Holistic Nurses Association (CHNA): https://www.chna.ca.
The CHNA supports the practice of holistic nursing across Canada through professional development, policy, and education and believes that complementary and integrative health care should be incorporated into all aspects of nursing and patient care within the Canadian health care system.

Canadian Interdisciplinary Network of Complementary Medicine Researchers (INCAM): https://iscmr.org/content.aspx?page_id=22&club_id=869917&module_id=372144.
This network facilitates research, knowledge, and education about CAM in Canada. Links to other associated networks and institutions are provided.

Canadian Nursing Association: https://www.cna-aiic.ca.
This website provides resources on professional practice and professional development.

Chinese Medicine and Acupuncture Association of Canada: https://www.cmaac.ca.
This organization aims to raise the profile and reputation of traditional Chinese medicine and acupuncture. The site includes the organization's history and a Canada-wide members' index.

College of Chiropractors of British Columbia: https://www.chirobc.com.
This website provides information from the governing body that regulates chiropractors in British Columbia.

College of Chiropractors of Ontario: https://cco.on.ca.
This website provides information from the governing body that regulates chiropractors in Ontario.

College of Nurses of Ontario: Ask Practice—Complementary Therapies: http://www.cno.org/Global/docs/prac/41021_CompTherapies.pdf.
This webpage presents several scenarios addressing questions that nurses have about providing complementary therapies as well as links to related practice standards and resources.

ConsumerLab.com: https://www.consumerlab.com.

The quality and quantity of ingredients in various brands of NHPs are independently tested by this organization. General use is free, but a small yearly fee is required to access the entire database.

M.D. Anderson Cancer Center — Complementary, Alternative, and Integrative Medicine: https://www.mdanderson.org/treatment-options/complementary-and-integrative-medicine.html.

The website of this cancer research and treatment centre (located in Texas, USA) provides information for both health care providers and the public about complementary medicine and how it can be integrated with allopathic medicine.

National Center for Complementary and Integrative Health: https://www.nccih.nih.gov.

The website of this research centre (located in Bethesda, Maryland, USA) provides information on various natural health products, research, training and grant opportunities, and ongoing clinical trials related to complementary and integrative health.

Natural Health Products: https://www.canada.ca/en/health-canada/services/drugs-health-products/natural-non-prescription.html.

This website explains Health Canada's role in regulating the sale of natural health products (NHPs) in Canada. It includes information on regulatory practices, definitions related to NHPs, and an index of various health-related issues.

Public Health Agency of Canada (PHAC): https://www.canada.ca/en/public-health.html.

PHAC focuses on efforts to prevent chronic diseases, injuries, and public health emergencies. The agency works closely with provinces and territories to keep Canadians healthy and reduce pressure on the health care system.

REFERENCES

A full reference list is available on the website for this book at https://evolve.elsevier.com/Canada/Potter/fundamentals/

37

Activity and Exercise

*Canadian content written by Jill Vihos, RN, MN, PhD,
with original chapter contributions by Jessica L. Bower, DNP, MSN, RN*

OBJECTIVES

Mastery of content in this chapter will enable you to:

- Define the key terms listed.
- Describe the role of the musculoskeletal and nervous systems in the regulation of activity and exercise.
- Describe physiological and pathological influences on body alignment and joint mobility.
- Describe how to maintain and use proper body mechanics.
- Describe the evidence that supports regular activity and exercise in patient care.
- Describe the benefits of implementing an exercise program for the purpose of health promotion.
- Describe the benefits of implementing exercise and activity during the acute, restorative, and continuing care of patients.
- Describe important factors to consider when planning an exercise program for patients across the lifespan and for those with specific chronic illnesses.
- Describe how to assess patients for activity tolerance.
- Identify the importance of intersectoral policies to promote physical activity by addressing the social determinants of health.
- Describe how to assess patients for complications related to immobility.
- Formulate nursing diagnoses for patients who experience impaired mobility and activity intolerance.
- Develop a nursing care plan for a patient with impaired mobility and activity intolerance.
- Describe the interventions for maintaining activity tolerance and mobility during the acute, restorative, and continuing care of patients.
- Evaluate the nursing care plan for maintaining activity and exercise for patients across the lifespan and with specific chronic illnesses.
- Describe how to use proper body mechanics and ergonomics to prevent musculoskeletal injuries.
- Explain the importance of no-lift policies for patients and health care providers.
- Describe equipment needed for safe patient handling and movement.
- Explain the impact of national patient safety resources, initiatives, and regulations in relation to patient handling and movement.

KEY TERMS

Activities of daily living (ADLs)
Activity tolerance
Antagonistic muscles
Antigravity muscles
Cartilage
Cartilaginous joint
Centre of gravity
Ergonomics
Exercise
Fibrous joint

Friction
Gait
Isometric contraction
Isotonic contraction
Joint
Ligaments
Mobility
Muscle tone
Pathological fractures
Posture

Proprioception
Range of motion (ROM)
Synarthrotic joint
Synchondrodial joint
Syndesmodial joint
Synergistic muscles
Synovial joint
Tendons

🌐 WEBSITE

http://evolve.elsevier.com/Canada/Potter/fundamentals/

CASE STUDY

Sandra (preferred pronouns: she/her) has been nursing for over 40 years. For more than 30 years of that time, prior to becoming a university nurse educator, she worked as a hospital staff nurse providing direct care to patients. Sandra worked primarily on medical and critical care units where patients required significant assistance with their activities of daily living. As is the case with most nurses, the wear and tear of lifting, turning, and transferring patients led to significant strain on her body, primarily on her back, knees, and feet.

When Sandra started her role as a nurse educator, her physical activity related to nursing consisted of demonstrating fundamental skills in the laboratory setting and providing assistance to students with their practice. During her fifth year of teaching that course, Sandra recognized that it was becoming increasingly difficult to position and transfer volunteer "patients." She began to question her health in response to becoming extremely tired and "sore" at the end of each day.

Upon reflection, Sandra realized that two factors were involved. The first was normal changes resulting from aging: the decrease in strength and endurance that occurs after age 40 among women. The second factor was her relatively sedentary lifestyle since leaving bedside nursing. After consultation with her primary health care provider, Sandra was assessed as experiencing functional decline from disuse. Recognizing from her nursing experience that she is at risk of losing independence with aging if she does not stay fit, Sandra determined action was necessary to address her current level of fitness.

In consultation with her health care provider, an exercise plan was established. Sandra's plan included using her gym membership (neglected for months and never attended routinely) at least three times per week for weight-bearing exercises, walking for no less than 30 minutes every day, and using stairs rather than the elevator at work.

To evaluate her plan for effectiveness, Sandra's anticipated outcomes include accomplishing teaching activities and daily routines effortlessly, with minimal backaches and with energy to spare.

Although Sandra was shocked to recognize that aging had affected her personal and professional life, the ingrained nursing habits of reflection and of establishing goals helped her feel confident that she could manage these changes.

Think about this case study as you read this chapter. There are review questions at the end of the chapter that relate to the case study.

Regular physical activity and exercise contribute to patients' physical and emotional well-being (Dames et al., 2021). This is a principle that you, as a nurse, should apply in the care of patients in all settings. *Functional decline* is the loss of a person's ability to perform **activities of daily living (ADLs)**, which are fundamental skills required to independently care for oneself, including mobility, eating, and bathing. The loss of ability to perform self-care may result not only from illness but also from deconditioning associated with inactivity, the negative effects of which can be seen over short periods of time. Deconditioning involves physiological changes following a period of inactivity, bed rest, or sedentary lifestyle. It is a risk for hospitalized patients who spend most of their time in bed, even when they can walk. As a result, nurses play an important role in helping to increase the overall activity of inpatients to minimize the risk of deconditioning.

A program of regular physical activity and exercise has the potential to enhance all dimensions of a patient's health (Box 37.1). This chapter provides you with knowledge of exercise and activity as it relates to health promotion, the acute phase of illness, and the restorative and continuing care of patients. Applying knowledge about exercise and activity will allow you to plan nursing strategies for individualized exercise and activity programs. Knowing the function of the musculoskeletal system in maintaining posture, balance, body mechanics, and movement, and implementing evidence-informed knowledge about safe patient handling are essential in protecting the safety of both the patient and the nurse (see Chapter 46).

SCIENTIFIC KNOWLEDGE BASE

Understanding the physiology and regulation of body mechanics, exercise, and activity helps nurses to provide individualized patient care.

Overview of Exercise and Activity

The coordinated efforts of the musculoskeletal and nervous systems maintain balance, posture, and body alignment during lifting, bending, moving, and performing ADLs. Proper balance, posture, and body alignment reduce the risk of injury to the musculoskeletal system, facilitate body movements, support physical mobility, and reduce muscle strain and excessive use of muscle energy (see Chapter 46).

Body Alignment. *Body alignment* refers to the relationship of one body part to another body part along a horizontal or vertical line.

BOX 37.1   Effects of Exercise

Cardiovascular System
Increased cardiac output
Improved myocardial contraction, thereby strengthening cardiac muscle
Decreased resting heart rate
Improved venous return

Pulmonary System
Increased respiratory rate and depth followed by a quicker return to resting state
Improved alveolar ventilation
Decreased work of breathing
Improved diaphragmatic excursion

Metabolic System
Increased basal metabolic rate
Increased use of glucose and fatty acids
Increased triglyceride breakdown
Increased gastric motility
Increased production of body heat

Musculoskeletal System
Improved muscle tone
Increased joint mobility
Improved muscle tolerance to physical exercise
Possible increase in muscle mass
Reduced bone loss

Activity Tolerance
Improved tolerance
Decreased fatigue

Psychosocial Factors
Improved tolerance to stress
Reports of "feeling better"
Reports of decrease in illness (e.g., colds, influenza)

Based on Power-Kean, K., Zettel, S., & El-Hussein, M. (2022). *Huether and McCance's understanding pathophysiology* (2nd Canadian ed.). Elsevier.

Correct alignment involves positioning in such a way that no excessive strain is placed on a person's joints, tendons, ligaments, or muscles, thereby maintaining adequate muscle tone and contributing to balance (see Chapter 46). **Muscle tone** is the internal state of muscle tension within an individual muscle or muscle groups.

Body Balance. Body balance is achieved when a **centre of gravity**—or point where weight is equally dispersed to maintain stability—is balanced over a stable base of support and is enhanced using proper posture (Patton, 2019). You can use balance to maintain proper body alignment and posture by taking two simple actions: (1) widening the base of support by separating your feet to a comfortable distance, and (2) bringing the centre of gravity closer to the base of support; do this by bending your knees and flexing your hips until you are squatting yet maintaining proper back alignment by keeping your trunk erect. For example, the nurse raises the height of a hospital bed when performing a procedure such as changing a dressing to prevent bending too far at the waist and shifting the base of support.

Friction. **Friction** is a force that occurs in a direction to oppose movement. It increases a patient's risk for skin and tissue damage and potential pressure injuries (see Chapter 47). Friction is reduced by following some basic principles:

- Avoid lifting or moving patients manually. Using a mechanical lift prevents friction.
- In situations when you must assist a patient to move manually, use a friction-reducing device such as a slider sheet, slide board, or transfer board to reduce friction.
- When possible, use some of the patient's strength and mobility to assist with transferring or moving the patient in bed. For instance, if patients can bend their knees as you assist them in moving up in bed, friction is decreased. Explain the procedure and tell the patient when to move (see Chapter 47).
- The greater the surface area of the object to be moved, the greater the friction. If a patient is unable to assist in moving up in bed, placing the patient's arms across their chest decreases surface area and reduces friction.

Exercise and Activity. **Exercise** is physical activity for the purpose of conditioning the body, improving health, and maintaining fitness, or it may be used as a therapeutic measure. When a person exercises, physiological changes occur in body systems (see Box 37.1). The exercise program designed for a patient depends on that individual's **activity tolerance**, or the kind and amount of exercise or activity that the individual is able to perform. Physiological, emotional, and developmental factors influence the patient's activity tolerance.

An active lifestyle is important for promoting and maintaining health and is also an essential treatment modality for chronic illnesses (Bullard et al., 2019). Regular physical activity and exercise enhance functioning of all body systems, including cardiopulmonary functioning (endurance), musculoskeletal fitness (strength, flexibility, and bone integrity), weight control and maintenance (body image), and psychological well-being (Dames et al., 2021).

The best program of physical activity includes a combination of exercises that produce different physiological and psychological benefits. Isotonic, isometric, and resistive isometric are three categories of exercise classified according to the type of muscle contraction involved. Isotonic exercises cause muscle contraction and changes in muscle length (**isotonic contraction**). Walking, swimming, dance aerobics, jogging, bicycling, and moving arms and legs with light resistance are examples of isotonic exercises. Isotonic exercises enhance circulatory and respiratory functioning; increase muscle mass, tone, and strength;

and promote osteoblastic activity (activity by bone-forming cells) to combat osteoporosis.

Isometric exercises involve tightening or tensing muscles without moving body parts (**isometric contraction**) (see Chapter 46). Isometric exercises are especially helpful to people who are recovering from injuries or procedures that limit range of motion. An example is quadriceps set exercises—pressing the knee toward the bed and holding—an exercise commonly done after knee surgery. Isometric exercises are ideal for patients who are unable to tolerate increased activity. A patient who is immobilized in bed can perform isometric exercises. Benefits of isometric exercises include minimized potential for muscle wasting by increasing muscle mass, tone, and strength, thus decreasing the potential for muscle wasting; increased circulation to the involved body part; and increased osteoblastic activity.

Resistive isometric exercises are those in which the individual contracts the muscle while pushing against a stationary object or resisting the movement of an object. A gradual increase in the amount of resistance and in the length of time that the muscle contraction is held will increase muscle strength and endurance. Examples of restrictive isometric exercises include the plank (for abdominal strengthening) and the wall push-up (for chest, triceps, and shoulder strengthening). The patient who is in a sitting position may do hip lifting, in which the hands push against a surface such as the seat of a chair to raise the hips. Resistive isometric exercises help to promote muscle strength and provide sufficient stress against bone to promote osteoblastic activity.

Regulation of Movement

Coordinated body movement involves the integrated functioning of the skeletal, muscular, and nervous systems. Because these three systems are highly integrated in mechanical support of the body, they are often considered a single functional unit.

Skeletal System. The skeletal system provides five functions in the body: support, protection, movement, mineral storage, and hematopoiesis (blood cell formation). In a discussion of body mechanics, two of these functions—support and movement—are most important (Patton, 2019). Bones provide the framework for support and contribute to shape, alignment, and positioning of body parts.

Bones are further characterized by firmness, rigidity, and elasticity. Firmness results from inorganic salts, such as calcium and phosphate, that form the bone matrix. Firmness is related to the bone's rigidity, which is necessary to keep long bones straight and enables bones to bear weight. In addition, bones have a degree of elasticity and flexibility that changes with age. For example, newborns have a large amount of cartilage and are highly flexible, but their bones are unable to support weight. Toddlers' bones are more pliable than those of older people and thus are better able to withstand falls. Older persons, especially women, are more susceptible to bone loss (resorption) and osteoporosis.

Bones protect vital organs (e.g., the skull around the brain; the ribs around the heart and lungs). They also aid in calcium regulation, store calcium, and release calcium into the body's circulation as needed. Patients with decreased calcium regulation and metabolism are at risk for developing osteoporosis and **pathological fractures** (fractures caused by weakened bone tissue) (Power-Kean et al., 2022) . Fractures from osteoporosis are more common than heart attack, stroke, and breast cancer combined. At least one in three women, and one in five men, will break a bone because of osteoporosis, and 80% of fragility fractures in postmenopausal women over age 50 are related to osteoporosis (Osteoporosis Canada, 2022).

In addition, the internal structure of bones contains bone marrow, which participates in red blood cell (RBC) production (hematopoiesis) and acts as a reservoir for blood. Patients with altered bone marrow function or diminished RBC production are usually weakened and fatigue easily, which decreases their mobility and places them at risk of falling.

Joints, ligaments, tendons, and cartilage permit strength and flexibility of the skeleton. Strength enables the skeletal system to support the body.

Joints. Joints or articulations are the connections between bones. Each joint is classified according to its structure and degree of mobility. Joints are classified as four types: synarthrotic, cartilaginous, fibrous, and synovial (Power-Kean et al., 2022). A person's flexibility is demonstrated through range of motion (ROM), which is the range of normal movement for a joint.

In a synarthrotic joint, bones are jointed by bones. No movement is associated with this type of joint, and the bony tissue that forms between the bones provides strength and stability. The classic example of this type of joint is the sacrum, in which vertebrae are joined (Figure 37.1, *A*).

The cartilaginous joint, or synchondrodial joint, has little movement but is elastic and uses cartilage to unite body surfaces. Cartilaginous joints are found when bones are exposed to constant pressure, such as the costosternal joints between the sternum and ribs (see Figure 37.1, *B*).

The fibrous joint, or syndesmodial joint, is a joint in which two bony surfaces are united by a ligament or membrane. The fibres of ligaments are flexible and stretch, permitting a limited amount of movement. For example, the paired bones of the lower leg (tibia and fibula) are fibrous joints (Power-Kean et al., 2022) (see Figure 37.1, *C*).

The synovial joint is a freely movable joint in which contiguous bony surfaces are covered by articular cartilage and connected by ligaments lined with a synovial membrane. Joining of the humeral radius and ulna by cartilage and ligaments forms a pivotal joint (see Figure 37.1, *D*). Other types of synovial joints are the ball-and-socket joints (e.g., hip joint) and the hinge joints (e.g., interphalangeal joints of the fingers).

Ligaments, Tendons, and Cartilage. Ligaments are white, shiny, flexible bands of fibrous tissue that support the skeletal system. Ligaments bind joints together and connect bones and cartilage. Ligaments are elastic and aid joint flexibility and support (Figure 37.2). In addition, some ligaments have a protective function. For example, ligaments between the vertebral bodies and the ligamentum flavum prevent damage to the spinal cord during movement of the back.

Tendons are white, glistening, fibrous bands of tissue that connect muscle to bone. Tendons are strong, flexible, and inelastic, and they occur in various lengths and thicknesses. The Achilles tendon (tendo calcaneus) is the thickest and strongest tendon in the body. It begins

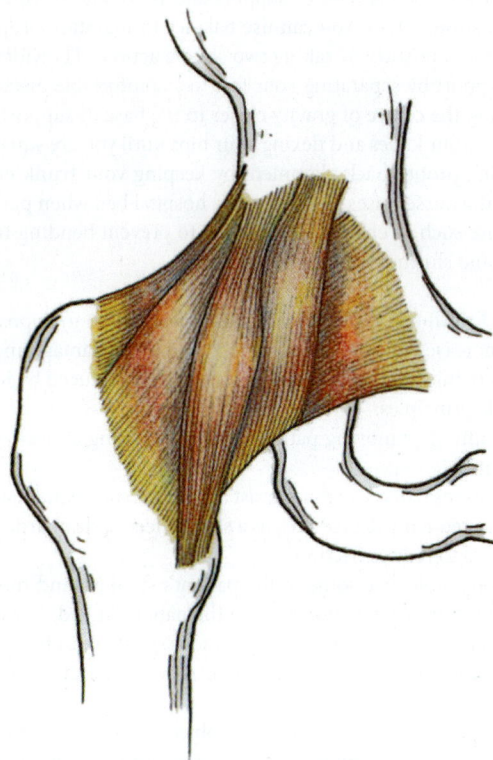

FIGURE 37.2 Ligaments of the hip joint.

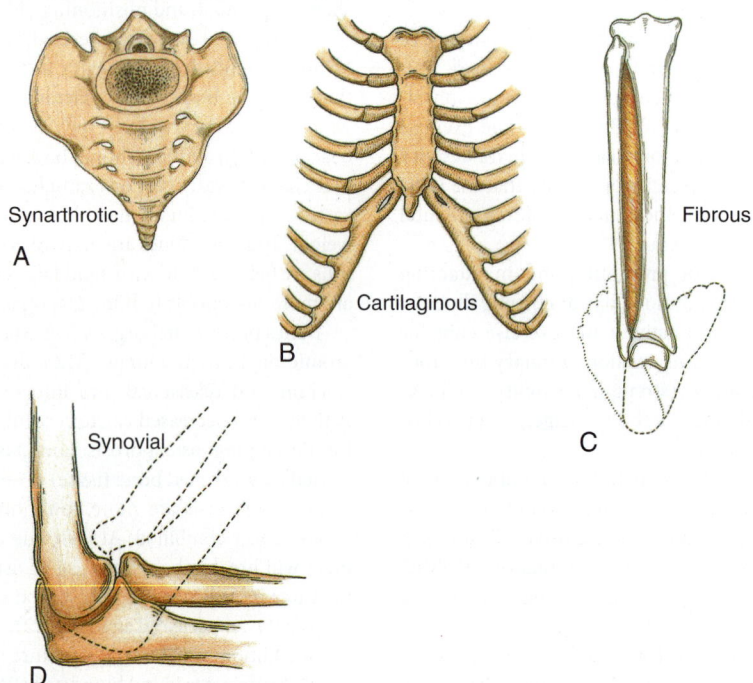

FIGURE 37.1 Joint types. **A,** Synarthrotic. **B,** Cartilaginous. **C,** Fibrous. **D,** Synovial.

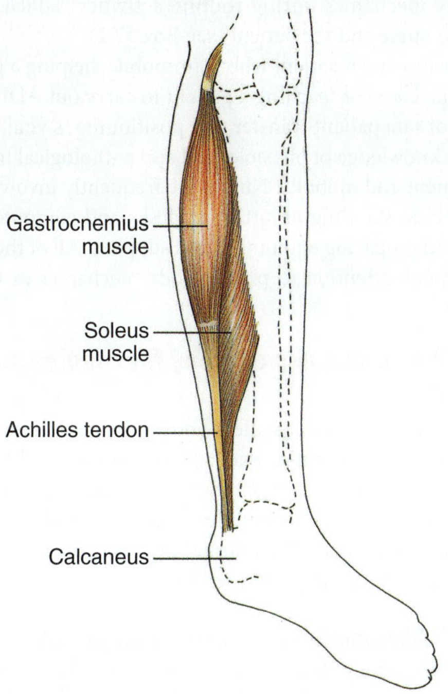

FIGURE 37.3 Tendons and muscles of the lower leg.

Gastrocnemius muscle

Soleus muscle

Achilles tendon

Calcaneus

near the middle of the posterior of the calf and attaches the gastrocnemius and soleus muscles in the calf to the calcaneal bone in the back of the foot (Figure 37.3).

Cartilage is nonvascular, supporting connective tissue with flexibility similar to that of firm plastic. The gristle-like nature of cartilage permits it to sustain weight and to serve as a shock absorber between articulating bones. It is located primarily in the joints and thorax, trachea, larynx, nose, and ear. The fetus has a large amount of temporary cartilage, which is replaced by bone developed during infancy. Permanent cartilage is unossified (not hardened), except in advanced age and in diseases such as osteoarthritis. Strength and flexibility do not result entirely from joints, ligaments, tendons, and cartilage. Adequate skeletal muscle is also necessary.

Skeletal Muscle. Muscles are made of fibres that contract when stimulated by an electrochemical impulse that travels from the nerve to the muscle across the neuromuscular junction. The electrochemical impulse causes the filaments (predominantly protein molecules of myosin and actin) within the fibre to slide past each other, with the filaments changing length.

Contraction of skeletal muscles allows people to walk, talk, run, breathe, and participate in physical activity. There are more than 600 skeletal muscles in the body. In addition to facilitating movement, these muscles determine the form and contour of our bodies. Most of our muscles span at least one joint and attach to both articulating bones. Adequate skeletal muscle is necessary for strength and flexibility (Patton, 2019). Muscle contractions can be categorized by functional purpose: moving, resisting, or stabilizing body parts. Muscle action necessary for active movement is referred to as *dynamic* or *isotonic contraction*. In contrast, static or isometric contraction causes an increase in muscle tension or muscle work but with no active movement of the muscle (e.g., instructing the patient in tightening and relaxing a muscle group, as in quadriceps set exercises or pelvic floor muscle exercises). Voluntary movement is a combination of isotonic and isometric contractions. For example, when the nurse lifts a patient up in bed, the patient's weight causes increased tension in the muscles of the nurse's

arms until the tension (isometric) is equal to the weight to be lifted and the weight of the lower arms. When this equilibrium is reached, continued stimulation of the muscles results in muscle shortening (isotonic) and bending of the elbows (active movement), and the patient is lifted off the bed.

Isometric contraction and exercise increases energy expenditure. As a nurse, you must recognize the energy expenditure (increased respiratory rate and increased work on the heart) associated with isometric exercises, because these types of exercises may be contraindicated in certain illnesses or conditions (e.g., myocardial infarction or chronic obstructive pulmonary disease [COPD]).

Muscle Groups. The antagonistic, synergistic, and antigravity muscle groups are coordinated by the nervous system and maintain posture and initiate movement. Antagonistic muscles, muscles that oppose the action of another muscle, facilitate movement at the joint. For example, during flexion of the arm, the active mover (the biceps brachii) contracts and its antagonist (the triceps brachii) relaxes. During extension of the arm, the active mover (the triceps brachii) contracts and the new antagonist (the biceps brachii) relaxes.

Synergistic muscles are two or more muscles that contract to accomplish the same movement. When the arm is flexed, the strength of the contraction of the biceps brachii is increased by contraction of the synergistic muscle, the brachialis.

Antigravity muscles work to stabilize joints. These muscles continuously oppose the effect of gravity on the body and permit a person to maintain an upright or sitting posture. In an adult, the antigravity muscles are the extensors of the leg—the gluteus maximus, the quadriceps femoris, and the soleus muscles—and the muscles of the back.

Skeletal muscles support posture and carry out voluntary movement. These muscles are attached to the skeleton by tendons, which provide strength and permit motion. The movement of the extremities is voluntary and requires coordination from the nervous system.

Nervous System. Movement and posture are regulated by the nervous system. The major voluntary motor area, located in the cerebral cortex, is the precentral gyrus, or motor strip. Motor fibres descend from the motor strip and cross at the level of the medulla. Motor fibres from the right motor strip initiate voluntary movement for the left side of the body, and the motor fibres from the left motor strip initiate voluntary movement for the right side of the body.

Transmission of the impulse from the nervous system to the musculoskeletal system is an electrochemical event and requires a neurotransmitter. *Neurotransmitters* are chemicals (e.g., acetylcholine) that transfer the electrical impulse from the nerve across the myoneural junction to stimulate the muscle, causing movement.

Movement can be impaired by disorders that alter neurotransmitter production, as in Parkinson's disease; alter transfer from the neurotransmitter to the muscle, as in myasthenia gravis; or alter activation of muscle activity, as in multiple sclerosis (Power-Kean et al., 2022).

Proprioception. Proprioception is the awareness of the position of the body and its parts (Power-Kean et al., 2022). Position is monitored by proprioceptors located on nerve endings in muscles, tendons, and joints. Posture, the position of the body when sitting or standing, is regulated by the nervous system and requires coordination of proprioception and balance. As a person carries out ADLs, proprioceptors monitor muscle activity and body position. For example, the proprioceptors on the soles of the feet contribute to correct posture during standing or walking. During standing, pressure is continuous on the bottom of the feet. The proprioceptors monitor the pressure, communicating this information through the nervous system to the antigravity muscles. The standing person remains upright until deciding to change position. As a person walks, the proprioceptors on the bottom of the feet monitor pressure changes. Thus, when the bottom of the moving foot comes in contact with the walking surface, the individual automatically moves the stationary foot forward. The proprioceptors allow people to walk without having to watch their feet.

Balance. A person must have adequate balance when standing, running, lifting, or performing ADLs. Balance is controlled by the nervous system, specifically by the cerebellum and the inner ear. The cerebellum coordinates all voluntary movement, particularly highly skilled movements, such as those required in skiing.

Within the inner ear are the semicircular canals, three fluid-filled structures that assist in maintaining balance. Fluid within the canals has inertia. When the head is suddenly rotated in one direction, the fluid remains stationary for a moment, whereas the canal turns with the head. This allows a person to change position suddenly without losing balance.

Principles of Body Mechanics, Safe Patient Transfer, and Positioning Techniques

Using principles of safe patient transfer and positioning during routine activities decreases work effort and places less strain on musculoskeletal structures (Box 37.2). Nurses can teach colleagues and patients' families how to transfer or position patients properly. Teaching a patient's family how to transfer the patient from bed to chair increases and reinforces the family's knowledge about proper body mechanics and safe transfer and positioning techniques. Using the principles of

---

BOX 37.2   Quality Improvement: Principles of Body Mechanics, Safe Patient Transfer, and Patient Positioning

- Mechanical lifts are essential when a patient is unable to assist.
- When transferring a patient, perform six check points:
  1. Three for the top: *Ears (1)* in line with *shoulders (2)*, shoulders in line with *hips (3)*.
  2. Three for the bottom: *Tighten stomach (1)* and *push your buttocks back (2)* while keeping your *body weight over the heels (3)*. Move your trunk forward, bending at the hips, not the waist.
  3. Elbows are tucked in to your sides.
  4. Use palms-up grip.
  5. Work in your comfort zone (area between shoulders and hips): Bend and tuck elbows into your sides, move hands from shoulders to hips.
  6. Weight transfer: Stand with a stable base of support, transfer weight side to side and front to back.
- When a patient is unable to assist, remember the following principles:
  - The wider the base of support, the greater the stability.
  - The lower the centre of gravity, the greater the stability.
  - Facing the direction of movement prevents abnormal twisting of the spine.
  - Dividing balanced activity between arms and legs reduces the risk of back injury.
  - Leverage, rolling, turning, or pivoting requires less work than lifting.
  - Use transfer sheets to reduce friction between the patient and the surface over which the patient is moved, to reduce the force required to reposition the patient.
  - Reducing the force of work reduces the risk of injury.
  - Maintaining good body mechanics reduces fatigue of the muscle groups.
  - Alternating periods of rest and activity helps reduce fatigue.
- When transferring a patient who is in the supine position with another health care provider, always work in the comfort zone of the taller person.

Adapted from Alberta Health Services. (2021). *Ergonomics training.* https://www.albertahealthservices.ca/careers/Page12772.aspx

---

proper body mechanics during routine activities reduces the risk of injury to the nurse and the patient (see Box 37.2).

Whether moving a patient who is immobile, helping a patient from the bed to the chair, or teaching a patient to carry out ADLs efficiently, knowledge of safe patient transfer and positioning is vital. Nurses also incorporate knowledge of physiological and pathological influences on body alignment and mobility. Nurses are frequently involved in activities that include standing or sitting at desks and computers to document care and preparing equipment and supplies. All of these activities require as much attention to proper body mechanics as to hands-on patient care.

Pathological Influences on Body Mechanics and Movement

Many pathological conditions affect body alignment, body movement, and the capacity for exercise and activity. These conditions include congenital abnormalities, degenerative diseases, and episodic illnesses affecting bones, joints, muscles, and the central nervous system. Chronic diseases affecting the internal organs can also affect an individual's capacity for activity and exercise.

Congenital Abnormalities. Congenital abnormalities affect musculoskeletal alignment, balance, and appearance. For example, osteogenesis imperfecta is an inherited disorder characterized by bones that are porous, short, bowed, and deformed; as a result, children with this disorder experience curvature of the spine and shortness of stature. Scoliosis is a structural curvature of the spine associated with vertebral rotation. Muscles, ligaments, and other soft tissues become shortened as a result. Balance and mobility are affected in proportion to the severity of abnormal spinal curvatures (Hockenberry & Wilson, 2019).

Disorders of Bones, Joints, and Muscles. Osteoporosis results in the reduction of bone density or mass. The cause is uncertain, and theories vary from hormonal imbalances to insufficient intake of nutrients (Power-Kean et al., 2022).

Joint mobility is altered by inflammatory and noninflammatory joint diseases and articular disruption. Inflammatory joint disease (e.g., arthritis) is characterized by inflammation or destruction of the synovial membrane and articular cartilage and the systemic signs of inflammation. Noninflammatory diseases have none of these characteristics, and the synovial fluid is normal (Power-Kean et al., 2022). Joint degeneration, which can occur with inflammatory and noninflammatory disease, is marked by changes in articular cartilage combined with overgrowth of bone at the articular ends. Degenerative changes commonly affect weight-bearing joints such as the hips and knees.

Articular disruption involves trauma to the articular capsules and ranges from mild, such as a tear resulting in a sprain, to severe, such as a separation leading to dislocation. Articular disruption also includes disorders such as developmental dysplasia of the hip (Hockenberry & Wilson, 2019).

Central Nervous System Damage and Disorders. Damage to any part of the central nervous system that regulates voluntary movement causes impaired body alignment and immobility (see Chapter 46). For example, a patient with a traumatic head injury experiences damage in the motor strip in the cerebrum. The amount of voluntary impairment is directly related to the amount of destruction of the motor strip. A patient with a complete spinal cord injury in the lumbar region has permanent damage below the level of the injury and retains control of trunk muscles, but not of the lower extremity muscles.

It is important to understand which type of voluntary and involuntary movement is present after damage to the central nervous system.

This information affects the type of interventions selected to maximize a patient's activity level.

Degenerative diseases of the central nervous system affect an individual's health and abilities over time. For example, Parkinson's disease or multiple sclerosis can affect an individual's control of movement and balance.

Musculoskeletal Trauma. Musculoskeletal trauma often results in bruises, contusions, sprains, and fractures. A *fracture* is a disruption of bone tissue continuity. Fractures most commonly result from direct external trauma. They also occur because of some deformity of the bone (e.g., with pathological fractures of osteoporosis). Fractures often result in a period of reduced mobility followed by a period of rehabilitation and are described in more detail in Chapter 46.

Other Chronic Diseases. Many chronic diseases of the internal organs also affect an individual's ability to be active and to exercise. Diseases of the heart, such as coronary artery disease and heart failure, can alter tissue perfusion, resulting in activity tolerance. Chronic diseases

of the lungs, such as asthma and COPD, can impair gas exchange, affecting activity tolerance. Diabetes, chronic renal impairment, and various cancers can all similarly affect one's ability to exercise.

NURSING KNOWLEDGE BASE

Application of knowledge about activity and exercise enables nurses to think critically about the holistic needs of patients. Nursing knowledge as it pertains to activity and exercise helps nurses to assess, identify, and intervene when patients have decreased activity tolerance or physical limitation that affects their mobility, ability to exercise, or both (see Chapter 46).

Deconditioning

In acute care settings, intervening to increase inpatients' activity and mobility levels as soon as possible to prevent deconditioning and other complications of immobilization is essential (Table 37.1). Nurses play a key role in assessing patients for complications associated with immobility and performing interventions such as ROM exercises and early

TABLE 37.1 Risks Associated With Deconditioning

Body System	Side Effects	Potential Complications	Nursing Actions
Respiratory	Decreased lung expansion Hypoventilation Impaired gas exchange Pulmonary secretion pooling	Atelectasis Pneumonia Hypoxemia Pulmonary edema Pulmonary embolism	Frequent respiratory system assessment, including rate, rhythm, depth, quality, effort of respiration, SpO_2, and auscultation of anterior and posterior lung fields Positioning in bed to facilitate maximum lung expansion Encouragement of deep-breathing and coughing exercises Encouragement of incentive spirometry Chest physiotherapy Daily ambulation
Circulatory	Venous pooling and peripheral edema in extremities as a result of decreased systemic vascular resistance Decreased cardiac output	Thrombus formation Emboli Orthostatic hypotension	Frequent circulatory system assessment, including pulse, blood pressure, skin colour, assessment of extremities for colour, sensation, movement, temperature, edema and peripheral pulses, and auscultation of heart sounds Application and ongoing assessment of compression stockings Passive range-of-motion exercises Assessment of blood pressure before ambulating, to prevent injury Daily ambulation
Integumentary	Decreased delivery of oxygen and nutrients to tissues Inflammation over bony prominences Shearing of skin during movement Tissue ischemia due to pressure between bony prominences and bed or chair	Skin breakdown Abrasions/excoriation Pressure injuries Infection	Frequent assessment of posterior skin surfaces to identify inflammation and skin breakdown Repositioning patients every 2–3 hours Assessment and management of skin to ensure integument is clean and dry Application of skin barriers to prevent skin breakdown
Musculoskeletal	Reduced muscle mass Decreased muscle strength Impaired joint mobility Decreased endurance	Fatigue Muscle atrophy Decreased stability and balance Joint contractures	Isotonic and isometric exercises Passive range-of-motion exercises Daily ambulation Application of splints to prevent joint contractures
Gastrointestinal	Decreased peristalsis Decreased fluid intake Decreased appetite	Abdominal distension Constipation Ileus Aspiration	Frequent abdominal assessment, including inspection, auscultation, and palpation Assessment of fluid intake and output Assessment of oral intake Assessment of daily bowel activity Daily ambulation High-protein diet

SpO_2, Peripheral capillary oxygen saturation.
Adapted from Gordon, S., Grimmer, K.A., & Barras, S. (2019). Assessment for incipient hospital-acquired deconditioning in acute hospital settings: A systematic literature review. *Journal of Rehabilitation Medicine, 51*(6), 397–404. doi:10.2340/16501977-2546; Jarvis, C., Browne, A. J., MacDonald-Jenkins, J., et al. (Eds.). (2018). *Physical examination & health assessment* (3rd Canadian ed.). Elsevier.

mobilization to prevent adverse outcomes (see Chapter 46). Extended or complicated hospitalizations among older persons commonly lead to significant decreases in muscle mass and functional decline, due to physiological changes that affect multiple body systems. Following hospital discharge, approximately 68% of older persons are below preadmission level of function and have a three times greater risk of readmission within 30 days if discharged in poor physical condition (Smith et al., 2020).

Physical benefits of inpatient mobilization include less delirium, pain, urinary discomfort, urinary tract infection, fatigue, deep vein thrombosis, and pneumonia, and improved ability to void (Gordon et al., 2019; Smith et al., 2020). Longer periods of hospitalization inevitably lead to more severe deconditioning, slower recovery, more functional decline, and longer length of hospital stay (Smith et al., 2020). These findings support the promotion of early mobility in hospitalized patients.

Safety Guidelines for Nursing Skills

Ensuring patient safety is an essential role of the nurse. To ensure patient safety, the nurse needs to communicate clearly with members of the health care team, assess and incorporate the patient's priorities of care and preferences, and use the best evidence when making decisions about patient's care. When performing the skills in this chapter, remember the following points to ensure safe patient handling and individualized patient-centred care:

- Mentally review the transfer steps before beginning the procedure; this ensures both your safety and that of the patient.
- Prior to transferring a patient, perform a functional assessment to determine the patient's mobility, strength, and the assistance that they are able to offer during transfer. Stand on the patient's weak side when assisting (Fairchild et al., 2018).
- Determine the amount and type of assistance required for transfer, including the type of transfer equipment and the number of personnel to safely transfer and prevent harm to the patient and health care providers.
- Raise the side rail on the side of the bed opposite where you are standing to prevent the patient from falling out of bed on that side.
- Arrange equipment (e.g., intravenous lines, feeding tube, indwelling catheter) in such a way that it does not interfere with the positioning or transfer process.
- Evaluate the patient for correct body alignment and pressure risks after the transfer.
- Make sure that all personnel understand how the equipment functions before it is used.
- Educate patients about how equipment functions, to reduce their anxiety and enlist their cooperation.

Safe Patient Handling

Nurses are exposed to the hazards related to lifting and transferring patients in many settings, such as inpatient nursing units, long-term care facilities, and the operating room. In most health care facilities, quality improvement programs and no-lift policies have been implemented. Manually lifting and transferring patients contributes to the high incidence of work-related musculoskeletal and back injuries in nurses and members of the health care team (Gomaa et al., 2020). Implementing evidence-informed interventions and ergonomics training programs can reduce the number of work-related injuries, which improves the health of the nurse and reduces indirect costs to the health care system (Lee et al., 2021).

Many provinces have implemented occupational health and safety legislation regarding lifting and moving loads. For instance, in Alberta the law requires that employers provide equipment and training and

that employees use that equipment and training (*Occupational Health and Safety Act Alberta* [Government of Alberta, 2020]). Health boards are implementing comprehensive safe patient-handling programs in all parts of Canada. Comprehensive safe patient-handling programs include the following elements (Veterans Health Administration [VHA], 2014):

- An ergonomics assessment protocol for health care environments
- Patient assessment criteria and algorithms for safe patient handling and movement
- Special equipment kept in convenient locations to help transfer patients
- Back-injury prevention and treatment resources for nurses
- An "after-action" review that allows the health care team to apply knowledge about moving patients safely in different settings
- A no-lift policy

It is the responsibility of the nurse not only to implement existing safe handling policies within the workplace but also to advocate for enhancements to safety. This includes identifying unsafe situations, such as broken equipment or the improper techniques of others. It involves reviewing literature and government policy to remain current on best practices. Nurses need to assume an active role in their workplaces to ensure that a culture of safety exists and that appropriate patient-handling equipment is readily available for use (Lee et al., 2021; Roy et al., 2021). The nurse must advocate for change within the workplace when safer options exist, for the benefit of all staff and patients.

Transfer Techniques. Nurses often provide care for immobilized patients whose position must be changed, who must be moved up in bed, or who must be transferred from a bed to a chair or from a bed to a stretcher. Body mechanics alone do not protect nurses from injury to their musculoskeletal systems when they move or transfer patients. Although nurses use many transfer techniques, knowledge of ergonomics and safe patient handling is crucial in maintaining caregiver and patient safety. **Ergonomics** is an applied science concerned with designing and arranging workplace settings in such a way that people interact more effectively with the objects they encounter in that environment.

Nurses must assess every situation that involves patient handling and movement, to minimize risk of injury. After completing the assessment, the nurse will use an algorithm (Figure 37.4) to guide decisions about safe patient handling (VHA, 2014). Skill 37.1 describes the steps commonly used in transferring patients safely and effectively. When transferring a patient, it is helpful to encourage maximum patient involvement. The nurse should use a patient's strength when lifting, transferring, or moving, when possible. Involving the patient has the additional benefit of increasing participation in self-care and can promote a sense of accomplishment.

Factors Influencing Activity and Exercise

Factors influencing activity and exercise include developmental changes, behavioural aspects, environmental issues, social determinants of health, cultural and ethnic influences, and family and social support. Nurses need to consider these areas of knowledge and incorporate them into the plan of care, whether the patient is seeking health promotion, acute care, or restorative and continuing care.

Developmental Changes. Throughout the lifespan, the body's appearance and functioning undergo change. The greatest change and impact on the maturational process are observed at both ends of the developmental spectrum.

Infants Through School-Aged Children. The newborn infant's spine is flexed and lacks the anteroposterior curves of the adult. The first

Algorithm ① Transfer to/from Seated Positions: *Bed to Chair, Chair to Chair, Chair to Exam Table*

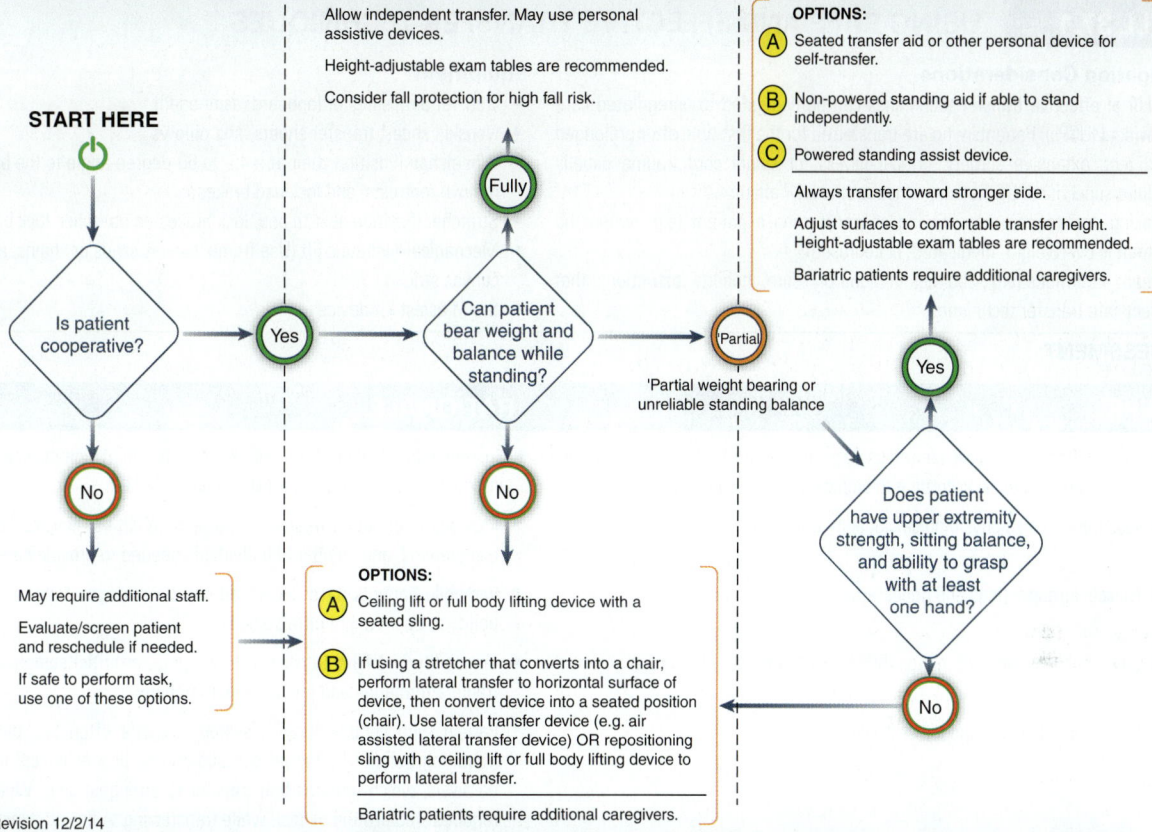

START HERE

Is patient cooperative?

- **Yes** → **Can patient bear weight and balance while standing?**
  - **Fully** → Allow independent transfer. May use personal assistive devices.

    Height-adjustable exam tables are recommended.

    Consider fall protection for high fall risk.
  - **Partial** ('Partial weight bearing or unreliable standing balance)
  - **No**
- **No**

OPTIONS:

A Seated transfer aid or other personal device for self-transfer.

B Non-powered standing aid if able to stand independently.

C Powered standing assist device.

Always transfer toward stronger side.

Adjust surfaces to comfortable transfer height. Height-adjustable exam tables are recommended.

Bariatric patients require additional caregivers.

Does patient have upper extremity strength, sitting balance, and ability to grasp with at least one hand?

- **Yes**
- **No**

(No branch of cooperative):

May require additional staff.

Evaluate/screen patient and reschedule if needed.

If safe to perform task, use one of these options.

OPTIONS:

A Ceiling lift or full body lifting device with a seated sling.

B If using a stretcher that converts into a chair, perform lateral transfer to horizontal surface of device, then convert device into a seated position (chair). Use lateral transfer device (e.g. air assisted lateral transfer device) OR repositioning sling with a ceiling lift or full body lifting device to perform lateral transfer.

Bariatric patients require additional caregivers.

Last Revision 12/2/14

A

Algorithm ② Lateral Transfer to/from Supine Positions: *Bed, Stretcher, Trolley, Procedure Table*

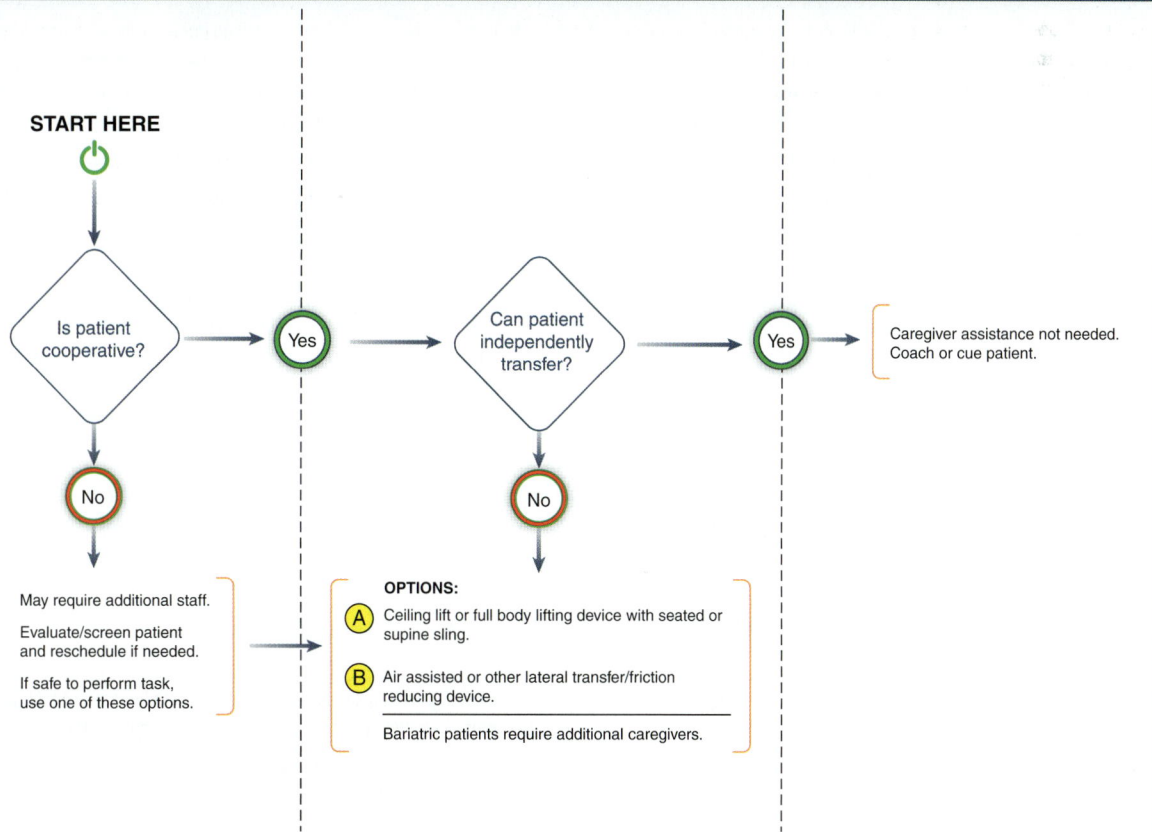

START HERE

Is patient cooperative?

- **Yes** → **Can patient independently transfer?**
  - **Yes** → Caregiver assistance not needed. Coach or cue patient.
  - **No**
- **No**

(No branch of cooperative):

May require additional staff.

Evaluate/screen patient and reschedule if needed.

If safe to perform task, use one of these options.

OPTIONS:

A Ceiling lift or full body lifting device with seated or supine sling.

B Air assisted or other lateral transfer/friction reducing device.

Bariatric patients require additional caregivers.

Last Revision 12/2/14

B

FIGURE 37.4 A, Veterans Health Administration (VHA) safe patient handling algorithm 1. **B,** VHA safe patient handling algorithm 2. (From VHA. [2014]. *Safe patient handling algorithms.* https://behealthyswhrcin.org/wp-content/uploads/2017/11/VHA-Safe-Patient-Handling-algorithms.pdf)

SKILL 37.1   USING SAFE AND EFFECTIVE TRANSFER TECHNIQUES

Delegation Considerations

The skill of effective transfer techniques can be delegated to unregulated care providers (UCPs). Patients who are transferred for the first time after prolonged bed rest, extensive surgery, critical illness, or spinal cord trauma usually require supervision by the nurse. Instruct the UCP about:

- Seeking assistance when moving or transferring a patient (e.g., when the patient is overweight, medicated, or confused).
- Patient limitations (e.g., changes in blood pressure, mobility restrictions) that affect safe transfer techniques.

Equipment

- Transfer belt, sling, or lapboard (as needed)
- Nonskid shoes, transfer sheets, and pillows
- Wheelchair (Position chair at a 45- to 60-degree angle to the bed, lock brakes, remove footrests, and lock bed brakes.)
- Stretcher (Position next to bed, lock brakes on stretcher, lock brakes on bed.)
- Mechanical/hydraulic lift (Use frame, canvas strips or chains, and hammock or canvas strips.)
- Stand-assist lift device

ASSESSMENT

STEPS	RATIONALE
1. Identify patient using two identifiers (e.g., name and birthday or name and medical record number) according to employer policy. Explain procedure.	• Ensures correct patient. Complies with The Joint Commission standards and improves patient safety (Joint Commission, 2022).
2. Assess the patient's physiological capacity to transfer:	• Provides information relative to patient's abilities, physical status, ability to comprehend, and number of individuals needed to provide safe transferring.
A. Muscle strength (legs and upper arms)	• Immobile patients have decreased muscle strength, tone, and mass. Affects ability to bear weight or raise body.
B. Joint mobility (range of motion [ROM]) and contracture formation	• Immobility or inflammatory processes (e.g., arthritis) sometimes lead to contracture formation and impaired joint mobility.
C. Paralysis or paresis (spastic or flaccid)	• Patient with central nervous system damage often has bilateral paralysis (requiring transfer by swivel bar, sliding bar, or mechanical lift) or unilateral paralysis, which requires belt transfer to strongest side. Weakness (paresis) requires stabilization of knee while transferring. A flaccid arm needs to be supported with a sling during transfer.
D. Bone continuity	• Patients with trauma to one leg or hip may be non–weight bearing during transfer. Amputees may use slide board to transfer.
3. Assess for weakness, dizziness, or orthostatic (postural) hypotension or risk for orthostatic hypotension (e.g., previously on bed rest, first time arising from supine position following surgical procedure, history of dizziness when arising).	• Determines risk of fainting or falling during transfer. Immobilized patients have decreased ability for the autonomic nervous system to equalize blood supply, resulting in drop of 20 mm Hg systolic or more in blood pressure when rising from sitting position (Lewis et al., 2023).
4. Assess activity tolerance, noting fatigue during activity.	• Determines ability of patient to help with transfer.
5. Assess proprioceptive function (awareness of posture and equilibrium), including ability to maintain balance while sitting in bed or on side of bed and tendency to sway toward one side.	• Determines stability of patient's balance for transfer and risk for falls.
6. Assess sensory status, including central and peripheral vision, adequacy of hearing, and presence of peripheral sensation loss.	• Determines influence of sensory loss on ability to make transfer. Visual field loss decreases patient's ability to see in direction of transfer. Peripheral sensation loss decreases proprioception. Patients with visual and hearing losses need transfer techniques adapted to deficits. Patients with a cerebrovascular accident (CVA) sometimes lose an area of visual field, which profoundly affects vision and perception.

CRITICAL DECISION POINT: *Patients with hemiplegia also often "neglect" one side of the body (inattention to or unawareness of one side of body or environment), which distorts perception of the visual field. If patient experiences neglect of one side, instruct them to scan all visual fields when transferring.*

7. Assess level of comfort (e.g., joint discomfort, muscle spasm) and measure level of pain on a 0–10 scale. Offer prescribed analgesic 30 minutes before transfer.	• Pain reduces patient's motivation and ability to be mobile. Pain relief before transfer can enhance patient participation.
8. Assess vital signs.	• Vital sign changes such as increased pulse and respiration and drop in blood pressure indicate activity intolerance (see Chapter 31).
9. Assess patient's cognitive status, including ability to follow verbal instructions, short-term memory, and recognition of physical deficits and limitations to movement.	• Determines patient's ability to follow directions and learn transfer techniques.

SKILL 37.1	USING SAFE AND EFFECTIVE TRANSFER TECHNIQUES—cont'd
STEPS	**RATIONALE**

CRITICAL DECISION POINT: *Patients with head trauma or cerebrovascular accident may have perceptual cognitive deficits that create safety risks. If the patient has difficulty comprehending, simplify instructions by providing one step at a time and maintain consistency.*

STEPS	RATIONALE
10. Assess patient's level of motivation, such as eagerness versus unwillingness to be mobile and perception of value of exercise.	• Altered physiological and psychological conditions reduce a patient's desire to engage in activity.
11. Assess patient's specific risk for falling or being injured during transfer (e.g., neuromuscular deficits, visual loss, motor weakness, fear of falling, or bone loss).	• Causes risk for tripping, losing balance.
12. Assess previous mode of transfer or currently assigned movement algorithm (if available).	• Determines mode of transfer and assistance required to provide continuity.
13. Assess patient's specific risk of falling or being injured when transferred (e.g., neuromuscular deficits, motor weakness, calcium loss from bones, cognitive and visual dysfunction, altered balance).	• Certain conditions increase risk of falling or potential injury.
14. Assess special transfer equipment needed for home setting and previous mode of transfer (if applicable).	• Prior teaching of family and support people, assessing home for safety risks and functionality, and providing applicable aids greatly enhance transfer ability at home.
15. Assess patient using employer algorithm to determine plan for safe patient handling and transfer.	• Determine patient's ability to assist with move. • Determine appropriate equipment and number of staff required to safely transfer patient (VHA, 2014).

PLANNING

1. Gather appropriate equipment.	
2. Determine number of people needed to assist with transfer by referring to proper algorithm. Do not start procedure until all caregivers are available.	• Ensures safe patient transfer.
3. Perform hand hygiene. Verify that bed brakes are locked.	• Reduces transmission of microorganisms. Promotes patient and caregiver safety.
4. Explain procedure to patient.	• Increases patient participation.

IMPLEMENTATION

1. Transfer patient.

A. Assisting a cooperative patient to sitting position in bed:

CRITICAL DECISION POINT: *Careful assessment of the patient's ability to assist in the following position technique is extremely important. Consider the use of a mechanical lift. Your role in helping the patient to a sitting position is to be a guide and to instruct. If the patient can bear weight and move to a sitting position independently, allow them to do so and offer assistance (VHA, 2014).*

(1) Raise bed to waist level. Place patient in supine position.	• Enables nurse to assess patient's body alignment continually.
(2) Face head of bed at a 45-degree angle and remove pillows.	• Proper positioning reduces twisting of nurse's body when moving patient. Pillows cause interference when patient is sitting up in bed.
(3) Place your feet in wide base of support, with one foot closer to the bed in front of the other foot.	• Improves balance and allows transfer of body weight as patient is moved to sitting position.
(4) Place your arm nearer head of bed under patient's shoulders, supporting their head and cervical vertebrae.	• Maintains alignment of head and cervical vertebrae and allows for even lifting of patient's upper trunk.
(5) Place other hand on bed surface.	• Provides support and balance.
(6) Raise patient to sitting position by shifting weight from front to back leg.	• Improves balance, overcomes inertia, and transfers weight in the direction patient is being moved.
(7) Push against bed using arm that is placed on bed surface.	• Divides activity between arms and legs and protects back from strain. By bracing one hand against the mattress and pushing against it as you lift the patient, you transfer weight away from your back muscles through your arm onto the mattress.

Continued

844   UNIT VIII   Basic Physiological Needs

SKILL 37.1   USING SAFE AND EFFECTIVE TRANSFER TECHNIQUES—cont'd

STEPS	RATIONALE

B. Assisting a cooperative patient who can partially bear weight to sitting position on side of bed:

(1) With bed flat and waist high, turn patient to a side-lying position with assistance of another caregiver if necessary. Patient needs to face nurse on side of bed that patient will be sitting on (see illustration, Step 1B[1]).

• Decreases amount of work needed by nurse and patient.

(2) Raise head of bed 30 degrees.

• Facilitates raising patient to sitting position and protects them from falling.

(3) Stand opposite patient's hips. Turn diagonally so you face patient and far corner of head of bed.

• Places nurse's centre of gravity nearer patient. Reduces twisting of nurse's body because nurse is facing direction of movement.

STEP 1B(1) Side-lying position.

STEP 1B(4) Proper foot placement.

(4) Place your feet apart with foot closest to bed in front of the other foot (see illustration for Step 1B[4]).

• Increases balance and allows transfer of body weight as nurse moves patient to a sitting position.

(5) Place your arm nearer head of bed under patient's shoulders, supporting head and cervical vertebrae.

• Maintains alignment of head and cervical vertebrae and allows for even lifting of patient's trunk.

(6) Place your other arm over patient's thighs (see illustration for Step 1B[6]).

• Supports hip and prevents patient from falling backward during procedure.

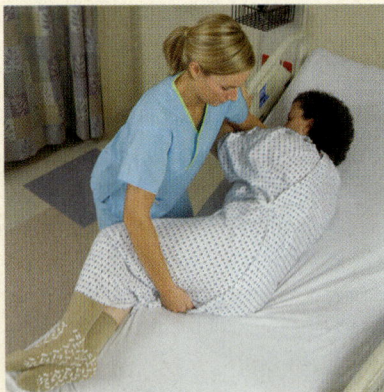

STEP 1B(6) Nurse places arm over patient's thighs.

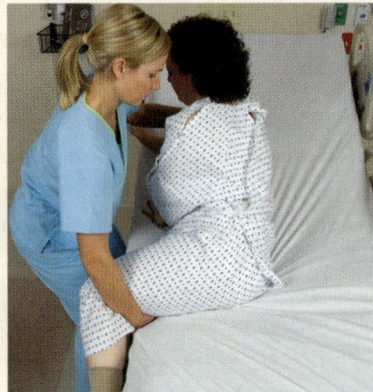

STEP 1B(7) Nurse shifts weight to rear leg and elevates patient.

(7) Move patient's lower legs and feet over side of bed. Pivot toward rear leg, allowing patient's upper legs to swing downward. At the same time, shift weight to back leg and elevate patient (see illustration for Step 1B[7]).

• Decreases friction and resistance. Weight of patient's legs when off bed allows gravity to lower legs, and weight of legs helps to pull them to sitting position.

SKILL 37.1	USING SAFE AND EFFECTIVE TRANSFER TECHNIQUES—cont'd

STEPS	RATIONALE

(8) Allow patient to dangle legs on side of bed for a few minutes. Have patient alternately flex and extend feet and move lower legs. Ask if patient feels dizzy. Have patient relax and take a few deep breaths until dizziness subsides and balance is gained.

- Determines ability to tolerate standing. Dizziness that lasts more than 60 seconds may indicate orthostatic hypotension; return patient to bed (Myszenski, 2017). Recheck blood pressure.

C. Transferring a cooperative patient who is partially weight bearing from bed to chair:

CRITICAL DECISION POINT: *Allow patient to transfer independently if able to fully bear weight. Stand by as needed to promote safe transfer (VHA, 2014). If patient has partial weight bearing with upper-body strength and caregiver must lift more than 115.9 kg (35 lb) of patient weight, use a stand-assist lift device and follow manufacturer instructions (Step 1C).*

STEP 1C Stand-assist device.

(1) Help patient to sitting position on side of bed (see Step 1B). Have chair placed next to bed at a 45-degree angle on patient's strong side. Allow patient to sit on side of bed (legs dangling) for a few minutes before transferring. Ask if patient feels dizzy. Do not leave unattended while patient is dangling legs.

- Positions chair within easy access for transfer. Placing chair on patient's stronger side allows patient to help with transferring. Dangling legs helps equilibrate blood pressure, reducing risk for dizziness or fainting when standing.

(2) Apply transfer belt or other transfer aids. Be sure it completely encircles patient's waist. Place the belt low and be sure it is snug. You may need to adjust belt once patient stands.

- Transfer belt maintains stability of patient during transfer and reduces risk for falling (Fairchild et al., 2018; VHA, 2014). Patient's arm needs to be in a sling if flaccid paralysis is present.

(3) Ensure that patient is wearing stable nonskid shoes. Weight-bearing or strong leg is forward, with weak foot back.

- Nonskid soles decrease risk of slipping during transfer. Always have patient wear shoes during transfer; bare feet increase risk of falls. Patient stands on stronger, or weight-bearing, leg.

(4) Spread feet apart.

- Ensures balance with wide base of support.

(5) Flex hips and knees, aligning knees with patient's knees (see illustration for Step 1C[5]).

- Flexing knees and hips lowers centre of gravity to object to be raised; aligning knees with those of patient allows for stabilization of knees when patient stands.

(6) Grasp transfer belt from underneath along patient's sides.

- Provides movement of patient at centre of gravity. Never lift patients with upper-extremity paralysis or paresis by or under arms (VHA, 2014).

Continued

STEPS	RATIONALE

STEP 1C(5) Nurse flexes hips and knees, aligning knees with patient's knees.

CRITICAL DECISION POINT: *Use a transfer belt or walking belt with handles in place of the under-axilla technique. The under-axilla technique is physically stressful for nurses and uncomfortable for patients (Fairchild et al., 2018).*

---

(7) Rock patient up to standing position on count of three while straightening hips and legs and keeping knees slightly flexed (see illustration for Step 1C[7]). Unless contraindicated, instruct patient to use their hands to push up, if applicable.

• Rocking motion gives patient's body momentum and requires less muscular effort to lift them.

STEP 1C(7) Nurse rocks patient to standing position.

(8) Maintain stability of patient's weak or paralyzed leg with knee.

• Often patient can maintain ability to stand on paralyzed or weak limb with support of knee to stabilize (Fairchild et al., 2018).

(9) Pivot on foot farther from chair.

• Maintains support of patient while allowing adequate space for patient to move.

SKILL 37.1 USING SAFE AND EFFECTIVE TRANSFER TECHNIQUES—cont'd

STEPS	RATIONALE

(10) Instruct patient to use armrests on chair for support and ease into chair (see illustration for Step 1C[10]).
- Increases patient stability.

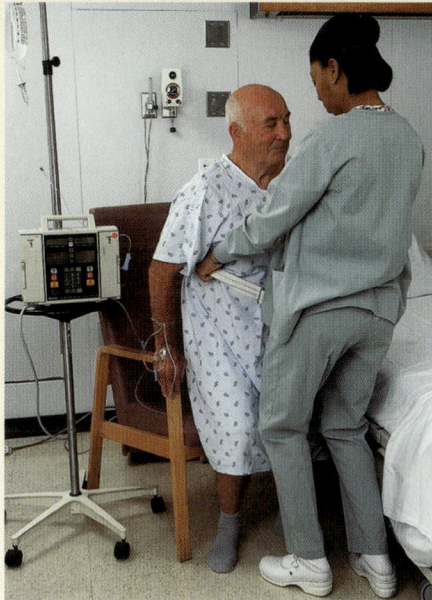

STEP 1C(10) Patient uses armrests for support.

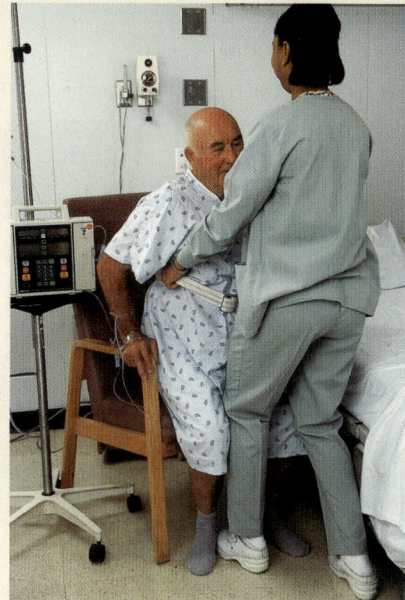

STEP 1C(11) Nurse eases patient into chair.

(11) Flex hips and knees while lowering patient into chair (see illustration for Step 1C[11]).
- Prevents injury to nurse from poor body mechanics.

(12) Assess patient for proper alignment for sitting position. Provide support for paralyzed extremities. A lapboard or sling supports the flaccid arm. Stabilize leg with bath blanket or pillow.
- Prevents injury to patient from poor body alignment.

(13) Praise patient's progress, effort, or performance.
- Continued support and encouragement provide incentive for patient perseverance.

D. Using mechanical lift and full-body sling to transfer an uncooperative patient who can bear partial weight or a patient who cannot bear weight and is either uncooperative or does not have upper-body strength to move from bed to chair:
- Mechanical lift devices prevent musculoskeletal injuries to health care workers (Lee et al., 2021; Roy et al., 2021).

(1) Position lift properly at bedside (see equipment instructions).
- Ensures safe elevation of patient off bed. (Before using lift, be thoroughly familiar with its operation.)

(2) Position chair near bed and allow adequate space to manoeuvre lift.
- Prepares environment for safe use of lift and subsequent transfer.

(3) Raise bed to high position with mattress flat. Lower side rail.
- Maintains nurse's alignment during transfer.

(4) Keep side rail up on side opposite from you.
- Maintains patient safety.

(5) Roll patient away from you.
- Positions patient for use of lift sling.

(6) Place sling under patient. Place lower edge under patient's knees (wide piece) and upper edge under patient's shoulders (narrow piece).
- Allows positioning of patient on mechanical/hydraulic sling. Places sling under patient's centre of gravity and greatest part of body weight.

(7) Roll patient to opposite side and pull body sling through.
- Completes positioning of patient on mechanical/hydraulic sling.

(8) Roll patient supine onto canvas seat.
- Sling needs to extend from shoulders to knees (hammock) to support patient's body weight equally.

(9) Remove patient's glasses if appropriate.
- Swivel bar is close to patient's head and can break eyeglasses.

(10) If using a transportable hydraulic lift, place horseshoe-shaped base of lift under side of bed (on side with chair).
- Positions hydraulic lift efficiently and promotes smooth transfer.

(11) Lower upper horizontal bar to sling level following manufacturer directions. Some lifts require valve to be locked.
- Positions lift close to patient. Locking valve prevents injury to patient.

Continued

SKILL 37.1   USING SAFE AND EFFECTIVE TRANSFER TECHNIQUES—cont'd

STEPS	RATIONALE
(12) Attach hooks on strap to holes in sling. Short straps hook to top holes of sling; longer straps hook to bottom of sling.	• Secures hydraulic lift to sling.
(13) Elevate head of bed.	• Positions patient in sitting position.
(14) Fold patient's arms over chest.	• Prevents injury to paralyzed arms.
(15) Use lift to raise patient off bed (see illustration for step 1D[15]).	• Moves patient off bed.

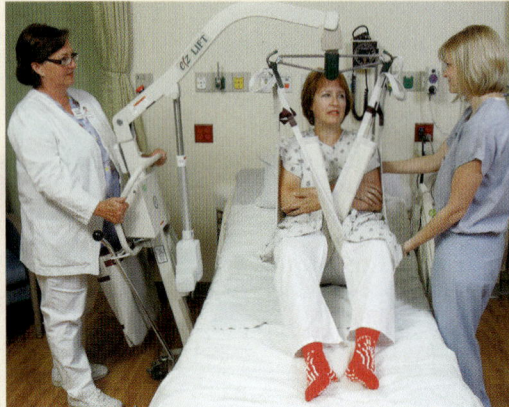

STEP 1D(15) Use mechanical lift to raise patient off bed.

STEPS	RATIONALE
(16) Use steering handle to pull lift from bed and manoeuvre to chair.	• Moves patient from bed to chair.
(17) Move lift to chair.	• Positions lift in front of chair.
(18) Position patient and lower slowly into chair following manufacturer guidelines (see illustration for Step 1D[18]).	• Safely guides patient into back of chair as seat descends.

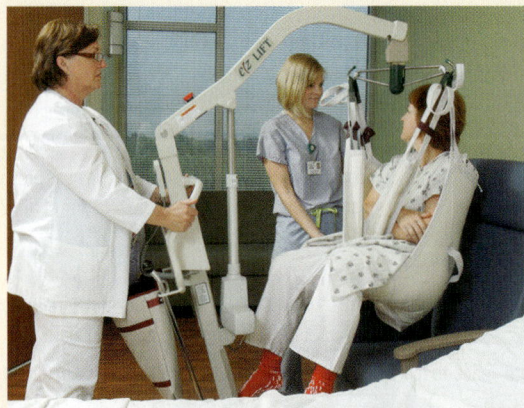

STEP 1D(18) Use mechanical lift to lower patient into chair.

STEPS	RATIONALE
(19) Remove straps and mechanical/hydraulic lift.	• Prevents damage to skin and underlying tissues from canvas or hooks.
(20) Check patient's sitting alignment and correct if necessary.	• Prevents injury from poor posture.
E. Transferring patient from bed to stretcher (bed at stretcher level):	
(1) Raise bed to height of stretcher.	• Bed and stretcher need to be at same level to allow patient to slide from bed to stretcher.
(2) Lower head of bed as much as patient can tolerate. Cross patient's arms on their chest. Ensure that bed brakes are locked.	• Prevents injury to arms during transfer.
(3) Lower side rails. Two caregivers stand on side where stretcher will be; third caregiver stands on other side.	• Minimizes caregivers' stretching. Prevents patient from falling out of bed and promotes safety.
(4) Two caregivers help patient roll onto side toward them (use of drawsheet is optional) with smooth, continuous motion.	• Positions patient for placing friction-reducing lateral transfer device.

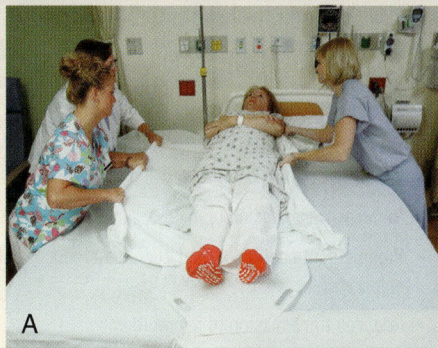

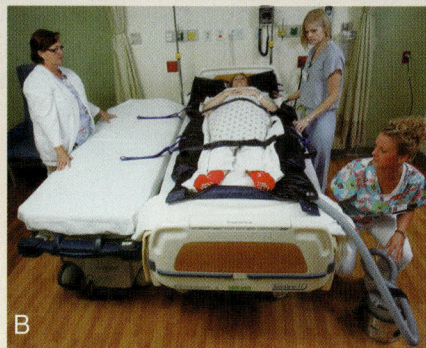

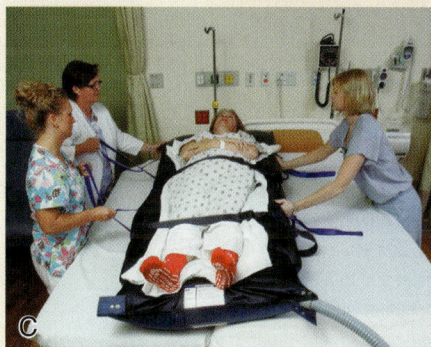

STEP 1E(5) **A,** Transfer of patient from bed to stretcher using slide board. **B,** Inflating air-assisted transfer device. **C,** Transfer of patient using air-assisted transfer device.

(5) Place slide board under drawsheet or follow manufacturer guidelines (see illustrations for Step 1E[5]). Gently roll patient back onto slide board.

(6) Align stretcher alongside bed. Lock wheels of stretcher once it is in place. Instruct patient not to move.

(7) All three caregivers place feet widely apart with one foot slightly in front of the other and grasp friction-reducing device.

(8) On count of three, two caregivers pull drawsheet or patient from bed onto stretcher while third person holds slide board in place. Using the friction-reducing slide board, shift weight from front to back foot (see illustration for Step 1E[8]). Position patient in centre of stretcher.

- Patient needs to be placed on transfer device properly to allow safe transfer.

- Positions stretcher in correct position for transfer and prevents patient from falling out of bed.

- Prepares for transfer. Wide base of support allows nurse to shift weight and minimizes back strain.

- Transfers patient smoothly and efficiently to the stretcher.

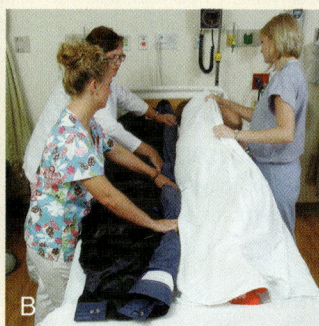

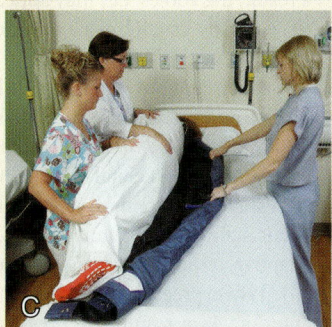

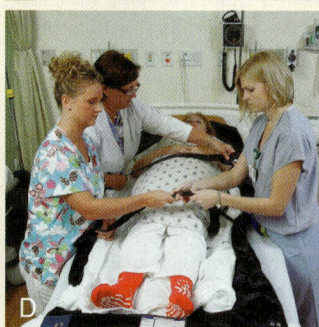

STEP 1E(8) **A,** Two caregivers position slide board under patient. **B,** Two caregivers place air-assisted device under patient. **C,** Patient rolls to opposite side while other caregiver unrolls air-assisted device. **D,** Secure safety straps.

SKILL 37.1   USING SAFE AND EFFECTIVE TRANSFER TECHNIQUES—cont'd

STEPS	RATIONALE
(9) Put up side rail of stretcher on side where caregivers are, roll stretcher away from side of bed, and put side rail up on that side.	• Side rails prevent patient from falling off stretcher.
(10) Cover patient with sheet or blanket.	• Promotes comfort and preserves patient dignity.
(11) Perform hand hygiene.	• Reduces transmission of microorganisms.
(12) Following transfer, evaluate patient's body alignment.	• Prompt identification of poor alignment reduces risks to patient's skin and musculoskeletal systems.
2. Perform hand hygiene.	• Reduces transmission of microorganisms.

EVALUATION

1. Evaluate vital signs. Ask if patient feels tired or dizzy.	• Evaluates patient's response to postural changes and activity.
2. Observe for correct body alignment and presence of pressure points on skin.	• Minimizes risk for immobility complications.
3. Ask if patient experienced pain during transfer; measure current pain level.	• Determines need for additional pain control or alteration of technique of transferring.
4. Use **teach back** to determine patient and family understanding about safe transfer techniques. State, "I want to be sure I explained how using the slide board prevents the risk for injury while we care for you. Can you explain to me the importance of using the slide board when we transfer you to a stretcher?" Revise instruction now or develop plan for revised patient teaching if patient is not able to teach back correctly.	• Evaluates what patient and family are able to explain or demonstrate.

UNEXPECTED OUTCOMES	RELATED INTERVENTIONS
Patient sustains injury on transfer	• Evaluate incident that caused injury (e.g., assessment inadequate, change in patient status, improper use of equipment). • Complete occurrence report according to institution policy.
Patient's level of weakness does not permit active transfer	• Obtain help from additional nursing personnel. • Increase bed activity and exercise to heighten tolerance.
Patient transfers well on some occasions, poorly on others	• Assess patient for factors that affect ability to transfer (e.g., pain, fatigue, confusion) before transfer. • Allow for a rest period before transferring, medicate for pain if indicated, or reorient patient.

RECORDING AND REPORTING

- Record procedure, including pertinent observations: weakness, ability to follow directions, weight-bearing ability, balance, ability to pivot, number of personnel needed to assist, and amount of assistance (muscle strength) required, in nurses' notes.
- Report any unusual occurrence to the nurse in charge. Report transfer ability and assistance needed to next shift or other caregivers. Report progress or transfer difficulties to rehabilitation staff (physiotherapist or occupational therapist).
- Document your evaluation of patient learning.

CARE IN THE COMMUNITY CONSIDERATIONS

- Teach family how to use safe patient-handling equipment, if necessary.
- Teach patient and family about the importance of safety while helping patients with mobility.

spinal curve occurs when the infant extends the neck from the prone position. As growth and stability increase, the thoracic spine straightens and the lumbar spinal curve appears, which allows sitting and standing.

The toddler's posture is awkward because of the slight swayback and protruding abdomen. As the child walks, the legs and feet are usually far apart and the feet are slightly everted. Toward the end of toddlerhood, posture appears less awkward, curves in the cervical and lumbar vertebrae are accentuated, and foot eversion disappears.

By the third year, the body is slimmer, taller, and better balanced. Abdominal protrusion is decreased, the feet are not as far apart, and the arms and legs have increased in length. The child appears more coordinated. The musculoskeletal system continues to grow and develop through adolescence (see Chapter 23).

Adolescence. Adolescent growth is often sporadic and uneven. As a result, the adolescent may appear awkward and uncoordinated. Adolescent girls usually grow and develop earlier than boys do. In girls, hips widen and fat is deposited in the upper arms, thighs, and buttocks. The adolescent boy's changes in shape are usually a result of long-bone growth and increased muscle mass (see Chapter 23).

Young to Middle-Aged Adults. A healthy adult also has the necessary musculoskeletal development and coordination to carry out ADLs. Normal changes in posture and body alignment in adulthood occur mainly in pregnant women. These changes result from the body's adaptive response to weight gain and the growing fetus (see Chapter 24). When pregnant, the woman's centre of gravity shifts toward the anterior. As a result, the pregnant woman leans back and is slightly swaybacked. Pregnant women frequently experience back pain.

Older Persons. In older persons, a progressive loss of bone mass occurs as a result of decreased physical activity, hormonal changes, and increased osteoclastic activity (activity by cells responsible for bone tissue absorption). Bone loss leads to weaker bones. Vertebrae become softer and long shaft bones become less resistant to bending. Changes in muscle tissue also occur as adults age, beginning as early as during the 20s for men and during the 40s for women. Muscle fibres shrink and have reduced tone and contractility. Strength and endurance change; fatigue occurs more readily, and overall energy may be reduced (Touhy et al., 2018).

Older persons may walk more slowly and appear less coordinated. They also may take smaller steps, keeping their feet closer together, which decreases their base of support. Thus, body balance may become unstable, and they are at greater risk for falls and injuries (see Chapter 25). It is important to encourage or plan physical activities for older persons. Exercise programs are important for socialization, independence, and maintaining core body strength. Physical exercise can improve endurance, coordination, and muscle stability and reduce risk for falls and injuries.

SAFETY ALERT Falls among older persons are a significant health concern in Canada. More than one-third of older persons experience falls. Falls are the leading cause of injury for older persons and can result in disability, persistent pain, loss of independence, reduced quality of life, and even death. In Canada, the direct health care costs for treating patients with falls are an estimated $2 billion annually (Healthcare Excellence, 2019). Use of fall risk assessment tools (Figure 37.5) and fall prevention initiatives (Box 37.3) can help to identify persons at risk for falls and implement prevention strategies

---

Behavioural Aspects. Physical activity benefits a person's overall holistic health and is reported to reduce stress (Goldstein et al., 2020). Patients are more likely to incorporate an exercise program into their daily lives if it is supported and assisted by family and friends, nurses, health care providers, and other members of the health care team. Nurses should take into consideration the patient's knowledge of exercise and activity, barriers to a program of exercise and physical activity, and current exercise habits.

Patients are more open to developing an exercise program if they are at the stage of being ready to change their behaviour. Prochaska and DiClemente's (1986) transtheoretical model of behaviour change has been the most utilized model of understanding and facilitating behaviour change since it was developed in the 1980s. It identifies five stages that individuals go through in implementing a lifestyle change: precontemplation, contemplation, preparation, action, and maintenance. Information on the benefits of regular exercise may be helpful to the patient in the contemplation stage. Patients' decisions to include a daily exercise routine in their lives may occur gradually with the provision of repeated information that is individualized to their needs and lifestyle (Box 37.4). Once the patient has reached the action stage, the nurse must develop, in collaboration with the patient, an exercise program that is customized to fit their needs. The nurse then must provide continued follow-up support and assistance until the exercise program becomes a daily routine.

It is vital for nurses to remember that personal choices and behaviours related to physical activity are shaped by the social determinants of health, including income and social status, employment and working conditions, physical environments, social support networks, biology and genetic endowment, education, access to health services, and healthy childhood development. Nurses must address potential barriers related to social, economic, and environmental factors to support patients and facilitate success with plans of care related to activity and exercise.

Environmental Issues

Health Policy. *A Common Vision for Increasing Physical Activity and Decreasing Sedentary Living in Canada: Let's Get Moving* (Public Health Agency of Canada [PHAC], 2020) is a framework that is informed and inspired by Indigenous perspectives, as well as input from many organizations, sectors, and leaders to guide policy to promote physical activity in Canada. The foundation, that physical activity for all, is guided by five principles: physical literacy, life course, population approach, evidence base, and motivation. The common vision is composed of six areas of focus for collaborative action: cultural norms, spaces and places, public engagement, partnerships, leadership and learning, and progress. The strategic initiatives require collaboration on behalf of organizations, communities, leaders, and governments to develop policy to address the biological, behavioural, social, psychological, technological, environmental, economic, and cultural factors that influence physical activity (Figure 37.6). Improving access, equity, and diversity; supporting physical literacy; encouraging play; and advocating supportive community design are initiatives to promote active living for all Canadians.

Work Sites. A common barrier for many patients is the lack of time needed to engage in a daily exercise program. Work sites have the potential to help their employees overcome the obstacle of time constraints by offering opportunities, reminders, and rewards for those committed to physical fitness (Burn et al., 2019). Signs could be used to encourage employees to use the stairs instead of elevators. Rewards such as free parking or discounted parking fees could be given to employees who walk from distant lots. For those who cycle or walk to work, establishing commuter groups can facilitate connections and support for new and continuing employees within agencies.

Schools. Sedentary behaviour and decreased physical activity are associated with childhood obesity (Liberali et al., 2021). Daily physical activity or physical education has been mandated in elementary schools across Canada. Children aged 5 to 11 years old should participate in at least 1 hour of moderate- to vigorous-intensity physical activity daily (Canadian Society for Exercise Physiology, 2021). Schools can provide a foundation for lifetime commitment to exercise and physical fitness by incorporating physical activity into a child's daily routine.

Community. The community's support of physical fitness can be instrumental in promoting the health of its members. Examples of community involvement to promote physical fitness are the provision of walking trails and track facilities in community parks and physical fitness classes offered by trained professionals. Success in implementing physical fitness programs depends on a collaborative effort between public health agencies, parks and recreational associations, provincial and local government agencies, health care agencies, and community members (Kelly et al., 2021).

Cultural and Ethnic Influences.
Culture plays an integral role in shaping environments to support physical activity. Cultural norms involve establishing social values and beliefs about physical activity (PHAC, 2020). Social norms that are supportive of physical activity are foundational in promoting physical activity as part of daily living—for example, walking rather than driving short distances to run errands, or taking the stairs rather than the elevator.

When nurses provide care for culturally diverse populations, it is important to assess individuals' perspectives of activity and how these are influenced by culture. Assess what motivates individuals to take up exercise and physical activity and what they see as appropriate, enjoyable, and beneficial. Variables that can influence participation, frequency, and duration when participating in exercise,

Alberta Health Services

Schmid Fall Risk Assessment Tool – Acute Care

To be completed on all patients upon admission, post-fall, and/or when the patient's status changes.
Score each area relating to patient's current status. Weights are in parenthesis.
Total weight at bottom.

Date of **Initial** Assessment: ____yyyy/mon/dd____   **Unit:** _____

**Select only one indicator for each category.

Mobility	Score	Score
(0) Ambulates with no gait disturbance		
(1) Ambulates or transfers with assistive devices		
(1) Ambulates with unsteady gait and no assistance		
(0) Unable to ambulate or transfer		

Mentation	Score	Score
(0) Alert oriented × 3		
(1) Periodic confusion		
(1) Confusion at all times		
(0) Comatose/unresponsive		

Elimination	Score	Score
(0) Independent in elimination		
(1) Independent with frequency or diarrhea		
(1) Needs assistance with toileting		
(1) Incontinence		

Prior Fall History (within past 6 months)	Score	Score
(1) Yes – Before admission (Home or previous inpatient care)		
(2) Yes – During this admission		
(0) No		
(0) Unknown		

Current Medications	Score	Score
(1) A score of I is given if the patient is on I or more of the following medications: Anti-convulsants/sedatives or psychotropics/hypnotics *(consider all medication side effects and role in fall risk)*		

	Score	Score
Total Score:		
Completed By: (signature/designation)		
Date: (yyyy/mon/dd)		

Total Score:
Score of 3 or more: Patient is at risk for falls and fall prevention interventions should be implemented–**see reverse side**

103511 ® Alberta Health Services. (2009/06)

FIGURE 37.5 Schmid Fall Risk Assessment Tool—Acute Care. (Nancy A. Schmid, MS, RN, NEA-BC.)

BOX 37.3	Unit Standard Fall Prevention Protocol

Use for all patients at risk for falls:
- Use appropriate orientation strategies.
- Use clear communication.
- Assist patients with sensory aids (i.e., hearing aids, glasses).
- Do comfort rounds every 2–3 hours (toileting needs, hydration, position changes).
- Teach patient and family about fall risk and prevention strategies.
- Ensure that call bell, personal items, and walking aids are within easy reach.
- Assess patient's understanding of the call bell system and determine if patient is able to use call bell.
- Remind patient to call for help when transferring, ambulating, and toileting.
- Assess whether patient is using assistive devices correctly.
- Have patient wear nonslip footwear for all transfers and ambulation.
- Clear barriers (e.g., clutter in room) prior to ambulating.

From Alberta Health Services. (2013). *Take action: Prevent a fall before it happens.* http://www.albertahealthservices.ca/assets/programs/ps-1051701-falls-prevention-guide.pdf

such as religious fasting periods, need to be considered. It is also important to know epidemiological statistics for specific chronic-disease entities that are associated with different cultural and ethnic groups (Box 37.5).

Family and Social Support

Social support can be used as a motivational tool to encourage and promote exercise and physical fitness. The patient can engage a friend or a significant other to participate in a "buddy system" whereby they walk together each day at a specified time. This companionship provides socialization and increases the enjoyment for some patients. It may lead to the development of a lifelong commitment to physical fitness. Parent engagement and support is essential when designing interventions to increase physical activity for children and adolescents. However, costs associated with access to recreational centres and organized sports can present a barrier for families. Facilitating access to safe facilities and opportunities for physical activity is a role that nurses can assume when supporting families to promote exercise and physical fitness (Khanom et al., 2020).

CRITICAL THINKING

Providing competent care requires a synthesis of knowledge, experience, and information gathered from patients; critical thinking attitudes; and intellectual and professional standards. Patients' conditions are always changing. Clinical judgements require nurses to anticipate the information necessary, analyze the data, and make decisions regarding patient care.

To understand activity tolerance and physical fitness and their impact on a patient, nurses must integrate knowledge from nursing and other disciplines, previous experiences, and information gathered from patients. As nurses begin the process of problem solving for patient care, a variety of concepts must be considered together to provide the best outcome for the patient. The foundation for planning and decision making is knowledge of the musculoskeletal system and of health alterations that create challenges for the patient in the area of activity, exercise, and body mechanics. In addition, nurses must stay current on and incorporate various guidelines, such as those supplied by Diabetes Canada (2018) and the *Canadian 24 Hour-Movement Guidelines: An*

BOX 37.4	General Strategies for Initiating and Maintaining an Exercise Program

There are five steps to beginning an exercise program:

Step 1: Assess Fitness Level
- Seek approval from a health care provider to begin. Are there any limitations to consider before determining the exercises in the fitness program?
- Record baseline fitness scores for aerobic and muscular fitness, flexibility, and body composition, such as the following: pulse rate before and after walking 1.6 km, how long it takes to walk 1.6 km, number of push-ups that can be done at a time, how far you are able to reach forward while seated on the floor with legs outstretched in front, waist circumference, and body mass index.

Step 2: Design the Fitness Program
- Consider fitness goals. Make goals attainable.
- Develop a balanced routine of aerobic activity and strength training.
- Start cautiously and progress slowly.
- Plan to include different activities.
- Try high-intensity interval training (HIIT).
- Build a program that includes different activities into a daily routine.
- Allow time for recovery.
- Record plan on paper to maintain adherence and assess progress.

Step 3: Assemble Equipment
- Choose athletic shoes designed for the chosen exercise.
- If choosing to exercise at home, try equipment at a fitness centre before purchasing.
- Consider fitness apps for smart devices to track distance, calories burned, or heart rate.

Step 4: Get Started
- Start slowly and build up a routine gradually.
- Divide exercise time throughout the day if time or fatigue is a barrier. Ten minutes of exercise three times a day instead of a single 30-minute workout may be better for some patients' schedules and medical conditions.
- Be creative and try a variety of activities.
- Listen to your body: if you feel pain, shortness of breath, or nausea, take a break. Avoid overexertion.
- Be flexible and give yourself permission to take days off if you are not feeling well.

Step 5: Monitor Progress
- Retake fitness assessment at 6 weeks and then every 3 to 6 months.
- If losing motivation: set new goals, exercise with a friend, or incorporate new activities.

Adapted from Mayo Clinic. (2021). *Healthy living fitness program: 5 steps to getting started.* http://www.mayoclinic.com/healthy-living/fitness/in-depth/fitness/art-20048269?pg=1

Integration of Physical Activity, Sedentary Behaviour, and Sleep developed by the Canadian Society for Exercise Physiology (2021).

Nurses' experiences and ability to think creatively enhance their approach to each new patient situation. For patients with limited exercise capacity or activity tolerance, nurses need to develop the nursing care plan to include interventions that maintain the present level of function with the goal of increasing the level of function. It is important to remember that patients have the capacity for improvement in spite of the impairments. Encouragement, support, commitment,

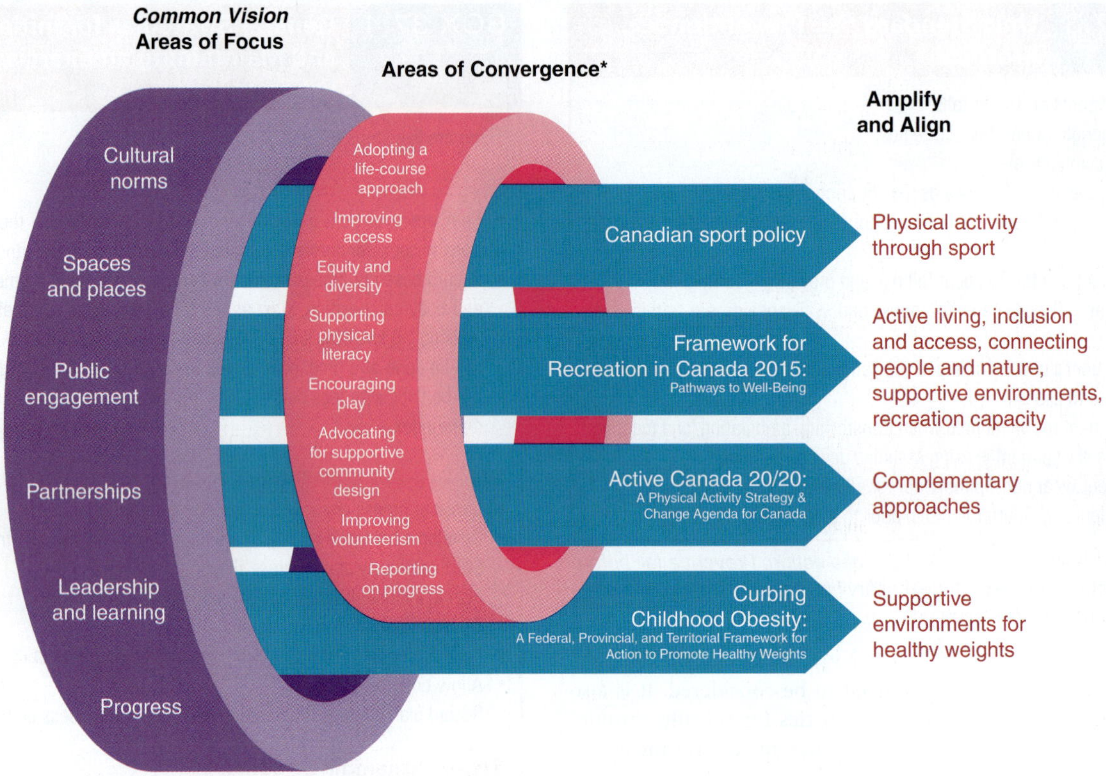

Common Vision Areas of Focus

Areas of Convergence*

Amplify and Align

Federal, Provincial and Territorial Ministers Responsible for Sport, Physical Activity and Recreation. (2015). Towards alignment: A collaborative agenda for recreation, sport and physical activity in Canada.

FIGURE 37.6 A common vision for increasing physical activity and reducing sedentary living in Canada framework. (© All rights reserved. Public Health Agency of Canada. [2018]. *A common vision for increasing physical activity and reducing sedentary living in Canada: Let's get moving.* Adapted and reproduced with permission from the Minister of Health, 2022.)

creativity, and perseverance are important attitudes in critical thinking for these patients.

Perseverance is necessary when caring for patients who depend on nurses for assistance with ambulation or exercise. In addition, responsibility for positioning often becomes repetitive, and nurses must recognize its importance (see Chapter 46). Perseverance is especially important in delegating these activities to other personnel and ensuring they are completed. Making certain that the task is performed correctly is also an essential nursing function. Difficulties with activity and mobility are often prolonged; creativity is necessary when designing interventions for improving activity tolerance and mobility skills.

❖ NURSING PROCESS

◆ Assessment

Assessment of body alignment and posture is completed with the patient standing, sitting, or lying down. Assess normal physiological changes in growth and development; deviations related to poor posture, trauma, muscle damage, or nerve dysfunction; and any learning needs of patients. Provide patients with opportunities to observe their posture and obtain important information about other factors that contribute to poor alignment, such as inactivity, fatigue, malnutrition, and psychological problems. To gather relevant information, ask questions related to the patient's exercise and activity tolerance. During assessment (Figure 37.7), consider all the elements that contribute to making appropriate nursing diagnoses.

Put the patient at ease so that unnatural or rigid positions are not assumed. When assessing body alignment of a patient who is immobilized or unconscious, remove pillows and positioning supports from the bed if not contraindicated, and place the patient in the supine position.

Patient Expectations

To ensure patient-centred care, assess a patient's expectations, values, and beliefs concerning activity and exercise and determine individual perceptions of what is normal or acceptable when developing a care plan. Perceived self-efficacy influences a person's willingness to engage in exercise. The outcomes people anticipate depend on their judgements of how well they will be able to perform in given situations (Bandura, 2006). Ask the patient to what extent they enjoy exercising and their belief in the ability to exercise. For example, pain and fatigue are factors that influence physical activity. When patients experience pain or fatigue following exercise, they may be unable to commit to exercise programs.

Body Alignment

Standing. Assessment of the standing patient includes the following: the head is erect and midline; body parts are symmetrical; the spine is straight with normal curvatures (cervical concave, thoracic convex, lumbar concave); the abdomen is comfortably tucked; the knees are in a straight line between the hips and ankles and slightly flexed; the feet are flat on the floor and pointed directly forward and slightly apart to maintain a wide base of support; and the arms hang comfortably at

BOX 37.5 CULTURAL ASPECTS OF CARE

Physical Activity

The Truth and Reconciliation Commission of Canada's (TRC) report exposed the impact of colonization on Indigenous culture, including lasting impacts of intergenerational trauma, loss of Indigenous culture and identity, and neglect of investment in infrastructure to facilitate healthy living conditions. Additionally, food insecurity has further affected health of individuals in Indigenous communities. Epidemiological studies indicate that physical inactivity is one of the risk factors associated with non–insulin-dependent diabetes mellitus (NIDDM). Historically, activity was a fundamental part of everyday life for all Canadians, as a mechanism for transportation, acquiring food, and labour. Rapid advances in technology are contributing to an increasingly sedentary lifestyle. In Canada, NIDDM is between 3.6 and 5.3 times more prevalent in the Indigenous population. Colonization has influenced traditional activity patterns of Indigenous people and has contributed to unhealthy living conditions arising from inadequate infrastructure and access to resources. Physical activity has been identified as playing an important role in the prevention and treatment of NIDDM, yet the Indigenous population has a disproportionate number of poor, unemployed, and disadvantaged individuals who lack access to recreation and leisure activities.

Implications for Practice

- Because physical inactivity is a modifiable risk factor for the development of NIDDM, prevention and treatment programs need to focus on activity and exercise and be tailored to the activity tolerance of the individual patient.
- Promotion of physical activity should be supported by recognizing that a symbiotic relationship exists between cultural values and traditional leisure pursuits. Patients with a strong spiritual connection to the land may enjoy outdoor or wilderness recreation.
- Actively collaborate with individuals and community groups when planning educational program initiatives to raise awareness of activity and exercise.
- Development of an exercise or prevention program, or both, should attempt to address social determinants of health to remove potential barriers, such as transportation and cost, to facilitate commitment to the program (Klepac Pogrmilovic et al., 2021).

Adapted from National Collaborating Centre for Aboriginal Health. (2013). *Physical activity fact sheet.* https://www.ccnsa-nccah.ca/495/Physical_Activity_Fact_Sheet.nccah?id=72; Public Health Agency of Canada. (2018). *A common vision for increasing physical activity and reducing sedentary living in Canada: Let's get moving.* https://www.canada.ca/en/public-health/services/publications/healthy-living/lets-get-moving.html#pa

the sides (Figure 37.8). The patient's centre of gravity is in the midline, and the line of gravity is from the middle of the forehead to a midpoint between the feet. Laterally, the line of gravity runs vertically from the middle of the skull to the posterior third of the foot (Wilson & Giddens, 2017). During assessment, the nurse needs to identify deviations from expected findings. Self-assessment of body alignment when standing is also important for the nurse, to optimize body mechanics for safe patient handling to prevent personal injury.

Mobility

Assessment of mobility helps the nurse to determine the patient's coordination and balance while the patient is walking, the ability to carry out ADLs, and the ability to participate in an exercise program. The assessment of **mobility**, the ability of the body to move freely and easily, has four components: ROM, gait, exercise, and activity tolerance.

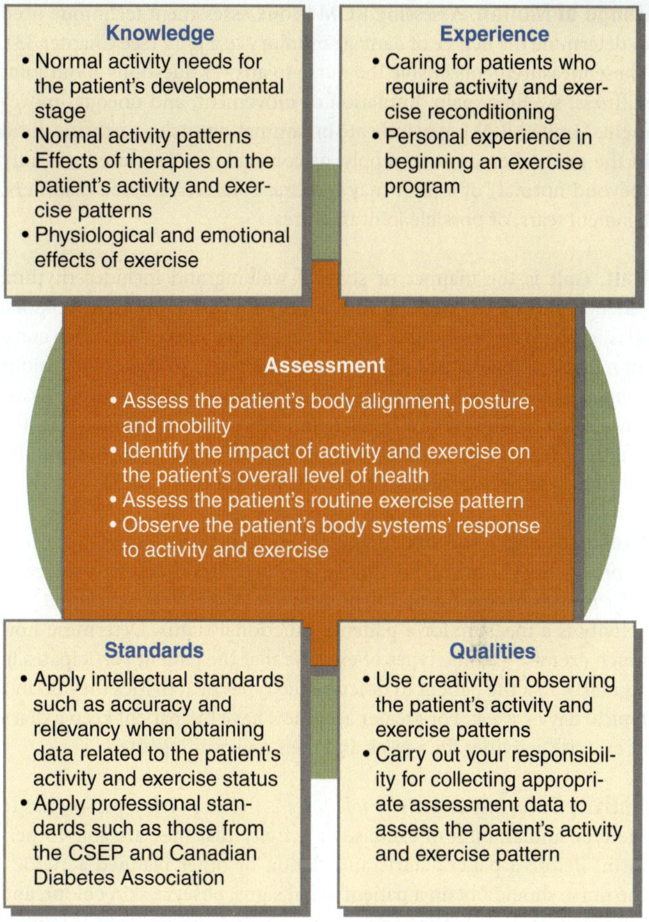

FIGURE 37.7 Critical thinking model for activity and exercise assessment. *CSEP,* Canadian Society for Exercise Physiology.

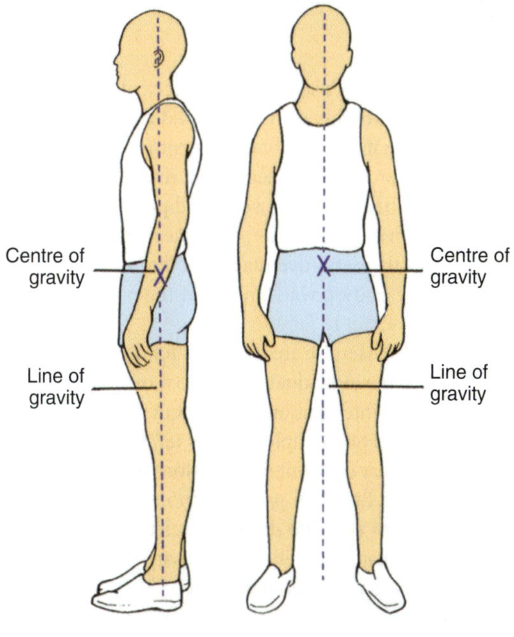

FIGURE 37.8 Correct body alignment when standing.

Range of Motion. Assessing ROM is one assessment technique used to determine the degree of damage or injury to a joint (see Chapter 33). These measurements enable the nurse to answer questions about joint stiffness, swelling, pain, limitation of movement, and unequal movement. Limited ROM may indicate inflammation such as arthritis, fluid in the joint, altered nerve supply, or contractures. Increased mobility (beyond normal) of a joint may indicate connective tissue disorders, ligament tears, or possible joint fractures.

Gait. Gait is the manner or style of walking and includes rhythm, cadence, and speed. Walking with a limp is a gait. Propulsive, scissors, spastic, steppage, and waddling are descriptive names for other common gaits. Assessing gait allows you as the nurse to draw conclusions about a patient's balance, posture, and ability to walk without assistance. Note conformity; a regular, smooth rhythm; symmetry in the length of leg swing; smooth swaying related to the gait phase; and a smooth, symmetrical arm swing (Wilson & Giddens, 2017).

Exercise and Activity. Regular exercise conditions the body, improves health, maintains fitness, and provides therapy to correct a deformity or restore the overall body to a maximal state of health. Daily activity is a measure for a patient's functional status. Determine how much exercise and the types of exercise that the patient participates in regularly. Ask the patient to describe the types of activities they do in a typical day or week. For greater accuracy, have the patient keep a diary of exercise activities for a week and then review it together.

Activity Tolerance. *Activity tolerance* is the response a person has to the type and amount of exercise or activity that they are able to perform. Before a patient starts ambulation or other planned activities, the nurse should obtain a patient's vital signs, observe skin colour, and ask about level of comfort and current energy level or sense of fatigue. Nurses need to assess activity tolerance when planning physical activity for health promotion and for patients with acute or chronic illness. This assessment provides baseline data about a patient's activity patterns and assists in determining which factors (physical, psychological, or motivational) are affecting activity tolerance. Box 37.6 lists factors that affect activity tolerance. Box 37.7 lists nursing assessment questions to ask.

◆ Nursing Diagnosis

Assessment of the patient's activity tolerance, physical fitness, body alignment, and joint mobility provides related clusters of data or defining characteristics that help the nurse identify a nursing diagnosis. Nurses must be accurate when identifying diagnoses. For example, a patient who reports being tired or weakened potentially could be diagnosed as having *activity intolerance or fatigue.* Defining characteristics are used to lead to the definitive diagnosis. For example, a finding of abnormal heart rate or dyspnea would lead the nurse to the diagnosis of *activity intolerance*, not to *fatigue.*

When activity and exercise are problems for a patient, nursing diagnoses often focus on the individual's ability to move. The diagnostic label should direct nursing interventions. This requires the correct selection of the related factors. For example, *activity intolerance related to excess weight gain* requires very different interventions than if the related factor is prolonged bed rest. Box 37.8 provides an example of how the diagnostic process leads to accurate diagnosis selection. The following are examples of nursing diagnoses related to activity and exercise:

- *Activity intolerance, potential to develop*
- *Health-seeking behaviours*
- *Readiness for enhanced self-care*
- *Risk for activity intolerance*

BOX 37.6   Factors Influencing Physical Activity Tolerance

Physiological Factors
Skeletal abnormalities
Muscular impairments
Endocrine or metabolic illnesses (e.g., diabetes mellitus or thyroid disease)
Hypoxemia
Decreased cardiac function
Decreased endurance
Impaired physical stability
Pain
Sleep pattern disturbance
Prior exercise patterns
Infectious processes and fever

Emotional Factors
Anxiety
Depression
Chemical addictions
Motivation

Developmental Factors
Age
Gender

Pregnancy
Physical growth and development of muscle and skeletal support

Modified from Lewis, S. L., Bucher, L., Heitkemper, M. M., et al. (2019). *Medical-surgical nursing in Canada* (4th ed.). Elsevier.

- *Ineffective activity planning*
- *Risk for ineffective activity planning*
- *Ineffective coping*
- *Impaired gas exchange*
- *Risk for injury*
- *Impaired physical mobility*
- *Imbalanced nutrition: more than body requirements*
- *Acute or persistent pain*
- *Risk for disuse syndrome*

◆ Planning

During planning, nurses need to synthesize information from multiple resources (Figure 37.9). The nurse's critical thinking ensures that the patient's care plan integrates all patient information. Best practice guidelines are especially important to consider when developing a care plan, as these documents establish scientifically based guidelines for selecting effective nursing interventions.

Concept maps assist in the planning of care. Figure 37.10 shows the relationship between a patient's medical diagnosis of heart failure and the identified nursing diagnosis.

Goals and Outcomes

Once the nurse has identified the nursing diagnoses, the nurse and the patient can set goals and expected outcomes to direct interventions. The plan includes consideration of pre-existing health concerns and of any risks of injury to the patient. It is especially important to have knowledge of the patient's home environment when planning therapies to maintain or improve activity, body alignment, and mobility. For some patients with alterations in joint mobility, family members may be the providers of care. It is important to include the patient's family in the care plan.

BOX 37.7 Nursing Assessment Questions

Nature of the Problem
- Tell me about the types of problems you are having with physical activities and exercise.
- How much do you exercise each day?
- Describe your typical day. What types of activities do you do?
- What types of exercise do you prefer?
- How long do you exercise at any given time?

Signs and Symptoms
- Do you have any muscle or joint pain during or after exercise?
- Do you have shortness of breath during any activity?
- Do you ever feel chest discomfort or pain during exercise or physical activity?

Onset and Duration
- Which activities cause you to become short of breath?
- How long does it take to resume normal breathing after exercise or physical activity?

Severity
- How far do you walk before the pain in your legs begins?
- On a scale of 0 to 10 (with 10 being the worst discomfort), rate your leg pain.
- Describe your shortness of breath as minimal, moderate, or severe after physical activities or exercise, or both.

Barriers to Exercise and Activity
- Do you have any chronic illnesses that affect your ability to carry out daily activities, such as grocery shopping, washing clothes, or daily walking?
- Do you have any physical limitations that prevent you from exercising on a daily basis?
- Do you have access to a community walking path or exercise equipment, or both?
- What prevents you from exercising 30 minutes each day?

Patient Values
- Tell me what you believe about the importance of regular exercise.
- How confident are you in being able to perform the exercises your health care provider has recommended?

Effect on Patient
- Has the lack of an exercise routine affected your weight?
- Do you feel more tired since you have not been able to exercise on a routine basis?
- Have you noticed any increase in shortness of breath when performing activities that require little exertion?

BOX 37.8 NURSING DIAGNOSTIC PROCESS
Impaired Physical Mobility

Assessment Activities	Defining Characteristics
Observe patient's gait.	Shuffled gait
	Uncoordinated gait
	Patient reports slower walking speed
Observe patient performing tasks such as eating, dressing, or recreational activities.	Uncoordinated movements
	Limited fine motor coordination
Measure range of joint motion.	Reduced joint motion in lower or upper extremities, or both
	Stiffness in joints
	Pain with movement
Measure patient's strength.	Has difficulty rising to sitting position or exiting bed

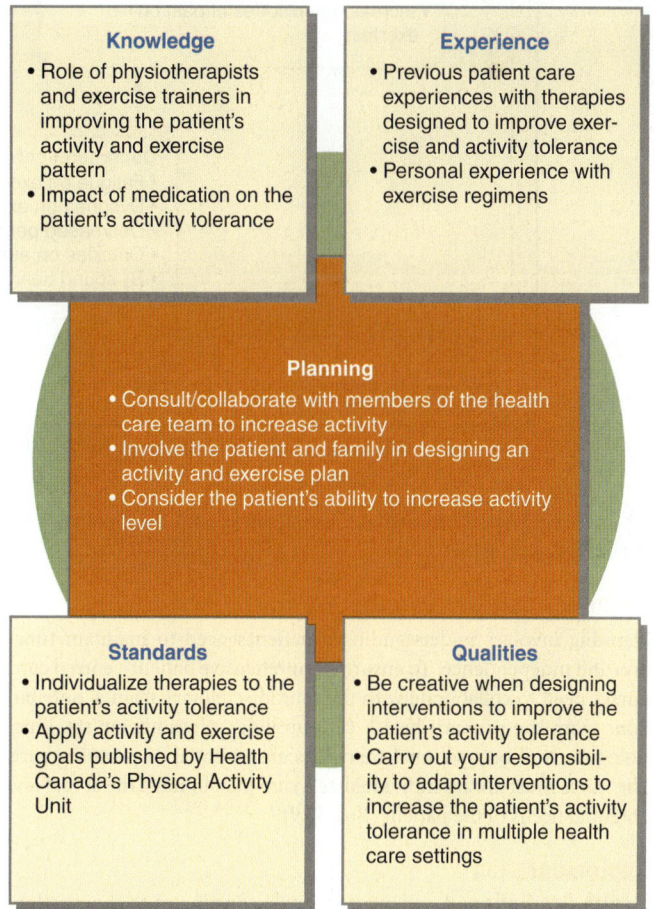

Knowledge
- Role of physiotherapists and exercise trainers in improving the patient's activity and exercise pattern
- Impact of medication on the patient's activity tolerance

Experience
- Previous patient care experiences with therapies designed to improve exercise and activity tolerance
- Personal experience with exercise regimens

Planning
- Consult/collaborate with members of the health care team to increase activity
- Involve the patient and family in designing an activity and exercise plan
- Consider the patient's ability to increase activity level

Standards
- Individualize therapies to the patient's activity tolerance
- Apply activity and exercise goals published by Health Canada's Physical Activity Unit

Qualities
- Be creative when designing interventions to improve the patient's activity tolerance
- Carry out your responsibility to adapt interventions to increase the patient's activity tolerance in multiple health care settings

FIGURE 37.9 Critical thinking model for activity and exercise planning.

Family caregivers play critical roles in the home environment, motivating and coaching patients to stay active. The general goal related to exercise and activity is to improve or maintain the patient's motor function and independence. The following are examples of outcomes for patients with deficits in activity and exercise (Ackley et al., 2020):
- Participates in prescribed physical activity while maintaining appropriate heart rate, blood pressure, and breathing rate
- States symptoms of adverse effects of exercise and reports onset of symptoms immediately
- Maintains normal skin colour; skin is warm and dry with activity
- Verbalizes an understanding of the need to increase activity gradually according to tolerance and symptoms
- Demonstrates increased tolerance to activity

Setting Priorities

Care planning is patient-centred, taking into consideration the patient's most immediate needs. Nurses need to determine the immediacy of any health problem by its effect on the patient's mental and physical health. For example, a patient may have chronic diseases such as diabetes and hypertension, which would be improved with an increase in exercise. However, if that same patient has recently

> concept map

Fatigue
- Patient reports decreased energy level
- Patient is unable to complete activities
- Patient limits activities with family

Impaired gas exchange
- Dyspnea with activity
- Respiratory rate >28 breaths/min at rest, SaO_2 80–85%
- Pallor
- Restless

Patient's chief medical diagnosis: Heart failure (NY class III)
Priority assessments: Levels of fatigue and dyspnea, exercise intolerance, chest pain

Acute pain
- Chest pain 6 on a scale of 0–10
- Increasing episodes of pain on exertion

Activity tolerance
- Patient reports increasing fatigue
- Increased chest pain on exertion
- Increased dyspnea on exertion

Decreased cardiac output
- Fatigue on exertion
- Dyspnea on exertion
- Decreased peripheral pulses <2+
- Crackles on auscultation
- S_3 sound heard on auscultation

——— Link between medical diagnosis and nursing diagnosis   - - - - Link between nursing diagnoses

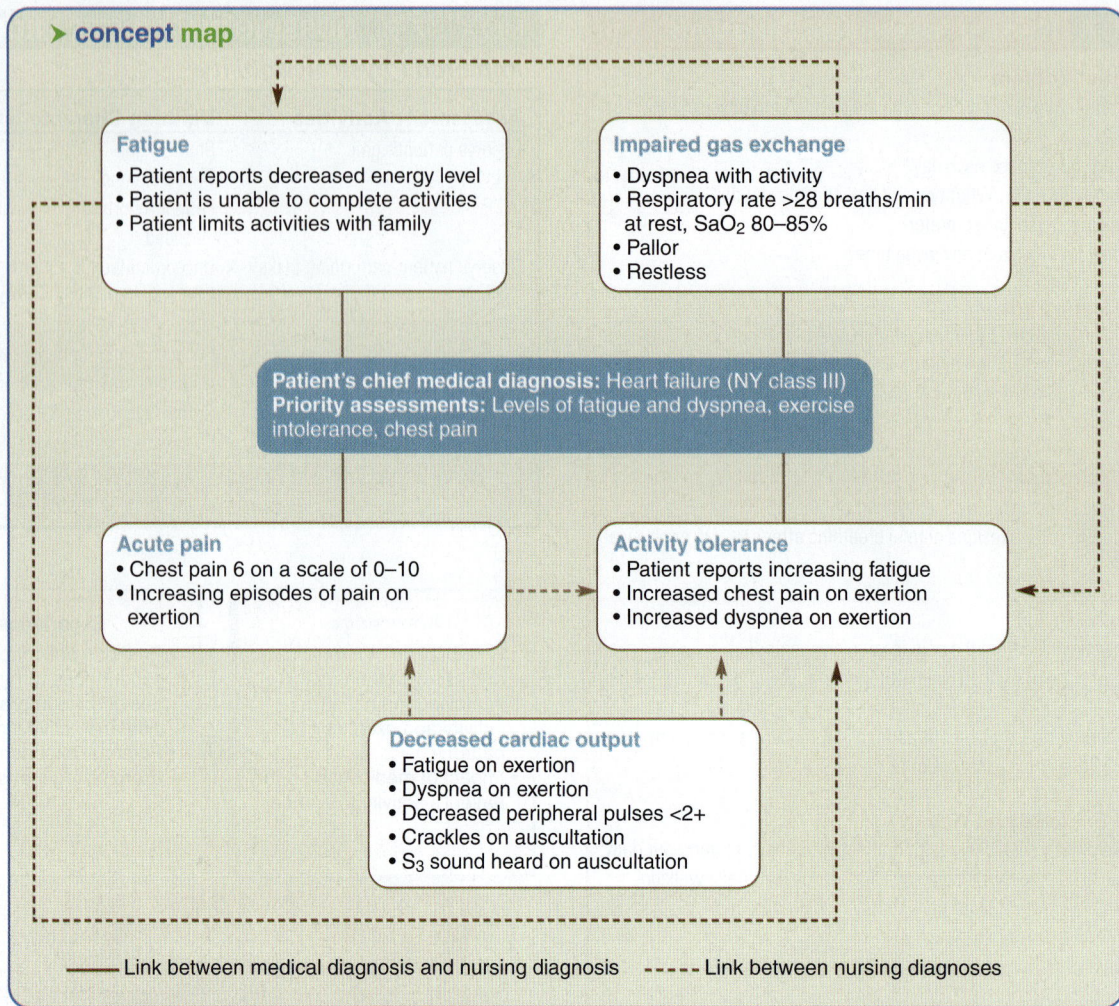

FIGURE 37.10 Concept map for a patient with heart failure and decreased activity.

experienced angina, immediate investigation and treatment of the angina is the priority.

Teamwork and Collaboration

Planning involves understanding a patient's need to maintain function and independence. To ensure comprehensive patient-centred care, nurses need to collaborate with the multidisciplinary team. Contributions from the primary health care provider, physiotherapists, kinesiologists, and occupational therapists are essential in planning care. The nurse must always individualize a care plan to meet the actual and potential needs of the patient (Box 37.9).

◆ Implementation

Health Promotion. A sedentary lifestyle contributes to the development of health-related challenges. As a nurse, you can promote health by encouraging patients to engage in a regular exercise program in any setting (Box 37.10). Discuss the recommendations for physical activity and fitness with the patient (Box 37.11). Design a program of physical activity in collaboration with the patient, taking into account age and developmental (see Box 37.11) and cultural factors. Collaborate with the patient's health care provider, physiotherapist, occupational therapist, and other members of the health care team to ensure patient-centred care.

Before starting an exercise program, teach patients to calculate their maximum heart rate by subtracting their current age in years from 220

and then determine their target heart rate by calculating 60% to 90% of this maximum rate, depending on their health care provider's recommendation. Patients should be taught to monitor their pulse during exercise and to exercise so that the heart rate is maintained within the target range.

Regardless of the exercise prescription implemented by the patient, warm-up and cool-down periods must be included in the program (Dames et al., 2021). The warm-up period usually lasts 5 to 10 minutes and may include stretching, calisthenics, and subsequent aerobic activity performed at a lower intensity. The warm-up period prepares the body and decreases the potential for injury. The cool-down period follows the exercise routine and usually lasts 5 to 10 minutes. The cool-down period allows the body to readjust to baseline functioning gradually and provides an opportunity to combine movement such as stretching with relaxation-enhancing mind–body awareness (Dames et al., 2021).

Many patients find it difficult to incorporate an exercise program into their daily routines because of time constraints. For these patients, it is beneficial to reinforce that exercise can be incorporated in small amounts—as little as 10 minutes at a time. Activities such as taking a short walk at lunch or walking to the corner store instead of driving can help increase total exercise. A more active lifestyle can involve taking the stairs instead of the elevator and parking farther from the entrance.

Other patients may benefit from a prescribed exercise and physical fitness program carefully designed to meet their needs and

BOX 37.9 NURSING CARE PLAN

Activity Intolerance

ASSESSMENT

Mrs. Mary Wertenberger is a 45-year-old homemaker. She has enrolled in a cardiovascular disease prevention (CDP) program prescribed by her health care provider and conducted by Eric Sieple, a registered nurse. Mrs. Wertenberger has several risk factors associated with cardiovascular disease. She expresses feelings of stress resulting from excessive demands on her time. Eric's assessment includes a discussion of Mrs. Wertenberger's current health conditions as well as a pertinent physical examination.

Assessment Activities	Findings and Defining Characteristics*
Ask Mrs. Wertenberger what prompted her health care provider to recommend a CDP program.	She responds, "I *gained 23 kg* over the past year. I become *fatigued* easily and lack the energy to keep up with even simple household chores. I don't want to leave the house anymore."
Ask Mrs. Wertenberger about her exercise and eating habits.	She responds, "I want to exercise but with the demands of child care and caring for my aging parents, I just don't feel like it. I feel pulled in every direction, that increases my stress, and then I want to eat, eat, eat!"
Perform baseline assessment.	Height: 160 cm Weight: *102 kg* Blood pressure: *152/90 mm Hg (at rest)* Pulse: 96 beats per minute (at rest) Breathing rate: 20 breaths per minute (at rest) Blood pressure: *164/96 mm Hg (climbing 10 steps)* Pulse: *120 beats per minute (climbing 10 steps)* Breathing rate: *36 breaths per minute (climbing 10 steps)*

*Defining characteristics are shown in italics.

NURSING DIAGNOSIS: Activity intolerance related to excessive weight gain, inactivity, and lack of cardiovascular fitness

PLANNING

Goals (Nursing Outcomes Classification)†	Expected Outcomes
	Health Beliefs
Mrs. Wertenberger will develop a plan of exercise that incorporates isotonic and isometric exercises.	Mrs. Wertenberger will state the physiological and psychological effects of exercise. Patient will commit to performing physical exercise at home.
	Activity Tolerance
Mrs. Wertenberger's activity tolerance will improve above baseline.	Mrs. Wertenberger will perform 20 minutes of exercise two times a week over the next 2 weeks. Mrs. Wertenberger will record exercise patterns three to four times over the next 2 weeks. Mrs. Wertenberger's level of fatigue associated with exercise will remain the same or decrease.
	Cardiovascular Pump Effectiveness
Mrs. Wertenberger's cardiopulmonary response to exercise will improve.	Mrs. Wertenberger's resting diastolic blood pressure will be below 80 mm Hg. Her systolic blood pressure will be below 140 mm Hg. Her resting heart rate will range between 75 and 85 beats per minute. Her respiratory rate will be 14 breaths/minute (at rest).

*Outcome classification labels from Moorhead, S., Swanson, E., Johnson, M., et al. (Eds.). (2018). *Nursing outcomes classification (NOC)* (6th ed.). Mosby.

INTERVENTIONS

Interventions (Nursing Interventions Classification)‡	Rationale
Exercise Promotion	
Provide Mrs. Wertenberger with information about the physiological benefits of a regular exercise program. Match instruction with her beliefs about the value of exercise.	Physical activity and exercise protect against the development of cardiovascular disease (CVD) and decrease other risk factors associated with CVD, such as obesity, hypertension, and hyperlipidemia (Joseph et al., 2020; Lacombe et al., 2019).
Provide Mrs. Wertenberger with information about the psychological benefits of a regular exercise program.	Physical activity and exercise increase self-esteem, feelings of enjoyment, self-confidence, and mood and decrease physical and psychological stress, anxiety, and depression (Goldstein et al., 2020).
Develop a progressive plan of exercise with Mrs. Wertenberger, such as 3 to 5 km or 20 minutes of brisk walking and quadriceps, biceps, and gluteal muscle isometric exercises three to four times per week.	Cross-training (a combination of exercise activities) provides variety to reduce boredom and increases potential for total body conditioning (Dames et al., 2021).

Continued

BOX 37.9   NURSING CARE PLAN—cont'd

Activity Intolerance

Interventions (Nursing Interventions Classification)‡	Rationale
Advise Mrs. Wertenberger to use an exercise log and to record the day, time, duration, and responses (pulse, feelings, shortness of breath, daily weight).	Keeping a log may increase adherence to exercise prescription.
Schedule weekly meetings with Mrs. Wertenberger for follow-up and review of exercise log, progress, and barriers.	Patients are more likely to increase physical activity and remain adherent to an exercise program if they are counselled by a health care provider (Dames et al., 2021).

‡Intervention classification labels from Butcher, H. K., Bulechek, G. M., McCloskey Dochterman, J. M., et al. (Eds.). (2019). *Nursing interventions classification (NIC)* (7th ed.). Mosby.

EVALUATION

Nursing Actions	Patient Responses and Findings	Achievement of Outcomes
Review Mrs. Wertenberger's exercise log at each visit.	She responds, "I make time to exercise because of this log. I hate missing a day and leaving a blank page; this represents failure. I want to succeed." Exercise log documents activity four times per week.	Mrs. Wertenberger reports enjoying exercise, as well as observing some personal benefits of exercise. The exercise log is facilitating adherence to the exercise prescription.
Record weight, blood pressure, and pulse.	Weight, 95 kg. Resting heart rate between 80 and 85 beats per minute. Blood pressure, 146/86 mm Hg.	Improved cardiovascular effects of exercise: • Heart rate is within normal range. • Blood pressure is lower but not at expected range. Monitor blood pressure as patient continues to lose weight.
Ask Mrs. Wertenberger if exercise is helping to lower fatigue level.	Mrs. Wertenberger responds, "At first, finding time to exercise was hard, but once I started feeling less tired and even less stressed, it was easy to integrate exercise into my daily activities."	Achieved improved activity tolerance with exercise.

BOX 37.10   Promoting Exercise

Nurses can do the following to help patients participate in exercise:
- Provide patients with information about the importance of exercise in preserving health.
- Encourage patients to pace activities and increase speed and intensity gradually to avoid pain.
- Administer prescribed anti-inflammatory medications 1 to 2 hours before starting an exercise program.
- Encourage patients to balance rest and activity and to get plenty of sleep.
- Teach patients how to use canes or walkers to assist with walking as needed.
- Encourage patients to choose smooth and even walking surfaces.
- Advise patients not to force joints past the point of resistance or pain.
- Instruct patients to check legs and feet daily for redness, swelling, blisters, or broken skin.
- Instruct patients to wear properly fitting shoes with nonslip soles.
- Encourage patients to walk with a companion or group so that exercise is socially rewarding.

expectations. A comprehensive exercise prescription incorporates a combination of aerobic exercise, stretching and flexibility exercises, and resistance training. Aerobic exercise includes such activities as walking, running, bicycling, aerobic dance, jumping rope, and cross-country skiing. Recommended frequency of aerobic exercise is three to five times per week, or every other day. For a patient who prefers to exercise every day, cross-training is recommended. For example, the patient may run one day and do yoga on the next day.

Stretching and flexibility exercises include active ROM exercises that allow for stretching of all muscle groups and joints. This form of exercise is ideal for warm-up and cool-down periods. Benefits include increased flexibility, improved circulation and posture, and an opportunity for relaxation.

Resistance training increases muscle strength and endurance and is associated with improved performance of daily activities and avoidance of injuries and disability. Formal resistance training includes weight training, but the same benefits can be obtained by performing ADLs such as pushing a vacuum cleaner, raking leaves, shoveling snow, and kneading bread. Some patients may use weight training to bulk up their muscles. However, the purpose of weight training from a health perspective is to develop tone and strength and to stimulate and maintain healthy bones (Brellinthin et al., 2019).

Body Mechanics. The Canadian Centre for Occupational Health and Safety (2019) has published numerous guidelines related to ergonomic standards for preventing musculoskeletal injuries in the workplace. More than half of all back pain in health care settings is associated with manual lifting tasks (Workers Health and Safety Centre, 2019). Back injuries are often the direct result of improper lifting and bending. The most common back injury is strain on the muscle group around the lumbar vertebrae. Injury to this area affects the ability to bend forward, backward, and from side to side. The ability to rotate the hips and lower back is also decreased. Body mechanics alone are not sufficient to prevent musculoskeletal injuries when lifting or transferring patients (Roy et al., 2021).

Before repositioning a patient, assess the weight to be moved and what assistance the patient can provide. Never attempt to lift a patient

BOX 37.11 Recommendations for Physical Activity

24-Hour Movement Guidelines for Children 5–11 and Youths 12–17 Years of Age
Preamble
- 24-hour movement guidelines are relevant for healthy children and youth, irrespective of gender, race, ethnicity, or socioeconomic status of the family.
- Children and youth are encouraged to have a balanced lifestyle with a daily balance of sleep, sedentary behaviours, and physical activities that support healthy development.
- Children and youth should participate in a range of physical activities, in a variety of environments (i.e., home, community, school; indoors and outdoors; land and water) and contexts (i.e., play, recreation, sport, active transportation, hobbies, and chores) across all seasons.
- Following guidelines for integrated physical activity, sedentary behaviour, and sleep is associated with better body composition, cardiorespiratory and muscle fitness, academic achievement and cognition, emotional regulation, prosocial behaviours, cardiovascular and metabolic health, and overall quality of life.
- Guidelines may be appropriate for children with a disability or medical condition; however, a health care provider should be consulted for additional guidance.

Guidelines
- At least 60 minutes of moderate- to vigorous-intensity physical activity daily involving a variety of aerobic activities
- Vigorous-intensity activities at least 3 days per week
- Activities that strengthen muscle and bone at least 3 days per week
- Several hours of a variety of structured and unstructured light physical activities
- Uninterrupted 9–11 hours of sleep per night (ages 5–13) and 8–10 hours per night (ages 14–17), with consistent bed and wake-up times
- No more than 2 hours per day of recreational screen time
- Limited sitting for extended periods
- Greater health benefits can be achieved by preserving sufficient sleep, greater time spent outdoors, and replacing sedentary behaviours and light physical activity with additional moderate to vigorous physical activity.

24-Hour Movement Guidelines for Adults 18–64 Years of Age
Preamble
- 24-hour movement guidelines are relevant to adults (aged 18–64), irrespective of gender, cultural background, or socioeconomic status.
- The guidelines may not be appropriate for adults who are pregnant or for persons living with a disability or medical condition.
- Adults should participate in a range of physical activities (i.e., weight bearing, non–weight bearing, sport and recreation) in a variety of environments (i.e., home, work, community; indoors and outdoors; land and water) and contexts (i.e., transportation, leisure, household) across all seasons.
- Long periods of sedentary behaviours should be limited.

- Healthy sleep hygiene (routines, behaviours, and environments) is conducive to sleeping well.
- Balanced activity, sedentary behaviour, and sleep can lower the risk of mortality, cardiovascular disease, hypertension, type 2 diabetes, several cancers, anxiety, depression, dementia, and weight gain while improving bone health, cognition, quality of life, and physical function.

Guidelines
A healthy 24 hours includes the following:
- Moderate to vigorous aerobic activities to accumulate to at least 150 minutes per week
- Muscle- and bone-strengthening activities using major muscle groups, at least 2 days per week
- 7–9 hours of good-quality sleep on a regular basis with consistent bed and wake-up times
- Limiting sedentary time to 8 hours or less, including no more than 3 hours of recreational screen time and breaking up long periods of sitting as much as possible

24-Hour Movement Guidelines for Adults Aged 65 and Older
Preamble
- 24-hour movement guidelines are relevant to adults aged 65 years or older, irrespective of gender, cultural background, or socioeconomic status.
- Guidelines may not be appropriate for adults aged 65 years or older who are living with a disability or mental condition and who should consult a health care provider for guidance.
- Long periods of sedentary behaviours should be limited.
- Healthy sleep hygiene (routines, behaviours, and environments) is conducive to sleeping well.
- Following guidelines is associated with health benefits including lower risk of mortality, cardiovascular disease, hypertension, type 2 diabetes, several cancers, anxiety, depression, dementia, weight gain, falls and fall-related injuries and improved bone health, cognition, quality of life, and physical function.

Guidelines
- Accumulate at least 150 minutes of moderate- to vigorous-intensity aerobic physical activity per week.
- Muscle- and bone-strengthening activities using major muscle groups at least 2 days per week
- Physical activities that challenge balance
- Several hours of light physical activities, including standing
- 7–8 hours of good-quality sleep on a regular basis, with consistent bed and wake-up times
- Limiting sedentary time to 8 hours or less, including no more than 3 hours of recreational screen time and breaking up long periods of sitting as often as possible

Adapted from Canadian Society for Exercise Physiology. (2020). *Canadian 24-hour movement guidelines: An integration of physical activity, sedentary behaviour, & sleep.* https://csepguidelines.ca

without assistance. When using mechanical lifts, a second person is always required to assist. Use mechanical lifts, friction-reduction devices, slide boards, and other handling aids available in the workplace (Alberta Health Services, 2022). Many health care agencies have a no-lift policy, in which manual lifting of the whole or a large part of the weight of the patient by a health care worker is prohibited, except in exceptional or life-threatening situations. Some agencies also have lift teams (Table 37.2).

Acute Care

Patients who are hospitalized should be encouraged to do stretching exercises, active ROM exercises, and low-intensity walking. Physiotherapists can also assist patients with isometric exercises. When patients cannot participate in active ROM, the nurse can maintain joint mobility and prevent contractures by implementing passive ROM into the plan of care. If needed, patients can be medicated for pain 30 minutes before exercise. An analgesic that makes the patient feel dizzy should not be used.

TABLE 37.2	Safe Patient Handling for Health Care Workers
Action	**Rationale**
When planning to move a patient, arrange for adequate help.	Ensures that caregiver has adequate assistance to prevent injury to self and patient.
Use patient-handling equipment and devices, such as height-adjustable beds, ceiling-mounted lifts, friction-reducing slide sheets, and air-assisted devices (Alperovitch-Najenson et al., 2020; Lee et al., 2021; Roy et al., 2021; Tullar et al., 2010).	These devices help to reduce the caregiver's muscular strain during patient handling.
Encourage patient to assist as much as possible.	This promotes patient's independence and strength and minimizes workload.
Take position close to patient (or object being lifted).	Keeps patient or object in same plane as lifter and close to caregiver's centre of gravity. Reduces horizontal reach and stresses on caregiver's back.
Tighten abdominal muscles and keep back, neck, pelvis, and feet aligned. Avoid twisting.	Reduces risk of injury to lumbar vertebrae and muscle groups. Twisting increases risk of injury.
Bend at knees; keep feet wide apart.	A broad base of support increases stability and maintains centre of gravity.
Use arms and legs (not back).	Leg muscles are stronger, larger muscles capable of greater work without injury.
Slide patient toward your body, using a pull sheet or slide board. When transferring a patient onto a stretcher or bed, a slide board is more appropriate.	Sliding requires less effort than lifting. A pull sheet minimizes shearing forces, which can damage patient's skin.
The person with the heaviest load coordinates efforts of the team involved by counting to three.	Simultaneous lifting minimizes the load for any one lifter.

Musculoskeletal System. Nurses can help maintain the musculoskeletal system in patients in acute care by encouraging the use of stretching and isometric exercises. The nurse should review the patient's chart and collaborate with physiotherapy and the health care provider to identify possible contraindications before initiating isometric exercises. A physiotherapist will design an isometric exercise program for the specific needs of a patient. The nurse's role is to follow that program and assist patients accordingly. For example, an exercise program includes isometric exercises of the biceps and triceps to prepare a patient for crutch walking. The patient should be instructed to stop the activity if pain, fatigue, or discomfort is experienced.

During isometrics, a patient tightens or contracts a muscle group for 10 seconds and then completely relaxes for several seconds. Repetitions are increased gradually for each muscle group until the isometric exercise is repeated 8 to 10 times. Patients should be instructed to perform the exercises slowly and increase repetitions as their physical condition improves. A patient needs to do isometric exercise for quadriceps and gluteal muscle groups, which are used for walking, four times per day until a patient is ambulatory.

Joint Mobility. The easiest intervention to maintain or improve joint mobility for patients and one that can be coordinated with other activities is the use of ROM exercises (see Chapter 46). In active ROM exercises, patients are able to move their joints independently. With passive ROM exercises, the nurse moves each joint in patients who are unable to perform these exercises themselves. The use of ROM exercises provides data to systematically assess and improve the patient's mobility.

Joints that are not moved periodically are at risk for *contractures*, a permanent shortening of a muscle followed by the eventual shortening of associated ligaments and tendons. Over time the joint becomes fixed in one position, and the patient loses normal use of it. Passive ROM exercises are the exercises of choice for patients who do not have voluntary motor control.

Some older persons who experience a decline in physical activity and changes in joints often have limited mobility and joint flexibility. A variety of recommended approaches can be used to help older persons use proper body mechanics and prevent injury.

Unless contraindicated, the nursing care plan includes exercising each joint through as nearly a full ROM as possible. Passive ROM

exercises should be initiated as soon as the patient loses the ability to move the extremity or joint. Chapter 46 details ROM exercises for each area and illustrates the motion of each joint.

Walking. Walking increases joint mobility and can be measured by length of time or distance walked. The nurse should measure distances walked in meters instead of charting "ambulated to nurses' station and back." Illness or trauma usually reduces activity tolerance, resulting in the need for help with walking or the use of assistive devices such as crutches, canes, or walkers. Patients who increase their walking distance before discharge improve their ability to independently perform basic ADLs, increase activity tolerance, and have a faster recovery after surgery.

Helping a Patient Walk

Helping a patient walk requires preparation. The patient's strength, coordination, baseline vital signs, and balance need to be assessed in order to determine the type of assistance needed. As the nurse helping a patient to walk, assess orientation and determine if there are any signs of distress. Postpone walking if you determine that the patient cannot walk safely. Evaluate the environment for safety before ambulation (e.g., removal of obstacles, a clean and dry floor, and the identification of rest points in case the patient's activity tolerance becomes less than expected or if the patient becomes dizzy). Have the patient wear supportive, nonskid shoes.

Help the patient to a position of sitting at the side of the bed and dangling the legs over the side of the bed for 1 to 2 minutes before standing. Dangling a patient's legs before standing is an intermediate step that allows assessment of the patient before changing positions to maintain safety and prevent injury to the patient. In some instances, the nurse will need to take the patient's blood pressure while the patient is sitting on the side of the bed.

Some patients experience orthostatic hypotension. *Orthostatic*, or *postural, hypotension* is defined as a drop in blood pressure that occurs with they change from a horizontal to vertical position (Lewis et al., 2023). Orthostatic hypotension is prevalent across all health care settings. Those at higher risk are patients who are immobilized, patients who are on prolonged bed rest, older persons, and patients with chronic diseases such as diabetes mellitus and cardiovascular disease (McDonagh et al., 2021). Signs and symptoms of orthostatic hypotension include dizziness, lightheadedness, nausea, tachycardia, pallor, and even fainting. Orthostatic hypotension usually stabilizes quickly, but if the patient develops dizziness lasting 60 seconds, the patient should be returned to bed (Myszenski, 2017).

Several methods are used to help a patient ambulate. Always provide support at the waist with a gait belt so that the patient's centre of gravity remains midline. A gait belt encircles the patient's waist snugly. The nurse holds the back of the belt behind the patient (Figure 37.11).

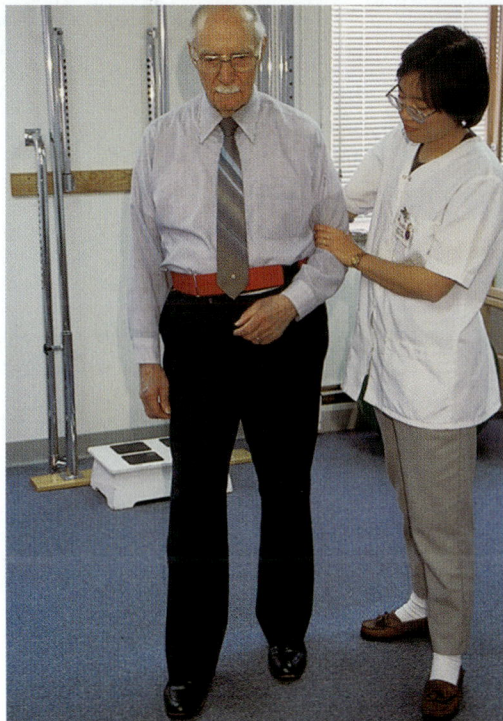

FIGURE 37.11 When helping a patient walk, the nurse uses a gait belt and walks slightly behind the patient's side. (From Sorrentino, S. A., Wilk, M. J., & Newmaster, R. [2009]. *Mosby's Canadian textbook for the support worker* [2nd ed., p. 439]. Elsevier.)

If the patient has a fainting (syncope) episode or begins to fall, assume a wide base of support with one foot in front of the other; this helps to support the patient's body weight (Figure 37.12, *A*). Extend one leg, let the patient slide against the leg, and gently lower the patient to the floor, protecting the head (see Figure 37.12, *B, C*). When the patient attempts to ambulate again, proceed more slowly, monitor for reports of dizziness, and take the patient's blood pressure before, during, and after ambulation.

Restorative and Continuing Care

Restorative and continuing care involves implementing activity and exercise strategies to assist the patient in regaining mobility and activity capacity after acute care is no longer needed. Restorative and continuing care also includes activities and exercises that restore and promote optimal functioning in patients with specific chronic illnesses, such as coronary heart disease (CHD), hypertension, COPD, and diabetes mellitus (Table 37.3). Remaining active while living with chronic diseases improves outcomes, including prevention of complications, improved function, and enhanced quality of life. Given the degree of physical compromise that individuals with one or more chronic diseases may experience, consultation with the patient's primary care provider, medical specialist, or both is prudent before implementation of an exercise plan. Some patients' chronic disease process may be so advanced that they are unable to participate in even the most modest of exercise programs.

Assistive Devices for Walking

In collaboration with other members of the health care team, such as physiotherapists, nurses can promote activity and exercise by teaching the proper use of canes, walkers, or crutches, depending on the assistive device most appropriate for the patient's condition.

Walkers. A walker is a lightweight, movable device that stands waist high and consists of a metal frame with handgrips, four widely placed sturdy legs, and one open side (Figure 37.13). Because it has a wide base of support, the walker provides great stability and security during walking. A walker can be used by a patient who has difficulties with balance. Walkers with wheels are useful for patients who have difficulty lifting and advancing the walker as they walk because of limited balance or endurance (Figures 37.14 and 37.15). To determine if the walker is

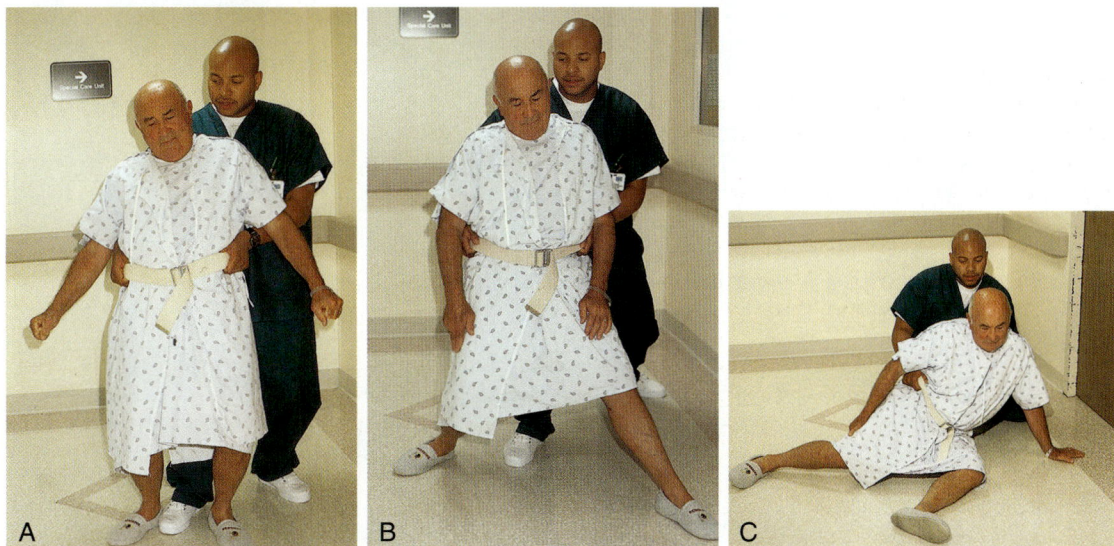

FIGURE 37.12 Safe patient handling during a fall. **A,** Stand with feet apart to provide a broad base of support. **B,** Extend one leg and let patient slide against it to the floor. **C,** Bend knees to lower body as patient slides to the floor.

TABLE 37.3	Physical Activity and Exercise—Recommendations From Diabetes Canada			
Definition and Recommended Frequency	**Intensity**	**Examples**	**Benefits**	

Aerobic Exercise

Exercise that involves continuous, rhythmic movements of large muscle groups normally lasting for at least 10 minutes at a time and depends primarily on aerobic energy-generating processes in the body (i.e., heart, lungs, cardiovascular system and oxidization or fuels in skeletal muscle). At least 150 minutes of moderate to vigorous intensity each week (e.g., 30 minutes, 5 days a week). Recommended for a minimum of 150 minutes per week (moderate intensity).

Moderate
50–70% of person's maximum heart rate

Light cycling
Brisk walking
Continuous swimming
Dancing
Water aerobics
Gardening
Domestic chores

Improved fitness, health, and body composition
Reduced complications of diabetes, such as lowered risk of heart disease
Improved diabetes lab values, including blood sugar, blood fats, and blood pressure

Vigorous
>70% of person's maximum heart rate

Running
Climbing stairs or hill-walking
Fast cycling or swimming
Aerobics
Most competitive sports and games

Resistance Exercise

Brief repetitive exercise using weights, weight machines, resistance bands, or one's own body weight (e.g., push-ups) to increase muscle strength and/or endurance.

2–3 times per week
Start with one set of 15–20 repetitions at moderate weight.
Progress to two sets of 10–15 repetitions.
Progress to three sets of 8 repetitions at heavier weight.

Exercise with weight machines
Weight-lifting

Maintaining or increasing lean muscle
Burning calories at rest throughout the day
Enhanced weight control and diabetes management

Adapted from Diabetes Canada. (2022). *Physical activity.* https://www.diabetes.ca/managing-my-diabetes/tools---resources/physical-activity; Sigal, R., Armstrong, M. J., Bacon, S. L., et al. (2018). *Physical activity and diabetes: Diabetes Canada clinical practice guidelines.* https://guidelines.diabetes.ca/cpg/chapter10

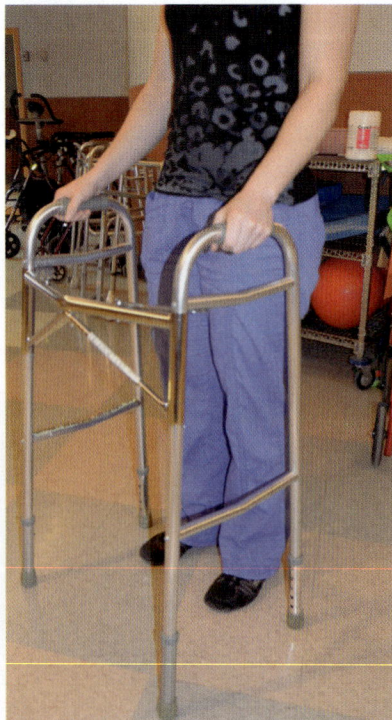
FIGURE 37.13 Patient using a standard walker.

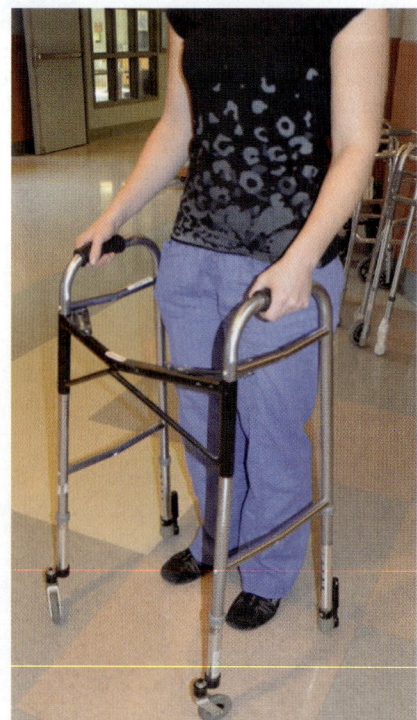
FIGURE 37.14 Patient using a two-wheeled walker.

FIGURE 37.15 Patient using a rollator walker.

FIGURE 37.16 Patient using a quad cane.

the correct size, instruct the patient to relax their arms at the side of the body and stand up straight. The top of the walker should line up with the crease on the inside of the patient's wrist. Elbows should be flexed about 15 to 30 degrees when standing inside the walker, with hands on the handgrips. To ambulate using a walker, the patient holds the handgrips on the upper bars, takes a step, moves the walker forward, and takes another step. Teach patients how to use walkers safely and how to avoid the risk of falling.

Canes. Canes are lightweight, easily movable devices made of wood or metal. They provide less support than a walker and are less stable. To determine the correct cane length for a patient, measure the distance from the patient's greater trochanter to the floor (Fairchild et al., 2018). Two common types of canes are the straight-legged cane and the quad cane. The straight-legged cane is more common and is used to support and balance a patient with decreased leg strength. The patient should keep the cane on the stronger side of the body. Teach the following three steps to promote maximum support when walking: First, instruct the patient to place the cane forward 15 to 25 cm, keeping body weight on both legs. Second, coach the patient to move the weaker leg forward to the cane so body weight is divided between the cane and the stronger leg. Third, have the patient advance the stronger leg past the cane so the cane supports the body weight and weaker leg. During walking the patient continually repeats these three steps. Assess the patient's knowledge to ensure that they know that two points of support, such as both feet or one foot and the cane, are on the floor at all times.

The quad cane provides the most support and is used when there is partial or complete leg paralysis or some hemiplegia (Figure 37.16). The patient is taught the same three steps that are used with the straight-legged cane.

Crutches. Crutches are often needed to increase mobility. A crutch is a wooden or metal staff. The use of crutches is often temporary (e.g., after ligament damage to the knee). However, some patients with paralysis of the lower extremities need them permanently.

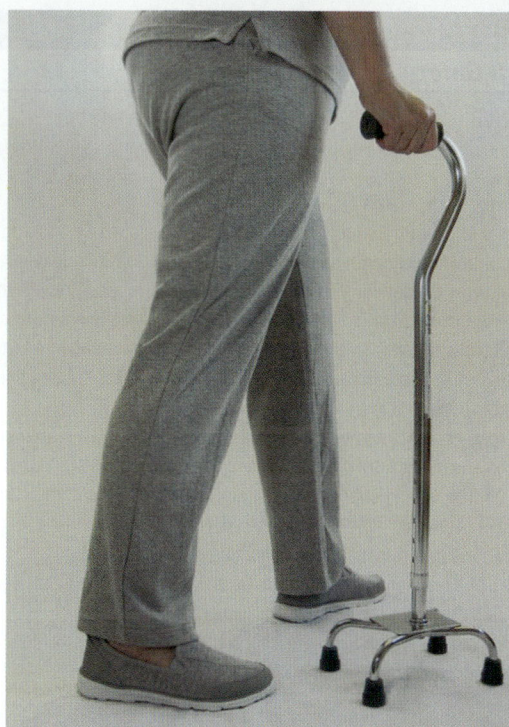

FIGURE 37.17 Double adjustable Lofstrand, or forearm, crutch.

The two types of crutches are the double adjustable, or forearm, crutch and the axillary wooden or metal crutch (which is the most common type) (Figure 37.17). The metal band and handgrip are adjusted to fit the patient's height. The axillary crutch has a padded curved surface at the top, which fits under the axilla. A handgrip

BOX 37.12 PATIENT TEACHING
Crutch Safety

Objective
- Patient will describe and demonstrate safe crutch walking.

Teaching Strategies
- Teach patient with axillary crutches about the dangers of pressure on the axillae, which occurs when leaning on the crutches to support body weight.
- Explain why the patient must use crutches that were measured for them.
- Show the patient how to routinely inspect crutch tips. Rubber tips should be securely attached to the crutches. When tips become worn out, they should be replaced. Rubber crutch tips increase surface friction and help prevent slipping.
- Explain that the crutch tips should remain dry. Water decreases surface friction and increases the risk of slipping.
- Explain that the patient should wear nonslip shoes and not wear an open gown or other long, flowing clothing to decrease the risk of falls.
- Show patient how to inspect the structure of the crutches.
- Cracks in a wooden crutch decrease its ability to support weight. Bends in aluminum crutches can alter body alignment.
- Provide patient with a list of medical supply companies in the community where repairs, new rubber tips, handgrips, and crutch pads can be obtained.
- Instruct patient to have spare crutches and spare tips readily available.

Evaluation
- Patient can describe principles of crutch safety.
- Patient correctly demonstrates proper use of crutches.

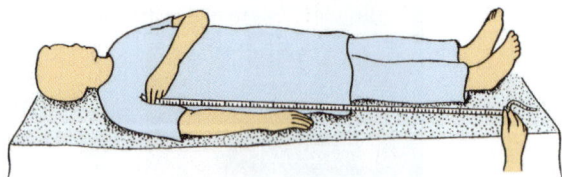

FIGURE 37.19 Verifying correct distance between crutch pads and axilla.

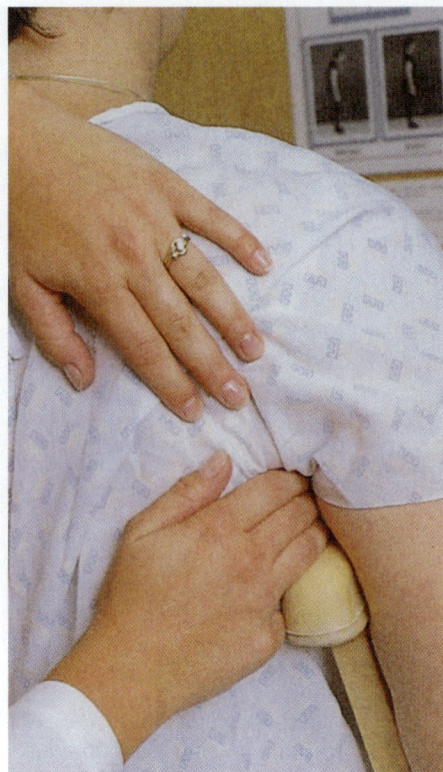

FIGURE 37.18 Measuring crutch length.

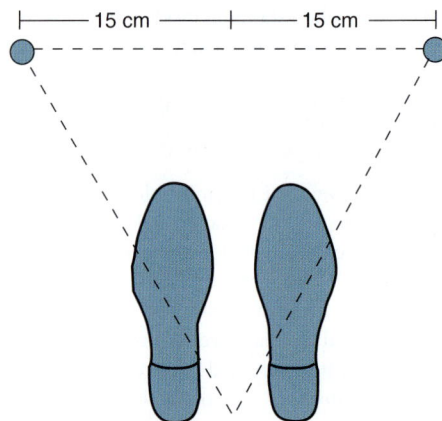

FIGURE 37.20 Tripod position, basic crutch stance.

in the form of a crossbar is held at the level of the palms to support the body. It is important to measure crutches for the appropriate length and to teach patients how to use their crutches safely to achieve a stable gait, ascend and descend stairs, and rise from a sitting position. Begin crutch instruction with guidelines for safe use (Box 37.12).

Measuring for Crutches. Measurement for the axillary crutch includes the patient's height, the angle of elbow flexion, and the distance between the crutch pad and the axilla. When crutches are fitted, the length of the crutch needs to be two to three fingerwidths from the axilla and the tips positioned approximately 5 cm lateral and 10 to 15 cm anterior to the front of the patient's shoes (Figure 37.18).

When fitting a patient with crutches, position the handgrips so the axillae are not supporting the patient's body weight. Pressure on the axillae increases the risk to underlying nerves, which sometimes results in partial paralysis of the arm. Determine the correct position of the handgrips with the patient upright, supporting weight by the handgrips with the elbows slightly flexed at 20 to 25 degrees. Elbow flexion may be verified with the goniometer. When determining the height and placement of the handgrips, verify that the distance between the crutch pad and the patient's axilla is approximately 5 cm (two or three fingerwidths) (Figure 37.19).

Crutch Gait. Patients assume a gait by alternately bearing weight on one or both legs and on the crutches. Determine the gait by assessing the patient's physical and functional abilities and the disease or injury that resulted in the need for crutches. This section summarizes the basic crutch stance and the four standard gaits: four-point alternating gait, three-point alternating gait, two-point gait, and swing-through gait.

The basic crutch stance is the tripod position, formed when the crutches are placed 15 cm in front of and 15 cm to the side of each foot (Figure 37.20). This position improves the patient's balance by providing a wider base of support. The body alignment of the patient in the tripod position includes an erect head and neck, straight vertebrae, and extended hips and knees. The axillae should not bear any weight. The patient assumes the tripod position before crutch walking.

Four-point alternating, or four-point, gait gives stability to the patient but requires weight bearing on both legs. Each leg is moved alternately with each opposing crutch, so three points of support are on the floor at all times (Figure 37.21, A).

Three-point alternating, or three-point, gait requires the patient to bear all of the weight on one foot. In a three-point gait the patient bears weight on both crutches and then on the uninvolved leg, repeating the sequence (see Figure 37.21, B). The affected leg does not touch the ground during the early phase of the three-point gait. Gradually the patient progresses to touch-down and full weight bearing on the affected leg.

The two-point gait requires at least partial weight bearing on each foot (see Figure 37.21, C). The patient moves a crutch at the same time as the opposing leg, so the crutch movements are similar to arm motion during normal walking.

Individuals with paraplegia who wear weight-supporting braces on their legs frequently use the swing-through gait. With weight placed on the supported legs, the patient places the crutches one stride in front and then swings to or through them while supporting their weight.

Crutch Walking on Stairs. When ascending stairs on crutches, the patient usually uses a modified three-point gait (Figure 37.22). The patient stands at the bottom of the stairs and transfers body weight to the crutches. The person then advances the unaffected leg between the crutches and the stairs. The patient then shifts weight from the crutches to the unaffected leg. Finally, the person aligns both crutches on the stairs. The patient repeats this sequence until they reach the top of the stairs.

A three-point sequence is also used to descend the stairs (Figure 37.23). The patient transfers body weight to the unaffected leg. The person then places the crutches on the stairs and begins to transfer body weight to the crutches, moving the affected leg forward. Finally, the patient moves the unaffected leg to the stairs with the crutches. The patient repeats the sequence until reaching the bottom of the stairs.

Because in most cases patients need to use crutches for some time, they need to be instructed to use them on the stairs before discharge. This teaching applies to all patients who are dependent on crutches, not just those who have stairs in their homes. Nurses will frequently collaborate with physiotherapists to provide instruction about crutch walking.

Sitting in a Chair With Crutches. As with crutch walking and crutch walking up and down stairs, the procedure for sitting in a chair involves phases and requires the patient to transfer weight (Figure 37.24). First the patient positions themselves at the centre front of the chair with the posterior aspect of the legs touching the chair. Then the patient holds both crutches in the hand opposite the affected leg. If both

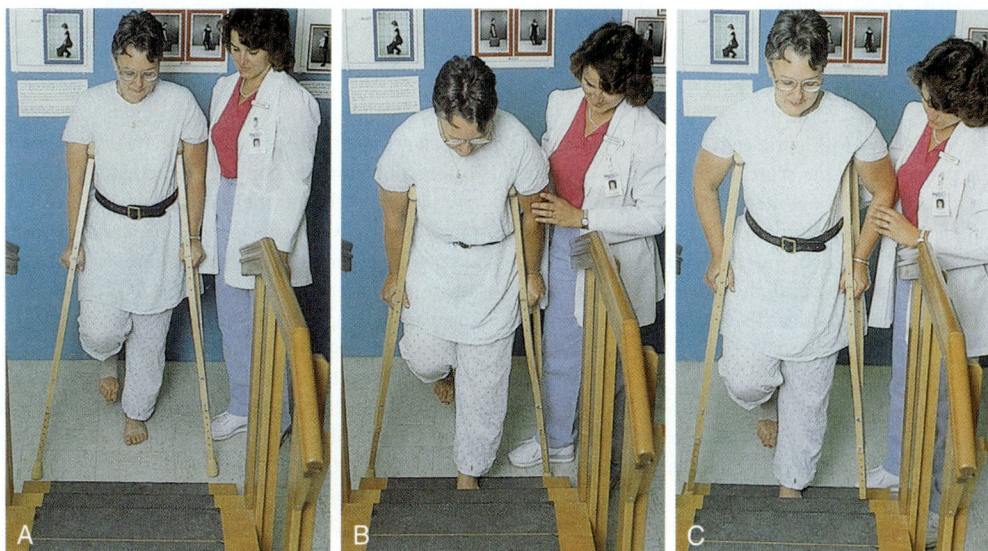

FIGURE 37.21 A, Four-point alternating gait. Solid feet and crutch tips show the order of foot and crutch tip movement in each of the four phases. *(Read from bottom to top.)* **B,** Three-point gait with weight borne on unaffected leg. Solid foot and crutch tips show weight bearing in each phase. *(Read from bottom to top.)* **C,** Two-point gait with weight borne partially on each foot and each crutch advancing with opposing leg. Solid areas indicate leg and crutch tips bearing weight. *(Read from bottom to top.)*

FIGURE 37.22 Ascending stairs. **A,** Weight is placed on crutch. **B,** Weight is transferred from crutches to unaffected leg on stairs. **C,** Crutches are aligned with unaffected leg on stairs.

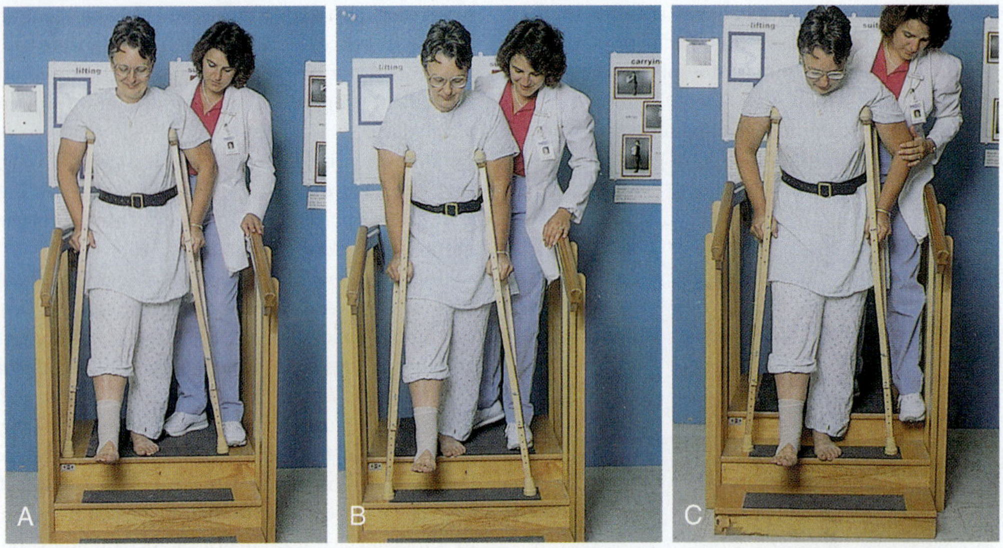

FIGURE 37.23 Descending stairs. **A,** Body weight is on unaffected leg. **B,** Body weight is transferred to crutches. **C,** Unaffected leg is aligned on stairs with crutches.

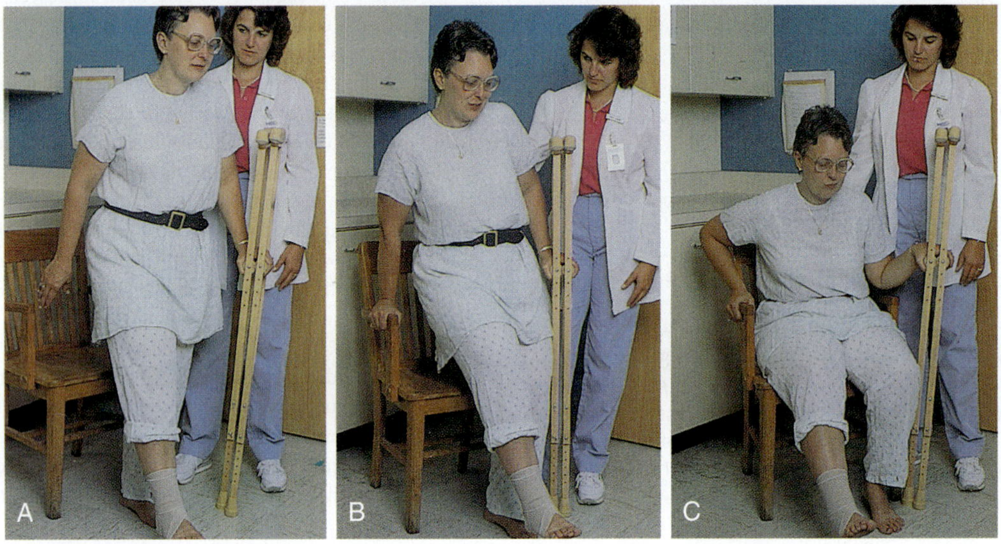

FIGURE 37.24 Sitting in a chair. **A,** Both crutches are held by one hand. Patient transfers weight to crutches and unaffected leg. **B,** Patient grasps arm of chair with free hand and begins to lower herself into chair. **C,** Patient completely lowers herself into chair.

legs are affected, as with a person with paraplegia who wears weight-supporting braces, the patient holds the crutches in the hand of their stronger side. With both crutches in one hand, the patient supports body weight on the unaffected leg and the crutches. While still holding the crutches, the patient grasps the arm of the chair with the remaining hand and lowers their body into it. To stand, the procedure is reversed, and the patient, when fully upright, assumes the tripod position before beginning to walk.

Restoration of Activity and Chronic Illness

Nurses design care plans to increase activity and exercise in patients with specific disease conditions and chronic illnesses such as CHD, hypertension, COPD, and diabetes mellitus.

Coronary Heart Disease. Research shows that activity and exercise play a role in secondary prevention or recurrence of CHD. Cardiac rehabilitation is an integral part of the comprehensive care of patients

who have been diagnosed with CHD. Nurses are involved in many aspects of cardiac rehabilitation and assist patients in developing exercise programs that fit their needs and levels of functioning. Increased physical activity appears to benefit individuals with myocardial infarction, angina pectoris, or heart failure, as well as those who have had a coronary artery bypass graft (CABG) or percutaneous transluminal coronary angioplasty (PCTA). Patients with CHD benefit from exercise and activity and can experience reduced mortality and morbidity, improved quality of life, increased psychological well-being, improved left ventricular function, increased functional capacity, decreased levels of blood lipids and apolipoproteins, and psychological well-being (Joseph et al., 2020; Lacombe et al., 2019).

Hypertension. Exercise has the effect of reducing systolic and diastolic blood pressure readings. Research shows that low- to moderate-intensity aerobic exercise (e.g., brisk walking, bicycling) is the most effective exercise for lowering blood pressure (Dames et al., 2021).

Chronic Obstructive Pulmonary Disease. Pulmonary rehabilitation helps patients reach an optimal level of functioning. Some patients are fearful of participating in exercise because of the potential of worsening dyspnea or difficulty breathing (Albarrati et al., 2020). This aversion to physical activity sets up a progressive deconditioning in which minimal physical exertion results in dyspnea. Pulmonary rehabilitation provides a safe environment for monitoring patients' progress with interventions that can improve respiratory muscle strength and increase exercise capacity (Chiu et al., 2020).

Diabetes Mellitus. Along with diet, glucose monitoring, and medication, exercise is an important component in the care of patients with diabetes mellitus. It is recommended that persons with diabetes have at least 150 minutes per week of aerobic exercise, in addition to at least two sessions per week of resistance exercise (Diabetes Canada, 2018). Endurance and resistance exercise appear to be equally effective in improving the control of metabolism in patients with type 2 and type 1 diabetes. Individuals with type 1 diabetes are encouraged to exercise because exercise leads to improved glucose control, cardiovascular fitness, and psychological well-being. Exercise lowers blood sugar levels, and the effects of exercise on blood sugar levels often last for at least 24 hours. The patient with type 1 diabetes should be instructed about certain risks and precautions regarding exercise. Instruction includes the need for a pre-exercise comprehensive physical examination; patients also should be instructed to perform low- to moderate-intensity exercises, to carry a concentrated form of carbohydrates (e.g., sugar packets, hard candy), and to wear a medical alert bracelet.

Exercise must occur on a regular basis to have the desired continued benefits in the management of blood glucose levels, lipids, and overall quality of life (Canadian Society for Exercise Physiology, 2021).

◆ Evaluation

Patient Expectations. For activity and exercise, nurses measure the effectiveness of nursing interventions by the success in meeting the patient's expected outcomes and goals of care. The patient is the only one who will experience the effectiveness and benefits of activity and exercise (Figure 37.25). Working closely with the patient will enable the nurse to identify goals and strategies that can be met realistically within the limits of the patient's priorities, capabilities, and health treatment (see Figure 37.25). The nurse should ask the patient questions such as "How well did you tolerate walking, and is that what you expected?" and "You have been walking regularly for a month now, how has it made you feel?" Continuous evaluation helps to determine whether new or revised therapies are required, and whether new nursing diagnoses have developed.

Patient Outcomes. To evaluate the effectiveness of nursing interventions in enhancing activity and exercise, nurses make comparisons with baseline measures that include pulse, blood pressure, oxygen saturation, strength, fatigue, and psychological well-being. Actual outcomes are compared with expected outcomes to determine the patient's health status and progression. The following is an example of questions a nurse might ask when a patient does not meet their expected outcomes:

- The last time we met you planned to walk outside for 20 minutes 3 days a week. However, you report that you are only able to walk twice a week right now. What do you think is preventing you from meeting your goal?
- You state that you experience leg pain after walking short distances. Describe your pain. Which pain-relieving measures have you tried?

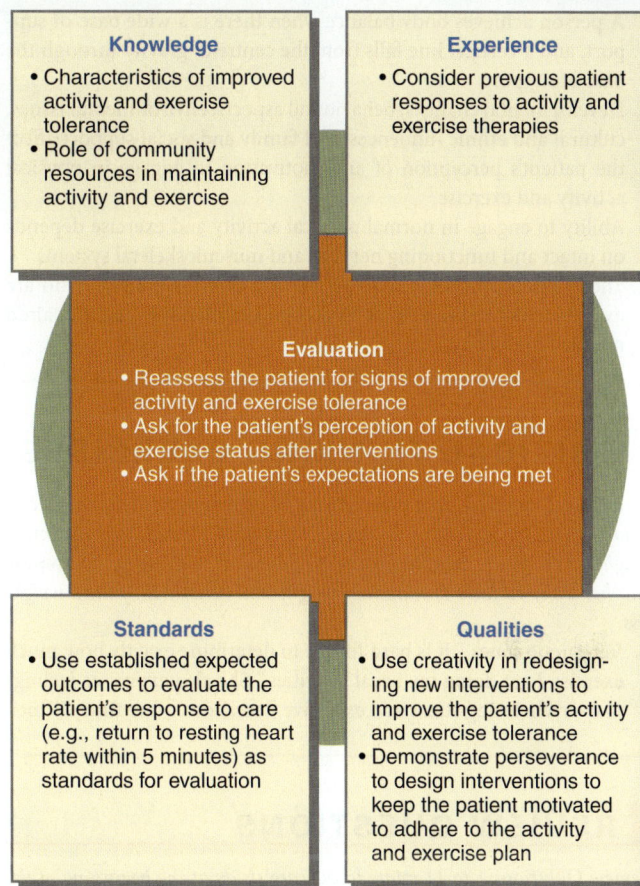

FIGURE 37.25 Critical thinking model for activity and exercise evaluation.

KEY CONCEPTS

- Exercise is physical activity for the purpose of conditioning the body, improving health, and maintaining fitness, or it may be used as a therapeutic measure.
- Deconditioning is a particular risk for hospitalized patients, who spend most of their time in bed even when they are able to walk.
- Body mechanics are the coordinated efforts of the musculoskeletal system and nervous system as the person moves, lifts, bends, stands, sits, lies down, and completes daily activities.
- Careful attention to body mechanics and use of appropriate equipment is critical in the prevention of musculoskeletal injuries.
- Activity tolerance is the kind and amount of exercise or work that a person is able to perform.
- Physiological, emotional, and developmental factors influence the patient's activity tolerance.
- 24-hour movement guidelines include a balance of physical activity, sedentary periods, and sleep to promote health.
- The best program of physical activity includes a combination of exercises that produce different physiological and psychological benefits.
- Coordinated body movement requires integrated functioning of the skeletal system, skeletal muscles, and nervous system.
- Coordination and regulation of muscle groups depend on muscle tone and activity of antagonistic, synergistic, and antigravity muscles.
- The nervous system controls balance through the functions of the cerebellum and inner ear function.

- A person achieves body balance when there is a wide base of support, and a vertical line falls from the centre of gravity through the base of support.
- Developmental changes, behavioural aspects, environmental issues, cultural and ethnic influences, and family and social support affect the patient's perception of and motivation to engage in physical activity and exercise.
- Ability to engage in normal physical activity and exercise depends on intact and functioning nervous and musculoskeletal systems.
- The nursing process is used to provide care for patients who are experiencing or are at risk for activity intolerance and impaired physical mobility.

- After identifying nursing diagnoses, nurses plan and implement interventions to increase activity and exercise, in collaboration with the patient, when possible.
- Range-of-motion (ROM) exercises incorporated into daily activities can include one or all of the body's joints.
- The nurse needs to apply proper algorithms when transferring and lifting patients.
- Assistive devices used to promote walking include canes, walkers, and crutches.

CRITICAL THINKING EXERCISES

Veronique (preferred pronouns: she/her) has experienced some success in losing weight. She states, however, "I feel like I should have lost more weight by now." She expresses concern about how to incorporate exercise into her daily routine to maintain weight and assist with future weight loss.

1. Veronique states, "It is hard for me to determine exactly how much exercise I get doing my usual activities." She also expresses feelings of overwhelming stress and excessive demands on her time. Which interventions would you suggest to Veronique to help assess her current level of exercise?
2. Recognizing the challenges Veronique has voiced in balancing the excessive demands on her time and incorporating an exercise program, develop some strategies to help her initiate and maintain daily exercise.
3. Develop a feedback method for Veronique, emphasizing her success in exercising and maintaining a healthy weight.

🌐 *Answers to Critical Thinking Exercises appear on the Evolve website.*

REVIEW QUESTIONS

Review Questions 1 to 11 relate to the case study at the beginning of the chapter.

1. Which of the following factors *most* motivated Sandra to participate in an exercise program?
   a. Receiving a pamphlet on exercise from her primary health care provider
   b. Self-reflection on her current state of activity and readiness to change behaviour
   c. Concern that she would be diagnosed with a chronic disease
   d. Receiving a prescribed exercise program from her primary health care provider
2. Functional decline was Sandra's primary concern, leading her to adopt an exercise plan. Functional decline, or the loss of ability to perform self-care or activities of daily living, may result from: *(Select all that apply.)*
   a. Consistent low- to moderate-intensity activity throughout the lifespan, which leads to musculoskeletal degeneration
   b. Episodes of acute illness and injury or chronic illness
   c. Deconditioning associated with inactivity
   d. "Overuse" of joints and muscles as a result of participating in aerobic activity for 150 minutes per week
3. In starting her exercise program, Sandra knows that positive effects of physical activity include:
   a. Improved myocardial contraction, leading to increased cardiac output, decreased alveolar ventilation, decreased basal metabolic rate, improved activity tolerance
   b. Decreased myocardial contraction, increased alveolar ventilation, decreased basal metabolic rate, improved activity tolerance
   c. Improved myocardial contraction, increased alveolar ventilation, increased basal metabolic rate, improved activity tolerance
   d. Decreased alveolar ventilation, decreased basal metabolic rate, decreased bone loss

4. Along with Sandra's exercise plan, she is aware that recommendations for an active week include: *(Select all that apply.)*
   a. Moderate to vigorous aerobic activities to accumulate to at least 150 minutes per week.
   b. Muscle- and bone-strengthening activities using major muscle groups, at least 2 days per week
   c. 5 to 6 hours of good-quality sleep on a regular basis with consistent bed and wake-up time
   d. No more than 5 hours of recreational screen time per day
   e. Breaking up long periods of sitting as much as possible
5. Sandra is aware that as she ages, her risk of developing osteoporosis increases. To prevent or mitigate the impact of osteoporosis, Sandra knows that she should:
   a. Engage in a range of isotonic exercise activity every week, eat foods high in calcium daily, and consult with her primary health care provider regarding vitamin D and calcium supplements.
   b. Avoid weight-bearing activities as they may contribute to fractures, engage in a range of isotonic exercises, and plan for extended sedentary periods daily to promote bone regeneration.
   c. Consult with her primary health care provider regarding daily vitamin D and calcium supplements; plan for extended sedentary periods daily to promote bone regeneration.
   d. Engage in weight-bearing exercises at least twice daily, plan for high-intensity aerobic activity to accelerate fitness goals, and take a calcium supplement once a week.
6. When teaching safe patient handling to students, Sandra consistently reinforces the importance of correct body alignment to promote stable balance and muscle tone, and to avoid excessive strain on joints, tendons, ligaments, and muscles. When transferring patients, correct alignment includes:
   a. Keeping ears in line with shoulders; shoulders in line with knees; relax stomach and keep weight on heels

b. Keeping nose in line with umbilicus; shoulders in line with knees; tighten stomach and push buttocks back while keeping weight on heels

c. Keeping ears in line with shoulders; shoulders in line with hips; tighten stomach and push buttocks back while keeping weight on heels

d. Keeping ears in line with shoulders; shoulders in line with hips; bend at waist to keep weight on toes

7. Sandra also reinforces the principles of proper body mechanics when transferring patients or carrying objects, which include: *(Select all that apply.)*
   a. Keep knees in a locked position.
   b. Bend at the waist to maintain a centre of gravity.
   c. Maintain a wide base of support.
   d. Hold objects away from the body for improved leverage.
   e. Encourage the patient to help as much as possible.

8. When teaching safe patient handling for transfers, Sandra educates students on which patient assessments to perform prior to transferring patients: What patient assessments should be performed?
   a. Patient's age, level of consciousness, mental health
   b. Patient's weight, level of consciousness, ability to assist
   c. Presence of medical equipment, presence of family members, patient's age
   d. Presence of family members, nutritional intake, patient's weight

9. Sandra emphasizes the importance of frequently assessing hospitalized patients for risks associated with immobilization leading to deconditioning. Priority assessments for patients at risk of deconditioning include:
   a. Respiratory, cardiovascular, skin integrity
   b. Repositioning, respiratory, peripheral pulses
   c. Pulse, blood pressure, range of motion
   d. Nutrient intake, deep breathing and coughing, muscle tone

10. .When conducting patient assessments, Sandra articulates the need to assess for potential complications of deconditioning that include:
    a. Hypothermia, diarrhea, and confusion
    b. Pneumonia, constipation, joint contractures
    c. Delirium, diarrhea, orthostatic hypertension
    d. Hypothermia, constipation, increased muscle tone

11. Sandra encourages her students to practise interventions to promote physical activity in patients who are immobile, including: *(Select all that apply.)*
    a. Passive range-of-motion exercises
    b. Incentive spirometry and deep breathing and coughing exercises
    c. Encouraging independent ambulation
    d. Demonstrating and assisting with isometric exercise to practise in bed

Answers: 1. b; 2. b, c; 3. c; 4. a, b; 5. a; 6. c; 7. c, e; 8. b; 9. a; 10. b; 11. a, b, d.

Rationales for Review Questions can be found on the Evolve website.

RECOMMENDED WEBSITES

Active Living Alliance for Canadians with a Disability: https://ala.ca
This organization is an alliance of individuals, agencies, and national associations that together promote, support, and enable Canadians with disabilities, across all settings and environments, to lead active and healthy lives.

Canadian Centre for Activity and Aging: http://www.uwo.ca/ccaa
This centre is a research and community resource institution whose mandate is to investigate the interrelationship of physical activity and aging and to develop strategies, based on research, to promote the independence of older persons.

Canadian Fitness and Lifestyle Research Institute: https://www.cflri.ca
The institute addresses the well-being of Canadians through research on and communication of information about physically active lifestyles to the public and private sectors.

Canadian Society for Exercise Physiology (CSEP): https://www.csep.ca
CSEP is the principal body for physical activity, health and fitness research, and personal training in Canada. It provides high-quality research, education, and training related to exercise physiology and science. It is the gold standard of health and fitness professionals and is dedicated to getting Canadians active safely by providing customized and specialized physical activity and fitness programs, as well as guidance and advice based on extensive training and evidence-informed research.

Public Health Agency of Canada: Health Promotion: https://www.phac-aspc.gc.ca/hp-ps/index-eng.php
The Public Health Agency of Canada maintains this website, which contains many useful health promotion resources and guides that will aid health care providers and community leaders in encouraging Canadians to take a more active role in improving their health.

REFERENCES

A full reference list is available on the website for this book at http://evolve.elsevier.com/Canada/Potter/fundamentals/

Quality and Patient Safety

Canadian content written by Chantal Backman, RN, MHA, PhD,
with original chapter contributions by Lynette Savage, BS, BSN, MS, PhD

OBJECTIVES

Mastery of content in this chapter will enable you to:

- Define the key terms listed.
- Describe the domains of quality of care.
- Explain the importance of "benchmarks" for public reporting of patient safety incidents.
- Describe methods to prevent and reduce safety risks.
- Describe strategies to maintain patient and staff safety.
- Describe the most common safety risks in health care.
- Recognize patient safety incidents and know how to respond effectively to minimize harm to the patient.
- Understand the importance of reporting safety incidents.
- Disclose patient safety incidents.

- Understand various approaches to improve quality and safety.
- Describe assessment activities designed to identify patients' physical, psychosocial, and cognitive statuses as they pertain to their safety.
- Identify relevant nursing diagnoses associated with risks to safety.
- Develop a nursing care plan for patients whose safety is threatened.
- Describe nursing interventions specific to patients' age for reducing safety risks.
- Describe methods to evaluate interventions designed to maintain or promote safety.
- Define the knowledge, skills, and attitudes necessary to promote safety in a health care setting.

KEY TERMS

Accessible care
Ambularm
Appropriate care
Bed-check
Cultural safety
Equitable
Harmful incident

Incident or occurrence report
Integrated care
Near miss
No-harm incident
Patient safety
Patient safety incident (adverse event)
Person-centred care

Quality of care
Restraint
Safe care
Workplace Hazardous Materials
    Information System (WHMIS)

🌐 WEBSITE

http://evolve.elsevier.com/Canada/Potter/fundamentals/

CASE STUDY

Mrs. Maureen (preferred pronouns: she/her), 80 years old, was brought by ambulance to the emergency department following a fall at home. She sustained an intracapsular fracture of her right hip at the femoral neck. She is waiting for emergency surgery. Ahmad (preferred pronouns: he/him), an RN in the emergency room, conducted a complete assessment of Mrs. Maureen. Following confirmation of the fracture by X-ray, the emergency department physician confirmed Mrs. Maureen as a candidate for surgery.

Upon arrival to the operating room, Melody (preferred pronouns: she/her), an RN, reassessed Mrs. Maureen and completed the surgical safety checklist with the operating room team. Melody realizes that the documentation stated that the fracture was on the left side. She completes a patient safety incident report. After surgery, Mrs. Maureen is stable and is transferred to the orthopedic unit. Judy (preferred pronouns: she/her), her assigned nurse (LPN), conducts a postoperative assessment. Mrs. Maureen's vital signs are stable, but she reports pain while voiding. Judy contacts the resident, who orders a urine analysis and some blood work. The results show that Mrs. Maureen has a urinary tract infection. Her hemoglobin level is 50 g/L. A blood transfusion is ordered. Mrs. Maureen is having difficulty managing her pain and shows signs of delirium.

Think about this case study as you read this chapter. There are review questions at the end of the chapter that relate to the case study.

Over the past several decades, quality and **patient safety** have become increasingly critical issues in health care. The Institute of Medicine's (IOM) report, *To Err Is Human: Building a Safer Health System* (IOM, 2000), was a pivotal publication that brought patient safety to the forefront of health care in the United States. In 2002, the Canadian National Steering Committee on Patient Safety published a report entitled *Building a Safer System*. That report outlined a national, integrated strategy for improving patient safety in the Canadian health care system.

Quality of care is defined as "the degree to which health care services for individuals and populations increase the likelihood of desired health outcomes and are consistent with current professional knowledge" (IOM, 2000). In Canada's health care systems, unintended patient harm happens every minute and 18 seconds, with a death occurring every 13 minutes and 14 seconds (Risk-Analytica, 2017). A report released by the Canadian Institute for Health Information (CIHI) indicated that in 2019–20, "1 in 18 hospital stays in Canada involved at least one harmful event (134 000 out of 2.5 million hospital stays)" (Horizant, 2022). These harmful events are divided into four main categories: 46% were related to health care and medications (e.g., developing bed sores or getting the wrong medicine); 30% were related to infections (e.g., surgical site infections); 20% were procedure related (e.g., bleeding after surgery); and 4% were patient accidents (e.g., falls) (CIHI, 2021). While most patients experience safe care, sometimes harmful events happen that affect patients. Many of these events are preventable (CIHI, 2021).

A **patient safety incident** (or **adverse event**) is "an event or circumstance that could have resulted, or did result, in unnecessary harm to a patient" (Health Standards Organization [HSO] & Canadian Patient Safety Institute [CPSI], 2020). There are three types of patient safety incidents defined by the Canadian Patient Safety Institute (CPSI):

- **Harmful incident**: an incident that resulted in patient harm (previously known as "preventable adverse event")
- **Near miss**: an incident that did not reach the patient (no harm resulted)
- **No-harm incident**: an incident that reached the patient, but no discernible harm resulted

The CPSI, the Health Standards Organization (HSO), and key stakeholders across Canada developed the *Canadian Quality and Patient Safety Framework for Health Services* (HSO & CPSI, 2020) to improve health care for all. In the framework, five goals were established to drive patient safety and quality improvement efforts in Canada. These are as follows:

1. **Person-centred care**: People using health services are equal partners in planning, developing, and monitoring care to make sure it meets their needs and to achieve the best outcomes.
2. **Safe care**: Health services are safe and free from preventable harm.
3. **Accessible care**: People have timely and **equitable** access to quality health services.
4. **Appropriate care**: Care is evidence-informed and person-centred.
5. **Integrated care**: Health services are continuous and well coordinated, promoting smooth transitions (HSO & CPSI, 2020; see also Box 38.2).

As part of the health care team, nurses are professionally responsible for engaging in activities that support cultural safety. The BC Patient Safety & Quality Council (2022) defines **cultural safety** as "an outcome based on respectful engagement that recognizes and strives to address power imbalances inherent in the health system." Cultural safety enables and promotes patient safety for all, including Indigenous peoples (including First Nations, Inuit, and Métis), Black people,

LGBTQ2 (including lesbian, gay, bisexual, transgender, queer or questioning and Two-Spirit) members, immigrants, members from visible minority groups, and many more diverse peoples. Cultural safety is defined by each individual's own health service experience (First Nations Health Managers Association & Canadian Foundation for Healthcare Improvement, 2021).

Considerable emphasis is being placed on improving the education of nursing students so that they become competent in promoting safe health care practices. The CPSI's *Safety Competencies Framework* (2nd ed.) includes the following key concepts for nurses and other health care providers: (1) patient safety culture, (2) teamwork, (3) communication, (4) safety, risk, and quality improvement, (5) optimizing human and system factors, and (6) recognizing, responding to, and disclosing patient safety incidents (CPSI, 2020).

Providing health care in a safe manner and in a safe community environment is essential for a patient's survival and well-being. By incorporating critical thinking skills when following the nursing process, nurses assume responsibility for assessing the patient and the environment for safety hazard, as well as for planning and intervening appropriately to maintain a safe environment. By paying attention to patient safety, nurses are functioning not only as providers of safe care but also as active participants in health promotion. Equally important is that nurses must ensure their own safety as they provide patient care.

In an effort to improve patient safety, many organizations focus on developing and monitoring key health care safety metrics as well as providing information to health care organizations and to the public. Health care organizations foster a patient-centred safety culture by doing the following:

- Continually focusing on performance-improvement programs
- Acting on risk-management findings and safety reports
- Providing current reliable technology
- Integrating evidence-informed practice into procedures
- Designing a safe work environment and atmosphere
- Providing continuing education and access to appropriate resources for staff (Box 38.1).

SCIENTIFIC KNOWLEDGE BASE

Factors Influencing Safety

Health care takes place in a high-risk and complex environment. While specialization allows a wider range of patient treatments and services, it also provides greater opportunities for things to

BOX 38.1	Resources Related to Safety and Safety Initiatives

- Healthcare Excellence Canada (formerly known as the Canadian Patient Safety Institute and the Canadian Foundation for Healthcare Improvement): https://www.healthcareexcellence.ca
- Accreditation Canada: https://accreditation.ca
- Government of Canada–Disease and Prevention Control Guidelines: https://www.canada.ca/en/public-health/services/reports-publications/disease-prevention-control-guidelines.html
- Public Health Agency of Canada: https://www.canada.ca/en/public-health.html
- The Joint Commission: https://www.jointcommission.org
- Agency for Healthcare Research and Quality: https://www.ahrq.gov
- Institute for Healthcare Improvement: https://www.ihi.org
- US Department of Veterans Affairs: VHA National Center for Patient Safety: https://www.patientsafety.va.gov

---

Goal 1: People-Centred Care
Actions:
1.1 Health services are provided with humility in a holistic, dignified, and respectful manner.
1.2 All aspects of care are co-designed with patients and providers.
1.3 Patients and providers have positive health service experiences.

Goal 2: Safe Care
Actions:
2.1 Safety culture is evident across the continuum of health services and settings.
2.2 Safe and effective care is provided and monitored.
2.3 Safe care is addressed as a public health concern.

Goal 3: Accessible Care
Actions:
3.1 Care, diagnostics, and services are accessible for all people in an equitable and timely manner.
3.2 Human resources are effectively matched to population needs.

Goal 4: Appropriate Care
Actions:
4.1 Health services are planned and delivered based on the needs of the population.
4.2 Appropriate care is actively promoted and monitored, and unwarranted variations are minimized.
4.3 Emerging treatments and technologies are systematically evaluated and implemented in health services.

Goal 5: Integrated Care
Actions:
5.1 Health services are planned and delivered based on the needs of the population.
5.2 Patient information is available to patients and providers across health services.

Excerpted from the Health Standards Organization & Canadian Patient Safety Institute. (2020). *The Canadian quality & patient safety framework for health services* (pp. 6–9). https://www.patientsafetyinstitute.ca/en/toolsResources/Canadian-Quality-and-Patient-Safety-Framework-for-Health-and-Social-Services/Documents/CPSI-10001-CQPS-Framework-English_FA_Online.pdf

---

go wrong and patient safety incidents to occur. Some factors that may influence safety include patient and health care provider factors, task factors, technology factors, and environmental factors (Carayon & Wood, 2010).

Patient and Health Care Provider Factors. Patient and health care provider factors are characteristics of individuals, such as health, age, weight, needs, mood, personality, knowledge and experience, intelligence, language, and cultural background. Some characteristics may vary depending on the situation (e.g., mood, fatigue, and stress).

Task Factors. Task factors are characteristics of the tasks that health care providers must perform; this includes the tasks themselves as well as their characteristics (e.g., workflow, time pressure, and workload).

Technology Factors. These factors refer to the technologies (and their quantity and quality) available within an organization. Such factors include (1) the number of technologies, (2) the types of technologies, (3) their availability, and (4) their location. The design of the technologies includes their integration with other technologies, propensity to breakdown, responsiveness, and other design characteristics.

Environmental Factors. Environmental factors are the features of the work environment. These features include lighting, noise, physical space, and layout. A safe environment reduces the risk for illness and injury and helps to contain the cost of health care by preventing extended lengths of treatment or hospitalization, or both; improving or maintaining a patient's functional status; and increasing a patient's sense of well-being. A safe environment affords protection to the staff as well, allowing them to function at an optimal level.

Physical hazards in the environment place patients at risk for accidental injury and death. In Canada, unintentional injuries were the fourth leading cause of death for individuals of all ages in 2020 (Statistics Canada, 2022) and were also a major cause of disability. Specific causes of injury and death include poisoning, suffocation, drowning, fires, burns, and machinery accidents. Among adults aged 65 and older, falls are the most common cause of unintentional injury (CIHI, 2019). Many physical hazards, especially those contributing to falls, can be minimized through adequate lighting, the reduction of obstacles, and the implementation of security measures.

Organizational Factors. Organizational factors are the structural, cultural, and policy-related characteristics of the institution (e.g., leadership characteristics, culture, policies, hierarchy, and span of control).

Karsh and colleagues (2006) explain that "none of these factors may be important to patient safety in and of itself; rather, it is typically the interaction between inputs that can influence patient safety. For example, lighting is not good or bad by itself, but lighting can be problematic for certain tasks or create glare on certain displays. Similarly, a technology such as computerized physician order entry may or may not influence patient safety; rather, it will have a positive or negative impact on safety depending on many factors such as (a) how well it is integrated into the physical environment and the workflow, (b) how much training is provided to end users, and (c) how end users perceive its ease of use and usefulness" (p. i60).

Systems Thinking and Quality Improvement

Systems in health care are highly complex and are "characterized by multiple actors, multiple choices, multiple hand-offs, . . . no ownership, no natural team and no one with hospital-wide authority to make changes and insure quality" (Leape, 1997). In Reason's Swiss cheese model (Reason, 1997), each slice of cheese represents a barrier put in place to try to make the health care system safer (Figure 38.1). Each safeguard inherently contains a number of weaknesses, which are represented by the holes in the cheese. The holes in the slices of cheese are continuously moving around, and often a subsequent barrier is able to stop a hazard from reaching the patient. But when the holes line up in certain combinations, hazards have the opportunity to sneak through the safeguards that have been put in place and find their way to the patient. The holes at the end of the system, which come into contact with the patient, are termed *active failures* and generally involve those directly involved in patient care (e.g., nurses, physicians).

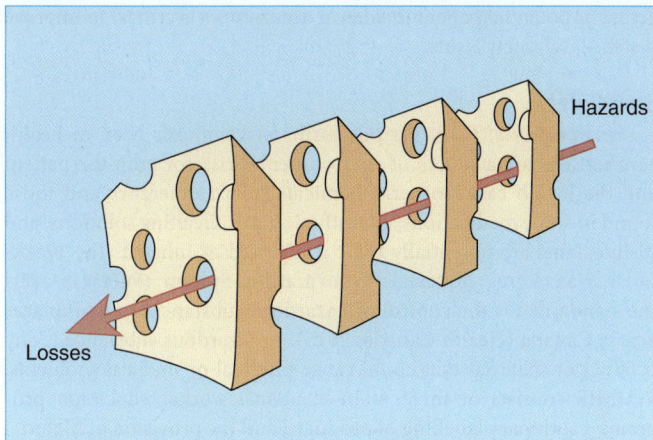

FIGURE 38.1 The Swiss cheese model of how defences, barriers, and safeguards may be penetrated by an accident trajectory. (From Reason, J. [2000]. Human error: Models and management. *British Medical Journal, 320*[7237], 768–770.)

The core principle of most "accident" frameworks is that multiple factors are involved in the accident, such as individual situational factors, workplace conditions, latent organizational and management decisions, or a combination of these factors. More complex processes and structures usually present greater potential for multiple factors and latent errors in the system. Health care providers who are directly in contact with patients most often identify the multiple failures that are cascading to cause the harm, but these individuals are fallible and, eventually, a patient may be harmed.

Reason (1997) states that only a systems approach (as opposed to an individual approach) will create a safer culture. His theory is strongly supported by evidence from other high-risk industries, which show the benefits of built-in defences, safeguards, and barriers. Defensive systems can either be "engineered" (referring to automated defensive systems such as automatic shut-downs [e.g., alarms, forcing functions, physical barriers]) or involve people dependent on defensive systems that rely on the skills and knowledge of the individual, such as pilots, surgeons, and anaesthetists. Policies and procedures are also defensive layers. For Reason (1997), the pivotal postincident question is why safeguards fail, rather than who caused the incident.

Safety Analysis or Safety Improvement Techniques. In the effort to ensure patient safety, many methods and techniques are applied, such as root cause analysis, failure mode and effect analysis, and Lean Six Sigma methodologies, to reduce or prevent errors. All of these methods provide different ways of analyzing and improving system design. But if nurses and other health care providers do not have training in systems thinking, any of those methods can lead to the wrong results.

Root cause analysis (RCA) is a retrospective approach used to find out what underlying features of a situation contributed to a patient safety incident. Adopting the idea that the immediate cause of an event is almost always the end result of multiple systems failures, RCA is used to seek to identify and understand all contributing causes in order to redesign the system to make it safer in the future.

Health care facilities often conduct a *failure mode and effect analysis (FMEA)* to identify problems with processes and products before they occur. FMEA is a prospective approach used to anticipate and prevent patient safety incidents through safe design. FMEA is an engineering approach—usually taken early in the development of a product—with the aim of imaginatively identifying potential failures and their effects. Knowledge from past failures may contribute to a designer's ability to foresee possible failures in their design. Designs are then adjusted to make failure less likely. FMEA is used to analyze every aspect of a system's design.

Human Factors. "Human factors" is a discipline dedicated to identifying and correcting incompatibility between people, their tools, and their environment. By identifying and correcting the elements leading to this incompatibility, an improvement in patient safety, efficiency, technology adoption, and user experience, as well as a reduction in the need for user training, can be achieved. To reiterate what James Reason, the eminent British psychologist and human factors expert, said, "we cannot change the human condition, but we can change the conditions under which humans work" (Reason, 1997).

Many organizations use human factor principles (e.g., forcing functions) to modify equipment (Cafazzo & St-Cyr, 2012). Forcing functions are built in the design of technologies to reduce or avoid errors and to ensure that the person will not miss key information or steps in a process. Furthermore, the goal of human factors engineering is to improve human performance. For example, by automating processes, fewer nurses are needed to collect the same information, the information is more complete and timely, the risk of data entry error is greatly reduced, and the need to retranscribe information from paper into a database has been eliminated (Backman et al., 2015). Despite the importance of human factors engineering in health care, the adoption and evaluation of these approaches have been slow in progressing. Some exceptions to this slow uptake include leading organizations such as Healthcare Human Factors group in Toronto, Ontario (https://humanfactors.ca) and the Armstrong Institute for Patient Safety and Quality at Johns Hopkins Hospital in Baltimore, Maryland (https://www.hopkinsmedicine.org/armstrong_institute/index.html).

Interdisciplinary Teamwork, Communication, and Feedback Skills. TeamSTEPPS® is a program that has been developed to provide health care providers with a range of strategies and techniques for improving teamwork (Agency for Healthcare Research and Quality [AHRQ], 2019). Effective teamwork does just not happen; it requires understanding of factors such as the characteristics of a successful team, how teams function, and ways to maintain good teamwork. Identifying the team members at the start of each episode of care is key in knowing the strengths and weaknesses of all team members. TeamSTEPPS is being widely incorporated into health care training and simulations.

NURSING KNOWLEDGE BASE

A nurse must be aware of common safety precautions and of the special risks to safety that are found in health care settings. A nurse must also be familiar with a patient's developmental level, mobility, sensory and cognitive statuses, and lifestyle choices.

Risks in Health Care Settings

Patient safety incidents occur when something that was planned as part of medical care does not work out, or when an inappropriate care plan was used. These incidents occur in all health care settings. Nurses must be aware of regulatory and organizational safety initiatives and individual patient risk factors. The AHRQ (2020) lists 20 tips to help prevent medical errors. The Joint Commission and the US Centers for Medicare and Medicaid Services emphasize error prevention and patient safety. Their "Speak Up" campaign encourages patients to take a role in preventing health care errors by becoming active, involved, and informed participants on the health care team. For example, patients are encouraged to ask health care workers if they have washed their hands before providing care. The five goals of the HSO and CPSI are specifically directed to reduce the risk of medical errors (Box 38.2). The goals highlight specific improvements in patient safety and ongoing problematic areas in health care. These evidence-informed recommendations require health care facilities to focus their attention on a series of specific actions. By aligning around five shared goals, the framework aims to focus action and resources to improve patient experiences and outcomes and reduce unwarranted care variation (HSO & CPSI, 2020).

When an actual or potential patient safety incident occurs, the nurse or health care provider who was involved must complete an incident report, also called an *occurrence report* in some settings. An **incident or occurrence report** is a confidential document that completely describes any patient incident occurring on the premises of a health care organization. Reporting allows an organization to identify trends or patterns throughout the facility and areas to improve. Focusing on the root cause of an event instead of the individual involved promotes a "culture of safety" that helps in specifically identifying what contributed to an error. The probability of an accident occurring declines when health care providers adhere to evidence-informed principles of safety (Taylor-Adams et al., 2008). It is important to note that reporting

actual or potential patient incidence occurrences is critical to improve system-level safety issues.

Staff Safety

Environmental Risk. Various forms of chemicals used in health care settings are a source of environmental risk for both the patient and the health care worker. Chemicals such as mercury and those found in some medications, anaesthetic gases, cleaning solutions, and disinfectants are potentially toxic if ingested or inhaled. The **Workplace Hazardous Materials Information System (WHMIS)** sets the standards for the control of hazardous substances in workplaces across Canada (Health Canada, 2015). A hazardous substance is any product or material that could cause physical or medical problems. WHMIS consists of three main elements: worker education programs, cautionary labelling of products, and the provision of Material Safety Data Sheets (MSDSs). Cautionary labels display the product's physical and health hazards and safety and first aid measures and identify the types of hazard that the product presents (Figure 38.2). MSDSs provide detailed information about the substance, any health hazards imposed, precautions for safe handling and use, and steps to take if the substance is released or spilled. Nurses must understand WHMIS labelling requirements and be aware of the location of MSDSs where they work.

Symbol	Name	Description
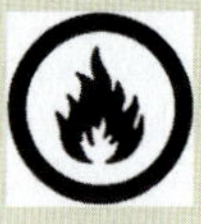	Flammable and combustible material	Product may catch fire when exposed to heat, sparks, or flame.
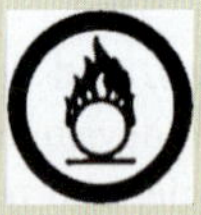	Oxidizing material	Product may cause a fire or explosion if exposed to combustible material.
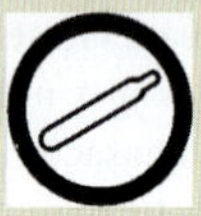	Compressed gas	Product is under high pressure. May explode or burst when heated, dropped, or damaged.
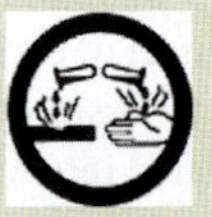	Corrosive material	Product can cause burns to eyes, skin, or respiratory system.
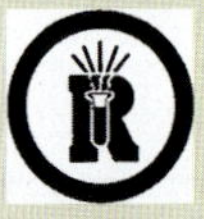	Dangerously reactive material	Product may react with light, heat, extreme temperatures, or vibration causing explosion, fire, or release of poisonous gases.
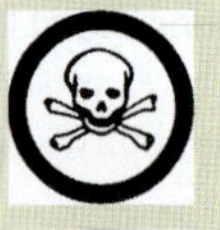	Poisonous and infectious material: immediate and serious toxic effects	Product may be fatal or cause serious or permanent damage if exposed to even once.
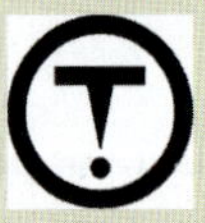	Poisonous and infectious material: other toxic effects	Product may cause cancer, birth defects, or other permanent damage if exposed to repeatedly.
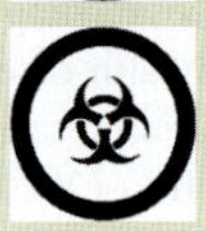	Poisonous and infectious material: biohazardous and infectious material	Product may cause disease, serious illness, or death.

FIGURE 38.2 Workplace Hazardous Materials Information System hazard symbols. (Adapted from Canadian Centre for Occupational Health and Safety. [2012]. *WHMIS labelling requirements.* https://www.ccohs.ca/topics/legislation/WHMIS)

Infection Prevention and Control. Controlling the spread of infection through the consistent use of routine practices helps maintain the safety of patients, staff, and visitors (see Chapter 34). The importance of these measures was illustrated during the outbreak of severe acute respiratory syndrome (SARS) in Toronto in 2003. The illness began with one individual admitted to an emergency department and spread to several patients and staff before its infectious nature was recognized and precautions were instituted. These measures have also been exemplified during the more recent worldwide COVID-19 pandemic.

Violence. Violence may be directed toward nurses from patients or patients' family members. Factors that can contribute to abusive situations include insufficient staffing levels, violation of patients' personal space due to lack of privacy, and provision of care that requires close physical contact (Canadian Nurses Association [CNA] & Canadian Federation of Nurses Unions [CFNU], 2015). Violence toward nurses can take the form of threats, intimidation, and physical behaviours, such as throwing objects. Nurses should seek assistance from co-workers to help them manage abusive situations (College of Nurses of Ontario [CNO], 2018). Incidents of workplace violence should be reported, as this is essential to the development of effective strategies to reduce such occurrences.

Patient Safety.
Specific risks to a patient's safety within the health care environment include falls, procedure-related accidents, and equipment-related accidents. The nurse assesses for these potential problem areas, considers the developmental level of the patient, and takes steps to prevent or minimize accidents.

Falls. Falls account for up to 90% of all reported incidents in hospitals. In addition to age, a history of previous falls, gait disturbance, balance and mobility difficulties, postural hypotension, sensory impairment, urinary and bladder dysfunction, use of medications, and certain medical diagnostic categories (e.g., cancer and cardiovascular, neurological, and cerebrovascular diseases) increase the risk of falling. One of the more common factors precipitating a fall is a patient's attempt to get out of bed to use the toilet.

Hip fractures are among the most serious fall-related injuries. Between April 2003 and March 2006, the rate of hip fracture in Canadian older persons during admission to hospital was close to 1 in 1 000 (CIHI, 2007). Older persons with a hip fracture may have a long period of recovery and may not be able to return to their previous level of functioning, even losing their ability to live independently (Parachute Canada, 2021a).

Falls that result in injuries can extend a patient's length of stay in the health care environment, placing the patient at greater risk for other complications. Nurses can implement multifaceted interventions to reduce the risk of falls, including assessment and communication about patient risks, staff assignments in close proximity, signage, improved patient hand-offs, nurse toilet and comfort safety rounds, and involving the patient and family (Spoelstra et al., 2012).

Procedure-Related Accidents. Procedure-related accidents are those that occur during therapy. They include medication and fluid administration errors, the improper application of external devices, and accidents related to the improper performance of procedures (e.g., incorrect urinary catheter insertion).

In a study of Canadian hospitals, Baker and colleagues (2004) found that 7.5% of patients were affected by medical errors during their hospital stay. The most common errors were related to surgical procedures and drug or fluid administration. In 15.9% of these cases, the errors resulted in the death of a patient. Etchells and colleagues (2008) stress that although medication errors cannot be avoided completely, systems can be designed to minimize the possibility and severity of errors. In order to reduce the likelihood of medication error, nurses must be aware of and stay current on "look-alike" names; nurses can post signs to this effect in medication rooms; and hospitals can choose to buy medication with labels that have tall-man lettering to reduce the risk of making errors (e.g., dimenhyDRINATE, and diphenhydramine [Institute for Safe Medication Practices (ISMP) Canada, 2016]). Nurses and health care facilities must build safety into processes of care and take a systems approach when making efforts to reduce medical errors (CNA & CFNU, 2019).

Nurses are able to prevent many procedure-related accidents by adhering to organizational policy and procedures and standards of nursing practice (Box 38.3). For example, proper preparation and administration of medications, use of patient and medication bar coding, and "smart" intravenous (IV) pumps can reduce medication errors (see Chapters 35 and 43). All nurses and other staff need to be aware that distractions and interruptions contribute to procedure-related accidents and need to be limited, especially during high-risk procedures such as medication administration. The potential for infection is reduced when surgical asepsis is used for sterile dressing changes or any invasive procedure such as insertion of a urinary catheter (see Chapter 34). Finally, correct use of safe patient handling techniques and equipment reduces the risk of injuries when moving and lifting patients (see Chapter 37).

BOX 38.3   Nine Life-Saving Patient Safety Solutions

- *Be aware of look-alike and sound-alike medication names.* Carefully review the medication orders of these drugs and use the 10 rights of medication safety.
- *Use patient identification.* Use two forms of patient identification, such as a hospital armband and medical record number.
- *Communicate during patient handover.* Communicate critical information, provide time for health care personnel to ask and resolve questions, and involve the patient and family during a handover process.
- *Perform correct procedure at correct body site.* Mark the operative site and take a "time out" to verify that it is the correct patient, operative site, and procedure before initiating the procedure.
- *Control concentrated electrolyte solutions.* Use the 10 rights of medication administration and follow the organization's protocols for these solutions.
- *Ensure medication accuracy at transitions in care.* Perform medication reconciliation at each health care transition. More specifically, during admission, transfer, and discharge, nurses should compare all medications a patient is taking against the medical order and against the patient's "home medication list."
- *Avoid catheter and tubing misconnections.* Nurses should be meticulous in the verification of the catheter and tubing connections, they should verify that the correct size catheter is in use, and they should verify that the correct connection tubing is being used. Nurses should label tubing and connections when a patient has multiple catheters.
- *Do not reuse single-use injection devices.* Nurses should never reuse needles, injection devices, or intravenous catheters.
- *Improve hand hygiene to prevent health care–associated infections.* Nurses should perform hand hygiene before and after each patient encounter and after contact with contaminated objects (even when gloves are worn). Family and visitors should be encouraged to perform hand hygiene before and after visits. (See Chapter 34 for more information on hand hygiene.)

Courtesy World Health Organization Collaborating Centre on Patient Safety Releases. (2007, May 2). *WHO launches nine patient safety solutions.* http://www.who.int/mediacentre/news/releases/2007/pr22/en/index.html

> **SAFETY ALERT** Always follow agency policy when using lifting devices, and do not use them alone. Student nurses should always work with qualified personnel when using these devices.

Equipment-Related Accidents. Accidents that are equipment related result from the malfunction, disrepair, or misuse of equipment, or from an electrical hazard. To avoid rapid infusion of IV fluids, all general-use and patient-controlled analgesic pumps need to have free-flow protection devices.

To avoid accidents, nurses should not operate monitoring or therapy equipment without adequate instruction. If faulty equipment is found, the nurse should place a tag on it to prevent it from being used on another patient and should promptly report any malfunctions. In health care settings, the clinical engineering staff are responsible for making regular safety checks of equipment.

Risks at Developmental Stages

A patient's developmental stage can present specific threats to safety. Patients throughout all developmental stages may be subject to abuse. Child abuse, domestic violence, and abuse of older persons are serious threats to safety. These topics are discussed in Chapters 24, 25, and 33.

Infants and Children. Unintentional injuries are the leading cause of death in Canadian children between the ages of 1 and 14 years; each year, 1 of every 230 children is hospitalized for treatment of unintentional injuries (Parachute Canada, 2016). The nature of the injuries sustained is related to normal growth and development. Small children are curious and trusting of their environment and do not perceive themselves to be in danger. The incidence of poisoning is highest in late infancy and toddlerhood because of children's increased level of oral activity and growing ability to explore the environment. Toddlers and preschoolers, who are attracted to water but do not perceive its dangers, are at a greater risk for drowning. Childhood injuries are also reflective of adults' perceptions of the causes of accidents and their ability to prevent them. For example, the incorrect use of vehicle restraints for children aged 5 to 14 places these children at greater risk of death from injuries sustained in motor vehicle accidents (the leading cause of death from injury in this age group) (Parachute Canada, 2016).

Adolescents. As children enter adolescence, they develop greater independence and begin to develop a sense of identity and their own values. Adolescents start to separate emotionally from their families, and peers generally have a stronger influence on them. The struggle for identity may cause a teenager to experience shyness, fear, and anxiety, with resulting dysfunction at home or school. In an attempt to relieve the tensions associated with physical and psychosocial changes, as well as peer pressures, adolescents may begin to act impulsively and engage in risk-taking behaviours such as smoking and substance use. In addition to the health risks posed by nicotine and other substances (e.g., alcohol, drugs, glue), the ingestion of such substances increases the incidence of accidents such as drowning and motor vehicle accidents.

Adults. Threats to an adult's safety are frequently related to lifestyle habits. For example, a patient who consumes excessive alcohol is at greater risk for motor vehicle accidents. A long-term smoker has a greater risk of cardiovascular and pulmonary diseases. Likewise, an adult experiencing a high level of stress is more likely to have an accident or illnesses such as headaches, gastrointestinal disorders, and infections.

Older Persons. The physiological changes that occur during the aging process increase a patient's risk for injury (Box 38.4). Changes in

---

BOX 38.4	Changes Associated With Aging That Increase the Risk of Accidents

Musculoskeletal Changes
Muscle strength and function decrease, joints become less mobile, bones are more brittle due to osteoporosis, postural changes (e.g., kyphosis) are common, and range of motion is limited.

Nervous System Changes
All voluntary or automatic reflexes slow to some extent, the ability to respond to multiple stimuli decreases, and sensitivity to touch is decreased.

Sensory Changes
Peripheral vision and lens accommodation decrease, lenses may develop opacity (cataracts), the stimuli threshold for light touch and pain increases, the transmission of hot and cold impulses is delayed, and hearing is impaired as high-frequency tones become less perceptible.

Genitourinary Changes
Nocturia and occurrences of incontinence increase with age.

Adapted from Touhy, T. A., & Jett, K. F. (2020). *Ebersole & Hess' toward healthy aging: Human needs and nursing response* (10th ed.). Elsevier.

---

vision, hearing, mobility, reflexes, circulation, and the ability to make quick judgements predispose older persons to falls (see Chapter 25). When a patient is hospitalized, confusion, multiple medical conditions, medications, immobility, urinary urgency, age-related sensory changes, postural instability, and an unfamiliar environment further contribute to the risk of falls (Meiner & Yeager, 2018). Certain disease states common to older persons, such as arthritis and cerebrovascular accidents, also increase the chances of injury. In 2017–18, unintentional falls were the most common cause of injury in adults aged 65 years and older, with 81% of injuries in this age group caused by falls (CIHI, 2019). Patients most often fall while transferring from beds, chairs, and toilets; while getting into or out of a bathtub; by tripping over carpet edges or doorway thresholds; by slipping on wet surfaces; and while descending stairs. Icy walkways and obstacles in the yard are also common causes of outdoor falls in older persons.

Individual Risk Factors

Other risk factors posing threats to safety are lifestyle, impaired mobility, sensory or communication impairment, and a lack of safety awareness.

Impaired Mobility. Impaired mobility due to muscle weakness, paralysis, or poor coordination or balance is a major factor in patient falls. Immobilization predisposes a patient to additional physiological and emotional hazards, which can in turn further restrict mobility and independence.

Sensory or Communication Impairment. Patients with visual, hearing, tactile, or communication impairment, such as aphasia or a language barrier, are at greater risk for injury. Such patients may not be able to perceive a potential danger or express their need for assistance (see Chapter 48).

Lack of Safety Awareness. Some patients are unaware of safety precautions, such as keeping medicine or poisons away from children or observing the expiration date on food products. A complete nursing assessment, including a home inspection, can help nurses identify a patient's level of knowledge regarding home safety so that deficiencies can be corrected with an individualized nursing care plan.

CRITICAL THINKING

Successful critical thinking requires a synthesis of a nurse's knowledge and experience, as well as of information gathered from patients, combined with professional standards. Clinical judgements require nurses to anticipate necessary information, analyze the data, and make decisions regarding patient care. Critical thinking is an ongoing process. During an assessment (Figure 38.3), the nurse should consider all critical thinking elements and information about the specific patient to make appropriate nursing diagnoses.

In the case of safety, a nurse integrates knowledge from nursing and other scientific disciplines with previous experiences in caring for patients who were at risk for or had an injury. This is combined with critical thinking attitudes such as responsibility and discipline, and any standards of practice that are applicable. Agency guidelines and professional nursing associations provide standards for nursing activities such as medication administration, fall-prevention steps, and infection control to guide nurses in the provision of safe care. One such set of standards is the Registered Nurses' Association of Ontario (RNAO) (2017) *Preventing Falls and Reducing Injury from Falls*. For example, while assessing a patient's home environment, the nurse needs to consider typical locations within the home where dangers commonly exist. For a patient who has a visual impairment, the nurse applies previous experience in caring for patients with visual changes to anticipate how to thoroughly assess the patient's needs. Critical thinking directs the nurse to anticipate what needs to be assessed and how to make conclusions about available data.

❖ SAFETY AND THE NURSING PROCESS

Nurses are responsible for incorporating critical thinking skills when using the nursing process, assessing each patient and their environment for hazards that threaten safety, and planning and intervening appropriately to maintain a safe environment. The nursing process provides a clinical decision-making approach to develop and implement an individualized plan of safe patient care.

◆ Assessment

To conduct a thorough patient assessment, nurses must consider possible threats to a patient's safety, including the patient's immediate environment, as well as any individual risk factors.

Health History. By conducting a health history, the nurse gathers data about the patient's level of wellness to determine if any underlying conditions exist that pose threats to safety. For example, nurses should give special attention to assessing the patient's gait, muscle strength and coordination, balance, and vision. A review of the patient's developmental status must be considered as assessment information is analyzed. A nurse must also review whether the patient has been exposed to any environmental hazards or is taking medications or undergoing procedures that pose risks. For example, the use of diuretics increases the frequency of voiding and may result in the patient having to use toilet facilities more often. This may then increase the likelihood of a fall, as these often occur when patients get out of bed quickly because of urinary urgency.

Patient's Home Environment. When caring for a patient in the home, a home hazard assessment is necessary. The nurse should walk through the home with the patient and discuss how the patient normally conducts daily activities. Key areas to inspect are the bathroom, kitchen, and areas with stairs. For example, when assessing the adequacy of the lighting, the nurse should inspect areas where the patient moves and works, such as outside walkways, steps, interior halls, and doorways. Getting a sense of the patient's routine helps the nurse recognize less obvious hazards.

Health Care Environment. When a patient is being cared for within a health care facility, a nurse must determine if any hazards exist in the immediate care environment. Does the placement of equipment or furniture pose barriers to ambulation? Does the positioning of the patient's bed allow the patient to reach items on a bedside table? Does the patient need assistance with ambulation? Is the patient aware of activity restrictions? Has the patient been taught to use the call bell, and is it within reach? Collaboration with clinical engineering staff is essential to make sure that equipment has been assessed and is in proper functioning condition.

Risk for Falls. Assessment of the patient's fall risk factors is essential in determining specific needs and targeting interventions to prevent falls. A fall assessment tool (Table 38.1) can help determine potential risks before accidents and injuries result. The tool shown in Table 38.1 is the Hendrich II Fall Risk Model. This tool is intended for use in acute care settings and takes into account the patient's ability to move independently

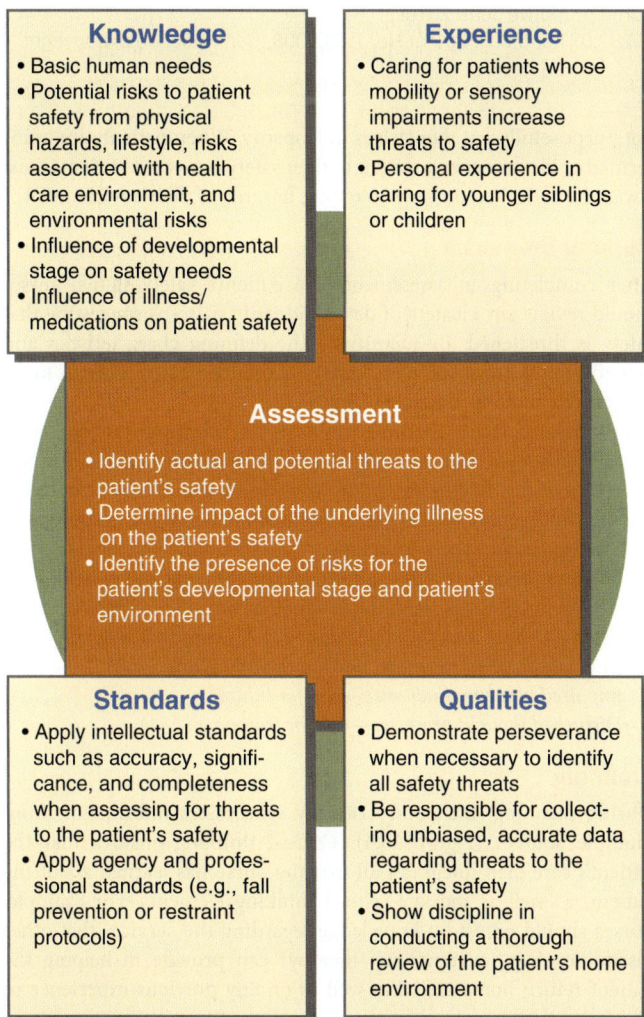

Knowledge
- Basic human needs
- Potential risks to patient safety from physical hazards, lifestyle, risks associated with health care environment, and environmental risks
- Influence of developmental stage on safety needs
- Influence of illness/medications on patient safety

Experience
- Caring for patients whose mobility or sensory impairments increase threats to safety
- Personal experience in caring for younger siblings or children

Assessment
- Identify actual and potential threats to the patient's safety
- Determine impact of the underlying illness on the patient's safety
- Identify the presence of risks for the patient's developmental stage and patient's environment

Standards
- Apply intellectual standards such as accuracy, significance, and completeness when assessing for threats to the patient's safety
- Apply agency and professional standards (e.g., fall prevention or restraint protocols)

Qualities
- Demonstrate perseverance when necessary to identify all safety threats
- Be responsible for collecting unbiased, accurate data regarding threats to the patient's safety
- Show discipline in conducting a thorough review of the patient's home environment

FIGURE 38.3 Critical thinking model for safety assessment.

TABLE 38.1   Hendrich II Fall Risk Model™

Risk Factor	Risk Point	Score
Confusion/Disorientation/Impulsivity	4	
Symptomatic Depression	2	
Altered Elimination	1	
Dizziness/Vertigo	1	
Gender (Male)	1	
Any Administered Antiepileptics (Anticonvulsants):	2	
Carbamazepine, divalproex sodium, ethotoin, ethosuximide, felbamate, fosphenytoin, gabapentin, lamotrigine, mephenytoin, methsuximide, phenobarbital, phenytoin, primidone, topiramate, trimethadione, valproic acid*		
Any Administered Benzodiazepines†:	1	
Alprazolam, chloridiazepoxide, clonazepam, clorazepate dipotassium, diazepam, flurazepam, halazepam, lorazepam, midazolam, oxazepam, temazepam, triazolam		
Get-Up-and-Go Test: "Rising from a Chair"		
If unable to assess, monitor for change in activity level, assess other risk factors, document both on patient chart with date and time.		
Ability to rise in a single movement—No loss of balance with steps	0	
Pushes up, successful in one attempt	1	
Multiple attempts but successful	3	
Unable to rise without assistance during test	4	
If unable to assess, document this on the patient chart with the date and time		
(A score of 5 or greater = High Risk)	Total Score	

Ongoing medication review updates:

*Levetiracetam (Keppra) was not assessed during the original research conducted to create the Hendrich Fall Risk Model. As an antiepileptic, levetiracetam does have adverse effects of somnolence and dizziness, which contribute to its fall risk and should be scored (effective June 2010).
†The study did not include the effect of benzodiazepine-like drugs since they were not on the market at that time. However, given their similarity in drug structure, mechanism of action, and drug effects, they should also be scored (effective June 2010).

as well as other factors that can increase the risk for falls, such as certain types of medications (Hendrich, 2016). Nurses should familiarize themselves with the fall assessment tool used in their clinical area as such tools vary among agencies. Patients should be assessed for their risk of falls on admission to the health care setting. An assessment should also be completed after a fall to determine why the fall occurred, as patients who have fallen are at much greater risk of falling again (Hendrich, 2016; RNAO, 2017). In many cases, family members can be significant resources in assessing a patient's fall risk. Families are often able to report on the patient's level of confusion and ability to ambulate.

Risk for Medical Errors. Nurses should always be alert to factors within the environment that create conditions in which medical errors are more likely to occur. Studies indicate that overwork and fatigue cause a significant decrease in alertness and concentration, leading to errors (Trinkoff et al., 2006). Nurses need to be aware of these factors and include checks and balances when working under stressful conditions. For example, verifying two patient identifiers (e.g., name and birthdate) in addition to checking the patient's identification bracelet before starting any procedure or administering any medication can reduce the risk for error.

As noted earlier, the National Steering Committee on Patient Safety (2002) made recommendations to improve the safety of Canada's health care system. At the core of these recommendations was the need to nurture a culture of safety within the system. The CPSI was established in 2003 to provide leadership in the development of such a culture.

Patient Expectations. Patients generally expect to be safe in their home and in the health care setting. However, a patient's viewpoint of what is safe may differ from the nurse's viewpoint. For this reason, any assessment must include the patient's understanding of their potential risk factors. This information will be important later if changes are needed in the patient's environment. Patients usually do

not purposefully put themselves in jeopardy. When patients are uninformed or inexperienced, threats to their safety can occur. Patients must always be consulted on ways to reduce hazards in their environment.

Nursing Diagnosis

After completing an assessment of a patient's safety status, nurses should review any clusters of data to identify patterns suggesting that safety is threatened. By identifying the defining characteristics and related factors from the data, nurses should be better able to make appropriate nursing diagnoses (Box 38.5).

The related factors become the basis for selecting nursing therapies. For example, *risk for injury related to impaired mobility* and *risk for injury related to barriers in the home environment* require different nursing interventions. The patient with altered mobility may require ambulatory aids and physiotherapy. When the related factor is barriers in the home, a nurse might recommend changes that will create a safer environment. At times, as in the example in Box 38.5, multiple related factors may apply. Examples of nursing diagnoses that may apply for patients whose safety is threatened are the following:

- *Impaired home maintenance—risk for injury*
- *Disturbed thought processes—risk for trauma*

Planning

During planning, the nurse critically synthesizes information from multiple sources (Figure 38.4). Critical thinking ensures that the patient's care plan integrates all that the nurse has learned about the patient, as well as the key critical thinking elements. For example, nurses should reflect on knowledge regarding the services that other disciplines (e.g., occupational therapy) can provide in helping the patient return home safely, as well as on any previous experience in which a patient benefited from safety interventions. These experiences can help nurses adapt approaches to suit new patients. Applying critical

BOX 38.5 NURSING DIAGNOSTIC PROCESS

Assessment Activities	Defining Characteristics	Nursing Diagnosis
Observe patient's mobility and body alignment.	Uncoordinated gait Poor posture	*Risk for injury related to impaired mobility, decreased vision, poorly lit home, and cluttered environment*
Ask patient about visual acuity.	Reports difficulty seeing at night Reports tripping over rugs and furniture	
Complete a home hazard appraisal.	Poorly lit home Rooms filled with small items Excessive amount of furniture for size of room Rugs not secure	

Knowledge
- Role of community resources in safety promotion
- Safety risks posed in use of home care therapies (e.g., home oxygenation, IV therapy)
- Safety interventions suited to patient's risks and condition

Experience
- Previous patient responses to planned nursing therapies to improve safety (e.g., what worked and what did not work)

Planning
- Select nursing interventions to promote safety according to the patient's developmental and health care needs
- Consult with occupational therapists and physiotherapists for assistive devices
- Select interventions that will improve the safety of the patient's home environment

Standards
- Establish interventions individualized to the patient's safety needs
- Apply agency and professional standards of providing interventions in a safe and appropriate manner

Qualities
- Use creativity to assist in designing interventions suited to patient needs and available resources
- Take risks to implement interventions that explore new resources or use current resources in new ways

FIGURE 38.4 Critical thinking model for safety planning.

thinking qualities such as creativity helps the nurse and the patient collaborate in planning interventions that are relevant and helpful, particularly when changes are being made in the home environment.

Goals and Outcomes. Planning and goal setting need to be done in collaboration with the patient, the family, and other members of the health care team (Box 38.6). The patient who is an active participant in reducing threats to safety will be more alert to potential hazards. Goals and outcomes must be measurable and realistic, with consideration to the resources available to the patient. The overall goal for a patient with a threat to safety is to remain free from injury. The following are examples of expected outcomes that focus on a patient's need for safety:

- Modifiable hazards will be reduced in the home environment by 100% within 1 month.
- The patient will not suffer a fall or injury.
- The patient will identify risks associated with visual impairment.

Setting Priorities. Nursing interventions are prioritized to provide safe and efficient care. For example, the patient described in the concept map in Figure 38.5 has several nursing diagnoses. The patient's mobility difficulty is an obvious priority because of its influence on skin integrity and the risk for falls. A nurse should plan individualized interventions based on the severity of risk factors and the patient's developmental stage, level of health, lifestyle, and culture (Box 38.7). Planning also involves understanding the patient's need to maintain independence within physical and cognitive capabilities. The nurse and the patient collaborate to establish ways of maintaining the patient's active involvement within the home and health care environment. Educating the patient and family is also an important intervention to reduce safety risks over the long term.

Continuity of Care. Patients need to learn how to identify and select resources within their community that enhance safety (e.g., block parent homes, local police departments, and neighbours willing to check on a patient's well-being). Collaboration with the patient and family and other disciplines such as social work, occupational therapy, and physiotherapy may become an important part of the plan of care. For example, a hospitalized patient may need to go to a rehabilitation facility to gain strength and endurance before being discharged home. Nurses need to ensure that the patient and family understand the need for these types of resources and are willing to make changes that will promote the patient's safety.

◆ Implementation

Nursing interventions are directed toward ensuring a patient's safety in all settings and include health promotion, developmental interventions, environmental interventions, and limiting specific risks to patient safety.

Health Promotion. To promote a patient's health, it is necessary for the individual to be in a safe environment and to practise a lifestyle that minimizes the risk of injury. Dames et al. (2021) have described passive and active strategies aimed at health promotion. *Passive strategies* are implemented through public health and government legislative interventions (e.g., sanitation and clean water laws). *Active strategies* are those in which the individual is actively involved through changes in lifestyle (e.g., wearing a seat belt or installing outdoor lighting) and participation in wellness programs. The nurse can participate by supporting legislation and working in community-based settings. Because environmental and community values have the greatest influence on

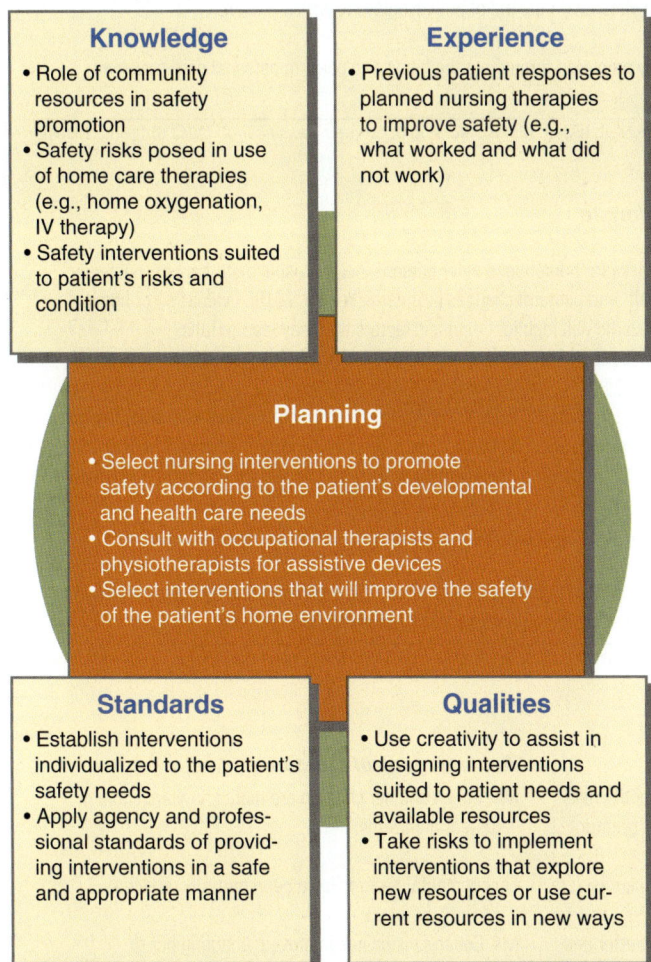

Risk for Injury

ASSESSMENT

The following is a scenario for developing a nursing care plan to mitigate against the risk of patient injuries. A visiting nurse is seeing Ms. Cohen, an 85-year-old woman, at her home. The patient has been recovering from a mild stroke affecting her left side. Ms. Cohen lives alone but receives regular assistance from her daughter and son, who both live within 16 km. The nurse's assessment includes a discussion of Ms. Cohen's health problem and how the stroke has affected her, as well as a pertinent physical examination.

Assessment Activities	*Findings and Defining Characteristics*
Ask Ms. Cohen how the stroke has affected her mobility.	She responds, "I bump into things, and I'm afraid I'm going to fall."
Conduct a home hazard assessment.	Cabinets in the kitchen are in disarray and full of breakable items that could fall out. Throw rugs are on floors; bathroom lighting is poor (40-watt bulb); bathtub lacks safety strips and grab bars; and home is cluttered with furniture and small objects.
Observe Ms. Cohen's gait and posture.	Ms. Cohen has kyphosis and has a hesitant, uncoordinated gait. She frequently holds walls for support.
Assess Ms. Cohen's muscle strength.	The left arm and leg are weaker than the right.
Assess visual acuity with corrective lenses.	Ms. Cohen has trouble reading and seeing familiar objects at a distance while wearing current glasses.

NURSING DIAGNOSIS: Risk for injury related to impaired mobility, decreased visual acuity, and physical environmental hazards

PLANNING

Goals (Nursing Outcomes Classification)*	*Expected Outcomes*
	Risk Control
Home will be free of hazards within 1 month.	Modifiable hazards in kitchen and hallway will be reduced in the home within 1 week. Revisions to bathroom will be completed in 1 month.
	Knowledge: Personal Safety
Patient and family will be knowledgeable of potential hazards for patient's age group within 1 week.	Patient and her daughter or son will identify risks and the steps to avoid them in the home at the conclusion of a teaching session next week.
	Fall Prevention Behaviour
Patient will express greater sense of feeling safe from falls in 1 month.	Patient will report improved vision with the aid of new eyeglasses within 1 week.
Patient will be free of injury within 2 weeks.	Patient will be able to safely ambulate throughout the home and perform personal care activities within 2 weeks.

*Outcome classification labels from Moorhead, S., Swanson, E., Johnson, M., & Maas, M. L (Eds.). (2018). *Nursing outcomes classification (NIC)* (6th ed.). Elsevier

INTERVENTIONS

Interventions (Nursing Interventions Classification)†	*Rationale*
Fall Prevention	
Review findings from home hazard assessment with patient and her daughter and son.	Fall risks for homebound older persons include visual disturbances, unsteady gait, and postural changes (Meiner & Yeager, 2018). Evaluation of home hazards will highlight extrinsic factors that may lead to falls.
Establish a list of priorities to modify. Have patient's son or daughter assist in installing bathroom safety devices.	Modification of environment reduces fall risk (McCullagh, 2006).
Install lighting (75-W bulbs, nonglare) throughout the home. Have patient's son or daughter install blinds over kitchen windows.	With aging, the pupil loses the ability to adjust to light, causing sensitivity to glare. Glare can make it difficult to clearly see a walking path (Meiner & Yeager, 2018).
Discuss with patient and daughter and son the normal changes of aging, effects of recent stroke, associated risks for injury, and how to reduce risks.	Education regarding management of hazards can reduce fear of falling (Touhy & Jett, 2020).
Encourage daughter or son to schedule patient's vision testing for new prescription within 2–4 weeks.	Improved visual acuity reduces incidence of falls (Dames et al., 2021).
Refer patient to a physiotherapist to assess need for assistive devices for kyphosis, left-sided weakness, and gait.	Exercise often improves gait, balance, and flexibility. Modifying gait problems by increasing lower extremity strength reduces fall risk.

†Intervention classification labels from Bulechek, G. M., Butcher, H. K., McCloskey Dochterman, J. M., et al. (Eds.). (2019). *Nursing interventions classification (NIC)* (7th ed.). Mosby.

EVALUATION

Nursing Actions	*Patient Response and Finding*	*Achievement of Outcome*
Ask patient and family to identify risks.	Ms. Cohen and her daughter and son are able to identify risks during a walk through the home and expressed a greater sense of safety as a result of changes made.	Ms. Cohen and her children are more knowledgeable of potential hazards.
Observe environment for elimination of hazards.	Throw rugs have been removed. Lighting has been increased to 75 watts, except in the bathroom and bedroom.	Environmental hazards have been partially reduced.
Reassess Ms. Cohen's visual acuity.	Ms. Cohen has new glasses and says she can read better and see distant objects more clearly.	Ms. Cohen's vision has improved, enabling her to ambulate more safely.
Observe Ms. Cohen's gait and posture.	Ms. Cohen's gait remains hesitant and uncoordinated; she reports that her daughter or son has not had time to take her to the physiotherapist.	The outcome of safe ambulation has not been totally achieved; continue to encourage Ms. Cohen and daughter or son to go to physiotherapy appointment.

> concept map

Nursing diagnosis: Risk for falls related to left-sided paralysis
• Imbalanced gait
• Receiving diuretic
• Urinary incontinence
• Fell at home 1 month ago

Nursing diagnosis: Risk for impaired skin integrity related to decreased sensation
• Sensory impairment left side
• Urinary incontinence
• Difficulty changing positions

Interventions
• Implement fall precautions
• Visit patient hourly to determine needs
• Avoid late evening fluids
• Schedule toileting and hygiene activities

Interventions
• Initiate skin care protocol
• Turn patient every 1.5 hours
• Offer urinal/toilet every 2 hours

Patient's chief medical diagnosis: 20 pack-year smoking history, left-sided paralysis from previous stroke, postoperative leg surgery
Priority assessments: Functional status, respiratory status, skin integrity

Nursing diagnosis: Impaired physical mobility related to left-sided paralysis
• Difficulty turning
• Reduced strength on left side
• Left-sided neglect

Nursing diagnosis: Ineffective airway clearance related to retained thick pulmonary secretions
• Abnormal lung sounds in both lobes
• Dyspnea
• Coughs with difficulty

Interventions
• Range of joint motion
• Schedule short walks
• Occupational therapy for bathing, dressing, and other ADLs

Interventions
• Teach cascade cough
• Increase fluids
• Assist patient with coughing and deep breathing every hour

—— Link between medical diagnosis and nursing diagnosis

FIGURE 38.5 Concept map for a patient with a cerebrovascular accident 3 months previously with left-sided paralysis, 2 days after right femoral–popliteal bypass. *ADLs,* Activities of daily living.

BOX 38.7 CULTURAL ASPECTS OF CARE

Cultural phenomena affecting health and safety include attitudes toward personal space, social organizations, communication, and environmental control. While conducting a home assessment for risks to safety, nurses must remember that they have entered the patient's territory and that the patient's attitude toward their residence and belongings must be appreciated. For example, some patients may be considered aloof and distant when it comes to personal space. It may be very difficult for them to have an outsider in their home who suggests changes regarding their personal belongings to reduce physical hazards. It is particularly difficult to determine a patient's attitude toward their home environment when the patient's primary language and that of the health care provider differ.

Another culturally sensitive issue involves the patient's sense of environmental control. Nurses must be aware of health beliefs and practices that will affect the outcome of interventions. For example, a reliance on family and religious organizations, as opposed to community resources, may affect the patient's adherence to nursing interventions and referrals.

Nurses must learn to ask questions sensitively and to show respect for different cultural beliefs. Adapting to different cultural beliefs and practices requires flexibility. Respect for the belief systems of others and the effects of those beliefs on the patient's well-being are critically important to competent health care. The nurse must have the ability and knowledge to communicate about and to understand health behaviours influenced by culture.

Implications for Practice

• Resistance to change long-standing habits can interfere with a cultural group's acceptance of injury-prevention practices. Nurses should include family members who have a strong influence, such as a dominant man or older woman, when providing safety education.
• Nurses should evaluate the use of traditional ethnic remedies or foods that contain lead, as these can increase a patient's risk for lead poisoning.
• Nurses should remember that living in rural areas and in manufactured housing places the patient at greater risk for fire-related injuries and death.
• Nurses should stress the importance of having fully functioning smoke detectors and a multipurpose fire extinguisher.
• Nurses should assess the patient's smoking and drinking habits. Residential fire deaths are often attributed to the use of cigarettes and alcohol.
• Patients who live in poverty and have low educational levels are at greater risk for injury and disease. Nurses should assist the patient and family in identifying community resources, such as the local health office or clinic.
• Nurses also need to be aware of family patterns and how the patient and family interact with each other. Family disruption and weak intergenerational ties can increase a patient's risk for injury from violent behaviour.

Adapted from Giger, J. N., & Davidhizar, R. (2002). The Giger and Davidhizar transcultural assessment model. *Journal of Transcultural Nursing, 13,* 185.

health promotion, community and home health nurses assess and recommend safety measures in the home, school, neighbourhood, and workplace.

Developmental Interventions. Accidents involving children are mostly preventable, thus parents need to be aware of specific dangers at each stage of growth and development. Accident prevention requires health education for parents and the removal of dangers whenever possible. Nurses are frequently in a position to educate parents about

reducing the risks of injuries for young children (see Chapter 23). Nurses working in prenatal and postpartum settings can incorporate safety into the care plan of the child-bearing family. Community health nurses can assess the home and show parents how to promote safety in their homes (Table 38.2). The following discussion highlights some specific risks at different developmental stages.

Infants, Toddlers, and Preschoolers. Small children must be protected from accidental poisoning. Strategies for prevention of the accidental ingestion of poisonous materials are outlined in Table 38.2.

TABLE 38.2	**Interventions to Promote Safety for Children and Adolescents**
Intervention	**Rationale**
Infants and Toddlers	
Ensure that infants sleep on their backs. Teach parents the mnemonic "back to sleep."	Sleeping on the back is associated with the lowest risk of sudden infant death syndrome (SIDS) (Canadian Paediatric Society [CPS], 2021).
Ensure that parents do not fill cribs with pillows, large stuffed toys, or comforters. Sheets should fit snugly.	Infants may become entwined in sheets and other bedding and suffocate (CPS, 2021).
Ensure that pacifiers are not attached to a string or ribbon and placed around a child's neck.	Strangulation may occur.
Ensure that all instructions for preparing and storing formula are being followed.	Proper formula preparation and storage prevents contamination. A formula may come in a concentrated form, or it may already be diluted and ready to use. Following directions ensures the proper concentration of the formula. Undiluted formula can cause fluid and electrolyte disturbances; overly diluted formula does not provide sufficient nutrients.
Ensure that only large, soft toys without small parts such as buttons are being used.	Small parts can become dislodged and choking and aspiration are possible.
Teach parents that playpens with mesh sides should not be left with a side down; spaces between crib slats should be <6 cm apart.	A child's head may become wedged in the lowered mesh side or between crib slats, and asphyxiation may occur.
Teach parents to never leave crib sides down or leave babies unattended on change tables or in infant seats, swings, strollers, or high chairs.	Infants and toddlers can roll or move and fall from change tables or out of accessories such as infant seats or swings.
Teach parents to discontinue using accessories such as infant seats and swings when the child becomes too active or physically too big.	When physically active or too big, the child can fall out of or tip over these accessories and suffer an injury.
Teach parents to never leave a child alone in the bathroom, in the tub, or near any water source (e.g., a pool).	Accidental drowning may occur.
Teach parents strategies to baby-proof the home: • Install safety locks on floor-level cabinets. • Use child-resistant caps. • Place small or sharp objects, medications, and cleaning agents out of children's reach. • Leave potentially poisonous materials in their original containers. • Remove poisonous plants from the home. Also ensure that parents are aware that poisoning can result from swallowing miniature button or disc batteries, commonly found in games, cameras, calculators, and watches.	Babies explore their world with their hands and mouth. Choking and poisoning may occur.
Teach parents to remove plastic bags from the cleaners or grocery store from the home.	Suffocation may occur if plastic covers the nose and mouth.
Ensure that electrical outlets are protected by covers.	Crawling babies may insert objects into outlets and experience an electrical shock.
Ensure that window guards are on all windows.	Guards prevent children from falling out of windows.
Ensure that keyless locks (e.g., deadbolts) have been installed on doors above a child's reach (even when they are standing on a chair).	Keyless locks prevent a toddler from leaving the house and wandering off. Death from exposure, car accidents, and drowning may occur if a toddler wanders away. Keyless locks allow for rapid exit in the case of fire.
Teach parents that children weighing <36 kg must always be in an age- and weight-appropriate car seat that has been installed according to the manufacturer's instructions. This includes car seats and booster seats. Children under 13 years should be in the back seat of the car. All passengers should wear their seat belts (CPS, 2020).	In case of a sudden stop or crash, an unrestrained child may suffer severe head injuries and death.
Encourage caregivers to learn cardiopulmonary resuscitation and the Heimlich manoeuvre.	Caregivers should be prepared to intervene in acute emergencies, such as choking.

Continued

TABLE 38.2	Interventions to Promote Safety for Children and Adolescents—cont'd
Intervention	**Rationale**
Preschoolers	
Encourage parents to teach children to swim at an early age, but always provide supervision near water.	Swimming is a useful skill that may some day save a child's life. However, all children need constant supervision near water.
Encourage parents to teach children how to cross streets and walk in parking lots. Instruct them to never run out into the street after a ball or toy.	Pedestrian accidents involving young children are common.
Encourage parents to teach children not to talk to, go with, or accept any item from a stranger. Children should also be taught not to go with a known adult unless they have their parent's permission (MissingKids.ca, 2019).	This precaution reduces the risk of exploitation and abduction.
Encourage parents to teach children basic physical safety rules, such as the proper use of safety scissors, never running with an object in their mouth or hand, and never attempting to use the stove or oven unassisted.	The risk of injury is lower if children are taught basic safety procedures.
Encourage parents to teach children not to eat items found in the street or grass.	Poisoning may occur.
Teach parents to remove doors from unused refrigerators and freezers and to instruct children not to play or hide in a car trunk or unused appliances.	If a child cannot freely exit from an appliance or car trunks, asphyxiation may occur.
School-Aged Children	
Encourage parents to teach children the safe use of equipment for play and work.	Children need to learn the safe, appropriate use of implements to avoid injury.
Encourage parents to teach children proper bicycle safety, including the use of a helmet and rules of the road.	These safety precautions may reduce injuries from falling off a bike or being hit by a car.
Encourage parents to teach children proper techniques for specific sports, as well as the need to wear proper safety gear (e.g., eyewear or mouth guards).	The use of proper sports techniques, the correct equipment, and protective gear prevents injuries.
Encourage parents to teach children not to operate electrical equipment while unsupervised.	If an electrical mishap were to occur, no one would be available to help.
Teach parents that children should never have access to firearms or other weapons. All firearms should be kept in locked cabinets.	Children are often fascinated by firearms and weapons and may attempt to play with them.
Encourage parents to teach children safe use of the Internet.	Children are vulnerable to being exploited by predators over the Internet.
Adolescents	
Encourage enrollment in driver's education classes.	Many injuries in this age group are related to motor vehicle accidents.
Provide information about the effects of using alcohol, drugs, or other substances (e.g., glue, aerosols, or gasoline).	Adolescents are prone to risk-taking behaviours and are subject to peer pressure.
Provide sex education, including safer sex practices, birth control, and abstinence.	Many adolescents begin sexual relationships. Pregnancy and sexually transmitted infections may result.
Refer adolescents to community and school-sponsored activities.	Adolescents need to socialize with peers yet need some supervision.
Encourage mentoring relationships between adults and adolescents.	Adolescents are in need of role models after whom they can pattern their behaviour.
Teach adolescents the safe use of the Internet.	Safe use of the Internet avoids overuse and possible exposure to inappropriate websites.

Adapted from Hockenberry, M., & Wilson, D. (2019). *Wong's nursing care of infants and children* (11th ed.). Mosby.

In any instance of accidental poisoning, guidelines for intervening (Box 38.8) should be adhered to. The poison control centre phone number should be visible on the telephone in homes with young children and on a parent's smartphone, and the centre should be called immediately if poisoning is suspected.

School-Aged Children. School-aged children increasingly explore their environment (see Chapter 23). They may travel to and from school on foot or by school bus, and they may have friends outside their immediate neighbourhood. They may also become more active in extracurricular activities. Parents, teachers, and nurses must instruct children in safe practices to follow at school and play. Table 38.2 lists nursing interventions to help guide parents in providing for the safety of school-aged children. Using examples when discussing safe practices is an effective way to teach school-aged children.

Because school-aged children participate in more activities outside their home and neighbourhood environments, they are at greater risk of injury from strangers. Children should be warned repeatedly not to accept candy, food, gifts, or rides from strangers and not to go anywhere with a known adult unless they have their parent's permission. In addition, children need to know what to do if a stranger approaches. Frequently, neighbourhoods have a "block parent" program. The owner of a block parent home ensures that an adult is home during the times when children are walking to and from school. If a stranger approaches a child, the child can run to that home (identified by a sign), and the adult will protect the child and call the proper authorities. A nurse may work with school systems or neighbourhoods to initiate such a system to protect children.

Sports safety is stressed in school sports, and parents and health care providers can reinforce these safety tips by insisting that children wear protective gear while participating in sports such as skateboarding and snowboarding. For example, schools provide hard batting helmets for baseball games, and parents should also provide this equipment when children are playing baseball in their own backyards.

Bicycle- and scooter-related injuries are a major cause of death and disability among children. Bikes should be in good working order and the proper size for the child. Children under the age of 10 years should

BOX 38.8   PROCEDURAL GUIDELINE
Interventions for Accidental Poisoning

Nurses should teach parents to call 911 or emergency services immediately if a child or an adult is unconscious, not breathing, or having convulsions or seizures due to poison contact or ingestion. If they think that their child has come in contact with poison and has mild or no symptoms, they should call their local poison control centre. Phone numbers for poison control centres across Canada can be accessed at https://safemedicationuse.ca/tools_resources/poison_centres.html (ISMP Canada, 2022).

Different types and methods of poisoning require different, immediate treatment:

- Swallowed poison—Remove the item from the child, and have the child spit out any remaining substance. Do not make the child vomit. Do not use syrup of ipecac.
- Skin poison—Remove the child's clothes and rinse the skin with lukewarm water for at least 15 minutes.
- Eye poison—Flush the child's eye by holding the eyelid open and pouring a steady stream of room-temperature water into the inner corner.
- Poisonous fumes—Take the child outside or into fresh air immediately. If the child has stopped breathing, start cardiopulmonary resuscitation (CPR) and do not stop until the child breathes on their own, or until someone can take over (American Academy of Pediatrics/Healthy Children.org, 2021).

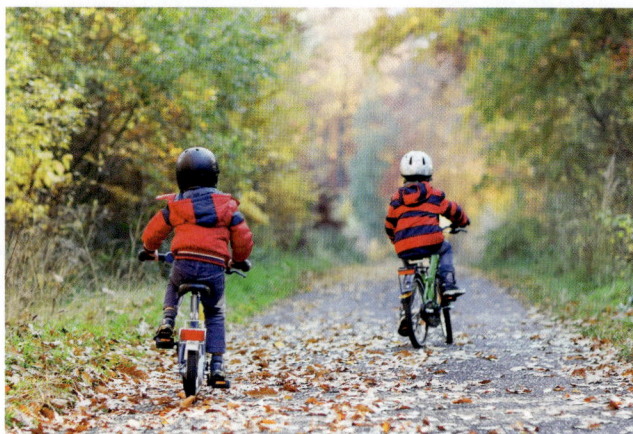

FIGURE 38.6 Proper bicycle safety equipment for school-aged children. (iStockphoto/romrodinka)

not be permitted to ride their bike on the road, as they have not yet developed the combined physical and cognitive skills to do this safely (Parachute Canada, 2022). They should also be cautioned not to engage in dangerous stunts or activities while bike riding. A properly fitted helmet should be worn, as it can decrease the risk of head injury by up to 85% (Parachute Canada, 2021b). Because most fatalities from bicycle accidents are related to head injuries, most provinces have implemented laws requiring that children wear bicycle helmets while cycling (Figure 38.6).

Adolescents. Risks to the safety of adolescents involve many factors outside the home environment, particularly their almost constant involvement with their peers (see Chapter 23). Adults serve as role models for adolescents and, through providing examples, setting expectations, and providing education, can help adolescents minimize risks to their safety. For example, adolescents who are considering getting a body piercing or tattoo need information about the risks for complications with these procedures and strategies for minimizing these risks.

This age group has a high incidence of suicide because of feelings of decreased self-worth and hopelessness. Nurses should be aware of the risks posed at this time and be prepared to teach adolescents and their parents measures to prevent accidents and injury (see Table 38.2).

When adolescents learn to drive, their environment expands, and so does their risk for injury. The potential for motor vehicle accidents is higher among teen drivers than in any other age group. Teens are more likely to speed, run red lights, and drive while intoxicated. The young driver must be taught to adhere to rules and regulations when using a car.

SAFETY ALERT Nurses should reinforce to new drivers and their parents the need to consistently wear safety belts and to never ride in a car with a driver who may be intoxicated. Assist parents and their teen in developing a plan of action to be used if the teen finds themselves with a driver who has been drinking or has used other substances.

Because adolescence is a time when mature sexual physical characteristics develop, adolescents may begin to have physical relationships with others. They need prompt, accurate instruction to prevent pregnancy and the spread of sexually transmitted infections (see Chapter 28).

Adults. Risks to young and middle-aged adults frequently result from lifestyle factors such as postpartum depression, high stress levels, inadequate nutrition, excessive alcohol intake, and problematic substance use (see Chapter 24). In our fast-paced society, there appears to be more expression of anger, which can quickly precipitate accidents (e.g., "road rage"). Adults need to have the opportunity to discuss the choices they have made in their life and the types of threats to safety that exist. Given information about threats to their well-being, adults may make the necessary modifications to their lifestyle practices. Useful resources are stress-management centres, employee-assistance programs, and health-promotion activities, which can be found in many communities and hospitals. In addition, neighbourhood centres, community clinics, and outpatient clinics are equipped to assist adults in modifying lifestyle habits that present risks to their health (e.g., smoking, overeating, lack of exercise, alcoholism).

Older Persons. Nursing interventions for older persons are designed to reduce the risk of falls and other accidents and to compensate for the physiological changes of aging (Box 38.9).

In older persons, diminished eyesight and impaired memory may result in an accidental overdose or missed doses of prescribed medications. The use of medication organizers that are filled once a week by the patient or family can help to prevent such errors. These organizers have the day and time on each box so that the patient knows when and what to take at any given time (Figure 38.7). They can be purchased at any drugstore at a very reasonable cost. Medication not in use or out of date should be taken to a pharmacy or municipal waste disposal depot for proper disposal (Government of Canada, 2014).

Burns and scalds are also more apt to occur with older individuals because they may become confused when turning the dials on a stove or other heating appliance. Nursing measures for preventing burns are designed to minimize the risk presented by impaired vision. Hot water faucets and dials can be colour-coded to make it easier for the adult to know what has been turned on. Lowering the thermostat setting on the water heater reduces the risk of scalding.

Older persons are more likely to have motor vehicle accidents because of three specific physiological changes. First, changes in visual acuity, depth perception, and peripheral vision prevent these persons

BOX 38.9 FOCUS ON OLDER PERSONS

Physiological Changes of Aging

- Older persons experience alterations in vision and hearing. Encourage yearly vision and hearing examinations and frequent cleaning of glasses and hearing aids as a means of preventing falls and burns.
- Older persons may have slower reaction times. Nurses should teach patient safety tips for avoiding motor vehicle accidents. Driving may need to be restricted to daylight hours or suspended altogether.
- Range of motion, flexibility, and strength are decreased. Nurses should encourage supervised exercise classes for older persons and teach them to seek assistance with household tasks as needed. Nurses should assess whether safety features, such as grab bars in the bathroom, are needed.
- Reflexes are slowed, and the ability to respond to multiple stimuli is reduced. Nurses should provide adequate, meaningful stimuli but prevent sensory overload.
- Nocturia and incontinence are more frequent in older persons. Nurses should institute a regular toileting schedule for the patient. A recommended frequency is every 3 hours. Diuretics are generally given in the morning; however, nurses should speak with the patient about their response to the drug to determine the best timing. Assistance should be provided, along with adequate lighting, to patients who need to use the bathroom at night.
- The family plays a significant role in the care of older persons. Often, family members serve as informal caregivers for older persons. In Canada in 2006, 30% of women and 22% of men between the ages of 45 and 54 provided informal care to an older person (Vanier Institute of the Family, 2010). Encourage the family to allow the older person to remain as independent as possible and to provide help for only those things that are necessary.
- The high prevalence of chronic conditions in older persons results in the use of a high number of prescription and over-the-counter medications. Coupled with age-related changes in pharmacokinetics, this presents a greater risk of serious adverse effects. Medications typically prescribed for older persons include anticholinergics, diuretics, anxiolytic and hypnotic agents, antidepressants, antihypertensives, vasodilators, analgesics, and laxatives, all of which may themselves pose risks or interact with other medications to increase the risk for falls. Review the patient's drug profile to ensure that any of the above noted drugs are used cautiously and assess the patient regularly for any adverse effects that may increase the risk for falls.

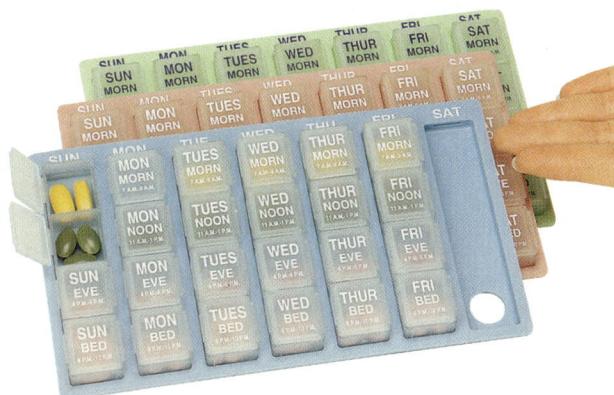

FIGURE 38.7 The One-Day-At-A-Time medicine organizer. (Courtesy Apothecary Products, Inc. Burnsville, MN.)

from quickly observing situations in which an accident is likely to occur. Second, decreased hearing acuity alters older persons' ability to hear emergency vehicle sirens or car and truck horns. Third, because of a decreased nervous system response, older persons may be unable to react as quickly as they once could to avoid an accident. A decline

in these skills may account for the most common types of accidents, including right-of-way and turning accidents. Nurses should educate these patients regarding safe driving practices (e.g., driving shorter distances or only in daylight, using side and rearview mirrors carefully, and looking back toward their "blind spot" before changing lanes). If hearing is compromised, patients might try keeping a window rolled down while driving or reducing the volume of the radio or music.

Eventually, counselling may be necessary to help a patient make the decision as to when to stop driving. This is not an easy decision as it can have implications for the patient's self-concept and self-esteem. It also has practical implications—the individual who has been accustomed to driving to daily activities will have to find alternative transportation. As a result, the patient may resist giving up their driver's licence and vehicle. Nurses can support the decision to stop driving by offering anticipatory guidance when an illness with progressive impairment is diagnosed, working with family members to determine how to approach the issue with the patient, and providing information about objective assessment of driver ability (Dobbs et al., 2015). When a patient makes this decision, nurses should help them locate resources in the community that provide transportation.

Pedestrian accidents can be reduced by persuading individuals to wear reflectors on garments when walking at night; to stand on the sidewalk and not in the street when waiting to cross; to always cross at corners and not in the middle of the block (particularly on a major street); to cross with the traffic light and not against it; and to look left, right, and left again before entering the street or crosswalk.

Environmental Interventions. Nurses can implement specific interventions aimed at maintaining a safe environment. Particularly important are measures for preventing fires and dealing with them if they do occur. Other environmental interventions are those that address basic needs, physical hazards, and the transmission of pathogens. Many communities now maintain registries with their public security agencies so that the community is aware if there is a vulnerable individual living either alone or with a family. Should there be an extended power outage, leaving some individuals vulnerable, such as a person requiring supplemental oxygen who may have limited tank time (as usually they use electricity-driven units in the home), the city or community has services organized to check on these individuals and, if necessary, transport them to shelters or other appropriate locations.

Other Environmental Interventions. Nurses can contribute to a safer environment by helping patients meet basic needs related to oxygen, humidity, nutrition, and temperature. To ensure that oxygen availability is not threatened, nurses should recommend to patients living at home that they have annual inspections of the heating system, chimney, and appliances. Carbon monoxide detectors are available for home use at a reasonable cost but should not be considered a replacement for the proper use and maintenance of fuel-burning appliances. To achieve a comfortable level of humidity in the home, patients can attach a humidifier to the furnace or, in the case of patients who have upper respiratory tract infections, use a room humidifier where they sleep. Nurses should teach basic techniques for food handling (e.g., handwashing and checking for spoilage) and preparation (e.g., keeping food refrigerated before serving) so that nutritional needs are met safely. It is also helpful for family members to write the date on packages of leftovers. Older persons who have difficulty preparing their own food may benefit from Meals on Wheels, an organization that provides fresh, nutritious meals in the home. Patient education for older persons and patients who enjoy outdoor activities should include ways to prevent and treat frostbite, hypothermia, heatstroke, and heat exhaustion (see Chapter 31).

Adequate lighting and security measures in and around the home, including the use of night-lights, exterior lighting, and good-quality locks on windows and doors, enable patients to reduce the risk of injury from crime. Local police departments and community organizations often have safety classes available to teach residents how to take precautions to minimize the chance of becoming involved in a crime. Some useful tips include always parking the car near a bright light or in a busy public area, carrying a whistle attached to the car keys, keeping car doors locked while driving, and always paying attention while driving, to notice if anyone starts to follow the car. Patients should be encouraged to join block associations and work closely with law enforcement personnel to reduce crime in their neighbourhoods.

To prevent the transmission of pathogens, nurses should teach aseptic practices. Patients and family members need to learn thorough hand hygiene practices (handwashing or the use of hand sanitizer) and when to use it (e.g., before and after caring for a family member, before food preparation, before preparing a medication for a family member,

and after contacting any body fluids). When patients require dressing changes or the use of syringes and needles, families should be shown how to properly dispose of contaminated items in the home, as most communities have regulations regarding the disposal of biohazardous waste.

Limiting Specific Risks to Patient Safety

A number of specific safety measures are applicable to patients in the home or health care settings. Nurses should take actions to help patients avoid injuries related to falls, the use of restraints and side rails, electrical hazards, and radiation. Special precautions are necessary to prevent injury in patients susceptible to having seizures.

Falls. Easy modifications in the home and health care environment can reduce the risk of falls (Table 38.3). A heavy or debilitated patient in a bed or wheelchair or on a toilet should be properly supported and secured. Side rails may be necessary (but improper use may be considered a patient restraint—see "Side Rails" section later in this chapter).

TABLE 38.3	Measures to Prevent Falls by Older Persons
Measure	**Rationale**
Stairs	
Install treads with a uniform depth of 22.5 cm and 22.5-cm risers (vertical face of steps).	If stairs are of uniform size, older persons do not need to continually adjust their vision.
Install uniform-textured or plain-coloured surfaces on each tread, and mark the edges of treads with a contrasting colour.	Uniform textures or colour helps to decrease vertigo. Marking the edges of treads provides obvious visual cues to end of stairs.
Ensure proper lighting of each tread. Block glare from the sun or a light bulb with translucent shades or a screen, or use lower-wattage or nonglare bulbs.	Older persons' vision is unable to adjust quickly to changes in lighting.
Ensure adequate headroom so that patients do not have to duck to negotiate stairs.	Sudden changes in head position may result in dizziness.
Remove protruding objects from staircase walls.	Decreased peripheral vision may prevent the patient from seeing an object.
Maintain outdoor walkways and stairs in good condition and free of holes, cracks, and splinters.	Decreased visual acuity can prevent the patient from seeing any structural defect.
Handrails	
Install a smooth but slip-resistant handrail at least 5 cm from wall.	A 5-cm distance allows the patient to grasp the handrail firmly for support.
Secure the handrail firmly so that the patient's weight is supported, especially at bottom and top of stairway.	Older persons have the greatest risk of falling at top and bottom of stairs because their centre of gravity is being shifted and balance is unstable.
Install grab rails in bathroom near the toilet and tub.	These measures enable the patient to have support while rising from a sitting to standing position.
Install an elevated toilet seat with armrests and nonslip strips.	
Floors	
Ensure that patients wear properly fitting shoes or slippers with a nonskid surface.	Such footwear reduces the chances of slipping.
Secure all carpeting, mats, and tiles; place nonskid backing under small rugs.	A sudden slip may cause dizziness and an inability to regain balance.
Place bath mats or nonskid, coloured strips on bathtub or shower stall floors and on the floor in front of the toilet.	Wet surfaces increase the risk of falling.
Secure electrical cords against the baseboards.	This measure prevents tripping.
Maintain proper illumination inside and outside where the patient moves and walks.	This measure reduces the risk of falling due to eye strain.
Health Care Facility Orientation	
Place disoriented patients in a room near the nurses' station.	Proximity provides for more frequent observation by nursing staff.
Supervise confused patients closely.	Confused patients often attempt to wander out of bed or the room.
Show the patient how to use the call light at the bedside and in the bathroom, and place it within easy reach.	The location and use of the call light are essential to patient safety.
Place bedside tables and overbed tables close to the patient.	This measure prevents the patient from searching or overreaching for items such as eyeglasses, dentures, a hearing aid, or the telephone.
Remove clutter from bedside tables, hallways, bathrooms, and grooming areas.	This measure eliminates potential hazards and promotes patient independence.

TABLE 38.3	Measures to Prevent Falls by Older Persons—cont'd
Measure	**Rationale**
Leave one side rail up and one down on the side where the oriented and ambulatory patient gets out of bed.	The patient can use the side rail for support when getting in and out of bed and to position self once in bed.
Transport	
Lock beds and wheelchairs when transferring a patient from a bed to a wheelchair or back to bed.	The locks provide stability and support during transfer.
Place side rails in the up position and secure safety straps around the patient when transporting them by stretcher.	This measure prevents the patient from rolling off the stretcher.

Adapted from Chang, J. T., Morton, S. C., Rubenstein, L. Z., et al. (2004). Interventions for the prevention of falls in older adults: Systematic review with meta-analysis of randomized clinical trials. *British Medical Journal, 328*, 680.

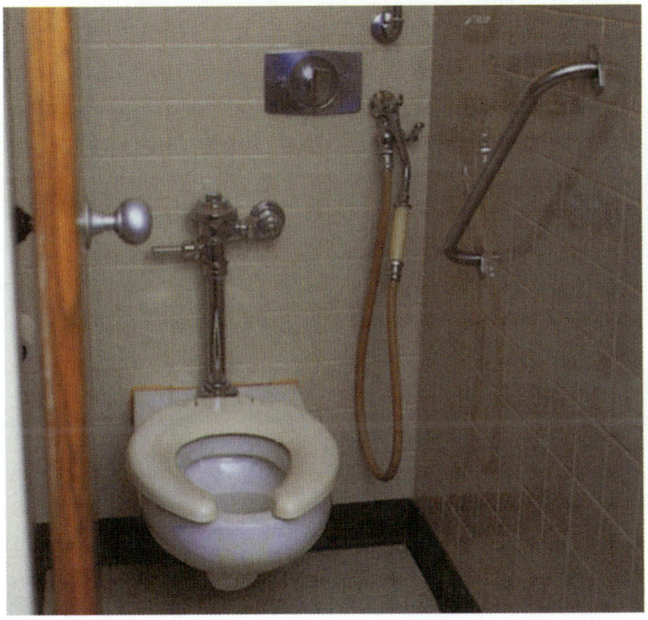

FIGURE 38.8 Safety bars beside a toilet and shower.

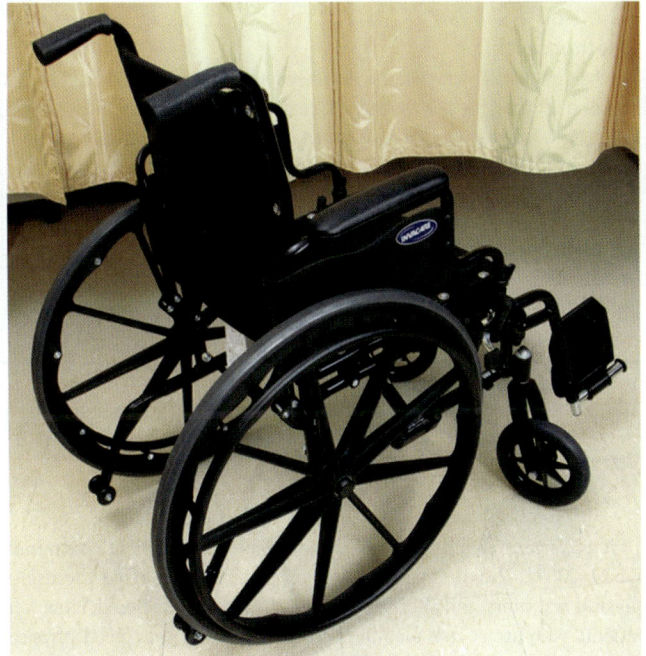

FIGURE 38.9 Wheelchair with safety locks and anti-tip bars.

Safety bars near toilets, locks on beds and wheelchairs, and call lights are additional safety features found in health care settings (Figures 38.8 and 38.9). Excess furniture and equipment should be removed. Weakened patients should wear rubber-soled shoes or slippers when walking or transferring. For patients who use assistive aids such as canes, crutches, or walkers, it is important to routinely check the condition of rubber tips and the integrity of the aid.

In the health care setting, injuries may occur when patients attempt to address self-care needs independently despite encouragement to call for assistance. One way to minimize the occurrence of such incidents is to check in on patients frequently during the day. A formal routine of nursing rounds, during which nurses visit patients every hour and provide necessary assistance, has been found to decrease the incidence of falls and increase patient satisfaction (Box 38.10).

Restraints. A restraint is a physical, chemical, or environmental means of controlling an individual's behaviour or actions (CNO, 2009). The use of restraints is controversial as they have caused injury and death. Nurses need to familiarize themselves with the legal aspects of restraint use. Nurses must also follow guidelines and standards provided by their provincial nursing governing body as well as policies and procedures set by their clinical practice setting. A least-restraint approach is recommended to ensure highest-quality care. This approach ensures that all alternative interventions are attempted before moving to the use of restraints, and that the form of restraint selected is the one that addresses a patient's needs in the least restrictive way (CNO, 2009).

It is imperative that nurses try alternative measures (Box 38.11), because the application of a restraint should always be a measure of last resort. The use of restraints must be guided by a patient's needs and requires a thorough assessment by the nurse and other members of the multidisciplinary team involved in the patient's care. A restraint-use algorithm provides evidence-informed guidelines for determining whether a restraint is appropriate and what interventions might be used (Figure 38.10).

The use of any type of restraint involves a psychological adjustment for the patient and family. If restraints must be used, the nurse must assist family members and the patient by explaining the purpose of the restraints, the patient's expected care while restrained, the precautions to be taken to avoid injury, and the temporary and protective aspects of restraints. Informed consent from family members may also be required before using restraints. The case study in Box 38.12 demonstrates family involvement in a decision about restraints.

BOX 38.10   RESEARCH HIGHLIGHT
Effects of Nursing Rounds

Research Focus

Hospitalized patients often require assistance with basic activities of daily living such as eating, toileting, and ambulating. Patients usually communicate their needs by use of a call light. Not meeting a patient's needs in a timely fashion decreases patient satisfaction and places them at greater risk for injury. The nurse plays a key role in the prevention of falls and injuries related to falls.

Research Abstract

Christiansen and colleagues (2018) wanted to know the impact of intentional rounding on patient and nursing outcomes and aimed to identify the barriers and facilitators surrounding implementation.

Methods

In their systematic literature review, they found 21 articles that met their inclusion criteria. Six studies reported a reduction in the number of falls, and another five studies reported a reduction in call bell use following the introduction of intentional rounding. Although results were positive, the overall quality of the studies was weak.

Implications for Practice

- Intentional rounding has demonstrated mixed results.
- A robust evaluation plan is needed to measure the impact of intentional rounding.

From Christiansen, A., Coventry, L., Graham, R., et al. (2018). Intentional rounding in acute adult healthcare settings: A systematic mixed-method review. *Journal of Clinical Nursing, 27*(9–10), 1759–1792. https://doi.org/10.1111/jocn.14370

BOX 38.11   Alternatives to Restraints

- Orient patients and families with the care environment; explain all procedures and treatments.
- Provide companionship and supervision; use trained sitters or adjust staffing.
- Offer diversionary activities, such as listening to music or having something to hold; enlist support and input from the family.
- Assign confused or disoriented patients to rooms near the nurses' station; observe these patients frequently.
- Use calm, simple statements and physical cues as needed.
- Use de-escalation, time-outs, and other verbal intervention techniques when managing aggressive behaviours.
- Provide appropriate visual and auditory stimuli (e.g., family pictures, a clock, or a radio).
- Remove cues that promote leaving (e.g., sight of elevators, stairs, or street clothes).
- Promote relaxation techniques and normal sleep patterns.
- Institute exercise and ambulation schedules as allowed by patients' conditions; consult a physiotherapist for mobility and exercise programs.
- Attend to the patient's toileting, food, and fluid needs.
- Camouflage intravenous lines with clothing, a stockinette, or a Kling dressing.
- Evaluate all medications the patients are receiving and ensure effective pain management.
- Reassess the physical status of patients, and review laboratory findings connected with their health.

Adapted from The Joint Commission (TJC). (2020). *Comprehensive accreditation manual for hospitals. Restraint and seclusion—enclosure beds, side rails and mitts.* https://www.jointcommission.org/standards/standard-faqs/hospital-and-hospital-clinics/provision-of-care-treatment-and-services-pc/000001668; American Nurses Association. (2021). Geriatric nursing resources for care of older adults. *Physical restraints.* https://hign.org/consultgeri/resources/protocols/physical-restraints

A physical restraint immobilizes a patient or a patient's extremity (CNO, 2009). The optimal goal with all patients is to avoid the use of physical restraints, and alternatives must always be considered. However, patients who are at risk for injury to self or others may need physical restraints temporarily. Physical restraints do not prevent falls and may actually increase the severity of an injury from a fall (RNAO, 2017).

Whenever patients are physically restrained, there is a natural tendency for them to try to remove the restraint, and this can lead to injury. Restrained patients can easily become entangled in a restraint device when attempting to get out of it. In some cases, death has resulted from strangulation or asphyxiation. As a result, long-term care facilities and many health care facilities have banned the use of the jacket (vest) restraint. The use of any physical restraint is also associated with serious complications, including pressure injuries, constipation, pneumonia, urinary and fecal incontinence, and urinary retention. Contractures, nerve damage, and circulatory impairment are also potential hazards. In addition, restrained patients can experience humiliation, fear, anger, and a loss of self-esteem.

SAFETY ALERT Routine assessment of a patient in a physical restraint is critical to prevent injury. The restraint must be moved and the patient repositioned at regular intervals, according to the agency's policy. Restraints should be used only after other alternatives have been tried, and the least restrictive method of restraint should be used. The use of restraints must be part of the patient's medical treatment. Restraints are considered a short-term intervention, and once they have been applied, regular assessments are needed to determine whether they should be continued. All assessments and interventions must be clearly documented according to the agency's policy.

For legal purposes, nurses must know the agency's policy and procedures for the appropriate use and monitoring of physical restraints. The use of a restraint must be clinically justified and be a part of the patient's prescribed medical treatment and care plan. A physician's order may be required, depending on provincial or territorial legislation and agency policy—in some settings, nurses may order restraints. Requirements for ordering restraints may vary depending on the circumstances of a patient's situation and the type of restraint needed; nurses must comply with the agency's policies. Assessment of patients who are restrained must be ongoing. Proper documentation, including the behaviours that necessitated the application of restraints, the procedure used in restraining, the condition of the body part restrained (e.g., circulation to the patient's hand), and the evaluation of the patient response, is essential. Restraints should be removed periodically and the patient should be assessed to determine if the restraints continue to be needed.

Skill 38.1 includes guidelines for the proper use and application of restraints. Use of restraints must meet the following objectives:
- Reduce the risk of patient injury
- Prevent the interruption of therapy, such as traction, IV infusion, nasogastric tube feeding, or Foley catheterization
- Prevent the confused or combative patient from removing life-support equipment
- Reduce the risk of injury to others by the patient

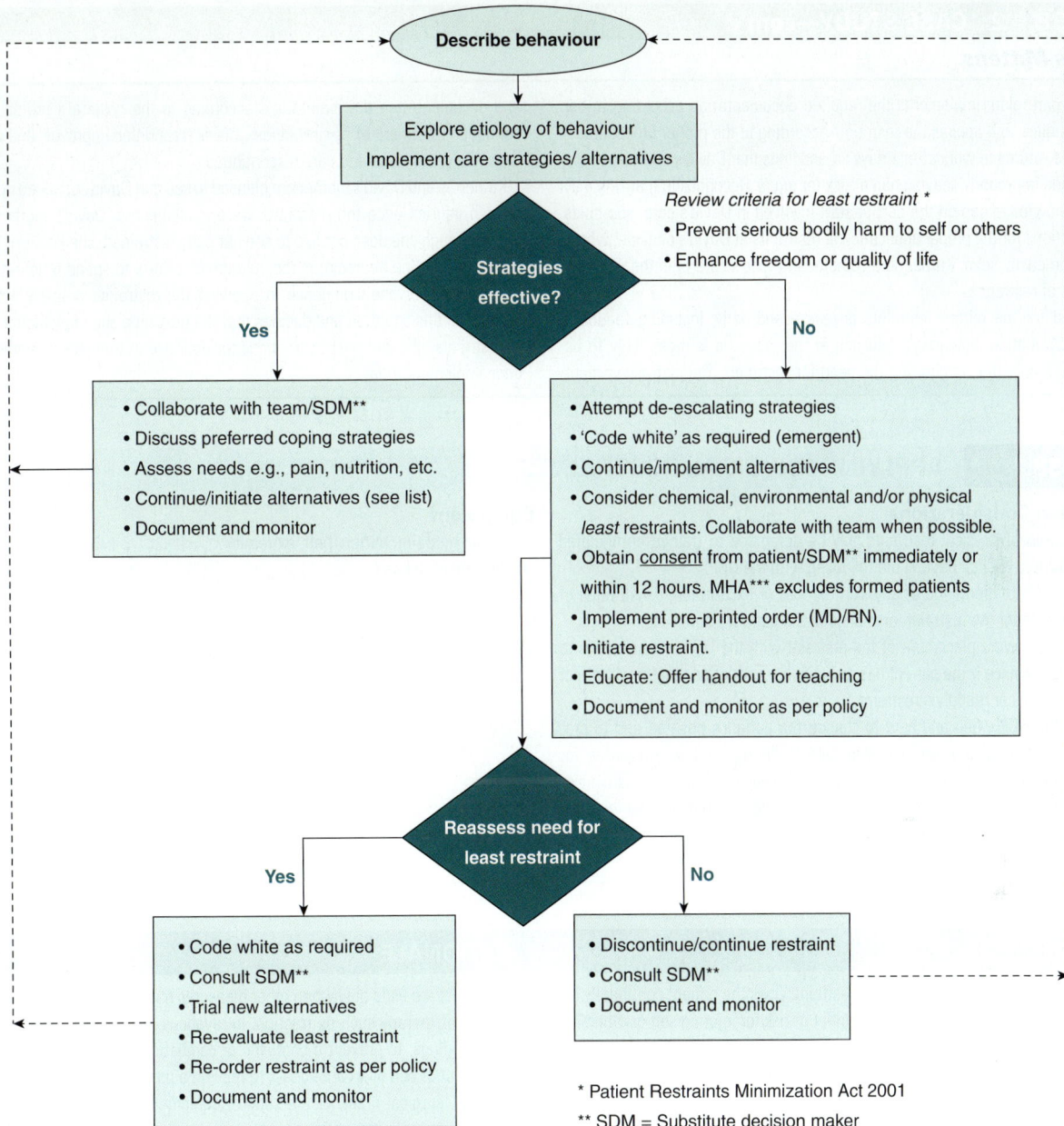

FIGURE 38.10 Alternative to restraints decision tree. (From Registered Nurses' Association of Ontario [RNAO]. [2012]. *Promoting safety: Alternative approaches to the use of restraints* [p. 116, Appendix N]. https://rnao.ca/sites/rnao-ca/files/Promoting_Safety_-_Alternative_Approaches_to_the_Use_of_Restraints_0. pdf. Copyright © the Ottawa Hospital, Department of Nursing Professional Practice.)

BOX 38.12 CASE STUDY

David's Mittens

Katherine has been caring for David, a 6-month-old boy who has been hospitalized for several weeks. David has a complex health condition and is currently experiencing severely dry, itchy skin associated with his illness. Katherine has noticed that anti-itch medications decrease David's discomfort but do not eliminate the itch entirely. As a result, he continues to scratch, and even with regularly trimmed nails, he has scratched himself hard enough to cause bleeding. David's mother plays with

him to distract him from the itch, and when he tries to scratch, she gently holds his hands. However, she cannot be with David at all times in the hospital. Another concern is that David scratches his skin while sleeping.

Katherine discusses the situation with David's mother, and they decide to use mitten restraints to protect David's skin. They agree to use the restraints when David sleeps and when he is awake and alone. Katherine notes this decision

BOX 38.12   CASE STUDY—cont'd

David's Mittens

in David's care plan, implements the required documentation according to her hospital's policy, and applies the restraints according to the proper procedure.

Katherine returns to work after 2 days off and finds that David's restraints have been applied improperly, leaving him at risk for injury. Recognizing that this may reflect a knowledge gap on the part of staff involved in David's care, she posts the instructions for the proper application of restraints at David's bedside, where they will be easily seen. Katherine also notes in David's care plan the need for proper use of restraints.

The need for the mitten restraints is reassessed daily, including feedback from David's mother. Volunteers visit him at the times he is most likely to be awake and alone, thus minimizing the need for restraints. Regular assessment

and documentation are maintained according to the hospital's protocol. With continued treatment of David's illness, his skin condition improves, and within 5 days, the mitten restraints are discontinued.

Katherine and David's mother are pleased to see that David sustained no further scratch injuries once the restraints were implemented. David's mother states that, although she does not like to see her baby restrained, she knows it is in his best interest. She appreciates the volunteers' efforts to spend time with David as well as everyone's diligence in applying the restraints properly. Katherine reflects on this situation and decides that the next time she implements the use of restraints, she will post instructions for their use at the bedside immediately upon implementation.

SKILL 38.1   APPLYING PHYSICAL RESTRAINTS

Delegation Considerations

The application of physical restraints may be delegated to trained unregulated care providers (UCPs). Review the following with the UCP:

- Ask the UCP to inform you of any skin redness or excoriation, constriction of circulation under the restraint, or change in the patient's breathing.
- Review the correct placement of the restraint with the UCP and ask them to request assistance if the patient has any mobility restrictions that might affect how to remove or reapply a restraint.
- Instruct the UCP when and how to change the patient's position and to provide range-of-motion exercises, skin care, toileting, and opportunities for socialization. However, nurses are always responsible for the assessment of a patient's safety needs, selection of appropriate alternative interventions, evaluation of the effectiveness of restraint, and ongoing assessment to prevent complications of restraint use.

Equipment

- Proper restraint: mitten, belt, extremity
- Padding (if needed)

PROCEDURE

STEPS	RATIONALE
1. Assess whether the patient needs a restraint. Does the patient continually try to interrupt needed therapy? Is the patient at risk for injuring self or others?	• Restraints are used only when other measures have failed to prevent the interruption of therapy such as traction, intravenous (IV) infusions, or nasogastric tube feedings; to prevent a confused or combative patient from self-injury by falling out of bed or a wheelchair; to prevent a patient from removing a urinary catheter, surgical drain, or life-support equipment; and to reduce the risk of injury to others by the patient.
2. Assess the patient's behaviour, such as confusion, disorientation, agitation, restlessness, combativeness, or inability to follow directions. Consult with a gerontological nurse specialist if available.	• If the patient's behaviour continues despite attempts to eliminate the cause of behaviour, use of physical restraint may be necessary.
3. Review the agency's policies regarding restraints. Consider the purpose, type, location, and duration of restraint. Determine whether signed consent for the use of restraint is needed.	• The least restrictive type of restraint must be ordered. A physician's order may be necessary—check provincial or territorial legislation and agency policy. Because restraints limit the patient's ability to move freely, the nurse must make clinical judgements appropriate to the patient's condition and the agency policy.
4. Review manufacturer's instructions before entering the patient's room. Determine the most appropriate size restraint.	• Nurses should be familiar with all devices used for patient care and protection. Incorrect application of a restraining device may result in patient injury or death.
5. Perform hand hygiene and gather equipment.	• Reduces transmission of microorganisms; promotes organization.
6. Introduce yourself to the patient and family. Assess their feelings about restraint use. Explain that restraint is temporary and designed to protect the patient from injury.	• Helps minimize patient anxiety during the application of the device and helps minimize family concern during the maintenance of restraint.
7. Inspect the area where the restraint is to be placed. Assess condition of skin underlying where the restraint is to be applied.	• Restraints may compress and interfere with functioning of devices or tubes. Inspection provides baseline assessment data regarding skin integrity.

Continued

SKILL 38.1   APPLYING PHYSICAL RESTRAINTS—cont'd

8. Approach the patient in a calm, confident manner. Check the patient's identification using two identifiers. Explain what you plan to do.

9. Adjust the bed to proper height and lower the side rail on the side of patient contact.

10. Provide privacy. Make sure the patient is comfortable and in proper body alignment. Drape patient as needed.

11. Pad the skin and bony prominences (if necessary) before applying restraints.

12. Apply the appropriate-size restraint, making sure it is not over an IV line or other device (e.g., dialysis shunt) and that it does not cover the patient's identification or allergy bracelet.

   A. **Belt restraint**: This device secures the patient to a bed or stretcher. Apply it over the patient's clothes or gown. Remove wrinkles from the front and back of the restraint while placing it around the patient's waist. Bring ties through slots in the belt. Avoid placing the belt across the chest or too tightly across the abdomen (see Step 12A illustration).

   B. **Extremity (ankle or wrist) restraint:** This restraint is designed to immobilize one or all extremities. Commercially available limb restraints are composed of sheepskin or foam padding (see Step 12B illustration). The limb restraint is wrapped around the wrist or ankle with the soft part toward the skin and is secured snugly in place with Velcro straps.

- Reduces patient anxiety and promotes cooperation.

- Allows nurse to use proper body mechanics and prevent injury.

- Privacy protects self-esteem. Proper body alignment promotes comfort and prevents contractures and neurovascular injury.

- Padding reduces friction and pressure on skin and underlying tissues.

- IV lines and other therapeutic devices may become occluded. The patient's ID and allergy information must always be visible and accessible.

- Restrains centre of gravity and prevents the patient from rolling off the stretcher or sitting up while on stretcher or from falling out of bed. Tight application may interfere with ventilation.

- Maintains immobilization of the extremity to protect the patient from injury from a fall or accidental removal of a therapeutic device (e.g., IV tube or Foley catheter). Tight application may interfere with circulation.

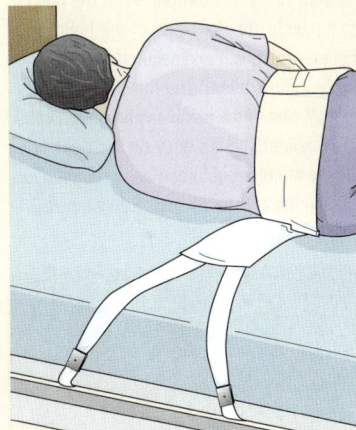

STEP 12A Belt restraint is tied to the bed frame and to an area that does not cause the restraint to tighten when the side rail is raised or lowered. (*From Sorrentino, S. A., & Remmert, L. [2021]. Mosby's textbook for nursing assistants [10th ed.]. Elsevier Inc.)*

STEP 12B Extremity restraint being applied to the wrist.

STEP 12C Mitten restraint.

STEP 12D Elbow restraint.

C. Mitten restraint: This thumbless mitten device is used to restrain the patient's hands (see Step 12C illustration). Place a hand in the mitten, being sure the mitten end is brought all the way over the wrist.

D. Elbow restraint: This piece of fabric with slots has tongue blades placed so that the elbow joint remains rigid (see Step 12D illustration).

E. Mummy restraint: The mummy restraint consists of a blanket or sheet. It is opened on the bed or crib with one corner folded toward the centre. The child is placed on the blanket with shoulders at the fold and feet toward the opposite corner (see Step 12E-1 illustration). With the child's right arm straight down against the body, the right side of the blanket is pulled firmly across the right shoulder and chest and secured beneath the left side of the body (see Step 12E-2 illustration). The left arm is placed straight against the body, and the left side of the blanket is brought across the shoulder and chest and locked beneath child's body on the right side (see Step 12E-3 illustration). The lower corner is folded and brought over the body and tucked or fastened securely with safety pins (see Step 12E-4 illustration).

- Prevents patients from dislodging invasive equipment, removing dressings, or scratching, yet allows greater movement than a wrist restraint.

- Commonly used with infants and children to prevent elbow flexion (e.g., when an IV line is in place).

- Maintains short-term restraint of small child or infant for an examination or treatment involving the head and neck. Effectively controls movement of torso and extremities.

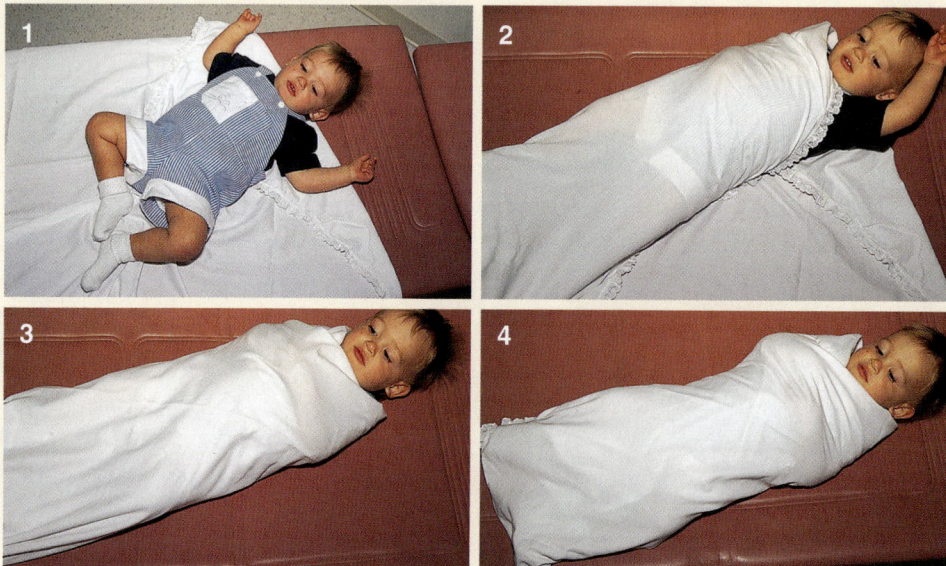

STEP 12E Mummy restraint.

Continued

SKILL 38.1 **APPLYING PHYSICAL RESTRAINTS—cont'd**

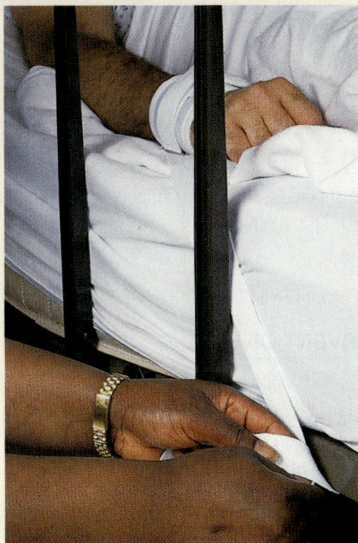

STEP 13 Tie restraint strap to the bed frame.

STEP 14 The Posey quick-release tie. (Courtesy J.T. Posey Co., Arcadia, CA.)

STEP 15 Place two fingers under the restraint to check tightness.

13. Attach restraints to the bed frame, which moves when the head of the bed is raised or lowered (see Step 13 illustration).	• Patient may be injured if restraint is secured to side rail and it is lowered.

CRITICAL DECISION POINT: *Do not attach end of restraint to side rails.*

14. Secure restraints with a quick-release tie (see Step 14 illustration). Do not tie in a knot.	• Allows for quick release in an emergency.
15. Insert two fingers under the secured restraint (see Step 15 illustration).	• A tight restraint may cause constriction and impede circulation. Checking for constriction prevents neurovascular injury.
16. The proper placement of the restraint, skin integrity, pulses, temperature, colour, and sensation of the restrained body part should be assessed at least every hour or according to the agency's policy.	• Frequent assessments prevent complications, such as suffocation, skin breakdown, and impaired circulation.
17. Restraints should be removed at regular intervals (see agency policy). If the patient is violent and noncompliant, remove one restraint at a time or have staff assist while removing the restraints. The patient should not be left unattended at this time.	• Provides opportunity to change patient's position and perform full range of motion, toileting, and exercise and to provide food or fluids.
18. Secure a call light or intercom system within the patient's reach.	• Allows patient, family, or caregiver to obtain assistance quickly.
19. Leave the bed or chair with wheels locked. The bed should be in its lowest position.	• Locked wheels prevent the bed or chair from moving if the patient attempts to get out. If the patient falls when the bed is in lowest position, the chances of injury are reduced.
20. Perform hand hygiene.	• Reduces transmission of microorganisms.

21. Reassess the patient's status and needs.

A. Inspect the patient for any injuries, including all hazards of immobility, while restraints are in use.	• Patient should be free of injury and not exhibit any signs of immobility complications.
B. Observe IV catheters, urinary catheters, and drainage tubes to ensure that they are positioned correctly and that therapy remains uninterrupted.	• Reinsertion can be uncomfortable and can increase the risk of infection or interrupt therapy.
C. Regularly reassess patient's need for continued use of the restraint (for medical or surgical reason) with the intent of discontinuing the restraint at the earliest possible time (see agency-specific policy).	• Use of restraints should be seen as a temporary measure and discontinued as soon as possible (CNO, 2009).
D. Provide appropriate sensory stimulation and reorient patient as needed.	• Use of restraints can further increase disorientation.

UNEXPECTED OUTCOMES	RELATED INTERVENTIONS
Patient has signs of impaired skin integrity	• Assess skin and provide appropriate therapy.
	• Notify the physician and reassess the need for continued use of the restraint.
	• Ensure correct application of restraint. Pad the skin under the restraint, and remove restraint more often.
Patient has altered neurovascular status in an extremity (cyanosis, pallor, coldness of skin, or complaints of tingling, pain, or numbness)	• Remove the restraint immediately, stay with the patient, and notify the physician.
	• Protect the extremity from further injury (e.g., pressure from tubing or encumbrance, positioning).
Patient is increasingly confused, disoriented, or agitated	• Identify the reason for this change in behaviour and attempt to eliminate the cause.
	• Attempt a restraint alternative.
Patient escapes from restraint device and suffers fall or injury	• Attend to the patient's immediate physical needs and inform the physician.
	• Reassess the type of restraint used, the correct application, and if alternatives can be used.

RECORDING AND REPORTING

- Record behaviours that place patient at risk for injury.
- Describe restraint alternatives attempted and patient's response.
- Record patient's and family's understanding of and consent to restraint application.
- Record type and location of the restraint and time applied.
- Record time of assessments and releases.
- Document the patient's behaviour after application of the restraint.
- Document specific assessments related to orientation, oxygenation, skin integrity, circulation, and positioning.
- Describe the patient's response when restraints were removed.

CARE IN THE COMMUNITY CONSIDERATIONS

- Plan care with family. If possible, use of an Ambularm may free patient from physical restraints.
- Instruct family members (or other caregivers) in the use of alternatives to restraints (see Box 38.11).
- A physical restraint may require a physician order. The restraint should not be sent home with the family unless the device is needed to protect the patient from injury. If physical restraints are necessary, the family members (or other caregivers) must be instructed in their proper application, the care needed while in restraints, and the complications to look for. Also inform caregivers whom to contact if any abnormal findings occur.
- A patient who needs to be restrained in bed should have a hospital bed and will require constant supervision in the home.

In keeping with current trends toward health promotion, improved assessment techniques and modifications of the environment are offered as alternatives to physical restraints. An **Ambularm** is a device worn on the leg that signals when the leg is in a dependent position, such as over the side rail or on the floor (Figure 38.11). The **Bed-Check** bed exit alarm system (Figure 38.12) uses a weight-sensitive sensor mat that can be placed on the patient's mattress or chair. This device sounds an audible alarm at the bedside when pressure is released off the sensor mat. Such devices are useful for patients who tend to climb out of bed unassisted but are in danger of falling. Other alarms can be placed on doors to alert staff or family members when a confused patient, prone to wandering, opens a door.

Another alternative form of restraint is the Posey Bed Enclosure (Figure 38.13), a soft-sided, self-contained enclosed bed. It allows for freedom of movement and thus reduces the side effects caused by physical restraints such as pressure injuries and loss of dignity. The Posey Bed Enclosure works well for patients who are restless and unpredictable, cognitively impaired, and at risk for injury if they were to fall or get out of bed, such as patients on anticoagulant therapy at risk for intracranial bleeding. The bed may also be a safer alternative to side rails.

A long-term care setting may be designed to include environmental restraints, such as locked nursing units. Residents with dementia may be at risk for injury if they wander away from their unit or building. A locked nursing unit can be designed to permit individuals the freedom

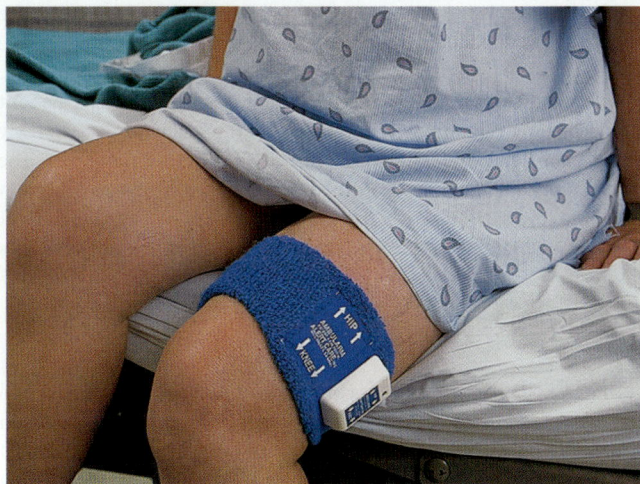

FIGURE 38.11 Patient wearing an Ambularm device.

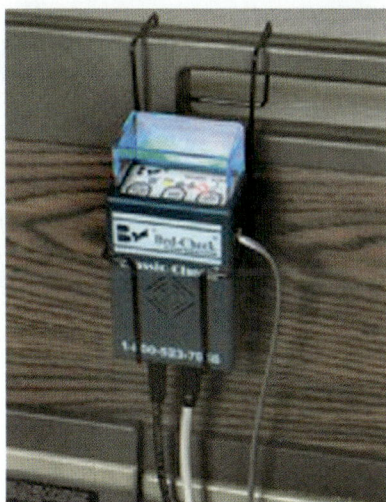

FIGURE 38.12 The Bed-Check bed exit alarm. (Courtesy Bed-Check Corp.)

FIGURE 38.13 The Posey Bed enclosure. (Courtesy J. T. Posey Co., Arcadia, CA.)

FIGURE 38.14 Side rails in the up position on a stretcher.

to wander safely around their unit and can include exits to secure, enclosed outdoor spaces when weather permits. A locked unit is still a form of restraint and should be implemented only after alternatives to restraint have proven unsuccessful.

In some situations, chemical restraints may be indicated. *Chemical restraint* is defined as "any form of psychoactive medication used, not to treat illness, but to intentionally inhibit a particular behaviour or movement" (CNO, 2009, p. 4). For example, it may be necessary to sedate a patient who is consistently pulling out a nasogastric tube. As with any other restraint, chemical restraints should be implemented only after nonrestraining measures (e.g., distraction, use of a sitter) have proven ineffective and with the informed consent of the patient or their substitute decision maker. Proper adherence to medication administration guidelines is vital to the safe use of chemical restraints, and the patient's response to and need for these medications must be assessed on a regular basis.

Side Rails. Side rails may help to increase a patient's mobility and stability when in bed or when moving from the bed to a chair. Side rails also help prevent the unconscious patient from falling out of bed or off a stretcher (Figure 38.14). However, raised side rails that cannot be opened by the patient are considered a restraint (CNO, 2009). Note that some

beds may have two-length side rails or four split rails. Two-length or two split side rails that are in the "up" position are considered a patient restraint, whereas two split side rails are not considered a restraint.

The use of side rails for a disoriented patient may cause more confusion and further injury. A confused patient who is determined to get out of bed may attempt to climb over the side rail or climb out at the foot of the bed, often resulting in a fall or injury. Nursing interventions to reduce a patient's confusion should first focus on the cause of the confusion. Frequently, a patient's attempt to explore their environment or to self-toilet is mistaken as confusion. A thorough assessment is essential. Whenever side rails are used, the bed should be maintained in the lowest position possible.

Electrical Hazards. Electrical equipment must be maintained in good working order and should be grounded. The third (longer) prong in an electrical plug is the ground. Theoretically, the ground prong carries any stray electrical current back to the ground—hence, its name. The other two prongs carry the power to the piece of electrical equipment. Improperly grounded or malfunctioning electrical equipment increases the risks of electrical injury and fire. Educating both the patient and the family can reduce the risk for electrical hazards in the home environment (Box 38.13).

BOX 38.13 PATIENT TEACHING

Prevention of Electrical Hazards in the Home

Objective
- Patient will recognize electrical hazards in the home and eliminate them.

Teaching Strategies
- Discuss grounding appliances and other equipment.
- Provide examples of common hazards: frayed cords, damaged equipment, and overloaded outlets.
- Discuss guidelines to prevent electrical shocks:
  - Use extension cords only when necessary, and use electrical tape to secure the cord to the floor where it will not be stepped on.
  - Do not run wires under carpeting.
  - Teach the patient to grasp the plug, not the cord, when unplugging items.
  - Teach the patient to keep electrical items away from water.
  - Teach the patient not to operate equipment with which they are unfamiliar.
  - Teach the patient to disconnect items before cleaning them.

Evaluation
- Have patient list electrical hazards existing in the home.
- Review with the patient the steps they will take to eliminate these hazards.
- Reassess the home after the patient has had an opportunity to eliminate the hazards.

If a patient receives an electrical shock in a health care setting, the nurse must immediately determine whether the patient has a pulse. If the patient has no pulse, cardiopulmonary resuscitation should be initiated and emergency personnel should be notified. If the patient has a pulse and remains alert and oriented, the nurse needs to quickly obtain vital signs and assess the skin for signs of thermal injury. The patient's physician must be notified. If an electrical shock occurs in the home, the nurse follows the same procedure but has the patient go to the emergency department and then notifies the patient's physician.

◆ Evaluation

Patient Care. The components of critical thinking should be applied to the evaluation step of the nursing process (Figure 38.15). The actual care delivered by the health care team is evaluated on the basis of expected outcomes. If the patient's goals have been met, the nursing interventions can be considered effective and appropriate. If not, the nurse must determine whether new risks to the patient have developed or whether previous risks remain. The patient and family need to participate in this process to find permanent ways to reduce risks to safety. Nurses need to continually assess the patient's and family's need for additional support services, such as home care, physiotherapy, counselling, and further teaching.

Patient Expectations

Nurses who have developed a good relationship with a patient whereby the patient feels safe and secure in the environment are more likely to have a patient with high levels of satisfaction regarding their care. Nurses must determine if patient expectations have been met. Is the patient satisfied with any changes made to the environment? Does the patient believe that their safety is ensured? If patient expectations have not been met, nurses must reassess not only the patient and the environment but also the patient's expressed desires.

▮ KEY CONCEPTS

- A safe environment is essential to promoting, maintaining, and restoring health.
- Nurses must maintain their own safety in order to provide safe care to patients.
- In the community, a safe environment is one in which basic needs are achievable, physical hazards are reduced, the transmission of pathogens is reduced, pollution is controlled, and sanitation is maintained.
- In a health care agency, a safe environment is one that minimizes falls, patient-inherent accidents, procedure-related accidents, and equipment-related accidents.
- A factor that reduces atmospheric oxygen is the presence of high carbon monoxide levels, which may result from an improperly functioning furnace.
- Prolonged exposure to extreme environmental temperatures can cause patient injury or even death.
- The reduction of physical hazards in the environment includes providing adequate lighting, decreasing clutter, and securing the home.
- The transmission of pathogens is reduced through medical and surgical asepsis, immunization, adequate food sanitation, insect and rodent control, and the appropriate disposal of human waste.
- Children less than 5 years of age are at the greatest risk for home accidents that may result in severe injury and death.
- The school-aged child is at risk for injury at home, at school, and while travelling to and from school.

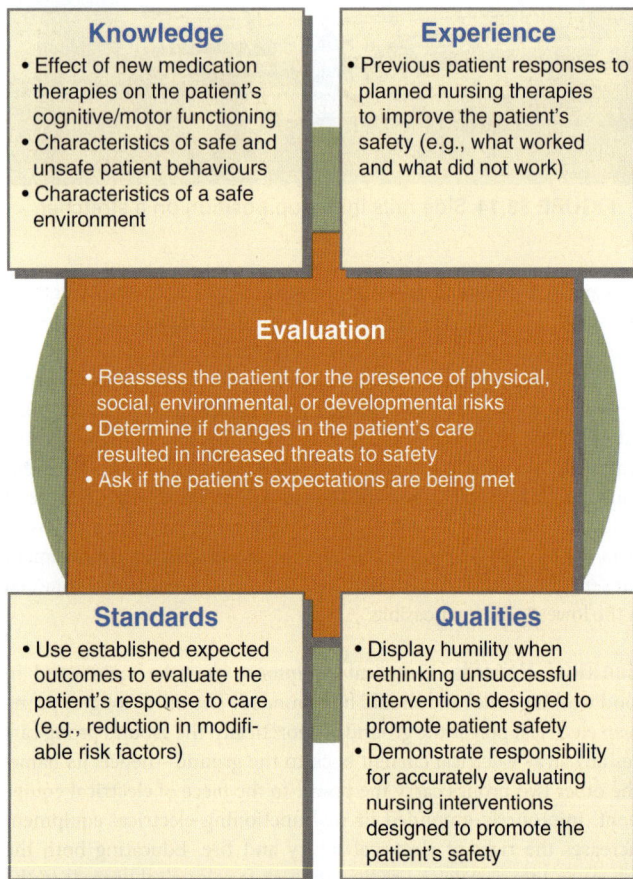

Knowledge
- Effect of new medication therapies on the patient's cognitive/motor functioning
- Characteristics of safe and unsafe patient behaviours
- Characteristics of a safe environment

Experience
- Previous patient responses to planned nursing therapies to improve the patient's safety (e.g., what worked and what did not work)

Evaluation
- Reassess the patient for the presence of physical, social, environmental, or developmental risks
- Determine if changes in the patient's care resulted in increased threats to safety
- Ask if the patient's expectations are being met

Standards
- Use established expected outcomes to evaluate the patient's response to care (e.g., reduction in modifiable risk factors)

Qualities
- Display humility when rethinking unsuccessful interventions designed to promote patient safety
- Demonstrate responsibility for accurately evaluating nursing interventions designed to promote the patient's safety

FIGURE 38.15 Critical thinking model for safety evaluation.

- Adolescents are at risk for injury from automobile accidents, suicide, and substance abuse.
- Threats to an adult's safety are frequently associated with lifestyle habits.
- Risks of injury for older patients are directly related to the physiological changes of the aging process; falls are the greatest cause of accidental injury in older persons.
- By incorporating critical thinking skills in the application of the nursing process, nurses assess the patient and the environment to determine risk factors for injury; cluster risk factors; formulate a

nursing diagnosis; and plan specific interventions, including patient education.
- Nursing interventions for promoting safety are individualized for developmental stage, lifestyle, and environment.
- Nursing interventions are developed to modify the environment for protection from falls, fires, poisoning, and electrical hazards.
- The expected outcomes include a safe physical environment, a patient whose expectations have been met and who is knowledgeable about safety factors and precautions, and a patient free of injury.

CRITICAL THINKING EXERCISES

1. Mrs. Santiago, who is 88 years old and has been functioning independently at home, was recently admitted to the hospital. Through your admission assessment, you learn that she experiences urinary frequency and urgency and occasional dizziness. When you perform the "Get-Up-and-Go" test, you find that she can get up on her own successfully after multiple attempts. Use the Hendrich II Fall Risk Model (see Table 38.1) to determine Mrs. Santiago's risk for a fall, and design specific interventions to ensure her safety in the hospital.

2. Mrs. Patel, a 76-year-old long-term care resident with Alzheimer's disease, has been refusing food and fluids for the past month. The family has agreed to the placement of a nasogastric tube to improve her fluid and nutritional statuses. Shortly after the first tube feeding

was started, Mrs. Patel became more restless, and she has been picking at the tube.
   a. What might be precipitating Mrs. Patel's behaviour of picking at the tube?
   b. What approaches can be used to eliminate interference with the treatment?
   c. If a restraint is necessary to avoid the disruption of therapy, what interventions are required to ensure the patient's safety while in restraints?

3. A family member of a patient reports that, just a few minutes ago, a lit cigarette dropped on the patient's mattress but that the small fire was put out. What actions are needed to ensure the safety of this patient?

🌐 *Answers to Critical Thinking Exercises appear on the Evolve website.*

REVIEW QUESTIONS

Review Questions 1 to 12 relate to the case study at the beginning of the chapter.

1. While completing the surgical safety checklist you notice that the consent form is for a hemi-arthroplasty of the left hip, although your patient states she fractured her right hip. What should your first action be?
   a. Ask the patient to tell you their name.
   b. Notify the surgeon and anaesthesiologist.
   c. Check to see if the patient has received any preoperative medications.
   d. Assume the patient is confused because she is older.

2. For your nursing care plan for Mrs. Maureen, which action would be appropriate given her urinary tract infection? *(Select all that apply.)*
   a. Encourage patient to void every 2–3 hours while awake.
   b. Restrict fluid intake to 1–2 litres per day.
   c. Monitor input and output daily.
   d. Patient verbalizes importance of performing perineal care at least twice a day.
   e. Foley catheter should be left in situ.

3. What is the main reason for Melody, RN, to complete a patient safety incident report for the documented fracture on the wrong side?
   a. To improve system-level safety issues
   b. To cover herself in case something goes wrong
   c. To track errors that happen in the emergency department
   d. To reprimand the RN who made the documentation error

4. What can Melody, RN, do to ensure Mrs. Maureen's safety post-surgery?
   a. Let Mrs. Maureen sleep because she is tired from her surgery.
   b. Confirm that she has a family member available to be at her side.
   c. Conduct hourly/intentional rounding.
   d. Encourage her to take all her pain medications.

5. What can Jody, LPN, do to prevent any falls? *(Select all that apply.)*
   a. Use physical restraints.
   b. Place both rails up when Mrs. Maureen is in bed.
   c. Ensure the chair and bed have wheels locked.
   d. Put the bed in its lowest position.

6. Mrs. Maureen's delirium is worsening. Jody reviews the patient's chart, and notices that Mrs. Maureen received a double dose of her pain medication. What are her next steps? *(Select all that apply.)*
   a. Call the attending physician or resident.
   b. Complete a patient incident report.
   c. Hold the next dose of pain medication.
   d. Assess her vital signs.

7. Jody, LPN, notes that medication and fluid administration errors are examples of:
   a. Patient-inherent accidents
   b. Procedure-related accidents
   c. Equipment-related accidents
   d. Environmental-related accidents

8. Jody, LPN, is aware that the physiological changes caused by aging increase the older patient's risk for:
   a. Falls
   b. Suicide
   c. Alcoholism
   d. Seizures

9. Jody, LPN, is concerned about the safety of Mrs. Maureen. As she is reflecting on what to do next, Jody knows that all of the following statements about restraints are TRUE, except:
   a. Restraints are used only after other alternatives have been tried.
   b. The least restrictive method of restraint should be used.
   c. Restraints are considered a long-term intervention.
   d. If a restraint is used, it must be part of the patient's medical treatment.
10. Jody, LPN, decides to provide teaching to Mrs. Maureen's family about safety in the home. She instructs them to: *(Select all that apply.)*
   a. Install grab rails in the bathroom near the toilet and tub.
   b. Place a bath mat on the shower stall floor.
   c. Make sure all carpeting, mats, and tiles are fixed.
   d. Ensure proper lighting.
11. Mrs. Maureen is becoming very agitated and confused. What of the following are acceptable alternatives to the use of restraints? *(Select all that apply.)*

   a. Attending to needs for toileting, food, and liquid
   b. Offering diversionary activities, such as music or something to hold
   c. Camouflaging IV lines with clothing or a stockinette
   d. Ensuring that a family member is with the patient at all times
12. Mrs. Maureen's condition is deteriorating and she can no longer weight-bear. What should Jody do?
   a. Keep her in bed as much as possible.
   b. Use a mechanical lift to move her from the bed to the chair.
   c. Hold Mrs. Maureen while she uses a walker.
   d. All of the above.

Answers: 1. a; 2. a, c, d; 3. a; 4. c; 5. c, d; 6. a, b, d; 7. b; 8. a; 9. c; 10. a, b, c, d; 11. a, b, c; 12. b.

🌐 *Rationales for the Review Questions appear on the Evolve website.*

RECOMMENDED WEBSITES

Canada Safety Council: https://canadasafetycouncil.org
The Canada Safety Council is a national, nongovernmental, charitable organization dedicated to providing safety education. Its mission is to reduce preventable deaths and injuries in public and private places throughout Canada.

DriveABLE: https://impirica.tech/driveable
This website is a useful resource for nurses working with patients who need to make a decision to stop driving. DriveABLE is an Alberta-based company that provides objective and evidence-informed approaches to assessing driver ability, as well as resources for supporting individuals and families through this process.

Healthcare Excellence Canada: https://www.healthcareexcellence.ca
Healthcare Excellence Canada (the amalgamation of both the Canadian Patient Safety Institute and the Canadian Foundation for Healthcare Improvement) is a new organization launched in spring 2021. Healthcare Excellence Canada's focus is on improving the quality and safety of health care for all Canadians. This website provides links to various topics relevant to promoting health care quality and patient safety.

Parachute: https://www.parachutecanada.org
Parachute is a national nonprofit organization dedicated to preventing injuries and saving lives. Parachute's injury-prevention program has become one of the leading injury-prevention groups in Canada.

Workplace Hazardous Materials Information System: https://www.hc-sc.gc.ca/ewh-semt/occup-travail/whmis-simdut/index-eng.php
This website is developed and maintained by Health Canada's WHMIS Division and includes policies and information related to WHMIS.

🌐 REFERENCES

A full reference list is available on the website for this book at http://evolve.elsevier.com/Canada/Potter/fundamentals/

Hygiene

*Canadian content written by Jaimee Feldstein, RN, MSN, PhD,
with original chapter contributions by Anne Griffin Perry, RN, MSN, EdD, FAAN*

OBJECTIVES

Mastery of content in this chapter will enable you to:

- Define the key terms listed.
- Describe common factors that influence personal hygiene practices.
- Explain the role that the nursing process and critical thinking play in the provision of hygiene care.
- Conduct a comprehensive assessment of a patient's total hygiene needs.
- Understand the importance of foot care for the diabetic patient.
- Describe conditions that place the patient at risk for conditions related to the hair, scalp, integument, feet, nails, eyes, ears, nose, mouth, and throat and discuss their related interventions.
- Describe how hygiene care for the older patient may differ from that for the younger patient.
- Describe an appropriate and safe infant hygiene routine.
- Describe the different approaches used in maintaining a patient's comfort and safety during hygiene care.
- Successfully perform hygiene for care of the integument, perineum, feet, hands and nails, mouth, eyes, ears, and nose.

KEY TERMS

Acne
Alopecia
Buccal mucosa
Cerumen
Complete bed bath
Cuticle
Dermis

Enucleation
Epidermis
Gingivitis
Halitosis
Lunula
Maceration
Mastication

Neuropathy
Partial bed bath
Perineal care
Periodontal disease
Stomatitis
Xerostomia

WEBSITE

http://evolve.elsevier.com/Canada/Potter/fundamentals/

CASE STUDY

You are a home health nurse visiting Martha (preferred pronouns: they/their), who is a morbidly obese 59-year-old individual living at home because Martha has limited mobility. Martha greets you while ambulating with a walker. Martha is also on home oxygen therapy for chronic obstructive pulmonary disease (COPD). Martha's past medical history includes diabetes mellitus, hypertension, and hyperlipidemia, for which she is on insulin therapy and oral antihypertensive and statin therapy. While talking casually to establish rapport, you take note of

Martha's unkempt hair and your sense of smell detects body odours, indicating lack of recent oral care and personal hygiene, including perineal care. The patient lives alone in an apartment with their dog. As you work with Martha you will need to do an assessment, plan ways to improve their hygiene, and perform an evaluation.

Think about this case study as you read this chapter. There are review questions at the end of the chapter that relate to this case study.

Personal hygiene affects an individual's comfort, safety, and physical and psychological well-being. Individuals who are well are capable of meeting their own hygiene needs, but those who are ill or have disabilities may require various levels of assistance. Many personal, social, environmental, and cultural factors can influence hygiene practices. In agency or home settings, nurses must determine a patient's ability to perform self-care and provide hygiene care according to the patient's needs and preferences. When providing care in the community setting, nurses can assist in helping the patient and family to adapt hygiene techniques, equipment, and approaches to their particular needs.

Because hygiene care requires close contact with a patient, therapeutic communication skills should be used (see Chapter 18) to build and promote a caring therapeutic relationship and to assist the nurse in providing patients with teaching or delivery of hygiene care. Other nursing activities can be integrated during hygiene care, including patient assessment and interventions, such as integumentary assessment, assessment of mood or affect, range-of-motion exercises, the application of dressings, and the inspection and care of intravenous (IV) sites. During hygiene care, nurses need to encourage and promote the patient's independence as much as possible, ensure privacy, convey respect, and maintain and support physical comfort and safety.

SCIENTIFIC KNOWLEDGE BASE

Proper hygiene care requires an understanding of the anatomy and physiology of the integument, oral cavity, eyes, ears, nose, hands, feet, and nails. The skin and mucosal cells exchange oxygen, nutrients, and fluids with underlying blood vessels. The cells require adequate nutrition, hydration, and circulation to resist injury and disease. Good hygiene techniques assist in promoting the normal structure and function of body tissues.

In addition, knowledge of pathophysiology is applied to provide skilled preventive hygiene care. As a nurse, you need to learn to recognize disease states that create changes in the integument, oral cavity, and sensory organs. For example, diabetes mellitus results in chronic vascular changes that impair healing of the skin and mucosa. In the early stages of untreated acquired immune deficiency syndrome (AIDS), fungal infections of the oral cavity are common. Stroke can result in paralysis of the trigeminal nerve, which eliminates the blink reflex, increasing the risk for corneal drying. In the presence of conditions such as these, hygiene practices are adapted to anticipate patient needs and minimize harmful effects. By integrating knowledge of anatomy, physiology, and pathophysiology during hygiene care, nurses can recognize abnormalities and initiate appropriate actions to prevent further injury.

The Skin

The skin is an active organ with the functions of protection, secretion, excretion, temperature regulation, and sensation (Table 39.1). The skin has three primary layers: epidermis, dermis, and subcutaneous (see Chapter 33). Bacteria commonly reside on the outer layer (the epidermis). These resident bacteria are normal flora (see Chapter 34); they do not cause disease but instead inhibit the multiplication of disease-causing microorganisms.

The skin can provide crucial information regarding a patient's health status and the functioning of other systems and organs (see Chapter 33).

The Feet, Hands, and Nails

The feet, hands, and nails often require special attention to prevent infection. Any injury or deformity to the foot, including growths or injuries to the overlying skin and nails, can be painful and thus interfere with a patient's normal ability to walk and weight-bear.

The hand, in contrast to the foot, is constructed largely for manipulation rather than support. Dexterity exists in the hand because of the wide range of movement between the thumb and fingers. Any condition that interferes with the movement of the hand (e.g., superficial or deep pain or joint inflammation) can impair a person's self-care abilities.

The nails are epithelial tissues that grow from the root of the nail bed, which is in the skin at the nail groove and hidden by the fold of skin called the cuticle. The visible part of the nail is the *nail body*. It has a crescent-shaped white area known as the lunula. Under the nail lies

TABLE 39.1	Function of the Skin and Implications for Care
Function and Description	**Implications for Care**
Protection The epidermis is relatively impermeable and protects the body from environmental stress (e.g., trauma, pathogens) and environmental factors (e.g., heat, cold).	Weakening of the epidermis occurs by scraping or stripping its surface (e.g., using dry razors, tape or dressing removal, or improper turning or positioning techniques resulting in shearing). Excessive dryness causes cracks and breaks in the skin and mucosa that allow bacteria to enter. Emollients soften the skin and prevent moisture loss, and hydration of the mucosa prevents dryness. Constant exposure of skin to moisture can cause maceration (softening), which interrupts dermal integrity and promotes ulcer formation and bacterial growth. Bed linen and clothing should be kept fresh and dry. Overuse of soaps, detergents, cosmetics, and deodorants can cause chemical irritation. Alkaline soaps neutralize the protective acid condition of skin. Cleaning the skin removes excess oil, sweat, dead skin cells, and dirt that can promote bacterial growth. Bath water should not be excessively hot or cold.
Sensation The skin contains sensory organs for touch, pain, temperature, and pressure.	Friction should be minimized to avoid the loss of the stratum corneum, which can result in the development of pressure injuries. Smoothing linen removes sources of mechanical irritation. To prevent accidental injury of the patient's skin, nurses should remove their own jewellery before giving care.
Temperature Regulation Body temperature is controlled by evaporation of perspiration, radiation, and conduction of heat from the body when blood vessels of the skin are vasodilated through lack of perspiration and vasoconstriction.	Factors that interfere with heat loss can alter temperature control. Wet bed linens or gowns interfere with convection, conduction, and evaporation. Excess blankets or bed coverings can interfere with heat loss through radiation and conduction and promote heat conservation.
Absorption and Secretion The skin allows limited excretion of some metabolic wastes and by-products such as minerals, sugars, and uric acid. Sebum lubricates and softens the skin and hair and decreases the amount of heat loss from the skin.	Perspiration and oil can harbour microorganisms. Bathing removes excess body secretions; however, excessive bathing can cause drying of the skin.

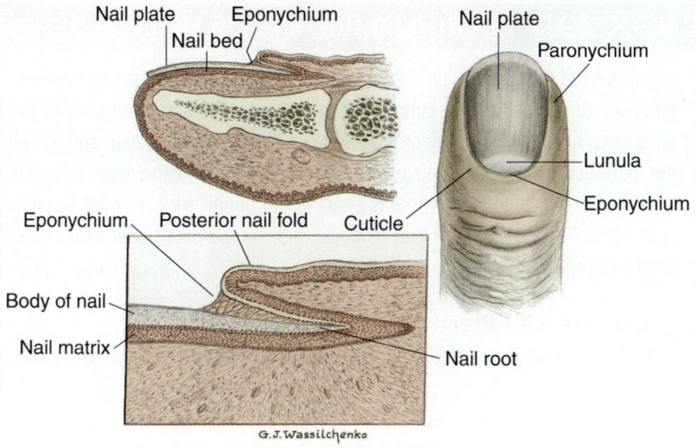

FIGURE 39.1 Anatomical structure of a normal nail.

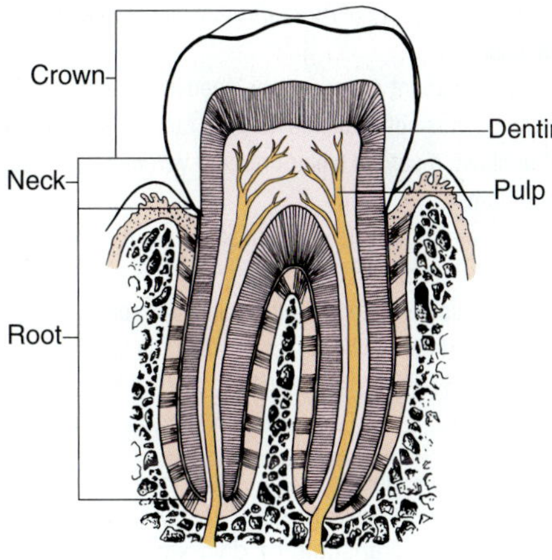

FIGURE 39.2 A normal tooth.

FIGURE 39.3 Hair follicles and relationship of follicles and their related structures to the epidermal and dermal layers of the skin. (From Lewis, S. M., Heitkemper, M. M., Dirksen, R. R., et al. [2019]. *Medical–surgical nursing in Canada: Assessment and management of clinical problems* [4th Canadian ed.]. Elsevier Canada.)

a layer of epithelium called the *nail bed* (Figure 39.1). In light-skinned individuals, a healthy nail is transparent, smooth, and convex, with a pink nail bed and translucent white tip. Some disease processes can cause changes in the shape, thickness, and curvature of the nail (see Chapter 33).

The Oral Cavity

The oral cavity extends from the lips to the anterior pillars of the tonsils. It is the structure for taste, mastication, and speech articulation. The **buccal mucosa** (oral mucosa) are normally light pink and moist. The floor of the mouth and the undersurface of the tongue are richly supplied with blood vessels, which allow for rapid absorption of sublingual medications (e.g., nitroglycerin). Any type of ulceration or trauma to the area can result in significant bleeding. The mouth also contains three pairs of salivary glands that start the digestive process by releasing enzymes, protect the mucosa from heat and chemical irritants, transmit taste information, and provide lubrication for the movement of food. Salivary secretion can be decreased by medications and disease processes.

There are 32 permanent teeth for chewing, or **mastication**. They are designed to cut, tear, and grind food so that it can be mixed with saliva and swallowed. A normal tooth consists of a crown, neck, and root (Figure 39.2). The periodontal membrane lies just below the gum margins, surrounds a tooth, and holds it firmly in place. Healthy teeth are free from cavities and are properly aligned.

Difficulty with chewing can develop when gum tissues become inflamed or infected or when teeth are lost or become loose. Regular oral hygiene is necessary to maintain the integrity of tooth surfaces and to prevent **gingivitis** (gum inflammation) and **periodontal disease**.

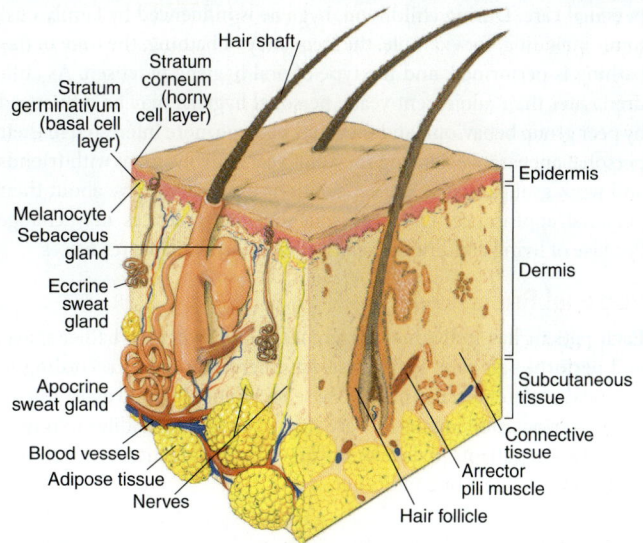

The Hair

Hair is produced by hair follicles located in the **dermis** (Figure 39.3). Hair growth, distribution, and pattern can indicate a person's general health status. Hormonal changes, emotional and physical stresses, aging, infection, and certain illnesses can affect hair colour and condition. The hair shaft itself is inert and cannot be directly affected by physiological factors. However, changes in its colour or condition are caused by hormonal or nutrient deficiencies of the hair follicle (see Figure 39.3).

The Eyes, Ears, and Nose

The eyes, ears, and nose require careful attention during the provision of hygiene. Chapter 33 describes the structure and function of these organs. Cleaning these sensitive sensory tissues should be done in a way that prevents injury and discomfort for the patient, such as being careful not to get soap in the patient's eyes. In addition, the time spent with a patient during hygiene provides an excellent opportunity to ask whether they have experienced any changes in vision, hearing, or sense of smell.

NURSING KNOWLEDGE BASE

Hygiene care is never routine; the care requires intimate contact with patients, and good communication skills are necessary to build and promote a therapeutic relationship. No two individuals perform hygiene in the same manner, thus it is important to individualize care from knowledge about the patient's unique hygiene practices and preferences.

While providing hygiene care, nurses can learn about patients' health promotion practices and needs, emotional needs, and needs pertaining to health care education. A patient's personal preferences for hygiene can be influenced by several factors.

Social Practices

Social groups influence hygiene preferences and practices, including the type of hygiene products used and the nature and frequency of personal care. During childhood, hygiene is influenced by family customs, including, for example, the frequency of bathing, the time of day bathing is performed, and the type of oral hygiene practised. As children enter their adolescent years, personal hygiene may be influenced by peer group behaviour, and they may become more interested in their personal appearance. During the adult years, involvement with friends and work groups shapes the expectations individuals have about their personal appearance. Older persons' hygiene practices may change because of living conditions, health status, and available resources.

Personal Preferences

Each patient has individual preferences about when to bathe, shave, and perform hair care. Patients select different products according to personal preferences and needs. These preferences should assist nurses in delivering individualized care for patients. In addition, nurses should assist patients in developing new hygiene practices when necessitated by an illness or condition.

Body Image

Patients' general appearance may reflect the importance that hygiene holds for them. Body image is a person's subjective concept of their physical appearance (see Chapter 27), and it can change frequently. When patients undergo surgery, illness, or a change in physical or mental health status or simply age, body image can alter dramatically. For this reason, nurses should make an effort to promote patients' hygienic comfort and appearance.

Body image affects the way in which hygiene is maintained. If the patient is neatly groomed, the nurse should consider the details of grooming when planning care and consult with the patient before making decisions about how hygiene care is to be provided. Patients who appear unkempt or uninterested in hygiene may require an assessment of their hygiene practices or of their mental status or require additional education about the importance of hygiene.

Socioeconomic Status

A person's economic resources can influence the type and extent of hygiene practices used. The nurse should be sensitive in considering whether a patient's economic status influences their ability to regularly maintain hygiene. When patients have the added challenge of a lack of resources, it can become difficult take a responsible role in health promotion activities such as basic hygiene.

When basic care items are not affordable, alternatives need to be considered. It is also important to assess whether the use of these products is an acceptable practice among patients' social or cultural group. For example, not all patients may choose to use deodorant or cosmetics.

Health Beliefs and Motivation

Knowledge about the importance of hygiene and its implications for well-being influences hygiene practices. However, knowledge alone is not enough. According to Gomes and colleagues (2020), individual characteristics such as personal factors (psychological, sociocultural, and biological) directly influence an individual's health promotion activities.

It is important to know, for example, whether patients perceive that they are at risk for dental disease, that dental disease is serious, and that brushing and flossing are effective in reducing this risk. When patients recognize that a risk is present and that reasonable action can be taken to reduce the risk, they are more receptive to counselling and teaching efforts.

Cultural Variables

Patients' cultural beliefs and personal values can influence hygiene care (Box 39.1). Individuals from diverse cultural backgrounds follow

---

BOX 39.1   Cultural Influences on Hygiene

Patients need a culturally competent plan for hygiene care. For some, hygiene practices are influenced by culture and are a potential source of conflict or stress in a hospital environment. Hygiene is a very personal matter and bathing, perineal hygiene, and hair care practices can be sensitive issues. Using knowledge from theoretical models enables the health care provider to provide culturally sensitive care that respects and incorporates the patient's cultural background.

Implications for Practice

- Maintain privacy, especially for women from cultures that value female modesty.
- Be aware that in some cultures, touch has many different meanings: touching the shoulder of a Japanese man can cause feelings of humiliation; some Asian women do not shake hands with other women or men; for some Indigenous people, touch can mean a prevention of harm.
- Be aware that to the patient of Asian descent, silence can be interpreted as a sign of respect.
- Provide gender-congruent caregivers as needed or requested. If a gender-congruent caregiver is not available, ask the family for assistance.
- Do not cut or shave a patient's hair or beard without prior discussion with the patient or family.
- Be aware that some cultures (e.g., Chinese, Filipino) discourage bathing for 7 to 10 days after childbirth.
- Bear in mind that some cultures (e.g., Chinese, Japanese, Korean, Hindu) consider the top parts of the body cleaner than the lower parts.
- Be aware that among Hindus and Muslims, the left hand is used for cleaning and the right hand is used for eating and praying.

Data from Giger, J. N., & Haddad, L. G. (2021). *Transcultural nursing: Assessment and intervention* (8th ed.). Mosby Elsevier; Purnell, L. D., & Fenkl, E. A. (2019). Transcultural diversity and health care. In *Handbook for culturally competent care*. Springer.

---

different self-care practices (see Chapter 11). Feelings of disapproval must not be conveyed when nurses are caring for patients whose hygienic practices are different from their own. For example, in some cultures, it is customary to bathe once a week; in North America, it is common to bathe or shower daily.

Physical Condition

Patients with certain types of physical limitations, disabilities, or pain often lack the physical energy, dexterity, and range of motion to perform hygiene care. A patient in traction or a cast or who has an IV line or other device connected to the body needs assistance with hygiene. Patients under the effects of sedation do not have the mental clarity or coordination to perform self-care. Chronic illnesses, such as cardiac disease, cancer, neurological disorders, and certain psychiatric conditions, may exhaust or incapacitate a patient. A weakened grasp resulting from arthritis, stroke, or muscular disorders can prevent a patient from using a toothbrush, washcloth, or comb.

CRITICAL THINKING

Successful critical thinking requires the synthesis of knowledge, experience, information gathered from patients, critical thinking qualities, and intellectual and professional standards. Clinical judgements require nurses to anticipate the information necessary to analyze data and make decisions regarding patient care. Patients' conditions are always changing, requiring ongoing critical thinking. During assessment, nurses must consider all contributing factors needed to make a nursing diagnosis (Figure 39.4).

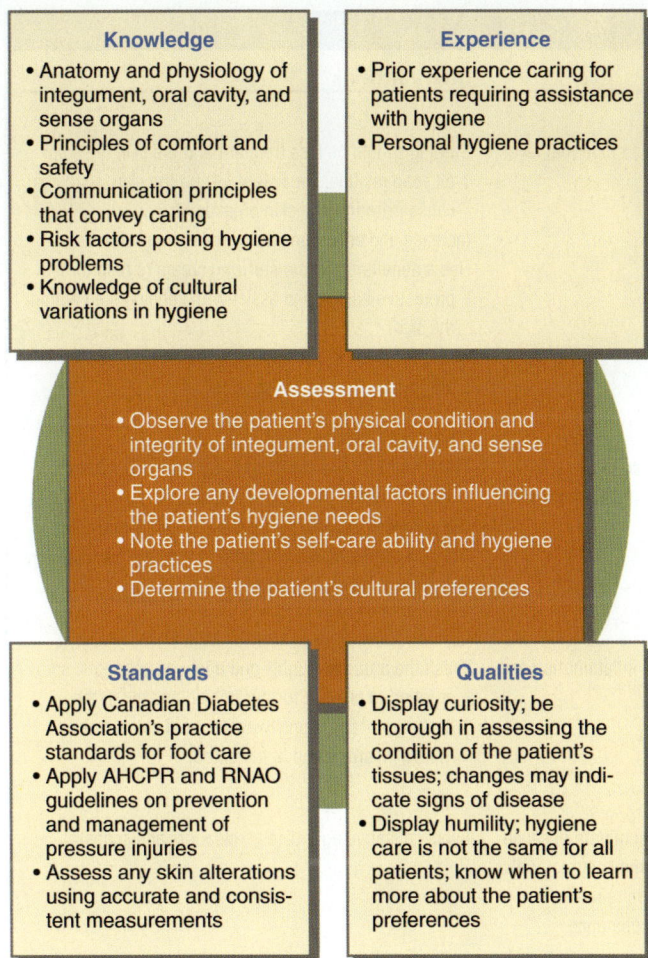

FIGURE 39.4 Critical thinking model for hygiene assessment. *AHCPR*, Agency for Health Care Policy and Research; *RNAO*, Registered Nurses' Association of Ontario.

Because hygiene care is so important for patients to feel comfortable, refreshed, and renewed, nurses should avoid making hygiene care a simple routine. Instead, nurses need to integrate knowledge from nursing and other disciplines, previous experiences, and information gathered from patients. In addition, attributes such as curiosity and humility are useful when designing a plan of care that will meet patients' hygiene needs. Agency and professional nursing standards and guidelines, such as those from the Registered Nurses' Association of Ontario (RNAO), can be used when planning care to meet the patient's hygiene needs.

❖ NURSING PROCESS

◆ Assessment

Important considerations for assessment include the patient's ability to perform self-care, usual hygiene practices, and preferences with special attention to balance, coordination, strength, range of motion, and activity tolerance. Nursing assessment is an ongoing process. It involves all phases of the nursing process, including goal setting, planning, intervention, and evaluation. Not all body regions need to be assessed before administering hygiene; however, routine assessment of a patient's condition is undertaken whenever patient care is provided. For example, during oral care, the condition of the teeth and mucosa can be inspected. If the patient has had a repeated symptom (e.g., dry skin or inflamed oral mucosa), it is important to conduct an assessment

before care is administered because variations in technique may be necessary.

Physical Examination. While assisting a patient with personal hygiene, carefully assess the integument, oral cavity structures, and the eyes, ears, and nose (see Chapter 33). Using the skills of inspection and palpation, look for alterations in the integrity and function of tissues. Assessment can also be used to determine the type and extent of hygiene care required and the need for specialized equipment (e.g., grab bars, tub chair, or lift). Special attention should be given to the structures most influenced by hygiene measures. Is the skin intact, especially over bony prominences? Is the skin dry from too much bathing or from other factors? Are calluses present on the feet, which may benefit from soaking? Is a coating of the tongue present, which necessitates frequent oral care? Over time, the nurse's assessment provides the baseline for determining whether hygienic measures maintain or improve the patient's condition.

The Skin. While inspecting the skin, thoroughly examine its colour, texture, thickness, turgor, temperature, and hydration. The skin should be smooth, warm, and supple and have good turgor. Pay special attention to the presence and condition of any lesions (see Chapter 33), and assess for dryness indicated by flaking, redness, scaling, and cracking. Certain common skin conditions affect how hygiene is administered (Table 39.2). Assess tattoos and body piercings for potential health risks such as skin irritation and infection, which are the most prevalent associated complications. Serious complications can include hepatitis B or C and HIV (Schreiber, 2019). Be alert to the possibility of hidden or unexpected piercings. Careful attention should be paid in assessing less obvious or difficult-to-reach skin surfaces, such as under the patient's breasts, under the patient's scrotum, or around the perineal tissues. Observed skin conditions should be documented and explained to the patient; teaching on proper skin care and specific hygiene techniques should also be discussed with the patient.

Certain conditions place patients at risk for impaired skin integrity (Box 39.2). Nurses must be particularly alert when assessing patients with reduced sensation, vascular insufficiency, or immobility. Both extremities should be assessed and patients should be assisted in turning so that skin surfaces can be fully viewed. The development of pressure injuries is a common complication that can extend hospital stays and threaten the well-being of long-term care patients. Tools such as the Braden Scale (Wei et al., 2020) are available to determine those patients who may be at risk for impaired skin integrity. When caring for patients with darkly pigmented skin, nurses should be aware of assessment techniques and skin characteristics unique to highly pigmented skin (Box 39.3).

The Feet and Nails. When assessing the feet, perform a thorough examination of all skin surfaces, including the areas between the toes and over the soles of the feet. The heels, soles, sides of the feet, and "knuckles" of the toes are prone to irritation from poorly fitting shoes. In addition, inspect the shape and size of the toes, as well as the shape of the foot. The toes are normally straight and flat. The feet should be in straight alignment with the ankle and tibia. Inspect the feet for lesions and note areas of dryness, inflammation, or cracking.

Assess the patient's gait. Painful foot disorders or decreased sensation can cause limping or an unnatural gait. Inquire whether the patient has foot discomfort and determine factors that aggravate the pain. Foot conditions may result from bone or muscular alterations or wearing poor-fitting footwear, rather than from skin disorders.

Patients with peripheral vascular disease, diabetes mellitus, and other diseases that affect peripheral circulation and sensation should be assessed for the adequacy of circulation to the feet (see Chapter 33). Inspection and daily foot care can help prevent the development

TABLE 39.2 | Common Skin Conditions

Characteristics	Implications	Interventions
Dry Skin Flaky, rough texture on exposed areas such as hands, arms, legs, or face	Skin may become infected if the epidermal layer is allowed to crack.	Bathing should be less frequent and the skin rinsed of all soap residue, because if left on the skin, soap can cause irritation and skin breakdown. Increase and encourage fluid intake, if permitted. Use a nonallergenic moisturizing cream to help form a protective barrier and assist with keeping fluid within the skin. Use creams to clean skin that is dry or if the patient is allergic to soaps or detergents.
Acne Inflammatory, papulopustular skin eruption, usually involving bacterial breakdown of sebum; appears on face, neck, shoulders, and back	Infected material within the pustule can spread if the area is squeezed or picked. Permanent scarring can result.	Wash hair and skin thoroughly each day with soap to remove excess oil and prevent secondary infections. Use cosmetics sparingly, as oily cosmetics and creams accumulate in pores and tend to worsen the condition. Use prescribed topical or oral antibiotics.
Skin Rashes Skin eruption that may result from overexposure to sun or moisture or from an allergic reaction (may be flat or raised, localized or systemic, pruritic or nonpruritic)	If skin is continually scratched, inflammation and infection may occur.	Wash the area thoroughly and apply an antiseptic spray or lotion to prevent further itching and aid in the healing process. Apply warm or cold compresses to relieve inflammation, if indicated.
Contact Dermatitis Inflammation of skin characterized by abrupt onset with erythema, pruritus, pain, and appearance of scaly oozing lesions (seen on face, neck, hands, forearms, and genitalia)	Dermatitis is often difficult to eliminate because the person is usually in continual contact with the substance causing the skin reaction, and it may be hard to identify this substance.	Avoid causative agents (e.g., cleaners and soaps).
Psoriasis A noncontagious, chronic skin condition characterized by an abnormal growth of keratinocytes (a type of skin cell) and an inflammatory reaction that results in the formation of thick, silvery, scaly, inflamed patches of skin; commonly seen on the scalp, knees, elbows, and chest	The cause of psoriasis is unknown, and no cure exists. It is often difficult to diagnosis as it has similar symptoms to eczema and atopic dermatitis.	Treatment options are aimed at reducing the extent and severity of the condition and improving quality of life. The patient should avoid trigger agents such as smoking, stress, excessive alcohol, and skin injury (e.g., sunburn).
Impetigo A bacterial skin infection characterized by red sores that can break open, ooze fluid, and develop a yellow-brown crust. The sores can occur anywhere on the body. It is one of the most common skin infections in children. While it can occur in adults, it is more common in children. Impetigo is contagious and can be spread to others through close contact or by sharing linens and clothing. Scratching can also spread sores to other parts of the body (HealthLink BC, 2018).	Impetigo is caused by one of two kinds of bacteria—strep (streptococcus) or staph (staphylococcus). It can occur in healthy intact skin, but more often bacteria enter the body when the skin has already been irritated or injured through other skin conditions, such as eczema, poison ivy, insect bites, burns, or cuts.	Impetigo is treated with antibiotics. For mild cases, a topical antibiotic (ointment or cream) is prescribed. For more serious cases, oral antibiotics may be prescribed.
Hand-Foot-and-Mouth Disease An illness caused by the enterovirus; manifests as sores or blisters in or on the mouth and on the hands, feet, and sometimes the buttocks and legs. The sores can be painful, and the illness usually lasts approximately 1 week. It is most common in children but can occur in adults and most often occurs in the summer or fall (HealthLink BC, 2021).	Symptoms may begin with fatigue, a sore throat, or a fever. Within 1–2 days, blisters or sores can appear. The virus spreads easily through coughing and sneezing, or through contact with infected stool or blister fluid.	Usually, medical treatment is not required. Interventions are focused on symptom management, which includes offering cool fluids, analgesics, and antipyretics.

TABLE 39.2	Common Skin Conditions—cont'd	
Characteristics	**Implications**	**Interventions**
Abrasion		
Scraping or rubbing away of epidermis that may result in localized bleeding and later weeping of serous fluid	Infection occurs easily because of the loss of this protective skin layer.	Caregivers should trim their fingernails and not wear jewellery when providing patient care. Clean the area and dry thoroughly and gently. Observe for retained moisture in dressings or bandages—excess moisture can increase the risk of infection. Lift—do not pull—when transferring or repositioning a patient. Consider the use of a lift, as needed, for immobile or heavy patients (see Chapter 46).

BOX 39.2 Risk Factors for Skin Impairment

Immobilization

When restricted from moving freely, patients' dependent body parts are exposed to pressure, reducing circulation to the affected body parts. Nurses should know which patients require assistance to turn and reposition.

Reduced Sensation

Patients with paralysis, circulatory insufficiency, or local nerve damage are unable to sense an injury to the skin. While bathing a patient, assess the status of sensory nerve function by checking for pain, tactile sensation, and temperature sensation.

Nutrition and Hydration Alterations

Patients with limited caloric and protein intake can develop thinner, less elastic skin, with a loss of subcutaneous tissue. This can result in impaired or delayed wound healing.

Secretions and Excretions on the Skin

Moisture on the skin's surface serves as a medium for bacterial growth and can cause irritation, soften epidermal cells, and lead to skin breakdown. The presence of perspiration, urine, fecal material, or wound drainage on the skin can also result in breakdown or infection, or both.

Vascular Insufficiency

Inadequate arterial supply to tissues and impaired venous return decrease the circulation to the extremities. Inadequate blood flow can cause ischemia and tissue breakdown. The risk of infection also exists because the delivery of nutrients, oxygen, and white blood cells to injured tissues is inadequate.

External Devices

An external device applied to or around the skin exerts pressure and friction on the skin. Assess all surfaces exposed to casts, cloth restraints, bandages and dressings, tubing, or orthopedic braces.

BOX 39.3 Skin Assessment and Implications for Practice

Identifying changes in skin colour is important in evaluating patients' risks for skin breakdown and pressure injuries (see Chapter 47). When a patient's natural skin contains more melanin, it is more difficult to determine hyperemia and cyanosis. Some hyperpigmentation areas are normal, such as slate grey nevus, which may be on the sacrum of African, Indigenous, and Asian patients. These areas should not be confused with skin colour changes such as hyperemia or cyanosis.

Implications for Practice

For dark-skinned patients, assess baseline skin tone by asking the patient or family to point out an area of baseline skin colour for that person. Assess the oral mucosa, over the cheekbones, and conjunctivae in the dark-skinned patient, and the nail beds and lips in light-skinned patients.

Assess localized skin changes:

- Colour darker than surrounding skin colour; purplish, bluish (cyanosis), eggplant
- Taut skin
- Shiny skin
- Induration (hardening of the tissues)
- Use natural light sources when possible because fluorescent light can give the skin a bluish tone
- Examine body sites with the least amount of melanin for underlying skin colour identification
   Assess for edema (nonpitting, pitting) (see Chapter 33).
   Assess skin temperature, using the back of the hand; if the patient's condition permits, do not use gloves when doing this assessment:
- Initially may feel warmer than surrounding skin
- Subsequently may feel cooler than surrounding skin

Data from MacDonald-Jenkins, J. (2018). Skin, hair, and nails. In C. Jarvis, A. Browne, J. MacDonald-Jenkins, et al. (Eds.), *Physical examination and health assessment* (3rd Canadian ed.). Elsevier.

of a foot ulcer. Foot ulcerations are a predisposing factor for lower extremity amputations in individuals with diabetes mellitus (Ferreira et al., 2018).

Palpation of the dorsalis pedis and posterior tibial pulses is used to determine whether adequate or reduced blood flow is reaching peripheral tissues. Edema and changes in skin colour, texture, and temperature can indicate whether patients require special hygiene care. Individuals with diabetes mellitus should also be assessed for **neuropathy**—degeneration of the peripheral nerves characterized by a loss

of sensation, which can lead to injury. Patients' sensation to light touch, pain, and temperature should be assessed.

Inspect the condition of the fingernails and toenails, looking for lesions, dryness, inflammation, and cracking (Table 39.3). The nail is surrounded by a cuticle, which slowly grows over the nail and must be regularly pushed back. The skin around the nail beds and cuticles should be smooth and without inflammation. Individuals should be asked whether they frequently polish their nails and use polish remover, because chemicals in these products can cause excessive nail

TABLE 39.3   Common Foot and Nail Conditions

Characteristics	Implications	Interventions
Callus A thickened portion of the epidermis consisting of a mass of horny, keratotic cells. It is usually flat, painless, and found on the undersurface of the foot or on the palm of the hand. It is caused by local friction or pressure.	The condition may cause discomfort when wearing tight shoes.	Advise the patient to wear gloves when using tools or objects that may create friction on palmar surfaces and to wear soft-soled shoes with insoles. Soak callus in warm water and magnesium sulphate (Epsom salts) to soften the cell layers. Apply cream or lotion to reduce reformation. Encourage the patient to see a podiatrist (ensure that the patient is aware of the associated cost).
Keratosis (corn) Corns are caused by chronic friction and pressure from ill-fitting or loose shoes. They are seen mainly on or between toes or over a bony prominence. A corn is usually cone shaped, round, and raised. Soft corns are macerated.	The conical shape compresses the underlying dermis, making it thin and tender. The pain worsens when tight shoes are worn. Corns can become soft and macerated by perspiration. The patient may suffer an alteration in gait resulting from pain.	Surgical removal may be necessary, depending on the severity of pain and size of the corn. The patient should avoid the use of oval corn pads, which can increase pressure on toes and reduce circulation. Use warm water soaks to soften the corns before gentle rubbing with a callus file or pumice stone (consult with health care provider or podiatrist). Wider and softer shoes are suggested.
Plantar Wart A fungating lesion caused by the papillomavirus that appears on the sole of the foot	Warts may be contagious, are painful, and can make walking difficult.	Treatment ordered may include applications of salicylic acid, electrodessication (burning with electrical spark), or freezing with solid carbon dioxide.
Athlete's Foot (Tinea Pedis) A fungal infection of the foot; scaliness and cracking of skin occur between the toes and on the soles of feet. Small blisters containing fluid may appear. The condition can be caused by wearing constricting footwear.	Athlete's foot can spread to other body parts, especially the hands. It is contagious and frequently recurs.	Feet should be well ventilated. Drying feet well after bathing and applying powder helps to prevent infection. Wearing clean socks or stockings reduces incidence. The health care provider may prescribe antifungal topical applications.
Ingrown Nail An ingrown toenail or fingernail grows inward into the soft tissue around the nail. An ingrown nail often results from improper nail trimming.	Ingrown nails can cause localized pain when pressure is applied and can lead to infection.	Treatment involves frequent hot soaks in an antiseptic solution and removal of the portion of nail that has grown into skin. Instruct the patient in proper nail-trimming techniques and provide a referral to a podiatrist. (Ensure that the patient is aware of the associated cost.)
Ram's Horn Nail An unusually long, curved, thickened nail	Attempts to cut ram's horn nails may result in damage to the nail bed with an increased risk of infection.	Refer the patient to a podiatrist. (Ensure that the patient is aware of the associated cost.)
Paronychia Inflammation of tissue surrounding the nail, after a hangnail or other injury. It occurs in individuals who frequently have their hands in water and is common in patients with diabetes.	Infection	Treatment can include hot compresses or soaks, or topical or oral antibiotics. Paronychia can be prevented by careful manicuring.
Foot Odour Results from excess perspiration, promoting microorganism growth.	The condition may cause discomfort because of excess perspiration and odour and increases patients' risk for infection.	Frequent washing, using foot deodorants and powders, and wearing clean footwear prevent or reduce foot odour.

dryness and discoloration. Disease can change the shape and curvature of the nails. Inflammatory lesions and fungus of the nail bed can cause thickened, horny nails, which can separate from the nail bed.

The Oral Cavity. All areas of the oral cavity need to be inspected carefully for colour, hydration, texture, and lesions (see Chapter 33). Patients who do not follow regular oral hygiene practices may have receding gum tissue, gingivitis, a coated tongue, discoloured teeth (particularly along the gum margins), dental caries, missing teeth, and halitosis (bad breath). Localized pain and infection are common symptoms of periodontal disease and certain tooth disorders.

Some patients in acute care settings require a complete oral assessment (Estes et al., 2018). The identification of risks for infection and other conditions can indicate the type and frequency of oral care. Proper oral care has been shown to decrease the risk of aspiration and nosocomial infections in ventilated patients (Galhardo et al., 2020). It is also well established that Gram-negative bacteria (e.g., *Pseudomonas aeruginosa*) found in dental plaque can result in pneumonia in hospitalized older persons. It is especially important to examine the oral cavity of patients receiving radiation or chemotherapy. Both treatments can reduce the amount of saliva, resulting in drying and **stomatitis** (inflammation of the oral mucosal tissues). The assessment serves as a basis for preventive care for patients as they undergo treatment.

The Hair. Before performing hair care, assess the condition of the hair and scalp. Healthy hair is clean, shiny, and untangled; the scalp is free of lesions. The hair of dark-skinned patients is usually thicker, drier, and curlier than that of lighter-skinned patients. Table 39.4 summarizes hair and scalp conditions that may be identified during the assessment. In community and home care settings, it is particularly important to inspect the hair for pediculosis capitis (head lice) so that the appropriate treatment can be provided. If head lice are suspected, guard against self-infestations by handwashing and using gloves or tongue blades to inspect the patient's hair. A loss of hair (**alopecia**) can result from the effects of chemotherapy medications, hormonal changes, or improper hair care practices or may be idiopathic. Patients at risk for scalp conditions are those who have experienced head trauma and those who practise poor hygiene.

The Eyes, Ears, and Nose. The condition and function of the eyes, ears, and nose need to be examined (see Chapter 33). Normally the eyes are free of infection and irritation. The sclerae are visible anteriorly as the white portion of the eye. The conjunctivae (the lining of the eyelids) are clear, pink, and without inflammation. The eyelid margins are in close approximation with the eyeball, and the lashes are turned outward. The lid margins are without inflammation, drainage, or lesions. The eyebrows are symmetrical.

TABLE 39.4	Conditions of Head and Body Hair and Scalp	
Characteristics	**Implications**	**Interventions**
Dandruff Scaling of the scalp is accompanied by itching. In severe cases, dandruff can be found on eyebrows.	Dandruff causes individuals embarrassment and if it enters the eyes, conjunctivitis may develop.	Shampoo regularly with a medicated shampoo. In severe cases, obtain a health care provider's advice.
Ticks Small, grey-brown parasites that burrow into the skin and suck the blood	Ticks transmit several diseases to individuals. The most common are Rocky Mountain spotted fever, tularemia, and Lyme disease.	Do not pull ticks quickly from the skin because their sucking apparatus remains and may cause infection. Ticks can be removed slowly with tweezers.
Pediculosis Capitis (Head Lice) Head lice require a source of human blood to survive. Transmission is by direct contact (e.g., head to head). The parasite is found near the scalp, attached to hair strands. Eggs look like oval particles, similar to dandruff. Bites or pustules may be observed behind the ears and at the hairline. Itching at the hairline is the most common symptom.	Contacts of patients (e.g., family members and classmates) should be examined and treated. Although no current evidence exists of transmission by shared articles, families may wish to wash bedding and combs in hot water. Dry-cleaning, or storing items in occlusive plastic bags for approximately 2 weeks is also effective (Cummings et al., 2018).	Check the entire scalp. Use a medicated shampoo to eliminate lice. Follow the product directions carefully; a repeat application is required 7–10 days later to ensure that surviving eggs are destroyed. Seek health care provider's advice if treatment is ineffective; a new medication may be required for effective chemical eradication. Some products can cause neurotoxicity and should not be used with children under 6 years of age. Do not use products containing lindane. This product has been withdrawn for use in some countries. Use a fine-toothed comb to assist with the manual removal of nits (the empty eggshell) and lice.
Pediculosis Corporis (Body Lice) Body lice differ from head lice in that they tend to cling to clothing and may not be easily seen. They suck blood and lay eggs on clothing and furniture.	The patient itches constantly. Scratches seen on the skin may become infected. Hemorrhagic spots may appear on skin where lice are sucking blood.	Ask the patient to bathe or shower thoroughly. After the skin is dried, apply a recommended pediculicide lotion. After 8–12 hours, have the patient take another bath or shower. Bag infested clothing or linen until laundered in hot water. Vacuum rooms thoroughly and throw away the bag after completion.
Pediculosis Pubis (Crab Lice) Crab lice parasites are found in pubic hair. Crab lice are greyish white with red legs.	Lice may be spread via bed linen, clothing, or furniture, or via sexual contact.	Clean pubic hair to remove body lice. Treatment of sexual partners is recommended.
Hair Loss (Alopecia) Alopecia occurs in individuals of all races. Balding patches are seen at the periphery of the hairline. Hair becomes brittle and broken. The condition can be caused by genetics, the use of hair curlers or hair picks, tight braiding, and some medications.	Patches of uneven hair growth and loss alter the patient's appearance and affect self-image.	Advise the patient to stop any hair care practices that might be further damaging the hair.

It is important to determine whether the patient wears contact lenses. This is especially significant for patients who enter hospitals or other agencies who are unresponsive or in a confused state. To determine whether a contact lens is present, stand to the side of the patient's eye and observe the cornea for the presence of a soft or rigid lens; if you do not see one, observe the sclera to detect whether a contact lens has shifted off the patient's cornea. An undetected lens can cause severe corneal injury if left in place too long.

Inspect the external ear structures (auricle, helix, and earlobe), and use an otoscope to inspect the external auditory canal and tympanic membrane. While performing hygiene measures, the nurse is most concerned with noting the presence of accumulated cerumen or drainage in the ear canal, local inflammation, tenderness on palpation, or the patient's report of pain (see Chapter 33).

Inspect the nares for signs of inflammation, discharge, lesions, edema, and deformity (see Chapter 33). The nasal mucosa is normally pink and clear and has little or no discharge. A clear, watery discharge may be the result of allergies. If the patient has any form of tubing exiting the nose (e.g., nasogastric tube), inspect the naris surfaces that come in contact with the tubing for tissue sloughing, localized tenderness, inflammation, and bleeding.

Developmental Changes. The normal process of aging influences the condition of body tissues and structures and, thus, the manner in which hygiene measures are performed. Chapter 48 addresses the changes in hearing, vision, and olfaction across the lifespan as a result of growth and development.

The Skin. Newborns' skin is relatively immature at birth. The epidermis and dermis are loosely bound together, and the skin is very thin. Friction against the skin layers can cause bruising, so newborns must be handled carefully during bathing. Any break in the skin can easily lead to infection.

Toddlers' skin layers are more tightly bound together. Thus, children have a greater resistance to infection and skin irritation. However, because of children's active play and the absence of established hygiene habits, greater attention is needed from parents and caregivers to provide thorough hygiene and to begin teaching good hygiene habits.

During adolescence, the growth and maturation of the integument increases. In girls, estrogen secretion causes the skin to become soft, smooth, and thicker, with increased vascularity. In boys, male hormones produce an increased thickness of the skin with some darkening in colour. Sebaceous glands become more active, predisposing adolescents to acne. Eccrine and apocrine sweat glands become fully functional during puberty. Adolescents usually begin to use deodorants, and more frequent bathing and shampooing become necessary to reduce body odours and eliminate oily hair. Sweating is usually more pronounced in boys.

The condition of adults' skin depends on hygiene practices and exposure to environmental irritants. Normally, the skin is elastic, well hydrated, firm, and smooth. When adults bathe frequently or are exposed to an environment with low humidity, the skin can become very dry and flaky.

With aging, the skin loses its resiliency and moisture, and sebaceous and sweat glands become less active. The epithelium thins, and elastic collagen fibres shrink, making the skin fragile and subject to bruising and breaking. These changes in the outer epidermis or stratum corneum (Bonté et al., 2019), warrant caution when turning and repositioning older persons. Typically, older persons' skin becomes drier and wrinkled. Because the skin may be excessively dry, older persons should avoid bathing daily and using very hot water or harsh soaps.

The Feet and Nails. When we stand, the feet provide support and absorb shock. With aging, they begin to show signs of wear and tear.

This may occur earlier if individuals have failed to wear comfortable, supportive footwear. The cushioning layer of fat on the soles of the feet becomes thin.

Chronic foot conditions are a common result of poor foot care, improperly fitting footwear, aging, and systemic disease. Older persons often have dry feet because of a decrease in sebaceous gland secretion, dehydration of epidermal cells, and poor condition of footwear. Callus formation and decreased sensation place the patient at a high risk for the development of foot ulcers (Boulton, 2019). Painful feet can be the result of congenital deformities, weak structure, injuries, and diseases such as diabetes, rheumatoid arthritis, or osteoarthritis. After 55 years of age, arthritis is a common cause of changes in the feet. Additional common foot conditions are hammer toes, hallux valgus (bunions), corns, and ingrown toenails.

Fungal infections can occur under toenails, causing dark yellow streaks or total discoloration. The nails can also become opaque, scaly, and hypertrophied. If foot or nail problems remain unresolved, patients can easily become disabled. Nurses must apply knowledge of typical changes in the feet and nails when anticipating the type of hygiene that patients will require.

The Oral Cavity. Infants begin teething at approximately 4 to 10 months of age (Miri-Aliabad et al., 2021). The first permanent (secondary) teeth erupt at about 6 years of age. From adolescence, when all of the permanent teeth are in place, through middle adulthood, the teeth and gums remain healthy if individuals avoid fermentable carbohydrates and sticky sweets. Regular dental care and hygiene practices such as brushing and flossing help to prevent caries and periodontal disease.

As individuals grow older, numerous factors can result in poor oral care. These include age-related changes of the mouth, chronic disease such as diabetes, physical disabilities involving hand grasp or strength affecting the ability to perform oral care, lack of attention to oral care, and prescribed medications that affect the buccal (oral) mucosa. Aging teeth become brittle, drier, and darker. Teeth can become uneven, jagged, and fractured. Gums lose vascularity and tissue elasticity, which can cause dentures to fit poorly. Many older persons are edentulous and wear complete or partial dentures. It is important to determine whether older patients wear dentures and the condition of underlying supportive gum tissue.

The Eyes, Ears, and Nose. Although the structure of the eyes does not have marked developmental changes, altered visual acuity can occur at several points during the aging process; for example, when children start school or when patients reach middle age, visual acuity may change. As patients age, they are also at risk for changes in visual clarity (e.g., caused by glaucoma or cataracts) and visual field losses (e.g., caused by macular degeneration or glaucoma).

Structures of the ears do not change as patients age; however, changes in hearing acuity or balance may occur with aging. In young children, changes in hearing acuity may result from a foreign object being placed in the ear—this may be a temporary change, resolved once the object is removed. Changes may also result from repeated ear infections or exposure to loud noise, such as when children or adolescents listen to loud music on headphones.

Older persons may have changes in the structure and function of the small bones in the inner ear that affect hearing acuity. Aging may result in increased cerumen production, which can also impede hearing acuity. In addition, the movement of fluid through the semicircular canals may change with age, and patients may experience positional dizziness or balance difficulties.

Although changes in the sense of smell can occur at any time, they seem to be more common in older persons. These changes may also affect taste and a patient's appetite.

New and acute changes in the structure and function of the eyes, ears, and nose must be fully assessed and evaluated. Timely evaluation of these changes may result in effective treatments or confirm that they are age related.

Use of Sensory Aids. When patients wear eyeglasses, contact lenses, artificial eyes, or hearing aids, nurses need to assess their knowledge and ask them to describe the methods that are used for routine care (Box 39.4). The information gathered is then compared with the proper care technique for these devices. Any differences between patient practice and standard practice may indicate a need for patient education.

Self-Care Ability. Patients with physical or cognitive impairments need assistance with all or some aspects of personal hygiene. Assessment of a patient's physical and cognitive statuses determines specifically which aspects of hygiene care can be performed independently, which require some assistance, and which require total assistance.

The assessment must include the measurement of the patient's muscle strength, flexibility and dexterity, balance, coordination, and activity tolerance—these qualities are needed to perform activities such as bathing, brushing teeth, and bending over to inspect the feet. The degree of assistance needed by the patient during hygiene care may also depend on vision, their ability to sit without support, their hand grasp strength, the range of motion in their extremities, or the presence of equipment such as an IV line, dressings, or traction. Painful conditions of the upper extremities pose special challenges. Self-care ability is assessed by asking the patient to perform activities such as brushing their teeth or combing their hair. The nurse needs to observe carefully as the patient carries out the activity and note whether the patient can perform the task thoroughly and correctly (Figure 39.5).

When a patient has self-care limitations, part of the assessment is to determine whether family or friends are available to assist. Assisting with hygiene measures can at times be unpleasant, so the assessment should include how the family members assist, how often this assistance is provided, and what their feelings are about being a caregiver. In addition, it is important to assess the home environment and its influence on the patient's hygiene practices. Does the home environment contain barriers that may affect the patient's self-care abilities? Water faucets that are too tight to easily adjust, bathtubs with high sides, and a bathroom too small to fit a wheelchair or walker in front of a sink are a few examples.

Hygiene Practices. An assessment of hygiene practices can reveal a patient's grooming preferences. For example, a patient may choose to groom their hair in a certain style or to trim nails a certain way. When a patient has a physical disability, special precautions may be needed to perform grooming without injury. Asking the patient to assist or teach how to perform preferred grooming practices gives the patient a greater sense of independence and helps the nurse to avoid causing the patient discomfort or injury.

Cultural Factors. A patient's cultural background is an influential factor when determining hygiene needs. Culture plays a role not only in hygiene practices and preferences but also in sensitivity regarding personal space (see Chapter 11). For example, some patients may view tasks associated with closeness and touch as being offensive or impolite. Nurses need to ask patients what would make them feel most comfortable during a bath. Instead of a full bath, perhaps a patient would prefer only a partial bath, with a family member performing the

---

BOX 39.4	Assessing a Patient's Use of Sensory Aids

Eyeglasses
Ask about purpose for wearing glasses (e.g., reading, distance, or both)
Ask about methods used to clean glasses
Ask about presence of symptoms (e.g., blurred vision, photophobia, headaches, irritation)

Contact Lenses
Determine type of lens worn
Ask about frequency and duration of time lenses are worn (including sleep time)
Ask about presence of symptoms (e.g., burning, excess tearing, redness, irritation, swelling, or sensitivity to light)
Ask about techniques used by patient to cleanse, store, insert, and remove lenses
Ask about use of eye drops or ointments
Determine whether patient has an emergency identification bracelet or card that alerts others to remove patient's lenses in case of emergency

Artificial Eye
Ask about method used to insert and remove eye
Ask about method for cleansing eye
Ask about presence of symptoms (e.g., drainage, inflammation, or pain involving the orbit)

Hearing Aid
Ask about type of aid worn
Ask about methods used to cleanse aid
Ask about patient's ability to change battery and adjust hearing aid volume

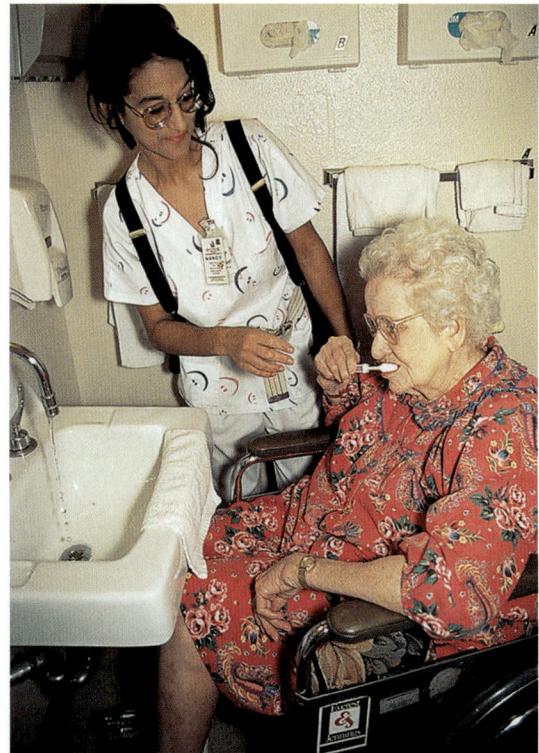

FIGURE 39.5 Observe the patient brushing teeth. Observation helps the nurse determine how much assistance the patient may need.

bathing of private body areas. The patient may also defer part of the hygiene care. If, in the nurse's judgement, hygiene is critical in order to prevent development or worsening of a health problem, such as skin breakdown, the nurse must take the time to understand the patient's concerns and negotiate a mutually satisfactory solution to the problem.

Patients at Risk for Hygiene Challenges. Some patients present risks that require more attentive and rigorous hygiene care (Table 39.5). These risks may result from adverse effects of medications, a lack of knowledge, an inability to perform hygiene, or a physical condition that potentially injures the skin or other structures. An immobilized patient who has a fever, for example, requires more frequent bathing to minimize perspiration on the skin, and more frequent turning and positioning to reduce the risk of skin breakdown.

Nurses need to anticipate whether a patient is predisposed to such risks and follow through with a complete assessment. For example, if a patient is receiving chemotherapy, the treatment has a risk of destroying the normal flora in the mouth, allowing for the overgrowth of opportunistic bacteria. Therefore, the oral examination should be more thorough and detailed, involving all surfaces of the tongue and mucosa. If a patient is diaphoretic, special attention should be given to body areas such as underneath the breasts and the perineal area, where moisture may collect and irritate skin surfaces. Nurses should anticipate problems created by these risks and provide appropriate preventive care. Their assessment should include a review of the patient's medical and surgical histories, medications, and specific risk factors.

Special Considerations in Hygiene Assessment. Depending on the type of hygiene the nurse is planning to provide, the nurse should conduct certain focused assessments. Before giving foot care, the nurse should assess the type of footwear worn by a patient. Children or young adults who frequently fail to wear socks may have excess perspiration that promotes fungal growth. Tight or poorly fitting shoes, socks, garters, or knee-high nylon stockings may cause skin irritation and

TABLE 39.5	Health Risks and Implications for Hygiene
Risks	**Hygiene Implications**
Oral	
Inability to use upper extremities due to paralysis, weakness, or restriction (e.g., cast or dressing)	Patient lacks upper extremity strength or dexterity needed to brush teeth.
Dehydration, inability to take fluids or food by mouth	Dehydration causes excess drying and fragility of the mucosa and increases the accumulation of secretions on the tongue and gums.
Presence of nasogastric or oxygen tubes; mouth breathers	These situations cause drying of the mucosa.
Chemotherapeutic drugs	Drugs kill rapidly multiplying cells, including normal cells lining the oral cavity. Ulcers and inflammation can develop.
Other medications (antihistamines)	These can cause a decrease in saliva production, which leads to thicker mucus and dryness of the oral mucosa (**xerostomia**).
Over-the-counter lozenges, cough drops, antacids, and chewable vitamins	Medications may contain large amounts of sugar. Repeated use increases sugar or acid content in mouth.
Radiation therapy to head and neck	Radiation therapy decreases function of the salivary glands, which can contribute to stomatitis (Pederson et al., 2018).
Oral surgery, trauma to mouth, placement of an oral airway	These situations cause trauma to the oral cavity with swelling, ulcerations, inflammation, and bleeding.
Immunosuppression; altered blood clotting	These conditions predispose to inflammation and bleeding gums.
Diabetes mellitus	Patients with diabetes are prone to dryness of the mouth, gingivitis, periodontal disease, and tooth loss.
Skin	
Immobilization	Dependent body parts are exposed to pressure from underlying surfaces. The inability to turn or change position increases the risk for pressure injuries.
Reduced sensation due to stroke, spinal cord injury, diabetes, local nerve damage	There is interruption in transmission of nerve impulses when excessive heat or cold, pressure, friction, or chemical irritants are applied to skin.
Limited protein or caloric intake and reduced hydration (e.g., caused by fever, burns, gastrointestinal alterations, poorly fitting dentures)	Limited caloric and protein intakes predispose to impaired tissue synthesis. The skin becomes thinner, less elastic, and smoother, with a loss of subcutaneous tissue. Poor wound healing may result. Reduced hydration impairs skin turgor.
Excessive secretions or excretions on the skin from perspiration, urine, watery fecal material, and wound drainage	Moisture is a medium for bacterial growth and can cause local skin irritation, softening of epidermal cells, and skin maceration.
Presence of external devices (e.g., casts, restraint, bandage, dressing)	A device can exert pressure or friction against the skin's surface.
Vascular insufficiency	Arterial blood supply to tissues is inadequate, or venous return is impaired, causing decreased circulation to the extremities. Tissue ischemia and breakdown may occur. The risk for infection is high.
Foot	
Inability to bend over or see clearly	Patient is unable to fully visualize the entire surface of each foot, impairing their ability to adequately assess condition of the skin and nails.
Eye Care	
Reduced dexterity and hand coordination	Physical limitations create an inability to safely insert or remove contact lenses.

interfere with circulation to the feet. Nurses should also assess whether patients wear clean footwear daily, because repeated use of soiled footwear can lead to infection. If patients have diabetes mellitus or another peripheral vascular disease, it is extremely important that they wear appropriate footwear. Extra-wide and extra-deep shoes accommodate bunions or hammer toes. Cushioned inner soles help redistribute pressure on the metatarsal head. Patients may need to be referred to a podiatrist and orthotic footwear specialist.

It is also important to assess patients' eating patterns before providing oral care. Patients should be asked whether difficulties are noted with chewing, swallowing, or the fit of their dentures, if any. Patients may have changed the type of food in their diet as a result of chewing difficulties. The presence of an ulcer or irritation may impair chewing and cause patients to avoid eating. This is common in older persons with poorly fitting dentures.

Patient Expectations. As is the case in any nursing assessment, it is important to know what patients expect from nursing care. For hygiene care, patients may simply expect to have hygiene preferences and practices applied in the health care setting. The nurse can assess the patient's expectations by asking questions such as "To make you most comfortable and feeling at home, how can I best perform your bath and personal care?" or "How can we help you care for your teeth, nails, and hair, now that you are at home?"

Understanding patients' expectations and applying them in practice is important in establishing a trusting relationship. Truly individualizing hygiene care shows respect for patients' needs. As the nurse learns what each patient expects, this information can be incorporated into the individual's plan of care (see "Planning" section later in this chapter).

◆ Nursing Diagnosis

Through assessment, nurses determine the condition of the skin, oral cavity, and other tissues, as well as a patient's need for and ability to meet personal hygiene needs. As nurses review all data gathered, they need to think about their knowledge pertaining to pre-existing conditions and then look for clusters of data suggesting a health problem trend. For example, an older person with degenerative arthritis can present with pain in the joints, weakness, mobility limitations in the dominant hand, and a generally unkempt appearance. A closer review of assessment data can reveal defining characteristics of an inability to wash body parts and difficulty turning and regulating a water faucet. The nursing diagnosis of *bathing/hygiene self-care deficit* is supported and becomes part of the plan of care. The accurate selection of nursing diagnoses requires critical thinking to identify actual or potential health problems. Assessment activities must be thorough in identifying all appropriate defining characteristics so that an accurate diagnosis can be made (Box 39.5).

The focus of nursing interventions depends on whether a patient has an actual alteration (e.g., impaired tissue integrity) or is at risk for a health problem (e.g., risk for impaired oral mucous membrane). The patient with an actual alteration requires extensive hygiene care, which is often more thorough than routine care. For example, if the patient has skin breakdown, the nurse must initiate care more frequently to keep intact skin surfaces clean and dry and to eliminate factors such as moisture or drainage that can worsen the condition of the skin. The nurse must also provide care to promote healing of injured skin surfaces (see Chapter 47). If the patient is at risk for a health problem, the nurse must institute preventive measures. In both cases, it may be beneficial to involve the wound-ostomy nurse in care planning. In the case of risk for impaired oral mucous membranes, it is important to keep the mucosa well hydrated, minimize foods irritating to tissues, and provide cleansing that soothes and reduces tissue inflammation.

The identification of related factors guides in the selection of nursing interventions. Diagnoses of *impaired oral mucous membrane related to malnutrition* and *impaired oral mucous membrane related to chemical trauma* require very different interventions. When malnutrition is a causal factor, the nurse needs to confer with a dietitian for appropriate dietary supplements and incorporate patient education into the plan. When mucosa are injured as a result of chemical trauma from chemotherapy, techniques for cleaning and hydrating inflamed tissues and eliminating sources of irritation are the focus of nursing care. Although many nursing diagnoses associated with hygiene challenges are possible, the following are a few of the more common diagnoses:

- *Impaired dentition*
- *Fatigue*
- *Ineffective health maintenance*
- *Risk for infection*
- *Deficient knowledge about hygiene practices*
- *Impaired physical mobility*
- *Impaired oral mucous membrane*
- *Self-care deficit, bathing/hygiene, dressing/grooming, toileting*
- *Chronic low self-esteem*
- *Risk for impaired skin integrity*
- *Ineffective tissue perfusion*

◆ Planning

During planning, nurses synthesize information from multiple resources (Figure 39.6). Professional nursing standards and evidence-informed clinical guidelines are especially important to consider when developing a care plan for the patient. For example, the clinical practice guidelines from Diabetes Canada (2020) offer valuable foot care guidelines for patients with diabetes. Critical thinking ensures that the patient's plan of care integrates knowledge about the individual

BOX 39.5 NURSING DIAGNOSTIC PROCESS

Assessment Activities	Defining Characteristics	Nursing Diagnosis
Observe patient's attempt to bathe self either in bed or at bathroom sink. (*Note:* Be sure positioning does not restrict potential movement.)	Unable to wash body or body parts	*Self-care deficit in bathing or hygiene related to upper extremity weakness and generalized fatigue*
Assess patient's upper extremity strength, range of motion, and coordination.	Restricted upper extremity range of motion and strength / Coordination adequate	
Ask patient about level of fatigue after bathing.	Reports fatigue and needs to rest after bathing	
Obtain vital signs before and after bathing.	Pulse elevated from 90 to 110 beats per minute, blood pressure stable, respirations elevated from 16 to 22 breaths per minute	

patient, including preferences, health status, equipment needed, assistance available, and previous experience in providing hygiene care. Certain patients have multiple nursing diagnoses. A concept map (Figure 39.7) shows graphically how numerous nursing diagnoses can be interrelated.

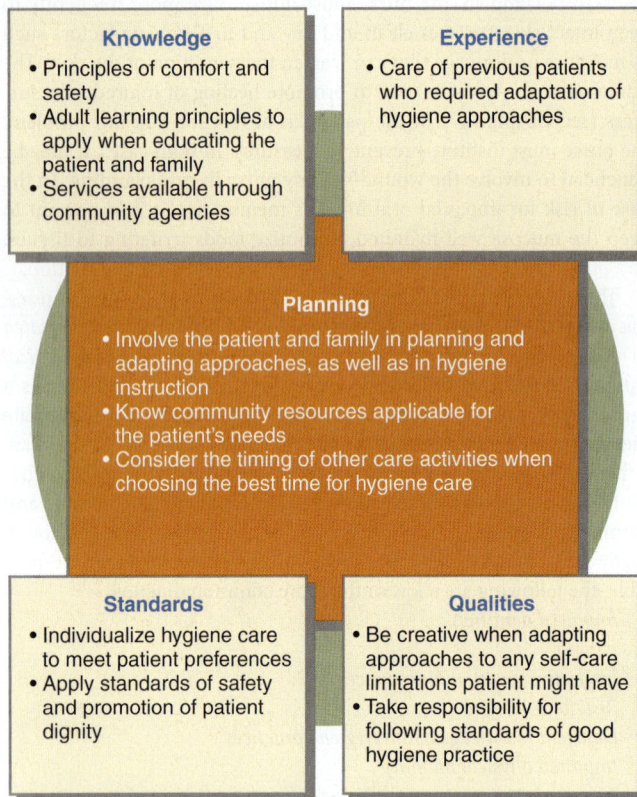

Knowledge
- Principles of comfort and safety
- Adult learning principles to apply when educating the patient and family
- Services available through community agencies

Experience
- Care of previous patients who required adaptation of hygiene approaches

Planning
- Involve the patient and family in planning and adapting approaches, as well as in hygiene instruction
- Know community resources applicable for the patient's needs
- Consider the timing of other care activities when choosing the best time for hygiene care

Standards
- Individualize hygiene care to meet patient preferences
- Apply standards of safety and promotion of patient dignity

Qualities
- Be creative when adapting approaches to any self-care limitations patient might have
- Take responsibility for following standards of good hygiene practice

FIGURE 39.6 Critical thinking model for hygiene planning.

Goals and Outcomes. The nurse and the patient work together to identify goals and expected outcomes and to develop an individualized care plan based on the patient's nursing diagnoses (Box 39.6). Goals are established with the patient's self-care abilities and resources in mind and focus on maintaining or improving the condition of the skin and mucosa, oral mucosa, or dental hygiene, for example. Outcomes should be appropriate, realistic, measurable, and achievable within patient limitations.

When providing patient hygiene, nurses care for a variety of patients with different self-care abilities and needs. For example, for a patient who has hemiparesis after a cerebrovascular accident, the nurse and the patient might develop the following goal: "Patient's musculoskeletal system remains free of breakdown or contractures." A series of realistic individualized expected outcomes would then be established to assist the patient in meeting this goal. These outcomes may include the following:

- Patient's skin is clean, dry, and intact without signs of inflammation.
- Patient's skin remains elastic and well hydrated.
- Patient's range of joint motion remains within normal limits on both affected and unaffected sides.

Setting Priorities. The patient's condition influences the plan for delivering hygiene. A seriously ill patient usually needs a daily bath because body secretions accumulate and can lead to skin breakdown. An older patient at home may require a visit from a home care aide to assist with a tub bath. Patients who are normally inactive during the day and have skin that tends to be dry may need to bathe only twice a week. Nurses must plan for necessary assistance for patients who are weakened or possess poor coordination. For example, a patient who has hemiparesis and has difficulty getting out of the tub should have a tub chair, handrails, or extra personnel available for help.

Timing is also important in planning hygiene. Being interrupted in the middle of a bath to undergo a diagnostic procedure can frustrate and embarrass the patient. After extensive diagnostic tests (e.g., a stress test), it may be best to delay hygiene and allow the patient to rest.

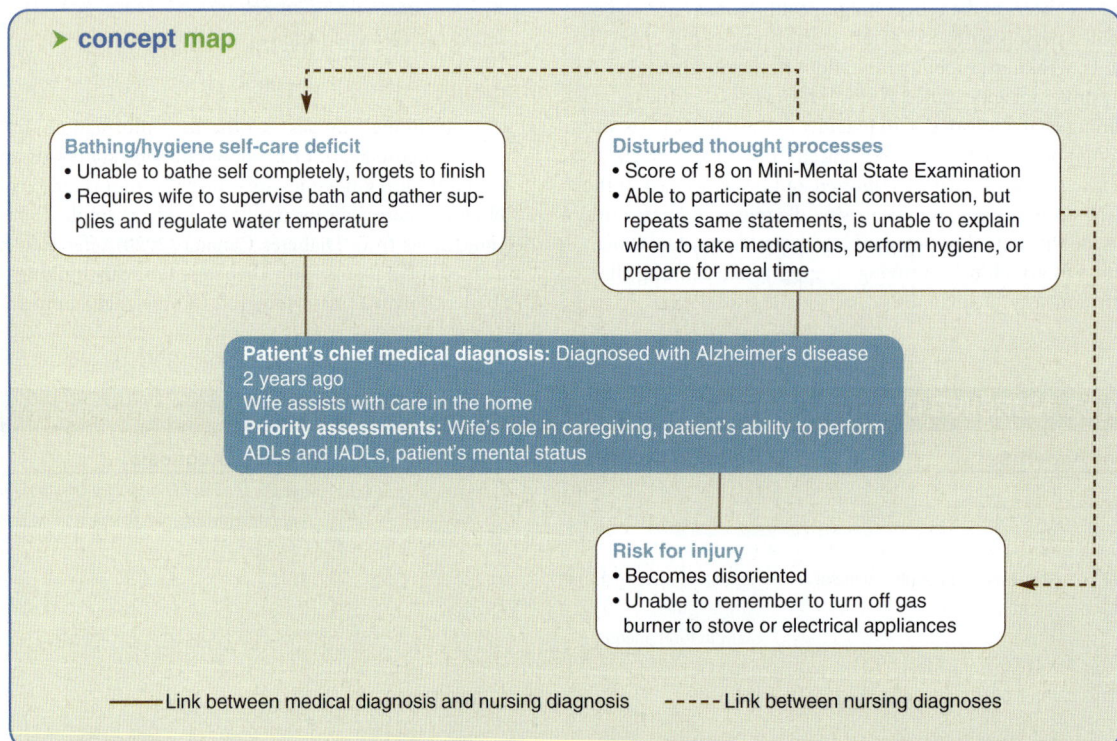

> **concept map**

Bathing/hygiene self-care deficit
- Unable to bathe self completely, forgets to finish
- Requires wife to supervise bath and gather supplies and regulate water temperature

Disturbed thought processes
- Score of 18 on Mini-Mental State Examination
- Able to participate in social conversation, but repeats same statements, is unable to explain when to take medications, perform hygiene, or prepare for meal time

Patient's chief medical diagnosis: Diagnosed with Alzheimer's disease 2 years ago
Wife assists with care in the home
Priority assessments: Wife's role in caregiving, patient's ability to perform ADLs and IADLs, patient's mental status

Risk for injury
- Becomes disoriented
- Unable to remember to turn off gas burner to stove or electrical appliances

——— Link between medical diagnosis and nursing diagnosis   - - - - Link between nursing diagnoses

FIGURE 39.7 Concept map for a patient with Alzheimer's disease and hygiene needs. *ADLs,* Activities of daily living; *IADLs,* instrumental activities of daily living.

Self-Care Deficit: Hygiene (Foot Care) Related to Visual Impairment and Knowledge Deficit

ASSESSMENT

Mr. James (preferred pronouns: he/him) is a 77-year-old who has had type 1 diabetes mellitus for 30+ years. He was recently admitted to the hospital for uncontrolled blood glucose levels. Examination of his feet reveals reddened areas over the bony prominences of the toes and calluses to the soles of the feet and to both heels. Mr. James's toenails are unkempt, yellow, and thickened. He states that he is unable to see well enough to trim his toenails because he has cataracts.

Assessment Activities	Findings and Defining Characteristics
Inspection	
Inspect the feet for dry, rough skin, fissures, calluses, lesions, blisters, inflammation, edema.	Redness over bony prominences of toes
Rationale: Daily inspection is especially important for those patients at increased risk for developing pressure injuries.	Calluses on soles of feet and heels
Prevention: Early recognition of risk factors associated with diabetic foot issues	
Inspect the toenails for discoloration, thickness, and any abnormal findings (e.g., ingrown toenails).	Unkempt, yellow, thickened toenails
Rationale: Monitor for signs of infections, redness, erythema for prevention and early recognition.	
Palpation	
Palpate the dorsalis pedis and posterior tibial pulses.	Pedal pulses weak bilaterally
Rationale: Decreased circulation due to neuropathy and vascular insufficiency can lead to the development of foot ulcers.	
Assess skin temperature and compare bilaterally.	Feet are cool to the touch bilaterally
Rationale: Decreased circulation increases patient's risk for development of diabetic foot ulcers.	
Palpate for edema, tenderness.	No edema or tenderness
Rationale: Bilateral dependent edema occurs with diabetic neuropathy.	
Assess sensation.	Decreased sensation bilaterally
Rationale: Neuropathy is a major risk factor for the development of foot ulcers.	
Assess range of motion.	Range of motion is within normal limits
Protection	
Assess type and condition of footwear.	Patient wears ill-fitting shoes that are well worn, have slippery soles, and are approximately 10 years old
	Socks are tight fitting around the ankles and have holes on the soles
Hygiene	
Inquire about present foot care practices.	Mr. James does not have any specific foot care practices, does not use moisturizing lotion, and has never visited a foot care specialist
Inspect feet for odour, cleanliness, excessive dryness or moisture, and condition of the nails.	Excessive dryness
	No odour is present
	Nails are unkempt, long, thickened, and discoloured

NURSING DIAGNOSIS: Self-care deficit: Hygiene (foot care) related to visual impairment and knowledge deficit.

PLANNING

Goals (Nursing Outcomes Classification)*	Intervention (Nursing Interventions Classification)†
Attain baseline of patient's current knowledge and practices regarding foot hygiene and access to resources.	Assess patient's knowledge and current foot care practices.
Increase patient's knowledge on the importance of foot hygiene.	Assess patient's ability to perform ADLs and IADLS.
	Provide instruction on the need for and the importance of daily inspection of the feet for signs of skin breakdown (e.g., redness, blisters, abrasions, ulcers), friction and calluses from ill-fitting footwear, and daily hygiene.
Eliminate underlying cause of redness over bony prominences and calluses.	Encourage patient to wear appropriate, well-fitting shoes and socks that are free from damage and not constricting.
Patient is able to describe and demonstrate proper technique for foot hygiene.	Demonstrate appropriate technique for foot inspection, hygiene, and application of moisturizing lotion.
Nails are clean and well-trimmed.	Toenails should be cut straight across to prevent ingrown toenails. Refer patient to foot specialist for nail care if necessary.

ADLs, Activities of daily living; *IADLs*, instrumental activities of daily living.

*Outcome classification labels from Moorhead, S., Swanson, E., Johnson, M., et al. (Eds.). (2018). *Nursing outcomes classification (NOC)* (6th ed.). Mosby/Elsevier.

†Intervention classification labels from Butcher, H. K., Bulechek, G. M., McCloskey Dochterman, J. M., et al. (Eds.). (2018). *Nursing interventions classification (NIC)* (7th ed.). Mosby/Elsevier.

EVALUATION

Patient's foot hygiene practices have improved. Feet are clean, skin integrity is maintained, feet are free from injury, and there is a decrease in dryness. Patient is seeing a foot care specialist every 3 to 4 weeks for nail care, callus removal, and foot assessment. Appropriate, well-fitting footwear is worn.

Continuity of Care. It is important to plan for care throughout the hospital stay, from admission to discharge, whether to a rehabilitation facility or back home. When a patient needs assistance as a result of a self-care limitation, the family becomes a valuable resource. Family members can usually assist with hygiene measures but may need support and guidance in adapting techniques to fit patient limitations. Nurses must be aware of equipment and procedures that were used while the patient was in the hospital or facility so that the patient and family are knowledgeable about the care, have the skill needed to provide the care, and have access to necessary equipment. In addition, various community resources may be needed. For example, if the nurse is involved in the care of a homeless patient, the nurse may need to be aware of the location of clothing distribution centres for basic hygiene supplies or a shelter where bathing facilities are available. Forming partnerships with social workers or staff in local area churches and schools can assist in ensuring that patients have the resources they need to maintain hygiene.

◆ Implementation

Providing hygiene is a very basic part of a patient's care. The nurse needs to use caring practices to help alleviate the patient's anxiety and promote comfort and relaxation while the nurse performs each hygiene measure. For example, while giving a patient a bath and changing a gown, the nurse needs to use a gentle approach in turning and repositioning the patient and use a soft, gentle voice while conversing with the patient, to help relieve any fears or concerns. For patients with symptoms such as pain or nausea, administering symptom-relief therapies before starting hygiene care can help prepare the patient for the procedure.

Another important part of implementation is assisting patients in administering their own hygiene. This includes educating patients on proper hygiene techniques and connecting patients with the community resources needed to enable them to perform hygiene care. The same patients at risk for hygiene challenges are those in greatest need of understanding their risks, knowing the implications, and having the information they need to make choices about when and how hygiene is performed.

Health Promotion. In primary health care settings, nurses educate and counsel patients and families on appropriate hygiene techniques. New parents need assistance in learning how to bathe their newborn. An older person needs to become informed about the importance of regular ear care to avoid hearing deficits resulting from accumulated cerumen. When assisting patients, nurses must maintain the standards for hygiene illustrated in this chapter and incorporate adaptations as needed to their patients' lifestyle, living arrangements, abilities, and preferences. Guidelines to assist nurses in providing education to patients about hygiene are presented in Box 39.7.

Acute and Restorative Care. Nursing knowledge and skills needed for performing hygiene care are consistent across all health care settings where acute and restorative care are provided. In addition, some of the skills in this section are applicable in areas of health promotion.

In health care settings where patients receive direct nursing care, a variety of scheduled hygiene measures are provided (Box 39.8). Times of providing such measures may change because of factors affecting the organization or the scheduling of care, such as planned diagnostic and treatment procedures, the patient's need for more hygiene, or the nurse's work assignment.

Bathing and Skin Care

Bathing and skin care are a part of total hygiene. The extent of a patient's bath and the methods used for bathing depend on their

---

BOX 39.7 | **Educating Patients About Hygiene Care**

- Make instructions relevant. After assessing a patient's knowledge, motivation, and health beliefs, provide information that relates to the patient's situation and will be most useful in resolving the patient's health problem. For example, when offering foot care instruction to a patient with diabetes mellitus, explain how the circulation to the feet can be impaired and how that poses a risk for poor healing and infection should the skin become cut or broken.
- Adapt teaching of techniques to the patient's personal bathing facilities. Not all patients will have the ideal situation that exists in a health care setting (e.g., easily accessible shower or a bedside table to place over a bed). Use the facilities or equipment that the patient has so that personal-care items are easy to reach, the patient's safety is ensured, and the patient feels comfortable when performing hygiene. For example, a young mother may feel more comfortable bathing an infant in a baby bath chair.
- Teach the patient steps to take to avoid injury. Almost any hygiene procedure can pose risks (e.g., cutting a nail too close to the skin, failing to adjust the water temperature of a bath, or using tap water for contact lens care). Any instruction you provide must clearly outline safety risks.
- Reinforce infection control practices. Damage to the skin, mucosa, eyes, or other tissues creates an immediate risk for infection. Be sure the patient understands the relationship between healthy and intact skin and tissues, hand hygiene practices, and the prevention of infection.

BOX 39.8 | **Hygiene Care Schedule in Acute and Long-Term Care Settings**

Early Morning Care

When nurses work the night shift, they may be required to provide basic hygiene to patients getting ready for breakfast, scheduled tests, or early morning surgery. Early morning care (often referred to as "A.M. care") includes offering a bedpan or urinal if the patient is not ambulatory, washing the patient's hands and face, and assisting with oral care.

Routine Morning Care

Before or after breakfast, care includes offering a bedpan or urinal to patients confined to bed; providing a bath or shower; giving perineal care; giving oral hygiene and foot, nail, and hair care; assisting with shaving, giving a back rub; changing the patient's gown or pyjamas; changing the bed linens; and straightening the patient's bedside unit and room. This is often referred to as "complete A.M. care."

Afternoon Care

Hospitalized patients often undergo many exhausting diagnostic tests or procedures in the morning. In rehabilitation centres, patients may participate in physiotherapy during the morning. Afternoon hygiene care includes washing the hands and face, assisting with oral care, offering a bedpan or urinal to those patients who are not ambulatory, and straightening bed linen.

Evening, or Hour-Before-Sleep, Care

Before bedtime, nurses can offer personal hygiene care that helps a patient relax to promote sleep. Evening care, or P.M. care, may include changing soiled bed linens, gowns, or pyjamas; assisting the patient in washing the face and hands; providing or assisting with oral hygiene; and offering a bedpan or urinal to nonambulatory patients.

physical abilities, their health problems, and the degree of hygiene required. If the patient is physically dependent or cognitively impaired, the nurse needs to increase skin assessment and provide skin care directed toward reducing the risk for skin breakdown. When bathing cognitively impaired patients, nurses must consider these patients' special needs and challenges (Box 39.9). These patients can easily become afraid, may use physical and verbal aggressive behaviours to avoid bathing, and may also display self-injurious behaviours (Konne et al., 2019).

A complete bed bath is used with patients who are totally dependent and require total hygiene care. It is an activity that can be exhausting for patients, even if the nurse provides all the care. Nurses must anticipate and assess whether patients are physically able to tolerate a complete bath. Observing for verbal and nonverbal cues provides a measure of their physical tolerance. A partial bed bath involves bathing only those body parts that would cause discomfort or odour if not cleaned, and those areas not easily reached by the patient. This includes perineal care. Aging or dependent patients in need of only partial hygiene and self-sufficient bedridden patients unable to reach all body parts receive partial bed baths. Nurses need to carefully assess patients to determine the amount of assistance required during hygiene care. Skill 39.1 outlines the procedures for bathing a bed-bound patient.

When administering a complete or partial bath, it is important to assess the condition of the skin to determine which type of cleaning product is necessary or whether the patient requires daily bathing. Patients with excessively dry skin are predisposed to skin impairment. The nurse may decide to skip a bath for a day or bathe only badly soiled areas. The use of a soap that contains emollients is another option. Lubricating the skin with lotion can also help reduce dryness.

The tub bath or shower can be used to give a more thorough bath than a bed bath. Safety is of primary concern because the surface of a tub or shower stall is slippery. In some settings, it is necessary to obtain

BOX 39.9 EVIDENCE-INFORMED PRACTICE

Bathing Patients Who Have Dementia or Alzheimer's Disease

Provide individualized and flexible patient-centred care:
- Obtain bathing history—what works, what doesn't work.
- Identify bathing preferences from the patient, other caregivers, or family.
- Determine the method that is least distressing to the patient (e.g., soaking feet in the bathtub; use of prepackaged commercial bath cleansing products [see Figure 39.8]; no-rinse shampoo cap—if hair washing causes the patient distress).
- If patient fears water, try using coloured water or drawing a bubble bath.
- Prepare the bath environment in advance, with adequate lighting and necessary supplies (soap, shampoo, towels, etc.).
- Minimize the time the patient is unclothed and ensure that the bathing environment is warm.
- Use distraction and negotiation instead of demands (e.g., give the patient a washcloth to keep hands occupied).
- Minimize noise in the bathing area or play the patient's favourite music softly in the background.
- Set priorities regarding which body parts need bathing and which parts can be "skipped" (e.g., separate hair washing from bathing).
- Assess whether the patient requires glasses or a hearing aid, which can assist with communication (remove aids as required during bathing after communicating your intent to the patient).
- Praise the patient's accomplishments.

Adapted from Alzheimer Society of Canada. (2021). *Personal care.* https://alzheimer.ca/en/help-support/im-caring-person-living-dementia/providing-day-day-care/personal-care/bathing; Konno, R., Kanzaki, H., Stern, C., et al. (2021). Assisted bathing of older people with dementia: A mixed methods systematic review protocol. *JBI Evidence Synthesis, 19*(2), 513–520. doi:10.11124/JBIES-20-00160

SKILL 39.1 BATHING A PATIENT

Delegation Considerations
Skills of bathing may be delegated to an unregulated care provider. Instructions about the following should be provided:
- The importance of not massaging reddened skin areas
- The clarification of early signs of impaired skin integrity
- The importance of reporting changes in the patient's skin
- Proper positioning of an in-dwelling catheter during perineal care
- The importance of reporting any perineal drainage, excoriation, or rash observed

Equipment
- Washcloths and bath towels
- Wash basin
- Bath blanket (warm, if possible)
- Cleaning solution (agency or patient specific)
- Personal hygiene items (unscented deodorant, powder, lotion)
- Clean hospital gown or patient's own pyjamas or gown
- Bed linen
- Linen bag
- Disposable gloves
- Disposable wipes
- Bedpan or urinal

PROCEDURE

STEPS	RATIONALE
General Instructions	
1. Review orders for specific safety measures concerning the patient's movement, positioning, or isolation precautions.	• Prevents accidental injury to the patient during bathing activities. • Determines level of assistance required by the patient.
2. Explain procedure and ask patient for suggestions on how to prepare supplies. Encourage and promote independence by asking the patient how much of the bath they wish to complete.	• Promotes patient's cooperation and participation. • Promotes patient's comfort and provides an opportunity to include cultural or personal hygiene preferences in hygiene care.

Continued

SKILL 39.1	**BATHING A PATIENT—cont'd**
STEPS	**RATIONALE**
3. Assess patient's ability to perform self-care and allow patient to perform as much of the bath as possible.	• Patient participates in plan of care. • Determines the amount of assistance required and the need for specialized equipment or additional personnel. • Encourages and promotes independence.
4. Assess patient's tolerance for activity, comfort level, cognitive ability, and musculoskeletal function.	• Determines patient's ability to perform self-care and level of assistance required. Also, determines type of bath to administer (e.g., tub bath or partial bed bath).

CRITICAL DECISION POINT: *Patients whose level of independence and mobility change frequently may require a varying amount of assistance during bathing.*

STEPS	RATIONALE
5. Assess patient's bathing preferences: frequency, type of hygiene products, and other factors related to patient preferences.	• Encourages and promotes patient participation.
6. Ask whether patient has noticed any irregularities or unusual marks on skin. Observe the skin throughout the procedure, paying particular attention to areas that were previously soiled or reddened or showed early signs of breakdown.	• Provides information to direct physical assessment of skin during bathing.
7. Begin complete or partial bed bath, or tub/whirlpool bath or shower.	
A. Complete or partial bed bath	
(1) Close room doors and draw the room divider curtain.	• Privacy ensures patient's mental and physical comfort.
(2) Prepare equipment and supplies.	• Reduces transmission of microorganisms and avoids interrupting the procedure or leaving the patient unattended to retrieve missing equipment.
(3) For nonambulatory patients, offer a bedpan or urinal. Provide a towel and washcloth for perineal care afterward.	• Patient will feel more comfortable after voiding. Prevents the interruption of bath.
(4) Perform hand hygiene. If patient's skin is soiled with drainage or body secretions, put on disposable gloves. Ensure that the patient is not allergic to latex.	• Reduces transmission of microorganisms.
(5) Place hospital bed at appropriate level, lower side rail closest to you. Assist patient in assuming a comfortable position, preferably supine. Bring or have the patient move toward the side closest to you.	• Raising the height of the bed to the appropriate position facilitates proper body mechanics. Maintains patient's comfort throughout procedure. Minimizes strain on back muscles because you do not have to reach across the bed.
(6) Loosen the top covers. Place bath blanket over the top sheet. Remove top sheet from under the blanket. If possible, have patient hold bath blanket while you withdraw sheet. Optional: Use the top sheet when a bath blanket is not available.	• Removal of top linens prevents them from becoming soiled or moist during the bath. Blanket provides warmth and privacy. The patient is not exposed unnecessarily.
(7) If top sheet is to be reused, fold it for replacement later. If not, dispose in linen bag, taking care not to allow linen to contact uniform.	• Proper disposal helps prevent transmission of microorganisms.
(8) Assist patient with oral hygiene. See Skill 39.3.	
(9) Remove patient's gown or pyjamas. If the patient has an intravenous (IV) line infusing and the gown has snaps, simply unsnap and remove the gown without disconnecting the IV tubing. If the gown does not have snaps, remove gown from the arm without IV line first; then lower the IV container or remove from the pump and slide the gown covering the affected arm over the tubing and container. Rehang IV container and check flow rate (see Step 7A[9] illustrations) or reset pump rate. Do not disconnect the tubing. If an extremity is injured or has reduced mobility, begin removal from the unaffected side. Ensure that the fresh gown has snaps.	• Provides full exposure of body parts during bathing. Undressing the unaffected side first allows easier manipulation of gown over the body part with reduced range of motion (ROM). • Manipulation of IV tubing and container may disrupt flow rate.

SKILL 39.1	BATHING A PATIENT—cont'd
STEPS	**RATIONALE**

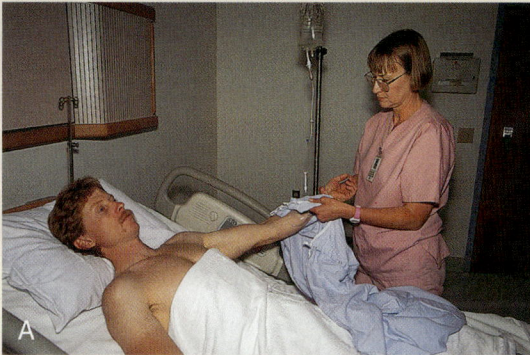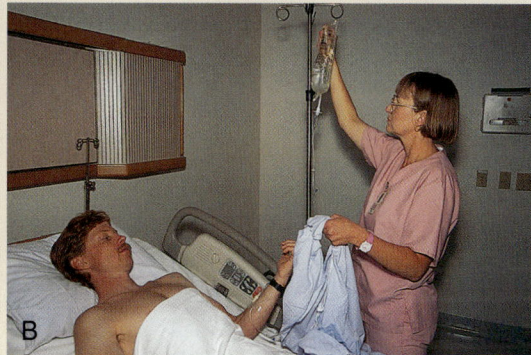

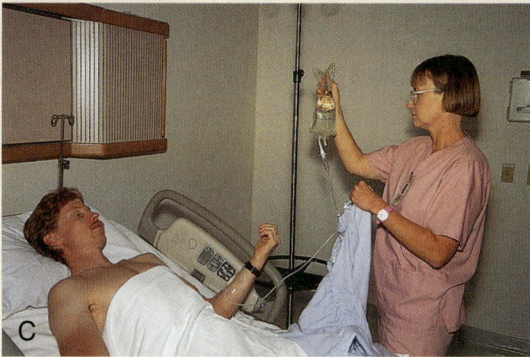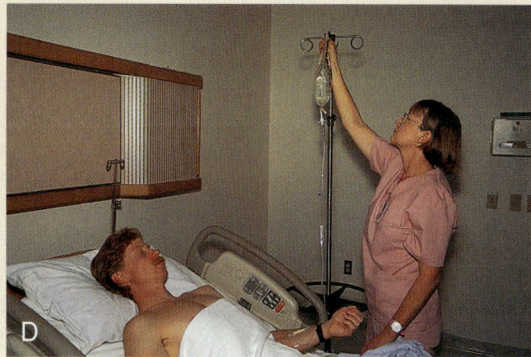

STEP 7A(9) **A,** Remove patient's gown. **B,** Remove IV bag from pole. **C,** Slide IV tubing through arm of patient's gown. **D,** Rehang IV bag and check flow rate.

CRITICAL DECISION POINT: *If available, be sure that patients with an IV line or upper extremity injury have a gown with snap or tie sleeves; this ensures easy access to the upper extremities during hygiene.*

CRITICAL DECISION POINT: *When an IV pump is used, it may be appropriate to manually adjust the IV flow rate to keep-vein-open (KVO) and remove the IV tubing from the pump (check agency policy). Once the gown has been removed, reset the pump to the prescribed IV flow rate (see Chapter 41).*

---

(10) Raise the side rail. Fill a wash basin two-thirds full with warm water. Have patient place fingers in water to test temperature tolerance. Change the water as necessary throughout the bath.

- Raising side rail maintains the patient's safety as you leave the bedside. Warm water promotes comfort, relaxes muscles, and prevents unnecessary chilling. Testing the temperature prevents accidental burns.

(11) Remove pillow, if allowed, and raise head of the bed 30–45 degrees. Place bath towel under the patient's head. Place a second bath towel over patient's chest.

- Removal of the pillow makes it easier to wash the patient's ears and neck. The placement of towels prevents soiling of the bed linen and bath blanket.

(12) Immerse washcloth in water and wring thoroughly. If desired, fold the washcloth around the fingers of your hand to form a mitt (see Step 7A[12] illustration).

- A mitt retains water and heat better than a loosely held washcloth and prevents splashing and cold edges from brushing against the patient.

Continued

SKILL 39.1   BATHING A PATIENT—cont'd

STEPS

RATIONALE

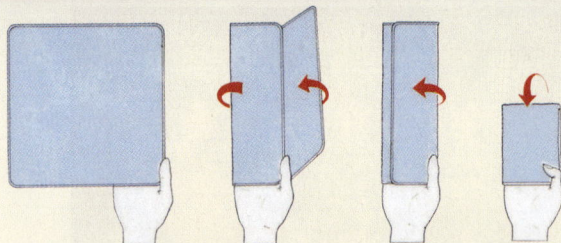

STEP 7A(12) Steps for folding washcloth to form a mitt.

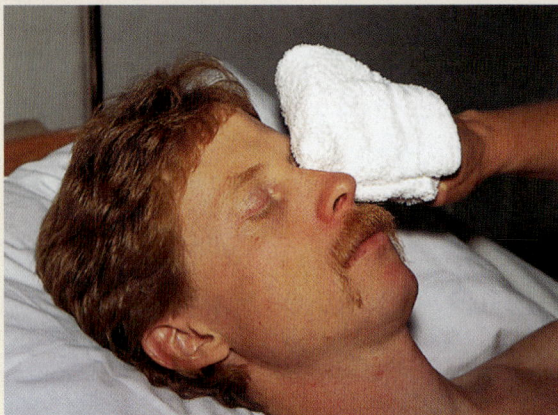

STEP 7A(13) Wash eye from inner to outer canthus.

(13) Inquire whether the patient is wearing contact lenses. Wash patient's eyes with plain warm water. Use a different section of mitt for each eye. Move mitt from inner to outer canthus (see Step 7A[13] illustration). Soak any crusts on eyelid for 2–3 minutes with damp cloth before attempting removal. Dry eyes thoroughly but gently.

(14) Ask whether patient prefers to use soap on their face. Wash, rinse, and thoroughly dry all areas of the face, neck, and ears. (Men may wish to shave at this point or after the bath.)

(15) Expose patient's arm that is farthest from you and place bath towel lengthwise under the arm.

(16) Bathe arm using long, firm strokes from distal to proximal areas (fingers to axilla). Raise and support arm as needed while thoroughly washing the axilla (see Step 7A[16] illustration).

- Soap irritates eyes. The use of separate sections of the mitt reduces infection transmission. Bathing the eye from inner to outer canthus prevents secretions from entering the nasolacrimal duct. Pressure can cause internal injury.

- Soap tends to dry the face, which is exposed to air more than other body parts.

- Prevents soiling of bed. Washing far side first eliminates contaminating clean areas once they are washed.

- Soap lowers the surface tension of the skin and facilitates removal of debris and bacteria when friction is applied during washing. Long, firm strokes stimulate circulation. Movement of the arm exposes the axilla and exercises the joint's normal ROM.

STEP 7A(16) Washing from fingers to axilla. (© Canstockphoto.com/Gina Sanders.)

(17) Rinse and dry arm and axilla thoroughly. If patient uses deodorant or talcum powder, apply it. Be sure to use unscented products where possible.

(18) Fold bath towel in half and lay it on the bed, beside the patient. Place a basin on the towel. Immerse patient's hand in water. Allow hand to soak for 3–5 minutes before washing hand and fingernails (see Skill 39.2). Remove basin and dry hand well.

(19) Cover the arm with bath blanket or towel. Repeat steps 15–18 for the other arm.

- Excess moisture causes skin maceration or softening. Deodorant controls body odour.

- Soaking softens cuticles and calluses of the hand, loosens debris beneath nails, and enhances the feeling of cleanliness. Thorough drying removes moisture from between fingers.
Note: Do not soak if the patient is diabetic or is cognitively impaired and unable to understand the procedure.

SKILL 39.1   BATHING A PATIENT—cont'd

STEPS	RATIONALE

CRITICAL DECISION POINT: *If a patient is at risk for falls, be sure the two side rails are up before obtaining fresh water or other supplies. Remember, side rails cannot be used as a restraint unless ordered.*

(20) Cover patient's chest with a bath towel, and fold bath blanket down to the umbilicus. With one hand, lift edge of towel away from patient's chest. With washcloth or mitted hand, bathe chest using long, firm strokes. Take special care to wash skinfolds under the patient's breasts. Keep patient's chest covered between wash and rinse periods. Dry well.

• Draping prevents unnecessary exposure of body parts. The towel maintains warmth and privacy. Secretions and dirt collect easily in areas of tight skinfolds. Skinfolds are susceptible to excoriation if not cleaned and dried properly.

(21) Place bath towel lengthwise over patient's chest and abdomen. (Two towels may be needed.) Fold blanket down to just above the pubic region.

• Prevents chilling and unnecessary exposure of body parts.

(22) With one hand, lift the bath towel. With mitted hand, bathe the abdomen, giving special attention to bathing the umbilicus and abdominal folds. Keep the abdomen covered between washing and rinsing. Dry well.

• Moisture and sediment that collect in skinfolds predispose skin to maceration and irritation.

(23) Cover patient's chest and abdomen with top of the bath blanket or bath towels. Expose far leg by folding blanket toward midline. Be sure the other leg and the perineum are covered.

• Maintains patient's warmth and comfort. Prevents chilling and unnecessary exposure.

(24) Place bath towel lengthwise under the far leg and, using firm strokes (unless contraindicated), wash, rinse, and dry thoroughly. Support the leg with one hand if the patient is unable to support it.

• Promotes venous return.

CRITICAL DECISION POINT: *Patients with a history of deep vein thrombosis (DVT) or hypercoagulation disorders should not have their lower extremities washed with long, firm strokes.*

(25) Clean the foot, making sure to bathe between toes. Clean and clip nails as per health care provider orders (see Skill 39.2). Dry well. If skin is dry, apply lotion.

• Secretions and moisture can accumulate between the toes. Lotion helps retain moisture and soften the skin.
• Patient's own nail clippers should be used to avoid the transmission of microorganisms.

CRITICAL DECISION POINT: *Do not massage any reddened area on the patient's skin as it can increase the risk of skin breakdown (Mitchell, 2018).*

(26) Repeat Steps 23–25 for the other leg and foot.

(27) Assist patient in assuming a prone or side-lying position (as applicable). Place the towel lengthwise along the patient's side. Put on disposable gloves if not done so already.

• Exposes back and buttocks for bathing. Prevents contact with microorganisms in body secretions.

(28) Wash, rinse, and dry patient's back from neck to buttocks using long, firm strokes (see Step 7A[28] illustration). Pay special attention to folds of the buttocks and the anus for redness or skin breakdown.
Give a back massage (see Chapter 32).
Change bath water if necessary and put on disposable gloves.

• Skinfolds near buttocks and anus may contain fecal secretions that harbour microorganisms.
• Prolonged pressure on the sacral area or other bony prominences may lead to the development of pressure injuries.
• Changing the water prevents the transfer of microorganisms from the anal area to genitalia.

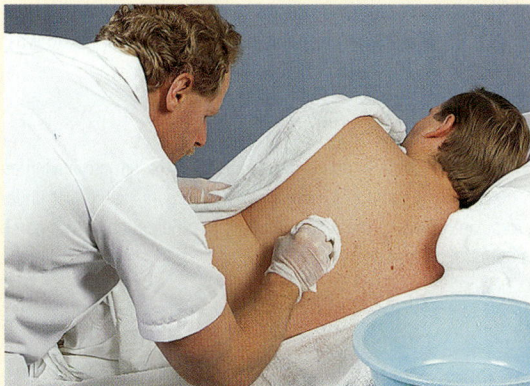

STEP 7A(28) Washing the patient's back.

Continued

| SKILL 39.1 | BATHING A PATIENT—cont'd |
| STEPS | RATIONALE |

(a) Perineal care for patients with female genitalia

(a1) Assist patient in assuming a dorsal recumbent position, if not contraindicated. Cover chest and upper extremities with a towel and lower extremities with a bath blanket. Expose only the genitalia. (If patient can wash, covering the entire body with a bath blanket may be preferable.) Clean the perineal area. Pay special attention to skinfolds. Patients at risk for infection of the genitalia, urinary tract, or reproductive tract include those with in-dwelling catheters or fecal or urinary incontinence. If fecal material is present, enclose in a fold of underpad and remove with disposable wipes.

- Provides easy access to genitalia.
- Patients capable of performing a partial bath usually prefer to wash their own genitalia.
- Secretions that accumulate on the surface of skin surrounding the genitalia act as a reservoir for infection.
- Cleaning reduces transmission of microorganisms from the anus to the urethra or genitalia.

(a2) Wash labia majora. Wipe from the perineum to the rectum. Repeat on the opposite side using a different section of the washcloth.

- Wiping from the perineum to the rectum reduces the chance of transmitting fecal organisms to the urinary meatus.

(a3) Separate the labia with your nondominant hand, exposing the urethral meatus and vaginal orifice. Wash downward from the pubic area toward the rectum in one smooth stroke (see Step 7A[28][a3] illustration). Use a separate section of cloth for each stroke. Cleanse thoroughly around the labia minora, clitoris, and vaginal orifice.

- This cleaning method reduces the risk of transferring microorganisms to the urinary meatus (cleaning from area of least contamination to most contamination, as secretions that collect around the labia minora facilitate bacterial growth). (For menstruating patients or patients with in-dwelling urinary catheters, clean with disposable wipes.)

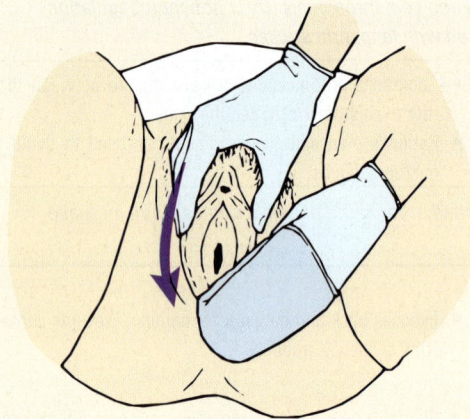

STEP 7A(28)(a3) Cleanse from perineum to rectum (front to back).

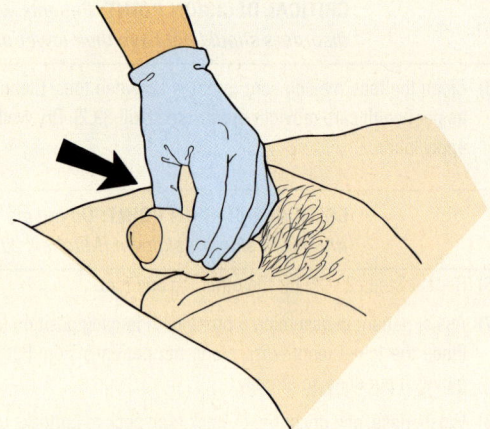

STEP 7A(28)(b2) Fully retract foreskin.

(a4) Assist patient to a comfortable position.

(a5) Remove disposable gloves and perform hand hygiene.

- Helps prevent the transmission of infection.

(b) Perineal care for patients with male genitalia

(b1) Lower the side rails and assist patient to a supine position. Note restriction in mobility. Patients at risk for infection of the genitalia, urinary tract, or reproductive tract include uncircumcised males and patients with in-dwelling catheters or fecal or urinary incontinence.

- Provides full exposure of male genitalia.
- Patients capable of performing a partial bath usually prefer to wash their own genitalia.

(b2) Gently raise the penis and place a bath towel underneath. Gently grasp the shaft of penis. If the patient is uncircumcised, retract the foreskin (see Step 7A[28][b2] illustration). If the patient has an erection, perineal care can be deferred until later.

- Gentle but firm handling reduces the chance of the patient having an erection. Secretions capable of harbouring microorganisms collect underneath the foreskin. Cleaning the penis can lead to an erection, which can embarrass both the patient and you.

SKILL 39.1 BATHING A PATIENT—cont'd

STEPS	RATIONALE
(b3) Wash tip of the penis at the urethral meatus first, using a circular motion. Clean from the meatus outward. Rinse and dry gently.	• The direction of the cleaning moves from areas of least contamination to most contamination, preventing microorganisms from entering the urethra.
(b4) Return foreskin to its natural position.	• Tightening of the foreskin around the shaft of the penis can cause local edema and discomfort.
(b5) Wash the shaft of the penis with gentle but firm downward strokes. Pay special attention to the underlying surface of the penis. Rinse and dry thoroughly.	• The underlying surface of the penis may have a greater accumulation of secretions.
(b6) Gently clean scrotum, making sure to wash underlying skinfolds. Rinse and dry thoroughly.	• Pressure on scrotal tissue can be painful to the patient. Secretions collect between skinfolds.
(b7) Inspect the surface of external genitalia after cleaning.	• Thick secretions may cover underlying skin lesions or areas of breakdown. Evaluation determines the need for additional hygiene.
(b8) If patient has bowel or urinary incontinence, apply a thin layer of skin barrier cream to the buttock, anus, and perineal area.	• Protects skin from excess moisture and toxins from urine and stool.
(b9) Assist patient to a comfortable position and cover with bath blanket.	
(29) Assist patient in dressing. Comb patient's hair. Some patients may want to apply makeup, or they may wish to shave at this point. Assist patient to a chair or wheelchair.	• Promotes patient's body image.
(30) Make the patient's bed (see Skill 39.5).	• Provides a clean environment.
(31) Remove soiled linen and place it in a linen bag. Clean and replace the bathing equipment. Replace the call light and personal possessions. Leave the room as clean and comfortable as possible.	• Helps prevent transmission of microorganisms. A clean environment promotes the patient's comfort. Keeping the call light and articles of care within reach promotes the patient's safety.
(32) Remove disposable gloves (if applied) and perform hand hygiene.	• Reduces the transmission of microorganisms.
B. Tub or whirlpool bath or shower (verify with agency policy whether a health care provider's order is needed and whether you need to remain in the room during the patient's bath)	
(1) Check tub or shower for cleanliness. Use cleaning techniques outlined in agency policy. Place rubber mat on tub or shower bottom. Place disposable bath mat or towel on the floor in front of the tub or shower.	• Cleaning helps prevent transmission of microorganisms. Mats prevent slipping and falling.
(2) Collect all hygienic aids, toiletry items, and linens requested by the patient. Place within easy reach of the tub or shower.	• Placing items close at hand prevents possible falls when patient reaches for equipment.
(3) Assist patient to the bathroom if necessary. Have patient wear a robe and slippers to bathroom.	• Assistance prevents accidental falls. Wearing a robe and slippers prevents chilling and provides for privacy and comfort.
(4) Demonstrate how to use the call signal for assistance.	• Bathrooms are equipped with signalling devices in case a patient feels faint or weak or needs immediate assistance. Patients prefer privacy during bathing, if safety is not jeopardized.
(5) Place an "occupied" sign on bathroom door.	• Maintains the patient's privacy.

Continued

SKILL 39.1   BATHING A PATIENT—cont'd

STEPS	RATIONALE
(6) Provide a shower seat or tub chair if needed (see Step 7B[6] illustration). Fill bathtub halfway with warm water. If patient's sensation is normal, ask patient to test the water, and adjust the temperature if the water is too warm. Explain which faucet controls hot water. If patient is taking a shower, turn it on and adjust the water temperature before the patient enters the shower stall.	• The use of assistive devices facilitates bathing and minimizes physical exertion. Adjusting water temperature prevents accidental burns. Older persons and patients with neurological alterations (e.g., spinal cord injury) are at high risk for burns as a result of reduced sensation.
(7) Instruct the patient to use safety bars when getting in and out of the tub or shower. Caution the patient against the use of bath oil in tub water.	• Prevents slipping and falling. Oil causes tub surfaces to become slippery.

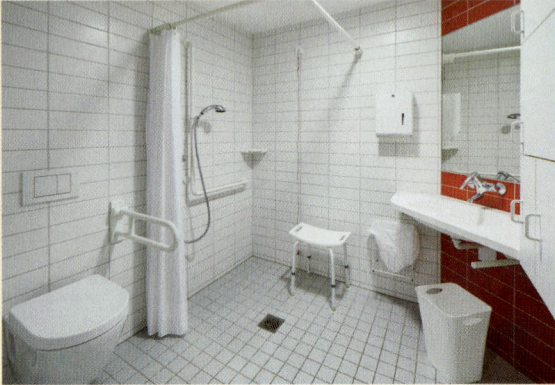

STEP 7B(6) Shower seat for patient safety. (iStockphoto/upixa.)

STEPS	RATIONALE
(8) Instruct patient not to remain in tub longer than 20 minutes. Debilitated patients should not be left alone while in the tub. Observe ROM during bath.	• Prolonged exposure to warm water may cause vasodilation and pooling of blood, leading to lightheadedness or dizziness. Measures joint mobility.
(9) Return to the bathroom when the patient signals, and knock before entering.	• Provides privacy.
(10) For the patient who is unsteady, drain the tub of water before patient attempts to get out of it. Place a bath towel over patient's shoulders. Assist patient in getting out of the tub as needed and assist with drying. If the patient is weak or unstable, have another person assist.	• Prevents accidental falls. Patient may become chilled as water drains.

CRITICAL DECISION POINT: *Weak or unstable patients need extra assistance in getting out of a tub. Planning for additional personnel is essential before attempting to assist a patient from the tub.*

STEPS	RATIONALE
(11) Observe patient's skin, paying particular attention to areas that were previously soiled or reddened or showed early signs of breakdown.	• Techniques used during bathing should leave skin clean and clear.
(12) Assist patient as needed in donning a clean gown or pyjamas, slippers, and robe. (In a home setting, the patient may don regular clothing.)	• Maintains warmth to prevent chilling.
(13) Assist patient to their room and to a comfortable position in a bed or chair.	• Maintains relaxation gained from bathing.
(14) Clean the tub or shower according to agency policy. Whirlpool baths may require special cleaning. Remove soiled linen and place it in a linen bag. Discard disposable equipment in the proper receptacle. Place an "unoccupied" sign on the bathroom door. Return supplies to the storage area.	• Helps prevent transmission of infection through soiled linen and moisture.
(15) Perform hand hygiene.	• Reduces transfer of microorganisms.

SKILL 39.1   BATHING A PATIENT—cont'd

UNEXPECTED OUTCOMES	RELATED INTERVENTIONS
Areas of excessive dryness, rashes, or irritation, or signs of pressure injury on patient's skin	• Review agency's skin care policy regarding special cleaning and moisturizing products. • Limit the frequency of complete baths. • Complete a pressure injury assessment (see Chapter 47). • Obtain a special bed surface if patient is at risk for or has skin breakdown.
Inflammation of skin and genitalia, with localized tenderness, swelling, and presence of foul-smelling discharge	• Bathe the area frequently to keep it clean and dry. • Obtain an order for a sitz bath. • Apply a protective barrier. • Notify the health care provider and apply prescribed antibacterial or antifungal ointment or cream.
Patient expresses perineal discomfort	• Increase the frequency of perineal care. • Assess the perineum for signs of excoriation, swelling, irritation, or discharge.
Patient unable to perform perineal care correctly	• Review perineal care with the patient. • Position the patient and have patient observe the cleaning procedure.
Patient becomes excessively fatigued and unable to cooperate or participate in bathing	• Reschedule bathing to a time when the patient is more rested. • Patients with cardiopulmonary conditions and breathing difficulties may require a pillow or elevated head of the bed during bathing. • Notify the health care provider about changes in the patient's fatigue level. • Schedule rest periods.
Patient seems unusually restless or complains of discomfort	• Consider analgesia before bathing. • Schedule rest periods before bathing.

RECORDING AND REPORTING
- Record condition of the skin and any significant findings (e.g., reddened areas, bruises, nevi, or joint or muscle pain).
- Report any evidence of alterations in skin integrity or increased wound secretions to the person in charge or the health care provider.
- Record the presence of any abnormal findings (e.g., the character and amount of discharge or condition of the genitalia) and record any related procedure you perform.
- Record the appearance of a suture line, if present.
- Report any break in a suture line or the presence of abnormalities to the person in charge or the health care provider.
- Record all procedures performed, the amount of assistance provided, the patient's reaction, and the extent of the patient's participation.

CARE IN THE COMMUNITY CONSIDERATIONS
- Assess the patient's tub and shower area for the need for safety devices (e.g., grab bars, bath mats).
- Assess the patient for the need for assistive bathing devices (e.g., shower chair, hand-held shower).
- Instruct caregivers to assess the patient's perineal area daily for signs of infection and skin breakdown.

OLDER PERSON CONSIDERATIONS
- Check the temperature of water carefully as the patient's sensitivity to temperature may be impaired.
- Continent patients may not require bathing every day, especially if dry skin is a problem.

a health care provider's order for a shower or tub bath. In some agencies, showers are equipped with a chair for patients with weakness or poor balance. Both tubs and showers should be equipped with grab bars for patients to hold on to during their entry and exit and when manoeuvring. Patients vary in how much assistance they need. Regardless of the type of bath the patient receives, the following guidelines should be used:

- *Provide privacy.* Close the door or pull the room curtains around the bathing area. While bathing the patient, expose only the areas being bathed.
- *Maintain safety.* Keep the side rails up while away from the patient's bedside. This is critical for dependent, debilitated, and unconscious patients. (*Note:* When side rails are used as a restraint, a health care provider's order may be needed. Check your agency's policy.) Place the call light within the patient's reach if you are leaving the room temporarily.
- *Maintain warmth.* The room should be kept warm because the patient is partially uncovered and may become chilled. Wet skin

causes an excess loss of heat through convection. Control drafts. Keep the patient covered, exposing only the body part being washed during the bath.
- *Promote independence.* Encourage the patient to participate in as many of the bathing activities as possible. Offer assistance when needed.
- *Anticipate needs.* Bring a new set of clothing and hygiene products to the bedside or bathroom.

Bag Baths. An innovative approach to the traditional bed bath was developed because of concern for patients who are predisposed to dry skin and risk for infection. When wash basins are not cleaned and dried completely after use, contamination with Gram-negative organisms may occur. Successive uses of the basin may cause a patient's skin to harbour more Gram-negative organisms. The "bag bath" (Figure 39.8) is a specially prepared package containing 10 washcloths that are pre-moistened with a mixture of water and a nonrinsable cleaner. The bag bath package is warmed in a microwave before use, and a different

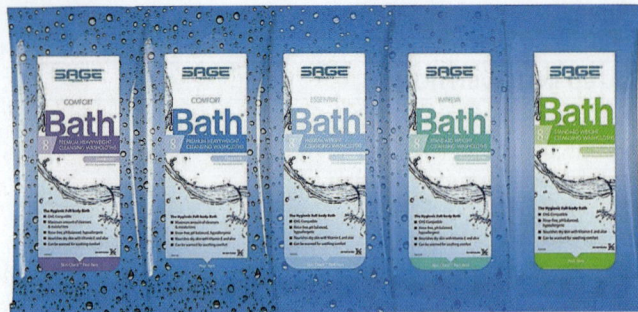

FIGURE 39.8 Commercial bath cleansing pack. (From Sage Products, Cary, IL. [2017]. http://shopsageproducts.com/no-rinse-bathing)

cloth is used for each part of the patient's body. With this technique, the skin air-dries because towel drying removes the emollient that is left behind after the water–cleaner solution evaporates. Health care personnel who have used the bag bath products report shorter bathing times and increased patient satisfaction and staff productivity (Paulela et al., 2018).

Perineal Care. Perineal care is usually part of a complete bed bath (see Skill 39.1). Patients most in need of perineal care are those at greatest risk for acquiring an infection (e.g., patients who have in-dwelling urinary catheters, patients who are recovering from rectal or genital surgery or childbirth, uncircumcised males, patients who are incontinent, or patients who are morbidly obese). In addition, patients who are having a menstrual period require good perineal care. Patients who are able to perform self-care should be encouraged to do so. Sometimes nurses may feel embarrassed when providing perineal care, particularly for patients of the opposite sex. Similarly, patients may feel embarrassed, but this should not cause nurses to overlook patients' hygiene needs. A professional, dignified, and sensitive approach can reduce embarrassment and put patients at ease.

If patients perform self-care, various conditions such as vaginal and urethral discharge, skin irritation, and unpleasant odours may go unnoticed. Nurses must be alert for complaints of burning during urination or localized tenderness, excoriation, or pain in the perineum. Nurses should also inspect their patients' bed linen for signs of discharge.

Back Rub. A back rub promotes relaxation, relieves muscular tension, stimulates circulation, and improves sleep. Massage is associated with a reduction in blood pressure and a reduction in pain, and it can decrease anxiety and depression (Dilaveri et al., 2020).

When providing a back rub, relaxation can be enhanced by reducing any noise and ensuring that the patient is comfortable. Because some individuals may dislike physical contact, it is important to ask the patient whether they would like a back rub and whether gentle or deep massage is preferred. The patient's medical record should be reviewed for any contraindications to massage (e.g., fractured ribs, burns of the skin, or heart surgery). Back rubs are an important strategy for reducing the incidence and prevalence of pressure injures. Box 39.10 outlines this strategy for reducing pressure injuries, along with the associated costs and nursing implications.

Foot and Nail Care. Foot and nail care should be incorporated into a person's regular hygiene routine. Routine care involves soaking to soften the cuticles, thorough cleansing, drying, and proper nail trimming. The exception involves patients with diabetes mellitus, who do not soak their feet because of the risk of infection. When

BOX 39.10   EVIDENCE-INFORMED PRACTICE

Reducing the Incidence and Prevalence of Pressure Injuries

According to a study by Kayser and colleagues (2018), the overall prevalence of pressure injuries in acute care settings is 7.2%. Pressure injuries cause patients stress, pain, and suffering; increased length of hospital stay; and increased workload for health care staff. A study from the United Kingdom found that the average individual cost of pressure injury treatment ranged from $1 500 for stage 1 to $18 000 for stage 4 ulcers (Mervis & Phillips, 2019). The goal of the Pressure Ulcer Awareness and Prevention (PUAP) program, created by Wounds Canada (2022), is to increase awareness of the high cost of pressure injuries through education and support, to improve clinical practice, and to create and improve current policies in health care facilities, to shift the focus from treatment to prevention of pressure injuries.

Nursing Implications

One of the key components of the nursing history and physical examination is the assessment of the integument for pre-existing conditions or risk assessment for potential breakdown in skin integrity. Risk assessment can be accomplished by using the Braden Scale for Assessment of Pressure Ulcer Risk (see Table 47.2) to identify those patients at risk so that strategies can be implemented to reduce their risk. Nurses are in a position to have an impact on the financial costs of pressure injuries to both the health care system and patients by completing thorough, daily skin assessment during hygiene care or independently for early recognition and early intervention.

Based on Kayser, S. A., VanGilder, C. A., Ayello, E. A., et al. (2018). Prevalence and analysis of medical device-related pressure injuries: Results from the International Pressure Ulcer Prevalence Survey. *Advances in Skin & Wound Care, 31*(6), 276–285; Mervis, J. S., & Phillips, T. J. (2019). Pressure ulcers: Pathophysiology, epidemiology, risk factors, and presentation. *Journal of the American Academy of Dermatology, 81*(4), 881–890; Wounds Canada. (2021). *Best practice recommendations.* https://www.woundscanada.ca/index.php?option= com_content&view=article&id=110&catid=12&Itemid=724

providing foot and nail care, patients may remain in bed or sit in a chair (Skill 39.2). In some settings or with specific patients, such as a person with diabetes mellitus, a health care provider's order is needed to trim the toenails. Before implementing this procedure, the nurse must check the agency's policy.

During the procedure, the nurse needs to take time to teach the patient and family members the proper techniques for cleaning and nail trimming. Measures to prevent infection and promote good circulation should be stressed. The patient needs to learn to protect their feet from injury, keep their feet clean and dry, and wear footwear that fits properly. The patient is instructed in the proper way to inspect all surfaces of the feet and hands for lesions, dryness, and signs of infection. It is important that patients be able to recognize any abnormalities and that they must report these conditions to their caregiver.

Patients with diabetes mellitus, peripheral vascular disease, or both are at risk for the development of foot ulcers as a result of poor peripheral blood supply to the feet and decreased sensation in the feet. These lesions are slow to heal because of compromised circulation over time and can result in amputation (Behroozian & Beckman, 2020). Appropriate patient teaching and daily foot care practices, along with early detection of diabetic foot ulcers, can decrease the risk of amputation (Diabetes Canada, 2020).

Patients with diabetes mellitus or peripheral vascular disease should be provided information regarding how circulation directly

SKILL 39.2   PERFORMING NAIL AND FOOT CARE

Delegation Considerations

The skill of nail and foot care for the nondiabetic patient can be delegated to a regulated or an unregulated care provider; however, this skill should not be delegated if the patient is diabetic. It is important to discuss the following:

- That nail clipping must be performed by the nurse
- Any special considerations for patient positioning

Equipment

- Wash basin
- Emesis basin
- Washcloth and bath towel
- Nail clippers (the patient's)
- Emery board or nail file
- Unscented lotion
- Disposable bath mat
- Paper towels
- Disposable gloves

PROCEDURE

STEPS	RATIONALE
1. Identify patients at risk for foot or nail conditions:	• Certain conditions increase the likelihood of foot or nail problems.
A. Older person	• Poor vision, lack of coordination, or inability to bend over contributes to difficulty in performing foot and nail care. Normal physiological changes of aging also result in nail and foot conditions (Muchna et al., 2018).
B. Diabetes mellitus	• Vascular changes associated with diabetes mellitus reduce blood flow to peripheral tissues. Breaks in skin integrity place a diabetic patient at high risk for a skin infection. Meticulous foot assessment and care reduce the diabetic patient's risk of debilitating foot conditions (Behroozian & Beckman, 2020).
C. Heart failure or renal disease	• Both conditions can increase tissue edema, particularly in dependent areas (e.g., feet). Edema reduces blood flow to neighbouring tissues.
D. Cerebrovascular accident (stroke)	• The presence of residual foot or leg weakness or paralysis results in altered walking patterns. An altered gait pattern increases friction and pressure on feet.
2. Assess patient's knowledge of foot and nail care practices.	• Determines patient's need for health teaching.
3. Ask patients about whether they use nail polish and polish remover frequently.	• Chemicals in these products can cause excessive dryness.
4. Assess patient's ability to care for nails or feet; consider visual alterations, fatigue, and musculoskeletal weakness.	• Demonstrates patient's knowledge of proper foot care. Determines the amount of assistance and teaching required.
5. Assess types of home remedies (e.g., aloe vera, herbal preparations) that the patient uses.	• Some preparations can cause injury to soft tissue; always consult a foot-care expert (Diabetes Canada, 2020).
A. Over-the-counter chemical preparations to remove corns or calluses	• Chemical preparations can cause burns and ulcerations.
B. Cutting or shaving of corns or calluses with razor blade or scissors	• Cutting of corns or shaving calluses may result in a break in skin integrity and increases the risk for infection.
C. Use of oval corn pads	• Oval pads may exert pressure on the toes, thereby decreasing circulation to surrounding tissues.
D. Application of adhesive tape	• The skin of older persons is thin and delicate and prone to tearing when adhesive tape is removed.
6. Assess type of footwear worn by patients: Are socks worn? Are shoes tight or ill fitting? Are garters or knee-high nylons worn? Is footwear clean?	• Some types of shoes and footwear may predispose patients to foot and nail problems (e.g., infection, areas of friction, ulcerations). In patients with diabetes mellitus, nonhealing plantar ulcerations have been identified as one of the primary causes of lower limb amputation (Diabetes Canada, 2020).
7. Observe patient's walking gait. Have the patient walk down a hall or in a straight line (if able).	• Structural as well as painful disorders of the feet can cause limping or an unnatural gait.
8. Assist an ambulatory patient to sit in a bedside chair. Help a bed-bound patient to a supine position with head of the bed elevated. Place a disposable bath mat on the floor under the patient's feet or place a towel on the mattress.	• Sitting in a chair facilitates immersing feet in the basin. The bath mat protects feet from exposure to soil or debris.

Continued

STEPS	RATIONALE
9. Obtain a health care provider's order for cutting nails if agency policy requires it.	• The patient's skin may be accidentally cut. Certain patients are more at risk for infection, depending on their medical condition.
10. Explain the procedure to the patient, including the fact that proper soaking requires several minutes.	• The patient must be willing to place their fingers and feet in the basin for 10–20 minutes. Patient may become anxious or fatigued.

CRITICAL DECISION POINT: *Patients with diabetes do not soak hands and feet. Soaking increases their risk of infection due to maceration of the skin.*

STEPS	RATIONALE
11. Perform hand hygiene. Arrange equipment on an overbed table.	• Reduces transmission of microorganisms. Easy access to equipment prevents delays.
12. Fill wash basin with warm water. Test water temperature.	• Warm water softens nails and thickened epidermal cells, reduces inflammation of the skin, and promotes local circulation. Proper water temperature prevents burns.
13. Place basin on bath mat or towel.	• Avoids spills; this maintains safety of the care provider and the patient.
14. Fill emesis basin with warm water, and place basin on paper towels on overbed table.	• Warm water softens nails and thickened epidermal cells.
15. Pull curtain around the bed or close the room door (if desired).	• Maintaining the patient's privacy reduces anxiety.
16. Inspect all surfaces of the fingers, toes, feet, and nails. Pay particular attention to areas of dryness, inflammation, or cracking. Also inspect the areas between toes, heels, and soles of feet.	• The integrity of feet and nails determines the frequency and level of hygiene required. Heels, soles, and sides of the feet are prone to irritation from ill-fitting shoes.

CRITICAL DECISION POINT: *Patients with peripheral vascular diseases or diabetes mellitus, older persons, and patients whose immune system is suppressed may require nail care from a specialist to reduce the risk of infection.*

STEPS	RATIONALE
17. Assess colour and temperature of toes, feet, and fingers. Assess capillary refill. Palpate radial and ulnar pulses of each hand and dorsalis pedis pulses of feet (see Chapter 33).	• Assesses the adequacy of blood flow to extremities. Peripheral vascular disease can contribute to poor wound healing. Patients who are immunocompromised or who have neuropathy or peripheral vascular disease are at increased risk of foot infections (Diabetes Canada, 2020).
18. Instruct patient to place their fingers in the emesis basin and place arms in a comfortable position. Assist patient in placing their feet in the basin.	• Prolonged positioning can cause discomfort unless normal anatomical alignment is maintained. • Patients with muscular weakness may have difficulty positioning their feet.
19. Allow patient's feet and fingernails to soak for 10–20 minutes (unless the patient has diabetes). Rewarm water after 10 minutes.	• Softening of corns, calluses, and cuticles ensures easy removal of dead cells and easy manipulation of cuticles.
20. Clean gently under the fingernails with an orange stick or the wooden end of a cotton-tipped swab while fingers are immersed (see Step 20 illustration). Remove fingers from the emesis basin, and dry thoroughly.	• The orange stick removes debris under nails that harbours microorganisms. Thorough drying impedes fungal growth and prevents maceration of the tissues.
21. Using nail clippers, clip fingernails straight across and even with the tops of fingers (see Step 21 illustration). Using a file, shape the nails straight across. If patient has circulatory problems, do not cut the nail; only file the nail.	• For infection-control purposes, use the patient's own nail clippers. Cutting straight across prevents splitting of the nail margins and the formation of sharp nail spikes that can irritate lateral nail margins. Filing prevents cutting the nail too close to the nail bed.
22. Push cuticle back gently with a wet facecloth. Thoroughly dry the hands.	• Reduces incidence of inflamed cuticles. Thorough drying impedes fungal growth and prevents maceration of the tissues.

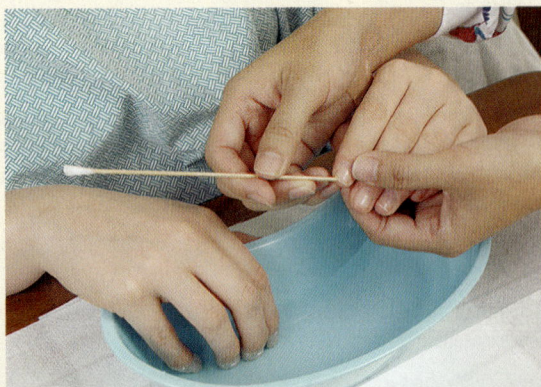
STEP 20 Clean fingernails with the end of a cotton-tipped swab or an orange stick.

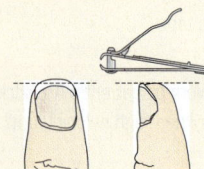
STEP 21 Using nail clippers, trim nails straight across.

SKILL 39.2   PERFORMING NAIL AND FOOT CARE—cont'd

STEPS	RATIONALE
23. Move the overbed table away from the patient.	• Provides easier access to the feet.
24. Put on disposable gloves, and scrub callused areas of the feet with a washcloth.	• Gloves help prevent transmission of fungal infection. Friction removes dead skin layers.
25. Clean gently under nails with an orange stick. Remove feet from basin, and dry them thoroughly.	• Removal of debris and excess moisture reduces chances of infection.
26. Clean and trim toenails using the procedures in Steps 21 and 22. Do not file the corners of toenails.	• For infection-control purposes, use the patient's own nail clippers. Shaping corners of toenails may damage tissues.
27. Apply lotion to feet and hands, and assist patient back to bed and into a comfortable position.	• Lotion lubricates dry skin by helping to retain moisture.
28. Remove disposable gloves and place in a receptacle. Clean and return the equipment and supplies to the proper place. Dispose of soiled linen in a hamper. Perform hand hygiene.	• Reduces the transmission of infection.
29. Inspect the nails and surrounding skin surfaces after soaking and nail trimming.	• Determines the condition of skin and nails. Allows caregiver to note any remaining rough nail edges.
30. Ask patient to explain or demonstrate nail care.	• Evaluates patient's level of learning techniques.
31. Observe patient's walk after toenail care.	• Evaluates the level of comfort and mobility achieved.

UNEXPECTED OUTCOMES	RELATED INTERVENTIONS
Inflammation and tenderness of cuticles and surrounding tissues	• Repeated soakings may be needed to relieve inflammation and loosen layers of cells from calluses or corns. • Patients with diabetes or peripheral vascular disease may require referral to a podiatrist. • Antifungal cream may be needed.
Localized areas of tenderness on feet, with calluses or corns at points of friction	• Change in footwear may be needed. • Refer to a podiatrist.
Appearance of ulcer between toes or other pressure areas on foot	• Notify health care provider. • Refer to a podiatrist. • Increase frequency of foot assessment and hygiene.

RECORDING AND REPORTING

- Document the procedure and any observations (e.g., breaks in the skin, inflammation, ulcerations) on the patient's record sheets using the forms provided by your agency or facility.
- Report any breaks in the skin or ulcerations to the person in charge or to the health care provider. These breaks are serious in patients with diabetes, peripheral vascular disease, and illnesses that impair circulation. Special foot care treatments may be needed.

CARE IN THE COMMUNITY CONSIDERATIONS

- If the patient has diabetes or decreased peripheral circulation, alternative therapies or foot soaking should be carried out only after consulting with a health care provider.
- An alternative therapy would be moleskin applied to areas of the feet that are experiencing friction—this is less likely to cause pressure than corn pads. Spot adhesive bandages can guard against friction, but they do not have padding to protect against pressure.
- If the patient is ambulatory, instruct them to soak their feet in a bathtub.
- If the patient's mobility is limited, a large basin or pan can be used for soaking.

affects the health and integrity of tissues of the feet and should be advised to use the following guidelines in a routine foot and nail care program:

- Inspect the feet daily, including the tops and soles of the feet, the heels, and the areas between the toes. Use a mirror to help inspect the feet thoroughly or ask a family member to check daily.
- Patients with diabetes mellitus should receive a thorough foot examination at least once a year. Patients with one or more high-risk foot conditions should be evaluated more frequently and referred to a specialist as necessary.
- Wash the feet daily using lukewarm water; *do not soak the feet.* If there is reduced sensation, a bath thermometer can be used at home to test the water temperature. Thoroughly dry the feet and in between toes.
- Do not cut corns or calluses or use commercial removers. Consult a physician, podiatrist, or certified foot nurse.
- If the feet perspire excessively, apply a nonallergenic foot powder.
- If dryness is noted along the sides of the feet, rub a nonallergenic lotion gently into the skin, wiping off any excess. *Do not apply lotion between the toes, as excessive moisture can result in infection.*
- Trim the toenails straight across and square; do not use scissors. Consult a podiatrist as needed.
- Do not use over-the-counter preparations or home remedies. Consult a physician, podiatrist, or certified foot nurse.

- Wearing constricting garments, such as elastic stockings, knee-high hose, and garters, and crossing the legs while sitting should be avoided, as these practices can cause impaired circulation to the lower extremities.
- Wear clean, dry socks or stockings daily. Change socks twice a day if feet perspire heavily. Socks should be free of holes or repairs that might cause pressure on the tissue.
- Do not walk barefoot.
- Wear properly fitted shoes with porous uppers if possible. The soles of shoes should be flexible and nonslipping. Shoes should be sturdy, closed in, and not restrictive to the feet. New shoes should be worn for short periods of time over several days to break them in, to avoid the formation of blisters. Patients with increased plantar pressure (e.g., due to erythema or callus) should use footwear that cushions and redistributes pressure. Patients with bony deformity (e.g., a bunion or Charcot's joint) may need extra-wide or extra-deep shoes with cushioned insoles.
- Do not wear high-heeled, open-toed, or pointed-toe shoes.
- Exercise regularly to improve circulation to the lower extremities. Walk slowly and elevate, rotate, flex, and extend the feet at the ankles. Dangle the feet over the side of the bed for 1 minute, then extend both legs and hold them parallel to the bed while lying supine for 1 minute, and, finally, rest for 1 minute.
- Do not apply hot water bottles or heating pads directly to the feet.
- Wash minor cuts immediately and dry them thoroughly. Use only mild cleaners. Antibiotics are not generally required for wounds with no signs of infection. Contact an interprofessional foot-care team to treat cuts or lacerations (Diabetes Canada, 2020).

Any patients who require regular, thorough foot care should have a caregiver or family member available to provide care when the patient is incapacitated. Patients with visual difficulties, physical constraints preventing movement, or cognitive challenges that impair their ability to assess the condition of the feet need caregiver or family assistance.

Oral Hygiene

Good oral hygiene helps to maintain the healthy state of the mouth, teeth, gums, lips, and tongue (Canadian Dental Association, 2022). Brushing cleans the teeth of food particles, plaque, and bacteria. It also massages the gums and relieves any discomfort resulting from unpleasant odours and tastes. Flossing helps to further remove plaque and bacteria from between the teeth to reduce gum inflammation and infection. Complete oral hygiene enhances well-being and comfort and stimulates the appetite.

Patients also benefit from a diet that excludes foods that contribute to plaque formation and tooth decay and that promotes healthy periodontal structures (Canadian Dental Association, 2022). Plaque-forming foods include carbonated beverages, breads, and starches. Oral hygiene done immediately after a meal further reduces plaque. Nurses can assist patients in maintaining good oral hygiene by teaching them the importance of correct techniques and a routine daily schedule.

Patients of all ages should be advised to have a dental checkup at least every 6 months. Education about common gum and tooth disorders and methods of prevention can motivate patients to follow good oral hygiene practices. Nurses need to provide assistance with oral hygiene for weakened or disabled patients. When patients have variations in oral mucosal integrity, hygiene techniques should be adapted to ensure thorough and effective care (Box 39.11).

Brushing and Flossing. Thorough tooth brushing at least four times a day (after meals and at bedtime) is basic to an effective oral hygiene program. If patients are unable to perform oral care four times per day, they should do it at least once during the day and always at night. All

---

BOX 39.11 FOCUS ON OLDER PERSONS

Dental Care

- Many older persons are edentulous (without teeth), and the teeth that are present are often diseased or decayed (Bakker et al., 2020).
- The periodontal membrane weakens, making it more prone to infection; periodontal disease can predispose older persons to systemic infection.
- The presence of chronic illnesses (e.g., diabetes mellitus, renal insufficiency, and cardiovascular diseases) increases older persons' risk for periodontal disease (Bakker et al., 2020).
- Dentures or partial plates may not fit properly, causing pain and discomfort; this, in turn, can affect digestive processes, the enjoyment of food, and nutritional status (Natapov et al., 2018).
- Weaker jaw muscles and shrinkage of the bony structure of the mouth may increase the work of chewing and lead to increased fatigue when eating (Natapov et al., 2018).
- Dry mouth can be caused by an age-related decline in saliva secretion, as well as by over 400 medications that are frequently used by older persons (Natapov et al., 2018).
- Poor nutritional status in some older persons can increase the risk for and severity of dental conditions (e.g., caries, periodontal disease, receding gums, and tooth degeneration) (Gupta et al., 2019).
- An inability or unwillingness to access dental care and the belief that tooth loss is a natural outcome of aging are reasons why some older persons do not seek dental care (Natapov et al., 2018).
- Financial limitations, low income, and lack of transportation also contribute to inadequate dental care of some older persons.

---

tooth surfaces should be brushed thoroughly with a fluoride toothpaste. A toothbrush should have a straight handle and a brush small enough to reach all areas of the mouth. A toothbrush with soft, rounded bristles should be used to stimulate gums without causing bleeding. Toothbrushes should be replaced every 3 months (Canadian Dental Association, 2022). Older patients with reduced dexterity and grip may require an enlarged handle with an easier grip or an electric toothbrush (Barouch et al., 2019). One simple way to make an enlarged brush handle is to pierce a soft rubber ball and push the brush handle through it or glue a short piece of plastic tubing around the handle. Commercially made foam rubber toothbrushes are useful for patients with sensitive gums. However, swabbing fails to clean teeth adequately because plaque accumulates around the base of the teeth. Foam rubber swabs should be used in moderation. Electric toothbrushes can be used, but nurses should consult their agency's policy to ascertain whether their use is permitted. Lemon-glycerine sponges should not be used because they dry mucous membranes and erode teeth enamel. "Moi-Stir" is a common brand-name salivary supplement that improves moisture and the texture of the tongue and mucosa.

When teaching patients about mouth care, the nurse should recommend that they not share toothbrushes with family members or drink directly from a bottle of mouthwash. Cross-contamination occurs easily. The use of disclosure tablets or drops to stain the plaque that collects at the gum line can be useful for showing patients how effectively they brush.

Patients can experience conditions that threaten the integrity of the oral mucosa. For example, mucosal changes associated with aging, use of chemotherapeutic drugs, or dehydration require a change in oral hygiene. More frequent mouth care and use of anti-infective agents are examples of ways nurses can revise approaches to meet patient needs. Unconscious patients and those with artificial airways (e.g., endotracheal or tracheal tubes) need more frequent and specialized oral hygiene. These patients have an increased risk of aspiration and, subsequently, aspiration pneumonia, and they also have more problems with dry and inflamed oral mucosa.

The amount of assistance needed by the patient when brushing the teeth may vary. Many patients can perform their own oral care and should be encouraged to do so. Nurses should observe patients when they are brushing their teeth to be sure proper techniques are being used. When assisting with or providing oral hygiene, the nurse must determine the amount of assistance needed and the individual's oral hygiene preferences (Skill 39.3).

Flossing. Dental flossing removes plaque and bacteria from between teeth. Flossing involves inserting waxed or unwaxed dental floss between all tooth surfaces, one space at a time. Flossing at least once a day is sufficient (Canadian Dental Association, 2022). To prevent bleeding, patients who are receiving chemotherapy or radiation or who are on anticoagulant therapy should use unwaxed floss and avoid vigorous flossing near the gum line. Applying toothpaste to the teeth before flossing allows fluoride to come in direct contact with tooth surfaces, aiding in cavity prevention. Because it is important to clean all tooth surfaces thoroughly, the nurse should not rush flossing. Placing a mirror in front of the patient helps the nurse to demonstrate the proper method for holding the floss and cleaning between the teeth. Flossing a patient's teeth is not realistic or appropriate in all care settings.

However, flossing may be done more frequently in rehabilitation and long-term care settings.

Patients With Special Needs. Some patients require special oral hygiene methods because of their level of dependence on the care provider or the presence of oral mucosa conditions. Unconscious patients are susceptible to drying of mucous-thickened salivary secretions because they are unable to eat or drink, frequently breathe through the mouth, and often receive oxygen therapy. Unconscious patients also cannot swallow salivary secretions that accumulate in the mouth. These secretions often contain Gram-negative bacteria that can cause pneumonia if aspirated into the lungs. While providing hygiene to unconscious patients, nurses must protect them from choking and aspiration. While cleaning the oral cavity, the nurse should never use their fingers to hold the patient's mouth open, as a human bite is highly contaminated. It may be necessary to perform mouth care at least every 2 hours for the unconscious patient. Research shows that the use of chlorhexidine with oral hygiene reduces the risk of ventilator-associated pneumonia (Rabello et al., 2018). The nurse needs to explain the steps of mouth care and the sensations the patient will feel and advise the patient when the procedure is completed (Skill 39.4).

Patients who receive chemotherapy, radiation, or nasogastric tube intubation or who have an infection of the mouth can suffer from

SKILL 39.3	PROVIDING ORAL HYGIENE

Delegation Considerations

The skill of oral hygiene can be delegated to an unregulated care provider (UCP). It is important to discuss the following with the UCP:

- How to adapt the procedure for a patient who is at risk of aspiration (e.g., those with an impaired level of consciousness or impaired swallowing, and those who are confused)
- To immediately report excessive patient coughing or choking during or after oral hygiene
- To report any bleeding of the oral mucosa or gums, lesions, or patient report of pain
- To report any concerns with dentures (e.g., ill-fitting or broken dentures)

Equipment

- Soft-bristled toothbrush
- Nonabrasive fluoride toothpaste or dentifrice
- Dental floss
- Water glass with cool water
- Normal saline or an essential oil antiseptic mouthwash (optional; follow patient's preference)
- Emesis basin
- Tongue blade
- Face towel
- Paper towels
- Disposable gloves

PROCEDURE

STEPS	RATIONALE
1. Determine patient's oral hygiene practices: **A.** Frequency of tooth brushing and flossing **B.** Type of toothpaste or dentifrice used **C.** Last dental visit **D.** Frequency of dental visits **E.** Type of mouthwash or moistening preparation, such as over-the-counter saliva substitutes or sugar-free gum with xylitol	• Allows caregiver to identify errors in technique, deficiencies in preventive oral hygiene, and patient's level of knowledge regarding dental care. • Mouthwash provides a pleasant aftertaste but can dry mucosa after extended use if it has an alcohol base.
2. Assess risk for oral hygiene conditions (see Table 39.5).	• Certain conditions increase the likelihood of impaired oral cavity integrity and the need for preventive care.
3. Assess patient's risk for aspiration: impaired swallowing, reduced gag reflex.	• An accumulation of secretions and dentifrice can increase the patient's risk for aspiration if the patient's ability to control oral secretions is impaired.
4. Assess patient's ability to grasp and manipulate a toothbrush. (For older persons, try a 30-second tooth brushing assessment.)	• A toothbrush test is useful in assessing dexterity and strength. Determines level of assistance required.
5. Prepare equipment at bedside.	• Avoids interrupting the procedure or leaving the patient unattended while retrieving missing equipment.
6. Perform hand hygiene and put on disposable gloves.	• Reduces the transmission of microorganisms.

Continued

SKILL 39.3   PROVIDING ORAL HYGIENE—cont'd

STEPS	RATIONALE
7. Inspect the integrity of lips, teeth, buccal mucosa, gums, palate, and tongue (see Chapter 33).	• Determines status of patient's oral cavity and the extent of need for oral hygiene.
8. Identify the presence of common oral conditions:	• Helps determine type of hygiene patient requires and information patient needs for self-care.
A. Dental caries—chalky white discoloration of a tooth or presence of brown or black discoloration	
B. Gingivitis—inflammation of gums	
C. Periodontitis—receding gum lines, inflammation, gaps between teeth	• Receding gums can occur with aging, and as a result, older patients require meticulous oral hygiene.
D. Halitosis—bad breath	
E. Cheilosis—cracking of the lips	
F. Stomatitis—inflammation of the oral tissues	• Patients receiving immunosuppressive chemotherapy (e.g., cancer chemotherapy) and patients with suppressed immune function are at risk for stomatitis (Pederson et al., 2018).
G. Dry, cracked, coated tongue	
9. Explain the procedure to the patient and discuss preferences regarding the use of hygiene aids.	• Some patients feel uncomfortable about having a caregiver care for their basic needs. Patient involvement with the procedure minimizes anxiety.
10. Raise the bed to a comfortable working position. Raise head of the bed (if patient's condition allows) and lower the side rail. Move the patient, or help patient move closer. A side-lying position can be used.	• Raising the bed and repositioning the patient prevents straining of muscles. A semi-Fowler position helps prevent patient from choking or aspirating.
11. Place paper towels on an overbed table, and arrange other equipment within easy reach.	• Prevents soiling of the tabletop. Equipment prepared in advance ensures a smooth, safe procedure.
12. Place a towel over patient's chest.	• Prevents soiling of bed linen and patient's clothing.
13. Apply toothpaste to brush, holding brush over the emesis basin. Pour a small amount of water over toothpaste.	• Moisture aids in the distribution of toothpaste over tooth surfaces.
14. The patient may assist by brushing. Hold toothbrush bristles at a 45-degree angle to gum line (see Step 14 illustration, part A). Be sure tips of bristles rest against and penetrate under gum line. Brush inner and outer surfaces of upper and lower teeth by brushing from gum to crown of each tooth. Clean biting surfaces of teeth by holding top of bristles parallel with teeth and brushing gently back and forth (see Step 14 illustration, part B). Brush sides of teeth by moving bristles back and forth (see Step 14 illustration, part C).	• Angle allows brush to reach all tooth surfaces and to clean under gum line where plaque and bacteria accumulate. Back-and-forth motion dislodges food particles caught between teeth and along chewing surfaces.

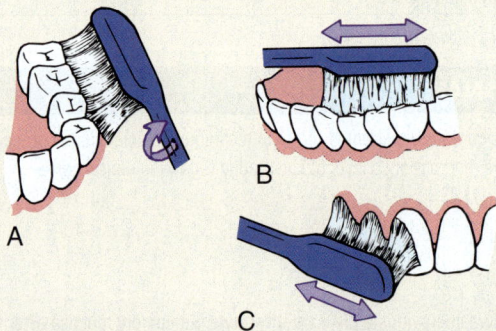

STEP 14 Directions for toothbrush placement. **A,** Gum line is brushed at a 45-degree angle. **B,** Parallel position is used for brushing biting surfaces. **C,** Lateral position is used for brushing sides of teeth.

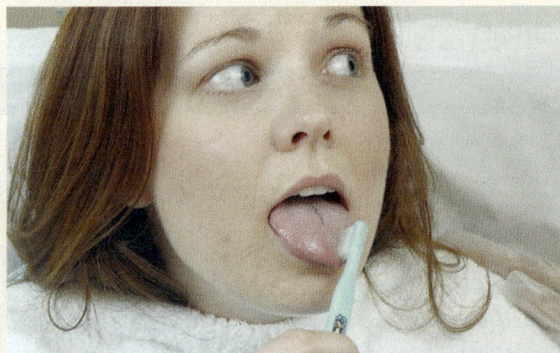

STEP 15 Assisting patient with brushing tongue.

STEPS	RATIONALE
15. Have patient hold brush at a 45-degree angle and lightly brush over surface and sides of tongue (see Step 15 illustration). Avoid initiating gag reflex.	• Microorganisms collect and grow on the tongue's surface and contribute to bad breath. Gagging may cause aspiration of toothpaste. Evaluates patient's ability to use correct technique.
16. Allow patient to rinse mouth thoroughly—taking several sips of water, swishing water across all tooth surfaces, and spitting into the emesis basin.	• Irrigation removes food particles.

SKILL 39.3   PROVIDING ORAL HYGIENE—cont'd

STEPS	RATIONALE
17. Allow patient to gargle and rinse mouth with mouthwash as desired.	• Mouthwash can be effective in reducing plaque and gingivitis (Canadian Dental Association, 2022).
18. Assist in wiping patient's mouth.	• Promotes sense of comfort.
19. Allow patient to floss.	• Reduces tartar between tooth surfaces.
20. Allow patient to rinse mouth thoroughly with cool water and spit into emesis basin. Assist in wiping patient's mouth.	• Irrigation removes plaque and tartar from the oral cavity.
21. Ask patient whether any area of oral cavity feels uncomfortable or irritated. Inspect the oral cavity.	• Pain can indicate a problem.
22. Assist patient to a comfortable position, remove emesis basin and bedside table, raise side rail, and lower bed to the original position.	• Provides for patient comfort and safety.
23. Wipe off overbed table, discard soiled linen and paper towels in appropriate containers, remove soiled gloves, and return equipment to the proper place.	• Proper disposal of soiled equipment helps prevent the spread of microorganisms.
24. Remove gloves and perform hand hygiene.	• Reduces the transmission of microorganisms.
25. Ask patient to describe proper hygiene techniques.	• Evaluates patient's learning.

UNEXPECTED OUTCOMES	RELATED INTERVENTIONS
Dryness and inflammation of oral mucosa	• Increase frequency of oral hygiene. • Increase patient's hydration (if permitted). • Apply water-soluble lubricant to the patient's lips.
Retraction of gum margins from teeth, localized areas of inflammation, and bleeding around gum margins	• Determine whether patient has an underlying bleeding tendency (e.g., anticoagulant therapy). • Report findings to the health care provider or person in charge. • Use a soft-bristled toothbrush. • Increase frequency of oral hygiene.
Signs of dental caries	• Refer patient to a dentist. • Teach patient oral hygiene techniques.

RECORDING AND REPORTING
• Record all procedures on a flow sheet provided by your agency or facility. Note the condition of the oral cavity in the patient care notes.
• Report any bleeding or the presence of lesions to the person in charge or the health care provider.

CARE IN THE COMMUNITY CONSIDERATIONS
• Teach the patient and caregiver to assess the oral cavity daily to determine any effects of medications on the oral cavity (e.g., reddened, inflamed gums).

SKILL 39.4   PERFORMING MOUTH CARE FOR AN UNCONSCIOUS OR DEBILITATED PATIENT

Delegation Considerations
Oral hygiene of an unconscious or debilitated patient can be delegated to an unregulated care provider (UCP). You must first assess the patient for the gag reflex and determine whether the person providing assistance can safely use oral suctioning for clearing the patient's oral secretions (see Chapter 40). When delegating tasks to a UCP, it is important to instruct them about the following:

• The proper way to position the patient for mouth care
• How to safely use oral suctioning for clearing oral secretions (see Chapter 41)
• To report any bleeding of the mucosa or gums, any painful reaction by the patient, or excessive coughing or choking

Equipment
• Antiseptic oral rinse (e.g., chlorhexidine gluconate)
• Small soft-bristled toothbrush
• Sponge swab (e.g., Toothette swab)
• Oral airway
• Padded tongue blade
• Face towel
• Paper towels
• Emesis basin
• Water glass with cool water
• Water-soluble lip lubricant
• Small-bulb syringe (optional)
• Suction equipment
• Disposable gloves

Continued

SKILL 39.4	PERFORMING MOUTH CARE FOR AN UNCONSCIOUS OR DEBILITATED PATIENT—cont'd

PROCEDURE

STEPS	RATIONALE
1. Assess patient's risk for oral hygiene challenges (see Table 39.5).	• Oral care is provided frequently to intubated patients who also have a nasogastric tube and who are at risk of aspiration, which can lead to pneumonia (Rabello et al., 2018).
2. Explain procedure to patient.	• Allows debilitated patient to anticipate procedure without anxiety. Unconscious patients retain the ability to hear.
3. Test for the presence of a gag reflex by touching the posterior pharyngeal wall with a tongue blade.	• Reveals whether patient is at risk for aspiration.

CRITICAL DECISION POINT: *Patients with an impaired gag reflex require oral care as well. You must determine the type of suction apparatus needed at the bedside to protect the patient's airway against aspiration.*

STEPS	RATIONALE
4. Raise bed to the appropriate height; lower head of the bed (if patient's condition permits) and then lower the side rail.	• Allows use of good body mechanics and reduces the risk of injury.
5. Pull curtain around the bed or close the room door.	• Provides privacy.
6. Perform hand hygiene and put on disposable gloves.	• Reduces the transfer of microorganisms. Gloves prevent contact with microorganisms in blood or saliva.
7. Place paper towels on an overbed table and arrange equipment. If needed, turn on a suction machine and connect tubing to the suction catheter.	• Prevents soiling of the tabletop. Equipment prepared in advance ensures a smooth, safe procedure.
8. Position patient on side (left lateral recumbent position) with head turned toward dependent side. Move patient close to the side of the bed. Raise the side rail.	• Turning the patient's head to the side allows secretions to drain from the mouth instead of collecting in the back of the pharynx. Prevents aspiration. Moving the patient close to the side of the bed facilitates proper body mechanics.
9. Place a towel under patient's head and an emesis basin under the chin.	• Prevents soiling of bed linen and patient's gown.
10. Carefully separate upper and lower teeth with padded tongue blade by inserting blade, quickly but gently, between back molars. Insert blade when patient is relaxed, if possible. Do not use force (see Step 10 illustration).	• Prevents patient from biting down on your fingers and provides access to oral cavity.

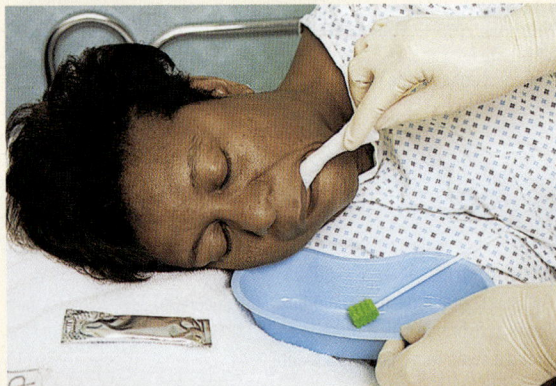

STEP 10 Separate upper and lower teeth with padded tongue blade.

STEP 14 Application of water-soluble moisturizer to lips.

CRITICAL DECISION POINT: *Never use fingers to separate the patient's teeth.*

STEPS	RATIONALE
11. Inspect condition of the oral cavity (see Chapter 33).	• Determines condition of the oral cavity and the need for hygiene.

SKILL 39.4	PERFORMING MOUTH CARE FOR AN UNCONSCIOUS OR DEBILITATED PATIENT—cont'd

STEPS	RATIONALE
12. Clean mouth using brush or sponge Toothette swabs moistened with chlorhexidine solution if patient condition can tolerate it; otherwise, moisten with water. Clean chewing and inner and outer tooth surfaces. Swab roof of mouth, gums, and inside cheeks. Gently swab or brush tongue, but avoid stimulating gag reflex (if present). Moisten clean swab or Toothette swab with water to rinse. (Bulb syringe may also be used to rinse.) Repeat rinse several times.	• Brushing action removes food particles between teeth and along chewing surfaces. Swabbing helps remove secretions and crusts from mucosa and moistens mucosa. Rinsing removes any debris and cleaning agent and provides for patient comfort.
13. Suction secretions as they accumulate, if necessary.	• Suction removes secretions and fluid that can collect in the posterior pharynx.
14. Apply a thin layer of water-soluble lubricant to lips (see Step 14 illustration).	• Lubricates lips to prevent drying and cracking.
15. Inform patient that procedure is completed.	• Provides meaningful stimulation to unconscious or less responsive patient.
16. Put on clean gloves, and inspect oral cavity.	• Determines efficacy of cleaning. Once thick secretions are removed, underlying inflammation or lesions may be revealed.
17. Ask debilitated patient whether mouth feels clean.	• Evaluates level of comfort.
18. Reposition patient in a comfortable position, raise side rail as appropriate or as ordered, and return the bed to original position.	• Maintains patient's comfort and safety. Raising all four side rails may be considered a restraint, and a health care provider's order is needed.
19. Clean equipment and return to its proper place. Place soiled linen in the proper receptacle.	• Proper disposal of soiled equipment helps prevent the spread of microorganisms.
20. Remove and discard gloves. Perform hand hygiene.	• Reduces transmission of microorganisms.
21. Assess patient's respirations on an ongoing basis.	• Ensures early recognition of aspiration.

UNEXPECTED OUTCOMES	RELATED INTERVENTIONS
Secretions or crusts remaining on oral mucosa, tongue, or gums	• Increase frequency of oral hygiene. • Try using a pediatric-size toothbrush—it may provide better hygiene if the oral cavity is difficult to access.
Localized inflammation of gums or mucosa	• Increase frequency of oral hygiene with a soft-bristle toothbrush. • Apply moisturizing gel on the oral mucosa. • Chemotherapy and radiation can cause stomatitis. To provide relief and promote oral hygiene, topical anti-inflammatories and anaesthetics may be prescribed (Galhardo et al., 2020).
Aspiration of secretions	• Suction oral airway. • Perform tracheal bronchial suctioning. • Notify the health care provider.

RECORDING AND REPORTING
• Record the procedure, including pertinent observations (e.g., the presence of bleeding gums, dry mucosa, ulcerations, or crusts on the tongue).
• Report any unusual findings to the person in charge or the health care provider.

CARE IN THE COMMUNITY CONSIDERATIONS
• The oral cavity should be irrigated with a bulb syringe.
• Mouth care should be given at least twice a day. Caregivers can buy nonprescription oral care solutions (e.g., chlorhexidine solutions) at most pharmacies.
• Have caregivers demonstrate positioning of the patient that will prevent aspiration.

stomatitis, an inflammation of the oral mucosa that can cause burning, pain, and a change in food tolerance. Gentle brushing and flossing are important in preventing bleeding of the gums. Patients should be advised to avoid using alcohol and commercial mouthwash and to stop smoking. Normal saline rinses (approximately 30 mL) used upon awaking in the morning, after each meal, and at bedtime can effectively clean the oral cavity. The rinses can be increased to every 2 hours, if

necessary. The physician or nurse practitioner may order a mild oral analgesic for pain control.

Patients with diabetes mellitus frequently have periodontal disease and should have regular, yearly (or more frequently if necessary) visits to the dental professional for oral health assessment and care. All tissues should be handled gently with a minimum of trauma. Patients should learn to follow rigid cleaning schedules, at least four times a day.

Denture Care. Patients should be encouraged to clean their dentures on a regular basis to avoid gingival infection and irritation. When patients become disabled, the care provider or family caregiver can assume responsibility for denture care (Box 39.12). Dentures are patients' personal property and need to be handled with care because they can be easily broken. They must be removed at night to give the gums a rest and prevent bacterial buildup. Dentures should be kept covered in water when they are not worn, to prevent warping, and they should always be stored in an enclosed, labelled cup and placed in a patient's bedside stand. Patients should be discouraged from removing dentures and placing them on a napkin or tissue because they could be easily thrown away.

Hair and Scalp Care

A person's appearance and feeling of well-being can often depend on the way their hair looks and feels. Illness or disability may prevent patients from maintaining daily hair care. Immobilized patients' hair soon becomes tangled. Dressings may leave sticky blood or antiseptic solutions on the hair. In the clinic and home care setting, nurses may encounter patients who have head lice. Proper hair care is important to a patient's body image. Brushing, combing, and shampooing are basic hair hygiene measures for all patients.

Brushing and Combing. Frequent brushing and combing helps to keep hair clean and distributes oil evenly along hair shafts and prevents hair from tangling. Patients should be encouraged to maintain routine hair care. However, patients with limited mobility or weakness and those who are confused require assistance. Patients in a hospital or long-term care facility appreciate the opportunity to have their hair brushed and combed before being seen by others.

When caring for patients from different cultures, it is important to learn as much as possible from them or their family about their preferred hair care practices. Cultural preferences affect how hair is combed and styled. Nurses should never trim or cut a patient's hair without the patient's consent.

BOX 39.12 PROCEDURAL GUIDELINE

Care of Dentures

Delegation Considerations

The skill of denture care can be delegated to an unregulated care provider (UCP). It is important to discuss the following with the UCP:

- To report any cracks found in the dentures
- To report any patient complaints of oral discomfort
- To report any signs of irritation, inflammation, or lesions

Equipment

- Soft-bristled toothbrush or denture toothbrush
- Denture cleaning agent or toothpaste
- Denture adhesive (optional)
- Glass of water
- Emesis basin or sink
- Washcloth
- Disposable gloves
- Denture cup (if dentures are to be stored after cleaning)

Procedure

1. Ask patient whether dentures fit and whether the gums or mucous membranes are tender or irritated.
2. Ask patient about preferences for denture care and products used. If patient is unable to care for own dentures, you must provide this care. Clean dentures for the patient during routine mouth care.
3. Fill emesis basin with tepid water or, if using sink, place washcloth in bottom of sink and fill sink with 2.5 cm of water.
4. Remove dentures. If patient is unable to do this independently, perform hand hygiene and put on gloves, grasp upper plate at front with thumb and index finger wrapped in gauze, and pull downward. Gently lift lower denture from jaw, and rotate one side downward to remove from patient's mouth. Place dentures in emesis basin or sink.
5. Apply cleaning agent to brush and brush surfaces of dentures (see Step 5 illustration). Hold dentures close to water. Hold the brush horizontally and

use a back-and-forth motion to clean biting surfaces. Use short strokes from the top of the denture to biting surfaces to clean outer and inner teeth surfaces. Hold the brush vertically and use short strokes to clean inner tooth surfaces. Hold the brush horizontally and use a back-and-forth motion to clean the undersurface of dentures.

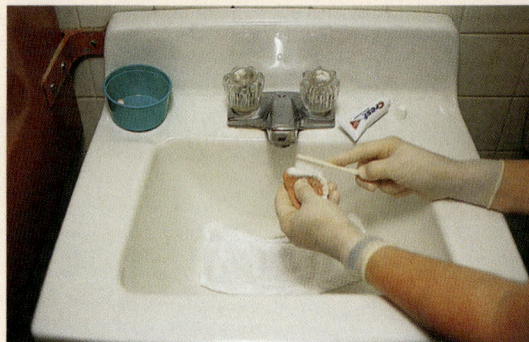

STEP 5 Brushing dentures.

6. Rinse thoroughly in tepid water.
7. Some patients use an adhesive to seal dentures in place. If so, apply a thin layer to the undersurface before inserting.
8. If patient needs assistance with the insertion of dentures, moisten the upper denture and press firmly to seal it in place. Then insert moistened lower denture. Ask whether dentures feel comfortable.
9. Dentures should be removed at night and the gums cleaned gently. Dentures should be stored in a denture container that is labelled with the patient's name and placed in the bedside table to prevent loss.
10. Remove and discard gloves and perform hand hygiene.

Long hair can easily become matted when patients are confined to bed, even for a short period. When lacerations or incisions involve the scalp, blood and topical medications can also cause tangling. Frequent brushing and combing keeps long hair neatly groomed. Braiding can help to avoid repeated tangles; however, braids should be unbraided periodically and the hair combed to ensure good hygiene. Braids made too tightly can result in bald patches. Nurses must always obtain permission from patients, if conscious, before braiding their hair.

To brush the hair, part it into two sections and separate each into two more sections; it is easier to brush smaller sections of hair. Brushing from the scalp toward the hair ends minimizes pulling. Moistening the hair with water frees tangles for easier combing.

Patients who develop head lice require special consideration in the way combing is performed. The lice are small, about the size of a sesame seed. Bright light or natural sunlight is necessary for the lice to be seen. Thorough combing is recommended and may remove nits (empty eggshells) if infestation is extensive. To remove head lice, the following steps are used:

- Put on a disposable gown and gloves.
- Use a grooming comb or hairbrush to remove any tangles.
- Divide the patient's hair in sections and fasten off the hair that is not being combed.
- Comb out from the scalp to the end of the hair (special fine-tooth combs are available in drugstores).
- Between each pass, dip the comb in a cup of water or use a paper towel to remove nits.
- After combing, look through the hair carefully for attached live lice.
- Catch live lice with a tweezers or comb.
- Move to the next section of hair after combing thoroughly.
- Instruct the family to clean the comb with an old toothbrush and dental floss and boil the comb (if possible). The ideal would be to discard the comb after each use, but some patients' financial situations may prevent the purchase of multiple combs.
- Instruct the family to comb and screen for lice daily.
- Instruct the family to separate the patient's clothes from other laundry and then wash them in hot water.

- Instruct caregivers on how to prevent the transmission of lice:
  - Do not share bed linens.
  - Avoid placing your bare hand on the patient's head.
  - Immediately wash your hands after providing hair care.
  - Separate all hair care products.

Shampooing. To promote and restore hair and scalp health, patients should be instructed to keep hair clean, combed, and brushed regularly. Patients may also need to know how to check for and remove parasites, such as lice (see Table 39.4). Nurses should inform patients that they need to notify their primary caregiver of changes in the texture and distribution of hair, which may indicate a serious systemic condition.

Frequency of shampooing depends on the patient's daily routines and the condition of their hair. Nurses should remind patients in hospitals or long-term care facilities that staying in bed, perspiring excessively, or undergoing treatments that leave blood or solutions in the hair may result in them needing more frequent shampooing.

For patients at home who have limited mobility, it can be challenging to find ways for them to shampoo their hair without causing injury to themselves. If patients are able to take a shower or bath, their hair can usually be shampooed without difficulty. A shower or tub chair may be used for ambulatory, weight-bearing patients who become fatigued or are prone to fainting. Hand-held shower nozzles enable patients to wash their hair in the tub or shower. Patients allowed to sit in a chair may choose to be shampooed in front of a sink or over a wash basin. However, bending is limited or contraindicated in certain conditions (e.g., eye surgery or neck injury). In these situations, the nurse needs to teach the patient and family members the degree of bending allowed.

If patients are unable to sit but can be moved, the nurse may transfer the patient to a stretcher for transportation to a sink or shower equipped with a hand-held nozzle. This equipment is commonly found in long-term care facilities. Again, the nurse needs to exercise caution when positioning the patient's head and neck, particularly for patients with any form of head or neck injury.

If patients are unable to sit in a chair or be transferred to a stretcher, shampooing must be done while the patient is in bed (Box 39.13).

BOX 39.13 PROCEDURAL GUIDELINE

Shampooing the Hair of a Bed-Bound Patient

Delegation Considerations

The skill of shampooing hair can be delegated to an unregulated care provider (UCP). It is important to discuss the following with the UCP:
- To follow any precautions necessary in positioning the patient
- To report any patient reports of neck pain
- To report condition of the scalp and hair

Equipment
- Bath towels
- Washcloths
- Shampoo
- Hair conditioner (if available)
- Water pitcher with warm water
- Plastic shampoo trough
- Wash basin
- Bath blanket
- Waterproof pad
- Clean comb and brush

- Hair dryer (if warranted by patient's condition)
- Disposable gloves (optional)

Procedure
1. Before washing the patient's hair, ensure that this procedure is not contraindicated for the patient. Certain medical conditions, such as head and neck injuries, spinal cord injuries, and arthritis, could place the patient at risk for injury during shampooing because of positioning and manipulation of the patient's head and neck.
2. Put on gloves if needed. Inspect the hair and scalp before initiating the procedure to determine the presence of any conditions that may require the use of special shampoos or treatments (e.g., for dandruff or the removal of dried blood).
3. Place waterproof pad under patient's shoulders, neck, and head (see Step 3 illustration). Position patient supine, with head and shoulders at top edge of the bed. Place a plastic trough under the patient's head and a wash basin at end of the trough. Be sure the trough spout extends beyond the edge of the mattress.

Continued

BOX 39.13 **PROCEDURAL GUIDELINE—cont'd**
Shampooing the Hair of a Bed-Bound Patient

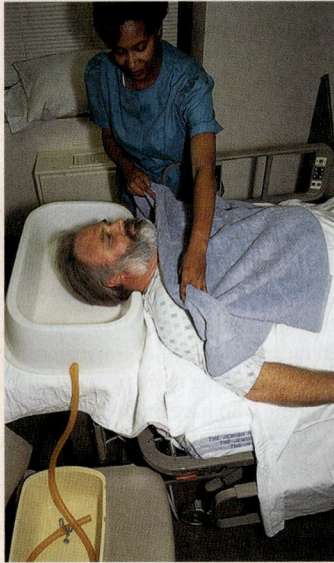

STEP 3 Pad has been placed under shoulders, neck, and head.

STEP 8 Pour water over hair.

4. Place rolled towel under patient's neck and bath towel over patient's shoulders.
5. Brush and comb patient's hair.
6. Obtain warm water.
7. Offer patient the option of holding a face towel or washcloth over the eyes.
8. Slowly pour water from a water pitcher over hair until it is completely wet (see Step 8 illustration). If hair contains matted blood, don gloves, apply peroxide to dissolve the clots, and then rinse the hair with saline. Apply small amount of shampoo.
9. Work up lather with both hands. Start at the hairline and work toward back of the neck. Lift head slightly with one hand to wash back of the head. Shampoo sides of the head. Massage scalp by applying pressure with fingertips, if not contraindicated.

10. Rinse hair with water. Make sure water drains into basin. Repeat rinsing until hair is free of soap.
11. Apply conditioner or cream rinse, if requested, and rinse hair thoroughly.
12. Wrap patient's head in bath towel. Dry patient's face with cloth used to protect eyes. Dry off any moisture along the neck or shoulders.
13. Dry patient's hair and scalp. Use a second towel if first one becomes saturated.
14. Comb hair to remove tangles, and dry with dryer if desired (not available in all agencies or facilities).
15. Apply oil preparation or conditioning product to hair, if desired by patient.
16. Assist patient to a comfortable position, and complete styling of hair.

A special shampoo trough can be positioned under the patient's head to catch water and suds. After shampooing, patients like having their hair styled and dried. Dry shampoos that reduce the need to wet the patient's hair are also available but are not highly effective. These dry shampoo preparations vary, and the application procedures, listed on the container, should be followed exactly. Also available are prepackaged shampoo cloths, which can be used to shampoo a patient in bed or in a chair. In some agencies, a health care provider's order is necessary to shampoo the dependent patient.

Shaving. Shaving facial hair can be done after a bath or shampoo. Some patients may prefer to shave their legs or axillae while bathing. When assisting a patient, the nurse should take care to avoid cutting the patient with a razor blade. Patients prone to bleeding (e.g., those receiving anticoagulants or high doses of aspirin; those with low platelet counts) must use an electric razor. Before using an electric razor, it is good to check for frayed cords and other electrical hazards, as well as the agency's policy regarding the use of these razors. Each razor blade or electric razor should be used on only one patient, to prevent spread of infection.

Before a razor blade is used for shaving, the skin must be softened to prevent pulling, scraping, or cuts. This is done by placing a warm washcloth over the patient's face for a few seconds, then applying shaving cream or lathering a mild soap to soften the skin. If the patient is unable to shave, the nurse may perform the task. To avoid causing discomfort or razor cuts, the nurse gently pulls the skin taut and uses short, firm razor strokes in the direction in which the hair grows (Figure 39.9). Short downward strokes work best to remove hair over the upper lip. A patient usually can explain the best way to move the razor across the skin. In dark-skinned patients, facial hair tends to be curly and can become ingrown unless shaved close to the skin.

Moustache and Beard Care

Patients with moustaches or beards require daily grooming. Keeping these areas clean is important because food particles and mucus can easily collect in the hair. If the patient is unable to carry out self-care, the nurse must perform this care for the patient. Beards can be gently combed out. A shaggy or unkempt moustache or beard can be trimmed, only with consent from the patient or family. For cultural or religious reasons, trimming or shaving off a moustache or beard cannot be performed without the patient's or family's consent.

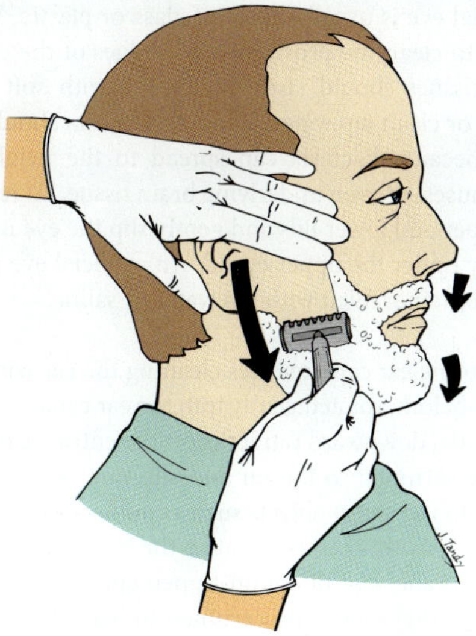

FIGURE 39.9 Shaving a patient. Shave in the direction of hair growth. Use longer strokes on the larger areas of the face. Use short strokes around the chin and lips. (From Sorrentino, S. A. [2004]. *Assisting with patient care* [2nd ed., p. 320, Fig. 17.5]. Mosby.)

Care of the Eyes, Ears, and Nose

Special attention is given to cleaning the eyes, ears, and nose during a routine bath and when drainage or discharge accumulates. This aspect of hygiene not only makes patients more comfortable, it also improves sensory perception (see Chapter 48). Care focuses on preventing infection and maintaining normal sensory function and requires approaches that consider patients' special needs.

Basic Eye Care. Cleaning the eyes involves simply washing them with a clean washcloth moistened in water. Soap may cause burning and irritation (see Skill 39.1). Direct pressure should never be applied over the eyeball because it may cause serious injury. When cleaning a patient's eyes, use a clean washcloth and cleanse from the inner to outer canthus. Use a different section of the washcloth for each eye. Unconscious patients often require more frequent eye care.

Secretions may collect along the lid margins and inner canthus when the blink reflex is absent or an eye does not close completely. It may be necessary to place an eye patch over the involved eye to prevent corneal drying and irritation. Lubricating eye drops may be given according to the health care provider's orders.

Eyeglasses. Glasses are made of hardened glass or plastic that is impact-resistant to prevent shattering. Nevertheless, because of their cost, extra care should be taken when cleaning glasses, and they should be protected from breakage or other damage when they are not worn. Glasses should be put in a case in a drawer of the bedside table when not in use and labelled with the patient's name.

Cool water is sufficient for cleaning glass lenses. A soft cloth is best for drying to prevent scratching the lens; paper towels can scratch a lens. Plastic lenses in particular are scratched easily, and special cleansing solutions and drying cloths are available for them. It is good to use whatever the patient's eye care specialist recommends.

Contact Lenses. A contact lens is a small, round, transparent, and sometimes coloured disc that fits directly over the cornea of the eye. Contact lenses are designed specifically to correct refractive errors of the eye or abnormalities in the cornea's shape. They are relatively easy to apply and remove.

BOX 39.14 PATIENT TEACHING

Contact Lens Care

Objectives
- Patient will be able to identify warning signs of corneal irritation and eye infection.
- Patient will be able to clean and care for contact lenses correctly.

Teaching Strategies

Encourage the patient to see a vision care specialist (ophthalmologist or optometrist) regularly:
- For low-risk patients: birth to 24 months: by age 3 months; age 2–5 years: prior to attending school; age 6–19 years: annually; age 20–64 years: every 1–2 years; and over age 65 years: annually
- The vision care specialist will determine the frequency for high-risk patients (British Columbia Doctors of Optometry, 2022).

Teach the patient the following facts about contact lens care:
- Special cleaning solutions should be used when cleaning and disinfecting contact lenses.
- Never use your fingernail on a lens to remove dirt or debris that does not loosen during washing with cleaning solutions.
- Follow recommendations of the lens manufacturer or your eye care practitioner when cleaning and disinfecting lenses.
- Remember the mnemonic RSVP: *r*edness, *s*ensitivity, *v*ision challenges, and *p*ain). If one of these symptoms occurs, remove the contact lenses immediately. If difficulties continue, contact a vision care specialist.
- Lenses become very slippery once cleaning solution is applied.
- If a lens is dropped on a hard surface, moisten your finger with the cleaning or wetting solution and gently touch the lens to pick it up. Then clean, rinse, and disinfect the lens.
- Lenses should be kept moist or wet when not worn.
- Use fresh solution daily when storing and disinfecting lenses.
- Do not wipe the lens with a tissue or towel.
- Thoroughly wash and rinse the lens storage case on a daily basis. Clean it periodically with soap or liquid detergent; rinse it thoroughly with warm water and air-dry it.
- To avoid a mix-up, always start with the same lens when removing or inserting lenses.
- Throw away disposable or planned replacement lenses after the prescribed wearing period.

Evaluation
- Ask the patient to identify the warning signs of corneal irritation and eye infection.
- Ask the patient to describe methods of improper contact lens handling that can lead to infection.
- Ask the patient to describe the techniques required to clean and store contact lenses.

Contact lenses are available in daily-wear, extended-wear, and disposable varieties. All lenses must be removed periodically to prevent ocular infection and corneal ulcers or abrasions. Patient education must include a discussion of proper lens care techniques to avoid microbial infections (e.g., keratitis) (Konne et al., 2019) (Box 39.14).

Daily-wear lenses should be removed overnight for cleaning and disinfecting; extended-wear lenses can be worn for up to 30 days without being removed. Disposable lenses are available in daily-wear and extended-wear varieties. Extended-wear disposable lenses are usually replaced every 1 to 2 weeks. Lenses should be replaced as often as recommended by the manufacturer (Konne et al., 2019). Pain, tearing, discomfort, and redness of the conjunctivae may be symptoms of lens overwear. The persistence of symptoms after lens removal may indicate serious ocular injury.

Contact lenses accumulate secretions and foreign matter while they are being worn. These materials deteriorate and then irritate the eye, causing distorted vision and the risk for infection. Contact lenses should be cleaned and thoroughly disinfected once removed. Patients should be cautioned to never use saliva, homemade saline, or tap water when cleaning lenses as these solutions may contain microorganisms that can cause serious infections.

Artificial Eyes. Patients with artificial eyes have had an **enucleation**, or removal, of an entire eyeball as a result of a tumour growth, severe infection, or eye trauma. Some artificial eyes are permanently implanted, whereas others can be removed for routine cleaning. Patients with an artificial eye usually prefer to care for their own eye. Nurses should respect the patient's wishes and assist by assembling needed equipment.

Patients may at times require assistance in prosthesis removal and cleaning. To remove an artificial eye, retract the lower eyelid and exert slight pressure just below the eye (Figure 39.10). This action causes the artificial eye to rise from the socket because the suction holding the eye in place has been broken. A small rubber bulb syringe or medicine dropper bulb may also be used to create a suction effect. The suction created by placing the bulb tip directly over the eye and squeezing lifts the artificial eye from the socket.

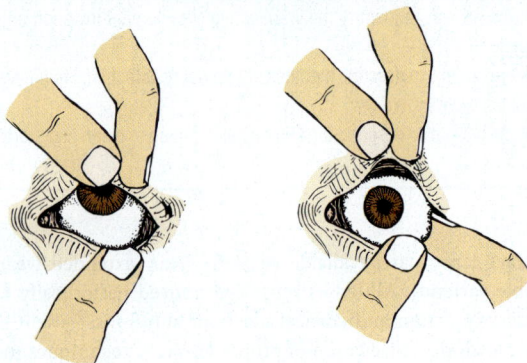

FIGURE 39.10 Removal of a prosthetic eye. To remove an artificial eye, retract the lower eyelid and exert slight pressure just below the eye. This action causes the artificial eye to rise from the socket because the suction holding the eye in place has been broken. A small, rubber bulb syringe or medicine-dropper bulb can also be used to create a suction effect. Place the bulb tip directly over the eye and squeeze it to create suction needed to lift the eye from the socket (not pictured).

The artificial eye is usually made of glass or plastic. Warm normal saline is used to clean the prosthesis. The edges of the eye socket and surrounding tissues should also be cleaned, with soft gauze moistened in saline or clean tap water. Signs of infection should be reported immediately because bacteria can spread to the neighbouring eye, underlying sinuses, or even underlying brain tissue. To reinsert the eye, retract the upper and lower lids and gently slip the eye into the socket, fitting it neatly under the upper eyelid. An artificial eye may be stored in a labelled container filled with tap water or saline.

Ear Care. Routine ear care involves cleaning the ear with the end of a moistened washcloth, rotated gently into the ear canal. When cerumen is visible, a gentle, downward retraction at the entrance of the ear canal may cause the cerumen to loosen and slip out. Nurses should warn patients never to use sharp objects such as bobby pins or paper clips to remove cerumen as this can traumatize the ear canal and rupture the tympanic membrane. Use of cotton-tipped applicators should also be avoided because they can cause cerumen to become impacted within the canal.

Children and older persons commonly have impacted cerumen. Excessive or impacted cerumen can usually be removed only by irrigation, which usually requires a health care provider's order. If a patient has a history of a perforated eardrum or if perforation is discovered during assessment, the procedure is contraindicated. Before irrigation, instill three drops of glycerine at bedtime to soften the cerumen and three drops of hydrogen peroxide twice a day to loosen the cerumen. Then irrigation with approximately 250 mL of warm water (at 37°C) into the ear canal mechanically washes away loosened cerumen. The use of cold or hot water can cause nausea or vomiting.

The patient may sit or lie on their side with the affected ear up. To irrigate the ear, place a small, curved basin under the affected ear to catch the irrigating solution, and use a bulb-irrigating syringe. The tip of the syringe should not occlude the ear canal, to avoid exerting pressure against the tympanic membrane. Direct a gentle irrigation at the top of the canal to loosen the cerumen from the sides of the canal. After the canal is clear, wipe off any moisture from the ear and inspect the canal for remaining cerumen.

Hearing Aid Care. Hearing aids are instruments made up of miniature parts working together as a system to amplify sound in a controlled manner. Aids receive normal low-intensity sound inputs and deliver them to the ear as louder outputs. The new class of hearing aids can reduce background noise interference. Computer chips placed in the aids allow for fine adjustments to a specific patient's hearing needs. Hearing aids are used by both hard-of-hearing individuals (those with a slight or moderate hearing loss) and deaf individuals (those with severe or profound hearing loss). While mechanical dysfunction of the external or middle ear causes conductive hearing loss, which could be due to impacted cerumen or a foreign body that obstructs the transmission of sound, sensorineural (perceptive) hearing loss indicates a pathology in the inner ear, cranial nerve VII damage, or presbycusis (gradual nerve degeneration that occurs with aging) (Dunya et al., 2021). The use of cochlear implants in children is growing rapidly. The findings of Kral and colleagues (2019) underscore the interconnectedness of brain function for auditory and linguistic functioning.

Three popular types of hearing aids are available. An *in-the-canal (ITC) aid* is the newest, smallest, and least visible hearing aid and fits entirely in the ear canal. It has cosmetic appeal, is easy to manipulate and place in the ear, does not interfere with wearing eyeglasses or using the telephone, and can be worn during most physical exercise. However, it requires an adequate ear diameter and depth for proper fit. It does not accommodate progressive hearing

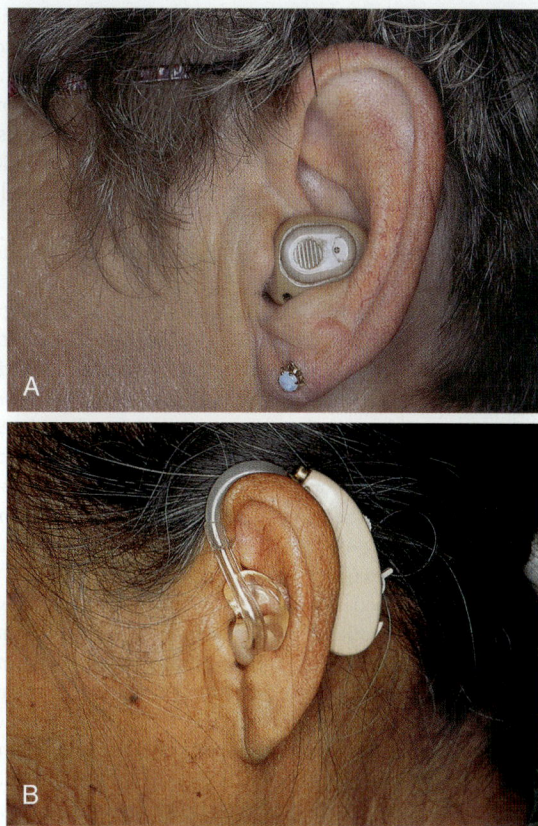

FIGURE 39.11 Two common types of hearing aids. **A,** In the ear. **B,** Behind the ear.

loss, and it requires manual dexterity to operate, insert, remove, and change the batteries. Also, cerumen tends to plug this model more than the other models.

An *in-the-ear (ITE, or intra-aural) aid* (Figure 39.11, *A*) fits into the external auditory canal and allows for better fine-tuning. It is more powerful and stronger than the ITC aid and therefore is useful for a wider range of hearing loss. It is easy to position and adjust and does not interfere with wearing eyeglasses. It is, however, more noticeable than the ITC aid and is not recommended for persons with moisture or skin conditions in the ear canal.

A *behind-the-ear (BTE, or postaural) aid* (see Figure 39.11, *B*) hooks around and behind the ear and is connected by a short, clear, hollow plastic tube to an ear mould inserted into the external auditory canal. It allows for fine-tuning. It is the largest of the three aids and is useful for patients with rapidly progressive hearing loss or manual dexterity difficulties and those who find partial ear occlusion intolerable. Disadvantages are that it is more visible, may interfere with wearing eyeglasses and using a phone, and is more difficult to keep in place during physical exercise. Box 39.15 reviews patient education guidelines for the care and use of a hearing aid.

Nasal Care. The patient can usually remove secretions from the nose by gently blowing into a soft tissue. The patient should be cautioned against harsh blowing; this can create pressure capable of injuring the eardrum, nasal mucosa, and even sensitive eye structures. Bleeding from the nares is a sign of harsh blowing.

If the patient is unable to remove nasal secretions, the nurse can assist by using a wet washcloth or a cotton-tipped applicator moistened in water or saline. The applicator should never be inserted beyond the length of the cotton tip. Excessive nasal secretions can also be removed by gentle suctioning.

BOX 39.15 Care and Use of Hearing Aids by the Patient

- Initially, wear a hearing aid for short periods; then gradually increase the wearing time to 10–12 hours.
- Once inserted, turn the aid slowly to one-third to one-half volume.
- Remember that a whistling sound indicates too high a volume, incorrect ear mould insertion, an improper fit of the aid, or a buildup of earwax or fluid.
- Adjust the volume to a comfortable level for talking at a distance of 1 m.
- Do not wear the aid under heat lamps, while using a hair dryer, or in very wet, cold weather.
- Keep in mind that batteries can last 70–85 hours—1 week with daily wearing of 10–12 hours.
- Remove or disconnect the battery when not in use.
- Replace ear moulds every 2–3 years.
- Routinely check the battery compartment: Is it clean? Are batteries inserted properly? Is the compartment shut all the way?
- Remember that dials on the hearing aid should be clean and easy to rotate, creating no static during adjusting.
- Keep the aid clean.
- Aids are usually cleaned with a soft cloth and warm soapy water; see the manufacturer's instructions.
- Avoid the use of hairspray and perfume while wearing the hearing aid; the residue from the spray can cause the aid to become oily and greasy.
- Do not submerse the aid in water.
- Routinely check the cord or tubing (depending on type of aid) for cracking, fraying, and poor connections.
- Follow up with an audiologist routinely to evaluate effectiveness of the current aid.
- Remember that the frequencies of newer computerized hearing aids can be easily adjusted.

Data from Eliopoulos, C. (2021). *Gerontological nursing* (9th ed.). Wolters Kluwer.

When patients have a nasogastric, feeding, or endotracheal tube inserted through the nose, the nurse should change the tape anchoring it when soiled or if it becomes loose. When tape becomes moist from nasal secretions, the skin and mucosa can easily become macerated. Friction from the tube can cause tissue sloughing. After carefully removing the tape, the nurse maintains hold of the tubing and thoroughly cleans and dries the nasal surface (see Chapter 43).

Patient's Room Environment

Attempting to make a patient's room as comfortable as possible is an important priority. The patient's room should be comfortable, safe, and large enough to allow the patient and several visitors to move about freely. Room temperature and ventilation are difficult to control; however, noise and odours can be controlled to create a more comfortable environment. Keeping the room neat and orderly also contributes to the patient's sense of well-being.

Maintaining Comfort. The nature of what constitutes a comfortable environment depends on the patient's age, severity of illness, and level of daily activity. Depending on the patient's age and physical condition, the room temperature should be maintained between 20°C and 23°C, if possible. Infants, older persons, and the acutely ill may need a warmer room. However, certain acutely ill patients (e.g., patients with head injuries) may benefit from cooler room temperatures to lower the body's metabolic demands to reduce intracranial pressure.

A good ventilation system keeps stale air and odours from lingering in the room. The acutely ill, infants, and older persons must be protected from drafts by ensuring that they are adequately dressed and covered with a lightweight blanket.

Good ventilation also reduces lingering odours caused by draining wounds, vomitus, bowel movements, and unemptied urinals. Room deodorizers can help remove many unpleasant odours but should be used with discretion in consideration of the patient's possible embarrassment. Before using room deodorizers, it is important to determine that the patient is not allergic or sensitive to the deodorizer itself. Vanilla, poured onto a gauze inside a basin, and placed under the bed, can work well to discreetly mask unpleasant odours. Bedpans and urinals should be emptied and rinsed promptly. Thorough hygiene measures are the best way to control body or breath odours.

Ill patients seem to be more sensitive to common hospital noises (e.g., IV pump alarms, suction apparatus, or stretchers exiting an elevator). The nurse should explain the source of any unfamiliar noise to the patient and family members. Until the patient is familiar with hospital noises, the noise level should be controlled as much as possible. This can also help the patient sleep (see Chapter 42).

Proper lighting is necessary for everyone's safety and comfort. A brightly lit room is usually stimulating, and a darkened room is best for rest and sleep. Room lighting can be adjusted by closing or opening drapes, regulating overbed lights, and closing or opening room doors. When entering a patient's room at night, the nurse should refrain from abruptly turning on an overhead light unless necessary.

Room Equipment. Although variations in hospital rooms exist across health care settings, a typical hospital room contains the following basic pieces of furniture: an overbed table, a bedside stand, chairs, and a bed (Figure 39.12). Long-term care and rehabilitation facilities may have similar equipment. The overbed table rolls on wheels and can be adjusted to various heights over the bed or a chair. The table provides an ideal working space for performing procedures. It also provides a surface on which to place meal trays, toiletry items, and objects frequently used by the patient. The bedpan and urinal should not be placed on the overbed table. The bedside stand is used to store the patient's personal possessions and hygiene equipment. A telephone (if supplied), water pitcher, and drinking cup are commonly found on top of the bedside stand.

Most hospital rooms contain an armless straight-backed chair or an upholstered lounge chair with arms. Straight-backed chairs are convenient to use when temporarily transferring the patient from the bed, such as during bed making. Lounge chairs tend to be more comfortable when a patient is willing and able to sit for an extended period.

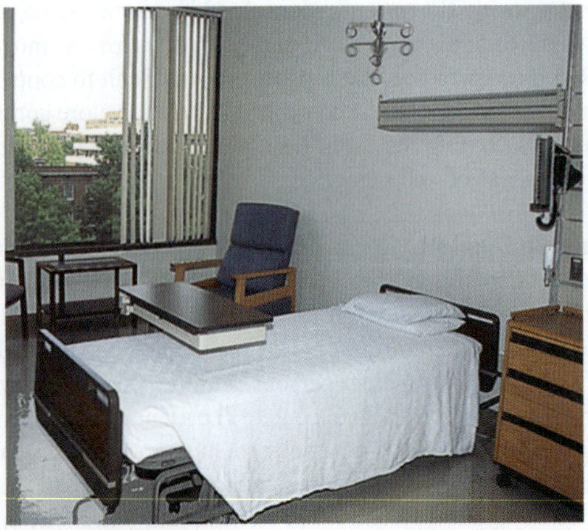

FIGURE 39.12 A typical hospital room.

Each room usually has an overbed light. Additional portable lighting can be used to provide extra light during bedside procedures. Other equipment usually found in a patient's room is a call bell, a television set (not available in all agencies and facilities), a wall-mounted blood pressure gauge, oxygen and vacuum wall outlets, and personal-care items. Special equipment designed for comfort or positioning patients includes foot boots, special mattresses, and bed boards (see Chapters 46 and 47). Nurses should check their agency's policy and the manufacturers' directions before using comfort and positioning equipment.

Beds. Seriously ill patients may remain in bed for a long time. Because a bed is the piece of equipment used most by a hospitalized patient, it should be designed for comfort, safety, and adaptability for changing positions. The typical hospital bed has a firm mattress on a metal frame that can be raised and lowered horizontally. Many hospitals are converting the standard hospital bed to one in which the mattress surface can be electronically adjusted for patient comfort. Different bed positions are used to promote patient comfort, minimize symptoms, promote lung expansion, and improve access during certain procedures (Table 39.6).

The position of a bed is usually changed by electrical controls incorporated into the patient's call light and in a panel on the side or foot of the bed (Figure 39.13). However, some facilities do have hospital beds that are manually controlled. It is important to become familiar with the use of the bed controls. Ease in raising and lowering a bed and in changing the position of the bed head and foot eliminates undue musculoskeletal strain on the care provider. Instructions should be provided to patients on the proper use of controls; they should be cautioned against raising the bed to a position that might cause harm.

Beds contain safety features such as locks on the wheels or casters, and alarms. Wheels should be locked when the bed is stationary to prevent accidental movement. Alarms should be turned on to protect patients at risk for falls when getting out of bed without assistance. Side rails protect patients from accidental falls. The headboard can be removed from most beds. This is important when the medical team must have easy access to the patient's head, such as during cardiopulmonary resuscitation.

Bed making. A patient's bed should be kept clean and comfortable. This requires frequent inspections to be sure linen is clean, dry, and free of wrinkles. When patients are diaphoretic, have draining wounds, or are incontinent, nurses should check frequently for soiled linen.

The bed is usually made in the morning after the patient's bath or while the patient is in the shower, sitting in a chair eating, or out of the room for procedures or tests. Throughout the day, bed linens should be straightened when they become loose or wrinkled. The bed linen should also be checked for food particles after meals and for wetness or soiling. Linens that are soiled or wet should be changed.

When changing bed linen, nurses need to follow the principles of medical asepsis by keeping soiled linen away from their uniform (Figure 39.14). Soiled linen is placed in special linen bags before discarding it in a hamper. To avoid air currents, which can spread microorganisms, bed linens should never be shaken. To avoid transmitting infection, soiled linen should not be placed on the floor. If clean linen touches the floor, it should be immediately removed.

During bed making, it is important to use proper body mechanics (see Chapter 37). The bed should always be raised to the appropriate height before changing linen so that the nurse does not have to bend or stretch over the mattress. The nurse should also move back and forth to opposite sides of the bed while putting on new linen. Body mechanics is also important when turning or repositioning the patient in bed.

TABLE 39.6	Common Bed Positions	
Position	**Description**	**Uses**
Fowler's 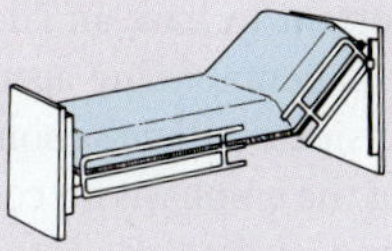	Head of bed raised to angle of 45 degrees or more; semi-sitting position; foot of bed may also be raised at knee	Is preferred while patient eats Is used during nasogastric tube insertion and nasotracheal suction Promotes lung expansion
Semi-Fowler's 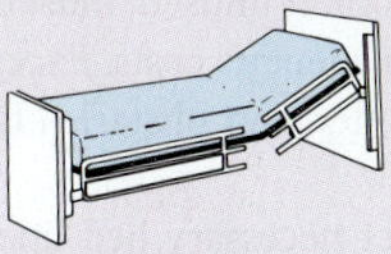	Head of bed raised approximately 30 degrees; inclination less than Fowler's position; foot of bed may also be raised at knee	Promotes lung expansion Is used when patients receive gastric feedings to reduce regurgitation and risk of aspiration
Trendelenburg's 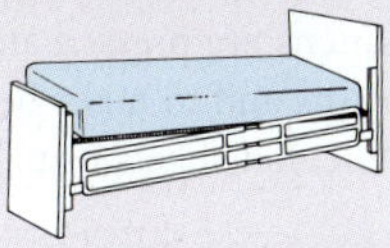	Entire bed frame tilted with head of bed down	Is used for postural drainage Facilitates venous return in patients with poor peripheral perfusion
Reverse Trendelenburg's 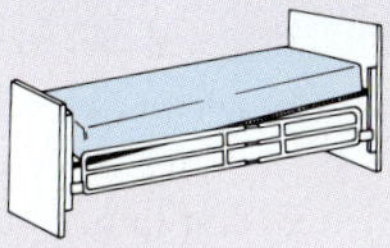	Entire bed frame tilted with foot of bed down	Is used infrequently Promotes gastric emptying Prevents esophageal reflux
Flat 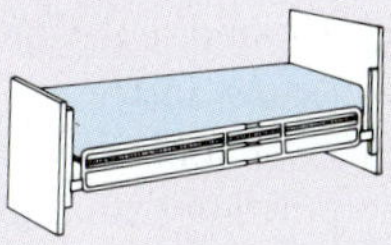	Entire bed frame horizontally parallel with floor	Is used for patients with vertebral injuries and in cervical traction Is used for patients who are hypotensive Is generally preferred by patients for sleeping

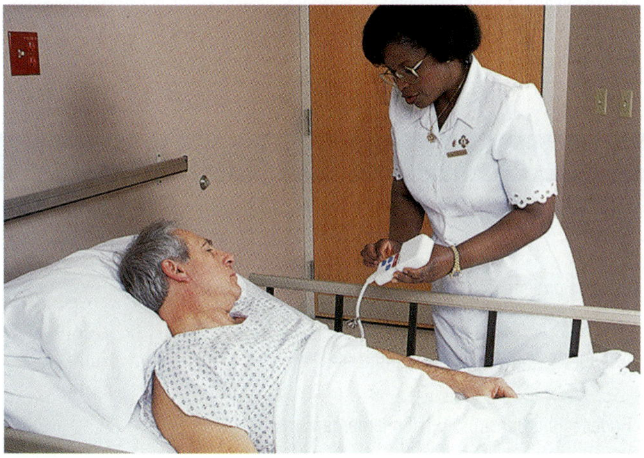

FIGURE 39.13 Instruct patient in use of call light and bed controls.

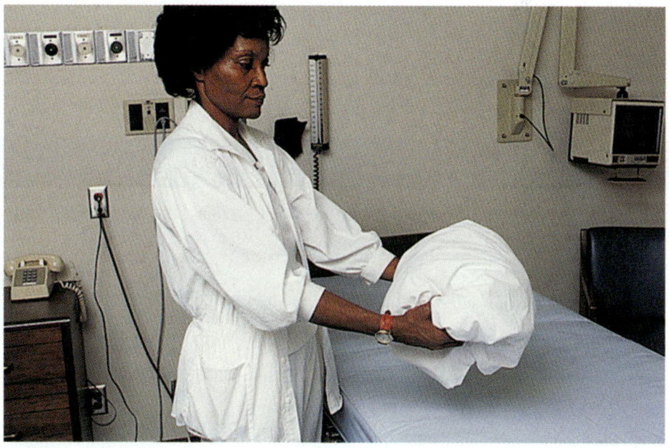

FIGURE 39.14 Holding linen away from the uniform prevents contact with microorganisms.

When patients are confined to a bed, organize bed-making activities to conserve time and energy (Figure 39.15 and Skill 39.5). The patient's privacy, comfort, and safety are all important. To help promote comfort and safety, use side rails to aid positioning and turning, keep a call light within the patient's reach, and maintain the proper bed position. After making a bed, always return it to the lowest horizontal position to prevent accidental falls should the patient get in and out of the bed alone.

When possible, a bed should be made while it is unoccupied (Box 39.16). Use clinical judgement regarding the best time to have the patient sit up in a chair while the bed is being made. When making an unoccupied bed, follow the basic principles for making an occupied bed.

An unoccupied bed can be open or closed. In an open bed, the top covers are folded back so that a patient can easily get into bed. In a closed bed, the top sheet, blanket, and bedspread are drawn up to the head of the mattress and under the pillows. A closed bed is prepared in a hospital room before a new patient is admitted to that room.

A surgical, recovery, or postoperative bed is a modified version of the open bed. The top bed linen is arranged for easy transfer of the

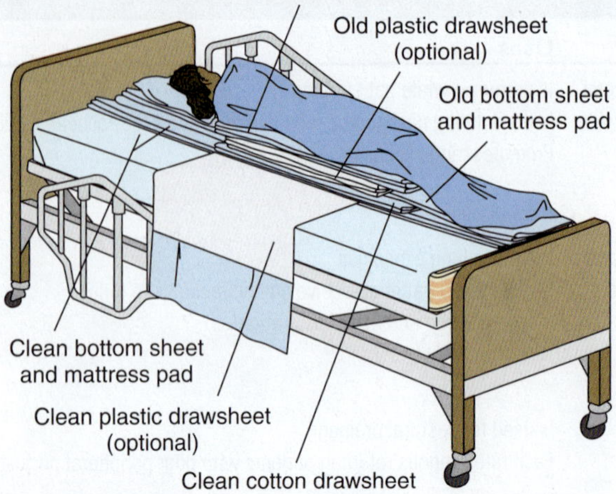

FIGURE 39.15 Equipment for making an occupied bed.

Labels (clockwise from top):
Old cotton drawsheet
Old plastic drawsheet (optional)
Old bottom sheet and mattress pad
Clean cotton drawsheet
Clean plastic drawsheet (optional)
Clean bottom sheet and mattress pad

patient from a stretcher to the bed. The top sheets and bedspread are not tucked or mitred at the corners. Instead, the top sheets are folded to one side or to the bottom third of the bed (Figure 39.16). This makes it easier to transfer the patient into the bed.

Linens. In any health care agency, it is important to have an adequate supply of linen to care appropriately for patients. Many agencies have "nurse servers," either within or just outside a patient's room, where a daily supply of linen is stored. Because of the emphasis on cost control in health care, it is important to not bring excess linen into a patient's room. Linen brought into a patient's room, if unused, must be discarded for laundering, which can increase an agency's costs. Excess linen lying around a patient's room creates clutter and obstacles for patient care activities.

Before bed making, it is important to collect necessary bed linen and the patient's personal items. In this way, the nurse has all equipment accessible to prepare the bed and room. Linens are pressed and folded to help prevent the spread of microorganisms and to make bed making easier. When fitted sheets are not available, flat sheets usually

SKILL 39.5	MAKING AN OCCUPIED BED

Delegation Considerations

The skill of making an occupied bed can be delegated to an unregulated care provider (UCP). It is important to discuss the following with the UCP:
- Any precautions or activity restrictions for the patient
- What to do if wound drainage, dressing material, drainage tubes, or IV tubing becomes dislodged or is found in the linens
- What to do if the patient becomes fatigued

Equipment

See Figure 39.15.
- Linen bag(s)
- Bottom sheet (flat or fitted)
- Drawsheet (optional)
- Top sheet
- Blanket
- Bedspread
- Waterproof pads or soaker pad (optional)
- Pillowcases
- Bedside chair or table
- Disposable gloves (optional)
- Towel
- Disinfectant

PROCEDURE

STEPS	RATIONALE
1. Assess potential for patient incontinence or excess drainage on bed linen.	• Determines the need for protective waterproof pads or extra bath blankets on the bed.
2. Check chart for orders or specific precautions concerning movement and positioning.	• Ensures patient safety and the use of proper body mechanics.
3. Explain procedure to the patient, noting that they will be asked to turn on their side and roll over the linen.	• Minimizes anxiety and encourages cooperation.
4. Perform hand hygiene and put on gloves. (Gloves are worn only if linen is soiled or if contact with body secretions is possible.)	• Reduces the transmission of microorganisms.
5. Assemble equipment and arrange it on a bedside chair or table. Remove unnecessary equipment such as a dietary tray or items used for hygiene.	• Assembling all equipment provides for a smooth procedure and assists in increasing the patient's comfort. Placing linen on a clean surface minimizes spread of infection.
6. Draw room curtain around bed or close room door.	• Maintains patient's privacy.
7. Adjust bed height to a comfortable working position. Lower any raised side rail on one side of the bed. Remove the call light.	• Minimizes strain on the back. It is easier to remove and put on linen evenly with the bed in a flat position. Provides easy access to bed and linen.
8. Loosen top linen at foot of the bed.	• Makes linen easier to remove.
9. Remove bedspread and blanket separately. If bedspread and blanket are soiled, place them in a linen bag. Keep soiled linen away from your uniform.	• Reduces the transmission of microorganisms.

| SKILL 39.5 | MAKING AN OCCUPIED BED—cont'd |
| STEPS | RATIONALE |

10. If blanket and bedspread are to be reused, fold them by bringing the top and bottom edges together. Fold the farthest side over onto nearer bottom edge. Bring top and bottom edges together again. Place folded linen over back of chair.

• Folding method facilitates replacement and minimizes wrinkles.

11. Cover patient with a bath blanket in the following manner: Unfold bath blanket over the top sheet. Ask patient to hold top edge of the bath blanket. If patient is unable to help, tuck top of bath blanket under the patient's shoulder. Grasp top sheet under bath blanket at patient's shoulders and bring sheet down to the foot of the bed. Remove the sheet and discard in a linen bag.

• A bath blanket provides warmth and keeps body parts covered during linen removal.

12. With assistance from another person, slide mattress toward the head of the bed.

• If mattress slides toward the foot of the bed when head of the bed is raised, it is difficult to tuck in linen. In addition, it is uncomfortable for the patient because the patient's feet may be pressed against or hang over the foot of the bed.

13. Position patient on the far side of the bed, turned onto their side and facing away from you. Be sure the side rail in front of the patient is up. Adjust pillow under the patient's head.

• Turning patient onto their side provides space for placement of clean linen. Side rail ensures the patient's safety, preventing forward falls from the bed surface, and helps the patient move.

14. Loosen bottom linens, moving from head to foot. With seam side down (facing the mattress), fanfold bottom sheet and drawsheet toward patient—first drawsheet, then bottom sheet. Tuck edges of linen just under patient's buttocks, back, and shoulders. Do not fanfold mattress pad if it is to be reused (see Step 14 illustration).

• Prepares for removal of all bottom linen simultaneously. Provides maximum workspace for placing clean linen. Later, when patient turns to the other side, soiled linen can be removed easily.

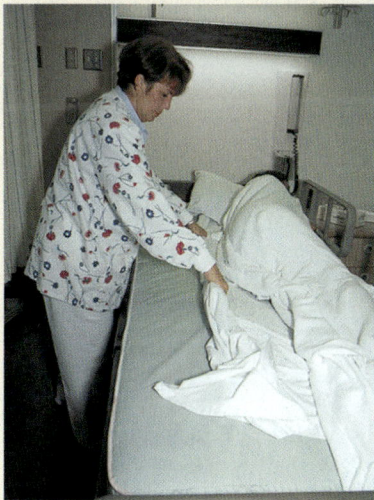
STEP 14 Old linen tucked under patient.

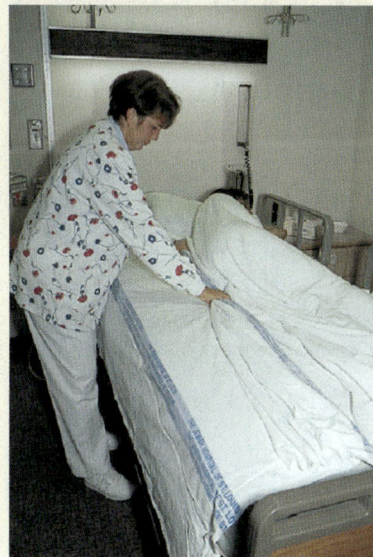
STEP 16B Clean linen applied to bed.

15. Wipe off any moisture on exposed mattress with towel and appropriate disinfectant.

• Reduces the transmission of microorganisms.

16. Put clean linen on exposed half of the bed:

A. Place clean mattress pad on bed by folding it lengthwise with centre crease in middle of the bed. Fanfold top layer over mattress. (If pad is reused, simply smooth out any wrinkles.)

• Putting on linen over the bed in successive layers minimizes energy and time used in bed making.

B. Unfold bottom sheet lengthwise so that centre crease is situated lengthwise along centre of bed. Fanfold sheet's top layer toward centre of bed alongside the patient. Smooth bottom layer of sheet over mattress and bring the edge over closest side of the mattress. Pull fitted sheet smoothly over mattress ends. Allow edge of flat unfitted sheet to hang about 25 cm over mattress edge. Lower hem of the bottom flat sheet should lie seam down and even with bottom edge of the mattress (see Step 16B illustration).

• Proper positioning of linen on one side ensures that adequate linen will be available to cover opposite side of the bed. Keeping seam edges down eliminates irritation to patient's skin.

Continued

SKILL 39.5   **MAKING AN OCCUPIED BED—cont'd**

STEPS	RATIONALE

17. Mitre bottom flat sheet at head of the bed (if fitted sheets are not in use):

  A. Face head of bed diagonally. Place your hand away from head of bed under top corner of the mattress, near mattress edge, and lift.

  B. With your other hand, tuck top edge of bottom sheet smoothly under the mattress so that side edges of sheet above and below the mattress would meet if brought together.

  C. Face side of the bed and pick up top edge of sheet at approximately 45 cm from top of mattress (see Step 17C illustration).

  D. Lift sheet and lay it on top of the mattress to form a neat triangular fold, with lower base of the triangle even with the mattress side edge (see Step 17D illustration).

- Mitred corner cannot be loosened easily even if the patient moves frequently in bed.

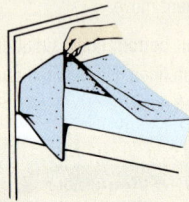

STEP 17C Pick up top edge of sheet.

STEP 17D Sheet on top of mattress in a triangular fold.

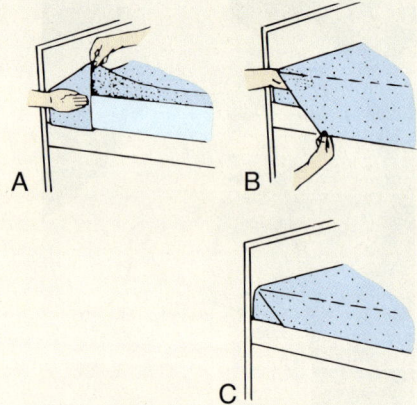

STEP 17E Lower edge of sheet tucked under mattress.

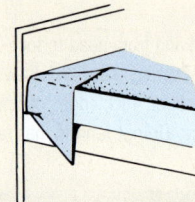

STEP 17F **A and B**, Triangular fold placed over side of mattress. **C**, Linen tucked under mattress.

  E. Tuck lower edge of sheet, which is hanging free below the mattress, under the mattress. Tuck with your palms down, without pulling triangular fold (see Step 17E illustration).

  F. Hold portion of sheet covering side of the mattress in place with one hand. With the other hand, pick up top of triangular linen fold and bring it down over side of the mattress (see Step 17F illustrations). Tuck this portion under the mattress (see Step 17F illustrations).

18. Tuck remaining portion of sheet under the mattress, moving toward foot of the bed. Keep linen smooth.

- Folds of linen are a source of irritation for the patient.

19. *(Optional)* Open drawsheet so that it unfolds in half. Lay centre fold along middle of bed lengthwise and position sheet so that it will be under the patient's buttocks and torso (see Step 19 illustration). Fanfold top layer toward the patient, with edge along the patient's back. Smooth bottom layer out over the mattress and tuck excess edge under the mattress (keep your palms down).

- Drawsheet is used to lift and reposition the patient. Placement under the patient's torso distributes most of the patient's body weight over the sheet.

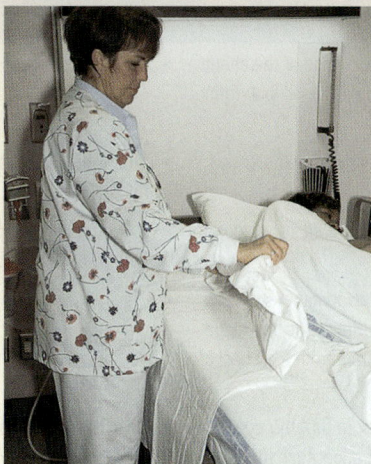

STEP 19 Optional drawsheet.

20. Place waterproof pad over drawsheet, with centre fold against the patient's side. Fanfold top layer toward the patient.

• Protects bed linen from being soiled.

21. Have patient roll slowly toward you, over the layers of linen. Raise side rail on working side and then go to the other side of the bed.

• Positions patient for removal and placement of linens. Maintains patient's safety and body alignment during turning.

22. Lower side rail. Assist patient in positioning on other side, over folds of linen (see Step 22 illustration). Loosen edges of soiled linen from under mattress.

• Exposes opposite side of bed for removal of soiled linen and placement of clean linen. Makes linen easier to remove.

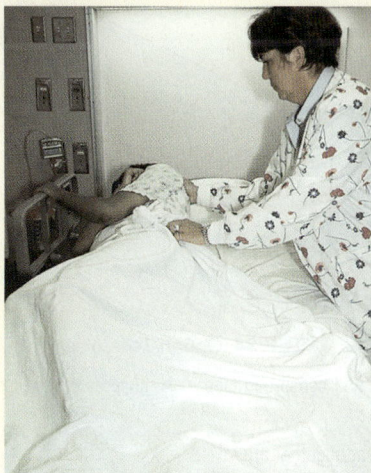

STEP 22 Assist patient to roll over folds of linen.

23. Remove soiled linen by folding it into a bundle or square, with soiled side turned in. Discard in linen bag. If necessary, wipe the mattress with antiseptic solution and dry mattress surface before putting on new linen.

• Reduces the transmission of microorganisms.

24. Pull clean, fanfolded linen smoothly over edge of mattress from head to foot of the bed.

• Smooth linen will not irritate patient's skin.

25. Assist patient in rolling back into supine position. Reposition pillow.

• Maintains patient's comfort.

26. Pull fitted sheet smoothly over mattress ends. Mitre top corner of bottom sheet (see Step 17). When tucking corner, be sure that sheet is smooth and free of wrinkles.

• Wrinkles and folds can cause irritation to the skin.

27. Facing side of the bed, grasp remaining edge of bottom flat sheet. Lean back; keeping your back straight, pull while tucking excess linen under the mattress. Proceed from head to foot of the bed. (Avoid lifting mattress during tucking to ensure fit.)

• Proper use of body mechanics while tucking linen prevents injury.

Continued

SKILL 39.5   MAKING AN OCCUPIED BED—cont'd

STEPS	RATIONALE
28. Smooth fanfolded drawsheet out over bottom sheet. Grasp edge of the sheet with your palms down, lean back, and tuck sheet under mattress. Tuck from middle to top and then to bottom.	• Tucking first at top or bottom may pull sheet sideways, causing poor fit.
29. Place top sheet over patient with centre fold lengthwise down middle of bed. Open sheet from head to foot and unfold over patient.	• Sheet should be equally distributed over bed by correctly positioning centre fold.
30. Ask patient to hold clean top sheet, or tuck sheet around patient's shoulders. Remove the bath blanket and discard in linen bag.	• Sheet prevents exposure of body parts. Having patient hold sheet encourages patient participation in care.
31. Place blanket on bed, unfolding it so that the crease runs lengthwise along the middle of the bed. Unfold blanket to cover the patient. The top edge should be parallel with edge of the top sheet and 15–20 cm from top sheet's edge.	• Blanket should be placed to cover patient completely and provide adequate warmth.
32. Place bedspread over the bed according to Step 31. Be sure that top edge of the bedspread extends about 2.5 cm above the blanket's edge. Tuck top edge of bedspread over and under top edge of the blanket.	• Gives the bed a neat appearance and provides extra warmth.
33. Make cuff by turning edge of top sheet down over top edge of the blanket and bedspread.	• Protects patient's face from rubbing against blanket or bedspread.
34. Standing on one side at foot of the bed, lift mattress corner slightly with one hand and tuck linens under mattress. Tuck top sheet and blanket under together. Be sure that linens are loose enough to allow movement of the patient's feet. Making a horizontal toe pleat is optional (see Step 34 illustration).	• Makes neat-appearing bed. Pressure injuries can develop on patient's toes and heels from feet rubbing against tight-fitting bed sheets.

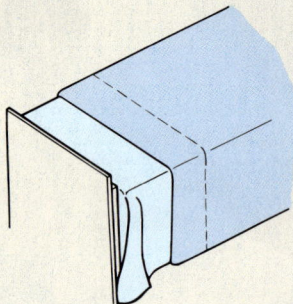

STEP 34 Optional toe pleat.

35. Make modified mitred corner with top sheet, blanket, and bedspread (see Box 39.16, Step 20 illustration):	• Ensures that top covers will not loosen easily.
A. Pick up side edge of top sheet, blanket, and bedspread together approximately 45 cm from foot of the mattress. Lift linen to form a triangular fold and lay it on the bed.	
B. Tuck lower edge of sheet, which is hanging free below mattress, under the mattress. Do not pull triangular fold.	
C. Pick up triangular fold and bring it down over mattress while holding linen in place alongside of the mattress. Do not tuck tip of triangle.	• Secures top linen but keeps even edge of blanket and top sheet draped over mattress.
36. Raise side rail. Make other side of bed; spread the sheet, blanket, and bedspread out evenly. Fold top edge of bedspread over the blanket and make cuff with top sheet (see Step 33); make modified mitred corner at foot of the bed (see Step 35).	• Side rail protects patient from accidental falls.
37. Change pillowcase:	
A. Have patient raise their head. While supporting the patient's neck with one hand, remove the pillow. Allow the patient to lower head.	• Support of neck muscles prevents injury during flexion and extension of neck.
B. Remove soiled case by grasping pillow at open end with one hand and pulling case back over pillow with the other hand. Discard case in linen bag.	• Pillows slide out easily, thus minimizing contact with soiled linen.

SKILL 39.5	MAKING AN OCCUPIED BED—cont'd
STEPS	**RATIONALE**
C. Grasp clean pillowcase at centre of closed end. Gather case, turning it inside out over the hand holding it. With the same hand, pick up the middle of one end of the pillow. Pull pillowcase down over pillow with the other hand.	• Eases sliding of pillowcase over pillow.
D. Be sure pillow corners fit evenly into corners of the pillowcase. Place pillow under the patient's head.	• Poorly fitting case constricts fluffing and expansion of the pillow and interferes with patient comfort.
38. Place call bell within the patient's reach and return the bed to a comfortable position.	• Ensures patient safety and comfort.
39. Open room curtains and rearrange furniture. Place personal items within easy reach on the overbed table or bedside stand. Return bed to a comfortable height.	• Promotes sense of well-being.
40. Discard dirty linen in a hamper or chute, remove gloves, and perform hand hygiene.	• Helps prevent the transmission of microorganisms.
41. Ask whether the patient feels comfortable.	• Ensures that bed linens are clean and smooth.
42. While you are performing this skill, inspect the patient's skin for areas of irritation.	• Folds in linen can cause pressure on the skin.
43. Observe the patient for signs of fatigue, dyspnea, pain, or discomfort throughout the skill.	• Provides data about patient's level of activity tolerance and ability to participate in other procedures.

UNEXPECTED OUTCOMES	**RELATED INTERVENTIONS**
Discomfort caused by linen fold	• Tighten sheets. • Change patient's position frequently.
Signs of breakdown of patient's skin	• Institute skin care measures to reduce risk of pressure injury (see Chapter 47). • Change patient's position frequently.

RECORDING AND REPORTING
• Making an occupied bed need not be recorded.

BOX 39.16 PROCEDURAL GUIDELINE
Making an Unoccupied Bed

Delegation Considerations
The skill of making an unoccupied bed can be delegated to an unregulated care provider (UCP).

Equipment
• Linen bag
• Bottom sheet (flat or fitted)
• Drawsheet (optional)
• Top sheet
• Blanket
• Bedspread
• Waterproof pads or soaker pad (optional)
• Pillowcases
• Bedside chair or table
• Disposable gloves (if linen is soiled)
• Washcloth
• Antiseptic cleanser

Procedure
1. Determine whether patient has been incontinent or excess drainage is on linen. Gloves will be necessary.
2. Assess activity orders or restrictions in mobility to plan whether patient can get out of bed for the procedure. If so, assist patient to bedside chair or recliner.
3. Raise bed to a comfortable working position. Lower the side rails on both sides of the bed.

BOX 39.16 PROCEDURAL GUIDELINE—cont'd
Making an Unoccupied Bed

4. Remove soiled linen and place in linen bag. Avoid shaking or fanning linen.
5. Reposition mattress and wipe off any moisture using a washcloth moistened in antiseptic solution. Dry thoroughly.
6. Put on all bottom linen on one side of bed before moving to opposite side.
7. Be sure fitted sheet is placed smoothly over mattress. To put on a flat unfitted sheet, allow about 25 cm to hang over mattress edge. The lower hem of the sheet should lie seam down, even with bottom edge of the mattress. Pull remaining top portion of sheet over top edge of the mattress.
8. While standing at head of the bed, mitre top corner of bottom sheet (see Skill 39.5, Step 17).
9. Tuck remaining portion of unfitted sheet under the mattress.
10. *Optional and agency or facility specific:* Put on a drawsheet, laying centre fold along middle of the bed lengthwise. Smooth drawsheet over the mattress and tuck excess edge under mattress, keeping palms down.
11. Move to opposite side of the bed and spread bottom sheet smoothly over edge of mattress from head to foot of the bed.
12. Put on fitted sheet smoothly over each mattress corner. For an unfitted sheet, mitre the top corner of bottom sheet (see Skill 39.5, Step 17), making sure corner is taut.
13. Grasp remaining edge of unfitted bottom sheet and tuck tightly under the mattress while moving from head to foot of the bed. Smooth folded drawsheet over the bottom sheet and tuck under mattress, first at middle, then at top, and then at bottom.
14. If needed, put on a waterproof pad or soaker pad over bottom sheet.
15. Place top sheet over bed with vertical centre fold lengthwise down middle of the bed. Open sheet out from head to foot, being sure top edge of the sheet is even with top edge of the mattress.
16. Make horizontal toe pleat (optional): Stand at foot of bed and fanfold sheet 5–10 cm across bed. Pull sheet up from bottom to make fold approximately 15 cm from bottom edge of the mattress (see Skill 39.5, Step 34).

17. Tuck in remaining portion of the sheet under foot of mattress. Place blanket over the bed with top edge parallel to top edge of sheet and 15–20 cm down from edge of sheet. (*Optional:* Put on additional bedspread over bed.)
18. Make cuff by turning edge of top sheet down over top edge of the blanket and bedspread.
19. Standing on one side at foot of the bed, lift mattress corner slightly with one hand, and with the other hand tuck top sheet, blanket, and bedspread under the mattress. Be sure the pleats are not pulled out.
20. Make modified mitred corner with top sheet, blanket, and bedspread. After triangular fold is made, do not tuck tip of triangle (see Step 20 illustration).

STEP 20 Modified mitred corner.

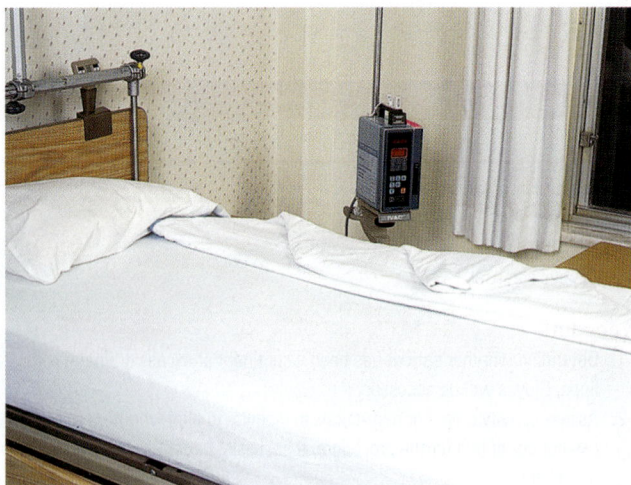

21. Go to other side of the bed. Spread sheet, blanket, and bedspread out evenly. Make cuff with top sheet and blanket. Make modified mitred corner at foot of the bed.
22. Put on clean pillowcase.
23. Place call light within patient's reach on a bed rail or pillow and return bed to height allowing for patient transfer. Assist the patient in getting into bed.
24. Arrange patient's room. Remove and discard supplies. Perform hand hygiene.

FIGURE 39.16 Surgical or recovery bed.

are pressed with a centre crease to be placed down the centre of the bed. The linen unfolds easily to the sides, with creases often fitting over the mattress edge. A complete linen change is not always necessary. The sheet, blanket, and bedspread may be reused for the same patient if they are not wet or soiled.

Disposal of linen must be done in such a way as to minimize the spread of infection (see Chapter 34). Agency policies provide guidelines for the proper way to bag and dispose of soiled linen. After a patient is discharged, all bed linens are sent to the laundry, the mattress and bed are cleaned by housekeeping staff, and new bed linen is applied.

◆ Evaluation
Patient Care. Evaluation of hygiene measures occurs both during and after each particular skill. For example, while bathing a patient, closely inspect the skin to determine whether drainage or other soiling has been effectively removed from the skin's surface. Once the bath is completed, ask the patient whether their comfort and relaxation have improved. When evaluating for the effectiveness of hygiene measures, observe for changes in the patient's behaviour. Does the patient assume a more relaxed position? Is the patient free of body odour? Is the patient able to fall asleep? Does the patient's facial expression convey a sense of comfort?

Frequently, it takes time for hygiene care to result in an improvement in a patient's condition. The presence of oral lesions, a scalp infestation, or skin excoriation often requires repeated measures and a combination of nursing interventions. Evaluate for improvement in the patient's condition over time and determine whether existing therapies are effective.

Throughout evaluation, consider the goals of care and evaluate whether expected outcomes are achieved. A critical thinking approach ensures that consideration is given to all factors when evaluating a patient's care (Figure 39.17). Knowledge base and experience provide important perspectives when analyzing observations made about a patient. For example, once the nurse has seen how dehydration of the oral mucosa clears with repeated hygiene, it helps them to recognize when progress in another patient is slow. The standards for evaluation are the expected outcomes established in the planning stage of the patient's care. If outcomes are not met, the care plan may need to be revised. Continual application of critical thinking and clinical judgement is necessary when considering all evaluation findings.

Patient Expectations. The final portion of the evaluation considers whether a patient's expectations have been met through hygiene care. The nurse might ask the patient, "Do you feel your bath and back rub helped to make you comfortable?" "Can you suggest ways in which we can improve your foot care?" "What further measures do you think are necessary to keep your mouth clean and refreshed?"

Patients' expectations are important guidelines in determining patient satisfaction. As the care provider, you must feel comfortable in addressing your patients' concerns and expectations. A caring approach can facilitate a discussion of these issues.

Patient Education About Infant Hygiene. An additional critical component to the nursing process and evaluation is education. While this chapter largely focuses on the care of the adult, the same principles of comfort and safety apply for infants. For nurses who are caring for a new parent and infant, infant hygiene is a critical piece of patient education.

It is recommended that infants not be bathed daily; instead, each day wipe the baby's face, neck, hands, and diaper area, in that order (see Box 39.17 for steps in infant bathing). Safety is of utmost importance when bathing an infant (see Box 39.18 for some infant hygiene recommendations). Always have at least one hand on the infant while in the tub. Also, never leave the infant alone while in the tub. If possible, the home's hot water tank should be set below 49°C. Cotton swabs, bath seats or rings, and bath oils should not be used. Cotton swabs can hurt

BOX 39.17 Infant Bathing Steps

1. Ensure that the room is warm: 22 to 27°C.
2. Use a sink, basin, or baby tub.
3. Lay out a blanket or towel.
4. Ensure that everything needed for the bath is within reach.
5. Use warm, not hot water.
6. Wash parts from cleanest to dirtiest. Start with the face, using only water, ending with the diaper area.
7. Use a mild unscented soap on visibly dirty areas.
8. Use mild unscented soap or baby shampoo on baby's hair, and rinse well.
9. Place infant on the towel and pat dry with careful attention to drying skin folds. Move quickly, because infants can become cold quickly.

Data from HealthLink BC. (2021). *Baby's best chance: Parents' handbook of pregnancy and baby care.* https://www.healthlinkbc.ca/pregnancy-parenting/babys-best-chance

BOX 39.18 Infant Hygiene and Safety Recommendations

Ears
Only the outer part of the ear should be cleaned, using a washcloth wrapped around your finger. Cotton swabs should not be used.

Oral Care
Wipe gums daily with a damp, clean cloth. Once the first teeth appear, use a soft baby toothbrush and a rice-sized dab of fluoride toothpaste in the morning and at bedtime.

Nails
Nails should be kept trimmed to keep the infant from scratching themselves. Trimming the infant's nails while they're asleep or calm, or following a bath when the nails are softer, is recommended.

Umbilical Cord Care
The umbilical area should be kept dry as much as possible. After bathing and diaper changes, wipe the area with a damp washcloth and dry well. When putting on a diaper, fold it down so that it lies below the cord.

After the cord falls off (around 5 to 15 days), clean the belly button for a few days. If the area around the cord is warm, red, or swollen, or has a foul-smelling discharge, or if the cord won't dry out, the health care provider should be called.

Genitals
Gently clean between the outer folds of the labia for infants with female genitalia. Don't pull on the foreskin of infants with male genitalia.

Data from HealthLink BC. (2021). *Baby's best chance: Parents' handbook of pregnancy and baby care.* https://www.healthlinkbc.ca/pregnancy-parenting/babys-best-chance

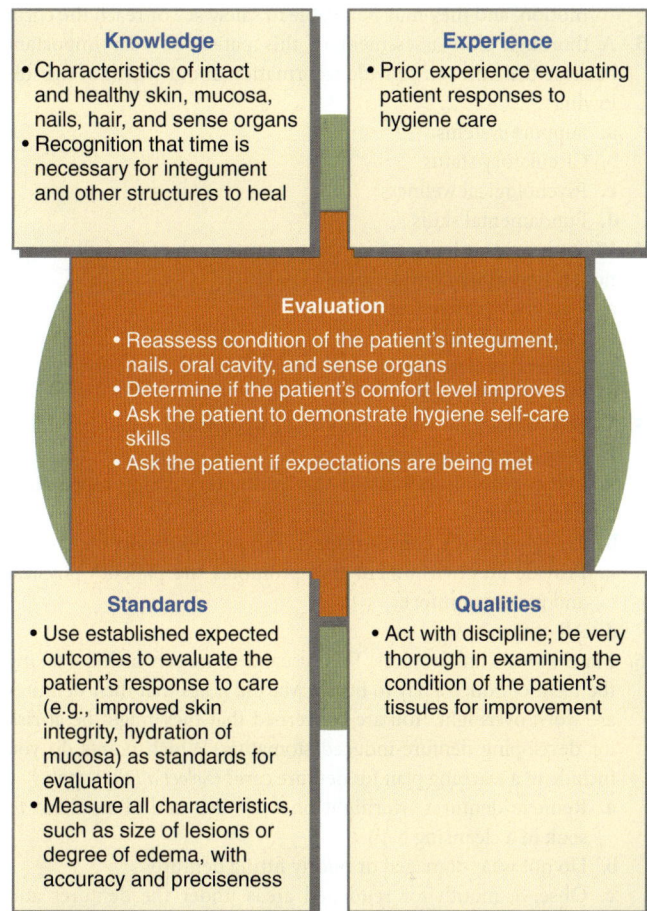

FIGURE 39.17 Critical thinking model for hygiene evaluation.

delicate areas like the ears. Bath seats or rings pose a drowning danger. Finally, bath oils will make the tub and the infant slippery and more vulnerable to slipping out of the caregiver's hands.

KEY CONCEPTS

- Nurses determine a patient's ability to perform self-care and provide hygiene care according to the patient's needs and preferences.
- During hygiene care, the nurse can integrate other activities such as physical assessment, wound care, and range-of-motion exercises.
- While providing daily hygiene needs, nurses use teaching and communication skills in developing a caring relationship with the patient.
- Various personal, sociocultural, socioeconomic, and developmental factors influence patients' hygiene practices.
- Patients' health beliefs predict the likelihood of their assuming health-promoting behaviour, such as the maintenance of good hygiene.
- Nurses might not assess all body regions before administering hygiene; however, routine assessment of the patient's condition is undertaken whenever care is given.
- Patients with reduced sensation, vascular insufficiency, and immobility are at greater risk for impaired skin integrity.
- Before carrying out basic hygiene measures, nurses must perform an assessment of each patient's physical and cognitive abilities, including muscle strength, flexibility and dexterity, balance, coordination, activity tolerance, and ability to comprehend. For patients suffering symptoms such as pain or nausea, administering symptom relief therapies before performing hygiene procedures better prepares the patient.
- Patients with diabetes mellitus require special nail and foot care.
- When administering oral care to unconscious patients, measures must be taken to prevent aspiration.
- A patient's room should be comfortable, safe, and uncluttered, to provide for patient comfort and safety.
- An evaluation of hygiene care is based on the patient's sense of comfort, relaxation, well-being, and understanding of hygiene techniques.

CRITICAL THINKING EXERCISES

1. Jack (he/him), a 19-year-old, remains in the hospital after a motorcycle accident in which he suffered multiple traumatic injuries. Jack has limited mobility due to casts to his left leg and arm. Discuss important factors to consider when administering hygiene care. Identify two nursing diagnoses and interventions, with rationales.
2. Marian (they/their), a 40-year-old, was admitted to the hospital for treatment of a malignant breast lesion. Marian is undergoing chemotherapy along with radiation treatment. During your assessment, Marian reports a loss of appetite, nausea and vomiting, and sores in their mouth. Marian is suffering from stomatitis. Identify two nursing diagnoses and interventions, with rationales.
3. Michelle (she/her), a 78-year-old, was transferred from an acute care hospital to a rehabilitation facility after a cerebrovascular accident. Michelle exhibits right hemiparesis and aphasia and is incontinent of urine and stool. During the initial assessment, you discover that Michelle has reddened areas on both heels, and her perineum and buttocks are excoriated. Identify two priority nursing diagnoses.

Discuss at least three factors that contributed to Michelle's impaired skin integrity.

Answers to Critical Thinking Exercises appear on the Evolve website.

REVIEW QUESTIONS

Review Questions 1 to 10 relate to the case study at the beginning of the chapter.

1. The patient's diabetes mellitus is considered when planning their care. In providing teaching on foot care, which of the following is most important to include?
   a. Daily inspection of their feet
   b. Application of lotion to the feet and between the toes daily
   c. Daily soaking of the feet in hot water
   d. Cutting the toenails in the shape of a curve
2. As part of your foot assessment, you notice that the patient has a corn on the sole of their foot. The patient reports that they have been trying to remove it from the bottom of their foot with a pair of scissors. Patient teaching should include which of the following?
   a. Increased circulation in the feet could cause severe bleeding if they were to injure the foot with the scissors.
   b. Peripheral vascular disease increases the risk of developing more corns.
   c. Diabetes mellitus places them at an increased risk for infection if there is an open wound on the foot.
   d. Their chronic disease and body habitus limits their range of motion, and they may be unable to safely see or reach the corn.
3. A thorough skin assessment of this patient is very important because the skin can provide information about which of the following?
   a. Support systems
   b. Circulatory status
   c. Psychological wellness
   d. Fundamental skills
4. When providing hair care for the patient, which of the following is not an important consideration?
   a. Caregiver preferences
   b. Family preferences
   c. Cultural preferences
   d. Patient preferences
5. Which of the following is important to consider when providing hygiene care for this patient?
   a. Use communication skills that promote a caring therapeutic relationship.
   b. Provide privacy, convey respect, and promote independence.
   c. Provide an environment that promotes the patient's physical and mental comfort.
   d. All of the above.
6. Martha wears full dentures. Their usual denture care includes taking the teeth out once a day to brush. Martha notes that their dentures are worn overnight. You are concerned that they might be at risk for developing denture-induced stomatitis. Which points do you include in a teaching plan for denture care? *(Select all that apply.)*
   a. Remove dentures overnight once a week and allow them to soak in a cleansing bath.
   b. Do not wear damaged or poorly fitting dentures.
   c. Observe mouth for reddened areas under the dentures and small red sores on the roof of the mouth.

d. See a dentist regularly.

e. Rinse dentures after meals.

f. Clean dentures every night with cleanser, rinsing well before replacing in their mouth at bedtime.

7. Because of Martha's body habitus, you have recommended several adaptive devices to assist with independent self-care while bathing, which include a shower chair, grab rails, and back sponges. What is the most important consideration when making recommendations to the patient about adaptive devices?

a. Cost of the device and supplies

b. The device ensures patient safety

c. The device maximizes independence

d. Ease of use of the device

8. Why would you include oxygenation as part of your hygiene assessment for this patient?

a. The nasal cannula can cause skin breakdown.

b. Excess moisture and condensation in the tubing is a hotbed for bacterial growth.

c. Continuous oxygen flow can cause nasal dryness and nosebleeds.

d. All of the above.

9. Martha expresses difficulty with perineal care and requests assistance as part of their care planning. Martha notes discomfort and burning in the perineal area but seems appears embarrassed about you assessing the area. What action should you take, initially?

a. Explain that because of these symptoms, you need to observe the perineal area.

b. Insist that only the nurse or home care worker complete their perineal care.

c. Honour the patient's request and don't assess the perineum, to avoid further embarrassment to the patient.

d. Ask if a family member can complete their perineal care.

10. Martha has limited mobility and sits for most of the day in a recliner chair. You notice they have a stage 1 pressure injury on the sacral area. When educating the patient on preventing further

breakdown of the current pressure injury and how to prevent other ones from forming, which following information would you NOT include?

a. Exercise the extremities both actively and passively.

b. Turn and reposition yourself every 2 hours.

c. Keep the skin moist and add extra linens under the sacral area.

d. Use pillows to elevate bony prominences.

Answers: 1. a; **2.** c; **3.** b; **4.** a; **5.** d; **6.** b; **7.** d; **8.** f; **9.** a; **10.** c.

Rationales for the Review Questions appear on the Evolve website.

RECOMMENDED WEBSITES

Alzheimer Society of Canada: https://www.alzheimer.ca
The Alzheimer Society of Canada website offers important information on Alzheimer's disease and other dementias, treatment, research, support, and services.

Canadian Dental Association: https://www.cda-adc.ca
The Canadian Dental Association website offers information on maintaining optimal oral health, including oral hygiene for older persons.

Diabetes Canada: https://www.diabetes.ca
The Diabetes Canada website offers information on the various types of diabetes, treatment, research, and services.

Public Health Agency of Canada: https://www.publichealth.gc.ca
This website is a valuable resource offering information on healthy living, disease, and injury prevention.

REFERENCES

A full reference list is available on the website for this book at http://evolve.elsevier.com/Canada/Potter/fundamentals/

Cardiopulmonary Functioning and Oxygenation

Canadian content written by Giuliana Harvey, RN, PhD, and Heather MacLean, RN, MN, CHSE, CCNE, CCSNE, with original chapter contributions by Carolyn J. Wright Boon, MSN, BSN

OBJECTIVES

Mastery of content in this chapter will enable you to:

- Define the key terms listed.
- Describe the structure and function of the cardiopulmonary system.
- Identify the physiological processes of cardiac output, myocardial blood flow, and coronary artery circulation.
- Diagram the electrical conduction system of the heart.
- Describe the relationship among cardiac output, preload, afterload, contractility, and heart rate.
- Identify the physiological processes involved in ventilation, perfusion, and exchange of respiratory gases.

- Describe the neural and chemical regulation of respiration.
- Describe the impact of a patient's level of health and their age, lifestyle, culture, and environment on cardiopulmonary oxygenation.
- Identify and describe clinical outcomes as a result of disturbances in conduction, altered cardiac output, impaired valvular function, myocardial ischemia, and impaired tissue perfusion.
- Identify and describe clinical outcomes of hyperventilation, hypoventilation, and hypoxemia.
- Identify nursing care interventions in the primary care, acute care, and restorative and continuing care settings that promote oxygenation.

KEY TERMS

Acute coronary syndrome
Afterload
Anemia
Arrythmias
Asystole
Atelectasis
Atrial fibrillation
Bronchoscopy
Cardiac index (CI)
Cardiac output
Cardiopulmonary rehabilitation
Cardiopulmonary resuscitation (CPR)
Chest physiotherapy (CPT)
Chest tube
Cor pulmonale
Cyanosis
Diaphragmatic breathing
Diffusion
Dyspnea
Dysrhythmias

Electrocardiogram (ECG)
Expiration
Hematemesis
Hemoptysis
Hemothorax
High-flow devices
Humidification
Hypercapnia
Hyperventilation
Hypoventilation
Hypovolemia
Hypoxia
Incentive spirometry
Inspiration
Low-flow devices
Myocardial contractility
Myocardial infarction (MI)
Myocardial ischemia
Nasal cannula
Nebulization

Non-ST-segment elevation myocardial infarction (NSTEMI)
Normal sinus rhythm (NSR)
Orthopnea
Pneumothorax
Postural drainage
Preload
Pulse oximeter
Pursed-lip breathing
Stable angina pectoris
ST-elevation myocardial infarction (STEMI)
Stroke volume
Subcutaneous emphysema
Unstable angina
Ventilation
Ventricular fibrillation
Ventricular tachycardia
Wheezing

🌐 WEBSITE

http://evolve.elsevier.com/Canada/Potter/fundamentals/

CASE STUDY

A 65-year-old patient of South Asian descent (preferred pronouns: she/her) was admitted after a myocardial infarction (MI) to the cardiac intensive care unit (CICU). Her first language is Punjabi, and she speaks minimal English. Her past medical history includes hypertension and type II diabetes. The patient is being transferred to the cardiac unit for further observation and management. The report the nurse received from the CICU indicates that the patient experienced an anterior–lateral MI. An echocardiogram indicates an ejection fraction of 35%, which confirms heart failure with respiratory complications. The nurse's assessment findings include the following:

- Neurological—Alert and oriented
- Cardiovascular—Heart sounds include the presence of S_1, S_2, and S_4, the cardiac rhythm shows a dysrhythmia, and jugular venous pressure is 5 cm.

- Respiratory—Short of breath on exertion and requires oxygen at 2 L via nasal prongs with ambulation; crackles are present at the bases bilaterally
- Gastrointestinal—Decreased appetite, bowel sounds present in four quadrants
- Genitourinary—Voiding independently
- Integumentary/Peripheral Vascular— +2 bilateral pedal edema
- Invasive—Two peripherally vascular access devices (PVAD) located in the right forearm and left antecubital fossa

Some of the patient's current medications include metoprolol, warfarin, aspirin, metformin, and Lipitor.

Think about this case study as you read this chapter. There are review questions at the end of the chapter that relate to the case study.

Oxygen is required to sustain life. The cardiac and respiratory systems function to supply the body's oxygen demands. Blood is oxygenated through the mechanisms of ventilation, perfusion, and transport of respiratory gases. Neural and chemical regulators control the rate and depth of respiration in response to tissues' changing oxygen demands.

SCIENTIFIC KNOWLEDGE BASE

Cardiovascular Physiology

Cardiopulmonary physiology involves delivery of (a) deoxygenated blood (blood that is high in carbon dioxide and low in oxygen) to the right side of the heart and to the pulmonary circulation and (b) oxygenated blood from the lungs to the left side of the heart and the tissues. The cardiac system delivers oxygen, nutrients, and other substances to the tissues and removes the waste products of cellular metabolism through the cardiac pump, the circulatory vascular system, and the integration of other systems (e.g., respiratory, digestive, and renal).

Structure and Function. The right ventricle pumps blood through the pulmonary circulation. The left ventricle pumps blood to the systemic circulation (Figure 40.1). The circulatory system exchanges respiratory gases, nutrients, and waste products between the blood and the tissues.

Myocardial Pump. The pumping action of the heart is essential to maintaining oxygen delivery. Coronary artery disease and cardiomyopathic (enlarged heart) conditions result in a diminished stroke volume (i.e., the volume of blood ejected from the ventricles) and decreased pump effectiveness. Hemorrhage and dehydration decrease pump effectiveness by decreasing the amount of blood ejected from the ventricles, thereby reducing circulating blood volume. The four chambers of the heart fill with blood during diastole and empty during systole.

The myocardial (cardiac muscle) fibres have contractile properties that enable them to stretch during filling. In a healthy heart, this stretch is proportionally related to the strength of contraction. As the myocardium stretches, the strength of the subsequent contraction increases; this is known as the *Frank–Starling (Starling's) law* of the heart. In the diseased heart, Starling's law does not apply because the stretch of the myocardium is beyond the heart's physiological limits. The subsequent contractile response results in insufficient ventricular ejection (volume), and blood begins to "back up" in the pulmonary (left heart failure) or systemic circulation (right heart failure).

Myocardial Blood Flow. To maintain adequate blood flow to the pulmonary and systemic circulation, myocardial blood flow must supply sufficient oxygen and nutrients to the myocardium itself. Blood flow through the heart is unidirectional. There are four heart valves

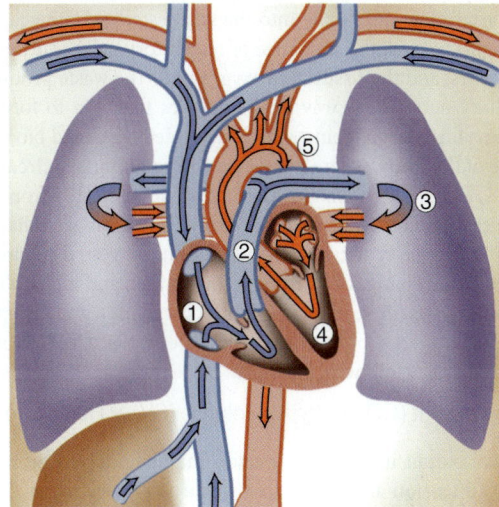

FIGURE 40.1 Schematic representation of blood flow through the heart. *Arrows* indicate direction of flow. *1,* The right atrium receives venous blood from the inferior and superior venae cavae and the coronary sinus. The blood then passes through the tricuspid valve into the right ventricle. *2,* With each contraction, the right ventricle pumps blood through the pulmonic valve into the pulmonary artery and to the lungs. *3,* Oxygenated blood flows from the lungs to the left atrium by way of the pulmonary veins. *4,* It then passes through the mitral valve and into the left ventricle. *5,* As the heart contracts, blood is ejected through the aortic valve into the aorta and thus enters the systemic circulation. (From Tyerman, J., & Cobbett, S. [Eds.]. [2023]. *Lewis's medical-surgical nursing in Canada: Assessment and management of clinical problems* [5th ed.]. Elsevier.)

that ensure this forward blood flow (see Figure 40.1). During ventricular diastole, the atrioventricular (mitral and tricuspid) valves open and blood passively flows from the higher-pressure atria into the relaxed ventricles. Toward the end of ventricular diastole, the atria contract, sending increased blood flow through the atrioventricular valves into the ventricles; this is known as "atrial kick." Ventricular pressure will continue to rise, thus causing the atrioventricular valves to close. This represents S_1, or the first heart sound. After ventricular filling, the systolic phase begins.

During the systolic phase, semilunar (aortic and pulmonic) valves open and blood flows from the ventricles into the aorta and pulmonary artery. As the ventricles empty, ventricular pressures decrease, allowing closure of the semilunar valves. Closure of these valves represents S_2, or the second heart sound. Patients with valvular disease may have backflow or regurgitation of blood through the incompetent valve, causing a murmur that is heard on auscultation (see Chapter 33 for further information about health assessment and physical examination).

Coronary Artery Circulation. Blood in the atria and ventricles does not supply oxygen and nutrients to the myocardium itself. The coronary circulation is the branch of the systemic circulation that supplies the myocardium with oxygen and nutrients and removes waste. The coronary arteries fill during ventricular diastole. The right and left coronary arteries arise from the aorta just above and behind the aortic valve through openings called the *coronary ostia* (coronary openings). The left coronary artery, the most abundant blood supply, feeds the left ventricular myocardium, which is more muscular and does most of the heart's work (Box 40.1).

Systemic Circulation. The arteries and veins of the systemic circulation deliver nutrients and oxygen to and remove waste from the tissues. Oxygenated blood flows from the left ventricle by way of the aorta and into large systemic arteries. These arteries branch into smaller arteries, into arterioles, and finally into the smallest vessels, the capillaries. At the capillary level, the exchange of respiratory gases, nutrients, and wastes occurs, and the tissues are oxygenated. The waste products exit the capillary network by way of the venules that join to form veins. These veins form larger veins, which carry deoxygenated blood to the right side of the heart, where it is returned to pulmonary circulation.

Blood Flow Regulation. The amount of blood ejected from the left ventricle each minute is the **cardiac output**. The normal cardiac output is 4 to 6 L/minute in the healthy 68-kg adult at rest. The circulating volume of blood changes according to the oxygen and metabolic needs of the body. For example, during exercise, pregnancy, and fever the cardiac output increases, but during sleep it decreases. Cardiac output is represented by the following formula:

Cardiac output (CO) = Stroke volume (SV) × Heart rate (HR)

Cardiac output in the older person may be affected by increased arterial wall tension and moderate myocardial hypertrophy due to an increased systolic blood pressure.

BOX 40.1 | **Coronary Arteries**

Right Coronary Artery
Right Atrium, Anterior Right Ventricle
Supplies
- Posterior aspect of septum (90% of population)
- Posterior papillary muscle
- Sinus and atrioventricular nodes (80–90% of population)
- Inferior aspect of left ventricle

Left Coronary Arteries
Left Anterior Descending Artery
Supplies
- Anterior left ventricular wall
- Anterior interventricular septum (septal branches supply conduction system, bundle of His, and bundle branches)
- Anterior papillary muscle
- Left ventricular apex
- Right ventricle

Circumflex Artery
Supplies
- Left atrium
- Posterior surfaces of left ventricle
- Posterior aspects of septum

Cardiac index (CI) is the adequacy of the cardiac output for an individual. It takes into account the body surface area (BSA) of the patient. The CI is determined by dividing the cardiac output by the BSA. The normal range is 2.5 to 4 L/min/m^3. Both cardiac output and the CI are measured with invasive pulmonary artery catheters.

Stroke volume is the amount of blood ejected from the left ventricle with each contraction. It can be affected by the amount of blood in the left ventricle at the end of diastole (preload), the resistance to left ventricular ejection (afterload), and myocardial contractility.

Preload is essentially the end-diastolic volume. The ventricles stretch when filling with blood. The more stretch on the ventricular muscle, the greater the contraction and the greater the stroke volume (Starling's law). In clinical situations, the preload and subsequent stroke volume can be manipulated by changing the amount of circulating blood volume. For example, in the patient with hemorrhagic shock, fluid therapy and replacement of blood increases volume, thus increasing the preload and stroke volume, which in turn increases cardiac output. If volume is not replaced, preload decreases, the cardiac output decreases, and, ultimately, the venous return to the right atrium decreases, further decreasing preload and cardiac output.

Afterload is the resistance to left ventricular ejection—the work that the heart must overcome to fully eject blood from the left ventricle. The diastolic aortic pressure is a good clinical measure of afterload. For example, in a patient with hypertension, the afterload is greater than normal, increasing the cardiac workload. Afterload in this situation can be manipulated by decreasing systemic blood pressure.

The invasive measurement and monitoring of these cardiopulmonary hemodynamics is usually performed in Critical Care Units. Some step-down or special care units may also have the capability to measure and monitor hemodynamics.

Myocardial contractility also affects stroke volume and cardiac output. Poor contraction decreases the amount of blood ejected by the ventricles during each contraction. Medications that can increase the force of myocardial contraction include digitalis preparations, epinephrine, and sympathomimetic medications (medications that mimic the effects of the sympathetic nervous system). Injury to the myocardial muscle, such as an acute myocardial infarction (AMI), can cause a decrease in myocardial contractility.

Heart rate affects blood flow because of the interaction between rate and diastolic filling time. With a sustained heart rate greater than 160 beats per minute, diastolic filling time decreases, decreasing stroke volume and cardiac output. The heart rate of the older person is slow to increase under stress and is likely related to lack of conditioning rather than age. While the size of the heart remains unchanged in the older person, the maximum coronary artery flow, stroke volumes, and cardiac output are reduced (Touhy et al., 2019). Exercise remains a health promotion strategy beneficial to maintaining health and cardiac function for all ages (Heart & Stroke Foundation of Canada [HSFC], 2022a).

Conduction System. The rhythmic relaxation and contraction of the atria and ventricles depend on continuous, organized transmission of electrical impulses. These impulses are generated and transmitted by way of the cardiac conduction system (Figure 40.2).

The heart's conduction system generates the necessary action potentials that conduct the impulses required to initiate the electrical chain of events resulting in the heartbeat. The autonomic nervous system influences the rate of impulse generation, the speed of transmission through the conductive pathway, and the strength of atrial and ventricular contractions. Sympathetic nerve fibres, which increase the rate of impulse generation and the speed of impulse transmission, innervate all parts of the atria and ventricles. The parasympathetic fibres originating from the vagus nerve decrease the rate and innervate

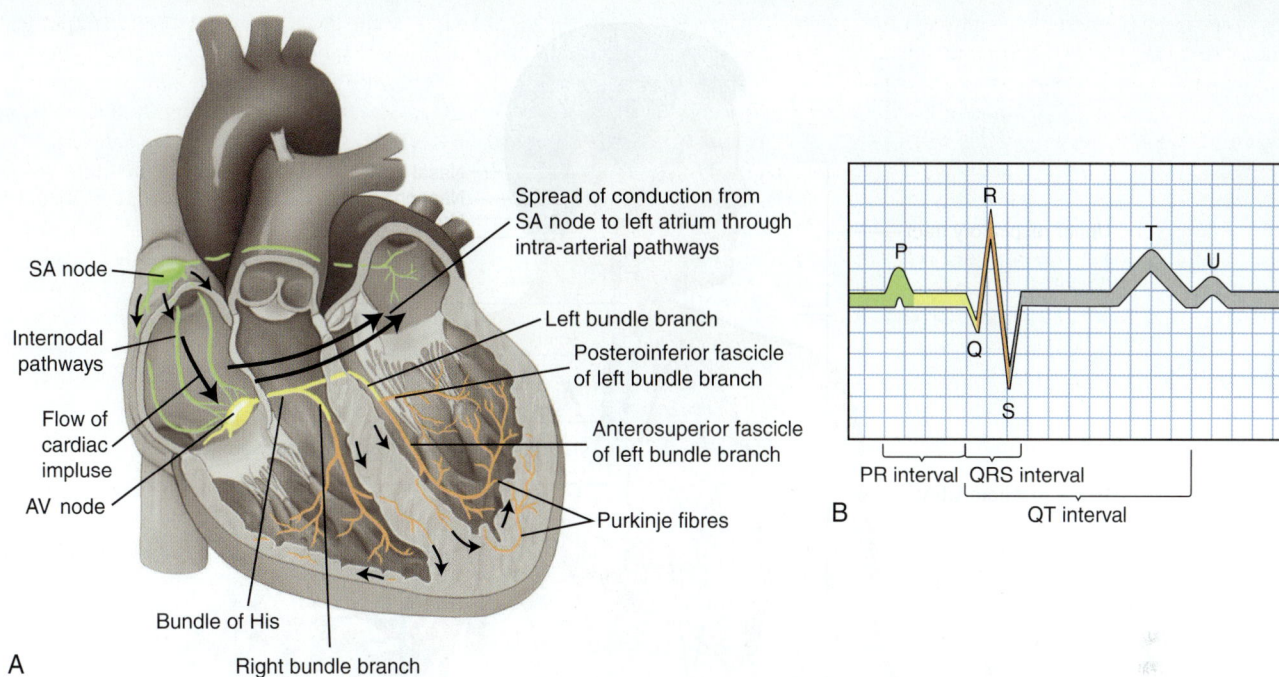

FIGURE 40.2 A, Conduction system of the heart. **B,** The normal electrocardiogram pattern. *AV,* Atrioventricular; *SA,* sinoatrial. (From Tyerman, J., & Cobbett, S. [Eds.]. [2023]. *Lewis's medical-surgical nursing in Canada: Assessment and management of clinical problems* [5th ed.]. Elsevier.)

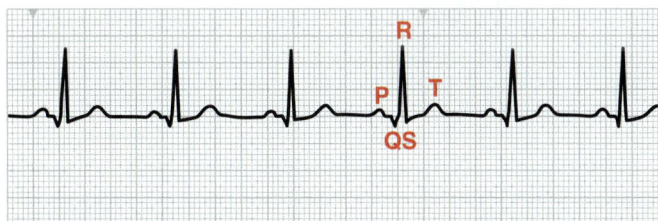

FIGURE 40.3 Normal electrocardiogram waveform. (From Tyerman, J., & Cobbett, S. [Eds.]. [2023]. *Lewis's medical-surgical nursing in Canada: Assessment and management of clinical problems* [5th ed.]. Elsevier.)

all parts of the atria and ventricles, as well as the sinoatrial (SA) and atrioventricular (AV) nodes.

The conduction system originates with the SA node, the "pacemaker" of the heart. The SA node is in the right atrium next to the entrance of the superior vena cava. Impulses are initiated at the SA node at an intrinsic rate of 60 to 100 beats per minute. The average resting adult rate is approximately 75 beats per minute.

The electrical impulses are then transmitted through the atria along intra-atrial pathways to the AV node. The AV node mediates impulses between the atria and the ventricles. The intrinsic rate of the normal AV node is 40 to 60 beats per minute. The AV node assists atrial emptying by delaying the impulse before transmitting it through the bundle of His and the ventricular Purkinje network. The intrinsic rate of the bundle of His and the ventricular Purkinje network is 20 to 40 beats per minute.

An **electrocardiogram (ECG)** reflects the electrical activity of the conduction system. An ECG monitors the regularity and path of the electrical impulse through the conduction system; however, it does not reflect muscular work of the heart. The normal sequence on the ECG is called **normal sinus rhythm (NSR)** (Figure 40.3).

NSR implies that the impulse originates at the SA node and follows the normal sequence through the conduction system. The P wave represents the electrical conduction through both atria. Atrial contraction follows the P wave. The PR interval represents the impulse travel time through the AV node, through the bundle of His, and to the Purkinje fibres. The normal length for the PR interval is 0.12 to 0.20 seconds (120–200 msec). An increase in the time (i.e., >0.20 seconds) indicates that there is a block in the impulse transmission through the AV node; a decrease (i.e., <0.12 seconds) indicates the initiation of the electrical impulse from a source other than the SA node.

The QRS complex indicates that the electrical impulse has travelled through the ventricles. Normal QRS duration is 0.06 to 0.10 seconds (60–100 msec). An increase in QRS duration indicates a delay in conduction time through the ventricles. Ventricular contraction usually follows the QRS complex.

The QT interval represents the time needed for ventricular depolarization and repolarization. The normal QT interval is 0.12 to 0.42 seconds (120–420 msec). Changes in electrolyte values, such as in hypocalcemia or during therapy with medications such as disopyramide, amiodarone, and sotolol, can increase the QT interval. Shortening of the QT interval occurs with digitalis therapy, hyperkalemia, and hypercalcemia.

Respiratory Physiology

Most cells in the body obtain their energy from chemical reactions involving oxygen and the elimination of carbon dioxide. The exchange of respiratory gases occurs between environmental air and the blood. There are three steps in the process of oxygenation: ventilation, perfusion, and diffusion.

Structure and Function. Conditions or diseases that change the structure and function of the lung can alter respiration. The respiratory muscles, pleural space, lungs, and alveoli (Figure 40.4) are essential for ventilation, perfusion, and exchange of respiratory gases. Gases are moved into and out of the lungs through pressure changes. Intrapleural pressure is either negative or less than atmospheric

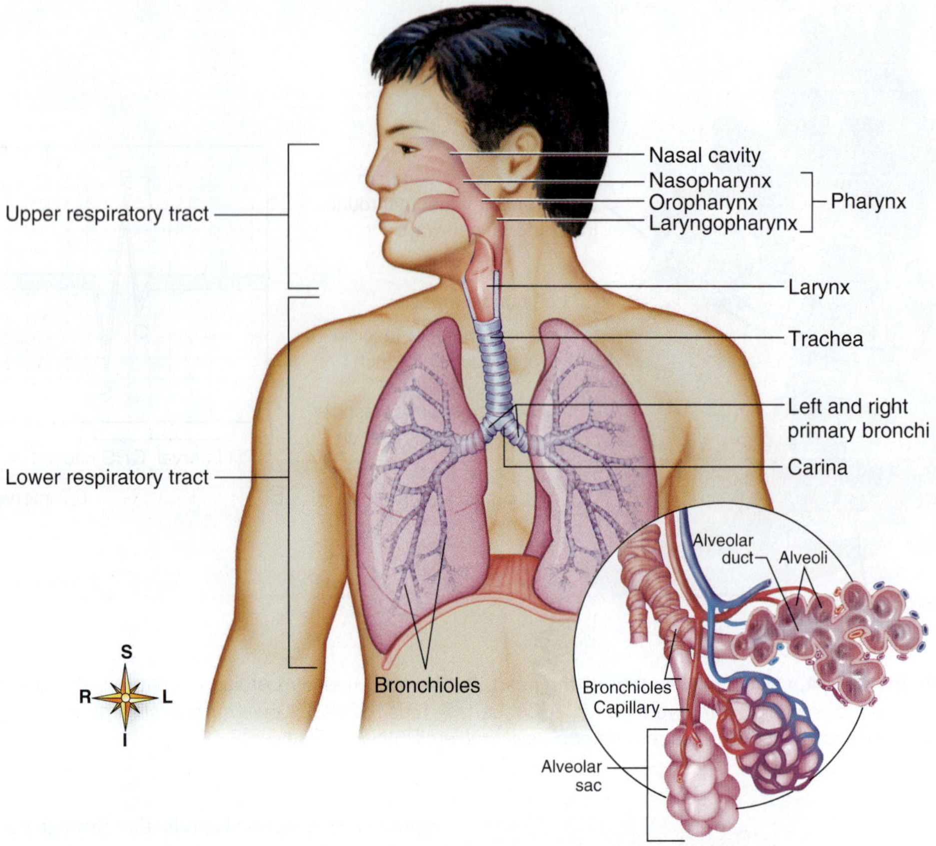

FIGURE 40.4 Structures of the pulmonary system. (From Power-Kean, K., Zettel, S., & El-Hussein, M. [2022]. *Huether and McCance's understanding pathophysiology* [2nd Canadian ed.]. Elsevier Inc.)

pressure, which is 760 mm Hg at sea level. For air to flow into the lungs, intrapleural pressure must become more negative, setting up a pressure gradient between the atmosphere and the alveoli. The diaphragm and external intercostal muscles contract to create a negative pleural pressure and increase the size of the thorax for inspiration. Together, relaxation of the diaphragm and contraction of the internal intercostal muscles allows air from the lung to escape. The coordination of the respiratory muscles is essential for effective respiration and gas exchange. The lung transfers oxygen from the atmosphere into the alveoli, where the oxygen is exchanged for carbon dioxide. The alveoli transfer oxygen and carbon dioxide to and from the blood through the alveolar membrane.

Ventilation is the process of moving gases into and out of the lungs. Ventilation requires coordination of the muscular and elastic properties of the lung and thorax, as well as intact innervation. The major inspiratory muscle of respiration is the diaphragm. It is innervated by the phrenic nerve, which exits the spinal cord at the fourth cervical vertebra. Perfusion relates to the ability of the cardiovascular system to pump oxygenated blood to the tissues and return deoxygenated blood to the lungs. Diffusion is responsible for moving the molecules from one area to another. For the exchange of respiratory gases to occur, the organs, nerves, and muscles of respiration must be intact and the central nervous system able to regulate the respiratory cycle.

Work of Breathing. Breathing is the effort required for expanding and contracting the lungs. In the healthy individual, breathing is quiet and accomplished with minimal effort. The amount of energy expended on breathing depends on the rate and depth of breathing, the ease with which the lungs can be expanded (compliance), and airway resistance.

Inspiration is an active process, stimulated by chemical receptors in the aorta. **Expiration** is a passive process that depends on the elastic-recoil properties of the lungs, requiring little or no muscle work. Elastic recoil is produced by elastic fibres in lung tissue and by surface tension in the fluid film lining the alveoli. Surfactant is a chemical produced in the lungs that maintains the surface tension of the alveoli and keeps them from collapsing. Patients with advanced chronic obstructive pulmonary disease (COPD) lose the elastic recoil of the lungs and thorax. As a result, the patient's work of breathing is increased. In addition, patients with certain pulmonary diseases can have decreased surfactant production and may, in turn, develop atelectasis. **Atelectasis** is the collapse of the alveoli that prevents normal gas exchange between carbon dioxide and oxygen.

Accessory muscles of respiration can increase lung volume during inspiration. Patients with COPD, especially emphysema, frequently use these muscles to increase lung volume. Prolonged use of the accessory muscles of respiration does not promote effective ventilation and causes fatigue. During assessment, one observes elevation of the patient's clavicles during inspiration.

Compliance is the ability of the lungs to distend or expand in response to increased intra-alveolar pressure. Compliance is decreased in diseases such as pulmonary edema, interstitial and pleural fibrosis, and congenital or traumatic structural abnormalities such as kyphosis or fractured ribs.

Airway resistance is the pressure difference between the mouth and the alveoli in relation to the rate of flow of inspired gas. Airway resistance can be increased by an airway obstruction, a small airway disease (such as asthma), and tracheal edema. When resistance is increased, the amount of air travelling through the anatomical airways is decreased.

Decreased lung compliance, increased airway resistance, active expiration, or the use of accessory muscles increases the work of breathing, resulting in increased energy expenditure. To meet this expenditure, the body increases its metabolic rate, and the need for oxygen, as well as for the elimination of carbon dioxide, increases. This sequence is a vicious cycle for a patient with impaired ventilation, causing further deterioration of respiratory status and the ability to oxygenate adequately.

Lung Volumes and Capacities. Spirometry is used to measure the volume of air entering or leaving the lungs. Variations in lung volumes may be associated with health states such as pregnancy, exercise, obesity, or obstructive and restrictive conditions of the lungs. The amount of surfactant, degree of compliance, and strength of respiratory muscles can affect pressures and volumes within the lungs.

Pulmonary Circulation. The primary function of the pulmonary circulation is to move blood to and from the alveolocapillary membrane in order for gas exchange to occur. The pulmonary circulation serves as a reservoir for blood so that the lung can increase its blood volume without large increases in pulmonary artery or venous pressures. The pulmonary circulation also acts as a filter, removing small thrombi before they can reach vital organs.

The pulmonary circulation begins at the pulmonary artery, which receives poorly oxygenated mixed venous blood from the right ventricle. Blood flow through this system depends on the pumping ability of the right ventricle, which has an output of approximately 4 to 6 L/minute. The flow continues from the pulmonary artery through the pulmonary arterioles to the pulmonary capillaries, where blood comes in contact with the alveolocapillary membrane and the exchange of respiratory gases occurs. The oxygen-rich blood then circulates through the pulmonary venules and pulmonary veins, returning to the left atrium.

Pressure and resistance within the pulmonary circulatory system are lower than that within the systemic circulatory system. The walls of the pulmonary vessels are thinner and contain less smooth muscle. The lung accepts the total cardiac output from the right ventricle and, except in cases of alveolar hypoxia or cor pulmonale, does not direct blood flow from one region to another. Cor pulmonale is a condition in which the right ventricle is enlarged, secondary to diseases of the lung, thorax, or pulmonary circulation.

Respiratory Gas Exchange. Respiratory gases are exchanged in the alveoli and the capillaries of the body tissues (Figure 40.5). Oxygen is transferred from the lungs to the blood, and carbon dioxide is transferred from the blood to the alveoli to be exhaled as a waste product. At the tissue level, oxygen is transferred from the blood to tissues, and carbon dioxide is transferred from tissues to the blood to return to the alveoli and be exhaled. This transfer is dependent on the process of diffusion.

Diffusion is the movement of molecules from an area of higher concentration to an area of lower concentration. Diffusion of respiratory gases occurs at the alveolocapillary membrane, and the rate of diffusion can be affected by the thickness of the membrane. Increased thickness of the membrane impedes diffusion because gases take longer to transfer across. Patients with pulmonary edema, pulmonary infiltrates, or a pulmonary effusion have an increased thickness of the alveolocapillary membrane, resulting in slowed diffusion, slowed exchange of respiratory gases, and impaired delivery of oxygen to tissues. The surface area of the membrane can be altered as a result of chronic disease (e.g., emphysema), acute disease (e.g., pneumothorax), or a surgical process (e.g., lobectomy). The alveolocapillary membrane can be destroyed or may thicken, changing the rate of diffusion. When fewer alveoli are functioning, the surface area is decreased.

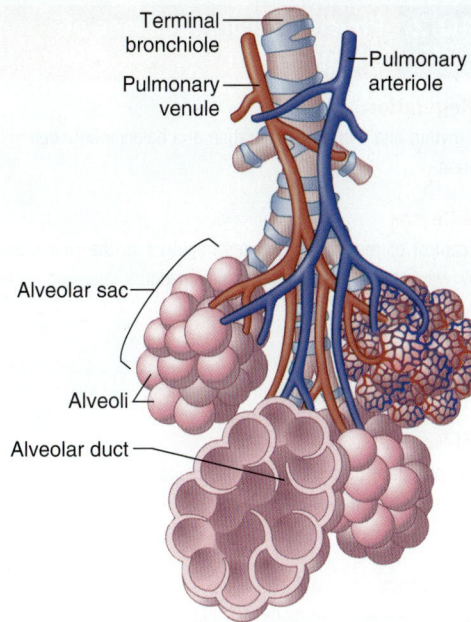

FIGURE 40.5 Alveoli. (From Power-Kean, K., Zettel, S., & El-Hussein, M. [2022]. *Huether and McCance's understanding pathophysiology* [2nd Canadian ed.]. Elsevier Inc.)

Oxygen Transport. The oxygen transport system consists of the lungs and cardiovascular system. Delivery depends on the amount of oxygen entering the lungs (ventilation), blood flow to the lungs and tissues (perfusion), rate of diffusion, and oxygen-carrying capacity. The capacity of the blood to carry oxygen is influenced by the amount of dissolved oxygen in the plasma, amount of hemoglobin, and tendency of hemoglobin to bind with oxygen. Only a relatively small amount of required oxygen, less than 1%, is dissolved in the plasma. Most oxygen is transported by hemoglobin, which serves as a carrier for oxygen and carbon dioxide. The hemoglobin molecule combines with oxygen to form oxyhemoglobin. The formation of oxyhemoglobin is easily reversible, allowing hemoglobin and oxygen to dissociate, which frees oxygen to enter tissues.

Carbon Dioxide Transport. Carbon dioxide diffuses into red blood cells and is rapidly hydrated into carbonic acid (H_2CO_3) because of the presence of carbonic anhydrase. The carbonic acid then dissociates into hydrogen (H^+) and bicarbonate (HCO_3^-) ions. The hydrogen ion is buffered by hemoglobin, and the HCO_3^- diffuses into the plasma (see Chapter 41). In addition, some of the carbon dioxide in red blood cells reacts with amino acid groups, forming carbamino compounds. This reaction can occur rapidly without the presence of an enzyme. Reduced hemoglobin (deoxyhemoglobin) can combine with carbon dioxide more easily than oxyhemoglobin, thus venous blood transports most of the carbon dioxide.

Regulation of Respiration. Regulation of respiration is necessary to ensure sufficient oxygen intake and carbon dioxide elimination to meet the body's demands (e.g., during exercise, infection, or pregnancy). Neural and chemical regulators control the process of respiration. Neural regulation includes the central nervous system control of respiratory rate, depth, and rhythm. Chemical regulation involves the influence of chemicals such as carbon dioxide and hydrogen ions on the rate and depth of respiration (Box 40.2).

Factors Affecting Oxygenation

Adequacy of circulation, ventilation, perfusion, and transport of respiratory gases to the tissues is influenced by four types of factors:

BOX 40.2 Physiological Processes of Oxygenation

Neural Regulation
Maintains rhythm and depth of respiration and balance between inspiration and expiration.

Cerebral Cortex
Voluntary control of respiration delivers impulses to the respiratory motor neurons by way of the spinal cord; accommodates speaking, eating, and swimming.

Medulla Oblongata
Automatic control of respiration occurs continuously.

Chemical Regulation
Maintains appropriate rate and depth of respirations according to changes in the blood's carbon dioxide (CO_2), oxygen (O_2), and hydrogen ion (H^+) concentration.

Chemoreceptors
Located in the medulla, aortic body, and carotid body. Changes in chemical content of O_2, CO_2, and H^+ stimulate chemoreceptors, which in turn stimulate neural regulators to adjust the rate and depth of ventilation to maintain normal arterial blood gas levels. Chemical regulation can occur during physical exercise and with some illnesses. It is a short-term adaptive mechanism.

TABLE 40.1 Physiological Processes Affecting Oxygenation

Process	Effect on Oxygenation
Anemia	Decreases oxygen-carrying capacity of blood
Toxic inhalant	Decreases oxygen-carrying capacity of blood
Airway obstruction	Limits delivery of inspired oxygen to alveoli
High altitude	Atmospheric oxygen concentration is lower and inspiratory oxygen concentration decreases
Fever	Increases metabolic rate and tissue oxygen demand
Decreased chest wall motion (e.g., from musculoskeletal impairments)	Prevents lowering of diaphragm and reduces anteroposterior diameter of thorax on inspiration, reducing volume of air inspired

(1) physiological, (2) developmental, (3) lifestyle, and (4) environmental. Developmental, lifestyle, and environmental factors will be presented in a later section.

Physiological Factors. Any condition that affects cardiopulmonary functioning directly affects the body's ability to meet oxygen demands. The general classifications of cardiac disorders are disturbances in conduction, impaired valvular function, myocardial hypoxia, cardiomyopathic conditions, and peripheral tissue hypoxia. Respiratory disorders include hyperventilation, hypoventilation, and hypoxia.

Other physiological processes affecting a patient's oxygenation are alterations that affect the oxygen-carrying capacity of blood, such as anemia; increases in the body's metabolic demands (e.g., pregnancy, fever, infection); and alterations that affect chest wall movement or the central nervous system (Table 40.1).

Decreased Oxygen-Carrying Capacity. Hemoglobin carries most of the oxygen to tissues. Anemia and inhalation of toxic substances decrease the oxygen-carrying capacity of blood by reducing the amount of available hemoglobin to transport oxygen. Anemia, a hemoglobin level lower than normal, is a result of decreased hemoglobin production, increased red blood cell destruction, blood loss, or a combination of these factors. Patients will experience fatigue, decreased activity tolerance, and increased breathlessness, as well as pallor (especially seen in the conjunctiva of the eye) and an increased heart rate.

Carbon monoxide is the most common toxic inhalant that decreases the oxygen-carrying capacity of blood. The affinity for hemoglobin to bind with carbon monoxide is greater than 200 times its affinity to bind with oxygen, creating a functional anemia. Because of the bond's strength, carbon monoxide is not easily dissociated from hemoglobin, making the hemoglobin unavailable for oxygen transport.

Decreased Inspired Oxygen Concentration. When the concentration of inspired oxygen declines, the blood has less oxygen-carrying capacity. Decreases in the fraction of inspired oxygen concentration (FiO_2) can be caused by an upper or lower airway obstruction limiting delivery of inspired oxygen to alveoli; decreased environmental oxygen, such as at high altitudes; or decreased inspiration as a result of an incorrect oxygen concentration setting on respiratory therapy equipment.

Hypovolemia. Hypovolemia is caused by conditions such as shock and severe dehydration resulting from extracellular fluid loss and reduced circulating blood volume. With a significant fluid loss, the body tries to adapt by increasing the heart rate and peripheral vasoconstriction to increase the volume of blood returned to the heart and, in turn, increase the cardiac output.

Increased Metabolic Rate. Increased metabolic activity causes increased oxygen demand. When body systems are unable to meet this increased demand, the level of oxygenation declines. An increased metabolic rate is a normal physiological response to pregnancy, wound healing, and exercise because the body is building tissue. Most people can meet the increased oxygen demand and do not display signs of oxygen deprivation. Fever increases the tissues' need for oxygen, and as a result, carbon dioxide production also increases.

If the febrile state persists, the metabolic rate remains high and the body begins to break down protein stores, resulting in muscle wasting and decreased muscle mass. Respiratory muscles such as the diaphragm and intercostal muscles are also wasted. The body attempts to adapt to the increased carbon dioxide levels by increasing the rate and depth of respiration. The patient's work of breathing increases, and the patient will eventually display signs and symptoms of hypoxemia. Patients with pulmonary diseases are at greater risk for hypoxemia and hypercapnia (a greater than normal amount of carbon dioxide in the blood). Assessment findings include an increased rate and depth of respiration, use of the accessory muscles of respiration, pursed-lip breathing, and decreased activity tolerance.

Conditions Affecting Chest Wall Movement. Any condition that reduces chest wall movement can result in decreased ventilation. If the diaphragm cannot fully descend with breathing, the volume of inspired air decreases, and less oxygen is delivered to the alveoli and, subsequently, to tissues.

Pregnancy. As the fetus grows during pregnancy, the greater size of the uterus pushes abdominal contents upward against the diaphragm. In the last trimester of pregnancy, the inspiratory capacity declines, resulting in dyspnea on exertion and increased fatigue.

Obesity. Morbidly obese patients have reduced lung volumes as a result of the heaviness of the lower thorax and abdomen, particularly when in the recumbent and supine positions. These patients have a reduction in compliance as a result of encroachment of the abdomen into the chest, increased work of breathing, and decreased lung volumes, and they may experience fatigue and have carbon dioxide retention. In some patients, an obesity–hypoventilation syndrome develops in which oxygenation is decreased and carbon dioxide is retained, resulting in daytime sleepiness. Morbidly obese patients may also develop obstructive sleep apnea, characterized by excessive daytime somnolence and loud snoring and apneic periods during sleep. The patient with obesity is also susceptible to pneumonia after surgery or an upper respiratory tract infection because the lungs cannot fully expand and pulmonary secretions are not mobilized in the lower lobes.

Musculoskeletal Abnormalities. Musculoskeletal impairments in the thoracic region reduce oxygenation. Such impairments may result from abnormal structural configurations, trauma, muscular diseases, and diseases of the central nervous system. Abnormal structural configurations impairing oxygenation include those that affect the rib cage, such as pectus excavatum (an indentation of the lower sternum), and those that affect the vertebral column, such as kyphosis, lordosis, or scoliosis.

Trauma. The person with multiple rib fractures can develop a flail chest, a condition in which fractures cause instability in part of the chest wall. The unstable chest wall allows the lung underlying the injured area to contract on inspiration and bulge on expiration, resulting in hypoxia. Chest wall or upper abdominal incisions may also decrease chest wall movement as the patient uses shallow respirations to minimize chest wall movement to avoid pain. Excessive or high doses of narcotic analgesics may depress the respiratory centre, further decreasing respiratory rate and chest wall expansion.

Neuromuscular Diseases. Diseases such as muscular dystrophy affect oxygenation of tissues by decreasing the patient's ability to expand and contract the chest wall. Ventilation is impaired, and atelectasis, hypercapnia, and hypoxemia can occur. Myasthenia gravis, Guillain-Barré syndrome, and poliomyelitis affect respiratory functioning and result in hypoventilation. Myasthenia gravis interferes with normal transmission of impulses from nerves to muscles, involving the whole body, including muscles of respiration. Guillain-Barré syndrome and poliomyelitis cause inflammation and paralysis of muscle groups. Guillain-Barré syndrome usually results in an ascending pattern of paralysis. Respiratory muscles become paralyzed as paralysis ascends to the thoracic region. Poliomyelitis may lead to general or local paralysis. Both disorders may reverse, but poliomyelitis usually results in more residual paralysis.

Central Nervous System Alterations. Diseases or trauma involving the medulla oblongata and spinal cord may result in impaired respiration. When the medulla oblongata is affected, neural regulation of respiration is damaged and abnormal breathing patterns may develop. If the phrenic nerve is damaged, the diaphragm may not descend, thus reducing inspiratory lung volumes and causing hypoxemia. Cervical trauma at C3 to C5 can result in paralysis of the phrenic nerve. Spinal cord trauma below the fifth cervical vertebra usually leaves the phrenic nerve intact but damages nerves that innervate the intercostal muscles, preventing anteroposterior chest expansion.

Influences of Chronic Disease. Oxygenation can be decreased as a direct consequence of chronic disease. It can also be decreased as a secondary effect, as with anemia. The physiological response to chronic hypoxemia is the development of a secondary polycythemia (increase in red blood cells). This adaptive response is the body's attempt to increase the amount of circulating hemoglobin to increase the available oxygen-binding sites.

Alterations in Cardiac Functioning

Illnesses and conditions that affect cardiac rhythm, strength of contraction, blood flow through the chambers, myocardial blood flow, and peripheral circulation cause alterations in cardiac functioning. Older persons experience reduced elasticity and recoil of blood vessels, and for those who have existing atherosclerosis or hypertension, there are significant implications that may occur (Touhy et al., 2019).

Disturbances in Conduction. An arrythmia or irregular heartbeat can be an early sign of an electrical cardiac conduction disorder. Some disturbances in conduction are a result of electrical impulses that do not originate from the SA node. These rhythm disturbances are called dysrhythmias, meaning a deviation from an otherwise normal sinus heart rhythm (Table 40.2). Dysrhythmias may occur as a primary

---

TABLE 40.2	Common Basic Cardiac Dysrhythmias
Rhythm Characteristics and Etiology	**Clinical Significance and Management**
Sinus Tachycardia Regular rhythm, rate 100–180 beats/min (higher in infants), normal P wave, normal QRS complex. Rate increase may be a normal response to exercise, emotion, or stressors such as pain, fever, pump failure, hyperthyroidism, and certain drugs and medications (e.g., caffeine, nitrates, epinephrine, nicotine).	Patient with damaged heart may not be able to sustain increased myocardial oxygen consumption by increased heart rate. Correct underlying causes; discontinue medications producing the adverse effect.

Sinus tachycardia

(From Wesley, K. [2017]. *Huzar's ECG and 12 lead interpretation* [5th ed.]. Mosby.)

TABLE 40.2   **Common Basic Cardiac Dysrhythmias—cont'd**

Rhythm Characteristics and Etiology	Clinical Significance and Management
Sinus Bradycardia	

Sinus Bradycardia

Regular rhythm, rate <60 beats/min, normal P wave, normal PR interval, normal QRS complex.

Rate decrease may be a normal response to sleep or in well-conditioned athletes; abnormal drops in rate may be caused by diminished blood flow to the sinoatrial (SA) node, vagal stimulation, hypothyroidism, increased intracranial pressure, or pharmacological agents (e.g., digoxin, propranolol, quinidine, procainamide).

No clinical significance unless associated with signs and symptoms of reduced cardiac output such as dizziness or syncope or presence of chest pain.

Bradycardia with hypotension and decreased cardiac output is treated with atropine; a pacemaker may be required.

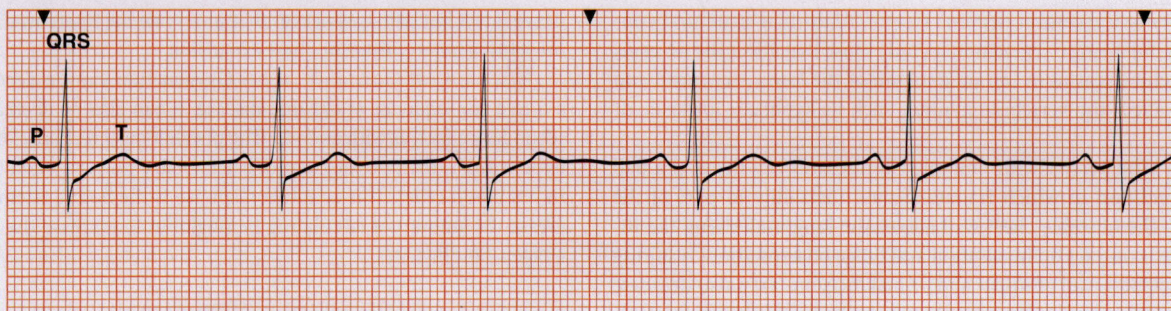

Sinus bradycardia

(From Wesley, K. [2017]. *Huzar's ECG and 12 lead interpretation* [5th ed.]. Mosby.)

Atrial Fibrillation (A-fib)

Chaotic, irregular atrial activity resulting in an irregular ventricular response. No identifiable P waves. Irregular ventricular response resulting in an irregular cardiac rate and rhythm. The rate is determined by the conduction of the multiple atrial impulses across the atrioventricular (AV) node.

Atrial fibrillation is caused by aging, calcification of the SA node, or changes in myocardial blood supply.

There is a loss of the atrial kick (portion of the cardiac output squeezed in the ventricles with a coordinated atrial contraction), pooling of blood in the atria, and development of microemboli. The patient may complain of fatigue, a fluttering in the chest, or shortness of breath if the ventricular response is rapid. A-fib is a commonly occurring dysrhythmia in the aging and older person. Anticoagulants such as warfarin may be used to reduce the risk of stroke. Warfarin is prescribed on the basis of the international normalized ratio (INR), thus dose adjustments are based on daily INR results.

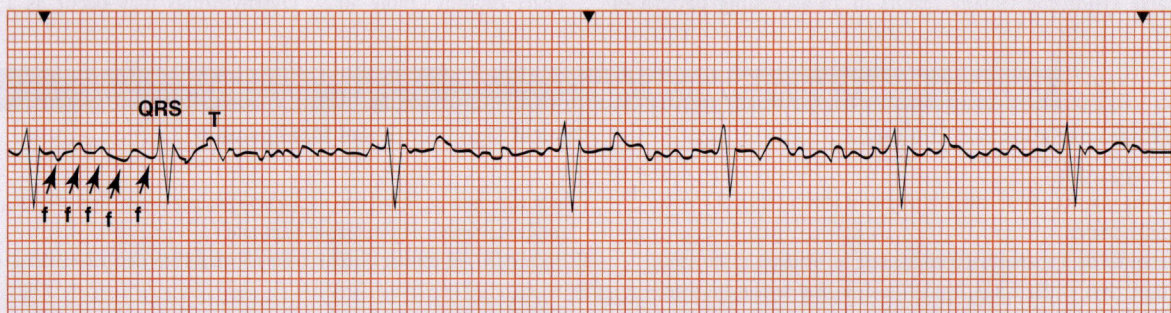

Coarse atrial fibrillation

(From Wesley, K. [2017]. *Huzar's ECG and 12 lead interpretation* [5th ed.]. Mosby.)

Ventricular Tachycardia (VT)

Rhythm slightly irregular, rate 100–200 beats/min, P wave absent, PR interval absent, QRS complex wide and bizarre, >0.12 seconds.

Results in a decreased cardiac output due to decreased ventricular filling time; may lead to severe hypotension and loss of pulse and consciousness.

Continued

TABLE 40.2 Common Basic Cardiac Dysrhythmias—cont'd

Rhythm Characteristics and Etiology	Clinical Significance and Management

VT is caused by changes in the normal pacemaker of the heart, such as decrease in blood flow, ischemia, or embolus.

If pulseless, interventions may include early defibrillation, cardiopulmonary resuscitation (CPR), intravenous access, and medications (American Heart Association [AHA], 2020).

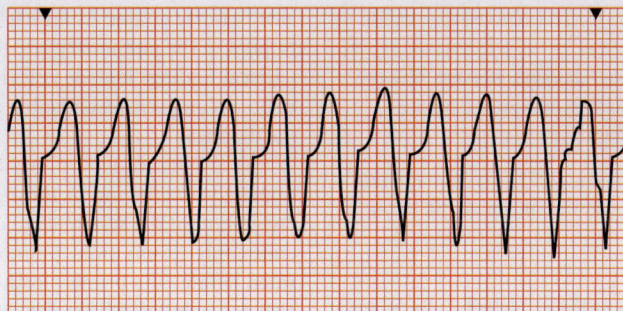

VT

(From Wesley, K. [2017]. *Huzar's ECG and 12 lead interpretation* [5th ed.]. Mosby.)

Ventricular Fibrillation

Uncoordinated electrical activity. No identifiable P, QRS, or T wave. Causes include sudden cardiac death, electrical shock, acute myocardial infarction, drowning, or trauma.

Acute loss of pulse and respiration. Early defibrillation, CPR, intravenous access, and medications may be used as initial interventions for ventricular fibrillation (AHA, 2020). The 2020 American Heart Association *Guidelines for CPR and ECC* reinforce the importance of early initiation of CPR by lay rescuers (AHA, 2020).

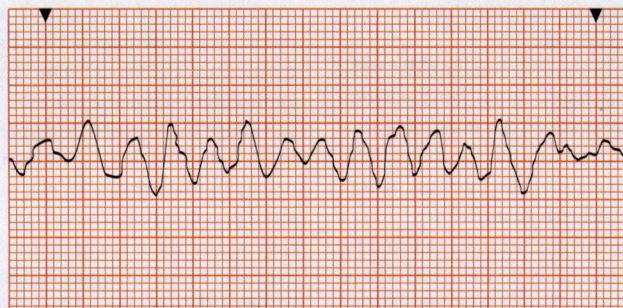

Coarse ventricular fibrillation

(From Wesley, K. [2017]. *Huzar's ECG and 12 lead interpretation* [5th ed.]. Mosby.)

Asystole

Classically referred to as a "flat line." There are no electrical impulses and therefore no QRS complex, no contraction, and no cardiac output. Possible causes are hypoxia, hyperkalemia and hypokalemia, pre-existing acidosis, drug overdose, and hypothermia.

The unresponsive patient will have no pulse, blood pressure, or respirations. The management of asystole consists of early medications, CPR, intravenous access, and correction of the underlying cause (AHA, 2020).

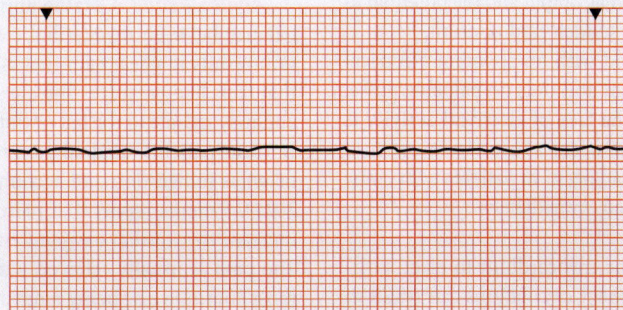

Ventricular asystole

(From Wesley, K. [2017]. *Huzar's ECG and 12 lead interpretation* [5th ed.]. Mosby.)

Adapted from Wesley, K. (2017). *Huzar's ECG and 12 lead interpretation* (5th ed.). Mosby.

<table>
<tr><td colspan="2">**BOX 40.3 | Automated External Defibrillator (AED)**</td></tr>
</table>

- An automated external defibrillator is a device used to administer an electrical shock through the chest wall to the heart.
- Survival rate is doubled when both CPR and the use of AED are combined.
- AEDs are simple to use, portable, and used when shock only is required.
- There have been more than 15 000 AEDs placed in communities across Canada since 2010.
- Once emergency medical response has been activated, less than 40% receive layperson-initiated CPR, and less than 12% have an AED applied.

CPR, Cardiopulmonary resuscitation.
From Heart and Stroke Foundation of Canada. (2022). *Restart a heart.* https://www.heartandstroke.ca/how-you-can-help/advocate/restart-a-heart

conduction disturbance; as a response to ischemia, valvular abnormality, anxiety, or drug toxicity; as a result of caffeine, alcohol, or tobacco use; or as a complication of acid–base or electrolyte imbalance (see Chapter 41). Such disturbances may be life-threatening and require treatment with medication or defibrillation (Box 40.3).

Dysrhythmias are classified by cardiac response and site of impulse origin. Cardiac response can be tachycardiac (>100 beats/min), bradycardiac (<60 beats/min), a premature (early) beat, or a blocked (delayed or absent) beat. Tachydysrhythmias and bradydysrhythmias can lower cardiac output and blood pressure. Tachydysrhythmias reduce cardiac output by decreasing diastolic filling time. Bradydysrhythmias lower cardiac output because of the decreased heart rate.

Atrial fibrillation is a common type of dysrhythmia in older persons. The electrical impulse in the atria is chaotic and originates from multiple sites. The rhythm is irregular because of the multiple pacemaker sites and the unpredictable conduction to the ventricles. The QRS complex is normal; however, it occurs at irregular intervals. Atrial fibrillation is often described as an irregularly irregular rhythm.

Abnormal impulses originating above the ventricles are referred to as *supraventricular dysrhythmias.* The abnormality on the waveform is the configuration and placement of the P wave. Ventricular conduction usually remains normal, and a normal QRS complex is observed.

Ventricular dysrhythmias represent an ectopic site of impulse formation within the ventricles. It is ectopic in that the impulse originates in the ventricle, not the SA node. The configuration of the QRS complex is usually widened and bizarre. P waves may or may not be present; often they are buried in the QRS complex. **Ventricular tachycardia** and **ventricular fibrillation** are life-threatening rhythms that require immediate intervention. Ventricular tachycardia is considered a life-threatening dysrhythmia because of the decreased cardiac output and the potential to deteriorate into ventricular fibrillation or sudden cardiac death.

Asystole is a lethal rhythm associated with no apparent electrical activity. The patient has no cardiac output and thus no palpable pulse. If the patient is on a cardiac monitor, the lack of electrical activity is noted by an absent rhythm. Asystole can occur as a primary event, it may follow ventricular fibrillation, or it can occur in patients with complete heart block. Asystole must be treated immediately.

Altered Cardiac Output. Failure of the myocardium to eject sufficient volume to the systemic and pulmonary circulations can result in heart failure. Heart failure is a growing epidemic, with approximately 600 000 Canadians living with the impact of the alteration in health (HSFC, 2022b). Primary coronary artery disease, cardiomyopathic conditions, valvular disorders, and pulmonary disease lead to myocardial pump failure.

Left-Sided Heart Failure. Left-sided heart failure is an abnormal condition characterized by impaired functioning of the left ventricle as a result of elevated pressures and pulmonary congestion. If left ventricular failure is significant, the amount of blood ejected from the left ventricle drops greatly, resulting in decreased cardiac output. Assessment findings may include decreased activity tolerance, breathlessness, dizziness, and confusion as a result of tissue hypoxia from the diminished cardiac output. As the left ventricle continues to fail, blood begins to pool in the pulmonary circulation, causing pulmonary congestion. Clinical findings include crackles on auscultation, hypoxia, shortness of breath on exertion and often at rest, cough, and paroxysmal nocturnal dyspnea.

Right-Sided Heart Failure. Right-sided heart failure results from impaired functioning of the right ventricle characterized by venous congestion in the systemic circulation. Right-sided heart failure more commonly results from pulmonary disease or from long-term left-sided failure. The primary pathological factor in right-sided failure is elevated pulmonary vascular resistance (PVR). As the PVR continues to rise, the right ventricle must generate more work, and the oxygen demand of the heart increases. As the failure continues, the amount of blood ejected from the right ventricle declines, and blood begins to "back up" in the systemic circulation. Clinically, the patient has weight gain, distended neck veins, hepatomegaly and splenomegaly, and dependent peripheral edema.

Impaired Valvular Function. Valvular heart disease is an acquired or congenital disorder of a cardiac valve characterized by stenosis and obstructed blood flow or valvular degeneration and regurgitation of blood. When stenosis occurs in the semilunar valves (aortic and pulmonic valves), the adjacent ventricles must work harder to move the ventricular volume beyond the stenotic valve. Over time, the stenosis can cause the ventricle to hypertrophy (enlarge), and if the condition is left untreated, left- or right-sided heart failure can occur. If stenosis occurs in the atrioventricular valves (mitral and tricuspid valves), the atrial pressure rises, causing the atria to hypertrophy. When regurgitation occurs, there is a backflow of blood into an adjacent chamber. For example, in mitral regurgitation, the mitral leaflets do not close completely. When the ventricles contract, blood escapes back into the atria, causing a murmur, or "whooshing" sound (see Chapter 33).

Myocardial Ischemia. **Myocardial ischemia** results when the supply of blood to the myocardium from the coronary arteries is insufficient to meet the oxygen demands of the organ. Common manifestations of this ischemia include stable angina pectoris and acute coronary syndrome, which consists of unstable angina and myocardial infarction.

Angina Pectoris. **Stable angina pectoris** is usually a transient imbalance between myocardial oxygen supply and demand. The condition results in chest pain that is aching, sharp, tingling, or burning or that feels like pressure. The chest pain may be left-sided or substernal and may radiate to the left or both arms, and to the jaw, neck, and back. In some patients, anginal pain may not radiate. The pain may be mistaken as indigestion and accompanied by dyspnea (Power-Kean et al., 2022). Patients report that pain is often precipitated by activities that increase myocardial oxygen demand (e.g., exercise, anxiety, or stress). The pain is usually relieved with rest and coronary vasodilators, the most common one being a nitroglycerine preparation.

Acute Coronary Syndrome. **Acute coronary syndrome (ACS)** is an overarching term that includes unstable angina, non-ST-segment elevation myocardial infarction (NSTEMI), and ST-segment (STEMI) myocardial infarction. ACS is an imbalance between the oxygen supply and demand to the myocardium. Causes of ACS include nonocclusive thrombosis on pre-existing plaque; coronary vasospasm; arterial narrowing from atherosclerosis; inflammation or infection; and secondary unstable angina from anemia, fever, or hypoxemia. **Unstable angina** or unpredictable chest pain has the potential to occur without an increase in myocardial demand and may be a precursor to a myocardial infarction (Power-Kean et al., 2022).

Myocardial infarction (MI) results from sudden decreases in coronary blood flow or an increase in myocardial oxygen demand without adequate coronary perfusion. MI can be classified as STEMI or NSTEMI. **ST elevation myocardial infarction (STEMI)** is a complete obstruction of blood flow in a coronary artery, whereas a **non-ST-segment elevation myocardial infarction (NSTEMI)** consists of a partial blockage of blood flow in a coronary artery (Power-Kean et al., 2022). Infarction occurs because of ischemia (which is reversible) and necrosis (which is not reversible) of myocardial tissue. The myocardium becomes cyanotic and cool after 8 to 10 seconds of reduced blood supply (Power-Kean et al., 2022). After 20 minutes of myocardial ischemia, cellular death occurs (Power-Kean et al., 2022).

Chest pain remains the most common symptom in both men and women but does not have to be present to indicate an MI (HSFC, 2022c). In fact, older persons or those diagnosed with diabetes may experience no pain or have silent infarctions (Power-Kean et al., 2022). It is also important to recognize that there are distinctions associated with symptoms of MIs experienced by men and women. In men, chest pain associated with MI is usually described as crushing, squeezing, or stabbing. The pain may be retrosternal and left precordial, and it may radiate from down the left arm to the neck, jaws, teeth, epigastric area, and back. The pain occurs at rest or on exertion, lasts more than 20 minutes, and is unrelieved by rest, position change, or sublingual nitroglycerine administration. The language women use to describe their pain may differ as they may describe it as pressure or tightness; this may influence their diagnosis and treatment (HSFC, 2022c). Women may experience other symptoms different from men's, such as fatigue, sleep difficulties, indigestion, and anxiety (HSFC, 2022c).

Sex and gender differences may exist in heart disease; for example, when it comes to heart disease women are "under-researched, under-diagnosed and under-treated, and under-supported during recovery" (HSFC, 2018, p. 2). Approximately 32 000 women die of heart disease and stroke in Canada each year; however, most women are unaware of the risk (HSFC, 2022d). A report by the Heart and Stroke Foundation of Canada (2018) states that "we still struggle to untangle and apply new knowledge about women and heart disease, and why some women—Indigenous women, ethnically diverse women, women living in poverty, and women in remote and rural locations—often face even greater inequities" (p. 2). HSFC (2018) also states that "Indigenous people of Canada-First Nations, Metis and Inuit are two times more likely to develop heart disease," with Indigenous women more likely to die from heart disease at a younger age than non-Indigenous women (p. 14).

There are both nonmodifiable and modifiable risk factors associated with coronary artery disease. For example, ethnicity is a nonmodifiable risk factor: people of African or South Asian background have a higher risk of heart disease (HSFC, 2022e). Other nonmodifiable risk factors include age, gender, family history, and personal circumstances related to healthy food, safe drinking water, and health services (HSFC, 2022e). Modifiable factors associated with coronary artery disease include hypertension, high blood cholesterol, diabetes, unhealthy weight, intake of too much alcohol, sedentary lifestyle, smoking, stress, and depression (HSFC, 2022e).

Alterations in Respiratory Functioning

Illnesses and conditions that affect ventilation or oxygen transport cause alterations in respiratory functioning. The three primary alterations are hyperventilation, hypoventilation, and hypoxia.

The goal of ventilation is to produce a normal arterial carbon dioxide tension ($PaCO_2$) between 35 and 45 mm Hg and maintain a normal arterial oxygen tension (PaO_2) between 80 and 100 mm Hg. *Hyperventilation* and *hypoventilation* refer to alveolar ventilation and not to the patient's respiratory rate. Arterial oxygen levels can be monitored using a noninvasive oxygen saturation monitor. The normal range is 95 to 100%. *Hypoxia* refers to a decrease in the amount of arterial oxygen.

Hyperventilation. **Hyperventilation** is a state of ventilation in excess of that required to eliminate the normal venous carbon dioxide produced by cellular metabolism. Anxiety, infections, drugs, or an acid–base imbalance can induce hyperventilation, as well as hypoxia associated with pulmonary embolus or shock. Acute anxiety can lead to hyperventilation and may cause loss of consciousness from excess carbon dioxide exhalation. Fever can cause hyperventilation. As a patient's body temperature increases, there is an increase in the metabolic rate, thereby increasing carbon dioxide production. The clinical response is an increased rate and depth of respiration.

Hyperventilation may also be chemically induced. Salicylate poisoning causes excessive stimulation of the respiratory centre as the body attempts to compensate for excess carbon dioxide. Amphetamines increase ventilation by raising carbon dioxide production. Hyperventilation can also occur as the body tries to compensate for metabolic acidosis by producing a respiratory alkalosis. For example, the diabetic patient who has gone into diabetic ketoacidosis is producing large amounts of metabolic acids. The respiratory system tries to correct the acid–base balance by overbreathing. Ventilation increases to reduce the amount of carbon dioxide available to form carbonic acid (see Chapter 41). Hemoglobin does not release oxygen to tissues as readily, and tissue hypoxia results. As symptoms worsen, the patient may become more agitated, which further increases the respiratory rate and can result in respiratory alkalosis.

Hypoventilation. **Hypoventilation** occurs when alveolar ventilation is inadequate to meet the body's oxygen demand or to eliminate sufficient carbon dioxide. As alveolar ventilation decreases, $PaCO_2$ is elevated. Severe atelectasis can produce hypoventilation. *Atelectasis* is a collapse of the alveoli that prevents normal respiratory exchange of oxygen and carbon dioxide. As alveoli collapse, less of the lung can be ventilated and hypoventilation occurs.

In patients with COPD, the inappropriate administration of excessive oxygen can result in hypoventilation. These patients have adapted to a high carbon dioxide level, and their carbon dioxide–sensitive chemoreceptors are essentially not functioning. Their stimulus to breathe is a decreased PaO_2. If excessive oxygen is administered, the oxygen requirement is satisfied and the stimulus to breathe is negated. High concentrations of oxygen (e.g., >24–28% [1–3 L/min]) prevent the PaO_2 from falling and obliterate the stimulus to breathe, resulting in hypoventilation. The excessive retention of carbon dioxide may lead to respiratory arrest.

Signs and symptoms of hypoventilation include mental status changes, dysrhythmias, and potential cardiac arrest. Treatment requires improving tissue oxygenation, restoring ventilatory function, treating the underlying cause of the hypoventilation, and achieving acid–base balance. If untreated, the patient's status can rapidly decline, leading to convulsions, unconsciousness, and death.

Hypoxia. **Hypoxia** is inadequate tissue oxygenation at the cellular level. This can result from a deficiency in oxygen delivery or oxygen utilization at the cellular level. Hypoxia can be caused by (a) a decreased hemoglobin level and lowered oxygen-carrying capacity of the blood; (b) a diminished concentration of inspired oxygen, which may occur at high altitudes; (c) the inability of the tissues to extract oxygen from the blood, as with cyanide poisoning; (d) decreased diffusion of oxygen from the alveoli to the blood, as in pneumonia; (e) poor tissue perfusion with oxygenated blood, as with shock; and (f) impaired ventilation, as with multiple rib fractures or chest trauma.

The clinical signs and symptoms of hypoxia include apprehension, restlessness, inability to concentrate, declining level of consciousness, dizziness, and behavioural changes. The patient with hypoxia is unable to lie down and appears fatigued and agitated. Vital sign changes include an increased pulse rate and increased rate and depth of respiration. The patient with a narcotic overdose, such as a heroin overdose, may display signs of hypoventilation. During early stages of hypoxia, the blood pressure is elevated unless the condition is caused by shock. As the hypoxia worsens, the respiratory rate may decline as a result of respiratory muscle fatigue.

Cyanosis, or blue discoloration of the skin and mucous membranes caused by the presence of desaturated hemoglobin in capillaries, is a late sign of hypoxia. The presence or absence of cyanosis is not a reliable measure of oxygenation status. Central cyanosis, observed in the tongue, soft palate, and conjunctiva of the eye, where blood flow is high, indicates hypoxemia. Peripheral cyanosis, seen in the extremities, nail beds, and earlobes, is often a result of vasoconstriction and stagnant blood flow. Cyanosis may be best observed in racialized persons by assessing mucous membranes and nailbeds (Medline Plus, 2021). Hypoxia is a life-threatening condition. Untreated, it can produce cardiac dysrhythmias that result in death. Hypoxia is managed by administration of oxygen and treatment of the underlying cause, such as airway obstruction.

NURSING KNOWLEDGE BASE

Developmental Factors

According to the Canadian Association of Schools of Nursing (CASN, 2022), foundational knowledge of human development expanding over the lifespan is an essential domain to consider when developing a plan of care. The developmental stage of the patient and the normal aging process can affect tissue oxygenation.

Infants and Toddlers. Infants and toddlers are at risk for upper respiratory tract infections as a result of frequent exposure to other children and exposure to second-hand smoke. In addition, during the teething process, some infants develop nasal congestion, which encourages bacterial growth and increases the potential for respiratory tract infection. Upper respiratory tract infections are usually not dangerous, and infants or toddlers recover with little difficulty.

School-Aged Children and Adolescents. School-aged children and adolescents are exposed to respiratory infections and respiratory risk factors such as second-hand smoke and cigarette smoking. A healthy child usually does not have adverse pulmonary effects from respiratory infections. A person who starts smoking in adolescence and continues to smoke into middle age, however, has an increased risk for cardiopulmonary disease and lung cancer.

Young and Middle-Aged Adults. Young and middle-aged adults are exposed to multiple cardiopulmonary risk factors: an unhealthy diet, lack of exercise, stress, over-the-counter and prescription drugs not used as intended, use of illegal drugs, and smoking. By reducing these modifiable factors patients may decrease their risk for cardiac or pulmonary diseases. During youth and middle age, lifelong habits and lifestyles are established. It is thus important to help these patients make good choices and informed decisions about lifestyle choices for the rest of their lives and about their health care practices.

Older Persons. The cardiac and respiratory systems undergo changes throughout the aging process (Box 40.4). These changes are associated with calcification of the heart valves, SA node, and costal cartilages. The arterial system develops atherosclerotic plaques. Osteoporosis leads to changes in the size and shape of the thorax.

The trachea and large bronchi become enlarged from calcification of the airways. The alveoli enlarge, decreasing the surface area available for gas exchange. The number of functional cilia is reduced, causing a decrease in the effectiveness of the cough mechanism, putting the older person at increased risk for respiratory infections (Touhy et al., 2019). Ventilation and transfer of respiratory gases decline with age because the lungs are unable to expand fully, leading to lower oxygenation levels.

Lifestyle Risk Factors

Lifestyle modifications that influence cardiopulmonary functioning are frequently difficult because a patient is being asked to change a habit or behaviour that may be enjoyed, such as cigarette smoking or eating certain foods; however, these changes can be achieved with encouragement, support, and time (Box 40.5). Risk factor modification is important and includes smoking cessation, weight reduction, a low-cholesterol and low-sodium diet, management of hypertension, and moderate exercise. Although it may be difficult to change long-term behaviour, assisting patients with healthy behaviours can slow or halt the progression of cardiopulmonary diseases.

Poor Nutrition. Nutrition affects cardiopulmonary function in several ways. Severe obesity decreases lung expansion, and the increased body weight increases oxygen demands to meet metabolic needs. The malnourished patient may experience respiratory muscle wasting, resulting in decreased muscle strength and respiratory excursion. Cough

---

BOX 40.4   FOCUS ON OLDER PERSONS

Changes to Cardiac and Respiratory Systems

- Cardiac problems differ from other chronic conditions in that, when they become acute, symptoms worsen rapidly and necessitate hospitalization, whereas other chronic conditions can be managed in the home (Touhy et al., 2019).
- In existing or developing atherosclerosis or hypertension, there may be increased consequences for older persons (Touhy et al., 2019).
- Mental status changes are often the first signs of respiratory problems and may include forgetfulness and irritability.
- Older persons may not complain of dyspnea until it affects the activities of daily living that are important to them.

- Changes in the older person's cough mechanism may lead to retention of pulmonary secretions, airway plugging, and atelectasis, if cough suppressants are not used with caution.
- Age-related changes in the structure of the chest and muscle strength can affect the older person's ability to cough, thus putting them at increased risk for respiratory infections (Touhy et al., 2019).
- For older persons who are sedentary, a compromised immune system may lead to respiratory complications. It is encouraged that older persons receive an annual influenza immunization and a single pneumococcal vaccine (Touhy et al., 2019).

❤ BOX 40.5   FOCUS ON PRIMARY HEALTH CARE

Positive Lifestyle Practices for Cardiopulmonary Health Promotion

As part of a primary health care focus, it is important to educate young to older persons about the following lifestyle practices that promote cardiopulmonary health:

- Maintain ideal body weight.
- Eat a low-fat, low-salt, low-sugar, calorie-appropriate diet.
- Engage in regular aerobic exercise 30 to 60 minutes daily.
- Use stress-reduction techniques.
- Reduce exposure to secondary infections.
- Do not smoke.
- Avoid exposure to second-hand smoke and other pollutants.

- Using recreational drugs (e.g., cannabis, cocaine, opioids) can increase the risk of stroke and of developing heart disease.
- Limit the use of alcohol.
- Have annual visits with a health care provider.
- Monitor blood pressure.
- Monitor cholesterol and triglyceride levels.
- Request an annual influenza vaccine, especially if at risk for development of influenza.
- Request a pneumococcal vaccine, if appropriate.

Adapted from Heart and Stroke Foundation of Canada. (2022). *Lifestyle risk factors*. https://www.heartandstroke.ca/stroke/risk-and-prevention/lifestyle-risk-factors

efficiency is reduced secondary to respiratory muscle weakness, putting the patient at risk for retention of pulmonary secretions. Diets high in fat increase cholesterol and atherogenesis in the coronary arteries.

Over 60% of adults in Canada are either overweight or obese (HSFC, 2022f). Patients who are morbidly obese, malnourished, or both are at risk for anemia. Diets high in carbohydrates may play a role in increasing the carbon dioxide load for patients with carbon dioxide retention. As carbohydrates are metabolized, an increased load of carbon dioxide is created and excreted via the lungs.

In Canada, hypertension continues to be the most prevalent risk factor for cardiovascular disease (Rabi et al., 2020). Health behaviour modification, such as the DASH-like diet, which consists of high amounts of fresh fruits, vegetables, dietary fibre, non-animal protein, low-fat dairy products, and reduced saturated fat in cholesterol, is recommended for both normotensive and hypertensive individuals (Hypertension Canada, 2022). Diets high in potassium may prevent and help improve control over hypertension. Additionally, it has been recommended that reducing intake of concentrated sugars such as those found in ultra-processed foods and beverages be considered for individuals with coronary heart disease (HSFC, 2022g). The HSFC (2020g) recommends that an individual's total intake of free sugars not exceed 10% (ideally less than 5%) of total daily calorie intake.

Inadequate Exercise. Exercise increases the body's metabolic activity and oxygen demand. The rate and depth of respiration increase, enabling the person to inhale more oxygen and exhale excess carbon dioxide. A physical exercise program has many benefits (see Chapter 37). People who exercise for 30 to 60 minutes daily have a lower pulse rate and blood pressure, decreased cholesterol level, increased blood flow, and greater oxygen extraction by working muscles. It is recommended that adults engage in 150 minutes of moderate to vigorous aerobic activity per week (HSFC, 2022h). By completing 10 minutes or more of aerobic activity at a time individuals can achieve this expectation (HSFC, 2022h).

Smoking. Cigarette smoking is associated with a number of diseases, including heart disease, chronic obstructive lung disease, and lung cancer. Smoking is a risk factor for heart disease, stroke, cancer, and respiratory disease. Inhaled nicotine causes vasoconstriction of peripheral and coronary blood vessels, increasing blood pressure, and decreasing blood flow to peripheral vessels. Women who take birth control pills and smoke cigarettes are at increased risk for cardiovascular conditions such as thrombophlebitis and pulmonary emboli.

Cigarette smoking is the leading cause of lung cancer death in Canada, accounting for more than 72% of all cases in Canada (Canadian Cancer Society, 2020a). The Registered Nurses' Association of Ontario (RNAO, 2017) has developed Best Practice Guidelines and recommendations for nurses to support and educate patients who use tobacco and thus improve clinical outcomes (RNAO, 2017). Lung cancer is the leading cause of cancer death in Canada for both men and women (Canadian Cancer Society, 2020b). It is estimated that 1 in 14 Canadian men and 1 in 15 Canadian women will develop lung cancer in their lifetime (Canadian Cancer Society, 2020b). The 5-year survival rate (2012–2014) for females with lung cancer is 22% and in males, 15% (Canadian Cancer Society, 2020b). Some studies that have found an increased risk of lung cancer with long-term use of recreational smoking of cannabis (Canadian Cancer Society, 2020a).

Excessive Substance Use. Excessive use of alcohol and other drugs can impair tissue oxygenation in two ways. First, the person who chronically abuses substances often has a poor nutritional intake. With the resultant decrease in intake of iron-rich foods, hemoglobin production declines. Second, excessive use of alcohol and certain other drugs can depress the respiratory centre, reducing the rate and depth of respiration and the amount of inhaled oxygen. Substance use by either smoking or inhaling, such as crack cocaine or inhaling fumes from paint or glue cans, causes direct injury to lung tissue that can lead to permanent lung damage and impaired oxygenation.

Stress. A continuous state of stress or severe anxiety increases the body's metabolic rate and the oxygen demand. The body responds to anxiety and other stresses with an increased rate and depth of respiration. Most people can adapt, but some, particularly those with chronic illnesses or acute life-threatening illnesses such as an MI, cannot tolerate the oxygen demands associated with anxiety (see Chapter 30).

Environmental Factors

The environment can also influence oxygenation. The incidence of pulmonary disease is higher in smoggy, urban areas than in rural areas. In addition, the patient's workplace may increase the risk for pulmonary disease. Some occupational pollutants are asbestos, talcum powder, dust, and airborne fibres. Asbestosis is an occupational lung disease that develops after exposure to asbestos. The lung in asbestosis is characterized by diffuse interstitial fibrosis, creating a restrictive lung disease. It can also cause pleural mesotheliomas and pleural plaques. Patients at risk for developing asbestosis include those working with textiles, fireproofing, or milling or in the production of paints, plastics, or some prefabricated construction. Patients exposed to asbestos who also smoke are at increased risk of developing lung cancer.

CRITICAL THINKING

Successful critical thinking requires a synthesis of knowledge, experience, information gathered from patients, critical thinking qualities, and intellectual and professional standards. Clinical judgements require nurses to anticipate the information necessary, analyze the data, and make decisions regarding the patient's care. During the assessment, nurses need to consider all elements that build toward making an appropriate nursing diagnosis (Figure 40.6).

To understand the oxygen demands of a patient and the ability of the patient's body to meet those demands, nurses need to integrate knowledge from nursing and other disciplines, previous experiences, and information gathered from patients. Professional standards, such as those developed by the HSFC, the Canadian Cardiovascular Society, the Canadian Lung Association, the Canadian Thoracic Society, and the Canadian Foundation for Infectious Diseases Society, provide valuable guidelines for the care and management of patients with altered oxygenation.

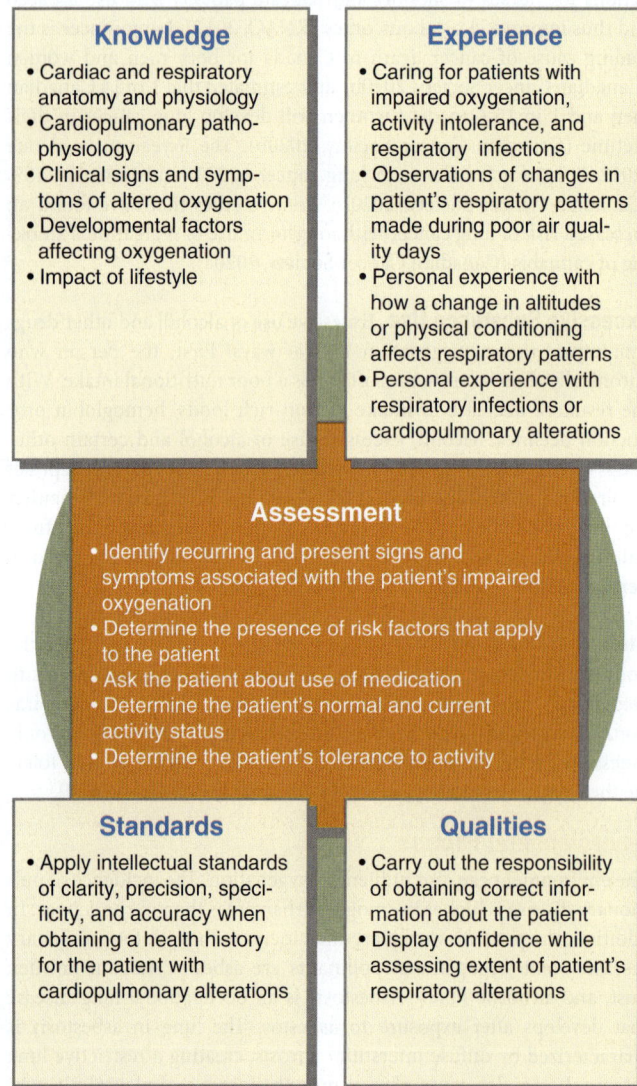

Knowledge
- Cardiac and respiratory anatomy and physiology
- Cardiopulmonary pathophysiology
- Clinical signs and symptoms of altered oxygenation
- Developmental factors affecting oxygenation
- Impact of lifestyle

Experience
- Caring for patients with impaired oxygenation, activity intolerance, and respiratory infections
- Observations of changes in patient's respiratory patterns made during poor air quality days
- Personal experience with how a change in altitudes or physical conditioning affects respiratory patterns
- Personal experience with respiratory infections or cardiopulmonary alterations

Assessment
- Identify recurring and present signs and symptoms associated with the patient's impaired oxygenation
- Determine the presence of risk factors that apply to the patient
- Ask the patient about use of medication
- Determine the patient's normal and current activity status
- Determine the patient's tolerance to activity

Standards
- Apply intellectual standards of clarity, precision, specificity, and accuracy when obtaining a health history for the patient with cardiopulmonary alterations

Qualities
- Carry out the responsibility of obtaining correct information about the patient
- Display confidence while assessing extent of patient's respiratory alterations

FIGURE 40.6 Critical thinking model for oxygenation assessment.

❖ NURSING PROCESS

◆ Assessment

The nursing assessment of a patient's cardiopulmonary functioning includes an in-depth history of the patient's normal and present cardiopulmonary function, past impairments in circulatory or respiratory functioning, and measures that the patient uses to optimize oxygenation. The history should include a review of medication, food, and other allergies, such as pet dander, mould, and environmental triggers.

Through physical examination of the patient's cardiopulmonary status, the extent of existing signs and symptoms is determined. A review of laboratory and diagnostic test results provides valuable data on respiratory and ventilatory parameters.

Health History. The health history should focus on the patient's ability to meet oxygen needs. The health history for cardiac function includes pain and characteristics of pain, dyspnea, fatigue, peripheral circulation, cardiac risk factors, and the presence of past or concurrent cardiac conditions. The health history for respiratory function includes presence of a cough, shortness of breath, wheezing, pain, environmental exposures, frequency of respiratory tract infections, pulmonary risk factors, past respiratory problems, current medication use, and smoking history or exposure to second-hand smoke.

Pain. Chest pain needs to be thoroughly evaluated with regard to location, duration, radiation, and frequency. Cardiac pain does not occur with respiratory variations and is most often on the left side of the chest; in men, it radiates to the left arm. Chest pain in women is much less definitive and may be a sensation of choking, breathlessness, or pain that radiates through to the back. Pericardial pain resulting from an inflammation of the pericardial sac is usually nonradiating and may occur with inspiration.

Pleuritic chest pain is peripheral and may radiate to the scapular regions. It is worsened by inspiratory manoeuvres, such as coughing, yawning, and sighing. Pleuritic pain is often caused from an inflammation or infection in the pleural space and is described as knifelike, lasting from a minute to hours and always in association with inspiration.

Musculoskeletal pain may be present following exercise, rib trauma, and prolonged coughing episodes. This pain is also aggravated by inspiratory movements and may easily be confused with pleuritic chest pain.

Fatigue. Fatigue is a subjective sensation in which the patient reports a loss of endurance. Fatigue in the patient with cardiopulmonary alterations is often an early sign of worsening of the chronic underlying process. To provide an objective measure of fatigue, the patient may be asked to rate the fatigue on a scale of 0 to 10, with 10 being the worst level of fatigue and 0 representing no fatigue.

Smoking. It is important to determine patients' direct and secondary exposure to cigarette smoke. Nurses should ask patients about any history of smoking, including the number of years smoked and the number of packages smoked per day. This is recorded as pack-year history. For example, if a patient smoked two packs a day for 20 years, the patient would have a 40-pack-year history (packages per day × years smoked).

It is also important to determine if the patient is exposed to second-hand smoke from family or co-workers. Exposure to second-hand smoke increases the patient's risk for chronic lung or cardiac diseases.

Dyspnea. **Dyspnea** is a clinical sign of hypoxia and manifests as breathlessness. It is the subjective sensation of difficult or uncomfortable breathing. Dyspnea is shortness of breath associated with exercise or excitement, but in some patients, dyspnea may be present without any relation to activity or exercise. Dyspnea is associated with many conditions, such as pulmonary diseases, cardiovascular diseases, neuromuscular conditions, and anemia. Dyspnea may occur in pregnant women in the final months of pregnancy. Environmental factors, such as pollution, cold air, and smoking, may also cause or worsen dyspnea.

Dyspnea can be associated with clinical signs such as exaggerated respiratory effort, use of the accessory muscles of respiration, nasal flaring, and marked increases in the rate and depth of respirations. The use of a visual analogue scale (VAS) can help patients make an objective assessment of their dyspnea. The VAS is a 100-mm vertical line with end points of 0 and 10. Zero is equated with no dyspnea and 10 is equated with the worst breathlessness the patient has experienced. Studies have validated the use of the VAS to evaluate a patient's dyspnea in the clinical setting (Pang et al., 2014). Nurses can evaluate the effectiveness of nursing interventions by monitoring a patient's assessment of their dyspnea.

If the patient has a history of dyspnea, it is important to determine the circumstances under which it occurred, such as with exertion, stress, or respiratory tract infection. The nurse should also determine whether the patient's perception of dyspnea affects the ability to lie flat. Orthopnea is a condition in which the person must use multiple pillows when lying down or must sit with their arms elevated and leaning forward to breathe. The number of pillows required for sleeping, such as two- or three-pillow orthopnea, usually quantifies the presence of orthopnea.

Cough. *Cough* is a sudden, audible expulsion of air from the lungs. The person breathes in, the glottis is partially closed, and the accessory muscles of expiration contract to expel the air forcibly. Coughing is a protective reflex to clear the trachea, bronchi, and lungs of irritants and secretions. The carina, the point of bifurcation of the right and left mainstem bronchus, is the most sensitive area for cough production. A cough is difficult to evaluate, and almost everyone has periods of coughing. Patients with a chronic cough tend to deny, underestimate, or minimize their coughing, often because they are so accustomed to it that they are unaware of how frequently it occurs.

Coughing is classified according to the time when the patient most frequently coughs. Patients with chronic sinusitis may cough only in the early morning or immediately after rising from sleep. This clears the airway of mucus resulting from sinus drainage. Patients with chronic bronchitis generally produce sputum all day, although greater amounts are produced after rising from a semi-recumbent or flat position. This is a result of the dependent accumulation of sputum in the airways and is associated with reduced mobility (see Chapter 46). When a patient has a cough, it is important to determine its frequency and whether it is productive or nonproductive. A productive cough results in sputum production, material coughed up from the lungs that may be swallowed or expectorated. Sputum contains mucus, cellular debris, and microorganisms, and it may contain pus or blood. When assessing a patient's cough, collect data about the type and quantity of sputum. Instruct the patient to try to produce some sputum; the patient should be careful not to simply clear the throat to produce a sample of saliva. Then inspect it for colour, consistency, odour, and amount (Box 40.6).

If hemoptysis (bloody sputum) is reported, determine if it is associated with coughing and bleeding from the upper respiratory tract, from sinus drainage, or from the gastrointestinal tract (hematemesis). In addition, the hemoptysis should be described according to amount, colour, and duration and whether it is mixed with sputum. When the patient reports bloody or blood-tinged sputum, diagnostic tests, such as examination of sputum specimens, chest X-ray examinations, bronchoscopy, and other X-ray studies, should be performed.

BOX 40.6	Sputum Characteristics
Colour	**Quantity**
Clear	Same as usual
White	Increased
Yellow	Decreased
Green	
Brown	**Consistency**
Red	Frothy
Streaked with blood	Watery
	Tenacious, thick
Changes in Colour	
Same colour throughout the day	**Presence of Blood**
Clearing with coughing	Occasional
Progressively darker	Early morning
	Bright or dark red
Odour	Blood tinged
None	
Foul	

Wheezing. Wheezing is characterized by a high-pitched musical sound caused by high-velocity movement of air through a narrowed airway. Wheezing may be associated with asthma, acute bronchitis, or pneumonia. Wheezing can occur on inspiration, expiration, or both. It is important to determine if there are any precipitating factors, such as respiratory infection, allergens, exercise, or stress.

Environmental or Geographical Exposures. Environmental exposure to many inhaled substances is closely linked to respiratory disease. Nurses should investigate exposures in a patient's home and workplace. The most common environmental exposures in the home are cigarette smoke, carbon monoxide, and radon. In addition, it is good to determine whether a patient who is a nonsmoker is passively exposed to smoke.

Carbon monoxide poisoning can result from a blocked furnace flue or fireplace. The patient may have vague complaints of general malaise, flu-like symptoms, and excessive sleepiness. Patients are particularly at risk in the late fall when they turn the heat on or begin to use the fireplace again. Radon gas, a radioactive substance that can damage lung tissue and cause lung cancer, enters homes through the ground. When homes are underventilated, this gas is not able to escape into the atmosphere and becomes trapped in the home.

An employment history should be obtained to assess exposure to substances such as asbestos, coal, cotton fibres, fumes, or chemical inhalants. This is particularly important with middle-aged and older persons, who may have worked in places without regulations to protect workers from carcinogens such as asbestos.

Exposure to pathogens may occur during travel. Schistosomiasis can be acquired in Asia, Africa, the Caribbean, and South America. This is infection of a human with a species of fluke found in fresh water that has been contaminated by human feces. Coccidioidomycosis is a fungal disease caused by inhalation of *Coccidioides immitis*, a windborne spore carried on dust particles.

Respiratory Infections. A health history should contain information about the patient's frequency and duration of respiratory tract infections. Although everyone occasionally experiences a cold, for some people it can result in bronchitis or pneumonia. On average, patients will have four colds per year. Nurses should determine if patients have had a recent pneumococcal or flu vaccine. Questioning older persons about receiving these vaccines is especially important, given their increased risk for respiratory disease (Touhy et al., 2019). Nurses should ask about any known exposure to tuberculosis (TB) and the results of the tuberculin skin test.

Allergies. When obtaining a respiratory system history, inquire about airborne allergens. The patient's allergic response may be watery eyes, sneezing, runny nose, or respiratory symptoms, such as cough or wheezing. Ask the patient specific questions about the type of allergens, response to these allergens, and successful and unsuccessful relief measures. In addition, determine the impact that environmental air quality and second-hand smoke exposure have on the patient's allergy and symptoms.

Safe nursing practice also includes obtaining information about food, medication, or insect-sting allergies. These data are usually obtained on initial history and physical examination. However, it is important to double-check this information with the patient, especially when obtaining information about respiratory allergens.

Health Risks. Familial risk factors, such as a family history of lung cancer or cardiovascular disease, need to be investigated. Documentation should include which blood relatives have had the disease and their present level of health or age at time of death. Other family risk factors include the presence of infectious diseases, particularly TB. It is important to determine who in the patient's household has been infected and the status of treatment.

Medications. The health history should also list medications the patient is using. These could include prescribed medications, over-the-counter medications, folk medicine, herbal medicines, alternative therapies, and illicit drugs and substances. Such medications may have adverse effects by themselves or through interactions with other drugs. A person using a prescribed bronchodilator drug, for example, may decide that using an over-the-counter inhalant will also be beneficial. Many of these contain ephedrine or ma huang, a natural chemical that acts like epinephrine. This product may react with the prescribed medication by potentiating or decreasing the effect of the prescribed medication. Patients taking warfarin for blood thinning will prolong the prothrombin time (international normalized ratio [INR]) results if they are taking gingko biloba, garlic, or ginseng with the anticoagulant. The drug interaction could precipitate a life-threatening bleed.

> **SAFETY ALERT** During history taking, ask patients to list all of the over-the-counter and herbal supplements that they are taking, including green tea, to ensure that medication interactions do not develop.

When patients are prescribed medications for which toxic levels can be monitored by blood analyses, nurses need to review these laboratory values. Common medications that can be monitored are digitalis preparations (digitalis levels), anticoagulants such as warfarin (Coumadin; INR level), and phenobarbital (phenobarbital levels). Toxic effects of these medications can impair cardiopulmonary functioning.

It is important to determine whether a patient uses illicit drugs. These drugs, particularly parenterally administered narcotics, which are often diluted with talcum powder, can cause pulmonary disorders resulting from the irritant effect of the powder on lung tissues.

As with all medication, nurses need to assess a patient's knowledge and ability to self-administer medications correctly (see Chapter 35). Of particular importance is the assessment of the patient's understanding of potential adverse effects of the medications. Patients should be able to recognize adverse reactions and be aware of the dangers in combining prescribed medications with over-the-counter drugs.

Physical Examination

The physical examination performed to assess the patient's level of tissue oxygenation includes evaluation of the cardiopulmonary system (see Chapter 33). Special consideration should be given when assessing the older person because changes in the cardiopulmonary system occur with the aging process (Table 40.3). These changes may result in changes in the patient's activity tolerance, level of fatigue, or transient changes in vital signs and may not be associated with a specific cardiopulmonary disease.

Inspection. Using inspection techniques, the nurse performs a head-to-toe observation of the patient for skin and mucous membrane colour, general appearance, level of consciousness, adequacy of systemic circulation, breathing patterns, and chest wall movement (Table 40.4). Any abnormalities should be investigated during palpation, percussion, and auscultation.

Inspection includes observations of the nails for clubbing. Clubbed nails, obliteration of the normal angle between the base of the nail and the skin, are seen in patients with prolonged oxygen deficiency, endocarditis, and congenital heart defects.

Chest wall movement is observed for retraction, sinking in of soft tissues of the chest between the intercostal spaces. The nurse should also observe for paradoxical breathing, asynchronous breathing, and the patient's breathing pattern (Table 40.5). In paradoxical breathing, the chest wall contracts during inspiration and expands during exhalation. Infants can experience sternal and substernal chest wall retractions with only a slight inspiratory effort because of the pliability of the chest wall. The anteroposterior diameter of the chest wall should be noted; conditions such as emphysema, advancing age, and COPD can cause the chest to assume a rounded shape.

Palpation. Palpation of the chest provides assessment data in several areas. It is used to document the type and amount of thoracic excursion, elicit any areas of tenderness, and identify tactile fremitus, thrills, heaves, and the cardiac point of maximal impulse (PMI). Palpation also aids in detecting abnormal masses or lumps in the axilla and breast tissue. Palpation of the extremities provides data about the peripheral circulation, the presence and quality of peripheral pulses, skin temperature, colour, and capillary refill (see Chapter 33).

The feet and legs should be palpated to assess for the presence or absence of peripheral edema. Patients with alterations in their cardiac function, such as those with heart failure or hypertension, often have pedal or lower extremity edema. Edema is graded from 1+ to 4+, depending on the depth of visible indentation after firm application of a finger (see Chapter 33).

Palpation of the pulses in the neck and extremities is performed to assess arterial blood flow (see Chapter 33). A scale of 0 (absent pulse) to 3+ (full, bounding pulse) is used to describe what is palpated. The normal pulse is graded at 2+, and a weak, thready pulse is graded as 1+.

Percussion. Percussion is used to detect the presence of abnormal fluid or air in the lungs. It also aids in determining diaphragmatic excursion (see Chapter 33).

Auscultation. Auscultation helps in identifying normal and abnormal heart and lung sounds (see Chapter 33). Auscultation of the cardiovascular system should include assessment for normal S_1 and S_2 sounds, the presence of abnormal S_3 and S_4 sounds (gallops), and murmurs or

TABLE 40.3	Assessment Findings in the Aging Cardiopulmonary System	
Function	**Pathophysiological Change**	**Key Clinical Findings**
Heart		
Muscle contraction	Thickening of the ventricular wall, increased collagen and decreased elastin in the heart muscle	Decreased cardiac output Diminished cardiac reserve
Blood flow	Heart valves become thicker and stiffer, more often in the mitral and aortic valves	Systolic ejection murmur
Conduction system	The SA node becomes fibrotic from calcification; the number of pacemaker cells in the SA node decreases	Increased PR, QRS, and Q-T intervals, decreased amplitude of the QRS complex
Arterial vessel compliance	Vessels become calcified, loss of arterial distensibility, decreased elastin in the vessel walls, more bends and twists (tortuous) in the vessels	Hypertension, with an increase in systolic blood pressure Fluctuation in blood pressure
Lungs		
Breathing mechanics	Decreased chest wall compliance, loss of elastic recoil Decreased respiratory muscle mass/strength	Prolonged exhalation phase Decreased vital capacity
Oxygenation	Increased ventilation–perfusion mismatch Decreased alveolar surface area Decreased carbon dioxide diffusion capacity	Decreased PaO_2 (arterial oxygen tension) Decreased cardiac output Slightly increased $PaCO_2$ (arterial carbon dioxide tension)
Breathing control/breathing pattern	Decreased responsiveness of central and peripheral chemoreceptors to hypoxemia and hypercapnia	Increased respiratory rate Decreased tidal volume
Lung defence mechanisms	Decreased number of cilia Decreased immunoglobulin A (IgA) production and humoral and cellular immunity	Decreased airway clearance Diminished cough reflex
Sleep and breathing	Decreased respiratory drive Decreased tone of upper airway muscles	Increased risk of aspiration and infection Decreased PaO_2 Snoring, obstructive sleep apnea

TABLE 40.4	Inspection of Cardiopulmonary Status			
Abnormality	**Cause**		**Abnormality**	**Cause**
Eyes			**Chest**	
Xanthelasma (yellow lipid lesions on eyelids)	Hyperlipidemia		Retractions	Increased work of breathing, dyspnea
Corneal arcus (whitish opaque ring around junction of cornea and sclera)	Hyperlipidemia in young to middle-aged adults, normal finding in older persons with arcus senilis		Asymmetry	Chest wall injury
			Skin	
Pale conjunctivae	Anemia		Peripheral cyanosis	Vasoconstriction and diminished blood flow
Cyanotic conjunctivae	Hypoxemia		Central cyanosis	Hypoxemia
Petechiae on conjunctivae	Fat embolus or bacterial endocarditis		Decreased skin turgor	Dehydration (normal finding in older persons, as a result of decreased skin elasticity)
Mouth and Lips				
Cyanotic mucous membranes	Decreased oxygenation (hypoxia)		Dependent edema	Associated with right-sided heart failure
Pursed-lip breathing	Associated with chronic lung disease		Periorbital edema	Associated with kidney disease
Neck Veins			**Fingertips and Nail Beds**	
Distension	Associated with right-sided heart failure		Cyanosis	Decreased cardiac output or hypoxia
			Splinter hemorrhages	Bacterial endocarditis
Nose			Clubbing	Chronic hypoxemia
Flaring nares	Air hunger, dyspnea			

From Solomon, B. S., Ball, J. W., Flynn, J. A., et al. (2019). *Seidel's guide to physical examination* (9th ed.). Elsevier.

TABLE 40.5   Assessment of Breathing Pattern

Pattern and Rate (Breaths/Minute)	Clinical Significance
Eupnea (12–20)	Normal rate in the adult
Tachypnea (>20)	Can result from anxiety or response to pain or fever, respiratory failure, shortness of breath, or a respiratory infection. May lead to respiratory alkalosis, paresthesia, tetany, and confusion
Bradypnea (<12)	Results from sleep, respiratory depression, drug overdose, or central nervous system lesion
Apnea (absence of respiration >15 seconds)	May be intermittent, such as in sleep apnea, or prolonged, as in a respiratory arrest
Kussmaul's respirations (usually >35, may be slow or normal)	Tachypnea pattern is associated with metabolic imbalance such as diabetic ketoacidosis, metabolic acidosis, or renal failure

rubs. Auscultation is also used to identify a bruit over the carotid arteries, abdominal aorta, and femoral arteries.

Auscultation of lung sounds involves listening for movement of air throughout all lung fields—anterior, posterior, and lateral. Adventitious breath sounds occur with collapse of a lung segment, fluid in a lung segment, or narrowing or obstruction of an airway. Auscultation is also used to evaluate the patient's response to interventions for improving the respiratory status.

Diagnostic Tests

There are a variety of diagnostic tests used to monitor cardiopulmonary functioning. Some of these tests can be obtained through screening, simple blood specimens, X-ray films, or other noninvasive means. One such screening mechanism is TB skin testing (Box 40.7). This is a simple test that is usually required annually for health care workers to monitor possible TB exposure. In contrast, invasive diagnostic tests, such as a thoracentesis, can be quite painful, depending on the patient's tolerance for pain.

Tables 40.6 and 40.7 and Box 40.8 summarize diagnostic testing used in the assessment and evaluation of patients with cardiopulmonary alterations. The nurse should explain the procedure and tell the patient what to expect, to reduce the patient's anxiety. The patient must understand the importance of following instructions, such as holding the breath as requested and not coughing during the procedure. After any procedure, the patient is monitored for signs of changes in cardiopulmonary functioning, sudden shortness of breath, pain, oxygen desaturation, and anxiety. The nurse needs to promote the patient's comfort and encourage the patient to rest after the test, because many patients find these tests to be tiring.

BOX 40.7   Tuberculosis Skin Testing

- Skin testing is used to determine past exposure to *Mycobacterium* tuberculosis.
- Tuberculosis skin testing (TST) is performed by administering an intradermal injection of 0.1 mL of tuberculin-purified protein derivative on the inner surface of the forearm. The injection produces a pale elevation of the skin (a wheal) 6–10 mm in diameter. Afterward, the injection site may be circled, and the patient is instructed not to wash off the circle.
- Tuberculin skin tests are read 48–72 hours after injection. If the site is not read within 72 hours, the patient must undergo another skin test.
- Positive results are indicated by a palpable, elevated, hardened, reddened area around the injection site, caused by edema and inflammation from the antigen–antibody reaction. The site is measured in millimetres. A positive test result occurs when the site is ≥10 mm.
- Reddened flat areas are *not* positive reactions and are not measured.
- TST in older persons (see Box 40.4) and those with altered immune function (e.g., HIV, patients receiving chemotherapy) is less reliable.

Patient Expectations

During assessment, nurses should ask patients what they expect from the encounter and what their priority is for management of their health. In identifying expectations, nurses involve patients in the decision-making process and allow them to participate in their care and know what will happen to them (Box 40.9). For example, if the nurse plans a smoking-cessation or weight-reduction program for a patient who is not ready for the change, both the nurse and the patient will become frustrated. It is important to establish short-term, realistic goals that

TABLE 40.6 Cardiopulmonary Diagnostic Blood Studies

Test and Normal Values	Interpretation
Complete Blood Count (CBC)	
Normal values for a CBC vary with age and gender.	A CBC determines the number and type of red and white blood cells per cubic millimetre of blood.
Cardiac Blood Studies	
CK (creatinine kinase) MB Levels rise 3–6 hours after infarction occurs. Peaks in 12–24 hours and then returns to normal within 2 days.	Cardiac enzymes are used to diagnose acute myocardial infarcts. CK-MB is specific to the myocardial cell and may quantify myocardial damage and timing of the onset of the infarction.
Myoglobin <90 ng/mL	Myoglobin is used for early evaluation of patients with suspected myocardial infarction and skeletal muscle damage. Increased levels indicate that cardiac muscle injury or death occurred approximately 3 hours after infarction.

Two cardiac-specific troponins released after a myocardial infarction:
    Cardiac troponin I (cTnI) <0.35 ng/mL
    Cardiac troponin T (cTnT) <0.1 ng/mL
	Cardiac troponins become elevated as early as 3 hours after myocardial injury.
	Often remains elevated for 7–10 days.
	Often remains elevated for up to 14 days.

B-type natriuretic peptide (BNP) BNP <100 ng/mL	BNP is a marker for heart failure and assists with identifying pulmonary or cardiac causes for shortness of breath. The more elevated the levels, the more severe the heart failure.
C-reactive protein <10 mg/L	C-reactive protein is used to detect inflammation if there is a high suspicion of tissue injury or infection in the body. It may also be used to assess for risk of developing coronary artery disease and stroke.
Serum Electrolytes	
Potassium (K^+) 3.5–5 mmol/L	Patients on diuretic therapy are at risk for hypokalemia (low potassium). Patients receiving angiotensin-converting enzyme inhibitors are at risk for hyperkalemia (elevated potassium).
Cholesterol	
Cholesterol <5.20 mmol/L	Contributing factors include sedentary lifestyle, intake of saturated fatty acids, and familial hypercholesterolemia.
Low-density lipoprotein (LDL)-cholesterol (bad cholesterol) <3.4 mmol/L	High LDL cholesterol (hypercholesterolemia) is caused by excessive intake of saturated fatty acids, dietary cholesterol intake, and obesity. Familial hypercholesterolemia and hyperlipidemia are also contributing factors, as are hypothyroidism, nephrotic syndrome, and diabetes mellitus.

High-density lipoprotein (HDL)-cholesterol (good cholesterol)
    Male: >0.75 mmol/L
    Female: >0.91 mmol/L
	Low HDL cholesterol is caused by cigarette smoking, obesity, lack of regular exercise, β-adrenergic blocking agents, genetic disorders of HDL metabolism, hypertriglyceridemia, and type 2 diabetes.

Triglycerides
    Male: 0.45–1.71 mmol/L
    Female: 0.40–1.52 mmol/L
	Obesity, excessive alcohol intake, diabetes mellitus, β-adrenergic blocking agents, and genetic predisposition cause hypertriglyceridemia.

Data from Pagana, K. D., Pagana, T. J., & Pike-MacDonald, S. A. (2019). *Mosby's Canadian manual of diagnostic and laboratory tests* (2nd ed.). Elsevier Canada.

build to a larger goal. For example, reducing the fat in the patient's diet might start out with replacing food such as whole milk with 2% milk and gradually introducing skim milk. A sudden change from whole to skim milk will most likely fail, because the change is too great. A plan for adding exercise to the patient's lifestyle could start with a commitment to exercise once a week for 20 minutes, or the patient could commit to a weight-reduction plan of 2 kg per month.

When addressing a patient's expectations, the nurse needs to remember that their goals and expectations may not always coincide with those of their patient. By addressing the patient's concerns and expectations, the nurse will establish a relationship that can address other health care goals and expected outcomes. Knowing the mindset of patients and respecting their wishes will go a long way toward helping patients make significant lifestyle changes to benefit their health.

◆ Nursing Diagnosis

Patients with an altered level of oxygenation can have nursing diagnoses that are primarily from a cardiovascular or pulmonary origin. Each nursing diagnosis is based on specific defining characteristics and the related etiology (Box 40.10). Nurses use the information gathered in the nursing assessment to identify and cluster the defining characteristics. The clustered defining characteristics support the nursing diagnosis.

Nursing diagnoses appropriate for the patient with alterations in oxygenation include, but are not limited to, the following:

- *Activity intolerance*
- *Risk for activity intolerance*
- *Ineffective airway clearance*
- *Anxiety*
- *Ineffective breathing pattern*
- *Decreased cardiac output*
- *Impaired comfort*
- *Impaired verbal communication*
- *Ineffective individual coping*
- *Fatigue*
- *Fear*
- *Risk for imbalanced fluid volume*

TABLE 40.7	Cardiac Function Diagnostic Tests
Test	**Significance**
12-Lead electrocardiogram (ECG)	Graphic recording of the electrical impulses generated by the heart, during the cardiac cycle. The test is used to detect abnormal electrical activity and the electrical position of the heart. The ECG includes 12 leads: I, II, III, AVR, AVL, AVF, and V1–6. It provides a 360-degree view of the heart.
Holter monitor	Portable ECG worn by the patient. The test produces a continuous ECG tracing over a period of time. Patients keep a diary of activity, noting when they experience rapid heartbeats or dizziness. Evaluation of the ECG recording along with the diary provides information about the heart's electrical activity during activities of daily living.
ECG exercise stress test	ECG is monitored while the patient walks on a treadmill at a specified speed and duration of time. Used to evaluate the cardiac response to physical stress. The test is not a valuable tool for evaluation of cardiac response in women because of increased false-positive findings among women.
Thallium stress test	An ECG stress test with the addition of thallium-201-injected IV. The test determines coronary blood flow changes with increased activity.
Electrophysiological study (EPS)	Invasive measure of intracardiac electrical pathways. Provides more specific information about difficult-to-treat dysrhythmias. EPS is used to assess the adequacy of antidysrhythmic medication.
Echocardiography	A transthoracic echo (TTE) is a noninvasive measure of heart structure and heart wall motion. It graphically demonstrates overall cardiac performance. Echocardiography can be performed via the esophagus and is referred to as *transesophageal echocardiography*, or TEE.
Scintigraphy	Radionuclide angiography. Used to evaluate cardiac structure, myocardial perfusion, and contractility.
Cardiac catheterization and angiography	Used to visualize cardiac chambers, valves, the great vessels, and coronary arteries. Pressures and volumes within the four chambers of the heart can also be measured.
Computed tomography angiography (CTA)	Noninvasive medical test that consists of a combination of a CT scan and an injection of contrast to create an image of the coronary vessels.
Cardiac magnetic resonance imaging	Considered to be the procedure of choice for evaluating pericardial disease, intracardiac masses and pericardiac masses, for imaging of right ventricle and pulmonary vessels, as well as assessing forms of congenital heart disease.

Data from Pagana, K. D., Pagana, T. J., & Pike-MacDonald, S. A. (2019). *Mosby's Canadian manual of diagnostic and laboratory tests* (2nd ed.). Elsevier Canada.

- *Impaired gas exchange*
- *Ineffective health maintenance*
- *Risk for infection*
- *Deficient (specify) knowledge*
- *Risk for impaired skin integrity*
- *Disturbed sleep pattern*
- *Ineffective tissue perfusion*
- *Impaired spontaneous ventilation*

◆ Planning

During planning, nurses use critical thinking skills to synthesize information from multiple sources (Figure 40.7). Critical thinking ensures that the nurse's plan of care integrates individualized patient needs. Professional standards are especially important to consider when developing a care plan. These standards often establish scientifically proven guidelines for selecting effective nursing interventions.

Goals and Outcomes. An individualized care plan is developed for each nursing diagnosis (Box 40.11). In collaboration with the patient, the nurse sets realistic expectations for care. Goals should be individualized and realistic with measurable outcomes.

Patients with impaired oxygenation require a nursing care plan directed toward meeting the actual or potential oxygenation needs of the patient. Individual outcomes are derived from patient-centred needs. For example, the goal of maintaining a patent airway can be evaluated by specific outcomes for the patient. These might include the following expected outcomes:

- Patient's lungs are clear to auscultation.
- Patient achieves maintenance and promotion of bilateral lung expansion.
- Patient coughs productively.
- Oxygen saturation is maintained or improved.

Often a patient with cardiopulmonary disease has multiple nursing diagnoses (Figure 40.8). In this case, the nurse needs to identify when goals or outcomes apply to more than one diagnosis. The presence of multiple diagnoses also makes priority setting a critical activity.

Setting Priorities. The patient's level of health, age, lifestyle, and environmental risks affect the level of tissue oxygenation. Patients with severe impairments in oxygenation frequently require nursing interventions in multiple areas. Nurses need to consider what the most important goal is during the limited amount of time a patient is seen in the hospital or primary care setting. For example, in an acute care setting, maintaining a patent airway has a higher priority than improving the patient's exercise tolerance. The need for a patent airway is an immediate need. In a second example, when caring for a patient who has an abdominal incision, pain control may have a greater priority than coughing and deep breathing. Again, in this situation, controlling the patient's pain ultimately will facilitate coughing and deep breathing.

However, in a community-based or primary setting, the priority may focus on smoking cessation, exercise, diet modifications, or a combination of these activities. Both the nurse and the patient need to be focused on the same goal and expected outcomes to be successful. In addition to being individualized, each goal should be realistic and attainable for the patient.

Collaborative Care. The time spent with the patient in any setting is limited. Therefore, nurses need to collaborate with family members, colleagues, and other specialists to accomplish the goals and outcomes that have been determined. Some patients may need to improve their exercise and activity tolerance; for some patients, their continuity of care may involve enrolling in a community-based cardiopulmonary rehabilitation program. Another patient may have the same health

BOX 40.8 Common Respiratory Tests and Methods

Oxygenation Tests

- *Pulse oximetry:* A **pulse oximeter** is a device used to indirectly measure pulse rate and oxygen saturation. A sensor is attached to the patient's finger, toe, nose, earlobe, or forehead (see figure). Accuracy is directly related to the perfusion of the probe area, a systolic blood pressure >90 mm Hg, and the hemoglobin level. The SpO_2 may be inaccurate in a patient wearing nail polish. Decreased levels correlate well with arterial oxygen levels and are used to trend oxygenation over time. Normal peripheral capillary oxygen saturation (SpO_2) values are greater than 95%. An SpO_2 below 70% is life-threatening. The SpO_2 value is one indicator that informs a respiratory assessment and is not the only indicator of respiratory function.

- *Arterial blood gas:* A radial or femoral artery is punctured to obtain arterial blood. Tests measure the oxygen concentration in the blood, the hydrogen ion concentration (pH), partial pressure of carbon dioxide ($PaCO_2$), and the partial pressure of oxygen (PaO_2). Normal values are as follows:
  - pH 7.35–7.45
  - $PaCO_2$ 35–45 mm Hg
  - PaO_2 80–100 mm Hg
  - SaO_2 95–100%

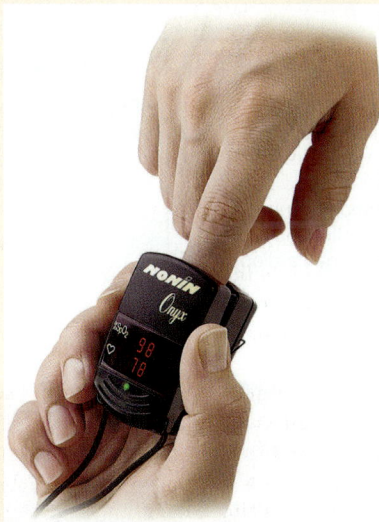

A

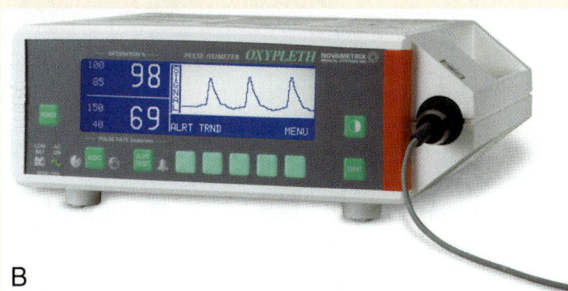

B

A, Portable pulse oximeter displays oxygen saturation (SpO_2) and pulse rate. **B,** A pulse oximeter displays the oxygen saturation and pulse rate as a digital reading. (From Tyerman, J., & Cobbett, S. [Eds.]. [2023]. *Lewis's medical-surgical nursing in Canada: Assessment and management of clinical problems* [5th ed.]. Elsevier.)

Pulmonary Function Tests

Pulmonary function tests measure lung volume (the amount of air moving into and out of the lungs) and capacity (how much air the lungs can hold). Respiratory therapists usually conduct these tests. The patient takes as deep a breath as possible and forcefully exhales into a mouthpiece attached to a machine. Pulmonary readings are recorded and compared with previous readings and with average normal values, which vary depending on the patient's age, gender, weight, height, and race. These tests are used to diagnose and monitor pulmonary disease and conditions (e.g., asthma, emphysema). They are also used to evaluate postoperative lung conditions.

Imaging

- *Chest X-ray examination:* Usually posteroanterior and lateral films are taken to adequately visualize all of the lung fields. A radiograph of the thorax is used to observe the lung fields for fluid, infiltrates (e.g., pneumonia), masses (e.g., lung cancer), fractures, pneumothorax, and other abnormal processes.

- *Computed tomography (CT) scan:* A CT scan provides visualization of fine detail of the lungs and other structures in the thorax. It is often used as part of the assessment of patients with pneumonia, lung masses, and suspected pulmonary emboli.

- *Ventilation/perfusion (nuclear medicine) lung scan:* This scan is used to detect pulmonary emboli. The results from two separate scans are compared: the perfusion scan uses an injected radioactive tracer to measure pulmonary blood flow, and the ventilation scan shows the pulmonary distribution of a different inhaled tracer. Mismatches (areas of ventilation without corresponding perfusion or blood flow) indicate pulmonary emboli.

Methods of Obtaining Respiratory Specimens for Analysis

Specimens are cultured so they can be used to detect the presence of blood, microbes, and abnormal cells. A variety of methods are used to obtain respiratory specimens.

- *Sputum tests:* Sputum is mucus from the respiratory system that is expectorated through the mouth. Sputum specimens are obtained when the patient coughs up sputum from the bronchi and trachea; specimens are easier to obtain in the morning when the secretions are coughed up upon awakening. Sputum tests include (a) *sputum culture and sensitivity (C& S)* test, used to identify a specific microorganism growing in the sputum and to identify medication resistance and sensitivities; (b) *sputum for acid-fast bacillus (AFB)*, a test used to screen for the presence of AFB for detection of TB by early-morning specimens on three consecutive days; and (c) *sputum for cytology*, used to identify abnormal lung cancer and differentiate the type of cancer cells (small cell, oat cell, large cell).

- *Bronchoscopy:* A narrow, flexible, fibre-optic scope is passed into the trachea and bronchi to enable visual examination of the tracheobronchial tree. The procedure is performed under conscious sedation to obtain fluid, sputum, or biopsy samples, and to remove mucous plugs or foreign bodies.

- *Thoracentesis:* This involves surgical perforation of the chest wall and pleural space with a needle to aspirate fluid for diagnostic or therapeutic purposes or to remove a specimen for biopsy. The procedure is performed using aseptic technique and local anaesthetic. The patient usually sits upright with the anterior thorax supported by pillows or an overbed table.

- *Nasopharyngeal aspirate or swab:* This swab is used to detect respiratory viruses. Aspirates are the best specimens from young children, whereas swabs can be used for obtaining samples from older children and adults.

Data from Pagana, K. D., Pagana, T. J., & Pike-MacDonald, S. A. (2019). *Mosby's Canadian manual of diagnostic and laboratory tests* (2nd ed.). Elsevier Canada.

BOX 40.9 CASE STUDY

Understanding Cardiac Rehabilitation: A Personal Story and Case Study

During my evening shift, a 48-year-old patient (preferred pronouns: he/him) was admitted to the cardiac medical unit with a late-presenting myocardial infarction (MI) and an associated tachyarrhythmia. He presented to the emergency department with mid-scapular pain. The patient did not associate the symptoms with a cardiac event. During the initial assessment of the patient, he was prepared and eager to return to work upon discharge from the hospital. The patient's perspective was not consistent with his partner's, who shared concerns about being overwhelmed with the dietary changes, new medications, and her partner's "denial" of the current diagnosis. In addition, his partner shared significant concerns about his frequent use of recreational cannabis. Later in the shift there was time to inquire about the patient and his partner's understanding of the cardiac rehabilitation program and their intention to use the resource. This was an opportune time to teach them about cardiac rehabilitation. They developed an understanding of this resource and began to recognize that it was more than just an exercise program. Together they understood that cardiac rehabilitation encompassed a holistic approach to wellness with members of an interprofessional team who have expertise in different areas of clinical practice. Cardiac rehabilitation offered this couple ongoing support and strategies for lifestyle changes to promote wellness.

Critical Thinking Questions

1. How do nurses assess patients' and families' readiness to learn?
2. What pertinent members of the interprofessional team support patients and families during cardiac rehabilitation? What are key elements of the conversation with patients and families regarding cardiac rehabilitation?
3. In addition to patients who have been diagnosed with an MI, what other patients might also benefit from cardiac rehabilitation? In your response, consider the patient in the case scenario shared at the beginning of this chapter.
4. How does the nurse inquire about this patient's use of recreational cannabis? What are the cardiac risks associated with his frequent use of cannabis?

BOX 40.10 NURSING DIAGNOSTIC PROCESS

Assessment Activities	Defining Characteristics	Nursing Diagnosis
Ask patient or family about patient's mood, attentiveness, memory, and activity level.	Confusion Decreased activity Fatigue Irritability Restlessness Sleepiness	*Impaired gas exchange related to decreased lung expansion*
Observe patient's respirations.	Dyspnea Impaired gas exchange related to collapsed alveoli Nasal flaring Tachypnea Use of accessory muscles	
Inspect skin and mucous membranes.	Diaphoresis Pallor Moist skin	
Auscultate chest.	Decreased respiratory excursion Abnormal, distant lung sounds	

care need but is unable to leave the home, and home physiotherapy is needed.

Collaboration with physiotherapists, nutritionists, and community-based nurses may be valuable for a patient with heart failure or chronic lung conditions and is an essential component of primary health care. These professionals work with the patient and the community to optimize resources to assist the patient in attaining the highest level of wellness. In addition, professionals can help to identify community resources and support systems for both the patient and family in preventing and managing symptoms related to cardiopulmonary diseases.

◆ Implementation

Nursing interventions for promoting and maintaining adequate oxygenation include independent nursing actions such as health-promotion

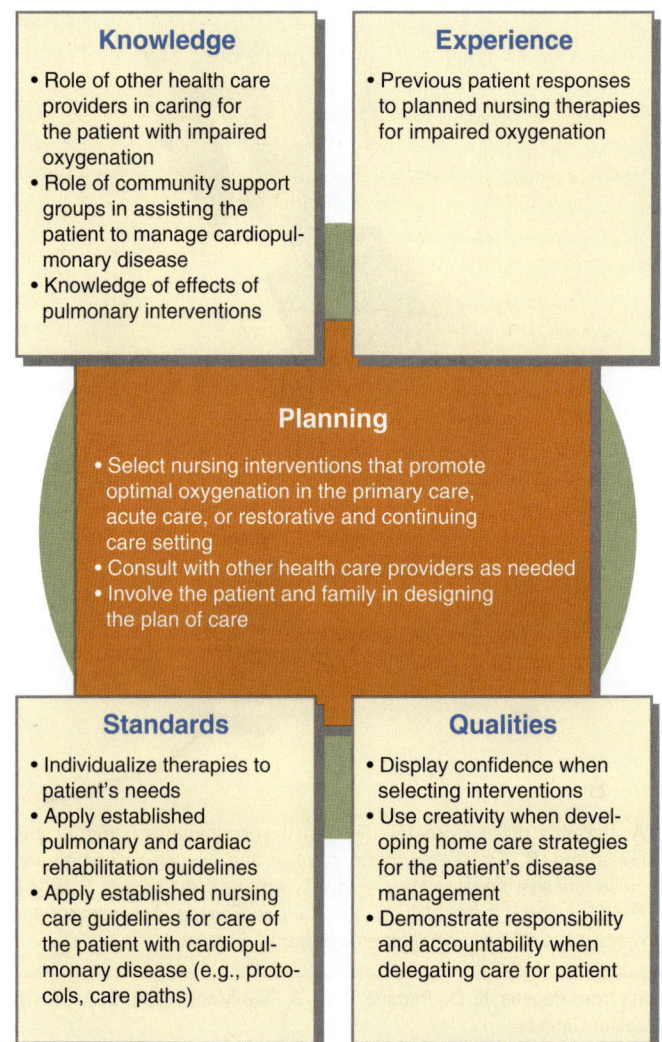

Knowledge
- Role of other health care providers in caring for the patient with impaired oxygenation
- Role of community support groups in assisting the patient to manage cardiopulmonary disease
- Knowledge of effects of pulmonary interventions

Experience
- Previous patient responses to planned nursing therapies for impaired oxygenation

Planning
- Select nursing interventions that promote optimal oxygenation in the primary care, acute care, or restorative and continuing care setting
- Consult with other health care providers as needed
- Involve the patient and family in designing the plan of care

Standards
- Individualize therapies to patient's needs
- Apply established pulmonary and cardiac rehabilitation guidelines
- Apply established nursing care guidelines for care of the patient with cardiopulmonary disease (e.g., protocols, care paths)

Qualities
- Display confidence when selecting interventions
- Use creativity when developing home care strategies for the patient's disease management
- Demonstrate responsibility and accountability when delegating care for patient

FIGURE 40.7 Critical thinking model for oxygenation planning.

◉ BOX 40.11 **NURSING CARE PLAN**

Ineffective Airway Clearance/Retained Secretions

ASSESSMENT

An older person with a history of chronic obstructive pulmonary disease (COPD) comes to the primary care office with complaints of continued coughing. They report having an intermittent productive cough that occasionally produces thick yellow sputum. Their vital signs are temperature 38.5°C, pulse 104 beats per minute, respirations 28 breaths per minute, and blood pressure 130/85 mm Hg, and SpO_2 is 84% on room air. They continue to smoke two to three cigarettes a day, an improvement from their previous 10 to 15 per day. The patient does not exercise and needs to complete self-care activities slowly, given the shortness of breath.

Assessment Activities	*Findings and Defining Characteristics*
Ask the patient how long they have had this cough.	The patient replies, "I have a morning cough every day, but this cough is different. It started about a week ago."
Ask the patient what is different about this cough.	The patient replies, "My ribs are getting sore. I can't cough up anything, my mouth is dry, and I have become more fatigued over the past week."
Observe the patient's skin and mucous membranes.	The skin and mucous membranes are dry.
Auscultate lung fields.	Abnormal lung sounds are in the upper lobes. The lower lobes are clear.
Ask the patient how many glasses of water they drink daily.	Over the last week they consumed two to three glasses a day.
Ask the patient to produce a sputum sample.	The patient is unable to produce a sputum sample for evaluation.

NURSING DIAGNOSIS: Ineffective airway clearance related to retained secretions and reduced fluid intake.

PLANNING

*Goals (Nursing Outcomes Classification)**	*Expected Outcomes*
	Respiratory Status: Airway Patency
Patient will be able to effectively clear secretions.	Lung sounds will be normal in 48 hours.
	Sputum will be thin, white, and watery.
	Respiratory rate will be within 20–24 breaths/min in 48 hours.
	Patient will be able to clear airway by coughing.
	Oral mucous membranes will be pink and moist.
Patient will increase oral hydration to 1 000 mL of water every 24 hours.	Patient will verbalize that their mouth is not dry.
	Patient will notice an increase in ease of sputum production.
	Patient will report that their sputum is thin, white, and watery.

*Outcome classification labels from Moorhead, S., Swanson, E., Johnson, M., et al. (Eds.). (2018). Nursing outcomes classification (NOC), (6th ed.). Mosby/Elsevier.

INTERVENTIONS

Interventions (Nursing Interventions Classification)†	*Rationale*
Airway Management	
Increase fluids to 1 000 mL in 24 hours if not contraindicated by cardiovascular disease.	Fluids help to liquefy secretions and promote ease of removal. Fluids will relieve oral mucosa and skin dryness.
Have patient deep-breathe and cough every 2 hours four to five times.	Retained secretions predispose patient to atelectasis and pneumonia.
Teach patient effective cough techniques.	Coughing techniques will help to clear the airway effectively and decrease fatigue from ineffective coughing.
Consider chest physiotherapy (CPT) if there is evidence of infiltrates on chest X-ray film.	Standards for CPT include sputum production >30 mL/day or infiltrates on chest X-ray film.

†Intervention classification labels from Butcher, H. K., Bulechek, G. M., McCloskey Dochterman, J. M., et al. (Eds.). (2018). Nursing interventions classification (NIC) (7th ed.). Elsevier.

EVALUATION

Nursing Actions	*Patient Response and Findings*	*Achievement of Outcome*
Ask the patient if they can deep-breathe and cough.	The patient reports, "It is easier to cough up my secretions now."	The patient is able to clear the airway by coughing.
Assess the chest for adventitious lung sounds.	The patient reports that they have not heard any wheezing or rattling in their chest.	Lungs clear to auscultation in all fields.
Assess respiratory rate.	No use of accessory muscles of respiration. Normal breathing pattern and respiratory rate.	Respiratory rate is between 20 and 24 breaths/min.
Assess patient's level of hydration.	Mucous membranes are moist. The patient reports, "My mouth isn't so dry anymore."	Oral mucous membranes are pink and moist.
Observe appearance of sputum.	Sputum is thin, white, and watery.	Sputum is thin, white, and watery.

➤ **concept map**

Risk for imbalanced body temperature
• Elevated body temperature >38.3°C
• Chills
• Diaphoresis
• Tachycardia

Impaired gas exchange
• Dyspnea
• Respiratory rate >28 breaths/min at rest
• Abnormal blood gases: PaO₂ 60, PaCO₂ 55, SaO₂ 80
• Tachycardia
• Confusion
• Decreased diaphragmatic excursion

Patient's chief medical diagnosis: Chronic obstructive pulmonary disease and pneumonia
Priority assessments: Oxygenation, airway clearance, fever control

Fatigue
• Respiratory rate >28 breaths/min
• Inability to complete ADLs
• Decreased activity tolerance, ambulation

Ineffective airway clearance
• Abnormal breath sounds > right lower lobe
• Dyspnea
• Orthopnea
• Yellow, thick sputum
• Restlessness

—— Link between medical diagnosis and nursing diagnosis ----- Link between nursing diagnoses

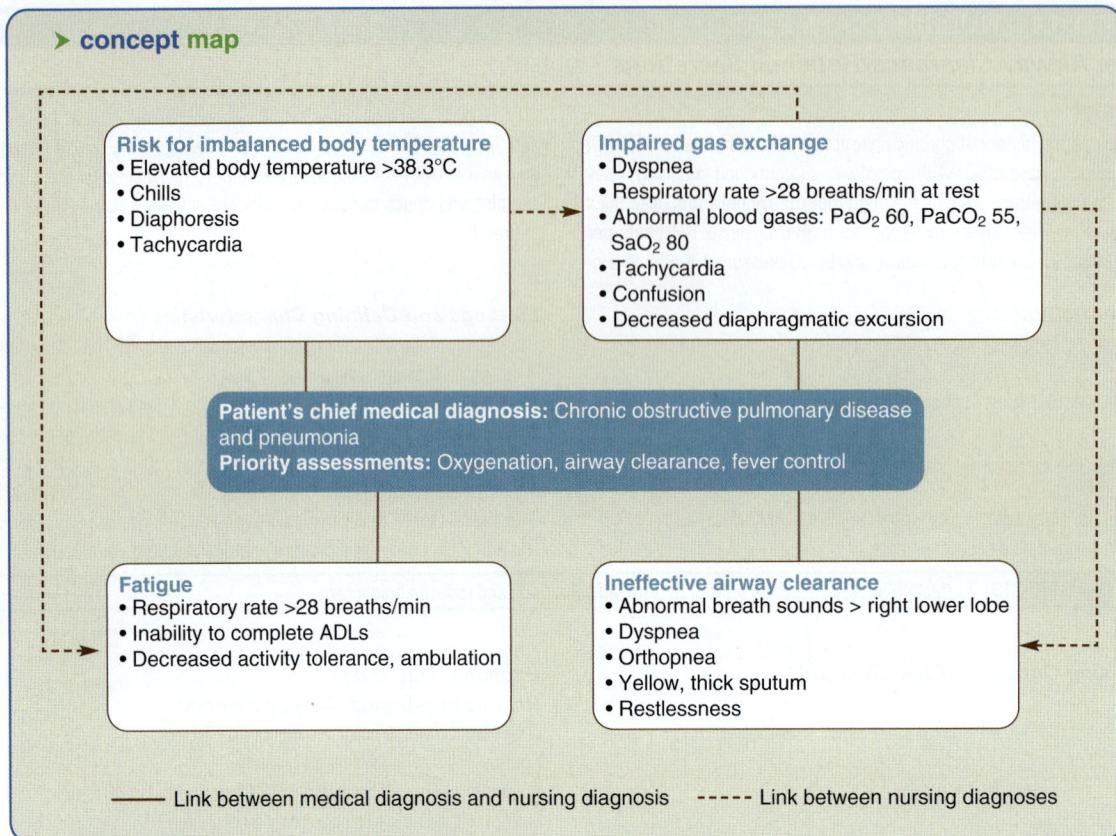

FIGURE 40.8 Concept map for a patient with chronic obstructive pulmonary disease and pneumonia. *ADLs,* Activities of daily living.

BOX 40.12 PATIENT TEACHING

Cardiovascular Disease

Objectives
• Patient will be able to describe the risk factors associated with cardiovascular disease.
• Patient will be able to demonstrate health promotion behaviours.

Teaching Strategies
• Explain to the patient about modifying risk factors, such as quitting smoking, reducing alcohol intake, being attentive to sugar intake, and modifying high-fat and high-carbohydrate diets.
• Inform the patient about other risk factors for cardiovascular disease, such as diabetes, obesity, physical inactivity, stress, and oral contraceptives.
• Discuss with the patient the importance of regular blood pressure and blood cholesterol monitoring (total cholesterol, high-density lipoprotein, low-density lipoprotein, and triglyceride levels).

• Educate the patient about low-fat, low-salt, and calorie-appropriate diets. Provide sample menus.
• Educate the patient about the benefits of exercising 30–60 minutes a day to help reduce weight and lower blood pressure. Help the patient develop an exercise program.

Evaluation
• Ask the patient to describe the modifiable and nonmodifiable risk factors for cardiovascular disease.
• Ask the patient to verbalize strategies for balanced nutrition.
• Obtain the patient's weight and blood pressure.
• Monitor the patient's serum cholesterol (total, high- and low-density lipids) and triglyceride levels.

and disease-prevention behaviours, positioning, and coughing techniques. Interdependent or dependent interventions include oxygen therapy, lung inflation techniques, hydration, medication administration, and chest physiotherapy (CPT).

Health Promotion

Maintaining the patient's optimal level of health is important in reducing the number and severity of respiratory symptoms. Prevention of respiratory infections is foremost in maintaining optimal health. Providing cardiopulmonary-related health information (Box 40.12 and

Box 40.13) is an important nursing responsibility and part of a primary health care model.

Vaccinations. Annual influenza vaccines are recommended for everyone 6 months and older (Centers for Disease Control [CDC], 2022a). Individuals with chronic illnesses (heart, lung, kidney, diabetes, or immunosuppressed), infants, older persons, and pregnant people should be immunized (CDC, 2022a). The vaccine is also recommended for people in close or frequent contact with anyone in high-risk groups. Vaccination should begin as soon as the vaccine

BOX 40.13 RESEARCH HIGHLIGHT

The Association Between Cannabis Use and Cardiac Dysthymias: A Systematic Review

Research Focus

Cannabis is considered to be the most commonly used drug, with approximately 3.8% of the global population (15–64 years of age) using cannabis at least once in the past year (Richards et al., 2020, p. 861). The implication of cannabis use has been correlated with an increase of heart rate and blood pressure immediately after use, which may precipitate cardiac dysrhythmia (Richards et al., 2020, p. 861).

Research Abstract

The purpose of the systematic review conducted by Richards and colleagues (2020) was to analyze the medical literature related to the association between cannabis use and cardiac dysrhythmias.

Methods

Peer-reviewed articles were analyzed from various databases that included Google Scholar, PubMed, and OpenGrey. The literature search included all human trials, case series, and case reports in any language and included both acute and chronic cannabis use. The researchers defined dysrhythmia as any irregular or regular rhythm with a rate greater than 100 beats per minute or less than 60 beats per minute. There were 67 articles that involved 3 804 080 human subjects that were included in the systematic review.

Results

The use of cannabis is correlated with an increased risk of cardiac dysrhythmias which, while rare, may be life-threatening (Richards et al., 2020, p. 866).

Implications for Practice

Based on this evidence nurses should do the following:

- Question the use of acute and chronic cannabis use in patients presenting with tachycardia, bradycardia, dysrhythmia, atypical ECG results, chest pain, or unexplained syncope (p. 866).
- Include questioning about cannabis use for adolescents and younger adults, who may minimize the risk related to cannabis use (p. 866).
- Educate older persons who are chronic or infrequent users of recreational or medical cannabis on the harmful association that may be "exacerbated" by underlying coronary arterial disease and risk factors (p. 866).

From Richards, J. R., Blohm, E., Toles, K. A., et al . (2020). The association of cannabis use and cardiac dysrhythmias: A systematic review. *Clinical Toxicology, 58*(9), 861–869. http://doi.org/10.1080/15563650.2020.1743847

becomes available, if possible, by October (CDC, 2022a). In Canada, it is estimated that, in a given year, an average of 12 200 hospitalizations and approximately 3 500 deaths occur due to influenza (Public Health Agency of Canada, 2021). After the vaccination, antibodies develop against the strains of the virus. When exposed to the influenza virus, the antibodies assist with preventing infection or reduce the severity of illness.

Pneumococcal vaccine is recommended for patients at increased risk of developing pneumonia, those with chronic illnesses or immunosuppression, those living in special environments such as long-term care facilities, and patients over the age of 65 years (CDC, 2022b). The CDC (2022b) recommends that adults who are between the ages of 19 and 64 and who smoke should also receive the pneumococcal vaccine.

Healthy Lifestyle Behaviour. Identification and elimination of risk factors for cardiopulmonary disease is an important part of primary health care. Nurses need to encourage patients to eat a healthy, low-fat, high-fibre diet; to monitor their cholesterol, triglyceride, high-density lipoprotein (HDL), and low-density lipoprotein (LDL) levels and reduce stress; to exercise; and to maintain a body weight in proportion to their height.

Elimination of use of cigarettes and other tobacco products, reduction in exposure to pollutants, monitoring of air quality, and adequate hydration are additional behaviours that promote health. Patients should be encouraged to examine their habits and to make changes to achieve their goals.

Exercise is a key factor in maintaining a healthy heart and lungs. Patients should be encouraged to exercise three to four times a week for 20 to 30 minutes. Aerobic exercise is necessary to improve lung function, strengthen muscles, and achieve better health. Walking is one of the most efficient ways of getting a good aerobic workout. Many shopping malls have programs that allow people to enter the mall before shops open and to use the enclosed area for walking. Some have measured and posted the distances to help people plan their activity and measure their progress. Patients should be taught how to take their pulse and pace themselves; it is better to walk 15 minutes every day than to walk to exhaustion to achieve a goal. Patients should plan a time interval and walk for the designated time. Gradually, they will notice that the distance increases as their endurance and fitness improve.

Patients with cardiopulmonary alterations need to minimize their risk for infection, especially during the winter months. Nurses need to teach patients to avoid large, crowded places; to keep their mouth and nose covered; and to be sure to dress warmly, including a scarf, hat, and gloves. This is especially important during the peak of the influenza season.

Patients with known cardiac disease and those with multiple risk factors should be cautioned to avoid exertion in cold weather. Shovelling snow is especially risky and in many patients can precipitate a cardiac event. Other activities, such as hanging holiday lights and decorations in the extreme cold, can precipitate chest pain and bronchospasm. Patients should be advised to avoid drinking alcohol before going out into cold weather because it blunts the respiratory drive when used in excess and may contribute to exposure to the cold by making the patient feel warm when the patient is really not protected from the cold.

Patients should also be taught to plan for the hot summer months. Activities should be limited to early in the day or late in the evening, when temperatures are lower. Patients should take care to maintain adequate hydration and sodium intake; this is especially true for patients taking diuretics. Caffeinated and alcoholic beverages should be limited or avoided completely, because they act as diuretics and can contribute to dehydration.

Environmental Pollutants. Avoiding exposure to second-hand smoke is essential to maintaining optimal cardiopulmonary function. Most businesses and restaurants now ban smoking or have separate areas designated as smoking areas. If patients are exposed to second-hand smoke in their home environment, counselling and support may be necessary to assist the smoker in successful smoking cessation or alterations in behaviour patterns, such as smoking outside.

Exposure to chemicals and pollutants in the work environment must also be considered. Patients such as farmers, painters, carpenters, and others who are exposed to pollutants benefit from the use of particulate filter masks to reduce inhalation of particles.

Acute Care

According to the Canadian Association of Schools of Nursing (CASN, 2022), one of the key competency domains for baccalaureate nurses is to consider interventions according to their abilities to monitor and manage complex patient needs. Patients with acute pulmonary illnesses require nursing interventions directed toward halting the pathological process (e.g., respiratory tract infection), shortening the duration and severity of the illness (e.g., hospitalization with pneumonia), and preventing complications from the illness or treatments (e.g., health care–associated infection resulting from invasive procedures).

Dyspnea Management. Dyspnea is difficult to quantify and to treat. Treatment modalities need to be individualized for each patient, and more than one therapy is usually implemented. The underlying process that causes or worsens dyspnea must be treated and stabilized initially, then four additional therapies—pharmacological measures, oxygen therapy, physical techniques, and psychosocial techniques—are implemented. Pharmacological treatments may include bronchodilators, steroids, mucolytics, and low-dose anti-anxiety medications. Oxygen therapy can reduce dyspnea associated with exercise. Physical techniques, such as cardiopulmonary reconditioning through exercise, breathing techniques, and cough control, can help to reduce dyspnea. Relaxation techniques, biofeedback, and meditation are physiological measures that the patient can use to help lessen the sensation of dyspnea.

Airway Maintenance. The airway is patent when the trachea, bronchi, and large airways are free from obstructions. Airway maintenance requires adequate hydration to prevent thick, tenacious secretions. Proper coughing techniques remove secretions and keep the airway open. A variety of interventions, such as suctioning, CPT, and nebulizer therapy, assist the patient in managing alterations in airway clearance.

Mobilization of Pulmonary Secretions. The ability of a patient to mobilize pulmonary secretions may make the difference between a short-term illness and a long recovery involving complications. Nursing interventions that promote mobilization of pulmonary secretions help the patient to achieve and maintain a clear airway, and encourage lung expansion and gas exchange.

Humidification. Humidification is the process of adding water to gas. Temperature is the most important factor affecting the amount of water vapour a gas can hold. The percentage of water in the gas in relation to its capacity for water is the *relative humidity*. Air or oxygen with a high relative humidity keeps the airways moist and helps loosen and mobilize pulmonary secretions. Humidification is necessary for patients receiving oxygen therapy at >4 L/minute. Bubbling oxygen through water can add humidity to the oxygen delivered to the upper airways, as with a nasal cannula or face mask. In the pediatric setting, oxygen tents are used to provide humidified oxygen in high concentrations. This device is beneficial for children who are diagnosed with croup, respiratory infections, and airway inflammation (Cobbett et al., 2020).

Nebulization. Nebulization is a process of adding moisture or medications to inspired air by mixing particles of varying sizes with the air. A nebulizer uses the aerosol principle to suspend a maximum number of water drops or particles of the desired size in inspired air. The moisture added to the respiratory system through nebulization improves clearance of pulmonary secretions.

Nebulization is often used for administration of bronchodilators and mucolytic agents.

When the thin layer of fluid that supports the mucous layer over the cilia is allowed to dry, the cilia are damaged and cannot adequately clear the airway. Humidification through nebulization enhances mucociliary clearance, the body's natural mechanism for removing mucus and cellular debris from the respiratory tract.

Chest physiotherapy. Chest physiotherapy (CPT) is a group of therapies used in combination to mobilize pulmonary secretions. These therapies include postural drainage, chest percussion, and vibration. CPT should be followed by productive coughing and suctioning of the patient who has a decreased ability to cough. CPT is recommended for patients who produce greater than 30 mL of sputum per day or have evidence of atelectasis by chest X-ray examination. This procedure can be safely used with infants and young children; however, conditions and diseases unique to children may at times contraindicate this procedure. CPT is used for a select group of patients. Box 40.14 describes the guidelines for determining if CPT is indicated for the patient.

Chest percussion involves striking the chest wall over the area being drained. The hand is positioned so that the fingers and thumb touch and the hands are cupped (Figure 40.9). Percussion on the surface of the chest wall sends waves of varying amplitude and frequency through the chest, changing the consistency and location of the sputum. Chest percussion is performed by striking the chest wall alternately with cupped hands (Figure 40.10). Percussion is performed over a single layer of clothing, not over buttons, snaps, or zippers. The single layer of clothing prevents slapping the patient's skin. Thicker or multiple layers of material dampen the vibrations.

BOX 40.14 Guidelines for Chest Physiotherapy

Nursing care and selection of chest physiotherapy (CPT) skills are based on specific assessment findings. The following guidelines are designed to help in physical assessment and subsequent decision making:

- Know the patient's normal range of vital signs. Conditions such as atelectasis and pneumonia requiring CPT can affect vital signs. The degree of change is related to the level of hypoxia, overall cardiopulmonary status, and tolerance of activity.
- Know the patient's medications. Certain medications, particularly diuretics and antihypertensives, cause fluid and hemodynamic changes. These changes may decrease the patient's tolerance of the positional changes of postural drainage. Steroid medications increase the patient's risk of pathological rib fractures and often contraindicate rib shaking.
- Know the patient's medical history. Certain conditions, such as increased intracranial pressure, spinal cord injuries, and abdominal aneurysm resection, contraindicate the positional changes of postural drainage. Thoracic trauma or surgery may also contraindicate percussion, vibration, and rib shaking. For adult and pediatric hospitalized patients without cystic fibrosis, chest physiotherapy is not recommended for the routine treatment of uncomplicated pneumonia, postoperative complications, and chronic obstructive pulmonary disease (COPD) (Strickland et al., 2013).
- Know the patient's level of cognitive function. Participation in controlled coughing techniques requires the patient to follow instructions. Congenital or acquired cognitive limitations may alter the patient's ability to learn and participate in these techniques.
- Be aware of the patient's exercise tolerance. CPT manoeuvres are fatiguing. When the patient is not used to physical activity, initial tolerance for the manoeuvres may be decreased. However, with gradual increases in activity and planned CPT, patient tolerance for the procedure will improve.

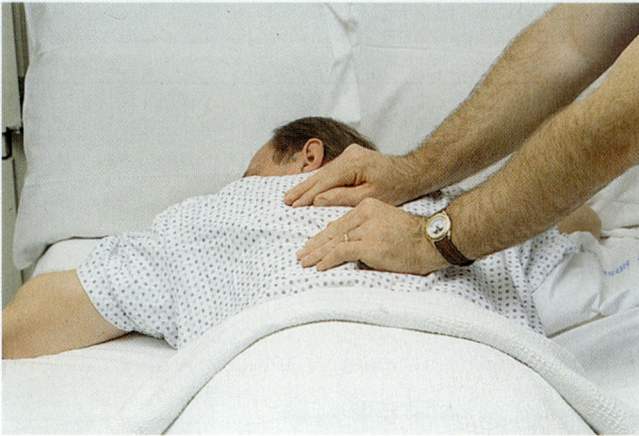

FIGURE 40.9 Hand position for chest wall percussion during chest physiotherapy.

FIGURE 40.10 Chest wall percussion, alternating hand clapping against the patient's chest wall.

Percussion is contraindicated in patients with bleeding disorders, osteoporosis, or fractured ribs. It is important to percuss the lung fields and not over the spine, abdomen, lower ribs, or breastbone, to prevent injury to the spleen, liver, or kidneys (Cystic Fibrosis Foundation, 2020).

Vibration is a fine, shaking pressure applied to the chest wall only during exhalation. This technique is thought to increase the velocity and turbulence of exhaled air, facilitating secretion removal. Vibration increases the exhalation of trapped air and may shake mucus loose and induce a cough.

Postural drainage is the use of positioning techniques that draw secretions from specific segments of the lungs and bronchi into the trachea. Coughing or suctioning normally removes secretions from the trachea. The procedure for postural drainage can include most lung segments (Table 40.8). Because patients may not require postural drainage of all lung segments, the procedure is based on clinical assessment findings. For example, patients with left lower lobe atelectasis may require postural drainage of only the affected region, whereas a child with cystic fibrosis may require postural drainage of all lung segments.

Suctioning Techniques. Suctioning is necessary when a patient is unable to clear respiratory tract secretions with coughing. The suctioning techniques include oropharyngeal and nasopharyngeal suctioning, orotracheal and nasotracheal suctioning, and suctioning of an artificial airway.

These techniques are based on common principles. In most cases, sterile technique is used for suctioning because the trachea is considered sterile. The mouth is considered clean; thus, the suctioning of oral secretions should be performed after suctioning of the oropharynx and trachea. Each type of suctioning requires the use of a round-tipped catheter with a number of side holes at the distal end of the catheter. Frequency of suctioning is determined by patient assessment and need. If secretions are identified by inspection or auscultation techniques, suctioning is required. Because sputum is not produced continuously or every 1 or 2 hours but occurs as a response to a pathological condition, there is no rationale for routine suctioning of all patients every 1 to 2 hours. In addition, suctioning reduces the amount of the available dead space in the oropharynx and trachea, often resulting in significant desaturation. It is important to monitor the patient to ensure adequate oxygenation. Too-frequent suctioning can put the patient at risk for development of hypoxemia, hypotension, arrhythmias, and possible trauma to the mucosa of the lungs (Lynn-McHale, 2011).

Oropharyngeal and Nasopharyngeal Suctioning. The oropharynx extends behind the mouth from the soft palate above the level of the hyoid bone and contains the tonsils. The nasopharynx is located behind the nose and extends to the level of the soft palate. Oropharyngeal or nasopharyngeal suctioning is used when the patient is able to cough effectively but is unable to clear secretions by expectorating or swallowing. The suction procedure is used after the patient has coughed (Skill 40.1). As the number of pulmonary secretions is reduced and the patient is less fatigued, the patient may be able to expectorate or swallow the mucus, and suctioning is no longer required.

Orotracheal and Nasotracheal Suctioning. Orotracheal or nasotracheal suctioning is necessary when the patient with pulmonary secretions is unable to manage secretions by coughing and does not have an artificial airway (see Skill 40.1). A catheter is passed through the mouth or nose into the trachea. The nose is the preferred route because stimulation of the gag reflex is minimal. The procedure is similar to nasopharyngeal suctioning, but the catheter tip is moved farther into the patient's trachea. The entire procedure from catheter passage to its removal should be done quickly, lasting no longer than 15 seconds (American Association of Respiratory Care [AARC], 2010). Unless in respiratory distress, the patient should be allowed to rest between passes of the catheter. If the patient is using supplemental oxygen, the oxygen cannula or mask should be replaced during rest periods.

Tracheal Suctioning. Tracheal suctioning is accomplished through an artificial airway such as an endotracheal tube or tracheostomy tube (see Skill 40.1). The suction catheter should be no greater than one-half the size of the internal diameter of the artificial airway (AARC, 2010). Secretion removal should be as atraumatic as possible. To avoid trauma to the mucosa of the lung, never apply suction pressure while inserting the catheter, and maintain suction pressure less than 150 mm Hg in adults (AARC, 2010). Apply suction intermittently *only* as the catheter is withdrawn. Rotating the catheter will enhance removal of secretions that have adhered to the sides of the endotracheal tube. Apply a mask and goggles and wear a barrier gown to prevent splashes with body fluids.

The practice of normal saline instillation (NSI) into artificial airways to improve secretion may be harmful and is not recommended.

TABLE 40.8   Positions for Postural Drainage

Lung Segment	Position of Patient
Adult	
Bilateral	High-Fowler's position

Apical Segments	
Right upper lobe—anterior segment	Supine with head of bed elevated 15–30 degrees

Left upper lobe—anterior segment	Supine with head elevated

Right upper lobe—posterior segment	Side lying with right side of chest elevated on pillows

Left upper lobe—posterior segment	Side lying with left side of chest elevated on pillows

Right middle lobe—anterior segment	Three-fourths supine position with dependent lung in Trendelenburg's position

Right middle lobe—posterior segment	Prone with thorax and abdomen elevated

Both lower lobes—anterior segments	Supine in Trendelenburg's position

Continued

TABLE 40.8	Positions for Postural Drainage—cont'd

Lung Segment	Position of Patient
Left lower lobe—lateral segment	Right side lying in Trendelenburg's position
Right lower lobe—lateral segment	Left lateral in Trendelenburg's position
Right lower lobe—posterior segment	Prone in Trendelenburg's position with abdomen and thorax elevated
Both lower lobes—posterior segments	Prone in Trendelenburg's position with abdomen and thorax elevated
Child	
Bilateral—apical segments	Sitting on nurse's lap, leaning slightly forward, flexed over pillow
Bilateral—middle anterior segments	Sitting on nurse's lap, leaning against nurse
Bilateral lobes—anterior segments	Lying supine on nurse's lap, back supported with pillow

SKILL 40.1   SUGGESTIONING

SKILL 40.1   SUCTIONING

Delegation Considerations

If the patient has been assessed and determined to be stable, the skill of performing suctioning of an established tracheostomy can be delegated to an unregulated care provider (UCP) when the patient has a permanent tracheostomy tube or is receiving oropharyngeal suctioning. Before delegating this skill, do the following:

- Discuss with the UCP any unique modifications of the skill, such as the need to reapply any supplemental oxygen equipment following the procedure.
- Discuss appropriate suction limits.
- Instruct the UCP to report any change in the patient's respiratory status, signs and symptoms of hypoxemia, secretion colour or volume, or unresolved coughing or gagging.
- Instruct the UCP to report any change in the patient's colour, vital signs, or pain level.

Equipment

Oropharyngeal suctioning
- Yankauer suction catheter
- Oral airway (if indicated)
- Two clean disposable gloves
- Portable or wall suction
- Mask, goggles, or face shield
- Connecting tube (1.8 m long)
- Water or normal saline (or as determined by agency policy)
- Cup or basin
- Pulse oximeter and stethoscope

Nasopharyngeal and nasotracheal suctioning
- Appropriate-size sterile suction catheter (smallest diameter that will remove secretions effectively)
- Connecting tube (1.8 m long)
- Two sterile gloves or one sterile and one clean disposable glove (refer to technique)
- Sterile basin
- Sterile water or normal saline (approximately 100 mL)
- Water-soluble lubricant
- Clean towel or paper drape
- Portable or wall suction
- Mask, goggles, or face shield
- Pulse oximeter and stethoscope

Tracheostomy suctioning
- Appropriate-size sterile suction catheter (smallest diameter that will remove secretions effectively)
- Connecting tube (1.8 m long)
- Two sterile gloves or one sterile and one clean disposable glove (refer to technique)
- Sterile basin
- Sterile water or normal saline (approximately 100 mL)
- Water-soluble lubricant
- Clean towel or paper drape
- Portable or wall suction
- Mask, goggles, or face shield
- Pulse oximeter and stethoscope

PROCEDURE

STEPS	RATIONALE
ASSESSMENT	
1. Perform hand hygiene and apply gloves and any other personal protective equipment (PPE) if exposure to airway secretions is present.	• Prevents transmission of microorganisms.
2. Identify patient using at least two identifiers according to agency policy. Compare identifiers with information on patient's medication administration record (MAR) or medical record.	• Ensures correct patient.
3. Assess for signs and symptoms of upper and lower airway obstruction, abnormal respiratory rate, adventitious sounds, nasal secretions, gurgling, drooling, restlessness, gastric secretions, or vomitus in mouth, and coughing without clearing secretions from airway.	• Physical signs and symptoms result from decreased oxygen to tissues, as well as pooling of secretions in upper and lower airways. A complete assessment is required before and after suction procedure.
4. Assess signs and symptoms associated with hypoxia and hypercapnia: decreased SpO_2, increased pulse and blood pressure, increased respiratory rate, apprehension, anxiety, decreased ability to concentrate, lethargy, decreased level of consciousness (especially acute), increased fatigue, dizziness, behavioural changes (especially irritability), dysrhythmias, pallor, and cyanosis.	• Physical signs and symptoms resulting from decreased oxygen to tissues indicate need for suctioning. Anxiety and pain consume oxygen and, in turn, worsen the signs of hypoxia.

Continued

STEPS	RATIONALE
5. Determine factors that normally influence upper or lower airway functioning:	
• Fluid status	• Fluid overload may increase amount of secretions. Dehydration promotes thicker secretions.
• Lack of humidity	• The environment influences secretion formation and gas exchange, necessitating airway suctioning when the patient cannot clear secretions effectively.
• Pulmonary disease, chronic obstructive pulmonary disease, pulmonary infection	• Increases patient's risk for retaining pulmonary secretions. Patients with respiratory infections are prone to increased secretions that are thicker and sometimes more difficult to expectorate.
• Anatomy	• Abnormal anatomy can impair normal drainage of secretions. For example, nasal swelling, a deviated septum, or facial fractures may impair nasal drainage. Tumours in or around the lower airway may impair secretion removal by occluding or externally compressing the lumen of the airway.
• Changes in level of consciousness	• Impairs patient's ability to cough independently or follow instructions to cough and clear airway.
• Decreased cough or gag reflex, dysphagia, presence of a feeding tube	• Increases patient's risk for aspiration and subsequent pulmonary infection.
• Allergies, sinus drainage	• Increases volume of secretions in pharynx.
6. Identify contraindications to nasotracheal suctioning: occluded nasal passages; nasal bleeding, epiglottitis, or croup; acute head, facial, or neck injury or surgery, coagulopathy, or bleeding disorder; irritable airway or laryngospasm or bronchospasm; gastric surgery with high anastomosis; myocardial infarction (AARC, 2004).	• These conditions are contraindications to nasal suctioning because passage of the catheter through the nasal route causes trauma to existing facial trauma or surgery, increases nasal bleeding, or causes severe bleeding in the presence of bleeding disorders. With epiglottitis, croup, laryngospasm, or irritable airway, the entrance of a suction catheter via the nasal route causes intractable coughing, hypoxemia, and severe bronchospasm, necessitating emergency intubation or tracheostomy. Hypoxemia may worsen cardiac damage in myocardial infarction (AARC, 2004).
7. Examine sputum microbiology data.	• Certain bacteria are easier to transmit or require isolation because of virulence or antibiotic resistance.
8. Assess for patient's or caregiver's knowledge, experience, and health literacy.	• Ensures patient or caregiver has the capacity to obtain, communicate, process, and understand basic health information and individualizes patient care.
9. Obtain prescriber's order if indicated by agency policy.	• Some institutions require a prescriber's order for tracheal suctioning.
PLANNING	
1. Remove and dispose of glove after assessment and perform hand hygiene. Prepare and organize equipment.	• Reduces transmission of microorganisms and ensures that the necessary equipment is obtained to implement intervention.
2. Explain the importance of coughing and encourage coughing during procedure.	• Facilitates secretion removal and may reduce frequency and duration of future suctioning.
3. Explain to patient how the procedure will help clear the airway and relieve breathing problems and that temporary coughing, sneezing, gagging, or shortness of breath is normal. Encourage patient to cough out secretions. Have patient practise coughing, if able. Splint surgical incisions, if necessary.	• Encourages cooperation and minimizes risks, anxiety, and pain.
4. Help patient to assume a position comfortable for you and for the patient (usually semi-Fowler's or sitting upright with their head hyperextended, unless contraindicated). Stand on patient's right if you are right-handed or on their left if you are left-handed.	• Reduces stimulation of gag reflex, promotes patient comfort and secretion drainage, and prevents aspiration. Hyperextension facilitates insertion of the catheter into the trachea. Position facilitates catheter insertion.
5. Place pulse oximeter on patient's finger. Take reading and leave pulse oximeter in place.	• Provides baseline oxygen level to determine patient's response to suctioning.
6. Place towel across the patient's chest.	• Reduces transmission of microorganisms by protecting gown from secretions.
IMPLEMENTATION	
1. Perform hand hygiene and apply PPE if not already applied during assessment and planning or if indicated.	• Reduces transmission of microorganisms.
2. Connect one end of connecting tubing to the suction machine and place the other end in a convenient location near the patient. Turn suction device on and set vacuum regulator to appropriate negative pressure: <150 mm Hg for adults has been recommended (AARC, 2004, 2010). *Appropriate pressure may vary, depending on the route of suctioning and the age of the patient; check agency policy.*	• Excessive negative pressure damages nasal pharyngeal and tracheal mucosa and induces greater hypoxia. Negative pressure should not exceed 150 mm Hg because high pressure increases the risk for airway trauma, hypoxemia, and atelectasis (AARC, 2004, 2010).

SKILL 40.1   SUCTIONING—cont'd

STEPS	RATIONALE
3. For all types of suctioning:	
A. Open suction kit or catheter using aseptic technique. If a sterile drape is available, place it across the patient's chest or on the overbed table. Do not allow the suction catheter to touch any nonsterile surfaces.	• Prepares catheter and helps prevent transmission of microorganisms. A sterile drape provides a sterile surface on which to lay the suction catheter between passes, if needed.
B. Unwrap or open sterile basin and place on bedside table. Fill basin or cup with approximately 100 mL of sterile normal saline solution or water (see Step 3B illustration).	• Normal saline or water is needed to flush catheter and tubing after each suction pass.

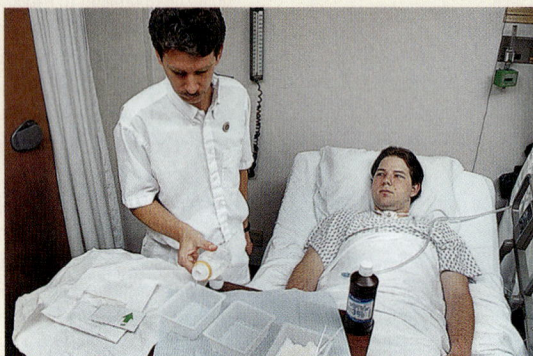

STEP 3B Pouring sterile saline into basin.

STEPS	RATIONALE
C. Turn on suction device. Set regulator to appropriate negative pressure. Perform hand hygiene.	
4. Suction airway.	
A. Oropharyngeal suctioning	
(1) Apply clean disposable gloves.	• Suction of oral cavity does not require use of sterile gloves. Suction may cause splashing of body fluids.
(2) Attach Yankauer to connecting tubing. Check that equipment is functioning properly by suctioning a small amount of water or normal saline from the cup or basin.	
(3) Remove oxygen mask if present. Keep oxygen mask near patient's face. Nasal cannula may remain in place (if present).	• Allows access to patient's mouth. Reduces chances of hypoxia.

CRITICAL DECISION POINT: *Be prepared to quickly reapply oxygen mask if SpO$_2$ falls or respiratory distress develops during or at the end of suctioning.*

STEPS	RATIONALE
(4) Insert Yankauer into the patient's mouth. With suction applied, move catheter around mouth, including pharynx and gum line, until secretions are cleared.	• Movement of catheter prevents suction tip from invaginating oral mucosal surfaces, thus potentially causing trauma.
(5) Encourage patient to cough and repeat suctioning if needed. Replace oxygen mask if used.	• Coughing moves secretions from lower to upper airways into mouth.
(6) Suction water from basin through catheter until catheter is cleared of secretions. Turn off suction.	• Clearing secretions before they dry reduces the probability of transmission of microorganisms and enhances delivery of preset suction pressures.
(7) Place catheter in a clean, dry area for reuse.	• Facilitates prompt removal of airway secretions when suctioning is needed in the future. Moist environment encourages microorganism growth.

CRITICAL DECISION POINT: *Do not store the catheter where it will come in contact with secretions or excretions, which promote bacterial growth. If the patient is capable of self-oral suctioning, place the catheter within reach.*

STEPS	RATIONALE
B. Nasopharyngeal and nasotracheal suctioning	
(1) Open lubricant. Squeeze a small amount onto open sterile catheter package without touching the package. Lubricant is *not* necessary for artificial airway suctioning.	• Prepares lubricant while maintaining sterility. Water-soluble lubricant is used to avoid lipoid aspiration pneumonia. Excessive lubricant can occlude the catheter.
(2) Apply a sterile glove to each hand, or apply a nonsterile glove to nondominant hand and a sterile glove to dominant hand.	• Reduces transmission of microorganisms and allows the nurse to maintain sterility of suction catheter.

Continued

SKILL 40.1   SUCTIONING—cont'd

STEPS	RATIONALE
(3) Pick up suction catheter with dominant hand without touching nonsterile surfaces. Pick up connecting tubing with nondominant hand. Secure catheter to tubing (see Step 4B[3] illustration).	• Maintains catheter sterility. Connects catheter to suction.

STEP 4B(3) Attaching catheter to suction.

STEPS	RATIONALE
(4) Check that the equipment is functioning properly by suctioning a small amount of normal saline solution from the basin.	• Ensures equipment function; lubricates catheter and tubing.
(5) Lightly coat distal 6–8 cm (2–3 inches) of catheter with water-soluble lubricant.	• Lubricates catheter for easier insertion.
(6) Remove oxygen delivery device, if applicable, with nondominant hand. *Without applying suction* and using dominant thumb and forefinger, gently insert catheter into naris during inhalation. **Never apply suction during insertion.**	• Application of suction pressure while introducing catheter into nasopharyngeal tissues increases risk of damage to mucosa. When advanced into trachea, suction could damage mucosa and increase risk of hypoxia.
(7) *Nasopharyngeal:* As the patient takes a deep breath, insert catheter following natural course of naris; slightly slant catheter downward and advance to back of pharynx. Do not force through naris. In adults, insert catheter about 16 cm (6.5 inches); in older children, 8–12 cm (3–5 inches); in infants and young children, 4–7.5 cm (1.5–3 inches) into trachea.	• Proper placement ensures removal of pharyngeal secretions. Ensure the catheter tip reaches the pharynx for suctioning. • If resistance is met during insertion, you may need to try the other naris. Do not force the catheter up the nares, because this will cause mucosal damage.
(a) Apply intermittent suction for no more than 15 seconds by placing and releasing nondominant thumb over catheter vent (AARC, 2010). Slowly withdraw catheter while rotating it back and forth between thumb and forefinger.	• Intermittent suction safely removes pharyngeal secretions. Suction time of >15 seconds increases risk for suction-induced hypoxemia (AARC, 2010).
(8) *Nasotracheal:* As patient takes a deep breath, advance catheter following natural course of naris, slightly slanted and downward to just above entrance into larynx and then the trachea. Allow patient to take a breath. Quickly insert catheter approximately 16–20 cm (6–8 inches) (in adult) into trachea (see Step 4B[8] illustration). Patient will begin to cough, then pull back catheter 1–2 cm (½ inch) before applying suction. *Note*: In older children, advance 16–20 cm (6–8 inches); in young children and infants, 8–14 cm (3–5½ inches).	• Ensures catheter will be inserted into trachea with minimal stress to patient.

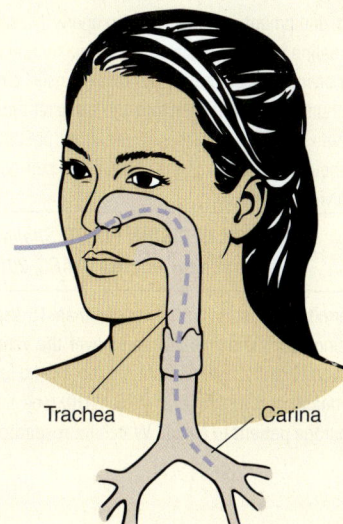

STEP 4B(8) Distance of insertion of nasotracheal catheter.

SKILL 40.1	SUCTIONING—cont'd
STEPS	**RATIONALE**

CRITICAL DECISION POINT: *Insert catheter during patient inhalation, especially if inserting catheter into the trachea, because the epiglottis is open. If there is difficulty passing the catheter, ask the patient to cough or say "ahh." Do not insert during swallowing or the catheter will most likely enter the esophagus. Never apply suction during insertion. The patient should cough. If the patient gags or becomes nauseated, the catheter is most likely in the esophagus and must be removed.*

(a) *Positioning option for nasotracheal suctioning:* In some instances, turning the patient's head to the right will help you suction the left mainstem bronchus; turning their head to the left will help you suction the right mainstem bronchus.	• Turning the patient's head to the side elevates the bronchial passage on the opposite side and facilitates passage of the catheter.

CRITICAL DECISION POINT: *Use nasal approach and perform tracheal suctioning before pharyngeal suctioning whenever possible. The mouth and pharynx contain more bacteria than the trachea does. If copious oral secretions are present before beginning the procedure, suction the mouth with an oral suction device.*

(b) Apply intermittent suction for 15 seconds or less (AARC, 2010) by placing and *releasing* your nondominant thumb over vent of the catheter and slowly withdrawing catheter while rotating it back and forth between your dominant thumb and forefinger. Encourage patient to cough. Replace oxygen device, if applicable.	• Intermittent suction and rotation of catheter prevent injury to mucosa. If the catheter "grabs" mucosa, remove your thumb to release suction. Suctioning longer than 10 seconds can cause cardiopulmonary compromise, usually from hypoxemia or vagal overload.

CRITICAL DECISION POINT: *Monitor the patient's vital signs and oxygen saturation during the procedure, note if the patient's pulse drops more than 20 beats per minute or increases more than 40 beats per minute, or oxygen saturation falls below 90% or 5% from baseline, in which case, cease suctioning.*

(9) Rinse catheter and connecting tubing with normal saline or water until cleared.	• Removes secretions from catheter. Secretions that remain in suction catheter or connecting tubing decrease suctioning efficiency.
(10) Assess for need to repeat suctioning procedure. Do not perform more than two passes with the catheter. Allow adequate time (at least 1 minute) between suction passes for ventilation and oxygenation (AARC, 2010). Ask patient to deep-breathe and to cough.	• Observe for alterations in cardiopulmonary status. Suctioning can induce hypoxemia, dysrhythmias, laryngospasm, and bronchospasm (AARC, 2010). Deep breathing reventilates and reoxygenates alveoli and reduces the risk for suction-induced hypoxemia. Repeated passes clear the airway of excessive secretions but can also remove oxygen and may induce laryngospasm.
C. Artificial airway (tracheostomy) suctioning	
(1) Apply one sterile glove to each hand, or apply a nonsterile glove to the nondominant hand and a sterile glove to the dominant hand.	• Reduces transmission of microorganisms and allows the nurse to maintain sterility of suction catheter.
(2) Pick up suction catheter with your dominant hand without touching nonsterile surfaces.	• Maintains catheter sterility. Establishes suction.
(3) Pick up connecting tubing with your nondominant hand. Secure catheter to tubing.	
(4) Check that equipment is functioning properly by suctioning a small amount of saline from the basin by occluding suction vent.	• Ensures equipment function; lubricates catheter and tubing.
(5) Without applying suction, gently but quickly insert catheter using your dominant thumb and forefinger into the artificial airway (it is best to time catheter insertion with inspiration) until patient coughs, usually 0.5–1 cm below the level of the tube. Then pull back 1 cm (½ inch) before applying suction.	• Application of suction pressure while introducing catheter into the trachea increases risk of damage to tracheal mucosa and greater hypoxia through removal of entrained oxygen present in the airways. The action of pulling back stimulates cough and removes the catheter from the mucosal wall so that the catheter is not resting against tracheal mucosa during suctioning.

CRITICAL DECISION POINT: *Shallow suctioning is recommended over deep suctioning, to prevent trauma to the tracheal mucosa (AARC, 2010).*

(6) Apply intermittent suction for no longer than 15 seconds by placing and releasing your nondominant thumb over the vent of the catheter; slowly withdraw catheter while rotating it back and forth between your dominant thumb and forefinger (AARC, 2010) (see Step 4C[6] illustration). Encourage patient to cough. Watch for respiratory distress.	• Intermittent suction and rotation of catheter prevent injury to tracheal mucosal lining. If catheter "grabs" mucosa, remove your thumb to release suction.

Continued

SKILL 40.1   **SUITIONING—cont'd**

STEPS   **RATIONALE**

STEP 4C(6) Suctioning tracheostomy.

CRITICAL DECISION POINT: *If the patient develops respiratory distress during suction procedure, immediately withdraw the catheter and supply additional oxygen and breaths as needed.*

---

(7) Encourage patient to deep-breathe, if able.

- Reoxygenates and re-expands alveoli. Suctioning can cause hypoxemia and atelectasis.

(8) Rinse catheter and connecting tubing with normal saline until clear. Use continuous suction.

- Removes catheter secretions. Secretions left in tubing decrease suction and provide an environment for microorganism growth. Secretions left in connecting tube decrease suctioning efficiency.

(9) Assess patient's cardiopulmonary status for secretion clearance and complications. Repeat once or twice more to clear secretions. Allow adequate time (at least 1 full minute) between suction passes for ventilation and reoxygenation. Perform oropharyngeal and nasopharyngeal (if necessary) suctioning to clear secretions (Steps 4A, 4B). Do not suction nose again after suctioning mouth.

- Suctioning can induce dysrhythmias, hypoxia, and bronchospasm and impair cerebral circulation or adversely affect hemodynamics (AARC, 2010).
- The upper airway is considered clean and the lower airway is considered sterile. Therefore, the same catheter can be used to suction from sterile to clean areas, but not from clean to sterile areas.

5. Complete procedure:

A. Disconnect catheter from connecting tubing. Roll catheter around fingers of your dominant hand. Pull glove off inside out so that the catheter remains in the glove. Pull off other glove over first glove in the same way to contain contaminants. Discard into appropriate receptacle. Turn off suction.

- Reduces transmission of microorganisms. Clean equipment should not be touched with contaminated gloves.

B. Remove towel and place in laundry or remove drape and discard in appropriate receptacle.

C. Reposition patient as indicated by condition. You may need to reapply clean gloves for patient's personal care (e.g., oral hygiene).

- Proper positioning based on patient's condition promotes comfort, encourages secretion drainage, and reduces risk of aspiration.

D. If indicated, readjust oxygen to original level.

- Helps patient's blood oxygen level return to baseline.

E. Discard remainder of normal saline into appropriate receptacle. If basin is disposable, discard into appropriate receptacle. If basin is reusable, rinse and place in soiled utility room.

- Solution is contaminated.

F. Remove goggles, mask, face shield, and gown and place in appropriate receptacles; perform hand hygiene.

- Reduces transmission of microorganisms.

G. Place unopened suction kit on suction machine table or at head of bed according to institution preference.

- Provides for immediate access of suction catheter and equipment in the event of an emergency or for the next suctioning procedure.

6. Compare patient's vital signs and SpO₂ saturation before and after suctioning.

- Identifies physiological effects of suction procedure to restore airway patency.

7. Ask patient if breathing is easier and if congestion is decreased. Auscultate lungs and compare respiratory assessment before and after suctioning.

- Provides subjective confirmation that airway obstruction is relieved with suctioning procedure.

8. Observe airway secretions.

- Provides data to document presence or absence of respiratory tract infection.

9. Remove PPE and discard into appropriate receptable.

- Reduces transmission of microorganisms.

EVALUATION

1. Compare patient's vital signs and cardiopulmonary assessment before and after suctioning.

- Identifies physiological effects of suction procedure to restore airway patency.

2. Ask patient if their breathing is easier and their congestion has decreased.

- Provides subjective confirmation that suction procedure has relieved airway.

3. Auscultate lungs and compare patient's respiratory assessment before and after suctioning.

- Provides objective information about any change in lung sounds.

4. Observe character of airway secretions.

- Provides data to document the presence or absence of respiratory tract infection or thickened secretions.

SKILL 40.1	SUCTIONING—cont'd	
STEPS	**RATIONALE**	

UNEXPECTED OUTCOMES	RELATED INTERVENTIONS
Worsening respiratory status	• Limit length of suctioning. • Determine need for more frequent suctioning, possibly of shorter duration. • Determine need for supplemental oxygen, supply oxygen between suction passes. • Notify health care provider.
Return of bloody secretions	• Determine amount of suction pressure used. It may need to be decreased. • Ensure suction is completed correctly by using intermittent suction and rotation of catheter. • Evaluate suctioning frequency. • Provide more frequent oral hygiene. • Determine other factors, such as prolonged bleeding time.
Unable to pass suction catheter through first naris attempted	• Try other naris or oral route. • Insert nasal airway, especially if suctioning through patient naris frequently. • Guide catheter along naris floor to avoid turbinates. • If obstruction is mucus, apply suction to relieve obstruction, but do not apply suction to mucosa. If obstruction is thought to be a blood clot, consult health care provider. • Increase lubrication of catheter.
Paroxysms of coughing	• Administer supplemental oxygen. • Allow patient to rest between passes of suction catheter. • Consult health care provider regarding need for inhaled bronchodilators or topical anaesthetics.
No secretions obtained	• Evaluate patient's fluid status. • Assess for signs of infection. • Determine need for chest physiotherapy. • Assess adequacy of humidification on oxygen delivery device.

RECORDING AND REPORTING

• Record the amount, consistency, colour, and odour of secretions and patient's response to procedure; document patient's pre-suctioning and post-suctioning cardiopulmonary status.

CARE IN THE COMMUNITY CONSIDERATIONS

• Nurses need to adhere to best practices for infection control while weighing cost-effectiveness in the setting of a chronic situation. If the patient has an established tracheostomy or requires long-term nasotracheal suctioning and infection is not present, clean suction technique is appropriate.
• Instruct the patient and family in infection-control measures for emptying the secretion jar. These secretions should be emptied in the toilet but they have a splash risk. Instruct the caregiver to apply a mask (shield if available) and gloves and bring the secretion jar as close to the toilet bowel as possible to decrease the risk of splash.

Clinical studies comparing suctioning after NSI with standard suctioning have not demonstrated any clinical or significant results (AARC, 2010).

The two current methods of suctioning are the open and closed methods. Open suctioning involves a sterile catheter that is opened at the time of suctioning. Sterile gloves are worn to perform the suction procedure. Closed suctioning involves a multiple-use suction catheter encased in a plastic sheath. Closed suctioning is most often used on patients who require mechanical ventilation to support their respiratory efforts, because it permits continuous delivery of oxygen while suction is performed, thus reducing the risk of oxygen desaturation. Although sterile gloves are not required in this procedure, at least nonsterile (i.e., disposable) gloves are recommended to prevent contact with splashes from body fluids.

Artificial Airways. An artificial airway is indicated for patients with a decreased level of consciousness or an airway obstruction and to aid in the removal of tracheobronchial secretions.

Oral Airway. The oral airway, the simplest type of artificial airway, prevents obstruction of the trachea by displacement of the tongue into the oropharynx (Figure 40.11). The oral airway extends from the teeth to the oropharynx, maintaining the tongue in the normal position. The correct-size airway must be used. Proper oral airway size is determined by measuring the distance from the corner of the mouth to the angle of the jaw just below the ear. The length is equal to the distance from the flange of the airway to the tip. If the airway is too small, the tongue is not held in the anterior portion of the mouth; if the airway is too large, it may force the tongue toward the epiglottis and obstruct the airway.

The airway is inserted by turning the curve of the airway toward the cheek and placing it over the tongue. When the airway is in the oropharynx, turn it so that the opening points downward. When correctly placed, the airway moves the tongue forward away from the oropharynx, and the flange, the flat portion of the airway, rests against the patient's teeth. Incorrect insertion merely forces the tongue back into the oropharynx.

Endotracheal and Tracheal Airway. An artificial airway is used for a patient with decreased level of consciousness or airway obstruction and aids in removal of tracheal bronchial secretions. The presence of an artificial airway places the patient at high risk for infection and airway injury. Sterile technique must be used in caring for and maintaining an artificial airway to help prevent health care–associated infections. Artificial airways need to be cared for and maintained in the correct position to prevent airway damage (Skill 40.2).

Endotracheal (ET) tubes are used as short-term artificial airways to administer mechanical ventilation, relieve upper airway obstruction, protect against aspiration, or clear secretions (Box 40.15). Only health care providers in critical care settings with special training may insert and maintain ET tubes. ET tubes are generally removed within 14 days; however, they may be used for a longer period of time if the patient is showing progress toward weaning from mechanical ventilation and extubation. If the patient requires long-term assistance from an artificial airway, a tracheostomy is considered. A surgical incision is made into the trachea, and a short artificial airway (a tracheostomy tube) is inserted.

Maintenance and Promotion of Lung Expansion. Nursing interventions to maintain or promote lung expansion include noninvasive

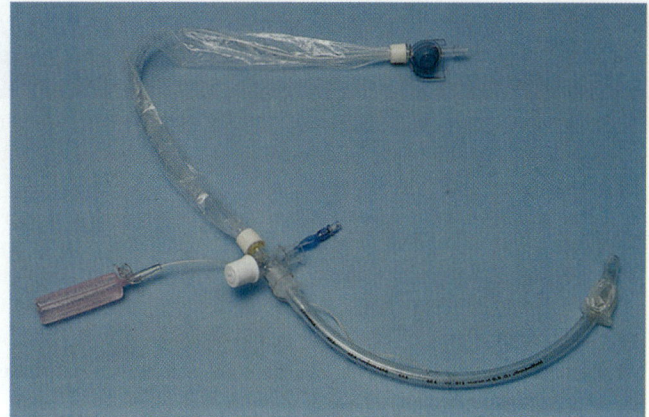

FIGURE 40.11 Artificial oral airways.

and invasive techniques. Noninvasive techniques are ambulation, positioning, and incentive spirometry. An invasive procedure is management of a chest tube.

Ambulation. Immobility is a major factor contributing to atelectasis and ventilator-associated pneumonia. Early ambulation has been

---

SKILL 40.2   CARE OF AN ARTIFICIAL AIRWAY (TRACHEOSTOMY)

Delegation Considerations
This skill should not be routinely delegated to an unregulated care provider (UCP). It is the nurse's responsibility to perform tracheal care, and often nurses must collaborate with the respiratory therapist. In some settings, patients who have well-established tracheostomy tubes may have the care delegated to UCPs. It is the nurse's responsibility to assess and ensure that proper artificial airway care is provided. In addition, UCPs may perform other aspects of the patient's care. The nurse must instruct the UCPs about the following:
- To report any changes in the patient's respiratory status, level of consciousness, confusion, restlessness, irritability, changes in vital signs (range to report), decreased pulse oximetry level (values to report), or change in level of comfort
- To report abnormal colour of tracheal stoma and drainage
- Emergency procedures in case the tracheostomy tube inadvertently becomes dislodged when ties are changed

Equipment
Tracheostomy care
- Towel
- Tracheostomy suction supplies
- Sterile tracheostomy care kit, if available, or three sterile 4 × 4 gauze pads
- Sterile cotton-tipped applicators
- Sterile tracheostomy dressing
- Sterile basin
- Small sterile brush (or disposable cannula)
- Tracheostomy ties (e.g., twill tape, manufactured tracheostomy ties, Velcro tracheostomy ties)
- Normal saline (NS)
- Scissors
- Pair of sterile and clean gloves
- Mask, goggles, face shield (if indicated)

PROCEDURE

STEPS	RATIONALE
ASSESSMENT	
1. Identify patient using at least two identifiers according to agency policy. Compare identifiers with information with patient's medication administration record (MAR) or medical record.	• Ensures correct patient.
2. Perform hand hygiene and apply gloves and any other personal protective equipment (PPE) if exposure to airway secretions is present.	• Helps prevent transmission of microorganisms.
3. Perform pulmonary assessment:	
A. Auscultate lung sounds.	• Provides baseline information.
B. Assess condition and patency of airway and surrounding tissues.	• Indicates if additional skin care to irritated areas is needed. Identifies potential pressure areas.
C. Note type and size of tube, movement of tube, and cuff size.	• Movement of tube predisposes the patient to tracheal trauma or tube dislodgement and may indicate the need for another size airway. Cuff size indicates the amount of air needed to properly inflate the cuff.
4. Assess for patient and caregiver's knowledge, experience, and health literacy.	

SKILL 40.2   CARE OF AN ARTIFICIAL AIRWAY (TRACHEOSTOMY)—cont'd

STEPS	RATIONALE
5. Perform hand hygiene, apply gloves, and other PPE as determined by patient condition and agency policy.	• Reduces transmission of microorganisms.
PLANNING	
1. Gather equipment and supplies. Position patient: usually supine or semi-Fowler's.	• Provides access to the site and facilitates completion of the procedure.
2. Explain procedure to the patient and caregiver.	• Reinforces information given to the patient and family and provides an opportunity for them to ask additional questions.
IMPLEMENTATION	
1. Perform hand hygiene, apply clean gloves and PPE (as indicated). Place towel across the patient's chest.	• Reduces transmission of microorganisms and protects linens and bedclothes.
2. Perform airway care.	
A. Tracheostomy care	
(1) Observe for signs and symptoms of need to perform tracheostomy care:	• A patient with a tracheostomy tube is at increased risk because of loss of natural airway protection of the upper airway.
(a) Soiled or loose ties or Velcro holder	
(b) Soiled or loose dressing	
(c) Nonstable tube	
(d) Excessive secretions	
(2) Suction tracheostomy (see Skill 40.1). Before removing gloves, remove soiled tracheostomy dressing and discard in glove with coiled catheter.	• Removes secretions so as not to occlude outer cannula while inner cannula is removed. Reduces need for patient to cough. Prevents aspiration of retained secretions. • Disposal method helps to contain microorganisms.
(3) Prepare equipment:	
(a) Perform hand hygiene. Open sterile tracheostomy kit. Open two 4 × 4 inch gauze packages using aseptic technique and pour normal saline (NS) on one package. Leave the second package dry. Open two packages of cotton-tipped swabs and pour NS on one package. Do not recap NS.	• Preparation and organization of equipment allow for efficient tracheostomy care and reconnecting of the patient to an oxygen source in a timely manner.
(b) Open sterile tracheostomy dressing package.	
(c) Unwrap sterile basin and pour approximately 2 cm (1 in) of NS into it.	
(d) Open small sterile brush package and place aseptically into sterile basin.	
(e) Prepare length of twill tape long enough to go around the patient's neck two times, approximately 60–75 cm (20–25 in) for an adult. Cut ends on diagonal. Lay aside in dry area.	• Cutting ends of the tie on a diagonal aids with inserting tie through eyelet.
(f) If using a commercially available tracheostomy tube holder, open package according to manufacturer's directions.	
3. Apply oxygen source loosely over tracheostomy if patient desaturates during procedure.	• Replenishes oxygen lost during suctioning (AARC, 2010).
4. Apply sterile gloves. Keep your dominant hand sterile throughout the procedure.	• Reduces transmission of microorganisms.
5. If a nondisposable inner cannula is used:	
A. While touching only the outer aspect of the tube, unlock and remove the inner cannula with your nondominant hand. Drop inner cannula into NS basin.	• Removes inner cannula for cleaning. NS loosens secretions from inner cannula.
B. Place tracheostomy collar or T tube over or near the outer cannula. (*Note:* T tube cannot be attached to all outer cannulas when the inner cannula is removed.)	• Maintains supply of oxygen to patient.
C. To prevent oxygen desaturation in affected patients, quickly pick up the inner cannula and use a small brush to remove secretions inside and outside cannula (see Step 5C illustration).	• A tracheostomy brush provides mechanical force to remove thick or dried secretions.
D. Hold inner cannula over basin and rinse with NS, using your nondominant hand to pour NS.	• Removes secretions from inner cannula.

Continued

STEP 5C Cleaning the tracheostomy inner cannula.

STEP 5E Reinserting the inner cannula.

   E. Replace inner cannula and secure "locking" mechanism (see Step 5E illustration). Reapply oxygen sources.
- Secures inner cannula and re-establishes oxygen supply.

6. If a disposable inner cannula is used:
   A. Remove cannula from manufacturer's packaging.
   B. While touching only the outer aspect of the tube, withdraw inner cannula and replace with a new cannula. Lock into position.
   C. Dispose of contaminated cannula in appropriate receptacle and apply oxygen source.
- Prevents unnecessary oxygen desaturation.

7. Using NS-saturated cotton-tipped swabs and 4 × 4 gauze, clean exposed outer cannula surfaces and stoma under faceplate, extending 5–10 cm (2–4 inches) in all directions from stoma (see Step 7 illustration). Clean in a circular motion from the stoma site outward, using your dominant hand to handle sterile supplies.
- Aseptically removes secretions from stoma site. Moving in an outward circle pulls mucus and other contaminants from the stoma to the periphery.

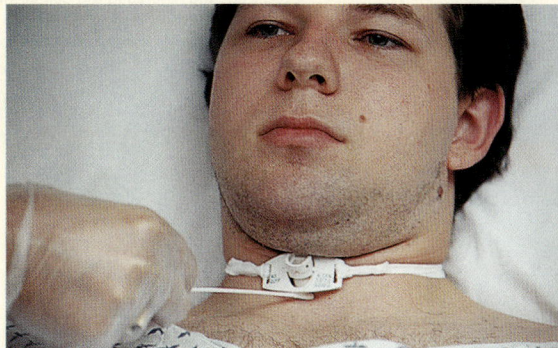

STEP 7 Cleaning around stoma.

8. Using NS-prepared cotton-tipped swabs and 4 × 4 gauze, clean outer tracheostomy tube flange and skin surfaces. Using dry 4 × 4 gauze, pat lightly at skin and exposed outer cannula surfaces.
- Dry surfaces prevent formation of moist environment conducive to growth of microorganisms and prevent skin excoriation.

9. Secure tracheostomy.
   A. Tracheostomy tie method:
      (1) Instruct assistant to apply gloves and hold the tracheostomy tube securely in place while ties are cut.
- Promotes hygiene, reduces transmission of microorganisms, and secures tracheostomy tube.

CRITICAL DECISION POINT: *The assistant must not release hold on the tracheostomy tube until new ties are firmly tied, to reduce risk of accidental extubation. If no assistant is present, do not cut old ties until new ties are in place and securely tied.*

SKILL 40.2   CARE OF AN ARTIFICIAL AIRWAY (TRACHEOSTOMY)—cont'd

STEPS	RATIONALE

(2) Take prepared tie and insert one end of tie through faceplate eyelet and pull ends even (see Step 9A[2] illustration).

STEP 9A(2) Replacing tracheostomy ties when an assistant is not available. Do not remove old tracheostomy ties until new ones are secure.

CRITICAL DECISION POINT: *Tracheostomy obturator should be kept at the bedside with a fresh tracheostomy to facilitate reinsertion of the outer cannula, if dislodged. An additional tracheostomy tube of the same size and kind should be kept on hand for emergency replacement (Morse et al., 2013).*

---

(3) Slide both ends of tie behind the patient's head and around their neck to other eyelet and insert one tie through second eyelet.

(4) Pull snugly.

(5) Tie ends securely in a double square knot, allowing space for only one loose or two snug fingerwidths in tie.

(6) Apply barrier cream, if ordered. Insert fresh 4 × 4 inch precut tracheostomy dressing under clean ties and faceplate (see Step 9A[6] illustration).

- Secures tracheostomy tube in place.
- One-finger slack prevents ties from being too tight when tracheostomy dressing is in place and prevents movement of the tracheostomy tube into the lower airway.
- Barrier cream helps prevent skin breakdown around the stoma (Karaca & Korkmaz, 2019). Absorbs drainage. Dressing prevents pressure on clavicle heads. Never cut a 2 × 2 or 4 × 4 inch gauze pad yourself because the cut edges fray and may increase the risk of infection (Wiegand, 2017).

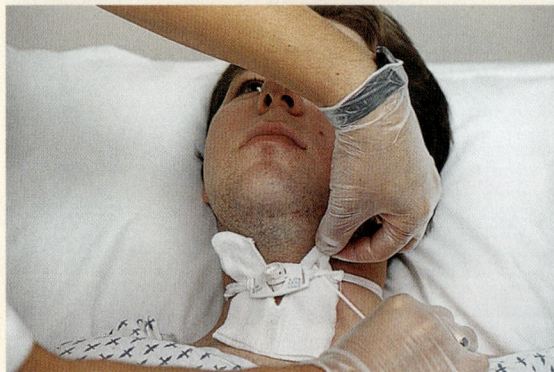

STEP 9A(6) Applying tracheostomy dressing.

B. Tracheostomy tube holder method:

(1) While wearing gloves, maintain a secure hold on tracheostomy tube. This can be done with an assistant, or, when an assistant is not available, by leaving the old tracheostomy tube holder in place until a new device is secure.

(2) Align strap under patient's neck. Ensure that Velcro attachments are positioned on either side of tracheostomy tube.

(3) Place narrow end of ties under and through faceplate eyelets. Pull ends even, and secure with Velcro closures.

- Prevents accidental displacement of tube.

Continued

SKILL 40.2	CARE OF AN ARTIFICIAL AIRWAY (TRACHEOSTOMY)—cont'd
STEPS	**RATIONALE**

STEPS	RATIONALE
(4) Verify that there is space for only one loose or two snug finger-width(s) under neck strap. Apply barrier cream, if ordered. Insert fresh 4 × 4 inch precut tracheostomy dressing under clean ties and face-plate.	• Barrier cream helps prevent skin breakdown around the stoma (Karaca & Korkmaz, 2019). • Never cut a 2 × 2 or 4 × 4 inch gauze pad yourself, because the cut edges fray and may increase the risk of infection (Wiegand, 2017).
10. Position patient comfortably and assess respiratory status.	• Promotes comfort. Some patients may require post-tracheostomy care suctioning.
11. Replace any oxygen delivery devices.	• Maintains oxygen therapy.
12. Remove and discard gloves and face shield. Replace cap on NS. Perform hand hygiene.	• Reduces transmission of infection. Once opened, NS can be considered free of bacteria for 24 hours, after which it should be discarded.

EVALUATION

STEPS	RATIONALE
1. Compare respiratory assessments before and after procedure.	• Identifies any changes in presence and quality of breath sounds after procedure.
2. Observe depth and position of tubes.	• Verifies that position of tube is correct.
3. Assess security of tracheostomy tube holder (e.g., tape or Velcro) by tugging at tube.	• Artificial airway should not move. Patient may cough.
4. Assess skin around mouth and oral mucosa and tracheostomy stoma for drainage, pressure, and signs of irritation.	• Skin breakdown or irritation should not be present.

UNEXPECTED OUTCOMES	RELATED INTERVENTIONS
Accidental decannulation of tracheostomy tube	• Call for assistance while remaining with the patient. • Replace old tracheostomy tube with a new spare tube of same size and kind kept at the bedside. • Prepare to manually ventilate a patient who develops respiratory distress.
Hard, reddened areas with or without excessive or foul-smelling secretions	• This indicates infection. Notify health care provider. • Increase frequency of tube care. • Remove inner cannula, if applicable, for cleaning and suctioning.
Insecure tube, artificial airway moves in or out, coughed out by patient	• Assess patient's respiratory status and observe for presence of mucous plugs. • Adjust or apply new ties.
Breakdown, pressure areas, or stomatitis	• Increase frequency of tube care. • Make sure skin areas are clean and dry.

RECORDING AND REPORTING

- Record respiratory assessments before and after care.
- Record tracheostomy care: type and size of tracheostomy tube, frequency and extent of care, patient tolerance, and any complications related to presence of the tube.

CARE IN THE COMMUNITY CONSIDERATIONS

- Instruct caregivers on how to obtain supplies.
- Instruct caregivers on signs and symptoms of respiratory distress, tube dysfunction, and respiratory and stoma infections.
- At home, clean technique is used with nonsterile gloves, and routine tracheostomy care should be done at least once a day after discharge from hospital.

---

correlated with increased general strength and lung expansion, thus respiratory therapists and physiotherapists should be involved in the patient's care. Early mobility and ambulation are particularly important for postoperative patients to prevent complications and promote airway clearance (Strickland et al., 2013).

Positioning. In the healthy, completely mobile person, adequate ventilation and oxygenation are maintained through frequent position changes during daily activities. Frequent changes of position are simple and cost-effective methods for reducing the risks of stasis of pulmonary secretions and decreased chest wall expansion.

The most effective position for patients with cardiopulmonary diseases is the 45-degree semi-Fowler's position, using gravity to assist in lung expansion and reduce pressure from the abdomen on the diaphragm. When the patient is in this position, the nurse

BOX 40.15	Highlights Related to the Care of an Endotracheal Tube (ET)

- Care of an ET tube is an advanced skill, thus requiring additional knowledge and preparation.
- Nurses with this advanced training may assist with the care of ET tubes by suctioning and securing the ET tube and changing the tape and commercially available devices.
- Sterile technique must be used when caring for a patient with an ET tube.
- A closed suctioning system is used to remove secretions through an ET tube.
- An oral airway should be immediately accessible in the event that the patient bites down and obstructs the ET tube.

needs to ensure that the patient does not slide down in bed, which could reduce lung expansion. A patient with unilateral lung disease (e.g., pneumothorax, atelectasis, pneumonia, thoracotomy, multiple trauma affecting one lung) should be positioned with the unaffected lung down ("good lung down"). This promotes better perfusion of the healthy lung, improving oxygenation. In the presence of pulmonary abscess or hemorrhage, the patient should be placed with the affected lung down to prevent drainage toward the unaffected (healthy) lung.

Incentive Spirometry. Incentive spirometry is a method of encouraging voluntary deep breathing by providing visual feedback to patients about inspiratory volume. Flow-oriented incentive spirometers consist of one or more plastic chambers containing freely moving coloured balls. The patient inhales slowly and with an even flow to elevate the balls and keep them floating as long as possible to ensure a maximally sustained inhalation. Volume-oriented incentive spirometry devices have a bellows that is raised to a predetermined volume by an inhaled breath. An achievement light or counter is used to provide visual feedback. Incentive spirometry is not recommended for routine prophylactic use in postoperative patients; instead, it is important to reinforce early ambulation and mobilization (Strickland et al., 2013).

Chest Tubes. Chest tubes are inserted to remove air and fluids from the pleural space, prevent air or fluid from re-entering the pleural space, and re-establish normal intrapleural and intrapulmonic pressures. A chest tube is a catheter inserted through the thorax to remove fluid or air. Chest tubes may be inserted at the bedside, in the emergency department, and in the operating room (Tyerman & Cobbett, 2023). Chest tubes are commonly used after chest surgery and chest trauma and for pneumothorax or hemothorax to promote lung re-expansion (Skill 40.3).

A pneumothorax is a collection of air in the pleural space. The loss of negative intrapleural pressure causes the lung to collapse. There are a variety of mechanisms associated with a pneumothorax. It may occur spontaneously or as a result of chest trauma, such as a stabbing or the chest striking the steering wheel in a motor vehicle accident. A pneumothorax may also result from the rupture of an emphysematous bleb on the surface of the lung (a large bulla resulting from the destruction caused by emphysema) or from an invasive procedure, such as insertion of a subclavian intravenous (IV) line.

A patient with a pneumothorax usually feels pain as atmospheric air irritates the parietal pleura. The pain may be sharp and pleuritic. Dyspnea is common and worsens as the size of the pneumothorax increases.

A hemothorax is an accumulation of blood and fluid in the pleural cavity between the parietal and visceral pleurae, usually as a result of trauma. It produces a counterpressure and prevents the lung from full expansion. A hemothorax can also be caused by the rupture of small blood vessels from inflammatory processes, such as pneumonia or TB. In addition to pain and dyspnea, signs and symptoms of shock can develop if blood loss is severe.

SKILL 40.3   CARE OF PATIENTS WITH CHEST TUBES

Delegation Considerations
This skill should not be delegated to an unregulated care provider (UCP). However, a UCP may assist with other aspects of the patient's care. It is important to inform the UCP of the following:
- Proper positioning of the patient with chest tubes to facilitate chest tube drainage and optimal function of the system
- How to ambulate and transfer a patient with chest drainage
- To report to the nurse any changes in vital signs, including oxygen saturation, chest pain, sudden shortness of breath, or excessive bubbling in the water-seal chamber
- To immediately report to the nurse a disconnection of the system, any change in type and amount of drainage, sudden bleeding, or sudden cessation of bubbling

Equipment
- Disposable chest drainage system (see Figure 40.12)
- Suction source and set-up (wall canister or portable)
- Disposable (nonsterile) gloves, face mask
- 2.5-cm (1-inch) waterproof adhesive tape or plastic zip-ties
- Sterile gauze sponges
- Petrolatum or Xeroform gauze, split chest-tube dressings, several 4 × 4 gauze dressings, large gauze dressings, 10-cm (4-inch) tape
- Two rubber-tipped (shodded) or toothless hemostats
- Stethoscope
- Pulse oximeter
- Sphygmomanometer

PROCEDURE

STEPS	RATIONALE
ASSESSMENT	
1. Identify patient using at least two identifiers, according to agency policy. Compare identifiers with information on the patient's medication administration record (MAR) or medical record. Review health care provider's order for chest tube placement.	• Ensures correct patient.
2. Assess significant medical history, review patient's medication record for anticoagulant therapy and known allergies.	• Medical history or injury may provide the reason for occurrence of pneumothorax, hemothorax, empyema, and/or pleural effusion. Anticoagulant therapy may increase procedure-related blood loss.
3. Assess for patient's or caregiver's knowledge, experience, and health literacy.	• Ensures patient or caregiver has the capacity to obtain, communicate, process, and understand basic health information and individualizes patient care.
4. Perform hand hygiene and complete respiratory assessment, vital signs, including SpO₂.	• Signs and symptoms should reflect improvement in respiratory distress and chest pain after insertion of the chest tube.

Continued

SKILL 40.3   CARE OF PATIENTS WITH CHEST TUBES—cont'd

STEPS	RATIONALE
5. Pulmonary status: Assess for respiratory distress, chest pain, breath sounds over affected lung area, and stable vital signs (see Chapter 31). Signs and symptoms of increased respiratory distress or chest pain include decreased breath sounds over the affected and nonaffected lungs, marked cyanosis, asymmetrical chest movements, presence of **subcutaneous emphysema** (air trapped in the subcutaneous tissue) around tube insertion site or neck, hypotension, and tachycardia.	• Notify health care provider immediately.
6. Assess vital signs, SpO$_2$, and level of orientation. Review patient's current hemoglobin and hematocrit levels.	• Changes in pulse and blood pressure may indicate infection, respiratory distress, or pain. Reflects blood loss and subsequent levels of oxygenation.
7. Pain: If possible, ask patient to rate level of pain on a scale of 0 to 10.	• Chest tubes can be painful and interfere with a patient's mobility, coughing and deep breathing, and rehabilitation.
8. For patients who have existing chest tubes, observe the following:	
A. Chest tube dressing and site surrounding tube insertion. Keep a box of sterile 4 × 4 inch gauze pads and petroleum gauze at the bedside.	• Ensures that dressing is intact and occlusive seal remains without air or fluid leaks and that area surrounding insertion site is free of drainage or skin irritation. The 4 × 4 inch gauze pads are used if the chest tube(s) becomes dislodged. Covering the site immediately and taping the dressing on three sides is essential. Notify health care provider immediately.
B. Check tubing for kinks, dependent loops, or clots.	• Maintains a patent, freely draining system, preventing fluid accumulation in the chest cavity. Presence of kinks, dependent loops, or clotted drainage increases the risk for infection, atelectasis, and tension pneumothorax.
C. Note the amount and type of drainage by marking the drainage level on the outside of the drainage-collection chamber in hourly or shift increments, or in increments established by health care provider or agency's policy.	• Reference point for future measurements. Drainage should decrease gradually and change from bloody to pink to straw coloured.
D. Check chest drainage system, which should be upright and below level of tube insertion.	• Facilitates drainage; the system must be in this position to function properly.
PLANNING	
1. Perform hand hygiene. Organize supplies and arrange at the bedside.	• Reduces transmission of infection.
2. Assist patient to appropriate position for insertion of the chest tube or assist to a position of optimal comfort during other chest tube care.	• Appropriate positioning is important for proper insertion of the chest tube. Position of optimal comfort, once tube is inserted, will allow for increase in physical activity, including deep breathing and coughing, and the use of the incentive spirometer.
IMPLEMENTATION	
1. Review health care provider's orders for care of chest tube and for chest tube placement.	• Insertion of a chest tube requires a health care provider's order.
2. Perform hand hygiene and don appropriate PPE.	• Reduces transmission of microorganisms.
3. Set up water-seal system (or dry system with suction).	• The water-seal system contains two or three compartments or chambers. Fluid drains into the first chamber. The second chamber contains the water seal, which allows air to escape because of the force of expiration but not to re-enter on inspiration. If suction is needed, a third chamber is used.
A. Set up water-seal system or dry system with suction according to manufacturer's guidelines.	• Reduces potential for contamination.
While maintaining sterility of drainage tubing, stand system upright and add sterile water or normal saline to appropriate compartment.	• Water seal camber acts as a one-way valve, so air cannot enter the pleural space (Sasa, 2019).
(1) Two-chamber system (without suction): Add sterile solution to water-seal chamber, bringing fluid to required level as indicated or ordered by health care provider.	• Depth of fluid dictates highest amount of negative pressure that can be present in the system.
(2) Three-chamber system (with suction): Add sterile solution to water-seal chamber. Add amount of sterile solution prescribed by health care provider to suction-control chamber, usually −20 cm H$_2$O pressure. Connect tubing from suction-control chamber to suction source. The suction-control chamber vent must not be occluded when using suction.	• Automatic control valve on dry suction-control device adjusts to changes in patient air leaks and fluctuation in suction source and vacuum to deliver prescribed amount of suction.
(3) Dry suction system: Fill water-seal chamber with sterile solution. Adjust suction-control dial to prescribed level of suction; suction ranges from −10 to −40 cm of water pressure. The suction-control chamber vent is never occluded when suction is used. On dry suction, **DO NOT** obstruct positive-pressure relief value. This allows air to escape.	

STEPS	RATIONALE
B. Set up waterless system according to manufacturer's guidelines.	• A waterless system is like a water-seal system except that sterile water is not required for suction. The suction-control chamber is replaced by a one-way valve located near the top of the system. The suction chamber contains a suction-control float ball that is set up by a suction-control dial (between −10 and −40 cm H_2O after suction is connected and turned on (Zisis et al., 2015). • Prevents atmospheric air from leaking into the system and the patient's intrapleural space. Provides opportunity to ensure an airtight system before connection to the patient.
4. Secure all tubing connections with tape applied in a double-spiral fashion using 2.5-cm (1-inch) adhesive tape or zip ties with a clamp (Pickett, 2017). Check system patency by: **A.** Clamping drainage tubing that will connect to the patient's chest tube **B.** Connecting tubing from float ball chamber to suction source **C.** Turning on suction to prescribed level	
5. Turn off suction source and unclamp drainage tubing before connecting patient to the system. The suction source is turned on again after the patient is connected.	• Having patient connected to suction when it is initiated could damage pleural tissue from a sudden increase in negative pressure. Coiled tubing prevents adequate drainage and may cause tension pneumothorax (Pickett, 2017; Wiegand, 2017).
6. If not administered during assessment, administer medication such as sedatives or analgesics as ordered (administer 30 minutes before the procedure). Provide psychological support to the patient.	• Reduces anxiety and pain during procedure.
7. Perform hand hygiene and apply clean gloves. Position patient for tube insertion so that the side in which the tube is to be inserted is accessible to the health care provider.	• Reduces transmission of microorganisms. • For pneumothorax, place patient in a lateral supine position. For hemothorax, place patient in semi-Fowler's position (Chotai & Mosenifar, 2018).
8. Assist health care provider with chest tube insertion by providing needed equipment, local analgesic, and with attaching drainage tube to chest tube (remove clamp). Turn on suction to the prescribed level.	
9. Tape or zip-tie all connections between the chest tube and drainage tube. (The chest tube is usually taped by the health care provider at the time of tube placement; check agency policy.)	• Secures chest tube to drainage system and reduces risk for air leak that causes breaks in airtight system (Chotai & Mosenifar, 2018).
10. Check systems for proper functioning. Health care provider orders chest X-ray film.	• Verifies intrapleural placement of the tube.
11. After tube placement, position the patient: **A.** Semi-Fowler's or high-Fowler's position to evacuate air (pneumothorax) (Chotai & Mosenifar, 2018) **B.** High-Fowler's position to drain fluid (hemothorax) (Chotai & Mosenifar, 2018)	• Permits optimum drainage of fluid, air, or both.
12. Check patency of air vents in the system. **A.** Water-seal vent must have no occlusion. **B.** Suction-control chamber vent is not occluded when suction is used. **C.** Waterless systems have relief valves without caps.	• Permits displaced air to pass into the atmosphere. • Provides safety factor of releasing excess negative pressure into the atmosphere. • Provides safety factor of releasing negative pressure.
13. Position excess tubing horizontally on the mattress next to the patient. Secure with the clamp provided so that it does not obstruct tubing.	• Prevents excess tubing from hanging over the edge of the mattress in a dependent loop. Drainage collected in the loop can occlude the drainage system, which puts the patient at risk for tension pneumothorax (Pickett, 2017; Weigand, 2017).
14. Adjust tubing to hang in a straight line from the chest tube to the drainage chamber.	• Promotes drainage and prevents fluid or blood from accumulating in pleural cavity.

CRITICAL DECISION POINT: *Frequent gentle lifting of the drain allows gravity to help blood and other viscous material to move to the drainage bottle. Patients with recent chest surgery or trauma need to have the chest drain lifted on the basis of assessment of the amount of drainage; some patients might need the chest tube drain lifted every 5–10 minutes until volume decreases. However, when coiled or dependent looping of tubing is unavoidable, lift the tubing every 15 minutes, at a minimum, to promote drainage (Pickett, 2017).*

15. Place two rubber-tipped hemostats (for each chest tube) in an easily accessible position (e.g., taped to top of the patient's headboard). These should remain with the patient when ambulating.	• Chest tubes are double-clamped under specific circumstances: (1) to assess for air leak, (2) to empty or quickly change disposable systems, (3) to assess whether the patient is ready to have the tube removed, or (4) if the chest tube becomes accidentally disconnected from the drainage system (Muzzy & Butler, 2015).

Continued

SKILL 40.3	CARE OF PATIENTS WITH CHEST TUBES—cont'd	
STEPS	**RATIONALE**	

CRITICAL DECISION POINT: *In the event of a chest tube disconnection or if the drainage system breaks, submerge the distal part of the tube 2–4 cm (1–2 in) below the surface of a 250-mL bottle of saline water or NS until a new chest tube unit can be set up (Harding et al., 2020).*

16. Dispose of sharps in a proper container, dispose of other used supplies, and perform hand hygiene.

17. Care of patient after chest tube insertion:

A. Perform hand hygiene and apply clean gloves. Assess vital signs, oxygen saturation, skin colour, breath sounds, rate depth, ease of respirations, and insertion site every 15 minutes for first 2 hours and then at least every shift (see agency policy).	• Provides immediate information about procedure-related complications such as respiratory distress and leakage.
B. For severe pain, administer medication with ordered analgesics, and use complementary pain relief measures (e.g., repositioning) as needed.	
C. Monitor colour, consistency, and amount of chest tube drainage every 15 minutes for the first 2 hours after insertion. Indicate level of drainage, fluid, date and time—write this on surface of the chamber.	
(1) From mediastinal tube, expect less than 100 mL/hr immediately after surgery and no more than 500 mL in the first 24 hours.	• Provides baseline for continuous assessment of type and quantity of drainage. Ensures early detection of complications.
(2) From posterior chest tube, drainage is grossly bloody during the first several hours after surgery and then changes to serous (Harding et al., 2020).	• A sudden gush of drainage may result from coughing or changing of patient's position. Acute bleeding indicates hemorrhage. Notify health care provider if there is more than 100–200 mL of bloody drainage in an hour (Wiegand, 2017).
(3) Expect minimal or no output from an anterior chest tube that is inserted for a pneumothorax (Wiegand, 2017).	• Acute bleeding indicates hemorrhage. Notify health care provider if there is more than 200 mL of bloody drainage in an hour (Harding et al., 2020; Pickett, 2017).

CRITICAL DECISION POINT: *Routine stripping or milking of the chest tube is not a recommended practice. Doing so can result in increased pressure in the thoracic cavity, causing damage to the lungs or the pleural tissues. If there is a visible clot in the tubing, gentle milking of the tubing (manual squeezing and releasing of parts of the tubing) may be indicated, but only if the patient is at risk of further harm from the clot, such as development of a tension pneumothorax (Wiegand, 2017).*

D. Observe chest dressing for drainage and determine whether it is still occlusive.	• Drainage around the tube may indicate blockage of the tube.

CRITICAL DECISION POINT: *If the dressing is not occlusive or is saturated with drainage, it may need to be changed. There is no standard for how chest tube dressing should be performed, such as a sterile versus nonsterile dressing change. Know the health care agency standards for this procedure. Some health care agencies require the use of petrolatum gauze around the chest tube, while others do not (Gross et al., 2016).*

E. Perform hand hygiene and apply clean gloves. Observe chest dressing for drainage and palpate around the tube for swelling and crepitus (subcutaneous emphysema) as noted by crackling.	• Indicates presence of trapping in subcutaneous tissues. Most occurrences of crepitus are minor, as small amounts are commonly absorbed. Large amounts are potentially dangerous—notify the health care provider (Pickett, 2017; Sasa, 2019).

CRITICAL DECISION POINT: *When patients develop subcutaneous emphysema (e.g., collection of air under the skin after chest tube placement), a crepitus (a crackling sensation) is felt with tactile fremitus on palpation. Subcutaneous emphysema can occur if tubing is blocked or kinked.*

F. Check tubing to ensure that it is free of kinks and dependent loops.	• Promotes drainage and prevents development of a tension pneumothorax.
G. Observe for fluctuation of water-seal chamber and drainage in tubing during inspiration and expiration. Observe for clots or debris in tubing.	• If fluctuation or tidalling stops, it means that either the lung is fully expanded or the system is obstructed. In a patient who is spontaneously breathing, fluid rises in the water-seal or diagnostic indicator (waterless system) with inspiration and falls with expiration. This indicates that the system is functioning properly (Wiegand, 2017).
H. Keep drainage system upright and below the level of the patient's chest.	• Promotes gravity drainage and prevents backflow of fluid and air into the pleural space.
I. Check for air leaks by monitoring bubbling in water-seal chamber. Intermittent bubbling is normal during expiration when air is being evacuated from the pleural cavity, but continuous bubbling during both inspiration and expiration indicates a leak in the system.	• Absence of bubbling may indicate that the lung is fully expanded in a patient with a pneumothorax. Check all connections and locate sources of air leak.

SKILL 40.3   CARE OF PATIENTS WITH CHEST TUBES—cont'd

STEPS	RATIONALE
J. Remove and dispose of gloves and used contaminated supplies in an appropriate biohazard container. Perform hand hygiene.	
18. Encourage patient to regularly take deep breaths and reposition as often as possible. Assist to semi- or high-Fowler's position and perform hand hygiene.	• Facilitates and maintains lung expansion as well as chest tube drainage.

EVALUATION

STEPS	RATIONALE
1. Observe patient for decreased respiratory distress and chest pain. Auscultate lungs and observe chest expansion.	• Determines status of lung expansion.
2. Monitor vital signs and SpO₂.	• Determines whether level of oxygenation has improved.
3. Determine patient's level of comfort on a scale of 1 to 10, comparing level with comfort before chest tube insertion and/or pain medication administration.	• Indicates need for analgesia. A patient with chest tube discomfort hesitates to take deep breaths and, as a result, is at risk for pneumonia and atelectasis.
4. Observe patient's ability to use deep-breathing exercises and reposition themselves while maintaining comfort.	• Indicates patient's ability to promote lung expansion and prevent complications. Patients need to be repositioned every 2 hours when a chest tube is in place (Wiegand, 2017).
5. Monitor continued functioning of system as indicated by reduction in amount of drainage, resolution of air leak, and complete re-expansion of the lung.	• Detects early signs of system complications or indicates possible removal of chest tube.

UNEXPECTED OUTCOMES	RELATED INTERVENTIONS
Substantial increase in bright red drainage	• Obtain vital signs and monitor drainage. • Assess patient's cardiopulmonary status and notify health care provider.
Sudden cessation of chest tube drainage	• Observe for a kink and possible clot in the chest drainage system. • Assess for mediastinal shift or respiratory distress (medical emergency) and notify health care provider.
Patient develops respiratory distress.	• Chest pain, decrease in breath sounds over affected and unaffected lungs, marked cyanosis, asymmetrical chest movements, presence of subcutaneous emphysema around tube insertion site or neck, hypotension, tachycardia and/or mediastinal shift are critical and indicate a severe change in patient status, such as excessive blood loss or tension pneumothorax. • Notify health care provider immediately, collect vital signs and SpO₂, prepare for chest X-ray, provide oxygen as ordered, ensure head of bed is elevated.
Air leak that is unrelated to patient's respirations	• Locate leak by clamping chest tube with two rubber-tipped (shodded or toothless) clamps close to the chest wall. If bubbling stops, the air leak is inside the patient's thorax or at the insertion site, and the health care provider should be notified. • If bubbling continues with the clamps near the chest wall, gradually move one clamp at a time down the drainage tubing away from the patient and toward the drainage chamber. When the bubbling stops, the leak is in the section of the tubing between the two clamps. If the leak occurs when the clamps are near the drainage system, then the leak is in the drainage system itself. If there is a leak in the tubing or the drainage system, the nurse can replace the tubing or the drainage system (Wiegand, 2017).
Chest tube is disconnected or dislodged	• Check connections and reattach chest tube using sterile technique (Chotai & Mosenifar, 2018). • Immediately apply pressure over chest tube insertion site. • Have an assistant obtain sterile petroleum gauze dressing. Apply as patient exhales, and secure dressing with a tight seal. Dressing with tape over three of four sides may allow for escape of air if there is residual pneumothorax. • Notify health care provider.

RECORDING AND REPORTING

• Record in patient care record the patency of chest tube; presence, type, and amount of drainage; presence of fluctuations; patient's vital signs, respiratory assessment, and chest dressing status; amount of suction and water seal; and level of comfort.

CARE IN THE COMMUNITY CONSIDERATIONS

• Patients with chronic conditions (e.g., uncomplicated pneumothorax, effusions, empyema) that require a chest tube may be discharged home with smaller mobile chest drains. These systems do not have a suction-control chamber and use a mechanical one-way valve instead of a water-seal chamber.

• Instruct patient in how to ambulate and remain active with a home chest tube drainage system.

• Provide patient with information on when to contact health care providers regarding changes in drainage system (e.g., chest pain, breathlessness, change in drainage).

FIGURE 40.12 Dry suction chest drainage system. (From Cobbett, S., Perry, A. G., Potter, P. A., et al. [Eds.]. [2020]. *Canadian clinical nursing skills & techniques.* Elsevier Canada.)

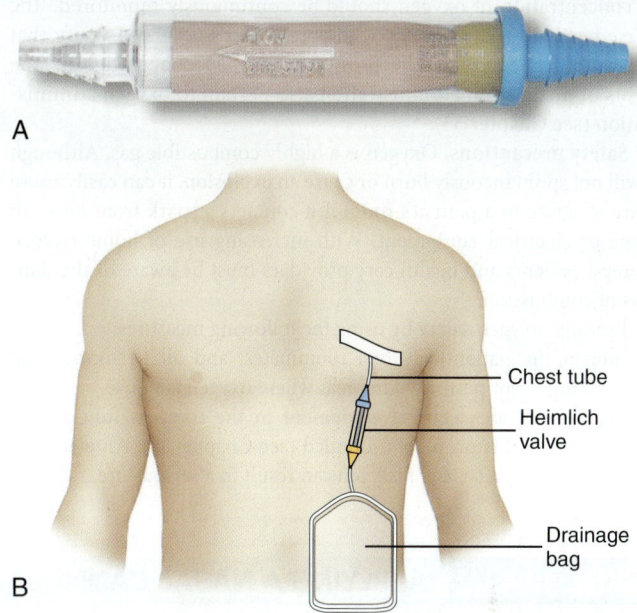

FIGURE 40.13 A, The Heimlich chest drain valve is a specially designed flutter valve that is used in place of a chest drainage unit for small, uncomplicated pneumothorax with little or no drainage and no need for suction. The valve allows for escape of air but prevents the re-entry of air into the pleural space. **B,** The valve is placed between the chest tube and the drainage bag, which can be worn under a person's clothes.

Disposable systems, such as an Atrium or Pleur-Evac chest drainage system, are one-piece moulded plastic units that provide for a single- or multiple-chamber closed drainage system (Figure 40.12). A single-chamber system allows air from a pneumothorax to bubble out of the water seal and escape through the air outlet, preventing air from re-entering the intrapleural space (Cobbett et al., 2020). A two- or three-chamber system drains both a hemothorax and a pneumothorax. The two-chamber system allows fluid to flow into a collection chamber and air to flow into the water seal chamber (Cobbett et al., 2020). A three-chamber system permits the drainage of fluid and air through controlled suction (Cobbett et al., 2020). The two- and three-chamber systems have two compartments—one for fluid or blood and a second for a water seal or a one-way valve (Cobbett et al., 2020). The three-chamber system has a third compartment for suction control, which may or may not be used (Cobbett et al., 2020).

There are two types of commercial drainage devices: water-seal and waterless systems. Although the principles of the waterless system are similar to those of the water-seal system, there are structural differences. The waterless system does not require fluid for setup, and the water seal is replaced by a one-way valve (Cobbett et al., 2020). The suction chamber, which does not depend on water, contains a float ball that is set by a control dial after the suction source is initiated (Cobbett et al., 2020). Dry suction chest drainage systems (see Figure 40.12) provide higher suction pressure levels. A self-compensating regulator controls dry suction units, and a dial is set to the prescribed suction control setting (Cobbett et al., 2020). Pressure is set between −10 cm H_2O and −40 cm H_2O and will be determined by the most responsible health care provider.

A Heimlich chest drain valve is a flutter value that is designed to replace a chest tube drainage unit. The Heimlich valve is used to remove air from the pleural space when there is little or no drainage present and thus no need for suction (Figure 40.13). A smaller chest tube (referred to as a *pigtail catheter*) may also be used for spontaneous pneumothoraxes, and these are less traumatic than large-bore chest tubes (Cobbett et al., 2020).

Special considerations. Chest tubes are not routinely clamped (Tyerman & Cobbett, 2023). Clamping a chest tube is only done under specific circumstances (see Skill 40.3) and is determined by a prescriber's orders or institution policy. The chest drainage unit must be handled carefully and the drainage device should be maintained below the patient's chest. If the tubing disconnects from the drainage unit, the patient is instructed to exhale as much as possible and to cough. This manoeuvre rids the pleural space of as much air as possible. The care provider needs to cleanse the tips of the tubing and reconnect them quickly. If the drainage unit is broken, the end of the chest tube can be quickly submerged in a container of sterile water to re-establish the seal. Clamping the chest tube may result in a tension pneumothorax. Air pressure builds in the pleural space, collapsing the lung and creating a life-threatening event.

Removal of chest tubes requires patient preparation. This includes administering pain medication 30 minutes prior to removal. Patients report various sensations during chest tube removal, the most frequent being burning, pain, and a pulling sensation.

Maintenance and Promotion of Oxygenation. Promotion of lung expansion and of mobilizing secretions and maintaining a patent airway assists the patient in meeting oxygenation needs. Some patients, however, also require oxygen therapy to keep a healthy level of tissue oxygenation.

Oxygen Therapy. Oxygen therapy is widely available and used in a variety of settings to relieve or prevent tissue hypoxia. Any patient with impaired tissue oxygenation can benefit from controlled oxygen administration. Oxygen is not a substitute for other treatment, however, and should be used only when indicated. Oxygen should be treated as a medication. It has dangerous adverse effects, such as atelectasis or oxygen toxicity. As with any medication, the dosage or concentration of oxygen should be continuously monitored. The nurse needs to routinely check the prescriber's orders to verify that the patient is receiving the prescribed oxygen concentration. The rights of medication administration also pertain to oxygen administration (see Chapter 35).

Safety precautions. Oxygen is a highly combustible gas. Although it will not spontaneously burn or cause an explosion, it can easily cause a fire to ignite in a patient's room if it contacts a spark from an open flame or electrical equipment. With increasing use of home oxygen therapy, patients and health care providers must be aware of the dangers of combustion.

Promote oxygen safety by using the following measures:
- Inform the patient, visitors, roommates, and all personnel that smoking is not permitted in areas where oxygen is in use.
- Ensure that all electrical equipment in the room is functioning correctly and is properly grounded (see Chapter 38). An electrical spark in the presence of oxygen can result in a serious fire.

- Locate the closest fire extinguisher.
- Know the fire procedures and the evacuation route for the area.
- Check the oxygen level of portable tanks before transporting a patient, to ensure that enough oxygen in the tank exists to complete the transport.

Supply of Oxygen. Oxygen is supplied to the patient's bedside either by oxygen tanks or through a permanent wall-piped system. Oxygen tanks are transported on wide-based carriers that allow the tank to be placed upright at the bedside. Regulators are used to control the amount of oxygen delivered. One common type is an upright flowmeter with a flow adjustment valve at the top. A second type is a cylinder indicator with a flow adjustment handle. In the home setting, oxygen therapy is also supplied in a variety of methods, including refillable cylinders.

SKILL 40.4   APPLYING A NASAL CANNULA OR OXYGEN MASK

Delegation Considerations
This skill cannot be delegated to an unregulated care provider (UCP). The nurse is responsible for assessing the patient and providing safe and accurate oxygen therapy, including adjustment of oxygen flow rate and evaluation of patient response. It is important to instruct the UCP about the following:
- Correct placement and adjustment of delivery device
- The type of equipment and the oxygen flow rate
- Unexpected outcomes associated with the oxygen delivery device (e.g., increased rate of breathing, decreased level of consciousness, increased confusion, pain, changes in vital signs) and the need to inform the nurse if any of these outcomes occur

Equipment
- Oxygen delivery device (e.g., nasal cannula or oxygen mask)
- Oxygen tubing
- Humidifier, if indicated
- Sterile water for humidification, if indicated
- Oxygen source
- Oxygen flowmeter
- Appropriate room signs

PROCEDURE

STEPS	RATIONALE
ASSESSMENT	
1. Identify patient using at least two identifiers according to agency policy. Compare identifiers with information on patient's medical administration record (MAR) or medical record.	- Ensures correct patient.
2. Inspect patient for signs and symptoms associated with hypoxia and presence of airway secretions. Observe for cognitive or behavioral changes, or both (e.g., apprehension, anxiety, confusion, fatigue, dizziness).	- Left untreated, hypoxia can produce cardiac dysrhythmias and death. Presence of airway secretions decreases the effectiveness of oxygen delivery.

CRITICAL DECISION POINT: *Patients with sudden changes in their vital signs, level of consciousness, or behaviour may be experiencing profound hypoxia. Patients who demonstrate subtle changes over time may have worsening of a chronic or existing condition or have a new medical condition.*

3. Obtain patient's most recent SpO$_2$ or arterial blood gas (ABG) values. Review patient's medical record for the medical order for oxygen, noting delivery method, flow rate, and duration of oxygen therapy.	- Provides objective baseline data to use to compare outcome of oxygen therapy. Ensures safe and accurate oxygen administration.
4. Assess for patient's or caregiver's knowledge, experience, and health literacy.	- Decreases patient's anxiety, which reduces oxygen consumption and increases patient cooperation.
PLANNING	
1. Perform hand hygiene.	- Reduces transmission of infection.
2. Prepare and organize equipment. Assist patient to a comfortable position, typically semi-Fowler's or high Fowler's.	
IMPLEMENTATION	
1. Attach oxygen delivery device (e.g., nasal cannula, mask) to oxygen tubing and adjusted to prescribed flow rate (see Step 1 illustration).	- Ensures correct oxygen delivery.

Continued

SKILL 40.4 APPLYING A NASAL CANNULA OR OXYGEN MASK—cont'd

STEPS	RATIONALE

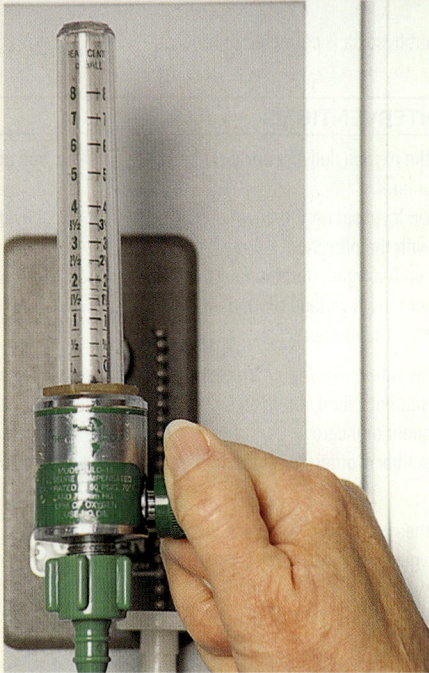

STEP 1 Adjusting flowmeter to prescribed oxygen flow rate.

STEP 2 Adjusting nasal cannula to fit patient and ensure comfort.

2. Place tips of the cannula into the patient's nares (see Step 2 illustration). If tips of the cannula are curved, they should point downward inside nostrils, then loop cannula tubing up and over the patient's ears. Adjust lanyard so that cannula fits snugly but not too tight and without pressure to the patient's nares and ears.

- Directs flow of oxygen into patient's upper respiratory tract. The patient is more likely to keep the device in place if it fits comfortably.

3. Maintain sufficient slack on oxygen tubing.

4. Observe for proper function of oxygen delivery device:

- Allows patient to turn their head without dislodging nasal cannula or causing mask to shift position.
- Ensures patency of delivery device and accuracy of prescribed oxygen flow rate.

   A. Nasal cannula: Cannula is positioned properly in the nares; oxygen flows through tips.

   B. Reservoir nasal cannula oxymizer: Fit as for nasal cannula. The reservoir is positioned under the patient's nose or worn as a pendant.

   C. Non-rebreathing mask: Apply mask over the patient's mouth and nose to form a tight seal. The valves on the mask close, so exhaled air does not enter the reservoir bag.

   D. Partial rebreathing mask: Apply mask over the patient's mouth and nose to form a tight seal. Ensure that the bag remains partially inflated.

   E. Venturi mask: Apply mask over the patient's mouth and nose to form a tight seal. Select appropriate flow rate.

   F. Simple face mask: Used for short-term oxygen delivery.

- Provides prescribed oxygen rate and reduces pressure on tips of nares.

- Oxygen-conserving cannula is indicated for long-term oxygen use.

- Does not allow exhaled air to be rebreathed. Valves on the mask side ports permit exhalation but close during inhalation to prevent inhaling room air.

- Allows exhaled air to mix with inhaled air. Ports on the side of the mask permit most of the expired air to escape; however, the bag remains partially inflated.
- Reduces buildup of carbon dioxide.

5. Verify settings on flowmeter and oxygen source for proper setup and prescribed flow rate. Check the cannula/mask every 4 hours or as agency policy dictates. If using humidification, ensure that the container is filled at all times.

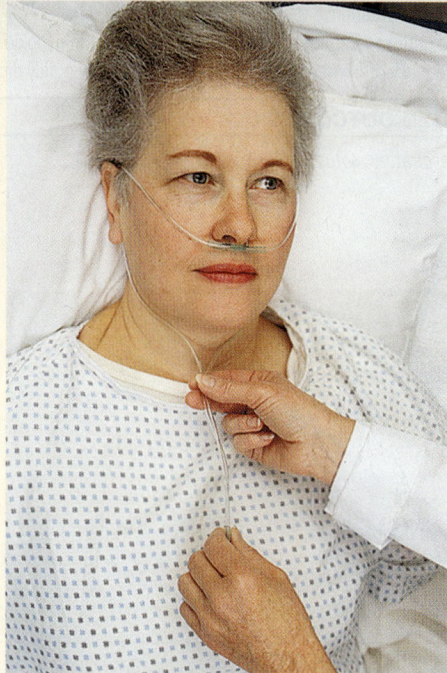

- Ensures delivery of prescribed oxygen flow rate and patency of the cannula/mask.
- Ensures patency of the cannula/mask and oxygen flow. Prevents inhalation of dehumidified oxygen.

CRITICAL DECISION POINT: *Pressure from face masks can result in medical device–related pressure injuries. Patients with sensitive skin (e.g., older persons, critically ill individuals) will need more frequent skin assessments in areas under and around the face mask.*

---

6. Observe patient's nares and superior surface of both ears for skin breakdown.

- Oxygen therapy can cause drying of nasal mucosa. Pressure on ears from cannula tubing or elastic can cause skin irritation.

7. Perform hand hygiene.

- Reduces transmission of microorganisms.

SKILL 40.4	APPLYING A NASAL CANNULA OR OXYGEN MASK—cont'd
STEPS	RATIONALE

EVALUATION

1. Monitor patient's response to changes in oxygen flow rate.
2. Inspect the patient for relief of symptoms associated with hypoxia.
3. Assess adequacy of oxygen flow each shift, or as agency policy dictates.

- Indicates that hypoxia is corrected or reduced.

UNEXPECTED OUTCOMES	RELATED INTERVENTIONS
Worsening respiratory status	• Check that the oxygen delivery device is patent, not kinked, and attached to the oxygen flowmeter. • Check oxygen level set on the flowmeter; determine if the delivered amount is consistent with the prescriber's order. • If not using wall oxygen, determine if the oxygen source contains enough oxygen to deliver the prescribed oxygen amount. • Notify health care provider.
Dry nasal and upper airway mucosa	• If oxygen flow rate is >4 L/min, determine the need for humidification. • Assess the patient's fluid status and increase fluids if appropriate. • Provide frequent oral care. • Obtain prescriber's order for treatment required to lubricate mucous membranes.
Skin breakdown over ears	• Adjust tightness of elastic strap as needed. • Use good hygiene and skin care around the ears. • Place soft, woven 4 × 4 gauze pads between elastic and ears. • Reposition elastic strap frequently.

RECORDING AND REPORTING

- Record oxygen delivery device and litre flow in the medical record. Document patient and family education. Report oxygen delivery device, litre flow, and response to changes in therapy to oncoming shift.

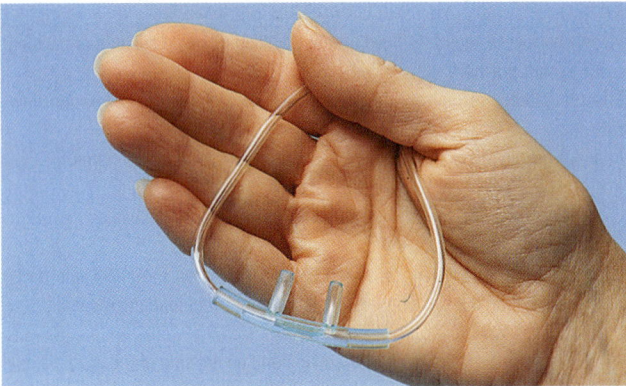

FIGURE 40.14 Nasal cannula.

TABLE 40.9	Approximate FiO₂ With Different Oxygen Delivery Devices	
Oxygen Delivery Device	Required Litre Flow (L/minute)	Approximate Percent Oxygen
Nasal cannula	1–2	24–28
	3–4	32–36
	5–6	40–44
Simple face mask	5–6	40
	6–7	50
	7–8	60
Venturi mask	4	24–28
	8	35–40
	12	50–60

In the hospital or home, oxygen tanks are delivered with the regulator in place. In the hospital, the respiratory care department usually connects the regulator to the oxygen source. Home care vendors are usually responsible for connecting the oxygen tank to the regulator for home use.

Methods of Oxygen Delivery. Oxygen delivery devices can be considered low-flow or high-flow systems. **Low-flow devices** such as nasal cannulas, simple face masks, and reservoir masks provide oxygen in concentrations that vary with the patient's respiratory pattern (Tyerman & Cobbett, 2023). **High-flow devices** deliver oxygen rates above the normal inspiratory flow rate and thus provide a fixed FiO₂ (fraction of inspired oxygen) regardless of the patient's inspiratory flow and breathing pattern (Tyerman & Cobbett, 2023). The Venturi mask is an example of a high-flow device.

Nasal cannula. A **nasal cannula** is a low-flow device used for oxygen delivery (Skill 40.4). The two nasal prongs, approximately 1.5 cm long, protrude from the centre of a disposable tube and are inserted into the nares (Figure 40.14). Oxygen is delivered via the cannulas with a flow rate of up to 6 L/minute. It is important to know what flow rate produces a given percentage of inspired oxygen concentration (FiO₂; Table 40.9). Nurses must also be alert for skin breakdown over the ears and in the nares from too tight an application of the nasal cannula. The use of humidity for low-flow devices may be dependent on the nurse's assessment, the environment, and the length of therapy (Tyerman & Cobbett, 2023).

FIGURE 40.15 Simple face mask.

FIGURE 40.16 Non-rebreather mask (note the one-way valve on exhalation port).

Oxygen masks. An oxygen mask is a device used to administer oxygen, humidity, or heated humidity. It is shaped to fit snugly over the mouth and nose and is secured in place with a strap.

The simple face mask (Figure 40.15) is used for short-term oxygen therapy. It fits loosely and delivers oxygen concentrations from 40 to 60%. The mask is contraindicated for patients with carbon dioxide retention because retention can be worsened.

The partial rebreathing mask and the non-rebreathing mask are low-flow devices with a reservoir bag. The partial rebreather mask provides an oxygen concentration of 40 to 60% with a minimum flow rate of 10 L/minute (Tyerman & Cobbett, 2023). The non-rebreather mask (Figure 40.16) provides a high concentration of oxygen at 60 to 90% with a minimum flow rate of 10 L/minute (Tyerman & Cobbett, 2023). Oxygen flows into the reservoir bag and mask during inhalation; one-way valves on the non-rebreather mask prevent expired air from flowing back into the bag. The nurse should frequently inspect the bag to make sure it is inflated. If it is deflated, the patient may be breathing large amounts of exhaled carbon dioxide. High-flow oxygen systems should be humidified (AARC, 2007).

The Venturi mask (Figure 40.17), a high-flow device, can be used to deliver oxygen concentrations of 24 to 60% with oxygen flow rates of 4 to 12 L/minute, depending on which flow-control meter is selected (see Table 40.9). This mask entrains room air to achieve a consistent and precise oxygen concentration. The Venturi mask is helpful for patients with COPD who require low, constant oxygen concentrations.

Home Oxygen Therapy. Indications for home oxygen therapy include a PaO_2 of 55 mm Hg or less or an SaO_2 of 88% or less on room air at rest, on exertion, or with exercise (Qaseem et al., 2011). Home oxygen therapy has a beneficial effect for patients with chronic cardiopulmonary diseases. This therapy improves patients' exercise tolerance and fatigue levels and, in some situations, assists in the management of dyspnea. When home oxygen is required, it is usually delivered by nasal cannula. When a patient has a permanent tracheostomy, however, a T tube or tracheostomy collar is necessary (AARC, 2007). Three types of oxygen are used: compressed oxygen, liquid oxygen (Figure 40.18), and oxygen concentrators. The advantages and disadvantages (Table 40.10) of each type are assessed, along with the patient's needs and community resources, before placing a certain delivery system in

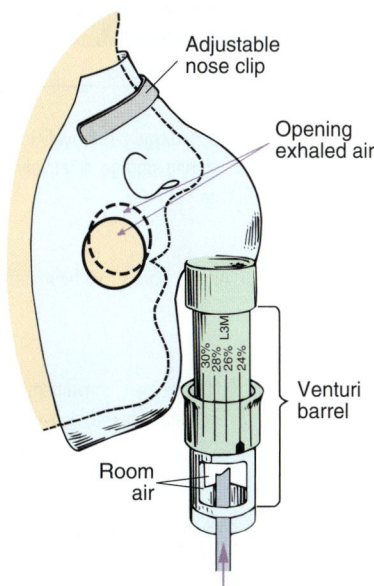

FIGURE 40.17 Venturi mask.

the home. In the home, the major consideration is the oxygen delivery source.

Patients requiring home oxygen need extensive teaching to be able to continue oxygen therapy at home efficiently and safely (Skill 40.5). This includes oxygen safety, regulation of the amount of oxygen, and how to use the prescribed home oxygen delivery system. It is important to coordinate the efforts of the patient and family, home care nurse, home respiratory therapist, and home oxygen equipment vendor. The social worker usually assists with arranging for the home care nurse and oxygen vendor.

Restoration of Cardiopulmonary Functioning. If a patient's hypoxia is severe and prolonged, cardiac arrest may result. A *cardiac arrest* is a

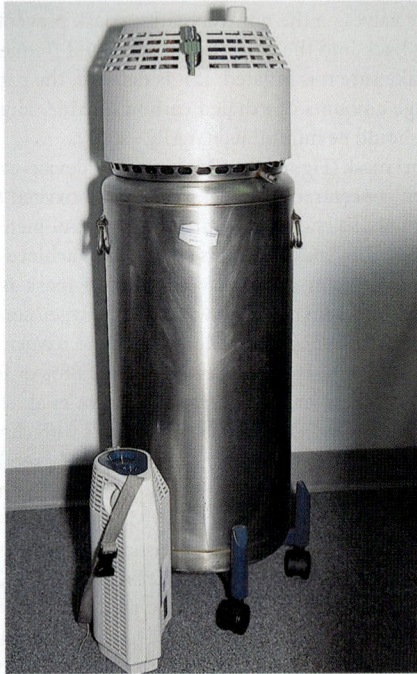

FIGURE 40.18 Primary and portable liquid oxygen source for ambulation.

sudden cessation of cardiac output and circulation. When this occurs, oxygen is not delivered to tissues, carbon dioxide is not transported from tissues, tissue metabolism becomes anaerobic, and metabolic and respiratory acidosis occurs. Permanent heart, brain, and other tissue damage occurs within 4 to 6 minutes.

Cardiopulmonary Resuscitation. Cardiac arrest is characterized by an absence of pulse and respiration. When a patient has had a cardiac arrest, cardiopulmonary resuscitation (CPR) must be initiated. CPR is a basic emergency procedure of artificial respiration and manual external cardiac massage. Most nursing students are required to have successfully completed a CPR course before their clinical experiences. The 2020 *American Heart Association Guidelines for CPR and ECC (Emergency Cardiovascular Care)* reinforce that CPR training should focus on lower socioeconomic, diverse racial, and ethnic populations because historically these populations have experienced lower rates of bystander CPR. In addition, to improve the rates of bystander CPR on women, CPR training should also emphasize gender-related barriers (American Heart Association [AHA], 2020). Women may be less likely to receive bystander CPR because of the fear associated with injury or being accused of inappropriate touching (AHA, 2020).

Emphasis is placed on ensuring that high-quality CPR is performed (AHA, 2020). Compressions must be provided at the appropriate rate and depth, the person administering CPR allowing for complete chest recoil after each compression, minimizing interruptions in compressions, avoiding excessive ventilation, and alternate compressor role at least every 2 minutes (AHA, 2020). The 2020 *American Heart Association Guidelines for CPR and ECC* reinforces the importance of early initiation of chest compressions and early defibrillation (AHA, 2020; Merchant et al., 2020). After resuscitation, health care providers may need to engage in debriefing to enhance their mental health and support self-care (AHA, 2020).

Restorative and Continuing Care

Restorative and continuing care may emphasize cardiopulmonary reconditioning as a structured rehabilitation program. Cardiopulmonary rehabilitation involves actively helping the patient to achieve and maintain an optimal level of health through controlled physical exercise, nutrition counselling, relaxation and stress management techniques, prescribed medications and oxygen, and adherence to this

TABLE 40.10	Home Oxygen Systems	
Primary Use	**Advantages**	**Disadvantages**
Compressed Gas Cylinders Stationary and portable intermittent therapy Used for exercise or sleep only	100% oxygen, relatively inexpensive, no loss of gas during storage, relatively portable, delivery of up to 15 L/min	Bulky, possibly unsightly, frequent refilling necessary with continuous use
Compressed Gas Small cylinder with compressed gas for easy portability	Allows from 1 to 5 hours of portable oxygen	Only lasts a few hours, E-cylinders not appropriate as sole source of oxygen
Liquid Oxygen Systems (see Figure 40.18) Used with active patients	100% oxygen, conveniently portable, portable units refilled at home, delivery of up to 6 L/min	Usually weekly delivery necessary for refill, evaporates if not used, potential for frostbite at connections and if liquid is spilled
Oxygen Concentrators Stationary system for patients requiring low-flow continuous oxygen and limited mobility	Provides large source of oxygen, inexpensive, delivery of 1–5 L/min, delivery up to 10 L/min with certain models	Oxygen concentration decreases as litre flow increases, power supply needed, electric bill increase, second system needed for portability

SKILL 40.5	USING HOME OXYGEN EQUIPMENT

Delegation Considerations

This skill should not be delegated to an unregulated care provider (UCP). However, once the patient is stable on home oxygen therapy, the UCP may perform certain aspects of care. The nurse is responsible for assessing the patient, checking the device setup, and providing safe and accurate oxygen therapy. The nurse must instruct the UCP about the following:

- Unique needs of the patient (e.g., home nasal cannula or mask) and any assistance needed in filling liquid canisters
- The type of equipment that the patient should have in the home and the oxygen flow rate
- Unexpected outcomes associated with the oxygen delivery device (e.g., increased rate of breathing, decreased level of consciousness, increased confusion, pain), and the need to inform the nurse if any occur

Equipment

- Nasal cannula, oxygen mask, or other prescribed delivery device (see Skill 40.4)
- Humidification device if oxygen delivery is >4 L/min
- Oxygen tubing
- Home oxygen delivery system with appropriate equipment
- "No Smoking/Oxygen in Use" sign for each entrance to the home

PROCEDURE

STEPS	RATIONALE

ASSESSMENT

1. Identify patient using at least two identifiers according to agency policy. Compare identifiers with information on patient's medication administration record (MAR) or medical record.
- Ensures correct patient.

2. Review health care provider's order for home oxygen equipment.
- A health care provider's order is required for home oxygen use.

3. Assess patient's or caregiver's knowledge, experience, and health literacy.
- Ensure that patient's caregiver has the capacity to obtain, communicate, process, and understand basic health information.

4. While patient is in the hospital, determine the patient's or caregiver's ability to use oxygen equipment correctly. In the home setting, reassess for appropriate use of equipment.
- Physical or cognitive impairments of the patient necessitate instructing a family member or significant other in how to operate home oxygen equipment. Ongoing assessment enables the nurse to determine specific components of skill that the patient or family easily complete.

5. Assess home environment for adequate electrical service if an oxygen concentrator is used.
- Oxygen concentrators require electricity to work. Continuous oxygen therapy must not be interrupted.

6. Assess the patient's and family's ability to observe for signs and symptoms of hypoxia.
- Hypoxia occurs at home despite use of oxygen therapy. Worsening of a patient's physical condition or another underlying condition, such as a change in respiratory status, can cause hypoxia.

7. Determine appropriate resources in the community for equipment and assistance, including maintenance and repair services, and medical equipment supplier.
- Ensures that there is readily available assistance for patients with home oxygen systems.

8. In case of power failure, determine appropriate backup system when using a compressor. Have a spare oxygen tank available.
- Many municipalities require that patients with home oxygen equipment notify emergency medical services (EMS) before bringing the equipment home. When there is a power outage, EMS calls the home, and in some cases the home is on a priority list for having power restored.

PLANNING

1. Explain the need for and use of home oxygen therapy.
- Improves adherence to the treatment regimen and decreases anxiety.

2. Provide resources to the family to investigate municipal requirements for home medical equipment involving oxygen.
- Many municipalities require that patients with home oxygen notify EMS before bringing equipment home.

IMPLEMENTATION

1. Perform hand hygiene.
- Reduces transmission of infection.

2. Place oxygen delivery system in a clutter-free environment that is well ventilated; away from walls, drapes, bedding, combustible materials; and at least 2.4 metres (8 feet) from heat source.
- Prevents injury from improper placement of oxygen equipment.

3. Demonstrate steps for preparation and completion of oxygen therapy.
- Demonstration is a reliable technique for teaching psychomotor skills and encourages the patient to ask questions.

    A. Compressed oxygen system

      (1) Turn cylinder valve counterclockwise two to three turns with a wrench. Store wrench with the oxygen tank.
- Turns on oxygen. Keeps wrench available.

      (2) Check cylinders by reading amount on the pressure gauge.
- Verifies adequate oxygen supply for patient use.

      (3) Store wrench with the oxygen tank or in another safe place near the tank.
- Storing wrench in a safe place ensures that it is available when needed.

SKILL 40.5   USING HOME OXYGEN EQUIPMENT—cont'd

STEPS	RATIONALE
B. Oxygen concentrator system	
(1) Plug concentrator into appropriate outlet.	• Provides power source.
(2) Turn on power switch.	• Starts concentrator motor.
(3) Alarm will sound for a few seconds.	• Alarm turns off when desired pressure inside the concentrator is reached.
C. Liquid oxygen system	
(1) Check liquid system by depressing the button at the lower right corner and reading the dial on the stationary oxygen reservoir or ambulatory tank.	• Verifies adequate oxygen supply.
(2) Collaborate with medical equipment provider to receive instruction on refilling ambulatory tank.	• Ambulatory tanks of liquid oxygen must be filled when empty.

CRITICAL DECISION POINT: *Fill ambulatory tanks only when they are empty. Liquid oxygen is stored at or below −183°C (−297°F) inside the reservoir, and the temperature inside the ambulatory tank is warmer. If cold oxygen from the reservoir mixes with warmer oxygen left in the ambulatory tank, the ambulatory tank may malfunction.*

STEPS	RATIONALE
(3) Refilling oxygen tank:	
(a) Wipe both filling connectors with a clean, dry, lint-free cloth.	• Removes dust and moisture from system.
(b) Turn off flow selector of ambulatory unit.	
(c) Attach ambulatory unit to stationary reservoir by inserting adapter from the ambulatory tank into adapter of the stationary reservoir.	• Secures connections.
(d) Open fill valve on ambulatory tank and apply firm pressure to top of the stationary reservoir (see Step 3C[3][d] illustration). Stay with unit while it is filling. You will hear a loud hissing noise. The tank fills in about 2 minutes.	• Prevents leaking of oxygen during filling process. If oxygen leaks during filling process, the connection between the ambulatory tank and reservoir will ice up and stick together.
(e) Disengage ambulatory unit from stationary reservoir when hissing noise changes and vapour cloud begins to form from stationary unit.	• Overfilling causes the ambulatory unit to malfunction from high pressure in the tank.
(f) Wipe both filling connectors with a clean, dry, lint-free cloth.	• Ice sometimes forms during filling. Wiping removes moisture from oxygen system.

STEP 3C(3)(d) Fill valve on ambulatory tank is open while applying firm pressure to top of ambulatory unit.

CRITICAL DECISION POINT: *If the ambulatory unit does not separate easily, valves from the reservoir and ambulatory unit may be frozen together. Wait until the valves warm to disengage (about 5–10 minutes). Do not touch any frosted areas because contact with skin may cause skin damage from frostbite.*

Continued

SKILL 40.5	USING HOME OXYGEN EQUIPMENT—cont'd	
STEPS		**RATIONALE**

STEPS	RATIONALE
4. Connect oxygen delivery device to oxygen system.	• Connects oxygen source to delivery system.
5. Adjust to prescribed flow rate (L/min).	• Ensures appropriate oxygen prescription.
6. Place oxygen delivery device on patient. Ensure patient has two sets of oxygen delivery devices and tubing.	• Delivers oxygen to patient. Extra devices are used when equipment is cleaned or in case of malfunction.
7. Perform hand hygiene.	• Reduces transmission of microorganisms.
8. Instruct patient and caregiver not to change oxygen flow rate.	• Provides prescribed amount of oxygen. Exceeding prescribed oxygen may be harmful (e.g., COPD).
9. Guide the patient and caregiver as they perform each step. Provide written material for reinforcement and review.	• Allows the nurse to correct errors in technique and discuss their implications.
10. Instruct the patient or caregiver to notify the health care provider if signs or symptoms of hypoxia or respiratory tract infection occur.	• Respiratory tract infections increase oxygen demand and may affect oxygen transfer from lungs to the blood. They may cause severe exacerbation of the patient's pulmonary disease.
11. Discuss emergency plan for power loss, natural disaster, and acute respiratory distress. Have patient or caregiver call 911 and notify the health care provider and home care agency.	• Ensures appropriate response and can prevent worsening of the patient's condition.
12. Instruct patient in safe home oxygen practices, including placing "No Smoking/Oxygen in Use" signs at each entrance to the home, not allowing smoking in the home, keeping oxygen tanks away from open flames, and storing tanks upright.	• Ensures safe use of oxygen in the home and prevents injury to the patient and family.
13. Monitor rate of oxygen delivery. All oxygen-delivery equipment should be checked at least daily by the patient or caregiver.	• Determines if the patient is regulating oxygen at prescribed rate.
14. Oxygen-delivery equipment must be maintained and serviced routinely according to the manufacturer's guidelines (AARC, 2007).	

EVALUATION

1. Monitor rate at which oxygen is being delivered during each home visit.	• Determines whether the patient or caregiver is regulating oxygen at the prescribed rate.
2. Ask the patient and caregiver about any problems or concerns about the home oxygen equipment.	• Determines the ability of the patient and family or caregiver to deal with stressors associated with home oxygen use.

UNEXPECTED OUTCOMES	RELATED INTERVENTIONS
Patient reports no oxygen flow	• Check tank pressure gauge. If level of oxygen is low, refill tank if portable, or provide an alternative source of oxygen, such as concentrator or H cylinder.
	• Notify home oxygen supplier of need for refill.
	• Reassure patient and family.
Unable to fill portable liquid oxygen from main source	• Check to see that portable tank is connected correctly.
	• Determine if valve is frozen.
	• Contact home oxygen supplier for service visit.
	• Provide an alternative oxygen source if necessary.
Patient has signs and symptoms associated with hypoxia	• Determine whether the oxygen delivery device and oxygen source are delivering oxygen properly.
	• Determine whether prescribed oxygen flow rate is set properly.
	• Assess the patient for changes in respiratory status, such as airway plugging, respiratory tract infection, or bronchospasm.

RECORDING AND REPORTING

• Record the patient's and family's ability to safely use the home oxygen equipment. Report the type of home oxygen equipment to be used and the patient's and family's understanding of how to use the equipment, knowledge of safety guidelines and unexpected outcomes, and ability to demonstrate proper use of the oxygen delivery device.

---

plan. As physical reconditioning occurs, the patient's symptoms of dyspnea, chest pain, fatigue, and activity intolerance should decrease. The patient's anxiety, depression, or somatic concerns also often decrease. The patient and the rehabilitation team define the goals of rehabilitation.

Hydration. Maintenance of adequate systemic hydration keeps mucociliary clearance normal. In patients with adequate hydration, pulmonary secretions are thin, white, watery, and easily removable with minimal coughing. Excessive coughing to clear thick, tenacious secretions is fatiguing and energy depleting. The best way to maintain thin secretions is to provide a fluid intake of 1 500 to 2 000 mL/day unless contraindicated by cardiac status. The colour, consistency, and ease of secretion expectoration can determine the adequacy of hydration.

Coughing Techniques. Coughing is effective for maintaining a patent airway. Coughing enables the patient to remove secretions from both the upper and lower airways. The normal series of events in the cough mechanism are deep inhalation, closure of the glottis, active contraction of the expiratory muscles, and glottis opening. Deep inhalation increases the lung volume and airway diameter, allowing the air to pass through partially obstructing mucous plugs or other foreign matter. Contraction of the expiratory muscles against the closed glottis causes a high intrathoracic pressure to develop. When the glottis opens, a large flow of air is expelled at a high speed, providing momentum for mucus to move to the upper airways, where it can be expectorated or swallowed.

The effectiveness of coughing is evaluated by sputum expectoration, the patient's report of swallowed sputum, or clearing of adventitious sounds by auscultation. Patients with chronic pulmonary diseases, upper respiratory tract infections, and lower respiratory tract infections should be encouraged to deep-breathe and cough at least every 2 hours while awake. Patients with a large amount of sputum should be encouraged to cough every hour while awake and every 2 to 3 hours while asleep until the acute phase of mucus production has ended. Coughing techniques include deep breathing and coughing for the postoperative patient, cascade, huff, and quad coughing.

With the *cascade cough,* the patient takes a slow, deep breath and holds it for 2 seconds while contracting expiratory muscles. Then the patient opens their mouth and performs a series of coughs throughout exhalation, thereby coughing at progressively lowered lung volumes. This technique promotes airway clearance and a patent airway in patients with large volumes of sputum.

The *huff cough* stimulates a natural cough reflex and is generally effective only for clearing central airways. While exhaling, the patient opens the glottis by saying the word "huff." With practice, the patient inhales more air and may be able to progress to the cascade cough.

The *quad cough* technique is used for patients without abdominal muscle control, such as those with spinal cord injuries. While the patient breathes out with a maximal expiratory effort, the patient or nurse pushes inward and upward on the abdominal muscles toward the diaphragm, causing the cough.

Breathing Exercises. Breathing exercises include techniques to improve ventilation and oxygenation. The three basic techniques are deep breathing and coughing exercises, pursed-lip breathing, and diaphragmatic breathing. Deep breathing and coughing exercises are routine interventions for postoperative patients (see Chapter 49).

Pursed-Lip Breathing. Pursed-lip breathing involves deep inspiration and prolonged expiration through pursed lips to prevent alveolar collapse. The patient is instructed to take a deep breath while sitting up and to exhale slowly through pursed lips, as if blowing through a straw. The patient then blows through a straw into a glass of water to learn the technique. Patients need to gain control of the exhalation phase so that it is longer than inhalation. The patient is usually able to perfect this technique by counting the inhalation time and gradually increasing the count during exhalation. In studies using pulse oximetry as a feedback tool, patients have been able to demonstrate an increase in their arterial oxygen saturation during pursed-lip breathing.

Diaphragmatic Breathing. Diaphragmatic breathing is more difficult and requires the patient to relax intercostal and accessory respiratory muscles while taking deep inspirations. The patient concentrates on expanding the diaphragm during controlled inspiration and is taught to place one hand flat below the breastbone and above the waist, and the other hand 2 to 3 cm below the first hand. The patient is asked to inhale while the lower hand moves outward during inspiration. The patient observes for inward movement as the diaphragm ascends. These exercises are initially taught with the patient in the supine position and then practised while the patient sits and stands. The exercise is often used with the pursed-lip breathing technique.

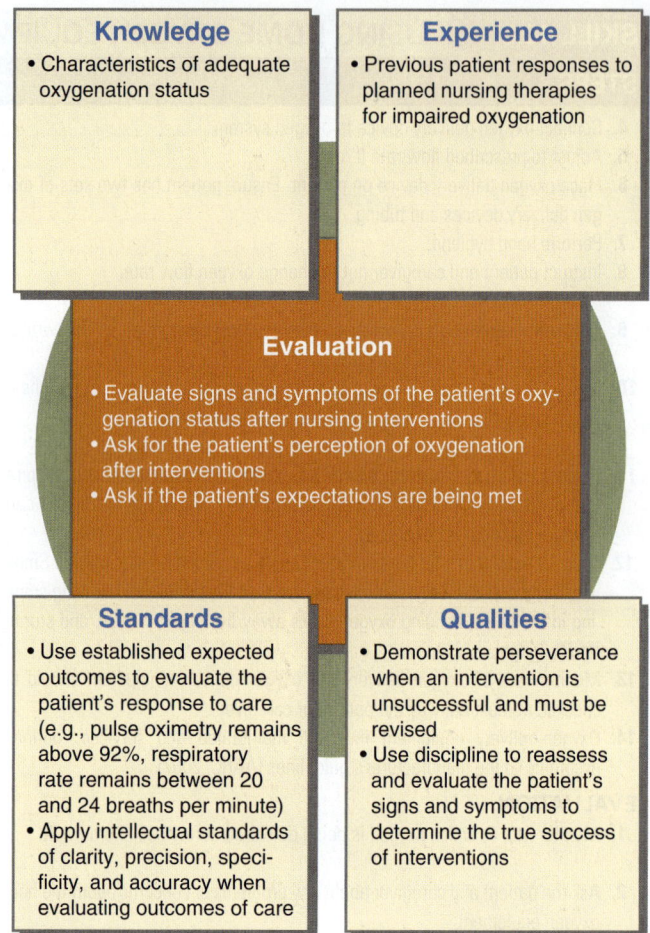

Knowledge	Experience
• Characteristics of adequate oxygenation status	• Previous patient responses to planned nursing therapies for impaired oxygenation

Evaluation

• Evaluate signs and symptoms of the patient's oxygenation status after nursing interventions
• Ask for the patient's perception of oxygenation after interventions
• Ask if the patient's expectations are being met

Standards	Qualities
• Use established expected outcomes to evaluate the patient's response to care (e.g., pulse oximetry remains above 92%, respiratory rate remains between 20 and 24 breaths per minute) • Apply intellectual standards of clarity, precision, specificity, and accuracy when evaluating outcomes of care	• Demonstrate perseverance when an intervention is unsuccessful and must be revised • Use discipline to reassess and evaluate the patient's signs and symptoms to determine the true success of interventions

FIGURE 40.19 Critical thinking model for oxygenation evaluation.

Diaphragmatic breathing is also useful for patients with pulmonary disease, for postoperative patients, and for pregnant people in labour to promote relaxation and provide pain control. The exercise improves efficiency of breathing by decreasing air trapping and reducing the work of breathing.

Evaluation

Nursing interventions and therapies are evaluated by comparing the patient's progress with the goals and expected outcomes of the nursing care plan. The nurse evaluates the actual care given to the patient by the health care team on the basis of the expected outcomes (Figure 40.19).

Patient Care. The patient is the only one who can evaluate their degree of breathlessness. The patient should be asked to rate breathlessness on a scale of 1 to 10, with 1 being no shortness of breath and 10 being severe shortness of breath. Arterial blood gas levels, pulmonary function tests, vital signs, ECG tracings, and physical assessment data provide objective measurement of the success of therapies and treatments. Outcomes are compared with expected outcomes to determine the patient's health status. Continuous evaluation helps to determine whether new or revised therapies are required and if new nursing diagnoses have developed and require a new plan of care.

When nursing measures directed toward improving oxygenation are unsuccessful, the nurse must immediately modify the nursing care plan. Nurses should not hesitate to notify the appropriate health care provider about a patient's deteriorating oxygenation status. Prompt notification can avoid an emergency situation, or even the need for CPR.

Patient Expectations. It is important to ask patients if their expectations of care have been met. For example, the nurse can ask the patient, "Do you feel as though you will be able to use the breathing techniques we have practised at home?" If the patient does not think this will work at home, then the patient's expectations for care management have not been met.

The nurse should ask the patient whether all questions and needs have been met. If not, the nurse needs to spend more time understanding what the patient wants and needs to meet their expectations. Working closely with the patient will enable the nurse to redefine those patient expectations that can be realistically met within the limitations of the patient's condition and treatment.

KEY CONCEPTS

- The primary function of the heart is to deliver deoxygenated blood to the lungs for oxygenation and to deliver oxygen and nutrients to the tissues.
- Preload, afterload, contractility, and heart rate alter cardiac output.
- Cardiac dysrhythmias are classified by cardiac activity and site of impulse origin.
- The primary function of the lungs is to transfer oxygen from the atmosphere into the alveoli and to transfer carbon dioxide out of the body as a waste product.
- Ventilation is the process of providing adequate oxygenation from the alveoli to the blood.
- Compliance, or the ability of the lungs to expand and contract, depends on the function of musculoskeletal and neurological systems and on other physiological factors.
- The process of inspiration (active process) and expiration (passive process) is caused by changes in intrapleural and intra-alveolar pressures and lung volumes.
- Respiration is controlled by the central nervous system and by chemicals within the blood.
- Decreased hemoglobin levels alter the patient's ability to transport oxygen.
- Impaired chest wall movement reduces the level of tissue oxygenation.
- Hyperventilation is a respiratory rate greater than that required to maintain normal levels of carbon dioxide.
- Hypoventilation causes carbon dioxide retention.
- Hypoxia occurs if the amount of oxygen delivered to tissues is too low.

- The health history and assessment include information about the patient's cough, dyspnea, fatigue, wheezing, chest pain, environmental exposures, respiratory infection, cardiopulmonary risk factors, and use of medications.
- Diagnostic and laboratory tests may be needed to complete the database for a patient with decreased oxygenation.
- Breathing exercises improve ventilation, oxygenation, and sensations of dyspnea.
- Nebulization delivers small drops of water or particles of medication to the airways.
- Chest physiotherapy includes postural drainage, percussion, and vibration to mobilize pulmonary secretions.
- Coughing and suctioning techniques are used to maintain a patent airway.
- Oxygen therapy is used to improve levels of tissue oxygenation and is delivered by a nasal cannula, various oxygen masks, or the use of an artificial airway.

CRITICAL THINKING EXERCISES

1. A patient is admitted to a medical unit after surgery for a tracheostomy. The patient begins to cough, they become short of breath, and their oxygen saturation is 88% on 2 L via nasal prongs. What are the nurse's priority actions?
2. A patient has been recently diagnosed with acute coronary syndrome. The patient just arrived from the emergency department to the cardiac unit. The lab results from the emergency department indicate that the troponin levels are normal. While returning from the bathroom, the patient informs the nurse that they are experiencing chest pain. What nursing interventions should the nurse implement? What pertinent information should the nurse share about the patient with the physician?
3. A patient has been admitted to the hospital with community-acquired pneumonia. The patient has a productive cough, their temperature is 38.9 °C, and the respiratory assessment reveals crackles and wheezes on auscultation of their chest. What additional assessments should the nurse complete? How do these assessment findings inform the nurse's care of the patient?
4. A patient is on a medical unit for a recent diagnosis of COPD. In the middle of the night the patient informs the nurse that they feel short of breath. The patient's respiratory rate is 34 breaths per minute and oxygen saturation is 84% on room air. How should the nurse support the patient during their experience of dyspnea?

Answers to Critical Thinking Exercises appear on the Evolve website.

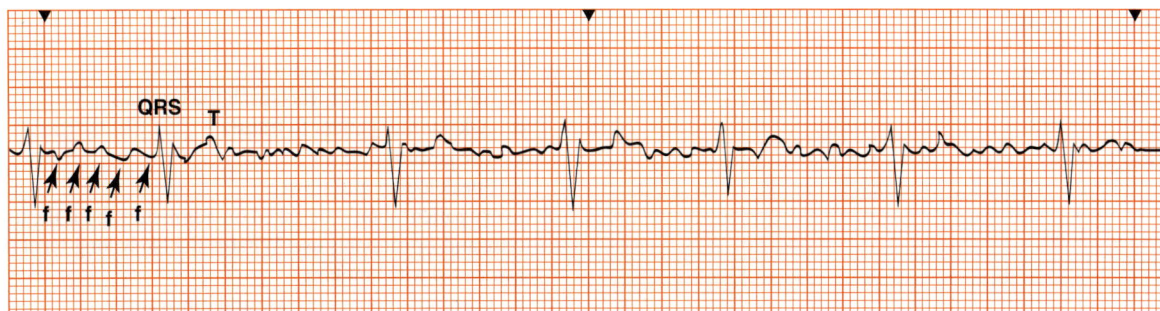

FIGURE Q.2 Coarse atrial fibrillation. (From Wesley, K. [2017]. *Huzar's ECG and 12 lead interpretation* [5th ed.]. Mosby.)

REVIEW QUESTIONS

Review Questions 1 to 10 relate to the case study at the beginning of the chapter.

1. Which assessment finding has the greatest implication for this patient's plan of care?
   a. Fatigued when ambulating
   b. Increased activity tolerance when ambulating
   c. Decreased breathlessness when ambulating
   d. Oxygen saturation of 95% on room air when ambulating

2. The telemetry monitor shows the following cardiac rhythm for the patient. Referencing Figure Q.2 (below), Which interventions are appropriate for this dysrhythmia? *(Select all that apply.)*
   a. Warfarin (Coumadin)
   b. Prepare for defibrillation
   c. Metoprolol (Lopressor)
   d. Apply nasal cannulas at 2 L/min
   e. Elevate the head of the bed
   f. Prepare for transcutaneous pacing
   g. Review the current partial thromboplastin time (PTT) lab value

3. The nurse documents these findings as part of the shift assessment:
   a. Temperature = 36.5 °C
   b. Heart rate = 110 beats per minute and irregular
   c. Respirations = 22 breaths per minute
   d. Blood pressure = 110/70 mm Hg
   e. Oxygen saturation = 92% on 2 L nasal prongs
   f. Reports feeling tired today
   g. Extremities cool to touch
   h. Short of breath while ambulating

   Highlight the assessment findings above that require follow-up by the nurse.

4. Which of the following risk factors are most applicable to this patient's health? *(Select all that apply.)*
   a. Postmenopausal
   b. Smoking
   c. Genetics
   d. Diabetes
   e. Diet
   f. Exercise
   g. Language barrier
   h. Hypertension
   i. Stress

5. The nurse assesses the patient and plans health teaching for them in preparation for discharge. Use an X for the health teaching below that is Indicated (appropriate or necessary), Contraindicated (could be harmful), or Nonessential (makes no difference or not necessary) before the patient's discharge at this time.

Health Teaching	Indicated	Contrain-dicated	Non-essential
a. Use ibuprofen for any pain being experienced.			
b. Take daily morning weights after voiding.			
c. Restrict sodium intake.			
d. Increase daily fluid intake to 8–10 cups.			

Health Teaching	Indicated	Contrain-dicated	Non-essential
e. Incentive spirometer must be used twice a day.			
f. Use adaptive devices as needed (e.g., sock aids, shoehorns).			
g. Follow up with worsening symptoms with health care provider.			
h. Record and track daily blood pressure.			

6. The patient informs the nurse that while at home they are not attentive to their diet and exercise. While the patient is in hospital, the family has brought in the occasional home-cooked meal; however, the patient has primarily been attentive to the hospital diet. The current assessment findings reveal the following:
   - Heart rate = 115 bpm
   - Blood pressure = 120/85 mm Hg
   - Urine output = 30 mL/hr
   - Respiratory rate = 22 per minute
   - Weight = 2 kg (5 lb) weight gain
   - Pedal edema +3
   - Course crackles to both lung fields
   - Reports "frequent waves of nausea"

   Choose the most likely options for the information missing from the statements below by selecting from the lists of options provided:
   Based on this patient's assessment data, the nurse determines that the patient's weight gain is due to _____(1)_____. The patient's nausea is caused by _____(2)_____ and the course crackles to the chest are related to _____(3)_____.

Answer Options for 1	Answer Options for 2	Answer Options for 3
Arrythmia	Ascites	Intravenous fluid
Diet	Aspirin	Sedentary lifestyle
Fluid overload	Coumadin	Poor ventricular function
Lack of exercise	Diabetes	Pedal edema

7. The nurse recognizes that the patient's language barrier may affect safety. Identify which resources would best minimize this safety risk. *(Select all that apply.)*
   a. Involve family
   b. Use a hospital translator
   c. Seek hospital staff who speak the language
   d. Ask another patient to translate
   e. Use gestures
   f. Speak louder and slower

8. Every patient should be asked on admission about the use of cigarette and/or cannabis use. What is the likely long-term risk factor associated with smoking?
   a. Cardiopulmonary disease and lung cancer
   b. Obesity and diabetes

c. Stress-related illnesses and pneumothorax

d. Hypotension and bradycardia

9. One significant complication from an MI may result in a temporary tracheostomy. During suctioning of a patient with a fresh tracheostomy who develops respiratory distress, what is the correct priority sequence of the following nursing actions? (Write the correct number from 1 to 5 in the spaces provided.)

a. ___ Immediately withdraw the suction catheter.

b. ___ Supply additional oxygen as needed.

c. ___ Take vital signs.

d. ___ Disconnect suction catheter.

e. ___ Remain with the patient until oxygen returns to baseline.

10. The nurse is preparing to clean the patient's tracheostomy. The nurse will clean the inner cannula with (1)_____ and will clean the stoma using a (2)_____ motion moving (3)_____.

Choose the most likely options from the list below for the information missing from this statement.

Answer options:

Alcohol

Circular

Inward

Normal saline

Outward

Zig-zag

Answers: 1. a; **2.** a, c; **3.** b, f, g, h; **4.** a, c, d, g, h; **5.** *Indicated:* b, c, g; *Contraindicated:* a, d; *Nonessential:* e, f, h; **6.** (1) fluid overload, (2) ascites, (3) poor ventricular function; **7.** a, b, c; **8.** a; **9.** a = 1, b = 2, c = 3, d = 4, e = 5; **10.** (1) normal saline, (2) circular, (3) outward.

🌐 *Rationales for the Review Questions appear on the Evolve website.*

RECOMMENDED WEBSITES

Canadian Cancer Society: https://www.canada.ca

Canadian Cardiovascular Society: http://www.ccs.ca/en

The Canadian Cardiovascular Society provides evidence-informed information and resources on cardiovascular health.

Canadian Thoracic Society: https://cts-sct.ca

The Canadian Thoracic Society provides evidence-informed information and resources regarding respiratory health.

Heart and Stroke Foundation of Canada: https://www.heartandstroke.ca

The Heart and Stroke Foundation is a national voluntary, nonprofit organization whose mission is to improve the health of Canadians by preventing heart disease and stroke through research, health promotion, and advocacy.

🌐 REFERENCES

A full reference list is available on the website for this book at http://evolve.elsevier.com/Canada/Potter/fundamentals/

Fluid, Electrolyte, and Acid–Base Balances

Written by Darlaine Jantzen, RN, MA, PhD, and Selena Hebig, BScN, RN, BSKin

OBJECTIVES

Mastery of content in this chapter will enable you to:

- Define the key terms listed.
- Describe the distribution, composition, movement, and regulation of body fluids.
- Describe the regulation and movement of major electrolytes.
- Describe the processes involved in regulating acid–base balance.
- Describe common fluid, electrolyte, and acid–base imbalances and identify related risk factors.
- Recognize risks factors for fluid imbalances specific to hospitalized persons.
- Choose appropriate clinical assessments for fluid, electrolyte, and acid–base balances.
- Interpret basic fluid, electrolyte, and acid–base laboratory values.

- Identify and discuss nursing interventions for patients with fluid, electrolyte, and acid–base imbalances.
- Explain the connection between fluid and electrolyte balance and fundamentals of care related to hydration, nutrition, and personal care.
- Identify the indications for infusion therapy, and procedure for, initiating, managing, and discontinuing intravenous infusions.
- Explain the purpose and nursing care related to central vascular access devices, including preventing and recognizing associated complications.
- Describe complications associated with intravenous therapy.
- Explain the purpose of, and procedure for, initiating a blood transfusion and interventions to manage transfusion reaction.

KEY TERMS

Active transport
Aldosterone
Anion gap
Anions
Antidiuretic hormone (ADH)
Arterial blood gas (ABG)
Autologous transfusion
Base excess
Buffer
Cations
Central vascular access devices (CVADs)
Colloid osmotic pressure
Colloids
Concentration gradient
Crystalloid
Dehydration
Diffusion
Dysnatremia
Edema
Electrolytes
Electronic infusion devices (EIDs)
Extracellular fluid (ECF)
Filtration
Fluid volume deficit (FVD)

Fluid volume excess (FVE)
Hemolysis
Homeostasis
Hydrostatic pressure
Hypercalcemia
Hyperchloremia
Hyperkalemia
Hypermagnesemia
Hypernatremia
Hypertonic
Hypocalcemia
Hypochloremia
Hypokalemia
Hypomagnesemia
Hyponatremia
Hypotonic
Hypovolemia
Infiltration
Insensible water loss
Interstitial fluid
Intracellular fluid (ICF)
Intravascular fluid
Ions
Isotonic

Metabolic acidosis
Metabolic alkalosis
Obligatory water loss
Osmolality
Osmolarity
Osmoreceptors
Osmosis
Osmotic pressure
Oxygen saturation
Peripheral intravenous catheter (PIVC)
Peripheral vascular access devices (PVADs)
Peripherally inserted central catheter (PICC)
Phlebitis
Respiratory acidosis
Respiratory alkalosis
Sensible water loss
Solutes
Solution
Solvent
Total parental nutrition (TPN)
Transcellular fluid
Transfusion reaction
Vascular access devices (VADs)

WEBSITE

http://evolve.elsevier.com/Canada/Potter/fundamentals/

Fluid, electrolyte, and acid–base balances within the body are essential for normal body function. These balances are maintained by ingestion, distribution, and excretion of water and electrolytes and by respiration. Within the body, these balances are maintained by the renal, pulmonary, and buffer systems. Imbalances may be caused by many factors, including altered intake, illness, or excessive losses, such as exercise-induced diaphoresis. These imbalances affect physiological processes at the cellular, tissue, and system levels of the body; therefore, understanding the mechanisms that contribute to fluid, electrolyte, and acid–base balances is essential to nursing practice.

SCIENTIFIC KNOWLEDGE BASE

This section provides a foundation for nurses' critical thinking and nursing practice. This is intended as a brief overview; anatomy and physiology textbooks expand on this information.

Water is the largest single component of the body. The average adult male weight is 60% water; however, this amount varies with age, gender, and body weight. A healthy, mobile, well-oriented adult can usually maintain normal fluid, electrolyte, and acid–base balances with renal, hormonal, and neural functions.

Distribution of Body Fluids

Body fluids are distributed in two distinct compartments, one containing intracellular fluid and the other containing extracellular fluid. **Intracellular fluid (ICF)**, or cytosol, includes all fluid within body cells, accounting for approximately 60% of the body's fluids (Marieb & Hoehn, 2019).

Extracellular fluid (ECF), all the fluid outside cells, is divided into three compartments: interstitial fluid, intravascular fluid, and transcellular fluids. **Interstitial fluid**, including lymph, is the fluid between the cells and outside the blood vessels. **Intravascular fluid** is blood plasma. **Transcellular fluid**, separated from other fluid by epithelium, includes cerebrospinal, pleural, peritoneal, and synovial fluids and the fluids in the gastrointestinal tract (Figure 41.1).

Composition of Body Fluids

Electrolytes are important **solutes** in all body fluids. An electrolyte, when dissolved in an aqueous solution, separates into **ions** and is able to carry an electrical current (Marieb & Hoehn, 2019). Positively charged electrolytes are **cations** (e.g., sodium [Na^+], potassium [K^+], calcium [Ca^{2+}]). Negatively charged electrolytes are **anions** (e.g., chloride [Cl^-], bicarbonate [HCO_3^-], sulphate [SO_4^-]). Electrolytes are vital to many body functions.

The body carefully regulates electrolyte concentration (Marieb & Hoehn, 2019). The value millimoles per litre (mmol/L) represents the amount of the specific electrolyte (solute) dissolved in a litre of fluid

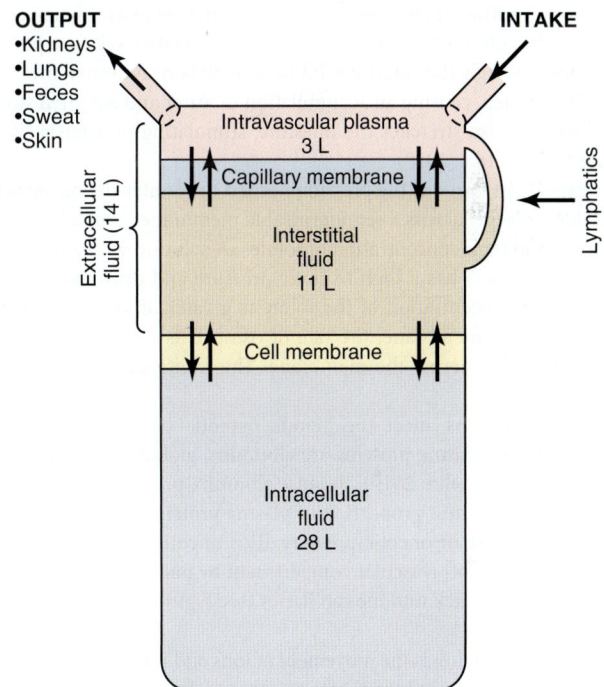

FIGURE 41.1 Body fluid distribution.

(**solution**). The solution in which a solute is dissolved is called a **solvent**. Electrolyte concentration within fluid compartments is influenced by electrical charge. During normal physiological processes, ions are exchanged for other ions with the same electrical charge.

Electrolytes are ingested, often in the form of bulk and trace minerals or salts, and then utilized for basic physiological processes, stored for future use, or excreted. These electrolytes are important for maintaining osmotic concentrations in body fluids. They are also necessary for enzyme reactions, nerve impulses, muscle contraction, and metabolism. In addition, some minerals contribute to the regulation of hormone production and strengthening of skeletal structures.

Movement of Water and Electrolytes

Fluids and electrolytes constantly shift between compartments, often across plasma membranes, to facilitate body processes such as tissue oxygenation, acid–base balance, and urine formation. The passage of molecules across the plasma membrane occurs through passive and active transport processes. Because cell membranes separating the body fluid compartments are selectively permeable, water can pass through them easily. However, most ions and other molecules pass through them more slowly. Passive transport processes include osmosis, diffusion, and filtration.

Osmosis. **Osmosis** is the movement of water through a semipermeable membrane from an area of lesser solute concentration to an area of greater solute concentration to equalize concentrations on both sides of the membrane (Figure 41.2). A semipermeable membrane allows water to pass through while remaining impermeable to most solutes. The rate of osmosis depends on the concentration of the solutes in the solution, temperature of the solution, electrical charges of the solutes, and differences between the osmotic pressures exerted by the solutions. The concentration of a solution is measured in osmols, which reflect the amount of a substance in solution in the form of molecules, ions, or both. Osmosis is an important concept when administering intravenous solutions, as their **osmolality** influences the potential benefits and risks. Another application of understanding osmosis is when considering the action of osmotic laxatives. These laxative salts are poorly absorbed through the intestinal lining and thus draw water into the intestinal lumen, causing an accumulation of water and softened stool. The swelling also stretches the intestine, stimulating peristalsis (Burchum & Rosenthal, 2019).

Osmotic pressure is the pressure needed to counter the movement of water (solvent) across a semipermeable membrane from a low concentration to high concentration of solutes. A solution with a high solute concentration has a high osmotic pressure and draws water into itself. If the concentration of the solute is greater on one side of the semipermeable membrane, the rate of osmosis is faster, and solvent rapidly transfers across the membrane. This continues until equilibrium is reached.

Plasma proteins affect the blood's osmotic pressure. The three main classes of plasma proteins are albumins, globulins, and fibrinogen (Marieb & Hoehn, 2019). Because albumin, produced in the liver, makes up the greatest proportion of plasma proteins, it exerts **colloid osmotic pressure** or oncotic pressure. This oncotic pressure tends to keep fluid in the intravascular compartment by pulling water from the interstitial space back into the capillaries (see Figure 41.2).

Diffusion. **Diffusion** is the movement of ions and molecules in a solution, often across a semipermeable membrane, from an area of higher concentration to an area of lower concentration (see a brief educational video on the Evolve website: Diffusion). The result is an even distribution of the solute in a solution. The rate of diffusion is affected by the molecule size, concentration, and temperature of a solution. The larger the molecule is and the cooler the solution is, the slower the rate of diffusion is. The difference between the two concentrations is known as a **concentration gradient**. Perfume permeating a room and a drop of food colouring moving through a glass of water are common examples of diffusion. Physiological examples include the movement of oxygen (O_2) and carbon dioxide (CO_2) between the alveoli and blood vessels in the lungs, neurotransmitters crossing the synaptic cleft, or the movement of lipids within the cell membrane. Some diffusion, still a passive transport process, is facilitated through a channel in the cell membrane (e.g., sodium, potassium, calcium) or with a carrier (Marieb & Hoehn, 2019).

Active Transport. **Active transport** processes facilitate the movement of molecules (solutes) across the plasma membrane across a concentration gradient, using chemical energy (adenosine triphosphate [ATP]). There are two types of active transport, primary and secondary. In primary active transport, a protein binds with a solute to carry it against a concentration gradient. There are three types of pumps: uniport, symport, and antiport (Marieb & Hoehn, 2019). The most-discussed primary active transport example, the sodium-potassium pump (Na^+/K^+ ATPase), is an antiport pump, as it transports solutes in opposite directions across the plasma membrane. Secondary active transport is more complex, as the sodium-potassium pump uses chemical energy to create a concentration gradient of sodium ions. Then, using the potential energy and a carrier protein, a sodium ion and a glucose molecule are transported back into the cell together (Figure 41.3).

Filtration. **Filtration**, the result of hydrostatic and colloid osmotic pressures, is a passive process whereby water moves into and out of the capillaries (Marieb & Hoehn, 2019). **Hydrostatic pressure** is the force exerted by fluids within a compartment. Hydrostatic pressure in the capillaries is higher at the arteriolar end (35 mm Hg) than at the venular end (15 mm Hg). While the colloid osmotic or oncotic pressure remains stable within the capillaries, the changing hydrostatic pressures in the capillaries result in a pressure gradient. The combined pressures and the pressure gradient result in a net filtration pressure (NFP), filtering up to 2 to 4 litres of water per day into the interstitial fluid (Figure 41.4). Problems occur when hydrostatic pressure is increased on the venous side of the capillary bed, as occurs in heart failure. The normal movement of water from the interstitial space into the intravascular space by filtration is then reversed. This results in an accumulation of excess fluid in the interstitial space, known as **edema**. In the introductory case study, this is the cause of Jiao's feet swelling. Filtration is also very important for urine formation as water and solutes are carried across the wall of the glomerular capillaries by hydrostatic or blood pressure. Falling blood pressure affects this process.

Fluid Homeostasis

Body fluids are regulated by fluid intake, hormonal controls, and fluid output in order to maintain **homeostasis**. Homeostasis is essential for survival. The primary hormones that regulate fluid are antidiuretic hormone, angiotensin II, aldosterone, and natriuretic peptides (Marieb & Hoehn, 2019).

Fluid Output Regulation. Fluid output occurs through four organs of water loss: the kidneys, the skin, the lungs, and the gastrointestinal tract. The kidneys are the major regulatory organs of fluid balance. They receive approximately 180 L of plasma to filter each day and produce 1 200 to 1 500 mL of urine (Table 41.1). Each day an **obligatory water loss** of approximately 500 mL is essential, regardless of intake. This is why a person with no fluid intake will die of dehydration within a matter of days. **Sensible water loss** includes water loss through urine and feces.

Insensible water loss is continuous, gradual loss of water from the respiratory and skin epitheliums (Marieb & Hoehn, 2019). This

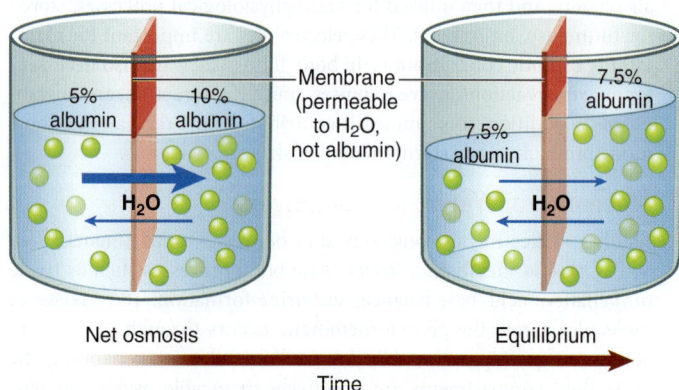

FIGURE 41.2 Osmosis.

FIGURE 41.3 Secondary active transport. A, An Na⁺/K⁺ (sodium/potassium) pump creates a concentration gradient of sodium ions. *Left,* Na⁺ ion binds to the Na⁺/K⁺ pump. *Right,* Adenosine triphosphate (ATP) hydrolysis fuels the transport of Na⁺ into the extracellular fluid (ECF), against their concentration gradient. **B,** A carrier protein uses the potential energy of the sodium ion gradient to power the transport of glucose. *Left,* From the ECF, an Na⁺ and a glucose molecule bind to another carrier protein. *Right,* The carrier protein transports the Na⁺ and glucose molecule into the cell—the Na⁺ with its concentration gradient, and the glucose against its concentration gradient. *ADP,* adenosine diphosphate; *P,* protein. (Redrawn from Amerman, E. C. [2016]. Human anatomy and physiology [p. 81, Fig. 3.11]. Pearson Education Inc.)

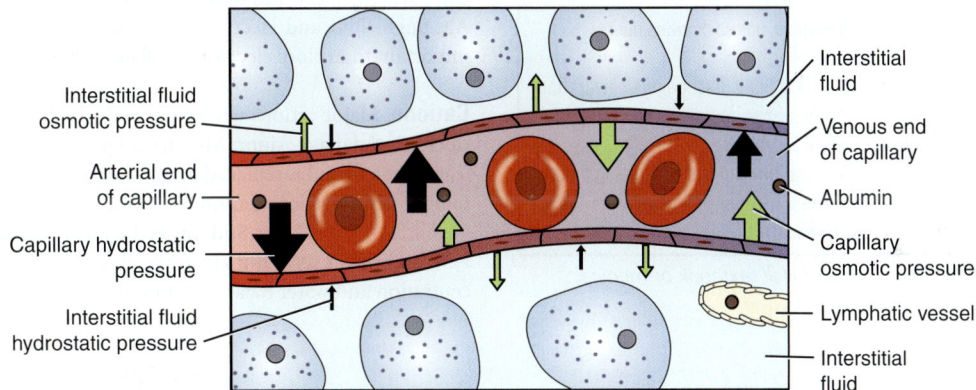

FIGURE 41.4 Capillary filtration. (From Copstead, L. C., & Banasik, J. L. [2013]. Pathophysiology [5th ed.]. Saunders.)

insensible water loss may increase in response to changes in respiratory rate and depth. Water loss from the skin is regulated by the sympathetic nervous system, which activates sweat glands. Fever may increase insensible water loss.

The gastrointestinal tract plays a vital role in fluid regulation. Every day, approximately 9 L of fluid is ingested or secreted into the small intestine and then absorbed into the enterocytes of the small intestine and from the large intestine. Only approximately 100 mL is lost through the feces, under normal conditions (Marieb & Hoehn, 2019). However, in the presence of a disease process, for example, diarrhea, the gastrointestinal tract may become the site of a large amount of fluid loss. This loss may have a significant impact on maintaining normal fluid homeostasis.

Fluid Intake Regulation. Fluid intake is regulated primarily through the thirst mechanism. The thirst control centre is located within the brain's hypothalamus. **Osmoreceptors** continually monitor the serum osmotic pressure, and when osmolality increases, even slightly (2–3%), the thirst centre is stimulated (Marieb & Hoehn, 2019). An increase in plasma sodium increases the osmotic pressure and stimulates the thirst mechanism. Increased plasma osmolality can occur with any condition that interferes with the oral ingestion of fluids or with the intake of hypertonic fluids. The thirst centre will also be stimulated if plasma volume decreases, and **hypovolemia** occurs, as in excessive vomiting and hemorrhage. In addition, stimulation of the renin–angiotensin–aldosterone mechanism, potassium depletion, psychological factors, and oropharyngeal dryness initiate the sensation of thirst.

The average adult's fluid intake is about 2 200 to 2 700 mL per day; oral intake accounts for 1 100 to 1 400 mL, solid foods for about 800 to 1 000 mL, and oxidative metabolism for 300 mL daily. Patients must be in an alert state to maintain their fluid intake independently. Infants, patients with neurological or psychological problems, and some older persons who are unable to perceive or respond to the thirst mechanism are at risk for **dehydration**.

Hormonal Regulation of Fluid

Antidiuretic hormone (ADH) is stored in the posterior pituitary gland and is released in response to changes in blood osmolality. The osmoreceptors in the hypothalamus are stimulated to release ADH when the osmolality increases. ADH promotes water conservation by acting directly on the renal tubules and collecting ducts to make them more permeable to water. This, in turn, causes water to return to the systemic circulation, which dilutes the blood and decreases its osmolality. As the body attempts to compensate, the patient will experience a temporary decrease in urinary output. When the blood has been sufficiently diluted, the osmoreceptors stop the release of ADH and urinary output is restored. ADH also stimulates the thirst centre to promote fluid intake (Figure 41.5).

Aldosterone is released by the adrenal cortex in response to increased plasma potassium or falling sodium levels or as part of the

TABLE 41.1	**Healthy Adult Average Fluid Intake and Output**	
	Normal (per Day)	**Prolonged Heavy Exercise (per Hour)**
Fluid Intake		
Fluids Ingested		
Oral	1 100–1 400 mL	280–1 100 mL/hr
Foods	800–1 000 mL	Highly variable
Metabolism	300 mL	16–50 mL/hr
TOTAL	2 200–2 700 mL	300–1 150 mL/hr
Fluid Output		
Skin (insensible and sweat)	500–600 mL	300–2 100 mL/hour
Insensible lungs	400 mL	20 mL/hr
Gastrointestinal	100–200 mL	Negligible, unless diarrhea during exercise
Urine	1 200–1 500 mL	20–1 000 mL/hr, depending on hydration status
TOTAL	2 200–2 700 mL	340–3 120 mL/hr
		Rehydration with Na^+-containing fluid necessary after prolonged vigorous exercise

Data from Hall, J. E. (2021). *Guyton and Hall textbook of medical physiology* (14th ed.). Elsevier.

renin–angiotensin–aldosterone system (RAAS) to counteract hypovolemia. To resolve hypovolemia, renin is released from the kidney in response to sympathetic nervous system stimulation and decreased renal blood flow, initiating a cascade of physiological and endocrine processes, one of which is the release of aldosterone. Aldosterone acts on the distal portion of the renal tubule to increase the reabsorption (saving) of sodium and the secretion and excretion of potassium and hydrogen.

Natriuretic peptides respond to increases in circulating blood volume. They are released from cardiac muscle cells and act on the peripheral vasculature, other hormones, and the kidney to facilitate diuresis. Natriuretic peptides increase sodium excretion and fluid loss while reducing thirst and blocking the release of ADH and aldosterone.

Regulation of Electrolytes

For normal cell function and human well-being, the body maintains a normal balance of electrolytes in the ECF and ICF, in spite of changes in intake and loss. This is accomplished primarily through electrolyte intake, absorption in the gastrointestinal tract, distribution, and excretion through the kidneys, feces, and sweat. Distribution is significant to overall electrolyte homeostasis, as some electrolytes, such as potassium, sodium, calcium, and phosphate, have very low plasma concentrations compared with cell and bone concentrations (Marieb & Hoehn, 2019). Although fluid and electrolyte balances are inextricably linked, it is important to explore electrolyte balance separately.

Cations. Major cations within the body fluids are sodium, potassium, calcium, and magnesium (Mg^{2+}). Cations interchange when one cation leaves the cell and is replaced by another. This occurs because cells tend to maintain electrical neutrality.

Sodium Regulation. Sodium is the most abundant cation (90%) in ECF and thus exerts the greatest influence on the ECF osmotic concentration and water balance. Sodium ions are also major contributors

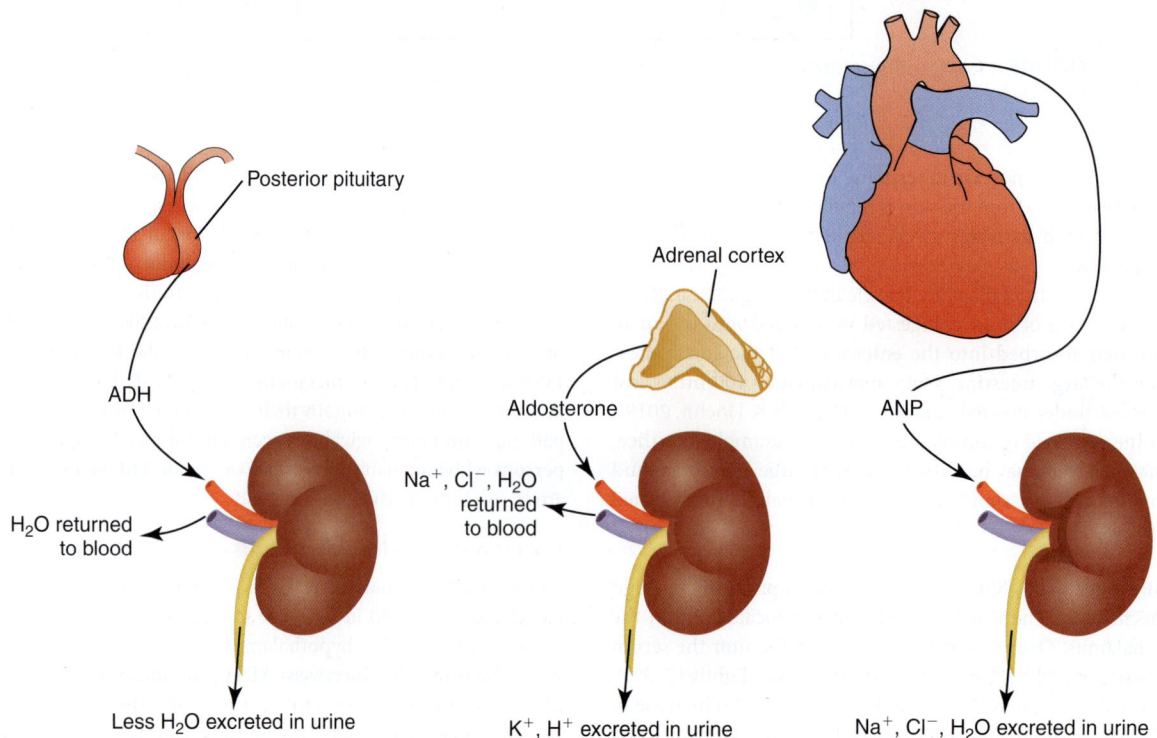

FIGURE 41.5 Hormone-influenced fluid excretion. *ADH*, Antidiuretic hormone; *ANP*, atrial natriuretic peptide; *Cl⁻*, chloride; *H⁺*, hydrogen ions; *H₂O*, water; *K⁺*, potassium; *Na⁺*, sodium.

to nerve impulse transmission, regulation of acid–base balance, and cellular chemical reactions. Normally, the intake and output of sodium is between 1.2 g and 3.3 g daily. With an increase in sodium intake and, therefore, an increase in ECF sodium content, water enters the ECF by osmosis. Therefore, increased sodium intake generally results in increased blood volume rather than significant changes in ECF sodium concentration.

The body continually responds to small changes in sodium content. A decrease in sodium in the ECF passing through the nephrons stimulates the RAAS to increase sodium reabsorption in the nephron. These actions indirectly increase water reabsorption as well (Marieb & Hoehn, 2019). The normal extracellular sodium concentration is 136 to 145 mmol/L. Sustained or severe problems with sodium concentration result in high sodium, above 145 mmol/L (hypernatremia), or low sodium, below 136 mmol/L (hyponatremia).

Potassium Regulation. Potassium is the major electrolyte and principal cation in the intracellular compartment. The majority (98%) of potassium content is in the ICF. Because the potassium concentration of ECF is relatively low, the cells expend energy to maintain the potassium content of ICF. Potassium is regulated by dietary intake and strongly affected by aldosterone, insulin, and epinephrine. Extracellular potassium concentration is affected by many complex mechanisms, including those of dietary intake and renal excretion. Renal excretion is regulated by changes in potassium concentration, changes in the acidity or alkalinity of a fluid (pH measurements), sodium reabsorption, and aldosterone levels. Aldosterone secretion is triggered by many factors; therefore, potassium balance is influenced by other factors, including changes in fluid volume, blood pressure, and acidosis (Marieb & Hoehn, 2019).

Potassium regulates many metabolic activities and is necessary for glycogen deposits in the liver and skeletal muscle, transmission and conduction of nerve impulses, normal cardiac conduction, and skeletal and smooth muscle contraction. The normal range for serum potassium concentrations is 3.5 to 5.1 mmol/L.

Calcium Regulation. Calcium is stored in bone, plasma, and body cells. Ninety-nine percent of calcium is located in bone, and only 1% is located in ECF. Approximately 50% of calcium in the plasma is bound to protein, primarily albumin, and 40% is free ionized calcium. The remaining small percentage is combined with nonprotein anions such as phosphate (PO_4^{3-}), citrate, and carbonate. Normal serum ionized calcium is 1.15 to 1.35 mmol/L. Normal total calcium is 2.10 to 2.50 mmol/L. Calcium is necessary for bone and teeth formation, blood clotting, hormone secretion, cell membrane integrity, cardiac conduction, transmission of nerve impulses, and muscle contraction.

Magnesium Regulation. Magnesium, the second most abundant intracellular cation, is essential for many intracellular activities, such as enzyme reactions. Magnesium, with a plasma concentration of 0.65 to 1.05 mmol/L, is important for bone structure and neuromuscular function, including skeletal and cardiac muscle excitability. Serum magnesium is regulated by dietary intake, renal mechanisms, and actions of the parathyroid hormone.

Anions. The three major anions of body fluids are chloride, bicarbonate, and phosphate ions.

Chloride Regulation. Chloride is the major anion in ECF. The transport of chloride follows sodium. Normal concentrations of chloride range from 98 to 106 mmol/L. Serum chloride is regulated by dietary intake and the kidneys. A person with normal renal function who has a high chloride intake will excrete a higher amount of urine chloride.

Bicarbonate Regulation. Bicarbonate is the major chemical base buffer within the body. The bicarbonate ion is found in ECF and ICF. The bicarbonate ion is an essential component of the carbonic

TABLE 41.2	Laboratory Normal Values for Adults
Item Measured	**Normal Value in Serum or Blood**
Osmolality	285–295 mmol/kg (SI units)
Blood urea nitrogen	3.6–7.1 mmol/L (SI units)
Creatinine	44–97 μmol/L (SI units) (female)
	53–106 μmol/L (SI units) (male)
Creatinine clearance	1.45–1.78 mL/sec (female)
	1.78–2.32 mL/sec (male)
Electrolytes	
Sodium (Na^+)	136–145 mmol/L (SI units)
Potassium (K^+)	3.5–5.1 mmol/L (SI units)
Chloride (Cl^-)	98–106 mmol/L (SI units)
Total CO_2 (CO_2 total content)	21–28 mmol/L (SI units)
Bicarbonate (HCO_3^-)	Arterial: 23–29 mmol/L (SI units)
	Venous: 21–28 mmol/L (SI units)
Total calcium (Ca^{2+})	2.10–2.50 mmol/L (SI units)
Ionized calcium (Ca^{2+})	1.15–1.35 mmol/L (SI units)
Magnesium (Mg^{2+})	0.65–1.05 mmol/L (SI units)
Phosphate	1.0–1.5 mmol/L (SI units)
Anion gap	16 ± 4 mmol/L (If potassium used in the calculation)
	12 ± 4 mmol/L (if potassium NOT used in calculation)
Arterial Blood Gases	
pH	7.35–7.45
$PaCO_2$	35–45 mm Hg (4.7–6 kPa)
PaO_2	80–100 mm Hg (10.7–133.3 kPa)
O_2 saturation (SaO_2)	95–100% (0.95–1.00)
Base excess	–2 to +2 mmol/L (SI units)

Laboratory values from Pagana, K., Pagana, T., & Pike-MacDonald, S.A. (2019). *Mosby's Canadian manual of diagnostic and laboratory tests* (2nd ed.). Elsevier.

acid–bicarbonate buffering system, which is essential to acid–base balance. The kidneys regulate bicarbonate. Normal arterial bicarbonate levels range between 23 and 29 mmol/L; venous bicarbonate is measured as carbon dioxide content, and the normal value is 21 to 28 mmol/L (Table 41.2).

Phosphate Regulation. Phosphorus is the major anion in the ICF; however, nearly all the phosphorus in the body exists in the form of phosphate. Phosphate's most important role is within the ICF, where it assists in the formation of high-energy compounds, such as ATP and nucleic acids, and in enzyme activity. Similar to magnesium and calcium, phosphate is used and stored in the skeleton. It also functions with calcium to develop and maintain teeth. Calcium and phosphate are inversely proportional; if one rises, the other falls. Phosphate also assists in acid–base regulation, promotes normal neuromuscular action, and participates in carbohydrate metabolism. Phosphate is normally absorbed through the gastrointestinal tract and is regulated by dietary intake, renal and intestinal excretion, and parathyroid hormone. The normal serum phosphorus level is 1.0 to 1.5 mmol/L.

Regulation of Acid–Base Balance

Acid–base balance exists when the rate at which the body produces and gains acids or bases, through cellular metabolism and gastrointestinal absorption, equals the rate at which acids or bases are excreted.

This balance results in a stable concentration of hydrogen ions (H^+) in body fluids that is expressed as the pH value. Hydrogen ions are primarily excreted by the kidneys. A normal hydrogen ion level is necessary to maintain cell membrane integrity and the speed of cellular enzymatic actions.

Arterial blood pH is inversely proportional to the hydrogen ion concentration (i.e., the greater the concentration, the more acidic the solution is and the lower the pH is; the lower the concentration, the more alkaline the solution is and the higher the pH is). The pH is also a reflection of the balance between carbon dioxide, which is regulated by the lungs, and bicarbonate, a base regulated by the kidneys. Normal pH is maintained by chemical buffers, and by buffer systems and regulatory mechanisms in the kidneys and lungs. A **buffer** is a substance or group of substances that can absorb or release hydrogen ions to stabilize pH, such as bicarbonate, phosphate, and proteins. The respiratory system, which controls the amount of carbon dioxide in the body, the hydrogen and bicarbonate ions, and therefore pH in the ECF, and the kidney are physiological buffer systems.

Buffers. Buffer systems are combinations of a weak acid and a weak base and are the short-term regulators of acid–base balance. The four main types of buffer systems are protein (amino acids, plasma proteins), hemoglobin (also a protein but unique in its buffering role), carbonic acid (H_2CO_3) and bicarbonate, and phosphate. Other types are the ammonia buffer system, a complex system that occurs in ICF, and the tubular system in the kidneys. All these buffers bind hydrogen ions until they can be permanently removed through the regulatory mechanisms in the lungs and the kidneys.

The carbonic acid–bicarbonate buffer system is used to evaluate acid–base balance, using the arterial blood gas (ABG) test. This system can be expressed as the following:

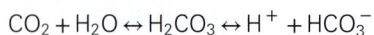

$$CO_2 + H_2O \leftrightarrow H_2CO_3 \leftrightarrow H^+ + HCO_3^-$$

Carbon dioxide + Water ↔ Carbonic acid
↔ Hydrogen ion + Bicarbonate

The carbonic acid–bicarbonate buffer system is the principal buffering system to react to change in the pH of ECF, and it reacts within seconds. Whenever carbon dioxide increases, an increase in hydrogen ions results, and whenever hydrogen ions are produced, more carbon dioxide results (Marieb & Hoehn, 2019). The lungs control the excretion of carbon dioxide, and the kidneys control the excretion of hydrogen and bicarbonate ions.

Another buffer system is the hemoglobin–oxyhemoglobin system within red blood cells (RBCs). This buffer system can have an immediate effect on pH because carbon dioxide diffuses readily into the RBCs and forms carbonic acid. The carbonic acid dissociates into hydrogen and bicarbonate ions, the latter of which diffuse into the plasma in exchange for chloride. The hydrogen ions attach to hemoglobin, whereas the carbon dioxide is carried to the lungs, where the reaction is reversed.

Regulatory Mechanisms. When the ability of buffer systems is exceeded, acid–base homeostasis is regulated by the lungs and the kidneys. The lungs adapt rapidly to an acid–base imbalance. Ordinarily, increased levels of hydrogen ions and carbon dioxide provide the stimulus for respiration. When the concentration of hydrogen ions is altered, the lungs react to correct the imbalance by altering the rate and depth of respiration. For example, when metabolic acidosis is present, respirations are increased, resulting in a greater amount of carbon dioxide being exhaled, which results in a decrease in the acidic level; when metabolic alkalosis is present, the lungs retain carbon dioxide by decreasing the respirations, thereby increasing the acidic level (Marieb & Hoehn, 2019).

The kidneys take from a few hours to several days to regulate acid–base imbalance. They regenerate or reabsorb bicarbonate in cases of acid excess and excrete it in cases of acid deficit. In addition, the kidneys use a phosphate ion to excrete hydrogen ions by forming phosphoric acid (H_3PO_4). Finally, the kidneys use the ammonia mechanism to regulate acid–base balance. In this mechanism, certain amino acids are chemically changed within the renal tubules into ammonia, which, in the presence of hydrogen ions, forms ammonium, which is excreted in the urine, thereby releasing hydrogen ions from the body (Marieb & Hoehn, 2019).

Disturbances in Electrolyte, Fluid, and Acid–Base Balances

Disturbances in electrolyte, fluid, or acid–base balance seldom occur alone and can disrupt normal body processes. For example, when body fluids are lost because of burns, illness, or trauma, the patient is also at risk for electrolyte imbalances. In addition, some untreated electrolyte imbalances (e.g., potassium loss) contribute to acid–base disturbances.

Fluid Disturbances. Fluid imbalances include volume imbalances, or disturbances in the amount of ECF, and osmolality imbalances, or disturbances in the concentration of body fluids (hyper- or hypo-osmolar imbalance). Isotonic deficit and excess exist when water and electrolytes are gained or lost in equal proportion. In contrast, osmolar imbalances are losses or excesses of only water, so the concentration (osmolality) of the serum is affected. It is important to recognize that maintaining fluid homeostasis is primarily related to circulatory volume. Hemodynamics respond quickly to changes in the intravascular compartment, followed more slowly by sodium and water balance mechanisms. Table 41.3 lists the common fluid isotonic and osmolality imbalances, the causes and signs, and related symptoms.

Fluid volume deficit is insufficient isotonic fluid in the extracellular compartment. Because this involves both intravascular and interstitial compartments, symptoms also relate to both compartments. Fluid volume excess is too much isotonic fluid in the extracellular compartment, and so symptoms also relate to intravascular and interstitial compartments, such as swollen fingers or ankles. Osmolar fluid imbalances involve a fluid imbalance accompanied by either elevated sodium (hypernatremia) or lower sodium (hyponatremia). Clinical dehydration, caused by reduced sodium and water intake, or loss of more water proportionately than salt, is a combined volume and osmolality imbalance. Serum sodium and osmolality values are required to diagnose hypertonic and hypotonic fluid volume deficits. Physical examination and lab values are important for diagnosing and treating these complex imbalances.

Electrolyte Imbalances. Many factors can disrupt electrolyte homeostasis, including acute infections causing diarrhea, metabolic disorders, altered electrolyte intake, sudden loss of electrolytes in the case of burns or acute vomiting, medications, and shifts in the distribution of electrolytes from cells or bones into the ECF. Table 41.4 provides a list of the causes, signs, and symptoms of electrolyte imbalances.

Sodium Imbalances. **Dysnatremia** (hypo- or hypernatremia) is complex and often presents with central nervous system symptoms, including headache, confusion, fatigue, reduced level of consciousness, or seizures (Bertschi, 2020). **Hyponatremia** is a lower-than-normal concentration of sodium in the blood (serum), which can occur with a net sodium loss or net water excess (see Table 41.3). It occurs frequently in seriously ill patients and is the most common electrolyte disturbance among older persons (Bertschi, 2020). Clinical indicators and treatment depend on the cause of hyponatremia and whether it is associated with a normal, decreased, or increased ECF volume. Sodium and

TABLE 41.3	Fluid Imbalances
Imbalance and Related Causes	**Signs and Symptoms**

Isotonic Imbalances—Water and Sodium Lost or Gained in Equal or Isotonic Proportions
Extracellular Fluid Volume Deficit—Body Fluids Have Decreased Volume but Normal Osmolality

Sodium and Water Intake Less Than Output, Causing Isotonic Loss:	*Physical examination:* Sudden weight loss (overnight), postural hypotension, tachycardia, thready pulse, dry mucous membranes, poor skin turgor, slow vein filling, flat neck veins when supine, dark yellow urine
Severely decreased oral intake of water and salt	
Increased GI output: vomiting, diarrhea, laxative overuse, drainage from fistulas or tubes	If severe: thirst, restlessness, confusion, hypotension; oliguria (urine output *below* 30 mL/hr); cold, clammy skin; hypovolemic shock
Increased renal output: use of diuretics, adrenal insufficiency (deficit of cortisol and aldosterone)	*Laboratory findings:* Increased hematocrit; increased BUN *above* 8.2 mmol/L (hemoconcentration); urine specific gravity usually *above* 1.030, unless renal cause
Loss of blood or plasma: hemorrhage, burns	
Massive sweating without water and salt intake	

Extracellular Fluid Volume Excess—Body Fluids Have Increased Volume but Normal Osmolality

Sodium and Water Intake Greater Than Output, Causing Isotonic Gain:	*Physical examination:* Sudden weight gain (overnight), edema (especially in dependent areas), full neck veins when upright or semi-upright, crackles in lungs
Excessive administration of Na^+-containing isotonic IV fluids or oral intake of salty foods and water	If severe: confusion, pulmonary edema
Renal retention of Na^+ and water: heart failure, cirrhosis, aldosterone or glucocorticoid excess, acute or chronic oliguric renal disease	*Laboratory findings:* Decreased hematocrit, decreased BUN *below* 2.9 mmol/L (hemodilution)

Osmolality Imbalances
Hypernatremia (Water Deficit; Hyperosmolar Imbalance)—Body Fluids Too Concentrated

Loss of Relatively More Water Than Salt:	*Physical examination:* Decreased level of consciousness (confusion, lethargy, coma), perhaps thirst, seizures if develops rapidly or is very severe
Diabetes insipidus (ADH deficiency)	
Osmotic diuresis	*Laboratory findings:* Serum Na^+ level *above* 145 mmol/L, serum osmolality *above* 295 mmol/kg
Large insensible perspiration and respiratory water output without increased water intake	
Gain of Relatively More Salt Than Water:	
Administration of tube feedings, hypertonic parenteral fluids, or salt tablets	
Lack of access to water, deliberate water deprivation, inability to respond to thirst (e.g., immobility, aphasia)	
Dysfunction of osmoreceptor-driven thirst drive	

Hyponatremia (Water Excess; Water Intoxication; Hypo-Osmolar Imbalance)—Body Fluids Too Dilute

Gain of Relatively More Water Than Salt:	*Physical examination:* Decreased level of consciousness (confusion, lethargy, coma), seizures if develops rapidly or is very severe
Excessive ADH (SIADH)	
Psychogenic polydipsia or forced excessive water intake	*Laboratory findings:* Serum Na^+ level *below* 136 mmol/L, serum osmolality *below* 285 mmol/kg
Excessive IV administration of D_5W	
Use of hypotonic irrigating solutions	
Tap-water enemas	
Loss of Relatively More Salt Than Water:	
Replacement of large body fluid output (e.g., diarrhea, vomiting) with water but no salt	

Combined Volume and Osmolality Imbalance
Clinical Dehydration (Extracellular Fluid Volume Deficit Plus Hypernatremia)—Body Fluids Have Decreased Volume and Are Too Concentrated

Sodium and Water Intake Less Than Output, With Loss of Relatively More Water Than Salt:	*Physical examination and laboratory findings:* Combination of those for ECV deficit plus those for hypernatremia (see previous signs)
All of the causes of ECV deficit (see previous causes) plus poor or no water intake, often with fever causing increased insensible water output	

ADH, Antidiuretic hormone; *BUN*, blood urea nitrogen; D_5W, 5% dextrose in water; *ECV*, extracellular fluid volume; *GI*, gastrointestinal; *IV*, intravenous; *SIADH*, syndrome of inappropriate secretion of antidiuretic hormone.
Laboratory values from Pagana, K., Pagana, T., & Pike-MacDonald, S. A. (2019). *Mosby's Canadian manual of diagnostic and laboratory tests* (2nd ed.). Elsevier.

TABLE 41.4 Electrolyte Imbalances

Imbalance and Related Causes	Signs and Symptoms
Hypokalemia—Low Serum Potassium (K⁺) Concentration ***Decreased K⁺ Intake:*** Excessive use of K⁺-free IV solutions ***Shift of K⁺ Into Cells:*** Alkalosis; treatment of diabetic ketoacidosis with insulin ***Increased K⁺ Output:*** Acute or chronic diarrhea; vomiting; other GI losses (e.g., nasogastric or fistula drainage); use of potassium-wasting diuretics; aldosterone excess; polyuria; glucocorticoid therapy	*Physical examination:* Bilateral muscle weakness that begins in quadriceps and may ascend to respiratory muscles, abdominal distension, decreased bowel sounds, constipation, dysrhythmias *Laboratory findings:* Serum K⁺ level *below* 3.5 mmol/L; ECG abnormalities: U waves, flattened or inverted T waves; ST segment depression
Hyperkalemia—High Serum Potassium (K⁺) Concentration ***Increased K⁺ Intake:*** Iatrogenic administration of large amounts of IV K⁺; rapid infusion of stored blood; excess ingestion of K⁺ salt substitutes ***Shift of K⁺ Out of Cells:*** Massive cellular damage (e.g., crushing trauma, cytotoxic chemotherapy); insufficient insulin (e.g., diabetic ketoacidosis); some types of acidosis ***Decreased K⁺ Output:*** Acute or chronic oliguria (e.g., severe ECV deficit, end-stage renal disease); use of potassium-sparing diuretics; adrenal insufficiency (deficit of cortisol and aldosterone)	*Physical examination:* Bilateral muscle weakness in quadriceps, transient abdominal cramps, diarrhea, dysrhythmias, cardiac arrest if severe *Laboratory findings:* Serum K⁺ level *above* 5.1 mmol/L; ECG abnormalities: peaked T waves; widened QRS complex; PR prolongation; terminal sine-wave pattern
Hypocalcemia—Low Serum Calcium (Ca²⁺) Concentration ***Decreased Ca²⁺ Intake and Absorption:*** Calcium-deficient diet; vitamin D deficiency (includes end-stage renal disease); chronic diarrhea; laxative misuse; steatorrhea ***Shift of Ca²⁺ Into Bone or Inactive Form:*** Hypoparathyroidism; rapid administration of citrated blood; hypoalbuminemia; alkalosis; pancreatitis; hyperphosphatemia (includes end-stage renal disease) ***Increased Ca²⁺ Output:*** Chronic diarrhea; steatorrhea	*Physical examination:* Numbness and tingling of fingers, toes, and circumoral (around mouth) region; positive Chvostek's sign (contraction of facial muscles when facial nerve is tapped); hyperactive reflexes; muscle twitching and cramping; carpal and pedal spasms; tetany; seizures; laryngospasm; dysrhythmias *Laboratory findings:* Total serum Ca²⁺ level *below* 2.1 mmol/L or serum ionized Ca²⁺ level *below* 1.15 mmol/L; ECG abnormalities: prolonged ST segments
Hypercalcemia—High Serum Calcium (Ca²⁺) Concentration ***Increased Ca²⁺ Intake and Absorption:*** Milk-alkali syndrome ***Shift of Ca²⁺ Out of Bone:*** Prolonged immobilization; hyperparathyroidism; bone tumours; nonosseous cancers that secrete bone-resorbing factors ***Decreased Ca²⁺ Output:*** Use of thiazide diuretics	*Physical examination:* Anorexia, nausea and vomiting, constipation, fatigue, diminished reflexes, lethargy, decreased level of consciousness, confusion, personality change, cardiac arrest if severe *Laboratory findings:* Total serum Ca²⁺ level *above* 2.5 mmol/L or serum ionized Ca²⁺ level *above* 1.35 mmol/L; ECG abnormalities: heart block, shortened ST segments
Hypomagnesemia—Low Serum Magnesium (Mg²⁺) Concentration ***Decreased Mg²⁺ Intake and Absorption:*** Malnutrition; chronic alcoholism; chronic diarrhea; laxative misuse; steatorrhea ***Shift of Mg²⁺ Into Inactive Form:*** Rapid administration of citrated blood ***Increased Mg²⁺ Output:*** Chronic diarrhea; steatorrhea; other GI losses (e.g., vomiting, nasogastric or fistula drainage); use of thiazide or loop diuretics; aldosterone excess	*Physical examination:* Positive Chvostek's sign, hyperactive deep tendon reflexes, muscle cramps and twitching, grimacing, dysphagia, tetany, seizures, insomnia, tachycardia, hypertension, dysrhythmias *Laboratory findings:* Serum Mg²⁺ level *below* 0.65 mmol/L; ECG abnormalities: prolonged QT interval
Hypermagnesemia—High Serum Magnesium (Mg²⁺) Concentration ***Increased Mg²⁺ Intake and Absorption:*** Excessive use of Mg²⁺-containing laxatives and antacids; parenteral overload of magnesium ***Decreased Mg²⁺ Output:*** Oliguric end-stage renal disease; adrenal insufficiency	*Physical examination:* Lethargy, hypoactive deep tendon reflexes, bradycardia, hypotension Acute elevation in Mg²⁺ levels: Flushing, sensation of warmth Severe acute hypermagnesemia: Decreased rate and depth of respirations, dysrhythmias, cardiac arrest *Laboratory findings:* Serum Mg²⁺ level *above* 1.05 mmol/L; ECG abnormalities: prolonged PR interval

ECG, Electrocardiogram; *ECV,* extracellular fluid volume; *GI,* gastrointestinal; *IV,* intravenous.
Laboratory values from Pagana, K., Pagana, T., & Pike-MacDonald, S. A. (2019). *Mosby's Canadian manual of diagnostic and laboratory tests* (2nd ed.). Elsevier.

chloride are not stored in the body; therefore, they must be consumed daily or provided through intravenous solutions in the ill. Children are particularly vulnerable to hyponatremia when receiving intravenous solutions; therefore, isotonic solutions are recommended, along with monitoring of sodium (Friedman, 2018). Chronic hyponatremia, with symptoms of malaise, fatigue, gait disturbances, falls, and changes in cognition, can be easily missed in older persons.

Hypernatremia is a greater-than-normal concentration of sodium in ECF that can be caused by excess water loss or overall sodium excess (see Table 41.3). When hypernatremia occurs, the body attempts to conserve as much water as possible through renal reabsorption.

Potassium Imbalances. **Hypokalemia** is one of the most common electrolyte imbalances (see Table 41.4). Hypokalemia, with potassium levels less than 3.5 mmol/L, results in cardiac arrhythmias, fatigue, and altered muscle activity throughout the body (Pagana et al., 2019). Because the normal amount of serum potassium is so small, little tolerance for fluctuations exists. The most common cause of hypokalemia is the use of potassium-wasting diuretics such as thiazide and loop diuretics.

Hyperkalemia is a greater-than-normal amount of potassium in the blood. Lethal cardiac arrhythmias result from potassium levels over 5.1 mmol/L, as well as skeletal muscle weakness and paralysis (see Table 41.4). The primary cause of hyperkalemia is renal failure, because any decrease in renal function diminishes the amount of potassium the kidney can excrete.

Calcium Imbalances. **Hypocalcemia** represents a drop in serum or ionized calcium. It can result from several illnesses, some of which directly affect the thyroid and parathyroid glands (see Table 41.4). Other causes include prolonged bed rest and renal insufficiency (in which the kidneys' inability to excrete phosphorus causes the phosphorus level to rise and the calcium level to decline). Signs and symptoms can be related to diminished functioning of the neuromuscular, cardiac, and renal systems.

Hypercalcemia is an increase in the total serum concentration of calcium or ionized calcium (see Table 41.4). Hypercalcemia is frequently a symptom of an underlying disease, such as malignancy or hyperparathyroidism, resulting in excess bone reabsorption with release of calcium (Marieb & Hoehn, 2019).

Magnesium Imbalances. Disturbances in magnesium levels are summarized in Table 41.4. Symptoms are the result of changes in neuromuscular excitability. **Hypomagnesemia**, a drop in serum magnesium below 0.65 mmol/L, occurs with malnutrition, malabsorption disorders, diarrhea, and alcohol withdrawal. This may cause neuromuscular symptoms, seizures, or cardiac arrhythmias. **Hypermagnesemia**, an increase in serum magnesium levels more than 1.05 mmol/L, depresses skeletal muscles and nerve function. Magnesium may inhibit acetylcholine, thereby causing a sedative effect.

Chloride Imbalances. **Hypochloremia** occurs when the serum chloride level falls below normal. Vomiting or prolonged and excessive nasogastric or fistula drainage can result in hypochloremia because of the loss of hydrochloric acid. The use of loop and thiazide diuretics also results in increased chloride loss as sodium is excreted. When serum chloride levels fall, metabolic alkalosis results as the body adapts by increasing reabsorption of the bicarbonate ion to maintain electrical neutrality.

Hyperchloremia occurs when the serum chloride level rises above normal, which usually occurs when the serum bicarbonate value falls or the sodium level rises. Hypochloremia and hyperchloremia rarely occur as single disease processes but are commonly associated with acid–base imbalance. No single set of symptoms is associated with these two alterations.

Acid–Base Balance. **Arterial blood gas (ABG)** analysis is the best way to evaluate acid–base balance and is based on the carbonic acid–bicarbonate buffer system. Measurement of ABGs involves analysis of six components: pH, $PaCO_2$, PaO_2, **oxygen saturation**, **base excess**, and bicarbonate (see Table 41.2). Deviation from a normal value will indicate that the patient is experiencing an acid–base imbalance. The definitions and values for ABG measures are provided in Table 41.5. Because accurate blood gas values require arterial blood analysis, they are drawn primarily in critical care and emergency settings. Jiao (see introductory case study) may have had ABGs drawn prior to or during her treatment in the ED.

TABLE 41.5	Arterial Blood Gas Measures	
Laboratory Measure	Normal Range in Adult Arterial Blood	Definition and Interpretation
pH	7.35–7.45	pH is a negative logarithm of the free H^+ concentration, a measure of how acid or alkaline the blood is. Values below 7.35 indicate abnormally acid; above 7.45 they indicate abnormally alkaline. Small changes in pH denote large changes in H^+ concentration and are clinically important.
$PaCO_2$	35–45 mm Hg (4.7–6 kPa)	$PaCO_2$ is partial pressure of carbon dioxide (CO_2), a measure of how well the lungs are excreting CO_2 produced by cells. Increased $PaCO_2$ indicates CO_2 accumulation in blood (more carbonic acid) caused by hypoventilation; decreased $PaCO_2$ indicates excessive CO_2 excretion (less carbonic acid) through hyperventilation.
HCO_3^-	23–29 mmol/L	Serum bicarbonate is excreted or retained by the kidneys to maintain a normal acid–base environment and is the principal buffer of the ECFs.
		A normal pH is maintained with a bicarbonate ratio 20 times that of the fluid concentration of carbonic acid (Marieb & Hoehn, 2019). Less than 23 mmol/L of bicarbonate usually indicates metabolic acidosis, whereas more than 29 mmol/L indicates metabolic alkalosis.
PaO_2	80–100 mm Hg (10–13.3 kPa)	PaO_2 is partial pressure of oxygen (O_2), a measure of how well gas exchange is occurring in the alveoli of the lungs. Values below normal indicate poor oxygenation of the blood.
SaO_2	95–100%	SaO_2 is the point at which hemoglobin is saturated by oxygen. Decreasing PaO_2 causes an increase in oxygen dissociation from hemoglobin. Oxygen saturation can be influenced by pH, $PaCO_2$, and body temperature. It drops rapidly when PaO_2 falls below 60 mm Hg (8 kPa).
Base excess	−2 to +2 mmol/L	Base excess reflects deviations from a serum pH of 7.4 (neutral). Base excess is observed buffering capacity minus the normal buffering capacity, a measure of how well the blood buffers are managing metabolic acids. Values below −2 (negative base excess) indicate excessive metabolic acids, usually the result of the elimination of too many bicarbonate ions; values above +2 indicate excessive amounts of bicarbonate.

Types of Acid–Base Imbalances

The four primary types of acid–base imbalance are respiratory acidosis, respiratory alkalosis, metabolic acidosis, and metabolic alkalosis (Table 41.6).

Respiratory Acidosis. Respiratory acidosis is marked by an increased $PaCO_2$, excess carbonic acid, and an increased hydrogen ion concentration (decreased pH). This occurs when respirations are not effective in excreting carbon dioxide, resulting in an increase in

hydrogen concentration. With respiratory acidosis, carbon dioxide crosses the blood–brain barrier, causing neurological changes, such as headaches, irritability, and, ultimately, impaired consciousness. Hypoxemia occurs simultaneously because of respiratory depression, resulting in further neurological impairment. Electrolyte changes such as hyperkalemia and hypercalcemia may accompany the acidosis. The renal system compensates by increasing bicarbonate and eliminating hydrogen ion. Jiao (see introductory case study) would have been at risk for respiratory acidosis because her heart failure resulted in fluid

TABLE 41.6   Acid–Base Imbalances

Imbalance and Related Causes	Signs and Symptoms
Respiratory Acidosis—Excessive Carbonic Acid Caused by Alveolar Hypoventilation	
Impaired Gas Exchange: Type B COPD (chronic bronchitis) or end-stage type A COPD (emphysema) Bacterial pneumonia Airway obstruction Extensive atelectasis (collapsed alveoli) Severe acute asthma episode *Impaired Neuromuscular Function:* Respiratory muscle weakness or paralysis from hypokalemia or neurological dysfunction Respiratory muscle fatigue, respiratory failure Chest wall injury or surgery causing pain with respiration *Dysfunction of Brainstem Respiratory Control:* Drug overdose with a respiratory depressant Some types of head injury	*Physical examination:* Headache, lightheadedness, decreased level of consciousness (confusion, lethargy, coma), dysrhythmias *Laboratory findings:* Arterial blood gas alterations: pH *below* 7.35, $PaCO_2$ *above* 45 mm Hg (6 kPa), HCO_3^- level normal if uncompensated or *above* 29 mmol/L if compensated
Respiratory Alkalosis—Deficient Carbonic Acid Caused by Alveolar Hyperventilation	
Hypoxemia from any cause (e.g., initial part of asthma episode, pneumonia) Acute pain Anxiety, psychological distress, sobbing Inappropriate mechanical ventilator settings Stimulation of brainstem respiratory control (e.g., meningitis, Gram-negative sepsis, head injury, aspirin overdose)	*Physical examination:* Lightheadedness, numbness and tingling of fingers, toes, and circumoral region, increased rate and depth of respirations, excitement and confusion possibly followed by decreased level of consciousness, dysrhythmias *Laboratory findings:* Arterial blood gas alterations: pH *above* 7.45, $PaCO_2$ *below* 35 mm Hg (4.7 kPa), HCO_3^- level normal if short lived or uncompensated or *below* 23 mmol/L if compensated
Metabolic Acidosis—Excessive Metabolic Acids	
Increase of Metabolic Acids (High Anion Gap): Ketoacidosis (diabetes, starvation, alcoholism) Hypermetabolic state (severe hyperthyroidism, burns, severe infection) Oliguric renal disease (acute kidney injury, end-stage renal disease) Circulatory shock (lactic acidosis) Ingestion of acid or acid precursors (e.g., methanol, ethylene glycol, boric acid, aspirin overdose) *Loss of Bicarbonate (Normal Anion Gap):* Diarrhea Pancreatic fistula or intestinal decompression Renal tubular acidosis	*Physical examination:* Decreased level of consciousness (lethargy, confusion, coma), abdominal pain, dysrhythmias, increased rate and depth of respirations (compensatory hyperventilation) *Laboratory findings:* Arterial blood gas alterations: pH *below* 7.35, $PaCO_2$ normal if uncompensated or *below* 35 mm Hg (4.7 kPa) if compensated, HCO_3^- level *below* 23 mmol/L
Metabolic Alkalosis—Deficient Metabolic Acids	
Increase of Bicarbonate: Excessive administration of sodium bicarbonate Massive blood transfusion (liver converts citrate to HCO_3^-) Mild or moderate ECV deficit (contraction alkalosis) *Loss of Metabolic Acid:* Excessive vomiting or gastric suctioning Hypokalemia Excess aldosterone	*Physical examination:* Lightheadedness, numbness and tingling of fingers, toes, and circumoral region; muscle cramps; possible excitement and confusion followed by decreased level of consciousness, dysrhythmias (may be caused by concurrent hypokalemia) *Laboratory findings:* Arterial blood gas alterations: pH *above* 7.45, $PaCO_2$ normal if uncompensated or *above* 45 mm Hg (6.0 kPa) if compensated, HCO_3^- *above* 29 mmol/L

COPD, Chronic obstructive pulmonary disease; *ECV,* extracellular fluid volume.
Laboratory values from Pagana, K., Pagana, T., & Pike-MacDonald, S. A. (2019). *Mosby's Canadian manual of diagnostic and laboratory tests* (2nd ed.). Elsevier.

compromising carbon dioxide excretion. Her reduced renal function would have limited the ability of her kidneys to compensate.

Respiratory Alkalosis.
Respiratory alkalosis is marked by decreased PaCO$_2$ and increased pH. Respiratory alkalosis can begin outside the respiratory system (e.g., anxiety with hyperventilation) or within the respiratory system (e.g., the initial phase of an asthma attack). Usually, the respiratory system corrects imbalances before compensatory changes are required.

Metabolic Acidosis.
Metabolic acidosis results from a decrease in serum bicarbonate or the production of organic or fixed acids. An analysis of serum electrolytes to detect an anion gap may be helpful in attempting to identify the cause of the metabolic acidosis. An anion gap reflects unmeasurable anions present in plasma and is calculated by subtracting the sum of chloride and bicarbonate from the amount of plasma sodium concentration. Compensation for metabolic acidosis initially involves an increase in respiratory rate and depth to eliminate carbon dioxide. If not quickly resolved, renal mechanisms are stimulated to increase hydrogen ion excretion, and to generate and release bicarbonate into the ECF.

Diabetic ketoacidosis (DKA) is characterized by hyperglycemia, high ketones, and metabolic acidosis. This diabetic emergency is caused by a total lack of insulin, in type 1 diabetes, causing severely elevated glucose levels. The body responds to the glucose deficit inside the cells by mobilizing fats, a process that results in increased ketone bodies. Together, these metabolic processes cause osmotic diuresis, acidosis, and hyperkalemia. Patients with type 2 diabetes are also at risk of developing metabolic acidosis from severe hyperglycemia, although the acidosis develops more slowly and is not associated with ketosis. The clinical response to these hyperglycemic emergencies is to administer insulin and intravenous fluids. It is critical to correct water and electrolyte imbalances and restore intravascular volume, based on individual assessments and diagnostics; however, an isotonic solution such as 0.9% saline or hypotonic 0.45% is recommended over the initial 24

to 48 hours (Lewis et al., 2023). Frequent monitoring of electrolytes, fluid balance, glucose, and ABGs is important in the treatment of DKA.

Metabolic Alkalosis.
Metabolic alkalosis is marked by the heavy loss of acid from the body or by increased levels of bicarbonate. The most common causes are vomiting and gastric suction, as well as potassium deficiency, hyperaldosteronism, and diuretic therapy (Marieb & Hoehn, 2019). The body attempts to compensate by increasing the excretion of bicarbonate and decreasing the rate and the depth of respirations. Symptoms associated with metabolic alkalosis are depressed respirations and tingling of the fingers and dizziness related to secondary low calcium (Lewis et al. 2023). In serious metabolic alkalosis, cardiac arrhythmias can occur.

KNOWLEDGE BASE OF NURSING PRACTICE

The essential functions of fluid, electrolyte, and acid–base balances are important aspects of the scientific knowledge base of nursing practice. Regardless of the area of practice, all nurses will be involved in assessment, planning, and interventions in relation to fluid, electrolytes, and acid–base balance. Identifying those persons most at risk for imbalances is important for promoting health and well-being (Table 41.7). Certain patients are particularly vulnerable to imbalances, including infants, older persons, hospitalized persons, and severely ill patients. Patients who are disoriented or immobile are also vulnerable to imbalances because they cannot respond independently to early symptoms. Prolonged or severe compromises may lead to irreversible chronic health problems.

Nurses play an essential role in assessing, intervening, educating, monitoring, and promoting quality of care relating to hydration and homeostasis (Holyrod, 2020). For example, nurses caring for Jiao (in the introductory case study) are conscientious in assessing her fluid intake, output, nutritional intake, and skin integrity related to fluid excess in her interstitial space, and they integrate these assessments into their nursing care.

TABLE 41.7	Risk Factors for Fluid, Electrolyte, and Acid–Base Imbalances
Age	*Very young:* ECV deficit, osmolality imbalances, clinical dehydration
	Older persons: ECV excess or deficit, osmolality imbalances
Environment	*Sodium-rich diet:* ECV excess
	Electrolyte-poor diet: Electrolyte deficits
	Hot weather: Clinical dehydration
	Hospitalization: Hyperosmolar dehydration
Gastrointestinal output	*Diarrhea:* ECV deficit, clinical dehydration, hypokalemia, hypocalcemia (if chronic), hypomagnesemia (if chronic), metabolic acidosis
	Drainage (e.g., nasogastric suctioning, fistulas): ECV deficit, hypokalemia; metabolic acidosis if intestinal or pancreatic drainage
	Vomiting: ECV deficit, clinical dehydration, hypokalemia, hypomagnesemia, metabolic alkalosis
Chronic diseases	*Cancer:* Hypercalcemia; with tumour lysis syndrome: hyperkalemia, hypocalcemia, hyperphosphatemia
	Diabetes: Microvascular complications, HHS, DKA,
	Chronic obstructive pulmonary disease: Respiratory acidosis
	Cirrhosis: ECV excess, hypokalemia
	Heart failure: ECV excess; other imbalances, depending on therapy
	Acute kidney injury: ECV excess, hyperkalemia, hypermagnesemia, hyperphosphatemia, metabolic acidosis
Trauma	*Burns:* ECV deficit, metabolic acidosis
	Crush injuries: Hyperkalemia
	Head injuries: Hyponatremia or hypernatremia
	Hemorrhage: ECV deficit, hyperkalemia if circulatory shock
Therapies	Diuretics and other medications (see Box 41.4)
	Infusion therapy: ECV excess, osmolality imbalances, electrolyte excesses
	Enteral and parenteral nutrition: Any fluid or electrolyte imbalance, depending on components of solution

DKA, Diabetic ketoacidosis; *ECV,* extracellular fluid volume; *HHS,* hyperosmolar hyperglycemic state.

❖ NURSING PROCESS

◆ Assessment

Patient care related to fluid, electrolyte, and acid–base balance begins with informed assessment. Using a systematic approach to collecting data and analyzing findings enables nurses to provide person-centred care. Nurses' clinical decisions are based on the quality of their assessments and clinical reasoning. By gathering data through a health history and physical examination, nurses can identify patients at risk of or experiencing imbalances. During assessment (Figure 41.6), nurses must consider all elements that contribute to making appropriate nursing diagnoses. Electronic documentation of nursing assessment is critical to safe patient care (see Chapter 16). Nurses should use critical thinking skills and document beyond the electronic health record dropboxes and standardized assessments, when necessary.

Patient Expectations. Assessment begins with establishing a trusting nurse–patient relationship and then eliciting the patient's needs, values, and preferences for a person-centred assessment. Often the patient's fluid, electrolyte, or acid–base disturbance is so serious that it prevents a review of patient expectations. However, if a patient is alert enough to discuss care, the nurse should explore with the patient their short-term needs (e.g., provision of comfort from nausea) and long-term needs

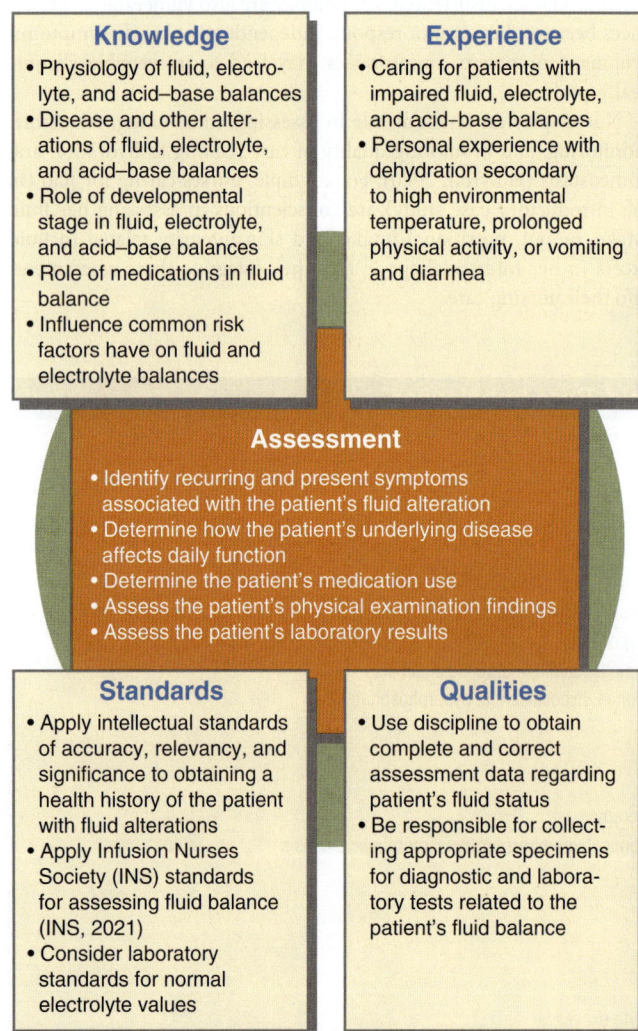

(e.g., understanding how to prevent alterations from occurring in the future). The nurse may also explore patient expectations with family and supportive friends. The patient's trust is strengthened through a competent response to sudden changes in condition and through clear communication with the patient, family members, or both.

Health History. The nursing assessment continues with a nursing health history, which is designed to reveal any risk factors or pre-existing conditions that may cause or contribute to a disturbance of fluid, electrolyte, and acid–base balances. Asking specific, focused questions will elicit the most useful data (Box 41.1).

Age. First, the patient's age is considered. An infant's proportion of total body water, approximately 75%, is greater than that of children or adults. Infants are at a greater risk for **fluid volume deficit (FVD)** and hyperosmolar imbalance because body water loss is proportionately greater per kilogram of weight, and therefore, they have smaller reserves. Assessment of fluid status for newborns is focused on output, often evaluated through number of voids, and assessment of fontanels. Mulder and Gardner (2015) stress that fluid loss is normal in the first few days of life, which contributes to a normal weight loss over the first 3 days of life.

Children ages 2 through 12 years have less stable regulatory responses to imbalance and when ill tend to have less tolerance for large changes. Children's frequent response to illnesses with fevers of higher temperatures and longer duration than those of adults, compounded by their more rapid respiratory rate, increases their insensible water loss. Adolescents have increased metabolic processes and water production because of the major rapid changes that occur during puberty. Adolescent girls experience changes in fluid balance with the hormonal changes associated with the menstrual cycle.

Aging has a significant impact on fluid, electrolyte, and acid–base balances and on older persons' capacity to compensate; therefore, nurses need to be able to identify the risk factors and work to prevent them (Box 41.2). With normal aging, the glomerular filtration rate is reduced because of a decrease in number and functional capacity of nephrons, along with reduced lung capacity because of a decrease in number of alveoli and loss of strength and elasticity in respiratory muscles (Lewis et al., 2023). Older persons have reduced aldosterone, which increases sodium excretion and may result in hyponatremia (Arai et al., 2014). Together these changes in normal aging contribute to an increased risk for fluid, electrolyte, and acid–base imbalances and reduced ability to excrete medication. Box 41.3 outlines evidence-informed nursing practice recommendations based on high-quality research (Arai et al., 2014; Armstrong et al., 2020; Bunn et al., 2015; El-Sharkawy et al., 2015a, 2015b, 2020; Minooee, 2021; Oates & Price, 2017; Shepherd, 2013; Wotton et al., 2008).

Reduced respiratory lung capacity impairs the ability of older persons to compensate for acid–base imbalances and maintain oxygen requirements. All these factors would inform nursing care for Jiao in the introductory case study.

Environmental Factors. Nurses also need to include certain environmental factors in the health history. Patients who have participated in vigorous exercise or are exposed to temperature extremes may have clinical signs of fluid and electrolyte alterations. Exposure to environmental temperatures exceeding 28°C to 30°C results in excessive sweating with weight loss. Excessive sweating with extreme exercise or exposure to high environmental temperatures can result in fluid deficits, hypernatremia, or clinical dehydration, because sweat is a hypotonic sodium-containing fluid.

Diet. The nurse should assess dietary intake (see Box 41.1) and recent changes in appetite or the ability to chew and swallow. It is good to explore if patients follow weight loss diets or gastrointestinal cleansing

---

Knowledge
- Physiology of fluid, electrolyte, and acid–base balances
- Disease and other alterations of fluid, electrolyte, and acid–base balances
- Role of developmental stage in fluid, electrolyte, and acid–base balances
- Role of medications in fluid balance
- Influence common risk factors have on fluid and electrolyte balances

Experience
- Caring for patients with impaired fluid, electrolyte, and acid–base balances
- Personal experience with dehydration secondary to high environmental temperature, prolonged physical activity, or vomiting and diarrhea

Assessment
- Identify recurring and present symptoms associated with the patient's fluid alteration
- Determine how the patient's underlying disease affects daily function
- Determine the patient's medication use
- Assess the patient's physical examination findings
- Assess the patient's laboratory results

Standards
- Apply intellectual standards of accuracy, relevancy, and significance to obtaining a health history of the patient with fluid alterations
- Apply Infusion Nurses Society (INS) standards for assessing fluid balance (INS, 2021)
- Consider laboratory standards for normal electrolyte values

Qualities
- Use discipline to obtain complete and correct assessment data regarding patient's fluid status
- Be responsible for collecting appropriate specimens for diagnostic and laboratory tests related to the patient's fluid balance

FIGURE 41.6 Critical thinking model for assessment of fluid, electrolyte, and acid–base balances.

BOX 41.1	Focused Nursing Assessment Questions

Nature of the Problem
- Are you currently under the care of a health care provider for management of any ongoing health problems, such as kidney or heart disease, diabetes, or blood pressure problems?
- Describe any new problems, such as vomiting, diarrhea, or a surgical procedure.

Signs and Symptoms
- In the past several weeks, have you lost or gained any weight?
- Do you feel thirsty, have a dry mouth or skin, or notice a lack of tears?
- Have you noticed a change in your urine output—decreased volume, dark colour, or concentrated appearance?
- Have you had any recent problems with vomiting or diarrhea? If so, for how long?
- Are you experiencing any problems with swelling of your hands, feet, ankles, or lower legs?
- Do you have difficulty breathing when you lie down at night?
- Have you noticed any dizziness, weakness, cramps, or unusual sensations, such as tingling?
- (Older persons) Have you had any falls in the past few weeks or months?

Severity
- How many times a day do you urinate?
- Do you continue to feel thirsty no matter how much fluid you drink?

- Are you experiencing these symptoms more at night than in the morning?
- Are you having difficulty concentrating or do you feel confused?
- How does this compare with what is normal or usual for you?

Predisposing Factors
- Do you work or exercise in a hot environment?
- How much do you usually drink every day? What type of fluids do you drink? How much alcohol do you drink in a typical week?
- Describe your normal diet. Are you following a weight loss program? Do you use supplements for weight loss, or a salt substitute? What kind of snacks do you eat?
- Have you had any recent changes in your appetite? Have you noticed any changes in the taste of your food? Do you have any difficulty swallowing or chewing?
- Do you take any over-the-counter or prescription medications or herbal remedies?

Effect on the Patient
- How have these symptoms affected you?
- Are you losing sleep, feeling irritable, or having difficulty performing your usual daily tasks?
- What treatments or solutions have you tried to resolve these symptoms?

BOX 41.2	FOCUS ON OLDER PERSONS

Factors Affecting Fluid, Electrolyte, and Acid–Base Balance

- Body composition changes, causing a decreased percentage of body weight as water (50%), reduced thirst response to increased serum osmolality, and other sensory deficits result in increased risk of extracellular fluid volume (ECV) deficit and hyperosmolar dehydration (Arai et al., 2014; El-Sharkawy et al., 2020).
- Some older people restrict fluid intake because of impaired mobility, concerns about bladder control, or loss of taste; this increases their risk of ECV deficit.
- Normal changes in skin elasticity alter skin turgor, even with normal fluid balance; therefore, this is not a reliable indicator of fluid volume deficit (FVD) or dehydration in older persons.
- Age-related changes in cerebral blood flow, the processing of thirst activation, decreased baroreceptor sensitivity to volume deficits, and reduced renal clearance of antidiuretic hormone (ADH) (vasopressin) all combine to decrease thirst and lower fluid intake.

- Baroreceptors become sluggish with age, often causing brief postural hypotension; have older persons arise slowly when taking orthostatic blood pressure measurements.
- Cardiovascular changes with aging often decrease the ability to adapt to a sudden increase in vascular volume, increasing risk of pulmonary edema with rapid infusion of isotonic intravenous fluids.
- Reduced renal function related to changes of normal aging make it more difficult to excrete a large acid load, increasing the risk of metabolic acidosis.
- Increased sensitivity to anticholinergic effects of medications causes dry mouth; use several different assessments for ECV deficit and dehydration rather than relying solely on dry mouth (Burchum & Rosenthal, 2019).
- The combined effects of normal aging, chronic diseases, and multiple medications often pose challenges to maintaining fluid and electrolyte balance.

regimes. When nutritional intake is inadequate, the body tries to preserve its protein stores by breaking down glycogen and fat stores. When excess free fatty acids are released, metabolic acidosis can occur because the liver converts free fatty acids to ketones, which are strong acids. With high-protein diets, ketosis can also occur. After fat and carbohydrate resources are depleted, the body begins to destroy protein stores. Hypoalbuminemia occurs with lack of amino acids in the diet and with liver dysfunction. In hypoalbuminemia, the serum colloid osmotic pressure is decreased, allowing fluid to shift from the circulating plasma to the interstitial fluid spaces. The nurse should also ask about complementary or alternative medicine (CAM) diet supplements or restrictions.

Lifestyle. Patients' history of using inhaled substances or alcohol consumption and of recreational drug use should be explored. These factors can alter the patient's fluid, electrolyte, and acid–base balance. Damage to the liver, kidneys, or lungs can alter compensatory mechanisms. For example, the excessive use of alcohol can

ultimately cause respiratory depression, which can result in respiratory acidosis.

Medication. The nurse should complete a best possible medication history (BPMH) or medication reconciliation (Institute for Safe Medication Practices [ISMP] Canada, 2015), including over-the-counter and herbal preparations (see Box 41.1 and Box 41.4). The nurse should evaluate the potential effects of medications to determine if specific laboratory values need to be assessed, using knowledge of physiology and pharmacology, and pharmacology references. The patient's knowledge of adverse effects and adherence to medication schedules should also be assessed. Nurses caring for Jiao in the introductory case study would have completed a medication reconciliation process to prevent medication errors.

Medical History

Acute Illness. DKA, head and chest trauma, gastrointestinal disturbances, sepsis, shock, and second- or third-degree burns are conditions

BOX 41.3   EVIDENCE-INFORMED PRACTICE

Preventing and Responding to Dehydration in Older Persons*

Evidence Summary

- Dehydration is the most common fluid and electrolyte challenge in older persons and has a very high mortality rate (Minooee, 2021).
- Older persons are at increased risk of illness and death from dehydration, overhydration, and salt overload.
- Reduced thirst sensation and diminished appetite contribute to dehydration in older persons. Older people also have diminished capacity to correct volume losses.
- Chronic dehydration contributes to constipation in older persons.
- Adequate hydration in older persons is recommended for the prevention of falls, possibly related to hypotension or postural hypotension.
- Dehydration is a risk factor for delirium. The risk for delirium can be reduced as much as 33% with each additional glass of water consumed (El-Sharkawy et al., 2015a).
- Signs and symptoms of dehydration can be easily confused with normal aging processes; therefore, assessment requires knowledge, skill, and commitment to acting on signs and symptoms.

Nursing Practice Guidelines

- Calculating fluid requirements should take into consideration individual characteristics, including weight, gender, environmental factors, physical activity, and comorbidities, such as renal and cardiac disease.
- Because older persons are more susceptible to dehydration and have a higher rate of mortality from dehydration, early detection of infection and disorders in fluid balance is very important (Shepherd, 2013).
- Identify risk factors for each older person from the following: age over 70 years, female, high or low body mass index, recent hospitalization, new admission to long-term care, situations causing increased insensible loss (pyrexia), decreased access or ability to request fluids, and situations causing decreased intake, such as swallowing disorder (dysphagia), physical frailty, and decreased sentience. Previous malnutrition, dehydration, polypharmacy, and having more than three medical conditions are significant risk factors.
- Establish an assessment, monitoring, and evaluation tool for identifying risk factors for older persons when initiating a caregiving relationship (e.g., on admission to long-term care; with home assessment of older persons; routine health care visits).
- Assessment of hydration status should include physiological measures (urine colour, blood pressure, pulse, and respiration) as well as observed intake patterns and treatments. Recommend blood testing to determine the cause and severity in suspected dehydration.
- Maintain fluid intake through documented planning using the nursing process in home, long-term care, and hospital settings, offering fluids every 1.5 hours (Minooee, 2021) to meet a daily fluid intake goal. Caffeinated beverages can be offered, in addition to water.
- Educate older persons and their family and friends on the importance of hydration.
- Diarrhea and vomiting are key causes of dehydration in older persons. Evaluate acute losses such as diarrhea and vomiting.
- Attend more diligently to fluid balance in the context of medical issues such as diabetes, with the use of diuretics, with decreased cognitive level or functional status, and with reduced level of consciousness.
- Minimize fasting for diagnostics and procedures (Minooee, 2021).
- Ensure availability of adequate fluids, including water, tea, coffee, milk, and other beverages, throughout the day and assist persons who are unable to access their own fluids. Replenish and refresh fluids through the day.
- Advocate for adequate staffing levels in long-term care and acute care facilities, as inadequate staffing is closely linked to increased mortality (Shepherd, 2013).
- Promote audits of hydration practices and barriers or obstacles in health care settings and identify benchmarks for improved practice.
- Ongoing management consists of daily fluid goals, comparing current intake with physiological needs, and monitoring actual consumption of fluids and fluid-rich foods.
- Incorporate the offer of fluids, hot or cold, into regular rounds, socializing, and aspects of care using the "little and often" approach. Offer assistive devices, such as drinking straws or feeder cups, as necessary.
- Fluid status documentation should include hydration, eating habits, weight, vital signs, and fluid preferences.

*Dehydration is defined variably. Shepherd (2013) defines dehydration as equal to or greater than 1% loss of body mass through fluid loss. See text and Tables 41.3 and 41.4 for exploration of dehydration and tonicity.

---

that place patients at high risk for fluid, electrolyte, and acid–base alterations. When obtaining a medical history, it is important to review any allergies. Treatment for fluid, electrolyte, and acid–base imbalances may involve exposure to latex in equipment and supplies. With newborns and infants, the nurse needs to assess the mother for known latex allergy to prevent inadvertent exposure to latex sensitization.

Burns. The burned patient can lose body fluids by many routes. The greater the body surface burned, the greater the fluid loss. Burns can result in a plasma-to-interstitial fluid shift. Plasma and interstitial fluids are also lost as burn exudate. Water vapour and heat are lost in proportion to the amount of skin that is burned away, increasing insensible losses. Blood leaks from damaged capillaries, adding to the loss of intravascular fluid volume. Sodium and water shift into the cells, further compromising ECF volume (Lewis et al., 2023). Cell damage is accompanied by a loss of serum proteins, and a release of potassium into the intravascular fluid.

Respiratory disorders. Many alterations in respiratory function predispose the patient to respiratory acidosis. For example, pneumonia or sedative overdose interferes with the elimination of carbon dioxide due to hypoventilation. As the carbon dioxide continues to build up in the bloodstream, the body's compensatory mechanisms can no longer adapt, and the pH decreases. Likewise, hyperventilation that occurs with conditions such as fever or anxiety can cause respiratory alkalosis when too much carbon dioxide is expelled with the increased respiratory rate.

Gastrointestinal disturbances. Gastroenteritis and nasogastric suctioning result in a loss of fluid, potassium, and chloride ions. Hydrogen ions are also lost, resulting in metabolic alkalosis. In contrast, loss of bicarbonate-rich intestinal or pancreatic fluids (diarrhea, fistulas) can cause metabolic acidosis and also hypokalemia. Timely education of infant and child caregivers is necessary to prevent clinical dehydration when the infant or child is experiencing diarrhea.

Trauma. Trauma resulting in hemorrhage causes FVD or hypovolemia. In addition, crush injuries causing cellular damage bring about a massive release of potassium into the intravascular fluid, causing hyperkalemia.

Head injury. Head injury can result in cerebral edema. Occasionally, this edema creates pressure on the pituitary gland and, as a result, ADH secretion is changed. Diabetes insipidus occurs when too little ADH is secreted and the patient excretes large volumes of diluted urine

BOX 41.4 Medications That Cause Fluid, Electrolyte, and Acid–Base Disturbances

- ACE inhibitors (e.g., captopril [Capoten]) and angiotensin II receptor blockers (e.g., Losartan [Cozaar]): Hyperkalemia
- Antidepressants, SSRIs (e.g., fluoxetine [Prozac]): Hyponatremia
- Calcium carbonate antacids: Hypercalcemia, mild metabolic alkalosis
- Corticosteroids (e.g., prednisone): Hypokalemia, metabolic alkalosis
- Diuretics, potassium-wasting (e.g., furosemide [Lasix], thiazides): ECV deficit, hyponatremia (thiazides), hypokalemia, hypomagnesemia, mild metabolic alkalosis
- Diuretics, potassium-sparing (e.g., spironolactone [Aldactone]): Hyperkalemia, mild metabolic acidosis
- Effervescent (fizzy) antacids and cold medications (high Na^+ content): ECV excess
- Laxatives: ECV deficit, hypokalemia, hypocalcemia, hypomagnesemia, metabolic acidosis
- Magnesium hydroxide (e.g., Milk of Magnesia): Hypermagnesemia
- Nonsteroidal anti-inflammatory drugs (e.g., ibuprofen [Advil]): Mild ECV excess, hyponatremia
- High-dose penicillins (e.g., carbenicillin): Hypokalemia, metabolic alkalosis; hyperkalemia with penicillin G (contains K^+)

ACE, Angiotensin-converting enzyme; *ECV*, extracellular fluid volume; *SSRI*, selective serotonin reuptake inhibitor.
Data from Burchum, J. R., & Rosenthal, L. D. (2019). *Lehne's pharmacology for nursing care* (10th ed.). Elsevier.

with a low specific gravity. Syndrome of inappropriate antidiuretic hormone (SIADH) results in water intoxication characterized by fluid volume expansion and hyponatremia, as well as hypotonicity of fluids as a result of high urine osmolality and low serum osmolality (Marieb & Hoehn, 2019).

Recent surgery. After surgery, patients can exhibit many acid–base changes. The more extensive the surgery and fluid loss are during the surgical procedure, the greater the body's response is to the surgical trauma. The patient who is reluctant to breathe deeply and cough may develop respiratory acidosis as a result of retained $PaCO_2$. The patient with nasogastric suction may develop metabolic alkalosis as a result of the loss of gastric acid, fluids, and electrolytes. In addition, the stress response of surgery may cause fluid shifts postoperatively when aldosterone, glucocorticoids, and ADH are increasingly secreted, causing sodium and chloride retention, potassium excretion, and decreased urinary output.

Chronic Illness. Chronic disease (e.g., diabetes mellitus, cancer, heart failure, or renal disease) can create fluid, electrolyte, and acid–base imbalances. The normal course of the patient's chronic disease is important to know in order to anticipate how fluid, electrolyte, and acid–base status may be affected.

Diabetes mellitus. Diabetes mellitus (DM)—both type 1 and type 2—and metabolic syndrome can lead to significant fluid and electrolyte disturbances. DKA is an acute complication of type 1 DM (most commonly) and results in hypovolemia (FVD), increased potassium, and metabolic acidosis. Hyperosmolar hyperglycemic state (HHS), an acute complication of type 2 DM, causes osmotic diuresis, leading to hypovolemia, and some electrolyte imbalances may also occur. Older persons with reduced thirst sensation are particularly vulnerable to HHS (Lewis et al., 2023). Nephropathy, a chronic complication of DM, is the leading cause of end-stage renal disease in Canada (Lewis et al., 2023).

Cancer. The types of fluid and electrolyte imbalances that are observed in a patient with cancer depend on the type and progression of the cancer and the related treatment. The potential electrolyte imbalances result from anatomical distortion and functional impairment from tumour growth or from tumour-related metabolic and endocrine abnormalities. Hypercalcemia can result when cancer cells secrete chemicals that prompt the release of calcium from the bone. Anorexia, stomatitis, and diarrhea, adverse effects of some chemotherapy or radiation, create risks for many imbalances.

Cardiovascular disease. In the patient with cardiovascular disease, diminished cardiac output reduces kidney perfusion, causing the patient to experience a decrease in urinary output. The patient will retain sodium and water, resulting in circulatory overload, and is at risk of developing pulmonary edema. Fluid and electrolyte imbalances associated with heart disease can be controlled with medications and with fluid and sodium restrictions.

Renal disorders. Kidney disease alters fluid and electrolyte balances by the abnormal retention of sodium, chloride, potassium, and water in the extracellular compartment. The plasma levels of metabolic waste products such as urea and creatinine are elevated because the kidneys are unable to filter and excrete the waste products of cellular metabolism. This elevation is toxic to cellular processes. Metabolic acidosis results when hydrogen ions are retained because of decreased renal function. Because of the renal disorder, the usual renal compensatory mechanisms, such as bicarbonate reabsorption, are not available; therefore, the body's ability to restore normal acid–base balance is limited.

The severity of fluid and electrolyte imbalance is proportional to the degree of renal failure. Acute kidney injury is reversible. Although chronic kidney disease is progressive, the patient may be treated successfully with dietary control of protein and salt intake, diuretic medications, and fluid restrictions. In end-stage renal disease, treatment with dialysis, transplantation, or both may be required.

Gastrointestinal disorders. Chronic gastrointestinal disorders can have a serious impact on fluid, electrolyte, and acid–base balances. Inflammatory bowel diseases, such as ulcerative colitis, regional enteritis, and celiac disease, are relatively common. Patients with liver failure may have several imbalances, including metabolic acidosis, ECF shifts in the case of ascites, and electrolyte disturbances. Key gastrointestinal assessments include the length of the illness, the presence of exacerbations if there is inflammatory bowel disease, and the type of treatment currently being administered. It is important to determine whether the patient has a history of acute illnesses such as diarrhea or vomiting. Any condition that results in the loss of gastrointestinal fluids predisposes the patient to the development of dehydration and a variety of electrolyte disturbances.

Physical Assessment. A thorough physical examination (see Chapter 31) is necessary because fluid and electrolyte imbalances or acid–base disturbances can affect all body systems. When conducting a physical examination, nurses need to incorporate knowledge regarding the signs and symptoms of fluid, electrolyte, and acid–base imbalances; disease processes that may affect these balances; developmental considerations; and common risk factors (see Table 41.7). For example, an examination of the oral cavity may reveal signs of dehydration. Table 41.8 outlines nursing assessment findings and links these to fluid, electrolyte, and acid–base imbalances; these findings can be used to inform the nurses caring for Jiao in the introductory case study. Nurses use orthostatic (postural) vital signs to assess the cardiovascular system as well as fluid volume (see Chapter 40). Orthostatic hypotension (a drop of systolic blood pressure [SBP] of 20 mm Hg or diastolic blood pressure [DBP] 10 mm Hg on standing for 3 minutes) may indicate FVD and can result in dizziness, syncope, or falls.

Assessing Fluid Intake and Output. Assessing fluid balance involves knowledge of normal fluid requirements and accurate measurement

TABLE 41.8   Focused Nursing Assessments and Relevant Imbalances

Assessment Technique	Assessment Findings (Adult)	Imbalances
Assess Daily Weight		
	Loss of 1 kg/24 hours or more	ECV deficit (FVD)
	Gain of 1 kg/24 hours or more	ECV excess (FVE)
Clinical Markers of Vascular Volume		
Blood pressure	Hypotension or orthostatic hypotension	ECV deficit
	Lightheadedness on sitting upright or standing	ECV deficit
Pulse rate and character	Rapid, thready	ECV deficit
	Bounding	ECV excess
Neck veins	Flat or collapsing with inhalation when supine	ECV deficit
	Distended when upright or semi-upright	ECV excess
Capillary refill	>2 seconds	ECV deficit (causing poor perfusion)
Lung auscultation	Crackles or wheezing	ECV excess
Urine output	<30–50 mL/hr	ECV deficit
Physical Assessment (Objective)		
Visual assessment (head to toe)	Edema in dependent areas (ankles or sacrum), fingers or around eyes	ECV excess
Mucous membranes	Dry tongue and oral membranes; decreased or absent tearing	ECV deficit
Skin assessment	Pinched skin fails to return to normal position within 3 seconds (poor skin turgor); not a reliable indicator in older persons	ECV deficit
Behaviour and Level of Consciousness		
	Restlessness, mild confusion	Severe ECV deficit
	Lethargy, confusion, coma	Hyponatremia, hypernatremia, hypercalcemia, acid–base imbalances
Cardiac and Respiratory		
Pulse rhythm and ECG (electrocardiogram)	Irregular pulse and ECG changes	K^+, Ca^{2+}, Mg^{2+}, and/or acid–base imbalances
Rate and depth of respirations	Increased	Metabolic acidosis (compensatory mechanism); respiratory alkalosis (cause)
	Decreased	Metabolic alkalosis (compensatory mechanism); respiratory acidosis (cause)
Neuromuscular Assessment		
Muscle strength bilaterally	Muscle weakness, especially quadriceps muscles	Hypokalemia, hyperkalemia
Reflexes and sensations	Decreased deep tendon reflexes	Hypercalcemia, hypermagnesemia
	Hyperactive reflexes, muscle twitching and cramps, tetany	Hypocalcemia, hypomagnesemia
	Numbness, tingling in fingertips, around mouth	Hypocalcemia, hypomagnesemia, respiratory alkalosis
	Muscle cramps, tetany	Hypocalcemia, hypomagnesemia, respiratory alkalosis
	Tremors	Hypomagnesemia
Gastrointestinal Assessment		
Inspection and auscultation	Edematous abdomen (ascites)	Third-spacing of fluid (shift in fluid)
	Decreased bowel sounds	Hypokalemia
Motility	Constipation	Hypokalemia, hypercalcemia
Thirst	Presence of thirst	Hypernatremia, severe ECV deficit

ECV, Extracellular fluid volume; *FVD,* fluid volume deficit; *FVE,* fluid volume excess.

techniques, and is critical to person-centred care in the acute care setting (Holroyd, 2020; McGloin, 2015). Inadequate fluid management, including inaccurate calculations of fluid balance, is considered a common barrier to safety, according to many reports (Holroyd, 2020). Therefore, the nurses caring for Jiao in the introductory case study establish methods for everyone involved in Jiao's care to record her fluid intake for each shift. Measuring and recording fluid intake and output over a 24-hour period is a fundamental aspect of fluid balance

assessment. A fluid balance chart (FBC) includes all intake (e.g., by mouth, intravenous solutions) and output (e.g., urine, nasogastric drainage) and the 24-hour balance (deficit or excess) or summary. An FBC should include the time of intake or output and accurate amounts (Holroyd, 2020). An FBC, used in conjunction with physical assessment, is an essential component of fluid monitoring across health care settings. Recognition of trends in intake and output is also important to recognizing and responding to problems promptly. Nurses can play a leadership role on the interprofessional team to promote, complete, and report accurate fluid status.

Daily weight is considered an accurate means to evaluate fluid balance and guide the interprofessional team, while a combination of weights and fluid balance is considered the most effective means (Crawford et al., 2018; Holroyd, 2020). For daily weights, such as with Jiao in the introductory case study, the patient should be weighed at the same time each day with the same scale after the patient voids. The patient should wear the same clothes (or clothes that weigh the same); if a bed scale is being used to weigh the patient, there should be the same number of sheets on the bed with each weighing. Patients with chronic health issues can learn to monitor their own fluid balance through weighing themselves daily, recording their weights, and reporting changes. Health care providers may direct patients with parameters and preferred action. Jiao (case study) will be using her daily weights on discharge. An increase in her weight would trigger contact with a health care provider, and potentially additional or changes to her medication. One kilogram of body weight gain over up to 7 days can be generally equated with 1 litre of fluid gain or loss (Holroyd, 2020). Refer to Table 41.8 for interpretation of significant findings.

Intake includes all liquids taken by mouth (e.g., gelatin, ice cream, soup, juice, and water) or through nasogastric or jejunostomy feeding tubes, intravenous fluids (including both continuous and intermittent intravenous fluids), and blood or its components. Some persons have swallowing difficulty so a thickened fluid diet may be required (see the Safety Alert in Chapter 43 [Nutrition]). The volume of fluid thickened is the same volume recorded for intake. For persons in institutional settings (e.g., long-term care, acute care), refer to agency standards for accurate volume for container size. A patient receiving tube feedings may receive numerous liquid medications and water may be used to flush the tube. Over a 24-hour period, these liquids can amount to significant intake and should always be recorded on the intake and output record. Output includes urine, diarrhea, vomitus, gastric suction, and drainage from postsurgical wounds or other tubes (see Chapter 49). Daily intake should equal output plus 500 mL (to cover for insensible fluid losses).

To measure output, ambulatory patients are instructed to save their urine in a calibrated receptacle that attaches to the rim of the toilet bowl. When a patient has an in-dwelling urinary catheter, drainage tube, or suction, output is recorded at predetermined times depending on the patient's condition and prescribers' orders. Patient and family cooperation is essential for accurate intake and output measurements. The patient and the family must be taught the purpose of the measurements, including oral intake. Electronic or paper forms are used to ensure consistent recording of intake and output by nurses or unregulated care providers. This recording must be accurate, and estimation is not acceptable for safe provision of care. Including fluid balance in handover reporting can improve consistency and quality of care for patients (Holroyd, 2020).

Laboratory Studies. Nurses need to review laboratory data, including serum and urinary electrolyte levels, hematocrit, blood creatinine level, blood urea nitrogen (BUN) levels, and urine specific gravity. Estimated glomerular filtration rate (eGFR), a calculation based on serum creatinine and demographic data, reflects renal function. While eGFR has been calculated on the basis of age, sex, and race, emerging evidence is informing work to find clinically feasible methods to estimate GFR excluding race (Zelnick et al., 2021). The eGFR is helpful for recognizing and monitoring renal disease, both acute and chronic. Serum electrolyte levels are measured to determine the hydration status, the electrolyte concentration of the blood plasma, and acid–base balance. The frequency with which these electrolyte levels are measured depends on the severity of the patient's illness. Serum electrolyte tests are routinely performed on any patient entering a hospital to screen for alterations and to serve as a baseline for future comparisons. Serum and urine osmolality are also used to assess fluid balance (Arai et al., 2014; El-Sharkaway et al., 2020). Other laboratory tests include brain natriuretic peptide (BNP) or atrial natriuretic peptide (ANP) to assist in diagnosing the cause of fluid volume excess. These are all diagnostic tests that may be conducted for Jiao from the introductory case study.

Arterial Blood Gases. To determine ABG levels, a sample of blood from an artery is taken to assess the patient's acid–base status and the adequacy of ventilation and oxygenation. Arterial blood is drawn from a peripheral artery (usually the radial artery) or from an arterial line, usually in critical care, operative, or emergency situations. After the specimen is obtained, care is taken to prevent air from entering the syringe because this will affect the ABG analysis. The syringe should be transported to the laboratory immediately. In the event of a delay of more than 20 minutes, the syringe is submerged in crushed ice for transport to the laboratory to reduce the metabolism of cells. Pressure is applied to the puncture site for at least 5 minutes to reduce the risk of hematoma formation.

Other Diagnostic Tests. A chest x-ray is commonly performed to assess patients for fluid in the lungs and to evaluate the heart and lung. An electrocardiogram is an important diagnostic test to assess cardiac status, and to determine cardiac rhythm abnormalities related to electrolyte imbalances (see Chapter 40). Microalbumin (MA), measured from a urine specimen, is a reliable test for renal disease. Microalbuminuria, greater than 2 mg/L, reflects early changes to the glomeruli and is a common screening test.

◆ Nursing Diagnosis

When caring for patients with suspected fluid, electrolyte, and acid–base imbalances, nurses use critical thinking to formulate nursing diagnoses. The assessment data that establish the risk for or the actual presence of a nursing diagnosis in these areas may be subtle, and patterns and trends emerge only when nurses conscientiously assess for them. Nurses must keep in mind that many body systems may be involved. Clustering of defining characteristics will lead nurses to select the appropriate diagnoses. For example, the nursing diagnosis *deficient fluid volume* is developed to demonstrate the nursing diagnostic process in Box 41.5.

An important part of formulating nursing diagnoses is identifying the relevant causative or related factor. Nursing interventions are chosen to treat or modify the related factor. *Fluid volume deficit related to loss of gastrointestinal fluids via vomiting* requires therapies different from those needed for *fluid volume deficit related to elevated body temperature.*

BOX 41.5 NURSING DIAGNOSTIC PROCESS
Deficient Fluid Volume (Adult)

Assessment Activities	Defining Characteristics
Assess blood pressure and pulse (orthostatic blood pressure)	Patient is hypotensive, with increased heart rate
Obtain daily weight measurements	Patient experiences sudden weight loss of up to 1 kg or more in 24 hours
Observe volume of urine output and measure intake and specific gravity	Decreased volume of output in comparison to intake; increased urine specific gravity is present
Assess skin turgor	Inelastic skin turgor noted
Ask if patient is thirsty or weak	Patient verbalizes thirst and weakness
Inspect mucous membranes for degree of moisture	Dry mucous membranes are noted

Possible nursing diagnoses for patients with fluid, electrolyte, and acid–base alterations include the following:
- *Fluid volume alteration*
- *Actual or risk of fluid volume deficit or hypovolemia*
- *Actual or risk of fluid volume excess or hypervolemia*
- *Electrolyte imbalance*
- *Impaired gas exchange*
- *Actual or risk of impaired skin integrity*
- *Ineffective therapeutic regimen management*
- *Lack of knowledge of fluid volume (or fluid regimen)*

◆ Planning

During the planning process, nurses synthesize information from multiple sources and to ensure that the patient's care plan integrates both scientific and nursing knowledge, the nurse's knowledge of the individual, and the patient's expectations (Figure 41.7).

Goals and Outcomes. The nurse develops an individual care plan for the nursing diagnoses (see Box 41.5 and Box 41.6). Goals or expectations for care set by the nurse and the patient should be individualized and realistic, with measurable outcomes, and developed

in a person-centred manner. For example, if the goal is to achieve and maintain homeostasis, the following related outcomes might be established:
- The patient will have normal fluid and electrolyte balance at discharge.
- The patient will be free of complications associated with the intravenous therapy.
- The patient will demonstrate fluid balance with moist, mucous membranes and good skin turgor.
- The patient will have serum electrolytes within the normal range within 48 hours.

Setting Priorities. The patient's clinical condition will determine which diagnosis takes priority. Many nursing diagnoses in the area of fluid, electrolyte, and acid–base balances are of highest priority because the consequences for the patient can be serious or even life-threatening. For example, in the concept map for a patient with gastroenteritis and dehydration (Figure 41.8), nausea and diarrhea caused a fluid volume deficit and electrolyte imbalances. Without treating the cause, the fluid, electrolyte, and acid–base imbalances will continue and progress.

Teamwork and Collaboration. Consultation with the patient's primary health care provider may assist in setting realistic time frames for the goals of care, particularly when the patient's physiological status is unstable. During planning, it is important to collaborate as much as possible with the patient, family, and other members of the interprofessional health care team. Family can be particularly helpful in identifying subtle changes in a patient's behaviour associated with imbalances (e.g., anxiety, confusion, or irritability).

For patients in acute care, discharge planning must begin early. The nurse must ensure that care can continue in the home or residential care setting with few disruptions. For example, when a patient is discharged on intravenous therapy, the nurse must determine the knowledge and skills of the person who is to assume caregiving responsibilities and make a referral for home intravenous therapy as soon as possible (Box 41.7). The nurse must also collaborate closely with other members of the health care team, such as the dietitian, pharmacist, and physician. In consultation with a dietitian, the nurse can recommend foods to increase intake of certain electrolytes or reduce intake as necessary (see Chapter 43). The pharmacist can help identify medications likely to cause electrolyte or acid–base disturbances and describe possible adverse effects of the patient's prescribed drugs. The physician directs the treatment of any fluid, electrolyte, or acid–base alteration.

Infusion Therapy Team. Managing fluid, electrolyte, and acid–base imbalances often involves infusion therapy or vascular access teams (VAT). The Infusion Nurses Society (INS) has developed standards of practice based on systematic review of the current evidence (Gorski et al., 2021). These standards, reviewed and published regularly, are a key source for standards to inform decision making (see Figure 41.7). Vascular access device (VAD) insertion, maintenance, and surveillance for quality improvement are conducted by individuals and teams with infusion therapy education, training, and validated competency (Gorski et al., 2021). Having a specialized team for VADs, including peripheral catheters, improves patient outcomes (e.g., reduced infections), comfort (e.g., reduced number of unsuccessful attempts to initiate a VAD), satisfaction, and persons' vessel health and preservation (Fiorini et al. 2019; Gorski et al., 2021). Evidence suggests that use of a VAT for VAD insertion reduces patients' experience of pain significantly (Fujioka et al., 2020).

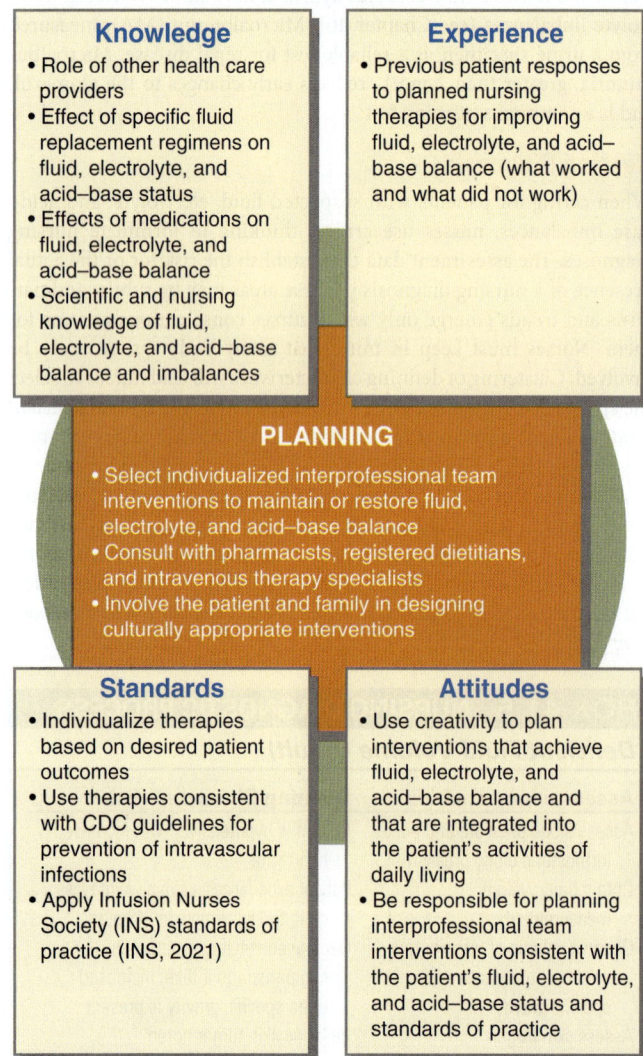

FIGURE 41.7 Critical thinking model for fluid, electrolyte, and acid–base balances planning. *CDC,* Centers for Disease Control and Prevention.

BOX 41.6 NURSING CARE PLAN

Fluid Volume Deficit

ASSESSMENT

Hilda Beck (pronouns: they/their) is a 72-year-old seen by their health care provider this morning after falling at home and telephoning a neighbour for assistance. They live alone in an apartment and have no chronic disease except for osteoarthritis of their hands. They have had diarrhea and vomiting for over 24 hours and have not eaten anything. Despite feeling slightly nauseated, they have tried to drink a little water, because they knew they needed fluid. Hilda is admitted for intravenous (IV) fluid therapy. X-ray films indicate they have no broken bones. Review of laboratory findings: hematocrit 55% (hemoconcentration caused by hypovolemia); sodium 148 mmol/L, and potassium 3 mmol/L. (Note: Hilda has hypokalemia in addition to extracellular fluid volume [ECV] deficit and hypernatremia [clinical dehydration].)

Assessment Activities	Findings/Defining Characteristics*
Ask Hilda to describe when their vomiting and diarrhea began and any accompanying signs and symptoms.	Hilda states that their gastrointestinal (GI) problems began suddenly yesterday and that they *get weak and lightheaded when they stand or sit upright*, which is why they fell. Hilda feels *weak* and has a *dry mouth*.
Ask about the current status of vomiting and diarrhea.	Hilda says they were still vomiting earlier this morning. They have not done so for the past 3 hours. They feel slightly nauseated. They have had three episodes of watery diarrhea this morning and more than six yesterday.
Assess Hilda's vital signs.	*Apical heart rate is 110 beats/min* with regular rhythm. Radial pulse is *weak; supine blood pressure (BP) is 90/58*. Temperature and respirations are within normal limits. Postural BP measurement is not taken since patient says that they *get lightheaded when they sit upright*.
Evaluate physical signs of ECV.	Neck veins are flat when they are supine; *100 mL of dark yellow urine* in past 4 hours; dry mucous membranes between cheek and gum; prolonged capillary refill time of 5 seconds.
Weigh the patient using a bed scale.	Weight is 55.5 kg. They state that usual weight at home is 58.5 kg (*3 kg weight loss*).

*Defining characteristics are shown in italics.

NURSING DIAGNOSIS: Deficient fluid volume related to increased output of GI fluids from vomiting and diarrhea

PLANNING

Goals (Nursing Outcomes Classification)[†]	Expected Outcomes
Fluid Balance	
Patient's fluid volume will return to normal by hospital discharge.	Heart rate and BP return to normal within 24 hours.
	Within 24 hours, Hilda does not report lightheadedness when sitting or standing.
	Urine colour becomes light yellow within 24 hours.
	Daily urine output equals intake of at least 1 500 mL by discharge.
Patient will describe how to manage fluid balance at home before hospital discharge.	Hilda describes how to replace GI fluid loss with fluids that contain sodium.
	Patient describes signs and symptoms indicating need to increase fluid and sodium intake.

[†]Outcome classification labels from Moorhead, S., Swanson, E., Johnson, M., et al. (2018). *Nursing outcomes classification (NOC)* (6th ed.). Mosby/Elsevier.

INTERVENTIONS

Interventions (Nursing Interventions Classification)[‡]	Rationale
Fluid/Electrolyte Management	
Provide Hilda with their favourite fluids at their preferred temperature.	Patient-centred care takes individual preferences into account. In contrast to popular belief, moderate amounts of caffeinated beverages are not likely to have an excessive diuretic effect (Shepherd, 2013).
Provide a pitcher and glass of water at the preferred temperature at their bedside; ensure they can access and pour from it easily; provide straw if they wish.	Weakness or chronic disease such as osteoarthritis of hands may make it difficult to manipulate a full water pitcher. Make fluid available in a form that is easy for the patient to access.
Administer IV therapy as prescribed, monitoring closely for early adverse effects of complications.	IV fluid replacement augments oral replacement when ECV deficit exists. Age-appropriate care is needed because of older persons' anatomical and physiological changes that affect volume delivery (Gorski et al., 2021).
Discuss different ways to prevent and treat dehydration at home. Provide written handout of information.	Patient education is enhanced when the nurse uses multiple senses during teaching sessions (see Chapter 21).

[‡]Intervention classification labels from Bulechek, G. M., Butcher, H. K., McCloskey Dochterman, J. M., et al. (2019). *Nursing interventions classification (NIC)* (7th ed.). Mosby.

BOX 41.6   NURSING CARE PLAN—cont'd

EVALUATION

Nursing Actions

Monitor vital signs, intake and output (I&O), daily weight, and orthostatic vital signs when no longer lightheaded.

Assess neck vein fullness when supine.

Assess mucous membranes.

Evaluate effectiveness of teaching regarding maintaining fluid balance at home.

Patient Response and Finding

T 37°C, RR 10, HR 72 beats/min, BP 120/78 sitting, 122/78 standing, denies lightheadedness

Intake 2 000 mL, output 2 000 mL of light yellow urine

Today's weight: 58.5 kg

Neck veins full when supine; mucous membranes moist

Hilda identified salty broth and commercial electrolyte replacement fluids for replacing GI fluid loss and indicated the need to increase their intake if their urine becomes dark yellow or they become lightheaded when sitting upright.

Achievement of Outcome

Vital signs have returned to normal range. There is no postural hypotension.

I&O measurements are balanced, urine is light yellow.

Daily weight has returned to their normal weight. Additional markers of ECV are normal.

Hilda describes effective home management of fluid balance.

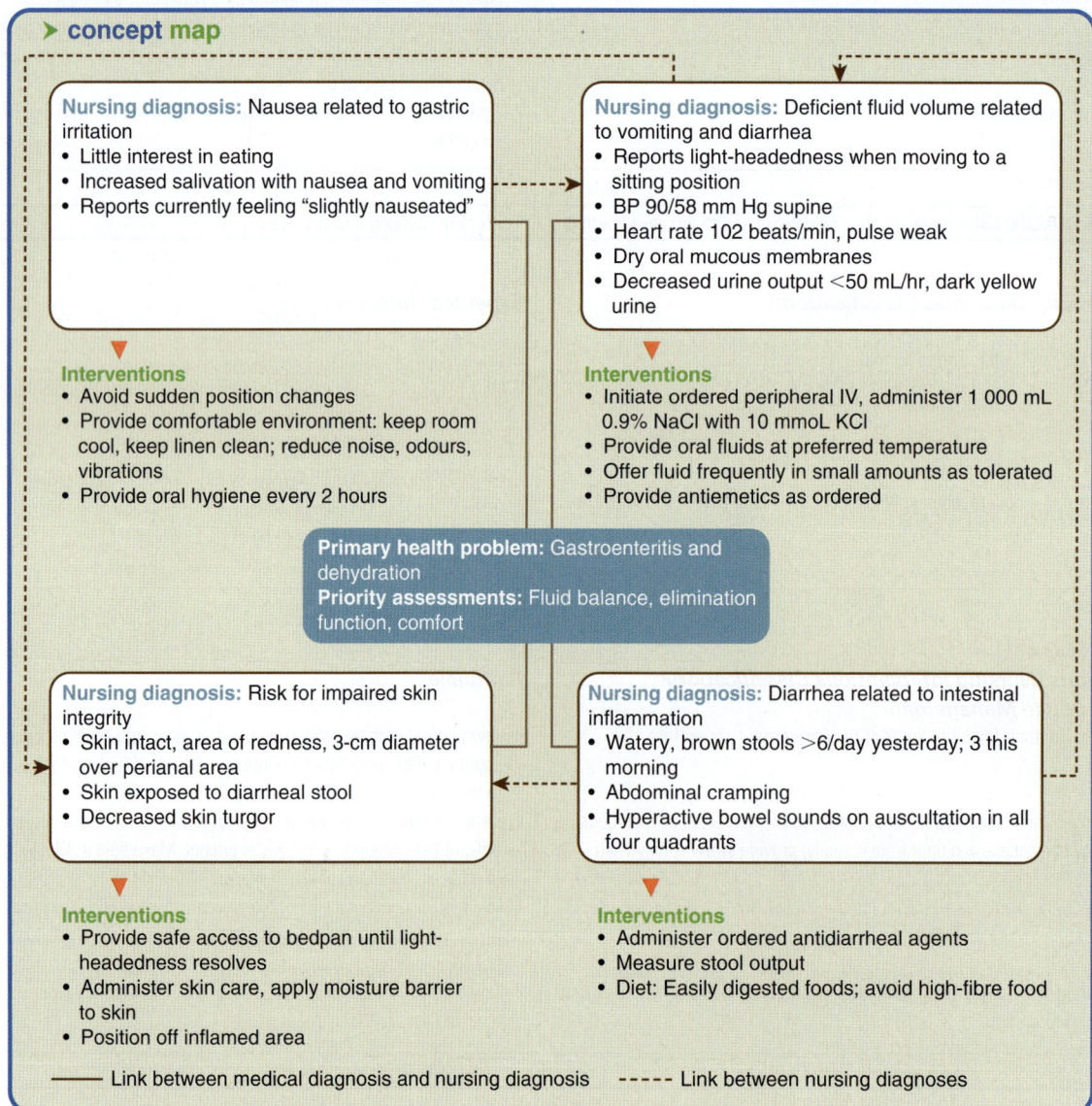

> **concept map**

Nursing diagnosis: Nausea related to gastric irritation
- Little interest in eating
- Increased salivation with nausea and vomiting
- Reports currently feeling "slightly nauseated"

Interventions
- Avoid sudden position changes
- Provide comfortable environment: keep room cool, keep linen clean; reduce noise, odours, vibrations
- Provide oral hygiene every 2 hours

Nursing diagnosis: Deficient fluid volume related to vomiting and diarrhea
- Reports light-headedness when moving to a sitting position
- BP 90/58 mm Hg supine
- Heart rate 102 beats/min, pulse weak
- Dry oral mucous membranes
- Decreased urine output <50 mL/hr, dark yellow urine

Interventions
- Initiate ordered peripheral IV, administer 1 000 mL 0.9% NaCl with 10 mmoL KCl
- Provide oral fluids at preferred temperature
- Offer fluid frequently in small amounts as tolerated
- Provide antiemetics as ordered

Primary health problem: Gastroenteritis and dehydration
Priority assessments: Fluid balance, elimination function, comfort

Nursing diagnosis: Risk for impaired skin integrity
- Skin intact, area of redness, 3-cm diameter over perianal area
- Skin exposed to diarrheal stool
- Decreased skin turgor

Interventions
- Provide safe access to bedpan until light-headedness resolves
- Administer skin care, apply moisture barrier to skin
- Position off inflamed area

Nursing diagnosis: Diarrhea related to intestinal inflammation
- Watery, brown stools >6/day yesterday; 3 this morning
- Abdominal cramping
- Hyperactive bowel sounds on auscultation in all four quadrants

Interventions
- Administer ordered antidiarrheal agents
- Measure stool output
- Diet: Easily digested foods; avoid high-fibre food

——— Link between medical diagnosis and nursing diagnosis   - - - - - Link between nursing diagnoses

FIGURE 41.8 Concept map for a patient with gastroenteritis and dehydration. *BP,* Blood pressure.

BOX 41.7 PATIENT TEACHING

Home Intravenous Therapy

Objective

- The patient, family caregiver, or both will demonstrate competence with administering intravenous (IV) therapy safely in the home.

Teaching Strategies

- Explain the purpose of IV therapy.
- Emphasize the risks involved when the IV system is not kept sterile.
- Be sure that the patient or family caregiver can manipulate the required equipment.
- Instruct them in hand hygiene and aseptic non-touch technique (ANNT) in the handling of all IV equipment.
- Teach them how to change IV solutions and tubing.
- Teach procedures for safe disposal in appropriate containers of all sharps and IV materials exposed to blood. Keep sharps containers away from children (see Chapter 35).
- Instruct patient and caregiver to apply pressure with sterile gauze if the catheter falls out until bleeding stops and then cover with sterile dressing.
- Instruct patient and caregiver about signs and symptoms of infiltration, phlebitis, and infection and reporting symptoms immediately.
- Instruct patient and family caregiver to report if the infusion slows or stops or if blood is seen in the tubing.

- Provide resources related to infusion therapy, such as monographs (for example, Institute for Safe Medication Practices [ISMP] Canada, 2016).
- Teach patient with family caregiver's assistance how to ambulate, perform hygiene, and participate in other activities of daily living without dislodging or disconnecting catheter and tubing:
  - For showering, protect the IV site and dressing from getting wet by covering it completely with plastic. If using an electronic infusion device, unplug around water.
  - Avoid pressure on the IV site and avoid trauma to the site when changing clothes.
  - Have patient avoid strenuous exercise of the arm with the IV catheter insertion.

Evaluation

- Ask patient and family caregiver the purpose of the infusion.
- Ask what they will do if the IV infusion stops.
- Ask patient and family caregiver to describe signs and symptoms of complications and the action they should take.
- Observe patient or family caregiver changing the IV container, tubing, and dressing and provide feedback.
- Observe the patient ambulating and participating in activities of daily living and provide feedback regarding protecting the IV catheter and equipment.

◆ Implementation

Health Promotion. Health promotion activities regarding fluid, electrolyte, and acid–base imbalances include patient education regarding fluid and electrolyte requirements, promotion of healthy environments affecting hydration, and advocating for secure access to safe water as a universal need and human right.

The establishment of healthy drinking habits begins in childhood. Evidence suggests that in school settings children do not meet their total fluid intake (TFI); therefore, nurses can have a role in reducing barriers to access to water, promoting free access to drinking water, and educating parents and teachers to be role models for optimal hydration (Bottin et al., 2019). Lower total water intake (TWI) is considered a risk factor for chronic illness; therefore, education across settings and populations to increase TWI is essential. Increasing TWI can be achieved through adding solid foods with high water content (e.g., fruits and vegetables) while reducing high osmolar load (e.g., high protein, high sodium) and by self-monitoring of water and beverage intake (e.g., volume consumed, body weight, urine colour) (Armstrong et al., 2020). Education to avoid overdrinking (e.g., excessive water intake) is also essential (Armstrong et al., 2020).

Patients and caregivers can be taught to recognize risk factors for imbalances and how to implement appropriate preventive measures. Health education for parents of infants regarding the serious imbalances that can result from gastrointestinal losses (emesis or diarrhea) helps them to recognize the risks and value of health care for restoring normal balance.

Even a healthy adult is at risk for developing imbalances when subjected to high temperatures. Nurses can advise people to increase water intake, maintain adequate ventilation, and refrain from excessive activity during heat waves. Box 41.3 provides guidelines for preventing dehydration in older persons. All patients with a chronic health alteration are at risk for developing changes in their fluid, electrolyte, and acid–base balances. They need to understand their own risk factors and the measures to be taken to avoid imbalances. For example, patients

with chronic kidney disease must avoid excess intake of fluid, sodium, potassium, magnesium, and phosphorus. Through diet education, these patients learn the types of foods to avoid and the suitable volume of fluid they are permitted daily (see Chapter 43). Patients with chronic health conditions need to be made aware of early signs and symptoms of fluid, electrolyte, and acid–base imbalances. A patient with heart disease should be instructed to obtain an accurate body weight each day at approximately the same time and to inform the health care provider of significant changes in weight from one day to another. Increase in weight, shortness of breath, orthopnea, and dependent edema are all associated with fluid retention.

Nurses engaged in health promotion can attend to environmental factors that influence the health of communities. Community needs assessments and quality improvement initiatives in relation to environmental determinants of health involve attention to safe drinking and access to safe water (see Chapter 4). Nurses need to understand this relationship between safe water and human health and advocate in particular for the rights of Indigenous people to safe, sustainable water supply (Allgood, 2009; Davidhizar et al., 2004; Sanderson et al., 2020). Globally, improved water quality and access to safe drinking water, though largely ignored, would have a significant impact on health, saving millions of lives (Allgood, 2009). While there have been successes in improving access to safe drinking water and reducing water contamination, household water treatment could bring about further advances in community health. These efforts relate strongly to nurses' advocacy role in health promotion of healthy fluid and electrolyte levels.

Acute Care. While fluid, electrolyte, and acid–base imbalances can occur in all settings, many patients are cared for in acute care settings. Persons in acute care, and also in long-term care, are particularly vulnerable to lapses in quality of care. Hydration and nutrition, both central to homeostasis, require diligent and person-centred nursing (Feo & Kitson, 2016; van Belle et al., 2020). Fundamental care has become devalued and, therefore, is being brought into focus for implementation of nursing care related to fluid, electrolyte, and acid–base balance.

Enteral Replacement of Fluids. Oral replacement of fluids and electrolytes is appropriate as long as the patient is not so physiologically compromised that oral fluids cannot be replaced rapidly. Patients unable to tolerate solid foods may still be able to ingest fluids. Nurses may use strategies to encourage fluid intake, such as frequently offering small sips of fluid, ice pops, and ice chips. Ice chips should be included in the intake and output measurements, at one-half the volume of the chips (i.e., 250 mL of ice chips = 125 mL). For children with mild gastroenteritis, diluted apple juice followed by preferred fluids is an effective alternative to electrolyte maintenance fluids, with fewer treatment failures (Freedman et al., 2016). Research over the past two decades supports the use of oral rehydration solutions (ORS), which has reduced mortality related to diarrhea around the world (Guarino et al., 2020; Leung & Hon, 2021). ORS are either glucose-electrolyte solutions or polymer-based solutions (e.g., made from rice, wheat, or maize). ORS should contain physiological concentrations of glucose and electrolytes, whereas carbonated drinks with a high carbohydrate content, low electrolyte content, and high osmolarity, and plain water are not recommended (Leung & Hon, 2021). Breastfeeding should be encouraged. A key nursing role is to encourage children and their caregivers regarding oral rehydration.

Oral replacement of fluids is contraindicated if the patient has a mechanical obstruction of the gastrointestinal tract, is at risk for aspiration, or has impaired swallowing. A feeding tube may be necessary, such as when the patient's gastrointestinal tract is healthy but the patient cannot ingest fluids (e.g., with impaired swallowing). Fluids can also be replaced through a gastrostomy or jejunostomy feeding tube or administered via a small-bore nasoenteral feeding tube. Maintaining adequate hydration for patients with enteral feeding involves an interprofessional team including dietitians, nurses, and other health care providers (Dunn, 2015). In caring for these patients, nurses need to assess for signs of dehydration and overhydration.

Restriction of Fluids. Patients who retain fluids and have **fluid volume excess (FVE)** require restricted fluid intake. Fluid restriction is often difficult for patients, particularly if they take medications that dry the oral mucous membranes or if they breathe through the mouth. The nurse should provide the rationale for fluid restrictions and the amount permitted, including ice chips, gelatin, or ice cream. In experiments, patients under fluid restrictions can lose 1 to 2% body mass within 13 to 24 hours and will experience thirst strongly, except for older persons, who often do not experience thirst (Arai et al., 2014; Shepherd, 2013).

The patient should be involved in decisions regarding the amount of fluid and the distribution of fluids over the day. Allowable fluids are often divided between diet services and nursing. Nurses must be attentive to the maximum allowed for the patient to drink independently and for medication administration (e.g., 500 mL/24 hours). Patients on fluid restriction can swallow a number of pills with as little as 30 mL of liquid. Patients on fluid restriction require mouth care frequently to moisten mucous membranes, decrease the chance of mucosal drying and cracking, and maintain comfort. While offering fluids is a natural response, person-centred care includes education, encouragement, and providing alternate comfort measures, including hard candies.

Interventions for Acid–Base Imbalances. Nursing interventions to promote acid–base balance support prescribed medical therapies and are aimed at reversing the acid–base imbalance. Such imbalances can be life-threatening and require rapid correction. In collaboration with the interprofessional team, the nurse must maintain a functional intravenous line and provide prescribed medications, such as insulin or sodium bicarbonate, and fluid and electrolyte replacement promptly.

Patients with acute acid–base disturbances often require repeated ABG analysis and close monitoring.

Parenteral Replacement of Fluids and Electrolytes. Fluid and electrolytes may be replaced through infusion directly into the circulatory system or intravenously, rather than via the digestive system. This is often referred to as *infusion therapy*. Parenteral replacement includes administration of **crystalloids**, **colloids**, and **total parenteral nutrition (TPN)**. TPN is a nutritionally adequate hypertonic solution consisting of glucose, other nutrients, and electrolytes. This solution is formulated to meet individual patient needs through interprofessional collaboration (e.g., dietitian, pharmacist, physician, nurse). See Chapter 43 for a full discussion of TPN and nutritional support.

For older persons, particularly frail adults, hydration using subcutaneous infusion has been shown to be safer with fewer adverse effects as compared to intravenous infusion in a systematic review by Danielsen et al. (2020). Although it is not commonly seen in many acute care settings, results of recent systematic review may lead to further use. For mild to moderate dehydration, or for those at risk of dehydration, requiring less than 1.5 L/24 hours, subcutaneous hydration has significant potential.

The goal of intravenous fluid administration is to maintain fluid, electrolyte, and energy demands when patients are limited in their intake and to prevent or correct fluid and electrolyte disturbances from excess losses. Intravenous fluid administration enables direct access to the vascular system, permitting the continuous infusion of fluids over a period of time. Intravenous fluid therapy must be continuously regulated to assess for changes in the patient's fluid and electrolyte balances. Knowledge of the correct ordered solution, the equipment needed, the procedures required to initiate an infusion, how to regulate the infusion rate and maintain the system, how to identify and correct problems, and how to discontinue the infusion is necessary for safe and appropriate therapy. Patient safety and quality improvement are continuously attended to in all infusion therapy–related care (Gorski et al., 2021). When providing infusion therapy to special populations such as infants and older persons, special competency is required. Consideration is given to anatomical and physiological differences, growth and development stage, and family preferences (Gorski et al., 2021).

Safe administration of intravenous fluids includes an evidence-informed knowledge base related to the solution prescribed, the patient-centred rationale, equipment selection based on best practice, and potential risks and complications (Table 41.9). Safe administration of intravenous fluids requires evidence-informed knowledge related to both vascular access and infusion therapy. Active patient engagement in the selection of device and site improves outcomes, promoting vessel health and preservation (Fiorini et al., 2019).

Types of solutions. The two main categories of intravenous fluids are crystalloids and colloids. Crystalloids are used most commonly and include dextrose, sodium chloride, and lactated Ringer's solutions (see Table 41.9). These solutions contain solutes that mix, dissolve, and cross semipermeable membranes. They vary in their tonicity. Colloids contain protein or starch, which does not cross semipermeable membranes and therefore remains suspended and distributed in the extracellular space, primarily the intravascular space, for up to several days. Colloids have been used to increase the osmotic pressure in the intravascular space to increase vascular volume in critical situations. Colloids are either semi-synthetic, such as dextran, pentastarch, or hetastarch, or human plasma derivatives, such as albumin, plasma proteins, or blood. Recent evidence suggests that crystalloids are as effective as colloids in many situations and are less costly (Lewis et al., 2018).

Vascular Access Devices. **Vascular access devices (VADs)** are catheters, cannulas, tubes, or devices designed for repeated access to the vascular system (Gorski et al., 2021). All VADS provide access to

TABLE 41.9	Intravenous Solutions	
Solution	**Concentration**	**Comments**
Dextrose in Water Solutions		*Dextrose* is the name used for glucose in intravenous solutions.
Dextrose 5% in water (D$_5$W)	Isotonic	Isotonic when first enters vein; dextrose enters cells rapidly, leaving free water, which dilutes ECF; most of water then enters cells by osmosis.
Dextrose 10% in water (D$_{10}$W)	Hypertonic	Hypertonic when first enters vein, dextrose enters cells rapidly, leaving free water, which dilutes ECF; most of water then enters cells by osmosis.
Saline Solutions		
0.225% sodium chloride (quarter normal saline; ¼ NS; 0.225% NaCl)	Hypotonic	Saline is sodium chloride in water. Expands ECV (vascular and interstitial) and rehydrates cells.
0.45% sodium chloride (half normal saline; ½ NS; 0.45% NaCl)	Hypotonic	Expands ECV (vascular and interstitial) and rehydrates cells.
0.9% sodium chloride (normal saline; NS; 0.9% NaCl)	Isotonic	Expands ECV (vascular and interstitial); does not enter cells.
3% or 5% sodium chloride (hypertonic saline; 3% or 5% NaCl)	Hypertonic	Draws water from cells into ECF by osmosis.
Dextrose in Saline Solutions		
Dextrose 5% in 0.45% NaCl sodium chloride (D$_5$ ½ NS; D$_5$0.45% NaCl)	Hypertonic	Dextrose enters cells rapidly, leaving 0.45% sodium chloride.
Dextrose 5% in 0.9% sodium chloride (D$_5$NS; D$_5$0.9% NaCl)	Hypertonic	Dextrose enters cells rapidly, leaving 0.9% sodium chloride.
Balanced Electrolyte Solutions		
Lactated Ringer's (LR)	Isotonic	Contains Na$^+$, K$^+$, Ca^{2+}, Cl$^-$, and lactate, which liver metabolizes to HCO$_3^-$. Expands ECV (vascular and interstitial); does not enter cells.
Dextrose 5% in lactated Ringer's (D$_5$LR)	Hypertonic	Dextrose enters cells rapidly, leaving lactated Ringer's.

ECF, Extracellular fluid; *ECV,* extracellular fluid volume.

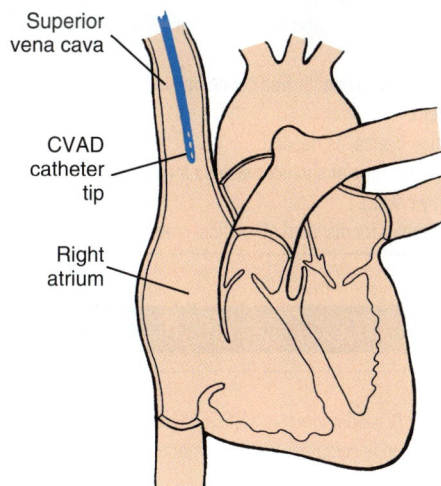

FIGURE 41.9 Central venous access devices (CVADs) deliver fluid into the superior vena cava near the heart.

FIGURE 41.10 Short-peripheral intravenous catheter (PIVC) with integrated extension set. (From Cobbett, S. L., Perry, A. G., Potter, P. A., et al. [Eds.] [2020]. *Canadian clinical nursing skills & techniques.* Elsevier. Photo courtesy Burl Jantzen.)

the venous system to deliver solutions and medications for diagnostic (e.g., contrast dye) or treatment purposes. These devices include **peripheral vascular access devices (PVADs)** and **central vascular access devices (CVADs).** PVAD catheters reside in the periphery in extremities, the external jugular vein, and scalp veins (neonates) and include both short and long peripheral intravenous catheters and midline catheters. CVADs' tips reside in the superior or inferior vena cava (Figure 41.9). Several factors are considered in determining whether to use peripheral or central devices, including anticipated duration of treatment, type of solution, and patients' characteristics (e.g., age, comorbidities, vessel health). The principle of selecting the least invasive and smallest device is followed, in collaboration with the patient, for vessel health and preservation (Fiorini et al., 2019; Gorski et al., 2021).

Peripheral venous catheters are referred to as *PVADs,* and also called *peripheral intravenous catheters* or *short peripheral venous catheters* (Figure 41.10). This language varies across jurisdictions and countries. In this chapter PVADs is used when discussing insertion devices to distinguish them from CVADs; however, when referring to the insertion, maintenance, and use of an intravenous catheter that resides in the peripheral vessels, we use the term **peripheral intravenous catheter (PIVC).** Nurses will also see the abbreviation PIV or PVC in referring to the same type of catheters.

Central venous catheters (CVCs), **peripherally inserted central catheters (PICCs),** tunnelled catheters (e.g., Hickman), nontunnelled, cuffed catheters, and implanted venous access ports are for long-term use (>15 days) or for administration of medications or solutions that are irritating to veins. A midline catheter, a catheter inserted in a peripheral vein in the upper arm and terminating at the axilla, is recommended for intermediate use (4–15 days) or when peripheral or central access is difficult or contraindicated (Gorski et al., 2021). Other reasons for using CVADs are presence of limited or poor peripheral veins, the need for good access to administer large volumes of fluid, and the need for reliable measurement of fluids. PICCs are quite common across settings. Adherence to aseptic non-touch technique (ANNT), evidence-informed assessment and care, correct dressing, and labelling are critical to the prevention of infection and effective monitoring of the PICC site and line. Nurses play an important role in the education of patients and families regarding VADs and in decisions regarding device selection for a proactive approach (Fiorini et al., 2019).

Peripheral vascular access devices: Nursing considerations. Comprehensive assessment is the first step in PIVC insertion (Skill 41.1, Steps 1 to 6, and 15; Box 41.8). Informed consent is required prior to performing vascular access and patients have the right to refuse treatment. Education regarding parenteral replacement of fluid and electrolytes or administration of follows principles of patient education (Chapter 21).

Insertion and management of a PIVC are now considered a routine nursing responsibility and skill (see Skill 41.1). Evidence-informed

SKILL 41.1   INSERTION OF A SHORT PERIPHERAL INTRAVENOUS CATHETER (PIVC)

Delegation Considerations

The skill of inserting a short peripheral intravenous catheter (PIVC) may be completed by other members of the health care team who have the appropriate education and the skill is within their governing body scope of practice. Assessment and care of short PIVC require effective communication and a collaborative health care team. Always refer to employer policy. The skill of inserting a short PIVC cannot be performed by unregulated care providers (UCPs) or by those who have not demonstrated competence in initiating intravenous therapy (Gorski et al., 2021, p. S26). However, it is important for UCPs to report to the nurse the following immediately:

- Signs and symptoms of complications (redness, swelling, leaking, bleeding, or drainage under the dressing, or patient expression of pain or discomfort)
- A loose, wet, or soiled dressing
- Low volume in an IV solution bag
- Any electronic infusion device alarms

Equipment

- Use a commercially prepared IV start kit or collect the following:
  - Single-use tourniquet, transparent semipermeable membrane (TSM) dressing with securement properties (preferred)
  - Antiseptic swab or wipe (chlorhexidine gluconate [CHG] and alcohol preferred; alternates include 2% CHG, povidone-iodine, or 70% alcohol)
  - 5 × 5–cm (2 × 2–inch) gauze pads
  - Tape
- Clean gloves (or sterile gloves if re-palpation of the vein is required after skin antiseptics).
- Commercially prepared 10-mL prefilled 0.9% normal saline (NS) syringe
- Single-use hair clippers or scissors for hair removal, if indicated
- Skin barrier swab, for sensitive skin.
- Appropriate short PIVC catheter with safety mechanism for venipuncture (see Figure 41.10)
- Short extension set with needle-free connector, if not using an integrated closed system catheter
- Vein visualization device, as needed
- Patient gown with snaps at shoulder seams, if available (makes removal during infusion therapy easier)
- Biomedical container for disposal of medical sharps

PROCEDURE

STEPS	RATIONALE

ASSESSMENT

1. Confirm clinical indication and prescription for short PIVC in patient's record.

- A prescription for IV medications is sufficient for short PIVC insertion. Verification that prescription is complete helps prevent medication errors.

2. Review patient allergies or skin sensitivities related to equipment required for insertion (e.g., latex, antiseptics, dressing adhesives, skin barrier solution).

- Prevents unnecessary complications or discomfort. Equipment used during short PIVC insertion may contain substances to which patient is allergic.

3. Review prescribed therapy, anticipated length of treatment, and patient characteristics to ensure the most appropriate VAD is selected (e.g., peripheral vascular access device [PVAD] or central vascular access device [CVAD])

- Infusions of continuous vesicants or solution with an osmolarity of greater than 900 mOsm/L are not recommended for PIVC.
- Patient assessment must include vascular characteristics, age, history of vascular access, comorbidities, and patient preferences (Fiorini et al., 2019; Piredda et al., 2017).

4. Consider most appropriate gauge of catheter required for infusion therapy or diagnostics.

- Use the smallest gauge PIVC with the fewest number of lumens. This promotes vein preservation, reduces risks of phlebitis, and causes the least discomfort. See Table 41.10.

5. Assess patient's knowledge of procedure, reason for prescribed therapy, arm placement preference, and risks related to short PIVC placement and that they must report signs and symptoms of complications immediately.

- Demonstrates learning and conforms with informed consent (Gorski et al., 2021); such assessment ensures safe delivery of care with a person-centred approach.

6. If administering IV fluids, assess for clinical factors or conditions that will respond to or be affected by administration of IV solutions (see Skill 41.2).

- Provides baseline to determine effectiveness of prescribed therapy. A systems approach is recommended to assess for fluid and electrolyte imbalances.

Continued

SKILL 41.1 INSERTION OF A SHORT PERIPHERAL INTRAVENOUS CATHETER (PIVC)—cont'd

IMPLEMENTATION

7. Perform hand hygiene.

8. Identify patient using at least two identifiers (e.g., name and birthday or name and medical record number) according to employer policy. Compare identifiers with information on patient's medical record and armband.

9. Provide patient education about rationale for infusion, including solution and medications prescribed; procedure for initiating PIVC; and signs and symptoms of complications (e.g., redness, pain tenderness, swelling, bleeding, drainage, or leaking at insertion site). Include rationale for device selection (e.g., short-term therapy, comfort). Obtain informed consent.

10. Change patient's gown or clothing to allow for easy removal. A gown with snaps at the shoulder may be used, if available.

11. Ensure patient is sitting or lying in a comfortable position that provides adequate light and positioning for vein assessment and PIVC insertion.

12. Perform hand hygiene. Collect and organize equipment on clean, clutter-free bedside stand or overbed table. Wipe surface with antiseptic wipe prior to use.

13. Apply tourniquet on upper arm or at least 10 cm (4 inches) above intended insertion site (see Step 13 illustration). Do not apply too tightly. Assess patient level of comfort and confirm presence of pulse distal to the tourniquet.

- Supports infection prevention and control by decreasing risk of microbial contamination.

- Ensures correct patient. Complies with Accreditation Canada's standards and improves patient safety (Health Standards Organization [HSO], 2019).

- Promotes person-centred care and patient safety.

- Reduces risk of inadvertently dislodging VAD or administration set when changing.

- Promotes comfort, relaxation, and vasodilation for the patient. Also enables good body mechanics to prevent nurse injury and to increase opportunity for a successful insertion.

- Reduces transmission of infection and contamination of equipment (Gorski et al., 2021). Easy access to equipment improves efficiency.

- The tourniquet provides dilation of the vein for ease of visualization or palpation; it should impede venous flow while maintaining arterial circulation. Caution should be used with older persons or patients with fragile skin. Apply over patient gown to prevent skin impairments or pulling of arm hair.

- Consider use of a blood pressure cuff for patient comfort. Inflate to approximately 50 mmHg to apply appropriate amount of pressure.

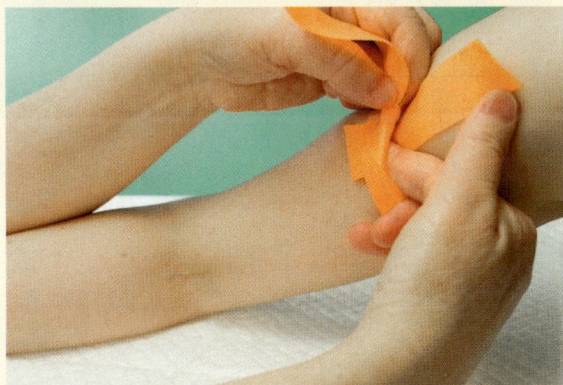

STEP 13 Application of tourniquet. (From Cobbett, S. L., Perry, A. G., Potter, P. A., et al. [Eds.] [2020]. *Canadian clinical nursing skills & techniques.* Elsevier. Photo courtesy Patrick Coble.)

14. Select the most appropriate vein and location by visual inspection and palpation (see Step 14 illustrations) using the following guidelines:
    - Veins should feel soft and bouncy and be adequate in size to accommodate selected catheter gauge.
    - Use the most distal site above the wrist in forearm (nondominant side preferred).
    - Do not use areas of flexion (e.g., antecubital fossa and hand) unless required for less than 24 hours or in an emergency situation.
    - Avoid using veins located in the hands unless for short-term use.
    - Do not use a site below a failed insertion attempt, unless completely healed.
    - Skin must be intact and free of signs of infection.
    - Ensure a minimum of 8 cm (3.2 in) or three fingers above the wrist.
    - Do not use an arm that has a fistula or a graft for dialysis.
    - Avoid using veins in the upper extremity on the affected side of breast surgery with axillary node dissection or lymphedema, after radiation, arteriovenous (AV) fistulas/grafts, or an affected extremity from a cerebrovascular accident (CVA) (Gorski et al., 2021).
    - Consider use of dry heat (warm blanket or compress) to enhance vasodilation of the vein, to improve visualization and ability to palpate vein.

- Promotes insertion success, vein preservation and decrease risk of phlebitis.
- Use of the hands can be very painful, limit patient's activities of daily living, and their ability to perform hand hygiene.
- Use of areas of flexion can cause patient discomfort and disrupt infusions. They are associated with significantly higher risks of infiltration and development of mechanical or bacterial phlebitis due to movement of the catheter and inability to maintain an occlusive dressing.
- Venipuncture below a failed PIVC may lead to infiltration or extravasation of infusates.
- Insertion attempt in an area of skin impairment increases risks of infection and patient discomfort.
- Insertion sites at the wrist are associated with increased risks of nerve damage.
- Using veins sites that may have impaired circulation or decreased sensation may increase risks of complication.
- Heat promotes comfort, decreases anxiety, and prevents vasoconstriction. Moist application increases risk of burns and cools rapidly and causes maceration of the skin.

SKILL 41.1 **INSERTION OF A SHORT PERIPHERAL INTRAVENOUS CATHETER (PIVC)—cont'd**

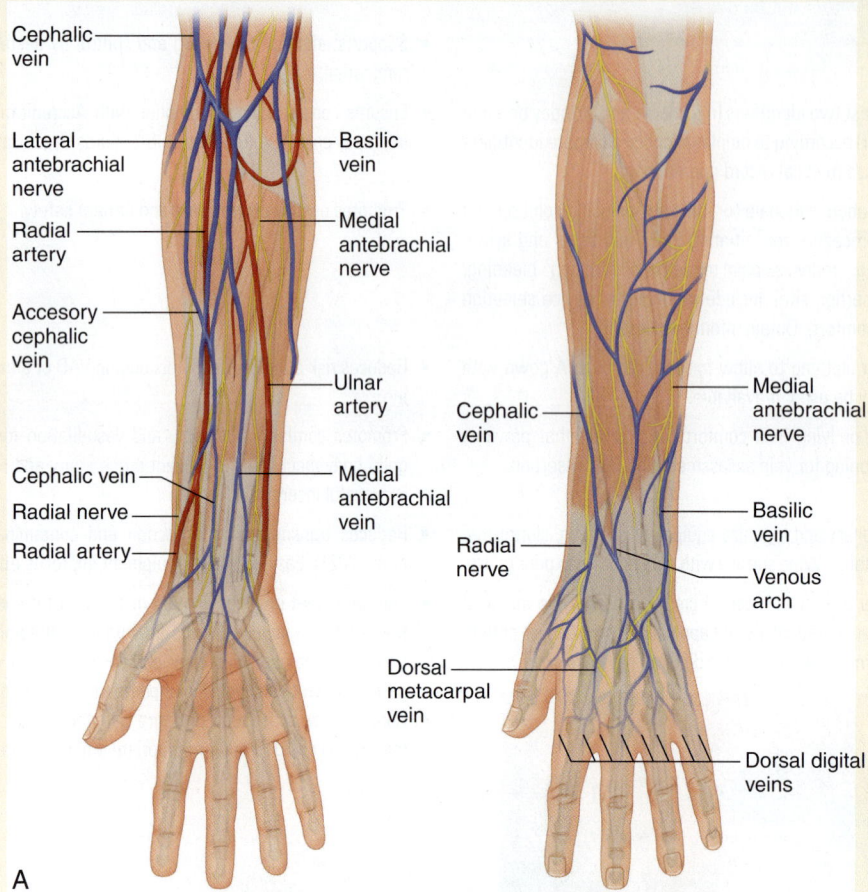

Cephalic vein
Lateral antebrachial nerve
Basilic vein
Radial artery
Medial antebrachial nerve
Accesory cephalic vein
Ulnar artery
Cephalic vein
Radial nerve
Medial antebrachial vein
Radial artery

Cephalic vein
Radial nerve
Medial antebrachial nerve
Basilic vein
Venous arch
Dorsal metacarpal vein
Dorsal digital veins

A

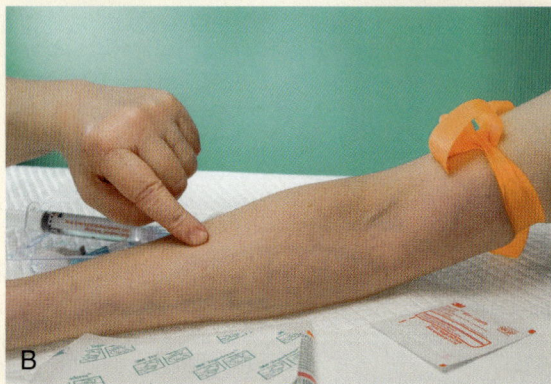

B

STEP 14 **A,** Vein map. **B,** Palpate vein and select site. (From Cobbett, S. L., Perry, A. G., Potter, P. A., et al. [Eds.] [2020]. *Canadian clinical nursing skills & techniques*. Elsevier. Photos: **A,** Canadian Vascular Access Association, **B,** Courtesy Patrick Coble.)

CRITICAL DECISION POINT: *Consider the use of vein visualization devices (if available in the agency) when no venous access is visible or easily palpated. Options may include near infrared light devices or ultrasound (requires additional education). Using vein visualization devices improves success of cannulation, decreases risks associated with traumatic or missed insertion attempts, and improves patient comfort (see Figures 41.11 and 41.12).*

15. Remove tourniquet and prepare supplies.

16. Select appropriate-size catheter; open and prepare sterile packages using aseptic non-touch technique (see Chapter 34).

• If assessment of vein has taken longer than 1 minute, remove tourniquet to avoid vein fatigue and patient discomfort.

• Use smallest-gauge peripheral catheter that will accommodate prescribed therapy and patient need (Gorski et al., 2021). Do not remove backing from sterile dressing until ready to secure PIVC. Leave IV in the sterile packaging until ready to insert, to maintain aseptic technique.

Continued

SKILL 41.1	INSERTION OF A SHORT PERIPHERAL INTRAVENOUS CATHETER (PIVC)—cont'd

17. Prime add-on device (short extension tubing with fused needle-free connector or separate needle-free connector) by attaching the prefilled 10 mL normal saline syringe. Slowly infuse the normal saline to remove all air and leave syringe attached to the device. Maintain aseptic non-touch technique at all times.

- Needle-free connectors protect health care workers by providing a needle-free system, therefore eliminating potential for needle-stick injuries (Gorski et al., 2021).
- Integrated IV catheter and extensions provide a closed system, ensuring decreased risks of blood exposure, and less manipulation of the catheter hub, decreasing risks of mechanical and bacterial phlebitis. Removing all air with normal saline or allowing blood to flow back in the integrated system prevents air from entering the patient's vein on PIVC insertion.

CRITICAL DECISION POINT: *If an integrated IV/extension set is not in use in the agency, short extension sets are recommended for use with PVAD for continuous and intermittent infusions. This reduces catheter manipulation and ease of IV administration set change, decreasing risks of contamination at catheter hub. All connections should be of a Luer-Lok type (Gorski et al., 2021).*

18. Prepare insertion site. If hair removal is required, use surgical clipper or scissors to trim hair. If site is visibly soiled, clean with antiseptic soap and water prior to application of antiseptic solution.

- Razors should not be used because they cause micro-cuts in the skin that can lead to increased risks of infection (Gorski et al., 2021). Removal of hair is very important to obtain adequate skin antisepsis, as is maintaining an occlusive dressing to prevent infection. Cleaning the skin prior to application of antiseptic solutions improves efficacy.

19. Perform hand hygiene and apply gloves.

- Decreases potential risk of microbial contamination and cross-contamination (Gorski et al., 2021).

CRITICAL DECISION POINT: *Gloves are not necessary to locate the vein but must be applied for VAD insertion using a non-touch technique where the site is not palpated after skin antisepsis (Gorski et al., 2021).*

20. Reapply tourniquet using the same technique for vein assessment (see Step 13).

- Assessment and insertion may be completed at the same application of the tourniquet, with more experienced inserters. Always be aware of the length of time the tourniquet is in place. It should not exceed 1 minute.

21. With your fingertip, palpate selected vein at intended insertion site by pressing downward. Note resilient, soft, bouncy feeling while releasing pressure.

- The fingertip is more sensitive and better for assessing vein location and condition.

CRITICAL DECISION POINT: *Vigorous friction and slapping or hard tapping of a vein, especially in older persons, can cause venous constriction or bruising and hematoma (Infusion Nurses Society [INS], 2021).*
CRITICAL DECISION POINT: *If vein palpation is necessary after performing skin antisepsis, use sterile gloves for palpation or perform skin antisepsis again, because touching cleaned area introduces microorganisms from your finger to site (Gorski et al., 2021).*

22. Clean insertion site with an antiseptic solution as follows (see Step 22 illustration):
- Solution of CHG and alcohol is preferred. Apply using a friction scrub in a back-and-forth motion for a minimum of 30 seconds. Solution must be allowed to completely air dry prior to PIVC insertion.
- Povidone iodine must remain on the skin for 1.5 to 2 minutes after application to completely dry and for adequate antisepsis.
- CHG without alcohol dry time is a minimum of 3 minutes for adequate antisepsis (INS, 2021).

- Solution of CHG and alcohol is preferred because it is a broad-spectrum biocide effective against Gram positive and Gram-negative bacteria and fungi. It has a quicker kill rate than other antimicrobials and has been shown to inhibit growth for at least 48 hours. The addition of alcohol decreases drying time on the skin.
- All antiseptic solutions must be applied according to instructions for use, to ensure adequate antisepsis to reduce risks of insertion site and systemic infections.
- Mechanical friction allows penetration of the solution to the epidermal layers of skin. Antiseptics must be allowed to fully dry to ensure efficacy. Do not wipe or blot, fan, or blow on skin to speed dry time.

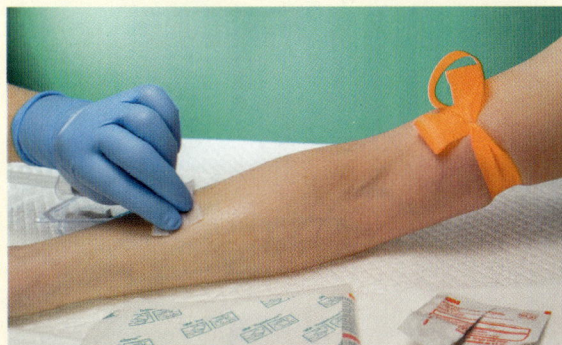

STEP 22 Clean venipuncture site. (From Cobbett, S. L., Perry, A. G., Potter, P. A., et al. [Eds.] [2020]. *Canadian clinical nursing skills & techniques.* Elsevier. Photo courtesy Patrick Coble.)

23. Stabilize vein with nondominant hand by placing fingers above and below intended insertion site, pulling skin taut (see Step 23 illustration).

• Stabilization of the vein for needle insertion is key to preventing rolling of the vein. Stretching the skin taut decreases drag during insertion.

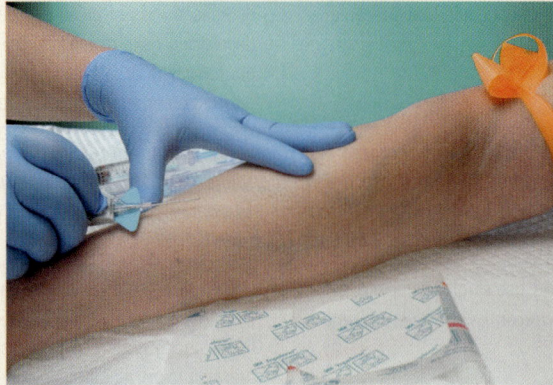

STEP 23 Stabilize vein. (From Cobbett, S. L., Perry, A. G., Potter, P. A., et al. [Eds.] [2020]. *Canadian clinical nursing skills & techniques*. Elsevier. Photo courtesy Patrick Coble.)

24. Perform venipuncture with bevel up, align catheter on top of intended insertion site at approximately a 10- to 15-degree angle, and puncture the skin and anterior vein wall (Gorski et al., 2021) (see Step 24 illustration). Observe for blood return in catheter (flashback). If the patient experiences any severe pain or paresthesias related to insertion, including electrical shock, tingling, burning, or numbness, remove PIVC immediately to prevent potential nerve damage.

• Ensure patient is aware to anticipate needle-stick and to remain as still as possible.
• Some manufactures require loosening of the catheter from the needle prior to insertion (follow specific instruction for use).
• Insert a PIVC at no more than a 30-degree angle, to reduce the risk of phlebitis (Gorski et al., 2021).

STEP 24 Perform venipuncture and observe for flashback. (From Cobbett, S. L., Perry, A. G., Potter, P. A., et al. [Eds.] [2020]. *Canadian clinical nursing skills & techniques*. Elsevier. Photo courtesy Patrick Coble.)

CRITICAL DECISION POINT: *Use each VAD only once for each insertion attempt.*

Continued

SKILL 41.1 INSERTION OF A SHORT PERIPHERAL INTRAVENOUS CATHETER (PIVC)—cont'd

25. Once blood return is observed in the catheter or flashback chamber, lower the angle parallel with the skin (see Step 25A illustration). Keeping skin taut, advance needle slightly farther into vein (see Step 25B illustration). Advance or thread catheter into the vein using the push-off tab and then release tourniquet (see Step 25C illustration). If catheter does not thread, do not reinsert the needle into the catheter.

- Lowering the angle after blood return decreases risk of puncturing the posterior vein wall.
- Advancing with skin taut will ensure the catheter and needle tip are inside the vein wall.
- Do not push using the catheter hub, as this contaminates the lumen. Using an integrated catheter/extension closed system eliminates this potential risk.
- Reinsertion of needle into the catheter can cause catheter to shear off and embolize into the vein.
- Advancing the entire stylet into the vein may penetrate wall of the vein, resulting in hematoma.
- Advancing catheter with finger on open hub causes contamination (Gorski et al., 2021).

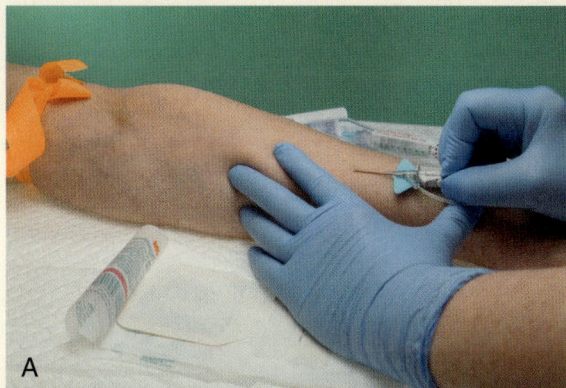

STEP 25 A, Lower catheter. **B,** Advance and thread. **C,** Thread catheter into vein using push-tab. (From Cobbett, S. L., Perry, A. G., Potter, P. A., et al. [Eds.] [2020]. *Canadian clinical nursing skills & techniques.* Elsevier. Photos courtesy Patrick Coble.)

CRITICAL DECISION POINT: *A single clinician should not make more than two attempts at initiating a PIVC and should limit total attempts to no more than four (CVAA, 2019; Gorski et al., 2021).*

SKILL 41.1   INSERTION OF A SHORT PERIPHERAL INTRAVENOUS CATHETER (PIVC)—cont'd

26. After successful insertion of catheter into the vein, engage safety mechanism to cover needle as per manufacturer's instructions and engage clamp if present (see Step 26 photo). If the PIVC has a blood control mechanism (e.g., clamp on integrated extension or filter in hub), this will stop blood flow until add-on extension or needle-free connector is attached (see Step 26 illustration). If PIVC does not have blood control, apply gentle but firm pressure above the insertion site to occlude blood flow, then attach add-on device. Avoid touching sterile connection ends. Dispose of sharps in biohazard container immediately after PIVC is secured.

- Safety engineered PIVC are designed to prevent needle-stick injuries, covering or enclosing sharp on removal.
- Blood control PIVC significantly decreases risk of blood exposure and enables attachment of add-on devices without risk of hub contamination.
- Digital pressure minimizes blood loss and allows attachment of extension set or needle-free connector.

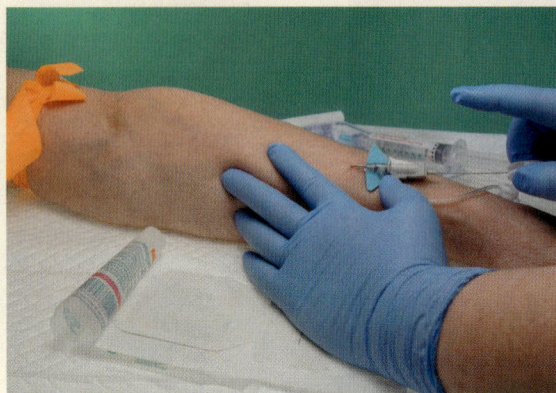

STEP 26 Engage safety mechanism. (From Cobbett, S. L., Perry, A. G., Potter, P. A., et al. [Eds.] [2020]. *Canadian clinical nursing skills & techniques*. Elsevier. Photo courtesy Patrick Coble.)

27. Apply sterile transparent securement dressing to cover and protect insertion site (see Step 27 illustration). Do not apply unsterile tape around the catheter, over the catheter hub, or under sterile dressing.
    A. Loop extension tubing alongside the dressing and secure with a piece of tape for patient comfort and additional securement. Do not obstruct PIVC site.
    B. Stretch netting or a tubular sleeve may be applied over the dressing to provide additional securement. Do not use rolled bandages.

- Occlusive, dry dressings prevent mechanical and bacterial phlebitis and loss of access.
- Dressing with securement properties or an addition of a stabilization device decreases risks of catheter dislodgement and movement. Tape on top of TSM dressing prevents moisture from being carried away from skin.
- *Optional:* A risk of medical adhesive-related skin injury (MARSI) is increased as result of age, joint movement, and edema; therefore, a skin protectant prior to dressing application may be considered (Gorski et al., 2021). TSM dressing allows for visualization of the insertion site and surrounding area for assessment of complications.
- Removal of tape from TSM dressing can tear dressing and cause catheter dislodgement.
- If a gauze dressing is required because of patient sensitivities to TSM dressing, assessment must be performed by palpation over the dressing, observing for any drainage and patient discomfort.
- Rolls of nonsterile tape can become contaminated with pathogenic bacteria, and thus increase risks of PIVC contamination, if applied under the sterile dressing.
- Rolled bandages can impair circulation or flow of infusion and obscure visualization for site assessment of complications.

STEP 27 Apply dressing. (From Cobbett, S. L., Perry, A. G., Potter, P. A., et al. [Eds.] [2020]. *Canadian clinical nursing skills & techniques*. Elsevier. Photo courtesy Patrick Coble.)

28. Attach primed add-on device (extension set or needle-free connector) with attached syringe to catheter (disengage clamp if present).

- Use aseptic non-touch technique when securing extension or needle-free connectors to catheter hub.
- Prompt connection maintains patency of vein and reduces backflow of blood. (Gorski et al., 2021).

Continued

29. Flush catheter using a push-pause or pulsatile technique to clear all visible blood from extension set and needle-free connector. Observe insertion site for swelling, with flush. If not using a commercially prepared prefilled syringe, leave 0.5–1.0 mL of normal saline in the flush syringe to prevent syringe-induced blood reflux in catheter (see Step 29 illustration).

- Clearing blood prevents risk of catheter occlusion and infection.
- If patient experiences discomfort or if swelling or leaking of fluid is observed during flush, this indicates that the catheter is no longer in the vein and must be removed immediately.

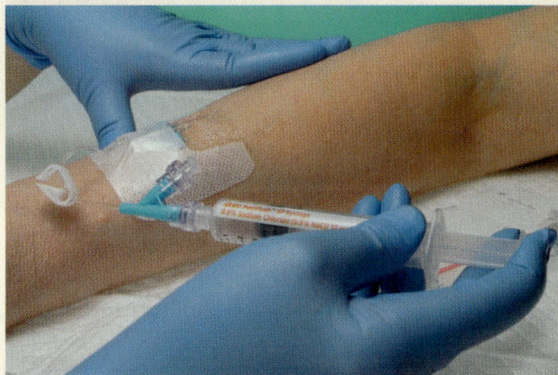

STEP 29 Flush PIVC. (From Cobbett, S. L., Perry, A. G., Potter, P. A., et al. [Eds.] [2020]. *Canadian clinical nursing skills & techniques*. Elsevier. Photo courtesy Patrick Coble.)

30. Close clamp.
   A. Remove flush syringe from needle-free connector, using appropriate clamping technique (see Step 30A illustration). (See Critical Decision Point.)
   B. Refer to Skill 41.2 if initiating infusion.

- Needle-free connectors come in many types and styles. It is important to know if the connector has neutral, negative, or positive displacement properties to determine if a specific clamping sequence is required to prevent reflux of blood into the PIVC on removal of the syringe.

STEP 30A Close clamp. (From Cobbett, S. L., Perry, A. G., Potter, P. A., et al. [Eds.] [2020]. *Canadian clinical nursing skills & techniques*. Elsevier. Photo courtesy Patrick Coble.)

CRITICAL DECISION POINT: *Needle-free connectors protect health care workers and decrease risk for needle-stick injuries. They have different internal mechanisms for fluid displacement and vary in the flush-clamp-disconnect sequence to prevent reflux of blood into the catheter on disconnection (Gorski et al., 2021). The sequence depends on the type of internal mechanism:*
- *Neutral displacement devices do not have a specified flush-clamp-disconnect sequence.*
- *For negative-pressure displacement devices, flush, clamp catheter, then disconnect syringe.*
- *For positive-pressure displacement, flush, disconnect syringe, then clamp catheter.*

31. Label dressing according to employer policy. Include date of insertion and initials (see Step 31 illustration).

- PIVC are changed on the basis of clinical assessment, thus it is important to know the insertion date to determine the length of time the PIVC has been in place and to alert the need for dressing change. Monitor for MARSI.

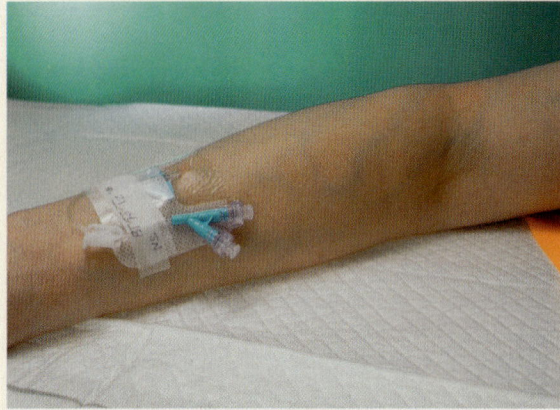

STEP 31 Label dressing. (From Cobbett, S. L., Perry, A. G., Potter, P. A., et al. [Eds.] [2020]. *Canadian clinical nursing skills & techniques.* Elsevier. Photo courtesy Patrick Coble.)

32. Dispose of any sharps in appropriate container, discard supplies, remove gloves, and perform hand hygiene.

- Reduces transmission of microorganisms; prevents accidental needle-stick injuries.

33. Review with patient the care and maintenance of PIVC and to report any signs and symptoms of complications immediately to a health care provider. Use teach-back to determine patient's and caregiver's understanding and develop a revised teaching plan if patient or caregiver is not able to teach back correctly.

- Promotes patient engagement in care of PIVC.
- Determines patient's and caregiver's level of understanding of instructional topic.

34. Document the following information in the patient chart or electronic health record (EHR):
- Date and time
- Indication for use
- Location of PIVC insertion
- Gauge, length, and type (e.g., Nexiva 22 g, 2.5 cm [1.0 in])
- Number of attempts
- Functionality of PIVC (i.e., flushes without resistance, no signs of complications)
- Local anaesthetic, if used
- Use of visualization technology, if used
- Patient response to procedure
- Patient education
- Signs and symptoms of IV-related complications, including interventions and patient response to treatments

35. Assess PIVC for patency and complications, dressing, and patient-specific concerns as per employer policy and procedure (see Skill 41.3).

- Frequent assessment helps prevent long-term damage, and early recognition leads to prompt treatment.

UNEXPECTED OUTCOMES	RELATED INTERVENTIONS
Catheter occlusion can occur from a bent catheter, positional catheter (catheter resting against catheter wall), kink or knot in extension tubing, clot formation, or precipitate formation from administration of incompatible medications or solutions.	• Determine cause and consider catheter removal. • Positional catheters can be repositioned to improve IV flow. • Remove occluded IV catheter. Occluded catheters should not be flushed, because an embolus can result from dislodging a clot.
Medical adhesive-related skin injury (MARSI)	• Monitor site for signs of injury and change dressing, using a different type of dressing, if indicated.
Phlebitis (i.e., vein inflammation): pain, redness, warmth, swelling, induration, or presence of palpable cord along course of vein (Gorski et al., 2021). Rate of infusion may be altered.	• Consider infusate, confirm need for vascular access. • Determine cause (e.g., chemical, mechanical). • *Chemical phlebitis:* Apply warm compress, elevate limb, consider slowing infusion rate, and determine if catheter removal is necessary (Gorski et al., 2021). • *Mechanical phlebitis:* Stabilize catheter, apply heat, elevate limb, continue to monitor, consider catheter removal if signs and symptoms persist (Gorski et al., 2021). • *Bacterial phlebitis:* Remove IV catheter (Gorski et al., 2021). • Document phlebitis using a standardized scale, including nursing interventions per employer policy and procedure (Table 41.11).

SKILL 41.1   INSERTION OF A SHORT PERIPHERAL INTRAVENOUS CATHETER (PIVC)—cont'd

Catheter-related infection can present as redness, swelling around or above IV site, pain, purulent drainage at insertion site, and body temperature elevations (Gorski et al., 2021).

Hematoma is bleeding under the skin caused by trauma to the vessel wall. It can occur during short-peripheral IV insertion if needle punctures are either adjacent vessels or posterior vein wall or can be seen with multiple venipuncture attempts.

Nerve injuries during short-peripheral IV insertion can occur. Be alert for patient complaints of paresthesias, including shock-like pain, tingling or pins and needles, burning, or numbness on insertion.

- Notify health care provider. Obtain prescription to culture drainage (Gorski et al., 2021).
- Remove IV catheter and culture purulent drainage from around IV site (Gorski et al., 2021).
- Remove IV catheter immediately and apply pressure and dry, sterile.
- Monitor for additional bleeding.
- Elevate extremity and monitor for circulatory, neurological, or motor dysfunction (Gorski et al., 2021).
- Notify health care provider of any signs and symptoms of nerve injury (Gorski et al., 2021).
- Immediately stop VAD insertion and remove device if patient complains of symptoms of paresthesias (Gorski et al., 2021).
- Continue to monitor neurovascular status (Gorski et al., 2021).

REPORTING

- Report the following to oncoming nursing staff: Location and gauge of VAD, site assessment, IV-related complications, status of VAD (e.g., saline lock or continuous infusion running).

CARE IN THE COMMUNITY CONSIDERATIONS

- Teach patient or caregiver to assess VAD site at least once per day or every 4 hours while awake during continuous infusions and to report any signs or symptoms of complications to their homes care or other health care provider (Gorski et al., 2021).
- Teach patient or caregiver to report any signs or symptoms of complications (e.g., redness, pain, tenderness, swelling, bleeding, drainage, or loose of soiled dressing), if flow rate slows or stops, or if patient sees blood in the IV administration set or on the dressing.
- Teach patient and family about hand hygiene and aseptic non-touch technique for all care related to VAD site and equipment.
- Teach caregiver to apply pressure with sterile gauze if catheter falls out and, if patient is on anticoagulant therapy, to tape sterile gauze in place for at least 20 minutes with pressure or until bleeding stops.
- Ensure that patient is able and willing to self-administer infusion therapy or that there is a reliable caregiver to provide infusion therapy care at home.
- Ensure that all sharps and equipment contaminated by blood are disposed of appropriately based on community standards. Some suppliers provide sharps containers for needle disposal. Teach patient and caregiver appropriate sharps disposal.
- Teach patient about activity restrictions (e.g., avoiding strenuous exercise of the arm with the IV line, protecting site while bathing or showering).

BOX 41.8   Safety Guidelines for Infusion Therapy

Ensuring patient safety is an essential role of the professional nurse. To ensure patient safety, communicate clearly with members of the health care team, assess and incorporate the patient's priorities of care and preferences, and use the best evidence when making decisions about a patient's care. When performing the skills in this chapter, remember the following points to ensure safe, person-centred care:

- Check that you have the necessary information, a prescription if required, and equipment available for the procedure before beginning.
- Before initiation of therapy, check patient identification using two patient identifiers and assess the appropriate route and rate of infusion and potential incompatibilities between infusing fluids and medications (Gorski et al., 2021).
- Determine if the patient has a latex allergy or latex sensitivity and use latex-free equipment and supplies if allergy or sensitivity is present (Gorski et al., 2021).

- Use special designated tubing for the brand of electronic infusion device (EID) and for blood transfusions and some medications.
- Review the steps of the procedure mentally before entering a patient's room (i.e., consider modifications that you may need to make for this specific patient and verify that the type of intravenous (IV) solution is appropriate for this patient).
- Maintain strict aseptic non-touch technique (ANNT) to prevent bloodstream infections (Gorski et al., 2021).
- If you contaminate a sterile object during the procedure, do not use it. Use a new sterile one.
- Use routine practices during procedures, and place all disposable blood-contaminated items and sharp items in designated puncture-resistant biohazard containers (Gorski et al., 2021).

education and skill development for nurses initiating PIVCs is essential for reducing complications rates (Gorski et al., 2021). Competency assessment and validation on an ongoing basis are required for nurses performing vascular access and should be documented according to agency policy (Gorski et al., 2021). Vascular visualization or ultrasound is used with difficult access and in special populations and is known to increase first-time insertion success (Gorski et al., 2021; Pitts & Ostroff, 2019). A key principle for PIVC insertion is to use the smallest gauge possible, generally gauge 20 or smaller (Gorski et al., 2021), because larger gauges are more likely to cause phlebitis (Table 41.10).

Nurses also play a role in the continual evaluation of the need for and appropriateness of a VAD, because prompt removal of unnecessary lines is key to preventing catheter-related bloodstream infections. The recommendations and discussion that follow here are general guidelines; nurses should be aware of and follow specific institutional and manufacturer's policies.

The management of PIVC requires careful monitoring of the site, patency, and dressing. The site should be assessed for patency and signs and symptoms of PIVC-related complications or catheter failure. Complications of PIVC include phlebitis, infiltration or extravasation, occlusion, infection, pain, leaking, and dislodgement (Marsh et al., 2020). Ray-Barruel and colleagues (2020) developed the I-DECIDED decision-making tool as the first comprehensive, evidence-informed, valid, and reliable PIVC assessment and decision tool (Box 41.9).

Scales to assess for phlebitis and infiltration are important tools for nurses initiating and managing PIVCs (Table 41.11 and Table 41.12). Phlebitis is the most frequent complication of short PIVC and is categorized as mechanical (catheter against the vein), chemical (solution or medication), or bacterial (contamination on

insertion or management) (Gunasegaran et al., 2018; Marsh et al., 2020). Infiltration and extravasation result from leakage of solution or medication into the surrounding tissue (Marsh et al., 2020). Pharmacological properties of the infusate, such as hyperosmolarity and pH or the ability to destroy cells, bring higher risk for causing extravasation. Nurses must follow agency policy for treating patients when this serious complication occurs.

Documentation of VAD insertion (see Skill 41.1) should include assessment, indication, date and time of insertion, number of attempts, type, length and gauge/size, site, patient's response, and patient's

TABLE 41.10	Recommendations for Short Peripheral Catheter Selection
Catheter Size (Gauge)	Clinical Indication
14, 16, 18	Trauma, surgery, rapid blood transfusions, and rapid fluid replacement
20	Continuous or intermittent infusions in adults; administration of blood transfusions in adults
22	Continuous or intermittent infusions in adults, children, newborns, and older persons; administration of blood or blood product in adults, children, newborns, or older persons
24	Continuous or intermittent infusions in adults, children, newborns, and older persons; administration of blood or blood product in adults, children, newborns, or older persons

Modified from Infusion Nurses Society (INS). (2021). *Policies and procedures for infusion therapy: Older adult* (4th ed.). Infusion Nurses Society (INS). (2021). *Policies and procedures for infusion therapy: Acute care* (6th ed.). Gorski, L. A., Hadaway, L., Hagle, M. E., et al. (2021). Infusion therapy standards of practice. *Journal of Infusion Nursing, 44*(Suppl 1), S1–S224. https://doi.org/10.1097/NAN.0000000 00000396

TABLE 41.11	Visual Infusion Phlebitis Scale
Score	Observation
1	Intravenous (IV) site appears healthy
2	One of the following is evident:
	Slight pain near IV site OR slight redness near IV site
3	Two of the following are evident:
	Pain at the IV site
	Erythema
	Swelling
4	All of the following signs are evident:
	Pain along path of cannula
	Induration
5	All of the following signs are evident and extensive:
	Pain along path of cannula
	Erythema
	Induration
	Palpable venous cord
6	All of the following signs are evident and extensive:
	Pain along path of cannula
	Erythema
	Induration
	Palpable venous cord
	Pyrexia

From Infusion Nurses Society. (2021). Infusion nursing standards of practice. *Journal of Infusion Nursing, 34*(1S), S138.

BOX 41.9   RESEARCH HIGHLIGHT

Validation Study for Peripheral Intravenous Catheter Decision-Making Tool

Research Focus

Although 70% of hospitalized persons have a vascular access device (VAD), a valid, evidence-informed tool for standardized assessment and timely removal of peripheral intravenous catheters (PIVCs) has not been developed and validated. Inadequate assessments contribute to higher complications with PIVC use and their remaining in use for no reason.

Research Abstract

An eight-step tool was developed on the basis of international vascular access guidelines, based on nine key principles and related assessments and decision steps represented by the mnemonic I-DECIDED[R]. Three phases of the study drew on the expertise of international vascular access experts and clinicians in three hospitals in Australia. In the first phase, the working group (Australia) conducted an initial face validity process, testing if the tool measures what it was designed to measure, followed by some wording changes. In the second phase, in which content validity was evaluated, 18 international experts and clinicians

determined that each principle and corresponding items strongly confirmed the tool, except for two principles (assessment of need for PIVC and patient knowledge needs at each shift). Reliability of the tool was evaluated in three hospitals in Australia for 34 pairs, showing high inter-rater reliability. The researchers reaffirmed the principle of assessing patient and family concerns based on evidence and encouraging patient collaboration in daily care decisions. While decision making is particular to each patient's situation, assessment informing decision making should be standardized and evidence informed.

Evidence-Informed Practice

- The I-DECIDED tool has been developed drawing on the expertise of an international expert group, following best practice guidelines, and its use is encouraged (see https://www.avatargroup.org.au/i-decided.html).
- A structured assessment and decision-making tool for PIVC helps prevent complications and promotes person-centred care, as well as a proactive approach to vessel health and preservation.

From Ray-Barruel, G., Cooke, M., Chopra, V., et al. (2020). The I-DECIDED clinical decision-making tool for peripheral intravenous catheter assessment and safe removal: A clinimetric evaluation. *BMJ Open, 10*(e035239). https://doi.org/10.1136/bmjopen-2019-035239

TABLE 41.12 Infiltration Scale

Grade	Clinical Criteria
0	No symptoms
1	Skin blanched
	Edema <2.54 cm (1 in) in any direction
	Cool to touch
	With or without pain
2	Skin blanched
	Edema 2.54–15.2 cm (1–6 in) in any direction
	Cool to touch
	With or without pain
3	Skin blanched, translucent
	Gross edema >15.2 cm (6 in) in any direction
	Cool to touch
	Mild–moderate pain
	Possible numbness
4	Skin blanched, translucent
	Skin tight, leaking
	Skin discoloured, bruised, swollen
	Gross edema >15.2 cm (6 in) in any direction
	Deep pitting tissue edema
	Circulatory impairment
	Moderate-to-severe pain
	Infiltration of any amount of blood product, irritant, or vesicant

From Groll, D., Davies, B., MacDonald, J., et al. (2010). Evaluation of the psychometric properties of the phlebitis and infiltration scales for the assessment of complications of peripheral vascular access devices. *Journal of Infusion Nursing, 33*(6), 385.

understanding. Documentation using standardized terminology in the electronic health record facilitates audit and comparison rates of complications (Marsh et al., 2020). Documentation upon removal should include assessment of the site and the VAD, decision making for removal, and care after removal (dressing).

Central vascular access devices: Nursing considerations. Nursing care of persons with a CVAD varies by type, purpose, and agency. The most common insertion sites for nontunnelled CVADs are the internal jugular and subclavian veins. Tunnelled cuffed catheters are tunnelled from the entry site, subcutaneously, to the preferred vein, where the catheter is inserted and advanced into the superior vena cava (Gorski et al., 2021). PICCs are inserted through a peripheral vein, such as the basilic, brachial, median cubital, or cephalic vein, and terminate in the lower third of the superior vena cava.

Nurses need to be able to recognize the following complications associated with CVADs: phlebitis, infiltration/extravasation, infection, occlusion, catheter damage, nerve injury, pneumothorax, arterial puncture, hemorrhage, cardiac tamponade, air embolus, and hemothorax. Nurses also need to be aware of strategies to prevent these complications when caring for patients with a CVAD. Evidence-informed and vigilant nursing care is important for insertion and in the maintenance of all CVADs. Nursing responsibilities for CVADs include careful assessment and monitoring, flushing, site care, and dressing changes to prevent catheter-associated bloodstream infection (CABSI). See Box 41.10 for evidence-informed practice for preventing CABSI. ANTT and diligent hand hygiene are essential for all aspects of care. Prior to insertion, chlorhexidine gluconate 2% in 70% isopropyl alcohol should be applied properly and allowed to dry. Maximal barrier precautions (including gown, mask, cap, and full

BOX 41.10 EVIDENCE-INFORMED PRACTICE

Preventing Catheter-Associated Bloodstream Infections (CABSI)

PICO Question: In hospitalized adult patients, which interventions for catheter insertion and care are best to prevent catheter–associated bloodstream infections (CABSI)?

Evidence Summary

CABSI is a serious complication of IV therapy that increases morbidity, hospital length of stay, and health care costs and, most importantly, has a negative impact on patients' well-being, recovery, and experiences. The highest risk of contamination is at insertion, but it also occurs when the lumen and plug are manipulated and needle-free connects are contaminated (Takashima et al., 2017). Dwell time for catheters also increases the risk of CABSI. Given the high prevalence of vascular access devices (VADs; both peripheral vascular access devices [PVADs] and central vascular access devices [CVADs]), prevention strategies would reduce hospital-acquired infections significantly (Chen et al., 2021). To prevent CABSI:

- Hand hygiene must be performed prior to any engagement with the VAD.
- Standard aseptic no-touch technique is required for catheter insertion and care, preventing the contamination of the catheter or site.
- Prior to catheter insertion, skin antisepsis is performed using a single-use applicator, sterile solution, and allowing for dry time (Gorski et al., 2021). An alcohol-based chlorhexidine is recommended. A crosshatch friction scrub technique is more effective at reducing bacterial load for skin antisepsis because it enables maximum contact between the skin and antiseptic, allowing the solution to reach deeper skin cell layers.
- CVAD insertion requires use of maximal sterile barrier precautions to avoid contamination and pathogen exposure. This includes using a mask, protective eyewear, cap, and the following sterile supplies: gown, gloves, and full-body drapes and towels (Gorski et al., 2021).
- Intact dressings protect the site from infection and catheter dislodgement. Transparent dressings are preferred and are changed every week, or immediately when loose, wet, or soiled (CVAA, 2019).

The Canadian Vascular Access Association's (CVAA, 2019) *Canadian Vascular Access and Infusion Therapy Guidelines* provides in-depth recommendations on the best dressings to use and for changing of needle-free connectors.

Central-line bundles are recommended to reduce risk of infection on insertion (Lee et al., 2018), including hand hygiene before catheter insertion; use of maximum sterile barrier precautions on insertion; chlorhexidine skin antisepsis before insertion and during dressing changes; avoidance of the femoral vein for central venous access for adults; and daily evaluation of line necessity, with prompt removal of nonessential lines.

Maintenance bundles are similar, with attention to hand hygiene, catheter hub asepsis, dressing change, and continued daily evaluation of PVAD need (Dumyati et al., 2014). The use of midline catheters would reduce CVAD use, thereby reducing CABSI (DeVries et al., 2019). Prophylactic antibiotic use is no longer recommended for ports (Choksi et al., 2020). Caspari and colleagues (2017) suggest that developing aids to quantify scrub time would increase adherence. Cyanoacrylate tissue adhesive has been approved for use with vascular access devices, and the benefits of this aid to device securement are now being recognized (Nicholson & Hill, 2019).

Application to Nursing Practice

- Advocate for monitoring of CABSI in your agency through standardized language use and electronic documentation following Infusion Nurses Society (INS) guidelines.
- Implement aseptic non-touch technique (ANTT) processes for all catheter insertion and maintenance processes.
- Consider implementation of prevention bundles if they are not in use in your agency.
- Engage in continuous education, training, and competency review, drawing on INS or CVAA infusion therapy and vascular access competencies.

drape) and ultrasound-guided procedure are key recommendations for insertion (Canadian Vascular Access Association [CVAA], 2019; Gorski et al., 2021). Nurses must ensure that the tip placement or location has been verified and documented before the CVAD is used. Finally, the date of insertion must be documented and, for PICCs, the measurement of the external segment.

Maintenance recommendations are aimed at maintaining patency and preventing complications, specifically catheter-related bloodstream infection (CR-BSI) or CLABSI. The manufacturer's stabilization device is preferred for PICCs and CVCs. Sterile, transparent, semipermeable membrane dressings are recommended (Gorski et al., 2021). CVAD dressings are assessed daily. The new dressing is labelled per agency policy. Transparent semipermeable dressing may be left intact for up to 5 to 7 days, unless they become wet, soiled, or loose. No dressing is required for a tunnelled catheter once the wound has healed, unless the patient prefers one.

The external segment of the CVAD (e.g., PICC) should be measured and results documented daily to ensure that the catheter remains in the correct placement. The insertion site should be inspected daily for tenderness, signs of infection, erythema, warmth, and edema, and assessment should include palpation. The chest and neck should be assessed for engorged veins and for difficulty with movement. The nurse should also assess the patient for signs of systemic infection, such as fever, chills, and hypotension.

Prior to accessing a CVAD, a vigorous mechanical scrub with 70% isopropyl alcohol with 5-second drying time or alcohol-based 2% chlorhexidine with 20-second drying time is recommended (Rickard et al., 2021). To prevent occlusion of the CVAD, the device is flushed and assessed for patency according to agency policy. Totally implanted vascular access devices, used for long-term treatment such as chemotherapy, are inserted surgically and are accessed by inserting a needle through the skin into the device. They can be used up to 2000 times and have the lowest incidence of infection.

Patient and family education is required for all patients with a CVAD. This should include care requirements and patient restrictions.

Administration of Intravenous Therapy

Types of solutions. Many prepared intravenous solutions are available for use (see Table 41.9). Solutions are classified as hypertonic, isotonic, or hypotonic. Osmolarity, reflecting the osmolar concentration in 1 L of solution (mOsm/L), is most often used to describe fluids outside the body. A solution with the same osmolarity as blood plasma is called isotonic. A hypertonic solution, with a higher osmotic pressure, such as 3% sodium chloride, pulls fluid from cells, causing them to shrink. An isotonic solution, with the same osmotic pressure as plasma, such as 0.9% sodium chloride, expands the body's fluid volume without causing a fluid shift from one compartment to another. A hypotonic solution, with an osmotic pressure lower than plasma, such as 0.45% sodium chloride, moves fluid into the cells, causing them to enlarge. Each of these actions occurs through osmosis.

In general, isotonic fluids are used most commonly for extracellular volume replacement (e.g., FVD after prolonged vomiting). The decision to use a hypotonic or hypertonic solution is based on the specific fluid and electrolyte imbalances. For example, the patient with a hypertonic fluid imbalance will in general receive a hypotonic intravenous solution to dilute the ECF and rehydrate the cells. All intravenous fluids should be given carefully, especially hypertonic solutions, because these pull fluid into the vascular space by osmosis, resulting in an increased vascular volume that can lead to pulmonary edema, particularly in patients with heart or renal failure. Certain additives, most commonly vitamins and potassium chloride, are frequently added to intravenous solutions.

SAFETY ALERT Under no circumstances should potassium chloride (KCl) be given by intravenous push. Direct intravenous infusion of KCl may cause death. If an intravenous fluid requires additives, a prescription must specify the required additives—for example, "1000 mL D51/2 NS with 20 mmol/L KCl at 125 mL/hour."

Patients with normal renal function who are receiving nothing by mouth (npo) should have potassium added to intravenous solutions. The body cannot conserve potassium, and even when the serum level falls, the kidneys continue to excrete potassium. Without oral or parenteral potassium intake, hypokalemia can develop quickly. Conversely, the nurse should verify that the patient has adequate renal function before administering an intravenous solution containing potassium, because hyperkalemia can develop quickly.

Equipment. Correct selection and preparation of intravenous equipment are necessary for safe and quick placement of an intravenous line. Intravenous cannulas are available in a variety of gauges. The larger the gauge, the smaller the diameter of the cannula. These cannulas are plastic tubing threaded over a needle. Once the cannula is inserted into the vein, the needle is withdrawn, leaving the cannula in place. Intravenous tubing or an intermittent infusion device, such as a needle-free connector, is then added.

SAFETY ALERT Intravenous pumps or volume-control (flow-control) devices ensure a prescribed rate of infusion. A prescribed rate of infusion is vital for children, patients with renal or cardiac failure, and critically ill patients. Electronic infusion devices must be used for medications that require precise rates of administration.

Insertion of a short peripheral intravenous catheter. A venipuncture is a technique in which a vein is punctured through the skin by a sharp, rigid stylet (e.g., butterfly needle or metal needle), a partially covered plastic catheter (over-the-needle catheter), or a needle attached to a syringe. Assessment of vessel characteristics allows for early recognition of risk for difficult cannulation, because vessel characteristics are more important than patient-related factors (Piredda et al., 2017). For these difficult cases, venipuncture should be performed by an experienced, skilled practitioner with the use of ultrasound or infrared light visualization (Gorski et al., 2021).

Venipuncture site. After the equipment is collected at the bedside, the nurse prepares to place the intravenous line by assessing the patient for a venipuncture site (see Skill 41.1). Common intravenous insertion sites are the hand and the arm (Figures 41.11 and 41.12). The use of the foot for an intravenous site is common with children but is avoided in the adult because of the danger of thrombophlebitis (Gorski et al., 2021).

Venipuncture is contraindicated in a site that has signs of infection, infiltration, or thrombosis. Arms on the side of a mastectomy, and extremities with an arteriovenous graft or fistula for dialysis should be avoided. It is important to place intravenous devices at the most distal point, when possible, as this allows for the use of proximal sites later if the patient needs a venipuncture site change. See Box 41.11 for guidelines concerning older persons.

Regulating the infusion flow rate. After the intravenous infusion is secured and the line is patent, the nurse must regulate the rate of infusion according to the prescription orders (Skill 41.2). An infusion rate that is too slow can lead to further cardiovascular and circulatory collapse in a critically ill patient. An intravenous fluid that is running too slowly can also clot more easily. An infusion rate that is too rapid can result in FVE. Fluids that run by gravity are adjusted through use of

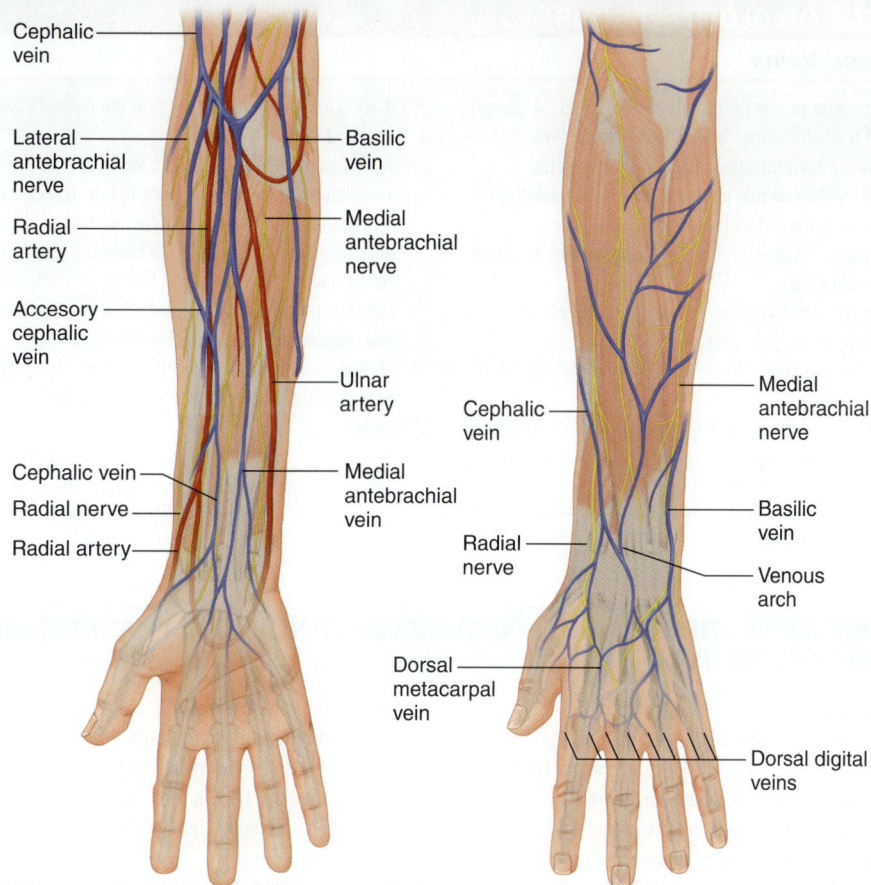

FIGURE 41.11 Common intravenous sites. (From Canadian Vascular Access Association.)

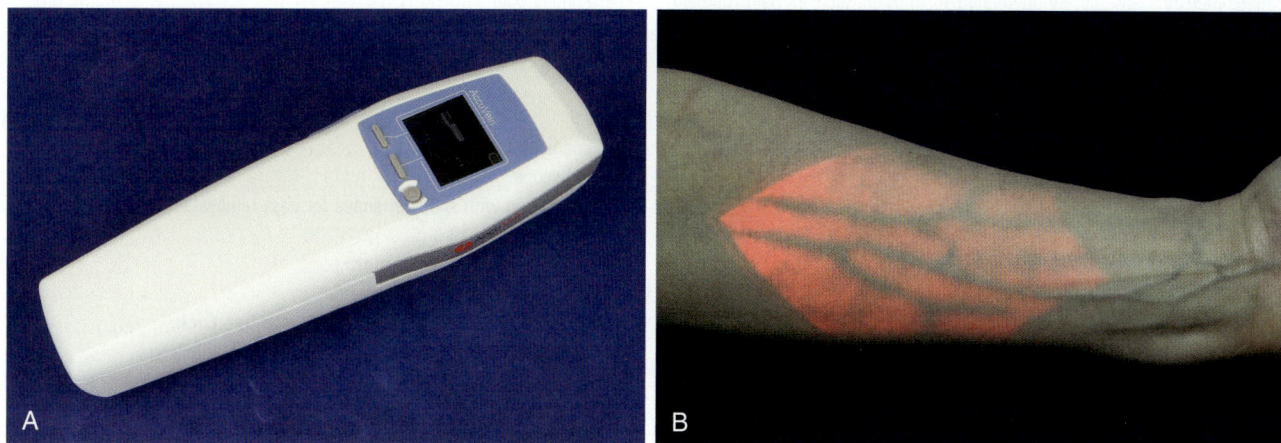

FIGURE 41.12 A, Vein finder. **B,** Veins illuminated. (Courtesy Darlaine Jantzen, RN, MA, PhD. Photo by Burl Jantzen.)

a flow control or regulator clamp. Fluids infused by an electronic infusion device or rate controller are regulated by a mechanical mechanism set at the prescribed rate. Regardless of the device in use, the patient requires close monitoring to verify the correct infusion of the intravenous solution and to detect any complication.

Electronic infusion devices (EIDs) or infusion pumps are necessary when administering low hourly volumes (e.g., less than 20 mL/hour) and for patients who are at risk for volume overload, such as neonatal, pediatric, and geriatric patients. In addition, when infusing high volumes of intravenous fluids (more than 150 mL/hour) to patients with impaired renal clearance, older persons, or children, or when infusing medications or intravenous fluids that require specific hourly volumes, EIDs permit accurate infusion. EIDs deliver the infusion via positive pressure and have become standard in most settings. Recent advances in infusion technology have resulted in a variety of devices available for use to ensure accurate delivery.

Many devices have operating and programming capabilities that allow for single- and multiple-solution infusions at different rates. A

BOX 41.11 FOCUS ON OLDER PERSONS

Protection of Skin and Veins

- Use the smallest gauge cannula or needle possible (e.g., 22 to 24 gauge). Veins are very fragile, and a smaller gauge allows better blood flow, to provide increased hemodilution of the intravenous fluids or medications.
- Avoid using the back of the hand for needle insertion, which may compromise the patient's need for independence and mobility.
- Impaired skin integrity may lead to susceptibility for tearing, venous sclerosis, and difficulty detecting complications.
- Avoid placement of an intravenous line in veins that are easily bumped, because less subcutaneous support tissue is present.
- If the patient has fragile skin and veins, use minimal or no tourniquet pressure.
- After applying a tourniquet, venous pressure rises rapidly, the vein is overstretched, and puncture with even a thin needle can rupture the wall of the vein.

- If using a tourniquet, place it over the patient's sleeve to decrease shearing of fragile skin.
- With loss of supportive tissue, veins tend to lie more superficially; lower the insertion angle for venipuncture to 5 to 15 degrees (Gorski et al., 2021).
- If the patient has lost subcutaneous tissue, the veins lose stability and will roll away from the needle. To stabilize the vein, apply traction to the skin below the projected insertion site.
- Nutritional deficiencies promote fluid to migrate into tissues surrounding vessels, making intravenous access more difficult.
- Multiple medication usage (e.g., anticoagulants, antibiotics, and steroids) increases the likelihood of fragile, transparent skin that bruises and bleeds easily.
- Dehydration related to a lower percentage of body weight as water and a diminished thirst mechanism contribute to difficult intravenous access.

SKILL 41.2 INITIATING, REGULATING, AND DISCONTINUING INTRAVENOUS INFUSIONS (IV)

Delegation Considerations

The skill of regulating IV infusions cannot be delegated to an unregulated care provider (UCP). The licensed practical nurses (LPN)/registered practical nurse (RPN) scope of practice varies by province and health authority. The skill of initiating and regulating IV infusions may be delegated to other health care team members. Always check employer policy. Caring for patients with IV infusions requires effective communication and a collaborative health care team. The nurse instructs the UCP to immediately report the following:

- When the IV solution bag is low and will require a new bag
- When the electronic infusion device is alarming
- Patient indicates any discomfort related to infusion such as pain, burning, bleeding, or swelling at the vascular access device (VAD) site

Equipment

Initiating and Regulating Infusion:
- Prescribed IV solution or medication
- Antiseptic swab(s) (70% alcohol or 2% chlorhexidine gluconate [CHG]/alcohol)
- Commercially prepared 10-mL prefilled 0.9% normal saline (NS) syringe(s)
- Clean gloves
- IV administration set (IV tubing), either macrodrip or microdrip, depending on prescribed rate; if using an electronic infusion device (EID), administration set must be compatible with the electronic device
- 0.2-micron filter if recommended for type of infusion
- EID and IV pole
- Watch with second hand to calculate drip rate
- Calculator, paper, and pencil
- Tape
- Label
- Biomedical sharps container
- Stethoscope
- Patient gown with shoulder snaps for easy removal with continuous infusion therapy (if available)

Changing IV Solution Container:
- Prescribed IV solution or medication

Discontinuing Infusion or Converting to Saline Lock:
- Antiseptic swab(s) (70% alcohol or 2% CHG/alcohol)
- Commercially prepared 10-mL prefilled 0.9% NS syringe(s)
- Clean gloves

PROCEDURE

STEP	RATIONALE
ASSESSMENT	
1. Review accuracy and completeness of health care provider prescription in patient's medical record for patient name and correct solution: type, volume, additives, infusion rate, and duration of infusion therapy. Follow the 10 rights of drug administration (see Chapter 35). If keep vein open (KVO) rate is prescribed, check employer policy regarding flow rate of KVO.	• Ensures delivery of correct IV solution and prescribed volume over prescribed time. • Prevents catheter clotting, thus preserving venous access while infusing a minimal amount of fluid. A prescription for KVO rate must specify an infusion rate as required by the rights of medication administration. Rates may vary from 0.5 mL/hr to 30 mL/hr, based on type of VAD, patient-specific therapy, and method of infusion (gravity or EID).

Continued

SKILL 41.2   INITIATING, REGULATING, AND DISCONTINUING INTRAVENOUS INFUSIONS (IV)—cont'd

2. Assess for clinical factors and conditions that will be affected by infusion therapy, including lab values, clinical markers of volume, allergies, and behaviour and cognition.

- Knowledge of infusion therapy modalities (e.g., peripheral VAD [PVAD], central VAD [CVAD], solution, medication, volume) is necessary to identify key assessments and treatment evaluation.

A. Body weight

- Changes in body weight can be an indication of fluid loss or gain.

B. Clinical markers of vascular volume:

(1) Urine output (decreased, dark yellow)

- Kidneys respond to extracellular volume (ECV) deficit by reducing urine production and concentrating urine. Kidney disease can also cause oliguria.

(2) Vital signs: blood pressure, respirations, pulse, temperature

- Changes in blood pressure may be associated with fluid volume status (fluid volume deficit [FVD]) seen in postural hypotension.
- Respirations can be altered in presence of acid–base balances.
- Temperature elevations increase need for fluid requirements (temperature 38.3°C [101°F] to 39.4°C [103°F] require at least 500 mL of fluid replacement within a 24-hr period) (Weinstein & Hagle, 2014).

(3) Distended neck veins (Normally veins are full when person is supine and flat when person is upright.)

- Indicator of fluid volume status: flat or collapsing with inhalation when supine with ECV deficit; full when upright or semi-upright with ECV excess.

(4) Auscultation of lungs

- Crackles or rhonchi in dependent parts of lung may signal fluid buildup caused by ECV excess.

(5) Capillary refill

- Indirect measure of tissue perfusion (sluggish with ECV deficit)

C. Clinical markers of interstitial volume:

(1) Skin turgor (pinch skin over sternum or inside of forearm)

- Failure of skin to return to normal position after several seconds indicates FVD.

(2) Dependent edema (pitting or nonpitting) (see Chapter 32)

- Edema is not usually apparent until 2–4 kg (4.4–8.8 lb) of fluid is retained. A weight gain of 1 kg (2.2 lb) is equivalent to retention of 1 L of body water (Holroyd, 2020).

(3) Oral mucosa membrane between cheek and gum (see Chapter 32)

- More reliable indicator than dry lips or skin. Dryness between cheek and gums indicates ECV deficit.

D. Thirst

- Occurs with hypernatremia and severe ECV deficit. Not a reliable indicator for older persons (Arai et al., 2014; El-Sharkawy et al., 2020).

E. Behaviour and level of consciousness:

(1) Restlessness and mild confusion

- Occurs with FVD or acid–base imbalance.

(2) Decreased level of consciousness (lethargy, confusion, coma)

- Occurs with severe ECV deficit.
- May occur with osmolality, fluid and electrolyte, and acid–base imbalances.

3. Identify patient risk for fluid and electrolyte imbalance given type of IV solution (e.g., newborn, history of cardiac or renal disease).

- Helps prioritize assessments. Volume control needs to be strict. Guides choice of infusion device.

4. Assess VAD function and patency just prior to administration (Gorski et al., 2021) (see Skill 41.3).

- Identifies complications that compromise integrity of VAD and may necessitate replacement of VAD. Reduces transmission of infection.
- Reduces risk of infiltration or extravasation (Gorski et al., 2021).

5. Assess IV system for patency from IV container to insertion site.

- Ensures delivery of prescribed volume over prescribed time.

6. Assess infusate for vesicant or irritant properties.

- Presence of a vesicant or irritant would prompt more frequent assessments and may require changing the VAD to a more suitable type, to prevent vessel damage (Gorski et al., 2021).

7. Assess patient's knowledge related to prescribed treatment, signs and symptoms of infusion related complications, and how to report them.

- Decreases anxiety and promotes cooperation and adherence to therapy. Prepares patient and caregiver by explaining procedure, its purpose, and what is expected of patient.

PLANNING

8. Have paper and pencil or calculator to calculate flow rate.

- Use mathematical calculations to obtain correct rate. Refer to medication math resources for assistance with calculations.

Continued

9. Check prescription to see how long each litre of fluid should infuse. If hourly rate (mL/hr) is not provided in prescription, calculate it by dividing volume by hours. For example:

$$mL/hr = \frac{Total\ infusion\ (mL)}{Hours\ of\ infusion}$$

$1000\ mL\ /\ 8\ hr = 125\ mL\ /\ hr$

or if 3 L is prescribed for 24 hours:

$3000\ mL\ /\ 24\ hr = 125\ mL\ /\ hr$

- Basis of calculation to ensure infusion of solution over prescribed hourly rate.

CRITICAL DECISION POINT: *It is common for health care providers to write an abbreviated IV prescription such as "D_5W with 20 mEq KCl 125 mL/hr continuous." This prescription implies that the IV should be maintained at this rate until a prescription has been written for the IV to be discontinued or changed to another prescription.*

10. *Infusion via EID:* Use hourly rate (mL/hr) to program pump.
- EID automatically delivers correct minute flow rate.

11. *Infusion via gravity:* Use hourly rate to calculate minute flow rate (gtt/mL). Know calibration (drop factor), in drops per millilitre (gtt/mL), of infusion set used by employer:
- Gravity infusion requires calculation of gtt/mL.

    A. Microdrip: 60 gtt/mL: Used to deliver rates less than 100 mL/hr.
    - Microdrip tubing universally delivers 60 gtt/mL. Used when small or very precise volumes are to be infused.

    B. Macrodrip: 10 to 15 gtt/mL (depending on manufacturer). Used to deliver rates greater than 100 mL/hr.
    - There are different commercial parenteral administration sets for macrodrip tubing. Used when large volumes or fast rates are necessary. Know drip factor for tubing being used.

    C. Select one of the following formulas to calculate minute flow rate (drops per minute) based on drop factor of infusion set:
    - Once you determine hourly rate, these formulas compute the correct flow rate.

    (i) mL/hr/60 min = mL/min

    Drop factor × mL/min = Drops/min

    or

    (ii) mL/hr × Drop factor/60 min = Drops/min

    D. Calculate minute flow rate for a bag 1 000 mL with 20 mEq KCl at 125 mL/hr.

    (i) **Microdrip:**
    - When using microdrip, millilitres per hour (mL/hr) always equals drops per minute (gtt/min).

    125 mL / hr × 60 gtt / mL = 7500 gtt / hr

    7500 gtt ÷ 60 min = 125 gtt / min

    (ii) **Macrodrip:**
    - Multiply volume by drop factor and divide product by time (in minutes).

    125 mL / hr × 15 gtt / mL = 1875 gtt / hr

    1875 gtt ÷ 60 min = 31 — 32 gtt / min

IMPLEMENTATION

12. Perform hand hygiene.
- Decreases potential risk of microbial contamination and cross-contamination (Gorski et al., 2021).

13. Identify patient using at least two identifiers (e.g., name and birthday or name and medical record number) according to employer policy. Compare identifiers with information on patient's medical record and armband.
- Ensures correct patient. Complies with Accreditation Canada's standards and improves patient safety (HSO, 2019).

Preparing IV Administration Set and Solution for Continuous or Intermittent Infusion

14. Prepare all infusions just prior to administration.
    A. Confirm IV solution using 10 rights of medication administration (see Chapter 35). Verify that solution information is correct by reviewing name of medication or solution, dosage and concentration, beyond-use and expiration dates, and sterility state.
- IV administration sets are changed at established intervals, when a VAD is changed or if there is suspected contamination.
- Administration set changes should be planned to coincide with the initiation of a new solution container/medication.
- For continuous infusions, change every 4–7 days or per agency policy.
- For intermittent infusions, administration sets are changed every 24 hours or per agency policy (CVAA, 2019).
- Reviewing label for accuracy reduces risk of medication errors (Gorski et al., 2021).

Continued

SKILL 41.2   INITIATING, REGULATING, AND DISCONTINUING INTRAVENOUS INFUSIONS (IV)—cont'd

B. Check solution for color and clarity. Check bag for leaks.

C. Open administration set (IV tubing), maintaining sterility. **Note:** EIDs sometimes have a dedicated administration set; follow manufacturer's instructions.

D. Place roller clamp about 2 cm to 5 cm below drip chamber and move roller clamp to "off" or "closed position.

E. Remove protective cap over spike port on infusion container or bag.

F. Remove protective cover from spike of administration set (IV tubing) using aseptic non-touch technique. Insert spike into port of IV bag using a twisting motion (see Step 14F illustration). If solution container is glass bottle, clean rubber stopper on glass-bottled solution with antiseptic swab and insert spike into rubber stopper of IV bottle. Bottles require vented tubing. If sterility of spike is compromised, discard IV administration set and open a new set.

- Sterility may be compromised if any of the following are observed:
  - Leaking of the container or bag
  - Discoloration of solution
  - Precipitate is visible
  - Solution is beyond use date or if expiration has passed
- Do not use if contamination is suspected.

- Prevent touch contamination, which allows microorganisms to enter infusion equipment and bloodstream.

- Close proximity of roller clamp to the drip chamber allows for more accurate regulation of flow rate. Moving clamp to "off" prevents accidental spillage of IV solution during priming.

- Provides access for insertion of IV administration set spike into solution using sterile technique.

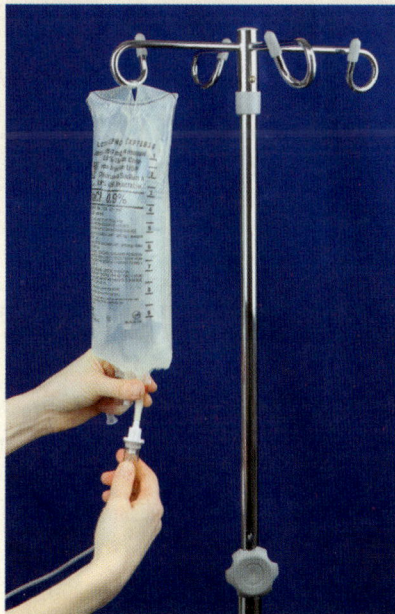

STEP 14F Prepare infusate bag and administration set. (From Cobbett, S. L., Perry, A. G., Potter, P. A., et al. [Eds.] [2020]. *Canadian clinical nursing skills & techniques.* Elsevier. Photo courtesy Burl Jantzen.)

G. Compress drip chamber and release, allowing it to fill one-third to one-half full.

- Creates suction effect; fluid enters drip chamber to prevent air from entering tubing.

H. Purge air from tubing by slowly opening the roller clamp (see Step 14H illustration). This will allow the IV solution to flow from the drip chamber to fill the tubing. If the administration set has in-line access ports, invert the port as the solution fills the tubing. This will ensure complete removal of air. When solution reaches the distal end of the tubing, close clamp. Label administration set with time and date, according to employer policy and procedure.

- Priming ensures that IV administration set is clear of air and filled with IV solution before connecting to VAD. Slowly filling tubing decreases turbulence and chance of bubble formation.Closing clamp prevents loss of solution.

- Labeling IV administration set identifies when administration set needs to be changed.

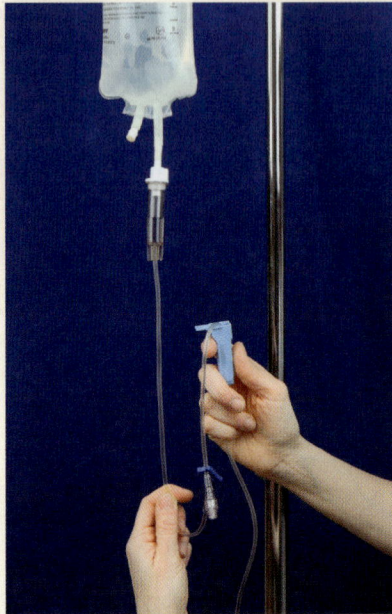

STEP 14H Purge air from administration set using roller clamp. (From Cobbett, S. L., Perry, A. G., Potter, P. A., et al. [Eds.] [2020]. *Canadian clinical nursing skills & techniques*. Elsevier. Photo courtesy Burl Jantzen.)

I. Confirm by visual inspection that tubing is clear of air and air bubbles. To remove small air bubbles, firmly tap tubing where they are located.

- Large air bubbles may act as emboli (Gorski et al., 2021).

Initiate Infusion

15. Perform hand hygiene and apply clean gloves.

- Promotes infection prevention and control.

16. Assess VAD function and patency (see Skill 41.3).

- Assessing just prior to initiating infusion reduces risk of infiltration and extravasation (see Table 41.12).

17. Scrub VAD needle-free connector with antiseptic swab for at least 15 seconds and let dry. Remove protective cap from administration set and connect via Luer-Lok to needle-free connector (see Step 17 illustration). Maintain aseptic non-touch technique at all times.

- Initiates flow of fluid through IV catheter, preventing clotting of VAD.

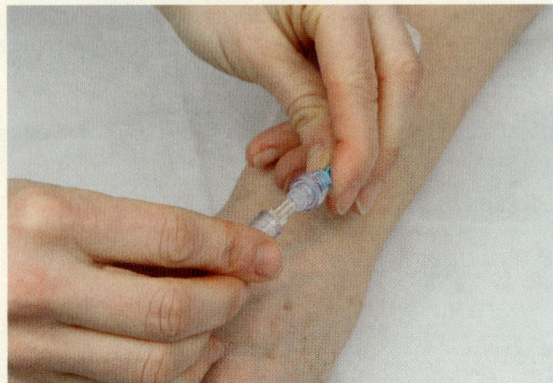

STEP 17 Attach administration set to scrubbed needle-free connector. (From Cobbett, S. L., Perry, A. G., Potter, P. A., et al. [Eds.]. [2020]. *Canadian Clinical nursing skills & techniques*. Elsevier. Photo courtesy Patrick Coble.)

Continued

SKILL 41.2	**INITIATING, REGULATING, AND DISCONTINUING INTRAVENOUS INFUSIONS (IV)—cont'd**

18. Regulate infusion via gravity

A. Place adhesive or fluid indicator tape on IV bag next to volume markings.

- Tape provides a visual cue as to whether fluids are being administered over correct time period.

B. Ensure that IV container is at least 76.2 cm (30 in) above IV site for adults and increase height for viscous fluids (INS, 2021).

- Pressure caused by gravity is necessary to overcome venous pressure and resistance from tubing and catheter.

C. Slowly open roller clamp on tubing until you can see drops in the drip chamber. Hold a watch with second hand at the same level as the drip chamber and count drip rate for 1 minute. Adjust roller clamp to increase or decrease rate of infusion.

- Regulates flow at prescribed rate.

19. Regulate infusion via EID

A. Load administration set into EID (see Step 19A illustration). Check manufacturer recommendations for correct IV container height.

- Ensures accuracy. Manufacturers may vary on the optimal distance between EID and IV solution container.

STEP 19A Loading primed administration set into EID. (Courtesy Darlaine Jantzen, RN, MA, PhD. Photo by Burl Jantzen.)

B. Regulate according to manufacturer's instructions.

C. Assess IV system from container to VAD insertion site when alarm signals.

- Alarm indicates situation that requires attention. Empty solution container, tubing kinks, closed clamp, infiltration, clotted catheter, air in tubing, or low battery can trigger EID alarm.

CRITICAL DECISION POINT: *An anti–free flow safeguard (preventing bolus infusion in the event of machine malfunction or when tubing is removed from machine) is an important element of an EID and is required. Always check and follow manufacturer's recommendations for specific device features.*

---

20. Teach patient purpose of EID if infusion therapy is delivered by EID, purpose of alarms, to avoid raising hand or arm that affects flow rate, and to avoid touching control clamp or EID.

- Information enables patient to protect IV site and informs patient about rationale for not altering control rate.

Changing IV Solution Container

21. Change solution container when prescription changes or when a small amount remains.

- Prevents waste of solution.
- Employer policy will specify maximum hang time for IV solution containers.

22. Perform hand hygiene.

- Reduces transmission of microorganisms.

23. Prepare new solution for changing. If using plastic bag, hang on IV pole and remove protective cover from IV administration set port. If using glass bottle, remove metal cap and metal and rubber disks.

- Permits quick, smooth, organized change from old to new container.

24. Close roller clamp on existing solution to stop flow rate. Remove IV administration set from EID if necessary to prevent contamination of new solution port or tubing spike (if used). Then remove old IV solution container from IV pole. Invert salutation container. Maintain aseptic non-touch technique.

- Prevents solution remaining in drip chamber from emptying while changing solutions. Prevents solution in bag from spilling.

25. Quickly remove spike from old solution container and insert spike into new container. Maintain aseptic non-touch technique.

- Reduces risk of solution in drip chamber becoming empty and maintains sterility.

CRITICAL DECISION POINT: *If any spike becomes contaminated by touching an unsterile object, discard and open a new administration set.*

26. Hang new container of solution on IV pole.

- Gravity helps with delivery of fluid into drip chamber.

27. Make sure that drip chamber is one-third to one-half full. If drip chamber is too full, level can be decreased by removing bag from IV pole, pinching off IV administration set below drip chamber, inverting container, squeezing drip chamber (see Step 27 illustration), releasing and turning solution container upright, and releasing pinch on tubing.

- Reduces risk for air entering IV administration set. If chamber is completely filled, you cannot observe or regulate drip rate.

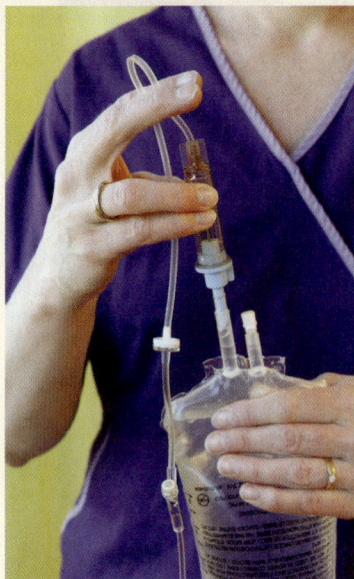

STEP 27 Pinch tubing, invert chamber, and squeeze drip chamber to remove a portion of the fluid. (Courtesy Darlaine Jantzen, RN, MA, PhD. Photo by Burl Jantzen.)

28. Regulate flow to prescribed rate by opening and adjusting roller clamp on IV administration set by opening roller clamp and programming and turning on EID.

- Maintains measures to restore fluid balance and deliver IV solution as prescribed.

29. Monitor infusion rate and VAD site for complications at least hourly (or per employer policy). Note volume of IV fluid infused and rate of infusion. Use watch to verify rate of infusion, even when using EID.

- Ensures delivery of prescribed volume over prescribed time and decreases risk for fluid and electrolyte imbalance.
- Flow controllers and pumps do not replace frequent, accurate nursing evaluation.
- EIDs can continue to infuse IV solutions after a complication has developed.

30. Evaluate patient's response to therapy (e.g., laboratory values, input and output [I&O], weights, vital signs, post-procedure assessments).

- Provides ongoing evaluation of patient's fluid status, including monitoring for FVE or FVD. Early recognition of complications leads to prompt treatment.

Discontinuing Infusion or Saline Lock

31. Check prescriber's order for discontinuation of intravenous therapy.

- Order is required for discontinuation of fluids or medication.

32. Perform hand hygiene and apply clean gloves

- Reduces transmission of microorganisms

33. Stop EID or close roller clamp to "off" position.

- Prevents fluid spillage.

34. Disconnect administration set from VAD needle-free connector. Attach a new, sterile cap to end of administration set (Gorski et al., 2021). Maintain aseptic non-touch technique.

- Specific clamping sequence is required to prevent reflux of blood into VAD catheter.
- Maintains sterility of administration set if required for intermittent use.

Continued

SKILL 41.2	INITIATING, REGULATING, AND DISCONTINUING INTRAVENOUS INFUSIONS (IV)—cont'd

35. Flush and lock VAD (see Skill 41.3).

- Decreases risk of intraluminal occlusion and clears infused medication from catheter (Gorski et al., 2021).

36. Remove and dispose of any used supplies; perform hand hygiene.

- Prevents transmission of infection.

37. Document the following in the nurses' notes in patient electronic health record (EHR) or chart:
- IV solution, rate of infusion in drops per minute (gtt/min) for infusions via gravity or millilitres per hour (mL/hr)
- Integrity and patency of system, including VAD according to employer policy
- Use of any EID or control device and identification number on that device, if required by employer policy
- Patient response (e.g., laboratory values, I&O, weights, vital signs, post-procedure assessments) to therapy and unexpected outcomes (e.g., signs and symptoms of FVE, FVD, or IV-related complications)
- Patient's and caregiver's level of understanding following instruction in nurses' notes in EHR or chart

UNEXPECTED OUTCOMES

1. *Solution does not infuse at prescribed rate*

A. *Sudden infusion of large volume of solution occurs; patient develops dyspnea, crackles in lung, dependent edema (edema in legs), and increased urine output, indicating FVE.*

B. *IV solution runs slower than prescribed.*

2. *IV patency is lost subsequent to IV solution container running empty.*

RELATED INTERVENTIONS

- Slow infusion rate: KVO rates must have specific rate prescribed by health care provider.
- Notify health care provider immediately.
- Place patient in high-Fowler's position.
- Anticipate new IV prescriptions.
- Anticipate administration of oxygen per prescription.
- Administer diuretics if prescribed.

- Check for positional change that affects rate, height of IV container, kinking of tubing, or obstruction.
- Check VAD site for complications.
- Consult health care provider for new prescription to provide necessary fluid volume.

- Discontinue present IV infusion and restart new short-peripheral catheter in new site.

REPORTING
- At change of shift or when leaving on break, report rate of and volume left in infusion to nurse in charge or next nurse assigned to care for patient.

CARE IN THE COMMUNITY CONSIDERATIONS
- Ensure that patient is able and willing to operate an EID and administer infusion therapy. If patient is unable to provide self-care, be sure that a reliable caregiver is available in the home.
- Discuss proper EID function with patient. Consider use of an ambulatory-type device. Observe patient operating infusion EID and administering infusion therapy.
- Teach patient and caregiver what EID alarms mean, methods to troubleshoot them, and how to disconnect the IV administration set from the EID pump in the event of pump failure.
- Ensure that patient's electrical outlets are properly grounded.
- Provide patient with a contact phone number to access 24 hours a day for problems.

variety of detectors and alarms respond to air in intravenous lines, completion of infusion, high and low pressure, low battery power, occlusion, and the inability to deliver at a preset rate.

SAFETY ALERT An anti–free-flow safeguard (preventing bolus infusion in the event of machine malfunction) is an important element of an electronic infusion device and is required. The manufacturer's recommendations for specific device features should always be checked.

Patency of the intravenous needle or catheter is routinely assessed (Skill 41.3). Gravity intravenous flow rates can also be affected by infiltration, a knot or kink in the tubing, the height of the solution, a restrictive intravenous dressing, and the position of the patient's extremity. An EID is sensitive to occlusions. If the patency of the PIVC is confirmed, the tubing and area around the insertion site should be inspected for anything that could obstruct the flow of intravenous fluids. A knot or kink in the tubing can decrease the flow rate or prompt occlusion alarms. The patient may also occlude the tubing by lying or sitting on it. The flow rate frequently resumes after the tubing is straightened. The height of the intravenous bag can also affect flow rates when an EID is not being used. Raising the bag usually increases the rate because of increased hydrostatic pressure.

SKILL 41.3 ASSESSMENT AND MAINTENANCE OF VASCULAR ACCESS DEVICES (VADS)

Delegation Considerations

Assessment and care of VADs require effective communication and a collaborative health care team. Always refer to employer policy. The skills required for caring and maintaining VADs cannot be performed by unregulated care providers (UCPs) or by those who have not demonstrated competence in such care (Gorski et al., 2021). However, it is important for UCPs to report to the nurse the following immediately:

- Signs and symptoms of complications (redness, swelling, leaking, bleeding, or drainage under the dressing, or patient expression of pain or discomfort)
- A loose, wet, or soiled dressing
- Any electronic infusion device alarms
- Patients with a CVAD experiencing shortness of breath

Equipment

Site Assessment, Patency, and Flushing:
- Clean gloves
- Antiseptic swabs: 2% chlorhexidine gluconate (CHG)/alcohol (preferred), 70% alcohol, or povidone-iodine
- 10-mL 0.9% sodium chloride prefilled syringe(s)—minimum one per VAD lumen

Needle-Free Connector Change:
- Clean gloves
- Needle-free connector(s)
- Antiseptic swabs: 2% CHG/alcohol (preferred), 70% alcohol, or povidone-iodine
- 10-mL 0.9% sodium chloride prefilled syringe(s)—minimum one per VAD lumen

PROCEDURE

STEPS	RATIONALE
ASSESSMENT	
1. Review patient chart for when to assess device based on type of VAD (peripheral VAD [PVAD] or central VAD [CVAD] , single or multi-lumen catheter). For CVADs, review documented external catheter length on insertion.	• Assessment and care depend on clinical setting, type of catheter, number of lumens, and purpose of therapy. • Comparing CVAD external segment measurements facilitates early recognition of dislodgement or migration (CVAA, 2019).
A. PVAD—Assess site and dressing at least once per shift, every 4 hours with continuous nonvesicant infusion, and at least every 30 minutes with vesicant infusion. Assess patency at least once per shift and immediately before starting an infusion or with needle-free connector change (CVAA, 2019).	
B. CVAD—Assess site and dressing at least once per shift. Assess patency at least every 7 days and immediately before starting an infusion or with needle-free connector change (CVAA, 2019).	
2. Review date of last needle-free connector change. Identify type of needle-free connector used.	• Needle-free connectors are changed every 4–7 days or if removed for any reason, presence of visible debris or blood, prior to drawing blood culture, or if contamination is suspected. This decreases the chance of occlusion and infection (CVAA, 2019). • Understanding the type of needle-free connector ensures appropriate flush-clamp-disconnect sequence based on the internal mechanism (e.g., positive, negative, or neutral displacement valve) (Gorski et al., 2021).
3. Assess clinical need for VAD.	• VADs should be assessed daily and removed if complications present unresolved or if no longer required for the plan of care.
4. Assess patient's knowledge of procedure and signs and symptoms of complications.	• Provides person-centred care by determining level of instruction needed.
IMPLEMENTATION **Assessment of VAD Site**	
5. Perform hand hygiene and apply clean gloves.	• Reduces spread of microorganisms, thereby helping to prevent infection.
6. Identify patient using at least two identifiers (e.g., name and birthday or name and medical record number) according to employer policy. Compare identifiers with information on patient's medical record and armband.	• Ensures correct patient. Complies with Accreditation Canada's standards and improves patient safety (HSO, 2019).
7. Inspect skin integrity at VAD insertion site, around dressing and along vein pathway.	• Identifies complications that compromise integrity and functionality of VAD, such as phlebitis, infiltration, and infection.
8. Palpate insertion site and along VAD pathway. Assess for any discomfort, tenderness, pain, tingling, or numbness.	• Identifies complications that compromise integrity and functionality of VAD, such as phlebitis, infiltration, and infection.
9. Inspect integrity of dressing and securement method. If applicable (e.g., PICC or midline) measure external length (CVAA, 2019).	• There is increased risk of infection or catheter dislodgement if dressing is compromised. • Dressings with securement properties or an addition of a stabilization device decrease risks of catheter dislodgement, movement, or mechanical phlebitis (Gorski et al., 2021). • Comparing CVAD external segment measurements facilitates early recognition of dislodgement or migration (CVAA, 2019).
10. If clamps are present on extension set, ensure they are engaged if VAD not in use.	• Reduces risk of occlusion and infection.

Continued

SKILL 41.3	ASSESSMENT AND MAINTENANCE OF VASCULAR ACCESS DEVICES (VADS)—cont'd

STEPS	RATIONALE
11. Verify that needle-free connector is secure and free of visible debris or blood.	• Prevents inadvertent disconnections and/or leaks, infection, and occlusion (Gorski et al., 2021).
12. Remove gloves and perform hand hygiene.	• Assists with infection prevention and control.
13. Document site condition, dressing and securement method, and patient report of pain or discomfort. Document measured external length, if applicable. Document any signs or symptoms of complications and patient teaching provided (CVAA, 2019).	

Assessment of VAD Patency

STEPS	RATIONALE
14. Perform hand hygiene.	• Assists with infection prevention and control.
15. Prepare and purge air from prefilled syringe(s) per manufacturer directions. Maintain aseptic non-touch technique at all times.	• Air is removed from all devices prior to connection to prevent air embolism (Gorski et al., 2021).

16. Vigorously scrub the needle-free connector surface with antiseptic swab and allow to air dry.	• Disinfecting with a new swab before each entry reduces intraluminal microbes and risk of infection. Scrub a minimum of 5–15 seconds. Allowing the solution to dry is important to allow proper disinfection.
	  • 2% CHG/alcohol swab requires 20-second dry time
	  • 70% alcohol requires 5-second dry time
	  • Povidone-iodine requires 6-minute dry time

17. Attach prefilled 10-mL 0.9% normal saline syringe to needle-free connector, maintaining aseptic non-touch technique. Disengage clamp if present.	• Use positive pressure techniques when assessing patency, flushing, and locking VADs to prevent blood reflux and occlusions. Commercially prepared prefilled flush syringes are designed to minimize blood reflux into catheter when compared to a traditional syringe (Gorski et al., 2021).
18. Flush with 1–2 mL and then gently aspirate for blood return. Avoid aspirating blood into the needle-free connector and/or flush syringe. Blood return should be free-flowing and with a colour and consistency of whole blood.	• Patency is confirmed by the ability to flush and aspirate blood return without resistance (CVAA, 2019). • Blood return is not always present in PVADs but must be present prior to vesicant administration (CVAA, 2019).
19. Using same attached syringe, flush catheter using push-pause or pulsatile technique (short 1-mL boluses). Do not forcibly flush against resistance.	• Patency is confirmed by the ability to flush and aspirate blood return without resistance (CVAA, 2019). • Flushing with appropriate volume using a pulsatile technique reduces risk of thrombotic catheter occlusion (Gorski et al., 2021).
20. While flushing, assess VAD for swelling, leaking, or discomfort or pain, or for changes in patient's taste and odour.	• These are signs and symptoms of complications that indicate VAD removal. Prefilled flush syringes can cause brief changes in taste and odour while flushing (CVAA, 2019).
21. Flush with appropriate volume according to agency policy. If using a traditional syringe for flushing (not a prefilled syringe), leave 0.5–1.0 mL at the end before disconnecting.	• Flushing with appropriate volume using a pulsatile technique reduces risk of thrombotic catheter occlusion (Gorski et al., 2021). • Commercially prepared prefilled flush syringes are designed to minimize blood reflux into catheter when compared to a traditional syringe. If using a traditional syringe for flushing, leaving a small amount of solution helps creates positive pressure to minimize reflux (Gorski et al., 2021).
22. Disconnect flush syringe from VAD using the appropriate clamping sequence. If a multi-lumen VAD is used, repeat Steps 15–20 to verify patency of each.	• Using the proper clamping sequence ensures positive pressure to minimize risk of occlusion.
23. Discard supplies and perform hand hygiene.	
24. Document VAD function, flushing without resistance and presence of blood on aspiration, and flush volume used. Document any signs or symptoms of complications and patient teaching provided (CVAA, 2019).	

Flushing and Locking VAD Post-Infusion or Medication Administration

STEPS	RATIONALE
Perform Steps 14–17 of this skill, as shown above.	• Flush all VADs when accessing, between incompatible solutions and/or medications, before and after blood sampling, and after disconnecting infusion. Flush with appropriate volume according to type of VAD and agency policy (CVAA, 2019).
25. Flush catheter using push-pause or pulsatile technique (short 1-mL boluses). Do not forcibly flush against resistance.	• Flushing with appropriate volume using a pulsatile technique reduces risk of thrombotic catheter occlusion and flushes medication from the intraluminal catheter space (Gorski et al., 2021).
26. While flushing, assess VAD for swelling, leaking, or discomfort or pain.	• These are signs and symptoms of complications that indicate VAD removal.

STEPS	RATIONALE
27. Flush with appropriate volume according to agency policy. If using a traditional syringe for flushing (not a prefilled syringe), leave 0.5–1.0 mL at the end before disconnecting.	• Flushing with appropriate volume using a pulsatile technique reduces risk of thrombotic catheter occlusion (Gorski et al., 2021). • Commercially prepared prefilled flush syringes are designed to minimize blood reflux into catheter when compared to a traditional syringe. If using a traditional syringe for flushing, leaving a small amount of solution helps creates positive pressure to minimize reflux (Gorski et al., 2021).
28. Disconnect flush syringe from VAD using the appropriate clamping sequence.	• Using the proper clamping sequence ensures positive pressure to minimize risk of occlusion.
29. Discard supplies and perform hand hygiene.	• Provides infection prevention and control and safety measures.
30. Document catheter type and location, VAD function (flushing without resistance), and flush volume used (per lumen if applicable). Document any signs or symptoms of complications and patient teaching provided.	• Informs care for the interprofessional team and supports continuing of care.

Changing Needle-Free Connector

STEPS	RATIONALE
31. Perform hand hygiene and apply clean gloves.	• Reduces transmission of microorganisms.
32. Using aseptic non-touch technique, attach prefilled 0.9% sodium chloride syringe to new sterile needle-free connector. Flush and prime connector to remove air. Leave prefilled syringe in place. Repeat for number of lumens required if multi-lumen catheter is used.	• Prevents risks of infection. • Priming with 0.9% sodium chloride prevents air from entering the circulatory system.
33. Close clamp on catheter if present. Remove existing needle-free connector from hub using aseptic non-touch technique.	• Reduces air entry into circulatory system, infection, and potential blood reflux into end of catheter.
34. Scrub catheter hub with antiseptic swab for and allow to air dry. Adhere to aseptic non-touch technique.	• Reduces risk of infection.
35. Attach primed needle-free connector to catheter hub and open clamp if present. Maintain aseptic non-touch technique at all times.	
36. Flush VAD and confirm patency using Steps 17–22 of this skill, as shown above.	
37. If using multi-lumen catheter, repeat Steps 33–36 in this skill for each lumen.	• All lumens require flushing to maintain patency following medication administration.
38. Discard supplies. Remove gloves and perform hand hygiene.	• Provides infection prevention and control, and safety measures.
39. Document catheter type and location, needle-free connector change (identify specific lumen if applicable), VAD function, and flush volume used (per lumen if applicable). Document any signs or symptoms of complications and patient teaching provided.	

UNEXPECTED OUTCOMES	RELATED INTERVENTIONS
Catheter occlusion can occur from a bent catheter, positional catheter (catheter resting against catheter wall), kink or knot in extension tubing, clot formation, or precipitate formation from administration of incompatible medications or solutions.	• Determine cause of occlusion. • Occluded catheters should not be flushed because an embolus can result from dislodging a clot.
Medical adhesive-related skin injury (MARSI) can present as redness, tears, or breakdown of the skin exposed to medical adhesive (Gorski et al., 2021).	• Use a different type of dressing if indicated.
Phlebitis (i.e., vein inflammation): pain, redness, warmth, swelling, induration, or presence of palpable cord along course of vein (Gorski et al., 2021). Rate of infusion may be altered.	• Confirm need for vascular access. Determine cause (e.g., chemical, mechanical, or bacterial). • Document phlebitis using a standardized scale, including nursing interventions per employer policy and procedure (see Table 41.11).
Catheter-related infection can present as redness, swelling around or above IV site, pain, purulent drainage at insertion site, and body temperature elevations (Gorski et al., 2021).	• Notify health care provider. Obtain prescription to culture drainage (Gorski et al., 2021). • Obtain blood cultures from peripheral and CVAD if prescribed. • Remove VAD (CVAD requires prescription) and replace with new VAD if still required for care.
Catheter dislodgement/migration	• For PIVCs, remove catheter and replace if still required for care. • For CVADs, consult agency policy and/or contact health care provider.

CARE IN THE COMMUNITY CONSIDERATIONS

- Outpatients or home care patients must be provided with education to perform daily assessments and report finding of complications to health care provider.
- Teach patient and family about hand hygiene and aseptic non-touch technique for all care related to VAD site and equipment.
- Teach patient about activity restrictions (e.g., avoiding strenuous exercise of the arm with the IV line, protecting site while bathing and showering).
- Teach patient and caregiver about how to recognize signs and symptoms of VAD-related complications, actions to take, how to report, and methods for preservation of VAD.

Flexion of an extremity, particularly at the wrist or elbow, or positioning can decrease flow rates. Although VAD placement in areas of flexion is discouraged, in emergencies it may be necessary. Immobilizing with an arm board provides some protection; however, this requires vigilant assessment, and careful positioning to enable visualization and to prevent pressure. However, an intravenous catheter should be re-sited rather than relying on a site that causes problems. Before discontinuing the infusion hampered by an extremity position, the nurse should start the infusion in another site, to verify that the patient has other accessible veins.

When using gravity, rather than an EID, sudden increases in flow can occur accidentally. Some intravenous catheters are positional in the patient's vein. Changes in flow rate are avoided by using an EID or volume-control device. If an EID is not available, vigilance is required to maintain a steady rate of infusion, preventing a rapid increase in vascular volume.

Maintaining the system. After the intravenous line is in place and the flow rate is regulated, the nurse must maintain the system. It is important to observe agency policy regarding maintenance of intravenous lines. Line maintenance is achieved by (1) keeping the system sterile; (2) changing solutions, tubing, and site dressings; and (3) assisting the patient with self-care activities so as not to disrupt the system.

Nurses play an important role in maintaining the integrity of both PVAD and CVAD systems to prevent infection from developing. Knowledge of potential sites for contamination informs nurses' practice. This begins with thorough hand hygiene before and after handling any component of the intravenous system.

The integrity of the intravenous system must always be maintained. Tubing must never be disconnected because it becomes tangled or because it might be more convenient in positioning or moving a patient or applying a gown. If a patient needs more room to manoeuvre, extension tubing can be added to an intravenous line. However, the use of extension tubing should be kept to a minimum, as each

connection of tubing provides an opportunity for contamination. Stopcocks are a source of contamination and should be replaced with a needle-free connector, when possible (Gorski et al., 2021). Whenever an intravenous line is disconnected from a stopcock, the port should be plugged with a sterile cap. A port should never remain exposed to air because of the risk of contamination. A new administration set should be exchanged with the subsequent fluid change.

Intravenous tubing also contains injection ports through which adapters can be inserted for medication injections. The INS recommends intravenous tubing (when the peripheral catheter site is changed). It may be used for up to 96 hours without increasing the chance of infection if it does not contain lipids, blood, or blood products (Gorski et al., 2021). Needle-free injection ports reduce the risk of needle-stick injury and reduce contamination, thereby promoting patient safety when connecting, accessing, or removing intravenous equipment. This risk is further minimized by using alcohol–chlorhexidine gluconate solution or povidone–iodine for cleaning the port both before and after use. Patients receiving intravenous therapy over several days will require a change of solutions. It is important to organize tasks so that this can be done in plenty of time before the solution empties and the cannula becomes clotted. Many agencies have policies regarding the "hang time" of intravenous fluids. Rickard and colleagues (2009) found no need to routinely replace intravenous fluid containers and recommend further research to establish set time points for replacing intravenous fluid containers. Skill 41.2 reviews steps for changing intravenous solutions.

The dressings over intravenous sites are applied to reduce the entrance of bacteria into the insertion site. The two forms of dressings are transparent and gauze. Transparent dressings reliably secure the intravenous device, allow continuous visual inspection of the intravenous site, become less easily soiled or moistened, and require less frequent changes than standard gauze. Intravenous dressings should be routinely changed per agency policy (Skill 41.4).

SKILL 41.4	CHANGING A SHORT-PERIPHERAL INTRAVENOUS CATHETER (PIVC) DRESSING

Delegation Considerations

The skill of changing a PIVC dressing may be delegated to other health care providers if they have had appropriate education and the skill is within their governing body scope of practice and is approved by employer policy. The skill of changing a PIVC dressing cannot be delegated to an unregulated care provider (UCP). The nurse instructs the UCP to report the following immediately:

- Report to the nurse if the dressing is visibly soiled, loose, or wet and if the patient indicates moistness or loosening of the PIVC dressing.
- Protect the PIVC dressing during hygiene and activities of daily living (ADLs).

Equipment

- Antiseptic swabs (2% chlorhexidine gluconate [CHG] with alcohol solution preferred, povidone-iodine, or 70% alcohol)
- Sterile transparent semipermeable membrane (TSM) dressing (with border preferred), or TSM dressing and added engineered stabilization device (ESD)
- Clean gloves

PROCEDURE

STEP	RATIONALE

ASSESSMENT

1. Review patient chart to determine type of dressing and when it was last changed. Dressing should be labelled to include date and time applied, insertion date.

   - TSM dressings are changed at least every 7 days, or immediately if dressing integrity is compromised. Gauze dressings are only used for patients with sensitivities. They are not recommended, as they prevent assessment of the site (Gorski et al., 2021)
   - If the dressing integrity is compromised, there is increased risk of infection or PVAD dislodgement.

2. Assess continuing need for device and remove if indicated (see Box 41.12).

3. Assess patient's understanding of the procedure, including the need to hold affected extremity still during dressing change.

   - Promotes cooperation and promotes active participation in person-centred care.

Continued

SKILL 41.4	CHANGING A SHORT-PERIPHERAL INTRAVENOUS CATHETER (PIVC) DRESSING—cont'd

IMPLEMENTATION

4. Perform hand hygiene

- Reduces transmission of infection and contamination of equipment.

5. Identify patient using at least two identifiers (e.g., name and birthday or name and medical record number) according to employer policy. Compare identifiers with information on patient's medical administration record (MAR) or medical record.

- Ensures correct patient. Complies with Accreditation Canada's standards and improves patient safety (HSO, 2019).

6. Organize equipment on a clean, clutter-free bedside stand or overbed table. Wipe surface with antiseptic wipe prior to use.

- Reduces transmission of infection and contamination of equipment (Gorski et al., 2021).

7. Perform hand hygiene and apply clean gloves.

8. Prior to removing dressing, assess the insertion site visually for complications related to PIVC (see Skill 41.3).

- Identifies complications that compromise integrity of PVAD and may necessitate its replacement.
- Presence of the following complications are indications for PVAD removal: redness, swelling, leaking, drainage, pain of discomfort.

9. Remove existing dressing. Stabilize catheter with nondominant hand (see Step 9 illustration). Remove dressing by pulling dressing away from the skin from proximal edge toward insertion site (Gorski et al., 2021). Repeat on all sides until dressing has been removed.

- Technique minimizes discomfort and injury to skin during removal.
- Stabilization of the catheter prevents loss of access.
- Removing dressing parallel to the skin in a lower and slow motion helps prevent medical adhesive-skin related injury (MARSI)
- Use alcohol swab on TSM dressing next to patient's skin to loosen dressing.

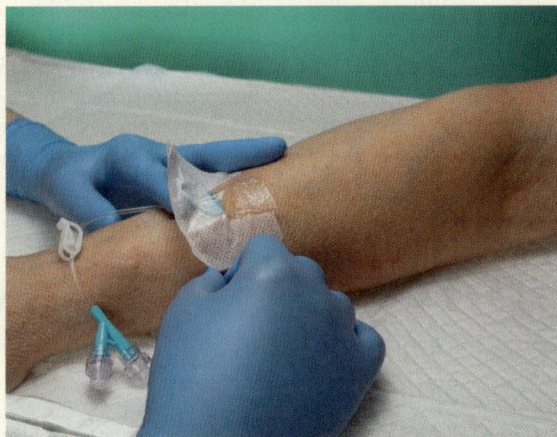

STEP 9 Remove transparent semipermeable membrane (TSM) dressing. (From Cobbett, S. L., Perry, A. G., Potter, P. A., et al. [Eds.]. [2020]. *Canadian clinical nursing skills & techniques*. Elsevier. Photo courtesy Patrick Coble.)

CRITICAL DECISION POINT: *Stabilize catheter throughout process while maintaining asepsis. If patient is restless or uncooperative, it is helpful to have another staff member help with procedure.*

10. Perform skin antisepsis to insertion site with CHG/alcohol swab using friction in back-and-forth motion for at least 30 seconds and allow to dry completely (minimum of 30 seconds). Alternative antiseptic solutions may be used for patient sensitivities (alcohol, povidone-iodine, CHG). Maintain aseptic non-touch technique at all times.

- Reduces incidence of catheter-related infections. Allow any skin antiseptic agent to fully dry for complete antisepsis and to prevent MARSI (Gorski et al., 2021).

11. *Optional:* Apply skin protectant to areas where an adhesive will attach to skin. Avoid area directly around insertion site. Allow to dry.

- Apply skin barrier solution to help protect skin integrity, prevent irritation from adhesive, and promote adhesion of dressing.

12. Apply sterile dressing over site (procedures differ; follow employer policy and manufacturer's guidelines) (see Skill 41.1, Step 28).

- Protects catheter insertion site and minimizes risk for infection. TSM dressing allows visualization of insertion site and surrounding area for assessment of complications (Gorski et al., 2021).

13. Remove and discard gloves and used equipment. Perform hand hygiene.

- Prevents transmission of microorganisms.

14. Secure extension tubing with tape. Do not tape over dressing.

- Prevents accidental dislodgement of PVAD. Provides safety and comfort for patient.

SKILL 41.4	CHANGING A SHORT-PERIPHERAL INTRAVENOUS CATHETER (PIVC) DRESSING—cont'd

15. Label dressing per employer policy. Information on label includes date of dressing change and initials.

16. Perform hand hygiene.

17. Evaluate function and patency of PIVC after dressing change (see Skill 41.3).

18. Document in patient's chart or in electronic health record (EHR) the time and date the PIVC dressing was changed, reason for change, type of dressing material used, patency of system, description of PIVC site, and patient tolerance.

- Communicates type of device and time interval for dressing change and site rotation.
- Reduces transmission of microorganisms.
- Validates that the PIVC is patent and functioning correctly. Manipulation of catheter and tubing may cause PIVC dislodgement.

UNEXPECTED OUTCOMES	RELATED INTERVENTIONS
PIVC is removed or dislodged accidentally.	• Restart new PIVC in other extremity or above previous insertion site if continued therapy is required.
Infusion of solutions or medications is not infusing at required or prescribed rates.	• Check PVAD and administration set tubing for bending, kinking, or dislodgement. • Check if infusion is dependent on patient's arm position. • Check and adjust height of infusion container. • Ensure there are no signs and symptoms of infiltration or extravasation at insertion site or surrounding PVAD location.

CARE IN THE COMMUNITY CONSIDERATIONS

- Educate patient and caregiver about the signs and symptoms of PIVC and infusion-related complications.
- Acknowledge for patient and caregivers that dressing change procedures in the community setting may be different from those in acute care, and provide rationale and reassurance.
- Observe patient and caregiver preforming hand hygiene.
- Ensure patient is aware to protect PIVC site during bathing or showing and that the site cannot be submerged in water. Instruct patient to cover the site with an occlusive plastic wrap or bag to keep the dressing dry and intact.
- Teach patient and caregiver what to do if dressing becomes compromised. If PIVC falls out or becomes dislodged, instruct to apply gauze with enough pressure to stop bleeding and to notify the health care provider.

To prevent the accidental disruption of an intravenous system, the nurse may need to assist the patient with hygiene, comfort measures, meals, and ambulation. Using a gown specifically made with snaps along the top sleeve seam helps facilitate changing the gown without disturbing the venipuncture site. Regular gowns are changed as follows:

1. Remove the sleeve of the gown from the arm without the intravenous line, maintaining the patient's privacy.
2. Remove the sleeve of the gown from the arm with the intravenous line.
3. Remove the intravenous solution container from its stand and pass it and the tubing through the sleeve. (If this involves removing the tubing from an intravenous electronic infusion device, use the roller clamp to slow the infusion to prevent the accidental infusion of a large volume of solution or medication.)
4. Place the intravenous solution container and tubing through the sleeve of the clean gown and hang it on its stand. (If the intravenous line is connected to an electronic infusion device, open the roller clamp. Turn on the pump.)
5. Place the arm with the intravenous line through the gown sleeve.
6. Place the arm without the intravenous line through the gown sleeve. (Breaking the integrity of an intravenous line to change a gown leads to contamination.)

Protective devices designed to prevent accidental dislodgement of an intravenous catheter can be used. The device fits comfortably around a patient's hand or arm and provides a plastic shield to cover the intravenous device. Protective devices extend the time a catheter remains in the vein and minimize repeated venipuncture.

The patient with an arm or a hand infusion is able to walk, unless contraindicated. A portable intravenous pole (a standard intravenous pole with wheels) is needed. The nurse helps the patient get out of bed and places the pole next to the involved arm. The patient should be instructed to hold on to the pole and push it while walking. The nurse needs to assess the equipment to make sure that the intravenous bag is at the proper height, the tubing is not tense, the flow rate is correct, and the tubing does not get contaminated. The patient should be instructed to report any blood in the tubing, a stoppage in the flow, or increased discomfort. Intravenous medications, especially antibiotics and potassium, can cause discomfort and burning sensations at the intravenous site. Although discomfort may be relieved by repositioning the extremity, the source of discomfort must always be carefully evaluated and may necessitate starting a new intravenous line in a larger vein.

Complications of intravenous therapy. An **infiltration** occurs when intravenous fluids enter the surrounding space around the venipuncture site (see Table 41.12). This manifests as swelling (from increased tissue fluid) and pallor and coolness (caused by decreased circulation) around the venipuncture site. Fluid may be flowing through the intravenous line at a decreased rate or may have stopped flowing. Pain may also be present and usually results from edema. This pain increases proportionately as the infiltration continues.

When infiltration occurs, the infusion must be discontinued, and if intravenous therapy is still necessary, a new catheter is inserted into a vein in another extremity. To reduce discomfort and edema, the extremity should be raised, which promotes venous drainage. Wrapping the extremity in a warm, moist towel for 20 minutes while keeping it elevated on a pillow also promotes venous return, increases circulation, and reduces pain and edema. This can be repeated three to four times per day until resolved. Infiltration of medications that cause extravasation require specific care, outlined by institutional policy.

Phlebitis is inflammation of the vein. Selected risk factors for phlebitis include the type of catheter material, chemical irritation of additives and medications given intravenously (e.g., antibiotics), the rate of the medication administration, the skill of the individual inserting the catheter, and the anatomical position of the catheter. Signs and symptoms may include pain, edema, erythema, increased skin temperature over the vein, and, in some instances, redness travelling along the path of the vein (Gorski et al., 2021). Dehydration may also be a contributing factor because of the increase in blood viscosity.

When phlebitis develops, the intravenous line must be discontinued, and a new line must be inserted in another vein. Warm, moist heat on the site of phlebitis can offer some relief to the patient. Phlebitis can be dangerous because blood clots (thrombophlebitis) can occur and, in some cases, may result in emboli. Such conditions can result in permanent damage to veins and in prolonging the patient's hospitalization.

Bleeding can occur around the venipuncture site during the infusion or through the catheter needle or tubing if these become inadvertently disconnected. Bleeding is common in patients who have received heparin or who have a bleeding disorder (e.g., leukemia or thrombocytopenia). If bleeding occurs around the venipuncture site and the catheter is within the vein, a pressure dressing may be applied over the site to control the bleeding. Bleeding from a vein is usually a slow, continuous seepage and is not serious.

Removal of peripheral intravenous catheters. Discontinuing an infusion is necessary after the prescribed amount of fluid or medication has been infused. If the PIVC is no longer required in the plan of care or if any complications (phlebitis, infiltration, loss of patency) occur, the PIVC should be removed. Refer to the Procedural Guideline in Box 41.12 for removal of a PIVC.

Safety and Quality Improvement.
As stated throughout this text, individual nurses and health care teams have important roles in ensuring patient safety and quality improvement. For individuals administering infusion therapy, competency assessment should include psychomotor skills, such as those outlined in this chapter, as well as application of knowledge, decision making, and ethical practice. Nurses contribute to quality improvement through using standardized documentation, fostering a culture of care, demonstrating accountability, and assisting in identifying clinical quality indicators and benchmarks (Gorski et al., 2021). Catheter failure documented in the electronic health record facilitates comparison of this important benchmark with international rates (Marsh et al., 2020). Because phlebitis is the most frequently measured and most prevalent complication of PIVCs, it should be the primary target in quality improvement initiatives (Marsh et al., 2020).

Blood Therapy.
The transfusion of blood or blood components includes the intravenous administration of whole blood or a component, such as plasma, packed red blood cells (RBCs), platelets, or cryoprecipitate. Other blood products, manufactured from human plasma, include albumin (5% or 25%), intravenous immune globulin (IVIG), Rh immune globulin (RHIG), and prothrombin complex concentrate (PCC). The primary objectives for blood product transfusions include the following: (1) to increase circulating blood volume after surgery, trauma, or hemorrhage; (2) to increase the number of RBCs and to maintain hemoglobin levels in patients with severe anemia; and (3) to provide selected cellular components as replacement therapy (e.g., clotting factors, platelets, albumin). Caring for patients receiving blood or blood products is a significant nursing responsibility. Thorough assessment, meticulous identification of the patient and transfusion, and careful monitoring are critical, as error could lead to dangerous and life-threatening events.

Blood Groups and Types. The most important grouping for transfusion purposes is the ABO system, which includes A, B, O, and AB blood types. The determination of blood groups is based on the presence or absence of A and B RBC antigens. Individuals with A antigens, B antigens, or no antigens belong to groups A, B, and O, respectively. The person with A and B antigens has AB blood. Individuals with type A blood naturally produce anti-B antibodies in their plasma. Similarly, individuals with type B blood naturally produce anti-A antibodies. An individual with type O blood has neither type A nor type B antigen and thus is considered a universal blood donor. Individuals with type AB blood produce neither antibody, which is why they can be universal recipients and receive any type of blood (Table 41.13). Rhesus, or Rh, factor is the second important consideration in blood typing. The Rh factor is an antigenic substance in the erythrocytes. A person with the factor is Rh positive, and a person without it is Rh negative. Blood must be matched for Rh factor as well as ABO grouping. Rh-negative people must receive only Rh-negative blood, whereas Rh-positive people can receive either Rh-negative or Rh-positive blood.

If incompatible or mismatched blood is transfused, a **transfusion reaction** occurs. The patient's, or recipient's, preformed antibodies (agglutinins) trigger RBC destruction. This response ranges from a mild response (e.g., faintness, dizziness) to severe anaphylactic shock or acute intravascular hemolysis, both of which can be life-threatening. Prompt intervention is required, including immediately stopping the transfusion, removing the tubing, and replacing the line with a normal saline infusion to maintain intravenous access. **Autologous transfusion**, or auto-transfusion, is the collection of a patient's own blood and is one approach to preventing transfusion reactions and decreasing the exposure to bloodborne infectious agents.

Blood Transfusions. When transfusing blood or blood components, assessment is required before, during, and after the transfusion, because of the risk of reactions and complications. Infusion of blood components or blood products requires a prescription from the primary health care provider. Prior to transfusion, the primary health care provider must obtain consent for transfusion, except in emergencies. The nurse then verifies that consent has been obtained, that it is current, and that the patient understands the reason for the blood transfusion. Patients with certain cultural backgrounds may abstain from blood transfusions (Box 41.13). The nurse should ask the patient if they have had a previous transfusion or a transfusion reaction. Before giving a transfusion, the nurse needs to explain the procedure and instruct the patient to report any adverse effects (e.g., chills, dizziness, or fever) once the transfusion begins. The nurse checks that the patient is properly identified (e.g., has ID armband), based on agency policy. This is critical to ensure that the patient is given the correct blood component, based on blood typing. Certain diagnostic tests are used to determine the need for blood component and the effectiveness of treatment, such as hemoglobin, platelet count, or coagulation values.

The nurse checks patient identification, component or product to be administered, the amount or volume, the rate of administration, and any other requirements, such as premedication (e.g., intravenous diuretic). Verification of the patient and the blood component should follow agency policy. When obtaining the blood component, the nurse checks the unit with patient documentation, with another person. If the patient has an intravenous line in place, the nurse needs to assess the venipuncture site and determine the appropriate gauge of the intravenous catheter. A large catheter, such as 18 to 22 gauge, is recommended for adults unless rapid infusion is required (16–18 gauge).

BOX 41.12 PROCEDURAL GUIDELINE

Removing a Short-Peripheral Intravenous Catheter (PIVC)

Delegation Considerations

The skill of removing a PIVC may be delegated to other health care providers if they have had appropriate education, it is within their governing body scope of practice, and it is approved by employer policy. The skill of removing a PIVC cannot be carried out by an unregulated care provider (UCP). The nurse instructs the UCP to report the following immediately:

- Report to the nurse any bleeding at the site after catheter has been removed.
- Report any complaints of pain by the patient or observation of redness at the site.

Equipment

- Clean gloves
- Sterile 5 × 5–cm (2 × 2–inch) or 10 × 10–cm (4 × 4–inch) gauze sponge or small adhesive dressing
- Tape

Procedure

1. Key assessments prior to removal of PIVC include identifying if the patient is on any anticoagulant or antiplatelet therapy or has a disorder that causes slow clotting.
2. Review accuracy and completeness of health care provider's prescription for discontinuation of PIVC, if required.
3. Perform hand hygiene and collect equipment.
4. Identify patient using at least two identifiers (e.g., name and birthday or name and medical record number) according to employer policy. Compare identifiers with information on patient's medication administration record (MAR) or medical record.
5. Perform hand hygiene and apply clean gloves. Palpate catheter site through intact dressing.
6. Assess patient's understanding of the reason for PVAD removal.
7. Explain procedure to patient before you remove the catheter.
8. If PIVC is connected to an administration set, turn administration set roller clamp to "off" position or turn electronic infusion device (EID) off and roller clamp to "off" position.
9. Carefully remove PIVC dressing as per Skill 41.4.

   Critical Decision Point: Never use scissors to remove the tape or dressing because you may accidentally cut the catheter.

10. Place clean, sterile gauze above insertion site and, using your dominant hand, withdraw catheter using a slow, steady motion and keeping the hub parallel to skin (see Step 10 illustration).

    Critical Decision Point: Do not raise or lift catheter before it is completely out of the vein, to avoid trauma or hematoma formation.

11. Apply pressure to site for a minimum of 30 seconds until bleeding has stopped. If patient has increased clotting, maintain pressure until hemostasis occurs.

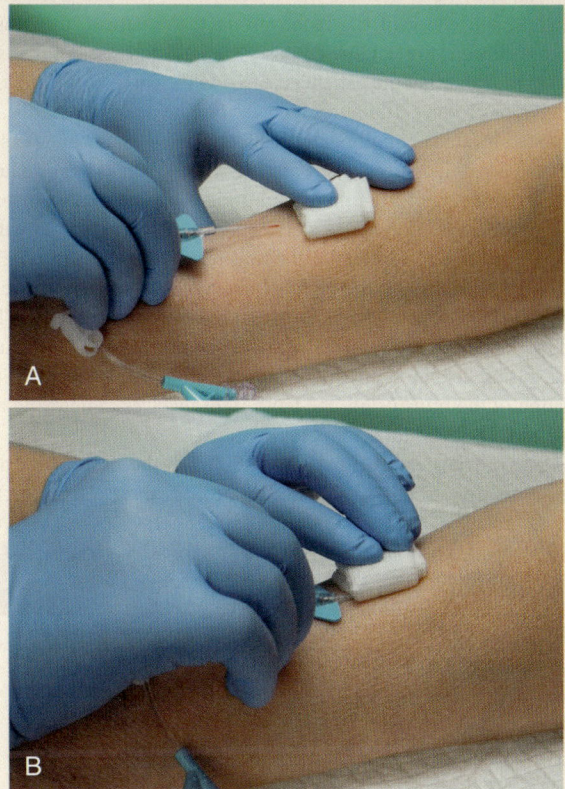

STEP 10 PIVC removal: **A,** Apply pressure and cover site. **B,** Remove catheter. From Cobbett, S. L., Perry, A.G., Potter, P. A., et al. [Eds.]. [2020]. *Canadian clinical nursing skills & techniques*. Elsevier. Photos courtesy Patrick Coble.)

12. Apply clean, folded gauze dressing over insertion site and secure with tape or a small adhesive dressing.
13. Inspect catheter for intactness after removal; note tip integrity and length.
14. Discard used supplies, remove gloves, and perform hand hygiene.
15. Document procedure in patient's medical record in electronic health record or chart.
16. Observe IV site for evidence of any complications, such as redness, pain, tenderness, swelling, bleeding, or drainage. Monitor for 24 to 48 hours after removal for postinfusion phlebitis.
17. Ensure patient understanding of a) purpose of the PIVC dressing, b) that it should remain in place for a minimum of 24 hours, and c) that they need to report any signs and symptoms of complication at insertion site to health care provider.

Blood administration tubing with a 70- to 260-micron filter is used, and the nurse needs to determine if the tubing is appropriate for the EID when using one. When priming blood administration tubing, 0.9% normal saline must be used to prevent hemolysis, or breakdown of RBCs. Timing of blood transfusion is extremely important. The infusion is begun within 30 minutes of accessing the blood component from the transfusion medical laboratory (TML) and is stopped after 4 hours. Bags and tubing are discarded in the biohazardous waste, according to agency policy.

Because of the danger of transfusion reactions, it is very important to use specific precautions and the 10 rights of medication administration (see Chapter 35) in administering blood or blood products. The nurse should first obtain the patient's baseline vital signs (temperature, blood pressure, pulse, respirations, and oxygen saturation) before the transfusion begins. This enables the nurse to determine when changes in vital signs occur, which can indicate that a transfusion reaction is developing. A thorough check of the blood product, the patient, the reason for the transfusion, the volume or dose, the rate, and site ensures safe administration and that the patient is receiving the correct type of blood component or product. The nurse then verifies the patient's identity, the documentation, blood component, and blood type with a second person. Verification is based on person-specific identifiers, such as name, date of birth, and unique medical number, and these are compared against the blood component label. A verbal statement of name and date of birth is used when possible. Additionally, the unit number and blood type on the blood component and the blood bank form must match. If even a minor discrepancy exists, the blood should not be given and the TML should be notified immediately. The nurse documents vital signs, time, and transfusion details on initiation and throughout the transfusion. On completion of the transfusion, the tenth right involves monitoring and documenting the patient response (evaluation).

The rate of transfusion is usually specified in the health care provider's orders. Initiation of a transfusion begins slowly (50 mL/hr) to

TABLE 41.13	ABO Compatibilities for Transfusion Therapy	
Component	**Compatibilities**	
Whole Blood	**Give Type-Specific Blood Only**	
Packed red cells (stored, washed, or frozen/washed)	*Donor*	*Recipient*
	O	O, A, B, AB
	A	A, AB
	B	B, AB
	AB	AB
Fresh-frozen plasma	*Donor*	*Recipient*
	O	O
	A	A, O
	B	B, O
	AB	AB, B, A, O
Platelets	RBC: ABO and Rh compatible *preferred*	
	Donor	*Recipient*
	O	O, A, B, AB
	A	A, AB
	B	B, AB
	AB	AB

ABO, Blood group consisting of groups A, AB, B, and O.

allow for the early detection of a transfusion reaction. The nurse needs to maintain the infusion rate, monitor for adverse effects, assess vital signs, and promptly record all findings. Vital signs are assessed and documented at 15 minutes and at the end of the transfusion, or as directed by agency policy. The nurse should observe for hives, fever or rigors, dyspnea, cough, or back or infusion site pain and note patient reports of unusual feelings. Upon completion, the administration tubing used for blood components should be discarded according to agency policy. If blood components or products are contraindicated, plasma expanders may be required in cases of sudden or extreme hypovolemia.

Transfusion Reactions and Complications. Noninfectious complications from transfusions are generally more common than infectious complications. Noninfectious complications such as allergic reactions (minor to severe), hemolytic transfusion reactions, and ABO transfusion reactions are a systemic response by the body to incompatible blood or blood component (e.g., white blood cells from donor blood). Causes may also include allergic sensitivity to the potassium or citrate preservative in the blood. Several types of acute reactions can result from blood transfusions (Table 41.14). Transfusion-related acute lung injury is the most serious transfusion reaction and requires critical care. If a transfusion reaction is anticipated or suspected, vital signs must be monitored more frequently (see Table 41.14).

A second category of transfusion reactions, infectious complications, includes diseases transmitted by infected blood donors who are asymptomatic. Because all units of blood collected must undergo serological testing and screening for human immunodeficiency virus (HIV) and hepatitis B virus, the risk of acquiring bloodborne infections from blood transfusions is reduced. Bacterial sepsis is more common in platelets.

Circulatory overload, or TACO, is a risk when a patient receives large volumes of whole blood or packed RBC transfusions for massive hemorrhagic shock or when a patient with normal blood volume receives blood. Patients particularly at risk for circulatory overload are older persons and those with cardiopulmonary diseases.

> **SAFETY ALERT** If a blood reaction is suspected, stop the transfusion immediately.

Blood transfusion reactions are life-threatening, but prompt nursing intervention can maintain the patient's physiological stability.
- Keep the intravenous line open by hanging 0.9% normal saline directly into the intravenous line and running the saline.
- Do not turn off the blood and simply turn on the 0.9% normal saline that is connected to the Y-tubing infusion set. This would cause blood

---

🌐 **BOX 41.13** **CULTURAL ASPECTS OF CARE**

Cultural Challenges in Blood Donation

Blood donation is critical to ensuring access to blood and blood components in both acute or emergent care and for the treatment of some chronic conditions (e.g., hemolytic anemia, sickle-cell disease). Some blood disorders affect minority and racialized populations disproportionately (Spratling & Lawrence, 2019). Therefore, increasing blood donation from communities where blood donors are underrepresented is needed in order to improve access to antigen-matched units through a diverse blood supply. Key findings of a systematic review (Spratling & Lawrence, 2019) identified knowing a blood recipient, understanding the benefit to their local community, recognizing the unique contribution for blood related to one's own race and ethnicity, and religious values such as "giving life" as facilitators in making blood donations. Medical mistrust and misunderstanding, awareness of racially discriminatory

experiments in recent history, and stories of wasted blood are barriers to blood donation (Spratling & Lawrence, 2019).

Implications for Practice
- Encourage positive community engagement through health education regarding blood donation.
- Create connections between donation and benefitting a colleague, friend, or community member.
- Communicate the need for blood among racialized and ethnic groups through local champions.
- It is important to establish and maintain trusting relationships or rebuild trust between health care providers and communities.

TABLE 41.14   Acute Adverse Effects of Transfusions

Adverse Effect	Cause	Clinical Manifestations	Management	Prevention
Transfusion Reactions—Caused by Immune Response to Blood Components				
Acute intravascular hemolytic	Infusion of ABO-incompatible whole blood, RBCs, or components containing 10 mL or more of RBCs. Antibodies in recipient's plasma attach to antigens on transfused RBCs, causing RBC destruction	Chills, fever, low back pain, flushing, tachycardia, tachypnea, hypotension, hemoglobinuria, hemoglobinemia, sudden oliguria (acute kidney injury), circulatory shock, cardiac arrest, death	Stop transfusion and save blood bag and administration set for follow-up. Keep IV site open with normal saline infused through new tubing. Maintain BP and treat shock as ordered, if present. Obtain blood samples *slowly* to avoid hemolysis; send for serological testing. Send urine specimen to laboratory. Give diuretics as prescribed to maintain urine flow. Insert in-dwelling urinary catheter or measure each voiding to monitor hourly urine output. Dialysis may be required if acute kidney injury occurs. ***Patient safety alert:*** *Do not transfuse additional RBC-containing components until transfusion service provides newly cross-matched units.*	Meticulously verify and document patient identification from sample collection to component infusion.
Febrile nonhemolytic (most common)	Antibodies against donor white blood cells	Sudden shaking chills (rigors), fever (rise in temperature 0.5°C [1°F] or more from start), headache, flushing, anxiety, muscle pain	Stop transfusion. Give antipyretics as prescribed; avoid using Aspirin in thrombocytopenic patients. ***Patient safety alert:*** *Do not restart transfusion.*	Consider leukocyte-poor blood products (filtered, washed, or frozen). Pretreat with antipyretics if prior history.
Mild allergic	Antibodies against donor plasma proteins	Flushing, itching, urticaria (hives)	Stop transfusion temporarily. Give antihistamine as directed. If symptoms are mild and transient, restart transfusion slowly. ***Patient safety alert:*** *Do not restart transfusion if fever, pulmonary symptoms, or hypotension develops.*	Treat prophylactically with antihistamines.
Anaphylactic	Antibodies to donor plasma, especially anti-IgA	Anxiety, urticaria, dyspnea, wheezing progressing to cyanosis, severe hypotension, circulatory shock, possible cardiac arrest	Stop transfusion. Have epinephrine ready for injection (0.4 mL of 1:1 000 solution subcutaneously or 0.1 mL of 1:1 000 solution diluted to 10 mL with saline for IV use). Provide BP support as ordered. Initiate CPR if indicated. ***Patient safety alert:*** *Do not restart transfusion.*	Transfuse extensively washed RBC products from which all plasma has been removed. Alternately use blood from IgA-deficient donor.
Other Acute Adverse Effects				
Circulatory overload	Blood administered faster than circulation can accommodate	*Dyspnea,* cough, crackles, or rales in dependent lobes of lungs; distended neck veins when upright	Turn down transfusion rate or stop transfusion. Place patient upright with feet in dependent position. Administer prescribed diuretics, oxygen, morphine. Phlebotomy may be indicated.	Adjust transfusion volume and flow rate on basis of patient size and clinical status. Have transfusion service divide unit into smaller aliquots for better spacing of fluid input.
Sepsis	Bacterial contamination of transfused blood components	Rapid onset of chills, high fever, severe hypotension, and circulatory shock. *May occur:* Vomiting, diarrhea, sudden oliguria (acute kidney injury), disseminated intravascular coagulation (DIC)	Stop transfusion. Obtain culture of patient's blood and send bag with remaining blood to transfusion service for further study. Treat as ordered: antibiotics, IV fluids, vasopressors, glucocorticoids.	Collect, process, store, and transfuse blood products according to blood-banking standards and infuse within 4 hours of starting time.

ABO, Blood group consisting of groups A, AB, B, and O; *BP,* blood pressure; *CPR,* cardiopulmonary resuscitation; *IgA,* immunoglobulin A; *IV,* intravenous; *RBC,* red blood cell.

remaining in the Y-tubing to infuse into the patient. Even a small amount of mismatched blood can cause a major reaction.

- Notify the primary health care provider immediately.
- Remain with the patient, observing signs and symptoms and monitoring vital signs as often as every 5 minutes.
- Prepare to administer emergency medications such as antihistamines, vasopressors, fluids, and steroids as per physician order or protocol.
- Prepare to perform cardiopulmonary resuscitation.
- Obtain a urine specimen and send it to the laboratory to determine the presence of hemoglobin as a result of RBC hemolysis.
- Save the blood container, tubing, attached labels, and transfusion record, and return them to the laboratory.

Restorative Care

After experiencing acute alterations in fluid, electrolyte, or acid–base balance, patients often require ongoing maintenance to prevent a recurrence of health alterations. Older persons and chronically ill patients require special considerations to prevent complications from developing.

Home Intravenous Therapy. Intravenous therapy is often continued in the home setting for patients who are discharged from the hospital and have not completed their prescribed treatment or who require long-term therapy. Ideally, a family member will be available at home if the patient suddenly cannot manage the intravenous system or if a problem develops. A home care nurse will work closely with the patient and family to ensure that a sterile intravenous system is maintained and that complications are avoided or recognized promptly. Refer to Box 41.7 for a summary of patient education guidelines for home intravenous therapy.

Nutritional Support. Most patients who have had electrolyte disorders or metabolic acid–base disturbances require ongoing nutritional support; therefore, patient education is included in all nursing assessment and interventions, preparing patients and families for care and prevention of complications. If patients are still responsible for meal preparation, particularly for necessary alterations, they should learn to understand the nutritional content of foods and to read the labels of commercially prepared foods, and they should work collaboratively with nurses to establish goals.

Medication Safety. Numerous medications and over-the-counter medications often influence fluid and electrolyte balances. Once patients return to home or in a residential care setting, medication safety remains an important aspect of their care. Patient and family education regarding patient medications is essential, particularly for those with polypharmacy and chronic illness. It is important to review all medications with patients, including potential medication interactions and adverse effects, and encourage them to consult with their local pharmacist regularly.

◆ Evaluation

Patient Expectations. Nurses routinely review with patients how well their concerns and expectations regarding fluid, electrolyte, or acid–base status have been addressed. Asking questions directed at presenting signs and symptoms and at anticipated responses to interventions is important to the nursing process. Additionally, using tools designed to evaluate patient-reported outcome measures (PROMs) and patient-reported experience measures (PREMs), which are standardized to integrate the patient's view, is important to the success of emerging health care systems. Often the patient's level of satisfaction with care also depends on the nurse's success in involving the person, their family, and their friends.

Patient Outcomes. The evaluation of a patient's clinical status is especially important if an acute fluid and electrolyte or acid–base imbalance exists. In some situations, the patient's condition can change very quickly, and the nurse must be able to recognize the signs and symptoms of impending problems by being aware of health alterations, the effects of medications and fluids, and the patient's presenting clinical status (see Figure 41.8). It is particularly important to evaluate the effectiveness of the interprofessional team interventions, review diagnoses, report outcomes, and remain open to revising the plan of care. This evaluation should include the patient's experience and goals, ongoing risk factors, clinical status, laboratory findings, and underlying or contributing problems.

The nurse needs to determine whether changes have occurred from the last patient assessment and analyze such changes. For example, have the physical signs and symptoms of the assessed condition begun to disappear or lessen in intensity? A patient's response to treatment of hyperkalemia would be evidenced by a decreasing serum potassium and a reduction in physical symptoms associated with hyperkalemia.

For patients with less acute alterations, evaluation likely occurs over a longer period. In this situation, the nurse's evaluation may be focused more on behavioural changes, such as the patient's ability to follow dietary restrictions and medication schedules. The family's ability to anticipate alterations and prevent problems from recurring may also be an important element of the evaluation. Beyond evaluating the patient's objective data, nurses are increasingly using subjective data collected from PROMs as a means for ensuring a person-centred approach to care (Schick-Makaroff & Mharapara, 2020). Supporting care of patients with fluid, electrolyte, and acid–base imbalances may include the integration of measurement tools to assess their quality of life, fatigue, physical function, and pain (see ICHOM, Chronic Kidney Disease, weblink at the end of the chapter for more information). Regardless of the tool, evaluation of care is incomplete without accessing the patient's reporting of their outcomes and their experience of care.

The patient's level of progress determines whether the nurse needs to continue or revise the care plan. If goals are not met, the nurse may need to consult with others on the interprofessional team to discuss additional methods, such as increasing the frequency of an intervention (e.g., provide more fluids to a dehydrated patient), introducing a new therapy (e.g., initiate insertion of an intravenous line), or discontinuing a particular therapy. This evaluation should also include daily reassessment of the need for a PIVC (Bourgault et al., 2021). Once outcomes have been met, the nurse can resolve the nursing diagnosis and focus on other priorities.

KEY CONCEPTS

- Body fluids are distributed in ECF and ICF compartments.
- A dynamic interplay of fluid and electrolyte intake and absorption, distribution, hormonal control, and output determines fluid and electrolyte balance.
- Volume disturbances include isotonic and osmolar deficits and excesses.
- Acid–base imbalances are buffered by chemical, biological, and physiological buffering, especially the lungs and kidneys.
- Chronic and serious illnesses increase the risk of fluid, electrolyte, and acid–base imbalances.
- Patients who are very young or very old are at greater risk for fluid, electrolyte, and acid–base imbalances.
- Assessment for fluid, electrolyte, and acid–base alterations includes the nursing health history, physical and behavioural assessments,

measurements of intake and output, daily weights, and specific laboratory data.

- Osmolar imbalances and extracellular fluid volume (ECV) deficit can be corrected by enteral or parenteral administration of fluid.
- Common complications of intravenous therapy are infiltration, phlebitis, infection, ECF excess, and bleeding at the infusion site.
- Blood transfusions are given to replace fluid volume loss from hemorrhage, treat anemia, or replace coagulation factors.
- Blood transfusions can be obtained from a donor, autologously, or through perioperative salvage.
- Administration of blood or blood products requires the nurse to follow a specific procedure in order to prevent and identify transfusion reactions quickly.
- In addition to transfusion reactions, the risks of transfusion include hyperkalemia, hypocalcemia, hypervolemia or circulatory overload, and infection.
- Treatment for electrolyte disturbances includes dietary and pharmacological interventions.
- The body's chemical buffering system responds first to acid–base abnormalities.
- The goals of therapy for acid–base imbalances are to treat the underlying illness and to restore the arterial blood pH to normal.
- With new technology emerging continually, nurses need to stay current on evidence to inform practice, particularly in relation to VADs.

CRITICAL THINKING EXERCISES

1. Jiao underwent a series of diagnostic tests in the ED. Which laboratory findings would you expect to be obtained, and which ones would you anticipate could be abnormal on the basis of her complaints? Which of these diagnostic tests would be most life-threatening?

2. The nurse is planning to insert a PIVC to administer medication to Jiao. What are the assessments the nurse needs to make prior to selecting a site and catheter? How will the nurse use these assessments to inform their decision?

3. If Jiao's respiratory status deteriorates because of a sudden infusion of the entire bag of infusate prior to the IV medication administration, she may need transfer to critical care. Jiao would likely be reporting difficulty breathing and have a respiratory rate of 40 breaths per minute. A nursing student asks the nurse caring for Jiao to interpret her last ABG results: pH = 7.30; PaO_2 = 70; $PaCO_2$ = 50; bicarbonate = 24 mmol/L. What interpretation will the nurse provide?

4. Jiao has a number of reasons for being at risk for fluid volume excess. What are these risks? How will the nurses caring for Jiao work to minimize the risks for fluid and electrolyte imbalances in the acute care setting? What are the indications for maintaining a fluid balance chart (FBC)?

5. Jiao's initial laboratory findings reveal a low hemoglobin level. The health care team is discussing the potential for a blood transfusion. What questions would you ask Jiao to solicit her preferences regarding blood transfusions? What are the key principles in providing care for Jiao in relation to blood products? How does a health promotion perspective inform the care of Jiao? What other options are available, and how realistic or viable are these options?

6. The nurse caring for Jiao is preparing her for discharge, where she will be expected to monitor her fluid balance. What does Jiao need to know to be able to do this accurately? Describe a teaching plan for this patient upon discharge.

⊕ *Answers to Critical Thinking Exercises appear on the Evolve website.*

REVIEW QUESTIONS

Review Questions 1 to 10 relate to the case study at the beginning of the chapter.

1. Regarding of the treatment for Jiao, what is the most critical electrolyte imbalance?
   a. Hypokalemia
   b. Hyperkalemia
   c. Hyponatremia
   d. Hypocalcemia

2. How does Jiao's age affect the seriousness of a fluid volume deficit?
   a. Older persons are the most at-risk group for harm from a fluid volume deficit.
   b. There are no risks related to her age or gender.
   c. Loss of skin integrity with aging increases risk of harm from fluid volume deficits.
   d. Older persons may develop fluid volume deficits slowly, masking severity.

3. Why do older persons, such as Jiao, more commonly experience fluid and electrolyte imbalances?
   a. They eat poor-quality food.
   b. They have a decreased thirst sensation.
   c. They have a more severe stress response.
   d. They have an overly active thirst response.

4. Which of the following are included in the output section of Jiao's fluid balance chart?
   a. Urine, vomitus, diarrhea, and drainage from wounds
   b. Diarrhea, gastric suction, and drainage from wounds
   c. Medications, juices, and water
   d. Urine, diarrhea, vomitus, gastric suction, and drainage from wounds or tubes

5. When deciding to remove Jiao's PIVC, what factors would the nurse consider first?
   a. Patient's poor knowledge of vascular access
   b. Dietary intake
   c. Use of PIVC for treatment plan
   d. Length of time in situ

6. If Jiao's condition deteriorates, the health care provider may consider inserting a CVAD. Where does a CVAD reside?
   a. Superior vena cava
   b. Heart
   c. Peripheral veins
   d. Radial artery

7. Which of the following is the first step for (PIVC) intravenous insertion?
   a. Performing hand hygiene
   b. Putting on nonsterile gloves
   c. Ensuring the 10 rights of medication administration
   d. Confirming the infusion rate

8. What are the indications of intravenous fluid infiltration?
   a. Phlebitis and coolness
   b. Edema and erythema
   c. Pallor and coolness
   d. Pain and erythema

9. How often should a PIVC catheter be replaced?
   a. Every 96 hours
   b. Every 72 hours
   c. When clinically indicated
   d. Every 48 hours

10. Following a renal diagnostic test, Jiao experiences a serious hemorrhage. Fifteen minutes after blood administration, she develops dyspnea, a cough, and a rapid heart rate. What does the nurse suspect is the cause?
    a. Sepsis
    b. Anaphylaxis
    c. Acute hemolytic reaction
    d. Circulatory overload

Answers: 1. b; **2.** d; **3.** b; **4.** b; **5.** d; **6.** c; **7.** a; **8.** a; **9.** c; **10.** d.

🌐 *Rationales for the Review Questions appear on the Evolve website.*

RECOMMENDED WEBSITES

Alliance for Vascular Access Teaching and Research (AVATAR): https://www.avatargroup.org.au
The AVATAR Group, an independent research group leading research related to vascular access, is based in Australia but works with international experts and nurse researchers. Their mission is to eliminate vascular access complications and improve patient care in all settings across the globe. The I-DECIDED[R] is available on this website: https://www.avatargroup.org.au/i-decided.html. A video related to the I-DECIDED[R] is available at https://www.youtube.com/watch?v=kMHOjWJWbsI

Association for Vascular Access: https://www.avainfo.org
The website for the Association for Vascular Access has many links to conferences and national and international organizations regarding vascular access.

Canadian Association of Nephrology Nurses and Technologists (CANNT): https://www.cannt.ca
This association exists to promote excellence in the care of patients with renal disease. They provide leadership through education, research, and dissemination of research. Nephrology nursing standards are available from the website and include standards for holistic patient care across areas of practice such as prevention, assessment, and nursing interventions.

Canadian Blood Services: Clinical Guide to Transfusion: https://professionaleducation.blood.ca/en/transfusion/clinical-guide-transfusion
Canadian Blood Services provides numerous resources, including professional education, best practices, and publications. The *Clinical Guide to Transfusion* is an online educational resource. The Blood Components chapter, along with Blood Administration and Adverse Reactions are extremely helpful.

Canadian Vascular Access Association (CVAA): https://www.cvaa.info
The Canadian Vascular Access Association provides leadership in advocating for safe, quality vascular access by promoting education, partnerships, knowledge, and research. The mission statement highlights the role of empowering and engaging members, with a vision for optimal patient outcomes. Of note, the CVAA journal is a partner with the *British Journal of Nursing*, where there is an IV therapy and vascular access supplement.

Diffusion Educational Video: https://www.youtube.com/watch?v=JnIkGtkO-Js
This brief video provides clarity regarding a complex and commonly misunderstood concept.

ICHOM (International Center for Health Outcome Measures): https://connect.ichom.org
To support person-centred care, health care providers use outcome measures and patient experience tools. This platform includes a number of standard sets, including one related to chronic kidney disease (CKD): https://connect.ichom.org/standard-sets/chronic-kidney-disease

Infusion Nurses Society (INS): https://www.ins1.org
This society is a global leader in intravenous therapy, playing a key role in synthesizing and disseminating the best evidence and publishing standards for infusion care. The society advances best practice through their publications, professional development opportunities, and advocacy.

Ontario Regional Blood Coordinating Network: https://www.transfusionontario.org
This government-funded network provides a number of services, including an educational service for registered nurses, called Bloody Easy Blood Administration. The online learning program requires registration; however, anyone can register and complete the module and an assessment test.

🌐 REFERENCES

A full reference list is available on the website for this book at http://evolve.elsevier.com/Canada/Potter/fundamentals/

42

Sleep

*Canadian content written by Claudette Taylor, RN, PhD, NP (Adult),
with original chapter contributions by Patricia A. Stockert, RN, BSN, MS, PhD*

OBJECTIVES

Understanding of the content in this chapter will enable you to:
- Define the key terms listed.
- Compare the characteristics of rest and sleep.
- Explain the effect of the 24-hour sleep–wake cycle on biological functions.
- Explain the mechanisms that regulate sleep.
- Describe the stages of a normal sleep cycle.
- Explain the functions of sleep and rest.
- Compare the sleep requirements of different age groups.
- Identify factors that normally promote sleep and factors that normally disrupt sleep.

- Describe the characteristics of common sleep disorders.
- Conduct a sleep history for a patient.
- Identify nursing diagnoses appropriate for patients with sleep alterations.
- Identify nursing interventions designed to promote normal sleep cycles for individuals of all ages.
- Describe ways to evaluate sleep therapies.
- Identify factors that contribute to obstructive sleep apnea.
- Identify proper sleep positions for infants.

KEY TERMS

Biological clocks

Cataplexy

Circadian rhythms

Emotional stress

Excessive daytime sleepiness (EDS)

Hypersomnolence

Hypnotics

Insomnia

Narcolepsy

Nocturia

Nonrapid eye movement (NREM) sleep

Obstructive sleep apnea (OSA)

Parasomnias

Polysomnogram

Rapid eye movement (REM) sleep

Rest

Sedatives

Sleep

Sleep apnea

Sleep architecture

Sleep deprivation

Sleep hygiene

WEBSITE

http://evolve.elsevier.com/Canada/Potter/fundamentals/

CASE STUDY

Ben (preferred pronouns: he/him) is a 13-year-old who attends junior high school. Lately, he has been abruptly falling asleep during class, which is an unusual behaviour for him. Ben's teacher is concerned about his behaviour and speaks to him about it. Ben assures his teacher that this behaviour will not continue. Unfortunately, a week later, Ben again falls asleep during class. Ben's teacher notifies his parents.

Think about this case study as you read this chapter. There are review questions at the end of the chapter that relate to the case study.

Sleep is essential for good health. Sleep is a basic necessity of life and is as important as air, food, and water (Newsom, 2022). Every individual requires sleep. For a variety of reasons, individuals are, on average, sleeping less. Continual sleep loss may have many, yet largely unknown, adverse outcomes for health and well-being. In the short term, insufficient sleep alters mood and decreases the ability to concentrate, make decisions, and participate in daily activities. In the long term, poor sleep has been associated with obesity, increased blood pressure, and heart disease (Han et al., 2019).

To help patients identify and treat their sleep pattern disturbances, nurses need to first understand the nature of sleep, the factors influencing sleep, and patients' sleep habits. Patients require an individualized approach to determine their personal habits and patterns of sleep, to address what is disrupting their sleep. Nursing interventions are often effective in resolving short- and long-term sleep disturbances.

Sleep provides healing, restoration, and metabolic recuperation (Borbély et al., 2016; Seingsukon et al., 2017). Achieving the most optimal sleep quality contributes to good health and assists with recuperating from illness. Ill patients often require more sleep and rest than healthy patients. The nature of the illness, however, often prevents some patients from getting adequate rest and sleep. Sleep can also be made difficult by the environment of a hospital or long-term care facility and the activities of health care providers. Some patients have pre-existing sleep disturbances, whereas other patients develop sleep problems as a result of illness or hospitalization.

SCIENTIFIC KNOWLEDGE BASE

Definition of Sleep

Sleep is a homeostatically regulated, universal, dynamic, highly organized, physiological, and behavioural state required by most living organisms to maintain health and well-being (Box 42.1) (Buysse, 2014; Carskadon & Dement, 2017; Mukherjee et al., 2015).

Physiology of Sleep

Sleep is a cyclical, physiological, and behavioural process that alternates with longer periods of wakefulness. Sleep physiology is controlled by three distinct processes: an *ultradian* process, a *homeostatic* process (process S), and a *circadian* process (process C). The ultradian process occurs within the sleep state and is characterized by the alteration of two sleep stages: nonrapid eye movement (NREM) sleep and rapid eye movement (REM) sleep. Process S and process C work together to regulate the timing and organization of sleep and wakefulness. Process S is dependent on the sleep–wake cycle, whereas process C functions to maintain a state of wakefulness (Achermann & Borbély, 2017; Borbély et al., 2016).

Circadian Rhythms. The biological functions of most living organisms are regulated by **circadian rhythms**. The term *circadian* is derived from the Latin words *circa*, which means "about," and *dien*, which means a day (Borbély et al., 2016; Turek & Zee, 2017). People experience cyclical rhythms as part of their everyday life. The sleep–wake cycle is the most familiar of the 24-hour circadian rhythms. Numerous biological and behavioural functions are influenced by circadian rhythms. Changes in body temperature, for example, exhibit circadian rhythmicity. Normally, a person's body temperature peaks in the afternoon, decreases gradually, and then drops sharply after a person falls asleep. The initial period of a person's sleep is characterized by high levels of growth hormones and increased blood glucose concentrations, blood pressure, and heart rate. Sensory acuity and mood are also maintained by the 24-hour circadian cycle (Van Cauter & Tasali, 2017). Factors that affect circadian rhythms and daily sleep–wake cycles include light, temperature, social activities, travel, and work routines. These environmental cues are called *zeitgebers* ("time-givers"). All individuals have **biological clocks** that synchronize their sleep–wake cycles, which explains why some individuals fall asleep at 9 P.M., whereas others go to bed at midnight. Different individuals also function at their best at different times of the day.

Hospitals or long-term care facilities usually do not adapt care to an individual's sleep–wake cycle preference. Typical hospital routines often interrupt sleep or prevent patients from falling asleep at their usual time. A person experiences poor sleep if their sleep–wake cycle

BOX 42.1	Behavioural Characteristics of Sleep

Recurrent
Involuntary
Reversible
Reduced responsiveness
Minimal movement
Species-specific posture

From Carskadon, M. A., & Dement, W. C. (2017). Normal human sleep: An overview. In M. H. Kryger, T. Roth, & W. C. Dement (Eds.), *Principles and practice of sleep medicine* (6th ed., pp. 15–24). Elsevier.

changes significantly. A serious illness is often indicated by reversals in the sleep–wake cycle, such as falling asleep during the day.

When the sleep–wake cycle is disrupted (e.g., by working rotating shifts), other physiological functions can also change. For example, the person may experience a decreased appetite and lose weight or may experience other common symptoms of sleep–wake cycle disturbances, such as anxiety, restlessness, irritability, and difficulty concentrating. Failure to maintain the usual sleep–wake cycle can negatively influence the individual's overall health.

Sleep Regulation. Sleep involves a sequence of physiological and behavioural states maintained by highly integrated central nervous system (CNS) activity, which is associated with changes in the autonomic nervous system and endocrine, cardiovascular, respiratory, gastrointestinal, renal, and musculoskeletal systems (Han et al., 2019; McGinty & Szymusiak, 2017). Each sequence of physiological states is identified by specific physiological responses and patterns of brain activity. Special instruments provide information about the structural and physiological aspects of sleep: for example, the electroencephalogram (EEG) measures electrical activity in the cerebral cortex, the electromyogram (EMG) measures muscle tone, and the electro-oculogram (EOG) measures eye movements (McGinty & Szymusiak, 2017).

Current theory suggests that sleep is a dynamic multiphase process. The body's major sleep centre is the hypothalamus. The hypothalamus secretes hypocretins (orexins) that promote wakefulness. The anterior pituitary gland also secretes hormones (e.g., growth hormone and prolactin) that promote sleep (McGinty & Szymusiak, 2017).

Researchers believe the ascending reticular activating system (RAS), located in the upper brainstem, contains special cells that maintain alertness and wakefulness. The RAS receives visual, auditory, pain, and tactile sensory stimuli. Activity from the cerebral cortex (e.g., emotions and thought processes) also stimulates the RAS. Arousal, wakefulness, and maintenance of consciousness result from neurons in the RAS that release serotonin and catecholamines, such as norepinephrine and dopamine (McGinty & Szymusiak, 2017; Siegel, 2017).

Whether a person remains awake or falls asleep depends on a balance of impulses received from higher centres (e.g., thoughts), peripheral sensory receptors (e.g., sound or light stimuli), and the limbic system (e.g., emotions) (Figure 42.1). As a person tries to fall asleep, the

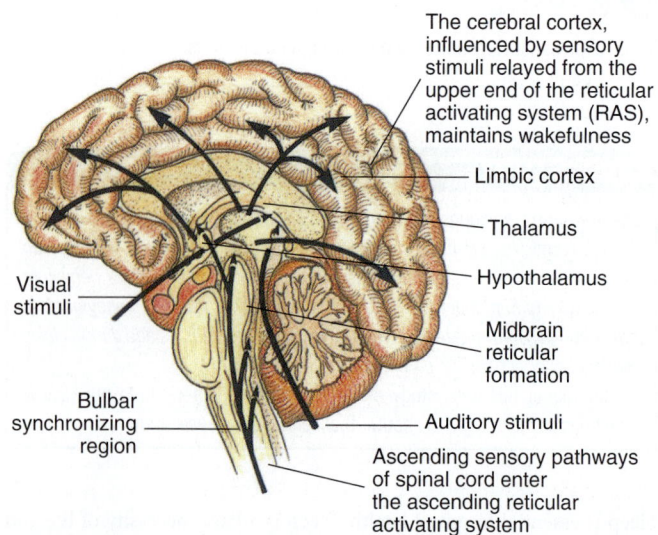

FIGURE 42.1 The reticular activating system and the bulbar synchronizing region control sensory input by intermittently activating and suppressing the brain's higher centres to control sleep and wakefulness.

BOX 42.2	Stages of the Sleep Cycle

Stage 1: Nonrapid Eye Movement (NREM)

This stage represents the lightest level of sleep.

The person is unresponsive but easily aroused by sensory stimuli, such as noise.

Physiological activity begins to decrease, accompanied by a gradual fall in vital signs and metabolism.

Muscle tone is present.

When awakened from this stage, a person feels as though they had been day-dreaming.

This stage lasts only a few minutes.

Accounts for about 2 to 5% of total sleep time in adults.

Stage 2: Nonrapid Eye Movement (NREM)

This stage is a period of sound sleep.

Relaxation progresses.

Body functions continue to slow.

Muscle tone remains present.

Eye movements are absent.

Accounts for the greatest proportion (45 to 55%) of total sleep time in adults.

Stage 3: Nonrapid Eye Movement (NREM)

This stage is the deepest period of sleep.

Individuals are difficult to arouse.

Muscles become completely relaxed.

Vital signs are significantly lower than during waking hours, but remain regular.

Parasomnias sometimes occur during this stage (e.g., sleepwalking, enuresis [bedwetting])

Accounts for 10% of total sleep time in adults and is more prominent during the first half of sleep.

If sleep loss has occurred previously, the sleeper will spend a considerable portion of the sleep period in this stage.

Rapid Eye Movement (REM) Sleep

Rapid eye movements are present.

Respirations are irregular and shallow.

Variable heart rate and blood pressure occur.

Vivid and elaborate dreams sometimes occur.

Dreaming occurs more frequently and is more complex than in NREM sleep.

This stage usually begins about 90 minutes after sleep has begun.

Loss of skeletal muscle tone occurs.

Gastric secretions increase.

The person is difficult to arouse.

The duration of REM sleep increases with each cycle.

REM sleep accounts for about 25% of total sleep time in adults.

From Carskadon, M. A., & Dement, W. C. (2017). Normal human sleep: An overview. In M. H. Kryger, T. Roth, & W. C. Dement (Eds.), *Principles and practice of sleep medicine* (6th ed., pp. 15–24). Elsevier.

eyes close and the body assumes a relaxed position and stimuli to the RAS declines. If the room is dark and quiet, the RAS further declines. At some point, an area of the brain called the *bulbar synchronizing region (BSR)* takes over, causing sleep.

Stages of Sleep. Changes in brainwave activity, muscle tone, body temperature, and eye movements are associated with different stages of sleep (Carskadon & Dement, 2017). Within sleep, two separate phases have been identified: **nonrapid eye movement (NREM) sleep** and **rapid eye movement (REM) sleep** (Box 42.2). During NREM sleep, a sleeper progresses through three stages (stages 1, 2, and 3) of increasingly deeper sleep. Stage 1, a light and drowsy sleep, occurs at the beginning of sleep and is the transitional stage between wakefulness and sleeping. Stage 2 is a deeper stage of sleep, although a sleeper may be easily aroused during this stage of sleep. Stage 3 involves even deeper sleep, and this stage is known as *delta sleep* or *slow-wave sleep* (SWS). Delta sleep or SWS sleep is thought to be the most restorative of all the sleep stages. REM sleep, also known as *paradoxical sleep*, follows NREM sleep and is not divided into stages. REM sleep shares some characteristics of NREM sleep and of wakefulness. REM sleep is "paradoxical" in the sense that, although a person is behaviourally asleep, the individual is physiologically active— brain activity is high, rapid eye movements are occurring, twitching of the extremities occurs, and males frequently develop erections (Siegel, 2017). The most characteristic feature of REM sleep is dreaming. REM sleep dreams are often vivid and emotional (Carskadon & Dement, 2017). REM sleep is the phase at the end of each sleep cycle.

Different factors promote or interfere with various stages of the sleep cycle. It is important for nurses to be aware of these factors and know about therapies that promote sleep and eliminate factors that disrupt it.

Sleep Cycle. The normal sleep pattern for an adult begins with a pre-sleep period during which the person is aware of only gradually developing sleepiness. This period normally lasts 10 to 30 minutes, but if a person has difficulty falling asleep, it can last an hour or longer. Once

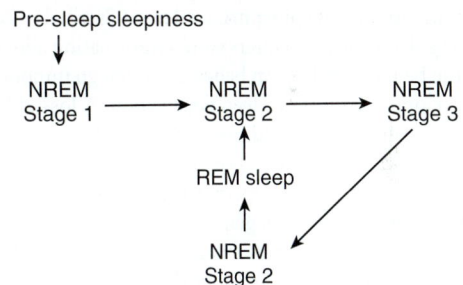

FIGURE 42.2 The stages of the adult sleep cycle. *NREM*, Nonrapid eye movement; *REM*, rapid eye movement.

asleep, the person usually passes through four to five complete sleep cycles per night, each consisting of three stages of NREM sleep and a period of REM sleep (Carskadon & Dement, 2017). Sleep begins when adults enter stage 1 NREM sleep. This stage usually persists for only a few minutes, and sleep may be easily interrupted by calling the person's name or by touching them. Stage 2 NREM sleep follows and continues for approximately 10 to 25 minutes. In stage 2, a person is not so easily awakened. Stage 2 NREM sleep then goes to stage 3 NREM, back to stage 2 NREM and then to REM sleep to complete the sleep cycle (Figure 42.2). NREM sleep and REM sleep continue to alternate throughout a night in this cyclical pattern (Carskadon & Dement, 2017). The number of sleep cycles depends on the total amount of time that a person spends sleeping.

The average length of the first cycle is 90 minutes, and subsequent cycles may last between 100 and 120 minutes. During the night, the NREM–REM sleep cycle is repeated four to five times, and with each subsequent cycle, less time is spent in stage 3 NREM sleep while the proportion of time spent in REM sleep increases. Of the total sleep time, 75 to 85% is spent in NREM sleep.

Not all people progress consistently through the stages of sleep. For example, a sleeper may move back and forth for short intervals between the NREM stages 2 and 3 before entering the REM stage. The amount of time spent in each stage varies over a person's lifespan. Newborns and children spend more time in deep sleep or SWS. This stage of sleep is highest in children, and for this reason it is often very difficult to wake young children from this particular stage of sleep. As individuals age, less time is spent in deep sleep (Carskadon & Dement, 2017).

Functions of Sleep

Although we spend a third of our time sleeping, many of the reasons why we sleep have yet to be understood. Many theories of why we sleep have been proposed, and all of these may be partially correct. For instance, it has been proposed that sleep allows for physiological and psychological restoration (Carskadon & Dement, 2017). During NREM sleep, biological functions slow. Normally, in daytime hours the heart rate of a healthy adult averages 70 to 80 beats per minute, or less, if the individual is in excellent physical condition. During sleep, the heart rate slows, beating 10 to 26 fewer times each minute, or 60 to 120 fewer beats each hour. Clearly, restful sleep is beneficial in preserving cardiac function. Other biological functions also decrease during sleep—for example, respirations, blood pressure, muscle tone, urine production, and hormone secretion (Carskadon & Dement, 2017). The body needs sleep for physiological restoration such as cell and tissue repair. Increased cell mitosis and increased protein synthesis have been observed during periods of NREM sleep.

REM sleep is necessary for brain tissue restoration and appears to be important for cognitive restoration. REM sleep is associated with changes in cerebral blood flow, increased cortical activity, increased oxygen consumption, and epinephrine release (Carskadon & Dement, 2017). During sleep, the brain filters stored information about the day's activities. The benefits of sleep on behaviour often go unnoticed until a problem develops as a result of sleep deprivation. A loss of REM sleep leads to feelings of confusion and suspicion.

Sleep is also believed to be important for immune function, renal function, regulation of body temperature, metabolism of glucose, and hormone secretion (Opp & Krueger, 2017).

In addition to physical functioning, sleep is essential for psychological and social functioning. Without sleep, individuals are irritable and anxious and often report high levels of stress.

Dreams. *Dreaming* is defined as a mental activity that occurs while individuals are asleep. Dreams can occur during both NREM and REM sleep. The majority of dreams take place in the REM sleep stage. REM sleep–related dreams are often vivid and elaborate, whereas NREM dreams are simpler and more realistic.

Studies of across-the-night changes in the characteristics of dreams suggest that dreams become more realistic as the night progresses. Dream content also appears to parallel cognitive and emotional development, as the recollection of dreams reported by children and adults is quite different (Stickgold & Wamsley, 2017).

Determinants of dreams, aside from age, include personality, physiological conditions (e.g., pregnancy), psychological conditions, pharmacological therapies, and situational factors. Personality also influences the quality of dreams; for example, a creative person tends to have elaborate and complex dreams, whereas a depressed person may dream of helplessness (Stickgold & Wamsley, 2017). Most people dream about their immediate concerns, such as an argument with a spouse or worries over work. Sometimes a person is unaware of the fears represented in bizarre dreams. Clinical psychologists can try to analyze the symbolic nature of dreams as part of a patient's psychotherapy. The ability to describe a dream and interpret its significance sometimes helps resolve personal concerns or fears.

Numerous theories have been proposed as to why individuals dream. For centuries, dreams have been seen as messages from the gods, and this belief is upheld by many cultures today. Sigmund Freud theorized that dreams were the expression of an individual's unconscious desires and that by exploring dreams, emotional problems could be cured (Stickgold & Wamsley, 2017).

Physical Illness

Any illness that causes pain, physical discomfort, or mood difficulties, such as anxiety or depression, often results in sleep challenges. Individuals who are ill frequently have trouble falling asleep or staying asleep. Illnesses can also force patients to sleep in unfamiliar positions. For example, when an arm or leg is in traction, patients have a difficult time finding a comfortable position for sleep.

Respiratory disease often interferes with sleep. While individuals sleep, their level of blood oxygen decreases. In healthy individuals, this decrease can be compensated for easily, whereas individuals with respiratory diseases often require supportive devices, practices, or therapies to assist them while they are sleeping. Symptoms associated with respiratory diseases may require individuals to alter their position to facilitate sleeping. For example, individuals with chronic obstructive lung disease, such as emphysema, are frequently short of breath and often require two or three pillows to sleep.

Cardiovascular disease interferes with sleep. Individuals with obesity are at greater risk for cardiovascular disease and, thus, for sleep disorders (Box 42.3). Chest pain, shortness of breath, diaphoresis, nausea, and palpitations, all symptoms associated with cardiovascular disease, frequently occur during the night and can disrupt sleep. Hypertension often causes early morning awakening and fatigue.

The sleep of individuals with musculoskeletal disorders such as osteoarthritis and rheumatoid arthritis may be disrupted by the pain that often accompanies these conditions (Doufas, 2017).

Nocturia, or urination during the night, disrupts sleep and the sleep cycle. This condition is most common in older people with reduced bladder tone or individuals who have cardiac disease, diabetes, or problems with elimination. After a person awakens repeatedly to urinate, returning to sleep is difficult.

Sleep Disorders

Sleep disorders are conditions that interfere with nighttime sleep. Currently, more than 80 sleep disorders have been identified in the literature. The American Academy of Sleep Medicine, which developed the International Classification of Sleep Disorders version 3 (ICSD3), classifies these disorders into eight major categories (Box 42.4).

Increasingly, evidence suggests that sleep disorders are related to serious medical conditions. Individuals with sleep disorders are at risk for developing hypertension, diabetes, cardiovascular and neurological diseases, and mental illnesses (Mukherjee et al., 2015). Sleep disorders can affect individuals of all ages, and the prevalence of these disorders increases with advancing age, with aging men being more vulnerable than aging women (Mander et al., 2017). Individuals with sleep disorders may experience difficulty falling asleep or staying asleep, daytime sleepiness, hypersomnolence, or abruptly falling asleep during the daytime (Cao & Guilleminault, 2017).

The insomnias are disorders related to difficulty falling asleep. Individuals with sleep-related breathing disorders have disordered respirations during sleep. Hypersomnia is a group of disorders that are not due to sleep-related breathing disorders and are caused by disturbances in circadian rhythms or in nocturnal sleep. The parasomnias are undesirable behaviours that usually occur during sleep. Circadian rhythm sleep disorders are caused by a misalignment between the timing of sleep and the societal norm or the desires of the individual.

BOX 42.3 RESEARCH HIGHLIGHT
Obesity, Sleep Disturbance, and Sleep Duration

Research Focus

Research has shown an association between obesity, sleep disturbances, and short sleep time. The prevalence of obesity has increased considerably over the past 25 years and is considered a global epidemic (Muscogiuri et al., 2019). *Obesity* refers to an excess of body fat and is a disorder that occurs when body fat excess impairs the health of individuals. Obesity is associated with an increased risk of many chronic diseases, including heart disease, diabetes, and hypertension (Anic et al., 2010; Ryan et al., 2014). Research has shown that obesity increases morbidity and mortality.

Obesity is a significant risk factor for sleep disturbances, particularly obstructive sleep apnea (OSA). OSA independently plays a role in the development of chronic conditions. Shorter sleep times have also been identified as playing a role in the development of obesity (Cooper et al., 2018).

Over the past several years, sleep duration in adults has decreased, on average, by 1.5 to 2 hours per night, and many individuals are reporting sleeping fewer than 6 hours per night. Researchers wanted to determine whether there was indeed a relationship between obesity and sleep disturbances and whether shorter sleep time increases the risk of obesity (Muscogiuri et al., 2019).

Research Abstract

Epidemiological studies suggest that obesity is the most significant risk factor for sleep disorders. The most prevalent type of obesity-related sleep disorder is OSA, which independently may increase the risk of chronic diseases including high blood pressure, insulin resistance, heart disease, and high cholesterol. Conversely, excessive consumption of unhealthy foods has been associated with short sleep times (<5 or 6 hours per night), which contributes to central obesity.

Implications for Practice

- During assessment of a patient's health problems, ask questions related to sleep quality and sleep patterns.
- If the patient indicates a problem with sleep, conduct a thorough sleep history.
- Reinforce good sleep hygiene habits.
- Encourage patients to notify their health care provider if they begin to experience sleep problems.
- Reinforce healthy eating habits.
- Encourage patients to seek the advice of other health care providers (e.g., dietitian, nutritionist).

From Muscogiuri, G., Barrea, L., Annunziata, et al. (2019). Obesity and sleep disturbance: The chicken or the egg? *Critical Reviews in Food and Science and Nutrition, 59*(13), 2158–2165. https://doi.org/10.1080/10408398.2018.1506979

In sleep-related movement disorders, the person experiences movements such as leg cramps or teeth grinding that disturb sleep. The "other sleep disorders category" contains sleep problems that do not fit into other categories.

Sleep laboratory studies are often used to diagnose a sleep disorder (Goldstein & Chervin, 2017). A **polysomnogram** involves the use of EEG, EMG, and EOG to monitor stages of sleep and wakefulness during nighttime sleep. The Multiple Sleep Latency Test (MSLT) provides objective information about sleepiness and selected aspects of sleep structure by measuring eye movements, muscle tone changes, and brain electrical activity during at least four napping opportunities spread throughout the day. The MSLT takes 8 to 10 hours to complete. Patients wear an Actigraph device on their wrist to measure sleep–wake patterns over an extended period of time. Actigraphy data provide information such as sleep time, number and duration of awakenings, and levels of activity and rest (Goldstein & Chervin, 2017).

Insomnia. Patients experience **insomnia** when they report problems falling asleep, staying asleep, and nonrestorative sleep with daytime consequences including fatigue and difficulty concentrating. Insomnia is the second most commonly expressed complaint reported in clinical practice after pain and the most common self-reported sleep-related problem (Wyatt & Crisostomo, 2008). Insomnia is more common in women, and its incidence increases with advancing age (Ong et al., 2017). Insomnia may indicate an underlying physical or psychological disorder (Reeve & Bailes, 2010). People experience short-term insomnia or chronic insomnia for a variety of reasons, including schedule changes (shift work, travel), situational crises, medications, dietary preferences, and illness (Sateia, 2014).

Insomnia is often associated with poor **sleep hygiene** and behaviours, including anxiety and depression, which may preclude initiating sleep and maintaining sleep. Management of insomnia depends on addressing the factors responsible for preventing a good night's sleep. Treatment may include nonpharmacological therapies such as relaxation therapy, cognitive-behavioural therapy, or pharmacological agents,

including over-the counter sleep aids (melatonin) and prescribed medications (hypnotics). Hypnotics are the least preferred method to manage insomnia because of their adverse effects (Sateia, 2014).

Behavioural and cognitive therapies have few adverse effects and have been demonstrated to be efficacious therapies in managing insomnia when they are adhered to (Buysse et al., 2017; Morin et al., 2017).

Sleep Apnea. **Sleep apnea** is a disorder in which people stop breathing for a period of at least 10 seconds while asleep (National Institute of Neurological Disorders and Stroke, 2022). There are two types of sleep apnea: obstructive sleep apnea and central sleep apnea. Central sleep apnea is caused by irregularities in the brain's normal signals to breathe. Most people with sleep apnea will have a combination of both types.

Obstructive sleep apnea (OSA) is a highly prevalent sleep disorder that is caused by relaxation of the soft tissues in the back of the throat. In OSA, the upper airway becomes partially or completely blocked, thereby diminishing the nasal airflow (hypopnea) or stopping it (apnea) for as long as 10 to 30 seconds. The person still attempts to breathe; chest and abdominal movements continue and often result in loud snoring and snorting sounds. When breathing is partially or completely diminished, each successive diaphragmatic movement becomes stronger until the obstruction is relieved. Apneic episodes are normally terminated by gasps, snorting, or brief periods of awakening. Structural abnormalities such as a deviated septum, nasal polyps, certain jaw configurations, or enlarged tonsils predispose an individual to OSA. The effort to breathe during sleep results in arousals from deep sleep, often to the stage 2 cycle. In severe cases, hundreds of hypopnea or apnea episodes occur every hour, resulting in severe interference with deep sleep.

The diagnosis of OSA is established by either a home sleep apnea test or a sleep test conducted in a lab setting. Once a diagnosis is confirmed, positive airway pressure (PAP) therapy is initiated to ensure a patent airway.

Risk factors for developing OSA include age, obesity, gender, ethnicity, smoking, alcohol use, and a positive family history. OSA is more common in Asians than in Whites. OSA affects men more than women,

---

BOX 42.4 Classification of Sleep Disorders

Insomnias
Chronic insomnia disorder
Short-term insomnia disorder
Other insomnia disorder

Sleep-Related Breathing Disorders
Obstructive Sleep Disorders
Obstructive sleep disorders, adults
Obstructive sleep disorders, pediatrics

Central Sleep Apnea Syndromes
Central sleep apnea syndrome with Cheyne-Stokes breathing
Central sleep apnea due to a medical disorder with Cheyne-Stokes breathing
Central sleep apnea due to high-altitude periodic breathing
Central sleep apnea due to a drug or substance

Primary Central Sleep Apnea
Primary sleep apnea of infancy
Primary sleep apnea of prematurity
Treatment-emergent central sleep apnea

Sleep-Related Hypoventilation Syndromes
Obesity hypoventilation syndrome
Congenital central alveolar hypoventilation syndrome
Late-onset central hypoventilation syndrome with hypothalamic dysfunction
Idiopathic central alveolar hypoventilation
Sleep-related medication related to a medical condition

Sleep-Related Hypoxemia Disorder
Central Disorders of Hypersomnolence
Narcolepsy type I
Narcolepsy type II
Idiopathic hypersomnia
Kleine-Levin syndrome
Hypersomnia due to a medical disorder
Hypersomnia due to a medication or substance
Hypersomnia associated with a psychiatric disorder
Insufficient sleep syndrome

Parasomnias
Parasomnias Usually Associated With NREM Sleep
Confusion arousals
Sleepwalking
Sleep terrors
Sleep-related eating disorder

Parasomnias-Associated REM Sleep
REM sleep behaviour disorder
Recurrent isolated sleep paralysis
Nightmare disorder

Other Parasomnias
Sleep-related hallucinations
Sleep-related eating disorder
Sleep-related enuresis (bedwetting)
Parasomnia due to drug or substance
Parasomnia due to a medical condition
Exploding head syndrome
Parasomnia, unspecified

Circadian Rhythm Sleep–Wake Disorders
Delayed sleep–wake disorder
Advanced sleep–wake disorder
Irregular sleep–wake disorder
Non–24-hour sleep–wake disorder
Shift work disorder
Jet lag disorder
Circadian sleep–wake disorder, not otherwise specified

Sleep-Related Movement Disorders
Restless legs syndrome
Periodic limb movements
Sleep-related leg cramps
Sleep-related bruxism (teeth grinding)
Benign sleep myoclonus of infancy
Sleep-related movement due to a medical condition
Sleep-related movement due to a medication or a substance

NREM, Non-rapid eye movement; *REM,* rapid eye movement.
Data from Sateia, M. J. (2014). Review: International classification of sleep disorders—Third edition: Highlights and modifications. *Contemporary Reviews in Sleep Medicine, 146*(5), 1390–1394. https://doi.org/10.1378/chest.14-0970

---

particularly obese men. OSA is a chronic disease that does not resolve unless the patient is counselled and motivated to lose weight and agrees to oral corrective surgery, if required (Patil et al., 2019).

Excessive daytime sleepiness (EDS) and fatigue are the most common complaints of individuals who have OSA. Those with severe OSA often report taking daytime naps and experience a disruption in their daily activities because of sleepiness. Feelings of sleepiness are usually most intense when waking up just after falling asleep and 12 hours after the mid-sleep period. In addition to reports of EDS, other symptoms of OSA are morning headaches, choking or gasping upon awakening, irritability, depression, difficulty concentrating, and decreased sex drive.

OSA causes a serious decline in the saturation level of arterial oxygen and contributes to high blood pressure (Newsom, 2022). Individuals with OSA are at risk for cardiac dysrhythmias, heart failure, pulmonary hypertension, angina, stroke, hypertension, and metabolic syndrome. In addition, if untreated, OSA may lead to coronary artery disease, mood disorders, daytime sleepiness, and a poorer quality of life (Redline, 2017).

Individuals who have OSA rarely achieve deep sleep because sleep is often fragmented. OSA may exact a heavy emotional toll on the individuals affected and their families. OSA may affect marital relationships and interactions within and outside the family, and frequently is an embarrassment to the patient (Newsom, 2022).

Treatment for OSA includes continuous positive airway pressure (CPAP). CPAP consists of a mask that fits over the nose and mouth through which air is continuously delivered into the airway to assist in keeping it open during sleep. Other treatments include addressing the underlying cardiac or respiratory complications and emotional difficulties that occur as a result of the symptoms of this disorder.

Narcolepsy. **Narcolepsy** is a rare, complex neurological sleep disorder for which there is no known cure. Narcolepsy is known to affect men and women of any age; however, it usually appears in adolescence. The clinical manifestations of narcolepsy are highly variable. Excessive daytime sleepiness is the most common complaint associated with narcolepsy. During the day, a person who has narcolepsy may suddenly feel an overwhelming wave of sleepiness and fall asleep (Cao & Guilleminault, 2017; Scammell, 2015). Narcolepsy is known to have a significant impact on REM sleep and is also known to intensify the emotions associated with this stage of sleep. Many individuals with narcolepsy experience hallucinations, vivid dreams, night terrors, sleepwalking, sleep paralysis, poor memory and concentration, or the feeling of being unable to move or talk just before waking or falling asleep. Cataplexy, or sudden bilateral (occasionally unilateral) loss of muscle tone accompanied by an overpowering urge to sleep, can occur at any time during the day and can last from a few seconds to as long as 30 minutes. These episodes are sporadic and can occur occasionally to several times per day. A history of cataplexy may be obtained by inquiring whether the loss of muscle tone occurs during the following: upon hearing or telling a joke, while laughing, or when angry. Other triggers are embarrassment, surprise, stress, or sexual arousal (Mignot, 2017). Some studies show a genetic link for narcolepsy (Mignot, 2017).

Narcolepsy may also affect energy levels, metabolism, appetite, and feelings of mental well-being. Individuals with narcolepsy can have intense cravings for carbohydrates, and greater than one-third of individuals with narcolepsy suffer from obesity.

Most people with narcolepsy tend to be diagnosed several years after onset of the condition, which means most of the symptoms associated with this disorder go untreated. Prior to diagnosis, individuals are frequently regarded as "different," antisocial, lacking in motivation, and uncooperative (Cao & Guilleminault, 2017).

There is no known cure for narcolepsy; therefore, treatment is targeted at symptom management. Traditionally, individuals with narcolepsy have been treated by two groups of medications: stimulants and antidepressants. Stimulants promote wakefulness and reduce the frequency of sleeping episodes. Modafinil is a wakefulness-promoting agent and has been shown to improve symptoms of fatigue and cognitive function (memory and concentration). Antidepressants suppress cataplexy and other REM-related symptoms (Cao & Guilleminault, 2017).

Nonpharmacological management should be initiated in all affected individuals. Education is an important component of the treatment plan for individuals with narcolepsy. Good sleep hygiene should be emphasized. The fundamental principles of sleep hygiene are listed in Box 42.5. Other management strategies include regular exercise, strategically timed daytime naps (if possible), a high-protein diet, deep breathing exercises, and chewing gum. Patients who have narcolepsy need to avoid factors that increase drowsiness (e.g., alcohol, heavy meals, exhausting activities, long-distance driving, and extended periods of sitting in hot, stuffy rooms).

BOX 42.5 Sleep Hygiene: Fundamental Principles

Avoid daytime naps.
Decrease consumption of caffeine, tobacco, and alcohol.
Exercise regularly, but not prior to bedtime.
Do not watch television, use the computer, or read while in bed.
Eat regular meals, do not go to bed hungry, and decrease consumption of liquids in the evening.
Maintain a regular sleep–wake schedule, even on weekends.
Maintain the bedroom as an environment solely for sleep.
Ensure a sleeping environment that is comfortable and quiet.

From Sleep Foundation. (2021). https://www.sleepfoundation.org/

Parasomnias. Parasomnias are undesirable sleep problems that occur while falling asleep, between sleep phases, or during transitions from sleep to wakefulness. The word *parasomnia* is derived from the Greek word *para* combined with the Latin word *somnus*, meaning event accompanying sleep. The parasomnia may range from abnormal sleep-related movements to emotions, perceptions, dreaming, or behaviours. Parasomnia may be the manifestation of an underlying physical or psychological disorder or may be caused by the ingestion of drugs or other substances (Cai & Bae, 2021). Parasomnias are more common in children than in adults (Verrier & Josephson, 2017).

Parasomnias that occur among older children include somnambulism (sleepwalking), night terrors, nightmares, nocturnal enuresis (bedwetting), body rocking, and bruxism (teeth grinding). When adults experience these symptoms, more serious disorders are often indicated. Specific treatment for these disorders varies; however, in all cases patients need to be supported and their safety maintained.

Shift Work. *Shift work sleep disorder (SWSD)* is a common sleep disorder experienced by individuals who work outside the traditional 9-to-5 workday. This disorder results from imposing a sleep–wake schedule that is contrary to the body's internal circadian clock. Most commonly associated with nighttime work, the health and economic consequences of this disorder are profound. Studies suggest that individuals who engage in shift work have a high risk of developing cardiovascular disease. The most common problems reported by shift workers are excessive sleepiness, fatigue, and insomnia. Not all individuals exposed to shift work develop this disorder (Jehan et al., 2017).

Sleep Deprivation. Sleep deprivation refers to insufficient sleep during a specific time period. The most common causes of sleep deprivation are lifestyle factors or work-related factors. One approach to understanding the functional significance of sleep is to consider the behavioural and physiological effects of sleep deprivation. Numerous studies on animal models subjected to periods of sleep deprivation have demonstrated that sleep deprivation results in changes in metabolism (weight loss despite increased food intake), impaired glucose metabolism, increased heart rate, skin lesions, decreased body temperature, and, with prolonged periods, death (National Heart, Lung and Blood Institute, 2022).

There are several types of sleep deprivation. Sleep deprivation may be observed as a reduction in sleep time so that sleep time does not meet the needs of the individual, prolonged wakefulness, and sleep disruption related to a pathophysiological process (e.g., cancer). The extent to which an individual experiences the effects of sleep deprivation depends on the physiological and behavioural requirements of the individual Moreover, the effects of sleep deprivation are cumulative, meaning a mild reduction in sleep time over a prolonged period may be detrimental to the individual.

Sleep deprivation may be experienced by individuals for a variety of reasons. Causes include illness (e.g., fever, difficulty breathing, or pain), emotional stress, certain medications, environmental disturbances (e.g., noise, unfamiliar surroundings, frequent nursing care), and variability in the timing of sleep due to shift work and travel. Factors contributing to sleep deprivation in hospitalized patients are outlined in Box 42.6.

A person's response to sleep deprivation is highly variable. Patients exhibit a variety of physiological and psychological symptoms (Box 42.7). The severity of symptoms is often related to the duration of sleep deprivation. The most effective treatment for sleep deprivation is the elimination or correction of factors that disrupt the sleep pattern.

BOX 42.6 Causes of Sleep Deprivation in Hospitalized Patients

Environmental Factors
Noise
Uncomfortable bed and pillows
Bright lights
Pathophysiological factors
Pain and discomfort
Use of invasive equipment such as intravenous lines, nasogastric tubes

Emotional Factors
Stress, worry
Lack of control
Lack of privacy
Anxiety about procedures and outcomes of investigations

BOX 42.7 Sleep Deprivation Symptoms

Physiological Symptoms
Ptosis, visual disturbances such as blurred vision
Clumsiness in fine motor skills
Decreased reflexes
Slowed response time
Decreased reasoning and judgement
Decreased auditory and visual alertness
Cardiac arrhythmias
Increased food intake
Decreasing satiety
Weight loss

Psychological Symptoms
Easily distracted
Confusion and disorientation
Forgetfulness
Increased sensitivity to pain
Irritability, withdrawal, apathy
Worry
Excessive sleepiness
Poor concentration
Agitation
Hyperactivity
Decreased motivation

Nurses play an important role in identifying individuals' treatable sleep deprivation problems.

NURSING KNOWLEDGE BASE

Sleep and Rest

When people are at **rest**, they usually feel mentally relaxed, free from anxiety, and physically calm. Rest does not imply inactivity, although rest is often thought of as the act of settling down in a comfortable chair or lying in bed. Usually, when individuals are at rest, they are in a state of mental, physical, and spiritual activity that leaves them feeling refreshed, rejuvenated, and ready to resume the activities of the day. Individuals have their own habits for obtaining rest and can adjust to new environments or conditions that affect their ability to rest. Rest may be obtained from reading a book, practising a relaxation exercise, listening to music, taking a long walk, or sitting quietly.

Illness and unfamiliar health care routines can easily affect the usual rest and sleep patterns of individuals entering a hospital or other health care facilities. Nurses may frequently care for patients on bed rest, which confines patients to bed in order to reduce the physical and psychological demands on their body. Patients may not necessarily feel rested because they may still have emotional worries that prevent complete relaxation. For example, concern over physical limitations or a fear of being unable to return to their usual lifestyle can cause patients to feel stressed and unable to relax. Nurses must always be aware of a patient's need for rest. Long periods without rest can lead to illness or to the worsening of an existing illness.

Normal Sleep Requirements and Patterns

Individual requirements for sleep duration and quality vary among individuals of all age groups. For example, one person may feel adequately rested after 6 hours of sleep, whereas another person may require 10 hours of sleep.

Newborns. During the first few weeks of life, newborns sleep about 16 hours a day, sleeping almost constantly during the first week. Sleep occurs equally across the day and night in newborns and is more strongly influenced by hunger than by light–dark cues. The sleep cycle of newborns is generally 40 to 50 minutes, with waking occurring after one to two sleep cycles. Sleep is classified as active sleep (REM sleep equivalent) or quiet sleep (NREM sleep equivalent). A third stage has also been identified and is known as *indeterminate sleep*. This sleep stage cannot be defined as either quiet sleep or active sleep by polysomnography. Newborn sleep cycles begin with active sleep; newborns spend the majority of their sleep time in this stage of sleep. The primary function of active sleep is thought to allow for the continued development of neural pathways.

Infants. By age 3 months, the amount of time the newborn spends in active sleep (REM sleep equivalent) diminishes, the required hours for sleep gradually decrease, and sleep–wake periods develop into a day/night cycle. By 6 months of age, infants enter sleep through NREM sleep. The ability to sleep during the night develops by 6 to 9 months of age. At this point, the infant's sleeping pattern is characterized by a nocturnal sleep period of 10 to 12 hours' duration, and two to three daytime naps, which collectively amount to 12 to 14 hours of total sleep time. Awakening commonly occurs early in the morning, although awakening during the night is not unusual because there are significant individual variations (Paavonen et al., 2020).

Toddlers. By 2 years of age, most children usually require 12 to 14 hours of sleep each day, which generally includes a nap in the afternoon and, for some, a morning nap as well. This amount of sleep is needed to re-energize the toddler and for continued growth and development. Lack of sleep makes a toddler feel tired and irritable. Awakening during the night is common for toddlers. A variety of factors may influence night waking, including dreams and a fear of being separated from their parents. During this period, the percentage of REM sleep continues to fall (Paavonen et al., 2020).

Preschoolers. A preschooler sleeps about 13 hours a night (about 20% of which is REM sleep). By 5 years of age, the preschooler rarely takes daytime naps, except in cultures where siestas are the custom (Hockenberry & Wilson, 2019). The preschooler usually has difficulty relaxing or quieting down after long, active days and may experience bedtime fears, waking during the night, or nightmares. Partial wakening, followed by a normal return to sleep, is frequent (Hockenberry & Wilson, 2019). In the waking period, the child may exhibit brief episodes of crying, walking aimlessly, unintelligible speech, sleepwalking, or bedwetting. Numerous factors may influence the sleep pattern of preschoolers, including day care and preschool schedules, family routines, and parental expectations as to the amount of sleep required for this developmental stage.

School-Aged Children. The amount of sleep needed varies during the school-age years. Both gender and ethnicity may explain the variability of sleep patterns in school-aged children. A longer sleep cycle has been observed in school-aged girls compared with their same-aged male counterparts. White children tend to have more NREM stage 1 sleep and less NREM stage 2 sleep than Black children. Most school-aged children sleep between 9 and 10 hours each night. Epidemiological studies of school-aged children have shown that shorter sleep times are associated with behavioural problems and symptoms of depression (Belmon et al., 2019).

Adolescents. Insufficient sleep is common among adolescents. There is no single reason for this sleep pattern. The demands of school (e.g., schedules, assignments, exams, and extracurricular activities), decreased parental influence, employment, and social media appear to play a significant role in the sleep patterns of adolescents (Newsom, 2022). Physiological (circadian and homeostatic) processes that regulate sleep and wakefulness are also thought to influence the sleep habits of adolescents. This shortened sleep time often results in EDS. As a result, adolescents may experience reduced performance in school, vulnerability to accidents, behaviour and mood issues, and increased use of alcohol or other substances. Some adolescents may experience poor sleep patterns because of underlying sleep disorders, including OSA, restless legs syndrome, and narcolepsy. Adolescents diagnosed with neurodevelopmental disorders such as autism spectrum disorder and attention-deficit disorder find it difficult to sleep well. Sufficient sleep is a challenge for adolescents living with mental health illness. Suicidal behaviour is more common among adolescents with poor sleep patterns (Newsom, 2022).

Young Adults. Most young adults average 6 to 8.5 hours of sleep per night. Approximately 20% of sleep time is REM sleep, which remains consistent throughout life. The stresses of a job, family relationships, and social activities frequently lead to both insomnia and the use of medications to aid sleep. Daytime sleepiness contributes to an increased number of accidents, decreased productivity, and interpersonal challenges in this age group. Pregnancy increases the need for sleep and rest. During the third trimester of pregnancy, women may experience insomnia, periodic limb movements, restless legs syndrome, and sleep-disordered breathing (Balserak & Lee, 2017).

Middle-Aged Adults. During middle adulthood, the total time spent sleeping at night begins to decline. The amount of stage 3 sleep begins to fall and continues to fall with advancing age. Insomnia is particularly common, probably because of the changes and stresses experienced in middle age. Anxiety, depression, and certain physical illnesses can cause sleep disturbances. Women who have menopausal symptoms often experience insomnia (Lee & Moe, 2011).

Older Persons. Aging results in several physiological and psychological changes, and alterations in sleep patterns frequently occur because of these changes. Studies suggest that poor sleep quality is a common complaint of older persons. Approximately 50% of older persons report difficulty sleeping. Aging is associated with changes in sleep architecture, or sleep pattern. Greater nighttime disturbances (increased awakenings at night), less slow-wave or deep sleep, increased frequency of daytime napping, and decreased total sleep time are changes in sleep architecture that occur with aging (National Institute of Aging, 2020).

Older women are at particular risk for sleep difficulties due to hormonal changes that accompany menopause (Baker et al., 2017). Hot flashes (episodes of warmth in the face and chest) occurring at night can cause difficulty sleeping and may lead to an increase in frequency of nighttime awakenings and, hence, less sleep time.

Numerous other factors are also related to the sleep problems reported by older men and women. These include the presence of comorbid physiological conditions (e.g., heart disease) and psychological conditions (e.g., depression), primary sleep disorders (e.g., insomnia), chronic pain, nocturia, use of multiple medications, and alterations in circadian rhythm expressions.

Factors Affecting Sleep

Often, several factors alter the quality and quantity of sleep, such as physiological, psychological, and environmental influences.

Medications and Substances. Many older persons take a variety of medications to control or treat chronic conditions, and these medications can seriously disrupt sleep. Daytime sleepiness, insomnia, and fatigue often result as a direct effect of commonly prescribed medications (Box 42.8). These medications may impair waking function and alter sleep patterns, which can be problematic for individuals (Cook, 2008a, 2008b). Antidepressants, antihistamines, and pain medications can cause daytime sleepiness or fatigue. Beta blockers have been associated with nightmares and vivid dreams. Diuretics can cause nocturia, thereby disrupting sleep. Medications prescribed for sleep can also be problematic as a result of their sedating effects during daytime hours (Kilduff & Mendelson, 2017). Other substances with addictive properties, such as nicotine and cannabis, can also result in disrupted sleep patterns (Gordon, 2019).

Lifestyle. A person's daily routine influences sleep patterns. An individual working a rotating shift (e.g., 2 weeks of day shifts followed by a week of night shifts) often has difficulty adjusting to the altered sleep schedule (Newsom, 2022). For example, the body's internal clock for bedtime is set at 11 P.M., but the work schedule instead forces sleep at 9 A.M. The individual is able to sleep only 3 or 4 hours because the body's clock perceives that the morning is the time to be awake and active. Difficulties with maintaining alertness during work time result in decreased and even hazardous performance. After several weeks of working a night shift, a person's biological clock usually does adjust. Other alterations in routines that disrupt sleep patterns are performing unaccustomed heavy work, engaging in late-night social activities, and changing the evening mealtime (Belenky et al., 2017; Van Dongen et al., 2017).

Usual Sleep Patterns. In the past century, the amount of sleep obtained nightly has decreased by more than 20% (Newsom, 2022), which indicates that many adults are sleep deprived and experience excessive sleepiness during the day. Sleepiness becomes pathological when it occurs at times when individuals need to or want to be awake. Individuals who experience temporary sleep deprivation as a result of an active social evening or a lengthened work schedule usually feel sleepy the next day. However, they are usually able to overcome these feelings despite the difficulty they experience in performing tasks and remaining attentive. Much more serious than temporary sleep deprivation is a chronic lack of sleep, which causes serious alterations in the

BOX 42.8   Medications and Their Effects on Sleep and Wakefulness

Hypnotics
Decrease NREM stage 3 sleep as well as REM sleep
Increase daytime sleepiness
Lead to poor memory and concentration
Depress respirations
May worsen sleep apnea in older persons

Diuretics
Nighttime awakenings caused by nocturia

Antidepressants
Cognitive impairment
Psychomotor impairment
Increase of NREM stage 1 sleep
Suppression of REM sleep
Decrease in total sleep time
Daytime sleepiness

Stimulants
Caffeine
Prevents the onset of sleep
Interrupts sleep during the night
Decreases the time spent in deep sleep
Interferes with REM sleep

Alcohol
Speeds onset of sleep
Reduces REM sleep
Interrupts sleep during the night and makes returning to sleep difficult

Beta-Adrenergic Blockers
Fatigue
Insomnia
Depression
Psychomotor impairment
Nightmares
Vivid dreams

Benzodiazepines
Alter REM sleep
Increase sleep time
Increase daytime sleepiness

Narcotics
Cause somnolence
Decrease amount of time spent in deep sleep stages
Suppress REM sleep
Depress respirations
Cause cognitive impairment
Cause psychomotor impairment

Nicotine
Increased sleep onset latency
Decreased sleep efficiency
Decreased in slow wave sleep

Cannabis
Increase in slow-wave sleep
Decreased REM sleep
Increase in REM latency
Strange dreams (with withdrawal)

Anticonvulsants
Decrease REM sleep time
May cause daytime drowsiness
May cause insomnia
Cause impaired cognition

Anti-Parkinsonian Drugs
May cause worsening of cognitive function, especially memory
Cause fatigue
Cause somnolence

NREM, Non-rapid eye movement; *REM*, rapid eye movement.

ability to perform daily functions. Sleepiness tends to be most difficult to overcome during the performance of sedentary (inactive) tasks. For example, single-vehicle accidents related to a driver falling asleep at the wheel occur most often between 2 A.M. and 5 A.M., as a result of the sleepiness that occurs when individuals are awake during what is their normal period of sleep (Philip et al., 2017).

Emotional Stress. Sleep is frequently disrupted by worry over personal problems or a personal situation. Emotional stress causes a person to be tense and often leads to frustration when sleep does not occur. Stress also causes a person to try too hard to fall asleep, to awaken frequently during the night, or to oversleep. Continued stress can lead to poor sleep quality and habits.

Older patients frequently experience personal losses, such as retirement, physical impairment, or the death of a loved one, all of which can lead to emotional stress. Older persons and other individuals who live with depressive mood difficulties may experience delays in falling asleep, the earlier appearance of REM sleep, frequent awakenings, increased total time in bed, feelings of having slept poorly, and early awakening (Newsom, 2022).

Environment. The physical environment in which a person sleeps can significantly influence the ability to fall asleep and remain asleep. Good ventilation is essential for restful sleep. The size, firmness, and position of the bed also affect the quality of sleep. If a person usually sleeps with another individual, sleeping alone often causes wakefulness. On the other hand, sleeping with a restless or snoring bed partner can disrupt sleep.

In hospitals and other inpatient facilities, noise creates a problem for patients. Noise in hospitals is usually new or strange and often loud, and patients wake easily. While in the hospital, the sleep of patients is often fragmented, with patients experiencing increased total wake times, increased nocturnal awakenings, and decreased REM sleep and total sleep time. Environment-induced noises (e.g., nursing activities) are sources of increased sound levels. Critical care units (CCUs) are sources of high noise levels as the result of staff consultations, monitor alarms, and equipment sounds (Pulak & Jensen, 2016). The environment is unpleasant for sleeping because of the proximity of patients, noise from confused and ill patients, the ringing of alarm systems and telephones, and disturbances caused by emergencies. Noise contributes to hearing impairment; delays in healing; impaired immune function; and increased blood pressure, heart rate, and stress.

The level of light in a room affects the ability to fall asleep. Some individuals prefer a dark room for sleep, whereas others, such as children or older persons, often prefer soft lighting during sleep. Individuals may also have trouble sleeping because of the temperature of a room. A room that is too warm or too cold often causes an individual to become restless.

Exercise and Fatigue. A person who is moderately fatigued usually achieves restful sleep, especially when the fatigue is the result of enjoyable work or exercise. Exercising that is completed at least 3 hours prior to bedtime allows the body enough time to cool down and maintain a state of fatigue that promotes relaxation (Newsom, 2022). However, excess fatigue resulting from exhausting or stressful work makes falling asleep difficult. Excess fatigue is a common problem for grade-school children and adolescents.

Food and Caloric Intake. Following good eating habits is important for proper sleep. Eating a large, heavy meal or a spicy meal at night often leads to indigestion that interferes with sleep. Insomnia can result from caffeine, alcohol, or nicotine consumed in the evening. Coffee, tea, cola, and chocolate contain caffeine that cause sleeplessness. Individuals who have insomnia can improve their sleep by drastically reducing or completely avoiding these substances (Newsom, 2022). Some food allergies cause insomnia. In infants, a milk allergy sometimes causes nighttime waking and crying, or colic.

Both weight loss and weight gain influence sleep patterns (Van Cauter & Tasali, 2017). Weight gain contributes to OSA because of the increased size of the soft tissue structures in the upper airway. Weight loss causes insomnia and decreased amounts of sleep. Certain sleep disorders are the result of the semi-starvation diets popular in a weight-conscious society.

CRITICAL THINKING

Successful critical thinking requires a synthesis of knowledge, including information gathered from individuals, past experience, critical thinking qualities, and intellectual and professional standards. In making clinical judgements nurses need to anticipate the required information, analyze the data, and make decisions regarding patient care. Adapting to the changing needs of a patient, based on sound decision making, constitutes critical thinking. During assessment (Figure 42.3), nurses need to consider all elements to make appropriate nursing diagnoses.

In the case of sleep, nurses integrate knowledge from disciplines such as nursing, pharmacology, and psychology. Nurses' experience with patients who have sleep problems, together with exploring research related to sleep, will aid in their understanding of effective forms of sleep therapies. Nurses need to use critical thinking qualities, such as perseverance, confidence, and discipline, to complete a comprehensive assessment and to develop a plan of care that can successfully manage the sleep problem. The framework for practice developed by the Canadian Nurses Association (2015) and standards of practice developed by each provincial and territorial nursing organization identify the nurse's role in patient care. In addition, evidence-informed geriatric nursing protocols for best practice, such as those in "Excessive Sleepiness" (Chasens et al., 2008), provide specific instructions for assessing and addressing the needs of older patients with sleep disorders. Moreover, clinical practice guidelines on the management of sleep disorders in the geriatric population (Praharaj et al., 2018) are an evidence-informed tool that nurses can reference for addressing the sleep requirements of this population.

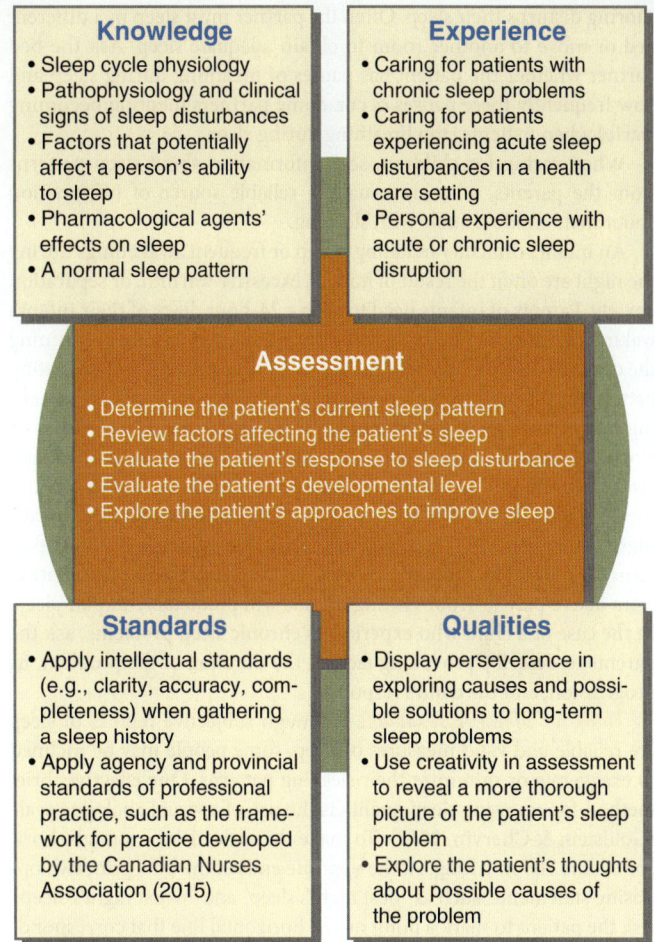

Knowledge
- Sleep cycle physiology
- Pathophysiology and clinical signs of sleep disturbances
- Factors that potentially affect a person's ability to sleep
- Pharmacological agents' effects on sleep
- A normal sleep pattern

Experience
- Caring for patients with chronic sleep problems
- Caring for patients experiencing acute sleep disturbances in a health care setting
- Personal experience with acute or chronic sleep disruption

Assessment
- Determine the patient's current sleep pattern
- Review factors affecting the patient's sleep
- Evaluate the patient's response to sleep disturbance
- Evaluate the patient's developmental level
- Explore the patient's approaches to improve sleep

Standards
- Apply intellectual standards (e.g., clarity, accuracy, completeness) when gathering a sleep history
- Apply agency and provincial standards of professional practice, such as the framework for practice developed by the Canadian Nurses Association (2015)

Qualities
- Display perseverance in exploring causes and possible solutions to long-term sleep problems
- Use creativity in assessment to reveal a more thorough picture of the patient's sleep problem
- Explore the patient's thoughts about possible causes of the problem

FIGURE 42.3 Critical thinking model for sleep assessment.

❖ NURSING PROCESS

◆ Assessment

Patients' sleep patterns are assessed by using the nursing history to gather information about factors that usually influence sleep. Because sleep is a subjective experience, only the patient is able to report whether it is sufficient and restful. If the patient is satisfied with the quantity and quality of sleep received, the nurse should consider it normal, and the nursing history is brief. If, however, a patient reports or suspects a sleep problem, the nurse needs to conduct a detailed history.

Sleep Assessment. Most individuals are able to provide a reasonably accurate estimate of their sleep patterns, particularly if any changes have occurred. In the nursing assessment, focus on understanding the characteristics of the patient's sleep problem and usual sleep habits so that your nursing care strategies to promote sleep are individualized. For example, if the nursing history reveals that a patient always reads before falling asleep, then offer reading material at bedtime.

Sources for Sleep Assessment. Usually, patients are the best resource for describing their sleep problems and how these problems differ from their usual sleep and waking patterns. The patient often knows the cause of their sleep challenges, such as a noisy environment or worry over a relationship. In addition, bed partners are often able to provide information on the patient's sleep patterns that assists in gaining insight to the nature of certain sleep disorders. For example, partners of patients with sleep apnea often complain that the patient's snoring disturbs their sleep. Often the partner must sleep in a different bed or move to another room to obtain adequate sleep. Ask the bed partner whether the patient has pauses of breathing during sleep and how frequently these pauses occur. Some partners mention becoming fearful when patients stop breathing during sleep.

When caring for children, seek information about sleep patterns from the parents, who are usually a reliable source of information about their child's trouble with sleeping.

An infant's difficulty in falling asleep or frequent awakenings during the night are often the result of hunger, excessive warmth, or separation anxiety. Parents of infants need to keep a 24-hour diary of their infant's waking and sleeping behaviour for several days to aid in determining the cause of the problem. Ask the parents to describe the infant's eating pattern and sleeping environment, both of which can influence sleeping behaviour. Older children often are able to verbalize the fears or worries that inhibit their ability to fall asleep. If children frequently awaken in the middle of bad dreams, parents may be able to identify the problem, although they may not be able to understand the meanings of the dreams. Ask parents to describe the typical behaviour patterns that foster or impair sleep. For example, excessive stimulation from active play or from visiting friends will predictably impair sleep. In the case of a child who experiences chronic sleep problems, ask the parents to describe provoking factors, the duration of the problem, its progression, and the child's responses.

Tools for Sleep Assessment. Although subjective reports of sleep are reliable and valid measures of sleep, some people may be inclined to exaggerate or minimize their sleeping patterns. One effective, brief method for assessing sleep quality is the use of a visual analogue scale (Goldstein & Chervin, 2017). To make the scale, draw a straight horizontal line 100 mm long. At the opposite ends of the line, print two opposing statements, such as "best night's sleep" and "worst night's sleep." Ask the patient to mark a point on the horizontal line that corresponds to their perception of the previous night's sleep. Measure the distance of the mark along the line in millimetres; this number is a numerical value for satisfaction with sleep. Use the scale repeatedly to show change over time. Such a scale is useful for assessing an individual's changes in sleep pattern over time.

Another brief subjective method to assess sleep is a numeric scale with a 0 to 10 sleep rating (Gabehart & Van Dongen, 2017; Goldstein & Chervin, 2017). Instruct the patient to first rate their sleep quantity, then their quality of sleep on a scale of 1 to 10, with 0 being the worst sleep and 10 being the best sleep.

Sleep History. When a patient reports having received adequate sleep, a sleep history is usually brief. The information needed for the nurse to plan care conducive to sleep includes the following: the usual bedtime, bedtime rituals, the preferred environment for sleeping, and the time the patient usually rises. When the nurse suspects a sleep problem, they should explore the quality and characteristics of sleep in greater depth by asking the patient to describe the nature of their sleep, including recent changes in their sleep pattern, sleep symptoms experienced during waking hours, use of sleep medications and other prescribed or over-the-counter medications, use of herbal products, diet, intake of substances such as caffeine or alcohol that influence sleep, and recent life events that may affect the patient's mental well-being.

Description of Sleeping Problems. When a patient reports a sleep problem, the nurse needs to conduct a more detailed history. A detailed assessment ensures that the appropriate therapeutic care is provided. Open-ended questions help a patient to describe the problem more fully. After the patient provides a general description of the problem, the nurse can ask some focused questions, which will usually reveal specific characteristics that are useful in planning therapies. The nurse needs to understand the nature of the sleep problem, its signs and symptoms, its onset and duration, its severity, any predisposing factors or causes, and the overall effect on the patient. The nurse should ask specific questions related to the sleep problem (Box 42.9). Proper questioning helps to determine the type of sleep disturbance and the nature of the problem. Box 42.10 gives examples of additional questions for the nurse to ask the patient when specific sleep disorders are suspected. The questions assist in selecting specific sleep therapies and the best time for implementation.

As an adjunct to the sleep history, the patient and the patient's bed partner can keep a sleep–wake diary for 1 to 4 weeks (Goldstein & Chervin, 2017). The patient completes the sleep–wake diary daily to provide information on day-to-day variations in sleep–wake patterns

---

BOX 42.9   Nursing Assessment Questions

Nature of the Problem
What type of problem are you having with your sleep?
Why do you think your sleep is inadequate?
Describe for me a recent typical night's sleep. How is this sleep different from what you are accustomed to?

Signs and Symptoms
Do you have difficulty falling asleep, staying asleep, or waking up?
Have you been told that you snore loudly?
Have you been told you stop breathing or gasp for breath during sleep?
Do you feel drowsy or fall asleep while reading, when watching television, while driving, or when participating in other daily activities?
Do you feel excessively sleepy or irritable?
Do you have trouble concentrating during waking hours?
Do you have headaches when awakening?
Does your child awaken from nightmares?

Onset and Duration
When did you notice the problem?
How long has this problem lasted?

Severity
How long does it take you to fall asleep?
How often during the week do you have trouble falling asleep?
How many hours of sleep a night did you get this week?
How does this amount of sleep compare to what is usual for you?
What do you do when you awaken during the night or when you awaken too early in the morning?

Predisposing Factors
What do you do just before you go to bed?
Have you recently had any changes at work or at home?
Describe your mood. Have you noticed any changes in your mood recently?
What recreational drugs do you take on a regular basis?
Are you taking any new prescription or over-the-counter medications?
Do you eat food (spicy or greasy foods) or drink substances (alcohol or caffeinated beverages) that interfere with your sleep?
Do you have a physical illness that interferes with your sleep?
Does anyone in your family have a history of sleep problems?

Effect on the Patient
How has the loss of sleep affected you?

BOX 42.10 Questions to Ask to Assess for Specific Sleep Disorders

Insomnia

Do you have difficulty falling asleep?

After you fall asleep, do you have difficulty staying asleep? How many times during a night's sleep do you awaken?

When you wake up in the morning, do you feel rested? What time do you wake up in the morning? What causes you to awaken early?

What do you do to prepare for sleep? What do you do to improve your sleep?

What do you think about as you try to fall asleep?

When did you notice you had problems sleeping?

How often do you have trouble sleeping?

Do you feel excessively tired or sleepy during the day?

Do you take naps during the daytime?

Do you have any problems with performing tasks (i.e., work-related or driving) during the daytime?

Sleep Apnea

Do you snore loudly? Does anyone else in your family snore loudly?

Has anyone (e.g., spouse, bed partner, roommate) ever told you that you stop breathing for short periods during your sleep?

Do you experience headaches after awakening?

Do you have difficulty staying awake during the day?

Narcolepsy

Do you sometimes fall asleep unexpectedly? (Friends or relatives may report these occurrences.)

Do you feel excessively tired or sleepy during the day?

Do you have trouble concentrating?

Have you ever had an episode of losing muscle control or falling to the floor after a laughing episode or when angry?

Have you ever had the feeling of being unable to move or talk just before falling asleep or upon awakening?

Do you have vivid dreams when going to sleep or waking up?

---

over extended periods. Entries in the diary can include 24-hour information about various waking and sleeping health behaviours, including evening and bedtime routines, the time the patient goes to bed, the amount of time it took for the patient to fall asleep, the number of awakenings during the night, total sleep time, sleep quality (did they feel rested in the morning), the time and length of daytime napping, mealtimes, type and amount of alcohol and caffeine consumed, current medications, and daytime activities. The partner helps to record the estimated times the patient falls asleep or awakens. Although the sleep diary can provide useful information, the patient needs to be motivated to participate in recording the entries.

Usual Sleep Pattern. What constitutes "normal sleep" is difficult to define because individuals vary in their perception of the adequate quantity and quality of sleep. It is the responsibility of all health care providers to inquire about sleep quality of all patients. Patients need to describe their usual sleep pattern in order to establish the significance of the changes caused by a sleep disorder. The following questions can be asked to determine a patient's sleep pattern:

1. What time do you usually go to bed each night?
2. What time do you usually fall asleep? Do you do anything special to help you fall asleep?
3. How many times do you awaken during the night? Why?
4. What time do you typically wake in the morning?
5. What is the average number of hours you sleep each night?

The patient's data are then compared with the predominant sleep pattern for other patients of the same age. On the basis of this comparison, the nurse can begin to assess for identifiable patterns, which may indicate a specific sleep disturbance, such as insomnia.

Patients with sleep problems frequently show patterns that differ drastically from their usual sleep pattern, or sometimes the change is relatively minor. Hospitalized patients usually need or want more sleep as a result of their illness; however, some patients require less sleep because they are less active. Some patients who are ill think that they need to try to sleep more than their usual amount of sleep, a perception that eventually makes sleeping difficult.

Physical and Psychological Illness. It is important to determine whether the patient has any pre-existing health conditions that interfere with sleep. Poor sleep quality has been associated with numerous physiological and psychological illnesses. Chronic diseases, such as chronic obstructive pulmonary disease, and painful disorders, such as arthritis, interfere with sleep. Sleep disturbance may occur because of the conditions themselves or because of medications taken to treat them. Several symptoms associated with these conditions, such as shortness of breath, pain, and nocturia, can potentially disrupt sleep. Psychiatric disorders can also interfere with sleep. For example, insomnia is common in individuals with schizophrenia, a chronic psychiatric disorder.

Insomnia is also common among individuals with depression. Anxiety disorders have also been associated with poor sleep (Oh et al., 2019). Hence, it is very important to assess patients' sleep pattern, medical and social history (e.g., alcohol, tobacco, and caffeine consumption), and medication usage, including a description of over-the-counter and prescribed drugs. The social history can provide useful information, such as a situational crisis that may be interfering with sleep. If a patient takes medications to aid sleep, the nurse should gather information about the type and amount of medication that the patient uses and assess the effectiveness of such medications and their effects on daytime function.

Current Life Events. During the assessment, the nurse needs to ask whether the patient is experiencing any changes in lifestyle that could disrupt sleep. A person's occupation often offers a clue to the nature of the sleep problem (Drake & Wright, 2017). Changes in job responsibilities, rotating shifts, or long hours contribute to a sleep disturbance. The nurse can question the patient about social activities, recent travel, or mealtime schedules to help clarify the sleep assessment.

Bedtime Routines. Patients should be asked what they do to prepare for sleep. For example, the patient may drink a glass of milk, take a sleeping pill, eat a snack, or watch television. The nurse should note the habits that are beneficial compared with those that disturb sleep. For example, watching television may promote sleep for one person, whereas watching TV may stimulate another person to stay awake. Sometimes pointing out that a particular habit is interfering with sleep helps patients to find ways to change or eliminate that habit.

Special attention must be paid to a child's bedtime rituals. Parents need to report whether it is necessary, for example, to read the child a bedtime story, rock the child to sleep, or engage in quiet play. Some young children need a special blanket or stuffed animal when going to sleep.

Bedroom Environment. During the assessment, the nurse should ask the patient to describe their preferred bedroom conditions. These preferences may be the lighting in the room, music or television in the background, or the need to have the bedroom door open or closed. Some children require the company of a parent to fall asleep. In a health care environment, environmental distractions often interfere with sleep, such as a roommate's television, an electronic monitor in the hallway, a noisy nurses' station, or another patient who cries out at night. It is important to identify strategies that the nurse or the patient can use to reduce the effects of the distractions or to control the environment (Newsom, 2022).

Behaviours of Sleep Deprivation. Some patients are unaware of how their sleep problems affect their behaviour. The patient should be observed for behaviours such as irritability, forgetfulness, confusion, lethargy, frequent yawning, and slurred speech. If sleep deprivation has lasted a long time, psychotic behaviour, such as delusions and paranoia, sometimes develop. For example, a patient may report seeing strange objects or colours in the room, or the patient may act afraid when a nurse enters the room.

Patient Expectations.

When a patient experiences a poor night's sleep, a vicious cycle of anticipatory anxiety may begin. The patient may fear that sleep will again be disturbed and will try harder and harder to sleep. When assessing a patient's sleep needs, the nurse needs to use a skilled, individualized, and caring approach, always asking the patient what they expect regarding their sleep, the interventions they currently use, and the success of these interventions. Patients should also be asked about what other interventions they may prefer, and how they could be implemented. It is important to understand the patient's expectations regarding their sleep pattern. When a patient asks for assistance because of sleep disturbance, the patient typically expects a nurse to respond promptly to assist them in improving their quantity and quality of sleep.

◆ Nursing Diagnosis

Nurses need to review their assessment in order to identify clusters of data that characterize a sleep pattern disturbance. When a sleep pattern disturbance is identified, it is important to be specific, as numerous factors may be the cause of these disturbances. By specifying the nature of a sleep disturbance and related factors, the nurse is able to develop with the patient the interventions particular to the patient's situation. For example, interventions developed for sleep apnea will differ from those developed to address sleep pattern disturbances related to psychological distress (e.g., anxiety, stress). Box 42.11 demonstrates how to use nursing assessment activities to identify and cluster defining characteristics to make an accurate nursing diagnosis related to sleep pattern disturbances.

Many factors can contribute to disturbed sleep patterns. It is important that the assessment identifies the probable cause of factors related to the sleep disturbance, such as a noisy environment, a situational crisis, or a high intake of caffeinated beverages in the evening. These causes become the focus of interventions for minimizing or eliminating the disturbance. For example, if a patient is experiencing insomnia as the result of a noisy health care environment, the nurse can use strategies to promote sleep, such as controlling the noise of hospital equipment, reducing interruptions, or keeping doors closed. If the insomnia is related to worry over a threatened marital separation, the nurse can introduce coping strategies and collaborate with other health care providers in offering support groups or other services available to support the patient (Carpenito, 2016). If the nurse incorrectly identifies the probable cause or related factors, the patient will not benefit from the strategies to minimize or eliminate the presumed sources of disruption.

Sleep problems affect patients in other ways. For example, the nurse may find that a patient with sleep apnea has conflicts with a spouse who is tired of and frustrated over the patient's snoring. In addition, the spouse may be concerned that the patient is breathing improperly and thus is in danger. The nursing diagnosis of *compromised family coping* indicates that the nurse needs to provide support to both the patient and the patient's spouse so that they both understand sleep apnea and obtain the medical treatment needed.

BOX 42.11   NURSING DIAGNOSTIC PROCESS

Insomnia

Assessment Activities	Defining Characteristics
Ask the patient to describe his their sleep pattern (past and present), the nature of the sleep problem, duration, etc.	The patient reports either a history or no history of sleep problems.
	The patient reports difficulty falling asleep, staying asleep, and awakening several times during the night.
	Once awakened, the patient reports difficulty returning to sleep.
	The patient reports the need to nap during the day because of daytime sleepiness.
	With the use of a visual analogue scale, the patient reports feeling fatigued following a night's sleep.
	The patient reports no regular bedtime routine and frequently remains in bed in the morning to "catch up" on the sleep lost the previous night.
Related Factors	
Pathophysiological	The patient reports frequent awakenings during the night, for example, due to problems breathing.
Treatment	The patient reports daytime sleepiness due to medication.
Situational (personal, lifestyle)	The patient reports difficulty falling asleep and staying asleep because of a personal crisis—for example, the loss of a patient's job; the patient reports problems sleeping related to a recent diagnosis of cancer.
Observe the patient's appearance.	The patient appears pale and has dark circles under their eyes.
Observe the patient's behaviour, and ask the patient's partner whether the patient is experiencing behavioural changes.	The patient is irritable and yawns frequently. The patient reports not feeling well-rested and having poor concentration.
	The partner describes times when the patient was lethargic and distracted.
	The patient and the patient's partner report napping during the day.
Determine whether the patient has experienced recent lifestyle changes.	The partner reports that the patient recently lost their job and is concerned about finding a new position.
	The patient reports being under tremendous stress because of a family member's illness.

The following are examples...

The following are examples of nursing diagnoses for patients with sleep problems:

- *Anxiety*
- *Ineffective breathing pattern*
- *Acute confusion*
- *Compromised family coping*
- *Ineffective coping*
- *Ineffective health maintenance*
- *Fatigue*
- *Ineffective protection*
- *Insomnia*
- *Disturbed sensory perception*
- *Sleep deprivation*

◆ Planning

Goals and Outcomes. During the planning of a strategy of care, nurses again synthesize information from multiple resources to develop an individualized plan of care (Figure 42.4 and Box 42.12). Nurses must consider standards of nursing practice and clinical practice guidelines when developing a plan of care. Clinical practice guidelines are evidence-informed recommendations developed by expert practitioners and arise from a synthesis of the best evidence of a particular topic (see Chapter 8).

As the nurse plans care for the patient with sleep problems, the nurse can create a concept map to help develop a holistic approach to patient-centred care (Figure 42.5). The concept map is created after identifying the relevant nursing diagnoses from the assessment database. In this example, the nursing diagnoses are linked to the patient's anxiety related to her mother's recent cancer diagnosis.

The concept map shows the relationships between the nursing diagnoses *anxiety, disturbed sleep pattern,* and *impaired social interaction.*

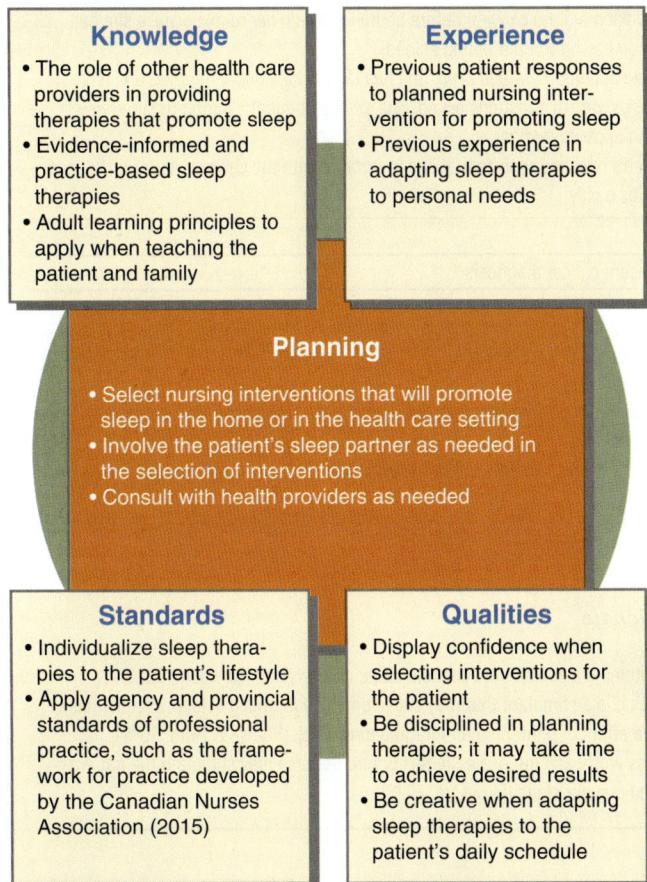

Knowledge
- The role of other health care providers in providing therapies that promote sleep
- Evidence-informed and practice-based sleep therapies
- Adult learning principles to apply when teaching the patient and family

Experience
- Previous patient responses to planned nursing intervention for promoting sleep
- Previous experience in adapting sleep therapies to personal needs

Planning
- Select nursing interventions that will promote sleep in the home or in the health care setting
- Involve the patient's sleep partner as needed in the selection of interventions
- Consult with health providers as needed

Standards
- Individualize sleep therapies to the patient's lifestyle
- Apply agency and provincial standards of professional practice, such as the framework for practice developed by the Canadian Nurses Association (2015)

Qualities
- Display confidence when selecting interventions for the patient
- Be disciplined in planning therapies; it may take time to achieve desired results
- Be creative when adapting sleep therapies to the patient's daily schedule

FIGURE 42.4 Critical thinking model for sleep planning.

This approach to planning care can assist the nurse in recognizing relationships between planned interventions. For this patient, interventions and successful outcomes for one nursing diagnosis affect the resolution of another nursing diagnosis.

When developing goals and outcomes, the nurse and the patient need to collaborate. As a result, the nurse will be more likely to set realistic goals and measurable outcomes. An effective plan includes outcomes that focus on the goal of improving the quantity and quality of sleep in the home over a realistic time period. Family members are often very helpful in contributing to the plan. A sleep promotion plan frequently requires many weeks to accomplish. The following is an example of a goal with patient outcomes:

Goal: The patient will control the environmental sources that disrupt sleep within 1 month.

Outcomes:

- The patient will identify factors in the immediate home environment that disrupt sleep within 2 weeks.
- The patient will report having a discussion with family members about environmental barriers to sleep within 2 weeks.
- The patient will report changes made in the bedroom to promote sleep within 4 weeks.
- The patient will report having fewer than two awakenings per night within 4 weeks.

Setting Priorities. The nurse needs to collaborate with the patient to establish the priority outcomes and interventions. It is important to remember that sleep problems are frequently the result of other health problems; management of these problems and their associated symptoms is the nurse's first priority. Once the symptoms are properly managed, the nurse can then focus on sleep therapies.

Collaborative Care. In collaboration with the patient and the patient's significant others, the nurse should ensure that any planned interventions, such as a change in sleep schedule or changes to the bedroom environment, are realistic and achievable. In a health care setting, the treatments or routines should be planned so that the patient is able to rest. For example, in the CCU, available electronic monitors can be used to track trends in vital signs without awakening the patient each hour. Other staff members should be informed of the plan of care so they can cluster activities at certain times to reduce the number of awakenings. In a long-term care facility, the plan of care involves better planning of rest periods around the activities of the other residents. Often, patients' roommates have very different schedules, and this must be considered.

The nature of the sleep disturbance determines whether referrals are necessary to additional health care providers. For example, if a sleep problem is related to a situational crisis or an emotional difficulty, the nurse may refer the patient to a psychiatric clinical nurse specialist or a clinical psychologist for counselling. When a patient has chronic insomnia, a referral to a sleep centre is beneficial. If the patient needs a referral for continued care in the community, the nurse should offer information about the sleep problem to the home care nurse. The success of sleep therapy depends on an approach that fits both the patient's lifestyle and the nature of the sleep disorder.

◆ Implementation

Nursing interventions that are designed to improve the quality of a person's rest and sleep focus largely on health promotion. Patients need adequate sleep and rest to maintain active and productive lives. During times of illness, rest and sleep promotion are important for recovery. Nursing care provided in acute care, restorative care, or continuing care settings differs from nursing care in the home setting. The primary differences are in the environment and the nurse's ability to support normal rest and sleep habits. The patient's age also influences the types

◎ BOX 42.12　NURSING CARE PLAN

Disturbed Sleep Pattern

ASSESSMENT

Andree (preferred pronouns: she/her) Smith is a 36-year-old lawyer who presents to the health care centre where you are working. Andree, accompanied by her husband, has come to the clinic because she is having problems sleeping. Andree and her husband have three children: two in school and one in preschool.

As you begin your assessment, Andree suddenly bursts into tears and tells you her mother has been recently diagnosed with breast cancer. Andree's assessment includes a thorough sleep history and a discussion on how this sleep problem is affecting her life. A physical examination is also conducted.

Assessment Activities

Sleep pattern (present and past)

*Findings and Defining Characteristics**

Andree reports difficulty falling asleep at night and awakening several times during the night. Andree states, *"I am so tired; I have no energy to do anything. I am irritable all of the time and I am having trouble concentrating at work."* Andree also reports that she has less patience with her children.

Relational Factors
Pathophysiological

Assess whether Andree has a history, a family history, or both of sleep problems.

Assess whether Andree has a history of medical or psychological disorders.

Andree reports no personal or family history of sleep problems.
Andree reports she has no history of any medical or psychiatric disorders.

Treatment

Assess Andree's use of medications (both over-the-counter and prescription), including names, dosage, and frequency.

Andree reports she recently started taking melatonin at bedtime to help her sleep. Aside from melatonin, Andree is on no other medication.

Situational (personal, home, community)

Ask Andree whether she has had any recent changes in her life.

Andree reports being highly anxious and states, *"Everything bothers me."* She also reports that she has *stopped* her routine of walking 2–4 km daily because she has no energy.

Situational (personal, lifestyle)

Ask Andree to describe her bedtime routine.

Andree reports she is going to bed between midnight and 1 A.M., which is 2 hours later than her usual bedtime. *It takes her an hour to fall asleep.* In the past, she received 7–8 hours of sleep each night, but now *it is closer to 5–6 hours.* She drinks two to three cups of coffee after dinner while surfing the Internet for information on her mother's condition. Andree also reports drinking a glass of wine before bedtime to help her relax because she has been having trouble falling asleep.

Observe Andree's appearance.
Assess Andree for signs of sleep problems.
Observe Andree's behaviour.
With Andree's permission, ask her husband whether Andree has exhibited any behavioural changes.

Andree appears *pale and tired.* She has *dark circles under her eyes* and is *slow to respond* to questions asked. She *yawns* frequently during the interview and appears restless.
Andree's husband reports that she is *irritable* with the children, is *forgetful,* and cries easily.

*Defining characteristics are in italic type.

NURSING DIAGNOSIS: Insomnia related to psychological stress from mother's recent cancer diagnosis.

PLANNING

Goals (Nursing Outcomes Classification)†
Sleep

Andree will achieve an improved sense of restorative sleep within 2 weeks.
Andree will report adherence to a regular bedtime routine within 1 week.
Andree will achieve a more normal sleep pattern within 2 weeks.
Within 2 weeks, Andree will report sleeping 7 hours nightly.

Expected Outcomes

Andree will report waking less during the night and feeling rested within 2 weeks.
Within 2 weeks, Andree will fall asleep within 30 minutes of going to bed.

†Outcomes from Ackley, B. J, Ladwig, G. B., Makid, M. B., et al. (2020) *Nursing diagnosis handbook* (12th edition). Elsevier.

INTERVENTIONS

Interventions (Nursing Interventions Classification)‡
Sleep Enhancement

Encourage Andree to establish a bedtime routine and a regular sleep pattern.
Instruct Andree to limit her consumption of caffeine and alcohol before bedtime.
Assist Andree in identifying ways to eliminate stressful concerns about work before bedtime (e.g., taking time before actual sleep time to read a light novel).

Rationale

Maintaining a consistent schedule helps induce sleep (Newsom, 2022).
Caffeine is a stimulant that may cause difficulty in falling asleep. Alcohol has the effect of lightening and fragmenting sleep (Roehrs & Roth, 2017).
Excess worry and intense activities before bedtime may stimulate the patient and prevent sleep (Newsom, 2022).

⊚ BOX 42.12 NURSING CARE PLAN

Disturbed Sleep Pattern—cont'd

Interventions (Nursing Interventions Classification)‡	Rationale
Adjust the sleep environment: have Andree control the noise, temperature, and light in the bedroom.	Develop an environment conducive to sleep (Morin et al., 2017; Newsom, 2022).
Exercise Promotion Encourage Andree to begin walking routinely during the day, but not 2 to 3 hours before bedtime.	Regular exercise increases activity levels and improves sleep quality. When exercise occurs just before bedtime, it can act as a stimulant that prevents sleep (Newsom, 2022).
Simple Relaxation Therapy Instruct Andree on how to perform muscle relaxation before bedtime.	Relaxation therapy can help to reduce anxiety, which interferes with sleep.

‡Intervention classification labels from Butcher, H. K., Bulechek, G. M., McCloskey Dochterman, J. M., et al. (2019). *Nursing interventions classification (NIC)* (7th ed.). Elsevier.

EVALUATION

Nursing Actions	Patient Response and Finding	Achievement of Outcome
Ask Andree whether she is able to fall asleep and stay asleep.	Andree responds, "It usually takes me 15 to 20 minutes to fall asleep, and I woke up once at night twice last week."	Andree reports she falls asleep within 30 minutes and wakes up less frequently during the night.
Ask Andree to describe her waking behaviours at work and home during the day.	Andree responds that she is able to concentrate on her work more. She reports she is less irritable with her children. She has restarted her walking routine.	Andree reports feeling more rested.
Observe Andree's waking nonverbal expressions and behaviour.	Andree sits in the chair without shifting position. She actively engages in conversation with you. She does not yawn during the interview. She is not as pale as she was previously and the circles under her eyes are almost gone.	Andree says she sleeps for an average of 7 hours a night.

of therapies that are most effective. Box 42.13 provides principles for promoting sleep in older patients.

Health Promotion. Nurses can help patients in community health and home settings to develop behaviours conducive to rest and relaxation. To develop good sleep habits at home, patients and their bed partners need to learn the techniques that promote sleep and the conditions that interfere with sleep (Box 42.14). Parents should also learn how to promote good sleep habits for their children. Patients benefit most from instructions that are formed on the basis of information about their homes and lifestyles, such as the types of activities that promote sleep for a shift worker or ways to make the home environment more conducive to sleep. Patients will then be more likely to apply information that is useful and relevant to their needs.

Environmental Controls. All patients require a sleeping environment with a comfortable room temperature, proper ventilation, minimal noise, a comfortable bed, and proper lighting (Newsom, 2022). Children and adults vary in their preferences for a comfortable room temperature. Parents should be instructed to position cribs away from open windows or drafts and to cover the infant with a light, warm blanket. Older persons often require extra blankets or covers.

Distracting noise should be eliminated so that the bedroom is as quiet as possible. In the home, the television, telephone, or the intermittent chiming of a clock can disrupt a patient's sleep. The family becomes an important part of the approach to reduce noise in the home, especially if the home is shared with several family members, all with different bedtime schedules. However, some patients are accustomed to sleeping with familiar inside noises, such as the hum of a fan. Commercial products that play soothing sounds, such as recordings of ocean waves or rainfall, can help to create a soothing environment for sleep.

The bed and mattress need to provide support and comfortable firmness. Bed boards can be placed under mattresses to provide additional support. Sometimes extra pillows can help to position a person comfortably in bed. For some patients, the position of the bed in the room also makes a difference.

Patients vary in their preference for the amount of light they can tolerate in the bedroom. Infants and older persons sleep best in softly lit rooms. Light should not shine directly on their eyes. Small table lamps can be used to prevent total darkness. For older persons, proper lighting reduces the chance of confusion and prevents falls while walking to the bathroom. Heavy shades, drapes, or slatted blinds are helpful if streetlights shine through windows, or if patients nap during the day.

Promoting Bedtime Routines. Bedtime routines help to relax patients in preparation for sleep (Centers for Disease Control and Prevention, 2016). Individuals should go to bed when they feel fatigued or sleepy. Going to bed while fully awake and thinking about other things often leads to insomnia and interferes with the perception of the bed as a stimulus for sleep. Newborns and infants sleep through so much of the day that a specific routine is hardly necessary. However, quiet activities, such as holding them snugly in blankets, singing or talking softly, and gentle rocking, help infants to fall asleep.

Parents need to reinforce short, predictable routines associated with preparing for bedtime. A bedtime routine that is used consistently (e.g., the same hour for bedtime, eating a snack, or pursuing a quiet activity) helps young children to avoid delaying sleep. Bedtime routines can include quiet activities such as reading stories, colouring, allowing children to sit in a parent's lap while listening to music, or listening to a prayer.

Adults need to avoid excessive mental stimulation just before bedtime. Reading a light novel, watching an enjoyable television program, or listening to music can help a person to relax. Relaxation exercises,

▶ concept map

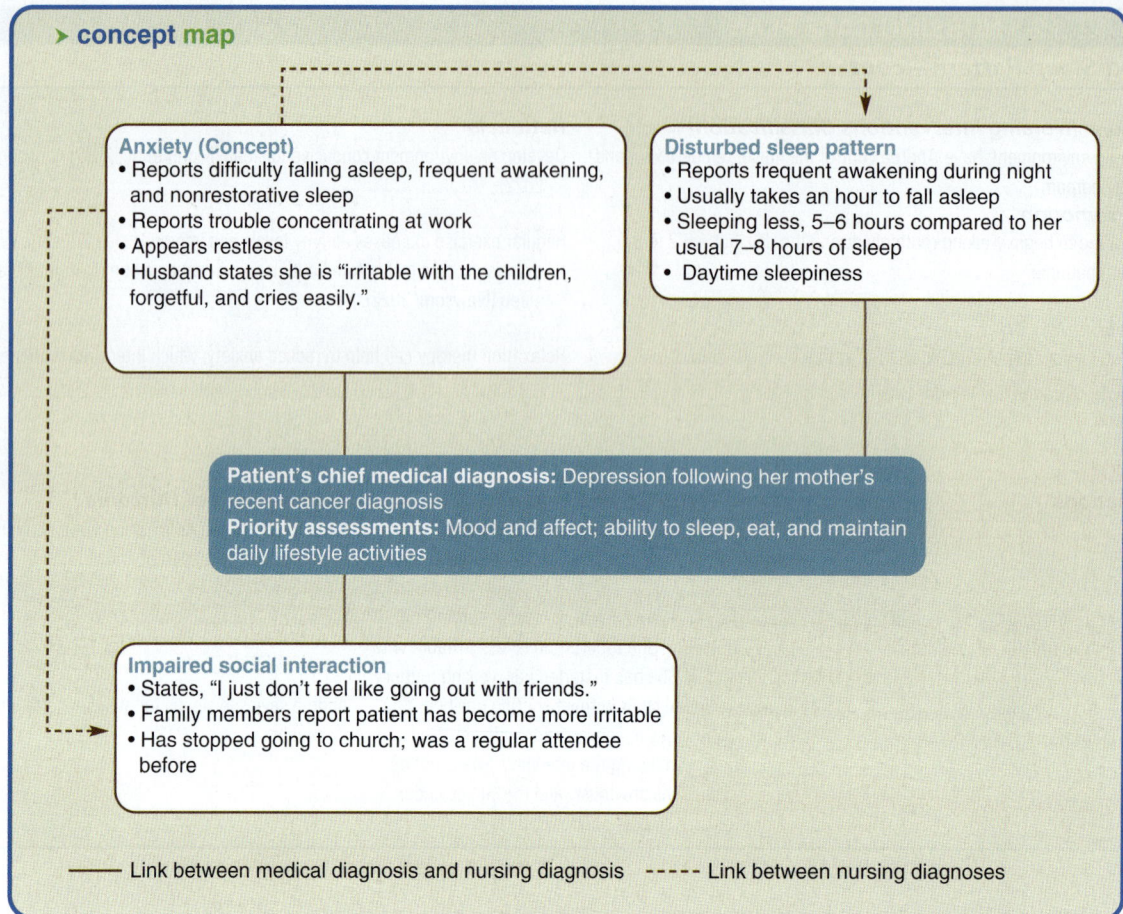

FIGURE 42.5 Concept map for a patient who has depression following the news of her mother's recent cancer diagnosis.

BOX 42.13 FOCUS ON OLDER PERSONS

Promoting Sleep

Sleep–Wake Pattern

- Maintain a regular bedtime and wake-up schedule, even on weekends or vacations (Newsom, 2022).
- Eliminate naps unless they are a routine part of the schedule.
- If naps are used, limit them to 20 minutes or less, twice a day, and avoid napping in the late afternoon or early evening.
- Go to bed when sleepy.
- Use a warm bath and relaxation techniques (reading, music, meditation, guided visual imagery) to promote sleep (Kavurmaci et al., 2020; Newsom, 2022).
- If unable to sleep within 15 to 30 minutes, get out of bed.
- Avoid work-related activities before bedtime.

Environment

- Sleep where you sleep best.
- Keep noise to a minimum; use soft music to mask noise if necessary.
- Use a night light and keep the path to the bathroom free of obstacles.
- Set the room temperature to your preference; use socks to promote warmth.
- For "clock watchers" remove the clock from the bedroom.
- Listen to relaxing music (Kavurmaci et al., 2020; Newsom 2022).

Medications

- Use sedatives and hypnotics as a last resort, and then only for the short term if absolutely necessary (Kilduff & Mendelson, 2017).
- Adjust medications being taken for other conditions, and assess for medication interactions that may cause insomnia or excessive daytime sleepiness (EDS).

Diet

- Limit intake of alcohol, caffeine, and nicotine in the late afternoon and evening (Haapasalo et al., 2018).
- Consume carbohydrates or milk as a light snack before bedtime.
- Decrease the intake of fluids 2 to 4 hours before sleep.

Physiological and Illness Factors

- Elevate the head of the bed and provide extra pillows as preferred.
- Use analgesics 30 minutes before bed to ease aches and pains.
- Use therapeutics to control symptoms of chronic conditions as prescribed (Doufas, 2017).

BOX 42.14 Sleep Hygiene Habits

Objective
- Patient will follow proper sleep hygiene habits at home.

Teaching Strategies
- Instruct the patient to try to exercise daily, preferably in the morning or afternoon, and to avoid vigorous exercise within 2 hours of bedtime.
- Caution the patient against sleeping long hours during weekends or holidays, to prevent disturbance of the normal sleep–wake cycle.
- Explain that the patient should not use the bedroom for intensive studying, snacking, TV watching, or other non-sleep activity, besides sex.
- Encourage the patient to try to avoid worrisome thinking when going to bed and to practise relaxation exercises.
- If the patient does not fall asleep within 30 minutes of going to bed, advise the patient to get out of bed and do some quiet activity until the patient feels sleepy enough to go back to bed.
- Advise the patient to limit consumption of caffeine and alcohol.
- Ask the patient to examine the sleeping environment. If noise or light is an issue, suggest the use of earplugs or eyeshades.
- Instruct the patient to avoid eating heavy meals 3 hours before bedtime; the patient may have a light snack before bedtime.

Evaluation
- Ask the patient to complete a sleep–wake and activity diary for 1 week, and compare it with the previous week's diary.
- Ask the patient to periodically complete a visual analogue or sleep rating scale to record perceptions of quality of sleep.

such as slow, deep breathing for 1 or 2 minutes, can help to relieve tension and prepare the body for rest (see Chapter 37). Guided imagery and praying also promote sleep for some patients.

At home, patients should be discouraged from trying to finish office work or to resolve family problems before bedtime. The bedroom is not a place to work, and patients need to always associate the bedroom with sleep. Working toward a consistent time for sleeping and wakening helps most patients to gain a healthy sleep pattern and to strengthen the rhythm of their sleep–wake cycle.

Promoting Safety. For any patient prone to confusion or falls, safety is critical. A small night light can assist the patient in orienting to the room environment before going to the bathroom. Beds set lower to the floor reduce the chance of a person falling when first standing. Patients should be instructed to remove clutter and small rugs from the path used to walk from the bed to the bathroom. If a patient needs assistance in ambulating from a bed to the bathroom, a small bell can be placed at the bedside to call family members. Sleepwalkers are unaware of their surroundings and are slow to react, which increases their risk of falls. Sleepwalkers should not be startled but instead gently awakened and led back to bed.

Infants' beds need to be safe. To reduce the chance of suffocation, pillows, stuffed toys, or the ends of loose blankets should not be placed in cribs. Loose-fitting plastic mattress covers are dangerous because infants can pull them over their face and suffocate. Parents should place infants on their back to prevent sudden infant death syndrome (SIDS) (Newsom, 2022).

Promoting Comfort. People fall asleep only after feeling comfortable and relaxed (Carpenito, 2016). Minor irritants often keep patients awake. Soft cotton nightclothes keep infants or small children warm and comfortable. Patients should be advised to wear loose-fitting nightwear. An extra blanket is sometimes all that is necessary to prevent a person from feeling chilled and thus being unable to fall asleep.

Patients need to void before retiring so they are not kept awake by a full bladder.

Establishing Periods of Rest and Sleep. Patients living at home should be encouraged to stay physically active during the day so that they will be more likely to sleep at night. Increasing daytime activity reduces the likelihood of having problems with falling asleep. In the home setting, nurses frequently care for patients with chronic debilitating disease. The nursing care plan includes having patients set aside afternoons for rest to promote optimal health. To provide uninterrupted rest periods, nurses should adjust patients' medication schedules, instruct patients to void before rest periods, and suggest turning off cell phones, electronic tablets, and other electronic devices.

Stress Reduction. The inability to sleep because of emotional stress can make a person feel irritable and tense. When patients feel emotionally upset, they should try not to force sleep. Otherwise, insomnia can develop, and bedtime is soon associated with the inability to relax. A patient who has difficulty falling asleep should be encouraged to get up and pursue a relaxing activity, such as reading, rather than staying in bed and thinking about sleep.

Preschoolers often have bedtime fears (e.g., fear of the dark or fear of strange noises) and frequently awaken during the night or have nightmares. When a child experiences a nightmare, the parent should enter the child's room immediately and talk to the child briefly about fears to provide a cooling-down period. One approach is to comfort the child and leave them in their own beds so that their fears are not used as an excuse to delay bedtime. Keeping a light turned on in the room will also help some children. The nurse should also bear in mind that cultural traditions can cause some families to approach sleep practices differently (Box 42.15).

Bedtime Snacks. Some individuals enjoy bedtime snacks, whereas others cannot sleep after eating. A dairy product snack, such as warm milk or cocoa, contains L-tryptophan and is often helpful in promoting sleep. A full meal before bedtime often causes gastrointestinal upset and can interfere with the ability to fall asleep.

Patients should be encouraged to avoid drinking or ingesting caffeine before bedtime. Because coffee, tea, cola, and chocolate act as stimulants, they can cause a person to stay awake or to awaken throughout the night (Newsom, 2022). Infants require special measures to minimize their nighttime awakenings for feeding. Children commonly need a middle-of-the-night bottle or to breastfeed at night. Hockenberry and Wilson (2019) recommend offering the last feeding as late as possible. Parents should be instructed not to give infants bottles in bed.

Pharmacological Approaches. Melatonin is a major hormone of the circadian system and plays an important role in promoting sleep (Buysse, 2014). Melatonin is a popular nutritional supplement to aid sleep. The recommended dosage is 0.3 to 1 mg taken 2 hours before bedtime (Newsom, 2022). Older persons who have decreased levels of melatonin find taking melatonin to be beneficial as a sleep aid (Lee-Chiong, 2008). The use of herbal supplements for the treatment of insomnia is not recommended because of the potential of drug-to-drug interactions. Patients should avoid using these treatments together (Krystal, 2017; Shochat & Ancoli-Israel, 2017) (see Chapter 36).

The use of nonprescription sleeping medications is not advisable. Patients need to learn the risks of taking such medications. Although these medications initially seem to be effective, over the long term, they can lead to further sleep disruption. Nurses can help patients to use behavioural and proper sleep hygiene habits to establish sleep patterns that do not require the use of medications.

Acute Care. Patients in an acute care setting frequently have their normal rest and sleep routines disrupted, which makes them more susceptible to periods of sleep deprivation. Sleep has a restorative function;

⊕ BOX 42.15 CULTURAL ASPECTS OF CARE

Co-Sleeping

Practices and patterns of sleep and rest vary among cultures. Culture and biology influence the development of sleep problems in children. Sleep patterns, bedtime routines, sleep aids, and sleep arrangements are a component of the cultural practices related to the use of space and the perception of comfortable distances for interactions with others. Sleep experts traditionally recommend having infants and children sleep in their own beds. Co-sleeping (i.e., the practice of infants and children sleeping with their parents) is a culturally preferred habit and is common in non-industrialized countries. Health care providers in Canada frequently discourage this practice because of safety issues. The dominant Canadian culture promotes independence in childhood. Because co-sleeping does not promote this independence, health care workers tend to discourage it. As a nurse, you need to be culturally sensitive when discussing co-sleeping practices with parents and developing sleeping plans for children.

Implications for Practice

- Complete a thorough sleep assessment of the child and the family.
- Discuss the risks of the child sleeping with the parents. During the discussion, remain culturally sensitive to and respectful of the parents' views.

- Co-sleeping affects the infant's normal sleep pattern by decreasing slow-wave sleep and increasing the number of nighttime arousals.
- Co-sleeping has been linked to an increased risk of sudden infant death syndrome (SIDS) under certain conditions, such as parental smoking and alcohol or drug use.
- Instruct parents who practise co-sleeping to avoid using alcohol or drugs that impair arousal. Decreased arousal prevents the parents from awakening if the child experiences problems.
- Co-sleeping should occur only with parents and not with another adult or child.
- Encourage the parents who co-sleep to use light sleeping clothes, to keep the room temperature comfortable, and to not bundle the child tightly or in too many clothes.

---

hence, in this setting, nursing interventions should focus on controlling factors in the environment that disrupt sleep, relieving physiological or psychological barriers to sleep, and providing uninterrupted rest and sleep periods for the patient. The nurse may accomplish this by organizing procedures to minimize the number of times the patient's sleep must be disrupted and by avoiding any unnecessary procedures during rest periods.

Environmental Controls. In a hospital setting, nurses can promote rest and sleep periods by reducing or eliminating environmental disturbances. When possible, the doors to patients' rooms should be closed. In semiprivate rooms, the curtains should be closed between patients. At night, the lights on a nursing unit should be dimmed. Noise levels can be reduced by conducting conversations and reports away from patient rooms and by keeping necessary conversations to a minimum, especially at night; reducing the volume of alarms, televisions, and other equipment; turning off bedside oxygen and other equipment not in use; and, when possible, avoiding noisy procedures until daytime hours (Carpenito, 2016). Patients' use of cell phones and laptop computers should be discouraged during rest periods, and their minimal use during the hospitalization period should be encouraged. Moreover, the nurse should limit visitors during rest periods.

Promoting Comfort. Compared with beds at home, hospital beds are often harder and of a different height, length, or width. Keeping beds clean and dry and in a comfortable position helps patients to relax. Pillows can be used for support (for painful limbs, splinting of surgical incisions). Some patients who have painful illnesses require special comfort measures, such as the application of dry or moist heat, use of supportive dressings or splints, or proper positioning before retiring (Figure 42.6).

Establishing Periods of Rest and Sleep. In a hospital or long-term care setting, it is sometimes difficult to provide patients with the time needed to rest and sleep. However, as stated earlier, nurses should plan their nursing care to avoid awakening patients for nonessential reasons. When possible, assessments, treatments, procedures, and routines should be scheduled for times when patients are awake. For

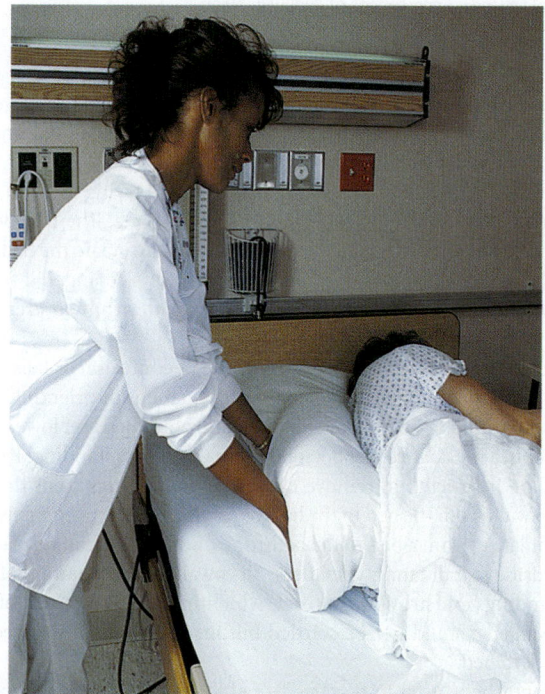

FIGURE 42.6 Positioning a patient for sleep.

example, if a patient's physical condition has been stable, nurses should avoid awakening the patient to check vital signs. Allowing patients to determine the timing and methods of delivery of personal care measures will promote rest. Bed baths and other routine hygiene measures should not be administered during the night simply because that timing may be most convenient for the nursing staff. Blood samples should be drawn at a time when the patient is awake. Unless maintaining a medication's therapeutic blood level is essential, medications should be given during waking hours. Nurses need to work with the radiology department and other support services to schedule diagnostic studies and therapies at intervals that allow patients time for rest. Nurses should always try to provide patients with 2 to 3 hours of uninterrupted sleep during the night (Hope et al., 2018).

When the patient's condition demands more frequent monitoring, activities should be scheduled to allow the patient to have extended rest periods. The nurse should plan activities in such a way both that health care personnel will avoid returning to the room every few minutes and that the patient will have up to an hour or more to rest quietly. For example, if a patient needs frequent dressing changes, is receiving intravenous therapy, and has drainage tubes from several sites, the nurse should not make a separate trip into the room to attend to each task. Instead, the nurse can use a single visit to change the dressing, regulate the intravenous system, and empty the drainage tubes. Nurses need to become patients' advocates for promoting optimal sleep, by postponing or rescheduling visits by family, asking consultants to reschedule visits, and questioning the frequency of certain procedures.

Promoting Safety. Patients with OSA are at risk for complications while in the hospital. Surgery and anaesthesia disrupt patients' normal sleep patterns. Postoperatively, these patients reach deep levels of REM sleep. This deep sleep causes muscle relaxation that can lead to OSA (Ehsan et al., 2016). Patients with OSA who are given opioid analgesics after surgery have an increased risk of developing airway obstruction because these medications suppress the normal arousal mechanisms. The nurse needs to monitor the patient's airway, respiratory rate, depth, and breath sounds frequently after surgery.

Nurses can recommend lifestyle changes to patients with OSA, including sleep hygiene improvements, alcohol moderation, smoking cessation, and a weight-loss program (Atwood et al., 2011). Such patients should be taught to prevent sleeping in the supine position by wearing a fanny pack or tight shirt with a tennis ball on the back, or by elevating the head of the bed 30 to 45 degrees (Atwood et al., 2011). As noted earlier, one of the most effective therapies is use of a nasal CPAP device at night, which requires a patient to wear a mask over the nose. The mask delivers room air at a high pressure and the air pressure prevents airway collapse. The CPAP device is portable and is effective particularly for OSA (Freedman, 2017).

Another treatment option is the use of an oral appliance. These appliances advance the mandible or tongue to relieve pharyngeal obstruction (Lettieri et al., 2017). In cases of severe sleep apnea, the tonsils, uvula, or portions of the soft palate are surgically removed. Success with surgical procedures is variable.

Stress Reduction. Patients who are hospitalized for extensive diagnostic testing often have difficulty resting or sleeping because of uncertainty about their state of health. Giving patients control over their health care can minimize uncertainty and anxiety. Providing information about the purpose of procedures and routines and answering questions will give patients the peace of mind they need to rest or to fall asleep. During the night shift, nurses can take time to sit and talk with patients who are unable to sleep and may be able to determine the factors preventing patients from sleeping. Back rubs help patients relax more thoroughly. If a sedative is indicated, the nurse should confer with the physician to ensure the lowest dosage is used initially. A sedative should be discontinued as soon as possible, to prevent a dependence that can seriously disrupt the normal sleep cycle. Nurses should be aware that the metabolism of medications in older persons is slower, making them more vulnerable to the adverse effects of sedatives, hypnotics, anti-anxiety drugs, and analgesics.

Restorative or Continuing Care. Nursing interventions implemented in the acute care setting are also used in the restorative or continuing care environment. Important considerations include controlling the environment, especially the noise level; establishing periods of rest and sleep; and promoting comfort. Nursing interventions related to the control of barriers to sleep are also implemented in these settings. Helping a patient achieve restful sleep in this environment sometimes takes a period of time.

Promoting Comfort. Comfort measures promote sleep and improve patients' sense of well-being. Nurses can promote comfort by offering a patient a warm bath or shower before bedtime. Other personal hygiene measures are mouth care and toileting (e.g., offering the bedpan or urinal). Back massages, soft music, and relaxation exercises also promote comfort. Proper positioning of the patient in bed is also very important. Using pillows to support limbs and other dependent body parts maintains skin integrity, thereby maintaining comfort (Milner & Belicki, 2010) (see Chapter 32).

Controlling Physiological Disturbances. Controlling the symptoms of patients with physical illnesses can promote sleep. For example, placing patients with respiratory disorders in an upright bed position and offering additional pillows may assist with their breathing. Teaching patients with chronic respiratory disorders (e.g., chronic obstructive pulmonary disease) pursed-lip breathing will decrease their respiratory rate and promote comfort and sleep. Humidified air, the use of supplemental oxygen, if appropriate, and other pharmacological therapies (i.e., bronchodilators) are also relevant considerations.

Patients with pain, nausea, and other symptoms may require nonpharmacological and pharmacological therapies to promote sleep (Doufas, 2017). Relaxation measures (e.g., music, guided imagery) are appropriate diversional therapies. Providing pain relief with analgesics is also appropriate. To promote patients' comfort and sleep, nurses need to collaborate with physicians and other health care personnel to determine the optimal plan for relief of patients' symptoms (Tang et al., 2021).

Pharmacological Approaches. Numerous pharmacological agents, both prescription and over-the-counter, are used to manage insomnia. Conversely, polypharmacy to manage insomnia is associated with disrupted sleep patterns, including increased nocturnal awakening and decreased REM sleep and total sleep time. Therefore, CNS stimulants, such as amphetamines, caffeine, nicotine, terbutaline, theophylline, and pemoline, need to be used sparingly and only under medical management (Chaudhary et al., 2019; Roehrs & Roth, 2017). In addition, withdrawal from CNS depressants, such as alcohol, barbiturates, tricyclic antidepressants (amitriptyline, imipramine, and doxepin), and triazolam, can cause insomnia. Nurses need to manage these medications carefully.

Medications that induce sleep are called hypnotics. Sedatives are medications that produce a calming or soothing effect (Kilduff & Mendelson, 2017). Hypnotics and sedatives can be used as sleep medications and will help in managing sleep problems, if used correctly. A patient who takes sleep medications needs to understand their proper use, their risks, and their possible adverse effects. Long-term use of anti-anxiety, sedative, or hypnotic agents, however, can disrupt sleep and lead to more serious problems.

One group of drugs considered to be relatively safe is the benzodiazepines. The benzodiazepines cause relaxation, anti-anxiety, and hypnotic effects by facilitating the action of neurons in the CNS that suppress responsiveness to stimulation, thereby decreasing levels of arousal (Kilduff & Mendelson, 2017). Unlike sedatives and hypnotics, benzodiazepines do not cause general CNS depression, and they also have a lower potential for abuse. These drugs are frequently prescribed because anti-anxiety effects occur at safe, nontoxic doses. In the older person, short-acting benzodiazepines, such as temazepam and triazolam, are preferred over long-acting agents (Kilduff & Mendelson, 2017).

Benzodiazepines need to be administered with caution in children younger than 12 years of age. These medications are contraindicated in infants younger than 6 months. Pregnant women need to avoid taking benzodiazepines because their use is associated with the risk of congenital anomalies. Nursing mothers do not receive these medications because they are excreted in breast milk. Initial doses are small, and increments are added gradually, on the basis of patient response, for a limited period of time. Patients should be warned not to take more than the prescribed dose, especially if the medication seems to become less effective after the initial use. If older patients who were continent, ambulatory, and alert suddenly become incontinent, confused, or demonstrate impaired mobility, the use of benzodiazepines needs to be considered as a possible cause. Regular use of any sleep medication often leads to drug tolerance. Rebound insomnia can be experienced after stopping the medication. Immediately administering a sleeping medication when a hospitalized patient complains of being unable to sleep will do the patient more harm than good. Alternative approaches need to be considered for promoting sleep. Routine monitoring of the patient's response to sleeping medications is also important.

Evaluation

The patient is an important source of information for evaluating outcomes related to sleep and rest. Each patient has a unique need for sleep and rest, and only the patient will know whether sleep problems have improved, and which interventions or therapies are most successful in promoting sleep (Figure 42.7). To evaluate the effectiveness of nursing interventions, the nurse makes comparisons with baseline sleep assessment data.

The nurse needs to determine whether expected outcomes have been met, using evaluative measures shortly after a therapy has been tried (e.g., by observing whether a patient falls asleep after noise has been reduced and the room has been darkened) and after a patient awakens from sleep (e.g., by asking a patient to describe the number of awakenings during the previous night). The patient and the patient's bed partner can usually provide accurate evaluative information. Over longer periods, assessment tools such as the visual analogue scale or the sleep rating scale can be used to determine whether sleep has progressively improved.

Nurses also need to evaluate the level of understanding that patients and their family members have gained after receiving instruction in sleep habits. Nurses can measure adherence to these practices during a home visit, when they are able to observe the environment. When expected outcomes are not met, the nursing measures or expected outcomes need to be revised on the basis of the patient's needs or preferences. When outcomes are not met, the nurse can ask questions such as "Do you feel as though you slept better when you exercised?" or "Do you feel rested when you wake up?"

When nurses successfully develop good relationships with patients and when they have developed therapeutic plans of care, subtle behaviours often indicate the patients' levels of satisfaction. The absence of signs of sleep problems, such as lethargy, frequent yawning, or position changes, may be noted. The nurse should ask the patient whether their sleep needs have been met, using such questions as "Are you feeling more rested?" or "Can you tell me if you feel we have done all we can to help improve your sleep?" If the patient's expectations have not been met, the nurse will need to spend more time trying to understand the patient's needs and preferences. Working closely with the patient and the patient's bed partner will enable the nurse to redefine the expectations that can be realistically met within the limits of the patient's condition and treatment.

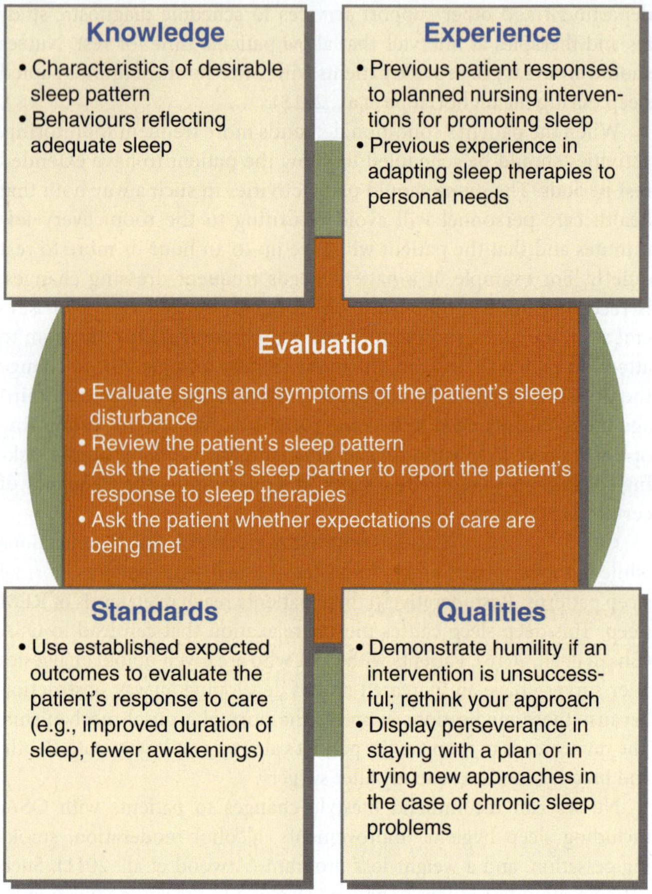

FIGURE 42.7 Critical thinking model for sleep evaluation.

KEY CONCEPTS

- Sleep provides physiological and psychological restoration.
- The 24-hour sleep–wake cycle is a circadian rhythm that influences physiological function and behaviour.
- The control and regulation of sleep depends on a balance between regulators within the central nervous system.
- During a typical night's sleep, a person passes through four to five complete sleep cycles. Each sleep cycle contains four nonrapid eye movement (NREM) stages of sleep and a period of rapid eye movement (REM) sleep.
- The most common type of sleep disorder is insomnia.
- The sleep pattern is frequently disrupted by the hectic pace of a person's lifestyle, emotional and psychological stress, and alcohol ingestion.
- If a patient's sleep is adequate, the nurse should assess the patient's usual bedtime, normal bedtime ritual, preferred environment for sleeping, and usual rising time.
- When a patient reports a sleep problem, the nurse needs to conduct a complete sleep history. Diagnosing sleep problems depends on identifying the factors that impair sleep.
- When planning interventions to promote sleep, the nurse needs to consider the characteristics of the patient's home environment and normal lifestyle.
- A regular bedtime routine of relaxing activities prepares a person physically and mentally for sleep.
- An environment with a darkened room, reduced noise, comfortable bed, and good ventilation promotes sleep.

- Important nursing interventions for promoting sleep in the hospitalized patient are controlling noise levels and establishing periods for uninterrupted sleep and rest.
- Control of pain or other disease symptoms is essential in promoting the ability to sleep.
- Long-term use of sleeping pills often leads to difficulty in initiating and maintaining sleep.

CRITICAL THINKING EXERCISES

1. Andree returns to the health care clinic with her husband, David, for a follow-up visit. She tells you that since she started her sleep hygiene plan she feels more rested but is still having some problems sleeping because of her husband's loud snoring. In addition to Andree's report of David's snoring, you note that he is overweight. On the basis of Andree's report of David's snoring, what additional assessment data should you gather from David?
2. On the basis of David's reported symptoms, what sleep condition do you suspect he might have?
3. What action would you take at this time?
4. Andree and David also tell you that they are concerned about their 15-year-old daughter. Her grades in school are getting worse, and she says she is always tired. What do you need to know about their daughter's sleep patterns?
5. What would you recommend to Andree and David about their daughter?

Answers to Critical Thinking Exercises appear on the Evolve website.

REVIEW QUESTIONS

Review Questions 1 to 7 relate to the case study at the beginning of the chapter.

1. The nurse is gathering a sleep history from Ben, who is being evaluated for narcolepsy. What symptom is the patient most likely to report?
   a. Sore throat
   b. Shortness of breath
   c. A good night's sleep
   d. Excessive daytime sleepiness
2. When preparing a plan of care to promote sleep for Ben, who has been diagnosed as having narcolepsy, which of the following priority nursing interventions would the nurse incorporate?
   a. Ensure that the patient follows hospital routines.
   b. Avoid awakening the patient for nonessential tasks.
   c. Give prescribed sleeping medications at dinner.
   d. Turn the TV volume down for late-night programming.
3. The nurse cautions Ben about the long-term use of sedatives and hypnotics because these medications are characterized by which of the following?
   a. They cause headaches and nausea.
   b. They are expensive and difficult to obtain.
   c. They cause severe depression and anxiety.
   d. They can lead to sleep disruption.
4. The nurse is providing health teaching for Ben regarding the use of herbal compounds, such as valerian, to aid sleep. Key information about the use of herbal compounds would include the following:
   a. It can cause urinary retention.
   b. It may cause diarrhea and anxiety.

   c. It may interfere with prescribed medications.
   d. It can lead to further sleep problems over time.
5. Ben also reports having vivid dreams. Based on the nurse's understanding of the sleep cycle, vivid dreaming occurs during which sleep phase?
   a. REM sleep
   b. Stage 1 NREM sleep
   c. Stage 4 NREM sleep
   d. Transition period from NREM to REM sleep
6. The nurse is developing a plan of care for a Ben, who is experiencing narcolepsy. Which of the following interventions is appropriate to include in the plan?
   a. Increase the amount of carbohydrates in the diet.
   b. Limit fluid intake 2 hours before bedtime.
   c. Preserve energy by limiting exercise to morning hours.
   d. Take one or two 20-minute naps during the day.
7. Which of the following nursing measures promotes sleep in school-aged children, like Ben?
   a. Encourage evening exercise.
   b. Encourage television viewing.
   c. Ensure that the room is dark and quiet.
   d. Encourage quiet activities before bedtime.
8. The nurse is providing instruction for a patient who is having difficulty falling asleep. The nurse identifies the need for further instruction when the patient says which of the following statements?
   a. I should avoid having drinks with caffeine before going to bed.
   b. If I can't get to sleep right away, I should get up and read a book.
   c. I should have an alcoholic drink before bedtime to help me relax.
   d. I should avoid exercising just before going to bed.
9. Which of the following interventions is appropriate to include in a care plan for improving sleep in the older person?
   a. Decrease fluids 2 to 4 hours before sleep.
   b. Exercise in the evening to increase fatigue.
   c. Allow the patient to sleep as late as possible.
   d. Take a nap during the day to make up for lost sleep.
10. Which statement made by a mother being discharged to home with her newborn indicates a need for further teaching?
    a. I won't put the baby to bed with a bottle.
    b. For the first few weeks, we are putting the cradle in our room.
    c. My grandmother told me that babies sleep better on their stomachs.
    d. I know I will have to get up during the night to feed the baby when he wakes up.

Answers: 1. d; 2. b; 3. d; 4. c; 5. a; 6. d; 7. d; 8. c; 9. a; 10. c.

Rationales for the Review Questions appear on the Evolve website.

RECOMMENDED WEBSITES

Canadian Lung Association: https://www.lung.ca
This website provides information on obstructive sleep apnea (OSA), including strategies to enhance living with OSA. Treatment modalities, such as continuous positive airway pressure (CPAP) devices, and general information about OSA are also presented on this website.

Canadian Sleep Society: https://css-scs.ca
This website provides a conduit for health care providers and researchers who are interested in sleep-related disorders, with an emphasis on sleep research performed in Canada. The site also provides information for the public on sleep-related topics and links to other sleep-related

organizations, to enhance the understanding of sleep and its related disorders.

National Sleep Foundation (US): https://www.thensf.org

This multilingual website, designed for both health care providers and the public, provides an exhaustive amount of information on a plethora of sleep-related topics—for example, restless leg syndrome, dementia, and menopause. The site provides access to sleep-related educational material and research reports, such as the 2011 annual Sleep in America poll that explores the impact of communication technology on sleep.

Public Health Agency of Canada: Sleep Apnea: https://www.canada.ca/en/public-health/services/chronic-diseases/sleep-apnea.html

REFERENCES

A full reference list is available on the website for this book at http://evolve.elsevier.com/Canada/Potter/fundamentals/

This website includes publications intended for health care providers and the general public that are related to sleep apnea and other sleep disorders. It also includes a link to *Fast Facts from the 2009 Canadian Community Health Survey—Sleep Apnea Rapid Response.* This survey, conducted by Statistics Canada, estimated the prevalence of sleep apnea in the Canadian population.

Veterans Affairs Canada (VAC): https://www.veterans.gc.ca

This website provides links to services, benefits, publications, and fact sheets relevant to Canadian veterans. Additionally, the site offers VAC information on many issues facing Canadian veterans, including the impact of post-traumatic stress disorder (PTSD) on sleep and strategies to help get a good night's sleep.

43

Nutrition

Written by Kathryn Weaver, RN, MN, PhD

OBJECTIVES

Mastery of content in this chapter will enable you to:

- Define the key terms listed.
- Explain the role of each major nutrient in proper nutrition.
- Explain the importance of maintaining a balance between energy intake and expenditure.
- List the end products of carbohydrate, protein, and fat metabolism.
- Explain the significance of saturated, unsaturated, polyunsaturated, and trans fats.
- Be aware of national position statements and recommendations regarding sugar consumption.
- Describe *Canada's Food Guide* and its value in planning nutritious meals for infants, adolescents, pregnant and lactating persons, and older persons.
- Explain how to interpret the nutritional value of foods using the nutrition facts table on food labels.
- Identify populations at increased risk of poor dietary intakes because their food environment or life circumstances do not support accessibility and availability of nutritious foods.
- Understand how to plan sample menus for cardiac diets, renal diets, lactose intolerance, gluten-free diets, and diabetes diets.
- Identify the role of the dietitian and speech-language pathologist in promoting healthy diets and preventing risks such as aspiration.
- Describe the major methods of nutritional assessment.
- Identify three major nutritional disorders, the patients who are at risk, and related nutrition therapy.
- Formulate a plan of care to help meet the specific nutritional needs of infants, toddlers, preschoolers, school-aged children, adolescents, adults, and older persons.
- Plan for the daily nutritional intake of pregnant persons.
- Identify the potential nutritional deficits associated with vegetarian diets, with special consideration to vegan and ovo-lactate diets.
- Identify any risks associated with genetically modified food.
- Explain how to set up a meal tray for the visually impaired patient.
- Describe diet counselling and patient teaching in relation to patient expectations.
- State the goals of enteral and parenteral nutrition.
- Describe the procedure for initiating and maintaining tube feedings and for avoiding related complications.

KEY TERMS

Amino acids
Anabolism
Anorexia
Anorexia nervosa
Anthropometry
Aquaporins
Aspiration
Basal metabolic rate (BMR)
Body mass index (BMI)
Bulimia nervosa
Carbohydrates
Catabolism
Cholesterol
Chyme
Complementary proteins
Complex carbohydrates
Dietary reference intakes (DRIs)
Diet culture
Dysphagia
Elemental formulas
Enteral nutrition
Enzymes
Essential amino acids
Fat-soluble vitamins

Fatty acids
Food security
Fortified foods
Free sugars
Functional foods
Genetically modified (GM) food
Gluconeogenesis
Glycemic index
Glycogenesis
Glycogenolysis
Hypervitaminosis
Ideal body weight (IBW)
Ketones
Lipid emulsions
Lipids
Macrominerals
Metabolism
Minerals
Modular formulas
Monounsaturated fatty acids
Nitrogen balance
Nonessential amino acids
Novel food
Nutrient density

Nutrients
Nutritional assessment
Nutritional screening
Obesogenic environment
Organic food
Parenteral nutrition
Peristalsis
Polymeric formulas
Polyunsaturated fatty acids
Refeeding syndrome
Resting energy expenditure (REE)
Saccharides
Saturated (fatty acids)
Simple carbohydrates
Specialty formulas
Trace elements
Trans fatty acids
Triglycerides
Unsaturated (fatty acids)
Vegetarianism
Vitamins
Waist circumference
Water-soluble vitamins

1097

🌐 **WEBSITE**

http://evolve.elsevier.com/Canada/Potter/fundamentals/

CASE STUDY*

A community palliative care nurse has been assigned to care for Arnold (preferred pronouns: he/him), an 80-year-old individual diagnosed with adenocarcinoma (cancer) of the stomach. Arnold's nutrition has played an important role in managing the demands of first, a chronic disease, and then a terminal illness diagnosis. Following the development of type 2 diabetes 20 years ago, he was heathy, having reduced his ingestion of fast foods, alcohol, and high-sugar beverages and increased his frequency of cycling, rowing, and hiking. Arnold was approximately 172.7 cm (5 feet, 8 inches) and weighed around 76.2 kg (168 lb) before the cancer was identified. Difficulty swallowing, regurgitation, and decreased appetite forced him to seek medical attention. Booked for surgery on an urgent basis, the surgery ended up being a quick open-and-close procedure because the cancer had metastasized. The surgeon asked Arnold before the surgery if he would want a gastrostomy (G-tube) inserted if they were unable to remove the tumour. Arnold agreed to the G-tube insertion, if necessary.

The nurse visiting twice a week taught Arnold and his spouse (preferred pronouns: she/her) how to care for the G-tube and manage enteral feedings. Early teaching ensured that Arnold and his spouse were aware of the importance of good hand hygiene, proper positioning during feedings, signs or symptoms indicating G-tube misplacement, and what to do if this happened. Arnold and his spouse were also taught to observe the insertion site for redness or leakage,

set up the feeding equipment, manage the infusion pump, and prevent tubing blockage. Because Arnold would be getting his diabetic medication through the tube, they were also taught this procedure.

As Arnold's weight slowly increased, he was deemed strong enough for radiation therapy. This therapy was initially successful in shrinking the tumour and its metastases. When the feeding tube was removed after about 2 months, Arnold could drink liquids and eat small amounts of chopped food. Arnold continued his active lifestyle, enjoying a good quality of life for 14 months before becoming ill again.

When the tumour grew and spread again, Arnold re-experienced difficulty eating. At this point, neither Arnold nor the physician was comfortable with having the G-tube reinserted. Arnold died within 2 months; his weight was 45.3 kg (under 100 lb).

During a follow-up visit with Arnold's spouse, the nurse asks her if she believes that Arnold would have allowed the G-tube to be inserted in the first place had he realized what the outcome would be. Arnold's spouse is adamant that he would do the same thing again, because he had 14 additional months of good-quality life that he would otherwise not have had without the G-tube.

Think about the case study as you read this chapter. There are review questions at the end of the chapter that relate to the case study.

*Written by Donna Bulman, PhD, RN, University of New Brunswick.

Proper nutrition and feeding safety—important to all Canadians—are a shared responsibility of government, industry, health providers, and consumers. Food supplies the energy required to accomplish everyday activities, building and repairing tissues, and regulating organs and systems while helping to prevent the contraction of certain diseases and aid in the recovery from other diseases. Food also holds symbolic meaning for many cultures and communities. Since the 1930s, Health Canada has worked collaboratively with federal partners, provinces, territories, and other stakeholders to enhance nutritional health and well-being through evidence-informed nutrition policies and standards. These efforts to advise about the safety and nutritional value of food have promoted environments that support Canadians in making healthy food choices (Health Canada, 2022a).

As nurses, we must pay as much attention to our patients' diets as to their illnesses, treatments, and therapies. In fact, diet can be a major treatment in illnesses, such as type 1 diabetes mellitus, a common health concern across Western nations, and nurses are key professionals responsible for educating patients and families about food choices and available technology (e.g., insulin pumps) that influence the course of the disease and assist in self-management. Along with type 1 diabetes, other conditions, such as type 2 diabetes, hypertension, and inflammatory bowel disease, require specialized nutritional support protocols that include diets low in sugars, cholesterol, or salt (Balestrieri et al., 2020; Diabetes Canada, 2022a; Heart and Stroke Foundation of Canada, 2022a).

Compared to citizens of other developed countries, the nutritional health of Canadians is good. This story may be changing, however, as Canadians face evolving demographic and economic issues that include a decline in resources available to rural and remote communities, the aging of the population, and the social isolation or marginalization of

certain groups of citizens. Recently, in Canada and around the world, the onset of the COVID-19 pandemic affected daily activities such as grocery shopping and social gatherings (Government of Canada, 2022a) and had greater severity for older persons, persons who belong to underrepresented minorities, and those living with underlying medical conditions (Butler & Barrientos, 2020). Among these vulnerable groups, dietary consumption of high amounts of saturated fat, refined carbohydrates, and sugars and low levels of fibre, unsaturated fats, and antioxidants has inhibited their adaptive immune systems, leading to greater COVID-19 pathology.

A decrease in international migration levels brought on by the COVID-19 travel restrictions (Statistics Canada, 2020) slowed 2019–2020 population growth in every province except Newfoundland and Labrador. Alongside this slight drop in population growth has been an increase in the number of older Canadians. Specifically, there were 6 835 866 people, or 18.0% of the population aged 65 and older, compared with 6 038 637 children aged 0 to 14 or 15.9% of the population in Canada on July 1, 2020 (Statistics Canada, 2020). Older persons are expected to account for one quarter of the Canadian population by 2059, while the share of children aged 0 to 14 will remain at 15 to 16% over the same period. In the territories, higher fertility and mortality rates account for more children than older persons; for instance, Nunavut has both the highest proportion of children aged 0 to 14 (31.7%) and the lowest share of adults aged 65 and older (4.0%) in the country.

Older persons who are choosing to stay in their own homes longer are at risk for poor nutrition associated with mobility impairments and social isolation. An Ontario study found that older Canadian adults living in subsidized housing self-reported their poverty rate as 14.9% and their food insecurity rate as 5.1%, or twice that of the general population of older persons in Canada (Pirrie et al., 2020). *Food insecurity* is the uncertainty of having a diet of sufficient quality or quantity (Health Canada, 2020a). Even those who self-reported being food secure described dietary habits that are consistent with a poor diet. For example, 42.7% reported eating high-fat or fast foods one to two times per week, and 33.4% did not eat fruits or vegetables every day. This trend is concerning because of the high rates of diabetes and hypertension in this population. Pirrie and colleagues (2020) hypothesized that the poor diet could be due in part to low health literacy and to lack of accessibility to nearby amenities such as grocery stores that offer healthy and affordable food. As a result of Canada's current agricultural policies, high-calorie and less nutritious foods are often cheaper to purchase than healthier foods like fresh fruits and vegetables. While it is important to have access to affordable nutritious food, "food swamps" (Pirrie et al., 2020), or neighbourhoods with greater access to foods high in fat and calories, often exist in areas of low socioeconomic status.

At the other end of the age continuum, the *2020 National Report Card on Child and Family Poverty in Canada* described child poverty rates as having flatlined in some regions, yet increasing in Atlantic Canada. To illustrate, the poverty rate for children under age 6 years is high in Nova Scotia (28.9%) in relation to the rest of Canada (19.2%), despite the introduction of the Canada Child Benefit in 2016 (Campaign 2000, 2020). Poverty rates are even worse among children from Indigenous and racialized communities, in immigrant families, or in families affected by disability (Campaign 2000, 2020). Specifically, 4 in 10 children live in Indigenous communities (Campaign 2000, 2020) and face significant obstacles to healthy eating that include a high prevalence of food insecurity situated within a larger context of historical colonization, assimilation policies, and forced removal from traditional lands (Gillies et al., 2020). Although school-based nutrition programs for Indigenous children may provide supportive social and physical environmental elements, more support is needed, such as incorporating culturally specific traditional foods and ways of learning and ensuring that school nutrition policies guide nutrition activities and engage families and community members.

Among adult Canadians, 22% identify as having a disability, with almost one third of these individuals who work living in poverty. This does not include the 13% of youth aged 15–24 years who live with a disability and are more likely to be neither in school nor working than are youth without a disability (Statistics Canada, 2018). A subsequent disability participation project (Abilities Centre & Canadian Disability Participation Project, 2020) reported that before the COVID-19 pandemic, case management was the only need considered to be "unmet" by 55% of a sample of 713 Canadians living with disabilities. However, during the pandemic, needs considered to be "unmet" by over 50% of respondents included emotional counselling (70%), access to food and groceries (53%), and access to medical equipment, supplies, and aids (58%). The situation has worsened for Canadian youth living with disabilities, whose usual employment within tourist and food service industries was compromised by COVID-19 lockdowns. In addition, in 2016, more than one quarter of racialized children (26%) and one third of immigrant children (35%) experienced poverty rates below the national average (Campaign 2000, 2020). Low socioeconomic status contributes to poorer health status through dietary profiles that are less consistent with national dietary guidelines.

Another alarming trend is the increase in overweight and obesity. In 2018, approximately 63.1% of adult Canadians reported height and weight that classified them as being overweight or obese—an increase from 61.9% in 2015 (Statistics Canada, 2019). Newfoundland and Labrador have the highest rates of obesity, whereas the lowest rate is in British Columbia (Elflein, 2022). Areas that have affordable and accessible healthy food options and relatively good walkability scores encourage children and adolescents to practise healthy eating and physical activity. In contrast, **obesogenic environments** are defined as the total influence of surroundings and opportunities on promoting obesity in individuals and populations (Mei et al., 2021). Economically disadvantaged areas are more likely to be obesogenic. A recent study found the prevalence of overweight and obesity at about 25–30% of children and youth in Ontario, with 2–3% being severely obese (Carsley et al., 2019). Boys aged 5 to 9 years had a higher prevalence of obesity than their female counterparts. Obesity in childhood has been associated with increased cardiovascular risk, obstructive sleep apnea, nonalcoholic fatty liver disease, impaired glucose tolerance, and increased exposure to bullying; the severity of childhood obesity has been linked to the severity of these negative outcomes (Carsley et al., 2019). Persons living with overweight or obesity in obesogenic environments are also vulnerable to the pressures of the surrounding **diet culture**, a belief system that labels certain body sizes as better than others, moralizes particular foods, and urges people to modify themselves to meet established standards (Dolan, 2018). The juxtaposition of obesogenic environment with diet culture has the potential to diminish a person's quality of mental health. As well, type 2 diabetes, which is an illness largely preventable through healthy eating and weight management (Diabetes Canada, 2022b) that in the past occurred mainly in older individuals, is now increasingly diagnosed in Canadian children. Among Indigenous children living in Ontario, the prevalence of diabetes was more than 50% greater than it is among non-Indigenous children (Shulman et al., 2020).

Together, the demographic and poverty trends interacting with both obesogenic environment and diet culture adversely affect the nutritional health of Canadians, and the resultant conditions border on epidemic proportions. It is critical that nurses acquire nutritional knowledge to apply to the complexities of diseases, diverse populations, and current demographics (age, gender, income level, and culture).

SCIENTIFIC KNOWLEDGE BASE

Nutrients: The Biochemical Units of Nutrition

The body requires fuel to provide energy for the chemical reactions that enable cellular growth and repair, organ function, and body movement. The energy requirement of a person at rest is called the **basal metabolic rate (BMR)**. This is the energy needed to maintain life-sustaining activities (breathing, circulation, heart rate, and temperature) for a specific period of time. The **resting energy expenditure (REE)** is a measurement that accounts for BMR plus energy to digest meals and perform mild activity. REE is a baseline of energy requirement accounting for approximately 60 to 75% of our daily needs. Factors of age, body mass, gender, fever, environmental temperature, pregnancy, lactation, starvation, stress, illness, injury, infection, activity level, thyroid function, or the use of certain drugs or medications may affect energy requirements or metabolism.

In general, when energy requirements are completely met by kilocalorie (kcal) intake in food, weight does not change. A kilocalorie (referred to as "calorie" by the general public) is the unit of energy required to raise 1 kilogram of water by 1°C. When the kilocalories ingested exceed energy demands over time, a person gains weight. If the kilocalories ingested fail to meet energy requirements, a person loses weight.

Nutrients are the elements supplied by food that are necessary for body processes and function. Energy needs are met from three categories of nutrients: carbohydrates, proteins, and fats. Other nutrients are water, vitamins, and minerals, which do not provide energy but contribute to metabolic processes, including acid–base balance. A nutrient is considered essential if the body cannot manufacture it in a sufficient quantity to meet metabolic demands.

Foods are described according to **nutrient density**, the proportion of essential nutrients to the number of kilocalories. High nutrient-density foods, such as fruits and vegetables, provide a large number of nutrients in relation to kilocalories. Low nutrient-density foods, such as alcohol or refined sugar, are high in kilocalories but nutrient poor.

Foods may also be described as functional, organic, or novel. **Functional foods** (Powers et al., 2019) have biologically active ingredients added that have demonstrated health benefits (e.g., probiotic yogourt, or pea fibre-fortified breads and pasta). **Fortified foods** have additional vitamins, minerals, or both to provide added health benefits (e.g., fortified soy beverages and fruit juice with calcium) or are enhanced with bioactive components through plant breeding, genetic modification, processing, or special livestock feeding techniques (e.g., eggs, milk, and meat with omega-3). **Organic foods** are vegetables, fruit, eggs, milk, and meat produced without synthetic (human-made) pesticides, herbicides, and fertilizers; genetically modified organisms (GMOs); antibiotics or growth hormones; or irradiation or ionizing radiation (a way to preserve food with radiation energy). Organic farmers may use natural pesticides approved for organic food production (Bialai, 2020). **Novel food** or **genetically modified (GM) food** contains the insertion of the genes of one organism into another organism, often to resist disease and develop desired characteristics, such as a hardier texture, higher nutritional value, or faster growth. According to Health Canada (2022b), the use of GM techniques does not introduce unique risks into the food supply; therefore, the potential for long-term effects from these foods are no different than it is for conventional foods that have been a safe part of the Canadian diet for a long time. Currently, over 140 GM foods are permitted for sale in Canada. There is no mandatory labelling of these foods; yet, voluntary method-of-production labelling is allowed because this helps consumers make informed choices and guides manufacturers in making claims about the use or nonuse of genetic engineering in their products.

Carbohydrates. **Carbohydrates** are the recommended source of energy in the diet. Each gram of carbohydrate produces 4 kcal and serves as the main source of fuel (glucose) for the brain, skeletal muscles during exercise, red and white blood cell production, and cell function of the renal medulla. Carbohydrates are obtained primarily from plant foods, except for lactose (milk sugar), and are classified according to their carbohydrate units, or **saccharides**.

Monosaccharides such as glucose (dextrose) or fructose (fruit sugar) are the building blocks of all other carbohydrates and cannot be broken down into a more basic carbohydrate unit. Disaccharides such as sucrose, lactose, and maltose are composed of two monosaccharides minus one unit of water. Both monosaccharides and disaccharides are classified as **simple carbohydrates** called *sugars*. **Free sugars** (the monosaccharides and disaccharides added to foods and beverages by the manufacturer, cook, or consumer) and sugars naturally present in honey, syrups, and fruit juice do not include the naturally occurring sources of sugars found in fruit, vegetables, and unsweetened milk. Polysaccharides are composed of many carbohydrate units and are classified as **complex carbohydrates**. They include *starch* (stored form of glucose in plants) and *glycogen* (stored glucose in animals and humans). Some polysaccharides cannot be digested because humans do not have enzymes capable of breaking them down. Insoluble fibres are not digestible and include cellulose, hemicellulose, and lignin. Soluble fibres include pectin, guar gum, and mucilage. Dietary fibre is important to disease prevention, as it decreases low-density lipoprotein (LDL) cholesterol associated with the development of heart disease (Soliman, 2019).

Carbohydrate-rich foods are ranked according to their **glycemic index**, the effect on blood glucose levels and insulin response (Diabetes Canada, 2022b). Carbohydrates that release glucose rapidly into the bloodstream (e.g., white bread, candy) have a high glycemic index. Carbohydrates that produce only small fluctuations in blood glucose (e.g., barley, lentils) have a low glycemic index and offer long-term health benefits of sustaining weight loss, prolonging physical endurance, and reducing risks associated with heart disease and diabetes.

Currently Canada does not have a quantitative guideline specific to total or added sugar intake as part of a healthy diet (Canadian Sugar Institute, 2022). Health Canada suggests choosing foods with little to no added sugars and avoiding sugar-sweetened drinks. The Heart and Stroke Foundation of Canada (2022b) and the World Health Organization (WHO, 2020) recommend consuming no more than 10% total calories per day from added sugars and ideally less than 5%. For an average 2 000 calorie-a-day diet, 10% is about 48 grams (or 12 teaspoons) of added (free) sugars. Sugars are often added to processed foods to improve their flavour, colour, texture, and shelf life. While foods containing natural sugars are an important part of a healthy diet because they also contain important nutrients, added sugars provide energy (calories) but no nutritional value on their own. Added sugar may be listed as glucose, fructose, dextrose, maltose, or sucrose on the ingredient listing on food labels. If any of these sugars are listed as the first or second ingredient on a food label, the food is likely high in sugar. One can of pop contains approximately 10 teaspoons of added sugar. Other foods often high in added sugar include energy drinks, fruit-flavoured drinks, sports drinks, hot chocolate, specialty coffees, baked goods, and desserts. Consuming too much sugar is associated with an increased risk of weight gain, overweight, obesity, heart disease, stroke, diabetes, high blood cholesterol, cancer, and dental cavities.

Proteins. Proteins are essential for synthesis (building) of body tissue in growth, maintenance, and repair. Collagen, hormones, enzymes, immune cells, DNA, and RNA are all composed of protein. In addition, blood clotting, fluid regulation, and acid–base balance require proteins. Nutrients and many pharmacological substances are transported in the blood by proteins.

The simplest form of protein is the *amino acid*. As with other nutrients, **essential amino acids** are those that the body cannot synthesize but must have provided in the diet. **Nonessential amino acids** can be synthesized by the body. **Amino acids** are linked together by peptide bonds to form larger protein molecules called *polypeptides*. Simple proteins such as albumin and insulin contain only amino acids or their derivatives. The combination of a simple protein with a nonprotein substance produces a more complex protein, such as lipoprotein, formed by combining a lipid (fat) and a simple protein.

Protein quality is determined by the balance of essential amino acids. Incomplete proteins lack a sufficient quantity of one or more essential amino acids and include cereals, legumes (beans, peas), and vegetables. A complete protein contains all of the nine essential amino acids in sufficient quantity to support growth and maintain nitrogen balance. Examples of foods that contain complete proteins are chicken, soybeans, fish, and cheese. Complete proteins are referred to as *high-quality proteins*. **Complementary proteins** are pairs of incomplete proteins that, when combined, supply the total amount of protein provided by complete protein sources.

Protein is the only major nutrient that contains nitrogen (it is 16% nitrogen) and is the only source of nitrogen for the body. Thus, nitrogen can be used to determine protein balance in the body. **Nitrogen balance** is achieved when the intake and output of nitrogen are equal. When the intake of nitrogen exceeds the output, the body is in positive nitrogen balance, which is required for growth, normal pregnancy, maintenance of lean muscle mass and vital organs, and wound healing. The nitrogen retained by the body is used for the building, repair, and replacement of body tissues. Negative nitrogen balance occurs when the body loses more nitrogen than it gains—for example, with severe infection, burns, fever, starvation, head injury, and trauma. The increased nitrogen loss is the result of body tissue destruction or loss of nitrogen-containing body fluids through urine, feces, sweat, and, at times, bleeding or vomiting. Nutrition during this period must provide nutrients to put patients into positive balance for healing.

Protein can be used to provide energy (4 kcal/g), but because of protein's essential role in growth, maintenance, and repair, adequate kilocalories should be provided in the diet from nonprotein sources. Protein is spared as an energy source when carbohydrate in the diet is sufficient to meet the energy needs of the body.

Fats. Fats (**lipids**) are the most calorically dense nutrient, providing 9 kcal/g. In addition to serving as fuel that supplies energy, fat cushions vital organs, lubricates body tissue, insulates, and protects cell membranes. Fats are composed of glycerol and fatty acids. **Triglycerides** circulate in the blood and are made up of three fatty acids attached to a glycerol. **Fatty acids** are composed of chains of carbon and hydrogen atoms with an acid group on one end of the chain and a methyl group at the other. Fatty acids can be **saturated**, in which each carbon in the chain has two attached hydrogen atoms, or **unsaturated**, in which an unequal number of hydrogen atoms are attached and the carbon atoms attach to each other with a double bond. **Monounsaturated fatty acids** have one double bond, whereas **polyunsaturated fatty acids** have two or more double carbon bonds. Most animal-based foods, such as cream, butter, cheeses, and fatty meats, as well as some vegetable oils such as coconut and palm kernel oil, and coconut milk, have high proportions of saturated fatty acids, whereas plant-based foods have higher amounts of monounsaturated and polyunsaturated fatty acids. The various types of fatty acids have significance for health and the incidence of disease, including heart disease, stroke, certain cancers, and diabetes. The WHO (WHO, 2020) recommends that total fat not exceed 30% of total energy intake, intake of saturated fats be less than 10% of total energy intake, and intake of trans fats be less than 1% of total energy intake. In addition, the WHO recommends shifting away from saturated fats and trans fats to unsaturated fats and toward the goal of eliminating industrially produced trans fats. The Heart and Stroke Foundation of Canada, Diabetes Canada, and the Canadian Cardiovascular Society all endorse these WHO recommendations.

Trans fatty acids contribute to the development of coronary artery disease (Antwi-Boasiako & Kersten, 2020). Formed by the partial hydrogenation of vegetable oils and mostly found in prepared foods, snack foods, and margarines, trans fats raise blood levels of so-called bad cholesterol (LDL cholesterol) while lowering blood levels of so-called good cholesterol (HDL cholesterol), which protects against heart disease (Health Canada, 2022c). Trans fatty acids have also been associated with type 2 diabetes (Neuenschwander et al., 2020), Alzheimer's disease and cognitive decline (Honda et al., 2019), infertility in men and women (Afshin et al., 2019; Skoracka et al., 2020), and prostate cancer in men (Liss et al., 2019). Increased research and consumer awareness have led to mandatory nutrition labelling of trans fats in Canada. On September 17, 2018, Health Canada banned the use of partially hydrogenated oils in foods (Canadian Food Inspection Agency, 2019a). It is now illegal for manufacturers to add partially hydrogenated oils to any foods sold in Canada. This ban is expected to help reduce the risk of heart disease among Canadians.

Cholesterol is a sterol that occurs naturally in animal foods but is also synthesized by the liver (Heart and Stroke Foundation of Canada, 2022a). Cholesterol deposits in blood vessel walls cause atherosclerosis, which is the underlying cause of coronary artery disease.

Water. Water is a critical component of the body because cell function depends on a fluid environment. Water makes up 60 to 70% of total body weight. The percentage of total body water is greater for lean people than for people with obesity because muscle contains more water than any other tissue except blood. Infants have the greatest percentage of total body water, and older people have the least. When deprived of water, a person cannot survive for more than a few days. Water helps regulate body temperature and acts as a solvent for nutrients and waste products. Water passes freely through membranes that separate body fluids inside (intracellular) and outside (extracellular) cells. Various water-transport proteins called **aquaporins** function as water-selective channels in many cells, altering the speed at which water crosses cell membranes and influencing conditions such as cataract formation, hypertension, and salivary gland function. Aquaporins are critical proteins regulating water fluid homeostasis in cells involved in inflammation (Meli et al., 2018). Fluid needs are met by ingesting liquids and solid foods high in water content, such as fresh fruits and vegetables. Water is also produced during digestion when food is oxidized. In a healthy individual, fluid intake from all sources equals fluid output through elimination, respiration, and sweating (see Chapters 37 and 40). An ill person can have an increased need for fluid (e.g., with fever or gastrointestinal losses) and also a decreased ability to excrete fluid (e.g., with cardiopulmonary or renal disease), which may lead to the need to restrict fluid intake.

Vitamins. **Vitamins** are organic substances essential to normal metabolism. The body is unable to synthesize most vitamins in the required amounts and depends on dietary intake. The quantity of vitamins in food is affected by food processing, storage, and preparation. Vitamin content is usually highest in fresh foods used quickly after minimal exposure to heat, air, or water. Certain vitamins function as antioxidants that neutralize substances called *free radicals*, which are thought to produce oxidative damage to body cells and tissues and to increase a person's risk for various cancers. Vitamins with antioxidant properties include water-soluble vitamin C and fat-soluble beta-carotene and vitamins A and E (Lazzarino et al., 2019).

Fat-Soluble Vitamins. The **fat-soluble vitamins** (A, D, E, and K) can be stored in the body. With the exception of vitamin D, these vitamins are provided only through dietary intake. Vitamin D is provided by both dietary intake and synthesis in the body with exposure to sunlight. Health Canada (Health Canada, 2020b) recommends that people over the age of 50 years take a daily vitamin D supplement of 400 international units (IU). The body can store fat-soluble vitamins; therefore, **hypervitaminosis** can result from megadoses (intentional or unintentional) of supplemental vitamins, excessive amounts of vitamins in fortified food, and excessive fish oils.

Water-Soluble Vitamins. The **water-soluble vitamins** are vitamins C and B complex (which consists of eight vitamins: thiamine, riboflavin, niacin, vitamin B_6, folate, vitamin B_{12}, pantothenic acid, and biotin). Another element, choline, is sometimes classified as a B vitamin. Water-soluble vitamins are easily destroyed by cooking and must be provided in the daily food intake. Although water-soluble vitamins are not stored in the body, toxicity may still occur with vitamin megadoses.

Minerals. **Minerals** are inorganic elements essential to the body as catalysts in biochemical reactions. Minerals become part of the structure of the body and its enzymes. For example, iron becomes attached to protein globin to form hemoglobin, which enhances oxygen-carrying capacity. Minerals are classified as **macrominerals** when the daily requirement is 100 mg or more and as microminerals or **trace elements** when less than 100 mg is needed daily. The macrominerals are calcium, sodium, potassium, phosphorus, magnesium, sulphur, and chloride. A higher sodium intake is associated with higher blood pressure, a risk factor for cardiovascular disease. Trace minerals include iron, iodine, fluoride, zinc, selenium, chromium, copper, manganese, molybdenum, and cobalt. Other trace minerals such as aluminum, cadmium, arsenic, and boron have possible but not clearly delineated nutritional functions. Arsenic, aluminum, and cadmium have toxic effects.

Anatomy and Physiology of the Digestive System

Digestion. Digestion of food consists of mechanical breakdown that results from chewing, churning, and mixing with fluid, as well as chemical reactions by which food is reduced to its simplest form. Each part of the gastrointestinal system has an important digestive or absorptive function (Figure 43.1).

Enzymes are an essential component of the chemistry of digestion. Enzymes are protein-like substances that act as catalysts to speed up chemical reactions. Most enzymes have one specific function and function best at a specific pH. The secretions of the gastrointestinal tract have vastly different pH levels. For example, saliva is relatively neutral, gastric juice is highly acidic, and the secretions of the small intestine are alkaline.

The mechanical, chemical, and hormonal activities of digestion are interdependent. Enzyme activity depends on the mechanical breakdown of food to increase the surface area for chemical action. Hormones regulate the flow of digestive secretions needed for enzyme supply. The secretion of digestive juices and the motility of the gastrointestinal tract are also regulated by physical, chemical, and hormonal factors. Action in the gastrointestinal tract is increased by nerve stimulation from the parasympathetic nervous system (e.g., the vagus nerve).

Digestion begins in the mouth, where chewing mechanically breaks down food. The food is mixed with saliva, which contains ptyalin (salivary amylase), an enzyme that acts on cooked starch to begin its conversion to maltose. The longer food is chewed, the more starch digestion occurs in the mouth. Proteins and fats are broken down physically but remain unchanged chemically because enzymes in the mouth do not react with these nutrients. Because simple sugars (monosaccharides) require no digestion, they may be absorbed from the mouth. Chewing reduces food particles to a size suitable for swallowing, and saliva provides lubrication to further ease swallowing of the food. The epiglottis is a flap of skin that closes over the trachea during swallowing to prevent aspiration. The tongue manoeuvres the mass of chewed food into the pharynx, which activates the swallowing reflex. Swallowed food

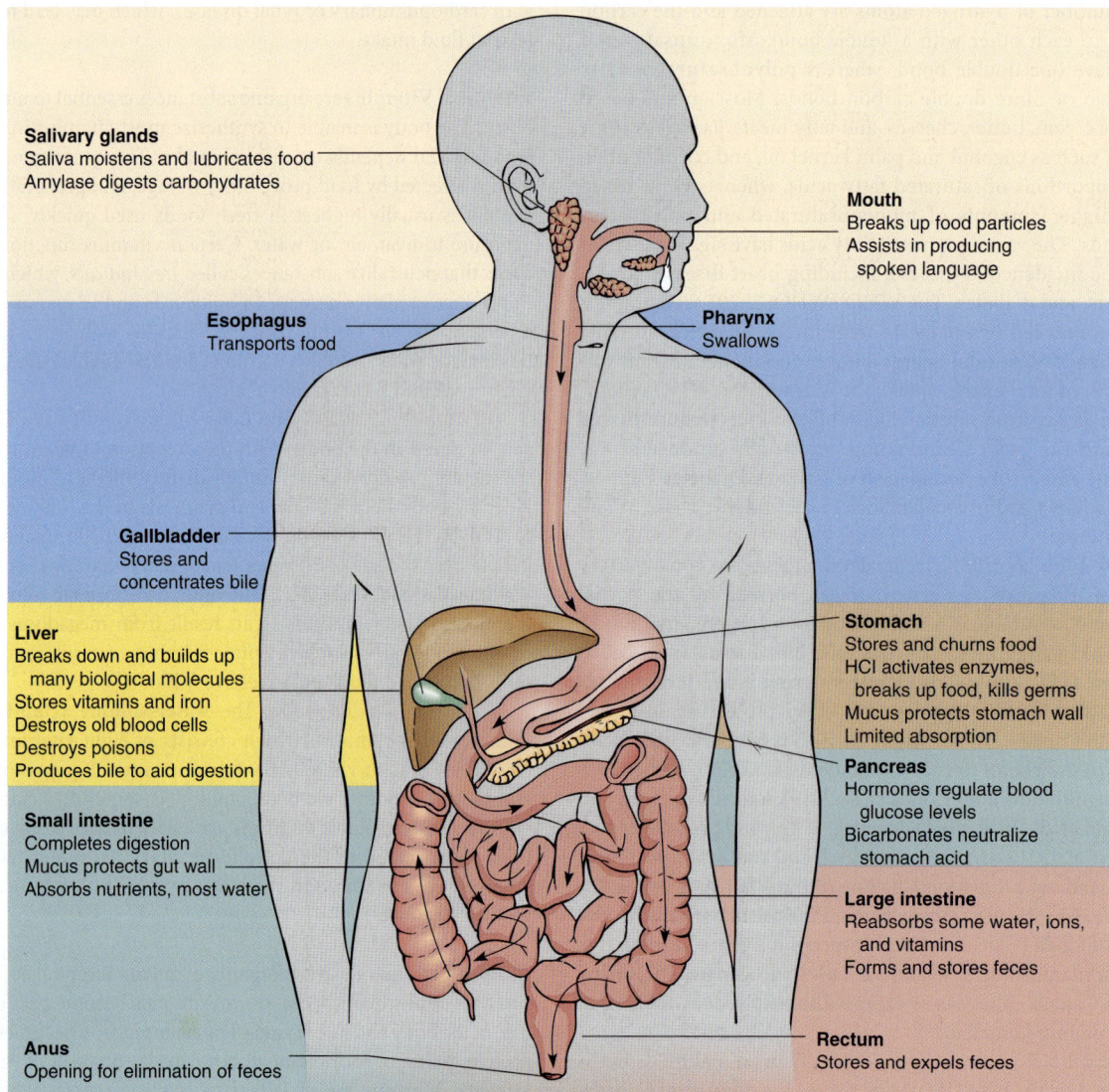

Salivary glands
Saliva moistens and lubricates food
Amylase digests carbohydrates

Mouth
Breaks up food particles
Assists in producing
    spoken language

Esophagus
Transports food

Pharynx
Swallows

Gallbladder
Stores and
concentrates bile

Stomach
Stores and churns food
HCl activates enzymes,
    breaks up food, kills germs
Mucus protects stomach wall
Limited absorption

Liver
Breaks down and builds up
    many biological molecules
Stores vitamins and iron
Destroys old blood cells
Destroys poisons
Produces bile to aid digestion

Pancreas
Hormones regulate blood
    glucose levels
Bicarbonates neutralize
    stomach acid

Small intestine
Completes digestion
Mucus protects gut wall
Absorbs nutrients, most water

Large intestine
Reabsorbs some water, ions,
    and vitamins
Forms and stores feces

Anus
Opening for elimination of feces

Rectum
Stores and expels feces

FIGURE 43.1 Summary of digestive system anatomy and organ function. *HCl,* Hydrochloric acid. (From Rolin Graphics.)

enters the esophagus and is moved along by wavelike muscular contractions (peristalsis) to the base of the esophagus, above the cardiac sphincter. Pressure from a bolus of food at the cardiac sphincter causes it to relax, allowing the food to enter the fundus (uppermost portion) of the stomach. Difficulty swallowing is referred to as dysphagia.

In the stomach, pepsinogen is secreted by chief cells and then converted by hydrochloric acid (HCl) to pepsin, a protein-splitting enzyme. Gastric lipase and amylase are produced to begin fat and starch digestion, respectively. The stomach's pyloric glands secrete gastrin, a hormone that triggers parietal cells to secrete intrinsic factor (IF) and HCl. IF is necessary for absorption of vitamin B_{12} in the ileum. HCl also destroys bacteria, increases the absorbability of iron and calcium, and maintains the pH of the gastric juice. The lining of the stomach is protected from autodigestion by a thick layer of mucus. Alcohol and aspirin are two substances directly absorbed through the lining of the stomach. The muscular walls of the stomach produce a churning action that continues mechanical digestion. The stomach acts as a reservoir where food remains for approximately 3 hours, within a range of 1 to 7 hours.

Food leaves the antrum, or distal stomach, via the pyloric sphincter and enters the duodenum as an acidic, liquefied mass called chyme. Chyme flows into the duodenum and is quickly mixed with bile, intestinal juices, and pancreatic secretions. Secretin and cholecystokinin (CCK) are hormones secreted by the mucosa of the small intestine. Secretin activates release of bicarbonate from the pancreas, raising the pH of chyme. CCK inhibits further gastrin secretion and initiates the release of additional digestive enzymes from the pancreas and gallbladder.

Bile is manufactured in the liver and stored in the gallbladder. Bile acts as a detergent, as it emulsifies fat to permit enzyme action while suspending fatty acids in solution. Pancreatic secretions contain six enzymes: amylase to digest starch; lipase to break down emulsified fats; and trypsin, elastase, chymotrypsin, and carboxypeptidase to break down proteins.

Peristalsis continues in the small intestine, mixing the secretions with the chyme. The mixture becomes increasingly alkaline, inhibiting the action of the gastric enzymes and promoting the action of the duodenal secretions. Epithelial cells in the inner walls of the small intestine secrete enzymes to facilitate digestion. These enzymes include sucrase, lactase, maltase, lipase, and peptidase. The major portion of digestion occurs in the small intestine, producing glucose, fructose, and galactose from carbohydrates; amino acids and dipeptides from proteins; and fatty acids, glycerides, and glycerol from lipids. Approximately 5 hours are required to pass food through the small intestine via peristalsis.

Absorption. The small intestine is the primary absorption site for nutrients. Its inner surface is lined with fingerlike projections called *villi*, which increase the surface area available for absorption. Nutrients are absorbed by means of passive diffusion, osmosis, active transport, and pinocytosis (Box 43.1).

The main source of water absorption is via the intestine. Approximately 7 L of gastrointestinal secretions and 1.2 L of oral intake, totalling 8.2 L of fluid, must be managed daily within the gastrointestinal tract. The small and large intestines reabsorb 8.1 L a day. The remaining 0.1 L is eliminated in feces. In addition to water, electrolytes and minerals are absorbed, and bacteria in the colon synthesize vitamin K and some B-complex vitamins. Finally, feces are formed in the colon for elimination.

Metabolism and Storage of Nutrients. Metabolism refers to all of the biochemical reactions within the cells of the body. Metabolic

---

BOX 43.1	Mechanisms for Intestinal Absorption of Nutrients

Mechanism Definition

Active Transport

In this energy-dependent process, particles move from an area of greater concentration to an area of lesser concentration. A special "carrier" is needed to move the particle across the cell membrane.

Passive Diffusion

The force by which particles move outward from an area of greater concentration to lesser concentration constitutes passive diffusion. The particles do not need a special "carrier" to move outward in all directions.

Osmosis

In this process, water moves through a membrane that separates solutions of different concentrations. Water moves to equalize the concentration pressures on both sides of the membrane.

Pinocytosis

Large molecules of nutrients are engulfed by the absorbing cell when the molecule attaches to the absorbing cell membrane.

Data from Nix, S. (2022). *Williams' basic nutrition and diet therapy* (16th ed.). Elsevier; Schlenker, E. D., & Gilbert, J. A. (2018). *Essentials of nutrition and diet therapy* (12th ed.). Mosby.

---

processes can be anabolic (building) or catabolic (breaking down). Anabolism is the production of more complex biochemical substances by synthesis of nutrients. Anabolism occurs when lean muscle is added to the body through diet and exercise. Amino acids are anabolized into tissues, hormones, and enzymes. Catabolism is the breakdown of biochemical substances into simpler substances. Starvation is an example of catabolism, when wasting of body tissues occurs. Normal metabolism and anabolism are physiologically possible when the body is in positive nitrogen balance, whereas catabolism occurs during physiological states of negative nitrogen balance.

Nutrients absorbed in the intestines, including water, are transported via the circulatory system to body tissues. Through the chemical changes of metabolism, nutrients are converted into a number of substances required by the body. Carbohydrates, protein, and fat undergo metabolism to produce chemical energy and to maintain a balance between anabolism and catabolism. To carry out the body's work, the chemical energy produced by metabolism is converted to other types of energy. For example, muscle contraction involves mechanical energy, nervous system function involves electrical energy, and the mechanisms of heat production involve thermal energy. All of these forms of energy originate in metabolism.

Nutrient metabolism consists of three main processes:
1. Catabolism of glycogen into glucose, carbon dioxide, and water (glycogenolysis)
2. Anabolism of glucose into glycogen for storage (glycogenesis)
3. Catabolism of amino acids and glycerol into glucose for energy (gluconeogenesis)

Glycogen, synthesized from glucose and stored in small reserves in liver and muscle tissue, provides energy during brief periods of fasting and maintains blood glucose levels as we sleep. Amino acids can be converted to fat and stored or catabolized into energy via gluconeogenesis. All body cells except red blood cells and neurons can oxidize fatty acids into ketones for energy in the absence of dietary carbohydrates (glucose). Some of the nutrients required by the body are stored in body tissues. The body's major form of reserve energy is fat, stored as adipose tissue.

Elimination. Chyme is moved by peristaltic action through the ileocecal valve into the large intestine, where it becomes feces. As feces move toward the rectum, water is absorbed into the intestinal mucosa. The longer the material stays in the large intestine, the more water is absorbed, causing the feces to become firmer. Exercise and fibre stimulate peristalsis. Feces contain cellulose and similar indigestible substances, sloughed epithelial cells from the gastrointestinal tract, digestive secretions, water, and microbes.

Dietary Guidelines

Dietary Reference Intakes. In 1997, the Food and Nutrition Board of the American National Institute of Medicine/National Academy of Sciences, in partnership with Health Canada, developed **dietary reference intakes (DRIs)** with respect to age, sex, pregnancy, and lactation (Health Canada, 2019b). The DRIs present evidenced-informed criteria for an acceptable range of minimum to maximum amounts of nutrients, vitamins, and minerals needed to avoid deficiencies or toxicities. The DRIs have four components: (1) the estimated average requirement (EAR), which is the recommended amount of a nutrient sufficient to maintain a specific body function for 50% of the population based on age and gender; (2) the recommended dietary allowance (RDA), which is the average needs of 97–98% of the population, not the exact needs of an individual; (3) the upper intake level (UL), which is the highest level believed to pose no risk of adverse health events but is not a recommended level of intake; and (4) the adequate intake (AI), which is the suggested intake for individuals based on observed or scientifically determined estimates of nutrient intakes and is used when insufficient evidence exists to set the RDA. Because this evidence is continually evolving, clinicians should consult current resources, such as Health Canada web pages, when determining a patient's specific nutrition needs or supplementation.

Food Guidelines. In 1942, Health Canada developed Canada's first food guide, *Canada's Official Food Rules*. Since then, the food guide has undergone changes in name, appearance, and content. However, its ultimate purpose—to inform daily food choices and promote optimal nutritional health—has not changed. The current guide, including Canada's Dietary Guidelines, launched in 2019, is based on evidence from the scientific bases (links between food, nutrients, and health), the Canadian context (what Canadians eat, their health status, and the environment in which they live), and the use of existing dietary guidance. It also considered input resulting from focus group research, public inquiries, media inquiries, trending nutrition topics on social media, meetings with professional associations, and other health stakeholders. In creating the new *Food Guide*, the Health Canada officials—many of them nutrition experts and researchers—did not meet with lobby stakeholder groups, including the beef, dairy, and juice industries, in order to reduce industry bias in the final dietary guidelines (Hui, 2019). The 2019 guidelines are consistent with current peer-reviewed systematic reviews and reports from leading scientific organizations and governmental agencies. The guidelines respond to challenges that Canadians have experienced in understanding and applying certain aspects of the food guide (e.g., healthy meals and snacks recommendations, the format not meeting the needs of all audiences). Regular intake of more plant-based foods (i.e., vegetables, fruit, whole grains, and plant-based proteins) and lower intake of processed meat (such as hot dogs, sausages, ham, corned beef, and beef jerky) and of foods that contain mostly saturated fat are emphasized. Patterns of eating more plant-based foods typically result in higher intakes of dietary fibre. Lower intake of processed meat decreases risk of colorectal cancer. Reducing high intakes of sugar-sweetened beverages and foods helps decrease the risk of dental decay and obesity.

Canada's food guide snapshot (Figure 43.2) shows the recommended proportion of protein foods, whole grain foods, vegetables, and fruit. Focus group research revealed that this was much easier to understand than portion sizes and number of daily servings. The guideline's recommendations are no longer food group– or portion-specific.

Included in *Canada's Food Guide* are specific suggestions for food choices. Consumers are to have plenty of vegetables and fruits (visually: half the plate), eat protein foods (visually: a quarter of the plate), and choose whole-grain foods (visually: a quarter of the plate). Among protein foods (e.g., legumes, nuts, seeds, tofu, fortified soy beverage, fish, shellfish, eggs, poultry, lean red meat including wild game, lower-fat

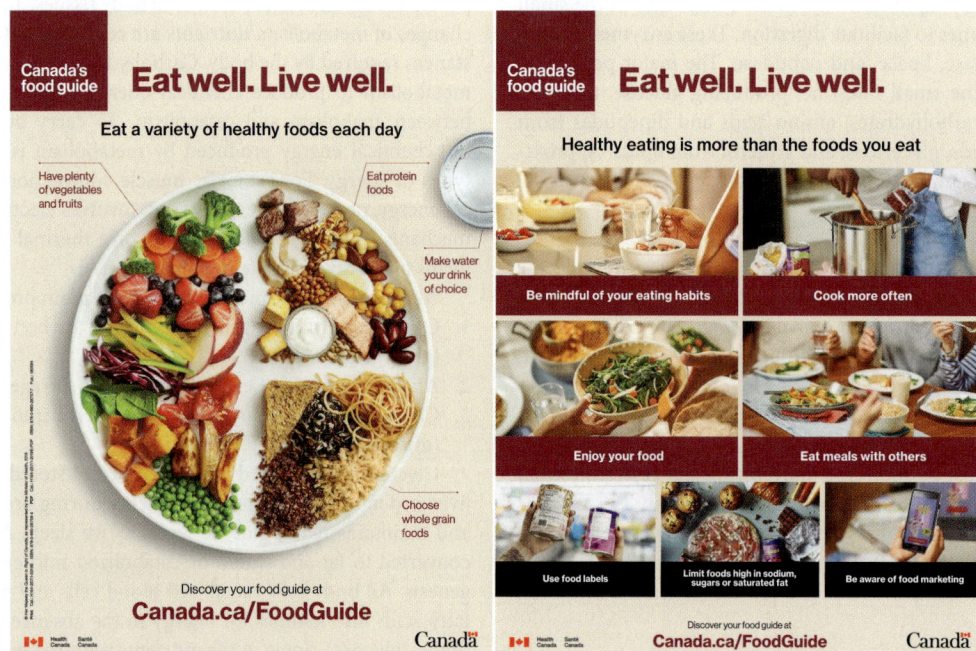

FIGURE 43.2 Food guide snapshot—*Canada's Food Guide.* (© All rights reserved. Canada's Dietary Guidelines. Health Canada, 2019. Modified, adapted and reproduced with permission from the Minister of Health, 2023.)

milk, lower fat yogourts, lower-fat kefir, and cheeses lower in fat and sodium), consumers are told to choose plant-based protein foods more often. Foods that contain mostly unsaturated fat should replace foods that contain mostly saturated fat to decrease LDL cholesterol, with the intention of promoting cardiovascular health. To help reduce the intake of free sugars, the majority of total sugars intake should come from nutritious foods, such as intact or cut fruit and vegetables, and unsweetened milk. If dried fruit is consumed, it should only be consumed with meals because it is sticky, often adheres to teeth, and contains sugars that can contribute to dental decay. Water should be the beverage of choice. Drinking water advisories are issued to protect the public from drinking water that is potentially unsafe, most notably in communities that are small, remote, or isolated.

Canada's food guide (Health Canada, 2022f) offers a high-level overview of not only what but also how Canadians should eat. Canadians are reminded to cook more often, eat meals with others, be mindful of their eating habits, and enjoy their food. The guidelines further advise the use of food labels, awareness of food marketing, and limiting foods high in sodium, sugars, or saturated fat. According to the Canadian Paediatric Society (Gowrishankar et al., 2020), recommended limits for sodium are less than 2 300 mg/day (ages 14 years and older). Such limits are geared toward addressing those characteristics of the diet most relevant to the promotion of health and reduction of chronic disease for Canadian populations.

Physical activity is also important in maintaining energy balance. It is recommended that adults spend at least 150 minutes per week carrying out moderate- to vigorous-intensity aerobic physical activity in bouts of 10 minutes or more. Children and youth should achieve at least 60 minutes of moderate to vigorous physical activity per day, low levels of sedentary behaviour, and sufficient sleep (Canadian Society for Exercise Physiology, 2020). In addition to following physical activity guidelines, other approaches such as reducing portion sizes (while maintaining proportionality) can help promote energy balance among adults. However, restricting intakes of nutritious foods can be a reason for concern because inadequate energy and nutrient intake can have a significant and lasting impact on health. Monitoring of weight status by a health care provider such as a nurse can help assess for unhealthy weights. Canadians are also advised to cut back on alcohol because of its links to liver disease and some types of cancer.

Examples of factors that influence the ability to make healthy eating decisions are limited employment opportunities and low incomes, lack of access to the land and resources, knowledge deficit of food practices, and the high prices of store-bought foods. Patterns of food consumption are further influenced by issues of **food security** (ability to acquire acceptable foods), preferences in body size, individual taste preferences, availability of particular species for food, knowledge of the nutritional deficits of store-bought food, and alteration of the natural environment. Health conditions such as anemia, dental caries, heart disease, obesity, and diabetes are related to such patterns.

It has been shown that the intake of traditional food among Indigenous peoples improves diet quality. These foods and the way they are obtained are intrinsically linked to culture, identity, way of life, and thus overall health. Examples of traditional foods of Indigenous people include large and small land mammals (moose, deer, elk, hare/rabbit, and caribou), sea mammals (seal and whale), fish (coastline fish such as salmon, cod, and arctic char; lake fish such as trout, walleye, whitefish, and northern pike; shellfish), birds (ducks, geese, and grouse), berries (blueberry, strawberry, raspberry, Saskatoon berry, and others), vegetables (corn, squash, fiddleheads, and mushrooms), beans, nuts (hazelnut), and other wild plants. Research has generally found that traditional food is safe to eat, although regional environmental risks should be considered. To supplement the 2019 *Dietary Guidelines*, healthy eating tools will be developed by Indigenous organizations for Indigenous peoples and will include tools distinct for individual Indigenous populations (Johnston, 2019).

Another population at increased risk for poor dietary intakes because their food environment or life circumstances do not support acceptance and availability of nutritious foods are newcomers to Canada, who may bring with them a food culture that they wish to preserve and share. Immigrants usually have fewer chronic conditions and tend to be healthier than the Canadian-born population when they first arrive in the country, owing to immigrants' food selection (Lu & Ng, 2019). However, changes resulting from living environment, unfamiliarity with grocery stores, availability of traditional foods, and lifestyle factors such as urbanization and language barriers impede immigrants' efforts to maintain their traditional dietary practices. In attempting to acquire the ingredients necessary for replicating familiar dishes, immigrants are limited to highly processed versions that are high in fat and sodium, therefore increasing their risk for chronic conditions. Through retrospective analysis of data collected from 140 South Asian adults who emigrated to Alberta, Subhan and Chan (2019) found central obesity (70%), hypercholesterolemia (27%), and hypertension (14%) were predominant health conditions, and they concluded that the diet quality of the majority of participants was inadequate. Long exposure to Canadian culture is associated with increased prevalence of obesity and growth stunting due to chronic malnutrition among immigrant children (Dondi et al., 2020). To date, Canada's *Food Guide* has not been modified to recognize the nutritional concerns of Asian Canadians or other immigrant groups.

Clearly, the *Food Guide* cannot stand alone as a tool to inform certain groups, including new immigrants and some Indigenous people, who ostensibly face more barriers to food literacy than other groups. Consideration should be given to addressing the determinants of health (e.g., biological, social, cultural, economic, and environmental factors and conditions that affect health) while making nutritional information more effective, understandable, and accessible for those at greater risk for poor health (Health Canada, 2019b). Health care providers and health policy makers, rather than food industry stakeholders, can play a significant role in operationalizing the dietary guidelines at individual and population levels (Bacon et al., 2019).

The Nutrition Label. The mandatory nutrition labelling of a nutrition facts table listing energy (calories) and 12 core nutrients (fat, saturated fat, trans fat, cholesterol, sodium, carbohydrate, fibre, sugars, protein, potassium, calcium, and iron) is required on most prepackaged foods in Canada. Recent improvements to the nutrition facts table (Figure 43.3) and lists of ingredients on food labels will make them easier for Canadians to understand and help them make informed choices. The food industry was given a 5-year transition period, ending on December 14, 2021, to make the necessary changes to their labels and to use up existing stocks of labels already printed. This deadline was extended until December 14, 2022, as a result of the challenges imposed by the COVID-19 pandemic. After December 15, 2022, the Canadian Food Inspection Agency will verify compliance and apply enforcement discretion in cases where noncompliant companies have detailed plans showing how and when they intend to meet the new requirements. Improvements to the nutrition facts table and list of ingredients on food labels include the following (Health Canada, 2022d):

1. Making the serving size more consistent, to make it easier to compare similar foods and more realistic to reflect the amount that Canadians typically eat in one sitting
2. Making the information easier to find and read by increasing the font size of serving size and calories, using black font text on white or neutral background, and adding a bold line under the calories
3. Revising the % daily values based on updated science

Nutrition Facts
Valeur nutritive
Per 1 cup (250 mL)
pour 1 tasse (250 mL)

Calories 110	% Daily Value* % valeur quotidienne*
Fat / Lipides 0 g	0 %
Saturated / saturés 0 g + Trans / trans 0 g	0 %
Carbohydrate / Glucides 26 g	
Fibre / Fibres 0 g	0 %
Sugars / Sucres 22 g	22 %
Protein / Protéines 2 g	
Cholesterol / Cholestérol 0 mg	
Sodium 0 mg	0 %
Potassium 450 mg	10 %
Calcium 30 mg	2 %
Iron / Fer 0 mg	0 %

*5% or less is **a little**, 15% or more is **a lot**
*5 % ou moins c'est **peu**, 15 % ou plus c'est **beaucoup**

FIGURE 43.3 Example of a nutrition facts table, showing labelling changes. (© All rights reserved. Changes to the Nutrition Facts Table. Health Canada, 2022 Adapted and reproduced with permission from the Minister of Health, 2022.)

4. Grouping sugars-based ingredients in brackets after the name "sugars" while adding a new % daily value for total sugars to help Canadians identify all of the sources of free sugars and to understand the proportion of free sugars compared to other ingredients
5. Updating the list of nutrients to:
   a. Add potassium, because of its importance for maintaining healthy blood pressure
   b. Remove vitamin A and vitamin C, because most Canadians get enough of these nutrients in their diets
6. Adding a footnote to the bottom of the table about % daily value to help consumers understand how much sugar and other nutrients (like sodium) are in their food. The label will explain that:
   a. 5% or less is a little
   b. 15% or more is a lot
7. Indicating the presence or potential presence of:
   a. Priority food allergens
   b. Gluten sources
   c. Added sulphites

This easy-to-read table, which appears on food labels in a consistent appearance, enables consumers to make informed food choices and compare products (see Figure 43.3).

Information that is provided voluntarily on food labels or in advertisements is often referred to as a *claim*. This may include specific claims such as "Product of Canada," "Low in fat," or "Fair trade." Thus, a claim is any representation that states, suggests, or implies that a food has particular characteristics relating to its origin, nutritional properties, production, processing, composition, or any other quality. In general, claims may be made about various aspects of a food, providing they are truthful, not misleading, nor likely to create an erroneous impression, and that they are in compliance with any specific requirements that exist for a given type of claim. Nutrient function claims are not made for a food per se; they may only be made regarding the energy value or nutrients in a food. For example, the nutrient function claim that "Milk helps build strong bones and teeth" is unacceptable, while "Milk is an excellent source of calcium, which helps build strong bones and teeth" is an acceptable claim. Certain claims, such as those relating to nutrient content; organic, kosher, or halal status; and certain disease risk-reduction claims, are subject to specific regulatory requirements in addition to the prohibitions in the *Food and Drugs Act* and *Safe Food for Canadians Act* (Canadian Food Inspection Agency, 2019b).

Health Promotion and Disease Prevention: A Call to Action From Dietitians. In 2011, the United Nations (UN) recommended monitoring the trends of noncommunicable diseases, scaling up measures to reduce risk factors (including unhealthy diet), strengthening health systems and services, and improving access to health care (Food and Agriculture Organization of the United Nations & WHO, 2019). Recently, the UN Food Systems Summit 2021 Working Group (Neufeld et al., 2020) proposed a definition of a healthy diet as one that promotes human health, prevents disease, safeguards planetary health by providing adequacy without excess of nutrients from foods that are nutritious and healthy, and avoids the introduction of health-harming substances through all stages of the value chain. Healthy diets are defined as affordable, culturally acceptable, and progressively changing toward systems that do not adversely affect local and regional ecologies. The UN Food Systems Summit 2021 Working Group has called for greater transparency and better management of commercial interests in research of the associations between food products and health outcomes. The goal is to eventually make recommendations that optimize human health outcomes based on individual characteristics and dietary patterns of populations. Responsibility for food safety is placed all along the value chain, including producers, processors, transporters, retailers, and consumers. To protect consumer health and fair-trade practices, the Working Group's challenge is engaging the food industry at all levels to understand their role in preventing food contamination through the application of good agricultural, manufacturing, and hygienic practices. Achieving sustainable food production and processing will require substantial changes in dietary practices across regions of the world—for example, reducing meat consumption where it is currently excessive. The evidence to inform the nature of those changes, and ways to ensure that the needs of vulnerable populations are not compromised, are economically feasible, and culturally acceptable, requires further investigation. For instance, foodborne illness may still be linked to poor hygiene conditions, close contact with animals, and limited access to clean water from market through household.

NURSING KNOWLEDGE BASE

Nutrition During Human Growth and Development

Infants Through School-Aged Children. Infancy is marked by rapid growth with high protein, vitamin, mineral, and energy requirements. According to the WHO, the average birth weight for male babies born full-term is 3.35 kg, or 7 pounds (lb) 6 ounces (oz); the average birth weight for female babies is 3.23 kg, or 7 lb 2 oz (De Pietro, 2021). A healthy birth weight for newborns ranges from 2.5 to 4.5 kg (Alberta Health Services, 2018). The infant usually doubles birth weight at 4 to 5 months and triples it at 1 year. An energy intake of approximately 110–120 kcal/kg/day is needed in the first 6 months, and 95–100 kcal/kg per day from 6 months to 1 year (Consolini, 2021). Commercial formulas and human breast milk each provide approximately 20 kcal/30 mL. A full-term newborn is able to digest and absorb simple carbohydrates, proteins, and a moderate amount of emulsified fat. Spitting up is a natural consequence of the baby's anatomy because the short esophagus and small stomach allow liquid to escape from the stomach easily (Mersch, 2019). Spitting up may occur during the first year, until the gastroesophageal sphincter (which opens to allow food to enter the stomach and gas to escape after meals) matures and the child learns to sit independently. Infants need 100 or more mL/kg per day of fluid because a large portion of their total body weight is water.

Breastfeeding. Health Canada, consistent with the WHO global recommendation for public health, recommends breastfeeding as the optimal method of infant feeding and the exclusive use of breast milk for the first 6 months of the infant's life, to be sustained for up to 2 years or longer with appropriate complementary feeding, for the nutrition, immunological protection, growth, and development of infants and toddlers (Public Health Agency of Canada [PHAC], 2019). Breastfeeding confers immunological and allergy protection to the infant during the period of breastfeeding, is economical and convenient (breast milk is always fresh and at the correct temperature), and provides an excellent opportunity for mother and infant to interact. Breast milk changes as a baby grows, is easier to digest than formula, helps protect against sudden infant death syndrome, and may also have a protective effect against obesity (Lyons et al., 2020). A daily vitamin D supplement of 400 IU is needed for breastfed infants (Alberta Health Services, 2019a). To ensure an infant's optimal vitamin D status, it is further suggested that breastfeeding parents also meet current recommended vitamin D intake during breastfeeding (Aghajafari et al., 2018). Other vitamin or mineral supplementation is not recommended for the first 6 months.

Breastfeeding initiation rates in Canada have increased from less than 25% in 1965 to 90% in 2015–16 (PHAC, 2021). Breastfeeding rates also varied across the country along a general west-to-east gradient, with the lowest rates occurring in Newfoundland and Labrador and the highest rates in British Columbia and the Yukon. Mothers living with lower income, lower education, history of trauma or substance use, social isolation, adolescent age, or immigrant status who participated in a Toronto program delivered under the Canada Prenatal Nutrition Program, reported being unprepared for the physical (e.g., pain), practical (e.g., cost of breastfeeding support and time pressures), and self-efficacy challenges (e.g., milk supply concerns and conflicting information) of breastfeeding (Francis et al., 2020). Provision of in-home support and services (e.g., nonjudgemental lactation consultant, electric breast pump) helped to address these breastfeeding challenges. Canadian health providers are encouraged to promote exclusive breastfeeding by creating an appropriate "baby-friendly" environment of awareness and support throughout the continuum of care from hospitals to community health services.

Formula. Commercially prepared infant formulas, cow's milk–based and iron fortified, are designed to contain the approximate nutrient composition of human milk. Protein in the formula is typically supplied as whey, soy, cow's milk base, casein hydrolysate, or elemental amino acids. The composition, processing, packaging, and labelling of all infant formulas are regulated under Canadian food and drug laws. Although it is now also possible to supplement commercial infant formula with probiotics for the treatment of infantile colic, a recent Cochrane review found no clear evidence that probiotics were effective at preventing infantile colic; yet daily crying time reduced with probiotic use compared to placebo (Ong et al., 2019).

Specialty formulas are indicated for infants with detected or suspected pathology. Health care providers caring for new mothers and their infants can address mothers' concerns about infant formulas and help them make informed choices when selecting the best substitute for human milk.

Regular cow's milk should not be used as the main dietary component during the first 12 months of life. Cow's milk does not provide optimal nutrient supply to the infant, introduces an excessively high intake of protein and fat during complementary feeding, and can increase risk for subsequent overweight or obesity (Marangoni et al.,

2019). Honey should not be used in the infant's diet, because it is a potential source of botulism toxin that can be fatal in children under 1 year of age (WHO, 2018a).

Introduction to Solid Food. Breast milk or formula provides sufficient nutrition for the first 6 months of the infant's life. However, Friel et al. (2018) concluded that there is not enough iron in breast milk to meet infant needs and they recommended introducing iron, given as either drops or in fortified foods, no earlier than 4 months and no later than 7 months, depending on the infant.

Cues indicating readiness for solid foods are the appearance of fine motor skills of the hand and fingers, hand-to-mouth movement, interest in adult food and self-feeding, increased milk consumption, ability to move food to the back of the mouth, and ability to sit alone in a highchair (Mayo Clinic Staff, 2021). Puréed smooth foods are typically the first semi-solid food to be introduced to an infant. The addition of foods should be governed by the infant's nutrient needs and physical readiness to handle different forms of foods and by the need to detect and control allergic reactions. New foods should be introduced one at a time, at least 3 to 4 days apart, to help determine if the baby is allergic. The new food should be prepared and served with little or no added salt or sugar. Commercial infant foods are not required, and they can be high in added sugar (Bernstein et al., 2020). The new food should be one single type of food, not a mixture of different foods (HealthLink BC, 2022).

Around the age of 6 months, open cups, rather than "sippy cups" with no-spill valves, are recommended to support the development of mature feeding skills by not holding the tongue tip down with each swallow (McNamee & Deleware, 2021). Caregivers need to be sensitive to the hunger and satiety cues of infants and young children. Responsive feeding allows the child to guide feeding and helps with encouraging self-feeding appropriate for the child's level of development.

It is important to consider that children are vulnerable to poor dietary intakes because their food choices are shaped by the foods that caregivers select and prepare. Household income, parental employment, and parental health affect the food choices available to children. In addition, food purchasing is influenced by convenience, commercial messages, and food marketing techniques that steer food choices in the direction of highly processed products (Health Canada, 2019b).

The growth rate slows during toddler years (ages 1 to 3 years). The toddler needs fewer kilocalories but an increased amount of protein in relation to body weight; consequently, appetite may decrease at about 18 months of age. Toddlers exhibit strong food preferences and can become picky eaters. Small, frequent meals consisting of breakfast, lunch, and dinner, with interspersed, nutrient-dense snacks, may improve nutritional intake (Ontario Dietitians in Public Health, 2019). Snacks work best mid-way between meals and should not be offered if the timing or quantity of snacking will interfere with the child's appetite for the next meal. Calcium and phosphorus are important for healthy bone growth. Whole milk should be used until the toddler reaches 2 years of age, to help ensure adequate intake of fatty acids for brain and neurological development. Young children who are breastfed or receiving breast milk should continue to receive a daily vitamin D supplement of 10 mcg (400 IU) until 2 years of age, when a vitamin D supplement is no longer recommended. Children's eating patterns should follow *Canada's Food Guide*. Toddlers who consume more than 720 mL of milk daily in lieu of other foods may develop milk anemia because milk is a poor source of iron.

The oral health of infants and children needs to focus on preventing cavities. Children who sleep with a bottle are at particular risk of developing early childhood tooth decay (ECTD), a severe type of tooth decay that can affect baby teeth, especially the upper front teeth. The sugars from the milk, juice, and drinks left in the mouth combine with bacteria in plaque to create an acid that damages the enamel of a tooth. The longer and more often food is left in the mouth, the greater the chance of developing ECTD. ECTD appears to be strongly associated with social determinants of health, including low household income and level of parental education or employment status. ECTD rates were higher in certain regions of Canada, including rural and remote northern communities, communities with a high proportion of Indigenous persons, other rural regions, and in the least affluent communities. In addition, Pierce and colleagues (2019) found associations between ECTD, the child's age at first dental visit, and parental beliefs about a child's oral health. Dental visits should begin within 6 months of the eruption of the first tooth or by 1 year of age at the latest. From the age of 3 years, twice-yearly dental inspections are recommended. Children under 3 years of age should have their teeth brushed by an adult, and parents need to supervise children less than 6 years of age during brushing (Canadian Dental Association, 2022).

For young children to develop healthy eating habits, a regular schedule of meals and snacks (i.e., three meals per day and two to three snacks) that offer a variety of foods prepared with little or no added salt or sugar is recommended. Nutritious, higher-fat foods are an important source of energy for young children. Dietary fat restriction is not recommended for children younger than 2 years of age because it may compromise a young child's intake of energy and essential fats and adversely affect growth and development. Frequent, nutrient-dense meals and snacks are important to meet a young child's needs for energy and nutrients. Continued breastfeeding should be encouraged, or up to 500 mL per day of homogenized (3.25% M.F.) cow's milk can be offered. Young children who are provided adequate nutrients and energy foods will self-select a nutritionally adequate diet. As with all age groups, fruit juice and sweetened beverages should be limited. Parents should encourage water to satisfy thirst. When caregivers act as role models they help instill lifelong healthy eating habits.

Preschoolers' (3 to 5 years old) dietary requirements are similar to those of toddlers. They consume slightly more than toddlers, and nutrient density is more important than quantity. Encouraging healthy eating is an important goal of parenting, and caregivers should try to use attractive food presentations and fun, educational initiatives rather than unhealthy food as a reward (Ontario Dietitians in Public Health, 2019). Because preschoolers have small stomachs, they need to eat small amounts of food more often throughout the day.

> **SAFETY ALERT** Foods such as hot dogs, hard candy, gum, cough drops, chewable vitamins, seeds, whole nuts, fish with bones, peanuts, marshmallows, grapes, raw vegetables, popcorn, and snacks on toothpicks or skewers have been implicated in choking deaths of preschoolers and toddlers and should be avoided for children younger than 4 years of age. Such foods should be prepared in a safe manner, for example, by dicing or cutting hot dogs or sausages lengthwise, grating raw carrots or hard fruits such as apples, removing pits from fruits, chopping grapes, thinly spreading nut butters on crackers or toast, and finely chopping fibrous or stringy foods such as celery, pineapple, or oranges (Ontario Dietitians in Public Health, 2019).

School-aged children, 6 to 12 years old, grow at a slower and steadier rate, with a gradual decline in energy requirements per unit of body weight. The school-aged child gains 3 to 5 kg in weight and 6 cm in height per year until puberty. Despite better appetites and more varied food intake, school-aged children's diets should be carefully assessed for adequate protein, vitamins, and minerals. School-aged children frequently fail to eat a proper breakfast and have an unsupervised food intake at school. Foods eaten during school hours represent approximately 26% of the total daily energy

consumed (Tugault-Lafleur & Black, 2020). Sugar-sweetened beverages contribute the largest proportion of sugar to the diets of 2- to 8-year-old children (21.8%) and 9- to 18-year-old youth (29.8%) compared with other sources of dietary sugar. Because overconsumption of sugared beverages displaces milk, which is rich in calcium and vitamin D, there is no reason to support the availability of these beverages in schools (Critch et al., 2020). Energy-adjusted intakes of vitamin A, vitamin D, vitamin B_{12}, calcium, and milk products were found to be substantially lower during school hours compared with non-school hours (Tugault-Lafleur et al., 2019). High amounts of fat, sugar, and salt can result from a liberal intake of commercially prepared snack foods. Recently, Grade 5 students from Ontario who participated in an 8-week food delivery program that included food literacy lesson plans demonstrated a significant improvement in fruit and vegetable intake (Woodruff et al., 2020). Consumption of fruits and vegetables is associated with reduced risk for chronic diseases, including cardiovascular disease, and all-cause mortality (Kim et al., 2019). Children who consumed fewer fruits and vegetables and skipped breakfast tended to be more vulnerable to obesity (Justamente et al., 2020).

Interventions to treat childhood obesity include multicomponent family-based behaviour-modification programs with supervised, structured exercise interventions, which have been found to improve blood pressure, inflammation, carotid artery intima media thickness, dysglycemia, dyslipidemia, and endothelial dysfunction in the short term. These interventions were not translated into long-term sustainable exercise or physical activity recommendations (McPhee et al., 2020). A review of school-based intervention studies with family involvement targeting dietary, physical activity, and sedentary behaviours among schoolchildren and their families identified the following effective interventions: teachers acting as role models actively involved in the delivery of the intervention, school policies supporting the availability of healthy food and beverage choices and limiting unhealthy snacks, increasing physical activity in the schoolyard during recess and in physical education classes, and encouraging parents via meetings and informative material to improve the home nutrition environment. Using incentives for children increased effectiveness. Programs that focused only on educational sessions and material for parents, without promoting relevant environmental and policy changes, were less effective. Cultural adaptations were recommended to increase the intervention's acceptance in specific or vulnerable population groups (Lambrinou et al., 2020).

Adolescents. Nutrition plays a critical role in transitioning from adolescence to healthy adulthood. During adolescence, physiological age is a better guide to nutritional needs than chronological age. Energy needs increase in order to meet the greater metabolic demands of growth. The daily requirement of protein also increases. Calcium and vitamin D are essential for the rapid bone growth that occurs in adolescence. Girls need a continuous source of iron to replace menstrual blood losses; boys need adequate iron for muscle development. In addition to meats and fish, fortified cereals, greens, nuts, dried fruits, and whole grains are iron-rich foods (Whitbread, 2022). Iodine supports increased thyroid activity, so adolescents' use of iodized table salt helps ensure adequate intake. B-complex vitamins are needed to support heightened metabolic activity.

Adolescents globally are consuming inadequate amounts of fruits and vegetables and alarmingly high levels of sodium and sugar. Less than half of adolescent girls in low- and middle-income countries reported eating dairy, fruits and vegetables, and meats. Even those who consumed fruits and vegetables daily did not meet the WHO dietary guidelines (Salam et al., 2019).

The adolescent's diet is influenced by factors other than nutritional needs, including concern about body image and appearance, desire for independence, and fad diets. Nutritional deficiencies may occur in adolescent girls as a result of dieting (Meija, 2019) and use of oral contraceptives (Bachrach, 2020). Adolescent girls may have inadequate intakes of calcium, vitamin B_6, vitamin B_{12}, folate, zinc, iron, magnesium, phosphorus, potassium, fibre, and vitamin A (Demory-Luce & Motil, 2022). The adolescent boy's diet may be inadequate in vitamin A and magnesium.

Snacks provide approximately 25% of teenagers' total dietary intake. Adolescents are encouraged to plan ahead to have healthy snacks available, to avoid the temptation of less healthy vending machine foods. Healthy options for snacking at school and work include apples, oatmeal, nut butter, canned fruit, canned tuna, plain popcorn, whole-grain crackers, and nuts, pumpkin seeds, or sunflower seeds (Health Canada, 2019b). Snacks like lower-fat yogourt or lower-fat cheese need to be kept in the refrigerator or in a cooler bag with an ice pack.

Adolescents often get their meals at fast-food restaurants, which offer larger portions of food, and the trend is that consumers are eating greater amounts (Elsevier, 2019). The consumption of fast foods has been associated with excess weight gain, which may be related to the higher energy and fat content of most of these foods. Many Canadian adolescents (79% of males and 63% of females 9 to 13 years old, and 92% of males and 50% of females 14 to 18 years old) report sodium intakes in excess of the upper intake level beyond which the risk of adverse health effects increases (Gowrishankar et al., 2020). Health promotion initiatives (e.g., reducing the availability of sugary drinks and junk foods in school cafeterias and vending machines) are being implemented in schools to develop supportive environments for healthier eating. In response, children aged 14 to 17 years who were eating lunch at school reported higher intakes of total fruits and vegetables, whole grains, fibre, vitamin C, and magnesium, and reported fewer calories from sugar-sweetened beverages compared with their peers who ate lunch off campus (Tugault-Lafleur & Black, 2020).

Canada's Food Guide (Health Canada, 2019b) directly encourages adolescents to work on building healthy eating habits through helping with grocery shopping, preparing meals and snacks (e.g., preparing breakfast the night before or bringing breakfast to early morning activities), being responsible for certain meals, and creating a grocery list. Adolescents are encouraged to eat meals with their families, eat without distractions (e.g., turn off the TV and put away phones, laptop computers, or other screens), and be aware of food marketing pressures. Finally, adolescents are urged to try including fruits and vegetables at every meal and to carry a reusable water bottle.

The onset of eating disorders such as **anorexia nervosa** or **bulimia nervosa** often occurs during early adolescence, when individuals are establishing independence and autonomy. Dieting and weight control are viewed as a defence for feelings of inadequacy or ineffectiveness. In later adolescence, when facing the task of separation–individualization, similar conflicts may arise (Weaver, 2018). Recognition of eating disorders, although more difficult to detect amid the pervasive diet culture, is essential for early intervention (Table 43.1).

Nurses who work with adolescents experiencing eating disorders need to be aware of the many implications that such a diagnosis can have on an adolescent. The ever-present threat to physical health must be carefully monitored. Beyond the illness and treatment, these youth experience difficult emotions and issues of identity, low self-esteem, and autonomy.

Sports and regular exercise necessitate dietary modification to meet the increased energy needs of adolescents. Carbohydrates, both simple and complex, are the main source of energy. Protein needs increase to 1.0 to 1.5 g/kg per day; fat needs do not increase. Athletes need to

TABLE 43.1	Potential Assessment for Eating Disorders

- Anorexia nervosa (AN) is the most predominant eating disorder for young women.
- AN presents as a body mass index (BMI) under 18.5 km/m^2 or less than fifth percentile in children or adolescents in relation to height, age, and developmental phase.
- The most common symptoms are obsessive fear of gaining weight, excessive preoccupation with being overweight, voluntary purging, and overexercising. The person is unable to rationally see their malnourished physical state. Death can result if weight continues to drop.
- Bradycardia with pulse under 50 beat per minute (bpm) indicates cardiovascular instability.
- Body temperature frequently drops below 36°C; the person may voluntarily induce hypothermia in order to shiver, consume energy, and lose more weight.
- Other signs may include pale conjunctives, dry tongue and skin, muscular weakness, peripheral edema, and hand calluses after self-induced vomiting.
- Physical consequences such as amenorrhea and osteopenia may occur.
- Pulse, blood pressure, and electrocardiogram (ECG) measurements can reveal cardiac complications. Blood is tested for liver, renal, and thyroid function, along with plasma ferritin, folate, and B_{12} vitamin.
- Bulimia nervosa is characterized by binge eating episodes and compensatory behaviours to prevent weight gain but, unlike with AN, the person may not be underweight, even when preoccupied by body shape image.
- Eating disorders are associated with other psychiatric conditions, especially mood disorders, anxiety disorders, post-traumatic stress disorder, substance use disorder, and personality or conduct disorder.

Based on Suciu, B., & Crisan, C. A. (2020). Feeding and eating disorders. In K. F. Shad & K. H. Dogan (Eds.), *Neurological and mental disorders*. InTechOpen. https://doi.org/10.5772/intechopen.92218. https://www.intechopen.com/books/neurological-and-mental-disorders/feeding-and-eating-disorders

ingest water before and after exercise to prevent dehydration, especially in hot environments. It is not necessary to supplement the diet with vitamins and minerals, but intake of iron-rich foods is required to prevent anemia (Burden & Pedlar, 2018) and foods high in calcium and vitamin D to prevent stress fractures (Knechtle et al., 2021).

Parents often have more influence over the adolescent diet than they believe they have. Effective strategies include limiting unhealthy foods kept at home and enhancing the appearance and taste of healthy foods. Making healthy foods more convenient and available and monitoring teen-targeted food-promotion strategies are ways to promote optimal nutritional health among adolescents (Truman & Elliott, 2019).

Pregnancy occurring within 4 years of menarche may place the pregnant person and fetus at risk because of the mother's anatomical and physiological immaturity. Most teenage girls do not want to gain weight, thus counselling adolescent pregnant persons on the nutritional needs associated with pregnancy may be difficult; suggestions are better tolerated than rigid directions. The diet of pregnant adolescents is often deficient in calcium, iron, and vitamins A and C. Prenatal vitamin and mineral supplements are recommended.

Young and Middle-Aged Adults. The demands for most nutrients are reduced as the growth period ends. Adults need nutrients for energy, maintenance, and repair, although their energy needs usually decline over the years. Obesity may become a problem as a result of decreased physical exercise, frequent dining out, and the increased

BOX 43.2 CASE STUDY

Nondiabetic Ketoacidosis Resulting From an Obesogenic Environment*

Tom (preferred pronouns: he, him), a 25-year-old, arrived at the emergency department (ED) with severe nausea, vomiting, and anorexia. In an attempt to lose weight, he had increased vigorous exercise and started the low-carbohydrate ketogenic diet several days earlier. Laboratory results showed elevated ketone, low pH, and normal blood glucose levels. He had no history of diabetes and consequently was diagnosed with nondiabetic ketoacidosis secondary to the ketogenic diet. Tom was admitted to a medical unit where, overnight, his potassium levels depleted due to excess vomiting, and his pH levels rose to 7.64. Nondiabetic ketoacidosis can be a life-threatening condition if it is left untreated (Alkhayat et al., 2020). As Tom's nurse, I provided around-the-clock antiemetics, intravenous (IV) potassium replacement, and hypotonic IV fluids. I provided ongoing support, as he was frightened about his state of illness. We discussed alternate healthy forms of weight loss, such as eating balanced, healthy meals with frequent exercise, rather than excessive dieting and exercising. Tom recognized that his dieting behaviours aimed for quick weight loss to achieve an unrealistic body standard as portrayed in the media. Following multiple days of treatment, he was discharged home. Afterward, I reflected on the fact that the creators of new diets often criticize traditional weight-loss dietary advice, and that nurses are challenged to give proper information to individuals, families, groups, and communities affected by the diet culture.

*Written by Morgan Rogers, BN, GN, University of New Brunswick.

ability to afford more luxury foods. Adults often engage in dieting behaviours to control or reduce their weight and to prevent diseases, such as high blood pressure, heart disease, type 2 diabetes, and certain cancers. The case study in Box 43.2 conveys a nurse's experiences caring for a young adult presenting with ketoacidosis as a consequence of following a ketogenic diet.

Poor oral hygiene and periodontal disease are potential risk factors for systemic diseases such as bacteremia, endocarditis, cardiopulmonary disease, and diabetes mellitus and for adverse outcomes in pregnancy (Lim et al., 2020). Women who use oral contraceptives may need extra vitamins. Iron and calcium intake also continues to be important.

Pregnancy. Nutrition during pregnancy influences birth weight and survival chances in infants. Generally, the fetus's needs are met at the expense of the pregnant person. If nutrient sources are not available or are unsafe (such as foods affected by the *Listeria* bacteria, which can cross through the placenta), both will suffer. Food poisoning during the first 3 months of pregnancy can cause a miscarriage. Later in the pregnancy, it can cause the baby to be born prematurely, a stillbirth, or very ill. Thus, it is paramount that pregnant persons are careful about what they eat and how they store, prepare, and cook their food. To lower the risk of food poisoning, pregnant persons should avoid eating hot dogs and non-dried deli meats straight from the package, dishes containing raw eggs or seafood, unpasteurized dairy products and fruit juices, raw sprouts, and pâtés and meat spreads that have to be refrigerated before use (Health Canada, 2021). The nutritional status of the pregnant person at the time of conception is important because significant aspects of fetal growth and development often occur before pregnancy is suspected.

The energy requirements associated with pregnancy are related to the pregnant person's body weight and activity levels. Pregnant persons need 100 kcal per day above the usual allowance during the first trimester and approximately 300 extra calories per day in the second and third trimesters. The additional nutrients should be obtained by adding a healthy extra snack or extra food to a meal. Some examples include fruit and yogurt, cereal with milk, an extra piece of toast at breakfast and milk at supper, spinach salad (made with spinach, hard-boiled egg, and walnuts), half an English muffin topped with Swiss cheese and sliced pear, or a bowl of cooked oatmeal made with ground almonds, applesauce, and cinnamon to taste (Health Canada, 2022e). A sample weekly menu is available at "My Menu Planner": https://www.unlockfood.ca/en/MenuPlanner.aspx. It is recommended by Health Canada that pregnant persons have at least 150 g of cooked fish each week to ensure omega-3 fats and other important nutrients and take a multivitamin containing 0.4 mg of folic acid and 16 to 20 mg of iron every day (Alberta Health Services, 2019b). Rigid recommendations about weight gain should be avoided because the quality of nutrition during pregnancy is more important than weight gain per se or than the number of kilocalories consumed per day.

Calcium intake is especially critical during the third trimester, when fetal bones are mineralized. Iron may be supplemented to provide for increased maternal blood volume, fetal blood storage, and maternal blood loss during delivery. Iodine needs increase 15 to 17% because of increased activity of the thyroid gland. Folic acid intake is particularly important for DNA synthesis and the growth of red blood cells; inadequate intake may lead to fetal neural tube defects and anencephaly (Centers for Disease Control and Prevention, 2022) or maternal preeclampsia (Serrano et al., 2018). Therefore, Health Canada (2022e) recommends that pregnant persons supplement their daily diet with 0.4 mg of folic acid and 16 to 20 mg of iron and that, when possible, folic acid be taken for at least three months before pregnancy. If it is determined that a pregnant person may benefit from a higher level of supplemental folic acid, a health care provider may wish to measure the person's red blood cell folate concentration to determine the most appropriate dose of folic acid.

It is important to keep variety in the daily diet while pregnant. Accordingly, pregnant persons are advised to eat plenty of fruits and vegetables; choose dark green and orange vegetables; choose whole-grain foods like bread, rice, and pasta; choose lean meats, dried peas, beans, tofu, and lentils; and have cooked fish each week. Dairy products like yogourt and cheese contribute to healthy bones for both the pregnant person and baby. Pregnant persons who do not drink milk are advised to drink fortified soy beverages (Health Canada, 2022e) and need to drink plenty of water. They should also avoid intake of artificial sweeteners, alcohol, excessive caffeine, and all medications not specifically ordered, as these substances pass through the placenta and affect the growing baby. Adequate fluid and fibre intake and moderate exercise help prevent constipation, which is commonly associated with pregnancy in response to the growing uterus, pregnancy hormones, and iron supplementation.

Lactation. Lactating persons need 500 kcal per day above the usual allowance because milk production increases energy requirements. The need for calcium remains the same as during pregnancy, but lactating persons who do not get enough vitamin A, thiamin, riboflavin, vitamin B_6, vitamin B_{12}, selenium, and iodine through diet alone may need to take supplements to ensure good breast milk quality (Butte & Stuebe, 2022). This is because both fat-soluble (vitamins A, D, K) and water-soluble vitamins (vitamins C, B_1, B_6, B_{12}, and folate) are secreted into breast milk, and their levels are reduced in breast milk when there is a maternal vitamin deficiency. Fluid intake should be adequate but need not be excessive. Caffeine, alcohol, and drugs are excreted in breast milk.

BOX 43.3 FOCUS ON OLDER PERSONS

Factors Affecting Nutritional Status

- Age-related gastrointestinal changes that affect digestion of food and maintenance of nutrition include changes in the teeth and gums, decreased bite force, reduced saliva production, atrophy of oral mucosal epithelial cells, increased taste threshold, decreased thirst sensation, reduced gag reflex, and decreased esophageal and colonic peristalsis (Dumic et al., 2019).
- Presence of other diseases, such as diabetes and cognitive impairments related to delirium, dementia, and depression, increase risk of poor nutrition (Tamura et al., 2020).
- Malnutrition in older persons has multiple causes, such as low income, low educational level, lack of physical functional level to meet activities of daily living, loss, dependency, loneliness, and lack of transportation (Besora-Moreno et al., 2020).

- Medications may have adverse effects, such as causing anorexia (loss of appetite), xerostomia (severe dryness of the mouth), early satiety, and impaired smell and taste perception (Mohn et al., 2018). Older persons are more likely to be prescribed medications than are younger individuals.
- Intake of calcium, vitamin D, and phosphorus may be deficient, increasing the risk for osteoporosis. Vitamin B_{12} may be deficient among older persons because of the high prevalence of gastrointestinal pathology and use of medications that alter vitamin B_{12} pharmacokinetics (Corcoran et al., 2019).
- Many nutrients interact with medications, and nurses should consult a drug handbook for information about specific interactions.

Most breastfeeding persons can drink a moderate amount of caffeine (i.e., 2–3 cups of a caffeinated beverage, such as coffee) per day without it affecting their infants; however, some young infants are sensitive to caffeine and become irritable or have difficulty sleeping, even with exposure to small amounts of caffeine (Butte & Stuebe, 2022). It takes a 60-kg person about 3 hours to eliminate from their body the alcohol in two servings of alcohol, each serving defined as 355 mL (12 ounces) of beer (4.5%), 120 mL (4 ounces) of table wine (12%), or 30 mL (1 ounce) of 100 proof whiskey (Drugs and Lactation Database, 2022).

Older Persons. Adults aged 65 years and older have a decreased need for energy because the metabolic rate slows with age. However, vitamin and mineral requirements remain unchanged from middle adulthood. Healthy eating maintains an older person's healthy weight, promotes and protects health and well-being, provides essential energy and nutrients, prevents and lowers the risk or slows the progression of chronic diseases (e.g., heart disease, type 2 diabetes), and prevents muscle and bone loss to reduce risk of falling or fractures (Health Canada, 2019b).

Many factors influence the nutritional status of older persons (Box 43.3). Income is significant because for those living on a fixed income, the amount of money available to buy food may be reduced. Health status is another important factor. The older person may be following a therapeutic diet; have difficulty eating because of physical symptoms, lack of teeth, or dentures; or be at risk for medication–nutrient interactions. Thirst sensation may diminish, leading to inadequate fluid intake or dehydration (see Chapter 41). Meats may be avoided because of the cost or difficulty to chew.

Older persons are encouraged to eat a variety of healthy foods to ensure they get enough different nutrients. *Canada's Food Guide* suggests that older persons choose fruits and vegetables, whole grains, and protein foods they enjoy. Frozen and canned options can be just as healthy and are easier to prepare. To accommodate for changes in sense of taste or smell, different spices and herbs can add more flavour, instead of salt. Choosing and preparing foods differently (e.g., cooking vegetables instead of eating them raw) can soften texture. Milk continues to be an important food for older persons to protect against osteoporosis (a decrease of bone-mass density). Although research has shown that older men lag behind women by approximately a decade in developing osteoporosis, it is recommended that both older men and women assess their risk of having a major fracture associated with osteoporosis, using available fracture-prediction tools that have been tested in the Canadian population (i.e., *WHO Fracture Risk Calculation Tool (FRAX®) for Canada, Canadian Association of Radiologist and Osteoporosis Canada (CAROC) Risk Assessment Tool*). To reduce risk of developing osteoporosis, lifestyle factors include regular

BOX 43.4 CASE STUDY

Balancing Nutrition Amidst Loneliness and a Global Pandemic*

George, an 83-year-old individual (preferred pronouns: he, him) living on Prince Edward Island, became widowed after losing his wife of 60 years. George's four children, who live in other Maritime provinces, supported him in learning to live alone. Initially, George had visitors often, and his daughters ensured that his freezer was stocked with easily prepared nutritious meals because George had never cooked. However, when the COVID-19 pandemic limited travel across provinces, George was challenged to prepare meals on his own. Getting groceries was difficult because George no longer drove; pandemic anxiety, limited transportation options, heavy bags, and long waiting in lines further deterred him. With minimal cooking knowledge, George often chose precooked, frozen, microwaveable meals or snacks. Although George had always enjoyed eating when the table was filled with loved ones and home-cooked meals that his wife prepared, he now felt cold and empty sitting alone, eating a warmed-up frozen dinner.

During a home care visit from a social worker and foot care nurse, George spoke of anxiety, disinterest in food and eating, and difficulty preparing meals. He discussed recent health changes of hypertension, increased A_1C, constipation, and decreased energy. George was helped to connect with a local service that delivered affordable daily nutritious meals. George was also connected with a companionship program for visiting and help with grocery shopping. The variety in meals and nutritious ingredients, along with the friendly social interaction, had positive impacts on George's mental and physical health. Soon after, George learned to use Facetime and ate meals virtually with his children! This case illuminates the precarious nutritional position of many older persons who sheltered in place to avoid exposure to COVID-19.

*Written by Katie Lamarche BN, RN, University of New Brunswick, Fredericton Downtown Community Health Centre.

weight-bearing and resistance-type exercise, as well as adequate vitamin and mineral intake (PHAC, 2022).

No matter where they live, older persons might struggle to have access to groceries. *Canada's Food Guide* recommends creating an emergency food supply by stocking their pantry with a variety of nonperishable food items (e.g., peanut butter, skim milk powder, canned fruits and vegetables, canned fish and legumes, and whole-grain pasta and oatmeal) to make a few meals for times when they are unable to get to the store. Box 43.4 depicts the effect of the COVID-19 pandemic on an older person's sense of food security and well-being.

Alternative Food Patterns

Many people follow special patterns of food intake that are based on religion (Table 43.2). For example, because of strong religious feelings against killing or eating cattle, certain groups do not eat meat. Individuals practising Muslim and Jewish faiths can eat meat only if it has been killed or prepared in certain ways governed by religious laws.

Food intake is also influenced by cultural background (Box 43.5), ethics, health beliefs, personal preference, or concern for the efficient use of land to produce food. Such special diets are not necessarily more or less nutritious than diets based on *Canada's Food Guide* or other nutritional guidelines, because good nutrition depends on a balanced intake of all required nutrients.

TABLE 43.2 Religion-Based Dietary Restrictions and Guidelines

Islam	Christianity	Hinduism	Judaism	Church of Jesus Christ of Latter-Day Saints (Mormons)
• Pork • Alcohol • Emulsifiers made from animal fats • Ramadan fasting sunrise to sunset for 1 month • Ritualized methods of animal slaughter required for meat ingestion	Holy-day observances may restrict meat. *Catholicism:* • Meat is not allowed on Fridays during Lent. • Fasting is expected on Good Friday and Ash Wednesday. *Eastern Orthodox Christians:* • Weekly fasts require abstention from alcohol, eggs, dairy, fish, meat, and olive oil. *Seventh-Day Adventists:* • Avoid fish, poultry, and other meat • Will eat some animal products, such as eggs and dairy • Avoid alcohol • A lacto-ovo-vegetarian diet is encouraged.	• Follow lacto-vegetarian diet • Do not eat meats, eggs, fish, or poultry • Do eat dairy • Onions, leek, scallion, chives, and garlic excluded • No prohibition on anything that does not cause any harm to self and others • Observe several fasting periods, some of which are limited to plant foods • New Moon days, holy days, and festivals require fasting.	• Pork • Shellfish (eat only fish with scales) • Rare meats • Blood (blood sausage, etc.) • Do not mix milk or dairy products with meat dishes • Must adhere to kosher food preparation methods • Observe 24 hours of fasting on Yom Kippur, a day of atonement • No leavened bread eaten during Passover (8 days) • No cooking on the Sabbath (Saturday)	• Alcohol • Tobacco • Caffeine • Limit meat • Eat respectfully and with appreciation through portion control, zero waste, and avoiding overindulgence

🌐 BOX 43.5 CULTURAL ASPECTS OF CARE

Nutrition

For most people, food patterns developed as a child through habits and culture interact to influence food intake. Food is the first thing parents give to their children, usually in the moments after birth. Love, education, protection, and advice are all offered; however, a tall glass of milk or a second helping of homemade casserole that can be immediately seen can make parents feel they have done something positive for their child. Thus, food and food habits serve as a focus of emotional association, with the sharing of food symbolizing a high degree of social intimacy and acceptance. Foods may be highly prized, reserved for special holidays, or mark social position.

Baby boomer parents may urge their children to have "one more bite"—seemingly equating food with love. As well, children are often rewarded for "being good" with a treat. They then associate the treat with "being good." In different cultures, certain foods are considered "heavy," "light," "foods for strength," "luxury," and so on. To illustrate, the theory of "hot" and "cold" foods predominates in traditional Asian medicine (Xie et al., 2020). Foods that can raise the body's inner heat, improve the circulation, and nourish the energy of the body are warm or hot foods; those that can calm the blood, clear toxins, and reduce heat are cold or cool foods. Classification of a food has nothing to do with spiciness but symbolically represents temperature. Some cultures believe that in order to keep harmony with nature, one must balance "cold," which represents menace and weakness, with hot, which characterizes warmth, strength, and reassurance.

In addition to culture influencing food intake and meanings of food, one's ethnicity may influence tolerance for specific foods. For example, the incidence of lactose intolerance around the world occurs in various ethnic or racial groups: Asian-Pacific, African, Indigenous North American, Mexican, Middle Eastern, and White individuals. This condition affects nutrient absorption, and calcium deficiency results. See Table 42.6 for food lists appropriate to lactose intolerance diets.

Implications for Practice
- Identify the meaning that certain types of food have for each patient.
- Lactose and other food intolerances unique to specific cultures require diet adaptation to meet nutrient, mineral, and vitamin daily-intake requirements.
- In some cultures, specific conditions require "hot" foods. Menstruation, cancer, pneumonia, earache, colds, paralysis, headache, and rheumatism are "cold" illnesses requiring "hot" foods (e.g., rice, grain cereals, alcohol, chocolate, pistachio nuts).
- Other conditions, such as pregnancy, fever, infections, diarrhea, rashes, ulcers, liver conditions, constipation, kidney conditions, and sore throats, are "hot" conditions requiring "cold" foods (e.g., beans, citrus fruits, dairy products, most fresh vegetables).
- An intimate, detailed knowledge of patients' different customs and beliefs, attitudes, and behaviours will help to determine why certain practices exist, how difficult it will be to change them, if necessary, and what techniques can be expected to be most helpful for initiating diet changes. Nutrition education that has proved disappointing could relate to the patient's retention of customs. Only changes in keeping with people's established food habits will be acceptable.
- It is wrong to use standards appropriate in industrialized societies as a measure of the nutritional adequacy of the diet of other and developing societies.

Adapted from Giger, J. N., & Haddad, L. (2020). *Transcultural nursing: Assessment and intervention* (8th ed.). Elsevier.

Vegetarian Diet. **Vegetarianism** is the consumption of a predominantly plant food diet. Vegetarian diets, in general, are low in saturated fat and cholesterol and high in fibre, folate, antioxidants such as vitamin C and E, potassium, and magnesium. Because of this, vegetarian diets may lower blood pressure, improve cholesterol levels, promote healthier weight, reduce incidence of type 2 diabetes (Heart and Stroke Foundation, 2022c), and prevent cancer (Madigan & Karhu, 2018).

Vegetarian diets may include the following:
1. *Semi or partial-vegetarian:* May eat some milk products, eggs, poultry, and fish while primarily consuming plant-based foods
2. *Pesco-vegetarian:* May eat fish, eggs, dairy products, grains, vegetables, fruits, legumes, seeds, nuts while avoiding meat and poultry
3. *Lacto-ovo-vegetarian:* Eating eggs, dairy products, grains, vegetables, fruits, legumes, seeds, nuts while avoiding meat, poultry, and fish
4. *Lacto-vegetarian:* Eating dairy products, grains, vegetables, fruits, legumes, seeds, nuts while avoiding meat, fish, poultry, and eggs
5. *Vegan:* Eating grains, vegetables, fruits, legumes, seeds, nuts while avoiding meat, fish, poultry, eggs, dairy, and honey

Appropriately planned vegetarian diets can help prevent colon cancer (Rose & Strombom, 2019). Specifically, vegan diets seem to confer lower risk for overall and for female-specific cancer, compared to other dietary patterns (Madigan & Karhu, 2018); lacto-ovo-vegetarian diets are linked to a lower risk of gastrointestinal tract cancers (American Institute for Cancer Research, 2021).

It may take planning across the lifespan to get enough protein, iron, zinc, calcium, vitamins D and B₁₂, and omega-3 fats from foods or supplements (Dietitians of Canada, 2019a). As a general rule, adults less than 65 years of age need approximately 0.8 grams of protein for every kilogram of body weight. This means that a 30-year-old person weighing 60 kg requires approximately (60 kg × 0.8) or 48 grams of protein daily. Adults over 65 years of age need more protein (1.0 gram of protein per kg of body weight) because the production of endogenous (used in the body) proteins from dietary proteins is impaired by reduced postprandial amino acid availability and decreased muscle blood flow (Richter et al., 2019). A range of plant protein products are needed because particular amino acids that are abundant in some foods may be limited in other foods and vice versa. By consuming a wide variety of foods, the amino acids "complement" each other to provide the essential amino acids in proper balance. *Canada's Food Guide* combines previous categories of "meat and alternatives" and "milk and milk products" into the new category of proteins that includes foods such as beans, lentils, nuts, seeds, lean meats and poultry, fish, shellfish, eggs, lower-fat milk and lower-fat dairy products. Canadians are instructed to "choose protein foods that come from plants more often." As stated earlier, plant-based protein foods can provide more fibre and less saturated fat than other types of protein foods. This can be beneficial for cardiovascular health. The guidelines also provide several recipes, many of which are vegan, such as tofu and vegetable stir fry, fresh avocado and bean lettuce wrap, and creamy hummus.

Recognizing that iron deficiency is the most common nutritional deficiency in children, it is essential that foods rich in iron are included for this population. Canadian adolescent girls and women of reproductive age who are vegetarian are at greater risk for low iron stores because the form of iron present in foods of plant origin is not well absorbed by the body (Rudloff et al., 2019); the rate of absorption can be increased by incorporating foods high in vitamin C, such as oranges and grapefruit and their juices, lemons, limes, kiwis, mangos, cantaloupe, potatoes, sweet peppers, broccoli, snow peas, and some green leafy vegetables (Dietitians of Canada, 2019a). Competitive athletes practising vegetarianism need almost twice the iron of nonvegetarian athletes and should have their iron checked periodically by their health care provider to determine if a supplement is needed (Wirnitzer,

2020). Vegan iron sources include firm or extra firm tofu, pinto and adzuki beans, almonds, and sesame seeds; iron is additionally found in fruits such as prunes, raisins, and apricots; dark green vegetables such as collards, okra, and bok choy; and blackstrap molasses (Dietitians of Canada, 2019b).

Calcium, zinc, and vitamin B₁₂ deserve special attention in vegetarian food guidelines. In addition to fortified soy drinks and products (e.g., soy yogourts, tofu), good vegan sources of calcium include navy beans and white beans; nuts and nut products like almonds and almond butter; seeds like sesame seeds and their butter (tahini); blackstrap molasses; vegetables such as bok choy, okra, collard greens, and turnip greens; and fruits like figs and fortified orange juice (Dietitians of Canada, 2018). Zinc is found in soy products; dried beans, peas, and lentils; nuts such as peanuts, pecans, and cashews; seeds such as pumpkin and flax; and whole grains and fortified cereals. Vegan diets do not provide vitamin B₁₂. It is recommended that vitamin B₁₂ be supplemented in people of all age groups who follow a strict vegan diet without consuming animal products. As well, Health Canada (Dietitians of Canada, 2019c) recommends that all people over the age of 50, regardless of type of diet, include foods fortified with vitamin B₁₂ (e.g., fortified nondairy milks, fortified meat alternatives, and breakfast cereals) in their daily food choices. Red Star nutritional yeast is the only brand of nutritional yeast in Canada fortified with vitamin B₁₂. It has a similar flavour to cheese and can be sprinkled on top of casseroles and in soups.

Vegan diets require a source of vitamin D when sun exposure is insufficient. Good sources of vitamin D include fortified soy and other fortified nondairy drinks and soft margarines (Dietitians of Canada, 2018). A vegetarian diet in childhood and adolescence requires good information and supervision by a pediatrician and, if necessary, an appropriately trained dietary specialist.

CRITICAL THINKING

Critical thinking requires gathering and synthesizing of knowledge, experience, and information from patients gained through intellectual and professional standards. Clinical judgements involve anticipating and analyzing required information, while being open to new ideas and multiple perspectives in decision making. Critical thinking is thus a dynamic process. During assessment (Figure 43.4), all elements that contribute to formulating appropriate nursing diagnoses are considered.

When assessing nutrition, the nurse integrates knowledge from nursing and other disciplines, previous experiences, information gathered from patients and families about food preferences, clinical observations, and dietary history. Professional standards, such as the DRIs and *Canada's Food Guide* (Health Canada, 2019b), provide guidelines for assessing and maintaining patient nutritional status. Other research-based standards from the Heart and Stroke Foundation of Canada, the Canadian Cancer Society, Canadian Society for Clinical Nutrition, and Diabetes Canada are available.

❖ NURSING PROCESS AND NUTRITION

Nurses are in an excellent position to recognize signs of poor nutrition and take steps to initiate change. Close contact with patients and their families enables nurses to make observations about physical status, food intake, weight changes, and responses to therapy.

◆ Assessment

Malnutrition is commonly overlooked in hospitalized patients. As many as 30–50% of patients show risk of malnutrition at admission, and malnutrition is a major contributor to increased morbidity and mortality, decreased quality of life, longer hospitalizations, more

Knowledge
- Normal nutrition parameters
- Anatomy and physiology of gastrointestinal system
- Cultural influences on nutrition
- Developmental factors affecting nutrition
- Effects of medications on nutritional status

Experience
- Caring for patients with altered nutrition
- Observation of nutritional practices of friends and family
- Personal assessment of nutritional practices

Assessment
- Identify the signs and symptoms associated with altered nutrition
- Gather data from patients regarding nutritional practices
- Determine patient's nutritional energy needs (REE 3 activity or illness factor)
- Obtain patient's dietary history

Standards
- Apply intellectual standards of accuracy, completeness, and significance when obtaining a health history for patients with altered nutrition
- Compare gathered data with established nutritional standards (e.g., dietary reference intake and *Eating Well With Canada's Food Guide*)

Qualities
- Be open-minded about the patient's nutritional practices when assessing nutritional status
- Display confidence when collecting data related to culture, socioeconomic status, physical functioning, dietary restrictions, and personal preferences as necessary for a complete nutritional assessment

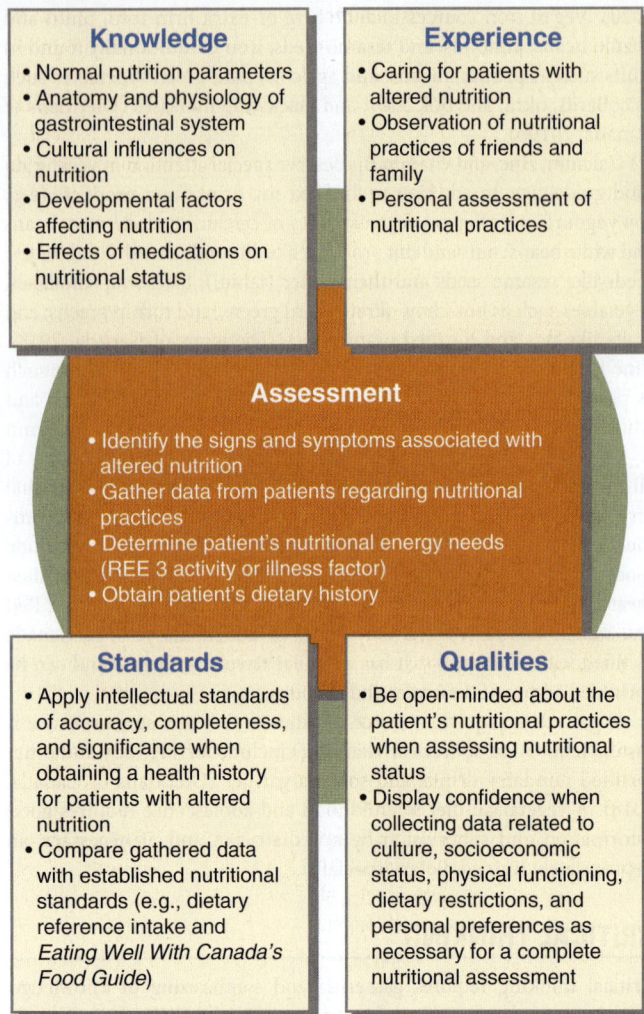

FIGURE 43.4 Critical thinking model for nutrition assessment. *REE,* Resting energy expenditure.

TABLE 43.3	Canadian Nutrition Screening Tool (CNST)		
Ask the Patient the Following Questions		**Yes**	**No**

1. Have you lost weight in the past 6 months without trying to lose this weight?
   - If the patient reports a weight loss but gained it back, consider it as a NO weight loss.
2. Have you been eating less than usual for more than a week?
   - Two "YES" answers indicate nutrition risk.
   - If the patient is uncertain regarding weight loss, ask if clothing is now fitting more loosely.
   - If the patient is unable to answer the questions, a knowledgeable informant can be asked to provide the information.

From Alberta Health Services. (2018). *Canadian Nutrition Screening Tool (CNST): Frequently asked questions.* https://www.albertahealthservices.ca/assets/info/nutrition/if-nfs-cnst-faq.pdf

to eat), sensory impairment (to consider ability to see, smell, and taste food), skin (to observe for signs of dehydration), clothes (to observe if clothes are too big, suggesting possible weight loss), hands (to determine adequacy of dexterity to open packaging or grasp cutlery), legs (to consider restricted mobility for community-dwelling individuals who must buy food or prepare meals), and urine output (to monitor for dehydration). As well, inadequate food intake (<50% of meals provided) needs to be identified and patients weighed weekly (Mahli, 2018).

Nutritional assessment goes beyond nutritional screening and involves anthropometry, laboratory tests, dietary and health history, clinical observation and physical examination, and patient expectations. Nutritional status is assessed when a condition exists that interferes with the patient's ability to ingest, digest, or absorb adequate nutrition. No single area or measurement accurately determines nutritional status. A patient's personal and social health context needs to be considered.

Anthropometry. **Anthropometry** is a measurement system of the size and makeup of the body. Patient height and weight are obtained for each admission. If height cannot be measured with the patient standing, the nurse should position the patient lying flat in bed as straight as possible with arms folded on the chest, and measure the patient lengthwise. If possible, the patient should be weighed at the same time each day, on the same scale, and with the same apparel. Serial measures over time provide more useful information than one-time measurement. An **ideal body weight (IBW)** provides an estimate of what a person should weigh. Rapid weight gain usually reflects fluid shifts. Five hundred mL of fluid equals 0.45 kg. For example, for a patient with renal failure or heart failure, a weight increase of 0.9 kg is significant, as it may indicate that the patient has retained a litre of fluid. Recent weight changes should be documented.

Body mass index (BMI) measures weight corrected for height and serves as an alternative to traditional height–weight relationships. Calculation of BMI is achieved by dividing the patient's weight in kilograms by height in metres squared: Weight (kg)/Height^2 (m^2). The BMI nomogram is available on Health Canada's website, at https://www.hc-sc.gc.ca/fn-an/nutrition/weights-poids/guide-ld-adult/bmi_chart_java-graph_imc_java-eng.php. A BMI measuring between 25 and 30 indicates overweight (Health Canada, 2019c). A BMI greater than 30 may begin to define obesity, a progressive,

frequent readmissions, and increased resource utilization—all leading to higher health care costs (Siegel et al., 2019). Bélanger and colleagues (2019) found 19.5% of a sample of 307 hospitalized Canadian children (median age of 5.3 years) were malnourished on admission, and nearly half of the patients studied lost weight during their hospital stay. The high prevalence of overall malnutrition suggests that initial screening using simple anthropometric measures should be conducted on hospital admission so that patients can receive appropriate nutrition-specific care.

Nutritional screening is a process of identifying characteristics associated with nutrition problems to identify those who would benefit from an individual nutritional care plan established by a nutrition specialist (e.g., dietitian, expert clinician) in consultation with an interprofessional team and monitored regularly throughout the hospital stay (Reber et al., 2019). The Canadian Nutrition Screening Tool (CNST) (Table 43.3) consists of two questions about weight loss and fluid intake. Two "YES" answers indicate increased nutritional risk.

Screening should be undertaken upon admission to a hospital ward and weekly thereafter at a basic level and should focus on the following areas: cognitive function (to consider impaired ability to recognize hunger and thirst, experience loss of appetite, or remember

relapsing chronic disease in which excess or abnormal fat (adipose) tissue impairs health (Wharton et al., 2020). Under this definition, body size and weight do not equal obesity. A patient could be classified as "normal weight" based on BMI, but still be diagnosed with obesity if they have excess or abnormal fat that impairs health (e.g., adiposity around organs). Conversely, a patient who has a high BMI and impaired health is distinguished from someone who may just be living in a larger body.

The BMI is a valid measurement of weight in relation to health; however, it is not recommended for use as the sole measurement of body composition or level of fitness because it does not differentiate between excess fat and muscle or bone and does not consider age, gender, or ethnicity (Armstrong, 2019). Care must further be taken when interpreting overweight and obesity results for Canadian childhood obesity, because cutoff points different from adult cutoffs have been used. The Canadian Task Force on Preventive Care, College of Family Physicians of Canada, Dietitians of Canada, Canadian Paediatric Society, and Community Health Nurses of Canada all recommend using the 2014 WHO growth charts (Growth Chart Canada, 2021).

The waist circumference (WC) measurement may help determine health risk. Overweight people who carry excess pounds around the waist are at greater risk for heart disease and stroke than those who carry it on their hips, thighs, and buttocks. The WC is measured at the part of the trunk located midway between the lower costal margin (bottom of lower rib) and the iliac crest (top of pelvic bone) while the person is standing, with feet slightly apart. The person doing the measuring should stand beside the individual and fit the tape snugly, without compressing underlying soft tissues. The circumference should be measured to the nearest 0.5 cm, at the end of a normal expiration. In men, a WC of 102 cm (40 inches) or greater places them at significant increased risk for heart disease and stroke. In women, this measurement is 88 cm (35 inches) or more. Using BMI and WC together is recommended to better identify the risk of obesity than using either BMI or WC alone, particularly in individuals with lower BMI (Wharton et al., 2020).

Canadian clinical practice guidelines on management of obesity in adults were developed by Obesity Canada and the Canadian Association of Bariatric Physicians and Surgeons. These guidelines (published in 2020) recommend that health care providers recognize obesity as a chronic disease, obtain patient permission to offer advice, and help treat this disease in an unbiased manner. A summary of the recommendations can be found in Wharton et al. (2020).

Laboratory and Biochemical Tests. No single laboratory or biochemical test can be used to diagnose malnutrition. Factors that may alter test results include fluid balance, liver function, kidney function, and the presence of disease. Common laboratory tests used to study nutritional status include measures of plasma proteins such as albumin, transferrin, prealbumin, retinol-binding protein, total iron-binding capacity, and hemoglobin. After feeding, the response time for changes in these proteins ranges from hours to weeks. The metabolic half-life of albumin is 21 days; transferrin, 7 days; prealbumin, 2 days; and retinol-binding protein, 12 hours. Prealbumin is preferred over albumin because of its shorter half-life, reflecting more rapid changes of the nutritional state. However, because inflammation inhibits visceral protein synthesis, the use of these proteins as biomarkers of nutritional status has been debated. Currently, the consensus is that laboratory markers could be used to complement a thorough nutrition-focused patient history and physical examination (Keller, 2019).

Nitrogen balance is important to establish serum protein status (see "Proteins" section). Nitrogen balance is calculated as nitrogen intake minus nitrogen loss from the body and is useful for evaluating protein metabolism because nitrogen is an essential part of protein building blocks —amino acids. Nitrogen output can be measured through laboratory analysis of a 24-hour urinary urea nitrogen level. In a study with patients admitted to a Neurological Intensive Care Unit, Kim and colleagues (2020) found that 80% of these patients were underfed in terms of nitrogen or protein balance. Their negative nitrogen balance (more nitrogen put out than taken in) on initial assessment was associated with poorer outcomes (e.g., more events of in-hospital mortality and poor functional outcome at 3 months). Negative nitrogen balance is present in catabolic states, such as starvation or physiological stress. In contrast, a positive (more nitrogen taken in than put out) 2–3 g nitrogen balance is ideal for anabolism.

Dietary History and Health History. The nurse gathers information about the patient's illness or activity level to determine energy needs and compare that information with food intake. Nursing assessment of nutrition also includes health status; age; cultural background (see Box 43.4); religious food patterns (see Table 43.2); socioeconomic status; personal food preferences; psychological factors; use of alcohol or illegal drugs; use of vitamin, mineral, or herbal supplements and prescription or over-the-counter drugs; and the patient's general nutrition knowledge. Polypharmacy (multiple concurrent medication use) is a significant predictor of nutritional status in older persons and requires careful assessment (Kose & Yasuno, 2020).

In addition to the general nursing health history, a diet history is needed to assess the patient's needs (Table 43.4). The dietary history focuses on the patient's habitual intake of foods and liquids, as well as information about preferences, ability to obtain food, and allergies. Eliciting the diet and health history requires careful and respectful exploration of the patient's perceived health status to identify any hidden areas of concern such as high use of alcoholic beverages. High use of alcoholic beverages is associated with vitamin deficiencies, sexual impotence, heart conditions, cancer, menstrual conditions, liver disease, difficulty keeping a healthy body weight, and greater long-term mortality (Dietitians of Canada, 2022).

Outpatients may keep a food diary spanning several days, which will enable more accurate calculation of nutritional intake and comparison to *Canada's Food Guide* and DRIs to see if dietary habits are adequate. Culturally sensitive food-frequency questionnaires may also be used to establish patterns over time.

Clinical Observation and Physical Examination. Clinical observation is key to nutritional assessment. Because improper nutrition affects all body systems, the nurse needs to observe the patient for signs of nutritional alterations during physical assessment (see Chapter 33). When the general physical assessment of the body systems is complete, pertinent areas can be rechecked to evaluate the patient's nutritional status. The clinical signs of nutritional status (Table 43.5) provide guidelines for observation during physical assessment.

The patient should be assessed for aspiration (choking) risk and dysphagia (difficulty when swallowing). Those at risk of aspiration may have decreased levels of alertness, decreased gag or cough reflexes, difficulty managing saliva, or a wet, gurgling voice. The warning signs of dysphagia include coughing during eating; change in voice tone or quality after swallowing; abnormal movements of the mouth, tongue, or lips; slow, weak, imprecise, inconsistent, or uncoordinated speech; abnormal gag reflex; delayed swallowing; incomplete oral clearance

TABLE 43.4 Obtaining a Dietary History (Acronym: FASTCHECK)

Components of a Dietary History	Areas to Assess and Questions to Ask
Food Practices	
Number, type, and location of meals eaten per day	How many meals do you eat? At what times do you usually eat? Are these scheduled meals or snacks? Where do you usually eat meals and snacks? With whom?
Food preferences	What types of food do you like?
Food-preparation practices	Who prepares the food?
Food-purchasing practices	Who purchases the food?
Allergies	Are you allergic to any foods? Specify these foods. What happens when you eat these foods? Specify the type of allergic response (e.g., hives, itching, anaphylaxis). What is done to treat allergies (e.g., EpiPen, oral antihistamines)?
Symptoms	
Indigestion, heartburn, gas, alterations in taste	What foods cause indigestion, gas, or heartburn? Does this occur each time you eat the food? Have you noticed any changes in taste? Did these changes occur with medications or following an illness?
Relief practices	What relieves the symptoms?

Tracking

Conduct a diet history by asking the patient to describe every item of food and drink ingested in a specific period. The easiest time period to recall is from the time one awakens to the time one goes to bed.

a. Using open-ended questions and systematic repetition, ask, "When you first woke up yesterday, what was the first thing you ate?" "How much of it did you have?" "What time was that?" "What did you eat or drink next?" "Do you have specific meals?" Also ask about foods and drinks as snacks between any meals and at bedtime.
b. Ask for specific types of foods and drinks: for example, "What kind of milk—whole, fat-free?" What kind of rice—brown, white?"
c. Record time and amounts of all food eaten.
d. Find out about methods of preparation (e.g., salt, fat) and ingredients in mixed dishes.
e. Record intake of drinks to assess the adequacy of fluid intake.
f. Determine if this intake is typical of most days.
g. Record type and amount of alcoholic beverages and nonfood items consumed.

Chewing and Swallowing	Do you wear dentures? Full or partial? Orthodontic devices? Are the dentures or devices comfortable? Assess the condition of the patient's teeth.
	Do you experience mouth pain or sores (e.g., cold sores, canker sores)?
	Do you have difficulty swallowing?
	Do you cough or gag when you swallow?
Hunger	
Appetite	Have you had a change in appetite?
	Have you noticed a change in weight?
	Was this change anticipated (e.g., were you following a weight-reduction diet)?
Satiety	Do you stop eating when feeling full?
	Do you pick at food between meals or eat substantially before bedtime?
Elimination Patterns	How often do you have bowel movements?
	Do you experience diarrhea with meals or specific foods? If yes, how do you manage the diarrhea?
	Do you experience constipation? If yes, how do you manage it?
Chemical Substances	
Medication use	What medications do you take?
Over-the-counter substances	Do you take any over-the-counter medications that your doctor does not prescribe? If yes, specify them.
Alcohol	How many servings of alcoholic beverages do you drink each day—one, two, three, five, ten, or more?
Supplements	Describe any nutritional or herbal supplements you use.
Knowledge	Do you believe your current diet is adequate for meeting your energy needs? If not, what would you like to change?

TABLE 43.5 Clinical Signs of Nutritional Status

Body Area	Signs of Good Nutrition	Signs of Poor Nutrition
General appearance	Alert; responsive	Listless, apathetic, cachectic appearance
Weight	Weight appropriate for height, age, body build	Obese or underweight appearance (special concern for underweight)
Posture	Erect posture; straight arms and legs	Sagging shoulders; sunken chest; humped back
Muscles	Well-developed, firm muscles; good tone; some fat under skin	Flaccid appearance, poor tone, underdeveloped tone; tenderness; edema; wasted appearance; inability to walk properly
Nervous system control	Good attention span; no irritability or restlessness; normal reflexes; psychological stability	Inattention; irritability; confusion; burning and tingling of hands and feet (paresthesia); loss of position and vibratory sense; weakness and tenderness of muscles (may result in inability to walk); decrease or loss of ankle and knee reflexes; absent vibratory sense
Gastrointestinal function	Good appetite and digestion; normal regular elimination; no palpable organs or masses	Anorexia; indigestion; constipation or diarrhea; liver or spleen enlargement
Cardiovascular function	Normal heart rate and rhythm; lack of murmurs; normal blood pressure for age	Rapid heart rate (above 100 beats/minute), enlarged heart; abnormal rhythm; elevated blood pressure
General vitality	Endurance; energy; good sleep habits; vigorous appearance	Easily fatigued; lack of energy; falling asleep easily; tired and apathetic appearance
Hair	Shiny, lustrous appearance; firmness; strands not easily plucked; healthy scalp	Stringy, dull, brittle, dry, thin, and sparse, depigmented appearance; strands that can be easily plucked
Skin (general)	Smooth and slightly moist skin with good colour	Rough, dry, scaly, pale, pigmented, irritated appearance; bruises; petechiae; subcutaneous fat loss
Face and neck	Uniform colour; smooth, pink, healthy appearance; no swelling	Greasy, discoloured, scaly, swollen appearance; dark skin over cheeks and under eyes; lumpiness or flakiness of skin around nose and mouth
Lips	Smoothness; good colour; moist (not chapped or swollen) appearance	Dry, scaly, swollen appearance; redness and swelling (cheilosis); angular lesions at corners of mouth; fissures or scars (stomatitis)
Mouth, oral membranes	Reddish pink, intact mucous membranes in oral cavity	Swollen, boggy oral mucous membranes
Gums	Pink; healthy appearance; no swelling or bleeding	Spongy gums that bleed easily; marginal redness, inflammation; receding gums
Tongue	Pink or deep reddish colour; lack of swelling; smoothness, presence of surface papillae; no lesions	Swelling, scarlet, and raw appearance; magenta colour, beefiness (glossitis); hyperemic and hypertrophic papillae; atrophic papillae
Teeth	Lack of cavities and pain; bright, straight appearance; not crowded; well-shaped jaw; clean appearance with no discolouration	Unfilled caries; absent teeth; worn surfaces; mottling (fluorosis); malpositioned appearance
Eyes	Bright, clear, shiny appearance; no sores at corner of membranes; eyelids moist and healthy pink colour; no prominent blood vessels or mound of tissue on sclera; no fatigue circles beneath eyes	Pale eye membranes (pale conjunctivae); redness of membrane (conjunctival infection); dryness; signs of infection; buildup of keratin debris in the conjunctiva (Bitot's spots), redness and fissuring of eyelid corners (angular palpebritis); dryness of eye membrane (conjunctival xerosis); dull appearance of cornea (corneal xerosis); soft cornea (keratomalacia)
Neck (glands)	Lack of enlargement	Thyroid enlargement
Nails	Firm, pink appearance	Spoon shape (koilonychia); brittleness; ridges
Legs, feet	Lack of tenderness, weakness, or swelling; good colour	Edema; tender calves; tingling; weakness
Skeleton	Lack of malformation	Bowlegs; knock knees; chest deformity at diaphragm; prominent scapulae and ribs

Based on Hood, W. A. (2020). Nutritional status assessment in adults technique. *Medscape*. http://emedicine.medscape.com/article/2141861-technique

or pocketing of food or medications; and regurgitation. In Canada, approximately half of all new stroke patients older than 65 years of age live with dysphagia for months after the stroke. Patients with dysphagia often do not show overt signs such as coughing when food enters the airway. Aspiration may be silent; this absence of any outward sign or distress is known as "silent aspiration," reported as occurring in 15–39% of subacute stroke patients (Fabricio et al., 2020). The greatest concern of health care providers who attend to patients with reports of dysphagia is the difficulty to diagnose aspiration in a clinical assessment. Early detection of dysphagia improves outcomes such as malnutrition, dehydration, pulmonary compromise, mortality, length of hospital stay, and overall health care expenditures (Attrill et al., 2018; Nyabanga et al., 2020).

The 2019 Canadian Stroke Rehabilitation Best Practice Guidelines (Teasell et al., 2020) recommend early assessment of all stroke patients by rehabilitation professionals with specialized training. Along with nurses, the core rehabilitation interprofessional team includes physiatrists, other physicians with expertise in stroke rehabilitation, occupational therapists, physiotherapists, speech-language pathologists, social workers, and dietitians. Nurses should implement aspiration precautions (Skill 43.1) and refer patients at risk of malnutrition, including those with dysphagia, to a dietitian for nutrition assessment and ongoing management.

SKILL 43.1   ASPIRATION PRECAUTIONS

Delegation Considerations

The assessment of aspiration risk and determination of positioning cannot be delegated to unregulated care providers (UCPs). However, UCPs may feed patients after receiving instructions about aspiration precautions. It is important to instruct UCPs about the following:

- Appropriate patient positioning to decrease aspiration risk
- Reporting of any onset of coughing, gagging, or pocketing of food

Equipment

- Personal protective equipment—mask
- Chair or electric bed (to allow patient to sit upright)
- Thickening agents as needed (commercial prethickened products or commercial thickening agent)
- Tongue blade
- Penlight

PROCEDURE

STEPS	RATIONALE
1. Give patients who are not alert within the first 24 hours post-stroke nothing by mouth (NPO) and monitor closely.	• Risk of aspiration is high (Iruthayarajah et al., 2018).
2. Patients should be screened for swallowing deficits as soon as they are alert and ready for trialling oral intake, using a valid screening tool by a speech-language pathologist (SLP) or appropriately trained expert in dysphagia. Face masks are worn with any patient contact.	• The SLP is qualified to assess and to advise on the safety of the patient's swallowing ability and the consistency of diet and fluids. An individualized management plan should be developed to address dysphagia, dietary needs, and specialized nutrition plans (Iruthayarajah et al., 2018).
3. Assess patients for signs and symptoms of dysphagia (e.g., cough, change in voice after swallowing). Video fluoroscopic swallow study or fibre-optic endoscopic examination of swallowing should be performed on all patients considered at risk for pharyngeal dysphagia or poor airway protection, based on results from the bedside swallowing assessment (Teasell et al., 2020).	• Patients at risk include those who have chronic obstructive pulmonary disease (COPD) or neurological or neuromuscular diseases and those who have had trauma to or surgical procedures of the oral cavity or throat.
4. Ask patient about any difficulties with chewing or swallowing foods with different textures.	• Certain types of food are more easily aspirated.
5. Elevate head of patient's bed so that hips are flexed at a 90-degree angle and head is flexed slightly forward, or help patient to the same position in a chair.	• Reduces risk of aspiration (Metheny, 2018).
6. The clinical bedside screening trial involves giving 3 to 10 mL of water, and if that is well tolerated, it is followed by a small cup (50–90 mL) of water.	• The water swallow test (WST) is a simple, inexpensive, and quick-to-perform screening test for aspiration in stroke patients (Ahmed et al., 2020; Ye et al., 2018). It yields a large false-negative rate and is not sensitive enough to detect silent aspirations or to differentiate between penetration or aspiration (Ahmed et al., 2020). In comparing the WST with the volume–viscosity swallow test (V-VST) using food boluses of different viscosities (e.g., water, nectar, pudding) at incrementally increased volumes (5, 10, and 15 mL) in patients with acute stroke, the V-VST provided more detailed information on the severity of dysphagia, compared with the WST (Ye et al., 2018).
7. For a patient who may feed self, explain that you are initially observing while the patient eats: A. Observe patient consume various consistencies of food and liquids, watching for signs of dysphagia. B. Note if patient becomes tired. C. Report signs and symptoms of dysphagia. D. Place identification on patient's record indicating that dysphagia is present.	• Self-feeding may reduce the risk of pneumonia (Teasell et al., 2020) and increases patient cooperation. • Referral to a dietitian and SLP is appropriate if patient has difficulty with a particular consistency. • Fatigue increases risk of aspiration. • Signs or symptoms indicate the need for further evaluation of swallowing by an SLP in collaboration with the radiology department, such as a fluoroscopic swallow study. A significant number of individuals who aspirate do not exhibit signs and symptoms of dysphagia (Teasell et al., 2020. • Alerts the health care team to the problem and helps the team develop and implement an individualized plan of care.
8. For patients who require supervision or assistance with eating because dysphagia and risk of aspiration have been identified, explain that you will assist them with their meal:	• Increases patient comfort.

SKILL 43.1   ASPIRATION PRECAUTIONS—cont'd

STEPS	RATIONALE
A. Perform hand hygiene.	• Reduces transmission of microorganisms.
B. As ordered or recommended by the feeding/swallowing team, add thickener to thin liquids to create the consistency of nectar, honey, or pudding.	• Thin liquids such as water and fruit juice are difficult to control in the mouth and are more easily aspirated (Nishinari et al., 2019). It is essential to follow the team's determination for consistency because best practices have not as yet been established.
C. Place 1/2 (2.5 g) to 1 teaspoon (5 g) of food on unaffected side of the mouth, allowing utensil to touch the mouth or tongue.	• Provides patient with tactile cues to begin eating.
D. Place hand on patient's throat to gently palpate swallowing event as it occurs. Swallowing twice is often necessary to clear the pharynx.	• Helps evaluate swallowing effort.
E. Provide verbal coaching and positive reinforcement while feeding patient: • Feel the food in your mouth. • Chew and taste the food. • Raise your tongue to the roof of your mouth. • Think about swallowing. • Close your mouth and swallow. • Swallow again. • Cough to clear airway.	• Verbal cueing keeps patient focused on swallowing. Positive reinforcement enhances patient's confidence in ability to swallow.
F. Observe for coughing, choking, gagging, and drooling of food; suction airway as necessary.	• These are indications that suggest dysphagia and risk for aspiration.
G. Provide rest periods as necessary during meal to avoid rushed or forced feeding.	• Avoiding fatigue decreases the risk of aspiration.
H. Using a penlight and tongue blade, gently inspect patient's oral cavity during and after the meal to detect pockets of food.	• Pockets of food in the mouth often indicate difficulty swallowing.
I. Ask patient to remain sitting upright for at least 30 minutes after the meal.	• Reduces the risk of gastroesophageal reflux, which causes aspiration (Metheny, 2018).
J. Help patient perform hand hygiene and mouth care. Provide education, assistance, and support to enable them to meet their oral hygiene needs, be able to select and use appropriate oral hygiene equipment, and recognize and manage difficulty of swallowing.	• Mouth care after meals helps control dental plaque and patient oral hygiene (Metheny, 2018).
K. Record intake and report any observations indicative of feeding and swallowing difficulties.	
L. Ensure return of patient's tray to appropriate place and perform hand hygiene.	• Reduces spread of microorganisms.
9. Weigh patient weekly at the same time on the same scale.	• Determines if weight is stable and reflects adequate caloric level.

UNEXPECTED OUTCOMES	RELATED INTERVENTIONS
Coughs, gags, food "stuck in throat," or left in mouth	• Patient may require a swallowing evaluation. • Initiate consultation with an SLP for swallowing exercises and techniques to improve swallowing and reduce risk of aspiration. • Notify the nurse in charge, health provider, and SLP of any symptoms that occurred during meal and which foods caused the symptoms.
Avoidance of certain textures of food *Weight loss*	• Change consistency and texture of food. • Discuss findings with the nurse in charge, health provider, SLP, or registered dietitian.

RECORDING AND REPORTING

• Document the following in the patient's chart: patient's tolerance of various food textures, amount of assistance required, position during meal, absence or presence of any symptoms of dysphagia, fatigue, and amount eaten.
• Report any coughing, gagging, choking, or swallowing difficulties to the nurse in charge or the health care provider.

SAFETY ALERT The importance of safety considerations (i.e., checking consistency of fluid, correct drinking utensil and volume of fluid, 90-degree head-of-bed elevation, supervision) for patients with impaired swallowing cannot be overstressed. During normal swallow, the larynx closes to provide airway protection from aspiration of liquid or solid matter. Healthy people can tolerate the dynamic and often fast flow of liquids during swallowing to cleanly direct liquids past the airway and into the esophagus. However, individuals with dysphagia find the flow of liquids difficult to control during passage through the pharynx. Laryngeal penetration involves entry of liquid or solid material into the laryngeal vestibule. Laryngeal penetration that fails to be expelled from the airway may be followed by aspiration of pharyngeal material if the laryngeal vestibule is not effectively cleared (Cvejic & Bardin, 2018).

One method of managing this challenge has been to thicken liquids so that they flow more slowly, which allows the individual time to coordinate safe swallowing. Liquids are thickened to various levels of viscosity with a range of starches and gums, including commercially prepared products, and typically range from the least viscous liquid (akin to the thickness of nectar) for mild dysphagia to increasingly thicker liquids (honey-like and spoon-thick or pudding consistency) for more severe dysphagia. Thicker liquids enhance the safety of swallowing and reduce the incidence of pneumonia. Consumption of thinner fluids may increase the total fluid intake and hydration; however, they also increase the incidence of aspiration pneumonia (Iruthayarajah et al., 2018). Although modifying diets by thickening liquids and modifying the texture of foods to reduce the risk of aspiration has become central to the current management of dysphagia, the effectiveness of this intervention has been questioned (O'Keeffe, 2018). Careful consideration is needed regarding when these diets might be recommended to patients and how discussions about modified diets should be conducted and how informed consent should be sought. Prescription of fluid thickness is patient-specific (Teasell et al., 2020).

Patients who have dysphagia are not to drink with a straw unless specifically advised by their therapist. When deemed safe to use, drinking straws reduce the volumes of discrete sips. Narrower straw diameters are associated with smaller bolus volumes (Pang et al., 2020). A straw may make it easier to get the liquid into the mouth and to take sequential sips without liquid spilling out of the mouth; yet, participants who drank from a cup ingested significantly more than those who used a straw. Pang and colleagues (2020) found no statistically significant difference in risk of penetration or aspiration of thin liquids between cup and straw usage in patients with mild oropharyngeal dysphagia. It is not known if individuals with more severe dysphagia demonstrate similar patterns of bolus size associated with straws.

Patient Expectations. Because patients rely on nurses and other health providers to identify health or nutrition problems, nurses must be knowledgeable about nutrition, nutritional screening, assessment, and referral to meet patient expectations and needs.

◆ Nursing Diagnosis

Assessment enables determination of any actual or potential nutrition problems. Assessment data are clustered together to inform a clinical judgement about individual, family, or community responses to problems and life processes. A problem may occur when overall intake is significantly decreased or increased, or when one or more nutrients are not ingested or absorbed. For example, a woman is seen at the community health clinic with a diagnosis of dysthymia (a chronic form of depression that is milder in severity than major depression) and with the profile shown in Box 43.6. Specific diagnoses are related to the actual nutritional problem (e.g., excessive intake) but may also involve problems that place the patient at risk for nutritional or health difficulties, such as physical inactivity.

BOX 43.6   NURSING DIAGNOSTIC PROCESS

Imbalanced Nutrition: More Than Body Requirements

Assessment Activities	Data and Defining Characteristics
Obtain height and weight	42-year-old patient with female genitalia Height: 162.5 cm Weight: 96.3 kg Body mass index (BMI) = 36.5
Obtain a food history	Lack of satiety High sugar and caffeine intake, two meals plus a large evening snack/day, two to three "hard" lemonade drinks per day
Fluid	Fluid intake is coffee with double cream and sugar, lemonade with alcohol, and juice, all high caloric and lacking nutrient density
Physical assessment	Short of breath on walking Large abdomen Blood pressure: 158/88 mm Hg Pulse: 90 beats/minute Respirations: 30 breaths/minute Reports low energy, fatigue, and intermittent feelings of hopelessness since their partner died 2 years ago
Laboratory values	Cholesterol and triglycerides elevated. All others within normal limits.
Medication	None
Social	Daily, prepares meals for and eats with their 10- and 13-year-old sons. Says "My sons are the only thing I have to look forward to. Without them, I would be sitting behind my desk at work all day and working, working, working (advertising executive). I know I am overweight and wheeze when I walk up the steps. I should be more active, but I just don't have the energy. My friends have stopped inviting me and my sons over to their house for meals and visits."

The nursing diagnostic statement is based on defining characteristics present in the assessment database. The suspected health problem related to the nursing diagnosis is stated. The following are examples of nursing diagnoses relevant to nutritional problems that may pertain to the 42-year-old individual with female genitalia being seen at the community health clinic (see Box 43.6):

- *Ineffective individual coping*
- *Health maintenance, ineffective*
- *Imbalanced nutrition: more than body requirements*
- *Fatigue*
- *Hopelessness*
- *Activity intolerance*
- *Risk for impaired cardiovascular function*
- *Social isolation*

◆ Planning

The planning for enhanced, optimal nutritional status requires a higher level of care than simply correcting problems. Information from multiple sources must be synthesized in an individualized approach responsive to the patient's needs (Figure 43.5). The nurse needs to consider all data sources when developing a nursing care plan (Box 43.7). It is crucial to refer to evidence-informed published standards.

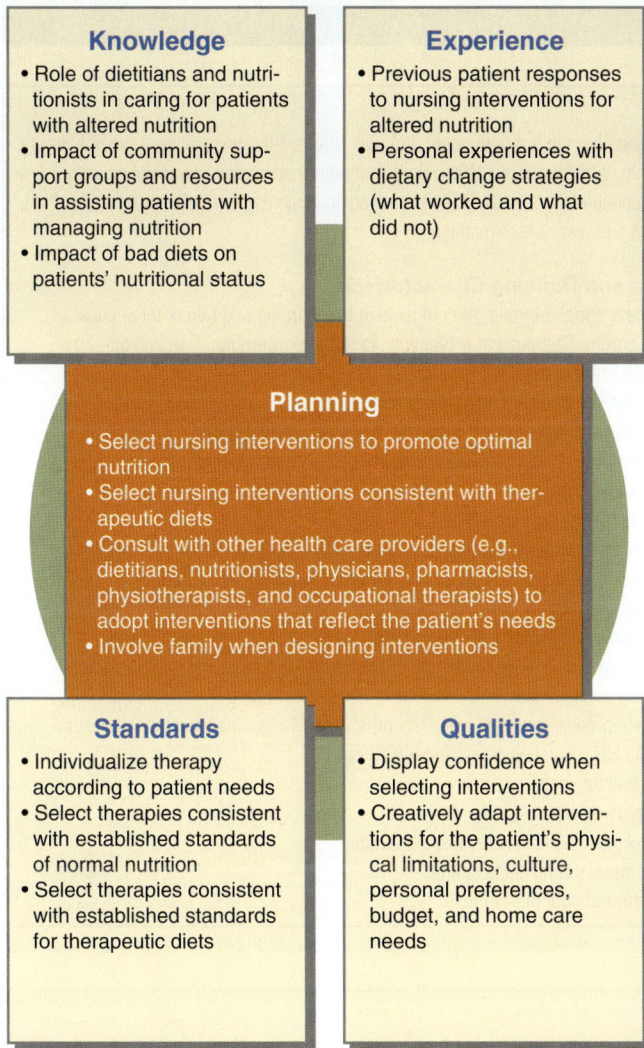

FIGURE 43.5 Critical thinking model for nutrition planning.

In clinical situations, patients have multiple related health problems. The concept map in Figure 43.6 shows the relationship of nursing diagnoses in a patient with diabetes.

Goals and Outcomes

Goals and outcomes and priorities of care reflect the patient's physiological, therapeutic, and individualized needs. Mutually planned goals negotiated between the patient, nurse, and dietitian help ensure success. An overall goal for an underweight patient might be "to achieve appropriate BMI height–weight range or be within 10% of ideal body weight." To accomplish this, the nurse can establish regular attainable goals such as moderate weight gain rather than one large overwhelming goal (Hooker et al., 2018). These smaller goals or outcomes can help the patient achieve the goal:

- Daily nutritional intake meets the minimal DRIs
- Patient may include a snack (nuts, dried fruits, and avocadoes) between meals and after dinner
- Patient gains 0.5 to 1 kg per week

The setting of goals and outcomes requires interprofessional input. A satisfactory care plan requires accurate exchange of information among the health care team.

Setting Priorities. By identifying patients at risk for nutritional problems, health care providers can help prevent or minimize those problems through timely interventions. Improving nutritional intake is a priority. With acute illness or surgery, food intake is often altered. The priority of care may be to provide optimal preoperative nutrition support for patients with malnutrition. Resumption of food intake postoperatively depends on the return of bowel function, the extent of the surgical procedure, and presence of complications (see Chapter 49).

Sometimes other priorities take precedence. For example, patients who have had throat surgery must be out of pain and comfortable before nutritional priorities can be addressed. It is also important to collaborate with the patient and family when setting care priorities so that all persons involved in the patient's care understand and support these priorities. Food purchase and preparation may involve the family, and the care plan may not succeed without their committed involvement.

Continuity of Care. In any health care setting, continuity of care, including nutritional interventions, is essential. Hospital discharge planning should extend nutritional interventions to the home or long-term care facility. In extended settings, the dietitian monitors the patient's nutritional status and intake and makes recommendations for changes.

When patients require long-term care or care at home, occupational therapists can help them to choose assistive devices, such as large-handled utensils and cups with a space for the nose. Food preparation areas can be rearranged to maximize the patient's function. Speech-language pathologists recommend appropriate dietary textures and feeding strategies and assist patients with swallowing exercises and techniques to reduce aspiration risk.

Diet Planning. Diet planning to manage specific illnesses such as diabetes, cardiac or renal disease, and conditions of lactose and gluten intolerance usually requires the patient to consult with a dietitian, nurse, and other interprofessional team members to develop knowledge and skills (Table 43.6).

Example of Diabetic Meal Planning. Patients who are diagnosed with diabetes cannot properly use and store glucose for energy. Glucose comes from fruit, milk, some vegetables, starchy foods, and sugar. To control blood glucose, patients need to eat a diet of healthy foods with a controlled amount of glucose, be active, and take insulin or oral antihyperglycemic agents, if needed.

Meal planning to control blood glucose levels is structured around eating three meals per day at regular times and spacing meals no more than 6 hours apart. Healthy snacks may be needed. Sweets such as sugar, regular pop, desserts, candies, jam, and honey are limited. High-fat food such as fried foods, chips, and pastries are limited because they may cause weight gain, which lessens blood glucose control and decreases heart health (Diabetes Canada, 2018). High-fibre foods help increase satiety and lower blood glucose and cholesterol levels. Persons living with diabetes are instructed to drink water rather than regular pop and fruit juice, which raise blood glucose. Regular physical activity improves blood glucose control.

Persons living with diabetes are to have at least three out of the four key categories at each meal: vegetables and fruit, grain products, milk and alternatives, and meat and alternatives (Diabetes Canada, 2018). Small amounts of fats help control weight and blood cholesterol. Carbohydrate counting focuses on foods that contain carbohydrate, as these raise blood glucose the most. The goal for grams of carbohydrate at each meal and snack are chosen in consultation with the registered dietitian and diabetic nurse educator to help reach or maintain a healthy weight. For accuracy in determining the carbohydrate content of food portions, patients are taught to use measuring cups and food scales and to check the nutrition label on food packages, food composition books,

◎ BOX 43.7   NURSING CARE PLAN

Imbalanced Nutrition: Less Than Body Requirements

ASSESSMENT

Belinda Wong, a nurse practitioner in a community health centre, is seeing 68-year-old Jan (preferred pronouns: she/her), who has a history of heart failure. Recently, Jan noticed a weight loss (15%). She has been taking an antidepressant (sertraline) for 3 months for an initial episode of depression related to losing her job 6 months ago. Jan was referred for counselling 3 months ago to help with depression. When Belinda inquired about Jan's financial situation, Jan responded that it was difficult living on an income from the Canada Pension Plan, but she was able to manage.

Assessment Activities	Data and Defining Characteristics
Ask Jan about her food intake during the last 2 days.	She says she drinks one glass of juice in the morning and two or three cups of coffee. She may eat a sandwich in the late afternoon. "I'm just not interested in food. It has no taste."
Assess Jan's knowledge base by asking her what she sees as strengths of her diet, about areas in which her diet is ineffective, and what resources she uses in guiding her meal planning.	She says she does not need to worry about being overweight and believes her diet is adequate for her needs, as she does not feel hungry. She says she thinks she should be eating more vegetables and drinking more milk. Her meal preparation is "quick and easy," which pleases her. She says she is "too tired to fuss over food."
Assess her use of medication.	She takes the following prescribed medications daily as instructed: sertraline, digoxin (cardiac glycoside), chlorothiazide (diuretic), and captopril (antihypertensive).
Ask Jan about social interaction.	Jan says she is lonely and does not get out much, although her psychologist recommended more socializing. Her friends were mostly at her workplace. They don't call her.
Weigh Jan and assess her posture.	This weight loss occurred over 6 months, down 11 kg. She has stooped posture. She has a low body mass index (BMI) of 17.
Observe Jan for signs of poor nutrition.	Dull, thinning hair
Dry, scaling skin
Pale conjunctivae and mucous membranes
Palpate her muscles and extremities.	2+ bilateral pitting ankle edema
Generalized poor muscle tone

NURSING DIAGNOSIS: *Imbalanced nutrition:* Less than body requirements related to a decreased ability to ingest food as a result of depression and loss of appetite associated with antidepressant use.

PLANNING

Goals (Nursing Outcomes Classification)*	Expected Outcomes
	Weight Control
Jan will progressively gain weight.	Patient will gain 0.5 to 1 kg/month until goal of 59 kg is reached.
	Nutritional Status: Nutrient Intake
Jan will consume adequate nourishment each day.	Patient will ingest 1 900 kcal/day, including 50 g of protein per day.
Jan will exhibit no signs of malnutrition.	Physical assessment and laboratory values will be within normal limits.

*Outcome classification labels are adapted from Moorhead, S., Swanson, E., Johnson, M., et al. (2018). *Nursing outcomes classification (NOC)* (6th ed.). Elsevier.

INTERVENTIONS

Interventions (Nursing Interventions Classification)†	Rationale
Nutritional Counselling	
Coordinate a plan of care with Jan, her family doctor, therapist, and dietitian.	Successful nutrition care planning involves an interprofessional approach (Pratt et al., 2020).
Individualize menu plans.	Encourages intake by incorporating food preferences and sharing records of meals (Chung et al., 2019).
Teach Jan about the value of consulting *Canada's Food Guide.*	Health Canada (2019b) recommendations for food selections provide optimal nutrition.
Nutritional Monitoring	
Monitor Jan monthly for weight gain, anemia, and serum albumin or prealbumin level.	Weight gain should be slow and progressive. Serum albumin of 335–480 mg/dL and prealbumin of 16–35 mg/dL are within normal limits (Keller, 2019).
Perform physical assessment of hair, eyes, mouth, skin, and muscle tone.	To monitor for improved nutritional status.
Nutritional Management	
Encourage Jan to eat small meals and increase dietary intake to help offset anorexia secondary to use of sertraline.	Sertraline is a selective serotonin reuptake inhibitor (SSRI) medication; diminished taste and anorexia are common effects of SSRIs. Frequent small meals help to reduce anorexia-associated weight loss.

BOX 43.7   NURSING CARE PLAN—cont'd

Interventions (Nursing Interventions Classification)†	*Rationale*
Encourage fluid intake early in the day.	Older persons need eight 250-mL glasses per day of fluid from beverage and food sources. Concentrating intake in the morning and early afternoon prevents nocturia.
Encourage fibre intake.	Fibre helps prevent constipation.
Encourage Jan to have congregate meals (lunch at senior centre) 5 times per week.	Eating with others encourages good nutrition and promotes socialization with peers (Health Canada, 2019b). Overcoming social isolation is helpful for older persons who do not exercise and eat nutritiously.

†Intervention classification labels adapted from Butcher, H. K., Bulechek, G., McCloskey Dochterman, J. M., et al. (Eds.). (2019). *Nursing interventions classification (NIC)* (7th ed.). Elsevier.

EVALUATION

Nursing Actions	*Patient Response and Finding*	*Achievement of Outcome*
Ask Jan to keep a food diary for 3 days.	Her diary reflects that she ate her main meal at the senior centre at noon, had fruit and grain products for breakfast, and had a sandwich with fruit and milk in the evening.	Jan is selecting more nutritionally rich foods, consistent with current guidelines.
Observe Jan's appearance.	Her skin is less pale, hair appears to be in better condition and styled. Ankle edema is present, but less than 1+.	Jan has improved physical parameters of nutrition; still needs follow-up.
Weigh Jan.	Weight gain of 2 kg in 4 weeks	Weight gain is steady; she is still below ideal body weight.
Ask Jan about appetite and energy level.	Jan responds that on days when she eats at the senior centre, her appetite seems better and she "wants to do more things." She notes that weekends are very lonely.	Weekday support for nutritional status appears effective. Jan needs to increase activity status and nutritional intake during weekends.

› concept map

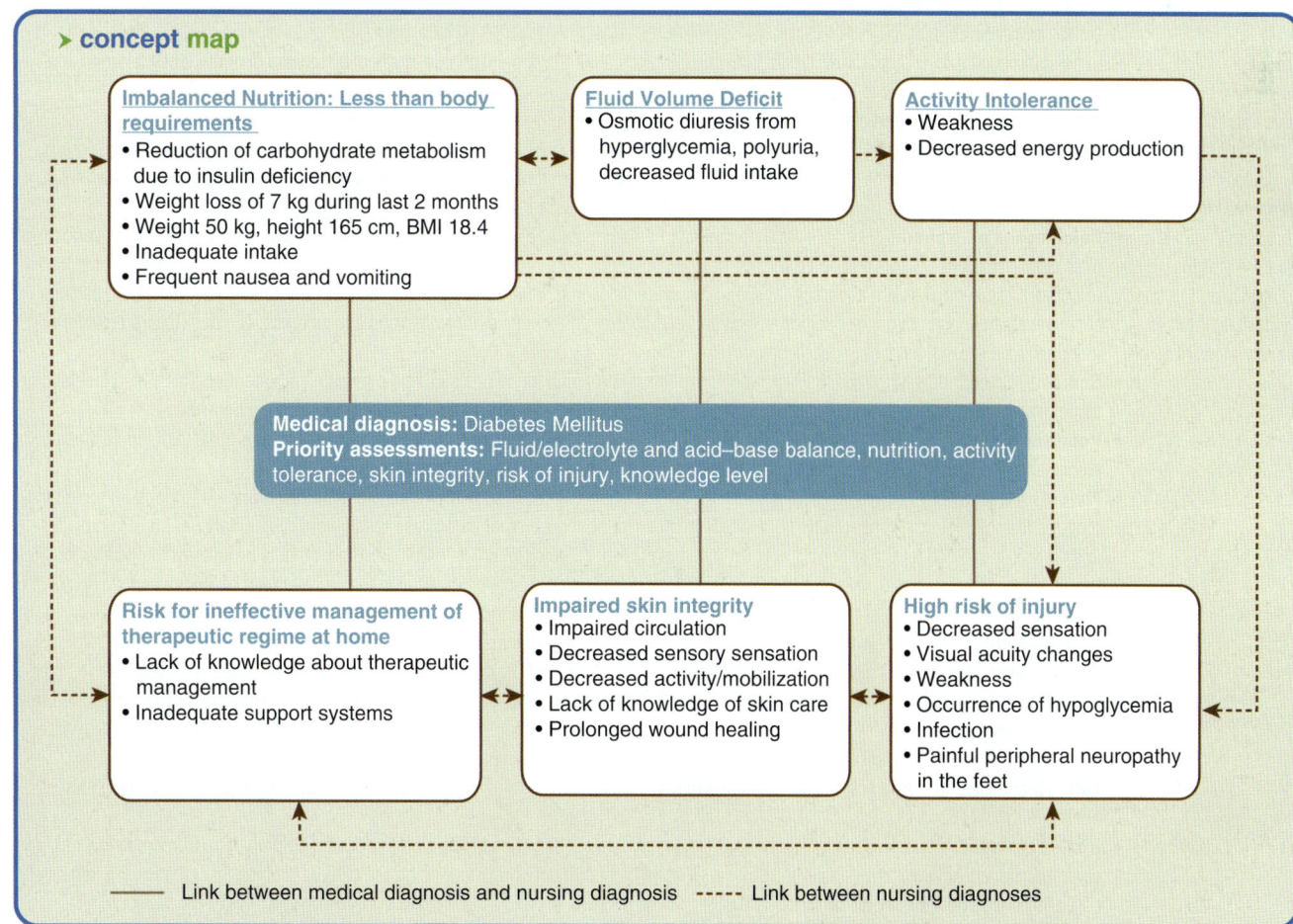

FIGURE 43.6 Concept map for patient with diabetes mellitus. *BMI,* Body mass index.

TABLE 43.6	Sample Menu Planning for Cardiac and Renal Diets and for Lactose and Gluten-Free Diets
Health Concern	**Menu Planning with Daily Servings and Examples**
Cardiac Goal is to reduce hypertension and overweight to prevent risk of stroke and heart attack	The **DASH diet**, similar to *Canada's Food Guide*, recommends a high level of vegetable and fruit intake. DASH food categories include vegetables; fruit; grains (mainly whole grains); low-fat or no-fat dairy foods; lean meats, poultry and fish; nuts, seeds and dry beans; and fats and oils. DASH daily servings and examples are as follows: • Vegetables: 4–5 servings 250 mL (1 cup) raw leafy vegetables 125 mL (½ cup) cooked vegetables 170 mL (6 oz) juice • Fruit: 4–5 servings 1 medium piece of fruit 63 mL (¼ cup) dried fruit 125 mL (½ cup) fresh, frozen or canned fruit • Grains (mainly whole grains): 7–8 servings 1 slice bread 250 mL (1 cup) ready-to-eat cereal 125 mL (½ cup) cooked rice, pasta or cereal • Low-fat or no-fat dairy foods: 2–3 servings 250 mL (1 cup) milk 250 ml (1 cup) yogourt 50 g (1½ oz) cheese • Lean meats, poultry and fish: 2 servings or less 85 g (3 oz) cooked lean meats, skinless poultry, or fish • Nuts, seeds and dry beans: 4–5 servings per week 1/3 cup (1.5 oz.) nuts 30 mL (2 tbsp) peanut butter 2 tbsp (1/2 oz.) seeds 1/2 cup cooked dry beans or peas • Fats and oils: 2–3 servings 5 mL (1 tsp) soft margarine 15 mL (1 tbsp) low-fat mayonnaise 30 mL (2 tbsp) light salad dressing 5 ml (1 tsp) vegetable oil
Renal Goal is to meet nutritional needs, reduce workload on the kidneys, preserve kidney function that is left (before starting dialysis), and control build-up of food wastes like urea.	There is no "special kidney diet" for everyone. Individual nutritional needs depend on age, medical history, amount of kidney function, activity level, and other factors. • **Fats**—Use monounsaturated and polyunsaturated fats such as olive oil, canola oil, and safflower oil. • **Protein**—Prior to starting dialysis, a low-protein diet (2 servings of 75–90 g protein foods per day) may be helpful. Once dialysis starts, more protein (about 3 servings of 75–90 g protein foods per day) is needed to replace muscle and tissue loss. Egg whites, egg white powder, or protein powder are considered good protein sources. • **Calcium and phosphorus**—Limit foods that contain large amounts of phosphorus, which can cause itchy skin or painful joints and loss of calcium from bones. Colas and soft drinks contain phosphorus. High- and moderate-phosphorus foods include milk products and protein foods such as seeds, nuts, dried peas, beans, and bran cereals. When dairy products cannot be incorporated into the daily diet, calcium supplements help prevent bone conditions, and vitamin D controls the balance of calcium and phosphorous. The health care provider or dietitian can discuss how best to get these nutrients. • **Sodium**—Do not add salt to food. Reducing sodium helps control high blood pressure and prevents fluid retention. Read food labels to find hidden salt, and avoid foods that contain a lot of salt, sodium, or MSG. Avoid salt substitutes that are high in potassium. • **Potassium**—Cardiac arrhythmias may result from a buildup of potassium. It is best to choose low-potassium fruits (e.g., apples, pears, plums, and blueberries) and vegetables (e.g., bean sprouts, cabbage, green beans, and lettuce). • **Fluids**—As kidney disease worsens, fluid intake may need to be limited, as too much fluid will lead to shortness of breath, an emergency that needs immediate medical attention. Soups, gelatin desserts, and ice cream are considered fluids. The primary health care provider and dialysis nurse will let the patient know how much to drink each day. Tips to keep from becoming thirsty include avoiding salty foods, freezing juice in an ice cube tray and eating it like a popsicle (these ice cubes are counted in the daily amount of fluids), and staying cool on hot days. • **Carbohydrates**—As a good source of energy, calories from carbohydrates may replace the calories from protein if a low-protein diet is recommended. Most fruits, breads, grains, and vegetables provide energy, as well as fibre, minerals, and vitamins. Fruits and vegetables containing large amounts of potassium may be limited. High-potassium fruits include oranges, nectarines, kiwis, raisins or other dried fruit, bananas, cantaloupe, honeydew melon, and prunes. Also limit or avoid asparagus, avocado, potatoes, tomatoes or tomato sauce, winter squash, pumpkin, and cooked spinach. • **Fats**—Monounsaturated and polyunsaturated fats (olive oil, canola oil, safflower oil) can be a good source of calories that help protect heart health. • **Iron**—People with advanced kidney failure also have anemia and usually need extra iron. Foods that contain extra iron are liver, beef, pork, chicken, lima and kidney beans, and iron-fortified cereals. The health care provider or dietitian will determine which foods with iron can be eaten, because of the kidney disease.

TABLE 43.6	Sample Menu Planning for Cardiac and Renal Diets and for Lactose and Gluten-Free Diets—cont'd
Health Concern	**Menu Planning with Daily Servings and Examples**
Lactose Intolerance	• *Lactose* is a sugar found in milk and milk products. Lactose intolerance happens when the body does not have enough lactase (enzyme needed to digest lactose). Without lactase, undigested lactose passes into the large intestine, where it is fermented by bacteria causing bloating, gas, cramping, nausea, diarrhea, and weight loss (in children).
	• Most people with lactose intolerance can tolerate some lactose in their diet. They are encouraged to eat small amounts of foods or beverages that have lactose with their meals. Lower lactose–containing foods eaten in small amounts (60–125 mL) can include cottage cheese; hard, aged cheese (cheddar, Swiss, Parmesan); yogourt; chocolate milk; and sour cream.
	• If these amounts cause discomfort, persons can try eating less or using lactose-free products or foods low in lactose, preferably fortified with calcium, such as lactose-hydrolyzed milk (e.g., Lactaid, Lacteeze) and soy and rice beverages. Lactase enzyme drops or tablets reduce the lactose in milk or dairy products.
	• Many foods that contain lactose are also important sources of calcium and vitamin D. Other sources of these nutrients are needed if lactose-containing foods are avoided. Examples of alternate sources of calcium are canned salmon (with the bones) and sardines, fortified soy and rice beverages, and calcium-fortified fruit juices. Lactose-free sources of vitamin D include fish, liver, and egg yolks. Lactose-free soy and rice beverages and nonhydrogenated margarine have been fortified with vitamin D. Persons are advised to talk to a registered dietitian if concerned that they are not getting enough calcium from food and to determine if they should take a calcium supplement.
Gluten-Free Goal is to treat celiac disease by avoiding foods that contain gluten	• *Gluten* is a protein found in grains such as wheat, barley, rye, and triticale. Gluten causes inflammation in the small intestines of people with celiac disease.
	• Foods that are naturally gluten-free include beans, seeds, and nuts in their natural, unprocessed form; fresh eggs; fresh meats, fish, and poultry (not breaded, batter-coated, or marinated); fruits and vegetables; and most dairy products. Various gluten-free products, such as bread and pasta, are available in grocery stores.
	• Grains and starches that are gluten-free include arrowroot, buckwheat, corn and cornmeal, flax, quinoa, rice, and gluten-free flours (rice, soy, corn, potato, and bean).
	• It is critical to avoid wheat and other products unless labelled "gluten-free." Health Canada's regulatory requirement for "gluten-free" foods does not refer to any specific threshold for gluten in products represented as "gluten-free"; however, Health Canada considers that levels of gluten protein below 20 parts per million generally do not represent health risks to consumers with celiac disease (Canadian Food Inspection Agency, 2019b).
	• Persons living with celiac disease must be alert to hidden sources of gluten. The list of ingredients on all labels must be read every time.

Cardiac diet: Heart and Stroke Foundation of Canada. (2020). *The DASH Diet to lower high blood pressure*. https://www.heartandstroke.ca/healthy-living/healthy-eating/dash-diet; ***Renal diet:*** Kidney Foundation of Canada. (2021). *Living with kidney failure*. https://kidney.ca/Support/Resources/Living-With-Kidney-Failure; ***Lactose intolerance diet:*** Dietitians of Canada. (2019). *Managing lactose intolerance*. https://www.unlockfood.ca/en/Articles/Allergies-and-Intolerances/Managing-Lactose-Intolerance.aspx; Canadian Digestive Health Foundation. (2021). *Lactose intolerance*. https://cdhf.ca/digestive-disorders/lactose-intolerant/what-is-lactose-intolerance/; ***Gluten-free diet:*** Canadian Celiac Association. (2021). *Getting started on the gluten-free diet*. https://www.celiac.ca/living-gluten-free/newly-diagnosed/; Canadian Celiac Association. (2021). *Living a healthy gluten free life*. https://www.celiac.ca/living-gluten-free/diet-nutrition/?gclid=EAIaIQobChMIh4TozZai8AIVZMyzCh0-fgy6EAMYAiAAEgLQHPD_BwE; Canadian Food Inspection Agency. (2019). *Gluten-free claims*. https://inspection.canada.ca/food-label-requirements/labelling/industry/allergens-and-gluten/eng/1388152325341/1388152326591?chap=2; Dietitians of Canada. (2021). *Eating well with celiac disease*. https://www.unlockfood.ca/en/Articles/Celiac-disease/Eating-well-with-celiac-disease.aspx

restaurant fact sheets, and pertinent websites. They are to write down what they eat and drink throughout the day (Diabetes Canada, 2018).

◆ Implementation

Chronic Disease, Nutrition, and Prevention.
Chronic diseases are long term and not contagious. One in three Canadian adults live with at least one of the following chronic diseases: cardiovascular disease, cancer, chronic respiratory disease, diabetes, and mood or anxiety disorders. The number of individuals living with these chronic diseases continues to increase because of the aging and growth of the Canadian population, and because people are living longer with their disease through advances in treatment and management (Branchard et al., 2018).

The WHO is coordinating a global action plan for how global health agencies can better work together to help countries advance their own health priorities across common sustainable development goals (WHO, 2018b). These include not only goals for good health and well-being but also goals to eliminate poverty and hunger; foster gender equality; and promote clean water, sanitation, affordable energy, decent work, industry and innovation, sustainable cities, and climate action—all of which are intertwined with good health. This plan is currently in draft form and open for public comments and feedback (Fletcher, 2019).

Health Promotion/Illness Prevention.
Nurses are in a key position to educate patients about proper nutritional habits that may promote health and prevent the development of many diseases. Early identification of potential or actual problems is the best way to avoid more serious health problems. Outpatient and community-based settings are key locations for nursing assessment of nutritional practices and status. Frequently, nurses are in a position to educate families about nutrition, inform them of community resources, and provide contact information so that families can direct questions to a dietitian or other professional nurse.

Insufficient income is the most significant barrier to healthy eating (French et al., 2019). Food selection and quantity are positively associated with income. In 2018, one in four children and youth under 18 years of age (23%) said they go to bed or to school hungry at least sometimes because there is not enough food at home; nearly three-quarters of the children in Nunavut (72%) and one-third of the children in the Northwest Territories (32%) lived in food-insecure households, compared with 16 to 23% among the remaining reporting provinces and territories (Vanier Institute, 2019). Elsewhere in the world, low-income preschoolers and toddlers had the lowest mean intake of fruits and milk and dairy products compared to middle- and high-income groups (Clark et al., 2020). Higher fruit and vegetable intake among children has been associated with higher education of parents and food availability at home (Łuszczki et al., 2019). At the same time, lower socioeconomic status and issues of cost, accessibility, and parental time commitment are associated with physical inactivity in Canadian children (ParticipACTION, 2020).

In March 2021, there were 1 303 997 visits to the food bank in Canada, an increase of 20% compared to 2019; 33.3% of those helped were under the age of 18 years (Food Banks Canada, 2021). The problem is worsened when children cannot access nutritional programs at schools: Canada is the only G8 country without a national school-based feeding program (Parker & Koeppel, 2020). Besides children, members of at-risk population groups for food insecurity include Indigenous people, lone-parent families, women, immigrants, and those over 65.

Although mandatory fortification of staple foods with micronutrients has helped to reduce income-related disparities (Mkambula et al., 2020), other interventions are needed to counter the threat to good nutrition and health from lack of purchasing power at individual and collective levels. For those on limited budgets, food preparation can be modified for substances that need to be used sparingly; for example, bean or cheese dishes can often replace meat. Menu planning a week in advance helps patients adhere to a specific diet, eat nutritiously, and stay within their budget. A nurse or dietitian may check menus for content. Often, simple tips can help, such as baking rather than frying to reduce fat intake, using lemon juice or spices to add flavour to low-sodium diets, and avoiding grocery shopping when hungry because it can lead to spontaneous purchases of foods not included in meal plans. Strategies to help financially disadvantaged groups improve their nutrition include collective kitchens and gardens (Bernard, 2018), coalitions with community-based organizations, antipoverty advocacy, and political commitment to policies of full employment (Government of Canada, 2022b). Also important are public-awareness forums (Government of Canada, 2018) and a rights-based approach to food security at the federal and provincial levels (Smith-Carrier, 2018), with support to families that have inadequate resources to meet their daily nutritional needs (Food Banks Canada, 2021). See Box 43.8 for an example of an innovative program that aims to increase food security for individuals, families, and communities.

> **SAFETY ALERT** Food safety is also an important public health issue. Food-borne illnesses can occur from poor hygiene practices and improper food storage or preparation. Nurses should educate patients about reducing the risks of food-borne illnesses (Table 43.7 and Box 43.9).

Acute Care. Many factors influence nutritional intake in acute care settings. Ill or debilitated patients often have loss of appetite (anorexia). The ketosis that accompanies starvation can further suppress appetite, as can the pain that results from surgical procedures and trauma. During hospitalizations, mealtimes are often interrupted, or the patient is too fatigued or uncomfortable to eat. Worry about families, finances, employment, or illness often interferes with getting an adequate diet. Medications may impair taste, cause nausea, interfere with absorption, or affect metabolism. Diagnostic testing may disrupt mealtimes or require a nothing by mouth (NPO) status. Patients who are NPO and receive only standard intravenous fluids for more than 7 days are at nutritional risk.

Nurses must continuously assess patient nutritional status and plan interventions that promote normal dietary intake, digestion, and metabolism of nutrients. Patients may have a gradual progression of dietary intake or need therapeutic diets to manage their illnesses (Box 43.10).

BOX 43.8   Focus on Food Security

Nutrition North Canada (NNC) is a federal government subsidy program that was launched on April 1, 2011, to provide residents of northern isolated communities in Saskatchewan, Manitoba, Ontario, Quebec, Labrador, Yukon, the Northwest Territories, and Nunavut with improved access to perishable nutritious food. The program is designed to reduce the high cost to consumers of food in the north where grocery costs are driven by transportation, the cost of maintaining stores, staff costs, spoilage and theft, high inventory costs, and retailer profit margins.

NNC works with stores across the north and food suppliers in southern Canada. NNC subsidizes (a) various perishable and nutritious food items (e.g., fruit, vegetables, milk, eggs, meat, and cheese) shipped by air to an eligible community and (b) traditional food commercially processed in the north (e.g., Arctic char, musk-ox, and caribou) shipped by air to an eligible community. Retail subsidies are applied against the total cost of an eligible product shipped by air to an eligible community. Customers in eligible communities can purchase subsidized food from registered northern retailers or directly from registered southern suppliers. To be eligible for NNC, a community must lack year-round road, rail, or marine access. In addition, the community must meet the territorial or provincial definition of a northern community, have a year-round population according to the national census, and have an airport, post office, or grocery store.

Based on a market-driven model, the subsidy is provided to retailers and suppliers registered with the program. In turn, these businesses are responsible for passing on the full subsidy to consumers. Communities receive either a "full subsidy" of between $1.20 and $16 per kilogram of eligible food shipped, or a "partial subsidy" of $0.05 per kilogram of eligible food shipped. NNC has succeeded in increasing the amount of perishable nutritious food available and in slightly reducing prices of eligible food in isolated northern communities. Even with the NNC subsidies, food is still too expensive for people to afford. Between April 2011 and March 2019, the average weekly cost of the Revised Northern Food Basket decreased by only 1.03%, or from $426.48 to $422.07 (Government of Canada, 2021)—more than double the cost of a roughly equivalent basket of food purchased in Toronto.

The NNC's current subsidization of products such as milk, bread, beans, and fresh and frozen fruits and vegetables, that although nutritious according to a Eurocentric diet, is questionable in the diets of Canadian Inuit people. In this way, the subsidy may ignore community needs and is discriminatory because of the lack of attention paid to the benefits of the diets historically consumed by Inuit populations. As well, bottled water is not subsidized, despite the fact that many of these communities are under boil-water advisories and cannot access clean drinking water. To avoid mimicking colonial governmentality, the NNC could consider the context in which it operates, consult with Inuit and Indigenous communities, and implement culturally sensitive policy (Cooper, 2020). Also, because the federal government does not currently have access to information on retailer profit margins, it cannot verify that the NNC subsidy is being fully passed on to consumers. In sum, further review is needed to gauge the NNC's effectiveness.

Based on Cooper, M. (2020). Nutrition North Canada riddled with problems: Subsidy program serving northern communities discourages food sovereignty. *The Manitoban,* April 13. https://www.themanitoban.com/2020/11/nutrition-north-canada-riddled-with-problems/40909/; Government of Canada. (2021). *Cost of the Revised Northern Food Basket in 2019–2020.* https://www.nutritionnorthcanada.gc.ca/eng/1610462030814/1610462073967; Leblanc-Laurendeau, O. (2019). *Food insecurity in northern Canada: An overview.* https://lop.parl.ca/sites/PublicWebsite/default/en_CA/ResearchPublications/202047E#:~:text=The%20high%20rates%20of%20food,change%20and%20environmental%20dispossession%20and

TABLE 43.7 Food Safety

Food-Borne Disease	Organism	Food Source	Symptoms*
Botulism	*Clostridium botulinum*	Improperly home-canned foods, smoked and salted fish, ham, sausage, shellfish	Symptoms vary from mild discomfort to death in 24 hours, initial nausea and dizziness progressing to motor (respiratory) paralysis
Escherichia coli	*Escherichia coli 0157:H7*	Undercooked meat and poultry, unpasteurized milk, and fresh fruits and vegetables that have been in contact with untreated water	Severe cramps, nausea, vomiting, diarrhea (may be bloody), fever, headache, renal failure. Appears 1–8 days after eating, lasts 1–7 days
Listeriosis	*Listeria monocytogenes*	Soft cheese, meat (hot dogs, pâté, lunch meats), unpasteurized milk	Diarrhea, fever, headache, pneumonia, meningitis, endocarditis. Can lead to miscarriage in pregnant persons or death of newborns. Gastrointestinal symptoms appear within 9–48 hours and invasive disease within 2–6 weeks
Perfringens enteritis	*Clostridium perfringens*	Cooked meats, poultry, gravy dishes held at room or warm temperature	Mild diarrhea, vomiting. Appears 8–16 hours after eating, lasts 1–2 days
Salmonellosis	*Salmonella*	Milk, custards, egg dishes, salad dressing, sandwich fillings, polluted shellfish, contaminated raw fruits and vegetables	Mild to severe diarrhea, cramps, vomiting. Appears 6–48 hours after ingestion, lasts 4–7 days
Shigellosis or bacillary dysentery	*Shigella dysenteriae*	Milk, milk products, seafood, salads ingestion, lasts 3–14 days	Mild diarrhea to fatal dysentery. Appears 7–36 hours after ingestion
Staphylococcus food poisoning	*Staphylococcus aureus*	Custards, cream fillings, improperly refrigerated meats, cheese, ice cream, potato salad, sauces, casseroles	Severe abdominal cramps, pain, vomiting, diarrhea, perspiration, headache, fever, prostration. Appears 1–6 hours after ingestion, lasts 1–2 days

*Symptoms are generally more severe for young children, older persons, pregnant people, and people with weakened immune systems. Children under 5 years of age carry 40% of the food-borne disease burden.

From Canadian Public Health Association. (2021). *Foodborne illnesses—What causes food poisoning?* https://www.cpha.ca/foodborne-illnesses-what-causes-food-poisoning; Centers for Disease Control and Prevention. (2019). *A–Z index for foodborne illness.* https://www.cdc.gov/foodsafety/diseases/index.html; Nix, S. (2022). *Williams' basic nutrition and diet therapy* (16th ed.). Mosby.

BOX 43.9 PATIENT TEACHING

Food Safety

Objectives
- Patient will verbalize measures to prevent food-borne illness.
- Patient will understand the primary types of illness and how they are transmitted.
- Patient will not experience food-borne illness.

Teaching Strategies
Populations particularly at risk are older and younger people and immunosuppressed individuals. Instruct patients on the following:
- Wash hands with warm, soapy water for at least 20 seconds before touching or eating food.
- Separate cutting boards. Use one board for produce and another for raw meat, poultry, fish, and seafood.
- Wash fresh fruits and vegetables thoroughly.
- Do not eat raw meats or drink unpasteurized milk.
- Do not buy or consume food that has passed the expiration date.
- Keep foods properly refrigerated at 4°C and frozen at −18°C.
- Wash dishes and cutting boards with hot, soapy water or use a bleach sanitizer of 5 mL bleach in 750 mL water.
- Thaw food, especially raw meat, poultry, fish or seafood, in the refrigerator.
- Cook food completely, using a clean thermometer to measure the temperature of meat, poultry, and fish. Keep a temperature chart that gives the safe cooking temperatures of foods handy to always know at what temperature each food is fully cooked. Insert the thermometer probe into the thickest part of the food to ensure accuracy.
- Refrigerate leftovers within 2 hours. Do not save for more than 4 days in the refrigerator.
- Wash dishcloths and towels regularly or use paper towels.
- Clean the inside of the refrigerator and microwave regularly to prevent microbial growth.
- Wash reusable grocery bags frequently.

Evaluation
- Ask patient to describe measures to prevent food-borne illnesses.
- Observe the patient for safe practices, if making a home visit.

From Dietitians of Canada. (2020). *Test the temperature—Use a thermometer for food safety.* https://www.unlockfood.ca/en/Articles/Food-safety/Test-the-temperature-%E2%80%93-Use-a-thermometer-for-food.aspx; Health Canada. (2019). *Food safety.* https://www.canada.ca/en/health-canada/topics/food-safety.html

Promoting Appetite. In providing an environment that promotes a patient's appetite, it is important to eliminate unpleasant odours, provide oral hygiene as needed to remove disagreeable tastes, and maintain patient comfort. Certain medications (e.g., insulin, glucocorticoids, and thyroid hormones) can affect dietary and nutrient intake and metabolism. Other medications (e.g., antifungal agents) can affect taste. Some psychotropic medications affect appetite, cause nausea, and alter taste. At times the nurse and dietitian can help the patient select foods to reduce the altered taste sensations or nausea. In other situations, medication may need to be changed.

Assisting Patients With Feeding

Many conditions, including cancer, stroke, and neuromuscular disorders, can cause feeding difficulties. The task of feeding requires nursing

---

BOX 43.10 Diet Progression and Therapeutic Diets

Clear Liquid
This diet is limited to broth, bouillon, coffee, tea, carbonated beverages, clear fruit juices, gelatin, or Popsicles.

Thickened Liquid
All liquids (e.g., juice, tea, coffee, water) must be thickened to the appropriate consistency (nectar, honey, or pudding) as recommended by the speech-language pathologist or feeding team when thin fluids cannot be safely swallowed and may be aspirated.

Full Liquid
To a clear- or thickened-liquid diet can be added smooth-textured dairy products, custards, refined cooked cereals, vegetable juice, puréed vegetables, or any fruit juices.

Puréed
This diet includes all of the above with the addition of scrambled eggs, puréed meats and vegetables, fruits (ripe bananas, mashed cooked fruits without the skins), or mashed potatoes and gravy.

Mechanical Soft
This diet includes all of the above with the addition of ground or finely diced meats, flaked fish, cottage cheese, cheese, rice, potatoes, pancakes, light breads, cooked vegetables, cooked or canned fruits, soups, or peanut butter.

Soft or Low Residue
Low-fibre, easily digested foods, such as pastas, casseroles, moist tender meats, canned cooked fruits and vegetables, desserts, cakes, and cookies without nuts or coconut, can be added.

High Fibre
This diet includes fresh uncooked fruits, steamed vegetables, bran, oatmeal, and dried fruits.

Low Sodium
A low-sodium diet is limited to 4 g (no added salt), 2 g, 1 g, or 500 mg sodium (severe sodium restriction), requiring selective food purchases.

Low Cholesterol
This diet is restricted to <200 mg/day cholesterol, in keeping with the National Cholesterol Education Program (NCEP) recommendations (Rohrs, 2019) and the Heart and Stroke Foundation of Canada (2022a).

Diabetic
In general, people with diabetes should follow a healthy diet recommended for the general population (Diabetes Canada, 2018; Gray & Threlkeld, 2019). See the section entitled "Example of Diabetic Meal Planning."

Regular
Dietary restrictions are not necessary unless specified.

---

knowledge and skilled intervention to protect patient safety, independence, and dignity.

Before Feeding. The nurse assesses the patient's risk for aspiration (see "Assessment" in this chapter and Skill 43.1). The patient should sit as upright as possible with head tilted slightly forward and may be supported by pillows, foam wedges, or rolled towels. A patient who is lying back or has the neck arched or hyperextended should not be fed because these positions create an open airway susceptible to aspiration. Glasses, hearing aids, and dentures should be functioning and in place. Clothing and bedding should be protected by items that should not be called "bibs." The nurse needs to check the suction apparatus at the bedside.

During Feeding. The patient is kept upright. To feed the patient, the nurse uses a rocking motion of utensil on the patient's tongue. To prevent aspiration, feeding recommendations are based on videofluoroscopic swallow study results (Teasell et al., 2020). If indicated by the feeding/swallowing team, the patient can take a drink between each mouthful of food to ease the process of eating. The nurse observes the patient for pouching of food. A metal teaspoon is usually best to use for feeding patients with bite reflexes.

The nurse needs to assess swallowing during feeding and give patients with dysphagia enough time to chew, allowing at least 5 to 10 seconds or longer for each bite or sip. The nurse should observe two completed swallows between mouthfuls. The patient's Adam's apple should move up and down. If the food is still present, the nurse can offer an empty spoonful to stimulate swallowing.

The nurse who is helping the patient to eat should sit in the patient's line of vision and provide appropriate prompting, encouragement, and direction, both verbally and nonverbally. The nurse needs to avoid hovering with the next spoonful of food, as this may cause a patient to

hurry and worsen any swallowing difficulties. Patience, attention, and time are essential. When possible, the nurse should try to heed special requests, such as for the food to be warmed up. Nurses can promote comfort and a sense of independence by providing opportunities for patients to direct the order and speed at which they want to eat. The nurse should give the patient as much choice as possible—for instance, by asking if the patient wants peas and potatoes together or separate on the spoon. The family can be asked about the patient's favourite foods. Because mealtime is usually a social activity, it is important that nurses and other health care providers talk to patients during meals. Nurses can use this opportunity to educate patients about therapeutic diets, medications, or adaptive devices.

Patients with visual deficits also need special assistance. If possible, the nurse should read aloud menu items and let the patient choose the meal. The patient should be told when the meal has arrived and where the tray is placed. Food needs to be positioned within the patient's visual field. If the patient wears glasses or contact lenses, they should be clean and in place. A dark tray or cloth can be placed under a light plate to define the plate edges, making it easier to locate the food. Patients with poor vision or blindness may be able to feed themselves if adequate information is given. The nurse can describe where certain foods are located on a plate (Figure 43.7) using either the clock-face method (e.g., "The meat is at 6 o'clock, mashed potatoes are at 9 o'clock, and the peas at 12 o'clock") or by saying items are at the top, bottom, right, or left side of the plate (Wisconsin Council of the Blind & Visually Impaired, 2019). Meat should be placed at 6 o'clock or at the bottom of the plate, as this is easiest for cutting. The patient should be told where the beverage is located in relation to the plate (e.g., "The glass of water is to the right or above 2 o'clock"). The nurse can ask the patient if they would like assistance with removing packaging from items. Hot drinks should be in non-spill containers; the nurse needs to tell the patient where they are placed.

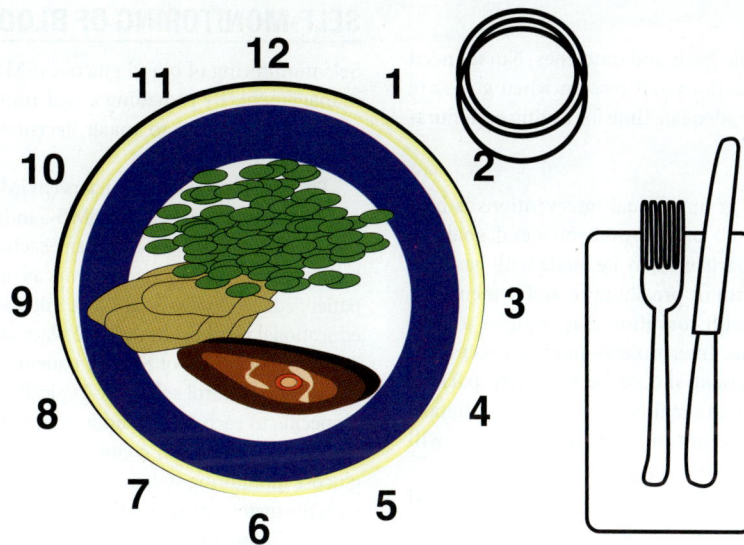

FIGURE 43.7 Using the clock-face method to identify contents and location of food on a plate.

BOX 43.11 CASE STUDY

*Working Through the Unexpected**

My 46-year-old patient (preferred pronouns: he/him) had just had a total bowel resection. Because of the large surgical interruption in the body's natural state, at our hospital we follow a strict protocol for reintroducing oral fluids, food, and medications. The patient remains NPO and on intravenous (IV) fluids until they produce flatus and bowel sounds in all four quadrants. During my initial postoperative assessment, this patient had no bowel sounds in any quadrant, which was expected following the surgery. I explained to him that the protocol for nutritional supplementation would begin with a clear fluid diet for 24 to 48 hours once his body was ready, and that progression through the protocol would be advanced by how his body responded. My patient didn't fully understand the ramifications of not following the protocol and, unfortunately, told his family he was starving. The family gave him something solid to eat. His body, following such an intense surgery, was not ready to handle the food, and he became nauseated and vomited what he had eaten as well as coffee-ground emesis. He required abdominal decompression. I placed a #16 Salem Sump nasogastric (NG) tube, which for several days was connected to low intermittent suction to alleviate abdominal distension. The patient also required replacement of his NG tube

losses 1:1 with an additional IV solution to maintain electrolyte balance. Blood work was done at least once daily to monitor electrolyte levels, hemoglobin, and any dehydration. When it became apparent that his recovery was taking longer than planned, we closely monitored his laboratory results for signs of decreased nutritional status, and we considered if total parental nutrition (TPN) would be necessary to supply his daily nutritional requirements. However, prior to needing to progress to TPN, we saw continuous improved laboratory results and heard faint bowel sounds in all four quadrants. We were able to remove the NG tube. We started him again on a clear fluid diet, which he tolerated well, so we advanced him to a full fluid diet, which he also tolerated well. He regained full bowel sounds and had flatus the following day. We were able to advance him to a regular diet. His lab work showed no nutritional deficits and he made a full recovery.

From this case, I hope undergraduate nurses will learn that meeting nutritional needs in patients following surgery is always different, and that decisions must be based on nursing expertise combined with knowledge of the patient's unique history, symptoms, and family support.

*Written by Ashley Kay, RN, BN, Dartmouth General Hospital, Nova Scotia.

When food intake is less than usual because of illness or fatigue, nutrient-dense items should be provided first. Small, frequent meals, five to six per day, may be required. Patients with decreased motor skills may retain more independence by using large-handled adaptive utensils, which are easier to grip and manipulate.

After Feeding. The patient should remain upright for 30 minutes after eating. The nurse should check again for pocketing of food. If the patient needs to lie down because of fatigue, the head of the bed can be raised to sitting-up level. Food intake should be documented. The nurse needs to identify if any particular food was eaten faster (e.g., a preference) or with difficulty (e.g., soft meat may need to be replaced with ground) and report and document any instances of choking and fatigue. After each meal, the patient should perform oral hygiene.

Restorative and Continuing Care

Patients discharged from a hospital with dietary prescriptions often need dietary education to plan meals that meet specific therapeutic requirements. Restorative care includes immediate postsurgical care and routine medical care pertinent to hospitalized and home care patients. The case study in Box 43.11 illustrates the need for nurses to educate visitors about a patient's nutritional status in order to avoid complications and enhance the patient's recovery following abdominal surgery.

After surgical intervention, particularly bowel resections and colon surgery, coordinated bowel motility temporarily ceases. This lack of coordinated propulsive action prevents effective transit of intestinal contents or tolerance of oral intake and leads to gas and fluid accumulation within the bowel. Motility typically returns within 1–3 days (Weledji, 2020).

◆ **Evaluation**

Care plans should reflect achievable goals and outcomes. Nurses need to evaluate outcomes of nursing actions and discern when goals are being met. They also need to allow adequate time for testing each nursing approach to a problem.

Patient Care. The effectiveness of nutritional interventions is best measured by meeting the expected patient outcomes and goals of care (Figure 43.8). Ongoing comparisons may be made with baseline measures of weight, serum albumin or prealbumin, and protein and kilocalorie intake. Changes in health condition may indicate a need to change the nutritional care plan. Interprofessional team members should be consulted, and the patient should be an active participant whenever possible. The patient's ability to incorporate dietary lifestyle changes with the least amount of stress or disruption will ensure success. When expected outcomes are not met, the interventions or outcomes are revised on the basis of the patients' needs and preferences.

Patient Expectations. Patients expect competent and accurate care. They expect nurses to alter the care plan if outcomes of nutritional therapies are unsuccessful. By working closely with patients, nurses can understand their expectations and try to meet them within the limits of their conditions and treatments.

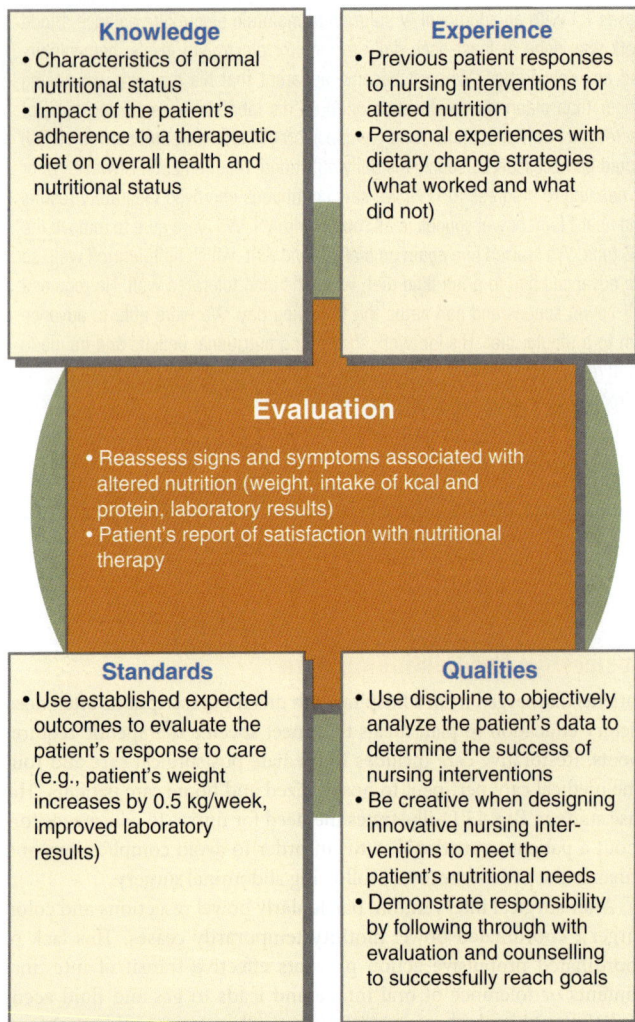

Knowledge
• Characteristics of normal nutritional status
• Impact of the patient's adherence to a therapeutic diet on overall health and nutritional status

Experience
• Previous patient responses to nursing interventions for altered nutrition
• Personal experiences with dietary change strategies (what worked and what did not)

Evaluation
• Reassess signs and symptoms associated with altered nutrition (weight, intake of kcal and protein, laboratory results)
• Patient's report of satisfaction with nutritional therapy

Standards
• Use established expected outcomes to evaluate the patient's response to care (e.g., patient's weight increases by 0.5 kg/week, improved laboratory results)

Qualities
• Use discipline to objectively analyze the patient's data to determine the success of nursing interventions
• Be creative when designing innovative nursing interventions to meet the patient's nutritional needs
• Demonstrate responsibility by following through with evaluation and counselling to successfully reach goals

FIGURE 43.8 Critical thinking model for nutritional evaluation.

SELF-MONITORING OF BLOOD GLUCOSE

Self-monitoring of blood glucose (SMBG) is a cornerstone of diabetes management. By providing a real-time blood glucose reading, SMBG enables the patient to make decisions regarding diet, exercise, and medication management.

Portable blood glucose meters (BGMs) are used at the hospital bedside and by patients who perform SMBG independently (Figure 43.9). Instructions for using a BGM accompany each product. Because errors in monitoring technique can cause errors in management strategies, thorough patient education is crucial. Once initial education has occurred, follow-up educational sessions should take place at each subsequent patient contact. To ensure accuracy of SMBG, patients must be taught to calibrate their BGM using control solutions. Typically, control solution for a glucometer is specific to each brand and is available from the manufacturer. Patients who are unsure which control solution is designated to work with their glucose monitoring system are advised to check the instructions that came with the meter, or look on the manufacturer's website.

The blood glucose level reported by a laboratory is sometimes higher than the measurement by the patient's home glucose monitor or the hospital's portable meter. This is because some meters measure capillary blood glucose from whole blood (via fingerstick), whereas laboratory venous samples yield plasma readings. Plasma samples, or venous samples, are 15–20% higher because plasma has a higher water content than that of whole blood, so there is more dissolved glucose in plasma than in whole blood (Gurung & Jialal, 2020). Most BGMs for home use report blood glucose only in terms of plasma glucose, to be more readily compared with laboratory values.

The chief advantage of SMBG is that it supplies immediate information about blood glucose levels that can be used to make adjustments in food intake, activity patterns, and medication dosages. It also produces accurate records of daily glucose fluctuations and trends, as well as alerting the patient to acute episodes of hyperglycemia and hypoglycemia (Figure 43.10). When the person with diabetes is ill, the blood glucose should be tested every 2 to 4 hours to determine the effects of this stressor on blood glucose level (Diabetes Canada, 2018). Blood glucose testing should be performed whenever hypoglycemia is suspected so that immediate action can be taken if necessary. If a patient is visually or

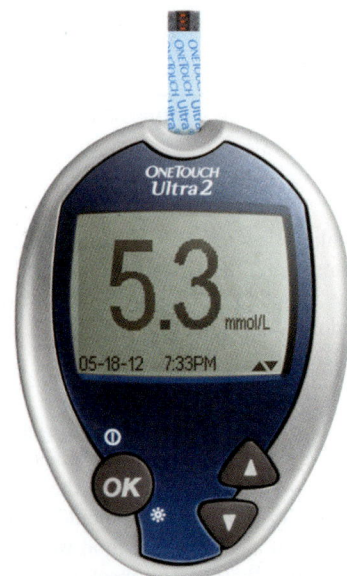

FIGURE 43.9 Blood glucose monitor. (Courtesy LifeScan, Inc., Milpitas, CA.)

cognitively impaired or has limited manual dexterity, the degree to which SMBG can be performed independently must be evaluated carefully.

SMBG is recommended as an essential part of daily diabetes management for all people using insulin or oral hypoglycemic agents (OHAs). The frequency of monitoring depends on several factors, including the patient's glycemic goals, type of diabetes, ability and willingness to perform the test independently, and treatment regimen. It is recommended that patients with type 1 diabetes test at least three times per day and include both preprandial and postprandial testing. Those using an insulin pump may test more frequently. People with type 2 diabetes treated with OHAs or through lifestyle changes alone have more variable and individualized testing regimens. For patients with type 2 diabetes treated with once-daily insulin and OHAs, monitoring at least once daily is recommended (Diabetes Canada, 2018). (See Skill 43.2 for a description of how to monitor blood glucose.)

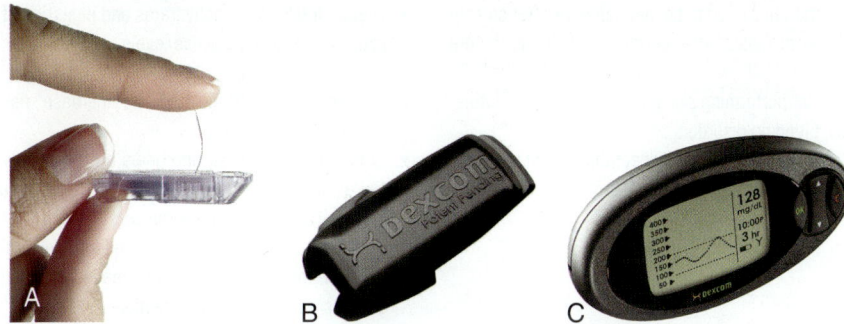

FIGURE 43.10 A tiny sensor **(A)** implanted under the skin transmits continuous reading to receiver **(B)**, to alert the wearer of any deviation from desired glucose target range. Readings are displayed and stored on the monitor **(C)**. (Courtesy DexCom, Inc.)

SKILL 43.2   BLOD GLUCOSE MONITORING

Self-testing of blood glucose level requires obtaining a large drop of blood by skin puncture. You can use a hand-held single-use lancet or an automatic lancet-holder device. The drop of blood is then applied on the specially prepared testing strip and inserted into a reflectance meter (see Figure 43.9). The meter provides an accurate measurement of blood glucose level in less than 60 seconds.

A variety of meters are on the Canadian market, such as the Glucometer II (Ames), Accu-Chek III (Boehringer Mannheim), Glucoscan 3000 (LifeScan), and OneTouch (LifeScan). Patients can purchase these meters at most pharmacies or from their diabetes educator. There are no standards of practice or certification requirements for distributors or users of portable glucose monitors outside of the hospital. However, Health Canada recommends following the instructions in the manual and test strip package insert carefully, washing hands using warm water to encourage blood flow before the test, drying hands well to avoid diluting the blood sample, using a new sterile lancet for each test, storing the meter and test strips in a cool, dry place like a bedroom, never in the bathroom, making sure test strips are stored in their original container at the temperature indicated and that they have not expired, and using a new test strip for each test (Health Canada, 2020c).

A wet-wash or dry-wipe method of testing is used. To perform a wet wash, the user flushes the blood-coated testing strip with water before inserting the strip into the glucose meter. The dry-wipe method requires the user to wipe off the blood-coated testing strip with a dry cotton ball before making a reading. Some products do not require blood to be flushed or wiped before a reading. The various methods allow measurement of blood glucose between 1.1 and 44.4 mmol/L. Most meters allow for alternative sites, such as the forearm, palm, and thigh.

New methods of obtaining glucose measurement (e.g., Dexcom G6, Medtronic Guardian Connect, and Freestyle Libre) that do not require finger-pricks are available on the Canadian market. Minimally invasive glucose meters have a very small, fine plastic sensor inserted through the abdomen, and they provide continuous readings of blood glucose levels. A biosensor is taped on the external abdomen (see Figure 43.10). Using a hand-held wireless meter or phone app, the patient activates the biosensor to transmit the blood glucose level at any time without puncturing the skin. Another model, the noninvasive glucose meter, punctures the skin not with a needle but with laser technology.

Diabetes Canada (n.d.) notes that available continuous glucose monitoring systems (CGMS) are the Dexcom G6 (https://www.dexcom.com/en-CA), Guardian™ Connect (https://www.medtronic.com/ca-en/diabetes/home/products/cgm-systems/guardian-connect.html), and the Medtronic MiniMed Paradigm REAL-Time System (https://www.medtronic.com/ca-en/diabetes/home/products/minimed-670g.html). A sensor is inserted under the skin and data are sent from the sensor to a transmitter, which displays the glucose value on an insulin pump continuously; values are updated every 5 minutes (see Figure 43.10). This system assists the patient and health care provider in identifying trends and tracking patterns. Thus it is particularly useful for managing insulin therapy, alerting the patient during episodes of hypoglycemia and hyperglycemia, and allowing prompt, immediate, and corrective action.

Delegation Considerations

The task of measuring blood glucose level after skin puncture (capillary puncture) can be delegated to an unregulated care provider (UCP) who is specifically instructed in performing the skill. The nurse must first assess the patient to determine that it is appropriate to delegate blood glucose monitoring. If the patient's condition changes frequently, this task should not be delegated. The nurse directs the UCP by

- Explaining appropriate sites to use for puncture and when to obtain glucose levels
- Reviewing expected levels and when to report to the nurse unexpected glucose levels

Equipment

- Personal protective equipment—mask, disposable gloves
- Antiseptic swab
- Cotton ball or tissue
- Sterile lancet or blood-letting device
- Heel-warming device (*optional*)
- Paper towel
- Blood glucose meter (e.g., OneTouch)
- Blood glucose test strips (brand determined by meter used)

Continued

PROCEDURE

STEPS	RATIONALE
1. Wear a mask upon all contact with a patient (see Chapter 34 for further information on infection prevention and control). Assess patient's understanding of purpose, how to perform test, and importance of glucose monitoring.	• Data set guidelines for nurse to develop teaching plan.
2. Determine whether specific conditions need to be met before or after sample collection (e.g., with fasting, after meals, after certain medications, before insulin doses).	• Dietary intake of carbohydrates and ingestion of concentrated glucose preparations alter blood glucose levels.
3. Determine whether risks exist for performing skin puncture (e.g., low platelet count, anticoagulant therapy, bleeding disorders).	• Abnormal clotting mechanisms increase risk for local ecchymosis and bleeding.
4. Assess area of skin to be used as puncture site. Inspect the patient's fingers, toes, and heel. Alternative sites are the earlobe, palm, arm, and thigh. Avoid using areas that have bruises and open lesions.	• Sides of fingers, toes, and heels are commonly selected because they have fewer nerve endings. Measurements at alternative sites are meter specific and may differ from measurements at traditional sites (Mathew & Tadi, 2021). The puncture site should not be edematous, inflamed, or recently punctured, because these factors cause increased interstitial fluid and blood to mix and also increase the risk for infection.
5. Review health provider's order for times and frequency of measurement.	• Health provider determines test schedule on basis of patient's physiological status and risk for glucose imbalance.
6. If diabetic patient performs test at home, assess patient's ability to handle skin-puncturing device. The patient may choose to continue self-testing while in hospital.	• Patient's physical health may change (e.g., vision disturbance, fatigue, pain, disease process), preventing patient from performing test.
7. Expected outcomes after completion of procedure:	
• Puncture site shows no evidence of bleeding or tissue damage.	• Hemostasis achieved. Lancet or needle did not puncture skin too deeply.
• Blood glucose level is normal.	• Normal fasting glucose level is 4 to 6 mmol/L, indicating good metabolic control.
• Patient demonstrates procedure.	• Patient demonstrates psychomotor learning.
• Patient explains test results.	• Patient validates knowledge.
8. Explain procedure and purpose to patient or family, or both. Offer opportunity to practise testing procedures. Provide resources and teaching aids for patient.	• Such explanations promote understanding and cooperation.
9. Perform hand hygiene before procedures. Put on fresh disposable gloves for each patient prior to lancet use.	• Hand hygiene and gloves reduce transfer of microorganisms.
10. Instruct patient to perform hand hygiene with soap and warm water, if patient is able.	• Hand washing promotes skin cleansing and vasodilation at selected puncture site. It establishes practice for patient when test is performed at home. Because of its ability to remove food residue from the hands and fingers, hand washing is superior to using alcohol pads to cleanse the test site.
11. Position patient comfortably in chair or in semi-Fowler's position in bed.	• This position ensures easy accessibility to puncture site. Patient will assume position when self-testing.
12. Remove test strip from container, then tightly seal cap. Check code on the test strip vial.	• Sealing cap protects unused strips from accidental discoloration caused by exposure to air or light. Code on test strip vial must match code entered into the glucose meter.
13. Turn on glucose meter, if necessary.	• Turning on activates meter.

CRITICAL DECISION POINT: *Some monitors are activated when the test strip is inserted and therefore do not have a specific on-off switch.*

SKILL 43.2   BLOOD GLUCOSE MONITORING—cont'd

STEPS	RATIONALE
14. Insert strip into glucose meter (refer to manufacturer's directions), and make necessary adjustments (see Step 14 illustration).	• Some machines must be calibrated; others require zeroing of timer. Each meter is adjusted differently.

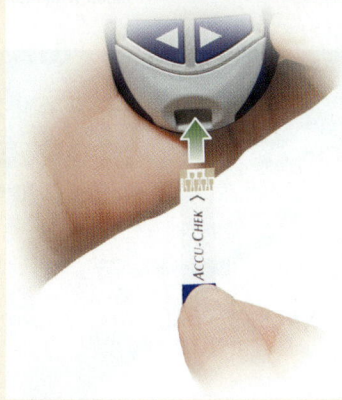

STEP 14 Load test strip into meter. (Courtesy Accu-Chek Glucometer.)

STEPS	RATIONALE
15. Remove unused glucose test strip from meter and place on paper towel or clean, dry surface with test pad facing up (see manufacturer's directions).	• Moisture on strip can alter accuracy of final test results.
16. Apply disposable gloves.	• Wearing gloves reduces risk for contamination by blood.
17. Choose puncture site. Puncture site should be vascular. In adults, select lateral side of finger; be sure to avoid central tip of finger, which has more dense nerve supply.	• Vascularity ensures free flow of blood after puncture.
18. Hold the finger that you will puncture in dependent position while gently massaging finger toward puncture site.	• Massage increases blood flow to area before puncture.
19. Clean site with antiseptic swab, and allow it to dry completely.	• The site must be allowed to dry because alcohol can cause blood to hemolyze.
20. Remove cover of lancet or blood-letting device. Hold lancet perpendicular to puncture site, and pierce finger or heel quickly in one continuous motion (do not force lancet).	• Cover keeps tip of lancet or needle sterile.
21. Some employers use lancet devices with an automatic blade retraction system. This reduces the possibility of self-sticks, preventing exposure to blood-borne pathogens. Place blood-letting device firmly against side of finger and push release button, causing needle to pierce skin (see Step 21 illustration).	• Blood-letting devices are designed to pierce skin to a specific depth, ensuring adequate blood flow. Perpendicular position ensures proper skin penetration.

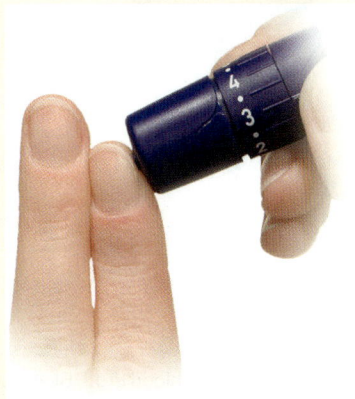

STEP 21 Prick side of patient's finger with lancet. (Courtesy Accu-Chek Glucometer.)

STEPS	RATIONALE
22. Wipe away first droplet of blood with cotton ball. (See manufacturer's directions for meter used.)	• First drop of blood may contain more serous fluid than blood cells.

Continued

STEPS	RATIONALE
23. Lightly squeeze puncture site (without touching) until a second large droplet of blood forms (see Step 23 illustration). Repuncturing is necessary if a large enough drop does not form to ensure accurate test results. (See manufacturer's direction regarding how blood is applied.)	• An adequate-sized droplet is needed to activate monitor and obtain accurate results. Excessive squeezing of tissues during blood sample collection may contribute to pain, bruising, scarring, hemolysis, and contamination of the blood with interstitial and intracellular fluid leading to inaccurate results.

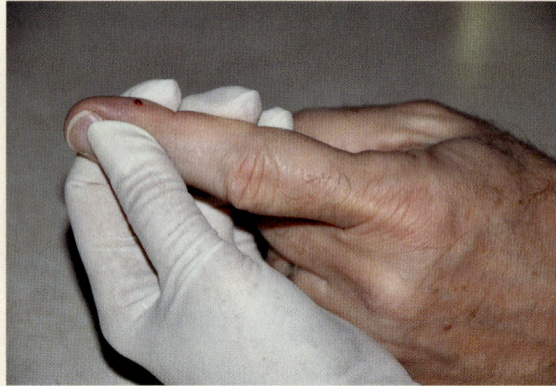

STEP 23 Squeeze puncture site until a large droplet of blood is expressed.

CRITICAL DECISION POINT: *Diabetic patients frequently have peripheral vascular disease. This makes it difficult to produce a large drop of blood after a fingerstick. To improve blood flow, be sure to hold patient's finger in dependent position before puncturing.*

---

24. Obtain test results.	• Exposure of blood to test strip for prescribed time ensures proper results.

CRITICAL DECISION POINT: *Some meters (such as OneTouch [LifeScan]) require blood sample to be applied to test strip already in the meter. Once the drop of blood is applied, the meter automatically calculates the reading.*

A. Be sure meter is still on. Bring test strip in the meter (in this example, an Accu-Check) to the drop of blood (see Step 24A illustration). The blood will be absorbed into the test strip (see manufacturer's instructions).	• Blood is absorbed into strip, and glucose device will show message on screen to signal that enough blood is obtained.

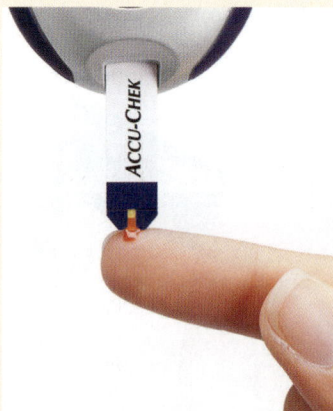

STEP 24A Touch the test strip to the blood drop. Blood is absorbed into the test strip. (Courtesy Accu-Chek Glucometer.)

CRITICAL DECISION POINT: *Do not scrape blood onto the test strips or apply blood to wrong side of test strip. This prevents accurate glucose measurement. Ensure enough blood is applied to completely fill the test window. Otherwise, a false reading or error message will be displayed.*

STEPS	RATIONALE

B. The blood glucose test result will appear on the screen (see Step 24B illustration). Some devices beep when measurement is completed.

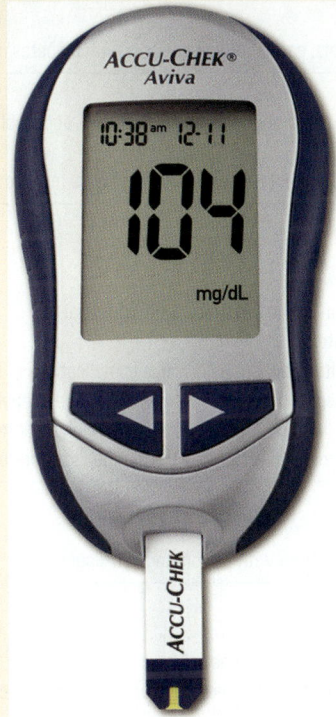

STEP 24B Results appear on meter screen. (Courtesy Accu-Chek Glucometer.)

STEPS	RATIONALE
25. Turn meter off. Dispose of test strip, lancet, and gloves in proper receptacle.	• Meter is battery powered. Proper disposal reduces risk for needlestick injury and spread of infection.
26. Discuss test results with patient.	• Discussion promotes participation and provides a teaching opportunity for continued self-monitoring of blood glucose testing.
27. Reinspect puncture site for bleeding or tissue injury.	• Site is possibly a source of discomfort and infection.
28. Compare glucose meter reading with normal blood glucose levels and previous test results.	• Comparison helps determine whether glucose level is normal.
29. Ask patient to discuss procedure.	• Discussion validates patient's level of learning.
30. Ask patient to explain test and results.	• Results of test may cause anxiety. Patient may misunderstand specific step of procedure.

UNEXPECTED OUTCOMES	RELATED INTERVENTIONS
Puncture site is bruised and continues to bleed	• Apply pressure. • Elevate hand above level of heart. • Notify health care provider.
Blood glucose level above or below target range	• Continue to monitor patient. • Check for medication orders regarding deviations in glucose level. • Administer insulin or carbohydrate source as ordered, depending on glucose level. • Notify health care provider.
Glucose meter malfunction	• Review instructions for troubleshooting glucose meter. • Repeat test. • Call the 1-800 company phone number found at the back of every blood glucose testing meter.
Patient misunderstanding of procedure and results	• Repeat instructions to patient. • Have patient demonstrate procedure.

Continued

| SKILL 43.2 | BLOOD GLUCOSE MONITORING—cont'd |
| STEPS | RATIONALE |

RECORDING AND REPORTING

- In nurses' notes or special flow sheet, record procedure, glucose level, and action taken for abnormal range.
- Describe response, including appearance of puncture site.
- Report abnormal blood glucose levels.
- Stress importance of timing the testing of blood glucose levels, particularly in patients with diabetes mellitus.

TEACHING CONSIDERATIONS

- Provide information on where a patient with diabetes mellitus can obtain testing samples, if applicable. When possible, teach with the same meter that the patient will use at home.
- Provide patient with information on what to do and whom to contact for assistance if glucose meter malfunctions.

PEDIATRIC CONSIDERATIONS

- Young children should be allowed to choose puncture site.
- Heel and great toe are common puncture sites in infants.
- Assess for localized complications in heels of premature infants who have blood drawn repeatedly.
- Heel warming facilitates obtaining a specimen from a neonate.
- Infection or abscess of the heel and necrotizing osteochondritis are the most serious complications of heelstick puncture in infants.
- To avoid osteochondritis, the puncture is made at the outer aspect of the heel and should not be deeper than 0.65 mm for premature newborns up to 1 kg (2 lbs), 0.85 mm for newborns weighing 1–2.5 kg (2–6 lbs), or 1.0 mm for infants from 3 to 6 months weighing between 2.5 and 9 kg (6–20 lbs) (Malinowski, 2020).
- Young children should be allowed with parent to demonstrate technique; technique can be incorporated in play activity for further understanding.

AGE-RELATED CONSIDERATIONS

- Warming fingertips may facilitate obtaining specimen.
- Some older persons have vision or dexterity problems that interfere with performing self-fingersticks.

CARE IN THE COMMUNITY CONSIDERATIONS

- Patients can use glucose meters routinely in their homes.
- Patients should be encouraged to attend a diabetic support group if it is needed.
- As visual acuity may affect a patient's ability to perform self-testing at home, there are new blood glucose testing meters that have talking ability (Ability411, 2021).

Based on Cobbett, S., Perry, A. G., Potter, P. A., et al. (Eds.). (2020). Chapter 9: Specimen collection. *Canadian clinical nursing skills and techniques.* Elsevier/Mosby.

ENTERAL TUBE FEEDING

Enteral nutrition refers to nutrients given via the gastrointestinal tract. When the patient cannot ingest food but is still able to digest and absorb nutrients, enteral tube feeding is indicated. Feeding tubes can be inserted through the nose or orally into the stomach or intestines (nasogastric-orogastric or nasointestinal-orointestinal tubes), surgically through a stoma (a surgically created opening) into the stomach or jejunum (gastrostomy or jejunostomy tubes), or endoscopically (percutaneous endoscopic gastrostomy [PEG] or jejunostomy [PEJ] tubes).

A registered nurse may insert nasogastric or orogastric tubes for abdominal decompression and for enteral feedings with an order from a physician (Wayne, 2018). Large-diameter (large-bore) sump tubing nasogastric tubes are most often used for both decompression and short-term enteral feeding, whereas small-bore, silastic tubing with an insertion stylet is used for longer-term feeding needs. Nasogastric tubes used for enteral feeding should be 6–12 Fr. The smaller the gauge, the higher the risk of blockage, while tubes over 12 Fr are more likely to cause discomfort (Best, 2019).

All other tubes must be inserted by a physician. In some settings (e.g., the Critical Care Unit), a large tube is used to start the tube feed, and if the patient tolerates it for the first 24 to 48 hours, a small-bore tube is then inserted. If the patient has a small-bore tube placed in the duodenum, the physician may elect to leave the sump tube in the stomach for gastric decompression and to prevent vomiting or aspiration. If enteral nutrition therapy is to be administered for less than 4 weeks, nasoenteral tubes may be used. Surgical or endoscopically placed tubes are preferred for long-term feeding

(>4 weeks) to reduce the discomfort of a nasal tube and to provide a more secure, reliable access. If enteral feed or medication cannot be administered into the stomach (for example, in the case of delayed gastric emptying or pyloric obstruction), enteral feed is administered into the small intestine—usually into the jejunum (Best, 2019).

Box 43.12 lists indications for enteral nutrition. The nurse inserts the nasoenteral tube (Skill 43.3), and the nurse or others, including caregivers in the home setting, can administer enteral tube feedings after placement has been confirmed. The best confirmation of proper tube placement is radiography (Adeyinka et al., 2022).

Enteral nutrition has been used successfully after surgery or trauma to provide fluids, electrolytes, and nutritional support. Gastric ileus may prevent nasogastric feedings, while nasointestinal or jejunostomy tubes allow successful postpyloric feeding of formula directly into the small intestine or jejunum or beyond the pyloric sphincter of the stomach (Best, 2019). Enteral feedings can be administered through a nasoenteric tube (Skill 43.4) or via a gastrostomy or jejunostomy tube (Skill 43.5).

Initiating Enteral Tube Feedings

Enteral formulas are usually one of four types. **Polymeric formulas** (1.0 to 2.0 kcal/mL) include milk-based blenderized foods prepared by hospital dietary staff or in the patient's home. The polymeric classification includes commercially prepared whole nutrient formulas. For this type of formula to be effective, the patient's gastrointestinal tract must be able to absorb whole nutrients. **Modular formulas** (3.8 to 4.0 kcal/mL) are single-macronutrient (e.g., protein, glucose, or lipids) preparations and are not nutritionally complete. This type of formula is added to other

BOX 43.12	Indications for Enteral Nutrition

Cancer
- Head and neck
- Upper gastrointestinal tract

Critical Illness or Trauma
- Respiratory failure with prolonged intubation or inadequate oral intake
- Patients in critical care with suspected or evidence of catabolism
- Trauma patients, especially those in a hypermetabolic state (e.g., burns)

Neurological and Muscular Disorders
- Brain neoplasm
- Stroke
- Cerebrovascular accident
- Neuromuscular disorders (e.g., amyotrophic lateral sclerosis, multiple sclerosis, Parkinson's disease)
- Dementia:

Patients with advanced dementia are offered quality-of-life diets; they risk injury with multiple insertions related to self-extubation of feeding tubes. Enteral feeding for end-stage dementia is controversial. Common reasons to initiate enteral feedings in these patients include prolonging survival, improving quality of life, preventing pressure injuries, and palliative care. However, expert consensus is that artificial hydration and nutrition should not be used solely to prolong life in people with advanced dementia when swallowing difficulties or disinclination to eat is a result of advancing disease (Ijaopo & Ijaopo, 2019). Decisions about artificial nutrition in people with dementia should be made on an individual basis after a comprehensive, interprofessional assessment that includes confirmation of advanced dementia and the absence of an acute, potentially reversible cause of the swallowing difficulty. It is paramount to involve the person's caregivers to manage their expectations and to ensure the wishes of the person with dementia are taken into account.
- Myopathy
- Parkinson's disease

Gastrointestinal Disorders
- Enterocutaneous fistula
- Inflammatory bowel disease
- Mild pancreatitis

Other Situations
- Respiratory failure with prolonged intubation
- Inadequate oral intake
- Continuous feedings
- Supine positioning:

Supine position is an indication for enteral feeding. Enteral feedings may be provided at the same rate as in the prone position, since most studies have reported the same residual in either position (Machado et al., 2020).

A 45-degree elevation is recommended, when possible, for supine patients to reduce their risk of aspiration and, if intubated, prevent ventilator-associated pneumonia (Rees Parrish & McCray, 2019).
- Cerebral vascular accident
- Local trauma
- Anorexia nervosa
- Difficulty chewing and swallowing
- Severe depression

SKILL 43.3	INSERTING A SMALL-BORE NASOENTERIC OR ORAL TUBE FOR ENTERAL FEEDING

Delegation Considerations

At most Canadian health care facilities, the nurse may insert a sump naso/orogastric tube without stylet according to primary health care provider orders, and under supervision until deemed competent to provide this skill autonomously. This skill should not be delegated to unregulated care providers or those without a certified competency.

Equipment
- Personal protective equipment—mask, gloves
- Nasogastric or nasointestinal (orogastric or orointestinal) tube (8 to 12 Fr) with guidewire or stylet
- Stethoscope
- 60-mL or larger Luer-Lok or catheter-tip syringe
- Entriflex nasogastric feeding tubes with safe enteral connections. (This weighted polyurethane feeding tube is designed for nasogastric and nasoduodenal feeding with a slimmer, lighter weighted tip for easier insertion. The feeding port is incompatible with Luer-Lok or intravenous [IV] connections, reducing the risk of accidental connection or inadvertent administration of IV-intended medications through the feeding tube).
- Hypoallergenic tape and tincture of benzoin or tube fixation device
- Scissors
- pH indicator strip (scale 0.0 to 11.0)
- Medication cup or container for aspirated fluid
- Glass of water and straw (not required for intubated patients)
- Water-soluble lubricant
- Emesis basin
- Absorbent pad
- Facial tissues
- Disposable gloves (multiple pairs needed)
- Suction equipment in case of aspiration
- Penlight to check placement of nasopharynx
- Tongue blade
- Disposable tape measure
- Felt-tip marker

Continued

SKILL 43.3	INSERTING A SMALL-BORE NASOENTERIC OR ORAL TUBE FOR ENTERAL FEEDING—cont'd

PROCEDURE

STEPS	RATIONALE
1. Assess patient's need for enteral tube feeding: NPO (nothing by mouth) status, functional gastrointestinal tract, inability to ingest sufficient nutrients. A. Review order for insertion of tube and enteral feeding schedule. 2. Masks must be worn for all patient contact. Explain procedure to patient. 3. Assess patency of nares. Have patient close each nostril alternately and breathe. Examine each naris for patency and skin breakdown. 4. Wearing gloves, assess the gag reflex by placing a tongue blade in patient's mouth, touching uvula to induce a gag response.	• Identifying patients who need tube feedings before they become nutritionally depleted may help to prevent complications related to malnutrition. • Procedures and tube feedings require a physician's order. • Patient can cooperate with the process. • Nares may be obstructed or irritated, or a septal defect may be present. • This assesses ability to swallow and determines whether patient is at risk for aspiration.

CRITICAL DECISION POINT: *Patients with impaired level of consciousness, or who are intubated and sedated, may also have impaired gag reflex, and their risk of aspiration is increased during this type of procedure and subsequent tube feedings. For patients who are intubated, sedated, or too ill to participate in the procedure, ensure that the patient's head is tilted toward the chest for enteral feeding tube insertion.*

STEPS	RATIONALE

5. Review patient's medical history for nasal problems (e.g., nosebleeds, oral or facial surgery, anticoagulation therapy, history of aspiration).
 	
6. Perform hand hygiene.
7. Auscultate abdomen for bowel sounds.
 	
8. Explain procedure to patient and how to communicate during insertion by raising index finger to indicate gagging or discomfort.
9. Stand on same side of bed as naris for insertion, and assist patient to high Fowler's position unless contraindicated. Place pillow behind patient's head and shoulders.
10. Place absorbent pad over patient's chest. Keep facial tissues within reach.
 	
11. Determine length of tube to be inserted and mark with tape:
   • Traditional method for placing the tube to the stomach has been to measure distance from tip of nose to earlobe and then to xiphoid process of sternum (NEX). However, the NEMU method (Nose→ Earlobe→ Mid-Umbilicus) is now used for children and adults (Patient Safety Movement Foundation, 2020).
   • Alternately, measure from the tip of the nose to ear to xiphoid process and subtract 10 cm from the measured length. Then add 5 cm if using the oral route. If using the nasal route, add an additional 10 cm (Morgan, 2021).
   • If placing the tube to small bowel (duodenum), follow employer-specific protocol; for example, the administration of 10 mg metoclopramide as a bowel motility agent, turning patient on right side, and injecting 200 cc of air to inflate the stomach.
12. Prepare nasogastric or nasointestinal tube for insertion according to manufacturer recommendation:
   A. Plastic tubes should *not* be iced.
13. Perform hand hygiene and put on gloves.
   A. If long-term tube, inject 10 mL of water from 30 mL or larger catheter-tip syringe into the tube and insert stylet/guidewire.
   B. Make certain that guidewire is securely positioned against weighted tip and that connections are snugly fitted together.
	• Nasoenteral tubes are not used in patients with recent nasal surgery, facial traumas, nosebleeds, or receiving anticoagulation therapy (Wayne, 2018).
	• Nasoenteral tubes are also contraindicated for patients with bowel ischemia or necrosis, active gastrointestinal bleeding, small or large bowel obstruction, and paralytic ileus (Adeyinka et al., 2022).
	• Hand hygiene reduces transfer of microorganisms.
	• Absence of bowel sounds may indicate decreased or absent peristalsis and increased risk for aspiration or abdominal distension.
	• Explanations reduce anxiety and help patient assist in insertion.
	
	• These actions facilitate manipulation of tube. Fowler's position reduces risk of aspiration and promotes effective swallowing.
	
	• Pad prevents soiling of gown. Insertion of tube may cause patient's eyes to tear.
	• For duodenal or jejunal placement, an additional 20 to 30 cm is required.
	• The traditional method of predicting tube length from NEX was found to be too short. Only guided tube placement or X-ray can eliminate risk of undetected esophageal placement (Taylor, 2020).
	
	• Tubes that are iced become stiff and inflexible, causing trauma to mucous membranes.
	
	• Hygiene and gloves reduce transmission of microorganisms.
	• Water releases a mechanism in the tip of the tube holding the guidewire in place to enable the guidewire to be removed following tube insertion.
	• Secure positioning and snug-fitting connections promote smooth passage of tube into gastrointestinal tract. Improperly positioned stylet can induce serious trauma (i.e., tracheal perforation, pneumothorax).

STEPS	RATIONALE
14. Cut tape 10 cm long or prepare tube fixation device. Split one end of tape lengthwise 5 cm.	• Tape is used to anchor tubing after insertion.
15. Dip tube with surface lubricant into glass of water. If tube is not prelubricated, use water-soluble lubricant.	• Activates lubricant to facilitate passage of tube into naris to gastrointestinal tract.
16. Insert tube through nostril to back of throat (posterior nasopharynx). Aim back and down toward ear.	• Natural contour facilitates passage of tube into gastrointestinal tract and reduces gagging by patient.
17. Have patient tilt head toward chest after tube has passed through nasopharynx.	• Tilting head forward closes off glottis and reduces risk of tube entering trachea. This technique is also used in patients who are intubated and sedated.

CRITICAL DECISION POINT: *Encourage a patient who is alert and communicating to swallow by giving small sips of water or ice chips when possible. For patients who are intubated and sedated, or unable to participate in the procedure, tilt patient's head toward the chest. Advance tube as patient swallows or as patient's head is tilted toward chest. Rotate tube 180 degrees while inserting.*

STEPS	RATIONALE
18. Emphasize the need to mouth-breathe and swallow during the procedure (when possible).	• Mouth-breathing and swallowing facilitate passage of tube and alleviate patient's fear during the procedure.
19. Advance tube each time patient swallows until desired length has been passed.	• Advancing tube while patient swallows reduces discomfort and trauma to patient.

CRITICAL DECISION POINT: *Do not force tube insertion. If resistance is met or patient starts to cough, choke, or become cyanotic, stop advancing the tube and pull tube back. It is important to note that heavily sedated, comatose, or paralyzed patients may not exhibit a cough or gag reflex during insertion and so this should not be used as the sole method of determining improper tube placement. It is also possible to slip a small-bore feeding tube into the trachea down past an endotracheal tube without loss of oxygenation; therefore, X-ray is the definitive step in determining tube placement.*

STEPS	RATIONALE
20. Check for position of tube in back of patient's throat with penlight and tongue blade.	• Tube may be coiled, kinked, or entering trachea. (Withdraw tube immediately if tube is coiled, respiratory status of patient changes, or patient begins to cough and skin colour changes. If distress is not present, withdraw tube fully and retry. Note whether tube was kinked; if so, it is likely to kink again in the same place.)
21. Perform measures to verify placement of tube, once desired length has been passed. Secure tube before X-ray examination, because it may become dislodged during procedure.	• Tube placement must be verified by X-ray examination before enteral feedings are initiated. Other tests that can be done at the bedside to ensure ongoing placement are as follows: • Observe for a change in length of the external portion of the feeding tube, as indicated by movement of the marked portion of the tube. • Review routine chest and abdominal radiography reports to look for notations about tube location. • Observe changes in volume of aspirate from the feeding tube—a large increase in volume may signal the upward dislocation of a small-bowel feeding tube in the stomach; persistent inability to withdraw fluid (or only a few drops of fluid) from the tube may signal upward displacement of a gastric tube into the esophagus. • Measure pH of feeding tube aspirates. • Encourage obtaining a radiograph to confirm tube position if the tube's position is in doubt (Wayne, 2018).

CRITICAL DECISION POINT: *Auscultation is* not *a reliable method for verification of tube placement because a tube inadvertently placed in the lungs, pharynx, or esophagus can transmit a sound similar to that of air entering the stomach (Boeykens, 2018; Metheny et al., 2019; Rigobello et al., 2020).*

STEPS	RATIONALE
22. After gastric aspirates are obtained (see Box 43.18), anchor tube to patient's nose and avoid pressure on nares. Mark exit site with indelible ink. Select one of the following options: **A.** Apply tape. **(1)** Apply tincture of benzoin or other skin adhesive on tip of patient's nose and tube and allow it to become "tacky."	• A properly secured tube allows the patient more mobility and prevents trauma to nasal mucosa. Mark tube at tip of naris; measure from line to end of tube; tape and secure to maintain position. • Skin adhesive helps tape adhere better and protects patient's skin.

Continued

SKILL 43.3   INSERTING A SMALL-BORE NASOENTERIC OR ORAL TUBE FOR ENTERAL FEEDING—cont'd

STEPS	RATIONALE
(2) Place the intact end of tape over bridge of patient's nose. Wrap each of the 5-cm strips around tube as it exits nose. Change position of tube at naris every 8 hours (q8h) (see Step 22A(2) illustration).	• Securing tape to nares prevents tissue necrosis. Changing tube position avoids erosion of naris.

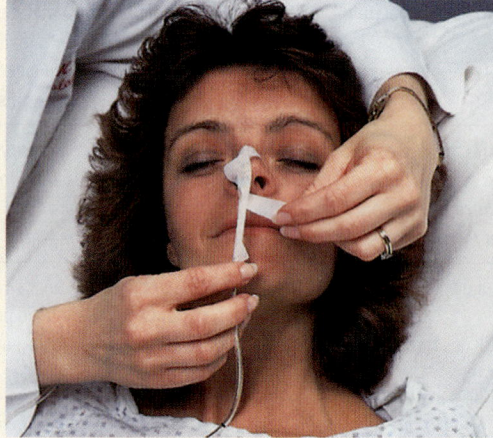

STEP 22A(2) Wrapping tape to anchor nasoenteral tube.

B. Apply tube fixation device, using nasal bridle or shaped adhesive patch. (1) Apply wide end of patch to bridge of nose. (2) Slip connector around tube as it exits nose (see Step 22B(2) illustration).	• Fixation device secures tube and reduces friction on nares (Lynch et al., 2018).

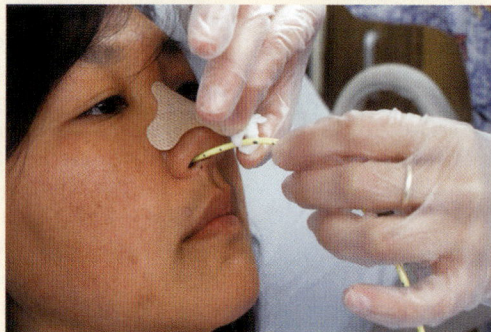

STEP 22B(2) Slipping connector around feeding tube.

23. A second anchoring of tube against cheek with gauze and transparent dressing may be advised to prevent tube from resting over bony points.	• Fastening the tube this way may help prevent it from being pulled by confused patients and avoids pressure points. However, the available evidence on interventions to reduce nasogastric tube dislodgement is of limited quantity and validity (Chauhan et al., 2021).
24. For intestinal placement, position patient on right side, when possible, until correct placement has been verified radiologically. Remove gloves. Perform hand hygiene, and assist patient to a comfortable position.	• Positioning patient on right side promotes passage of the tube into the small intestine (duodenum or jejunum).

CRITICAL DECISION POINT: *Leave stylet/guidewire in place until correct position is ensured by X-ray film. Never attempt to reinsert partially or fully removed stylet/guidewire while feeding tube is in place.*

Clinically sound judgement is required for nasogastric insertion and placement verification. The use of an electromagnetic tracking system displays the placement pathway, enabling continuous position confirmation at the bedside with no inadvertent placements into the lungs documented (Jacobson et al., 2019). A meta-analysis to compare the performance of electromagnetic-guided versus endoscopic placement found no difference between these two groups in terms of procedure success rate, reinsertion rate, number of attempts, placement-related complications, tube-related complications, insertion time, total procedure time, patient discomfort, recommendation scores, length of hospital stay, mortality, and total costs (Wei et al., 2020).

SKILL 43.3	INSERTING A SMALL-BORE NASOENTERIC OR ORAL TUBE FOR ENTERAL FEEDING—cont'd

STEPS	RATIONALE
25. Obtain X-ray film of abdomen.	• X-ray examination verifies placement of tube (Metheny et al., 2019).
26. Perform hand hygiene, apply clean gloves, and administer oral hygiene (see Chapter 39). Cleanse tubing at nostril.	• Oral hygiene promotes patient comfort and integrity of oral mucous membranes.
27. Remove gloves, dispose of equipment, and perform hand hygiene.	• These actions reduce transmission of microorganisms.
28. Inspect patient's naris and oropharynx for any irritation after insertion.	• If tube insertion was difficult, irritation of naris or oropharynx may have occurred.
29. Ask patient whether they feel comfortable.	• Patient's level of comfort is evaluated. (This may be a challenge if a language barrier exists or if the patient has dementia or is confused.)
30. Observe patient for any difficulty breathing or for coughing or gagging.	• Improper position of the tube may cause these symptoms or increase symptoms in patients who have heart failure, pneumonia, asthma, and other cardiac or respiratory conditions.
31. Auscultate lung sounds.	• Abnormal lung sounds can be an early sign of aspiration.
32. Assess for feeding tube placement at 4-hour intervals to ensure that the tube has remained in the desired location.	To repeat from Step 21 • Observe for change in length of the external portion of the feeding tube. • Observe changes in volume of aspirate from the feeding tube. • Measure pH of feeding tube aspirates. • Encourage obtaining a radiograph to confirm tube position if the tube's position is in doubt.
33. Assess for intolerance to feedings every 4 hours.	Monitor abdominal discomfort, nausea/vomiting, and gastric residual volumes (GRVs) based on any relevant employer policy to use GRV as a criterion for confirming intestinal intolerance and determining continuation or interruption of enteral nutrition (Tatsumi, 2019).

UNEXPECTED OUTCOMES	RELATED INTERVENTIONS
Aspiration of stomach contents into the respiratory tract (immediate response), evidenced by coughing, dyspnea, cyanosis, auscultation of crackles or wheezes	• Position patient on side. • Suction nasotracheally and orotracheally. • Consult physician immediately to order chest X-ray.
Aspiration of stomach contents into respiratory tract (delayed response), evidenced by dyspnea, fever, auscultation of crackles or wheezes	• Consult physician to obtain order for chest X-ray. • Prepare for possible initiation of antibiotics.
Development of bacterial aspiration pneumonia from contaminated saliva for patients NPO or being fed enterally	• Limited oral hydration leads to dry mouth and increased concentration of oral bacteria. It is imperative that scrupulous oral hygiene be maintained, which includes using a soft tooth brush to clean teeth, gums, roof of mouth, and cheeks. Patients who are discharged home or maintain self-care, as well as their families, must be counselled regarding this risk. Patients who are unable to contribute to their oral hygiene should have an oral cleansing program provided by using chlorhexidine oral swabs twice daily, especially for chronically intubated patients. It is important to place these patients in a semi-recumbent position (head up 45 degrees), as long as it is not contraindicated (Kollmeier & Keenaghan, 2021).
Displacement of feeding tube to another site (e.g., from duodenum to stomach, which may occur when patient coughs or vomits)	• Confirm that mark on tube (made at initial insertion) is at exit site. • Remeasure distance from naris to mid-umbilicus, and compare with baseline measurement from insertion. • Aspirate gastrointestinal contents and measure pH (Chauhan et al., 2021). • Discuss findings with physician. • Reconfirm placement by X-ray film (optional). • If tube is displaced, prepare to remove it, and insert and verify placement of new tube. • If there is a question of aspiration, obtain chest X-ray film.

CRITICAL DECISION POINT: *To prevent clogging of feeding tube, flush feeding tube before and after enteral medication administration and q6h and prn using 30 mL of sterile water. Giving oral medications and free water administration are also done using sterile water, because a number of cases have been reported of tap water contamination among hospitalized patients (Morgan, 2020). Try to find an alternative route for medication administration when small-bore tubes (especially the temporary nasogastric silastic tubes) are used because they frequently clog.*

Continued

SKILL 43.3	INSERTING A SMALL-BORE NASOENTERIC OR ORAL TUBE FOR ENTERAL FEEDING—cont'd

STEPS	RATIONALE
Clogging of feeding tube	• To prevent feeding tube clogging that results from medication, use liquid forms of medication whenever possible. When the solid form of dosage is used, make sure there is no contraindication to crushing the tablets (i.e., sustained-release cardiac meds should *not* be crushed as this will adversely affect the patient's heart rate and blood pressure) and that capsules can be opened; dissolve tablets or capsules well, and administer each medication separately. Flush after each medication and after all medications are administered (Tadlock et al., 2018).
	• Aspirate gastric contents with 60-mL syringe to assess patency of tube.
	• Irrigate tube with water. Research supports water as the best choice for initial declogging efforts and recommends that nurses use sterile water for declogging (Tillott et al., 2020).
	• Use of beverages such as carbonated soda and cranberry juice is not recommended because of the risk of worsening the clog and lack of evidence of efficacy. The use of pancreatic enzyme/sodium bicarbonate solution to treat a clogged enteral feeding tube requires a prescriber's order (Nursing Pharmacy Liaison Committee, 2020).
	• Do *not* use a small-barrel syringe (i.e., 20 cm or less) because smaller syringes have greater psi (pounds per square inch) and injection of air or liquid under high pressure (above 40 psi) may cause tube rupture (Drummond Hayes & Drummond Hayes, 2018).
Irritation of naris and nasal mucosa	• Provide hygiene and remove and replace tube. (*Note:* This action requires a physician's order.)
	• Consider removing tube and inserting it into the other naris (physician order required).

RECORDING AND REPORTING

• Record and report type and size of tube placed, location of distal tip of tube (mark and measure), patient's tolerance of procedure, pH value, and confirmation of tube position by X-ray examination.

SKILL 43.4	ADMINISTERING ENTERAL FEEDINGS VIA NASOENTERIC TUBE

Delegation Considerations

Administration of enteral tube feeding via nasoenteric tube is an agency-specific procedure that may or may *not* be delegated to unregulated care providers (UCPs) after the nurse verifies tube placement. The nurse is responsible for patient assessment. Depending on the employer's protocol, the nurse directs the UCPs to

• Ensure that the patient is sitting upright in a chair or in bed.
• Infuse the feeding slowly.
• Report any difficulty infusing the feeding or any discomfort voiced by the patient.

Equipment

• Personal protective equipment—mask, gloves
• Disposable feeding bag and tubing or ready-to-hang system
• 30-mL or larger Luer-Lok or catheter-tip syringe
• Stethoscope
• pH indicator strip (scale 0 to 14)
• Infusion pump (required for intestinal feedings): use pump designed for tube feedings
• Prescribed enteral feedings
• Disposable gloves
• Equipment to obtain blood glucose by fingerstick

PROCEDURE

STEPS	RATIONALE
1. Assess patient's need for enteral tube feedings: impaired swallowing, tracheostomy, decreased level of consciousness, head or neck surgery, facial trauma, surgical procedures involving upper alimentary canal.	• Identify patients who need tube feedings before they become nutritionally depleted.
2. Evaluate patient's nutritional status (see Table 43.4). Obtain baseline weight and laboratory values (e.g., albumin, transferrin, prealbumin). Assess patient for fluid volume excess or deficit, electrolyte abnormalities, and metabolic abnormalities, such as hyperglycemia.	• Enteral feedings are intended to restore or maintain a patient's nutritional status. Fluid volume assessment provides objective data to measure effectiveness of feedings.

SKILL 43.4   **ADMINISTERING ENTERAL FEEDINGS VIA NASOENTERIC TUBE—cont'd**

STEPS	RATIONALE
3. Verify physician's order for formula, rate, route, and frequency and for laboratory data and bedside assessments, such as fingerstick blood glucose measurement.	• Tube feedings, laboratory tests, and bedside tests must be ordered by the physician.
4. Explain procedure to patient.	• Well-informed patients tend to be cooperative and comfortable.
5. Masks must be worn for all patient contact. Perform hand hygiene.	• Use of mask and hand hygiene reduces transmission of microorganisms.
6. Auscultate for bowel sounds before feeding.	• Absence of bowel sounds may indicate decreased ability of gastrointestinal tract to digest or absorb nutrients.
7. Prepare feeding container to administer formula:	
A. Check expiration date on formula and integrity of container.	• Tube feedings administered within the designated shelf life from a container without cracks or breaks reduce the patient's risk of acquiring tube feeding–borne gastrointestinal infections.
B. Have tube feeding formula at room temperature.	• Cold formula may cause gastric cramping and discomfort because the liquid is not warmed by the mouth and esophagus.
C. Perform hand hygiene and apply gloves.	
D. Shake formula container well and fill feeding container with formula (see Step 7D illustration). Open stopcock on tubing and fill with formula to remove air.	• Filling the tubing with formula prevents excess air from entering. • Tubing must be free of contamination in order to prevent bacterial growth.

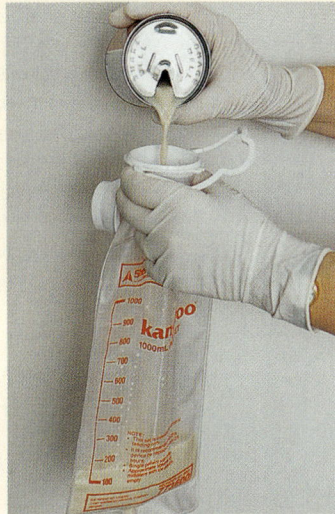

STEP 7D Pouring formula into feeding container.

   E. Connect tubing to container, as needed, or prepare ready-to-hang container.

CRITICAL DECISION POINT: *Tube feedings are infused by feeding pumps and the tubes do not fit intravenous (IV) pumps.*

---

8. For intermittent feeding, have syringe ready, and ensure formula is at room temperature.	• Cold formula may cause gastric cramping.
9. Place patient in high Fowler's position or elevate head of bed at least 45 degrees.	• Elevating the patient's head helps prevent aspiration.
10. Verify tube placement (see Box 43.15). Consider the results from pH testing together with the aspirate's appearance.	• Colour may help differentiate gastric from intestinal placement. Most intestinal aspirates are stained by bile to a distinct yellow colour and most gastric aspirates are not so stained. The aspirate's colour must be considered in combination with other assessment data (Metheny et al., 2019).

Continued

STEPS	RATIONALE
11. Check pH of aspirate; confirm measurement of length of tube from naris to tip of connection port; ensure original mark is in the same position.	• Aspirates from initially placed nasogastric tubes with a pH of 1–5.5 are reliable to differentiate if the tube is in or outside the stomach, but the lower the pH, the more convincing is the evidence that the aspirate is from the stomach instead of the respiratory tract (Metheny et al., 2019).
12. When available, check CO_2 at the distal end of naso- or orogastric (NG/OG) tubes.	• Carbon dioxide detectors may be helpful in distinguishing between gastric and pulmonary placement of a NG tube, but are not sufficiently accurate to use as a single confirmatory method (Metheny et al., 2019). Based on available research, more than one method of monitoring the placement of NG/OG tubes at the bedside should be used; an abdominal radiograph should be obtained if there is any doubt that the tube ends in the stomach.

CRITICAL DECISION POINT: *Auscultation is not a reliable method for verification of placement because a tube inadvertently placed in lungs, pharynx, or esophagus can transmit sound similar to that of air entering stomach (Metheny et al., 2019).*

---

13. Check for gastric residual.
   A. Draw 30 mL of air with syringe. Connect to end of feeding tube. Flush tube with air.
   B. Pull back evenly to aspirate gastric contents (see Step 13B illustration).
	• Residual volume indicates whether gastric emptying is delayed. Continue feeding at the defined rate as long as GRV is not greater than 500 mL and there are no clinical signs of intolerance. Enteral nutrition should be delayed for critical care patients if gastric aspirate volume is above 500 mL/6 hr (Singer et al., 2019). For pediatric patients, the amount of residual volume will be less. Depending on agency policy and physician or dietitian decision, if residual volume exceeds 500 mL, feedings may be withheld. Further research is needed to recommend the frequency of the need to monitor GRVs. To this end, a Cochrane Intervention Review is investigating the clinical efficacy and safety of monitoring GRV during enteral nutrition (Yasuda et al., 2019). One event of elevated residual volume should not prompt cessation of enteral tube feeding but instead should prompt the nurse to monitor for signs and symptoms of intolerance (Pham et al., 2019).

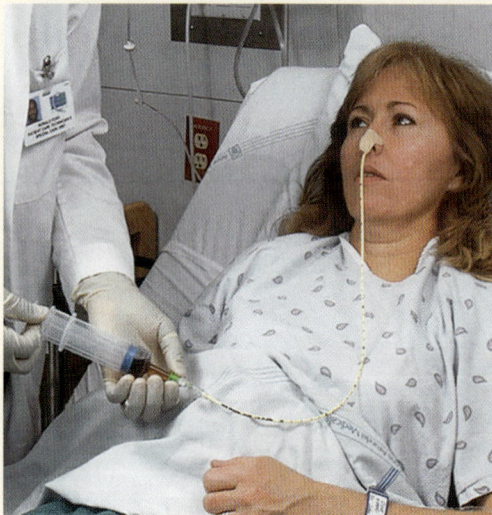

STEP 13B Check for gastric residual (small-bore tube).

Please note that if checking for gastric residual when a small-bore tube is in place, consult agency policy. Soft, small-bore tubes may collapse when GRV is checked, making assessment of residuals falsely low.

Remember that tube location is important. A tube in the small bowel would have ongoing secretions and much more residual.

   C. Return aspirated contents to stomach if specified by agency policy.

14. Flush tubing with 30 to 50 mL of water at room temperature.

15. Label feeding tube bag. Complete and post nutrition label on bag to indicate type of formula, rate, time, and date.

• Return of aspirate is also a controversial topic that requires further research (Yasuda et al., 2019).
• Ensure tube is clear and patent. Check agency policy because drinking water (tap, bottled, and well water) may contain chemical contaminants.

STEPS

RATIONALE

16. Initiate feeding:
  A. Syringe or intermittent feeding:
   (1) Pinch proximal end of the feeding tube.
   (2) Remove plunger from syringe and attach barrel of syringe to end of tube.
   (3) Fill syringe with measured amount of formula (see Step 16A[3] illustration). Release tube and hold syringe high enough to allow it to empty gradually by gravity, and refill; repeat until prescribed amount has been delivered to the patient.

- Pinching prevents air from entering patient's stomach.

- Gradual emptying of tube feeding by gravity from syringe or feeding bag reduces risk of abdominal discomfort, vomiting, or diarrhea induced by bolus or too-rapid infusion of tube feedings.

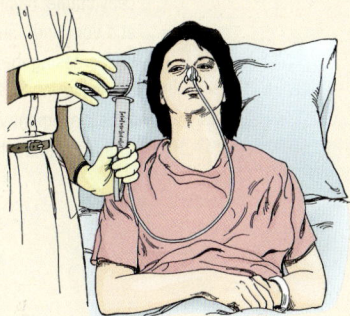

STEP 16A(3) Fill syringe with formula.

   (4) If feeding bag is used, hang feeding bag on an IV pole (see Step 16A[4] illustration). Fill bag with prescribed amount of formula, and allow bag to empty gradually over at least 30 minutes, depending on the amount of feeding.

- A feeding pump is used to infuse the formula. An IV pump must not be used for enteral feedings.

STEP 16A(4) Administration via feeding bag.

   (5) Document tube assessment for placement, formula infusing, and infusion rate; elevate head of bed at least 45 degrees.

Continued

SKILL 43.4   ADMINISTERING ENTERAL FEEDINGS VIA NASOENTERIC TUBE—cont'd

STEPS	RATIONALE

B. Continuous-drip method (see Step 16B illustration):

    (1) Prime and hang feeding bag and tubing.

    (2) Connect distal end of tubing to the proximal end of the feeding tube.

    (3) Connect tubing through infusion pump and set rate (see Step 16B illustration).

    (4) Do not hang any longer than a 4-hour supply, to decrease risk of food spoilage potentially resulting in gastrointestinal irritation or infection.

- Continuous feeding method is designed to deliver a prescribed hourly rate of feeding. This method reduces risk of abdominal discomfort. ***Patients who receive continuous-drip feedings should have residuals checked as per employer policy.*** Frequency of checking gastric residuals varies, and research has not clearly determined the need. GRV monitoring leads to unnecessary interruptions of enteral nutrition delivery with subsequent inadequate feeding (Yasuda et al., 2019). Although in nursing practice, GRVs are usually checked every 4 hours × 48 hours post-initiation of new continuous feed, consideration is being given to (a) stopping the GRV checks if the patient is clinically stable, has no apparent tolerance issues (abdominal distension, nausea, and vomiting), and has shown clear evidence of tolerance for 48 hours, and (b) increasing the time interval between GRV checks to more than 6 to 8 hours (Rees Parrish & McCray, 2019).
- Tube placement verification is difficult with continuous feeding because pH of formula affects the stomach pH.

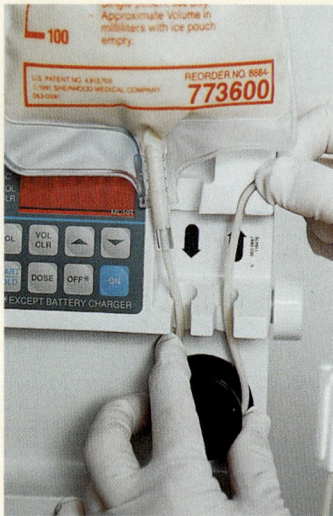

STEP 16B Prime and connect tubing through infusion pump.

17. Advance the rate of tube feeding gradually (see Box 43.13).

- Tube feedings should be advanced gradually to prevent diarrhea and gastric intolerance to formula.

18. After intermittent infusion or at end of continuous infusion, flush nasoenteral tubing with water. On average, 30 mL of water is used, but the amount can vary from 10 mL to over 30 mL. Repeat every 4 to 6 hours. Remove gloves and perform hand hygiene.

- Flushing maintains patency of feeding tube and provides patient with a source of water to help maintain fluid and electrolyte balance.

CRITICAL DECISION POINT: *It may be necessary to consult with a dietitian to recommend a total free water requirement per day. This avoids the potential of fluid overload.*

---

19. When tube feedings are not being administered (e.g., they may be held prior to tests or procedures such as extubation), cap or clamp the proximal end of the feeding tube.

- Closing the end of the tube prevents air from entering stomach between feedings and prevents contamination.

20. Rinse bag and tubing with water whenever feedings are interrupted or every 8 hours.

- Rinsing bag and tubing clears old tube formula and reduces bacterial growth.

21. Change bag and tubing every 24 hours.

- Changing bag and tubing reduces patient's exposure to bacterial growth occurring in those items.

22. Measure amount of aspirate (residual) every 8 to 12 hours.

- These measurements help evaluate tolerance of tube feeding.

23. Monitor fingerstick blood glucose level every 6 hours until maximum administration rate is reached and maintained for 24 hours.

- These levels alert the nurse to patient's tolerance of glucose. Remember that if feedings are stopped, monitor for any drop in glucose level—especially if patient is on an insulin therapy.

24. Monitor intake and output every 8 hours and compute 24-hour totals.

- Intake and output are indications of fluid balance or fluid volume excess or deficit.

25. Weigh patient daily until maximum administration rate is reached and maintained for 24 hours; then weigh patient three times per week.

- Weight gain is an indicator of improved nutritional status; however, sudden gain of more than 1 kg in 24 hours usually indicates fluid retention.

26. Observe patient's respiratory status.

- Increased respiratory rate may indicate aspiration of tube feeding.

27. Observe return of normal laboratory values.

- Improving laboratory values (e.g., albumin, transferrin, and prealbumin) indicate improved nutritional status.

SKILL 43.4   ADMINISTERING ENTERAL FEEDINGS VIA NASOENTERIC TUBE—cont'd

UNEXPECTED OUTCOMES	RELATED INTERVENTIONS
(In addition to those identified in Skill 43.1) *Gastric residual exceeding 200 to 500 mL (see agency policy)*	• See Step 13 for further information about residual volumes. If established by agency policy, withhold feeding and notify physician. • According to Canadian Clinical Nurse Specialist Brenda Morgan (2020), if GRV is <300 mL, return aspirated residual to patient via the feeding tube. Discard aspirate if >300 mL. • Maintain patient in semi-Fowler's position, or have head of bed elevated at least 30 to 45 degrees. • Perform physical assessment. • Assess glycemic control.
Diarrhea three times or more in 24 hours	• Notify physician. • Confer with dietitian. • Institute skin-care measures. • Diarrhea could relate to the speed and method of administration and the type of enteral nutrition formula (Tatsumi, 2019). • Look for other causes of the diarrhea (e.g., antibiotics; consider change in antibiotics only for patients receiving antibiotics).
Nausea and vomiting	• Notify physician. • Check patency of tube. • Aspirate for residual, keeping in mind that GRV remains the most common factor in defining feed intolerance, despite the lack of evidence to support this (Tume & Valla, 2018). • Auscultate for bowel sounds.

RECORDING AND REPORTING
• Record amount and type of feeding and patient's response to tube feeding, patency of tube, and any side effects.
• Report patient's tolerance and adverse effects.

CARE IN THE COMMUNITY CONSIDERATIONS
• Teach patient or primary caregiver how to determine correct placement of feeding tube using pH strips.
• Inform patient or primary caregiver of signs associated with pulmonary aspiration and delayed gastric emptying.
• Describe signs and symptoms associated with feeding tube complications and advise when to call physician.

SKILL 43.5   ADMINISTERING ENTERAL FEEDINGS VIA GASTROSTOMY OR JEJUNOSTOMY TUBE

Delegation Considerations

Administration of enteral tube feeding via a gastrostomy or jejunostomy tube is a procedure that—depending on employer policy—can be delegated to an unregulated care provider (UCP) after the nurse verifies tube placement. UCPs should never test the position of the tube or give the first dose of a tube feeding.
• Ensure that the patient is sitting upright in a chair or in bed and instruct the UCP to infuse the feeding slowly.
• Instruct the UCP to report any difficulty infusing the feeding or any discomfort voiced by the patient.

Equipment
• Personal protective equipment—mask, gloves
• Disposable feeding container or ready-to-hang bag
• 30-mL or larger Luer-Lok or catheter-tip syringe
• Formula
• Infusion pump: Use pump designed for tube feedings
• pH indicator strips (scale 0 to 14)
• Medication cup or container for aspirated fluid
• Stethoscope
• Disposable gloves
• Equipment to obtain blood glucose by fingerstick

PROCEDURE

STEPS	RATIONALE
1. Assess patient's need for enteral tube feedings (see Skill 43.3 and Skill 43.4): impaired swallowing, decreased level of consciousness, surgical procedures involving upper alimentary tract, need for long-term enteral nutrition.	• This assessment identifies patients who need tube feedings before they become nutritionally depleted. Enteral feeding preserves the function and mass of the gut, promotes wound healing, diminishes hypermetabolism in burn injuries, and may decrease infection in critically ill patients (Singh, 2019).
2. Obtain baseline weight and laboratory values (blood glucose, albumin, transferrin, prealbumin).	• Enteral feedings are intended to restore or maintain nutritional status. Baseline weight and laboratory values provide objective data to measure effectiveness of feedings.

Continued

SKILL 43.5	ADMINISTERING ENTERAL FEEDINGS VIA GASTROSTOMY OR JEJUNOSTOMY TUBE—cont'd
STEPS	**RATIONALE**
3. Verify physician's order for formula, rate, route, and frequency.	• Tube feedings must be ordered by a physician.
4. Masks must be worn for all patient contact. Perform hand hygiene.	• Mask and hand hygiene reduces transmission of microorganisms.
5. Explain procedure to patient.	• Well-informed patients are more cooperative and at ease than patients who are ill-informed.
6. Auscultate for bowel sounds before feeding. Consult physician if bowel sounds are absent.	• Absence of bowel sounds may indicate decrease in or absence of peristalsis and increased risk of aspiration or abdominal distension.
7. Assess gastrostomy or jejunostomy site for breakdown, irritation, or drainage.	• Infection, pressure from tube, or drainage of gastric secretions can cause skin breakdown.
8. Perform hand hygiene and apply gloves.	
9. Prepare feeding container to administer formula:	
A. Have tube feeding formula at room temperature.	• Cold formula may cause gastric cramping and discomfort because the liquid is not warmed by mouth and esophagus.
B. Connect tubing to container, as needed, or prepare ready-to-hang bag.	• Tubing must be free of contamination in order to prevent bacterial growth.
C. Shake formula well. Fill container and tubing with formula.	• Placement of formula through tubing prevents excess air from entering gastro-intestinal tract.
10. For intermittent feeding, have syringe ready and ensure formula is at room temperature.	• Cold formula may cause gastric cramping.
11. Elevate head of bed to 45 degrees.	• Elevating patient's head helps prevent aspiration.
12. Apply gloves and verify tube placement.	
A. *Gastrostomy tube:* Attach syringe and aspirate gastric secretions; observe their appearance and check pH. Usual practice is to return aspirated contents to stomach unless the volume exceeds 100 mL or the specified amount on several consecutive occasions. Check employer policy regarding stopping the feeding and notifying the physician.	• Fluid from gastric tube of patient who has fasted for at least 4 hours usually has a pH of 1 to 4, especially when patient is not receiving a gastric-acid inhibitor. Continuous administration of tube feedings may elevate pH (McLaren & Arbuckle, 2020). Gastric residual may indicate whether gastric emptying is delayed. Returning gastric residual volume may increase the risk of tube blockage and infection, whereas discarding gastric residues may increase the risk of fluid and electrolyte imbalance (Wen et al., 2019).
B. *Jejunostomy tube:* Aspirate intestinal secretions, observe their appearance, and check pH.	• Presence of intestinal fluid indicates that the end of the tube is in the small intestine (i.e., the duodenum or jejunum). In general, the intestinal residual is very small (10 mL or less). If fluid appears acidic on pH test, if fluid looks like gastric fluid, or if the residual volume is large (more than 10 mL), displacement of the tube into the stomach may have occurred.
13. Flush with 30 mL of room temperature water.	
14. Initiate feedings:	• Gastrostomy and jejunostomy feedings are usually given continuously to ensure proper absorption. However, initial feedings may be given by bolus to assess patient's tolerance to formula. See Box 43.13 for guidelines to advance enteral feedings.
A. Syringe feedings:	
(1) Pinch proximal end of gastrostomy or jejunostomy tube.	• Pinching prevents excessive air from entering the patient's stomach and prevents leakage of gastric contents.
(2) Remove plunger and attach barrel of syringe to end of tube; then fill syringe with formula.	
(3) Release tube and elevate syringe. Allow syringe to empty gradually by gravity. Refill until prescribed amount has been delivered to patient.	• Gradual administration of tube feedings by gravity reduces the risk of diarrhea induced by bolus tube feedings.
B. Continuous drip method:	• Continuous-feeding method is designed to deliver a prescribed hourly rate of feeding. This method reduces the risk of diarrhea and risk of abdominal discomfort. Patients who receive continuous-drip feedings should have residuals checked as per employer policy and tube placement verified every 4 hours. It is usual to measure GRVs every 4 hours in critically ill patients; however, there is no evidence to support monitoring GRVs of critical care patients receiving enteral nutrition (Rees Parrish & McCray, 2019).
	• GRVs are usually reduced in noncritically ill patients after the first 48 hours of being fed.

SKILL 43.5	**ADMINISTERING ENTERAL FEEDINGS VIA GASTROSTOMY OR JEJUNOSTOMY TUBE—cont'd**

STEPS	**RATIONALE**

STEPS	**RATIONALE**
(1) Verify that volume in container is sufficient for length of feeding (4 to 8 hours, check manufacturer's recommendations).	
(2) Hang container on IV pole, and clear tubing of air.	• Hanging the container allows for gravity-based flow of formula, which prevents accumulation of air in the patient's stomach.
(3) Thread tubing into pump according to manufacturer's directions.	
(4) Connect tubing to end of gastrostomy or jejunostomy tube.	
(5) Begin infusion at prescribed rate.	
15. Administer water via feeding tube as ordered with or between feedings.	• Water helps patients maintain fluid and electrolyte balance.
16. Flush tube with 30 mL of sterile or cool boiled water every 4 to 6 hours and before and after administering medications via feeding tube.	• Flushing maintains patency of tube and provides patient with some free water. Small jejunal tubes are prone to clogging and are difficult to replace (McLaren & Arbuckle, 2020).
17. When tube feedings are not being administered, cap or clamp the proximal end of the gastrostomy or jejunostomy tube.	• Closing the end of the tube prevents excess air from entering the gastrointestinal tract between feedings and prevents leakage of gastric contents.
18. Rinse container and tubing with water after all intermittent feedings.	• Rinsing clears formula from tubing and reduces bacterial growth in container and tubing. The container and tubing should be changed every 24 hours.
19. Assess skin around tube exit site. Before site has healed, clean with normal saline. A small precut gauze dressing may be applied to exit site and secured with tape. The dressing is assessed for drainage and changed daily and as needed. Once site has healed, cleanse the skin around the tube daily with warm water and mild soap. A fully healed tubing exit site is left open to air. If patient received nasogastric feedings before tube insertion and then undergoes a procedure, tube is not used for first 4 to 6 hours after procedure. (Patient will be NPO status the night before the procedure. Post-procedure documentation—as per agency policy—will indicate when to use tube.) Feeding will resume at previous nasogastric rates once it is safe to begin feeding.	• Report any drainage, redness, swelling, or displacement of the tube to the physician. Leakage of gastric drainage may cause skin irritation. • Post-procedure monitoring is performed to check for bleeding.
20. Dispose of supplies and perform hand hygiene.	• Hygiene prevents transmission of microorganisms.
21. Evaluate patient's tolerance to tube feeding. Measure the amount of aspirate every 8 to 12 hours.	• Measurements help evaluate tolerance of tube feeding.
22. Monitor fingerstick blood glucose level every 6 hours until maximum administration rate is reached and maintained for 24 hours.	• Alerts nurse to patient's tolerance of glucose.
23. Monitor intake and output every 24 hours.	• Intake and output are indications of fluid volume balance.
24. Weigh patient daily until maximum administration rate is reached and maintained for 24 hours; then weigh patient three times per week.	• Weight gain indicates improved nutritional status; however, a sudden gain of more than 1 kg in 24 hours usually indicates fluid retention.
25. Observe return of normal laboratory values.	• Improved laboratory values (albumin, transferrin, prealbumin) indicate improving nutritional status.
26. Inspect stoma site for impaired skin integrity.	• Enteral tubes can cause pressure and excoriation at the stoma site. In addition, gastric secretions irritate patient's skin.

UNEXPECTED OUTCOMES	**RELATED INTERVENTIONS**
Aspiration of formula when gastric emptying is delayed or formula is administered too rapidly and produces vomiting	• Position patient in side-lying position. • Suction airway. • Notify physician. • Obtain chest X-ray film.
Skin breakdown around gastrostomy or jejunostomy site	• Institute skin care practices. • Use pressure relief measures around tube. • Provide appropriate wound care (see Chapter 47).

RECORDING AND REPORTING

• Record amount and type of feeding and patient's response to tube feeding, patency of tube, stoma site, and skin integrity, and document any side effects.
• Report to incoming nursing staff type of feeding, status of feeding tube, patient's tolerance, and adverse effects.

Continued

SKILL 43.5 | ADMINISTERING ENTERAL FEEDINGS VIA GASTROSTOMY OR JEJUNOSTOMY TUBE—cont'd

CARE IN THE COMMUNITY CONSIDERATIONS

Teaching patient or primary caregiver how to determine correct placement of feeding tube

- Aspirate and check pH.
- Measure tube length.

Signs associated with pulmonary aspiration and delayed gastric emptying

- Advise patient or primary caregiver to be alert for increased or laboured breathing.
- Instruct to report shortness of breath.
- Instruct to report enlarged or tender abdomen.
- Instruct to be alert for residuals exceeding 200 mL (Shepherd Center, 2018).

Reinforcing signs and symptoms associated with feeding tube complications and when to call physician

- Shortness of breath
- Laboured breathing
- Cramping, vomiting
- Diarrhea two to three times per day
- Constipation
- Tube occlusion
- Tube length increase of 3 to 5 cm or dislodgement

BOX 43.13 | Advancing the Rate of Tube Feeding

Intermittent

1. Start formula at ordered concentration.
2. If based on physician order and agency policy, infuse bolus of formula over at least 20 to 30 minutes via syringe or feeding container.
3. Begin feedings with no more than 150 to 250 mL at one time. Increase incrementally by 50 mL per feeding per day for adults to achieve needed volume and calories in six to eight feedings. Rates for pediatric patients may increase by 5 to 10 mL per 8 to 24 hours. (*Note:* Concentrated formulas at full strength may be infused at slower rates until tolerance is achieved.)

Continuous

1. Start formula at ordered concentration full strength for isotonic formula (concentration of its nutrients is the same as the concentration of plasma—the fluid component of blood—at approximately 300 mOsm/kg water) or at ordered concentration. Usually, hypertonic formulas are also started at full strength but at a slower rate because hypertonic formulas create a pressure gradient that draws water into the intestine and may cause diarrhea and cramping.
2. Begin infusion at designated rate.
3. Advance rate slowly (e.g., 10 to 20 mL/hour per day, depending on patient's age) to target rate if tolerated (tolerance indicated by absence of nausea and diarrhea and by low gastric residuals).

BOX 43.14   PROCEDURAL GUIDELINE

Discontinuing Enteral Feedings via Nasogastric Tube

Equipment

- Personal protective equipment—mask
- Clean gloves, facial tissues, towel or absorbent pad, disposable bag

Procedure

1. Check the physician's order to discontinue nasogastric tube.
2. Educate patient about what to expect during the procedure:
   A. Patient may experience irritation of nose and throat, as well as watering of the eyes.
   B. Encourage patient to exhale as the tube is being removed, to promote comfort and ease of removal.
3. Perform hand hygiene and apply mask and gloves.
4. Assist patient to sit up in high Fowler's position, if possible (to protect patient from drainage). Encourage patient participation.
   A. Place towel over patient's chest.
   B. Provide tissues to patient.
5. Disconnect tube from pump and from patient's gown.
6. Ask patient to take a deep breath and exhale slowly; pinch tube and withdraw it slowly.
7. Provide oral care to patient; provide skin care around patient's nares.
8. Document procedure and total fluid balances.

---

foods for meeting the patient's individual nutritional needs. **Elemental formulas** (1.0 to 3.0 kcal/mL) contain predigested nutrients that are easier for a partially dysfunctional gastrointestinal tract to absorb. Finally, **specialty formulas** (1.0 to 2.0 kcal/mL) are designed to meet specific nutritional needs in certain illnesses (e.g., liver failure, pulmonary disease, or human immunodeficiency virus [HIV] infection).

Tube feedings are typically started at full strength at slow rates (Box 43.13). The hourly rate is increased every 12 to 24 hours if there are no signs of intolerance (nausea, cramping, vomiting, diarrhea).

Studies have demonstrated a beneficial effect of enteral feedings compared with parenteral (intravenously administered) nutrition. Feeding by the enteral route may reduce sepsis, blunt the hypermetabolic response to trauma, and maintain intestinal structure and function (Tatsumi, 2019). To remove the tube, the procedure outlined in Box 43.14 is used.

Preventing Complications

A serious complication associated with enteral feeding is aspiration of enteral formula into the tracheobronchial tree. Such aspiration irritates the bronchial mucosa, resulting in decreased blood supply to affected pulmonary tissue (Adeyinka et al., 2022). This leads to necrotizing infection, pneumonia, and potential abscess formation. The high glucose content serves as a bacterial growth medium, thereby promoting infection. Adult respiratory distress syndrome is also frequently associated with pulmonary aspiration. Common conditions that increase the risk of aspiration include coughing, nasotracheal suctioning, an artificial airway, decreased level of consciousness, and lying flat during and after feeding.

Small-bore feeding tubes create less discomfort for patients and are currently most often used (Figure 43.11). For adults, most of these tubes are 8 to 12 Fr and 91 to 109 cm long. A stylet is often used during insertion of a small-bore tube to stiffen it. The stylet is removed when the correct position of the feeding tube is confirmed.

At present, the most reliable method for verification of placement of small-bore feeding tubes is X-ray examination (Box 43.15). Measuring the pH of secretions withdrawn from the feeding tube may also help

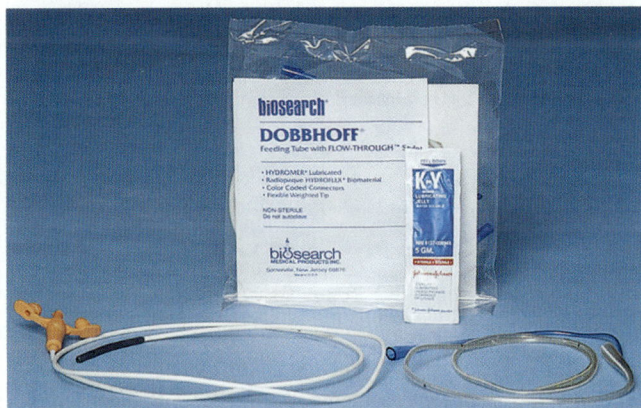

FIGURE 43.11 Enteral tubes, small bore.

differentiate the location of the tube (Box 43.16). Patients who take acid inhibitor medications usually have an acidic pH value ranging from 4.0 (after 4 hours of fasting) to 6.0 (with continuous enteral nutrition infusion). In contrast, intestinal aspirate has a pH of 7.8 to 8.0. More precise indicators are needed to help differentiate the source of tube feeding aspirate (Rigobello et al., 2020).

Major complications of enteral nutrition are outlined in Table 43.8. Of special note, severely malnourished patients are at risk for electrolyte disturbances from **refeeding syndrome** (metabolic disturbances that occur as a result of reinstituting nutrition) because cations such as potassium, magnesium, and phosphate move intracellularly during enteral nutrition or parenteral nutrition therapy. There can be situations where enteral nutrition is not effective in nourishing the body, and the nurse's role is to support a patient in a different way. Recall the chapter-opening case about Arnold, the older person living with type 2 diabetes and stomach cancer, where it was not acceptable to reinsert a gastroscopy tube after the tumour grew back.

LARGE-BORE TUBE AND NASOGASTRIC OR OROGASTRIC SUCTIONING

Gastric decompression is the use of suction to drain the stomach to relieve blockage of the intestinal tract, to wash out stomach contents when a person has taken poisonous material, or after surgery (Wayne, 2018).

After surgery, the objectives for drainage are the following:
- Reduce abdominal distension
- Speed the return of bowel function
- Reduce the chance of wound dehiscence and hernia

BOX 43.15 RESEARCH HIGHLIGHT
Accuracy in Determining Placement of Feeding Tubes

Research Focus

Two possible adverse outcomes of enteral nutrition are (1) accidental placement of a nasoenteral feeding tube into the lung and (2) pulmonary aspiration of gastric contents.

Research Abstract

The precise incidence of accidental tube misplacements into the lung is unknown, but estimates of close to 5% have been cited. Patients at highest risk are those with a decreased level of consciousness; those who are confused, uncooperative, or agitated; those who have an endotracheal tube; those who have undergone recent extubation; and those with poor gag reflex. A feeding tube accidentally inserted into the lung may end in the tracheobronchial tree or may perforate into the pleural space. In either event, efforts are made to detect the misplacement before the introduction of tube feedings because inadvertent infusion of formula into the lung promotes tissue consolidation, pneumonia, and respiratory failure. The most accurate method for checking feeding tube placement is X-ray examination; the most effective nonradiological method is aspirating fluid from the feeding tube, measuring its pH, and describing its appearance. Although observing for respiratory distress is helpful in alert patients (especially when firm large-diameter tubes are used), it is of little benefit in those who have a decreased level of consciousness and when small-bore tubes are used. Risk factors for pulmonary aspiration in tube-fed patients include feeding into the stomach in the presence of gastric atony (which results in high gastric residual

volumes), poor gag reflexes, mechanical ventilation, and flat positioning in bed. Bedside methods used to detect pulmonary aspiration are not well defined.

Evidence-Informed Practice

- Radiography is the most reliable method available to confirm correct feeding tube location, especially when small-bore tubes are initially inserted. When the radiographic method is not feasible, there is evidence to support the measurement of CO_2 levels at the distal end of the tube, although this method cannot determine where the tip of the tube ends in the gastrointestinal tract—esophagus, stomach, or small bowel (Boeykens, 2018).
- Another method involves testing the feeding tube aspirate's pH and observing its appearance. A properly obtained pH of 0 to 5.5 is a good indication of gastric placement; a pH of 6 or higher could indicate placement in the lung or intestine, in which gastric pH is usually high. Intestinal fluid is usually bile-stained (dark golden yellow); gastric fluid is usually grassy green, off-white to tan, or clear and colourless.
- A supplementary method to confirm placement consists of marking the feeding tube with indelible ink at the exit site from the naris or lip at the time of radiography. The nurse must confirm this mark before feeding or administering medication through the tube. The measurement from naris to tip of tube must also be recorded. The exit-point mark is not a foolproof indication of correct tube placement, inasmuch as the tube's distal tip can move from its original position while the external portion remains intact.
- The auscultatory method should *not* be used to determine tube location.

From Boeykens, K. (2018). Verification of blindly inserted nasogastric feeding tubes: A review of different test methods. *Journal of Perioperative & and Critical Intensive Care Nursing, 4*(3), https://www.longdom.org/open-access/verification-of-blindly-inserted-nasogastric-feeding-tubes-a-review-of-different-test-methods-2471-9870-10000145.pdf; Metheny, N. A., Krieger, M. M., Healey, F., et al. (2019). A review of guidelines to distinguish between gastric and pulmonary placement of nasogastric tubes. *Heart Lung, 48*(3), 226–235. https://doi.org/10.1016/j.hrtlng.2019.01.003; Wayne, G. (2018). *Nasogastric intubation.* https://nurseslabs.com/nasogastric-intubation/

BOX 43.16   PROCEDURAL GUIDELINE

Obtaining Gastrointestinal Aspirate for pH Measurement, Large- and Small-Bore Feeding Tubes: Intermittent and Continuous Feeding

Critical Decision Point: Obtaining gastrointestinal aspirate for pH measurement to verify placement is crucial, whether a large- or small-bore tube is used and whether the tube will be used for decompression or feeding. *Note:* An X-ray examination to verify tube placement must be completed before enteral feedings are initiated.

Delegation Considerations

The skill of measuring pH in gastrointestinal aspirate should *not* be delegated to unregulated care providers.

Equipment

- Personal protective equipment—mask, gloves
- 60-mL syringe
- pH test paper (scale of 0 to 11)
- Absorbent pad
- Small medication cup
- Disposable gloves

Procedure

1. Perform hand hygiene and apply mask. Perform measures to verify placement of tube:
   A. For intermittently fed patients, test placement immediately before feeding (usually a period of at least 4 hours will have elapsed since previous feeding). More frequent checking has been associated with increased clogging of small-bore tubes. To avoid clogging, flush tube with 30 mL of water after aspirating for the residual volume. Sterile saline flushes may be ordered if the patient is hyponatremic (Morgan, 2020).
   B. For continuously tube-fed patients, check agency policy. If the patient is tolerating the feedings without incident and other indicators of correct location are present (the mark on the tube at the exit site has remained in its original position, and the most recent X-ray films confirm correct position of tube), it is reasonable to continue feedings. **If risk of tube displacement is high and the tube has moved, consider the need for an X-ray film to verify placement** (Metheny et al., 2019). Plan to test pH at times when feeding may be withheld (e.g., during diagnostic testing, during chest physiotherapy, or to avoid medication interaction).
   C. Wait at least 1 hour after medication administration by tube or mouth.
2. Apply disposable gloves.
3. Draw 30 mL of air, or an equivalent amount for infants and children, into syringe, then attach syringe to end of feeding tube. Flush tube with the 30 mL of air to clear out formula or medications before attempting to aspirate fluid. It will probably be more difficult to aspirate fluid from the small intestine than from the stomach. Repositioning the patient from side to side may be helpful. More than one bolus of air through the tube may be needed.

4. Draw back on syringe and obtain 5 to 10 mL of gastric aspirate. Observe appearance of aspirate (see illustration Step 4A). Gently mix aspirate in syringe. Then expel a few drops into a clean medicine cup. Dip the pH strip into the fluid or apply a few drops of the fluid to the strip (see illustration Step 4B). Compare the colour of the strip with the colour on the chart provided by the manufacturer.
   A. The pH of gastric fluid usually ranges from 1 to 5.
      - There is lack of consensus on the best pH cut-point, as values of ≤4.0, ≤5.0, and ≤5.5 have been cited in various guidelines (Metheny et al., 2019).
   B. The pH of intestinal fluid is usually higher than 6.
   C. Patients with continuous tube feeding may have a pH of 5 or higher.
   D. The pH of pleural fluid from the tracheobronchial tree is generally higher than 6.

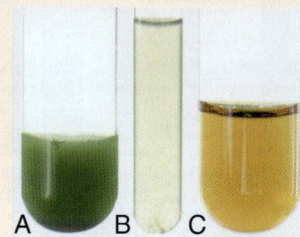

STEP 4A Gastrointestinal contents. **A,** Stomach. **B,** Stomach. **C,** Intestinal. (Courtesy of Dr. Norma A. Metheny, Professor, St. Louis University School of Nursing.)

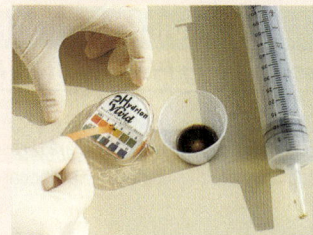

STEP 4B Comparing pH strip with colour chart.

5. Remove gloves and discard supplies. Perform hand hygiene.

Critical Decision Point: If after repeated attempts it is not possible to aspirate fluid from a tube that was originally confirmed by X-ray examination to be in the desired position, the tube is considered correctly placed if (1) no risk factors for tube dislocation exist, (2) the tube has remained in the original taped position and the tube's measurement remains constant, and (3) the patient is not experiencing difficulty. If in doubt, repeat radiographic examination of patient to confirm placement.

TABLE 43.8   Complications of Enteral Tube Feeding

Problem	Possible Cause	Intervention
Pulmonary aspiration	Regurgitation of formula	Verify tube placement
	Feeding tube displaced	Reposition tube and verify tube placement
	Patient in supine position	Elevate head of bed 45 degrees during feedings and for 2 hours afterward
	Deficient gag reflex	Reassess for return of normal gag reflex; until then, place patient on aspiration precautions and place patient in supine position
	Gastroesophageal reflux disease	Verify tube placement
	Delayed gastric emptying	Lower rate of delivery to increase tolerance

TABLE 43.8	Complications of Enteral Tube Feeding—cont'd	
Problem	**Possible Cause**	**Intervention**
Diarrhea	Hyperosmolar formula or medications	Deliver formula continuously, deliver at lower rate, dilute formula, or change to isotonic enteral nutrition (physician order required and may consult with dietitian)
	Allergy to elixir ingredients (sorbitol)	Liquid medications are often sweetened with sorbitol; consider this as possible cause of diarrhea
	Antibiotic therapy	Antibiotics may destroy normal intestinal flora; health care provider may change medication; treat symptoms with antidiarrheal agents
	Bacterial contamination	Do not hang formula longer than 4–8 hours in bag; wash bag out well when refilling; change tube feeding bags every 24 hours; use aseptic practices
		Check expiration dates
	Malabsorption	Check for pancreatic insufficiency; use low-fat, lactose-free formula and continuous feedings
Constipation	Lack of fibre	Select a formula containing fibre
	Lack of free water	Add water as needed as flushes*
	Medications	Evaluate adverse effects; suggest stool softener or bulk-forming laxative
	Inactivity	Monitor patient's ability to ambulate; collaborate with health care provider for activity order or physiotherapy
Tube occlusion	Pulverized medications given per tube	Irrigate with 30 mL water before and after each medication per tube*
		Ideally, each medication should be given separately
	Insufficient tube irrigation	Dilute crushed medications if not liquid
	Sedimentation of formula	Shake cans well before administering (read label)
	Reaction of incompatible medications or formula	Read pharmacological information on compatibility of drugs and formula
Tube displacement	Coughing, vomiting	Replace tube and confirm placement before restarting tube feeding
	Tube not taped securely	With placement verification, check that tape is secure (nasoenteral)
Abdominal cramping, nausea, or vomiting	High osmolality of formula	Suggest an isotonic formula, or dilute current formula
		Suggest use of lactose-free formula
		Stop feeding if there is a risk of gastrointestinal tract obstruction
		Use greater proportion of carbohydrate
		Warm formula to room temperature
	Rapid increase in rate or volume	Lower rate of delivery to increase tolerance
	Delayed gastric emptying	If the gastric residual is >250 mL after a gastric residual volume check, a promotility agent should be considered
		A full assessment should be conducted to find out reason for high level
	Lactose intolerance	Suggest use of lactose-free formula
	Intestinal obstruction	Stop feeding if there is a risk of gastrointestinal tract obstruction
	High-fat formula used	Use greater proportion of carbohydrate
	Cold formula used	Warm formula to room temperature
Delayed gastric emptying	Diabetic gastroparesis	Consult with health care provider regarding medication for increasing gastric motility
	Prematurity	Check for residual (see agency policy)
	Inactivity	Consult health care provider regarding advancing tube to intestinal placement
		Monitor medications and pathological conditions that may affect gastrointestinal motility
Serum electrolyte imbalance	Excess gastrointestinal losses	Monitor serum electrolyte levels daily
	Dehydration	Provide free water as per dietitian's recommendation
	Cirrhosis	Know of links with specific pathological condition
	Heart failure, edema	Monitor patient's weight
	Diabetes mellitus	Monitor glucose tolerance and type of feedings
Increased respiratory quotient	Overfeeding of carbohydrates	Balance kilocalorie needs provided from fat, protein, and carbohydrate with greater proportion of fat in formula (to decrease CO_2 production)
Fluid overload	Refeeding syndrome in malnutrition	Restrict fluids if necessary, and use either a specialized formula or a diluted enteral formula at first
	Excess free water or diluted (hypotonic) formula	Monitor levels of serum proteins and electrolytes
		Use a more concentrated formula with fluid volume excess that does not carry a risk of refeeding syndrome
Hyperosmolar dehydration	Hypertonic formula with insufficient free water	Slow rate of delivery, dilute, or change to isotonic formula

*Check first for fluid restrictions that would affect volume of water given. A physician's order is required to add free H_2O; this will be patient-specific.

The two types of tubes most commonly used for gastric decompression are the Levine and Salem sump tube. The tubes are large: 16 to 18 Fr may be inserted for adults, while sizes suitable for children vary from size 5 Fr for younger children to size 12 Fr for older children (Wayne, 2018) (Skill 43.6 and Box 43.17).

Medication

It is recommended that medications *not* be administered via large-bore tube while suctioning is required. If a large-bore tube must be used, then suctioning should be withheld for at least 30 minutes after medication is administered. Nurses need to consult with the pharmacist and refer to employer policy.

PARENTERAL NUTRITION

Parenteral nutrition is a form of specialized nutrition support in which nutrients are provided intravenously. Safe administration of this form of nutrition depends on appropriate assessment of nutrition needs, meticulous management of the central venous catheter (CVC) or central venous access device (CVAD), and careful monitoring to prevent

SKILL 43.6	INSERTING A LARGE-BORE NASOENTERIC OR OROGASTRIC TUBE FOR GASTRIC SUCTIONING

Delegation Considerations

This skill requires problem-solving and knowledge application unique to a professional nurse. For this reason, this skill should *not* be delegated to unregulated care providers.

Equipment

- Personal protective equipment—mask, gloves
- Nasogastric or nasointestinal (orogastric or orointestinal) tube (12 to 18 Fr)
- Stethoscope
- 60-mL or larger Luer-Lok or catheter-tip syringe
- Hypoallergenic tape and tincture of benzoin or tube fixation device
- Scissors
- pH indicator strip (scale of 0 to 14)
- Glass of water and straw (not required for intubated patients)
- Water-soluble lubricant
- Emesis basin
- Absorbent pad
- Facial tissues
- Disposable gloves (multiple pairs needed)
- Suction equipment in case of aspiration
- Penlight to check placement of nasopharynx
- Tongue blade
- Disposable tape measure
- Felt-tip marker
- Suction device for continuous or intermittent suctioning

PROCEDURE

STEPS	RATIONALE
1. Assess the need for large-bore tube (i.e., for gastric suctioning or lavage). **A.** Review physician's order for type of tube and enteral feeding schedule.	• Identify patients who require gastric drainage or flushing. • ***Procedure and tube feedings require a physician's order.***
2. Perform hand hygiene and apply mask. Assess patency of nares. Have patient close each nostril alternately and breathe. Examine each naris for patency and skin breakdown.	• Nares may be obstructed or irritated, or septal defect may be present.
3. Assess the gag reflex. Place tongue blade in patient's mouth, touching uvula to induce a gag response.	• Assessing gag reflex identifies patient's ability to swallow and determines risk for aspiration.

CRITICAL DECISION POINT: *Patients with impaired consciousness or who are intubated and sedated may also have impaired gag reflex, and their risk of aspiration is increased during this type of procedure and subsequent tube feedings. For a patient who is intubated, sedated, or too ill to participate, ensure that their head is tilted toward the chest for enteral feeding tube insertion.*

4. Review patient's medical history for nasal problems (e.g., nosebleeds, oral or facial surgery, anticoagulation therapy, history of aspiration).	• Nasoenteral tubes are contraindicated in patients who have undergone recent nasal surgery, have sustained facial traumas, have nosebleeds, or are receiving anticoagulation therapy (Wayne, 2018). Caution is exercised while performing any endonasal procedure where disruption of the anterior cranial base is possible.
5. Perform hand hygiene (before auscultating abdomen).	• Hygiene reduces transfer of microorganisms.
6. Auscultate patient's abdomen for bowel sounds.	• Absence of bowel sounds may indicate decrease in or absence of peristalsis and increased risk for aspiration or abdominal distension.

STEPS	RATIONALE
7. Explain procedure to patient and how to communicate during intubation by raising index finger to indicate gagging or discomfort.	• Information reduces anxiety and helps patient assist in insertion. Being alert and communicating help patients tolerate the procedure better.
8. Stand on same side of bed as naris for insertion and assist patient to high Fowler's position unless that position is contraindicated. Place pillow behind patient's head and shoulders.	• Fowler's position allows easier manipulation of tube, reduces risk of aspiration, and promotes effective swallowing.
9. Place absorbent pad over patient's chest. Keep facial tissues within reach.	• Pad prevents soiling of gown. Insertion of tube may cause patient's eyes to tear.
10. Determine length of tube to be inserted, and mark with tape. Traditional method: Measure distance from tip of nose to earlobe to mid-umbilicus (see Step 10 illustration).	• Length approximates distance from nose to stomach in 98% of patients. For duodenal or jejunal placement, an additional 20 to 30 cm is required.

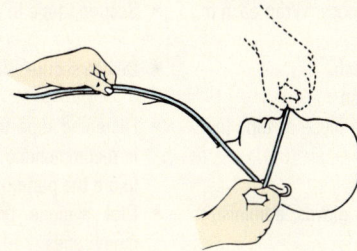

STEP 10 Length of tube to be inserted is equal to distance from tip of nose to earlobe to mid-umbilicus.

STEPS	RATIONALE
11. Prepare nasogastric or nasointestinal tube for intubation.	
12. Perform hand hygiene and put on gloves.	• Hygiene and gloves reduce transmission of microorganisms.
13. Cut tape 10 cm long or prepare tube fixation device. Split one end of tape lengthwise 5 cm.	• To be used to anchor tubing after insertion.
14. Dip tube with surface lubricant into glass of water. If tube is not self-lubricating, water-soluble lubricant should be used.	• Activates lubricant to facilitate passage of tube into naris to gastrointestinal tract. Do not use petroleum-based products because of the risk of aspiration into the lung and resultant chemical pneumonitis.
15. Insert tube through nostril to back of throat (posterior nasopharynx). Aim back and down toward ear.	• Natural contour facilitates passage of tube into gastrointestinal tract and reduces gagging by patient.
16. Have patient tilt head toward chest after tube has passed through nasopharynx.	• Tilting head forward closes off glottis and reduces risk of tube's entering trachea. This technique is also used in patients who are intubated and sedated.

CRITICAL DECISION POINT: *Encourage patients who are alert and communicating to swallow by giving small sips of water or ice chips when possible. For patients who are intubated, sedated, or unable to participate, tilt head toward chest. Advance the tube as patient swallows or as head is tilted toward chest. Rotate tube 180 degrees while inserting.*

STEPS	RATIONALE
17. Emphasize the need to mouth-breathe and swallow during the procedure (when possible).	• Mouth-breathing and swallowing facilitate passage of tube and alleviate patient's fears during the procedure.

CRITICAL DECISION POINT: *Do not force tube insertion. If resistance is met or patient starts to cough, choke, or become cyanotic, stop advancing the tube and pull tube back.*

STEPS	RATIONALE
18. Check for position of tube in back of throat with penlight and tongue blade.	• Tube may be coiled, kinked, or entering trachea. (Withdraw tube immediately if tube is coiled, if respiratory status of patient changes, or if patient begins to cough and skin colour changes; if distress is not present, withdraw tube fully and retry. Note whether tube was kinked; if so, it is likely to kink again in the same place.)
19. Perform measures to verify placement of tube, by measuring pH.	• *Note:* Tube placement must be verified by X-ray examination before enteral feeds are initiated. Another test that can be done at the bedside to ensure ongoing placement is to measure pH of aspirated gastric fluids.
A. Examine gastric contents and yield.	• Respiratory and gastric contents may look similar, but aspirating gastric contents yields a greater amount, whereas aspirating respiratory contents may yield only a few millilitres.

Continued

SKILL 43.6	INSERTING A LARGE-BORE NASOENTERIC OR OROGASTRIC TUBE FOR GASTRIC SUCTIONING—cont'd
STEPS	RATIONALE

CRITICAL DECISION POINT: *Auscultation is not considered a reliable method for verification of tube placement because a tube inadvertently placed in the lungs, pharynx, or esophagus can transmit a sound similar to that of air entering the stomach (Boeykens, 2018).*

20. After gastric aspirates are obtained, anchor tube to patient's nose and avoid pressure on nares. Mark exit site on tube with indelible ink. Select one of the following options to secure tube:
   A. Apply tape
      (1) Apply tincture of benzoin or other skin adhesive on tip of patient's nose and tube and allow it to become "tacky."
      (2) Place intact end of tape over bridge of patient's nose. Wrap each of the 5-cm strips around tube as it exits nose.
   B. Apply tube fixation device, using shaped adhesive patch.
      (1) Apply wide end of patch to bridge of patient's nose.
21. Fasten end of nasogastric tube to patient's gown with a piece of tape (not safety pin).

22. Remove gloves. Perform hand hygiene and apply clean gloves; administer oral hygiene (see Chapter 39). Cleanse tubing at nostril.
23. Remove gloves, dispose of equipment, and perform hand hygiene.
24. Inspect naris and oropharynx for any irritation after insertion.
25. Ask patient whether they feel comfortable.

26. Observe patient for any difficulty breathing, for coughing, or for gagging.

27. Auscultate lung sounds.
28. Connect tube to suction device as ordered.

- A properly secured tube allows the patient more mobility and prevents trauma to nasal mucosa. Mark tube at tip of naris; measure from mark to end of tube; tape and secure to maintain position.
- Skin adhesive helps tape adhere better and protects skin.
- Securing tape to nares prevents tissue necrosis.
- Device secures tube and reduces friction on nares.
- Fastening tape to gown reduces traction on the naris if tube moves. Tape is recommended because safety pins may become unfastened and possibly injure the patient.
- Oral hygiene promotes patient comfort and integrity of oral mucous membranes.
- Hygiene reduces transmission of microorganisms.
- If tube insertion was difficult, irritation of naris or oropharynx may have occurred.
- Patients' level of comfort is evaluated. (This may be a challenge if a language barrier exists or if the patient has dementia or is confused.)
- Improper position of the tube may cause these symptoms or increase symptoms in patients who have heart failure, pneumonia, asthma, and other cardiac or respiratory conditions.
- Abnormal lung sounds can be an early sign of aspiration.
- May be ordered as a continuous or intermittent suction and at various pressures (e.g., 80 mm Hg). In some circumstances, tubes are placed by surgeon but contraindicated or strict protocols for flush or suction (i.e., post-esophagectomy).

BOX 43.17   PROCEDURAL GUIDELINE

Providing Suction

Equipment
- Personal protective equipment (PPE)—mask, gloves
- Suction device, connecting tubing (connector as required)

Procedure
1. Check the physician's order for type and amount of suction. Suctioning may be ordered as continuous or intermittent. The amount must be ordered by the physician.
2. To reduce patient's anxiety, educate patient about the procedure.
3. Wash hands thoroughly to limit spread of microorganisms and apply PPE.
4. Set up suction device as per employer policy.
5. Set type and amount of suction as ordered.
6. Monitor patient and suction system regularly. Provide data for overall care. Monitor for bleeding or blockage:
   Patient: Note abdominal distension, nausea, feeling of discomfort, bowel sounds, electrolyte levels.
   Device: Note kinks, blockages, flow, and settings.
   Drainage: Note amount, colour, and consistency.
7. Secure tubing as described in Skill 43.3, Step 22A(2). Keep tubing lower than stomach to facilitate drainage. Secure tubing to prevent inadvertent pulling or removal.
8. Measure output at least every 8 hours or as per institution or agency policy.
9. Document as per institution or agency protocol.

or treat metabolic complications. Parenteral nutrition is administered in a variety of settings, including the patient's home. Regardless of the setting, the nurse adheres to the same principles of asepsis and infusion management to ensure safe nutrition support.

Patients who are unable to digest or absorb enteral nutrition benefit from parenteral nutrition. Patients in highly stressed physiological states, such as sepsis, head injury, or burns, are also candidates for parenteral nutrition therapy. Box 43.18 lists other indications for parenteral nutrition. Clinical and laboratory monitoring by an interprofessional team is required throughout parenteral nutrition therapy. The need for continued parenteral nutrition is re-evaluated regularly, with the goal of eventually using the gastrointestinal tract. Disuse of the gastrointestinal tract has been associated with villus atrophy and generalized cell shrinkage. Translocation of bacteria from the local gut to systemic regions has been noted in relation to gastrointestinal cell shrinkage; such translocation can result in Gram-negative septicemia.

Lipid emulsions provide supplemental kilocalories and prevent deficiencies of essential fatty acids. These emulsions can be administered through a separate peripheral catheter, through the CVC by Y-connector tubing (see Chapter 41), or as an admixture to the parenteral nutrition solution. The addition of lipid emulsion to the parenteral nutrition solution is called a *3-in-1 admixture* and is administered over a 24-hour period. The admixture should not be used if oil droplets are observed or if an oil or creamy layer is observed on the surface of the admixture. This observation indicates that the emulsion has broken into large lipid droplets that can cause fat emboli if administered. Lipid emulsions are white and opaque; thus, care should be taken to avoid confusing enteral formula with parenteral lipids.

Contraindications to giving lipids are hyperlipidemia, lipid nephrosis, severe liver failure, and egg allergy.

BOX 43.18 Indications for Parenteral Nutrition

Nonfunctional Gastrointestinal Tract
- Massive small bowel resection or gastrointestinal surgery
- Paralytic ileus
- Intestinal obstruction
- Trauma to abdomen, head, or neck
- Severe malabsorption
- Intolerance of enteral feeding (established by trial)
- Chemotherapy, radiation therapy, bone marrow transplantation

Extended Bowel Rest
- Enterocutaneous fistula
- Inflammatory bowel disease exacerbation
- Severe diarrhea
- Moderate to severe pancreatitis

Preoperative Total Parenteral Nutrition
- Preoperative bowel rest
- Treatment for comorbid severe malnutrition in patients with nonfunctional gastrointestinal tracts
- Severely catabolic patients when gastrointestinal tract is nonusable for more than 4 to 7 days

Initiating Parenteral Nutrition

Patients with short-term nutritional needs often receive intravenous solutions of less than 10% dextrose in a peripheral vein in combination with amino acids and lipids. Peripheral solutions are not as calorically dense and are therefore less irritating to the peripheral veins, and their use is usually temporary. Administering parenteral nutrition with greater than 10% dextrose requires a CVC (Figure 43.12) that is placed into a high-flow central vein (such as the superior vena cava) by a physician using sterile technique (see Chapter 41).

Nurses who have special training insert peripherally inserted central catheters (PICCs) that are started in a vein of the forearm or upper arm and threaded into the subclavian vein or the superior vena cava (Figure 43.13).

After central catheter or PICC placement is verified by chest X-ray examination or radiographically confirmed and documented, the catheter is flushed with saline or heparin. The physician may suture the CVC in place. A PICC is usually stabilized with sterile strips of tape and a sterile dressing. The types of dressings to be applied vary and a variety of policies and protocols are adhered to. The nurse who is new to the nursing unit can check the appropriate dressing protocol and policy before proceeding. Wing-to-tip of the PICC should be measured and documented daily. With a tube suspected to be migrating 2 cm or more, all fluids should be stopped and radiography repeated for placement verification. Also, to verify placement, the PICC line may be

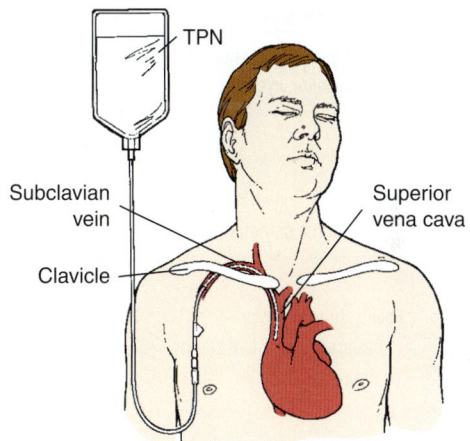

FIGURE 43.12 Parenteral nutrition via central venous catheter (CVC). *TPN,* Total parenteral nutrition. (From *Mosby's dictionary of medicine, nursing, and health professionals* [11th ed.], 2021. Mosby.)

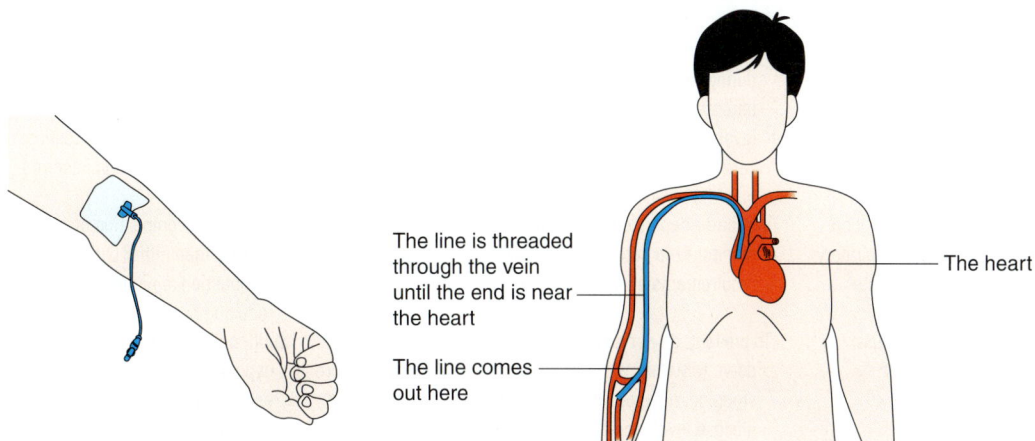

FIGURE 43.13 Peripherally inserted central catheter (PICC) line insertion.

flushed by specially trained nurses and, if noted to be occluded, special procedures (e.g., alteplase) are carried out to ensure line patency.

Before beginning any parenteral infusion, the nurse verifies the physician's order and inspects the solution for particulate matter or a break in the lipid emulsion. An infusion pump is always used. An initial rate of 40 to 60 mL/hour may be recommended. In some institutions, the solutions are infused separately at a specified rate until the therapy is no longer required. In this instance, each solution would have a separate infusion pump. Parenteral nutrition in the hospital is infused 24 hours a day. The parenteral infusion is refrigerated until needed, while the lipids are stored at room temperature.

The rate is gradually increased until the patient's complete nutrition needs are supplied. Patients who receive parenteral nutrition at home frequently administer the entire daily solution over 12 hours at night. This allows the patient to disconnect from the infusion each morning, flush the central catheter, and have independent mobility during the day.

Preventing Complications

Complications of parenteral nutrition include mechanical complications from insertion of the CVC, infection, and metabolic alterations (Table 43.9). Pneumothorax occurs when a puncture in the pulmonary system results in accumulation of air in the pleural cavity and subsequent impairment in breathing. Pneumothorax is usually accompanied by symptoms of sudden sharp chest pain, dyspnea, and coughing. In relation to parenteral nutrition, pneumothorax most often occurs during CVC placement.

Electrolyte abnormalities should be corrected before starting parenteral nutrition. Calorie goals should be reached gradually. It is important to base caloric and protein needs on the patient's current weight to avoid overfeeding.

The goal is for patients to switch from parenteral nutrition to enteral nutrition or oral feeding. Specified weights and intakes are recorded. Once patients are meeting one-third to one-half of their kilocalorie needs per day, parenteral nutrition is usually decreased to half the original volume. Enteral nutrition feedings should then be increased to meet the patient's needs. When 75% of daily energy needs are consistently met with tube feeding, parenteral nutrition may be discontinued. Patients who make the transition from parenteral nutrition to oral feedings typically have early satiety and decreased appetite. Calorie and protein counts are recommended when patients begin taking soft foods. Parenteral nutrition should be gradually decreased in response to increased oral intake. If oral intake is inadequate, small, frequent meals may prove helpful. Some institutions will discontinue lipid emulsion first, then continue parenteral infusion until requirements are met.

TABLE 43.9	Complications of Parenteral Nutrition (PN)		
Problem	**Signs and Symptoms**	**Intervention**	**Rationale**
Air embolism	Tachypnea, apnea, wheezing, hypotension, cyanosis	Turn patient to left lateral decubitus position, instruct patient to perform Valsalva manoeuvre (holding one's breath and "bearing down"), and lower head of bed. Cap the open end of catheter or tape perforation in catheter wall. Administer oxygen; notify health care provider.	The Valsalva manoeuvre increases venous pressure to prevent air from entering the bloodstream during catheter insertion and when catheter is disconnected or cap is changed. Maintaining integrity of closed system prevents air emboli.
Catheter occlusion	No flow or sluggish flow through the catheter	Temporarily stop infusion and flush with saline or heparin. If effort to flush is unsuccessful, attempt to aspirate clot; if still unsuccessful, follow protocol for use of thrombolytic agent (e.g., alteplase).	Alteplase has been shown to be effective in restoring catheter patency.
Catheter sepsis	Fever, chills, glucose intolerance, positive blood culture	Change catheter site dressing if it becomes wet or contaminated, use sterile mask and gloves when changing dressing or tubing, catheter caps, or PN containers. Change infusion tubing regularly (usually every 24 hours). Assess insertion sites for signs and symptoms of infection (see Chapter 34). Do not hang a single container of PN for more than 24 hours or a container of lipids more than 12 hours; use an inline 0.22-mcg filter when possible.	A filtered tubing is required to remove bacteria. With 3-in-1-admixture TPN, filtration is not possible because of large lipid molecules.
Electrolyte imbalance	Monitor Na, Ca, K, Cl, PO_4, Mg, and CO_2 levels	See Chapter 41 for signs of deficiency or toxicity. Monitor intake, output, and electrolytes, especially potassium, magnesium, and phosphorous levels during the first week of parenteral therapy. Check total parenteral nutrition (TPN) for supplemental electrolyte levels at regular intervals—often weekly. Notify health care provider of imbalances. Supplemental vitamin K must be given as ordered throughout therapy.	Adequate hydration and balance of electrolytes are essential for normal function of cells and organs. Vitamin K can be synthesized by microflora found in the jejunum and ileum with normal use of the gastrointestinal tract; however, because PN circumvents gastrointestinal use, exogenous vitamin K must be administered.
Hypercapnia	Increased O_2 consumption, increased CO_2, respiratory quotient >1.0, minute ventilation	Ventilator-dependent patients are at risk; to prevent, monitor parameters, provide 30–60% of energy requirements as fat per physician's order.	Because the combustion of fat yields less carbon dioxide than either carbohydrate or protein combustion, a higher-fat diet may be preferable for reducing hypercapnia.
Hypoglycemia	Diaphoresis, shakiness, confusion, loss of consciousness	To prevent, do not discontinue PN abruptly but taper rate down to within 10% of infusion rate 1 to 2 hours before stopping. If hypoglycemia is suspected, test blood glucose level, and administer intravenous (IV) bolus of 10% dextrose per physician order if necessary.	Sudden discontinuation of the solution can cause hypoglycemia. Patients with diabetes are especially at risk.

TABLE 43.9 Complications of Parenteral Nutrition (PN)—cont'd

Problem	Signs and Symptoms	Intervention	Rationale
Hyperglycemia	Thirst, headache, lethargy, increased urination	Monitor blood glucose level daily until it is stable and then as ordered or as needed. PN is initiated slowly and tapered up to maximal infusion rate. If patient has diabetes mellitus, additional insulin may be required during therapy.	Prevent and correct hyperglycemia because its development during PN has been independently associated with higher rates of mortality and hospital complications (Ma et al., 2018).
Hyperglycemic hyperosmolar nonketotic dehydration or coma	Hyperglycemia (>500 mg/dL), glycosuria, serum osmolarity >350 mOsm/L, confusion, azotemia, headache, severe signs of dehydration (see Chapter 41), hypernatremia, metabolic acidosis, convulsions, coma	To prevent, monitor blood glucose, blood urea nitrogen, serum osmolarity, glucose in urine, and fluid losses; administer insulin as ordered; replace fluids as needed; maintain consistent infusion rate; and provide 30% of daily energy needs as fat. Patients at risk are those who are hypermetabolic, those receiving steroids, older persons, diabetic patients, those who have impaired renal or pancreatic function, and those who are septic.	Too-rapid administration of hypertonic dextrose can result in an osmotic diuresis and dehydration (see Chapter 41). Thus, if an infusion falls behind schedule, the nurse should not increase the rate in an attempt to catch up.
Refeeding syndrome	Cardiac dysrhythmias, heart failure, respiratory distress, convulsions, coma, or death	Watch malnourished or cachectic patients for low serum (extracellular) levels of electrolytes and edema.	Ingestion of concentrated glucose increases the basal metabolic rate and is accompanied by increases in endogenous insulin production, which causes cations (potassium, magnesium, and phosphorus) to move intracellularly. The shifting of electrolytes and fluid increases cardiac workload, heart rate, and oxygen consumption, which strains the respiratory system.
Pneumothorax	Severe dyspnea, cyanosis, radiographic confirmation	Complication that occurs upon catheter insertion may evolve slowly afterward. Monitor patient for first 24 hours for pulmonary distress.	Enables pneumothorax to be detected early and monitors for enlargement.
Thrombosis of central vein	Unilateral edema of neck, shoulder, and arm; pain	Notify health care provider. Prevention of catheter-related thromboses includes proper positioning of the catheter and preventing infections. Thromboprophylaxis for patients with a central venous catheter is not presently recommended.	The use of catheter-directed thrombolysis in patients with extensive central catheter-related deep vein thrombosis remains a case-by-case decision, best guided by consultation with a thrombosis expert or interventional radiologist (Thrombosis Canada, 2021).

KEY CONCEPTS

- Nurses need current, culturally sensitive nutritional knowledge to apply to the complexities of health care, illness, and the changing needs of Canada's diverse populations and demographics.
- A balanced diet featuring carbohydrates, fats, proteins, vitamins, minerals, and water provides the essential nutrients for normal physiological functioning throughout the lifespan.
- Through digestion, food is broken down into its simplest form for absorption. Digestion and absorption occur mainly in the small intestine.
- Recommendations for nutrient intakes, called dietary reference intakes (DRIs), are based on amounts of vitamins, minerals, and other substances like fibre that people require in order to prevent deficiencies and lower their risk of developing chronic conditions such as cancer, diabetes, and heart disease. Checking the nutrition facts table that lists calories and 12 key nutrients on most packaged foods, as well as eating a variety of foods, can help Canadians make informed food choices and get the nutrients important to their health.
- Guidelines for dietary change advocate reduced intake of saturated and trans fats, sodium, and refined sugars, as well as an increased intake of complex carbohydrates and fibre.
- Nutritional screening helps identify patients at risk of malnourishment. Because improper nutrition can affect all body systems, nutritional assessment includes total physical assessment.
- Interprofessional collaboration is essential to helping a patient achieve optimal nutrition.
- Special diets alter the composition, texture, digestibility, and residue of foods to suit the patient's particular needs.
- Nurses in clinical practice settings may provide nutritional support to patients who are unable to ingest food orally because of health issues or to maintain adequate nutrition intake. Within the bounds of relevant employer policies, nurses are responsible for inserting the nasogastric tube, monitoring its placement, administering feedings, and reducing complications.

CRITICAL THINKING EXERCISES

In considering the needs of Arnold and his spouse (from the chapter-opening case study), reflect on the following questions:

1. Given that the terminal diagnosis made at the time of the surgery, do you believe the G-tube insertion was warranted? Why or why not?
2. What teaching was required on the part of the nurse (e.g., hand hygiene, proper positioning during feedings, monitoring for signs or symptoms of G-tube misplacement and site redness or leakage, managing the infusion pump, preventing tubing blockage, and administering medication through the tube)? How was support provided to Arnold and his spouse?
3. What do you think the G-tube nutrition ultimately meant to Arnold and his spouse?

Answers to Critical Thinking Exercises appear on the Evolve website.

REVIEW QUESTIONS

Review Questions 1 to 8 relate to the case study at the beginning of the chapter.

1. Arnold was most at risk for malnutrition before the G-tube was inserted for feedings because:
   a. A part of his stomach had been surgically removed to confirm the diagnosis of adenosarcoma.
   b. He had cut down on the amounts of fat, sodium, and cholesterol since being diagnosed with diabetes.
   c. As an older person, he experienced age-related gastrointestinal changes, such as reduced saliva production, increased taste threshold, and decreased peristalsis.
   d. He was taking an oral medication that had a potential adverse effect of hypoglycemia to treat diabetes.

2. When learning to manage type 2 diabetes, Arnold would have learned that a function of carbohydrates in his diet was to:
   a. Enable chemical reactions
   b. Promote growth and repair of tissues
   c. Supply energy
   d. Maintain water balance

3. Through his education for diabetes, Arnold would also have learned that carbohydrates: *(Select all that apply.)*
   a. Are readily supplied through adequate servings of fruits, vegetables, and the dairy group
   b. Are simple sugars that should be avoided because they cause a rapid spike in glucose levels
   c. Are needed to provide 60 to 80% of daily calories
   d. Are classified as polysaccharides when they include starch and glycogen, and fibre.

4. When a patient like Arnold is unable to take fluid or food by eating normally over an extended period of time, which of the following alternatives is better?
   a. Giving liquid nutrients through a tube leading from the mouth or nose to the stomach or intestine
   b. Giving solutions through a tubing in a peripheral vein
   c. Giving continuous tube feedings regulated via an electric feeding pump
   d. Giving feedings through a tube inserted through the skin and tissue of the abdomen

5. When Arnold was living at home with his spouse, what did he and his caregivers have to do to determine the patency of the enteral tube?
   a. Arrange for Arnold to have an X-ray performed periodically.
   b. Auscultate Arnold's abdomen for bowel sounds before each feeding.
   c. Instill air into the tube to check for placement and patency before each feeding.
   d. Check the placement marking at the insertion site at the abdominal wall.

6. Situation: Arnold needed metformin 100 mg bid for type 2 diabetes. What was the best way for Arnold to receive this?
   a. Take it by mouth with a small sip of water. Maintain a 45-degree head elevation for 30 minutes.
   b. Crush the tablet and mix it with water so it could be put directly into the tubing while the feeding was running to ensure medication distribution.
   c. Switch to a less viscous feeding formula by diluting the formula itself with water to avoid clogging the tubing.
   d. Crush the tablet, mix it with water, and flush the tubing with 30 mL of water before and after putting the medication into the tubing.

7. Arnold tolerated the G-tube feeding for months. However, then he began to no longer tolerate the tube feedings. All of the following, EXCEPT WHICH ONE, are signs of intolerance to a tube feeding?
   a. Nausea
   b. Diarrhea
   c. Abdominal cramping
   d. Abdominal distension
   e. Very low gastric residual volumes

8. The community palliative care nurse is visiting Arnold and his spouse. Arnold is at the end of life. His spouse has continued to care for him and sit at his bedside. Arnold is semi-conscious, dehydrated, free of pain, constipated, without distress, and expected to die in a day or two. Which of the following is an appropriate patient outcome or an appropriate intervention for Arnold and his spouse?
   a. Arnold will be free of constipation.
   b. Arnold will remain free of pain and distress.
   c. Administer an antiemetic to prevent vomiting and further dehydration.
   d. Tell the spouse to offer Arnold sips of water to relieve the dehydration.

Answers 1. c; 2. c; 3. a, d; 4. d; 5. d; 6. d; 7. e; 8. b.

🌐 *Rationales for the Review Questions appear on the Evolve website.*

RECOMMENDED WEBSITES

Diabetes Canada: https://www.diabetes.ca
This web page provides information about signs and symptoms for various types of diabetes, tips for living with diabetes, and useful clinical practice guidelines.

Dietitians of Canada: https://www.dietitians.ca
Dietitians of Canada is an association of food and nutrition professionals committed to the health and well-being of Canadians. This website contains numerous resources about nutrition and links to other resources and research conferences.

Health Canada: *Canada's Food Guide:* https://www.hc-sc.gc.ca/fn-an/index-eng.php
This web page provides information about using *Canada's Food Guide* to assist with healthy eating.

Health Canada: Food and Nutrition: https://www.hc-sc.gc.ca/fn-an/index-eng.php
This web page provides information for the public about food, nutrition, food safety issues, allergy alerts, food policy and legislation, and other nutrition issues.

Heart and Stroke Canada: https://www.heartandstroke.ca
Public education about heart and stroke warning signs and prevention strategies for healthy eating, increasing physical activity, and reducing stress are found on this site.

National Eating Disorder Information Centre (NEDIC): http://www.nedic.ca
This website provides information, resources, and support for individuals, families, and professionals regarding eating disorders and weight preoccupation.

Office of Nutrition Policy and Promotion (ONPP): https://www.hc-sc.gc.ca/ahc-asc/branch-dirgen/hpfb-dgpsa/onpp-bppn/index-eng.php
The Office of Nutrition Policy and Promotion promotes the nutritional health and well-being of Canadians. This web page contains current information about nutrition and Canadian nutrition policy.

Public Health Agency of Canada (PHAC): https://www.canada.ca/en/public-health.html

The activities of the Public Health Agency of Canada focus on preventing disease and injuries, responding to public health threats, and promoting behaviours that affect health, pregnancy, wellness, infant care, older-person care, and more.

REFERENCES

A full reference list is available on the website for this book at http://evolve.elsevier.com/Canada/Potter/fundamentals/

44

Urinary Elimination

Canadian content written by Laura Robbs, RN, MN, NSWOC, WOCC(C), NCA,
Nicholas Joachimides, RN, BScN, IIWCC, NSWOC, MClSc, MSc, CHE, CpedN(c),
Carly Lindsay, RN, BNSc, MClSc-WH, NSWOC, WOCC(C), and
Najwa Shbat, RN, BScN, NSWOC, NCA, with original chapter contributions by
Lenetra Jefferson, PhD, MSN, BSN, LMT, and Kathleen F. Hunter, RN, NP, PhD, GNC(C), NCA

OBJECTIVES

Mastery of content in this chapter will enable you to:

- Define the key terms listed.
- Describe the process of urination.
- Identify factors that commonly influence urinary elimination.
- Compare common alterations in urinary elimination.
- Identify two modalities of renal replacement therapy.
- Obtain a nursing health history for a patient with urinary elimination problems.
- Identify nursing diagnoses appropriate for patients with alterations in urinary elimination.
- Obtain urine specimens.
- Describe characteristics of normal and abnormal urine.
- Describe the nursing implications of common diagnostic tests of the urinary system.
- Describe nursing measures to promote normal micturition and to reduce episodes of incontinence.
- Insert a urinary catheter.
- Describe nursing measures to reduce urinary tract infections.
- Irrigate a urinary catheter.

KEY TERMS

Bacteremia
Bacteriuria
Bladder training
Catheter-associated UTI (CAUTI)
Catheterization
Cystitis
Dysuria
Hematuria

Incontinence-associated dermatitis (IAD)
In-dwelling catheterization
Intermittent catheterization
Micturition
Nephrostomy
Nocturia
Pelvic floor muscle exercises (PFMEs)
Postvoid residual (PVR)

Pyelonephritis
Renin
Suprapubic catheterization
Urinary diversion
Urinary incontinence (UI)
Urinary retention

🌐 WEBSITE

http://evolve.elsevier.com/Canada/Potter/fundamentals/

CASE STUDY

Harjit (preferred pronouns: he/him) is an active and fit 80-year-old man. In the past year, Harjit has noticed that he needs to urinate more often during the day, and he also wakes up more often at night to urinate. Harjit has also noticed that he rushes to the bathroom when he gets the urge to urinate and sometimes leaks urine on the way. His family doctor referred him to a urologist, and he was diagnosed with prostate enlargement.

Unfortunately, Harjit slipped on black ice when going for his daily walk. As a result, he fractured his hip, requiring a surgical repair in an acute care hospital. After his surgery, Harjit was not able to empty his bladder and it was found that he was retaining urine. As a result, Harjit's physician ordered an in-dwelling catheter to be inserted.

Think about this case study as you read this chapter. There are review questions at the end of the chapter that relate to the case study.

Normal elimination of urinary wastes is a basic function. Many illnesses and conditions, both acute and chronic, can affect the urinary function. Nurses play a key role in the assessment of urinary tract function, promotion of continence, and management of incontinence and optimal bladder emptying. Understanding the reasons for urinary elimination problems and finding evidence-informed solutions acceptable to patients are essential nursing functions.

SCIENTIFIC KNOWLEDGE BASE

Urinary elimination depends on the coordinated function of the kidneys, ureters, bladder, and urethra. Kidneys remove wastes (excess water and by-products of metabolism) from the blood to form urine. Ureters transport urine from the kidneys to the bladder. The bladder

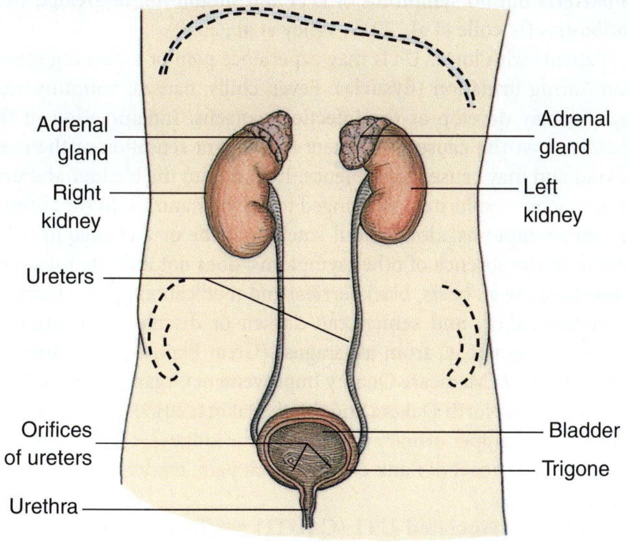

Adrenal gland
Right kidney
Ureters
Orifices of ureters
Urethra
Adrenal gland
Left kidney
Bladder
Trigone

FIGURE 44.1 Organs of the urinary system.

stores urine until the urge to urinate develops. Micturition (urination) occurs when a complex neural response allows the bladder to contract, the urethral sphincter to relax, and urine to leave the body through the urethra (Figure 44.1).

Upper Urinary Tract

Kidneys. The kidneys lie on either side of the vertebral column behind the peritoneum and against the deep muscles of the back. The kidneys extend from the twelfth thoracic vertebra to the third lumbar vertebra. Normally, the left kidney is higher than the right one because of the anatomical position of the liver.

Waste products of metabolism that collect in the blood are filtered in the kidneys. Blood reaches each kidney by a renal (kidney) artery that branches from the abdominal aorta. The *nephron* is the functional unit of the kidney, where waste products are removed, and urine is formed. Nephrons also play a crucial role in fluid and electrolyte balance.

A cluster of blood vessels forms the capillary network of the *glomerulus* of the nephron, which is the initial site of filtration of the blood and the beginning of urine formation. The glomerular capillaries permit filtration of water, glucose, amino acids, urea, creatinine, and major electrolytes. Large proteins and blood cells normally do not filter through the glomerulus. The presence of proteins (proteinuria) or blood (hematuria) in urine is a sign of glomerular injury.

The glomerulus filters approximately 125 mL of plasma per minute (180 L/day). Most (99%) of the filtrate is reabsorbed into the plasma, with the remaining 1% excreted as urine. The reabsorption process maintains fluid and electrolyte balance (Huether, 2019). Normal urine production ranges from 1 to 2 L/day and is affected by many factors, including fluid intake and body temperature (Huether, 2019). An output of less than 30 mL/hr may indicate renal alterations.

The kidneys play a role in other functions, including producing red blood cells (RBCs), blood pressure regulation, and bone mineralization. Erythropoietin stimulates the bone marrow to increase the rate of production of red blood cells (Huether, 2019). Patients with chronic alterations in kidney function cannot produce sufficient quantities of this hormone and are therefore prone to anemia (Huether, 2019).

Renin, another hormone produced by the kidneys, plays a role in blood pressure control by regulating renal blood flow via the renin–angiotensin–aldosterone system (RAAS). Renin is released from the juxtaglomerular cells when blood pressure decreases, converting

angiotensinogen (a substance synthesized by the liver) into angiotensin I. Angiotensin I is converted to angiotensin II in the lungs. Angiotensin II causes vasoconstriction and stimulates aldosterone release from the adrenal cortex. Aldosterone causes retention of water, which increases blood volume. The kidneys also produce prostaglandin E_2 and prostacyclin, which are important in maintaining renal blood flow through vasodilation. These mechanisms increase arterial blood pressure and renal blood flow (Huether, 2019).

The kidneys play a role in calcium and phosphate regulation by producing a substance that converts vitamin D into its active form. The disruption of these other regulatory functions in patients with kidney impairment can lead to bone disease from impaired calcium resorption, hypertension, and anemia.

Ureters. Urine enters the renal pelvis from the collecting ducts and travels to the bladder through the ureters. The *ureters* are tubular structures that enter the urinary bladder obliquely through the posterior wall at the ureterovesical junction (the juncture of the ureters and the bladder). Peristaltic waves cause urine to enter the bladder in spurts rather than steadily. Contraction of the bladder compresses the ureters at the junction during micturition to prevent the reflux of urine.

An obstruction within a ureter, such as a kidney stone (renal calculus), can result in distension of the ureter (hydroureter) and backup of urine to the pelvis of the kidney (hydronephrosis), potentially causing long-term renal impairment.

Lower Urinary Tract

Bladder. The urinary *bladder* is a hollow, distensible muscular organ lined with uroepithelium that stores and excretes urine. It is composed of the lower trigone base lying between the ureter and urethral openings, and the upper dome of the detrusor muscle. When empty, the bladder lies behind the symphysis pubis in the pelvic cavity. It rests against the anterior wall of the rectum in men and against the anterior walls of the cervix and vagina in individuals with female genitalia.

The bladder expands as it becomes filled with urine. During filling, pressure remains low as the relaxed bladder is normally highly compliant. When the bladder is full, it expands and extends above the symphysis pubis. Contraction of the detrusor expels urine from the body. In a pregnant individual, the developing fetus pushes against the bladder, reducing its capacity and causing a feeling of fullness.

Urethra. Urine travels from the bladder through the urethra (a fibromuscular tube) and passes outside of the body through the urethral meatus. The urethra transverses the pelvic floor muscles, a layer of skeletal muscle that stabilizes the urethra and forms part of the continence mechanism. Circular smooth muscle and striated sphincter muscle (also known as the *external sphincter*, or *rhabdosphincter*) in the urethra also contribute to closure between voids and aid in continence. In individuals with female genitalia, the urethra is approximately 5 cm long (Newman et al., 2021a). This short length predisposes patients with female genitalia to infection. The male urethra is about 20 cm long (Newman et al., 2021b).

Act of Urination

Urination, also known as *micturition* or *voiding*, is the process of bladder emptying. Micturition requires simultaneous contraction of the bladder and relaxation of the outlet. The pontine micturition centre (PMC), located in the brainstem, coordinates the mechanical process of micturition. When activated, it stimulates urination by producing bladder muscle contraction and urethral sphincter relaxation. The neural circuitry that controls voiding and continence involves pathways at various levels of the brain, the spinal cord, and the peripheral nervous system and is under the mediation of multiple neurotransmitters. The mechanisms of storing and eliminating urine depend on the coordinated activity of the two functional units of the lower urinary tract: the urinary bladder and urinary outlet (Rahman & Siddik, 2021).

When the urinary bladder becomes distended, the stretch receptors of the bladder wall transmit signals to notify the brain, which results in awareness of bladder fullness or desire to urinate. The higher brain determines the appropriateness of initiating the voiding reflex by communicating with the PMC to either provoke or suppress the voiding reflex. When it is not socially acceptable to void, the higher brain suppresses the PMC by transmitting inhibitory signals, and the urge to urinate disappears, which allows delaying voiding until finding a socially acceptable place and time (Rahman & Siddik, 2021). At an appropriate time and place, the brain withdraws the suppression of the PMC, which allows initiating a micturition reflex. The individual may voluntarily contract the pelvic floor muscles to keep the external urethral sphincter closed and suppress the voiding reflex (Rahman & Siddik, 2021).

Sensory nerves from the bladder and urethra carry afferent signals through the spinal reflex arc and up the spinal cord to the pontine micturition centre in the brainstem. Efferent signals move back down, inhibiting sympathetic fibres of the hypogastric nerve innervating the bladder and Onuf's nucleus in the sacral spinal cord where motor neurons innervating the rhabdosphincter are located, resulting in relaxation of the sphincter and contraction of the detrusor muscle. Before full maturation of the nervous system in infants occurs, bladder evacuation happens through non-neural mechanisms and, at later stages of development, by primitive reflex pathways at the spinal cord level. As the child matures, voluntary control over the bladder emptying develops, allowing for the suppression of the voiding reflex (Rahman & Siddik, 2021). In adults, the first urge to void is usually felt when the bladder is half full of urine, with a strong urge at 500 mL.

Common Alterations in Urinary Elimination

Most patients with urinary problems have disturbances in the act of micturition that involve a failure to store urine, a failure to empty urine, or both. Disturbances may be acute or chronic and result from infection, an overactive bladder, impaired contractility, obstruction to urine outflow, or inability to control micturition voluntarily due to mechanical or neural dysfunction.

Urinary Tract Infections. Urinary tract infection (UTI) can involve the lower urinary tract, causing cystitis, urethritis, and prostatitis in patients with male genitalia. Patients with female genitalia are more susceptible to infection because of the short urethra and the proximity of the rectum to the urethral meatus. UTIs are generally considered a disease of individuals with female genitalia; however, UTIs affect individuals with female genitalia throughout the lifespan, and specific populations of individuals with male genitalia (including infants and older men) are also susceptible. Epidemiologically, pyelonephritis is more common in those with female genitalia but carries increased morbidity when it does occur in those with male genitalia (Albracht et al., 2021). Causes of UTI can include obstruction of the urinary tract (e.g., benign prostatic hyperplasia in individuals with male genitalia, or pelvic organ prolapse in individuals with female genitalia), incomplete bladder emptying, and abnormal anatomy. Older persons, patients using antibiotics, and patients with progressive underlying disease or decreased immunity are also at increased risk. UTI can spread to the upper tract, causing kidney infection (**pyelonephritis**) and possibly long-term kidney damage. Bacteria can also spread to the bloodstream (**bacteremia**), leading to urosepsis. It is important to know that not all **bacteriuria** (bacteria in the urine) causes infection. *Asymptomatic* bacteriuria is the presence

of bacteria but no symptoms of UTI and should not be treated with antibiotics (Nicolle et al., 2019; Wiley et al., 2020).

Patients with lower UTIs may experience pain or a burning sensation during urination (**dysuria**). Fever, chills, nausea, vomiting, and malaise may develop as the infection worsens. Inflammation of the bladder (**cystitis**) causes a frequent and urgent sensation of the need to void and may cause incontinence. Irritation to the bladder and urethral mucosa results in blood-tinged urine (hematuria). In the absence of other symptoms, cloudy, foul-smelling urine or a change in urine colour, in the absence of other symptoms, does not indicate infection. Some foods (e.g., beets, blackberries) and medications (e.g., rifampin, phenazopyridine, and senna) can darken or discolour the urine or cause an odour (e.g., from asparagus) (Great Plains Quality Innovation Network & Medicare Quality Improvement Organization for Kansas, Nebraska, North Dakota and South Dakota, 2019). If the infection spreads to the upper urinary tract (i.e., to the kidneys, causing pyelonephritis), rapid onset of flank or lower back pain, tenderness, fever, and chills can occur.

Catheter-associated UTI (CAUTI) results in increased length of hospital stay, morbidity, and mortality for patients. The trend in Canada is to reduce unnecessary use of in-dwelling catheters in all settings and remove them as soon as clinically indicated. Commonly accepted indications for insertion of a urinary catheter are listed in Box 44.1. Catheters should never be inserted for nursing convenience. CAUTIs are often polymicrobial and caused by multiple-drug-resistant uro-pathogens (Bonkat et al., 2021). Bacteria ascend the catheter tubing, and shortly after a catheter is inserted, a biofilm starts to form as organisms adhere to the catheter surface. As long as the catheter remains in the bladder, the biofilm remains and matures. Urease-producing bacteria can cause encrustation with a crystalline biofilm. The duration of catheterization is the most important risk factor for the development of a CAUTI (Bonkat et al., 2021), hence the focus on avoiding unnecessary catheterization and timely removal.

Urinary Incontinence and Other Lower Urinary Tract Symptoms. **Urinary incontinence (UI)** is defined as any complaint of involuntary loss of urine (Abrams et al. 2018). It often occurs along with other lower urinary tract symptoms, including storage (e.g., daytime frequency, nocturia, urgency), voiding (e.g., intermittent or slow stream, hesitancy), and postmicturition symptoms (e.g., postmicturition dribble). There are many types of UI, described in Table 44.1. In Canada, it is estimated that nearly 10% of the Canadian population has daily moderate-to-severe incontinence, with an estimated cost of 8.5 billion dollars to individuals, employers, and the health care system (Taylor & Cahill, 2018). The psychosocial impact ranges from minor lifestyle changes to stigma, embarrassment, and self-imposed social isolation (Taylor & Cahill, 2018).

> **SAFETY ALERT** Continued episodes of incontinence create the potential for skin breakdown. The immobilized patient who experiences frequent incontinence is especially at risk for pressure injuries (see Chapter 47). Timely and meticulous skin care is essential.

Nocturia. **Nocturia** is a prevalent and bothersome lower urinary tract symptom defined as the need to get up at night on a regular basis to urinate and the number of times urine is passed during the main sleep period. To count as a nocturnal void, a sleep period must precede and follow the urinary episode (Hashim et al., 2018). Having woken to pass urine for the first time, each urination must

BOX 44.1 Indications and Contraindications for Use of an In-Dwelling Urinary Catheter in Individuals With Male and Female Genitalia

Indications
- Postoperative urinary retention (per facility removal policy)
- Bladder outlet obstruction (e.g., gross hematuria, benign prostatic hyperplasia in individuals with male genitalia, pelvic organ prolapse in individuals with female genitalia, urethral strictures)
- Acute urinary retention requires immediate attention.
- Need for accurate measurements of urine output in critically ill patients for which urine cannot be measured in any other way
- Individuals who require prolonged immobilization (e.g., potentially unstable thoracic or lumbar spine, multiple traumatic injuries such as pelvic fractures)
- Continuous bladder irrigation for clot retention or intravesical medication infusion
- Administration of medications into the bladder (e.g., chemotherapy to treat bladder cancer)
- To improve comfort for end-of-life care, if needed
- Perioperative use in selected surgical procedures:
  - Urological/gynecological/perineal procedures and other surgeries on contiguous structures of the genitourinary tract
  - Anticipated prolonged duration of surgery (catheter should be removed in the recovery unit once patient is awake)
  - Patients anticipated to receive large-volume infusions or diuretics during surgery
  - Operative patients with urinary incontinence
  - Need for intraoperative hemodynamic monitoring of fluids

Contraindications
- For perceived comfort in patients with urinary or fecal incontinence
- As a means for obtaining urine for tests when patients can voluntarily void
- Prolonged postoperative use without appropriate indications

From Newman, D., Quallich, S., Hull, M., et al. (2021). Insertion of an indwelling urethral catheter in the adult male. *Urologic Nursing*, 41(2), 86–96; Newman, D., Quallich, S., Hull, M., et al. (2021). Insertion of an indwelling urethral catheter in the adult female. *Urologic Nursing*, 41(2), 76–85.

be followed by sleep or the intention to sleep (Hashim et al., 2018). Prevalence of nocturia increases with age and is seen in multiple conditions, including an overactive bladder, prostate enlargement (men), excess urine production at night (nocturnal polyuria) associated with peripheral edema in heart failure, obstructive sleep apnea, and loss of arginine vasopressin (antidiuretic hormone) circadian rhythm. Polyuria can also occur in metabolic imbalances such as hyperglycemia and hypercalcemia.

Regardless of the cause, it is important to learn whether the patient wakes at night to void or voids because they are awake. Assessment includes evaluating lower urinary tract symptoms, postvoid residual urine, and a bladder diary with 24-hour urine output (time and volume of each void). Getting up at night for any reason other than the need to urinate is not considered nocturia, although it may appear as such on voiding diaries. Treatment options may include reducing fluid intake in the evening, elevating the feet for 1 to 2 hours before bedtime to encourage the return of fluid from the lower extremities, medication to reduce the volume of urine produced overnight, or medication to relax the bladder muscle.

SAFETY ALERT Micturition syncope is a type of situational syncope that is reflex mediated and triggered by micturition and defecation, leading to a slow heart rate and hypotension resulting in transient loss of consciousness. Dehydration, fatigue, and medical illness are thought to play a role. To avoid injury, at-risk patients should be cautioned to sit when voiding and not to stand up suddenly.

Urinary Retention. Urinary retention is the marked accumulation of urine in the bladder due to the bladder's inability to empty. Normally, urine production slowly fills the bladder and prevents activation of stretch receptors until the bladder distends to a certain extent. The micturition reflex then occurs, and the bladder empties. With urinary retention, the bladder becomes unable to respond to the micturition reflex and thus is unable to empty. Urine continues to collect in the bladder, causing feelings of pressure, discomfort, tenderness over the symphysis pubis, restlessness, and diaphoresis. As retention progresses, overflow incontinence may occur. Pressure in the bladder builds to a point at which the urethral sphincter is unable to hold back urine, and a small volume escapes. Urinary retention results from an underactive or acontractile detrusor muscle or urethral obstruction. Acute urinary retention can occur postpartum or following urogenital surgery because of medication adverse effects (e.g., anticholinergic adverse effects) or from fecal impaction. Postoperative urinary retention (POUR) is a type of acute urinary retention that can result from general, spinal, and regional anaesthetics; by suppressing micturition control and reflexes at the central nervous and peripheral nervous systems, it blocks neural transmission in the sacral spinal cord. Reducing the effects of POUR can be achieved through timely intervention. However, if it is left untreated, it can have lasting effects on the patient. Chronic urinary retention can occur in individuals with male genitalia with prostate enlargement and in individuals with female genitalia who have pelvic organ prolapse or urethral stricture, or in conditions that alter motor and sensory innervation of the bladder.

Key signs of acute urinary retention are the absence of urine output over several hours, bladder distension, restlessness, diaphoresis, and moderate-to-extreme abdominal discomfort. A patient under the influence of anaesthetics or analgesics may feel only pressure, but an alert patient experiences severe pain as the bladder distends beyond its normal capacity. A person with chronic urinary retention may not be aware of the overfull bladder and may experience the repeated inability to empty the bladder despite the ability to pass some urine (D'Ancona et al., 2019). In severe urinary retention, the bladder may hold a litre or more of urine, well over the normal capacity of 400–600 mL. Intermittent catheterization may be needed to empty the bladder and reduce the risk of overflow incontinence and UTI.

SAFETY ALERT Bladder distension can trigger autonomic dysreflexia in individuals with spinal cord injury above the T6 level. Dysregulation of the autonomic nervous system triggers an uncoordinated autonomic response that could result in potentially life-threatening hypertension. Immediate recognition and correction of the disorder (irrigating or changing the Foley catheter) can be life-saving. Patients with traumatic spinal injuries and autonomic dysreflexia have a higher death rate (Eldahan & Rabchevsky, 2018).

Urinary Diversions. A urinary stoma to divert the flow of urine from the kidneys directly to the abdominal surface is a urinary diversion. It can be created for several reasons, including cancer of the bladder, trauma, radiation injury to the bladder, fistulas, and chronic cystitis. A urinary diversion may be temporary or permanent. The patient with an incontinent urinary diversion must wear an ostomy appliance

TABLE 44.1	Types of Urinary Incontinence	
Definition	**Causes/Risk Factors**	**Common Interventions**
Transient urinary incontinence (UI): Urine loss resulting from causes outside of or affecting the urinary system that resolves when the underlying causes are treated	TOILETED acronym (Ermer-Seltun & Engberg, 2022): • **T**hin, dry urethral epithelium • **O**bstruction • **I**nfection • **L**imited mobility • **E**motional/psychological issues • **T**herapeutic medications • **E**ndocrine disorders • **D**elirium	Identify and treat the underlying cause. *Conservative:* Supportive measures such as fluid and bowel management, toileting assistance, containment pads if required *Pharmacological:* Medication review and appropriate adjustment by the prescriber. Individuals with atrophic vaginitis may benefit from low-dose vaginal estrogen.
Urge UI: Report of involuntary loss of urine associated with urgency, frequency, or nocturia (D'Ancona et al., 2019). Can be part of overactive bladder (OAB) syndrome	Central nervous system disorders related to detrusor overactivity (dementia, cerebrovascular accident, Parkinson's disease, multiple sclerosis), increasing age, outflow obstruction, particularly in persons with an enlarged prostate (D'Ancona et al., 2019)	*Conservative:* Fluid and bowel management, caffeine reduction, pelvic floor muscles exercises (PFMEs), scheduled voiding regimes, urge suppression and bladder retraining *Pharmacological:* Bladder antimuscarinic agents (e.g., oxybutynin, tolterodine, solifenacin, fesoterodine) or β_3-adrenoreceptor agonist agent (mirabegron) *Surgical/Invasive:* Injection of botulinum toxin into bladder, sacral nerve stimulation
Stress UI: Report of involuntary loss of urine on effort or physical exertion, including sporting activities, or on sneezing or coughing (D'Ancona et al., 2019)	Most common in individuals with female genitalia (poor sphincter closure or urethral hypermobility) but can occur in individuals with male genitalia after radical prostatectomy. Risk factors in individuals with female genitalia include obesity, number of deliveries, weakness of the pelvic floor, heavy lifting, and prior hysterectomy.	*Conservative:* Lifestyle strategies (weight loss, fluid and bowel management, smoking cessation, caffeine reduction), PFMEs, pessary *Pharmacological:* Serotonin-norepinephrine reuptake inhibitor (SNRI) in individuals with female genitalia (duloxetine) *Surgical:* In individuals with female genitalia, urethral bulking, tapes and slings, colposuspension; artificial sphincter in individuals with male genitalia
Mixed UI: Urine loss that has features of both stress and urge incontinence		Combinations of urgency and stress UI interventions
UI associated with chronic retention of urine (previously overflow UI): Involuntary loss of urine when the bladder does not completely empty with a high residual urine volume or a palpable nonpainful bladder remaining after voiding Residual volume greater than 300 mL for more than 6 months is indicative of chronic urinary retention (Sheldon & Santos, 2022).	Bladder outlet obstruction from prostate enlargement, or pelvic organ prolapse (POP) in individuals with female genitalia or fecal impaction Poor contractility of the bladder (detrusor) muscles seen in neurological conditions (e.g., diabetes, spinal cord injury). Spinal lesions C2–T12 can result in a hyperreflective bladder with loss of coordination between bladder contraction (dyssynergia). Lesions below S1 can lead to a hypotonic or atonic bladder and poor emptying (Huether, 2019).	*Conservative:* Fluid and bowel management, scheduled voiding regimens (e.g., timed voiding), double voiding, intermittent catheterization, in-dwelling urinary catheter (last resort) *Pharmacological:* Outlet obstruction in men: α_1-antagonists (tamsulosin, terazosin), 5α-reductase inhibitors (dutasteride, finasteride) *Surgical:* Prostate surgery, intraurethral stent, botulinum toxin to detrusor
Functional UI: Urine loss due to inability to reach the toilet	Cognitive, physical function, or mobility impairments	*Conservative:* Timed toileting (scheduled or prompted voiding), containment products (e.g., pads, condom catheter)—supplementary but not a substitute for toileting assistance
Neurogenic bladder dysfunction Lower urinary tract dysfunction caused by an underlying disease or disorder of the nervous system. Symptoms can include urge incontinence, frequency, and retention.	Dysfunction is caused by disease or disorders directly affecting the central nervous system, such as stroke, spinal cord injuries, cerebral palsy, traumatic brain injury, multiple sclerosis, Parkinson's disease, dementia, and Guillain-Barre syndrome.	The goal is to preserve continence and renal function while improving the quality of life. Clean intermittent catheterization combined with antimuscarinic agents, β_3-agonist, α-blockers to decrease bladder outlet resistance. Sacral neuromodulation. Pudendal neuromodulation immediately after spinal cord injury (Gray, 2022)

continuously because no sphincter control exists to regulate urine flow. Local irritation and skin breakdown occur when urine comes in contact with the skin for long periods. Figure 44.2 illustrates three approaches to urinary diversion.

The ileal conduit involves separating a loop of intestinal ileum with its blood supply intact. The ureters are implanted into the isolated segment of the ileum, with the remaining ileum reconnected. The isolated ileal segment can then be used as a conduit for continuous urine drainage. The orthotopic neobladder is an internal pouch created with the ileum and is reconnected to the urethra. Patients will void via the urethra but may need to perform intermittent catheterization. The Indiana pouch is a continent internal pouch created from the ileum. A portion of the Indiana pouch is connected to the abdominal wall and acts as a continent nipple, and intermittent catheterization is needed for emptying (Lenis et al., 2020).

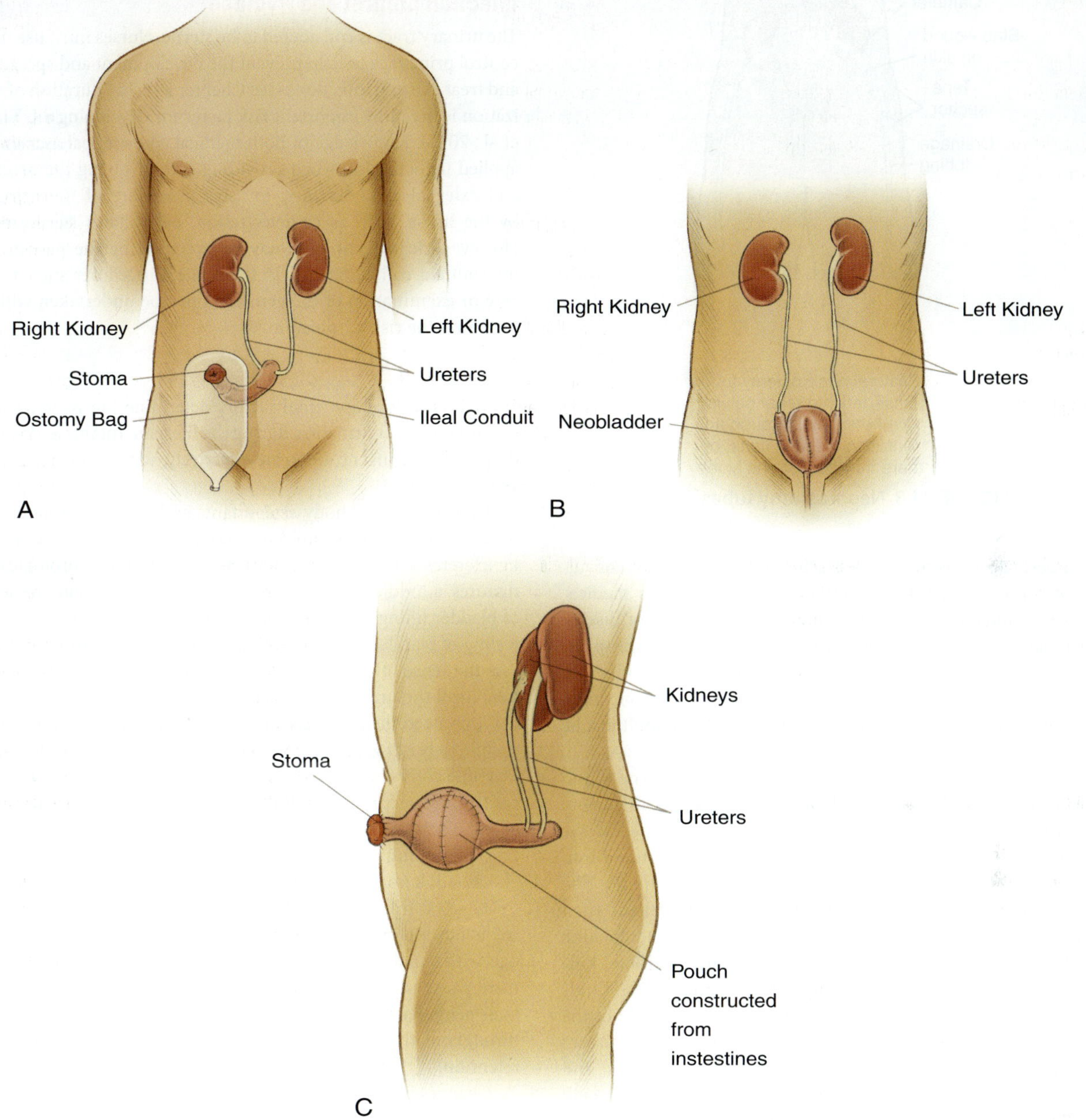

FIGURE 44.2 Types of urinary diversions: **A,** Ileal conduit. **B,** Orthotopic neobladder. **C,** Indiana pouch. (From Bladder Cancer Canada. [2021]. *The bladder is gone—now what?* https://bladdercancercanad a.org/en/diversion-types)

The disadvantage of an ileal conduit or internal reservoir is that if urine outflow becomes obstructed, irreversible damage to the kidneys can occur secondary to chronic infections or hydronephrosis.

A *ureterostomy,* although rarely done, involves bringing the end of one or both ureters to the abdominal surface. More commonly, neph-rostomy tubes are inserted; this procedure involves inserting a tube directly into the renal pelvis to provide urinary drainage. Nephrostomy tubes can be inserted bilaterally (Figure 44.3).

It is essential that the stoma's pouching system fits correctly, that the patient (or caregiver) is capable of changing the pouching system easily, and that skin around the stoma remains protected and intact. Unprotected skin that comes in contact with urine will quickly become macerated and break down, causing pain, infection, increased hospital stays, and the potential breakdown of the stoma. All patients must be referred to a nurse specialized in wound, ostomy and continence

(NSWOC) for preoperative stoma siting and assessment and should be followed closely for several months postoperatively. The patient should also be referred to the Ostomy Canada Society, an invaluable source of advice and networking.

A urinary diversion poses threats to a patient's body image, and adjustment to it takes time. Although a normal lifestyle is possible with a stoma, adjustment can be difficult, and each person will cope differently.

Renal Failure. Irreversible damage to the glomeruli or renal tubules causes a decline in kidney function and leads to end-stage renal disease. In end-stage disease, there is severely reduced or absent urine output from the bladder, as well as metabolic disturbances that result in uremic syndrome, including increased nitrogenous wastes in the blood, altered regulatory functions causing marked fluid and electrolyte

Catheter

Stab wound
on skin

Tape
anchor

Drainage
tubing

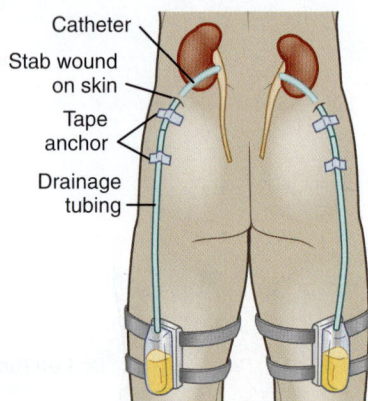

Bilateral nephrostomy tubes
inserted into renal pelvis;
catheters exit through an
incision on each flank, or
there may be just one kidney

FIGURE 44.3 Nephrostomy tubes.

abnormalities, nausea, vomiting, headache, coma, and risk of convulsions. The condition may be managed conservatively with medications and a regimen of dietary and fluid restrictions. Severe disease requires renal replacement therapy, either dialysis or organ transplantation. Dialysis may take one of two forms: peritoneal or hemodialysis. Both dialysis modalities can be applied for a short or long time; however, specialized equipment and nurses with specific training must be available.

Peritoneal dialysis is an indirect method of cleaning the blood of waste products and excess fluid using osmosis and diffusion. The peritoneum functions as a semipermeable membrane for the procedure. A sterile electrolyte solution (dialysate) is instilled into the peritoneal cavity by gravity via a surgically placed catheter. The dialysate is left in the cavity for a prescribed time interval and then drained out by gravity. Hemodialysis involves using a machine equipped with a semipermeable filtering membrane (artificial kidney) that removes accumulated waste products and excess fluids from the blood. Dialysate fluid is pumped through one side of the filter membrane (artificial kidney) while the patient's blood passes through the other side. The processes of diffusion, osmosis, and ultrafiltration clean the patient's blood, which is returned through a specially placed vascular access device such as an arteriovenous fistula or hemodialysis catheter. Organ transplantation replaces a patient's diseased kidney with a healthy one from a living or cadaver donor of compatible blood and tissue type. Special medications (immunosuppressives) are administered for life to prevent the body from rejecting the transplanted organ. Unlike dialysis, successful organ transplantation offers the patient the potential for restoration of normal kidney function.

NURSING KNOWLEDGE BASE

Urinary elimination is a basic human function that is usually a private process. Nurses are often the first to become aware that a patient has elimination problems and must be alert to cues, prepared to discuss relevant assessment and treatment options, and provide counselling and support. These skills require a sound base of scientific knowledge related to anatomy and physiology and an understanding of concepts such as infection control and hygiene, normal growth and development, and psychosocial and cultural considerations.

Infection Control and Hygiene

The urinary tract is considered to be sterile. Nurses must use infection-control principles to help prevent the development and spread of UTIs and treat existing infections (see Chapter 34). The duration of catheterization is the most important risk factor for developing a UTI (Bonkat et al., 2021). Knowledge of both medical and surgical asepsis must be applied meticulously when providing care involving the urinary tract and external genitalia. Any invasive procedure of the urinary tract by the nurse, such as catheterization, necessitates sterile technique. However, clean technique may be practised by the patient for self-intermittent catheterization in the home. Procedures such as perineal care or examination of the genitalia must be undertaken with care to minimize the risk of infection.

Growth and Development

Growth and developmental factors determine the patient's ability to control the act of urination during the lifespan. Infants and young children cannot concentrate urine effectively, with urine appearing light yellow and clear.

Relative to their body size, infants and children excrete large volumes of urine. For example, a 6-month-old infant who weighs 6 to 8 kg excretes 400 to 500 mL of urine daily. As the neurological system matures, a toddler 2 to 3 years of age is able to associate the sensations of bladder filling and urination. A child must be able to recognize the feeling of bladder fullness, hold urine for 1 to 2 hours, and communicate the sense of urgency to an adult. Many toddlers may then be able to control the urethral sphincter, and toilet training can begin. Young children need their parents' understanding, patience, and consistency. A child may not gain full control of micturition until 4 or 5 years of age. Daytime control of micturition is easier to accomplish than nighttime control and occurs earlier in the child's development, usually by 2 years of age. Occasional daytime accidents or nocturnal enuresis (bedwetting) may continue until 5 years of age.

The adult normally voids 1 500 to 1 600 mL of urine daily or approximately 500 mL every 4 hours. During pregnancy, increased urinary frequency is common, and susceptibility to UTIs increases. In individuals with female genitalia, child-bearing and hormonal changes during menopause may contribute to urinary difficulties. In individuals with male genitalia, prostate enlargement can begin in the 40s and continue throughout the lifespan, resulting in urinary frequency and urinary retention.

Changes in kidney and bladder function also occur with aging. The kidney's ability to concentrate urine or reabsorb water and sodium declines. Alterations in kidney function include a reduction in glomerular filtration rate, from 125 mL/min in younger adults to 60 to 70 mL/min in adults 80 years of age. The older person often experiences nocturia caused by excessive 24-hour urine production, excessive nighttime urine production, or inadequate bladder capacity (Palmer, 2022). Detrusor contractility also decreases, contributing to less effective emptying, elevated **postvoid residual (PVR)** (the volume remaining in the bladder after a void), and increased susceptibility to UTI. A decrease in urethral closure pressure in those with female genitalia, which is generally associated with a decline in estrogen levels, can contribute to an increase in incontinence (Ermer-Seltun & Engberg, 2022). Older persons with male genitalia commonly experience incomplete bladder emptying associated with prostatic enlargement.

Psychosocial and Cultural Considerations

Nurses must consider that urinary elimination problems may result in alterations of sexuality and self-concept (including body image, self-esteem, roles, and identity). The embarrassment associated with elimination problems may delay or prevent seeking help (Agochukwu-Mmonu et al., 2020). Individuals with incontinence often blame themselves for their condition and go to great lengths, including self-imposed social isolation, to keep others from finding out about it. Therefore, as a routine part of care, nurses must initiate a discussion by asking patients if they are experiencing any issues related to urinary elimination or bladder control. It is also important to determine how bothersome symptoms are for each patient before planning care. Research has shown that self-management of urinary incontinence through a booklet or the Internet can effectively motivate patients (Bokne et al., 2019).

Sociocultural factors may influence the patient's expectation of the degree of privacy and location for attending to urinary needs. The nurse's approach to a patient's elimination needs must consider cultural, social, and gender habits. If a patient prefers privacy, the nurse should try to prevent interruptions as the patient voids. A patient with less need for privacy should also be treated with understanding and acceptance. It is important to ensure that the patient is comfortable when they are trying to void. In some cultures, people prefer to squat over a receptacle rather than sit on one. Culture dictates when and where it is appropriate to urinate. In some cultures, a woman with urinary needs should be assisted only by another woman.

CRITICAL THINKING

Critical thinking during the assessment of urinary elimination requires the integration of evidence-informed knowledge from nursing and other disciplines, experiential knowledge, and an understanding of the patient's perceptions of the alterations in elimination and their impact. Critical thinking also involves an understanding of relevant cultural, environmental, and personal factors, including the unique goals of every patient. Empathy, teaching, and ongoing support are needed to assist the patient in meeting these goals and maintaining improvement. In Canada, little research has been undertaken to understand urinary symptoms and problems among Indigenous groups, in spite of the prevalence of risk factors such as diabetes in these populations. Moving forward, partnerships with Indigenous people need to be formed to better understand and address urinary health needs.

Professional standards provide valuable directions for the treatment and management of elimination problems. When planning and implementing care for patients with alterations in urinary elimination, nurses need to use standards developed by professional organizations, such as Nurses Specialized in Wound Ostomy and Continence Canada, Canadian Nurse Continence Advisors Association, the Canadian Continence Foundation, the United Ostomy Association of Canada, and the Urology Nurses of Canada.

❖ NURSING PROCESS AND ALTERATIONS IN URINARY FUNCTION

◆ Assessment

To identify a urinary elimination problem and gather data for a care plan, nurses obtain information by collecting a health history, performing a focused physical assessment, assessing the patient's urine, and reviewing information from diagnostic tests and examinations. Nurses use critical thinking to synthesize this information as assessment proceeds (Figure 44.4). Adequate assessment should result in the formulation of nursing diagnoses appropriate for alterations in urinary elimination. In addition, nurses should be alert to individual needs related to normal aging that predispose older persons to specific elimination problems (Box 44.2).

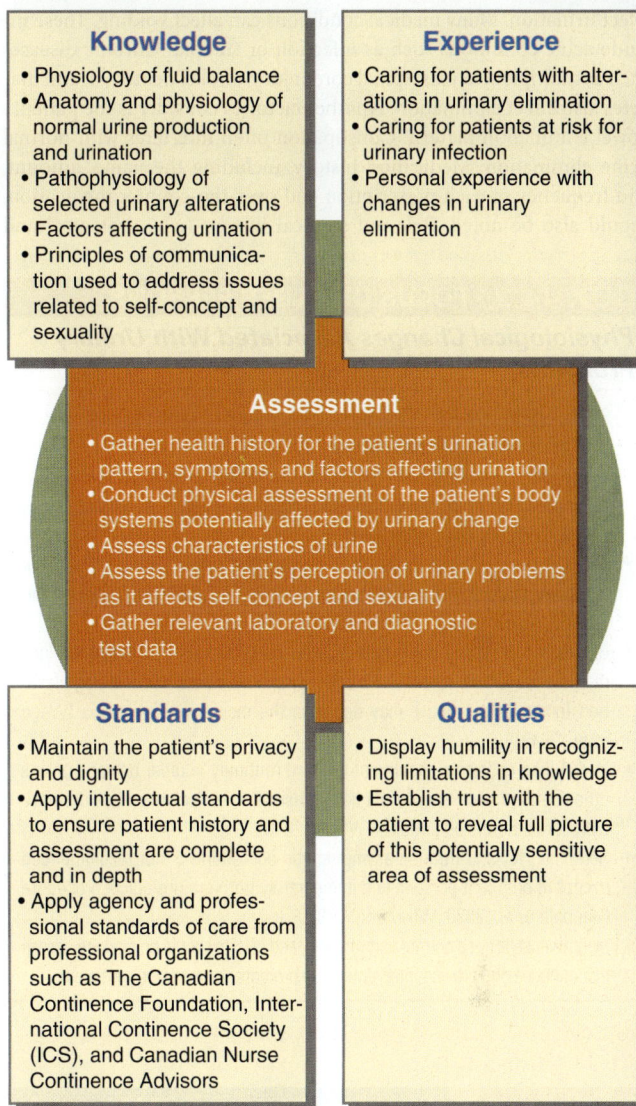

Knowledge
- Physiology of fluid balance
- Anatomy and physiology of normal urine production and urination
- Pathophysiology of selected urinary alterations
- Factors affecting urination
- Principles of communication used to address issues related to self-concept and sexuality

Experience
- Caring for patients with alterations in urinary elimination
- Caring for patients at risk for urinary infection
- Personal experience with changes in urinary elimination

Assessment
- Gather health history for the patient's urination pattern, symptoms, and factors affecting urination
- Conduct physical assessment of the patient's body systems potentially affected by urinary change
- Assess characteristics of urine
- Assess the patient's perception of urinary problems as it affects self-concept and sexuality
- Gather relevant laboratory and diagnostic test data

Standards
- Maintain the patient's privacy and dignity
- Apply intellectual standards to ensure patient history and assessment are complete and in depth
- Apply agency and professional standards of care from professional organizations such as The Canadian Continence Foundation, International Continence Society (ICS), and Canadian Nurse Continence Advisors

Qualities
- Display humility in recognizing limitations in knowledge
- Establish trust with the patient to reveal full picture of this potentially sensitive area of assessment

FIGURE 44.4 Critical thinking model for urinary elimination assessment.

Health History. The nursing health history includes reviewing the patient's urinary elimination pattern and lower urinary tract symptoms. This information is used to identify urinary alterations and to assess factors that may affect voiding.

Pattern of Urination. The patient should be asked about usual daily voiding patterns and any recent changes. Information about voiding symptoms such as hesitancy (Table 44.2) and the overall urination pattern, including average time between voids and episodes of urgency and incontinence, is important to a nursing assessment and establishes a baseline for comparison.

A bladder diary is an important diagnostic tool (Figure 44.5), particularly because many adults are not aware of how often they void throughout the day. The patient or the caregiver records times of urination and leakage, estimates of the amount lost (dribbled, wet pad, wet clothing), and types and amount of fluids ingested. Recording factors that precipitated urination or leakage, such as a strong urge or a cough, is particularly helpful. A 3-day (72-hour) voiding diary helps in evaluating lifestyle habits (e.g., fluid intake) in relation to the voiding pattern and symptoms (Kershaw & Jha, 2021).

Factors Affecting Urination. The nurse must consider the patient's medical history, surgical history, and current environment that may affect urination. Many medical conditions can affect voiding. These include acute conditions such as infection or trauma. Chronic diseases such as multiple sclerosis, spinal cord injury, stroke, dementia, and diabetes also affect elimination. Another factor to consider is the patient's bowel elimination pattern. Constipation often interferes with normal urine elimination. Medication history, including the name, amount, and frequency of each prescription and over-the-counter medication, should also be noted. Relevant surgical history (e.g., urological and gynecological interventions, pelvic radiation) should be considered because surgery may cause scarring and disruption of neurological pathways. The presence or history of an in-dwelling catheter should be noted because of the potential for infection, catheter blockage, or skin care problems. Environmental barriers in the home or health care setting also should be evaluated. The nurse needs to assess the patient's mobility and ability to dress or undress and use the toilet independently. Such aids as elevated toilet seats, grab bars, or a portable commode may be needed.

One of the most important parts of the assessment is the impact of alterations in elimination on the patient's lifestyle and quality of life. The effect of urinary incontinence, in particular, can be substantial; it is important to discuss changes the patient has made to cope with the condition. It is also important to note whether the patient has previously seen a health care provider for help with or advice on urination.

Physical Assessment. A physical examination (see Chapter 33) provides nurses with data to determine the presence and severity of urinary elimination problems. The primary structures reviewed are the skin and mucosal membranes of the perineum, urethral and vaginal orifices, bladder (by palpation), and rectum.

Skin and Mucosal Membranes. The nurse assesses the condition of the skin and mucosal membranes. Problems with urinary elimination are often associated with fluid and electrolyte disturbances. By assessing skin turgor and the oral mucosa, the nurse is assessing the patient's hydration status. Urinary incontinence increases the risk of skin breakdown (see Chapter 47).

Kidneys. Flank pain usually develops if the kidneys become infected or inflamed. The nurse can assess for flank tenderness early in the disease by percussing the costovertebral angle (the angle formed by the spine and the twelfth rib). Auscultation is performed to detect the presence of a renal artery bruit (sound resulting from turbulent blood flow through a narrowed artery).

BOX 44.2   FOCUS ON OLDER PERSONS

Physiological Changes Associated With Urinary Problems

- Physiological changes in the lower urinary tract occur in the continent as well as the incontinent older person.
- Dilute urine discourages bacterial growth; therefore, older persons should be encouraged to increase their fluid intake to at least six glasses a day unless medically contraindicated.
- There is not sufficient evidence to support the use of cranberry juice or cranberry products in reducing urinary tract infections (NSWOCC, CNCA, UNC & IPAC, 2020).
- Restriction of fluids 2 hours before sleep, combined with elevating the legs to allow for venous return and bladder emptying before bedtime (leg elevation for at least 1 hour), may decrease the incidence of nocturia (Wagg et al., 2013).
- In-dwelling catheters should not be used routinely in older persons unless other options have been trialled. The risk of infection increases dramatically for catheterized patients (WOCN, 2016).
- Screening for and treating asymptomatic bacteriuria is not recommended except in pregnant persons and immediately before a urological procedure (Godbole et al., 2020; Wiley et al., 2020).
- Incontinence is not a normal part of aging, and efforts should be made to assess incontinence and provide interventions to promote the return to continence.

TABLE 44.2   Common Symptoms of Urinary Alterations

Symptom	Common Causes or Associated Factors
Incontinence: Involuntary loss of urine	See Table 44.1
Urgency: Report of a sudden, compelling desire to pass urine which is difficult to defer (D'Ancona et al., 2019)	Overactive bladder syndrome that is neurogenic, sensory, or idiopathic; calculi or tumour; urinary tract infection (UTI)
Dysuria: Report of pain, burning, or other discomforts during voiding (D'Ancona et al., 2019)	Bladder inflammation; urethral trauma; UTI; inflammation of the urethra, sphincter, or both
Frequency: Voiding more than eight times in 24 hours	Increased fluid intake, bladder infection or inflammation, increased pressure on the bladder (pregnancy, psychological stress), incomplete emptying, small bladder capacity, overactive bladder syndrome, polyuria
Hesitancy: Report of delay in initiating voiding (when the individual is ready to pass urine) (D'Ancona et al., 2019)	Hypotonic bladder, anxiety, urethral stricture, obstruction associated with prostate enlargement
Polyuria: Report that urine excretion volume over 24 hours is noticeably larger than previous excretion (D'Ancona et al., 2019)	Excess fluid intake, diabetes mellitus or diabetes insipidus (hyperglycemia), diuretic use, nocturnal polyuria, postobstructive diuresis
Oliguria: Diminished urinary output relative to intake (usually 400 mL/24 hr)	Dehydration, renal failure, increased antidiuretic hormone (ADH) secretion
Nocturia: The number of times urine is passed during the main sleep period (D'Ancona et al., 2019)	Excessive fluid intake before bed (especially coffee or alcohol), renal disease, overactive bladder, heart failure with peripheral edema, prostate enlargement, sleep apnea
Dribbling: Leakage of urine despite voluntary control of urination	Stress incontinence, overflow from urinary retention, postvoid pooling of urine in the urethra (individuals with male genitalia)
Hematuria: Report of passage of visible blood mixed with urine	Kidney or bladder neoplasms, renal disease, infection of kidney or bladder, trauma, calculi, bleeding disorders, UTI
Elevated postvoid residual urine	Neurogenic bladder, prostate enlargement, trauma, pelvic organ prolapse, inflammation or stricture of the urethra

Bladder Diary DAY 1

TIME	AMOUNT URINATED		URGENCY?		LEAKAGE		DRINKS	
	How many times	How much	Yes	No	How many times	How much	Which drink	How much
EXAMPLE:	3 times	A little / Some / (A lot)			once	(A little) / Some / A lot	water	1 cup
6-8 am								
8-10 am								
10-12 pm								
12-2 pm								
2-4 pm								
4-6 pm								
6-8 pm								
8-10 pm								
10-12 pm								
12-2 am								
2-4 am								
4-6 am								

A little   Some   A lot

Bladder Diary DAY 2

TIME	AMOUNT URINATED		URGENCY?		LEAKAGE		DRINKS	
	How many times	How much	Yes	No	How many times	How much	Which drink	How much
EXAMPLE:	3 times	A little / Some / (A lot)			once	(A little) / Some / A lot	water	1 cup
6-8 am								
8-10 am								
10-12 pm								
12-2 pm								
2-4 pm								
4-6 pm								
6-8 pm								
8-10 pm								
10-12 pm								
12-2 am								
2-4 am								
4-6 am								

A little   Some   A lot

FIGURE 44.5 Sample urinary diary. (From Canadian Continence Foundation. [2016]. http://www.canadiancontinence.ca/pdfs/Bladder-Diary.pdf)

Nurses with advanced examination skills learn to palpate the kidneys during an abdominal examination. The kidneys' position, shape, and size can reveal renal swelling.

Bladder. In adults, the bladder rests below the symphysis pubis and is difficult to palpate. When distended, the bladder rises above the symphysis pubis at the midline of the abdomen and may extend to just below the umbilicus. On inspection, a swelling or convex curvature of the lower abdomen may be noted. The nurse should lightly palpate the lower abdomen. The partially filled bladder normally feels smooth and rounded. As light pressure is applied to the bladder, the patient may feel the urge to urinate, tenderness, or even pain. Percussion of a full bladder yields a dull note.

The Perineum of Patients With Female Genitalia. When examining the patients with female genitalia, the nurse requests that they assume a dorsal recumbent position to fully expose the genitalia. The perineum is inspected for skin integrity and for the presence of incontinence-associated dermatitis or other skin alternations. The nurse needs to inspect the vaginal orifice carefully for signs of inflammation and describe any drainage.

Also, the urethral meatus should be assessed and the presence of any discharge, inflammation, or lesions noted. Normally, the meatus is pink and appears as a small, slit-like opening below the clitoris and above the vaginal orifice. It may recede well into the vaginal vault with aging, making catheterization difficult. Discharge from the meatus is normally not present. If it is present, specimens of urethral discharge should be obtained before the patient voids.

Speculum examination and assessment of pelvic floor strength in patients with female genitalia are advanced skills. On speculum examination, the vagina is assessed for pelvic organ prolapse, vaginal atrophy, and atrophic vaginitis, a common result of estrogen depletion after menopause. Signs of atrophy include dry, thin, pale mucosa with loss of rugae; a urethral caruncle (red urethral meatus) or red labia and vaginal walls indicate inflammation associated with vaginitis (Flint & Davis, 2021). Pelvic floor muscle strength can be digitally assessed in individuals with female genitalia by gently inserting a lubricated, gloved finger into the vagina. The examiner asks the patient to squeeze around the finger as firmly as possible and then hold the contraction for up to 10 seconds. Digital assessment is very useful in helping the patient to identify the pelvic floor muscles correctly.

The Perineum of a Patient With Male Genitalia. The male urethral meatus normally appears as a small opening at the tip of the penis. The nurse should inspect the meatus for any discharge, inflammation, or lesions. If the foreskin needs to be retracted in uncircumcised men to see the meatus, it must be replaced to avoid constriction of the glans. Disposable gloves should be worn when retracting the foreskin. Pelvic floor muscle strength can be digitally assessed in men by gently inserting a lubricated, gloved finger into the rectum and asking the patient to squeeze around it.

Assessment of Urine.

Assessment of urine involves measuring the patient's fluid intake and urine output and observing characteristics of the urine.

Intake and Output. It is important to assess the patient's average daily fluid intake. If an accurate measurement of fluid intake is needed from the patient who is at home, the nurse can ask them to show a commonly used glass or cup on which the intake estimate is based. In a health care setting, a patient's fluid intake is measured either when the prescriber orders intake and output measurements or when nursing judgement warrants a more precise measurement (see Chapter 41). A change in urine volume is a significant indicator of fluid alterations or kidney disease. While caring for the patient, the nurse assesses urine volume by measuring the output with each void (using a urine hat, bedpans, or urinals) (Figure 44.6). Special receptacles (urometers) are attached between in-dwelling catheters and drainage bags and are a convenient means of accurately measuring urine volume (Figure 44.7). A urometer holds 100 to 400 mL of urine. After measuring urine with a urometer, the nurse drains the cylinder into the urinary drainage bag or into a receptacle for disposal. Urometers are indicated when precise hourly measurements of urine are needed.

When urine from a drainage bag is measured, the urine should be drained into a plastic graduated receptacle for a more precise measurement of output (Figure 44.8). Each patient should have a graduated receptacle for their exclusive use to prevent potential cross-contamination.

Nurses should report any extreme increase or decrease in urine volume. An hourly output of less than 30 mL for more than 2 hours is cause for concern. Similarly, consistently high volumes of urine (polyuria), over 2 000 to 2 500 mL daily, should be reported to a physician.

Characteristics of Urine. During the assessment, the patient's urine is inspected for colour, clarity, and odour.

Colour. Normal urine ranges from a pale straw colour to amber, depending on its concentration. Urine is usually more concentrated in the morning or with fluid-volume deficits. As a person drinks more fluids, urine becomes less concentrated.

Bleeding from the kidneys or ureters causes dark red urine; bleeding from the bladder or urethra causes urine to become bright red. Various medications and foods also change urine colour and will cause a false positive on a urinalysis. For example, phenazopyridine, a urinary analgesic, colours the urine bright orange. Eating beets, rhubarb, or blackberries may cause red urine. Special dyes used in intravenous

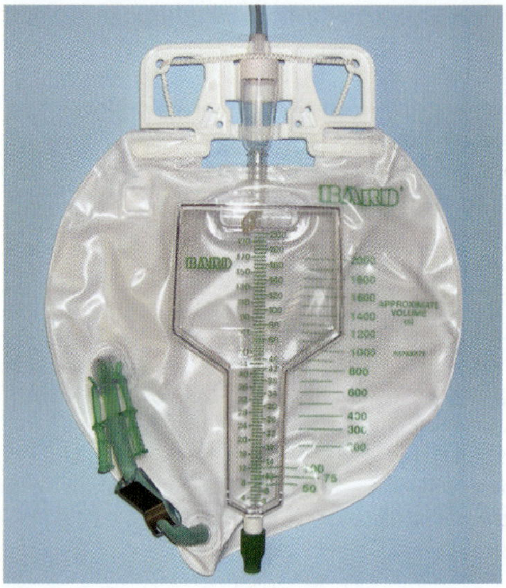

FIGURE 44.7 Urometer. (Courtesy Michael Gallagher, RN, BSN, OSF, Saint Francis Medical Center, Peoria, IL.)

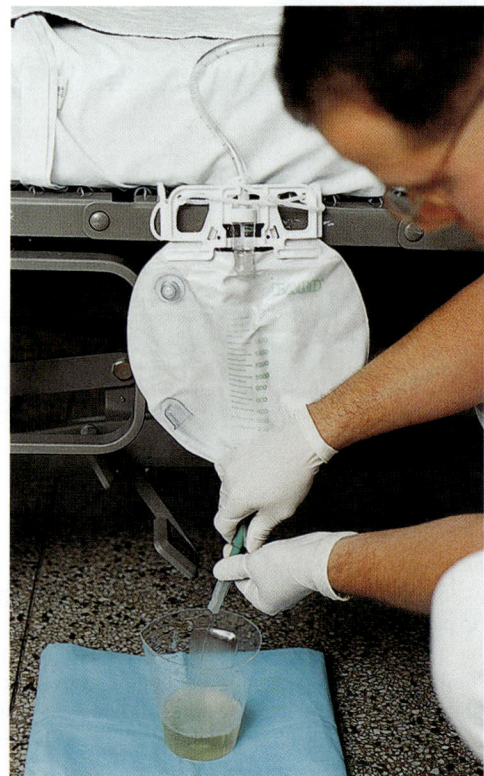

FIGURE 44.8 Urine drainage bag.

FIGURE 44.6 Urine hat.

diagnostic studies also discolour the urine. Dark amber urine may result from high concentrations of bilirubin caused by liver dysfunction or vitamin B. The nurse should document and report any abnormal colour or sediment, especially if the cause is unknown.

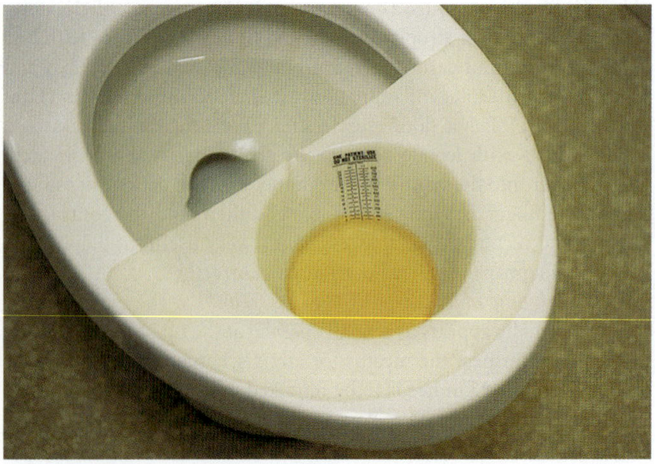

Clarity. Normal urine appears transparent at voiding but may become cloudy if left standing. In patients with renal disease, urine may appear cloudy or foamy because of high protein concentrations. Urine also will appear thick and cloudy as a result of bacteria. Patients with urinary diversions such as an ileal conduit or orthotopic neobladder will always produce a small amount of mucus. An increase in mucus production is a symptom of UTI within this patient population (Lee et al., 2020).

Odour. Urine has a characteristic odour. The more concentrated the urine, the stronger the odour. Stagnant urine has an ammonia odour, which is common in patients who are repeatedly incontinent. A sweet or fruity odour occurs from acetone or acetoacetic acid (by-products of incomplete fat metabolism) seen with diabetes mellitus or starvation.

Urine Testing. It is common to collect urine specimens for laboratory testing (Table 44.3). The type of test being completed determines the method of collection. All specimens are labelled with the patient's name, the date, and the time of collection. Specimens should be transported to the laboratory quickly to ensure the accuracy of test results. Agency infection control policies require adherence to standard precautions or routine practices by all personnel during the handling of specimens (see Chapter 34).

Specimen collection. For specimen collection, the nurse collects random, clean-voided or midstream (Skill 44.1), sterile (Figure 44.9), and timed specimens.

Urine collection in children. Collecting specimens from infants and children is often difficult. School-aged children and adolescents are usually able to cooperate, although they may be embarrassed. Preschool children and toddlers have difficulty voiding on request. Offering a young child fluid 30 minutes before requesting a specimen may help. The nurse must use terms for urination that the child can understand. A young child may be reluctant to void in unfamiliar receptacles. A potty chair or specimen hat placed under the toilet seat is usually effective. Special collection devices must be used for infants and toddlers who are not toilet trained. The caregiver should be consulted to assist; this will help comfort the child and ease the procedure. Clear plastic, single-use bags with self-adhering material can be attached over the child's urethral meatus. Specimens should never be obtained by squeezing urine from the diaper material as other contaminates can cause the results to be inaccurate.

Common Urine Tests

Urinalysis. The laboratory performs a urinalysis on a specimen obtained through any of the previously described methods. Table 44.4 lists normal values for a urinalysis. The specimen should be examined as soon as possible after it is collected, preferably within 2 hours. For protein, the first voided specimen in the morning is preferred to ensure a uniform concentration of constituents (Pagana et al., 2019). For a quick screening, the nurse can perform specific portions of the urinalysis with special reagent strips. The strip is dipped into the urine and observed for a colour change in the time interval designated on the package. The use of dipsticks to diagnose UTIs should be avoided because they may provide misleading information (Godbole et al., 2020; Nurses Specialized in Wound, Ostomy and Continence Canada [NSWOCC], Canadian Nurse Continence Advisors [CNCA], Urology Nurses of Canada [UNC], & Infection Prevention and Control Canada [IPAC], 2020).

Specific gravity. The *specific gravity* is the weight or degree of concentration of a substance compared with an equal amount of water. A urine specimen is poured into a special dry, clean cylinder. The weighted urinometer is suspended in the cylinder of urine. The concentration of dissolved substances in the urine aids in the determination of a patient's fluid balance. This measurement is always done as part of a complete urinalysis. Nurses working in a Critical Care Unit may be responsible for doing periodic measurements of specific gravity of urine as part of a comprehensive assessment of particular patients.

If questions regarding the accuracy of specific gravity measurements arise, a urine osmolality test should be obtained. Although both tests measure urine concentration, the osmolality test is more accurate because it measures the total number of particles in a solution (see Chapter 41).

Urine culture. For a urine culture, a sterile or clean-voided sample of urine is required. Because urine is an excellent medium for bacterial growth and bacteriological changes may alter test results, facilities

TABLE 44.3	Urine Testing
Collection Type (Use of Specimen)	**Nursing Considerations**
Random specimen (routine urinalysis or collection for other tests such as urine electrolytes)	Can be collected during normal voiding from an in-dwelling catheter or a urinary diversion collection bag and collected in a clean specimen cup.
Clean-voided or midstream specimen (culture and sensitivity)	See Skill 44.1. Collected in a sterile specimen cup.
Catheter specimen (culture and sensitivity and other tests)	If the patient has an in-dwelling catheter, a specimen can be collected using aseptic technique through the special port (see Figure 44.9) found on the side of the catheter. When symptomatic CAUTI is suspected and the specimen is for culture and sensitivity, the catheter should be changed before specimen collection and initiation of antibiotics, as biofilm has likely formed on the old catheter (Godbole et al., 2020; Nicolle, 2014). Clamp the tubing below the port, allowing fresh, uncontaminated urine to collect in the tube. After wiping the port with an antimicrobial swab, insert a sterile syringe tip and withdraw at least 3 to 5 mL of urine. Using the sterile aseptic technique, transfer urine to a sterile container (see Chapter 34).
Timed urine specimens (for measuring levels of adrenal cortical steroids or hormones, creatinine clearance, or protein quantity tests)	The time required between collections may be 2, 12, or 24 hours. The timed period begins after the patient urinates and ends with a final voiding at the end of the time period. The patient voids into a clean receptacle. The urine is transferred to the special collection container, which may contain special preservatives. Each specimen must be free of feces and toilet tissue. Missed specimens make the entire collection inaccurate. Check agency policy and with the laboratory for specific instructions.

CAUTI, Catheter-associated urinary tract infection.

SKILL 44.1 COLLECTING A MIDSTREAM (CLEAN-VOIDED) URINE SPECIMEN

Delegation Considerations

Collecting a midstream (clean-voided) urine specimen may be delegated to unregulated care providers (UCPs). If appropriate, an alert patient who is physically able may be instructed to collect the specimen. It is the nurse's responsibility to ensure that this specimen is obtained correctly and in a timely manner. Be aware of agency policy regarding specimen collection.

Instruct the UCP to inform a nurse of the following:

- When the specimen was obtained
- Whether the patient was unable to initiate a stream or had pain or burning on urination
- Whether the collected specimen is dark, bloody, or cloudy; is odorous, or contains mucus

Equipment

- Soap or cleaning solution, washcloth, towel, and handwashing basin
- Commercial kit for clean-voided specimen or individual supplies as listed
- Sterile cotton balls or sterile gauze pads
- Antiseptic solution (e.g., chlorhexidine or povidone-iodine) or sterile normal saline or water, as approved by agency; check for patient allergy, and if an allergy exists, provide an alternative
- Sterile water
- Sterile specimen collection cup or jar
- Sterile and nonsterile (disposable) gloves
- Bedpan, bedside commode, or specimen hat
- Completed specimen label
- Completed laboratory requisition form

PROCEDURE

STEPS	RATIONALE
1. Assess voiding status of the patient:	
A. When the patient last voided	- May indicate readiness to void.
B. Level of awareness or developmental stage	- Reveals patient's ability to cooperate during procedure.
C. Mobility, balance, and physical limitations	- Determines level of assistance needed in acquiring specimen.
2. Assess the patient's understanding of the purpose of the test and method of collection.	- Information allows for clarification and promotes patient cooperation.
3. Explain procedure to patient:	
A. Reason midstream specimen is needed	
B. Ways patient and family can assist	- Helps patient understand the procedure.
C. Ways to obtain specimens free of feces	- Feces change the characteristics of urine and may cause abnormal values.
4. Provide fluids to drink a half-hour before collection unless contraindicated (i.e., fluid restriction) if the patient does not feel the urge to void.	- Improves the likelihood of the patient being able to void.
5. Identify patient and perform hand hygiene.	- Ensures accuracy of specimen collection. Decreases likelihood of transfer of microorganisms.
6. Provide privacy for the patient by closing the door or bed curtain.	- Privacy allows patient to relax and produce specimen more quickly.
7. Give patient or family members soap, washcloth, and towel to clean perineal area.	- Patient may prefer to wash their own perineal area. Cleaning prevents contamination of specimens as the urine passes from the urethra.
8. Apply nonsterile gloves and assist non-ambulatory patients with perineal care. Assist patient with female genitalia onto the bedpan. Raise head of bed.	- Provides easy access to the perineal area to collect the specimen. A semi-sitting position may ease voiding.
9. Using surgical asepsis, open sterile kit (see Step 9 illustration) if using one or prepare sterile supplies. Apply sterile gloves after opening sterile cup, placing cap with sterile inside surface up; do not touch inside of container or cap (see Chapter 34).	- The sterile technique is essential to maintain sterility of equipment and specimen. Sterile gloves prevent the transmission of microorganisms. A contaminated specimen is the most frequent reason for inaccurate reporting of urine cultures and sensitivities.

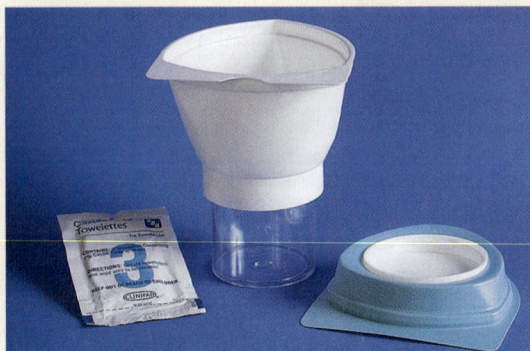

STEP 9 Commercial midstream urine collection kit.

Continued

10. Pour antiseptic solution over cotton balls or gauze pads unless kit contains prepared gauze pads in antiseptic solution.

- Cotton balls or gauze pads will be used to further clean the perineum.

11. Assist or allow the patient to independently clean perineum and collect specimen:

A. Patient with female genitalia

(1) Spread labia with thumb and forefinger of nondominant hand.

- Provides access to urethral meatus.

(2) Clean area with cotton ball or gauze and approved solution, moving from front (above urethral orifice) to back (toward anus; see Step 11A[2] illustration). Using a fresh swab each time, repeat front-to-back motion three times (begin left side, then right side, then centre).

- Clean from area of least contamination to area of greatest contamination to decrease bacterial levels.

(3) If agency policy indicates, rinse area with sterile water, and dry with cotton ball or gauze.

- Prevents contamination of specimen with antiseptic solution.

(4) While you or the patient continue holding labia apart, patient should initiate stream; after stream is achieved, pass container into stream and collect 30 to 60 mL (see Step 11A[4] illustration).

- Initial stream flushes out microorganisms that accumulate at the urethral meatus and prevents transfer into the specimen.

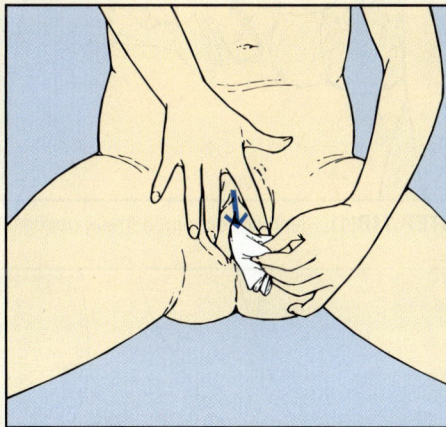

STEP 11A(2) Cleaning technique (female genitalia).

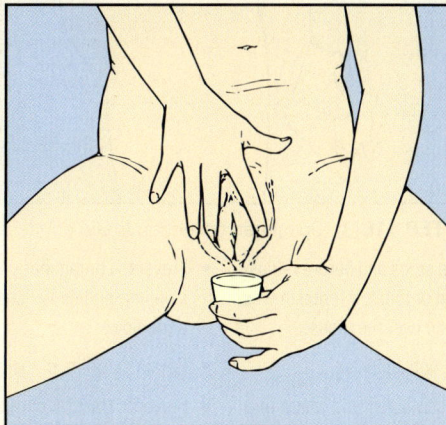

STEP 11A(4) Specimen collection (female genitalia).

B. Patient with male genitalia

(1) Hold patient's penis with one hand or have the patient hold their penis; using circular motion and antiseptic swab or cotton ball with approved solution, clean end of penis, moving from centre to outside (see Step 11B[1] illustration). In uncircumcised individuals, the foreskin should be retracted before cleaning.

- Clean from area of least contamination to area of greatest contamination to decrease bacterial levels.

(2) If agency procedure indicates, rinse area with sterile water and dry with a cotton ball or gauze.

- Prevents contamination of specimen with antiseptic solution.

(3) After the patient has initiated urine stream, pass specimen collection container into stream and collect 30 to 60 mL (see Step 11B[3] illustration).

- Initial stream flushes out microorganisms that accumulate at the urethral meatus and prevents transfer into specimen.
- The amount required to be collected may vary from agency to agency, depending on collection equipment and laboratory procedures.

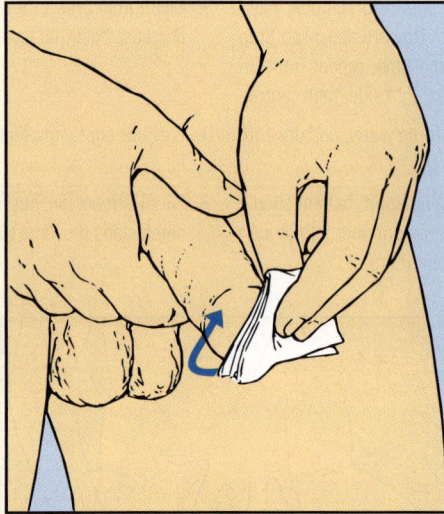

STEP 11B(1) Cleaning technique (male genitalia).

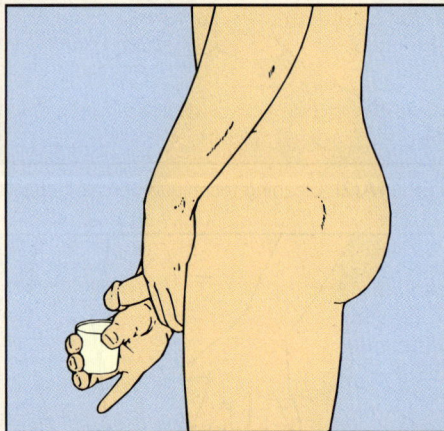

STEP 11B(3) Specimen collection (male genitalia).

12. Remove specimen container before the flow of urine stops and before releasing labia or penis. Patient finishes voiding in bedpan or toilet. If foreskin was retracted for specimen collection, it must be replaced over the glans.

- Prevents contamination of specimen with skin flora. If foreskin is not replaced, swelling and constriction may occur, causing pain and possible obstruction of urine flow.

13. Replace cap securely on specimen container (touch outside only).

- Retains sterility of inside of the container and prevents spillage of urine.

14. Clean any urine from the exterior surface of the container, and place in a plastic specimen bag.

- Prevents transfer of microorganisms to others.

15. Remove bedpan (if applicable), assist patient to a comfortable position, and provide handwashing basin if needed.

- Promotes relaxing environment.

16. Label specimen and attach laboratory requisition.

- Prevents inaccurate identification that could lead to errors in diagnosis or treatment.

Continued

COLLECTING A MIDSTREAM (CLEAN-VOIDED) URINE SPECIMEN—cont'd

> **CRITICAL DECISION POINT:** *If patient is menstruating, indicate this information on the laboratory requisition.*

17. Remove gloves, dispose of them in a proper receptacle, and perform hand hygiene.	• Reduces transmission of infection.
18. Transport specimen to the laboratory within 15 to 30 minutes or refrigerate immediately.	• Because bacteria grow quickly in urine, urine should be sent to the laboratory within 30 minutes. Check agency policy on refrigeration if transport is delayed. (Pagana et al., 2019).

UNEXPECTED OUTCOMES	RELATED INTERVENTIONS
Urine specimen is contaminated with feces or toilet paper	• Repeat instruction to the patient or assist patient in obtaining a new specimen. • Obtain a new specimen. • Consider using an in-and-out catheterization to obtain a specimen.
Specimen is accidentally discarded	• Repeat specimen collection.

RECORDING AND REPORTING
- Record date and time urine specimen was obtained in nurses' notes.
- Notify health care provider of any significant abnormalities.

CARE IN THE COMMUNITY CONSIDERATIONS
- If the patient is required to collect specimens as an outpatient, a clean technique may be used. Provide proper instruction for collection.
- Appropriate equipment must be given to the patient and family.
- Information on storing the specimen until the time of delivery to the health care provider's office or hospital laboratory must be provided.

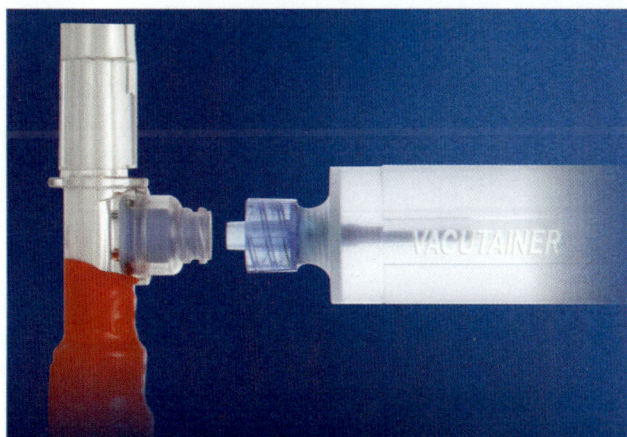

FIGURE 44.9 Urine specimen collection. Aspiration from a collection port in drainage tubing on an in-dwelling catheter (needleless technique). (Courtesy and © Becton, Dickinson and Company.)

may require that urine samples for culture and sensitivity be stored in a refrigerator until pickup.

Usually, it is approximately 24 to 48 hours before the laboratory can report findings of bacterial growth. While results are pending, a broad-spectrum antibiotic may be ordered as soon as a culture has been obtained. The test for sensitivity determines which specific antibiotics are effective. The results of a urine culture may show that another antibiotic would be more effective. In this case, a new antibiotic is ordered.

Diagnostic Examinations. The urinary system is amenable to accurate diagnostic study by several radiographic techniques. The two approaches for visualization of urinary structures (direct and indirect techniques) can be simple or complex and may necessitate extensive nursing intervention. These procedures are subdivided into invasive or noninvasive categories (Table 44.5).

Many of the nursing responsibilities related to diagnostic examinations of the urinary tract are common to more than one type of procedure. Common responsibilities before an examination include the following:

- Witnessing a signed consent (if agency policy allows)
- Administering bowel preparation medications (check agency policy)
- Ensuring that the patient receives the appropriate pretest diet (clear liquids) or nothing by mouth (NPO), as needed
  Common post-procedure interventions may include the following:
- Assessing intake and output
- Observing characteristics of urine (colour, clarity, presence of blood)

Patient Expectations. Patients depend on their caregivers to recognize and promptly meet their needs. Nurses need to use a skilled and caring approach, be creative in using a variety of assessment techniques, and serve as patient advocates. A caring nurse will meet the patient's needs in a way that is acceptable and individualized to the patient and the family situation. Patients with alterations in urinary elimination expect nurses to be respectful of privacy needs and sensitive to the impact of urinary impairments on sexuality and self-concept. The nurse and patient should develop the care plan together whenever possible and establish mutually acceptable goals. Cultural practices and personal preferences also must be considered.

◆ **Nursing Diagnosis**

A thorough assessment of the patient's urinary elimination function reveals data patterns that allow the nurse to make relevant and accurate nursing diagnoses. The diagnosis may focus on a specific alteration or an associated problem, such as impaired skin integrity related to urinary incontinence. Identification of defining characteristics leads the nurse to select an appropriate diagnosis. In addition, specifying related factors for each diagnosis enables selection of individualized nursing interventions (see Chapter 15). A sample of diagnostic reasoning is found in Box 44.3. Nursing diagnoses common to patients with alterations in urine elimination include the following:

- *Disturbed body image*
- *Pain (acute, chronic)*

TABLE 44.4   Routine Urinalysis

Measurement (Normal Value)	Interpretation
Routine Laboratory Value	
pH (4.6–8.0, average 6.0)	pH indicates acid–base balance. Urine that stands for several hours becomes alkaline. An acid pH helps protect against bacterial growth.
Protein (none or up to 8 mg/100 mL)	Protein is not normally present in urine. It is seen in renal disease because damage to glomeruli or tubules allows the protein to enter the urine.
Glucose (none)	Diabetic patients have glucose in their urine as a result of the inability of tubules to reabsorb high glucose concentrations (180 mg/100 mL). Ingestion of high concentrations of glucose may cause some glucose to appear in the urine of healthy people.
Ketones (none)	Patients whose diabetes mellitus is poorly controlled experience a breakdown of fatty acids. Ketones are end products of fat metabolism. Patients with dehydration, starvation, or excessive aspirin usage also may have ketonuria.
Blood (up to two red blood cells [RBCs])	Damage to glomeruli or tubules may allow RBCs to enter the urine. Trauma, disease, or surgery of the lower urinary tract also may cause blood to be present. In individuals with female genitalia, blood in a routine urine specimen may indicate contamination with menstrual fluid.
Specific gravity (1.010–1.025)	Specific gravity measures concentration of particles in urine. High specific gravity reflects concentrated urine, and low specific gravity reflects diluted urine. Dehydration, reduced renal blood flow, and increased antidiuretic hormone (ADH) secretion elevate specific gravity. Overhydration, early renal disease, and inadequate ADH secretion reduce specific gravity.
Microscopic Examination	
White blood cells (WBCs) (0–4 per low-power field)	Greater numbers may indicate urinary tract infection (UTI).
Bacteria (none)	Bacteria indicate UTI. (Patient may or may not have symptoms.)
Casts (none)	Casts are cylindrical bodies whose shapes take on the likeness of objects within the renal tubule. Types include hyaline, WBCs, RBCs, granular cells, and epithelial cells. Their presence is always an abnormal finding and indicates renal alterations.

Data from Pagana, K. D., Pagana, T. J., & Pike-MacDonald, S. (2019). *Mosby's Canadian manual of diagnostic and laboratory tests* (2nd ed.). Elsevier Inc.

- *Self-care deficit, toileting*
- *Impaired skin integrity*
- *Impaired urinary elimination*
- *Urinary incontinence (transient, urge, stress, mixed, functional, UI associated with chronic retention of urine [formerly overflow])*
- *Urinary retention (acute vs. chronic)*

Common symptoms that contribute to a nursing diagnosis of impaired urinary elimination, such as frequency, urgency, and nocturia, were described in Table 44.2. Each of these symptoms is associated with multiple underlying disorders. Nurses need to assimilate what has been learned from personal history-taking, physical assessment, and diagnostic tests to determine a nursing diagnosis and an appropriate care plan.

◆ Planning

During planning, nurses integrate the knowledge gained from assessment and the knowledge related to resources and available therapies to develop an individualized care plan (Box 44.4). The patient's needs should be matched with clinical and professional standards recommended in the literature (Figure 44.10). Building a relationship of trust with the patient is important because implementing the care plan involves interaction of a very personal nature.

Goals and Outcomes. The care plan for alterations in urinary elimination must include realistic and individualized goals along with relevant outcomes. The nurse and patient must collaborate in setting goals and outcomes. A general goal might be normal urinary elimination, but the individual goal may differ depending on the problem. The goals may be short term or long term. For example, for a patient with urinary retention after surgery, the short-term goal may be "Patient will have normal voiding with complete bladder emptying within 24 hours." Relevant expected outcomes for this goal may include the following:

- Patient will void within 6 hours (Gray et al., 2020).
- Urinary output of 300 mL or greater will occur with each voiding.
- Patient's bladder will not be distended on palpation.
- Patient will not continually feel an urge to void.

Conversely, the patient with stress incontinence may have a long-term goal that involves weeks of pelvic floor muscle exercises (PFMEs; also known as *Kegel exercises*) to achieve urinary control: "Patient will achieve improved urinary continence within 12 weeks after the start of pelvic floor muscle exercise program." Goals must be reasonably achievable for the patient and be relevant to the patient's situation.

Setting Priorities. Urinary elimination is a personal and intimate activity. The nurse must establish a relationship with the patient that promotes open discussion. A supportive and collaborative environment helps to make the patient's priorities apparent and fosters a mutual understanding of realistic goals.

When a patient has multiple nursing diagnoses (Figure 44.11), the nurse must recognize the primary health problem and its influence on other conditions. In the example of the patient with cognitive impairment, the resultant incontinence creates several risks. Focusing on

TABLE 44.5 Diagnostic Examinations

Name of Procedure	Purpose and Method of Procedure	Special Nursing Considerations
Noninvasive Procedures		
Abdominal roentgenogram (plain film; kidney, ureter, bladder [KUB], or flat plate)	To determine the size, shape, symmetry, and location of the kidneys; diagnose urinary calculi; preliminary X-ray imaging before IVP	No special preparation or precautions; bowel preparation is required if preliminary X-ray imaging is before IVP.
Computerized axial tomographic (CT) scan	A computerized X-ray procedure is used to obtain detailed images of structures within a selected plane of the body. The computer reconstructs a cross-sectional image and thus allows the health care provider to view pathological conditions such as tumours and obstructions.	Bowel preparation as per agency or health care provider preference. Prepare patient for the procedure (e.g., a patient will be placed into a large machine and need to lie still; feelings of claustrophobia occur in some patients).
Intravenous pyelogram (IVP)	To view the collecting ducts and renal pelvis and outline the ureters, bladder, and urethra using dye, which is excreted through the urine. A dye is injected intravenously. The patient's ability to empty the bladder is assessed through a postvoiding X-ray film.	Bowel preparation will be completed as per agency or health care provider preference. Only clear liquids are permitted until after the test is completed. After the test, fluid intake is encouraged to dilute and flush the dye from the patient. Observe for late symptoms of an allergic reaction (e.g., rash, throat tightness, difficulty breathing).
Retrograde pyelogram	Series of X-ray films provide detailed anatomical views of the ureter, ureteropelvic junction, renal pelvis, and calyces. A ureteral catheter is placed in the lower ureteral segment. Then, contrast material is injected or infused into the upper urinary tract.	Same as for IVP
Retrograde urethrogram (RUG)	To obtain oblique X-ray films of the male urethra by instilling a small volume of iodine-bound contrast material into the urethra from a retrograde direction	
Renal (kidney) scan	To determine renal blood flow, anatomical structure of the kidneys, and excretory function using a radioisotope	Usually, no bowel preparation is needed, but check agency policy. After the test, the only precaution is rinsing the bedpan or urinal after use and flushing the urine, because urine will contain a minute amount of radioisotope. Rinse fluid carefully using a double flush.
Renal ultrasonography	To identify gross renal structures and structural abnormalities in the kidney using high-frequency, inaudible sound waves	No bowel preparation is needed.
Bladder ultrasonography	To identify structural abnormalities of bladder or lower urinary tract. It is also used to estimate the volume of urine in the bladder and to measure postvoid residual volume.	Patient may be asked to drink fluids before the ultrasonography, to cause bladder distension for better results. To measure postvoid residual volume, ultrasonography should be performed within 10 minutes of voiding (Ballsteadt & Woodbury, 2022). No special care is necessary after either study.
Invasive Procedures		
Endoscopy	Use of an endoscope allows for direct visualization, specimen collection, or treatment of the interior of the kidney (nephroscopy), ureter (ureteroscopy), bladder (cystoscopy), and urethra (cystourethroscopy). This procedure is commonly performed with local anaesthesia but can be done with conscious sedation or general anaesthesia.	Signed consent is obtained. If ordered, bowel preparation is completed. Follow agency policy for preoperative preparation and checklist (see Chapter 49). After the patient's return, assess vital signs and the characteristics of urine, monitor intake and output, encourage ingestion of fluids, and observe for fever, dysuria, and pain in the suprapubic region.

Continued

TABLE 44.5	Diagnostic Examinations—cont'd	
Name of Procedure	**Purpose and Method of Procedure**	**Special Nursing Considerations**
Arteriogram (angiography)	Used primarily to visualize the renal arteries or their branches to detect narrowing or occlusion. A catheter is placed in one of the femoral arteries and introduced up to the level of the renal arteries. Radiopaque contrast is injected through the catheter while X-ray images are taken in rapid succession.	Signed consent is required. Follow agency preprocedure checklist. After the procedure, monitor vital signs frequently until the patient is stable; bed rest is maintained for a prescribed time interval; fluids are encouraged to flush the contrast from the system. Monitor the affected extremity for neurocirculatory function (pulse, skin temperature, sensation, and movement), and observe catheter site for bleeding, swelling, increased tenderness, or hematoma formation. The health care provider must be notified immediately of any post-procedure abnormality.
Uroflowmetry and urodynamic testing	Uroflowmetry measures the rate of urine expelled and is noninvasive. The patient voids into a urine flowmeter. Complete urodynamics determines bladder and sphincter function in the case of urinary obstruction or urinary incontinence. A catheter is inserted, the urine is drained, and sterile water or contrast liquid is used to fill the bladder. Pressure readings are taken and compared with the patient's reported sensations.	Explain need for the patient to report all sensations during the test. After the test, assess the patient for sensations of sweating, pain, nausea, bladder fullness, or a strong urge to void.

Data from Pagana, K. D., Pagana, T. J., & Pike-MacDonald, S. (2019). *Mosby's Canadian manual of diagnostic and laboratory tests* (2nd ed.). Elsevier Inc.

BOX 44.3   NURSING DIAGNOSTIC PROCESS

Assessment Activities	Defining Characteristics	Nursing Diagnosis
Assess the timing and precipitating factors of urinary leakage.	Patient states that they have "loss of urine" whenever they sneeze, cough, or laugh. Patient states that they have been having leakage problems for several years.	*Stress urinary incontinence related to decreased pelvic muscle tone and urethral sphincter trauma, as evidenced by urine leakage associated with increased intra-abdominal pressure, use of containment products, and previous vaginal deliveries*
Observe patient behaviour and management and coping strategies.	Patient is wearing a mini menstrual pad continuously. Patient is reluctant to interact with others and tries not to cough or laugh. They may squeeze or cross their legs when coughing or laughing.	
Review medical history.	Patient is menopausal and has had three vaginal births. Review birth weights of their children.	

management of incontinence will often help to resolve more than one nursing diagnosis. Although physical care needs may appear to have higher priority, psychological needs related to self-esteem or sexuality may be of higher priority to the patient. Attention to the patient's perceived needs may be the most satisfactory and successful approach to accomplishing all of the goals. Reinforcement and praise of good health habits can improve adherence to the care plan.

Continuity of Care. The care plan incorporates health-promotion activities and therapeutic interventions for patients. Preventive interventions may be required for patients at risk for urinary conditions. It is important to consider the patient's home environment and normal elimination routines when planning therapies. Consultation with other health care providers and with the patient's family is often necessary. For example, the physiotherapist can design an exercise plan to increase strength and endurance so that the patient can ambulate to the bathroom safely. The need for home care services should be explored and appropriate referrals made. The family may need to alter the home environment to make it easier and safer for the patient to use the bathroom. A referral to an NSWOC or a nurse continence advisor would be appropriate.

◆ Implementation

Implementation is the action phase of the nursing process. Nurses carry out the independent and collaborative activities needed to assist the patient in achieving the desired outcomes and goals. Independent activities are those determined by nurses using their own judgment, such as teaching self-care activities to the patient. Collaborative activities are those ordered by the prescriber that nurses carry out, such as medication administration.

Health Promotion. The focus of health promotion is to assist the patient in understanding and participating in self-care practices that will preserve and protect healthy urinary system function. In a recent Canadian study, less than half of those people with urinary symptoms sought health care for these symptoms (Shaw et al., 2020). Over one

◎ BOX 44.4 NURSING CARE PLAN
Mixed Urinary Incontinence

ASSESSMENT

Kay, a home care nurse, is seeing Emily, a 75-year-old widow (preferred pronouns: she/her) at home. Emily was referred by her physician because of arthritis and early dementia. She has had three urinary tract infections in the past year. She lives alone, but her daughter lives less than a 10-minute drive away. Kay's assessment includes a discussion of Emily's current health problems.

Assessment Activities	*Findings and Defining Characteristics*
Ask Emily about how she is coping with her arthritis.	She responds, "It slows me down. The pain medication is helping, but it takes me longer to get out of my chair and get anywhere." Emily begins to cry and states, "You can see the plastic cover on my chair. I'm so embarrassed; sometimes, I can't get out of the chair fast enough, and I lose my water. I've been wearing those diapers lately."
Ask Emily to describe how long she has had trouble controlling her urine and whether she has ever sought help.	Emily says that she has had trouble with dribbling for more than 10 years, but she didn't think anything could be done because of her age. But, over the past few years, it has gotten worse. With little warning, she has to rush to the bathroom and is often wet on the way. She also leaks when she coughs.
Ask Emily about any changes, such as new medication, that may have contributed to her worsening symptoms.	Emily says that she has not started any new medications.
Ask Emily to complete a bladder diary for 3 days when she is likely to be at home most of the time, and provide a receptacle so that she can measure several of her voids. Establish a diary format she understands and can work with.	Emily completes the diary for only 2 days because she finds it difficult to write everything down and often forgets to do this task.
Assess bladder diary findings and usual bowel patterns. Discuss patterns with Emily, so she becomes aware of her usual bladder and bowel routines and is able to participate in her care planning.	The diary findings discussed are as follows: 1. Largest volume void is 200 mL and longest interval between voids is 1.25 hours. Voiding two times in the night 2. Two episodes of incontinence occur on the way to the bathroom. Emily records that she gets a sudden urge to void but is "very wet" on the way to the bathroom. 3. Emily also records that she can feel her urine dribbling while coughing. 4. Fluid intake is low, averaging 800 mL per 24 hours. 5. Patient usually has two to three bowel movements per week.

NURSING DIAGNOSIS: *Mixed urinary incontinence.* The patient has symptoms of urge incontinence: frequency associated with severe urgency and nocturia. She also describes episodes of stress incontinence. Her impaired mobility makes it more difficult to get to the bathroom in time. The patient may also be at risk for a urinary tract infection (UTI) due to reduced fluid intake.

PLANNING

*Goals (Nursing Outcomes Classification)**	*Expected Outcomes*
Patient will review bladder diary and think about aspects of their elimination pattern that may be amenable to change.	Enhanced understanding of bladder function
Patient will report reduced episodes of incontinence within 1 month and longer intervals between voids.	Reduced episodes of urinary incontinence
Patient will increase fluid intake to help ensure adequate hydration and prevent urinary tract infection.	Adequate hydration

*Outcome classification labels from Moorhead, S., Swanson, E., Johnson, M., et al. (Eds.). (2018). Nursing outcomes classification (NOC) (6th ed.). Mosby.

INTERVENTIONS

Interventions (Nursing Interventions Classification)	*Rationale*
Urinary Incontinence Care	
Discuss "normal" bladder habits with the patient and their actual patterns of intake and output, based on the bladder diary.	The success of conservative therapies for urinary incontinence (UI), such as pelvic floor muscle exercises (PFMEs), requires motivation and ongoing commitment and self-care. The patient must be an active part of assessment and care planning. Provide written reminders for individuals who have memory issues. Prompted voiding, either alone or as part of a behavioural modification program, improves continence in older, care-dependent people (Burkhard et al., 2020).

Continued

◎ BOX 44.4   NURSING CARE PLAN—cont'd

Interventions (Nursing Interventions Classification)

Refer to a continence specialist to assess pelvic floor strength, to establish baseline, and to teach patient appropriate muscles to tighten. Instruct patient to practice PFMEs at least twice a day. The continence specialist will also assess for urogenital atrophy. Examples of nursing continence specialists in Canada include nurse continence advisors (NCAs) and nurses specialized in wound, ostomy and continence (NSWOC). There are also physiotherapists who specialize in rehabilitation of the pelvic floor muscles in individuals with male genitalia and those with female genitalia.

Work with patient to establish a manageable bladder training program, asking the patient to void at regular, prespecified intervals throughout the day based on maximum intervals in bladder diary (1.25 hours). Gradually increase the interval by 15 to 30 minutes per week as tolerated until an acceptable pattern is achieved. Patient will need prompting and support from caregivers to undertake this.

Discuss safety issues related to the patient's nocturia and the possibility of acquiring a bedside commode.

Encourage the patient to increase noncaffeinated fluid intake gradually to approximately 1 500 mL during the day, with fluid intake restricted after suppertime.

Rationale

Cognitively intact and motivated older persons can learn PFMEs when able to identify the correct musculature. There is evidence that PFMEs are effective for cure or improvement of incontinence and improvement in quality of life. The effect applies in individuals with female genitalia with stress UI, urge UI, and mixed UI, though the effect in mixed UIs is lower than in individuals with female genitalia with pure stress UI (Burkhard et al., 2020).

Persons with early dementia may be helped with written instructions and reminders from caregivers.

Urogenital atrophy is a contributor to UTI in older individuals with female genitalia that can be treated with low-dose vaginal estrogen.

Bladder training reduces frequency and urgency in individuals with female genitalia with overactive bladder syndrome but may be more successful when pelvic floor muscle strength has improved.

Older persons who get up at night to urinate are more likely to experience a fall. Because older persons are also at increased risk for bone fractures, it is important to identify persons with nocturia and to ensure that appropriate safety precautions are taken.

Adequate hydration will help prevent UTI and maintain dilute urine. Avoiding fluids before bedtime may reduce nocturia.

EVALUATION

Nursing Action	Patient Response and Finding	Achievement of Outcome
Ask patient to complete a bladder diary at regular intervals (monthly or every 2 months) to compare to the baseline diary. Provide written instructions.	Three months after initiating conservative treatment, patient responds, "I'm dry most of the time now."	Emily has reduced her episodes of incontinence and increased the interval between voids. She is now voiding every 3 hours on average and is up one or two times at night. She reports that she feels better because she is getting more sleep.

third felt UI was normal, and over 90% believed old age to be a possible cause. Targeted health promotion and education can improve how people perceive bladder problems and help-seeking. Nurses must maintain an open, caring attitude and provide bladder health education to those seeking information. There is evidence that continence education can improve continence status. An international randomized trial demonstrated a sustainable improvement in incontinence symptoms among untreated older individuals with female genitalia exposed to a group continence promotion workshop compared to those exposed to a healthy aging workshop (Tannenbalm et al., 2019).

Patient Education. The success of therapies aimed at solving or minimizing urinary elimination problems depends in part on successful patient education. Although many patients may need to learn about all aspects of urinary elimination, the nurse should first focus the teaching on the patient's specific elimination problems. For example, patients who practise poor hygiene benefit most from learning about the normal sterility of the urinary tract and ways to prevent infection. Patients also learn the significance of symptoms of urinary alterations so that early preventive health care can be initiated.

Nurses can easily incorporate teaching while providing nursing care. For example, when attempting to increase a patient's fluid intake, a good time to discuss the benefits of this action is while giving fluids with medications or meals. Teaching about perineal hygiene may be appropriate while giving a bath or performing catheter care.

Promoting Regular Micturition. Maintaining regular patterns of urinary elimination can help prevent many urination difficulties. Patients with urinary incontinence commonly void frequently throughout the day to avoid accidental urine loss. However, frequent voiding (e.g., at hourly intervals) may contribute to creating a small-capacity bladder. Conversely, patients who hold their urine for long periods (more than 8 hours) may develop a hypotonic bladder with incomplete emptying. Nurses should reinforce the importance of voiding regularly (approximately every 3 to 4 hours) to help maintain a normal bladder capacity (400 to 500 mL). Because constipated stool in the rectum may compress the urethra and impede emptying, nurses should emphasize the importance of regular bowel movements and encourage measures to enhance regularity, including diets rich in fibre (see Chapter 45).

Many nursing measures have been designed to promote normal voiding in patients at risk for urination difficulties and with established urination problems. Nurses can initiate many of these measures independently.

Stimulating micturition reflex. The patient's ability to void depends on feeling the urge to urinate, controlling the urethral sphincter, and relaxing during voiding. Nurses can help a patient learn to relax and stimulate the micturition reflex by enabling the patient to assume the normal position for voiding. A person with female genitalia is better able to void in a squatting or sitting position. If the patient is unable to use toilet facilities, the nurse can help the patient into a sitting position

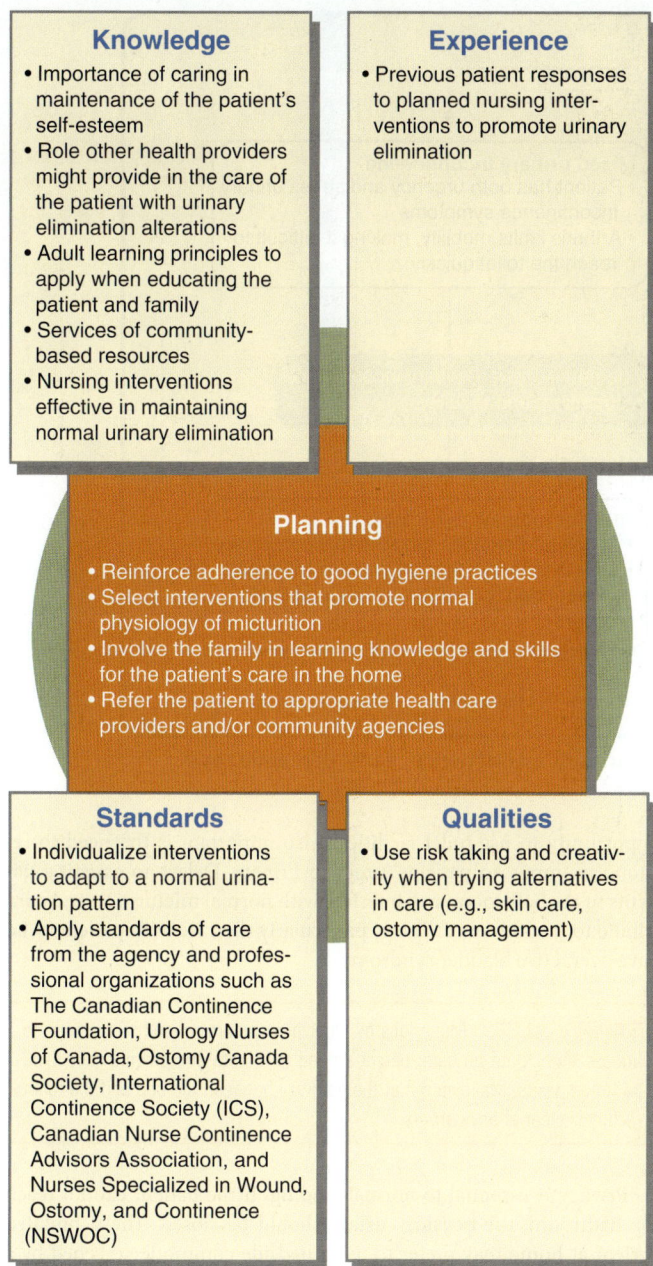

Knowledge
- Importance of caring in maintenance of the patient's self-esteem
- Role other health providers might provide in the care of the patient with urinary elimination alterations
- Adult learning principles to apply when educating the patient and family
- Services of community-based resources
- Nursing interventions effective in maintaining normal urinary elimination

Experience
- Previous patient responses to planned nursing interventions to promote urinary elimination

Planning
- Reinforce adherence to good hygiene practices
- Select interventions that promote normal physiology of micturition
- Involve the family in learning knowledge and skills for the patient's care in the home
- Refer the patient to appropriate health care providers and/or community agencies

Standards
- Individualize interventions to adapt to a normal urination pattern
- Apply standards of care from the agency and professional organizations such as The Canadian Continence Foundation, Urology Nurses of Canada, Ostomy Canada Society, International Continence Society (ICS), Canadian Nurse Continence Advisors Association, and Nurses Specialized in Wound, Ostomy, and Continence (NSWOC)

Qualities
- Use risk taking and creativity when trying alternatives in care (e.g., skin care, ostomy management)

FIGURE 44.10 Critical thinking model for urinary elimination planning.

on a bedpan or bedside commode. A smaller slipper bed pan may be easier for the patient to use. A person with male genitalia voids more easily in a standing position. If the patient cannot reach toilet facilities, they may stand at the bedside and void into a urinal (a metal or plastic receptacle for urine). A urinal for patients with female genitalia, with an elongated spout, may be helpful to patients with limited mobility (Figure 44.12).

Providing certain sensory stimuli also may promote relaxation and voiding. The sound of running water helps many patients void. Stroking the inner thigh may stimulate sensory nerves and promote the micturition reflex. The nurse can also pour warm water over the patient's perineum to create the urge to urinate. If urine output is being measured, the nurse must first measure the volume of water that will be poured over the perineal area.

Maintaining elimination habits. Many patients follow routines to promote normal voiding. In a hospital or long-term care facility, nursing routines may conflict with those of patients. When a patient is admitted to hospital or another care setting, the nurse should obtain information on usual voiding patterns when taking the nursing history. Integrating patients' habits into the care plan fosters normal voiding and will assist in preventing problems related to urination.

Maintaining adequate fluid intake. Patients with urinary incontinence often reduce fluid intake because they believe that this will help keep them dry. In reality, maintaining an adequate fluid intake of 1 500 to 2 000 mL promotes continence because concentrated urine can irritate the bladder mucosa. Fluid intake should not include caffeinated beverages, which have a diuretic effect. The patient should be reminded that many vegetables and fruits have a high fluid content and can contribute to daily fluid intake. At the patient's home, it may be helpful to establish a schedule for drinking fluids (e.g., with meals or medications). Fluids should be minimized after supper to minimize nocturia.

The nurse can teach the patient to avoid use of foods, substances, and fluids that may cause worsening of lower urinary tract symptoms:
- Tobacco (smoker's cough aggravates stress urinary incontinence)
- Alcohol (acts as a diuretic)
- Substances containing caffeine, such as coffee, tea, and chocolate (may worsen urgency and urgency incontinence, increases frequency)
- Carbonated beverages
- Artificial sweeteners (e.g., Aspartame)

Promoting Complete Bladder Emptying. Under normal circumstances, a small amount of urine (50 mL) remains in the bladder after voiding (residual urine) because the urinary sphincters close. Thus, people normally remain continent and dry. People with residual urine are able to remain dry when their urethral closure pressure is sufficient to prevent leakage. However, urinary incontinence may occur when too much residual urine is in the bladder or when the urinary sphincters are too weak to maintain closure pressure. As well as contributing to incontinence, residual urine can be a medium for bacterial growth.

Patients should be encouraged to take their time while voiding and try again when they feel they have not emptied their bladders fully (double voiding). Those with consistently elevated PVRs (>100 mL) may require intermittent catheterization. Portable bladder scanners offer a noninvasive means of assessing PVRs. Box 44.5 describes the procedure for using a bladder scanner.

Preventing Infection. One of the most important considerations for a patient with alterations in urinary elimination is the need to prevent infection of the urinary system. Good perineal hygiene that includes cleaning the urethral meatus after each voiding or bowel movement is essential. Patients with limited dexterity due to conditions such as arthritis or stroke can benefit from the use of a squirt bottle filled with warm water to rinse the perineum after defecation. Hand hygiene remains one of the most effective aspects of preventing infection.

Patients should be encouraged to drink sufficient fluids to maintain a urine output of at least 1 200 mL per day. Patients need to consume sufficient fluid based on their weight (25–35 mL/kg/day); for example, if an individual weighs 60 kg, they should be drinking 2 100 mL/day. Drinking adequate fluid helps to dilute the urine and create a downward drainage effect (NSWOC, CNCA, UNC, IPAC, 2020). Urine is normally acidic and tends to inhibit the growth of microorganisms.

Catheters and Incontinence Products. Many measures can be used in health care settings to decrease the incidence of urinary alterations. The use of a urinary catheter requires a prescriber order and should only be implemented when the criteria for insertion of an in-dwelling urinary catheter (see Box 44.1) have been met. Incontinence alone is

> concept map

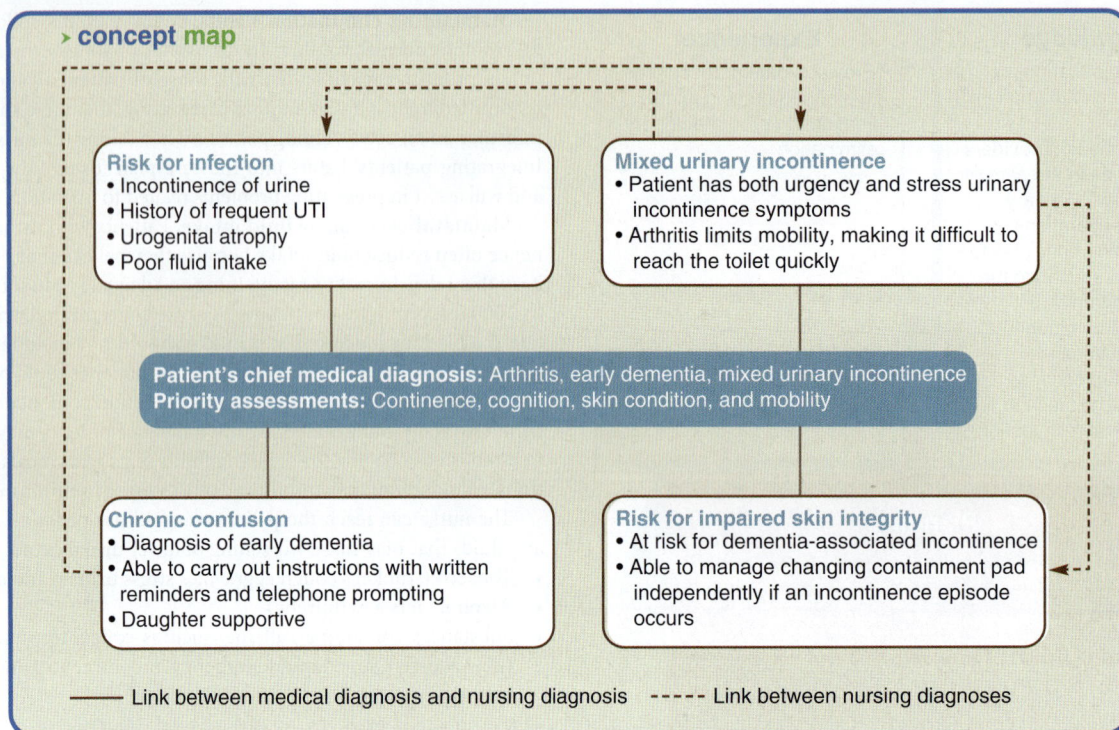

Risk for infection
- Incontinence of urine
- History of frequent UTI
- Urogenital atrophy
- Poor fluid intake

Mixed urinary incontinence
- Patient has both urgency and stress urinary incontinence symptoms
- Arthritis limits mobility, making it difficult to reach the toilet quickly

Patient's chief medical diagnosis: Arthritis, early dementia, mixed urinary incontinence
Priority assessments: Continence, cognition, skin condition, and mobility

Chronic confusion
- Diagnosis of early dementia
- Able to carry out instructions with written reminders and telephone prompting
- Daughter supportive

Risk for impaired skin integrity
- At risk for dementia-associated incontinence
- Able to manage changing containment pad independently if an incontinence episode occurs

——— Link between medical diagnosis and nursing diagnosis   - - - - Link between nursing diagnoses

FIGURE 44.11 Concept map for patient with mixed urinary incontinence, early dementia, and recurrent urinary tract infection (UTI).

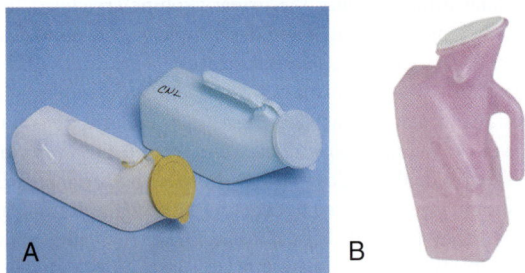

FIGURE 44.12 Types of urinals for patients with (**A**) male and (**B**) female genitalia. (**B,** Courtesy Briggs Medical Service Co.)

not a reason to insert a urinary catheter. Patients experiencing incontinence should be managed with an individualized combination of incontinence containment products and conservative and pharmacological interventions prior to any consideration of catheterization.

Special Considerations in Acute Care. Conservative interventions listed in Table 44.1 are discussed in detail in the next section. Many are appropriate to implement in acute care. Toileting strategies should be implemented, and continence aids such as urinals should be used first to avoid unnecessary use of incontinence containment products (pads or briefs) or in-dwelling urinary catheters. In-dwelling catheters should only be inserted when absolutely indicated. In acute care, continued use of an in-dwelling catheter should be reassessed daily (Leis & Soong, 2017). Nurses have a key role to play in reassessment and reminders to remove catheters that are no longer needed.

Maintaining Elimination Habits. Patients usually require time to void. Requesting a urine specimen on demand does not contribute to relaxation and normal voiding habits. Patients should be given at least 30 minutes to provide a specimen. Patients normally void upon awakening or before meals; therefore, the nurse should offer them the

opportunity to use toilet facilities. Also important is the need to respond promptly to patients' urges to urinate. Delays in assisting patients to the bathroom may interfere with normal micturition and contribute to incontinence. This is particularly the case with patients who have overactive bladder syndrome.

> **SAFETY ALERT** Many falls by older persons are related to the urge to urinate. Anticipate an older person's need to urinate and provide scheduled bathroom visits. Make sure that the pathway between the bed and the toilet facility is clear of any barriers.

Privacy is essential to normal voiding. If the patient cannot reach the bathroom, the bedside curtain should be closed. The debilitated patient at home may prefer to use a bedside commode screened by a partition or room divider. Young children are often unable to void in the presence of people other than their parents.

When possible, nurses should encourage the continued use of special measures that a patient uses to void. The patient may be able to relax and void more easily while reading or listening to music. Having a cup or glass of fluids also may promote urination.

Catheterization. Catheterization of the bladder involves introducing a narrow tube through the urethra and into the bladder to allow a continuous flow of urine into a drainage receptacle. Indications for in-dwelling urethral catheterization, which is to be avoided if possible, were provided earlier in the chapter, in Box 44.1, along with a discussion about CAUTI prevention. Intermittent catheterization is used to empty the bladder in people who are unable to empty their bladder completely. Intermittent catheterization can be used to collect a sterile urine specimen, but only in patients who are unable to provide a midstream specimen. Bladder catheterization carries the risk of CAUTI, blockage, and trauma to the urethra, so it is preferable to rely on other measures for either specimen collection or the management of incontinence (Newman et al., 2021a, 2021b).

BOX 44.5 PROCEDURAL GUIDELINE

Using a Bladder Scanner to Measure Postvoid Residual

Delegation Considerations:

In some provinces, the skill of measuring bladder volume by a portable ultrasound bladder scanner can be delegated to an unregulated care provider (UCP). Nurses must be aware of the legislation in their practice jurisdiction. However, it is important to establish competency in bladder scan measurements because reliability between different care provider readings can be poor. The regulated nurse must first determine the timing and frequency of the bladder scan measurement and interpret the measurements obtained. The nurse is also responsible for assessing the patient's ability to toilet before measurement of postvoid residual (PVR) and assessing the abdomen for distension if urinary retention is suspected. When using a device:

- Follow manufacturer recommendations for use of the device.
- Measure PVR volumes within 10 minutes after the patient voids.
- Report and record bladder scanner volumes.

Equipment:

- Bladder scanner
- Ultrasound gel
- Cleaning agent for scanner head, such as an alcohol pad
- Clean gloves (optional)

Steps:

1. Identify the patient using two identifiers (e.g., name and birthday or name and medical record number) according to agency policy.
2. Perform hand hygiene. Discuss the procedure with the patient. If the measurement is for PVR, ask the patient to void, and measure and record voided urine volume. (Apply gloves if the patient requires assistance with voiding). The scan measurement should be within 10 minutes of voiding.
3. Help patient to the supine position with their head slightly elevated. Raise bed to appropriate working height. If side rails are raised, lower side rail on working side.
4. Expose the patient's lower abdomen.
5. Turn on the scanner per manufacturer guidelines.
6. Set the gender designation per manufacturer guidelines. People without a uterus should be designated as "male" for use of the bladder scanner.
7. Wipe the scanner head with an alcohol pad or other cleanser and allowed to air-dry.
8. Palpate the patient's symphysis pubis (pubic bone). Apply a generous amount of ultrasound gel (or, if available, a bladder scan gel pad) to the midline abdomen 2.5 to 4 cm (1 to 1.5 inches) above the symphysis pubis. The ultrasound gel ensures adequate transmission and thus accurate measurement.
9. Place the scanner head on the gel, ensuring that the scanner head is oriented per manufacturer guidelines (see Step 9 illustration).

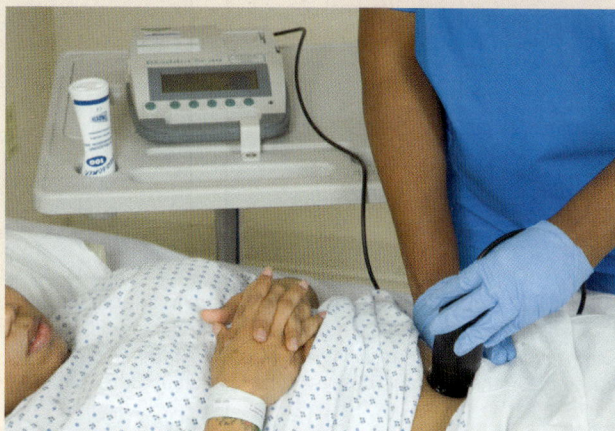

STEP 9 Point scanner head slightly downward toward the bladder.

10. Apply light pressure, keep the scanner head steady, and point it slightly downward toward the bladder. Press and release the scan button.
11. Verify accurate aim (refer to manufacturer guidelines). Complete the scan and print the image (if needed) (see Step 11 illustration).

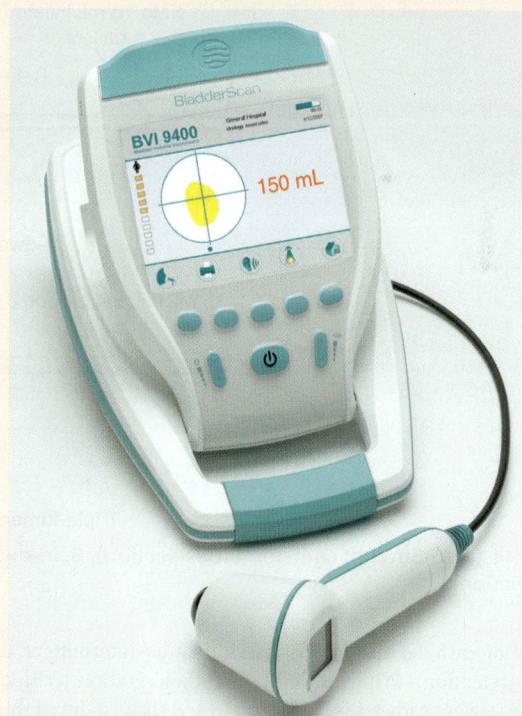

STEP 11 Bladder scan image (*Courtesy Verathon, Inc.*)

12. Remove ultrasound gel from the patient's abdomen with a paper towel.
13. Remove ultrasound gel from scanner head and wipe with an alcohol pad or other cleanser; let air dry.
14. Help the patient to a comfortable position. Lower bed and place side rails accordingly.
15. Dispose of soiled towels and pads. Perform hand hygiene.

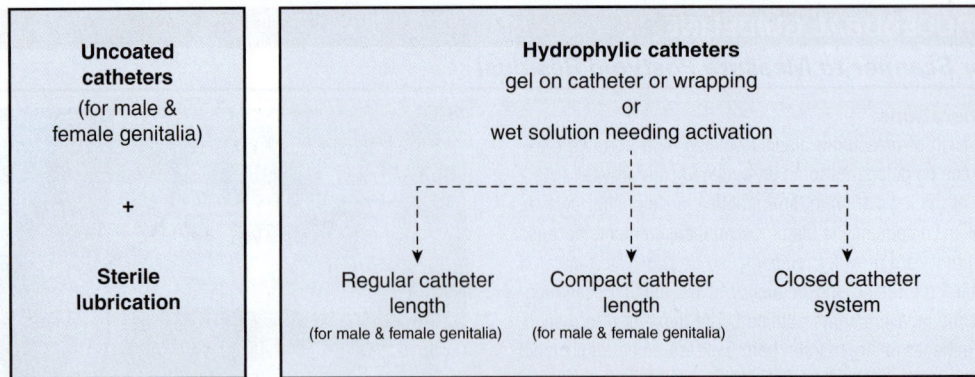

FIGURE 44.13 Types of intermittent catheters available in Canada. (Adapted from Nurses Specialized in Wound, Ostomy and Continence Canada, Canadian Nurse Continence Advisors, Urology Nurses of Canada, and Infection Prevention and Control Canada. [2020]. *Clean intermittent urethral catheterization in adults: Canadian best practice recommendations for nurses* [p. 23, Figure 2]. http://nswoc.ca/wp-content/uploads/2020/05/Clean-Intermittent-Urethral-Catheterization-Adults-for-Nurses-BPR-May2020-lr-1.pdf)

FIGURE 44.14 A, Straight catheter (cross-section), **B,** In-dwelling (Foley) retention catheter (cross-section). **C,** Triple-lumen catheter (cross-section).

Types of catheterization. Catheters may be intermittent or indwelling (retention). With **intermittent catheterization** technique, a single-use straight catheter (see Figure 44.14, *A*) is introduced through the urethra just long enough to drain the bladder. The straight catheter has a single lumen with a small opening about 1.3 cm from the tip. Urine drains from the tip, through the lumen, and into a receptacle. Intermittent catheterization is performed by the patient or by a nurse. It is common in patients who have incomplete bladder emptying due to neurogenic conditions (e.g., spinal cord injury).

Intermittent catheters come as either uncoated or hydrophilic (Figure 44.13). Uncoated catheters require the use of sterile lubrication, while hydrophilic catheters are coated with gel on the catheter or wrapping, or they may have a wet solution needing activation. Hydrophilic catheters come in many options, including different sizes and lengths available in both regular and compact for both the patient with male or

the patient with female genitalia. Closed systems include the catheter, prelubrication, and a collection bag.

In the hospital, intermittent catheterization is sterile, to reduce the risk of health care–associated infections. In the community, some patients are known to reuse their catheters after cleansing; this reuse is no longer recommended, as all intermittent catheters available in Canada are manufactured for single use only (NSWOCC, CNCA, UNC & IPAC, 2020).

The *coude catheter* is a type of catheter that has a curved tip and is used for patients with male genitalia who have an enlarged prostate that partly obstructs the urethra. It is less traumatic during insertion because it is stiffer and easier to control than the straight-tip catheter. However, the use of this type of catheter requires additional consideration. The nurse needs to read the manufacturers' instructions as there is a small notch on the funnel, which should be facing upward for insertion. The nurse should check with the prescriber for any additional special considerations.

An in-dwelling (or Foley) catheterization (Figure 44.14, *B*) is performed by inserting a catheter through the urethra, and the catheter is retained for longer periods in the bladder by means of a small balloon that anchors it against the bladder neck. In acute care, the catheter remains in place until daily review of its need indicates it should be removed. Some acute care settings have catheter-removal prompt systems to remind the nurse to assess if the catheter is still needed and to get a prescriber's order to remove it if no longer appropriate. Patients with long-term catheters need to have an individualized routine for changing, established on the basis of agency policy and pattern of blockage. A blocked catheter should be changed as soon as possible. In-dwelling catheters have either two lumens (the most common type; one lumen drains urine and the other carries sterile water to inflate or deflate the balloon) or three lumens (the third lumen allows for irrigation). The triple-lumen catheter (see Figure 44.14, *C*) is used for continuous bladder irrigation. They can be used on a short- or long-term basis.

Catheters are manufactured in many different materials (latex, silicone, Teflon) and come in many different diameters. Guidelines on how to make appropriate decisions regarding catheter selection are provided in Box 44.6.

Catheter insertion. For urethral catheterization of any type, a prescriber's order is required. The nurse must use strict aseptic technique (see Chapter 34). Organizing equipment before beginning the procedure prevents interruptions. The steps for inserting in-dwelling and single-use straight catheters are nearly the same. The difference lies in the procedure taken to inflate the in-dwelling catheter balloon and secure the catheter. Skill 44.2 lists the steps for inserting in-dwelling and single-use straight catheters in individuals with male genitalia and those with female genitalia.

Closed drainage systems. After inserting an in-dwelling catheter, the nurse needs to maintain a closed urinary drainage system to minimize the risk of infection. Urinary drainage bags are plastic and can hold about 1 000 to 1 500 mL of urine. The drainage bag should never be raised above the level of the patient's bladder. The bag should hang on the bed frame or wheelchair without touching the floor. Urine in the bag and tubing can become a medium for bacteria, and infection is likely to develop if urine flows back into the bladder. Therefore, the bag should not be hung on the bed's side rails because it can be raised above the level of the bladder accidentally. When the patient ambulates, the drainage bag must be held below the patient's waist.

If the catheter must be disconnected from the drainage tubing, both tips should be cleaned with an alcohol swab before being reconnected to minimize the transfer of microorganisms into the tubing.

Most drainage bags contain an anti-reflux valve to prevent urine in the bag from re-entering the drainage tubing and contaminating the patient's bladder. A spigot at the base of the bag is used to empty the bag. The spigot should always be clamped, except during emptying, and tucked into the protective pouch on the side of the bag (see agency policy). To ensure that the drainage system remains unobstructed, the nurse should check for kinks or bends in the tubing, avoid positioning the patient on the drainage tubing, and observe for clots or sediment that may occlude the collecting tubing.

Routine catheter care. Patients with in-dwelling catheters have a number of special care needs. Nursing measures are directed at maintaining patient comfort, preventing infection, and maintaining an unobstructed flow of urine.

Perineal hygiene. A buildup of secretions or encrustation at the catheter insertion site is a source of irritation and potential infection. Nurses should provide perineal hygiene (see Chapter 39) at least twice

---

BOX 44.6 Guidelines for Appropriate Catheter Size Selection: Intermittent and In-dwelling

- The catheter size should be determined according to the size of the patient's urethral canal. When the French system is used, the larger the gauge number, the larger the catheter size. In general, an 8- to 10-Fr gauge is required for children, 10 to 12 Fr for adult patients with female genitalia, and 12 to 16 Fr for adult patients with male genitalia (Cottenden et al., 2013). Choose a catheter size large enough to allow free drainage yet small enough to reduce the risk of trauma (NSWOCC, CNCA, UNC & IPAC, 2020).
- After urological procedures (prostatectomy), a 20- to 24-Fr three-lumen in-dwelling catheter may be used to allow clot drainage and irrigation.
- The expected time required for in-dwelling catheterization will determine the catheter material selection (Teflon- or silicone-coated latex, 100% silicone, hydrophilic-coated latex).
- Plastic catheters are suitable only for intermittent catheterization because of their inflexibility. Some intermittent catheters are hydrophilic (add water to make lubricious) or prelubricated to decrease friction and discomfort on insertion.
- Latex in-dwelling catheters come with or without a coating (silicone, Teflon, or silver). Be aware of patient allergies to any of these materials. Latex catheters may become encrusted more quickly than other materials (WOCN, 2016).
- Urinary catheters come in varying sizes, configurations, and construction materials. Therefore, the choice of catheter depends on the circumstances for use (Newman, 2022). Balloon size is also important to consider when selecting an in-dwelling catheter. Balloon sizes range from 3 mL (pediatric) to large postoperative volumes (30 mL). In adults, the 10-mL size allows for optimal drainage, whereas the 30-mL size is used to control postoperative hematuria (Newman, 2022).
- Only sterile water should be used to inflate the balloon in in-dwelling catheters because saline may crystallize in the balloon port, clogging it and preventing balloon deflation and catheter removal (Newman, 2022).
- Urine leakage around the in-dwelling catheter may be due to bladder spasms secondary to constipation or fecal impaction, the use of a large catheter balloon (30 mL) or a large catheter (>18 Fr) that causes irritation, the presence of a urinary tract infection, kinking of the catheter, or trauma at the bladder neck from traction on the balloon. A decrease in lumen size, the use of anticholinergic medication, or a referral to a urologist may be warranted.

---

daily, after a bowel movement, or as needed for a patient with an in-dwelling catheter. Soap and water or skin cleansers are effective in reducing the number of microorganisms around the urethra and help to maintain skin health and patient comfort. The nurse should take care not to accidentally advance the catheter upward into the bladder during cleaning as this action risks introducing bacteria into the bladder.

Catheter care. In addition to routine perineal hygiene, many institutions recommend that patients with catheters receive special care three times a day and after defecation or bowel incontinence to help minimize discomfort and infection (Skill 44.3).

Fluid intake. All patients with catheters should have a daily fluid intake of at least 2 000 to 2 500 mL. Encouraging self-management in patients with a long-term catheter can improve their fluid intake, which can be met through oral intake or intravenous infusion. A high fluid intake produces a large volume of urine that flushes the bladder and keeps the catheter tubing free of sediment.

Preventing infection. The most important strategy in preventing the onset of infection is performing hand hygiene between patients. Maintaining a closed urinary drainage system is also important

SKILL 44.2   INSERTING AND REMOVING A STRAIGHT (INTERMITTENT) OR IN-DWELLING CATHETER

Delegation Considerations

Catheterization is usually not delegated to unregulated care providers (UCPs). However, in some settings, agency policy may permit this skill to be delegated to UCPs who have been properly instructed. UCPs routinely assist with positioning the patient and maintaining patient privacy and comfort, empty urine from the collection bag, and provide perineal care. If a UCP is performing the skill, instruct them to inform a nurse of the following:

- Patient discomfort or fever
- Abnormal colour, odour, or amount of urine in drainage bag

Equipment

Catheterization kit containing the following sterile items:

- Gloves (extra pair optional)
- Drapes, one fenestrated
- Lubricant
- Antiseptic cleaning solution
- Cotton balls
- Forceps
- Prefilled syringe with sterile water to inflate the balloon of an in-dwelling catheter
- Catheter of correct size and type for procedure (i.e., intermittent or in-dwelling)
- Sterile drainage tubing with collection bag and multipurpose tube holder or tape, safety pin, and elastic band for securing tubing to bed if the patient is bed-bound (for an in-dwelling catheter)
- Receptacle or basin (usually bottom of catheterization tray)
- Specimen container
- Blanket

PROCEDURE

STEPS	RATIONALE
1. Review patient's medical record, including prescriber's order and nurses' notes.	• Determines purpose of inserting catheter: preparation for surgery, urinary irrigations, collection of sterile specimens, measurement of residual urine, and size and style of catheter. Assess for allergies and any pertinent past medical and urological history (e.g., urethral stricture, benign prostatic hyperplasia, pelvic organ prolapse, prior bladder, prostate, urethral or pelvic surgery). If the patient with male genitalia has an artificial urinary sphincter, contact urology (Newman et al., 2021a).
2. Close bedside curtain or door.	• Offers privacy, reduces embarrassment, and aids in relaxation during the procedure.
3. Assess the status of the patient:	
A. Ask patient when they last voided, or check intake and output flow sheet, or palpate bladder.	• Determines time of last voiding or potential for bladder fullness.
B. Level of awareness or developmental stage	• Reveals the patient's ability to cooperate and the level of explanation needed.
C. Mobility and physical limitations of patient	• Affects the way that the patient can be positioned.
D. Patient's anatomy and age	• Determines catheter size: 8 to 10 Fr is generally used for children, 10 to 12 for adult patients with female genitalia, 12 to 16 for adult patients with male genitalia.
E. Distended bladder	• Causes pain. Can indicate need to insert catheter if patient is unable to void independently.
F. Perform hand hygiene. Apply clean gloves. Inspect perineum for erythema, drainage, and odour.	• Reduces infection. Determines condition of the perineum.
G. Note any pathological condition that may impair passage of catheter (e.g., enlarged prostate in individuals with male genitalia, pelvic organ prolapse in individuals with female genitalia).	• Obstruction prevents the passage of the catheter through the urethra into the bladder. Use of coude catheter may be required for those with an enlarged prostate.
H. Allergies	• Procedure risks exposure to antiseptic, tape, latex, and lubricant. Betadine allergies are common, but may not be known to the patient.
4. Assess patient's knowledge of the purpose for catheterization.	• Reveals need for patient instruction.
5. Explain procedure to patient.	• Promotes cooperation.
6. Arrange for extra nursing personnel to assist as necessary.	• Patient may be unable to assume positioning for the procedure.
7. Perform hand hygiene.	• Reduces transmission of microorganisms.
8. Raise bed to appropriate working height.	• Promotes use of proper body mechanics.
9. Facing patient, stand on the left side of the bed if right-handed (on the right side of the bed if left-handed). Clear the bedside table and arrange equipment.	• To insert a catheter successfully, you must assume a comfortable position with all equipment easily accessible.
10. Raise side rail on the opposite side of the bed and lower side rail on the working side.	• Promotes patient safety.

Continued

SKILL 44.2	INSERTING AND REMOVING A STRAIGHT (INTERMITTENT) OR IN-DWELLING CATHETER—cont'd

11. Place waterproof pad under patient.

• Prevents soiling of bed linens.

12. Position patient:

   A. Patient with female genitalia

   (1) Assist to dorsal recumbent position (supine with knees flexed). Ask patient to relax thighs so that the hips can be rotated externally.

   • Provides good visualization of perineal structures. Support legs with pillows to reduce muscle tension and promote comfort.

   (2) Assist to side-lying (modified left lateral) position with upper leg flexed at hip if unable to assume dorsal recumbent position. If this position is used, you must take extra precautions to cover rectal area with drape to reduce chance of cross-contamination.

   • This alternative position is used if patient cannot abduct legs at hip joint (e.g., if patient has arthritic joints). Support patient with pillows if necessary to maintain position.

   B. Patient with male genitalia

   (1) Assist to supine position with thighs slightly abducted.

   • Comfortable position for patient that aids in visualization.

13. Drape patient:

   • Avoids unnecessary exposure of body parts and maintains patient's comfort.

   A. Patient with female genitalia (see Step 13A illustration)

   (1) Drape with bath blanket. Place blanket in diamond fashion over patient, with one corner at patient's midsection, side corners over each thigh and abdomen, and last corner over perineum.

   B. Patient with male genitalia (see Step 13B illustration)

   (1) Drape upper trunk with bath blanket and cover lower extremities with bed sheets, exposing only genitalia.

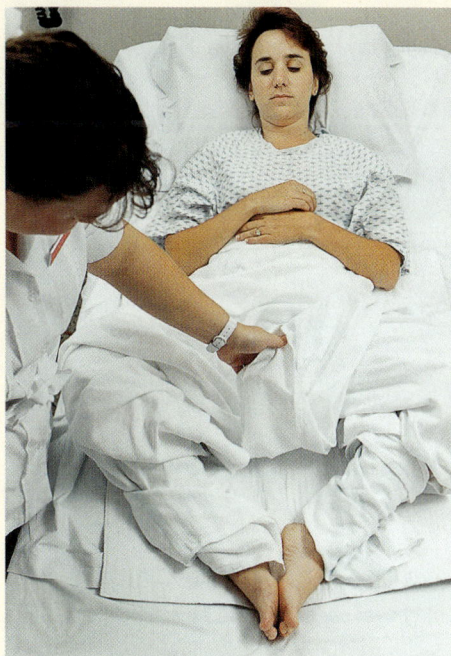

STEP 13A Draping technique (patient with female genitalia).

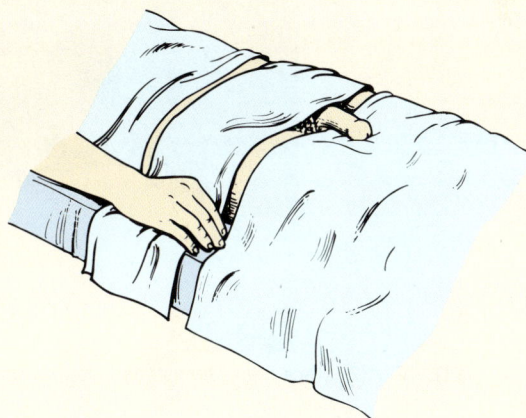

STEP 13B Draping technique (patient with male genitalia).

14. Wearing disposable gloves, wash perineal area with soap and water as needed; dry thoroughly. Remove and discard gloves; perform hand hygiene.

• Reduces microorganisms near the urethral meatus and allows further opportunity to visualize perineum and landmarks.

15. Position lamp to illuminate perineal area (have an assistant hold flashlight, if necessary).

• Permits accurate identification and good visualization of urethral meatus.

16. Open package containing drainage system; place drainage bag over the edge of the bottom bed frame, and bring drainage tube up between side rails and mattress.

• Prepares system for eventual connection with catheter.

CRITICAL DECISION POINT: *This step is necessary only when an in-dwelling catheter is being inserted and a drainage system is not part of the catheterization kit.*

---

17. Open catheterization kit according to directions, keeping bottom of container sterile.

• Prevents transmission of microorganisms from table or work area to sterile supplies. The materials in the kit are arranged in sequence of use.

18. Place plastic bag that contained kit within reach of work area to use as a waterproof bag to dispose of used supplies.

- Allows you to handle sterile supplies without contamination.

19. Apply sterile gloves (see Chapter 34).

CRITICAL DECISION POINT: *If underpad is the first item in the catheterization kit, place pad plastic side down under patient, touching only the edges so as to maintain sterility. Then apply sterile gloves.*

---

20. Organize supplies on sterile field. Open inner sterile package containing catheter. Pour sterile antiseptic solution into correct compartment containing sterile cotton balls. Open packet containing lubricant.
Remove specimen container (lid should be placed loosely on top) and prefilled syringe from collection compartment of tray, and set them aside on sterile field.

- Maintains principles of surgical asepsis and organizes work area.
- *Note:* Do not preinflate the balloon, because it is no longer recommended (Newman et al., 2021a, 2021b).

21. Lubricate 2.5 to 5 cm of catheter for individuals with female genitalia and 12.5 to 17.7 cm for individuals with male genitalia.

- Makes insertion of the catheter easier by decreasing friction.

CRITICAL DECISION POINT: *Some catheters have plastic sheaths over them that must be removed before lubrication. (Be sure to read manufacture instructions.) In some cases, the prescriber may order local anaesthetic lubricant.*

---

22. Apply sterile drape:

A. Patient with female genitalia

(1) Allow top edge of drape to form a cuff over both gloved hands. Place drape on bed between patient's thighs. Slip cuffed edge just under buttocks, taking care not to touch contaminated surface with gloves.

- Outer surface of drape covering hands remains sterile. Sterile drape against sterile gloves is sterile.

(2) Pick up fenestrated sterile drape and allow it to unfold without touching any unsterile objects. Apply drape over perineum, exposing labia and being sure not to touch contaminated surface (see Step 22A[2] illustration).

- Maintains sterility of work surface.

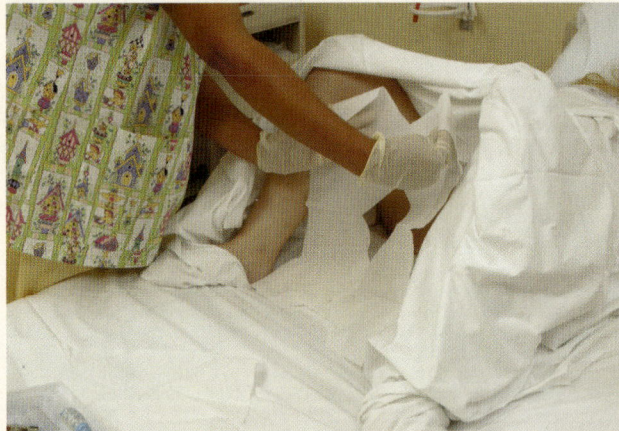

STEP 22A(2) Place sterile fenestrated drape (with opening in centre) over perineum with labia exposed.

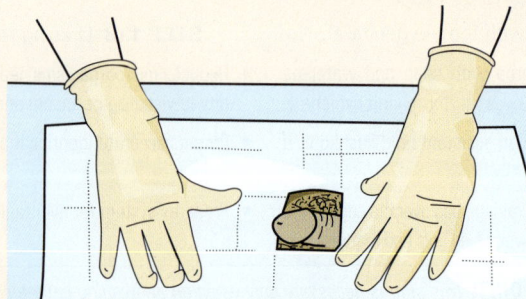

STEP 22B(1) Draping patient with male genitalia with fenestrated drape.

Continued

SKILL 44.2	INSERTING AND REMOVING A STRAIGHT (INTERMITTENT) OR IN-DWELLING CATHETER—cont'd

B. Patient with male genitalia

(1) Two methods are used for draping, depending on preference.
First method: Apply drape over thighs and under penis without completely opening fenestrated drape.
Second method: Apply drape over thighs just below penis. Pick up fenestrated sterile drape, allow it to unfold without touching any unsterile objects, and drape it over penis with fenestrated slit resting over penis (see Step 22B[1] illustration).

- Maintains sterility of work surface.

23. Place sterile tray and contents on sterile drape. Open specimen container.

- Provides easy access to supplies during catheter insertion. Maintains aseptic technique during procedure.

24. Clean urethral meatus:

A. Patient with female genitalia

(1) With nondominant hand, carefully retract labia to fully expose urethral meatus. Maintain position of nondominant hand throughout procedure.

(2) Using forceps held in sterile dominant hand, pick up cotton ball saturated with antiseptic solution, and clean perineal area, microwiping from clitoris toward anus (front to back). Using a new cotton ball for each area, wipe along the far labial fold, near labial fold, and directly over centre of urethral meatus (see Step 24A[2] illustration).

- Full visualization of urethral meatus is provided. Full retraction prevents contamination of urethral meatus during cleaning.
- Cleaning reduces number of microorganisms at urethral meatus. Use of a single cotton ball for each wipe prevents transfer of microorganisms. Cleaning for each of the three areas proceeds from area of least contamination to that of most contamination. Dominant hand remains sterile.

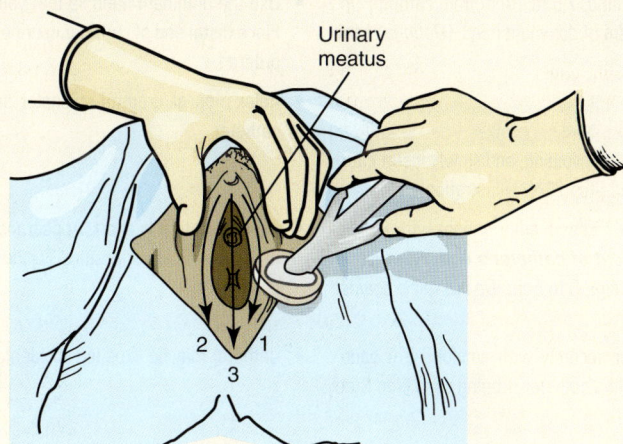

Urinary meatus

STEP 24A(2) Cleaning the perineum of a patient with female genitalia. (*Note:* If either hand touches the labia, the hand that touches it is considered to be contaminated.)

CRITICAL DECISION POINT: *If the labia close during cleaning, then the cleaning procedure must be repeated because the area has become contaminated.*

B. Patient with male genitalia

(1) If patient is not circumcised, retract foreskin with nondominant hand. Grasp penis at shaft just below glans. Retract urethral meatus between thumb and forefinger. Maintain nondominant hand in this position throughout procedure.

(2) With sterile dominant hand, pick up cotton ball with forceps and clean penis. Move in a circular motion from urethral meatus down to base of glans. Repeat cleaning three more times, using a clean cotton ball each time (see Step 24B[2] illustration).

- If foreskin is accidentally released or if penis is dropped during cleaning, the process must be repeated because the area has become contaminated.
- Cleaning reduces number of microorganisms at urethral meatus and proceeds from area of least contamination to that of most contamination. Dominant hand remains sterile.
- Some kits may include presoaked iodine swabs; follow agency policy.

SKILL 44.2   INSERTING AND REMOVING A STRAIGHT (INTERMITTENT) OR IN-DWELLING CATHETER—cont'd

STEP 24B(2) Cleaning technique (patient with male genitalia).

CRITICAL DECISION POINT: *If the foreskin does not remain retracted during cleaning, then the cleaning procedure must be repeated because the area has become contaminated.*

---

25. Pick up catheter with gloved dominant hand, 7.5 to 10 cm from catheter tip. Hold end of catheter loosely coiled in palm of dominant hand. (*Optional:* May grasp catheter with forceps.)

26. Insert catheter:

    A. Patient with female genitalia

    (1) Ask patient to bear down gently as if voiding, and slowly insert catheter through urethral meatus (see Step 26A[1] illustration)

    (2) Advance catheter a total of 5 to 7.5 cm in adult patient with female genitalia or ***until urine flows out of catheter's end.*** When urine appears, advance catheter another 2.5 to 5 cm. *Do not force against resistance.*

    (3) Release labia and hold catheter securely with nondominant hand. Slowly inflate balloon if in-dwelling catheter is being used (see Step 26A[3] illustrations; see Step 29).

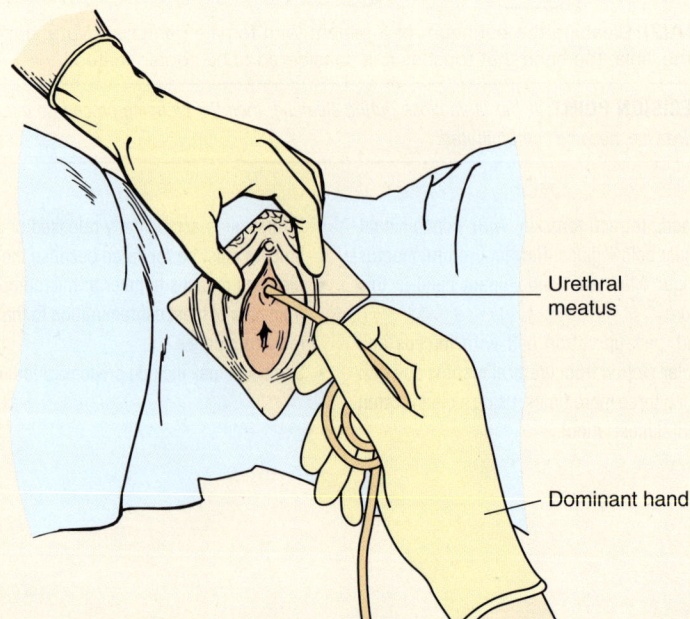

• Use the dominant hand so that you can manipulate the catheter more readily. Place distal end of catheter in urine tray receptacle if straight catheterization is ordered.

• Relaxation of urethral sphincter and pelvic floor muscle aids in insertion of catheter.

• Female urethra is short. Appearance of urine indicates that the catheter tip is in bladder or lower urethra. Further advancement of catheter ensures bladder placement.

• Catheter may be expelled accidentally by bladder or sphincter contraction.

Urethral meatus

Dominant hand

STEP 26A(1) Inserting catheter into the urinary meatus of a patient with female genitalia.

Continued

SKILL 44.2 | **INSERTING AND REMOVING A STRAIGHT (INTERMITTENT) OR IN-DWELLING CATHETER—cont'd**

To drainage bag

STEP 26A(3) Inflating balloon (in-dwelling catheter).

CRITICAL DECISION POINT: *If no urine appears, check whether catheter is in vagina. If misplaced, leave catheter in vagina as landmark indicating where not to insert, and insert another through urethral meatus.*

B. Patient with male genitalia

(1) Lift penis to position perpendicular to patient's body and apply light traction (see Step 26B[1] illustration).

• Straightens urethral canal to ease catheter insertion.

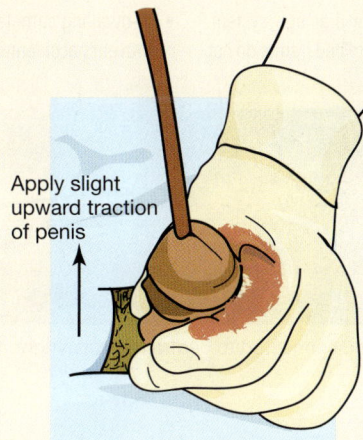

Apply slight upward traction of penis

STEP 26B(1) Position penis perpendicular to body for catheter insertion.

(2) Educate the patient regarding diaphragmatic breathing techniques (Newman et al., 2021a).

• These breathing techniques help to relax the pelvic floor and prevent urethra contraction, promoting easier insertion of the catheter and minimizing discomfort (Newman et al., 2021a).

(3) Advance catheter 17 to 22.5 cm in adult patient with male genitalia or *until urine flows out of catheter's end.* If resistance is felt, withdraw catheter; do not force it through urethra. When urine appears, advance catheter another 2.5 to 5 cm to the bifurcation ("Y" juncture). *Do not use force against resistance.*

• The adult male urethra is long. It is normal to meet resistance at the prostate. When resistance is felt, you should hold the catheter firmly without forcing it. After a few seconds, the muscle relaxes and the catheter is advanced. Appearance of urine indicates that the catheter tip is in bladder or urethra. Advancement of the catheter to the bifurcation ensures proper placement.

(4) Lower penis and hold catheter securely in nondominant hand. Place end of catheter in urine tray. Inflate balloon if in-dwelling catheter is being used (see Step 29).

• Catheter may be expelled accidentally by bladder or urethral contraction. Collection of urine prevents soiling and provides output measurement.

SKILL 44.2	INSERTING AND REMOVING A STRAIGHT (INTERMITTENT) OR IN-DWELLING CATHETER—cont'd

(5) Reduce (or reposition) the foreskin if the patient is uncircumcised.

- Paraphimosis (retraction and constriction of the foreskin behind the glans penis) secondary to catheterization may occur if foreskin is not reduced.

27. Collect urine specimen as needed. Fill specimen cup or jar to desired level (20 to 30 mL) by holding end of catheter over the cup with your dominant hand.

- Allows sterile specimen to be obtained for culture analysis.

28. Allow bladder to empty fully (about 800 to 1 000 mL) unless institution policy restricts maximal volume of urine to drain with each catheterization. Check institution policy before beginning catheterization.

- Monitor the patient's condition; if the vital signs change or bleeding occurs, temporarily stop the flow of urine and continue when the patient's condition warrants. Retained urine may serve as a reservoir for growth of microorganisms.

CRITICAL DECISION POINT: *If a single-use straight catheter was inserted, withdraw it slowly but smoothly until it is removed.*

---

29. Inflate balloon fully per manufacturer's recommendation (can be found printed on the lumen) and then release catheter with nondominant hand and pull gently.

- Inflation of balloon anchors the catheter tip in place above the bladder outlet to prevent the catheter's removal. Note size of balloon on catheter. Most commonly, a 5-mL balloon is used, but a 30-mL balloon may be ordered in some cases. A prefilled syringe may be included with the kit. Use only the amount included. Do not overinflate the balloon. A 5-mL balloon should be inflated with the supplied amount (10 mL) to allow symmetrical expansion.

CRITICAL DECISION POINT: *If resistance to inflation is noted or if patient complains of pain, the balloon may not be entirely within the bladder. Stop inflation, aspirate the fluid injected into the balloon, and advance the catheter a little more before attempting to inflate the balloon again.*

---

30. Attach end of in-dwelling catheter to collecting tube of drainage system. Drainage bag must be below level of bladder. Attach bag to bed frame; do not place bag on bed's side rails (see Step 30 illustration).

- In-dwelling catheters drain the bladder by gravity. Attaching to the bed frame prevents accidental pulling of the catheter when a bed rail is lowered.

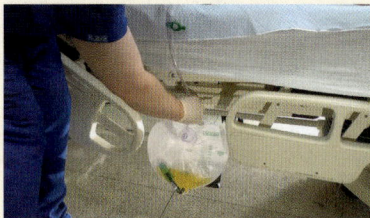

STEP 30 Drainage bag below level of bladder, connected to bedframe. (Copyright *Mosby's Clinical Skills: Essentials Collection*)

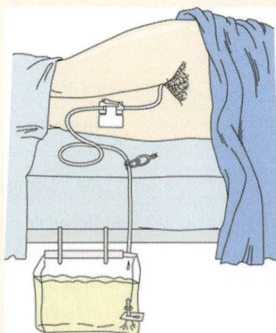

STEP 31A(1) Tape catheter to inner thigh (patient with female genitalia) and coil extra tubing on bed and attach to sheet. (From Sorrentino, S. A., Remmert, L. N., & Wilk, M. J. [2018]. *Mosby's Canadian textbook for the support worker* [4th ed.]. Elsevier.)

Continued

SKILL 44.2	INSERTING AND REMOVING A STRAIGHT (INTERMITTENT) OR IN-DWELLING CATHETER—cont'd

STEP 31B(1) Tape catheter to lower thigh (patient with male genitalia) and coil extra tubing on bed and attach to sheet. (From Sorrentino, S. A., Remmert, L. N., & Wilk, M. J. [2018]. *Mosby's Canadian textbook for the support worker* [4th ed.]. Elsevier.)

31. Anchor catheter:

   A. Patient with female genitalia

      (1) Secure catheter tubing to inner thigh or abdomen with a strip of nonallergenic tape (or multipurpose tube holders with a Velcro strap or a catheter securement device). Allow for slack so that movement of thigh does not create tension on catheter (see Step 31A[1] illustration).

   • Anchoring catheter to inner thigh reduces pressure on urethra, thus reducing possibility of tissue injury (Yates, 2018).

   B. Patient with male genitalia
   (1) Secure catheter tubing to top of thigh or lower abdomen (with penis directed toward chest). Allow for slack so that movement does not create tension on catheter (see Step 31B[1] illustration).

   • Anchoring catheter to lower abdomen reduces pressure on urethra at junction of penis and scrotum, thus reducing possibility of tissue injury. Unsecured catheters may cause traction and pressure that leads to severe tissue erosion and damage to the urethral sphincter and urethra, particularly in patients with male genitalia (Yates, 2018).

   C. Example of catheter securement device (see Step 31C illustration)

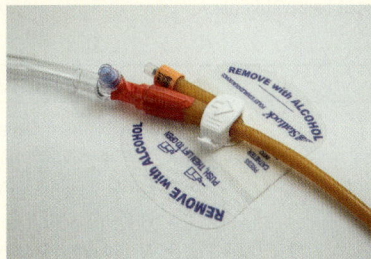

STEP 31C Example of a catheter securement device. (Courtesy Laurence Fernandez.)

32. Assist patient to comfortable position. Wash and dry perineal area as needed.
   • Maintains comfort and security.

33. Remove gloves and dispose of equipment, drapes, and urine in proper receptacles.
   • Reduces transmission of microorganisms.

34. Perform hand hygiene.
   • Reduces transmission of microorganisms.

35. Palpate bladder.
   • Determines whether distension has been relieved.

36. Ask about patient's comfort.
   • Determines whether patient's sensation of discomfort or fullness has been relieved.

37. Observe character and amount of urine in drainage system.
   • Determines whether urine is flowing adequately.

38. Ensure that no urine is leaking from catheter or tubing connections.
   • Prevents injury to patient's skin.

39. Removal of in-dwelling Foley catheter:

   A. Review medical order for removal of catheter. In cases of genitourinary surgery, it is especially important to obtain an order.
   • Premature removal of catheter in patients who have undergone genitourinary surgery could injure the patient.

SKILL 44.2	INSERTING AND REMOVING A STRAIGHT (INTERMITTENT) OR IN-DWELLING CATHETER—cont'd

B. Perform hand hygiene, put on clean gloves, and provide privacy.
- Procedure requires use of medical asepsis.

C. Prepare the patient:
- Prepares patient, to minimize anxiety.

  (1) Provide an explanation of procedure.

  (2) Position patient with waterproof pad under buttocks and cover with bath blanket, exposing only genital area and catheter. Position patients with female genitalia in dorsal recumbent position and patients with male genitalia in supine position.
- Shows respect for patient dignity by only exposing genital area and catheter.

  (3) Remove catheter securement device and free drainage tubing.

D. If needed, provide hygiene of genital area with soap and water.
- Antiseptic skin cleaners have not been proven to decrease risk for catheter-associated urinary tract infection (WOCN, 2016).

E. Move syringe plunger up and down to loosen, and then withdraw plunger to 0.5 mL. Insert hub of syringe into inflation valve (balloon port). Allow balloon fluid to drain into syringe by gravity. Make sure that entire amount of fluid is removed by comparing removed amount to volume needed for inflation.
- Partially inflated balloon can traumatize urethral wall during removal. Passive drainage of catheter balloon will prevent formation of ridges in balloon. These ridges can cause discomfort or trauma during removal.

F. Pull catheter out smoothly and slowly. Examine it to ensure that it is whole. The catheter should slide out easily. Do not use force. If you note any resistance, repeat Step 39E to remove remaining water. Notify health care provider if balloon does not deflate completely.
- Promotes patient comfort and safety.

G. Wrap contaminated catheter in waterproof pad. Unhook collection bag and drainage tubing from bed.
- Reduces transmission of microorganisms.

H. Reposition patient as necessary. Provide hygiene as needed. Lower level of bed and position side rails accordingly.

I. Empty, measure, and record urine present in drainage bag. Discard in appropriate receptacle. Remove and discard gloves. Perform hand hygiene.
- Records urinary output. Reduces transmission of microorganisms.

J. Encourage patient to maintain or increase fluid intake (unless contraindicated).
- Maintains normal urine output.

K. Initiate voiding record or bladder diary. Instruct patient to report when urge to void occurs and that all urine needs to be measured. Make sure that patient understands how to use collection container.
- Evaluates bladder function.

L. Ensure easy access to toilet, commode, bedpan, or urinal. Place urine "hat" on toilet seat if patient is using toilet. Place call bell within easy reach.

UNEXPECTED OUTCOMES | RELATED INTERVENTIONS

Urethral or perineal irritation or discomfort
- Observe for leaking catheter; replace if necessary.
- Assess whether in-dwelling catheter is anchored properly.
- Perform perineal hygiene and catheter care more frequently.

Fever or odour, burning sensations, or blood in collection bag.
- Obtain a new sterile specimen from the catheter port.
- Notify prescriber.

Urinary retention and inability to void after catheter is removed
- Provide adequate fluid intake and ensure patient privacy.
- If patient is unable to void within 6 hours after catheter removal, notify prescriber.

RECORDING AND REPORTING
- Report and record date and time, type and size of catheter inserted, amount of water used to inflate the balloon, characteristics of urine, amount of urine, reasons for catheterization, specimen collection if appropriate, and patient's response to procedure and education provided (Newman et al., 2021a).
- Initiate intake and output record.
- If catheter is definitely in bladder and no urine is noted within 1 hour, absence of urine should be reported to prescriber immediately.

CARE IN THE COMMUNITY CONSIDERATIONS
- Patients who are at home may use a leg bag during the day and switch to a large-volume bag at night so that sleep can be uninterrupted. Attach the large-volume bag to the spigot at the bottom of the leg bag.
- Patients may catheterize themselves at home, using a clean technique.

| **SKILL 44.3** | **IN-DWELLING CATHETER CARE** |

Delegation Considerations

Perineal care is often part of routine hygiene care that is delegated to unregulated care providers (UCPs). Proper assessment and care of the perineal area requires professional clinical judgement. If the patient has had trauma or surgical procedures that involve the perineal area, care of this area should not be delegated.

- Instruct the UCP to report any patient discomfort, perineal pain, perineal discharge, or odour to a nurse. The UCP should also report on the condition of the catheter and drainage tubing (e.g., leaks, encrustations, or any discoloured or foul-smelling urine).

Equipment

- Catheter care kit or individual supplies
- Disposable gloves
- Cotton balls or large swabs
- Clean washcloth and towel
- Warm water and soap
- Antiseptic swab or cloth (if agency policy directs)
- Bath blanket
- Waterproof absorbent pad

PROCEDURE

STEPS	**RATIONALE**
1. Assess for episode of bowel incontinence or patient discomfort or provide care as per agency routine regarding hygiene measures (see Chapter 39).	• Accumulation of secretions or feces causes irritation to perineal tissues and acts as a source of bacterial growth.
2. Explain procedure to patient. Offer the able patient an opportunity to perform self-care.	• Reduces anxiety and promotes cooperation. Embarrassment may motivate patient to perform their own hygiene.
3. Close door or bedside curtain.	• Maintains patient privacy.
4. Perform hand hygiene.	• Reduces transmission of infection.
5. Position patient.	
A. Patient with female genitalia	• Ensures easy access to perineal tissues.
(1) Dorsal recumbent position	
B. Patient with male genitalia	
(1) Supine or Fowler's position	
6. Place waterproof pad under patient.	• Prevents soiling of bed linens.
7. Drape bath blanket over patient so that only perineal area is exposed.	• Prevents unnecessary exposure of body parts.
8. Apply gloves.	
9. Remove anchor device to free catheter tubing.	
10. With nondominant hand:	
A. Patient with female genitalia	
(1) Gently retract labia to expose urethral meatus and catheter insertion site fully, maintaining position of hand throughout procedure.	• Provides full visualization of urethral meatus. Full retraction prevents contamination of urethral meatus during cleaning.
B. Patient with male genitalia	
(1) Retract foreskin if not circumcised, and hold penis at shaft just below glans, maintaining position throughout procedure.	• If foreskin is accidentally released or penis is dropped during cleaning, the process must be repeated because the area has become contaminated.
11. Assess urethral meatus and surrounding tissue for inflammation, swelling, and discharge. Note amount, colour, odour, and consistency of discharge. Ask patient if any burning or discomfort has been experienced.	• Determines presence of local infection and status of hygiene.
12. Clean perineal tissue:	
A. Patient with female genitalia	
(1) Use clean cloth and perineal cleanser. Clean around urethral meatus and catheter. Moving from pubis toward anus, clean labia minora. Use a clean side of the cloth for each wipe. Finally, clean around anus. Dry each area well.	• Reduces the number of microorganisms at the urethral meatus. Use of a clean cloth prevents transfer of microorganisms.
B. Patient with male genitalia	
(1) While spreading urethral meatus, clean around catheter first, and then wipe in circular motion around meatus and glans.	• Cleaning moves from area of least contamination to that of most contamination.
13. Reassess urethral meatus for discharge.	• Determines whether cleaning is complete.
14. While stabilizing the catheter with the nondominant hand, use a towel and perineal cleanser to wipe in a circular motion along the length of the catheter for 10 cm (see Step 14 illustration).	• Reduces presence of secretions or drainage on exterior surface of catheter. • Some agencies may use antiseptic swab or cloth to wipe off tubing. Check policy.

SKILL 44.3   IN-DWELLING CATHETER CARE—cont'd

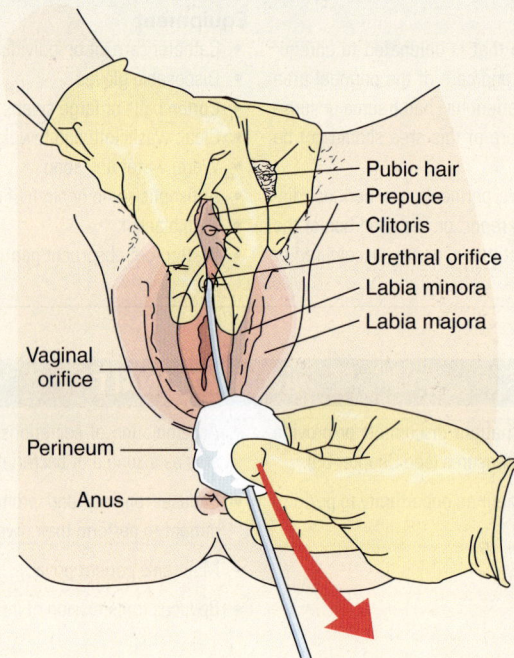

STEP 14 Cleaning catheter during catheter care. (Based on Wound Ostomy and Continence Nurses Society. [2016]. *Care and management of patients with urinary catheters: A clinical resource guide.* [WOCN®]. https://www.wocn.org)

15. In patient with male genitalia, reduce (or reposition) the foreskin.   • Prevents trauma to the head of the penis.

16. Re-anchor catheter tubing.   • Prevents trauma to the urethra.

17. Place patient in a safe, comfortable position.   • Promotes comfort.

18. Dispose of contaminated supplies, remove gloves, and perform hand hygiene.   • Reduces spread of infection.

UNEXPECTED OUTCOMES	RELATED INTERVENTIONS
Urethral discharge	• Increase frequency of in-dwelling catheter care. • Notify prescriber. • Assess for urethral trauma. • Monitor urine output.

RECORDING AND REPORTING
• Report and record the presence and characteristics of drainage, the condition of the perineal tissue, and any discomfort reported by the patient.
• If infection is suspected, report findings to prescriber.

CARE IN THE COMMUNITY CONSIDERATIONS
• If patient is discharged with an in-dwelling catheter in place, the patient and family should be taught catheter care as well as educated about the signs and symptoms that should be reported to a nurse or prescriber. A referral for home care may be needed.

(Wound Ostomy and Continence Nurses Society [WOCN], 2016). A break in the system can lead to the introduction of microorganisms. Locations at risk are the catheter insertion site, the drainage bag, the spigot, the tube junction, and the junction of the tube and the bag (Figure 44.15).

In addition, the nurse should monitor the patency of the system to prevent the pooling of urine within the tubing. Bacteria can travel up drainage tubing to grow in pools of urine. If this urine flows back into the patient's bladder, an infection will likely develop. The patient should be observed for symptoms of UTI, and any changes in their condition need to be documented. Suggested methods to prevent infections in catheterized patients are provided in Box 44.7.

Catheter irrigations and instillations. Sometimes it may be necessary to irrigate an in-dwelling urinary catheter using a triple-lumen catheter and sterile solution to maintain patency after urogenital

surgery or prevent blood clots from occluding the catheter. This is usually done by continuous closed-bladder irrigation. Occasionally, an intermittent closed irrigation may be ordered if the catheter is occluded and it is deemed harmful to remove the catheter (e.g., after urological surgery). A prescriber may order bladder instillations for select bladder medications, with instruction as to how long the medication stays in the bladder. Unnecessary catheter irrigation should be avoided (Lo et al., 2014). If a catheter becomes occluded by sediment and encrustation, it should be changed to avoid flushing debris containing bacteria into the bladder. Bladder irrigations or washouts to "unblock" such catheters that break the closed urinary drainage system increase risk of UTI.

Maintenance of a closed system is essential during continuous or intermittent irrigations (Skill 44.4) and instillations. Therefore, an order from a prescriber is required for all irrigations and instillations.

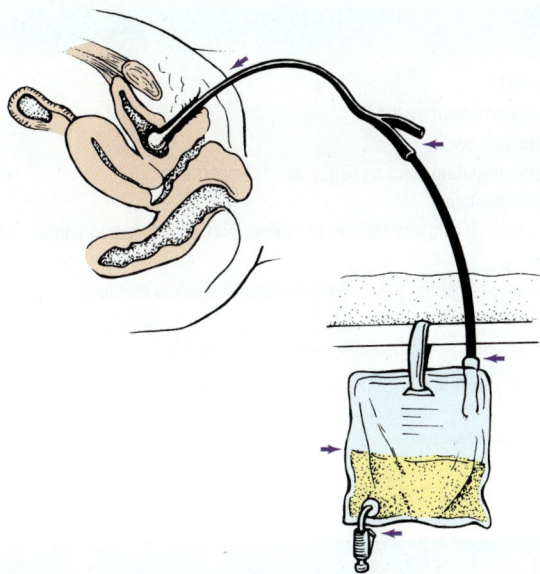

FIGURE 44.15 Potential sites for introduction of infectious organisms into a urinary drainage system.

Removal of In-Dwelling Catheter. When removing an in-dwelling catheter, the nurse needs to promote normal bladder function and prevent trauma to the urethra. Timely removal of in-dwelling catheters that are no longer required is a key intervention in reducing the incidence of CAUTI (WOCN, 2016). The patient may experience some discomfort when voiding after the initial removal of the catheter. Until the bladder regains full tone, the patient may experience urinary frequency or retention. Ongoing reports of dysuria and frequency may indicate an infection. The patient's urinary function is assessed by noting the first voiding after catheter removal and by documenting the time and amount of voiding during the next 24 to 48 hours. If there is no output within 6 hours of catheter removal the nurse should check fluid intake and notify the prescriber (Gray et al., 2020). If there is no output within 6 hours of catheter removal or if the patient experiences discomfort, it may become necessary to reinsert the catheter or perform an intermittent catheterization as per prescriber order. The nurse should record the time and amount of voids, including incontinence, on a bladder record. An ultrasound bladder scanner can assist with monitoring PVR urine. If amounts are small, frequent assessment for bladder distension, abdominal pain, dribbling, incontinence, and any sensation of incomplete emptying is necessary

Alternatives to Urethral Catheterization. Alternatives for urinary drainage can be used to avoid the risks associated with catheters inserted through the urethra: absorbent containment products, suprapubic catheterization, and condom catheters.

Incontinence Containment Products. Both disposable and washable absorbent pads are available in many absorbencies and styles. These include insert pads designed for individuals with male or female genitalia to wear with underwear, all-in-one briefs, pull-ups, and underpads (DeMarinis at al., 2017). Absorbent pads for urine are designed with multiple layers to absorb urine. Some people may need a combination of products to manage incontinence. Incontinence pads are helpful to contain urine leakage but they are not a replacement for assisting patients to the toilet. Menstrual products should not be used for urinary incontinence because incontinence containment products are made to absorb more fluid and neutralize the urine to prevent skin breakdown.

Suprapubic Catheterization. Suprapubic catheterization involves surgical placement of a catheter through the abdominal wall above the symphysis pubis and into the urinary bladder (Figure 44.16). For individuals needing long-term catheterization, a suprapubic rather than urethrally inserted catheter may be an option for comfort, although CAUTI can still occur (WOCN, 2016). A physician performs the procedure under local or general anaesthesia. The catheter is anchored in place with sutures, a commercially prepared body seal, or both. Once the track is healed, nurses may be authorized to change this type of device. Urine drains into a urinary drainage bag. Maintenance of the tubing and drainage bag is the same as for an in-dwelling catheter. The suprapubic catheter is relatively painless and reduces the incidence of infection commonly seen with in-dwelling catheters. Studies comparing the use of this method of urinary drainage have shown mixed results. While infection rates may be slightly lower, the long-term complications are similar (WOCN, 2016). Sediment, clots, encrustations, or the abdominal wall itself can block the suprapubic catheter. Adequate fluid intake will help minimize the risk of blockage by sediment or infection due to stagnation. The suprapubic catheter must remain patent at all times. Nurses must monitor the patient's intake and output carefully, monitor the appearance of urine, and observe for signs of infection (e.g., fever and chills). Nurses also should administer skin care around the insertion site.

Condom catheters. The second alternative to catheterization is the condom catheter (external urinary catheter; Box 44.8). This may

SKILL 44.4   **CLOSED CATHETER IRRIGATION**

Delegation Considerations

Closed catheter irrigation is usually not delegated to unregulated care providers (UCPs). Closed catheter irrigation is usually done in patients with complications such as gross hematuria or after urological surgery.

- UCPs may assist with other aspects of patient care, such as positioning the patient and measuring intake and output.
- Instruct the UCP to report any complaints of pain, discomfort, or fever to a nurse.
- Instruct the UCP to report the presence of clots in the output or a change in output to a nurse.

Equipment

- Closed intermittent method:
  - Antiseptic swab
  - Sterile irrigation solution bag at room temperature
  - Sterile container
  - Luer-lock needleless syringe to access port (check manufacturer requirements)
  - Clamp to temporarily occlude catheter as irrigant is instilled
- Closed continuous method:
  - Sterile irrigation solution bag at room temperature
  - Irrigation tubing and clamp
  - IV pole
  - Antiseptic swab
  - Bath blanket

PROCEDURE

STEPS	RATIONALE
1. Assess prescriber's order for the type of irrigation (continuous or intermittent) and irrigation solution to use.	• Ensures proper selection of equipment.
2. Assess colour of urine and presence of mucus or sediment.	• Determines whether patient is bleeding, has infection, or is sloughing tissue.
3. Determine type of catheter in place:	
A. Triple lumen (one lumen to inflate balloon, one to instill irrigation solution, one to allow outflow of urine).	• Triple lumen is for closed continuous irrigation.
B. Double lumen (one lumen to inflate balloon, one to allow outflow of urine).	• Double lumen may be in place for closed intermittent irrigation/instillation.
4. Determine patency of drainage tubing.	• Ensures that drainage tubing is not kinked, clamped incorrectly, or looped.
5. Assess amount of urine in drainage bag (may want to empty drainage bag before irrigation).	• If drainage bag is not empty, you will need to subtract urine volume from the amount drained to determine whether all irrigant has returned.
6. Explain procedure and purpose to patient.	• Helps patient relax and cooperate during procedure.
7. Perform hand hygiene and apply disposable gloves for closed methods.	• Prevents transmission of microorganisms.
8. Provide privacy by pulling bed curtains closed. Fold back covers so that the catheter is exposed. Cover patient's upper torso with bath blanket.	• Promotes patient comfort.
9. Assess lower abdomen for bladder distension. (If a portable bladder scanner is available, it can be used to assess bladder volume.)	• Detects whether catheter is malfunctioning or blocking urinary drainage.
10. Position patient in dorsal recumbent or supine position.	• Promotes patient comfort and provides easy access to catheter.
11. Closed intermittent irrigation (with double-lumen catheter):	
A. Prepare prescribed sterile solution in sterile graduated cup.	• Ensures that irrigating fluid remains sterile.
B. Draw sterile solution into syringe by using aseptic technique.	

CRITICAL DECISION POINT: *Avoid cold solution as irrigant because it may cause bladder spasm and discomfort.*

STEPS	RATIONALE
C. Clamp in-dwelling catheter just distal to injection (specimen) port.	• Occlusion of catheter allows irrigant to be instilled into catheter.
D. Clean injection port with antiseptic swab (same port used for specimen collection).	• Reduces transmission of infection.
E. Insert needless syringe tip through port.	
F. Slowly inject fluid into catheter and bladder.	• Slow, continuous pressure reduces trauma to the bladder wall.

CRITICAL DECISION POINT: *If catheter does not irrigate easily, stop the irrigation. The catheter may be occluded or tip may be placed in the urethra and not in the bladder. Contact prescriber, as the catheter may need to be removed or replaced.*

Continued

SKILL 44.4 **CLOSED CATHETER IRRIGATION—cont'd**

G. Withdraw syringe, remove clamp, and allow solution to drain into drainage bag. If instillation was ordered by prescriber, keep clamped to allow solution to remain in bladder for ordered time.

• Allows drainage by gravity. Some medications stay in the bladder for a specific time. Do not leave unattended.

CRITICAL DECISION POINT: *If solution is to remain in bladder, do not forget to clamp tubing at the end of the instillation period.*

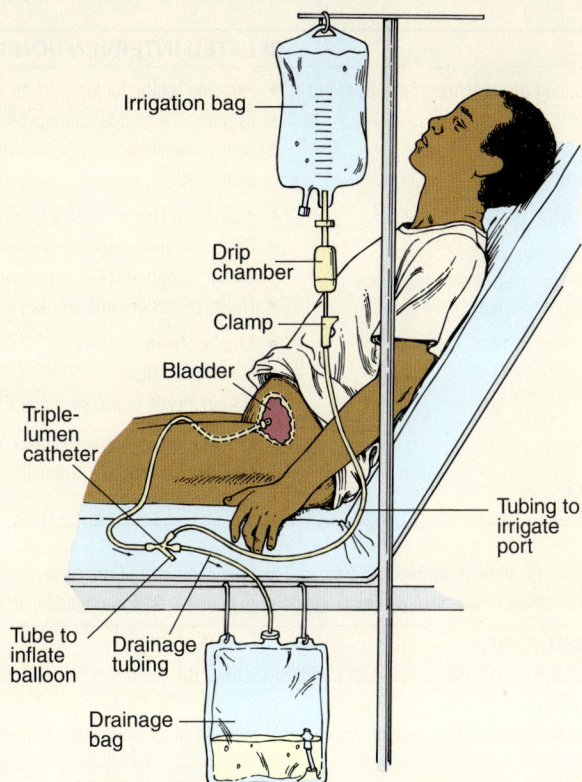

STEP 12 Closed continuous bladder irrigation.

12. Closed continuous irrigation (with triple-lumen catheter) (see Step 12 illustration).

A. Using the aseptic technique, insert tip of sterile irrigation tubing into bag of sterile irrigating solution.

• Prevents entrance of microorganisms.

B. Close clamp on tubing and hang bag of solution on IV pole.

C. Open clamp and allow solution to flow through (prime) tubing, keeping end of tubing sterile. Close clamp.

• Removes air from tubing.

D. Wipe off irrigation port of triple-lumen catheter with antiseptic swab, and then attach to irrigation tubing.

• Third lumen provides means for irrigation solution to enter bladder. System must remain sterile.

E. Be sure that drainage bag and tubing are securely connected to the drainage port of the triple-lumen catheter.

• Ensures that urine and irrigation solution will drain from bladder.

F. For intermittent flow, clamp tubing on drainage system, open clamp on irrigation tubing, and allow prescribed amount of fluid to enter bladder (100 mL is normal for adults). Close irrigation clamp and then open drainage tubing clamp. (*Optional:* Leave clamp closed for time ordered. See previous Critical Decision Point.)

• Fluid instills through catheter into bladder, flushing system. Fluid drains out after irrigation is completed.

G. For continuous drainage, calculate drip rate and adjust the clamp on irrigation tubing accordingly. Be sure that the clamp on drainage tubing is open and check volume of drainage in drainage bag. Ensure that drainage tubing is patent, and avoid kinks.

• Ensures continuous, even irrigation of catheter system.
• Prevents accumulation of solution in bladder, which may cause bladder distension and possible injury.

SKILL 44.4	**CLOSED CATHETER IRRIGATION—cont'd**

13. When irrigation is complete, dispose of contaminated supplies, remove gloves, and perform hand hygiene.	• Prevents spread of infection.
14. Calculate fluid used to irrigate bladder and catheter and subtract from total output.	• Determines accurate urinary output, ensures accurate measurement of irrigation fluid to calculate actual output
15. Assess characteristics of output: viscosity, colour, and presence of matter (e.g., sediment, clots, blood).	• Evaluates results of irrigation.

UNEXPECTED OUTCOMES	**RELATED INTERVENTIONS**
Irrigating solution does not return or is not flowing at prescribed rate, possible occlusion of catheter	• Examine tubing for kinks, clots, or urine sediment. • Evaluate for bladder distension. • Notify prescriber if irrigant is retained, if patient reports pain, or if bladder is distended.
Bright red bleeding with irrigation	• Assess for shock (check vital signs, skin colour, and moisture). • Closed intermittent—stop irrigation. • Closed continuous—leave flowing. • Notify prescriber immediately.
Increased cloudiness of urine, fever	• Monitor fever. • Notify prescriber. • Obtain sterile urine specimen if ordered by the prescriber.
Increase in pain	• Examine tubing for kinks, clots, or urine sediment. • Evaluate for bladder distension. • Notify prescriber.

RECORDING AND REPORTING
• Record type and amount of irrigation solution used, amount returned as drainage, and the character of drainage.
• Record and report any findings such as reports of fever, pain, sudden bleeding, inability to instill fluid into bladder, or presence of blood clots.

CARE IN THE COMMUNITY CONSIDERATIONS
• If patient is discharged with an in-dwelling catheter and requires bladder irrigations, either the patient or the patient's family must be properly instructed in how to perform this task, or a referral is made to home care.
• Teach patient and family to observe urine colour, clarity, odour, amount, and signs of obstruction or urinary tract infection.

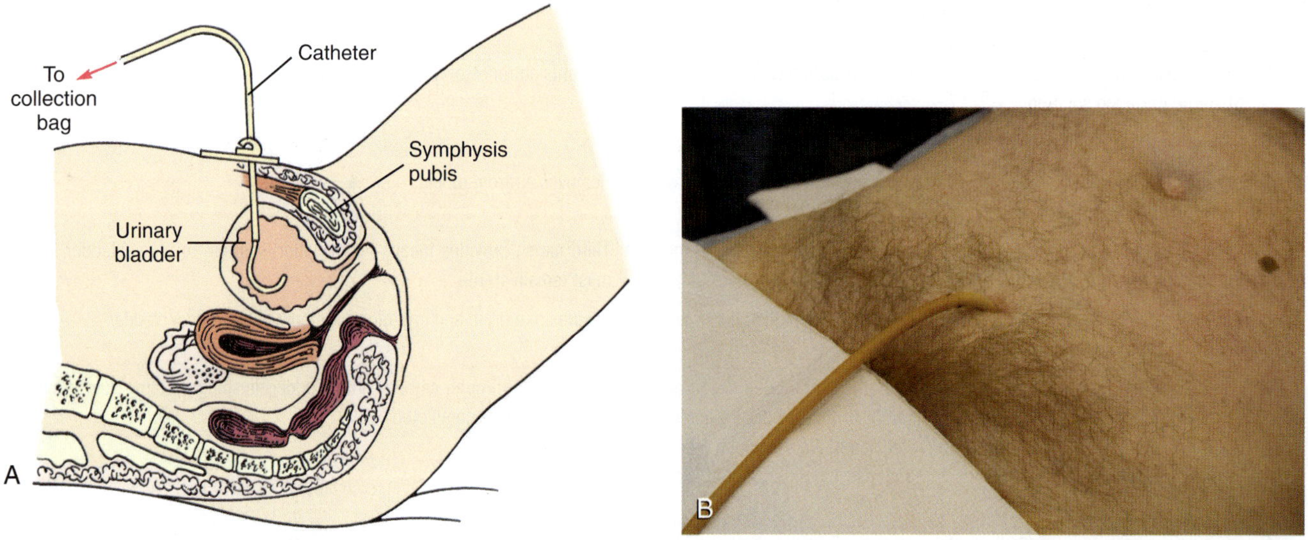

FIGURE 44.16 A, Placement of suprapubic catheter above the symphysis pubis. **B,** Suprapubic catheter without a dressing.

BOX 44.8 PROCEDURAL GUIDELINE
Applying a Condom Catheter

Delegation Considerations:
The application of a condom catheter can be delegated to unregulated care providers (UCPs). The registered nurse is responsible for assessing the condition of the penis over time and should inform the UCP to notify the registered nurse of any signs of skin irritation or tissue swelling.

Equipment:
- Condom catheter (may be self-adhesive or provided with elastic adhesive tape)
- Collection bag
- Basin with warm water
- Towel and washcloth
- Disposable gloves
- Scissors

Procedure:
1. Check prescriber's order.
2. Perform hand hygiene.
3. Assess urinary elimination patterns, the patient's ability to urinate voluntarily, and continence.
4. Assess the patient's mental status to determine appropriate teaching related to condom catheter care.
5. Assess condition of penis and scrotum. Ensure that the foreskin of the uncircumcised patient with male genitalia is not retracted.
6. Assess the patient's knowledge of the purpose of the condom catheter.
7. Explain procedure to patient.
8. Raise bed to working height and raise far upper side rail.
9. Using sheet, drape patient so that only genitals are exposed.
10. Prepare condom catheter and drainage system (see manufacturer's directions).
11. Apply gloves and provide perineal care.
    A. If necessary, clip hair at base of penile shaft.
12. Apply skin preparation to penile shaft and allow to dry.
13. Holding penis in nondominant hand, apply condom by rolling smoothly onto penis. *Note:* Leave a 2.5-cm to 5-cm space between tip of penis and end of catheter (see Step 13 illustration).

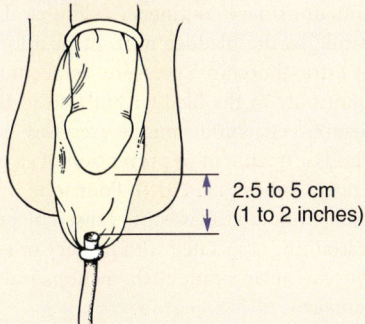

STEP 13 Distance between end of penis and tip of catheter.

14. Secure condom catheter:
    A. If self-adhesive catheter is used, follow the manufacturer's directions.
    B. If elastic adhesive is used, wrap the strip of adhesive over the condom catheter to secure it in place, using a spiral technique (see Step 14B illustration). *Note:* Adhesive tape must never be used.

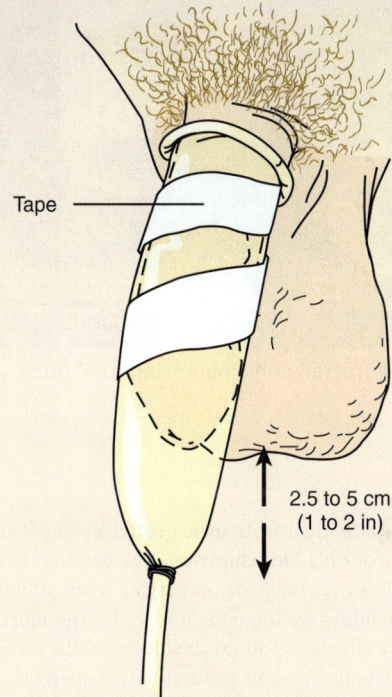

STEP 14B Elastic tape is applied in spiral fashion to secure the condom catheter to the penis.

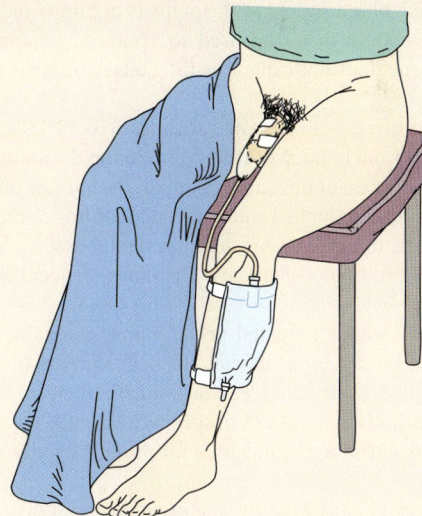

STEP 15 Attach condom catheter to leg bag.

15. Attach catheter to leg drainage bag (see Step 15 illustration). If using large drainage bag, attach to lower bed frame.
16. Make patient comfortable.
17. Observe urinary drainage, drainage tube patency, condition of penis, and tape placement.

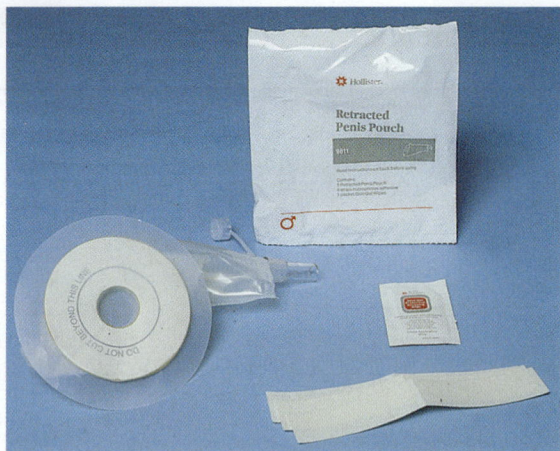

FIGURE 44.17 Retracted penis pouch external urinary device.

be appropriate for individuals with male genitalia and who have complete and spontaneous bladder emptying. The condom is a soft, pliable sheath that slips over the penis. It may be worn at night only or continuously, depending on the patient's needs. The most common is the self-adhesive silicone condom sheath or sheath with brush-on adhesive, although some are still secured with a strip of elastic tape (Geng et al., 2016). Latex products are also still available; the nurse needs to ensure that the patient does not have a latex allergy if one is used. Care must be taken to ensure that whatever type or size of condom is used, blood supply to the penis is not impaired. Standard adhesive tape should never be used to secure a condom catheter because this tape does not expand with changes in penis size and is painful to remove.

Condom catheters are associated with less risk of UTI, but infections may result from buildup of secretions around the urethra, trauma to the urethral meatus, or pressure buildup in the outflow tubing. Condom catheters must be applied and changed according to the manufacturer's directions to prevent abrasion, dermatitis, ischemia, necrosis, edema, and maceration of the penis. Therefore, frequent skin assessment is vital.

For a person with a retracted penis, maintaining a conventional condom catheter may prove difficult. To help alleviate this problem, special externally applied devices are available that are secured by hydrocolloid strips (Figure 44.17), or specially designed underwear can be used. The manufacturer's guidelines for product application should be consulted.

Maintenance of Skin Integrity. **Incontinence-associated dermatitis (IAD)** is a type of irritant dermatitis and moisture-associated skin damage within the adult population that is caused by prolonged exposure to urine or stool on the skin. The presentation of IAD can range from intact skin with blanchable erythema, maceration, swelling, and bullae to erosions and denudation leading to cutaneous wounds. IAD may be patchy or continuous and have poorly demarcated edges. Patients will report discomfort and describe pain as burning, itching, or tingling. Secondary cutaneous candidiasis (yeast) commonly occurs with IAD and presents as pustules and satellite lesions. IAD should not be confused with stage 1 pressure injuries (Beeckman, 2017).

Perineal care should occur as soon as possible after the incontinence episode to avoid prolonged skin exposure. Perineal skin care should be focused on the principles of cleansing and protecting the skin. Cleansing should be completed with a pH-balanced cleanser; soap and water should be avoided. Protecting the skin with moisture barrier perineal-specific creams, pastes, lotions, or films will form a barrier between the outer layer of the skin (stratum corneum) and the incontinence. Topical antifungal creams or powders can be used for secondary cutaneous infections (Beeckman et al., 2015).

Conservative Management to Promote Continence. In acute, rehabilitation, restorative, and continuing care settings, several approaches have shown success in improving bladder control. They include lifestyle changes, pelvic floor muscle exercises, bladder retraining, and toileting schedules for management of urgency, stress, and mixed urinary incontinence. Intermittent self-catheterization may be an option for individuals with poor bladder emptying. In clinical practice, nonsurgical and nonpharmacological therapies are trialled first because they usually carry the least risk of harm (Burkhard et al., 2020). Because the success of conservative therapies necessitates changes in daily lifestyle and ongoing adherence, it is important that the patient be provided with support and follow-up to enhance motivation.

Lifestyle Modification. Several lifestyle factors have been associated with urinary incontinence. Smoking has been associated with increased risk of incontinence in some studies, although the link is not completely clear (Kawahara et al., 2020). Extra weight, particularly in obese and moderately obese individuals, is believed to increase intrapelvic pressure (Balalau et al., 2021). Caffeine has a weak diuretic effect and may contribute to urinary incontinence (Balalau et al., 2021). Nurses can play an important role in educating, counselling, and supporting the patient to enable lifestyle modification that reduces the risk factors for incontinence.

Pelvic Floor Muscle Exercises and Training. The pelvic floor muscles consist of the levator ani and the coccygeus muscle. They provide an important function for urinary continence (Chiu et al., 2018). The pelvic floor musculature (PFM) spans the opening in the bony pelvis and combines with connective tissue to provide structural support for the pelvic organs. The pelvic floor muscles act as a hammock of support to maintain urinary continence (Chiu et al., 2018). A well-toned PFM maintains the bladder neck in position to ensure that any increase in intra-abdominal pressure, as occurs with coughing, is transmitted not only to the bladder but also to the bladder neck to maintain closure. Pelvic floor muscle exercises are considered an important method of treatment or prevention of stress or mixed urinary incontinence (Chiur et al., 2018). Poor tone in the pelvic floor muscles can result from muscle wasting caused by prolonged immobility, frequent straining associated with urinary or fecal elimination, stretching of muscles during childbirth, menopausal muscle atrophy, or traumatic damage.

Pelvic floor muscle exercises (PFMEs), formerly known as *Kegel exercises*, are used to improve function of the pelvic floor, improving urethral stability (Burkhard et al., 2020). Pelvic floor muscle training (PFMT) appears to speed the recovery of continence following radical prostatectomy in patients with male genitalia, and if done in the early postpartum period improves urinary incontinence in patients with female genitalia for up to 12 months (Burkhard et al., 2020). Patients begin these exercises by trying to suppress passing flatus rectally to teach them the correct muscles to contract. The

BOX 44.9 PATIENT TEACHING

Pelvic Floor Muscle Exercises

Objectives

The patient will achieve continence or experience fewer episodes of incontinence due to increased pelvic floor muscle tone and strength.

Teaching Strategies

- Explain the method used to identify proper muscle contraction by having the patient try to stop the passage of flatus. Patients with female genitalia can check contraction by inserting a finger into the vagina; Patients with male genitalia can look for a slight movement of the penis.
- After the correct muscle group is identified, instruct the patient to lie down with knees bent and apart or sit.
- Instruct the patient to contract the pelvic floor muscle gradually and hold the contraction for up to 10 seconds without tensing the muscles of the legs, buttocks, back, or abdomen. Remind the patient to breathe during the exercise.
- Instruct the patient to relax the muscle gradually for an equal time period between each contraction.
- The patient should perform 10 repetitions three times a day.
- Patients with mild cognitive impairment or early-stage dementia should be supported by written reminders and prompting from caregivers.
- Teach the patient and the caregiver to periodically keep a 24- to 72-hour urinary diary to identify changes in patterns of urinary elimination.

Evaluation

- Ask the patient if they have practised the exercises and how often practice occurs.
- Specialized continence clinicians assess muscle tone during vaginal (patient with female genitalia) or rectal (patient with male genitalia) examination by asking the patient to perform the contraction.
- Monitor the patient's urinary diary.
- Ask the patient and the caregiver about the degree of satisfaction related to the control achieved over urinary elimination.

exercises are then practised at nonvoiding times (Box 44.9). Patients should be alert and motivated to perform the exercises. They also should be aware that it may take 12 to 16 weeks to notice appreciable change, but that maintaining the exercises is important in order to obtain a positive outcome. PFMT involves a systematic program, led by a specialist physiotherapist or specialized continence nurse, for patients with poor pelvic floor tone who need additional coaching and biofeedback.

Bladder Training. Bladder training is a program of patient education and a scheduled voiding regimen with gradually adjusted voiding intervals (Burkhard et al., 2020). The goal of bladder training is to correct faulty habit patterns of frequent urination, improve control over bladder urgency, prolong voiding intervals, increase bladder capacity, reduce incontinent episodes, and restore patient confidence in controlling bladder function (Burkhard et al., 2020). For bladder training to be successful, patients must be alert, motivated, and physically able to follow a training program. Patients with urinary retention are not suitable candidates for bladder training. The program includes education, scheduled voiding, and positive reinforcement. The first step in bladder training is establishing a baseline. The patient or caregiver completes a urinary diary to assess maximum voiding intervals. It is not uncommon for patients with frequency or an overactive bladder to void small amounts hourly or more often. An initial training schedule for such a patient might involve a voiding schedule of every 75 minutes while awake, increasing every 1 to 3 weeks by 15-minute increments toward a 3-hour schedule. The rate of incremental changes will depend on the patient's progress and on their ability to adhere to a rigid schedule. Urge suppression techniques are helpful, such as counting backward from 100 when the urge to void is felt and performing pelvic floor muscle contractions. The nurse must be aware that the patient who has experienced an incontinence episode in public will be particularly hesitant to deter voiding for even brief periods.

Prompted Voiding, Timed Toileting, and Habit Retraining. Timed toileting, habit retraining, and prompted voiding are potentially useful strategies for patients with cognitive or physical impairment, or both, who rely on caregiver assistance. Timed toileting and habit retraining involves assessing a patient's normal pattern of voiding to establish a toileting schedule that preempts incontinence or reduces the number of incontinence episodes. Several randomized controlled studies have confirmed a positive effect on continence outcomes for prompt voiding compared to standard care (Burkhard et al., 2020). Such interventions are labour intensive, which may limit their feasibility. When combined with positive reinforcement, this approach is also called *prompted voiding*. Prompted voiding implies that caregivers, rather than the patient, initiate the decision to void (Burkhard et al., 2020). This is best suited for daytime use in settings where caregivers can follow the protocol and with patients who do not require more than one person to assist with transfer and who show improvement in an initial 3-day trial.

Intermittent Self-Catheterization. Some patients with chronic disorders such as spinal cord injury learn to perform self-catheterization. The patient must be physically able to manipulate equipment and assume a position for successful catheterization (NSWOCC, CNCA, UNC & IPAC, 2020). The nurse must teach the patient the structure of the urinary tract, the clean versus sterile technique, the importance of adequate fluid intake, and the frequency of self-catheterization. An individual is advised to catheterize at a frequency to achieve a catheterized volume no greater than 500 mL per catheterization, unless otherwise directed by their health care provider. This typically equates to four to six catheterizations in 24 hours for an individual who is dependent on catheterization for all urine output (NSWOCC, CNCA, UNC & IPAC, 2020).

Pharmacological Strategies. Medication therapy, either alone or in combination with other therapies, can help address issues of urinary incontinence and retention. The major categories of medication are presented in Table 44.6.

> **SAFETY ALERT** α-Adrenergic blockers may cause postural hypotension and increase the patient's risk of falling and injury. Instruct patients taking these medications to plan their nighttime toileting and to get out of bed slowly.

TABLE 44.6	Medications Used to Treat Urinary Incontinence and Retention			
Classification	**Action**	**Generic Name**	**Adverse Effects**	**Contraindications, Effects, or Alerts/ Comments**
Urge incontinence: Antimuscarinics (anticholinergics)	• Anticholinergic/ antimuscarinic • Inhibits effect of acetylcholine on smooth muscle antispasmodic	Fesoterodine, Oxybutynin (including immediate release [IR]) Propiverine (including IR), Solifenacin, Tolterodine (including IR), Trospium (including IR)	Dry mouth is the most common adverse effect, although constipation, blurred vision, fatigue and cognitive dysfunction may occur. Once daily (extended release) formulations are associated with lower rates of adverse events compared to IR formulations.	Narrow-angle glaucoma Gastrointestinal obstruction Ulcerative colitis Myasthenia gravis Retention elevated residual. Long-term antimuscarinic treatment should be used with caution in older patients, especially those who are at risk for or have cognitive dysfunction.
β_3- Adrenoreceptor agonist	Stimulates β_3 adrenoreceptors to promote detrusor (bladder) relaxation	Mirabegron	The most common adverse effects include hypertension, nasopharyngitis, and UTI.	Not for use in those with systolic BP >180 mm Hg or diastolic BP >110 mm Hg
Urinary incontinence (UI) associated with chronic retention of urine (previously from prostatic hyperplasia): α-Adrenergic blockers	Block α receptors to relax bladder neck or proximal urethra and reduce symptoms of obstructive voiding	Terazosin Doxazosin Tamsulosin	Postural hypotension, syncope, and fainting	Patients taking antihypertensives will require dosage titration.
Stress or urge incontinence in postmenopausal individuals with female genitalia: Low-dose, topical (vaginal) hormone replacement therapy	Reduces irritation and atrophic vaginitis. Can reduce symptoms of overactive bladder and stress incontinence as well as reducing the frequency of UTIs	Low-dose estrogen creams, tablets, or rings	Sore breasts Spotting (rare with a low dose)	In patients with a history of breast cancer, the treating oncologist should be consulted.
Nocturia: Antidiuretic hormone analogues	To treat primary nocturnal enuresis (bedwetting) in children and nocturnal polyuria in adults by decreasing urine output through replacing arginine vasopressin (antidiuretic hormone)	Desmopressin	Hyponatremia	Caution required for use in frail older persons. The use of desmopressin carries a risk of developing hyponatremia. Do not use desmopressin for long-term control of UI.

BP, Blood pressure; *UTI*, urinary tract infection.
Data from Burkhard, F.C., Bosch, J. L. H. R., Cruz, F., et al. (2020). *European Association of Urology guidelines on urinary incontinence in adults.* https://uroweb.org/wp-content/uploads/EAU-Guidelines-on-Urinary-Incontinence-2020.pdf

◆ **Evaluation**

Patient Care. The patient is the best source of evaluation of outcomes and responses to nursing care (Figure 44.18). However, nurses will also evaluate the effectiveness of nursing interventions through comparisons with baseline data. The nurse should evaluate for changes in the patient's voiding pattern, the presence of urinary tract alteration, and the patient's physical condition. Actual outcomes are compared with expected outcomes to determine the patient's health status. Continuous evaluation enables the nurse to determine whether new or revised therapies are required or if any new nursing diagnoses have developed.

Patient Expectations. If, as a nurse, you have developed a trusting relationship with a patient, indications of the patient's degree of satisfaction with their care will be evident. The patient may smile or nod in appreciation. However, you need to confirm whether the patient's expectations have been met to full satisfaction. You may need to ask specifically about the patient's degree of urinary control and comfort. If simply asked, "How are you feeling today?" the patient may reply with a noncommittal "Okay." You need specific information about how well an intervention has met the patient's need in order to continue or revise the care plan. You can also assist the patient in redefining unrealistic expectations when impairment in function is not likely to be altered as completely as they might like.

Knowledge
- Clinical signs of normal micturition
- Characteristics of normal urine
- Behaviours that demonstrate learning

Experience
- Previous patient responses to planned nursing interventions to promote urinary elimination

Evaluation
- Reassess the patient's urination pattern and signs and symptoms of alterations
- Inspect the character of the patient's urine
- Have the patient and family demonstrate any self-care skills
- Have the patient discuss feelings regarding any permanent changes in elimination
- Ask patient if expectations are being met

Standards
- Use expected outcomes established in patient's plan of care
- Use established expected outcomes from professional organizations to evaluate the patient's response to care

Qualities
- Be accountable and responsible for onset of any complications related to care
- Demonstrate perseverance when necessary because some interventions (e.g., pelvic floor exercises) may take weeks to months to effect any change
- Adapt and revise approaches if interventions are ineffective

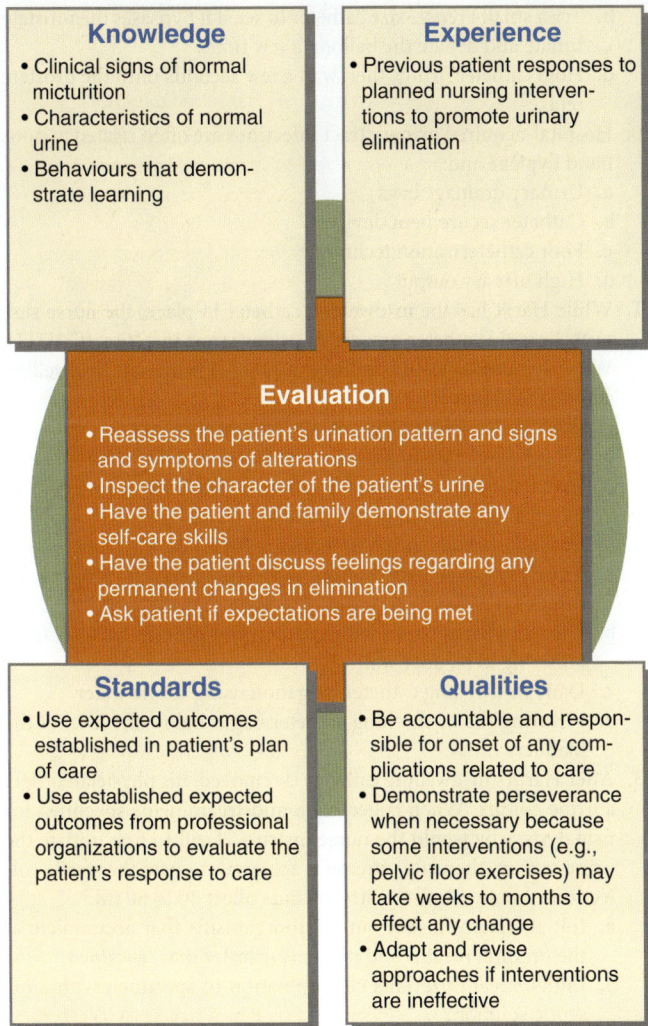

FIGURE 44.18 Critical thinking model for urinary elimination evaluation.

KEY CONCEPTS

- The act of micturition, or voiding, is influenced by complex interactions between the bladder, spinal cord, and brain, involving autonomic (involuntary) and somatic (voluntary) nerves. Symptoms common to urinary disturbances include urgency, frequency, dysuria, polyuria, oliguria, and difficulty in starting the urinary stream.
- When collected properly, a clean-voided urine specimen does not contain bacteria from the urethral meatus.
- Methods of promoting the micturition reflex assist patients in sensing the urge to urinate and urethral sphincter relaxation.
- An increased fluid intake results in increased urine formation, which reduces the risk of urinary tract infections.
- An in-dwelling urinary catheter remains in the bladder for an extended period. It has potential for biofilm formation, making the risk of infection greater than with intermittent catheterization.
- Closed catheter irrigation may be needed to maintain catheter patency and prevent blood clots, especially after urological surgery.
- A catheter drainage system should be a closed system positioned to allow free drainage of urine by gravity.
- Incontinence is classified as transient, urge, stress, mixed, and functional. Each type can be addressed through a variety of nursing interventions and prescribed treatments.

- Nurses need to follow specific guidelines for in-dwelling catheter insertion to reduce the occurrence of catheter-associated urinary tract infections. In acute care, nurses have an important role in advocating for the removal of in-dwelling catheters if these are no longer needed.

CRITICAL THINKING EXERCISES

1. A 77-year-old patient (preferred pronouns: she/her) has had problems with urgency and urge incontinence for the past 2 years. The episodes are becoming increasingly frequent. She has been attempting to deal with the incontinence by using an absorbent pad in her underwear, but she feels as though everyone knows about her incontinence. The embarrassment of urinary odours often keeps her at home. She has given up attending daily mass at church.
   a. How can you help this patient regain control of her urinary elimination?
   b. What nursing diagnoses apply to this patient?
   c. For one of the diagnoses, provide one goal or outcome and two nursing interventions.

2. A 37-year-old patient with female genitalia has been admitted with back pain radiating downward into their groin. The patient has also noticed blood in their urine for a week, but was hoping it would go away. The patient is scheduled to undergo an intravenous pyelogram (IVP) in 4 hours.
   a. What is the purpose of the IVP?
   b. What nursing care is needed before this patient goes to the radiography department?
   c. Provide at least two nursing responsibilities for care of a patient who has undergone an IVP.

3. A 70-year-old patient (preferred pronouns: she/her) has physical limitations related to rheumatoid arthritis. Her daughter, with whom she lives, has brought her to her family practitioner's office. You are the family nurse practitioner in the practice. As you assess the patient, you ask her how she is coping. She begins to answer but then starts to cry and says, "I know when I have to go to the bathroom, but I often don't make it in time." Her daughter asks you for suggestions on how to manage, as she has noticed that her mother's perineal skin is reddened and sore. What assessments need to be completed before planning interventions for this patient's care?

Answers to Critical Thinking Exercises appear on the Evolve website.

REVIEW QUESTIONS

Review Questions 1 to 14 relate to the case study at the beginning of the chapter.

1. How could this onset of urinary incontinence affect Harjit?
   a. The patient may feel the incontinence is part of getting older and decide not to seek help.
   b. The patient may worry that the incontinence could cause urinary tract infections.
   c. The patient is not bothered at all by these changes in his urinary function and control.
   d. The patient feels that all these symptoms are related to not being circumcised at birth.

2. Prostate enlargement can contribute to lower urinary tract issues in which of the following ways?
   a. By causing stress urinary incontinence
   b. By causing urinary frequency and possibly retention

    c. By causing a change in the colour and odour of urine

    d. By increasing the acidity of the urine

3. Nocturia is "the number of times urine is passed during the main sleeping period." What factors can contribute to nocturia?

    a. Weak pelvic floor muscles after radical prostatectomy

    b. Obesity and the number of vaginal deliveries

    c. Peripheral edema and obstructive sleep apnea

    d. Long-time use of an in-dwelling urinary catheter

4. The normal urine output for an adult like Harjit is:

    a. 1 000 mL/day

    b. 1 500 to 1 600 mL/day

    c. 3 000 to 3 200 mL/day

    d. 4 000 mL/day

5. Harjit has to rush to the bathroom when he experiences an urge to urinate and he leaks urine on the way. This is most likely urge incontinence. Which factors can contribute to urge incontinence?

    a. Prostate cancer and radical prostatectomy surgery

    b. Obesity, number of deliveries, ethnicity

    c. Kidney failure treated with peritoneal dialysis

    d. Central nervous system disorders and outflow obstruction

6. What history should the nurse consider that could be contributing to Harjit's lower urinary tract symptoms of urgency, frequency, and nocturia?

    a. Whether he has had micturition syncope associated with dehydration

    b. Whether he had issues with toilet training and bedwetting as a young child

    c. Whether he had radical prostatectomy surgery for prostate cancer

    d. Whether he has an elevated postvoid residual volume due to an enlarged prostate

7. The nurse asks Harjit to complete a 3-day bladder diary. How could a bladder diary assist the nurse in the diagnosis and treatment of incontinence?

    a. To evaluate lifestyle habits (e.g., fluid intake) in relation to the voiding pattern and symptoms

    b. To determine fluid and fibre intake and to assess and treat constipation

    c. To evaluate mobility and ability to dress or undress and use the toilet independently

    d. To evaluate how the alterations in elimination affect lifestyle and quality of life

8. What size of in-dwelling catheter would be best for Harjit?

    a. 12 to 16 Fr gauge

    b. 8 to 10 Fr gauge

    c. 20 to 24 Fr gauge

    d. 30 Fr gauge

9. When inserting an in-dwelling urinary catheter, the nurse feels resistance as the catheter meets Harjit's prostate. Which of the following is an appropriate nursing intervention?

    a. Firmly apply pressure to the catheter until it bypasses the prostate

    b. Try a small French-size catheter to see if it bypasses the prostate

    c. Inflate and deflate the balloon a few times

    d. Hold catheter firmly, then wait a few seconds until the prostate relaxes

10. Hospital-acquired urinary tract infections are often related to poor hand hygiene and:

    a. Urinary drainage bags

    b. Catheter securement devices

    c. Poor catheterization technique

    d. High urinary output

11. While Harjit has the in-dwelling catheter in place, the nurse suspects he had a catheter-associated urinary tract infection (CAUTI). What symptoms would indicate a CAUTI when an in-dwelling catheter is in place?

    a. Burning on voiding/dysuria and urinary urgency

    b. Cloudy, foul-smelling urine or a change in urine colour

    c. Urinary incontinence and bright red blood in the urine

    d. Fever, chills, vomiting, and malaise

12. What is a key intervention in reducing CAUTIs?

    a. Timely removal of in-dwelling catheters that are no longer indicated

    b. Diet supplementation with cranberry to prevent bacteria from adhering to bladder wall

    c. Daily in-dwelling catheter irrigation using sterile water

    d. Ensuring the in-dwelling catheter bag is below the level of the bladder

13. After Harjit's in-dwelling catheter is removed, his physician orders a urine culture. When collecting a midstream urine specimen for urinalysis, why would the nurse instruct Harjit to first initiate the urine stream, then after stream is achieved, to pass the sterile collection container into the stream and collect 30 to 60 mL?

    a. Initial stream flushes out microorganisms that accumulate at the urethral meatus and prevents transfer into specimen.

    b. Initial stream prevents contamination of specimen with antiseptic solution.

    c. Initial stream prevents contamination of specimen with skin flora.

    d. Initial stream retains sterility of inside of container and prevents spillage of urine.

14. The day Harjit is being discharged home, he shares with his nurse that he still is having to rush to the bathroom to urinate and he can leak urine on the way. What would be an appropriate lifestyle modification that the nurse could discuss with Harjit to help with this urge incontinence?

    a. Decrease his total fluid intake to 1 000 mL per day

    b. Avoid caffeine and to strengthen his pelvic floor muscles

    c. Use a condom catheter and a leg bag

    d. Urinate every hour to avoid leakage of urine

Answers: 1. a; **2.** b; **3.** c; **4.** b; **5.** d; **6.** d; **7.** a; **8.** a; **9.** d; **10.** c; **11.** d; **12.** a; **13.** a; **14.** b.

🌐 *Rationales for the Review Questions appear on the Evolve website.*

RECOMMENDED WEBSITES

Canadian Continence Foundation: https://www.canadiancontinence.ca

The Canadian Continence Foundation is a national, nonprofit organization that serves the education needs of people experiencing incontinence. The foundation implements and promotes professional education and research to advanced treatment and management of incontinence.

Canadian Nurse Continence Advisors Association (CNCA): https://www.cnca.ca

This national association is mandated to enhance the specialty of nurse continence advisors (NCA) in Canada by promoting education, research, and clinical practice.

Continence Products Advisor: https://www.continenceproductadvisor.org

This website provides noncommercial, evidence-informed information for consumers and health care providers on continence products, including a wide variety of devices and equipment to support continence.

fur7International Continence Society (ICS): https://www.ics.org
This organization is an international society with a global focus to improve quality of life for those affected by urinary, bowel, and pelvic floor disorders. ICS addresses education, research, and advocacy regarding incontinence.

Kidney Foundation of Canada: https://www.kidney.ca
This national volunteer organization is committed to reducing the burden of kidney disease through funding research, providing education and support, promoting access to health care, and increasing public awareness about kidney health and organ donation.

Nurses Specialized in Wound, Ostomy and Continence Canada: https://nswoc.ca
Nurses Specialized in Wound, Ostomy and Continence Canada (NSWOCC) is a not-for-profit association for over 500 nurses specializing in the nursing care of patients with challenges in wound, ostomy, and continence.

NSWOCC acts in the public interest for nurses specialized in wound, ostomy and continence (NSWOC) to give national leadership in wound, ostomy, and continence, promoting high standards for NSWOC practice, education, research, and administration to achieve quality specialized nursing care.

Ostomy Canada Society: https://www.ostomycanada.ca
Ostomy Canada Society is a nonprofit volunteer organization dedicated to all people with an ostomy and to their families, helping them to live life to the fullest through support, education, collaboration, and advocacy.

Urology Nurses of Canada: https://www.unc.org
This national not-for profit association has a mandate to enhance the specialty of urological nursing in Canada by promoting education, leadership, research, and clinical practice. The activities of the Urology Nurses of Canada are designed to enrich members' professional growth and development.

REFERENCES

A full reference list is available on the website for this book at http://evolve.elsevier.com/Canada/Potter/fundamentals/

45

Bowel Elimination

Canadian content written by Barbara G. Anderson, RN, MN, with original chapter contributions by Jane Fellows, MSN, CWOCN-AP

OBJECTIVES

Mastery of content in this chapter will enable you to:

- Define the key terms listed.
- Explain the role of gastrointestinal organs in digestion and elimination.
- Describe the integrated processes of oral pharyngeal swallowing and breathing.
- Describe the functions of the large intestine.
- Explain the physiological aspects of normal defecation.
- Discuss the psychological and physiological factors that influence the elimination process.
- Describe the common physiological alterations in elimination.
- Assess a patient's pattern of elimination.
- List the nursing diagnoses related to alterations in elimination.
- Describe the nursing implications for common diagnostic examinations of the gastrointestinal tract.
- List the nursing measures that promote normal elimination.
- List the nursing measures included in bowel training.
- Describe the nursing measures required for patients with a bowel diversion.
- Use critical thinking in the provision of care to patients with alterations in bowel elimination.

KEY TERMS

Bolus

Bowel incontinence

Bowel retraining

Cathartics

Chyme

Colitis

Colostomy

Constipation

Defecation

Diarrhea

Effluent

Enema

Fecal immunochemical test (FIT)

Feces

Fibre

Flatulence

Flatus

Gastrocolic reflex

Hemorrhoids

Ileostomy

Impaction

Lactose intolerance

Laxatives

Masticate

Nurse specialized in wound, ostomy, and continence (NSWOC)

Paralytic ileus

Peristalsis

Peristaltic contractions

Rectal suppository

Stoma

Valsalva manoeuvre

🌐 WEBSITE

http://evolve.elsevier.com/Canada/Potter/fundamentals/

CASE STUDY

Olivia (preferred pronouns: she/her) is a 67-year-old retired registered practical nurse (RPN) living in Ontario who has been experiencing chronic constipation.

This case study will summarize three episodes of care: an inpatient medical/surgical unit hospital admission in 2018, an outpatient geriatric clinic visit in 2018, and an inpatient medical/surgical unit hospital admission in 2020.

Episode One: In 2018, Olivia came to the emergency department for repeated vomiting of bile emesis that started early in the day. Following a computed tomography (CT) scan, a bowel obstruction caused by a fecal impaction was diagnosed and Olivia was admitted to a medical/surgical unit.

Olivia required the insertion of a nasogastric (NG) tube and the administration of total parenteral nutrition (TPN) through a peripherally inserted central line. She was treated with laxatives and the administration of cleansing enemas repeatedly over 14 days, which finally cleared her bowel. Her bowel function returned after 10 days, and on day 14 she was discharged. On discharge, a referral was made to a gastroenterologist for an assessment and colonoscopy, as well as a referral for an assessment and follow-up in a geriatric outpatient clinic. Continence issues are a component of a comprehensive geriatric assessment.

Episode Two: A clinical nurse specialist/nurse continence advisor (CNS/NCA) assessed Olivia in the outpatient geriatric clinic for chronic constipation and bowel incontinence 3 months after her discharge from acute care.

Episode Three: Olivia was admitted once again as an inpatient to a medical/surgical unit in 2020, following a diagnosis of colon cancer after a colonoscopy. She will undergo a new pouching colostomy.

Think about this case study as you read this chapter. There are review questions at the end of the chapter that relate to the case study.

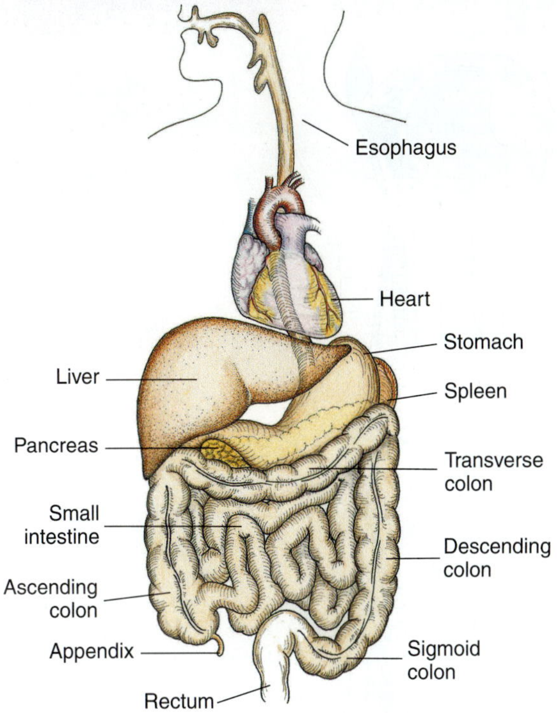

FIGURE 45.1 Organs of the gastrointestinal tract (with the heart as a reference point).

Bowel elimination is crucial to human function and hence critical for nurses to understand in the care of their patients. The gastrointestinal (GI) system is a remarkable structure that allows the ingestion of food and absorption of nutrients and, ultimately, the elimination of waste.

Regular elimination of bowel waste is essential for normal body functioning. Alterations in bowel elimination are often early indications of problems within either the GI tract or another body system.

To manage the bowel elimination problems of patients, as a nurse, you must understand the normal elimination process and the factors that promote, impede, or cause alterations in elimination. Of particular concern in managing bowel elimination is supportive nursing care that is respectful of the patient's privacy and emotional needs.

SCIENTIFIC KNOWLEDGE BASE

The purposes of the GI tract are to ingest food, break down the ingested food into absorbable forms (digestion), absorb fluid and nutrients, prepare food for both absorption and use by the body's cells, and provide temporary storage of feces. The GI tract is a series of hollow, multilayered, muscular organs that are lined with mucous membranes (Figure 45.1). The mucosal and muscle layers are innervated by the intrinsic enteric nervous system comprising sensory, interneuronal, and motor fibres. The rate of rhythmic contractions is specific to each organ and is controlled by the pacemaker cells in the muscle layers. The central nervous system receives input from the GI tract through sensory fibres, which travel in the vagus and sympathetic nerves. Extrinsic sympathetic and parasympathetic motor nerves terminate on the enteric nervous system and act to modulate the activity of the intrinsic enteric nervous system. The GI tract begins at the mouth and continues through to the anus. The mouth, esophagus, and stomach receive food, and initial digestion occurs. The duodenum, jejunum, and ileum are where most digestion and absorption occurs. Finally, the cecum, colon, and rectum store and then eliminate waste. The salivary glands, liver, and pancreas are accessory organs that aid digestion. The GI tract also functions as a specialized immune system, preventing bacteria and viruses of the nonsterile lumen from entering the bloodstream (Power-Kean et al., 2023).

Mouth

The mouth is the point of entry into the GI tract. The mouth mechanically and chemically breaks down nutrients into usable sizes and forms. The teeth **masticate** food, breaking it down into a soft, moist ball (a **bolus**) suitable for swallowing. Saliva, which is produced by the salivary glands in the mouth, dilutes and softens the food in the mouth for easier swallowing and commences digestion of carbohydrates. In addition, mucus from the salivary glands lubricates the passage of the bolus through the pharynx and down the esophagus during swallowing.

Swallowing begins with the lips closing and the tongue curling with its tip and then the back being pressed to the roof of the mouth (Figure 45.2). The action of swallowing tips the bolus into the pharynx. The pharyngeal cavity is common to both the GI tract and the respiratory tract. The swallowed bolus must cross the nasopharynx, and the soft palate must elevate toward the nasopharynx to prevent material from entering the back of the nose. To prevent aspiration, the vocal cords in the glottis close, the epiglottis moves downward to seal off the trachea, and breathing is inhibited in the central nervous system. The bolus enters the esophagus through the relaxed upper esophageal sphincter. This complex process is under striated muscle control and requires an intact nervous system (Power-Kean et al., 2023).

Esophagus

The esophagus provides a conduit to the stomach through the chest cavity. The esophagus is a straight tube about 25 cm in length. Smooth muscle layers of the esophagus provide the peristaltic contractions to move food along its length. Its mucous membranes secrete mucus that aids in the lubrication of food. Sphincters on either end of the esophagus prevent air from entering the esophagus and stomach during breathing and reflux of stomach contents into the esophagus (Power-Kean et al., 2023).

The bolus travels down the relaxed esophagus mainly by gravity to the lower esophageal sphincter, which is opened by the initiation of swallowing in the pharynx and upper esophageal sphincter. A wave of **peristaltic contractions** propels the bolus into the stomach. Peristaltic contractions relax over the bolus and contract behind the bolus, thus moving contents through the length of the GI tract. If the bolus moves slowly or is stuck, a local reflex will relax the area ahead of the bolus and produce a powerful contraction behind the bolus. In the esophagus, this action is known as *secondary peristalsis*. Tertiary contractions of the esophagus are frequently simultaneous and are produced by irritation of the mucosa by gastric contents. These contractions can be extremely painful and may mimic cardiac chest pain (Power-Kean et al., 2023).

Stomach

The stomach performs several tasks: storage of swallowed food and liquid, mixing of food with liquid and gastric digestive juices, and the controlled emptying of its contents through the pyloric sphincter into the small intestine. The stomach is a baglike structure located in the upper quadrant of the abdomen.

Peristaltic and mixing contractions of the stomach are controlled by the intrinsic pacemaker activity of the smooth muscle cells. The stomach is innervated by the enteric nervous system and connections to the parasympathetic and sympathetic nervous systems. The emptying of the stomach is regulated by neural and hormonal mechanisms.

The stomach produces two key GI hormones: gastrin and ghrelin. Gastrin stimulates gastric acid secretion. Ghrelin is newly discovered and has growth hormone–releasing activity and stimulates food intake and digestion while reducing energy expenditures. Gastrin and somatostatin regulate the secretion of acid and pepsin in the stomach.

The stomach also secretes hydrochloric acid (HCl) and the intrinsic factor. HCl facilitates the digestion of protein and is antibacterial. The intrinsic factor is essential in the absorption of vitamin B_{12}. Mucus protects the stomach mucosa from acidity and enzyme

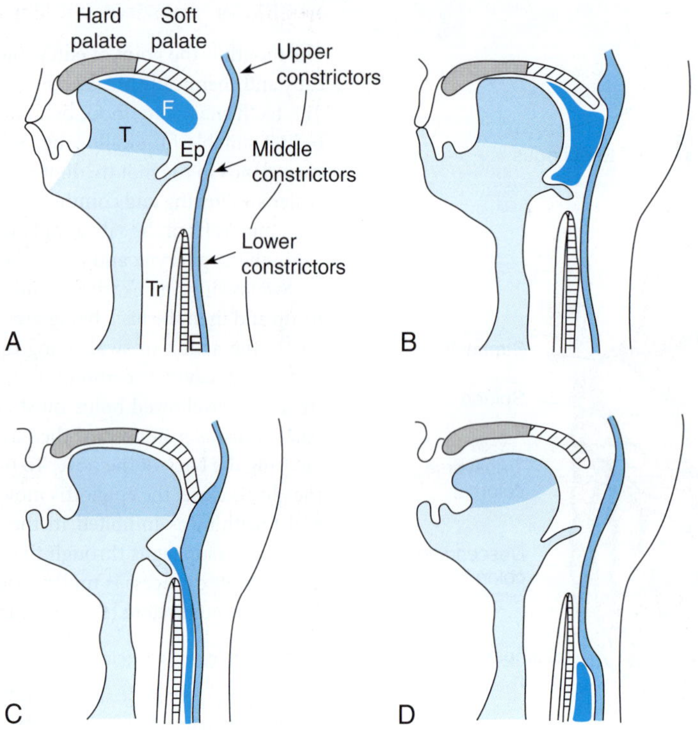

FIGURE 45.2 Oral and pharyngeal events during swallowing. **A,** The bolus (*F*) is propelled into the pharynx by placement of the tongue (*T*) on the hard palate. **B,** Further propulsion is caused by movement of the more distal regions of the tongue against the palate. Contraction of the upper constrictors of the pharynx and the soft palate separates the oropharynx from the nasopharynx. **C,** Contraction of the pharynx and relaxation of the cricopharyngeal muscle propel the bolus through the upper esophageal sphincter. Upward movement of the glottis and downward movement of the epiglottis (*Ep*) seal off the trachea (*Tr*), and the respiratory drive is inhibited in the central nervous system. **D,** The bolus is now in the esophagus (*E*) and is propelled into the stomach by a peristaltic contraction. (From Johnson, L. R. [2013]. *Gastrointestinal physiology* [7th ed., p. 28]. Mosby.)

activity (Power-Kean et al., 2023). The rate at which the stomach empties depends on the content of the dissolved and partially digested bolus (**chyme**). Water diffuses from both the stomach and the small intestine and is emptied rapidly. Carbohydrates are emptied only slightly more slowly, particularly if they are not strongly acidic. Proteins empty even more slowly and in smaller amounts as determined by the acidity of the chyme. Fats are emptied the slowest of all. The controlled emptying allows the pancreatic secretions and bile to neutralize the chyme and secrete enzymes for luminal digestion (Power-Kean et al., 2023).

Small Intestine

The small intestine consists of the duodenum, jejunum, and ileum. The duodenum is about 22 cm long and connects the stomach to the jejunum. The duodenum also contains the opening for the common bile duct and main pancreatic duct. The jejunum and ileum are over 7 m long and are folded closely to fit in the abdomen (Power-Kean et al., 2023).

The duodenum continues to process the chyme from the stomach. The chyme that enters the duodenum is acidic and contains partially digested protein, carbohydrates, and unemulsified fats. The presence of these substances stimulates the release of the hormones secretin and cholecystokinin from the duodenal mucosa. Secretin stimulates the pancreas to secrete bicarbonate to neutralize the acid. Cholecystokinin stimulates the pancreas to secrete the following enzymes: (1) amylases, which convert carbohydrates to disaccharides; (2) proteases, which further hydrolyze proteins into smaller peptides; and (3) lipases, which hydrolyze triglycerides into fatty acids and monoglycerides. The presence of fats in the duodenum further stimulates cholecystokinin release, which causes the gallbladder to contract, which in turn releases bile to emulsify the fats. Any blockage of the release of these enzymes prevents the digestion of fats and proteins and results in large, fatty, and foul-smelling

stools. Undigested fats and proteins reach the colon and are responsible for the changes in fecal appearance (Power-Kean et al., 2023).

The second section of the small intestine, the jejunum, is approximately 2.7 m long. Its primary function is the absorption of carbohydrates and proteins. The ileum, which is approximately 3.7 m long, specializes in the absorption of water, certain vitamins, iron, fats, and bile salts. Most nutrients and electrolytes are absorbed in the small intestine, specifically by the duodenum and the jejunum.

If the small intestine function is impaired, the digestive process is greatly altered. For example, conditions such as inflammation, surgical resection, or obstruction can disrupt contractile activity, reduce the area of absorption, or block the passage of chyme. As a result, electrolyte and nutrient deficiencies can develop (Power-Kean et al., 2023).

Large Intestine

The lower GI tract is called the large intestine because it is larger in diameter than the small intestine; however, at 1.5 to 1.8 m in length, it is much shorter. The large intestine is the primary organ of bowel elimination and is divided into the cecum, the colon, and the rectum (Figure 45.3).

Chyme from the terminal ileum enters the cecum of the large intestine, propelled by waves of peristalsis through the ileocecal sphincter, a circular muscle layer that regulates ileal emptying and prevents regurgitation of fecal contents.

The colon is divided into the ascending, transverse, descending, and sigmoid colons. The colon's muscular tissue allows it to accommodate and eliminate large quantities of waste and gas (**flatus**). The colon has three functions: absorption, secretion, and elimination. Each day, a large volume of water and significant amounts of sodium and chloride are absorbed by the colon (Power-Kean et al., 2023).

Two types of muscle contractions occur in the colon: slow-mixing contractions and mass **peristalsis** (or mass movement). Slow-mixing

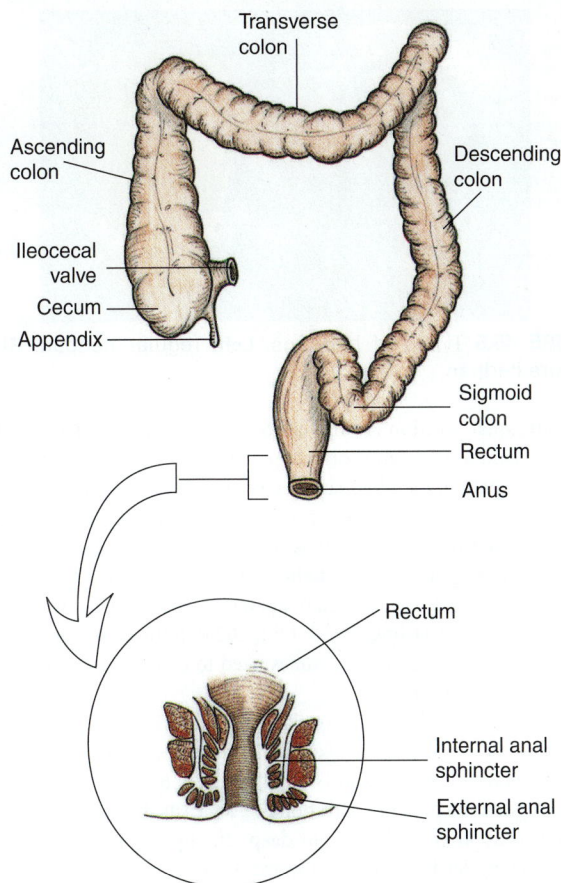

FIGURE 45.3 Divisions of the large intestine.

contractions move contents through the colon and expose the chyme to the mucosa, where active absorption of sodium and chloride causes water absorption and dries the chyme to feces. Intestinal content is the main stimulus for the slow-mixing contractions. Mass peristalsis movements then push the feces toward the rectum. The ingestion of food is the main stimulus for mass peristalsis, which is known as the gastrocolic reflex. In adults, these mass movements occur only three or four times each day (Power-Kean et al., 2023).

When the slow-mixing contractions increase and the mass peristalsis diminishes, water continues to be absorbed and the feces dry out, resulting in constipation. Conversely, when the mixing movements are decreased and the mass peristalsis is increased, the water has less time to be absorbed, and the stool will be watery (diarrhea) (Power-Kean et al., 2023).

The secretory function of the colon aids in electrolyte balance. Bicarbonate is secreted in exchange for chloride. Approximately 4 to 9 mmol of potassium is also excreted daily. Extreme alterations in colon function (e.g., diarrhea) can cause severe electrolyte disturbances (Power-Kean et al., 2023). The rectum is the final portion of the large intestine. Normally, the rectum is empty of waste products, or feces, until just before defecation. The rectum contains vertical and transverse folds of tissue that may help to temporarily hold fecal contents during defecation. Each fold contains an artery and vein that can become distended from pressure during straining. This distension can result in the formation of hemorrhoids (Power-Kean et al., 2023).

The volume of fluids absorbed by the GI tract is high. Oral fluid intake is approximately 1.2 L per day; an additional 7 L of fluid enters from the blood as the result of the secretion of digestive enzymes by the mucosa, liver, gallbladder, and pancreas, and by osmosis as the

numbers of molecules in the lumen increase by digestion. Absorption from the small and large intestine amounts to 8.1 L per day, leaving 100 mL to be excreted in the feces. Therefore, maintaining fluid and electrolyte balance is a key function of the GI system (Power-Kean et al., 2023).

Anus and Rectum

The means of preserving continence and defecation is complex and multifaceted, entailing the incorporation of somatic and visceral mechanisms, under the control of the central nervous system (Oliveira et al., 2020). These mechanisms involve the flawless coordination among the brain, spinal cord, enteric neurons, the muscle of the colon, the rectum, anus, and pelvic floor (Oliveira et al., 2020). Feces and flatus are expelled from the rectum through the anal canal and the anus. Contraction and relaxation of the internal anal sphincter are under autonomic (unconscious) control, whereas the external anal sphincter is under somatic neural (conscious) control. The anal canal is richly supplied with sensory and motor nerve fibres to help control continence. Additionally, the maintenance of the acute anorectal angle formed by the puborectalis and levator ani (pelvic floor) muscles may play a role in continence, but not necessarily the key role that was previously assumed (Oliveira et al., 2020).

When feces enter the rectum, the internal anal sphincter relaxes, and this enables the anal canal to determine if the contents are solid or liquid. This action occurs concurrently with the reflexive contraction of the external sphincter. Additionally, this contraction can be accompanied by a voluntary squeeze of the sphincter muscles. The rectum is able to hold feces until their presence stimulates stretch receptors in the mucosa, producing an urge to defecate. The patient then seeks out an appropriate place to defecate, assumes a squatting position to straighten the anorectal angle, and voluntarily relaxes the external sphincter. Bearing down tenses abdominal muscles. The pelvic floor muscles relax and the feces enter the lower rectum. Involuntary propulsive contractions continue until the rectum is emptied. When the last of the feces passes, the external anal sphincter reflexively closes (Oliveira et al., 2020).

NURSING KNOWLEDGE BASE

Process of Defecation

The physiological factors critical to bowel function and defecation include the acute anorectal angle; reflexes that cause the external anal sphincter to contract when the internal anal sphincter relaxes; pressure in the anal canal at rest facilitated by the internal anal sphincter and voluntary action of the external anal sphincter; sensory response of the rectum to filling with feces; absorption of fluid from the intestine to create formed stool consistency; complete evacuation of the rectum; and physical and cognitive abilities to get to the bathroom when needed. Stool consistency affects rectal sensation, emptying, and anal continence (Oliveira et al., 2020). Normal defecation should be painless, resulting in the passage of a soft, formed stool.

Defecation begins with contractions in the left colon, moving the stool toward the anus. When a stool reaches the rectum, the distension causes relaxation of the internal anal sphincter and signals an awareness of the need to defecate. At the time of defecation, the external sphincter relaxes and abdominal muscles contract to increase intrarectal pressure and force the stool out (Oliveira et al., 2020).

Position During Defecation. Instead of straining, patients should be taught about the optimal position to facilitate defecation. Squatting is the normal position during defecation. Toilets are designed to facilitate this posture, by allowing the person to lean forward, exert

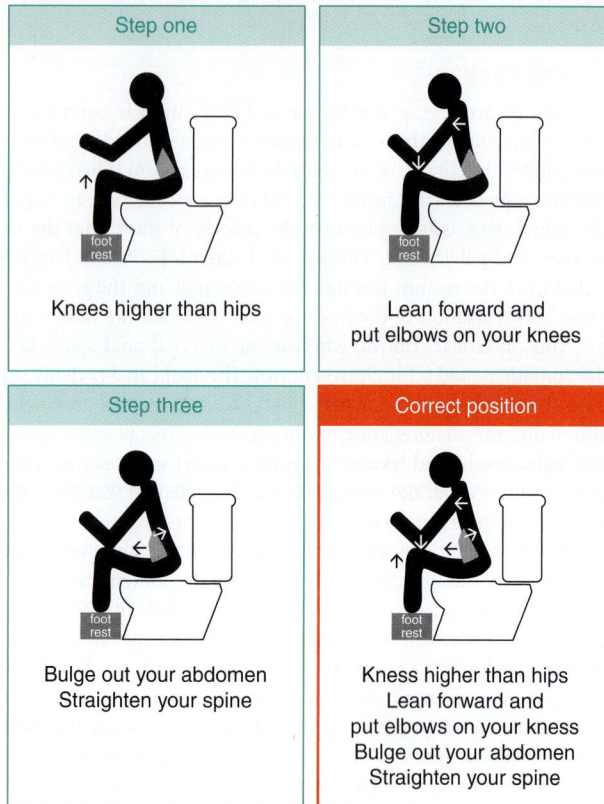

Correct position for opening your bowels

Step one	Step two
Knees higher than hips	Lean forward and put elbows on your knees

Step three	Correct position
Bulge out your abdomen Straighten your spine	Kness higher than hips Lean forward and put elbows on your kness Bulge out your abdomen Straighten your spine

FIGURE 45.4 Correct position for opening the bowels during defecation. (Redrawn by permission of Ray Addison, Nurse Consultant in Bladder and Bowel Dysfunction, and Wendy Ness, Colorectal Nurse Specialist. Produced by Norgine Pharmaceuticals Limited, 2003.)

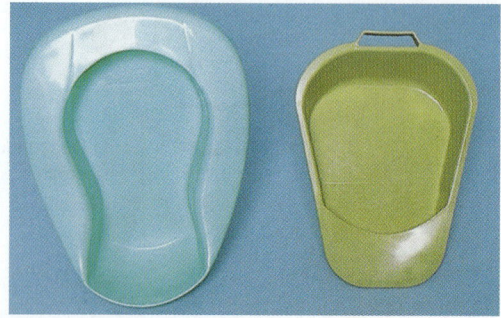

FIGURE 45.5 Types of bedpans. **Left,** regular bedpan. **Right,** fracture bedpan.

intra-abdominal pressure, and contract the thigh muscles. Bulging out the abdomen—rather than contracting the abdominal muscles—more effectively opens the bowels (Figure 45.4). For patients who are immobilized in bed, defecation is often difficult. In a supine position, it is impossible to contract the muscles used during defecation. If the patient's condition permits, the head of the bed should be raised to 30 to 60 degrees; this action assists the patient to a sitting position on a bedpan, promoting defecation (Klingman & Loft, 2020).

Promotion of Normal Defecation. Several interventions can stimulate the defecation reflex, affect the character of feces, or increase peristalsis to help patients evacuate bowel contents normally and without discomfort.

Sitting Position. Nurses might need to assist patients who have difficulty sitting because of muscular weakness and mobility challenges. Regular toilets are too low for patients who are unable to lower themselves to a sitting position because of joint- or muscle-wasting diseases. Elevated toilet seats require less effort to sit or stand; however, they can create difficulties in achieving a squat position. In many provinces and territories, elevated toilet seats can be acquired through a service agency for minimal or no cost. The community nurse will complete a home assessment that considers the patient's abilities and any needed equipment or assistive devices to facilitate bowel management.

Positioning on Bedpan. Encouraging patients to use a toilet or bedside commode best supports a bowel movement because of an adequate squat position (Klingman & Loft, 2020). The nurse needs to perform hand hygiene and confirm patient identification prior to positioning the patient on a bedpan. Personal protective equipment (PPE) is worn for transmission-based precautions (e.g., contact). Patients restricted to bed must use bedpans for defecation. The nurse needs to determine if the patient is able to help in positioning on a bedpan; otherwise, providing or removing a bedpan is more readily facilitated with two care providers (Klingman & Loft, 2020). Sitting on a bedpan can be extremely uncomfortable. Nurses need to help patients to position themselves comfortably.

Two types of bedpans are available (Figure 45.5). The regular bedpan, made of metal or hard plastic, has a curved, smooth upper end and a tapered lower end and is approximately 5 cm deep. A fracture pan, designed for patients with body or leg casts, has a shallow upper end and is approximately 1.3 cm deep. The upper end (wide end) of the pan fits under the buttocks toward the sacrum, and the lower end (tapered end) fits just under the upper thighs. The pan should be high enough so that feces enter the pan. The nurse should not force the bedpan under the patient's hips. A metal bedpan should be warmed with water first, then dried.

Nurses need to ensure that patients' privacy is maintained during bowel elimination. The call light and a supply of toilet paper should be within easy reach. When the patient finishes, the nurse should respond to the call signal immediately and remove the pan. The patient likely will require assistance with wiping. To remove the pan, the nurse can ask the patient to roll off to the side or to raise their hips. The pan should be held steady to avoid spilling. It is important to avoid pulling the pan from under the patient's hips; these actions can pull the patient's skin and cause tissue injury, such as shearing (see Chapter 47). After the pan is removed, while wearing gloves, the nurse cleans the anal and perineal areas and assists the patient with hand hygiene. After assessing the stool, the nurse should immediately empty the bedpan's contents into the toilet or in a special receptacle in the utility room. The bedpan should be rinsed thoroughly. Care must be taken to avoid splashing the contents or the rinse. Avoiding spillage is of critical importance when using universal infection control precautions. The patient uses the same bedpan each time. The nurse should refer to organizational policy for the sanitizing bedpans. Some organizations have disposable macerator products. The nurse charts the characteristics of the feces.

When positioning a patient on a bedpan, the nurse needs to use the proper method to prevent muscle strain and discomfort. This means never trying to lift a patient onto a bedpan. A patient should never be placed on a bedpan and then left with the bed flat unless demanded by activity restrictions. When the bed is flat, the hips remain hyperextended.

Figure 45.6 shows proper and improper positions on a bedpan. The best method is to ensure that the patient is positioned high in bed. The patient's head is raised about 30 degrees to prevent hyperextension of

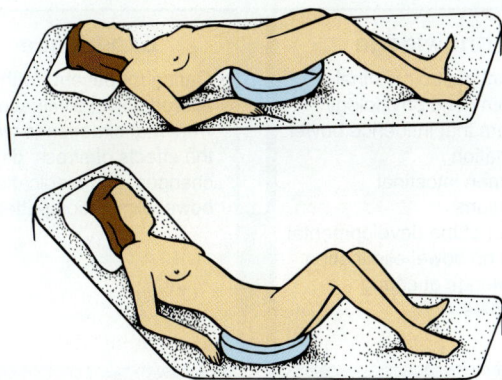

FIGURE 45.6 Positions on a bedpan. **Top,** Improper positioning of patient. **Bottom,** Proper positioning of the patient reduces back strain.

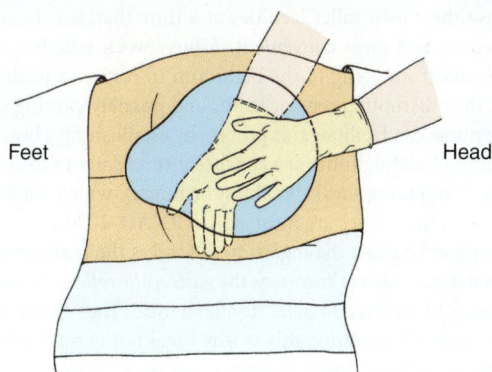

FIGURE 45.7 Positioning an immobilized patient on a bedpan.

the back and to provide support to the upper torso. The patient then raises their hips by bending the knees and lifting the hips upward. The nurse places their hand, palm up, under the patient's sacrum, resting the elbow on the mattress and using it as a lever to help in lifting, while slipping the pan under the patient. Patients who have had abdominal surgery are hesitant to exert strain on suture lines and may have difficulty positioning themselves on a bedpan. To prevent abrasions, the nurse should not force the pan along the patient's skin. Nurses must always wear gloves when handling a bedpan.

If the patient is immobile or if it is unsafe to allow the patient to exert such effort, as the patient's nurse you can assist the patient to roll onto the bedpan by using the following steps:

1. Lower the head of the bed flat and assist the patient to roll onto one side, backside toward you.
2. Place the bedpan firmly against the buttocks, down into the mattress with the open rim toward the patient's feet (Figure 45.7).
3. Keeping one hand against the bedpan, place your other hand around the patient's far hip. Ask the patient to roll back onto the pan, flat in bed. Do not shove the pan under the patient.
4. When the patient is positioned comfortably, raise the head of the bed 30 degrees.
5. Place a rolled towel or small pillow under the lumbar curve of the patient's back for added comfort.
6. Ask the patient to bend their knees to assume a squatting position, unless contraindicated (Klingman & Loft, 2020). Avoid raising the knee gatch, to prevent contractures.

Factors Affecting Normal Bowel Elimination

Many factors influence the process of bowel elimination. Knowledge of these factors enables nurses to anticipate measures required to maintain a normal pattern of bowel elimination.

Diet. The food a person eats influences bowel elimination. Regular daily food intake helps to maintain a routine pattern of peristalsis in the colon. Fibre, the indigestible residue in the diet, provides the bulk of fecal material. Dietary fibre is classified as insoluble and soluble fibre. Insoluble fibre is found in whole grains, wheat bran, and vegetables and does not dissolve in water. It is effective in preventing constipation. Soluble fibres are found in some beans, certain fruits and vegetables, and wheat bran. Soluble fibre forms a gel when mixed with water and is not as effective in preventing constipation. Low dietary fibre and poor fluid intake are common predisposing factors to constipation, resulting in a stool consistency that is dry, hard, and difficult to pass (Registered Nurses' Association of Ontario [RNAO], 2020).

Ingestion of a high-fibre diet or taking a fibre supplement can improve the likelihood of a regular bowel elimination pattern if other factors are normal. However, because fibre retains fluid in the GI tract, when additional fibre is ingested, adequate fluid intake is essential; inadequate fluid intake can lead to serious constipation or impaction. Recommended daily fluid intake for adults is at minimum 1.5 L.

Intolerance to certain foods can cause problems with bowel elimination. For example, lactose intolerance is the inability to digest lactose, the predominant sugar in milk. When lactose cannot be absorbed, it acts as an osmotic laxative, resulting in pain, abdominal distension, flatulence, and diarrhea (Fassio et al., 2018). Individuals who have lactose intolerance must learn how much lactose their body can tolerate. For example, some individuals can drink one glass of milk without effect, but not two.

Fluid Intake. An inadequate fluid intake or disturbances that result in fluid loss (such as vomiting) can affect the character of feces. Fluid liquefies intestinal contents to ease their passage through the colon. Reduced fluid intake slows the passage of food through the intestine and can result in hardening of the stool. Unless a medical contraindication exists, an adult should drink six to eight glasses (1 500 to 2 000 mL) of noncaffeinated fluid daily (RNAO, 2020). Equally important is to avoid consuming large amounts of caffeinated beverages, such as tea and coffee, as they can be irritating to the bowel and dehydrating. Some patients find that artificial sweeteners can be a bowel irritant as well (Cowie et al., 2014).

Older persons tend to have an insufficient intake of fluids and are more at risk of developing constipation. Sometimes, older persons reduce their fluid intake in an attempt to reduce micturition (see Chapter 44). In addition, in some individuals an increased ingestion of milk or milk products may slow peristalsis and cause constipation (Fassio et al., 2018).

Physical Activity. Physical activity promotes peristalsis, whereas immobilization depresses peristalsis. Thus, early ambulation is encouraged as a patient's illness begins to resolve or as soon as possible after surgery, to promote maintenance of peristalsis and thereby normal bowel elimination. Maintaining the tone of skeletal muscles used during defecation is important. Weakened abdominal and pelvic floor muscles impair the ability to increase intra-abdominal pressure and to control the external sphincter. Muscle tone may be weakened or lost as a result of long-term illness or neurological disease that impairs nerve transmission. Patients who experience these changes in the abdominal and pelvic floor muscles are at increased risk for constipation (Sibanda et al., 2018).

Personal Bowel Elimination Habits. Personal bowel elimination habits can affect bowel function. Most individuals benefit from being able to use their own toilet facilities at a time that, for them, is both most effective and most convenient. A busy work schedule may prevent a person from going to the bathroom in response to the urge to defecate, thus disrupting regular habits and possibly causing constipation. The nurse can facilitate this process by establishing a bowel protocol, including toileting times at a consistent time daily 15 to 20 minutes following a triggering meal (breakfast or lunch), which capitalizes on when gastrocolic reflexes are most active (RNAO, 2020).

As discussed earlier, the ingestion of food is the main stimulus for mass peristalsis, which is known as the *gastrocolic reflex*. This reflex frequently leads to the need to defecate after a meal. The reflex is strongest when the stomach is empty; this is why breakfast is referred to as the "triggering meal" for a bowel movement for most people.

Privacy. The patient's privacy must be maintained during bowel elimination. In hospital or long-term care settings, where patients may be in ward accommodation, maintaining visual, auditory, and olfactory privacy is important. Ignoring the call to have a bowel movement will result in weaker future defecation signals (Sibanda et al., 2018).

Privacy and sensitivity must also be attended to when discussing bowel elimination with patients. Patients may be cautious about discussing bowel elimination because they are embarrassed to broach the subject. It is the nurse's responsibility to ask about bowel elimination problems and to create a therapeutic climate for the patient to voice their concerns (Bliss & Norton, 2010).

CRITICAL THINKING

Successful critical thinking requires a synthesis of knowledge, experience, information gathered from patients, critical thinking attitudes, and intellectual and professional standards. Clinical judgements require nurses to anticipate the information necessary, analyze the data, and make decisions regarding patient care. During the assessment (Figure 45.8), nurses must consider all elements that build toward making appropriate diagnoses and determining the contributing factors to a patient's issues.

To assess a patient's bowel elimination, nurses must integrate their knowledge from nursing and other disciplines to better understand a patient's response to bowel elimination interruptions. As emphasized earlier, patients often respond to disruptions in bowel elimination with embarrassment. Sensitivity on the nurse's part is essential.

❖ NURSING PROCESS AND BOWEL ELIMINATION

◆ Assessment

Assessment for bowel elimination patterns and abnormalities includes a nursing health history, a physical assessment of the abdomen, inspection of fecal characteristics, and a review of relevant test results. In addition, the nurse needs to determine the patient's perception of the problem and goals for treatment, medical history, pattern and types of fluid and food intake, chewing ability, medications, and recent illnesses and stressors.

Health History. The nursing health history provides a review of the patient's usual bowel patterns and habits. What a patient defines as "normal" may differ from factors and conditions that typically promote normal bowel elimination. The nurse can determine the patient's bowel elimination problems by first identifying the normal and abnormal patterns and habits and then understanding the patient's perception of what is normal and abnormal regarding bowel elimination. Much of the nursing health history can be organized around the factors that affect bowel elimination:

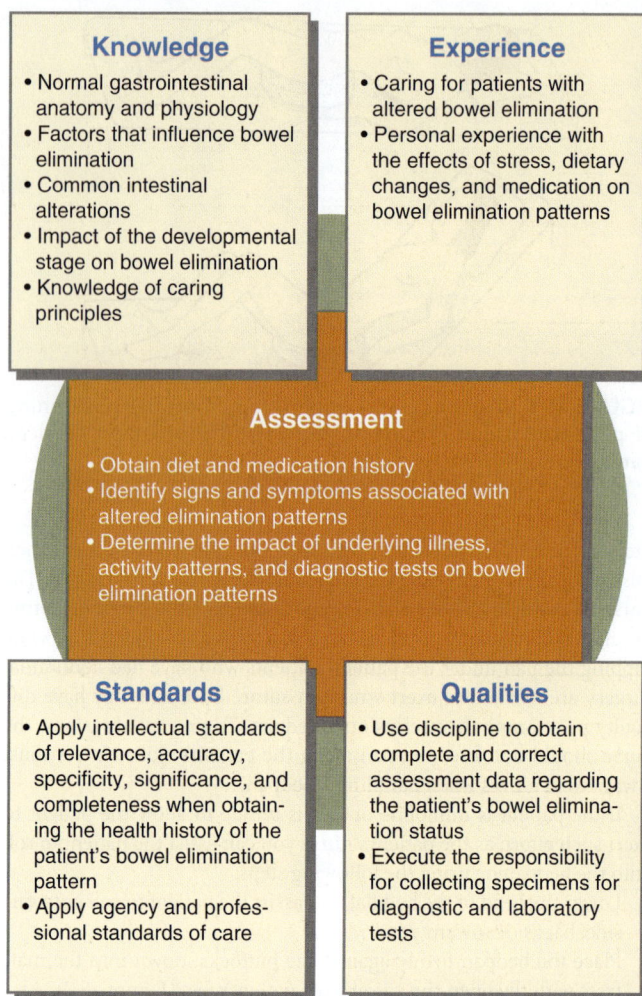

Knowledge
- Normal gastrointestinal anatomy and physiology
- Factors that influence bowel elimination
- Common intestinal alterations
- Impact of the developmental stage on bowel elimination
- Knowledge of caring principles

Experience
- Caring for patients with altered bowel elimination
- Personal experience with the effects of stress, dietary changes, and medication on bowel elimination patterns

Assessment
- Obtain diet and medication history
- Identify signs and symptoms associated with altered elimination patterns
- Determine the impact of underlying illness, activity patterns, and diagnostic tests on bowel elimination patterns

Standards
- Apply intellectual standards of relevance, accuracy, specificity, significance, and completeness when obtaining the health history of the patient's bowel elimination pattern
- Apply agency and professional standards of care

Qualities
- Use discipline to obtain complete and correct assessment data regarding the patient's bowel elimination status
- Execute the responsibility for collecting specimens for diagnostic and laboratory tests

FIGURE 45.8 Critical thinking model for bowel elimination assessment.

- *Determination of the patient's usual bowel elimination pattern:* The frequency and time of day of the patient's bowel eliminations should be noted. Have the patient or caregiver complete a bowel elimination diary for a week to enable an accurate assessment of the typical bowel elimination pattern.
- *The patient's description of the usual stool characteristics:* The patient's description should indicate whether the stool is normally watery or formed, soft or hard; the typical colour; whether the stool floats or sinks; and whether blood is present. Ask the patient to describe the usual shape of the stool and the number of stools per day. The Bristol Stool Form Scale is a helpful clinical tool used to show patients how to determine the nature of their usual stools (Figure 45.9).
- *Identification of routines followed to promote normal bowel elimination:* Examples of routines to promote bowel elimination are drinking hot liquids, eating specific foods, or taking time to defecate at a certain time of the day.
- *Assessment of the use of laxatives, suppositories, or enemas:* It is important to assess whether the patient uses enemas, laxatives, suppositories, or bulk-forming food additives in order to have a bowel movement. Ask the patient how often such an aid is used.
- *Assessment of cognitive abilities:* The nurse must determine the patient's ability to understand the questions posed. The nurse may need to conduct a brief mental status examination. In situations of concern, obtaining a corroborating history is critical.

The bristol stool form scale

Type 1	Separate hard lumps, like nuts (hard to pass)
Type 2	Sausage-shaped but lumpy
Type 3	Like a sausage but with cracks on its surface
Type 4	Like a sausage or snake, smooth and soft
Type 5	Soft blobs with clear-cut edges (passed easily)
Type 6	Fluffy pieces with ragged edges, a mushy stool
Type 7	Watery, no solid pieces ENTIRELY LIQUID

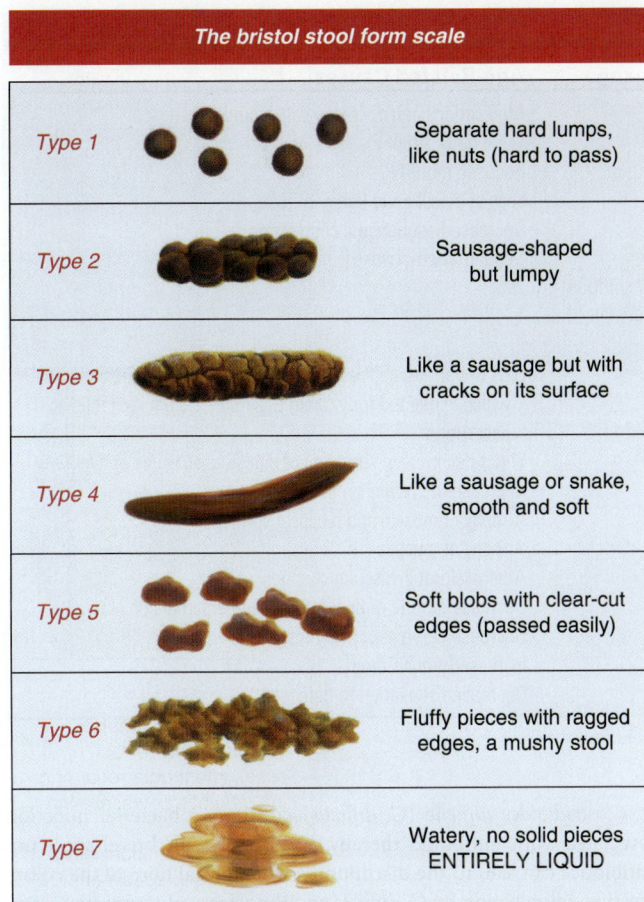

FIGURE 45.9 The Bristol Stool Form Scale. Copyright 2000 Rome Foundation, Inc. All Rights Reserved. Reprinted with permission from the Rome Foundation; all rights reserved.

- *Changes in appetite:* Note any changes in the patient's normal eating patterns and any change in weight (i.e., the amount lost or gained). If a change of weight has occurred, ask whether the weight change was planned, such as weight loss as a result of a low-calorie diet.
- *Diet history:* Determine the patient's dietary preferences. Assess the intake of fruits, vegetables, cereals, and breads and whether mealtimes are regular or irregular. In the case of the patient who is frail and living alone, determine whether acquiring food requires assistance (e.g., financial help, food preparation assistance, or transportation to a grocery store with a full selection of fresh fruits and vegetables).
- *Description of daily fluid intake:* Determine the type and amount of fluid consumed in a typical day. The patient might need to estimate the amount by using common household measurements.
- *History of surgery or illnesses affecting the GI tract:* This information can help to explain symptoms and to assess the patient's potential for maintaining or restoring a normal bowel elimination pattern. A patient's family history of GI cancer is also relevant to the nursing assessment.
- *Medication history:* Ask for a list of the patient's current medications. The medication history must include both prescribed and over-the-counter medications (e.g., laxatives, antacids, iron supplements, and analgesics) that might alter defecation or fecal characteristics. The community nurse should ask to see the medications.
- *Emotional state:* The patient's emotional state can significantly alter the frequency of defecation. During assessment, observe and ask directly about the patient's emotions and the presence of stress.

- *History of exercise:* Ask the patient to describe the type and amount of daily exercise and if there have been any recent changes to this activity level.
- *History of pain or discomfort:* Ask whether the patient has a history of abdominal or anal pain or pain with defecation. The quality, radiation, triggers, and location of pain may help to identify the source of the problem.
- *Environment and adaptive aids:* Patients have many different living arrangements. Where patients live may affect their toileting habits. If the patient is sharing living quarters, how many bathrooms are available? Does the patient have their own bathroom, or does the patient need to share the facilities and thus adjust the time the bathroom is used to accommodate other persons? If the patient lives alone, are they capable of ambulating to the toilet safely? If the patient is not independent in bowel management, who assists the patient and how? Does the patient use a bedpan, commode, or urinal? Does the patient wear incontinence products? Does the patient use a raised toilet seat or require grab bars?
- *Mobility and dexterity:* The patient's mobility and dexterity need to be evaluated to determine whether the patient needs assistive devices or personal assistance.
- *Presence and status of bowel diversions:* If the patient has an ostomy, assess the frequency of fecal drainage, the character of the feces, the appearance and condition of the stoma (e.g., the colour, the presence of swelling, and signs of irritation), the type of fecal collection device used, and the methods used to maintain the ostomy's function.

Physical Assessment. The physical assessment (see Chapter 33) is used to evaluate a patient's body systems and functions that are likely to be affected by the presence of bowel elimination problems.

Mouth. The nurse's inspection of the mouth includes examining the patient's teeth, tongue, and gums. Poor dentition or poorly fitting dentures influence the ability to chew (see Chapter 43). Sores in the mouth can make eating not only difficult but also painful. A dry mouth may indicate dehydration (Jarvis & Wilson-Keates, 2019).

Abdomen. All four abdominal quadrants should be inspected for contour, shape, symmetry, and skin colour. Masses, peristaltic waves, scars, venous patterns, stomas, and lesions should be noted. Normally, peristaltic waves are not visible; however, observable peristalsis can be a sign of intestinal obstruction.

Abdominal distension appears as an overall outward protuberance of the abdomen. Distension may be caused by obesity, intestinal gas, fluid in the peritoneal cavity, ovarian cyst, pregnancy, feces, or a large tumour (Jarvis & Luctkar-Flude, 2019). A distended abdomen feels tight and the skin appears taut, as if stretched (Jarvis & Luctkar-Flude, 2019).

Auscultation is performed before palpation and percussion to avoid affecting bowel sounds. The abdomen is auscultated with the stethoscope to assess bowel sounds in each quadrant for 5 minutes (see Chapter 33). While auscultating, the nurse should note the character and frequency of the bowel sounds. An increase in pitch or a tinkling sound may be heard when the abdomen is distended. Bowel sounds are high-pitched, occurring irregularly anywhere from 5 to 30 times per minute. It is not necessary to count bowel sounds; rather, assess whether they are normal, hyperactive, or hypoactive (Jarvis & Luctkar-Flude, 2019). Abnormal bowel sounds have two distinct patterns. Hyperactive sounds are noisy, high-pitched, cascading, tinkling sounds that signal increased motility and may signal a bowel obstruction.

Sounds may be hypoactive or absent after abdominal surgery (ileus) or with inflammation or infection of the peritoneum (Jarvis & Luctkar-Flude, 2019). The absence of bowel sounds following surgery may

TABLE 45.1	Normal Age-Related Changes in the Gastrointestinal Tract	
Portion of Gastrointestinal Tract	**Functional or Physiological Change**	**Age-Related Causes**
Mouth	Difficulty chewing and oral dryness	Medications can decrease saliva production
		Taste buds atrophy
Esophagus	Increased incidence of acid reflux	Reduced motility
		Loss of muscle and ligament tone
		Decreased esophageal contractions
Stomach	Decrease in acid secretions	Degeneration of gastric mucosa
	Not able to accommodate large amounts of food	
	Increased risk of peptic ulcer disease, anemia, and stomach cancer	
	Decrease in mucosal thickness	Loss of parietal cells also leads to loss of the intrinsic factor, which is needed for vitamin B$_{12}$, iron, calcium, and folic acid absorption
Small intestine	Decreased nutrient absorption	Slight decrease in secretion of digestive enzymes and motility
		Decrease in protein synthesis
		Atrophy of muscle and mucosal surfaces
Large intestine	Increased risk of diverticuli	Atrophy of mucosa
	Increased occurrence of constipation	Atherosclerotic vascular changes
	Missed defecation signal	Decrease in tone of anal internal and external sphincters
		Decrease nerve supply to rectal area
		Increased transit time
		Decreased sensation to defecate

Data from Meiner, S. E., & Yeager, J. J. (2019). *Gerontologic nursing* (6th ed.). Elsevier.

suggest an ileus before there are signs and symptoms, such as vomiting or abdominal pain.

Percussion is used to detect lesions, fluid, or gas in the abdomen. Familiarity with the five percussion notes (see Chapter 33) enables identification of the underlying abdominal structures. Gas or flatulence creates a tympanic note. Masses, tumours, and fluid are dull to percussion.

The nurse should gently palpate the abdomen for masses or areas of tenderness (see Chapter 32). During this procedure, the nurse needs to encourage the patient to relax. Tensing of the abdominal muscles interferes with palpating underlying organs or masses (Jarvis & Luctkar-Flude, 2019).

Rectum. The area around the anus is inspected for lesions, discolorations, inflammation, and hemorrhoids. Abnormalities should be carefully recorded (see Chapter 32) (Jarvis & Luctkar-Flude, 2019).

Factors Related to Altered Patterns of Bowel Elimination

Age-Related Changes. Normal age-related changes affect bowel elimination (Table 45.1). In addition, many issues associated with aging can significantly alter bowel elimination, including polypharmacy, poor nutrition, life stressors, and comorbidities (Meiner & Yeager, 2019).

Older persons also lose muscle tone in the perineal floor and decreased anal sphincter tone, as well as decreased autonomic nerve supply to the rectal area. Although the integrity of the external sphincter may remain intact, older persons may have difficulty controlling bowel evacuation and are at risk for incontinence. In addition, older persons may have a slowing of the nerve impulses to the anal region: some individuals are less aware of the need to defecate and, as a result, develop irregular bowel movements and are at risk for constipation (Meiner & Yeager, 2019).

Infectious Disease. Microbial agents, including viruses, bacteria, and protozoa, can infect the GI tract. These infections can cause diarrhea and inflammatory or ulcerative changes in the small or large intestine. Most infections are spread by the oral–fecal route, through contaminated food or water.

Clostridioides difficile (*C. difficile*) colitis is a bacterial infection associated with antibiotic therapy. Treatment with broad-spectrum antibiotics can lead to the disruption of the normal flora of the colon, creating colonization by *C. difficile* and the release of toxins that damage the mucosa and cause inflammation. The infection manifests with mild to moderate diarrhea and lower abdominal cramping. *C. difficile* is a leading cause of morbidity and mortality in several countries, including Canada (Balsells et al., 2019). The systematic review by Balsells and colleagues (2019) highlights the universal impact of disease of *C. difficile*, research priorities, and the need for ongoing vigilance in controlling *C. difficile* in the health care sector and in the community. Stool specimen collection for the testing of *C. difficile* or its toxins should be done as soon as possible after the onset of diarrhea. Treatment includes immediate discontinuation of the antibiotic and in cases where symptoms are severe, treatment is aimed at eradication of *C. difficile* (Power-Kean et al., 2023).

The primary mode of transmission for *C. difficile* within health care facilities is by person-to-person spread. Contact precautions should be implemented for patients with acute diarrhea suspected or confirmed to be caused by *C. difficile* infection. Patients should be placed on contact precautions, preferably in a single room, until the diarrhea is resolved or its cause is determined not to be infectious. Hand hygiene using soap and water after glove removal must be performed when a dedicated staff handwashing sink is available. If a handwashing sink is not available, hand hygiene must be performed using an alcohol-based hand rub that has an alcohol concentration between 60 and 90% (Power-Kean et al., 2023). Hand hygiene is performed frequently after patient care, contact with the patient's environment, and removing gloves at point of care; just prior to leaving the patient's room; after handling fecal matter; and after handling bedpans and commodes (Provincial Infectious Diseases Advisory Committee [PIDAC], 2013).

The rotavirus is an example of a viral infection and is responsible for most nonbacterial food-borne epidemic gastroenteritis in all age groups. The virus is shed both before and for days after clinical illness. Very few infectious virions are actually needed to cause disease.

Rotavirus infection begins after about 24 hours' incubation and presents with mild to moderate fever and vomiting, followed by watery stools. Treatment is focused on preventing dehydration. A rotavirus vaccine is available (Power-Kean et al., 2023).

Norovirus is one of the leading causes of viral gastroenteritis globally and often results in significant morbidity, mortality, and costs to the health care systems (Gaythorpe et al., 2018). Petrignani and colleagues (2018) reported on a systematic review discussing long-term health impacts and serious complications of norovirus infection. Outbreaks of the highly contagious Norwalk virus are common in Canadian schools, hospitals, day care centres, and long-term care facilities. The Norwalk virus has been described as "the winter vomiting disease" and rapidly spreads to staff, students, and patients. When the Norwalk virus is detected, standard infection control procedures need to be implemented rapidly, accompanied by further precautions, such as isolation of the affected units, strict handwashing protocols, the wearing of gloves and gowns, and a thorough washing down of the affected units. When an outbreak occurs, the institution is frequently closed to visitors, and infected staff are required to remain off duty until they are symptom-free for 48 hours. In healthy individuals, symptoms last from 12 to 60 hours. The very young, older persons, and those who are immunocompromised are at higher risk of serious complication and death (Gaythorpe et al., 2018).

Irritable Bowel Syndrome. Irritable bowel syndrome (IBS) is a functional GI disorder with chronic intestinal symptoms that cannot be explained by structural or biochemical abnormalities. The symptoms of IBS can include abdominal pain, altered bowel function, flatulence, bloating, nausea, anorexia, diarrhea, or constipation. The hallmark symptom is abdominal pain that is relieved by defecation and accompanied by a change in the frequency or consistency of stools (Power-Kean et al., 2023).

IBS is related to diet, stress, and psychological factors, and its onset may be triggered by a GI infection. The precise pathophysiology of IBS is not understood. Management is multimodal, based on the patient's most troublesome symptoms and includes counselling, dietary fibre modifications, and medications (such as bulking polymer agents, probiotics, and antidepressants) (Fukudo et al., 2021). For additional management recommendations a helpful resource is the evidence-informed clinical practice guidelines for irritable bowel syndrome (Fukudo et al., 2021). The nurse can support the patient with IBS by offering coaching on stress management and on maintaining a high-fibre diet (Power-Kean et al., 2023).

Inflammatory Bowel Disease. Inflammatory bowel disease (IBD) is thought to be an autoimmune disease. Significant morbidity and related health care costs are associated with IBD (Vachon & Scott, 2020). There are two main types of IBD, ulcerative colitis (UC) and Crohn's disease (CD). UC typically affects only the large intestine, while CD can affect any part of the GI tract, from the mouth to anus. The cause of UC and CD is thought to be multifactorial; these factors are just now starting to be understood. Patients experience a range of symptoms associated with inflammation of the gut, including abdominal pain, fever, vomiting, diarrhea, rectal bleeding, anemia, and weight loss. There is currently no known cure, but symptoms can be managed through use of anti-inflammatory steroids or immunosuppressants to reduce inflammation, dietary changes to try and remove environmental triggers, and (in severe cases) surgery to remove damaged portions of the bowel. Vachon and Scott (2020) provide up-to-date information on treating IBD, including disease categorization, specific medication options for each category, as well as monitoring treatment and medication effectiveness.

Diabetes. Patients with diabetes frequently report constipation, diarrhea, abdominal distension, bloating, and abdominal pain. In patients with diabetes, pathophysiological changes may include the following: smooth muscle structure and function, the density of the interstitial cells of Cajal in the small intestine, and autonomic and enteric neuropathies (Piper & Saad, 2017). Hyperglycemia can directly reduce or slow gastric contractions and the GI emptying rate. GI symptoms are more prevalent in patients with poor glycemic control. Symptoms can be improved with individualized dietary changes, including reducing fats and increasing daily fibre intake (deMolitor, 2019).

Pain. Normally, the act of defecation is painless. However, several conditions can result in discomfort, including hemorrhoids, rectal surgery, rectal fistulas, and abdominal surgery. In these instances, to avoid pain, the patient often suppresses the urge to defecate. As a result, constipation and impaction may develop.

Pelvic Floor Trauma. Trauma to the pelvic floor muscles from pregnancy, labour and delivery, and aging can affect bowel elimination in individuals with female genitalia.

As pregnancy advances, the size of the fetus increases and pressure is exerted on the rectum. A temporary obstruction created by the fetus impairs the passage of feces. Slowing of peristalsis during the third trimester often leads to constipation. A pregnant person's frequent straining during defecation or delivery can result in the formation of permanent hemorrhoids. Damage to the perineum extending to the anal sphincters during labour can also alter sphincter integrity (Blomquist et al., 2020).

Older persons with female genitalia, particularly those who have borne children, frequently develop loss of tone and weakening of the ligaments and muscles of the anterior and posterior vaginal walls. This condition can lead to cystocele (the dropping of the bladder into the vagina), rectocele (the pouching of the feces-filled rectum into the vagina), and sometimes complete prolapse of the uterus out of the vagina. All of these conditions alter the anorectal angle and may inhibit complete evacuation (Oliveira et al., 2020). Nurse continence advisors (i.e., registered nurses who are specially educated in continence care) treat these conditions by educating patients about high-fibre diets and teaching pelvic floor muscle exercises, often referred to as *Kegel exercises* (Cowie et al., 2014).

Acute Illness, Surgery, and Anaesthesia. The GI system may be affected by any acute illness. Changes in the patient's fluid status, mobility patterns, nutrition, and sleep cycle can affect regular bowel habits. Surgical interventions on the GI tract affect bowel elimination, as will surgery on other systems, such as the musculoskeletal and cardiovascular systems.

The general anaesthetic agents used during surgery cause temporary cessation of peristalsis (see Chapter 49). Inhaled anaesthetic agents block the parasympathetic impulses to the enteric nervous system, and the stress of surgery stimulates the sympathetic nervous system. The anaesthetic's action slows or stops the integrated contractions. Pain-control medication that contains opioids has the adverse effect of slowing mass peristalsis (or mass movement) and increasing the slow-mixing contractions and fluid absorption from the colon. Thus, following surgery, abdominal discomfort from intraluminal gas and constipation are frequent, and the surgeon's postoperative orders typically include bowel routine with laxatives and enemas if bowel movements do not occur within 2 to 3 days. Thus, nurses need to note whether and when the first bowel movement post-surgery occurs, because the patient may require treatment for constipation. Early postoperative ambulation stimulates the evacuation of flatus, stimulates peristalsis, and alleviates abdominal pain (Lewis et al., 2023).

The patient who receives local or regional anaesthesia is less at risk for bowel elimination alterations because bowel activity may be affected minimally or not at all. Any surgery that involves direct manipulation of the bowel temporarily stops peristalsis. This condition, called

paralytic ileus, usually lasts for more than 2 or 3 days. If the patient remains inactive or is unable to eat after surgery, return of normal bowel function may be further delayed (Lewis et al., 2023).

Enteral Feeding. Patients receiving enteral feeding will experience changes in bowel elimination. When the absorptive area of the small intestine is reduced, patients may receive nutrition through enteral feeding administered by tube into the GI tract. Enteral feeding contains nutrients that do not need further digestion to be rapidly absorbed by the diminished area of the intestine.

Patients receiving their nutrition through enteral feeding may experience diarrhea. This can be due to the feed running too quickly, medications, or an active infection (Lewis et al., 2023). It is important to rule out *C. difficile* (Lewis et al., 2023). Conversely, a patient could experience problems with constipation. This is usually related to the type of formula used, and a change to a high-fibre formula may resolve the constipation (Lewis et al., 2023). Again, medications the patient is taking must be examined for their effects on the GI system (Lewis et al., 2023).

Medications That Affect Elimination. Medication may have certain expected actions on the bowel; for example, some medications promote defecation, and others control diarrhea. In addition, medications prescribed for acute and chronic conditions may have secondary effects on the patient's bowel elimination patterns (Table 45.2).

Laboratory Tests. Laboratory and diagnostic examinations yield useful information concerning bowel elimination problems (Table 45.3). Laboratory analysis of fecal contents can detect pathological conditions, such as tumours, bleeding, and infection.

Fecal Specimens. Nurses are directly responsible for ensuring that fecal specimens are accurately obtained, properly labelled in appropriate containers, and transported to the laboratory on time. Institutions provide special containers for fecal specimens. Some tests require specimens to be placed in chemical preservatives.

Medical aseptic technique should be used during collection of stool specimens (see Chapter 34). Because approximately 25% of the solid portion of a stool is bacteria from the colon, disposable gloves should be worn when handling fecal specimens.

Hand hygiene, as well as standard precautions and routine practices, is necessary for anyone who might come in contact with the specimen. The patient can often obtain the specimen if properly instructed. The nurse should explain to the patient that feces cannot be mixed with urine or water. For this reason, the patient must defecate into a clean, dry bedpan or a special container placed under the toilet seat (Pagana et al., 2019).

Tests performed by the laboratory for occult (microscopic) blood in the stool and stool cultures require only a small sample. About 2.5 cm of formed stool or 15 to 30 mL of liquid diarrhea stool is collected. Tests for measuring the output of fecal fat require a 3- to 5-day collection of stool. All fecal material must be saved throughout the test period.

After obtaining a fecal specimen, the nurse needs to label and tightly seal the container, complete the laboratory requisition forms, and record the specimen collections in the patient's medical record. The nurse should avoid delays in sending specimens to the laboratory because some tests, such as measurements for ova and parasites, require the stool to be warm. Stool specimens for enteric pathogens and *C. difficile* require refrigeration. When stool specimens are allowed to stand at room temperature, bacteriological changes occur that can alter the test results (Pagana et al., 2019).

Screening Tests. The **fecal immunochemical test (FIT),** which is a test used to detect blood in stool that cannot be seen with the naked eye by submitting one to three bowel movements, replaces the guaiac-based fecal occult blood test (gFOBT). Most colorectal cancer screening programs in Canada screen using the FIT (Canadian Cancer Society, 2022). Nurses are encouraged to visit the Cancer Care Ontario

TABLE 45.2 Medications and the Gastrointestinal System

Medication	Action
Opioids	Increase the mixing action of segmentation contractions and slow the propulsive contractions, often resulting in constipation, nausea, vomiting, or anorexia (Sealock et al., 2021).
Anticholinergics (such as atropine)	Inhibit gastric acid secretion and depress gastrointestinal motility. Although anticholinergics are useful in treating hyperactive bowel disorders, they can cause constipation (Sealock et al., 2021).
Antibiotics	Frequently produce diarrhea by disrupting the normal bacterial flora in the gastrointestinal tract. Antibiotic use has been shown to promote infection with the highly contagious *Clostridioides difficile*, which has a high mortality rate in older persons (RNAO, 2020). See the Choosing Wisely Canada (2020) recommendation and supporting evidence. Concurrently taking a specific probiotic supplement that mixes *Lactobacillus acidophilus, L. casei*, and L. *rhamnosus* strains has been shown to reduce the incidence of diarrhea and to reduce the risk of *C. difficile* infections (McFarland et al., 2018).
Nonsteroidal anti-inflammatory drugs (NSAIDs) (such as acetylsalicylic acid)	Prostaglandin inhibitors are used to treat arthritis pain but can also promote gastrointestinal irritation that can range from dyspepsia to life-threatening hemorrhage (Sealock et al., 2021).
Histamine₂ (H₂) antagonists (such as ranitidine) Proton pump inhibitors (such as omeprazole)	Reduce the secretion of hydrochloric acid and are commonly used to treat many acid-related disorders. These medications suppress gastric acid secretion and may also predispose patients to GI infections (Sealock et al., 2021).
Iron	Can cause dark stools and can lead to constipation (Sealock et al., 2021).
Aluminum and calcium-containing medications	Adverse gastrointestinal effects include constipation, obstruction, nausea, vomiting, and flatulence (Sealock et al., 2021).
Patients may experience constipation, as a result of medications they are taking	Medications that cause constipation include anticholinergics, antidepressants, antiemetics, antihistamines, antihypertensives, anti-Parkinson agents, antipsychotics, antacids containing aluminum, analgesics, NSAIDs, histamine-2 blockers, hypnotics, diuretics, sedatives, iron supplements, and opioids (RNAO, 2020). See Appendix P in the RNAO guideline, *A Proactive Approach to Bladder and Bowel Management in Adults*, for a list of medication categories that can cause constipation. See the Government of Canada's Drug Product Database (https://health-products.canada.ca/dpd-bdpp/index-eng.jsp) to search the uses and adverse effects of specific medications.

TABLE 45.3	Laboratory and Diagnostic Tests for Bowel Function
Measurement	**Interpretation**
Laboratory Tests	
Total bilirubin	Increased levels of bilirubin may result from hepatobiliary diseases, obstructions in the bile duct, and hemolytic anemias.
Alkaline phosphatase (ALP)	Elevated levels of alkaline phosphatase may indicate obstructive hepatobiliary diseases, hepatobiliary carcinomas, and bone disorders.
Amylase, blood	Elevated levels of amylase may indicate abnormalities of the pancreas, such as inflammation, gastrointestinal (GI) disease (necrotic bowel, perforated bowel, duodenal obstruction, or peptic ulcer), tumours, acute cholecystitis, and diabetic ketoacidosis.
Carcinoembryonic antigen (CEA)	Carcinoembryonic antigen is elevated in the presence of cancer, Crohn's disease, peptic ulcer, inflammation of the GI tract (colitis, cholecystitis, pancreatitis, diverticulitis), or hepatobiliary organs (e.g., cirrhosis).
Direct Visualization	
Endoscopy	A colonoscopy is a routine examination for persons 50 years of age and older. The rectum, colon, and small bowel are visualized directly during the procedure. Normally, the GI tract is free of polyps, tumours, inflammation, ulcers, hernias, obstruction, and ulcerations. If a lesion, such as a polyp, is identified, the prescriber removes the growth or a portion of the growth and sends it to pathology for analysis. If bleeding is present, the prescriber may attempt to coagulate the source. In some cases, identification of an abnormality may indicate the need for follow-up surgery for the patient.
Indirect Visualization	
X-ray with contrast medium	An X-ray may show the presence of acute abnormalities in the GI tract. A series of X-rays will allow for indirect visualization of the entire tract. The presence of tumours, ulcerations, inflammation, or other abnormalities may indicate the need for further diagnostic testing and medical or surgical intervention.

Data from Pagana, K. D., Pagana, & T. J., Pike-MacDonald, S. A. (Eds.). (2019). *Mosby's Canadian manual of diagnostic and laboratory tests* (2nd Canadian ed.). Elsevier.

website (https://www.cancercareontario.ca) or another similar provincial website and the Canadian Cancer Society website (https://www.cancer.ca) for the most up-to-date recommendations regarding screening, risk factors, warning signs, and follow-up. For example, Cancer Care Ontario recommends FIT screening for people at average risk (Cancer Care Ontario, 2019a). The recommendation is for screening with an FIT every 2 years for people with symptoms. A colonoscopy within 8 weeks of an abnormal FIT result is recommended (Cancer Care Ontario, 2019b). Consult the *ColonCancerCheck (CCC) Guide to Average Risk Screening with the Fecal Immunochemical Test (FIT)* that is available in Ontario (Cancer Care Ontario, 2019a) for specific details.

Fecal characteristics. Inspection of fecal characteristics (Table 45.4) reveals information about the nature of bowel elimination alterations. Several factors can influence each characteristic. A key to assessment is knowing whether any recent changes have occurred. The patient can best provide this information during the health history assessment.

Diagnostic Examinations. A variety of radiological and diagnostic tests may be ordered for the patient who experiences altered bowel elimination (Box 45.1). GI structures may be visualized using either a direct or indirect approach. Each test has a prescribed preparation routine for emptying the GI area under study to facilitate visualization. Many facilities use light sedation or procedural sedation during these procedures. Nurses need to be sure they understand the safety precautions involved in the use of this form of anaesthesia. In many institutions, special training is required. A crash cart must be present at the bedside, and the patient must be monitored continuously with pulse oximetry and frequent vital signs, usually every 15 minutes during and immediately following the procedure. Nurses need to check employer policy regarding the use of sedation for these examinations (Pagana et al., 2019).

Diagnostic Tests. Diagnostic examinations that involve visualization of GI structures often require that portions of the bowel be empty. The patient receives a prescribed bowel preparation before the test. Usually, the patient is asked to use Pico-Salax®

(https://www.pico-salax.ca/about-pico-salax.html) as a bowel preparation medication. Pico-Salax® has replaced polyethylene glycol because the 4-L volume was too large for patients to consume. Other medications, cathartics, or enemas may also be used. In addition, the patient is not allowed to eat or drink after midnight of the day preceding examinations such as a colonoscopy, endoscopy, or other testing that requires visualization of the lower GI tract. Following the diagnostic procedure, the patient may experience changes in bowel elimination, such as increased gas or loose stools. These changes will stop when the patient resumes a normal eating pattern (Pagana et al., 2019). Bowel preparations can cause complications in older persons, such as dehydration and electrolyte imbalances (Davis, 2019).

◆ Nursing Diagnosis

Nursing assessment of the patient's bowel function reveals data that may indicate an actual or potential bowel elimination problem or a problem resulting from bowel elimination alterations. The concept map in Figure 45.10 depicts how the nursing diagnosis of constipation may be related to other diagnoses. In this example, a patient with cancer has developed constipation as a result of activity intolerance and imbalanced nutrition. Both conditions are a result of the patient's pain. Nursing diagnoses (Herdman et al., 2021) that may apply to patients with bowel elimination problems include the following:

- *Impaired bowel incontinence*
- *Constipation*
- *Risk for constipation*
- *Perceived constipation*
- *Diarrhea*

Richmond and Wright (2006) developed a constipation risk assessment scale (Figure 45.11). In a subsequent report (Richmond & Wright, 2008), these authors published reliability and validity of their constipation risk assessment scale.

A patient's associated conditions, such as body-image changes or skin breakdown, require interventions unrelated to bowel function

TABLE 45.4   Characteristics of Stool

Characteristic	Normal	Abnormal	Cause of Abnormality
Colour	Brown	White or clay	Absence of bile pigment, such as in obstructive jaundice. Stool with visible mucus or pus may suggest an infection, inflammatory bowel disease, or cancer.
		Black or tarry (i.e., melena)	Ingestion of iron or bismuth preparations or upper gastrointestinal bleeding with blood partially digested (a distinct malodor)
		Bright red	Lower gastrointestinal bleeding, hemorrhoids
		Pale yellow, greasy stool	Indicates increased fat content (steatorrhea) Malabsorption of fat
		Mucus or pus	Spastic constipation, colitis, excessive straining
		Bloody mucus	Blood in feces, inflammation, infection, hemorrhoids
Odour	Pungent; affected by food type	Noxious change	Blood in feces or infection
Consistency	Soft, formed	Liquid	Diarrhea, reduced absorption
		Hard	Constipation
Frequency (and any recent change)	Daily or two to three times weekly	More than three times a day or less than once a week	Hypomotility or hypermotility (multifactorial)
Shape	Resembles diameter of rectum	Narrow, pencil shaped	Anal or distal rectal carcinoma
Constituents	Undigested food, dead bacteria, fat, bile pigment, cells lining intestinal mucosa, water	Blood, pus, foreign bodies, mucus, worms	Internal bleeding, infection, swallowed objects, irritation, inflammation
		Excess fat	Malabsorption syndrome, enteritis, pancreatic disease, surgical resection of intestine

Data from Jarvis, C., Browne, A., MacDonald-Jenkins, J., et al. (Eds.). (2019). *Physical examination and health assessment* (3rd Canadian ed.). Elsevier Canada.

impairment. In some instances, however, nurses need to direct as much attention to the associated condition as to the bowel elimination problem.

Nurses' ability to identify the correct nursing diagnosis depends not only on the thoroughness of assessment but also on recognition of defining characteristics and factors that can impair bowel elimination (Box 45.2). The nurse needs to determine the patient's risk and then institute measures to ensure maintenance of normal bowel function.

Common Bowel Elimination Problems. Nurses may care for patients who have or are at risk for bowel elimination problems because of emotional stress (anxiety or depression), inflammatory diseases, prescribed therapy, disorders impairing defecation, or physiological changes in the GI tract, such as surgical alteration of intestinal structures.

Constipation. Constipation is a symptom, not a disease (Table 45.5). The signs of constipation vary among patients but usually include difficult or infrequent bowel movements (fewer than three per week (RNAO, 2020). Common signs are abdominal pain and distension and a sensation of fullness and pressure in the rectum. Straining during defecation is also an associated sign. When intestinal motility slows, the fecal mass becomes exposed over time to the intestinal walls and most of the fecal water is absorbed. Little water is left to soften and lubricate the stool. Passage of a dry, hard stool may cause rectal pain (Bardsley, 2017). Constipation is a common concern during acute hospital admissions for older persons.

Constipation can be a significant hazard to health, resulting in serious complications, including a bowel obstruction. The Valsalva manoeuvre involves a drawing in of the chest muscles on a closed glottis with a tightening of the abdominal muscles at the same time, causing an increase in intra-abdominal pressure. This can occur with straining to initiate a bowel movement. The Valsalva manoeuvre may cause harm and should be avoided in patients who have a head injury, cardiac conditions, hemorrhoids, or liver cirrhosis and in those who have had recent eye or abdominal, gynecological, or rectal surgery (Lewis et al., 2023). The effort to pass a stool can cause sutures to separate, thereby

reopening the wound. The muscles used to strain during a bowel movement may also cause transient ischemic attacks and syncope, particularly in frail older persons (Touhy et al., 2019). The Valsalva manoeuvre can be avoided by exhaling through the mouth during straining.

Constipation can also occur in conjunction with the treatment of urinary conditions, as an adverse effect of the medication but also because individuals with urinary incontinence may reduce their fluid intake to reduce the frequency of their need to urinate.

Impaction. Fecal **impaction** results from unrelieved constipation and can lead to overflow incontinence. Fecal impaction is a collection of hardened feces that are wedged in the rectum and cannot be expelled. In cases of severe impaction, the mass can extend into the sigmoid colon. Patients who are immobile and dehydrated or have impaired rectal sensation, depression, delirium, and dementia are most at risk for impaction.

An obvious sign of impaction is the inability to pass a stool for several days, despite the repeated urge to defecate. A continuous oozing of diarrhea stool may develop when the liquid portion of feces located higher in the colon seeps around the impacted mass. Loss of appetite (anorexia), nausea or vomiting, abdominal distension and cramping, and rectal pain may accompany the condition. If the nurse suspects an impaction, they can gently perform a digital examination of the rectum and palpate for the impacted mass (Cowie et al., 2014).

Diarrhea. Diarrhea is an increase in the number of stools (several bowel movements per day) and the passage of liquid, unformed feces. Diarrhea can be acute or chronic. Diarrhea can be caused by infectious organisms (as discussed earlier), food intolerances, medications (including chemotherapy), or intestinal disease. Intestinal contents pass through the small and large intestine too quickly to allow the usual absorption of fluid and nutrients. Irritation within the colon can result in an increased mucus secretion. As a result, feces become watery and the patient may be unable to control the urge to defecate (Power-Kean et al., 2023).

Excess loss of colonic fluid can result in serious fluid, electrolyte, or acid–base imbalances. Older persons are particularly susceptible to complications associated with diarrhea (see Chapter 41). Repeated

BOX 45.1 Radiological and Diagnostic Tests

Flat Plate Radiography
- A simple X-ray film of the abdomen that requires no preparation

Computerized Tomography Scan
- An X-ray examination of the body from many angles that uses a scanner and is analyzed by a computer
- The preparation may be either nothing by mouth (NPO) or no preparation.
- The patient must be informed of the need to lie very still. If claustrophobia is a problem, light sedation may be used.

Ultrasound Imaging
- Technique used to visualize the abdomen and organs within
- High-frequency sound waves echo off body organs to create a picture.
- The preparation depends on the organ to be visualized and may include either fasting or no preparation.

Upper Gastrointestinal Barium Swallow (Esophagogram)
- An X-ray examination that uses an opaque contrast medium (e.g., barium) to visualize the structure and motility of the upper gastrointestinal tract, including the pharynx, esophagus, and stomach
- The patient must be restricted to NPO (nothing by mouth) for at least 8 hours before the examination.
- The patient must remove all jewellery and other metallic objects.
- After the test, the patient must increase intake of fluids to facilitate passage and elimination of the barium. Cathartics are recommended.

Lower Gastrointestinal Barium Enema
- A series of X-ray examinations that uses an opaque contrast medium to visualize the lower gastrointestinal tract
- The preparation includes a bowel preparation or cathartic to empty any remaining stool particles.

Upper Gastrointestinal Endoscopy
- An endoscopic examination of the upper gastrointestinal tract that allows a more direct visualization via a fibreoptic-lighted endoscope
- The preparation is similar to that of the upper gastrointestinal barium swallow.
- Light sedation is required.

Colonoscopy
- An endoscopic examination of the rectum and colon that uses a long, flexible tube (i.e., a colonoscope) inserted into the rectum
- Bowel must be clean and free of fecal material.
- Light sedation is required.

Sigmoidoscopy
- An examination of the interior of the sigmoid colon
- Preparation is similar to that of a colonoscopy.
- Light sedation is required.

Magnetic Resonance Imaging
- A noninvasive examination that uses magnetic and radio waves to produce a picture of the inside of the body
- It provides better contrast between normal and pathological tissue than an ultrasound.
- The preparation is NPO 4 to 6 hours before examination.
- No metallic objects are allowed in the room, including metal objects on clothes.

From Pagana, K. D., Pagana, T. J., & Pike-MacDonald, S. A. (2019). *Mosby's Canadian manual of diagnostic and laboratory tests* (2nd Canadian ed.). Elsevier Inc.

passage of diarrhea stools exposes the skin of the perineum and the buttocks to irritating intestinal contents; therefore, meticulous skin care and containment of fecal drainage is needed to prevent skin breakdown (see Chapter 47) (Power-Kean et al., 2023).

The aims of treatment are to remove the precipitating conditions and to slow peristalsis. Medications that are opiumlike (such as loperamide) are used to decrease GI motility and stimulate water and electrolyte absorption. Loperamide should not be given until a definitive bacterial cause has been identified, including the cause of diarrhea from travelling. Antidiarrheal medications should not be used with patients who have blood in their stool or a high fever, because they could risk worsening the disease. Antibiotics are used only when enteric pathogens have been identified (Power-Kean et al., 2023).

Communicable food-borne pathogens can also cause diarrhea. The risk of food-borne illnesses can be greatly reduced by thorough handwashing after using the bathroom and before and after preparing foods, and by properly storing and preparing fresh produce and meats. When diarrhea is the result of a food-borne virus, the goal is usually to rid the system of the pathogen, not to slow peristalsis.

Incontinence. Bowel incontinence is the inability to control the passage of feces and gas from the anus. Bowel incontinence is devastating to patients and has a significant effect on functional, social, and psychological well-being (Massirfufulay et al., 2019). The possible embarrassment of soiling clothes can lead to self-imposed social isolation (Cowie et al., 2014). Contributing factors to bowel incontinence include diet, fluid intake (in particular, caffeine), alcohol use, and nicotine use (Cowie et al., 2014). Physical conditions that impair anal sphincter function, compliance, or control can cause incontinence. Additionally, patients without the cognitive awareness of the urge to defecate are at risk for incontinence (Cowie et al., 2014). Conditions that create frequent, loose, large-volume, watery stools are predispositions for bowel incontinence (Massirfufulay et al., 2019). Bowel incontinence can be successfully managed and treated with nursing interventions (Box 45.3).

Flatulence. In most healthy individuals, 100 to 200 mL of gas is present in the GI tract. Gas in the upper GI tract may increase from the swallowing of air. Gas production in the colon occurs from bacteria digesting cellulose in the colon.

As gas accumulates in the lumen of the intestines, the bowel wall stretches and distends, resulting in flatulence. Flatulence is a common cause of abdominal fullness, pain, and cramping. Normally, intestinal gas escapes through the mouth (belching) or the anus (passing of flatus). For a person eating a normal diet, 50 to 500 mL of gas is passed 10 to 15 times a day. However, if intestinal motility is reduced as a result of the effects of opiates, general anaesthetics, abdominal surgery, or immobilization, flatulence can become severe enough to cause abdominal distension and severe, sharp pain (Lewis et al., 2023).

Hemorrhoids. Hemorrhoids are dilated, engorged veins in the lining of the rectum. They are either external or internal. External hemorrhoids are clearly visible as protrusions of skin. If the underlying vein is hardened, a purplish discoloration (i.e., thrombosis) may be visible. This condition causes increased pain, and the hemorrhoid may need to be excised. Internal hemorrhoids have an outer mucous membrane. Increased venous pressure as a result of pregnancy, heart failure, chronic liver disease, or straining at defecation can cause hemorrhoids. The presence of hemorrhoids is frequently accompanied by fecal soiling of undergarments and irritation of the distended veins by overly vigorous cleaning of the anus. Meticulous cleaning following a bowel movement may reduce the possibility of irritation (Lewis et al., 2023).

◆ Planning

During the planning of care, the nurse synthesizes information from multiple resources (Figure 45.12). Critical thinking ensures that the

> concept **map**

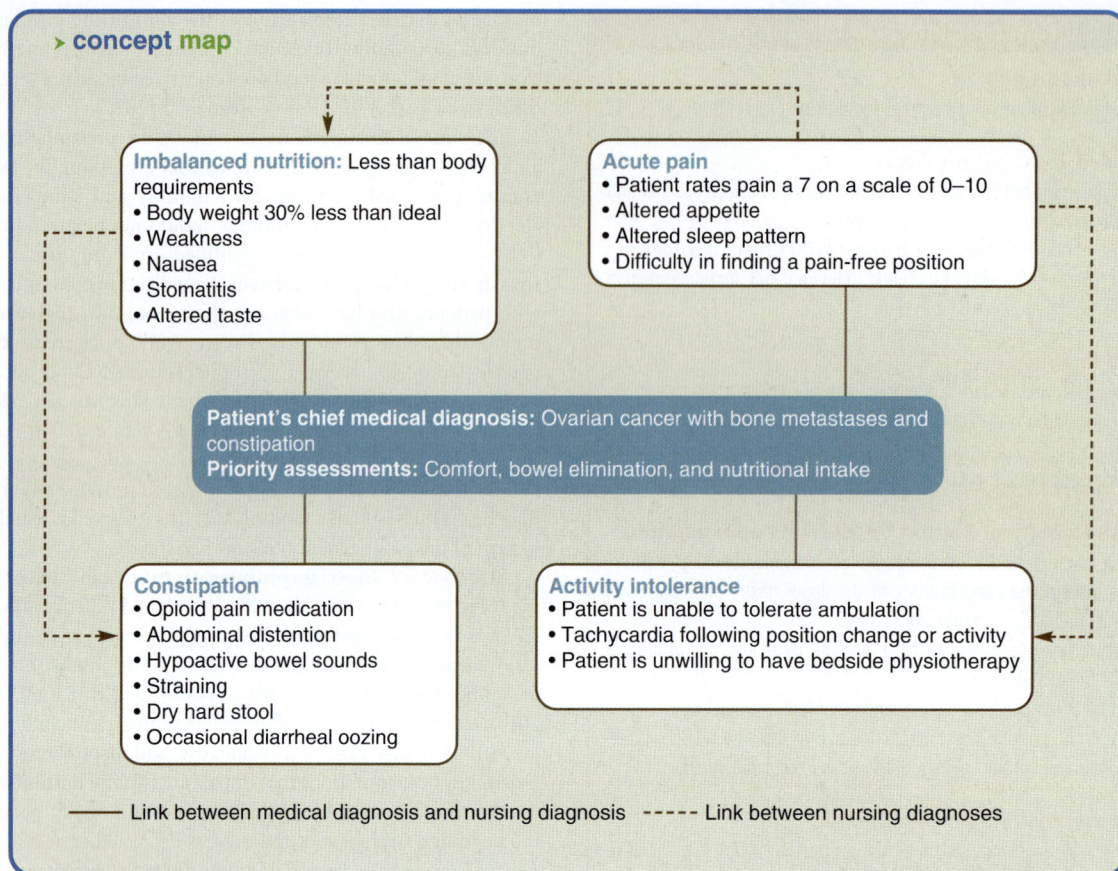

Imbalanced nutrition: Less than body requirements
• Body weight 30% less than ideal
• Weakness
• Nausea
• Stomatitis
• Altered taste

Acute pain
• Patient rates pain a 7 on a scale of 0–10
• Altered appetite
• Altered sleep pattern
• Difficulty in finding a pain-free position

Patient's chief medical diagnosis: Ovarian cancer with bone metastases and constipation
Priority assessments: Comfort, bowel elimination, and nutritional intake

Constipation
• Opioid pain medication
• Abdominal distention
• Hypoactive bowel sounds
• Straining
• Dry hard stool
• Occasional diarrheal oozing

Activity intolerance
• Patient is unable to tolerate ambulation
• Tachycardia following position change or activity
• Patient is unwilling to have bedside physiotherapy

——— Link between medical diagnosis and nursing diagnosis   - - - - Link between nursing diagnoses

FIGURE 45.10 Concept map for a patient who has ovarian cancer with bone metastases and constipation.

plan of care integrates all that the nurse knows about the patient and the clinical problem. Nurses must rely on professional standards. The guidelines on incontinence (see Chapter 44) can assist nurses in protecting the patient's skin, promoting continence, and reducing the embarrassment associated with incontinence. In addition, the Registered Nurses' Association of Ontario (RNAO, 2016) and Wounds Canada (Norton et al., 2017) have guidelines on the reduction of pressure injuries; these guidelines can assist the nurse in developing care plans for patients with bowel incontinence (see Chapter 47).

McNichol and colleagues (2018) conducted a literature review of incontinence-associated dermatitis (IAD), recommending a mnemonic, ACT (**a**ccess, **c**leanse, **t**reat), to help clinicians consider strategies for both preventing and managing IAD. Francis (2018) has provided a guide to clinicians to help differentiate between IAD from containment products and a pressure injury. Nurses are expected to not routinely use incontinence containment products (including briefs or pads) for older persons (Choosing Wisely Canada, 2020) but rather to explore toileting options, if possible. Where it is necessary to use incontinence containment products, it is imperative to provide cleansing and a product change as soon as possible following a bowel movement in order to protect the patient's skin.

Goals and Outcomes. The nurse and the patient establish goals and outcomes by incorporating the patient's bowel elimination habits or routines as much as possible and by reinforcing routines that promote health. The nurse must also consider pre-existing health concerns. For example, if the patient is at risk for the worsening of heart failure, an outcome of increased fluid intake must be tailored to the patient's

cardiac function and ability to safely handle the increased fluid. For another example, if the patient's bowel habits caused the elimination problem, the nurse can help the patient learn new bowel habits. The overall goal of returning the patient to a normal bowel elimination pattern may include the following outcomes:
• The patient practises regular defecation habits.
• The patient lists the proper fluid and food intake needed to achieve regular bowel elimination.
• The patient implements a regular exercise program.
• The patient reports daily passage of soft, formed brown stool.
• The patient does not report any discomfort associated with defecation.

Setting Priorities. Defecation patterns vary among individuals. For this reason, the nurse and the patient must work together closely to plan effective interventions (Box 45.4). A realistic time frame to establish a normal defecation pattern for one patient might differ from that for another patient. For the patient who has a new ostomy as the result of newly diagnosed cancer, the priority of coping with cancer and its treatment may precede the patient's need to independently manage the bowel diversion. For another patient, however, when a bowel diversion is necessary, coping with the changes in body image may become a high priority for both the patient and the patient's family.

Continuity of Care. When patients are disabled or debilitated by illness, nurses need to include the patient's caregiver in the plan of care. Caregivers may have the same bowel elimination habits as the patient. Thus, teaching both the patient and the patient's caregiver is

<u>**Circle risk factors in table and total**</u>

Gender:

Male	1
Female	2

Mobility:

Independently mobile	0
Dependent on walking aids/assistance from others	1
Restricted to bed/chair	2
Spinal cord injury/spinal cord compression	3

Fibre intake:

5 pieces fruit/veg or more consumed daily	0
3 or 4 pieces fruit/veg consumed daily	1
2 pieces fruit/veg or less consumed daily	2

Bran products consumed daily	Yes	0
	No	2

Fluid intake:

10 cups/glasses or more consumed daily	0
6 to 9 cups/glasses consumed daily	1
5 cups/glasses or less consumed daily	2

Personal beliefs:

Does patient believe they are prone to constipation?   Yes/No

Has laxatives ever been used for constipation?   Yes/No____

Current bowel habit: _____   _____

Section sub total [ ]

Ward patients only:

Does patient have difficulty evacuating bowels in hospital toilets?

	No	0
	Yes	2

Patients requiring commode/bedpan:

Does patient anticipate problems using a commode or bedpan?

	No/Not applicable	0
	Yes	2

Section sub total [ ]

Conditions which increase risk of constipation.

From medical notes, patient history and blood results, assess presence of the following:

Physiological conditions

Metabolic disorders:

Hypokalaemia/uraemia/lead poisoning	2

Pelvic conditions:

Hysterectomy/ovarian tumour/uterine prolapse/pregnancy	3

Neuromuscular disorders:

Parkinson's disease/Multiple sclerosis/Systemic sclerosis/Hirschsprung's disease/Cerebrovascular accident/Spina bifida/Rheumatoid arthritis/Cerebral tumour	3

Endocrine disorders:

Diabetes mellitus/Hypothyroidism/Hypopituitarism/Hypercalcaemia	3

Colorectal/abdominal disorders:

Irritable bowel syndrome/Crohn's disease/Diverticulitis/Ulcerative colitis/Colorectal tumour/Anorectal stricture /Anorectal fissure/Anorectal prolapse/Haemorrhoids/Hernias	3

Psychological conditions

Psychiatric illness:

Depression/Anorexia nervosa/Bulimia nervosa	2

Learning disabilities or dementia

(as evidenced by lack of understanding of speech or situations)	2

Section sub total [ ]

Medications which increase risk of constipation.

Is patient presently taking any of the following medications on a regular basis?

Antiemetics	2	**Analgesics:**	
Calcium channel blockers	2	Non-opioid analgesia	3
Iron supplements	2	OR continuous opioid therapy	5

Anticholinergic containing medication:			
Anticonvulsants	2	**Cytotoxic chemotherapy:**	
Antidepressants	2	Cytotoxic chemotherapy	3
Antiparkinson drugs	2	OR Vinca alkaloid agents	5
Antispasmodics	2		

Section sub total [ ]

Total score [ ]

FIGURE 45.11 Constipation risk assessment scale. (From Richmond, J. P., & Wright, M. E. [2006]. Development of a constipation risk assessment scale. *Journal of Orthopaedic Nursing, 10*, 186–197 [Figure 3, p. 194].)

an important part of the care plan. Other health team members, such as dietitians and enterostomal therapist (ET) nurses, can be valuable resources. When patients require surgical intervention, a critical pathway may be used to coordinate the activities of the interprofessional health care team.

The patient who has alterations in bowel elimination will require intervention from many members of the health care team. Certain tasks, such as assisting patients onto the bedpan or bedside commode, are appropriate to delegate to unregulated care providers (UCPs). The nurse needs to remind the UCP to report any abnormal findings or difficulties encountered during the bowel elimination process. Nonnursing personnel perform many of the diagnostic tests used to evaluate the GI system. Nurses must maintain ongoing communication with these caregivers to ensure that the patient's safety, needs, wants, and concerns are addressed.

◆ **Implementation**

The success of nursing interventions depends on improving the patient's and the caregivers' understanding of bowel elimination. In the home, hospital, or long-term care facility, patients capable of learning can be taught effective bowel habits.

The patient and the patient's caregiver need to be taught about proper diet, adequate fluid intake, and factors that stimulate or slow peristalsis, such as emotional stress. The patient should also learn the importance of establishing regular bowel routines, participating in regular exercise, and taking appropriate measures when bowel elimination problems develop.

Management of Bowel Elimination. One of the most important habits nurses can encourage patients to establish is a daily bowel routine that includes adequate fluid and food intake as well as regular exercise. The urge to defecate usually occurs within an hour following a meal, after breakfast being the most common time for most individuals. Having access to a bathroom, privacy, and a comfortable seated position are all factors in the routine. Many patients have their established routines for defecation at home, which can become disrupted if they are ill. In a hospital or long-term care facility, nurses need to ensure that treatment routines do not interfere with a patient's bowel elimination routine. The provision of privacy is important to maintain. When a patient shares the room with other patients, the curtain should be pulled around the area so the patient can relax, with the knowledge that interruptions will not occur. The call light should always be placed

BOX 45.2   NURSING DIAGNOSTIC PROCESS

Assessment Activities	Defining Characteristics	Nursing Diagnosis
Inspect the abdomen for shape, symmetry.	Distended abdomen	*Diarrhea related to gastrointestinal disorder*
Auscultate for bowel sounds.	Bowel sounds are hyperactive and audible without a stethoscope.	
Percuss for general tympany.	Hyperresonance is present with gaseous distension.	
Assess frequency of stools.	Patient reports having more than three loose bowel movements a day, accompanied by muscle cramps.	
Assess hydration status.	Loss of skin turgor and dry mucous membranes.	
Have patient describe the pain, cramping, or any associated factors.	Pain is colicky in nature and spasmodic.	
Evaluate the perianal area for redness and irritation.	Breakdown of perianal tissues	

From Ackley, B., Ladwig, G., Makic, M., et al. (2020). *Nursing diagnosis handbook: An evidence-based guide to planning care* (12th ed.). Elsevier; Jarvis, C., Browne, A., MacDonald-Jenkins, J., et al. (Eds.), (2019). *Physical examination and health assessment* (3rd Canadian ed.). Elsevier Canada.

within the patient's reach. Bathroom doors should be closed, although the nurse may stand close by in case the patient needs assistance.

Maintenance of Proper Fluid and Food Intake. Daily fluid intake should be between 1 500 and 2 000 mL per day of noncaffeinated beverages. Dietary fibre intake should be from 25 to 30 g per day. In choosing a diet to promote normal bowel elimination, nurses need to consider the frequency of defecation, the characteristics of the feces, and the types of foods that impair or promote defecation. The patient with frequent constipation or impaction requires an increased intake of high-fibre foods and more fluids. The patient needs to understand that diet therapy is only one factor to consider and may not give immediate relief from discomfort such as constipation. Many evidence-informed interventions are available to reduce the risk of constipation (see Table 45.5).

If diarrhea is a concern, the patient can eat foods with a low-fibre content, such as applesauce, bananas, and rice, to reduce gastric upset or abdominal cramping. Diarrhea caused by illness can be debilitating. If the patient cannot tolerate foods or liquids orally, intravenous therapy (with potassium supplements) is necessary. The patient then returns to a normal diet slowly, often beginning with fluids. Excessively hot or cold fluids stimulate peristalsis, thereby causing abdominal cramps and further diarrhea. As the tolerance to liquids improves, solid foods are ordered. Following a severe diarrheal episode, milk products may need to be withheld until the enterocyte population has matured. Milk products may have the effect of perpetuating the diarrhea.

Promotion of Regular Exercise. A daily exercise program helps prevent bowel elimination problems. Walking, riding a stationary bicycle, or swimming stimulates peristalsis. Patients who are sedentary at work

are most in need of regular exercise. For patients with mobility challenges, such as arthritis, a passive exercise program may be helpful.

For a patient who is temporarily immobilized, the nurse should attempt ambulation of the patient as soon as possible. If the condition permits, the nurse can assist a postoperative patient in walking to a chair on the evening of the day of surgery. The patient should walk farther each day.

Exercises can help bedridden patients to more comfortably use a bedpan. The patient can practise the following exercises:

- Lie supine; tighten the abdominal muscles as though pushing them to the floor. Hold them tight to the count of three; relax. Repeat 5 to 10 times as tolerated.
- Flex and contract the thigh muscles by raising one knee slowly toward the chest. Repeat for each leg at least five times and increase the frequency as tolerated.

Bowel Retraining. The patient with incontinence is unable to maintain bowel control. A **bowel retraining** program can help some patients achieve normal defecation, especially those who still have some neuromuscular control.

The training program involves setting up a daily routine. By attempting to defecate at the same time each day and by using measures that promote defecation, the patient gains control of the bowel reflexes. The program requires time, patience, and consistency. The patient's physical readiness and ability to benefit from bowel training needs to be determined before undertaking such a program. A successful program includes the following:

- Assessing the patient's normal bowel elimination pattern and recording times when the patient is incontinent
- Choosing a time based on the patient's pattern to initiate defecation-control measures by assisting the patient to the toilet at the designated time
- Offering a hot drink (e.g., tea), fruit juice (e.g., prune juice), or another fluid that normally stimulates peristalsis for the patient before the selected defecation time
- Instructing the patient to avoid medications such as analgesics, which may increase constipation
- Providing privacy and setting a time limit for the defecation (15 to 20 minutes)
- Instructing the patient to lean forward at the hips while sitting on the toilet, to apply manual pressure with the hands over the abdomen, and to bear down but not to strain to stimulate the colon to empty
- Refraining from making critical remarks or conveying frustration if the patient is unable to defecate
- Providing regular meals with adequate fluids and fibre (RNAO, 2020)
- Maintaining normal exercise within the patient's physical ability

Hemorrhoids. Many patients experience discomfort from alterations in their bowel elimination. Pain results when hemorrhoid tissues are directly irritated. The primary goal for the patient with hemorrhoids is to have soft-formed, painless bowel movements. Proper diet, fluids, and regular exercise improve the likelihood of the stools being soft. If the patient becomes constipated, passage of hard stools may cause bleeding and irritation. Local heat provides temporary relief to swollen hemorrhoids. A sitz bath is the most effective means of heat application.

Maintenance of Skin Integrity. The patient with diarrhea or bowel incontinence is at risk for skin breakdown when fecal contents remain on the skin. Liquid stool is usually acidic and contains digestive enzymes. Irritation from repeated wiping with toilet tissue aggravates the breakdown of skin. Bathing the skin after soiling helps but may result in more breakdown unless the skin is thoroughly dried.

TABLE 45.5 Modifiable Contributing Factors Associated With Constipation and Recommended Best Practice for Prevention and Treatment

Modifiable Contributing Factors	Best Practice for Prevention and Example Interventions to Consider
Physiological • Type and amount (less than 1500–2000 mL per day) of fluid intake • Intake of caffeinated beverages and sugar substitutes • Insufficient fibre intake (less than 25–30 g per day) • Poor dietary habits, including high intake of animal fats (RNAO 2020; Touhy et al., 2019)	• Assess and seek information about physiological factors related to constipation • Encourage healthy fluid intake of 1500–2000 mL per day (unless clinical contraindications, e.g., heart failure) • Gradually introduce dietary fibre intake of 25–30 g per day • *Canada's Food Guide:* https://food-guide.canada.ca/en/ • Dietitian referral for dietary improvements (RNAO 2020; Touhy et al., 2019)
Functional • Decreased physical activity and mobility • Sedentary lifestyle, including lengthy bed rest and deconditioning • Balance • Positioning for toileting • Toileting routine (usual routine, changes) • Habitual suppression of urge to defecate • Irregular defecation habits (RNAO 2020; Touhy et al., 2019)	• Assess and seek information about functional abilities related to constipation • Encourage individualized physical activity • OT/PT consult for mobility, physical activity, toileting positioning, balance, and toileting equipment • Promote toileting "squat" positioning • Promote regular and consistent toileting daily, following a triggering meal to maximize the gastrocolic reflex • Habit retraining (RNAO 2020; Touhy et al., 2019)
Cognitive Ability • Self-care, social, interactional, and interpretive abilities (Wells & Dawson, 2000) • Recognition and recall • Identifying the urge to defecate • Remembering how to respond • Locating the toilet • Comprehension and expression • Understanding reminders • Asking for assistance • Voluntary and purposeful movement • Spatial orientation • Attention deficits and conversation • Remembering how to respond	• Assess and seek information about cognitive self-care social, interactional, and interpretive abilities related to constipation • Do not routinely use incontinence containment products (including briefs or pads) for older persons (Choosing Wisely Canada, 2020) • Provide reminders and cues • Signage for toilet location • Provide toileting assistance • OT consult for sitting balance
Psychosocial • Avoidance of the urge to defecate • Depression • Emotional stress	• Assess and seek information about psychosocial factors related to constipation • Address social distress related to toileting, such as isolation and embarrassment • Do not routinely recommend antidepressants as a first-line treatment for mild depressive symptoms in adults (Choosing Wisely Canada, 2020)
Living Environment • Privacy • Home/Institution • Recent environmental changes • Disruptions in daily activities • Use of restraints (physical and chemical)	• Assess and seek information about living environment factors related to constipation • Provide for privacy • Orientation to environment • Orientation to routines • Minimize use of restraints • Do not recommend antipsychotic medicines as the first choice to treat symptoms of dementia (Choosing Wisely Canada, 2020)
Pharmacological • Number and type of medications • Prolonged and overuse of laxatives	• Assess and obtain information about pharmacological factors related to constipation • Medication review • Medication reconciliation (MedRec) (Institute for Safe Medication Practices [ISMP] Canada, 2000–2021) • Address chronic use of laxatives • Consult clinical pharmacist, primary care provider, community pharmacist Resources: • See Appendix P in the RNAO (2020) *A Proactive Approach to Bladder and Bowel Management in Adults* guideline document for a list of medication categories that can cause constipation. • The RNAO guideline also provides a web link to the Government of Canada's Drug Product Database (https://health-products.canada.ca/dpd-bdpp/index-eng.jsp) to search the uses and adverse effects of specific medications.

OT, Occupational therapist; *PT,* physiotherapist.
Data from Choosing Wisely Canada (2020). *Nine tests and treatments to question in nursing.* https://choosingwiselycanada.org/nursing/; Institute for Safe Medication Practices (ISMP) Canada. (2000–2021). *Medication reconciliation (MedRec).* https://www.ismp-canada.org/medrec/; Registered Nurses' Association of Ontario (RNAO). (2020). *A proactive approach to bladder and bowel management in adults* (4th ed.). https://rnao.ca/sites/rnao-ca/files/bpg/Bladder_and_Bowel_Management_FINAL_WEB.pdf; Touhy, T. A., Jett, K. F., Boscart, V., et al. (Eds.). (2019). *Ebersole and Hess' gerontological nursing & healthy aging* (2nd Canadian ed.). Elsevier Canada; Wells, D. L., & Dawson, P. (2000). Description of retained abilities in older persons with dementia. *Research in Nursing and Health, 23*(2), 158–166. https://doi.org/10.1002/(SICI)1098-240X(200004)23:2%3C158::AID-NUR8%3E3.0.CO;2-L

BOX 45.3 RESEARCH HIGHLIGHT

The Prevalence, Incidence, and Correlates of Fecal Incontinence Among Older People Residing in Long-Term Care Facilities: A Systematic Review

Research Focus

Massirfufulay and colleagues (2019) conducted a systematic review to describe the prevalence, incidence, and correlates of bowel incontinence among long-term care residents.

Research Abstract

The authors conducted a systematic review that included studies conducted in both nursing and residential care facilities, with participants who were 60 years of age and older. The authors defined double incontinence as both bladder and bowel incontinence, isolated bowel incontinence with no bladder incontinence, and all bowel incontinence as anyone with bowel incontinence (whether isolated or double).

Methods and Results

The authors completed a search of CINAHL and MEDLINE databases up to December 31, 2017, for studies that reported the prevalence and/or incidence and correlates of bowel incontinence. Of 278 citations identified, 23 studies met the inclusion criteria for the review. Of the 23 studies that the authors included, 12 were identified as high-quality, 5 medium-quality, and 6 low-quality studies. Associated most frequently with bowel incontinence were cognitive impairment, limited functional ability, urinary incontinence, reduced mobility, advanced age, and diarrhea.

Implications for Practice

The authors concluded that bowel incontinence is prevalent in older persons living in long-term care facilities, noting that it is an issue amenable to management. There are multiple factors that need to be considered when considering interventions. The nurse should consider all modifiable contributing factors when planning interventions to improve or manage bowel incontinence experienced by older persons living in both nursing and residential care facilities.

From Massirfufulay, K. M., Saga, S., & Blekken, L. E. (2019). The prevalence, incidence, and correlates of fecal incontinence among older people residing in care homes: A systematic review. *JAMDA: Journal of Post-Acute and Long-Term Care Medicine, 20*(8), 956–962. https://doi.org/10.1016/j.jamda.2019.03.033

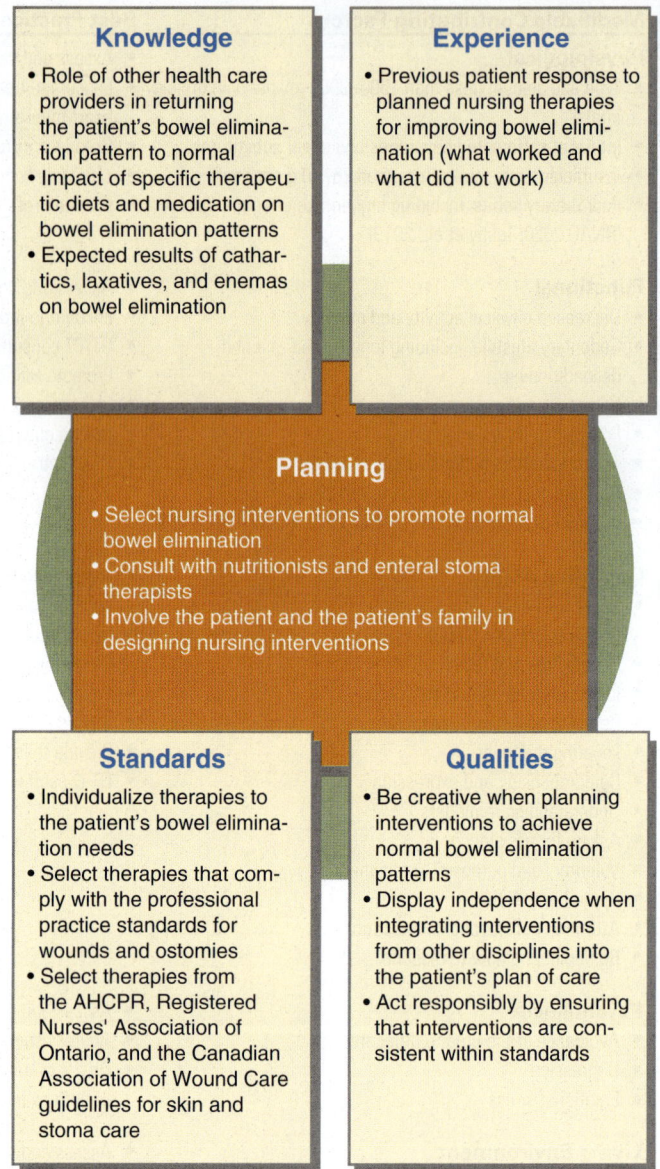

Knowledge
- Role of other health care providers in returning the patient's bowel elimination pattern to normal
- Impact of specific therapeutic diets and medication on bowel elimination patterns
- Expected results of cathartics, laxatives, and enemas on bowel elimination

Experience
- Previous patient response to planned nursing therapies for improving bowel elimination (what worked and what did not work)

Planning
- Select nursing interventions to promote normal bowel elimination
- Consult with nutritionists and enteral stoma therapists
- Involve the patient and the patient's family in designing nursing interventions

Standards
- Individualize therapies to the patient's bowel elimination needs
- Select therapies that comply with the professional practice standards for wounds and ostomies
- Select therapies from the AHCPR, Registered Nurses' Association of Ontario, and the Canadian Association of Wound Care guidelines for skin and stoma care

Qualities
- Be creative when planning interventions to achieve normal bowel elimination patterns
- Display independence when integrating interventions from other disciplines into the patient's plan of care
- Act responsibly by ensuring that interventions are consistent within standards

FIGURE 45.12 Critical thinking model for bowel elimination planning. *AHCPR,* Agency for Health Care Policy and Research.

When caring for an incontinent patient who is unable to ask for assistance, the nurse should check often for defecation. The anal areas can be protected with barrier cream that holds moisture in the skin to prevent drying and cracking. Yeast infections of the skin can develop easily. Several powdered antifungal agents are effective against yeast. Baby powder or cornstarch should not be used because they have no medicinal properties and they frequently cake on the skin, which makes them difficult to remove.

Medications. Medications may be used to initiate and facilitate bowel elimination. Cathartics, laxatives, and occasionally an enema are used to control constipation, whereas antidiarrheal preparations assist the patient in resolving diarrhea. These medications are available over the counter and as prescriptions. Patients must be cautioned not to use these over-the-counter medications on a prolonged basis without consulting their health care provider.

Laxatives are defined as products that stimulate evacuation of the formed stool from the rectum, whereas cathartics are defined as products that evacuate unformed and usually watery fecal material from the entire colon. Laxatives are thus milder in action than cathartics. When used correctly, laxatives and cathartics safely maintain normal bowel elimination patterns; however, chronic use of cathartics causes the large intestine to lose muscle tone and to become less responsive to stimulation by laxatives. Laxative overuse can also cause serious diarrhea that can lead to dehydration and electrolyte depletion. Mineral oil, a common laxative, decreases fat-soluble vitamin absorption. Laxatives can influence the efficacy of other medications by altering the transit time (i.e., the time the medication remains in the GI tract and is available for absorption).

> **SAFETY ALERT** Excessive use of laxatives, enemas, or bulk-forming agents increases the patient's risk for diarrhea and abnormal bowel elimination and destroys the patient's normal defecation reflex. In addition, the patient may develop an altered absorption of nutrients, fluid and electrolyte imbalances, and generalized weakness. When these symptoms occur in chronically ill or older patients, they may result in an increased risk for falls and other injuries.

BOX 45.4 NURSING CARE PLAN
Constipation

ASSESSMENT

Javier is a nurse who visits Larry (preferred pronouns: he/his) at his home on a cattle ranch. Larry lives 40 km from town. He is 22 years old and had surgery 6 days ago for repair of a broken right leg. Larry tells Javier, "I just don't feel good."

Assessment Activities	Findings and Defining Characteristics
Ask Larry about his recent bowel elimination patterns over the last 5 days.	Larry has not had a bowel movement since he left the hospital 4 days ago and he feels like his abdomen is tight and sore.
Review Larry's medication.	Larry has been prescribed opioids for pain. He is taking them regularly, as prescribed.
Review Larry's dietary intake over the past day.	Larry has eaten eggs, bacon, and toast for breakfast and soup for lunch. For supper, Larry had chicken, rice, and corn. He drinks about six cups of coffee each day, no water, but will drink a cola.
Ask about any nausea or vomiting.	Larry has not felt nauseated.
Auscultate the abdomen.	Decreased bowel sounds are auscultated throughout all four abdominal quadrants.
Palpate the abdomen.	While Javier is palpating Larry's abdomen, Larry tells Javier, "It really hurts." On palpation, the left lower quadrant is tender and firm.

NURSING DIAGNOSIS: Constipation related to opiate-containing pain medication and decreased fibre intake.

PLANNING

Goals (Nursing Outcomes Classification)*	Expected Outcomes
Bowel Elimination	
Larry will establish normal defecation.	Larry will drink at least 1 500 mL of fluid over the next 8 hours.
Larry will express relief from constipation.	Larry will report passage of soft stool without straining within 24 hours.
Nutritional Status: Food and Fluid Intake	
Larry will identify measures to prevent constipation.	Larry will increase the fibre content of his diet.
Larry will increase the amount of daily exercise.	

*Outcome classification labels from Ackley, B., Ladwig, G., Makic, M., et al. (2020). *Nursing diagnosis handbook: An evidence-based guide to planning care* (12th ed.). Elsevier.

INTERVENTIONS

Interventions	Rationale
Constipation or Impaction Management	
Encourage fluid intake of fruit juice, water, and other appropriate fluids.	Adequate fluid intake is necessary to prevent hard, dry stool. Water is a natural stool softener.
Encourage activity within the limits of Larry's mobility regimen.	Even minimal activity (such as leg lifts) increases peristalsis.
Add bran flakes or bran to the diet.	The number of bowel movements is increased with consumption of bran.
Provide bowel medications as ordered.	Medications can soften the stool and prevent straining.
Provide a private atmosphere for bowel elimination.	Patients should feel relaxed when moving their bowels.

EVALUATION

Nursing Actions	Patient Response and Findings	Achievement of Outcome
Ask Larry to identify foods high in fibre.	Larry is able to correctly identify high-fibre foods. Review of the 24-hour diet diary shows that Larry is selecting high-fibre, low-fat foods.	Larry is making excellent progress in introducing high-fibre and low-fat foods into his diet.
Ask Larry to plan menus to increase fibre.	Review of the 24-hour diet diary shows meals planned that have high-fibre content. Larry reviews his shopping list, which includes bran, oat, and fruit products.	Larry is knowledgeable about fibre content and purchases foods that are high in fibre.
Ask Larry about increased activity.	Larry states that he has not changed his level of activity.	Larry has not increased his level of activity and needs to continue to work on increasing his physical activity.
Observe Larry's subsequent stool for characteristics such as consistency and colour.	Stools occur now every 24 to 48 hours. Larry states he does not "feel regular." The abdomen is soft and nondistended. Stools are formed and hard, and Larry reports straining.	Larry has not achieved passage of a regular, formed stool.

TABLE 45.6	Common Types of Laxatives and Cathartics		
Agents and Brand Names	**Action**	**Indications**	**Risks**
Bulk Forming			
Methylcellulose	The high-fibre content absorbs water and increases solid intestinal bulk.	These agents are the least irritating, most natural, and safest cathartics. These agents are the medications of choice for treating chronic constipation (e.g., during pregnancy or as the result of a low-residue diet).	These agents can cause obstruction if not mixed with at least 240 mL of water or juice and swallowed quickly.
Psyllium	These agents stretch the intestinal wall to stimulate peristalsis.	These agents may also be used to relieve mild, watery diarrhea.	Use caution with bulk-forming laxatives that also contain stimulants. These agents are not used in patients for whom large fluid intake is contraindicated.
Emollient			
Docusate sodium Docusate calcium	Stool softeners are detergents that lower the surface tension of feces, allowing water and fat to penetrate. They may increase the secretion of water by the intestines.	These agents are used for short-term therapy to relieve straining on defecation. These agents would be beneficial for patients who have hemorrhoids, have undergone perianal surgery, are pregnant, or are recovering from myocardial infarction.	These agents are of little value for treatment of chronic constipation.
Saline			
Magnesium citrate or citrate of magnesia	These agents contain a salt preparation that is not absorbed by the intestines.	These agents are used only for acute emptying of the bowel (e.g., as a preparation for endoscopic examination, in cases of suspected poisoning, or to treat acute constipation).	These agents are not used for long-term management of constipation.
Magnesium hydroxide	The osmotic effect increases pressure in the bowel to act as stimulant for peristalsis.		These agents are contraindicated for patients with kidney dysfunction (to avoid a toxic buildup of magnesium).
Sodium phosphate enema	Sodium phosphate		Phosphate salts are not used for patients on fluid restriction or for renal patients (because of risk of hyperphosphatemia due to the accumulation of phosphorus).
Stimulant Cathartics			
Bisacodyl	These agents irritate the intestinal mucosa to increase motility.	These agents may be used to prepare the bowel for diagnostic procedures.	These agents may cause severe cramping.
Castor oil	These agents decrease absorption in the small bowel and colon.		These agents are not for long-term use.
Phenolphthalein	Phenolphthalein and danthron may cause pink or red urine.		
Lubricants			
Mineral oil	These agents coat the fecal contents, which allows for easier passage of the stool.	These agents are used to prevent straining on defecation (e.g., for patients who have hemorrhoids and for those who are recovering from perianal surgery).	These agents decrease the absorption of fat-soluble vitamins (A, D, E, and K).
	These agents reduce water absorption in the colon.		These agents can cause a dangerous form of pneumonia if aspirated into the lungs. Mineral oil, when taken with emollients, can increase the risk for fat emboli.

Data from Sealock, K., Seneviratne, C., Lilley, L. L., et al. (2021). *Lilley's pharmacology for Canadian healthcare practice* (4th Canadian ed.). Elsevier Canada.

Cathartics and laxatives. A patient is often unable to defecate normally because of pain, constipation, or impaction. Cathartics and laxatives provide the short-term action of emptying the bowel. They are also used in bowel evacuation for patients undergoing GI tests and abdominal surgery. Although the terms *cathartic* and *laxative* are often used interchangeably, cathartics have a stronger effect on the intestines. Five types of laxatives and cathartics are available (Table 45.6).

Cathartics and laxatives are available in oral, tablet, and powder suppository dosage forms (see Chapter 35). Although the oral route is most commonly used, cathartics that are prepared as suppositories are more effective because of their stimulant effect on the rectal mucosa. Cathartic suppositories such as bisacodyl (Dulcolax) can act within 30 minutes. Older persons who use Dulcolax often have a strong, sudden urge to defecate.

Electrolyte Balance and Antidiarrheal Agents. For patients with diarrhea, frequent passage of liquid stools becomes a concern. When a person has secretory diarrhea, cells at the base of the villi secrete massive amounts of fluid into the lumen of the small intestine. However, the tip of the villi can still absorb sugars and fluids. Therefore, diarrhea can quickly lead to serious electrolyte imbalances, particularly in infants and children (see Chapter 41). Therefore, the first course of action is to immediately replace fluids by mouth. Fluids with adequate electrolyte content (e.g., Pedialyte and Gastrolyte) are a wise choice. In developing countries without a safe water supply or during epidemics of infectious diarrhea (e.g., cholera), millions of lives have been saved by using a cheap, safe, and simple method of replacing water and salts lost through diarrhea. This method, known as *oral rehydration therapy (ORT)*, involves mixing a very low-cost package of salts (sodium, potassium chloride, citrate or bicarbonate, and glucose) with boiled water.

Many patients will use over-the-counter agents, such as Imodium, to relieve common diarrhea. However, the most effective antidiarrheal agents are prescriptive opiates, such as codeine phosphate, opium tincture (Paregoric), and diphenoxylate (Lomotil). Opiates inhibit the peristaltic waves that move feces forward but also increase the segmental contractions that mix intestinal contents and expose the contents to the mucosal absorbing surface. The further effect of opiates on increasing the absorption of sodium and water also dries out the feces. As a result, more water is absorbed by the colonic mucosa. These antidiarrheal agents should be used with caution because opiates may be addictive.

Rectal Suppositories. A rectal suppository may be used to stimulate defecation for a patient having difficulty initiating a bowel movement. Rectal suppositories are solid, bullet-shaped preparations designed for easy insertion into the rectum. The suppository dissolves at body temperature and gradually spreads over the lining of the lower bowel (rectum). Glycerin suppositories are used to lubricate the stool in the rectum, facilitating evacuation. Stimulant suppositories like Dulcolax contain medication that is absorbed into the bloodstream from the rectum and stimulates the mucosa, increasing peristalsis.

Enemas. An enema is the instillation of a solution into the rectum and sigmoid colon. The primary reason for using an enema is to promote defecation by stimulating peristalsis. The volume of fluid instilled breaks up the fecal mass, stretches the rectal wall, and initiates the defecation reflex. Enemas are also used as a vehicle for administering medications that exert a local effect on rectal mucosa.

The most common use for an enema is temporary relief of constipation. Other indications include removing impacted feces; beginning a program of bowel training; and emptying the bowel before diagnostic tests, surgery, or childbirth.

Cleansing enemas. Cleansing enemas promote the complete evacuation of feces from the colon. They act by stimulating peristalsis through the infusion of a large volume of solution or through local irritation of the colon's mucosa. Solutions used in cleansing enemas include tap water, normal saline, low-volume hypertonic saline, and soapsuds solution. Each solution exerts a different osmotic effect to move fluids between the colon and the interstitial spaces beyond the intestinal wall. Infants and children should receive only normal saline because they are at risk for fluid imbalance.

A prescriber may order a high- or low-cleansing enema. The terms *high* and *low* refer to the height from which, and hence the pressure

with which, the fluid is delivered. High enemas are given to cleanse the entire colon. After the enema is infused, the patient is asked to turn from the left lateral position to the dorsal recumbent position and to the right lateral position. The position change ensures that fluid reaches all of the large intestine. A low enema cleanses only the rectum and the sigmoid colon.

Tap water. Tap water is hypotonic and exerts a lower osmotic pressure than that of fluid in interstitial spaces. After infusion into the colon, tap water escapes from the bowel lumen into the interstitial spaces. The net movement of water is low. The infused volume stimulates defecation before large amounts of water leave the bowel. Tap water enemas should not be repeated because water toxicity or circulatory overload can develop if large amounts of water are absorbed.

Normal saline. Physiologically, normal saline is the safest solution to use because it exerts the same osmotic pressure as that of fluids in the interstitial spaces surrounding the bowel. The volume of infused saline stimulates peristalsis. Unlike tap water enemas, saline enemas do not create the danger of excess fluid absorption.

Hypertonic solutions. Hypertonic solutions infused into the bowel exert osmotic pressure that pulls fluids out of the interstitial spaces. The colon fills with fluid, and the resultant distension promotes defecation. Patients unable to tolerate large volumes of fluid benefit most from this type of enema, which is, by design, low volume. Patients with contraindications for this type of enema are patients who are dehydrated and young infants. A hypertonic solution of 120 to 180 mL is usually effective. The commercially prepared Fleet Enema is the most commonly used hypertonic solution.

Soapsuds. Soapsuds may be added to tap water or saline to create the effect of intestinal irritation to stimulate peristalsis. Only pure castile soap is safe to use. A liquid form of castile soap is included in most soapsuds enema kits. Harsh soaps or detergents can cause serious bowel inflammation.

Oil-Retention Enemas. Oil-retention enemas lubricate the rectum and colon. The feces absorb the oil and become softer and easier to pass. To enhance the action of the oil, the patient retains the enema for several hours, if possible.

Other Types of Enemas. Carminative enemas provide relief from gaseous distension. Use of a carminative enema improves the ability to pass flatus. An example of a carminative enema is MGW solution, which contains 30 mL of magnesium, 60 mL of glycerin, and 90 mL of water.

Medicated enemas contain medications. An example is sodium polystyrene sulphonate (Kayexalate), which is used to treat patients with dangerously high serum potassium levels. This medication contains a resin that exchanges sodium ions for potassium ions in the large intestine. Another medicated enema is neomycin solution, which is an antibiotic used to reduce bacteria in the colon before bowel surgery.

Enema Administration. Enemas are administered in either commercially packaged, disposable units or with reusable equipment prepared before use. Sterile technique is unnecessary because the colon normally contains bacteria; however, gloves should be worn to prevent the transmission of fecal microorganisms.

The nurse should explain the procedure to the patient, including the position to assume, precautions to take to avoid discomfort, and the length of time necessary to retain the solution before defecation. If the patient is to receive the enema at home, the procedure must be explained to a caregiver.

Often the prescriber orders "enemas until clear." This order means that the enema is to be repeated until the patient passes fluid that is clear and contains no fecal material. As many as three enemas may be necessary, but the nurse should caution the patient against using more than three enemas. Excess enema use seriously depletes fluids and electrolytes. If the enema fails to return a clear solution after three times (check employer policy on the maximum number of enemas permitted) or if the patient seems to not tolerate the rigours of repeated enemas, the prescriber should be notified.

Giving an enema to a patient who is unable to contract the external sphincter can pose difficulties. In these cases, the enema should be given with the patient positioned on the bedpan. Giving the enema with the patient sitting on the toilet is unsafe because the curved rectal tubing can abrade the rectal wall. Skill 45.1 outlines the steps for enema administration.

> **SAFETY ALERT** A rectal check is done prior to instilling an enema. For patients with an impaction, the fecal mass may be too large to be passed voluntarily. If enemas fail, the nurse may consider breaking up the fecal mass with their finger and removing it in sections (Box 45.5). The procedure will be very uncomfortable for the patient. Excess rectal manipulation may cause irritation to the mucosa, bleeding, perforation of the bowel wall, and stimulation of the vagus nerve, which results in a reflex slowing of the heart rate. Because of the procedure's potential complications, a prescriber's order is necessary for a nurse to remove a fecal impaction.

Surgical Management of Bowel Elimination

Inserting and Maintaining a Nasogastric Tube. A patient's condition or situation may warrant special interventions to decompress the GI tract. Such conditions include surgery, infections of the GI tract, trauma to the GI tract, and the absence of peristalsis.

A nasogastric (NG) tube is a pliable tube that is inserted through the patient's nasopharynx into the stomach. The tube has a hollow lumen that allows removal of gastric secretions and introduction of solutions into the stomach. NG intubation has several purposes (Table 45.7).

The Levin and Salem sump tubes are the most common tubes used for stomach decompression. The Levin tube is a single-lumen tube with holes near the tip. A sump tube may be connected to either a drainage bag or an intermittent suction device to drain stomach secretions.

The Salem sump tube is preferable for stomach decompression. This tube has two lumina: one for removal of gastric contents (Figure 45.13) and one to provide an air vent. A blue "pigtail" is the air vent that connects with the second lumen. When the sump tube's main lumen is connected to suction, the air vent permits free, continuous drainage of secretions. The air vent should never be clamped off, connected to suction, or used for irrigation.

Bowel Diversions. In Canada, approximately 13 000 people undergo ostomy surgeries every year, and an estimated population of 70 000 Canadians live with an ostomy (Vancouver United Ostomy Association Chapter, 2019). Certain diseases cause conditions that prevent the normal passage of feces through the rectum. The treatment for these disorders may result in the need for a stoma, which is a temporary or permanent artificial opening in the abdominal wall. The opening may be either an ileostomy, a surgical opening in the ileum, or a colostomy, a surgical opening in the colon. The ends of the intestine are brought through the abdominal wall to create the stoma (RNAO, 2019).

A nurse specialized in wound, ostomy, and continence (NSWOC) (Wound, Ostomy, and Continence Nurses Society Task Force, 2018) is a nurse who is specifically trained to care for wound, ostomy, and continence management. A health care provider with specialized knowledge and skill (NSWOC or surgeon) provides preoperative stoma site marking for bowel diversions, to select the optimal site in order to mitigate postoperative complications (Canadian Society of Colon and Rectal Surgeons [CSCRS] & Nurses Specialized in Wound, Ostomy

and Continence Canada [NSWOCC], 2020; McKenna et al., 2016). NSWOC Canada (NSWOCC) is a not-for-profit association of nurses who specialize in wound, ostomy, and continence (https://nswoc.ca). NSWOCs offer a multimodal program to decrease postoperative complications, as well as to improve patient safety, satisfaction, and recovery time (Miller et al., 2017).

The standard bowel diversion creates a stoma, or the patient can undergo reconstructive surgery that uses the native sphincter for bowel continence. The reconstructive surgery includes either a continent stoma procedure, which is now rarely done, or the ileoanal pouch anastomosis, which is described later in the chapter.

Ostomies. The location of the ostomy determines the consistency of the stool. An ileostomy bypasses the entire large intestine. As a result, stools are frequent and liquid. The same is true for a colostomy of the ascending colon (Figure 45.14). A colostomy of the transverse colon, in general, results in a more solid, formed stool (see Figure 45.14). The descending colostomy and sigmoid colostomy emit a near-normal stool (see Figure 45.14). The location of a colostomy is determined by the patient's medical problem and general condition. Colostomies have three types of construction: loop colostomy, end colostomy, and double-barrel colostomy.

Loop colostomy. A loop colostomy is usually performed in a medical emergency when closure of the colostomy is anticipated. Loop colostomies are usually temporary large stomas constructed in the transverse colon. The surgeon pulls a loop of bowel onto the abdomen. The loop ostomy has two openings through the one stoma (see Figure 45.14). The proximal end drains stool, whereas the distal portion drains mucus (Gallagher & Harding, 2019).

End colostomy. The end colostomy consists of one stoma formed from one end of the bowel with the distal portion of the GI tract either removed or sewn closed (known as *Hartmann's pouch*) and left in the abdominal cavity. For many patients, end colostomies are a result of surgical treatment for colorectal cancer. In such cases, the rectum might also be removed. Patients with diverticulitis who are treated surgically often have a temporary end colostomy with a Hartmann's pouch (Figure 45.15).

Double-barrel colostomy. In a double-barrel colostomy (in contrast to the loop colostomy), the bowel is surgically severed and the two ends are brought out onto the abdomen (see Figure 45.14). The double-barrel colostomy consists of two distinct stomas: the proximal functioning stoma and the distal nonfunctioning stoma.

Kock continent ileostomy. The Kock continent ileostomy is created using the patient's small intestine to create a pouch. This procedure is occasionally used in the treatment of ulcerative colitis. The pouch has a continent stoma, which is a nipple-type valve that is drained with an external catheter. The patient places the external catheter intermittently in the stoma and empties the pouch several times a day. The stoma is covered with a protective dressing or a stoma cap (RNAO, 2019).

Psychological Considerations. A stoma can cause serious body-image changes, particularly when it is permanent. Ayaz-Alkaya (2019) conducted a review of the literature to summarize empirical evidence related to psychosocial health in individuals with a stoma. The author concluded that psychosocial issues identified in their review included poor body-image perception and self-respect, depression, sexual difficulties, and lower psychosocial adaptation and made a recommendation for further research to be conducted to study the efficacy of interventions (Ayaz-Alkaya, 2019). An important factor in the patient's reactions is physiological challenges, such as the character of the fecal secretions and the ability to control them. The patient's self-esteem can be impaired by the presence of foul odors, spillage, or leakage of liquid stools and the inability to regulate bowel movements.

| **SKILL 45.1** | **ADMINISTERING A CLEANSING ENEMA** |

Delegation Considerations

The skill of administering an enema can be delegated to unregulated care providers (UCPs). Nurses have the responsibility to assess the patient for specific considerations, such as their safety, the need for alternative positioning and comfort, and the presence of stable vital signs, as well as a rectal check prior to the procedure. In addition, nurses have the responsibility to determine the patient's response to the enema. If the enema is a medicated enema, it cannot be delegated to a UCP. If delegating this task to a UCP:

- Inform and assist the UCP in the proper way to position patients who have mobility restrictions, such as patients with arthritis or severe fatigue.
- Instruct the UCP how to position patients who have therapeutic equipment present, such as drains, intravenous catheters, or traction.
- Instruct the UCP about the specific signs and symptoms that will appear in patients not tolerating the procedure and about when the procedure must be stopped. For example, these signs and symptoms may include abdominal pain more than a pressure sensation, abdominal cramping, abdominal distension, or rectal bleeding.

Equipment

- Clean gloves
- Water-soluble lubricant
- Waterproof, absorbent pads
- Bath blanket
- Toilet tissue
- Bedpan, bedside commode, or access
- Washbasin, washcloths, towel
- Intravenous (IV) pole
- Enema bag administration
- Enema container
- Tubing and clamp (if not already attached to the enema container)
- Appropriate size rectal tube: 22 to 30 Fr
- Correct volume of warmed solution: 750 to 1 000 mL
- Prepackaged enema
- Prepackaged enema container with rectal tip

PROCEDURE

STEPS	**RATIONALE**
1. Assess status of the patient: last bowel movement, normal bowel patterns, presence of hemorrhoids, mobility, external sphincter control, and abdominal pain.	• Assessment is used to determine the factors indicating a need for an enema and influences the type of enema used.
2. Assess the patient for presence of increased intracranial pressure, glaucoma, or recent rectal or prostate surgery.	• These conditions contraindicate the use of an enema.
3. Check the patient's medical record to clarify the rationale for the enema.	• The nurse needs to determine the purpose of the enema administration, either as a preparation for a special procedure or for relief of constipation.
4. Review the prescriber's order for the enema.	• A prescriber's order is required. The order determines the number and type of enemas to be given.
5. Determine the patient's level of understanding of the purpose of the enema.	• The patient's current level of understanding allows the nurse to plan for appropriate teaching measures.
6. Perform hand hygiene. Collect appropriate equipment.	• Proper hand hygiene reduces the transmission of microorganisms.
7. Correctly identify the patient and explain the procedure.	• Explaining the procedure promotes patient cooperation and reduces anxiety.
8. Assemble the enema bag with the appropriate solution and rectal tube.	
9. Perform hand hygiene and apply gloves.	• Proper hand hygiene reduces the transmission of microorganisms.
10. Provide privacy by closing the curtains around the bed or by closing the door.	• Privacy reduces embarrassment for the patient.
11. Raise the bed to an appropriate working height; raise the side rail on the patient's left side.	• Raising the bed and use of the side rail promote good body mechanics and patient safety.
12. Assist the patient into a position lying on the left side with right knee flexed (i.e., left lateral recumbent position).	• The left lateral recumbent position allows the enema solution to flow downward by gravity along the natural curve of the sigmoid colon and rectum, thus improving retention of the solution.

CRITICAL DECISION POINT: *Patients who have poor sphincter control will have difficulty retaining the enema solution. If the patient is suspected of having poor sphincter control, position the patient on a bedpan.*

13. Place a waterproof pad under the hips and buttocks.	• A waterproof pad prevents soiling of the bed linen.
14. Cover the patient with a bath blanket, exposing only the rectal area, with the anus clearly visible.	• The bath blanket provides warmth, reduces exposure of body parts, and allows the patient to feel more relaxed and comfortable.

Continued

SKILL 45.1   **ADMINISTERING A CLEANSING ENEMA—cont'd**

15. Place the bedpan or commode in an easily accessible position. If the patient will be expelling contents in the toilet, ensure the toilet is available. (If the patient will be walking to the bathroom to expel the enema, place the patient's slippers and bathrobe in an easily accessible position.)

- A bedpan or commode should be nearby in case the patient is unable to retain the enema solution.

16. Administer the enema:

A. Enema bag

(1) Add warmed solution to the enema bag: warm the tap water as it flows from faucet, place the saline container in a basin of hot water before adding saline to the enema bag, check the temperature of the solution with a bath thermometer or by pouring a small amount of solution over your inner wrist.

- Hot water can burn intestinal mucosa. Cold water can cause abdominal cramping and is difficult to retain.

(2) Raise the container, release the clamp, and allow the solution to flow long enough to fill the tubing.

- Raising the container removes air from the tubing.

(3) Reclamp the tubing.

- Reclamping prevents further loss of the solution.

(4) Lubricate 6 to 8 cm (2–3 inches) of the tip of the rectal tube with lubricating jelly.

- The lubricating jelly allows smooth insertion of the rectal tube without risk of irritation or trauma to the mucosa.

(5) Gently separate the buttocks and locate the anus. Instruct the patient to relax by breathing out slowly through the mouth.

- Exhaling promotes relaxation of the external anal sphincter.

(6) Insert tip of the rectal tube slowly by pointing the tip in the direction of the patient's umbilicus (see Step 16A[6] illustration) for about 7 to 10 cm.

- Careful insertion prevents trauma to the rectal mucosa from an accidental lodging of the tube against the rectal wall. Insertion beyond the proper limit can cause bowel perforation.

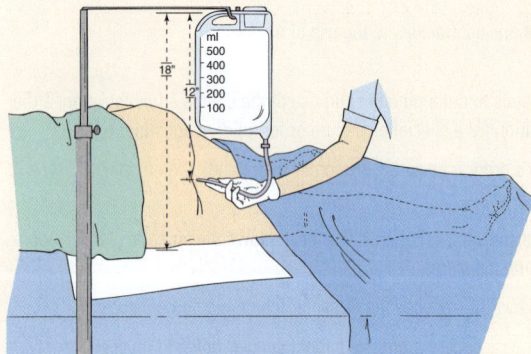

STEP 16A(6) Insertion of a rectal tube into the rectum.

CRITICAL DECISION POINT: *If the tube does not pass easily, do not force it. Consider allowing a small amount of fluid to infuse and then try reinserting the tube slowly.*

---

(7) Hold the tubing in the rectum constantly until the end of the fluid instillation.

- Bowel contractions can cause expulsion of the rectal tube.

(8) Open the regulating clamp and allow the solution to enter slowly with the enema container at the patient's hip level.

- Rapid instillation can stimulate evacuation of the rectal tube.

(9) Raise height of the enema container slowly to the appropriate level above the anus: 30 to 45 cm for a high enema, 30 cm for a regular enema, 7.5 cm for a low enema (see Step 16A[6] illustration). Instillation time varies depending on the volume of solution administered.

- Raising the height slowly allows for continuous, slow instillation of the solution. Raising the container too high causes rapid instillation and possible painful distension of the colon.

(10) Lower the container or clamp tubing if the patient complains of cramping or if fluid escapes around the rectal tube.

- Temporary cessation of instillation prevents cramping but may prevent the patient from retaining all the fluid, thus altering the effectiveness of the enema.

(11) Clamp the tubing after all solution is instilled.

- Clamping prevents entrance of air into the rectum.

Continued

SKILL 45.1 ADMINISTERING A CLEANSING ENEMA—cont'd

B. Prepackaged disposable container

(1) Remove the plastic cap from the rectal tip. The tip is already lubricated, but more jelly can be applied as needed.
- Lubrication provides for smooth insertion of rectal tube while avoiding rectal irritation or trauma.

(2) Gently separate the buttocks and locate the anus. Instruct the patient to relax by breathing out slowly through the mouth.
- Breathing out promotes relaxation of the external rectal sphincter.

(3) Insert the tip of the bottle gently into the rectum about 7 to 10 cm.
- Gentle insertion prevents trauma to the rectal mucosa.

(4) Squeeze the bottle until all the solution has entered the rectum and colon. Instruct the patient to retain the solution until the urge to defecate occurs, usually within 2 to 5 minutes.
- Hypertonic solutions require only small volumes to stimulate defecation.

17. Place layers of toilet tissue around the tube at the anus and gently withdraw the rectal tube.
- The use of toilet paper provides the patient with comfort and cleanliness.

18. Explain to the patient that the feeling of distension is normal. Ask the patient to retain the solution for as long as possible while lying quietly in bed.
- The enema solution distends the bowel. The length of retention varies depending on the type of enema and the patient's ability to contract the rectal sphincter. Longer retention promotes more effective stimulation of peristalsis and defecation.

19. Discard the enema container and tubing in the proper receptacle, or rinse thoroughly with warm soap and water if the container is to be reused.
- Proper handling of the used enema container and tubing reduces transmission and growth of microorganisms.

20. Assist the patient to the bathroom or help to position the patient on a bedpan.
- The normal squatting position promotes defecation.

21. Observe the character of the feces and solution (caution the patient against flushing the toilet until you can inspect the feces).
- The character of the expelled feces determines the efficacy of the enema.

CRITICAL DECISION POINT: *When enemas are ordered "until clear," observe the contents of the solution passed. Return is "clear" when no solid fecal material exists, but solution may be coloured.*

---

22. Assist patient as needed to wash the anal area with warm soap and water (if providing perineal care, use gloves).
- Fecal contents can irritate the skin. Proper hygiene promotes the patient's comfort.

23. Remove and discard gloves and perform hand hygiene.
- Proper hand hygiene reduces transmission of microorganisms.

24. Inspect the colour, consistency, and amount of stool and fluid passed.
- The colour, consistency, and amount of stool determine whether the stool is evacuated or fluid is retained. Note any abnormalities, such as the presence of blood or mucus.

25. Assess the condition of the abdomen; cramping, rigidity, or distension can indicate a serious problem.
- The condition of the abdomen determines whether distension is relieved. Excess volume can distend or perforate the bowel.

Unexpected Outcomes

Rigidity and distension of the abdomen

Abdominal pain or cramping

Bleeding

Related Interventions

- Stop the enema administration if fluid is still being instilled.
- Notify the prescriber and obtain vital signs.

- Slow the rate of instillation.

- Stop the enema administration.
- Notify the prescriber and obtain vital signs.

RECORDING AND REPORTING
- Record the type and volume of the enema given and the characteristics of the results.
- Report to the prescriber if the patient failed to defecate.

CARE IN THE COMMUNITY CONSIDERATIONS
- For patients who require enemas for bowel preparation at home, instruct the patient's caregiver not to exceed the recommended fluid volume levels or the recommended number of enemas. Emphasize to family members the need for slow administration of warmed fluid.

From Klingman, L., & Loft, M. (2020). Chapter 35: Bowel elimination and gastric intubation. In A. G. Perry, P. A. Potter, W. Ostendorf, et al. (Eds.). *Canadian clinical nursing skills and techniques* (pp. 946–973). Elsevier Inc.

BOX 45.5   PROCEDURAL GUIDELINE
Digital Removal of Stool

Delegation Considerations:
The digital removal of stool should not be delegated to unregulated care providers (UCPs).

Equipment:
- Vital sign equipment/stethoscope
- Bath blanket
- Waterproof pad
- Clean gloves (two pair of gloves)
- Lubricant
- Towel
- Washcloth
- Soap and water
- Bedpan

Procedure:
1. Check the patient record for a prescriber's order for manual disimpaction and use of anaesthetic lubricant. Determine if the patient is at risk for rectal bleeding (i.e., receiving anticoagulant therapy or has a past history of rectal surgery).
2. Perform hand hygiene and patient identification prior to the procedure. Explain the procedure to the patient.
3. Take baseline vital signs prior to the procedure. Perform abdominal inspection, auscultate all four quadrants for bowel sounds, and palpate for distension or masses. Help the patient to lie on the left side with knees flexed and back toward you.
4. Drape the trunk and lower extremities with a bath blanket and place a waterproof pad under the buttocks. Keep a bedpan next to the patient.
5. Apply two pair of disposable gloves and lubricate the index finger of your dominant hand with a lubricant.
6. Gently insert the gloved index finger into the rectum and advance the finger slowly along the rectal wall toward the umbilicus.
7. Gently loosen the fecal mass by massaging around it. Work the finger into the hardened mass.
8. Work the feces downward toward the end of the rectum. Remove small pieces at a time and discard into the bedpan.
9. Reassess the patient's vital signs and look for signs of fatigue. Stop the procedure if the heart rate drops significantly or if the heart rhythm changes. Monitor for 1 hour post-procedure.
10. Continue to remove feces and allow the patient to rest at intervals.
11. After completion, wash and dry the buttocks and anal area.
12. Remove the bedpan and dispose of the feces. Remove gloves by turning them inside out, and then discard.
13. Assist the patient to the toilet or position the patient on a clean bedpan if the urge to defecate develops.
14. Perform hand hygiene. Record results of the removal of the impaction by describing the fecal characteristics.
15. Follow the procedure with enemas or cathartics as ordered by prescriber.
16. Reassess the patient's bowel sounds, palpate the abdomen, and reassess vital signs, as well as level of comfort.

From Klingman, L., & Loft, M. (2020). Chapter 35: Bowel elimination and gastric intubation. In A. G. Perry, P. A. Potter, W. Ostendorf, et al. (Eds.). *Canadian clinical nursing skills and techniques* (pp. 946–973). Elsevier Inc.

TABLE 45.7   Purposes of Nasogastric Intubation

Purpose	Description	Type of Tube
Decompression	Removal of secretions and gaseous substances from the gastrointestinal tract to prevent or relieve abdominal distension	Salem sump, Levin, Miller-Abbott
Feeding (i.e., gavage; see Chapter 43)	Instillation of liquid nutritional supplements or feedings into the stomach for patients unable to swallow fluid	Duo, Dobhoff, Levin
Compression	Internal application of pressure by means of an inflated balloon to prevent internal esophageal or gastrointestinal hemorrhage	Sengstaken-Blakemore
Lavage	Irrigation of the stomach in cases of active bleeding, poisoning, or gastric dilation	Levin, Ewald, Salem sump

FIGURE 45.13 Gastric contents. **A,** Stomach. **B,** Stomach. **C,** Intestinal. (Courtesy Dr. Norma Metheny, St. Louis University, School of Nursing. St. Louis, MO.)

Care of Ostomies. Patients with temporary or permanent bowel diversions have unique bowel elimination needs. Individuals with an ostomy wear a pouch or appliance to collect the **effluent** (the stool discharged from an ostomy) from the stomas (RNAO, 2019). These patients must use meticulous skin care to prevent liquid stool from irritating the skin around the stoma (Figure 45.16).

Irrigating a Colostomy. Colostomy irrigation is one of the management options for the person with a sigmoid or descending colostomy (WOCN Society Clinical Guideline, 2018). Although this practice is not as common as it once was, some patients may be instructed to irrigate their left-sided colostomies in order to regulate colon emptying. Other patients do not want to spend the additional 60 to 90 minutes in the bathroom every day, and they empty their pouch only as necessary (Vancouver United Ostomy Association Chapter, 2019).

Specific equipment for irrigating a colostomy should be used. An enema set should never be used to irrigate a colostomy. A special cone-tipped irrigator (Figure 45.17) is used. This device prevents both bowel penetration and backflow of the irrigating solution. Patients usually sit on the toilet and place an irrigating sleeve over the stoma. The end of this sleeve extends into the bowl of the toilet. The prescriber orders the amount and type of solution. For adults, the amount ranges from 500 to 700 mL of tap water. The solution is instilled slowly through the lubricated cone tip. Irrigation should take 5 to 10 minutes. The patient then removes the cone tip and waits 30 to 45 minutes for the solution and feces to drain out of the irrigation sleeve. Once the drainage stops, the patient applies a stoma cap or a pouch. If a patient chooses

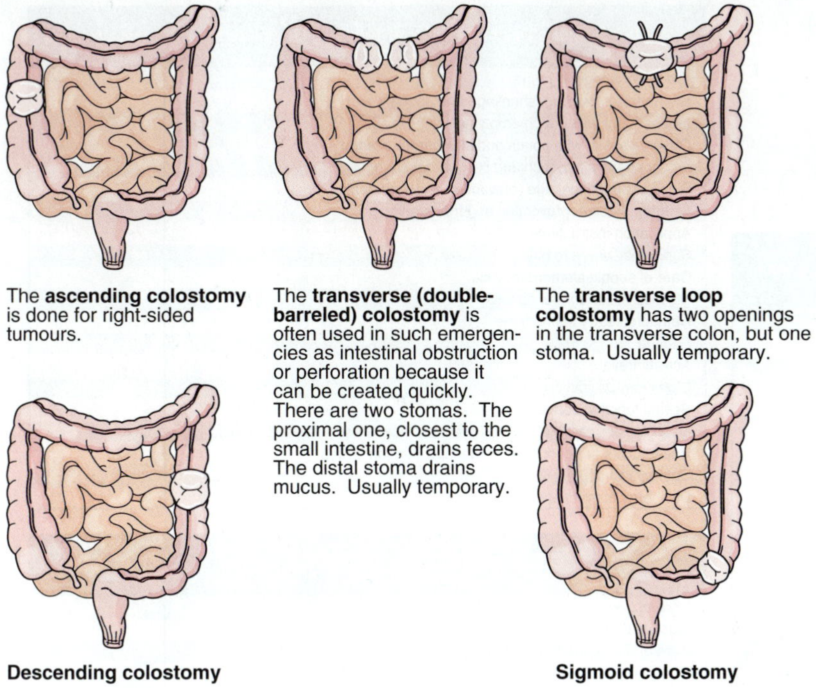

The **ascending colostomy** is done for right-sided tumours.

The **transverse (double-barreled) colostomy is** often used in such emergencies as intestinal obstruction or perforation because it can be created quickly. There are two stomas. The proximal one, closest to the small intestine, drains feces. The distal stoma drains mucus. Usually temporary.

The **transverse loop colostomy** has two openings in the transverse colon, but one stoma. Usually temporary.

Descending colostomy

Sigmoid colostomy

FIGURE 45.14 Different types of colostomies. (From Monahan, F. D., Neighbors, M., Sands, J. K., et al. [2007]. *Phipps' medical-surgical nursing: Health and illness perspectives* [8th ed., p. 1262, Fig. 43.10]. Mosby/Elsevier.)

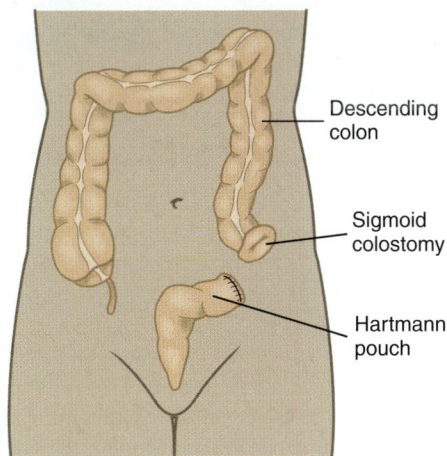

Descending colon

Sigmoid colostomy

Hartmann pouch

FIGURE 45.15 Sigmoid colostomy. Distal bowel is oversewn and left in place to create a Hartmann pouch. (Lewis, S. L., Bucher, L., Heitkemper, M., et al. [Eds.]. [2019]. *Medical-surgical nursing in Canada: Assessment and management of clinical problems* [4th Canadian ed., Fig. 45.10]. Elsevier Canada.)

to irrigate the colostomy, the timing of the irrigation can be individualized to the patient's lifestyle.

Pouching Ostomies. Ostomies require a pouch to collect fecal material. An effective pouching system protects the skin, contains fecal material, remains odour-free, and is comfortable and inconspicuous. A person wearing a pouch should feel secure in participating in any activity.

Many pouching systems are available. To ensure that a pouch fits well and meets the patient's needs, a number of factors need to be considered: the location of the ostomy; the type and size of the stoma; the amount and consistency of the effluent; the size and contour of the abdomen; the condition of the skin around the stoma; skin sensitivities or allergies; the physical activities of the patient; cognitive abilities for

learning; the patient's personal preference, age, and dexterity; and the cost of the equipment. The staff nurse collaborates with the NSWOC to ensure that the correct pouching system is used. For example, a referral to an NSWOC would be appropriate to plan the care of a patient who has a high-output ostomy that requires a pouch modification.

A pouching system consists of a pouch and a skin barrier (Figure 45.18). Pouches come in one- and two-piece systems that are disposable or reusable. Some pouches have the opening precut by the manufacturer; others require the stoma opening to be custom cut to the patient's specific stoma size.

Skin barriers include wafers, pastes, powders, and liquid film that are applied to the skin around the stoma. Wafer skin barriers, which are permanently attached to the ostomy pouch, are called *one-piece pouch systems*. In a *two-piece system*, the pouch can be detached from the skin barrier for emptying or changing. This system allows the skin barrier to remain around the patient's stoma for several days, thus minimizing the chance of skin damage from too-frequent removal of the skin barrier from the peristomal skin (Figure 45.19). When using a two-piece pouching system, the skin barrier and pouch must be the same corresponding size and from the same manufacturer. The pouch from one manufacturer will not fit correctly on the skin barrier from another manufacturer. The nurse needs to ensure the patient understands that an ostomy pouch made for collecting fecal matter (i.e., a pouch specifically for a colostomy or ileostomy) must be used and not a pouch for collecting urine.

Patients need to be instructed to measure the stoma size carefully when selecting and cutting out the opening on the wafer skin barrier. A good skin barrier protects the skin, prevents irritation from repeated removal of the pouch, and is comfortable for the patient to wear. Skill 45.2 describes the steps for applying one type of pouch system.

Nutritional Considerations for Patients With Ostomies. Nutritional therapy is important for patients with ostomies. During the first weeks after surgery, many prescribers recommend low-fibre diets,

Appendix E: Sample Ostomy Teaching Record

OSTOMY TEACHING RECORD

Client: _____

Address: _____

Before Surgery: Teaching Completed	Date & Initial
Date of surgery	
Type of surgery/ostomy	
Reason for surgery	
E.T. Nurse visit	
Stoma site selection and marking	
Stoma location and appearance	
Given teaching booklets about surgery	
Given samples of pouching system	
Purpose of pouch and skin barrier	
Knowledge of others with an ostomy	
Viewed ostomy video	

After Surgery: While in Hospital Teaching Completed	Date & Initial
Stoma (size, swelling, shrinkage and appearance)	
Type of drainage while in hospital	
Observe/assist with pouch emptying	
Independent with pouch emptying	
Observe/assist with release of gas from pouch	
Independent with release of gas from pouch	
Observe/assist with pouch and skin barrier change	
Discuss odour control options	
Signs of pouch leakage (prevention and treatment)	
Viewed ostomy video and given teaching booklet (if not done pre-op)	
Who to call if problems occur after discharge from hospital	

After Surgery: Discharged Home Teaching Completed	Date & Initial
Type of drainage at home	
Stoma (size, swelling, shrinkage and appearance)	
Independent with pouch emptying	
Observe/assist with pouch and skin barrier change	
Independent with pouch and skin barrier change	
Signs of pouch leakage (prevention and treatment)	
Skin breakdown (prevention and treatment)	
Application instructions	
Supply list/where to buy	
Care of supplies/emergency kit	
Discuss odour control options	
Nutrition/dietary instructions	
Bathing	
Activity/travel	
Clothing modifications	
Sexual function concerns	
Financial Assistance (A.D.P., Private Insurance, Social Assistance, Disability)	
United Ostomy Association of Canada Support Group	
Ostomy visitor	
Discharge instructions	

Colostomy: Teaching Completed	Date & Initial
Care of perineal wound (if present)	
Mucous drainage per rectum (if rectum left in place)	
Care of a mucous fistula (if present)	
Colostomy irrigation information	
Trial of a colostomy irrigation (optional)	
Constipation/diarrhea/gas	

Ileostomy: Teaching Completed	Date & Initial
Care of perineal wound (if present)	
Mucous drainage per rectum (if rectum left in place)	
Sodium loss and replacement	
Potassium loss and replacement	
Obstruction and management	
Fluid imbalance and treatment	
Medication	

FIGURE 45.16 Sample ostomy teaching record. *A.D.P.,* Assistive Devices Program; *E.T.,* enterostomal therapist. (From ET NOW, Red Cross Care Partners, Waterloo, Ontario, Canada.)

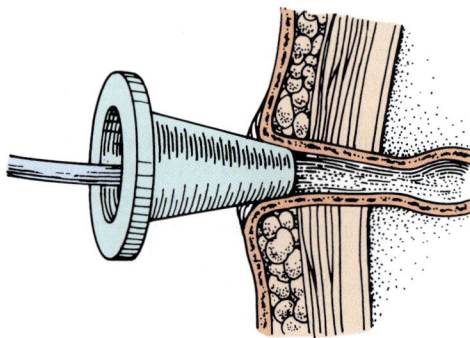

FIGURE 45.17 Ostomy irrigation cone inserted into the stoma.

particularly for ileostomy patients, because the small bowel requires time to adapt to the diversion. Low-fibre foods include bread, noodles, rice, cream cheese, eggs (not fried), strained fruit juices, lean meats, fish, and poultry. As ostomies heal, patients can eat almost any food. High-fibre foods, such as fresh fruits and vegetables, help to ensure a more solid stool, which is needed to achieve success at irrigation. Blockage must be avoided. The stoma's surgical construction can affect the likelihood of blockage.

Patients with an ileostomy should eat slowly and chew their food completely. Drinking 10 to 12 glasses of water daily also helps to prevent blockage. High-fibre foods that may cause problems include stringy meats; mushrooms; popcorn; some fruits, such as cherries; and some seafood, such as shrimp and crab. Ostomy patients may benefit from avoiding foods that cause gas and odour, such as broccoli, cauliflower, dried beans, and Brussels sprouts.

◆ Evaluation

Patient Care. The effectiveness of care depends on success in meeting the goals and expected outcomes of care. Optimally, the patient will be able to have regular, pain-free defecation of soft, formed stools. The patient is the only person who is able to determine whether the bowel elimination problems have been relieved and which therapies were most effective (Figure 45.20). The patient will also be able to demonstrate information learned regarding establishment of a normal bowel elimination pattern. The patient will be able to demonstrate any skills learned, such as ostomy protocols and skin protection. The patient will be able to accomplish normal defecation by manipulating components of daily living, such as diet, fluid intake, and exercise. The patient will have minimal reliance on artificial means of defecation, such as enemas and laxative use.

FIGURE 45.19 A, Mechanical injury to the peristomal skin. **B,** Candidiasis damage to the peristomal skin. (Permission to use these copyrighted photos has been granted by the owner, Hollister Incorporated.)

Clamp Clip Wire closure

A Narrow valve

B C

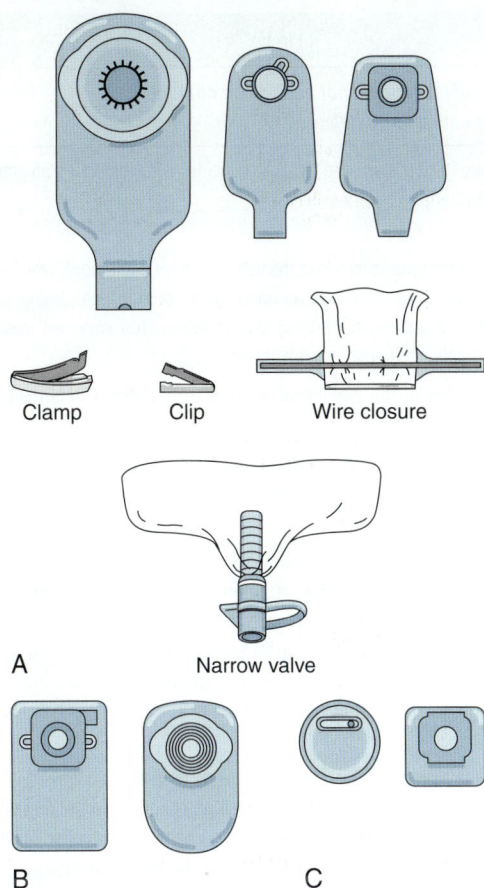

FIGURE 45.18 Common ostomy pouch products, closures, and patches. **A,** Drainable pouches and pouch closures. **B,** Nondrainable pouches. **C,** Patches for regulated colostomies. (From Monahan, F. D., Neighbors, M., Sands, J. K., et al. [2007]. *Phipps' medical-surgical nursing: Health and illness perspectives* [8th ed., p. 1264]. Mosby Elsevier.)

Patient Expectations. If the nurse has been successful in establishing a therapeutic relationship with the patient, the patient will feel more comfortable in discussing the intimate details often associated with bowel elimination. Patients often expect nurses to answer all their questions regarding diagnostic tests and the preparation for those tests. Patients will be concerned about discomfort and exposure. Fear of losing control of their bowel elimination is especially worrisome to many patients. The patient will also not be as fearful of embarrassment as the nurse assists the patient with their bowel elimination needs. The patient will relate a feeling of comfort and freedom from pain as bowel elimination needs are met within the limits of the patient's condition and treatment.

SKILL 45.2 POUCHING AN OSTOMY

Delegation Considerations
The skill of pouching a newly established ostomy should not be delegated to unregulated care providers (UCPs). Pouching of a well-established ostomy can be delegated to a UCP. The nurse must do the following:
- Assist the caregiver in selecting the appropriate pouch and skin barrier.
- Inform the caregiver of the signs of stomal and peristomal skin changes that should be reported to a nurse.
- Ask the caregiver to monitor and report the characteristics and volume of the ostomy output and report changes in volume or consistency to a nurse for further assessment.

Equipment
- Clear drainable colostomy (or ileostomy) pouch in the correct size for a two-piece system or custom cut to fit a one-piece system with an attached skin barrier
- Pouch closure device, such as a clamp or clip if needed
- Clean gloves
- Gauze pads and washcloths
- Towel or disposable waterproof barrier
- Basin with warm tap water
- Scissors and pen
- Adhesive remover (optional)

PROCEDURE

STEPS	RATIONALE
1. Perform hand hygiene and patient identification steps.	
2. Apply gloves. Observe the skin barrier and pouch for leakage and the length of time in place. Depending on the type of pouching system used (e.g., an opaque pouch), you may need to remove the pouch to fully observe the stoma. Clear pouches permit viewing of the stoma without their removal.	• Leakage may indicate the need for a different type of pouch or sealant.

CRITICAL DECISION POINT: *Intact skin barriers with no evidence of leakage do not need to be changed daily and can remain in place for 3 to 5 days (depending on manufacturer's guidelines).*

3. Observe the stoma for colour, swelling, trauma, and healing; the stoma should be moist and reddish-pink. Assess the type of stoma. Stomas can be flush with the skin or can be a budlike protrusion on the abdomen.

- Stoma characteristics are one factor to consider when selecting an appropriate pouching system.

4. Measure the stoma at each pouching change. Follow the pouch manufacturer's directions and measuring guide to determine which pouch to use on the basis of the patient's stoma size. The opening around the appliance should be no greater than 2 mm larger than the stoma.

- The size of the stoma determines the correct size of equipment, which prevents trauma to the stoma. Too large an opening can permit fecal drainage to ooze from under the appliance, causing skin irritation. Too small an opening can cause the appliance to cut into the stoma.

5. Observe the abdominal incision (if present).

- The relationship of the abdominal incision to the stoma determines proper placement of the pouch.

6. Observe the effluent from the stoma and record intake and output. Empty the pouch if it is more than one-third to one-half full. Ask the patient about skin tenderness. Remove gloves and perform hand hygiene.

- Effluent from the stoma is caustic. If effluent comes in contact with the sensitive peristomal skin, the risk of skin breakdown increases. Pouches must be emptied because the weight of the pouch may disrupt the seal of adhesive on the skin.

7. Assess the abdomen for the best type of pouching system to use. Consider the following:
   A. Contour and peristomal plane
   B. Presence of scars, incisions
   C. Location and type of stoma

- The characteristics of the abdomen determine the pouching system selection and the need for additional equipment. For a stoma to have an adequate seal with an ostomy appliance, the stoma must be placed within the abdominal rectus muscle, away from abdominal creases and folds, away from the bony understructures, and surrounded by at least 5 cm of smooth surface on all sides.

8. Assess the patient's self-care ability to determine the best type of pouching system to use.

- Patients who have difficulty using their hands or who have limited vision may find a one-piece system or a precut pouch and skin barrier more desirable to use; others prefer being able to keep the skin barrier in place for several days, changing just the pouch, and therefore prefer the two-piece system.

9. After removing the skin barrier and pouch, assess the skin around the stoma, noting scars, folds, skin breakdown, and the peristomal suture line, if present. Keep the pouch loosely attached to the stoma to collect any drainage while the system is being changed.

- Assessing the skin around the stoma determines the need for barrier paste to increase adherence of the pouch to the skin or to fill in irregularities.

CRITICAL DECISION POINT: *If the skin around the stoma is discoloured, weeping, itchy, or sore, refer the patient to an ostomy specialist (Fellows & Cobbett, 2020).*

10. Determine the patient's emotional response to and knowledge and understanding of an ostomy and its care.

- Understanding the patient's perspective assists in determining both the extent to which the patient is able to participate in care and the patient's need for teaching and the clarification of information.

11. Explain the procedure to the patient; encourage the patient's interaction and questions.

- Explaining the procedure reduces the patient's anxiety and encourages the patient's participation.

12. Perform hand hygiene and patient identification. Assemble the equipment and close the room curtains or door.

- Proper hand hygiene reduces the transmission of infection. Organizing the equipment optimizes the use of time and conserves the patient's and nurse's energy. Privacy reduces embarrassment for the patient.

13. Position the patient either standing or in a semi-reclining position and draped. If seated, position the patient either on or in front of the toilet.

- When the patient is semi-reclined, fewer wrinkles ease the application of the pouching system; draping maintains the patient's dignity.

14. Perform hand hygiene and apply disposable gloves.

- Proper hand hygiene reduces transmission of microorganisms.

15. Place the towel or disposable waterproof barrier under the patient.

- The towel or waterproof barrier protects the bed linen.

16. Completely remove the used pouch and skin barrier by gently pushing the skin away from the barrier. An adhesive remover may be used to facilitate removal of the skin barrier.

- Working gently reduces trauma; jerking irritates the skin and can cause tears.

17. Clean the peristomal skin gently with warm tap water using gauze pads or a clean washcloth; do not scrub the skin; dry completely by patting the skin with gauze or a towel.

- Avoid the use of soap because it leaves a residue on the skin that interferes with pouch adhesion to the skin. Skin must be as dry as the skin barrier; the pouch does not adhere to wet skin. If blood appears on the gauze pad, do not be alarmed; the stoma, if rubbed, may ooze some blood from the cleaning process. The stoma's surface is a highly vascular mucous membrane. Bleeding into the pouch is abnormal.

Continued

SKILL 45.2   POUCHING AN OSTOMY—cont'd

18. Measure the stoma for the correct size of pouching system needed, using the manufacturer's measuring guide (see Step 18 illustration).

   • Measuring the stoma ensures accuracy in determining the correct pouch size needed. The stoma shrinks and does not reach its usual size for 6 to 8 weeks.

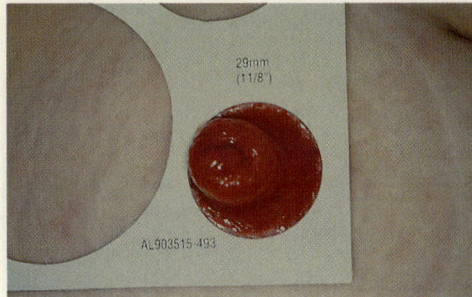

STEP 18 Measuring a stoma.

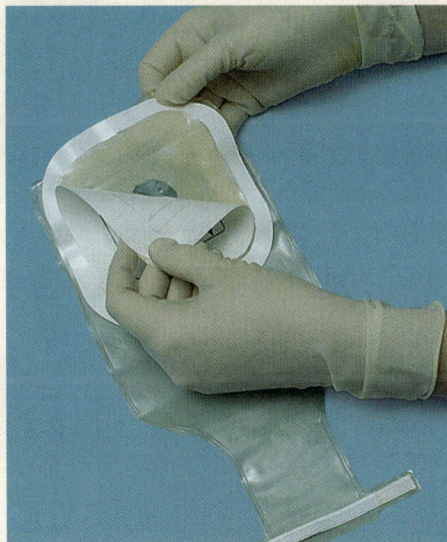

STEP 19 Preparing an ostomy pouch.

19. Select the appropriate pouch for the patient on the basis of patient assessment. For a custom cut-to-fit pouch, use an ostomy guide to cut an opening on the pouch 2 mm larger than the stoma before removing the backing. Prepare the pouch by removing the backing from the barrier and adhesive (see Step 19 illustration). For an ileostomy, apply a thin circle of barrier paste around the opening in the pouch; allow to dry.

   • The barrier paste facilitates the seal and protects the skin. The size of the pouch opening keeps drainage off the skin and reduces the risk of damage to the stoma during peristalsis or physical activity. The pouch and skin barrier are changed whenever leaking occurs. They can also be changed before or after a tub bath or shower. The stool is alkaline, which is an irritant on the skin; fecal bacteria can colonize on the skin and increase the risk of infection. Change the pouch and skin barrier when the patient is comfortable; before a meal is better because this timing avoids increased peristalsis and the chance of evacuation during the pouch change.

CRITICAL DECISION POINT: *If the patient has a large volume of liquid stool from an ileostomy, consider using a high-output pouch that will contain the volume of effluent and reduce the frequency of pouch emptying.*

---

20. Apply the skin barrier and pouch. If creases occur next to the stoma, use a barrier paste to fill in; let dry 1 to 2 minutes.

CRITICAL DECISION POINT: *If the patient has a surgical incision near the stoma, the skin barrier may need to be trimmed to fit.*

A. For a one-piece pouching system:

   (1) Use skin sealant wipes on the skin directly under the adhesive skin barrier or pouch; allow to dry. Press the adhesive backing of the pouch or skin barrier smoothly against the skin, starting from the bottom and working up and around the sides.

Continued

SKILL 45.2   POUCHING AN OSTOMY—cont'd

(2) Hold the pouch by the barrier, centre it over the stoma, and press down gently on the barrier; the bottom of the pouch should point toward the patient's knees (see Step 20A[2] illustration).

(3) Maintain gentle finger pressure around the barrier for 1 to 2 minutes.

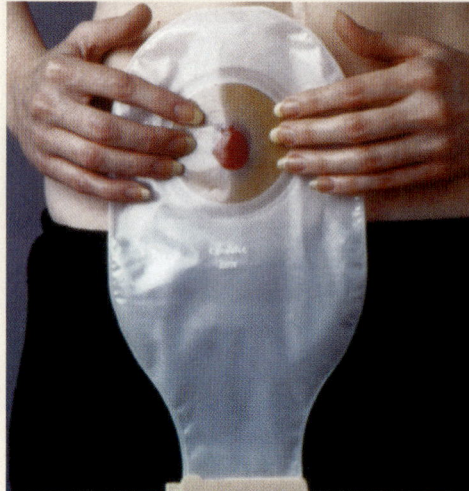

STEP 20A(2) Applying a one-piece pouch. (Courtesy ConvaTec, Princeton, NJ.)

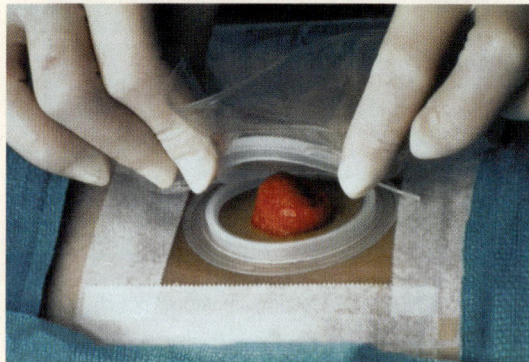

STEP 20B(1) Application of a barrier-paste flange; separate inner surface and position. (Courtesy ConvaTec, Princeton, NJ.)

B. For a two-piece pouching system:

(1) Apply the flange (the barrier with adhesive) as in steps above for a one-piece system (see Step 20B[1] illustration). Then snap on the pouch and maintain finger pressure.

- The flange creates a wrinkle-free, secure seal and decreases irritation from the adhesive on skin.

C. For both pouching systems, gently tug on the pouch in a downward direction.

- Tugging on the pouch determines whether the pouch is securely attached.

21. Apply a nonallergenic paper tape around the pectin skin barrier in a "picture frame" method. Half of the tape should be on the skin barrier and half on the patient's skin. Some patients prefer a belt attached to the pouch for extra security in place of the tape.

- "Picture framing" the pectin skin barrier adds to the security of keeping the pouch system attached securely.

CRITICAL DECISION POINT: *If the patient chooses to wear a belt, ensure that it is not fastened too tightly, by placing two fingers between the belt and the patient's skin.*

---

22. Fold the bottom of drainable open-ended pouches up once and close using a closure device such as a clamp (or follow the manufacturer's instructions for closure).

- Proper closure maintains a secure seal to prevent leaking.

23. Properly dispose of the old pouch and the soiled equipment.

24. Remove gloves and perform hand hygiene.

- Proper hand hygiene reduces transmission of microorganisms.

Continued

SKILL 45.2 POUCHING AN OSTOMY—cont'd

25. Change a one- or two-piece pouch every 3 to 7 days unless it is leaking; a pouch can remain in place for tub bath or shower; after a bath or shower, pat the adhesive dry.
- Avoid unnecessary trauma to the skin from too-frequent changes. Drying the adhesive ensures adhesion of the pouch.

26. Ask whether the patient feels discomfort around the stoma.
- The patient's perception of discomfort determines the presence of skin irritation.

27. While the pouch is removed and the skin is being cleaned, note appearance of the skin around the stoma and the existing incision (if present). Reinspect the condition of the skin barrier and adhesive.
- Assessing the skin and existing incision determines the condition of the tissues and the progress of healing. The condition of the skin barrier and adhesive can indicate the presence of leaks.

28. Observe the patient's nonverbal behaviours as the pouch is applied. Ask whether the patient has any questions about the pouching.
- Nonverbal behaviours indicate the patient's emotional response to the stoma and their readiness for learning. The patient's questions determine the level of understanding of the procedure.

UNEXPECTED OUTCOMES	RELATED INTERVENTIONS
Damage of the peristomal skin	Assess for the following conditions and report their occurrence to the prescriber for treatment: • Mechanical damage (see Figure 45.19, A) due to inappropriate skin care or incorrect tape removal) • Chemical damage due to the effluent coming into contact with the peristomal skin or a skin reaction to the adhesive • Damage due to a fungus (e.g., candidiasis; see Figure 45.19, B), usually caused by excessive skin moisture
Necrosis of stoma (purple or black discoloration, dryness, failure to bleed, or sloughing of tissue)	• Assess the circulation to the stoma. • Observe for excessive edema or tension on the bowel suture line (if present). • Immediately report this finding to the prescriber.

RECORDING AND REPORTING
- Chart the type of pouch and skin barrier applied.
- Record the amount, appearance, and texture of the stool; the condition of the peristomal skin; and the condition of any sutures.
- Report any of the following to the charge nurse or the prescriber, or both:
  - Any abnormal appearance of the stoma, the suture line, the peristomal skin, the character of output, or the absence of bowel sounds
  - No flatus in 24 to 36 hours and no stool by the third day
- Document abdominal distension, excessive tenderness, and the nature of bowel sounds.
- Record the patient's level of participation and need for instruction.

CARE IN THE COMMUNITY CONSIDERATIONS
- Evaluate the patient's home toileting facilities. Note the presence of adequate toileting facilities.
- Caution the patient that most ostomy pouches and barriers cannot be flushed down the toilet; they clog the plumbing system. Dispose of used ostomy pouch according to employer policy and local sanitation regulations.

Manufacturer websites: https://www.coloplast.ca; https://www.convatec.ca; http://www.hollister.ca/en-ca
From Fellows, J., & Cobbett, S. L. (2020). Chapter 36: Ostomy care. In A. G. Perry, P. A. Potter, W. Ostendorf, et al. (Eds.). *Canadian clinical nursing skills and techniques* (pp. 974–988). Elsevier Inc.

KEY CONCEPTS
- The mechanical breakdown of food elements, gastrointestinal motility, and selective absorption and secretion of substances by the large intestine influence the character of feces.
- Food high in fibre content and an increased fluid intake keep feces soft.
- Ongoing use of cathartics, laxatives, and enemas affects and delays the reflexes of normal defecation.
- Vagal stimulation, which slows the heart rate, may occur during straining while defecating, receiving enemas, and during digital removal of an impacted stool.
- The greatest danger from diarrhea is developing an imbalance of fluids and electrolytes.
- The location of an ostomy influences the consistency of the stool.
- Assessment of bowel elimination patterns should focus on bowel habits, factors that normally influence defecation, recent changes in bowel elimination, and a physical examination.
- Indirect and direct visualization of the lower gastrointestinal tract requires cleansing of the bowel before the procedure.
- When selecting a diet to promote normal bowel elimination, the nurse needs to consider the frequency of defecation, the fecal characteristics, and the effect of foods on gastrointestinal function.

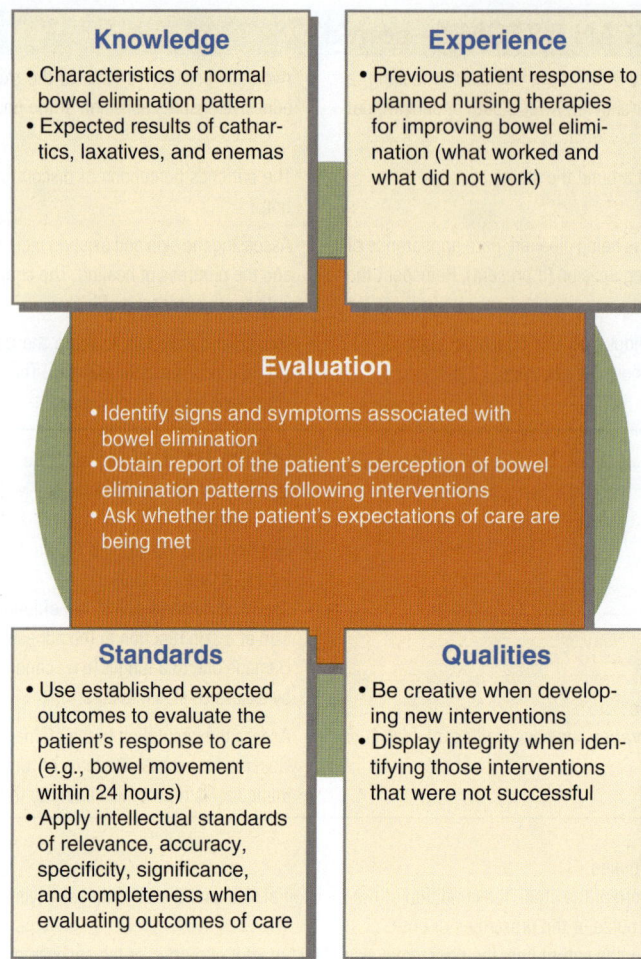

Knowledge
- Characteristics of normal bowel elimination pattern
- Expected results of cathartics, laxatives, and enemas

Experience
- Previous patient response to planned nursing therapies for improving bowel elimination (what worked and what did not work)

Evaluation
- Identify signs and symptoms associated with bowel elimination
- Obtain report of the patient's perception of bowel elimination patterns following interventions
- Ask whether the patient's expectations of care are being met

Standards
- Use established expected outcomes to evaluate the patient's response to care (e.g., bowel movement within 24 hours)
- Apply intellectual standards of relevance, accuracy, specificity, significance, and completeness when evaluating outcomes of care

Qualities
- Be creative when developing new interventions
- Display integrity when identifying those interventions that were not successful

FIGURE 45.20 Critical thinking model for bowel elimination evaluation.

- Proper positioning on a bedpan allows the patient to assume a position similar to squatting without experiencing muscle strain.
- Nasogastric intubation decompresses the gastric contents by removing secretions and gaseous products from the gastrointestinal tract.
- The purposes of gastric decompression are to keep the gastrointestinal tract free of secretions, to reduce nausea and gas, and to decrease the risk of vomiting and aspiration.

- Proper selection and use of an ostomy pouching system are necessary to prevent damage to the skin around the stoma.
- Dangers during digital removal of stool include traumatizing the rectal mucosa and promoting vagal stimulation.
- Skin breakdown can occur after repeated exposure to liquid stool.

CRITICAL THINKING EXERCISES

1. In care episode one, Olivia is admitted to a medical/surgical unit for a bowel obstruction. She has experienced worsening constipation problems all her adult life, with hard, pellet-like stools that she strains to pass. She has been trying to manage her bowel issues on her own by using over-the-counter laxatives. There is a family history of colon cancer, both her mother at age 60 and her brother at age 58. What additional pieces of assessment data do you need?

2. In care episode two, Olivia is assessed in an outpatient geriatric clinic. She has continued to experience problems with hard stools. She has been trying to manage her bowel issues on her own by taking over-the-counter laxatives and a probiotic. When she takes laxatives, she reports that she has two bowel accidents a day. The stools are often hard at first, followed by watery stools. She has no warning and no control when the urge to defecate occurs. She needs immediate access to a toilet. It is so unpredictable that she is no longer comfortable leaving home, which is limiting her social activity.

Her beverage of preference is diet cola, consuming four to six cans a day. She has reduced her dietary fibre intake because she feels it is making her bowel incontinence worse. She walks her dog twice a day for 20 minutes. She feels that walking helps her with managing her stress. What additional pieces of assessment data do you need? What points of information do you think the clinical nurse specialist/nurse continence advisor will include in Olivia's teaching plan?

3. In care episode three, Olivia is admitted as an inpatient to a medical/surgical unit in 2020 following a diagnosis of colon cancer after a colonoscopy. She will have a new pouching colostomy. What referrals would you recommend and why? Olivia and her caregiver need to learn what the colostomy means for her future bowel elimination needs. What do you tell them?

Answers to Critical Thinking Exercises appear on the Evolve website.

REVIEW QUESTIONS

Review Questions 1 to 11 relate to the case study at the beginning of the chapter.
Care Episode One:

1. In thinking about Olivia's nutritional needs during her first hospitalization for a bowel obstruction, the nurse needs to understand that most nutrients and electrolytes are absorbed in which of the following areas:
   a. Stomach
   b. Duodenum
   c. Ileum
   d. Cecum
2. What is one of the greatest concerns in caring for Olivia related to the nasogastric tube?
   a. Dehydration
   b. Maintaining comfort
   c. Constipation
   d. Nutritional therapy
3. During inspection of Olivia's abdomen, the nurse notes that it is visibly distended. The nurse should proceed with the client's abdominal assessment by next performing:
   a. Palpation
   b. Percussion
   c. A rectal check
   d. Auscultation
4. A cleansing enema is ordered for Olivia to try to clear the fecal impaction. What amount of solution should be instilled?
   a. 150 to 200 mL
   b. 200 to 400 mL
   c. 400 to 750 mL
   d. 750 to 1 000 mL
5. During the enema, Olivia complains of pain. The nurse notes rectal bleeding and blood in the return fluid. What action should the nurse take?
   a. Stop the instillation.
   b. Slow the rate of instillation.
   c. Stop the instillation, notify the prescriber, and obtain vital signs.
   d. Tell the patient to breathe slowly and relax.

6. The nurse is preparing Olivia for discharge from hospital following her bowel obstruction. What resource would the nurse use to advise Olivia on bowel cancer screening?
   a. ColonCancerCheck; Colorectal Screening Program, Cancer Care Ontario
   b. Screening for Colorectal Cancer, Government of Canada
   c. Ask the attending physician
   d. Refer the patient to her primary health care provider for advice
Care Episode Two:
7. In considering Olivia's risk factors for constipation, the nurse would identify which of the following? *(Select all that apply.)*
   a. Restriction of fluid intake that includes both caffeine and artificial sweetener
   b. Restriction of dietary fibre intake
   c. Regular exercise
   d. Toileting for a bowel movement at inconsistent times
   e. Managing stress
8. In considering the factors related to Olivia's bowel incontinence, which of the following situations results in diarrhea that occurs with a fecal impaction?
   a. A clear liquid diet
   b. Irritation of the intestinal mucosa
   c. Seepage of stool around the impaction
   d. Inability of the patient to form a stool
9. Identify and prioritize the interventions the nurse should include in Olivia's plan of care. *(Select all that apply.)*
   a. Toileting for a bowel movement at a consistent time each day following a triggering meal
   b. Increase fluid intake to at least four to five 237-mL (8-ounce) glasses of water over the course of the day, replacing cola with water
   c. Increase physical activity
   d. Gradually increase dietary fibre with the goal over time to achieve about 25 mg of fibre per day
   e. Incorporate additional stress-management strategies.
Care Episode Three:
10. What term is given to the stool discharged from an ostomy?
   a. Effluent
   b. Stool
   c. Colonic fluid
   d. Mucus
11. What term describes a nurse who is trained to care for ostomy patients?
   a. Nurse specialized in wound, ostomy and continence (NSWOC)
   b. Nurse practitioner
   c. Ostomy practitioner
   d. GI therapist

Answers: 1. b; **2.** b; **3.** d; **4.** d; **5.** c; **6.** a; **7.** a, b; **8.** c; **9.** a, b, d; **10.** a; **11.** a.

Rationales for the Review Questions appear on the Evolve website.

RECOMMENDED WEBSITES

Canadian Cancer Society: https://www.cancer.ca
This website is a source for general information about all types of cancers, as well as Canadian statistics of the prevalence, mortality, and survival rates for specific cancers.

Canadian Digestive Health Foundation: https://www.cdhf.ca
The Canadian Digestive Health Foundation (CDHF) supports research and education in the management and cure of digestive diseases and disorders.

Canadian Nurse Continence Advisors: https://www.cnca.ca
This website has both provider and patient resources including education and research about urinary and bowel incontinence.

Colorectal Cancer Canada: https://www.colorectalcancercanada.com
Colorectal cancer is the second most common cause of cancer deaths in Canada. Colorectal Cancer Canada is a nonprofit organization that supports individuals with colorectal cancer, their families, and caregivers.

Diabetes Canada: https://www.diabetes.ca
This website has resources to assist patients in improving glycemic control.

Government of Canada: Norovirus: https://www.canada.ca/en/public-health/services/food-poisoning/norovirus.html
While Canada's food supply is generally very safe, sometimes the food we eat can carry viruses, like noroviruses, that make us sick. Noroviruses are a group of viruses that cause gastroenteritis in people.

Health Canada: *Canada's Food Guide:* https://food-guide.canada.ca/en/guidelines/

Canada's Food Guide is based on the best available scientific evidence. It promotes healthy eating and overall nutritional well-being, and supports improvements to the Canadian food environment.

Registered Nurses' Association of Ontario (RNAO) Best Practice Guidelines:

- *Supporting Adults Who Anticipate or Live With an Ostomy:* https://rnao.ca/bpg/guidelines/ostomy
  This Best Practice Guideline provides nurses and interprofessional team members with evidence-informed recommendations for the most effective strategies to support adults who anticipate or live with an ostomy.

- *A Proactive Approach to Bladder and Bowel Management in Adults:* https://rnao.ca/bpg/guidelines/proactive-approach-bladder-and-bowel-management-adults
  This Best Practice Guideline provides evidence-informed recommendations for effective strategies to support adults living with urinary incontinence, fecal incontinence, or constipation. The guidelines can help improve quality of care and lead to positive health outcomes.

University of Utah, Constipation Management APP: https://webapps.med.utah.edu/constmgmt/
This website provides a simple application for constipation and its management.

🌐 REFERENCES

A full reference list is available on the website for this book at http://evolve.elsevier.com/Canada/Potter/fundamentals/

46

Mobility and Immobility

*Canadian content written by Jill Vihos, RN, BScN, MN, PhD,
with original chapter contributions by Kimberly Diane Baxter, DNP, APRN, FNP-BC*

OBJECTIVES

Mastery of content in this chapter will enable you to:

- Define the key terms listed.
- Describe physiological and pathological influences on body alignment and joint mobility.
- Identify changes in physiological and psychosocial function that are associated with immobility.
- Assess for expected and impaired body alignment and mobility.
- Formulate appropriate nursing diagnoses for impaired mobility.
- Develop individualized nursing care plans for patients with impaired mobility.
- Compare and contrast active and passive range-of-motion (ROM) exercises.
- Describe essential techniques when assisting with active and passive ROM exercises, assisting a patient to move up in bed, repositioning a patient, assisting a patient to a sitting position, and transferring a patient from a bed to a chair or from a bed to a stretcher.
- Describe interventions for improving or maintaining patients' mobility.
- Evaluate the nursing care plan for maintaining body alignment and mobility.

KEY TERMS

Activity tolerance
Anthropometric measurements
Atelectasis
Bed rest
Body alignment
Body mechanics
Chest physiotherapy (CPT)
Disease atrophy
Disuse osteoporosis
Embolus
Ergonomic assistive devices
Exercise
Footdrop
Friction

Full-body slings
Gait
Hemiparesis
Hemiplegia
Hypostatic pneumonia
Immobility
Instrumental activities of daily living (IADLs)
Joint contracture
Joints
Ligaments
Mobility
Muscle atrophy
Negative nitrogen balance

Orthostatic hypotension
Osteoporosis
Paraplegia
Pathological fractures
Posture
Pressure injury/injuries
Quadriplegia
Range of motion (ROM)
Shear
Tendons
Thrombus
Trochanter roll
Urinary stasis

WEBSITE

http://evolve.elsevier.com/Canada/Potter/fundamentals/

CASE STUDY

Kate (preferred pronouns: she/her) is a 36-year-old individual who has multiple sclerosis and was admitted to the neurology unit 3 days ago for exacerbation of symptoms. She came to the emergency department with a chief concern of weakness, difficulty balancing, and extreme pain, with loss of muscle function in her legs. Kate was diagnosed with multiple sclerosis 3 years ago. She is married and has two children, ages 7 years and 4 years. Prior to admission, she adhered closely to her medication regimen and continued her very active lifestyle, enjoying outdoor activities with her family. Since hospital admission 3 days ago, Kate's muscle function in her lower extremities has deteriorated significantly and she is unable to leave her bed and cannot walk.

Think about this case study as you read this chapter. There are review questions at the end of the chapter that relate to the case study.

Mobility refers to the ability to move easily and independently. To maintain optimal mobility, musculoskeletal and nervous system function must be intact. Illnesses, surgery, injuries, pain, and aging can temporarily or permanently impair mobility. Nurses must assess for hazards created by immobility and know how to care for patients who are immobile in order to prevent complications. This care includes positioning patients to maintain optimal body alignment and safely moving patients when they cannot do so independently. Integration of evidence-informed practice related to mobility is essential for providing comprehensive nursing care.

SCIENTIFIC KNOWLEDGE BASE

Nature of Movement

Movement is a complex process that requires coordination between the musculoskeletal and nervous system. As a nurse, you will assess how a patient's physical and psychological condition affects body movement. Body mechanics are the coordinated efforts of the musculoskeletal and nervous systems to maintain balance, posture, and body alignment during lifting, bending, moving, and performing activities of daily living (ADLs). Knowing how patients initiate movement and understanding your own movements requires a basic understanding of body mechanics. Lifting techniques historically used in nursing practice can cause debilitating injuries to nurses and other health care providers (Lee et al., 2021). In Canada, government legislation and employer policies require nurses to use evidence-informed guidelines regarding body alignment, balance, gravity, and friction when implementing nursing interventions such as positioning patients, assessing a patient's risk for falls, and selecting the safest way to move or transfer patients (Alberta Health Services, 2021; Shaw et al., 2021) (see Chapter 37).

Alignment and Balance. The terms body alignment and posture are analogous and refer to the positioning of the joints, tendons, ligaments, and muscles while standing, sitting, and lying. Collectively, joints, tendons, and ligaments are stabilizing and supporting structures of the musculoskeletal system. Joints are structures, or articulations, that connect two or more adjacent parts of the skeleton to facilitate movement. Ligaments are bands of tough, fibrous tissue that surround joints and connect bone to bone to reinforce joint stability to limit extreme movement of joints. Tendons are bands of fibrous connective tissue that attach muscle to bone.

Being in correct body alignment means that the individual's centre of gravity is stable. Correct body alignment reduces strain on musculoskeletal structures, minimizes the risk of injuries and falls, aids in maintaining adequate muscle tone, and contributes to balance. Balance is enhanced with correct body posture and when the body's centre of gravity is kept low within a wide base of support (see Chapter 37).

Balance is required for maintaining a static position (e.g., sitting), moving (e.g., walking), and performing ADLs. Disease, injury, pain, physical development (e.g., age), life changes (e.g., pregnancy), medications (e.g., in which dizziness or drowsiness is an adverse effect), and deconditioning (as a result of prolonged immobility) can compromise the ability to remain balanced. Impaired balance is a major threat to mobility and physical safety and contributes to a fear of falling and self-imposed activity restrictions (see Chapter 37).

Gravity and Friction. *Weight* is the force exerted on a body by gravity. The force of weight is always directed downward, which is why an unbalanced object falls. Unsteady patients fall when their centre of gravity becomes unbalanced; the gravitational pull of their weight moves outside their base of support.

Friction is a force that occurs in a direction opposing movement. The greater the surface area of the object to be moved, the greater the friction. A larger object produces greater resistance to movement. The force exerted against the skin while the skin remains stationary and the bony structures move is called shear. An example of shear is when the head of a hospital bed is elevated beyond 60 degrees and gravity pulls a patient so that the bony skeleton moves toward the foot of the bed while the skin remains against the sheets. The blood vessels in the underlying tissue are stretched and damaged, resulting in impeded blood flow to the deep tissues. Ultimately, pressure injuries often develop within the undermined tissue; the surface tissue appears less affected. To reduce friction when a patient is unable to assist in moving up in bed, nurses use ergonomic assistive devices such as friction-reducing transfer sheets and full-body slings (Schoenfisch et al., 2019). Full-body slings are used to mechanically lift a patient off the surface of a bed, thereby preventing friction, tearing, or shearing of the patient's skin and protecting the nurse and other staff from injury.

Whenever possible, nurses should use some of the patient's strength when lifting, transferring, or moving the patient. The procedure should be explained to the patient and the patient told when and what body parts to move. The result should be a synchronized movement in which the patient can participate and in which friction is decreased. A patient's participation in self-care may promote their sense of accomplishment.

Pathological Influences on Mobility

Pathological conditions affect mobility, including congenital and acquired impairments, degenerative and episodic conditions, and disease processes. Although a complete description of each is beyond the scope of this chapter, four categories of pathological influences are presented here: postural abnormalities, impaired muscle development, central nervous system damage, and direct trauma to the musculoskeletal system.

Postural Abnormalities. Congenital or acquired postural abnormalities affect the efficiency of the musculoskeletal system, as well as body alignment, balance, and appearance. During assessment, the nurse observes body alignment and range of motion (ROM; see Chapter 37). Postural abnormalities can cause pain, impair alignment or mobility, or both. Knowledge about the characteristics, causes, and treatment of common postural abnormalities (Table 46.1) is necessary for moving, transferring, and positioning a patient. Some postural abnormalities may limit ROM. Nurses intervene to maintain a patient's maximum ROM in unaffected joints and then often collaborate with physiotherapists to design interventions to strengthen affected muscles and joints, improve the patient's posture, and adequately use affected and unaffected muscle groups. Referral to or collaboration with a physiotherapist and occupational therapist may enhance nursing interventions for a patient with a postural abnormality.

Impaired Muscle Development. Injury and disease can lead to numerous alterations in musculoskeletal function. For example, the muscular dystrophies are a group of familial disorders that cause degeneration of skeletal muscle fibres. Patients with muscular dystrophies experience progressive, symmetrical weakness and wasting of skeletal muscle groups, with increasing disability and deformity (McCance & Huether, 2019).

Damage to the Central Nervous System. Damage to any component of the central nervous system that regulates voluntary movement results in impaired body mobility. Trauma from a head injury, ischemia from a stroke or cerebrovascular accident (CVA), hemorrhage, tumour, or bacterial infection such as meningitis can damage the cerebellum

Abnormality	Description	Cause	Possible Treatments*
Torticollis	Inclining of head to the affected side, in which the sternocleidomastoid muscle is contracted	Congenital or acquired condition	Surgery, heat, support, or immobilization, depending on cause and severity, gentle range of motion
Lordosis	Exaggeration of anterior convex curve of lumbar spine	Congenital condition Temporary condition (e.g., pregnancy)	Spine-stretching exercises (based on cause)
Kyphosis	Increased convexity in curvature of thoracic spine	Congenital condition Rickets, osteoporosis Tuberculosis of the spine Gerontological changes	Spine-stretching exercises, sleeping without pillows, use of bed board, bracing, spinal fusion (based on cause and severity)
Kypholordosis	Combination of kyphosis and lordosis	Congenital condition	Similar to methods used in kyphosis or lordosis (based on cause) Immobilization and surgery (based on cause and severity)
Scoliosis	Lateral "S"- or "C"-shaped curvature of spinal column with vertebral rotation, unequal heights of hips and shoulders	Sometimes a consequence of numerous congenital, connective tissue, and neuromuscular disorders Poliomyelitis Spastic paralysis Unequal leg length	Approximately half of children with scoliosis require surgery. Nonsurgical treatment is with braces and exercises.
Kyphoscoliosis	Abnormal anteroposterior and lateral curvature of spine	Congenital condition Poliomyelitis Cor pulmonale	Immobilization and surgery (based on cause and severity)
Congenital hip dysplasia	Hip instability with limited abduction of hips and, occasionally, adduction contractures (head of femur does not articulate with acetabulum because of abnormal shallowness of acetabulum)	Congenital condition (more common with breech deliveries)	Maintenance of continuous abduction of the thigh so that head of femur presses into centre of acetabulum Abduction splints, casting, surgery
Knock-knee (genu valgum)	Legs curved inward so that knees come together as person walks	Congenital condition Rickets	Knee braces, surgery if not corrected by growth
Bowlegs (genu varum)	One or both legs bent outward at knee, which is normal until 2 to 3 years of age	Congenital condition Rickets	Slowing rate of curving if not corrected by growth With rickets, increase of vitamin D, calcium, and phosphorus intake to normal ranges
Clubfoot	95%: medial deviation and plantar flexion of foot (equinovarus) 5%: lateral deviation and dorsiflexion (calcaneovalgus)	Congenital condition	Casts, splints such as Denis–Browne splint, and surgery (based on degree and rigidity of deformity)
Footdrop	Inability to dorsiflex and evert foot because of peroneal nerve damage	Congenital condition Trauma Improper position of patient who is immobilized	None (cannot be corrected) Prevention through physiotherapy Bracing with ankle–foot orthotic
Pigeon-toes (metatarsus adductus or metatarsus varus)	Internal rotation of forefoot or entire foot, common in infants, often accompanied by developmental dysplasia of the hip	Congenital condition Habit	Growth, wearing reversed shoes, casting, bracing

*Severity of the condition and its cause will dictate treatment, which must be individualized.
Based on McCance, K. L., & Huether, S. E. (2019). *Pathophysiology: The biologic basis for disease in adults and children* (8th ed.). Mosby.

or the motor region in the cerebral cortex. Damage to the cerebellum causes problems with balance, and motor impairment is directly related to the amount of destruction of the motor region. For example, a person with a right-sided cerebral hemorrhage with necrosis has destruction of the right motor strip that results in left-sided **hemiplegia** (muscle paralysis) or **hemiparesis** (muscle weakness). Trauma to the spinal cord also impairs mobility. For example, a complete transection of the spinal cord results in a bilateral loss of voluntary motor control below the level of the trauma, because motor fibres are cut. Injury above the first thoracic vertebra results in **quadriplegia** (also known as

tetraplegia) (four-limb paralysis), and injury below that level results in **paraplegia** (two-limb paralysis).

Direct Trauma to the Musculoskeletal System. Direct trauma to the musculoskeletal system can result in bruises, contusions, sprains, and fractures. A *fracture* is a disruption of bone tissue continuity. Fractures most commonly result from direct external trauma but can also occur as a consequence of some deformity of the bone (e.g., **pathological fractures**, or bone fractures that result from disease rather than injury, such as osteoporosis, Paget's disease, metastatic cancer, or osteogenesis imperfecta). Young children are usually able to form new bone more easily than adults and, as a result, have few complications after a fracture. Treatment often includes positioning the fractured bone in proper alignment and immobilizing it to promote healing and restore function. Even this temporary immobilization can result in some **muscle atrophy** (loss of muscle tissue), loss of tone, and joint stiffness. After the fracture has healed, physiotherapy may be required to regain functional losses.

NURSING KNOWLEDGE BASE

Mobility–Immobility

Fully understanding mobility requires more than an overview of the physiology and regulation of movement by the musculoskeletal and nervous systems. Nurses must also know how to apply these scientific principles in the clinical setting in order to determine the safest way to move patients and understand the effect of immobility on a patient's physiological, psychological, and developmental health status.

Factors Influencing Mobility–Immobility. To determine how to move patients safely, nurses need to assess a patient's ability to move. As stated earlier, *mobility* refers to a person's ability to move about freely. **Immobility** refers to the inability to move about freely. Mobility and immobility are best understood as the end points of a continuum, with many degrees of partial mobility in between. Some patients move back and forth on this continuum, but for other patients, immobility is absolute and continues indefinitely. The terms *bed rest* and *impaired physical mobility* are frequently used when discussing patients on the mobility–immobility continuum.

Bed rest is an intervention that restricts patients to bed for therapeutic reasons. Although not common, health care providers may prescribe this intervention. The general objectives of bed rest are as follows:

- To reduce physical activity and the oxygen needs of the body
- To reduce pain, including postoperative pain, and the need for large doses of analgesics
- To promote safety for patients recovering from the effects of anaesthetics or who are sedated
- To allow patients who are ill or debilitated to rest
- To allow patients who are exhausted the opportunity for uninterrupted rest

The duration of bed rest depends on the illness or injury and the patient's prior state of health.

The effects of muscular deconditioning associated with lack of physical activity are often apparent within days. The individual of average weight and height without a chronic illness on bed rest loses muscle strength from baseline levels at a rate of 3% a day. Deconditioning can occur to any individual regardless of age. Immobility is also associated with cardiovascular, skeletal, and other organ changes. The term **disease atrophy** describes the tendency of cells and tissue to reduce in size and function in response to prolonged inactivity resulting from bed rest, trauma, casting of a body part, or local nerve damage (McCance & Huether, 2019). *Impaired physical mobility* is defined by the North American Nursing Diagnosis Association as a state in which the individual experiences or is at risk of experiencing limitation of physical movement (Ackley et al., 2020).

Periods of immobility due to disability or injury or prolonged bed rest can cause major physiological, psychological, and social effects. These effects can be gradual or immediate and vary from patient to patient. The greater the extent and the longer the duration of immobility, the more pronounced are the consequences. The patient with complete mobility restrictions is continually at risk for side effects of immobility. When possible, it is imperative that patients, especially older persons, have limited bed rest and that their activity is more than movement from bed to chair. Loss of walking independence increases hospital stays, need for rehabilitation services, or long-term care placement. In addition, the deconditioning related to reduced walking increases the risk for patient falls (Xu et al., 2018).

Systemic Effects of Immobility. Exercise has positive outcomes for all major systems of the body (see Chapter 37). When there is an alteration in mobility, each body system is at risk for impairment. The severity of the impairment depends on the patient's overall health, degree and length of immobility, and age. For example, persons with chronic illness develop pronounced effects of immobility.

Metabolic Changes. Changes in mobility alter endocrine metabolism, calcium resorption, and functioning of the gastrointestinal system. The endocrine system, made up of hormone-secreting glands, maintains and regulates the following: (1) response to stress and injury; (2) growth and development; (3) reproduction; (4) homeostasis; and (5) energy production, use, and storage.

When injury or stress occurs, the endocrine system triggers a series of responses aimed at maintaining blood pressure and preserving life. The endocrine system is important in maintaining homeostasis. Tissues and cells live in an internal environment that the endocrine system helps regulate through maintenance of sodium, potassium, water, and acid–base balance. The endocrine system also helps regulate energy metabolism. Thyroid hormone increases the basal metabolic rate (BMR), and energy becomes available to cells through the integrated action of gastrointestinal and pancreatic hormones (McCance & Huether, 2019).

Immobility disrupts normal metabolic functioning, decreasing the metabolic rate. This decrease in BMR alters the metabolism of carbohydrates, fats, and proteins; causes fluid, electrolyte, and calcium imbalances; and produces gastrointestinal disturbances, such as decreased appetite and slowing of peristalsis. However, in response to hypermetabolic processes (i.e., infection, fever, wound healing), patients who are immobilized may have an increased BMR because of increased cellular oxygen requirements (McCance & Huether, 2019).

A deficiency in calories and protein is characteristic of patients with a decreased appetite secondary to immobility. The body is constantly synthesizing proteins and breaking them down into amino acids to form other proteins. When the patient is immobile, the body excretes more nitrogen (the end product of amino acid breakdown) than protein ingested, resulting in **negative nitrogen balance**. Weight loss, decreased muscle mass, and weakness result from tissue catabolism (tissue breakdown) (McCance & Huether, 2019). Another metabolic change associated with immobility is calcium resorption (loss) from bones. Immobility causes the release of calcium into circulation. Normally, the kidneys can excrete the excess calcium. However, if the kidneys are unable to respond appropriately, hypercalcemia results. Pathological fractures occur if calcium resorption continues as a patient remains on bed rest or continues to be immobile (McCance & Huether, 2019).

Impaired gastrointestinal functioning can result from decreased mobility. Difficulty in passing stools (constipation) is a common symptom, although pseudodiarrhea may result from a fecal impaction (accumulation of hardened feces). This finding is not normal diarrhea, but rather liquid stool passing around the area of impaction. Left untreated, fecal impaction can result in a mechanical bowel obstruction that may partially or completely occlude the intestinal lumen, blocking normal propulsion of liquid and gas. The resulting fluid in the intestine produces distension and increases intraluminal pressure.

Over time, intestinal function becomes depressed, dehydration occurs, absorption ceases, and fluid and electrolyte disturbances worsen.

Respiratory Changes. Regular aerobic exercise is known to enhance respiratory functioning. In contrast, lack of movement and exercise places patients at higher risk for respiratory complications. Patients who are immobile are at a high risk of developing pulmonary complications such as **atelectasis** (collapse of alveoli) and **hypostatic pneumonia** (inflammation of the lung from stasis or pooling of secretions). Both conditions decrease oxygenation, prolong recovery, and add to the patient's discomfort (Lewis et al., 2023). In atelectasis, secretions block a bronchiole or a bronchus, and the distal lung tissue (alveoli) collapses as the existing air is absorbed, producing hypoventilation. The site of the blockage determines the severity of atelectasis. A lung lobe or even a whole lung may collapse. At some point in the development of these complications, there is a proportional decline in the patient's ability to cough productively. Ultimately, the distribution of mucus in the bronchi increases, particularly when the patient is in the supine, prone, or lateral position. Mucus accumulates in the dependent regions of the airways. Hypostatic pneumonia frequently results because mucus is an excellent medium for bacterial growth.

Cardiovascular Changes. Immobilization also affects the cardiovascular system, frequently resulting in orthostatic hypotension, increased cardiac workload, and thrombus formation.

Orthostatic hypotension is a drop of blood pressure greater than 20 mm Hg in systolic blood pressure and of 10 mm Hg in diastolic blood pressure. Symptoms include dizziness, light-headedness, nausea, tachycardia, pallor, or fainting when the patient changes from a lying or sitting position to a standing position (Ball et al., 2019). In the immobilized patient, decreased circulating fluid volume, pooling of blood in the lower extremities, and decreased autonomic response occur. These responses are especially evident in older persons.

As the workload of the heart increases, its oxygen consumption does as well. Therefore, the heart works harder and less efficiently during periods of prolonged rest. As immobilization increases, cardiac output falls, further decreasing cardiac efficiency and increasing workload.

Patients who are immobile are also at risk for thrombus formation. A **thrombus** is an accumulation of platelets, fibrin, clotting factors, and the cellular elements of the blood attached to the interior wall of a vein or artery, sometimes occluding the lumen of the vessel (Figure 46.1). Three factors contribute to venous thrombus formation: (1) loss of integrity of the vessel wall (e.g., injury during surgical procedures), (2) alterations in blood flow (e.g., slow blood flow in calf veins associated with bed rest), and (3) alterations in blood constituents (e.g., a change in clotting factors or increased platelet activity). These three factors are sometimes referred to as *Virchow's triad* (McCance & Huether, 2019). A dislodged venous thrombus, called an **embolus**, may travel through the circulatory system to the lungs and impair circulation and oxygenation. Venous emboli that travel to the lungs are called *pulmonary emboli* and may be life-threatening. More than 90% of all pulmonary emboli begin in the legs or pelvis (Copstead-Kirkhorn & Banasik, 2018). As a nurse, you will practice in numerous situations where deep vein thrombosis must be prevented, especially during perioperative care.

Musculoskeletal Changes. Immobility affects the musculoskeletal system by causing temporary or permanent impairment that may lead to permanent disability. Muscle effects resulting from restricted mobility include loss of endurance, strength, and muscle mass, as well as decreased stability and balance. Skeletal effects of immobility include impaired calcium metabolism and impaired joint mobility.

Muscle effects. Because of protein breakdown, a patient loses lean body mass when immobile. Reduced muscle mass makes it difficult for patients to sustain activity. If immobility continues and the patient does not exercise, there is further loss of muscle mass.

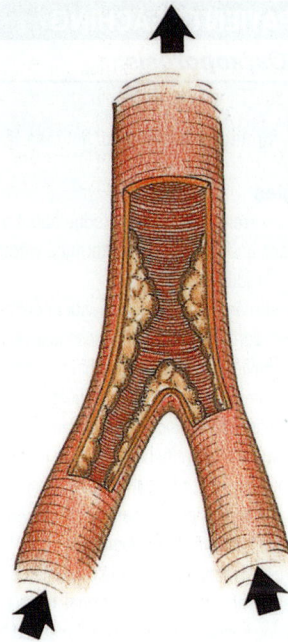

FIGURE 46.1 Thrombus formation in a vessel.

Prolonged immobility often leads to *disuse atrophy*, the reduction in normal size of muscle fibres after prolonged bed rest, trauma, casting, or local nerve damage. Loss of endurance, decreased muscle mass and strength, and joint instability (see "Skeletal Effects" in next section) put patients at risk for falls.

Skeletal effects. Immobilization causes two skeletal changes: impaired calcium metabolism and joint abnormalities. Because immobilization results in bone resorption, the bone tissue is less dense and **disuse osteoporosis** results, putting the patient at risk for pathological fractures. Bone resorption also causes calcium to be released in the blood, resulting in hypercalcemia.

Osteoporosis (or porous bone) is a disease characterized by loss of bone mass and deterioration of bone tissue that can lead to increased risk of fractures. Osteoporosis is a major health concern in Canada. Eighty percent of fractures in women over 50 are related to osteoporosis. Fragility fractures are responsible for increased mortality and morbidity in older persons (Brown et al., 2021). Although primary osteoporosis is different in origin from the osteoporosis that results from immobility, nurses must recognize that immobilized patients are at high risk for accelerated bone loss if they have primary osteoporosis. Interventions for preventing disability in immobilized patients with primary osteoporosis include early patient evaluation, and consultation with and referral to health care providers, dietitians, occupational therapists, and physiotherapists. Patient teaching should focus on limiting the severity of the disease through diet and activity (Box 46.1).

Immobility can also lead to joint contractures. A **joint contracture** is an abnormal and possibly permanent condition characterized by fixation of a joint. Flexor muscles for joints are stronger than extensor muscles and therefore contribute to the formation of contractures. Disuse, atrophy, and shortening of the muscle fibres cause joint contraction. When a contracture occurs, the joint cannot obtain full ROM. Contractures may leave a joint or joints in a nonfunctional position (Figure 46.2) and can be permanent. Interventions to prevent development of contractures in patients who are immobile are essential for nurses and health care providers to carry out.

Footdrop is the inability to dorsiflex and evert the foot because of peroneal nerve damage. It is a common and debilitating contracture

Objective
- Patient will identify strategies to prevent or limit the severity of osteoporosis.

Teaching Strategies
- Assess the patient's current state of knowledge about osteoporosis, including the disease processes and self-care, to determine whether information needs to be reinforced or introduced.
- Provide the patient (and caregiver, if present) with information about common risk factors (e.g., smoking, caffeine, alcohol). Assess learner readiness to engage in change of lifestyle behaviours and adapt teaching to individual patients.
- Provide patient and caregiver with dietary education, including current recommended dietary allowances for calcium and vitamin D, and review foods high in calcium and vitamin D. To identify how patients access supplements and recommended foods, integrate questions in order to assess social determinants of health, to explore potential barriers such as income, physical environments, social supports, and access to health services (Orsted et al., 2017). Explore patient's cultural preferences or beliefs regarding use of supplements and eating recommended foods. Collaborate with the interprofessional team to address the patient's challenges to accessing supplements and recommended foods, as necessary.
- Provide the patient and caregiver with activity education, including appropriate types of weight-bearing exercises as recommended by the health care provider or physiotherapist to prevent injury or fractures.
- Provide the patient and caregiver with information about safety, fall prevention, and strategies to create a safe home environment. Collaborate with the interprofessional team to determine if home assessment is required, as well as support for assistive devices or home modifications.
- Teach the patient and caregiver how to self-administer prescribed medications. Engage the patient and caregiver in return demonstrations to assess their understanding and determine if home supports are required.

Evaluation
- Patient and caregiver openly discuss lifestyle and risk factors and identify supports they can access if they are ready to change risk behaviours.
- Patient and caregiver identify foods high in calcium and vitamin D. If access is a barrier for patients, strategies to facilitate access can include collaborating with social workers to identify sources of financial support and working with patients to identify community resources, such as food distribution programs and community kitchen programs.
- Patient and caregiver demonstrate appropriate weight-bearing exercises.
- Patient and caregiver identify safety strategies to prevent falls.
- Patient and caregiver demonstrate appropriate knowledge about medications.
- Patient and caregiver express positive but realistic feedback regarding the effects of disease.

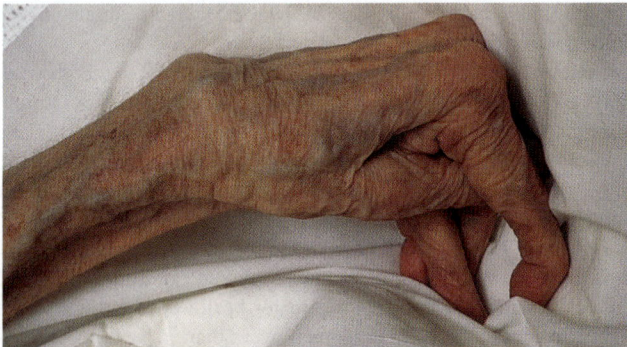

FIGURE 46.2 A contracture of the joints in the fingers. (From Sorrentino, S. A., & Wilk, M. J. [2018]. *Mosby's Canadian textbook for the support worker* [4th ed.]. Mosby.)

(Figures 46.3 and 46.4) that causes the foot to be permanently fixed in plantar flexion. Ambulation becomes difficult because the patient cannot dorsiflex the foot and is unable to lift their toes off the ground. Footdrop can be associated with a variety of etiologies, including prolonged bed rest, peroneal nerve damage, peripheral neuropathy, and CVAs (strokes).

Urinary Elimination Changes. Immobility also alters a patient's urinary elimination. In the upright position, gravitational force facilities flow of urine out of the renal pelvis and into the ureters and bladder. When the patient is recumbent or flat, the kidneys and the ureters are in a level position. Urine formed by the kidney must enter the bladder unaided by gravity. Peristaltic contractions of the ureters are insufficient to overcome gravity. Consequently, the renal pelvis may fill before urine enters the ureters. This condition, called **urinary stasis**, increases the risk of urinary tract infection and renal calculi (see Chapter 44). *Renal calculi* are calcium stones that lodge in the renal pelvis and pass through the ureters. Patients who are immobile are at risk for calculi because of both urinary stasis and altered calcium metabolism leading to hypercalcemia.

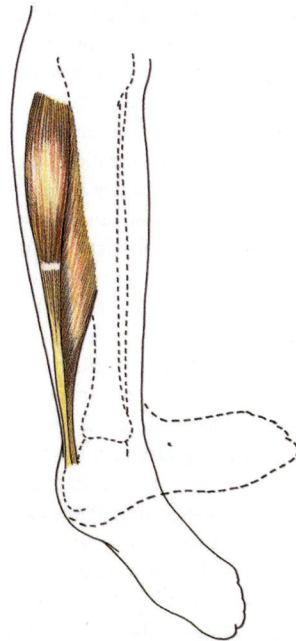

FIGURE 46.3 Footdrop. The ankle is fixed in plantar flexion. Normally, the ankle is able to flex (*dotted line*), which eases walking.

As the period of immobility continues, oral fluid intake can decrease, and this increases the risk for dehydration. As a result, urinary output may decline around the fifth or sixth day after immobilization and the urine is often highly concentrated. Concentrated urine increases the risk for calculi formation and infection. Patients who are immobile may have limited access to bathing equipment and be unable to perform adequate perineal hygiene, leading to increased risk for urinary tract contamination by *Escherichia coli* bacteria.

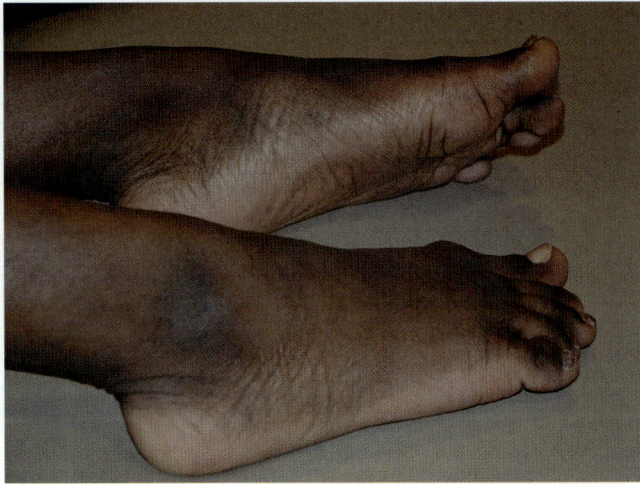

FIGURE 46.4 Patient with bilateral footdrop.

Patients who are immobile may be unable to use the bathroom or a bedside commode. Voiding on a bedpan or using a urinal does not provide the usual sensory stimulation to void and does not allow gravity to act on the bladder sphincter. Consequently, patients may be unable to void or completely empty their bladder. This situation leads to residual urine in the bladder, which increases the risk for infection. Complete urinary retention requires catheterization. Both intermittent catheterization and in-dwelling catheters increase the risk of developing urinary tract infection.

Integumentary Changes. Immobility is a major risk factor for developing pressure injuries. Preventing a pressure injury is much less expensive for health care facilities and causes patients less distress than treating one; therefore, preventative nursing interventions are imperative (Norton et al., 2017).

A **pressure injury** is localized damage to the skin, underlying soft tissue, or both as a result of prolonged ischemia (decreased blood supply in the tissues). The injury can present as intact skin or an open ulcer (pressure injury) and may be painful. A pressure injury is characterized initially by inflammation and usually forms over a bony prominence. Ischemia develops when the pressure on the skin is greater than the pressure inside the small peripheral blood vessels supplying blood to the skin. Adequate blood flow is necessary to supply oxygen and nutrients for tissue metabolism and the elimination of metabolic wastes. Pressure affects cellular metabolism by decreasing or totally eliminating tissue circulation.

People who are conscious have voluntary muscle control and normal perception of pressure to perceive decreased circulation to tissue. They change positions regularly to increase circulation to tissue, thus preventing formation of pressure injuries. To avoid the development of pressure injuries in individuals with impaired sensation or mobility, they may require assistance to regularly reposition themselves. Areas of skin covering bony prominences (i.e., scapulae, elbows, coccyx, heels) are most at risk for skin breakdown. Nurses must be aware of these areas and assist patients with frequent position changes, whether patients are lying down or sitting.

SAFETY ALERT Implement a comprehensive skin care program to prevent skin breakdown in all patients, from newborns to older persons. Effective skin care programs include accurate and consistent assessment and documentation as well as interventions to protect the skin (e.g., turning the patient every 2 hours and using mechanical devices such as lifts when you need to move the patient to reduce friction and shear [Norton et al., 2017]).

Psychosocial Effects of Immobility. Immobilization can contribute to decreased social interaction, social isolation, sensory deprivation, loss of independence, and role changes (Boscart et al., 2023; Norton et al., 2017). These, in turn, may lead to emotional reactions, behavioural responses, sensory alterations, and changes in coping. Every patient responds to immobility differently.

Immobility may lead to depression in some patients because of changes in role, self-concept, and other factors. *Depression* is an affective disorder characterized by exaggerated feelings of sadness, melancholy, dejection, worthlessness, emptiness, and hopelessness out of proportion to reality. Depression can result from worrying about present and future levels of health, finances, and family needs. Because immobilization removes the patient from a daily routine, individuals may worry about disability. Worrying can quickly increase the patient's depression, leading to withdrawal. By assessing behavioural changes throughout a patient's restricted mobility, nurses are better equipped to identify changes in self-concept, recognize early signs of depression, develop nursing interventions, and collaborate with the interprofessional team to ensure that proper supports are provided for the patient.

Developmental Changes. Immobility often leads to developmental changes in very young children and in older persons. The immobilized young or middle-aged adult who has been healthy may experience few, if any, developmental changes. However, exceptions exist, and patients must be fully assessed for developmental implications.

Infants, Toddlers, and Preschoolers. The newborn's spine is flexed and lacks the anteroposterior curves of the adult. As the baby grows, musculoskeletal development permits support of weight for standing and walking. Posture is awkward because the head and upper trunk are carried forward. Because body weight is not evenly distributed along a line of gravity, posture is off balance, and falls occur often. When the infant, toddler, or preschooler is immobilized, it is usually because of trauma or the need to correct a congenital skeletal abnormality. Prolonged immobilization can delay the child's gross motor skills, intellectual development, musculoskeletal development, or a combination of these growth areas. Nurses caring for immobilized children should plan activities that provide physical and psychosocial stimuli. Frequent skin assessment of pediatric patients who are immobilized is essential. In acute care settings, equipment-related factors can contribute to development of pressure injuries. A comprehensive assessment should include pressure injury risk assessment and head-to-toe skin assessment, with close attention to areas under splints, braces, traction devices, and tracheostomies (Norton et al., 2017).

Adolescents. The adolescence stage is usually initiated by a tremendous growth spurt (see Chapter 24). Growth is frequently uneven. Prolonged immobilization may alter adolescent growth patterns. When the activity level is reduced because of trauma, illness, or surgery, the adolescent may lag behind peers in gaining independence. Social isolation and self-concept are concerns for this age group when immobilization occurs.

Adults. An adult who has correct posture and body alignment feels good, looks good, and generally appears self-confident. The healthy adult also has the necessary musculoskeletal development and coordination to carry out ADLs. When periods of prolonged immobility occur, however, all physiological systems are at risk. In addition, the role of the adult may change with regard to the family or social structure. The adult may lose their identity and self-concept associated with a job.

Older Persons. A progressive loss of total bone mass (strength), muscle strength, and aerobic capacity occurs in older persons. Some of the possible causes of this loss are decreased physical activity, hormonal changes, and bone resorption. Older persons may walk more

<table>
<tr></tr>
</table>

BOX 46.2	Functional Decline in Hospitalized Immobile Older Persons

For many older persons, admission to the hospital often results in functional decline despite the treatment for which they were admitted. Some older persons have difficulties with mobility and can quickly regress to a dependent state. Rapid intervention of an interprofessional health care team is required to maintain the patient's functional capacity.

- Usual aging is associated with decreased muscle strength and aerobic capacity, which becomes exacerbated if a patient's nutritional state is poor.
- A nutritional assessment needs to be included in the plan of care for the older person experiencing immobility.
- Anorexia and insufficient assistance with eating food lead to malnutrition, which contributes to the known challenges associated with immobility.
- Improved nutrition increases the patient's ability to perform physical reconditioning exercises.
- There is a direct relationship between the success of older persons' rehabilitation and their nutritional status.

Adapted from Boscart, V., McCleary, L., Taucar, L.S., et al. (2023). *Ebersole & Hess' gerontological nursing and healthy aging in Canada* (3rd ed.). Elsevier Inc.

slowly, take smaller steps, and appear less coordinated. Adverse effects of prescribed medications can include altering of a sense of balance or changes in blood pressure, which increase older persons' risks for falls and injuries (see Chapter 25). The outcomes of a fall include possible injury, hospitalization, loss of independence, and psychological effects.

Older persons may experience functional-status changes secondary to hospitalization and altered mobility status (Box 46.2). Immobilization of older persons increases their physical dependence on others and accelerates functional losses (Fazio et al., 2020). Immobilization of some older persons results from a degenerative disease, neurological trauma, or chronic illness. In others, immobilization can occur suddenly, such as after a stroke. When providing nursing care for an older person, nurses should develop a care plan that encourages the patient to perform as many self-care activities as possible, thereby maintaining the highest level of mobility and functionality. Nurses may inadvertently contribute to a patient's immobility by providing unnecessary help with activities such as bathing and transferring.

CRITICAL THINKING

Critical thinking requires nurses to synthesize knowledge, experience, patient data, and professional standards. Each of these sources must be integrated into the nurse's diagnosis and care plan for the patient with impaired mobility (Figure 46.5). Over the past decade, most health care facilities in Canada have established standards of practice related to moving and transferring patients, as well as the prevention of falls and pressure sores.

❖ NURSING PROCESS

Nurses must apply the nursing process and use a critical thinking approach to develop individualized care plans for patients with mobility impairments or risk for immobility. The aim of the care plan is to improve the patient's functional status, promote self-care, maintain psychological well-being, and reduce the hazards of immobility.

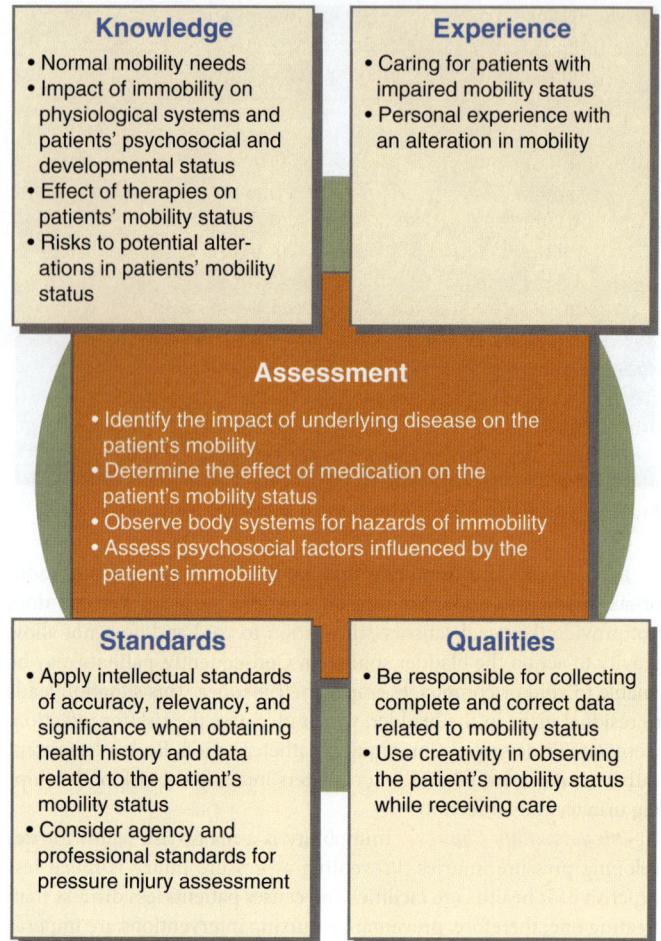

Knowledge
- Normal mobility needs
- Impact of immobility on physiological systems and patients' psychosocial and developmental status
- Effect of therapies on patients' mobility status
- Risks to potential alterations in patients' mobility status

Experience
- Caring for patients with impaired mobility status
- Personal experience with an alteration in mobility

Assessment
- Identify the impact of underlying disease on the patient's mobility
- Determine the effect of medication on the patient's mobility status
- Observe body systems for hazards of immobility
- Assess psychosocial factors influenced by the patient's immobility

Standards
- Apply intellectual standards of accuracy, relevancy, and significance when obtaining health history and data related to the patient's mobility status
- Consider agency and professional standards for pressure injury assessment

Qualities
- Be responsible for collecting complete and correct data related to mobility status
- Use creativity in observing the patient's mobility status while receiving care

FIGURE 46.5 Critical thinking model for mobility assessment.

◆ Assessment

Nursing assessment with a focus on mobility and immobility must incorporate the following:

1. A patient's normal mobility status
2. The effects of diseases or conditions on mobility
3. The patient's risk for mobility alterations as a result of treatments

During assessment, nurses critically analyze findings and collaborate with patients and the interprofessional team to ensure that patient-centred clinical decisions are made.

Patient Expectations. Usually, the nurse will assess a patient's degree of mobility and immobility during the health history interview and physical examination. The nurse must include the patient as a partner in designing the plan of care and assess how the patient perceives any limitations in mobility. Has the patient had a disability for an extended period of time, or is the patient well adapted to the use of an assist device or even a wheelchair? Is the limitation in mobility sudden and unexpected, causing the patient to be fearful or full of questions? Nurses must have respect for the patient's preferences, values, and needs during assessment and when designing a plan of care (Ackley et al., 2020).

Mobility. Assessment of patient mobility focuses on ROM, gait, exercise and activity tolerance, and body alignment. When unsure of the patient's abilities, the nurse begins assessment of mobility with the patient in the most supportive position and moves to higher levels of mobility according to the patient's tolerance.

Generally, the nurse starts assessing movement while the patient is lying, then proceeds to assessing sitting positions in bed, transfers to chair, and, finally, gait. This sequence of assessment helps to protect the patient's safety.

Range of Motion. **Range of motion (ROM)** is the maximum amount of movement available at a joint in one of the four planes of the body: medial, sagittal, frontal, or transverse. The *medial plane* is a line through the axis of the body, separating the body into equal halves, a left side and a right side. The *sagittal plane* is any plane parallel to the medial plane. The *frontal plane* passes through the body from side to side and divides the body into front and back. The *transverse plane* is a horizontal line that divides the body into upper and lower portions. The anatomical position is used as a reference when describing the parts of the body as they relate to each other (Figure 46.6).

Ligaments, muscles, and the nature of the joint control joint mobility in each of the planes. Joint movements are described using the following terms and examples provided in Table 46.2:

- *Flexion and extension:* Flexion is decreasing the angle between two adjoining bones (bending of the joint); extension is increasing the angle between two adjoining bones (extending the joint).

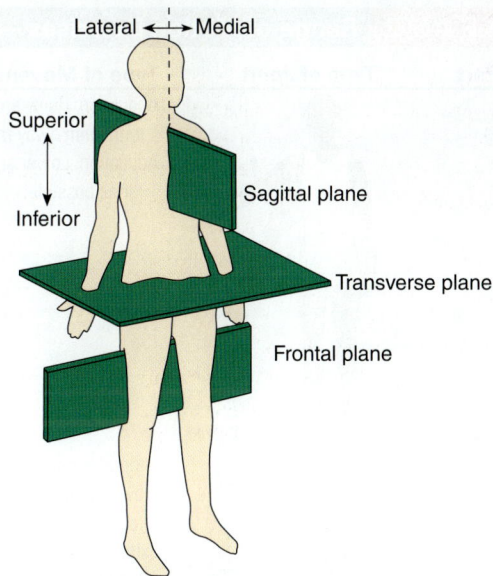

FIGURE 46.6 Planes of the body.

TABLE 46.2	Range-of-Motion Exercises			
Body Part	**Type of Joint**	**Type of Movement**	**Range (Degrees)**	**Primary Muscles**
Neck, cervical spine	Pivotal	Flexion: Bring chin to rest on chest.	45	Sternocleidomastoid
		Extension: Return head to erect position.	45	Trapezius
		Hyperextension: Bend head back as far as possible.	10	Trapezius
		Lateral flexion: Tilt head as far as possible toward each shoulder.	40–45	Sternocleidomastoid
		Rotation: Turn head as far as possible along transverse plane to look to each side.	180	Sternocleidomastoid, trapezius
Shoulder	Ball and socket	Flexion: Raise arm from side position forward to position above the head.	180	Coracobrachialis, biceps brachii, deltoid, pectoralis major
		Extension: Return arm to position at side of the body.	180	Latissimus dorsi, teres major, triceps brachii
		Hyperextension: Move arm behind body, keeping elbow straight.	45–60	Latissimus dorsi, teres major, deltoid

Continued

TABLE 46.2   Range-of-Motion Exercises—cont'd

Body Part	Type of Joint	Type of Movement	Range (Degrees)	Primary Muscles
		Abduction: Raise arm to side to position above head with palm away from head.	180	Deltoid, supraspinatus
		Adduction: Lower arm sideways and across body as far as possible.	320	Pectoralis major
		Internal rotation: With elbow flexed, rotate shoulder by moving arm until thumb is turned inward and toward back.	90	Pectoralis major, latissimus dorsi, teres major, subscapularis
		External rotation: With elbow flexed, move arm until thumb is upward and lateral to head.	90	Infraspinatus, teres major, deltoid
		Circumduction: Move arm in full circle. (Circumduction is a combination of all movements of the ball-and-socket joint.)	360	Deltoid, coracobrachialis, latissimus dorsi, teres major
Elbow	Hinge	Flexion: Bend elbow so that lower arm moves toward its shoulder joint and the hand is level with the shoulder.	150	Biceps brachii, brachialis, brachioradialis
		Extension: Straighten elbow by lowering hand.	150	Triceps brachii
Forearm	Pivotal	Supination: Turn lower arm and hand so that the palm is up.	70–90	Supinator, biceps brachii
		Pronation: Turn lower arm so that the palm is down.	70–90	Pronator teres, pronator quadratus

TABLE 46.2 | **Range-of-Motion Exercises—cont'd**

Body Part	Type of Joint	Type of Movement	Range (Degrees)	Primary Muscles
Wrist	Condyloid	Flexion: Move palm toward inner aspect of forearm.	80–90	Flexor carpi ulnaris, flexor carpi radialis
		Extension: Move fingers and hand posterior to midline.	80–90	Extensor carpi radialis brevis, extensor carpi radialis longus, extensor carpi ulnaris
		Hyperextension: Bring dorsal surface of hand back as far as possible.	80–90	Extensor carpi radialis brevis, extensor carpi radialis longus, extensor carpi ulnaris
		Abduction (radial deviation): Place hand with palm up and extend wrist laterally toward the thumb.	Up to 30	Flexor carpi radialis, extensor carpi radialis brevis, extensor carpi radialis longus
		Adduction (ulnar deviation): Place hand with palm up and extend wrist medially toward the fifth finger.	30–50	Flexor carpi ulnaris, extensor carpi ulnaris
Fingers	Condyloid hinge	Flexion: Make a fist.	90	Lumbricals, interosseous volaris, interosseous dorsalis
		Extension: Straighten fingers.	90	Extensor digiti quinti proprius, extensor digitorum communis, extensor indicis proprius
		Hyperextension: Bend fingers back as far as possible.	30–60	Extensor digitorum
		Abduction: Spread fingers apart.	30	Interosseous dorsalis
		Adduction: Bring fingers together.	30	Interosseous volaris
Thumb	Saddle	Flexion: Move thumb across palmar surface of hand.	90	Flexor pollicis brevis
		Extension: Move thumb straight away from hand.	90	Extensor pollicis longus, extensor pollicis brevis
		Abduction: Extend thumb laterally (usually done when placing fingers in abduction and adduction).	30	Abductor pollicis brevis
		Adduction: Move thumb back toward hand.	30	Adductor pollicis obliquus, adductor pollicis transversus
		Opposition: Touch thumb to each finger of the same hand.		Opponeus pollicis, opponeus digiti minimi

Continued

TABLE 46.2		Range-of-Motion Exercises—cont'd		
Body Part	**Type of Joint**	**Type of Movement**	**Range (Degrees)**	**Primary Muscles**
Hip	Ball and socket	Flexion: Move leg forward and up.	90–120	Psoas major, iliacus, sartorius
		Extension: Move leg back beside other leg.	90–120	Gluteus maximus, semitendinosus, semimembranosus
		Hyperextension: Move leg behind the body.	30–50	Gluteus maximus, semitendinosus, semimembranosus
		Abduction: Move leg laterally away from the body.	30–50	Gluteus medius, gluteus minimus
		Adduction: Move leg back toward medial position and beyond, if possible.	30–50	Adductor longus, adductor brevis, adductor magnus
		Internal rotation: Turn foot and leg toward other leg.	90	Gluteus medius, gluteus minimus, tensor fasciae latae
		External rotation: Turn foot and leg away from other leg.	90	Obturatorius internus, obturatorius externus
		Circumduction: Move leg in a circle.		Psoas major, gluteus maximus, gluteus medius, adductor magnus
Knee	Hinge	Flexion: Bring heel back toward back of thigh.	120–130	Biceps femoris, semitendinosus, semimembranosus, sartorius
		Extension: Return leg to the floor.	120–130	Rectus femoris, vastus lateralis, vastus medialis, vastus intermedius
Ankle	Hinge	Dorsiflexion: Move foot so that toes are pointed upward.	20–30	Tibialis anterior
		Plantar flexion: Move foot so that toes are pointed downward.	45–50	Gastrocnemius, soleus

TABLE 46.2 Range-of-Motion Exercises—cont'd

Body Part	Type of Joint	Type of Movement	Range (Degrees)	Primary Muscles
Foot	Gliding	Inversion: Turn sole of foot medially.	10 or less	Tibialis anterior, tibialis posterior
		Eversion: Turn sole of foot laterally.	10 or less	Peroneus longus, peroneus brevis
Toes	Condyloid	Flexion: Curl toes downward.	30–60	Flexor digitorum, lumbricalis pedis, flexor hallucis brevis
		Extension: Straighten toes.	30–60	Extensor digitorum longus, extensor digitorum brevis, extensor hallucis longus
		Abduction: Spread toes apart.	15 or less	Abductor hallucis, interosseous dorsalis
		Adduction: Bring toes together.	15 or less	Adductor hallucis, interosseous plantaris
		Adduction: Bring toes together.	15 or less	Adductor hallucis, interosseous plantaris

- *Hyperextension:* This is movement of a body part beyond its normal resting extended position.
- *Dorsiflexion and plantar flexion:* Dorsiflexion is the flexion of the ankle moving toes and foot upward; plantar flexion of the ankle is bending of the toes and foot downward.
- *Abduction and adduction:* Abduction is movement of an extremity away from the midline of the body; adduction is movement of an extremity toward the midline of the body.
- *Eversion and inversion:* Eversion is the turning of a body part away from the midline; inversion is the turning of a body part toward the midline.
- *Pronation and supination:* Pronation is movement of a body part so that the front or ventral surface faces downward; supination is movement of a body part so that the front or ventral surface faces upward.
- *Internal and external rotation:* Internal rotation is rotation of the joint inward; external rotation is rotation of the joint outward.
- *Circumduction:* This is the circular movement of a limb in a cone-shaped manner (e.g., shoulder).

Assessment of ROM is important as a baseline measure to determine a patient's mobility status and to later compare and evaluate whether loss in joint mobility has occurred as a result of clinical changes or treatments. ROM assessment includes examining the patient for stiffness, swelling, pain, limited movement, and unequal movement. Patients with restricted mobility require ROM exercises to reduce the hazards of immobility, such as contractures. Limited ROM often indicates inflammation such as arthritis, fluid in the joint, or altered nerve supply. Increased mobility (beyond normal ROM) of a joint sometimes indicates connective tissue disorders, ligament tears, or possible joint fractures.

ROM exercises may be active (the patient is able to move all joints through their ROM unassisted), passive (the patient is unable to move independently, and the nurse moves each joint through its ROM), or somewhere in between (see Table 46.2). To assess the type of ROM

exercise a patient can perform, the nurse must first review the medical plan of care to determine whether active ROM exercises are appropriate. Then, the patient's ability to engage in active ROM exercise is assessed. Passive ROM exercises are prescribed for patients who are unable to move because of paralysis, sedation, or generalized weakness. Passive ROM exercises improve joint mobility, prevent contractures, and help prepare the patient for ongoing rehabilitation exercises (Smith et al., 2016). With a patient who is weak, the nurse may provide support while the patient performs most of the movement, or the patient may be able to move some joints actively while the nurse passively moves others (Box 46.3). The nurse's assessment will help to determine the patient's need for assistance, teaching, or reinforcement. In general, exercises should be as active as health and mobility allow. Assessment data from patients with limited joint movements vary on the basis of the area affected.

Gait. The term **gait** is used to describe a particular manner or style of walking. It is a coordinated action that requires the integration of sensory function, muscle strength, proprioception, balance, and a properly functioning central nervous system (vestibular system and cerebellum). The gait cycle begins with the heel strike of one leg and continues to the heel strike of the other leg. Assessing a patient's gait helps nurses to draw conclusions about balance, posture, safety, and ability to walk without assistance, all of which affect the risk of falling. Here are a few ways to assess a patient's gait:

1. Observe the patent entering the room, and note speed, stride, and balance.
2. Ask the patient to walk across the room, turn, and come back.
3. Ask the patient to walk heel-to-toe in a straight line. This may be difficult for older patients, even in the absence of disease, so stay at the patient's side during the walk.

Exercise and Activity Tolerance. **Exercise** is physical activity for conditioning the body, improving health, and maintaining fitness. It can be used as therapy to correct a deformity or to restore the overall body to a maximal state of health. When a person exercises,

BOX 46.3 How to Perform Passive Range-of-Motion Exercises

1. Perform hand hygiene.
2. Identify the patient using two unique identifiers (e.g., chart, wrist band).
3. Explain the procedure and its purpose to the patient. Provide additional information, as needed.
4. Assess the patient's health status, including pain, to determine the patient's activity tolerance and need for analgesia.
5. Assist the patient into a comfortable position in a bed or chair.
6. Perform range-of-motion exercises, working from head to toe:
   a. Head and neck: flexion, extension, rotation, lateral flexion
   b. Shoulder: flexion, extension, abduction, adduction, internal rotation, external rotation
   c. Elbow: flexion, extension, supination, pronation
   d. Wrist: flexion, extension, adduction, abduction, rotation
   e. Hand, fingers, and thumb: flexion, extension, adduction, abduction, opposition, circumduction of thumb
   f. Hip: flexion, extension, abduction, adduction, internal rotation, external rotation*
   g. Knee: flexion, extension
   h. Ankle: plantar flexion, dorsiflexion, inversion, eversion
   i. Feet and toes: flexion, extension

*Contraindicated in patients who have undergone total hip arthroplasty.
Adapted from Smith, N., Caple, C., & Pravikoff, D. (2016). Range-of-motion exercises, passive. CINAHL Nursing Guide, EBSCO Publishing. *Nursing practice and skill-CEU.* CINAHL AN: T703878.

physiological changes occur in body systems (see Chapter 37). Nurses assess a patient's exercise history by asking what exercise the patient normally engages in and the amount of exercise performed daily and weekly. For example, if a patient walks, what distance does the person typically walk, and how often? If a patient does not exercise regularly, the nurse will want to focus on their activity tolerance.

Activity tolerance is the type and amount of exercise or work that a person is able to perform without undue exertion or possible injury. Assessment of a patient's activity tolerance is necessary when planning activities for the patient, such as walking, ROM exercises, or ADLs. Activity tolerance assessment includes data from physiological, emotional, and developmental domains (see Chapter 37).

After a prolonged period of inactivity, the nurse should monitor the patient for symptoms such as dyspnea, fatigue, or chest pain. If these symptoms develop, the nurse must assess for a change in vital signs (heart rate and blood pressure). A weak or debilitated patient is unable to sustain even slight changes in activity because of the increased demand for energy. Simple tasks such as eating or moving in bed often result in extreme fatigue. When the patient experiences decreased activity tolerance, the nurse must assess the time needed by the patient to recover. Decreasing recovery time indicates improved activity tolerance.

People who are depressed, worried, or anxious are frequently unable to tolerate exercise. Patients who are depressed tend to withdraw from activity rather than participate in it. Patients who worry or are anxious expend a great amount of mental energy and often report feeling fatigued. Because of this, they may experience physical and emotional exhaustion.

Developmental changes also affect activity tolerance. As the infant enters the toddler stage, the activity level increases and the need for sleep declines. The child entering preschool or primary grades expends mental energy in learning and may require more rest after school or before strenuous play. The adolescent going through puberty may require more rest because much of the body's energy is expended for growth and hormone changes (see Chapter 24).

Pregnancy causes fluctuations in energy tolerance, especially during the first and third trimesters. Hormonal changes and fetal development use body energy, and expectant mothers may be unable or unmotivated to carry out physical activities. During the last trimester, fetal development consumes a great deal of the mother's energy, and the size and location of the fetus may limit the mother's ability to take a deep breath, resulting in less oxygen being available for physical activities.

Activity changes continue through adulthood and are primarily related to employment and lifestyle choices. As the person grows older, activity tolerance changes. Muscle mass is reduced, posture changes, and bone composition changes. Changes in the cardiopulmonary system, such as decreased maximum heart rate and decreased lung compliance, affect the intensity of exercise. With progressing age, some older persons still exercise but do so at a reduced intensity. The more inactive a patient becomes, the more pronounced these activity changes are.

Body Alignment. Nursing assessment of body alignment is done with the patient lying, sitting, or standing. Objectives of body alignment assessment include the following:
- Determining normal physiological changes in body alignment resulting from growth and development for each individual patient
- Identifying deviations in body alignment caused by incorrect posture
- Providing opportunities for patients to observe their posture
- Identifying learning needs of patients for maintaining correct body alignment
- Identifying trauma, muscle damage, or nerve dysfunction
- Obtaining information about other factors contributing to poor alignment, such as fatigue, malnutrition, and psychological issues

The first step in assessing body alignment is to put the patient at ease so that the person does not assume an unnatural or rigid position. When assessing the body alignment of a patient who is immobilized or unconscious, pillows and positioning supports should be removed from the bed and the patient placed in the supine position.

Standing. When the patient is standing, the nurse assesses the following for correct body alignment:
- The head is erect and midline.
- When observed posteriorly, the shoulders and hips are straight and parallel.
- When observed posteriorly, the vertebral column is straight.
- When observed laterally, the head is erect and the spinal curves are aligned in a reversed "S" pattern. The cervical vertebrae are anteriorly convex, the thoracic vertebrae are posteriorly convex, and the lumbar vertebrae are anteriorly convex.
- When observed laterally, the abdomen is comfortably tucked in and the knees and ankles are slightly flexed. The person appears comfortable and does not seem conscious of the flexion of knees or ankles.
- Arms hang comfortably at the sides.
- Feet are placed slightly apart to achieve a base of support, and the toes are pointed forward.
- When observed posteriorly, the centre of gravity is in the midline, and the line of gravity is from the middle of the forehead to a midpoint between the feet. Laterally, the line of gravity runs vertically from the middle of the skull to the posterior third of the foot (Figure 46.7).

Sitting. Characteristics of correct alignment of the sitting patient include the following (Figure 46.8):
- The head is erect, and the neck and vertebral column are in straight alignment.

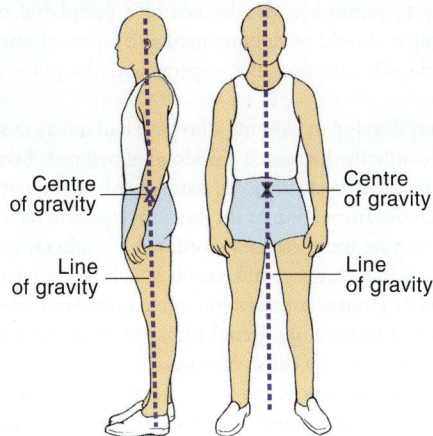

FIGURE 46.7 Correct body alignment when standing.

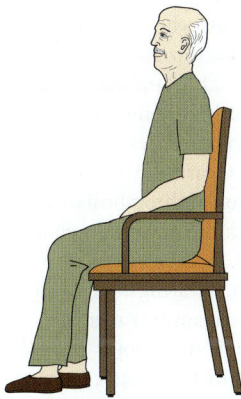

FIGURE 46.8 Correct body alignment when sitting. The patient's feet are flat on the floor, the calves do not touch the chair, and the back is straight and against the back of the chair. (From Sorrentino, S. A., & Wilk, M. J. [2018]. *Mosby's Canadian textbook for the support worker* [4th ed]. Mosby.)

- Body weight is evenly distributed on the buttocks and thighs.
- Thighs are parallel and in a horizontal plane.
- Both feet are supported on the floor or on wheelchair footrests. With patients of short stature, a footstool can be used to ensure ankles are comfortably flexed.
- A 2.5- to 5-cm space is maintained between the edge of the seat and the popliteal space on the posterior surface of the knee. This space ensures that no pressure is on the popliteal artery or nerve to decrease circulation or impair nerve function.
- The patient's forearms are supported on the armrest, in their lap, or on a table in front of the chair.

Assessing alignment when the patient is sitting is important if the patient has muscle weakness, muscle paralysis, or nerve damage. Diminished sensation impairs the patient's ability to perceive pressure or decreased circulation. Proper alignment while sitting reduces the risk of musculoskeletal system damage.

Lying. People who are conscious have voluntary muscle control and normal perception of pressure. Because their ROM, sensation, and circulation are within normal limits, they change positions when they perceive muscle strain and decreased circulation when lying down.

Assessment of body alignment for a patient who is immobilized or bedridden is done with the patient in the lateral position. All positioning supports should be removed from the bed except for the pillow under the head, and the body is supported with an adequate mattress (Figure 46.9). This position allows for full view of the spine and back

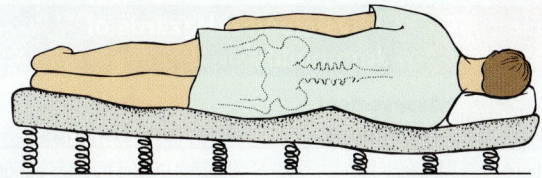

FIGURE 46.9 Lateral lying position for assessment of body alignment.

and provides other baseline body alignment data, such as whether the patient can remain positioned without aid. The vertebrae should be aligned, and the position should not cause discomfort. Patients with impaired mobility (e.g., traction or arthritis), decreased sensation (e.g., hemiparesis following a CVA), impaired circulation (e.g., diabetes), or lack of voluntary muscle control (e.g., spinal cord injury) are at risk for damage when lying down.

Immobility

Physiological Assessment. Assessment of the patient for physiological hazards of immobility is done while performing a head-to-toe physical assessment (see Chapter 33). Additionally, the examiner should assess relationships between the patient's immobility and psychosocial health, developmental stage, and the social determinants of health (Orsted et al., 2017). Physiological hazards of immobility that may be identified during a nursing assessment are summarized below and in Table 46.3.

Metabolic system. When assessing metabolic functioning, nurses use **anthropometric measurements** (measures of height, weight, and skin fold thickness) to evaluate muscle atrophy. In addition, the nurse may need to analyze intake and output records to determine whether intake equals output or if a fluid imbalance exists (see Chapter 41). Dehydration and edema can increase the rate of skin breakdown in a patient who is immobilized. Monitoring laboratory data such as electrolytes, serum protein (albumin and total protein) levels, and blood urea nitrogen can help in determining metabolic functioning.

Assessment of wound healing and monitoring of food intake and elimination patterns will help to identify altered gastrointestinal functioning and determine if there are potential metabolic concerns. If a patient who is immobile has a wound, the rate of healing indicates how well nutrients are being delivered to tissues. Normal progression of healing indicates that metabolic needs of injured tissues are being met. Anorexia occurs commonly in patients who are immobilized. The patient's food intake should be assessed before the meal tray is removed to determine the amount eaten. The patient's dietary patterns and food preferences are assessed at the onset of immobilization, to help prevent nutritional imbalances.

Respiratory system. A respiratory assessment is performed at least every 2 hours for patients with restricted activity. The nurse needs to inspect chest wall movements during the full inspiratory–expiratory cycle. If a patient has an atelectatic area, chest movement may be asymmetrical. The entire lung region should be auscultated to identify diminished breath sounds, crackles, or wheezes. Auscultation is focused on the dependent lung fields because pulmonary secretions tend to collect in lower regions. The nurse needs to perform a complete respiratory assessment to identify the presence of secretions and to determine nursing interventions necessary for optimal respiratory function.

Cardiovascular system. Cardiovascular assessment of the patient who is immobile includes blood pressure monitoring, evaluation of apical and peripheral pulses, and observation for signs of venous stasis (e.g., edema and poor wound healing). All patients should have their vital signs monitored during the first few attempts at sitting or standing.

TABLE 46.3		Physiological Hazards of Immobility
System	**Assessment Techniques**	**Abnormal Findings**
Metabolic	Inspection	Delayed wound healing, abnormal laboratory data
	Inspection	Muscle atrophy
	Anthropometric measurements (mid-upper arm circumference, triceps skinfold measurement)	Decreased amount of subcutaneous fat
	Inspection, palpation	Generalized edema
Respiratory	Inspection	Asymmetrical chest wall movement, dyspnea, increased respiratory rate
	Auscultation	Crackles, wheezes, decreased air entry
Cardiovascular	Auscultation	Orthostatic hypotension
	Auscultation, palpation	Increased heart rate, third heart sound, weak peripheral pulses
	Inspection, palpation	Dependent edema in feet and legs (if seated) and in sacrum (if lying)
Musculoskeletal	Inspection, palpation	Decreased range of motion, erythema, asymmetrical diameter in calf or thigh
	Inspection, palpation	Joint contracture
	Inspection	Activity intolerance, muscle atrophy, joint contracture
Elimination	Inspection	Decreased urine output, cloudy or concentrated urine, decreased frequency of bowel movements
	Palpation	Distended bladder and abdomen
	Auscultation	Decreased bowel sounds
Skin	Inspection, palpation	Impaired skin integrity

When monitoring orthostatic blood pressure, the nurse must move the patient gradually during position changes from supine to sitting or standing and assess for dizziness. First, with the patient in a supine position, the nurse obtains baseline blood pressure and pulse measurements. Next, the nurse assists the patient to a position sitting at the side of the bed. The patient should remain sitting for 3 minutes before the blood pressure and pulse are taken. The nurse should not leave the patient and continually monitor the patient for dizziness or lightheadedness. If the patient has no dizziness or drop in blood pressure (≥20 mm Hg systolic or 10 mm Hg diastolic), the nurse assists the patient to a standing position and retakes the blood pressure and pulse immediately and again after 3 minutes of standing. The patient should be monitored for dizziness throughout this procedure. The longer the period of immobility, the greater the risk of hypotension when the patient stands (McCance & Huether, 2019).

Frequent and peripheral pulse assessment are performed on patients who are immobile. Recumbent positions increase cardiac workload and result in an increased pulse rate. In some patients, particularly older persons, the heart may not tolerate the increased workload and cardiac failure may develop. A third heart sound, heard at the apex with the bell of the stethoscope, can be an early indication of heart failure. Monitoring of peripheral pulses helps the nurse to evaluate the heart's ability to pump blood. Absence of a peripheral pulse in the lower extremities should be documented and reported immediately to the patient's health care provider, especially if the pulse was present previously.

Edema may develop in patients who have had injury or whose heart is unable to handle the increased workload of bed rest. Because edema moves to dependent body regions, assessment of the patient who is immobile includes inspection of the sacrum, legs, and feet. If the heart is unable to tolerate the increased workload, peripheral body regions, such as the hands, feet, nose, and earlobes, will be colder than central body regions. The nurse assesses for other sources of edema beyond heart failure and immobility. Renal impairment and certain medications, such as steroids, can cause edema.

Deep vein thrombosis (DVT) is a hazard of restricted mobility. To assess for a DVT, the patient's elastic stockings or sequential compression devices (SCDs) are removed every 8 hours (or according to employer policy) and the calves observed for redness, warmth, and tenderness. Homans' sign, or calf pain on dorsiflexion of the foot, is contraindicated in patients when a DVT is suspected, as vigorous dorsiflexion may dislodge the thrombus.

Daily measurement of bilateral calf circumference is an assessment for DVT. The nurse marks a point on each calf 10 cm from the mid-patella. The circumference is measured each day, using the mark for placement of the tape measure. Unilateral increases in calf diameter can be an early indication of thrombosis. Because DVTs can also occur in the thigh, daily thigh measurements should be taken if the patient is prone to thrombosis. In many patients, DVTs can be prevented by doing active exercise and wearing compression devices, in conjunction with prescribed anticoagulant treatment.

If a patient has a DVT, an embolus can dislodge and travel through the circulatory system to the lung, causing a pulmonary embolism (PE). The signs and symptoms of PE vary depending on the size of the embolus and, hence, the extent of occlusion of the pulmonary vasculature. A massive PE can cause sudden and profound shock, including hypotension, tachycardia, tachypnea, hypoxia, and chest pain. Individuals can die within hours if the PE is not identified and treated quickly (McCance & Huether, 2019).

Musculoskeletal system. Nurses need to assess patients who are immobile for musculoskeletal abnormalities, such as decreased muscle tone and strength, loss of muscle mass, reduced ROM, and contractures. Anthropometric measurements (weight, body mass index [BMI], skin fold measurements) may indicate loss of muscle mass.

During assessment of ROM, the nurse can palpate muscle tone by asking the patient to relax and then passively moving each limb at several joints while palpating for resistance or rigidity. Muscle strength is assessed by having the patient assume a stable position and then performing manoeuvres to assess strength of the major muscle groups (see Chapter 37). Assessment of ROM is important as a baseline to compare later measurements and evaluate whether a loss in joint mobility has occurred. ROM can be measured with a goniometer.

Disuse osteoporosis cannot be identified by physical assessment. However, patients on prolonged bed rest, postmenopausal women, patients taking steroids, and people with increased serum and urine calcium levels have a greater risk for bone demineralization. The nurse should consider the risk of disuse osteoporosis when planning nursing interventions. Although some falls result in injury, others occur because of pathological fractures secondary to osteoporosis. Patients who are at risk for osteoporosis should have their diet assessed for calcium intake .

Integumentary system. Early identification of high-risk patients and of their risk factors can help prevent pressure injuries. The patient's skin must be continually assessed for breakdown and colour changes.

The nurse needs to know a patient's normal skin colouring in order to assess for colour changes, in both light- and dark-skinned patients (Jarvis, 2019). Using the Braden Scale Assessment (see Table 47.2), the nurse can identify patients at high risk for impaired skin integrity or early skin changes (Orsted et al., 2017). The skin should be observed often during routine care (e.g., when the patient is turned, during hygiene measures, and when providing for elimination needs). Skin assessment should occur every 2 hours (Norton et al., 2017) and is based on patients' mobility, hydration, and physiological status. Prompt identification of skin changes facilitates early intervention.

Elimination system. To determine the effects of immobility on elimination, the patient's total intake and output is assessed each shift and every 24 hours. The amounts should be compared over time to determine that the patient is receiving the correct amount and type of fluids orally or parenterally (see Chapter 41). Inadequate intake and output or fluid and electrolyte imbalances increase the risk for renal system impairment, ranging from recurrent infections to kidney failure. Dehydration also increases the risk for skin breakdown, thrombus formation, respiratory infections, and constipation.

Immobility impairs gastrointestinal peristalsis. Assessment of bowel elimination includes an analysis of a patient's dietary choices and fluid intake, review of medications, monitoring of the frequency and consistency of bowel movements, and an abdominal examination (Jarvis, 2019). With accurate assessment, the nurse can intervene before constipation and fecal impaction occur.

Psychosocial Assessment. Many alterations in psychological, sociocultural, cognitive, and developmental functioning are related to immobility. Nursing care must focus on all of these dimensions. Often the focus of immobility is on the early visible physical manifestations, such as skin impairment, but the psychosocial and developmental aspects of immobility should not be overlooked.

Abrupt changes in cognition may have a physiological cause, such as surgery, a medication reaction, a PE, or an acute infection. For example, confusion is a primary symptom of compromised older persons with an acute urinary tract infection or fever. Identifying confusion is an important component of the nurse's assessment. Acute confusion in older persons is not normal and should be thoroughly examined (Boscart et al., 2023; Registered Nurses' Association of Ontario [RNAO], 2016).

Common reactions to immobilization are boredom, feelings of isolation, depression, and anger. The patient's history should be explored to identify mental health concerns, risk for social isolation, support systems, and resources. Families are a key resource for providing information about behaviour changes. The nurse should listen to family members if they report emotional changes. Examples of change that may indicate psychosocial concerns are a cooperative patient who becomes less cooperative, or an independent patient who asks for more help than is necessary. The nurse should investigate reasons for such alterations. Identifying how the patient usually copes with loss is vital (see Chapter 26). A change in mobility status, whether permanent or not, may cause a grief reaction.

Because psychosocial changes usually occur gradually, it is important to observe the patient's behaviour on a daily basis. If behavioural changes occur, the cause or causes should be determined and the changes evaluated as short or long term. Identifying the cause helps the nurse to design appropriate nursing interventions. For example, a fear of falling often limits the bariatric or older person's mobility; fear may be related to past experiences of falling and not being able to get up (Van Seben et al., 2019). Interventions include encouraging the patient to lean forward before standing, rather than standing straight up, and teaching the patient how to get up and down from the floor, with assistance if needed.

Unexplained changes in the sleep–wake cycle should be identified and corrected. Nurses can prevent or minimize most stimuli that interrupt the sleep–wake cycle (e.g., nursing activities, a noisy environment, or discomfort). However, the effects of some medications such as analgesics, sleeping pills, or cardiovascular medications can also cause sleep disturbances (see Chapter 42).

Developmental Assessment. Nurses need to include a developmental assessment of patients who are immobilized, to ensure that the patients' holistic needs are met. When caring for a young child, the nurse needs to determine whether the child can meet expected developmental tasks. The child's development may regress or be slowed because of immobilization. After identifying a child's developmental needs, the nurse should design nursing interventions that maintain expected development and provide physical and psychological stimuli. The nurse should also assure the parents that developmental delays are usually temporary (see Chapter 23).

Immobilization of a family member changes the family's functioning. The family's response to this change may lead to problems, stress, and anxieties. When children see parents who are immobile, they may have difficulty understanding what is occurring and with coping.

Immobility can have a significant effect on the older person's levels of health, independence, and functional status. Nursing assessment enables the nurse to determine the older person's ability to meet needs independently and to adapt to developmental changes such as declining physical functioning and altered family and peer relationships. A decline in developmental functioning needs prompt investigation to determine why the change occurred and what can be done to return the patient to an optimal level of functioning as soon as possible. Activities that reduce immobility and promote participation in ADLs are vital to preventing functional decline (Cohen et al., 2019). Assessment should also include the patient's home, community, and social determinants of health to identify factors that are risks to the patient's mobility and safety (see Chapter 38).

Patient Expectations. It is important to explore patient expectations by asking patients to explain what they know about their mobility status, what questions they and their families have, and how the immobility is affecting their goals. Nurses must work collaboratively with patients, their families, and the interprofessional team to establish realistic, achievable, and measurable goals to facilitate optimal health for patients who are affected by immobility.

◆ Nursing Diagnosis

A patient who is partially or completely immobilized may have one or more nursing diagnoses. Two diagnoses most directly related to mobility problems are *impaired physical mobility* and *risk for disuse syndrome*. The diagnosis of *impaired physical mobility* is used for the patient who has some limitation but is not completely immobile. The diagnosis of *risk for disuse syndrome* should be considered for the patient who is immobile and at risk for multisystem pathophysiology because of inactivity. The list of potential diagnoses is extensive, because immobility affects multiple body systems:

- *Activity intolerance*
- *Ineffective airway clearance*
- *Ineffective breathing pattern*
- *Ineffective individual coping*
- *Risk for disuse syndrome*
- *Risk for fluid volume deficit*
- *Impaired gas exchange*
- *Risk for infection*
- *Risk for injury*

BOX 46.4   RESEARCH HIGHLIGHT
The Meaning of Mobility

Research Focus

It is widely known that decreased mobility contributes to physical and psychological impairment. Little is known, however, about the significance of mobility to other residents and to nurses in long-term care facilities. The purpose of this study was to determine nurses' and residents' perceptions of mobility in order to develop strategies that would support mobility in the adult living in a long-term care facility.

Research Abstract

In this exploratory, qualitative study by Bourret and colleagues (2002), residents and nursing staff made up focus groups in three long-term care facilities. A total of 20 residents and 15 nurses participated in the study. When asked about the importance of mobility, both groups identified it as key to quality of life. Older persons equated mobility with freedom, choice, and independence. Nurses

valued mobility and associated it with freedom and autonomy. Both nurses and residents viewed having to wait for assistance as an impediment to mobility. Nurses identified further obstacles such as heavy workload and lack of time. Residents focused on physical barriers such as steep ramps, crowded elevators, and the negative attitudes of staff.

Evidence-Informed Practice

- Mobility is central to patients' quality of life and well-being.
- Nurses play a key role in assessing and assisting patients with their mobility needs.
- Nurses should focus on minimizing obstacles to mobility.
- Nurses should coordinate with other health care providers to meet patients' mobility needs.
- Nurses need to use creative strategies to encourage mobility in older persons.

From Bourret, E., Bernick, L., Cott, C., et al. (2002). The meaning of mobility for residents and staff in long-term care facilities. *Journal of Advanced Nursing, 37*(4), 338–345.

- *Risk for impaired skin integrity*
- *Disturbed sleep pattern*
- *Social isolation*
- *Ineffective (peripheral) tissue perfusion*
- *Impaired urinary elimination*
- *Risk for impaired metabolic imbalance syndrome*
- *Risk for venous thromboembolism*
- *Impaired physical mobility*
- *Impaired skin integrity*
- *Risk for dysfunctional gastrointestinal motility*

Selection of a nursing diagnosis is based on assessment. Assessment reveals clusters of data to determine whether a patient is *at risk*, or if an *actual* problem-focused diagnosis exists. For a problem-focused diagnosis, observable assessment data will reveal a *related factor* or *causative factor* for the diagnosis. Using the diagnosis *impaired physical mobility related to bed rest*, the problem is *impaired physical mobility*, and the related factor is *bed rest*. Identifying the related factor enables nurses to select interventions used to manage or eliminate the related factor.

Accurate identification of nursing diagnosis is important to planning patient-centred goals and subsequent nursing interventions. For example, *impaired physical mobility related to bed rest* requires different interventions from those for *impaired physical mobility related to pain in the left shoulder*. Nurses need to identify and cluster defining characteristics that support the nursing diagnosis selected (Box 46.4). The diagnosis related to reluctance to initiate movement requires slightly different interventions from those for a diagnosis related to pain (i.e., interventions aimed at keeping the patient as mobile as possible to encourage ROM exercises and self-care activities in contrast to assisting the patient with comfort measures to promote patient movement). In both situations, the nurse explains how activity enhances healthy body functioning.

Immobility may also lead to complications, such as PEs or pneumonia. If these conditions develop, the nurse will need to collaborate with the health care provider or nurse practitioner for prescribed therapy to intervene.

◆ Planning

During planning, nurses synthesize assessment data and information from resources such as professional standards, guidelines for prevention of falls and pressure injuries, evidence-informed research, and past

BOX 46.4   NURSING DIAGNOSTIC PROCESS

Assessment Activities	Defining Characteristics	Nursing Diagnosis
Measure range of motion (ROM) during exercises of extremities.	Patient has limited ROM with left shoulder.	*Impaired physical mobility related to left shoulder pain*
Pain assessment	Patient has impaired coordination while attempting to perform ROM with left shoulder.	
Observe patient use left shoulder in activities of daily living.	Patient is reluctant to attempt movement with left shoulder.	
Ask patient about perception of pain.	Patient complains of sharp pain in shoulder.	
Ask patient about endurance and activity tolerance.	Patient reports decreased muscle strength in left shoulder.	

experience with similar patients (Figure 46.10). Collaboration with the interprofessional team, including respiratory therapists, occupational therapists, and physiotherapists, is important when developing care plans for patients who are immobile. The patient is a full partner in designing the plan of care, and this input must be reflected when establishing the goals and outcomes of care.

Goals and Outcomes. In collaboration with patients, nurses develop an individualized care plan for each nursing diagnosis (Box 46.5). Goals should be individualized, realistic, and measurable, focusing on prevention of problems or risks to body alignment and mobility.

Nurses develop goals and expected outcomes to help patients achieve their highest level of mobility and reduce the hazards of immobility. For example, a patient who has left-sided paralysis after a stroke may have two long-term goals. The first, directed toward improved mobility, is "Patient uses walker to ambulate safely around the home and grocery store." A parallel goal, directed toward the hazards of immobility, is "Patient's skin will remain intact." Both of these goals are essential to restoring the patient's maximum mobility. Because

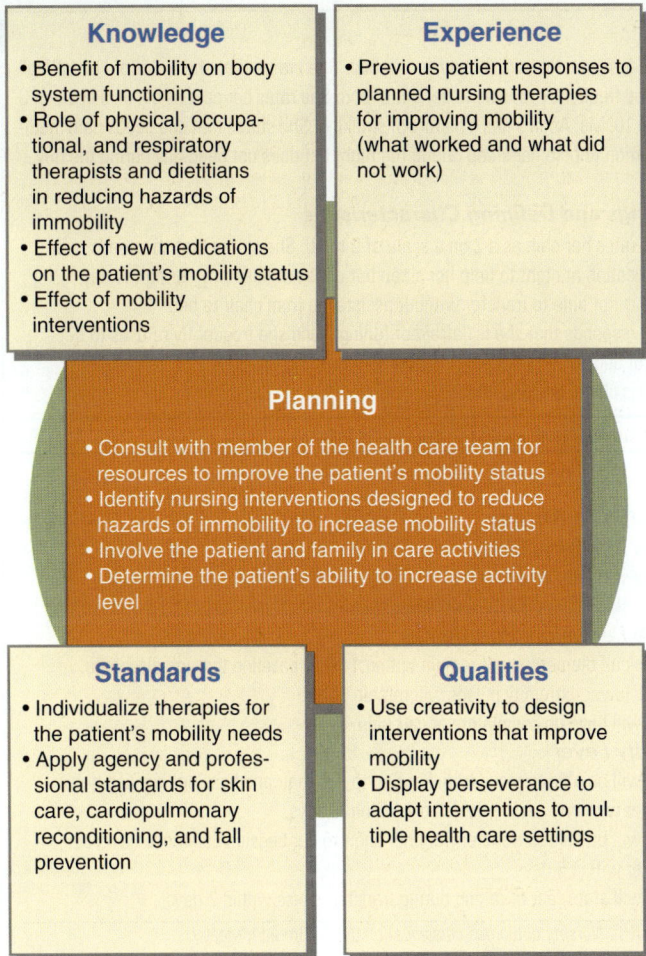

FIGURE 46.10 Critical thinking model for immobility planning.

Knowledge
- Benefit of mobility on body system functioning
- Role of physical, occupational, and respiratory therapists and dietitians in reducing hazards of immobility
- Effect of new medications on the patient's mobility status
- Effect of mobility interventions

Experience
- Previous patient responses to planned nursing therapies for improving mobility (what worked and what did not work)

Planning
- Consult with member of the health care team for resources to improve the patient's mobility status
- Identify nursing interventions designed to reduce hazards of immobility to increase mobility status
- Involve the patient and family in care activities
- Determine the patient's ability to increase activity level

Standards
- Individualize therapies for the patient's mobility needs
- Apply agency and professional standards for skin care, cardiopulmonary reconditioning, and fall prevention

Qualities
- Use creativity to design interventions that improve mobility
- Display perseverance to adapt interventions to multiple health care settings

sensation is impaired, both the patient and caregivers must be aware of the patient's need to have the skin free of pressure. Expected outcomes for the goal of maintaining skin integrity include the following:
- Patient's skin colour and temperature return to normal baseline within 20 minutes of position change.
- Patient's skin remains dry and intact.

Setting Priorities. The impact that a health problem has on a patient's mental and physical health determines the immediacy of any problem. Nurses need to set priorities when planning care to ensure that immediate needs are met first. This is important when patients have multiple diagnoses (Figure 46.11). Interventions should be planned according to the severity of risks to the patient. The plan should be individualized according to the patient's developmental stage, level of health, and lifestyle.

Potential complications should not be overlooked. Many times, actual conditions such as pressure injuries and disuse osteoporosis get addressed after they develop. Nurses must be vigilant in monitoring the patient and reinforcing interventions aimed at preventing complications of impaired mobility to the patient, their family, and other caregivers.

Teamwork and Collaboration. Care of the patient experiencing alterations in mobility requires a team approach. The interventions planned for the patient may be done directly by the nurse or delegated to unregulated care providers (UCPs). UCPs can reinforce leg exercises,

use of the incentive spirometer, and coughing and deep breathing. They may also turn and position patients, apply elastic stockings, and assess leg circumferences and height and weight.

When delegating skills associated with care of the patient who is immobile, nurses need to be vigilant in performing routine assessments to identify any developing complications early. The nurse is also responsible for informing the UCP when patients are at risk for immobility hazards so that complications can be prevented. For example, although turning and positioning of a patient who is comatose may be delegated, the nurse must ensure that it is done correctly and that the position is changed frequently enough to reduce the risk for poor alignment and future injury to the skin and musculoskeletal system. The frequency of turning is based on patient assessment for risk of developing pressure injuries (see Chapter 47).

Nurses collaborate with other health team members, such as physiotherapists or occupational therapists, when considering a patient's mobility needs. For example, physiotherapists are a resource for planning ROM or strengthening exercises, and occupational therapists are a resource for planning ADLs that patients need to modify or relearn. Wound care specialists and respiratory therapists are often involved in patient care, especially with patients who are experiencing complications related to their immobility. The nurse can consult with a registered dietitian when the patient is experiencing nutritional challenges and consult a social worker or psychologist to assist with coping or other psychosocial issues.

Discharge planning begins when a patient enters the health care system. In anticipation of the patient's discharge from an institution, it is important to make appropriate referrals or consult a case manager to ensure that the patient's needs are met at home. The patient's home environment should be considered when setting goals and planning therapies to maintain or improve body alignment and mobility. Referrals should be made early in the care process for ongoing care and therapy at home to help the patient remain mobile or further regain mobility at home.

◆ **Implementation**

Health Promotion. Health promotion activities include a variety of interventions that can be divided into education, prevention, and early detection. Examples of health promotion activities that address mobility and immobility include prevention of work-related injury, fall prevention measures, exercise, and early detection of bone or joint abnormalities.

Prevention of Work-Related Musculoskeletal Injuries. Injuries occur as a result of overexertion, which can result in back injuries and other musculoskeletal conditions. Back injuries are often the direct result of improper lifting and bending. The most common back injury is strain on the lumbar muscle group, which includes the muscles around the lumbar vertebrae. Injury to these areas affects the ability to bend forward, backward, and from side to side and limits the ability to rotate the hips and lower back. Staff use of ergonomic programs in health care facilities can reduce costs, injuries to employees, and missed work days (Lee et al., 2021; Roy et al., 2020).

Nurses and other health care staff are especially at risk for injury to lumbar muscles when lifting, transferring, or positioning immobilized patients. Nurses need to be aware of employer policies and protocols that protect staff and patients from injury. When transferring a patient, the nurse must always perform a functional assessment of the patient to determine the assistance the nurse will need (see Chapter 37). Current evidence supports use of mechanical or other ergonomic assistive devices as the safest way to reposition patients who are unable to do these activities themselves. Many agencies have instituted no-lift policies (see Chapter 37).

Impaired Physical Mobility

ASSESSMENT

Barbara (preferred pronouns: she/her), an 84-year-old patient, has been admitted for rehabilitation after a total hip arthroplasty for osteoarthritis 5 days ago. The wound is clean, dry, and intact. Staples are to be removed in 9 days. She is weight bearing as tolerated (WBAT). She is not able to safely transfer independently from a chair to the bed. She states that she is "afraid of falling" and frequently refuses to get out of bed. She rates her pain as a 2 on a scale of 0 to 10. Ms. Adams has a history of smoking. She states that she needs pain medication to help her sleep during the night but does not need any during the day.

Assessment Activities	Findings and Defining Characteristics
Assess Barbara's pain level. Ask her to rate her pain on a scale from 0 to 10.	Patient rates her pain as a 2 on a scale of 0 to 10. She states that she needs pain medication at night to help her sleep but does not need any during the day.
Assess Barbara's ability to transfer.	Patient is not able to transfer without assistance from chair to bed.
Ask Barbara how her surgery has affected her mobility.	Patient responds that she is "afraid of falling," and she frequently refuses to get out of bed.
Assess Barbara's wound status.	Wound is clean, dry, and intact.

NURSING DIAGNOSIS: Impaired physical mobility related to musculoskeletal impairment from surgery and a fear of falling.

PLANNING

Goals (Nursing Outcomes Classification)*	Expected Outcomes
Patient will be free from skin breakdown by discharge.	**Tissue Integrity: Skin** Patient's skin will remain intact. Patient's skin will be free of erythema.
Patient will exhibit no evidence of deep vein thrombosis (DVT) by discharge.	**Tissue Perfusion: Peripheral** Patient's calf diameters will remain within 1 cm of baseline through discharge. Patient's lower extremity pulses will remain equal. Patient will have no complaints of calf pain.
Patient will be able to safely transfer with assistive device by discharge.	**Mobility Level** Patient will be able to move from her bed to her chair and back again using her walker with one-person assistance within 5 days. Patient will be able to transfer from her chair to her bedside commode using her walker within 5 days. Patient will state fear of falling during transfer is less within 2 days.

*Outcome classification labels from Moorhead, S., Swanson, E., Johnson, M., et al. (Eds.). (2018). *Nursing outcomes classification (NOC)* (6th ed.). Mosby.

INTERVENTIONS

Interventions (Nursing Interventions Classification)†	Rationale
Circulatory Care	
Administer low-dose anticoagulant as prescribed.	Administration of low-dose anticoagulant has been shown to reduce risk for vein thrombosis.
Apply graduated compression stockings as prescribed and remove them each shift for hygiene.	Application increases venous tone, improving venous return and reducing venous stasis.
Reinforce antiembolic exercises while awake.	Exercises promote venous return.
Assist patient out of bed slowly.	Moving slowly will decrease the likelihood of orthostatic hypotension. Moving the patient slowly will also avoid the perception by the patient of being rushed, which may cause the patient to become fearful.
Skin Surveillance	
Instruct patient to shift position every 1 to 1.5 hours while awake.	Position changes should occur every 1 to 1.5 hours or more frequently if needed. This reduces the risk of pressure injury development.
When patient is recumbent, place patient in a 30-degree lateral position.	The 30-degree lateral position reduces pressure from the sacral area and reduces the risk of skin breakdown (Norton et al., 2017).
Use pressure-relieving devices such as pillows, wedges, specific splints, or other medical aids to keep patient's heels off bed. Use whole-body devices such as alternating pressure and constant low-pressure mattresses.	Small blood vessels of the heel make overlying skin more susceptible to ischemia when subject to prolonged pressure due to immobility. Use of a pressure-relieving device under the lower legs raises the heels to reduce pressure so that tissue blood flow is maintained (Norton et al., 2017).
Positioning	
Explain positioning procedure to patient.	Reduces anxiety.
Refer patient to physiotherapy for transfer training.	Helps to strengthen muscles used in transfer.
Encourage patient to assist in transfer and positioning.	Promotes independence.
Teach patient safe positioning after total hip replacement—for example, no hip flexion >90 degrees, do not cross legs, do not lie on affected side, and when in bed use a pillow between the knees.	Minimizes risk of dislocation of hip. Patient education is important for continued rehabilitation and healing.

†Intervention classification labels from Butcher, H. K., Bulechek, G. M., McCloskey Dochterman, J. M., et al. (Eds.). (2019). *Nursing interventions classification (NIC)* (7th ed.). Mosby.

BOX 46.5 NURSING CARE PLAN—cont'd
Impaired Physical Mobility

EVALUATION

Nursing Actions	Patient Response and Finding	Achievement of Outcome
Ask Barbara if her mobility has improved postoperatively. Observe patient transfer from bed to chair, noting range of motion, comfort, and confidence.	Patient is able to transfer from the chair to the bed with assistance.	Patient has achieved goal of transferring with assistance.
Observe Barbara's skin integrity at each shift.	Patient's wound remains clean, dry, and intact. No breakdown is noted on extremities or the sacral area.	Patient has achieved outcome that skin will remain intact.
Perform circulatory assessment of extremities at every shift.	Patient's calf diameters remain within 1 cm of baseline. Swelling, pain, redness, and warmth are not evident.	DVT is not evident.
Ask Barbara to rate her fear of falling on a scale of 0 to 10.	Patient rates fear of falling a 7 on a scale of 0 to 10. Patient is getting out of bed every shift.	Outcome of decrease in fear of falling has not been totally achieved. Continue to encourage patient.

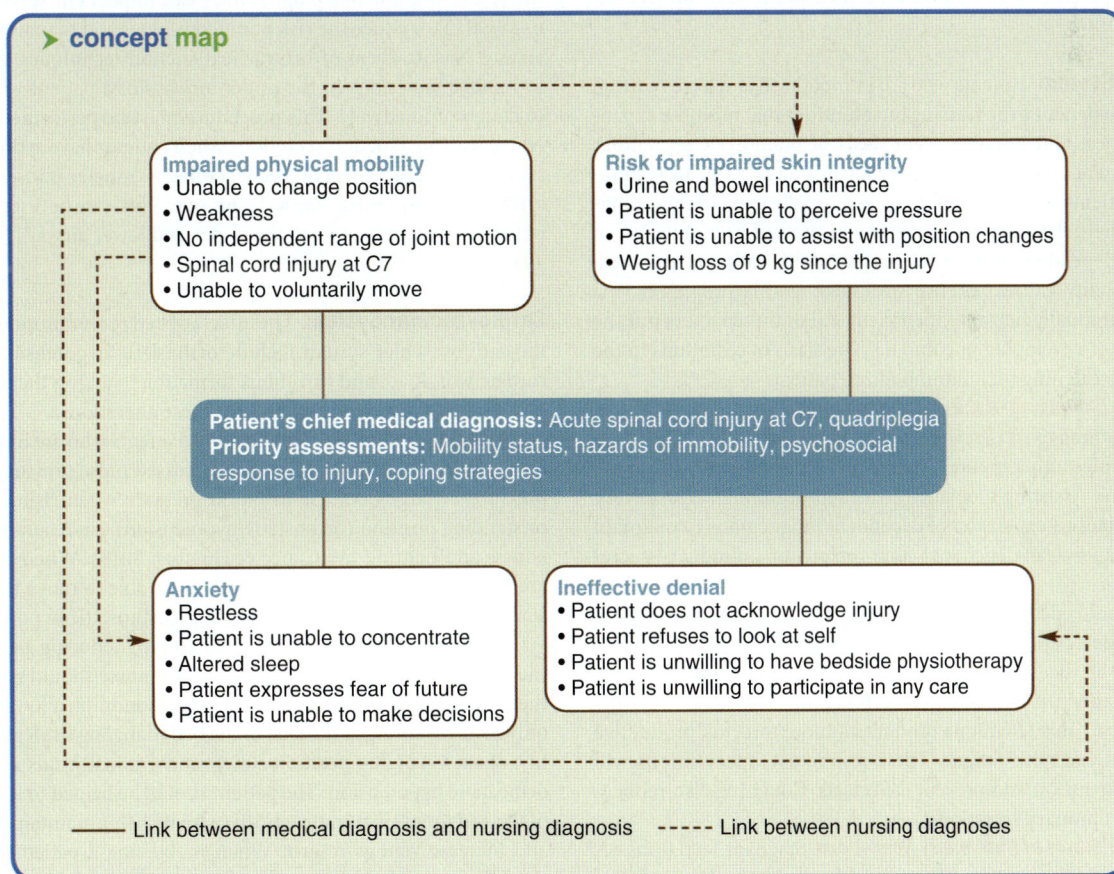

FIGURE 46.11 Concept map for patient with quadriplegia related to an acute spinal cord injury at C7.

Exercise. Although many diseases and physical challenges cause or contribute to immobility, exercise programs enhance feelings of well-being and improve endurance, strength, and health (see Chapter 37). Exercise reduces the risk of developing a number of health problems, such as cardiovascular disease, diabetes, and osteoporosis. The Self-Management Resource Center (2022) chronic-disease self-management program encourages appropriate exercise for maintaining and improving strength, flexibility, and endurance. All patients should be encouraged to find a type of exercise that meets their lifestyle and particular health-related needs. Nurses can collaborate with a physiotherapist to design individualized exercise programs for patients who have challenges with mobility.

Acute Care

In the acute care setting, interventions are used to reduce the hazards of immobility. Nurses should know proper positioning and transferring techniques to safely move patients (see Chapter 37).

Patients in acute care settings who experience altered physical mobility may experience health challenges associated with the side effects of immobility, such as impaired respiratory status, orthostatic hypotension, and impaired skin integrity. Nurses need to design interventions to reduce the impact of immobility on body systems and prepare the patient for the restorative phase of care.

Metabolic System. Because the body needs protein to repair injured tissue and rebuild depleted protein stores, the patient who is immobilized should be on a high-protein, high-calorie diet. A high-calorie intake provides sufficient fuel to meet metabolic demands and replace subcutaneous tissue. The nurse should ensure that the patient is taking vitamins B and C and supplements when necessary. Supplementation with vitamin C is needed for skin integrity and wound healing; vitamin B complex assists in energy metabolism.

If the patient is unable to eat, nutrition must be provided parenterally or enterally. Enteral feedings include delivery through a nasogastric, gastrostomy, or jejunostomy tube of high-protein, high-calorie solutions with complete requirements of vitamins, minerals, and electrolytes (see Chapter 43). *Total parenteral nutrition* refers to delivery of nutritional supplements through a central or peripheral intravenous catheter.

Respiratory System. Patients who are immobilized and have reduced ventilation can benefit from nursing interventions that promote expansion of the chest and lungs, prevent stasis of pulmonary secretions, maintain a patent airway, and promote adequate exchange of respiratory gases. Patients who are immobile need to fully expand their lungs to maintain their elastic recoil property and prevent accumulation of secretions in dependent areas of the lungs. Additionally, patients with restricted mobility can experience weakness; as this progresses, the cough reflex gradually becomes inefficient. All of these factors put the patient at risk of developing pneumonia. The stasis of secretions in the lungs is life-threatening for an immobilized patient.

Promoting Expansion of the Chest and Lungs. Frequent repositioning, deep-breathing exercises, incentive spirometry, controlled coughing, and chest physiotherapy are nursing interventions used to promote lung expansion. Assisting the patient with repositioning at least every 2 hours promotes re-expansion of dependent lung regions to maintain elastic recoil and clear dependent lung regions or pulmonary secretions.

Nurses should encourage patients to deep-breathe and cough every 1 to 2 hours. Alert patients can be taught to deep-breathe or yawn every hour or to use an incentive spirometer (see Chapter 40). The nurse can instruct the patient to take in three deep breaths and cough with the third exhalation. This technique produces a more forceful, productive cough without excessive fatigue. These respiratory interventions will aid alveolar expansion and prevent atelectasis. Coughing also reduces the stasis of pulmonary secretions.

Preventing Stasis of Pulmonary Secretions. Stagnant secretions accumulating in the bronchi and lungs may lead to growth of bacteria and subsequent development of pneumonia. Changing the patient's position every 2 hours can aid in reducing stagnation of secretions. Through frequent position changes, dependent lung areas are rotated, mobilizing secretions.

Adequate fluid intake is essential for patients who are immobile. Unless there is a medical contraindication, an adult needs to drink at least 1 100 to 1 400 mL of noncaffeinated fluids daily. This maintains expected mucociliary clearance. In patients free from infection and with adequate hydration, pulmonary secretions will appear thin, watery, and clear. The patient can easily remove the secretions by coughing. Without adequate hydration, the secretions are thick and

difficult to remove. Offering fluids that patients prefer on a regularly timed schedule also helps with bowel and urine elimination and aids in maintaining circulation and skin integrity.

Chest physiotherapy (CPT) (percussion and positioning) is an effective method for preventing stasis of pulmonary secretions. CPT techniques help the patient to drain secretions from specific segments of the bronchi and lungs into the trachea so that the patient can cough and expel the secretions. Respiratory assessment findings can be used to identify areas of the lungs requiring CPT (see Chapter 40).

Maintaining a Patent Airway. Patients who are immobilized are generally weakened. If weakness progresses, the cough reflex gradually becomes inefficient. The stasis of secretions in the lungs may be life-threatening because hypostatic pneumonia can easily develop. The dislodging and mobilizing of the stagnant secretions reduce the risk of pneumonia. Assessment findings that indicate pneumonia include productive cough with greenish-yellow sputum, fever, pain on breathing, crackles and wheezes, and dyspnea. Nurses should actively work with patients to deep-breathe and cough every 1 to 2 hours as described earlier, in the section "Promoting Expansion of the Chest and Lungs."

In the patient who is immobilized, an obstructed airway is usually the result of a mucous plug. Nurses can implement several therapies (e.g., CPT) to reduce the risk of mucous plugs and to maintain a patent airway. Nasotracheal or orotracheal suction techniques may be used to remove secretions in the upper airways of a patient who is unable to cough productively. This procedure must be performed aseptically. Nurses can also suction secretions when patients have artificial airways such as an endotracheal or tracheal tube. A catheter is inserted into the artificial airway using sterile technique. This can be used to remove pulmonary secretions from the upper and lower airways (see Chapter 40).

Cardiovascular System. The effects of bed rest or immobilization on the cardiovascular system include orthostatic hypotension, increased cardiac workload, and thrombus formation. Nursing therapies should be designed to minimize or prevent these alterations.

Reducing Orthostatic Hypotension. Patients who are immobile usually have increased pulse rate and decreased pulse pressure and blood pressure. A large decrease in blood pressure when rising to a sitting or standing position (orthostatic hypotension) can result in lightheadedness and fainting (McCance & Huether, 2019). When patients who are on bed rest or have been immobile are able to move to a sitting or standing position, they often experience orthostatic hypotension.

Interventions should be directed toward reducing or eliminating the effects of orthostatic hypotension. The nurse should attempt to get the patient moving as soon as the physical condition allows, even if this only involves sitting at the side of the bed (dangling the legs) or moving to a chair. Changing position slowly and gradually aids in preventing orthostatic hypotension. The patient should be helped to sit on the side of the bed for a few minutes, as this activity helps maintain muscle tone and increase venous return. When mobilizing a patient for the first time, the nurse should always perform a functional assessment using a safe patient-handling algorithm (see Chapter 37). This is a precautionary step that prevents the nurse and patient from experiencing injury and allows the patient to do as much of the transfer as possible.

Reducing Cardiac Workload. Cardiac workload is increased by immobility. A nursing intervention that reduces cardiac workload involves instructing patients to avoid using the Valsalva manoeuvre when moving up in bed, defecating, or lifting household objects. During a Valsalva manoeuvre, the person holds their breath and strains, which increases intrathoracic pressure, thus decreasing venous return and cardiac output. When the strain is released, venous return and cardiac output immediately increase and systolic blood pressure and pulse pressure rise. These pressure changes produce a reflex bradycardia and a possible decrease in blood pressure that may cause sudden cardiac death in patients with heart disease. The patient should be reminded to breathe out while defecating, lifting, or moving side to side or moving up in bed.

Preventing Thrombus Formation. The most cost-effective way to address the risk of DVT is through prevention (prophylaxis). It begins with identifying patients at risk and continues throughout the time patients are immobile or otherwise at risk. This requires collaboration between nurses and health care providers. By performing frequent patient assessments, nurses can identify risk factors. Interventions used to reduce the risk of thrombus formation in patients who are immobilized include leg exercises, encouraging fluids intake, position changes, and patient teaching of preventive measures. Intervention begins when the patient becomes immobile. Preoperative patients should be given this information before surgery (see Chapter 49).

Prophylaxis also includes anticoagulation, mechanical prevention with graduated compression stockings, and intermittent pneumatic compression devices. These interventions require a prescription. Anticoagulants most often prescribed include unfractionated heparin (UFH) (usually given as 5000 units two or three times daily), low-molecular-weight heparins (LMWH) (e.g., tinzaparin, enoxaparin, and dalteparin), and vitamin K antagonists (e.g., warfarin).

Bleeding is a potential adverse effect of anticoagulant medications because anticoagulants suppress clot formation. The nurse must continually assess the patient for signs of bleeding, such as bruising, hematuria, coffee ground–like vomitus or gastrointestinal aspirate, guaiac-positive stools, and bleeding gums. Most patients receiving prophylactic doses of anticoagulants do not experience adverse effects, the risk of bleeding is present.

Sequential compression devices (SCDs) and intermittent pneumatic compression (IPC) devices are used to prevent blood clots in the lower extremities. These consist of sleeves or stockings made of fabric or plastic that are wrapped around the leg and secured with Velcro (Box 46.6). The sleeves are then connected to a pump that alternately inflates and deflates the stocking around the leg. A typical cycle is inflation for 10 to 15 seconds and deflation for 45 to 60 seconds. Inflation pressures average 40 mm Hg. Use of SCDs or IPCs on the legs decreases venous stasis by increasing venous return through the deep veins of the legs. For optimal results, use of SCD or IPC devices is begun as soon as possible and maintained until the patient becomes fully ambulatory. Wearing graduated compression stockings can help prevent DVT, but patients must receive the right size, and the SCD or IPC must be used correctly. Comprehensive nursing care includes removing the SCD or IPC every shift to verify skin integrity and assess skin for pressure points. Additionally, peripheral neurovascular assessment of the extremity, including extremity colour, sensation, movement, temperature, palpation of distal pulses, and assessment for edema, must be performed by the nurse every shift.

Elastic stockings (sometimes called *thromboembolic device [TED] hose* or thigh-high antiembolic stockings) aid in maintaining external pressure on the muscles of the lower extremities and thus promote venous return (Box 46.7). When considering applying elastic stockings, the nurse must first assess the patient's suitability for wearing them. Stockings should not be applied if any local condition affects the leg (e.g., any skin lesion, gangrenous condition, or recent vein ligation) because application may compromise circulation. To determine correct stocking size, the nurse measures the patient's legs with a tape measure. The stockings must be applied properly and be removed and reapplied at least once per shift. The nurse must assess circulation at the toes to ensure that the hose are not too tight. The stockings should always be clean and dry; it may be useful for the patient to have two pairs.

Proper positioning used with other therapies (e.g., heparin or elastic stockings) reduces a patient's risk of thrombus formation because

---

BOX 46.6 PROCEDURAL GUIDELINE

Application of Sequential Compression Stockings

Delegation Considerations

The skill of applying sequential compression stockings (SCSs) can be delegated to unregulated care providers (UCPs). The nurse is responsible for assessing circulation in the extremities; therefore, when application of the SCSs is delegated, it is important to instruct the UCP to do the following:

- Notify the nurse if the patient complains of pain in the leg.
- Notify the nurse if discoloration develops in the extremities.

Equipment

- Tape measure, sequential compression stockings, stockinette, hygiene supplies

Procedure

1. Assess patient for the need for sequential compression stockings.
2. Obtain baseline assessment data about the status of circulation, pulse, and skin integrity on the patient's lower extremities before initiating application of sequential compression stockings.
3. Measure the patient for proper-size stocking by measuring around the largest part of the patient's thigh. Review the manufacturer's directions regarding measuring for proper fit.
4. Perform hand hygiene. Provide hygiene to lower extremities if needed.
5. Place a protective stockinette over the patient's leg.

6. Wrap the stocking around the leg, starting at the ankle, with the opening over the patella (see Step 6 illustration).
   A. Attach the stockings to the insufflator and verify that the intermittent pressure is between 35 and 45 mm Hg.

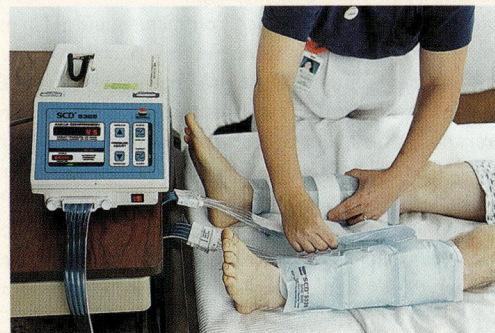

STEP 6 Application of sequential compression stocking.

7. Record date and time of stocking application, and stocking length and size in electronic medical record.
8. Record condition of skin and circulatory assessment.
9. Monitor skin integrity and circulation to the patient's lower extremities as prescribed or according to the manufacturer's guidelines.

BOX 46.7 PROCEDURAL GUIDELINE

Application of Elastic Stockings

Delegation Considerations

The skill of applying elastic stockings can be performed by unregulated care providers (UCPs). The nurse is responsible for assessing circulation to the lower extremities; therefore, when application of the stockings is delegated, it is important to instruct the UCP to report if the patient develops leg pain or discoloration.

Equipment

- Tape measure, elastic stockings, hygiene supplies

Procedure

1. Assess the need for elastic stockings and condition of the patient's skin.
2. Observe for conditions that might contraindicate use of stockings.
3. Perform hand hygiene. Provide hygiene to lower extremities if needed.
4. Use tape measure to measure the patient's legs to determine proper stocking size (measure according to manufacturer's directions). Elastic stockings come in two lengths: knee length and thigh length.
5. Apply stockings:
   A. Turn elastic stocking inside out up to the heel. Place one hand into the sock, holding heel. Pull top of sock with the other hand inside out over foot of sock.
   B. Place patient's toes into the foot of the elastic stocking, making sure that sock is smooth (see Step 5B illustration).

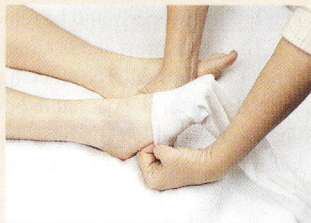

STEP 5B

C. Slide remaining portion of sock over the patient's foot, being sure that the toes are covered. Make sure the foot fits into the toe and heel position of the sock (see Step 5C illustration).

D. Slide top of sock up over patient's calf until sock is completely extended. Be sure sock is smooth and no ridges or wrinkles are present, particularly behind the knee (see Step 5D illustration).

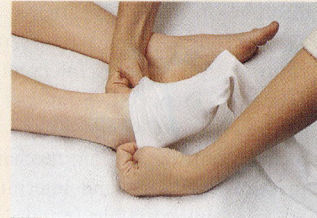

STEP 5C

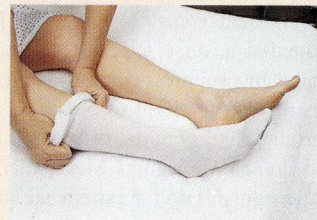

STEP 5D

6. Instruct patient not to roll socks partially down.
7. Record date and time of stocking application, and stocking length and size in the electronic medical record.
8. Record condition of skin and circulatory assessment.

---

compression of the leg veins is minimized. When positioning patients, the nurse must use caution to prevent pressure on the posterior knee and deep veins in the lower extremities. Patients should be taught to avoid the following: crossing their legs, sitting for prolonged periods of time, wearing clothing that constricts the legs or waist, putting pillows under their knees, and massaging their legs.

ROM exercises can reduce the risk of contractures and aid in preventing thrombi. Activity causes contraction of the skeletal muscles, which in turn exerts pressure on the veins to promote venous return, thereby reducing venous stasis. Specific exercises that help prevent thrombophlebitis are ankle pumps, foot circles, and knee flexion. Ankle pumps, sometimes called *calf pumps,* include alternating plantar flexion and dorsiflexion. To perform foot circles, the patient rotates the ankle. Patients should be encouraged to make letters of the alphabet with their feet every 1 to 2 hours. Knee flexion involves alternately extending and flexing the knee. These exercises are sometimes referred to as *antiembolic exercises* and should be done hourly while the patient is awake.

Suspected DVT should be reported immediately to the patient's health care provider. The nurse needs to elevate the patient's leg but avoid pressure on the suspected thrombus area. The family, patient, and all health care personnel should be instructed to not massage the area because of the danger of dislodging the thrombus.

Musculoskeletal System. Exercise to prevent muscle atrophy and joint contractures helps maintain musculoskeletal function. If a patient is unable to move part or all of their body, the nurse can perform passive ROM exercises for all immobilized joints while bathing the patient and at least two or three more times a day (see "Restorative Care" section). If one extremity is paralyzed, the patient can be taught to put each joint independently through its ROM. Patients on bed rest should have active ROM exercises incorporated into their daily schedules. Nurses teach patients to integrate exercises during ADLs.

Some orthopedic conditions require frequent passive ROM exercises to restore the injured joint's function after surgery, such as a total knee arthroplasty. This is beneficial when the patient must gradually increase the degree and duration of flexion and extension. Patients with such conditions may use automatic equipment (continuous passive motion [CPM]) for passive ROM exercises (Figure 46.12). The CPM machine moves an extremity to a prescribed angle for a prescribed period. An interprofessional approach is used when CPM therapy is prescribed. In most institutions, physiotherapists are responsible for first-time administration and adjustment of CPM machines. It is important to assess the patient's pain level and administer analgesia as needed before using CPM.

Elimination System. The nursing interventions for maintaining optimal urinary functioning are directed at keeping the patient well hydrated and preventing urinary stasis, calculi, and infections without causing bladder distension.

Adequate hydration (i.e., at least 1 100 to 1 400 mL of noncaffeinated fluids per day) helps prevent development of renal calculi and urinary

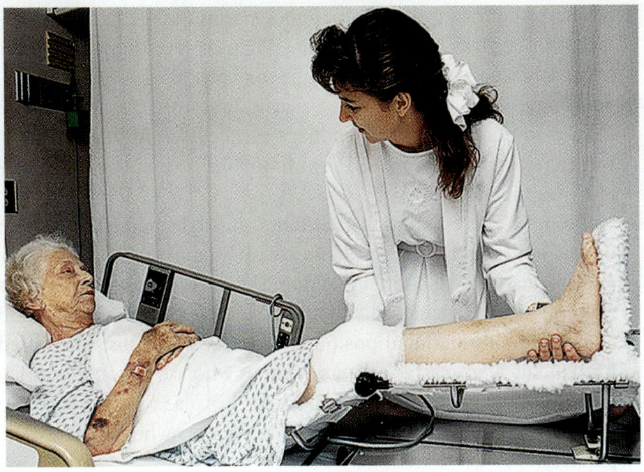

FIGURE 46.12 Continuous passive motion machine.

tract infections. The patient who is well hydrated should void large amounts of dilute urine that are approximately equal to fluid intake. If the patient is incontinent, the care plan can be modified to include toileting aids and a hygiene schedule so that the increased urinary output does not cause skin breakdown.

To prevent bladder distension, the nurse needs to assess the frequency and amount of urinary output. A patient who continually dribbles urine and whose bladder is distended may have overflow incontinence. If the patient does not have voluntary control of bladder elimination, bladder training may be necessary. If the patient experiences bladder distension, the nurse may be required to insert a straight catheter or an in-dwelling Foley catheter (see Chapter 44).

The frequency and consistency of bowel movements must be recorded. A diet rich in fluids, fruits, vegetables, and fibre can facilitate normal peristalsis. If a patient is unable to maintain regular bowel patterns, stool softeners, cathartics, or enemas may be needed (see Chapter 45).

Integumentary System. The major risk to the skin from restricted mobility is the formation of pressure injuries. Early identification of high-risk patients helps prevent pressure injuries from occurring. Thus, nursing interventions aimed toward preventing pressure injuries are imperative (Norton et al., 2017).

Interventions aimed at prevention include continuous assessment using a standardized tool, positioning, skin care, and the use of therapeutic devices to relieve pressure. The immobilized patient's position should be changed according to the patient's activity level, perceptual ability, treatment protocols, and daily routines. Although turning the patient every 1 to 2 hours is recommended for preventing pressure injuries, it may also be necessary to use devices for relieving pressure on the skin. The amount of time that a patient sits uninterrupted in a chair should be limited to 1 hour or less, although this time interval should be individualized. Patients need to be repositioned frequently because uninterrupted pressure leads to skin breakdown.

Pressure-relieving mattresses, such as reactive mattresses that reduce pressure and active mattresses that relieve pressure, can be implemented with patients who are immobile, to redistribute pressure and prevent pressure injury. However, patients must still be repositioned at least every 2 hours, and skin must be assessed for skin integrity (Lovegrove et al., 2020). When patients are sitting in chairs, nurses must teach patients who are able to shift their weight to do so every 15 minutes. Patients who are chair-bound should have a device for the chair that reduces pressure; however, doughnut-shaped devices should not be used (Norton et al., 2017). If a pressure injury does develop, treatment should commence immediately. Wounds Canada's *Best Practice Recommendations for the*

Prevention and Management of Pressure Injuries and *Best Practice Recommendations for the Prevention and Management of Wounds* provide guidelines based on best practices for preventing and treating pressure injuries (Norton et al., 2017; Orsted et al., 2017).

Psychosocial Changes. As stated earlier, prolonged immobilization can affect a patient's psychosocial well-being. Nurses must assess patients' health history and psychosocial status. Patients with a history of depression are at greater risk for developing psychosocial changes during bed rest or immobilization.

The nurse needs to observe the patient's ability to cope with restricted mobility. If the nursing care plan is not improving coping patterns, a clinical nurse specialist, counsellor, social worker, spiritual advisor, or other consultant may be consulted. Their recommendations should be incorporated into the care plan.

Providing routine and informal socialization is an intervention used to promote psychosocial health of patients who are immobile. Nursing activities should be planned to enable patients to talk and interact with staff. If possible, the patient should be placed in a room with others who are mobile and interactive. If a private room is required, staff members and family should be asked to visit throughout the shift to provide meaningful interaction.

Nurses can provide stimuli to maintain a patient's orientation. Use of a calendar and a clock; providing a newspaper, books, radio, or television; and encouraging visits from friends and family may reduce the risk of social isolation and delirium (RNAO, 2016). Spending time in the room talking and listening to the patient also helps reduce isolation.

Nurses can involve patients in their care by encouraging them to perform as many ADLs as independently as possible. Patients should continue to perform personal grooming independently. This type of activity preserves the patient's dignity and gives the patient a sense of accomplishment.

In institutional health care settings, nursing care activities should not be scheduled between 2200 hours and 0700 hours, to minimize interruptions of sleep. For example, the nurse may administer medications and assess vital signs at the time when the patient is turned or receives special skin care.

Developmental Changes in Children. Ideally, pediatric patients with mobility challenges continue expected development. Nursing interventions that provide mental and physical stimulation can facilitate expected development when mobility is limited. Nurses need to incorporate play activities into the care plan. For example, completing puzzles helps a child to develop fine motor skills, and reading helps the child to develop cognitively. Parents should be encouraged to stay with a child who is hospitalized. A child who is immobilized should be placed with children of the same age who are not immobilized, unless a contagious disease is present. A child should be allowed to participate in nursing interventions such as dressing changes and cast care. The nurse needs to assess for significant changes from normal behavioural patterns and consult with a clinical nurse specialist, counsellor, or other health care provider who specializes in children's care, when needed.

Positioning Devices and Techniques. Patients with impaired function of the nervous, skeletal, or muscular system and with general weakness often require help to attain proper body alignment while in bed or sitting. Skin integrity should be assessed regularly for pressure points or skin breakdown when using positioning devices.

Several positioning devices are available for maintaining good body alignment for patients:

- *Pillows:* They provide support, elevate body parts, and can splint incisional areas, reducing postoperative pain during activity or coughing and deep breathing. Before using a pillow, determine whether it is the proper size. A thick pillow under the patient's head increases cervical flexion, leading to strain on joints and muscles of the neck and upper back, and compression of blood vessels and nerves that supply the neck. A thin pillow under body prominences may be inadequate to protect skin and tissue from damage caused by pressure. When additional pillows are unavailable, or if they are an improper size, use folded sheets, blankets, or towels as positioning aids.

- *Wedge (or abductor) pillow:* This is a triangular-shaped pillow made of heavy foam used to maintain the legs in abduction after total hip replacement surgery.
- *Foot boot:* This device prevents footdrop by maintaining the feet in dorsiflexion. Foot boots are made of rigid plastic or heavy foam (Figure 46.13). They keep the foot flexed at the proper angle and the weight of the bed sheets off the toes. Remove the foot boots two or three times a day to assess skin integrity and joint mobility.
- *Trochanter roll:* This prevents external rotation of the hips when the patient is in a supine position. A **trochanter roll** is formed by folding a cotton bath blanket lengthwise to a width that will extend from the greater trochanter of the femur to the lower border of the popliteal space (Figure 46.14). The blanket is placed under the

buttocks and then rolled counterclockwise until the thigh is in neutral position or in inward rotation. When correct alignment of the hip is achieved, the patella faces directly upward.

- *Sandbags:* These are sand-filled plastic tubes or bags that can be shaped to body contours. Sandbags can be used in place of or in addition to trochanter rolls. They immobilize an extremity or maintain body alignment.
- *Hand rolls:* These maintain the thumb in slight adduction and in opposition to the fingers. A hand roll maintains the hand, thumb, and fingers in a functional position, thus preventing contractures (Figure 46.15). Evaluate the hand roll to make sure that the hand is indeed in a functional position. Hand rolls are most often used for patients whose arms are paralyzed or who are unconscious. Do not use rolled washcloths as hand rolls, because they do not keep the thumb well abducted, especially in patients who have a spastic paralysis.
- *Hand–wrist splints:* These are individually moulded for the patient to maintain proper alignment of the thumb (slight adduction) and the wrist (slight extension). Use splints only on the patient for whom the splint was made (Figure 46.16) and follow the splint schedule (e.g., wear for 2 hours, remove for 2 hours).

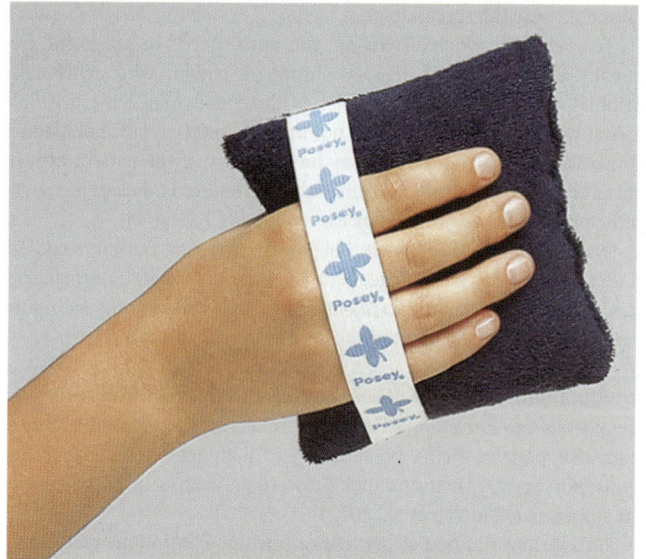

FIGURE 46.13 Foot boot.

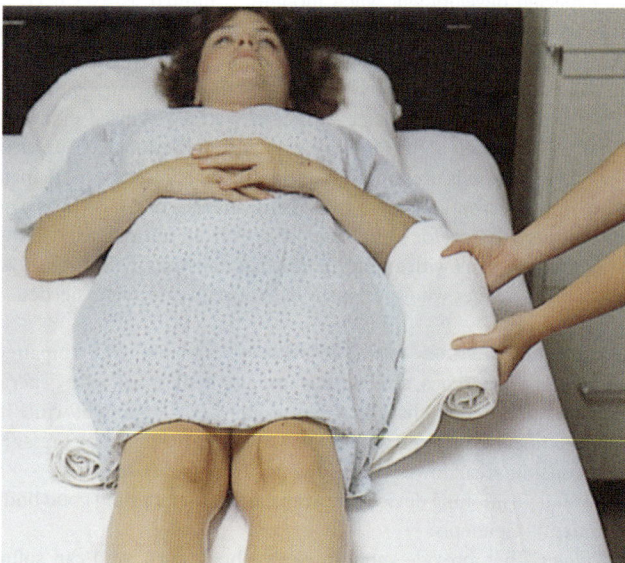

FIGURE 46.15 Hand roll. (Courtesy J. T. Posey, Arcadia, CA.)

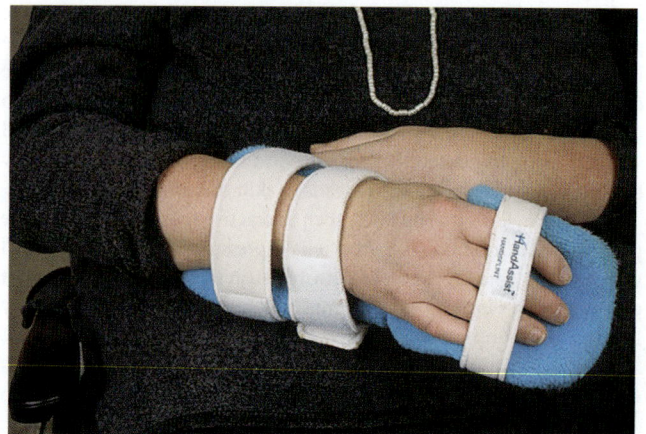

FIGURE 46.14 Trochanter roll.

FIGURE 46.16 Hand–wrist splint. (From Sorrentino, S. A., & Wilk, M. J. [2018]. *Mosby's Canadian textbook for the support worker* [4th ed.]. Mosby.)

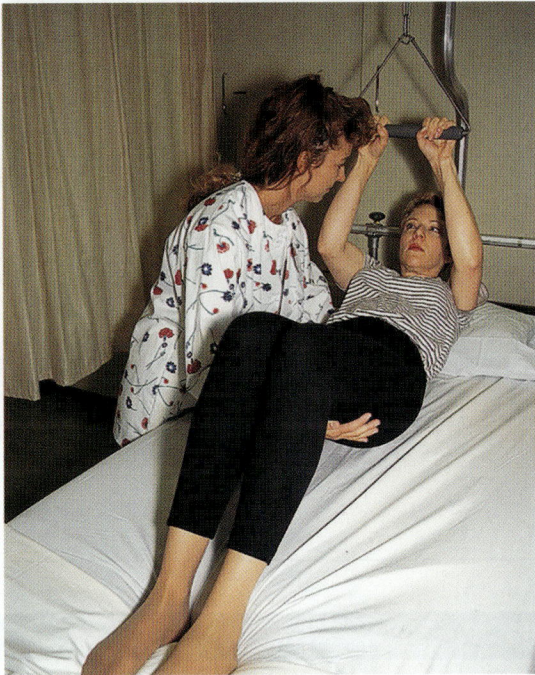

FIGURE 46.17 Patient using a trapeze bar.

- *Trapeze bar:* This is a triangular device that descends from a securely fastened overhead bar attached to the bed frame. A trapeze bar allows the patient to use their upper extremities to raise the trunk off the bed, to assist in transfer from the bed to a wheelchair, or to perform arm exercises (Figure 46.17). It is a useful device for increasing independence, maintaining upper body strength, and decreasing the shearing action from sliding across or up and down in bed.

Although each procedure for positioning has specific guidelines, there are universal steps to follow for patients who require positioning assistance (Skill 46.1). Following the guidelines reduces the risk of injury to the musculoskeletal system when a patient is lying or sitting. When joints are unsupported, their alignment is impaired. Joints must be positioned in a slightly flexed position, or their mobility is decreased. During positioning, the nurse must also assess bony prominences (pressure points; see Figure 47.2). When actual or potential pressure areas exist, nursing interventions involve removal of the pressure, thus decreasing the risk for development of pressure injuries and further trauma to the musculoskeletal system. For these patients the 30-degree lateral position is used.

Supported Fowler's Position. In the supported Fowler's position, the head of the bed is elevated 45 to 60 degrees and the patient's knees are slightly elevated without pressure to restrict circulation in the lower legs; the patient is sitting up in bed. The head of the bed should not be elevated more than 60 degrees because this position increases shearing force on the patient's back and heels. The patient's illness and overall condition influence the angle of head and knee elevation and the length of time that the patient should remain in the supported Fowler's position. Supports must permit flexion of the hips and knees and proper alignment of the normal curves in the cervical, thoracic, and lumbar vertebrae. The following are common trouble areas for the patient in the supported Fowler's position (see Skill 46.1 for preventive measures):

- Increased cervical flexion, because the pillow at the head is too thick and the head thrusts forward
- Hyperextension of the knees, allowing the patient to slide to the foot of the bed

- Pressure on the posterior aspect of the knees, decreasing circulation to the feet
- External rotation of the hips
- Arms hanging unsupported at the patient's sides
- Unsupported feet or pressure on the heels
- Unprotected pressure points at the sacrum and heels
- Increased shearing force on the back and heels when the head of the bed is raised greater than 60 degrees

Supine Position. The supine position is a back-lying position. In the supine position, the relationship of body parts is essentially the same as in good standing alignment except that the body is in the horizontal plane. Pillows, trochanter rolls, and hand rolls or arm splints are used to increase comfort and reduce injury to the skin or musculoskeletal system. The mattress should support the cervical, thoracic, and lumbar vertebrae. Shoulders are supported, and the elbows are slightly flexed to control shoulder rotation. A foot support is used to prevent foot-drop and maintain proper alignment. The following are some common trouble areas for patients in the supine position (see Skill 46.1 for preventive measures):

- Increased cervical flexion because the pillow at the head is too thick and the head thrusts forward
- Head flat on the mattress
- Shoulders unsupported and internally rotated
- Elbows extended
- Thumb not in opposition to the fingers
- Hips externally rotated
- Unsupported feet
- Unprotected pressure points at the occipital region of the head, vertebrae, coccyx, elbows, and heels

Prone Position. The patient in the prone position is lying chest down. Often the head is turned to the side. If a pillow is under the head, it should be thin enough to prevent cervical flexion or extension and maintain alignment of the lumbar spine. Placing a pillow under the lower leg permits dorsiflexion of the ankles and some knee flexion, which promotes relaxation. If a pillow is unavailable, the ankles should be in dorsiflexion over the end of the mattress. Although the prone position is seldom used in practice, nurses should consider this as an alternative, especially for patients who normally sleep in this position. The prone position has emerged as a standard treatment for patients with moderate to severe acute respiratory distress syndrome (Morata et al., 2021). Specialty beds that safely position acutely ill patients in the prone position are available.

Nurses should assess for and correct any of the following potential trouble points for patients in the prone position (see Skill 46.1 for preventive measures):

- Neck hyperextension
- Hyperextension of the lumbar spine
- Plantar flexion of the ankles
- Unprotected pressure points at the chin, elbows, hips, knees, and toes

Side-Lying Position. In the side-lying (or lateral) position, the patient is resting on the side with the major portion of body weight on the dependent hip and shoulder. A 30-degree lateral position is recommended for patients at risk for pressure injuries. Trunk alignment should be the same as in standing. For example, the structural curves of the spine should be maintained, the head should be supported in line with the midline of the trunk, and rotation of the spine needs to be avoided. The following trouble points are common in the side-lying position (see Skill 46.1 for preventive measures):

- Lateral flexion of the neck
- Spinal curves out of normal alignment
- Shoulder and hip joints internally rotated, adducted, or unsupported

- Lack of support for the feet
- Lack of protection for pressure points at the ear, shoulder, anterior iliac spine, trochanter, and ankles
- Excessive lateral flexion of the spine if the patient has large hips and a pillow is not placed superior to the hips at the waist

Modified Left Lateral Recumbent Position. The modified left lateral recumbent position differs from the lateral position in the distribution

of the patient's weight. In left lateral recumbent position, the weight is placed on the anterior ilium, humerus, and clavicle. Trouble points common in this position include the following (see Skill 46.1 for preventive measures):

- Lateral flexion of the neck
- Internal rotation, adduction, or lack of support to the shoulders and hips

SKILL 46.1 — MOVING AND POSITIONING PATIENTS IN BED

Delegation Considerations

The skills of moving and positioning patients in bed can be delegated to unregulated care providers (UCPs). The nurse is responsible for assessing the patient's level of comfort and for any potential hazards. Instruct the UCP about:

- Any moving and positioning limitations unique to the patient
- Individual needs for body alignment (e.g., patient with spinal cord injury)
- Scheduled times to reposition patient throughout shift
- When to request assistance (e.g., if the patient has a spinal cord injury, when the patient is unable to assist the nurse, has a lot of equipment, or is confused)

Equipment

- Pillows
- Appropriate safe patient-handling assistive device (e.g., friction-reducing transfer sheet)
- Positioning devices as required (e.g., trochanter roll, extra pillows, hand rolls)
- Side rails

ASSESSMENT

STEPS	RATIONALE
1. Identify patient using two identifiers (e.g., name and birthday or name and medical record number), according to employer policy.	• Ensures correct patient. Complies with the Joint Commission (2022) standards and improves patient safety.
2. Assess patient's body alignment and comfort level while patient is lying down.	• Provides baseline data for later comparisons. Determines ways to improve position and alignment.
3. Assess for risk factors that may contribute to complications of immobility:	• Increased risk factors require more frequent repositioning.
• Paralysis: Hemiparesis resulting from cerebrovascular accident (CVA); decreased sensation	• Paralysis impairs movement and causes muscle tone changes; sensation is often affected. Because of difficulty in moving and poor awareness of the involved body part, the patient is unable to protect and position the affected body part (Lewis et al., 2023).
• Impaired mobility: Traction or arthritis or other contributing disease processes	• Traction or arthritic changes of affected extremity result in decreased range of motion (ROM).
• Impaired circulation	• Decreased circulation to skin and underlying tissues predisposes the patient to pressure injuries.
• Age: Very young, older persons	• Premature and young infants require frequent turning because their skin is fragile. Normal physiological changes associated with aging predispose older persons to greater risks for developing complications of immobility (LeBlanc et al., 2017).
• Sensation: Decreased from CVA, paralysis, neuropathy	• Because of poor awareness of body part or reduced sensation, patient is unable to protect and position body part from pressure.
• Level of consciousness and mental status	• Determines need for special aids or devices. Patients with altered levels of consciousness may not understand instructions or be able to help during positioning.
• Assess condition of patient's skin.	• Provides a baseline to determine effects of positioning.
4. Assess patient's physical ability to help with moving and positioning:	• Enables nurse to use patient's mobility, coordination, and strength. Determines need for additional help. Ensures patient's and nurse's safety (Alberta Health Services, 2021; Matz et al., 2019).
• Age	• Some older persons may move more slowly and with less strength.
• Disease process	• Cardiopulmonary disease may require the patient to have the head of the bed elevated.
• Strength, coordination	• Determines amount of assistance provided by patient during position change.
• ROM	• Limited ROM may contraindicate certain positions.
5. Assess health care provider's prescription before positioning. Clarify whether any positions are contraindicated because of the patient's condition (e.g., spinal cord injury; respiratory difficulties; certain neurological conditions; presence of incisions, drain, or tubing).	• Placing patient in an inappropriate position could cause injury.
6. Perform hand hygiene.	• Reduces transfer of microorganisms.

SKILL 46.1	MOVING AND POSITIONING PATIENTS IN BED—cont'd
STEPS	**RATIONALE**

7. Assess for the presence of tubes, incisions, and equipment (e.g., traction).	• Alters positioning procedure and affects patient's ability to independently change positions.
8. Assess ability and motivation of the patient, family members, and primary caregiver to participate in moving and positioning the patient in bed, in anticipation of discharge to home.	• Determines ability of patient and caregivers to assist with positioning.

PLANNING

1. Collect appropriate equipment. Based on functional assessment of the patient, get assistance as needed. Close door to the room or bedside curtains.	• Having an appropriate number of people to position the patient prevents patient and nurse injury. Provides for patient privacy.
2. Perform hand hygiene.	• Reduces transfer of microorganisms.
3. Adjust level of bed to a comfortable working height. If two or multiple nurses are involved in positioning, raise height of the bed to the comfort zone of the tallest nurse.	• Raises level of work to centre of gravity and provides for patient's and nurse's safety. • For the tallest nurse, adjusting bed to their working height prevents exaggerated bending at the waist, which can lead to injury when repositioning.
4. Remove all pillows and devices used for positioning.	• Reduces interference with positioning.
5. Explain procedure to patient.	• Decreases anxiety and increases patient cooperation.

IMPLEMENTATION

1. Assist patient in moving up in bed.
   A. Can patient assist?
     (1) Fully able to assist, nurse assistance not needed; nurse stands by to assist.
     (2) Partially able to assist; patient can assist with nurse using positioning cues or aids (e.g., friction-reducing transfer sheet).
	• Determines degree of risk in repositioning patient and technique required to safely assist patient.

CRITICAL DECISION POINT: *Before lowering head of the bed to flatten bed, account for all tubing, drains, and equipment to prevent dislodgement or tipping if caught in the mattress or bed frame as bed is lowered.*

B. Assist patient in moving up in bed using friction-reducing transfer sheets (two or more nurses).	• This is not a one-person task. Helping a patient move up in bed without help from other co-workers or without the aid of assistive devices is not recommended or considered safe for the patient or the nurse. If the patient is unable to fully assist, refer to Step C.
(1) Position patient supine with head of bed flat or in Trendelenburg position in bed if this is tolerated. A nurse stands on each side of the bed.	• Enables nurse to assess body alignment. Reduces pull of gravity, friction, and possible shear on patient's skin. With the bed in Trendelenburg position, gravity helps with moving patient proximally in bed.
(2) Lower side rails. Remove pillow from under the head and shoulders, and place pillow at head of bed.	• Prevents striking of patient's head against head of the bed.
(3) Turn patient side to side to place repositioning device under patient. Ensure patient's shoulders and hips are on the repositioning device being used.	• Reduces surface area and friction. • Supports patient's body weight and reduces friction during movement.
(4) Return patient to supine position. Instruct patient to lie flat on back, cross arms on chest, and bend their knees. If the patient is unable to bend their knees, place a pillow under their lower legs to decrease friction during repositioning.	• Even distribution of patient's weight makes lifting and positioning easier.
(5) Fanfold repositioning device (e.g., friction-reducing transfer sheet) on both sides, with each nurse grasping firmly (palms up) near the patient.	• Provides strong handles to grip transfer sheet without slipping. Palms-up grip is safe and effective as it promotes use of the more powerful biceps muscles.

(6) Nurses or workers assume a six-checkpoint position (Alberta Health Services, 2021):
     (a) "3 for the top"—ears over shoulders and shoulders over hips
     (b) "3 for the bottom"—tighten stomach and push buttocks back while keeping body weight over the heels. Reposition trunk forward by bending at the hips and not at the waist.
     (c) Elbows tucked in
     (d) Safe effective grip (palms up)
     (e) Comfort zone (bend elbows and tuck elbows into sides, move hands to shoulders and to hips)
     (f) Weight transfer—stable base, transfer side to side and front to back
	• Promotes optimal body mechanics.
	 • Maintains three natural curves of the spine.
	 • Stable and flexible base helps maintain balance and centre of gravity during transfer.
	 • Keeps load close.
	 • Facilitates use of more powerful quadriceps and biceps muscle groups.

Continued

SKILL 46.1 MOVING AND POSITIONING PATIENTS IN BED—cont'd

STEPS	RATIONALE
(7) Grasp top sheet at the patient's shoulder and hip level (palms up). Place feet shoulder-width apart and point foot nearest head of the bed in the direction of the move (forward–backward stance; see Step 1B[7] illustration).	• Facing the direction of movement prevents twisting of nurse's body while moving the patient. • A stable base of support increases balance. This stance enables the nurse to shift body weight as the patient is repositioned up in bed, thereby reducing force needed to move load.

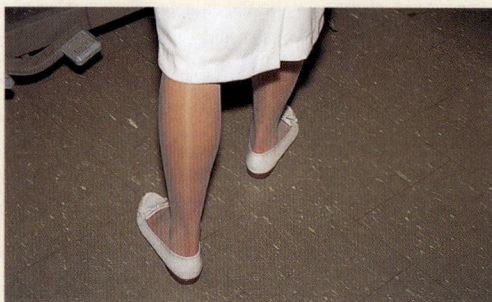

STEP 1B(7) Position of feet: feet placed apart in a forward-to-backward stance.

(8) Instruct patient to flex neck, tilting chin toward chest.	• Prevents hyperextension of neck when moving patient up in bed.
(9) Instruct patient to assist moving by bending knees and pushing with feet on bed surface.	• Reduces friction. Increases patient mobility. Decreases workload.
(9) The primary nurse counts "1-2-3 slide." Instruct patient to push with their heels and elevate trunk while breathing out on the command word "slide," thus moving toward head of bed.	• Prepares patient for repositioning. Reinforces assistance in moving up in bed. Increases patient cooperation. Breathing out avoids Valsalva manoeuvre.
(10) On command "slide," rock and shift weight from back to front leg. At the same time, the patient pushes with their heels and elevates trunk.	• Rocking enables the nurse to improve balance and overcome inertia. Shifting weight counteracts the patient's weight and reduces the force needed to move load. The patient's assistance reduces friction and workload.
(11) Tuck in top sheet of friction-reducing transfer sheet after repositioning. If using transitory slider sheet, remove it from under patient.	• Patient will slide if slider set remains under patient.

2. Position patient in one of the following positions using correct body alignment to protect pressure areas. Begin with patient lying supine and reposition in bed following Step 1B.

   A. Position patient in supported Fowler's position (see Step 2A illustration).

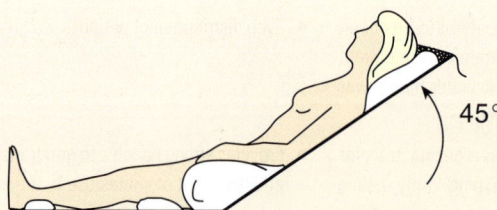

STEP 2A Supported Fowler's position.

(1) With patient supine, elevate head of bed 45 to 60 degrees if not contraindicated.	• Increases comfort, improves ventilation, and increases patient's opportunity to socialize or relax.
(2) Rest patient's head against the mattress or on a small pillow.	• Prevents flexion contractures of cervical vertebrae.
(3) Use pillows to support patient's arms and hands if the patient does not have voluntary control or use of hands and arms.	• Prevents shoulder subluxation from effect of downward pull of unsupported arms, promotes circulation by preventing venous pooling, and prevents flexion contractures of arms and wrists.
(4) Position pillow at patient's lower back.	• Supports lumbar vertebrae and decreases flexion of vertebrae.

SKILL 46.1   MOVING AND POSITIONING PATIENTS IN BED—cont'd

STEPS	RATIONALE
(5) Place a small pillow under patient's thigh.	• Prevents hyperextension of knee and occlusion of popliteal artery caused by pressure from body weight.
(6) Position patient's heel in heel boots or other heel pressure relief devices.	• Heel pressure relief devices are more effective than pillows for consistently reducing pressure from the mattress on the heels. When pillows are used, they must be repositioned each time the patient moves or is repositioned.

CRITICAL DECISION POINT: *To keep feet in proper alignment and prevent footdrop, use foot support devices. A foot cradle may also be used for patients with poor peripheral circulation as a means of reducing pressure on the tips of the patient's toes.*

STEPS	RATIONALE
B. Position patient with hemiplegia in supported Fowler's position.	
(1) Elevate head of bed 45 to 60 degrees. Adjust head of bed according to patient's condition. For example, those with increased risk of pressure injuries remain at a 30-degree angle (semi-Fowler's).	• Increases comfort, improves ventilation, and increases patient's opportunity to relax.
(2) Position patient in sitting position as straight as possible.	• Counteracts tendency to slump toward affected side. Improves ventilation and cardiac output and decreases intracranial pressure. Improves patient's ability to swallow and helps to prevent aspiration of food, liquids, and gastric secretions.
(3) Position patient's head on a small pillow with the chin slightly forward. If patient is totally unable to control head movement, avoid hyperextension of the neck.	• Prevents hyperextension of neck. Too many pillows under the head may cause or worsen neck flexion contracture.
(4) Provide support for involved arm and hand on overbed table in front of patient. Place arm away from patient's side and support elbow with pillow.	• Paralyzed muscles do not automatically resist pull of gravity as they do normally. As a result, shoulder subluxation, pain, and edema may occur.
• Position *flaccid* hand in a normal resting position with the wrist slightly extended, arches of hand maintained, and fingers partially flexed. You may use a hand grip or section of a rubber ball cut in half; clasp patient's hands together.	
• Position *spastic* hand with wrist in neutral position or slightly extended; fingers should be extended with palm down. It may be difficult to position spastic hands without the use of specially made splints for the patient (discuss with occupational therapist).	
(5) Flex patient's knees and hips by using a pillow or folded blanket under their knees.	• Ensures proper alignment. Flexion prevents prolonged hyperextension, which could impair joint mobility.
(6) Support patient's feet in dorsiflexion with firm pillow or therapeutic boots or splints.	• Prevents footdrop. Stimulation of ball of the foot by a hard surface has a tendency to increase muscle tone in a patient with extensor spasticity of lower extremity. Therapeutic boots or splints are manufactured with thick padding to cushion the heel and prevent pressure injuries.
C. Position patient in supported supine position.	
(1) Be sure patient is comfortable on their back with head of bed flat.	• Some patients' physical conditions will not tolerate a supine position.
(2) Place a small rolled towel under the lumbar area of the patient's back.	• Provides support for lumbar spine.
(3) Place a pillow under patient's upper shoulders, neck, or head.	• Maintains correct alignment and prevents flexion contractures of cervical vertebrae.
(4) Place trochanter rolls or sandbags parallel to lateral surface of the patient's thighs if patient is immobile.	• Reduces external rotation of hip.
(5) Position patient's heels in heel boots or other heel pressure relief device (check employer policy).	• Heel pressure relief devices are more effective than pillows for consistently reducing pressure from the mattress on the patient's heels. Reducing pressure on heels prevents possible pressure sores.

Continued

SKILL 46.1	MOVING AND POSITIONING PATIENTS IN BED—cont'd
STEPS	**RATIONALE**

(6) If needed, support feet in dorsiflexion with foot support devices (check employer policy).

- Maintains dorsiflexion and prevents footdrop.

(7) Place pillows under pronated forearms, keeping upper arms parallel to patient's body (see Step 2C[7] illustrations).

- Reduces internal rotation of shoulder and prevents extension of elbows. Maintains correct body alignment.

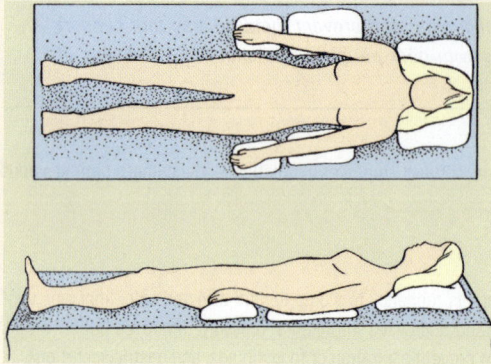

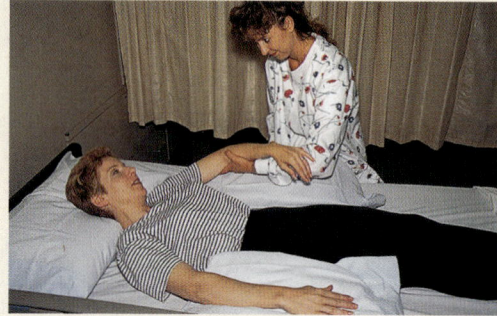

STEP 2C(7) Supine position with pillows in place.

(8) Place hand rolls in patient's hands. Consider occupational therapy referral for use of hand splints, if necessary.

- Reduces extension of fingers and abduction of thumb. Maintains thumb slightly adducted and in opposition to fingers.

D. Position hemiplegic patient in supine position.

(1) Assess patient to determine that the person is comfortable on their back with the head of bed flat.

- Some patients' physical conditions do not tolerate supine position.

(2) Place folded towel or small pillow under shoulder of affected side.

- Decreases possibility of pain, joint contracture, and subluxation. Maintains mobility in muscles around shoulder to permit normal movement patterns.

(3) Keep affected arm away from body with elbow extended and palm up. (An alternative is to place arm out to the side, with the elbow bent and hand toward head of the bed.)

- Maintains mobility in arm, joints, and shoulder to permit normal movement patterns. (Alternative position counteracts limitation of ability of arm to rotate outward at shoulder [external rotation]. External rotation must be present to raise arm overhead without pain.)

CRITICAL DECISION POINT: *Position the affected hand in one of the recommended positions for flaccid or spastic hand.*

---

(4) Place a folded towel under the hip of patient's involved side.

- Diminishes effect of spasticity in entire leg by controlling hip position.

(5) Flex affected knee 30 degrees by supporting it on a pillow or folded blanket.

- Slight flexion breaks up abnormal extension pattern of leg. Extensor spasticity is most severe when the patient is supine.

(6) If needed, support feet in dorsiflexion with foot support devices (check employer policy).

- Maintains foot in dorsiflexion and prevents footdrop. Foot support devices prevent stimulation to ball of the foot by a hard surface, which has a tendency to increase muscle tone in a patient with extensor spasticity of lower extremity.

E. Position patient in prone position. This requires two staff members to safely position patient.

- In certain patients with pulmonary conditions such as acute respiratory distress syndrome, use of a prone position can help improve oxygenation.

(1) With a repositioning device under the patient and one nurse standing on each side of the bed, reposition patient toward one side of the bed. Ensure that side rail on opposite side is up for safety.

- Prepares patient for positioning.

(2) With patient supine, the primary nurse grasps the top sheet at the patient's shoulder and hip level using a safe, effective grip (palms up, elbows tucked into sides) and assumes a position to use a front-to-back weight transfer.

- Promotes use of stronger biceps muscles. Front-to-back weight transfer promotes nurses' safety by preventing rotation of spine that can lead to injury.

(3) The secondary nurse positions to perform a back-to-front weight transfer and places hands on the patient's shoulder and hip to provide directional guidance only.

SKILL 46.1	MOVING AND POSITIONING PATIENTS IN BED—cont'd
STEPS	**RATIONALE**

(4) Primary nurse counts "1-2-3 slide," and on command word "slide" primary worker performs a front-to-back weight transfer while the secondary worker uses a back-to-front weight transfer. Nurses use a combined slide-and-turn motion so that the patient first slides toward the primary worker and is then turned onto their side. At the end of the move, the patient will be facing the secondary nurse.

(5) Roll patient over arm positioned close to the body, with elbow straight and hand under hip. Position patient on their abdomen in centre of the bed.

- Positions patient correctly so that alignment can be maintained.
- Diminishes effects of spasticity in entire leg by controlling hip position. Slight hip flexion breaks up abnormal extension pattern of leg; extensor spasticity is most severe when the patient is supine.

(6) Turn patient's head to one side and support their head with a small pillow (see Step 2E[6] illustration).

- Reduces flexion or hyperextension of cervical vertebrae.

(7) Place small pillow under patient's abdomen below level of diaphragm (see Step 2E[7] illustration).

- Reduces pressure on breasts of some patients and decreases hyperextension of lumbar vertebrae and strain on lower back. Improves breathing by reducing mattress pressure on diaphragm.

(8) Support patient's arms in flexed position, level at shoulders.

- Maintains proper body alignment. Support reduces risk of joint dislocation.

(9) Support patient's lower legs with pillows to elevate toes (see Step 2E[9] illustration).

- Prevents footdrop. Reduces external rotation of hips. Reduces mattress pressure on toes.

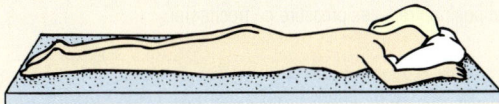

STEP 2E(6) Prone position, head supported with pillow.

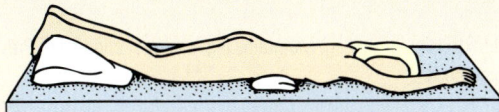

STEP 2E(7) Prone position, pillow under patient's abdomen and feet.

STEP 2E(9) Prone position with pillows supporting lower legs.

***

CRITICAL DECISION POINT: *Increase frequency of position changes if pressure areas begin to appear, joint mobility becomes impaired or worsened, or patient complains of discomfort. Consult with physiotherapist and occupational therapist as needed. Use 30-degree lateral position to help prevent pressure injuries.*

***

F. Position patient with hemiplegia in prone position.

(1) Move patient toward unaffected side.

- Creates room for proper patient alignment in centre of bed when patient is rolled onto their abdomen.

(2) Roll patient onto their side.

(3) Place pillow on patient's abdomen.

- Prevents sagging of abdomen when patient is rolled over; decreases hyperextension of lumbar vertebrae and strain on lower back.

(4) Roll patient onto abdomen by positioning involved arm close to patient's body, with elbow straight and hand under hip. Roll patient carefully over arm.

- Prevents injury to affected side.

(5) Turn patient's head toward involved side.

- Promotes development of neck and trunk extension, which is necessary for standing and walking.

(6) Position involved arm out to side, with elbow bent, hand toward head of bed, and fingers extended (if possible).

- Counteracts limitation of the arm's ability to rotate outward at the shoulder (external rotation). External rotation must be present to raise arm over head without pain.

(7) Flex patient's knees slightly by placing a pillow under their legs from knees to ankles.

- Flexion prevents prolonged hyperextension, which could impair joint mobility.

(8) Keep patient's feet at right angle to legs by using a pillow high enough to keep their toes off the mattress.

- Maintains feet in dorsiflexion.

Continued

SKILL 46.1   **MOVING AND POSITIONING PATIENTS IN BED—cont'd**

STEPS	RATIONALE

G. Position patient in 30-degree lateral (side-lying) position.

(1) Lower head of bed completely or as low as the patient can tolerate.

• Provides position of comfort for patient and removes pressure from bony prominences on back and buttocks.

(2) Position patient in supine position at side of bed opposite direction toward which patient is to be turned. Reposition upper trunk, supporting shoulders first, followed by repositioning of lower trunk, supporting hips. Raise side rails and move to opposite side of bed.

• Provides room for patient to turn to side.

(3) Prepare to turn patient onto their side. Flex patient's knee that will not be next to the mattress. Place one hand on the patient's hip and one hand on the patient's shoulder.

• Positioning will set up leverage for easy turning.

(4) Roll patient onto side toward you.

• Rolling decreases trauma to tissues. In addition, patient is positioned so that leverage on the hip makes turning easy.

(5) Place pillow under patient's head and neck.

• Maintains alignment. Reduces lateral neck flexion. Decreases strain on sternocleidomastoid muscle.

(6) Bring patient's shoulder blade forward.

• Prevents patient's weight from resting directly on their shoulder joint.

(7) Position both arms in a slightly flexed position. The upper arm is supported by a pillow level with the shoulder; the other arm, by the mattress.

• Decreases internal rotation and adduction of the shoulder. Supporting both arms in a slightly flexed position protects the joint and improves ventilation because the chest is able to expand more easily.

(8) Place your hands under the patient's hips and bring dependent hip slightly forward so that angle from hip to mattress is approximately 30 degrees.

• The 30-degree lateral position reduces pressure on trochanter.

(9) Place tuck-back pillow behind patient's back. (Make by folding pillow lengthwise. The smooth area is slightly tucked under the patient's back.)

• Provides support to maintain patient on their side.

(10) Place pillow under semiflexed upper leg level at hip from groin to foot (see Step 2G[10] illustrations).

• Flexion prevents hyperextension of the leg. Maintains leg in correct alignment. Prevents pressure on bony prominence.

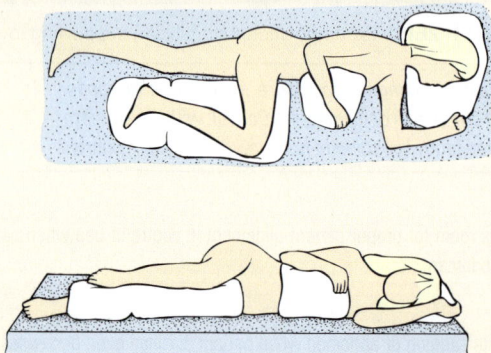

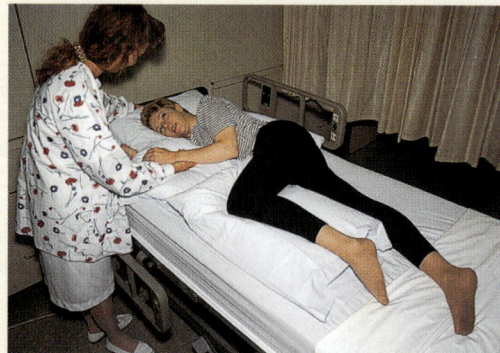

STEP 2G(10) Side-lying position with pillows in place.

(11) Support patient's feet in dorsiflexion with foot support devices (check employer policy).

• Maintains dorsiflexion of foot. Prevents footdrop. Foot support devices prevent stimulation to the ball of the foot by a hard surface, which has a tendency to increase muscle tone in a patient with extensor spasticity of lower extremity.

H. Position patient in left lateral recumbent (semiprone) position (one nurse).

(1) Lower head of bed completely.

• Provides for proper body alignment while patient is lying down.

(2) Assess patient's level of comfort in the supine position.

• Some patient's physical conditions do not tolerate supine position.

(3) Position patient in supine position on side of bed opposite the direction the patient is to be turned. Reposition patient's upper trunk, supporting the shoulders first; reposition lower trunk, supporting hips. Raise side rails and move to opposite side of bed.

• Prepares patient for positioning.

SKILL 46.1   MOVING AND POSITIONING PATIENTS IN BED—cont'd

STEPS	RATIONALE
(4) Move to other side of bed and roll patient on their side. Position patient in lateral position and lying partially on abdomen, with dependent shoulder lifted out and arm placed at patient's side.	• Patient is rolled only partially onto abdomen.
(5) Place a small pillow under the patient's head.	• Patient is rolled only partially onto their abdomen.
(6) Place pillow under patient's flexed upper arm, supporting arm level with shoulder.	• Maintains proper alignment and prevents lateral neck flexion. Prevents internal rotation of shoulder.
(7) Place pillow under patient's flexed upper leg, supporting leg level with hip.	• Prevents internal rotation of hip and adduction of leg. Flexion prevents hyperextension of leg. Reduces mattress pressure on knees and ankles.
(8) Support patient's feet in dorsiflexion with foot support devices (check employer policy) (see Step 2H[8] illustration).	• Maintains foot in dorsiflexion. Prevents footdrop. Foot support devices prevent stimulation to ball of foot by hard surface, which has tendency to increase muscle tone in patient with extensor spasticity of lower extremity.

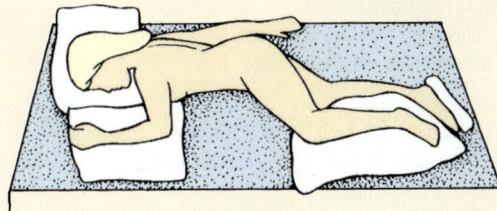

STEP 2H(8) Left lateral recumbent (semiprone) position with pillows in place.

CRITICAL DECISION POINT: *Supervise and aid UCPs when a prescription is to logroll a patient. In patients who have suffered a spinal cord injury or are recovering from neck, back, or vertebral column surgery, the spinal column must be maintained in straight alignment to prevent further injury.*

I. Logrolling patient (three to five nurses).	
(1) Place patient in supine position on side of bed opposite the direction to be turned.	• Prepares patient for turning onto their side.
(2) Place small pillow between patient's knees.	• Prevents tension on the spinal column and adduction of the hip.
(3) Cross patient's arms on their chest and bend knee on the opposite side the patient will be turned toward.	• Prevents injury to arms. • Facilitates weight transfer when logrolling.
(4) Position two nurses on side of bed to which the patient will be turned. Position third nurse on the other side of bed (see Step 2I[4] illustration).	• Distributes weight equally among nurses. • For patients with spinal cord injury or vertebral column trauma, stabilizing the patient's head and neck facilitates synchronous movement of the vertebral column when logrolling and prevents injury to the patient.

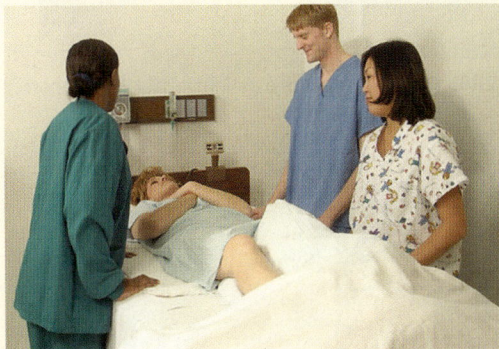

STEP 2I(4) Position nurses on each side of patient.

Continued

SKILL 46.1	MOVING AND POSITIONING PATIENTS IN BED—cont'd
STEPS	RATIONALE

SAFETY ALERT: If a patient has a spinal cord injury, or actual or suspected vertebral column fracture, a fourth nurse must be positioned at the head of the bed to stabilize the patient's head and neck to ensure synchronous movement of the entire vertebral column when logrolling. If needed, use a fifth nurse on the same side as the third nurse.

(5) The nurse on the opposite side of the bed passes the edge of the transfer sheet to the nurses on the side of the bed to which the patient is to be turned. These nurses fanfold or roll the sheet and then grasp the sheet using a safe, effective grip (palms up, elbows at sides) and position themselves to do a front-to-back weight transfer.

- Provides strong handles to grip the transfer sheet or pull sheet without slipping.
- Using palms up, elbows at sides facilitates maximum use of the stronger biceps muscles.
- Safety of the nurse is facilitated by using a front-to-back weight transfer, as this action prevents rotation of the spine that can lead to injury.

(6) The nurse on the opposite side of the bed positions open-palmed hands on the patient's shoulder and hip to provide directional guidance only. For the nurses on the side that the patient is to be turned: the first nurse grasps the transfer sheet at the patient's shoulders and lower back, and the second nurse grasps the transfer sheet at the patient's hips and lower thighs.

(7) The nurse on the opposite side of the bed counts "1-2-3 roll," and on the command word "roll" the two nurses perform a front-to-back weight transfer, while the nurse on the opposite side of the bed gently guides the patient using a back-to-front weight transfer. At the completion of the move, the patient will be facing the two nurses (see Step 2I[7] illustration).

- Maintains proper alignment in the patient by moving all body parts at the same time, preventing tension or twisting of the spinal column.

(8) The nurse on the opposite side of the bed places pillows along the length of the patient (see Step 2I[8] illustration).

- Pillows keep the patient aligned.

(9) Gently lean the patient as a unit back toward the pillows for support (see Step 2I[9] illustration).

- Ensures continued straight alignment of spinal column, preventing injury.

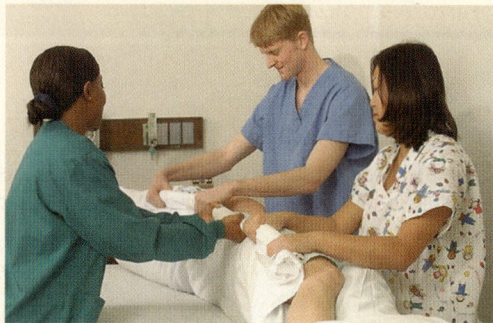

STEP 2I(7) Move patient as a unit, maintaining proper alignment.

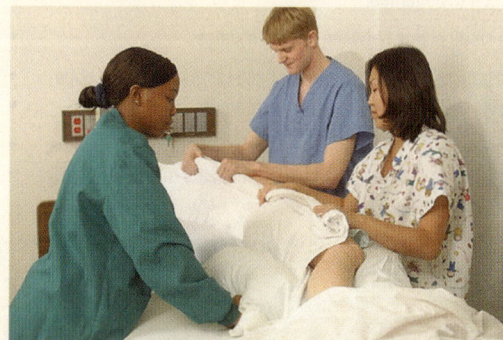

STEP 2I(8) Place pillows along patient's back for support.

STEP 2I(9) Gently lean patient as a unit against pillows.

SKILL 46.1	MOVING AND POSITIONING PATIENTS IN BED—cont'd
STEPS	**RATIONALE**
3. Perform hand hygiene.	• Reduces transmission of microorganisms.

EVALUATION

1. Evaluate patient's level of comfort and ability to assist in position change.	• Patients with reduced activity tolerance and increased levels of pain may find position changes very tiring and will need post-position change interventions to restore their level of comfort.
2. After each position change, evaluate patient's body alignment and assess pressure areas. Observe for areas of erythema or breakdown involving skin.	• Prompt identification of poor alignment reduces risks to the patient's skin and musculoskeletal systems.

UNEXPECTED OUTCOMES	RELATED INTERVENTIONS
Joint contractures develop or worsen (Cause: Improper positioning results in shortening of muscles)	• Consult physiotherapy or occupational therapy or both. • Ensure that activity and ROM prescriptions are implemented consistently.
Skin erythema and breakdown (Cause: Inadequate frequency of repositioning)	• Increase frequency of turning and repositioning. • Place turning schedule above patient's bed. • Implement other activities per employer skin care policy or protocol (e.g., assess more frequently, consult dietitian, place patient on pressure-relieving mattress).
Patient avoids moving	• Administer analgesia as prescribed by health care provider to ensure patient's comfort before moving if patient is in pain. • Allow pain medication to take effect before positioning. • Provide patient education about benefits of moving.

RECORDING AND REPORTING

- Document repositioning or turning and any relevant observations during procedure (e.g., condition of skin, joint movement, patient's ability to assist with positioning) in nurses' notes.
- Report observations at change of shift.
- Document your evaluation of patient learning.

CARE IN THE COMMUNITY CONSIDERATIONS

- Teach family about the importance of body mechanics for themselves and the patient.
- Teach family how to use safe patient-handling equipment, if necessary.
- Teach patient and family about the signs of skin breakdown and the importance of safety during positioning patients with decreased sensation or mobility.

- Lack of support for the feet
- Lack of protection for pressure points at the ilium, humerus, clavicle, knees, and ankles

Transfer Techniques. Nurses often provide care for patients who must be assisted to change positions, who must be moved up in bed, or who must be transferred from a bed to a chair or from a bed to a stretcher. Use of proper body mechanics will enable you as a nurse to position, move, or transfer patients safely and also protect you from injury to the musculoskeletal system (see Chapter 37). Although many transfer techniques are used, the following general guidelines should be followed in any transfer procedure:

- Raise the side rail on the side of the bed opposite you to prevent the patient from falling out of bed.
- Elevate the level of the bed to a comfortable working height.
- Assess the patient's mobility and strength to determine what assistance the patient can offer during transfer.
- Determine the need for assistance from other care providers or mechanical lifts.
- Explain the procedure to the patient and describe what is expected of the patient.
- Assess for correct body alignment and pressure areas after each transfer.

> **SAFETY ALERT** Recognition of your own personal strengths and limits is crucial. Moving a patient who is completely immobilized by yourself is dangerous and not allowed in many agencies. If you are attempting transfer or moving techniques for the first time, you should request help to reduce the risk of injury to yourself and to the patient.

Repositioning Patients. When repositioning a patient, a safe transfer is the first priority. Patients require various levels of assistance to move up in bed, move to the side-lying position, or sit up at the side of the bed. For example, a young, healthy woman may need only a little support as she sits at the side of the bed for the first time after childbirth, whereas an older person may need help from one or more nurses to do the same task one day after abdominal surgery.

The nurse must always enlist the patient's help to the fullest extent possible. To determine what the patient is able to do alone and how many people are needed to help move the patient in bed, the nurse needs to assess the patient to determine whether the illness, injury, or treatment contradicts exertion (e.g., cardiovascular disease, spinal cord injury, vertebral column surgery).

Next, the nurse must perform a functional assessment of the patient (Table 46.4). A functional assessment includes the following:

- Determine whether the patient is able to communicate their needs and comprehend and follow directions.
- Assess the patient's vision and hearing.
- Assess the patient's medical status, including conditions and limitations that will affect the move, attachments or appliances, pain and fatigue, and medications that will affect the move.
- Assess the patient's hand grip strength.
- Assess the patient's ability to raise their hips when knees are bent and feet are on the bed (bridging).
- Assess the patient's ability to roll side to side in bed.

If the patient is deficient in any of these assessments, at least two nurses are required to safely transfer and reposition the patient in bed. As the patient's nurse, you must then determine the comfort level of the patient and evaluate personal strength and knowledge of the procedure.

Finally, determine whether the patient is too heavy or immobile for you to complete the procedure alone (see Skill 46.1). Use of mechanical transfer devices may be warranted (Figure 46.18), and employer lifting and transferring policies must be followed.

Assessment criteria and tools have been developed to help nurses gather data and to assess and plan for the safe transfer of patients. An example of a safe patient handling functional assessment record form is shown in Table 46.4.

Restorative Care

The goal of restorative care for the patient who is immobile is to maximize functional mobility and independence and reduce residual functional deficits such as impaired gait and decreased endurance. The focus in restorative care is on not only ADLs that relate to physical self-care but also **instrumental activities of daily living (IADLs)**. IADLs are activities that are necessary to be independent in society beyond eating, grooming, transferring, and toileting. They include such skills as shopping, preparing meals, banking, and taking medications.

In restorative care, nurses use many of the interventions described in the "Health Promotion" and "Acute Care" sections in this chapter, but the emphasis is on working collaboratively with patients and their significant others and with other health care providers. The goal is to enhance the patient's quality of life by helping the patient return to maximal functional ability in both ADLs and IADLs.

Intensive specialized rehabilitation such as occupational or physiotherapy is common. If the patient is in a health care facility they will likely go to the therapy department two to three times a day. Nurses work collaboratively with these professionals and reinforce exercises and teaching. For example, after a stroke, a patient will likely receive gait training from a physiotherapist, speech rehabilitation from a speech therapist, and training from an occupational therapist on getting dressed and preparing food. Working with the interprofessional team to develop a plan of care, the nurse can reinforce and further enhance the patient's mobilization. The therapy may not be able to restore total functional health, but it may help the patient adapt to limited mobility and related complications.

Restorative interventions are focused on the regaining of mobility. According to evidenced-informed protocols, common restorative interventions used by nurses include promotion of exercises for maintaining or regaining joint mobility and teaching of the use of assistive devices for walking (Box 46.8). Items frequently used to help a patient adapt to mobility limitations include walkers, canes, wheelchairs, and assistive devices such as raised toilet seats, reaching sticks, special silverware, and adaptive clothing with Velcro closures.

TABLE 46.4	Safe Patient Handling Functional Assessment Record	
Question	**Yes/ No/Not Applicable**	**Comments**
Patient Health Information		
Communication		
Is patient able to communicate needs?		
Are vision and hearing adequate? List aides if used.		
Cognitive Status		
Is patient able to recall instructions?		
Is patient able to judge capabilities in moving?		
Emotional/Behaviour Status		
Is patient cooperative and predictable in behaviour?		
Is patient's mood stable?		
Medical Status		
Conditions/Limitations that will affect move		
Does patient have attachments or appliances?		
Does patient have pain or fatigue?		
Is patient on medication that will affect move?		
Functional Assessment		
Can patient grip, push, and pull hands? Right Left		
In supine position, can patient raise their hips with their knees bent and feet on bed?		
Can patient roll side to side in bed? Right Left		
Can patient get into a sitting position at the side of the bed and maintain sitting position for 15 seconds?		
Can patient straighten at least one leg and hold it for 3 seconds? Right Left		
Can patient get into a standing position?		If "no," a mechanical lift is required.
Is patient able to bear body weight for 15 seconds?		If "no," a mechanical lift is required.
Is patient predictable and reliable in physical and mental performance?		If "no," a mechanical lift is required.
Are all caregivers able to perform the task?		

Adapted from Alberta Health Services. (2021). *Ergonomics training: It's your move.* https://ahamms01.https.internapcdn.net/ahamms01/Content/AHS_Website/modules/iym/presentation_html5.html

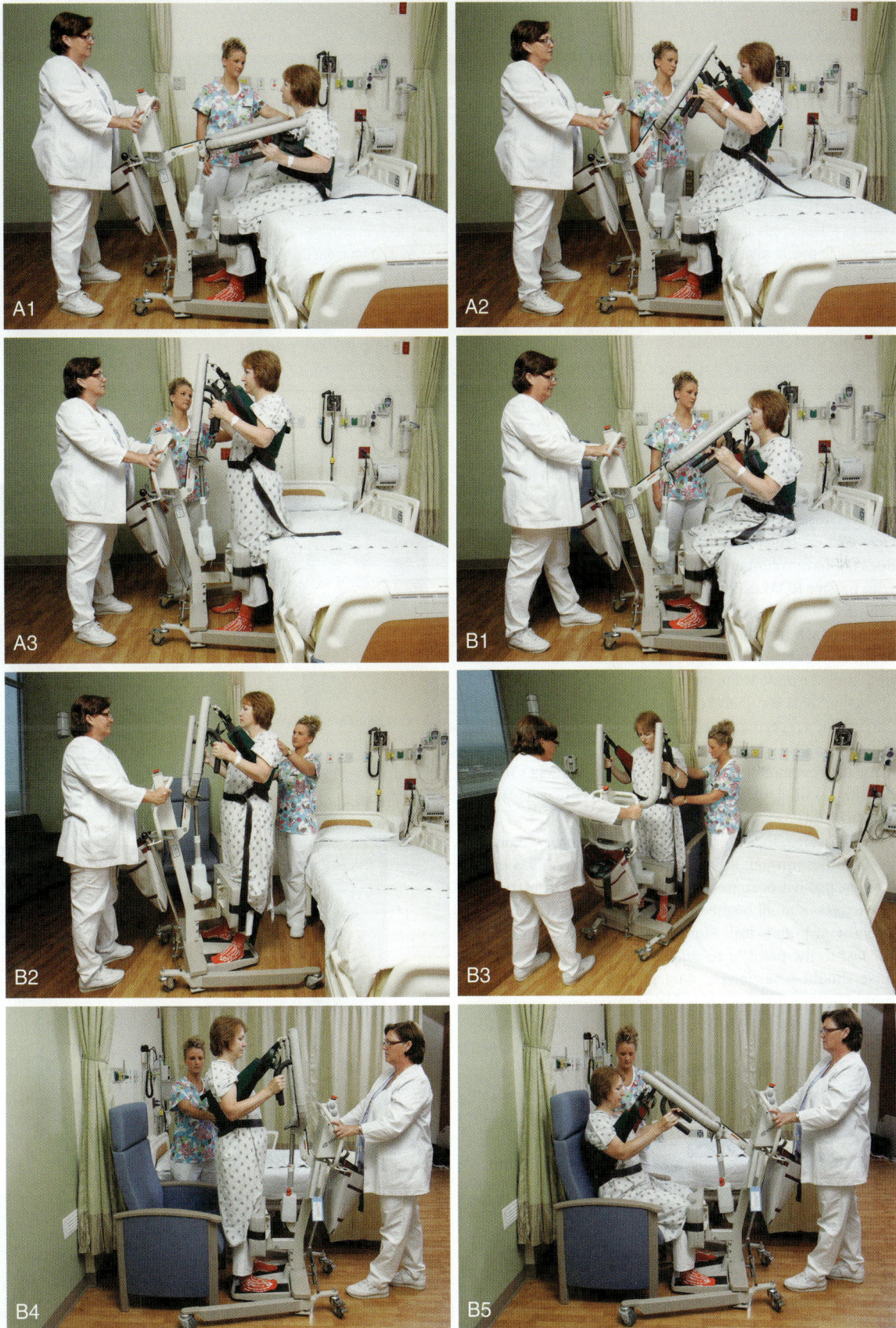

FIGURE 46.18 Using a motorized lift for patient transfer. **A1,** Safety straps are secured appropriately when using a motorized lift to help a patient move to standing position. **A2,** Patient grasps handles as the nurse enables motorized lift. **A3,** Patient is in standing position with feet on the floor and is ready to ambulate to a chair with nurses' help. **B1,** When the patient is unable to walk, the nurse secures safety straps, and platform of the motorized lift is used. **B2,** Patient in upright position. **B3,** Positioning patient in front of chair. **B4,** Explaining to patient the need to hold on to the handles as motorized lift begins to lower patient into chair. **B5,** Guiding patient into chair.

Range-of-Motion (ROM) Exercises. To ensure adequate joint mobility, the nurse needs to teach the patient about ROM exercises. Walking also increases joint mobility. Occasionally, patients need to use assistive devices such as crutches or walkers to help them walk. When the patient does not have voluntary motor control, nurses should assist the patient with passive ROM exercises.

Patients with restricted mobility are unable to perform some or all ROM exercises independently. Such patients include those with limited movement in one extremity and those who are completely immobilized. ROM exercises should be provided to maintain maximum joint mobility.

To ensure that patients routinely receive ROM exercises, the nurse should schedule them at specific times, perhaps with another nursing activity, such as during the patient's bath. This will enable the nurse to systematically reassess mobility while improving the patient's ROM. In addition, during bathing, the extremities and joints are usually put through complete ROM.

Unless contraindicated, the care plan should include movement of the patient's extremities through the fullest ROM possible. ROM exercises may be active, passive, or somewhere in between (active assisted). Passive ROM exercises should begin as soon as the patient's ability to move the extremity or joint is lost. Movements are carried out slowly and smoothly, just to the point of resistance; ROM should not cause pain. The nurse should *never force a joint beyond its capacity.* Each movement should be repeated five times during the session.

When performing passive ROM exercises, the nurse stands at the side of the bed closest to the joint being exercised. Passive ROM exercises are performed using a head-to-toe sequence and moving from larger to smaller joints. If an extremity is to be moved or lifted, the nurse can place a cupped hand under the joint to support it (Figure 46.19), support the joint by holding the adjacent distal and proximal areas (Figure 46.20), or support the joint with one hand and cradle the distal portion of the extremity with the remaining arm (Figure 46.21). See Table 46.2 for detailed ROM exercises and illustrated motion for each joint.

◆ Evaluation

Patient Care. To evaluate outcomes and response to nursing care, the effectiveness of all interventions must be measured. Actual outcomes are compared with the outcomes selected during planning. The nurse evaluates specific interventions designed to promote body alignment, improve mobility, and protect the patient from the hazards of immobility. Patient and family instruction to prevent future risks to body alignment and to identify immobility hazards is also evaluated (Figure 46.22). Evaluation enables the nurse to determine whether new or revised therapies are required and if new nursing diagnoses have developed.

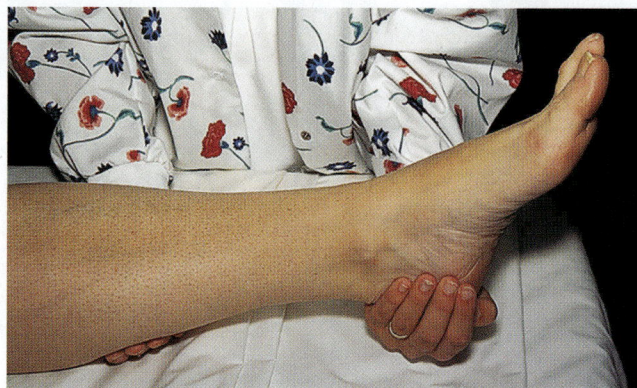

FIGURE 46.19 Using a cupped hand to support a joint.

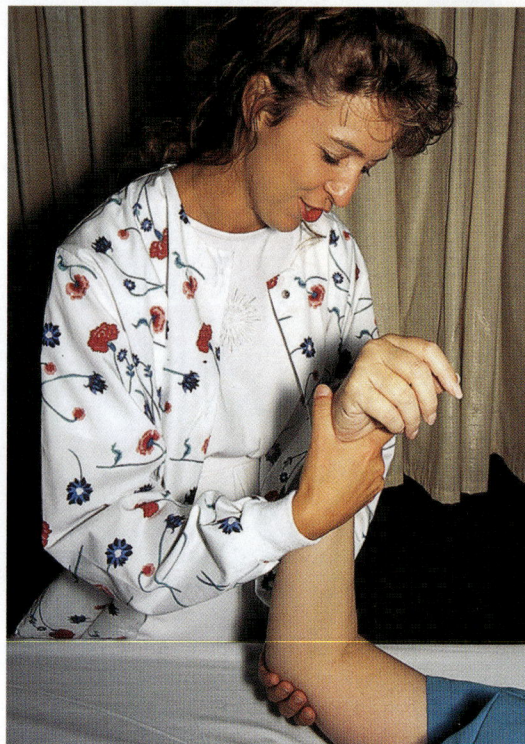

FIGURE 46.20 Supporting the joint by holding the distal and proximal areas adjacent to the joint.

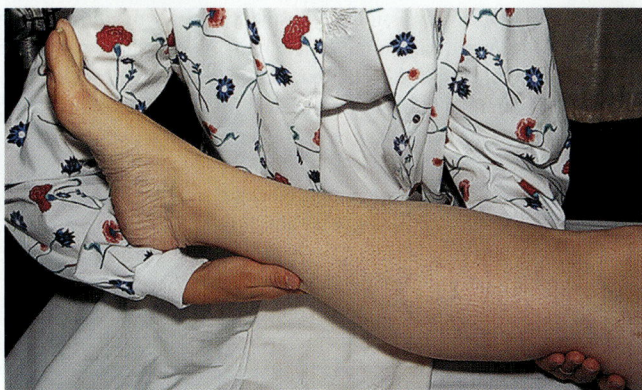

FIGURE 46.21 Cradling the distal portion of an extremity.

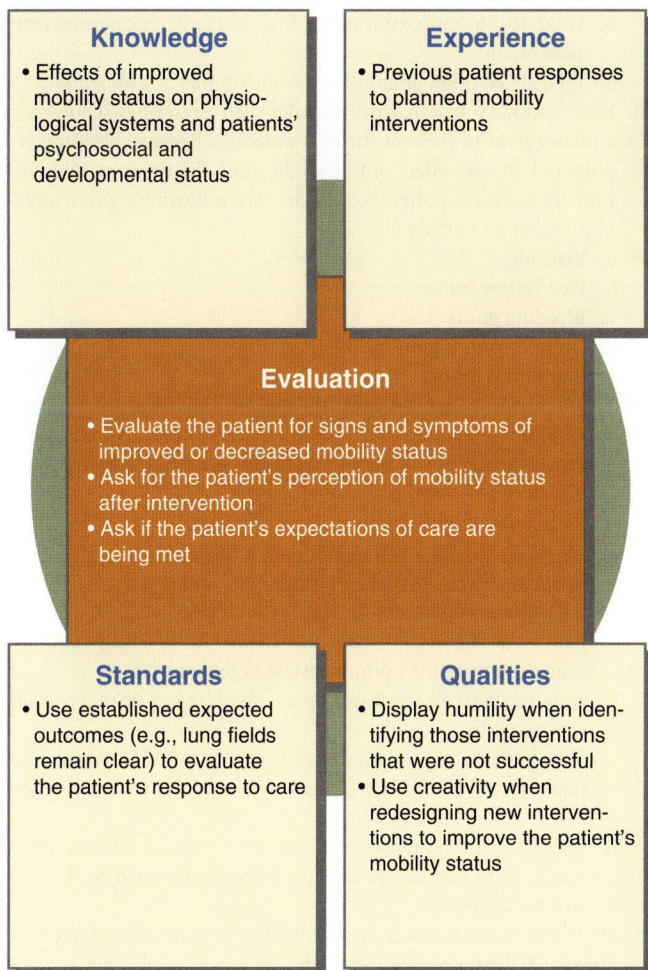

Knowledge
• Effects of improved mobility status on physiological systems and patients' psychosocial and developmental status

Experience
• Previous patient responses to planned mobility interventions

Evaluation
• Evaluate the patient for signs and symptoms of improved or decreased mobility status
• Ask for the patient's perception of mobility status after intervention
• Ask if the patient's expectations of care are being met

Standards
• Use established expected outcomes (e.g., lung fields remain clear) to evaluate the patient's response to care

Qualities
• Display humility when identifying those interventions that were not successful
• Use creativity when redesigning new interventions to improve the patient's mobility status

FIGURE 46.22 Critical thinking model for immobility evaluation.

Patient Expectations. Patients who are immobile and dependent on others for some or all of their needs are at risk of becoming overly dependent or doing too much themselves too early. Finding the balance between independence and dependence is a difficult task. Desire for control over mobility is unique for each patient. For the patient who is completely dependent on others for care, control over how and when things are done may be very important. Important questions that nurses must consider regarding patient expectations include the following: Do patients feel they are treated with dignity? Do caregivers treat them as adults? Are they given opportunities to make meaningful choices? For patients who are immobile, it is essential to collaborate on a mutually acceptable plan of care.

KEY CONCEPTS

• Body mechanics are the coordinated efforts of the musculoskeletal and nervous systems as the person moves, lifts, bends, stands, sits, lies down, and completes daily activities.
• Balance is assisted through nervous system control by the cerebellum and inner ear.
• Range-of-motion (ROM) exercises include one or all of the body joints and can be active or passive.
• Body alignment is the condition of joints, tendons, ligaments, and muscles in various body positions.
• Balance is achieved when a wide base of support is present, the centre of gravity falls within the base of support, and a vertical line falls from the centre of gravity through the base of support.
• Developmental stages influence body alignment and mobility; the greatest impact of physiological changes on the musculoskeletal system is observed in children and older persons.
• The risk of disabilities related to immobilization depends on the extent and duration of immobilization and the patient's overall level of health.
• Immobility may result from illness or trauma or may be prescribed for therapeutic reasons (bed rest).
• Immobility presents hazards in the physiological, psychological, and developmental dimensions.
• The nursing process and critical thinking synthesis are used to provide care for patients who are experiencing or are at risk for the side effects of impaired body alignment and immobility.
• After identifying nursing diagnoses, nurses plan and implement interventions to prevent or minimize the hazards and complications of impaired body alignment and immobilization.
• Patients with weakness and impaired function of the nervous, skeletal, or muscular system often require nursing assistance to attain proper body alignment while in bed or sitting and to transfer from a bed to a chair.
• Positioning devices help patients maintain good body alignment while lying or sitting.
• Assistive devices to promote walking include canes, walkers, and crutches.

CRITICAL THINKING EXERCISES

1. You are caring for a 57-year-old patient who had bilateral total knee replacements for osteoarthritis 2 days ago. The patient is beginning to transfer to a chair with help. The patient is 45 kg overweight and has a history of deep vein thrombosis. The patient has compression stockings, continuous passive range of motion, and a saline lock. Make a list of potential nursing diagnoses.
2. When you are conducting a home visit for a 75-year-old woman, the patient's granddaughter runs in and says, "Did you show the nurse the sore on your leg that you got from falling yesterday?" What questions about mobility are important to ask the patient? How do you begin your assessment?
3. You are caring for a 68-year-old man who is immobilized after spinal cord trauma from a motor vehicle accident. What potential complications would you assess for in this patient?

Answers to Critical Thinking Exercises appear on the Evolve website.

REVIEW QUESTIONS

Review Questions 1 to 13 relate to the case study at the beginning of the chapter.

1. As the nurse caring for Kate, you will assess for physiological risks of immobility that include:
   a. Increased respiratory rate, muscle atrophy, skin breakdown
   b. Decreased respiratory rate, joint contractures, decreased heart rate
   c. Decreased respiratory rate, increased basal metabolic rate, increased muscle tone
   d. Increased respiratory rate, joint contractures, increased muscle tone

2. During the time that Kate is unable to mobilize, priority nursing assessments will include the following areas:
   a. Metabolic, genitourinary, gastrointestinal
   b. Respiratory, cardiovascular, integumentary
   c. ADLs, genitourinary, integumentary
   d. IADLs, musculoskeletal, metabolic

3. As a result of Kate's limited mobility, complications of immobility are a concern. During assessment, the nurse notes that Kate has difficulty breathing while lying flat. Which of the following assessment data support a possible pulmonary condition related to impaired mobility? *(Select all that apply.)*
   a. BP is 128/84 mm Hg
   b. Respirations are 26/min on room air
   c. HR is 114 beats/min
   d. Crackles over lower lobes heard on auscultation
   e. Pain reported as 3 on a scale from 0 to 10 after medication

4. After 4 days, Kate is still unable to walk. On assessment, the nurse identifies the following as a sign associated with immobility:
   a. Decreased peristalsis
   b. Decreased heart rate
   c. Increased blood pressure
   d. Increased urinary output

5. By conducting comprehensive, holistic assessments, the nurse identifies the following nursing diagnosis for Kate: *(Select all that apply.)*
   a. Ineffective breathing pattern
   b. Increased activity tolerance
   c. Risk for infection
   d. Risk for interrupted family processes
   e. Risk for ineffective individual coping

6. To maintain a patent airway in patients who are immobile, which of the following nursing interventions should be implemented? *(Select all that apply.)*
   a. Isometric exercises
   b. Administration of a low-dose anticoagulant
   c. Nasotracheal or orotracheal suction, as needed
   d. Use of an incentive spirometer every 2 hours while awake

7. Kate's primary health care provider prescribes elastic stockings, or thromboembolic device hose. When applying the elastic stockings on Kate, the nurse teaches Kate that the purpose of the elastic stockings is to _____.
   a. Increase blood pressure
   b. Promote venous return to the heart
   c. Prevent pressure injuries
   d. Assist with range of motion exercises

8. One week after admission to hospital, Kate is diagnosed with hospital-acquired pneumonia. Kate remains unable to walk, with partial mobility in bed. Her primary health care provider prescribes sequential compression devices (SCD). When assessing to confirm that the SCDs have been applied correctly, proper application is confirmed when: *(Select all that apply.)*
   a. Initial patient measurement is made around the calves.
   b. Inflation pressure averages 40 mm Hg.
   c. The patient's leg is placed in the SCD sleeve, with back of knee aligned with popliteal opening on the sleeve.
   d. The activation light indicates the SCD is functioning.

9. During the time that SCD is prescribed for Kate, the nurse will complete which of the following shift assessments?
   a. Vital signs, daily weight, nutritional assessment
   b. Vital signs, peripheral vascular assessment of the legs, skin integrity of the lower legs
   c. Waist-to-hip ratio, vital signs, thigh circumference, respiratory assessment
   d. Vital signs, thigh circumference, nutritional assessments

10. Kate's primary health care provider also prescribes a low-dose anticoagulant to prevent thrombophlebitis. Because bleeding is a potential adverse effect of this medication, the nurse should continually assess the patient for which of the following signs of bleeding? *(Select all that apply.)*
    a. Bruising
    b. Pale yellow urine
    c. Bleeding gums
    d. Coffee ground–like emesis
    e. Light brown stool

11. When planning care for Kate, which of the following nursing measures will best facilitate the resumption of activities of daily living?
    a. Encouraging use of an overhead trapeze for positioning and transfer
    b. Frequent family visits
    c. Assisting Kate to a wheelchair once a day
    d. Ensuring there is a prescription for physiotherapy

12. Patient-centred outcomes for Kate will include:
    a. Pain is maintained at 5 on a scale from 0 to 10, family visiting is limited to promote optimal rest, skin remains intact
    b. Adherence to all treatments prescribed by her primary health care provider
    c. Skin remains dry and intact, lower extremity pulses remain palpable, family presence is facilitated, Kate is able to transfer from bed to chair with assistance
    d. Daily nutritional intake will increase with Kate consuming all meals, Kate will accept maximum assistance with ADLs, skin will remain intact

13. Preventative measures to reduce the risk of Kate developing musculoskeletal complications include:
    a. Integration of foods high in omega 3 fatty acids
    b. Prophylactic therapy with muscle relaxants
    c. Assisting with range-of-motion exercises throughout the day
    d. Application of elastic stockings

Answers: 1. a; **2.** b; **3.** b, c, d; **4.** a; **5.** a, c, d, e; **6.** c, d; **7.** b; **8.** b, c, d; **9.** b; **10.** a, c, d; **11.** a; **12.** c; **13.** c.

🌐 *Rationales for the Review Questions appear on the Evolve website.*

RECOMMENDED WEBSITES

(American) Association of Rehabilitation Nurses: https://www.rehabnurse.org

This website provides an extensive list of links to resources for nurses working with patients with actual or potential impairments or disabilities. It provides information about both prevention and treatment. Although the content has an American orientation, it is also useful to Canadian nurses.

Canadian Physical Activity Guidelines: https://csepguidelines.ca

The Canadian Society of Exercise Physiologists provides guides to physical activity for all age groups and has developed guidelines specific to persons with spinal cord injuries. The guidelines provided through this website are a good source of consumer education on the benefits of activity.

Osteoporosis Canada: https://www.osteoporosis.ca

Osteoporosis Canada is a national organization that works toward educating and supporting individuals and communities in the prevention and treatment of osteoporosis. This website provides numerous links to evidence-informed resources on osteoporosis.

Registered Nurses' Association of Ontario (RNAO) Best Practice Guidelines: *Preventing Falls and Reducing Injury from Falls*: https://rnao.ca/bpg/guidelines/prevention-falls-and-fall-injuries

The RNAO has developed a series of practice guidelines based on the consensus of nurse experts across a variety of practice, academic, and research agencies. This site provides information on preventing falls and reducing risk for falls among adults age 18 years and older across the continuum of care..

Wounds Canada: https://www.woundscanada.ca

Wounds Canada is a nonprofit organization dedicated to advancing wound prevention and care for Canadians. Wounds Canada develops and provides educational resources and programs and supports research to promote best practices that inform clinicians, support persons living with wounds, and advise policymakers. Their *Foundations of Best Practice for Skin and Wound Management* can be found at the following URL: https://www.woundscanada.ca/docman/public/health-care-professional/bpr-workshop/165-wc-bpr-prevention-and-management-of-wounds/file.

REFERENCES

A full reference list is available on the website for this book at http://evolve.elsevier.com/Canada/Potter/fundamentals/

47

Skin Integrity and Wound Care

Canadian content written by Rosemary Kohr, RN, BA, BScN, MScN, PhD, Tertiary Care Nurse Practitioner Certificate, with original chapter contributions by Janice C. Colwell, RN, MS, CWOCN, FAAN

OBJECTIVES

Mastery of content in this chapter will enable you to:

- Describe the key terms listed.
- Identify the risk factors that contribute to pressure injury formation.
- Recognize the stages of pressure injury.
- Describe the etiology and key components of venous, arterial, diabetic, and malignant wounds.
- Explain the normal process of wound healing.
- Describe the differences between wounds that heal by primary and secondary intention.
- Describe the complications of wound healing.

- Explain the factors that impede or promote wound healing.
- Describe the differences in nursing care for acute and chronic wounds.
- Describe the types of dressings appropriate for moist wound healing.
- Complete an assessment for a patient with impaired skin integrity.
- List nursing diagnoses associated with impaired skin integrity.
- Develop a nursing care plan for a patient with impaired skin integrity.
- List appropriate nursing interventions for a patient with impaired skin integrity.
- State evaluation criteria for a patient with impaired skin integrity.

KEY TERMS

Abrasion	Fistula	Puncture
Approximated	Friction	Purulent
Blanching	Granulation tissue	Sanguineous
Collagen	Hematoma	Secondary intention
Darkly pigmented skin	Hemorrhage	Serosanguineous
Debridement	Hemostasis	Serous
Dehiscence	Hyperemia	Shear
Drainage evacuators	Induration	Slough
Epithelialization	Laceration	Sutures
Eschar	Nonviable tissue	Tissue ischemia
Evisceration	Periwound	Wound
Exudate	Pressure injury	Wound contraction
Fibrin	Primary intention	

WEBSITE

http://evolve.elsevier.com/Canada/Potter/fundamentals/

CASE STUDY

For many patients, the wound is only a part of the story. For example, consider the following scenario:

You are caring for Kathy, a 65-year-old woman (preferred pronouns: she/her) who lives with her recently retired husband and who has a 30-year history of diabetes mellitus. She currently takes insulin, but her diabetes is poorly controlled because of her inability to adhere to a 1 200-calorie diabetic diet and her "hit-or-miss" approach to testing her serum glucose on a regular basis. She is 32 kg overweight.

For the last 10 years, she has reported decreased sensation in her lower extremities. She does not practise good foot care; she cuts her own toenails and, at home, goes barefoot or wears socks. She regularly soaks her feet in an Epsom-salt footbath because she "read this was good for your feet."

She was admitted to the hospital for elective repair of an abdominal aneurysm. The surgery went well, but postoperatively Kathy had difficulty ambulating or performing coughing and deep-breathing exercises. On her second postoperative day, she developed pneumonia, which required intravenous antibiotics. During

Continued

the course of her pneumonia, Kathy stated she was "too tired" to walk or get up to use the commode or toilet. She required an adult continence product as she was now incontinent of urine and stool. She complained of pain when repositioned and would generally reposition herself on her back. Two weeks after her surgery, Kathy developed a large, draining sacral wound, which is now 6 cm in diameter. The base of the wound can be visualized down to bone. In

addition, she has a small (3 × 4 cm) area covered with a hard black eschar on her left heel. Skin assessment also reveals areas of prolonged redness over pressure points, especially on the right heel and over both hips.

Think about this case study as you read this chapter. There are review questions at the end of the chapter that relate to the case study.

When planning care for Kathy in the case study above, a concept map is useful for individualizing care for her because she has multiple health conditions and related nursing diagnoses (Figure 47.1). This map assists in using critical thinking skills to organize complex patient assessment data and related nursing diagnoses with the patient's chief medical diagnosis. As the nurse identifies linkages between nursing diagnoses and patient's medical diagnosis, the concept map also links potential interventions with the patient's health care needs and goals.

Skin, the body's largest organ, constitutes 15% of the total adult body weight (Wysocki, 2016). It protects against disease-causing organisms; senses pain, temperature, and touch; and synthesizes vitamin D. Injury to the skin poses risks to safety and triggers a complex healing response.

As a nurse, one of your most important responsibilities is to monitor skin integrity and prevent skin breakdown. Understanding normal

wound healing helps in planning, implementing, and assessing interventions that maintain skin integrity and optimize wound healing.

SCIENTIFIC KNOWLEDGE BASE

Skin

The skin has two layers: the epidermis and the dermis (Figure 47.2). These two layers are separated by a membrane, often referred to as the *dermal–epidermal junction*. The epidermis, or top layer, also consists of several layers. The stratum corneum is the thin, outermost layer of the epidermis, consisting of flattened, keratinized cells. The cells originate from the innermost epidermal (or basal) layer. These cells divide, proliferate, and migrate toward the epidermal surface.

After cells reach the stratum corneum, they flatten and die. This constant movement ensures replacement of surface cells sloughed

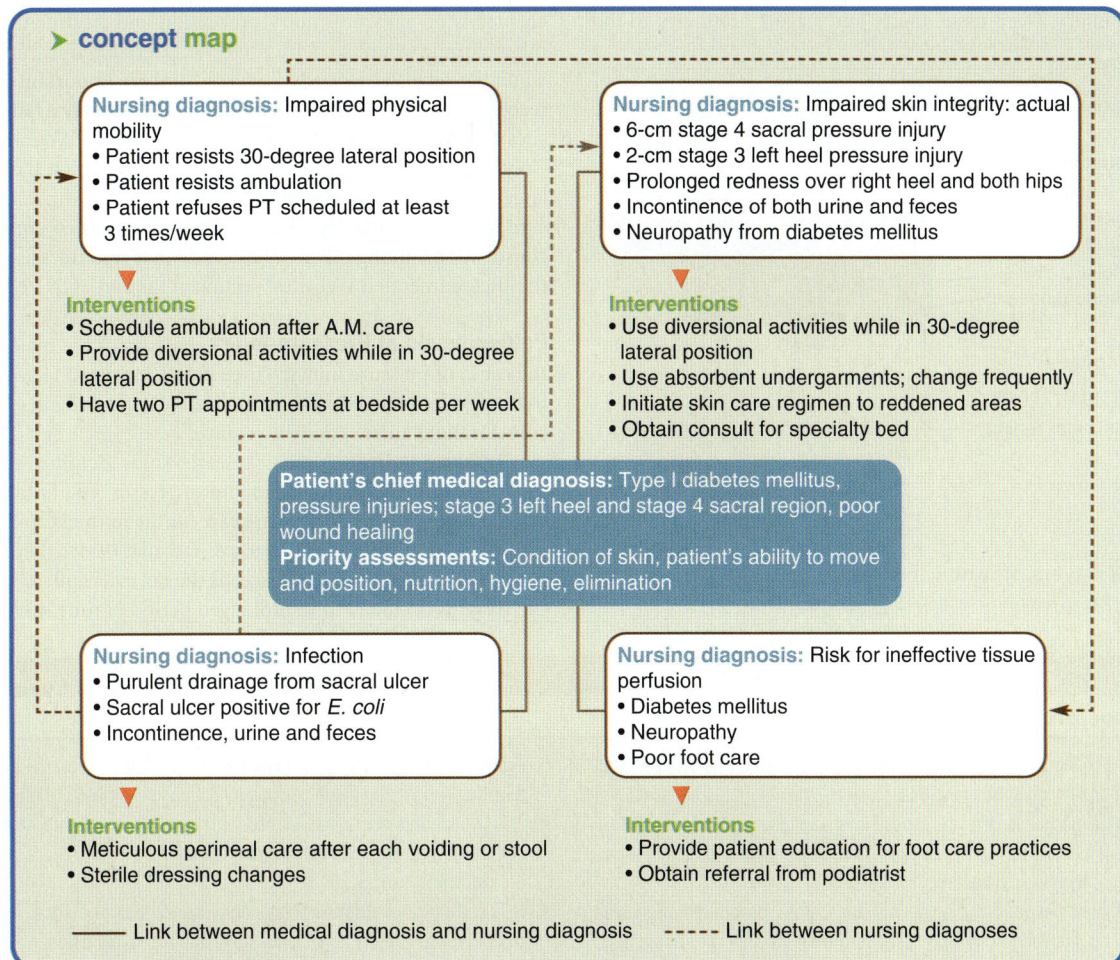

FIGURE 47.1 Concept map for a patient with a chronic wound. *PT,* Physiotherapy.

during normal desquamation or shedding. The stratum corneum protects underlying cells and tissues from dehydration and prevents the entrance of certain chemical agents. The stratum corneum allows the evaporation of water from the skin and permits the absorption of certain topical medications.

The dermis, the inner layer of the skin, provides tensile strength, mechanical support, and protection to the underlying muscles, bones, and organs. It differs from the epidermis in that it contains mostly connective tissue and few skin cells. Collagen (a tough, fibrous protein), blood vessels, and nerves are in the dermal layer. Fibroblasts, which are responsible for collagen formation, are the only distinctive cell type within the dermis.

Understanding skin structure helps nurses to maintain skin integrity and promote wound healing. Intact skin protects the patient from chemical and mechanical injuries. When the skin is injured, the epidermis functions to resurface the wound and restore the barrier against invading organisms while the dermis responds to restore the structural integrity (collagen) and the physical properties of the skin. Age alters skin characteristics and makes skin more vulnerable to damage. Box 47.1 provides a summary of the changes in aging skin.

Pressure Injury

Pressure ulcer, pressure sore, decubitus ulcer, and *bedsore* have long been used as terms describing impaired skin integrity related to unrelieved, prolonged pressure. However, this terminology has been changed to *pressure injury,* and staging now uses numbers rather than Roman numerals (National Pressure Injury Advisory Panel [NPIAP], 2017). This change reflects the fact that not all impaired skin integrity results in a pressure injury. Deep tissue injury and stage 1 are injury to the

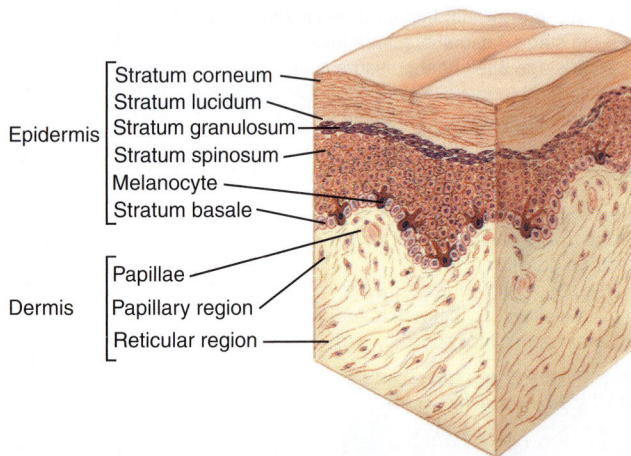

FIGURE 47.2 Layers of skin. (From Applegate, E. [2011]. *The anatomy and physiology learning system* [4th ed.]. Saunders.)

tissue without breaking the skin, although at high risk of further damage. The pressure injury guidelines developed by the Registered Nurses' Association of Ontario (RNAO) (RNAO, 2016a) provide consistency with the NPIAP standards. A **pressure injury** is localized to skin and underlying tissue, usually over a bony prominence, as a result of pressure, shear, or friction, or a combination of these factors and is affected by moisture, nutrition, perfusion, and comorbidities (Figure 47.3).

Pressure injuries have a high prevalence rate in all health care settings. While it is a challenge to arrive at accurate figures, the classic study by Woodbury and Houghton (2004) estimates that one in four individuals within the Canadian health care system—including acute care, complex continuing care, home care, and long-term care—has some issue with skin integrity, and reflects inadequate clinician observation. The consistent "take-home" message is that many chronic wounds are preventable and, with appropriate management, healable.

The impact of pressure injury and other chronic wounds on quality of life is significant, as normal activities may be restricted because of pain, odour, or treatments. Costs associated with chronic wound care can substantially increase the burden on the health care system. It has been estimated that chronic wounds' cost to the Canadian health care system is approximately $3.9 billion annually—approximately 3% of total health care expenditures. Given the increase in the aging population and the fact that chronic illnesses such as diabetes are on the rise, it is reasonable to predict an increase in costs related to chronic wound care in the decades to come (WOUNDS National Stakeholder Roundtable Report, 2012).

Thus, it is essential that attention be paid to the causes of pressure injury as well as to the healing process of wounds. The focus of this chapter is on pressure injury prevention and treatment options, but other chronic wounds, such as diabetic, arterial, venous, and malignant wounds, will also be briefly discussed and are important for nurses to recognize and treat. Additional resources are readily available on websites for Wounds Canada, Nurses Specialized in Wound, Ostomy & Continence Canada (NSWOCC), and RNAO, which has produced a large number of evidence-informed Best Practice Guidelines for pressure injuries, venous leg ulcers, diabetic foot ulcers, continence, and constipation, among others. These and other resources are provided in the "Recommended Websites" section at the end of this chapter.

Pathogenesis of Pressure Injury. Pressure is the major element in the cause of pressure injury. Three pressure-related factors contribute to the development of pressure injuries: (1) pressure intensity, (2) pressure duration, and (3) tissue tolerance.

Pressure Intensity. A classic research study identified capillary closing pressure as the minimal amount of pressure required to collapse a capillary (e.g., when the pressure exceeds the normal capillary pressure range of 15 to 32 mm Hg) (Burton & Yamada, 1951). Therefore, if pressure applied over a capillary exceeds the normal capillary pressure and the vessel is occluded for a prolonged period of time, **tissue ischemia**,

BOX 47.1 FOCUS ON OLDER PERSONS

Skin-Associated Issues

- Age-related changes, such as reduced skin elasticity, decreased collagen, and thinning of underlying muscle and tissues, cause the older person's skin to be easily torn via mechanical trauma, especially shearing forces (Wysocki, 2016).
- Concomitant medical conditions and polypharmacy, common in the older person, interfere with wound healing.
- The attachment between the epidermis and dermis becomes flattened in older persons, allowing skin to be easily torn from mechanical trauma (e.g., tape removal).

- Aging causes a diminished inflammatory response, resulting in slow epithelialization and wound healing (Doughty & Sparks-Defriese, 2016).
- The hypodermis decreases in size with age. Older patients have little subcutaneous padding over bony prominences, so they are more prone to skin breakdown (Wysocki, 2016).
- Reduced nutritional intake, commonly seen in older persons, increases the risk of pressure injury development and impaired wound healing (Gould et al., 2015).

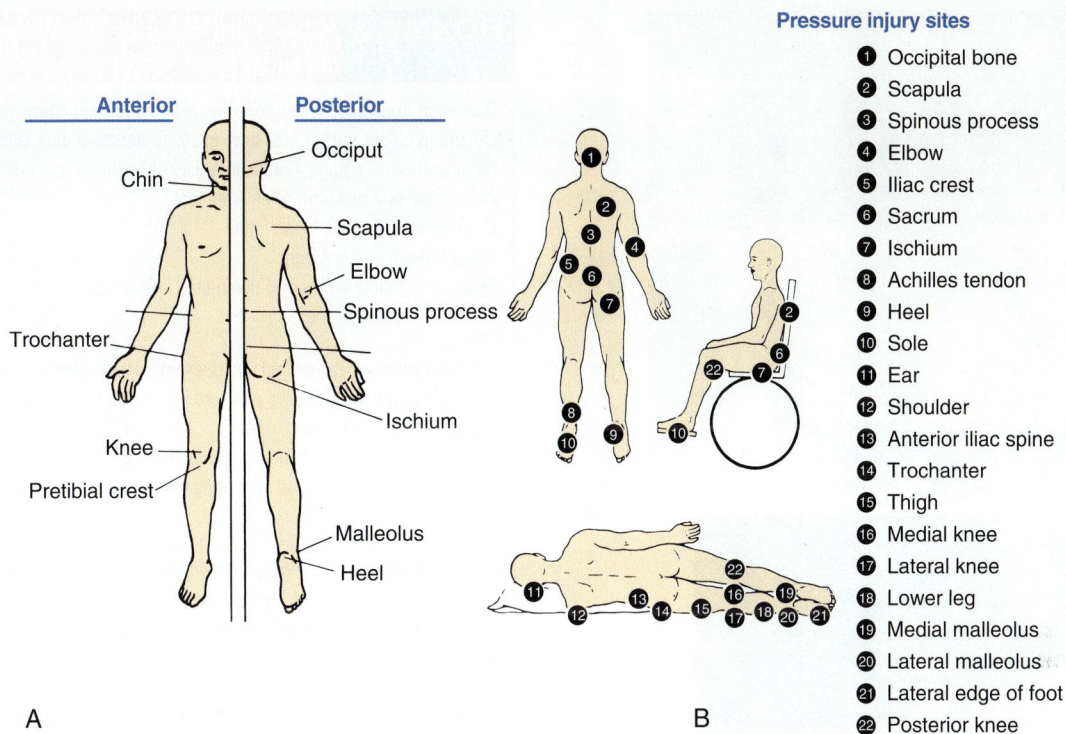

Pressure injury sites
1. Occipital bone
2. Scapula
3. Spinous process
4. Elbow
5. Iliac crest
6. Sacrum
7. Ischium
8. Achilles tendon
9. Heel
10. Sole
11. Ear
12. Shoulder
13. Anterior iliac spine
14. Trochanter
15. Thigh
16. Medial knee
17. Lateral knee
18. Lower leg
19. Medial malleolus
20. Lateral malleolus
21. Lateral edge of foot
22. Posterior knee

FIGURE 47.3 A, Bony prominences most frequently underlying pressure injury. **B,** Common pressure injury sites. (Adapted from Trelease, C. C. [1988]. Developing standards for wound care. *Ostomy/Wound Management, 20,* 46.)

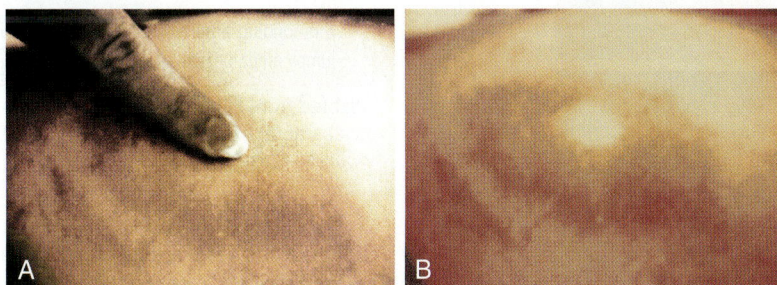

FIGURE 47.4 A, Reactive hyperemia. **B,** Blanching erythema: blanches with fingertip pressure.

or reduction in blood flow, can occur. If the patient has decreased sensation and thus does not have the cue of discomfort to prompt shifting (off-loading) pressure, tissue death may result. The clinical presentation of obstructed blood flow occurs when the nurse evaluates areas of pressure. After a period of tissue ischemia, if pressure is relieved and blood flow returns, the skin turns red. The effect of this redness is vasodilatation (blood vessel expansion), called **hyperemia** (redness) (Figure 47.4, *A*). The area of hyperemia is evaluated by pressing a finger over the affected area. If the area blanches (turns lighter in colour) (see Figure 47.4, *B*) and the redness returns when you remove your finger, hyperemia is transient and is an attempt to overcome the ischemic episode; thus, it is called *blanching hyperemia* (Pieper, 2016). If, however, the erythematous area does not blanch *(nonblanching erythema)* (Figure 47.5) when you apply pressure, deeper tissue damage is probable.

Blanching occurs when the normal red tones of light-skinned patients are absent. Blanching does not occur in patients with darkly pigmented skin. The definition derived by the Task Force on the Implications for Darkly Pigmented Intact Skin in the Prediction and Prevention of Pressure Ulcers (Bennett, 1995) still stands today (Edsberg et al., 2016). **Darkly pigmented skin** is defined as skin that "remains

unchanged (does not blanch) when pressure is applied over a bony prominence, irrespective of the patient's race or ethnicity." Characteristics of intact dark skin that will alert nurses to the potential for pressure injuries are found in Box 47.2.

Pressure Duration. Two considerations are related to duration of pressure. Low pressures over a prolonged time period and high-intensity pressure over a short period of time both cause tissue damage. Extended pressure occludes blood flow and nutrients and contributes to cell death (Pieper, 2016). Clinical implications of pressure duration include evaluating the amount of pressure (check the skin for reactive hyperemia) and the amount of time that a patient tolerates pressure (check to be sure that after removing pressure, the affected area blanches).

Tissue Tolerance. The ability of tissue to endure pressure depends on the integrity of both the tissue and supporting structures. The extrinsic factors of shear, friction, and moisture affect the ability of the skin to tolerate pressure: the greater the degree to which these factors are present, the more susceptible the skin will be to damage from pressure. Another factor related to tissue tolerance pertains to the ability of the underlying skin structures (blood vessels, collagen) to assist in

BOX 47.2   **Characteristics of Dark Skin at Risk of Skin Breakdown**

Dark skin tones, especially darkly pigmented skin, may not demonstrate change in colour with a pressure injury. To assess a dark-skinned patient for the presence of a stage 1 pressure injury, the following should be considered:
Assess the skin in a well-lit environment.
Use natural light or halogen light.
Avoid using florescent light.
Assess the following (assess noninjured skin areas first):

Colour
- Colour remains unchanged and does not blanch when pressure is applied.
- If patient previously had a pressure injury, that area of skin might be lighter than the original colour.
- Localized areas of inflammation may take on an eggplant (purplish-blue or violet) colour rather than appearing reddened.

Temperature
- Circumscribed area of intact skin may be warm to touch. As tissue changes colour, intact skin feels cool to touch.
- Inflammation is detected by making comparisons to surrounding skin.

Appearance
- Edema may occur with induration and appear taut and shiny.
- Injured skin with a stage 1 pressure injury might show low resilience. Document tissue resilience: tissue on palpation is boggy or mushy when compared to surrounding skin.

Palpation
- Surrounding area may be sensitive or tender to touch or may be hard or lumpy on palpation.

Adapted from Nix, D. P. (2016). Skin and wound inspection and assessment. In R. A. Bryant & D. P. Nix (Eds.), *Acute and chronic wounds: Current management concepts* (5th ed.). Elsevier.

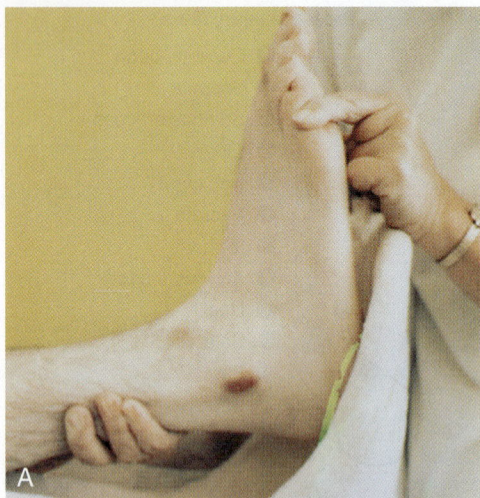

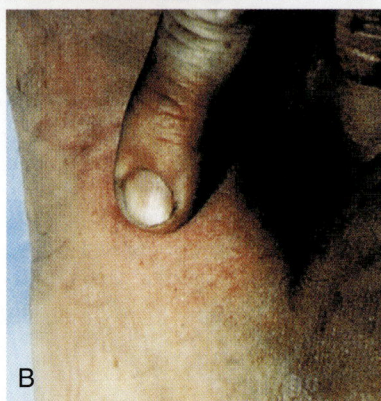

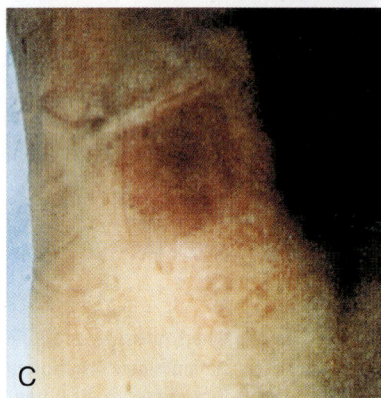

FIGURE 47.5 A, Reactive hyperemia. **B** and **C,** In nonblanching erythema, the area is much darker than the surrounding skin and does not blanch with fingertip pressure. (Pires, M., & Muller, A. [1991]. Detection and management of early tissue pressure indicators: A pictorial essay. *Progressions, 3*[3], 3.)

redistributing pressure. Systemic factors such as poor nutrition, age, and low blood pressure affect tissue tolerance to externally applied pressure.

NURSING KNOWLEDGE BASE

Prediction and Prevention of Pressure Injury

A major aspect of nursing care is the maintenance of skin integrity. Consistent, planned skin care interventions are critical to ensuring high-quality care. Nurses need to take every opportunity to observe and assess their patients' skin for impaired skin integrity.

Risk Factors for Pressure Injury Development. A variety of factors predisposes a patient to pressure injury. These factors are often directly related to disease, such as a decreased level of consciousness, the after-effects of trauma, or the presence of a cast, or are secondary to an illness, such as decreased sensation after a cerebrovascular accident.

The use of a pressure injury risk assessment tool, such as the Braden Scale (Braden & Bergstrom, 1988; discussed later), provides an initial assessment to determine appropriate interventions and ongoing regular assessment to evaluate skin status and treatment efficacy.

Impaired Sensory Perception. Patients with altered sensory perception of pain and pressure are at more risk of impaired skin integrity than are patients with normal sensation. Patients with impaired sensory perception of pain and pressure may not feel increased, prolonged pressure or pain and are at high risk of developing a pressure injury.

Impaired Mobility. Patients unable to independently change positions are at risk for pressure injury development. For example, patients with spinal cord injuries have decreased or absent motor and sensory perception and are unable to reposition themselves.

Alteration in Level of Consciousness. Patients who are confused or disoriented or with changing levels of consciousness may not be able to understand the sensation of pressure and respond by repositioning independently. As well, they may not be able to communicate discomfort or pain. Patients in a coma cannot perceive pressure and are unable to move voluntarily to relieve pressure.

Shear. **Shear** is the force exerted parallel to the skin and results from both gravity pushing down on the body and resistance (friction) between the patient and a surface (Pieper, 2016). For example, shear force occurs when the head of the bed is elevated and the skeleton starts to slide but the skin is fixed because of friction with the bed (Figure 47.6). In addition, shear force occurs when a patient is transferred from the bed to a stretcher and the patient's skin is pulled across the bed. When shear is present, the skin and subcutaneous layers adhere to the surface of the bed, while layers of muscle and the bones slide in the direction of body movement. The underlying tissue capillaries are stretched and angulated by the shear force. As a result, necrosis occurs deep within the tissue layers, causing undermining of the dermis. Heels are particularly vulnerable to injury from shear as patients are often repositioned in bed without the heels being supported.

Friction. The force of two surfaces moving across one another, such as the mechanical force exerted when skin is dragged across a coarse surface such as bed linens, is called **friction** (Wound, Ostomy and Continence Nurses Society [WOCN], 2016). Unlike shear injuries, friction injuries affect the epidermis, or top layer of the skin. The denuded skin appears red and painful and is sometimes referred to as a "sheet burn." A friction injury occurs in a patient who is dragged over the bed surface instead of being lifted slightly during position changes.

Moisture. The presence and duration of moisture on the skin increases the risk of ulcer formation. Moisture reduces the skin's resistance to other physical factors such as pressure and shear force. Prolonged moisture softens skin, which makes it more susceptible to damage. Immobilized patients, who are unable to take care of their own hygiene needs, depend on nurses to keep their skin dry and intact. Skin moisture originates from wound drainage, excessive perspiration, and fecal or urinary incontinence.

Nutrition. Adequate nutritional intake is essential for not only wound healing but also wound prevention (Kennerly et al., 2015). In particular, high-protein oral nutritional supplementation is necessary in patients whose prealbumin or albumin, hemoglobin, and serum zinc stores are low (Litchford et al., 2014; Posthauer et al., 2015; RNAO, 2016a).

For patients weakened or debilitated by illness, nutritional therapy is especially important. A patient who has undergone surgery (see Chapter 49) and is well nourished still requires at least 1 500 kcal/day for nutritional maintenance. Alternatives such as enteral feedings and parenteral nutrition (see Chapter 43) are available for patients unable to maintain normal food intake.

Normal wound healing also requires proper nutrition (Table 47.1). Deficiencies in any of the essential nutrients result in impaired or delayed healing (Stotts, 2016a). Physiological processes of wound healing depend on availability of protein, vitamins (especially A and C), and trace minerals such as zinc and copper. **Collagen** is a protein formed from amino acids acquired by fibroblasts from protein ingested in food. Vitamin C is necessary for the synthesis of collagen, and

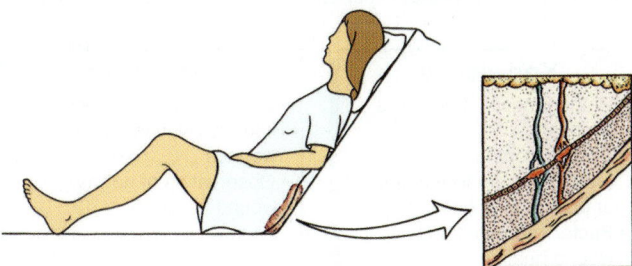

FIGURE 47.6 Sketch of shear force exerted against the sacral area.

TABLE 47.1 Role of Selected Nutrients in Wound Healing

Nutrient	Role in Healing	Recommendations	Sources
Calories	Fuel for cell energy "protein protection"	35–40 kcal/kg/day, or enough to maintain positive nitrogen balance	
Protein	Fibroplasia, angiogenesis, collagen formation, and wound remodelling, immune function	1.0–1.5 g/kg/day, or enough to maintain positive nitrogen balance	Poultry, fish, eggs, beef
Vitamin C (ascorbic acid)	Collagen synthesis, capillary wall integrity, fibroblast function, immunological function, antioxidant	100–1 000 mg/day Need long time before clinical scurvy from vitamin C deficiency develops Low toxicity	Citrus fruits, tomatoes, potatoes, fortified fruit juices
Vitamin A	Epithelialization, wound closure, inflammatory response, angiogenesis, collagen formation Can reverse steroid effects on skin and delayed healing	1 600–2 000 retinol equivalents per day Supplement if deficient 20 000 units × 10 days	Green leafy vegetables (spinach), broccoli, carrots, sweet potatoes, liver
Vitamin E	No known role in wound healing, antioxidant	None	Fish, oysters, liver, dark meat, eggs, legumes
Zinc	Collagen formation, protein synthesis, cell membrane and host defences	15–30 mg Correct deficiencies No improvement in wound healing with supplementation unless zinc deficient Use with caution: large doses can be toxic May inhibit copper metabolism and impair immune function	Vegetables, meats, legumes
Fluid	Essential fluid environment for all cell functions	30–35 mL/kg/day Increase by another 10–15 mL/kg if patient is on an air-fluidized bed	Use noncaffeine, nonalcoholic fluids without sugar Water is best: 6–8 glasses/day

Adapted from Ayello, E. A., Thomas, D. R., & Litchford, M. A. (1999). Nutritional aspects of wound healing. *Home Health Nurse, 17*(11), 719; and Stotts, N. A. (2016). Nutritional assessment and support. In R. A. Bryant & D. P. Nix (Eds.), *Acute and chronic wounds: Current management concepts* (5th ed.). Mosby.

vitamin A reduces the negative effects of steroids on wound healing. Zinc is used for epithelialization and collagen synthesis, and copper for collagen fibre linking.

Calories provide the energy to support wound healing. Protein needs, especially, are increased. A balanced nutrient intake is critical for wound healing, including protein, fat, carbohydrates, vitamins, and minerals. Serum proteins are biochemical indicators of malnutrition (Stotts, 2016a). Although serum albumin is the most frequently measured of these laboratory parameters, it is not sensitive to rapid changes in nutritional status. The best measure of nutritional status is prealbumin because it reflects not only what the patient has ingested but also what the body has absorbed, digested, and metabolized (Stotts, 2016a).

Tissue Perfusion. Oxygen fuels the cellular functions essential to the healing process; therefore, the ability to perfuse the tissues with adequate amounts of oxygenated blood is critical to wound healing (Doughty & Sparks-Defriese, 2016). Patients with shock or peripheral vascular diseases, such as diabetes, are at risk of poor tissue perfusion due to poor circulation. Oxygen requirements depend on the phase of wound healing; for instance, chronic tissue hypoxia is associated with impaired collagen synthesis and reduced tissue resistance to infection.

Infection. Wound infection prolongs the inflammatory phase, delays collagen synthesis, prevents epithelialization, and increases the production of proinflammatory cytokines, which leads to additional tissue destruction (Stotts, 2016b). Indications that a wound infection is present are the presence of pus; a change in odour, volume, or the character of wound drainage; redness in the surrounding tissue; fever; or pain (Box 47.3).

Pain. Uncontrolled pain can affect the patient's ability to tolerate movement and can decrease tissue perfusion because of rapid, shallow breathing and tensed muscles. In addition, the patient's appetite may be diminished because of nausea from pain, and if the restorative powers of sleep are not accessible, the individual may feel hopeless and depressed from the unrelenting nature of both the wound and the persistent pain (Jenkins, 2020; Kohr & Gibson, 2008).

Age. Physiological changes occur with aging. These changes will affect the healing trajectory of a wound. For example, decrease in the functioning of macrophages leads to a delayed inflammatory response, delayed collagen synthesis, and slower epithelialization.

Psychosocial Impact of Wounds. The patient's psychological response to any wound is part of the nursing assessment. Body-image changes often impose a great stress on the patient's adaptive

mechanisms. In addition, body-image changes influence self-concept (see Chapter 27) and sexuality (see Chapter 28). Nurses must ensure that the patient's personal and social resources for adaptation are a part of the assessment. Factors that affect the patient's perception of the wound include the presence of scars, drains (drains are often necessary for weeks or even months after certain procedures), odour from drainage, and temporary or permanent prosthetic devices.

CRITICAL THINKING

Successful critical thinking requires a synthesis of knowledge, experience, information gathered from patients, critical thinking attitudes, and intellectual and professional standards. Clinical judgement involves anticipating the information necessary, analyzing the data, and making decisions regarding patient care. Critical thinking is always changing. During assessment, it is important to consider all elements that build toward making appropriate nursing diagnoses (Figure 47.7).

When caring for patients who have impaired skin integrity and chronic wounds, nurses must integrate knowledge from nursing and other disciplines, previous experiences, and information gathered from

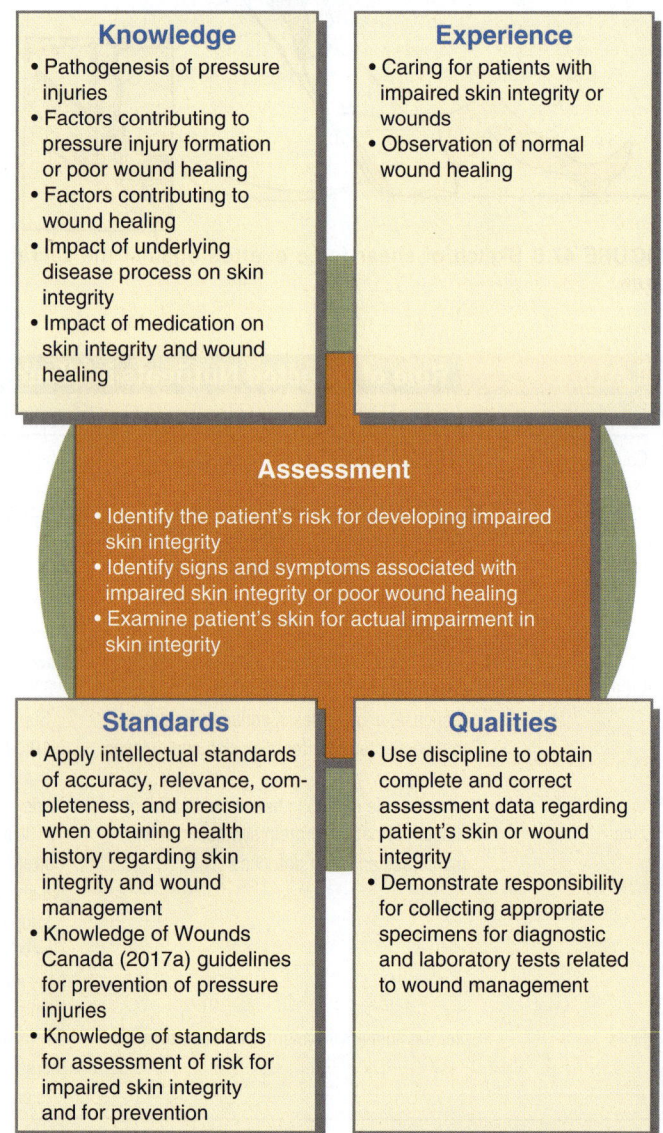

Knowledge
- Pathogenesis of pressure injuries
- Factors contributing to pressure injury formation or poor wound healing
- Factors contributing to wound healing
- Impact of underlying disease process on skin integrity
- Impact of medication on skin integrity and wound healing

Experience
- Caring for patients with impaired skin integrity or wounds
- Observation of normal wound healing

Assessment
- Identify the patient's risk for developing impaired skin integrity
- Identify signs and symptoms associated with impaired skin integrity or poor wound healing
- Examine patient's skin for actual impairment in skin integrity

Standards
- Apply intellectual standards of accuracy, relevance, completeness, and precision when obtaining health history regarding skin integrity and wound management
- Knowledge of Wounds Canada (2017a) guidelines for prevention of pressure injuries
- Knowledge of standards for assessment of risk for impaired skin integrity and for prevention

Qualities
- Use discipline to obtain complete and correct assessment data regarding patient's skin or wound integrity
- Demonstrate responsibility for collecting appropriate specimens for diagnostic and laboratory tests related to wound management

FIGURE 47.7 Critical thinking for skin integrity and wound care assessment.

BOX 47.3	Classic Signs of Wound Infection

- Pain and tenderness at the wound site
- Erythema (reddening of the surrounding tissue)
- Edema (swelling), **induration** (increased firmness of the tissue)
- Inflammation of wound edges
- Purulent discharge
- Warmth in surrounding tissue
- Fever, chills
- Foul odour
- Elevated white blood cell count
- Delayed healing

Chronic Wounds

These show the above signs and symptoms as well as the following:
- Increased exudates
- Bright red discoloration of granulation tissue
- New areas of slough or breakdown on the wound surface
- Undermining (dead space under the edges of the wound)

patients to understand the risks to skin integrity and wound healing. Knowledge of normal musculoskeletal physiology, the pathogenesis of pressure injuries, normal wound healing, and the pathophysiology of underlying diseases provides nurses with a scientific basis for care. Wounds Canada (formerly Canadian Association of Wound Care) (Orsted et al., 2017) and the RNAO (2016a) provide evidence-derived guidelines for assessment of the risk of impaired skin integrity, prevention measures, and interventions to promote wound healing, as well as other standards of practice that nurses should use in planning care. Past experience with patients at risk of impaired skin integrity or with patients with wounds increases the experiential knowledge base helping nurses to identify interventions.

Finally, as a nurse, you need to ensure that you remain attentive during assessment to obtain comprehensive and correct assessment data. As identified previously, a *continuum* exists to wound healing that implies change over time. You need to be aware that the patient and the skin or wound condition will not remain static, so you should reassess on a regular basis and adjust your plan of care accordingly. Knowledge and experience regarding wound healing will assist you in taking advantage of all the available and appropriate treatment options.

Assessment for tissue pressure damage involves visual and tactile inspection of the skin. The nurse's baseline assessment will determine the patient's normal skin characteristics and any potential or actual areas of breakdown (see Figure 47.3). The nurse needs to take into account the specific characteristics of a patient's skin, including pigmentation and effects of aging or medication (Bennett, 1995; Gould et al., 2015). Assessment characteristics of darkly pigmented skin appear in Boxes 47.4 and 47.5.

🌐 BOX 47.4 CULTURAL ASPECTS OF CARE

Skin Colour Impact

As a nurse, your ability to detect cyanosis and other changes in skin colour in patients is an important clinical skill. However, this detection can become a challenge in dark-skinned patients. Cyanosis is a slightly bluish greyish slate-like or dark purple discoloration of the skin due to tissues near the skin surface having low oxygen saturation. Colour differentiation of cyanosis varies according to skin pigmentation. In dark-skinned patients, you need to know the individual's baseline skin tone. You should not confuse the normal hyperpigmentation of congenital dermal melanocytosis seen on the sacrum of African, Indigenous, and Asian individuals as cyanosis. Observe the patient's skin in non-glare daylight. The Gaskin's Nursing Assessment of Skin Color (GNASC) is a useful assessment tool for identifying changes in skin colour that increase the patient's risk of pressure injuries.

Implications for Practice
- Cyanosis is difficult but possible to detect in the dark-skinned patient.
- Be aware of situations that produce changes in skin tone, such as inadequate lighting.
- Examine body sites with the least melanin, such as under the arm, for underlying colour identification.
- Evaluate pigmented skin for colour-specific changes in skin tone.

Adapted from Gaskin, F. C. (1986). Detection of cyanosis in the person with dark skin. *Journal of National Black Nurses' Association, 1,* 52; Myers, J. (2015). Challenges of identifying eczema in darkly pigmented skin. *Nursing Children and Young People, 27*(6), 24–28; National Pressure Injury Advisory Panel (NPIAP). (2019). *Pressure injury stages.* https://npiap.com/page/PressureInjuryStages; Henderson, C. T., Ayello, E. A., Sussman, C., et al. (1997). Draft definition of stage I pressure ulcers: Inclusion of persons with darkly pigmented skin. *Advances in Wound Care, 10*(5), 16–19.

Particular attention must be paid to areas located over bony prominences or under casts, traction, splints, braces, collars, or other orthopedic devices. Oxygen tubing around noses and ears should be inspected. The frequency of pressure checks depends on the schedule of appliance application and the skin's response to the external pressure (Figure 47.8).

When hyperemia is noted, the nurse must document the location, size, and colour and reassess the area after 1 hour (Figure 47.9, *A*). When abnormal reactive hyperemia is suspected, the nurse can outline the affected area with a marker to make reassessment easier.

BOX 47.5 Nursing Assessment Questions

Skin Integrity
Sensation
- Do you have any loss of feeling in your feet or legs or anywhere else?
- Do you feel more (or less) sensitive to heat or cold?

Mobility
- Do you have any physical conditions, injury, or paralysis that limits your mobility?
- Can you easily change your position?
- Is it painful to move?

Continence
- Do you have any problems with urine or bowel continence?
- Do you need help when you use the toilet?
- How often do you need to use the toilet? During the day? During the night?

Presence of a Wound
- How did this wound happen?
- When did this wound occur?
- When did you last receive a tetanus shot?
- What happened to this wound since it occurred? Is it getting better? Or worse?
- What treatments, activities, or care have slowed or helped the wound healing process? Are there other things we could be doing to improve things?
- Is the wound painful? If so, can you describe the pain (burning, stabbing, sharp, dull) or is it itchy? What have you been doing to manage this? Is it working?
- What would you like, in terms of the goal for yourself, in relation to this wound and its healing?

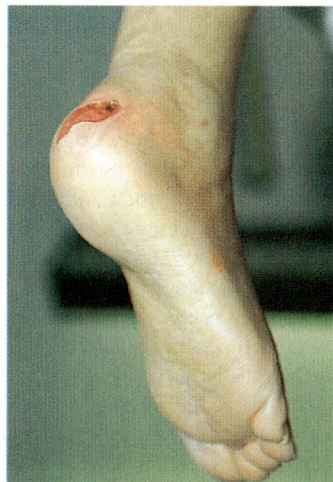

FIGURE 47.8 A pressure injury on the heel caused by pressure exerted by the mattress.

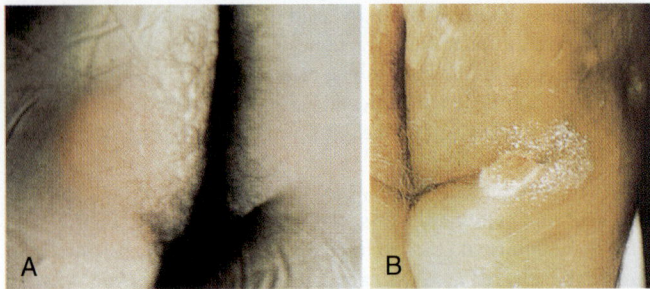

FIGURE 47.9 **A,** Hyperemia on ischial tuberosity. **B,** Ulcer. (Pires, M., & Muller, A. [1991]. Decision and management of early tissue pressure indicators: A pictorial essay. *Progressions, 3*[3], 3.)

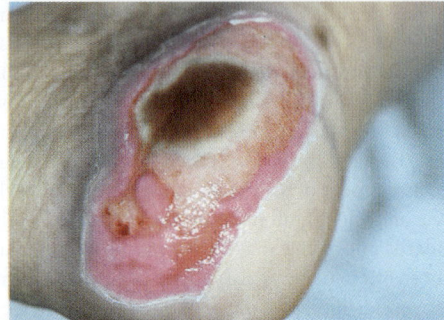

FIGURE 47.10 Pressure injury with tissue necrosis.

These signs are early indicators of impaired skin integrity, but damage to the underlying tissue is sometimes more progressive (see Figure 47.9, *B*). Palpation with the fingertips will help in assessing and identifying induration or other damage to skin and underlying tissues.

The nurse should gently palpate the reddened tissue, observing for blanching as normal skin tones return in patients with light-toned skin. In addition, the nurse palpates for induration, noting size in millimetres or centimetres of the induration around the injured area. Changes in the temperature of the surrounding skin and tissues should also be noted.

❖ NURSING PROCESS

◆ Assessment

Skin integrity is subject to change over time. Baseline and continual assessment data support critical information about the patient's skin integrity and the increased risk of developing pressure injuries. The specific factors, such as continence status or mobility, help focus the nursing assessment (see Box 47.5).

Skin

The neurologically impaired patient, the chronically ill patient in long-term care, the patient with diminished mental status, and patients in the Critical Care Unit (CCU) or oncology, hospice, or orthopedic departments all have an increased potential of developing pressure injuries. Nurses need to recognize the importance of ongoing assessment and prompt treatment, should skin breakdown occur.

Risk Assessment

By identifying and promptly treating at-risk patients, nurses can spare patients with little risk of pressure injury development the unnecessary and sometimes costly preventive treatments and related risks of complications (Skill 47.1). Prevention and treatment of pressure injuries are *major* nursing priorities, no matter what the health care setting. Evidence exists that a program of prevention guided by consistent risk assessment simultaneously reduces the institutional incidence of pressure injuries by as much as 60% and decreases the costs of prevention at the same time (Braden, 2001). The Braden Pressure Ulcer Risk Assessment Scale has been identified by Wounds Canada and the RNAO Best Practice Guidelines as a reliable and valid risk assessment tool across all health care sectors and is the most commonly used tool (Orsted et al., 2017; RNAO, 2016a). However, an

assessment tool is exactly that—a tool to assist nurses in planning intervention strategies and evaluation of a patient's skin on an ongoing basis. No assessment tool can replace your clinical judgement as a nurse (RNAO, 2016a).

Braden Scale

The Braden Scale (Table 47.2) was developed on the basis of risk factors in a long-term care population (Bergstrom et al., 1987). It is the most widely used risk assessment tool in North America to assess patients for risk of skin breakdown. There are six subscales: sensory perception, moisture, activity, mobility, nutrition, and friction and shear. While the total score provides a prediction of risk of skin breakdown, it is important to pay particular attention to the subscales. When a subscale result is low, interventions should be initiated, relevant to that indicator (Guest et al., 2018). Remember, the *lower* the score, the *higher* the risk; the total score ranges from 6 to 23, and a lower total score indicates a higher risk of pressure injury development (Braden & Bergstrom, 1989). The cutoff score for onset of pressure injury risk with the Braden Scale in the general adult population is 18 (Ayello & Braden, 2002). The Braden Scale is highly reliable and has been widely used to identify patients at greatest risk of developing pressure injuries (Bergstrom et al., 1987; Braden & Bergstrom, 1994; Orsted et al., 2017).

Classification of Pressure Injury

Nurses need to assess pressure injury at regular intervals using systematic variables to evaluate wound healing, plan appropriate interventions, and evaluate progress. One method used for assessment of a pressure injury is a staging system. Staging systems for pressure injury are based on the description of the depth of tissue destroyed. Accurate staging requires knowledge of the skin layers. A major drawback of a staging system is that a wound covered with necrotic tissue cannot be staged because the necrotic tissue is covering the depth of the wound (Figure 47.10). The necrotic tissue must be debrided or removed to expose the wound base to allow for assessment.

In 2007, the National Pressure Injury Advisory Panel (NPIAP) proposed a four-stage classification system with an additional deep tissue injury descriptor (NPIAP, 2016) (Table 47.3). In 2016, the NPIAP revised the staging definitions, including changing the terminology from *pressure ulcer* to *pressure injury*. While this may seem confusing, it addresses the problem of deep tissue injury and stage 1, which appear as intact skin, not as an ulcer. In addition, as stated earlier, the use of Roman numerals (I, II, II, IV) has been changed to numbers (1, 2, 3, 4)

| SKILL 47.1 | ASSESSMENT FOR RISK OF PRESSURE INJURY DEVELOPMENT | ⏵ |

Delegation Considerations

Assessment of patients for risk of pressure injury should not be delegated to unregulated care providers (UCPs); however, prevention strategies should be included in their work plan. Check with your institution's policy in this regard.

Prevention

- Document changes to patient's skin, such as redness, blistering, abrasions, or cuts.
- Keep patient's skin dry: clean well after incontinence (urine or stool) or exposure to other body fluids.
- Reposition patient according to frequency established in nursing care plan or agency policy.
- Avoid trauma to patient's skin from tape, pressure, friction, or shear.

Equipment

- Use a risk assessment tool: Braden Scale (used in this skill) or other tool, according to agency policy.
- Documentation record

PROCEDURE

STEPS	RATIONALE
1. Identify at-risk individuals needing prevention and specific risk factors.	• Identification determines factors that increase the patient's risk of developing pressure injuries (Braden, 2001; RNAO, 2016a).
A. Use a validated risk assessment tool (e.g., the Braden Scale).	• Consistent, reliable, comparable assessments are ensured (NPIAP, 2016; RNAO, 2016a; WOCN, 2017a).
B. Assess the patient on admission to the hospital, long-term care facility, home care program, or other health care facility.	• A baseline assessment is provided.
C. Inspect the condition of the patient's skin at least once a day (see Box 47.5) and examine all bony prominences, noting skin integrity. (Check agency policy for reassessment and reassess at periodic intervals.) If redness or discoloration is noted, palpate area of redness for blanchable erythema.	• Routine skin assessments will help identify changes in patient's risk of pressure injuries. • Nonblanchable erythema or discoloration in the patient's skin may be an early indicator of skin injury (Pieper, 2016).

CRITICAL DECISION POINT: *In dark-skinned patients, the discoloration appears as a deepening of the normal colour (see Box 47.2). Darkly pigmented skin does not always show direct changes in colour (Bennett, 1995; NPIAP, 2016).*

STEPS	RATIONALE
D. Observe all assistive devices, such as braces or casts, and medical equipment, such as nasogastric and enteral tubes and catheters, for pressure points.	• Presence of medical equipment may cause pressure and skin breakdown in sensitive regions, such as nostrils, ears, or other bony prominences.
2. Determine patient's ability to respond meaningfully to pressure-related discomfort (sensory perception).	• Patients with completely, very, or slightly limited ability to respond to pressure-related discomfort cannot communicate discomfort; they will have a limited ability to feel pain and thus risk developing pressure injuries.
3. Assess the degree to which patient's skin is exposed to moisture.	• Exposure to excessive moisture increases the risk of skin breakdown due to changes in skin pH and maceration of skin.
4. Evaluate the patient's activity level.	• The patient who is bedfast, chairfast, or only walks occasionally limits repositioning and pressure off-loading due to physical inactivity.
A. Determine patient's ability to change and control body position (mobility).	• Potential for friction and shear injury increases when the patient is completely dependent on others for position change.
B. Determine patient's preferred positions.	• Habitual positioning (e.g., lying on one side or the other) may result in skin breakdown as the patient may resist repositioning to different areas.
5. Assess patient's usual food and fluid intake pattern (nutrition and hydration).	• A patient who never eats a complete meal, rarely eats a complete meal, or has limited fluid intake is at risk of skin breakdown.
A. Review weight pattern and nutritional laboratory values.	• Decreased nutritional status is linked with pressure ulcer formation and poor wound healing (Kennerly et al., 2015; RNAO, 2016a; Wong et al., 2019).
B. Complete a fluid intake assessment.	• Fluid imbalance, either dehydration or edema, can increase the patient's risk of pressure injuries.
6. Evaluate for the presence of friction and shear.	• The patient who has spastic limbs, requires maximum assistance in moving, or slides against sheets when moved is at an increased risk of skin damage.
7. Document the risk assessment on admission, on a regular basis according to institutional policy, and if any change in status occurs (Sibbald et al., 2006).	• The documentation provides a baseline to track risk of development of pressure injuries and allow planning of interventions.

SKILL 47.1 ASSESSMENT FOR RISK OF PRESSURE INJURY DEVELOPMENT—cont'd

STEPS	RATIONALE
A. Observe the Braden Scale scores: as they become lower, predicted risk becomes higher. Existing skin breakdown increases the risk by one level.	• Scores: 15–16, mild risk 13–14, moderate risk 10–12, high risk <10, very high risk • Existing skin breakdown indicates that risk factors are already present and require attention.
B. Link risk assessment to preventive protocols.	• Prevention protocols will target problem areas to assist in prevention of skin breakdown (Gadd & Morris, 2014; Guest et al., 2018).
C. Institute mild-risk interventions (score of 15–16). Plan of care should include frequent turning; maximum remobilization; off-load heel pressure; use of pressure-reducing support surface; and managing moisture, nutrition, and friction and shear.	• The risk of skin breakdown is decreased.
D. Institute moderate-risk interventions (score of 13–14). Plan of care should include interventions for mild risk (Step 7C), as well as use of foam wedges to position the patient in the 30-degree lateral position.	• The increased risk of skin breakdown is decreased with appropriate interventions.
E. Institute high-risk interventions (score of 10–12). Plan of care should include interventions for moderate risk (Step 7D), as well as instructions to turn the patient with small shifts in weight.	• The factors that contribute to skin breakdown are identified, and appropriate interventions are planned.
F. Institute very high-risk interventions (score of <10). Plan of care should include interventions for high risk (Step 7E) as well as use of a pressure-relieving surface, which still requires frequent repositioning of patient.	• Plan interventions to decrease the effects of immobility, decreased sensory perception, moisture, friction, shear, decreased activity, and nutritional issues in a high-risk individual.
8. Provide education to patient and family regarding pressure injury risk.	• Patient and family understand and participate as much as possible in the interventions designed to reduce pressure injury risk.
9. Evaluate measures to reduce pressure injury development.	• Evaluation on a regular basis provides opportunity to assess and adjust interventions.
A. Observe patient's skin for areas at risk.	• Patient's response to risk-reduction interventions is determined over time.
B. Observe tolerance of patient for positioning.	• Frequent change in position further reduces patient's risk of developing pressure injuries.
C. Monitor success of a toileting program or other measures to reduce the frequency of incontinence of urine or stool.	• Avoiding moisture from urine or stool on patient's skin reduces risk of skin breakdown.
D. Evaluate laboratory nutrition values.	• Value of nutritional supplements in improving nutritional status is determined.

UNEXPECTED OUTCOMES	RELATED INTERVENTIONS
No blanching when skin is firmly pressed, purple discoloration, or significant colour change	• Reassess frequency of turning schedule. • Implement agency's skin care protocols. • Consider support surface to reduce pressure injury risk.

RECORDING AND REPORTING
• Record patient's risk score and subscores.
• Record appearance of skin (at pressure points, etc.).
• Describe position, turning intervals, pressure-relieving devices, and other prevention strategies.
• Report any need for additional consultations (e.g., wound care specialist or dietitian) for the high-risk patient.

CARE IN THE COMMUNITY CONSIDERATIONS
• Instruct caregiver to use the 30-degree lateral position. This position reduces pressure over the trochanter.
• Pressure-relief manoeuvres need to be individualized for patient needs and the home environment. Provide the family with resources to access equipment.

TABLE 47.2   Braden Scale for Predicting Pressure Sore Risk

Patient's Name _____ Evaluator's Name _____ Date of Assessment _____

Characteristic	Score: 1	Score: 2	Score: 3	Score: 4
Sensory Perception Ability to respond meaningfully to pressure-related discomfort	1. Completely limited Unresponsive (does not moan, flinch, or gasp) to painful stimuli due to diminished level of consciousness or sedation. OR Limited ability to feel pain over most of body surface.	2. Very limited Responds only to painful stimuli. Cannot communicate discomfort except by moaning or restlessness. OR Has a sensory impairment that limits the ability to feel pain or discomfort over half of body.	3. Slightly limited Responds to verbal commands but cannot always communicate discomfort or need to be turned. OR Has some sensory impairment that limits ability to feel pain or discomfort in one or two extremities.	4. No impairment Responds to verbal commands. Has no sensory deficit that would limit ability to feel or voice pain or discomfort.
Moisture Degree to which skin is exposed to moisture	1. Constantly moist Skin is kept moist almost constantly by perspiration, urine, etc. Dampness is detected every time patient is moved or turned.	2. Moist Skin is often, but not always, moist. Linen must be changed at least once a shift.	3. Occasionally moist Skin is occasionally moist, requiring an extra linen change approximately once a day.	4. Rarely moist Skin is usually dry. Linen only requires changing at routine intervals.
Activity Degree of physical activity	1. Bedfast Confined to bed.	2. Chairfast Ability to walk severely limited or nonexistent. Cannot bear own weight or must be assisted into chair or wheelchair.	3. Walks occasionally Walks occasionally during day but for very short distances, with or without assistance. Spends majority of each shift in bed or chair.	4. Walks frequently Walks outside the room at least twice a day and inside room at least once every 2 hours during waking hours.
Mobility Ability to change and control body position	1. Completely immobile Does not make even slight changes in body or extremity position without assistance.	2. Very limited Makes occasional slight changes in body or extremity position but unable to make frequent or significant changes independently.	3. Slightly limited Makes frequent though slight changes in body or extremity position independently.	4. No limitations Makes major and frequent changes in position without assistance.
Nutrition Usual food intake pattern	1. Very poor Never eats a complete meal. Rarely eats more than one-third of any food offered. Eats two servings or less of protein (meat or dairy products) per day. Takes fluids poorly. Does not take a liquid dietary supplement. OR Is NPO or maintained on clear liquids or IVs for more than 5 days.	2. Probably inadequate Rarely eats a complete meal and generally eats only about half of any food offered. Protein intake includes only three servings of meat or dairy products per day. Occasionally will take a dietary supplement. OR Receives less than optimum amount of liquid diet or tube feeding.	3. Adequate Eats over half of most meals. Eats a total of four servings of protein (meat, dairy products) each day. Occasionally will refuse a meal but will usually take a supplement if offered. OR Is on a tube feeding or total parenteral nutrition regimen that probably meets most nutritional needs.	4. Excellent Eats most of every meal. Never refuses a meal. Usually eats a total of four or more servings of meat and dairy products. Occasionally eats between meals. Does not require supplementation.
Friction and Shear	1. Problem Requires moderate to maximum assistance in moving. Complete lifting without sliding against sheets is impossible. Frequently slides down in bed or chair, requiring frequent repositioning with maximum assistance. Spasticity, contractures, or agitation leads to almost constant friction.	2. Potential problem Moves feebly or requires minimum assistance. During a move, skin probably slides to some extent against sheets, chair, restraints, or other devices. Maintains relatively good position in chair or bed most of the time but occasionally slides down.	3. No apparent problem Moves in bed and in chair independently and has sufficient muscle strength to lift up completely during move. Maintains good position in bed or chair at all times.	
TOTAL SCORE				

NPO, Nothing by mouth.

for simpler documentation. Where pressure injury is observed, documentation needs to occur. *Staging* describes the pressure injury depth at the point of assessment. Thus, once staged, the wound as it heals (or deteriorates) is identified as (for example) a *healing* stage 3 pressure injury (Nix, 2016). While this is a recent change in documentation naming, it does not change the descriptions of the actual pressure injury (NPIAP, 2016; Box 47.6).

When assessing patients with darkly pigmented skin, proper lighting is important to accurately assess the skin (see Box 47.2). Either natural light or a halogen light is recommended. This prevents the blue tones that fluorescent light sources produce on darkly pigmented skin, which interfere with accurate assessment (Bennett, 1995).

For a wound with nonviable tissue, the amount (percentage) and appearance (colour) of viable and nonviable tissue need to be included. This information is important to develop a plan of care based on the healing ability of the wound.

Granulation tissue is red, moist tissue composed of new blood vessels, the presence of which indicates progression toward healing.

TABLE 47.3	Guidelines for Staging Pressure Injury

The following criteria can be used as a visual aid to help identify and appropriately stage pressure injury. The definitions were derived from work done by the National Pressure Injury Advisory Panel and published in February 2007; revision April 2016 and 2019.

Suspected Deep Tissue Injury

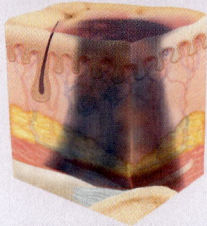

Intact or nonintact skin with localized area of persistent nonblanchable deep red, maroon, purple discoloration or epidermal separation revealing a dark wound bed or blood-filled blister. Pain and temperature change often precede skin colour changes. Discoloration may appear differently in darkly pigmented skin. This injury results from intense or prolonged pressure and shear forces at the bone–muscle interface. The wound may evolve rapidly to reveal the actual extent of tissue injury, or it may resolve without tissue loss.

Stage 1

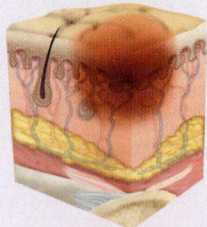

Intact skin with a localized area of nonblanchable erythema, which may appear differently in darkly pigmented skin. Presence of blanchable erythema or changes in sensation, temperature, or firmness may precede visual changes. Colour changes do not include purple or maroon discoloration; these may indicate deep tissue pressure injury.

Stage 2

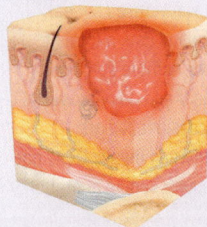

Partial-thickness loss of skin with exposed dermis. The wound bed is viable, pink or red, and moist and may also present as an intact or ruptured serum-filled blister. Adipose (fat) is not visible and deeper tissues are not visible. Granulation tissue, slough, and eschar are not present. These injuries commonly result from adverse microclimate and shear in the skin over the pelvis and shear in the heel. This stage should not be used to describe moisture-associated skin damage (MASD), including incontinence-associated dermatitis (IAD), intertriginous dermatitis (ITD), medical adhesive–related skin injury (MARSI), or traumatic wounds (skin tears, burns, abrasions).

Stage 3

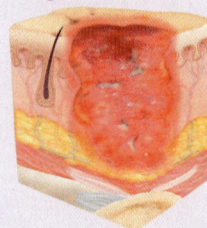

Full-thickness loss of skin, in which adipose (fat) is visible in the ulcer and granulation tissue and epibole (rolled wound edges) are often present. Slough, eschar, or both may be visible. The depth of tissue damage varies by anatomical location; areas of significant adiposity can develop deep wounds. Undermining and tunnelling may occur. Fascia, muscle, tendon, ligament, cartilage, and bone are not exposed.

Continued

TABLE 47.3	Guidelines for Staging Pressure Injury—cont'd
Stage 4 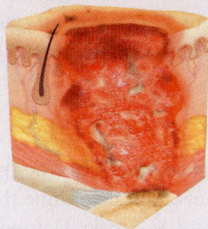	Full-thickness skin and tissue loss with exposed or directly palpable fascia, muscle, tendon, ligament, cartilage, or bone in the ulcer. Slough, eschar, or both may be visible. Epibole (rolled edges), undermining, tunnelling, or a combination of these often occur. Depth varies by anatomical location.
Unstageable 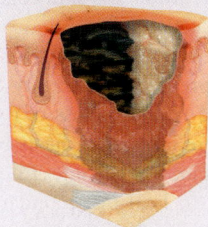	Full-thickness skin and tissue loss in which the extent of tissue damage within the ulcer cannot be confirmed because it is obscured by slough or eschar. If slough or eschar is removed, a stage 3 or stage 4 pressure injury will be revealed. Stable eschar (i.e., dry, adherent, intact without erythema or fluctuance) on the heel or ischemic limb should not be softened or removed.

Used with permission from the National Pressure Injury Advisory Panel (NPIAP). Copyright 2022 NPIAP.

BOX 47.6 National Pressure Injury Advisory Panel Staging Guidelines

Suspected Deep Tissue Injury
Please refer to Table 47.3 for a description of a suspected deep tissue injury.

Further Description
Deep tissue injury may be difficult to detect in individuals with dark skin tones. Evolution may include a thin blister over a dark wound bed. The wound may further evolve and become covered by thin eschar. Evolution may be rapid, exposing additional layers of tissue, even with optimal treatment.

Stage 1
Please refer to Table 47.3 for a description of a stage 1 pressure injury.

Further Description
The area may be painful, firm, soft, warmer, or cooler as compared with adjacent tissue. Stage I may be difficult to detect in individuals with dark skin tones. The stage may indicate at-risk persons (a heralding sign of risk).

Stage 2
Please refer to Table 47.3 for a description of a stage 2 pressure injury.

Further Description
The stage presents as a shiny or dry, shallow ulcer without slough or bruising. (Bruising indicates suspected deep tissue injury.) This stage should not be used to describe skin tears, tape burns, perineal dermatitis, maceration, or excoriation.

Stage 3
Please refer to Table 47.3 for a description of a stage 3 pressure injury.

Further Description
The depth of a stage 3 pressure injury varies by anatomical location. The bridge of the nose, ear, occiput, and malleolus do not have subcutaneous tissue, and stage 3 pressure injury can be shallow. In contrast, areas of significant adiposity can develop extremely deep stage 3 pressure injury. The bone or tendon is not visible or directly palpable.

Stage 4
Please see Table 47.3 for a description of a stage 4 pressure injury.

Further Description
The depth of a stage 4 pressure injury varies by anatomical location. The bridge of the nose, ear, occiput, and malleolus do not have subcutaneous tissue and these ulcers can be shallow. Stage 4 injuries can extend into muscle or supporting structures (e.g., fascia, tendon, or joint capsule) or both, making osteomyelitis possible. Exposed bone or tendon is visible or directly palpable.

Unstageable
Please refer to Table 47.3 for a description of an unstageable pressure injury.

Further Description
Until enough slough or eschar is removed to expose the base of the wound, the true depth and, therefore, stage cannot be determined. Stable (dry, adherent, intact without erythema or fluctuance) eschar on the heels serves as "the body's natural (biological) cover" and should not be removed. The staging system was defined by Shea in 1975 and provides a name to the amount of anatomical tissue loss. The original definitions were confusing to many clinicians and led to inaccurate staging of wounds associated with or due to perineal dermatitis and those due to deep tissue injury.

Used with permission from the National Pressure Injury Advisory Panel (NPIAP). Copyright 2022 NPIAP.

Soft yellow or white tissue is characteristic of slough (a stringy substance attached to the wound bed), which will need to be removed before the wound is able to heal. Black or brown necrotic tissue is eschar, which usually needs to be removed before healing can proceed. Sharp debridement of a wound, to remove nonviable tissue, can be performed only by a nurse who has the appropriate knowledge, skill, and clinical judgement and agency or institution policy and procedure in place.

Measuring wound dimensions provides a good indicator of wound healing progress (Nix, 2016). Consistent measurement of length × width is appropriate to track progress. Measurement is taken using the analogue clock system: patient's head, and thus the "top" of the wound is at 12 o'clock, bottom of the wound is at 6 o'clock, and so on. While a disposable ruler is likely most readily available, mobile technology has developed automated and accurate wound measurement tools, which provide better consistency of measurement (Biagioni et al., 2021). Depth is obtained by using a sterile cotton-tipped applicator to gently probe for tunnelling and undermining in the wound bed.

Wound exudate describes the amount, colour, consistency, and odour of wound drainage and is part of the wound assessment. Excessive exudate usually indicates presence of an infection. The periwound condition needs to be included in the assessment. The periwound skin is evaluated for redness, warmth, maceration, or edema (swelling). Any of these factors indicate wound deterioration.

Wound Classifications

A wound is a disruption of the integrity and function of tissues in the body (Bryant & Clark, 2016). It is imperative to understand that *all wounds are not created equal*. Understanding the etiology (causes) of a wound is important because the treatment for the wound varies, depending on the underlying disease process. Some treatments are even harmful to certain wounds, so nurses need to obtain a complete history, including the etiology of the wound.

Wound classification systems vary. A system may describe the status of skin integrity, cause of the wound, severity or extent of tissue injury or damage, cleanliness of the wound (Table 47.4), or descriptive qualities of wound tissue, such as colour (Figure 47.11). Wound classifications enable nurses to understand the factors associated with a wound and implications for healing.

Process of Wound Healing

Wound healing comprises integrated physiological processes. The tissue layers involved and their capacity for regeneration determine the mechanism for repair of any wound (Doughty & Sparks-Defriese, 2016). Two types of wounds are those with tissue loss, and those without. A clean surgical incision is an example of a wound with little tissue loss. The surgical wound heals by primary intention. The skin edges are approximated, or closed, and the risk of infection is low.

Healing occurs quickly, with minimal scar formation, as long as infection and secondary breakdown are prevented (Doughty & Sparks-Defriese, 2016). In contrast, a wound involving loss of tissue, such as a burn, pressure injury, or severe laceration, heals by secondary intention. The wound is left open until it becomes filled by scar tissue. It takes longer for a wound to heal by secondary intention; thus, the chance of infection is greater. If scarring from secondary intention is severe, loss of tissue function is often permanent (Figure 47.12).

All chronic wounds described in this chapter are discussed in detail in the RNAO Best Practice Guidelines, which are readily available online at https://www.rnao.org.

Wound Repair

Partial-thickness wounds are shallow wounds involving loss of the epidermis (top layer) and possibly partial loss of the dermis. Epidermal wounds, such as a clean surgical wound or an abrasion, heal by regeneration. However, full-thickness wounds extending into the dermis (involving both layers of tissue) heal by scar formation because deeper

TABLE 47.4 Wound Classification

Description	Causes	Implications for Healing
Onset and Duration		
Acute		
A wound that proceeds through an orderly and timely reparative process that results in sustained restoration of anatomical and functional integrity	Trauma, a surgical incision	Wounds are usually easily cleaned and repaired. Wound edges are clean and intact.
Chronic		
Wound that fails to proceed through an orderly and timely process to produce anatomical and functional integrity	Vascular compromise, chronic inflammation, or repetitive insults to the tissue (Doughty & Sparks-Defriese, 2016)	Continued exposure to insult impedes wound healing.
Healing Process		
Primary Intention		
Wound that is closed	Surgical incision, wound that is sutured or stapled	Healing occurs by epithelialization; heals quickly with minimal scar formation.
Secondary Intention		
Wound edges are not approximated	Pressure wounds, surgical wounds that have tissue loss	Wound heals by granulation tissue formation, wound contraction, and epithelialization.
Tertiary Intention		
Wound is left open for several days, then wound edges are approximated	Wounds that are contaminated and require observation for signs of inflammation	Closure of wound is delayed until risk of infection is resolved (Doughty & Sparks-Defriese, 2016).

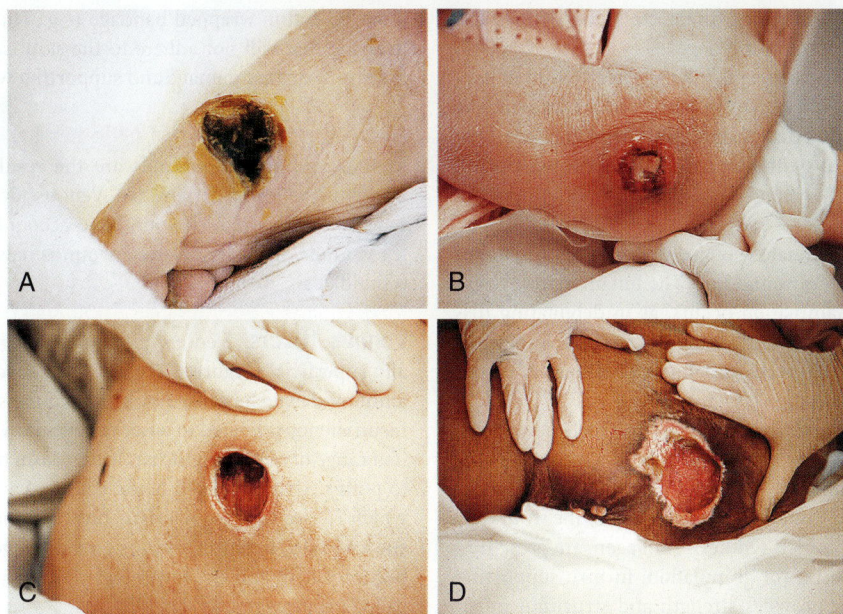

FIGURE 47.11 Wounds classified by colour assessment. **A,** Black wound. **B,** Yellow wound. **C,** Red wound. **D,** Mixed-colour wound. (Courtesy Scott Health Care—A Molnlycke Company. Philadelphia, PA.)

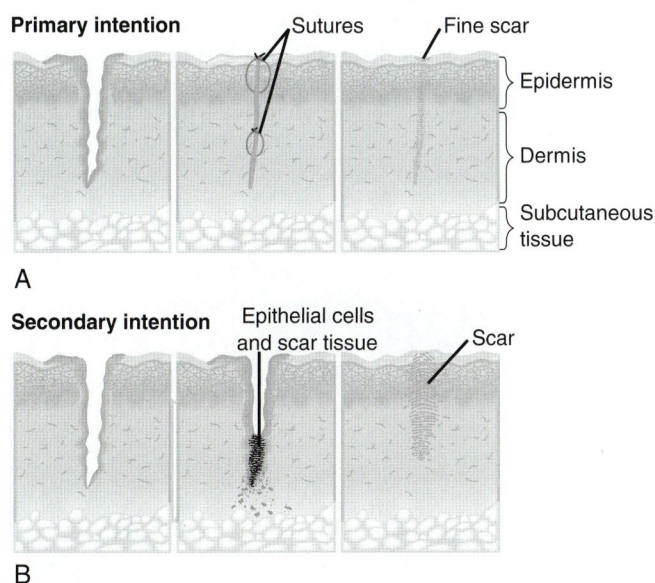

FIGURE 47.12 A, Wound healing by primary intention such as a surgical incision. Wound healing edges are pulled together and approximated with sutures or staples, and healing occurs by connective tissue deposition. **B,** Wound healing by secondary intention. Wound edges are not approximated, and healing occurs by granulation tissue formation and contraction of the wound edges. (Bryant, R. A., & Nix, D. P. [Eds.]. [2016]. *Acute and chronic wounds: Nursing management* [5th ed.]. Elsevier. Used with permission.)

structures do not regenerate. Pressure injuries are an example of full-thickness wounds.

Partial-Thickness Wound Repair. Three components make up the healing process of a partial-thickness wound: inflammatory response, epithelial proliferation (reproduction) and migration,

and re-establishment of the epidermal layers. Tissue trauma causes the *inflammatory response*, which, in turn, causes redness and swelling to the area, as well as a moderate amount of serous exudate. Normally, this response is limited to the first 24 hours after wounding. Epithelial cells begin to regenerate, providing new replacement cells. This *epithelial proliferation and migration* start at the wound edges and the epidermal cells lining the epidermal appendages, allowing for quick resurfacing. Epithelial cells begin migrating across the wound bed soon after wounding. A wound left open to air can resurface within 6 to 7 days, whereas a wound that is kept moist can resurface in 4 days. The difference in the healing rate is related to the fact that epidermal cells only migrate across a moist surface. In a dry wound, the cells migrate down into a moist level before migration can occur (Doughty & Sparks-Defriese, 2016). New epithelium is only a few cells thick and must undergo *re-establishment of the epidermal layers*. The cells slowly re-establish normal thickness and appear as dry pink tissue.

Full-Thickness Wound Repair. Inflammatory, proliferative, and remodelling phases are involved in the healing process of a full-thickness wound. Note the differences between partial- and full-thickness wounds.

Inflammatory Phase. The *inflammation stage* is the body's reaction to wounding, beginning within minutes of injury and, in full-thickness wounds, lasting approximately 3 days. During **hemostasis**, injured blood vessels constrict, and platelets gather to stop bleeding. Clots form a **fibrin** matrix that later provides a framework for cellular repair. Damaged tissue and mast cells secrete histamine, resulting in vasodilation of surrounding capillaries and exudation of serum and white blood cells into damaged tissues. This results in localized redness, edema, warmth, and throbbing. The inflammatory response is beneficial, and attempting to cool the area or reduce the swelling has no value, unless the swelling occurs within a closed compartment (e.g., ankle or neck).

Leukocytes (white blood cells) reach the wound within a few hours. The primary white blood cell is the neutrophil, which begins to ingest bacteria and small debris. The second important leukocyte is the monocyte, which transforms into macrophages.

The macrophages are the "garbage cells" that clean a wound of bacteria, dead cells, and debris by phagocytosis. Macrophages continue the process of clearing the wound of debris and release growth factors that attract fibroblasts, the cells that synthesize collagen (connective tissue). Collagen appears as early as the second day and is the main component of scar tissue.

In a clean wound, the inflammatory phase accomplishes control of bleeding and establishes a clean wound bed. The inflammatory phase is prolonged if too little inflammation occurs, as in debilitating diseases such as cancer or after the administration of steroids. Too much inflammation also decreases the speed of healing, as arriving cells compete for available nutrients.

Proliferative Phase. The *proliferative phase,* in which new blood vessels appear as reconstruction progresses, lasts from 3 to 24 days. The main activities during this phase are filling of the wound with granulation tissue, contraction of the wound, and resurfacing of the wound by epithelialization. Fibroblasts, which synthesize collagen, are present in this phase, providing the matrix for granulation, in turn supporting re-epithelialization. Collagen provides strength and structural integrity to a wound. During this period, the wound contracts to reduce the area that requires healing (**wound contraction**). Lastly, epithelial cells migrate from the wound edges to resurface. In a clean wound, when the proliferative phase is complete, the vascular bed has been re-established and the area filled with replacement tissue (collagen/granulation tissue) and the surface has been repaired (**epithelialization**). Impairment of healing during this stage usually results from systemic factors such as age, anemia, hypoproteinemia, and zinc deficiency.

Remodelling. *Maturation,* the final stage of healing, can take up to 2 years to occur, depending on the depth and extent of the wound. The collagen scar continues to reorganize and gain strength for several months. Usually, scar tissue contains fewer pigmented cells (melanocytes) and has a lighter colour than normal skin. Healed wounds are at risk for pressure injury as they usually do not have the tensile strength of the tissue they replace.

Skin Tears

Aging skin is at a greater risk of developing skin tears because of the thinning of the epidermis. Dehydration, poor nutrition, prolonged use of corticosteroids, impaired sensory perception, and cognitive impairment are all risk factors for skin breakdown. Nurses need to be very careful when moving older patients in bed or transferring them from bed to gurney for tests, for example. Skin tears and bruising are common concerns in this population (Figure 47.13). Any open area on the skin creates the potential for infection (portal of entry for bacteria). Using tape or adhesive dressings on fragile skin can also precipitate skin tears. The use of simple, high-quality gauze pads held in place with

a woven cotton wrapped bandage (e.g., Kling wrap) or a soft silicone dressing that will not adhere to the skin is effective in protecting the area from further damage and supporting wound healing.

Venous and Arterial Wounds

Venous and arterial wounds are the result of poor circulation and occur in the lower extremities. Venous ulcers are the most common type of lower extremity wound and account for approximately 80% of leg wounds. In addition, these wounds have a recurrence rate of 70% (Gould et al., 2016).

Venous Ulcers. Venous ulcers are irregular in shape and generally superficial (Figure 47.14, *A*). These wounds usually have a large amount of exudate caused by edema in the surrounding tissue. Venous insufficiency is related to weak vein walls in the legs; furthermore, limited range of motion in the ankle decreases the ability of the calf muscle to pump. Serum and red blood cells leak into the surrounding tissue, which causes the characteristic brownish hemosiderin staining of tissue and skin. In chronic venous insufficiency, the edema in the tissue becomes firm and the lower legs develop a wooden-like appearance, called *lipodermatosclerosis.*

Treatment of Venous Leg Ulcers. It is important that nurses assess the ankle-brachial pressure index before using compression therapy to prevent, treat, or diminish edema in the lower legs (Bernatchez et al., 2022; RNAO, 2016a). Because venous leg ulcers are often hard-to-heal wounds, patients may have tried a variety of products, such as lanolin in topical moisturizers, topical antibiotics, or others. These products may create allergic-contact dermatitis, and it is best to avoid using anything but the simplest, natural products to clean, debride, moisten, and cover these ulcers. Normal saline, autolytic debriding agents,

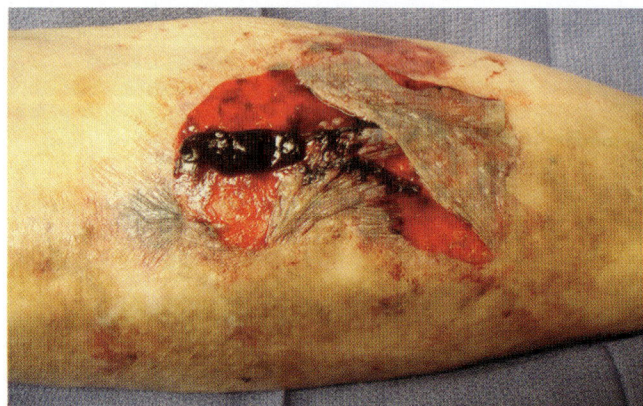

FIGURE 47.13 Skin tear. (Courtesy Rose Hamm. Cain, J. E. [2009]. *Mosby's PDQ for wound care* [p. 18]. Mosby.)

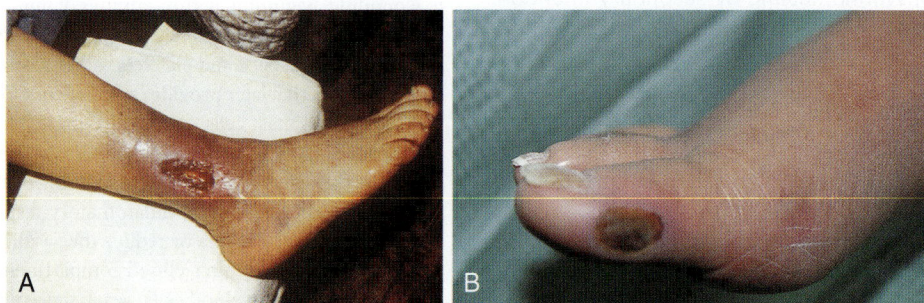

FIGURE 47.14 A, Venous leg ulcer. **B,** Arterial lower limb wound. (Bryant, R., & Nix, D. [2016]. *Acute and chronic wounds: Current management concepts* [5th ed., Plates 34 and 35]. Elsevier.)

preservative-free hydrogels, and soft silicone dressings can be used. Products to avoid are those with preservatives, chemicals in the dressing, and fragrances. Edema control is essential, but many patients are not willing to try or maintain compression therapy. A wound care specialist with training in compression therapy can be helpful in assisting nurses to determine (1) whether the patient has adequate blood flow to allow for compression and (2) different types of compression treatments that may be better suited to certain patients and their goals, especially as lifestyle modifications are usually required to heal venous ulcers.

Arterial Ulcers. Arterial ulcers (also called *ischemic ulcers*) are caused by inadequate blood flow to the lower extremity (unlike venous ulcers, which are caused by poor blood return). Arterial ulcers have a "punched-out" appearance that is both deeper and smaller than venous ulcers. They are often located on the feet, over the tips of the toes, or on the toe joints, but may be found on other locations on the lower leg (see Figure 47.14, *B*). Arterial wounds may be necrotic (black, crusted) in appearance or have very pale wound beds. The legs of a patient with arterial disease are often thin and have shiny, taut, and hairless skin with an almost translucent appearance.

Because of the nature of this disease, arterial wounds are quite resistant to healing and could be considered "maintenance" wounds, where the goal is to provide comfort and protection from infection. These wounds are not good candidates for debridement because poor blood flow will limit ability to heal. The best option for nonhealing wounds such as most arterial wounds is to keep these wounds clean and dry. A solution of povidone (Betadine) (10% in a 1% solution) is commonly used to decrease bacterial load in the wound and promote drying of the tissues. The povidone solution can be applied using gauze pads soaked in the solution (covered with simple clean dressing and changed daily) or painted on and left open to the air. Care should be taken to cleanse and inspect the wound area, particularly between the toes, to ensure there are no hidden areas of concern.

Diabetic Ulcers

In Canada, approximately 12.5 million people are living with diabetes or prediabetes (where blood sugar is higher than normal range), according to Diabetes Canada (2020). The Indigenous population has much higher percentages of individuals with diabetes than the general population, often with more disastrous outcomes owing to factors ranging from gaps in health care access to disadvantages related to the determinants of health (Halseth, 2019). Diabetes is a disease that requires major lifestyle changes, including careful monitoring of blood glucose. Complications related to poorly controlled diabetes can have serious results: renal failure, which may require dialysis; diabetic neuropathy, which may lead to limb amputation (Figure 47.15); and retinal neuropathy, which leads to blindness. People with diabetes have compromised healing potential. Any break in the skin can cause long-term problems because these wounds resist healing. Forty-five percent of lower-extremity amputations occur in individuals with diabetes. One lower-limb amputation of a nontraumatic nature (e.g., diabetes related) will result in a second limb amputation within 3 years and death within 5 years (Tentolouris et al., 2004). These are sobering statistics and reinforce how important it is for nurses to provide education, as well as careful assessment and early intervention, to patients with diabetes.

Diabetic ulcers occur because of neuropathic changes related to diabetes. They most commonly are found over bony prominences located on the plantar surface of the foot, over the metatarsal heads, and beneath the heels. These changes include sensory neuropathy, loss of protective sensation (e.g., a decrease in the ability to feel pain or temperature change); autonomic neuropathy, or absence of sweating

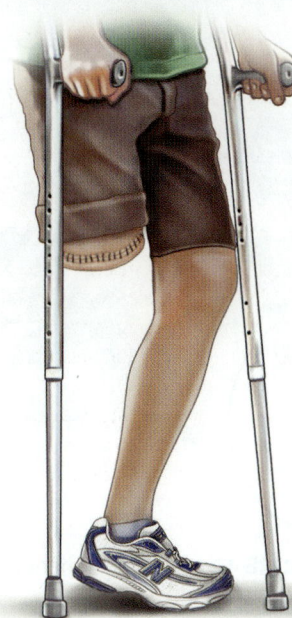
FIGURE 47.15 Person with above-knee amputation.

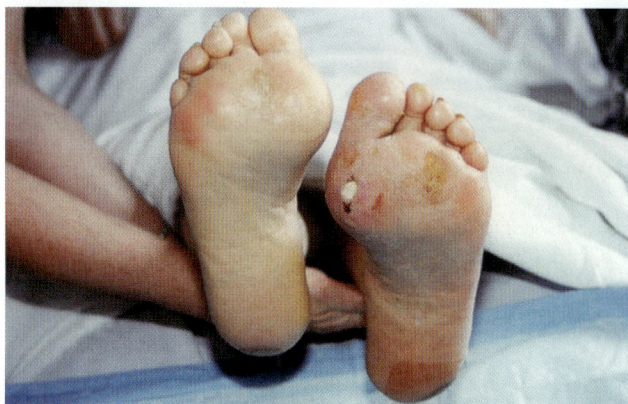
FIGURE 47.16 Diabetic foot with callus and packing in wound. (Bryant, R., & Nix, D. [2016]. *Acute and chronic wounds: Current management concepts* [3rd ed., Plate 38]. Elsevier. Reprinted with permission.)

leading to dry skin with fissures, cracks, and calluses over pressure points (heels and ball of the foot); and motor neuropathy, resulting in changes in muscle contractions leading to high arches and cocked-up "hammer" toes. These contribute to pressure points, creating calluses (Figure 47.16).

Assessment. A simple monofilament test is quick and effective to determine the extent of plantar neuropathy (Figure 47.17) (Chicharro-Luna et al., 2020). However, in patients with diabetes, it can be assumed that peripheral neuropathy is a risk; nurses should provide education and conduct close inspection and palpation of the feet and lower legs. Prevention starts with patient teaching regarding appropriate footwear, including wearing hard-soled shoes indoors; testing water temperature before bathing or showering; and good foot care, available from a certified foot-care nurse or chiropodist.

Diabetic Wound Treatment. If the diabetic wound can heal, then necrotic tissue and callus buildup must be debrided to establish a clean

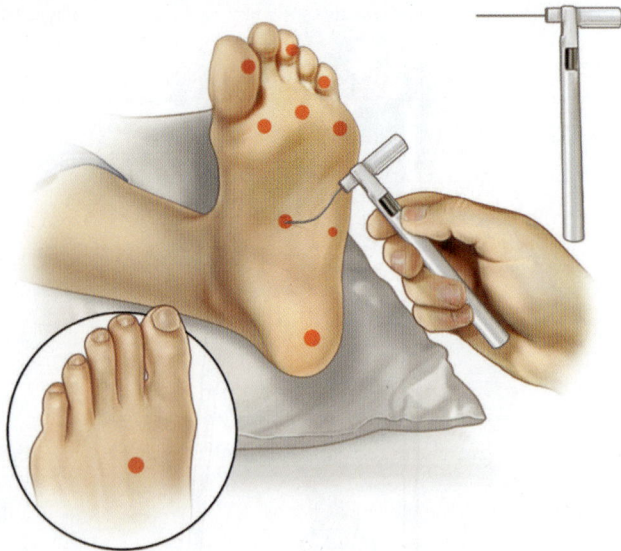

FIGURE 47.17 Monofilament test.

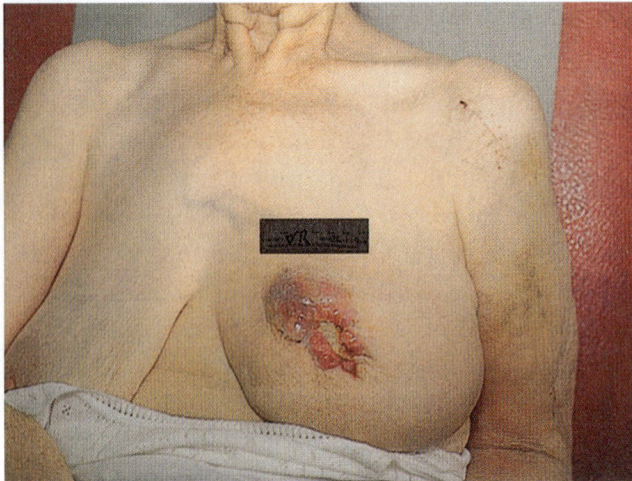

FIGURE 47.18 Malignant breast tumour. (Bale, S., & Jones, V. [2005]. *Wound care nursing: A patient-centred approach* [2nd ed., p. 195, Fig. 9.16]. Mosby. Reprinted with permission.)

wound bed and diminish pressure. Sharp or surgical debridement should be performed only by a qualified health care provider (RN or MD) with appropriate skills and knowledge and supported by agency or institution policy regarding sharp and surgical debridement. Incorrect sharp or surgical debridement can significantly harm the patient. Diabetic wounds may be prophylactically treated with some form of topical antimicrobial dressing. If the patient reports pain at the wound site, particularly persistent pain, osteomyelitis (bone infection) should be suspected. The nurse needs to ensure that the health care provider primarily responsible for the patient is aware of this so that appropriate action can be taken.

Malignant or Fungating Wounds

Cancer tumours may extrude through the skin as swollen masses with numerous fissures that drain purulent, often very malodorous exudate, that sometimes bleed when cleaned or touched. Typical sites for fungating wounds are the side of the face or neck and the breast or groin area (Figure 47.18). These wounds are not only painful at dressing

change but also often embarrass the patient because of their odour and unsightliness. They are malignant wounds that will not heal, but the tumours may be reduced in size with radiation or chemotherapy.

Care of the malignant or fungating wound requires attention to environmental and extrinsic issues such as odour, drainage, and appearance of the wound. Wound odour is related to bacteria, so when it is present, the nurse needs to consider topical antifungal or antimicrobial dressings such as metronidazole (Flagyl) or silver dressings. While charcoal dressings are also available to provide odour management, they are not always effective once they are wet. To avoid trauma to the wound bed, use of adhesive dressings should be avoided and instead atraumatic dressings used, such as soft silicone (which allows for moisture vapour transfer) or hydrofibre (which gels when wet) to decrease pain at dressing changes. Barrier products such as dimethicone-based creams will provide supportive care and protect the periwound skin. Minimizing the frequency of dressing changes as well as using "low-profile," nonbulky dressings will enhance quality of life.

Acute and Surgical Wounds

As a nurse, you may be in situations in which you are assessing a wound, either at the time of injury before treatment, or after therapy, when the wound is relatively stable. Each situation requires you to make different observations and to take different actions. Regardless of the setting, it is important that you obtain information regarding the cause and history of the wound (see Box 47.5).

Emergency Setting, or Acute, Wounds. Nurses see wounds in any setting, including the clinic, emergency department, youth camps, or their own backyard. When a patient's condition is judged to be stable because of the presence of spontaneous breathing, a clear airway, and a strong carotid pulse (see Chapter 40), the wound should be inspected for bleeding. The type of wound determines criteria for inspection. For example, a patient presenting with an abrasion would not likely require the nurse to look for signs of internal bleeding, but in the event of a puncture wound, they would check for any internal bleeding.

An abrasion is superficial with little bleeding and is considered a partial-thickness wound. The wound often appears "weepy" because of plasma leakage from damaged capillaries. A laceration, which is a jagged, unintentional (i.e., nonsurgical) wound, sometimes bleeds more profusely, depending on the wound's depth and location. For example, minor scalp lacerations tend to bleed profusely because of the rich blood supply to the scalp. Lacerations greater than 5 cm long or 2.5 cm deep cause serious bleeding. Puncture wounds bleed in relation to the depth and size of the wound; for example, a nail puncture does not cause as much bleeding as a knife wound. The primary dangers of puncture wounds are internal bleeding and infection.

The wound should be inspected for contaminate material. Most traumatic wounds are dirty. Soil, broken glass, shreds of cloth, and foreign substances clinging to penetrating objects sometimes become embedded in the wound.

The next step is to assess the size (including depth) of the wound. A deep laceration requires suturing. A large, open wound may expose bone or tissue that needs to be protected.

When the injury is a result of trauma from a dirty penetrating object, the nurse needs to determine when the patient last received a tetanus toxoid injection. Tetanus bacteria reside in soil and in the gut of humans and animals. A tetanus antitoxin injection is necessary if the patient's last one was more than 5 years ago.

Stable Setting, or Surgical Wounds. When the patient's condition is stabilized (e.g., after surgery or treatment), the wound is assessed to determine its healing progress. If the wound is covered by a dressing and the dressing is intact and not saturated with drainage, the nurse should leave it intact unless serious complications are suspected. Only the dressing and external drains are inspected.

Dressings contaminated with external drainage (e.g., feces or urine) need to be changed, as well as saturated dressings with leakage to periwound tissue. When changing dressings, care should be taken to avoid accidental removal or displacement of underlying drains. Because removal of dressings may be painful, the nurse should assess the patient's need for an analgesic, and once ordered, make sure it is given at least 30 minutes before exposing the wound.

Wound Appearance. When assessing wound appearance, the nurse checks whether the wound edges are closed. A surgical incision healing by primary intention should have clean, well-approximated edges. A puncture wound is usually a small, circular wound with the edges coming together toward the centre. Crusts from exudate often form along wound edges.

If the wound edges are separated, the nurse inspects the condition of tissue at the wound base, looking for complications such as dehiscence and evisceration. The outer edges of a wound normally appear inflamed for the first 2 to 3 days, but this slowly disappears. Within 7 to 10 days, a normally healing wound resurfaces with epithelial cells, and edges close.

Table 47.5 lists assessment characteristics for abnormal wound healing in primary and secondary wounds. If an infection develops, the area directly surrounding the wound becomes inflamed and swollen.

Skin discoloration usually results from bruising of interstitial tissues or hematoma formation. Blood collecting beneath the skin first takes on a bluish or purplish appearance. Gradually, as clotted blood is broken down, shades of brown and yellow appear.

Character of Wound Drainage. The amount, colour, odour, and consistency of drainage should be noted. The amount of drainage depends on the location and extent of the wound. For example, drainage is minimal after a simple appendectomy. In contrast, a large abscess may have moderate drainage for several days. When an accurate measurement of the amount of drainage within a dressing is needed, the nurse can weigh the dressing and compare it with the weight of the same dressing when clean and dry. The general rule is that 1 g of drainage equals 1 mL of drainage volume. Another method of quantifying wound drainage

is to chart the number of dressings used and frequency of changes. An increase or decrease in number or frequency of dressings will indicate a relative increase or decrease in wound drainage.

The colour and consistency of drainage vary depending on the type of drainage, including serous, sanguineous, serosanguineous, and purulent (Table 47.6). If drainage has a pungent or strong odour, infection should be suspected.

The wound's appearance is described according to the characteristics observed. An example of accurate recording follows:

Abdominal incision is 5 cm in width, in RLQ (right lower quadrant); wound edges well approximated without inflammation or exudate. 1.2 cm diameter circle of serous drainage present on one 4 × 4 gauze changed every 8 hours.

Drains. If a large amount of drainage is anticipated, a drain is often inserted in or near a surgical wound. Some drains are sutured in place. *Exercise caution when changing the dressing around drains, regardless of whether they are sutured, to prevent accidental removal.*

TABLE 47.6	Types of Wound Drainage
Type	**Appearance**
Serous	Clear, watery plasma
Purulent	Thick, yellow, green, tan, or brown
Serosanguineous	Pale, red, watery: mixture of clear and red fluid
Sanguineous	Bright red: indicates active bleeding

TABLE 47.5	Assessment of Abnormal Healing in Primary and Secondary Intention Wounds	
Primary Intention Wounds	**Secondary Intention Wounds**
Wound's incision line poorly approximated	Pale or fragile granulation tissue; granulation tissue bed is excessively dry or moist
Drainage present more than 3 days after closure	Exudate present
Inflammation decreased in first 3 to 5 days after injury	Necrotic or sloughy tissue present in wound base
No epithelialization of wound edges by day 4	Epithelialization not continuous
No healing ridge by day 9	Fruity, earthy, or putrid odour present
	Presence of fistula(s), tunnelling, undermining

Adapted from Nix, D. (2016). Skin and wound inspection and assessment. In R. A. Bryant & D. P. Nix (Eds.), *Acute and chronic wounds: Current management concepts* (5th ed.). Elsevier.

A Penrose drain lies under a dressing; at the time of placement, a pin or clip is placed through the drain to prevent it from slipping farther into a wound (Figure 47.19). It is usually the nurse's responsibility to pull or advance the drain as drainage decreases to permit healing deep within the wound site.

When assessing the number of drains, drain placement, character of drainage, and condition of collecting equipment, the nurse first observes the security of the drain and its location with respect to the wound. Next to note is the character of drainage. If a collecting device is available, the drainage volume should be measured. Because a drainage system needs to be patent, the nurse needs to look for drainage flow through the tubing, as well as around the tubing. *A sudden decrease in drainage through the tubing may indicate a blocked drain, which may require surgical revision. Contact the physician in this case.* When a drain is connected to suction, the system needs to be assessed to ensure that the pressure ordered is being exerted. Evacuator units such as a Hemovac or Jackson-Pratt (Figure 47.20) exert a constant low pressure as long as the suction device (bladder or bag) is fully compressed.

These types of drainage devices are often referred to as *self-suction*. If the evacuator device is unable to maintain a vacuum on its own, the surgeon should be notified, who will then order a secondary vacuum system (such as wall suction). If fluid accumulates within the tissues, optimal wound healing will not progress, increasing risk of infection.

Wound Closures. Surgical wounds are closed with staples, sutures, or wound closures. A frequent skin closure is the stainless steel staple. The staple provides more strength than nylon or silk sutures and causes less irritation to tissue. However, the nurse should look for irritation around staple or suture sites and note whether closures are intact. Normally, for the first 2 to 3 days after surgery, skin around sutures or staples is edematous. Continued swelling indicates that closures are too tight. Overly tight suture material may cut into the skin, which can lead to wound separation or wound dehiscence. Early suture removal reduces formation of defects along the suture line and minimizes chances of unattractive scar formation.

Tissue adhesive such as Dermabond forms a strong bond across apposed wound edges, which allows normal healing to occur below. It can be used to replace small sutures for incisional repair. The product is applied across the approximated wound edges, which are then held together until the solution dries, providing an adhesive closure. Although surgeons generally use it for small superficial lacerations, some may use it on larger wounds, where subcutaneous sutures are needed (Januchowski & Ferguson, 2014; Majeed et al., 2020).

Palpation of the Wound. When inspecting a wound, it is important to observe for swelling or separation of wound edges. Wearing sterile gloves, lightly press the wound edges to detect localized areas of tenderness or drainage collection. If pressure causes fluid to be expressed, the character of the drainage should be noted. The patient is normally sensitive to palpation of wound edges; however, extreme tenderness may be indicative of infection.

Wound Cultures. If purulent or suspicious-looking drainage is detected, a specimen of the drainage may need to be obtained for culture (see Chapter 34). A wound culture sample should never be collected from old drainage. Resident colonies of bacteria from the skin grow within exudate and are not always the true causative organisms of wound infection. First, the wound is cleaned with normal saline to remove skin flora. Aerobic organisms grow in superficial wounds exposed to the air, and anaerobic organisms tend to grow within body cavities. Follow agency policy or protocol for specimen collection (Box 47.7). Swab the cleanest, healthiest looking tissue to obtain results consistent with the infectious condition of the wound. It is also appropriate to swab any areas with undermining. See Figure 47.21 for a description of how to swab a wound.

Gram stains, which result in more appropriate treatment earlier in the course of infection than do cultures, are often also performed, but they do not usually require any additional specimens. The gold standard of wound culture is tissue biopsy, obtained by a physician or nurse with specialized training (Stotts, 2016b).

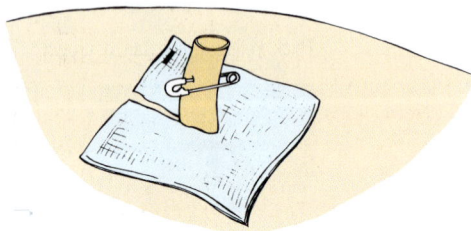

FIGURE 47.19 Penrose drain.

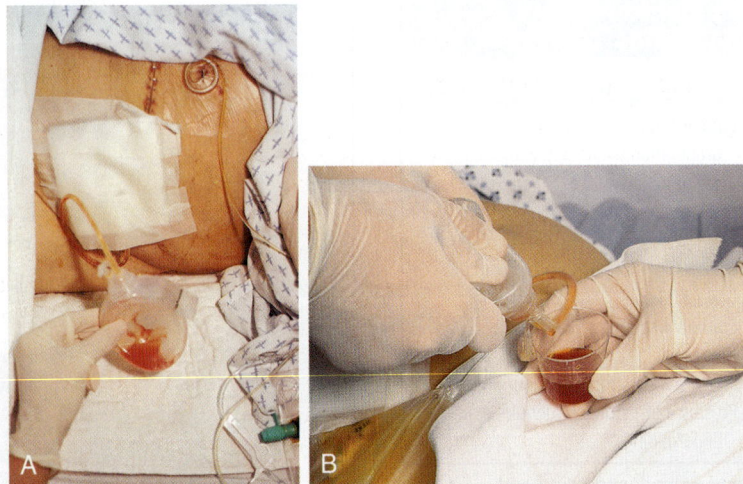

FIGURE 47.20 Jackson-Pratt drainage device. **A,** Drainage tubes and reservoir. **B,** Emptying drainage reservoir.

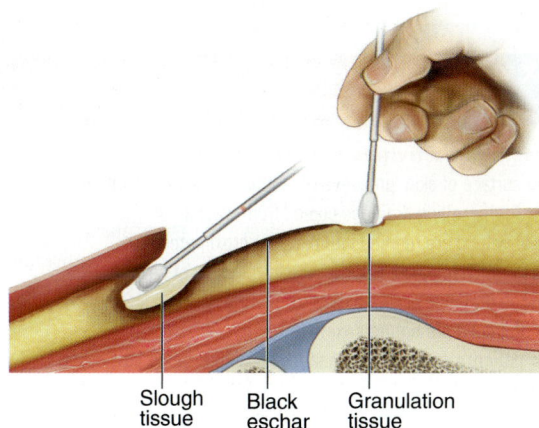

FIGURE 47.21 Swabbing technique. Swab wound from healthiest looking tissue to obtain results consistent with infectious condition of wound. It is also appropriate to swab any areas with undermining. (Illustration by Nancy A. Bauer. From Bauer, N. A. [2007, revised]. *RNAO best practice guideline: Assessment and management of stage I–IV pressure ulcers* [p. 100]. Author.)

Complications of Wound Healing

Hemorrhage. **Hemorrhage**, or bleeding from a wound site, is normal during and immediately after initial trauma. Hemostasis occurs within several minutes unless large blood vessels are involved or the patient has poor clotting function. Hemorrhages that occur after hemostasis indicate a slipped surgical suture, a dislodged clot, infection, or erosion of a blood vessel by a foreign object (e.g., a drain). Hemorrhage occurs externally or internally.

Internal bleeding is detected by looking for distention or swelling of the affected body part, a change in the type and amount of drainage from a surgical drain, or signs of hypovolemic shock. A **hematoma** is a localized collection of blood underneath the tissues. It appears as a swelling, a change in colour, sensation, or warmth, or a mass that often takes on a bluish discoloration. A hematoma near a major artery or vein is dangerous because pressure from the expanding hematoma obstructs blood flow.

External hemorrhaging is obvious. The dressings covering the wound need to be observed for bloody drainage. If bleeding is extensive, the dressing soon becomes saturated, and frequently blood drains from under the dressing and pools beneath the patient. *Observe all*

wounds closely, particularly surgical wounds, in which the risk of hemorrhage is greatest during the first 24 to 48 hours after surgery or injury.

Infection. Wound infection is the second most common health care–associated infection (see Chapter 34). However, infection may not be revealed through a lab culture due to poor culture technique or administration of antibiotics. In fact, all chronic wounds are considered contaminated with bacteria. What differentiates contaminated wounds from infected wounds is the amount of bacteria present. It is generally agreed that infected wounds have more than 100 000 (10⁵) organisms per gram of tissue (Stotts, 2016b). The chances of wound infection are greater when the wound contains necrotic tissue, when contaminants are in or near the wound, and when blood supply and local tissue defences are reduced.

Bacterial infection inhibits wound healing. Some contaminated or traumatic wounds show signs of infection early, within 2 to 3 days. A surgical wound infection may not develop until day 4 or 5. The patient has a fever, tenderness and pain at the wound site, and an elevated white blood cell count. The edges of the wound appear inflamed. If drainage is present, it is odorous and purulent and is a yellow, green, or brown colour, depending on the causative organism.

Dehiscence. When a wound fails to heal properly, the layers of skin and tissue separate. This most commonly occurs before collagen formation (3 to 11 days after injury). **Dehiscence** is the partial or total separation of wound layers. A patient at risk of poor wound healing (e.g., poor nutritional status, infection, or obesity) is at risk of dehiscence. Patients with obesity have a higher risk because of the constant strain placed on their wounds and the poor healing qualities of adipose tissue (Pierpont et al., 2014; Sandy-Hodgetts et al., 2018). Dehiscence involves abdominal surgical wounds and may occur after a sudden strain, such as coughing, vomiting, or sitting up (Figure 47.22). Patients often report feeling as though something has given way. *When an increased amount of serosanguineous drainage from a wound occurs, be alert for the potential for dehiscence.* A strategy to prevent dehiscence is to provide support to the area, using a folded thin blanket or pillow placed over an abdominal wound when the patient is coughing. This splints and supports healing tissue when coughing increases intra-abdominal pressure.

Evisceration. With total separation of wound layers, **evisceration** (protrusion of visceral organs through a wound opening) sometimes occurs. It is an emergent condition that requires surgical repair. *When evisceration occurs, quickly place sterile towels soaked in sterile saline over the extruding tissues to reduce the chance of bacterial invasion and drying of the tissues and contact the physician.* If the organs protrude through the wound, blood supply to the tissues is compromised. The patient should not receive anything by mouth (NPO). Observe for signs and symptoms of shock, and prepare the patient for emergency surgery.

Fistulas. A **fistula** is an abnormal passage between two organs or between an organ and the outside of the body. Most fistulas form as a result of poor wound healing or complication of disease, such as Crohn's disease. Trauma, infection, radiation exposure, and diseases such as cancer will prevent tissue layers from closing properly and will allow the fistula tract to form. Fistulas increase the risk of infection and fluid and electrolyte imbalances from fluid loss. Chronic drainage of fluids through a fistula also predisposes a patient to skin breakdown (Box 47.8).

◆ Nursing Diagnosis

Through assessment, clusters of data reveal whether an actual or a risk of *impaired skin integrity* exists. Assessment data may

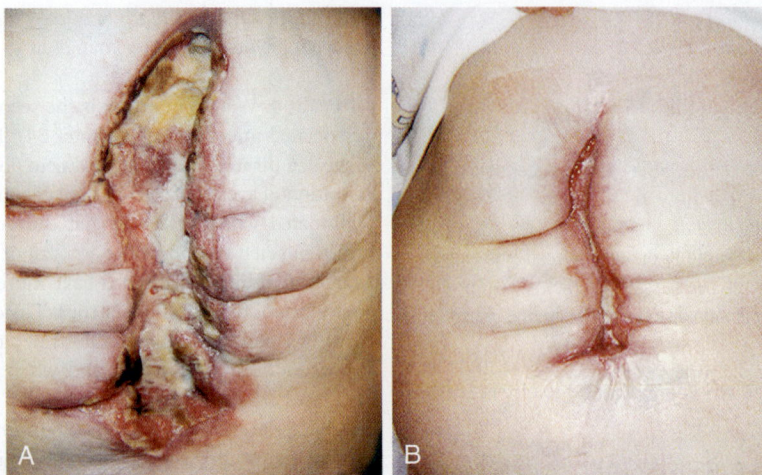

FIGURE 47.22 A, Dehisced wound before wound V.A.C. therapy. **B,** Dehisced wound after wound V.A.C. therapy. (Courtesy Kinetic Concepts, Inc. San Antonio, TX.)

BOX 47.8	Risk of Skin Breakdown From Body Fluids

Low Risk
Saliva
Serosanguineous drainage

Moderate Risk
Bile
Stool
Urine
Ascitic fluid
Purulent exudate

High Risk
Gastric drainage
Pancreatic drainage

BOX 47.9	Impaired Skin Integrity Related to a Contaminated Wound

Assessment Activities That Define Characteristics
Inspect surface of skin: presence of wound, break in skin integrity.
Yellow, foul-smelling drainage comes from wound.
Edges of wound are red and warm, not approximated.
Sutures remain in place. Inspect wound for signs of healing.
Brown-red drainage occurs 5 days after surgery.
Edges of wound are not approximated.
Obtain patient's temperature, heart rate, white blood cell count, and serum albumin level.
Patient is febrile, heart rate is 125 beats per minute, leukocyte (white blood cell) count is 12 000/mm³, and serum albumin level is less than 3.5 mg/100 mL.

---

support more than one diagnostic label. For example, a postoperative patient has purulent drainage from a surgical wound and reports tenderness around the area of the wound. These data support a nursing diagnosis of *impaired skin integrity related to a contaminated wound* (Box 47.9). After completing an assessment of the patient's wound, the nurse will be able to develop nursing diagnoses that will direct supportive and preventive care. Multiple nursing diagnoses are associated with impaired skin integrity and wounds:

- *Risk of infection*
- *Imbalanced nutrition: less than body requirements*
- *Acute or chronic pain*
- *Impaired physical mobility*
- *Impaired skin integrity*
- *Risk of impaired skin integrity*
- *Ineffective tissue perfusion*
- *Impaired tissue integrity*

Some patients are at risk of poor wound healing because of previously defined factors that impair healing. Thus, even though the patient's wound appears normal, the nurse would identify nursing diagnoses, such as *impaired nutrition* or *ineffective tissue perfusion,* that direct nursing care toward support of wound repair.

The nature of a wound can cause problems unrelated to wound healing. *Alteration in comfort* and *impaired mobility* are conditions that have implications for the patient's eventual recovery. For example, a large abdominal incision can cause enough pain to interfere with the patient's ability to turn in bed effectively.

◆ Planning

After identifying nursing diagnoses, the nurse needs to develop a plan of care for the patient who is at risk or who has actual impaired skin integrity. During planning, the nurse synthesizes information from multiple resources (see Figure 47.7). Critical thinking ensures that the patient's plan of care integrates everything the nurse knows about the individual, as well as key critical thinking elements. Professional standards of practice are especially important to consider when developing a plan of care (Kottner et al., 2019). As the patient's nurse, ask yourself what aspects of care you are able to perform without medical orders, what aspects of care you can delegate to other regulated and unregulated health care providers, and what are the patient goals.

Goals and Outcomes

Nursing care is based on the patient's identified needs and priorities. As a nurse, your first step is to ensure you are on the same path with the patient, regarding goals and expected outcomes. In addition, you need to consider whether the wound is likely to heal. For example, a pressure injury with unrelieved pressure, along with the patient's possible poor nutritional intake, is unlikely to heal. In addition, patients in terminal stages of illness may not have the physiological resources to heal, despite optimal environmental supports. Thus, it is important to plan interventions according to risk of skin breakdown, type and severity of the wound, and underlying causes and complications, such as infection, incontinence, poor nutrition, and peripheral vascular diseases, which affect wound healing.

A goal frequently identified is to see wound improvement within a 2-week period. The outcomes of this goal could include the following:

- Higher percentage of granulation tissue in the wound base
- No further skin breakdown in any body location
- An increase in caloric intake of 10%

These outcomes are reasonable if the overall goal for the patient is to heal the injury. Other goals of care for patients with wounds include preventing infection, maintaining skin integrity, comfort, and health promotion.

Setting Priorities

Priorities in wound care are based on comprehensive patient assessment, goals and expectations, and established outcomes. These priorities also depend on whether the patient's condition is stable or acute (emergent). An acute wound needs immediate intervention, whereas in the presence of a chronic, stable wound, other factors, such as pressure relief, may have greater priority. No matter what the situation, preventive interventions such as good skin care, appropriate positioning, moisture management (e.g., incontinence), and elimination of friction and shear are priorities. Promotion of skin health is also essential and includes patient and family education (Box 47.10). No matter what the setting, existing skin breakdown, from skin tears to large chronic wounds, requires ongoing attention because it is frequently the reason for both hospitalization and decrease in quality of life for patients. Patient and family preferences, daily activities, and the

---

BOX 47.10   RESEARCH HIGHLIGHT

Evaluation of Patient Education Materials on Pressure Injury Prevention in Hospitals and Health Services

Research Focus

There is a gap in the literature surrounding the potential benefits of improving patient understanding of pressure injuries (PIs). Limited research has been conducted on access and reliable information in PI educational materials. The aim of the study was to assess the availability and accuracy of online patient education on PI prevention through a content analysis of the educational materials.

Research Abstract

Pressure injuries (PIs) are a common quality indicator for hospital care, and preventing PIs often requires patient engagement; as such, Australian consensus research has recommended that high-quality education materials be made to patients for PIs via hospital networks. The purpose of this study was to assess the availability and accuracy of patient education materials on PIs in publicly available hospital websites in Victoria, Australia.

Two independent coders assessed 212 websites for content on PI prevention and management, analyzing availability and accuracy of PI definitions, risk factors, preventive strategies, referral, visual tools, consumer endorsement, information for family and caregivers, and translation in community languages. A greater proportion of hospitals did not have any patient education materials on PI prevention publicly available, with private hospitals (compared with public) and metropolitan hospitals (compared to rural) more likely to have materials available on their sites. The available materials contained accurate messages regarding PI-defining characteristics and risk factors for PIs, although there was considerable variability in the availability of other information. Our findings suggest a significant deficit in the availability of educational materials for acute care patients and their families. There is a need for evidence-informed, consumer-endorsed, uniform materials on all hospital websites to prevent development of PIs in acute care.

Objectives of the Study

- Determine availability of PI patient online education in hospital settings
- Identify accuracy of information regarding definitions, risk factors, preventive strategies, referral, visual tools, consumer endorsement, information for family and caregivers, and translation in community languages

Methods

The researchers analyzed available PI educational materials located on the web pages of health services and hospitals in one region of Australia. They then examined relationships between availability of materials and a variety of factors, including private versus public hospitals and rural versus urban settings, using separate chi-square tests. A qualitative content analysis was conducted to evaluate the accuracy of information about PI prevention and management.

Results

The results showed more than half of the 212 hospital websites accessed (66.5%) did not contain any information for patients on prevention and management of PIs, indicating that only 34.5% had these materials. Private hospitals were more likely to have patient information about PIs on their website (45 out of 83) than public hospitals (26 out of 103). Similarly, metropolitan hospitals were more likely to have PI materials on their websites (57 of 120) than were rural hospitals (14 of 92), and the association between the location type and PI educational material availability was statistically significant.

While all identified educational materials contained some form of definition or explanation and included preventative strategies, which were accurate, many lacked other basic information, such as messages encouraging collaboration with health care providers, information for caregivers, and visual tools. Furthermore, few presented information on community or consumer endorsement or the availability of this information in other community languages.

The findings suggest that more than half of the hospitals lack educational materials designed for patients to prevent and manage PIs. The current data suggest that hospital websites are lacking uniform accessible educational materials for patients. This gap likely contributes to the lack of knowledge about PIs and creates a barrier for patients and their families to participate in patient-focused decision making. This study adds significance to the body of knowledge regarding knowledge translation and patient-focused care.

Implications for Practice

Future research should include a focus on health literacy. Findings from this study can help improve educational material content as well as consider how health care providers and hospitals could reconsider their roles and actions as educators for patients and families experiencing PIs.

From Team, V., Bouguettaya, A., Richards, C., et al. (2020). Patient education materials sn pressure injury prevention in hospitals and health services in Victoria, Australia: Availability and content analysis. *International Wound Journal, 17*(2), 370–379.

healing potential of the wound need to be included in the collaborative setting of priorities.

Collaborative Care

Wound care is not just a nursing responsibility; it is a team effort, including a physiotherapist, occupational therapist, dietitian, pharmacist, and physician, as well as the patient, family, and nurse. With early discharge from health care settings, it is important to consider what resources are required to plan for the patient's ongoing care. Anticipating wound care needs and related equipment and resources, such as referral to a home care agency or outpatient wound care clinic, supports not only wound healing but also the patient's independence.

Patients and their families often are expected to continue wound management after discharge (Box 47.11). Patients, families, and caregivers need education in and knowledge of wound care so that they understand the importance of good nutrition, pressure off-loading (particularly when sitting in a recliner chair for long periods of time), and how different wound dressings are used. The nurse's role, no matter the health care setting, is to work with the patient and family to develop and support their understanding and involvement to optimize wound healing as much as possible. Nurses need to keep in mind the patient's and family's ability to manage dressing changes and other aspects of care that will be important to support best outcomes, as well as how the home care nurse can provide support.

◆ Implementation: Preventing Skin Breakdown

Health Promotion. Prevention is the most effective intervention for problems with skin breakdown. Prompt, early identification of patient risk factors aids in the prevention of pressure injuries. Use of a risk assessment tool, such as the Braden Scale (see Table 47.2), is a first step in identifying a patient's risk of skin breakdown. Table 47.7 provides nursing interventions based on risk factors identified in the Braden Scale. If risk factors are identified, nurses must follow up with interventions. The three major areas of nursing interventions for prevention of skin breakdown are (1) skin care, including hygiene and moisture management; (2) mechanical loading and support devices, including positioning and use of therapeutic surfaces; and (3) education (Mitchell, 2018; RNAO, 2016a).

Topical Skin Care. Skin assessments (see Box 47.5) should be done at a minimum of once a day; however, high-risk patients may require more frequent skin assessments, such as every shift. In addition, the patient's skin must be kept clean and dry. Assessment and skin hygiene are two major defences for preventing skin breakdown. To clean the skin, use of soaps and hot water should be avoided. Instead, the nurse should use cleansers with nonionic surfactants that are

TABLE 47.7	A Quick Guide to Pressure Injury Prevention
Risk Factor	**Nursing Interventions**
Decreased sensory perception	Assess pressure points for signs of nonblanching reactive hyperemia.
	Provide a pressure-redistribution surface.
Moisture	Assess need for incontinence management.
	After each incontinent episode, clean area with no-rinse perineal cleaner and protect skin with a moisture-barrier ointment.
Friction and shear	Reposition patient by using a drawsheet to lift patient off the surface. Ensure heels are also supported.
	Provide a trapeze to facilitate movement.
	Position patient at a 30-degree lateral turn and limit head elevation to 30 degrees.
Decreased activity or mobility	Establish and post an individualized turning schedule.
	Ensure functionality of pressure off-loading devices for wheelchair, bed.
Poor nutrition	Assess teeth or dentures; ensure good mouth care.
	Provide adequate nutritional and fluid intake; assist with intake, as necessary.
	Consult dietitian for nutritional evaluation.

BOX 47.11	Home Care Recommendations for Ulcer or Wound Assessment

Assessment and documentation of the wound should occur at least weekly, unless evidence of deterioration (including infection) exists, in which case reassess both the wound and the patient's overall management immediately. In the home setting, it is essential to include the patient and family in monitoring the progress of the wound.

Psychosocial Assessment and Management
- Assess the patient's resources (e.g., availability and skill of caregivers, finances, equipment). A successful treatment program requires adequate caregiver and equipment resources.
- Evaluate the caregiver's ability to comprehend and implement the treatment requirements.
- Evaluate the caregiver's ability to physically manage (level of strength and endurance) wound treatment.
- Consider economic factors that may limit the supply and availability of equipment, as well as provide caregiver relief.
- Use an approach that focuses on the psychosocial and physical factors affecting wound care (House, 2015).

Wound Care Dressings
- Consider caregiver time and ability when selecting a dressing.

- Consider a dressing that, while more expensive per unit, may decrease frequency of dressing change (which is more cost-effective than a cheaper dressing requiring more frequent dressing change).
- Dressings for healable wounds should provide moisture management without macerating or drying out the wound bed, decrease bioburden, and support wound debridement.

Infection Control
- All wounds are colonized; thus, the focus in the home is to avoid introduction of contamination into the wound, either by instruments, dressings, or technique at dressing change (Sibbald et al., 2003).
- Depending on the status of the wound (surgical/acute or chronic), secondary dressings may be clean or sterile, but the contact layer dressing should be from a sterile (unopened) package.
- The aseptic "no-touch" technique is generally used. This technique is a method of changing surface dressings without touching the wound or the surface of any dressing that might be in contact with the wound. Adherent dressings should be grasped by the corner and removed slowly, whereas gauze dressings can be pinched in the centre and lifted off (Sonoiki et al., 2020).
- Place soiled dressings in a plastic bag and securely fasten bag closure. Disposal of contaminated dressings in the home should be done in a manner consistent with local regulations and home care agency policies.

gentle to the skin (Orsted et al., 2017; RNAO, 2016a). Many types of products are available for skin care. Nurses need to be familiar with what is most appropriate for the specific needs of the patient.

After cleaning the skin and making sure it is completely dry, a small amount of moisturizer is applied to keep the epidermis lubricated but not oversaturated. It is important to control, contain, or correct incontinence, perspiration, and wound drainage (Bryant & Clark, 2016).

To aid in preventing and managing incontinence, clinicians find the RNAO *Best Practice Guidelines on Promoting Continence Using Prompted Voiding* helpful, although the Canadian Urological Association (CUA) has also developed Canadian guidelines, accessible on the CUA website. Patients with fecal incontinence who are also receiving enteral tube feeding present a management challenge. In instances such as this, it may be helpful to obtain the expertise of an advanced practice nurse with a focus on wound care or management of incontinence.

When patients have an episode of incontinence, the affected area should be gently cleaned (a no-rinse perineal cleanser is a good option) and dried, and an occlusive barrier cream applied to the exposed area. The barrier cream will protect skin from excessive moisture and bacteria found in the urine or stool. The barrier cream should not interfere with the function of the adult continence brief. Methods for controlling or containing incontinence vary. While medication and surgery are possible treatments, along with catheters or fecal continence systems, behavioural techniques should be considered with the patient, such as prompted or timed voiding. The guidelines mentioned earlier (RNAO and CUA) are excellent resources to help nurses consider these options with their patients, when possible.

Before initiating use of absorbent incontinence pads and briefs, the nurse should explore the use of the behavioural techniques mentioned above. These products are only part of the treatment plan for incontinence. Only products that wick moisture away from the patient's skin should be used (Bryant & Clark, 2016; Wounds Canada, 2017a). Underpads need to be used with caution, because some of these pads do not wick the drainage away from the patient's skin and will cause skin damage. In addition, patients who are provided with low air loss or other specialty pressure-relief bed surfaces require specifically designed continence pads for these bed surfaces.

Positioning.
Positioning interventions reduce pressure and shearing force to the skin. Elevating the head of the bed to 30 degrees or less will decrease the chance of pressure injuries developing from shearing forces (RNAO, 2016a). A *Cochrane Review* of studies examining repositioning related to pressure injury prevention (Gillespie et al., 2014) indicated that there were limited reliable results as to timed repositioning (e.g., 2, 3, 4, or 6 hours). However, repositioning is essential for preventing skin breakdown and supporting healing (Fletcher, 2017). Nurses need to be aware of patients' activity level, perceptual ability, and daily routines (Fletcher, 2017; RNAO, 2016a) when determining the best possible plan for the individual. When repositioning a patient, the nurse can use pillows, foam wedges, or other devices to protect bony prominences (RNAO, 2016a). The RNAO guidelines recommend a 30-degree lateral position, which prevents positioning directly over a bony prominence. The nurse should use a sheet under the patient when needing to change their position, and lift, rather than drag, the patient. The patient's heels must be supported whenever moving patients in bed. Physiotherapists (PTs) and occupational therapists (OTs) are a great resource because they are skilled at assessment and treatment modalities for both seating and positioning for beds, chairs, and wheelchairs.

> **SAFETY ALERT** Incorrect positioning of an immobile patient may create a shearing injury. When repositioning the patient, obtain assistance. With at least one other caregiver, place a drawsheet under the patient, and then, grasping the sides of the sheet, use it to lift the patient up and toward the new position. Remember to ensure the heels are not dragging on the bed, as this may contribute to shearing and friction injuries.

If the patient can sit in a chair, the duration should be limited. For example, if the care plan is to reposition every 2 hours, then sitting should also be less than 2 hours. In the sitting position, the pressure on the ischial tuberosities is greater than when lying down. Patients with some independent mobility should be encouraged to shift weight every 15 minutes when sitting, which provides short-term relief on the ischial tuberosities (RNAO, 2016a). Seating surfaces should be high-density foam, gel, or air cushion to redistribute weight away from the ischial areas. The PT or OT can help the nurse assess and ensure that cushions are correctly inflated and positioned. Rigid and doughnut-shaped cushions are contraindicated because they reduce blood supply to the area, which results in wider areas of ischemia (RNAO, 2016a).

After repositioning, the patient's skin should be reassessed. See Box 47.2 for identifying characteristics that indicate early signs of tissue ischemia in darkly pigmented skin. For patients who have light-toned skin, the nurse should check for normal reactive hyperemia and blanching.

Reddened areas should never be massaged. Massaging reddened areas damages capillaries in the underlying tissues and increases the risk of pressure injury formation to those areas (RNAO, 2016a).

Support Surfaces (Therapeutic Beds and Mattresses).
A *support surface* (i.e., mattresses, integrated bed system, mattress replacement, overlay or seat cushion, or seat cushion overlay) is a specialized device for pressure redistribution designed to manage tissue loads, microclimate, and other therapeutic functions (NPIAP, 2007/2019). A variety of support surfaces exist, including specialty beds and mattresses that reduce the hazards of immobility to the skin and musculoskeletal system. However, none of them eliminates the need for meticulous nursing care, and no single device eliminates the effects of pressure on the skin.

When selecting support surfaces, the nurse must thoroughly assess the patient's needs. Knowledge about support surface characteristics (Table 47.8) will help in decision making, along with consultations with the PT and OT.

No matter what the setting (e.g., hospital, home), nurses need to fully explain to patients and families why and how these specialty surfaces are to be used (Box 47.12). Some common errors made when this information is not provided include the following: placing the wrong side of the support surface toward the patient, not plugging in or turning on powered support surfaces, using inappropriate absorbent underlay or bedding, failing to do "hand checks," and improper inflation (too much or too little) for some support surfaces. Hand checks are done by placing the hand under the support surface (or, if an overlay, between it and the standard mattress or cushion), at the pressure point, with the palm facing up and fingers flat. There should be at least 2.5 cm of support surface between the patient's pressure point and the caregiver's hand. If not, the support cushion or bed surface does not provide adequate support.

Education.
Education of the patient and caregivers is an important nursing function (Orsted et al., 2017). Nurses need to consider their patient's language, educational level, and learning needs, especially older patients or those for whom English is not their first language.

TABLE 47.8 Support Surfaces

Categories and Definitions	Mechanism of Action	Indications	Examples of Manufacturers in Canada*
Low-Air-Loss Available in a mattress placed directly on the existing bed frame or an overlay placed directly on top of an existing surface	Pressure redistribution Provides a flow of air to assist in managing the heat and humidity of the skin	Prevention or treatment of skin breakdown	Arjo-Huntleigh EHOB Hill-Rom Quart Healthcare
Nonpowered Any support surface not requiring or using external sources of energy for operation. Examples: foam, interconnected air-filled cells	Pressure redistribution Air moves to and from cells as body position changes	Prevention or treatment of skin breakdown	Arjo-Huntleigh EHOB Hill-Rom Quart Healthcare
Air-Fluidized Beds Surfaces that change load distribution properties when powered and when patient is in contact with the surface	Provides pressure redistribution via a fluidlike medium created by forcing air through beads, as characterized by immersion and envelopment	Prevention or treatment of skin breakdown May also be used to protect newly flapped or grafted surgical sites and for patients with excessive moisture	Arjo-Huntleigh Hill-Rom
Lateral Rotation Provides passive motion to promote mobilization of respiratory secretions and provides low-air-loss therapy	Features a support surface that provides rotation about a longitudinal axis, as characterized by degree of patient turn, duration, and frequency	Treatment and prevention of pulmonary complications associated with immobility	Arjo-Huntleigh Hill-Rom Quart Healthcare

*Refer to company website for specific product information and current product availability.

BOX 47.12 PATIENT TEACHING
Pressure-Redistribution Surfaces

Objectives
- Patient and family will describe their understanding of the purposes and basic operations of the pressure-redistribution surfaces.

Teaching Strategies
- Explain reasons for the pressure-redistribution surface.
- Explain proper body mechanics while using the pressure-redistribution surface.
- Educate patient and family about the use and care of the pressure-redistribution surface.
- Explain additional pressure-redistribution measures.

Evaluation
- Patient and family will state the basic purposes for the pressure-redistribution surface.
- Patient and family will describe the function of the pressure-redistribution surface.
- Patient and family will demonstrate proper use of the pressure-redistribution surface.

Appropriate educational tools should be used, including web-based videos and written materials when teaching patients, family, and caregivers how to prevent and treat skin breakdown. Materials can be accessed from reputable government, educational, and national organizations such as Wounds Canada and NSWOCC (see "Recommended Websites" section). The wound care industry also provides excellent educational materials, although some may be product specific. Nurses can readily access any of these sites by conducting an Internet search.

It is important to understand the impact of the experience of a chronic wound for patients and their caregivers (Lusher, 2020; Orsted et al., 2017; RNAO, 2016a). Through research, clinicians are beginning to explore the concerns and issues faced by patients and their frail older spouses caring for their loved ones with pressure injuries (Aloweni et al., 2019; Goldberg & Beltz, 2010; Koschwanez et al., 2013). Interventions need to meet the psychosocial needs of patients and their caregivers (Erfurt-Berge et al., 2019; Orsted et al., 2017; RNAO, 2016a).

Management of Pressure Injury. Treatment of patients with pressure injury requires a holistic, team approach (Gould et al., 2020; RNAO, 2016a). Expertise of other members of the interprofessional health care team (physician, physiotherapist, occupational therapist, dietitian, pharmacist) is essential for supportive measures such as adequate nutrients and redistribution of pressure (Skill 47.2).

Optimizing wound healing requires monitoring of the wound, but unless infection is suspected or present, wounds heal best when undisturbed. Many current wound dressings are designed to remain in place for up to a week or even longer, and this approach supports healing in chronic, noninfected wounds (Orsted et al., 2017; RNAO, 2016a). However, nurses still need to regularly assess and document the wound: its location, stage, size, tissue type, exudate, and surrounding skin condition (Nix, 2016).

The use and documentation of a systematic approach to assessment of pressure injury leads to better decision making and optimal outcomes (Hebert, 2018; Hess, 2018). Using a tool helps link the assessment to outcomes so that an evaluation of the plan of care follows objective criteria (Hess, 2018). For example, the Bates-Jensen Wound Assessment Tool (BWAT) contains 13 items to assess wound characteristics, which

SKILL 47.2	TREATING PRESSURE INJURIES	

Delegation Considerations

The skill of treating pressure injuries cannot be delegated to unregulated care providers (UCPs). In some practice settings, nurses can delegate *nonsterile* dressing application for chronic, established wounds when a nurse has evaluated and designated the protocol. The *assessment* of the wound remains within the scope of the nurse, however, even if the dressing change is delegated. Instruct nursing assistive personnel to do the following:

- Report changes in skin integrity to a nurse immediately.
- Report pain, fever, or wound drainage to a nurse immediately.
- Report any potential contamination to the existing dressing (e.g., patient incontinence or other bodily fluids; dressing becomes dislodged).

Equipment

- Disposable gloves (clean)
- Plastic bag for dressing disposal
- Disposable measuring tape
- Cotton-tipped applicators (sterile)
- Topical cleaning agent
- Dressing of choice (see Table 47.9)
- Hypoallergenic tape (if needed)
- Documentation record
- Measurement tool to record ongoing wound progress

PROCEDURE

STEPS	RATIONALE

1. Assess patient's level of comfort using a scale of 1 to 10 and the need for pain medication.
2. Determine if patient has allergies to topical agents.
3. Review order for topical agent or dressing.
4. Close room door or bedside curtains. Position patient to allow dressing removal.
5. Perform hand hygiene, and apply clean gloves. Remove dressing, and place in plastic bag.

- Pain management enables better tolerance for dressing change.
- Topical agents cause localized skin reactions.
- Administration of proper medication and treatment is ensured.
- Privacy is provided; area is accessible for dressing change.
- Transmission of microorganisms is reduced; accidental exposure to body fluids is prevented.

6. Assess pressure injury or wound. All pressure wounds need individual assessments (see Step 6 illustration).

- Consistent assessment will provide the basis for evaluating wound progress (RNAO, 2016a).

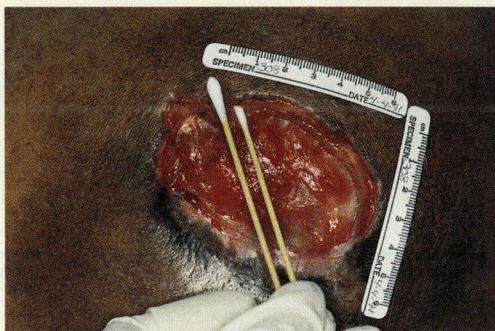

STEP 6 Measuring wound depth (Steps B, C, and D.)

A. Note colour, type, and percentage of tissue present in the wound base.
B. Measure width and length of the wound(s). Determine width by measuring the dimension from left to right and the length from top to bottom.
Wound measurement uses the analogue clock. Facing the patient, the head is at 12 o'clock, which is the 'top'/head of the wound.
C. Measure depth of wound using sterile cotton-tipped applicator (see Step 6 illustration).

- Determining tissue type assists in dressing selection.
- Wound size will change as healing progresses; therefore, longest and widest areas of the wound will change over time. Measuring width and length by measuring the same area will provide a consistent measurement (Nix, 2016).
- Depth is important to determine wound volume. Although surface area adequately represents tissue loss in stage 2 wounds, volume more adequately represents tissue loss in stage 3 and 4 wounds (RNAO, 2016a).

D. Measure depth of undermining using sterile cotton-tipped applicator to gently probe under skin edges (see Step 6 illustration).

- Undermining represents loss of underlying tissue (subcutaneous and muscle) to a greater extent than the skin. Undermining indicates progressive tissue loss.

7. Assess periwound skin for maceration, redness, and denuded areas.

- Deterioration of skin around a wound indicates infection, excessive wound exudate, or skin stripping from adhesive removal.

8. Change to sterile gloves, if needed (check agency policy).

- Avoid potential contamination of wound from external source. Refer to institutional policy regarding use of clean or sterile gloves.

9. Clean wound thoroughly with warmed normal saline, tap water, or cleaning agent.

- Wound debris must be removed to support healing tissue (Brown, 2018; RNAO, 2016a).

SKILL 47.2	TREATING PRESSURE INJURIES—cont'd	
STEPS		**RATIONALE**

10. Apply topical agents, as prescribed.

    A. Enzymatic debridement, as prescribed. Carefully read instructions.

        (1) Apply thin, even layer of ointment over necrotic areas of ulcer only, where eschar has been scored, if required. Protect periwound skin.

- A thick layer of ointment is not necessary; a thin layer absorbs and is more effective (Bryant & Nix, 2016). Check manufacturer's directions for frequency of application.

        (2) Apply secondary nonadherent gauze dressing directly over wound.

- Wound is protected. Bacteria are prevented from entering wound.

        (3) Tape securely in place.

- Dressing is kept in place. Use tape or adhesive that will not irritate skin.

    B. Hydrogel

        (1) Cover surface of ulcer with thin layer of hydrogel using applicator or gloved hand.

- A moist wound environment is maintained.

        (2) Apply secondary nonadherent gauze dressing or transparent dressing over wound, and adhere to intact skin.

- Wound base is covered and hydrogel–wound interface is maintained.

    C. Calcium alginate or hydrofibre

        (1) Lightly pack wound with alginate or hydrofibre using applicator or gloved fingers.

- Wound moisture is maintained while excess drainage is absorbed.

        (2) Apply secondary dressing of nonadherent gauze, absorbent pad, or foam over alginate. Tape in place.

- Alginate is held against wound surface.

11. Remove gloves, dispose of soiled supplies. Perform hand hygiene.

- Transmission of microorganisms is reduced.

12. Assess wound at each dressing change or sooner if the wound or patient's condition deteriorates (Nix, 2016). Utilize agency's tool for wound assessment.

- Not all patients with wounds will follow a healing trajectory, due to comorbidities. Consistent assessment provides a record of healing progress, deterioration, or stalled wound.

13. Compare wound assessment to identified plan of care, and discuss with health care team if there is increase in size of wound, increased presence of pain, foul-smelling drainage, or increase in devitalized tissue.

- Wound care is an interprofessional activity and requires involvement of the team of health care providers as well as the patient and family.

> **CRITICAL DECISION POINT:** *A clean pressure wound should show evidence of approximately 30% healing within 2 to 4 weeks. Do not use the pressure injury staging system to measure healing. The system measures depth of wound, not healing (WOCN, 2016).*

14. Complete wound documentation required for one of the wound assessment instruments per agency's protocol.

- Assessments compared over time will determine progress toward wound healing.

UNEXPECTED OUTCOMES

RELATED INTERVENTIONS

Maceration of skin surrounding wound

- Reduce exposure of surrounding skin to topical agents and moisture.
- Use a dimethicone barrier wipe or cream on periwound skin or silicone border dressing.
- Use a dressing that will wick exudate away from periwound skin.

Deepening of wound and increased drainage

- Notify health care team regarding possible wound infection.
- Obtain necessary wound cultures as required.
- Obtain additional consults (e.g., wound care specialist).

RECORDING AND REPORTING

- Record assessment of wound (including measurement) in patient's record.
- Describe type of topical agent used, dressing applied, and patient's response.
- Report any deterioration in wound appearance (including odour).

CARE IN THE COMMUNITY CONSIDERATIONS

- Assess ability of patient or family to manage dressing changes and provide education (demonstrate and ensure that family, patient, or both can show or describe how to manage dressings and support).
- Patients need to dispose of contaminated dressings in the home in a manner consistent with local regulations (WOCN, 2016).
- Discuss need for a home pressure-redistribution surface or bed.

are then rated by the nurse, using a Likert-type scale (score of 1 indicates the healthiest and 5 indicates the least healthy attribute for each characteristic). Tools such as the BWAT may seem overly detailed and time consuming, but when used accurately and regularly, they provide a method of ensuring reliable documentation of evaluating whether the goals of the wound management plan are effective.

Many organizations use electronic documentation systems, including wound care documentation. These approaches are rapidly replacing "paper and pen" versions of documentation and assessment, and often provide options for wound photography and automated wound measurement as well as embedded best practice recommendations (Jacob et al., 2020; Kulikov et al., 2019; Nair, 2018).

Wound Management. Maintenance of a physiological local wound environment is the goal of effective wound management (Bryant & Nix, 2016). To maintain a healthy wound environment, nurses need to pay attention to the following directives: prevent and manage infection, clean the wound, remove nonviable tissue, manage exudate, maintain the wound in a moist (not wet) environment, and protect the wound. A wound will not move through the phases of wound healing if the wound is infected or if underlying causes are not addressed. Prevention of wound infection includes wound irrigation, cleaning, and removal of nonviable tissue.

Cleaning a Wound. Only noncytotoxic wound cleaners, such as normal saline or commercial wound cleaners, should be used to clean wounds. Noncytotoxic cleaners will not damage or kill fibroblasts and healing tissue (Bryant & Nix, 2016). Cytotoxic solutions, used full strength, are not recommended to cleanse or irrigate *healable* wounds. These are bleach (sodium hypochlorite or *Dakin's* solution), acetic acid (vinegar), povidone-iodine (Betadine), chlorhexidine, and hydrogen peroxide, and they are *not* to be used in clean granulating wounds because they inhibit wound healing (Orsted et al., 2017; RNAO, 2016a).

For a number of years there has been a recommendation to use potable tap water in cleaning and irrigating wounds. From the research literature, there appears to be no particular risk related to using tap water from safe (municipal) water sources (Queirós et al., 2014). However, when using tap water in rural areas or from unknown sources, or if there could be potential contamination from the delivery system (e.g., rusted faucet or pipes), it is better to err on the side of caution and use sterile water or normal saline as the cleanser of choice.

Irrigation. Irrigation is a common method of delivering the wound cleaning solution to the wound. Studies have shown that there is an optimal effective range of irrigation pressures that ensure adequate removal of bacteria (RNAO, 2016a; Rodeheaver, 2012). To ensure an irrigation pressure within the correct range of 8–15 psi and avoid trauma to the wound bed, the nurse should use a 30- to 35-cc syringe with a 18- to 19-gauge angiocatheter or a 100-mL saline squeeze bottle (Bryant & Nix 2016).

Debridement. **Debridement** is the removal of nonviable, necrotic tissue and is necessary to rid the injury of a source of infection, to enable visualization of the wound bed, and to provide a clean base for healing. However, a dry necrotic heel ulcer is an exception. According to the RNAO (2016a) guidelines, stable, dry, black eschar on heels should not be debrided if no evidence of infection (e.g., pain, purulence, or erythema) appears. The method of debridement—mechanical, autolytic, chemical, or sharp or surgical—will depend on which is most appropriate to the patient's condition and care goals (Orsted et al., 2017; RNAO, 2016a). During the debridement process, increases in wound exudate, odour, and size are likely to be observed. Pain that may occur with debridement should be assessed and effectively managed (Orsted et al., 2017; RNAO, 2016a).

Mechanical debridement, or a "wet-to-dry" saline gauze dressing, is *not* considered appropriate, as it is nonselective in its removal of both devitalized and viable tissue (Orsted et al., 2017). Biological debridement is the use of maggot therapy, which is as effective as surgical debridement, but currently limited in accessibility. Sterile maggots are used in a wound because they ingest the dead tissue and do not impede granulation (Sun et al., 2016). Topical enzymes in chemical or enzymatic debridement induce changes in the substrate, resulting in the breakdown of necrotic tissue (Carter et al., 2016). Depending on the type of enzyme used, the preparation either digests or dissolves tissue. Care must be taken to apply enzymes only to the wound bed, never periwound tissue.

Current best practice treatment options are autolytic and sharp or surgical debridement (the gold standard). In autolytic debridement, synthetic dressings allow the eschar and fibrinous slough within the wound to be self-digested by the action of enzymes present in wound fluids (Orsted et al., 2017). Dressings that support moisture at the wound surface (e.g., hydrogel or hydrocolloid) maintain a moist wound bed ("moist like your eyeball"), which allows the movement of epithelial cells and facilitates wound closure; however, a wound that has excessive exudate (drainage) provides an environment that supports bacterial growth, macerates the periwound skin, and slows the healing process (Orsted et al., 2017). If exudate is excessive, an absorptive dressing (e.g., calcium alginate, hydrofibre, or foam) should be used, and volume, consistency, and odour of drainage evaluated to determine whether infection may be present.

Sharp or surgical debridement is the most efficient way to reach vitalized tissue at the base of a wound and is also used when sepsis can be localized and excised. Surgical debridement with a scalpel, scissors, or other sharp instrument should be performed only by health care providers with the knowledge, skill, and competence to perform the procedure, usually physicians and advanced practice nurses (e.g., nurse practitioners). As a nurse, your regulating authority (e.g., College of Nurses) and your agency or institution policy mandate whether you are able to perform sharp or surgical debridement.

It is important to remember that the wound will not heal, regardless of the use of topical therapy (Bryant & Nix, 2016), unless the underlying causative factors (e.g., malnourishment, shear, friction, pressure, and moisture) are controlled or eliminated. In addition, as the wound goes through the phases of healing, the treatment plan will need to be altered. For example, in the management of a wound with slough and necrotic tissue, the nurse may initially use a hydrocolloid dressing to autolytically debride the wound. Because the hydrocolloid dressing interacts with the wound to gradually liquefy and debride the slough/necrotic tissue, it should be left intact—up to 1 week if possible. Once the wound is free of necrotic, sloughy tissue, the nurse would discontinue the hydrocolloid dressing and choose a different type of dressing after assessing the wound base characteristics (e.g., Is there drainage? Increased bacteria? Ongoing slough/necrotic tissue?). Continued reassessment is key to supporting the wound as it moves through the phases of wound healing. It cannot be stressed enough how important it is for you, as the nurse, to explain the process of wound healing to the patient and family.

Growth Factors. Growth factors regulate most of the key actions of cells during wound healing (Schultz, 2016). Through extensive studies of the molecular regulation of healing, researchers now better understand the role of various growth factors involved in wound healing, including epidermal growth factor, platelet-derived growth factor, fibroblast growth factor, and transforming growth factor. Depending on the setting, the nurse may be responsible for use of this treatment modality.

Nutritional Status. Nutritional assessment and support of the patient with a wound is a vital component in normal cellular integrity and tissue repair (Molnar et al., 2016; Stotts, 2016a; Weiss et al., 2016). Inadequate nutrition must be addressed with early intervention to support healing. The Canadian Malnutrition Task Force (2017) recommends nutritional assessment within 24 hours of hospital admission. The patient's mouth and skin should be assessed for signs of nutritional deficiencies (see Chapter 43). Reassessments reflect changes in status and effects of interventions (Litchford et al., 2014). Box 47.13 defines parameters for clinically significant malnutrition (Agency for Health Care Policy and Research [AHCPR], 1994; Cederholm et al., 2015).

Protein Status. Patients with a potential for or actual decreased serum albumin levels or poor protein intake need a nutritional evaluation to ensure proper caloric intake (Laporte et al., 2015; Orsted et al., 2017). A patient can lose as much as 50 g of protein per day from an open, weeping pressure injury. Although the recommended intake

BOX 47.13   AHCPR* Recommendations for Nutritional Assessment and Management of Pressure Injury

Assessment of Clinically Significant Malnutrition

Serum albumin is less than 3.5 mg/100 mL.
Total lymphocyte count is less than 1 800/mm³.
Body weight has decreased more than 15%.

Interventions

- Involve dietitian to prevent malnutrition and ensure adequate dietary intake.
- Maintain serum albumin level greater than 3.5 mg/100 mL.
- Maintain total lymphocyte count greater than 1 800/mm³.
- Perform an abbreviated nutritional assessment, according to institutional policy and as defined by the subjective global assessment at least every 3 months for patients who are unable to take food by mouth or who experience an involuntary change in weight.
- Encourage dietary intake or supplementation if a patient with a pressure injury is malnourished. If dietary intake continues to be inadequate, impractical, or impossible, use nutritional support (usually tube feeding) to place the patient into positive nitrogen balance (approximately 30 to 35 calories/kg/day and 1.25 to 1.50 g of protein/kg/day) according to the goals of care.
- Give vitamin and mineral supplements if deficiencies are suspected or confirmed.

*Qaseem, A., Humphrey, L. L., Forciea, M. A., et al.; Clinical Guidelines Committee of the American College of Physicians. (2015). Treatment of pressure ulcers: A clinical practice guideline from the American College of Physicians. *Annals of Internal Medicine, 162*(5), 370–379. https://doi.org/10.7326/M14-1568.
AHCPR, Agency for Health Care Policy and Research.

of protein for adults is 0.8 g/kg/day, a higher intake of protein up to 1.8 g/kg/day is necessary for healing. Increased protein intake helps rebuild epidermal tissue. Increased caloric intake helps replace subcutaneous tissue. Vitamin C promotes collagen synthesis, capillary wall integrity, fibroblast function, and immunological function.

Hemoglobin. Low hemoglobin decreases delivery of oxygen to the tissues and leads to further ischemia. When possible, hemoglobin should be maintained at 12 g/100 mL.

Dressings

For surgical wounds that heal by primary intention, it is common to remove dressings as soon as drainage stops. In contrast, when a wound is healing by secondary intention, the dressing material provides an optimal healing environment.

Purposes of Dressings. A dressing serves several purposes:

- Protects wound from microorganism contamination
- Aids in hemostasis
- Promotes healing by absorbing drainage and supports autolytic debridement
- Supports or splints the wound site
- Protects the patient from seeing the wound (if perceived as unpleasant)
- Promotes thermal insulation of the wound surface
- Provides a moist environment for the wound bed

In a normally healing wound, when wound drainage is minimal, the healing process forms a natural fibrin seal that eliminates the need for a dressing. Wounds with extensive tissue loss always need a dressing.

A pressure dressing is applied with elastic bandages, exerts localized downward pressure over an actual or potential bleeding site, and eliminates dead space in underlying tissues so that wound healing progresses normally. Pressure dressings need to be checked to be sure that they do not interfere with circulation to a body part. Skin colour, pulses

in distal extremities, the patient's comfort, and changes in sensation should be assessed. Pressure dressings are not routinely removed.

Specific dressings cover and protect certain types of wounds, such as large wounds, wounds with drainage tubes or suction catheters in the wound, wounds that need frequent changing, and fistulas. For these wounds, pouches or special wound collection systems cover the wound and collect wound drainage. Some of these devices have a plastic flange on the front of the wound pouch, which enables changing wound packing without removing the wound pouch from the skin.

Understanding the method of action and purpose of the dressing selection facilitates wound healing (Bryant & Nix, 2016). When you know the characteristics of the wound, and the function of the dressings, choosing the correct type of dressing is clear. For example, a wet, draining wound requires a dressing that absorbs drainage and wicks it away from the wound and periwound, whereas a wound requiring removal of slough or crust would need an occlusive (hydrocolloid) dressing for autolytic debridement.

A primary function of a dressing on a healing wound is to protect the fragile wound bed. Most traditional surgical dressings have three layers: a contact or primary layer, an absorbent layer, and an outer protective or secondary layer. The contact dressing covers the incision and part of the adjacent skin. Fibrin, blood products, and debris adhere to the contact dressing's surface. A dressing that does not adhere to the wound bed, such as soft silicone, will not stick to the suture line. Use of dry gauze or improper removal of the dressing will disrupt the healing epidermal surface. If a dressing sticks to the surgical incision, the dressing needs soaking with saline solution or water to release it from the incisional area and prevent trauma to the wound bed.

Types of Dressings. Wet-to-dry and wet-to-moist dressings are still often ordered, despite extensive research literature over the past 50 years that has clearly identified *moist wound healing* dressings as the optimal dressing choice to manage and support healing within the wound. As clinical researchers develop more appropriate dressings, it is essential to understand the reason why wet-to-dry and wet-to-moist dressings are neither current best practice nor supported in the research literature.

The basic premise behind the wet-to-dry dressing is to put a wet dressing (gauze and normal saline) on a wound, allow it to dry out, and then pull off the now-dry dressing, thereby mechanically debriding the wound. This is not effective, however, since the action is nonselective, so healthy granulating tissue is removed along with any necrotic or sloughy tissue. In addition, this is inevitably painful to the patient; given the current availability of nontraumatic dressings, this is contrary to optimal patient care.

Wet-to-moist dressings involve the use of a saline-soaked gauze that is not left to dry out on the wound, but rather kept moist on the wound through frequent dressing changes. Research has shown that frequency of dressing changes has a negative impact on wound healing (the disruption of fragile granulation tissue, cooling down the wound bed). As well, the dressing that is moistened with normal saline becomes a hypertonic environment that pulls fluid out of the wound bed in a way that leaves a slurry of blood and proteins on the surface of the wound, which, if not kept constantly moist, dries out (becoming a wet-to-dry dressing).

However, since these approaches are still used in some situations, as a nurse, you need to know the steps to follow when applying this type of dressing to a wound. It is strongly recommended that you consider alternatives (and there are many) to this approach, since it is not effective in promoting wound healing. You are encouraged to discuss the rationale for moist wound healing for the patient in question with the other care providers, in order to support evidence-informed best practices (Ovington, 2001).

Dressings vary by type of material and mode of application (wet or dry) (Skill 47.3). They need to be easy to apply, comfortable, and made

SKILL 47.3 APPLYING DRY AND MOIST DRESSINGS

Delegation Considerations

The skill of applying dry and moist dressings to the new acute wound (generally a surgical wound) cannot be delegated to unregulated care providers (UCPs). In some settings, nurses can delegate aspects of wound care, such as changing of dressings using *clean* techniques for chronic wounds. The *assessment* of the wound remains within the scope of the nurse, however, even if the dressing change is delegated. Instruct nursing assistive personnel to do the following:

- Report pain, fever, bleeding, or wound drainage to a nurse immediately.
- Report any potential contamination to the existing dressing (e.g., patient incontinence or other bodily fluids; dressing becomes dislodged). While surgeons often have specific orders for postsurgical (acute) wounds, it is important to support wound healing using best practice. Ensuring the wound is protected from potential contamination, observing for signs of infection, and attention to the patient's need for analgesic prior to dressing change are all important considerations.

Equipment

- Sterile gloves
- Variety of gauze dressings and pads
- Irrigation kit
- Cleaning solution
- Sterile solution
- Clean, disposable gloves
- Tape, ties, or bandages, as needed
- Waterproof bag
- Extra gauze dressings, or abdominal pads

PROCEDURE

STEPS	RATIONALE
1. Perform hand hygiene. Obtain information about wound characteristics (e.g., size, location, history of wound progress or management).	• Transmission of microorganisms is reduced. Plan for proper type and amount of supplies needed. Know when assistance ("an extra pair of hands") is needed to apply and affix dressing.
2. Assess patient's level of comfort. If analgesic has been ordered, assess need and provide if required.	• Removal of a dry dressing is painful; some patients require pain medication.
3. Review orders for dressing change procedure. Be prepared to adjust dressing depending on wound progress.	• Orders indicate type of dressing or applications to use; wounds change over time, so previous dressing may not be appropriate to current state of wound.
4. Explain procedure to patient, respond to questions. Instruct patient not to touch wound area or opened dressing supplies.	• Explanation decreases anxiety. Sudden, unexpected movement on the patient's part may result in contamination of wound and supplies.
5. Close room or cubicle curtains and windows.	• Privacy is provided; airborne microorganisms are reduced.
6. Position patient comfortably, drape with bath blanket to expose only wound site.	• Wound is accessible; unnecessary exposure is minimized.
7. Place disposable bag within reach of work area. Fold top of bag to make cuff (see Step 7 illustration).	• Soiled dressings can easily be disposed of. Bag's outer surface is not soiled.

STEP 7 Disposable waterproof bag placed near the dressing site.

8. Apply face mask and protective eyewear, if needed.	• Transmission of pathogens to exposed tissues is reduced. Mask and eyewear protect from splashes.
9. Put on clean, disposable gloves; remove tape, bandage, or ties.	• Transmission of infectious organisms from soiled dressings to hands is prevented.
10. Remove tape: pull parallel to skin toward dressing; remove remaining adhesive from skin.	• Pulling tape toward dressing reduces stress on suture line or periwound skin.

SKILL 47.3	APPLYING DRY AND MOIST DRESSINGS—cont'd
STEPS	**RATIONALE**

11. With gloved hand, carefully remove gauze dressings one layer at a time, taking care not to dislodge drains or tubes.	• Appearance of drainage is sometimes upsetting to patient. Removal of one layer at a time reduces the chance of accidental removal of underlying drains.
A. If dressing sticks on a wet-to-dry dressing, do not moisten it; instead, gently free dressing, and alert patient of potential discomfort.	• Wet-to-dry dressing should debride wound (Ramundo, 2016). Do not wet the dressing to remove it. However, reassess and select other method of debridement.

CRITICAL DECISION POINT: *Never use a wet-to-dry dressing in a clean granulating wound. Use only for debridement and only if other debridement options are unavailable (Ramundo, 2016).*

12. Observe character and amount of drainage on dressing and appearance of wound.	• Estimate of drainage amount and appearance of wound assist in determining progress.
13. Fold dressings with drainage contained inside and remove gloves inside out. With small dressings, remove gloves inside out over dressing (see Step 13 illustration). Dispose of gloves and soiled dressings in disposable bag. Perform hand hygiene.	• Transmission of microorganisms is reduced. Hands do not come into contact with material on gloves.
14. Open sterile dressing tray or individually wrapped sterile supplies. Place on bedside table (see Step 14 illustration).	• Sterile dressings remain sterile while on or within sterile surface. Preparation of supplies prevents break in technique during dressing change.

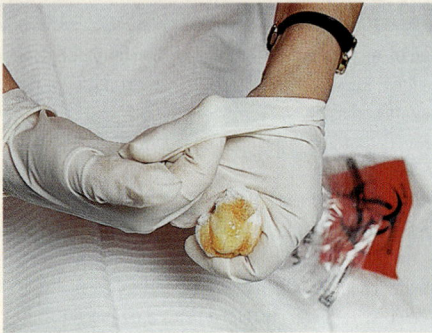

STEP 13 Removal of disposable gloves over contaminated dressing.

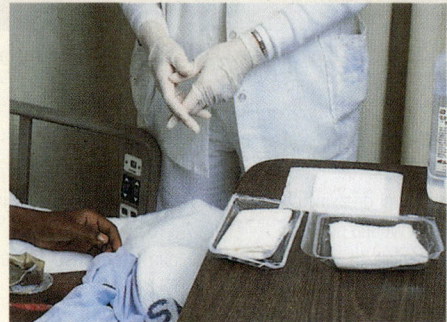

STEP 14 Sterile dressing equipment.

15. If required, clean or irrigate wound:	
A. Pour prescribed solution into sterile irrigation container or use single-use bottle of normal saline.	
B. Using syringe or single-use bottle, irrigate wound at 10–15 psi	• 10–15 psi will effectively remove loose debris without damage to the granulating tissue of the wound bed.
C. Continue until the irrigation flow is clear.	• Use patient positioning to assist in irrigation (e.g., side-lying).
D. Dry surrounding skin.	

CRITICAL DECISION POINT: *Some wound cleansers are available in spray bottles with "stream." Use "spray" setting to loosen debris and stream function to irrigate. Do not irrigate sinus tracks or wounds where the base of the wound cannot be determined.*

16. Apply dressing:	
A. Dry dressing	
(1) Perform hand hygiene. Apply sterile gloves.	• Sterile supplies can be handled without contamination.
(2) Inspect wound for appearance, drains, drainage, and integrity.	• Wound healing status is indicated.
(3) Clean wound with solution: Use warmed (body temperature) solution when possible	• Cold or room temperature solution can affect growth factor and impede healing.
(a) Clean from least contaminated area to most contaminated area.	• Contamination of previously cleaned area is prevented.
(4) Gently pat periwound area to dry.	• Protection and absorption of wound drainage is provided.
(5) Apply appropriate type of dressing to cover the wound.	• Wound is protected from external environment.
(6) Apply topper (cover) dressing if required.	• Topper dressing prevents strikethrough of wound drainage and provides a surface to tape the dressing in place.
B. Moist dressing	
(1) Perform hand hygiene. Apply clean gloves.	
(2) Remove old dressings, discard in secure garbage container.	

Continued

SKILL 47.3	APPLYING DRY AND MOIST DRESSINGS—cont'd
STEPS	**RATIONALE**

(3) Assess surrounding skin (see Step 16B[3] illustration). Discard gloves.

- Surrounding skin assessment provides an evaluation of wound management.

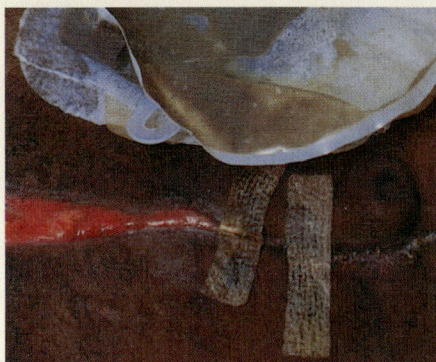

STEP 16B(3) Exposure of wound facilitates assessment of wound and surrounding skin.

(4) Perform hand hygiene. Apply sterile gloves as required.

(5) Clean wound base with warmed-to-body-temperature (if possible) normal saline or commercially prepared wound cleaner. Assess wound base.

(6) Moisten gauze with prescribed solution. Gently wring out excess solution. Unfold.

(7) Apply gauze as a single layer (see Step 16B[7] illustration) directly onto the wound surface. If wound is deep, gently and lightly "pack" dressing into wound base by hand or with forceps until all wound surfaces are in contact with the gauze. If tunnelling is present, use a cotton-tipped applicator to place gauze into tunnelled area. Ensure that only ONE piece of ribbon gauze is used in a tunnelling wound. Document the length of ribbon dressing; also document the number of dressings used in packing the wound (see Step 16B[7] illustration).

- Handling of sterile supplies can occur without contamination.
- Cleaning removes wound debris for adequate assessment.
- Gauze needs to be moist to allow for absorption of wound debris.
- Inner gauze needs to be moist, not dripping wet, to absorb drainage and adhere to debris. Excessively moist dressings result in moisture-associated skin damage (maceration) in the periwound skin (Gray & Weir, 2007). The wound needs to be loosely packed to facilitate wicking of drainage into absorbent outer layer of dressing.
- Care must be taken to document packing placed in a wound to avoid possible dressing being left in the wound when the dressing is changed.

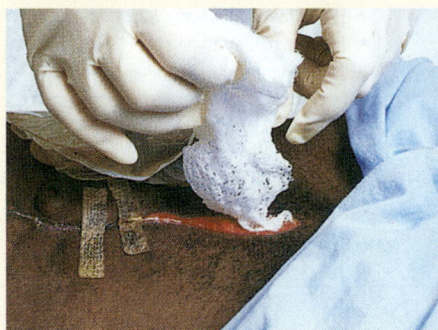

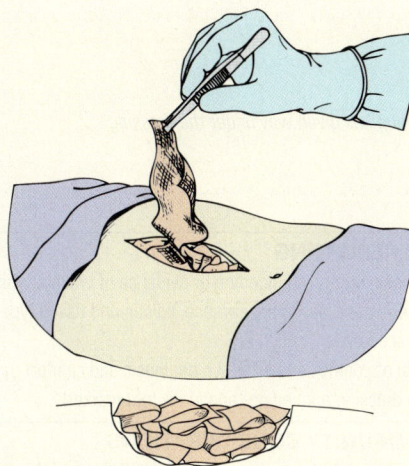

STEP 16B(7) Packing wound with single layer of gauze.

(8) Cover with sterile dry gauze and topper dressing.

17. Secure dressing.

  A. Tape: Apply nonallergenic tape to secure dressing in place.

  B. Montgomery ties (see Figure 47.23)

    (1) Expose adhesive surface of tape on end of each tie.

    (2) Place ties on opposite sides of dressing.

    (3) Place adhesive directly on skin or use skin barrier.

- Topper dressing prevents strikethrough of wound drainage and provides a surface to tape the dressing in place.
- The goal for securing a dressing is to keep the dressing in place and intact without causing damage to underlying and surrounding skin.
- Protect periwound skin from breakdown through frequent dressing changes.
- Skin barrier (Stomahesive) protects intact skin from stretch and tension of adhesive tape.

SKILL 47.3	APPLYING DRY AND MOIST DRESSINGS—cont'd	
STEPS	**RATIONALE**	

C. For dressings on an extremity, secure dressing with rolled gauze or an elastic net (see Step 17C illustration)

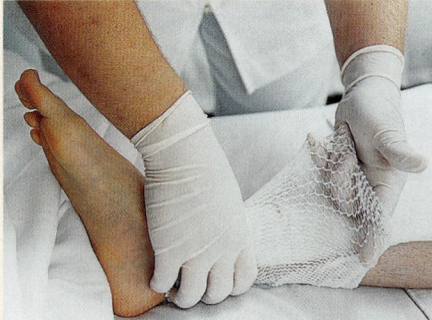

STEP 17C Elastic net securing a lower extremity dressing.

18. Remove gloves and dispose of them in bag. Remove any mask or eyewear.	• Transmission of infection is reduced.
19. Dispose of supplies; perform hand hygiene.	• Transmission of infection is reduced.
20. Assist patient to comfortable position.	• Patient's sense of well-being is promoted. Comfort is enhanced.

UNEXPECTED OUTCOMES	RELATED INTERVENTIONS
Wound appears inflamed, tender, with or without drainage	• Monitor patient for signs of infection (e.g., increased temperature or white blood cell count). • Obtain wound culture. • Notify health care provider.
Wound drainage increases	• Increase frequency of dressing changes. • Notify health care provider, who may consider drain placement to facilitate wound drainage.
Wound bleeds during dressing change	• Observe colour. If drainage is bright red and excessive, you will need to apply pressure. • Inspect along dressing and underneath patient to determine amount of bleeding. • Obtain vital signs, as needed. • Notify health care provider.
Sensation that "something has given way under the dressing"	• Observe wound for increased drainage or separation of sutures. • Protect wound. Cover with sterile moist dressing. • Instruct patient to lie still. • Notify health care provider.

RECORDING AND REPORTING

• Immediately report brisk, bright-red bleeding or evidence of wound dehiscence or evisceration to health care provider.
• Report wound and periwound tissue appearance, colour, and tissue type and presence and characteristics of exudate, type, and amount of dressings used, and tolerance of patient to procedure.
• Record patient's level of comfort and effective analgesic and comfort measures.
• Write date and time dressing applied on tape in ink (not marker).

CARE IN THE COMMUNITY CONSIDERATIONS

• More expensive specialty dressings are sometimes used because they have longer wear-time and often have antimicrobial properties.
• Assess ability of patient and family to manage dressing changes independently, and teach as possible.
• Patients need to dispose of contaminated dressings in the home in a manner consistent with local regulations.

of materials that promote wound healing. Wounds Canada (2017b) has "Product Picker" guidelines that nurses can use in selecting dressings that respond to the need of the wound, based on the goal for the wound: to heal, to protect from infection, to provide comfort, or to maintain current status (e.g., nonhealing wound). As with an unfamiliar medication, if you are using a dressing you are not familiar with, you should look it up to learn its properties and how to use it correctly (Box 47.14; see also Table 47.9).

Woven Gauze Dressings. In the past, woven gauze dressings were commonly used to provide coverage for wounds; however, research has demonstrated that their efficacy in wound healing is limited and they may actually impede wound healing because of the irritation from small gauze debris unintentionally left in the wound (Orsted et al., 2017). *Nonwoven* gauze nonetheless remains useful as packing material (e.g., Nu-gauze) and is available in different textures and in various lengths and sizes; the 4 × 4 and ribbon dressings are the most

- Use a dressing that will continuously provide a moist ("like your eyeball") environment. Wet-to-dry dressings should be avoided.
- Perform wound care using topical dressings as determined by a thorough assessment. No specific studies have proven to be an optimal dressing type for pressure wounds.
- Choose a dressing that keeps the surrounding intact (periwound) skin dry while keeping the wound bed moist.
- Choose a dressing that controls exudate but does not desiccate the wound bed.
- Consider caregiver time, ease of use, availability, and cost when selecting a dressing.
- Eliminate wound dead space by loosely filling all cavities with dressing material.

WOCN, Wound, ostomy, and continence nurses.
Adapted from Wound, Ostomy and Continence Nurses Society. (2016). *Guideline for prevention and management of pressure injuries (ulcers).* WOCN Clinical Practice Guidelines Series. Author.

common. Ensure that the "packing" is not jammed into the wound: it should be packed *lightly* to prevent abscess development but mainly to support the healthy closure of the wound (from the inside outward). For example, in a dry base wound, a nonwoven gauze moistened with hydrogel; in a wet/contaminated base wound, hypertonic sodium ribbon (goes in dry); and in an infected wound bed, cadexomer iodine or silver or medical-grade honey dressing (Orsted et al., 2017; Sibbald et al., 2006). A simple gauze "island" dressing can be used to cover a clean wound with minimal drainage. The "island" refers to the gauze pad surrounded by a lightly adhesive fabric. Acute surgical wounds are often packed with saline-moistened nonwoven gauze and the dressing changed at frequent intervals, usually determined by the surgeon.

Transparent Film Dressings. Self-adhesive, transparent film dressings are particularly useful in securing intravenous (IV) lines and other tubing, since these dressings provide an occlusive barrier. Transparent films should not be used as dressings for skin tears or to protect areas of skin subject to breakdown. Because they are occlusive, there is limited moisture–vapour transfer, causing interstitial fluid from the skin tear to remain in the wound and on periwound skin, thus creating potential for maceration and deterioration of the tissues. In addition, transparent

TABLE 47.9　Wound Care Dressings

CLASS		LOCAL WOUND CARE			CARE CONSIDERATIONS
	Description	Tissue Debridement	Infection	Moisture Balance	Indications and Contraindications
1. Films and membranes	Occlusive adhesive sheet. Impermeable to H_2O molecules and bacteria	+	−	−	Limited moisture vapour transmission rate. Not for draining or infected wounds.* Best use: to affix IV or other drains/tubing where occlusive barrier is important.
2. Nonadherent contact layer	Sheets of low adherence to tissue. Nonmedicated tulles, silicone, and petrolatum-based woven dressings	−	−	−	Allows moisture–vapour transfer: drainage evaporates off the wound. Requires a cover (absorbent) dressing. Choose silicone-woven dressings when possible (tulle and petrolatum-based products have limited moisture–vapour transfer capacity).
3. Hydrogels	Polymers with high H_2O content. Available in gels, solid sheets, or impregnated gauze	++	−	+	Should not be used on draining wounds. Solid sheets should not be used on infected wounds.
4. Hydrocolloids	May contain gelatin, sodium, carboxymethylcellulose, polysaccharides, or pectin, or a combination of these. Sheet dressings are occlusive and have polyurethane film outer layer	+++	+/−	++	Should be used with care on fragile skin. Should not be used on heavily draining or infected wounds.* Create occlusive barrier to protect the wound from outside contamination. Characteristic odour may accompany dressing change and should not be confused with infection.
5. Calcium alginates	Sheets or fibrous ropes of calcium sodium alginate (seaweed derivative). Have hemostatic capabilities	++	+	+++	Should not be used on dry wounds. Avoid packing into narrow, deep sinuses because of low tensile strength. Bioresorbable.
6. Composite dressings	Multilayered, combination dressings to increase absorbency and autolysis	+	−	+++	Use on wounds on which dressing may stay in place for several days.*
7. Foams	Nonadhesive or adhesive polyurethane foam. May have occlusive backing. Sheets or cavity packing. Some have fluid lock.	−	−	+++	Use on moderate to heavily draining wounds. Occlusive foams should not be used on heavily draining or infected wounds.*
8. Charcoal	Contains odour-absorbent charcoal within product	−	−	+	Some charcoal products are inactivated by moisture. Ensure that dressing edges are sealed.

TABLE 47.9	Wound Care Dressings—cont'd				
CLASS		**LOCAL WOUND CARE**			**CARE CONSIDERATIONS**
	Description	**Tissue Debridement**	**Infection**	**Moisture Balance**	**Indications and Contraindications**
9. Hypertonic	Sheet, ribbon, or gel impregnated with sodium concentrate.	+	+	++	Gauze ribbon should not be used on dry wounds. May be painful on sensitive tissue. Gel may be used on dry wounds.
10. Hydrophilic fibres	Sheet or packing strip of sodium carboxymethylcellulose. Converts to a solid gel when activated by moisture (fluid lock).	+	−	+++	Best for moderate amount of exudate. Should not be used on dry wounds. Avoid packing into narrow deep sinuses because of low tensile strength.
11. Antimicrobials	Medical-grade honey, silver, cadexomer iodine, Gentian violet/methylene blue—with vehicle for delivery: sheets, gels, alginates, foams, or paste	+	+++	+	Broad spectrum against bacteria. Not to be used on patients with known hypersensitivities to any product components.
12. Other devices	NPWT applies localized negative pressure to surface and margins of wound. Dressings consist of polyurethane or polyvinyl alcohol materials.	−	+	+++	Pressure-distributing wound dressing actively removes fluid from the wound and promotes wound edge approximation. Advanced skill required for patient selection for this therapy.
13. Biological	Living human fibroblasts provided in sheets at ambient or frozen temperatures. Extracellular matrix. Collagen-containing preparations. Hyaluronic acid. Platelet-derived growth factor.	−	−	−	Should not be used on wounds with infection, sinus tracts, excessive exudate, or on patients known to have hypersensitivity to any of the product components. Cultural issues related to source. Advanced skill required for patient selection for this therapy.

NPWT, Negative pressure wound; +, appropriateness of the dressing for tissue debridement, infection, and moisture balance; −, dressing is not considered beneficial in these areas. Use with caution if critical colonization is suspected.
From Registered Nurses' Association of Ontario. (2011, revised 2016). *RNAO best practice guideline: Assessment and management of stage I–IV pressure ulcers* (pp. 102–103). Author.

film dressings can be difficult to remove and can cause unnecessary trauma to fragile periwound tissue. When removing a transparent film dressing, use the "lateral pull" technique. Stabilize the dressing with one hand while gently pulling laterally at the edge of the film with your other hand and continue slowly around the dressing to remove it. This will break the adhesive seal with minimal damage to the skin.

Absorbent Clear Acrylic Dressings. As the name suggests, these dressings provide visibility of the wound. The dressing is specifically designed to absorb drainage from the wound (usually a skin tear) and provides a layer with one-way moisture–vapour transfer. This dressing is water-resistant (so the patient can shower) and can be left in place for extended wear time.

Nonadherent Contact Layer Dressings. Nonadherent contact layer dressings protect fragile granulating tissue while allowing the interstitial fluid and moisture from the wound to evaporate. This provides a moist "like your eyeball" environment that promotes healing. The contact layer remains undisturbed while a secondary cover dressing can be changed when saturated or soiled. Early forms of contact layer dressings were tulle (paraffin) or petrolatum jelly, which tend to prevent moisture–vapour transfer. The newer, less greasy tulle or silicone contact layers are more effective in this regard. Contact layer dressings are placed over the open wound and generally draped across the intact periwound skin, although some are cut to fit the wound. For effective wound healing, the contact layer remains in place for a number of days, while the secondary cover dressing is changed as needed.

Soft Silicone Dressings. Soft silicone dressings are designed to float above the wound surface, since silicone is hydrophobic. Thus, the wound bed can proceed in the healing cascade without interruption and without causing trauma to the wound bed or periwound skin on removal. Silicone dressings now range from contact layer to absorbent surgical dressings for draining wounds. These dressings are *atraumatic* (decrease pain at dressing change) and are useful in dealing with fungating wounds or any wound where the periwound skin is fragile, such as in pediatric or older patients.

Hydrocolloid Dressings. Hydrocolloid dressings are designed for autolytic debridement when there is minimal drainage, no evidence of infection, and slough in the wound bed. Hydrocolloid dressings have a complex formulation of colloidal, elastomeric, and gel components that interact with the wound environment to liquefy slough, while not affecting the "good" tissue in the wound bed. These dressings are adhesive and occlusive and should be left on the wound for (usually) 5–7 days. This type of dressing is most useful on shallow to moderately deep wounds. Hydrocolloid dressings should not be used in heavily draining wounds or in full-thickness or infected wounds. Because of how hydrocolloids interact with the wound bed matter, when the dressing is removed, residue in the wound bed may be confused with pus (colour, odour) until the wound is cleaned. A barrier wipe must be used to protect the periwound, since a hydrocolloid dressing is adherent. As well, these dressings should be used with caution where the periwound tissue is fragile or friable.

Hydrogel Dressings. Hydrogel dressings donate moisture to the wound bed (hence, the term *hydro,* indicating "water"). They may be sheet or in tubes, basically water- or glycerin-based amorphous gel. This type of dressing hydrates dry wound beds and helps to soften slough and eschar. A small amount of hydrogel can be mixed to assist in application of cadexomer iodine (e.g., Iodosorb). Hydrogels should not be used on draining wounds; sheets should not be used on infected wounds. When using hydrogel from a tube, the gel should not be squirted directly into the wound; rather, use a sterile gauze dressing or sterile implement (e.g., tongue depressor) to apply the gel so that potential contamination of the tube from matter in the wound is avoided.

Foam Dressings. Foam dressings are composed of nonadhesive or adhesive polyurethane foam and are provided in a variety of shapes and sizes. The main purpose of a foam dressing is to absorb drainage, and it can be left intact for up to 7 days. Foam dressings are designed to wick drainage off the wound or periwound through moisture–vapour transfer, which helps prevent maceration. Non-border foam dressings can be cut to fit around drainage tubes.

Calcium Alginate and Hydrofibre Dressings. Calcium alginate dressings are manufactured from seaweed and are available in sheet and rope form. The alginate forms a thickened, stronger surface when wet. These highly absorbent dressings are useful in highly draining wounds but require an appropriate cover dressing. Calcium sodium alginate products (e.g., Kaldostat) also provide hemostasis where bleeding is an issue. Alginate dressings should be removed when saturated.

Hydrofibre dressings are used in similar situations to alginates. They are composed of sodium carboxymethylcellulose and available in sheets or ribbon. The main advantage of the hydrofibre dressing is that when exposed to fluid, it becomes a solid gel. This is particularly useful when the wound bed or wound edge is friable, for example, in malignant fungating wounds.

Neither of these dressings should be used on or in dry wounds. Secondary dressing (usually some form of absorbent pad) is required.

Composite Dressings. Composite dressings are a multilayered combination of two different dressing types, designed to provide both absorption and autolysis. Composite dressings can remain in place for up to 3 days.

Topical Treatment for Infected Wounds.

Superficially infected wounds require topical dressings to deal with the bacteria within the wound and surrounding tissue (Sibbald et al., 2013). Deep tissue infection requires the addition of antibiotic therapy, which can be determined from wound swab cultures (Cadogan et al., 2011). Topical dressings effective as antibacterials include hypertonic sodium (e.g., Mesalt), slow-release iodine (e.g., Iodosorb, Inadine), Gentian violet/ methylene blue (e.g., Hydrofera Blue), medical-grade honey, and silver antimicrobials (any "AG" product). The nurse must be familiar with the products to know how (and when) they should be used.

Hypertonic Dressings. Hypertonic dressings are available in ribbon, sheet, or gel form and are designed to be changed every 24–48 hours. Do not wet the dressing. Hypertonic dressings contain high sodium concentration, pulling out interstitial fluid and decreasing edema. This improves blood flow to tissues surrounding the wound, and the sodium creates a negative environment for bacterial growth. Wounds change over time, so when there is minimal drainage, the hypertonic saline dressing should be discontinued.

Cadexomer Iodine. Cadexomer iodine dressings target bacteria in wounds. Products are available in sheets or a tube and provide a slow-release version of iodine in a starch matrix. The dressing will show that is working when the wound colour changes: brownish-orange when applied and it gradually changes to cream-coloured as the iodine is absorbed, usually over 72 hours. The dressing must be left intact for 3 days. Changing more frequently interferes with effectiveness of the product. Caution is required in using large amounts of cadexomer iodine (see product monograph for limits), and use in breastfeeding

women and patients with thyroid conditions or shellfish allergy should be avoided.

Silver Dressings. Silver dressings are antimicrobial (similar to cadexomer iodine). They are effective against approximately 150 different pathogens, including fungal infections, methicillin-resistant *Staphylococcus aureus* (MRSA), and vancomycin-resistant enterococci (VRE). Silver dressings come in sheet, ribbon, rope, woven, gel, and foam formats and sometimes require a secondary dressing. Silver dressings are activated by moisture, which is usually present in critically colonized or infected wounds. Dry wounds tipping into infection can benefit from silver gel dressings or a scant amount of hydrogel prior to application of the silver dressing. Depending on the product, the antimicrobial effect of silver is 3 to 7 days (check product information). Sensitivity to silver dressings has not been reported, but as the silver is activating, patients may experience slight stinging in the wound, which usually dissipates.

Honey (Medical-Grade Leptosperum Honey). Honey has long been known to have antimicrobial properties. It is a particularly effective treatment option for infection. It changes the wound bed pH, creating a negative environment for bacterial proliferation. It produces a low concentration of hydrogen peroxide, which kills bacteria and does not damage healing tissue. In addition, by killing bacteria, wound odour is decreased. The medical-grade format of Manuka honey is available as colloid, alginate, gel, and paste. It is particularly useful post-abscess (incision and drainage) wounds, since gel format can be applied directly to the wound (without packing material) and a ribbon dressing at the surface only, with a simple absorbent cover dressing. The wound can be irrigated and more medical-grade gel honey introduced to the wound. Wounds treated with honey will have an increase in drainage initially and may require more frequent dressing changes.

Gentian Violet/Methylene Blue (Hydrofera Blue). Gentian violet/methylene blue/hydrofera blue–impregnated dressing pulls bacteria from the wound where it is killed in the dressing, rather than downloading antibacterial product into the wound bed. It provides broad-spectrum bacteriostatic coverage against microorganisms such as MRSA, VRE, and *Candida*. The available dressings are in a foam-type format in squares and tubes, which are useful for deeper, narrow wounds. Colour change in the dressing indicates effectiveness, as the purple colour will become white. The dressing must remain moist. The dressing can be lifted and checked at 24 hours; subsequent dressings can remain intact (and re-moistened if needed) for up to 72 hours. As with every dressing one is not familiar with, check the product monograph or website for complete information on use.

Negative Pressure Wound Therapy. Negative pressure wound therapy (NPWT) involves use of a machine that applies localized negative pressure to the surface and margins of the wound, pulling up the base of the wound and enhancing healing rates. It can be very effective, particularly for wounds in which rapid healing is viable, and will enhance patients' quality of life. Over the past few years, smaller, mobile versions of NPWT have become available for many different types of wounds. NPWT is a relatively expensive method, but in the appropriate situation, significantly increases wound healing, thus decreasing the requirement for health care resources, including hospitalization. Usually these dressings are changed three times a week.

NPWT is also used to enhance the viability of split-thickness skin grafts. Placing it over the graft intraoperatively decreases the ability of the graft to shift and evacuates fluids that build up under the graft (Frantz et al., 2016).

Changing Dressings.

Wounds change (or should change) over time. As a nurse, you should anticipate this when preparing to change a dressing. You can still have similar dressings as previously used, within close proximity; in the hospital, you should only bring in dressing supplies you will be using, since unused dressings will likely be considered contaminated and discarded. Be familiar with the location of any drains or tubing and any specific supplies required. Being unprepared is not only a waste of time but can also result in a break in aseptic technique (see Chapter 34), accidental dislodging of a drain, and unnecessary patient discomfort.

As a nurse, your judgement is required in modifying the dressing change procedure. Dressings are designed for particular wound requirements (e.g., moisture or infection management). If the character of a wound has changed, provide clear communication with the physician or wound specialist or nurse who documents your interventions, even though you do not require a medical order to change a dressing. If a specific order is written, it is your responsibility to assess the current status of the wound in relation to the order. You need to communicate any change to the wound or dressing requirements to the physician or wound specialist and discuss available options, based on evidence-informed best practice.

An order to "reinforce dressing prn" (add dressings without removing the original) is common immediately after surgery, when the surgeon does not want accidental disruption of the suture line or bleeding. The medical or operating room record usually indicates whether drains are present and from what body cavity they drain. After the first dressing change, document in the patient care plan the location of drains, type (and number) of dressing materials, and other pertinent information related to care of the wound.

Clean or Sterile Technique. The body of literature about sterile versus clean dressing techniques is growing. The RNAO guidelines (RNAO 2011/2016, 2016b) recommend sterile dressings, good hand hygiene, and clean gloves changed between each of the patient's wounds or when soiled. For surgical wounds, preliminary research indicates no difference in the healing rate of wounds when a clean rather than a sterile dressing change technique is used (Kent et al., 2018). Although aseptic or sterile technique is often used for surgical wound care, the most important aspect of this approach is to ensure as clean a field as possible with the use of sterile dressing packs, sterile scissors and forceps, and sterile dressings and gloves.

Preparing for Dressing Change (in Any Care Setting). To prepare a patient for a dressing change, the nurse will need to do the following:

- Administer required analgesics so that peak effects occur during the dressing change.
- Describe steps of the procedure to lessen patient anxiety.
- Gather all supplies required for the dressing change.
- Recognize normal signs of healing.
- Answer questions about the procedure or the wound.

Patient and caregiver education on wound healing and how to change the dressing are important, particularly in the home care setting. The nurse needs to demonstrate dressing changes to the patient and family and then provide an opportunity for them to practise changing a dressing when the nurse is present and able to provide feedback and encouragement. In acute care, by the time the patient is ready to be discharged, wound healing has usually progressed past the point when complications such as dehiscence or evisceration might occur.

Packing a Wound. When packing a wound, the nurse must first assess the size, depth, and shape of the wound, then assess for tunnelling and undermining of the wound. These wound characteristics will help determine the size and type of dressing material needed to pack the wound. Wounds created from incision and drainage of abscess may not require any packing if under 5 cm in depth (O'Bright, 2017). Various dressing materials, such as alginates, are used to pack wounds. If nonwoven gauze is the appropriate dressing material, the nurse needs to saturate the gauze with the ordered solution, wring it out, unfold it,

and lightly pack it into the wound. The entire wound surface needs to be in light contact with part of the moist gauze dressing (see Skill 47.3). As stated in the RNAO guidelines (2011/2016), "keeping the wound moist and the surrounding intact skin dry" (p. 43) will prevent maceration and help maintain a moist wound environment, and when using a dressing "*loosely* pack any sinus tract or cavity to eliminate dead space" (p. 77).

It is important to use a light touch when packing. The purpose of packing a tunnel or sinus tract is to keep edges from coming together and forming dead space where abscess may occur. Over-packing the wound causes pressure on the tissue in the wound bed, decreasing blood flow to the area and preventing healing and wound closure (Kerr et al., 2006). The amount of packing placed in the wound should be documented to ensure there is no chance for any packing material to be left in the wound when the dressing is changed.

Securing Dressings. Tape, ties, a secondary dressing, or gauze net may be used to secure the primary wound dressing. The choice depends on wound size and location, presence of drainage, frequency of dressing changes, and patient's level of activity. Equally important is the potential for skin stripping if tape is applied and removed frequently from the same area of skin. Patients with chronic wounds tend to have fragile skin prone to breakdown. Thus, it is important to pay attention to methods used in affixing dressings.

If tape must be used, the nurse needs to ensure that periwound skin is not excoriated or at risk of breakdown and that the patient has no allergy or sensitivity to tape. Nonallergenic paper and silicone tapes are available to minimize skin reactions. Skin that is sensitive to regular adhesive tape becomes severely inflamed and denuded and, in some cases, even sloughs when the tape is removed. A barrier wipe (e.g., NoSting®) should be used to protect periwound skin and provide additional "tack" to help tape adhere but not damage underlying skin. Skin under the tape should be assessed at each dressing change. If skin does not remain intact or is irritated, alternatives such as silicone tape or Montgomery ties (Figure 47.23) should be considered.

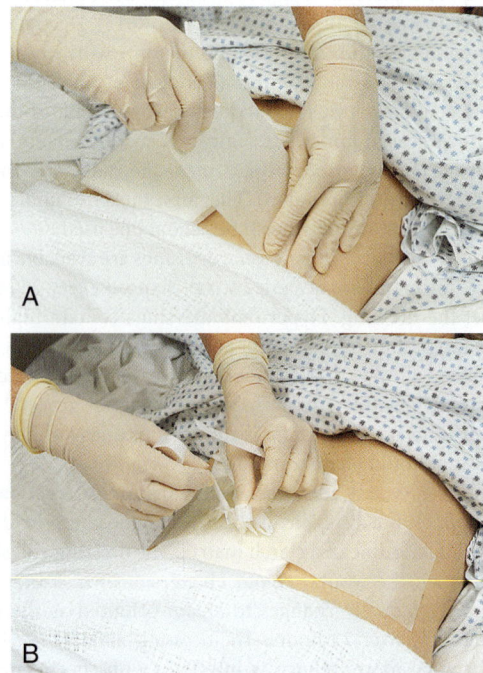

FIGURE 47.23 Montgomery ties. **A,** Each tie is placed at side of dressing. **B,** Securing ties encloses dressing.

Tape is available in various widths. The nurse needs to choose the size that sufficiently secures the dressing. Strips of 7.6-cm adhesive tape will likely ensure that a large dressing does not continually slip off. When applying tape, the skin must be dry so that the tape will adhere to several centimetres of skin on both sides of the dressing in a "window-pane" fashion. If needed, tape can be placed across the middle of the dressing. When securing the dressing, the nurse presses the tape gently, exerting pressure away from the wound. With tension occurring in both directions away from the wound, skin distortion and irritation is minimized. Tape should never be applied over irritated or broken skin. Alternatives, such as gauze wrap or burn-net dressings, may be more appropriate.

To remove tape safely, a lateral pull approach is used. The nurse loosens the tape ends and gently pulls the outer end parallel with the skin surface toward the wound. The nurse applies light pressure to the skin away from the wound while loosening and removing the tape. Lateral pull helps release the tape adhesive. If tape covers an area of hair growth, it will be less painful for the patient if the tape is gently pulled in the direction of hair growth. Adhesive remover is not recommended since it is drying to the skin. Gentle removal, with patience, is the best approach.

When frequent dressing changes are required, particularly for large abdominal or chest wounds, the nurse must avoid repeated removal of tape by using dressings secured with pairs of reusable Montgomery ties (see Figure 47.23). Each section consists of a long strip; half contains an adhesive backing to apply to the skin, and the other half folds back and contains a cloth tie to fasten across a dressing and untie at dressing changes.

Comfort Measures. The wound environment may be painful, depending on the extent of tissue injury and the patient's medical health issues. Nurses can minimize discomfort during wound care using several techniques. Providing analgesic medications 30 to 45 minutes before dressing changes (depending on a drug's time of peak action) reduces discomfort. Using a gentle touch when removing tape, cleaning the wound, and manipulating dressings and drains will minimize patient pain and discomfort. In addition, nurses need to consider ways to prop or position the patient with pillows or foam wedges, particularly in complex, time-consuming dressing changes.

Surgical or Traumatic Wound Considerations

Basic Skin Cleaning for Surgical or Traumatic Wounds. Surgical or traumatic wounds are cleaned by applying noncytotoxic solutions with sterile gauze or through irrigation. The following three principles are important when cleaning an incision or the area surrounding a drain:

1. Clean in a direction from the least contaminated area, such as from the wound or incision to the surrounding skin (Figure 47.24) or from an isolated drain site to the surrounding skin (Figure 47.25).
2. Use gentle friction when applying solutions locally to the skin.
3. When irrigating, allow the solution to flow from the least to most contaminated area (Skill 47.4).

Never use the same piece of gauze to clean across an incision or wound twice. Use gauze to clean the periwound skin, not the open wound. Open wound beds are damaged by the abrasive contact of gauze.

Cleaning Skin and Drain Sites. If an open drain leaks onto surrounding skin, the nurse must ensure that the drainage is removed from the skin to avoid maceration or excoriation of tissue from potentially caustic drainage. The drain itself may also need to be regularly cleaned to avoid a buildup of possible contaminated material. Barrier wipe is applied to skin around the drain site to protect it from maceration.

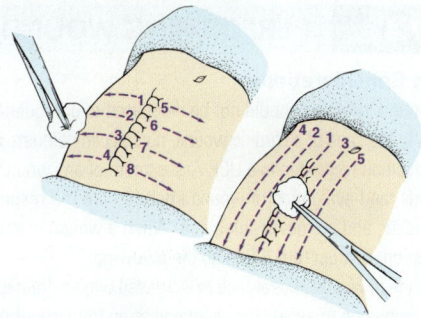

FIGURE 47.24 Methods for cleaning a wound site.

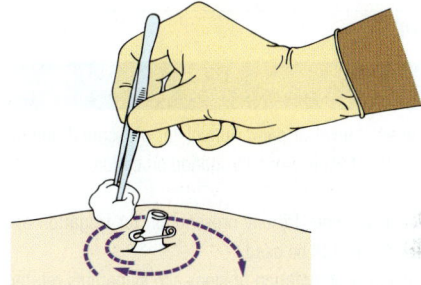

FIGURE 47.25 Cleaning a drain site.

Drain sites are a source of contamination because moist drainage harbours microorganisms. If a wound has a dry incisional area and a moist drain site, the nurse should use two separate swabs or gauze pads, one to clean from the top of the incision toward the drain and one to clean from the bottom of the incision toward the drain. To clean an isolated drain site, clean around the drain, moving in circular rotations outward from a point closest to the drain. In this situation, the skin near the site is more contaminated than the site itself. To clean circular wounds, use the same technique as in cleaning around a drain.

Irrigation. Irrigation is a method of cleaning wounds. Usually, a syringe or commercial product is used to flush the area with a constant low-pressure flow of noncytotoxic solution (usually saline). The gentle washing action of the irrigation cleans a wound of exudate and debris. Irrigation is particularly useful for open, deep wounds. A common refrain regarding irrigation is *Irrigate, irrigate, irrigate . . . and then irrigate some more.* However, it is important to check that the irrigant is not left pooled in the wound bed (usually by repositioning the patient to allow gravity to assist in drainage).

Wound Irrigation. Irrigation of an open wound requires sterile technique. Generally, a 30- to 35-cc syringe with either an 18- to 19-gauge device (angiocatheter) or a wound irrigation tip that delivers approximately 8–15 psi of pressure is required to remove loose slough and debris from the wound but will not harm granulating tissue. Selection of syringe size may also depend on the extent of irrigation required. The smaller the diameter of the syringe, the greater the pressure exerted (RNAO, 2016a). One must always irrigate a wound with the syringe tip over but not in the drainage site. Fluid needs to flow directly into the wound and not over a contaminated area before entering the wound. Skill 47.4 lists steps for wound irrigation. Wounds should not be irrigated when the base cannot be determined (e.g., tunnelling sinus) or into a body cavity.

Sutures. A surgeon closes a wound by bringing the wound edges as close together as possible to reduce scar formation. Proper wound

SKILL 47.4 PERFORMING WOUND IRRIGATION

Delegation Considerations

The skill of wound irrigation should not be delegated to unregulated care providers (UCPs). In the case of a chronic wound, nurses can delegate cleaning of the wound with clean technique to a UCP. Assessment of any wound, care of acute new wounds, and evaluation of wound irrigation are the responsibility of the nurse, however, and are never delegated. When a wound is stable or requires clean irrigation, instruct the UCP to do the following:

- Report change in wound appearance or increased wound drainage to the nurse.
- Use clean technique to avoid cross-contamination from irrigation syringes and equipment.

Equipment

- Irrigant or cleaning solution (volume 1.2 to 2 times the estimated wound volume)
- Irrigation delivery system, depending on amount of pressure desired:
  - Sterile 30- to 35-cc irrigation syringe with sterile soft angiocatheter or 18- to 19-gauge needle (RNAO, 2016a) or hand-held shower, if appropriate.
- Disposable gloves and sterile gloves (check agency policy)
- Waterproof underpad, if needed
- Dressing supplies
- Disposable waterproof bag
- Gown, if risk of spray
- Goggles, mask, or both if risk of spray

PROCEDURE

STEPS	RATIONALE
1. Assess patient's level of pain. Administer prescribed analgesic 30 to 45 minutes before starting wound irrigation procedure.	• Discomfort may be related directly to the wound or indirectly to muscle tension or immobility. Increased comfort permits patient to move more easily and be positioned to facilitate wound irrigation.
2. Review medical record for any prescription for irrigation of open wound and type of solution to be used.	• Open wound irrigation requires medical order, including type of solution to use.
3. Assess recent documentation of signs and symptoms related to patient's open wound.	• Data are used as baseline to indicate change in condition of wound (Orsted et al., 2017)
A. Condition of skin and wound	
B. Elevation of body temperature	• Elevated temperature may indicate response to infection.
C. Drainage from wound (amount, colour)	• Amount will decrease as healing takes place.
D. Odour	• Strong odour may indicate infection.
E. Consistency of drainage	• Leukocytes produce thick drainage.
4. Explain procedure of wound irrigation and cleaning.	• Information will reduce patient's anxiety.
5. Perform hand hygiene.	• Transmission of microorganisms is reduced.
6. Position patient comfortably to permit gravitational flow of irrigating solution through wound and into collection receptacle. Position patient so that wound is vertical to collection basin.	• Directing solution from top to bottom of wound and from clean to contaminated area prevents further infection. Positioning patient during planning stage provides bed surfaces for later preparation of equipment.
7. Warm irrigation solution to approximate body temperature.	• Warmed solution increases comfort and reduces vascular constriction response in tissues.
8. Form cuff on waterproof bag and place it near bed.	• Cuffing helps to maintain large opening, thereby permitting placement of contaminated dressing without touching refuse bag itself.
9. Close room door or bed curtains.	• Privacy is maintained.
10. Apply gown, goggles, or mask, if needed.	• Gown, goggles, and mask protect from splashes or sprays of blood and body fluids.
11. Put on disposable gloves, remove soiled dressing, and discard in waterproof bag. Discard gloves.	• Transmission of microorganisms is reduced.
12. Prepare equipment; open sterile supplies.	
13. Put on sterile gloves (check agency policy).	
14. Irrigate wound with wide opening:	
A. Fill 35-mL syringe with irrigation solution.	• Flushing wound helps remove debris and facilitates healing by secondary intention.
B. Attach 19-gauge needle or angiocatheter.	• Angiocatheter provides ideal pressure for cleaning and removal of debris.
C. Hold syringe tip 2.5 cm above upper end of wound and over area being cleaned.	• Holding the tip above the wound prevents syringe contamination. Careful placement of the syringe prevents unsafe pressure of the flowing solution.
D. Using continuous pressure, flush wound; repeat Steps 14A, 14B, and 14C until solution draining into basin is clear.	• Clear solution indicates that all debris has been removed.
15. Irrigate deep wound with very small opening:	
A. Attach soft angiocatheter to filled irrigating syringe.	• Catheter permits direct flow of irrigant into wound. Expect wound to take longer to empty when opening is small.
B. Lubricate tip of catheter with irrigating solution; then gently insert tip of catheter and pull out about 1 cm.	• Tip is not in fragile inner wall of wound.
C. Using slow, continuous pressure, flush wound.	

CRITICAL DECISION POINT: *Caution: Splashing may occur during this step.*

Continued

SKILL 47.4   PERFORMING WOUND IRRIGATION—cont'd

STEPS	RATIONALE
D. Pinch off catheter just below syringe while keeping catheter in place. **E.** Remove and refill syringe. Reconnect to catheter and repeat until solution draining into basin is clear.	• Sterile solution will not be contaminated.
16. Clean wound with hand-held shower:	• Method is useful for patients able to shower with assistance or independently. Shower may be accomplished at home. A shower table is helpful for bed-bound or acutely ill patients.
A. With patient seated comfortably in shower chair, adjust spray to gentle flow; water temperature should be warm. **B.** Cover showerhead with clean washcloth, if needed. **C.** Shower for 5 to 10 minutes with showerhead 30 cm from wound.	

CRITICAL DECISION POINT: *Wound infection is evidenced by foul odour, purulent discharge, inflammation more than 3 cm beyond wound edge, if a nondraining wound begins to drain, or if the patient is febrile. Consider using antimicrobial dressings. Culture a wound if systemic antibiotics are required (Orsted et al., 2017).*

STEPS	RATIONALE
17. Obtain cultures, if needed, after cleaning with nonbacteriostatic saline.	• Routine culturing of open wounds is not recommended. Use correct swab culture technique (Orsted et al., 2017; RNAO, 2016a). If required, quantitative bacterial cultures (tissue biopsy or wound fluid by needle aspiration) should be performed.
18. Pat dry wound edges with gauze; dry patient, if shower or whirlpool is used.	• Maceration of surrounding tissue is prevented if excess moisture is dried.
19. Apply appropriate dressing (see Skill 47.3 and Box 47.14).	• Protective barrier and healing environment for wound are maintained.
20. Remove gloves and, if worn, mask, goggles, and gown.	• Transfer of microorganisms is prevented.
21. Dispose of equipment and soiled supplies. Perform hand hygiene.	• Transmission of microorganisms is reduced.
22. Assist patient to comfortable position.	
23. Assess type of tissue in the wound bed.	• Wound healing progress is identified and type of wound cleaning needed is determined.
24. Inspect dressing periodically.	• Patient's response to wound irrigation and need to modify plan of care are determined.
25. Evaluate skin integrity.	• Determines further wound breakdown.
26. Observe patient for signs of discomfort.	• Patient's pain should not increase as a result of wound irrigation.
27. Observe for presence of retained irrigant.	• Retained irrigant is a medium for bacterial growth, and subsequent infection may occur.

UNEXPECTED OUTCOMES	RELATED INTERVENTIONS
Wound does not appear to heal	• Ensure underlying causes are treated. • Consider obtaining wound culture. • Notify physician or wound specialist, who may change dressing type, and care plan.
Wound drainage increases	• Apply dressing designed to absorb drainage and wick from wound bed. • Consider critical colonization or infection. Obtain culture if systemic antibiotics are recommended.

RECORDING AND REPORTING
• Record wound irrigation and patient response on progress notes.
• Immediately report to health care provider or wound specialist any evidence of fresh bleeding, sharp increase in pain, retention of irrigant, or signs of shock.
• At change of shift, report expected and unexpected outcomes that have occurred.

CARE IN THE COMMUNITY CONSIDERATIONS
• Determine if tap water is potable (e.g., treated municipal water supply) and home is adequately clean. If patient or caregiver is to irrigate wound, change dressing, or both, explain method, demonstrate it, and have them explain and show it to you.
• If cost or conditions warrant, teach the patient or caregiver how to make saline solution. Determine safety (of handling boiling water). Normal saline can be made by using 10 mL of salt in 1 L of boiling water and should be discarded after 24–48 hours.

---

closure involves control of bleeding and minimal trauma and tension to tissues.

Sutures are threads or metal used to sew body tissues together. The patient's history of wound healing, the site of surgery, the tissues involved, and the purpose of the sutures determine choice of suture material. For example, if the patient has had repeated surgery for an abdominal hernia, wire sutures may be used to provide greater strength for wound closure. In contrast, a small laceration of the face calls for use of very fine polyester sutures to minimize scar formation.

Sutures are available in a variety of materials, including silk, steel, cotton, linen, wire, nylon, and polyester. Steel staples are a common type of outer skin closure that cause less trauma to tissues than do sutures, while providing extra strength. Tape closures such as Steri-Strips applied over the wound to keep the edges closed are also used, although adhesive glue is now commonly used as well.

Sutures are placed within tissue layers in deep wounds as well as superficially, as the final means for wound closure. Deep sutures are usually an absorbable material that will disappear over time; however, sutures are foreign bodies and thus are capable of causing local inflammation. The surgeon tries to minimize tissue injury by using the finest suture possible and the smallest number necessary.

Suture Removal. Policies vary within institutions as to who is able to remove sutures. If it is appropriate for the nurse to remove them, an order is required. Special scissors with curved cutting tips or special staple removers slide under the skin closures for suture removal (Figure 47.26). If the suture line appears to be healing better in certain locations than in others, the surgeon may choose to have only some sutures removed (e.g., every other one).

To remove staples, simply insert the tips of the staple remover under each wire staple. While slowly closing the ends of the staple remover together, squeeze the centre of the staple with the tips, freeing the staple from the skin (see Figure 47.26).

To remove sutures, first check the type of suturing used (Figure 47.27). With intermittent suturing, the surgeon ties each individual suture made in the skin. Continuous suturing, as the name implies, is a series of sutures with only two knots, one at the beginning and one at the end of the suture line. Retention sutures are placed more deeply than skin sutures, and nurses may or may not remove them, depending on agency policy.

How the suture crosses and penetrates the skin determines the method for removal. Never pull the visible portion of a suture through underlying tissue. Sutures on the skin's surface harbour microorganisms and debris, but the portion of the suture beneath the skin is sterile. Pulling the contaminated portion of the suture through tissues may lead to infection. Suture materials should be clipped as close to the skin edge on one side as possible and the suture pulled through from the other side (Figure 47.28).

Drainage Evacuation. When drainage interferes with healing, drainage evacuation is achieved by using either a drain alone or a drainage tube with continuous suction. Special skin barriers need to be applied, including hydrocolloid dressings, similar to those used with ostomies (see Chapter 45), around drain sites. The skin barriers are soft material applied to the skin with adhesive. Drainage flows on the barrier but not directly on the skin.

Drainage evacuators (Figure 47.29) are convenient, portable units that connect to tubular drains lying within a wound bed and exert a safe, constant, low-pressure vacuum to remove and collect drainage. To set the suction on a drainage evacuator with the drainage port open, the lever on the diaphragm is raised. One pushes straight down on the lever to lower the diaphragm. Closure of the port prevents escape of air and creates vacuum pressure. The nurse needs to ensure that suction is exerted and connection points between the evacuator and tubing are intact. After the evacuator collects drainage, its volume and character should be assessed every shift and as needed. When the evacuator fills, the nurse measures output by emptying the contents into a graduated cylinder and immediately resets the evacuator to apply suction.

Bandages and Binders. A simple gauze dressing is often not enough to immobilize or provide support to a wound. Binders and bandages applied over or around dressings provide extra protection and therapeutic benefits by doing the following:

- Creating pressure over a body part (e.g., an elastic pressure bandage applied over an arterial puncture site)
- Immobilizing a body part (e.g., an elastic bandage applied around a sprained ankle)
- Supporting a wound (e.g., an abdominal binder applied over a large abdominal incision and dressing)

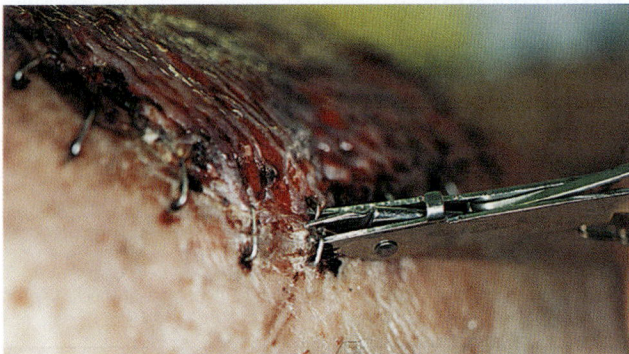

FIGURE 47.28 Removal of intermittent suture. **A,** Cut the suture as close to the skin as possible, away from the knot. **B,** Remove the suture and never pull the contaminated stitch through the tissues.

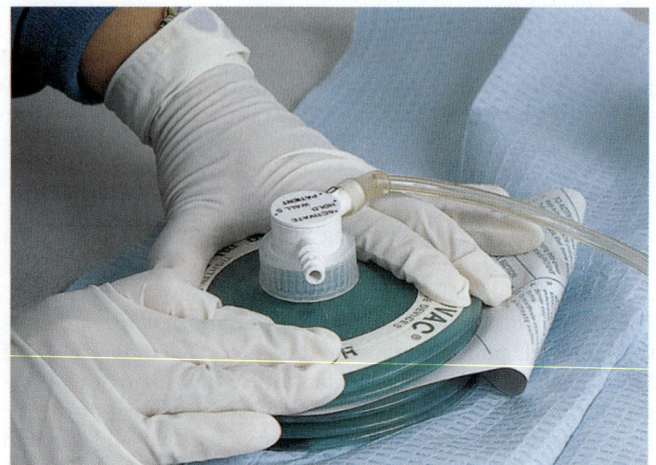

FIGURE 47.26 Staple remover.

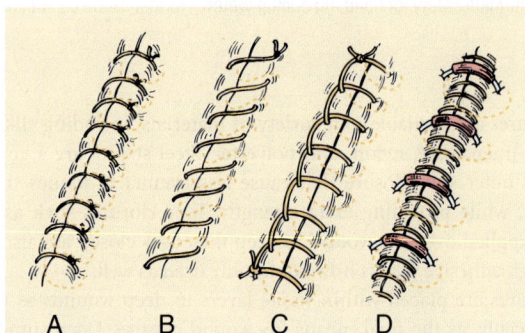

FIGURE 47.27 Examples of suturing methods. **A,** Intermittent. **B,** Continuous. **C,** Blanket continuous. **D,** Retention.

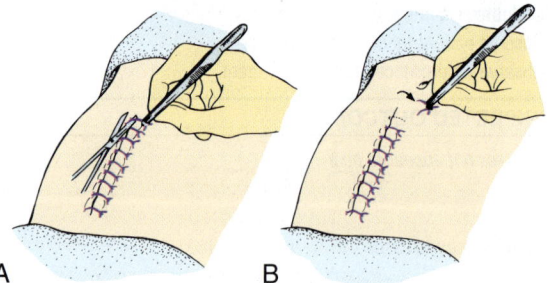

FIGURE 47.29 Drainage evacuator.

- Reducing or preventing edema (e.g., a well-supporting bra to minimize breast discomfort after birth of a baby)
- Securing a splint (e.g., a bandage applied around hand splints for correction of deformities)
- Securing dressings (e.g., elastic webbing applied around leg dressings after a vein stripping)

Bandages are available in rolls of various widths and materials, including gauze, elasticized knit, elastic webbing, flannel, and muslin. Gauze bandages are lightweight and inexpensive, conform easily to the contours of the body, and permit air circulation to prevent skin maceration. Elastic bandages conform well to body parts but also exert pressure.

Principles for Applying Bandages and Binders. Correctly applied bandages and binders do not cause injury to underlying and nearby body parts or create discomfort for the patient. For example, a chest binder should not be so tight as to restrict chest wall expansion. Before applying a bandage or binder, the nurse is responsible for the following:

- Inspecting the skin for abrasions, edema, discoloration, or exposed wound edges
- Covering exposed wounds or open abrasions with a sterile dressing
- Assessing condition of underlying dressings and changing them, if soiled
- Assessing skin of underlying areas that will be distal to the bandage for signs of circulatory impairment (coolness, pallor or cyanosis, diminished or absent pulses, swelling, numbness, and tingling) to provide a means for comparing changes in circulation after bandage application

After applying a bandage, the nurse must assess, document, and immediately report changes in circulation, skin integrity, comfort level, and body function (e.g., ventilation, movement). The bandage may need to be readjusted once it is applied. The nurse should explain to the patient that the binder may feel relatively firm or tight. Nurses must always assess a bandage carefully to make sure the application follows the written order and is providing therapeutic benefit. Any soiled bandages need to be replaced.

Binder Application. Binders are especially designed for the body part to be supported. Most binders are made of elastic or cotton. The most common types of binders are the abdominal binder and breast binder (Skill 47.5). Well-fitting bras are more common now than breast binders, although both methods provide support after breast surgery or exert pressure to reduce lactation in a woman after childbirth.

Abdominal binders. An abdominal binder supports large abdominal incisions that are vulnerable to tension or stress as the patient moves or coughs. An abdominal binder is secured with safety pins, Velcro strips, or metal stays.

Bandage Application. Rolls of bandage secure or support dressings over irregularly shaped body parts. Each roll has a free outer end and a terminal end at the centre of the roll. The rolled portion of the bandage is its body, and its outer surface is placed against the patient's skin or dressing. Skill 47.6 describes the steps for applying an elastic bandage.

The Whole Person, the Whole Team

Skin management and wound care require involvement of the entire health care team because the factors that create skin breakdown, such as pressure and nutrition, are assessed and treated by experts within the health care team: physiotherapist, occupational therapist, dietitian, nurse, physician, social worker, and pharmacist. In addition, the wound belongs to the patient. Nurses need to recognize the individual's situation and goals on both the development and healing potential of a wound.

Case Study. John Purata (preferred pronouns: he/him) is an 84-year-old patient who has returned from hospital to his home in a long-term care facility where you are looking after the ulcer on his sacrum, developed in acute care after hip replacement surgery. Mr. Purata has been too tired to get up for meals, and his nutritional intake has declined. Although he is on a pressure-relief surface, Mr. Purata tends to lie on his back. You have mentioned to him the importance of repositioning to assist in healing the wound, but he merely closes his eyes and tells you he is fine the way he is. When you and the other staff in the long-term care facility try to get him up to walk, Mr. Purata is hesitant and requires a great deal of coaching and encouragement to walk even a few steps. He then says he is too tired to go further and asks to go back to bed. He is frequently lying in bed, with eyes closed and the lights dim. His daughter and son are concerned that he seems to have lost his "get up and go" attitude. The wound is not improving, and you are concerned.

- What are the key issues that need to be addressed?
- What members of the health care team need to be involved?
- What would be realistic goals for Mr. Purata?
- How would you develop a plan of care for this patient?

◆ Evaluation

Nursing interventions for reducing and treating pressure injuries are evaluated by determining the patient's response to nursing therapies and whether the patient achieved each goal (Figure 47.30). To evaluate outcomes and responses to care, nurses measure the effectiveness of interventions. The optimal outcomes are to prevent injury to the skin and tissues, reduce injury to the skin and underlying tissues, and restore skin integrity (Coleman & Nielsen, 2019).

Because each patient has different risk factors for impaired skin integrity, nurses need to individualize nursing interventions. Patients with minimal mobility impairments or relatively stable health status may only need a few measures.

Nurses will assess patients with impaired skin integrity on an ongoing basis for factors that contribute to skin breakdown. This includes a comprehensive skin assessment and a wound assessment using a validated risk assessment tool. Assessment provides the foundation for the plan of care and is critical for monitoring the effectiveness of the plan (Nix, 2016).

As a nurse, you need to include the patient and the caregiver in the assessment process. Determine what they know about impaired skin integrity and develop a plan of care to provide education. Chronic wounds such as pressure injuries take time to heal, and it is likely that the patient will be in the home or long-term care setting with the pressure injury.

If the identified outcomes are not met for a patient with impaired skin integrity, questions to ask include the following:

- Was the etiology of the skin impairment addressed? Were pressure, friction, shear, and moisture components identified; did the plan of care decrease the contribution of each of these components? Were other factors, such as underlying chronic disease, also addressed?
- Was wound healing supported by providing the wound base with a moist, protected environment?
- Were issues such as nutrition assessed and a plan of care developed that provided the patient with the calories to support healing?

Nurses evaluate the need for additional referrals to other experts in wound management, such as occupational therapists, dietitians, and wound care specialists. Care of the patient with a pressure injury or other chronic wound requires an interprofessional team approach.

SKILL 47.5   APPLYING AN ABDOMINAL OR BREAST BINDER

Delegation Considerations

The skills of applying a binder (abdominal or breast) can be delegated to unregulated care providers (UCPs). The nurse remains responsible for wound assessment and evaluation of wound care interventions. Complete an assessment of the patient's ability to breathe deeply, cough effectively, and move independently; assess skin for irritation or abrasion; assess the incision or wound and dressing; and assess the patient's comfort level before a binder or sling is applied for the first time. When delegating the skill of applying a binder, instruct the UCP to do the following:

- Immediately report any change in the patient's respiratory status.
- Report an increase in wound drainage.
- Report changes in skin integrity under or adjacent to the binder.
- Remove the binder at prescribed intervals.

Equipment

- Disposable gloves, if wound drainage is present
- Abdominal binder:
  - Correct size cloth or elastic straight binder
  - Safety pins (6 to 8), unless Velcro closure or metal fasteners are attached
- Breast binder:
  - Correct size binder
  - Safety pins (approximately 12), unless Velcro closure is attached

PROCEDURE

STEPS	RATIONALE
1. Observe patient with need for support of chest or abdomen. Observe ability to breathe deeply and cough effectively.	• Baseline assessment determines patient's ability to breathe and cough. Impaired ventilation of lungs can lead to alveolar atelectasis and inadequate arterial oxygenation.
2. Review medical record, if a medical prescription for particular binder is required, and reasons for application.	• Application of supportive binders may be used on nursing judgement. In some situations, physician input is required.
3. Inspect skin for actual or potential alterations in integrity. Observe for irritation, abrasion, skin surfaces that rub against each other, or allergic response to adhesive tape used to secure dressing.	• Actual impairments in skin integrity can be worsened with application of a binder. Binder can cause pressure and excoriation.
4. Inspect any surgical dressing.	• Dressing replacement or reinforcement precedes application of any binder.

CRITICAL DECISION POINT: *Dressing should be clean and dry, and incision or wound should be entirely covered by dressing.*

STEPS	RATIONALE
5. Assess patient's comfort level, using analogue scale of 0 to 10 (see Chapter 32), noting any objective signs and symptoms of pain.	• Data will determine effectiveness of binder placement.

CRITICAL DECISION POINT: *Expect patient in moderate to severe pain to have diaphoresis, tachycardia, and elevated blood pressure.*

STEPS	RATIONALE
6. Gather necessary data regarding size of patient and appropriate binder.	• Proper fit of binder will be ensured.
7. Explain procedure to patient.	• Increases patient understanding and cooperation.
8. Teach skill to patient or caregiver.	• Anxiety is reduced and continuity of care after discharge is ensured.
9. Perform hand hygiene and apply gloves (if likely to contact wound drainage).	• Transmission of microorganisms is reduced.
10. Close curtains or room door.	• Patient's comfort and dignity are maintained.
11. Apply binder:	
A. Abdominal binder:	
(1) Position patient in supine position with head slightly elevated and knees slightly flexed.	• Muscular tension on abdominal organs is minimized.
(2) Fanfold far side of binder toward midline of binder.	• Patient's time in uncomfortable position is reduced.
(3) Instruct and help patient to roll away from you toward raised side rail while firmly supporting abdominal incision and dressing with hands.	• Pain and discomfort are reduced.
(4) Place fanfolded ends of binder under patient.	• Placement and centring of binder are accomplished with minimal discomfort.
(5) Instruct or assist patient to roll over folded ends.	
(6) Unfold and stretch ends out smoothly on far side of bed.	• Skin integrity and comfort are maintained.
(7) Instruct patient to roll back into supine position.	• Chest expansion and adequate wound support are facilitated when binder is closed.
(8) Adjust binder so that supine patient is centred over binder using symphysis pubis and costal margins as lower and upper landmarks.	• Support from binder is centred over abdominal structures, which reduces incidence of decreased lung expansion.

Continued

SKILL 47.5   APPLYING AN ABDOMINAL OR BREAST BINDER—cont'd

CRITICAL DECISION POINT: *Cover any exposed areas of an incision or wound with sterile dressing.*

(9) Close binder. Pull one end of binder over centre of patient's abdomen. While maintaining tension on that end of binder, pull opposite end of binder over centre and secure with Velcro closure tabs, metal fasteners, or horizontally placed safety pins.	• Continuous wound support and comfort are provided.
B. Breast binder:	
(1) Assist patient in placing arms through binder's armholes.	• Binder placement process is made easier for patient.
(2) Assist patient to supine position in bed.	• Supine positioning facilitates normal anatomical position of breasts; facilitates healing and comfort.
(3) Pad area under breasts, if necessary.	• Skin contact with undersurface is prevented.
(4) Using Velcro closure tabs or horizontally placed safety pins, secure binder at nipple level first. Continue closure process above and then below nipple line until entire binder is closed.	• Horizontal placement of pins may reduce risk of uneven pressure or localized irritation.
(5) Make appropriate adjustments, including individualizing fit of shoulder straps and pinning waistline darts to reduce binder size.	• Support to patient's breasts is maintained.
(6) Instruct and observe skill development in self-care related to reapplying breast binder.	• Self-care is an integral aspect of discharge planning. Skin integrity and comfort-level goals are ensured.
12. Remove gloves and perform hand hygiene.	• Cross-infections are prevented.
13. Assess patient's comfort level, using analogue scale of 0 to 10, noting any objective signs and symptoms.	• Effectiveness of binder placement is determined. Binders should not increase discomfort.
14. Adjust binder, as necessary.	• Comfort and chest expansion are promoted.
15. Observe site for skin integrity, circulation, and characteristics of the wound. (Periodically remove binder and surgical dressing to assess wound characteristics.)	• Binder should not result in complication to skin, wound, or underlying organs.
16. Assess patient's ability to breathe properly.	• Any impaired ventilation and potential pulmonary complications are identified.
17. Identify patient's need for assistance with activities such as combing hair.	• Mobility of upper extremities may be limited, depending on severity and location of incision.

UNEXPECTED OUTCOMES / RELATED INTERVENTIONS

UNEXPECTED OUTCOMES	RELATED INTERVENTIONS
Patient's pain increases	• Remove binder and assess wound. • Reapply binder using less pressure.
Patient develops impaired skin integrity under the binder	• Remove binder. • Initiate skin care measures to heal affected site.

RECORDING AND REPORTING
• Report any skin irritation at between-shift report.
• Record application of binder, condition of skin, circulation, integrity of dressing, and patient's comfort level.
• Report ineffective lung expansion to physician immediately.

CARE IN THE COMMUNITY CONSIDERATIONS
• Abdominal and breast binders can be washed and air-dried.
• Instruct caregiver to avoid excessive pressure with binder application.

SKILL 47.6   APPLYING AN ELASTIC BANDAGE

Delegation Considerations
The application of an elastic bandage can be delegated to unregulated care providers (UCPs). The nurse is responsible for wound assessment and the evaluation of the wound. In addition, the nurse should assess for adequate circulation to the extremity distal to the elastic bandage (e.g., pulse, skin temperature, capillary refill). When delegating this skill to a UCP, inform them of any restrictions that the patient might have (e.g., unable to independently raise leg or independently roll over). Also instruct the UCP to report the following:
• Any change in the skin colour of the patient's injured extremity
• Any increases in the patient's pain

Equipment
• Correct width and number of bandages
• Safety pins, clips, or adhesive tape
• Disposable gloves, if wound drainage is present

SKILL 47.6　APPLYING AN ELASTIC BANDAGE—cont'd

PROCEDURE

STEPS	RATIONALE
1. Perform hand hygiene and apply gloves, if needed. Inspect skin for alterations in integrity as indicated by abrasions, discoloration, chafing, or edema. (Look carefully at bony prominences.)	• Altered skin integrity contraindicates the use of elastic bandages.
2. Inspect surgical dressing. Remove gloves and perform hand hygiene.	• Surgical dressing replacement or reinforcement precedes application.
3. Observe adequacy of circulation (distal to bandage) by noting surface temperature, skin colour, and sensation of body parts to be wrapped.	• Comparison of area before and after application of bandage is necessary to ensure continued adequate circulation. Impairment of circulation may result in coolness to touch when compared with opposite side of body, cyanosis or pallor of skin, diminished or absent pulses, edema or localized pooling, and numbness or tingling of part.
4. Review medical record for specific orders related to application of elastic bandage. Note area to be covered, type of bandage required, frequency of change, and previous response to treatment.	• Specific prescription may direct procedure, including factors such as extent of application (e.g., toe to knee, toe to groin) and duration of treatment.
5. Identify patient's and primary caregiver's present knowledge level of skill, if bandaging will be continued at home.	• Planning and teaching should be individualized.
6. Explain procedure to patient.	• Increased knowledge promotes cooperation and reduces anxiety.
7. Teach skill to patient or primary caregiver.	• Anxiety is reduced and continuity of care after discharge is ensured.
8. Perform hand hygiene and apply gloves if drainage is present.	• Transmission of microorganisms is reduced.
9. Close room door or curtains.	• Patient's comfort and dignity are maintained.
10. Help patient to assume comfortable, anatomically correct position.	• Alignment is maintained, and musculoskeletal deformity is prevented.

CRITICAL DECISION POINT: *Bandages applied to lower extremities are applied before patient sits or stands. Elevation of dependent extremities for 20 minutes before bandage application will enhance venous return.*

STEPS	RATIONALE
11. Hold the roll of elastic bandage in your dominant hand and use the other hand to lightly hold beginning of bandage at distal body part. Continue transferring roll to your dominant hand as bandage is wrapped.	• Appropriate and consistent bandage tension is maintained.

CRITICAL DECISION POINT: *Toes or fingertips should be visible for follow-up circulatory assessment.*

STEPS	RATIONALE
12. Apply bandage from distal point toward proximal boundary using a variety of turns to cover various shapes of body parts.	• Bandage is applied in a manner that conforms evenly to body part and promotes venous return.
13. Unroll and very slightly stretch bandage.	• Uniform bandage tension is maintained.
14. Overlap turns by one-half to two-thirds width of bandage roll.	• Uneven bandage tension and circulatory impairment are prevented.
15. Secure first bandage with clip or tape before applying additional rolls.	
16. Apply additional rolls without leaving any uncovered skin surface. Secure last bandage applied.	• Wrinkling and loose ends are prevented.
17. Remove gloves, if worn, and perform hand hygiene.	• Transmission of microorganisms is reduced.
A. Assess distal circulation when bandage application is complete and at least twice during 8-hour period.	• Early detection and management of circulatory impairment ensure healthy neurovascular status.
B. Observe skin colour for pallor or cyanosis.	
C. Palpate skin for warmth.	
D. Palpate pulses and compare bilaterally.	
E. Ask if patient is aware of pain, numbness, tingling, or other discomfort.	• Neurovascular changes indicate impaired venous return.
F. Observe mobility of extremity.	• Joint immobility is determined; if bandage is too tight, movement will be restricted.
18. Have patient demonstrate bandage application.	• Return demonstration documents learning.

UNEXPECTED OUTCOMES	RELATED INTERVENTIONS
Impaired circulation distal to elastic bandage	• Release bandage.
	• Palpate extremity and assess pulse, temperature, and capillary refill.
	• Reapply dressing with less pressure.
Break in skin under elastic bandage	• Remove bandage.
	• Reapply bandage with less pressure.
Inability of patient to change dressing	• Determine barriers to applying bandage.
	• Explore options (e.g., different type of dressing).

Continued

SKILL 47.6 APPLYING AN ELASTIC BANDAGE—cont'd

RECORDING AND REPORTING

- Document condition of the wound, integrity of dressing, application of bandage, circulation, and patient's comfort level.
- Report any changes in neurological or circulatory status to the nurse in charge or physician.

CARE IN THE COMMUNITY CONSIDERATIONS

- Instruct patient or caregiver not to secure bandages too tightly, which interferes with circulation.
- Elastic bandages that are used to reduce swelling are best applied to the feet in the morning, before getting out of bed.
- Always remove an elastic bandage daily and inspect the area.

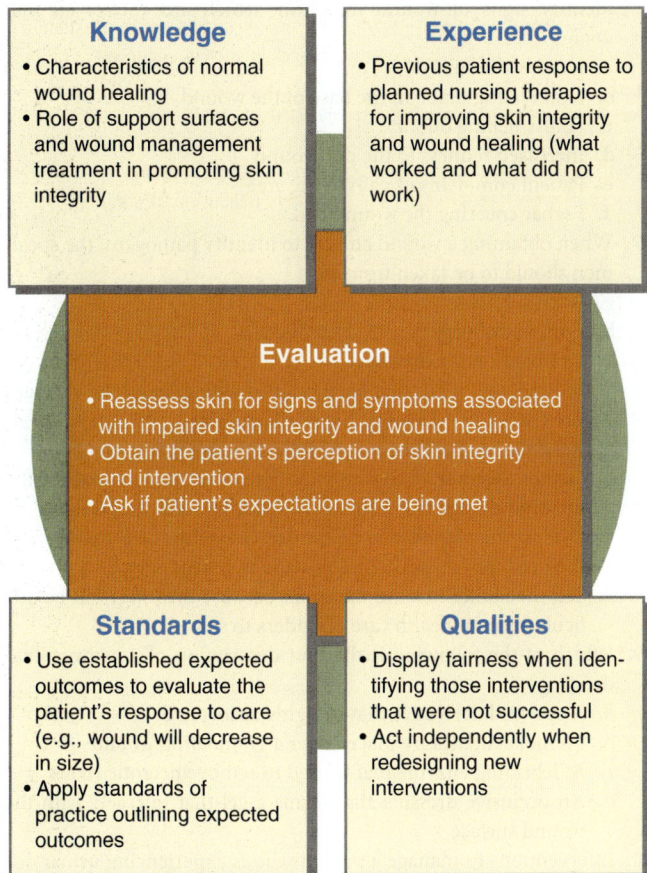

Knowledge
- Characteristics of normal wound healing
- Role of support surfaces and wound management treatment in promoting skin integrity

Experience
- Previous patient response to planned nursing therapies for improving skin integrity and wound healing (what worked and what did not work)

Evaluation
- Reassess skin for signs and symptoms associated with impaired skin integrity and wound healing
- Obtain the patient's perception of skin integrity and intervention
- Ask if patient's expectations are being met

Standards
- Use established expected outcomes to evaluate the patient's response to care (e.g., wound will decrease in size)
- Apply standards of practice outlining expected outcomes

Qualities
- Display fairness when identifying those interventions that were not successful
- Act independently when redesigning new interventions

FIGURE 47.30 Critical thinking model for skin integrity and wound care evaluation.

KEY CONCEPTS

- Prevention of skin breakdown is a major nursing focus for all patients, irrespective of their age or the health care setting.
- Patients should be assessed for risk of skin breakdown with the use of a validated risk assessment tool, such as the Braden Scale, on admission to care and at regularly scheduled intervals—more frequently if health status changes.
- Low or at-risk score in any subscale of the assessment tool should be addressed and monitored.
- Changes in mobility, sensory perception, level of consciousness, and nutrition, as well as the presence of moisture, increase the risk of developing pressure injuries.
- Preventive skin care is aimed at controlling external pressure on bony prominences and keeping the skin clean, well lubricated, hydrated, and free of excess moisture.
- Proper positioning (the 30-degree rule) reduces the effects of pressure and guards against shearing force.
- Wound assessment requires a description of the appearance of the wound base, size (length × width × depth), presence of exudate, and the periwound skin condition.
- Moist wound-healing approaches are based on evidence and support the healing cycle of wounds.
- Wounds require pressure off-loading, adequate nutrition and hydration, blood flow, and an absence of infection to heal.
- Arterial, venous, and diabetic wounds are often the result of impaired peripheral circulation to the extremities.
- Wound irrigation should be at room or body temperature and provide 4 to 15 psi of pressure to avoid damaging fragile granulating tissue.
- Therapeutic beds and mattresses redistribute the effects of pressure; selection is based on assessment data to identify the best bed for individual needs.
- Cleaning and topical agents used to treat wounds vary according to the condition of the wound bed. Assessment of the wound will enable the nurse to select proper skin care agents.
- Nutritional interventions are directed at improving wound healing through increasing protein and calorie levels, as required.
- When extensive tissue loss occurs, a wound heals by secondary intention.
- The chances of wound infection are greater when the wound contains dead or necrotic tissue, when foreign bodies lie on or near the wound, and when the blood supply and tissue defences are reduced.
- The principles of wound first aid include control of bleeding, cleaning, and protection.
- Dressings with effective moisture–vapour transfer rates support transfer of drainage via wicking and help prevent external bacterial contamination.
- A moist environment ("moist like your eyeball") supports wound healing.
- When cleaning wounds or drain sites, clean from the least to most contaminated area, away from wound edges.
- A bandage or binder should be applied in a manner that does not impair circulation or irritate the skin.

CRITICAL THINKING EXERCISES

A patient (preferred pronouns: she/her) is 76 years old, at postoperative day 7 after a total hip replacement. Her hip incision at postoperative day 4 is red and oozing foul-smelling, tan-coloured drainage. Significant medical history includes arthritis and mild hypertension.

Because of surgical pain at the incision site, she has been reluctant to transfer from bed to chair. Now on postoperative day 7, she tells you the incision is sore, and also tells you she feels a painful, burning sensation in the sacral region. She is continent of urine and stool but requires assistance to get to the bathroom or commode chair. You observe that she has difficulty lifting herself to the side of the bed when preparing for bed-to-chair transfers.

1. The staples from the surgical incision were removed and an order was written for a moist saline gauze dressing to be applied to the area three times a day. Would this be the approach that best supports wound healing? Provide a rationale and suggest alternative approaches. When the dressing is removed, what are the critical factors to assess?

2. A head-to-toe skin assessment is done per institutional policy on a daily basis. At the most recent assessment, redness was noted over the sacral area, and on direct examination, a small area of denuded tissue was noted. The involved area has minimal depth and a red, moist base. How would you describe the impairment in skin integrity in your charting?

3. What will you include in your plan of care to address the impairment in skin integrity in the sacral area?

4. The patient will be discharged tomorrow. What issues must be assessed regarding her care before discharge? Explain why those issues are of importance.

🌐 *Answers to Critical Thinking Exercises appear on the Evolve website.*

REVIEW QUESTIONS

Review Questions 1 to 10 relate to the case study at the beginning of the chapter.

1. Your patient, Kathy, has type 2 diabetes. When you review her history, you identify a number of issues which lead you to consider nursing care that will focus on:
   a. Increasing knowledge regarding diabetes management
   b. Providing pamphlets on healthy eating
   c. Identifying the patient's goals
   d. Increasing the patient's mobility
   e. Ensuring the patient gets enough rest

2. Kathy has several pressure injuries. Kathy developed a large draining sacral wound, which is now 6 cm in diameter. The base of the wound can be visualized down to bone. At which stage is this pressure injury?
   a. Stage 1
   b. Stage 2
   c. Stage 3
   d. Stage 4
   e. Unstageable (Stage X)

3. Kathy has reddened areas on her right heel and both her hips. When you touch these areas with your fingertip, you notice that these areas do not blanch. What does this indicate?
   a. A local skin infection requiring antibiotics
   b. This patient has sensitive skin and requires special bed linen
   c. A stage 1 pressure injury that requires pressure off-loading

   d. Reactive hyperemia, a reaction that causes the blood vessels to dilate in the injured area

4. Patients with pressure injuries require which of the following?
   a. Repositioning at least every 4 to 6 hours
   b. Bed rest and a quiet environment
   c. Frequent dressing changes
   d. Nutritional assessment from a dietitian

5. There is serous drainage from the patient's sacral wound. Serous drainage is defined as:
   a. Fresh bleeding
   b. Thick and yellow
   c. Clear, watery plasma
   d. Beige to brown and foul-smelling

6. When you observe Kathy's sacral wound several days later, you identify signs of wound infection, which are: *(Select all that apply.)*
   a. Increased drainage
   b. Granulating tissue in the base of the wound
   c. Foul-smelling odour
   d. Increased redness to the periwound
   e. Patient complains of pain to the area
   f. Eschar covering the wound bed

7. When obtaining a wound culture to identify pathogens, the specimen should to be taken from the:
   a. Necrotic tissue
   b. Wound drainage
   c. Drainage on the dressing
   d. Wound after it has first been cleaned with appropriate cleaner

8. Before changing a dressing, the nurse should:
   a. Read the medical orders and follow them exactly
   b. Gather together all the supplies that might be required for the dressing change and remove the dressing from the wound
   c. Discuss the plan to change the dressing with the patient, assess the need for analgesia, and provide it, if necessary
   d. Tell the family to leave the room because dressings can be difficult for non–health care providers to see

9. Which of the following is the best description of a hydrocolloid dressing?
   a. A seaweed derivative that is highly absorptive
   b. Premoistened gauze placed over a granulating wound
   c. A debriding enzyme that is used to remove necrotic tissue
   d. An occlusive dressing that forms a gel that interacts with the wound surface

10. Interventions to manage a patient who is experiencing urinary or fecal incontinence include:
   a. Keeping the buttocks exposed to air at all times
   b. Use of large absorbent diapers that are changed when saturated
   c. Utilization of a perineal cleanser, followed by application of a moisture barrier cream or ointment
   d. Frequent cleaning, application of an ointment, and coverage of the areas with a thick, absorbent towel

Answers: 1. c; **2.** d; **3.** c; **4.** a; **5.** c; **6.** a, c, d, e; **7.** d; **8.** c; **9.** d; **10.** c.

🌐 *Rationales for the Review Questions appear on the Evolve website.*

RECOMMENDED WEBSITES

Connecting Learners with Knowledge: Learning Together: https://www.clwk.ca/get-resource/wound-management-guideline/

This website provides a number of useful tools and educational videos for clinicians with a role in wound care. This site is an excellent resource for clinical knowledge and practice specific to products. It was developed and is supported by the British Columbia Provincial Nursing Skin & Wound Care Committee.

European Pressure Ulcer Advisory Panel: https://www.epuap.org

Created in 1996, this group of health care providers and wound care experts works to lead and support all European countries in the efforts to prevent and treat pressure injuries. The mission statement is "to provide the relief of persons suffering from or at risk of pressure ulcers, in particular through research and the education of the public." Numerous links to European wound care organizations appear on the website.

National Pressure Injury Advisory Panel (NPIAP): https://www.npiap.com

The NPIAP provides interprofessional leadership for improved patient outcomes in pressure injury prevention and management through education, public policy, and research.

Nurses Specialized in Wound, Ostomy and Continence Canada (NSWOCC): https://nswoc.ca/

NSWOCC is an association of nurses with a specialty in wound, ostomy, and continence care. This association promotes education, research, and standards for WOC nursing practice. Nurses with the NSWOCC designation have obtained additional post-baccalaureate level certification to offer care to patients with the following conditions: abdominal stomata (openings), fistulas, draining wounds, and selected disorders of the integumentary (skin), gastrointestinal, and genitourinary systems. This organization also offers affiliate programs for nurses who do not have baccalaureate-level nursing education.

Registered Nurses' Association of Ontario (RNAO) Best Practice Guidelines: https://rnao.ca/bpg

This website provides links to the RNAO Best Practice Guidelines, including the revised version of *Risk Assessment and Prevention of Pressure Ulcers* and *Assessment and Management of Stage I to IV Pressure Ulcers*, now called *Assessment and Management of Pressure Injuries for the Interprofessional Team* (3rd edition), which can be downloaded for no cost as a pdf file or purchased through RNAO.

The South West Regional Wound Care Program: https://swrwoundcareprogram.ca

This website, also known as "The Toolkit," contains skin, wound, and ostomy care–related resources for health care providers and members of the public, primarily intended for those within the Southwest catchment of Ontario. Similar to the other sites provided here, this website is open access and provides a wealth of information on best practices in wound care, including information for patients.

World Wide Wounds: http://www.worldwidewounds.com

World Wide Wounds is an online, peer-reviewed journal with a focus on current research and evidence-informed practice issues related to wound care.

Wound Care Management: https://www.lhsc.on.ca/wound

This website is a clinical resource, based on evidence-informed best practices for wound care. The site includes numerous links to online resources, including those for typical wounds and dressing options.

Wound, Ostomy and Continence Nurses (WOCN) Society: https://www.wocn.org

The WOCN Society is a professional nursing society based in the United States that supports the practice and delivery of expert health care to patients with wounds, ostomies, and incontinence.

Wounds Canada (formerly Canadian Association of Wound Care (CAWC): https://www.woundscanada.ca

Wounds Canada is an interprofessional national organization dedicated to prevention, treatment, evaluation, and scholarship regarding wound care across the continuum of care. This website has quick reference guides and best practice articles available for downloading on all aspects of wound care practice, as well as information on upcoming seminars, conferences, and scholarship funding opportunities.

🌐 REFERENCES

A full reference list is available on the website for this book at http://evolve.elsevier.com/Canada/Potter/fundamentals/

48

Sensory Alterations

Canadian content written by Annette M. Lane, MN, PhD, and Sandra P. Hirst, RN, PhD, GNC(c), with original chapter contributions by Jill Parsons, RN, PhD

OBJECTIVES

Mastery of content in this chapter will enable you to:

- Describe the key terms listed.
- Differentiate among the processes of reception, perception, and reaction to sensory stimuli.
- Describe the relationship of sensory function to an individual's level of wellness.
- Describe common causes and effects of sensory alterations.
- Describe common sensory changes that normally take place as individuals age.
- Conduct an assessment of an individual's sensory status.

- Develop a plan of care for individuals with sensory alterations.
- Identify interventions for preventing sensory deprivation and controlling sensory overload.
- Describe conditions in the health care setting or patient's home that nurses can adjust to promote meaningful sensory stimulation.
- Explain ways to maintain a safe environment for patients with sensory deficits.
- Identify the benefits of working with an interprofessional team.
- Evaluate the effects of the nursing process when caring for patients with sensory alterations.

KEY TERMS

Age-related macular degeneration (AMD)
Aphasia
Audiologist
Auditory
Carpal tunnel syndrome
Cataracts
Central auditory processing disorders
Cerumen
Conductive hearing loss
Delirium
Diabetic retinopathy
Expressive aphasia
Glaucoma
Global aphasia

Gustatory
Health promotion
Hyperesthesia
Kinesthetic
Myopia
Olfactory
Otitis media
Otolaryngologist
Ototoxic
Perception
Presbycusis
Presbyopia
Proprioceptive
Receptive aphasia

Refractive error
Retinal detachment
Sensorineural hearing loss
Sensory deficit
Sensory deprivation
Sensory overload
Stereognosis
Strabismus
Tactile
Tinnitus
Tympanic membrane
Vertigo
Visual
Xerostomia

🌐 WEBSITE

http://evolve.elsevier.com/Canada/Potter/fundamentals/

CASE STUDY

Judy (preferred pronouns: she/her) is a 70-year-old who is widowed and lives alone. She is active in the community and has a number of friends. For the last several years, Judy has noticed problems with vision in her left eye. Her vision is blurred and she has trouble with reading and night driving. Judy now needs to rely on her neighbour to drive her to volunteer commitments. She is feeling depressed and lonely as she awaits cataract surgery.

Her cousin, Suzanne, has come from another province to spend some time with Judy. Having significant hearing loss, Suzanne understands what it is like to lose, or partially lose, a sense that is so vital in daily living.

As a beginning nurse, you are accompanying the community health nurse on a home visit to assess Judy. You wonder what you will assess in terms of Judy's sight and her home. Although your assessment only pertains to Judy, through conversation with both Judy and Suzanne, you are learning about the challenges of living with sight loss and hearing loss. (Please see the Nursing Care Plan in Box 48.9 later in this chapter).

Think about this case study as you read this chapter. There are review questions at the end of the chapter that relate to the case study.

People rely on a variety of sensory stimuli to give meaning and order to events occurring in their environment. The senses help form the perceptual base of our world (Boscart et al., 2023). Stimulation comes from many sources inside and outside the body, particularly through the senses of sight (**visual**), hearing (**auditory**), touch (**tactile**), smell (**olfactory**), and taste (**gustatory**). The body also has a **kinesthetic** sense that enables a person to be aware of the position and movement of body parts without seeing them. **Stereognosis** is a sense that allows a person to recognize an object's size, shape, and texture. Meaningful stimuli allow a person to learn about the environment and are necessary for healthy functioning and normal development.

Sensory alterations have been perceived by many as inevitable with aging and, therefore, are overlooked and not treated (Mick et al., 2020). However, sensory alterations can occur at any age and can have multiple causations. They can also have a substantial detrimental effect on the individual's ability to care for themselves in their home, maintain independence, and learn and adopt necessary self-care practices (Mick et al., 2020; Peelle, 2019). Individually, hearing and vision loss are associated with depression, cognitive decline, delirium, functional decline, and falls (Humes et al., 2020). More serious is dual sensory impairment, such as both vision and hearing loss. Such impairment restricts one's capacity to participate fully in a range of social environments without some means of assistance (Guthrie et al., 2018) and increases depression and anxiety (Simning et al., 2019). With age and as the prevalence of chronic disease increases, sensory acuity often declines for taste, smell, and texture perception, and this can have an influence on food perception, preference, and food intake (Boesveldt et al., 2018; Mueller-Schotte et al., 2019; Risso et al., 2020).

Many patients seeking health care have pre-existing sensory alterations (e.g., cataracts) or more than one sensory alteration (e.g., both hearing and visual deficits). Others may develop sensory alterations because of medical treatment (e.g., hearing loss from antibiotic use). In other cases, there can be environmental causes resulting in sensory deficits, such as hearing loss due to frequent exposure to occupational noise. The health care environment itself can cause sensory alterations. For example, a hospital unit is often a place of unfamiliar sights, sounds, and smells that can lead to sensory overload resulting in delirium. In contrast, being hospitalized can also lead to sensory deprivation in some individuals due to the lack of meaningful contact with familiar supports, such as family and friends.

As a nurse, you must be able to recognize the factors that can lead to sensory alterations, know how those factors can be prevented or minimized, understand the implications of sensory alterations, and work with the patient in facilitating their independence and self-care needs.

SCIENTIFIC KNOWLEDGE BASE

Normal Sensation

The nervous system continuously receives thousands of bits of information from sensory nerve receptors, relays the information through appropriate channels, and integrates the information into a meaningful response. Sensory stimuli reach the sensory receptors and can elicit an immediate reaction or present information to the brain to be stored for future use. The nervous system must be intact for sensory stimuli to reach appropriate brain centres and for the individual to perceive the sensation. After interpreting the significance of a sensation, the person can then react to the stimulus (Tables 48.1 and 48.2).

TABLE 48.1	Normal Hearing	
Function	**Anatomy and Physiology**
The Ear Transmits to the brain an accurate pattern of all sounds received from the environment, the relative intensity of these sounds, and the direction from which they originate.	The auditory system is composed of three major parts: external or outer ear, middle ear, and inner ear (see Figure 48.1, *B*).
External Ear The purpose of the hair follicles and the cerumen is to protect against the entry of foreign matter into the canal and lubricate the canal to inhibit growth of bacteria and fungi. The external auditory canal shelters the tympanic membrane and maintains the elasticity of the tympanic membrane by maintaining a relatively constant temperature and humidity.	The external ear is composed of the auricle (or pinna) and the external auditory canal. The pinna directs and funnels sound waves into the external auditory canal and then to the eardrum (**tympanic membrane**). The outer one-third of the canal is lined with hair follicles and glands that secrete cerumen or ear wax.
Middle Ear The function of the middle ear is to transmit sound from the external auditory canal to the inner ear. The functions of the tympanic membrane are to cause the ossicles to vibrate in order to transmit sound waves to the inner ear and to protect the middle ear.	The middle ear consists of the tympanic membrane, the ossicles, and the oval window. The tympanic membrane is located at an oblique angle at the end of the auditory canal. The ossicles are three small bones (malleus, incus, and stapes). They are often nicknamed *hammer*, *anvil*, and *stirrup*, respectively. Movement of the stapes in the oval window creates vibrations in the fluid of the inner ear.
Inner Ear When vibrations at the oval window are transmitted to the inner ear they distort and move the fluid and hair cells in the labyrinth. The inner ear converts sound waves for the transmission and interpretation by the brain regarding body position, sound, and movement. The impulses are then transmitted along the eighth cranial nerve to the brain.	The inner ear contains three interconnected bony structures: cochlea, vestibule, and semicircular canals. They are often called the *labyrinth* because of their winding canal system. They contain fluid and tiny hair cells.

TABLE 48.2	Normal Vision
Function	**Anatomy and Physiology**
The Eye	
Transmits to the brain an accurate pattern of light reflected from solid objects in the environment and transformed into colour and hue.	The external parts of the eye include the eyebrows, eyelids, eyelashes, conjunctiva, cornea, sclera, and tear ducts. The internal structures include the sclera, cornea, choroid, ciliary body, iris, pupil, lens, and retina (see Figure 48.1, *A*). Light rays enter the convex cornea and begin to converge. Fine adjustment of light rays occurs as they pass through the pupil and through the lens. The ciliary muscles change the shape of the lens to focus the light on the retina. The retina has a pigmented layer of cells to enhance visual acuity. The sensory retina contains the rods and cones—photoreceptor cells sensitive to stimulation from light. Photoreceptor cells send electrical impulses by way of the optic nerve to the brain.

Reception, perception, and reaction are the three components of any sensory experience. Reception begins with stimulation of a receptor nerve cell, which is usually designed for only one type of stimulus, such as light, touch, or sound. In the case of specialized senses, the receptors are grouped close together or located in specialized organs (McCance & Huether, 2019), such as the taste buds of the tongue or the retina of the eye (Figure 48.1, *A*). When a nerve impulse is created, it travels along pathways to the spinal cord or directly to the brain. For example, sound waves stimulate hair cell receptors within the organ of Corti (located in the inner ear), which causes impulses to travel along the eighth cranial nerve to the acoustic area of the temporal lobe (see Figure 48.1, *B*). Sensory nerve pathways usually cross over to send stimuli to opposite sides of the brain.

The actual **perception** or awareness of unique sensations depends on the receiving region of the cerebral cortex, where specialized brain cells interpret the quality and nature of sensory stimuli. When the person becomes conscious of the stimuli and receives the information, perception takes place. Perception includes integration and interpretation of the stimuli on the basis of the person's experiences. A person's level of consciousness influences how well stimuli are perceived and interpreted. Any factors lowering consciousness impair sensory perception.

If sensation is incomplete, such as blurred vision, or if the person has a cognitive impairment, they may misinterpret the stimuli and may react inappropriately (e.g., become aggressive). It is impossible to react to all the multiple stimuli entering the nervous system. The brain prevents sensory bombardment by discarding or storing sensory information. A person will usually react to stimuli that are most meaningful or significant at the time. After continued reception of the same stimulus, however, a person stops responding, and the sensory experience goes unnoticed. For example, a person concentrating on reading a good book may not be aware of music in the background. This adaptability phenomenon occurs with most sensory stimuli, except for those of pain.

Sensory Deficits

A loss in the normal function of sensory reception and perception is a **sensory deficit**. The growing prevalence of sensory deficits is of concern, particularly with the increase in the number of people reaching 65 years and over (Canadian Institute for Health Information [CIHI], 2017).

When senses are impaired, the sense of self is affected. Initially, a person may withdraw by avoiding communication or socialization with others in an attempt to cope with the sensory loss. It becomes difficult for the person to interact safely with the environment until new skills are learned. When a deficit develops gradually or when considerable time has passed since the onset of an acute sensory loss, the person may learn to rely on unaffected senses. When one sense is impaired, people depend on their other intact senses. However, individuals with dual sensory impairments, for example, vision and hearing loss,

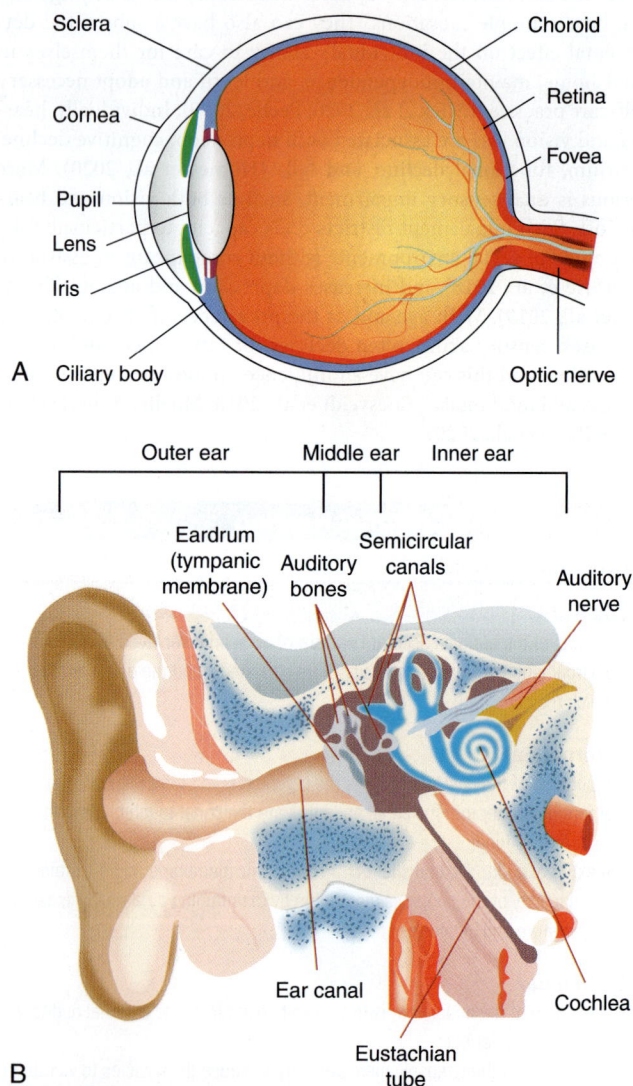

FIGURE 48.1 Anatomy of the eye and ear. **A,** Anatomy of the eye. **B,** Anatomy of the ear. (**A,** National Eye Institute, https://medialibrary.nei.nih.gov/; **B,** https://www.allamericanhearing.com/i-wonder-if-i-have-a-hearing-loss/anatomy-of-the-ear/)

have increased difficulty compensating (Davidson & Guthrie, 2019), although those who receive sensory rehabilitation services may experience good health and independence (Urqueta Alfaro et al., 2020).

Patients with sensory deficits may change their behaviour in effective or ineffective ways. For example, one patient with a hearing impairment may turn the unaffected ear toward the speaker to hear better, whereas another patient may avoid people to avoid the embarrassment of not being able to understand their speech.

Visual Deficits. Most vision loss in Canada is caused by cataracts, age-related macular degeneration (AMD), glaucoma, and diabetic retinopathy (Aljied et al., 2018; Canadian National Institute for the Blind [CNIB], 2022a).

Age-Related Macular Degeneration. Age-related macular degeneration (AMD) is the leading eye disease causing vision loss in Canadians over the age of 50 (Fighting Blindness Canada, 2022). It is incurable. It is a condition in which the macula (located in the centre of the retina) results in a gradual or sudden loss of central vision. First signs may include blurring of reading matter, distortion or loss of central vision, and distortion of vertical lines (Figure 48.2, *B*).

Cataract. Every individual will develop cataracts if they live long enough. Cataracts usually develop gradually and without pain, resulting in blurring, decreased vision, and glare. Cloudy or opaque areas in part of or the entire lens interfere with passage of light through the lens

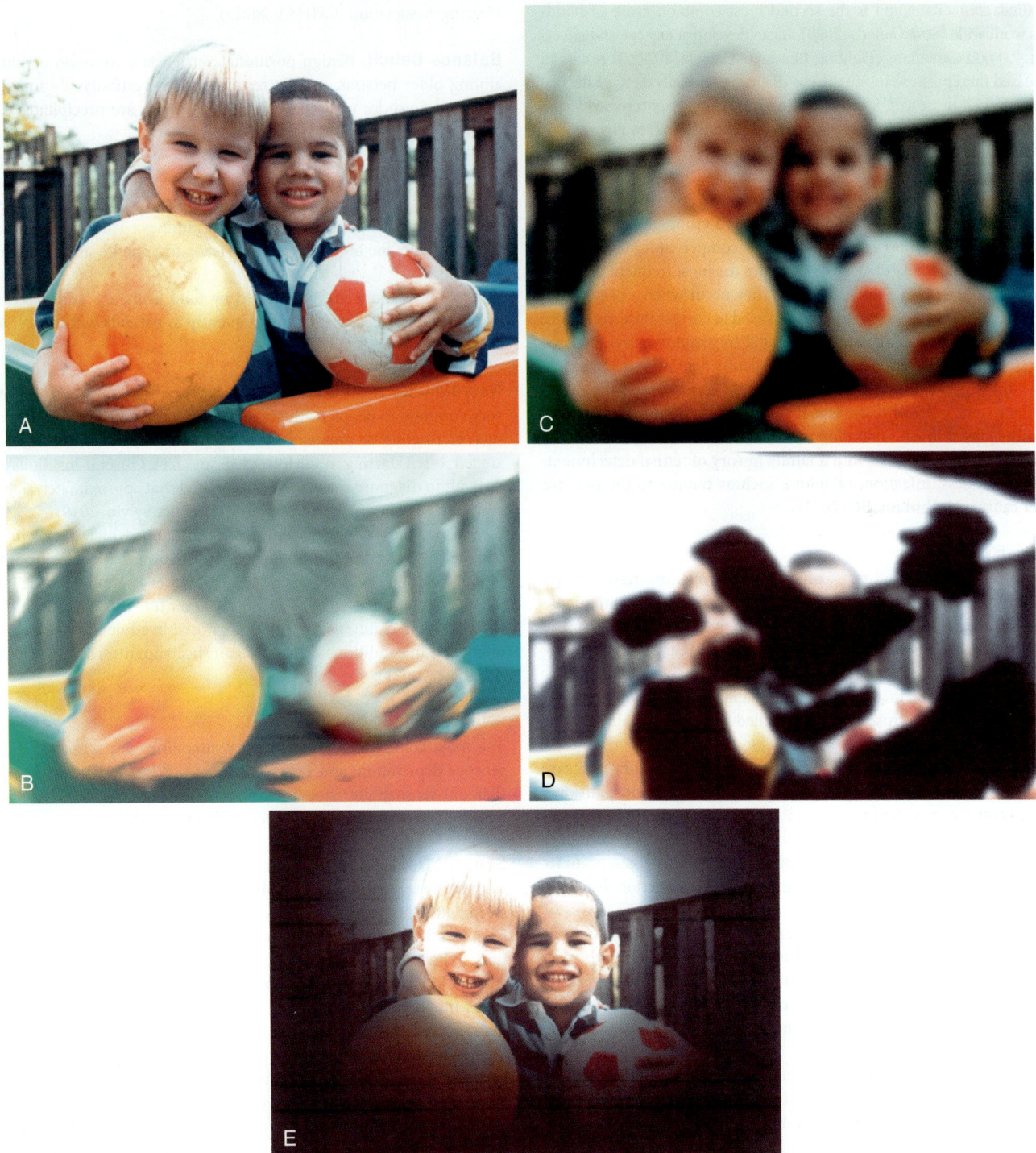

FIGURE 48.2 Visualizations when eye disease is present. **A,** Normal vision. **B,** Age-related macular degeneration. **C,** Cataract. **D,** Diabetic retinopathy. **E,** Glaucoma. (National Eye Institute, https://medialibrary.nei.nih.gov/)

(see Figure 48.2, *C*). Although associated with aging, cataracts can also be caused by diabetes, injury, or medications, especially steroids.

Diabetic Retinopathy. Diabetic retinopathy is the result of pathological changes that occur in the blood vessels of the retina, resulting in decreased vision or vision loss caused by hemorrhage and macular edema. It is the leading cause of vision loss in working-age Canadians (Fighting Blindness Canada, 2020). Long-term or poorly managed diabetes can lead to progressive damage to the blood vessels that feed the retina. These blood vessels leak into the retina, resulting in severe vision loss or blindness (see Figure 48.2, *D*).

Glaucoma. Glaucoma is the second most common cause of blindness worldwide (Seva Canada, 2020). It can develop at any age and affects over 400 000 Canadians (Fighting Blindness Canada, 2021). It results in increased fluid pressure inside the eye that can eventually damage the optic nerve. Left untreated, it can result in visual field loss, decreased visual acuity, a halo effect seen around objects, and blindness (see Figure 48.2, *E*). Glaucoma can be idiopathic in origin or may be caused by eye injury, inflammation, tumours, diabetes, or medications such as steroids.

Dry Eyes. Dry eyes occur more frequently with aging. This condition results in a gritty feeling, pain, itching, blurred vision, light sensitivity, redness, and sometimes excessive tears as a compensatory response.

Refractive Errors. Refractive errors are the most frequent yet most easily correctible source of vision loss. They occur when a person's vision is reduced and corrective lenses are used to correct the error. There are three types of refractive error: myopia (nearsightedness), hyperopia (farsightedness), and presbyopia (difficulty reading small print).

Retinal Detachment. Retinal detachment occurs when the retina develops small holes or tears. This may occur with thinning of the retina with aging or from separation of the vitreous from the retina and is more common in persons with a family history of retinal detachment. Nearsightedness, infection, or injury, such as trauma to the eye, are other causes (HealthLink BC, 2021a).

Hearing Deficits

Conductive Hearing Loss. Conductive hearing loss results when sound waves are not effectively transmitted through the outer and middle ear to the inner ear. Common causes are partial or total blockage of the ear canal, such as blockage caused by colds, allergies, and ear infections.

Presbycusis. Presbycusis is a common progressive hearing disorder in older persons that results in the inability to hear high-pitched sounds, making speech seem more muffled and unclear (HealthLink BC, 2020).

Central Auditory Processing Disorders. Central auditory processing disorders involve damage to the auditory centres and pathways in the central cortex. Some causes include traumatic brain injury, tumours, and heredity.

Cerumen Accumulation. Buildup of cerumen (earwax) can occur in the external auditory canal. Hard cerumen causes conduction deafness. This is more common in older people.

Ménière's Disease. Ménière's disease is a disorder of the inner ear characterized by hearing loss, tinnitus (background noises in the ear, hissing or ringing sounds, or discrete tones or pulses), and vertigo (sudden loss of balance). It likely is caused by increased fluid in the inner ear. This disorder usually begins in people between the ages of 20 and 50 years.

Otitis Media. Otitis media is an infection of the middle ear that is common in infants and children. Recurrent or chronic otitis media can cause damage to the eardrum or middle ear, resulting in permanent hearing loss.

Otosclerosis. Otosclerosis is a hereditary condition, resulting in hardening of the ossicles in the middle ear and gradual and progressive hearing loss that is usually accompanied by tinnitus.

Sensorineural Hearing Loss. Sensorineural hearing loss results from damage to the inner ear (cochlea) or hearing nerve in the brain, or the hair cells in the cochlea or of the nerve cells between the inner ear and central auditory cortex. Adult sensorineural hearing loss can be caused by excessive noise levels; certain medications; viruses; and metabolic, vascular, and other systemic alterations (Hain, 2022).

Tinnitus. Tinnitus affects about 10 to 15% of the population. It is often described as a ringing, buzzing, or pulsating sound in the ear. It can be intermittent or constant, have one or more tones, and vary in volume. It does not always include hearing loss (Canadian Hard of Hearing Association [CHHA], 2021a).

Balance Deficit.
Benign positional vertigo is a common condition among older persons, usually resulting from vestibular dysfunction. Frequent episodes of vertigo or disequilibrium are precipitated by a change in the position of the head.

Taste Deficits.
Xerostomia is a decrease in salivary production that leads to thicker mucus and dry mouth. It may result from the adverse effects of medications such as antihistamines. This condition can interfere with the ability to eat and leads to appetite and nutritional problems.

Taste alterations are manifested by food aversions and decreased caloric intake. These can occur frequently in patients with cancer and as people age.

Neurological Deficits.
Peripheral neuropathy is a disorder that is very common in people with diabetes and in older persons. Sensations such as tingling or pins and needles, numbness, weakness, and pain are felt, often starting in the lower legs and feet. Onset is insidious and difficult to diagnose early on. It is estimated that approximately 50% of diabetics have peripheral neuropathy (Hicks & Selvin, 2019).

Sensory processing disorder is a condition in which the brain has trouble receiving and responding to information that comes from the senses. Common sounds may be painful or overwhelming for the individual or light touch may be considered painful. This condition tends to be found in children but can be diagnosed in adults. This disorder is often seen in conditions such as autism spectrum disorder (MyHealth.Alberta.ca, 2021).

Sensory Alterations

The most common types of sensory alterations are sensory deficits, sensory deprivation, and sensory overload. When a patient has more than one sensory alteration, the ability to function and relate effectively within the environment can be seriously impaired.

Sensory Deprivation.
The reticular activating system in the brainstem mediates all sensory stimuli to the cerebral cortex. Even in deep sleep, individuals are able to receive stimuli. Sensory stimulation must be of sufficient quality and quantity to maintain a person's awareness. When a person experiences an inadequate quality or quantity of stimulation, sensory deprivation occurs. Sensory deprivation involves either the lack of sensory stimuli in the environment or an inability to interpret stimuli (Hirst & Stares, 2020).

A decrease in stimuli can occur when patients are placed in isolation. Isolation precautions are used for patients who test positive for transmissible organisms. When placed in isolation, the person is confined to one room, and the number of people entering the room, as well as the person's contact with the outside world, is reduced. Nurses are required to follow transmission-based precautions, which include frequent hand hygiene and the use of masks and gloves. Most organisms are transmitted via the hands of caregivers. Masks may prevent

BOX 48.1　Effects of Sensory Deprivation

Cognitive

Reduced capacity to learn

Inability to think or to problem solve

Poor task performance

Disorientation/confusion

Bizarre thinking

Increased need for socialization, altered mechanisms of attention

Affective

Boredom

Restlessness

Increased anxiety

Emotional lability (e.g., rapid mood swings)

Panic

Increased need for physical stimulation

Perceptual

Alterations in

Visual/motor coordination

Reduced colour perception

Less tactile accuracy

Changes in ability to perceive size and shape

Changes in spatial and time judgement

From Potter, P., Perry, A., Stockert, P., et al. (2021). *Fundamentals of nursing* (10th ed.). Elsevier.

visualization of caregivers' faces, and gloves will alter the sense of touch. Patients who are moved into isolation are at risk of developing delirium. **Delirium** is a serious, potentially preventable complication (Hayhurst et al., 2020). It is an acute, short-term disturbance of consciousness that may last a few hours or become permanent if not detected and treated. Delirium is a neuropsychiatric disorder that is characterized by a loss of attention and accompanied by cognitive change, perceptual disturbance, or change in level of consciousness (Hayhurst et al., 2020; Maldonado, 2018).

Sensory deprivation has many serious effects (Box 48.1). The symptoms can easily cause nurses and health care providers to believe that a patient is psychologically ill and confused, is suffering from severe electrolyte imbalance, or is under the influence of psychotropic drugs. Nurses can help prevent sensory deprivation by being aware of the contributing factors and identifying patients who are at risk. Nurses need to take prompt action to reduce or eliminate the risk factors and treat the resultant behavioural changes (Burke, 2022).

Sensory Overload. When a person receives multiple sensory stimuli and cannot perceptually disregard or selectively ignore some stimuli, **sensory overload** occurs. Excessive sensory stimulation prevents the brain from appropriately responding to or ignoring certain stimuli. Because of the multitude of stimuli leading to overload, the person no longer perceives their environment in a way that makes sense. Overload prevents meaningful response by the brain; the person's thoughts race, attention moves in many directions, and anxiety and restlessness may occur. As a result, overload causes a state similar to that produced by sensory deprivation. However, in contrast to deprivation, overload is individualized. The amount of stimuli necessary for healthy function varies with each individual. A person's tolerance to sensory overload may vary by level of fatigue, attitude, and emotional and physical well-being.

The acutely ill patient may easily be affected by sensory overload. The patient in constant pain or who undergoes frequent monitoring of vital signs or lacks sleep is at risk. Multiple stimuli can combine to cause overload, even if the patient is receiving a comforting word and nurses are attempting to decrease their stress. Admission to a Critical Care Unit (CCU) can be a precipitating factor for sensory overload and delirium (Al Mutair et al., 2020). Lights are always on, and sounds can be heard from monitoring equipment, staff conversations, equipment alarms, and the activities of people in the unit.

The behavioural changes associated with sensory overload can easily be confused with mood swings or simple disorientation. Symptoms such as racing thoughts, scattered attention, restlessness, and anxiety need to be observed. Gestures such as pulling at the sheets or tubing or plucking at unseen things in the air are often exhibited. Constant reorientation, control of excessive stimuli, and, if possible, providing care in blocks of time are important components of the patient's care. Providing clocks and calendars, dimming of lights, family support, and clear communication can help prevent sensory overload and delirium in patients (Burke, 2022).

NURSING KNOWLEDGE BASE

Factors Influencing Sensory Function

Many factors influence sensory function, including the patient's age, the quantity and quality of stimuli, family support, environment, medications, culture and ethnicity, and various chronic illnesses. While each of these factors is described here separately, there is rarely one factor responsible for sensory alteration. Most often there are multiple factors present that interact, causing changes in sensory functioning, such as in a newborn baby in the Neonatal Intensive Care Unit (NICU). Not only does the environment influence the senses, but the medical condition of the infant and their developmental level or physical maturity may impair the child's sensory functioning. Sensory alteration also affects the child's medical condition.

Age. Infants and children are at risk for visual and hearing impairment because of a number of genetic, prenatal, and postnatal conditions. Periodically screening babies with risk indicators facilitates early detection of developmental delays and provides an opportunity for treatment through stimulation (Araujo et al., 2020).

Sixty percent of children diagnosed with learning difficulties have unrecognized vision challenges, and nearly 20% of school-age children have vision problems (Sangha, 2019). Certain eye conditions can lead to visual impairment. **Strabismus** (crossed eyes) usually begins in infancy or childhood. School children with significant strabismus can experience self-image challenges. Strabismus is often treated by surgically adjusting the tension on the eye muscles. Amblyopia (lazy eye) is poor vision in an eye that did not develop normal sight during early childhood. The main causes of amblyopia are strabismus, refractive errors, or cloudiness of the eye tissues (Mayo Clinic, 2021a).

With aging comes an increase in the incidence of sensory loss. Sensory losses in older age affect all of the sensory organs. This means that aging adults may experience changes in how they enjoy pastimes such as reading, watching television, or talking with friends. Even the enjoyment of eating may be diminished by age due to changes in taste sensation (Hirst & Stares, 2020).

The incidence of vision loss is also more prevalent with aging. The four most common causes of blindness increase with age. At age 65, one in nine Canadians have irreversible vision loss. At age 75 years, this number increases to one in four Canadians (Canadian Association of Optometrists, 2018a). Individuals who have vision loss are more likely than those without vision problems to:

- Be admitted to a long-term care facility, 3 years earlier
- Experience twice the number of falls
- Experience three times the incidence of depression
- Have four times as many hip fractures
- Have double the mortality rate (Canadian Association of Optometrists, 2018a).

Presbyopia is a normal visual change that occurs in individuals over 40 years of age. It is caused by age-related stiffening of the lens of the eye, resulting in an inability of the lens to change shape to allow focusing (accommodation) clearly on close objects, such as reading a newspaper (Singh & Tripathy, 2021). Other visual difficulties normally associated with aging include reduced visual fields, increased glare sensitivity, impaired night vision, reduced accommodation and depth perception, and reduced colour discrimination (Hirst & Stares, 2020) (Box 48.2). Colours with short wavelengths, such as blues, pinks, beiges, and greens, become more difficult to distinguish, while colours with long wavelengths, such as reds, oranges, and yellows, are easier to discriminate (Boscart et al., 2023). The visual changes can occur gradually, and in many cases older people may not notice their vision deteriorating until it significantly interferes with their ability to engage in regular or everyday activities, or when they realize that the vision loss is taking place.

About 3 in every 1 000 Canadian infants are born severely deaf, with the same number born with significant hearing loss (Canadian Paediatric Society, 2022). Hearing loss in babies, children, and adults has many causes, and each hearing loss is unique to the individual (CHHA, 2021b). Aging is the number one cause of hearing loss. Hearing changes include decreased hearing acuity, speech intelligibility, pitch discrimination, and hearing threshold (Box 48.3). Older persons hear low-pitched sounds best but have difficulty hearing conversation over background noise. Speech sounds are garbled, and reception of and reaction to speech are delayed. Older people have difficulty discriminating particular consonants (*z, t, f, g*) and high-frequency sounds (e.g., *s, sh, ph, k*) (presbycusis). A challenge with age-related hearing loss is that some individuals may not even be aware of their deficit, or what they may have considered age-related changes are, in fact, abnormal changes. A serious concern for persons with a hearing deficit is that they may be inappropriately labelled as cognitively impaired (Boscart et al., 2023).

The olfactory system, which gives us the ability to detect odours in the environment, declines with age, owing to normal physiological aging changes (Lafreniere & Parham, 2019). Diminished sense of smell results from a reduction in the number of olfactory sensory neurons and bulb cells. Changes include a reduction in olfactory nerve fibres by the age of 50 years, reduced taste discrimination, and reduced sensitivity to odours. More than half of people 65 years of age and older report a change in sense of smell. This can result in decreased enjoyment of eating and drinking, as well as pose a safety risk for not detecting harmful odours in the environment.

Diminished sense of taste with aging likely results from a reduction in the function or number of taste buds, along with decreased saliva production. Smoking, poor oral hygiene, nasal polyps, and radiation therapy may also contribute to diminished taste sensation (National Institute on Aging, 2020). Changes in sensory perception can affect the enjoyment of food and dietary choices and can lead to malnutrition in older people (National Institute on Aging, 2020).

Proprioceptive changes with advancing years include increased difficulty with balance, spatial orientation, and coordination, contributing to falls (Ferlinc et al., 2019). Proprioceptive dysfunction can be caused by vestibular dysfunction and neuropathy, or by any factor that affects the reception, transmission, perception, or interpretation of proprioceptive stimuli (Ferlinc et al., 2019). Older persons experience tactile changes, including declining sensitivity to pain, pressure, and temperature. Factors affecting tactile changes are numerous and include trauma, infection, metabolic or vascular changes, and degenerative diseases (U.S. National Library of Medicine, MedlinePlus, 2021).

Nurses must be careful not to assume automatically that a patient's sensory impairment is related to advancing age. Nurses must conduct a careful assessment to determine the true cause(s).

Stimuli. As mentioned earlier, the presence or absence and the quantity of stimuli can affect the individual's cognitive and mental status. Sensory deprivation and sensory overload can occur. Meaningful stimuli reduce the incidence of sensory deprivation and may help to alleviate sensory overload. In a patient's home or a long-term care facility, meaningful stimuli may include pets, music, television, family photographs, a calendar, and a clock. The presence of others can offer positive stimulation.

Family Support. The amount and quality of contact with family members and significant others can influence the degree of isolation a patient feels. The absence of visitors during hospitalization or residency in a long-term care facility can also affect sensory status. This is a common problem in hospital settings where visitation is restricted. The ability to discuss fears or concerns with loved ones is an important coping mechanism for most people. Therefore, the absence of meaningful conversation can cause a person to become sensorially deprived, and nurses may not be alerted to this problem until behavioural changes occur.

Environment. A person's work environment can increase the risk for sensory alterations. Individuals who are exposed to loud noises at work or who have occupations that involve the risk of exposure to chemicals or flying particles should be screened for hearing and visual problems. In one Canadian study, 54% of men and 49% of women working in a vulnerable environment (defined as working in a loud environment, not being required to wear hearing protection, and rarely using such protection) had experienced tinnitus (Ramage-Morin & Gosselin, 2018). An estimated 11 million Canadians (43%) have worked in noisy environments, and over 6 million of them (56%) were classified as being vulnerable to workplace noise according to Ramage-Morin and Gosselin (2018). Noise exposure over time, coupled with the loss of blood supply to the cochlea with aging, will result in hearing loss. Harmful noise levels occur in the workplace and in recreational

BOX 48.2	Aging Changes to Vision That Affect Visual Ability

Peripheral vision decreases
Pupils shrink in size
Ciliary muscles that change the shape of the lens become less flexible
Cornea becomes more opaque and yellowed
Tear production decreases
Lens becomes thickened and cloudy

BOX 48.3	Aging Changes to Hearing That Affect Hearing Ability

Increased rigidity of the ossicles
Decreased elasticity of the tympanic membrane
Increased cerumen production
Decreased number of neurons and blood vessels
Loss of hair cells in inner ear

environments. Poor noise control, inadequate hearing protection, and lack of education about the risks of hearing loss are contributing factors. Those who work with vibrating power tools, such as farmers, lawn care workers, and people who work around machinery, are at risk for occupation-related hearing loss (Lawson, 2020).

Genova and colleagues (2020) reported in their review of the literature that occupations that require repetitive manual work involving flexion and extension at the wrist, forceful grip with the hand, or vibrations of the hand and arm can cause pressure on the median nerve, resulting in carpal tunnel syndrome. This is a condition characterized by swelling or inflammation of the wrists. This inflammation creates pressure on the nerve as it passes through the narrow area (the carpal tunnel) in the wrist. The patient can experience numbness, tingling, pain, and a reduction of the grip strength and function of the affected hand (Genova et al., 2020; Wang, 2018).

Older farmers and ranchers and other outdoor workers must deal with the effects of aging as well as the hazards in their work environment. They are subject to noise injury from the equipment, leading to hearing loss. Fatigue, reduced vision, arthritis, and slower reaction time that occur with aging can increase these workers' risk for injury. Older agricultural workers working with toxins (pesticides and herbicides) may experience loss of vision or sense of touch.

As discussed earlier, the hospital environment can place a patient at risk for sensory alterations from exposure to environmental stimuli or a change in sensory input, due to immobility because of bed rest, disability, or physical circumstances (e.g., casts or traction), or when placed in isolation. Infants in NICUs experience an overload of sensory stimuli from the bright lights, excessive noise, and painful procedures. This sensory overload alters their physiological responses and can lead to decreased social interaction, altered rest and sleep patterns, restlessness, irritability and crying, as well as overall reduction in auditory response and motor development (Khan & Khan, 2021) (Box 48.4).

Children have unique developmental, biological, and behavioural characteristics that make them particularly vulnerable to environmental hazards, including toxins such as mercury, lead, pesticides, second-hand smoke, and moulds. Their metabolism is rapid, they drink more water per body volume than adults, and they breathe more rapidly, taking in more air per body volume than adults. Exposure to such toxins can result in developmental and behavioural disabilities, impaired hearing, numbness or pain, impaired sensation, impaired coordination, and other symptoms, depending on the toxin and the nature of the exposure (Persico et al., 2020; Yang & Massey, 2019).

Medications. Aging changes and the high prevalence of chronic disease in older persons increase the likelihood of this population taking multiple medications, either those prescribed by a health care provider or taken by self-medication. Multiple medications can pose considerable risks to the individual (Wastesson et al., 2018). *Self-medication* is defined as the use of nonprescription or prescription drugs without the advice or supervision of a medical practitioner (Rajamma et al., 2021). Generally, the medicine is suggested or shared by a relative or friend.

Medications can contribute to numerous adverse effects and combination toxicity. Hearing loss may occur as an adverse effect of prescription medications, such as thiazide diuretics and certain antibiotics. Overuse of laxatives, which are available over the counter, can lead to bowel dependency.

Ethnicity. Certain sensory deficits have been found to occur at higher rates in certain genders and ethnicities. Regarding vision loss, some findings that are based on ethnicity include the following:

- White Canadians have somewhat higher rates of overall vision loss compared to racialized groups.

BOX 48.4 RESEARCH HIGHLIGHT

An Observational Study of Sound Exposure in a Single-Room Configured Neonatal Unit (SENSE)

Research Focus

To measure sound exposure in a single-room setting on a neonatal unit, and assess findings specific to present day sound level recommendations.

Methods

Sound meters were placed inside 51 incubators and open cots and within the environment of each occupied single room. One-second incremental monitoring of decibels on an A-weighted scale (dBA) was recorded over 2 days.

Results

All continuous sound pressure levels were significantly higher than the recommended 45 dBA for incubators and open cots. Maximum sound levels were significantly higher than the recommended 65 dBA, reaching up to 126.7 dBA inside the incubator and 124.7 dBA inside the open cot. Incubators had a higher total percentage of time above 45 dBA than open cots for both day (99.84% vs. 75.59%) and night (98.66% vs. 59.56%).

Sound levels surpassed the recommended maximum exposure levels identified by the American Academy of Pediatrics. The long-term effects of such sensory exposure on preterm infants' neurodevelopment is unknown.

Implications for Practice

Nurses need to pay attention to factors contributing to increased sound levels in neonatal units.

From Best, K., Hughes, I., New, K., et al. (2020). An observational study of sound exposure in a single-room configured neonatal unit (SENSE study). *Journal of Neonatal Nursing, 26*(6), 344–351. https://doi.org/10.1016/j.jnn.2020.05.002

- Older (aged 60+) racialized women have the highest rates of cataract, while older racialized males have the lowest rates.
- Men from racialized populations have high rates of glaucoma.
- White Canadians are more likely to have vision loss from AMD than Black Canadians; the reverse is true for refractive errors.
- Chinese Canadians have double the rate of AMD compared to White Canadians and may have twice the rate of diabetic retinopathy.
- Chinese Canadian children are more likely to experience nearsightedness than children who are White.
- Indigenous Canadians have very high rates of type 2 diabetes and related complications (Crowshoe et al., 2018).
- Asian and Inuit populations have much higher rates of closed-angle glaucoma than in the general population (Reiff Ellis, 2022).

Vision loss affects women slightly more than men (Shaqiri et al., 2018); however, this may reflect the greater longevity of women. More research needs to be conducted to identify whether gender and ethnicity are the causative factors or whether other factors such as lifestyle, poverty, inadequate nutrition, genetics, access to treatment, or environment are the causative or associative factors.

CRITICAL THINKING

Critical thinking involves synthesizing knowledge and information gathered from patients, experience, and intellectual and professional standards. During assessment (Figure 48.3), nurses consider all critical thinking elements that help them make appropriate nursing diagnoses. Falcó-Pegueroles et al. (2021) discussed how critical thinking skills are essential for all nurses. Critical thinking is a complex, dynamic process formed by attitudes and strategic skills, with the aim of achieving safe,

Knowledge

- Pathophysiology of specific sensory deficit
- Factors that potentially may alter sensory function
- Effects of sensory deprivation or overload
- Communication principles used to interact with patients with sensory deficits

Experience

- Caring for patients with sudden and long-term sensory alterations
- Personal experience with temporary or permanent sensory deficit

Assessment

- Patient's health promotion practices
- Health history regarding extent of risks for and existing sensory deficits
- Review of potential factors that may affect the patient's sensory function
- Extent of lifestyle and self-care alterations
- Patient's expectations regarding sensory alterations

Standards

- Apply intellectual standards of clarity, precision, accuracy, and depth when assessing the patient's sensory function
- Apply agency and professional guidelines when assessing sensory function

Qualities

- Show confidence in your ability to provide a safe level of care
- Use curiosity to clarify and explore the nature of signs and symptoms to rule out causes other than sensory change

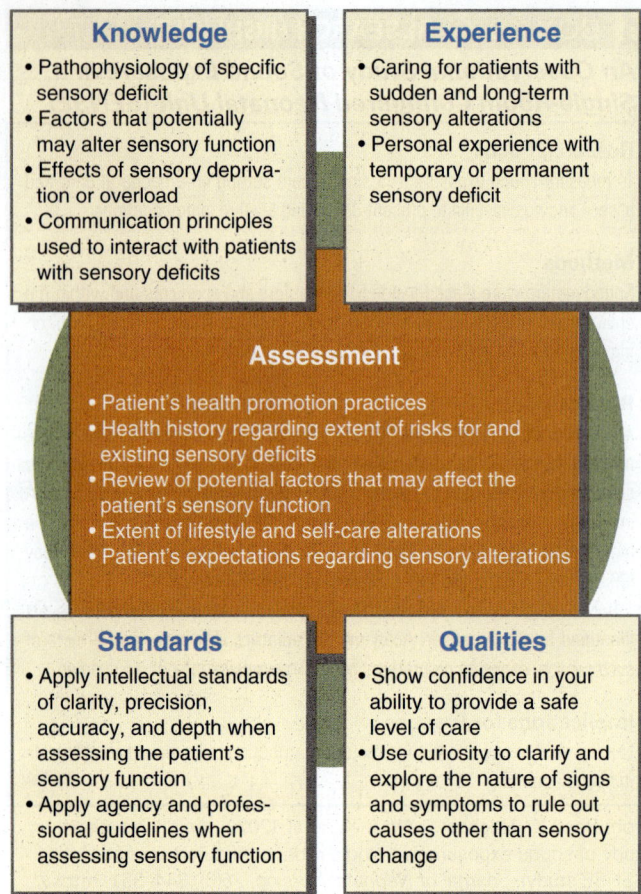

FIGURE 48.3 Critical thinking model for sensory alterations assessment.

high-quality patient care. Critical thinking requires interpreting and synthesizing information to make decisions in planning and delivering nursing care.

Care for patients with sensory alterations requires integration of knowledge from several areas: normal anatomy and physiology of the sensory and nervous systems, the pathophysiology of sensory deficits and factors that affect sensory function, therapeutic communication principles, and normal aging changes. This information enables nurses to conduct appropriate assessments, anticipate what to recognize when a patient describes a sensory problem, and recognize abnormalities. For example, knowing that someone with glaucoma will have tunnel vision (i.e., they can see clearly at the centre of their visual field but cannot see the periphery) will help the nurse recognize that when the person is sitting down for a meal they may not see the location of the cup or other dining utensils that would be outside the centre of their vision.

Previous experience in caring for patients with sensory deficits enables you as a nurse to recognize limitations in function in each new patient and how those limitations might affect the patient's ability to carry out daily activities. For example, after caring for a patient with a hearing impairment, you will be able to conduct a more effective assessment of the next patient.

Standards of care and practice, such as those from the Canadian Ophthalmological Society, the Registered Nurses' Association of Ontario (RNAO), the Canadian Gerontological Nursing Association, and the Canadian National Institute for the Blind (CNIB), provide criteria for screening sensory conditions and for establishing standards for competent, safe, and effective care and practice. Using critical thinking, nurses can conduct a thorough assessment and then plan,

implement, and evaluate care that will enable the patient to function safely and effectively.

❖ NURSING PROCESS

◆ Assessment

When assessing patients with or at risk for sensory alterations, nurses must consider how the patient's particular illness may lead or has led to sensory changes. As well, all the factors that may influence sensory function must be considered. For example, if the patient has a hearing impairment, the nurse's communication style needs to be adjusted and assessment is focused on relevant criteria related to hearing deficits. Nurses collect a history that assesses the patient's current sensory status and the degree to which a sensory deficit affects the patient's lifestyle, psychosocial adjustment, developmental status, self-care ability, and safety. The assessment must also focus on the quality and quantity of environmental stimuli.

The location of the patient assessment is important. There should be privacy with no distractions. The nurse should sit at the same eye level as the patient, to create a supportive atmosphere and reduce the power differential between the nurse and the patient. To understand the nature of a communication problem, the nurse must know whether a patient has trouble speaking, understanding, naming, reading, or writing. Patients who have existing sensory deficits often develop alternative ways of communicating.

A deaf or hearing-impaired patient may read lips, use sign language, listen with the help of a hearing aid, or read and write notes. Visually impaired patients may be unable to observe facial expressions and other nonverbal behaviours that clarify the content of spoken communication. Instead, they rely on voice tones and inflections to detect the emotional tone of communication. Nurses need to face such patients, allowing them to see the nurse's face and mouth movements clearly. If the person has a visual impairment, the nurse should speak clearly with a moderate rate of speech and pause to determine understanding. Lighting should be sufficient. If the patient cannot hear the nurse well, the patient will watch the nurse's mouth movements in order to understand the nurse's questions. The nurse should not sit with a window behind them as this creates glare for the patient, who then cannot see facial features and mouth movements.

Patients with **aphasia** have varied degrees of inability to speak, interpret, or understand language. **Expressive aphasia**, a motor type of aphasia, is the inability to name common objects or express simple ideas in words or writing. For example, a patient understands a question but is unable to express an answer. Sensory or **receptive aphasia** is the inability to understand written or spoken language; a patient is able to express words but is unable to understand questions or comments of others. **Global aphasia** is the inability to understand language or communicate orally.

The temporary or permanent loss of the ability to speak can be extremely traumatic to an individual. The nurse should assess for alternate communication methods and whether they cause anxiety. The nurse needs to determine whether the patient has developed a sign-language system or symbols to communicate their needs.

A family member who is identified as a caregiver or a support person to the patient should be included in the nurse's interview, either at the same time as the interview with the patient or in a separate interview. If it is suspected that the patient is not providing accurate information about their health or cannot provide adequate information, a separate interview with a family member should be held. The nurse may need to clarify the patient's health problems or medications or the family member's perception of how the patient is coping or managing daily activities. If the family member is a caregiver to the patient, the nurse may need to interview this individual to discover the person's coping ability and stress level as caregiver.

Use of Assistive Devices. Nurses need to assess for the use of assistive devices (e.g., hearing aids or glasses) and the sensory effects for patients. This includes learning how often the devices are used daily, the patient's or family caregiver's method for cleaning devices, and the patient's knowledge of what to do when a problem with the device develops. Just because the patient has an assistive device, the nurse should not assume that it works or that the patient uses it or benefits from it.

Many people are reluctant to wear a hearing aid (Ritter et al., 2020). Several factors may determine a person's likelihood of wearing a hearing aid: perceived need for improved hearing, attitude toward the hearing impairment, and motivation to seek solutions. Cost may also be a concern for having hearing assessed and for purchasing a hearing aid if the patient is not covered by a provincial health plan. Although provinces and territories have plans that may pay a portion or all of the cost of hearing aids, it is important that older persons ask their retailers what products are covered by government support (CHHA, 2021c).

Sensory Alterations History. The nursing health history includes assessment of the nature and characteristics of sensory alterations or any problem related to an alteration. The history begins with asking the patient to describe the sensory deficit, as in the examples provided in Box 48.5. The patient's ethnic or cultural background needs

to be considered because certain sensory deficits are more common in certain groups. It is also important to ensure that patients are able to communicate in the examiner's language, in order to be able to answer questions and describe their condition accurately.

Knowledge about the onset and duration of the sensory alteration can be helpful. The nurse can then learn how long the patient has taken measures to adjust to the alteration. It is also useful to assess the patient's self-rating for a sensory deficit, by simply saying, for example, "Rate your hearing as excellent, good, fair, poor, or bad." Then, from the patient's self-rating, the nurse can explore the patient's perception of a sensory loss. This provides an in-depth look at how the patient's quality of life has been affected.

Screening. The World Health Organization (WHO) (2022) estimates that globally, 2.2 billion people have a near or distance vision impairment. In at least 1 billion of these cases, vision impairment could have been prevented. Vision loss is costly in Canada. It is estimated that the economic costs of blindness and partial sight loss is close to 16 billion dollars per year, with costs to the health care system being just over 8.5 billion (Vision 2020, 2020).

Visual impairment is common during childhood. The most common visual problem is a refractive error such as nearsightedness. Parents must know signs suggesting visual impairment (e.g., failure to react to light and reduced eye contact from the infant) and should be instructed to report these signs to a health care provider immediately. Vision screening of school-aged children and adolescents can aid in detecting problems early.

For vision assessment, a number of age-specific tools are available from the Canadian Paediatric Society and are often found on provincial and territorial websites; for example, Manitoba (Manitoba Education and Training Inclusion Support Branch, 2019) has released its own screening manual. The vision screening manual contains a variety of vision test results, vision history forms, a pinhole mask, and vision cards for distance and near vision testing for children in kindergarten to Grade 12. (See Box 48.6 for vision screening guidelines.)

Children at risk for hearing impairment include those with a family history of childhood hearing impairment, perinatal infection (rubella, herpes, cytomegalovirus), low birth weight, chronic ear infection, and Down syndrome. Nurses should advise pregnant persons of the

---

BOX 48.5 Nursing Assessment Questions

Nature of the Problem
- What problem are you having with your vision or hearing?
- What have you tried to correct the vision or hearing difficulty?
- Do you use any devices to improve your vision or hearing?
- How effective are your glasses or hearing aids?

Signs and Symptoms
- Ask a patient with visual alterations: Do you require books with large print or on audiotape? Are you able to prepare a meal or write a cheque? Do you notice any eye irritation or drainage?
- Ask a patient with hearing alterations: Which types of sounds or tones do you have difficulty hearing? Do people tell you that they have to "shout" for you to hear them? Do people ask you not to talk so loud? Do you have a ringing, crackling, or buzzing in your ears? Is there pain—sharp, dull, burning, itching? Have you noticed any redness, swelling, or drainage? Any signs of infection?

Onset and Duration
- When did you notice the problem? How long has it lasted?
- Does it come and go, or is it constant?
- What makes the problem better or worse?

Predisposing Factors
- Do you work or participate in any activities that have the potential for vision or hearing injury? If so, how do you protect your hearing and vision?
- Do you have a family history of cataracts, glaucoma, macular degeneration, or hearing loss?
- When was your last vision or hearing examination?

Effect on Patient
- What effect has your vision or hearing impairment had on your work, family, or social life?
- Have changes in your vision or hearing affected your feelings of independence?
- How does your vision or hearing challenge make you feel about yourself?
- Do you have problems with routine care of glasses, contact lenses, or hearing aids?

BOX 48.6 Recommended Vision Screening Guidelines for Infants, Children, Youth, and Adults

- From 6 to 9 months of age, infants should have a minimum of one eye examination (Canadian Ophthalmological Society, 2019).
- From 2 to 5 years of age, preferably at 3 years of age, a full eye exam should be conducted (Canadian Ophthalmological Society, 2019).
- For children and youth aged 6 to 19, yearly examinations are suggested (Canadian Association of Optometrists, 2018b).
- Healthy adults with no risk factors or vision problems should have an eye examination every 5 years. High-risk individuals, such as those with diabetes, a family history of eye-related issues, or anyone with a history of eye problems should have an examination every 3 years. Those over 50 years of age who are at high risk should have an examination every 2 years.
- Low-risk individuals between 56 to 65 years of age should have an eye examination at least every 3 years. The frequency of eye examinations at 65 years of age is either every 2 years (Canadian Association of Optometrists, 2022) or yearly (BC Doctors of Optometry, 2022). High-risk individuals between the ages of 50 and 60 years of age should have examinations every 2 years, and those over 60 should have a yearly eye examination (Canadian Association of Optometrists, 2022).

importance of early prenatal care, avoidance of using ototoxic drugs, and testing for syphilis or rubella.

Children with chronic middle ear infections, a common cause of impaired hearing, should receive periodic auditory testing. Parents must be warned of the related risks (e.g., exposure to smoke, previous history of ear infections, siblings with otitis media, attending day care) and advised to seek medical care when their child has symptoms of earache or respiratory infection (Newbould et al., 2020).

Many teenagers and young adults already have permanent hearing loss caused by exposure to excessive noise from electronic listening devices, automobile stereo systems, and concerts. According to Gopal and colleagues (2019), recreational hearing loss, through, for example, personal audio systems, may be the most significant risk factor for music-induced hearing loss in adolescents. Parents and children need to take precautions when involved in activities associated with high-intensity noise.

The guidelines for hearing screening for adults are less prescriptive than those for vision. In general, if a patient works or lives in an environment where the noise level is high, routine screening is highly recommended and may be mandated by occupational health and safety measures in the workplace. Nurses in occupational settings can assess for symptoms of tinnitus and make prompt referrals. Early detection may prevent hearing disabilities. As the prevalence of hearing loss increases with age, individuals over 60 years of age should have a hearing test every 2 years. If hearing loss is identified, hearing examinations should be performed yearly (HealthLink BC, 2021b). Nurses should encourage patients to follow through with recommendations for hearing aids.

There are a number of bedside assessment tools that can be used to assess hearing impairment. The screening version of the Hearing Handicap Inventory for the Elderly (HHIE-S) is a 5-minute, 10-item questionnaire designed to assess how a patient perceives the emotional and social effects of hearing loss. The greater the handicapping effect from the hearing loss, the higher the score (Heffernan et al., 2020). The Minimum Data Set (MDS) assessment (used within long-term care facilities) can be used at admission and on a regular basis to detect conductive, sensorineural, or mixed hearing loss (McCreedy et al., 2018).

A health history can also reveal any recent changes in a patient's behaviour. Often friends or family are the best resources for this information because the patient may be unaware of any change. Details will be revealed by asking the following questions:

- Have you noticed any change in the person's hearing (e.g., television being turned louder)?
- Has your family member or friend shown any recent mood swings (e.g., outbursts of anger, nervousness, fear, or irritability)?
- Have you noticed the person avoiding social activities?
- Has the person fallen recently?

It is important to remember that many adults are sensitive about admitting losses and may hesitate to share information.

The nurse should also rely on personal observation of the patient to detect sensory alterations. Some useful observations indicating hearing loss are the following: the patient seems inattentive to others, responds to questions inappropriately, believes people are talking about them, has trouble following clear directions, asks to have something repeated, has monotonous voice quality and speaks unusually loudly or softly, has the television set to an unusually loud volume, and leans their head to one side when being spoken to (Mayo Clinic, 2021b).

Acknowledging a need to improve hearing is a person's first step. Nurses can give patients useful information on the benefits of wearing a hearing aid. A wide variety of aids are available that may not only successfully enhance a person's hearing but can also be cosmetically acceptable. It is also important to have a family member or friend available to assist with hearing aid adjustment (Box 48.7).

BOX 48.7 Troubleshooting Hearing Aid Malfunction

Objectives
- Patient and family member will identify source of malfunction in hearing aid.
- Patient and family member will demonstrate hearing aid care.

Teaching Strategies
- Show patient and family member locations on hearing aid device where damage (e.g., cracks, fraying) is likely to occur: ear mould or case, earphone, dials, cord, and connection plugs.
- Demonstrate battery replacement and stress the importance of having an extra set of unused batteries available.
- Review method to check volume: turn dial to maximum gain and then check. Is voice clear?
- Consult manufacturer's directions for specific care measures for cleaning battery case and ear mould.
- Review factors to report to hearing aid laboratory: static, distortion of sound, poor volume quality.

Nurses are often consulted for guidance when changes in vision and hearing occur. Consequently, a nurse's knowledge of screening techniques is important. It is also important that nurses are familiar with the normal aging process, as well as the signs and symptoms of common diseases so that appropriate suggestions for referral can be made.

Factors other than sensory deprivation or overload may cause impaired perception (e.g., medications or pain). The patient's medication history should be assessed, which comprises prescribed and over-the-counter medications, as well as herbal products and caffeine. Information regarding the frequency, dose, method of administration, and last time these medications were taken should be included. Nurses should conduct a thorough pain assessment when pain is suspected to be causing perceptual problems.

Mental Status. Mental status assessment is an important component of any evaluation of sensory function. This is particularly important as visual impairment is a risk factor for cognitive decline (Zheng et al., 2018). Visual impairment can be associated with hallucinations. Approximately 16% of individuals with AMD will develop Charles Bonnet syndrome (Niazi et al., 2020), a syndrome characterized by visual hallucinations, ocular pathology causing visual deterioration, and preserved cognitive status. Affected individuals are fully aware that the hallucinations are not real. They are reluctant to report these experiences, fearing that they may be diagnosed with a dementia (Russell et al., 2018).

Observing the patient during history-taking, physical examination, and nursing care provides valuable data for evaluation of a patient's mental status. An assessment of mental status is valuable particularly if sensory deprivation or overload is suspected. The nurse should observe the patient's physical appearance and behaviour, measure the patient's cognitive ability, and assess the patient's emotional status. The Mini-Mental State Examination (MMSE) is an example of a tool that can be used to measure disorientation, altered conceptualization and abstract thinking, and change in problem-solving abilities (Folstein et al., 1975) (see Chapter 33). For example, a patient with severe sensory deprivation may not be able to carry on a conversation, remain attentive, or display recent or past memory.

If the patient resides in their own home, it is good to check for cleanliness in the home, spoiled food on the counter or in the fridge, misplaced items, inappropriate dress, and losing the way to the store or other locations they used to frequent.

Physical Assessment. To identify sensory deficits and their severity, nurses need to assess vision, hearing, olfaction, taste, and the ability to discriminate light touch, temperature, pain, and position. Chapter 33 describes assessment techniques in detail. Table 48.3 summarizes assessment techniques for identifying sensory deficits. The data will be more accurate if the examination room is private, quiet, and comfortable for the patient.

Ability to Perform Self-Care. Patients' functional abilities in their home environment or health care setting, including feeding, dressing, grooming, and toileting, should be assessed. For example, the nurse can assess whether a patient with altered vision can find items on a meal tray and can read directions on a prescription. Dual sensory loss, or vision or hearing loss alone, contributes to a decline in an individual's ability to complete instrumental activities of daily living (Mueller-Schotte et al., 2019). The nurse should determine a visually impaired patient's ability to perform daily routines such as reading bills, writing cheques, or driving a vehicle at night. Does a patient's loss of balance prevent rising from a toilet seat safely? Any impairment in the ability to perform self-care has implications for planning discharge from a health care setting and for providing resources within the home. Vision loss in older people increases the risk of falls (Saftari & Kwon, 2018) and the likelihood of moving to a long-term care facility.

TABLE 48.3	Assessment of Sensory Function	
Assessment	**Behaviour Indicating Deficit (Children)**	**Behaviour Indicating Deficit (Adults)**
Vision Ask patient to read newspaper, magazine, or lettering on menu. Measure visual acuity with Snellen chart (see Chapter 33) or the Vision Screening Tool. Assess visual fields and depth perception. Assess pupil size and accommodation to light. Ask patient to identify colours on colour chart or crayons. Observe patient conducting activities of daily living (ADLs).	Self-stimulation, including eye rubbing, body rocking, sniffing or smelling, arm twirling; hitching (using legs to propel while in sitting position) instead of crawling	Poor coordination, squinting, underreaching or overreaching for objects, persistent repositioning of objects, impaired night vision, accidental falls
Hearing Perform conventional assessment, including whisper and tuning fork (see Chapter 33). Perform audiometry, if indicated. Observe patient conversing with others. Assess patient's perception of hearing ability and history of tinnitus. Inspect ear canal for hardened cerumen.	Frightened when unfamiliar people approach, no reflex or purposeful response to sounds, failure to be awakened by loud noise, slow or absent development of speech, greater response to movement than to sound, avoidance of social interaction with other children	Blank looks, decreased attention span, lack of reaction to loud noises, increased volume of speech, positioning of head toward sound, smiling and nodding of head in approval when someone speaks, use of other means of communication such as lip-reading or writing, complaints of ringing in ears
Touch Assess patient for sensitivity to light touch (see Chapter 33) and temperature. Check patient's ability to discriminate between sharp and dull stimuli. Assess whether patient can distinguish objects (coin or safety pin) in the hand with eyes closed. Ask whether patient feels unusual sensations.	Inability to perform developmental tasks related to grasping objects or drawing, repeated injury from handling of harmful objects (e.g., hot stove, sharp knife)	Clumsiness, overreaction or underreaction to painful stimulus, failure to respond when touched, avoidance of touch, sensation of pins and needles, numbness
Smell Ask patient to close eyes and identify several nonirritating odours (e.g., coffee, vanilla).	Difficult to assess until child is 6 or 7 years old, difficulty discriminating noxious odours	Failure to react to noxious or strong odour, increased body odour, decreased sensitivity to odours
Taste Ask patient to sample and distinguish different tastes (e.g., lemon, sugar, salt). Have patient drink or sip water and wait 1 minute between each taste. Ask patient if recent weight change has occurred.	Inability to tell whether food is salty or sweet, possible ingestion of strange-tasting things	Change in appetite, excessive use of seasoning and sugar, complaints about taste of food, weight change
Position Sense Perform conventional tests for balance and position sense (see Chapter 33).	Clumsiness, extraneous movement, excessive arm swinging in children with hyperactivity or learning difficulty Inability to sit or stand as per expected milestones	Poor balance and spatial orientation, shuffling gait, reduced response to brace self when falling, slow and deliberate movements, a history that includes falls

Health Promotion Habits. Nurses must assess the daily routines that patients follow to maintain sensory function. What type of eye and ear care is incorporated into daily hygiene? For those individuals who participate in sports or recreational activities or who work in a setting where ear or eye injury is a possibility (e.g., chemical exposure or constant exposure to loud noise), it is good to determine if safety glasses or hearing protective devices (HPDs) are worn. Do patients who use assistive devices such as eyeglasses, contact lenses, or hearing aids know how to care for them (see Chapter 39)? Are the devices used? Are they in proper working order?

Hazards. A patient with sensory alterations is at risk for injury if the living environment is unsafe. For example, a patient with visual impairment cannot see potential hazards clearly. A patient with proprioceptive problems may lose their balance easily and fall. The condition of the home, the rooms, and the front and back entrances can be problematic for the patient with sensory alterations. Some of the more common hazards are the following:

- Uneven, cracked walkways leading to front or back door
- Doormats with slippery backing
- Extension and telephone cords in the main route of walking traffic
- Loose area rugs on hardwood floors or tiles; runners placed over carpeting
- Bathrooms without shower or tub grab bars
- Water faucets unmarked to designate hot and cold
- Bathroom floor with slippery surface
- Absence of smoke detectors in rooms
- Unlit stairways, lack of handrails
- Floors cluttered with material and excessive furniture, including footstools
- Kitchen equipment (e.g., ranges, irons, toasters) with hard-to-read settings

Patients living with visual impairment may also be unable to read medication labels and syringe gauges. Therefore, the nurse should ask the patient to read a label to determine whether they can adequately see the instructions. If a patient has a hearing impairment, the nurse should check to see whether the sounds of a doorbell, telephone, smoke alarm, and alarm clock are easy to discriminate.

In the hospital environment, caregivers often forget to rearrange furniture and equipment to keep paths from the bed and chair to the bathroom and entrance clear. Walking into a patient's room and looking for safety hazards must be a routine part of nursing care. Check frequently for the following:

- Is the call light within easy, safe reach?
- Are intravenous (IV) poles on wheels and easy to move?
- Are footstools against the bed?
- Are suction machines, IV pumps, or drainage bags positioned so that a patient can rise from a bed or chair easily?

◆ Nursing Diagnosis

After assessment, nurses review all available data and look for patterns and trends suggestive of a health problem relating to sensory alterations (Box 48.8). For example, a patient's advanced age, inattentiveness during conversations, and self-rating of hearing as "poor" are all defining characteristics for the nursing diagnosis *disturbed sensory perception (auditory)*. Nurses need to validate their findings to ensure accuracy of the diagnosis. For example, the diagnosis *disturbed thought processes* could mistakenly be made if the nurse does not confirm the patient's hearing deficit and perception of poor hearing.

As well, the factor that likely causes the patient's health problem must be determined. In the previous example, impacted cerumen is the cause of the patient's hearing alteration. The etiology or related factor of

---

BOX 48.8 NURSING DIAGNOSTIC PROCESS

Assessment Activities	Defining Characteristics	Nursing Diagnosis
Assess patient's visual acuity.	Has reduced ability to see objects clearly. Needs brighter light to read. Has trouble distinguishing edges of stairs. May have fallen or have had a recent fracture.	*Risk for injury related to visual impairment from cataract formation*
Visit home setting and inspect for any hazards that may pose risks to patient.	Lighting in rooms, hallways, and stairwells is very dim. Carpet in living room is old, and edges are curled up. Steps lead up to front entrance of home.	
Review medical record from clinic visit.	Bilateral cataracts	

---

a nursing diagnosis is a condition that can be affected by nursing interventions. The etiology must be accurate; otherwise, nursing therapies will be ineffective. For a patient with impacted cerumen, regular irrigation of the ear canal has the potential to improve auditory perception (Michaudet & Malaty, 2018). In contrast, if the patient's auditory alteration is related to hearing loss from nerve deafness, nursing interventions for alternative communication methods will be necessary.

The patient may also have health care concerns for which sensory alteration is the etiology, such as with the diagnosis *risk for injury*. People with vision loss have an approximately 27% greater incidence of falls compared to those without vision loss (Ehrlich et al., 2019). Nurses may also select nursing diagnoses by recognizing the way that sensory alterations affect a patient's ability to function (e.g., self-care deficit). In addition, most patients present to health care providers with multiple diagnoses. In the example of the concept map in Figure 48.4, a patient with retinal detachment has the nursing diagnosis *disturbed sensory perception*, which can lead to risk for falls and fear. Nurses must recognize patterns of data that reveal health problems created by the patient's sensory alteration. Examples of nursing diagnoses that might apply to patients with sensory alterations are the following:

- *Impaired adjustment*
- *Impaired verbal communication*
- *Risk for injury*
- *Impaired physical mobility*
- *Self-care deficit—for example, bathing, oral hygiene*
- *Situational low self-esteem*
- *Risk for falls*
- *Social isolation*

◆ Planning

During planning, nurses use critical thinking skills to synthesize information from multiple sources (Figure 48.5), including knowledge gained from the assessment and knowledge of how sensory deficits affect normal functioning. In this way, nurses can recognize the extent of a patient's deficit and know the type of interventions most likely to be helpful. Also to consider are the roles that other health care providers can play in planning care and the available community resources

> concept map

Disturbed sensory perception: visual
• Unable to see clearly in right eye
• Floaters seen in visual field of right eye
• Talks about fear of vision not returning

Risk for falls
• Visual acuity reduced
• Patient is over age 65
• Patient lives alone
• Lighting levels low in hallways and staircases of home

Patient's chief medical diagnosis: Retinal detachment of right eye after blunt injury to forehead
Priority assessments: Vision, ability to perform ADLs and IADLs, general affect and mood, conditions in home environment

Fear
• Patient afraid to drive
• Expresses concern vision will not return to normal
• Reports inability to remain attentive at work
• Frequently checks vision and ability to see objects in immediate environment

——— Link between medical diagnosis and nursing diagnosis   ----- Link between nursing diagnoses

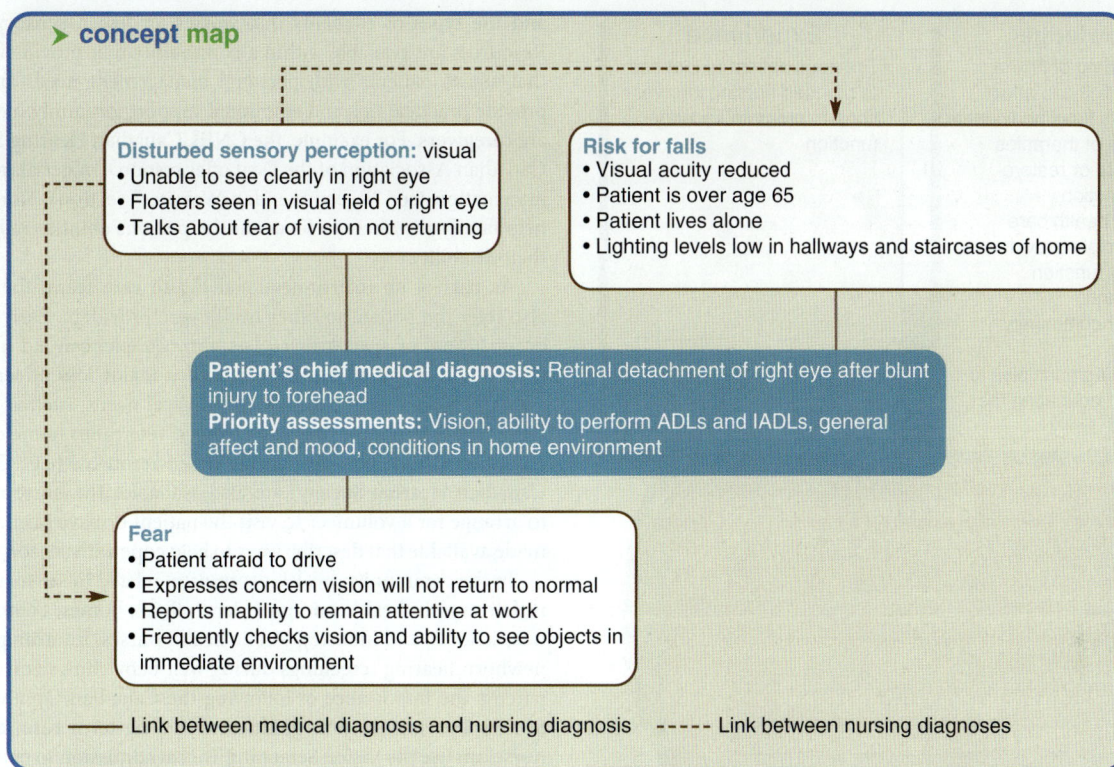

FIGURE 48.4 Concept map for patient with retinal detachment. *ADLs,* Activities of daily living; *IADLs,* instrumental activities of daily living.

(e.g., CNIB) that may be useful. These resources and the nurse's previous experience in caring for patients with sensory alterations can be invaluable when planning nursing approaches.

When applying critical thinking to planning care, professional standards can be particularly useful. These standards, in the form of clinical pathways or clinical practice guidelines, often recommend interventions based on research evidence for the patient's condition. For example, patients who have visual deficits and are hospitalized may be placed on a fall-prevention protocol that will incorporate research-based precautions to ensure patient safety.

Goals and Outcomes. During planning, as a nurse you will develop an individualized plan of care for each nursing diagnosis (Box 48.9). With the patient, develop a realistic plan that incorporates what you know about the patient's sensory challenges and the extent to which sensory function can be maintained or improved. If maintenance or improvement is not realistic, preventing injury and learning alternative ways of maintaining independence are key. Goals and outcomes should be realistic and measurable. A goal of care for a patient with an actual or potential sensory alteration may be this: "The patient will regain improvement in hearing acuity within 2 weeks." Associated outcomes for this goal might be the following:

• The patient will report using communication techniques for improved reception of messages within 2 weeks.
• The patient will successfully demonstrate the technique for cleaning the hearing aid within 1 week.
• The patient will self-report improved hearing acuity.

Setting Priorities. Priorities of care must be set with regard to the type and extent of sensory alteration that affects a patient. For example, a patient who enters the emergency department after experiencing eye trauma may have priorities of reducing anxiety and preventing further

injury to the eye. In contrast, a patient who is being discharged from an outpatient surgery department following cataract removal may have the priority of learning about any self-care requirements. In both cases, however, safety is always a top priority. The patient can also help prioritize aspects of care. For example, patients may wish to learn ways to communicate more effectively or to participate in favourite hobbies, given their sensory limitation.

Some sensory alterations are short term (e.g., a patient suffering sensory or perceptual alterations as a result of sensory overload in a CCU) (Box 48.10). Appropriate interventions are thus likely to be temporary (e.g., frequent reorientation or introduction of pleasant stimuli, such as holding a hand). Sensory alterations such as permanent visual loss require long-term goals of care for patients to adapt. Sometimes it becomes necessary for the patient to make major changes in self-care activities, communication, or socialization. Patients who have sensory alterations at the time of entering a health care setting often already have strategies they developed to adapt their lifestyle to their sensory limitations. Nurses need to allow persons with sensory impairment to control whatever part of their care they can.

◆ **Implementation**

Nursing interventions involve the patient and family. The most effective interventions enable the patient with sensory alterations to function safely with existing deficits and to continue a normal lifestyle as much as possible. Learning to adjust to sensory impairments can occur at any age with proper support and resources.

When developing a plan of care, it is important to consider all resources available to patients. The family can play a key role in providing meaningful stimulation and learning ways to help the patient adjust to any limitations. Family members should understand how a patient's sensory impairment affects their daily activities. Family and friends can be more supportive when they understand sensory deficits

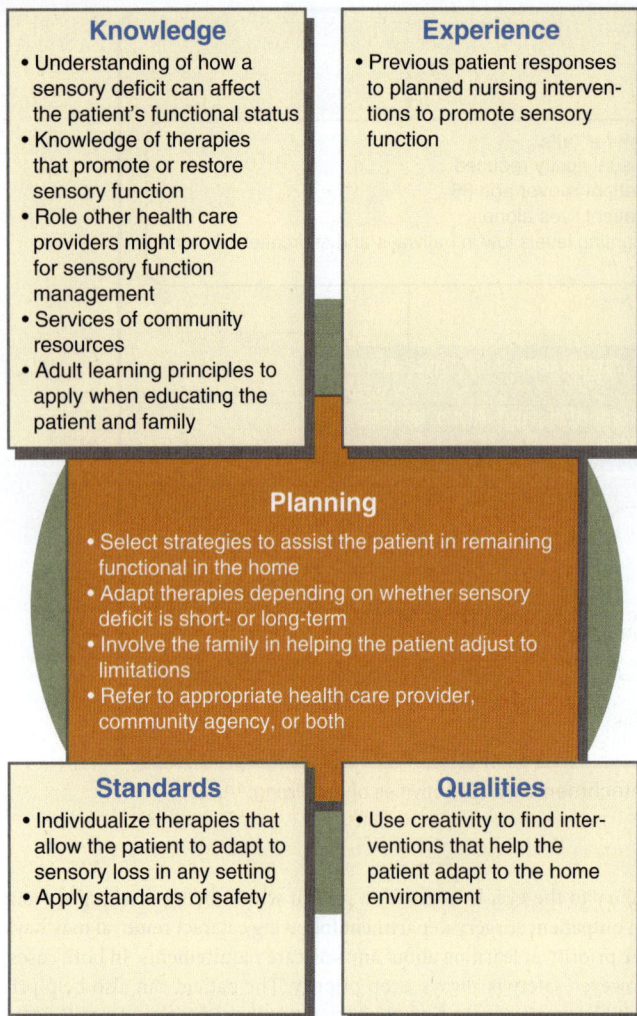

Knowledge
- Understanding of how a sensory deficit can affect the patient's functional status
- Knowledge of therapies that promote or restore sensory function
- Role other health care providers might provide for sensory function management
- Services of community resources
- Adult learning principles to apply when educating the patient and family

Experience
- Previous patient responses to planned nursing interventions to promote sensory function

Planning
- Select strategies to assist the patient in remaining functional in the home
- Adapt therapies depending on whether sensory deficit is short- or long-term
- Involve the family in helping the patient adjust to limitations
- Refer to appropriate health care provider, community agency, or both

Standards
- Individualize therapies that allow the patient to adapt to sensory loss in any setting
- Apply standards of safety

Qualities
- Use creativity to find interventions that help the patient adapt to the home environment

FIGURE 48.5 Critical thinking model for sensory alterations planning.

and the types of elements that worsen or lessen sensory problems. Resources are available within a community that provide information that assists patients with personal management needs and can also provide practical tips and emotional support for family members who are caregivers. For example, the CNIB, Canadian Hearing Society, and Canadian Association of the Deaf offer resource materials and product information (see "Recommended Websites" section). Nurses need to help family members to focus on the person's abilities rather than on their disability.

As part of an interprofessional health care team, the nurse may also refer the patient to other health care providers. Early referrals to occupational or speech therapists, for example, can aid in a patient's recovery. If a patient has experienced a major loss of sensory function and is also unable to manage medical needs, such as medication self-administration or dressing changes, referral to home care may be an option. Numerous community-based resources (e.g., CNIB or the Canadian Hearing Society) are also available. The nurse may be able to arrange for a volunteer to visit the patient or have printed materials made available that describe ways to help cope with sensory challenges.

In the community, **health promotion** related to sensory alterations is delivered in health care providers' offices, homes, community centres, schools, and industry. Public health nurses, for example, conduct newborn hearing screenings during well-baby clinics and reinforce to parents the importance of following the Canadian Ophthalmological Society eye examination guidelines. In long-term care facilities, the nurse can use the Vision Screening Tool at admission to provide a baseline and then annually to assess for changes in vision. In school health programs, the nurse can stress the importance of maintaining the health of eyes and ears. Occupational health nurses play a key role in preventing injury, such as ensuring that safety standards are followed.

Preventive Safety. Trauma is a common cause of blindness in children. Penetrating injuries from propulsive objects such as firecrackers, slingshots, rubber bands, or rocks, and penetrating wounds from sticks, scissors, or toys are just a few examples. Parents and children require education about ways to avoid eye trauma. Safety equipment can easily be found in most sports shops and large department stores and online.

◎ **BOX 48.9 NURSING CARE PLAN**

Disturbed Sensory Perception

ASSESSMENT

As mentioned in the case study at the beginning of this chapter, Judy is a 70-year-old widow who lives alone. As a beginning nurse, you accompany the community health nurse to the visit. Judy tells you and the community health nurse that her vision has become progressively blurred over the last several years. She comments that she is having her neighbour drive her places she needs to go.

Assessment Activities	Findings and Defining Characteristics
Ask Judy to describe her vision changes.	Judy states, "My left eye seems to have a film over it that makes my vision blurred. I am having difficulty reading. I also have difficulty with night driving; the headlights are large and blurred."
Ask Judy to describe any life changes that have occurred since the change in vision.	Judy indicates that she has always managed her home and done volunteering. She says she is losing her independence because she has to have someone drive her, and she is now hesitant to use stairs at home.
Assess Judy's visual acuity.	Judy cannot read the Snellen chart with the left eye.
Ask Judy the results of the visit to the ophthalmologist.	Judy states that she was told she has a cataract in the left eye and a cataract beginning in her right eye; surgery is planned on her left eye.
Conduct a home hazard assessment.	The home is cluttered, the lighting is dim, and the stairs going into the house have no handrails.

NURSING DIAGNOSIS: *Risk for injury.*

Continued

BOX 48.9 NURSING CARE PLAN—cont'd

PLANNING

Goals (Nursing Outcomes Classification)*

Judy will maintain independence in a safe home environment.

Judy will make the best use of existing visual function.

Expected Outcomes

Safe Home Environment

Judy will verbalize changes made to protect and maintain visual acuity for indoor and outdoor activities in 2 weeks. A safety check of her home will show removal of safety hazards in 1 week.

Judy will explain plans for alternative transportation to work and social activities in 1 week.

Sensory Function: Vision

Judy will use visual aid devices in 1 week.

*Outcome classification labels from Moorhead, S., Swanson, E., Johnson, M., et al. (Eds.). (2018). *Nursing outcomes classification (NOC)* (6th ed.). Mosby/Elsevier.

INTERVENTIONS

Interventions (Nursing Interventions Classification)†

Environmental Management

Teach Judy how to improve the safety of her environment, such as making sure her home is free of clutter, footstools, and electrical cords, and to avoid rearranging furniture.

Teach Judy to use a light over the shoulder for reading and writing.

Encourage use of a magnifier for Judy to use to read the newspaper and mail and advise her on where to purchase it.

Encourage her to make an appointment with an ophthalmologist within the next 4 weeks.

Emotional Support

Encourage Judy to express feelings regarding loss of vision and lifestyle changes.

Family Involvement Promotion

Confer with Judy on selecting a family member, friend, or community resource person who can provide transportation until after the eye condition has been corrected.

Rationale

Keeping the area clutter free reduces the risk of injury (Gell et al., 2020; Morrice et al., 2021).

People with cataracts see better with brighter and wider illumination (Mayo Clinic, 2022).

Devices will provide magnification to improve visual acuity (Boscart et al., 2023).

Older persons need a routine eye examination annually or as recommended (Boscart et al., 2023).

People with vision loss experience a greater risk of depression compared with those without vision loss (Nollett et al., 2019).

An alternative means of transportation will foster safety.

†Intervention classification labels are from Butcher, H. K., Bulechek, G. M., McCloskey Docherterman, J., et al. (2019). *Nursing interventions classification (NIC)* (7th ed.). Mosby.

EVALUATION

Nursing Actions	Patient Response and Finding	Achievement of Outcome
Ask Judy to describe the changes that have made the home environment safer.	Judy responds that the family has removed the clutter, and handrails have been placed at the entryway. Lighting has been placed behind her chair, and 100-watt lights are in the living room.	Judy reports feeling safer walking up and down the stairs and moving about in her home. The home hazards have been reduced.
During a home visit, observe the home environment for safety hazards.		
Observe Judy's verbal and nonverbal responses to the lifestyle adaptations.	Judy says, "I feel safer when walking in my home."	
As Judy uses a magnifier, have her read a medication label.	Judy is able to read the name of her medication and dosage correctly.	Better use is made of current vision.
Ask Judy if she is able to maintain a degree of independence with the environmental and lifestyle modifications.	Judy states, "I am more independent at home, and until surgery, I do not mind someone driving for me."	Judy has attained some degree of independence.
Ask Judy to identify source of transportation.	Judy says a family member has agreed to drive her for shopping and to her surgery.	Judy has transportation through the weeks required for the surgical experience.

In Canada, the use of facial protection (e.g., visors) in minor hockey is mandated (Hockey Canada, 2022).

Since the required use of hockey visors in amateur sport, there has been a steady decline in the incidence of eye injuries in hockey. The biggest barrier that remains today is the stigma associated with using visors and face masks. Parents should play an active role in encouraging their children to wear eye protection on the ice (CNIB, 2022b).

Adults are at risk for eye injury while working in jobs involving exposure to chemicals or flying objects. The Canadian Centre for Occupational Health and Safety has guidelines for safety in the workplace. Employers are required to have employees wear eye goggles or use equipment such as HPDs to reduce the risk of injury. Eyewash stations should be provided where a worker is exposed to potential contact with a biological or chemical substance (Canadian Centre for Occupational Health and Safety, 2017). Nurses in occupational health settings can reinforce use of protective devices and ensure that features such as eyewash stations are in close proximity to the risk for injury.

To prevent hearing loss, individuals need to avoid exposure to continuously high noise levels and brief, loud impulse noise. The potential for hearing loss increases as the decibel level rises. Various provincial jurisdictions mandate occupational noise exposure limits (Ramage-Morin & Gosselin, 2018). HPDs should be worn by patients who must work around noise. Earplugs and earphones are useful in blocking high-decibel sounds.

Another means of hearing-loss prevention involves regular immunization of children against diseases capable of causing hearing loss (e.g., rubella, mumps, and measles). Public health nurses, nurse practitioners, and nurses who work in physicians' offices, schools, and community clinics should reinforce the importance of early and timely immunization. When a child or an adult develops any type of health condition, caution should be used in prescribing drugs that are ototoxic.

Adaptations for Visual Loss.

When a patient experiences changes in visual acuity, peripheral vision, adaptation to the dark, or depth perception, safety becomes a concern. With reduced peripheral vision, a patient cannot see panoramically because the outer visual field is less discrete. This creates a special hazard for driving or walking in crowded areas. Adults with reduced adaptation to the dark require three times as much light to see objects as they did as young adults. With reduced depth perception, a person cannot see how far away objects are located, making walking down stairs or over uneven surfaces dangerous.

Driving can also be a safety hazard. Reduced peripheral vision may prevent a driver from seeing a car in an adjacent lane. Reduced adaptation to the dark and sensitivity to glare make driving at night a significant risk. Although vision is a primary consideration for safety, other factors exist as well. For older persons, decreased reaction time, reduced hearing, and decreased strength in the legs and arms may further compromise driving skills. Safety tips for those who continue to drive include driving in familiar areas, not driving during rush hour, avoiding major highways for local drives, using rear-view and side-view mirrors when changing lanes, and avoiding driving at dusk or at night. Older drivers with visual impairment are 40% more likely to have caused a collision than those without visual impairment. In 2015, auto collisions were the second greatest cause of accidental death in 65- to 79-year-olds in Canada, behind falls (Yao et al., 2019).

In Ontario, drivers over the age of 80 are required to renew their licence every 2 years. The renewal process involves a vision test, a written test, a group educational session, and, for some applicants, a driving test (Government of Ontario, 2022). British Columbia requires a driver's retest for individuals approaching their eightieth birthday.

Drivers need to complete a medical examination, vision test, and road test (ICBC, 2022).

Visual alterations can make conducting normal activities of daily living more difficult. Because of reduced depth perception, patients can trip on throw rugs, runners, or stairs. Flooring or carpeting should be kept in good repair. The patient should be advised to use low-pile carpeting. Thresholds between rooms should be level with the floor. Clutter should be removed to ensure clear pathways for walking. Furniture should be arranged so that the patient can move about easily without fear of tripping or running into objects. Any stairwell should have a securely fastened handrail extending the full length of the stairs.

Front and back entrances to homes, work areas, and stairwells need to be properly lit. Light fixtures need higher-wattage bulbs with wider illumination. Although less energy efficient, incandescent lighting may be preferred over fluorescent lighting because of the flickering of fluorescent lights. However, there are ways in which flickering of fluorescent lighting can be reduced (CNIB, 2019). The CNIB website offers suggestions for lighting and other modifications for visually impaired persons. A light switch should be located at the top and bottom of stairwells. It is also important that lighting on the stairs does not cast shadows. The nurse should ensure that the patient is able to see the edge of each step clearly, especially the first and last steps. When possible, steps inside and outside the home should be replaced with ramps.

When a patient is unable to see visual contrasts, a number of interventions can be helpful. Sometimes settings on electrical appliances and equipment are only highlighted in black and white or shades of grey. Coloured tape, paint, nail polish, or raised label dots can be used to colour-code appliance dials. Colour can also be useful to highlight the edge of stairs. Applying a broad strip of coloured tape at the stair edge can help a person better see the edges. The nurse can tour the home with the patient to find opportunities for colour-coding. Telephones with large numbers or "picture phones" may be helpful to connect with significant others.

The nurse should also ensure that the patient is able to self-administer medications safely. Labels on medication containers should be in large print. A friend or spouse should always be familiar with dosage schedules. Using a magnifying glass or having family members read prescription medication labels for the patient may be helpful. Several auxiliary communication aids are currently available, including Braille embossers and audible prescription labelling systems (Wong et al., 2020). People who are visually impaired may have some difficulty manipulating eyedroppers. Eye-drop dispensers are available and often allow people with vision loss to independently administer their drops.

The pupil's ability to adjust to light diminishes with age, resulting in the older person becoming more sensitive to glare. Nurses can suggest ways for the patient to minimize glare, such as selecting satin and non-glossy finishes for walls and countertops in the home, selecting a tile pattern for flooring, and choosing sheer curtains, tinted windows, or adjustable shades to reduce outdoor light. Wearing sunglasses outside can reduce the glare of direct sunlight.

The ability to read is important to everyone. Therefore, patients should be encouraged to use their glasses whenever possible (e.g., during procedures and patient instruction), which helps patients remain oriented, maintain some control, and retain their dignity. Patients with reduced visual acuity may need more than corrective lenses. A pocket magnifier can help a patient read most printed material. Telescopic lens eyeglasses are smaller, are easier to focus, and have a greater range. Books and other publications are also available in larger print. If a patient has legal or other important documents they wish to read, standard copying machines with enlarging capabilities can be used to print the documents. Closed-circuit television magnifying units or portable or desktop video magnifiers using solid-state digital technology enlarge written characters. Minimum and maximum magnification varies from 12 to 60 times the original, depending on the screen size. As well, many word-processing programs allow print to be enlarged, as do e-reader tablets. Audio-recorded books are available and can be readily purchased in bookstores or online or borrowed from public libraries or the CNIB.

With aging, a person experiences a change in colour perception. Nurses can offer suggestions of ways the patient may decorate a room and paint hallways or stairwells so that differentiations can be made in surfaces and objects in a room.

The patient with recent visual impairment often requires help with walking. The presence of an eye patch, frequently instilled eye drops, and the swelling of eyelid structures following surgery are just a few factors that can cause a patient to need more assistance than usual. A sighted guide can give confidence to the visually impaired person and ensure safe mobility. The CNIB has resources on their site that are specific to vision loss and provide information on how to support an individual with visual impairment. For example, the CNIB (2022b) offers the following tips:

- Ask the patient if they want assistance when walking.
- If assistance is accepted, offer an elbow or arm.
- Give a detailed description of surroundings.
- Pause before curbs or stairs and inform the individual of what is coming.
- Inform the individual where they are located in relation to objects.

While walking the patient, describe the course of movement and ensure that obstacles have been removed. A patient with visual impairment should never be left standing alone in an unfamiliar area. For patients who undergo eye surgery, it is important to teach family members techniques for assisting with ambulation. For those patients who are blind, mobility training is available from the CNIB. Guide dogs may also prove useful (CNIB, 2022c). A patient who spends considerable time in bed should have a call light nearby. Necessary objects should be placed in front of the patient to prevent falls caused by reaching over the bedside. Side rails may also be useful to provide added security. At night, a night-light reduces the time required for the eyes to adapt to the dark and enables the patient to see well enough to function without keeping the regular light on.

The nurse should face the patient when speaking, use simple sentences, and speak more slowly and at a normal volume (Boscart et al., 2023). It is wise to note on the intercom button and the patient's chart if the patient is deaf or blind. A patient lacking the ability to speak cannot call out for assistance. Patients should have message boards or the call light easily available.

Adaptations for Reduced Hearing. To maximize residual hearing function, the nurse works closely with the patient to suggest ways to modify the environment. Telephones and televisions can be amplified. Alarm clocks that shake the bed or activate a flashing light are useful devices. An innovative way to enrich the lives of those with a hearing impairment is recorded music. Some patients with severe hearing loss can hear music recorded in the low-frequency sound cycles. Closed captioning, in which audio content and non-speech information, such as the identity of speakers and sound effects, are described using words or symbols, is available for many television programs.

Important environmental sounds may best be heard if amplified or changed to a lower-pitched, buzzer-like sound. Lamps are available that respond with light to sounds such as doorbells, burglar alarms, smoke detectors, and babies crying. These lamps can be purchased from hearing aid dealers, telephone companies, appliance stores, and online. Signalling devices allow the person with hearing loss to have greater independence. Family members or anyone who calls the

patient regularly should learn to let the telephone ring for longer periods. Amplified receivers for telephones and telephone communications devices use a computer and a printer to transfer words over the telephone for people who are hearing impaired. Both sender and receiver must have the special device to complete a call. Telecommunication relay services (TRS) are available from most telephone companies. A telephone operator service translates voice to text and vice versa. Video relay services (VRS) are also available. VRS enables individuals with hearing disabilities who use American Sign Language to communicate with voice telephone users through video equipment rather than through typed text. Video equipment links the VRS user with an operator so that they can see and communicate with each other in signed conversation (Government of Canada, 2022). On their website, the Canadian Hard of Hearing Association provides a list of hearing assistive technology available in Canada at this time.

When beginning a conversation with a patient who has a hearing deficit, it helps to reduce any background noise by turning off or lowering the volume of any television, appliance, or radio (Box 48.11). It is also helpful to have conversations in settings where the acoustics are better, which aids in controlling and muffling extraneous background noises. In a group setting, forming a semicircle in front of the patient helps them see who is speaking next, thereby fostering group involvement. The patient with a hearing impairment may be able to speak normally. However, the deaf patient's inability to hear self-spoken words may cause serious speech alterations. Patients may use sign language (American or Quebec Sign Language), lip-read, write with a pad and pencil, or learn to use a computer, electronic tablet, or smartphone for communication. Special communication boards that contain common terms used in nursing care (e.g., pain, bathroom, dizzy, or walk) help patients express their needs.

BOX 48.11 Communication Methods for Patients With Hearing Impairment

- Get the patient's attention. Do not startle the patient when entering the room. Do not approach a patient from behind. Be sure the patient knows you wish to speak.
- Face the patient and stand or sit on the same level. Be sure your face and lips are illuminated to promote lip-reading. Keep hands away from the mouth.
- If the patient wears glasses, be sure they are clean so that your gestures and face can be seen.
- If the patient wears a hearing aid, make sure it is in place and working.
- Speak slowly and articulate clearly. Older persons may take longer to process verbal messages.
- Use a normal tone of voice and inflections of speech. Do not speak with something in your mouth.
- When you are not understood, rephrase rather than repeat the conversation.
- Use visible expressions. Speak with your hands, your face, and your eyes.
- Do not shout. Loud sounds are usually higher pitched and may impede hearing by accentuating vowel sounds and concealing consonants. If it is necessary to raise your voice, speak in lower tones.
- Speak toward the patient's best or unaffected ear. Use written information to enhance the spoken word.
- Do not restrict a deaf patient's hands. Ensure that IV lines are not secured to both of the patient's hands if the preferred method of communication is sign language.
- Avoid speaking from another room or while walking away.
- Record a hearing impairment in the medical record.

Patient instruction is one aspect of communication. Patients can learn by listening to audio recordings or the sound portion of a televised teaching session. Patients with hearing impairment may benefit from written instructional materials and visual teaching aids (e.g., posters and graphs).

If a patient has any of the following ear conditions, a hearing aid cannot be used: visible congenital or traumatic deformity of the ear, active drainage in the last 90 days, sudden or progressive hearing loss within the last 90 days, acute or chronic dizziness, unilateral sudden hearing loss within the last 90 days, visible cerumen accumulation or a foreign body in the ear canal, pain or discomfort in the ear, or an audiometric air–bone gap of 15 decibels or greater. All but the last of these can be detected on physical examination. Referrals to or recommendations that the patient see an otolaryngologist or audiologist for further counselling should be made (Newsted et al., 2020).

Another option for those with severe to profound hearing loss is a cochlear implant. This is a small, complex electronic device that can help provide a sense of sound to a person who is profoundly deaf or severely hard of hearing. The implant consists of an external portion that sits behind the ear and a second portion that is surgically placed under the skin. An implant does not restore normal hearing. Instead, it can give a deaf person a useful representation of sounds in the environment and helps the person understand speech. A Pocket Talker can also be used to augment spoken volume.

Adaptations for Reduced Taste and Olfaction. Nurses can easily promote the sense of taste by using measures to enhance remaining taste perception.

Good oral hygiene keeps the taste buds well hydrated. Taste perception is heightened if foods are well seasoned, differently textured, and eaten separately. Flavoured vinegar or lemon juice can add tartness to food. The nurse can ask the patient what foods appeal most to taste. If taste perception is improved, food intake and appetite will also improve. A patient can learn to check dates on food packages and the colour and texture of food. Leftovers should be kept in labelled containers with the preparation date.

A reduced sensitivity to odours means that the patient may be unable to smell leaking gas, a smouldering cigarette or fire, or spoiled food. The patient should use smoke and carbon monoxide detectors and other alternative precautions, such as checking ashtrays or placing cigarette butts in water. Pilot gas flames should be checked visually or professionally on a regular basis.

Stimulation of the sense of smell with aromas such as brewing coffee, cooking garlic, and baking bread can heighten taste sensation. Blending or mixing foods should be avoided because these actions make it difficult to identify tastes. Smell can be improved by strengthening pleasant olfactory stimulation. A patient's environment can be made more pleasant with smells such as cologne, mild room deodorizers, fragrant flowers, and sachets, although the patient must be assessed for allergies or sensitivities before using these items. Certain aromas may cause patients to lose their appetite.

Removal of unpleasant odours improves the quality of a person's environment. Nurses should keep a patient's room clean, empty bedpans or urinals after use, remove and dispose of soiled dressings, and keep bathroom doors closed.

Adaptations for Reduced Tactile Sensation. Patients with reduced tactile sensation usually have the impairment over a limited portion of their bodies. Nurses can stimulate existing function by using touch therapeutically. If the patient is willing to be touched, hair brushing, and touching of the arms or shoulders are ways of increasing tactile contact. When sensation is reduced, firm pressure may be necessary

for the patient to feel the nurse's hand. Turning and repositioning can also improve the quality of tactile sensation. When invasive procedures are being performed, it is important to use touch by holding the patient's hands and keeping them warm and dry.

If a patient is overly sensitive to tactile stimuli (hyperesthesia), nurses must minimize irritating stimuli. Keeping bed linens loose to minimize direct contact with the patient and protecting the skin from exposure to irritants are helpful measures. If the patient has numbness and tingling or pain in the hands, as with carpal tunnel syndrome, special wrist splints may be worn to dorsiflex the wrist to relieve the nerve pressure. For those patients who use computers, special keyboards and wrist pads are available to decrease the pressure on the median nerve, aid in relief of pain, and promote healing.

Patients with reduced tactile sensation risk injury because they are unable to sense pressure on bony prominences or the need to change position. These patients rely on nurses for timely repositioning, moving tubes or devices they may be lying on, and turning them to avoid skin breakdown. When the patient is less able to sense temperature variations, nurses should be extra cautious when applying heat and cold therapies and preparing bathwater. Nurses must check the condition of the patient's skin frequently.

The Braden Scale (see Chapter 47) (Braden & Bergstrom, 1988) is a validated tool for assessing pressure injury risk for patients in various nursing settings (Huang et al., 2021; Theeranut et al., 2021). Those identified as at risk are monitored closely to implement preventive and treatment strategies as indicated.

When patients have reduced sensation in their extremities, they are also at risk for injury from exposure to temperature extremes. Nurses should caution them on the use of water bottles or heating pads (see Chapter 47). The temperature of bathwater should always be checked before stepping into the tub.

> **SAFETY ALERT** To create a safe environment, the nurse begins by looking at the results of the home and therapeutic environment assessment (see Chapter 38).

Adaptations to the Environment. The patient with recent sensory impairment requires a complete orientation to the immediate environment. Reorientation to the institutional environment may be provided by ensuring that name tags on uniforms are visible, addressing the patient by name, explaining where the patient is (especially if patients are transported to different areas for treatment), and using conversational cues to time or location. Nurses can reduce the tendency for patients to become confused by offering short, simple, repeated explanations and reassurance. Family members and visitors can also help orient patients to the hospital surroundings.

Patients with serious visual impairment must feel comfortable in knowing the boundaries of the immediate environment. They may want to touch the boundaries of a room or objects to gain a sense of their surroundings. The patient may need to walk through a room and feel the walls to establish a sense of direction. Nurses can help by describing furniture or equipment within the room. As it takes time to absorb a room's arrangement, the patient may need further reorientation, with the nurse explaining the location of key items (e.g., call light, telephone, and chair).

It is important to keep all objects in the same position and place. Simply moving a chair aside may create a dangerous safety hazard. The nurse needs to ask the patient if any item should be arranged to make ambulation easier. Traffic patterns should be kept clear, and use of furniture with sharp edges should be avoided. The patient who is blind needs extra time to perform tasks and a detailed description of how to perform an activity.

Patients confined to bed are at risk for sensory deprivation. Normally, movement gives an integrated awareness of the self through vestibular and tactile stimulation. A person's sensory perception is influenced by movement patterns. The limited movement of bed rest changes how a person interprets the environment; surroundings seem different, and objects seem to assume shapes different from normal. A person who is on bed rest requires routine stimulation through range-of-motion exercises, positioning, and participation in self-care activities (as appropriate). Comfort measures such as washing the patient's face and hands and providing back rubs can help improve the quality of stimulation and lessen the chance of sensory deprivation. Planning time to talk with patients is also essential. The nurse should explain unfamiliar environmental noises and sensations. As well, a calm, unhurried approach during contact with a patient gives the nurse quality time to help reorient and familiarize the patient with care activities. The patient who is well enough to read will benefit from having a variety of reading materials.

Promoting Self-Care. The ability to perform self-care is essential for self-esteem. People with chronic conditions who are supported to perform self-care report a higher quality of life, independence, and greater self-esteem, along with lower levels of depression, anxiety, and fatigue (Auld et al., 2018; Matarese et al., 2018). Frequently, family members and nurses believe that patients with sensory impairments require assistance when, in fact, they can help themselves. Useful guidelines are available to assist patients with visual or tactile impairment so that they can help themselves with daily living activities. For example, a meal tray can be set up as though food on the tray and condiments and drinks around the tray are numbers on the face of a clock. The visually impaired patient can easily become oriented to the items after the nurse or family member explains each item's location.

The patient with visual impairment may need assistance in reaching toilet facilities safely. Safety bars should be installed near the toilet. It may be helpful to have the bar be a different colour than the wall for easier visibility. Towels should never be placed on safety bars because they may interfere with a person's grasp. Toilet paper should be within easy reach. The use of sharply contrasting colours, especially red, on drawers and other places helps promote functional independence. Choosing clothes that match can be an issue, but techniques such as hanging clothes together on a hanger or marking them with similar labels can make it easier for the patient to choose what they want to wear. The patient's preference must always be considered when helping to arrange or buy clothes.

If tactile sense is diminished, the patient can dress more easily with zippers or Velcro strips, pullover sweaters or blouses, and elasticized waists. If a patient has partial paralysis and reduced sensation, the affected side should be dressed first.

Patients with proprioceptive challenges may lose balance easily. Floor mats should have rubberized, skid-proof bottoms; they should be checked and replaced as needed. Bathrooms should have nonskid surfaces in the tub and shower. Grab bars should be installed either vertically or horizontally in tubs and showers, depending on how the patient is able to grasp or hold on to the bar. Nurses can instruct family members to supervise ambulation and sitting, make frequent checks to prevent falls, and help caution the patient against leaning forward.

Any sensory impairment can have a significant influence on body image, and it is important for the patient to feel well-groomed and attractive. Some patients may need assistance with basic grooming. Others may need assistance with medication selection, clothing identification, and learning to manage routine procedures, such as blood pressure and glucose monitoring. A variety of aids are available to help individuals with varying types of sensory deficits. It is important to assist patients in maintaining a degree of independence and in having as much control over the management of their care and lifestyle as possible.

◆ Evaluation

Evaluation of Patient Care. It is essential to determine whether care measures maintain or improve patients' ability to interact and function within their environment. Only patients themselves will know if their sensory abilities are improved and which interventions or therapies are most successful in facilitating a change in their performance (Figure 48.6). Nurses can collaborate with family members to determine if a patient's ability to function within the home has improved. To evaluate the effectiveness of nursing interventions, nurses use critical thinking and make comparisons with the baseline sensory assessment data to evaluate if sensory alterations have changed.

If, as a nurse, you have developed a good relationship with a patient and have a therapeutic plan of care, you may notice subtle behaviours that indicate the level of the patient's satisfaction. Note whether the patient responds appropriately, such as by smiling. As well, observe whether the patient interacts more and is not asking to have information repeated. Ask the patient, for example, "Can you tell me if you feel we have done all we can do to help improve your ability to hear?" If the patient's expectations have not been met, then you need to spend more time understanding the patient's needs and specific preferences. Ask the patient, "What else can the health care team do to meet your

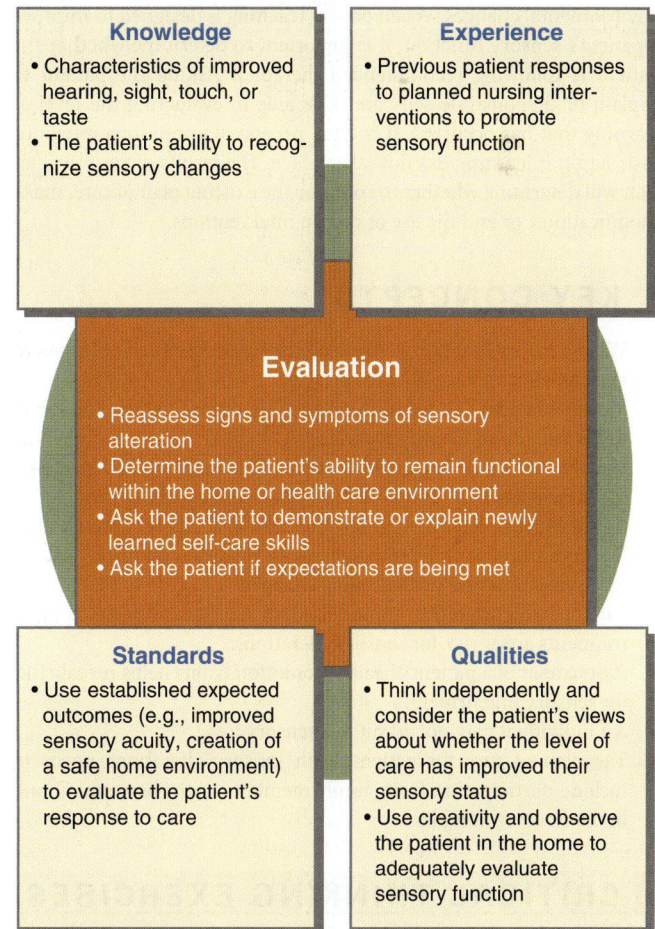

Knowledge
- Characteristics of improved hearing, sight, touch, or taste
- The patient's ability to recognize sensory changes

Experience
- Previous patient responses to planned nursing interventions to promote sensory function

Evaluation
- Reassess signs and symptoms of sensory alteration
- Determine the patient's ability to remain functional within the home or health care environment
- Ask the patient to demonstrate or explain newly learned self-care skills
- Ask the patient if expectations are being met

Standards
- Use established expected outcomes (e.g., improved sensory acuity, creation of a safe home environment) to evaluate the patient's response to care

Qualities
- Think independently and consider the patient's views about whether the level of care has improved their sensory status
- Use creativity and observe the patient in the home to adequately evaluate sensory function

FIGURE 48.6 Critical thinking model for sensory alterations evaluation.

needs?" Working closely with the patient and family will enable you to redefine expectations that can be realistically met within the limits of the patient's condition and therapies. Interventions are effective when goals and expectations have been met.

Patient Outcomes. As the nurse, you determine if expected outcomes have been met. The nature of the sensory alteration influences the way you evaluate the outcome of care. Look back on the goals and interventions for nursing care. Discuss goals and interventions with the patient, family, and interprofessional team members and reflect on their perspectives of meeting these goals. What went well? What could have been improved? What still needs to be done? What is the patient's perception of the nursing care? For example, you use proper communication techniques with a patient with a hearing deficit and then evaluate whether the patient has gained the ability to hear or interact more effectively. When expected outcomes have not been achieved, it may be necessary to change interventions or alter the patient's environment. Family members may need to be involved in support of the patient. You may also consult with the interprofessional team (e.g., physician, occupational therapist, audiologist) for suggestions to achieve unmet needs. The patient must be involved in all evaluation and planning activities.

If nursing care has been directed at improving sensory acuity, evaluate the integrity of the sensory organs and the patient's ability to perceive stimuli. Any interventions designed to relieve problems associated with sensory alterations are evaluated on the basis of the patient's ability to function normally without injury. When you attempt to directly or indirectly (through education) alter the patient's environment, evaluation is directed at observing whether the patient makes environmental changes. When patient teaching is designed to improve a patient's sensory function, it is important to determine whether the patient is following recommended therapies. Asking the patient to explain or demonstrate self-care skills aids in evaluating the level of learning that has occurred. It is often necessary to reinforce previous instruction if learning has not taken place. The results of your evaluation will determine whether to continue the existing plan of care, make modifications, or end the use of certain interventions.

KEY CONCEPTS

- When sensory function is impaired, the sense of self can be impaired and can affect one's ability to socialize.
- Multiple factors can result in sensory alterations, which are sometimes difficult to identify separately.
- Uncorrected vision impairment can lead to falls, fractures, depression, social isolation, behavioural changes, and cognitive impairment.
- Aging usually results in a gradual decline of acuity in all senses.
- It is important to differentiate between medical conditions or disease symptoms and normal aging changes.
- Patients who are older, immobilized, or confined in isolated environments are at risk for sensory alterations.
- Assessment of a patient's health promotion habits helps reveal risks for sensory impairment.
- An individual may not admit to a sensory loss.
- The plan of care for patients with sensory alterations needs to include participation from family members in the assessment and in the intervention plan.

CRITICAL THINKING EXERCISES

1. Arthur (preferred pronouns: he/him) is a 54-year-old farmer who is having a physical examination. Overall, his health is good. His spouse reports that over the past year she has noticed bruising on his arms and legs and burns on his arms. He says he has no idea how they got there and that they do not hurt. What assessment data are needed? What is your nursing diagnosis? Are there several? What specific interventions may be needed?

2. Mona (preferred pronouns: she/her), 79 years old, is visiting the nurse practitioner clinic for a routine checkup for the first time. You notice that she needed help reading the paper forms requesting information on her health history. She also told you she is having increased difficulty driving at night. What questions would you ask and what screening would you do regarding her visual difficulties, in addition to your full assessment?

3. You have an opportunity to speak with a group of parents and students regarding prevention of hearing impairment. What information would you share with this varied age group to promote healthy hearing?

4. You are a nurse in a long-term care facility. It is suspected that Elise (preferred pronouns: she/her) may have methicillin-resistant *Staphylococcus aureus* (MRSA). As a precaution, you place her on isolation in her room until the test results arrive. She has been on isolation for 4 days now. She has been displaying angry behaviour, not recognizing staff, and asking when she can return home. What would your assessment include? What type of interventions can you and your colleagues carry out for Elise?

Answers to Critical Thinking Exercises appear on the Evolve website.

REVIEW QUESTIONS

Review Questions 1 to 10 relate to the case study at the beginning of the chapter.

1. In your home visit with Judy, you observe how she gets up from her chair and moves around her living room. You are aware that the sense that enables Judy to be aware of the position and movement of body parts without seeing them is:
   a. Tactile
   b. Auditory
   c. Gustatory
   d. Kinesthetic

2. As you consider Judy's vision challenges, or those of other individuals with visual impairment, you reflect on the sense that allows a person to recognize an object's size, shape, and texture. That sense is:
   a. Tactile
   b. Gustatory
   c. Kinesthetic
   d. Stereognostic

3. When you are assessing the level of difficulty that Judy is having with sight, you ask her what she is able do for herself and what activities she is still doing. You are aware that while she awaits surgery, she may be at risk for sensory:
   a. Deficits
   b. Stimuli
   c. Deprivation
   d. Overload

4. Of all the assessments you need to conduct to ensure Judy is safe when she returns home from her cataract surgery, which one of the following would be the lowest priority?
   a. Environmental—identifying hazards in home
   b. Cognitive tests for impairment
   c. Ability to read labels of medication
   d. Her mood—risk for depression

5. Suzanne describes to you her challenges with hearing loss prior to getting a hearing aid. She tells you that the most effective question the nurse asked when obtaining a current history of her hearing loss was which of the following?
   a. "How long have you been deaf?"
   b. "Do you also have vision problems?"
   c. "Why don't you pay attention to me while I speak?"
   d. "How does your hearing now compare with your hearing a year ago?"

6. During your conversation with Suzanne, she also outlines some important do's and don'ts in relation to communicating with individuals who are hearing impaired. An important "do" is:
   a. Use a normal tone of voice.
   b. Avoid using hands when you speak, because of distraction.
   c. Speak toward the affected ear in order to enhance hearing.
   d. Speak louder to make sure the individual hears you.

7. For individuals like Suzanne, who are hearing impaired, environmental adaptations can enhance their quality of life and safety. Which of the following is not an effective environmental adaptation?
   a. Amplification of telephones and television
   b. Closed captioning on the television
   c. High-pitched amplifiers
   d. Lamps that turn on when a doorbell rings

8. As you reflect on the challenges faced by Judy and Suzanne, you recall that sensory deficits happen when a problem with sensory reception or perception occurs. As a result, individuals may:
   a. Rely solely on one sense
   b. Respond normally to stimuli
   c. Withdraw socially to cope with the loss
   d. Function safely within their environment

9. In thinking about those who have sensory alterations, such as Judy and Suzanne, you are aware that the most important priority of care is:
   a. Safety
   b. Regaining full perception
   c. Comfort
   d. The individual's ability to communicate

10. In working with individuals who have sensory alterations, whether visual (Judy) or hearing (Suzanne), an important goal of care is to:
   a. Ensure that they follow your instructions
   b. Promote self-care
   c. Teach family members to assist them whenever possible
   d. Promote dependence

Answers: 1. d, **2.** d, **3.** c, **4.** b, **5.** d, **6.** a, **7.** c, **8.** c, **9.** a, **10.** b.

🌐 *Rationales for the Review Questions appear on the Evolve website.*

RECOMMENDED WEBSITES

Canadian Association of the Deaf: https://www.cad.ca
A nonprofit organization to protect the rights, needs, and concerns of deaf people in Canada.

Canadian Fall Prevention Education Collaborative and Canadian Fall Prevention Curriculum: http://canadianfallprevention.ca
The centre offers a platform for sharing current evidence, programs, and events related to fall and injury prevention for older persons.

Canadian Hard of Hearing Association: https://www.chha.ca/chha
The Canadian Hard of Hearing Association is a nonprofit organization dedicated to empowering all Canadians living with a hearing loss through education, public awareness, services, and advocacy.

Canadian Hearing Society: https://www.chs.ca
The Canadian Hearing Society provides services that prevent hearing loss and promote the independence of deaf and hearing-impaired people.

Canadian Helen Keller Centre: https://www.chkc.org
The Canadian Helen Keller Centre (CHKC) provides training programs to individuals who are deaf-blind to help them increase and maintain their independence and autonomy, access services in the community, and decrease isolation. The website provides links relevant to deaf-blindness and communicating with people who are deaf-blind.

Canadian National Institute for the Blind (CNIB): https://www.cnib.ca
CNIB is a national, voluntary organization that offers information and support to people with vision loss.

CNIB: Guide Dogs: https://www.cnib.ca/en/programs-and-services/live/cnib-guide-dogs?region=ab

Canadian Ophthalmological Society: https://www.cos-sco.ca
This website is for eye physicians and surgeons in Canada. It provides information on vision health and when you should see an ophthalmologist.

SeeHear Canada: https://www.seehear.ca
SeeHear screens hearing and vision for both elementary-aged children in their schools and adults in their workplaces.

Voice for Deaf and Hard of Hearing Children: https://www.voicefordeafkids.com
This nonprofit organization provides support and education for the general public on deaf and hard of hearing children.

🌐 REFERENCES

A full reference list is available on the website for this book at http://evolve.elsevier.com/Canada/Potter/fundamentals/

49

Care of Surgical Patients

Canadian content written by Claudette Taylor, PhD, NP,
with original chapter contributions by Sharon Ferguson Beasley, PhD, MSN, RN, CNE

OBJECTIVES

Mastery of content in this chapter will enable you to:

- Describe the three phases of perioperative nursing.
- Describe the differences between the three phases of perioperative nursing.
- Explain the importance of a nursing assessment to determine if a patient has risk factors for surgery.
- Explain why comorbid condition may increase a patient's risk for postoperative complications.
- Explain the reasons why exercises in the postoperative period are required.

- Demonstrate postoperative exercises: diaphragmatic breathing, coughing, turning, and leg exercises.
- Design a preoperative teaching plan.
- Explain how a nurse uses sound clinical judgement when making an intraoperative assessment and how it promotes patient safety.
- Describe preparing the patient for surgery.
- Explain the nurse' role in the intraoperative period.
- Explain the differences and similarities in caring for ambulatory (day) surgical patients and caring for inpatient surgical patients.

KEY TERMS

Abdominal gas
Ambulatory surgery
Antiembolism stockings
Atelectasis
Bariatric
Cholecystectomy
Circulating nurse
Clinical pathways
Conscious sedation
Convalescence

Dehiscence
Dermatomes
General anaesthesia
Informed consent
Intermittent sequential compression stockings
Latex sensitivity
Local anaesthesia
Malignant hyperthermia
Paralytic ileus

Perioperative nursing
Postanaesthesia Recovery Score (PARS)
Postanaesthesia Recovery Score for Ambulatory Patients (PARSAP)
Preoperative teaching plan
Procedural sedation
Regional anaesthesia
Same-day surgery
Scrub nurse

🌐 WEBSITE

http://evolve.elsevier.com/Canada/Potter/fundamentals/

CASE STUDY

Amanda (preferred pronouns: she/her), 38 years old, arrives in the emergency department reporting pain, rated 8/10, in her right upper quadrant. Amanda describes this pain as dull and constant. She has vomited twice since arriving in the department. Amanda appears pale, her tongue is dry, and she admits she has been sick since having a spicy chicken dinner with French fries, two nights ago. Present vital signs include temperature of 38.5°C, pulse rate of 100, respiratory rate of 24 breaths per minute, and blood pressure of 142/88. Amanda's weight is 120 kg, and her body mass index (BMI) is 34.

Upon completion of blood work and an ultrasound, the emergency room physician diagnoses Amanda with cholecystitis with the presence of large gallstones. A surgeon is consulted, and surgery is planned for this evening. Amanda is transferred to the surgical ward until her surgery. In the meantime,

the registered nurse begins to prepare Amanda for surgery by preparing Amanda's preoperative plan of care. Amanda's assessment reveals the following information:

- Medical history: hypertension; generalized anxiety disorder
- Surgical history: none
- Medications: birth control pill; anxiety pill; antihypertensive pill (Medication Reconciliation Form to be obtained from the pharmacy)
- Allergies: penicillin (rash); no food, environmental, or latex allergies
- Social: lives with partner of 2 years; smoker (2 packs/per day), occasional alcohol and cannabis use; has no medication coverage; presently unemployed

Think about this case study as you review this chapter. There are review questions at the end of the chapter that relate to the case study.

Perioperative nursing care includes care given before (preoperative), during (intraoperative), and after (postoperative) surgery. Surgical procedures generally take place in a hospital, although some minor surgical procedures can be conducted in a physician's office. Perioperative nursing is based on nurses' understanding of several important principles, including the following:

- Excellence in perioperative practice
- Interprofessional teamwork
- Effective and therapeutic communication and collaboration with the patient, the patient's family, and the surgical team
- Effective and efficient patient assessment and intervention in all phases
- Advocacy on behalf of the patient and the patient's family
- Understanding of cost containment
- Understanding of patient safety

As a nurse, you must act as an advocate for your patient, communicate with compassion, thoroughly document patient care, and emphasize patient safety in all phases of care. The nursing process provides a basis for perioperative nursing, with the nurse individualizing strategies so that the patient receives continuity of care from admission into the health care system through convalescence. By using the nursing process, nurses can help to anticipate patient needs and minimize complications. The World Health Organization (WHO) has produced the *Surgical Safety Checklist* (WHO, 2009) to facilitate patient safety throughout the operative procedure.

The continuing care of the surgical patient has shifted from hospital-based to home-based convalescence, with the patient and family assuming increased responsibility. As the length of hospital stays decreases, the educational needs of the patients and their families increase. Patients are sent home often with complex medical or surgical conditions that require education and follow-up. Preoperative patient teaching has been demonstrated to be effective for ensuring positive surgical outcomes (Hovsepian et al., 2017).

HISTORY OF SURGICAL NURSING

Surgery gave physicians the means to treat conditions that were difficult or impossible to manage solely through medicinal applications. Early surgeons had little knowledge of the principles of asepsis, and anaesthesia techniques were primitive and unsafe. Indeed, the early surgeon's success was based on speed. The discovery of anaesthesia, in the 1840s, revolutionized surgery. Anaesthesia provided a combination of analgesia, muscle relaxation, and amnesia, which allowed the time for surgical procedures to be extended. The value of handwashing and the development of germ theory in the 1860s (Pasteur) and 1870s (Koch) triggered the study of aseptic technique, which reduced postoperative infections and mortality. Joseph Lister (1827–1912) (after whom the term "listerism" was later coined) focused on practising antisepsis during the performance of operations. Initially, antisepsis was one way to protect patients from pathogens in the environment. After experimenting with carbolic acid dressings and continuous carbolic acid sprays during surgical operations, Lister, in 1867, described a reduced incidence of gangrene and mortality. He eventually abandoned carbolic acid by 1890, when Koch demonstrated heat to be more effective than chemicals for sterilizing instruments (Al Hasan et al., 2019). Together, Pasteur, Lister, and Koch helped provide a scientific basis to help prevent infection in hospitals.

Asepsis and the techniques associated with it ensured that the patient did not acquire in-hospital infections. Germ theory influenced nursing practice through the creation of carefully delineated procedures designed to preserve asepsis (Kisacky, 2017). Nurses working in the first operating rooms (ORs) cleaned the rooms and equipment, prepared the solutions and dressings, performed technical tasks such as obtaining supplies, administered anaesthetics as graduates, and occasionally accompanied patients to the surgical ward to deliver nursing care.

In Canada, OR nursing became part of training at the Montreal General Hospital in 1890 ("Nurses life in the Montreal General Hospital," 1892). Toronto General Hospital, St. Michael's Hospital in Toronto, and Winnipeg General Hospital quickly followed suit. OR nursing in the early twentieth century became organized around the technology of surgery. Nurses ensured that the aseptic conditions of the surgical environment were maintained by all personnel and, along with physicians, became the first specialists in anaesthesia. As sterile ORs developed, OR nursing became a specialty separate from anaesthesia and surgical nursing. Two roles emerged: the sterile scrub nurse, who handled the instruments and passed them to the surgeon, and the circulating nurse, who ensured that all sponges used in operations were accounted for outside the patient's body and that aseptic conditions were maintained. OR nursing was confined to activities in and around the OR and was a well-established field of practice by the 1920s.

During the Second World War, a proliferation of courses that focused on OR nursing developed. These post-diploma courses subsequently enabled nurses to join the military, where they were highly valued as working with trauma patients (Huijuan et al., 2020). During the Second World War, the expertise of nurses in caring for soldiers with traumatic injuries accelerated. "The primary purpose of dressings shifted from one of limiting blood loss in the field to one of preventing infection and accelerating healing—while also shifting the level of knowledge and expertise to perform dressing changes and treat the underlying wounds" (Toman, 2007, p. 135).

The trend of including OR experience in training continued into the 1960s. However, during the 1970s, a change occurred in nursing education, whereby nurses were expected to acquire a broad knowledge base. As a result, many schools eliminated OR experience from the curriculum, believing that it focused only on manual skills (Sandelowski, 2000). What was not recognized was the important role that OR nurses play in ensuring patients' comfort and safety and continuity of care before, during, and after their surgical journey.

In 1956 in the United States, the Association of Operating Room Nurses (AORN) was formed. The organization developed standards of nursing practice that outlined the perioperative nurse's scope of responsibility. AORN was the first nursing organization to develop structure, process, and outcome standards as defined by the American Nurses Association. AORN has since changed its name to the Association of periOperative Registered Nurses; however, AORN is still used as its acronym. The organization continues to be a driving force for the practice of perioperative nursing and works closely with Canadian associations. Perioperative nurses care for patients during preoperative, intraoperative, and postoperative periods. They work collaboratively with surgeons, anaesthetists, registered nurse first assistants, nurses, and other health care providers.

In Canada, the Operating Room Nurses Association of Canada (ORNAC) was founded in 1983. The mission of this professional organization is to be a leader of evidence-informed perioperative nursing (ORNAC, 2021). ORNAC sets the standards for Canadian perioperative nursing practice. ORNAC's values are (1) knowledge—education and research are essential components that guide practice; (2) collaboration—with nurses within the specialty, organizations, agencies, and other disciplines; (3) respect—for the worth, quality, diversity, and importance of patients and of each other; (4) professionalism and accountability—to advance the specialty; and (5) continuous quality improvement—to achieve excellence. Opportunities exist in conjunction with the Canadian Nurses Association (CNA) for registered nurses to obtain perioperative nursing certification. To advance nursing standards in the field, the National Association of Perianesthesia Nurses of Canada (NAPANc, 2018) has published the fourth edition of its standards. Areas covered include, for example, nursing process, ethics, continuing competence, and research. In addition to NAPANc, there are provincial associations for perioperative nursing. For example, the Ontario PeriAnesthesia Nurses Association (OPANA) was founded in 1985 to represent all nurses in Ontario who are involved in the care of patients pre- and postanaesthesia. These nursing environments are usually same-day (ambulatory) care, postanaesthetic care units, and preadmission units. The vision of OPANA is that of a respected nursing practice that promotes high-quality patient care throughout the perianaesthesia road to recovery. Perianaesthesia nursing is considered a specialty area of nursing practice.

Same-Day (Ambulatory) Surgery

A more recent change in the surgical field is the advent of same-day surgery, also referred to as *ambulatory surgery* or *short-stay surgery*. In ambulatory or same-day surgery, the patient is admitted on the day of surgery, has the surgery, and then goes home the same day. These services are provided within a hospital setting. More than half of all surgical procedures are conducted on an outpatient basis, including ophthalmic, gastroenterological, gynecological, otorhinolaryngological, orthopedic, cosmetic and restorative, and general procedures, and the incidence of same-day surgery has greatly increased. The process of admitting patients and then observing them overnight (23-hour admission) can also occur.

There are several potential benefits for the patient who has same-day surgery. Anaesthesia medications that metabolize rapidly with few after-effects allow for shorter operative times. Nurses recognize the benefit of early postoperative ambulation and encourage patients to assume an active role in recovery. Same-day surgery also results in shorter hospital stays, as patients are usually discharged the day of surgery. This reduces the possibility of developing hospital-acquired infections, which occur when patients become colonized with bacteria found in the hospital setting. Procedures such as tumour biopsies, gallbladder removal (cholecystectomy), and appendectomy can now be done using laparoscopic procedures. Because of the small incision required, a laparoscopic appendectomy involves a hospital stay of only a few to 24 hours and a recovery period of a week. In contrast, a traditional open appendectomy required a right lower quadrant abdominal incision and involved a hospital stay of 3 to 5 days and a recovery period of at least 2 weeks (Rosen et al., 2017). Thus, many surgeons use laparoscopic procedures for a variety of surgical interventions, thereby decreasing the length of surgery and hospitalization, as well as associated costs, and minimizing risks to their patients. Laparoscopic approaches are just one form of the increasingly used minimally invasive surgical (MIS) techniques. For example, specialized instruments and cameras as well as medical imaging equipment can be used for procedures such as total hip arthroscopy (DeCook, 2019), vascular surgery, or minimally invasive brain surgery. There is also robotic–laparoendoscopic single-site surgery with instruments dedicated to this approach, such as the da Vinci SI surgical system (Autorino et al., 2013). Construction of new OR suites is increasingly providing dedicated rooms for MIS, and OR nurses are being educated about their role related to the techniques as well as intraoperative patient care.

Same-day surgery requires that nurses provide extensive preoperative and postoperative teaching and assess the patient's available support systems and readiness for self-care. For example, discharge education should include potential complications and what to do about them; instructions on care of incision sites and any drains, diet and activity, and pain management; and telephone numbers for contacting the health care provider, if needed. Surgical day care nurses frequently call patients at home on the day after surgery to inquire about how recovery is progressing. As well, home care nurses must refer the patient to appropriate community agencies for services such as physiotherapy and wound care, if required. Currently, apps are being developed for the web and for cell phone use. These apps are being used to help prepare patients mentally and physically for surgery, as well as provide education regarding the surgical procedure and postoperative care.

Role of Registered Nurse First Assistant (RNFA). The RNFA is an experienced perioperative nurse who has completed advanced education that provides additional knowledge along with advanced technical skills. The RNFA works collaboratively with surgeons and other members of the surgical team (Registered Nurses' Association of Ontario [RNAO], 2022). The Operating Room Nurses Association of Canada (ORNAC, 2021) has been advocating for the RNFA role since late 1980s, and the role was formally recognized in Canada in 1994.

Introduction of Anaesthetist's Assistant (AA). Recently, AAs have been introduced into the OR environment. The AAs set up equipment used for anaesthesia and assist with all aspects of the anaesthetic care plan, such as assisting with intubation and regional anaesthesia as well as satellite procedures like diagnostic imaging. AAs work under the direct supervision of an anaesthetist. Admission requirements, for example, to the Michener Institute, for an AA credentialing program are to have a respiratory therapist diploma or BScN with a minimum of 2 years' critical care experience.

SCIENTIFIC KNOWLEDGE BASE

Classification of Surgery

Surgical procedures are classified according to seriousness, urgency, and purpose (Table 49.1). A procedure may fall into more than one classification. For example, surgical removal of a disfiguring scar is minor in seriousness, elective in urgency, and reconstructive in purpose. Frequently, the classes overlap. An urgent procedure is also considered major in seriousness. As well, the same operation may be performed for different reasons on different patients. For example, a gastrectomy may be performed as an emergency procedure to resect a bleeding ulcer or as an urgent procedure to remove a cancerous growth. The classification indicates to nurses the level of care a patient might require. Hospitals have a system for prioritizing the booking of surgeries based on their classification.

The American Society of Anesthesiologists (ASA) assigns classification on the basis of a patient's physical status (PS) independent of the proposed surgical procedure (Table 49.2). In a Canadian study, Sankar and colleagues (2014) found that the ASA-PS scale has moderate interrater reliability and is a valid marker of a patient's preoperative health status. ASA-PS class I and class II patients are acceptable for ambulatory surgery. Patients in classes IV and V require inpatient surgery because they are at higher risk for complications (e.g., cardiac or pulmonary complications). The ASA classification system is used in Canadian hospitals.

NURSING KNOWLEDGE BASE

Nursing knowledge offers important contributions for the care of the perioperative patient. For example, nursing research has shown the benefit of preoperative education in promoting positive patient outcomes after surgery. Structured preoperative teaching that includes, for example, the ORNAC (2021) standards as well as a return demonstration of postoperative exercises has been shown to improve outcomes

TABLE 49.1 Classification of Surgical Procedures

Type	Description	Examples
Seriousness		
Major	Involves extensive reconstruction or alteration in body parts; poses great risks to well-being	Coronary artery bypass, colon resection, removal of larynx, resection of lung lobe
Minor	Involves minimal alteration in body parts; often designed to correct deformities; involves minimal risks compared with major procedures	Cataract extraction, facial plastic surgery, tooth extraction
Urgency		
Elective	Usually is optional and may not be necessary for health	Bunionectomy, facial plastic surgery, breast reconstruction, removal of wart
Urgent	Is necessary for patient's health; may prevent additional health problems from developing (e.g., tissue destruction or impaired organ function); not necessarily emergency	Excision of cancerous tumour, removal of gallbladder for stones, vascular repair for obstructed artery (e.g., coronary artery bypass)
Emergency	Must be done immediately to save life or preserve function of body part	Repair of perforated appendix, repair of traumatic amputation, control of internal hemorrhaging
Purpose		
Diagnostic	Surgical exploration that allows physician to confirm diagnosis; may involve removal of tissue for further diagnostic testing	Exploratory laparotomy (incision into peritoneal cavity to inspect abdominal organs), breast biopsy
Ablative	Excision or removal of diseased body part	Amputation, removal of appendix, cholecystectomy
Palliative	Relieves or reduces intensity of disease symptoms; will not produce cure	Colostomy, debridement of necrotic tissue, removal of brain tumour
Reconstructive or restorative	Restores function or appearance to traumatized or malfunctioning tissues	Internal fixation of fractures, scar revision
Procurement for transplant	Removal of organs, tissues, or both from a person pronounced dead for purpose of transplantation into another person. Sometimes there are living donors such as one person donating a kidney to another.	Kidney, heart, or liver transplant
Constructive	Restores function lost or reduced as a result of congenital anomalies	Repair of cleft palate, closure of atrial septal defect in heart
Cosmetic	Performed to improve personal appearance	Blepharoplasty to correct eyelid deformities; rhinoplasty to reshape nose

such as pain severity, pulmonary function, length of stay, and patients' levels of anxiety.

Significant evidence-informed knowledge is also available for proper wound care interventions. Nursing research has contributed to what is known about the characteristics of wound healing and the types of applications most likely to be beneficial (see Chapter 47).

Within the OR setting, increased knowledge based on research has improved the standards for infection control and patient safety. For example, surgical hand scrubs (see Chapter 34) can now be performed without the use of brushes, as a result of research that has shown the efficacy of alcohol-based hand rubs (Macinga et al., 2014). Evidence-informed practice changes within the OR improve the quality of care for surgical patients and, ultimately, improve patient outcomes.

CRITICAL THINKING

Successful critical thinking requires a synthesis of knowledge, information gathered from patients, nursing experience, critical thinking qualities, and intellectual and professional standards. To make clinical judgements, nurses need to anticipate the information necessary, analyze the data, and make decisions regarding patient care. A patient's condition is always changing. During assessment (Figure 49.1), nurses must consider all of the elements that contribute to making appropriate nursing diagnoses.

When caring for the perioperative patient, nurses make clinical care decisions by integrating knowledge of anatomy, physiology, pathophysiology, and the surgical stress response with previous experiences in caring for surgical patients and information gathered from the patient,

such as medical and surgical history, potential for surgical risk, and coping resources. Nurses' use of critical thinking qualities, such as perseverance, is needed to develop a plan of care that provides successful perioperative care (e.g., airway management, infection control, pain management, and discharge planning). Professional standards and guidelines developed by, for example, the Association of periOperative Registered Nurses (AORN, 2021), National Association of Peri-Anesthesia Nurses of Canada (NAPANc, 2018), American Society of PeriAnesthesia Nurses (ASPAN, 2019), Ontario PeriAnesthesia Nurses Association (OPANA, 2018), and Operating Room Nurses Association of Canada (ORNAC, 2021), as well as agency policies, provide valuable information for perioperative management and evaluation of processes and outcomes.

❖ NURSING PROCESS IN THE PREOPERATIVE SURGICAL PHASE

Surgical patients enter the health care setting in different stages of health. A patient may enter the hospital on a predetermined day feeling relatively healthy and prepared to face elective surgery. In contrast, a victim of a motor vehicle collision may face emergency surgery with no time to prepare. The ability to establish rapport and maintain a professional relationship with the patient is an essential component of the preoperative phase. Nurses must do this quickly but compassionately and effectively.

The surgical patient may undergo tests and procedures to confirm or rule out health problems requiring surgery. Usually patients scheduled for same-day surgery have tests done several days before surgery.

TABLE 49.2	Physical Status (PS) Classification of the American Society of Anesthesiologists (ASA)			
ASA PS Classification	**Definition**	**Adult Examples, Including, but Not Limited to:**	**Pediatric Examples, Including, but Not Limited to:**	**Obstetric Examples, Including, but Not Limited to:**
ASA I	A normal healthy patient	Healthy, non-smoking, no or minimal alcohol use	Healthy (no acute or chronic disease), normal BMI percentile for age	
ASA II	A patient with mild systemic disease	Mild diseases only without substantive functional limitations. Current smoker, social alcohol drinker, pregnancy,* obesity (30<BMI<40), well-controlled DM/HTN, mild lung disease	Asymptomatic congenital cardiac disease, well controlled dysrhythmias, asthma without exacerbation, well controlled epilepsy, non-insulin dependent diabetes mellitus, abnormal BMI percentile for age, mild/moderate OSA, oncologic state in remission, autism with mild limitations	Normal pregnancy,* well controlled gestational HTN, controlled preeclampsia without severe features, diet-controlled gestational DM.
ASA III	A patient with severe systemic disease	Substantive functional limitations; One or more moderate to severe diseases. Poorly controlled DM or HTN, COPD, morbid obesity (BMI ≥40), active hepatitis, alcohol dependence or abuse, implanted pacemaker, moderate reduction of ejection fraction, ESRD undergoing regularly scheduled dialysis, history (>3 months) of MI, CVA, TIA, or CAD/stents.	Uncorrected stable congenital cardiac abnormality, asthma with exacerbation, poorly controlled epilepsy, insulin dependent diabetes mellitus, morbid obesity, malnutrition, severe OSA, oncologic state, renal failure, muscular dystrophy, cystic fibrosis, history of organ transplantation, brain/spinal cord malformation, symptomatic hydrocephalus, premature infant PCA <60 weeks, autism with severe limitations, metabolic disease, difficult airway, long term parenteral nutrition. Full term infants <6 weeks of age.	Preeclampsia with severe features, gestational DM with complications or high insulin requirements, a thrombophilic disease requiring anticoagulation.
ASA IV	A patient with severe systemic disease that is a constant threat to life	Recent (<3 months) MI, CVA, TIA or CAD/stents, ongoing cardiac ischemia or severe valve dysfunction, severe reduction of ejection fraction, shock, sepsis, DIC, ARD or ESRD not undergoing regularly scheduled dialysis	Symptomatic congenital cardiac abnormality, congestive heart failure, active sequelae of prematurity, acute hypoxic-ischemic encephalopathy, shock, sepsis, disseminated intravascular coagulation, automatic implantable cardioverter-defibrillator, ventilator dependence, endocrinopathy, severe trauma, severe respiratory distress, advanced oncologic state.	Preeclampsia with severe features complicated by HELLP or other adverse event, peripartum cardiomyopathy with EF <40, uncorrected/decompensated heart disease, acquired or congenital.
ASA V	A moribund patient who is not expected to survive without the operation	Ruptured abdominal/thoracic aneurysm, massive trauma, intracranial bleed with mass effect, ischemic bowel in the face of significant cardiac pathology or multiple organ/system dysfunction	Massive trauma, intracranial hemorrhage with mass effect, patient requiring ECMO, respiratory failure or arrest, malignant hypertension, decompensated congestive heart failure, hepatic encephalopathy, ischemic bowel or multiple organ/system dysfunction.	Uterine rupture
ASA VI	A declared brain-dead patient and whose organs are being removed for donor purposes			

BMI, Body mass index; *CAD*, coronary artery disease; *COPD*, chronic obstructive pulmonary disease; *CVA*, cerebrovascular accident; *DIC*, disseminated intravascular coagulation; *DM*, diabetes mellitus; *ECMO*, extracorporeal membrane oxygenation; *EF*, ejection fraction; *ESRD*, end-stage renal disease; *HELLP*, hemolysis, elevated liver enzymes, low platelet count syndrome, *HTN*, hypertension; *OSA*, obstructive sleep apnea; *PCA*, post-conceptional age; *TIA*, transient ischemic attack.

NOTE: The addition of an "E" to the physical status class indicates emergency surgery, such as ASA-IE, ASA-IIE, and so on.

*Although pregnancy is not a disease, the *parturient*'s physiological state is significantly altered from the woman who is not pregnant, hence the assignment of ASA 2 for a woman with uncomplicated pregnancy.

Reprinted with permission from (*ASA physical status classification system*, 2020) of the American Society of Anesthesiologists. A copy of the full text can be obtained from ASA, 1061 American Lane, Schaumburg, IL, 60173-4973 or online at https://www.asahq.org.

Knowledge
- Anatomy and physiology of affected body systems
- Surgical risk factors
- Type of surgical procedure to be performed
- Surgical stress response
- Infection control practices

Experience
- Caring for patients who have had surgery
- Personal experience with surgery

Assessment
- Physical examination focused on the patient's history and planned surgery
- Assessment of factors that pose surgical risks for the patient
- Patient's previous experience with surgery
- Patient's coping resources
- Results of preoperative diagnostic tests

Standards
- Apply intellectual standards of specificity, accuracy, and completeness
- Apply agency and professional standards of practice (e.g., AORN, American Society of PeriAnesthesia Nurses (ASPAN) and ORNAC)

Qualities
- Use discipline in collecting a complete patient history
- Use perseverance to ensure a comprehensive assessment

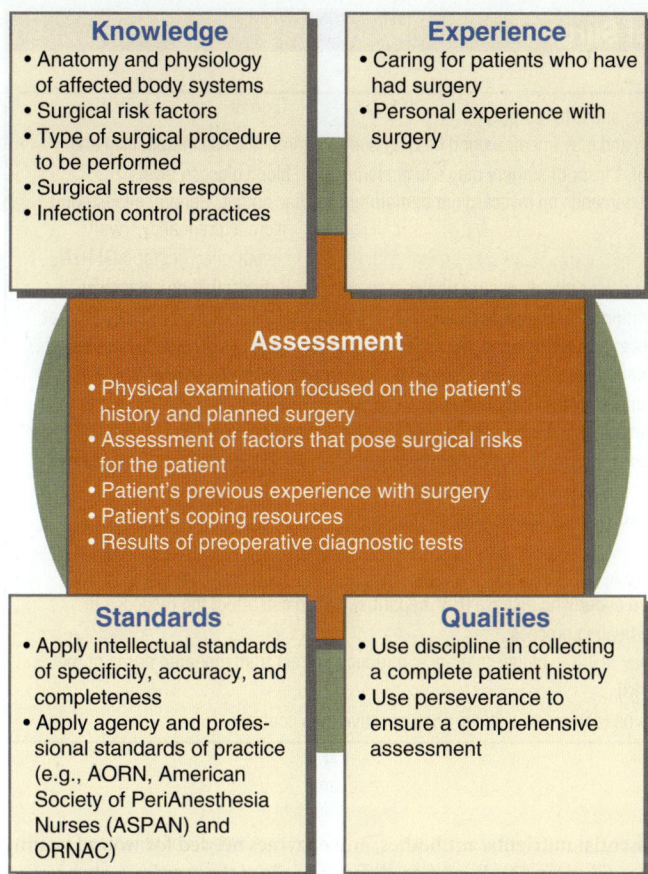

FIGURE 49.1 Critical thinking model for surgical patient assessment. *AORN*, Association of Perioperative Registered Nurses; *ORNAC*, Operating Room Nurses Association of Canada.

Testing done the day of surgery is usually limited to such tests as glucose monitoring for the patient with diabetes and electrocardiography testing for patients with heart conditions. Nurses must be familiar with the tests, their purpose, and how to monitor results. Anaesthetists also want to review these tests prior to the patients' surgical procedure.

The patient meets many members of the interprofessional team, including surgeons, anaesthesiologists, physiotherapists, and nurses. All play a role in the patient's care and recovery. Family members may attempt to provide support through their presence but face many of the same stressors as the patient. Nurses must communicate effectively with the patient and family because *the nurse–patient relationship is the foundation of care* (see Chapter 18). Nurses need to assess the patient's physical, emotional, and spiritual well-being and cultural heritage; recognize the degree of surgical risk; coordinate diagnostic tests; identify nursing diagnoses and nursing interventions; and establish outcomes in collaboration with the patient and their family. Pertinent data and the care plan are communicated among the members of the surgical team.

◆ Assessment

The assessment of the surgical patient is intended to establish the patient's baseline preoperative function to assist in preventing and recognizing possible postoperative complications. Assessment of the surgical patient can be extensive. Ambulatory surgical programs require that patient data be completed several days in advance. Since patients are admitted only hours before the surgical event, nurses must organize and verify data obtained preoperatively to implement a perioperative care plan. This occurs not only with the ambulatory care patient but

also with the patient who will require a more prolonged hospital stay. Increasingly, patients are admitted on the day of surgery, even for such major procedures as open-heart surgery and bowel surgery.

Most assessments begin in a preadmission clinic before admission for surgery. The purpose of the preadmission is to prepare the patient physically and emotionally for surgery (OPANA, 2018). Patients may answer a self-report inventory and the nurse may complete an initial physical examination, draw blood or complete other laboratory tests, begin teaching, identify potential risks, and answer questions. This process streamlines the care required for the patient on the day of surgery. In the immediate preoperative period, nurses assess the patient's understanding of previous teaching and individualize patient and family care.

The physician usually performs a comprehensive history and physical examination with follow-up by the preadmission nurse. In this case, the nurse needs to review assessments and testing already completed and to highlight significant information (e.g., the patient being on diuretics). The focus is on key measurements for all body systems to ensure that no obvious health problems are overlooked and that the patient has understood education previously provided. Even though the surgeon will screen the patient before scheduling surgery, preoperative assessment occasionally reveals an abnormality that delays or cancels surgery. For example, the patient may have a cough and low-grade fever on admission. This may indicate the onset of infection, and the surgeon will need to be notified immediately.

Nursing Health History. The nurse should conduct an initial interview to collect a patient history similar to that described in Chapter 33. If a patient is unable to relate all the necessary information, the nurse should rely on family members as resources.

Medical History. A review of the patient's medical history should include past illnesses and the primary reason for currently seeking medical care. The patient's current medical record and medical records from past hospitalizations are excellent sources of data.

Pre-existing illnesses can influence the choice of anaesthetic agents used and the patient's ability to tolerate surgery and reach full recovery (Table 49.3). Patients must be carefully screened for medical conditions that may increase the risk for complications during or after surgery. For example, a patient who has a history of heart failure may experience a further decline in cardiac function both intraoperatively and postoperatively. Intravenous (IV) fluids may need to be administered at a slower rate, or a diuretic may need to be given if blood transfusions are required.

Risk Factors. Various conditions and factors increase a person's risk when undergoing surgery. Knowledge of risk factors enables nurses to take necessary precautions in planning care.

Age. Infants are at risk during surgery because of their immature physiological status. During surgery, nurses and physicians are especially concerned with maintaining an infant's normal body temperature. The infant's shivering reflex is underdeveloped, and often wide temperature variations occur. Anaesthesia adds to the risk because anaesthetics can cause vasodilation and heat loss.

During surgery, an infant has difficulty maintaining a normal circulatory blood volume. The total blood volume of an infant is considerably less than that of an older child or an adult. Therefore, even a small amount of blood loss can be serious. A reduced circulatory volume makes it difficult for the infant to respond to increased oxygen demands during surgery. In addition, the infant is highly susceptible to complications associated with dehydration. However, if blood or fluids are replaced too quickly, overhydration may occur. Other important

TABLE 49.3   Medical Conditions That Increase Risks of Surgery

Type of Condition	Reason for Risk
Bleeding disorders (thrombocytopenia, hemophilia)	Increase risk of hemorrhaging during and after surgery
Diabetes mellitus	Increases susceptibility to infection and may impair wound healing due to altered glucose metabolism and associated circulatory impairment. Stress of surgery may cause increases in blood glucose levels.
Heart disease (recent myocardial infarction, dysrhythmias, heart failure) and peripheral vascular disease	Stress of surgery causes increased demands on myocardium to maintain cardiac output. General anaesthetic agents depress cardiac function.
Obstructive sleep apnea	Administration of opioids increases risk of airway obstruction postoperatively. Patients will desaturate as revealed by drop in oxygen saturation by pulse oximetry.
Upper respiratory infection	Increases risk of respiratory complications during anaesthesia (e.g., pneumonia and spasm of laryngeal muscles)
Liver disease	Alters metabolism and elimination of medications administered during surgery and impairs wound healing and clotting time because of alterations in protein metabolism
Fever	Predisposes patient to fluid and electrolyte imbalances and may indicate underlying infection
Chronic respiratory disease (emphysema, bronchitis, asthma)	Reduces patient's means to compensate for acid–base alterations (see Chapter 41). Anaesthetic agents reduce respiratory function, increasing risk for severe hypoventilation.
Immunological disorders (leukemia, HIV, bone marrow depression, and use of chemotherapeutic agents or immunosuppressive medications)	Increase risk of infection and delayed wound healing after surgery
Abuse of street drugs	Patients who abuse drugs may have underlying disease (HIV, hepatitis), which can affect the response to anaesthesia and surgery and the healing process.
Chronic pain	Regular use of pain medications may result in higher tolerance, a reduced effect from repeated doses of the same analgesic class (RNAO, 2013). Increased doses of analgesics may be required to achieve postoperative pain control.

and unique aspects of a child's surgical care are airway management, treatment of seizures, management of temperature alterations, identification and treatment of emergence delirium and delayed emergence from anaesthesia, treatment of pain and agitation, and availability of age-appropriate emergency equipment and medications.

Older patients are also at risk for complications. With advancing age, a patient's physical capacity to adapt to the stress of surgery is hampered. A recent Canadian study examined 257 older patients who underwent emergency general surgery. More than 50% experienced an in-hospital complication following surgery, the most common being cardiac events, surgical infection or sepsis, and postoperative bleeding (Lees et al., 2015). Despite the risk, the majority of patients undergoing surgery are older persons. Table 49.4 summarizes the physiological factors that place older patients at risk during surgery.

Nutrition. Normal tissue repair and resistance to infection depend on adequate nutrients. Surgery intensifies this need. After surgery, a patient requires at least 1 500 kcal/day to maintain energy reserves. Increased protein, vitamins A and C, and zinc facilitate wound healing (see Chapters 43 and 47). A malnourished patient is prone to poor tolerance of anaesthesia, negative nitrogen balance, delayed blood clotting mechanisms, infection, poor wound healing, and the potential for multiple organ failure. If a patient is having elective surgery, attempts to correct nutritional imbalances should be made before the surgery. However, if a malnourished patient must undergo an emergency procedure, efforts to restore nutrients will occur after surgery.

Obesity. Obesity increases surgical risk by reducing respiratory and cardiac functions. Hypertension, coronary artery disease, diabetes mellitus, and heart failure are common in the **bariatric** (obese) population. Embolus, **atelectasis** (partial or total collapse of the alveoli), and pneumonia are also more frequent postoperative complications in the obese patient. The patient may have difficulty resuming normal physical activity after surgery. The patient with obesity is susceptible to poor wound healing and wound infection because of the structure of fatty tissue, which contains a poor blood supply. This slows delivery of essential nutrients, antibodies, and enzymes needed for wound healing (see Chapter 47). It is often difficult to close the surgical wound of an obese patient because of the thick adipose layer. A patient with obesity is also at risk for **dehiscence** (opening of the suture line).

Immunocompetence. For the patient with cancer, radiation therapy may be given preoperatively to reduce the size of the cancerous tumour so that it can be removed surgically. Radiation has some unavoidable effects on normal tissue, such as excess thinning of skin layers, destruction of collagen, and impaired vascularization of tissue. Ideally, the surgeon waits 4 to 6 weeks after completion of radiation treatments to perform surgery. Otherwise, the patient may face serious problems with wound healing. In addition, chemotherapeutic medications used for cancer treatment, immunosuppressive medications used to prevent rejection after organ transplantation, and steroids used to treat a variety of inflammatory conditions increase the risk for infection.

Fluid and Electrolyte Imbalances. The body responds to surgery as a form of trauma. As a result of the adrenocortical stress response, sodium and water are retained and potassium is lost within the first 2 to 5 days after surgery. The severity of the stress response influences the degree of fluid and electrolyte imbalances. The more extensive the surgery, the greater is the stress response. A patient who is hypovolemic or who has serious preoperative electrolyte alterations is at significant risk during and after surgery. For example, an excess or depletion of potassium increases the chance of dysrhythmia. If the patient has preexisting renal, gastrointestinal, or cardiovascular abnormalities, the risk for fluid and electrolyte alterations is even greater.

Pregnancy. The perioperative care plan must address the needs of both the pregnant person and the developing fetus. Surgery is performed on a pregnant patient only on an emergency basis. All the pregnant person's major systems are affected during pregnancy. For example, cardiac output significantly increases, as does respiratory tidal volume to accommodate the increase in metabolic rate. Gastrointestinal motility decreases, hormone levels increase, and energy levels decrease with advancing pregnancy. Laboratory and hemodynamic values change.

TABLE 49.4	Physiological Factors That Place the Older Person at Risk During Surgery	
Alterations	**Risks**	**Nursing Implications**
Cardiovascular System		
Degenerative change in myocardium and valves	Reduced cardiac reserve and arrhythmias	Assess baseline vital signs. Recognize the longer time period required for heart rate to return to normal after stress on the heart and evaluate the occurrence of tachycardia accordingly.
Rigidity of arterial walls and reduction in sympathetic and parasympathetic innervation to heart	Alterations may predispose patient to postoperative hemorrhage or an increase in systolic and diastolic blood pressure	Maintain adequate fluid balance to minimize either dehydration or circulatory overload. Assess vital signs frequently. Assess wound drainage.
Increase in calcium and cholesterol deposits within small arteries; thickened arterial walls	Predispose patient to clot formation in lower extremities	Instruct patient on techniques for performing leg exercises and proper turning. Apply elastic stockings, or intermittent sequential compression stockings.
Integumentary System		
Decreased subcutaneous tissue and increased fragility of skin	Prone to pressure injuries and skin tears	Assess skin at least every 4 hours; pad all bony prominences during surgery. Turn or reposition at least every 2 hours (see Chapter 47).
Pulmonary System		
Stiffening and reduction in size of the rib cage	Reduced vital capacity. Could retain secretions	Instruct patient in proper technique for coughing and deep breathing.
Reduced range of movement in diaphragm	Residual capacity (volume of air left in lung after normal breath) increases, reducing amount of new air brought into lungs with each inspiration	When possible, have patient ambulate and sit in chair frequently.
Stiffened lung tissue and enlarged air spaces	Alteration reduces blood oxygenation	Obtain baseline oxygen saturation; measure as indicated throughout the perioperative period.
Renal System		
Reduced blood flow to kidneys	Increased risk of shock when blood loss occurs	For patients hospitalized before surgery, determine baseline urinary output for 24 hours.
Reduced glomerular filtration rate and excretory times	Limits ability to eliminate medications or toxic substances	Assess for adverse response to medications.
Reduced bladder capacity	Voiding frequency increases, and a larger amount of urine stays in the bladder after voiding. Sensation of need to void may not occur until bladder is filled.	Instruct patient to notify nurse immediately when sensation of bladder fullness develops. Keep call light and bedpan within easy reach. Toilet every 2 hours, or more frequently if indicated.
Neurological System		
Sensory losses, including reduced tactile sense	Decreased ability to respond to early warning signs of surgical complications such as delirium	Inspect bony prominences for signs of pressure that patient may not sense. Orient patient to surrounding environment. Observe for nonverbal signs of pain.
Decreased reaction time	Confusion after anaesthesia. Delirium is a disturbance of attention and awareness that develops over a short period of time (Kaya, 2018). Delirium manifests in three subtypes: hyperactive, hypoactive, and mixed (Kirpinar, 2018). Older patients undergoing surgery are at high risk for delirium. Delirium can be caused by medications such as narcotics, or by physiological reasons such as infection or dehydration.	Allow adequate time for patient to respond, process information, and perform activities. Use Best Practice Guidelines (BPGs) on screening and caregiving strategies for older persons with delirium, dementia, and depression (RNAO, 2003/2010, 2010/2016). Institute fall precautions (RNAO, 2017b).
Metabolic System		
Lower basal metabolic rate	Reduced total oxygen consumption	Ensure adequate nutritional intake when diet is resumed but avoid intake of excess calories.
Reduced number of red blood cells and hemoglobin levels	Ability to carry adequate oxygen to tissues is reduced	Administer blood products if required. Monitor blood test results.
Change in total amounts of body potassium and water volume	Greater risk for fluid or electrolyte imbalance occurs	Monitor electrolyte levels and supplement as necessary.
Impaired thermoregulatory mechanisms	Cold operating rooms; exposure of body parts during procedure, intravenous (IV) fluids, medications	Ensure careful, close monitoring of patient temperature; provide warm blankets; monitor cardiac function; warm IV fluids.

Fibrinogen levels increase, making pregnant patients more susceptible to the development of deep vein thrombosis because of increased coagulability. Hemoglobin and hematocrit levels decrease, mostly as a result of the effects of hemodilution (increased circulating volume). The white blood cell (WBC) count is elevated when the person is near term and postpartum without the presence of infection. However, infection always must be ruled out in the presence of an elevated WBC count. General anaesthesia is administered with caution because of the increased risk for fetal death and preterm labour. Psychological considerations for the pregnant person and their family are essential.

Previous Surgeries. Although previous surgery does not necessarily present as a risk factor, a patient's past experience with surgery can highlight many potential issues. The nurse should ask the patient to recall the previous type of surgery, level of discomfort, extent of disability, and overall level of care provided. Any complications that the patient experienced must be addressed. It is also important to assess patients for nausea and vomiting with previous surgeries, as research has shown these can be troublesome symptoms that are not always adequately medicated (Wilson et al., 2016) and can increase the risk for aspiration. Prior anaesthesia records may be a useful source of information if previous complications such as malignant hyperthermia occurred. This information helps nurses to anticipate the patient's preoperative and postoperative needs. Previous surgery also may influence the level of physical care required after a surgical procedure. For example, a patient who has had a previous thoracotomy for resection of a lung lobe has a greater risk for postoperative pulmonary complications than does a patient with intact, normal lungs.

Perceptions and Understanding of Surgery. The surgical experience affects not only the patient, but also the entire family. The nurse must therefore prepare both the patient and the family. Identifying a patient's and family's knowledge, expectations, and perceptions enables the nurse to plan teaching and to provide individualized emotional support measures.

Each patient may feel fearful when entering the surgical setting. Some fears are due to past hospital experiences, warnings received from friends and family, or lack of knowledge. The nurse must assess the patient's understanding of the planned surgery and its implications. For example, the nurse needs to determine whether the patient undergoing a breast biopsy recognizes that they will have a biopsy performed, not a mastectomy. The nurse might ask questions such as "Tell me what you think will happen before and after surgery," or "Explain what you know about your surgery." If a patient is misinformed or unaware of the reason for surgery, the nurse must confer with the physician before the patient is sent to the surgical suite. It is also good to determine whether further explanations are needed related to routine preoperative and postoperative procedures. When a patient is well prepared and knows what to expect, the patient's knowledge is reinforced, and accuracy and consistency are maintained.

Medication History. If a patient regularly uses prescription or over-the-counter medications, the surgeon or anaesthesiologist may temporarily discontinue the medications before surgery or adjust the dosages. Certain medications have special implications for the surgical patient, creating greater risks for complications or interacting negatively with anaesthetic agents (Table 49.5). For example, nurses must instruct patients in a preadmission unit to ask the physician whether usual medications should be taken on the morning of surgery. Patients also should be asked whether any herbal preparations are used, because many patients do not view herbs as medications and may omit them from their medication history (see Chapter 36). Certain herbs may interfere with the action of other medications (a pharmacist must be consulted). For hospitalized patients, prescription medications taken preoperatively are automatically discontinued postoperatively unless the prescriber reorders them. It is important for the nurse to be aware of the patient's previous medications that likely will need to be resumed postoperatively (e.g., antihypertensives).

Allergies. Nurses must assess for allergies to medications that may be given during a phase of the surgical experience. In addition, it is critical to assess for latex, food, and contact allergies (e.g., allergies to tape, ointments, or solutions). A patient may be too young or have too few exposures to medications to know whether they have any allergies. The type of allergic response is also very important to assess. Allergies need to

TABLE 49.5	Medications With Special Implications for the Surgical Patient
Medication Class	**Effects During Surgery**
Antibiotics	Antibiotics can potentiate action of anaesthetic agents. For example, if taken within 2 weeks before surgery, aminoglycosides (gentamicin, tobramycin, neomycin) may cause mild respiratory depression due to depressed neuromuscular transmission.
Antidysrhythmics	Antidysrhythmics can reduce cardiac contractility and impair cardiac conduction during anaesthesia.
Anticoagulants	Anticoagulants alter normal clotting factors and thus increase risk of hemorrhaging. They should be discontinued before surgery. Aspirin (ASA) is a commonly used medication that can alter clotting mechanisms. Many older patients take ASA, and the nurse should be alert to whether they have discontinued use presurgery. Most surgeons will have the patient stop taking ASA 4 to 5 days before the surgery.
Anticonvulsants	Long-term use of certain anticonvulsants (e.g., phenytoin [Dilantin] and phenobarbital) can alter the metabolism of anaesthetic agents.
Antihypertensives	Antihypertensives may interact with anaesthetic agents to cause bradycardia, hypotension, and impaired circulation. Some may inhibit synthesis and storage of norepinephrine in sympathetic nerve endings.
Corticosteroids	With prolonged use, corticosteroids cause adrenal atrophy, which reduces the body's ability to withstand stress. Before and during surgery, dosages may be temporarily altered.
Insulin	Diabetic patients' need for insulin after surgery is altered. Stress response and intravenous administration of glucose solutions can increase dosage requirements after surgery. Decreased nutritional intake can decrease dosage requirements.
Diuretics	Diuretics potentiate electrolyte imbalances (particularly potassium) after surgery.
Nonsteroidal anti-inflammatory drugs (NSAIDs)	NSAIDs inhibit platelet aggregation and may prolong bleeding time, increasing susceptibility to postoperative bleeding.
Herbal therapies: ginger, gingko, ginseng	Some herbal therapies have the ability to affect platelet activity and increase susceptibility to postoperative bleeding. Ginseng may increase hypoglycemia with insulin therapy.

be delineated from unpleasant adverse effects. For example, the patient may state that codeine causes nausea (an adverse effect), or that it causes hypotension and confusion (an allergy). When asking a patient about allergies, the nurse needs to realize that the term *allergy* can be confusing for some patients. Asking a patient whether they have ever "had a problem with a medication or substance" may be a helpful approach.

It is critical that the patient be asked specifically about latex allergies because a latex-free environment must be provided for patients with latex allergies. Nurses must ensure that a list of the patient's allergies is noted appropriately in the patient's medical record or the electronic chart, as well as in any other places designated by institutional policy, such as an allergy band.

Smoking Habits.
The patient who smokes is at greater risk for postoperative pulmonary complications than one who does not. The chronic smoker already has an increased amount and thickness of mucous secretions in the lungs. General anaesthetics increase airway irritation and stimulate pulmonary secretions, which are retained as a result of reduction in ciliary activity during anaesthesia. After surgery, the patient who smokes has greater difficulty clearing the airways of mucous secretions and needs education on the importance of postoperative deep breathing and coughing (see Chapter 40). In addition, smoking can compromise blood flow to the heart, which can affect the response to surgery. Nurses play a key role in reducing smoking and can refer to nursing Best Practice Guidelines (BPGs) on smoking cessation (RNAO, 2017a), when appropriate. During the postoperative period, nicotine replacement therapy may be required to support the patient who smokes.

Alcohol Ingestion and Substance Use and Abuse.
Habitual use of alcohol and illegal drugs predisposes the patient to adverse reactions to anaesthetic agents. The patient also may experience a cross-tolerance to anaesthetic agents, necessitating higher-than-normal amounts. In addition, the physician may need to increase postoperative dosages of analgesics. Patients with a history of excessive alcohol ingestion also may be malnourished, which may contribute to delayed wound healing. These patients are at risk for liver disease, portal hypertension, and esophageal varices (predisposing the patient to bleeding disorders). The patient who habitually uses alcohol and is required to remain in the hospital for longer than 24 hours is also at risk for acute alcohol withdrawal and its more severe form, delirium tremens.

Family Support.
It is important for nurses to determine the extent of the patient's support from family members or friends. Because blood relations do not always define family, it is best to have the patient identify their sources of support (see Chapter 20). Surgery can result in temporary or permanent disability that requires added assistance during recovery. The patient usually cannot immediately assume the same level of physical activity enjoyed before surgery. Often a patient returns home with dressings to change or exercises to perform. With same-day surgery, patients and families assume responsibility for postoperative care. The family is an important resource for the patient with physical limitations and can provide the emotional support needed to motivate the patient to return to a previous state of health. In addition, the family may better remember preoperative and postoperative teaching.

The nurse should ask whether family members or friends could provide support. The patient may want someone present when the nurse provides instructions or explanations. Family presence should be encouraged, when feasible, especially for patients having ambulatory surgery. Often a family member can become the patient's coach, offering valuable support during the postoperative period, when the patient's participation in care is vital.

Occupation.
The nurse should assess the patient's occupational history to anticipate the possible effects of surgery on recovery and eventual work performance. Any restrictions should be explained before a patient returns to work, such as lifting, use of the extremities, or climbing stairs. When a patient is unable to return to their job, the nurse should confer with a social worker or occupational therapist to refer the patient to job-training programs or to help the patient seek economic assistance.

Preoperative Preparation for Pain Assessment and Management.
Surgical manipulation of tissues, treatments, and positioning on the OR table may result in postoperative pain for the patient. Pain is a very personal experience and requires an individualized care plan. Preoperatively, the nurse should prepare the patient and family for the assessment and management of pain (see Chapter 32), including the patient's and the family's expectations for pain management after surgery. The nurse should begin education regarding pain management as soon as possible (Box 49.1). The preoperative assessment should

---

BOX 49.1 RESEARCH HIGHLIGHT

A Randomized Controlled Trial of an Individualized Preoperative Education Intervention for Symptom Management After Total Knee Arthroplasty

Research Focus

The aim of this study was to determine the effect of preoperative educational intervention on postsurgical pain and nausea.

Research Abstract

Total knee replacement is a common surgical procedure performed to reduce pain and immobility usually caused by osteoarthritis. Pain and nausea are common symptoms for patients after this procedure. Although previous research studies have examined educational interventions for pain prevention and treatment in this population, none of the studies focused on analgesic pain management and antiemetic therapy. This Canadian study aimed to determine the effect of an individualized preoperative educational intervention on interference, due to pain, with activities on postoperative day 3, and the effect of this educational intervention on nausea, pain, and analgesic and antiemetic administration on postoperative days 1, 2, and 3. Topics covered in the intervention included the importance of pain management to promote activity, communicating with health care providers, asking for analgesics and antiemetics, misbeliefs about taking medications, and nonpharmacological measures.

Methods

The sample of 143 participants was randomized to the intervention group or to standard care. Those in the standard group got the usual teaching. Those in the intervention group received the usual teaching plus a booklet on symptom management, an individual teaching session, and a follow-up support call.

Results

The results revealed that there were no differences between the two groups. Participants had severe nausea and pain and yet received antiemetics and analgesics in insufficient doses. The authors concluded that more than individualized teaching is required to reflect a change in symptom management. They suggest that further research is needed on modifying factors in the hospital system to bring about change in symptom management.

From Wilson, R., Watt-Watson, J., Hodnett, E., et al. (2016). A randomized controlled trial of an individualized preoperative education intervention for symptom management after total knee arthroplasty. *Orthopaedic Nursing, 35*(1), 20–28. [Seminal Research].

introduce to the patient the use of a pain instrument to rate the presence and severity of pain postoperatively (see Chapter 32). Several instruments for both pediatric and adult patients are available. Frequent pain assessments with the patient are necessary to alert the nurse to treat the pain and assess the adequacy (outcome) of pain interventions.

Review of Emotional Health. Surgery is psychologically stressful. The patient may be anxious about the surgery and its implications. Patients often feel that they are powerless over their situation. Family members may perceive the patient's surgery as a disruption of their lifestyle. Hospitalization and the recovery period at home may be lengthy. The family is usually concerned about the patient returning to a normal, productive life. When the patient has chronic illness, the family may be fearful that surgery will result in further disability or may be hopeful that the patient will improve. To understand the impact of surgery on a patient's and a family's emotional health, the nurse should assess the patient's feelings about surgery, self-concept, body image, and coping resources.

It is often difficult to assess feelings thoroughly when ambulatory surgery is scheduled; nurses usually have less time to establish a relationship with patients. In some day surgical programs, the nurse may visit with a patient in the home or on the telephone before surgery. If visiting in a hospital room, the nurse should choose a time for discussion after admitting procedures or diagnostic tests have been completed. The nurse should explain to the patient that it is normal to have fears and concerns. The patient's ability to share feelings partially depends on the nurse's willingness to listen, be supportive, and clarify misconceptions.

If the patient feels powerless, the nurse should attempt to determine the reason. The medical diagnosis may generate apprehension of increased dependence and loss of physical or mental function. The thought of being "put to sleep" under anaesthesia may create concern about loss of control. Most patients want to retain the power to make decisions about treatment. Nurses must assure patients of their right to ask questions and seek information.

A patient may be angry about the need for surgery. For example, a young person may feel that it is unfair to have a disorder that typically affects older people. Surgery may occur at a time when it is inconvenient or potentially disruptive. The patient occasionally may express anger verbally at the nurse or the physician. Being argumentative or overly demanding, refusing to cooperate, and criticizing the health care team's efforts to provide care are manifestations of the patient's anger and anxiety.

Body Image. Surgical removal of any diseased body part may leave permanent disfigurement or alteration in body function. Loss of certain body functions (e.g., with a colostomy or ureterostomy) may compound patients' fears. Nurses should assess for the body-image alterations that patients perceive will result from surgery. Patients will respond differently depending on their culture, self-concept, and degree of self-esteem (see Chapter 27). Excision of breast tissue, colostomy, ureterostomy, hysterectomy, or removal of the prostate gland may affect patients' perceptions of their sexuality.

Nurses should encourage patients to express their concerns about sexuality. The patient facing even temporary sexual dysfunction requires understanding and support. Discussions about the patient's sexuality should be held with the patient's sexual partner so that both individuals can gain a shared understanding of how to cope with limitations in sexual function.

Coping Resources. When reviewing the patient's coping resources, it is important to ask them about specific family members and friends who may provide support. Once they are identified, these individuals should be included in any patient teaching and interventions aimed at

managing stress and anxiety. If the patient has had previous surgery, the nurse should determine what behaviours helped to resolve any tension or nervousness. The nurse may instruct the patient on relaxation exercises that can help control anxiety.

Culture. Patients come from diverse cultural and religious backgrounds that affect the way they perceive and react to their surgical experience. If cultural, ethnic, and religious differences are not acknowledged and incorporated into the perioperative care plan, desired surgical outcomes may not be achieved. Therefore, learning about a patient's cultural and ethnic heritage can help nurses provide effective perioperative care. Although it is important to recognize and plan for differences based on culture, nurses also must recognize that members of the same culture are individuals and may not hold these shared beliefs. Box 49.2 highlights some cultural care aspects in the perioperative period.

Patient Expectations. Patients rely on their caregivers for information, comfort, pain control, adequate monitoring, and performance of interventions that ensure their safety throughout the surgical

---

🌐 BOX 49.2 CULTURAL ASPECTS OF CARE

Providing Culturally Sensitive Care to Patients Undergoing Surgery

Providing individualized education and perioperative nursing care to patients of various cultural, religious, and ethnic groups can be challenging. Using a variety of resources available within a health care agency, whether in written from or from the Internet, will help nurses to provide culturally sensitive care (Giese et al., 2017).

Implications for Practice

- Preoperative assessment should include a cultural assessment with questions regarding such topics as primary language spoken, feelings about surgery and pain, pain management, expectations, support system, and feelings toward self-care with postoperative implications (e.g., Does the patient relate to a concept of pain? Does the patient have feelings about the gender of the caregiver? Does the patient follow customs that give family members control over decisions? Does the patient have religious convictions that affect perioperative care, such as opposition to the administration of blood products?).
- Use the services of a professional interpreter, if necessary, to communicate with a patient. Use sensitivity if a professional interpreter is needed to communicate with a patient, because some patients may have difficulty sharing personal health information with people who are younger than themselves or are of a specific gender.
- Use pictures or phrase cards with various languages to communicate with a patient whose language is different from yours; these cards can be used to assess pain, comfort, temperature, need to void, and so forth.
- Provide preoperative and postoperative educational materials in a variety of languages.

Resources

Cultural Competence Guidelines for the Delivery of Primary Health Care in Nova Scotia (2011): https://novascotia.ca/dhw/diversity/documents/CulturalCompetenceGuidelines_Summer08-Nova-Scotia.pdf

Cultural Competence: Staff of the College of Physicians and Surgeons of the Nova Scotia (2013): From a URL formerly found at http://robertswright.ca/upload/385169/documents/9D72177FDED76DFC.pdf

Promoting Cultural Competence in Nursing. (2018). Canadian Nurses Association: https://hl-prod-ca-oc-download.s3-ca-central-1.amazonaws.com/CNA/2f975e7e-4a40-45ca-863c-5ebf0a138d5e/UploadedImages/documents/Position_Statement_Promoting_Cultural_Competence_in_Nursing.pdf

experience. Nurses need to have a caring attitude, advocate for the patient, be skilled in surgical assessment and interventions, and anticipate the patient's needs throughout the perioperative period. Nurses must understand the patient's expectations in order to develop an individualized care plan. Does the patient expect full pain relief or simply to have pain reduced? Does the patient expect to be independent immediately after surgery, or do they expect to be fully dependent on nursing staff or on family members? These are only a few of the questions that need to be asked of the surgical patient to establish a care plan congruent with their needs and expectations.

Physical Examination. Nurses should conduct a partial or complete physical examination, depending on the patient's preoperative condition (see Chapter 33). Assessment focuses on findings related to the patient's medical history and on body systems that likely will be affected by the surgery.

General Survey. The nurse should first observe the patient's general appearance. Gestures and body movements may reflect weakness caused by illness. The patient may appear malnourished. Height, body weight, and history of recent weight loss are important indicators of nutritional status.

Preoperative vital signs, including blood pressure while sitting and standing, provide important baseline data with which alterations that occur during and after surgery can be compared. Some institutions request that blood pressure be obtained in both arms for comparison. Anxiety and fear commonly cause elevations in heart rate and blood pressure. As the effects of the anaesthesia diminish after surgery, vital sign findings are compared with the preoperative baseline. Preoperative assessment of vital signs is also important to rule out fluid and electrolyte abnormalities (see Chapter 31).

An elevated temperature before surgery is a cause for concern. If the patient has an underlying infection, the surgeon may choose to postpone surgery until the infection has been treated. An elevated body temperature increases the risk for fluid and electrolyte imbalances after surgery.

Head and Neck. The condition of oral mucous membranes is one indicator of the patient's level of hydration. A dehydrated patient is at risk for developing serious fluid and electrolyte imbalances during surgery. Inspection of the soft palate and nasal sinuses can reveal sinus drainage, indicative of respiratory or sinus infection. Cervical lymph node enlargement may reveal local or systemic infection.

The jugular veins should be inspected for distension. Excess fluid within the circulatory system or failure of the heart to contract efficiently may lead to jugular vein distension and reveal a risk for cardiovascular complications during surgery.

During the examination of the oral mucosa, loose or capped teeth must be identified because they could become dislodged during endotracheal intubation. Dentures must be noted so that they can be removed before surgery, especially if general anaesthesia is required.

Integument. The nurse should carefully inspect the skin, especially over bony prominences, such as the heels, elbows, sacrum, and scapula. During surgery, a patient must lie in a fixed position, often for several hours. As a result, the patient may have an increased risk for pressure injuries (see Chapter 47), especially if the patient is older and skin is thin and dry and has poor turgor. Chronic use of steroids also increases the patient's susceptibility to skin tears. In addition, the overall condition of the skin reveals the patient's level of hydration.

Thorax and Lungs. Assessment of the patient's breathing pattern and chest excursion aids in assessing ventilatory capacity. A decline in ventilatory function places the patient at risk for respiratory complications. For example, a patient who has high abdominal surgery will have difficulty breathing deeply because of a painful abdominal incision.

Auscultation of breath sounds will indicate whether the patient has pulmonary congestion or narrowing of airways.

Existing atelectasis or moisture in the airways will be aggravated during surgery. Serious pulmonary congestion may cause postponement of the surgery. Certain anaesthetics can cause laryngeal muscle spasm; thus, if wheezing in the airways is heard on auscultation preoperatively, the patient is at risk for further airway narrowing during surgery and after extubation (removal of the endotracheal tube). The physician should be made aware of these findings.

Heart and Vascular System. The nurse should assess the character of the apical, radial, and peripheral pulses; the capillary refill; and the colour and temperature of the patient's extremities. If peripheral pulses are not palpable, a Doppler instrument should be used to assess their presence. Acceptable capillary refill occurs in less than 3 seconds. Measurement of capillary refill and assessment of peripheral pulses are particularly important for the patient undergoing vascular surgery or orthopedic surgery (see Chapter 33).

Abdomen. The abdomen should be assessed for size, shape, symmetry, and presence of distension. Assessment of preoperative bowel sounds is useful as a baseline. The nurse also should ask the patient whether they have regular bowel movements and inquire about the colour and consistency of stools.

Neurological Status. Preoperative assessment of neurological status is imperative for all patients who will be receiving general anaesthesia. The baseline neurological status assists with the assessment of ascent from anaesthesia. During the health history and physical assessment, the nurse observes the patient's level of orientation, alertness, and mood, noting whether the patient answers questions appropriately and can recall recent and past events. A patient who will have surgery for neurological disease (e.g., brain tumour or aneurysm) may demonstrate an impaired level of consciousness or altered behaviour.

If the patient is scheduled for spinal anaesthesia, preoperative assessment of gross motor function and strength is important. Spinal anaesthesia causes temporary paralysis of the lower extremities. The nurse should be aware if a patient enters surgery with weakness or impaired mobility of the lower extremities so that, when the spinal anaesthetic wears off, full motor function is not expected to return.

Diagnostic Screening. Before a patient has surgery, the surgeon may order diagnostic tests as determined by the patient's history and physical assessment. Table 49.6 lists common diagnostic tests performed

TABLE 49.6	Common Diagnostic Tests Performed Preoperatively Based on Patient History
History	**Tests**
Hepatic disease	International normalized ratio (INR); activated partial thromboplastin time (aPTT); liver enzymes, such as serum aspartate aminotransferase; alkaline phosphatase
Cardiovascular disease	Blood urea nitrogen (BUN), creatinine, complete blood count (CBC), chest X-ray, electrocardiogram (ECG)
Pulmonary disease	CBC, chest X-ray, ECG, blood gases
Central nervous system disease	White blood cell (WBC) count, electrolytes, BUN, creatinine, glucose, electroencephalography (EEG)
Medications	
Diuretics	Electrolytes, and perhaps BUN and creatinine
Steroids	Electrolytes, glucose
Anticoagulants	INR, aPTT

preoperatively based on the patient's medical history. The tests ordered are also determined by the procedure itself. For procedures where blood loss is expected (e.g., hip and knee replacements), a type and cross-match would be indicated preoperatively. The surgeon will designate the number of blood units to have available during surgery. Table 49.7 outlines the purpose and normal values for the more common blood tests. If diagnostic tests reveal severe health problems, the surgeon may cancel surgery until the condition stabilizes. Nurses are responsible for the preparation of patients for diagnostic studies and for coordinating completion of the tests. Nurses also review diagnostic results as they become available, not only to alert physicians to these findings and to assist with planning appropriate therapy, but also to integrate these findings into nursing decisions related to patient care.

If a patient has a history of heart disease, an electrocardiogram (ECG) is usually ordered. The ECG measures the electrical activity of the heart to assess the heart rate, rhythm, and other factors. A chest X-ray (an examination of the condition of the heart and lungs) is usually required for thoracic surgery or if the patient has certain medical conditions.

Pulmonary function testing and arterial blood gas analysis may be performed on patients with pre-existing lung disease. Blood glucose levels and glycosylated hemoglobin (HbA1c) are measured on patients with diabetes. HbA1c measures the amount of hemoglobin A1c in the blood, which reflects the patient's average blood glucose level over the long term (Pagana et al., 2019).

Autologous infusions are an option for some patients who choose to donate their own blood before surgery. Although Canadian Blood Services screens all blood donors and blood products for infections such as human immunodeficiency virus (HIV) and hepatitis, some patients are more comfortable donating their own blood. The donation usually must be made several weeks before the scheduled surgery. Because of the short time frame now from preadmission to the day of surgery, autologous infusions may not always be possible as there may not be enough time to complete the process. Autotransfusion via the use of a

TABLE 49.7	Diagnostic Screening for Surgical Patients
Measurement and Normal Values	**Interpretation**

Complete Blood Count (CBC)
Red blood cells (RBCs):
  Men: $4.7–6.1 \times 10^{12}$/L;
  Women: $4.2–5.4 \times 10^{12}$/L
Hemoglobin (Hgb):
  Men: 140–180 mmol/L;
  Women: 120–160 mmol/L
Hematocrit (Hct):
  Men: 0.42–0.52;
  Women: 0.37–0.47
White blood cells (WBCs):
  Adults and children >2 years: $5–10 \times 10^{9}$/L
	Peripheral venous sample of blood measures RBCs, WBCs, Hgb, and Hct. May reveal infection, low blood volume, and potential for oxygenation problems. Surgeon may order blood replacement.

Serum Electrolytes *Sodium (Na):* 136–145 mmol/L *Potassium (K):* 3.5–5.0 mmol/L *Chloride (Cl):* 98–106 mmol/L *Bicarbonate (HCO₃):* 22–26 mmol/L	Peripheral venous sample of blood reveals significant fluid and electrolyte imbalances preoperatively. Attention is given to Na, K, and Cl levels. Intravenous (IV) fluid replacement may be indicated preoperatively.
Coagulation Studies *International normalized ratio (INR):* 0.8–1.20 *Activated partial thromboplastin time (aPTT):* 30–40 seconds *Platelets:* $150–400 \times 10^{9}$/L	INR, aPTT, and platelet counts reveal clotting ability of blood. These studies are used to indicate patients at risk for bleeding tendencies or thrombus formation.
Serum Creatinine *Men:* 53–106 mcmol/L *Women:* 44–97 mcmol/L	Ability of kidneys to excrete creatinine, a by-product of muscle metabolism, indicates renal function. Elevated level can indicate renal failure.
Blood Urea Nitrogen (BUN) 3.6–7.1 mmol/L	Ability of kidneys to excrete urea and nitrogen indicates renal function. BUN becomes elevated if patient is dehydrated. Preoperative IV fluid replacement may be needed.
Glucose *Fasting:* 4.0–6.0 mmol/L	Finger stick or peripheral blood sample. Patients may require treatment of low or high levels preoperatively and postoperatively. Elevated blood sugar levels are usually the result of a deficiency in insulin secretion (type 1 diabetes), insulin action, or combination of both (type 2 diabetes).

Adapted from MacDonald, S., et al. (2023). *Pagana's Canadian manual of diagnostic and laboratory tests* (3rd ed.). Elsevier Inc.

cell-saver device during surgery may be possible if physicians anticipate large blood loss (e.g., open heart surgery).

◆ Nursing Diagnosis

Nurses cluster patterns of defining characteristics gathered during assessment to identify nursing diagnoses for the surgical patient (Box 49.3). The patient with pre-existing health problems is likely to have a variety of risk diagnoses. For example, a patient with pre-existing bronchitis who has abnormal breath sounds and a productive cough will be at risk for ineffective airway clearance. In addition, a patient who undergoes a surgical procedure is at risk for developing infection at the surgical site, the IV site, or in the bloodstream (sepsis). A diagnosis of risk for infection will require the nurse's attention from admission through convalescence.

The related factors for each diagnosis establish directions for nursing care that will be provided during one or all of the surgical phases. For example, the diagnosis of risk for infection related to an invasive procedure will require different interventions from those if the related factor is inadequate immune response. Preoperative nursing diagnoses enable the nurse to take precautions and actions ensuring that the care provided during the intraoperative and postoperative phases is consistent with the patient's needs.

Nursing diagnoses made preoperatively will also focus on the potential risks a patient may face after surgery. Preventive care is essential so that the surgical patient can be managed effectively. The following are common nursing diagnoses relevant to the surgical patient:

- *Ineffective airway clearance*
- *Risk for allergy response to latex*
- *Anxiety*
- *Disturbed body image*
- *Risk for ineffective thermoregulation*
- *Ineffective breathing pattern*
- *Ineffective coping*
- *Fear*
- *Risk for deficient fluid volume*
- *Risk for infection*
- *Risk for perioperative positioning injury*
- *Deficient knowledge (specify)*
- *Impaired physical mobility*
- *Acute pain*
- *Powerlessness*
- *Impaired skin integrity*
- *Disturbed sleep pattern*
- *Delayed surgical recovery*

◆ Planning

During planning, nurses once again synthesize information from multiple resources (Figure 49.2). For example, knowledge pertaining to adult learning principles, coupled with the patient's unique needs, will ensure a well-designed preoperative teaching plan. Critical thinking ensures that the patient's care plan integrates the nurse's knowledge, previous experience, and established standards of care. Previous experience in caring for surgical patients helps nurses anticipate how to approach patient care (e.g., complications to prevent and anticipate, and methods to reduce anxiety). Professional standards and evidence-informed practices are especially important to consider when developing a care plan, as they provide a scientific basis for selecting effective nursing interventions. Nurses need to develop an individualized care plan for each nursing diagnosis (Box 49.4). The nurse and the patient together can set realistic expectations for care.

Successful planning requires the involvement of both the surgical patient and the family in establishing the care plan. Early patient involvement minimizes surgical risks and postoperative complications. A patient who is well informed about the surgical experience is less likely to be fearful and can prepare to participate in the postoperative recovery phase so that outcomes can be met. Diagnosis, interventions,

---

BOX 49.3 NURSING DIAGNOSTIC PROCESS

Assessment Activities	Defining Characteristics	Nursing Diagnosis
Ask patient to describe previous surgical experiences.	Patient mentions a traumatic prior experience with surgery	*Fear related to knowledge deficit and previous surgical experience*
Ask patient about preoperative education and preparation before admission.	Unaware of preoperative testing	
Observe patient's nonverbal behaviour.	Patient's behaviour indicates fear and tension	
Assess vital signs.	Increased heart rate	

Based on Ackley, B. J., Ladwig, G. B., Makic, M. B., et al. (2020). *Nursing diagnosis handbook: An evidenced based guide to planning care* (12th ed.). Elsevier.

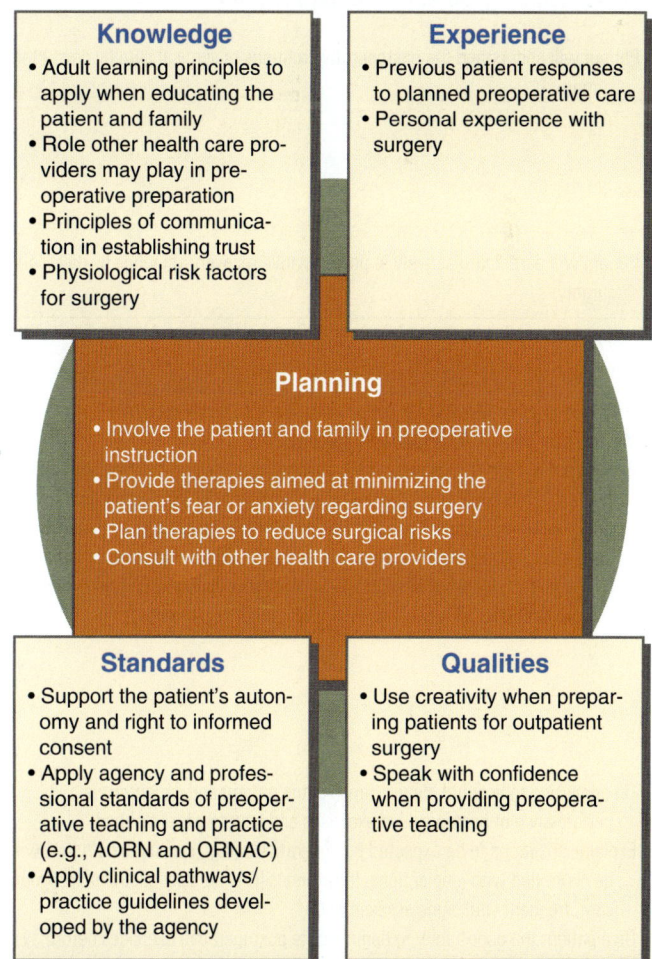

Knowledge
- Adult learning principles to apply when educating the patient and family
- Role other health care providers may play in preoperative preparation
- Principles of communication in establishing trust
- Physiological risk factors for surgery

Experience
- Previous patient responses to planned preoperative care
- Personal experience with surgery

Planning
- Involve the patient and family in preoperative instruction
- Provide therapies aimed at minimizing the patient's fear or anxiety regarding surgery
- Plan therapies to reduce surgical risks
- Consult with other health care providers

Standards
- Support the patient's autonomy and right to informed consent
- Apply agency and professional standards of preoperative teaching and practice (e.g., AORN and ORNAC)
- Apply clinical pathways/practice guidelines developed by the agency

Qualities
- Use creativity when preparing patients for outpatient surgery
- Speak with confidence when providing preoperative teaching

FIGURE 49.2 Critical thinking model for surgical patient planning. *AORN,* Association of periOperative Registered Nurses; *ORNAC,* Operating Room Nurses Association of Canada.

◎ BOX 49.4   NURSING CARE PLAN

Deficient Knowledge Regarding Preoperative and Postoperative Care Requirements

ASSESSMENT

Elisa (preferred pronouns: she/her) is an 80-year-old woman scheduled to be admitted in 5 days for elective bowel resection. Joe (preferred pronouns: he/him) is the nurse in the clinic surgery service assigned to prepare Elisa for surgery.

During his initial discussion with Elisa, Joe observes her to be alert and oriented. Elisa has severely reduced visual acuity but is able to hear Joe's questions clearly.

Assessment Activities

Ask the patient about previous surgeries and her experience with them.

Ask the patient what she has been told regarding her surgery.

Ask the patient what she has been told regarding preoperative preparation and what to expect postoperatively.

Assess the patient's ability to read typical font type.

Assess the patient's family and support system for preoperative and postoperative assistance.

Findings and Defining Characteristics

She responds, "I had surgery over 20 years ago, and I was in the hospital for 10 days."

She states that her surgeon explained the procedure using a picture of the bowel and indicating the location of the part to be removed.

She states that she received information from the surgeon's office regarding medicines to stop taking and those she should take on the morning of surgery, her diet before surgery and when to stop eating, and whom to call with questions. She does not recall receiving information regarding what to expect postoperatively.

She is unable to read the text font on the newspaper; she can read the headlines with her glasses.

She states that her daughter will be coming into town on the day of surgery to help her after surgery.

NURSING DIAGNOSIS: Deficient knowledge regarding preoperative and postoperative care requirements related to lack of exposure to information.

PLANNING

Goals (Nursing Outcomes Classification)*

Patient will understand the postoperative routines of surgical care by day before surgery.

Patient will participate actively in postoperative recovery activities by day 1 after surgery.

Expected Outcomes

Knowledge of Treatment Procedures

Patient will discuss monitoring routines after surgery by morning of surgery in the preoperative period.

Patient will be able to describe importance of postoperative exercises by morning of surgery, including turn, cough, and deep breathing; incentive spirometer; and leg exercises.

Patient will be able to describe schedule for activity and nutritional management postoperatively by day 1 after surgery.

Patient will successfully perform postoperative exercises by morning of surgery in the preoperative period.

*Outcome classification labels from Moorhead, S., Swanson, E., Johnson, M., et al. (Eds.). (2018). *Nursing outcomes classification (NOC)* (6th ed.). Mosby/Elsevier.

INTERVENTIONS

Interventions (Nursing Interventions Classification)†

Teaching in the Preoperative Period

Provide patient and her daughter with hospital website and YouTube instructions that explain preoperative and postoperative routines. Supply instruction booklet designed for the visually impaired. Make a follow-up call to patient and to her daughter to give them an opportunity to ask questions and voice concerns. Document all phases of education—preoperative before admission, day of surgery, and postoperative—provided to patient in her record.

Rationale

Preadmission education can require less teaching time and better performance of exercises on admission. Knowing what to expect can help to reduce anxiety in patients who are undergoing surgery. Carr and colleagues (2005) conducted a study with women undergoing major gynecological surgery, to explore the impact of anxiety and depression on pain experience over time following surgery. The results revealed that preoperative anxiety was predictive of postoperative anxiety as well as higher pain scores and that nurses need to identify these patients so that interventions can be implemented. In addition, the authors suggested that patients may benefit from specific information, such as length of stay or what the pain will be like.

On admission to hospital, demonstrate to the patient and daughter the performance of postoperative exercises and how to get out of bed.

Demonstration is an effective method to reinforce didactic instruction.

Explain sensations to be expected postoperatively (e.g., incisional pain that will be controlled with medications, intravenous [IV] line, nasogastric tube, wound care, frequent vital signs assessments).

Teaching about sensory aspects (what the patient sees, feels, smells) should be structured.

Give patient the opportunity to demonstrate postoperative exercises before surgery.

Return demonstration indicates patient learning and provides an opportunity to reinforce instruction.

Continued

BOX 49.4 NURSING CARE PLAN—cont'd

Interventions (Nursing Interventions Classification)†	Rationale
Correct any unrealistic expectations that the patient or daughter may have regarding surgery.	Unrealistic expectations, when unmet, can contribute to a patient's anxiety. Psychological preparation for surgery reduces anxiety.

†Intervention classification labels from Butcher, H. K., Bulechek, G. M., McCloskey Dochterman, J. M., et al. (Eds.). (2019). *Nursing interventions classification (NIC)* (7th ed.). Mosby.

EVALUATION

Nursing Actions	Patient Response and Finding	Achievement of Outcome
Ask patient to describe typical monitoring and care activities after surgery. Document evaluation of patient's understanding and demonstration of learned activities in the patient's record.	Patient is able to verbalize typical monitoring and care after surgery. She states that the instruction booklet and YouTube instructions were both helpful.	The patient has a good understanding of the typical postoperative course.
Observe patient's demonstration of postoperative exercises.	Patient is able to demonstrate leg exercises and deep-breathing and coughing exercises.	Patient is able to demonstrate the postoperative exercises her daughter showed her.
Explore with the patient and daughter if they have any remaining fears or concerns.	Both the patient and her daughter deny any fears or concerns at the present time.	Informational and psychological needs of the patient and her daughter have been met.

and outcomes are established to ensure recovery or maintenance of the preoperative state.

Goals and Outcomes. The preoperative care plan is based on individualized nursing diagnoses. This plan is reviewed and modified during the intraoperative and postoperative periods. Outcomes established for each goal of care provide measurable behavioural evidence to gauge the patient's progress toward meeting the stated goals.

The following example provides a goal of care and expected outcomes relevant for the preoperative surgical patient:

- Patient is able to verbalize the significance of postoperative exercises.
- Patient verbalizes prevention of lung congestion and pneumonia as reasons for deep-breathing and coughing exercises.
- Patient verbalizes promotion of blood flow to prevent leg clots as reason for postoperative leg exercises.
- Patient verbalizes rationale for early ambulation, as it improves lung function, assists with return of bowel function, and promotes recovery.

Note: Incentive spirometry as a treatment is used much less now or not at all in the hospital setting. A review by Liu and colleagues (2019) concluded that incentive spirometry may be beneficial for patients undergoing thoracic surgery to prevent postoperative complications, such as pneumonia. The authors recommended randomized clinical trials to confirm its effectiveness. Postoperative physiotherapy regimens with or without incentive spirometry appeared to be effective following thoracic surgery, compared to no physiotherapy. In Restrepo and colleagues' (2011) update on the American Association of Respiratory Care Clinical Practice Guidelines related to incentive spirometry, the authors made several recommendations, one of which is that incentive spirometry alone is not recommended for routine use in pre- and postoperative care. The guideline also suggests that deep-breathing exercises provide the same benefit as incentive spirometry in the pre- and postoperative setting.

Setting Priorities. Using clinical judgement, nurses should prioritize nursing diagnoses and interventions based on the assessed unique needs of each patient. Patients who need emergency surgery may experience changes in their physiological status that require the nurse to reprioritize quickly. For example, if a patient's blood pressure begins to drop, hemodynamic stabilization becomes a priority over

education. Generally, when the preoperative situation is more controlled, the approach to each patient needs to reflect an understanding of the implications of the patient's age, physical and psychological health, educational level, and cultural and religious practices. Increasingly, patients are preparing advanced medical directives to indicate their wishes regarding any unexpected aggressive medical treatment that might arise.

◆ Implementation

Preoperative nursing interventions provide the patient with an understanding of the surgery and prepare the patient not only physically and psychologically for surgical intervention but also to be an active participant in the recovery process.

Informed Consent. Surgery cannot be legally or ethically performed until a patient understands the need for a procedure, the steps involved, the risks, the expected results, and alternative treatments. The surgeon is responsible for explaining the procedure and obtaining the **informed consent**. Often, the consent is signed in the physician's office or in the preadmission unit. If, as a nurse, you are involved in obtaining the signature, you must ensure before signing that the patient understands the procedure. If the patient is unclear about the procedure, the consent should not be signed and the physician should be notified (see Chapter 10).

Preoperative Teaching. Education is an important aspect of the patient's surgical experience. Preoperative teaching reflects a patient's expected postoperative course of events and has a positive influence on the patient's recovery.

Nurses in preadmission clinics may contact patients up to 1 week before surgery to answer the patient's questions and reinforce explanations. Preoperative information and instructions may include telephone calls, mailings from the physician's office or hospital, preoperative teaching guidelines and checklists, and the use of hospital websites or **clinical pathways** (Figure 49.3).

Pritchard (2011) has discussed the importance of giving appropriate information to patients preoperatively. Information needs to be tailored to address patients' individual needs; this targeted information, then, is meaningful to the patient. Establishing a relationship with patients facilitates understanding of their specific situation so that information given addresses their concerns. Pritchard (2011) suggests

FIGURE 49.3 Preoperative patient instructions for a clinical pathway for a total hip arthroplasty. The first day of a 6-day pathway highlights what the patient can expect before surgery. *DVT*, Deep venous thrombosis; *NVS*, neuro vital signs; *PVA*, peripheral vascular assessment. (Courtesy The Ottawa Hospital, Ottawa, ON.)

Patient _____   Chart No. _____

Day of Surgery Post-op / Post Anesthetic Care Unit (PACU)

Date: yyaa _____ mm _____ dj _____

Critical Path	Patient Outcomes
Oxygen saturation monitoring (SpO$_2$) and oxygen administration per oxygen titration protocol. **Vital signs (VS), assessment, treatment, and teaching per PACU standards of care.** **Additional Orders** • Bedrest • NPO to clear fluids prn • Pillow between knees • In/out catheterization as ordered • May transfer to ward when PACU discharge criteria is achieved	**Pain Control** • Indicates adequate pain control. Pain equal or less than 3 at rest, equal or less than 5 with activity; pain not preventing movement; patient satisfied with pain control. • Achieves PACU discharge criteria for transfer to ward

Patient progress corresponds with clinical pathway

☐ Yes ☐ No   Signature: _____ , Initial _____ Time: _____   NTV – circle above, VC _____

D = 8-12 h day shift	**E** = evening shift, if applicable	**N** = 8-12 h night shift

Variance Codes (VC)	**186**	Activity variance	**NTV**	Non-Tracked Variance
	492	Not discharged by end of pathway – continued need for acute care	**OFF**	Ordered off clinical pathway
	510	Not discharged by end of pathway – non-medical reason		

CHART
FIGURE 49.3, cont'd

Patient _____   Chart No. _____

Day of Surgery Post-op Ward

Date: yyaa _____   mm _____   dj _____

Critical Path	**Patient Outcomes**
Assessments/Treatments • VS, PVA/NVS, SpO$_2$, pain q4h × 24 hrs • Monitor dressing q4 hours • Pillow between legs at all times • Pain management per Acute Pain Service (APS) or Orthopedic orders as applicable • Oxygen per Oxygen Titration Protocol	**Assessments/Treatments** • Minimal oozing on dressing **Pain Control** • Indicates adequate pain control. Pain equal or less than 3 at rest, equal or less than 5 with activity; pain not preventing movement; patient satisfied with pain control.
Activity • Deep breathing and coughing (DB & C) • Up in chair × 1 _____ initial if able • Mobilize if able • Activity as tolerated • **Verify orders for Weight bearing status and hip precautions**	**Activity** • Completes transfer with assistance • Demonstrates understanding of positioning while in bed
Nutrition • Diet as ordered	**Nutrition** • Able to tolerate diet as ordered
Elimination • Monitor bowel sounds and elimination	**Elimination** • Patient has bowel sounds • Patient able to void

Patient Teaching
• Reinforce:
  – DB & C
  – Ankle pumping exercises
  – Pillow positioning to maintain good alignment
• Pain management
• Hip precautions
• Weight bearing status
• Bowel management
• Ensure patient has Total Hip Arthroplasty booklet
	Prevention of DVT
	• Performs ankle pumping exercises
	• Prophylaxis medication started
	
	Patient Teaching
	• Demonstrates:
	  – DB & C
	  – Pillow positioning and leg alignment
	  – Ankle pumping exercises
	  – Understanding of hip precautions
	  – Understanding of pain management
	  – Understanding of weight bearing status
	  – Use of mobility aids

Discharge Planning • Review discharge plan and consult appropriate health-care provider if potential problems identified – Possible discharge tomorrow if discharge criteria met	

Patient progress corresponds with clinical pathway

D ☐ Yes ☐ No   Signature: _____ ,   Initial _____   Time: _____   NTV – circle above, VC _____

E ☐ Yes ☐ No   Signature: _____ ,   Initial _____   Time: _____   NTV – circle above, VC _____

N ☐ Yes ☐ No   Signature: _____ ,   Initial _____   Time: _____   NTV – circle above, VC _____

D = 8-12 h day shift	**E** = evening shift, if applicable	**N** = 8-12 h night shift

Variance Codes (VC)	**186**	Activity variance	**NTV**	Non-Tracked Variance
	492	Not discharged by end of pathway – continued need for acute care	**OFF**	Ordered off clinical pathway
	510	Not discharged by end of pathway – non-medical reason		

FIGURE 49.3, cont'd

Patient _____ Chart No. _____

Post-op Day 1

Date: yyaa _____ mm _____ dj _____

Critical Path	**Patient Outcomes**

Assessments/Treatments
- VS with SpO$_2$, PVA/NVS q shift
- Pain assessment q4h
- Discontinue saline lock if IV access no longer required
- Monitor dressing q4h
- Discontinue bulky dressing and change to strip dressing
- Pillow between legs at all times
- Pain management as per APS or Orthopedic orders as applicable
- Wean off APS pain modality if applicable
- Oxygen per Oxygen Titration Protocol. Wean if possible.

Activity
- **Verify orders for Weight bearing status and hip precautions**
- DB & C
- Exercise program with Physiotherapy
- Up in chair × 3:
  at _____ initial _____   at _____ initial _____
  at _____ initial _____
- Ambulate
- Gait training on stairs if applicable

Nutrition
- Diet as ordered

Elimination
- Monitor bowel sounds and elimination

Patient Teaching
- Reinforce:
  – DB & C
  – Ankle pumping exercises
  – Pillow positioning to maintain good alignment
- Pain management
- Hip precautions
- Weight bearing status
- Bowel management
- Ensure patient has Total Hip Arthroplasty booklet

Discharge Planning
- Review discharge plan

Discharge
- Consider for possible discharge today if discharge criteria met
- If unable to discharge today, discuss discharge plan with patient

Assessments/Treatments
- Minimal oozing on dressing

Pain Control
- Indicates adequate pain control. Pain equal or less than 3 at rest, equal or less than 5 with activity; pain not preventing movement; patient satisfied with pain control.

Wound
- Minimal oozing
- Incision dry and intact
- Edges well approximated

Activity
- Completes transfer with assistance progressing to independent
- Ambulates with assistance progressing to independent
- Performs exercises according to self-directed exercise program
- Ambulates in stairs as needed

Nutrition
- Able to tolerate diet as ordered

Elimination
- Voiding well
- Patient has bowel sounds

Patient Teaching
- Demonstrates:
  – DB & C
  – Pillow position and leg alignment
  – Ankle pumping exercises
  – Understanding of hip precautions
  – Understanding of pain management
  – Understanding of weight bearing status
  – Use of mobility aids

Discharge Criteria for Early Discharge Pathway
- Post-op x-ray arranged
- No evidence of DVT
- No discharge/redness/swelling from incision
- Ambulates independently/safely with mobility devices
- Manages stairs as needed
- Time to Up and Go Test score less than or equal to 30 seconds
- **Patient and family verbalizes/understands:**
  – Post discharge care   – Pain management
  – Signs and symptoms of DVT   – Bowel management
  – Emergency resources   – Hip precautions
  – Wound care   – Exercise program
  – Equipment recommendations for home safety

Patient progress corresponds with clinical pathway	**D** = 8-12 h day shift	**E** = evening shift, if applicable	**N** = 8-12 h night shift

D ☐ Yes ☐ No   Signature: _____ ,   Initial _____   Time: _____   NTV – circle above, VC _____

E ☐ Yes ☐ No   Signature: _____ ,   Initial _____   Time: _____   NTV – circle above, VC _____

N ☐ Yes ☐ No   Signature: _____ ,   Initial _____   Time: _____   NTV – circle above, VC _____

Variance Codes (VC)	**186**	Activity variance	**NTV**	Non-Tracked Variance
	492	Not discharged by end of pathway – continued need for acute care	**OFF**	Ordered off clinical pathway
	510	Not discharged by end of pathway – non-medical reason		

CP 04 A (4 – 6)   **CHART**   © THE OTTAWA HOSPITAL – L'HÔPITAL D'OTTAWA

FIGURE 49.3, cont'd

Patient _____   Chart No. _____

Post-op Day 2

Date: yyaa _____   mm _____   dj _____

Critical Path	Patient Outcomes

Critical Path

Assessments/Treatments
- VS, PVA/NVS q shift
- Pain assessment q4h
- Discontinue saline lock if IV access no longer required
- Pain management as per Orthopedic orders
- Discontinue Oxygen Titration Protocol

Activity
- **Verify orders for Weight bearing status and hip precautions**
- Continue exercise program
- Up in chair × 3 minimum:
  at _____ initial _____   at _____ initial _____
  at _____ initial _____
- Ambulate
- Gait training on stairs if applicable

Nutrition
- Diet as ordered

Elimination
- Monitor bowel sounds and elimination

Patient Teaching
- Reinforce:
  – DB & C
  – Ankle pumping exercises
  – Pillow positioning to maintain good alignment
- Pain management
- Hip precautions
- Weight bearing status
- Bowel management
- Ensure patient has Total Hip Arthroplasty booklet

Discharge
- Consider for possible discharge today if discharge criteria met
- If unable to discharge today, discuss discharge plan with patient

Patient Outcomes

Assessments/Treatments
- Patient hemodynamically stable

Pain Control
- Indicates adequate pain control. Pain equal or less than 3 at rest, equal or less than 5 with activity; pain not preventing movement; patient satisfied with pain control.

Wound
- Minimal oozing

Activity
- Ambulates independently using assistive devices
- Ambulates on stairs as needed
- Transfers independently using appropriate mobility devices

Nutrition
- Able to tolerate diet as ordered

Elimination
- Patient has bowel sounds
- Patient able to void

Patient Teaching
- Demonstrates:
  – DB & C   – Use of mobility aids
  – Pillow position and leg alignment   – Ankle pumping exercises
  – Understanding of hip precautions   – Understanding of pain management
  – Understanding of weight bearing status

Discharge Criteria
- Post-op x-ray done
- No evidence of DVT
- No discharge/redness/swelling from incision
- Ambulates independently/safely with mobility devices
- Manages stairs as needed
- Time to Up and Go Test score less than or equal to 30 seconds
- **Patient and family verbalizes/understands:**
  – Post discharge care   – Pain management
  – Signs and symptoms of DVT   – Bowel management
  – Emergency resources   – Hip precautions
  – Wound care   – Exercise program
  – Equipment recommendations for home safety

Patient progress corresponds with clinical pathway	**D** = 8-12 h day shift	**E** = evening shift, if applicable	**N** = 8-12 h night shift

D ☐ Yes ☐ No   Signature: _____ ,   Initial _____   Time: _____   NTV – circle above, VC _____

E ☐ Yes ☐ No   Signature: _____ ,   Initial _____   Time: _____   NTV – circle above, VC _____

N ☐ Yes ☐ No   Signature: _____ ,   Initial _____   Time: _____   NTV – circle above, VC _____

Variance Codes (VC)	186	Activity variance	NTV	Non-Tracked Variance
	492	Not discharged by end of pathway – continued need for acute care	OFF	Ordered off clinical pathway
	510	Not discharged by end of pathway – non-medical reason		

FIGURE 49.3, cont'd

Patient _____ Chart No. _____

Post-op Day 3

Date: yyaa _____   mm _____   dj _____

Critical Path	Patient Outcomes
Assessments/Treatments • VS with PVA/NVS q shift • Pain assessment q4h • Discontinue saline lock • If incisional drainage notify physician • Pain management as per Orthopedic orders **Activity** • **Verify orders for Weight bearing status and hip precautions** • Continue exercise program • Up in chair × 3 minimum: at _____ initial _____ at _____ initial _____ at _____ initial _____ • Ambulate • Gait training on stairs if applicable **Nutrition** • Diet as ordered **Elimination** • Monitor bowel sounds and elimination **Patient Teaching** • Reinforce: – DB & C – Ankle pumping exercises – Pillow positioning to maintain good alignment • Pain management • Hip precautions • Weight bearing status • Bowel management • Ensure patient has Total Hip Arthroplasty booklet **Discharge Planning** • If unable to discharge today, continue care as per post-op day 3 pathway until discharged **Discharge** • Discharge by 10 a.m. once discharge criteria met unless otherwise indicated by physician	**Pain Control** • Indicates adequate pain control. Pain equal or less than 3 at rest, equal or less than 5 with activity; pain not preventing movement; patient satisfied with pain control. **Activity** • Ambulates independently using assistive devices • Transfers independently using appropriate mobility devices • Ambulates on stairs as needed **Nutrition** • Able to tolerate diet as ordered **Elimination** • Patient has bowel sounds • Patient is voiding **Patient Teaching** • Demonstrates: – DB & C – Pillow position and leg alignment – Ankle pumping exercises – Understanding of hip precautions – Understanding of pain management – Understanding of weight bearing status – Use of mobility aids **Discharge Criteria** • Post-op x-ray done • No evidence of DVT • No discharge/redness/swelling from incision • Ambulates independently/safely with mobility devices • Manages stairs as needed • Time to Up and Go Test score less than or equal to 30 seconds • **Patient and family verbalizes/understands:** – Post discharge care – Pain management – Signs and symptoms of DVT – Bowel management – Emergency resources – Hip precautions – Wound care – Exercise program – Equipment recommendations for home safety

Patient progress corresponds with clinical pathway	**D** = 8-12 h day shift	**E** = evening shift, if applicable	**N** = 8-12 h night shift

D ☐ Yes ☐ No Signature: _____, Initial _____ Time: _____ NTV – circle above, VC _____

E ☐ Yes ☐ No Signature: _____, Initial _____ Time: _____ NTV – circle above, VC _____

N ☐ Yes ☐ No Signature: _____, Initial _____ Time: _____ NTV – circle above, VC _____

Variance Codes (VC)	186	Activity variance		NTV	Non-Tracked Variance
	492	Not discharged by end of pathway – continued need for acute care		OFF	Ordered off clinical pathway
	510	Not discharged by end of pathway – non-medical reason			

CP 04 A (6 – 6)   **CHART**   © THE OTTAWA HOSPITAL – L'HÔPITAL D'OTTAWA

FIGURE 49.3, cont'd

that the use of standard information sheets, such as preoperative information sheets, is not sufficient to address patients' information needs or to reduce their preoperative anxiety.

Including family members in preoperative preparation is advised. Family members need to be aware of the normal expectations after discharge from the hospital. They also may recognize untoward events that may unfold once the patient is home. If anxious relatives do not understand routine postoperative events, their anxiety will likely heighten the patient's fears and concerns. Preoperative preparation of family members can help to minimize anxiety and misunderstanding.

Nurses should provide patients with information about sensations typically experienced after surgery. Preparatory information helps patients anticipate the steps of a procedure and thus helps them form realistic images of the surgical experience. When events occur as predicted, patients are better able to cope and attend to them. For example, in the OR, the anaesthesiologist may apply ointment to patients' eyes to prevent corneal damage. Warning patients about sensations of blurred vision will reduce their anxiety on awakening from surgery. Sensations that may be described include expected pain at the surgical site, tightness of dressings, dryness of the mouth, or a sore throat resulting from an endotracheal tube.

Anxiety and fear are barriers to learning, and both emotions are heightened as surgery approaches. The nurse should assess the surgical patient's readiness and ability to learn. If the patient is capable of and receptive to learning, information should be presented in a logical sequence, beginning with preoperative events and advancing to intraoperative and postoperative routines. The following discussion addresses aspects of patient knowledge that demonstrate a patient's understanding of the surgical experience.

Patient Cites Reasons for Preoperative Instructions and Exercises. If given a rationale for preoperative and postoperative procedures, the patient is better prepared to participate in their own care. Every preoperative teaching program includes explanation and demonstration of postoperative exercises: diaphragmatic breathing, coughing, turning, and leg exercises. These exercises are designed to prevent postoperative complications (Skill 49.1). Physiotherapists, as part of the interprofessional team, can facilitate patient mobility postoperatively.

If the patient is measured for elastic stockings or sequential compression devices, the nurse must teach about the purpose of these devices and the nursing care that will be required after their application (see Chapter 46).

After explaining each exercise, the nurse should demonstrate it. Nurses act as a coach, guiding the patient through each exercise. For example, as a nurse, you need to assess whether the patient is sitting properly and help the patient place their hands in the proper position during breathing. You then allow the patient time for independent practice.

Patient States the Time of Surgery. The patient and family should be told the approximate time that surgery will begin. If the hospital has a busy OR schedule, it is best to let them know whether other procedures are scheduled before the patient's. The surgeon usually informs the patient and family of the anticipated length of surgery. Unanticipated delays may occur for many reasons. The family needs to be aware that delays do not necessarily indicate a problem.

Patient Knows Where the Postoperative Unit Is and Where the Family Will Be During Surgery and Recovery. The unit to which the patient is admitted before surgery may be different from the postoperative unit. The family needs to know where the patient will be taken after surgery. The nurse also should explain where the family can wait and where the surgeon will attempt to find family members after surgery. Many institutions have implemented programs in which the circulating nurse gives periodic reports to the family in the waiting room when prolonged surgeries are involved. If the patient will be taken to a special unit postoperatively, it helps to orient the patient and family

members to the unit's environment before surgery. Programs designed to connect with the family also have been developed in day-surgery areas (Andrews, 2009).

Patient Discusses Anticipated Postoperative Monitoring and Therapies. The patient and family need to know about postoperative events. If they understand the frequency of postoperative vital sign monitoring before surgery occurs, they will be less apprehensive when nurses do this. Nurses can also explain whether the patient is likely to have IV lines, monitoring lines, dressings, or drainage tubes or whether they will require ventilator support.

Patient Describes Surgical Procedures and Postoperative Treatment. After the surgeon has explained the basic purpose of the surgical procedure, the patient may ask the nurse additional questions to clarify any misunderstandings. Pre-established teaching standards, such as those integrated in clinical pathways for preoperative and postoperative care (Figure 49.4), give nurses an excellent guide for instruction. A good starting point is to ask what the patient has been told. If the patient has limited understanding about the surgery, the nurse can provide additional explanations. If necessary, the surgeon can be asked to re-inform the patient.

Patient Describes Postoperative Activity Resumption. The type of surgery a patient undergoes affects the speed with which normal physical activity and regular eating habits can be resumed. Nurses should explain that it is normal to progress gradually in both activity and eating. If the patient tolerates activity and diet well, activity levels will progress more quickly.

Patient Describes Pain-Relief Measures. Typically, one of the patient's fears is pain. The family is also concerned for the patient's comfort. Pain after surgery is to be expected. The nurse should inform the patient and family of interventions available for pain relief (e.g., analgesics, positioning, splinting, and relaxation exercises; see Chapter 32). The patient needs to know the schedule for analgesic medications, their route of administration, and their effects.

Patients having surgery may avoid taking pain-relief medications for fear of becoming dependent on them. Nurses should encourage the patient to use analgesics as needed and explain to the patient that the risks of becoming dependent are minimal. The patient needs to understand that unless the pain is controlled, it will be difficult to participate in postoperative therapy such as mobilization. The patient should be encouraged to inform a nurse before the pain becomes a constant discomfort. If a patient waits until pain becomes excruciating, an analgesic may not provide relief at the dose prescribed. Patients who will have patient-controlled analgesia (PCA) after surgery should be taught how to push the button when they begin to feel discomfort and should understand that use of PCA will not cause overmedication (see Chapter 32). The patient should also understand the length of time it takes for the medication to begin working. Information from preoperative assessment will be helpful to the nurse when teaching about pain-relief measures. Pain reporting and expectations regarding pain management based on a patient's cultural beliefs are areas that need to be explored both individually and systematically through research (Douglas, 1999; Ramer et al., 1999). For example, Lovering (2006) conducted a collaborative inquiry project in Saudi Arabia to examine cultural attitudes and beliefs in patients and staff about the causes, treatment, and experiences of pain.

Patient Expresses Feelings Regarding Surgery. If the patient is admitted to the hospital during the preoperative surgical phase, frequent visits by staff, diagnostic testing, and physical preparation for surgery consume a lot of time; as a result, the patient has few opportunities to reflect on the upcoming surgical experience. Nurses must recognize the patient as a unique individual. The patient and family need time to express their feelings about the surgery. The patient's level of anxiety influences the frequency of discussions. While delivering bedside care, the nurse can encourage

SKILL 49.1	DEMONSTRATING POSTOPERATIVE EXERCISES	◗

Delegation Considerations

The skill of demonstrating postoperative exercises should not be delegated to unregulated care providers (UCPs). However, other aspects of patient care may be delegated. When using UCPs be sure to do the following:

- Educate the UCP to encourage patients to practise exercises regularly, following instruction.
- Instruct the UCP to inform the nurse if patients are unwilling to perform these exercises.

Equipment

- Pillow or wrapped blanket (used to splint surgical incision during coughing)
- Positive expiratory pressure (PEP) device might be used

PROCEDURE

STEPS	RATIONALE
1. Assess the patient's risk for postoperative respiratory complications. Review the medical history to identify presence of chronic pulmonary conditions (e.g., emphysema, chronic bronchitis, asthma), any condition that affects chest wall movement, history of smoking, and presence of reduced hemoglobin.	• General anaesthesia predisposes the patient to respiratory challenges because the lungs are not fully inflated during surgery and the cough reflex is suppressed, so that mucus collects within airway passages. After surgery, the patient may have reduced lung volume and require greater efforts to cough and breathe deeply; inadequate lung expansion can lead to atelectasis and pneumonia. The patient is at greater risk for developing respiratory complications if other chronic lung conditions are present. Smoking damages ciliary clearance and increases mucous secretion. Reduced hemoglobin level can lead to inadequate oxygenation.
2. Assess patient's ability to cough and breathe deeply by having the patient take a deep breath and observing movement of shoulders and chest wall. Measure chest excursion during deep breath. Ask patient to cough after taking a deep breath.	• Reveals maximum potential for chest expansion and ability to cough forcefully; serves as baseline to measure ability to perform exercises after surgery.
3. Assess risk for postoperative thrombus formation. (Older patients, those with active cancer, and those immobilized for more than 3 days are most at risk.) Observe for localized tenderness along the distribution of the venous system, swollen calf or thigh, calf swelling more than 3 cm compared with asymptomatic leg, pitting edema in symptomatic leg, and collateral superficial veins. If any of these signs are present, notify the physician. The most common test for diagnosing deep venous thrombosis (DVT) is ultrasound. A D-dimer test may also be done (National Heart Lung and Blood Institute [NHLBI], 2022).	• Venous stasis, decreased perfusion, and vein trauma exist simultaneously for thrombus formation to occur (Lewis et al., 2023). After general anaesthesia, circulation is slowed, thus increasing the risk for clot formation. Immobilization results in decreased muscular contraction in the lower extremities, which promotes venous stasis.
4. Assess the patient's ability to move independently while in bed.	• Determines existence of any mobility restrictions.
5. Explain postoperative exercises to the patient, including their importance to recovery and physiological benefits.	• Information helps the patient to understand the significance of exercises and can motivate learning. People tend to learn new skills when benefits can be gained.

6. Demonstrate exercises.
  A. Diaphragmatic breathing
    (1) Assist the patient to a comfortable sitting position on side of bed or in a chair or to standing position.
    (2) Stand or sit facing the patient.
    (3) Instruct the patient to place the palms of their hands across from each other, down and along the lower borders of the anterior rib cage. Place tips of third fingers lightly together (see Step 6A[3] illustration). Demonstrate for the patient.
	
	• Upright position facilitates diaphragmatic excursion.
	
	• Allows the patient to observe the breathing exercise.
	• Position of hands allows the patient to feel movement of the chest and abdomen as the diaphragm descends and lungs expand.

STEPS	RATIONALE

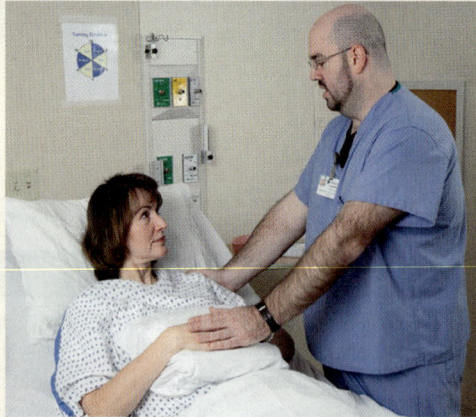

STEP 6A(3) Deep-breathing exercise—placement of hands on upper abdomen during inhalation.

(4) Have the patient take slow, deep breaths, inhaling through the nose and pushing the abdomen against their hands. Tell the patient to feel the middle fingers separate during inhalation. Demonstrate.

- Taking slow, deep breaths prevents panting or hyperventilation. Inhaling through the nose warms, humidifies, and filters air.

(5) Explain that the patient will feel normal downward movement of the diaphragm during inspiration. Explain that abdominal organs descend and the chest wall expands.

- Explanation and demonstration focus on normal ventilatory movement of the chest wall. The patient develops understanding of how diaphragmatic breathing feels.

(6) Avoid using auxiliary chest and shoulder muscles while inhaling and instruct the patient in the same manner.

- Using auxiliary chest and shoulder muscles increases useless energy expenditure.

(7) Have the patient hold a slow, deep breath for a count of three and then slowly exhale through the mouth as if blowing out a candle (with pursed lips). Tell the patient that middle fingertips will touch as the chest wall contracts.

- Allows for gradual expulsion of all air and helps prevent airway collapse by facilitating maintenance of positive airway pressure.

(8) Repeat breathing exercise three to five times.

- Allows the patient to observe a slow, rhythmic breathing pattern.

(9) Have the patient practise the exercise. Instruct the patient to take 10 slow, deep breaths every hour while awake during the postoperative period until mobile.

- Repetition of the exercise reinforces learning. Regular deep breathing helps prevent postoperative complications.

B. Positive expiratory pressure (PEP) device

- The PEP device creates pressure in the lungs and keeps airways from closing. It helps move mucus up.

(1) Perform hand hygiene.

- Reduces transmission of microorganisms.

(2) Set PEP device to the setting ordered. PEP allows exhalation against resistance, therefore increasing airway pressure (Strickland et al., 2013). There is no high-level evidence to support the routine use of PEP, except in patients with cystic fibrosis (Strickland et al., 2013).

- The higher the setting, the more effort will be required by the patient. Ideally, it should deliver 10–20 cm H_2O during passive expiration (American Association for Respiratory Care [AARC], 2003; Cincinnati Children's Hospital Medical Center, 2018).

(3) Instruct the patient to assume semi-Fowler's or high-Fowler's position, and place nose clip on the patient's nose.

- Promotes optimal lung expansion and expectoration of mucus (AARC, 2003).

(4) Have the patient place their lips around the mouthpiece. The patient should take a full breath and then exhale two to three times longer than inhalation. Pattern should be repeated for 10 to 20 breaths.

- Ensures that all breathing is done through the mouth and that the device is used properly.

(5) Remove device from the mouth and have the patient take a slow, deep breath and hold for 3 seconds.

- Promotes lung expansion before coughing.

(6) Instruct the patient to exhale in quick, short, forced exhalations or "huffs."

- "Huff" coughing, or forced expiratory technique, promotes bronchial hygiene through increased expectoration of secretions.

C. Controlled coughing

(1) Explain the importance of maintaining an upright position.

- Position facilitates diaphragm excursion and enhances thorax expansion.

(2) Demonstrate coughing. Take two slow, deep breaths, inhaling through the nose and exhaling through the mouth.

- Deep breaths expand the lungs fully so that air moves behind mucus and facilitates the effects of coughing.

(3) Inhale deeply a third time and hold breath to count of three. Cough fully for two or three consecutive coughs without inhaling between coughs. (Tell the patient to push all air out of lungs.)

- Consecutive coughs help remove mucus more effectively and completely than one forceful cough.

CRITICAL DECISION POINT: *Coughing may be contraindicated after brain or eye surgery.*

Continued

SKILL 49.1   DEMONSTRATING POSTOPERATIVE EXERCISES—cont'd

STEPS	RATIONALE

(4) Caution the patient against simply clearing the throat instead of coughing. Explain that coughing will not cause injury to the incision when done correctly.

(5) If surgical incision will be abdominal or thoracic, teach the patient to place one hand over the incisional area and the other hand on top of it. During breathing and coughing exercises, the patient presses gently against the incisional area to splint or support it. Placing a pillow over the incision is optional (see Step 6C[5] illustration).

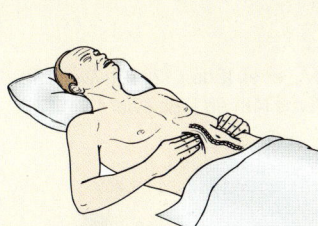

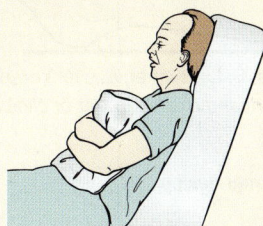

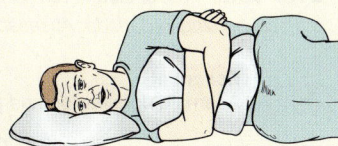

• Clearing the throat does not remove mucus from deep in airways. Postoperative incisional pain makes it harder for the patient to cough effectively.

• Surgical incision cuts through muscles, tissues, and nerve endings. Deep breathing and coughing exercises place additional stress on the suture line and cause discomfort.

• Splinting the incision with hands provides firm support and reduces incisional pulling. (Some patients prefer to have a pillow to place over the incision.)

STEP 6C(5) Techniques for splinting incision. (From Lewis, S. L., Bucher, L., Heitkezmper, M. M., et al. [Eds.]. [2019]. *Medical-surgical nursing in Canada: Assessment and management of clinical problems* [4th Canadian ed.]. Elsevier.)

(6) The patient continues to practise coughing exercises, splinting imaginary incision. Instruct the patient to cough two to three times every 2 hours while awake.

(7) Instruct the patient to examine sputum for consistency, odour, amount, and colour changes.

D. Turning
(Note that turning properly applies when patient is in hospital, as well as once patient returns home.)

(1) Instruct the patient to assume supine position and move to side of the bed if permitted by surgery. Have the patient move by bending their knees and pressing their heels against the mattress to raise and move the buttocks (see Step 6D[1] illustration). Top side rails on both sides of the bed should be raised.

(2) Instruct the patient to place their right hand over the incisional area to splint it.

• Value of deep coughing with splinting is stressed to expectorate mucus effectively with minimal discomfort.

• Sputum consistency, odour, amount, and colour changes may indicate presence of pulmonary complication, such as pneumonia.

• Positioning begins on side of the bed so that turning to the other side will not cause the patient to roll toward the bed's edge.

• Supports and minimizes pulling on the suture line during turning.

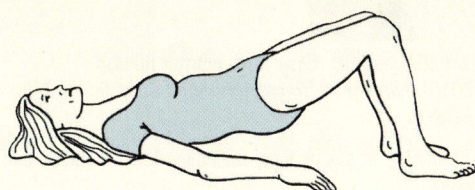

STEP 6D(1) Buttocks lift.

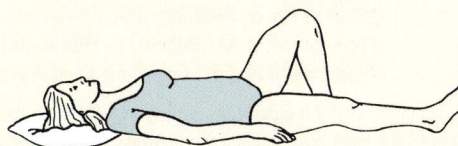

STEP 6D(3) Leg position for turning.

(3) Instruct the patient to keep the right leg straight and flex the left knee up (see Step 6D[3] illustration). If back or vascular surgery was performed, the patient will need to logroll or will require assistance with turning.

(4) Have the patient grab the right side rail with their left hand, pull toward right, and roll onto their right side.

(5) Instruct the patient to turn every 2 hours while awake.

E. Leg exercises
Patients do these in hospital and also once they are at home.

(1) Have the patient assume supine position in bed. Demonstrate leg exercises by performing passive range-of-motion exercises and simultaneously explaining exercise.

(2) Rotate each ankle in a complete circle. Instruct the patient to draw imaginary circles with their big toe (see Step 6E[2] illustration). Repeat five times.

(3) Have patient alternate dorsiflexion and plantar flexion of both feet. Direct the patient to feel their calf muscles contract and relax alternately (see Step 6E[3] illustrations, parts A and B). Repeat five times.

• A straight leg stabilizes the patient's position. A flexed left leg shifts weight for easier turning.

• Pulling toward side rail reduces effort needed for turning.

• Reduces risk of vascular and pulmonary complications.

• Provides normal anatomical position of lower extremities.

• Leg exercises maintain joint mobility and promote venous return to prevent thrombi.

• Stretches and contracts gastrocnemius muscles.

SKILL 49.1	DEMONSTRATING POSTOPERATIVE EXERCISES—cont'd
STEPS	**RATIONALE**

Desirable
Foot circles

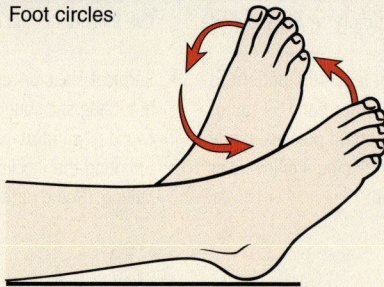

STEP 6E(2) Foot circles. (From Lewis, S. L., Bucher, L., Heitkemper, M. M., et al. [Eds.]. [2019]. *Medical-surgical nursing in Canada: Assessment and management of clinical problems* [4th ed.]. Elsevier.)

Essential
Alternate dorsiflexion and plantar flexion

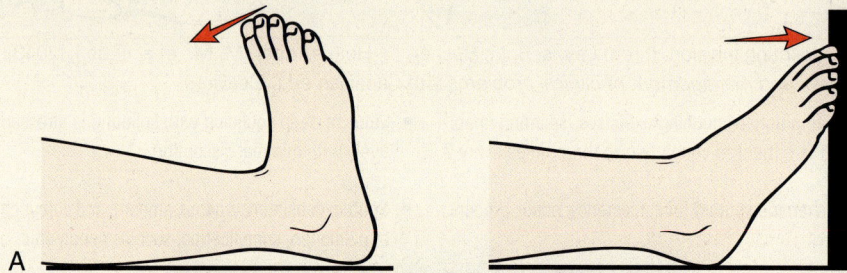

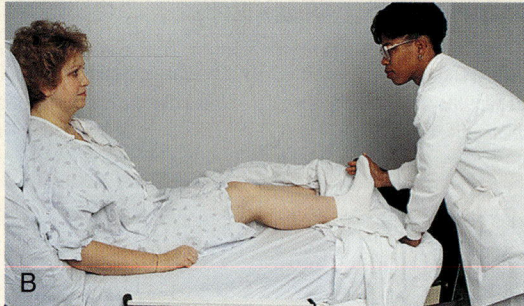

A

B

STEP 6E(3) **A,** Alternate dorsiflexion and plantar flexion. **B,** Patient pushes feet to perform plantar flexion. (From Lewis, S. M., Bucher, L., Heitkemper, M. M., et al. [Eds.] [2019]. *Medical-surgical nursing in Canada: Assessment and management of clinical problems* [4th ed.]. Elsevier.)

(4) Have patient perform quadriceps setting by tightening the thigh and bringing the knee down toward the mattress, then relaxing (see Step 6E[4] illustration). Repeat five times.

• Contracts muscles of upper legs, maintains knee mobility, and enhances venous return.

(5) Have the patient alternately raise each leg straight up from the bed surface, keeping legs straight, and then have the patient bend their leg at the hip and knee (see Step 6E[5] illustration). Repeat five times.

• Promotes contraction and relaxation of quadriceps muscles.

Quadriceps (thigh) setting

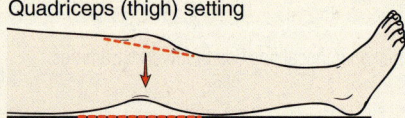

STEP 6E(4) Quadriceps (thigh) setting. (From Lewis, S. M., Bucher, L., Heitkemper, M. M., et al. [Eds.]. [2019]. *Medical-surgical nursing in Canada: Assessment and management of clinical problems* [4th ed.]. Elsevier.)

Hip and knee movements

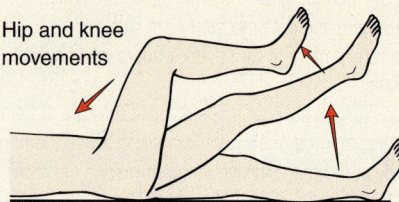

STEP 6E(5) Hip and knee movements. (From Lewis, S. L., Bucher, L., Heitkemper, M. M., et al. [Eds.]. [2019]. *Medical-surgical nursing in Canada: Assessment and management of clinical problems* [4th ed.]. Elsevier.)

Continued

SKILL 49.1	DEMONSTRATING POSTOPERATIVE EXERCISES—cont'd	
STEPS	**RATIONALE**	

STEPS	RATIONALE
7. Have the patient practise exercises at least every 2 hours while awake. Instruct the patient to coordinate turning and leg exercises with diaphragmatic breathing and coughing exercises. 8. Observe the patient's ability to perform all exercises independently.	• Repetition of sequence reinforces learning. Establishes routine for exercises that develops habit for performance. Sequence of exercises should be leg exercises, turning, breathing, and coughing. • Ensures that the patient has learned correct techniques. Documents the patient's education and provides data for instructional follow-up.

UNEXPECTED OUTCOMES	RELATED INTERVENTIONS
Inability to perform exercises correctly after surgery	• Assess for the presence of anxiety, pain, and fatigue. • Teach the patient stress reduction techniques, pain management strategies, or both. • Repeat the teaching, using additional demonstration or repeat demonstration at a time when family members or friends are present.
Unwillingness to perform exercises postoperatively because of incisional pain of thorax or abdomen (deep breathing, coughing, and turning) or because of surgery involving lower abdomen, groin, buttocks, or legs (leg exercises, turning)	• Instruct the patient to ask for pain medication 30 minutes before performing postoperative exercises or to use patient-controlled analgesia (PCA) immediately before exercising. • Report to the surgeon inadequate pain relief and the need to change analgesic or increase dose.

RECORDING AND REPORTING
• Record the exercises demonstrated and whether the patient can perform them independently.
• Report any problems the patient has in practising exercises to the nurse assigned to the patient on the next shift for follow-up.

expression of concerns. Family members may wish to discuss their concerns without the patient present so that their fears will not frighten the patient and vice versa. Establishing a trusting and therapeutic relationship with the patient and family allows this to happen.

Acute Care. Activities in the acute care setting during the preoperative phase focus on interventions to prepare the patient physically for surgery. This situation occurs less frequently now, as many patients enter hospital on the day of surgery.

Physical Preparation. The degree of preoperative physical preparation depends on the patient's health status and on the surgery to be performed. A seriously ill patient receives more supportive care in the form of medications, IV fluid therapy, and monitoring than does a patient facing a minor elective procedure. Nurses should explain the purpose of all procedures.

Maintenance of normal fluid and electrolyte balances. The patient requiring surgery is vulnerable to fluid and electrolyte imbalances as a result of inadequate preoperative intake, excessive fluid losses during surgery, and the physiological effect of third spacing (redistribution of intravascular fluid into interstitial space) in the initial postoperative period (see Chapter 41). A patient traditionally took nothing by mouth (NPO) after midnight on the morning of surgery to keep the stomach empty and thus reduce the risk of vomiting and aspiration. Recommendations for preoperative fasting have been published by the Canadian Anesthesiologists' Society (2022) and by the American Society of Anesthesiologists (ASA, 2011). They recommended fasting from clear liquids at least 2 hours before elective procedures requiring general anaesthesia, regional anaesthesia, or sedation/analgesia. The nurse should remove fluids and solid foods from the patient's bedside and post a sign over the patient's bed to alert hospital personnel and family members about fasting restrictions. The patient may be instructed to take specific medications (e.g., cardiovascular medications, anticonvulsants, or antibiotics) with a sip of water. A patient who is at home on the evening before surgery

must understand the importance of the specific fasting period that has been ordered. Patients can rinse their mouths with water or mouthwash and brush their teeth immediately before surgery as long as they do not swallow water. The nurse must notify the surgeon and anaesthesiologist if the patient has eaten or consumed fluids during the fasting period.

During surgery, normal mechanisms for controlling fluid and electrolyte balances, including respiration, digestion, circulation, and elimination, are disturbed. The surgical procedure may cause extensive losses of blood and other body fluids. The surgical stress response aggravates any fluid and electrolyte imbalances. The patient's preoperative diet should include foods high in protein, with sufficient carbohydrates, fat, and vitamins. If a patient cannot eat because of gastrointestinal alterations or impairments in consciousness, an IV route for fluid replacement is started. The physician assesses serum electrolyte levels to determine the type of IV fluids and electrolyte additives to administer. Patients with severe nutritional imbalances may require supplements containing concentrated protein and glucose (see Chapter 43).

Reduction of risk of surgical wound infection. The risk of developing a surgical wound infection is determined by the amount and type of microorganisms contaminating a wound, the susceptibility of the host, and the surgical wound itself. All three factors interact to cause infection. Antibiotics may be ordered in the preoperative period and may be administered prophylactically. Antibiotics are given orally or intravenously that cover aerobic and anaerobic bacteria and reduce the risk of surgical wound infection. The optimal time of for antibiotic prophylaxis is within 1 hour of surgical time (Piscioneri, 2021). Microorganisms grow and multiply on the skin, and without proper skin preparation, the risk of postoperative wound infection is high. Many surgeons instruct patients to bathe or shower the evening before surgery. Some physicians may request that patients bathe or shower more than once, whereas others may ask patients to give special attention to cleaning the proposed operative site; this attention could include the

Patient(e) _____   Chart No. – N° du dossier _____

Post-op Day 1 — Jour 1 post-opératoire

Date: yyaa _____   mm _____   dj _____

Critical Path	**Patient Outcomes**

Assessments/Treatments

- VS, NVS, Pain q4h → q shift, SpO$_2$
- Monitor dressing / Hemovac
- Monitor Intake & Output
- Pain management as per APS
  - Discontinue APS modality as per weaning guideline if patient meets criteria
  - If single dose intrathecal only: discontinue from APS 24 hours following time of injection

Activity

- DB&C
- Exercise program
- Pivot transfer with walker
- Confirm weight bearing status
- Up in chair x 2 _____ initial, _____ initial
- Ambulate x 1 with assistance: _____ initial
- Assistive devices, specify: _____

Nutrition

- Diet as ordered

Elimination

- Catheter as ordered

Patient Teaching

- Reinforce exercise program
- Proper pillow positioning
- Hip precautions
- If on Low Molecular Weight Heparin – start self injection teaching and provide booklet
- Ensure patient has Total Hip Arthroplasty patient information booklet
- Pain management

Pain Control

- Adequate pain control achieved: Pain ≤ 3 rest, ≤ 5 activity; pain not preventing movement; satisfied with pain control

Activity

- Completes transfer with assistance
- Performs exercises according to self directed exercise program

Prevention of DVT

- Demonstrates appropriate exercises & positioning for prevention of DVT
- Verbalizes understanding of anticoagulant therapy

Patient Teaching

- Verbalizes understanding of "Total Hip Arthroplasty" instructions and exercise program
- Understands basics of self injection if applicable
- Demonstrates:
  - Proper positioning
  - Understanding of weight-bearing status

Patient progress corresponds with clinical pathway

Physiotherapy:

☐ Yes ☐ No Signature: _____   Time: _____   NTV – circle above, VC _____

Nursing:

D ☐ Yes ☐ No Signature: _____, Initial _____   Time: _____   NTV – circle above, VC _____

E ☐ Yes ☐ No Signature: _____, Initial _____   Time: _____   NTV – circle above, VC _____

N ☐ Yes ☐ No Signature: _____, Initial _____   Time: _____   NTV – circle above, VC _____

D = 8-12 h day shift	**E** = evening shift, if applicable	**N** = 8-12 h night shift

Variance Codes (VC)	**186**	Activity variance	**510**	Not discharged by end of pathway – non-medical reason
	653	Consult not sent by Day 3	**NTV**	Non-Tracked Variance
	492	Not discharged by end of pathway – continued need for acute care	**OFF**	Ordered off clinical pathway

© THE OTTAWA HOSPITAL – L'HÔPITAL D'OTTAWA   CHART – DOSSIER   CP 4A (3 – 7)

FIGURE 49.4 Clinical pathway for a total hip arthroplasty, primary/revision and hip resurfacing. It highlights what the patient can expect on the first day after surgery. (Courtesy The Ottawa Hospital, Ottawa, ON.)

use of an antibacterial soap. Depending on the surgical procedure, a patient may also need to shower on the morning of surgery. If the surgical procedure involves the head, neck, or upper chest area, the patient may be required to shampoo their hair. Cleaning and trimming of fingernails and toenails also may be necessary.

The need for hair removal is less common now and depends on the amount of hair, the location of the incision, and the surgical procedure planned. Hair removal can damage and cause breaks in the patient's skin, which may allow for the entry of microorganisms. Hair removal with a clipper or shaver before surgery is not necessary. To investigate the utility of hair removal, Kowalski and colleagues (2017) conducted a randomized study of 1 700 patients to determine if hair removal prior to surgery decreased surgical infection rates. Patients were randomized to either the shaved group or the nonshaved group. The authors found no significant difference in infection rate between the shaved group (6.12%) and the nonshaved group (6.32%).

Short hospital stays can reduce the chance of a hospital-acquired infection occurring. Respiratory, urinary tract, and wound infections can all be acquired during hospitalization. Thus one advantage of ambulatory surgical procedures is that the patient usually returns home once the surgery has been completed, avoiding a hospital stay that could expose them to infection.

Precautions for patient requiring infection-control procedures. If a patient requires surgery but also has an infectious process, the OR must be notified in advance to ensure appropriate preparation. For example, patients with tuberculosis would be placed in a reverse airflow OR suite and subsequently in a reverse airflow room in the postanaesthesia care unit (PACU). Patients with methicillin-resistant *Staphylococcus aureus* (MRSA) may have their surgery performed at the end of the day so that the surgical suite can be cleaned afterward. These patients on transfer to the PACU are placed in an isolation room. Many hospitals now require that all "same-day admit" patients be screened for MRSA and vancomycin-resistant enterococci (VRE).

Prevention of bowel incontinence. The patient may receive a bowel preparation (e.g., a cathartic or enema) if the surgery involves the lower gastrointestinal system or lower abdominal organs. Manipulation of portions of the gastrointestinal tract during surgery results in absence of peristalsis for 24 hours or longer. Enemas and cathartics, such as GoLYTELY, clean the gastrointestinal tract to prevent intraoperative incontinence and postoperative constipation. An empty bowel reduces the risk for injury to the intestines and minimizes contamination of the operative wound if a portion of the bowel is incised or opened accidentally, or if colon surgery is planned (see Chapter 45).

Promotion of rest and comfort. Rest is essential for normal healing. Anxiety about the impending surgery can easily interfere with the patient's ability to relax or sleep. As well, the underlying condition requiring surgery may be painful, further impairing rest.

If the patient is admitted to the hospital before the day of surgery, the nurse should attempt to make the patient's environment quiet and comfortable. Sometimes the patient is ordered an anxiolytic agent for the night before surgery. Anxiolytic agents such as benzodiazepines (e.g., alprazolam [Xanax]) act on the cerebral cortex and limbic system to relieve anxiety and promote sleep (Kilduff & Mendelson, 2017).

An advantage of ambulatory surgery or same-day surgical admissions is that the patient is able to sleep at home the night before surgery. They are likely to get more rest in a familiar environment. The nonhospitalized patient also may have medication ordered by the physician if apprehension about surgery interferes with a good night's rest.

Preparation on the Day of Surgery. Nurses must complete a number of interventions before releasing the patient for surgery.

Hygiene. Basic hygiene measures provide additional comfort before surgery. The patient may want to bathe before surgery. Because the patient cannot wear personal nightwear to the OR, the nurse must provide a clean hospital gown. If the patient has been NPO for the last several hours, their mouth may be very dry. The nurse may offer the patient mouthwash and toothpaste, again with the caution not to swallow any water.

Hair and cosmetics. During surgery with general anaesthesia, the patient's head is positioned to introduce an endotracheal tube into the airway (see Chapter 40). This procedure may involve manipulation of the patient's hair and scalp. To avoid injury, the patient should be asked to remove hairpins or clips before leaving for surgery. Hairpieces or wigs also should be removed. Long hair can be braided. The patient will wear a disposable hat before entering the OR.

During and after surgery, the anaesthesiologist and nurses will assess skin and mucous membranes to determine the patient's level of oxygenation and circulation. Therefore, all makeup (lipstick, powder, blush, nail polish) should be removed to expose normal skin and nail colouring. Pulse oximetry is capable of recording accurate measurements through most nail polish colours, but removal is still considered good practice. Contact lenses, false eyelashes, and eye makeup also must be removed. The patient's glasses can be stored or given to the family immediately before the patient enters the OR.

Removal of prostheses. It is easy for any type of prosthetic device to become lost or damaged during surgery. The patient must remove all prostheses, including partial or complete dentures, artificial limbs, artificial eyes, and hearing aids. If a patient has a brace or a splint, the nurse may need to determine whether it should remain with the patient.

Many patients are embarrassed at having to remove dentures, wigs, or other devices that enhance their personal appearance. Privacy should be offered as these personal items are removed. Patients may be allowed to keep personal items until they reach the preoperative area. For safekeeping, dentures must be placed in special containers labelled with the patient's name and other identification required by the agency. In many institutions, nurses must make an inventory of all prosthetic devices or personal items and lock them away according to agency policy. It is also common practice for nurses to give prostheses to family members or to keep items like dentures at the patient's bedside. Documentation in the nursing notes, the surgical checklist, or per agency policy should reflect these actions.

Safeguarding valuables. If a patient has any valuables, the nurse should give them to family members or secure them for safekeeping. Many hospitals require patients to sign a release form that frees the institution of responsibility for any lost valuables. Valuables usually can be stored and locked in a designated location. Often patients are reluctant to remove wedding rings or religious medals. A wedding band can be taped in place. However, if there is a risk that the patient will experience swelling of the hand or fingers (related to mastectomy, hand surgery, or fluid shifts), the wedding band should be removed. For safety, metal items, such as for pierced areas, should also be removed. The location of valuables is documented per hospital policy.

Preparing the bowel and bladder. The patient may require an enema or cathartic on the morning of surgery to ensure that the colon is empty. If so, it should be given at least 1 hour before the patient is scheduled to leave for surgery, allowing time for the patient to defecate without rushing. The nurse should instruct the patient to void just before leaving for the OR and before giving preoperative medications. An empty bladder prevents a patient from becoming incontinent during surgery. This is important during abdominal surgery, when it may be necessary for the surgeon to manipulate the bladder. An empty bladder also makes abdominal organs more accessible during surgery. The last time of voiding is charted. If the patient is unable to void, this should be noted on the preoperative (pre-procedure) checklist. An indwelling urinary catheter may be placed if the surgery is long or the incision will be in the lower abdomen.

Vital signs. The nurse must measure a final preoperative set of vital signs. The anaesthesiologist uses these values as a baseline during surgery. If preoperative vital signs are abnormal, surgery may need to be postponed. The physician should be notified of any abnormalities before sending the patient to surgery.

Documentation. Before the patient goes to the OR, the nurse needs to check the contents of the medical record to ensure that pertinent laboratory results are present. Any abnormal findings in laboratory results, such as low potassium, should be reported. Consent forms need to be checked for accuracy of information. A preoperative or preprocedural checklist (Figure 49.5) provides nurses with guidelines to ensure that nursing interventions are completed. Nurses should also check the nursing notes to ensure that documentation of care is current. This is especially important if the hospitalized patient experienced unexpected problems on the night before surgery. The OR should be alerted through notation of any positioning challenges for the patient, such as difficulty flexing knees, or of any sensory impairment.

Performing special procedures. A patient's condition may warrant special interventions before surgery. The patient may need IV infusions started or a nasogastric tube inserted before leaving the patient unit for surgery. These procedures also may be done once the patient is in the preoperative area or in the OR.

Administering preoperative medications. The advent of ambulatory surgery has reduced the use of preoperative medications. However, the anaesthesiologist or surgeon may order preanaesthetic medications ("on-call medications," "pre-ops") to reduce the patient's anxiety, the amount of general anaesthesia required, the risk of nausea and vomiting and resultant aspiration, and respiratory tract secretions.

The nurse should provide all nursing care measures before giving the patient preoperative medications at the prescribed time. The consent form needs to be signed before the administration of these medications. In addition, the patient should be helped to void. Because the medications cause sedation, the patient should not be allowed to leave the bed or stretcher until personnel arrive to transport them to the OR. The patient should be warned to expect drowsiness and a dry mouth.

> **SAFETY ALERT** Explain to the patient the effects of any preoperative medications. Remind the patient to remain in bed or on the stretcher. Raise the side rails and keep the bed or stretcher in the low position. Place the call light within easy reach of the patient.

Latex sensitivity or allergy. As the incidence and prevalence of latex sensitivity and allergy have increased, the need to recognize potential sources of latex is critical. Guidelines developed through Canadian and American health care organizations are also available for the management of latex allergies and safe latex use in health care facilities (Sussman & Gold, 2006). The American Association of Nurse Anesthesiology (AANA) developed guidelines in 1993 for managing latex allergies, and these were revised in 2014 and reaffirmed in 2018 (AANA, 2018). This document is an excellent resource for all health care personnel.

The OR and PACU can contain innumerable products that have latex in them. Some common sources are gloves, IV tubing, syringes, and rubber stoppers on bottles and vials. Latex is also present in objects that may be overlooked, such as adhesive tape, disposable electrodes, endotracheal tube cuffs, protection sheets, and ventilator equipment. However, many hospitals have moved to latex-free products. Persons most at risk are people with a previous sensitivity to latex or rubber products, people with neural tube defects such as spina bifida, patients with a history of multiple surgeries, health care providers, and those with a history of contact dermatitis or atopic immunological reactions (OPANA, 2018).

Symptoms of a latex reaction can include local effects ranging from urticaria and flat or raised red patches to vesicular, scaling, or bleeding eruptions. Acute dermatitis also may occur. Rhinitis and rhinorrhea are other common symptoms in both mild and severe latex reactions. Immediate hypersensitivity reactions can be life-threatening, with the patient exhibiting focal or generalized urticaria, edema, bronchospasm, and mucous hypersecretion, which can compromise respiratory status. Vasodilatation compounded by increased capillary permeability can lead to circulatory collapse and eventual death.

Protocols exist for providing care for patients with a latex allergy or sensitivity. Patients with this allergy should be identified preoperatively. Latex-free kits are available; they include latex-free equipment (e.g., a latex-free Ambu bag) and follow the patients throughout their hospitalization. Although latex kits are available, the move to latex-free products has decreased their use. It is recommended that the patient with a latex allergy be scheduled as the first case of the day in the OR (OPANA, 2018). The patient can then be safely accommodated by using appropriate latex-free items during the perioperative period and recovery. Box 49.5 lists precautions for patients with latex sensitivity or allergy.

Surgical safety checklist. The World Health Organization (WHO, 2009) has a surgical safety checklist, a tool designed by experts in surgery, anaesthesia, and nursing, that can be used to foster communication between surgeons and nurses about a patient's condition and risk factors at critical time points: during sign-in, time-out (surgical phase), and sign-out. This checklist is endorsed by the Canadian Patient Safety Institute (2018).

Eliminating wrong site and wrong procedure surgery. Whenever an invasive surgical procedure is to be performed, the nurse and the surgeon must ensure that the site has been marked by the surgeon (see agency policy). Indelible ink may be used to mark left and right distinction, multiple structures (e.g., fingers), and levels of the spine. The nurse also must verify the patient and the procedure to be performed. In addition, once the patient reaches the OR, they are introduced to the surgical team. The patient is asked to describe what procedure is being performed and to indicate the site for the surgery. The consent form is verified.

◆ Evaluation

Patient Care. The nurse in the preoperative area will be the source for evaluating outcomes during the preoperative period (Figure 49.6). With regard to the preoperative patient's care plan, limited time is available to evaluate the outcomes. The patient's current status is compared with expected outcomes to determine whether new or revised interventions or nursing diagnoses need to be implemented.

Because interventions continue during and after surgery, evaluation of many goals and outcomes do not occur until after surgery. For example, the nurse will not be able to evaluate the success in preventing postoperative wound infection or promoting return of normal physiological function until a few days after surgery. If the patient is having ambulatory surgery, they will return home; therefore, the effectiveness of certain interventions is evaluated at follow-up appointments.

Patient Expectations. Determining whether the patient's expectations have been met regarding preoperative teaching may be difficult. Nurses are evaluating patients in a hurried atmosphere because there are many things that need to be accomplished in a short amount of time. The patient's surgery may be an emergency, or performance of various procedures may make it difficult for nurses to find time for evaluation. It is important that nurses remember to attend to the patient's emotional needs (privacy, fear, anxiety), as well as to their physical needs. The patient should be given an opportunity to state whether expectations have been met. If expectations have not been

The Ottawa Hospital | L'Hôpital d'Ottawa

PRE PROCEDURE CHECKLIST
FEUILLE DE VÉRIFICATION PRÉ-INTERVENTION

Nurse to initial each column – L'infirmière doit parapher chaque colonne	Yes Oui	No Non	N/A S/O
Addressograph plate – Plaque d'adressographe			
Precautions if yes, check – Précautions si oui, cochez : ☐ contact(es) ☐ airborne – aériennes ☐ droplet – gouttelettes ☐ other – autre :			
Identity bracelet verified – Bracelet d'identité vérifié			
Allergies status confirmed, bracelet on prn-Statut d'allergies confirmé, bracelet mis prn			
Weight – Poids : ☐ kg ☐ lbs			
Consent CON 17 completed as per policy Admin. no. (00291) – Consentement CON 17 rempli selon la politique Admin n° (00291)			
Blood and blood products consent CON 66 completed as per policy Admin. no. (00045) Consentement à recevoir du sang ou des produits sanguins CON 66 rempli selon la politique Admin n° (00045)			
Consult notes/Medical history – Notes de consultation/Antécédents médicaux ☐ on chart – au dossier ☐ on – sur OACIS			
Patient Admission History – Antécédents du patient à l'admission (NUR 71 A) ☐ on chart – au dossier ☐ on – sur OACIS			
Medication Administration Records (MAR) – Fiches d'administration des médicaments (FAM)			
Teeth – Dents : ☐ capped – couronne ☐ loose – branlante			
Removed – Enlevé(s) : ☐ dentures dentiers ☐ bridge pont ☐ glasses lunettes ☐ contacts verres de contacts ☐ makeup/nail polish maquillage/vernis à ongles ☐ jewellery/body piercing bijoux/perçage corporel			
Hearing aid – Appareil auditif : ☐ removed – enlevé ☐ in ear – dans l'oreille (case must be labelled and sent to OR – L'étui doit être étiquetté et envoyé au bloc opératoire)			
Communication barrier – Conflit de communication If yes, Interpreter to accompany patient to OR – Si oui, l'interprète doit accompagner le patient au bloc opératoire			
Skin integrity problem – Problème de l'intégrité de la peau Site :			
Surgical implants – Implants chirurgicaux Site :			
Pacemaker/Internal defibrillator – Stimulateur cardiaque/Défibrillateur interne			
Antibiotics ordered – Antibiotiques ordonnés ☐ Sent to OR with patient – Envoyés au bloc avec le patient ☐ Given/started on unit – Administré/débuté à l'unité			
Diagnostic testing completed as per orders or pathway – Examens diagnostiques complets selon ordonnances ou plan			
Blood glucose by point of care testing (POCT) – Glycémie par tests aux points de service			
Pregnancy test – Examen de grossesse Done prn – Fait prn : ☐ + ☐ -			
CPR & Plan of Treatment – RCR et plan de traitement (SPO 238 on front of chart – au devant du dossier)			
NPO since – À jeun depuis :			
Family/SDM have been notified of procedure time ☐ Patient refused ☐ No family available Person Notified (name) Telephone number Date/Time notified			

PRINTED NAME-NOM EN LETTRES MOULÉES	SIGNATURE	INIT	DATE (yyaa-mm-dj)	TIME HEURE

ORA 06 (04/2015) Cat.: 412550   CHART-DOSSIER

FIGURE 49.5 Preprocedure checklist. *CPR,* Cardiopulmonary resuscitation; *NPO,* nothing by mouth; *OR,* operating room; *prn,* as needed; *SDM,* substitute decision maker. (Courtesy The Ottawa Hospital, Ottawa, ON.)

BOX 49.5 EVIDENCE-INFORMED PRACTICE

Latex Precautions

1. Survey the patient care area and remove any products containing latex (e.g., examination gloves, rubber sheets, or blood pressure cuff).
2. Place a latex precautions label on the patient's chart and latex precautions signs on the door to the patient's room and on the transport cart.
3. Use only nonlatex gloves. Order an adequate supply.
4. Review the supplies to be used for the patient and substitute with latex-free supplies as necessary.
5. Review the medications to be administered and verify that they are latex-free. Include the following steps:
   a. Notify the pharmacy of the need for latex precautions.
   b. Verify that all prescribed medications are latex-free.
   c. Place a sign in the area where medications (including mixing solutions) are kept, indicating that the patient is on latex precautions.
   d. Use latex-free syringes.
6. Review the intravenous supplies to be used and verify that they are latex-free. Include the following steps:
   a. Use latex-free solutions.
   b. Use latex-free tubing.
   c. Use latex-free syringes, including those for patient-controlled analgesia.
   d. Use latex-free tape.
7. Verify that bedding and support garments are latex-free (e.g., mattress protectors, antiembolism stockings, and binders).
8. Verify that dressings and tape are latex-free.
9. Notify the family and visitors of the use of latex precautions.
10. Routinely survey the patient care area to verify that latex products are not present (e.g., examination gloves, balloons).
11. Before transfer to another area or agency, notify care providers of the need for latex precautions.
12. Provide education programs about latex allergy to health care providers, patients, and family or caregivers. This education should include the following:
    a. Definition of latex allergy
    b. Exposures to latex
    c. Latex avoidance
    d. Signs and symptoms of a reaction to latex
    e. Emergency treatment of a reaction to latex

Adapted from Australasian Society of Clinical Immunology and Allergy. (2010). Clinical Guidelines (Nursing): *Latex—management of a patient at risk of or with a known latex allergy.* The Royal Children's Hospital Melbourne. https://www.rch.org.au/rchcpg/hospital_clinical_guideline_index/Latex_management_of_a_patient_at_risk_of_or_with_a_known_latex_allergy/

met, the nurse needs to work closely with the patient to redefine expectations that can be realistically met within the time limits imposed by the particular setting.

TRANSPORT TO THE OPERATING ROOM

Personnel in the OR notify the nursing division or ambulatory surgery area when it is time for the patient's surgery. In many hospitals, an orderly or transporter brings a stretcher for transporting the patient. The transporter checks the patient's identification bracelet against the patient's chart to ensure that the right person is going to surgery. Because the patient may have received preoperative medications, the

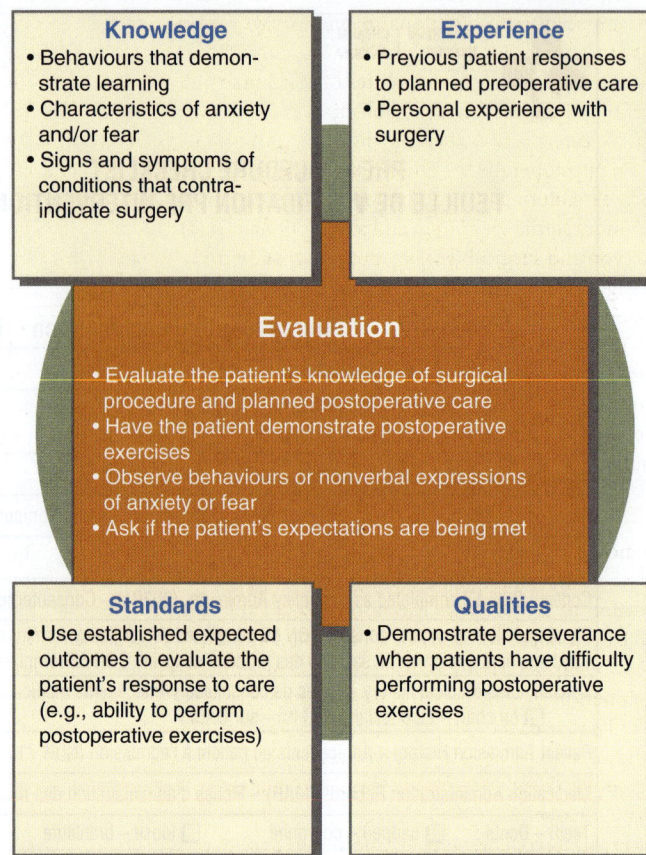

Knowledge
- Behaviours that demonstrate learning
- Characteristics of anxiety and/or fear
- Signs and symptoms of conditions that contraindicate surgery

Experience
- Previous patient responses to planned preoperative care
- Personal experience with surgery

Evaluation
- Evaluate the patient's knowledge of surgical procedure and planned postoperative care
- Have the patient demonstrate postoperative exercises
- Observe behaviours or nonverbal expressions of anxiety or fear
- Ask if the patient's expectations are being met

Standards
- Use established expected outcomes to evaluate the patient's response to care (e.g., ability to perform postoperative exercises)

Qualities
- Demonstrate perseverance when patients have difficulty performing postoperative exercises

FIGURE 49.6 Critical thinking model for surgical patient evaluation.

nurses and transporter assist the patient when transferring from bed to stretcher to prevent falls. The ambulatory surgery patient may ambulate to the OR if able to do so and not medicated. The nurse should provide the family with an opportunity to visit before the patient is transported to the OR, then direct the family to a waiting area. In some hospitals, the family may be allowed to wait with the patient in the OR holding area until the patient is transported into the OR.

After the patient leaves the nursing unit, the bed and the room are prepared if the patient is returning to the same nursing unit. For recording vital signs, many institutions now have automated blood pressure machines. In addition, with bedside monitoring equipment, patient information can be scanned at the bedside and entered into the electronic chart. Other materials required at the bedside include the following:

- Emesis basin
- Clean gown
- Washcloth, towel, and facial tissues
- IV pole and, often, IV pump
- Suction equipment (if needed)
- Oxygen equipment (if needed)
- Extra pillows for positioning the patient comfortably
- Bed pads to protect bed linens from drainage
- Bed raised to stretcher height with bed linens pulled back and furniture moved to accommodate the stretcher and equipment (such as IV lines)

INTRAOPERATIVE SURGICAL PHASE

Care of the patient during surgery requires careful preparation and knowledge of the events that occur during the surgical procedure.

The nurse usually functions in one of two roles in the OR: as circulating nurse or as scrub nurse. The circulating nurse must be a registered nurse. Responsibilities of this nurse include reviewing the preoperative assessment, establishing and implementing the intraoperative care plan, evaluating the care, and providing for continuity of care postoperatively. The circulating nurse assists with procedures, such as endotracheal intubation, as needed. In addition, this nurse monitors sterile technique and a safe OR environment and assists the surgeon and surgical team by providing additional supplies, verifying sponge and instrument counts, and maintaining accurate and complete written records.

The scrub nurse may be a registered nurse or a registered practical nurse. This nurse maintains a sterile field during the surgical procedure, assists with applying sterile drapes, hands the surgeons instruments and other sterile supplies, and completes sponge and instrument counts.

Preoperative (Holding) Area

In most hospitals, the patient enters a holding area outside the OR. The nurse in the holding area validates the patient's identification and the location of the surgery. The nurse also verifies that appropriate data have been obtained, assesses a patient's readiness both physically and emotionally, and reinforces teaching. Nurses in the holding area are members of the OR staff and wear surgical scrub suits, hats, and footwear in accordance with infection control policies. In some ambulatory surgical settings, a perioperative primary nurse admits the patient, circulates for the operative procedure, and manages the patient's recovery and discharge.

In the preoperative area, the nurse or the anaesthesiologist may insert an IV catheter into the patient's arm to establish a route for fluid replacement and IV medications. A large-bore (18-gauge) IV catheter is used for easy infusion of fluids and blood products if necessary. The nurse also applies a blood pressure cuff. The cuff will remain in place throughout the surgery so that the anaesthesiologist can assess blood pressure readings. The nurse usually reviews the preoperative checklist, and the anaesthesiologist may perform a patient assessment at this time.

If any preoperative medications have been given, the patient will begin to feel drowsy. The temperature in the holding area and adjacent OR suites is usually cool, and the patient should be offered an extra blanket. The patient's stay in the holding area is usually brief.

Admission to the Operating Room

Nurses transfer the patient to the OR via a stretcher. Usually, the patient is still awake and will notice nurses and physicians wearing surgical masks, gowns, and eyewear. The staff carefully transfer the patient to the OR table, after ensuring that the stretcher and table are locked in place. After the patient is on the table, a safety strap is fastened around the patient. The nurse supports the patient by explaining procedures and encouraging the patient to ask questions. Sights and sounds in the surgical suite may seem frightening to patients.

❖ NURSING PROCESS IN THE INTRAOPERATIVE SURGICAL PHASE

◆ Assessment

In the holding area, the nurse conducts a focused preoperative assessment to verify that the patient is ready for surgery and to plan intraoperative care. Because patients will not be able to speak for themselves while under general anaesthesia, this preoperative assessment in the OR is important for the patient's safety.

> **SAFETY ALERT** Verification of the patient's name by patient response compared with chart and ID bracelet is completed before sedation. The chart is reviewed for consent forms, allergies, medical history, physical assessment findings, test results, and verification of preoperative medications. The nurse verifies with the patient the planned surgical procedure and the surgical site before anaesthesia is administered. Some agencies ask the patient to mark the surgical site. The nurse ensures that the patient's prosthetic devices and valuables have been removed.

Nurses review the preoperative care plan to establish an intraoperative care plan and assess the patient's psychological comfort.

◆ Nursing Diagnosis

Nurses review preoperative nursing diagnoses and modify them to individualize the care plan in the OR.

◆ Planning

Goals and Outcomes. Patient-centred outcomes of preoperative care extend into the intraoperative phase. For example, one goal would be to maintain skin integrity. An expected outcome would be that the patient will have intact skin and show no signs of redness.

◆ Implementation

A primary focus of intraoperative care is to prevent injury and complications related to anaesthesia, surgery, positioning, and equipment used. The perioperative nurse serves as an advocate for the patient during surgery and protects the patient's dignity and rights at all times.

Physical Preparation. After safely securing the patient on the OR table, the nurse applies monitoring devices to the patient before surgery. Patients receiving general and regional anaesthesia undergo continuous ECG monitoring during surgery. Small plastic electrodes are placed on the chest and extremities to record electrical activity of the heart. A monitor in the OR displays the heart's electrical activity. Pulse oximetry will be used to monitor oxygen saturation. An electrical cautery grounding pad is applied to the skin. Antiembolism stockings or intermittent sequential compression stockings may be applied intraoperatively (especially during long surgeries) or postoperatively according to agency policy (see Chapter 46). The nurse documents device application and patient tolerance to procedures.

Introduction of Anaesthesia. Patients undergoing surgical procedures receive one of four types of anaesthesia: general, regional, local, or procedural sedation.

General Anaesthesia. General anaesthesia is a state of total unconsciousness resulting from anaesthetic agents (Merchant et al., 2016). Modern anaesthetic agents are much easier to reverse and allow the patient to recover with fewer untoward effects. General anaesthesia results in an immobile, quiet patient who does not recall the surgical procedure. An anaesthesiologist gives general anaesthetics by IV and inhalation routes through the three phases of anaesthesia: induction, maintenance, and emergence. Surgery that requires general anaesthesia involves major procedures with extensive tissue manipulation or the desire for analgesia, muscle relaxation, immobility, and control of the autonomic nervous system.

Induction includes the administration of anaesthetic agents and endotracheal intubation. The maintenance phase includes positioning the patient, preparing the skin for incision, and the surgical procedure itself. Appropriate levels of anaesthesia are maintained during this phase. During emergence, anaesthetics are decreased and the patient begins to awaken. Because of the short half-life of current medications, emergence often begins to occur in the OR.

The duration of anaesthesia depends on the length of surgery. The greatest risks from general anaesthesia are the adverse effects of anaesthetic agents, including cardiovascular depression or irritability, respiratory depression, and hepatic and renal damage.

Regional Anaesthesia. Induction of **regional anaesthesia** results in loss of sensation in an area of the body. The method of induction influences the portion of sensory pathways that are anaesthetized. No loss of consciousness occurs with regional anaesthesia, but the patient may be sedated. The anaesthesiologist gives regional anaesthetics by infiltration and local application. Administration techniques include nerve blocks, intrathecal (spinal) or epidural anaesthesia, and IV regional anaesthesia. With epidural anaesthesia, a spinal needle is progressed into the epidural space, whereas with intrathecal anaesthesia, it is into the subarachnoid space. Both epidural and intrathecal anaesthesia affect motor, sensory, and sympathetic nerves. With intrathecal anaesthesia, the onset of anaesthesia is faster and the amount of medication required is much less than with epidural anaesthesia.

Infiltrative anaesthetics do involve risks, particularly in the case of intrathecal (spinal) anaesthesia. Because the level of anaesthesia may rise, which means that the anaesthetic agent moves upward in the spinal cord, breathing may be affected. This migration of the anaesthetic agent depends on the medication type, amount, and patient position. If the level of anaesthesia rises, respiratory paralysis may develop, requiring resuscitation. Elevation of the upper body prevents respiratory paralysis. The patient may experience a sudden fall in blood pressure, which results from extensive vasodilation caused by the anaesthetic block to sympathetic vasomotor nerves and pain and motor nerve fibres. The patient requires careful monitoring during and immediately after surgery.

Because the patient is responsive and capable of breathing voluntarily, it is not necessary for the anaesthesiologist to use an endotracheal tube. OR personnel can gain a false sense of security because of the patient's relative alertness. Nurses must remember that burns and other trauma can occur on the anaesthetized part of the body without the patient's being aware of these injuries. Therefore, nurses must observe the position of the extremities and the condition of the skin frequently.

Local Anaesthesia. **Local anaesthesia** involves loss of sensation at the desired site (e.g., a growth on the skin or the cornea of the eye). The anaesthetic agent (e.g., lidocaine) inhibits nerve conduction until the drug diffuses into the body's circulation. It may be injected locally or applied topically. The patient experiences a loss in pain and touch sensation at the site. Local anaesthesia is commonly used for minor procedures performed in ambulatory surgery. Physicians may infiltrate the operative area with local anaesthetics to promote postoperative pain relief. For example, peripheral nerve blocks produce anaesthetic effect both at and distal to the site of injection (Abdel-Aziz & Adams, 2017).

Procedural sedation. **Procedural sedation** (also referred to as **conscious sedation**) is routinely used for procedures that do not require complete anaesthesia but rather a depressed level of consciousness. Sedation is a state of reduced excitement achieved by the administration of a sedative agent (Merchant et al., 2016). The Ramsay Sedation Scale (RSS modified) can be used as a guide to levels of sedation (Stone, 2017). With this sedation, procedures that need to be performed can be more acceptable to the patient. The patient must independently retain a patent airway and airway reflexes and must be able to respond appropriately to physical and verbal stimuli (Merchant et al., 2016). Ketamine has become popular for procedural sedation.

Advantages of procedural sedation include adequate sedation and reduction of fear and anxiety with less risk than with general anaesthesia

and a more rapid recovery. Sedation does not reduce sensation of pain; therefore, other treatments may be required to reduce pain. A variety of diagnostic and therapeutic procedures are appropriate for procedural sedation (burn dressing changes, some cosmetic surgery, pulmonary biopsy and bronchoscopy, colonoscopy, and many others). Nurses assisting with the administration of local anaesthesia and procedural sedation must demonstrate competency in the care of these patients. Knowledge of anatomy, physiology, cardiac dysrhythmias, procedural complications, and pharmacological principles related to the administration of individual agents is essential. Nurses also must be able to assess, diagnose, and intervene in the event of untoward reactions and demonstrate skill in airway management and oxygen delivery. Resuscitation equipment must be readily available when local anaesthesia or procedural sedation is used. AORN (2021) has guidelines on care of the patient receiving anaesthesia and care of patients receiving moderate sedation or analgesia.

Positioning the Patient for Surgery. When general anaesthesia is being used, the nursing personnel and surgeon often do not position the patient until the stage of complete relaxation is achieved. The choice of position is usually determined by the surgical approach. Ideally, the patient's position provides good access to the operative site and sustains adequate circulatory and respiratory function. It should not impair neuromuscular structures. The patient's comfort and safety must be considered.

Normal range of joint motion is maintained in an alert person by pain and pressure receptors. If a joint is extended too far, pain stimuli provide a warning that muscle and joint strain is too great. In a patient who is anaesthetized, normal defence mechanisms cannot guard against joint damage, muscle stretch, and strain. The muscles are so relaxed that it is relatively easy to place the patient in a position that the individual normally could not assume while awake. The patient then remains in a given position, often for several hours. Although it may be necessary to place a patient in an unusual position, attempts should be made to maintain correct alignment and protect the patient from pressure, abrasion, and other injuries. Attachments to the operating table allow protection and padding of extremities and bony prominences. Positioning should not impede normal movement of the diaphragm or interfere with circulation to body parts. If restraints are necessary, the area to be restrained should be padded to prevent skin trauma.

Documentation of Intraoperative Care. During the intraoperative phase, the nursing staff continues the preoperative care plan. Strict asepsis must be followed to minimize the risk of surgical wound infection. IV fluid infusion and monitoring of urinary and nasogastric output are examples of actions that nurses will take to maintain the patient's fluid balance. Throughout the surgical procedure, an accurate record is kept of patient care activities and procedures performed by OR personnel. Documentation of intraoperative care provides useful data for the nurse who will care for the patient postoperatively.

◆ Evaluation

Interventions implemented during the intraoperative phase are evaluated throughout the surgical procedure.

Patient Care. Nurses perform intraoperative evaluation of the patient. Blood pressure, heart rate and rhythm, and oxygen saturation are monitored continuously. Temperature is measured during and upon completion of the surgical procedure. Intake and output is carefully recorded. The skin is inspected under the grounding pad and at areas where pressure from positioning may have been exerted.

Patient Expectations. Nurses should frequently question patients not undergoing general anaesthesia about pain, numbness, perceived room temperature, and overall comfort. The circulating nurse provides updates to family members in the waiting room.

POSTOPERATIVE SURGICAL PHASE

After surgery, a patient's care can become complex as a result of physiological changes that may occur. Patients who have undergone general anaesthesia are more likely to face complications than those who have had only local anaesthesia or procedural sedation. The patient who has had general anaesthesia usually has undergone extensive surgery as well. In contrast, an ambulatory surgical patient who has had local anaesthesia with no sedation and has stable vital signs may be discharged immediately. A patient who has undergone regional or general anaesthesia usually is transferred to the PACU to be stabilized before discharge to the nursing unit or back to the ambulatory surgery area.

To assess a patient's postoperative condition, nurses must apply critical thinking while relying on information from the preoperative nursing assessment, knowledge regarding the surgical procedure performed, and reports on events occurring during surgery. This information helps nurses detect any changes and make decisions about the patient's care. A variation from the patient's norm may indicate the onset of surgery-related complications. Along with the anaesthesiologist or anaesthetist assistant, the circulating nurse may accompany the patient to the PACU and report to the nurse to provide continuity of care.

A patient's postoperative course involves two phases: the immediate recovery period and postoperative convalescence. For an ambulatory surgical patient, recovery normally lasts only 1 to 2 hours, and convalescence occurs at home. For a hospitalized patient, recovery may last a few hours, and convalescence occurs in the hospital over one or more days, depending on the extent of the surgery and the patient's response to it.

Immediate Postoperative Recovery

Before the patient arrives in the PACU, the PACU nurse obtains data from the surgical team in the OR regarding the patient's general status and the need for special equipment and nursing care. Careful planning allows the nursing staff to consider placement of patients in the PACU. For example, patients who have undergone spinal anaesthesia are aware of their surroundings and may benefit from being in a quieter part of the PACU, away from patients who need frequent monitoring. The patient with a serious infection such as tuberculosis should be isolated from other patients. Standard precautions or routine practices for infection control are used for all patients (see Chapter 34). Nurses must be familiar with agency and professional protocols related to preventing respiratory infection transmission (Public Health Ontario, 2012).

When the patient is admitted to the PACU, the nursing staff can inform family members. Usually, nurses would advise family members to remain in the designated waiting area so that they can be found when the surgeon arrives to explain the patient's condition. The surgeon is responsible for describing the patient's status, the results of the surgery, and any complications that may have been encountered. Nurses can be a valuable resource to the family if complications arose during the operative phase.

When the patient enters the PACU (Figure 49.7), nurses and members of the surgical team confer about the patient's status. The surgical team's report includes a review of anaesthetic agents administered so that nurses can anticipate both how quickly a patient should regain consciousness and their analgesic needs. A report on IV fluids or blood products administered during surgery alerts nurses to the

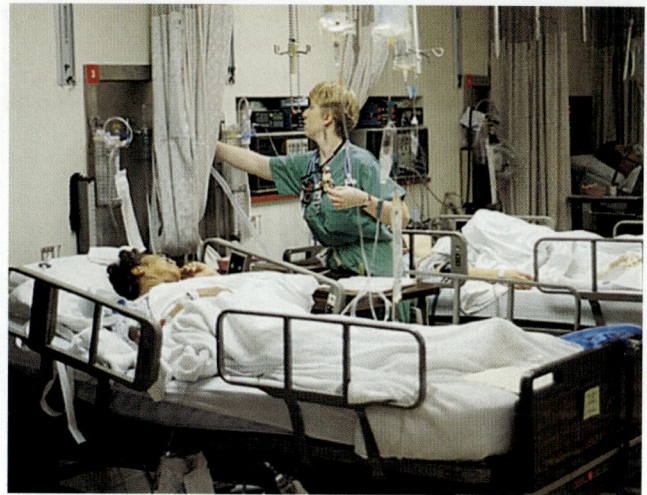
FIGURE 49.7 Postanaesthesia care unit.

patient's fluid and electrolyte balances. The surgeon often reports any special concerns (e.g., whether the patient is at risk for hemorrhaging or infection). The anaesthesiologist discusses whether there were complications during surgery, such as excessive blood loss or cardiac irregularities. Frequently, this report takes place while PACU nurses are admitting the patient. A nurse will attach the patient to monitoring equipment such as the noninvasive blood pressure monitor, ECG monitor, and pulse oximeter. Patients usually receive some form of oxygen in this immediate recovery period. The nurse takes vital signs when the patient arrives and confirms these with the surgical team.

After reviewing events in the OR, the PACU nurse conducts a complete assessment of the patient's status. This assessment should be performed rapidly and thoroughly and be targeted to the needs of the postsurgical patient. Standards of perianaesthetic nursing practice, such as those of NAPANc (2018), which are used by OPANA, function as a guide for agencies in outlining the urgent nature and components of the admission assessment as well as ongoing monitoring of patient status. A systems approach to assessment is discussed in a later section outlining the nursing process in postoperative care. Nursing care in the PACU focuses on monitoring and maintaining respiratory, circulatory, neurological, and fluid and electrolyte status; assessing wound status; and assessing and managing pain (see "Nursing Process in Postoperative Care"). After receiving hand-off communication from the OR, the PACU nurse conducts a complete systems assessment during the first few minutes of PACU care (Box 49.6).

Discharge From the Postanaesthesia Care Unit

Nurses evaluate readiness for discharge from the PACU by comparing vital sign stability with the preoperative data. Other outcomes for discharge are body temperature control, good ventilatory function, orientation to surroundings, absence of complications, minimal pain and nausea, controlled wound drainage, adequate urine output, and fluid and electrolyte balances. Patients who had more extensive surgery that required anaesthesia of longer duration usually recover more slowly. Many PACU staff use an objective scoring system that helps to delineate when patients may be discharged. The Aldrete score, or the **Postanaesthesia Recovery Score (PARS)**, is the most widely used scoring tool (Table 49.8). The patient must receive a composite score of 8 to 10 before discharge from the PACU. Some agencies have modified this scoring system; for example, some remove movement of extremities and add presence of pain, and some agencies require that the patient have a composite score of 10 before discharge from the PACU. If the

BOX 49.6 Initial Postanaesthesia Care Assessment: Parameters to Assess

Initial assessment in the PACU includes the following:

- Integration of data received at hand-off for transfer of care
- Vital signs
- Respiratory status—airway patency, breath sounds, type of artificial airway, mechanical ventilator settings, oxygen saturation, and end-tidal CO_2 values
- Intake and output
- Pain/sedation/comfort assessment (including psychoemotional status), presence of nausea or vomiting
- Neurological function: level of consciousness (may use Glasgow Coma scale), pupillary response (if indicated)
- Position of the patient
- Condition and colour of skin, status of any suspected pressure areas
- Patient safety needs (positioning to prevent aspiration)
- Neurovascular status: peripheral pulses and sensation of extremity or extremities
- Condition of surgical dressings or suture line, drains, tubes, receptacles
- Amount, appearance, and type of drainage
- Muscular response and strength/mobility
- Fluid therapy—location of intravenous (IV) lines, patency of IV lines, amount and type of solution (crystalloids or blood products) infused, next fluid to be administered
- Procedure-specific assessments, such as expected drainage amount, specific positioning aids for orthopedic surgery.

Adapted from Glick, D. (2020). Overview of post-anesthetic care for adult patients. *UpToDate.* https://www.uptodate.com/contents/overview-of-post-anesthetic-care-for-adult-patients; Rothrock, J. C. (2019). *Alexander's care of the patient in surgery* (16th ed.). Elsevier.

TABLE 49.8 Postanaesthetic Recovery Score or Modified Aldrete Score

Parameter	Task	Score
Activity	Able to move four extremities voluntarily or on command	2
	Able to move two extremities voluntarily or on command	1
	Unable to move extremities voluntarily or on command	0
Respiration	Able to breathe deeply and cough freely	2
	Dyspnea or limited breathing	1
	Apneic	0
Blood pressure	± 20% of preanaesthetic level	2
	± 20–49% of preanaesthetic level	1
	± 50% of preanaesthetic level	0
Consciousness	Fully awake	2
	Arousable on calling	1
	Not responding	0
Oxygen saturation	SpO_2 >94% on room air	2
	Needs O_2 inhalation to maintain SpO_2 >94%	1
	SpO_2 <94% even with extra O_2	0
Total		

Adapted from Aldrete, J. A., & Kroulik, D. (1970). A post-anesthetic recovery score. *Anesthesia and Analgesia, 49,* 924–934; Aldrete, J. A. (1998). Modifications to the post-anesthesia score for use in ambulatory surgery. *Journal of PeriAnesthesia Nursing, 13*(3), 148.

patient's condition is still poor after 2 to 3 hours, the stay in the PACU lengthens or the surgeon may transfer the patient to a Critical Care Unit (CCU). More recently, some agencies have been using the Post-Anesthesic Discharge Scoring System (PADSS).

When the patient is ready to be discharged from the PACU, the PACU nurse may call the nursing unit to report the patient's status, including vital signs, respiratory status, the type of surgery and anaesthesia performed, any complications that occurred during surgery or in the PACU, blood loss, level of consciousness, general physical condition, type and amount of fluids received, and presence of IV lines, drainage tubes, and dressings. The nurse also should review physician orders that require attention. The PACU nurse's report helps the nurse in the acute patient care area to anticipate special patient needs and obtain necessary equipment. Any outstanding family issues are also addressed.

Orderlies or other personnel, who might include nurses, transport the patient on a stretcher. Usually the PACU nurse does not accompany the patient to the surgical unit, but a verbal report will be given to the acute care nurse reviewing the patient's condition and course of care. Some institutions have policies related to which patients must be accompanied by a nurse, such as those who have experienced recent seizure activity or who have had upper airway surgery. Staff members assist in safely transferring the patient to a bed (see Chapter 37).

Recovery in Ambulatory Surgery

The thoroughness and extent of postoperative recovery care depend on the ambulatory patient's condition, type of surgery, and anaesthesia.

There are two phases of postanaesthesia recovery. During phase I, nurses focus on helping the patient safely transition from a totally anaesthetized state to one requiring less acute interventions. After patients become stable and no longer require such intensive monitoring, nurses transfer them to phase II recovery. During phase II, nurses focus on continuing the recovery process, addressing the patient's needs, and preparing the patient and family for discharge from phase II (NAPANc, 2018).

With new anaesthetic agents and techniques, patients experience a more rapid awakening in the OR (Apfelbaum et al., 2002; Fredman et al., 2002; Saar, 2001). Therefore, some ambulatory surgery patients may bypass phase I. This is known as *fast tracking* (Rice et al., 2015; White et al., 2003). Phase II recovery may consist of a room equipped with medical recliner chairs, side tables, and footrests. Kitchen facilities for preparing light snacks and beverages are usually located in the area, along with bathrooms. Aldrete (1998) has added five more areas of functional assessment for the ambulatory surgery patient, which constitute the Postanaesthesia Recovery Score for Ambulatory Patients (PARSAP) (Table 49.9). The phase II environment is designed to promote both the patient's and the family's comfort and well-being until discharge. Nurses continue to monitor patients but not at the same intensity as during phase I. In phase II recovery, nurses initiate postoperative teaching with patients and family members (Box 49.7).

Ambulatory surgical patients are discharged to home when they meet certain criteria. A patient being monitored by PARSAP must achieve a score of 18 or higher before being discharged. An exception may be allowed if the patient was unable to walk or move their extremities before surgery (Aldrete, 1998). Postoperative nausea and vomiting may occur once the patient is home, even if the symptoms were not present at the time of discharge. Attention must be paid to these symptoms, because they affect patient recovery, whether in the hospital or at home for ambulatory surgical patients (Lichtor & Chang, 2012). An option for therapy includes the prophylactic use of the medication ondansetron (McQuaid, 2021).

TABLE 49.9 Postanaesthesia Aldrete Recovery Score for Ambulatory Patients

Original Criteria	Modified Criteria	Point Value
Colour	*Oxygenation*	
Pink	SpO$_2$ >92% on room air	2
Pale or dusky	SpO$_2$ >90% on oxygen	1
Cyanotic	SpO$_2$ < 90% on oxygen	0
Respiration		
Can breathe deeply and cough	Breathes deeply and coughs freely	2
Shallow but adequate exchange	Dyspneic, shallow or limited breathing	1
Apnea or obstruction	Apnea	0
Circulation		
Blood pressure within 20% of normal	Blood pressure ± 20 mm Hg of normal	2
Blood pressure within 20 to 50% of normal	Blood pressure ± 20 to 50 mm Hg of normal	1
Blood pressure deviating >50% from normal	Blood pressure more than ± 50 mm Hg of normal	0
Consciousness		
Awake and alert and orientated	Fully awake	2
Arousable but readily drifts back to sleep	Arousable on calling	1
No response	Not responsive	0
Activity		
Moves all extremities	Same	2
Moves two extremities	Same	1
No extremities	Same	0

Data from Aldrete, J. A., & Kroulik, D. (1970). A post-anesthetic recovery score. *Anesthesia and Analgesia, 49*, 924–934; Aldrete, J. A. (1995). The post-anesthesia recovery score revisited. *Journal of Clinical Anesthesia, 7*(1), 89. Reprinted from Butterworth IV, J. F., Mackey, D. C., & Wasnick, J. D. (Eds.). (2018). Chapter 56: Postanesthesia care (p. 1294, Table 56.2). *Morgan & Mikhail's clinical anesthesiology* (6th ed.). McGraw-Hill Education.

Written postoperative instructions and prescriptions are reviewed with the patient and the family, and the nurse should ensure that they verbalize understanding of these instructions. The patient is discharged to the care of a responsible adult.

Postoperative Convalescence

Inpatients are kept in the PACU until their condition stabilizes; they are then transported to the postoperative nursing unit. Ambulatory surgery patients will return home. Nursing care focuses on returning the patient to a relatively functional level of wellness as soon as possible. The speed of convalescence depends on the presurgical general state of health, the type or extent of surgery, the risk factors involved, and any postoperative complications.

❖ NURSING PROCESS IN POSTOPERATIVE CARE

Nursing care in the PACU is focused on managing pain and monitoring and maintaining respiratory, circulatory, fluid and electrolyte, and neurological status. Other important assessments include temperature, skin and incision or wound status, and genitourinary and gastrointestinal function. Nurses in the surgical unit continue to assess these critical factors until the patient's discharge from the acute care facility.

BOX 49.7 PATIENT TEACHING

Postoperative Instructions for Ambulatory Surgical Patients

Objectives
- Patient will verbalize resources to contact for assistance.
- Patient will describe signs and symptoms of postoperative problems.
- Patient will list the name and dose of medications to self-administer.
- Patient will describe guidelines related to specific surgery.

Teaching Strategies
- Provide instruction sheet with physician's or nurse's telephone number, surgery centre's number, and follow-up appointment date and time. Allow patient and family to ask questions.
- Explain to family members the signs and symptoms of infection for which to observe.
- Explain name, dose, schedule, and purpose of medications. Provide medication information leaflets.
- Explain activity restrictions, diet progression, and any special wound care related to specific surgery. Provide instruction sheet with clear, focused explanations.

Evaluation
- Ask patient to describe signs indicating potential problems and normal convalescence.
- Ask patient to explain when and how to call health care providers such as the home care nurse.
- Make sure patient records follow-up appointment in diary or on an electronic device.
- Ask patient and family members to describe the signs and symptoms of infection.
- Ask patient to verbalize name of medication, dose, and when to take.
- Ask patient to demonstrate proper activity or movement and wound care.

❖ Assessment

After patient assessment upon arrival to the PACU, the nurse repeats evaluation of vital signs and other key observations at least every 15 minutes or more frequently, depending on the patient's condition and unit policy. This assessment usually continues until discharge from the PACU. Once the patient is returned to the surgical unit, the nurse admitting the patient takes vital signs immediately in order to compare them with the PACU findings. Vital sign monitoring in the surgical nursing unit initially should be at least hourly for 4 hours and then every 4 hours, unless complications develop. Frequency of assessment should always be based on the patient's current condition, which can change rapidly, especially during the postoperative period.

Nurses need to thoroughly document their assessment, including circulatory and respiratory status, level of consciousness, temperature, condition of dressings and drains, pain and comfort level, skin warmth and colour, ability to move extremities, IV fluid status, and urinary output measurements. Patient data can be entered on flow sheets, by electronic documentation, or as written progress notes. The initial findings are a baseline for comparing any postoperative changes.

Once the patient returns to the acute care area, the nurse's focus is on completing the assessment, meeting the patient's immediate needs, and providing an opportunity for the family to be with the patient. The call light and emesis basin should be within the patient's reach. The nurse can explain the purpose of postoperative procedures or equipment and the patient's status. The family should know that the patient will fall in and out of sleep for most of the rest of the day, owing to the effects of general anaesthesia and pain medication. The family also should be reminded that frequent assessments are to be expected and that limited sensation and movement in the patient's extremities may remain for a few hours if the patient had intrathecal (spinal) or epidural anaesthesia.

Respiration. Major concerns for the nurse caring for patients post-anaesthesia and after surgery are hypoventilation, hypoxemia, and airway obstruction. Certain anaesthetic agents may cause respiratory depression. Thus, nurses must be especially alert for shallow, slow breathing and a weak cough. Airway patency, respiratory rate, rhythm, depth of ventilation, symmetry of chest wall movement, breath sounds, and colour of mucous membranes must all be assessed. If breathing is unusually shallow, placing a hand near the patient's nose or mouth allows the nurse to feel exhaled air. Pulse oximetry should reflect 92 to 100% saturation. Some agencies now have directives that allow nurses to administer oxygen at 3 L/minute via nasal prongs if the patient has a saturation of less than 92%.

The patient often has an oral or nasal airway (see Chapter 40) inserted in the OR after removal of the endotracheal tube, to maintain a patent airway until the patient can protect their airway. As the patient awakens in the PACU, they will spit out the airway or the nurse will ask them to spit it out. The patient's ability to do so signifies the return of a normal gag reflex.

One of the nurse's greatest concerns is airway obstruction. A number of factors can contribute to obstruction, including weak pharyngeal or laryngeal muscle tone from anaesthetics; secretions in the pharynx, bronchial tree, or trachea; and laryngeal or subglottic edema (da Silva de Sousa et al., 2020). Signs of airway obstruction include snoring, nasal flaring, and use of accessory muscles to breathe (da Silva de Sousa et al., 2020). In the postanaesthetic patient, the tongue causes the majority of airway obstructions. Ongoing assessment of airway patency is crucial. Patients are often kept in a side-lying position until airways are clear.

In the acute care area, nurses continue to assess respiratory status and breath sounds. Older patients, smokers, and patients with a history of respiratory disease are prone to developing complications such as atelectasis or pneumonia. The patient is also assessed for any signs of shortness of breath with activity.

Circulation. The patient is at risk for cardiovascular complications resulting from actual or potential blood loss from the surgical site, adverse effects of anaesthesia, electrolyte imbalances, and depression of normal circulatory regulating mechanisms. Careful assessment of heart rate and rhythm, along with blood pressure, reveals the patient's cardiovascular status. A rhythm strip is usually obtained postoperatively, compared with any preoperative ECG tracings, and mounted on the PACU record. The vital signs are monitored at least every 15 minutes throughout the PACU recovery phase. Preoperative vital signs are compared with postoperative values. The physician should be notified if the patient's blood pressure drops progressively with each check or if the heart rate changes or becomes irregular.

The nurse assesses circulatory perfusion by noting capillary refill, pulses, and the colour and temperature of the nail beds and skin. If the patient has had vascular surgery or has casts or constricting devices that may impair circulation, the nurse should assess peripheral pulses and capillary refill distal to the site of surgery. For example, after surgery to the femoral artery, the posterior tibial and dorsalis pedis pulses are assessed. The nurse should also compare pulses in the affected extremity with those in the nonaffected extremity.

A common early circulatory problem is hemorrhage. Blood loss may occur externally through a drain or incision, or internally. Either type of hemorrhage may result in a fall in blood pressure; elevated heart and respiratory rates; thready pulse; cool, clammy, pale skin;

and restlessness. Often, the first sign of hemorrhage is restlessness. Signs such as thready pulse and clammy skin are noted much later, after significant blood loss has occurred. To prevent deterioration of the patient, the surgeon must be notified of significant changes, from baseline, of heart rate, blood pressure, and respirations. The nurse must maintain IV fluid infusion and may need to increase IV replacement fluids. The patient's vital signs are monitored every 15 minutes or more frequently until their condition stabilizes. Oxygen may need to be continued. Volume replacement and medications to promote perfusion to vital organs such as the brain may be considered. In the initial postoperative period, isotonic solutions such as 0.9% normal saline and Ringer's lactate are used (Neal, 2019).

Plasma expanders (colloids) may be used instead of blood transfusions. Colloids may be made from blood products (i.e., albumin), but artificial colloids, such as hetastarch, may also be used (Neal, 2019). Colloids may be used in hypovolemic shock; however, a large randomized trial demonstrated no improvement in mortality with their administration (Neal, 2019).

Temperature Control. The OR and recovery room environments are kept extremely cool. The patient's anaesthetically depressed level of body function results in a lowering of metabolism and a fall in body temperature. When patients begin to awaken, they usually complain of feeling cold and uncomfortable. The length of time spent in the OR and laminar flow rooms contributes to heat loss. Surgeries that require an open body cavity also contribute to heat loss. Older persons and pediatric patients are at higher risk for developing conditions associated with hypothermia. Hypothermia can cause cardiac irregularities, hypotension, and coagulopathy (Butterworth et al., 2018).

In rare instances, **malignant hyperthermia**, a genetically determined condition and a life-threatening complication of anaesthesia, develops. Due to the release of intracellular calcium, muscle contractions occur throughout the body. Other symptoms can be tachypnea, cardiac arrhythmias, unstable blood pressure, cyanosis, and skin mottling. An elevated temperature, a sign of the condition, occurs late. It is often seen during the induction phase of anaesthesia and is managed by discontinuing the anaesthetic agent causing the condition, administering oxygen, and starting dantrolene (Glahn et al., 2020). Fluid resuscitation is required. Without prompt detection and treatment, it can be fatal.

For all patients, temperature is monitored closely in the acute care area. Because an elevated temperature may be the first indication of an infection, nurses need to evaluate the patient for a potential source of infection, including the IV site (if present), the surgical incision or wound, and the respiratory and urinary tracts. The physician must be notified, because further evaluation, including blood, sputum, and urinary cultures, likely will be needed. In older patients, fever may not be seen with infection (Litwack, 2006).

Fluid and Electrolyte Balances. Because of the surgical patient's risk for fluid and electrolyte abnormalities, nurses need to assess the patient's hydration status and monitor cardiac and neurological function for signs of electrolyte alterations (see Chapter 41). Laboratory values are monitored and compared with the patient's baseline values.

One of the nurse's important responsibilities is monitoring the rate and maintaining the patency of IV infusions. The patient's only source of fluid intake immediately after surgery is through IV catheters. Nurses must inspect the catheter insertion site to ensure that the catheter is properly positioned within a vein so that fluid flows freely. Nurses need to record the IV infusions received as well as any sources of oral intake once peristalsis returns. All sources of output are measured, including urine, drainage from surgically placed drains, gastric drainage, and drainage from wounds, and any insensible loss from diaphoresis is noted. Daily weights may be assessed postoperatively if the patient has a known cardiac or renal history (e.g., heart failure). It is important to compare preoperative and postoperative weights and to be consistent in the scale used, the amount of clothing worn by the patient, and the time of day to obtain accurate weight measurement. *Accurate recording of intake and output is crucial.* It is also important to be aware of the amount of fluids received in the intraoperative and immediate postoperative period. For example, if large amounts of fluid were received during surgery, the patient may exhibit signs of fluid retention, such as pedal edema or abnormal breath sounds.

Neurological Functions. The patient is often drowsy in the PACU. As anaesthetic agents are metabolized, the patient's reflexes return, muscle strength is regained, and a normal level of orientation returns. A patient should at least be oriented to self and to the hospital before discharge from the PACU. Gag reflexes (see Chapter 33), hand grips, and movement of the patient's extremities are assessed. If the patient has had surgery involving a portion of the neurological system, a more thorough neurological assessment needs to be conducted, including assessing pupil size and reaction.

Patients who had regional anaesthesia begin to experience a return in motor function before tactile sensation. The patient's sensation is checked along dermatomes (segmental skin areas innervated by specific segments of the spinal cord). Knowing where anaesthesia was introduced, the nurse is able to check the distribution of the spinal nerves affected (see Chapter 33). Typically, the nurse assesses the dermatome level by touching the patient bilaterally and documenting where they feel touch. The sense of touch can be tested using a paper clip, for example. Assessment of extremity strength, movement, and sensation continues to be important if spinal or epidural anaesthesia has been given, although the patient should remain in the PACU until sensation and voluntary movement of the lower extremities have been re-established.

Skin Integrity and Condition of the Wound. In the PACU, nurses assess the condition of the patient's skin, noting rashes, petechiae, abrasions, or burns. A rash may indicate a medication sensitivity or allergy. Abrasions or petechiae may result from a clotting disorder or from inappropriate positioning that injures skin layers. Burns may indicate that an electrical cautery grounding pad was incorrectly placed on the patient's skin. Burns or serious injury to the skin should be documented in an incident report (see Chapter 16). The nurse should also make a note if the patient complains of any burning or pain in the eye that could indicate a corneal abrasion.

After surgery, most wounds are covered with a dressing that protects the site and collects drainage. Nurses need to observe the amount, colour, odour, and consistency of drainage on dressings. Serosanguineous drainage is the most common type of drainage occurring immediately after surgery. The amount of drainage is estimated by noting the number of saturated gauze sponges. If drainage appears on the outer surface of a dressing, another way to assess drainage is by drawing a circle around the outer perimeter of the drainage on the dressing and dating it with the time noted. This way, nurses can easily note if drainage is increasing (see Chapter 47).

The nurse on the surgical nursing unit usually will have the first opportunity to view and thoroughly assess and document the status of the incision or wound. Initially, it is important to note if wound edges are approximated and no active bleeding or drainage is present. The wound needs to be assessed for redness, swelling, signs of infection, and slipped sutures or staples. Wound assessment is especially

important because it forms the baseline for continued monitoring during the patient's hospital stay.

Pressure injuries can occur in the patient undergoing surgery. Older patients may have several risk factors, such as nutritional or cardiovascular deficiencies or diabetes, that predispose them to these injuries (Posthauer et al., 2014). It is important to assess the patient's mobility level. If the patient is unable or unwilling to turn, pressure injuries can occur. Nurses should use the Braden Scale to determine the patient's risk of developing pressure injuries (RNAO, 2016). Preventive measures such as a turning schedule and pressure-reduction devices can be instituted (see Chapter 47).

Genitourinary Function. Depending on the surgery, a patient may not regain voluntary control over urinary function for 6 to 8 hours after anaesthesia. An epidural or spinal anaesthetic may prevent the patient from feeling bladder fullness. The nurse should palpate the lower abdomen just above the symphysis pubis for bladder distension or use a bladder scanner to identify the amount of urine in the bladder. If the patient has a urinary catheter, there should be a continuous flow of urine—30 to 50 mL/hour in adults. The colour and the odour of the urine should be observed. Surgery involving portions of the urinary tract normally causes bloody urine for at least 12 to 24 hours, depending on the type of surgery. The nurse needs to conduct ongoing assessment of genitourinary function.

Gastrointestinal Function. Anaesthetics slow gastrointestinal motility and may cause nausea. Normally, during the immediate recovery phase, faint or absent bowel sounds are auscultated in all four quadrants. The abdomen is inspected for distension that may be caused by an accumulation of gas. In a patient who has had abdominal surgery, distension will develop if internal bleeding occurs; however, this is a late sign of bleeding. Distension also may occur in the patient who develops a paralytic ileus as a result of handling of the bowel in surgery.

Nurses need to closely monitor the patient's initial oral intake for potential aspiration or the presence of nausea and vomiting. Assessment also includes checking every 4 to 8 hours for return of peristalsis. Routinely, nurses auscultate the abdomen to detect return of normal bowel sounds; 5 to 30 loud gurgles per minute over each quadrant indicates that peristalsis has returned. High-pitched tinkling sounds accompanied by abdominal distension suggest that the bowel is not functioning properly. The nurse should ask the patient if they are passing gas (flatus). This is an important sign indicating normal bowel function. If a nasogastric tube is in place, the nurse needs to assess the patency of the tube (see Chapter 45), the colour and amount of any drainage, and (if ordered) the level of suction required.

Pain and Comfort. Pain management is included in the overall aim of ensuring patient comfort. Comfort is also achieved through nursing measures such as bathing and providing clean bedding. As patients awaken from general anaesthesia, the sensation of pain becomes prominent. Pain can be perceived before full consciousness is regained. Acute incisional pain can cause patients to become restless and may be responsible for temporary changes in vital signs. It is difficult for patients to begin coughing and undertaking deep breathing exercises when they experience pain. The patient who had regional or local anaesthesia may not experience pain initially because the incisional area is still anaesthetized.

Assessment of the patient's discomfort and evaluation of pain-relief therapies are essential nursing functions. Pain scales are an effective method for nurses to assess postoperative pain, evaluate response to analgesics, and objectively document pain severity (see Chapter 32). In addition, Best Practice Guidelines provide guidance for decision making (RNAO, 2013). By frequently assessing pain, nurses can evaluate the effectiveness of interventions (e.g., positioning, analgesics) throughout the patient's recovery. The nurse's caring presence at the bedside promotes communication between the nurse and the patient, which, in turn, enables effective pain management.

Patient Expectations. The nurse assesses the patient's and family's expectations and perceived progress in the recovery and convalescence phases. Ongoing assessment of expectations regarding pain control, comfort level, dietary intake, activity level, and readiness for discharge is also performed. The nurse determines the patient's and the family's expectations regarding needs at home and incorporates these into the care plan.

◆ Nursing Diagnosis

Nurses determine the status of health problems identified from preoperative nursing diagnoses and cluster new relevant data to identify new diagnoses. Previously defined diagnoses, such as *impaired skin integrity*, may continue as a postoperative condition. The nurse may identify new risk factors leading to identification of nursing diagnoses. For example, an older patient who has undergone major abdominal surgery and who has a pre-existing condition of reduced hip mobility resulting from arthritis will likely have the diagnosis of *impaired physical mobility*. The surgery itself may add risk factors for the patient. Nurses also must consider the needs of the patient's family when making diagnoses. For example, difficulties of the family coping with the patient's condition require nursing intervention. Early dialogue with the family can aid in identifying any challenges.

◆ Planning

Because of the critical nature of the immediate postoperative period, nursing care in the PACU involves close monitoring of the patient and frequent assessments to ensure a return to stable physiological and cognitive function. During the convalescent phase, the nurse uses current physical assessment data and analysis of the preoperative nursing health history for planning the patient's care. The surgeon's postoperative plan and the institution's clinical pathways are also guidelines. Typical postoperative plans include the following:

- Frequency of vital sign monitoring and other assessments such as oxygen saturation
- Types of IV fluids and rates of infusion
- Postoperative medications (especially those for pain and nausea)
- Resumption of preoperative medications as condition allows (some oral medications will be converted to the IV route with appropriate dose adjustment). Some institutions provide a medication reconciliation and orders form to be used in the postoperative period.
- Fluids and food allowed by mouth
- Level of activity that the patient is allowed to resume
- Position that the patient is to maintain while in bed
- Intake and output
- Laboratory tests and diagnostic studies
- Special directions (e.g., surgical drains to suction, tube irrigations, dressing changes)
- Patient teaching and discharge planning
- Behaviour changes

Goals and Outcomes. Nurses consider the effects of the stress of surgery and the limitations it produces when establishing goals, patient outcomes, and nursing interventions for the patient. Measurable outcomes with indicators help to ensure timely and appropriate recovery from surgery. For example, the patient at risk for impaired physical mobility should have specific outcomes that include targeted

ambulation (e.g., steps to take and distance down hallway) and range of joint movement. After each outcome is met, the patient ultimately will achieve the goal of independent mobility at a preoperative level or better. The nurse needs to carefully consider all goals of care established during the preoperative surgical phase. The following is an example of goals and outcomes for the postoperative period:

- Patient achieves a return of normal physiological function after surgery.
- Patient's vital signs return to preoperative baseline.
- Patient's airway is patent, respirations are even, and the patient is experiencing no distress.
- Patient's temperature returns to baseline. Patient's fluid and electrolyte levels remain balanced.
- Patient verbalizes feeling of increased strength and ability to move.

Setting Priorities. In the PACU, priorities of care include the assessment and stability of the patient's airway; interventions for an impaired airway; assessment of the patient's respiratory, circulatory, neurological, and fluid and electrolyte status; and pain control. As the patient progresses on the acute care unit, priorities should focus on advancement of patient activity. The patient generally will have multiple nursing diagnoses. Nurses may re-establish priorities several times as the patient's health status changes.

Continuity of Care. In the recovery phase, nurses collaborate on the care plan with staff from respiratory therapy, physiotherapy, occupational therapy, dietary, social work, home care, and other areas to meet the patient's needs. The goal of all these disciplines is to assist the patient to return to the best possible level of functioning with a smooth transition to home. The family's role in the care plan to foster recovery is also essential.

◆ Implementation

Health Promotion. Primary causes of postoperative complications include the surgical wound, the effects of prolonged immobilization during surgery and convalescence, preoperative risks such as age (Box 49.8), and the influence of anaesthesia and analgesics. Nursing interventions in the postoperative period are directed at preventing complications so that the patient returns to the highest level of functioning possible. Failure of the patient to become actively involved in recovery adds to the risk for complications (Table 49.10). Virtually any body system can be affected. Nurses must consider the interrelationship of all systems and therapies provided.

Maintaining Respiratory Function. To prevent respiratory complications, pulmonary interventions should be started early. The benefits of thorough preoperative teaching are realized when patients are able to participate actively. When the patient awakens from anaesthesia, the nurse may need to assist them in maintaining a patent airway. The following measures are used to maintain airway patency:

- Position the patient on one side with the face downward and the neck slightly extended to facilitate a forward movement of the tongue and the flow of mucous secretions out of the mouth. A small, folded towel supports the head. Another positioning technique to promote a patent airway involves slightly elevating the head of the bed and slightly extending the patient's neck, with the head turned to the side. In some patients, the PACU nurse may need to perform a jaw thrust manoeuvre or chin lift continuously to maintain the airway. The patient should never be positioned with their arms over or across the chest because this reduces maximum chest expansion.
- Suction artificial airways and the oral cavity for mucous secretions (see Chapter 40). Care must be taken to avoid eliciting the gag reflex, which could cause vomiting.

BOX 49.8 FOCUS ON OLDER PERSONS

Risks of Surgery

- Advances in medical technology and therapies enable patients to live longer (Canadian Hospice Palliative Care Association, 2020). Consequently, nurses are caring for many more surgical patients of advanced age and are required to know age-related factors that affect the outcomes of a surgical procedure. Hypothermia and acute postoperative complications including frailty, pneumonia, embolism may be seen in seen in older persons (Lin et al., 2016).
- A smaller margin of physiological reserve makes the older person less able to compensate during the perioperative period for changes that can occur due to infection, hemorrhage, alterations in blood pressure, and fluid and electrolyte abnormalities.
- Older patients are at greater risk for postoperative delirium after procedures such as hip replacement and cardiac surgery (Harris et al., 2019; OPANA, 2018). A rapid decline in cognitive function, fluctuations in awareness and orientation, disturbed sleep–wake cycle, and personality and mood changes characterize the typical presentation. Delirium may be the first indicator of infection, fluid or electrolyte imbalances, or deteriorating respiratory or hemodynamic status. Postoperative delirium is associated with extended lengths of hospital stay, loss of independence, increased morbidity and mortality, and increased health care costs. Delirium may present as hyperactive, hypoactive, or mixed (Kirpinar, 2018).
- Altered and unexpected medication responses are often related to different pharmacokinetics in the older person. Thus, when caring for the perioperative older patient, nurses must be alert to the possibility of a high risk for adverse medication events with the administration of anaesthetic agents and postoperative analgesics, especially narcotics. "Start lower and go slow" should be the guiding principle when medicating older persons, because of their slower medication-clearance capability (RNAO, 2007; American Geriatrics Society Expert Panel, 2015).

The following measures promote expansion of the lungs:

- Encourage diaphragmatic breathing exercises every hour while patients are awake. Maximal inspirations lasting 3 to 5 seconds open up the alveoli.
- Encourage early ambulation. Walking causes patients to assume a position that does not restrict chest wall expansion and stimulates an increased respiratory rate.
- Help patients who are restricted to bed to turn on their side every 1 to 2 hours while awake and to sit when possible. Turning permits expansion of the lungs. Sitting causes lowering of abdominal organs, thus facilitating diaphragmatic movement and lung expansion.
- Keep the patient comfortable. A patient who is comfortable will be able to participate in the postoperative regimen. Assess, document, treat, and evaluate the patient's pain on a regular basis.

The following measures promote removal of pulmonary secretions if they are present:

- Encourage coughing exercises every 2 hours while patients are awake, and maintain pain control to promote a deep, productive cough. Coughing may be contraindicated for patients who have had eye or intracranial surgery, because of the potential increase in intraocular or intracranial pressure.
- Provide oral hygiene to facilitate expectoration of mucus. The oral mucosa becomes dry when patients are NPO or are placed on limited fluid intake.
- Initiate orotracheal or nasotracheal suction for patients who are too weak or unable to cough (see Chapter 40).
- Administer oxygen as ordered and monitor oxygen saturation with a pulse oximeter.

Preventing Circulatory Complications. Measures directed at preventing circulatory complications avert circulatory stasis. Some patients are at greater risk of venous stasis because of the nature of their surgery or medical history. The following measures promote normal venous return and circulatory blood flow:

TABLE 49.10 Postoperative Complications	
Complication	**Cause**
Respiratory System	
Atelectasis: Collapse of alveoli with retained mucous secretions. Signs and symptoms include elevated respiratory rate, dyspnea, fever, crackles auscultated over involved lobes of lungs, productive cough, decreased oxygen saturation.	Inadequate lung expansion. Anaesthesia, analgesia, and immobilized position prevent full lung expansion. There is greater risk in patients with upper abdominal surgery who have pain during inspiration and repress deep breathing.
Pneumonia: Inflammation of alveoli. It may involve one or several lobes of lung. Development in lower dependent lobes of lung is common in immobilized surgical patient. Signs and symptoms include fever, chills, productive cough, chest pain, purulent mucus, and dyspnea as well as decreased oxygen saturation.	Poor lung expansion with retained secretions or aspirated secretions.
Hypoxemia: Inadequate concentration of oxygen in arterial blood. Signs and symptoms include restlessness, decreased mental alertness, dyspnea, high or low blood pressure, tachycardia or bradycardia, diaphoresis, and cyanosis.	Respirations are depressed by anaesthetics or analgesics. Increased retention of mucus with impaired ventilation occurs because of pain or poor positioning.
Pulmonary embolism: Embolus blocking pulmonary arterial blood flow to one or more lobes of lung. Signs and symptoms include dyspnea, sudden chest pain, cyanosis, tachycardia, and drop in blood pressure.	Same factors lead to formation of thrombus or embolus. Immobilized surgical patient with pre-existing circulatory or coagulation disorders is at risk.
Circulatory System	
Hemorrhage: Loss of large amount of blood externally or internally in short period of time. Signs and symptoms include hypotension, weak and rapid pulse, cool and clammy skin, rapid breathing, restlessness, and reduced urine output.	Slipping of suture or dislodged clot at incisional site. Patients with coagulation disorders are at greater risk. Blood loss with fractures can also occur.

TABLE 49.10	Postoperative Complications—cont'd
Complication	**Cause**
Hypovolemic shock: Inadequate perfusion of tissues and cells from loss of circulatory fluid volume. Signs and symptoms are the same as for hemorrhage.	In surgical patient, hypovolemic shock is usually caused by hemorrhage.
Thrombophlebitis: Inflammation of vein often accompanied by clot formation. Veins in legs are most commonly affected. Signs and symptoms include swelling and inflammation of involved site and aching or cramping pain. Vein feels hard, cordlike, and sensitive to touch.	Venous stasis is aggravated by prolonged sitting or immobilization. Trauma to vessel wall and hypercoagulability of blood increase risk of vessel inflammation.
Thrombus: Formation of clot attached to interior wall of a vein or artery, which can occlude the vessel lumen. Signs and symptoms include localized tenderness along distribution of the venous system, swollen calf or thigh, calf swelling more than 3 cm compared with asymptomatic leg, pitting edema in symptomatic leg, collateral superficial veins, and decrease in pulse below location of thrombus (if arterial).	Venous stasis (see discussion of thrombophlebitis) and vessel trauma. Venous injury is common after surgery of legs, abdomen, pelvis, and major vessels. Patients with pelvic and abdominal cancer or traumatic injuries to the pelvis or lower extremities are at high risk for thrombus formation.
Embolus: Piece of thrombus that has dislodged and circulates in bloodstream until it lodges in another vessel, commonly in the lungs, heart, brain, or mesentery.	Thrombi form with increased coagulability of blood (e.g., polycythemia).
Gastrointestinal System	
Paralytic ileus: Nonmechanical obstruction of the bowel caused by physiological, neurogenic, or chemical imbalance associated with decreased peristalsis.	Handling of intestines during surgery can lead to loss of peristalsis for a few hours to several days.
Abdominal distension: Retention of air within intestines and abdominal cavity during gastrointestinal surgery. Signs and symptoms include increased abdominal girth, tympanic percussion over abdominal quadrants, and patient complaints of fullness, "gas pains," and referred shoulder pain.	Slowed peristalsis from anaesthesia, bowel manipulation, or immobilization. During laparoscopic surgeries, influx of air for procedure causes distension.
Nausea and vomiting: Symptoms of improper gastric emptying or chemical stimulation of vomiting centre. Patient complains of gagging or feeling full or sick to stomach.	Abdominal distension, fear, severe pain, medications, eating or drinking before peristalsis returns.
Genitourinary System	
Urinary retention: Involuntary accumulation of urine in bladder as a result of loss of muscle tone. Signs and symptoms include inability to void, restlessness, and bladder distension. It appears 6 to 8 hours after surgery.	Effects of anaesthesia and narcotic analgesics. Local manipulation of tissues surrounding bladder as well as edema interfere with bladder tone. Poor positioning of patient impairs voiding reflexes.
Urinary tract infection: An infection of the urinary tract as a result of bacterial or yeast contamination. Signs and symptoms include dysuria, itching, abdominal pain, possible fever, cloudy urine, white blood cells, and leukocyte esterase positive on urinalysis.	Most frequently a result of catheterization of the bladder.
Integumentary System	
Wound infection: An invasion of deep or superficial wound tissues by pathogenic microorganisms. Signs and symptoms include warm, red, and tender skin around incision; fever and chills; and purulent material exiting from drains or from separated wound edges. Infection usually appears 3 to 6 days after surgery.	Infection is caused by poor aseptic technique or contaminated wound or surgical site before surgical exploration. For example, with a bowel perforation, the patient is at increased risk for a wound infection because of bacterial contamination from the large intestine.
Wound dehiscence: Separation of wound edges at suture line. Signs and symptoms include increased drainage and appearance of underlying tissues. This usually occurs 6 to 8 days after surgery.	Malnutrition, obesity, preoperative radiation to surgical site, old age, poor circulation to tissues, and unusual strain on suture line from coughing or positioning cause dehiscence.
Wound evisceration: Protrusion of internal organs and tissues through incision. Usually occurs 6 to 8 days after surgery.	See discussion of wound dehiscence. Patient with dehiscence is at risk for developing evisceration.
Skin breakdown: Result of pressure or shearing forces. Surgical patients are at increased risk if alterations in nutrition and circulation are present, resulting in edema and delayed healing.	Prolonged periods on the operating room (OR) table and in the bed postoperatively can lead to pressure breakdown. Skin breakdown results from shearing during positioning on the OR table and improper pulling of the patient up in bed.
Nervous System	
Complex pain situations: These might include situations in which pain is unresponsive to standard treatment or where there are multiple sources of pain.	The source may be related to, for example, surgical site or concomitant injuries or pathology.

- Encourage patients to perform leg exercises at least every hour while awake. Exercise may be limited in an affected extremity involving vascular repair or realignment of fractured bones and torn cartilage.
- Apply elastic antiembolism stockings or sequential compression stockings as ordered by the physician (see Chapter 46). The antiembolism stockings should be removed at least once per shift. Perform a thorough assessment of the skin of the lower extremities at this time.
- Encourage early ambulation. Some patients are expected to ambulate on the evening of surgery, depending on the severity of the surgery and their condition. Even if a patient has an epidural catheter or a PCA device, ambulation should be encouraged. The degree of activity allowed progresses as the condition improves. Before ambulation, assess the patient's vital signs. Abnormalities may contraindicate ambulation. If vital signs are at baseline, first help the patient to sit on the side of the bed. Patient complaints of dizziness are a sign of postural hypotension. Rechecking the patient's blood pressure will help to determine whether ambulation is safe. Assist with ambulation by standing at the patient's side and ensuring that he or she can stand safely and walk steadily. The first few times out of bed, patients may be able to walk only a few metres. This should improve each time. Evaluate tolerance to activity by periodically assessing the pulse rate as the patient ambulates.
- Avoid positioning patients in a manner that interrupts blood flow to their extremities. While in bed, patients should not have pillows or rolled blankets placed under their knees. Compression of the popliteal vessels can cause thrombi. When patients sit in chairs, their legs should be elevated on footstools. A patient should never be allowed to sit with one leg crossed over the other.
- Administer anticoagulant medications as required. Physicians often order prophylactic doses of anticoagulants, such as heparin or Fragmin (dalteparin), for patients at greatest risk for thrombus formation.
- Promote adequate fluid intake. Adequate hydration prevents concentrated buildup of formed blood elements, such as platelets and red blood cells. When the plasma volume is low, these elements may gather and form small clots within blood vessels.

Achieving Rest and Comfort. A surgical patient's pain increases as the effects of anaesthesia diminish. The patient becomes more aware of the surroundings and more perceptive of discomfort. The incisional area may be only one source of pain. Irritation from **abdominal gas**, drainage tubes, tight dressings or casts, and the muscular strains caused from positioning on the OR table can cause discomfort.

It is common to administer narcotic analgesics immediately after surgery. Initial analgesic doses are usually given by IV infusion in the PACU and are titrated to ensure that the patient is comfortable. After an anaesthetized patient is awake and aware, a PCA may be used. This is given by IV or subcutaneous infusion or via an epidural, often with Dilaudid or morphine. The PCA system allows patients to administer their own analgesics from a specially prepared pump (see Chapter 32). If patients are able to gain a sense of control over their pain, they usually have fewer postoperative problems. Currently, the Ambit pump is being used at some institutions for ambulatory patients who have had, for example, shoulder or knee surgery. Patients can administer a bolus, and they are usually operating them at home for 1–2 days. Some patients receive epidural analgesia that may be continued during the recovery period (see Chapter 32). Increasingly, patients are being prescribed a combination of opioid and nonopioid analgesics to decrease opioid-related adverse effects (Mujukian et al., 2019) in the postoperative period. For example, as soon as peristalsis returns, patients may be given a combination of acetaminophen and a nonsteroidal anti-inflammatory medication.

In the acute care area, nurses continually assess the patient, obtain vital signs, and complete a pain assessment. Patients who will have PCA after surgery should be taught how to push the button when they begin to feel pain, and they should understand that use of PCA will not cause them to overmedicate. Patients should be taught to administer PCA prior to activities that may increase pain, such as mobilization. If the patient has a PCA system and is trying to use it more frequently than the amount programmed, the nurse should investigate their pain further and contact the physician or the advanced practice nurse on the acute pain service to increase, for example, the amount of medication received. PCA provides a useful monitor of the effectiveness of pain medication. As oral intake is tolerated, the nurse facilitates changing the patient's pain medication from IV to oral administration. It is important to ensure adequate pain coverage when the patient is switched from an IV to an oral route (Chou et al., 2016). Sometimes patients are given a subcutaneous injection of analgesia before being transferred to the acute care area, to ensure pain control over this time period. Intramuscular injections of analgesics are seldom used. The importance of nonpharmacological interventions should not be overlooked (Rabow et al., 2021). The nurse should assess which care measures may contribute to pain and use nonpharmacological measures to treat it. An example would be to lower the head of the bed and use a pillow for incisional splinting while turning a patient with recent abdominal surgery. Nurses can also use other methods of promoting pain relief, such as positioning, back rubs, distraction, or imagery. Ice packs may be ordered for patients undergoing joint replacement surgery (see Chapter 32).

Pain can slow recovery significantly. The patient becomes reluctant to cough, breathe deeply, turn, ambulate, or perform necessary exercises. Nurses should assess the patient's pain thoroughly (see Chapter 32). It should not be assumed that the pain is from the surgery. When the patient asks for pain medication, it is important to determine the location, intensity, and character of the pain. During the first 24 to 48 hours after surgery, the nurse should provide analgesics on a regular basis around the clock to improve pain control (RNAO, 2013). If pain medications are not relieving discomfort, the nurse should notify the physician or the acute pain service after completing a thorough assessment. In addition, the postoperative nurse needs to recognize the potential complications of analgesics and know what to do if they occur.

Acute Care

Temperature Regulation. Temperature regulation is important in the postoperative period. Patients are often cool after surgery, so the PACU nurse should provide warmed blankets in the immediate postoperative period. If the patient's temperature is 35.6°C or below, a warming device such as the Bair Hugger may be used. Increasing body warmth causes the patient's metabolism to rise and circulatory and respiratory functions to improve.

Shivering may not be a sign of hypothermia but rather an adverse effect of certain anaesthetic agents. Meperidine (Demerol) may be given in small increments to decrease shivering. Deep breathing and coughing help to expel retained anaesthetic gases.

Malignant hyperthermia is a potentially lethal condition that can occur in patients who receive general anaesthesia (OPANA, 2018). It should be suspected when there is unexpected tachycardia and tachypnea; jaw muscle rigidity; body rigidity of limbs, abdomen, and chest; or hyperkalemia. Temperature elevation is a late sign. The PACU nurse will immediately administer dantrolene sodium ordered by the physician.

Infection is another possible cause of temperature elevation. The following interventions decrease the risk of postoperative infections: encouraging deep breathing and coughing, assisting with early ambulation, removing in-dwelling urinary catheters and IV catheters once the patient is voiding and drinking, and providing aseptic care of the surgical wound. Cultures are obtained from patients suspected of having infections (see Chapter 47).

Maintaining Neurological Function. Orientation to the environment is important in maintaining the patient's mental status. The nurse needs to reorient the patient, explain that surgery has been completed, and describe procedures and nursing measures. The patient who was properly prepared before surgery is less likely to be anxious when nurses provide care. Any change in level of consciousness should be promptly reported to a physician.

Maintaining Fluid and Electrolyte Balances. An important nursing responsibility is maintaining patency and prescribed rate of IV infusions and monitoring fluid and electrolyte balances in the postoperative period. As the patient begins to take and tolerate oral fluids, the IV rate will be decreased. When an ambulatory surgical patient awakens and is able to tolerate fluids by mouth without gastrointestinal upset, the IV catheter is removed. When the patient no longer needs a continuous IV infusion, the IV line may be saline locked to preserve the site for antibiotics or other use (see Chapter 41). The patient also may receive blood products or artificial volume expanders, depending on blood loss during and after surgery.

Promoting Normal Bowel Elimination and Adequate Nutrition. Normally a patient who has had general anaesthesia does not receive fluids to drink in the PACU because of bowel sluggishness, the risk of nausea and vomiting, and grogginess from general anaesthesia. To minimize nausea, the patient should avoid sudden movement. For patients identified as being at high risk for the development of nausea and vomiting, or patients who must not vomit (e.g., eye surgery), a combination of antiemetics may be recommended (McQuaid, 2021). If the patient has a nasogastric tube, it is important to note the position of the tube and observe for drainage. If suction is required, the nurse needs to verify that it is maintained at the required level (see Chapter 45). Occlusion of a nasogastric tube results in accumulation of gastric contents within the stomach.

The patient likely will begin taking ice chips or sips of fluids once they are returned to the acute care unit. If these are tolerated, a clear liquid meal usually will be ordered. Interventions to prevent gastrointestinal complications will promote return of normal elimination and faster return of normal nutritional intake. It takes several days for a patient who has had surgery on gastrointestinal structures (e.g., a colon resection) to resume a normal diet. Normal peristalsis may not return for 2 to 3 days. In contrast, the patient whose gastrointestinal tract is unaffected directly by surgery can resume dietary intake after recovering from the effects of anaesthesia. The following measures promote return of normal elimination:

- Maintain a gradual progression in dietary intake. For the first few hours after surgery, the patient receives only IV fluids. If bowel sounds are active and the physician orders a normal diet for the first evening after surgery, begin by providing clear liquids, such as water, ginger ale, broth, or tea, after nausea subsides. Overloading the patient with large amounts of fluids may lead to distension and vomiting. If the patient tolerates liquids without nausea, advance the diet as ordered. Patients who have had abdominal surgery are usually NPO for the first 24 to 48 hours after the procedure. As peristalsis returns, provide clear liquids, followed by full liquids, a light diet of solid foods, and, finally, the patient's usual diet. Encourage intake of foods high in protein and vitamin C.
- Promote ambulation and exercise. Physical activity stimulates a return of peristalsis. The patient who suffers abdominal distension and "gas pain" may obtain relief while walking.
- Maintain an adequate fluid intake. Fluids keep fecal material soft for easy passage. Fruit juices and warm liquids are especially effective.
- Administer fibre supplements, stool softeners, and rectal suppositories such as Dulcolax (bisacodyl) as ordered. If constipation or distension develops, the physician may attempt to stimulate peristalsis with cathartics or enemas, but caution must be exercised in their use. Always report bowel sounds to the physician when communicating the patient's bowel pattern postsurgery.

It is also important to promote adequate food intake by stimulating the patient's appetite:

- Remove sources of noxious odours and provide small servings of nonspicy foods.
- Assist the patient to a comfortable position during mealtime. The patient should sit, if possible, to minimize pressure on the abdomen.
- Provide desired servings of food. For example, a patient may be more willing to face their first meal when servings are not large.
- Provide frequent oral hygiene. Adequate hydration and cleaning of the oral cavity eliminate dryness and bad tastes.
- Provide meals when the patient is rested and free from pain. Often a patient loses interest in eating if mealtime has been preceded by exhausting activities, such as ambulation, coughing and deep breathing exercises, or extensive dressing changes. When a patient has pain, the associated nausea often causes a loss of appetite.

Promoting Urinary Elimination. The depressant effects of anaesthetics and analgesics impair the sensation of bladder fullness. If bladder tone is reduced, the patient has difficulty starting urination. However, patients should void within 8 to 12 hours after surgery. Because a full bladder can be painful and often causes restlessness in recovery, it may become necessary to insert a catheter. If the patient has an in-dwelling urinary catheter, the goal should be to have it removed as soon as possible because of the high risk for development of a health care–associated infection.

Patients who undergo surgery of the urinary system frequently have an in-dwelling urinary catheter inserted to maintain free urinary flow until voluntary control of urination returns. The following measures promote normal urinary elimination (see Chapter 44):

- Help the patient to assume normal positions during voiding. The patient with male genitalia may need assistance to stand to void. Bedpans make voiding difficult. A patient with female genitalia will have better results if they are able to use a toilet or a bedside commode.
- Check the patient frequently for the need to void. A patient restricted to bed needs assistance in handling and using bedpans or urinals. Often the patient acquires a sudden feeling of bladder fullness and urgency to void and will need help quickly.
- Assess for bladder distension. If a patient does not void within 8 hours of surgery or if bladder distension is present, it may be necessary to insert a straight in-and-out urinary catheter. A physician's order is needed for this. Continued difficulty in voiding may necessitate an in-dwelling catheter, although the risk for a urinary tract infection increases.
- Monitor intake and output. Urine output should be at least 30 mL/hour for adults. If the urine is dark, concentrated, and low in volume, the physician should be notified. A patient can easily become dehydrated as a result of fluid loss from the surgical wound. Measure intake and output for several days after surgery until normal fluid intake and urinary output are achieved.

Promoting Wound Healing. A surgical wound undergoes considerable stress during convalescence. Inadequate nutrition, impaired circulation, and metabolic alterations increase the risk for delayed healing (see Chapter 47). Strain on sutures from coughing, vomiting, distension, and movement of body parts can disrupt the wound layers. Nurses need to protect the wound and promote healing. A critical time for wound healing is 24 to 72 hours after surgery, after which time a seal is established. If a wound becomes infected, it usually occurs 3 to 6 days after surgery. Nurses must use the aseptic technique during dressing changes and wound care (see Chapters 34 and 47). Surgical drains must remain patent so that accumulated secretions can escape from the wound bed. Ongoing observation of the wound aids in identifying early signs and symptoms of infection.

Maintaining and Enhancing Self-Concept. The appearance of wounds, bulky dressings, and extruding drains and tubes can threaten a patient's self-concept. The effects of surgery, such as disfiguring scars, may create permanent changes in the patient's body image. If surgery leads to impairment in body function, the patient's role within the family can change significantly.

Nurses should observe patients for alterations in self-concept. Patients may show revulsion toward their appearance by refusing to look at incisions, carefully covering dressings with bedclothes, or refusing to get out of bed because of tubes and devices. The fear of not being able to return to a functional role in the family may cause patients to avoid participating in the care plan.

The family becomes an important part of efforts to improve the patient's self-concept. The nurse can explain the patient's appearance and encourage the family to be accepting of the patient's concerns and promote the patient's independence. If the condition is permanent, the family and patient will go through a grieving process. The nurse can be very supportive throughout this process. The following measures help to maintain the patient's self-concept:

- Provide privacy during dressing changes or inspection of the wound. Keep room curtains closed around the bed when changing and applying dressings and drape the patient so that only the dressing or incisional area is exposed.
- Maintain the patient's hygiene. Wound drainage and antiseptic solutions from the surgical skin preparation dry on the patient's skin surface and cause irritation. When patients return to the unit, they should be given a postoperative bath and provided oral hygiene. In addition, a complete bath on the first day after surgery can make the patient feel renewed. When the patient's gown becomes soiled by wound drainage, offer a clean gown and washcloth. Keep the patient's hair clean and neatly combed. Offer frequent oral hygiene. Room deodorizers may be useful if the odour from drainage seems particularly troublesome to the patient and the family.
- Prevent drainage devices from overflowing. Contents of drainage collections are measured every 8 hours or 12 hours for output recording and are emptied as they become full. Maintain a pleasant environment; self-concept is heightened by the patient being in comfortable surroundings. Store or remove unused supplies and keep the patient's bedside orderly and clean.
- Offer opportunities for the patient to discuss feelings about their appearance. A patient who avoids looking at an incision may need to discuss fears or concerns. A patient having surgery for the first time is often more anxious than one who has had multiple surgeries. When the patient chooses to look at an incision for the first time, the area should be clean. Eventually, the patient should be able to care for the incision site by applying simple dressings or cleaning the affected area.
- Provide the family with opportunities to discuss ways to promote the patient's self-concept. Encouraging independence can be difficult for a family member who has a strong desire to assist the patient in any way. By knowing about the appearance of a wound or incision, family members can be supportive during dressing changes. The topic or tone of a conversation can also help family members support a patient who is dwelling on fears and concerns. Family members should not avoid discussing the future. However, they need help to know when it is appropriate to discuss future plans. Then the patient and family can work together to discuss realistic plans for the patient's return home.

BOX 49.9 FOCUS ON PRIMARY HEALTH CARE

Recovery at Home

Regardless of the length of time the patient spends in the hospital, it is essential that nurses ensure that the patient and family have the appropriate information and skills needed to continue a successful recovery at home. However, time is often very limited, especially with the move toward preadmission units and short hospital stays. A comprehensive approach is needed to ensure continuity of care from hospital to home. A patient is often expected to continue dressing care, follow any activity restrictions, continue medication therapy, and observe for signs and symptoms of complications upon returning home. In addition, the patient needs someone to be present for the first 24 hours to ensure that no delayed reaction from the anaesthesia occurs, such as difficulty breathing. A referral to home care assists patients who are unable to perform self-care activities. Close association with home care services is required for some patients if dressing changes or physiotherapy is needed. It is useful to have a case management nurse in attendance at discharge to convey what tasks a patient can perform effectively. Berg and colleagues (2013) conducted a qualitative study of 31 patients in Sweden recovering from day surgery. The results indicated that patients need knowledge regarding what is considered a normal recovery and how to care for themselves after surgery.

Restorative and Continuing Care. The nurse, the patient, and the family work to prepare the patient for discharge. Education regarding wound care, activity level, diet, medications, and specifics related to the type of surgery is an ongoing process throughout hospitalization. After discharge, some patients will need assistance from home care services with tasks such as wound care (Box 49.9). For patients with ambulatory surgery, focused education within the limited time in care is essential. Including the family or a significant person provides a resource for the patient once they are at home (see Box 49.7). With both ambulatory and hospitalized patients, nurses make patients aware of a wide variety of educational materials, including those from the hospital website. For example, educational materials with many pictures should be used for patients who have limited reading ability. Materials should be sensitive to various cultures and religions. However, the provision of materials does not ensure understanding. Verification, return demonstration, and ongoing clarification are required.

◆ **Evaluation**

Patient Care. Nurses evaluate the effectiveness of care provided to the surgical patient on outcomes after nursing interventions. In all surgical settings, nurses consult with the patient and family to gather evaluation data. The nurse can evaluate the outcomes of the patient who had ambulatory surgery by telephoning the patient's home, asking specific questions to determine whether complications have developed and whether the patient understands restrictions or medications. This call is usually placed 24 hours after surgery, which enables the nurse to evaluate the progress of recovery.

In an acute care setting, evaluation of the patient is ongoing. If a patient fails to progress as expected, the nurse needs to revise the patient's care plan according to the priorities of the patient's needs. Every effort is made to assist the patient in returning to as healthy and functional state as possible. Nursing evaluation also includes determining the extent to which the patient and the family have learned self-care measures.

Patient Expectations. With shorter hospital stays and ambulatory surgery, it is especially important to evaluate patient expectations early in the postoperative process. Pain relief is usually a priority. Asking the patient if everything possible has been done to alleviate pain, including with nonpharmacological measures, can determine whether the patient's needs have been met. Timeliness of response to the patient's needs, such as scheduled times for pain medication and prompt answering of a call light, may increase patient satisfaction. The patient usually wants to be discharged from acute care as soon as possible and when indicated by the physician. In some institutions, for continuity of care, the electronic chart is started in the preadmission unit, then follows the patient to day surgery unit, then to the OR, then the PACU.

Good communication among members of the interprofessional team ensures that patient needs are met and that discharge plans are in place and enhances the patient's satisfaction with care.

KEY CONCEPTS

- Perioperative nursing is nursing care provided to the surgical patient before, during, and after surgery.
- Surgery is classified by level of severity, urgency, and purpose.
- The preoperative period may be several days or only a few hours long.
- Preoperative assessment of vital signs and physical findings provides an important baseline with which to compare postoperative assessment data.
- Nursing diagnoses of the surgical patient may pose implications for nursing care during one or all phases of surgery.
- Primary responsibility for obtaining informed consent rests with the patient's surgeon.
- Structured preoperative teaching has a positive influence on a patient's postoperative recovery.
- Basic to preoperative teaching is an explanation of all preoperative and postoperative activities and demonstration of postoperative exercises.
- In ambulatory surgery, nurses must use the limited time available to educate patients, assess their health status, and prepare them for surgery.
- A routine preoperative (preprocedure) checklist can be used as a guide for final preparation of the patient before surgery.
- Many responsibilities of nurses within the OR focus on protecting the patient from potential harm.
- All medications taken before surgery are automatically discontinued after surgery unless a physician reorders the medications.
- Family members or other supportive networks are important in assisting patients with any physical limitations and in providing emotional support during postoperative recovery and ongoing care at home.
- Assessment of the postoperative patient centres on the body systems most likely to be affected by anaesthesia, immobilization, and surgical trauma.
- Accurate pain assessment and intervention are necessary for healing.
- Nurses in the postoperative surgical unit provide the discharge education required so that the patient and the family can manage at home.

CRITICAL THINKING EXERCISES

1. An 82-year-old patient is admitted for surgery on a fractured hip caused by a fall. What postoperative complications are typical in the older patient undergoing this type of surgery?
2. A 52-year-old patient is about to undergo thoracic surgery. The patient has smoked one pack of cigarettes per day for 30 years.

What type of pulmonary preventive measures would you expect this patient to need postoperatively?
3. A patient was admitted for same-day surgery for an inguinal hernia repair. What discharge criteria would be used for this patient, and what discharge instructions would they require?
4. Your patient is scheduled for abdominal hysterectomy at 2:00 p.m. Based on NPO guidelines, what fasting schedule should you implement in collaboration with the surgeon and the anaesthesiologist?
5. You are doing preoperative teaching for a patient undergoing a minimally invasive surgical technique. Identify one advantage of this type of surgery.

Answers to Critical Thinking Exercises appear on the Evolve website.

REVIEW QUESTIONS

Questions 1 to 13 relate to the case study at the beginning of the chapter.

1. Based on her BMI measurement, Amanda is obese. She is therefore at risk for poor wound healing and for wound infection postoperatively because:
   a. Ventilatory capacity is reduced.
   b. Fatty tissue has a poor blood supply.
   c. Risk for dehiscence is increased.
   d. Resuming normal physical activity is delayed.
2. The nurse should ask Amanda preoperatively for the name and dose of all prescription and over-the-counter medications taken before surgery because these medications:
   a. May cause allergies to develop
   b. Are automatically ordered postoperatively
   c. May create greater risks for complications or interact with anaesthetic agents
   d. Should be taken on the morning of surgery with sips of water
3. Amanda, who smokes two packs of cigarettes per day, is most at risk postoperatively for which of the following?
   a. Infection
   b. Pneumonia
   c. Hypotension
   d. Cardiac dysrhythmias
4. Family members should be included when the nurse teaches Amanda preoperative exercises so that they can:
   a. Supervise Amanda at home
   b. Coach Amanda postoperatively
   c. Practise with Amanda while waiting to be taken to the operating room
   d. Assist the nurse by getting Amanda to do her exercises every 2 hours
5. In the postoperative period, measuring Amanda's input and output helps assess which of the following?
   a. Renal and circulatory function
   b. Patient comfort
   c. Neurological function
   d. Gastrointestinal function
6. In the PACU, one measure taken to maintain airway patency is to:
   a. Suction the pharynx and bronchial tree
   b. Give oxygen through a mask at 10 L/minute
   c. Position the patient so that the tongue falls forward
   d. Sit the patient in high-Fowler's position
7. Which one of the following measures promotes normal venous return and circulatory blood flow?
   a. Suctioning artificial airways and the oral cavity
   b. Monitoring fluid and electrolyte status during every shift

   c. Having the patient deep-breathe and cough

   d. Encouraging the patient to perform leg exercises at least once an hour while awake

8. A patient with an international normalized ratio (INR) or an activated partial thromboplastin time (aPTT) greater than normal is at risk postoperatively for:

   a. Anemia

   b. Bleeding

   c. Infection

   d. Cardiac dysrhythmias

9. When engaging Amanda in deep-breathing and coughing exercises, it is important to have her sitting because this position:

   a. Is more comfortable

   b. Facilitates expansion of the thorax

   c. Increases the patient's view of the room and is more relaxing

   d. Helps the patient to splint with a pillow

10. In the postoperative period, if Amanda experiences unexpected tachycardia and tachypnea; jaw muscle rigidity; body rigidity of limbs, abdomen, and chest; or hyperkalemia, the nurse should suspect which of the following?

    a. Infection

    b. Hypertension

    c. Pneumonia

    d. Malignant hyperthermia

11. In the postoperative period, which of the following actions should the nurse encourage Amanda to do? *(Select all that apply.)*

    a. Deep-breathing and coughing

    b. Read as many books as possible

    c. Use the incentive spirometer hourly throughout the day

    d. Use a pillow when moving to splint the incision

12. Preoperatively, what information should the nurse provide to Amanda? *(Select all that apply.)*

    a. The importance of early ambulation

    b. She will experience pain after surgery and most likely she will have a PCA pump that she can use to control her pain within defined limits.

    c. She will be discharged the day of her surgery.

    d. She will be wearing antithrombotic leggings after surgery to prevent blood clots from encouraging.

    e. She will most likely have an incision in her right upper abdomen.

13. What type of procedure will Amanda have to treat her illness?

    a. A laparoscopic cholecystectomy

    b. A traditional cholecystectomy

Answers: 1. b; **2.** c; **3.** b; **4.** b; **5.** a; **6.** c; **7.** d; **8.** b; **9.** b; **10.** d; **11.** a, c, d; **12.** a, b, d, e; **13.** b.

🌐 *Rationales for the Review Questions appear on the Evolve website.*

RECOMMENDED WEBSITES

Canadian Anesthesiologists' Society: https://www.cas.ca
This website offers patient information about anaesthesia and provides guidelines for using anaesthesia.

National Association of PeriAnesthesia Nurses of Canada: http://www.napanc.cs
Perianaesthesia nurses are registered nurses with advanced knowledge in the care of patients during all phases of perianaesthesia, including, for example, nurses in postanaesthetic care units, same-day surgery, and diagnostic imaging. The aim of this organization is to advance education for perianaesthesia nurses across Canada.

Ontario PeriAnesthesia Nurses Association: https://www.opana.org
This website provides position statements on and standards of perianaesthesia nursing practice.

Operating Room Nurses Association of Canada: https://www.ornac.ca
This website provides practice standards for Canadian operating room nurses, as well as information on certification with the Canadian Nurses Association (CNA).

🌐 REFERENCES

A full reference list is available on the website for this book at http://evolve.elsevier.com/Canada/Potter/fundamentals/

Laboratory Values

Sarah Ibrahim, RN, MN, PhD, CHSE

The tables in this appendix list some of the most common tests, their normal values, and possible etiologies of abnormal values. Laboratory values are expressed in the Système International d'Unités (SI) units, which are used in Canada. Conventional units, used in the United States, are presented after the SI units in parentheses. Laboratory values may vary with different techniques and in different laboratories. Possible etiologies are presented in alphabetical order. SI abbreviations and other symbols appearing in the tables are defined as follows:

<	=	less than
>	=	greater than
≥	=	greater than or equal to
≤	=	less than or equal to
AU	=	arbitrary unit
cm H$_2$O	=	centimetres of water
dL	=	decilitre
EU	=	Ehrlich unit
fL	=	femtolitre
g	=	gram
IU	=	international unit
k	=	kilo
kPa	=	kilopascal
L	=	litre
mcg	=	microgram (one millionth [10^{-6}] of a gram)
mcIU	=	micro–international unit (one millionth [10^{-6}] of an international unit)
mcL	=	microlitre
mcmol	=	micromole
McU	=	microunit
mEq	=	milliequivalent
mg	=	milligram (one thousandth [10^{-3}] of a gram)
mL	=	millilitre
mm	=	millimetre
mm Hg	=	millimetre of mercury
mmol	=	millimole
mOsm	=	milliosmole
mU	=	milliunit (one hundredth [10^{-2}] of a unit)
ng	=	nanogram (one billionth [10^{-9}] of a gram)
nmol	=	nanomole (one billionth [10^{-9}] of a mole)
pg	=	picogram (one trillionth [10^{-12}] of a gram)
pmol	=	picomole (one trillionth [10^{-12}] of a mole)
U	=	unit

TABLE A.1 — Serum, Plasma, and Whole Blood Chemistries

Test	Normal Values (SI Units [Conventional Units])	POSSIBLE ETIOLOGY Higher Values	POSSIBLE ETIOLOGY Lower Values
Acetone • Quantitative • Qualitative	 <200 mcmol/L (<1.16 mg/dL) Negative (negative)	DKA, high-fat diet, low-carbohydrate diet, starvation	—
Alanine aminotransferase (ALT; formerly known as serum glutamate pyruvate transferase [SGPT])	5–35 U/L (same as in SI units)	Liver disease, shock	—
Albumin	35–55 g/L (3.5–5.5 g/dL)	Dehydration	Malnutrition, pregnancy, liver disease, protein-losing nephropathies, third-space losses, inflammatory disease, familial idiopathic dysproteinemia

Continued

TABLE A.1 Serum, Plasma, and Whole Blood Chemistries—cont'd

Test	Normal Values (SI Units [Conventional Units])	POSSIBLE ETIOLOGY Higher Values	Lower Values
Aldolase	<8.0 mU/L (3–8.2 Sibley-Lehninger U/dL)	Muscular disease, muscular dystrophy, dermatomyositis, polymyositis, muscle injury, muscular trauma, gangrenous/ischemic processes, hepatocellular disease, hepatitis, cirrhosis, MI, infection	Hereditary fructose intolerance, late muscular dystrophy, muscle wasting disease, renal disease
α_1-Antitrypsin	0.85–2.13 g/L (85–213 mg/dL)	Acute and chronic inflammatory disorders, infections (i.e., thyroid infections), malignancy, stress	Chronic lung disease (early onset of emphysema), neonatal respiratory distress syndrome, cirrhosis (in children), end-stage cancer, malnutrition, nephrotic syndrome, protein-losing enteropathy, hepatic failure
α-Fetoprotein	0–40 mcg/L (<40 ng/mL)	Cancers of testes, lymphoma, stomach, colon, breasts, and ovaries; liver cell necrosis (i.e., cirrhosis, hepatitis); carcinoma of liver; fetal death; fetal distress or congenital abnormalities; neural tube defects (i.e., anencephaly, spina bifida) or multiple pregnancies in pregnant persons	In pregnant persons, fetal trisomy 21 (Down syndrome) or fetal wastage
Ammonia	6–47 mcmol/L (10–80 mcg/dL)	GI bleeding and obstruction with mild liver disease, genetic metabolic disorder of urea cycle, hemolytic disease of newborn, hepatic encephalopathy and hepatic coma, portal hypertension, Reye syndrome, primary hepatocellular disease, asparagine intoxication, severe heart failure or congestive hepatomegaly	Essential or malignant hypertension, hyperornithinemia
Amylase	25–125 U/L	Acute and chronic pancreatitis, GI disease, acute cholecystitis, mumps (salivary gland disease), perforated ulcers, ruptured ectopic pregnancy, renal failure, DKA, pulmonary infarction	Acute alcoholism, cirrhosis of liver, extensive destruction of pancreas
Aspartate aminotransferase (AST) (formerly known as serum glutamic oxaloacetic transferase [SGOT])	0–35 U/L (same as SI units)	Acute hepatitis, liver disease, MI, skeletal muscle disease, acute hemolytic anemia, acute pancreatitis	Acute renal disease, chronic renal dialysis, DKA, beriberi, pregnancy
B-type (brain-type) natriuretic peptide	<100 mcg/L (<100 ng/mL)	Cor pulmonale, heart failure, heart transplant rejection, hypertension, MI	—
Bicarbonate	23–29 mmol/L (23–29 mEq/L)	Use of mercurial diuretics, aldosteronism, compensated respiratory acidosis, metabolic alkalosis	Acute kidney injury, compensated respiratory alkalosis, diarrhea, metabolic acidosis, starvation, chronic use of loop diuretics
Bilirubin			—
• Total	3–22 mcmol/L (0.2–1.3 mg/dL)	**Direct Bilirubin:** Gallstones, extrahepatic duct obstruction (tumour, inflammation, gallstone, scarring, surgical trauma), extensive liver metastasis, cholestasis from medications, Dubin-Johnson syndrome, Rotor syndrome	
• Indirect	3.4–12 mcmol/L (0.2–0.8 mg/dL)		
• Direct	1.7–5.1 mcmol/L (0.1–0.3 mg/dL)	**Indirect Bilirubin:** Erythroblastosis fetalis, transfusion reaction, sickle cell anemia, hemolytic jaundice, hemolytic anemia, pernicious anemia, large-volume blood transfusion, resolution of large hematoma, hepatitis, cirrhosis, sepsis, neonatal hyperbilirubinemia, Crigler-Najjar syndrome, Gilbert syndrome	
		Increased Urine Levels of Bilirubin: Gallstones, extrahepatic duct obstruction (tumour, inflammation, gallstone, scarring, surgical trauma), extensive liver metastasis, cholestasis from medications, Dubin-Johnson syndrome, Rotor syndrome	

TABLE A.1   Serum, Plasma, and Whole Blood Chemistries—cont'd

Test	Normal Values (SI Units [Conventional Units])	POSSIBLE ETIOLOGY	
		Higher Values	Lower Values
Blood gases*			
• Arterial pH	7.35–7.45 (same as SI units)	Alkalosis	Acidosis
• Venous pH	7.35–7.45 (same as SI units)	Alkalosis	Acidosis
• Partial pressure of carbon dioxide in arterial blood (PaCO$_2$)	35–45 mm Hg (same as SI units)	Compensated metabolic alkalosis, respiratory acidosis	Compensated metabolic acidosis, respiratory alkalosis
• Partial pressure of oxygen in arterial blood (PaO$_2$)	80–100 mm Hg (same as SI units)	Administration of high concentration of oxygen	Chronic lung disease, decreased cardiac output
• Partial pressure of oxygen in venous blood (PvO$_2$)	40–50 mm Hg (same as SI units)		
Calcium	Adult: 2.10–2.750 mmol/L (8.4–10.6 mg/dL) Total calcium: <1.65 or >3.25 mmol/L (13 mg/dL)	Hyperparathyroidism, nonparathyroid PTH-producing tumour (e.g., lung or renal carcinoma), metastatic tumour to bone, Paget's disease of bone, prolonged immobilization, milk-alkali syndrome, vitamin D intoxication, lymphoma, granulomatous infections such as sarcoidosis and tuberculosis, Addison's disease, acromegaly, hyperthyroidism	Hypoparathyroidism, renal failure, hyperphosphatemia secondary to renal failure, rickets, vitamin D deficiency, osteomalacia, hypoalbuminemia, malabsorption, pancreatitis, fat embolism, alkalosis
Calcium, ionized	Adult: 1.15–1.35 mmol/L (4.6–5.1 mg/dL) Ionized calcium: <0.80 mmol/L or >1.58 mmol/L (7 mg/dL)	—	—
Carbon dioxide (CO$_2$ content)	21–28 mmol/L (21–28 mEq/L)	COPD, metabolic alkalosis, severe vomiting, high-volume gastric suction, use of mercurial diuretics	Chronic use of loop diuretics, DKA, metabolic acidosis, renal failure, shock, starvation
Chloride	98–106 mmol/L (98–106 mEq/L)	Dehydration, excessive infusion of normal saline solution, metabolic acidosis, renal tubular acidosis, Cushing's syndrome, kidney dysfunction, hyperparathyroidism, eclampsia, respiratory alkalosis	Overhydration, SIADH, heart failure, vomiting or prolonged gastric suction, chronic diarrhea or high-output GI fistula, chronic respiratory acidosis, metabolic alkalosis, salt-losing nephritis, Addison's disease, diuretic therapy
Cholesterol	<5.2 mmol/L (<200 mg/dL) age dependent	Familial hypercholesterolemia, familial hyperlipidemia, hypothyroidism, uncontrolled diabetes mellitus, nephrotic syndrome, pregnancy, high-cholesterol diet, xanthomatosis, hypertension, MI, atherosclerosis, biliary cirrhosis, extrahepatic biliary, stress, nephrotic syndrome renal disease	Malabsorption, malnutrition, advanced cancer, hyperthyroidism, cholesterol-lowering medication, pernicious anemia, hemolytic anemia, sepsis/stress, liver disease, acute MI
• High-density lipoproteins (HDL)	>0.91 mmol/L (>35 mg/dL)		
• Low-density lipoproteins (LDL)	<3.4 mmol/L (<130 mg/dL)		
Cholinesterase (RBC)	5–10 U/L (same as SI units)	Reticulocytosis, hyperlipidemia, nephrosis, diabetes	Poisoning from organic phosphate insecticides, hepatocellular disease, individuals with congenital enzyme deficiency, malnutrition and other forms of hypoalbuminemia
Copper	11–22 mcmol/L (70–140 mcg/dL)	Cirrhosis, contraceptive use by patient with female genitalia	Wilson's disease
Cortisol		Adrenal adenoma, Cushing's syndrome, hyperthyroidism, pancreatitis, stress, ectopic ACTH-producing tumours, obesity	Addison's disease, adrenal insufficiency, hypopituitary states, hypothyroidism, liver disease
• 0800 hours	170–635 nmol/L (6–23 mcg/dL)		
• 1600 hours	<84–413 nmol/L (3–53 mcg/dL)		
Creatine		Active rheumatoid arthritis, biliary obstruction, hyperthyroidism, renal disease, severe muscle disease	Diabetes mellitus
Creatine kinase (CK)		Diseases or injury affecting the heart muscle, skeletal muscle, and brain	—
• Male	20–215 U/L (same as SI units)		
• Female	20–160 U/L (same as SI units)		
Creatine kinase isozyme of heart (CK-MB [CK-2])		Acute MI, cardiac aneurysm surgery, cardiac defibrillation, myocarditis, ventricular arrhythmias, cardiac ischemia: Any disease or injury to the myocardium causes CK-MB to spill out of the damaged cells and into the bloodstream, producing elevations in CK-MB levels	—
• Male	20–215 mcg/L (same as SI units)		
• Female	20–160 mcg/L (same as SI units)		

Continued

TABLE A.1   Serum, Plasma, and Whole Blood Chemistries—cont'd

Test	Normal Values (SI Units [Conventional Units])	POSSIBLE ETIOLOGY Higher Values	Lower Values
Creatine kinase mass fraction	0–6%	—	—
Creatinine		Severe renal disease, rhabdomyolysis, acromegaly, gigantism	Diseases with decreased muscle mass (e.g., muscular dystrophy, myasthenia gravis)
• Male	53–106 mcmol/L (0.6–1.2 mg/dL)		
• Female	44–97 mcmol/L (0.5–1.1 mg/dL)		
Ferritin (serum)		Hemochromatosis, hemosiderosis, megaloblastic anemia, hemolytic anemia, alcoholic/inflammatory hepatocellular disease, inflammatory disease, advanced cancers, chronic illnesses such as leukemias, cirrhosis, chronic hepatitis, or collagen-vascular diseases	Iron-deficiency anemia, severe protein deficiency, hemodialysis
• Male	20–200 mcg/L (20–200 ng/mL)		
• Female	20–150 mcg/L (20–150 ng/mL)		
Folic acid (folate)	11–57 mmol/L (5–25 ng/mL)	Pernicious anemia, vegetarianism, recent massive blood transfusion	Malnutrition, malabsorption syndrome, pregnancy, folic acid deficiency (megaloblastic) anemia, hemolytic anemia, malignancy, liver disease, chronic renal disease
Gamma-glutamyltranspeptidase (GGT)		Liver diseases (e.g., hepatitis, cirrhosis, hepatic necrosis, hepatic tumour or metastasis, hepatotoxic medications, cholestasis, jaundice), MI, alcohol ingestion, pancreatic disease, Epstein-Barr virus	—
• Male	8–38 U/L (same as SI units)		
• Female	5–27 U/L (same as SI units)		
Glucose, fasting	3.9–6.1 mmol/L (70–110 mg/dL)	Diabetes mellitus, acute stress response, Cushing's syndrome, pheochromocytoma, chronic renal failure, glucagonoma, acute pancreatitis, diuretic therapy, corticosteroid therapy, acromegaly	Insulinoma, hypothyroidism, hypopituitarism, Addison's disease, extensive liver disease, insulin overdose, starvation
Glucose, 2-hr oral glucose tolerance testing (OGTT)		Diabetes mellitus	Hyperinsulinism
• Fasting	4–6 mmol/L (70–110 mg/dL)		
• 1 hr	<11.1 mmol/L (<200 mg/dL)		
• 2 hr	<7.8 mmol/L (<140 mg/dL)		
Haptoglobin	0.5–2.2 g/L (50–220 mg/dL)	Collagen-rheumatic diseases, infection (e.g., pyelonephritis, urinary tract infection, pneumonia), tissue destruction (e.g., MI), nephritis, ulcerative colitis, neoplasia, biliary obstruction	Hemolytic anemia, transfusion reactions, prosthetic heart valves, primary liver disease, hematoma, tissue hemorrhage
Homocysteine		Cardiovascular disease, cerebrovascular disease, cystinuria, folate deficiency, malnutrition, peripheral vascular disease, vitamin B_6 or B_{12} deficiency	—
• 0–30 years	4.6–8.1 mcmol/L (same as SI units)		
• 30–59 years			
• Male	6.13–11.2 mcmol/L (same as SI units)		
• Female	4.5–7.9 mcmol/L (same as SI units)		
• >59 years	5.8–11.9 mcmol/L (same as SI units)		
Insulin	43–186 pmol/L (6–26 microU/mL)	Insulinoma, Cushing's syndrome, acromegaly, fructose or galactose intolerance	Diabetes mellitus, hypopituitarism
Iron		Hemosiderosis or hemochromatosis, iron poisoning, hemolytic anemia, massive blood transfusions, hepatitis or hepatic necrosis, lead toxicity	Insufficient dietary iron, chronic blood loss (irregular menses, uterine cancer, GI cancer, inflammatory bowel disease, diverticulosis, urological tract [hematuria] cancer, hemangioma, arteriovenous malformation), inadequate intestinal absorption of iron, pregnancy (late), iron-deficiency anemia, neoplasia
• Male	13–31 mcmol/L (75–175 mcg/dL)		
• Female	5–29 mcmol/L (28–162 mcg/dL)		

TABLE A.1   Serum, Plasma, and Whole Blood Chemistries—cont'd

Test	Normal Values (SI Units [Conventional Units])	POSSIBLE ETIOLOGY Higher Values	Lower Values
Total iron-binding capacity (TIBC)	45–73 mcmol/L (250–410 mcg/dL)	Estrogen therapy, pregnancy (late), polycythemia vera, iron-deficiency anemia	Malnutrition, hypoproteinemia, inflammatory diseases, cirrhosis, hemolytic anemia, pernicious anemia, sickle cell anemia
Lactic acid (venous blood)	0.6–2.2 mmol/L (5–20 mg/dL)	Shock, tissue ischemia, carbon monoxide poisoning, severe liver disease, genetic errors of metabolism, diabetes mellitus (nonketotic)	—
Lactic dehydrogenase (LDH)	45–90 U/L (same as SI units)	MI, pulmonary disease (e.g., embolism, infarction, pneumonia, heart failure), hepatic disease (e.g., hepatitis, active cirrhosis, neoplasm), RBC disease, skeletal muscle disease and injury, renal parenchymal disease, intestinal ischemia and infarction, neoplastic states, testicular tumours (seminoma, dysgerminomas), lymphoma and other reticuloendothelial system (RES) tumours, advanced solid tumour malignancies, pancreatitis, diffuse disease or injury (e.g., heat stroke, collagen disease, shock, hypotension)	—
Lactic dehydrogenase (LDH) isoenzymes			
• LDH_1	0.17–0.27 (17–27%)	MI, pernicious anemia, strenuous exercise	—
• LDH_2	0.27–0.37 (27–37%)	Exercise, pulmonary embolus, sickle cell crisis	—
• LDH_3	0.18–0.25 (18–25%)	Malignant lymphoma, pulmonary embolus	—
• LDH_4	0.03–0.08 (3–8%)	Systemic lupus erythematosus, pancreatitis, pulmonary infarction, renal disease	—
• LDH_5	0.0–0.05 (0–5%)	Heart failure, hepatitis, pulmonary embolus and infarction, skeletal muscle damage, strenuous exercise	—
Lipase	0–160 U/L (same as SI units)	Pancreatic diseases, biliary diseases, renal failure, intestinal diseases, salivary gland inflammation or tumour, peptic ulcer disease	—
Magnesium	0.65–1.05 mmol/L (1.2–2.1 mEq/L)	Renal insufficiency, ingestion of magnesium-containing antacids or salts, Addison's disease, hypothyroidism	Chronic alcoholism, hyperparathyroidism, hyperthyroidism, hypoparathyroidism, malnutrition, severe malabsorption, chronic renal tubular disease
Myoglobin	1.0–5.3 nmol/L (<90 ng/mL)	MI, myositis, malignant hyperthermia, muscular dystrophy, skeletal muscle ischemia or trauma, rhabdomyolysis, seizures	Polymyositis
Osmolality	285–295 mmol/kg (280–295 mOsm/kg)	Hypernatremia; hyperglycemia; hyperosmolar nonketotic hyperglycemia; ketosis; azotemia; dehydration; mannitol therapy; ingestion of ethanol, methanol, or ethylene glycol; uremia; diabetes insipidus; renal tubular necrosis; severe pyelonephritis	Overhydration, SIADH secretion, paraneoplastic syndromes associated with carcinoma (lung, breast, colon)
Oxygen saturation		Increased inspired oxygen, polycythemia hyperventilation	Anemia, mucous plug, bronchospasm, atelectasis, pneumothorax, pulmonary edema, acute respiratory distress syndrome (ARDS), restrictive lung disease, atrial or ventricular cardiac septal defects, emboli, inadequate O_2 in inspired air (suffocation), severe hypoventilation states, such as oversedation or neurological somnolence
• Arterial	95–100% (same as SI units)		
• Venous	60–80% (same as SI units)		

Continued

TABLE A.1   Serum, Plasma, and Whole Blood Chemistries—cont'd

Test	Normal Values (SI Units [Conventional Units])	POSSIBLE ETIOLOGY	
		Higher Values	Lower Values
pH	*See* Blood gases		
Phenylalanine		Phenylketonuria	—
Phosphatase, acid	<30 U/L (<3.0 U/L)	Prostatic carcinoma, benign prostatic hypertrophy, prostatitis, multiple myeloma, Paget's disease, hyperparathyroidism, metastasis to the bone, multiple myeloma, sickle cell crisis, thrombocytosis, lysosomal disorders (e.g., Gaucher's disease), renal diseases, liver diseases (such as cirrhosis), rape or sexual intercourse	—
Phosphatase, alkaline (ALP)	40–160 U/L (same as SI units)	Primary cirrhosis, intrahepatic or extrahepatic biliary obstruction, primary or metastatic liver tumour, metastatic tumour to the bone, healing fracture, hyperparathyroidism, osteomalacia, Paget's disease, rheumatoid arthritis, rickets, intestinal ischemia or infarction, MI, sarcoidosis	Hypophosphatemia, hypophosphatasia, malnutrition, milk-alkali syndrome, pernicious anemia, scurvy (vitamin C deficiency)
Phosphorus, phosphate	1.0–1.5 mmol/L (3.0–4.5 mg/dL)†	Hypoparathyroidism, renal failure, increased dietary or IV intake of phosphorus, acromegaly, bone metastasis, sarcoidosis, hypocalcemia, acidosis, rhabdomyolysis, advanced lymphoma or myeloma, hemolytic anemia	Inadequate dietary ingestion of phosphorus, chronic antacid ingestion, hyperparathyroidism, hypercalcemia, chronic alcoholism, vitamin D deficiency (rickets), treatment of hyperglycemia, plasminogen, hyperinsulinism (childhood), malnutrition, alkalosis, Gram-negative sepsis
Potassium	3.5–5.1 mmol/L (3.5–5.1 mEq/L)	Excessive dietary intake, excessive IV intake, acute or chronic renal failure, Addison's disease, hypoaldosteronism, aldosterone-inhibiting diuretics (e.g., spironolactone, triamterene), crush injury to tissues, hemolysis, transfusion of hemolyzed blood, infection, acidosis, dehydration	Deficient dietary intake, deficient IV intake, burns, GI disorders (e.g., diarrhea, vomiting, villous adenomas), diuretics, hyperaldosteronism, Cushing's syndrome, renal tubular acidosis, licorice ingestion, alkalosis, insulin administration, glucose administration, ascites, renal artery stenosis, cystic fibrosis, trauma, surgery, or burns
Prostate-specific antigen (PSA)	0–4 mcg/L (0–4 ng/mL)	Benign prostatic hypertrophy, prostate cancer, prostatitis	—
Proteins		Burns, cirrhosis (globulin fraction), dehydration	Congenital agammaglobulinemia, increased capillary permeability, inflammatory disease, liver disease, malabsorption, malnutrition
• Total	64–83 g/L (6.4–8.3 g/dL)		
• Albumin	35–50 g/L (3.5–5 g/dL)		
• Globulin	23–34 g/L (2.3–3.4 g/dL)		
• Albumin/globulin ratio	1.5 : 1–2.5 : 1 (same as SI units)	Multiple myeloma (globulin fraction), shock, vomiting	Malnutrition, nephrotic syndrome, proteinuria, renal disease, severe burns
Pseudocholinesterase (serum)	8–18 U/mL (same as SI units)	Reticulocytosis, hyperlipemia, nephrosis, diabetes	Poisoning from organic phosphate insecticides, hepatocellular disease, individuals with congenital enzyme deficiency, malnutrition and other forms of hypoalbuminemia

TABLE A.1	Serum, Plasma, and Whole Blood Chemistries—cont'd		
		POSSIBLE ETIOLOGY	
Test	**Normal Values (SI Units [Conventional Units])**	**Higher Values**	**Lower Values**
Renin • Upright position, sodium depleted (sodium-restricted diet) • Upright position, sodium replaced (normal-sodium diet)	20–39 years: 2.9–24 mcg/L/hr (2.9–24 ng/mL/hr) >40 years: 2.9–10.8 mcg/L/hr (2.9–10.8 ng/mL/hr) 20–39 years: 0.1–4.3 mcg/L/hr (0.1–4.3 ng/mL/hr) >40 years: 0.1–3 mcg/L/hr (0.1–3 ng/mL/hr)	Essential hypertension, malignant hypertension, renovascular hypertension, chronic renal failure, sodium-losing GI disease (vomiting or diarrhea), Addison's disease, renin-producing renal tumour, Bartter syndrome, cirrhosis, hyperkalemia, hemorrhage	Primary aldosteronism, steroid therapy, congenital adrenal hyperplasia
Sodium	136–145 mmol/L (136–145 mEq/L)	Corticosteroid therapy, dehydration, impaired renal function, increased dietary or IV intake, primary aldosteronism	Addison's disease, decreased dietary or IV intake, DKA, diuretic therapy, excessive loss from GI tract, excessive perspiration, water intoxication
Testosterone • Male • Female	9.5–30 nmol/L (275–875 ng/dL) 0.8–2.6 nmol/L (23–875 ng/dL)	Idiopathic sexual precocity, pinealoma, encephalitis, congenital adrenal hyperplasia, adrenocortical tumour, testicular or extragonadal tumour, hyperthyroidism, testosterone resistance syndromes Ovarian tumour, adrenal tumour, congenital adrenocortical hyperplasia, trophoblastic tumour, polycystic ovaries, idiopathic hirsutism	Klinefelter's syndrome, cryptorchidism, primary and secondary hypogonadism, trisomy 21, orchiectomy, hepatic cirrhosis —
Thyroid-stimulating hormone (TSH)	0.4–4.8 mIU/L (0.4–4.8 mIU/mL)	Primary hypothyroidism (thyroid dysfunction), thyroiditis, thyroid agenesis, congenital cretinism, large doses of iodine, radioactive iodine injection, surgical ablation of thyroid, severe and chronic illnesses, pituitary TSH-secreting tumour	Secondary hypothyroidism, hyperthyroidism, suppressive doses of thyroid medication, factitious hyperthyroidism
Thyroxine (T_4), total • Adult male • Adult female • Adult >60 years	51–154 nmol/L (4–12 mcg/dL) 64–154 nmol/L (5–12 mcg/dL) 64–142 nmol/L (5–11 mcg/dL)	Primary hyperthyroid states (e.g., Graves' disease, Plummer disease, toxic thyroid adenoma), acute thyroiditis, familial dysalbuminemic hyperthyroxinemia, factitious hyperthyroidism, struma ovarii TBG increase (e.g., as occurs in pregnancy, hepatitis, congenital hyperproteinemia)	Hypothyroid states (e.g., cretinism, surgical ablation, myxedema), pituitary insufficiency, hypothalamic failure, protein malnutrition and other protein-depleted states (e.g., nephrotic syndrome), iodine insufficiency, nonthyroid illnesses (e.g., renal failure, Cushing's disease, cirrhosis, surgery, advanced cancer)
Thyroxine (T_4), free	13–27 pmol/L (1.0–2.1 ng/dL)	Primary hyperthyroid states (e.g., Graves' disease, Plummer disease, toxic thyroid adenoma), acute thyroiditis, factitious hyperthyroidism, struma ovarii	Hypothyroid states (e.g., cretinism, surgical ablation, myxedema), pituitary insufficiency, hypothalamic failure, iodine insufficiency, nonthyroid illnesses (e.g., renal failure, Cushing's disease, cirrhosis, surgery, advanced cancer)
Triglycerides • Male • Female	0.45–1.71 mmol/L (40–150 mg/dL) 0.40–1.52 mmol/L (35–135 mg/dL)	Glycogen storage disease (von Gierke disease), familial hypertriglyceridemia, apoprotein C-II deficiency, hyperlipidemias, hypothyroidism, high-carbohydrate diet, poorly controlled diabetes, nephrotic syndrome, chronic renal failure	Hyperthyroidism, malabsorption syndrome, malnutrition, abetalipoproteinemia

Continued

TABLE A.1	Serum, Plasma, and Whole Blood Chemistries—cont'd		
		POSSIBLE ETIOLOGY	
Test	**Normal Values (SI Units [Conventional Units])**	**Higher Values**	**Lower Values**
Tri-iodothyronine (T$_3$)	1.1–2.9 mmol/L (70–190 ng/dL)	Primary hyperthyroid states (e.g., Graves' disease, Plummer disease, toxic thyroid adenoma), acute thyroiditis, factitious hyperthyroidism, struma ovarii, pregnancy, hepatitis, congenital hyperproteinemia	Hypothyroid states (e.g., cretinism, surgical ablation, myxedema), pituitary insufficiency, hypothalamic failure, protein malnutrition and other protein-depleted states (e.g., nephrotic syndrome), iodine insufficiency, nonthyroid illnesses (e.g., renal failure, Cushing's disease, cirrhosis, surgery, advanced cancer), hepatic diseases
Tri-iodothyronine (T$_3$) uptake	24–34 AU (24–34%)	Hyperthyroidism, hypoproteinemia (e.g., protein malnutrition, protein-losing enteropathy, nephropathy), familial dysalbuminemic hyperthyroxinemia, nonthyroid conditions (e.g., renal failure, Cushing's disease, cirrhosis, surgery, advanced cancer), factitious hyperthyroidism, struma ovarii	Hypothyroid states (e.g., cretinism, surgical ablation, pituitary insufficiency, hypothalamic failure, myxedema), hepatitis and cirrhosis, pregnancy, congenital hyperproteinemia
Troponin T (cTnT)	<0.1 mcg/L (<0.1 ng/mL)	Cardiac muscle damage (resulting from MI, myocarditis, or pericarditis), chronic renal failure, multiorgan failure, severe heart failure	—
Troponin I (cTnI)	<0.35 mcg/L (<0.35 ng/mL)		—
Urea nitrogen, blood (blood urea nitrogen [BUN], serum urea nitrogen)	2.9–8.2 mmol/L (8–23 mg/dL)	Prerenal causes, hypovolemia, shock, burns, dehydration, heart failure, MI, GI bleeding, excessive protein ingestion (alimentary tube feeding), excessive protein catabolism, starvation, sepsis, renal disease (e.g., glomerulonephritis, pyelonephritis, acute tubular necrosis), renal failure, nephrotoxic medications, ureteral obstruction from stones, tumour, or congenital anomalies, bladder outlet obstruction from prostatic hypertrophy or cancer or bladder/urethral congenital anomalies, postrenal azotemia	Liver failure, overhydration because of fluid overload in the SIADH secretion, negative nitrogen balance (e.g., malnutrition, malabsorption), pregnancy, nephrotic syndrome
Uric acid		Increased ingestion of purines, genetic inborn error in purine metabolism, metastatic cancer, multiple myeloma, leukemias, cancer chemotherapy, hemolysis, rhabdomyolysis (e.g., heavy exercise, burns, crush injury, epileptic seizure, MI)	Wilson disease, Fanconi's syndrome, lead poisoning, yellow atrophy of liver
• Male	240–501 mcmol/L (4.0–8.5 mg/dL)		
• Female	160–430 mcmol/L (2.7–7.3 mg/dL)		
Vitamin B$_{12}$	118–701 pmol/L (160–950 pg/mL)	Leukemia, polycythemia vera, severe liver dysfunction, myeloproliferative disease	Pernicious anemia, malabsorption syndromes (e.g., inflammatory bowel disease, sprue, Crohn's disease), intestinal worm infestation, atrophic gastritis, Zollinger-Ellison syndrome, large proximal gastrectomy, resection of terminal ileum, achlorhydria, pregnancy, vitamin C deficiency, folic acid deficiency
Zinc protoporphyrin (ZPP)	0–69 mcmol ZPP/mol heme	Lead poisoning, vanadium exposure, iron deficiency, anemia of chronic illness, sickle cell anemia, sideroblastic anemia	—

*Because arterial blood gases are influenced by altitude, the values for PaCO$_2$, PaO$_2$, and PvO$_2$ decrease as altitude increases. The lower values are normal for an altitude of 1.6 km (1 mile).
†Values for older persons are significantly lower than those for younger adults.
ACTH, Adrenocorticotropic hormone; *COPD,* chronic obstructive pulmonary disease; *DKA,* diabetic ketoacidosis; *GI,* gastrointestinal; *IV,* intravenous; *MI,* myocardial infarction; *PTH,* parathyroid hormone; *RBC,* red blood cell; *SIADH,* syndrome of inappropriate antidiuretic hormone, *TBG,* thyroxine-binding globulin.

TABLE A.2	Hematology		

Test	Normal Values (SI Units [Conventional Units])	POSSIBLE ETIOLOGY	
		Higher Values	Lower Values
Activated coagulation time or automated clotting time (ACT)	70–120 sec (same as SI units)	Heparin administration, clotting factor deficiencies, cirrhosis of the liver, Coumarin administration, lupus inhibitor	Thrombosis
Activated partial thromboplastin time (aPTT)	25–40 sec* (same as SI units)	Congenital clotting factor deficiencies (e.g., von Willebrand's disease, hemophilia, hypofibrinogenemia), cirrhosis of liver, vitamin K deficiency, DIC, heparin administration, Coumarin administration	Early stages of DIC, extensive cancer (e.g., ovarian, pancreatic, colon)
D-dimer	<3.0 nmol/L (<0.4 mcg/mL)	DIC, primary fibrinolysis, during thrombolytic or defibrination therapy, deep-vein thrombosis, pulmonary embolism, arterial thromboembolism, sickle cell anemia with or without vaso-occlusive crisis, pregnancy, malignancy, surgery	—
Erythrocyte count† (RBC count) [altitude dependent])		Erythrocytosis, congenital heart disease, severe COPD, polycythemia vera, severe dehydration (e.g., severe diarrhea or burns), hemoglobinopathies, thalassemia trait	Anemia, hemoglobinopathy, cirrhosis, hemolytic anemia (as in erythroblastosis fetalis, hemoglobinopathies, medication-induced reactions, transfusion reactions, paroxysmal nocturnal hemoglobinuria), hemorrhage, dietary deficiency, bone marrow failure, prosthetic valves, renal disease, normal pregnancy, rheumatoid/ collagen-vascular diseases (e.g., rheumatoid arthritis, lupus, sarcoidosis), lymphoma, multiple myeloma, leukemia, Hodgkin's disease
• Male	$4.7–6.2 \times 10^{12}$/L		
• Female	$4.2–5.4 \times 10^{12}$/L		
Erythrocyte sedimentation rate (ESR), Westergren Method		*Moderate increase:* Acute hepatitis, MI, rheumatoid arthritis, chronic renal failure (e.g., nephritis, nephrosis), malignant diseases (e.g., multiple myeloma, Hodgkin's disease, advanced carcinomas), bacterial infection, inflammatory diseases, necrotic diseases, diseases associated with increased protein levels, severe anemias (e.g., iron deficiency or vitamin B_{12} deficiency)	Sickle cell disease, spherocytosis, hypofibrinogenemia, polycythemia vera
• Male	≤15 mm/hr (same as SI units)		
• Female	≤20 mm/hr (same as SI units)		
Fibrin split (degradation) products	<10 mg/L (<10 mcg/mL)	DIC, heart or vascular surgery, thromboembolism, thrombosis, advanced malignancy, severe inflammation, postoperative states, massive trauma, deficiency in protein S and protein C, antithrombin III deficiency	Anticoagulation therapy
Fibrinogen	5.8–11.8 mcmol/L (200–400 mg/dL)	Acute inflammatory reactions (e.g., rheumatoid arthritis, glomerulonephritis), trauma, acute infection such as pneumonia, coronary heart disease, stroke, peripheral vascular disease, cigarette smoking, pregnancy	Liver disease (hepatitis, cirrhosis), DIC, fibrinolysis, congenital afibrinogenemia, advanced carcinoma, malnutrition, large-volume blood transfusion
Hematocrit (altitude dependent)†		Erythrocytosis, congenital heart disease, polycythemia vera, severe dehydration (e.g., severe diarrhea, burns), severe COPD	Anemia, hemoglobinopathy, cirrhosis, hemolytic anemia, hemorrhage dietary deficiency, bone marrow failure, prosthetic valves, renal disease, normal pregnancy, rheumatoid/collagen-vascular diseases (e.g., rheumatoid arthritis, lupus), lymphoma, multiple myeloma, leukemia, Hodgkin's disease
• Male	0.42–0.52 volume fraction (42–52%)		
• Female	0.37–0.47 volume fraction (37–47%)		
Hemoglobin, glycosylated or glycated (hemoglobin A_{1c} [HbA_{1c}])	4–5.9% (adult without diabetes)	Newly diagnosed diabetes, poorly controlled diabetes, nondiabetic hyperglycemia, patients with splenectomy, pregnancy	Hemolytic anemia, chronic blood loss, chronic renal failure

Continued

TABLE A.2 Hematology—cont'd

Test	Normal Values (SI Units [Conventional Units])	POSSIBLE ETIOLOGY	
		Higher Values	Lower Values
International normalized ratio (INR)	0.9–1.1	Same as for PT	—
Mean corpuscular hemoglobin (MCH) [Hb/RBC]	27–31 pg (same as SI units)	Macrocytic anemia	Microcytic anemia, hypochromic anemia
Mean corpuscular hemoglobin concentration (MCHC) [Hb/Hct]	27–31 g/dL (same as SI units)	Spherocytosis, intravascular hemolysis, cold agglutinins	Iron-deficiency anemia, thalassemia
Mean corpuscular volume (MCV) [Hct/RBC]	76–100 fL (76–100 mm^3)	Pernicious anemia (vitamin B$_{12}$ deficiency), folic acid deficiency, antimetabolite therapy, alcoholism, chronic liver disease	Iron-deficiency anemia, thalassemia, anemia of chronic illness
Partial thromboplastin time (PTT)	60–70 sec (same as SI units)	Congenital clotting factor deficiencies, cirrhosis of liver, vitamin K deficiency, DIC, heparin administration, Coumarin administration	Early stages of DIC, extensive cancer (e.g., ovarian, pancreatic, colon)
Platelet count (thrombocytes)	150–400 × 10^9/L (150 000–400 000/mm^3)	Malignant disorders (leukemia, lymphoma, solid tumours such as of the colon), polycythemia vera, rheumatoid arthritis, iron-deficiency anemia or following hemorrhagic anemia	Hypersplenism, hemorrhage, immune thrombocytopenia (e.g., idiopathic thrombocytopenia, neonatal, post-transfusion, or medication-induced thrombocytopenia), leukemia and other myelofibrosis disorders, thrombotic thrombocytopenia, Graves' disease, inherited disorders (e.g., Wiskott-Aldrich, Bernard-Soulier, Zieve syndromes), DIC, systemic lupus erythematosus, pernicious anemia, hemolytic anemia, cancer chemotherapy, infection
Prothrombin time (PT; Protime)	11–12.5 sec	Liver disease (e.g., cirrhosis, hepatitis), hereditary factor deficiency, vitamin K deficiency, bile duct obstruction, Coumarin ingestion, DIC, massive blood transfusion, salicylate intoxication	—
Red cell distribution width (RDW)	11–14.5% (same as SI units)	Iron-deficiency anemia, B$_{12}$ vitamin or folate-deficiency anemia, hemoglobinopathies (e.g., sickle cell disease or protein C disease), hemolytic anemias: fragmentation increases RDW variation, posthemorrhagic anemias	—
Reticulocyte count (manual)	0.5–2% total number of RBCs	Hemolytic anemia (e.g., immune hemolytic anemia, hemoglobinopathies, hypersplenism, trauma from a prosthetic heart valve), hemorrhage (3 to 4 days later), hemolytic disease of the newborn, treatment for deficiency in iron, vitamin B$_{12}$, or folate	Pernicious anemia and folic acid deficiency, iron-deficiency anemia, aplastic anemia, radiation therapy, malignancy, marrow failure, adrenocortical hypofunction, anterior pituitary hypofunction, chronic diseases
Sickle cell solubility	0%	Sickle cell anemia	
WBC count[†]	3.5–12.0 × 10^9/L (3 500–12 000/mm^3)	Infection; leukemic neoplasia or other myeloproliferative disorders; other malignancy, trauma, stress, or hemorrhage; tissue necrosis; inflammation; dehydration; thyroid storm; steroid use	Medication toxicity, bone marrow failure, overwhelming infections, dietary deficiency (e.g., vitamin B$_{12}$ deficiency, iron deficiency), congenital bone marrow aplasia, bone marrow infiltration (e.g., myelofibrosis), autoimmune disease, hypersplenism
WBC differential			
• Band neutrophils	0–1 × 10^9/L (0–9%)	Acute infections	—
• Basophils	0.01–0.05 × 10^9/L (15–50/mm^3; 0.5–1%)	Basophilia, myeloproliferative disease (e.g., myelofibrosis, polycythemia rubra vera), leukemia	Basopenia, acute allergic reactions, hyperthyroidism, stress reactions

TABLE A.2	Hematology—cont'd		
Test	Normal Values (SI Units [Conventional Units])	POSSIBLE ETIOLOGY Higher Values	Lower Values
• Eosinophils	0.00–0.25 × 10⁹/L (50–250/mm³; 1–4%)	Eosinophilia, parasitic infections, allergic reactions, eczema, leukemia, autoimmune diseases	Eosinopenia, increased adrenosteroid production
• Lymphocytes	1.5–3.0 × 10⁹/L (1 500–3 000/mm³; 20–40%)	Lymphocytosis, chronic bacterial infection, viral infection (e.g., mumps, rubella), lymphocytic leukemia, multiple myeloma, infectious mononucleosis, radiation, infectious hepatitis	Lymphocytopenia, leukemia, sepsis, immunodeficiency diseases, lupus erythematosus, later stages of human immunodeficiency virus infection, medication therapy: adrenocorticosteroids, antineoplastics; radiation therapy
• Monocytes	0.3–0.5 × 10⁹/L (300–500/mm³; 2–8%)	Monocytosis, chronic inflammatory disorders, viral infections (e.g., infectious mononucleosis), tuberculosis, chronic ulcerative colitis, parasites (e.g., malaria)	Monocytopenia, aplastic anemia, hairy cell leukemia, medication therapy: prednisone
• Neutrophils	3.0–5.8 × 10⁹/L (3 000–5 800/mm³; 55–70%)	Neutrophilia, physical or emotional stress, acute suppurative infection, myelocytic leukemia, trauma, Cushing's syndrome, inflammatory disorders (e.g., rheumatic fever, thyroiditis, rheumatoid arthritis), metabolic disorders (e.g., ketoacidosis, gout, eclampsia)	Neutropenia, aplastic anemia, dietary deficiency, overwhelming bacterial infection (especially in older persons), viral infections (e.g., hepatitis, influenza, measles), radiation therapy, Addison's disease, medication therapy: myelotoxic agents (as in chemotherapy)

*For patients receiving anticoagulant therapy, aPTT is 1.5–2.5 times the control value in seconds; PT is 1.5–2.0 times the control value in seconds.
†Components of complete blood count (CBC).
COPD, Chronic obstructive pulmonary disease; DIC, disseminated intravascular coagulation; MI, myocardial infarction; RBC, red blood cell; WBC, white blood cell.

TABLE A.3	Serology–Immunology		
Test	Normal Values (SI Units [Conventional Units])	POSSIBLE ETIOLOGY Higher Values	Lower Values
Antinuclear antibody (ANA)	Negative at 1:40 dilution (same as SI units)	SLE, rheumatoid arthritis, periarteritis (polyarteritis) nodosa, dermatomyositis, polymyositis, scleroderma, Sjögren's syndrome, Raynaud's phenomenon, other immune diseases, leukemia, infectious mononucleosis, myasthenia gravis, cirrhosis, chronic hepatitis	—
Anti-DNA antibody	Negative <70 U/mL (same as SI units)	Collagen-vascular diseases, other autoimmune diseases, such as rheumatic fever; chronic hepatitis, infectious mononucleosis, biliary cirrhosis	—
Anti-RNP (ribonucleoprotein)	Negative (negative)	Mixed connective tissue disease (MCTD), SLE, discoid lupus scleroderma	—
Anti-Sm (Smith)	Negative (negative)	SLE	—
Anti-streptolysin-O titre (ASO titre)	≤160 Todd units/mL (same as SI units)	Streptococcal infection, acute rheumatic fever, bacterial endocarditis, acute glomerulonephritis, scarlet fever, streptococcal pyoderma	—
C-reactive protein (CRP)	<10 mg/L (<1.0 mg/dL)	Acute, noninfectious inflammatory reaction, collagen-vascular diseases, tissue infarction or damage, bacterial infections such as postoperative wound infection, urinary tract infection, or tuberculosis, malignant disease, bacterial infection, increased risk for cardiovascular ischemic events	—
Carcinoembryonic antigen (CEA)	<5 mcg/L (5 ng/mL)	Cancer (gastrointestinal, breast, lung, pancreatic, hepatobiliary), inflammation (colitis, cholecystitis, pancreatitis, diverticulitis), cirrhosis, Crohn's disease, peptic ulcer	—

Continued

TABLE A.3   Serology–Immunology—cont'd

Test	Normal Values (SI Units [Conventional Units])	POSSIBLE ETIOLOGY	
		Higher Values	**Lower Values**
Complement assay components • Total • C3 • C4	 30–75 kU/L (30–75 U/mL) 0.75–1.75 g/L (75–175 mg/dL) 0.22–0.45 g/L (22–45 mg/dL)	Rheumatic fever (acute), MI (acute), ulcerative colitis, inflammatory illnesses, stress, and trauma, cancer	Hereditary angioedema, severe liver diseases such as hepatitis or cirrhosis, autoimmune disease (SLE, glomerulonephritis, lupus nephritis, rheumatoid arthritis [severe and active], Sjögren's syndrome), serum sickness, renal transplant rejection (acute), protein malnutrition, anemia, malnutrition, infection such as Gram-negative sepsis or bacterial endocarditis, glomerulonephritis
Direct antihuman globulin test (DAT) or direct Coombs' test	Negative (negative) (no agglutination)	Hemolytic disease of the newborn, incompatible blood transfusion reaction, lymphoma, autoimmune hemolytic anemia, mycoplasmal infection, infectious mononucleosis, hemolytic anemia after heart bypass, adult hemolytic anemia (idiopathic)	—
Fluorescent treponemal antibody absorption (FTAAbs)	Negative (nonreactive)	Syphilis	—
Hepatitis A antibody	Negative (negative)	Hepatitis A	—
Hepatitis B surface antigen (HBsAg)	Negative (negative)	Hepatitis B	—
Hepatitis C antibody	Negative (negative)	Hepatitis C	—
Immunoglobulins (Igs) • IgA	 0.85–3.85 g/L (85–385 mg/dL)	Chronic liver diseases (e.g., primary biliary cirrhosis), chronic infections, inflammatory bowel disease	Ataxia, telangiectasia, congenital isolated deficiency, hypoproteinemia (e.g., nephrotic syndrome, protein-losing enteropathies), medication immunosuppression (steroids, dextran), AIDS
• IgD	Minimal	Chronic infection, connective tissue disease	—
• IgE	Minimal	Anaphylactic shock, atopic disease (allergies), parasite infections	—
• IgG	5.65–17.65 g/L (565–1 765 mg/dL)	Chronic granulomatous infections (e.g., tuberculosis, Wegener granulomatosis, sarcoidosis), hyperimmunization reactions, chronic liver disease, multiple myeloma, autoimmune diseases, intrauterine devices	Wiskott-Aldrich syndrome, agammaglobulinemia, AIDS, hypoproteinemia (e.g., nephrotic syndrome, protein-losing enteropathies), medication immunosuppression (steroids, dextran), non-IgG multiple myeloma, leukemia
• IgM	0.55–3.75 g/L (55–375 mg/dL)	Waldenström macroglobulinemia, chronic infections (e.g., hepatitis, mononucleosis, sarcoidosis), autoimmune diseases (e.g., SLE, rheumatoid arthritis), acute infections, chronic liver disorders (e.g., biliary cirrhosis)	Agammaglobulinemia, AIDS, hypoproteinemia (e.g., nephrotic syndrome, protein-losing enteropathies), medication immunosuppression (steroids, dextran), IgG or IgA multiple myeloma, leukemia
Monospot or Mono-Test	Negative (<1:28 titre)	Infectious mononucleosis, chronic EBV infection, chronic fatigue syndrome, Burkitt lymphoma, some forms of chronic hepatitis	—
Rheumatoid factor (RA factor)	Negative or <60 IU/mL by nephelometric method	Rheumatoid arthritis, other immune disease (e.g., SLE, Sjögren's syndrome, scleroderma), chronic viral infection, subacute bacterial endocarditis, tuberculosis, chronic active hepatitis, dermatomyositis, infectious mononucleosis, leukemia, biliary cirrhosis, syphilis, renal disease	—
RPR (rapid plasma reagin) test	Negative or nonreactive (same as SI units)	—	—

TABLE A.3	Serology–Immunology—cont'd		
		POSSIBLE ETIOLOGY	
Test	**Normal Values (SI Units [Conventional Units])**	**Higher Values**	**Lower Values**
Thyroid antibodies	Titre <9 IU/mL	*Chronic thyroiditis (Hashimoto thyroiditis):* Antimicrosomal antibodies attack the microsome in the thyroid cells. The immune complex creates an inflammatory and destructive process in the gland, which is mediated through the complement system. *Rheumatoid arthritis, rheumatoid-collagen disease:* The association with other autoimmune diseases is well known. The mechanism of this association, however, is not well known. *Pernicious anemia:* APCAs have been associated with the presence of antimicrosomal antibodies. *Thyrotoxicosis, hypothyroidism, thyroid carcinoma:* Microsomes leak out of the thyroid as a result of the presence of these destructive diseases; they stimulate the immune system to produce antimicrosomal antibodies. *Myxedema:* Antithyroid microsomal antibodies destroy the thyroid cell, which results in hypofunction of the gland.	—
VDRL (Venereal Disease Research Laboratory) test	Negative or nonreactive (same as SI units)	Syphilis	—

AIDS, Acquired immune deficiency syndrome; APCAs, antiparietal cell antibodies; EBV, Epstein–Barr virus; IV, intravenous; MI, myocardial infarction; SLE, systemic lupus erythematosus.

TABLE A.4	Urine Chemistry			
			POSSIBLE ETIOLOGY	
Test	**Specimen**	**Normal Values (SI Units [Conventional Units])**	**Higher Values**	**Lower Values**
Acetone (ketones)	Random	Negative (negative)	Diabetes mellitus, high-fat and low-carbohydrate diets, starvation states	—
Aldosterone	24 hr	17–70 nmol/24 hr (2–26 mcg/24 hr)	*Primary aldosteronism:* Aldosterone-producing adrenal adenoma (Conn disease), adrenal cortical nodular hyperplasia, Bartter syndrome. *Secondary aldosteronism:* Hyponatremia, hyperkalemia, diuretic ingestion resulting in hypovolemia and hyponatremia, laxative abuse, stress, malignant hypertension, poor perfusion states (e.g., heart failure), decreased intravascular volume (e.g., cirrhosis, nephrotic syndrome), renal arterial stenosis, pregnancy and oral contraceptives, hypovolemia or hemorrhage, Cushing's disease	Renin deficiency, steroid therapy, Addison's disease, patients on high-sodium diet, hypernatremia, antihypertensive therapy, aldosterone deficiency
Amylase	24 hr	25–125 U/L (same as SI units)	Acute pancreatitis, chronic relapsing pancreatitis, peptic ulcer penetrating into the pancreas, GI disease, acute cholecystitis, parotiditis (mumps), ruptured ectopic pregnancy, renal failure, diabetic ketoacidosis, pulmonary infarction, after endoscopic retrograde pancreatography	—

Continued

TABLE A.4   Urine Chemistry—cont'd

Test	Specimen	Normal Values (SI Units [Conventional Units])	POSSIBLE ETIOLOGY Higher Values	Lower Values
Bence-Jones protein	Random	Kappa total light chain: <0.68 mg/dL Lambda total light chain: <0.40 mg/dL Kappa/lambda ratio: 0.7–6.2	Multiple myeloma (plasmacytoma), chronic lymphocytic leukemia, lymphoma, metastatic colon, breast, lung, or prostate cancer, amyloidosis, Waldenström macroglobulinemia	—
Bilirubin	Random	3–22 mcmol/L (0.2–1.3 mg/dL)	Gallstones, extrahepatic duct obstruction (tumour, inflammation, gallstone, scarring, surgical trauma), extensive liver metastasis, cholestasis from medications, Dubin-Johnson syndrome, Rotor syndrome	—
Calcium	24 hr	2.10–2.7 mmol/day (8.4–10.6 mg/dL)	*Hyperparathyroidism, nonparathyroid PTH-producing tumour (e.g., lung or renal carcinoma):* PTH or a similar hormone mobilizes calcium stores from the bone to the blood. *Metastatic tumour to bone, Paget's disease of bone, prolonged immobilization:* Bone destruction or thinning causes calcium to leak from the bone and into the blood. *Milk-alkali syndrome:* With increased ingestion of milk products or antacids (which contain calcium), the serum calcium level can be elevated. *Vitamin D intoxication:* Vitamin D works synergistically with PTH to increase serum calcium level. *Lymphoma, granulomatous infections such as sarcoidosis and tuberculosis:* These diseases are associated with enhanced levels of vitamin D, which works synergistically with PTH to increase serum calcium level. *Addison's disease:* Glucocorticosteroids inhibit vitamin D activity. When steroid activity is decreased, vitamin D action is enhanced. Vitamin D works synergistically with PTH to increase serum calcium levels. Acromegaly, hyperthyroidism	*Hypoparathyroidism:* PTH acts to increase serum calcium levels. If PTH levels are reduced, serum calcium levels decline. *Renal failure, hyperphosphatemia secondary to renal failure:* Excess anions, present in patients with renal failure, bind serum calcium. *Rickets, vitamin D deficiency:* Vitamin D acts synergistically with PTH. PTH acts to increase serum calcium levels. Without that synergism, calcium levels decline. *Osteomalacia, hypoalbuminemia, malabsorption:* Less calcium is available to the blood. *Pancreatitis, fat embolism:* Pancreatitis is associated with saponification (binding of calcium to fats) of the peripancreatic tissue. This reduces calcium levels in the blood. *Alkalosis:* High pH in the blood drives the calcium to intracellular spaces. Blood levels decline.
Catecholamines • Epinephrine • Norepinephrine	24 hr	<590 mmol/day (<100 mcg/24 hr) <109 nmol/day (<20 mcg/24 hr) <590 nmol/day (<100 mcg/24 hr)	Pheochromocytomas, neuroblastomas, ganglioneuromas, ganglioblastomas, severe stress, strenuous exercise, acute anxiety	—
Chloride	24 hr	98–106 mmol/L (98–106 mEq/L)	Dehydration, excessive infusion of normal saline solution, metabolic acidosis, renal tubular acidosis, Cushing's syndrome, kidney dysfunction, hyperparathyroidism, eclampsia, respiratory alkalosis	Overhydration, syndrome of inappropriate secretion of antidiuretic hormone, heart failure, vomiting or prolonged gastric suction, chronic diarrhea or high-output GI fistula, chronic respiratory acidosis, metabolic alkalosis, salt-losing nephritis, Addison's disease, diuretic therapy, hypokalemia, aldosteronism
Coproporphyrin • Male • Female	24 hr	 15–167 nmol/24 hr (10–109 mcg/24 hr) 5–86 nmol/24 hr (3–56 mcg/24 hr)	Lead poisoning, oral contraceptive use, poliomyelitis	—

TABLE A.4 Urine Chemistry—cont'd

Test	Specimen	Normal Values (SI Units [Conventional Units])	POSSIBLE ETIOLOGY Higher Values	Lower Values
Creatine	24 hr		Diseases or injury affecting the heart muscle, skeletal muscle, and brain	—
• Male		20–215 U/L (same as SI units)		
• Female		20–160 U/L (same as SI units)		
Creatinine	24 hr		Diseases affecting renal function, such as glomerulonephritis, pyelonephritis, acute tubular necrosis, urinary tract obstruction, reduced renal blood flow (e.g., shock, dehydration, heart failure, atherosclerosis), diabetic nephropathy, nephritis, rhabdomyolysis, acromegaly, gigantism	Debilitation, decreased muscle mass (e.g., muscular dystrophy, myasthenia gravis)
• Male		53–106 mcmol/L (0.6–1.2 mg/dL)		
• Female		44–97 mcmol/L (0.5–1.1. mg/dL)		
Creatinine clearance			Exercise, pregnancy, high–cardiac output syndromes	Impaired kidney function (e.g., renal artery atherosclerosis, glomerulonephritis, acute tubular necrosis), conditions causing decreases in GFR (e.g., heart failure, cirrhosis with ascites, shock, dehydration)
• Male		1.78–2.32 mL/sec (107–139 mL/min)		
• Female		1.45–1.78 mL/sec (87–107 mL/min)		
Estriol	24 hr		Feminization syndromes, precocious puberty, ovarian tumour, testicular tumour, adrenal tumour, normal pregnancy, hepatic cirrhosis, liver necrosis, hyperthyroidism	A failing pregnancy, Turner's syndrome, hypopituitarism, primary and secondary hypogonadism, Stein-Leventhal syndrome, menopause, anorexia nervosa
• Female				
• Ovulatory phase		13–54 mcg/24 hr (104–370 nmol/L)		
• Luteal phase		4–100 mcg/24 hr (15–37 nmol/L)		
• Pregnancy		First trimester: 0–800 mcg/24 hr (0–2 900 nmol/L) Second trimester: 800–1 200 mcg/24 hr (2 900–4 400 nmol/L) Third trimester: 5 000–12 000 mcg/24 hr (18 000–180 000 nmol/L)		
• Menopause		1.4–19.6 mcg/24 hr (5.2–72.5 nmol/L)		
• Male		1–11 mcg/24 hr (18–67 nmol/L)	—	—
Glucose	Random	Random: negative Fasting: <6.1 mmol/L (70–11 mg/dL)	Diabetes mellitus, acute stress response, Cushing's syndrome, pheochromocytoma, chronic renal failure, glucagonoma, acute pancreatitis, diuretic therapy, corticosteroid therapy, acromegaly	Insulinoma, hypothyroidism, hypopituitarism, Addison's disease, extensive liver disease, insulin overdose, starvation
Hemoglobin	Random		Erythrocytosis, congenital heart disease, severe chronic obstructive pulmonary disease, polycythemia vera, severe dehydration (e.g., severe diarrhea, burns)	—
• Male		140–180 mmol/L (14–18 g/dL)		
• Female		120–160 (12–16 g/dL)		
5-Hydroxyindole-acetic acid (5-HIAA)	24 hr	10–40 mcmol/day (2–8 mg/24 hr)	Carcinoid tumour of the appendix, bowel, lung, breast, or ovary; noncarcinoid illness, cystic fibrosis, intestinal malabsorption	Depression, migraine
Ketone bodies	Random	Negative (negative)	Poorly controlled diabetes mellitus, starvation, alcoholism, weight-reduction diets, prolonged vomiting, anorexia, high-protein diets, glycogen storage diseases, febrile illnesses in infants and children, hyperthyroidism, severe stress or illness, excessive aspirin ingestion	—
Lead	24 hr	<0.48 mcmol/day (<10 mcg/day)	Lead exposure	—
Metanephrine	24 hr	12–60 pg/mL	Pheochromocytoma	—

Continued

TABLE A.4 Urine Chemistry—cont'd

Test	Specimen	Normal Values (SI Units [Conventional Units])	POSSIBLE ETIOLOGY Higher Values	Lower Values
Myoglobin	Random	1.0–5.3 nmol/L (<90 ng/mL)	Myocardial infarction, skeletal muscle inflammation (myositis), malignant hyperthermia, muscular dystrophy, skeletal muscle ischemia, skeletal muscle trauma, rhabdomyolysis seizures	Polymyositis
pH	Random	4.6–8.0 (average, 6.0)	Alkalemia, urinary tract infections, gastric suction, vomiting, renal tubular acidosis	Acidemia, diabetes mellitus, starvation, respiratory acidosis
Porphobilinogen	Random 24 hr	Negative (negative) 0–6.6 mg/24 hr (0–2 mg/24 hr)	Acute intermittent porphyria, congenital erythropoietic porphyria, hereditary coproporphyria, variegate porphyria, lead poisoning	—
Potassium	24 hr	25–100 mmol/day (25–100 mEq/L/day)	Chronic renal failure, renal tubular acidosis, starvation, Cushing's syndrome, hyperaldosteronism, excessive intake of licorice, alkalosis, diuretic therapy	Dehydration, Addison's disease, malnutrition, vomiting, diarrhea, malabsorption, acute renal failure
Protein (dipstick)	Random	Negative (negative)	Heart failure, nephritis, nephrosis, physiological stress	—
Protein (qualitative) • At rest • During exercise	24 hr	0–8 mg/dL 50–80 mg/24 hr (0.05–0.08 g/day) <250 mg/24 hr (<0.25 g/day)	Nephrotic syndrome, glomerulonephritis, malignant hypertension, diabetic glomerulosclerosis, polycystic kidney disease, systemic lupus erythematosus, Goodpasture's syndrome, heavy-metal poisoning, bacterial pyelonephritis, nephrotoxic medication therapy, trauma, macroglobulinemia, multiple myelomas, pre-eclampsia, heart failure, orthostatic proteinuria, severe muscle exertion, renal vein thrombosis: Congestion of the kidneys is associated with proteinuria.	—
Sodium, blood	24 hr	136–145 mmol/L (136–145 mEq/L)	Increased dietary intake, excessive sodium in intravenous fluids	Cushing's syndrome, hyperaldosteronism
Specific gravity	Random	1.005–1.030 (usually, 1.010–1.025)*	Dehydration, pituitary tumour or trauma, decreased renal blood flow (as in heart failure, renal artery stenosis, or hypotension), glycosuria and proteinuria, water restriction, fever, excessive sweating, vomiting, diarrhea	Overhydration, diabetes insipidus, renal failure, diuresis
Uric acid • Male • Female		240–501 mcmol/L (4.0–8.5 mg/dL) 160–430 mcmol/L (2.7–7.3 mg/dL) (250–750 mg/24 hr)	Increased ingestion of purines, genetic inborn error in purine metabolism, metastatic cancer, multiple myeloma, leukemias, cancer chemotherapy, hemolysis, rhabdomyolysis	Idiopathic, chronic renal disease, acidosis (ketotic [diabetic or starvation] or lactic), hypothyroidism, toxemia of pregnancy, hyperlipoproteinemia, alcoholism, shock or chronic blood volume depletion states, Wilson disease, Fanconi's syndrome, lead poisoning, yellow atrophy of liver
Urobilinogen	24 hr	0.5–4.0 mg/24 hr (0.5–4.0 Ehrlich units/24 hr)	Hemolytic anemia, pernicious anemia, hemolysis because of medications, hematoma, excessive ecchymosis	Biliary obstruction, cholestasis
Uroporphyrins • Male • Female	24 hr	10–53 nmol/24 hr (8–44 mcg/24 hr) 10–26 nmol/24 hr (4–22 mcg/24 hr)	Acute intermittent porphyria, congenital erythropoietic porphyria, hereditary coproporphyria, variegate porphyria, lead poisoning	—
Vanillylmandelic acid	24 hr	<35 mcmol/day (<6.8 mg/24 hr)	Pheochromocytomas, neuroblastomas, ganglioneuromas, ganglioblastomas, severe stress, strenuous exercise, acute anxiety	—

*Values decrease with age.
GFR, Glomerular filtration rate; GI, gastrointestinal; PTH, parathyroid hormone.

TABLE A.5	Gastric Analysis		

| Test | Normal Values (SI Units [Conventional Units]) | POSSIBLE ETIOLOGY | |
		Higher Values	Lower Values
Basal			
Total acidity	15–45 mmol/L (15–45 mEq/L)	Gastric and duodenal ulcers, Zollinger-Ellison syndrome	Gastric carcinoma, severe gastritis
Post-stimulation			
Free hydrochloric acid	10–130 mmol/L (10–130 mEq/L)	—	—
Total acidity	20–150 mmol/L (20–150 mEq/L)	—	—

TABLE A.6	Fecal Analysis		

| Test | Normal Values (SI Units [Conventional Units) | POSSIBLE ETIOLOGY | |
		Higher Values	Lower Values
Blood*	Negative (negative)	Anal fissures, hemorrhoids, inflammatory bowel disease, malignant tumour, peptic ulcer	—
Colour			
• Brown		Various shades, depending on diet	—
• Clay		Biliary obstruction or presence of barium sulphate	—
• Tarry		More than 100 mL of blood in GI tract	—
• Red		Blood in large intestine	—
• Black		Blood in upper GI tract, or iron medication	—
Fecal fat	7–21 mmol/day (2–6 g/24 hr)	Cystic fibrosis, malabsorption secondary to sprue, celiac disease, Whipple's disease, Crohn's disease (regional enteritis), or radiation enteritis, maldigestion secondary to obstruction of the pancreatobiliary tree (e.g., cancer, stricture, gallstones), short-gut syndrome secondary to surgical resection, surgical bypass, or congenital anomaly	—
Mucus	Negative (negative)	Mucous colitis, spastic constipation	—
Pus	Negative (negative)	Chronic bacillary dysentery, chronic ulcerative colitis, localized abscesses	—
Urobilinogen	51–372 mcmol/100 g of stool (30–220 mg/100 g of stool)	Hemolytic anemias	Complete biliary obstruction

*Ingestion of meat may produce false-positive results. Patient may be placed on a meat-free diet for 3 days before the test.
GI, Gastrointestinal.

TABLE A.7	Cerebrospinal Fluid Analysis		

| | Normal Values (SI Units [Conventional Units]) | POSSIBLE ETIOLOGY | |
Test		Higher Values	Lower Values
Blood	Negative (negative)	Intracranial hemorrhage	—
Cell count (age dependent)			
• White blood cells (WBCs)	0–5×10^6 WBCs/L (0–10 cells/mcL)	Inflammation or infections of CNS	—
• Red blood cells (RBCs)	0		—
Chloride	116–122 mmol/L of CSF (116–122 mEq/L of CSF)	Uremia	Bacterial infections of CNS (meningitis, encephalitis)
Glucose	2.8–4.2 mmol/L of CSF (50–75 mg/dL of CSF) or 60–70% of blood glucose level	Diabetes mellitus, viral infections of CNS	Bacterial infections and tuberculosis of CNS
Protein			
• Lumbar	0.15–0.45 g/L (15–45 mg/dL)	Guillain-Barré syndrome, poliomyelitis, traumatic tap	—
• Cisternal	0.15–0.25 g/L (15–25 mg/dL)	*Cerebral neoplasm, brain abscess, cerebral hemorrhage, cancer metastasis to the brain:* These pathological conditions are associated with disruption in the blood–brain barrier, which results in increased uptake of radionuclide in the cerebral cortex. *Acute cerebral infarction:* In the first few days to weeks after a stroke, the scan may appear normal. After a few weeks, however, the blood–brain barrier has been disrupted and cortical uptake occurs. This appearance is pathognomonic of stroke. *Subdural hematoma:* The cortex/ subcortical tissue and meninges may become distorted and lateralized. Cerebral thrombosis, cerebrovascular occlusive disease, hematoma, arteriovenous malformation, aneurysm, CSF leakage, hydrocephalus	
• Ventricular	0.05–0.15 g/L (5–15 mg/dL)	Acute meningitis, brain tumour, chronic CNS infections, multiple sclerosis	—
Pressure	100–200 mm Hg H_2O (same as SI units)	Hemorrhage, intracranial tumour, meningitis	Head injury, spinal tumour, subdural hematoma

CNS, Central nervous system; *CSF,* cerebrospinal fluid.
Note: The content of this appendix is based on the values presented in Pagana, K. D., Pagana, T. J., & Pike-MacDonald, S. A. (2019). *Mosby's Canadian manual of diagnostic and laboratory tests* (2nd Canadian ed.). Elsevier.

INDEX

Page numbers followed by "f" indicate figures, "t" indicate tables, and "b" indicate boxes.

Enzymes, 1212
in digestion, 1102
EOL care. *See* End-of-life care
Eosinophils, for infection, 687t
Ephedra, 829t
Epidemiology, 69–70
of infection control, 708
Epidermis, 902, 902t, 1292, 1292f
Epidural analgesia, 596
Epidural catheters, 596–597, 597f
Epidural route, for medications, 732
Epidural space, 597, 597f
Epigenesis, 352
Epigenetics, 357
Epiglottis, 1102–1103, 1211
Epithelialization, 1306
Epp Report, 5
Equality, equity *versus*, 7f
Equianalgesic chart, 594
Equipment
in health assessment and physical
examination, 609, 610b
in implementation process, 220
in intravenous therapy, 1050, 1050b
in patient's room, 942–950, 942f,
944f
Equipment-related accidents, 878
Equitable, safety and, 873
Equity, 174–175
equality *versus*, 7f
Erasure, 400
Erectile dysfunction, 484, 484t
Ergonomic assistive devices, 1248
Ergonomics, 840
Erikson's psychosocial theory of
development (1963), 457
Erikson's theory of eight stages of life,
352, 353t, 354f
Erythema, 618
Erythrocyte sedimentation rate
(ESR), for infection, 687t
Eschar, 1302–1304
Escherichia coli, 677, 678t, 1252
food safety in, 1127t
Esophagus, digestive role of, 1211
ESR. *See* Erythrocyte sedimentation
rate
Essential amino acids, 1100
Essential fatty acids (EFAs), in
integrative health practices,
819t–821t
Estimated average requirement
(EAR), 1104
Estimated glomerular filtration rate
(eGFR), 1031
Estrogen, 389
Ethical criteria, for nursing
judgement, 92
Ethical decision-making framework,
115, 115f
Ethical dilemma, 114–115
how to analyze an, 115b
Ethical knowing, 294–296
Ethical theory, 112–114
Ethics, 110–114
accountability and, 111
advocacy and, 111–112
analysis and nursing, 114–116
Code of Ethics, 111
definition of, 109
futile care, 116–117
issues in nursing practice, 116–118
nursing and, 111–112
in nursing practice, 119b
in practical nursing in Canada, 66

Ethics *(Continued)*
responsibility and, 111
safety issues related to work
environment and, 118
safe care, working with a health
care team to promote, 118
social networking and safety, 118
theories and principles of, 112–114
applied ethics, 113
autonomy, 113
beneficence, 113
bioethics, 113–114
biomedical ethics, 113–114
consequentialism, 113
deontology, 113
descriptive moral, 112–113
feminist ethics, 114
justice, 114
metaethics, 112–113
nonmaleficence, 114
normative ethics, 113
relational ethics, 114
utilitarianism, 113
Ethnic identity, self-concept and,
457–458
Ethnicity
and gender roles in young adults,
399
sensory function and, 1347
Ethnocultural diversity, in Canada,
143, 144b
Ethylene oxide gas, in disinfection
and sterilization, 692t
Etiology, 199–200, 199t–200t, 200f
Eupnea, 545
Eustress, 509–510
Euthanasia, 130
Evaluation, 296
of body temperature, 538
in communication within the
nursing process, 288–289, 289b
in community health nursing,
56–57
criteria for, 93
critical thinking and, 223, 224f
critical thinking model
for self-concept, 468b–469b,
471, 471f
for sexuality, 488b, 489–490, 490f
in fluid, electrolyte, and acid-base
balance, 1070
goals and expected outcomes of, 228
in nursing and teaching processes,
333t, 340–341
in nursing care, 223
in nursing leadership, 181
in nursing process, 74, 188
process of, 223–228
care plan revision, 227
collecting evaluative data, 225,
226f
discontinuing care plan, 227
documenting findings, 227
identifying criteria and
standards, 224–225
interpreting and summarizing
findings, 225–226,
226t–227t
modifying care plan, 227–228
in safety, 898, 898f
in transfer techniques, for
immobilized patients, 842t
in urinary elimination, 1206, 1207f
work of other staff members, 222
Evaluative data, collecting, 225, 226f

Evaluative measures, 225, 226f
Evaporation, 525
EVD. *See* Ebola virus disease
Evening primrose oil, 827t–828t
Eversion, 1255t–1259t, 1259
Evidence
CNA definition of, 98
collection of, 100–101
critique the, 101–102
integrate the, 102
non-research, 99
researching the, 100–102
sources of, 101t
Evidence-informed articles, elements
of, 101
Evidence-informed decision making,
16, 98
processes involved, 100f
relationship between research and
quality improvement and,
98–99, 99t
support for, 102
Evidence-informed knowledge,
critical thinking and, 86
Evidence-informed practice, 98–108.
e1, 27, 98b
applying research findings in, 107
CNA definition, 98
ethical issues in research and,
106–107, 106b
evaluate the design or change, 102
history of nursing research and,
102–103
integrate the, 102
nursing knowledge development,
99, 99t, 100f, 100b
nursing research and, 103, 103f
relationship between decision
making, research and quality
improvement and, 98–99, 99t
research designs and, 104–105
research synthesis and, 105–106, 106t
researching, 100–102, 101t
steps for successful, 100b
Evisceration, in wound healing, 1311
Evolution, of Canadian health care
delivery system, 20–22
early health care, 20–22
indigenous health care, 22
Examination tables, 610
Excessive daytime sleepiness (EDS),
1078
Excitement stage, sexual response
cycle and, 478
Excoriation, 631
Excretion, as skin impairment risk
factor, 907b
Executive skills, 323
Exercise and physical activity. *See also*
Activity and exercise
in adolescents, 1109
body temperature and, 526
heart rates and, 544t
for immobility, 1267
inadequate, affecting
cardiopulmonary functioning,
967
for older persons, 426–427, 426f
promotion, 1226
respiration and, 546b
sleep and, 1083
for stress management, 518
in young adulthood, 403
Exercise program, initiating and
maintaining an, 853b

Exhaustion stage, in general
adaptation syndrome, 507
Exogenous infection, 682
Exophthalmos, 626
Exostosis, 633
Exosystem, 356
Expected outcomes
associated with death and grief,
445b–446b
guidelines for writing, 205–206
measurable, 206
mutual, 206
of nursing process, 203, 205, 205t
observable, 206
patient-centered, 205
realistic, 206
for self-esteem improvement,
468b–469b
singular, 205
time-limited, 206
Experience, critical thinking and, 89
Experimental research, 104, 104b
Expiration, 958
diaphragmatic and chest wall
movement during, 545f
Explanations, asking, in
nontherapeutic communication
techniques, 287
Exploratory descriptive designs, 105
Expressive aphasia, 288, 1348
Expressive functioning, 319, 319b
Extended family, 311b, 316–317
Extension, 1255, 1255t–1259t
External devices, as skin impairment
risk factor, 907b
External ear, anatomy and physiology
of, 1341t
External rotation, 1255t–1259t, 1259
External sphincter, 1163
External structure, of family, 315f,
316–317
Extracellular fluid (ECF), 1015
Extract, 727t
Extraocular movements, assessment
of, 628, 628f
Extrauterine life, transition from
intrauterine to, 365–367
Extremity restraint, 892t
Exudates, 681
Eye contact
to enhance a patient's self-esteem,
464f
in nonverbal communication,
277–278
Eye drops, administration of, 762t
Eye ointment, administration of, 762t
Eye poison, interventions for, 886b
Eyebrows, assessment of, 626
Eyeglasses, 911b, 939
Eyelids, assessment of, 626–627
Eyes
anatomy and physiology of, 1342f
assessment of, 625–628
basic care, 939–940
bathing techniques for, 939–941
changes with aging, 418t, 910–911
common problems in, 626b
defence mechanisms of, 681t
external eye structures, 626–627
conjunctivae and sclerae, 627
eyebrows, 626
eyelids, 626–627
lacrimal apparatus, 627, 627f
position and alignment of, 626
pupils and irises, 627, 627f

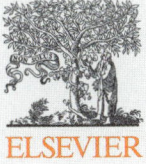

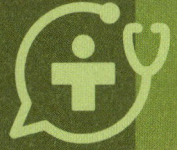

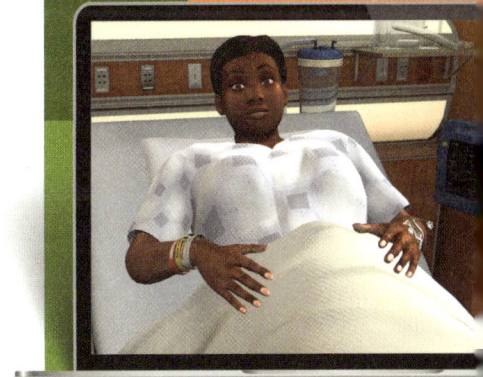

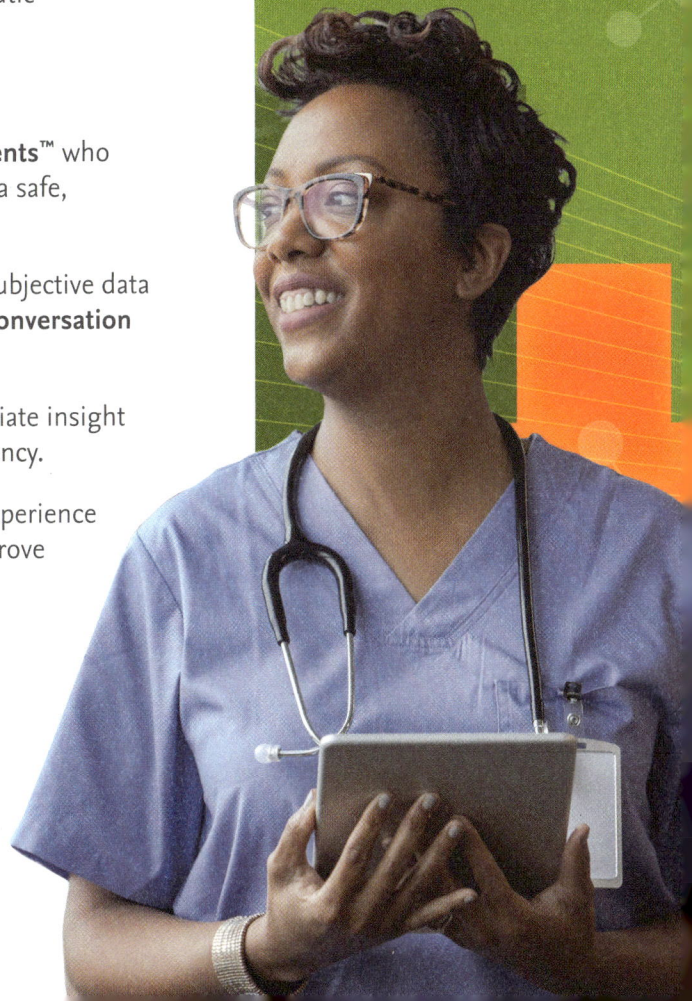

SPECIAL FEATURES